Medical-Surgical Nursing
A Nursing Process Approach

Medical-Surgical

Nursing

A Nursing Process Approach

Barbara C. Long, MSN, RN

Associate Professor Emeritus of Medical-Surgical Nursing
Frances Payne Bolton School of Nursing
Case Western Reserve University
Cleveland, Ohio

Wilma J. Phipps, PhD, RN, FAAN

Professor Emeritus of Medical-Surgical Nursing
Frances Payne Bolton School of Nursing
Case Western Reserve University
Cleveland, Ohio

Virginia L. Cassmeyer, PhD, RN, CS

Associate Professor
School of Nursing
University of Kansas
Kansas City, Kansas

THIRD EDITION

*with **725** illustrations and **9** color plates*

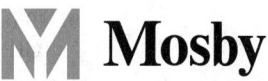

Mosby

St. Louis   Baltimore   Boston   Chicago   London   Philadelphia   Sydney   Toronto

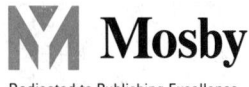

Mosby
Dedicated to Publishing Excellence

Publisher: Alison Miller
Editor: Terry Van Schaik
Developmental Editor: Janet Livingston
Project Manager: John Rogers
Book Designer: Susan Lane

THIRD EDITION

Printed in the United States of America

Mosby–Year Book, Inc.
11830 Westline Industrial Drive
St. Louis, Missouri 63146

Library of Congress Cataloging in Publication Data

Medical-surgical nursing : a nursing process approach / [edited by]
    Barbara C. Long, Wilma J. Phipps, Virginia L. Cassmeyer. —4th ed.
        p.   cm.
    Includes bibliographical references and index.
    ISBN 0-8016-6672-4
    1. Nursing. 2. Surgical nursing. I. Long, Barbara C.
II. Phipps, Wilma J., 1925-   . III. Cassmeyer, Virginia.
    [DNLM: 1. Nursing Care. 2. Nursing Process. 3. Surgical Nursing.
WY 150 M48933]
RT41.E87   1993
610.73—dc20
DNLM/DLC
for Library of Congress   92-49614
                                                              CIP

    94 95 96 97 GW/VH 9 8 7 6 5 4 3 2

Contributors

Terri Abraham, *MSN, RN, CCRN*
Nurse Manager, ICU
St Mary's Hospital
Richmond, Virginia

Martha L. Allen, *MSN, RN*
Head Nurse, Medical ICU
University Hospitals of Cleveland
Clinical Instructor in Medical-Surgical
    Nursing
Frances Payne Bolton School of Nursing
Case Western Reserve University
Cleveland, Ohio

Dorothy R. Blevins, *MSN, RN*
Associate Professor
Kent State University School of Nursing
Kent, Ohio

Mary Jo Boehnlein, *MSN, RN, CNA*
Director Operating Room, Recovery
    Room, and Ambulatory Surgery
Mount Sinai Medical Center
Cleveland, Ohio

Frances R. Chester, *BSN, RN, MPA, CPQA*
Quality Management/Risk Management
    Specialist
Weston, Hurd, Fallon, Paisley and Howley
Cleveland, Ohio

Elizabeth Cameron Eckstein, *MSN, RN*
Infection Control Nurse
Cleveland VA Medical Center
Cleveland, Ohio

H. Fred Farley, *MSN, RN*
Vice President of Nursing
Arnot Ogden Memorial Hospital
Elmira, New York

Sally M. Featherstone, *MN, RN, CS*
Director, Psychiatric Nursing
Barnes Hospital at Washington University
    Medical Center
St. Louis, Missouri

Diane E. Fritsch, *MSN, RN CCRN*
Clinical Nurse Specialist, Trauma
    Critical Care Nursing Service
MetroHealth Medical Center
Cleveland, Ohio

Greer Glazer, *PhD, RN*
Associate Professor of Nursing
Kent State University
Kent, Ohio

Rosemarie Hogan, *MSN, RN*
Assistant Dean of Nursing
Frances Payne Bolton School of Nursing
Case Western Reserve University
Cleveland, Ohio

Maura A. Hopkins, *MSN, RN*
Assistant Director of Nursing
    Specialty Services
Kaiser Permanente Medical Center
Santa Rosa, California

Donald D. Kautz, *MSN, RN, CS, CRRN*
Doctoral Candidate
University of Kentucky College of Nursing
Lexington, Kentucky

Deborah Goldenberg Klein, *MSN, RN,*
    CS, CCRN
Clinical Nurse Specialist
    Trauma/Critical Care Nursing Service
MetroHealth Medical Center
Clinical Instructor, Acute and Critical
    Care Nursing
Frances Payne Bolton School of Nursing
Case Western Reserve University
Cleveland, Ohio

Denise M. Kresevic, *MSN, RN, CS*
Clinical Nurse Specialist
University Hospitals of Cleveland
Clinical Instructor in Medical-Surgical
    Nursing
Frances Payne Bolton School of Nursing
Case Western Reserve University
Cleveland, Ohio

Mary Kay Lehman, *MSN, RN*
Doctoral Candidate
    Case Western Reserve University
Instructor in Medical-Surgical Nursing
Frances Payne Bolton School of Nursing
Case Western Reserve University
Cleveland, Ohio

Ruth A. Lincoln, *MSN, RN, RNC*
Advanced Clinical Nurse
University Hospitals of Cleveland
Clinical Instructor in Medical-Surgical
    Nursing
Frances Payne Bolton School of Nursing
Case Western Reserve University
Cleveland, Ohio

Gail Osterfield, *MSN, RN*
Assistant Professor of Nursing
Kent State University
Kent, Ohio

Carol G. Phipps, *MSN, RN*
Head Nurse, Preadmission Assessment
    and Teaching Center
University Hospitals of Cleveland
Cleveland, Ohio

Dora A. Rice, *MSN, RN, CIC*
Infection Control Nurse
Cleveland VA Medical Center
Cleveland, Ohio

Rebecca Anne Roberts, *MSN, RN, ET*
Clinical Nurse Specialist
University Hospitals of Cleveland
Clinical Instructor in Medical-Surgical
    Nursing
Frances Payne Bolton School of Nursing
Case Western Reserve University
Cleveland, Ohio

Grace A. Rotter, *MSN, RN, CIC*
Clinical Quality Manager
Cleveland VA Medical Center
Clinical Instructor in Community Health
    Nursing
Frances Payne Bolton School of Nursing
Case Western Reserve University
Cleveland, Ohio

Elizabeth Anne Schenk, *MSN, RN*
Vice President of Nursing
Heather Hill Inc.
Munson, Ohio

Susan Moeller Schneider, MSN, RN
Oncology Clinical Nurse Specialist
University Hospitals of Cleveland
Clinical Instructor of Medical-Surgical
  Nursing
Frances Payne Bolton School of Nursing
Case Western Reserve University
Cleveland, Ohio

Barbara J. Sibley, MA, MS, ND, RN, RNC
Former Advanced Clinical Nurse
Psychiatric Mental Health Nursing
University Hospitals of Cleveland
Cleveland, Ohio

Carol E. Smith, PhD, RN
Professor, School of Nursing
University of Kansas
Kansas City, Kansas

Roberta A. Stokes, MSN, RN, CHN,
  CNN, CS
Nurse Educator, Transition Care Unit
Cleveland Clinic Foundation
Cleveland, Ohio

Kathryn Sabo Thompson, MSN, RN
Project Leader, Special Care Unit
University Hospitals of Cleveland
Cleveland, Ohio

M. Eileen Walsh, MSN, RN
Assistant Professor, School of Nursing
Medical College of Ohio
Coordinator, Cardiovascular Risk
  Intervention Programs
H.L. Morse Center
Toledo, Ohio

Judith H. Watt-Watson, MScN, RN
Clinical Associate, Professor
School of Nursing, University of Toronto
Toronto, Ontario, Canada

E. Ronald Wright, PhD
Associate Professor of Nursing and Biology
Case Western Reserve University
Cleveland, Ohio

Nancy Fugate Woods, PhD, RN, FAAN
Professor and Chair
  Parent and Child Nursing
University of Washington
Seattle, Washington

Mary A. (Sandy) Wyper, PhD, RN
Assistant Professor of Nursing
Kent State University
Kent, Ohio

Lynne C. Yurko, BSN, RN
Unit Manager, Burn Intensive Care Unit
MetroHealth Medical Center
Cleveland, Ohio

REVIEWERS

The publisher and authors wish to acknowledge the assistance of the following reviewers:

Molly J. Allison, *BSN, MSN*
Angelo State University

Betty Aubuchon, *RN, PhD*
Southern Illinois University at Edwardsville

Janice E. Bachtell, *PhD, RN*
Northern Virginia Community College

Lois K. Baker, *RN, PhD, CPNP*
Cedarville College

Esther Bay, *MSN, CCRN, CS*
Henry Ford Community College

Mary Ellen Beebe, *BSN, MN, MSN*
Lakeshore Technical College

Mary Ruth Beeber, *BSN, MAN*
Gannon University

Clara W. Boyle, *BS, MS, EdD*
San Jose State University
Deanza College

Daryle L. Brown, *BSN, MA, MED, EdD*
Pace University

Carole Broxson, *BSN, MSN*
Sinclair Community College

Karen D. Carpenter, *PhD, RN, CCRN*
University of South Carolina-Coastal Carolina
  College

Janet A. Conway, *RN, PhD*
Cedarville College

Peggy Craik, *BSN, MSN, MBA*
University of Mary Hardin-Baylor

Sheila Cunningham, *BSN, MSN*
Neumann College

Lorraine Delehanty, *BSN, MSN*
Lakewood Community College

Chris Gehlbach, *BSN, MSN*
Sauk Valley Community College

Barbara A. Hagerich, *MSN, RN*
Mercy Regional Health System

Dorothy Susan Hayes, *ADN, BS*
Madisonville Health Technology Center

Elizabeth L. Hughes, *MSN, RN, CDE*
Barnes Hospital

Patricia A. Jablonski, *RN, MSN*
Hudson Valley Community College
Albany Medical Center

Kay Setter Kline, *RN, BA, BSN, MSN, PhD*
Grand Valley State University

Dianna Koerner, *BSN, MS, MN*
Fort Hays State University

Pamela D. Korte, *BSN, MSN*
Monroe Community College

Mary LeGrand, *RN, BSN*
Barnes Hospital

Laura Jean Looper, *RN, BA, MA*
College of Marin

JoAnn Lowdon, *RN, BA, MALS*
Blue Ridge Community College

Sandra E. Marra, *RN, MSN, MA*
West Virginia University

Edwina A. McConnell, *RN, PhD*
Texas Tech University-Health Sciences Center

Carolyn Y. Middendorf, *MN, RN*
Washburn University

Betty Jean Oeding, *BSN, MSN*
College of the Desert

Helen Ortega, *RN, C, MS*
Napa Valley College

Anna G. Pierce, *RN, PhD*
Columbia University

Susanne Ptak, *BS, GN, MA*
Orange County Community College

Susan A. Reed, *MSN, RNCS*
Fort Howard Veterans Administration Medical
  Center

Jean L. Reese, *BSN, MN, PhD*
University of Iowa

M. Gaie Rubenfeld, *RN, MS*
Eastern Michigan University

Nancy L. Rubinski, *BS, MA*
Muskegon Community College

Anna Louise Scandiffio, *RN, MS*
Veterans Affairs Medical Center

Elaine Schmidt, *RN, MSN*
Indiana Vocational Technical College

Sally E. Schuster, *BSN, MSN*
Gannon University

Catherine Seibold, *BS, BSN, MSN*
Gannon University

Marlene Kay Seller, *RN, BSN, MN*
Labette Community College

Carolbeth Snyder, *BSN, RNC*
Wake Technical Community College

Pamela L. Sonney, *RN, MSN, FNP, C*
Wake Technical Community College

Constance R. Uphold, *PhD, ARNP, RN-C*
University of Florida

Janis Waite, *RN, MSN*
Illinois Central College

Kathleen S. Whalen, *BSN, MN*
Community College of Denver

Lois White, *RN, PhD*
Del Mar College

Preface

Medical-surgical nursing practice encompasses the nursing care of adults who are at risk for or who are experiencing pathophysiologic disorders. The study of medical-surgical nursing, therefore, includes knowledge of pathophysiologic disorders (including medical therapy), methods of prevention, and nursing activities (thought processes and actions) to assist persons to achieve their optimal health. If "everything" the nurse should know to achieve these ends were included in one text, the book itself would be too extensive for the student, not only in scope but also in physical size. To facilitate learning, the authors of this text have chosen to focus on the *essential* information required by students in their first medical-surgical nursing course. Content covered in great detail in other nursing texts, such as fundamentals of nursing or care of children, is summarized briefly (if appropriate) or omitted.

Nursing Process continues to be the approach used in this text, most especially in the latter units that discuss pathophysiologic disorders. Greater emphasis has been placed in this third edition in correlating the content of the *Implementation* sections with that of *Data analysis: nursing diagnoses;* this change should facilitate student learning.

Throughout the book the recipients of nursing services are referred to as *patients* rather than *clients*. Although *client* is widely used in the nursing community, the article "Complexities and Clarity in Nurse-Client and Nurse-Patient Relationships" by L. Nowakowski, which appeared in the July-August 1985 issue of the *Journal of Professional Nursing*, makes a real distinction between who is a client and who is a patient. Using her framework, we decided that *patient* was a better term to use in this book. We found Nowakowski's criteria for differentiating between clients and patients to be thought provoking and helpful, and we recommend the article to the reader.

ORGANIZATION

The first five units of the book focus on general information required for medical-surgical nursing practice regardless of underlying functional problems or pathologies. Unit One introduces the student to the *nature of medical-surgical nursing,* reviewing important concepts of health and illness, nursing process, ethics in nursing practice, and quality assurance. Unit Two focuses on *health promotion,* including discussions of cultural influences affecting patient responses, special needs of the elderly, and stress management. Unit Three describes the nature of and care required

for persons with *common problems* encountered in medical-surgical nursing practice; fluid and electrolyte imbalances; acid-base imbalances; shock; pain; cancer; sleep disorders; substance abuse; chronic illness; and loss, dying, and death. Content related to *infection* is grouped in Unit Four. The chapter on biologic defense mechanisms provides the underlying theory for the following chapters on infection control, sexually transmitted diseases, and AIDS. Unit Five provides information on the care of patients during the perioperative period.

The next six units discuss specific problems of functional areas: gas transport (Six), metabolic and endocrine (Seven), digestion or elimination (Eight), sexual and reproductive (Nine), cognition, sensation and motion (Ten), and defense and protection (Eleven). The overall organization of chapters in these units is as follows:

REVIEW OF ANATOMY AND PHYSIOLOGY
PREVENTION AND HEALTH EDUCATION

MAJOR HEALTH PROBLEMS

Etiology/Epidemiology
Pathophysiology
Nursing Process
Assessment
    Data analysis: nursing diagnoses
    Planning: expected patient outcomes
    Implementation
        Assisting with achievement of therapeutic goals
        Interventions to achieve patient outcomes
    Evaluation

The final unit discusses care of persons in special environments of care: emergencies and disasters in the community, critical care units, and home care.

NEW TO THIS EDITION

Changes in this edition include *new chapters* on cultural influences on health and illness prevention, promotion of health in the elderly, sleep disorders, AIDS (now a separate chapter), organ transplantation, and home care of the ill adult. Fluid and electrolyte imbalances have been separated from acid-base imbalances into two chapters. Content on the liver has been separated out and placed in the metabolic and endocrine unit because of the liver's major metabolic functions. Content on biliary and pancreatic problems has been placed in the digestion unit.

Reflecting today's patient population, content on the care of the *elderly* has been increased. Content on elderly persons now includes a new chapter "Promotion of Health in the Elderly." Assessment, interventions, and common complications in elderly persons are summarized in new highlighted boxes throughout the text. A section on "Physiologic Changes with Aging" is included in chapters with reviews of anatomy and physiology.

Etiology of specific disorders is discussed more fully in the text, and the *pathophysiology* content has been expanded in many instances to indicate the bases of observed symptoms. Rationales for nursing interventions have been added when indicated. The implementation sections have two divisions: activities that promote achievement of therapeutic goals and activities directed specifically toward achievement of patient outcomes. This organization should help the student understand the differences between interdependent and independent nursing actions.

Also new to this edition is increased emphasis on the national health objectives, rights of disabled persons, and the right to die with dignity. The *National Health Objectives for Year 2000* are introduced in Chapter 5: Health Promotion: Nutrition and Exercise and then highlighted in appropriate chapters. Information on the *Americans with Disabilities Act* is discussed in Chapter 14: Chronic Illness. The topics of *Advance Directives* and *Living Wills* are discussed in Chapter 15: Loss, Dying, and Death and are referred to in appropriate chapters.

ADDITIONAL FEATURES

Tables of medical information provide a quick *review* for the student. The use of *boxes* for highlighting important information has been continued based on positive input from readers and reviewers. Boxes have been numbered in this edition to facilitate box identification. Recurring boxes throughout the text are specially designed so they are easy to locate and present patient teaching, guidelines for care, and nursing research. Selected *nursing care plans* have been included to serve as models for students developing their own care plans. Other pedagogic features include chapter objectives, chapter outlines, summaries of chapter content, and study questions. Normal laboratory values, abbreviations in common usage, and recommended daily dietary allowances can be found in the appendices.

TEACHING-LEARNING PACKAGE

For the third edition of our text we are pleased to offer an extensive number of ancillary products for instructors and students to use in class and clinical settings.

Instructor's Resource Manual

Includes topical outlines for each chapter and suggested ways of presenting content. Also features tips for special class and clinical activities. An extensive Test Bank with an answer key assists instructors in formulating test questions. Transparency masters of key illustrations supplement overhead transparencies. Student Review Sheets are included as an additional resource.

Overhead Transparencies

Packet includes 100 transparency acetates for classroom use. Important figures and diagrams have been chosen for inclusion in the packet.

CompuTest 3

Computerized Test Bank for use with IBM PC. Includes multiple-choice questions and a user's manual so that instructors can add, delete, or rearrange test items from any part of the text.

Student Learning Guide

Enables students to make maximum use of review time by presenting objectives, self-assessment activities, and decision-making tools.

ACKNOWLEDGMENTS

We are pleased to welcome Virginia L. Cassmeyer as a new editor. Dr. Cassmeyer has been a contributor to this book since the first edition. We are grateful for the expert contributions by our chapter authors. We thank the readers who wrote to us with ideas or suggestions and trust that they will be pleased with changes that have been made. New illustrations are the work of Nancy Burgard of Cleveland. The preparation of parts of the manuscript was by Sondra Patrizi.

We greatly appreciate the strong support we have received from editors and project managers at Mosby–Year Book, Inc., particularly Linda Duncan, Terry Van Schaik, Janet Livingston, and John Rogers. We could not have completed this third edition without them.

Barbara C. Long
Wilma J. Phipps
Virginia L. Cassmeyer

Contents

Unit Four

Infection

Unit Six

Gas Transport Problems

Unit Seven

Metabolic and Endocrine Problems

Unit Eight

Problems with Digestion or Elimination

Unit Nine

Sexual and Reproductive Problems

Unit Ten

Problems of Cognition, Sensation, and Motion

Unit Eleven

Problems of Defense and Protection

41   The Patient with Immunologic Problems   1427

Barbara C. Long
E. Ronald Wright

42   The Patient with an Organ/Tissue Transplant   1446

Virginia L. Cassmeyer

43   The Patient with Dermatologic Problems   1469

Barbara C. Long

44 The Patient with Burns 1500

Deborah Goldenberg Klein
Diane E. Fritsch
Lynne C. Yurko

Unit Twelve

Special Environments of Care

45 Problems Encountered in Emergencies and Disasters 1537

Barbara C. Long

Appendixes

Color Plates following p. 1478

Medical-Surgical Nursing Practice

Unit One

1

Perspectives of Medical-Surgical Nursing

Barbara C. Long

After studying this chapter, the learner should be able to:

- Differentiate the practice of medical-surgical nursing from other nursing disciplines.
- Differentiate health promotion and prevention of illness, and the three levels of prevention.
- Identify stages of disease development.
- Differentiate independent and interdependent nursing functions.
- Describe five steps of nursing process.
- Identify ethical issues that may occur in the practice of medical-surgical nursing.

SCOPE OF MEDICAL-SURGICAL NURSING

Medical-surgical nursing practice encompasses the nursing care of adults who are at risk for or who are experiencing pathophysiologic disorders. In most health care centers children are separated from adults because of their different needs, and the specialty practice of pediatric nursing has developed with the focus on the nursing care of children. Thus medical-surgical nursing practice has developed primarily as the nursing care of persons (1) who have attained physical/developmental maturity, (2) who are at risk for or who have expressed variations in their personal norms of physical functioning, and (3) who may require therapeutic medical or surgical intervention.

In the past *medical care* was the general term for the care given sick persons by professionals; the term is now used to denote the care given by members of the medical profession (physicians). The trend in American society is toward a health orientation; therefore, *health care* is the more acceptable term for the care provided by all health care professionals. The term *health care* is broader in that it includes assisting people to stay well in addition to providing care when they are ill. The care of the sick remains a primary responsibility of health care professionals, and this care is still provided primarily in health care institutions such as acute care hospitals or long-term care centers. There is an increased use, however, of ambulatory care, primary care, and family care centers as well as other types of health care services, in part because it is more economic to keep people well than to provide care when they are sick.[33]

Nurses are one group of health care professionals. In addition to participating in health promotion, nurses are actively involved in prevention of disease and health education for persons who are at high risk for acquiring specific diseases. Health promotion, disease prevention, and care of persons with specific pathophysiologic disorders require a knowledge base of the following:

1. Health and illness
2. Factors influencing the occurrence and course of specific disorders
3. Common responses to the disorders
4. Nursing interventions that assist the person to achieve optimal health or to die with maximum comfort and dignity

HEALTH AND ILLNESS

Health and illness are complex concepts, and they are interpreted in different ways by different individuals or groups. Both health and illness are multidimensional concepts; that is, there are multiple aspects to be considered and multiple factors that may be of influence.

Definitions of Health

During the early centuries health was defined in terms of that which was normal or natural. Therefore, anything abnormal or against nature was considered not healthy and to be avoided; for example, lepers were called "unclean." Treatment of diseases consisted of amulets or spells to drive out the evil or unnatural spirits causing the abnormality. "Leeching" was a popular treatment and consisted of applying leeches (blood-sucking worms) to suck out the tainted blood. Wounds were treated by cautery to burn out the evil forces that would prevent healing. Even in more modern times, "tonics," which often included a laxative, were taken frequently by people to stay healthy.

In later years health was defined primarily as freedom from disease. During the middle of the 20th century the concept of *mental health* was introduced, meaning the ability of the individual to cope successfully with stress in a functional manner. In 1974 the World Health Organization (WHO) defined health more broadly: complete physical, mental, and social well-being and not merely the absence of disease and infirmity. This definition introduced the concept of the subjective as well as the objective physical or behavioral responses.

The various views about health usually contain one or more of the following perspectives:

Biologic or clinical: absence of pathologic condition
Psychologic: well-being and self-actualization
Sociologic: ability to meet social responsibilities and role functions
Adaptive: adaptation to a changing environment

Patients and health care providers may have different views of health and may therefore be working toward different goals that may or may not be in conflict. For example, people who "feel well" and who hold the view that health is a sense of well-being may not be willing to follow-up on screening tests even when a disease may be suspected by the clinician.

Health is a dynamic, ever-changing state. It reflects the person's level of functioning in various physiologic, psychologic, and sociocultural dimensions. People can simultaneously be functioning at a high level in one aspect, such as nutrition, but at a low level in another aspect, such as oxygenation or self-esteem. Nursing is concerned with holistic health, the effect of functioning of the subcomponents on total functioning. Thus each patient is assessed in various dimensions, with consideration given for the person's overall functioning and sense of well-being. Each person has different genetic factors and is exposed to different environmental factors. There is therefore *no one* nursing approach for all persons who are at risk for or who have a specific illness, disease, or injury. The approach used by nurses to provide care to a specific patient depends on the pertinent factors unique to that patient.

Health Promotion and Prevention

The goal of nursing is to assist people to achieve optimal health, the highest level of functioning that is achievable for each person. This includes activities that promote health and prevent illness.

Health promotion

Health promotion refers to activities directed toward helping persons maintain or achieve a high level of functioning and feeling of well-being. The nursing activities include teaching, counseling, and motivating persons to develop life-styles that include adequate nutrition, exercise, and rest or relaxation. Persons functioning at a high level have an increased capacity to withstand physical and emotional stressors. (See Chapter 5 for further information on health promotion.)

Table 1-1 Levels of prevention

Level	Definition	Examples
Primary	Prevention of disease	Immunization, environmental sanitation, accident prevention, anticipatory counseling and guidance (for example, premarital counseling)
Secondary	Early detection and treatment of disease	Screening for tuberculosis, diabetes, glaucoma Breast or testes self-examination Outpatient mental health programs
Tertiary	Prevention of disabilities, rehabilitation	Prevention of complications of immobility Cardiac rehabilitation programs

Health promotion activities are carried out whenever the opportunities occur. Thus health teaching and counseling are instituted not only with well persons but also when persons are hospitalized. For example, teaching about adequate nutrition can be done while assisting a patient to select items from a hospital menu.

Prevention

Prevention refers to activities directed toward protecting persons from potential or actual threats to health and the subsequent consequences.[27] In other words, prevention means inhibiting the development of disease, slowing down the progression of disease, and protecting the body from further harmful effects. There are three different levels of protection: primary, secondary, and tertiary (Table 1-1).

Primary prevention

Primary prevention includes specific protective measures against disease or trauma, such as immunizations against diphtheria or measles, environmental sanitation, and protection against occupational hazards (for example, wearing safety glasses to prevent eye injuries). Early successes in primary prevention have been the result of activities directed at preventing the occurrence of infectious diseases such as polio or smallpox through immunization and typhoid fever through purification of water. More recently dental caries have been prevented by fluoridation of water supplies.

The major health problems today are chronic diseases and accidental injuries and their sequelae, both of which require modification of deeply rooted behaviors such as use of alcohol, tobacco and drugs, and poor nutritional and exercise patterns. Health promotion activities are considered a form of primary prevention.

Secondary prevention

Secondary prevention includes early detection and prompt intervention to stop the disease at an early stage, decrease the intensity, or prevent complications. This is accomplished by screening for diseases such as diabetes, carcinoma in situ, tuberculosis, or glaucoma. The purpose is to detect early symptoms about which the patient is unaware or lacks knowledge, so that prompt intervention is effective for control or cure. Screening for contacts of persons with sexually transmitted diseases and treating the infected person to prevent spread of the disease are other examples of secondary prevention.

Tertiary prevention

Tertiary prevention consists of activities that prevent or limit disabilities and help restore the person with a disability to an optimal level of functioning (for example, rehabilitation). Tertiary prevention begins in the early period of recovery from an illness and includes activities such as moving and turning immobile patients to prevent respiratory complications or decubiti, encouraging leg exercises to prevent muscle weakness, and encouraging or assisting with range-of-motion exercises to prevent contractures.

Rehabilitation programs for persons with cardiac disease or with disabilities resulting from a cerebral vascular accident (stroke) are initiated before the patient is discharged from the hospital. Chapter 14 discusses the concept of rehabilitation in more detail. Preventive measures for specific disorders are described in the appropriate chapters of this text.

At Risk Status

Some persons are considered to have a greater possibility of becoming ill or acquiring a specific disease because of the presence of certain factors. These persons are considered to be *at risk* and the specific factors are termed *risk factors*. For example, a woman over age 35 with a family history of breast cancer who had her first menstrual period before age 12 and who has never had a child would be considered at high risk for developing breast cancer because several of the known risk factors for breast cancer are present. This woman may not develop breast cancer; however, a greater than normal probability exists that she might.

Some risk factors, such as age and genetic factors, cannot be altered, whereas other factors, such as smoking or diet, are under the control of the person. To alter the risk factor, persons need to receive information related to the specific health threats. People frequently test the validity of health information by asking laypersons and professionals about the specific risks. Knowing about the risks does not always result in altered behavior, since some people receive satisfaction from the risk behaviors and deny the risk for themselves, even in the presence of contradictory information, saying, in effect, "It won't happen to me." Frequently there is no direct causal relationship, therefore the behaviors are easy for some persons to dismiss. There are also no immediate tangible rewards for engaging in the

Table 1-2 Environmental factors affecting health

Type	Examples	Possible effects
Chemical	Lead, arsenic	Poisoning
	Cholesterol	Myocardial infarction
Physical	Automobiles	Accidents
	High noise level	Deafness
	Heat	Burns, heatstroke
	Cold	Frostbite, hypothermia
	Radiation	Cancer
Biologic	Bacteria, virus, fungi	Infections
Psychosocial	Stress	Ulcers, hypertension

desired behaviors. Some persons therefore deliberately choose to continue engaging in the risk behaviors.

To promote health behaviors that decrease the at risk status, people first have to receive the information. Then positive reinforcement for altering behavior is more effective than negative comments about the at risk behaviors. Group sessions (such as weight loss groups or smoker's groups) may be helpful when participants reinforce each other's positive behaviors. Finally, health care professionals should be *role models*, demonstrating the desired health behaviors.

Illness

Although the terms *illness* and *disease* are sometimes used interchangeably, the terms do not relate to the same concepts. A person with a chronic disease such as diabetes may say, "I feel well." Illness is a more abstract term than disease and is essentially the opposite of wellness. Both illness and wellness have a strong subjective component, that of feeling ill or that of feeling well. Illness implies malfunctioning, a lower level of functioning.

Humans are constantly responding and adapting to changes in the external and internal (body) environments. A variety of chemical, physical, biologic, and psychosocial factors in the external environment can influence a person's functioning (Table 1-2). Defense mechanisms, either biologic (Chapter 16) or psychologic (Chapter 6), serve to protect the person from environmental factors that may cause harm. Illness results when defense mechanisms become inadequate or inappropriate.

A relatively stable internal environment is necessary for cellular growth and functioning. The process of maintaining this relatively constant environment is the process of *homeostasis* or *dynamic equilibrium*. The term *dynamic equilibrium* is more descriptive, because it implies fluctuations within a normal range rather than a static condition. Maintaining a dynamic equilibrium involves an adequate exchange of oxygen and carbon dioxide through respiration, an adequate nutrient supply to meet basal metabolic needs, and a normal balance of fluids and electrolytes. Variations above or below normal ranges lead to illness and disease.

Disease

Diseases are specific pathologic conditions with characteristic signs and symptoms. Diseases may involve a specific organ or body part or may affect the body as a whole. Functioning of the part or body system may be impaired. The body has many integrated defense mechanisms and compensatory responses that maintain functioning for a period of time when a threat to the system occurs, but if the causative factors or stressors persist, altered structure or functioning results. Terms commonly used when discussing specific diseases are listed in Table 1-3.

Diseases have a natural life history, usually progressing through stages. The time factor varies; acute diseases have a sudden onset and are usually of short duration, whereas chronic diseases often have a gradual or indefinite onset and have a longer duration. In the first stage of development of a disease, the *presymptomatic* or *subclinical stage*, pathogenic changes have started to occur but no detectable signs or symptoms are apparent. Examples of this stage are the formation of atheromatous plaques in the coronary vessel or early malignant growth.[20] The second stage, the *clinical stage*, is characterized by the presence of signs and symptoms. It is at this stage that the person may seek help. The third stage, the *rehabilitation stage*, occurs with chronic diseases and is characterized by residual disabilities. During this stage the person must learn how to adapt to changes in life-style that result from the disability and learn how to prevent further disability.

Illness Behavior and Sick Role

When people perceive that they are ill, they may take action for relief of symptoms; they may decide to take no action; or they may vacillate between action and no action. Persons who decide to take action may seek help from a friend or family member, from a "folk-specialist" (someone of their cultural group who is frequently consulted about illness), from a professional such as a minister, or from a health care professional. Nonhealth care persons may either deal with the problems themselves or refer the patient to someone else. Often these people act as gatekeeper in helping make the decision when and from whom the sick person should seek help. Persons who perceive they are ill but take no action do so for a variety of reasons (Box 1-1). Low income persons are more apt to seek assistance when they are ill if the health care provider or agency is within the community and easily accessible. Some persons know they should take action but some reason holds them back and thus they vacillate between action and no action.

Some persons are labeled as "noncompliant" because they do not follow the directions of the health care provider. Noncompliance may be defined as the failure of the person to participate in carrying out the plan of care after initially indicating the intention to comply or because of the presence of factors that prevent action.[14] Failure to carry out an action may result from some of the same reasons as failure to seek health care rather than a deliberate action of noncompliance.

When illness becomes legitimized by the physician during the clinical stage, the patient assumes the *sick role* and is exempted from normal social roles and responsibilities as required by the type and severity of the illness (see Chapter 3). The social expectation is that the sick person seeks help and wants to get well. The sick role permits the patient to assume a dependent relationship that facilitates receiving the required health care. Many persons

Table 1-3   **Terminology used with diseases**

Category	Term	Definition
Duration	Acute	Disease with sudden onset and short duration
	Chronic	Disease of long duration; onset may be insidious or may follow an acute disorder
Characteristics	Incidence	Frequency of occurrence of a disease
	Onset	Beginning of a disease
	Course	Pattern of development and resolution
	Duration	Length of time disease is present
	Prognosis	Ultimate outcome
Factors	Epidemiology	Rate and influencing factors of disease occurring in given populations
	Etiology	Cause of disease
	Pathophysiology	Physiologic mechanisms and effects of disease processes
Phenomena	Signs	Observable changes in body function (objective)
	Symptoms	Indication of disease perceived by the patient (subjective)
	Syndrome	Cluster of signs and symptoms that collectively indicate altered functioning
Results	Spontaneous resolution	Healing that occurs with little or no treatment
	Therapeutic intervention	Treatment directed toward a cure or alleviation of signs and symptoms
Statistics	Morbidity	Number of persons having the disease in a given population
	Mortality	Number of persons who die from the disease

find the sick role undesirable and have difficulty with the enforced dependency, although they see it as necessary to achieve the desired end, that is, wellness. They find it helpful if they are kept informed and allowed to make decisions if they are able and desire to do so. The patient is expected to relinquish the sick role and assume increasing independence during the recovery and rehabilitation stage.

MEDICAL-SURGICAL NURSING PRACTICE

Types of Nursing Practice

Nursing actions can be divided into two types—independent and interdependent. *Independent* nursing actions are those which the nurse takes after analysis of data pertaining to those aspects of the patient's health that are amenable to nursing intervention. Providing quality care for persons at risk for or experiencing pathophysiologic disorders requires a systematic approach. In recent years the term *nursing process* has become synonymous with the systematic approach used in providing nursing care.

Interdependent nursing practice consists of activities carried out in collaboration with other health care professionals, such as physicians, nutritionists, and social workers. Nurses participate in team planning with other health care professionals. Nurses are the health care professionals who have the greatest patient contact. They are therefore in a position to assist other professionals by providing additional data through monitoring and by carrying out prescribed treatments patients are unable to do for themselves, sometimes termed a *dependent* function. As patients are able to assume greater responsibility for their own care, *self-care activities* are promoted.

Knowledge Base

The ability to plan and implement nursing care, monitor the patient's condition, and carry out treatments effectively requires a sound knowledge base not only about people and factors pertaining to their health but also about the patho-

---

1-1

Selected reasons for not seeking health care

Denial that symptoms are present
Symptoms not viewed as important
Fear of consequences (for example, pain, cancer, death)
Fear of health care professionals or health care agencies
Lack of knowledge concerning which symptoms require medical care
Lack of availability of transportation
Lack of money for transportation or health care
Disabilities that hinder getting to health care agency

---

physiologic disorders per se. The following types of knowledge about diseases can be useful in planning and providing patient care: epidemiology and etiology, pathophysiology, signs and symptoms of disease, and medical therapy.

Knowledge of epidemiologic and etiologic factors helps to identify the populations at risk. *Epidemiology* is the study of the incidence, distribution, and determinants of diseases and injuries in human populations. In other words, epidemiology is concerned with the extent of specific diseases or injuries in specific groups of people and the factors that influence that distribution.[20] *Etiology* refers to the specific causes of a disease. Most diseases have *multiple causality*; that is, multiple factors are working and interacting together that lead to disease occurrence. This is an important point when teaching about prevention of disease, since avoidance of only one factor may not prevent disease occurrence.

Pathophysiology is the study of the effect of disease (pathology) on body organs and systems and on total body functioning. A *pathophysiologic* disorder is one in which

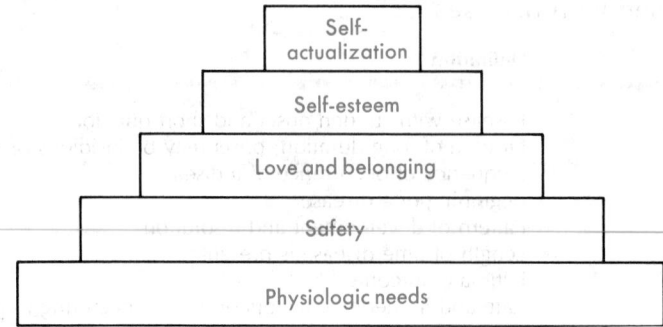

Fig. 1-1 Maslow's hierarchy of needs.

there is altered physiologic functioning, as differentiated from a *pathopsychologic* disorder in which there is altered mental functioning. Knowledge of the physiologic effects of pathology and the nature of the compensatory or adaptive responses facilitates understanding of patient responses for the purposes of monitoring the patient's status for maladaptive responses and teaching the patient about the disease.

Knowledge of the signs and symptoms and medical therapies of common diseases facilitates monitoring for presence and course of diseases, supporting and teaching the patient, and carrying out therapies patients cannot do for themselves.

Frameworks for Nursing Practice

The focus of nursing practice depends on the nurse's philosophical framework. In earlier years of professional nursing, the medical model was the primary approach. Thus when a systematic approach to data collection was first initiated, *body systems* was a framework that was commonly used. For example, data that pertained specifically to the respiratory system were collected, then analyzed to identify respiratory problems.

Another framework that has been used in the practice of medical-surgical nursing is *human needs*. Maslow describes a hierarchy of needs in which physiologic needs are the most basic, followed by safety, love and belonging, self-esteem, and self-actualization (Fig. 1-1). The needs are ranked in ascending order from the needs that are basic to survival to those that focus on development of self (growth-motivated needs). In principle, the more basic needs are satisfied first. For example, a person who is having difficulty breathing (physiologic need for oxygen) attends to that need before dealing with a feeling of loss of worth as a person (self-esteem). In most situations, however, the needs in the hierarchy exist simultaneously to different extents. Lower level needs have to be met, at least partially, before seeking gratification of higher order needs. For example, a person may omit a meal to carry out an activity that increases self-esteem. New needs usually emerge gradually except when danger is present or when the person is acutely ill.

The use of human needs as a framework for nursing care consists of collecting and analyzing data that pertain to each of the need categories. The concept of hierarchy of needs is useful during planning of care by helping to set priorities; for example, survival needs would usually take priority over growth needs.

Several theoretic frameworks have been developed specifically for nursing practice and serve as a reference to guide nurses in assessment and implementation of nursing care. The concepts are abstract to allow for broad application. All the frameworks are applicable to the care of patients with medical-surgical disorders. Some of the more commonly used frameworks include Rogers' Life Process model, Roy's Adaptation model, Orem's Self-care Agency model, and Johnson's Behavioral Systems model. The manner in which data are organized and used differs with the conceptual framework, but the underlying process used by the nurse is the same.

NURSING PROCESS

The systematic approach used to carry out nursing's independent functions is frequently termed *nursing process*. It is a way of thinking and acting based on the scientific method rather than on intuition. It provides organization and direction of nursing activities, a means for predicting outcomes and evaluating results, and a method for establishing standards of nursing care.

Nursing process provides a framework for (1) identification of health care needs amenable to nursing care, (2) determination of patient goals (outcomes) and nursing actions, (3) implementation of nursing actions, and (4) evaluation of results of nursing actions. This systematic process is usually divided into either four or five steps; the overall process is the same regardless of the number of steps. The five-step process is as follows:

1. Assessment: collecting patient data of pertinence to nursing
2. Data analysis: using the collected data to identify the patient's health care needs that can be influenced by nursing care (nursing diagnoses)
3. Planning: determining priorities, expected patient outcomes, and specific nursing actions
4. Implementation: carrying out the planned nursing actions necessary to accomplish the defined goals
5. Evaluation: determining the extent to which the goals have been achieved

Nurses who use a four-step approach include data analysis

Table 1-4   **Types of data**

Type	Definition	Methods	Examples
Subjective	Statements by the person concerning thoughts or feelings (psychologic, physical) that cannot be validated	Interview, interaction	Statements about pain, nausea, itching Statements about fears, desires, beliefs, attitudes, values
Objective	Data perceptible by the external senses that can be validated by others	Inspection, auscultation, palpation, percussion, olfaction	Vomiting, scratching, auditory breath sounds, palpable lymph nodes, breath odor

as part of assessment; thus the four steps become assessment, planning, implementation, and evaluation.

Nursing process is discussed in great detail in fundamentals of nursing texts and in some books devoted to the topic; thus only a brief summary is presented here.

Assessment

An initial assessment is made when the person first enters the hospital or health care agency. However, since health is a dynamic, ever-changing state, assessment must be a continuous, ongoing process.

Data may be collected from a primary source (patient) or from secondary sources (family, friends, patient records, health team members). The data may be subjective or objective (Table 1-4). The differentiation is important. *Subjective* data are necessary for providing understanding of the patient's experience and sense of illness or well-being, but since these data cannot be validated, they are subject to wide interpretation. For example, one person may describe a specific pain intensity as "severe," whereas another person may describe the same pain intensity as "mild." *Objective* data are verifiable and measurable; for example, each person palpating the same lymph node can describe it as 2×3 cm in size, oval shaped, and freely movable. Subjective data are collected either by a nursing history or during patient/family interactions. Objective data are obtained by means of a head-to-toe physical examination or by physical inspection carried on during nursing care activities. Data specific to patients with medical-surgical disorders are described in later chapters of the text. Differentiation is made between subjective and objective data.

Data Analysis: Nursing Diagnosis

The second step of nursing process is making conclusions from the collected data. The process of data analysis may be referred to as *diagnosis*; however, so as not to confuse the process with the end product, the term *nursing diagnosis* in this discussion is limited to the end product of data analysis.

Some form of organizing framework for the data is required to facilitate data analysis. The theoretic framework used by the nurse in practice may identify categories useful for data analysis. Gordon[13] has identified eleven *functional health patterns* (see Box 1-2) that contribute to health, quality of life, and achievement of human potential. These patterns are interrelated, interactive, and interdependent; thus all patterns need to be assessed for function or dys-

---

1-2

Gordon's functional health patterns

Health perception—Health management
Nutritional—Metabolic
Elimination
Activity—Exercise
Sleep—Rest
Cognitive—Perceptual
Self-perception—Self-concept
Role relationship
Sexuality—Reproductive
Coping—Stress tolerance
Value—Belief

From Gordon M: *Manual of nursing diagnosis 1991-1992*, St. Louis, 1991, Mosby–Year Book.

---

function. The health patterns can be used as a guiding framework for data collection, regardless of the conceptual framework for nursing practice used by the practitioner.

The North American Nursing Diagnosis Association (NANDA) has developed a taxonomy in which the NANDA nursing diagnoses are grouped under the nine headings of exchanging, communicating, relating, valuing, choosing, moving, perceiving, knowing, and feeling.

General conclusions

Four general conclusions can be drawn from analysis of patient data (Fig. 1-2):

1. Data is insufficient; more data must be gathered before conclusions can be made.
2. The person or family is functioning at optimal level and is not at high risk; no interventions are required.
3. The person or family is functioning well, but health risk factors are high; a high risk for dysfunction is present, such as "Infection, high risk for."
4. The person or family is functioning inadequately and actions are desirable.

When dysfunctions are identified, one of three approaches may be taken. First, the person or family may have already identified the dysfunction and may have taken appropriate actions; therefore no further help is needed. Second, action is needed that is better carried out by another health professional; the nurse makes the appropriate referral. In the third option, nursing interventions are indicated and the nurse then determines the nursing diagnosis.

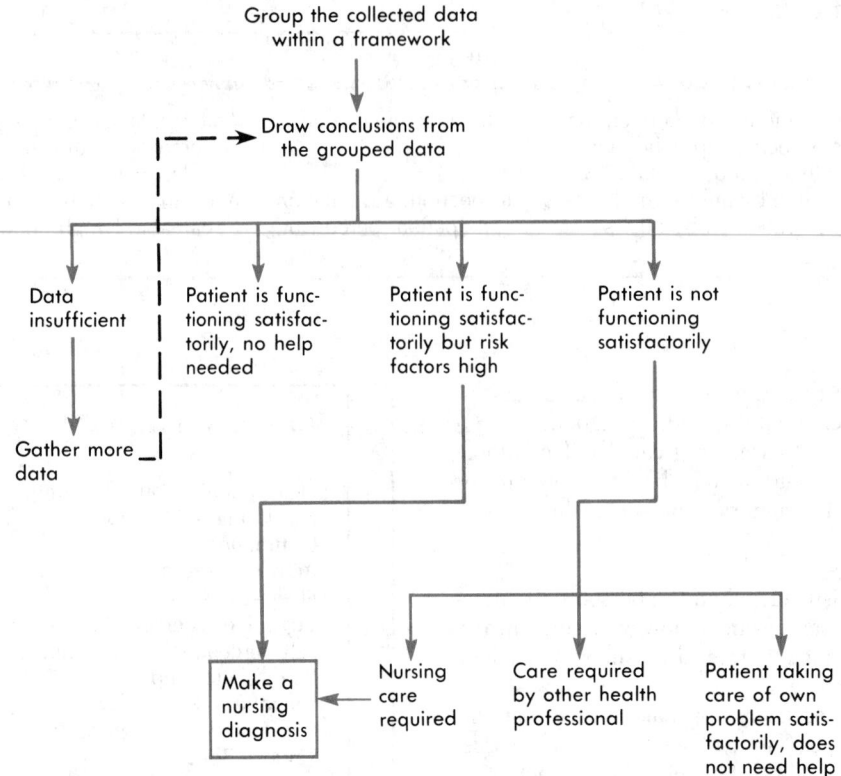

Fig. 1-2   Process of data analysis.

Nursing diagnosis

Although nursing diagnosis has been defined in various ways, most definitions include the following characteristics:

1. A statement or conclusion
2. An actual or high-risk health problem
3. Identified from a nursing assessment
4. The legal and educational domain of nursing

Nursing diagnoses are therefore different from medical diagnoses. The domain of medical practice is the identification of disease (medical diagnosis) and the treatment of these diseases. In 1980, the Congress of Nursing Practice of the American Nurses' Association defined nursing as "the diagnosis and treatment of *human responses to actual or potential health problems.*"[33] Thus a disease cannot be considered a nursing diagnosis, but how a person *responds* to dysfunction, such as by activity intolerance, anxiety, incontinence, and so forth, is the domain of nursing.

Some nursing actions, however, do *not* ensue from nursing diagnoses. Recall that nursing actions may be of two types, independent and interdependent or collaborative. Making a nursing diagnosis and carrying out actions appropriate for the identified nursing diagnoses are nursing's independent actions. Monitoring activities to collect data for the physician (collaborative action) is not an action that ensues from nursing diagnoses.

Nursing diagnoses statements are not limited to dysfunction (patient problems). The goal of nursing is optimal health of the person/family; support and assistance may be needed to help persons *maintain* certain health practices.

For example, one woman sought assistance from a nurse to help her work through her feelings about caring for her dying mother. The woman was coping satisfactorily but needed support from the nurse to maintain coping. Most accepted nursing diagnoses identified to date relate primarily to problems or high-risk problems. It is anticipated that in the future more diagnoses will be developed that are intended to help persons move toward optimal levels of health.

A nursing diagnosis statement consists of two parts: (1) a pattern of functioning or health problem, and (2) the factors that influence or are related to the functioning (etiologic or related factors). In addition, each diagnosis has defining characteristics, such as a cluster of signs and symptoms, that serve as criteria for diagnostic judgment. Gordon[13] refers to the three components as the PES format: health problem (P), etiologic or related factors (E), and defining characteristics or cluster of signs and symptoms (S). The third component (S) is not listed in the diagnosis statement but can be found in reference materials.

An example of a nursing diagnosis is as follows:

> Constipation related to decreased activity following surgery and to low fluid intake

The phrase "related to" is used to cite the etiologic factors rather than "due to," as an indication of relatedness but not necessarily to show cause and effect.

Nursing diagnoses approved by NANDA are listed in Box 1-3. These diagnoses are used throughout this text.

1-3

NANDA-accepted nursing diagnoses

Activity intolerance
Activity intolerance, high risk for
Adjustment, impaired
Airway clearance, ineffective
Anxiety
Aspiration, high risk for
Body image disturbance
Body temperature, altered, high risk for
Bowel incontinence
Breastfeeding, effective
Breastfeeding, ineffective
Breastfeeding, interrupted
Breathing pattern, ineffective
Cardiac output, decreased
Caregiver role strain
Caregiver role strain, high risk for
Communication, impaired verbal
Constipation
Constipation, colonic
Constipation, perceived
Coping, defensive
Coping, family: potential for growth
Coping, ineffective family: compromised
Coping, ineffective family: disabling
Coping, ineffective individual
Decisional conflict (specify)
Denial, ineffective
Diarrhea
Disuse syndrome, high risk for
Diversional activity deficit
Dysfunctional Ventilatory Weaning Response
  (DVWR)
Dysreflexia
Family processes, altered
Fatigue
Fear
Fluid volume deficit (1)
Fluid volume deficit (2)
Fluid volume deficit, high risk for
Fluid volume excess
Gas exchange, impaired
Grieving, anticipatory
Grieving, dysfunctional
Growth and development, altered
Health maintenance, altered
Health seeking behaviors (specify)
Home maintenance management, impaired
Hopelessness
Hyperthermia
Hypothermia
Inability to sustain spontaneous ventilation
Incontinence, functional
Incontinence, reflex
Incontinence, stress
Incontinence, total
Incontinence, urge
Infant feeding pattern, ineffective
Infection, high risk for
Injury, high risk for
Knowledge deficit (specify)
Management of therapeutic regimen (individuals), in-
  effective

Mobility, impaired physical
Noncompliance (specify)
Nutrition, altered: less than body requirements
Nutrition, altered: more than body requirements
Nutrition, altered: high risk for more than body re-
  quirements
Oral mucous membrane, altered
Pain
Pain, chronic
Parental role conflict
Parenting, altered
Parenting, altered, high risk for
Peripheral neurovascular dysfunction, high risk for
Personal identity disturbance
Poisoning, high risk for
Post-trauma response
Powerlessness
Protection, altered
Rape-trauma syndrome
Rape-trauma syndrome: compound reaction
Rape-trauma syndrome, silent reaction
Relocation stress syndrome
Role performance, altered
Self care deficit, bathing/hygiene
Self care deficit, dressing/grooming
Self care deficit, feeding
Self care deficit, toileting
Self-esteem disturbance
Self-esteem, chronic low
Self-esteem, situational low
Self-mutilation, high risk for
Sensory/perceptual alterations (specify) (visual, audi-
  tory, kinesthetic, gustatory, tactile, olfactory)
Sexual dysfunction
Sexuality patterns, altered
Skin integrity, impaired
Skin integrity, impaired, high risk for
Sleep pattern disturbance
Social interaction, impaired
Social isolation
Spiritual distress (distress of the human spirit)
Suffocation, high risk for
Swallowing, impaired
Thermoregulation, ineffective
Thought processes, altered
Tissue integrity, impaired
Tissue perfusion, altered (specify type) (renal, cere-
  bral; cardiopulmonary, gastrointestinal, peripheral)
Trauma, high risk for
Unilateral neglect
Urinary elimination, altered patterns
Urinary retention
Violence, high risk for: self-directed or directed at
  others

Planning

Planning nursing care involves several steps:
1. Setting priorities when several nursing diagnoses have been identified
2. Determining goals (outcomes) of care for each nursing diagnosis
3. Selecting specific nursing actions

Setting priorities

When several nursing diagnoses have been identified, it must be determined which diagnoses take priority. One approach is the basic needs approach. Nursing diagnoses that pertain to physiologic and safety needs usually take precedence over love and belonging or self-esteem needs.

Priorities can also be determined by considering threats to the integrity of the individual. The following priority system can be used:

First   Immediate life-threatening problems (for example, lack of oxygen)
Second   Threats to physiologic or psychologic integrity for which the person is at *high risk*
Third   Threats to physiologic or psychologic integrity for which the person is at *low risk* (but which may occur if action is not taken)
Fourth   Health maintenance

This system does not deny the importance of health maintenance but emphasizes that when health problems are present, these problems are attended to first.

Setting of priorities does not mean numbering each nursing diagnosis from 1 to N in order of importance. It means that when a large number of nursing diagnoses have been identified, the most important diagnoses are selected to be principally addressed.

Goal setting

The next step in planning is to determine the goals or desired patient outcomes to be achieved. *Mutual nurse-patient goal setting* is implemented whenever possible so that there is congruency between what both the nurse and the patient expect as a result of nursing interventions. The role of the nurse is to facilitate the patient's recovery and future health maintenance; thus both must be moving toward the same goals.

Goals (expected patient outcomes) are stated as *observable patient behaviors*: behavior (or signs) that is observed in the patient if the goal is met. For example, the statement "prevent skin breakdown" is a poor goal, since it indicates nursing action and does not indicate a patient outcome to be met. The same idea stated in observable patient-outcome terms is "skin on sacral area remains intact, no redness is observed." To evaluate whether this goal had been met, the sacral area is inspected for signs of redness or breakdown in skin integrity.

Patient outcomes are written according to the following criteria: have measurable verbs, be specific in content and time, and be attainable.[5] Examples of verbs that are *not* measurable are "understands," "knows," or "appreciates." Time is included when appropriate; for example, "Walks around room 6/24, to nurses station 6/25, and to lounge 6/26." The more specifically the expected outcomes are written, the easier is the evaluation. The expected patient outcomes serve as the criteria for evaluation.

Health care agencies participate in quality assurance review (see Chapter 2). During the process of quality assurance review, *standards* are developed and outcome criteria are identified. Some of these outcome criteria are useful guidelines in determining expected patient outcomes.

Goals are derived primarily from the first part (the pattern of functioning) of the nursing diagnosis statement.

Example:

Nursing diagnosis   Activity intolerance: decreased muscle strength (legs) related to decreased activity
Long-term goal   Leg muscles test at full baseline strength
Short-term goal   Patient raises legs 2 inches above bed against resistance within 3 days

Long-term goals describe what patient behaviors are expected for resolution of the nursing diagnosis. Short-term goals describe expected patient behaviors indicating that action is headed in the right direction toward resolution, that is, they are short steps to be achieved toward reaching the long-term goal.

Selection of nursing actions

Usually several alternative actions can be chosen to reach a desired outcome or goal. Selection of actions is usually guided by the second part (etiologic factors) of the nursing diagnosis. For example, different nursing actions are selected for a nursing diagnosis of "Sleep pattern disturbance: insomnia related to fear of surgery" than are selected for a nursing diagnosis of "Sleep pattern disturbance: insomnia related to persistent cough."

The action alternatives are identified and choices are made depending on the specific patient situation. Patient input is sought when feasible. When a nurse follows a preset plan of action for any given nursing diagnosis, patient care is not individualized and there is less potential for accomplishment of the desired outcomes. The determination of action alternatives is based on knowledge from experts, suggestions from the patient, observations of actions of others, suggestions from other health care providers, and the nurse's own creativity. Actions are based on scientific principles.

Selection of action is based on the following guidelines:
- The greatest possibility of success
- The least risk
- The least discomfort
- The least intrusiveness for the patient

Once the course of action has been selected, the *frequency* of action must also be determined. For example, the frequency of deep breathing and coughing exercises selected as an activity would be planned at different intervals for different patients based on risk factors such as obesity and smoking habits identified through analysis of the data.

Implementation

Nursing interventions for persons who are at risk for or who have pathophysiologic disorders are directed toward *restoring* optimal health and *maintaining* optimal health (see Box 1-4). Although the major focus of the care of the person who is ill may be health restoration, health maintenance interventions may be carried out concurrently to help the person maintain optimal functioning wherever possible.

Guidelines for Care

1-4

Patients at risk for or who have a pathophysiologic disorder

Health restoration

Assisting with achievement of therapeutic goals
    Monitoring for signs of healing or complications
    Carrying out prescribed medical therapies that
        the patient is unable to do for self
Promoting functioning of those mechanisms nec-
    essary for optimal health, for example, oxygen-
    ation, nutrition, elimination
Promoting comfort and activities of daily living
    (ADL)
Modifying the environment to enhance healing
    and wellness
Counseling and teaching
    Promoting coping and adaptation to changes in
        health care
    Teaching the patient to care for self

Health maintenance

Monitoring for changes in health status
Teaching the patient and family or friends
    The nature of the illness or disease
    Signs and symptoms indicating presence of dis-
        ease or complications to be reported to phy-
        sician
    Health promotion activities (nutrition, activity,
        etc.)
    Specific preventive measures
    Rationale for medical therapies
    Name, dosage, actions, and side effects of pre-
        scribed medications
    Availability of community resources
    Need for continual monitoring or follow-up
        care, as necessary

1-5

Possible reasons for not achieving patient goals

Database	Incomplete; changes in data
Nursing diag- **nosis**	Inaccurate data analysis; inaccu- rate statement
Goals	Unrelated to nursing diagnosis; nonspecific; unrealistic
Nursing ac- **tions**	Unrelated to nursing diagnosis or goal(s); nonspecific, therefore poorly implemented; inade- quate in degree of action taken

nent record. In others the data are recopied onto other sheets in the permanent record. Flow sheets are used extensively in special care areas such as intensive care units, where continual monitoring of several parameters is necessary.

Different formats may be used to record nursing interventions and patient responses. Forms or narrative notes may be used for charting significant data pertaining to each nursing diagnosis. The important point is that, regardless of the format used by the health care agency, activities that were carried out must be documented to clarify the nursing care provided and to serve as a data base for evaluation of the effectiveness of the care provided.

Evaluation

The last step of nursing process consists of determining whether the desired outcomes are met, analyzing the effectiveness of nursing interventions, and planning for subsequent care. The method of evaluation consists of collecting data from the patient based on the criteria established as patient goals (outcomes). Thus the more specifically the goals are stated in observable patient behaviors, the easier the task of evaluation. For example, a nursing diagnosis of "Constipation, related to inadequate fluid intake" could have a goal of "Stool soft and formed." Evaluation then consists of inspecting the stool. If it is soft and formed, the goal is achieved and the patient's constipation is corrected.

Some of the reasons why goals are not achieved are listed in Box 1-5.

Once the possible reason for the lack of goal achievement is identified, revisions are made and the process is repeated. As can be noted, nursing care is an ongoing and dynamic process that requires constant assessment and evaluation.

ETHICAL DILEMMAS IN MEDICAL-SURGICAL NURSING

An ethical dilemma arises when, based on moral considerations, one of two opposing actions can be taken and the person perceives the possibility of either response. Evidence can be presented to support either action, but the evidence on both sides is inconclusive.[8]

Numerous ethical dilemmas arise in medical-surgical nursing practice. The dilemmas are not solely the domain of medical-surgical nursing but occur to a large extent

---

The interventions selected for a specific patient will be determined by the identified nursing diagnoses and the specific pathophysiologic disorders present or for which the person is at risk. Possible nursing interventions are described in appropriate chapters in this text.

Because the goal of nursing care is the patient's optimal health, self-care is stressed to the extent possible; the patient is usually ultimately responsible for on-going health maintenance. Thus teaching, supporting, and motivating are major nursing strategies. If self-care is impossible or inappropriate, the nurse then compensates for the patient's inability by performing the actions. Monitoring is an ongoing strategy; the type and degree usually depend on the illness or disease.

Recording (documentation)

Actions that have been taken and the patient's response to the actions need to be documented. Responses to monitoring activities are most easily recorded on *flow sheets*. The flow sheets provide a means of quick comparison of a specific monitoring parameter over time. Data such as vital signs, fluid intake and output, activity, and urine tests are recorded as they are gathered. In some institutions these sheets subsequently become part of the patient's perma-

during the care of these patients. These dilemmas may include, but are not limited to, the following:

1. Withholding information from the patient
2. Providing informed consent
3. Use of invasive techniques
4. Selection of patients for scarce therapies (such as organ transplantation)
5. Withholding or withdrawing treatment/nourishment
6. Quality of life versus prolongation of life
7. Right to commit suicide with terminal illness
8. Euthanasia
9. Definitions of death

Nursing students have an opportunity to discuss the ethical issues and to obtain feedback and support from instructors and fellow students. Because ethical dilemmas are complex and do not have one conclusive action, the professional nurse may be frequently faced with unresolved issues. Mechanisms have been developed to assist nurses to cope with conflicts that ensue. Team conferences may be held under the leadership of a nurse ethicist who has advanced preparation in ethics. Interdisciplinary conferences may also be instituted. Support may be given on an individual basis with the nurse ethicist.

Some ethical issues are discussed in appropriate chapters of this text. The reference list for this chapter includes some resources from the literature that may be helpful.

SUMMARY

1. Medical-surgical nursing focuses on the care of adults who are at risk for or who have medical-surgical disorders.
2. Health promotion refers to activities directed toward helping persons to maintain or achieve a high level of functioning and feeling of well-being.
3. Prevention refers to activities directed toward protecting persons from potential or actual threats to health and the subsequent consequences.
4. Primary prevention includes protective measures against disease or trauma. Secondary prevention includes early detection and treatment to decrease the intensity or to prevent complications. Tertiary prevention consists of activities that prevent or limit disabilities and help promote rehabilitation.
5. Persons at risk are those considered to have a greater possibility of becoming ill or acquiring a certain disease. Factors that place the person at risk are termed risk factors.
6. Illness can be considered the opposite of wellness and implies a lower level of functioning. Disease is a pathologic process having a characteristic set of signs and symptoms. Diseases may be acute or chronic.
7. The stages of disease progression are (1) presymptomatic or subclinical stage in which changes are occurring but no signs or symptoms are present; (2) the clinical stage, characterized by signs and symptoms; and (3) the rehabilitation stage (in chronic diseases), characterized by residual disabilities.
8. The sick role exempts the person from normal social roles and responsibilities and permits the person to assume a dependent relationship that facilitates receiving the required medical care.
9. Independent nursing actions are those which the nurse takes after analysis of data pertaining to those aspects of the person's health that are amenable to nursing intervention. Interdependent or collaborative nursing actions are those taken by the nurse in assisting other health care professionals.
10. Epidemiology is the study of the incidence, distribution, and determinants of diseases and injuries in human populations. Etiology refers to the study of specific causes of diseases.
11. Pathophysiology is the study of the effect of disease on body organs and systems and on total body functioning.
12. Signs are objective evidence and symptoms are subjective evidence of disease or dysfunction.
13. The five steps of nursing process are assessment, data analysis, planning, implementation, and evaluation.
14. Gordon's 11 functional health patterns are useful for data collection and analysis regardless of the conceptual model.
15. Two types of assessment are initial and ongoing; baseline observations are those that are made initially for future comparison.
16. Nursing diagnosis is a statement of an actual or potential health problem identified from nursing assessment and which is the legal and educational domain of nursing.
17. Nursing diagnosis statements consist of two parts: pattern of functioning and etiology; each diagnosis also has defining characteristics such as a cluster of signs and symptoms.
18. Goals are determined from the pattern of functioning and nursing actions from the etiologies.
19. Priorities for care can be set on the basis of life-threatening problems, high risk, low risk, and health maintenance.
20. Expected patient outcomes (goals) are written as observable patient behaviors.
21. Nursing actions are selected on the basis of the greatest possibility of success with the least risk, discomfort or intrusiveness to the patient.
22. Evaluation consists of collecting patient data based on criteria established in the expected patient outcomes.
23. Numerous ethical dilemmas occur in medical-surgical nursing practice, including withholding of information or therapies, use of invasive techniques, and issues associated with death.
24. Nurse ethicists can assist practicing nurses to cope with conflicts resulting from ethical dilemmas.

STUDY QUESTIONS

- What are some practices you follow that promote health or prevent disease? What practices do you follow that are deterrents to health? How difficult would it be for you to change your behavior?
- How do the three levels of prevention differ?
- What theoretic framework do you use in the practice of

nursing? Can you correlate Gordon's functional health patterns with your framework for data analysis?
- How do the different parts of a nursing diagnosis assist you in planning nursing care?
- Read some of the chapter references that cite specific ethical dilemmas. To what extent do you think these dilemmas might provide conflicts to you in the care of these patients?

REFERENCES AND SELECTED READINGS

1. Alfaro R: *Application of nursing process: a step-by-step guide*, Philadelphia, 1986, JB Lippincott.
2. Allen CV: *Comprehending the nursing process: a workbook approach*, Norwalk, CT, 1991, Appleton & Lange.
3. American Nurses' Association: *Ethics in nursing*, Kansas City, MO, 1988, The Association.
4. American Nurses Association Committee on Ethics: *Guidelines on withholding or withdrawing food and fluids*, Kansas City, Mo, 1988, The Association.
5. Carpenito LJ: *Handbook of nursing diagnosis ed 4*, Hagerstown, MD, 1991, JB Lippincott.
*6. Carpenito LJ: *Nursing care plans and documentation: nursing diagnoses and collaborative problems*, Hagerstown, MD, 1991, JB Lippincott Co.
*7. Cassells J, Redman B: Preparing students to be moral agents in clinical nursing practice, *Nurs Clin North Am* 24:463-473, 1989.
8. Davis AJ, Aroskar MA: *Ethical dilemmas and nursing practice*, ed 3, Norwalk, CT, 1991, Appleton & Lange.
9. Edelman C, Mandle CL: *Health promotion throughout the life span*, St Louis, 1986, Mosby–Year Book.
10. Fowler MD, Levine-Ariff J: *Ethics at the bedside: a source book for the critical care nurse*, Hagerstown, MD, 1987, JB Lippincott.
11. Friedman E, editor: *Making choices: ethics issues for health care professionals*, Chicago, 1986, American Hospital Association.
12. Gillick MR: Common-sense models of health and disease, *N Engl J Med* 313(11):700-703, 1985.
13. Gordon M: *Manual of nursing diagnosis 1991-1992*, St Louis, 1991, Mosby–Year Book.
*14. Gordon M: *Nursing diagnosis: process and application*, ed 2, St Louis, 1987, Mosby–Year Book.
15. Greenberg JS: Health and wellness: a conceptual differentiation, *J Sch Health* 55:403-406, 1985.
16. Griffith-Kenney JW, Christensen PJ: *Nursing process, application of theories, frameworks and models*, ed 2, St Louis, 1986, Mosby–Year Book.
*17. Iwerson E: Dilemmas in practice: life at what cost? *Am J Nurs* 88:639-640, 1988.
*18. Iyer P, Camp N: *Nursing documentation: a nursing process approach*, St Louis, 1991, Mosby–Year Book.
19. Kim MJ, McFarland GK, McLane AM: *Pocket guide to nursing diagnoses*, ed 4, St Louis, 1991, Mosby–Year Book.
20. Mausner JS, Kramer S: *Epidemiology: an introductory text*, ed 2, Philadelphia, 1985, WB Saunders.
21. McFarland GK, McFarlane EA: *Nursing diagnosis and intervention: planning for patient care*, St Louis, 1989, Mosby–Year Book.
*22. Mitchell C: Dilemmas in practice: steadying the hand that feeds, *Am J Nurs* 87:293-296, 1987.
*23. Mumma CM: Withholding nutrition: a nursing perspective, *Nurs Adm Q* 10(3):31-38, 1986.
*24. Muyskens JL: Dilemmas in practice: acting alone, *Am J Nurs* 87:1141-1146, 1987.
*25. Otte DM, Allen KS: Ethical principles in the nursing care of terminally ill adults, *Oncol Nurs Forum* 14(5):87-91, 1987.
*26. Pauly-O'Neill S: Dilemmas in practice: questioning the use of invasive technology, *AJN* 91(1):19-20, 1991.
27. Pender NJ: *Health promotion in nursing practice*, ed 3, Norwalk, Ct, 1987, Appleton & Lange.
28. Prohaska TR, et al: Health practices and illness cognition in young, middle aged, and elderly adults, *J Gerontol* 40:569-578, 1985.
29. Silva M: *Ethical decision making in nursing*, Norwalk, CT, 1989, Appleton & Lange.
*30. Thomasma DC: Ethics and professional practice in oncology, *Sem Oncol Nurs* 5(2):89-94, 1989.
31. Thomasma DC: The range of euthanasia, *Am Coll Surg Bull* 73(8):3-13, 1988.
32. Webster JA: The wellness mode: feeling good about you, *AORN J* 41:713-718, 1985.

Classic

33. American Nurses Association: *Nursing: a social policy statement*, No. NP-63, Kansas City, Mo, 1980, The Association.
34. Maudinger MO, Jauron GD: Developing a nursing diagnosis, *Nurs Outlook* 23:94-98, 1975.

*Recommended for student reading.

2

Quality Management in Nursing

Frances R. Chester
Mary Lou Monahan

After studying this chapter, the learner should be able to:

- Define quality management.
- Identify three reasons why quality management is an important aspect of the practice of nursing.
- Describe the steps of the American Nurses' Association (ANA) model of quality assurance.
- State the difference between standards and criteria.
- Name five mechanisms involved in implementing quality management programs.
- Describe the use of quality indicators as one means for monitoring quality of care.

IMPETUS FOR QUALITY MANAGEMENT

Nursing is committed to professional excellence in providing the highest quality of care possible. Implicit in this commitment is the responsibility to evaluate the quality and appropriateness of that care. However, it has only been in the last 21 years that attempts have been made to develop an extrinsic, systematic approach to monitor and improve care. The impetus for this change has come from a variety of sources: (1) legislation; (2) changes in third-party reimbursement; (3) economic factors; and (4) the nursing profession itself. *Until recently this process was known as quality assurance; it is now called quality management.* ✳

Legislation

Since the passage of Medicare/Medicaid legislation in 1965, the federal government has become the largest source of third-party health care payment. Because of this increasing financial commitment, Congress and government officials at all levels are under pressure to ensure: (1) that the services rendered are necessary; (2) that they meet professionally recognized standards of care; and (3) that they contain costs.

Third-Party Reimbursement

To establish some system of accountability for expenditures, Congress created a system for reviewing health care expenses as part of Public Law 92-603, the Social Security Amendments of 1972. This legislation established a nationwide network of professional standards review organizations (PSROs) for review of patient care financed by the federal government. Private insurance carriers such as Blue Cross also established standards for review of the care for which they have been asked to make payment.

These efforts were essentially ineffectual and by 1981 more stringent fiscal measures were passed by Congress in the Omnibus Reconciliation Act, which imposed cost-sharing requirements on Medicare beneficiaries and made substantial reductions in federal contributions to Medicaid. Changes in the Social Security Act in 1982 mandated prospective Medicare payments using the 467 Diagnosis Related Group (DRG) categories. Both of these later legislative changes have resulted in cost-containment strategies that have increasingly raised questions of whether the quality of health care has diminished because of the increased emphasis on reducing costs.

Economic Factors

Because health care costs have assumed an increasing share of the gross national product (GNP) in the past two decades, consumers and legislators have increased scrutiny of the components of this cost. Reviewing the cost of illness raises vital questions about the relation of quality of care to cost. For example, the principle of "high cost/low benefit" is defined by poor quality of health care in terms of overdiagnosis or overtreatment, which can lead to excessive health care expenditures even in the absence of any *iatrogenic* or untoward consequences. *Poor quality in the form of misdiagnosis, mistreatment, or inadequate nursing care can increase mortality or morbidity, length of hospital stay, and loss of earnings, and, therefore, this poor quality can increase the costs of health care to individuals and to society.*

2-1

American Nurses' Association standards of nursing practice

Standard I: The collection of data about the health status of the client/patient is systematic and continuous. The data are accessible, communicated, and recorded.

Standard II: Nursing diagnoses are derived from health status data.

Standard III: The plan of nursing care includes goals derived from the nursing diagnoses.

Standard IV: The plan of nursing care includes priorities and the prescribed nursing approaches or measures to achieve the goals derived from the nursing diagnoses.

Standard V: Nursing actions provide for client/patient participation in health promotion, maintenance, and restoration.

Standard VI: Nursing actions assist the client/patient to maximize health capabilities.

Standard VII: The client's/patient's progress or lack of progress toward goal achievement is determined by the client/patient and the nurse.

Standard VIII: The client's/patient's progress or lack of progress toward goal achievement directs reassessment, reordering of priorities, new goal setting, and revision of the plan of nursing care.

From American Nurses' Association Standards of Nursing Practice, Kansas City, Mo., 1973, The Association. Reprinted by permission of the American Nurses' Association.

The current economic situation that exists with health care costs growing at an unacceptable rate, budgetary cutbacks, and DRG reimbursement has implications for nursing. More than ever before, the nursing profession must demonstrate the value and benefits of its service if it wishes to retain government and consumer support.

Professional Standards

Last but certainly not least, the nursing profession itself places as its highest goal the delivery of quality health care. The American Nurses' Association (ANA) published *Standards of Nursing Practice*[26] in 1973 for the purpose of ensuring quality health care to the public (see Box 2-1). However, primary responsibility for implementing these standards rests with the individual nurse in the practice setting. Individual nurses must be familiar with both general and specific standards pertinent to the patient population for whom they are responsible (for example, the standards of care for the orthopedic patient). These standards identify elements of nursing care that must be met to ensure that quality care is delivered and to provide a baseline for measuring that quality.

Other professional standards that apply to the nurse in the practice setting are nurse practice acts, medical practice acts, and standards set by the Joint Commission on Accreditation of Healthcare Organizations (JCAHO).[11] Almost every state has a nurse practice act and a medical practice act. Both of these are external sources of standards for nursing practices. Together they define and delineate, from a legal standpoint, the content and practice of nursing.

Nurse practice acts define nursing practice and identify those activities that fall within the province of nursing. *Medical practice acts* further delineate nursing practice by defining those areas that are the exclusive province of the physician. Such exclusions limit the activities in which nurses may engage. Neither act sets actual standards for practice; rather, they define general areas of activity for both professions and establish the legal relationship of the nurse to society and to related professions.

The JCAHO is a voluntary, nongovernmental organization that, since its incorporation in 1951, has established standards for operation of hospitals and other health facilities. It conducts surveys and accreditation programs to promote high-quality care and to ensure that patients receive the optimum benefits that medical science has to offer. It emphasizes organization and administration of functions for efficient patient care. Compliance with JCAHO standards is recognized by issuance of certificates of accreditation.

The governing body of the JCAHO, the Board of Commissioners, consists of 24 persons appointed by its four member organizations: The American College of Physicians, the American College of Surgeons, the American Hospital Association, and the American Medical Association. Effective January 1993 a nurse-at-large member will be added to the governing body.

JCAHO accreditation is voluntary and is not the same as licensure or certification by state or local authorities. However, accreditation has come to be recognized as a benchmark of quality and is used by some regulatory agencies as one criterion for licensure or certification and by some insurance agencies as a condition for honoring reimbursement claims. In addition to its standards for organization of the nursing service department, a standard on quality of professional services was added in 1976, and delineates the characteristics of a patient care evaluation program. Since 1988, this standard required an ongoing, planned, and systematic process for evaluating the quality and appropriateness of patient care. This process is composed of the following 10 steps:

1. Assign responsibility for monitoring and evaluation activities
2. Delineate the scope of care provided by the nursing department
3. Identify the most important aspects of care provided by the nursing staff
4. Identify indicators (and appropriate clinical criteria) for monitoring the important aspects of care
5. Establish thresholds (levels, patterns, trends) for the indicators that trigger evaluation of the care
6. Monitor the important aspects of care by collecting and organizing the data for each indicator
7. Evaluate care when thresholds are reached to identify either opportunities to improve care or problems
8. Take actions to improve or to correct identified problems
9. Assess the effectiveness of the actions and document the improvement in care
10. Communicate the results of the monitoring and evaluation process to relevant individuals, departments, or services and to the organizationwide quality management program

Although the monitoring and evaluation process does not identify every case of suspected substandard care, it does help the nursing staff identify situations on which its attention could be most productively focused. An annual appraisal is conducted of the nursing quality management program to evaluate its effectiveness and revise the indicators as necessary.

DEFINITION OF QUALITY MANAGEMENT

Quality management can be described on two levels. In its strictest sense, it is a set of techniques for assuring the maintenance and improvement of standards and the efficiency and effectiveness of nursing care; more broadly, it is an effort to control nursing practice. As such, it involves relationships between nurses and consumers and between nurses and governmental bodies.

Quality management can be defined as a process that involves evaluating the degree of excellence of the observable and measurable characteristics of delivered nursing care. The purpose of quality management is always twofold. *First,* it determines the extent to which predetermined standards are being met by a particular nursing program. *Second,* these findings are used to make decisions about changes that are to be implemented by persons carrying out the program of care. *Both* must be in place if nursing is to ensure its accountability to the consumer. Although the specific target of each evaluation may differ depending on the information about quality that is desired, the purpose of the evaluation is always the same.

Nurses who are engaged in the delivery of health services cannot escape inclusion of quality management reviews in their practice responsibilities. Indeed, some proficiency in evaluation must be part of the modern nurse's basic repertoire.

The quality management process is not mysterious. Most nurses are well on their way to expertise in this area by virtue of their basic education and experience. Nurses who are expert in the care of specific patient populations (for example, patients with cardiac disease) possess the knowledge necessary to determine desired health processes and outcomes for that population. These nurses are well acquainted with nursing interventions to be used in assisting patients toward health and wellness. They are also aware of the observable changes that will occur at certain intervals in the course of healing.

Most nurses are not expert, however, in the methods used to conduct these evaluations. The following section describes the steps in the quality management review process.

QUALITY MANAGEMENT PROCESS

A variety of techniques have been proposed to perform the quality management review. Presented here is the problem-solving model used by the ANA. Its eight steps include the following:

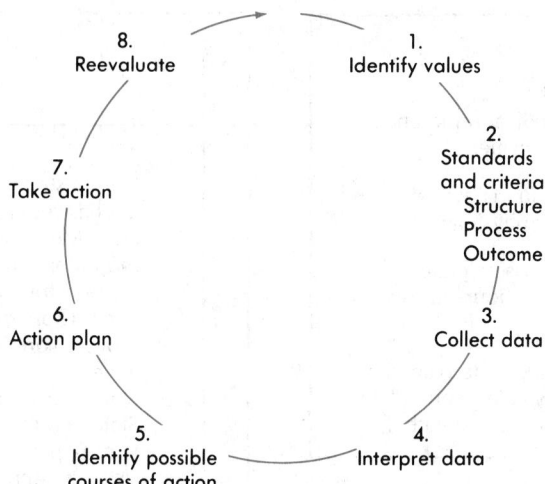

Fig. 2-1 American Nurses' Association model for quality assurance review. (From American Nurses' Association: *Quality assurance for nursing care*, Kansas City, Mo, 1976, The Association. Reprinted by permission of the American Nurses' Association.)

1. Identify values
2. Identify standards and criteria
3. Measure degree of attainment of standards and criteria
4. Interpret strengths and weaknesses
5. Identify possible courses of action
6. Select a course of action
7. Take action
8. Reevaluate

Each of these steps is discussed and illustrated with a clinical example (Fig. 2-1).

Topics for quality management reviews are generally placed in some order of priority based on their frequency of occurrence and their real or potential impact on patient care. Impact is usually gauged by whether efficiency or effectiveness of patient care is affected. *Efficiency* is generally defined in terms of accomplishing a task with a minimum of resources (time, money, personnel); *effectiveness* is defined in terms of accomplishment of predetermined goals. The focus for the evaluation may be the nurse, the unit or institution, the nursing care, or a combination of the three.

If the focus of the evaluation is the nurse, it can include the actions of a single nurse or of all the nurses in a department, and any area of nursing activity can be examined. For example, is the nursing staff satisfied with the primary nursing program instituted 3 months ago? What criteria do the nursing staff use to determine the frequency of vital sign monitoring in the immediate postoperative period? Are the nursing standards for administration of intravenous therapy being adhered to?

If the nursing unit or institution is the focus of the quality management review, it might examine the administrative structure, the physical plant and equipment, or staffing. For example, a review could be implemented to determine whether required educational records for nurses in the critical care units are up to date. Or a review could

be undertaken in conjunction with the environmental services department to determine if an appropriate number of wheelchairs and IV poles are available and whether they are all functional.

When nursing care or a nursing care problem is the focus of the review, it is generally best to limit the scope to a certain population (for example, patients with certain diagnoses, surgical procedures, nursing care problems, or degree of illness) so that the project is manageable in terms of all the variables to be considered.

It is critical to remember that the perspective of the consumer must be considered in any evaluation. In selected instances, such as using patient outcomes or in attempting to validate patient care plans with patients themselves, consumer input is essential.

Steps in a Quality Management Review
Step 1: Identify values

Before the implementation of the quality management model there must be an examination of the *societal, professional,* and *individual values* that guide the health care in the respective agency. The very word *quality* implies that someone somewhere has determined that certain outcomes have more value than others. As applied to nursing care, the individual nurse, nursing unit, hospital, and community interacts to influence the development of criteria to be used in the review process.

To cite some obvious examples, in most Catholic hospitals a high value is placed on human life from the moment of conception; therefore, in a Catholic institution abortions are not performed. A prevailing societal or cultural value may influence another hospital to favor a youth orientation. The emphasis in health care at that institution may, therefore, be oriented toward teen and young adult programs as opposed to geriatric programs. Whatever the setting, the set of values must be identified and understood if the quality assurance review is to be fair and accurate.

2-2

Example of standards and outcomes

Patient goal Adequate pain medication to enable mobilization and pulmonary hygiene.

Structure	Pain medication is available and ordered by physician.
Process	Nursing staff assess patient at least every 4 hours for discomfort.
Outcome	Patient has adequate pain control, and is able to ambulate, cough, and deep breathe.

Step 2: Identify structure, process, outcome, standards, and criteria

A *standard* is the desirable or achievable level or range of performance of a certain criterion, or a framework against which performance is compared. An example of a standard is, "Every patient will have an admission assessment by a registered nurse." A *criterion measure* is that variable believed to be the indicator of the quality of care, for example, "The assessment form will be completed by the admitting nurse within 8 hours of admission."

The *standards for nursing practice* are generally developed by *clinical nursing leaders* in the institution, *using their professional expertise* as well as *professional research and literature*. The standards are made operational by construction of the criterion elements. These criteria, which are the actual evaluation criteria, are generally developed by a quality assurance committee, the nursing practice committee, or some similar group.

The actual criteria that are developed can be of three types: structure, process, and outcome (Box 2-2). *Structure criteria describe the environmental elements, setting, and conditions within which the nurse-patient relationship occurs.* It includes the philosophy and objectives of the institution; its fiscal resources, equipment, physical facilities, management structure, accreditation, and licensure; and the quality and characteristics of the professional and technical employees. Examples of structure criteria include, "Hospital beds must be 3 feet apart." All patients must sign the required consent form before any invasive or surgical procedure." "The current license number of each registered nurse must be on file in the main nursing office."

Process criteria describe the nature and sequence of nursing care activities. For example, process criteria might describe the nursing plan for a patient who demands pain medication every 1½ hours, although he has made a contract with his primary nurse that he will not do so. A teaching plan for a diabetic patient is another example.

Outcome criteria focus on the results of the processes of health care. Many experts consider them the ultimate indicators of the quality of patient care. For the patient the outcome is measurable in terms of change in health, knowledge, or functional status. Examples of outcome criteria for the person with an ostomy are listed in Box 2-3.

2-3

Outcome criteria for the person with a colostomy or ileostomy

The patient or significant other can do the following:
1. Demonstrate how to measure the stoma for an appliance. (The stoma shrinks as healing occurs. Measure the stoma before purchasing more appliances.)
2. Demonstrate proper application of the appliance. (Application includes appliance removal, skin care, and reapplying an appliance.)
3. State plans for follow-up care.
4. State community resources available for obtaining permanent appliances and financial assistance, and list support groups. (Include the name of one surgical supply house, and the telephone number of the Ostomy Association, the Visiting Nurses Association, or some other home care support group).
5. State need to observe stoma and skin around it for redness, bleeding, or excoriation.
6. Patient or significant other has information packet, which has been reviewed with the nurse.

After the criteria are written, they are validated, generally by "consensus among peers." The rationale for this validation step is to ensure that all criteria are correct and relevant and reflect nursing practice at the particular institution. Usually, nurses most expert in the selected clinical area are chosen to do the review.

The final step in the criteria writing process is the establishment, by the quality management committee and the "nurse experts," of a specific and observable level of performance for each criterion measure. For example, for the outcome criterion, "Patient or significant other is able to demonstrate proper technique in insulin administration," at least 90% compliance might be expected. However, for the outcome criterion, "Patient is able to apply own stoma appliance," the committee may decide that 80% compliance is appropriate, because many of the patients are elderly, are not completely independent in activities of daily living by the time of discharge, and are frequently discharged to nursing homes.

Step 3: Measure degree of attainment of standards and criteria

Many methods are available to collect data to assess the attainment of the standards and criteria. The degree to which the actual practice exceeds, meets, or falls below the validated criteria provides the data necessary to evaluate the strengths and weaknesses of the nursing care program. Data collection methods might include *questionnaires, staff interviews, patient interviews, self-assessment questionnaires, performance evaluations, utilization reviews, patient care audits, patient or staff complaints,* and *direct observation.* Whatever the method selected, the data should be easily accessible, and questions of efficiency and accuracy should be considered.

Table 2-1

Outcome criteria for person with colostomy	Level of performance (percentage of compliance)*	Identified problems, strengths, and weaknesses
Patient or significant others can do the following:		
Demonstrate how to measure the stoma for an appliance.	85%	One patient was blind; no documentation on two patients.
Demonstrate proper application of the appliance.	85%	Two patients stated it would have been helpful to have a mirror provided; one patient was blind.
State plans for follow-up care.	60%	Forty percent of patients were being transferred to an extended care facility
State community resources available for purchase of permanent appliances, for financial assistance, and support groups.	80%	Twenty percent of charts audited had one of these components missing.
State need to observe stoma and skin around it for redness and excoriation.	75%	No documentation of this being done on 25% of charts.
Patient or significant other has ostomy informational booklet, which has been reviewed with nurse.	100%	

*Expected compliance in these areas is 100%.

Specific questions that the quality management review committee needs to answer at this point include:

1. Who will collect the data?
2. What will be the source of the data?
3. Where will the data be collected?
4. When will the data be collected?
5. How will the data be collected?

The answers to these questions will assist the committee in deciding whether the review can be accomplished as planned given the inherent requirements for efficiency and accuracy. As a final check, the committee should be certain that each criterion measure is written so that a decision can be easily made as to whether or not the standard has been met.

Once the data is collected, the results are tabulated, and it is determined whether the percentage of yes and no answers corresponds to the previously established level of performance (for example, percentage of compliance) for each criterion. If the level of performance does not achieve the expectations, the criterion for this evaluation item has not been met.

Table 2-1 illustrates one method for keeping track of a multicriterion evaluation process.

Step 4: Interpret strengths and weaknesses

The degree to which the levels of performance have been met serves as the basis for describing the strengths and weaknesses of the nursing care program. However, it is essential that certain subtle factors are not overlooked before final judgments are made. Consider the following: One *outcome criteria for a patient with a pacemaker is, "The patient or significant other is able to take a pulse."* A retrospective nursing audit was performed on patients with pacemakers to determine whether the outcome was being met. On nursing unit A, 95% of the patients could take their pulse, whereas on nursing unit C, only 65% of the patients could. Careful inspection of the patient data revealed that, in

general, patients on unit C were older, had fewer significant others, and were frequently discharged to extended care facilities. Comparing the two units using this information provided insights into reasons for the differences in the units that would have been missed if the evaluator had not questioned why the figures from the two units were so different.

Step 5: Identify possible courses of action

After identifying the strengths and weaknesses, possible courses of action to correct the weaknesses are developed. The goal of the action plan is elimination of the weaknesses and reinforcement of the strengths of the existing program. Consideration should be given to how best to motivate the nursing staff to implement the desired changes. Generally the best results are obtained when those staff most affected by the quality management review are involved in the planning of subsequent courses of action.

Solutions to the identified problems can be numerous and can include administrative changes, further clinical research into the problem, continuing education, changes in practice, environmental changes, a reward system for improved compliance, or even the organization of peer pressure. Each of the possible solutions has advantages and disadvantages, and the peer group has to weigh each one.

Step 6: Select a course of action

After examining the alternatives, the peer group selects the course of action, based on such considerations as the identified problem, available resources, and organizational structure. How the course of action is implemented varies among institutions. Different institutions make varying decisions about how the plan for change is presented to the administration and how the change is to be implemented. In the case of a nursing practice change, at one institution the director of nursing may wish to make the final decision and at another institution the director of

Quality management review topic: learning needs of the patient with a colostomy or ileostomy

Step 1: Identify values

Patient and family education and patient involvement in care are high priorities at this institution. Nurses on the surgical units were concerned that ostomy patients, in particular, were not receiving adequate discharge information.

Step 2: Identify criteria

The outcome criteria (revised in 1990) for the person with a colostomy or ileostomy were selected as the evaluation criteria (see Box 2-3).

Step 3: Collect data

Charts of 30 patients with the discharge diagnosis of some type of ostomy were selected at random from patients discharged in the previous 6 months. Review of patients records using the outcome criteria for the person with a colostomy or ileostomy revealed incomplete teaching plans and no record of the patients having received any type of information booklets. (The rule is, "If it isn't documented, it hasn't been done.")

Step 4: Interpret data

The quality management committee was certain that the patients had received more information than was documented in the record. But where was such documentation to be found? It was also apparent to the committee that some of the criterion elements required updating.

Step 5: Identify possible courses of action

It was observed that the documentation system for discharge planning for these patients needed to be more efficient, yet more thorough. The surgical nursing staff suggested that the outcome criteria sheet be printed on a Nurse's Note Sheet. Another suggestion was to use a large stamp containing elements of the teaching plan, which could be checked off as completed. A group of experienced nurses was formed, who, with the assistance of the clinical nurse specialist, rewrote and assisted in the validation process for the outcome criteria.

Step 6: Write the action plan

The quality management committee met with the surgical nursing staff and concluded that the best choice was to have the outcome criteria overprinted on the Nurse's Note Sheet. The appropriate administrative approval was obtained.

Step 7: Implement the action plan

One member of the quality management committee was assigned to oversee the production of the new forms. After they were obtained, the unit nursing staff took the responsibility for introducing them and explaining their purpose to the other staff members. An evaluation was planned for 4 months later.

Step 8: Reevaluate

Four months after the implementation, the surgical nursing staff conducted a repeat review. There was 100% compliance with each criterion element.

---

nursing may only wish to be informed of the findings, delegating to the committee responsibility to make appropriate changes.

Step 7: Take action

Improving the quality of nursing care implies change, and sooner or later some action must be taken. Implementation of selected action generally includes time frames, persons responsible for overseeing each step of the plan, and selection of a date for reevaluation. This action step is critical to the success of the quality management review.

Step 8: Reevaluate the process

We have added this step to the original ANA model. The rationale for its addition is to illustrate that *once a corrective action or other type of action is taken, the action is monitored* *to ascertain if it is effective in solving the problem.* Therefore, once an action is taken, the cycle begins over again. See Box 2-4 for a clinical example of a quality management review.

MONITORING ACTIVITIES AND INSTRUMENTS

In addition to problem-focused quality management reviews, a variety of methods have been devised for ongoing assessment of the nursing care program. Some of the more frequently used methods are described here.

Incident Reports

Whenever an untoward event occurs involving a patient, nurse, or visitor, an incident report must be completed. Generally these are compiled by the hospital and/or the hospital insurance carrier. Increases in certain types of incidents, such as medication errors or patient falls, is a signal to the quality assurance committee that a review of either of these two areas may be indicated.

Quality Indicators (Monitors or Screens)

Recently the JCAHO has mandated that quality indicators be monitored on an ongoing basis. Each department in an institution determines its own quality indicators.

Quality indicators are those items that a health care agency believes are indicators of quality patient care. For example, quality indicators used by a nursing service would depend on the patient population being served and on *high-risk, high-volume events* that need monitoring. In *medical-surgical nursing*, quality indicators might include the following: (1) *number of patient falls,* (2) *ratio of medication errors to the total doses administered,* and (3) *the number of pressure sores (decubitus ulcers). For each of the quality indicators a threshold of acceptance is set. In the case of falls this threshold might be not more than one patient fall per nursing unit each month.*

By setting the threshold for acceptance a determination can be made as to how well the quality indicator is being met. It is important to establish in advance how and at what intervals data will be collected for each quality indicator.

The appropriateness of each quality indicator needs to be assessed on a *regular basis.* If a particular indicator is no longer high risk or high volume, consideration is given to deleting it. *The important thing to remember is that quality indicators should not be stagnant but should change as circumstances change.*

Nursing Audit

The nursing audit compares predetermined criteria with the documentation found in the patient record. There are two types of audit: retrospective and concurrent. A *retrospective audit is a critical examination of nursing actions, with a view toward improvement in practice. A retrospective review is performed after the patient has been discharged.* The reviewer has the advantage of using data from the patient's entire stay, from admission to discharge, and of evaluating the results for a large numbers of comparable patients. One advantage of a retrospective audit is that sometimes practitioners gain impressions from single cases in which they are personally involved. These impressions, however, may not be borne out by later systematic study of a large number of cases.

A concurrent audit is a critical examination of the patient's progress toward a desired health status (outcome) and patient care management activities (processes) while the care is in progress. Patient questionnaires, interviews, and observation of care as it is being given, and review of the patient record are possible sources of data for a concurrent review. Concurrent review has the advantage of providing opportunities for making changes in the ongoing care program. Retrospective and concurrent reviews each have their own advantages, and may be used singly or together in a quality management review. The term *nursing audit* is used less frequently; it is being replaced by the term *evaluation study.*

Peer Review

Nursing peer review occurs when nurses establish standards and criteria and evaluate the quality of each other's patient care. The peer review process may be performed within a single unit or by specialty, for example, orthopedic nurses. Clinical nurse specialists also frequently have a peer review group that they use to monitor their practice.

Patient Satisfaction Questionnaire

A patient satisfaction questionnaire is generally used when written data regarding a patient's perceptions of his or her hospitalization are needed, for example, by hospital management or a nurse researcher. Many hospitals routinely distribute these questionnaires to all patients and request that they complete them. Other hospitals have patient ombudsmen who visit patients, question them regarding their hospitalization experience, answer any questions they may have, and intervene in their behalf, if necessary.

Staff Satisfaction Surveys

Staff satisfaction surveys, either questionnaires or interviews, are used by the administration to assess general employee satisfaction or to elicit responses to certain program changes, such as the way nursing care is delivered.

Utilization Review

The utilization review program was mandated by the JCAHO in 1978. Its primary goal is the appropriate allocation of hospital resources. This program does not focus primarily on nursing, but it does provide data that may require nursing involvement in a more thorough evaluation.

Infection Control Reports

Because nurses are involved in the direct care of patients, they may at times be included in infection surveillance and infection control programs. Even when the nursing staff is not involved directly, they should be familiar with the monthly report of nosocomial infections on their respective unit. Questions can be raised about nursing procedures and practices that may affect the infection rate on the unit.

ETHICAL ISSUES

Several other issues are being raised as part of the quality management process. These issues relate to confidentiality of patient information and ethical problems encountered as part of the quality management process. Both of these are discussed below.

Confidentiality and the Quality Management Process

Confidentiality of data is an issue frequently associated with quality management. The availability and use of evaluative data about a patient or groups of patients has always been of concern to health professionals. The increasing use of *computerized data* about patients has generated enormous concern for potential *threats to privacy.* Most quality management studies can be conducted without the recording of patients' names and are reported in terms of *aggregate data.* Review of care provided to an individual patient requires constant vigilance to ensure protection of the patient's identity.

Ethics and Quality Management

Ethical problems can and do influence the quality management concerns of nurses. Certainly there are traditional areas of mutual interest: patient education, informed consent, and unnecessary surgery or procedures. But ethical problems probably occur much more frequently than is apparent through patient care evaluation, particularly because quality management has focused largely on technical aspects of care—whether appropriate tests are ordered, whether surgical complications were prevented or managed, and whether patient records list the steps taken in treatment.

For several reasons, quality management will need to focus more on *ethical decision making* in the future.

First, the rapidly increasing opportunities in patient care will provide more options for patients and providers. A heart transplant for one patient, for example, may mean that a heart must be sacrificed in a "brain dead" patient who is on a ventilator. *Balancing individual rights* with *social good* will become more frequent and more difficult in the future.

Second, as resources continue to diminish, problems of *distributive justice* will arise. It is possible that in the future some type of health care *rationing* could exist. Who should receive this service? How much service should they receive? Who should pay? As public policymakers attempt to reduce all care choices to cost-benefit analyses, nurses must be aware of the limitations of these calculations and the inability of accounting for human pain and suffering mathematically.

Third, nurses as well as other health professionals must participate in these ethical decisions or risk losing their unique influence entirely. For example, in cases of the comatose, terminally ill patient, peer review would focus not only on the clinical aspects of death but also on the human dimension. Did the patient have a "living will" or a durable power of attorney? Were the wishes of the patient or significant others followed? Did the health care provider confer with the patient and/or family to keep them totally informed? Were the providers guided by the wishes of the patient and family? Did the provider seek competent, objective, and relevant third-party opinions?

None of the decisions can be made irrespective of federal or state laws? But there are questions of quality that lie within the realm of quality management activity. In addition to questions of nontreatment, other *ethical dilemmas* must be recognized, analyzed, and resolved within a quality assurance framework. One approach suggests that decisions themselves are less important than the approach taken by the participants. In analyzing problems did they use accurate and necessary information? Was the reasoning logical? Did the decision-maker account for the values and rights of the individual? Use of the systematic quality assurance process has much to offer in this area in the future.

FUTURE TRENDS

The application of *total quality management* (TQM) concepts and the principles of *continuous quality improvement* (CQI) are becoming important and successful strategies in health care organizations as they cope with the changes in the industry. TQM is a conceptual approach different from quality management. It calls for continuous improvement in the total process that provides care, not simply in the improved actions of the individual nurse. Improvement is based upon both outcome and process.

TQM demands that the change be based on the needs of the patient, not the values of the providers. It requires the meaningful participation of all health care personnel that a patient may come in contact with and a rapid and thoughtful response from top management to suggestions made by participating personnel. An example of TQM is a product utilized for the patient's colostomy causing a skin reaction. Follow-up would include determining if other patients are also having skin reactions and if the vendor supplying the product has received other reports of reactions. Top management may then make the decision to have the product discontinued for patient care based on the nurse's findings and a report from the vendor.

CQI does not replace *quality management* but complements and enhances existing efforts. The efforts range from improved patient care, employee morale, patient satisfaction, and outcomes to decrease costs and duplication of services.

SUMMARY

1. Nursing's commitment to professional excellence includes monitoring the quality of care given.
2. Four factors have influenced quality management in nursing. These are (1) legislation, (2) changes in third-party reimbursement, (3) economic factors, and (4) professional standards.
3. The ANA Standards of Nursing Practice include 8 standards to be followed by all nurses in giving care.
4. The Joint Commission on the Accreditation of Health Care Organizations (JCAHO) is a voluntary organization that accredits hospitals and other health care organizations.
5. The JCAHO publishes an Accreditation Manual, which includes a standard of quality of professional services. This standard forms the basis for evaluating patient care.
6. The ANA quality management model consists of 8 steps:
   a. Identify values.
   b. Identify structure, process, outcome, standards, and criteria.
   c. Measure the degree of attainment of standards and criteria.
   d. Interpret strength and weaknesses.
   e. Identify possible courses of action.
   f. Select a course of action.
   g. Take action.
   h. Reevaluate.
7. Outcome criteria pertinent to a specific patient population must be developed as part of the quality management process and before an evaluation of the quality of nursing care can be made.
8. Outcome criteria should be measurable in terms of change in health, knowledge, or functional status of the patient.
9. Structure criteria describe the setting and conditions in which the nurse-patient relationship occurs.

10. Process criteria describe the nature and sequence of nursing care activities.
11. Quality management is an ongoing process in which the results of the evaluation of patient care are interpreted to caregivers so that needed improvements in care can be made.
12. Quality indicators are items that a health care agency believes are indicators of quality of care.
13. *Total quality management* and *continuous quality improvement* is an ongoing process that places primary emphasis on improving collaborative practice approaches and requiring evaluation on the interdependent outcomes of those combined efforts.

STUDY QUESTIONS

- Identify one clinical problem and the steps you would use to assess it using the ANA model.
- Identify four nursing process standards for a patient with impaired mobility.
- Identify the quality management model used in a hospital in which you have clinical experience.
- Investigate the impact of the quality management program on the quality of patient care in a hospital in which you have clinical experience.

REFERENCES AND SUGGESTED READINGS

1. American Nurses' Association: Task force on nursing practice standards and guidelines: working paper, *J Nurs Qual Assur* 5(3):1-17, 1991.
2. Andrews SL: QA vs. QI: the changing role of quality in health care, *JQA* 13(1):14-15, 38, 1991.
3. Arikian MA, Kingery C, Beall K, Abbott R: Education and QA: a model for continuous improvement in skin integrity, *J Nurs Qual Assur* 5(1):1-7, 1990.
4.* Batslden PB: Building knowledge for quality improvement in healthcare: an introductory glossary, *JQA* 13(5):8-12, 1991.
5. Bliersbach C: Quality improvement: one-third of the quality equation, *JQA* 13(5):58-61, 1991.
6. Brannon D: Quality assurance feedback as a nursing management strategy, *Hospital Health Services Adm* 34(4):547-555, 1989.
7. Connington ME, Dupuis P: *Unit-based nursing quality assurance*, Rockville, Md, 1990, Aspen Publishers.
8.* Crockett D, Sutcliffe S: Staff participation in nursing quality assurance, *Nurs Manage* 17(10):41-42, 1986.
9.* Fralic MF, Kowalski PM, Llewellyn FA: The staff nurse as quality monitors, *Amer J Nurs* 91(4):41-42, 1991.
10. Goldmann RC: Nursing process components as a framework for monitoring and evaluation activities. *J Nurs Qual Assur* 4(4):17-25, 1990.
11. Joint Commission on Accreditation of Healthcare Organizations: *Accreditation manual for hospitals*, Chicago, 1991, The Commission.
12. Jones KR: Maintaining quality in a changing environment, *Nurs Econ* 9(3):159-164, 1991.
13. Kravlovec OJ, Huttner CA, Dixon MD: The application of total quality management concepts in a service-line cardiovascular program, *Nurs Admin Q* 15(2):1-8, 1991.
14. Lynn ML, Osborn DP: Deming's quality principles: a health care application, *Hospital Health Services Adm* 36(1):111-120, 1991.
15. McLaughlin CP, Kaluzny AD: Total quality management in health: making it work, *Health Care Manage Rev* 15(3):7-14, 1990.
16. Omachonu VK: Quality of care: new criteria for evaluation, *Health Care Manage Rev* 15(4):43-50, 1990.
17.* Osinski EG: Developing patient outcomes as a quality measure of nursing care, *Nurs Manage* 18(10):28-29, 1987.
18. Ott MJ: Quality assurance: monitoring individual compliance with standards of nursing care, *Nurs Manage* 18(5):57-64, 1987.
19. Redfern SJ: Measuring the quality of nursing care: a consideration of different approaches, *J Adv Nurs* 15(11):1260-71, 1990.
20. Sinioris ME: TQM: the new frontier for quality and productivity improvement in health care, *JQA* 12(4):14-17, 1990.
21. Slee VN: Quality management nee quality assurance, *JONA* 21(5):9-12, 1991.
22.* Taylor AG, Hudson K, Keeling A: Quality nursing care: the consumers' perspective revisited, *J Nurs Qual Assur* 5(2):23-31, 1991.
23. Tucker SM, Canobbio MM, Paquette EV, Wells MF: *Patient care standards: nursing process, diagnosis, and outcome*, ed. 5, St Louis, 1992, Mosby–Year Book.

Classic

24. Aduddell P, Weeks L: A cost effective approach to quality assurance, *Nurs Econ* 1:279-82, 1984.
25. American Nurses' Association: *Quality assurance for nursing care*, Kansas City, Mo, 1976, The Association.
26.* American Nurses' Association: *Standards of nursing practice*, Kansas City, Mo, 1973, The Association.
27. Bergman R: Evaluation of nursing care: could it make a difference? *Int J Nurs Stud* 19:53-60, 1982.
28.* Blake B: Quality assurance: an ethical responsibility, *Supervisor Nurs* 12:32-38, 1981.
29.* Brown BJ: Quality assurance update, *Nurs Adm Q* 7(3):1-93, 1983.
30. Bulman T: Ambulatory care: a practical way to quality assurance, *Nurs Manage* 16(12):19-24, 1985.
31.* Curtis B, Simpson L: Auditing: a method for evaluting quality of care, *J Nurs Adm* 15(10):14-21, 1985.
32. Davis K: Nursing and the health care debates, *Image* 15:67, 1983.
33. Donabedian A: Criteria, norms and standards of quality: What do they mean? *Am J Public Health* 71:409-412, 1981.
34. Ferguson D, Brunner N: Balancing priorities to attain quality care, *Nurs Manage* 13:67-69, 1982.
35. Griffith N, Megel M: Quality assurance: an educational approach, *Nurs Outlook* 29:670-673, 1981.
36. Howe M: Developing instruments for measurement of criteria: a clinical nursing perspective, *Nurs Res* 29:100-103, 1980.
37. Inzinga M: Legislative issues and health care trends: quality assurance, *Nurs Adm Legislative Update* 8:80-85, 1984.
38.* Lane G, Cronin K, Peirce A: Teaching diploma students how to utilize the ANA quality assurance model, *J Nurs Educ* 21(9):42-44, 1982.
39.* Maciorowski L, Larsen E, Keane A: Quality assurance evaluate thyself, *J Nurs Adm* 15:38-42, 1985.
40. Marriner A: The research process in quality assurance, *Am J Nurs* 79:2158-2161, 1979.
41.* Moore K: What nurses learn from nursing audit, *Nurs Outlook* 27:254-258, 1979.

*Recommended for student reading.

42. Padilla G, Grant M: Quality assurance programme for nursing, *J Adv Nurs* 7:135-145, 1982.

43. Phaneuf M: *The nursing audit*, ed 2, New York, 1976, Appleton-Century-Crofts.

44. Smeltzer C, Fettman B, Rajki K: Nursing quality assurance: a process, not a tool, *J Nurs Adm* 13(1):5-9, 1983.

45. Westfall UE: Nursing diagnosis: its use in quality assurance, *Top Clin Nurs* 5(4):78-88, 1984.

46. Williamson J, et al: *Teaching quality assurance and cost containment in health care*, San Francisco, 1982, Jossey-Bass, Inc., Publishers.

Health Promotion and Illness Prevention

Unit Two

3

Cultural Influences on Health and Illness

Barbara J. Sibley

After studying this chapter, the learner should be able to:

- Have an awareness of one's self as a member of a cultural group.
- Respect similarities and differences in others.
- Inquire about other's values, traditions, preferences, and expectations before acting.
- Demonstrate ability to plan, mediate, and implement nursing care that brings about the most harmony between a patient's culture and recommended health behaviors.
- Serve as advocate on behalf of the cultural needs of patients and families to relevant components of the health care system.
- Distinguish between the concepts of culture, ethnicity, nationality, and race.
- Describe and give examples of at least two other theories of disease in addition to Western biomedicine.

The following example illustrates how a brief interaction between a nurse and a patient of different cultural backgrounds can lead to serious misunderstandings in the health care system:

> Fran brought her Italian-born father to the emergency room because he had suddenly developed chest pains. While Fran was at the registration desk, a young American-born nurse quickly asked him a few routine questions. When Fran returned, the nurse expressed surprise that Fran's father said he had been having pains for several days and had been seen by his physician. Fran turned to her father and reminded him (in English) that this was not true and asked him why he had said it. He responded, "She spoke so fast I didn't quite understand her question very well, and I thought those were the answers she wanted."

Let us now examine the concept of culture and learn how to become more culturally sensitive so that the best possible nursing care can be provided.

DEFINITIONS OF CULTURE

The word and concept of culture used throughout this chapter refers to culture in its broadest sense. Therefore, not only art, music, and literature are included (as the word culture is used in the narrower sense) but also all aspects of daily life, ways of thinking, and self-expression. We are born not *with* a culture but *into* a culture. From birth onward, we are aware when and by whom we are handled. We know by tone of voice what is said to us, we feel how we are clothed, and we taste what we are fed. As we grow, our culture becomes more apparent to us through our language; religion; family history; social, economic, and geographic background; customs; and how we view the world.

Everyone has a culture, whether it is well assimilated into mainstream America as portrayed in the popular media or recently arrived from overseas. All of us come from families who at one time immigrated from other countries. Even the prehistoric ancestors of Native American Indians immigrated from the Far East to what is now the United States.

Culture itself is invisible, but it underlies all behavior. It provides a context for people to think and act, constraints to help guide behavior, and alternative solutions to problem solving. Without culture, we are not human, because that is what separates us from the other primates.[22]

Box 3-1 provides some useful definitions for terms frequently used when discussing culture and health.

CULTURAL AND BIOLOGIC TRAITS

Box 3-2 provides some examples of cultural and biologic traits found in individuals. These traits are observable, describable, and/or behavioral manifestations of one's cultural and biologic background. Cultural and biologic traits are divided into four major categories:

1. Physical appearance (body), such as inherited features, posture, and grooming, are objective and relatively easy to observe.

2. Psychologic orientation, mental characteristics (mind) begins as genetic potential but includes attributes and abilities acquired over time. These characteristics are more subtle and take longer for a nurse to identify through additional observation and conversation with the patient.

3. External influences (social and physical environment) include all external impacts on a person since birth, such as family, social, economic, community, nutritional, and climatic conditions. When combined, they exert a profound effect on a person's socialization. The more significant of these are learned by further conversation with the patient and/or family.

4. Internal synthesis of body, mind, and environment

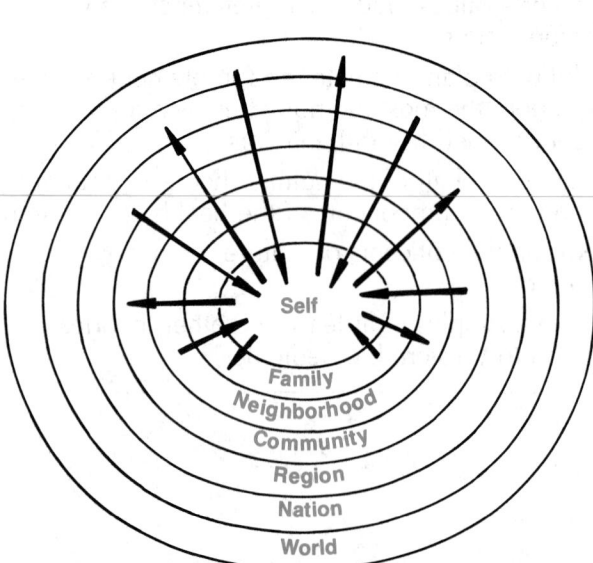

Fig. 3-1   Levels of cultural and societal influences interacting between an individual self and the social environment.

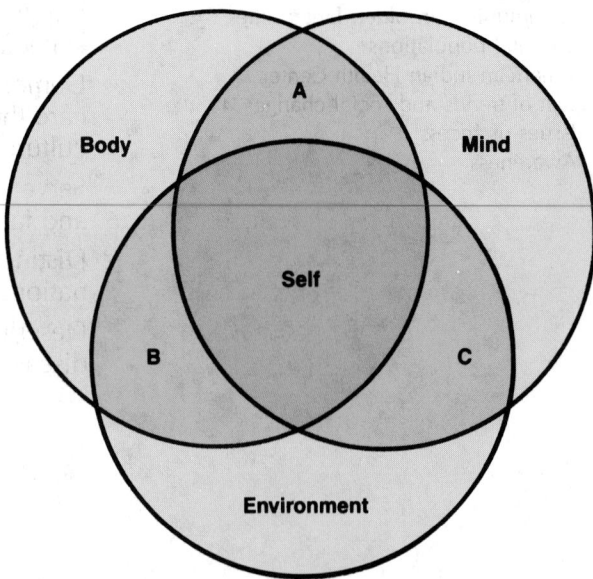

Fig. 3-2   Interrelationships between the body, mind, and environment to form the self.

(self) is a summation of the person's response to the social and physical environment to this point in time, given the attributes of his or her mind and body. Included are one's self concept, achievements, preferences, social values, and world view. Together the mind, body, and environment produce a distinct and unique individual called the *self*.

Figure 3-1 illustrates major levels of external influences that affect an individual because of indirect or direct contact with the social and physical environment. The self is shown in the center. Arrows in the diagram, indicating influences, move in both directions as individuals and groups at different levels deliberately or inadvertently work

to bring about change in the various cultural, social, and political systems around them.

Figure 3-2 shows how interrelationships between the body, mind, and environment form the self. Different disciplines in the social and natural sciences focus on different segments of the overlapping circles. Biologists, physiologists, geneticists, and pathologists, for example, are primarily interested in the composition and functioning of the human body. Psychologists, counselors, educators, and others focus on how the mind works in individuals or groups. Sociologists, political scientists, geographers, and historians are examples of persons who concentrate on

---

3-1 Definitions about culture and health

Anthropology   The study of humankind, from prehistory to present, that consists of a historic, biologic, cultural, linguistic, geographic, and/or biologic point of view.

Biology   The study of all living things; in this context, it is the study of anatomy, physiology, and pathology of the human body.

Biocultural   Includes both biologic and cultural variables.

Biomedicine   Medical practice and research that primarily emphasizes pathophysiology of the human body (with less consideration of the patient's own experience of illness, as found in the biopsychosocial and holistic models of health care).

Biopsychosocial   The study of a person or group that combines biologic, psychologic, and sociologic variables and needs; similar to holistic.

Culture   Learned behavior of a person or group that involves language, origin, history, religion, dress, diet, traditions, world view, etc.; similar to ethnicity.

Cross-cultural nursing or transcultural nursing   Nursing care that focuses on cultural aspects of patients, especially when the culture is different from the nurses providing the care.

Subculture   A recognizable segment of a larger cultural group that shares some characteristics of the larger group but with unique features of its own.

Cultural sensitivity   A learned skill in which a person has an awareness of and appreciation for another's cultural uniqueness. Same as ethnosensitivity.

Epidemiology   Study of diseases and illness and their transmission in groups and populations of people.

Ethnology   A study that analyzes the cultures of a group or groups of people.

Ethnicity   Subset of culture; a smaller group that identifies itself (and is seen by others) as distinct because of learned characteristics, such as language, traditions, appearance, and geographic origin.

Ethnocentrism   A belief that one's own culture (ethnicity) is superior to any others.

Ethnomedicine   A comparative study of medical systems across cultures or subcultures; similar to medical anthropology.

Ethnosensitivity   Same as cultural sensitivity.

Folk culture   The culture of a smaller, more traditional group; similar to ethnic.

Folk medicine   Knowledgeable and respected practitioners. Traditional system of caring for ill members of a community.

Holistic Health Care   A balanced view of human health that includes psychologic, social, and cultural components along with the biologic ones.

Nationality   A people from a place with specified political and geographic boundaries, which are changeable; several different ethnic groups can be found within one nation.

Norms   Commonly shared customs and standards of behavior that are acceptable within a given group of people.

Psychology   The study of human behavior, the function of the mind and the senses, including perception.

Psychosocial   The psychologic and social components, background, and needs of a person or group.

Race   Inherited biologic and physical characteristics of a population or individual that is representative of a particular group. Only three major races are usually described worldwide: Caucasian, Black, and Oriental.

Religion   System of beliefs, usually about a higher power or powers, that has specified rules and sanctions to encourage conformity; often a significant factor of a cultural group.

Shaman   A practitioner of folk medicine in a local community.

Sociology   Study of social structures and interactions of groups of people, usually in large Western communities.

Sociocultural   Refers to the social and cultural components, background, and needs of a person or group.

Western   That which originated in Western Europe, in contrast to nonwestern, eastern (oriental), folk, native, and indigenous.

Values   Shared desirable ideals and goals of individuals and groups.

3-2

Cultural and biologic traits of an individual

Physical appearance (body)
Age and developmental stage
Sex and gender identity
Size, height, weight
Skin color
Hair color, configuration, presence/absence
Race (self-identified, perceived by others)
Posture, facial expression
Grooming, personal hygiene
Dress: style, condition
Presence of physical disability
Other characteristics not listed above

Mental characteristics. Psychologic orientation (mind)
Cognitive ability, intelligence
Level of consciousness
Emotional disposition, temperament
Aptitude, ability
Sensory acuity (visual, auditory)
Personal traits
Mental health
Other characteristics not listed above

External influences (social and physical environment)
Family history, ancestry, geographic origin
Strength of family unit, lines of authority
Role in family, birth order
Languages, communication patterns
Expectations and behavioral norms for age, sex, role
Format (rituals) for major life events (birth, marriage, illness, death)
Economic and work opportunities, access to resources

Housing, living arrangements
Dominant religion, other religions
Theories of disease causation
Availability, quality, variety of health care services
Political, governmental structure
Dietary customs, access to food
Community resources in education, art, music, recreation
Geographic and climatic features
Other influences not listed above

Internal synthesis of body, mind, and environment (self)
Self-concept, self-perception, expectations of self
Beliefs, values, spirituality, religious affiliation
Affect, mood, congruity between words and affect
Attitudes toward health and self care; health history, utilization of health services
Personal goals, short and long term
Work role, economic contribution to self, others
Areas of accomplishment, achievement, sources of pride
Knowledge base, utilization of educational opportunities
Response to stress, coping strategies, ability to adapt
Language usage: formal, slang, dialect
Food preferences, dietary restrictions
Interests in applied and fine arts, crafts, hobbies, music, literature
Reading ability and preferences
Other characteristics not listed above

---

social or natural systems external to the individual. Many disciplines overlap, such as social workers who are concerned not only about physical and mental health, but also support systems available within the family and community. Anthropologists study people in all categories but tend to specialize in one or two major segments.

Medicine concentrates primarily on the body, but a subspecialty, psychiatry, attends to the mind and mental health.

A major distinction between the professions of medicine and nursing is that medicine is chiefly interested in examining the body and its pathology, making a diagnosis, and prescribing treatment. Nursing, on the other hand, addresses the *health and well being of an individual within the social and cultural environment.* Because of this holistic perspective, nursing attends to any and all aspects shown in Box 3-2 and Figure 3-2.

In Figure 3-2, segments labeled *A*, *B*, and *C* represent the overlap of each of the major components with one of the other two. For example, segment *A* includes the domain

of both the body and the mind. Within this category are concepts such as body image and the flight/fight reaction. In segment *B*, where the body and the environment overlap, such categories as nutrition and pollution-generated illness are found. Finally, segment *C*, the combination of mind and environment, is an area that includes topics such as educational achievement or depression from job loss.

PURPOSE FOR LEARNING ABOUT A PERSON'S CULTURE

Why should nurses take the time and energy to pay attention to their patients' cultural background, along with tending to their medical and comfort needs?

The main reason is that it proves to be easier both for the nurse and for the patient. Initially, it takes a little more time to make a cultural assessment, but the insights gained by the nurse provide a more accurate picture of the patient's social and cultural background. Therefore, the nurse can expect an increased likelihood of patient compliance with agreed upon recommended behaviors. Nurse anthropologists Tripp-Reimer, Brink, and Saunders state:

cultural assessments elicit shared beliefs, values and customs that have relevance to health behaviors; they are performed to identify patterns that may assist or interfere with a nursing intervention or planned treatment regimen.[48]

CONCEPTS OF CULTURE, ETHNICITY, NATIONALITY, AND RACE

As previously stated, culture is learned through social contact from birth onward and is an integral part of each person throughout his or her lifespan.

Ethnicity refers to a subset of culture; a smaller, more cohesive group that is identified with a particular set of characteristics, involving distinctive language, music, dress, and dietary preferences, among others. A description of an ethnic group could also include race, but *ethnicity is applied accurately only to learned traits.*

Nationality refers to a *geographic location of a country* with politically drawn boundary lines. However, the concept becomes blurred when more than one ethnic group lives within a single country, or when boundary lines change through wars and treaties, leaving ethnic identity unchanged.

Race is *genetic.* However, *beliefs and perceptions about race are learned,* creating confusion about the distinction between race and culture. The concept and definition of race are both simple and complex. Labels are used to indicate which of the three major racial groups (Black, Caucasian, and Oriental) a person belongs. However, the racial labels in themselves do not say anything about behavior, economic level, and other sociocultural attributes. Nor do they indicate the richness or variety within these groups. Beyond major physical features such as skin and hair color, racial labels do not include any other components that make an individual what he or she is at a given point in time.

Studies of personality traits, disorders, and even genetic markers have shown that there are often more differences *within* a single arbitrary racial group than there are *between* groups.[30] These research studies make the isolated use of race as a social concept meaningless. However, among many people a racial label still carries deep emotional overtones that have been passed on through families and communities. The emotions may be full of pride or fear, but in either case the emotions need to be acknowledged so that communication gaps between people can be honestly addressed.

Negative racial stereotyping is not uncommon, but when it is engaged in by a nurse in response to a colleague or a patient, it diminishes the other person's confidence and trust. With colleagues, this loss interferes with team work and cooperation. With patients, it results in reduced sharing of information required to do good nursing care.

The United States has been called a "melting pot" for many ethnic groups that immigrated to this country. When ethnic groups also have been Caucasians, blending with the dominant White mainstream through assimilation and acculturation has been relatively easy and inconspicuous.[45] However, for Orientals and Blacks, their racial characteristics are still visible, even when most other learned cultural features are similar to the predominant White mainstream.

Recently, a movement to reconstruct and preserve some of the unique features of many ethnic groups has occurred, with perhaps a secondary goal of retrieving some of the remembered (if not practiced) associated positive values.

Having defined the concepts of culture, ethnicity, nationality, and race as applied to groups, we now need to acknowledge individual differences among representatives of each of those categories. Although generalizations are useful, it is essential to find out if a particular patient fits the common pattern for his or her group. The patient can be asked, "Are you like all others of your racial group, nationality, or race? If the answer is "no, I am not," the nurse is reminded that he or she has no reason to expect the patient to be just like all the others of his or her group.

A community is defined as *diverse* if its members include representatives from several different groups that have a variety of backgrounds, values, languages, appearances, or other identifiable features. An individual also can be in several diverse cultural and social roles at the same time. For example, a particular woman can be a wife, mother, sister, daughter, neighbor, bank teller, choir member, and shopper all in the same week. In each role, cultural expectations for her behavior, dress, demeanor, and language vary. She knows what these are, because she has learned these cultural roles subtly over many years.

A final note on diversity comes from a well-known nurse anthropologist, Agnes Aamodt, who said: "Sameness can be deadening. Diversity is one of my reasons for being."[1]

TOWARD CULTURAL SENSITIVITY

An orthopedic nurse does not have to break a leg to appreciate the pain, loss of independence, job interruption, postponement of activities, and general frustration that a patient in a leg cast experiences. However, a healthy respect for how this event has temporarily changed a patient's life contributes to the best nursing care for that person at that time.

Likewise, a nurse does not have to have first-hand experience with the cultures of each of her or his patients. However, development of cultural sensitivity involves an appreciation of how an illness is perceived by a patient, as well as its impact on his or her life and the lives of the families.

It is helpful to keep in mind that persons from another culture may seem very different to a nurse. However, from the patient's point of view, the health care system and some of the nurses are the ones seen as strange. An understanding nurse can be very helpful in guiding patients and families through the system.

The initial step in becoming a more culturally sensitive nurse is an awareness of how culture influences values, thoughts, feelings, and actions.

It is also necessary for a nurse to acknowledge any negative feelings and fears he or she may have about certain groups and explore why this may be so. For example:

Where have these feelings and fears come from?

Is discomfort based on lack of familiarity?

Have judgments been made based on another group's

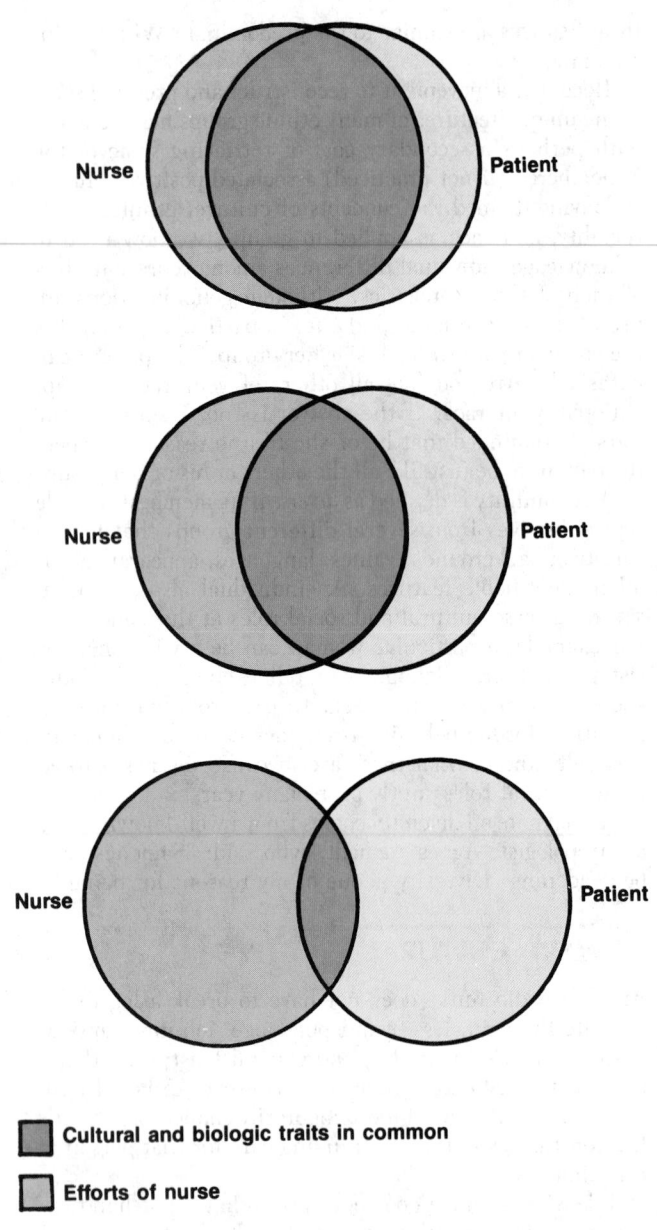

Cultural and biologic traits in common

Efforts of nurse

Fig. 3-3   As the cultural and biologic similarities between nurse and patient decrease, the effort of the nurse needs to increase to bridge their differences.

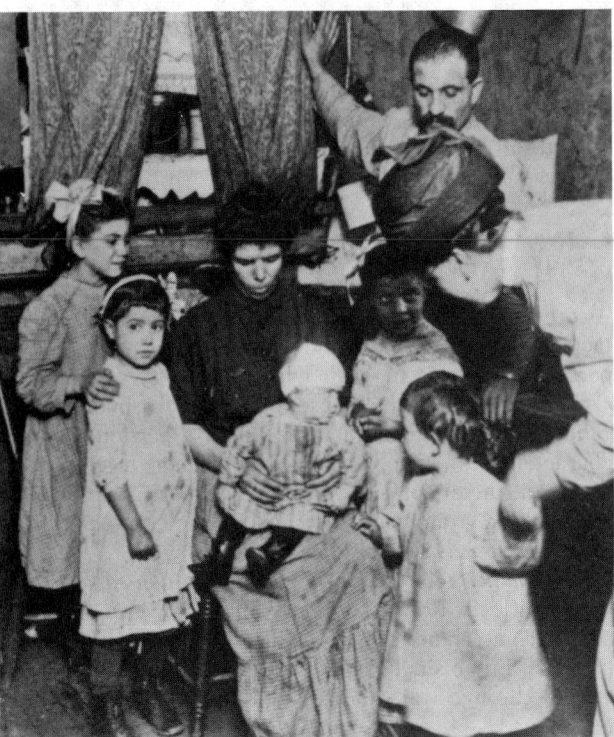

Fig. 3-4   Visiting nurse is checking on the health of a family recently arrived from Europe circa 1915. (From University Hospitals of Cleveland archives.)

minimal (or excessive) access to economic success or perhaps unacceptable behaviors found in some members of the group?

Are these negative impressions generalized to a broader, undeserving population?

Take some time to discuss your feelings with classmates, instructors, family, and maybe your neighbors. In doing so, you learn how to be less judgmental and more open to others.

A model for *ethnosensitivity training* has been adapted from Peace Corps experience for use by physicians entering family practice. It can be valuable for nurses as well. A series of developmental stages are encountered as one becomes more culturally sensitive. Beginning with an ethnocentric (my culture is better than your culture) feeling of fear, the learner progresses through feelings of denial, superiority, minimization, and relativism. With increased awareness, the student eventually acquires empathy and finally integration as an ethnosensitive person.[3,4]

The more similar the nurse and patient are to each other, the more cultural traits and values they are likely to share. Conversely, the fewer the traits shared, the more necessary it is for the nurse to observe and inquire what is important and meaningful to the patient. Figure 3-3 illustrates this concept. If a nurse who is young, White, urban, and female is caring for a patient who is also young, White, urban, and female, chances are they share many experiences, values, and tastes. However, if either the patient or the nurse were middle-aged, Black, from a small town, and male, fewer characteristics are shared. In this example, the nurse would need to have greater self awareness as well as greater sensitivity to the culture of the patient before assuming shared or unshared values and goals.

Sensitivity to other cultures is not new to nursing. Figure 3-4 shows a visiting nurse in about 1915 making a home visit to a family recently arrived to the United States from western Europe. Figure 3-5, also from about 1915, provides an example of nurses teaching infant care to a group of adolescent girls in an urban hospital. The photograph also indicates an example of cultural differences over time. *Historical time* (sensitivity to persons of different ages and different historical experiences) is also helpful when providing nursing care. These photographs can be compared with other photographs in this chapter to see

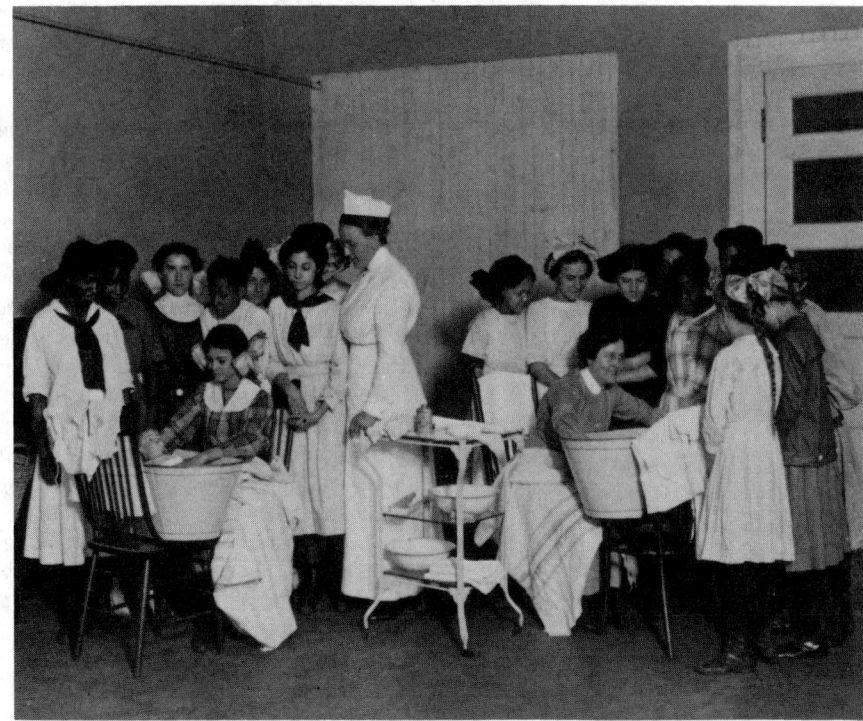

Fig. 3-5   Nurses are providing classes in infant care to adolescent girls circa 1915. (From University Hospitals of Cleveland archives.)

how the appearance (e.g., dress, hairdo) changes over time. These illustrations provide cues about the changes in the culture of nursing over the years.

PERCEPTIONS OF ILLNESS AND DISEASE CAUSATION

All cultures have distinct ways of taking care of their members over a lifespan. How each group responds to staying well, becoming ill, coping with life-threatening events, seeking treatment, and dying is of general interest to health professionals and is a special field of study for nurse anthropologists, medical anthropologists, and sociologists. Nurse anthropologists (some of whom are cited throughout this chapter) have examined the phenomenon of *cross-cultural nursing* and the *concept of caring.** Medical anthropologists have written extensively about medical care and its relationship to the needs of the people being served, usually by comparing practices in different cultures. Often a better understanding of the Western medical model can be obtained by exploring models in non-western communities.[33,35,41]

Systems for health care in different cultures vary considerably in content, but what they have in common is a set of beliefs, practitioners (such as lay and local healers, shamans, doctors, and nurses), family support networks, rituals, and patterns of behavior to assist in recovery. In addition, there is usually some kind of institution and a

means of expressing the value of assistance received, whether by gifts, loyalty, direct cash payment, or third-party reimbursement.

The use of explanatory models, as described by Kleinman,[40] is helpful in reviewing the rationale given for illness episodes. He lists five major questions that a model can address:

1. Etiology (origin or cause of the illness)
2. Time and mode of onset of symptoms
3. Pathophysiology (the disease process)
4. Course of sickness (including both degree of severity and type of sick role—acute, chronic, impaired)
5. Treatment

Explanatory models are as diverse as their holders. According to Kleinman, one of the reasons some patients tend to be noncompliant is that their model of illness is very different from that of their physician. If the physician is not addressing the patient's questions or comes with a different cognitive base, they may be exchanging words, but not meanings with the same personal significance. Kleinman cites the following example:

> Mrs. Smith is a 45-year-old Caucasian American housewife with chronic low back pain who has sought out the help of a noted orthopedic surgeon at a university hospital. Her conceptualization of her illness is that it has a definite relationship to psychological and social stress as well as to physical exertion. She believes it important to understand what is wrong and to participate in planning her course of treatment. She places considerable value on the quality and time spent communicating with her doctors. She was disappointed with the care she received from this orthopedic surgeon, primarily be-

cause he spent little time with her, did not offer her a detailed explanation of what was wrong, and told her that all she had to concern herself with was taking the medicines and carrying out the program of rest and graduated exercises he prescribed. Interviews with this doctor revealed that he did not recognize explaining to patients as essential and played down the role of psychosocial stress, which he believed fell outside the purview of surgical treatment.

Mrs. Smith failed to comply with her regimen and soon discontinued care completely. She later consulted a chiropractor, whom she characterized in positive terms as meeting the expectations she had of a care-giver. She reported symptom improvement under his care, whereas she had experienced no such improvement while undergoing treatment from the orthopedist.[40]

It is useful at this point to distinguish the difference among the concepts of illness, disease, and sickness, as clarified by Twaddle.[49] An *illness is what a person feels*, and includes such symptoms as pain, dizziness, nausea, or shortness of breath. A *disease is what a physician diagnoses* after using techniques like direct examination, tests, radiologic findings, and consultation with other professionals. *Sickness is a label by society* applied to someone who does not have to fulfill his or her usual role because of the illness or disease. The *sick role* is permitted by society when the seriousness of the problem is recognized. Other persons assist with functions normally performed by the sick person. The use of the sick role can also be abused, as when a person describes symptoms to avoid performing normal duties, to receive compensation, or to find other secondary gains.

Folk and Traditional Care

Many manifestations of health care and healing in the United States do not involve physicians, nurses, or hospitals. Television evangelists, for example, offer forms of faith healing and Christian spiritualism. Another example of folk beliefs about illness is described in an article by Bailey about hypertension among African Americans in Detroit:

> African Americans' ethnomedical beliefs and practices are currently a composite, containing elements from a variety of sources: European folklore, Greek classical medicine, modern scientific medicine, and particularly African folklore. These diverse threads are tied together by the tenets of fundamentalist Christianity, elements from the vodun religion of Haiti, and the added spice of sympathetic magic. It should be noted that this health belief system is not exclusively confined to African Americans, but is shared by segments of the Anglo American population.[2]

Harwood[38] describes a study of health practices among Puerto Ricans living in New York City. Their disease causation and therapeutic system originated in ancient Greece and is found today in many Latin (Spanish-speaking) cultures. This theory views health as a balance between four *bodily humors: blood, phlegm, black bile, and yellow bile*. When not in balance, the body becomes *too hot, too cold, too wet, or too dry*. Foods, medicines, and herbs likewise are classified as hot or cold. To restore balance, hot foods are given for a cold illness and vice versa. For example, arthritic pain can come from plunging hands into cold water and is helped by such items as garlic or aspirin, both

classified as hot. If a health care giver is unfamiliar with the patient's hot-cold system, the "wrong" medicine or foods could be prescribed by the physician, but not be accepted by the patient. The patient is labeled noncompliant, but the patient faults the health care system for choosing an inappropriate remedy. More recent descriptions of the use of hot and cold in relation to disease are readily available, including one by Kay and Yoder[13] in a study among Mexican-American women.

The concept of "nerves" is another illustration of an illness state conditioned by social, cultural, and sometimes gender factors. Davis and Low[7] suggest when women's social roles are threatened during rapid social change, a case of nerves provides respite from the stress. In Latin American cultures, for example, women could take time out and be nurtured until they adapted to new and threatening circumstances, such as a family member going to war, extreme poverty, or rejection by a suitor. Although primarily described as an illness among women, the similar concept of a nervous breakdown has been applied to both sexes. It is an illness that requires at least family, if not medical, attention.

These examples are only a few of many found among residents of the United States, depending on their cultural traditions and history. Native healers, shamans, and lay practitioners are trusted by the people they serve and are familiar with their clients' traditions and histories. They offer assistance that is harmonious with local beliefs and expectations and may also encourage social conformity.

Theories of non-Western disease causation are summarized by Moore et al[43]: sorcery, breach of taboo, disease-object intrusion, spirit intrusion, and soul loss. Evidence of these theories is still present in many communities in the United States. Such beliefs are taken seriously by members of these communities, but because they are considered outside modern Western medical practice, they are often ignored in the contemporary health care system. An examination of these cultural and religious beliefs provides clues to explain why members of some groups avoid the Western biomedical system or fail to adhere to it.

Predetermination

Some diseases are inherited, providing a predetermined condition through genetic composition. Examples include cystic fibrosis and hemophilia. Sickle cell anemia is another genetically determined disease. It is found in higher percentages among the Black population. The origin of sickle cell anemia has been traced to Africa, where a linked characteristic provided resistance to malaria. Thus those with the trait survived at higher rates and were able to pass on this advantage to their offspring. No longer an advantage, the illness at times causes extreme pain and a limited life span for those who have it.

Other predetermined health concerns include developmental problems, such as incomplete embryologic formation of the roof of the mouth (cleft palate) or of the spinal column (spina bifida). Developmental diseases also include scoliosis found primarily among children, and dementia and Alzheimer's disease, among the elderly.

Disorders such as diabetes and heart disease have genetic components, but are also influenced by cultural and behavioral considerations like diet and exercise.

Some people associate their diseases with predetermination, in that they believe it is their fate or God's will that they suffer their particular illnesses.

Germ Theory of Disease

In the mid 1800s, the French chemist Louis Pasteur discovered that tiny microbes were responsible for fermentation and recognized other bacilli that caused diseases in animals and people. His observations revolutionized medical practice, because some infectious diseases that had killed thousands could now be controlled or cured. This germ theory of disease also provided a rationale for Florence Nightingale's efforts to sanitize health care practices for the British army during the Crimean War and later for citizens in her native England.

The germ theory of disease (also called the theory of specific etiology) is appropriate for infectious diseases. The presence of germs (bacteria or microorganisms) however, is only one factor in the disease process, as the discussion of stress and other disease causation theories indicate.

Western Biomedicine

With the germ theory and other discoveries, the mind set of modern Western medicine (from western Europe) became primarily one of cause (etiology) and cure. This biomedical model is still the basis for most practice and teaching in medical schools in this country. Advanced technology is used to provide physicians with increasingly accurate and refined data so they can make better diagnoses and prescribe proper treatment.

The medical profession prides itself in being objective, scientific, unemotional, and detached and often avoids subjective interpretations from its patients. Medical practitioners have divided the body and its systems into specialties and subspecialities. Along with specialization has come a sense of superiority about its own beliefs, and disdain and rejection of other approaches, especially those labeled non-Western. Unfortunately, this mind set, according to Moore et al.

> has impeded the acceptance of an ecological view founded on the more general notion that disease results from adaptive failure (and has) slowed the search for a broader range of causal factors that may eventually lead to effective treatment of chronic disease such as cancers.[43]

Some Western medical practitioners realize they need to reconsider the whole patient again, and a more humanistic approach can be found in fields like family medicine.

Stress and the General Adaptation Syndrome

In 1956, long after the germ theory, Hans Selye summarized his thinking about stress in his classic work *The Stress of Life*. According to Selye, the person became ill when exposed to stressors like tension, fatigue, and temperature extremes. Thus, not everyone exposed to disease organisms got sick, but only those whose systems were made vulnerable by stress. Selye identified specific diseases of adaptation, notably hypertension, gastric and duodenal ulcers, certain rheumatic problems, allergies, and cardiovascular and renal problems. He offered the general adaptation syndrome as an alternative to the biochemical medical model because the biochemical medical model focused on the body's response to drugs, rather than on the body's own defense mechanisms[46] (See Chapter 6).

Behavioral and Environmental Factors

Studies in public health and epidemiology have shown that disease patterns often involve a behavioral component. For instance, measles inoculation in the United States was not only encouraged, but also was required of school children for admission to kindergarten. These preventive measures worked so well in reducing the incidence of the disease that many communities became careless in maintaining the requirement. Thus after a new generation grew up only partially protected by the vaccine, measles became epidemic in several American colleges.

In some communities, people have no funding or access to inoculations against childhood diseases, resulting in children at risk for major health problems.

Substances in the environment have been associated with several diseases, such as allergic hypersensitivity, cancer, asbestosis, black lung, brown lung, blood poisoning, and probably some birth defects. Chemicals and toxins in the air, water, and food chain, coming from industrial waste, work places, agriculture, automobiles, and people's homes are being investigated. Attention is given to intercept some of these toxins, although not without economic consequences or controversy.

Epidemiologic studies of cancer mortality thoughout the United States and elsewhere have generated data via cancer registries. From these registries, cancer mapping is used to locate which geographic and environmental regions and which economic groups, sexes, and races have the highest rates of the disease.

Two other culturally influenced factors related to cancer death rates are also under investigation. These are behavioral factors (diet, smoking, alcohol use, and access to health care) and reproductive factors (a woman's age at first full-term delivery, number of children, and the total number of months of lactation). Results from this research are publicized with the goal of reducing cancer risk factors for future generations. An examination of each cancer case in isolation from environmental and cultural perspectives would not reveal these culturally influenced risk factors.

High-risk behavior is also linked with many other disease and health problems. Examples are use of tobacco products, dietary excesses, use of alcohol and street drugs, abuse of prescription medications, and driving motor vehicles carelessly while drunk or without using a seat belt. In addition, avoidance of routine health maintenance and not responding to early warning signs are behaviors associated with higher health risks.

Self care, self-help groups, and lay initiatives in health care are ideas that have grown in recent years. This is partially in response to the impersonal and large-scale high technology of our present health industry. Self-help groups teach members to take responsibility for their own health. The models are based on prevention, with an interest in holistic health. Nurses support a person's desire to be actively involved in their health care and healing. Dossey[9] provides an example by suggesting nurses awaken their patients' inner healer by engaging in exercises in imagery before undergoing surgical procedures. She states that the process lessens anxiety, reduces the need for medication, and results in quicker healing.

Discussion

When health is threatened, cultural characteristics of a group are major factors influencing choices made for seeking assistance. First, a person usually confers with family and friends for advice, and maybe tries a home remedy. This is the initial step in the illness referral system. If no improvement occurs, a local lay or professional healer may be sought. If no relief is forthcoming with this effort, Western medical staff and institutions may be approached.

Once within the system however, a person may still turn to other options in addition to Western medical practice. For instance, a patient who insists on the latest surgical and high technologic treatment may also ask family members to say some extra prayers for him. Thus he would be utilizing beliefs in two major systems, medical and religious, at the same time.

What one believes determines which symptoms to describe, which labels to use, and what treatment to seek from available alternatives. According to the medical anthropologists Good and Good,[36] healing is viewed across meaning systems (popular, religious, folk, professional) that result in constructing culturally specific illness realities.

CULTURAL CONCEPTS APPLIED TO HEALTH AND ILLNESS

Concept of Self and World View

Some research on the concept of self has come from the cross-cultural study of psychiatry. For example, Fabrega states:

> The disease of schizophrenia can be said to alter and disturb an individual's customary sense of self, sense of boundaries between self and others (of the behavioral environment), and the ability of the self to relate meaningfully to the cultural world. [The author cites Hallowell in noting that self-accountability and self-awareness are fundamental to functioning in a society. Hallowell further notes] a distinction between the subjective (pertaining to the self) and the objective (things not pertaining to self) as a necessary requirement of being human.[10]

Florsheim[11] examines the concept of self from both Western and Eastern (India) perspectives. He states that the Eastern self is fluid and interdependent whereas the Western self is more solid and autonomous.

The concept of self is fundamental to all people but varies according to the individuals's cultural and symbolic system. It is another way of noting how people see themselves fitting into a larger order.

The concept of self is relevant in health care, and examples are found among persons with physical disabilities. How they view themselves may be partially influenced by how they are viewed and treated by others.[20] Self-concept becomes especially meaningful in cases of severe brain injury. When a patient is in a coma and lacks cognitive ability, he or she may be assisted by artificial means to survive indefinitely. Mwaria[17] has written about families of such patients, and notes that they find themselves in socially ambiguous and isolated positions. In trying to define their own concept of self, they wonder if it also applies to their comatose relative as well. This, in turn, affects their decisions about maintaining life-support systems.

Symbols and Meanings

What does it mean to a person to be helpless in bed, to be dependent, to have little control over events that are happening? All cultures contain an emotional loading or symbolism for certain words, objects, and behaviors. An examination of a few in the health field are relevant. For instance, if someone hears the word cancer, or sees many people wearing white lab coats and using high-technology equipment, he or she can become very anxious or frightened. In this state, the meanings of these symbols evoke strong emotions that can interfere with the ability to be attentive or rational.

Likewise, the failing heart has a distressing meaning for a patient. The failure takes on a new and more hopeful meaning if heart transplantation becomes an option. Yet, a third but ambivalent meaning appears when the patient realizes that a heart will not be available unless another person dies first.

Many people have a need, whether it is religious, philosophical, or just human, to seek meaning in adversity. The need for family support and a change in religious commitment may become more intense during health crises.

When discussing their illness with their physicians, people select symptoms that have meaning for them, but these symptoms may not be the same ones chosen by the physician to make a diagnosis. Communication discontinuities such as this indicate meanings and symbolism vary according to one's perspective.[36]

Shame and Face

The concepts of both shame and face are especially familiar to persons knowledgeable with Oriental or Middle-Eastern cultures. Shame appears in Western cultures in a mild version, found in the expression, "shame on you!" Shame can be brought on by one's self or incurred by others through improper or unacceptable words or behavior. It is something to avoid because it brings embarrassment to one's self, one's family, and perhaps to one's community.

Face refers to one's dignity and how to treat others. In a culture where face is important, when a person uses poor judgment, has a disagreement, or makes a mistake, he or she is allowed a way to recover without embarrassment, thus saving face. A person can be helped to save face by being offered alternatives, a graceful way out, or an opportunity to try again.

If a conflict arises between family members who prefer being seen as harmonious in the health care setting, the disagreement can be overlooked to help the family save face. When patients want to ask questions of their physician or nurse, they might hesitate, fearing shame on themselves for appearing ignorant, or feeling shame for the health professional if he or she is unable to provide an answer.

Sick Role and Expectations from Self and Others

The concept of the *sick role* is mentioned again to address some cultural variations. Sickness is a sign of weakness for one person, an occasion for family support and solidarity for another, or an indication that one has violated a social norm for a third. A patient may be expected to assume a helpless role or be urged to be strong. A patient's family may expect him or her to maintain a more dependent state at a time when nurses are encouraging greater independence in preparation for discharge. In such cases, nurses are challenged to elicit family cooperation and participation in discharge teaching.

Gender Identification and Role

A person's gender identity and role may conform to the expected social norm and cause no notice. However, if an individual has a sexual identification different from his or her anatomy, prefers a partner of the same sex, or chooses a nontraditional social role, special sensitivity is necessary for the nurse to carry out appropriate care without being judgmental.

Because sexual orientation is established in children by about age 6,[15] the nontraditional adult patient has probably been dealing with a variety of social conflicts for a number of years. He or she may or may not have achieved internal harmony or acceptance from family members. Partners of homosexual patients may expect the same visitation rights as partners of heterosexual patients and they should be accorded the same courtesy and privileges.

As society in the United States keeps changing, nurses can expect to see and perhaps experience more role options for both sexes. More women are becoming the major bread-winners for their families, and more men are spending time at home caring for children. In the process, women have acquired higher incidences of heart attacks and ulcers as they take on stress at work, and men have acquired new somatic and/or psychologic problems related to their adjustment to a domestic role.[8] Nurses need to be alert to manifestations of sex role shifts as they care not only for their patients but also for themselves.

Direct Nursing Care Factors
Discussion

The nursing role is a unique one. Nurses not only share management of private bodily functions with total strangers, but also ask them to express very personal feelings and fears. Each person's culture provides ground rules and boundaries for communication, closeness, and touch. Nurses may need to violate these rules to provide essential care. An awareness of different boundaries can facilitate care delivery and generate less anxiety for patients. The best source for learning about rules of an unfamiliar cultural group is the patient or a relative because they are the experts about their own customs.

Verbal communication

Some individuals share their feelings with strangers easily and tell nurses things they hesitate to mention to family members. Others withhold comments until their families arrive, and even then may not share much. Dodd[34] discusses verbal and nonverbal intercultural communications.

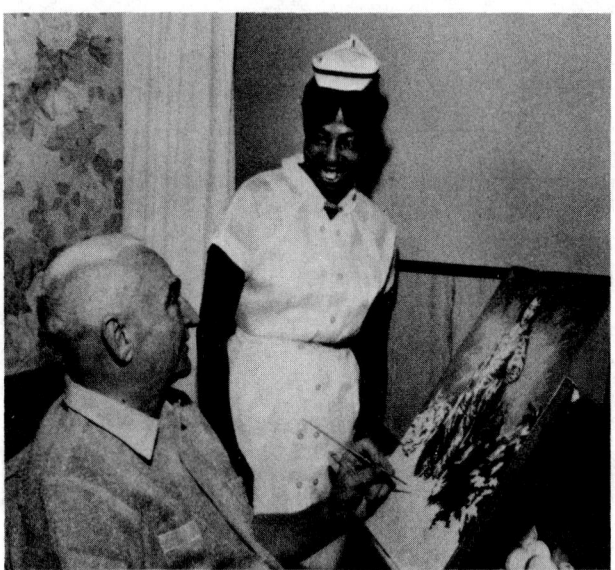

Fig. 3-6 Although from different generations, sexes, races, and backgrounds, this nurse and patient share a creative moment together circa 1960. (From University Hospitals of Cleveland archives.)

His works are helpful in describing many kinds of communication, including those in the following discussion.

Body language and nonverbal cues

The term kinesics refers to a means of communicating without using words, such as body position, facial expressions, gestures, and body movement. These cues can provide significant data for nurses. The sigh, the turning of the head, the joyous smile, and the winces of pain are nonverbally expressed and also may be nonverbally absorbed by nurses, as they watch for responses to their ministrations. *The Silent Language* written by Hall[37] in 1973 is still useful for increasing sensitivity on this topic. Figure 3-6 shows an example of nonverbal communication beween people of different generations, sexes, cultural backgrounds, and races as they share a creative moment together.

Personal space and use of touch

The *study of spatial relationships between people* is called *proxemics* and is obviously significant in the health care field. Some individuals are used to a high degree of intimacy and closeness, but others are deeply offended by the same degree of contact. As with other means of communication, it is desirable to confirm expectations involving touch and to assist a patient to anticipate when touching is necessary. Figure 3-7 shows that touching works both ways; a nurse examines a patient while the patient explores the inviting attachment on the stethoscope.

Expression and tolerance of pain

Zatzick and Dimsdale[29] summarized the literature on cultural differences in response to levels of pain. They conclude that no consistent experimental evidence exists to

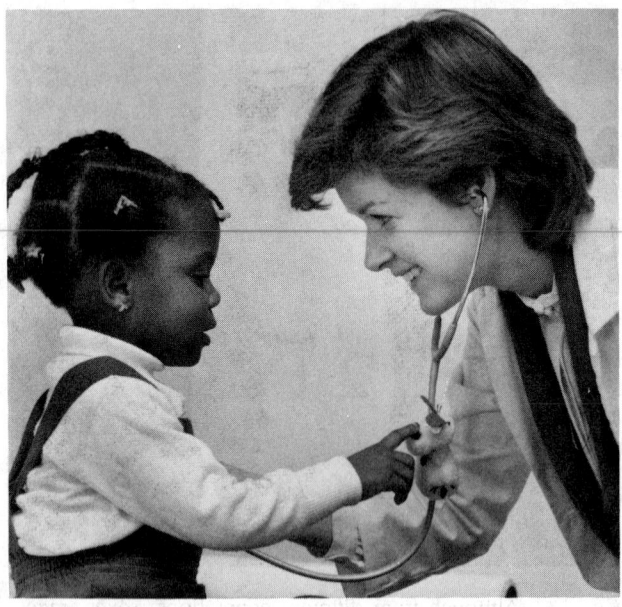

Fig. 3-7 Touching works both ways as this nurse examines her asthma patient circa 1980. (Courtesy of Colin Klein, University Hospitals of Cleveland.)

suggest cultural differences in *pain threshold*. However, they do suggest different degrees of *pain tolerance* or behavioral manifestations of the pain experience in different racial or ethnic groups. Some groups encourage a stiff upper lip or even denial of pain, whereas others expect expressiveness and moaning, grunting, or crying when in pain. In some groups, the response to pain or to embarrassment is laughter, but it is important to understand that this kind of laughter does not mean that something is funny.

Rejection of medication, surgery and blood products

Religious prohibitions may raise issues in the performance of certain medical procedures. For example, members of the Jehovah's Witness community do not ordinarily accept blood transfusions. Therefore, alternatives are necessary in case of surgery or trauma. Christian Scientists usually resist recommendations for surgery and medications, depending instead on healthful living and communication with God for assistance. Members of this faith also observe that not every case of surgical or medical intervention is successful, which indicates to them that the biomedical community has an incomplete understanding of the healing process.

Use of transplants

The status of transplantation is well described and illustrated in an article by Swerdlow[24] in *National Geographic*. He refers to a new kind of kinship between donor family and recipient. There are many controversial political, economic, and social issues about the availability and use of organs. In response to a 1984 Congressional act to outlaw the buying or selling of organs, the United Network for

Organ Sharing has received the federal mandate for management of organ sharing.[21] Some professionals express concern about equitable distribution of organs across cultural and ethnic groups, as well as geographic boundaries. See Chapter 42 for more information on transplantation.

Dietary considerations

Food availability and preferences can have a significant impact on a person, especially when he or she is ill. Although diet may need to be regulated for strictly medical reasons, cultural considerations are also important.

A person's religion may prohibit certain foods (pork for orthodox Jews), and his or her genetic composition may influence refusal of other foods (milk for persons with lactase deficiency, especially Blacks). In addition, a philosophic orientation may result in rejection of certain categories of food (meat for vegetarians).

Role of family and friends

Families from some communities expect many members to visit the patient as a way of assisting the patients's progress toward regaining health. Nurses can learn to weigh the importance of the patient's need for rest versus the need to feel love and support when deciding to enforce or relax visitation policies. To avoid becoming involved in family tensions and conflict, it is helpful to ask families to designate a representative with whom most information can be exchanged.

Patients from other families or cultures may not want to be seen by anybody when ill, and may request that visitors be limited to one or two special people until they feel much better.

NURSING ATTENTION TO THE CULTURAL DIMENSION

According to Affonso as cited in Tripp-Reimer, Brink, and Saunders,

> Cultural assessments provide meaning to behavior which might otherwise be judged in a negative way or continue to be confusing to the nurse.[48]

The authors state that a cultural assessment involves a

> shared negotiation or contract between client and professional in which each is treated as an equal bringing important and relevant materials to the interview.

When using a culturally sensitive approach, nurses see patients and their familes as experts about their own cultural background. It is the nurse's obligation to inquire further when the patient or family indicates a value, belief, or practice that may interfere with acceptance of routine Western medical practice, hospital policies, or nursing care. Suggested areas for inquiry, in the form of cultural and biologic traits, are shown in Box 3-2 at the beginning of this chapter.

Making an Assessment

Tripp-Reimer, Brink, and Saunders[48] state that most patients do not need thorough cultural assessments. Cultural questions are included in many routine nursing assessment tools. Sufficient information may be obtained by finding out dietary preferences, religious affiliation, family patterns, ethnic identification, and health care practices. If, however, a patient does not understand, or is not cooperative or compliant, a further examination of cultural factors may be necessary.

If so, the following questions may be helpful in assessing the patient's perspective and his or her definition of the situation.

1. What do you call your illness?
2. When did it start? Why do you think it started then?
3. What do you think caused it?
4. How have you been taking care of yourself? Did you consult someone else about what to do for your illness? If so, who did you consult? What did the person recommend?
5. How long do you think your illness will last? Is it a serious illness? What problems has your illness caused you?
6. Is there anything else you would like to tell me?

A cultural assessment is a *nonjudgmental clarification of patient and/or family concerns and beliefs.* Such findings need not be accepted as the nurse's own, and the nurse and patient may agree to disagree. They may discuss and negotiate the best way to serve the patient's preferences while not threatening the patient's fundamental medical and nursing care.

It is the professional's obligation to separate normative data from patient specific data; that is, whether a particular patient fits the normal pattern for his or her group. If not, find out what is unique about that individual and take that information into consideration when providing nursing care.

If a patient talks about or engages in behavior that is illegal, nonjudgmental acceptance does not apply. Such behavior needs to be brought to the attention of the appropriate authorities. For example, action is required when the nurse becomes aware of evidence of abuse and/or neglect of others (usually children, but sometimes the elderly), or if the nurse suspects the use of illegal substances, such as cocaine or marijuana while in the hospital.

Selecting Nursing Diagnoses

The North American Nursing Diagnosis Association (NANDA) approved list for 1990 contains 100 nursing diagnoses. Of these, over one-half have a significant psycho/social/cultural focus. This is another illustration of the attention the nursing profession places on holistic health care in a sociocultural context.

Among the many nursing diagnoses that incorporate cultural components, the following have been selected as particularly applicable for patients whose culture differs significantly from the nurses providing the care:

- Coping, ineffective family: compromised—Inadequate or incorrect information or understanding, preoccupation by significant person with personal reactions, temporary family disorganization and role changes, crises, prolonged disability of significant person
- Noncompliance—Patient value system (health beliefs, cultural influences, spiritual values), client-provider relationships, treatment side effects, cognitive/perceptual alterations
- Personal identity disturbance—Confusion, changes in lifestyle, trauma, changes in social involvement
- Spiritual distress—Separation from religious/cultural ties, conflict between spiritual beliefs and prescribed health regimen
- Family process, altered—Situation transition/crisis, Development transition/crisis

These and many other nursing diagnoses can be helpful in guiding the diagnostic part of the nursing care planning process.

Planning Care

The care plan for a patient with a predominantly cultural nursing diagnosis may specify further inquiry into the patient's beliefs and values, especially when confusion or noncompliance exists. The care plan may list knowledge deficits that need to be addressed in patient and family teaching. Alterations in routine practices may be suggested to accommodate preferences and anxieties that have been expressed by the patient or family. Family meetings may be requested by the nurse to exchange information and to increase mutual understanding of the patient's problems, prognosis, and future needs.

Nurses are often asked to be creative in assisting patients regain their health. The domain of a patient's cultural background is no exception. Health care providers have greater opportunities to practice this skill as populations become more mobile and cross-cultural contact becomes more commonplace. Figure 3-8 shows a group of nurses with diverse cultural and biologic characteristics meeting together to plan care for their unit of hospitalized patients. As this group learns more about themselves and how to work together and with each other, they become increasingly valuable to their equally diverse patient population.

Serving as Advocate

After making an assessment, identifying diagnoses, and planning care, the next step is action. The nurse has a major role as an advocate on behalf of the patient to the rest of the health care system. This role is based on a greater understanding of the patient's cultural needs. The needs may be as simple as alerting dietary service to provide a meatless menu for a patient who is a vegetarian, or as complex as arranging for a translator for a patient or family who do not speak English and need assistance communicating with the health care team.

Another manifestation of the advocate role is to become a negotiator, or cultural broker, to mediate between what is permissible and acceptable to the patient and what can be tolerated within the policies and procedures of the health care system. An example is allowing family to come after visiting hours to accommodate a family member's irregular work schedule.

The nursing care plan may also recommend consultation with other health team members. The nurse can then present unfamiliar aspects of the patient's background to others so that the team's combined efforts can be maximized on the patient's behalf.

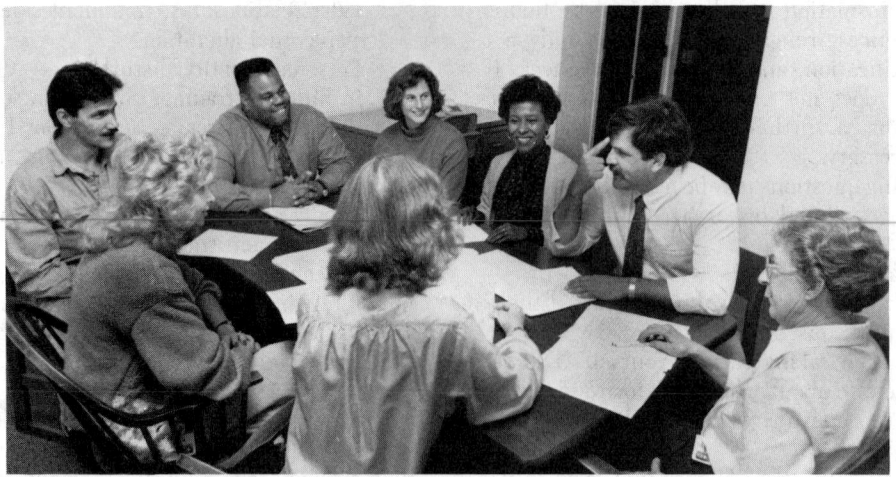

Fig. 3-8 Diverse group of nurses works together to plan care on the unit for their equally diverse patient population.

EXAMPLES OF NURSING CARE IN SPECIALIZED CULTURAL SETTINGS

Many groups of people in need of nursing care are in special subcultures by virtue of their age, location, developmental level, ethnic background, sensory abilities, or other distinguishing features. Openness to education on the part of the nurse and the people being served is necessary for getting needed services to the populations of these isolated communities. A few subcultures listed in the following discussion suggest opportunities for nursing students to consider when seeking further educational or employment opportunities.

Frontier Nursing Service

An early example of a nurse-managed system for special care is the Frontier Nursing Service, founded in 1925 by Mary Breckenridge.[31] Since then, this organization has been attending to families, especially mothers and babies, in the Appalachian hills of Kentucky. Formerly traveling by horseback, the nurses now use jeeps to reach their clients in the remote communities.

Nursing Homes

For many years, nursing homes have been locations for nursing activities. Although many homes have established a less restrictive environment for their residents, they are also becoming more aware of cultural traditions among the staff. Culture exists not only with the other people, but also within institutions themselves. A culturally sensititve nurse can learn to respect the need for stability on the part of the staff, while advocating change to provide a more restraint-free environment for the residents.[6]

Services for the Disabled

Persons with disabilities in speech, hearing, vision, or ambulation belong to unique subcultural communities, whether organized or not. Some are established to meet persons' needs for special environments. These populations provide a challenge for nurses by extending their talents to those whose physical or mental skills cannot be taken for granted.

Hispanic Populations

Opportunities exist in many regions of the United States for those interested in providing health care services to Spanish-speaking communities. For example, many persons of Puerto Rican background live in New York City and Connecticut. Cuban immigrants reside in Florida, and many persons with ties in Mexico migrate to California, Texas, and Colorado. A bilingual health care provider is helpful, especially a person who is familiar with special health care features, such as the concept of "nerves" or the hot-cold phenomenon (see discussion on p. 36).

Communities in Older, Larger Cities

Nurses have served patients in the inner cities for many years. Lillian Wald and Lavinia Dock helped establish what was to become the Henry Street Settlement, in New York City in 1893. According to Kelly:

> Each nurse was carefully oriented to the customs of the immigrants she served and was able to demonstrate the value of understanding the family and the environment in giving good nursing care.[39]

Modern counterparts of these early workers are found in organizations such as Visiting Nurse Associations, neighborhood clinics, and home care agencies.

Many large cities include a significant Black population. These communities, often in the older central portions of cities, have special needs for health care services. Hospitals in these locations also may be older, underfunded, understaffed, and busy. Their emergency rooms often provide routine family health care that was served by the family doctor of an earlier era. Free-standing outpatient clinics are a partial solution to reach these communities. Books such as Stack's *All Our Kin*[47] and Wilson's *The Truly Disadvantaged*[28] provide insight and information to help understand the perspective from which many of these patients come. This is particularly helpful when a nurse has no first-hand experience with these populations.

Oriental Populations

Other populations of special interest because of their cultural heritage include those with origins in such counties as China, Japan, Korea, and Vietnam. In the past, many immigrants from the Orient settled on or near the west coast of the United States, but now representatives of these countries can be found in many states, including Vietnamese shrimp fishers in Texas and factory employees in Iowa.

Nurses giving care to these populations will find it helpful to recall the concepts of "shame" and "face" discussed earlier. For example, when the nurse asks the patient if he or she understands what has been taught, the patient may smile and nod, indicating "yes", even when he or she doesn't understand. In oriental cultures it would be impolite to indicate that the nurse had not been understood because this would cause the nurse to lose "face."

American Indian Health Center

The American Indian Health Center located in Tuba City, Arizona, provides outpatient care and hospitalization for Native Americans, primarily from the southwest. Cultural pattern differences between the biomedical model of the United States Government that finances the Center and the tribal members can be quite large. Social problems related to reservation status and limited economic opportunities are often manifested as high-risk health behaviors that offer a special challenge to nurses providing care to these populations.

IMPACT OF RECENT TRENDS AND SOCIAL CHANGES

A discussion about cultural influences on health and illness is incomplete without reference to several major social, cultural, economic, and political issues involving health care delivery. These too, are the products of the cultural climate of the times and none are resolved easily or quickly. An awareness of some of these concerns helps nurses see their professional role within the larger context of the society around them.

Issues of Access

Who can get health care and who cannot? Is health care racist? These questions were addressed by Osborne in 1978[44] but are far from resolution today. The issues were updated and reviewed in a nursing journal by Funkhouser and Moser in 1990.[12] These authors discuss the historic and cultural patterns that may serve to explain, but not excuse, the difference in health service available to many Blacks and other minorities, compared to that available to the dominant white population.

Another limitation of access involves cost. Health decision making, which traditionally had been privately discussed between patient and physician, now often includes insurers, employers (who choose the insurers), the courts, and governmental policy makers. The ability to pay for health care is a real fact of life in the 1990s. It is also devastating to increasing numbers of underinsured, un-

insured, and unemployed populations. The National League for Nursing has issued a position statement regarding access to nursing services.[18] The nursing profession needs to be politically aware so that patients are cared for in a cost-effective manner.

With a better-educated, assertive, and consumer-oriented public, health care personnel are finding that people are shopping around and asking more questions, as well as taking more responsibility for their own health care decisions. Likewise, the depersonalization of the health care industry has been one of the factors responsible for the increase in lawsuits by patients who are dissatisfied with the outcomes of their care.

Awareness

While the health system is asked to do more with less, a movement is growing for health promotion, disease prevention, and a healthier life-style. More people are reducing their smoking and drinking, exercising more, eating more sensibly, and seeking preventive health care. The decreased incidence of morbidity from myocardial infarction reflects a culturally induced behavioral change.

An extension of caring more for the self is caring more for the environment, as described by Smith and Whitney.[23] Both local and global issues are raised by concerned citizens about reduction of health risks to populations from various environmental sources. In addition, people are concerned about reduction of further risks to the health of the planet itself so that it will be safe for the use of future generations.

SUMMARY

1. All persons have a culture and are affiliated with various cultural and subcultural groups over their lifespans.
2. Awareness of cultural values of others makes nursing care easier for both nurses and their patients and families.
3. Cultural sensitivity (ethnosensitivity) is an acquired skill and can be learned along with other skills to become a more effective nurse.
4. Racial characteristics are inherited but because cultural beliefs and perceptions about race are learned, they may interfere with open communication and acceptance between persons from different racial groups.
5. Ethnicity refers to a distinctive subcultural group that considers itself unique because of its language, religion, foods, and traditions.
6. Religious beliefs of patients may prevent them from accepting certain diets, medical procedures, and other care judged as routine by the dominant health care community.
7. An illness is what a person feels, a disease is what a physician diagnoses, and sickness is a label from society.
8. Western biomedicine is only one way of viewing health, illness, and disease causation. Alternatives include various folk traditions, stress theories, the holistic approach, and developmental and environmental considerations.
9. Everyone speaks a silent language when their body

and expressions provide nonverbal cues indicative of their feelings, moods, and attitudes.

10. Over half of the NANDA-approved nursing diagnoses have a significant psycho/social/cultural focus, providing many opportunities to apply cultural sensitivity to direct nursing care.

11. Nurses can serve as cultural brokers to negotiate appropriate care and services for their patients with the rest of the health care system.

12. Many opportunities exist for nursing in specialized cultural and subcultural settings, such as in services for the disabled, the elderly, those in the inner cities, and immigrants from other countries.

13. Cultural biases and fears may be involved in decision-making regarding allocation of resources to serve special population groups.

STUDY QUESTIONS

• Discuss the impact of internal and external forces (heredity versus environment) on the formation of a person. Give examples of each from your own experience.

• Discuss the different cultural roles you fill in the course of a week. What are the norms for behavior, language, and dress for each role?

• List some commonly held beliefs about a cultural or ethnic group of your acquaintance. Seek out a representative of that group and learn how many of those beliefs actually apply to that particular person.

• Check a current newspaper or magazine for an article about a controversial health care issue. Bring it into class and listen to different viewpoints about the topic from your classmates.

• Discuss some of the differences between the culture of nursing and the culture of medicine from a current and historic point of view.

REFERENCES AND SELECTED READINGS

1. Aamodt AM: Care and culture: *An introspective commentary.* In Barbee EL, editor: *The anthropology of nurse anthropologists,* San Francisco, 1991, Council on Nursing and Anthropology.
2. Bailey EJ: Hypertension: An analysis of Detroit African American health care treatment patterns, *Human Organization* 50:287-296, 1991.
3. Bennett MJ: Towards ethnorelativism: A *developmental model of intercultural sensitivity.* In Paige RM, editor: *Cross-cultural orientation: New conceptualizations and applications,* Lanham, Md, 1986, University Press of America.
4.* Borkan JM, Neher JO: A developmental model of ethnosensitivity in family practice training, *Fam Med* 23:212-17, 1991.
5. Brink PJ: *Notes of a nurse anthropologist.* In Barbee EL, editor: *The anthropology of nurse anthropologists,* San Francisco, 1991, Council on Nursing and Anthropology.
6.* Cutchins CH: Blueprint for restraint-free care, *Am J Nurs* 91(7):36-42, 1991.
7. Davis DL, Low SM: *Gender, health, and illness: The case of nerves,* New York, 1989, Hemisphere Publishing.
8.* Dickstein LJ, et al: Men's changing social roles in the 1990s:

Emerging issues in the psychiatric treatment of men, *Hosp Community Psychiatry* 42:701-705, 1991.
9.* Dossey B: Awakening the inner healer, *Am J Nurs* 91(8)30-34, 1991.
10. Fabrega H: The self and schizophrenia: A cultural perspective, *Schizophrenia Bulletin* 15:277-290, 1989.
11. Florsheim P: Cross-cultural views of self in treatment of mental illness: Disentangling the curative aspects of myth from the mythic aspects of cure, *Psychiatry* 53:304-15, 1990.
12.* Funkhouser SW, Moser DK: Is health care racist?, *Advances Nurs Sci* 12(2):47-55, 1990.
13. Kay M, Yoder M: Hot and cold in women's ethnotherapeutics: The American Mexican west, *Soc Sci Med* 25:347-355, 1987.
14. Leininger MM: Transcultural care diversity and universality: A theory of nursing, *Nurs Health Care* 6:209-212, 1985.
15. Levine SB: *Sex is not simple,* Columbus, Ohio, 1988, Ohio Psychology Publishing Company.
16. Morse JM: Concepts of caring and caring as a concept, *Advances Nurs Sci* 13:1-14, 1990.
17. Mwaria CB: The concept of self in the context of crisis: A study of families of the severely brain-injured, *Soc Sci Med* 30:889-893, 1990.
18. National League for Nursing, *Position statement: Consumer access to nursing services,* New York, 1990, National League for Nursing.
19.* Peoples J, Bailey G: *Humanity: An introduction to anthropology,* ed 2, St Paul, 1991, West Publishing.
20. Phillips MJ: Damaged goods: Oral narratives of the experience of disability in American culture, *Soc Sci Med* 30:849-857, 1990.
21. Rapaport FT, Waltzer WC, Anaise D: How can one balance duty to all cultures and ethnic groups with effective procurement and equitable distribution of organs for clinical transplantation?—New evidence of the key importance of local primacy for a successful organ donation effort, *Transplantation Proceedings* 22:1007-1009, 1990.
22. Reminick RA: Personal communication, August, 1991.
23.* Smith MN, Whitney GM: *Caring for the environment: The ecology of health.* In Chinn P, editor: *Anthology of caring,* New York, 1991, National League for Nursing.
24.* Swerdlow JL: A new kind of kinship, *National Geographic* 180(3):64-91, 1991.
25. Swinney JE: Letters to the editor, *Advances in Nurs Sci* 13(3):vi-viii, 1991.
26.* Tripp-Reimer T, Afifi LA: Cross-cultural perspectives on patient teaching, *Nurs Clin North Am* 24:613-619, 1989.
27. Tripp-Reimer T, Brink PJ: *Cultural brokerage.* In Bulecheck G, McCloskey M, editors: *Nursing interventions: Treatments for nursing diagnoses,* Philadelphia, 1985, WB Saunders.
28.* Wilson WJ: *The truly disadvantaged: The inner city, the underclass, and public policy,* Chicago, 1987, University of Chicago Press.
29. Zatzick DF, Dimsdale JE: Cultural variations in response to painful stimuli, *Psychosomatic Medicine* 52:544-57, 1990.
30.* Zuckerman M: Some dubious premises in research and theory on racial difference, scientific, social, and ethical issues, *American Psychologist* 45:1297-1303, 1990.

Classic

31.* Breckenridge M: *Wide neighborhoods: A story of the Frontier Nursing Service,* New York, 1952, Harper & Row.
32. Byerly EL, Molgaard CA: *Social institutions and disease transmission: The new age gathering.* In Chrisman N, Maretzki T, editors: *Clinically applied anthropology,* Cheney, Wash, 1982, Eastern Washington University.
33. Chrisman NJ, Maretzki TW: *Clinically applied anthropology: Anthropologists in health science settings,* Dordrecht, Holland, 1982, D Reidel Publishing.

---

*Recommended for student reading.

34. Dodd CH: *Dynamics of intercultural communication,* Dubuque, Iowa, 1982, Wm C Brown.

35. Eisenberg L: Disease and illness: Distinctions between professional and popular ideas of sickness, *Culture, Medicine and Psychiatry,* 1:9-23, 1977.

36. Good BJ, Good MD: *The meaning of symptoms: A cultural hermeneutic model for clinical practice.* In Eisenberg L, Kleinman A, editors: The relevance of social science for medicine, Dordrecht, Holland, 1981, D Reidel Publishing.

37.* Hall ET: *The Silent Language,* New York, 1973, Anchor Press.

38. Harwood A: The hot-cold theory of disease: Implications for treatment of Puerto Rican patients, *J Am Med Assn* 216:1153-1158, 1971.

39.* Kelly LY: Dimensions of professional nursing, ed 4, New York, 1981, Macmillan Publishing.

40. Kleinman A: *Patients and healers in the context of culture: an exploration of the borderland between anthropology, medicine, and psychiatry,* Berkeley, Calif, 1980, University of California Press.

41. Kleinman A: The cultural meanings and social uses of illness: A role for medical anthropology and clinically oriented social science in the development of primary care theory and research, *J Fam Prac,* 16:539-45, 1983.

42.* Leininger MM: *Transcultural nursing: Concepts theories and practices,* New York, 1978, John Wiley & Sons.

43. Moore LG, et al: *The biocultural basis of health: Expanding views of medical anthropology,* Prospect Heights, Ill, 1980, Waveland Press.

44.* Osborne OH: Aging and the black diaspora: *The African, Caribbean and African-American experience.* In Leininger M, editor: *Transcultural nursing: Concepts theories and practices,* New York, 1978, John Wiley & Sons.

45. Reminick RA: *Theory of ethnicity: an anthropologist's perspective,* Lanham, Md, 1983, University Press of America.

46. Selye H: *The stress of life,* New York, 1956, McGraw-Hill Book.

47.* Stack C: *All our kin: Strategies for survival in a black community,* New York, 1974, Harper & Row.

48.* Tripp-Reimer T, Brink PJ, Saunders JM: Cultural Assessment: Content and Process, *Nurs Outlook* 32(2):78-82, 1984.

49. Twaddle AC: *Sickness and the sickness career: Some implications.* In Eisenberg L, Kleinman A, editors: *The relevance of social science for medicine,* Dordrecht, Holland, 1981, D Reidel Publishing.

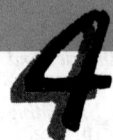

4

Promotion of Health in the Elderly

Ruth Lincoln

After studying this chapter, the learner should be able to:

- Distinguish between primary and secondary changes of aging.
- Describe psychosocial aspects of aging.
- Compare health concerns of elderly adults with those of younger adults.
- Describe health promotion strategies for the older adult.
- Describe special precautions for the hospitalized elderly.

This chapter discusses the characteristics of the elderly from a health perspective. Major health needs of the elderly and the role of the nurse in assisting the elderly with health promotion and health problems are addressed. The chapter focuses on assisting elderly persons to improve the quality of their lives.

The number of persons over age 65 in the United States is increasing dramatically. The elderly population, at 30 million in 1990, is predicted to be at 39 million in 2010 and at 66 million by 2030. Accounting for 4% of the population in 1900, the percentage of elderly will increase 23% by the year 2030. The largest growth is occurring among those over the age of 85 years.[13]

The elderly account for the highest proportion of those with chronic illness and functional disability. Improving the quality of life, rather than searching for means to increase longevity, becomes of utmost importance. According to the most recent publication on national health objectives by the U.S. Department of Health and Human Services, the major goal for the 1990s is to increase the span of healthy life for all Americans.[13]

CONCEPTS OF AGING

Although 65 years of age is usually considered the beginning of late adulthood, tremendous individual variation exists. Age is more a sociocultural concept than a physiologic or chronologic one.

Theories of Aging

Biologic aging theory focuses on cellular aging; changes in replicating cells, loss or injury to cells, and changes in noncellular materials or regulatory systems that "program" aging. One cellular theory postulates that a limited number of cell divisions occur under the influence of a biologic clock or program. Another explanation maintains that aging is a random chemical process, influenced by damage from free radicals. Radiation "hits" lead to cellular mutations, which cause aging as they accumulate over the years.

Physiologic theories of aging relate the aging process to a decline in the immune system. Either the immune system succumbs as aging progresses or an autoimmunity develops. As immune competence decreases, the incidence of infections, cancer, and autoimmune diseases rises.

Another physiologic theory maintains that "cross-linking" occurs in collagen cells. As the cross-linkages accumulate, organs deteriorate from impaired function.[11]

None of these theories has been accepted as the final truth about aging. Researchers continue to seek the answer to the question: What causes the body to age?

Physiologic Aging

In late adulthood, physiologic function does not correlate with chronologic age. Adult years are not characterized by specific events at particular ages, with the exception of menopause. Some biologic variables remain constant throughout the lifespan (for example, fasting blood sugar, blood pH). However, the normal range for some electrolytes and enzymes is different for the elderly than for younger adults (Table 4-1). Other body functions begin a gradual decline after age 30, continuing into the late decades (Fig. 4-1). Certain generalizations can be made, however:

1. The older the age group, the greater the variability among individuals.
2. The rate of decline varies among body functions.
3. Changes previously thought to be associated with aging have been shown to result from lack of physical conditioning or from disease.

Primary and Secondary Aging

Primary aging refers to biologic changes that are universal, gradual, intrinsic, and inevitable. Graying hair and wrinkles are examples of primary aging changes. *Secondary aging* refers to pathophysiologic conditions. These may be more prevalent in the elderly but are not universal. More importantly, secondary changes are treatable and sometimes reversible. In the past, many conditions that were attributed to old age have been proven to be pathologic. Some of these are senility, arthritis, loss of hearing, muscle weakness, and incontinence. The 93-year-old man who complained to his doctor about his gimpy right leg is an example

Table 4-1   Reference ranges that are appreciably different in old age*

	Range for adults	Range for elderly
Albumin	37-51 g/L	33-49 g/L
Globulin	19-33 g/L	20-41 g/L
Potassium	3.6-4.7 mmol/L	3.6-5.2 mmol/L
Urea	3.2-7.2 mmol/L	3.9-9.9 mmol/L
Creatinine	62-123 μmol/L	52-159 μmol/L
	(0.7-1.4 mg/dl)	(0.6-1.8 mg/100 m/L)
Uric acid (men)	4.0-7.6 mg/dl	3.1-7.8 mg/dl
Uric acid (women)	2.6-6.2 mg/dl	2.1-7.7 mg/dl
Calcium (men)	2.25-2.60 mmol/L	2.19-2.59 mmol/L
Calcium (women)	2.18-2.55 mmol/L	2.18-2.68 mmol/L
Alkaline phosphatase (men)	19-75 IU/L	22-81 IU/L
Alkaline phosphatase (women)	14-67 IU/L	22-83 IU/L
Erythrocyte sedimentation rate (women)	0-7 mm/h	6-69 mm/h
Leukocyte count	4000-11,000/mm³	3100-8900/mm³

*Ranges given are likely to vary slightly from those of many American laboratories, which often do not adjust ranges for gender or age.
Modified from Hazzard W, et al: *Principles of Geriatric Medicine*, New York, 1990, McGraw-Hill.

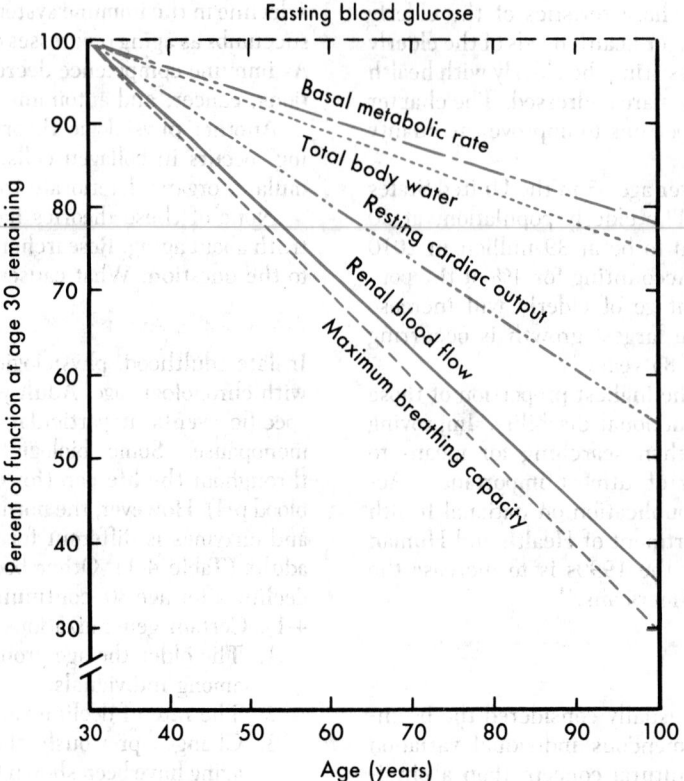

Fig. 4-1 Biologic concepts of aging. (From Shock NW: *Biologic concepts of aging.* In Simon A, Epstein LJ, editors: *Aging in modern society*, Washington, DC, 1968, American Psychiatric Association. Reprinted by permission.)

of primary versus secondary aging. The doctor said, "You're old; you have to put up with aches and pains." The old man retorted, "Tell that to my left leg."

The nurse working with the elderly must know the common aging changes. Assessment should include baseline function, prediction of functional changes, and discrimination between primary and secondary aging. Because the elderly often believe the myths regarding what they "must put up with," they need to be encouraged to seek medical treatment for their chronic and acute conditions. Some symptoms, such as weakness and fatigue, are helped by diet and exercise.

Sexuality

Both men and women maintain interest in sexual activity into the late adulthood years. More women cease having sexual activity after age 65 than do men. The primary reasons for the cessation are lack of acceptable sexual partner for widows or an ailing husband for married women (rather than lack of interest).[31]

Cultural attitudes toward the elderly influence both sexes. Older men and women are frequently thought of as sexually unattractive and lacking in ability to engage in sex. However, Masters and Johnson[36] have found that although sexual responses are slower, the elderly still have the same phases of excitement, plateau, orgasm, and resolution as younger persons. Men, in particular, can expect

adequate sexual performance up to and beyond the eighth decade (see Chapter 34).

Sexual problems occur more frequently for the elderly. Women may have dyspareunia as a result of vaginal thinning and decreased lubrication. These factors are caused by postmenopausal steroid starvation. Men tend to be affected by secondary impotence related to performance anxiety and low self-esteem. Diabetes, alcohol, and medications for hypertension are other prominent causes of impotence.

Masters and Johnson report a condition known as "widower's syndrome."[36] Following an extended period of sexual inactivity, a man cannot achieve or maintain an erection. An equivalent condition occurs in women: the vagina constricts and undergoes atrophic changes. The conclusion is that those who do not engage in sexual activity lose the ability.

Sexuality is more than the physical act of intercourse. Elderly persons continue to need human companionship and the sharing of love and affection. Nurses need to be aware of the components of sexuality and how the elderly may be affected by chronic illness, loss of a partner, and need for touch. Being sensitive to family dynamics is just as important for a newly married couple in their seventies as for a young couple.[31] Through counseling the nurse can explain aging changes, suggesting vaginal lubrication for women and extra physical stimulation for men. Changes in sexual position and styles of lovemaking are appropriate for those with disabling diseases. Nurses have a vital role in enabling elderly persons to express their needs for love and affection.

Unfortunately, the elderly are susceptible to sexually transmitted disease, though not in the same numbers as younger adults. Acquired immune deficiency syndrome (AIDS) is becoming increasingly prevalent in the elderly as the epidemic spreads among all age groups. The "at risk" categories differ for elderly (for example, not as many are intravenous drug abusers).[29] However, other risk factors are present: the decline in the ability of the immune system to ward off infections makes them more susceptible to organisms from sexually transmitted diseases. Women in particular are more vulnerable because of the friable vaginal lining that occurs with aging. "Safe sex" education and counseling for those at risk should not be overlooked just because the person is over 65 years of age.[29]

Psychosocial Aging

Aging has long been associated with deterioration in function rather than an expansion of abilities. New evidence is accumulating to support multifactor systems theories to account for the richness and variety encountered among older adults.

Reed proposes the view that adult development is a progressive, not a decremental, phenomenon.[38] She emphasizes the role of person–environment interactions in successful aging and views aging behavior not as decremental, but as "trade-offs." Important concepts are that adults:

1. Have a clearer perception of themselves and others not clouded by the context of the situation
2. Are better equipped to engage in complex and meaningful interactions with others
3. Conceptualize problems better and delegate less complex details to others
4. Are better able to predict future consequences
5. Develop more realistic solutions to problems
6. Are increasingly capable of transforming conflicts into meaningful experiences.

The "trade-offs" for the older adult are a decreased intellectual dexterity, decreased flexibility in thinking, and loss of ability to remember details. These may appear as deficiencies to young adults but actually help the elderly provide a stabilizing force for society.

A positive outlook on aging is crucial to the nurse's capacity to evaluate the abilities of the elderly in any setting. An 84-year-old woman admitted to the hospital from a nursing home is not the equivalent of a regressed child. She should be regarded as an experienced adult, integrally related to the environment, no matter what her functional level.

Nurses are challenged to facilitate well-being among adults who have developed useful modes of functioning as they age. Strategies are not appropriate if they are based on physical strength, deftness of function, and speed of recall. The developmental tasks of late adulthood are summarized in Box 4-1. Box 4-2 discusses research on the effect of restricted activity in the elderly.

Intellectual Function

Intellectual function curves stay relatively stable throughout a person's lifespan (Fig. 4-2). Research has shown that many components of cognitive function remain intact in the elderly. Problem solving, verbal ability, recognition, and memory span are examples of areas in which normal elderly persons scored well.[33] Only when the tests were timed and speed was important did results decline.

The implications for the nurse are clear when devising teaching strategies for the elderly. Older adults are capable of learning. They retain content best when it is related to something familiar, is sequenced, and plenty of time is allowed to learn each facet.

Health Problems

Chronic diseases are a major health problem and are much more common among the elderly population (see Box 4-3). Estimates show that 85% of the elderly have one or more chronic diseases. Heart disease and hypertension are the most prevalent, with 50% of persons over the age of 65 years having observable signs of heart disease. Gastrointestinal disorders, rheumatism, and arthritis affect large numbers of the elderly. Visual problems, atherosclerosis, lung disease, and hypertension appear to be associated with lower socioeconomic status.

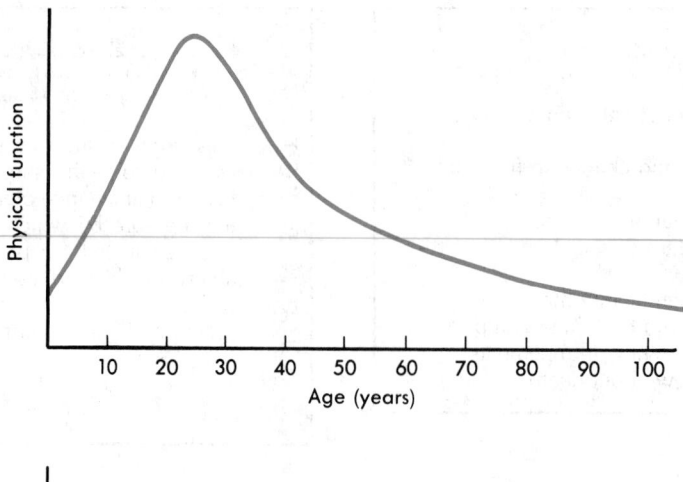

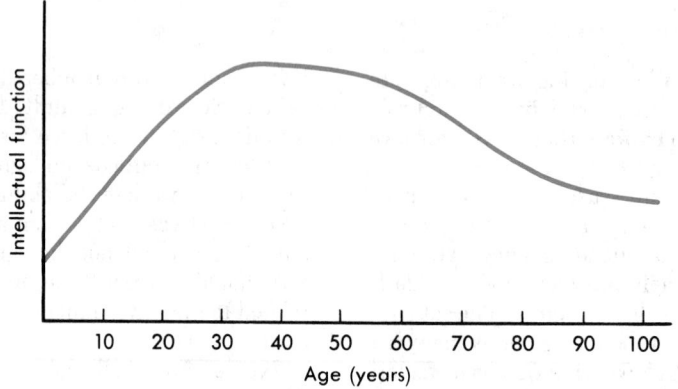

Fig. 4-2   Comparison of physical and intellectual function over life span.

4-3	**Major health problems of late adulthood**
	Heart disease
	Hypertension
	Cancer
	Renal disease
	Chronic obstructive pulmonary disease
	Acute pulmonary disease (pneumonia, pulmonary edema)
	Vascular disease (cerebrovascular accident, peripheral vascular disease)
	Arthritis
	Skin disorders
	Accidents
	Alcoholism

The figures on prevalence of health problems may be misleading. The important issues are: what is normal functioning and how disabling are the chronic conditions?

Despite chronic disease, 83% of persons over the age of 65 have little difficulty carrying out activities of daily living. Only 5% live in nursing homes, although 35% will be in a nursing home at one time or another. Another 5% are homebound.

The following factors are important to remember when evaluating the physical capacities of the elderly:

1. Organ systems have a great compensatory ability, despite loss of cells and tissue through aging (such as in the brain, kidney, heart, and liver).
2. Compensatory mechanisms may fail when the organism is stressed through illness and disease (for example, renal failure can occur with urinary tract infection).
3. The body takes a longer time to return to normal following a stressful event.
4. Once a stressful event has occurred, the individual may not return to baseline function.
5. The immune system is decreasingly effective as the individual ages, causing increased susceptibility to infection. The elderly are much more prone to pneumonia, skin infections, urinary tract infection, and sepsis.
6. The symptomatology of a particular disease is often atypical in the elderly (for example, a myocardial infarction without severe crushing chest pain, an infection without a fever, a gastrointestinal hemorrhage without severe stomach pain).
7. The most typical sign that an individual has had a change in physical well-being is sudden onset of confusion.

Stress situations may produce more pronounced reactions in the elderly and require a longer period of readjustment. The Holmes-Rahe Stress Scale, which is concerned with social readjustment in adults, has been

Table 4-2   Social readjustment rating scale (life change units)

Life event	Mean value	Life event	Mean value
Death of spouse	100	Son or daughter leaving home	29
Divorce	73	Trouble with in-laws	29
Marital separation	65	Outstanding personal achievement	28
Jail term	63	Wife beginning or stopping work	26
Death of close family member	63	Begin or end school	26
Personal injury or illness	53	Change in living conditions	25
Marriage	50	Revision of personal habits	24
Fired at work	47	Trouble with boss	23
Marital reconciliation	45	Change in work hours or conditions	20
Retirement	45	Change in residence	20
Change in health of family member	44	Change in schools	20
Pregnancy	40	Change in recreation	19
Sex difficulties	39	Change in church activities	19
Gain of new family member	39	Change in social activities	18
Business readjustment	39	Mortgage or loan less than $10,000	17
Change in financial state	38	Change in sleeping habits	16
Death of close friend	37	Change in number of family get-togethers	15
Change to different line of work	36	Change in eating habits	15
Change in number of arguments with spouse	35	Vacation	13
Mortgage over $10,000	31	Christmas	12
Foreclosure of mortgage or loan	30	Minor violations of the law	11
Change in responsibilities at work	29		

From Holmes T, Rahe H-*J Pyschosom Res* 11:213, 1967.

criticized for lack of applicability to the elderly (see Table 4-2). The reader may find it helpful to compare the stressful events listed in Table 4-2 with the stressful life changes for the elderly in Box 4-4.

PREVENTION AND HEALTH EDUCATION
Primary Prevention

The goal of health care for the elderly is to keep people functioning at the optimal level for their age. Health promotion is just as important for the elderly person as for the young person. Nurses in any health care setting have an ideal opportunity to assist elderly persons with health promotion.

Even in the acute care setting where the focus is on illness, the nurse should identify priority needs and introduce an educational program designed to enhance the person's life style after hospitalization.

The four main areas the nurse should address are *health habits* (smoking and drinking), *exercise, nutrition,* and *immunizations.* This section also addresses general principles in teaching the elderly.

Health habits

Nursing assessment in any setting should include questions regarding smoking and alcohol use. Smoking cessation can have positive health benefits for a person at any age. Reduced incidence of respiratory infections and improved ventilatory capacity are two of these. A smoking history should tell not only packs per day, but also the meaning of smoking to the individual, habits connected with smoking (for example, eating and drinking, reading, answering the phone) and attempts made to stop in the past. The nurse can help the elder to analyze his or her smoking

Stressful life changes for the elderly

Loss of driver's license
Multiple relocations
Hemiplegia
Sensory deficits
Hospitalization
Institutionalization
Mechanical speech difficulties
Loss of children and friends
Dispersal of significant belongings
Incompetency proceedings
Inheritance conflicts
Birth of grandchildren
Moving to a nursing home
Inadequate health insurance coverage

behavior to find ways to cut down or quit. Encourage the use of special programs, such as SmokeEnders or Smokestoppers.

Alcohol abuse is a largely unrecognized problem among the elderly. The signs and symptoms are similar to other secondary aging processes; tremors, sleep difficulties, gait abnormalities, depression, and malnutrition. The elderly person and his or her family may deny the seriousness of the problem, and health professionals may neglect to assess the individual for alcohol abuse.

Elderly persons have a decreased tolerance for alcohol because of a declining ability of the liver to detoxify and metabolize it. Loneliness and depression may intensify the feelings that lead to drinking. Heavy drinking contributes to confusion, injuries from falls, self-neglect, and malnutrition.[8]

Table 4-3 Benefits of exercise

System	Benefit
Cardiovascular	Increased maximum oxygen consumption
	Increased cardiac output
	Reduced mean blood pressure
Pulmonary	Reduced loss of Vo_2 maximum
Musculoskeletal	Increased bone mineral content
	Decreased loss of calcium
	Preservation of lean muscle mass
Regulatory system	Increased basal metabolic rate
	Increased hemoregulation
Nervous system	Decreased sleeplessness
	Decreased anxiety

From Schilke J: Slowing the aging process with physical activity, *J Gerontol Nurs* 17(5):5-9, 1991

4-5 Causes of malnutrition in the elderly

Acute and chronic illness
Limited financial resources
Psychologic factors such as boredom and lack of companionship while eating
Loss of teeth
Faulty eating patterns
Fads and notions regarding certain foods
Lack of energy to prepare foods
Lack of knowledge of appropriate nutrition
Decreased digestive enzymes

4-6 Immunizations for the elderly

Pneumococcal 23-valent vaccine; given one time
Influenza vaccine; given annually in the fall
Tetanus vaccine, for penetrating injuries, or booster; given every 10 years.[26]

The nurse should always be alert to symptoms that hint of alcohol abuse and ask questions regarding drinking habits. Teach patients about aging changes that aggravate the effect of alcohol and inform them about community agencies that are available to assist with alcohol problems. Many of these agencies have chapters of Alcoholic Anonymous. For more information on alcohol abuse see Chapter 13.

Exercise

An exercise program has many benefits for the older person, whether or not they have engaged in exercise in the past. Exercise increases endurance, strengthens the muscles, and enhances the cardiovascular system. Table 4-3 shows the benefits to the body systems.

A variety of exercise programs are recommended depending on the interests of the older person. The best and simplest is a walking program. Walking 30 to 60 minutes three times a week can improve fitness quickly and easily.

Other forms of exercise that may appeal to the older person are swimming, water exercise, bicycling, gardening, dancing, and many other sports. Whatever the type of program, the following guidelines are important:

1. Seek the advice of a physician before starting a strenuous exercise program.
2. Do not exercise to the point of dyspnea or pain.
3. Stop if signs of activity intolerance appear; dizziness, nausea, palpitations, or fatigue.[26]

When advising elderly persons about an exercise program, the nurse should instruct them in taking their pulse rate and teach them to aim for 75% to 85% of the maximum heart rate.[26] Aerobic exercise, which increases oxygen uptake and strengthens the cardiovascular system, should be performed three or more times weekly for maximum benefit.

Nutrition

Nutritional requirements of elderly persons differ from those of younger adults. The physical changes associated with aging, changes in the gastrointestinal tract, the digestive enzymes, and metabolism all affect nutritional status. Social factors may have as much impact on the individual's nutrition as physical changes. Some of these are loneliness, difficulty obtaining food, difficulty in preparing food, and social isolation. Malnutrition is common (see Box 4-5). The following are the nutritional needs of elderly persons:

Calories should be reduced by 5% per decade between age 55 to 75; 7% after 75 years of age.

Carbohydrate levels should be maintained, but should be obtained from fruits, vegetables, cereals, and breads. Only moderate amounts of foods with refined sugars (e.g., candy, cake, cookies) should be consumed.

Protein consumption should be reduced, especially red meats and high-fat dairy products. Fish, poultry, and combinations of plant foods should be increased.

Fat levels should be maintained, but fats should make up no more than 25% to 30% of daily caloric intake.

Vitamin supplements are not necessary unless dietary intake is poor. Absorption and storage capacity of vitamins decline. Vitamin D deficiency occurs occasionally.

Mineral supplements are not needed unless a physician diagnoses deficiencies. Those over 85 years of age are often deficient in calcium and zinc.

Water consumption should not change, but dehydration is common among elderly. Six to seven glasses of fluid should be taken per day.[17]

Immunizations

Persons over the age of 65 should be advised to have yearly immunizations against influenza and a one time immunization against pneumonia as part of the annual physical examination (see Box 4-6). As the immunologic system ages, the elderly person becomes more susceptible to acute communicable diseases. The reserve capacity to recover

---

4-7

Recommended health screening

Complete physical examination

Women (breast examination)
Self	Monthly
Professional	Annually
Mammogram	Annually until age 70, then discretionary
Pap and pelvic	Annually

Men (penis, scrotum, testicles)
Self	Monthly
Professional	Annually

Rectal examination

Both men and women	Annually
Proctosigmoidoscopy every 3-5 years after results of two consecutive annual tests negative	
Stool for occult blood	Annually

Dental examination

	Every 6-12 mon
Oral screen for cancer	Every 6-12 mon

Modified from Pastorino C, Dickey T: Health promotion for elderly, *Orthop Nurs* 9(6):36, 1990.

---

from stress declines as well. High-risk individuals are those with chronic disorders of the pulmonary and cardiovascular systems. Immunizations for influenza change annually as different strains of the influenza virus are identified. The best advice is to have patients check with their physician. Some communities offer influenza immunizations through the local health department.

Health education

The elderly adult learner presents an interesting challenge to the nurse in any setting. The same teaching–learning principles apply to the older person as to a younger adult, with some additional guidelines. As with any adult learner, the environment must be comfortable and familiar, so as not to distract from the learning process. For the elderly person, this means the nurse must take particular care to ensure that the patient is warm, relaxed, and free from pain and other discomforts. The older adult may have a hearing or vision impairment that inhibits the learning process, and the nurse must take these into consideration when planning teaching methods.

The nurse should teach the content of any teaching plan in several short sessions. Focus on single elements of the topic, reinforcing previous learning. This is especially true if the person has a short attention span or is distracted by the treatments and equipment in the environment.

One problem the nurse may overlook in the elderly patient is low literacy.[16] When a patient has cognitive and sensory impairments, the lack of good reading and vocabulary skills may hamper well-intentioned educational efforts. Low literacy provokes several reactions. The person may say she or he understands the teaching, when in fact he or she did not, resulting in withdrawal from the situation or disregarding complicated instructions. The following are hints for teaching patients with low literacy:

1. Use simple one or two syllable words.
2. Use large print materials.
3. Use pictures with colors and symbols.
4. Divide teaching sessions into segments.
5. Reinforce previous learning.
6. Give positive rewards for mastering content (for example, praise, attention, touch)
7. Involve other family members in the teaching process.[16]

Secondary Prevention
Health screening

Health screening is as important for the elderly as for the younger adult. The elderly person should have an annual physical examination. Box 4-7 lists the recommended screening procedures for both sexes.

Medications

The elderly use a highly disproportionate amount of medications compared with the younger adult. Most elderly take three or more therapeutic agents, and drug reactions and interactions are far more prevalent. Table 4-4 shows the pharmacokinetic changes that occur in the elderly.

Four problems affect the elderly as they take medications: *drug interactions, adverse reactions, drug and food interactions,* and *medication errors.* Each category is detailed in the following discussion.

Drug interactions

Some medications interact with others, causing harmful effects. Table 4-5 shows some of the possible combinations that are problems for the elderly.

Adverse reactions

Medications that cause no problems for middle-aged adults may be harmful for the elderly because of the physiologic changes mentioned previously. Table 4-6 shows typical medications taken by the elderly and the most common adverse reactions.

Table 4-4 **Pharmacokinetic changes in the elderly**

Process	Change	Possible result
Absorption	Decrease in HCL in stomach	Inadequate absorption of weak acid drugs
	Delay in gastric emptying	Prolonged exposure of drug to mucosa leads to possible overdosage and toxicity
Distribution	Decrease in cardiac output	Slower circulation of drug to desired sites of action and elimination
	Decrease in body muscle mass	Onset and duration of action of many drugs changes
	Increase in body fat	Fat-soluble drugs have delayed onset of action
	Decrease in body water	More sensitive to water-soluble drugs
	Decrease in serum albumin	Increase in amount of free-active (usually protein bound) drugs Increased potential for drug interactions
	Slowing of active transport systems	Delayed drug action
	Increased sensitivity to CNS drugs	Possible seizures, excitation, certain drugs (barbiturates) cause confusion
Biotransformation	Impaired liver function	Elevated plasma levels of drugs because of a decrease in first pass effect and in biotransformation Elevated levels of active metabolites of drugs
Excretion	Impaired kidney function	Elevated plasma levels of drugs

From Gray M: Polypharmacy in the elderly, *Orthop Nurs* 9(6):49, 1990.

Table 4-5 **Drug interactions and their potential results**

Drug A	Drug B	Potential results
Digoxin	Furosemide	Reduced potassium produced by B could increase risk of arrhythmia produced by A
Warfarin	Aspirin	Protein displacement of A by B could increase risk of bleeding
Tetracycline	Antacid	Absorption impairment of A by B could reduce the antibiotic efficacy of A

From Hershey L, Whitney C: *Drugs and the elderly.* In Kart C, Metress E, Metress S, editors: *Aging, health, and society,* Boston, 1988, Jones & Bartlett.

Table 4-6 **Typical medications and their effects**

Medication	Effect on elderly
Tranquilizers	CNS effects (sleepiness)
Aminoglycoside antibiotics	Ototoxicity, nephrotoxicity[14]
Anticoagulants	Risk of bleeding
Phenothiazines	Risk of tardive dyskinesia
Beta blockers	Light-headedness, slowed heart rate
Digoxin	Confusion

Modified from Hershey L, Whitney C: *Drugs and the elderly.* In, Kart C, Metress E, Metress S, editors: *Aging, health and society,* Boston, 1988, Jones & Bartlett.

Beta blockers can be particularly problematic for elders because these commonly prescribed agents depress cardiac contractility, leading to lethargy and dyspnea. Elderly persons are more prone to orthostatic hypotension, hypoglycemia, thyroid dysfunction, arthritic changes, and depression, all of which are possible side effects of beta blockers.[23]

Drug and food interactions

Some foods may inhibit or change the effect of a particular medication more dramatically in elderly than middle-aged persons. Levodopa taken by patients with Parkinson's disease has a reduced effect if taken with a high-protein meal. The antidepressants in the monoamine oxidase inhibitor (MAO) group are affected by red wine, blue cheese, and herring, causing malignant hypertension.[17]

Medication errors

Medication errors are common among the elderly. Some of the typical ones when the person is taking own medication are omitting prescribed drugs, taking drugs at the wrong times, and taking medications without fully knowing why they are prescribed. *In studies of medication errors, the persons most likely to err were those who took the most medications, those who lived alone, and those who were relatively less well-educated.*[17]

Facilitating learning about medications

First, the nurse should make a detailed and thorough assessment whenever he or she comes in contact with the elderly. Questions included in medication history are found in Box 4-8.

Education is based on the strengths and deficits found in the medication history. If the patient does not know the name of the drug, but remembers the pink "heart" pill, the nurse emphasizes the pink Lanoxin pill for the heart

4-8	**Patient medication history**

General questions

What medications do you take every day?

What are they used for?

Have you taken any other medications during the last month? last year?

What do you take for pain? How often?

What do you take to help you sleep? How often?

What do you take for constipation? How often?

Do you take any vitamins and health food preparations?

What medications do you share with your family? Friends?

What alcoholic beverages do you consume? How often? How much?

Do you smoke? How often?

Have you used any home remedies to treat this problem? Any other problem?

Adverse/allergic responses

Have you ever had an allergic response to medication?

Can you describe how it affected you?

Did you have this reaction in a hospital? At home?

What was done when you had this reaction?

Questions about taking medications

When do you take your medications? (time of day and number of times)

What happens if you miss a medication?

Are there any medications you take differently than the prescription says?

Do you have trouble reading the regular labels?

Do you have trouble removing the cap on the medication?

Do you have trouble in pouring or drawing up medication?

Do you have trouble swallowing any of your medications?

Care of medications

Where do you store your medications?

What happens with left over medications?

Do you purchase medications in large quantities?

Obtaining prescription medications

Have your medications been prescribed by more than one doctor?

Where do you get your prescriptions filled?

Psychosocial aspects

With whom do you live?

Have you ever omitted medications because they were too expensive?

How do you pay for your medications?

Modified from Gray M: Polypharmacy in the elderly, *Orthop Nurs* 9(6):49, 1990.

when discussing the medication. When administering medications in the acute care setting, the nurse is obligated to repeat the name, dose, and desired effect of the drugs. Through repetition, even persons with cognitive and learning impairments start to gain name recognition for their medications.

Whenever possible, patients should be allowed to take their own medications in the hospital setting. Self-medication allows the nurse to assess the patient's understanding of the drugs and the timing of them. It also provides an opportunity to observe side effects, such as lethargy or hypotension.

When teaching the patient how to take medications at home, the nurse must allow sufficient time for adequate learning. The following hints assist the nurse:

1. Teach in several short sessions spread over 1 to 2 days rather than one crammed session as the patient is being discharged.
2. Simplify medication schedules; for example, use colored stickers for different bottles.
3. Use large print instructions.
4. Coordinate times for medications with the person's daily schedule, for example with meals, when reading paper, before or after brushing teeth.
5. Use pictures for a person who cannot read well, for example, use a drawing of a clock with hands showing the medication time.
6. Use special containers as reminders for a forgetful person. For example, egg cartons labelled with days/times or a medication box with compartments (found in drugstores and pharmacies).
7. Emphasize important reminders; take with food, take all the medication.
8. Remind the elder to carry a list of medications with them and show it to any physician, at any clinic, or when coming to the hospital.[34]

MAJOR HEALTH PROBLEMS OF THE ELDERLY

Although many elderly persons maintain independent lifestyles, they are usually affected by one or more health problems. The number of problems increases proportionately as the person ages. This section addresses the systems most likely to show effects of primary and secondary aging. The nursing process is the framework for each system.

COGNITIVE PERCEPTUAL PROBLEMS

The elderly differ from their younger counterparts in several aspects of cognitive and perceptual function. *The most dramatic changes occur in the central nervous system; the peripheral motor neurons and the autonomic nervous system remain relatively constant throughout the life span.*

4-9	Aging changes
	Decreased brain weight
	Diminished enzyme activity
	Slowed reflexes
	Decreased sensory receptors for temperature, pain, and tactile discrimination
	Weakening of interneuron connections
	Increased response time
	Chronic hypoxia

The changes listed in Box 4-9 affect complex processes such as learning, memory, language, and mentation. Although loss of memory is not considered a primary aging change, many older persons have progressively increasing problems with short-term memory. Pain and temperature, taste, and touch are all dulled to some extent as one ages. Hearing and vision become less acute as the elder experiences *presbyopia* and *presbycusis* (see Chapter 38). Long-distance vision is less acute, as well as is night vision, and tolerance for glare decreases. The older person has more difficulty hearing high tones and discriminating speech in noisy situations.

Nursing Process
Assessment
Subjective data

Orientation: obtain information about long- and short-term memory, judgment, abstract thinking, insight, loss of vision and hearing, changes in ability to recognize hot and cold, and pain.

Objective data

Determine the patient's ability to discriminate between hot and cold objects, and *hearing and visual losses.* See Box 4-10 for the many variables that can be associated with confusion in the elderly.

Although delirium (temporary) is the more common form of confusion, the nurse should be aware that *chronic dementia* may be present. The most common dementia is *Alzheimer's disease,* which afflicts 50% to 60% of those who have organic brain disease (see Chapter 37). This devastating condition progressively affects the memory until the patient no longer remembers how to eat, dress, or toilet and is unable to recognize loved ones' faces. *The patient and family need great support and encouragement when the patient with Alzheimer's disease is hospitalized for an acute illness.*

Using a modified mental status examination (Box 4-11), the nurse can efficiently determine the amount of orientation and judgment the elder retains.

Data analysis: nursing diagnoses

Nursing diagnoses are determined from analysis of patient data. Possible nursing diagnoses for persons with cognitive perceptual problems may include, but are not limited to, the following:

Diagnostic title	Possible etiologies
Thought processes, altered	Acute confusional states, chronic dementia (Alzheimer's disease), stress
Sensory/perceptual alteration	CVA, dementia, diabetes, neuromuscular diseases

Planning: expected patient outcomes

Expected patient outcomes for the person with a cognitive perceptual problem may include, but are not limited to, the following:
1. Maintains orientation
2. States that he or she understands procedures and routines
3. Remains free from harm during hospitalization

Implementation
Interventions to achieve patient outcomes
Promoting orientation

Imagine a relatively independent 72-year-old woman who comes to the hospital with pneumonia. She is stripped of her belongings, taken to a strange room, jabbed with needles, and barraged by questions from strangers. A needle is placed in a vein for antibiotics; her hands are restrained to keep her from pulling it out. Her glasses and hearing aid are in the drawer. She compensates adequately until nightfall. Then she cannot distinguish shapes or outlines. She becomes quite agitated, thrashing about. A sedative does not help her. Suddenly she cries out, loosens her wrists, gets out of bed, and falls. The many stressors have overtaxed her hypoxic brain and she has become confused and delirious.

The nurse can prevent or at least minimize these common effects by following a few simple measures. Give patients detailed, repeated explanations of where they are and what is being done to them. Place glasses and hearing aid on the patient while he or she is awake. Maintaining adequate hydration and pain control is often sufficient to clear a confused state. *A friend or relative staying through the night could eliminate the need for restraints, and an antihistamine that causes drowsiness is preferable to a sedative for sleep.*[39]

When caring for confused patients, the nurse should endeavor to maintain as structured an environment as possible. Fitting the patient's usual routine to that of the hospital may be difficult, but any adaptations that can be made helps maintain the elder's orientation. Competing stimuli should be kept to a minimum. The following general guidelines may prove helpful when caring for a confused or demented patient:
1. Use the first name of the patient and ask the patient to call you by your first name.
2. Give simple one-step directions, repeat as necessary.
3. Encourage any remaining social skills.
4. Promote reminiscence and life review.

<table>
<tr><td>

4-10

Variables associated with confusion in the elderly

Physiologic
Pulmonary disease
Cardiovascular disease
Anemia
Infections
Trauma
Dehydration
Electrolyte imbalance
Hypoglycemia/hyper-
glycemia

Medications
Sedatives/hypnotics
Narcotic analgesics
Antihypertensives
Antiarrhythmics
Anticonvulsants
Diuretics
Digitalis
Tagamet

Environmental
Strange equipment
Unfamiliar surroundings
Restraints
Tubings (IV, Foley)
Strange people

Sensory limitation
Decreased vision
Decreased hearing
Sensory overload
Sensory deprivation

Emotional stressors
Loss of health
Loss of loved ones
Loss of home
Loss of cherished pos-
sessions
Loss of pets
Expectations of sick role

Modified from Roberts B, Lincoln R: Cognitive disturbances in hospitalized and institutionalized elders (abstract), *Nurs Res* 35(2):126-127, 1986.

</td><td>

4-11

Mental status examination

Orientation
    What day is it?
    What season is it?
    What is the holiday closest to today? (past or future)

Long-term memory
    How old are you?
    What is your birth date?
    What happened at Pearl Harbor? *or*, What happened to President Kennedy?

Short-term memory
    What was the last meal you ate?

Abstract thinking
    What is 2 plus 2? 5 minus 3?

Insight
    What do you think is wrong with you?

Judgment
    What would you do if you spilled your tray on the floor? *or*, What would you do if you had to go to the bathroom?

From Lincoln R: University Hospitals of Cleveland, 1986.

</td></tr>
</table>

5. Use distraction for negative behavior (never scold or argue).
6. Decrease physical stressors such as pain or full bladder.
7. Allow rest or "time-out" periods that alternate with physically active periods.
8. Speak slowly and distinctly in one- or two-syllable words.
9. Avoid tranquilizers and sedatives as much as possible.
10. Reduce extraneous stimuli such as TV, radio, or large groups of people.[7]

Promoting communication

The ability to communicate is often impaired in patients with cognitive deficits. *Those who know what the nurse is asking but have trouble following directions need physical guidance, such as laying out the articles for the bath. Persons who have difficulty understanding what is being said need verbal prompts and someone to show them the desired behavior. When attention disorders are present, the nurse may need to prompt the patient frequently.*[12]

Reducing agitation

Agitation in an elderly demented patient can be one of the most difficult behaviors for the nurse to manage. Agitated patients may pull out intravenous lines, disrupt dressings, remove catheters, fall out of bed, wander about, and generally create problems. Helpful strategies for the agitated elder may also be useful in preventing agitation.

Looking for the possible meaning of the behavior gives clues to interventions. Removal of clothing may indicate a need for toileting. Respond to kicking and biting by removing as much stimuli as possible, including other persons in the environment. If the person is agitated at bath time, the nurse should leave and return when the patient is less agitated. The same advice is true for giving medications. A minimum of physical and chemical restraints should be used.[27]

Using touch

Touch is of great value in caring for confused patients.[32] Even the most demented person, who has lost the ability to understand verbal communication, can recognize the tender healing touch of a compassionate nurse. Elderly persons who have been alone or institutionalized may suffer most from lack of physical contact. The nurse who uses touch for comfort, protection, and affection finds this an important part of the care of all elderly.

Maintaining sensory function

The eyes of older people adjust more slowly to changes in light. Bright lights or sunlight may be almost unbearable; therefore, blinds may need to be partially drawn. Many elderly persons see poorly in the dark; night lights are used to reduce confusion and to prevent accidents among those who get up during the night. Many older persons require glasses or contact lenses. These visual aids must be protected from damage or loss and need to be kept clean for best use.

The major changes that affect the hearing of elderly adults are difficulties with speech discrimination, loss of ability to hear high-pitched tones, and problems with background noises. Nurses should make certain that any hearing aids are functioning correctly and are used when the patient is awake.

Pocket talkers are available for the hearing impaired. When speaking, talk slowly and face the patient with good lighting so the patient can see your face as you talk.

Evaluation

Questions to consider include the following:
1. Has the patient regained or maintained orientation to the surroundings?
2. Can the patient state understanding of treatment regime?
3. Has the patient remained free from injury during hospitalizations?
4. Is the patient able to hear and see well enough to communicate with others?

MUSCULOSKELETAL PROBLEMS

One of the most common problems of secondary aging is joint and muscle disease (see Box 4-12). *Osteoarthritis, rheumatism,* and *osteoporosis are prevalent among the elderly.* As joints stiffen and muscle tone decreases, the individual may develop an awkward, halting gait. The ability to rise from a chair or to get in and out of cars or buses becomes difficult. Impaired gait, cardiovascular changes, sensory deficits, and osteoporosis make the elderly susceptible to falls. The factors contributing to falls are listed in Box 4-13. Falls account for 23% of deaths and injuries in people over the age of 65.

Nursing Process
Assessment
Subjective data

Obtain information from the patient about limitations of joint and muscle movement, ability to walk, turn, and go up stairs. Learn about problems the patient has with bathing, dressing, toileting, grooming, eating, and carrying out household tasks.

Objective data

Check patient for muscle tone and strength, joint flexibility, range-of-motion, and gait, and whether the patient uses assistive aids such as a cane, walker, or crutches.

4-12	Aging changes of musculoskeletal system
	Decreased lean muscle mass
	Increased body fat
	Decreased muscle strength
	Demineralization of bones
	Decreased joint mobility

4-13	Factors associated with falls	
	Intrinsic	**Extrinsic**
	Limited mobility	Poor lighting
	Decreased vision	Unfamiliar environment
	Confused mental state	Loose slippers
	Orthostatic hypotension	Cluttered equipment
	Decreased ability to	and furniture
	maintain equilibrium	

Data analysis: nursing diagnoses

Nursing diagnoses are determined from analysis of patient data. Possible nursing diagnoses for the person with musculoskeletal problems may include, but are not limited, to the following:

Diagnostic title	Possible etiologies
Mobility, impaired physical	Arthritis, osteoporosis, neuromuscular diseases, stroke
Self-care deficit	Same as above

Planning: expected patient outcomes

Expected patient outcomes for the person with musculoskeletal problems may include, but are not limited to, the following:
1. Walks in the hall with assistance at least three times daily.
2. Transfers from the bed to the chair with one assistant.
3. Washes own face, hands, and trunk.
4. Feeds self after tray is set up.
5. Transfers independently to the bedside commode, using quad cane.
6. Is safe from harm and injury.

Implementation
Assisting with achievement of therapeutic goals

Physical therapists and occupational therapists are involved early in the hospitalization to arrange a program of care that maintains as much independence for the patient as possible. Sometimes providing a cane or walker and raising a toilet seat is all that is necessary to maintain functional independence. In other cases, assistive devices, such as long-handled spoons and reachers, facilitate a person's dressing and feeding self.

Interventions to achieve patient outcomes
Promoting mobility

The elderly often have fragile bones and joints from osteoarthritis and osteoporosis. Use caution when working with the person. Do not lift an elderly person under the armpits when assisting to move, stand, walk, or transfer from one surface to another. Support the person's trunk and joints as the person is moved. Transfer and lifting sheets are helpful and may allow one caregiver to move or transfer the patient without additional help.

Active and passive range-of-motion exercises are as important for the elderly person as for the younger adult. Because elders may have more limitations of joint motion, great care must be taken not to move the joint past the point of resistance or pain.

Progressive activity, such as getting the patient out of bed soon after admission, and progressive ambulation are essential aspects of nursing care that help maintain independence and function. The term *dysfunctional syndrome* as applied to the elderly *refers to a loss of function through imposed bedrest and altered nutrition patterns during hospitalization.*[19] This decline occurs despite improved medical health and is attributable to a lack of aggressive measures designed to maintain the person's baseline function.

Prevention of dysfunctional syndrome includes early ambulation, arrangements for indepencence in toileting, dining in a central location in a social situation, and encouraging independence in bathing, grooming, and dressing. Fulfilling the goal of functional independence necessitates ingenuity and patience on the part of the nurse. It involves spending more time allowing the elder to do for herself or himself instead of doing it for them. This may require increased staffing.

Preventing injury

Nurses have often used restraints on the elderly person with the mistaken idea that injurious falls can be prevented with these devices. *The restraints themselves are often more dangerous than any falls that may be prevented. When patients are held down with waist belts and extremity restraints, decreased functional capacity, loss of independence, incontinence, and decreased musculoskeletal and cardiovascular tone can result.* Far worse, however, is the psychologic impact resulting from using restraints. *Anger, fear, humiliation, embarrassment, discomfort, and demoralization are some of the undesirable effects documented when restraints are used.*[3]

Removing restraints from patients in long-term care facilities is part of the requirements of the Omnibus Budget Reconciliation Act of 1987. In facilities where this has been achieved, *falls* have been *reduced by 30%,* and less danger of strangulation and injury from restraints have occurred.[3]

Nursing strategies to maintain patient safety are complex and must be individually determined. *Nurses should assess the needs of each patient and determine the relative risks of "tying down" over risk of falling.* Family members can play a significant role in understanding the patient's needs as well as participating in the care of the elder.

Changes can be made *in the environment* to protect patients. Some of these changes *are low beds, half side-rails, carpeted or cushioned floors, bed alarms,* and *chairs adapted to accommodate patients of various heights and weights.*[5]

If all attempts fail to maintain safety of the elder and restraints become necessary as a last resort, the following measures should be taken:

1. Use the least amount of restraint possible; for example, wrist versus chest restraints.
2. Reevaluate the need for the restraint every 4 to 8 hours.
3. Monitor the patient closely for chafing, redness, tenderness, and circulation under the restraint.
4. Follow manufacturer's directions carefully when applying restraints.

5. Remember that the patient needs increased nursing care while restrained; for example, offering bedpan / urinal, feeding, and turning.
6. *Remove the restraint every 2 hours to exercise the part restrained.*
7. Always explain the need for the restraint to the patient, no matter how much cognitive impairment may be present; for example, for his or her protection and not for punishment.
8. Continue to seek alternatives and remove the restraint as soon as possible.

Preventing orthostatic hypotension

Orthostatic hypotension is a special problem of some elderly that increases the risk of falling. This condition is caused by an inadequate baroreceptor response to sudden changes of position or changes during the digestive process. When the person gets out of bed, rises from a hot bath, or eats a large meal, blood pressure may drop precipitously, causing the patient to become faint and fall.

The nurse should *teach the following measures to prevent orthostatic hypotension:*

1. Sleep with the head of bed elevated 8 to 12 inches.
2. Get up slowly from lying position in three stages: sit up, dangle feet over side of bed, then stand up.
3. Do not bend all the way to the floor or stand up quickly.
4. Postpone grooming activities, such as shaving and bathing, to 1 hour after arising.
5. Wear support hose at night.
6. Get out of a hot bath slowly.
7. Wait for an hour or so after a meal to engage in strenuous activity.
8. Be cautious with position changes 1 hour after taking antihypertensive medications.
9. Use a rocking chair to increase circulation.
10. Avoid the Valsalva maneuver.[1]

Evaluation

Questions to consider include the following:

1. Is the patient able to transfer independently?
2. Is the patient walking further each day?
3. Is the patient able to feed self, dress self, bathe self, toilet self?
4. Is joint mobility maintained?
5. Is patient safety maintained?

CARDIOPULMONARY PROBLEMS

One of the most pronounced changes that occurs as a person ages is the decline in pulmonary function. Although the changes in the cardiovascular system are not as dramatic, some differences exist between the older and the younger adult (see Box 4-14).

Nursing Process
Assessment
Subjective data

Seek information from the patient about fatigue, especially with normal routines, breathlessness, palpitations, swollen ankles, need to sleep with several pillows, persis-

---

4-14

Aging changes of respiratory and cardiovascular system

Respiratory system

Decreased elasticity of lungs and chest wall
Decreased recoil of lungs
Increased residual lung volume
Decreased forced expiratory volume
Decreased oxygen pressure (PO_2) (PO_2 decreases about 4 mm Hg/decade)

Cardiovascular system

Decreased elasticity of blood vessels
Decreased cardiac output
Possible blocking of blood vessels by fatty deposits (atherosclerosis)
Increased peripheral vascular resistance leading to increased blood pressure
Slowed circulation
Decreased efficiency of valves in veins of lower extremities

---

tent cough, falls with dizziness, chest pain, confusion, and medication history.

Objective data

Check the patient's vital signs, orthostatic blood pressure, edema, use of accessory breathing muscles, condition of legs and feet, capillary refill, temperature of hands and feet, and peripheral pulses.

Data analysis: nursing diagnoses

Nursing diagnoses are determined from analysis of patient data. Possible nursing diagnoses for the person with cardiopulmonary problems may include, but are not limited to, the following:

Diagnostic title	Possible etiologies
Breathing pattern, ineffective	Chronic obstructive pulmonary disease (COPD), sedentary lifestyle, bronchitis, pneumonia
Cardiac output, decreased	Congestive heart failure (CHF), stress
Activity intolerance	Sedentary lifestyle, immobility

Planning: expected patient outcomes

Expected patient outcomes for the person with cardiopulmonary changes may include, but are not limited to, the following:

1. Walks the length of the room without dyspnea.
2. Maintains normal respiratory rate.
3. Accomplishes own ADL with a minimum of fatigue.

Implementation

Interventions to achieve patient outcome
Decreasing fatigue

The primary focus of the nurse in caring for the patient with an ineffective breathing pattern or activity intolerance is coping with the residual effects of fatigue. Energy-saving techniques are valuable for the patient who becomes breathless with exertion or who has chronic fatigue.

1. Sit rather than stand for grooming or household chores.
2. Take frequent rest periods between activities.
3. Avoid extremes of temperature.
4. Wear loose clothing and use long-handled reachers.
5. Have friends or family help with household chores.
6. Plan meals in advance and organize cooking activities.
7. Sit down while preparing meals.
8. Practice relaxation exercises.
9. Remove self from stressful situations.

Facilitating learning

Smoking and exposure to secondary passive smoke are the biggest risk factors in developing pulmonary disease at any age. The nurse can promote a smoke-free environment by encouraging smokers to stop smoking and referring them to programs such as SmokeEnders. Even the elderly patient can enjoy improved health with the cessation of smoking.[17]

The nurse should teach the patient to report any unusual signs or symptoms. Cardiopulmonary disease often has an atypical presentation in the elderly. Therefore symptoms that seem insignificant may indicate a serious problem. Some *symptoms to watch for are chronic indigestion, heartburn, confusion, tingling or numbness in the extremities, shortness of breath,* and *edema not alleviated by elevating the feet.* Frequent blood pressure checks are important. Other tips are to avoid tight garters and crossing legs and to engage in a suitable exercise program (see primary prevention on p. 51).

Medications should be reviewed frequently, because the elderly are more prone to side effects and drug interactions, especially when taking heart medications.

Evaluation

Questions to consider include the following:

1. Can the patient walk a prescribed distance without dyspnea?
2. Is normal respiratory rate maintained?
3. Can ADL be accomplished successfully with a minimum of fatigue?

GASTROINTESTINAL PROBLEMS

The changes in the gastrointestinal system can affect the mouth, teeth, and gums; the esophagus and stomach; and the large and small intestines (see Box 4-15).

Nursing Process
Assessment
Subjective data

Inquire about the patient's appetite, dysphagia, choking, condition of teeth and gums, types of foods and liquids taken, symptoms following meals, problems with constipation, indigestion, and bowel habits.

Objective data

Assess the condition of the patient's mouth and mucous membranes, presence of gag reflex, and chewing and swallowing ability. Perform an abdominal assessment.

4-15	Aging changes of gastrointestinal systems	
	Decreased motility	Decreased salivation
	Decreased enzymal activity	Decreased taste
	Atrophied musculature	Decreased sphincter tone
	Decreased absorption	Decreased metabolism

Data analysis: nursing diagnoses

Nursing diagnoses are determined from an analysis of patient data. Possible nursing diagnoses for the patient with gastrointestinal problems may include, but are not limited to, the following:

Diagnostic title	Possible etiologies
Nutrition, less than body requirements	Poorly fitting dentures, tooth loss, lack of sensation, hiatal hernia, loss of taste or smell, anorexia
Constipation	Lack of muscle tone, reliance on use of laxatives/enemas, lack of bulk in diet, low fluid intake

Planning: expected patient outcomes

Expected patient outcomes for the patient with gastrointestinal problems may include, but are not limited to, the following:

1. Maintains/regains weight.
2. States satisfaction with diet.
3. Has normal bowel movements and patterns.

Implementation

Interventions to achieve patient outcomes

Maintaining/regaining weight

For the person who tends to choke, check the fit of dentures, suggest slower eating with smaller bites, and alternating liquids with solids.

If the patient has a poor appetite, determine high-protein, high-calorie foods that appeal to him or her; offer small frequent meals. Persons with a hiatal hernia and/or esophageal reflux can be helped by avoiding cold liquids, sitting up for 1 to 2 hours after meals, and taking small doses of antacids and H_2 antagonists such as cimetidine or ranitidine. Teach the patient to keep the head raised during sleep by elevating the head of the bed on 3-inch blocks.[6]

Preventing aspiration

To prevent aspiration in a patient with decreased sensation in the mouth and throat, try giving soft foods such as custard, gelatin, and applesauce rather than liquids. Give small bites and wait between mouthfuls. Ask the patient to keep the head bent forward. Put the utensil in the patient's hand, giving verbal directions, to promote independence. If patient needs help, sit beside him or her and tell him/her each food that will be fed.[17]

Promoting alternative feeding methods

For patients who are unable to chew or swallow, two main feeding alternatives are available. The easiest and least complicated is the percutaneous enterostomal gastrostomy (PEG) (see Chapter 31). Under local anesthesia, a small tube is placed directly into the stomach through the abdominal wall and stitched in place. After 24 hours, the tube is used to give enriched formula feedings either continuously or in several bolus feedings. Another alternative is a Dobhoff tube placed through the nose into the stomach through which feedings can be given. Patients must be observed closely for the possibility of aspiration, the head is kept elevated during feeding, and small amounts are given at first to test tolerance. One complication of tube feedings is diarrhea. This can be managed by slowing down the feeding and giving high-fiber formulas. The dietitian or nutritionist can be consulted about the type of tube feeding.[6]

Relieving constipation

More than 700 constipation remedies exist, and some studies report that over 50% of the elderly use laxatives regularly. In many cases, the use of cathartics may cause rather than cure constipation. Laxatives hinder the absorption of vitamins and may upset the patient's electrolyte balance.

Teaching should focus on developing or maintaining normal habits. Because of decreased sphincter control, removing laxatives from the patient's routine may be difficult, but normal patterns can be resumed with use of stool softeners and bulk-forming agents, such as Metamucil. Patient should be advised to use natural substances to help aid elimination, such as prunes and prune juice. Adding bran to cereal or other foods is sometimes helpful. The elderly often neglect to drink enough fluids for fear of incontinence or because limited mobility creates problems getting to the toilet. Sometimes by merely increasing the intake of water, the person can relieve constipation.

When trying to regain normal bowel habits, the patient should go to the bathroom after breakfast and other meals to take advantage of the gastrocolic reflex. Sometimes using a mild glycerine suppository may stimulate the bowels. The elderly person should be encouraged to keep trying to regain normal habits; sometimes the process takes several weeks, after years of laxative abuse. Use enemas only as a last resort. If the stool is very hard and impacted, use an oil retention enema before the cleansing enema to soften the stool. Use greater caution when giving cleansing enemas to the elderly than to younger adults. The rectal mucosa may be very friable and easily traumatized. The elderly are much more prone to electrolyte imbalances and can become very weak and hypokalemic following administration of multiple enemas.

Evaluation

Questions to consider include the following:

1. Is the patient's weight being maintained or increasing?
2. Is the patient stating satisfaction with diet?
3. Are the bowel patterns more normal?
4. Does the patient state satisfaction with amount and frequency of bowel movements?

4-16	Aging changes of the integumentary system	
	Graying hair	Decreased elasticity of skin
	Loss of connective tissue	
	Decreased vascularity	Loss of subcutaneous fat
	Liver spots	
	Senile purpura	Decreased skin turgor
	Decreased seborrheic secretions	Tooth loss
		Malodorous breath
	Seborrheic keratoses	Receding gums
	Decreased venous circulation	Hardened nails
		Corns, calluses

INTEGUMENTARY PROBLEMS

The primary aging changes that occur in the integumentary system are the ones most noticeable to the lay person and are commonly associated with "growing old" (see Box 4-16).

The skin changes occur as the basal membrane flattens and epidermal turnover rate diminishes. These changes cause a decrease in the barrier function of the skin, making it more susceptible to irritants and allergens. As the hair follicles decrease and melanocytes become less active, the hair becomes gray and thin. Decreased sweat production and decreased subcutaneous fat lead to altered thermoregulation, making the elderly more prone to hypothermia in the winter and heat exhaustion in the summer. Wrinkling is due to loss of elasticity and decreased subcutaneous fat. Fingernails and toenails become brittle and thick, with many deformities resulting from trauma and circulatory impairment.[17]

Nursing Process
Assessment
Subjective data

Obtain information from the patient about dry skin, pruritus, skin and nail infections, tooth loss and decay, gum disease, bathing patterns, use of emollients, skin-care habits, mouth-care habits, and foot problems.

Objective data

Assess the patient for dryness of skin, skin turgor (test over sternum, not on forearm), rashes and skin lesions, condition of hair, nails, gums, and mouth, and capillary refill.

Data analysis: nursing diagnoses

Nursing diagnoses are determined from analysis of patient data. Possible nursing diagnoses for the person with integumentary system problems may include, but are not limited to, the following:

Diagnostic title	Possible etiologies
Skin integrity, impaired	Dehydration, immobility, shearing, poor venous circulation, incontinence
Oral mucus membranes, altered	Gingivitis, stomatitis, tooth loss

Planning: expected patient outcomes

Expected patient outcomes for the person with integumentary problems may include, but are not limited to, the following:
1. Skin and mucous membranes remain intact.
2. No signs of infection are present.
3. Feet remain healthy.

Implementation
Interventions to achieve patient outcomes
Maintaining skin integrity

Dryness and itching. The elderly are especially prone to very dry, itching skin, called "senile pruritus." The best treatment is frequent use of creams and emollients. Elderly persons do not need daily baths, but they should include more sponge baths in their routine and decrease the use of soap. Liquid cleansers made for sensitive skin are often recommended in place of soap. Hot showers or baths should be avoided, and skin should be patted instead of rubbed dry. Perfumed creams and perfumes containing alcohol can be drying and irritating to already compromised skin texture.

Skin tumors. Both benign and malignant skin tumors are common in the elderly, especially those individuals who have prolonged exposure to the sun. Elderly persons should be advised to see a doctor if they have any changes in their skin, especially changes in moles or pigmented areas. The major concern is that a skin lesion might be a *malignant melanoma*. If found early these tumors can be removed with no further complications. Teaching should include daily inspection of skin, wearing protective clothing for work or leisure activities out-of-doors, and avoiding exposure to the ultraviolet rays of the sun. When out in the sun, the elderly should wear a sun screen lotion with a skin protection factor of at least 15.

Preventing pressure sores and shearing lesions

Elderly patients who are bed bound for all or part of the day are especially susceptible to *pressure sores* and *shearing lesions*. Pressure sores are ischemic areas of breakdown that occur when fragile tissue is compressed between a bony prominence (sacrum, heels, scapulae) and a firm surface such as a mattress or a chair. Shearing lesions arise from loss of outer layers of skin, resulting from friction when a person is moved or turned in bed. Treatment of deep pressure sores can cost thousands of dollars. Nurses can help prevent this serious complication.

Prevention requires meticulous attention to relief of pressure through turning schedules and pressure-reducing devices. Maintaining clear, dry skin, adequate hydration (up to 2400 ml/day) and supplemental nutrition for the malnourished is equally critical to prevention of pressure sores.

Promoting proper foot care

Elderly persons have more corns, calluses, bunions, hammer toes, and horny toenails than younger persons. They are taught to wear protective footwear, clean and inspect feet daily, and guard against frostbite and burns. For difficult toenails or other foot problems, a podiatrist should be consulted. Diabetic patients should never cut their own toenails but should have a professional attend to foot care.[24]

Preventing intravenous therapy injury

Elderly persons create special problems for the phlebotomist and intravenous therapist. Their veins are fragile and inelastic, making it difficult to enlarge them with a tourniquet. Hematomas form quickly. Sometimes anatomic markings are not in the usual places. When choosing a vein, use the network on the back of the forearm, the cephalic vein on the thumb side of the hand, and the basilar vein on the posterior arm.[10]

Select as small a cannula as possible, protect the skin with proper skin preparation, and use the indirect method of entering the vein. Maintain traction on the skin during insertion. Always remove the needle gently so as not to damage the vein.[10]

Maintaining mucous membranes and dental health

Tooth decay is not a serious problem among the elderly; they are much more afflicted by peridontal disease. Peridontal disease is responsible for most tooth loss after age 35.[2] Gingivitis (gum disease) and periodontitis (bone disease) occur when plaque develops in gum crevices, then the bacterial growth causes receding gums and invasion of the bone.[17]

For sore receding gums, broken teeth, ill-fitting dentures, or malodorous breath, the nurse should refer the patient to a dentist or oral health clinic. Other helpful measures include:

1. Frequent mouth care for patients who are using oxygen, are taking nothing by mouth, or are immunosuppressed.
2. Use of emollients to lips and nares for patients who are using oxygen or nasogastric and Dobhoff tubes
3. Frequent suctioning of secretions for those who cannot handle secretions themselves
4. Treatment of yeast (thrush) infections

Evaluation

Questions to consider include the following:

1. Is skin integrity maintained?
2. Are there any signs of infection or pressure sores?
3. Is skin on the feet intact?
4. Are the mucous membranes intact?
5. Does the patient have access to regular dental care?

URINARY PROBLEMS

Although aging leads to decreased kidney function, most elderly can maintain normal voiding. Incontinence is always a result of pathologic process and not of primary aging, (see Box 4-17).

Nursing Process
Assessment
Subjective data

Obtain information from the patient about usual urinary patterns, any changes in habits, pain, hesitancy, burning, urgency, and loss of control. If incontinence exists, assess

---

4-17	**Aging changes of urinary system**

Reduced renal blood flow
Decreased glomerular filtration rate
Decreased bladder muscle tone

---

amount, frequency, type of management, and loss of control with sneezing, coughing, or movement.

Objective data

Observe the patient's urine for color, consistency, amount, and presence of blood. If cloudy, or if sediment is present, send urine for culture and sensitivity.

Data analysis: nursing diagnoses

Nursing diagnoses are determined from analysis of patient data. Possible nursing diagnoses for the person with urinary problems may include, but are not limited to, the following:

Diagnostic title	Possible etiologies
Incontinence, functional	Altered environment, sensory, cognitive, or mobility deficits

Planning: expected patient outcomes

Expected patient outcomes for the person with urinary elimination problems may include, but are not limited to, the following:

1. Increased time between voidings.
2. Decreased number of incontinent episodes.

Implementation
Interventions to achieve patient outcomes
Minimizing functional incontinence

Elderly persons are especially susceptible to functional incontinence. Factors affecting this condition are urinary infections, inability to get to the bathroom, and altered fluid intake caused by illness and hospitalization. Use of restraints and attachment of multiple tubes often hinder the ability of the person to accomplish independent toileting. The presence of cognitive impairment and limited mobility complicates the situation.

The nurse can assist the patient getting to the bathroom independently through modification of the environment. This may involve moving furniture and equipment to clear a path to the bathroom or arranging for a bedside commode to be placed near enough to the patient's bed for easy use. Sometimes providing a cane or walker is all that is necessary, as well as giving the patient some privacy. If special equipment presents a hindrance, the nurse can teach the patient how to manipulate intravenous tubing or machinery or urge the patient to call for assistance.

It is important for the nurse to remember that incontinence is embarrassing and shameful for the patient. The patient should be treated in a matter-of-fact manner, never scolded, and helped to avoid future incidents. The nurse may tell the patient that urinary control in the hospital is much more difficult where the surroundings are unfamiliar and assure the patient that when he or she returns home, continence may be regained or improved.

Continuous intravenous fluids, having nothing orally because of diagnostic studies, and altered eating schedules may interfere with voiding patterns. Whenever possible, fluids should be encouraged, up to 2 L/day, with the bulk of the liquids given between 8 AM and 7 PM. Limiting the fluids at night helps prevent incontinent episodes during sleeping hours. If the patient is restrained or hindered by intravenous or other tubings, he or she should be offered opportunities to void before and after meals and at bedtime. Urinary tract infections are common and should be treated with the appropriate antibiotics.

Some elderly men can only void when standing. Others may have urinary frequency and hesitancy because of an enlarged prostate, which is common in older men. Assistance should be provided as necessary to handle these difficult problems. Maintaining as much independence as possible is important in keeping the elderly person from losing functional capacity.

Promoting urinary elimination

Foley catheters may be placed in some patients to monitor and accurately record urinary output. After the catheter is removed, the elderly patient may have trouble regaining bladder control, especially if mild incontinence was present previously.

The best approach for urinary retention following catheter removal is to do a straight catheterization every 6 to 8 hours until the person is able to void voluntarily. This is much preferable to reinserting the indwelling catheter. For the person who is incontinent, teaching Kegel strengthening exercises may help tone the pelvic floor muscles. The patient should be reassured that most incontinence ceases after a routine of fluids and voiding has been re-established.

For any elderly person who has problems with incontinence, it is important for the nurse to determine what type of incontinence is present. In many cases, stress and urge incontinence are exaggerated by functional incontinence. *Urinary incontinence is never a normal part of aging.* The nurse may be the first person to discover the patient's problem, and referrals for incontinence studies can be a vital part of the nursing care.

Evaluation

Questions to consider including the following:
1. Have the number of incontinent episodes decreased?
2. Is the patient able to toilet independently?
3. Does the patient state that control of incontinent episodes is to his or her satisfaction?

OTHER PHYSIOLOGIC PROBLEMS

DEHYDRATION

Dehydration is a common problem among the elderly and is a frequent cause of admission to the hospital.

Nursing Process
Assessment
Subjective data

Seek information from the patient about usual fluid intake, types of fluids preferred, thirst, ability to handle fluid containers, swallowing ability, usual pattern of consumption, changes in intake related to illness, and medications that affect intake and output (diuretics, laxatives).

Objective data

Assess the patient for skin turgor, texture, fragility, and temperature; condition of mucous membranes; weakness, and orientation.

Data analysis: nursing diagnoses

Nursing diagnoses are determined from analysis of patient data. Possible diagnoses for the patient with dehydration may include, but are not limited to, the following:

Diagnostic title	Possible etiologies
Fluid volume deficit or Fluid volume deficit, high risk for	Dysphagia, congestive heart failure, medications, dementia, depression, stroke, hypertension, use of diuretics, inability to obtain fluids, fear of incontinence, fever, diarrhea, renal failure

Planning: expected patient outcomes

Expected patient outcomes for the person with dehydration may include, but are not limited to, the following:
1. Takes 2000 ml of fluid in 24 hours.
2. Intake is greater than output for 48 hours.
3. Skin and mucous membranes are intact and moist.
4. Urine is light amber color and is clear.

Implementation
Interventions to achieve patient outcomes
Promoting hydration

The nurse can take several steps to promote hydration: encourage fluid intake of 7 to 8 glasses a day; offer a variety of fluids, especially juices; weigh the patient daily; keep accurate intake and output records; and provide cups and pitchers that the person can handle.

Facilitating learning

Instruct the patient in the importance of maintaining adequate fluid intake. Teach which fluids are best: soups and fruit juices may have high sodium content; milk increases phlegm; alcohol depresses the CNS; coffee, tea, and colas contain caffeine, which is a stimulant; soft drinks and gelatins are high in sugar.[18]

Evaluation

Questions to consider include the following:
1. Is the volume of fluids adequate?
2. Is the intake greater than the output?
3. Are skin and mucous membranes moist, pink, and intact?
4. What are the color and consistency of urine?

PAIN

Nursing Process
Assessment

Assessment of pain in the elderly person is more complex than in the younger adult. Pain may appear in atypical forms. Conditions that normally cause pain in young persons may not do so in the elderly.

The nurse assesses for location, quality, intensity, onset, duration, and physical manifestations of pain in the same manner as for any patient. In addition, the nurse must attend to the impact of pain on activities of daily living, gait, and behavior.

Factors that affect pain in the elderly are different than those affecting younger persons. Impaired vision and hearing, problems expressing oneself, ability to concentrate, and cognitive changes may interfere with assessment. More attention must be paid to nonverbal expressions, as well as soliciting comments from family members.[14]

The belief system of the elderly person affects his or her expression of pain. Some believe that pain is a normal part of the aging process and must be endured stoically. If the person fears loss of autonomy, she or he may deny having pain. A fear of serious illness may lead to denial of pain. Some ethnic groups believe showing pain is not acceptable, whereas others may be more vocal when they experience pain (see Chapter 3).

An atypical presentation of pain is much more common in the elderly. For example, one half of patients with myocardial infarctions have no pain. Diseases usually associated with severe pain, such as peptic ulcer, appendicitis, and pneumonia, may only provoke mild pain in older persons. Some abdominal emergencies present as chest pain at first. Depression masks pain and pain may be difficult to assess, especially if the patient is also cognitively impaired.

Taking all these factors into consideration, the nurse must establish rapport with the elderly person by taking plenty of time and phrasing questions in several different ways. For the asphasic patient, a pain chart with a drawing of a body to which the patient may point may be helpful. Patients may be asked to rate their pain using a pain scale numbered 1 to 10, with 10 being the most severe pain ever felt and 1 for the least severe pain (see Chapter 10 for more information). Showing concern for the patient and his or her suffering rather than dismissing the pain as "part of growing old" assists immeasurably in gathering accurate data.

Data analysis: nursing diagnoses

Nursing diagnoses are determined from an analysis of patient data. Possible nursing diagnoses for the person with pain may include, but are not limited to, the following:

Diagnostic title	Possible etiologies
Pain	Pathophysiologic changes, trauma/diagnostic tests, immobility, improper positioning, disability

Planning: expected patient outcomes

Expected patient outcomes for the person with pain may include, but are not limited to, the following:
1. States pain is decreased.
2. Exhibits fewer nonverbal signs of pain.
3. Is more independent in ADL.

Implementation
Interventions to achieve patient outcomes
Alleviating/minimizing pain

In the care of the elderly, the nurse should consider a variety of modifications in managing pain that differ from those used with the younger adult. Elderly persons are more prone to mild arthritis and fibrositis. The incidence of osteoporosis, especially involving the spine and femur, is very high in elderly women. Great care must be taken to protect the joints, back, and shoulders when transferring, moving, and turning. Where one nurse could handle a younger adult, two persons may be needed to move the older patient in bed or to help him or her walk.

Protective adipose tissue under the skin disappears with age, and the volume of circulating blood, particularly to the small outer arteries, may be diminished. This affects the ability to withstand cold without discomfort. Several layers of light-weight clothing are warmer than fewer heavy layers when the person is cold. Many elderly persons wish to wear socks and additional clothing in bed. Provision must be made to prevent drafts in the room while maintaining good air circulation.

Elderly patients may tolerate smaller doses of pain medications than younger adults (see secondary prevention, p. 53). *Bizarre reactions to pain medications may occur, such as hallucinations, delirium, aggravated pain, and agitation.* Great caution should be used in starting and/or changing dosages of narcotics to prevent reactions and interactions. The nonsteroidal antiinflammatory medications are gaining in popularity for treating pain from arthritis and neuralgias. These drugs create fewer side effects, and elderly patients tolerate them better (see Chapter 40 for more information about these medications).

Evaluation

Questions to consider include the following:
1. Does the patient show less evidence of pain?
2. Does the patient rate pain between 2 and 3?
3. Is the patient able to do ADL more independently?

SPECIAL CONSIDERATIONS

SLEEP PATTERN DISTURBANCE

Elderly persons have less Stage 4 (deep) sleep and more periods of wakefulness than younger adults. Rapid eye movement (REM) sleep is often interrupted, causing sleepiness and a pattern of napping throughout the day. The nurse should recognize that elderly persons do not necessarily need more sleep than younger adults, but that the sleep is obtained in shorter periods throughout the day rather than just at night.

A variety of measures are helpful for sleeplessness. A glass of warm milk at bedtime and a soothing back rub, as well as following usual nighttime routines, help prepare the patient for sleep. Keep a low nightlight on, lower the bed, and provide adequate supervision at night to prevent accidents. If the person is likely to get up for toileting, place a bedside commode next to the bed and teach the person how to use it safely. Sedatives interfere with REM sleep and may cause increased confusion. An antihistamine that causes drowsiness is the sleeping medication of choice.

DIAGNOSTIC TESTS

Diagnostic tests should be judiciously spaced to prevent overtaxing the elderly individual. Routine preparations for tests may need to be modified to prevent exhaustion or dehydration. Elderly persons may become weak or dizzy from test preparations such as multiple enemas or the withholding of food. Do not leave weak patients unattended on a treatment table. Advise persons who are dizzy to sit up slowly and to remain sitting on the edge of the table for a few moments before standing. The dizziness is caused by the slow compensation of inelastic blood vessels.

Place pads under the normal curves of the back and under bony prominences in elderly patients who must lie on treatment or operating room tables for lengthy periods because they develop pressure sores rapidly. If the patient is placed in the lithotomy position, place both legs in (and remove both from) the stirrups at the same time to prevent pull on unresilient muscles.

ANESTHESIA AND SURGERY

For the patient who is undergoing surgery, age in itself is not a risk factor. The risk factors for the elderly are the presence and severity of any underlying disease, such as congestive heart failure, renal disease, ischemic heart problems, or chronic obstructive lung disease.[11] The surgeon and anesthesiologist study the patient carefully to determine how much risk is involved. Their recommendations are made according to the type of surgery and concerns about cardiopulmonary function.

During the preoperative period, the nurse assists the patient in restoring fluids that have been lost through dehydration, bowel disease, or blood loss. In addition, the nurse provides basic preoperative teaching. Teaching is particularly important for an elderly person with cognitive deficits and who may need extra time and patience to understand the procedures that have been planned. Family members may be concerned that the person's age makes him or her a poor risk. They need careful detailed explanations of the surgery and the intraoperative procedures.

When choosing anesthesia for the elderly, the anesthesiologist is most likely to use a regional anesthetic. If general anesthesia is necessary, then shorter-acting anesthetic agents are best. With underlying cardiopulmonary disease, the risks are greater for aspiration, shock, pulmonary edema, and myocardial infarction.[11]

Postoperatively the elderly are more prone to confusion and sleepiness. Other problems are *hypothermia, respiratory depression, fluctuations in blood pressure, and renal failure.*

Postoperative nursing care focuses careful attention to vital signs, being alert to early signs of shock or hypertension. Warm blankets are even more important for the elderly than for the younger adult. Monitor urinary output, BUN, and creatinine carefully. The person who is confused may require frequent reorientation and repetition of instructions. Having a familiar family member at the bedside helps the elderly patient who is frightened and confused. Although they should be used as little as possible, restraints may be necessary in the early postoperative period to keep the person from tugging at intravenous lines, nasogastric tubes, and oxygen tubes. Attendance by a significant other may eliminate the need for restraints.

The postoperative course may be longer for the elderly patient. As the functional reserve capacity is decreased, the individual may be more susceptible to urinary and pulmonary infections. Return to baseline function requires more effort on the part of both the nurse and the patient. If the patient is discharged while still below his or her normal function level, relatives or home nursing services will be needed to meet the patient's needs until full recuperation is accomplished (see Chapter 47 for more information on home care).

DIABETES

Elderly persons are more susceptible to abnormalities in glucoregulation than are younger persons. In the elderly, the presenting signs are not an elevated blood sugar but microvascular changes that go undetected until signs and symptoms of complications, such as neuropathy, nephropathy, or retinopathy, occur. The fasting blood sugar may be normal; a glucose-tolerance test is needed for a definite diagnosis. Factors that lead to a decline in glucose tolerance in the elderly are obesity, deconditioning, decreased muscle mass, poor diet, coexisting diseases, and medications.[11]

The diagnosis is often made when the patient is under care for some other condition such as an infection, workup for surgery, or other complicating illness. Non-insulin-dependent diabetes is seen most often in obese patients over 50 years of age who have had significant glucose intolerance for several years before being detected.

The goal of medicine is not vigorous treatment of the hyperglycemia but rather adequate control in the hope of minimizing organ complications. About half of elderly diabetics need sulfonylurea drugs and fewer than half require insulin.[11] The nurse teaches the patient the significance of weight loss (80% of elderly diabetics are overweight), aerobic exercise, and good foot and skin care. See Chapter 28 for more information about diabetes.

PSYCHOSOCIAL CHANGES
General Care

In dealing with psychosocial changes the nurse assesses the physiologic changes, the diseases present, and the person's emotional makeup and apparent adjustment to the particular situation. Older persons frequently talk at length about their families and the past; their conversations may give clues to interests that should be encouraged and to problems confronting them. Plans should be made to

---

4-18

Community support services for older persons

Senior citizen centers	Social, nutritional, educational, and counseling services
Geriatric day care centers	Assistive daytime nursing care, and social, nutritional, and rehabilitative services may be available
Adult foster home care	Care in private home for the older person who is unable to live alone
Meals on Wheels	Meals delivered to the person's home
Homemaking service	Household chores, shopping, and so on
Transportation service	Arranged pickup by public transportation system
Home health service	Skilled home nursing care
Legal services	Will, settlement of estate
Respite care	Short-term care to support primary caregiver, provided by hospitals, extended care facilities, or Visiting Nurse's Association
Counseling services	Private, governmental, public services for patient and caregivers
Support groups	Private, nonprofit groups related to specific diagnosis
Rehabilitation services	Physical and occupational therapy in home or hospital

---

4-19

Nursing Research

Frierson R: Suicide attempts by the old and very old, *Arch Intern Med* 151(1):141-144, 1991.

A study of suicide attempts was made among 95 elderly patients (age 60 to 90) and evaluated by a consult service after a suicide attempt. The subjects differed significantly when compared with younger age groups who attempted suicide, but the younger age groups were similar to the elderly who successfully committed suicide. Recommendations are increased detection and treatment of depression and alcoholism, early psychiatric referral, limited access to firearms, and strategies to decrease social isolation.

---

help them maintain as much independence as possible despite their limitations. Community resources are available to assist older persons maintain independence and meet their social needs (see Box 4-18).

Elderly patients are often lonely and appreciate just talking with others. Volunteers may provide a service by visiting with the elderly. Many patients appreciate visits with a member of the clergy. When visiting with elderly persons, it should be remembered that, although they commonly talk about events and activities in their own past, they usually are interested in the activities of younger persons and of the world around them.

The need to be useful is important to all persons. There are many tasks in which even the elderly person who is ill may be able to participate. At home, the elderly may be able to help with the dishes or with meal preparation. They may be interested in crafts or making useful items. The older person may be quite slow, and great care must be taken not to show impatience, which may discourage further participation.

Depression is not uncommon in the elderly, and the elderly may be suicidal. Nurses need to be alert to signs of depression and thoughts of suicide, especially in older persons who are lonely and may not have a social support system. Box 4-19 describes a recent study of suicide in the elderly and makes several recommendations of which nurses should be aware.

Elderly persons are usually aware of death as an imminent possibility and sometimes see it as a welcome event. The issue should not be avoided. If the patient shows genuine concern about impending death, the nurse can encourage discussion of feelings (Chapter 15). The family may also need opportunities to discuss their feelings about death.

Discharge Planning

Following hospitalization the younger adult most frequently returns home to an independent lifestyle, whereas the older adult must be evaluated for ability and resources to manage at home. Some of the factors to consider are:

1. Has patient been functioning independently before hospitalization?
2. If patient is independent, has function returned to baseline?
3. Are appropriate caregivers or support persons at home?
4. Are other dependent disabled persons in the home?
5. What is the health of the primary caregiver?
6. How capable are the caregivers emotionally, physically, mentally?
7. What financial resources are available for home care, such as supplies and equipment?

The patient who has declining function and requires

increasing amounts of assistance with activities of daily living usually has three choices for discharge placement:

1. Home, with family caregiver
2. Home with family and/or professional nursing services or other assistance (see Chapter 47)
3. Nursing home or extended care facility

The nurse often becomes the coordinator for the discharge planning for the elderly patient who needs assistance after discharge. For the patient returning home, the nurse must teach transfer techniques, physical care, use of special equipment, and knowledge of medications. If the patient needs home nursing services, the nurse makes the appropriate referral, listing all the patient's needs. Social work services are necessary for the patient who must be transferred to an extended care facility or needs financial assistance.

In the case of the patient who may need institutional care, the nurse has a key role. First, the patient's functional abilities must be delineated thoroughly to determine if placement is really necessary. Then the nurse and social worker help the family choose the appropriate facility by giving them a list of available places and teaching them how to evaluate each one. This is frequently a difficult task for family members, who may feel guilty about removing the patient from the home. The nurse gives emotional support during the decision-making process to both the family and the patient, who may view the decision negatively because he or she is losing autonomy.

The nurse may be caught in a controversy between the patient's wishes to return home and the wishes of the family and physician to institutionalize the patient. It is not unusual for the patient to deny the amount of care needed. In such a situation, ethical principles must be carefully considered.

Patient autonomy may need to be weighed against the greatest good for the greatest number (the family). The process involves listing alternatives, predicting consequences, and selecting the solution based on those consequences. For example, a positive consequence results if a patient with declining physical function is returned home. However, harm could occur from a fall, and continued physical decline might result (negative consequence). Therefore the protected environment of the nursing home would be a positive consequence, and the family would be relieved from the burden of care.[15]

Each case must be decided individually with as much input from all parties as possible. The nurse is obligated to support the process and the chosen solution, no matter what her or his personal values. In many cases the options are limited, and the solution brings sadness to all involved.

Terminating Treatment

The nurse is frequently involved in decisions about initiating or withholding treatments for the elderly person who is terminally ill. No simple legislated answers exist to the questions, "Who should have treatment?" or "Is withholding fluids and food a form of passive euthanasia?" Some states have legal provision for a *living will,* but even this document does not guarantee that the patient's wishes will be followed in the event he or she is incompetent or unable to make known his or her desires.

Some experts recommend that *a durable power of attorney for health care* be obtained while the person is mentally competent. Then when the patient becomes ill or incapacitated, the person with the durable power of attorney can act on the patient's behalf and assure that the patient's wishes are carried out.

When a patient has no living will or durable power of attorney, the health team must consider the following factors when making decisions regarding withholding of treatments:

1. Did the patient express any wishes when competent?
2. What are the wishes of the family?
3. Does the giving of treatment represent a disproportionate burden to others?
4. What is the quality of life for the individual?[15]

The nurse can act as advocate for the patient by interviewing family members, supporting the decision-making process, and encouraging the parties involved to make the decisions without haste. Wishes the patient expresses while competent should be carefully documented in the patient's record.

Patient Self-Determination Act

Congress passed the Patient Self-Determination Act (PSDA) in 1990 so that the patient's wishes about prolongation of life are known to health care institutions. This act, which went into effect on December 1, 1991, provides that all health care institutions receiving Medicare or Medicaid funds must ask patients on admission if they have a *living will* or a *durable power of attorney for health care.* The patient's answer must be recorded in the patient's medical record.

In some institutions the admissions office personnel obtain this information, in others the nurse admitting the patient is responsible for obtaining the information.

An estimated 20% of patients answer yes to whether they have a living will or durable power of attorney.[9] Those who say yes are asked to provide a copy of the documents for their medical record.

Laws about living wills and durable power of attorney for health care vary from state to state. Therefore patients must receive, in writing, an explanation of the law in their state and the specific institution's policy about refusing treatment and advance directives for end-of-life decisions.

The PSDA also requires that health-care facilities provide in-service for staff members and programs for the community about the PSDA and right-to-die laws in their states. In addition, members of the staff may not alter a patient's care based on whether she or he has a living will or durable power of attorney.

Nurses need to keep informed about laws in their own states because many have legislation pending on end-of-life decisions.

The following recommendations from Bosek and Fitzpatrick may be helpful when discussing these issues with a patient:

> When discussing living wills or durable power of attorney for health care, focus on the patient's autonomy and his right to make his own decisions, not on death or dying. Reassure him that you haven't brought up the subject because you expect him to need life-support measures soon, but because no one can predict when a medical crisis will occur.[4]

STANDARDS FOR GERIATRIC NURSING PRACTICE

The American Nurse's Association has developed standards for geriatric nursing practice that embody those interventions considered to be based on knowledge derived from nursing, the natural, behavioral, and applied sciences, and the humanities. The standards address themselves to the following nursing actions:

1. Observing and interpreting signs and symptoms of normal aging, as well as pathologic changes, and intervening appropriately.
2. Differentiating between pathologic social behavior and the usual lifestyle of the aged person.
3. Demonstrating an appreciation for the heritage, values, and wisdom of older persons.
4. Supporting and promoting physiologic functioning in the aged.
5. Providing protective and safety measures and supporting the aged during stressful situations.
6. Using methods to promote effective communication and socialization of aged persons with individuals, family, and others, thus increasing sensory stimulation.
7. Helping the older person adapt to the physical and psychosocial limitations of his environment, yet fulfill his needs.
8. Assisting with the obtaining and use of helpful mechanical devices for improving function.
9. Resolving personal attitudes about aging, dependence, and death to provide assistance in meeting these crises with dignity and comfort.

SUMMARY

1. Persons in late adulthood focus on life accomplishments and look toward life's end, while maintaining autonomy and dignity.
2. Elderly adults often have more than one chronic illness, with the incidence increasing with age.
3. Nursing care must be tailored according to the specific physical, psychologic, sexual, and social effects of any disease or illness on the individual.
4. Nurses need to be cognizant of the differences between primary and secondary aging changes in elderly.
5. Nursing care should be predicated on the belief that late adulthood is a time of diversity, richness, and increasing complexity.
6. Health promotion is as important for older age groups as for younger persons in maintaining a high quality of life.
7. The strengths of the older person should be given the same consideration as their disabilities when devising health care strategies.
8. Many conditions have the initial symptom of confusion in the elderly.
9. The elderly are more susceptible to falls, but restraints are not an adequate intervention.
10. The elderly are often malnourished because of physiologic and social aging changes.
11. Constipation is a secondary aging change and can be controlled with diet and habit training.
12. Urinary incontinence is a secondary aging change. The most common form is functional incontinence.
13. Hearing and vision defects affect the ability of the elderly to communicate adequately.
14. The elderly experience many minor discomforts, but some do not have pain as a typical symptom of disease.
15. Dehydration is diagnosed for many elderly when admitted to the acute-care setting.
16. Helping the elderly with discharge planning is a major nursing role.
17. Supporting decision-making in an ethical context is a challenge for the nurse who works with aged persons.
18. The purpose of the Patient Self-Determination Act (PSDA) that went into effect on December 1, 1991, is to ensure that the patient's wishes about prolongation of life be respected.
19. Geriatric nursing standards provide a context of care for the nurse.

STUDY QUESTIONS

- Talk with and observe persons over 65 years of age. How do you and they differ in terms of physical development and major concerns in your lives?
- Review the eating patterns of an elderly person of your acquaintance; compare his or her food intake with your understanding of an adequate diet. If there are inadequacies, what are some possible reasons?
- From what you have read in newspapers and heard discussed, what would you select as major problems of elderly people in your community?
- What services are available for the elderly in your community?
- Compare your grandparents or other elderly relatives with other elderly acquaintances for differentiation in primary and secondary aging.

REFERENCES AND SELECTED READINGS

1.* Aronson L, Carlson-Wolfe N, and Schoener S: Pressures that fall on rising, *Geriatr Nurs* 12:(2)58-60, 1991.
2.* Berg R, Cassells J: *The second fifty years*, Washington, DC, 1990, National Academy Press.
3.* Blakeslee J, et al: Making the transition to restraint-free care, *J Gerontol Nurs* 17(2):4-8, 1991.
4.* Bosek MSD, Fitzpatrick J: Legally speaking—finding the right words, *RN* 54(11):66-67, 1991.
5. Brower T: Alternatives to restraints, *J Gerontol Nurs* 17(2):18-20, 1991.
6. Esberger K: Guide to gastrointestinal problems of elders, *Geriatr Nurs* 12(2):74-75, 1991.
7. Gilmore G, Whitehouse P, Wykle M: *Memory, aging, and dementia*, New York, 1987, Springer Publishing.
8. Gray M: Polypharmacy in the elderly, *Orthop Nurs* 9(6):49, 1990.
9. Greve P: Legally speaking—Advance directives—what the new law means to you, *RN* 54(11):63-66, 1991.
10.* Hadaway L: Intravenous tips, *Geriatr Nurs* 12(2):78, 1991.
11. Hazzard W, et al: *Principles of geriatric medicine*, New York, 1990, McGraw-Hill.

*Recommended for student reading.

12. Heacock P, et al: Caring for the cognitivity impaired, *J Gerontol Nurs* 17(3):22-26, 1991.

13. US Dept of Health and Human Services: *Healthy People 2000: National health promotion and disease preventions: 1991 objectives,* Washington, DC, 1990, US Government Printing Office.

14. Herr K, Mowby P: Pain assessment in the elderly, *J Gerontol Nurs* 17(4):13-19, 1991.

15.* Hogstel M: Safety or autonomy, *J Gerontol Nurs* 17(3):5-10, 1991.

16. Hussey L: Overcoming the clinical barriers of low literacy and medication noncompliance among elderly, *J Gerontol Nurs* 17(3):27-29, 1991.

17. Kart C, Metress E, Metress S: *Aging, health, and society,* Boston, 1988, Jones & Bartlett Publishers.

18.* Kositzke J: A question of balance: dehydration in the elderly, *J Gerontol Nurs* 16(4):7-9, 1990.

19. Landefeld S, Palmer R, Kresevic D: Dysfunctional syndrome, *GAS Abstracts,* 1990.

20. Lang N, et al: *Quality of health care for older people in America,* Kansas City, Mo, 1990, American Nurses' Association.

21. McCaffery M, Beebe A: *Pain: clinical manual for nursing practice,* St. Louis, 1989, Mosby–Yearbook.

22. Melers C: Antibiotics: Old drugs, new information, *Geriatr Nurs* 12(2):61-63, 1991.

23. Newbern V: Beta blockers, *Geriatric Nurs* 12(2):119-121, 1991.

24. Osterman H, Stuck R: The aging foot, *Orthop Nurs* 9(6):43, 1990.

25. Palmore E, et al: *Normal aging III,* Durham, NC, 1985, Duke University Press.

26. Pastorino C, Dickey T: Health promotion for the elderly, *Orthop Nurs* 9(60):36, 1990.

27. Roper J, Shapiro J, Chang B: Agitation in the demented patient, *J Gerontol Nurs* 17(3):17, 1991.

28.* Schilke J: Slowing the aging process with physical activity, *J Gerontol Nurs* 17(6):5-9, 1991.

29. Scura K, Whipple B: Older adults as an HIV positive risk group, *J Gerontol Nurs* 16(1):6-10, 1990.

30. Talashek M, Tichy A, Epping H: Sexually transmitted disease in elderly, *J Gerontol Nurs* 16(4):33, 1990.

31. Travis S: Older adults' sexuality and remarriage, *J Gerontol Nurs* 13:9, 1987.

32.* Vortherms R: Clinically improving communication through touch, *J Gerontol Nurs* 17(5):6-9, 1991.

Classic

33. Birren J, Schale K: *Handbook of the psychology of aging,* New York, 1977, Van Nostrand Reinhold.

34. Boyce M: *Guidelines for printed materials for older adults,* Battle Creek, Mich, 1981, Michigan Health Council.

35. Butler R: *Why survive? Being old in America,* New York, 1975, Harper & Row.

36. Masters W, Johnson V: *Human sexual response,* Boston, 1966, Little, Brown, & Co.

37. Murray R, Zentner J: *Nursing assessment and health promotion through the lifespan,* Englewood Cliffs, NJ, 1979, Prentice-Hall.

38. Reed P: Implications of the life-span developmental framework for wellbeing in adulthood and aging, *Adv Nurs Sci* 6(1):18-25, 1983.

39. Wolanin MO, Phillips L: *Confusion: Prevention and care,* St Louis, 1981, Mosby–Yearbook.

Audiovisual Resources

Feeding techniques for adult dysphagic patients, Chicago, Rehabilitation Institute of Chicago. (Video tape)

Into aging, ed 2, Thorofare, NJ, 1991, Slack Publishers. (Boxed simulation game)

Peege, Princeton, NJ, Phoenix Films. (Film)

Presentation of illness in the elderly, Philadelphia, 1988, JB Lippincott. (Video tape)

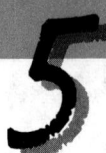

Health Promotion: Nutrition and Exercise

Barbara C. Long

After studying this chapter, the learner should be able to:

- Describe factors affecting health-promoting behaviors and approaches to facilitate health promotion.
- Differentiate nutrient standards, food guides, and dietary guidelines in terms of purpose.
- Describe seven dietary guidelines recommended by Department of Health and Human Services/U.S. Department of Agriculture.
- Differentiate saturated, monounsaturated, and polyunsaturated fats, and cholesterol in terms of definition and recommendations for health.
- Use the daily food guide to evaluate adequacy of nutrient intake.
- Explain approaches to facilitate weight loss and weight gain.
- Describe the effects and benefits of exercise and recommendations for physical fitness programs.

Year 2000 national health objectives priority areas

Health promotion
  Physical activity and fitness
  Nutrition
  Tobacco
  Alcohol and other drugs
  Family planning
  Mental health and mental disorders
  Violent and abusive behavior
  Educational and community-based programs

Health protection
  Unintentional injuries
  Occupational safety and health
  Environmental health
  Food and drug safety
  Oral health

Preventive services
  Maternal and infant health
  Heart disease and stroke
  Cancer
  Diabetes and chronic disabling conditions
  HIV infection
  Sexually transmitted diseases
  Immunization and infectious diseases
  Clinical preventive services

Surveillance and data systems

From US Dept of Health and Human Services and Public Health Service: *Healthy People 2000: National health promotion and disease prevention objectives*, Washington, DC, 1991.

Health promotion and disease prevention have become major aspects of health care in the United States. In 1979 the Surgeon General presented a document that described a national public health agenda for the first time. This was followed in 1980 by the *1990 Health Objectives* that set forth measurable objectives in areas of health status, risk reduction, public and professional awareness, health services and protective measures, and surveillance and evaluation. Although progress was noted, many of the objectives were not being met by the late 1980s.[37] Therefore a new set of objectives, *Year 2000 National Health Objectives*, has been developed with four major sections: *health promotion*, health protection, preventive services, and surveillance and data systems[35] (Box 5-1). Note that the first two categories of health promotion are *physical activity* and *fitness* and *nutrition*.

Because the goal of nursing is to assist people to achieve optimal health (Chapter 1), nurses are among the leaders of health professionals working toward meeting the national health objectives. The American Nurses' Association (ANA) has placed new emphasis on health promotion, health teaching, and self-care.[22] Nurses are well prepared as health teachers and health advocates. Therefore health promotion is one aspect of medical-surgical nursing.

HEALTH PROMOTION IN MEDICAL-SURGICAL NURSING PRACTICE

Health promotion can be defined as activities directed toward helping persons maintain or achieve a high level of functioning and well-being. Health promotion is an integral part of nursing care for all types of patients and clients in all types of environments of care. In ambulatory care centers, health promotion assumes a major focus. In acute care centers the major focus is assisting patients to regain their health (illness care). However, health care must also be considered; that which is healthy must be promoted or maintained.

Health promotion strengthens the person's capacity to withstand physical and emotional stress. Thus the person who is in an excellent nutritional state, has good physical endurance, and copes well with stress is at less risk of developing a pathophysiologic disorder, and has resources to use in regaining optimal functioning more quickly if illness or disease does occur.

Factors Affecting Health-Promoting Behaviors

Why do some persons take actions that promote a high level of functioning, whereas others do not? Pender[26] has identified factors that (1) affect the individual's perceptions, (2) modify behaviors, and (3) influence the likelihood of health-promoting actions (Figure 5-1).

Individual perceptions

Motivation to participate in health-promoting behaviors is influenced by the person's perceptions about health and perceptions about self:
1. Perceptions about health
   a. Value placed on health by the person
   b. Desire for the highest achievable health level versus that for maintaining status quo
   c. Evaluation of present health status
   d. Perceived benefits of the health-promoting behaviors
2. Perceptions about self
   a. Perceived control over own behavior (internal versus external control)
   b. Desire for mastery of the environment
   c. Self-concept
   d. Self-esteem

Thus persons who do not value health or see a need to improve their health status, who are not self-motivated, or who have a poor self-concept are less likely to engage in health-promoting behaviors. Nursing approaches in these situations include helping these persons identify their values and explore feelings about themselves with emphasis placed on identifying strengths. Helping these persons set their own goals (thus exerting internal control) greatly increases the likelihood of achieving desired behaviors.

Modifying factors

Pender[26] has identified categories of modifying factors: demographic (age, sex, ethnicity, education, income), biologic, interpersonal, situational, and behavioral variables. The specific effect of demographic variables on health-promoting behaviors is not clearly established and requires further research.

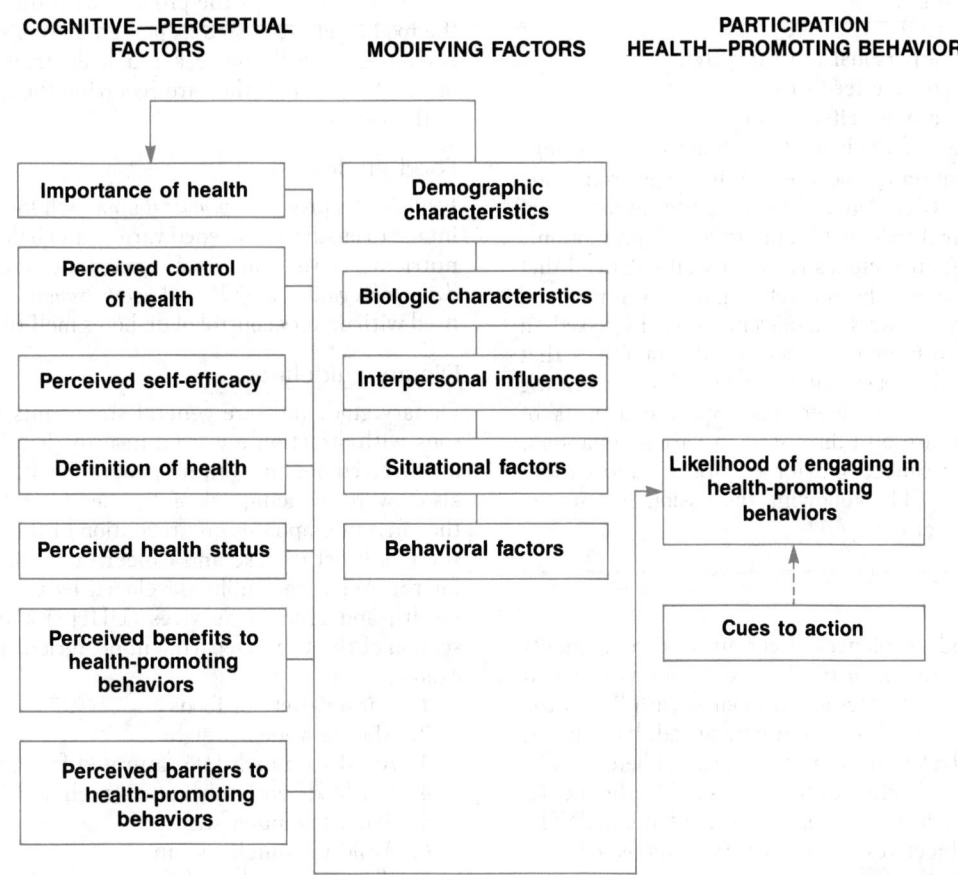

Fig. 5-1   Pender's health promotion model. (From Pender NJ: *Health promotion in nursing practice*, ed 2, East Norwalk, Ct, 1987, Appleton & Lange.)

The major interpersonal factors influencing health-promoting behaviors are the *influence of family or friends* and the *family patterns of health care*. Persons more likely to participate are those who have support for the health-promoting behaviors from family or friends and who have been raised in a family in which health-promoting behaviors are valued. Health teaching is enhanced when the patient's support persons are included in the teaching.

Situational factors include the availability of opportunities to engage in health-promoting behaviors. For example, facilitation of a nutritionally balanced weight control program is enhanced by the availability of fruits and vegetables rather than vending machines with candy and potato chips. Nurses can assist patients in exploring alternative ways of achieving their goals.

Health-promoting actions

The probability that a person will engage in health-promoting actions is influenced by actual or perceived barriers to action, such as cost, time, or ability, and the presence of cues to action.[26] Nursing approaches include assisting the person in differentiating between perceived and actual barriers and promoting behaviors directed toward overcoming actual barriers.

Cues to action include hearing about activities that promote health either in interactions with others or through the mass media. Nursing strategies include health teaching of patients or encouraging patients to read, to listen to radio, or to watch television programs that emphasize health promotion. Nurses also need to be instrumental in the development of these health-teaching tools.

Additional strategies that may be used to motivate persons and help them develop positive health behaviors include modeling, self-confrontation, and behavior modification. The nurse who carries out positive health behaviors, such as exercising regularly, serves as a *model* that others may emulate. Modeling positive health behaviors is an important nursing role function that, unfortunately, is not carried out to the degree that it should if health promotion is truly valued. *Self-confrontation* includes helping persons identify inconsistencies in health beliefs, values, or behaviors; dissatisfaction with these inconsistencies that follow the awareness may lead to behavioral changes.[26]

Behavior modification, or operant conditioning, consists of changing the behavior by means of a cognitive plan that is made by the person with the health care professional and rewards positive behaviors. Positive reinforcement of desired behaviors increases the likelihood of desirable behavior repetitions. The person is involved throughout the process. Behavior modification is accomplished over a period of time by the following self-actions:

1. Setting own goals
2. Self-monitoring
3. Developing a personal reward system
4. Obtaining positive feedback
5. Developing a new self-concept
6. Developing and implementing an activity program

Behavior modification has been useful in weight reduction programs (p. 82). (See Pender[26] for in-depth discussion of these and other methods that facilitate health promotion.)

Health promotion includes eating a well-balanced diet with emphasis on weight control, regular exercise, and reduction of stress. Stress management is discussed in Chapter 6. Health promotion also includes practices that decrease the risk of disease, such as not smoking and eating a low-fat, low-salt, high-fiber diet. Specific aspects of health promotion are also discussed in various chapters, such as those for cancer and for respiratory and cardiovascular disorders. The following discussion focuses on nutrition and exercise.

NUTRITION

Food excesses and imbalances of certain food components are of as much concern in the United States as nutrient deficiencies. Dietary factors are associated with five of the ten leading causes of death in American adults: cancer, heart disease, stroke, liver disease, and diabetes. (The other five causes of adult deaths are suicide, homicide, accidents, chronic lung disease, and HIV infection.)[35] The specific dietary objectives of the *Year 2000 National Health Objectives* include the following[35]:

1. Reduce the number of overweight adults (age 20 and older) to no more than 20% of the adult population.
2. Reduce dietary fat intake to less than 30% of calories and saturated fat intake to less than 10% of calories.
3. Increase daily intake of complex carbohydrates and fiber-containing foods to 5 or more servings for fruits and vegetables (including legumes), and 6 or more servings for grain products.
4. Decrease salt and sodium intake so that:
   More than 65% of home meals are prepared without adding salt
   More than 80% of persons avoid using salt at the table
   More than 40% of adults regularly purchase foods modified or lower in sodium

These topics are discussed in the following pages.

Nutritional Guidelines

There are three types of nutritional guidelines for health promotion: nutrient standards, food guides, and dietary guidelines.

Nutrient standards

Dietary standards are designed for the maintenance of good nutrition of practically all healthy people in the United States.[36] *Recommended dietary allowances* (RDAs), which are listed in Appendix C, are the accepted nutrient standards for proteins, vitamins, and minerals. The RDAs differ for age groups of children, men, and women based on weight and height. Labels found on many food products now include comparisons of the product with the RDAs. Because the food labels are listed as percentages of the total RDAs, persons can easily make a rough estimate for their own use to determine if they are receiving the desired quantity of the nutrients.

Food guides

Food guides provide a *practical* approach for organizing food intake to ensure the needed variety and balance of required nutrients. Two examples of food guides are the *Basic Four daily food guide* (p. 79) and *food exchange lists* commonly used with dietary control of diabetes mellitus (Chapter 28).

Dietary guidelines

Dietary guidelines are general statements to provide persons with direction toward a healthy diet. The guidelines are directed not only toward general health promotion, but also toward reducing risk of disease. Therefore they reflect the current emphases on prevention of the major diseases, such as heart disease and cancer. The dietary guidelines for the American public developed by the Department of Health and Human Services (DHHS) and the nutrition section of the U.S. Department of Agriculture[33] are a good example:

1. Eat a variety of foods
2. Maintain ideal weight
3. Avoid too much fat, saturated fat, and cholesterol
4. Eat foods with adequate starch and fiber
5. Avoid too much sugar
6. Avoid too much sodium
7. If you drink alcohol, do so in moderation

These seven guidelines are presented in the following discussion.

Eat a variety of foods

The greater the variety of foods ingested, the more likely the person receives the required nutrients. Good nutritional status exists when the necessary nutrients (protein, fat, carbohydrate, minerals, vitamins, and water) are consumed in sufficient amounts and are used appropriately by the body to meet needs. All persons need the same nutrients throughout life.

All nutrients are equally important, although they are not required in equal amounts. The nutrients providing energy (protein, fats, carbohydrates) and water are required in much larger quantities than vitamins that regulate body processes. The differences in the quantities of various nutrients required by an individual are much greater than the change in amounts of any one nutrient over the life cycle. Growth, basal metabolic needs, and physical activity are the major factors responsible for changing nutrient needs. Disease, trauma, variations in metabolism (normal and or abnormal), medications, and treatments can also affect needs. The major effects of good nutrition include the following:

Growth and development of tissues/organs

Source of energy for metabolic processes and physical activity

Table 5-1   Height and weight tables for adults with desirable weights for persons age 25 and over

Men*					Women*†			
Height		Small frame (lb)	Medium frame (lb)	Large frame (lb)	Height		Small frame (lb)	Medium frame (lb)	Large frame (lb)
ft	in				ft	in			
5	2	112-120	118-129	126-141	4	10	92-98	96-107	104-119
5	3	115-123	121-133	129-144	4	11	94-101	98-110	106-122
5	4	118-126	124-136	132-148	5	0	96-104	101-113	109-125
5	5	121-129	127-139	135-152	5	1	99-107	104-116	112-128
5	6	124-133	130-143	138-156	5	2	102-110	107-119	115-131
5	7	128-137	134-147	142-161	5	3	105-113	110-122	118-134
5	8	132-141	138-152	147-166	5	4	108-116	113-126	121-138
5	9	136-145	142-156	151-170	5	5	111-119	116-130	125-142
5	10	140-150	146-160	155-174	5	6	114-123	120-135	129-146
5	11	144-154	150-165	159-179	5	7	118-127	124-139	133-150
6	0	148-158	154-170	164-184	5	8	122-131	128-143	137-154
6	1	152-162	158-175	168-189	5	9	126-135	132-147	141-158
6	2	156-167	162-180	173-194	5	10	130-140	136-151	145-163
6	3	160-171	167-185	178-199	5	11	134-144	140-155	149-168
6	4	164-175	172-190	182-204	6	0	138-148	144-159	153-173

From Metropolitan Life Insurance Co., New York.
*Height for men with shoes with 1-in heels; height for women with shoes with 2-in heels.
†For women 18-25 years old, subtract 1 lb for each year under 25.

Tissue healing and repair
Resistance to infection

One method to ensure a good variety of foods is to follow the guidelines of the Basic Four food groups: milk products, meat/protein, vegetables/fruits, and bread/cereal (see p. 79).

Maintain ideal weight

Weight control is a major concern of many Americans; at least one out of every four Americans follows a weight-reducing diet at any given time.[36] *Ideal body weight* (IBW) is difficult to identify because of individual variations, such as sex, age, genetic framework, and metabolic needs. Two men of the same age may weigh the same, but one may be an athlete and have large amounts of muscle with little fat, whereas the other may have considerable fat. However, height and weight tables are practical guides for determining a *general* weight range (Table 5-1). The height and weight table must be used with caution because it is based on "averages" and the "average person" does not exist.

The terms *overweight* and *obesity* must be differentiated and may be described in different ways. However, *overweight* generally refers to weight between the high point and 20% above IBW established by height and weight standards. *Obesity* is described as *more than 20% above the* height and weight standards. *Massive obesity* places the person at a high risk for numerous disorders; this condition is discussed in Chapter 31. Overweight, as contrasted to massive obesity, has not yet been demonstrated as placing the person at risk for disease.[36] Many persons, however, do not feel at their optimal level of fitness and self-esteem when they are overweight. Thus, health promotion usually includes helping persons maintain their IBW by restricting energy input (high-calorie foods) while increasing energy output (physical activity) (see p. 83).

Underweight is described as 20% below the accepted weight and height standards. Unplanned weight loss may be an early sign of a medical disorder and medical evaluation should be sought. Some weight loss may be due to inadequate calorie intake or failure to increase calorie intake when physical activity is increased. Undernutrition leads to nutritional deficits that affect growth and development, metabolism, and the body's protective mechanisms. *Hospitalized patients are at risk for malnutrition* for several reasons. First, stress and increased metabolic rates from certain disorders deplete nutrient stores. Secondly, the patient is less active and may be relatively immobile. Thirdly, the patient may not be ingesting the required nutrients because of anorexia, nausea/vomiting, missed meals because of tests or surgery, or prescribed restrictive diets. Ongoing assessment of the patient's nutrient status is important. Protein-calorie malnutrition, a severe form of undernutrition, is discussed in Chapter 31.

Avoid too much fat, saturated fats, and cholesterol

We need fat in our foods, particularly to supply essential amino acids, especially linoleic acid that cannot be synthesized in the body. The body synthesizes fats from amino acids, but food provides an additional supply. Excess fats that the body cannot use are deposited in the tissue, adding to body weight. In addition, research strongly supports a relationship between dietary fat and the incidence of cancer, especially cancer of the breast, colon and rectum, and prostate.[2]

The American public is becoming better informed about the effects of high levels of serum cholesterol as a risk factor for coronary heart disease. High serum triglycerides are additional risk factors (Chapter 25). A 1990 survey found that 65% of adults reported having had their cho-

5-2

Definition of terms pertaining to fats and cholesterol

Lipids A group of fatty substances that are insoluble in water.

Triglycerides Simple lipids that are composed of one molecule of glycerol linked to three molecules of fatty acids.

Saturated fats Fatty acids that have no double bonds in the carbon chains: the fatty acid is filled (saturated) with hydrogen atoms; of animal origin.

Monounsaturated fats Fatty acids that have one double bond (one less hydrogen atom); of plant origin (for example, olive oil).

Polyunsaturated fats Fatty acids that have two or more double bonds (fewer hydrogen atoms); of plant origin (for example, vegetable oils).

Lipoproteins The form in which fats are carried in the blood stream: the unsoluble fat is wrapped in a water-soluble protein; may be low or high density.

Cholesterol A steroid that is found in animal fats and body tissues; most cholesterol is synthesized in the body; carried in blood stream primarily attached to low-density lipoproteins; of animal origin only.

5-3

Foods high in sodium

Salt-preserved foods: ham, bacon, sausage, hot dogs, cold cuts

Salted or smoked fish

Salted snacks: crackers, popcorn, pretzels, potato chips, nuts

Spices/condiments: meat tenderizer, bouillon cubes, celery salt, garlic salt, MSG, pickles, olives, Worcestershire sauce, soy sauce

Cheese

---

lesterol levels tested; however, only 24% stated that they were trying to lower their cholesterol levels through dietary means.[1] The National Cholesterol Education Program (NCEP) of the National Heart, Lung, and Blood Institute lists the following guidelines for adults:

1. Have cholesterol level measured every 5 years
2. Know your cholesterol level
3. Take steps to lower the cholesterol level, if elevated

NCEP established recent guidelines that define serum cholesterol of above 200 mg/dl as undesirable because of the increased risk for coronary heart disease.[30]

The phrase "avoid too much fat, saturated fat, and cholesterol" is vague; therefore more direction is needed. The 1991 nutritional guidelines by NCEP (and consistent with *Year 2000 National Objectives* and with guidelines set by other health agencies) are as follows:

Total fat	Average no more than 30% of calories
Saturated fatty acids	Less than 10%
Monounsaturated	10% to 15%
Polyunsaturated	Up to 10%
Cholesterol	Less than 300 mg/day

The different types of fats are defined in Box 5-2. Note that the more hydrogen is found in the fatty acid, the more it is saturated. Although saturated fats are of animal origin, unsaturated oils can be hardened commercially by injection of hydrogen gas to saturate them, producing margarines. About 40% of fats are visible in foods; the remainder is hidden, especially in red meats. Note also that cholesterol is not a fat but is related in that it is carried in the serum attached to fatty acids. Cholesterol is essential as a precursor to body steroids, for the development of bile acids, and as a component of cell membranes. Excess serum cholesterol not excreted contributes to the formation of atheromatous plaques in linings of blood vessels, especially the coronary arteries. This leads to blocking of the blood vessels. The recommended cholesterol intake of less than 300 mg/day is about one-half to one-third the amount in the usual American diet.[36] Recommended foods with lower cholesterol are listed on p. 82.

Eat foods with adequate starch and fiber

Starch is a polysaccharide (complex carbohydrate) found primarily in cereal grains, legumes, and vegetables (especially potatoes). It is the most important source of carbohydrate because it contains more nutrients than sugars. Carbohydrates are an important energy source for the body. The suggested *National Objectives for the Year 2000* include increasing the daily intake for grain products and legumes to 6 *or more daily servings*.

Dietary fiber contains cellulose and some noncellulose polysaccharides. Cellulose is not digestible therefore it remains in the gastrointestinal tract, providing bulk to help stimulate peristalsis in the intestines. The noncellulose polysaccharides absorb water to add to the bulk. Noncellulose substances also bind dietary cholesterol, preventing its absorption. Dietary fiber, therefore, is important to promote normal bowel elimination and to decrease dietary cholesterol absorption. In addition dietary fiber has been shown to have an inverse association with colon cancer; that is, a high intake of dietary fiber decreases the risk for colon cancer.[2] Sources of dietary fiber include whole grains (wheat, rye, oats) used in cereals and breads, bran, fruits, and vegetables.

The current intake of dietary fibers in the United States is about 10 to 15 g daily. The National Cancer Institute recommends *increasing daily fiber intake to 20 to 30 g* with an upper limit of 35 g to avoid adverse effects.[2] The suggested *National Objectives for the Year 2000* are to increase daily servings of *fruits and vegetables to 5 or more* and *grain/legumes products to 6 or more*. These suggested servings will provide 20 to 30 g of dietary fiber.[28]

Avoid too much sugar

Excess amounts of sugar add to caloric intake without supplying nutrients; they also contribute to formation of dental caries. In general, sugars in American diets average about 20% of daily calories.[36] Persons who diet by cutting

5-4	**Effect of some drugs on nutritional status**
Aspirin	Malabsorption of folate
	Excretion of vitamin C
Barbiturates	Malabsorption of thiamin, vitamin B_{12}
	Excretion of vitamin C
Corticosteroids	Malabsorption of calcium, zinc, phosphorus
Hydralazine	Excretion of pyridoxine
Methotrexate	Malabsorption of vitamin B_{12}, folate, fat
Mineral oil	Malabsorption of fat-soluble vitamins, calcium, phosphorus
Neomycin	Malabsorption of major nutrients
Oral contraceptives	Possible decreased absorption of vitamin C, B complex vitamins, magnesium, zinc
Penicillin	Loss of potassium
Tetracycline	Malabsorption of calcium, iron, magnesium, pyridoxine
	Excretion of vitamin C, riboflavin, niacin, folic acid
Thiazides	Excretion of potassium, magnesium, zinc, riboflavin

5-5	**Medications to be taken with food**	
Aminophylline	Nitrofurantoin
Chlorothiazide	(Macrodantin)
(Diuril)	Phenylbutazone
Ferrous sulfate	(Butazolidin)
Indomethacin	Phenytoin (Dilantin)
(Indocin)	Prednisolone
Metronidazole	Reserpine (Serpasil)
(Flagyl)	Triamterene (Dyrenium)

out sugar but continue to consume fats, deceive themselves because fats provide almost double the amount of calories. Use of artificial sweeteners does not necessarily reduce calories because the artificial sweeteners do not relieve the desire for "something sweet," and the person then may turn to fats to achieve the feeling of satiety.[36] Substituting complex carbohydrates for some of the sugars provides for greater intake of essential nutrients and feelings of satiety.

Avoid too much sodium

Sodium, a major body electrolyte (Chapter 7), can affect blood pressure levels. Although the cause of hypertension is unknown, a decreased sodium intake can help decrease blood pressure in persons with hypertension. Sodium in the form of salt-cured or salt-pickled foods has been associated with the increased incidence of gastric cancer.[2] Foods that are high in sodium are listed in Box 5-3. Most American diets are high in sodium, and dietary recommendations suggest that sodium intake be decreased to promote health. The suggested *National Objectives for the Year 2000* include the following:
- Increase to at least 50% of the proportion of households that purchase foods low in sodium, prepare foods without adding salt, and do not add salt at the table.

If you drink alcohol, do so in moderation

Alcohol is high in calories but low in nutrients. Excess alcohol intake leads to medical disorders and possible alcohol abuse (Chapter 13). Persons who drink excessively often do not eat balanced meals and therefore experience malnutrition. A large percentage of automobile accidents (a major public health problem) are caused by persons who

have been drinking alcohol. All health guidelines suggest that if you drink alcohol, you should do so in moderation.

Food-Drug Interactions

Some medications may affect nutritional status if taken over a period of time (see Box 5-4). Conversely, food can interfere with absorption of oral medications.

Drugs are absorbed more readily if the gastrointestinal tract is free of food. Drugs taken with water when the stomach is empty move rapidly into the small intestines, where much drug absorption takes place. Fatty foods delay gastric emptying for as long as 2 hours; therefore, drugs that are absorbed in the small intestine have delayed absorption if taken with a meal high in fats. Food particularly delays the absorption of antimicrobial drugs, specifically the tetracyclines, the penicillins, and the sulfonamides. However, medications that have a gastric irritant effect may be enhanced if taken with food (see Box 5-5).

Drugs that are normally slightly acidic, such as aspirin or barbiturates, usually ionize and are absorbed in the stomach. If the stomach pH increases, such as by milk or antacids, the rate and extent of absorption of these drugs decreases. Alteration in stomach acidity may also break down the protective coating of spansules or enteric-coated tablets, resulting in premature release of contents. Acidic liquids, such as lemon, pineapple, or cranberry juices or dry ginger ale may inactivate acid-unstable drugs, such as ampicillin, potassium, penicillin G, cloxacillin, and erythromycin.

Food components can interact with oral medication by the chemical or physical binding of one substance on another, thus interfering with absorption of either the food component or the drug. Tetracycline becomes bound with calcium, aluminum, or magnesium ions when taken with milk or antacids. This decreases absorption of tetracycline. Foods containing tyramine (cheeses, wines) may interact with monoamine oxidase (MAO) inhibitors, such as phenelzine (Nardil) or tranylcypromine (Parnate), which are depressants, causing hypertensive reactions.

Nursing Process
Assessment

To assess nutritional status, it is necessary to determine the supply of available nutrients, the sources available for metabolic processes, body size, and physical signs. Data are obtained primarily by patient interview, by observing the patient's general appearance, and by physical examination.

Subjective data

Data to be collected to determine nutritional status include the following:

Food intake
   Typical day food/fluid pattern (type, amount)
   Recent changes in amount and type of intake
   Recent changes in appetite
Eating ability
   Dentures (fit, comfort)
   Problems with chewing or swallowing
Weight
   Usual and current weight
   Patient's perception of weight level
      If overweight/underweight: lifetime patterns, feelings about weight, reasons for recent change
Food supplements, medications, drugs (types, duration)

Food intake

When collecting data about nutrition, it is especially important to phrase the questions so that patients describe what they typically eat rather than what they think they should. For example, the question, "Do you usually drink orange juice for breakfast?" implies (1) that breakfast is a desirable or expected behavior and (2) that orange juice is essential. Thus the patient may answer. "Yes," believing that is the expected answer, when in fact neither orange juice nor breakfast is usually eaten. A better approach is to say, "Tell me what you typically eat and drink in a day. What do you usually eat or drink first?" Questioning should elicit a picture of total food consumption for a day including all snacks. Designation by meals or snacks is not really necessary and may bias answers by implying value judgments.[24]

Identification of amount consumed is as important as the type of food. Often people find this difficult to estimate. Persons familiar with cooking may be able to estimate in terms of tablespoons or cups. For the hospitalized patient the equipment or portions on the tray can be used as a basis for comparison.

Changes in appetite or in the amount or type of food or fluids ingested may be the result of illness (for example, anorexia, nausea, vomiting, or pain), self-imposed dietary regimens, or emotional or physical stress.

Additional data

If nutritional intake is identified as inadequate, additional data facilitates analysis and planning:
1. Food and fluid likes and dislikes
2. Financial resources
3. Facilities and ability for purchasing, storing, and preparing food
4. Problems with prescribed diets

Objective data
Height and weight

Height and weight are easily measured and are important data to obtain and use. The most reliable weight measurement is in the morning after voiding and before eating or drinking fluids. The patient's weight and height are compared with a table of recommended values (see Table 5-1, p. 75). Interpretation of the table requires knowing

Table 5-2 Estimating body frame from height/wrist ratio

Sex	Frame size		
	Small	**Medium**	**Large**
Male	r > 10.4	r = 9.6 to 10.4	r < 9.6
Female	r > 10.9	r = 9.9 to 10.9	r < 9.9

frame size, which is determined by comparing height with wrist circumference. Measure the wrist distal to the styloid process on the right hand.[7] The height/wrist ratio (r) formula is as follows:

$$r = \frac{\text{Height (cm)}}{\text{Wrist circumference (cm)}}$$

Compare the ratio (r) with Table 5-2 to determine frame size.

Physical examination data

The time elapsing between the lack of nutrient supply and the actual appearance of clinical signs that are obvious on physical examination can be as little as a week or as long as several years. Data from a head-to-toe physical examination that suggest malnutrition may include the following:

Hair: lack of shine, thin and sparse, easily plucked
Eyes: pale conjunctiva, fissures at corner of eyelids
Lips: redness, dry, scaly, edema, fissures at corners of lips
Tongue: swollen, smooth, raw, scaly, enlarged papillae
Teeth: cavities, loose or missing teeth
Gums: bleed easily, spongy
Skin: lack of subcutaneous fat, dryness, petechiae
Nails: brittle, ridged, spoon shaped
Muscles: decreased muscle tone, tenderness, difficulty walking

Body mass index

A relative index of body fatness can be determined by calculating the body mass index (BMI) using the following formula:

$$\text{BMI} = \frac{\text{Weight (kg)}}{\text{Height (m)}^2}$$

Divide the number of pounds by 2.2 to determine weight in kg. Divide the number of inches by 39.37 to determine height in meters; then multiply this number by itself to square it. For example, the BMI calculation of a person who weighs 125 lbs and is 5 ft 3 in tall is as follows:

$$125 \div 2.2 = 56.8 \text{ kg}$$

5 ft 3 in = 63 in; 63 ÷ 39.37 = 1.6; 1.6 × 1.6 = 2.56

Therefore, the BMI would be 56.8 ÷ 2.56 = 22.18 kg/m²

For health maintenance, the BMI range for adults is 20 to 25 kg/m².[36] A person above that range, especially above 30 kg/m², is at risk. The person in the sample calculation is not at a health risk for overweight at the present time.

Table 5-3   Daily food guide for adults

Food group (servings/day)	Amount/serving	Nutrients supplied
Milk		
2 or more	1 c milk 40 g (1½ oz) cheese 1¾ c ice cream 1 c yogurt	Protein, calcium, phosphorus, riboflavin, other vitamins and minerals (except iron and vitamin C)
Meat protein		
2 or more	60 to 75 g (2 to 3 oz) lean meat, poultry, fish 2 eggs 1 c cooked beans, peas, lentils 4 Tbsp peanut butter	Protein, fat, B complex vitamins, (plant products lack vitamin B_{12})
Vegetables/fruits		
4 or more total		
1 dark green or deep yellow at least every other day	½ c broccoli, kale, carrots, squash, spinach, sweet potatoes, turnip or mustard greens, apricots, cantaloupe, pumpkin	Vitamin A
1/day (vitamin C sources)	½ c citrus fruits/juices, cabbage, broccoli, brussels sprouts, peppers, strawberries, tomatoes	Vitamin C
2 to 3/day (other)	½ c medium potato or apple, other vegetables or fruits	All fruits/vegetables: vitamins, minerals (low sodium), fiber
Bread/cereal		
4 or more (whole grain or enriched)	1 slice bread 30 g (1 oz) dry cereal ½ to ¾ c cooked cereal, rice, pasta	Complex carbohydrates, protein, iron, thiamin, riboflavin, niacin

Skinfold measurement

Body fat can be estimated by skinfold measurements. Calipers are used to measure skinfolds by compressing the skin and subcutaneous fat, not muscle, into a fold at specific body sites (for example, biceps, triceps, subcapsular, and suprailiac areas).

Data analysis: nursing diagnoses
Analysis of food intake

Food guides developed to help people choose the kinds and amounts of food to eat for health can be used for rapid evaluation of adequacy of the diet eaten at home or food intake in the hospital. Many different food guides are available, since to be effective they must be devised for a specific country or culture and feature the foods readily available and acceptable to the people being evaluated.

A daily food guide used in the United States is shown in Table 5-3. The guide groups staple food items rich in protein, vitamins, and minerals into four major classes according to their major nutrient contributions. Recommendations are made for the number and size of servings to be selected from each food group. To evaluate a diet quickly, one checks to see if the recommended types of food and servings are included in the usual dietary pattern.

Because foods are mixtures of nutrients, the protein, vitamin, and mineral requirements are substantially met when the daily intake includes the recommended servings

from each group. The calorie level of the basic diet is low, but it is approximately sufficient for adult basal metabolism. Adequacy of energy intake is best judged by evaluation of body weight. In this method of evaluation, fats, oils, and sweets are not tabulated because they provide primarily energy.

Each food group contributes particular nutrients to the total diet. The absence of any one food group from the diet or particular types of food should alert the nurse that the person has a potential nutrition problem. Box 5-6 is an example of an analysis of food intake using the daily food guide.

The daily food guide can also be used for evaluating vegetarian diets. Many people are vegetarians and their reasons vary (for example, religion, food cost, philosophy). The diets vary as well. Generally the lactoovovegetarian (includes milk products and eggs) diet is nutritionally sound when a variety of foods is included. Persons on more restricted vegetarian (vegan) diets should be considered at nutritional risk and candidates for more detailed study (refer to dietitian). One potential problem with the vegan diet is vitamin B_{12} insufficiency unless fortified cereal or a dietary supplement is taken. The young adult who has changed to a vegan diet may use body stores of B_{12} for a time (a 5-year store is possible), but is at potential risk, especially if intake of folacin in vegetables is high, masking the signs of megaloblastic anemia.

5-6

Assessment of a diet history

45-year-old woman with obesity and hypertension; meals eaten at home

7 AM
1 c cooked oatmeal
2 tsp sugar
1 c skim milk (fortified)
3 c coffee, plain

10:15 AM
2 c coffee, plain

1 PM
Sandwich
  2 slices white bread, enriched
  ½ tsp margarine
  ½ tsp mayonnaise
  60 g (2 oz) meatloaf or luncheon meat
4 cookies (fig bars, gingersnaps)
3 c coffee, plain

4 PM
7 cookies
½ c unsweetened fruit (canned, frozen, or fresh)
2 c tea, plain

10 PM
8 soda crackers
60 g (2 oz) American cheese
360 ml (12 oz) cola (sweet)
½ c homemade bread-and-butter pickles

Midnight
2 aspirin
1 c tea, plain

Assessment

Food group	Servings
Milk	
Skim milk	1
Cheese	1
Meat-protein	
Meatloaf	1
Fruits, vegetables	
Fruit	1
Vegetable	1
Bread, cereal	
Oatmeal	2
Bread, enriched	2
Crackers	2
Sweets	
Cookies	11
Cola (360 ml [12 oz])	
Pickles, cucumber	
Fats	
Margarine	
Mayonnaise	

Evaluation

Choice from milk group adequate. Meat intake low. Fruit and vegetable intake low; choice of items rich in vitamin C or A happenstance. Bread intake is 6 servings. Intake of sweets, particularly cookies, high. Use of pickles and soda crackers questionable, since patient reports that low-sodium diet was prescribed for her several years ago.

Dietitian was asked to check caloric value. Intake is 1500 to 1600 calories/day, which includes 800 calories from basic food items; remainder from sweets and fat. Protein levels adequate, although source of protein could be improved.

To the reader: Identify nutritional risks for this person; identify appropriate interventions and behavioral goals for her.

From Neville, J: *Assessment of nutritional status and dietary counseling.* In Phipps, et al: *Medical-surgical nursing: concepts and clinical practice,* ed 4, St Louis, 1991, Mosby–Year Book.

Nursing diagnoses

Nursing diagnoses are determined from analysis of patient data. Possible nursing diagnoses for the person with a nutritional imbalance include the following:

Diagnostic title	Possible etiologies
Knowledge deficit	Lack of information
Nutrition, altered: high risk for more than body requirements	Dysfunctional eating behaviors
Nutrition, altered: more than body requirements	Dysfunctional eating behaviors, lack of exercise
Nutrition, altered: less than body requirements	Dysfunctional eating behaviors, anorexia, decreased intake because of tests or surgery

Planning: expected patient outcomes

Expected patient outcomes to promote good nutritional status may include, but are not limited to, the following:
1. Describes desired servings for each food group to meet basic nutritive needs.
2. Maintains weight within desired weight ranges.
3. Describes modifications in dietary intake to correct existing or potential nutritional deficits or excesses.

Implementation
Interventions to achieve patient outcomes
Facilitating patient teaching

Good nutrition can be promoted by giving positive reinforcement for selection of balanced meals from hospital

5-7

Types of diet modifications

Protein	Increased with losses from tissue catabolism, bleeding, exudates
	Decreased for chronic renal failure or hepatic coma
	Elimination of specific proteins (for example, allergies or malabsorption of gluten)
Fats	Increased to provide essential calories in concentrated form
	Decreased for pain with gallbladder disease
	Modified for disorders of digestion or absorption, lipid metabolism, or to alter serum lipid levels
Carbohydrates	Increased for weight gain
	Decreased for weight loss or diabetes mellitus
	Changed from simple to complex carbohydrates in diabetes mellitus
	Elimination of specific carbohydrates with disorders of carbohydrate intolerance (for example, lactase deficiency)
Vitamins	Increased for vitamin deficiency
	Provided in an alternate form to enhance absorption or use
Minerals	Sodium restriction with hypertension, fluid retention, kidney disease
	Potassium and calcium increased or decreased for lack or excess
	Provided by prescription for deficiency
Liquid, soft, pureed	Postoperative, diseases of gastrointestinal tract, difficulty with chewing or swallowing
Elimination diets	Food allergies

menus. Teaching patients with specific knowledge deficits includes identification of the patient's motivation to learn. Patients with extensive lack of knowledge about food preparation, particularly with ways of preparing nutritionally balanced meals at low cost, may profit from the services of a dietitian.

The daily food guide (Table 5-3) is a useful tool for teaching persons a method of evaluating their own food intake. The dietitian may be helpful in developing a specific food guide for persons whose cultural patterns or personal preferences (for example, vegetarians) do not fit the standard food guides.

Persons who have been prescribed a dietary modification may need interpretation of the rationale for the diet and assistance in planning acceptable meals using the prescribed dietary plan (see Box 5-7). The dietitian usually initiates the discussion of a new home-going diet, but the nurse serves as interpreter to the patient by providing explanations about the diet and feedback on how to make changes in current dietary patterns to meet the dietary prescription. Because the patients are the ones who must implement the dietary changes, they need to internalize the need for a behavior change. This takes active participation in all phases of the learning process. The person who does the cooking (if not the patient) also needs to be involved in the learning process. Dietary changes are more likely to be implemented if the changes can be easily adjusted to the family's usual meal plans.

Facilitating weight loss

Diet. Diet is the most important method of weight reduction. Weight loss for some persons may be achieved by eating three regular, balanced meals a day that include the four basic food groups and avoiding fried foods, sweets, and between-meal snacks. Other persons achieve better results with planned, frequent small meals. Some obese persons omit breakfast but then snack frequently and thus ingest more calories and fewer required nutrients. Therefore, *changes in eating patterns* are usually required for permanent weight loss.

Persons consuming high levels of calories before weight-reduction diets are likely to be successful in achieving rapid weight loss, because the calorie deficit between need and the recommended diet is large. There is a difference in weight loss patterns between men and women. If both a man and a woman are instructed to adhere to a 1000-calorie intake, the man should lose at a faster rate, not because he is more cooperative but because his calorie deficit is greater.[24]

Rapid weight loss is usually the result of loss of fluid rather than fat. Thus after an initial successful loss of weight on a weight-control diet, a plateau is reached when weight appears to remain constant or decrease only slightly. This can be discouraging to the person who is following the prescribed approach. Reinforcement to continue the regimen is usually needed at this point.

Diets are planned on an individual basis, with the caloric intake planned at a level below the person's caloric need for maintaining weight. The calorie intake should come from complex carbohydrates and proteins. A protein intake of about 1 g/kg of ideal body weight should be maintained. Fats must be decreased. Salt-free diets are of no long-term value for weight reduction, because the weight loss relates to water loss, and the weight returns when salt is added to the diet.

Fasting diets are controversial. Rapid weight loss may be necessary in some instances; however, weight gain following the fasting period is a common occurrence. Most fasting programs use a high-protein liquid; some commercial products use hydrolyzed collagen that is low in nutritional value. Close medical supervision is imperative for fasting diets because risks are high (such as ketosis, metabolic acidosis, hypokalemia, hepatic impairment, renal insufficiency, and death).

Table 5-4   Guidelines for decreasing dietary fats and cholesterol

Food groups	Use	Decrease
Meat	Fish, skinned poultry, lean cuts of meat	Fatty meats, sausages, hot dogs, cold cuts
Milk products	Skimmed or 1% milk, low-fat cheeses, and yogurt	Whole milk, whole milk yogurt, natural cheeses, sour cream
	Egg whites	Egg yolks
Fruits	All fruits	
Vegetables	All vegetables	Butter or sauces added to vegetables
Bread/cereal	Low-fat crackers and cookies, angel food cake, homemade baked goods with limited unsaturated fats	High fat crackers and cookies, commercially baked goods, foods made with saturated fats
	Whole grain breads/cereals; rice, pasta	Breads/cereals without whole grain: egg noodles
Fats/oils	Canola, corn, safflower, sesame, soybean, and sunflower oils	Coconut and palm kernel oil; butter, saturated fat, bacon fat
	Seeds and nuts	Coconut

From Expert Panel: Report of the National Cholesterol Education Program Expert Panel on detection, evaluation, and treatment of high blood cholesterol in adults, *Arch Intern Med* 148:36-69, 1988.

Fad diets should generally be avoided, although they usually induce rapid weight loss in a relatively easy way. However, nutrients will be lost (marked protein catabolism with losses of nitrogen, phosphorus, calcium, potassium, sodium, and water). Weight then returns to the original level after termination of the diet, because the person's general pattern of eating has not been changed.

Exercise. Exercise is an essential component of any weight control program. It promotes expenditure of energy and makes body appearance more pleasing to the person and thus desirable to maintain. Although the actual number of calories used are few, the combination of diet and exercise promotes loss of fat rather than lean tissue. It is important that the exercise program be agreeable to the person so that it becomes a pattern of behavior to be continued throughout life (see p. 83).

Behavior modification for weight control. Behavior modification (p. 73) for weight control consists of changing the pattern of eating and exercising. Without changes in eating behaviors and exercise participation, overweight persons usually return to their original weight after dieting.

Self-control is important in learning to change eating habits to facilitate weight loss and to maintain desirable body weight. Setting one's own goals and developing a personal reward system can facilitate motivation to participate in the desirable behaviors. Self-monitoring by means of planning the menus and keeping food diaries increases the person's awareness of the foods consumed. (Many persons are unaware of the number of calories consumed, especially by "nibbling.")

Reinforcement from others is a major factor in the success of a weight control program. The effectiveness of weight control groups, such as Weight Watchers, is based on this concept.

Facilitating weight gain

Persons who are underweight or have inadequate nutritional stores need encouragement to eat the right nutrients and calories. Motivating a person with anorexia to eat can be a challenge. Interventions that can correct the cause leads to improved appetite. Determining the person's likes and dislikes, providing an environment conducive to eating, and providing several small meals rather than three large meals a day may facilitate an adequate nutritional intake.

If the patient can eat, a high-calorie, high-protein diet is indicated to provide energy and amino acids for tissue building. The diet is essentially a normal one with added protein and supplementary high-caloric feedings. High-protein diets are contraindicated if a patient has liver disease because protein catabolism takes place in the liver. For persons with protein-calorie malnutrition, enteral and parenteral feedings are frequently necessary (see Chapter 31).

Facilitating control of dietary fats and cholesterol

As cited previously (p. 76), adults should know their cholesterol levels and should take measures to decrease the level if it is greater than 200 mg/dl. The usual American diet is 10% to 15% of kcal *higher* in total fats (10% higher in saturated fats, 5% higher in monounsaturated fats, and slightly higher in polyunsaturated fats) than the recommended levels. The cholesterol level of the average American diet is *two to two and one-half times* that of the recommended level of less than 300 mg/day[11]. Therefore, it is necessary for all people to modify these intakes to the recommended levels (p. 76). Guidelines for decreasing fats and cholesterol are listed in Table 5-4.

Maintaining a low-saturated fat, low-cholesterol diet is not always easy because it involves deleting some well-liked foods, such as high-fat cheeses and cold cuts. Learning to eat a diet that is lower in saturated fats and cholesterol, as with other types of permanent diet changes, requires a change in eating behavior patterns (behavior modification, p. 73). People need to know the differences among the types of fats, cholesterol and fat content of foods, and how to read food labels.[21] For example, many producers of plant-based products advertise that their product has zero cholesterol; this is in fact true, but one must remember that cholesterol comes only from animal products. The advertised product may be high in saturated fats, which the body can then use to produce cholesterol.

5-8	**Benefits of aerobic exercise**

Sense of well-being
Enhanced coping with stress
Decreased anxiety or depression
More restful sleep
Maintenance of physiologic functioning at optimum level
Enhanced weight control
Decreased risk of osteoporosis
Decreased risk factors for coronary artery disease
Better control of hypertension and diabetes mellitus
Decreased risk of colon cancer
Assistance with reduction of addictive behavior (for example, smoking, overeating, or drinking)

5-9	**Physiologic effects of exercise**

Musculoskeletal system
    Maintains muscle strength
    Maintains joint flexibility
    Maintains endurance (tolerance to continue an activity)
    Increases mineral content of bones
Neurosensory system
    Maintains coordination
    Maintains orientation to environment
Circulatory system
    Maintains a more constant average work load on heart
    Maintains normal blood pressure regulatory adjustment to transient position changes
    Promotes venous return through contraction of muscles
Respiratory system
    Contributes to ease of breathing
    Provides stimulus to deep breathing and aeration of alveoli
    Provides movement of secretions
Gastrointestinal system
    Maintains elimination through muscle activity and visceral reflex patterns
    Encourages the person to heed defecation reflex
Urinary system
    Promotes urine formation
    Promotes complete emptying of bladder

EXERCISE

Regular physical activity can help individuals feel well, cope with stress, enhance normal body functioning, and decrease risk factors for some diseases. Physical activity and fitness is the first listed category of health promotion in the *Year 2000 national health objectives*. When the 1990 objectives for physical activity and fitness were evaluated, it was found that the actual numbers of adults who participated in moderate daily activity or in vigorous exercise at least 3 times a week were far below the desired levels.[27] Much health teaching and active promotion of exercise and fitness are necessary, therefore, if the following objectives for the Year 2000[35] are to be met:

Increase to more than 30% the proportion of people older than age 6 who engage regularly, preferably daily, in light to moderate activity for at least 30 minutes per day.

Increase to more than 20% the proportion of people older than age 18 who engage in vigorous physical activity for more than 20 minutes, 3 or more days a week.

Although a positive trend has developed toward increased exercise in recent years, many adults live a sedentary life-style. People are aware that activity or mobility is necessary for health but many still do not take the effort to increase their activity level. Persons who do not value exercise as a means of maintaining optimal health often find excuses for not participating in a planned exercise program on an on-going basis. Exercise does imply effort; if exercise is not valued, the effort is not made.

Benefits of Exercise

A program of regular exercise can have both psychologic and physiologic benefits (see Box 5-8). A physically fit person also generally has greater endurance and faster recovery time (return to resting rate), which can contribute to more rapid recovery from illness.

Exercise is important *regardless of age*. Some elderly persons believe they are too old to begin an active fitness program, but these programs are possible even for persons with chronic illness. The fitness program is individually planned and based on the person's interests, capabilities, and limitations.

Physically, exercise enhances cardiovascular fitness, endurance, muscle strength, flexibility, and weight control. It has positive effects on the musculoskeletal, neurosensory, circulatory, respiratory, gastrointestinal, and urinary systems (see Box 5-9).

Exercise Programs
Classification of exercise

Exercises may be classified as aerobic or anaerobic. *Aerobic* exercises are those activities that are supported by aerobic metabolism (the breakdown of carbohydrates and fats to carbon dioxide and water in the presence of oxygen, that is, the Krebs cycle). Aerobic exercises are characterized by activities that involve large muscle groups and that are performed in a rhythmic and continuous nature for more than 15 minutes. Examples of aerobic exercises include brisk walking, jogging, bicycling, swimming, skating, cross-country skiing, and aerobic dancing.

Anaerobic exercises involve anaerobic metabolism (the breakdown of glucose to lactic acid in the absence of oxygen). This occurs with high-intensity activities in which the available oxygen is used up and the anaerobic pathways are then used to provide the necessary additional energy. Anaerobic types of exercises include weight lifting and competitive sports, such as football, soccer, basketball, baseball, volleyball, and hockey. Greater benefits to overall physical fitness and well-being are achieved with aerobic rather than with anaerobic exercises.

Table 5-5   **Target pulse rates with exercise**

Category	Pulse target zone	Pulse return after exercise
Healthy active adults	70% to 85% of maximum heart rate (220 minus age)	Less than 120 in 5 min
Obese, low physical conditioning	50% to 60% of maximum heart rate	Less than 100 in 10 min / Baseline level in 10 min
Cardiac disease, following bed rest	No more than 20 beats above baseline	Baseline level in 5 min

Table 5-6   **Complications of immobility**

System	Physiologic effect	Dysfunction/pathology	Nursing intervention (preventive)
Cardiovascular	Pooling of venous blood in legs Decreased venous return to heart Decreased cardiac output	Thrombophlebitis Pulmonary embolus Postural hypotension Decreased tolerance for activity when initiated	Range-of-motion: active and passive Isometric exercises of legs Turn frequently Avoid pressure on major blood vessels Slow mobilization
Respiratory	Pooling of secretions from decreased movement Decreased stimulation to cough Decreased depth of ventilation	Hypostatic pneumonia Atelectasis	Turn and move frequently Active range-of-motion Deep breathing and coughing
Gastrointestinal	Decreased peristalsis Change in eating/drinking habits Change in position to eliminate (bedpan)	Constipation	Increase fluid intake Good dietary intake of fiber foods Active movement in bed Use of stool softener or suppositories
Urinary	Increased calcium from bone destruction Alkaline urine Urinary stasis	Urinary calculi Urinary retention Urinary tract infection	Increase fluid intake Decrease calcium intake Use commode rather than bedpan if possible
Musculoskeletal	Muscle atrophy and shortening Fibrosis or bony ankylosis of joints Loss of bone matrix with release of calcium	Muscle weakness Contractures Osteoporosis	Active range-of-motion Isometric and isotonic exercises Positioning of joints to facilitate use
Neurologic	Decreased stimuli	Decreased orientation	Social contacts Diversionary materials
Skin	Friction, pressure, or shearing forces Decreased circulation from pressure Break in skin integrity Maceration from perspiration or urinary incontinence	Abrasions Decubitus ulcers	Frequent assessment Protection of vulnerable areas (foam or alternating pressure mattresses, sheepskin, flotation pads, elbow or heel pads) Turn frequently

Recommendations for physical fitness programs

Persons with a personal or family history of cardiovascular disease or who are over 35 years of age should have a physical examination before beginning an exercise program. A program is then planned on the basis of the person's tolerance and interests (it should be enjoyable).

Tolerance is evaluated by assessing pulse rate (Table 5-5). For example, a healthy, active 50-year-old person should aim at maintaining a pulse rate during exercise of 70% to 85% of 170 beats per minute (220 minus 50), that is, within a range of 119 to 145. The pulse is then assessed for the time it takes to return to normal. Tolerance to activity of hospitalized patients who are starting to ambulate (aerobic exercise) after inactivity is assessed in the same manner; that is, the pulse rate should not increase greater than 20 beats per minute over the patient's baseline pulse rate and should return to baseline level within 5 minutes after ambulating.

Exercising should be done on a regular basis; one of the national health goals for the year 2000 is 20 minutes of exercise three times a week by all persons.[28] All persons should start each exercise period with deep diaphragmatic breathing and stretching exercises. Stretching exercises improve flexibility and help prevent injuries. Duration of the exercise period, which depends on the person's conditioning, is usually about 15 to 60 minutes per period. The exercises should be performed at just under the anaerobic threshold (identified by a tightness or "burning" sensation in the muscles and shortness of breath). Pulse and respirations should be increased but talking should still be possible. It is best to start out slowly and gradually extend the program as conditioning improves. If the pulse target zone is exceeded or if the recovery period is extended, the exercise is too strenuous. With *inactivity* there is a loss of 20% conditioning within 2 to 3 weeks and up to 50% loss by 1 month.[38]

Types of exercises

Isometric exercise. With isometric exercises, opposing muscles are contracted, thus increasing the tone of the muscle fibers but not changing muscle length or moving the joints. The purpose of these exercises is to maintain muscle strength and tone. There is very little effect on cardiovascular or respiratory conditioning, although isometric exercises may not be easily tolerated by persons with coronary artery disease. Examples of isometric exercises for hospitalized patients are quadriceps-setting exercises and gluteal sets (Chapter 20) to maintain muscle strength in the thighs and buttocks for walking.

Persons doing isometric exercises should be taught to *exhale while exerting effort.* Many persons tend to hold their breath while bearing down (Valsalva maneuver). This increases intrathoracic pressure, causing a decrease in venous return to the heart. When the breath is then released, the intrathoracic pressure decreases, causing a large surge of blood return to the heart and increasing the cardiac work load. Exhaling while exerting effort can prevent the Valsalva effect.

Isotonic exercises. With isotonic exercises, muscle length changes and joint movements occur. There is less muscle tension than with isometric exercises. Isotonic exercises maintain and increase muscle strength. Aerobic exercises are one form of isotonic exercises. Some types of isotonic exercises for the hospitalized patient include moving and turning in bed, ambulating, and moving arms and legs against light resistance.

Facilitating exercise

Getting started is probably the biggest hurdle in developing a regular exercise program. The following are some suggestions:

1. Identify types of physical activity that are most preferable. If you like what you are doing, then you are more apt to continue doing it. Exercise should be pleasurable.
2. Develop a weekly plan that sets *specific time periods* for the activity, which is based on desires and daily schedule. For example, it may be easier to exercise before or immediately after work or during a lunch period. Once you are at home and relaxed, it is often more difficult to get up and get going. Scheduled exercises are more likely to be carried out than just planning three times a week.
3. Begin the activity for short periods at a low level, then increase time and effort toward the desired goal. If you do too much initially and ache or become overtired, you are more apt to give up the activity.
4. Share the activity with others; you are more likely to continue the activity if other persons are involved. Doing exercises at home alone on a regular basis requires considerable willpower to continue for any period of time. Get a friend to walk with you; the time goes faster and is more enjoyable if socialization occurs concurrently. Some community agencies have scheduled aerobic classes such as low-impact aerobics or water exercises that are fun. If you pay for the class, you are more likely to attend to get your money's worth.
5. Set small goals toward meeting the long-term goal. Achievement of small goals increases feelings of self-esteem. Reward yourself when you achieve each goal, such as each time you add an additional mile to your walk.
6. If for some reason, such as illness, you have had to stop your exercise program, start back with the activity at a lower level than when you ended. Muscle strength and tone are lost with only a short absence of activity. Then work toward achieving your desired level.

Activity or exercise should be incorporated into one's life-style, attaining the same importance as eating or sleeping. Physical activity performed on a regular basis gives a sense of well-being that is part of feeling healthy. And feeling healthy contributes to longer life.

Immobility

Immobility may be accompanied by a number of complications that can involve any or all of the major systems of the body (Table 5-6). It is important that those caring for the patient whose mobility is impaired be aware of these potential complications and be skilled in interventions designed to help prevent them. The patient is encouraged to be as active as possible within the activity limitations by moving and turning in bed and by carrying out active range-of-motion, isometric, and isotonic exercises.

SUMMARY

1. Factors influencing health-promoting behaviors include perceptions about health and self, demographic factors, influence of family or friends, family patterns of health care, availability of opportunities to engage in health-promoting behaviors, and actual or perceived barriers to health-promoting actions.
2. Health-promoting strategies include health teaching, modeling, self-confrontation, and behavior modification.
3. Three types of nutritional guidelines are nutrient standards (recommended dietary allowances), food guides (the Basic Four and food exchange lists), and dietary guidelines.
4. A recommended dietary guideline includes (1) eating a variety of foods; (2) maintaining ideal weight; (3) avoiding too much fat, saturated fat, and cholesterol; (4) eating foods with adequate starch and fiber; (5) avoiding too much sugar; (6) avoiding too much sodium; and (7) consuming alcohol in moderation.
5. Overweight refers to weight between ideal body weight and 20% above ideal body weight (IBW). Obesity is more than 20% above the height-weight standards. Underweight is 20% below the height-weight standards.
6. Guidelines for cholesterol awareness and actions include having cholesterol measured every 5 years, knowing your cholesterol level, and taking steps to lower the elevated cholesterol level. A dietary intake of less than 300 mg cholesterol is recommended.
7. Dietary fiber provides bulk to help stimulate intestinal peristalsis, binds dietary cholesterol to prevent absorption, and is a factor in reducing risk for cancer of the colon. An intake of 20 to 30 g of dietary fiber is recommended.
8. Recommendations for decreasing sodium intake include eating foods low in sodium, preparing foods without adding salt, and not adding salt at the table.
9. Medications may affect nutritional status; food can, in turn, affect absorption of oral medications.
10. The dietary food guide is useful for a quick dietary assessment and for use in health teaching.
11. Methods of weight reduction include diet, exercise, and behavior modification.
12. Exercise enhances cardiovascular fitness, endurance, muscle strength, flexibility, weight control, sense of well-being, sleep, and ability to cope with stress. Exercise also has a positive effect on the body systems, decreases risk factors of coronary artery disease, provides better control of hypertension, and assists in reducing addictive behaviors.
13. Aerobic exercises are those that involve large muscle movements in a continuous and rhythmic manner for more than 15 minutes. Anaerobic exercises are high intensity activities that use up available oxygen and are supported by anaerobic pathways.
14. Activity tolerance of healthy active adults is assessed by a pulse rate 70% to 85% of maximum heart rate (220 minus age) that returns to normal within 5 minutes.
15. Isometric exercises are those that include muscle contraction without joint movement. Isotonic exercises include muscle contraction with joint movement.
16. Persons doing isometric exercises should exhale while exerting effort to prevent Valsalva maneuver.

STUDY QUESTIONS

- Select a health behavior that you do not follow. How does this behavior relate to your definition of health? What factors can you identify that may be barriers to the desired behaviors?
- In what ways do your eating behaviors differ from the seven recommended dietary guidelines? What measures could you take to meet or maintain each of the guidelines?
- Why would it be ineffective to tell an overweight person he/she should lose weight?
- How often do you engage in 15 minutes or more of aerobic activities each week? What changes, if any, could you make to meet recommendations for health promotion?

REFERENCES AND SELECTED READINGS

1. *Americans aware of cholesterol dangers*, April 10, 1991, Cleveland, The Plain Dealer.
2. Butrum RR, Clifford CK, Lanza E: NCI dietary guidelines: rationale, *Am J Clin Nutr* 48:888-895, 1988.
3.* Cerato PL: How safe are modified fasts, *RN* 52(11):79-81, 1989.
4. Clark JB, Queener SF, Karb VB: *Pharmacologic basis of nursing practice*, ed 3, St Louis, 1990, Mosby–Year Book.
5.* Clark SR: Compliance and health behavior, *Top Clin Nurs* 7(4):39-46, 1986.
6. Cornacchia HJ, Barrett S: *Consumer health: a guide to intelligent decisions*, ed 4, St Louis, 1989, Mosby–Year Book.
7.* Curtas S, Chapman G, Meguid MM: Evaluation of nutritional status, *Nurs Clin North Am* 24:301-312, 1989.
8. Dychtwald K, Flower J: *Age wave: the challenges and opportunities of an aging America*, Los Angeles, 1989, Jeremy P Tarcher.
9. Dychtwald K, MacLean J: *Wellness and health promotion for the elderly*, Rockville, Md, 1986, Aspen Systems.
10. Ebersole P, Hess P: *Toward healthy aging: human needs and nursing response*, ed 3, St Louis, 1989, Mosby–Year Book.
11. Expert Panel: Report of the National Cholesterol Education Program Expert Panel on detection, evaluation, and treatment of high blood cholesterol in adults, *Arch Intern Med* 148:36-69, 1988.
12. Factors related to cholesterol screening and cholesterol level awareness, *MMWR* 39(37):633-637, 1990.
13. Getchell B: *Fit: a personal guide*, ed 2, Indianapolis, 1986, Benchmark Press.
14. Haskell WL, Montoye HJ, Orenstein D: Physical activity and exercise to achieve health-related physical fitness components, *Public Health Rep* 100(2):202-210, 1985.
15. Hospital malnutrition still abounds, *Nutr Rev* 46:315-317, 1988.

*Recommended for student reading.

16. Johnson C, Greenland P: Effects of exercise, dietary cholesterol, and dietary fat on blood lipids, *Arch Intern Med* 150:137-140, 1990.

17. Krause MV, Mahan LK: *Food, nutrition, and diet therapy*, ed 8, Philadelphia, 1991, WB Saunders.

18. Marwick C: Changes brewing for food labels as national concern about diet and health continues to grow, *JAMA* 262:752-755, 1989.

19.* Massachusetts Medical Society Committee on Nutrition: Fast-food fare: consumer guidelines, *New Eng J Med* 321:752-533, 1989.

20. McCain GH: Sources of health information for consumers and health practitioners, *Fam Community Health* 9(2):46-50, 1986.

21.* McCann BS: Promoting adherence to low-fat, low-cholesterol diets: review and recommendations, *J Am Dietetic Assoc* 90:1408-1414, 1990.

22. Molloy D: Now is the time to advocate wellness, *Am Nurse* April 4, 1991.

23. National Research Council: *Recommended dietary allowances*, ed 10, National Academy Press, Washington, DC, 1989, The Council.

24. Neville J: *Assessment of nutritional status and dietary counseling.* In Phipps WJ, et al, editors: *Medical-surgical nursing: concepts and clinical practice*, ed 4, St Louis, 1991, Mosby—Year Book.

25. Nowak RK, Schultz KO: A comparison of two methods for determination of body frame size, *J Am Dietetic Assoc* 87:339-341, 1987.

26.* Pender NJ: *Health promotion in nursing practice*, ed 2, Norwalk, Ct, 1987, Appleton & Lange.

27. Progress toward achieving the 1990 national objectives for physical fitness and exercise, *MMWR* 38(26):449-453, 1989.

28. Public Health Service: *Promoting health-preventing disease: Year 2000 objectives for the nation, draft for public review and comment*, Washington, DC, 1989, US Dept of Health and Human Services.

29. Public Health Service: *Healthy people 2000: national health promotion and disease prevention objectives*, Washington, DC, 1990, US Dept of Health and Human Services.

30. Schectman G, et al: Dietary intake of American reporting adherence to low-cholesterol diet (NHANES II), *Am J Public Health* 80:698-703, 1990.

31. Stoto MA, Behrens R, Rosemont C, editors: *Healthy people 2000: citizens chart the course*, Washington, DC, 1990, National Academy Press.

32. *Surgeon General's report on nutrition and health*, Washington, DC, 1988, US Dept of Health and Human Services.

33. US Dept of Agriculture, Human Nutrition Information Service: *Nutrition and your health: dietary guidelines for Americans; eat a variety of foods*, Washington DC, 1986, US Superintendent of Documents.

34. US Dept of Agriculture and the US Dept of Health and Human Services: *Nutrition and your health: dietary guidelines for Americans*, ed 2, Washington, DC, 1985, US Superintendent of Documents.

35. US Dept of Health and Human Services and Public Health Service: *Healthy People 2000: national health promotion and disease prevention objectives, 1991*, Washington, DC, US Government Printing Office.

36. Williams SR: Essentials of nutrition and diet therapy, ed 5, St Louis, 1990, Mosby—Year Book.

37. Year 2000 national health objectives, *MMWR* 38(37):629-633, 1989.

Classic

38. Cantu RC: *Toward fitness: guided exercise for those with health problems*, New York, 1980, Human Sciences Press.

39. Cantu RC: Health maintenance through physical conditioning, Littleton, Mass, 1981, PSG Publishing.

40. Cooper KH: *The aerobics way*, New York, 1977, M Evans & Co. Inc.

41. Stefee P: Malnutrition in hospitalized patients, *JAMA* 244:2630-2635, 1980.

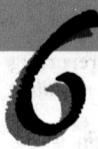

6

Stressors, Stress, and Stress Management

Virginia L. Cassmeyer
Barbara C. Long
May Wykle

After studying this chapter, the learner should be able to:

- Define adaptation.
- Differentiate between stressors and stress response.
- Explain the relationship of dealing with stressors to optimal functioning and growth.
- Describe the neuroendocrine response to stressors.
- Describe behavioral responses to stressors.
- Define coping.
- Describe types of coping strategies.
- Identify assessment parameters of anxiety.
- Describe interventions for persons with anxiety.
- Describe approaches to crisis intervention.
- Describe methods of stress management.

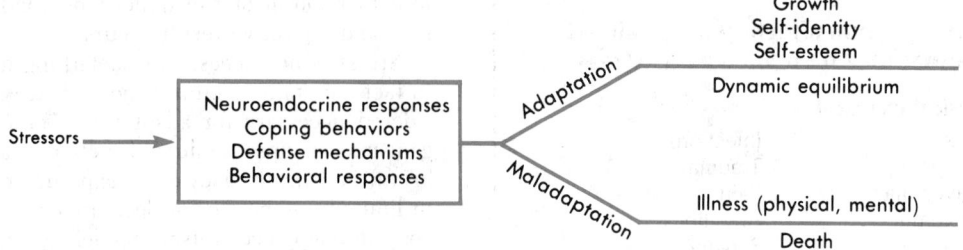

Fig. 6-1   Responses to stressors may lead to adaptation or maladaptation.

Promotion of health involves activities that facilitate a sense of well-being. This implies a feeling of "ease," which is accomplished in part by coping effectively with internal or external stressors. Nurses can help patients learn how to cope with stressors in positive ways and thus prevent or diminish the effects of the stressors and the stress response. This chapter discusses various concepts of adaptation, stressors, stress response, and stress management.

ADAPTATION

Humans can be conceptualized as open systems that respond to stimuli from the internal and external environments. This process of interaction can be termed *adaptation.* In this context, adaptation has neither positive nor negative values. However, many prefer to use the term in a positive sense, to mean the process of interaction with the environment that promotes homeostasis or dynamic equilibrium and growth. The process that leads to inadequate functioning is then termed *maladaptation.*

Human beings adapt biologically, psychologically, emotionally, and socially. The goal of biologic adaptation is survival or stability of internal processes. When the ability to maintain this equilibrium is lost, pathophysiologic disorders result. Psychologic and emotional adaptation is directed toward preservation of self-identity and self-esteem. The person adapting in these modes is mentally healthy, whereas maladaptation leads to mental illness. Social adaptation depends on the sociocultural expectations of the society of which the person is a member. A maladaptive or socially deviant behavior in one society may be acceptable in another.

Although any changing environmental stimuli can initiate the need for adaptation, stressors create major adaptive demands for individuals. As shown in Figure 6-1, the neuroendocrine responses, coping behaviors, defense mechanisms, and behavioral responses are major strategies available for meeting adaptive demands associated with stressors. Nurses work with persons in adaptation at many levels including:

1. Helping to identify and remove stressors requiring adaptive demands.
2. Supporting healthy strategies that help to meet the adaptive demands of stressors.
3. Helping persons use higher level defense mechanisms.

4. Helping persons deal with the psychologic responses to stressors.
5. Helping persons develop alternative coping behaviors or behavioral responses to stressors.
6. Helping persons deal with the illnesses that result if adaptation is not effective.

STRESSORS/STRESS AS CONCEPTS

The ability of the human body to initiate and sustain a response to stressors is one of the major protective mechanisms that allows individuals to exist in a hostile environment. Both the healthy and ill—those in the hospital, in extended care facilities, or in their own homes—are exposed to stressors. Because stressors are so ubiquitous, the individual must possess mechanisms to deal with them.

Stressors

Before exploring the responses to stressors, the concept of stressors will be discussed. A *stressor* can be defined as a noxious or threatening stimulus that can elicit a stress response. A stressor may be actual or potential, biophysical-chemical, or psychosocial-cultural. Although most of the stressors that are experienced by patients in the hospital are negative stimuli and severe in nature, stressors can be positive stimuli, such as marriage, physical exercise, or the birth of a child. Stressors also can be nonsevere, everyday hassles. Important in the definition of stressors is that, although some of the more severe stimuli would probably be perceived as a stressor for anyone, individuals differ as to which stimuli are stressors.

Many different studies have shown that stressors can be biologic, physical, chemical, social, developmental, cultural, or psychological stimuli.[28,32,40] Stressors can range from the daily hassles of an alarm clock that doesn't go off on time, to an approaching deadline, to the onset of the common cold in a relatively healthy person, to major burns over 50% of the body. The stressors that the nurse deals with vary depending on the patient population. The nurse in an outpatient setting, in home health care, or in discharge planning may focus more on daily hassles and primary health care problems. The nurse working with patients during the acute or critical stages of illness may deal with more severe stressors.

Box 6-1 lists some common stimuli affecting hospitalized adults that may be perceived as stressors. This list is not inclusive, but does contain stressors that might be more

<table>
<tr><td colspan="2">

6-1

Common stimuli affecting hospitalized adults that may be perceived as stressors

Biophysical-chemical

Hypoxia	Infections
Hypercapnia	Trauma
Hypoglycemia	Pain
Hypovolemia	Any illness
Hypotension	Surgery
Decreased cardiac output	Immobilization
Alcohol	Restraints
Caffeine	Constant light
All drugs	Noise
X-ray contrast media	Sleep deprivation
Anesthesia	Discomfort
Blood transfusions	Fatigue
Weakness	Burns

Psychosociocultural

Anger	Anxiety
Fear	Uncertainty
Loss	Dependency
Isolation	Invasion of privacy
Sensory overload	Sensory deprivation
Role changes	Financial burdens
Guilt	Language barriers
Loss of control	Exposure of body
Stigma of diagnosis	Unpleasant sights and sounds
Unfamiliar sounds	Change in body image

From Phipps WJ, et al: *Medical-surgical nursing: concepts and clinical practice*, ed 4, St Louis, 1991, Mosby—Year Book.

</td></tr>
</table>

universally found in acute and critical care settings. The list can be used by the nurse during assessment of a patient. One of the first steps of care is to identify the potential stressors.

Stress

The term *stress* has been used for many years to denote mental strain, for example, "He's under stress." Every person has some definition for the word stress. For the purpose of this chapter *stress* is defined as:

An integrated body response, including intellectual, behavioral, emotional, and physiologic components, to a stimuli that is perceived on a conscious or unconscious level as noxious or threatening. The response serves as a protective mechanism. It is elicited to allow the individual to adapt to or adjust to noxious or threatening stimuli and is graded. The response varies depending on the type, strength, and duration of the stimuli and is modified by characteristics of the person.

The response to stressors may have either negative or positive results or both. For example, a person may experience pain (a stressor). The pain may cause anorexia, which may lead to nutrient imbalance and inactivity, which may lead to the side effects of immobility. These are negative results. On the other hand, the presence of pain may guide the person to seek medical intervention. This may

lead to removal of the underlying condition causing the pain and a positive result occurs.

Stress is not necessarily something to be avoided, and in fact a certain amount of normal stress (*eustress*) is considered necessary for adaptation. For example, microorganisms can upset cellular function, leading to disequilibrium and death. However, exposure to microorganisms in limited numbers or of decreased strength can help the body develop mechanisms to defend against subsequent exposures. Similarly, exposure to daily hassels helps develop useful coping methods that facilitate dealing with new stressors. Coping with biologic or psychosocial stressors in an adaptive manner aids optimal functioning and growth. Maladaptation leads to dysfunction and pathophysiologic or psychopathologic disorders.

RESPONSES TO STRESSORS

Integrated Psychobiologic Response

People respond to stressors as a *unified whole*, that is, compensatory or defense mechanisms are initiated to help the individual cope with the stressor biologically and psychologically. Some of the evoked responses are biologic, others are behavioral, and both frequently occur simultaneously. For example, anxiety can cause sweaty palms, pale skin, and frequent voiding, as well as decreased attention span, decreased ability to follow directions, or immobility. For the purpose of learning, however, it is easier to separate physiologic responses from behavioral responses.

The scientist with whom the concepts of stress and stressor are most closely associated is Hans Selye. When he was a medical student, Selye observed in diverse persons with various diseases similar signs and symptoms that he labeled as the *syndrome of just being sick*.[67] When he first observed this syndrome, he questioned whether the underlying mechanism could be identified. Years later, while involved in experimental studies designed to discover a new hormone, he noted that injections of a tissue extract, which supposedly contained the hormone, resulted in enlargement of the adrenal cortex, ulcers of the gastrointestinal tract, and atrophy of the lymph nodes and thymus gland.[65] Although Selye[67] at first ascribed these changes to the hypothetical hormone supposedly in the tissue extract, he later found that injections of any extracts, as well as other stimuli, such as cold and x-rays, caused the same response.

General Adaptation Syndrome

Selye labeled this nonspecific response to various agents the general adaptation syndrome (GAS).[65,67] GAS became known as the stress syndrome and was viewed as having three stages: alarm reaction, resistance, and exhaustion. The first two stages are repeated continuously throughout life as persons encounter stressors. The exhaustion stage occurs when resistance cannot be sustained, and altered functioning then results.

Alarm reaction stage. During the initial alarm stage (shock), the "fight or flight" response is initiated. The individual prepares to counteract the stressor or remove himself or herself from the stressor. If the shock is too severe, a "freeze" response occurs; the person is overwhelmed by the stressor and cannot fight or flee. During

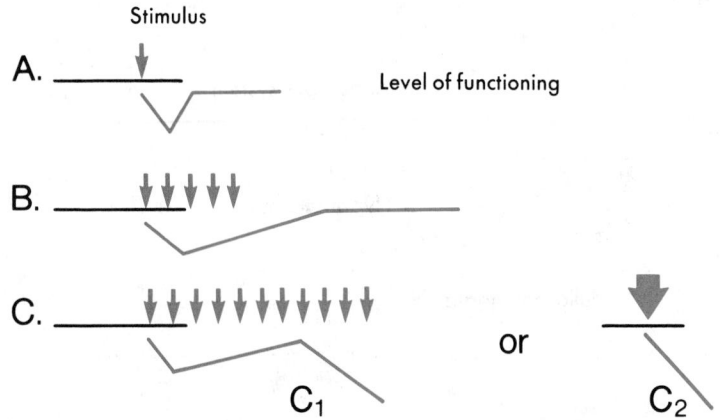

Fig. 6-2   General adaptation syndrome. **A,** Alarm reaction with return to prestressed level. **B,** Continued application of stimulus leads to resistance stage; return to prestressed level may occur when stimulus is removed. **C,** Depletion of resources with continued stimuli or strong damaging stimulus leads to exhaustion.

the alarm reaction stage, the neuroendocrine mechanisms are activated. If the compensatory mechanisms are sufficient to deal with the stressor, the individual returns to the prestressed level (Fig. 6-2, A).

Resistance stage. Continual and prolonged application of the stressor leads to the resistance stage. During this stage, continued adrenocortical activity facilitates adaptation. Energy is required to maintain a high level of resistance. If the stressor is maintained a sufficient time, stress-related pathophysiologic disorders may result. If adaptation is successful and the stressor removed, the person may return to the prestressed level (Fig. 6-2, B).

Exhaustion stage. If the original stressor is so damaging that defense mechanisms are ineffective or if the stressor is not removed and energy to maintain resistance is depleted, the exhaustion stage occurs (Fig. 6-2, C). Examples of extreme stressors are arterial bleeding, pressure on the hypothalamus, overwhelming infection, blockage of a major branch of the coronary artery, or sudden death of a spouse. Unless the primary biologic condition can be controlled promptly, death may ensue.

Selye[65] proposed that the hormones produced during GAS were responsible for the diseases of adaptation. The stress response or GAS involves the sympathetic branch of the autonomic nervous system and the pituitary and adrenal glands. Selye also described the local adaptation syndrome (LAS), which is the response to a locally applied stimulus. The inflammatory process is an example of LAS.

Selye's work built on the work of Walter Cannon, who in 1935 described the stresses and strains of homeostasis. Some major criticisms of Selye's work must also be noted. First, in his early work, Selye did not acknowledge that psychologic events could serve as stressors. His later writings did acknowledge this fact.[63] The work of various persons as early as the 1950s[50] revealed that the GAS could be elicited in response to psychologic stimuli.

Another criticism of Selye's work was the idea that

stimuli that serve as stressors were stressors for everyone. The work of Lazarus[57] and Cox[47] pointed out that a stimulus must be perceived as a stressor before the GAS response is elicited.

The meaning of the stressor for the individual is one of the major factors influencing the stress response. Stressors creating a change that is viewed negatively have a high probability of an increased stress response. For example, a woman who places great value on her body as a means of personal and sexual gratification will likely experience a greater response to removal of a breast than a woman who places less significance on her bodily appearance.

The individual's *perception* of the stressor (and hence the meaning that is interpreted) is influenced by cognitive ability, verbal skills, past experiences, interpersonal relationships, significant others' responses, and feelings of control. A sense of control over the stressor helps to decrease the response. For example, patients who know in advance some measures to decrease postoperative pain (that is, have control over the pain) usually adapt more effectively in the postoperative period. Persons who have developed a repertoire of coping skills can select one that facilitates adaptation to a new stressor. Thus persons who have had to cope with numerous intense stressors in the past are often able to cope effectively when crises occur.

When health status is poor, less energy is available to deal with environmental stimuli, and responses to stressors may be affected. Nutritional deficits especially place the person at higher risk of maladaptive responses (see Chapter 5).

Another important factor in relation to psychologic and emotional influences on physiologic stressors is that in some experiments[60,61] where physical stressors were induced while controlling or minimizing the discomfort, suddenness, or unpleasantness of the stimuli, the GAS was not elicited. This may mean that all stressor stimuli must have a psychosocial-cultural component.

One last criticism of Selye's work relates to his description of the stress response as nonspecific. This character-

Stressors

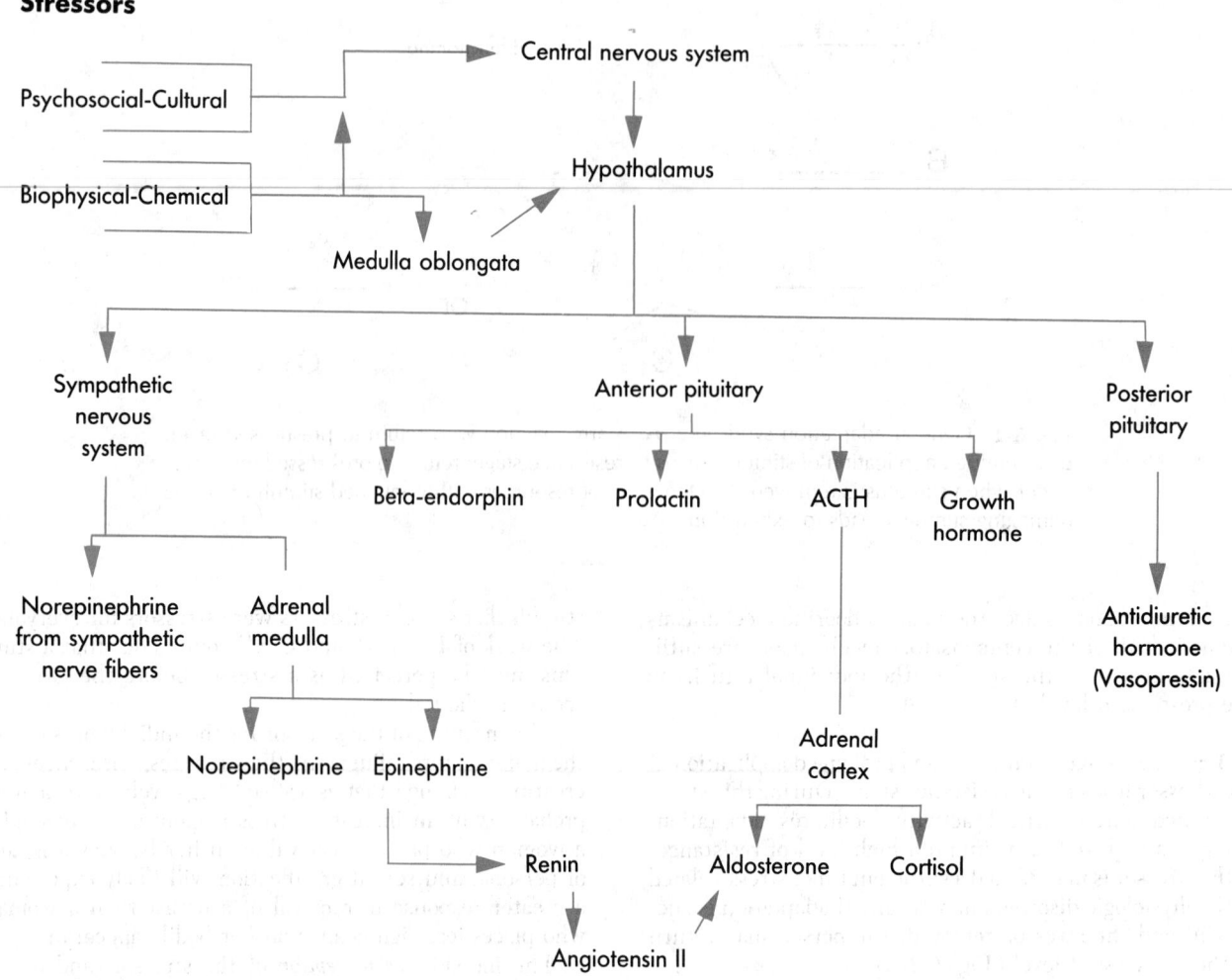

Fig. 6-3   Physiologic components involved in the neuroendocrine response to stressors.

istic meant that the same response occurred regardless of the stressor. Current data do not support this assumption. In animal studies,[59] different hormonal and neurochemical responses occur in response to different stressors. Despite these criticisms, Selye's work still provides the basis of the physiologic response that can be elicited by stressors and an appreciation of the various stimuli that may serve as stressors in many persons.

Neuroendocrine Response to Stressors

The physiologic components involved in the stress response include the central nervous system, the hypothalamus, the sympathetic nervous system, the anterior and posterior pituitary gland, and the adrenal cortex and medulla. These physiologic components and their secretions (hormones and catecholamines) are responsible for the neuroendocrine response to stressors. As discussed earlier in this chapter, not all of these components are necessarily involved in the response to every stressor; but to provide holistic nursing care, the nurse must know the effects of response to stressors of each of these components of the neuroendocrine response.

The physiologic components of the neuroendocrine

stress response are shown in Figure 6-3. Stressors, either perceived at the level of the *central nervous system* or on an unconscious level by *baroreceptors, chemoreceptors,* or *glucoreceptors,* which transfer information to the *medulla oblongata,* serve as the *afferent input.* This information is eventually forwarded to the *hypothalamus,* which coordinates the response. The hypothalamus activates the *sympathetic nervous system* and the *anterior* and *posterior pituitary glands.* The *adrenal medulla* is activated when the sympathetic nervous system is stimulated.

The hypothalamus stimulates the anterior pituitary gland by releasing hormones such as corticotropin-releasing hormone (CRH), growth hormone-releasing hormone (GHRH), or prolactin-releasing hormone (PRH) or by inhibiting its secretion of inhibiting hormones. For example, dopamine acts as a prolactin-inhibiting hormone (PIH) and thus prolactin secretion is increased when dopamine secretion is decreased.

Adrenocorticotropin hormone (ACTH), which is released from the anterior pituitary gland, stimulates the release of cortisol from the adrenal cortex. The adrenal cortex also releases the hormone aldosterone in response to ACTH secretion. However, the major controller of al-

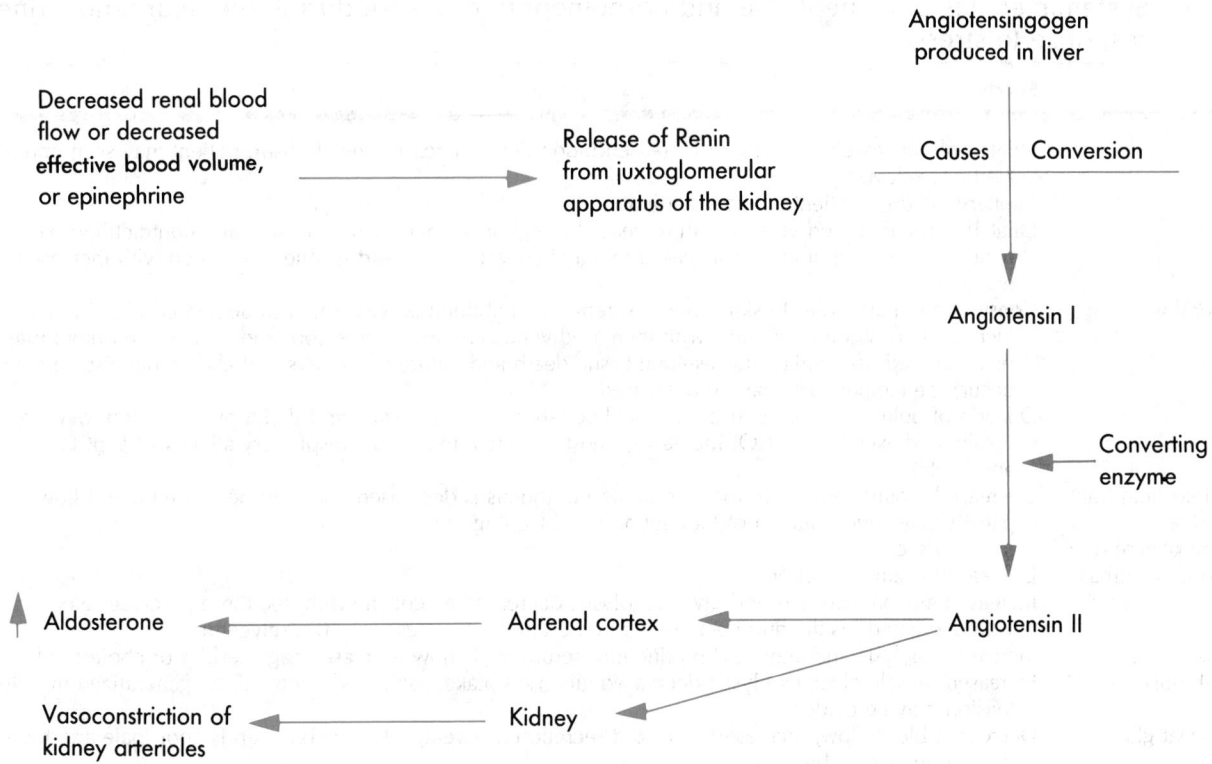

Fig. 6-4   Renin-angiotensin-aldosterone system.

dosterone secretion is the renin-angiotensin system, which is shown in Figure 6-4.

Another endocrine gland activated by the hypothalamus is the posterior pituitary gland. The posterior pituitary gland, when stimulated, releases antidiuretic hormone (ADH) or vasopressin. The effects of stimulation of the sympathetic nervous system, anterior and posterior pituitary glands, and adrenal cortex and medulla are mediated by the catecholamines and hormones released by the nervous system or the glands.

Catecholamines

The catecholamines, epinephrine and norepinephrine, act by stimulating receptors unique for them. The receptors are located on various cells throughout the body. The catecholamine receptors are divided into two major classes, alpha (α) and beta (β), with two subclasses of each major class. The activation of these receptors by endogenous or exogenous catecholamines results in selected physiologic actions.

Stimulation of α_1 receptors is primarily associated with excitation or stimulation, and stimulation of α_2 receptors is primarily associated with relaxation or inhibition. Stimulation of β_1 receptors is primarily associated with stimulation of cardiac activity, and stimulation of β_2 receptors is associated with all other effects associated with beta receptors such as bronchial dilation.

During the neuroendocrine response to stressors, both norepinephrine and epinephrine are released. Norepinephrine binds primarily to α receptors, whereas epinephrine activates both α and β receptors. The effects of

catecholamines during the stress response then are due to a combination of the actions of both catecholamines and activation of several different receptors. The effects seen with the release of catecholamines during the stress response are summarized in Table 6-1.

Cortisol

Cortisol is released from the adrenal cortex under the control of CRH and ACTH. Cortisol has major effects on metabolism and fluid and electrolyte balance and has antiinflammatory and immunosuppressant effects. It enhances the activity of other hormones. Detailed information of the effects of cortisol on the body are presented in Box 6-2.

Aldosterone

Aldosterone is released from the adrenal cortex primarily in response to activation of the renin-angiotensin system as diagrammed in Figure 6-4. Some aldosterone is released in response to ACTH from the anterior pituitary gland. Aldosterone acts on the distal kidney tubule cells and causes reabsorption of sodium and water and excretion of potassium and hydrogen ions. Aldosterone helps to maintain vascular volume and blood pressure.

Antidiuretic hormone

Antidiuretic hormone (ADH) or vasopressin is released during the neuroendocrine response to stressors. ADH acts on the kidneys to increase water reabsorption. Water is reabsorbed in response to the osmotic gradient established by the difference in osmolality of the tubular fluid and the

Table 6-1 Systemic effects of epinephrine and norepinephrine release during the neuroendocrine response to stressors

Organ	Effects
Brain	Dilated blood vessels resulting in increased blood flow; increased metabolism; patient may seem more alert or restless
Eyes	Pupilary dilation; patient appears startled
Heart	Dilated coronary blood vessels with increased blood flow; increased heart rate and contractility; patient's cardiac output and stroke volume may increase if the heart is able to keep up with increased demand
Peripheral vascular system	Constriction of arterioles to skin, mucosa, renal, and abdominal viscera, with decreased blood flow; increased constriction of veins with increased venous return; skin is cool and pale; urine output may be decreased; ischemia with resultant tissue death and failure of kidneys and abdominal viscera may occur; toe temperature may be decreased
Lungs	Dilation of pulmonary vascular bed; bronchodilation; increased rate and depth of respiration; oxygen uptake and excretion of CO_2 increases; and the patient may show respiratory alkalosis ($\downarrow$ pCO_2 and $\uparrow$ pH)
Gastrointestinal tract (GI)	Decreased motility and secretion; production of mucus is decreased and with decreased blood flow patient may have irritation of GI tract and GI bleeding
Exocrine pancreas	Decreased secretions
Endocrine pancreas	Decreased insulin secretion
Liver	Increased gluconeogenesis and glycogenolysis; decreased glycogen synthesis; these processes along with decreased insulin and decreased glucose uptake may result in hyperglycemia
Adipose tissue	Increased lipolysis and fatty acid production; serum may show increased triglycerides or cholesterol
Skeletal muscle	Increased muscle glycogenolysis; decreased glucose uptake, increased contractility; generalized muscle tension may be evident
Skin, sweat glands	Decreased blood flow, increased localized secretion of sweat; piloerection; skin is cool, pale and moist; goose bumps may be evident

From Phipps WJ, et al: *Medical-surgical nursing: concepts and clinical practice*, ed 4, St Louis, 1991, Mosby—Year Book.

medullary interstitial fluid. ADH controls the osmolality of body fluid. ADH in high concentration can result in arteriole vasoconstriction and can help to increase blood pressure.

Other pituitary hormones

Endogenous opiates (B-endorphins) are released as part of the neuroendocrine response to stressors. Release of endogenous opiates in stressful situations may account for the analgesic effect experienced by trauma patients.

Growth hormone is released from the anterior pituitary during the neuroendocrine response to stressors. Hypoglycemia and strenuous exercise are two stressors associated with an increase in growth hormone. Growth hormone helps to provide nutrients for the energy needs during the stress response. It helps to maintain the blood glucose level, and increases lipolysis, free fatty acid levels, and ketone formation, which provide nutrients for various tissues, such as skeletal and cardiac muscles.

Prolactin[24] is released in the presence of certain stressors. The function of prolactin in relation to dealing with stressors is unknown.

The overall affects of the release of the hormones and catecholamines during a neuroendocrine response to stressors, if the response is effective, are summarized in Box 6-3.

Coping

Coping refers to processes or skills that individuals use to deal with events, circumstances, or situations that are out

Types of coping strategies

Category	Examples
Action	Taking walks, washing floors, gardening
Cognitive	Problem solving
Intrapsychic	Religion, activities to search for meaning of stress
Interpersonal	Use of support persons, talking it over with someone
Emotional	Use of defense mechanisms, such as denial

of the ordinary and thus become stressors. Coping strategies are overall plans of action for overcoming stressors.[2] Thus coping is a general behavioral response to stressors.

People cope with stressors in one or more ways (see Table 6-2). Actions to cope with stressors may be adaptive or maladaptive, depending on the achieved level of functioning. Some persons respond to most stressors in one characteristic mode; however, this limits their ability for adaptation when new stressors occur that interfere with this coping mode. For example, persons who generally respond to stressors by physical activity are severely hampered when an illness (stressor) occurs that decreases physical mobility. Persons who have developed several coping strategies are better able to cope effectively with new stressors.

<table>
<tr><td>

6-2

Systemic effects of cortisol release during the neuroendocrine response to stressors

Metabolic effects

Maintains blood glucose by:
  Increasing gluconeogenesis
  Decreasing glucose uptake by many body cells, particularly muscle
Increases protein catabolism, which provides substrate for glucose formation
Promotes lipolysis to provide alternative nutrient sources

Fluid and electrolyte effects

Promotes sodium and water retention
Promotes potassium excretion

Antiinflammatory/immunosuppressive effects

Decreases eosinophils, basophils, monocytes, and lymphocytes in the circulation
Increases neutrophil (polymorphonuclear leukocytes) by movement from bone marrow and circulatory pools
Decreases leukocyte accumulation at inflammatory sites
Inhibits release of inflammatory substances (kinins, prostaglandins, leukotrienes)
Degrades collagen
Decreases scar tissue formation
Decreases lymphoid tissue mass, participation of T-lymphocytes in cellular-mediated immunity, and production of interleukin 1 and 2

Miscellaneous effects

Maintains emotional stability
Increases red blood cell formation
Possibly increases platelet formation
Increases gastric acid and pepsin production
Is permissive for other hormones and catecholamines (cortisol is necessary for the full functioning of some other hormones and catecholamines), particularily in relation to blood pressure control, cardiac output, and metabolic effects of epinephrine and norepinephrine.

From Phipps WJ, et al: *Medical-surgical nursing: concepts and clinical practice,* ed 4, St Louis, 1991, Mosby–Year Book.

</td></tr>
</table>

<table>
<tr><td>

6-3

Overall effects of an effective stress response

Increased glucose and fatty acids for energy
Increased oxygen uptake
Increased excretion of CO_2
Maintenance of blood volume and cardiac output
Increased muscle activity
Increased mental alertness

</td></tr>
</table>

primitive kind are avoided. Defense mechanisms become pathologic when they are overused.

A defense mechanism is effective when it succeeds in easing intrapsychic tensions. When lower level defense mechanisms fail, a more pathologic process evolves, and the person exhibits psychiatric symptoms. All defense mechanisms are unconscious with the exception of suppression. Two defense mechanisms, denial and repression, are frequently manifested by the hospitalized patient and are discussed in more detail in the following section.

Denial

One of the defense mechanisms used frequently in dealing with illness is denial. This mechanism occurs during the early stages of crisis after the initial stressful impact. Denial of the illness helps the person deal with increased tension by protecting the ego (self) from reality. The pattern used by the person is similar to games played by children when they close their eyes and believe no one can see them. "It's not there because I don't see it." That which cannot be perceived is therefore not painful.

During denial intolerable thoughts are disowned. The ego gets rid of unwelcome facts (such as an illness) while still retaining its faculty for reality testing. The person manifests denial by disowning any body changes. For example, patients with coronary disease may deny they have had heart attacks and blame their discomfort on indigestion. Patients may even deny the severity of the pain and act as though the pain were not present.

Denial works well for the person who has been independent and has a self-image of a strong, self-made individual or who views sickness as a sign of weakness. Denial can be complete or partial and includes a "splitting" of thoughts, feelings, and actions; for example, the patient may own the thoughts but deny the feelings.

Approaches that may be useful when working with the person exhibiting denial include the following:

1. Explore fears and anxieties underlying the denial.
2. Avoid direct confrontation of denial.
3. Assist person in controlling selected aspects of care.
4. Provide reassurance of the person's worth as a human being despite being in a dependent state.
5. Reinforce behaviors indicating reality acceptance.
6. Set limits kindly but firmly when denial behavior interferes with treatment.

Regression

Regression is a defense mechanism often seen in persons who are ill, because regression facilitates acceptance of the

Defense Mechanisms

Defense mechanisms are unconscious processes used by individuals in adjustment to life stressors. They evolve during personality development and serve to protect the personality, satisfy emotional needs, maintain harmony between conflicting tendencies, and reduce tension or anxiety by modifying reality to make it more acceptable. Defense mechanisms are compromise solutions.

There are two levels of defense mechanisms: those that are considered more primitive and those that are of a higher level (see Box 6-4). Defense mechanisms are used by mentally healthy people as well as by those who are neurotic or psychotic. In the mentally healthy, defense mechanisms are used less frequently, and those mechanisms of a more

6-4

Defense Mechanisms

Higher level: less primitive mechanisms

Repression	Ideas painful to consciousness are forced into the unconscious.
Suppression	Thoughts or desires are consciously inhibited.
Sublimation	Energy of repressed tendencies is transformed and directed to socially acceptable goals.
Identification	Person assumes the personal qualities or elements of the personality of another.
Compensation	Person makes up, covers up, or disguises real or fancied inadequacies in another area.
Displacement	An emotion is transferred or displaced from its original object to a more acceptable substitute that is less threatening.
Rationalization	Plausible explanations are given to account for a belief or behavior motivated from unconscious sources.

Lower level: more primitive mechanisms

Denial	Intolerable thoughts, feelings, or wishes are disavowed; person refutes external elements of reality that are unpleasant or painful.
Regression	Person reverts to a pattern of behavior belonging to an earlier stage of development.
Conversion	Painful emotional experience is repressed and later is expressed in the form of a physical symptom.
Projection	That which is emotionally unacceptable within the self is rejected and attributed to others.
Introjection	Person absorbs the emotional attitudes, wishes, ideals, or personality of others into oneself; the aspirations and self-restraints of others are incorporated into the personality.
Reaction formation	Person adopts attitudes and behavior that are opposites of the impulses to which the individual is reacting.

patient role. Regression makes a dependency relationship possible because of the individual's reversion to behavior patterns of an earlier level of development. Illness necessitates patients placing themselves in the hands of competent others. They often become self-centered and concerned only with their own needs and interests. These interests focus on what is happening to the person and on their acceptance or rejection by care givers. Often regression helps patients promote conservation of energy.

Approaches that may be useful when working with the person exhibiting regression include the following:

1. Explore the observable behavior with the patient.
2. Discuss the patient's goals.
3. Discuss the patient's unreadiness to attain goals and revise as appropriate.

Specific Behavioral Responses

Stressors and the stress response lead to behaviors that are either adaptive or maladaptive. Persons who display adaptive behavior are those who make appropriate use of their coping mechanisms and do not exhibit symptoms of psychologic disturbance. Those with maladaptive behavior are at the end of the spectrum (Fig. 6-5); their psychiatric symptoms are a way of dealing with the increased stress. (For further information on maladaptive behavior consult a psychiatric–mental health text.) Anxiety and other common behaviors resulting from the stress of illness are discussed in the following section.

Anxiety

Anxiety is a psychologic response to stressors with both physiologic and psychologic components. It is a feeling of dread or uneasiness from an unrecognized source. Anxiety results when a person perceives a threat to the self either physically or psychologically (such as to self-esteem, body image, or identity).

Anxiety is manifested in different levels ranging from mild to severe.[62] In Box 6-5, note the changes in the way the person relates to the environment associated with the different levels of anxiety. Awareness, which is heightened with mild anxiety, begins to decrease until the panic stage, in which perceptions of the environment become distorted. Persons can vacillate among the several levels of anxiety. The level of anxiety engendered and its manifestations depend on the person's maturity, understanding of need, level of self-esteem, and coping mechanisms.

Anxiety is a psychologic response that cannot be seen; it is only implied by the individual's actions. The state of *anxiousness* manifested by behavioral changes is communicated interpersonally. Highly anxious persons can transmit the sense of anxiousness to others; for example, a very anxious patient can heighten a family member's anxiety and vice versa.

Although the ego attempts to deal with anxiety through the use of defense mechanisms, certain degrees of anxiety are reflected in behaviors resulting from a discharge of energy necessary to restore equilibrium. These responses range from behavior that is adaptive to behavior that is considered, by our social standards, maladaptive (see Fig. 6-5). The types of behavioral reactions that occur are influenced by psychosociocultural factors, basic personality development, past experiences, values, and economic status. Because anxiety is so common, assessment criteria, nursing diagnoses, outcomes, and interventions are discussed in detail in the Nursing Process section of this chapter.

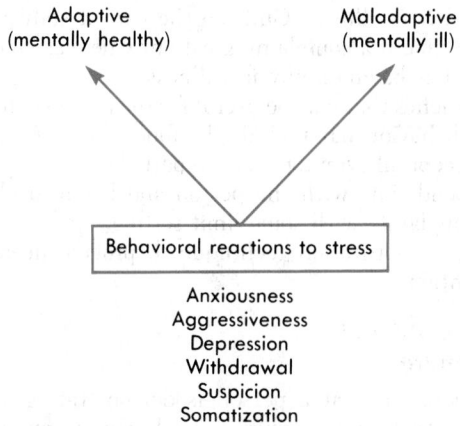

Fig. 6-5   Behavioral responses of persons experiencing anxiety from stress, such as illness, range from adaptive to maladaptive behavior.

6-5	Levels of anxiety	
	Level	**Behavior patterns**
	Mild anxiety	Increased alertness
		Quick eye movements
		Increased hearing ability
		Increased awareness
	Moderate anxiety	Decreased awareness of environmental details
		Focus on selected aspects of self (or illness)
	Severe anxiety	Disturbances in thought patterns
		Incongruency of thoughts, feelings, and actions
		Perceptual field greatly decreased
	Panic	Distorted perceptions of environment
		Inability to see or understand situation
		Unpredictable responses
		Random motor activity

Aggressive behavior

Whenever self-concept is threatened, individuals may respond by aggression, a way that makes them feel less helpless and more powerful. Aggression is one way of handling anxiety. People are often angry at the loss of health status and question what is happening to them. They become irritable and uncooperative and may project their anger on others and become demanding. Expression of anger in socially acceptable ways prevents anger from being turned inward, causing depression.

Approaches that prove to be useful when working with a person exhibiting aggressive behavior include the following:

1. Provide opportunities for the person to express feelings and the reasons for the feelings.
2. Accept expressions of hostility without retaliation or making the person feel guilty.
3. Anticipate the demands of the patient.
4. Maintain eye contact with the patient.
5. Approach patient in calm, direct manner without any signs of aggression.
6. Decrease environmental stimuli.
7. Set limits.
8. Provide outlets, if possible, for increased psychomotor activity within the confines of the hospital unit.
9. Chemical or physical restraints are used only if all other measures fail and the person becomes harmful to others or to self.

Depressed behavior

Depression is a normal response to illness, once the illness has been accepted. The person may describe feelings of sadness or unhappiness. Some common signs of depressed behavior include the following:

1. Decreased interaction with others
2. Lack of interest in activities or environment
3. Voiced concern about illness and amount of care required
4. Expressed wish for or concerns about dying

5. Dependent behavior
6. Decreased activity
7. Complaints of fatigue or inability to sleep
8. Crying spells

Any expressions about suicide should be taken seriously and the person referred for immediate counseling.

Approaches useful when working with a person exhibiting depressed behavior include the following:

1. Approach the patient in a serious mood.
2. Convey by action and communication an understanding of what the person must be feeling.
3. Help the person express feelings.
4. Convey acceptance of the right to feel sad.
5. Listen to the person so that the anger can be turned outward.

Withdrawn behavior

Withdrawal is commonly noted during illness. It permits the person to conserve mental and physical energy needed to deal with stressors and to promote repair and restoration. Withdrawn patients usually do not pose many problems and are apt to be labeled "good" patients. They demand little from others and thus may be overlooked. Withdrawn patients regress more easily to earlier levels of behavior at which they can accept the patient role. They may have feelings of low self-worth.

Approaches that may be useful when working with the withdrawn person may include the following:

1. Spend time with the person, even if you are both silent, to increase the person's self-worth.
2. Provide gentle encouragement to talk, express feelings, and relate to others.

Suspicious behavior

A sense of powerlessness or lack of control as a result of stressors and the stress response and anxiety may lead to

Table 6-3 Signs of anxiety

Type	Observations
Physiologic	
Skin	Pale or ashen, moist
Pupils	Dilated
Respirations	Deeper; may or may not be faster
Pulse	Increased rate and strength
Body temperature	Slightly increased
GI tract	Anorexia, nausea, constipation
Urinary tract	Frequency of urination with moderate stress response, oliguria with severe stress response
Motor system	Restlessness, frequent hand movements with moderate stress response; immobility with severe stress response
Behavior	Decreased attention span
	Decreased ability to follow directions
	Increased acting out
	Increased somatization
Interaction	Increased number of questions
	Constant seeking of reassurance
	Frequent shifting of topics of conversation
	Avoidance of focusing on feelings
	Focus on equipment or procedures

suspicious behavior. Suspicious patients have difficulty with trust and may have had previous experiences in which they learned to distrust others. They are often suspicious of the health care staff, the health care routines, the medicine, and the procedures. Whispered conversations by others within the person's hearing may reinforce feelings of suspiciousness that others are talking about the person.

Approaches that may be useful when working with persons exhibiting suspicious behavior may include the following:

1. Let the person talk about concerns but do not insist.
2. Keep promises made to the person to promote trust.
3. Avoid an overzealous approach, which may make the person more suspicious.
4. Provide explanations of procedures and routines so the person knows what to expect.
5. Avoid whispering or talking about the person within his or her hearing.

Somatic behavior

A familiar reaction to illness is one that can be called *flight into illness*. Patients somaticize their concerns; that is, they have learned to express anxiety through complaints about a variety of physical symptoms. They may be preoccupied with body functions and feelings of pain. Vague complaints of backache, headache, or fatigue are expressed to legitimize the *attention needed*. Staff often become angry at patients who use somatic behavior because of the frequent vague symptomatic complaints. Staff members feel "caught" if they minimize the symptoms, because there is always the possibility that the complaints are truly con-

nected with an illness. Guilt on the part of staff prevails for some time if a complaining patient who was ignored is diagnosed as having a physical illness.

Approaches that may be useful for the person exhibiting somatic behavior may include the following:

1. Accept all symptoms and report them.
2. Spend time with the person and listen to physical complaints with some limit setting.
3. Use a saturation technique to provide needed attention.

Nursing Process
Assessment

The conclusion that a person is demonstrating anxious behavior can be made when several signs of anxiety are present. With mild anxiety the signs are fewer and less prominent. Signs of anxiety are more overt in persons who are experiencing severe anxiety or panic.

Subjective data

Subjective data may include the following[12,21]:

1. States feeling apprehensive, uncertain, fearful, out of control, helpless, or anxious
2. States fears of unspecific consequences
3. States feeling overexcited, rattled, distressed, or jittery
4. States feeling tired and having difficulty sleeping

Data from the initial nursing history and the situation (such as proposed surgery, diagnostic tests) may provide clues to possible etiologies.

Objective data are listed in Table 6-3; observations are made about the person's behavior and interaction in addition to the physiologic signs. The physiologic signs result from the stimulation of the sympathetic nervous system and the adrenal medulla. Restlessness and an increased awareness of the environment are early signs of anxiety. The person focuses more on the self as anxiety increases. Physiologic signs usually begin with moderate anxiety and are more prevalent and intense during severe anxiety and panic.

Data analysis: nursing diagnoses

The nursing diagnosis of *anxiety* is best qualified whenever possible by citing the anxiety level (mild, moderate, severe, or panic, as noted in Box 6-5). Possible *etiologies* include the following[21]:

Threat to self-concept
Threat of death
Threat to or change in health status, socioeconomic status, role functioning, environment, or interaction patterns
Situational and maturational crises
Interpersonal transmission and contagion
Unmet needs

Planning: expected patient outcomes

The expected patient outcomes depend on the behaviors demonstrated by the anxious person; the outcomes indicate a decrease in the exhibited behaviors. Expected patient outcomes for the anxious person may include, but are not limited to, the following:

1. The person states feeling more relaxed and less anxious.
2. The person states sleep is improved.
3. Vital signs return to usual norms.
4. Elimination is regular.
5. Diaphoresis is decreased.
6. Muscles are relaxed and the person rests quietly.
7. The person demonstrates increased ability to follow directions.
8. The person demonstrates effective coping skills.

Implementation

Interventions for the person experiencing stressors and the stress response may include general interventions to reduce the effects of the stressor and the stress response, crises intervention for panic, specific support approaches, and additional stress management therapies.

General interventions to achieve patient outcomes

Nursing actions support the body's mechanisms for handling stressors and provide an environment that permits the person to mobilize defenses.

Supporting protective mechanisms

Rest is absolutely essential with severe stressors and the stress response to maintain energy supply for metabolic functions essential for life. The person is kept comfortably warm but never overly warm, because overheating causes vasodilation and counteracts the arteriolar constriction necessary to ensure an adequate blood supply to vital organs.

Even a minor stress response can cause annoying discomforts such as backache, generalized muscle tension, and headache. These discomforts can act as additional stressors, and comfort measures such as back rubs, position changes, and back support to relax the muscles are indicated. Pain should be alleviated as much as possible, and noise and disturbance should be kept to a minimum. During a severe stress response, oral food and fluids may need to be withheld until nausea subsides and gastrointestinal tract activity returns to normal.

Providing structure

Structure decreases anxiety and is helpful for the person experiencing mild or moderate anxiety. Explanations are one method of providing structure. Each new experience should be explained to patients and, if possible, related to familiar experiences. The higher the level of anxiety, the more simple should be the explanations.

If patients are to have treatments or tests, they need to be given some idea of what will be done, the preparation involved, and the reasons why the procedure is necessary. To remove water pitchers and inform patients that they cannot have any more water until after x-ray examinations can generate many anxious thoughts: "What x-ray examination?" "I wonder when it is?" "What will it be like?" "It must be something special if I can't have any water." Lack of knowledge as a cause of anxiety reflects the nurse's lack of consideration for patients' rights.

Explanations should be given in the patient's own terms, at appropriate times, and repeated as necessary. If the patient is very anxious, repeated explanation may be necessary, since extreme anxiety reduces intellectual function. It is useless to give explanations to patients who are severely anxious or sedated or to those who have high temperatures or severe pain. Repetition is often required for older persons and children because they may have short attention spans or poor recent memory.

Time spent in giving explanations to relatives is not wasted. Not only does it relieve their anxieties, which may be transmitted to the patient, but it also saves having to untangle misinformation. Often the family is helpful in interpreting necessary instructions to the patient in a manner that the patient understands and accepts.

Promoting exploration of feelings

In most instances a large part of the nurse's work is to encourage patients to express anxieties, to help patients see the fear in their situations, to help them seek outlets for their fears and tensions, and to allay these negative feelings whenever possible. Nurses provide opportunities for the patient to talk, but they should not probe. There is a difference between prying into a patient's thoughts and beliefs and eliciting information that aids in the understanding of behavior and in planning for care. Without seeming unduly curious, one can usually find some topic of personal interest to the patient that provides an opening. A picture on the bedside table may create such an example. Nurses who listen with sincere interest and without making judgments about the patient may begin to gain insight into the patient as a person. More important, the patient may begin to speak about personal fears.

As soon as the patient begins to talk about feelings, the nurse should proceed with conversation, taking cues from what the patient offers. The nurse who feels inadequate or anxious may cut off the conversation. For instance, if a patient says, "You know, I don't think I'll ever get to see my little boy again," a common response is, "Oh, don't say that, certainly you will; you're going to be all right," when the patient may very well not be all right. Would it not be better to respond, "What makes you feel this way?" Such a response helps the patient explore the subject and leaves opportunity for the patient to examine this concern. The nurse who is willing to listen to patients, to be guided by their reactions, and to work with them rather than to make decisions for them will give them needed emotional support. Solving patient's problems, even if it were possible, is not the aim of nursing. Indeed, it would tend to make patients less healthy psychologically.

The art of meaningful communication involves more than just listening; it includes moving the conversation so that the patient's attempts to communicate are assisted. Observing the patient for facial changes and general body movements provides opportunities for the nurse to discover from the individual the full meaning of the situation. For example, consider the patient who sucks in air while talking. The mouth becomes drier and drier as the tongue seems to stick in the mouth. These patients are not at ease and show anxiety even though their words may be quite innocuous. A simple statement such as, "Your mouth seems very dry. Would a glass of water help?" allows the nurse to clarify observations. Such an approach gives the patient a chance to tell what is being felt and to gain understanding by talking about it.

The nurse helps patients examine those problems that they are able to bring into awareness. Underlying problems should be handled by people trained in psychotherapy. A nurse needs to recognize normal anxiety reactions and to report exaggerated reactions that may indicate the need for psychiatric referral.

When any patient's anxiety increases to a high level, the nurse may need to sit with the patient. The nurse's presence is often reassuring. If possible, the patient is helped to recognize the anxiety by the nurse asking, "Are you uncomfortable?" or "What are you feeling?" In severe anxiety and panic, being there is most important, and touch may be used as a means of reassurance. Some severely anxious persons, however, view touching as an intrusion of their personal boundary, and the nurse needs to keep this in mind. When the patient is able to talk, the nurse helps the patient to describe what is happening, what has happened, and what is expected to happen.

Supporting coping mechanisms

There is no one specific or best way to cope with any given situation. What is useful to one individual may be inappropriate for another. The nature of the stressor, the developmental level of the individual, the social and cultural environment, and the physical and interpersonal resources available all influence the style and effectiveness of coping strategies.

It is most useful to help a person to cope in ways that are congruent with previously established styles. Data must therefore be collected to identify the person's usual coping strategies. One method is by asking the question, "What do you usually do when things get tough?" Weisman suggests seven simple questions that may obtain a great deal of information about coping strategies[70]:

1. What problems, if any, do you see this illness creating?
2. How do you plan to deal with them?
3. When faced with a problem you must do something about, what do you do?
4. How does it usually work out?
5. To whom do you turn when you need help?
6. What has happened in the past when you have asked for help?
7. What kinds of problems usually tend to upset you or get you down?

These questions establish perception of the current problems, present and usual ways of dealing with problems, sources and responses to help, and recurrent problems that affect coping.

Stress management includes reinforcing appropriate coping mechanisms and helping the person explore alternative strategies if existing coping mechanisms are inappropriate.

Facilitating problem solving

Some persons solve problems in a haphazard manner while others are very structured in their approach to problem solving. Problem solving can be a means for coping

Nursing Research 6-6

Monro BH, et al: Effect of relaxation therapy on post-myocardial infarction patient's rehabilitation, *Nurs Res* 37:231-235, 1988.

This experimental study involved 57 subjects (27 experimental, 30 control) who were participants in a cardiac rehabilitation program. The study was designed to measure whether practicing Benson's relaxation techniques resulted in improvement in psychosocial functioning as measured by Sickness Impact Profile, aerobic conditioning level (MET Level), systolic and diastolic blood pressure, or heart rate. The study also explored the influence of behavioral style on the outcome measures.

The major finding was that diastolic blood pressure was reduced and maintained over a 3-month period. Systolic blood pressure was also reduced, but the reduction was not statistically significant. Subjects in this study showed improvement in psychosocial functioning, aerobic conditioning, and heart rates, but the practice of the relaxation techniques did not enhance these improvements. Behavioral style was not related to outcome measures.

The lack of significant findings for some of the outcome measures may have been related to the nonspecificity of the measures. For example, the measure of behavior style did not contain many items regarding hostility and anger, which may be the most important factors of personality type related to coronary risk. The measure used to evaluate psychosocial functioning focused on illness rather than overall psychosocial functioning.

with stressors and the stress response and is more effective if the problem-solving steps are consciously followed. The steps include the following:

1. Gathering data
2. Identifying the problem (or effect of stressor)
3. Identifying factors affecting the problem or stressor
4. Determining goals
5. Exploring alternative ways and consequences to achieve the goals
6. Implementing actions
7. Evaluating effectiveness of actions

If the stressor has been identified, the nurse first assists the patient in exploring feelings and reactions associated with the stressor. Often persons are not consciously aware of what they are feeling and therefore may select inappropriate actions. Persons vary in their ability to identify problems and in their desire to discuss personal feelings, although it is widely accepted that talking does help. If the patient is urged indiscriminately to talk about problems, the relationship becomes superficial and mechanical. The identification of the consequences of actions is often omitted but is an important component if problem solving is to be effective.

Problem solving reduces ambiguity and feelings of loss of control. Persons who do not generally employ conscious problem solving as a means of coping with stressors may benefit from learning about problem solving as a strategy for coping with stress.

6-7

Progressive relaxation

1. Assume a comfortable position in a quiet room
2. Begin by focusing on easy breathing
3. Tense specific muscle groups (see step 5) for 5 to 7 seconds, then relax quickly
4. Concentrate for 10 seconds on the sensations of the relaxed muscles
5. Follow a sequence, repeating each muscle group, tensing two or three times:
   a. Hand and arm: clench fist, pull elbow tightly, wrinkle nose, purse lips, smile with teeth tightly clenched
   b. Face: wrinkle forehead, close eyes tightly, wrinkle nose, purse lips, smile with teeth tightly clenched
   c. Neck; pull chin to chest
   d. Trunk: pull shoulder blades together, tighten stomach and buttocks
   e. Leg and foot: push down with leg, point toes upward (dorsiflexion) dominant leg first
6. Repeat process in any areas in which increased tension has been identified

---

Teaching relaxation techniques

Relaxation exercises are developed from the concept that the stress response with anxiety does not and cannot exist when the muscles of the body are relaxed. Relaxation exercises do not "cure" the stressors or the stress response but do help to minimize effects of the stress response and give the person a sense of control. A daily program of relaxation exercises has an effect on physiologic responses to stressors (for example, lowering of elevated blood pressure or elevated blood sugars) and in psychologic responses to stressors (for example, decreased level of anxiety) (See Research Box 6-6). They are also helpful on a short-term basis when anxiety is present.

There are four basic components of relaxation techniques:

1. *Quiet environment:* deleting all possible noise and distractions
2. *Comfortable position:* sitting with no undue muscle tension
3. *Passive attitude:* emptying all thoughts from the conscious mind
4. *Mental device:* focusing on a sound, word, phrase, mental image, object, or breathing pattern to shift the mind from logical, externally oriented thoughts

The important factor is that the person empties the mind of all thoughts and concentrates on the mental device. It is natural for the mind to wander. When this occurs, the person simply redirects the mind back to the mental device. Each relaxation session should take approximately 20 minutes.

There are several approaches to performing relaxation exercises. Two approaches that can be carried out by nursing instructions to patients, without use of special equipment and without physician's orders, are *progressive relaxation* and *Benson's relaxation response.*

Progressive relaxation consists of tensing and relaxing muscle groups and focusing on the feelings of relaxation (Box 6-7). The systematic application of progressive relaxation has three major effects, which are as follows[45]:

Progressive relaxation

1. Muscle groups are relaxed more and more with each practice.
2. Each of the major muscle groups is relaxed one after the other. As a new muscle group is added, the previously relaxed portions also relax.

3. More total body relaxation is experienced as the person moves into the relaxation phase. The relaxed state is maintained beyond the relaxation period.

Benson's relaxation response omits the muscle tensing. It is particularly helpful for muscle relaxation in patients who are experiencing pain or discomfort. It is important to remain with the patient to coach and encourage the relaxation.[41]

Benson's relaxation response

1. Assume a comfortable sitting position in a quiet room.
2. Close eyes.
3. Relax body muscles (that is, "let go").
4. Concentrate on breathing. Repeat a word or sound such as "one" or "um-m" after each exhalation.
5. Continue for about 20 minutes.
6. Open eyes.
7. Take time to adjust to surroundings before moving.

For some acute stressors, such as those experienced by hospitalized adults, the nurse may use abridged forms of relaxation techniques that can be implemented more rapidly. Effective abridged relaxation techniques include deep breathing or squeezing and relaxing the hands.

Implementing music therapy

Music therapy is an intervention available for patients to help achieve relaxation and to promote coping with stressors and the stress response. Music therapy has been used successfully in various environments including intensive care units, dentists offices, and surgery units.[15,37] Music therapy has been used with patients who have acute and chronic health problems.

When using music therapy, the patient's preference must be considered, because the type of music that is relaxing and pleasant for one person may be irritating and unpleasant for another. Instrumental music is better than vocal music because words often evoke various emotional responses. Additionally, music is best listened to using headphones, which helps to decrease other stimuli. The patient should be able to control the volume.

Music therapy is easily applied. All that is required are a source of music (tapes, CDs) and a machine. Cassette tapes and players are most frequently used because the tapes can be individualized, these materials are least expensive, and the most portable. Last, this equipment could

Table 6-4   Antianxiety agents

Generic name	Trade name	Usual adult dosage	Elderly dosage
Benzodiazepines			
Alprazolam	Xanax	0.25-0.5 mg tid	0.25 mg bid/tid
Chlordiazepoxide	Librium	5-25 mg qid	5 mg bid/qid
	Libritabs		
Clorazepate	Tranxene	7.5-15 mg bid/qid	7.5-15 mg qd
Diazepam	Valium	2-10 mg bid/qid	2-2.5 mg qd or bid
Halazepam	Paxipam	20-40 mg tid/qid	20 mg qd or bid
Lorazepam	Ativan	1-3 mg bid/tid	0.5-1 mg bid
Oxazepam	Serax	10-30 mg tid/qid	10-15 mg tid
Prazepam	Centrax	10 mg tid or 20-40 mg at bedtime	5 mg bid/tid or 15 mg at bedtime
Nonbenzodiazepines			
Hydroxyzine HCl	Atarax	25-100 mg tid/qid	Same as adult dosage
Meprobamate	Equanil	400 mg bid/tid or 600 mg bid	Same as adult dosage
	Meprospan		
	Miltown		

be available in a variety of clinical settings. Nurses need no special skills to apply this intervention, and patients can use it without any need to practice this intervention, as is true for many other relaxation interventions. All that is needed from the patient's perspective is an enjoyment of music.

Providing antianxiety medications

In some instances, the patient may be prescribed an antianxiety medication to reduce the anxiety symptoms. The antianxiety agents may be divided into two groups, the benzodiazepines and the nonbenzodiazepines (Table 6-4). Note that the dosage of benzodiazepines is less for elderly persons who metabolize the drugs slowly, resulting in a prolonged depressant effect. Dosage should also be reduced for persons with impaired liver or kidney function.

The benozodiazepines are the most frequently prescribed antianxiety agents. These drugs act by inhibiting transmission of stimuli from the limbic system of the brain (septum, amygdala, and hippocampus). Side effects include drowsiness, dizziness, and weakness.

Antianxiety agents produce muscle relaxation and a sense of well-being. The drugs are prescribed for short-term relief of anxiety but not for anxiety from daily stressors. Long-term therapy leads to increased tolerance and dependence; larger doses are then needed to produce the desired effects and drug abuse may ensue.

Persons taking antianxiety agents are cautioned not to drink alcohol or take other CNS depressants during therapy because of serious complications, even death, as a result of synergistic effects. People also need to be cautious when driving or working around heavy machinery because of possible dizziness.

Crisis intervention

Awareness of what occurs during a crisis helps the nurse understand the accompanying behavior. When the ego is met with overwhelming anxiety created by biologic, physiologic, or social threats to the self, a crisis ensues. The ego is not able to cope successfully with the sudden disequilibrium, and the person needs assistance to use the situation as a growth experience.

A crisis occurs when a person is unable to use customary methods of coping when faced for a time with what seems to be an unsurmountable obstacle to an important life goal. A period of disorganization ensues, a period of upset during which many abortive attempts at solutions are made.

Phases of crisis

Shontz describes several phases or stages that occur during crisis.[68] These stages are similar to the stages of death and dying as described by Kübler-Ross.

1. *Initial impact.* During this phase the person experiences shock and depersonalization as reality is clearly perceived. Functioning is organized and automatic with individual centering and docility.

2. *Realization.* In the second phase the existing self-structure collapses. Reality seems overwhelming, and the person experiences high anxiety, panic, and helplessness. There is inability to plan, reason, or understand the situation.

3. *Defensive retreat.* The third phase is one of regression in which an attempt is made to establish previous identity, to return to better times. Reality is avoided, and denial and wishful thinking may help to relieve the anxiety. When challenged, the ego reacts with anger and the person may experience rage and disorientation. Thinking is situation-bound, and change is resisted.

4. *Acknowledgement.* This is the "yes" stage, "It has happened to me." The individual experiences depression and self-depreciation. Reality imposes itself again and looms large in relating the event to one's life. Without intervention the person may become more disorganized, depressed, and suicidal.

5. *Adaptation.* This is the stage when change occurs if help is adequate. New identity appears along with hope and renewed sense of personal worth. Anxiety is subse-

quently decreased and satisfaction is increased as a result of the stabilization and reorganization. Functional improvement is noted without actual change in disability status.

The model just offered is a useful approach for explaining what a person experiences during an illness crisis, even though reactions to crisis are individual. People are not equally vulnerable to all categories of stressors, but there is thought to be some commonality in the reactions. Knowledge about the commonalities can facilitate plans for nursing intervention.

Intervention

The essential element of crisis intervention is the intensive nature of support required to help the ego maintain its integrity and its ability to use coping mechanisms. Crisis, according to Caplan,[44] is self-limiting. Early intervention can prevent maladaptive behavior, and the individual can emerge a stronger person. Acute illness or catastrophic illness often precipitates a crisis reaction. The outcome of a crisis is governed by the kind of interaction that takes place between the individual and key figures in the environment during the time of crisis.

Often because of changes in society, previous guidelines for behavior in stressful situations render the individual helpless. In crisis the individual is helped to find ways to facilitate efforts to enlarge on the experience. A state of disequilibrium produces a felt need to reduce anxiety. The following balancing factors have been identified as being necessary to resolve the problem and to avert crisis:

1. A realistic perception of the event
2. Adequate situational support (staff and family)
3. Adequate coping mechanisms[2]

When one or more of these balancing factors are absent, the result is an increase in axiety, with immobilization and an inability to avert the crisis (Fig. 6-6).

In crisis, help should be immediate. Staying with the person, talking through the situation, and encouraging catharsis facilitate recognition and expression of feelings and subsequent relief of guilt. Strengthening coping mechanisms is crucial in preventing the formation of symptoms. Personal growth is facilitated by using problem-solving skills and a hierarchy of needs framework to help the person set priorities.

Specific support approaches

Persons who are having difficulty coping because of severe or multiple stressors may be referred for individual or group counseling. A person may need assistance and support from the nurse in seeking out and initiating counseling.

Therapeutic groups consist of persons who are experiencing common stressors. Peer support is given because the participants share the common experience. Persons often are able to express their feelings more easily when they know that the group members understand what they are experiencing. Approaches found helpful in solving the common problems are also shared. Therapeutic groups may be self-help groups or be directed by health professionals. Examples of therapeutic groups are Al-Anon (for family member of alcoholics), Parents Without Partners, Reach

to Recovery (postmastectomy), "ostomy" groups, bereavement groups, and the American Cancer Society's "I Can Cope" program.

Additional stress management therapies

In dealing with some stressors, particularly chronic stressors or diseases associated with stressors and the stress response, the nurse may use some stress management therapies requiring special training or equipment. These are implemented over a long-term basis and usually in outpatient settings. Stress management therapists help people design and implement a structured program of change to enable the individual to control and deal more effectively with stressors and the stress response. Some of the therapies include biofeedback, autogenic training, behavioral change programs, and systematic desensitization.

Biofeedback

Biofeedback is a system of learning voluntary control over autonomically regulated body functions so that an individual is able to monitor the physiologic stress response and to replace it with a nonstressful response. For example, if after a stressful day you notice soreness and muscle tension in your shoulders, you can sit quietly and concentrate on relaxing the shoulder muscles to feel the tension slip away.

With biofeedback, machinery is used to "train" the person to monitor certain parameters. For example, muscle activity can be monitored with an electromyograph (EMG) and the stimuli converted into a visual or auditory signal. Using this biofeedback, the person can learn how to replace muscle tension with muscle relaxation. Machines can also be used to measure skin temperature or sweat activity, and a similar feedback approach is used. The person is then weaned from the machine to produce the desired effects without machinery. A comprehensive biofeedback program includes feedback from multiple systems and sites.

Autogenic training

Autogenic training teaches cognitive behavioral change together with physiologic behavioral change through passive concentration to decrease sympathetic nervous system activity. The person repeats a statement verbally with the physiologic state that is being practiced. The physiologic states are heaviness and warmth of extremities, calm and regular heartbeat and breathing, abdominal warmth, and cooling of forehead.[49] The methods are similar to that of transcendental meditation.

Behavioral change programs

Some specific stress-related behaviors, such as smoking or overeating, may be eliminated by behavioral conditioning. The programs consist of the following:

1. Self-monitoring to identify characteristics and situations associated with the behaviors
2. Identifying outcome criteria in precise behavioral terms
3. Developing a formal contract with the therapist stating short-term goals with rewards and frequency of evaluation

The overall goal is a change in the person's behavior. Be-

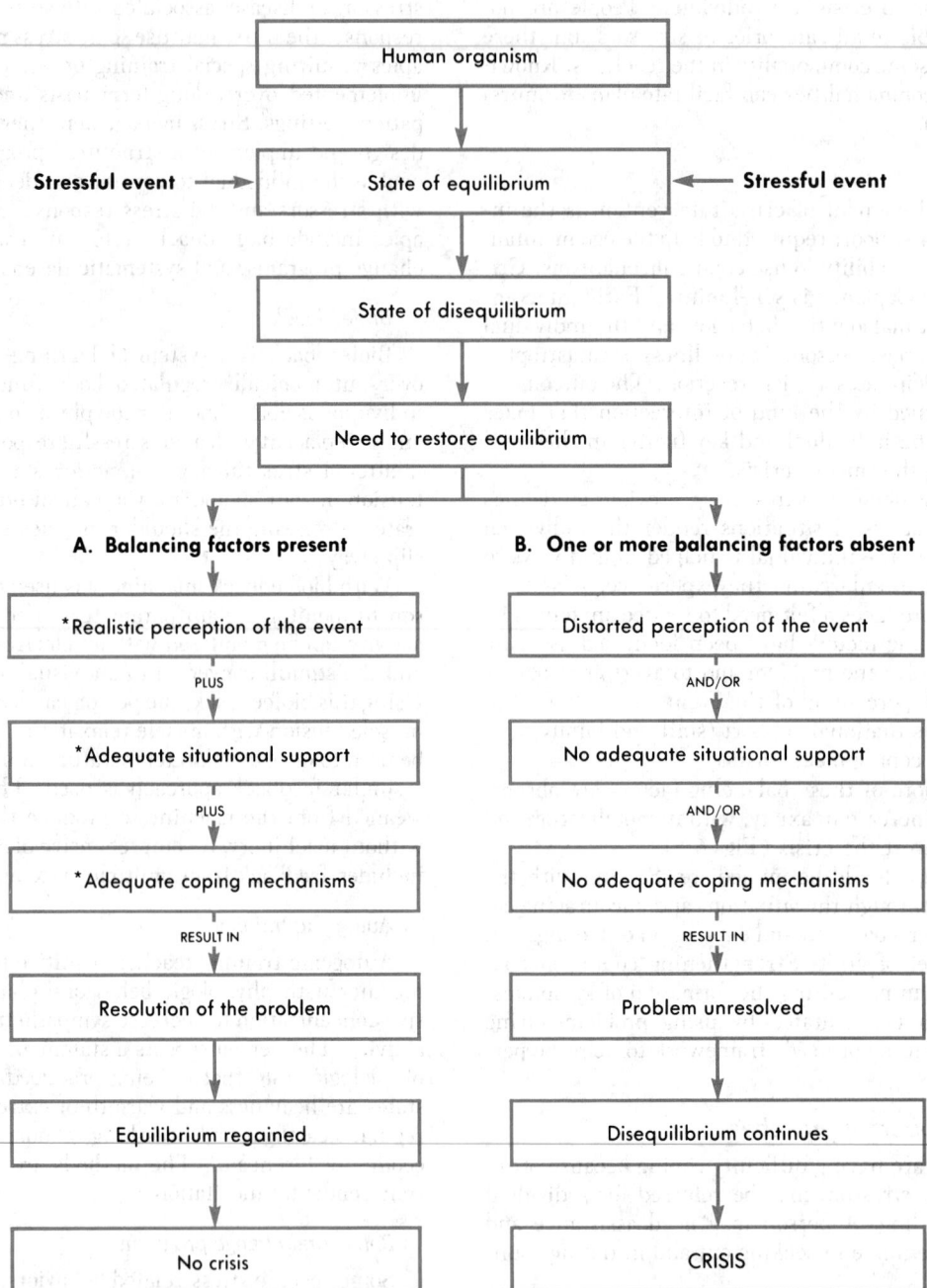

Fig. 6-6   Paradigm: effect of balancing factors in stressful event. (From Aguilera DC: *Crisis intervention: theory and methodology,* ed 6, St Louis, 1989, Mosby–Year Book.)

havioral change programs are most effective with highly motivated persons; they must sincerely *want* to change the behavior.

Systematic desensitization

Systematic desensitization provides specific stressors (such as those related to phobias) in increasing doses while the individual practices relaxation skills. The person is first taught effective relaxation skills. Stimuli eliciting the anxiety are then presented in increasing intensity, starting at a minimal level while the person uses the relaxation techniques. Then the person is instructed to relax while imagining the situation in more threatening circumstances. The principle of systematic desensitization is to train the person to behave (relax) in a manner opposite to anxiety behavior (tension). A low initial stimulus that increases in intensity gives the person a sense of control over and of coping with the undesirable stimulus, thus decreasing the anxiety.

Evaluation

The evaluation depends on the exact patient outcomes. Questions to consider include the following:
1. Does the person appear more relaxed?
2. Is the person sleeping for 6 to 8 hours at night?
3. Are the patient's vital signs back to baseline?
4. Does the patient appear able to follow directions well?

SUMMARY

1. Adaptation is a process of interaction with the environment that promotes homeostasis and growth. Maladaptation leads to inadequate functioning.
2. Responses to stressors include neuroendocrine response, coping behaviors, defense mechanisms, and specific behavioral responses.
3. Response to stressors is influenced by the type of stimuli, the meaning of the stressor, perception of stressor, sense of control, coping resources, and health status.
4. The general adaptation syndrome consists of three stages: alarm reaction, resistance, and exhaustion. The first two stages occur frequently throughout life; death may ensue from exhaustion.
5. The physiologic stress response consists of stimulation of the sympathetic nervous system, adrenal medulla, anterior and posterior pituitary glands, and the adrenal cortex.
6. The neuroendocrine response to stress is integrated by the hypothalamus.
7. Norepinephrine released by the sympathetic nervous system and the adrenal medulla primarily causes vasoconstriction of blood vessels of the skin; mucous membrane, and abdominal and pelvic organs shifting blood to blood vessels of the heart, lung, and brain, which were dilated by the action of epinephrine.
8. In addition to dilating selected blood vessels, epinephrine increases cardiac function, dilates bronchial smooth muscles, and alters metabolism to provide substrates for energy needs.

9. Cortisol, acting in concert with catecholamines, growth hormone, and glucagon, helps to mobilize substrates for energy.
10. Cortisol may also serve a major function by its antiinflammatory and immunosuppressive actions by dampening the stress response to prevent overactivity.
11. Water and sodium balance, osmolality, and blood volume are protected by the action of aldosterone and ADH, which are released during the neuroendocrine response to stressors.
12. Types of coping strategies include action, cognitive, intrapsychic, interpersonal, or emotional strategies.
13. Defense mechanisms are unconscious mechanisms used by individuals in adjustment to life stressors. Mentally healthy persons use defense mechanisms occasionally, avoiding more primitive mechanisms.
14. Some specific behavioral responses to stressors include anxiety, aggressive behavior, depressed behavior, withdrawn behavior, suspicious behavior, and somatic behavior.
15. Anxiety results when a person perceives a threat to the self, either physically or psychologically.
16. Anxiety may be mild, moderate, severe, or a state of panic. When anxiety increases, awareness of the environment decreases and physiologic signs increase.
17. Rest and relief of discomfort conserve energy for coping with stressors and the stress response; providing explanations provides structure, which helps to decrease anxiety. Exploration of feelings helps to relieve tension associated with the stress response, and problem solving reduces feelings of loss of control associated with the stress response.
18. Relaxation is the opposite of the tension associated with the stress response; it also gives the person a sense of control. Basic components of relaxation techniques are quiet environment, comfortable position, passive attitude, and a mental device to remove externally oriented thoughts.
19. The most frequently prescribed antianxiety agents are the benzodiazepines. Alcohol or other CNS depressants should be avoided when taking antianxiety agents.
20. Crisis occurs when anxiety overwhelms the self and the person is unable to use coping mechanisms. Crisis is self-limiting. Balancing factors necessary to resolve crises include a realistic perception of the event, adequate situational support, and adequate coping mechanisms.
21. Stress management therapies include biofeedback, autogenic training, behavioral change programs, and systematic desensitization.

STUDY QUESTIONS

- Should you try to lead a life that is free from stressors? Explain.
- Think back over several situations when you were experiencing the stress response. What type of physical symptoms did you experience? What is the physiologic reason for each symptom that you experienced? Where the symptoms always the same? If not, state why.

- In what way(s) do you cope with stressors? What other coping strategies might be useful for you?
- Try one or both of the relaxation techniques described in this chapter. Describe the sensations experienced during relaxation. How did you feel after completing the exercise? What types of difficulties did you have in carrying out the relaxation exercises? Identify a patient situation from your experience where you think relaxation exercises might have been a useful nursing intervention.

REFERENCES AND SELECTED READINGS

1. * Agras S: *Panic: facing fears, phobias, and anxiety,* New York, 1985, WH Freeman.
2. * Aguilera DC: *Crisis intervention: theory and methodology,* ed 6, St Louis 1989, Mosby–Year Book.
3. Beck C, Rawlins R, Williams S: *Mental health—psychiatric nursing: a holistic life-cycle,* ed 2, St Louis, 1987, Mosby–Year Book.
4. * Benner P, Wrubel J: *The primacy of caring: stress and coping in health and illness,* Menlo Park, Calif, 1989, Addison Wesley.
5. Berne RM, Levy MN: *Physiology,* ed 2, St Louis, 1988, Mosby–Year Book.
6. * Billings CV: Come here, nurse! *Am J Nurs* 86:915-916, 1986.
7. * Crockett MS: How a disabled, depressed patient learned to break an unhappy cycle, *Am J Nurs* 86:294-297, 1986.
8. * Dossey B: Awakening the inner healer, *Am J Nurs* 91:30-34, 1991.
9. Ebersole R, Hess R: *Toward healthy aging: human needs and nursing response,* ed 3, St Louis, 1990, Mosby–Year Book.
10. Gaillard RC, Al-DamLeiji S: Stress and the pituitary adrenal axis, *Baillieres Clin Endocrinol Metab* 1:319-354, 1987.
11. * Glod C: Psychopharmacology and clinical practice, *Nurs Clin North Am* 26:375-399, 1991.
12. Gordon M: *Manual of nursing diagnosis 1991-1992,* St Louis, 1991, Mosby–Year Book.
13. Granner D: Hormones of the adrenal medulla. In Murray RK, et al, editors: *Harper's biochemistry,* 21, New York, 1988, Lange Medical Books.
14. Groeï MW, Shekleton ME: *Basic pathophysiology: a holistic approach,* ed 3, St Louis, 1989, Mosby–Year Book.
15. Guzzetta C: Effect of relaxation and music therapy on patients in a coronary care unit with presumptive acute myocardial infarction, *Heart Lung* 18:609-616, 1989.
16. * Harris B: Drugs and depression, *Am J Nurs* 86:292-293, 1986.
17. * Hillhouse J, Adler C: Stress, health, and immunity: a review of the literature and implications for the nursing profession, *Holistic Nursing Practice* 1991:5(4):22-31.
18. * Hornberger CA: *Perceived stressors, perceived stress response, and level of cardiac reactivity in wellness sample,* University of Kansas School of Nursing, Kansas City, 1989 (unpublished master's thesis).
19. Johnson D: Metabolic and endocrine alterations in the multiple injured patient, *Crit Care Nurs Q* 11(2):35-41, 1988.
20. Karb V, Queener SF, Freeman JB: *Handbook of drugs for nursing practice,* St Louis, 1989, Mosby–Year Book.
21. Kim MJ, McFarland GK, McLane AM: *Pocket guide to nursing diagnosis,* ed 3, St Louis, 1989, Mosby–Year Book.
22. Kuhn MM: *Pharmacotherapeutics: a nursing process approach,* ed 2, Philadelphia, 1991, FA Davis.

23. * Lindsay AM, Carrieri VK: Stress response, In Linday AM, Carrieri VK, West CM, editors: *Pathophysiological phenomenon in nursing: human responses to illness,* Philadelphia, 1986, WB Saunders.
24. McCance K, Huether SE: *Pathophysiology: the biologic base for disease in adults and children,* St Louis, 1990, Mosby–Year Book.
25. McEwen B, Brinton RE: Neuroendocrine aspects of adaptation, *Prog Brain Res* 72:11-26, 1987.
26. McKenry LM, Salerno E: *Mosby's pharmacology in nursing,* ed 17, St Louis, 1989, Mosby–Year Book.
27. Mellion MB: Exercise therapy for anxiety and depression: what are the specific considerations for clinical application? *Postgrad Med* 77(3):91-95, 1985.
28. Meyer D: *Development of an instrument to measure perceived environmental stressors of surgical intensive care patients,* University of Kansas, Kansas City, 1985 (unpublished master's thesis).
29. * Minot SR: Depression: what does it mean? *Am J Nurs* 86:283-287, 1986.
30. Moos R: *Coping with physical illness,* ed 2, New York, 1985, Plenum Publishing.
31. Munro BH, et al: Effect of relaxation therapy on post-myocardial infarction patient's rehabilitation, *Nurs Res* 37, 231-235, 1988.
32. * Owen PL: A dozen tasks vie for your attention at the same time, with no respite in sight—what can you do to keep stress at bay? *Am J Nurs* 86:52-53, 1986.
33. Pender NJ: Effects of progressive muscle relaxation training on anxiety and health locus of control among hypertensive adults, *Res Nurs Health* 8(1):67-72, 1985.
34. * Roberts J, et al: Coping revisited: the relation between appraised seriousness of an event, coping responses and adjustment to illness, *Nurs Pap* 19:45-54, 1987.
35. Robinson L: Stress and anxiety, *Nurs Clin North Am* 25:935-943, 1990.
36. Shoemaker W, et al, editors: *Textbook of critical care,* ed 2, Philadelphia, 1989, WB Saunders.
37. Stevens K: Patients' perception of music during surgery, *J Adv Nurs* 15:1045-1051, 1990.
38. Symposium on anxiety disorders, *Psychiatr Clin North Am* 8(1):1-179, 1985.

Classics

39. Axelrod J, Reisine T: Stress hormones: their interaction and regulation, *Science* 224:452-453, 1984.
40. Ballard KS: *Identification of environmental stress for patients in the surgical intensive care unit,* University of Kansas, Kansas City, 1979 (unpublished master's thesis).
41. Benson H: *The relaxation response,* New York, 1975, William Morrow.
42. Cannon WD: Stresses and strains of homeostasis, *Am J Med Sci* 189:1-14, 1935.
43. Cannon WB: *The wisdom of the body,* New York, 1963, WW Norton.
44. Caplan G: *Principles of preventative psychiatry,* New York, 1964, Basic Books.
45. Carlson CE, editor: *Behavioral concepts and nursing interventions,* ed 2, Philadelphia, 1978, WB Saunders.
46. * Clarke M: Stress and coping: constructs for nursing, *J Adv Nurs,* 9:3-13, 1984.
47. Cox T: *Stress,* New York, 1978, Macmillan Press.
48. Curtis J, Detert R: *How to relax,* Palo Alto, Calif, 1981, Mayfield Publishing.
49. Danskin D, Crow M: *Biofeedback: an introduction and guide,* Palo Alto, Calif, 1981, Mayfield Publishing.
50. Hetzel BS, et al: Changes in urinary 17-hydroxy-corticoste-

*Recommended for student reading.

roid excretion during stressful life situations in man, *J Clin Endocrinol* 15:1057-1068, 1955.

51. Hoff LA: *People in crisis: understanding and helping,* Menlo Park, Calif, 1984, Addison-Wesley.

52. Hyman RB, Woog P: Stressful life events and illness onset: a review of crucial variables, *Res Nurs Health* 5:155-163, 1982.

53.* Jasmin SA, Hill L, Smith N: Keeping your delicate balance: the art of managing stress, *Nurs 81* 11(6)52-57, 1981.

54.* Jupp H, et al: Group cognitive/anxiety management, *J Adv Nurs* 9:573-580, 1984.

55. Kogan HN, Betrus P: Self-management: a nursing mode of therapeutic influence, *Adv Nurs Sci* 6:55-73, 1984.

56. Lazarus R: *Patterns of adjustment,* New York, 1976, McGraw Hill.

57. Lazarus R: *Psychological stress and the coping process,* New York, 1966, McGraw Hill.

58. Lazarus RS, Folkman S: *Stress, appraisal and coping,* New York, 1984, Springer Publishing.

59. Lenox RH, et al: Specific hormonal and neurochemical responses to different stressors, *Neuroendocrinology* 30:300-308, 1980.

60. Mason JW: A re-evaluation of the concept of nonspecificity in stress theory, *J Psychiatric Res* 8:323-333, 1971.

61. Mason J: *Specificity in the organization of neuroendocrine response profiles.* In Seeman P, Brown GM, editors: *Frontiers in neurology and neuroscience research,* First International Symposium of the Neuroscience Institute, University of Toronto, 1974.

62. Peplau H: *A working definition of anxiety.* In Burd S, Marshall M, editors: *Some clinical approaches to psychiatric nursing,* New York, 1963, Macmillan Publishing.

63.* Selye H: *Stress in health and disease,* Sevenoaks, 1976, Butterworth.

64.* Selye H: *Stress without distress,* New York, 1975, New American Library.

65. Selye H: The general adaptation syndrome and the diseases of adaptation. *J Clin Endocrinol* 6:117-230, 1946.

66. Selye H: *The stress of life,* rev ed, New York, 1976, McGraw-Hill.

67. Selye H: The stress syndrome, *Am J Nurs* 65:97-99, 1965.

68. Shontz F: *The psychological aspects of physical illness and disability,* New York, 1975, Macmillan Publishing.

69.* Sutterley DC: Stress and health: a survey of self-regulation modalities, *Top Clini Nurs* 1(1): 1-29, 1979.

70.* Weisman A: *Coping with cancer,* New York, 1979, McGraw-Hill.

Common Problems Encountered in Medical-Surgical Nursing

Unit Three

7

Fluid and Electrolyte Imbalances

Mary Kay Lehman
Barbara Soltis

After studying this chapter, the learner should be able to:

- Describe the mechanisms for maintaining fluid and electrolyte balance.
- Describe the mechanisms and effects of fluid deficit and excess.
- Describe the mechanisms and effects of deficits and excesses of sodium, potassium, calcium, and magnesium.
- Identify data indicating fluid or electrolyte imbalances.
- Develop a nursing care plan for a patient with a fluid and electrolyte imbalance.

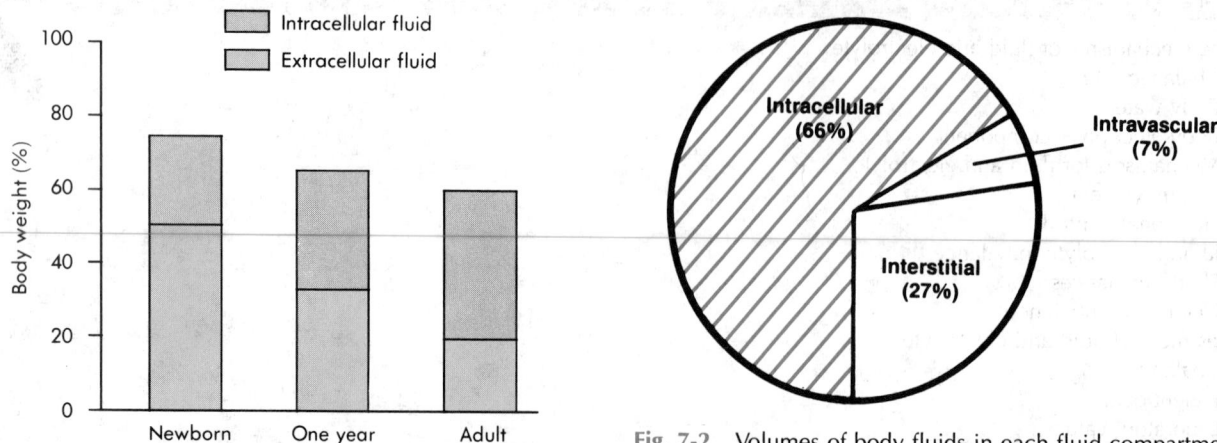

Fig. 7-1 In the newborn more than half of total body fluid is extracellular. As the child grows, proportions gradually approximate adult levels.

Fig. 7-2 Volumes of body fluids in each fluid compartment.

The *internal environment* is a term used to describe body water and the constituent electrolytes and other dissolved substances that sustain all the physiologic processes that maintain life. The amount and distribution of water in the various body compartments, as well as the type and amount of electrolytes and nonelectrolytes dissolved in the water, are kept in an extremely delicate balance by a number of control mechanisms. These mechanisms are so effective that normal values have been established for all constituents of the internal environment in healthy individuals. Knowledge of these normal values is used for detection and correction of imbalances that occur during illness.

The assessment and maintenance of a patient's fluid and electrolyte balance is a major nursing responsibility. This chapter describes some basic information about water and electrolytes in the body and the causes and effects of common fluid and electrolyte imbalances. The last part of the chapter discusses nursing measures employed to prevent, identify, and alleviate these imbalances and to relieve discomfort.

BASIC MECHANISMS OF FLUID AND ELECTROLYTE BALANCE

Body Water

A large percentage of body weight is composed of water containing dissolved particles of organic and inorganic substances vital to life. A newborn infant's weight is approximately 75% water, whereas a young adult male's is about 60% and a female's 50% (Fig. 7-1). The percentage of body weight that is water gradually declines with age. Because fat contains little water, the more obese an individual is, the smaller the percentage of weight that is water. Both obese and aged persons have increased risk of morbidity and mortality in situations involving fluid loss because they have less fluid reserve on which to draw.

Fluid distribution

Fluid and electrolytes are found in the body either within the cell (*intracellular*) or outside the cell (*extracellular*)

(Table 7-1). The extracellular fluid (ECF) is contained in two compartments: the *interstitial* fluid (fluid between the cells) and *intravascular* fluid (fluid in the blood vessels). The largest percentage of body water is located in the billions of individual body cells (Fig. 7-2).

Fluid balance

Body fluid is constantly being lost and must be replaced for normal processes to continue. With an average daily intake of food and liquids, the healthy body easily maintains compartmental balance. The body receives water from ingested food and fluids and through metabolism of both foodstuffs and body tissues. Solid foods, such as meat and vegetables, contain 60% to 90% water. Table 7-2 shows the approximate daily intake for an average adult. Note that the normal daily replacement of water equals the normal daily loss. Easily measurable intake (liquid) and easily measurable output (urine) are also approximately equal. These figures therefore serve as guides for determining normal fluid balance and emphasize the great need for recording patient fluid intake and output accurately.

Two vital processes demand continual expenditure of water: the removal of body heat by vaporization of water through the skin and lungs, and the excretion of urea and other metabolic wastes by the kidneys. The volume of water used in these processes varies greatly with external influences such as temperature and humidity.

Body Electrolyte Component
Types of body electrolytes

All body fluids contain chemical compounds. Chemical compounds in solution may be classified as electrolytes or nonelectrolytes on the basis of their ability to conduct an electric current in solution. *Electrolytes in solution break up into charged particles called ions.* Sodium chloride in solution exists as positively charged sodium ions, Na^+, and negatively charged chloride ions, Cl^-. *Positively charged ions are called cations. Negatively charged ions are called anions.* Proteins are special types of charged molecules. They have a charge that depends on the pH of the body fluids. At normal

Table 7-1   Body fluid distribution

Compartment	Description	Fluid
Intracellular	Fluid within cells	Intracellular fluid (ICF)
Extracellular	Fluid outside cells	Extracellular fluid (ECF)
Intravascular	Fluid within blood vessels	Plasma
Interstitial	Fluid in tissues (between cells or in body spaces)	Examples: interstitial fluid, lymph, cerebrospinal fluid, intraocular fluid, GI secretions, urine, sweat, exudates

Table 7-2   Normal fluid intake and loss in an adult eating 2500 calories per day (approximate figures)

Intake		Output	
Route	**Amount of gain (ml)**	**Route**	**Amount of loss (ml)**
Water in food	1000	Skin	500
Water from oxidation	300	Lungs	350
Water as liquid by mouth	1200	Feces	150
		Kidney	1500
TOTAL	2500	TOTAL	2500

Table 7-3   Normal electrolyte content of body fluids*

	Extracellular		
Electrolytes (anions and cations)	**Intravascular (mEq/L)**	**Interstitial (mEq/L)**	**Intracellular (mEq/L)**
Sodium (Na^+)	142	146	15
Potassium (K^+)	5	5	150
Calcium (Ca^{++})	5	3	2
Magnesium (Mg^{++})	2	1	27
Chloride (Cl^-)	102	114	1
Bicarbonate (HCO_3^-)	27	30	10
Protein ($Prot^-$)	16	1	63
Phosphate ($HPO_4^=$)	2	2	100
Sulfate ($SO_4^=$)	1	1	20
Organic acids	5	8	0

*Note that the electrolyte level of the intravascular and interstitial fluids (extracellular) is approximately the same and that sodium and chloride contents are markedly higher in these fluids, whereas potassium, phosphate, and protein contents are markedly higher in intracellular fluid.

plasma pH (7.4) the proteins exist with a net negative charge. Nonelectrolytes such as urea, dextrose, and creatine remain molecularly intact and are essentially uncharged.

Each electrolyte has specific functions. *The general functions of all electrolytes are to (1) promote neuromuscular irritability, (2) maintain body fluid volume and osmolality, (3) distribute body water between fluid compartments, and (4) regulate acid-base balance.*

Distribution of body electrolytes

The three fluid compartments contain similar electrolytes, but the concentration of the electrolytes in each compartment varies greatly (Table 7-3). Electrolytes move between compartments, but most of the exchange occurs between *interstitial* and *intravascular* fluids.

Differences in individual ion concentrations occur in various *extracellular* fluids. For instance, gastric secretion is acid; hence the concentration of hydrogen ions is high. Pancreatic secretion, on the other hand, is more alkaline than plasma and contains a high concentration of bicarbonate. Gastric and pancreatic secretions and bile all contain high concentrations of sodium ions. Knowing the common electrolytes found in various body fluids is helpful in preventing depletion of necessary substances and in noting early signs of imbalance.

Electrolyte balance

In health the ratio of cations to anions in each of the body fluids and the concentration of the various ions in these fluids are relatively constant. Dietary intake, and in some instances, intravenous infusions are the routes by which an individual obtains a supply of electrolytes to replace daily losses and to keep the body in electrolyte balance. Electrolyte loss is mainly through the kidneys, with smaller losses through the skin and lungs and relatively minimal losses through the bowel. The kidneys selectively excrete certain electrolytes, retaining those needed for normal body fluid composition. Hormonal influences affect the kidneys' selective function. For example, the adrenocortical hormone aldosterone favors sodium reabsorption and the excretion of potassium.

Mechanisms for Fluid and Electrolyte Movement

Fluids, electrolytes, gases, and small molecules move freely through the semipermeable membranes that separate compartments. This movement occurs constantly as oxygen and nutrients are carried to cells and wastes are removed from cells by the blood. In spite of the constant movement of water and dissolved particles *(solutes)* back and forth, the actual amount of water and concentration of solutes in each compartment remain relatively unchanged when the body is functioning normally. *The mechanisms by which water and solutes move are osmosis, diffusion, and filtration.*

Osmosis

Osmosis is the movement of a solvent (water) through a semipermeable membrane from an area of lower concentration of

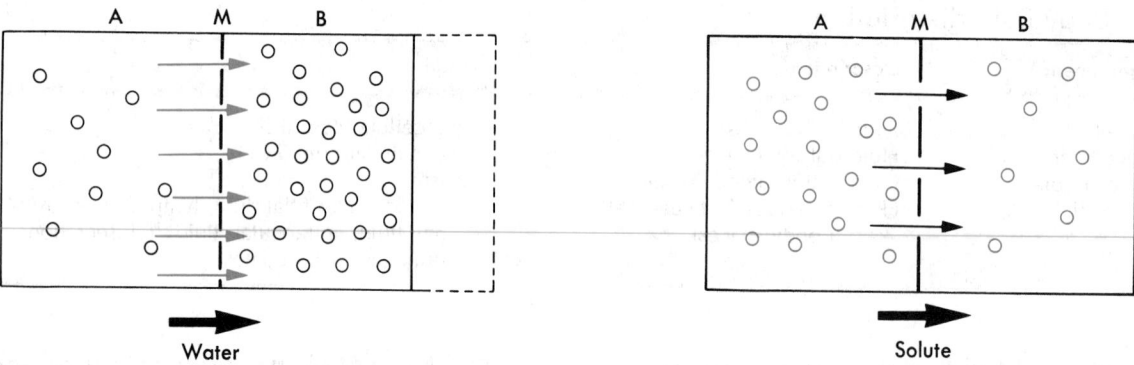

Fig. 7-3 Osmosis: water moves from area of lesser solute concentration *(A)* through a semi-permeable membrane *(M)* to area of greater solute concentrations *(B)* until concentration of solute on both sides of the membrane is equal. Compartment B will have to expand (as shown by dotted lines) to accept the additional water.

Fig. 7-4 Diffusion: Solute moves through membrane *(M)* from area of greater concentration *(A)* to area of lesser concentration *(B)* until concentration on both sides is equal.

Table 7-4 Factors influencing hormone release and effects on fluid and electrolyte balance

Hormone	Factors promoting or inhibiting hormone release	Effect
Aldosterone	**Promotes hormone release**	
	Increased serum potassium	Reabsorption of sodium and water: increased blood volume, hypertension
	Decreased serum sodium	Excretion of potassium: hypokalemia
	Decreased blood volume	Excretion of hydrogen ions: alkalosis
	Inhibits hormone release	
	Increased serum sodium	Excretion of sodium and water: decreased blood volume, hypotension
	Decreased serum potassium	
	Increased blood volume	Potassium retention; hyperkalemia
	Spironolactone (diuretic)	Retention of hydrogen ions: acidosis
Antidiuretic hormone (ADH)	**Promotes hormone release**	
	Hyperosmolar plasma	Reabsorption of water in renal tubules
	Low blood volume	
	Pain, stress	
	Drugs: narcotics, anesthetics	
	Inhibits hormone release	
	Hyposmolar plasma	Blocking of water reabsorption: loss of water via kidneys
	Increased blood volume	
	Alcohol ingestion	
Parathormone	**Promotes hormone release**	
	Decreased serum calcium	Loss of calcium from bone
		Increased absorption of calcium from GI tract
		Decreased renal excretion of calcium, increased excretion of phosphate
	Inhibits hormone release	
	Increased serum calcium	Decreased absorption of calcium from GI tract
	Increased calcium and vitamin D in diet	Increased renal excretion of calcium, decreased loss of phosphate

solute to an area of higher concentration (Fig. 7-3). The water moves to dilute the more highly concentrated solution until an equilibrium is reached on both sides of the semipermeable membrane. *The concentration of solute in any one compartment is called osmotic pressure or osmolality and is determined by the total number of dissolved particles per unit of solvent.*

Because of their large size, *protein molecules* normally have *little movement between compartments.* Their presence, especially in the intravascular fluid, creates a pressure called *colloid osmotic* or *oncotic* pressure, which *functions to hold water within the compartment.*

Diffusion

Diffusion is the movement of a solute from an area of greater concentration to an area of lesser concentration (Fig. 7-4). This is known as *movement down a concentration gradient.* Diffusion includes dispersion of solute throughout the fluid within a compartment, as well as movement of the solute through a membrane that separates two compartments until its concentration is equal on both sides of the membrane. The semipermeable walls of blood vessels and cells contain tiny pores through which small molecules and electrolytes diffuse freely.

Large molecules such as glucose are too large to pass through membrane pores and are assisted in crossing the membrane by *carrier substances;* this process is known as *facilitated diffusion.*

Filtration

Filtration pressure is another means by which water and diffusible particles are moved through a membrane. Movement occurs because the weight or pressure of the fluid is greater on one side of the membrane than on the other. Filtration pressure is discussed later in this chapter in relation to normal exchange of water and solutes across capillary membranes (p. 118).

Hormonal Control

Three hormones play a particularly vital role in maintaining fluid and electrolyte balance as follows:
1. *Antidiuretic hormone* (ADH)
   a. Is produced in the hypothalamus and stored and released from the posterior pituitary gland
   b. Acts on the renal tubules to retain water and to decrease urinary output
2. *Aldosterone*
   a. Is secreted by the adrenal cortex
   b. Acts on the renal tubules to reabsorb sodium and to excrete potassium
   c. Increases circulatory volume by reabsorbing water along with sodium
3. *Parathormone*
   a. Produced by the parathyroid glands
   b. Promotes absorption of calcium from the intestine
   c. Promotes release of calcium from bone
   d. Increases the excretion of phosphate ions by the kidneys

Table 7-4 lists the factors that stimulate or inhibit release of these hormones.

FLUID AND ELECTROLYTE IMBALANCE

Almost all medical-surgical conditions threaten fluid and electrolyte balance. There may be deficits or excesses of water or of any electrolyte. Actually several imbalances occur simultaneously because of the interrelationship of body fluids and their electrolytes. For clarity, *imbalances of body fluid and of each ion are considered separately.*

Fluid Imbalances

Osmolality is determined by the total number of particles dissolved in a unit of solvent. The osmolality of body fluid is measured in milliosmols or thousandths of an osmol because the number of particles in solution is relatively small. Normal osmolality of body fluids is approximately 300 mOsm/L. Solutions relate to normal osmolality in the following ways:
1. *Isosmolar:* same osmolality as body fluids
2. *Hyposmolar:* less osmolality than body fluids
3. *Hyperosmolar:* Greater osmolality than body fluids

When the body gains or loses fluid in excess of normal fluid balance, the intercompartmental fluid movement that occurs depends on whether the extracellular fluid becomes hyperosmolar or hyposmolar,[2] or remains isosmolar. The effects of different types of fluid imbalances are illustrated in Table 7-5.

Fluid loss

There are a number of ways in which body fluids and electrolytes contained therein are lost or made unavailable for normal fluid and electrolyte balance, as summarized in the list below.

Losses of fluid and electrolytes

Skin: diaphoresis, oozing from severe wounds or burns
GI tract: profuse salivation, vomiting, diarrhea, GI drainage, enemas
Kidneys: diuretics, polyuria
Hemorrhage
Trapping of fluids: wound swelling, edema, ascites, intestinal obstruction

The GI tract secretes approximately 8 L of fluid daily (Fig. 7-5); therefore, large amounts of fluid may be lost through

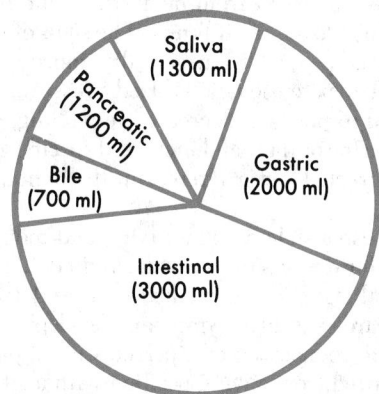

Fig. 7-5   Fluid volume of gastrointestinal secretions.

Table 7-5 **Fluid imbalances**

Fluid imbalance	Pathophysiology	Signs and symptoms	Therapy
Isosmolar fluid deficit	Decreased body water and electrolytes; extracellular fluid remains isosmolar but volume decreases	Hypotension, increased pulse and respirations, cool skin, delayed vein filling, shock, decreased urinary output	Replacement of water and sodium: oral intake of salty fluids; IV of normal saline
Hyperosmolar fluid deficit	Decreased body water more than decreased electrolytes; water moves out of cells to dilute extracellular fluid (cellular dehydration)	Thirst; skin flushed, dry, poor turgor; dry coated tongue; increased body temperature; increased hemoglobin and hematocrit levels; apprehension, restlessness	Water taken orally, if possible; IV of 5% dextrose in water; additional water given with tube feedings
Hyposmolar fluid excess (water intoxication)	Excess body water without excess electrolytes; water moves into cells causing cells to swell	Behavior changes, confusion, incoordination; sudden weight gain; warm moist skin; lethargy, convulsions	Water restriction; for severe signs, 3% to 5% sodium chloride IV
Isosmolar fluid excess (edema)	Excess body water and sodium; excess fluid moves into extracellular spaces	Edema of dependent body parts: pitting edema over bony prominences; swollen, tight, shiny skin Pulmonary edema: dyspnea; wheezing cough with frothy sputum; cyanosis	Elevation of dependent part; treatment of underlying condition; diuretics, reduced salt intake; treatment of pulmonary edema

the GI tract. Loss of both water and solutes leads to *isosmolar* fluid deficit with resulting circulatory collapse. Loss of water in excess of solutes leads to a *hyperosmolar* fluid deficit with resulting dehydration.

Isosmolar volume deficit: extracellular fluid deficit

Sodium ions constitute most of the osmolality of extracellular fluid. If both water and sodium are lost, the result is isosmolar volume loss; the extracellular fluid becomes depleted, and circulating blood volume is decreased (see Table 7-5). The body attempts to maintain circulation vital to tissue perfusion by initiating several compensatory mechanisms (see Box 7-1). If adequate blood volume cannot be maintained by these mechanisms, cardiac output is decreased and blood pressure drops. If volume depletion occurs rapidly, shock may ensue.

Isosmolar loss can result from hemorrhage, profuse diaphoresis, and large losses of GI fluids. The signs of volume depletion include: poor skin turgor, dry mucous membranes, postural hypotension, low blood pressure, tachycardia, increased respiration, decreased vein filling, weight loss, decreased urine output, and increased specific gravity. Treatment is directed toward replacing both fluids and electrolytes.

Nurses are responsible for identifying and monitoring patients at risk for developing isosmolar fluid deficit. Taking postural vital signs is one method used to detect this deficit before cardiovascular symptoms develop. *Postural vital signs* are the comparison of a person's blood pressure and pulse measured from a lying position with a sitting or standing position. A drop in blood pressure of 10 torr or more with an increase in pulse rate indicates postural hypotension and signals a state of isosmolar fluid depletion.

If plasma proteins are lost from the body, as occurs in hemorrhage, or if they are shifted from the blood to the interstitial fluid, as occurs in burns, the blood volume drops rapidly because fluid from interstitial spaces cannot be mobilized to maintain it, and shock follows (see Chapter 9). Whole blood, plasma, or plasma expanders usually must be given to these patients to replace the protein loss before extensive fluid therapy is effective.

Hyperosmolar fluid deficit

When water is lost from the body in excess of sodium and other electrolytes or when water intake is inadequate to replace normal losses, the extracellular fluid becomes hyperosmolar (see Table 7-5). Water moves out of the cells by osmosis to dilute the extracellular compartment and *cellular dehydration* results. As both extracellular and intracellular fluids decrease, cell function is impaired because food, oxygen, and waste products are inadequately diffused.

Imbalances may originate in either the *fluid* or the *solute portion of the ECF.* There may be (1) *decreased intake of water,* (2) *excess loss of water without proportional loss of solutes,* (3) *increased solute intake without sufficient water,* and (4) *excess accumulation of solutes secondary to a particular disease condition.*

Any person who does not have fluids available to drink, who cannot take fluids independently, or who does not respond to thirst will be likely to develop a water deficit.

When solutes are *taken in without sufficient water,* such as occurs when *high-protein tube feedings are given,* the extracellular fluid becomes *hyperosmolar.* The kidneys attempt to remove excess solute by excreting large amounts of urine; this is known as *osmotic diuresis.*

Thirst and weight loss are early symptoms of water deficit and become more pronounced as the deficit in-

<table>
<tr><td>

7-1

Compensatory mechanisms to maintain circulation

Mechanism 1

Decreased intravascular fluid increases the plasma colloid osmotic pressure.
Interstitial fluid is pulled back into the blood vessel to equalize pressure (Starling's law of the capillaries, p. 118).
Blood volume is increased.

Mechanism 2

Blood flow through kidneys is decreased because of the decreased blood volume.
Aldosterone is released from adrenal cortex resulting in sodium retention and potassium excretion.
Sodium retention increases the reabsorption of water because of osmolality.
Urinary excretion is decreased and extracellular fluid is increased.
Blood volume is increased.

</td><td>

7-2

Signs of acute water intoxication

Changes in behavior: confusion, incoordination, convulsions

Hyperventilation

Sudden weight gain

Warm, moist skin

Increased intracranial pressure: slow bounding pulse with an increase in systolic and decrease in diastolic blood pressures

Peripheral edema, usually not marked

</td></tr>
</table>

creases. Body temperature begins to rise as less water is available for temperature regulation. When cells are not able to continue providing water to replace ECF losses, signs of collapse of the circulatory system appear. Dry mouth and throat cause difficulty with speech.

Dehydration may be *encountered in patients who have dysphagia (difficulty swallowing)*, are *unaware that they are thirsty (confused, disoriented)*, *hyperventilate excessively*, or have *severe diarrhea or diabetes insipidus*. Treatment consists of water replacement. Intravenous infusion of 5% dextrose in water is given to the patient who cannot take oral fluids. Water is given along with or between tube feedings.

In addition to providing fluids and participating in the treatment of conditions underlying water loss, nurses use measures to decrease discomfort and ensure patient safety. *Mouth care* is especially important to *relieve dryness of mucous membranes and remove debris on lips and teeth. Safety measures* such as side rails on beds are necessary for patients who have developed restlessness, confusion, lethargy, or other mental changes as a result of water deficit. *Monitoring intake and output* and *changes in the patient's weight* and *vital signs* will *indicate whether the patient's condition* is *improving or deteriorating.*

A state of *adequate hydration* will be *evidenced by mental alertness, moist mucous membranes, and urinary output that is approximately equal to fluid intake.*

Fluid excess

Fluid that is retained in the body in excess of normal is termed overhydration. There may be an excess of water without an increase in electrolytes (hyposmolar fluid excess) or an increase in both water and electrolytes (isotonic fluid excess).

Hyposmolar fluid excess (water intoxication)

If an excess of water is present without an increase in sodium or protein, *water enters the cells* through *osmosis,*

causing them to swell. This is referred to as *water intoxication* (dilution syndrome) (see Table 7-5). This form of overhydration can occur when the water intake is greater than the kidney's ability to excrete it.

Water excess can *occur in the following situations:*

1. *Excess secretion of ADH as seen in acute stress such as trauma, surgery, pain, fear, acute infections, anesthetics, analgesics (morphine, meperidine), and cerebral lesions*
2. *Low renal blood flow, as seen in congestive heart failure, cirrhosis of the liver, acute renal insufficiency, and Addison's disease*
3. *Large amount of water given rectally as occurs with repeated enemas*
4. *Frequent and continuous amounts of water taken orally, especially in the seriously ill patient who drinks sodium-free liquids rather than eating solid foods*
5. *Absorption of irrigating fluids during transurethral resection of the prostate*

Water excess can be caused by ingestion of large amounts of tap water, a behavior called *psychogenic polydipsia.* The ingestion of frequent sips of tap water by one who is not able to tolerate food or other fluids because of illness can also lead to water excess.

Because brain cells are particularly sensitive to the increase in intracellular water, the most common signs are manifestations of changes in the patient's *mental status.*

In acute water intoxication there is swelling of the cells, which may develop rapidly and dramatically. Signs of water intoxication are listed in Box 7-2.

When the condition develops more slowly, there may be apathy, sleepiness, anorexia, nausea, and vomiting. A low serum sodium concentration is a usual finding.

The principal intervention for water intoxication is water restriction. In severe cases of hyposmolarity, when the serum sodium is critically depressed (<116 mEq/L), administration of furosemide (Lasix) and infusion of 3% to 5% hypertonic saline may be used. The saline will raise the sodium level while the diuretic will cause water loss. Administration of saline without diuretics will not maintain the sodium level because sodium will continue to be excreted by the kidneys. Furosemide inhibits some of this urinary sodium excretion and assists in preventing hypervolemia.

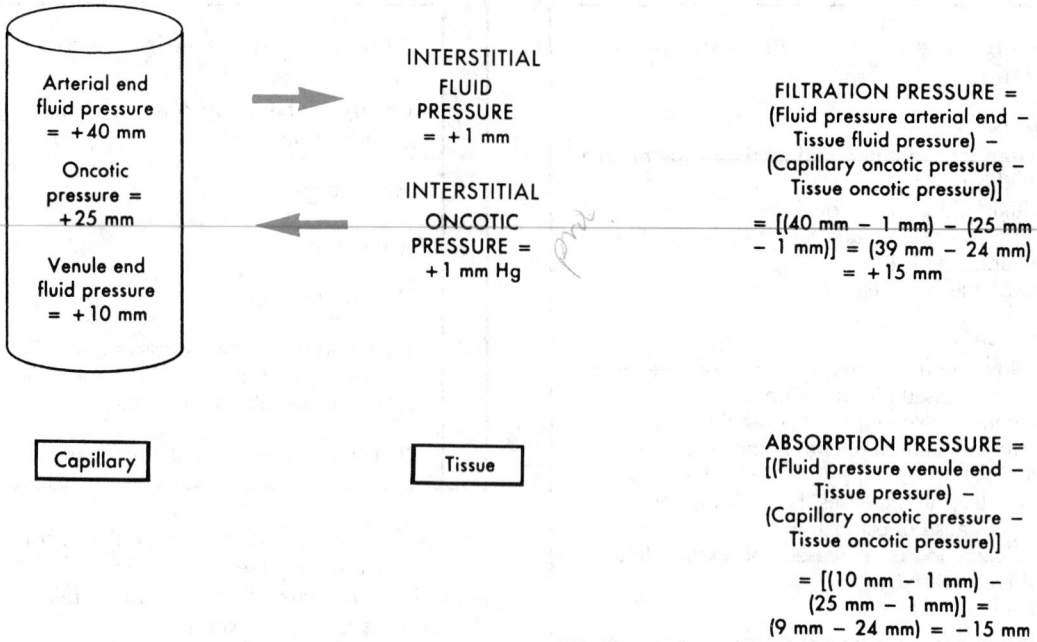

Fig. 7-6 Starling's law of capillaries. An equilibrium exists between forces filtering fluid out of capillary and forces absorbing fluid back into capillary. Note that fluid pressure within capillary is greater than fluid pressure in tissue. This differential (fluid pressure gradient) serves as a filtering force. Note also that oncotic pressure (colloid osmotic pressure) is greater within capillary. This serves as an absorbing force.

During treatment hourly intake and output measurements are necessary. Infusions should be given by use of a controlled infusion device to prevent too rapid administration. Daily weights, serum sodium levels, and neurological status should also be assessed.

Providing for the safety of patients with this imbalance is a priority nursing function, because of the confusion and other mental changes that exist. Any *patient who is receiving a large amount of water orally, rectally, or intravenously needs to be monitored carefully for signs of water intoxication, especially if a condition of excess ADH prevails.*

Isosmolar fluid excess (edema)

If an *excess of body water* is present with an accompanying *increase in sodium (isosmolar fluid), the excess fluid is retained in the extracellular compartment and leads to the formation of edema* (see Table 7-5). *Edema is the accumulation of fluid in the interstitial spaces.* A negative interstitial fluid pressure occurs in normal tissue, and cells are held in close approximation to facilitate the exchange of gases, nutrients, and waste products between the cells and capillaries. If fluid accumulates in the interstitial space and is not removed, either by direct return to the blood vessel or through the lymph system, a positive interstitial fluid pressure develops, and cells are pushed farther apart. If a finger is pressed over an edematous area, the indentation made by the finger may remain briefly as the fluid is pushed to another area; this is called *pitting edema.* The fluid refills the interstitial space in the "pit" area within a few seconds.

In the healthy individual, *edema does not develop immediately with the initial inflow of fluid into the interstitial spaces because of the body's compensatory mechanisms, that* is, the existing negative interstitial fluid pressure and the removal by the lymph system of excess fluids and proteins that accumulate in the interstitial spaces.

Capillary dynamics

A review of normal capillary dynamics aids in understanding the various factors that can cause edema to develop. *Two types of pressure influence the flow of fluid across a capillary membrane: fluid pressure* (resulting from the hydrostatic force of fluid) and *colloid osmotic pressure* or *oncotic pressure* (pressure resulting from the presence of proteins that do not diffuse across the membrane wall). *Fluid pressure within the capillary is much greater than fluid pressure in the interstitial space;* this force *filters fluid out of the capillary.* Because a larger number of protein molecules is found in plasma than in interstitial fluid, the oncotic pressure within the capillary serves as a force to *reabsorb* fluid into the capillary.

According to *Starling's "law of the capillaries,"* pressures that *promote movement of fluid out of the capillary are greatest at the arteriole end,* whereas *pressures promoting fluid movement back into the capillary are greatest at the venule end.* An exchange of fluid occurs across the capillary membrane with an overall equilibrium between the forces filtering fluid out of the capillary and the forces absorbing fluid back into the capillary (Fig. 7-6).

Pathophysiology of edema

Edema was defined as an accumulation of fluid in the interstitial spaces creating a positive fluid pressure. Thus *edema can be produced* by the following:

1. *Increase in capillary fluid pressure*

Table 7-6   Causes of edema according to underlying physiologic mechanism

Fluid pressure	Oncotic pressure

Increased capillary fluid pressure
Increased venous pressure
Vein obstruction
  Varicose veins
  Thrombophlebitis
  Pressure on veins from casts, tight bandages, or garters
Increased total volume with decreased cardiac output
  Congestive heart failure
  Fluid overloading
 	
Sodium and water retention: increased aldosterone from:
Decreased renal blood flow
  Congestive heart failure
  Renal failure
Increased production of aldosterone
  Cushing's syndrome
Aldosterone added to system
  Corticosteroid therapy
Inability to destroy aldosterone
  Cirrhosis of liver
	Decreased capillary oncotic pressure
	Loss of serum protein
	Burns, draining wounds, fistulas
	Hemorrhage
	Nephrotic syndrome
	Chronic diarrhea
	
	Decreased intake of protein
	Malnutrition
	Kwashiorkor
	
	Decreased production of albumin
	Liver disease
	
	Increased interstitial oncotic pressure
	Increased capillary permeability to protein
	Burns
	Inflammatory reactions
	  Trauma
	  Infections
	Allergic reactions (hives)
	
	Blocked lymphatics: decreased removal of tissue fluid and protein
	Malignant diseases
	Surgical removal of lymph nodes
	Elephantiasis

2. *Decrease in capillary oncotic pressure*

3. *Increase in interstitial oncotic pressure* (Table 7-6)

The same mechanisms that create edema in the interstitial spaces can create fluid collection in *potential fluid spaces. These are spaces between two membranes that normally contain only traces of fluid. The main potential fluid* spaces are *intrapleural* (lung and chest wall), *pericardial* (heart and pericardial sac), *peritoneal* (intestines and abdominal wall), and *joint spaces.* Large amounts of fluid also collect in areas of trauma, burn, and surgical wounds. *When fluid is abnormally accumulated in any of these places, the condition is referred to as third-spacing of fluids.* The symptoms of fluid collection in these spaces are usually caused by the pressure of the collected fluid against adjoining organs or structures. *Large amounts of fluid may collect in the peritoneal space (ascites). This fluid is high in protein and electrolytes. Accumulation of large amounts of fluid in all body tissue is called anasarca.*

Overloading of vascular system

A major cause of increased capillary fluid pressure is overloading of the vascular system. This *overloading results in an increase in the hydrostatic pressure of the blood,* in turn *resulting in generalized tissue edema.* More important, if the increase in hydrostatic pressure is great enough to push large amounts of fluid into the alveoli of the lungs, it rapidly leads to death from "drowning" in one's own fluids *(pulmonary edema).* The *hydrostatic pressure* in the *pulmonary vessels* normally is much lower than that in the general circulation, and therefore any increase is reflected rapidly in the lungs.

Overloading of the vascular system may be caused by giving too much fluid within a short period of time to a person who cannot dispose of the surplus because of circulatory or renal disease. Elderly people tolerate increases in blood volume poorly, because, with inelastic vessels, only relatively small increases in volume are needed to markedly increase hydrostatic pressure. Monitoring the central venous pressure is one method used to determine if overloading is occurring.

Overloading the vascular system also may be caused by increasing the oncotic (pull) pressure of the intravascular fluid by giving proteins so rapidly that the body cannot dispose of those that are in excess of its need. This overloading causes fluids to be pulled into the intravascular compartment from other body fluid compartments. The blood volume increases rapidly, neutralizing the oncotic pressure but increasing the hydrostatic pressure of the vascular system and the oncotic pressure of the interstitial fluid compartment. Fluid is then pushed into the tissues. *Overloading is a danger when fluids such as plasma, plasma expanders, albumin, or blood are given to any patient regardless of age or state of health.*

Treatment of edema

Edema is often treated with diuretics. Some diuretics, such as the *thiazides, block sodium reabsorption and consequently water reabsorption by the renal tubules. Other diuretic agents are partially or completely unabsorbable by the renal tubules*

Table 7-7   Common diuretics and their effect on fluid and electrolyte balance

Generic name	Trade name	Method of administration	Peak effect	Probable effects on fluid and electrolyte balance
Thiazides				
Chlorothiazide	Diuril	Oral	4 hr	Hyponatremia
				Hypokalemia
				↓ ECF volume
				Hyperglycemia
				Hyperuricemia
Hydrochlorothiazide	Esidrix HydroDiuril	Oral	3-4 hr	Hypomagnesemia
Loop diuretics (act mainly on ascending loop of Henle)				
Furosemide	Lasix	IM or IV	½ hr	Hypokalemia
		Oral	2-4 hr	Hyperuricemia
				↓ ECF volume
Ethacrynic acid	Edecrin	Oral	2-4 hr	Hyponatremia
		IV	½ hr	
Bumetanide	Bumex	Oral	½-1 hr	Hypokalemia
				Hypouricemia
		IM	40 min	Hyponatremia
				Hypocalcemia
		IV	5 min	Hypochloremia
Aldosterone antagonist (opposes potassium-losing action of aldosterone)				
Spironolactone	Aldactone	Oral	72 hr	Hyperkalemia
				Hyponatremia
Potassium-conserving action				
Triamterene	Dyrenium	Oral	4-8 hr	Hyperkalemia
Osmotic agent				
Mannitol	Osmitrol	IV infused over 24-hr period	—	Hyponatremia
				Hypochloremia
				↑ ECF volume

and tend to carry sodium and water with them into the urine. When diuretics are given, a large amount of fluid is lost from the vascular compartment, increasing its oncotic pressure and causing fluid to be pulled back into it from the tissues. *Potassium is usually lost along with sodium and water.* Table 7-7 shows some diuretics and their effects.

Reducing the salt intake also may reduce edema because the remaining supply of sodium seems to be needed to maintain the isotonicity of the blood and thus is not available for holding water. If edema is caused by venous stasis, elevating dependent body parts and applying supportive stockings help promote venous return.

Edema caused by decreased intravascular oncotic pressure is treated by correcting protein deficiencies and administering colloidal solutions such as albumin.

Electrolyte Imbalances

Serum electrolytes are measured in milliequivalents per liter (mEq/L), indicating the chemical combining activity of an electrolyte. For example, 1 mEq of the cation sodium is available to combine with 1mEq of an anion such as chloride or bicarbonate. The concentration of cations in blood serum or plasma is the same as the concentration of anions when expressed in terms of milliequivalents. This is more useful than measuring electrolytes in milligrams per 100 ml, which is only an indication of the amount of an electrolyte by weight and thus gives no information about the relationship between cations and anions. *No single electrolyte can be out of balance without causing some others to be out of balance.*

Sodium, potassium, and *calcium* are all *essential* for the *passage of nerve impulses.* Whenever the concentrations of any of these cations are increased or decreased in body fluids, the increase or decrease is reflected in the stimulation of muscles by nerves. The muscles may become weak and atonic because of inadequate stimulation, or they may become somewhat spastic because of excess stimulation. For example, a decrease in calcium concentration in body fluids causes the stimulus to be increased and results in muscle spasms. GI and cardiac symptoms, so often produced by electrolyte imbalances, result in part from changes in neural stimulation on the muscles of these systems.

With *cation imbalances,* the *distribution of body fluids* is *frequently upset.* Abnormal collections of fluid probably cause some of the GI symptoms such as nausea, vomiting, and diarrhea. Decreased amounts may cause anorexia, dyspepsia, and constipation. It is thought that edema of ce-

7-3	**Causes and symptoms of sodium deficit**

Causes	**Symptoms**
Loss of GI fluids	Headache
Vomiting	Muscle weakness
Diarrhea	Fatigue
GI or biliary drain-	Apathy
age	Postural hypotension
Fistulas	Nausea/vomiting
Loss through skin	Abdominal cramps
Diaphoresis	**Severe prolonged**
Large open lesions	**deficit**
(burns)	Shock
Shifting of body fluids	Mental confusion
Massive edema	Coma
Ascites	
Burns	
Small bowel ob-	
struction	

7-4	**Causes and symptoms of sodium excess**

Causes
More water than sodium is lost from the body
An abnormally large intake of sodium
   Taking too many salt tablets
   IV saline infused too rapidly
   Foods—prepared/frozen/canned, smoked/
     dairy products in large amounts

Symptoms
Dry, sticky mucous membranes
Low urinary output
Firm, rubbery tissue turgor
Severe prolonged excess
   Manic excitement
   Tachycardia
   Death

rebral tissues may be responsible for headache, convulsions, and coma.

Sodium

Sodium deficit (hyponatremia)

The normal concentration of sodium in the blood is 138 to 145 mEq/L. A low sodium level in the blood (*hyponatremia*) can indicate either a deficit of sodium or an excess of water. Whenever sodium is lost from the body fluids, *the osmotic pressure of the ECF decreases* and *water diffuses into the cell, where there is greater osmotic pressure*. The *plasma volume* is *then decreased*, and *symptoms of hypovolemia may be present*. In response to this reduction of the sodium concentration in the extracellular fluid, potassium moves out of the intracellular fluid. Therefore, the patient with sodium imbalance is also likely to have a potassium imbalance.

Sodium depletion results most often from the loss of GI secretions. It can also occur from losses through the skin and in the shifting of body fluids so that the sodium is not accessible for use.

Anyone who is perspiring profusely because of environmental conditions, exercise, or fever is losing large amounts of both sodium and water. If salt is not replaced with water, such as by drinking salty fluids, water intoxication occurs. The ability of the cells to depolarize and repolarize normally is impaired in sodium deficit. The causes and symptoms of sodium deficit are summarized in Box 7-3.

Treatment of shock, if present, is the first concern. Saline solution, usually 0.9% sodium chloride, *is given intravenously* at a *rapid* rate. Plasma expanders may also be infused.

If other electrolytes (potassium, calcium, bicarbonate) have been depleted, these also need to be replaced. Treatment that alleviates the underlying cause will prevent further sodium loss. Salt or salty foods are added to the diet for sodium depletion, which develops slowly or follows profuse perspiration (diaphoresis) or vomiting.

Safety measures, such as the use of side rails on the bed, supervision of ambulation, and frequent observation, are necessary if the patient becomes weak or confused or experiences marked hypotension.

Sodium excess (hypernatremia)

A serum sodium level greater than 145 mEq/L is known as *hypernatremia*. There are actually *two kinds of sodium excess, edema* and *hypernatremia*. When there is a *sodium* and *water excess, edema exists;* when there is an *excess of sodium in relation to water* in the *extracellular compartment, hypernatremia exists*. The causes and symptoms of sodium excess are listed in Box 7-4.

As seen in Table 7-8, *hypernatremia does not necessarily indicate an excess of total body sodium.*

If fluids are greatly limited or if excess salt is taken into the body and retained because of poor renal function, sodium may be concentrated in body fluids. Excess intravascular sodium causes fluid to be withdrawn from interstitial spaces. Extracellular fluids become hyperosmolar and draw water from the cells, causing cellular dehydration. If fluids are not given to dilute the sodium and if excretion of sodium is not increased, severe fluid and electrolyte disturbances occur, causing manic excitement, tachycardia, and eventual death.

Water alone is given to treat sodium excess. If cardiac and renal function is normal, a liberal amount of water is administered orally, or 5% dextrose in water is given intravenously. In the absence of normal cardiac and renal function, hydration must be carried out with caution to prevent fluid overloading in the patient.

Diuretics are of *value* in *removing sodium. If sodium excess is severe*, with or without excess water retention, and *does not respond to other treatment, renal dialysis may be necessary.*

Potassium

Potassium is the major cation of the cells. During the *formation of new tissue (anabolism)* or *when glucose is converted to glycogen, potassium enters the cell.* With *tissue breakdown (catabolism), potassium leaves the cell.* This occurs with

Table 7-8   Comparison of serum sodium levels with total body sodium*

Condition	Serum sodium	Total body sodium
Prolonged sweating	Low (hyponatremia)	Low
Diuretics and low sodium diets	Low	Low
Addison's disease	Low	Low
Edema (cardiac, renal, hepatic disease)	Low or normal	High
Excretion of dilute urine, early stages of gastrointestinal sodium loss	Normal	Low
Excess oral or IV sodium intake	High (hypernatremia)	High
Water and sodium loss with water loss > sodium loss	High	Low

*Note that a low or high serum level does not necessarily correspond with total body sodium.

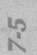

Causes and symptoms of hypokalemia

Causes
Decreased potassium intake
Increased potassium loss
   Increased aldosterone activity
   GI losses
   Potassium-losing diuretics
   Loss from cells as in trauma, burns
Conditions causing very large urine output
Potassium shift into cells
   Treatment of acidosis
   Metabolic alkalosis
Symptoms
Muscle weakness
Anorexia, nausea/vomiting
Diminished deep tendon reflexes, lethargy
Cardiac dysrhythmias
ECG changes
Severe or prolonged deficit
   Flaccid paralysis
   Kidney damage
   Paralytic ileus
   Cardiac/respiratory arrest

---

trauma, dehydration, or starvation. The normal serum level of potassium is 3.5 to 5.0 mEq/L.

Potassium deficit (hypokalemia)

A *serum potassium level below 3.5 mEq/L is known as hypokalemia.* The body's mechanism for conserving potassium is not as effective as that for conserving sodium, and the kidneys may excrete potassium even when the body needs it. *Whenever sodium is being retained in the body through reabsorption by the kidney tubules, potassium is excreted.* Thus *whenever aldosterone secretion is increased,* such as in *stress, potassium is excreted. Potassium depletion,* therefore, *is common* in *many diseases* and *injuries* and *during therapy such as surgery. Potassium* may also be *lost through the urine* as a *result of certain diuretics* such as the thiazides and furosemide (Lasix).

The patient who has a balanced diet withheld for several days, is dehydrated, or is given large amounts of parenteral fluids with no replacement of potassium develops potassium depletion. Dilution of extracellular potassium by the administration of 5% dextrose without potassium supplements and potassium loss caused by catabolism of body proteins account for many electrolyte imbalances in the postoperative patient.

The practice of giving multiple enemas is becoming less common because it is now known that some of the enema fluid is absorbed and dilutes the potassium in the interstitial compartment, upsetting the balance between compartments. Solutions for hyperosmolar enemas may damage cells in the bowel mucosa, causing potassium loss.

Potassium has *a direct effect on cardiac and skeletal muscle function.* The patient with *potassium deficit* shows *characteristic electrocardiographic changes* of *flattened or inverted T waves with a prolonged Q-T interval* (see Chapter 24). The most *striking symptom of hypokalemia* is *muscle weakness.* Digitalis toxicity can occur in patients taking digitalis if they develop hypokalemia. With severe hypokalemia, the patient may die unless potassium is administered promptly. The causes and symptoms of hypokalemia are summarized in Box 7-5.

The *safest way to administer potassium is orally.* Fresh fruits (especially oranges and bananas) or foods high in protein are good sources of potassium (Box 7-6). A potassium salt may be prescribed orally; if given in liquid form, it should be given in fruit or vegetable juice or chilled to increase palatability. When potassium is given intravenously, it must be diluted, and the rate of flow must be monitored closely to prevent hyperkalemia and atrial arrest. The usual rate of infusion should not exceed 20 mEq of potassium per hour. Potassium is never given in a bolus or IV push.

Potassium excess (hyperkalemia)

A *serum potassium level greater than 5.0 mEq/L is termed hyperkalemia.* This condition does not occur as frequently as hypokalemia, especially if renal function is normal.

As previously stated, *whenever there is severe tissue damage, potassium is released from the cells into the extracellular fluids.* Because shock usually accompanies this damage,

---

7-6

Foods rich in potassium

Fruits	**Vegetables**
(including juices)	Asparagus
Apricots	Dried beans
Bananas	Broccoli
Grapefruit	Cabbage
Melon	Carrots
Cantaloupe	Celery
Honeydew	Mushrooms
Dried fruits	Dried peas
Figs, dates, raisins	Potatoes
Oranges	White, sweet
	Spinach
Protein foods	Squash
Beef	
Chicken	**Beverages**
Liver	Cocoa
Pork	Cola drinks
Veal	Dry, instant tea
Turkey	and coffee
Milk	
Nuts, peanut	
butter	

*Most raw vegetables contain potassium, much of which is lost in cooking.

7-7

Causes and symptoms of hyperkalemia

Causes

Potassium intake (parenteral or oral) in excess of
  kidneys' ability to excrete
Renal failure
Adrenal insufficiency
Potassium enters bloodstream, from injured cells
  with extensive trauma
Metabolic acidosis

Symptoms

Nausea, vomiting
Diarrhea, colic
Cardiac dysrhythmias
ECG changes
Numbness, tingling
Severe or prolonged excess*
  Flaccid paralysis
  Cardiac arrest
  Anuria

*Prolonged potassium excess results in symptoms similar to those of hypokalemia.

---

renal function is reduced, and a high blood potassium level results. There is great danger in giving extra potassium to any patient with poor renal function. If the patient is dehydrated or has lost vascular fluid, glucose and water or plasma expanders usually are given until renal function returns. Untreated adrenal insufficiency also is a contraindication for giving potassium.

The *patient with hyperkalemia develops spasticity of muscles* because of their overstimulation by nerve impulses. The patient *complains of nausea, colic, diarrhea, and skeletal muscle spasms.* The muscles later become weak because the overstimulation produces an accumulation of lactic acid and because potassium is lost from the muscle cells.

If the condition is not controlled, overstimulation of the cardiac muscle causes the heartbeat to become irregular and eventually stop. ECG evidence of potassium elevation includes tall, peaked, symmetric, or tented T waves with a short Q-T interval. As the blood potassium level increases further, the QRS spreads and atrial arrest occurs. Box 7-7 shows the causes and symptoms of hyperkalemia.

If the patient who has hyperkalemia needs a blood transfusion, *fresh* blood must be used. Cells in blood that has been stored for several days tend to release potassium during storage. A transfusion of stored blood may further increase the patient's serum potassium level.

When hyperkalemia occurs, the patient is allowed nothing orally, and infusion of 10% glucose with 50 units of insulin is often given to induce transfer of potassium from the serum to the intracellular fluid. If the patient is in a state of acidosis (p. 137), correction of the situation results in movement of potassium back to the cell.

Kayexalate, a cation exchange resin, can be given orally or rectally. It results in the release of sodium and binding of potassium, with the potassium then excreted in the stool. If the patient is in renal failure or if the serum potassium is dangerously high, hemodialysis is necessary. The patient is placed on absolute bed rest until the potassium blood level is returned to normal.

Calcium

There is a considerable amount of calcium in the human body, most of it located in the bony skeleton and a small amount dissolved in body fluids. Serum calcium level must be maintained at a level of 4.5 to 5.8 mEq/L to maintain vital functions of neuromuscular irritability and blood clotting. Calcium is present in the blood in two forms, free ionized calcium and calcium bound to protein. Only ionized calcium is physiologically active. Both *parathyroid hormone* and *vitamin D* are necessary for normal absorption of calcium from the GI tract, for reabsorption of calcium from bone to maintain the normal serum calcium level, and for prevention of excess calcium loss in urine.

Calcium deficit (hypocalcemia)

A *decrease in serum calcium level below 4.5 mEq/L is termed hypocalcemia.* Some conditions lead to excessive calcium binding, such as the infusion of large amounts of blood containing citrate (citrate is a blood preservative and binds calcium) and alkalosis (more calcium is bound in an alkaline medium). When these conditions are present, the patient begins to show signs of calcium deficit, because, although the total amount of blood calcium is not changed, there is less physiologically active (unbound, ionized) calcium available.

Causes and symptoms of hypocalcemia

Causes
Excess binding of calcium ions
  Large amount of citrated blood
  Alkalosis
Dietary deficiency of calcium
Low protein diet
Chronic renal failure
Pancreatic disease
Disease of small bowel
Draining intestinal fistulas
Deficiency of parathyroid hormone or vitamin D
Increased magnesium
Overuse of antacids and laxatives

Symptoms
Osteoporosis, pathologic fractures
Tingling around nose, mouth, ears, fingers, toes
Muscle spasm of feet and hands
Tetany
Nausea, vomiting
Diarrhea
Cardiac dysrhythmias, cardiac arrest
Calcium deposits in body tissues

Causes and symptoms of hypercalcemia

Causes
Loss from bone
  Immobilization
  Metastatic bone cancer
  Multiple myeloma
Excess intake
  Dietary
  Antacids containing calcium
Increased absorption
  Increased parathyroid hormone
  Increased vitamin D

Symptoms
Thirst, polyuria
Renal stones
Decreased deep tendon reflexes
Lethargy, coma
Cardiac dysrhythmias, cardiac arrest
Decreased muscle tone
Decreased GI motility

Patients with pancreatic disease or disease of the small intestine may fail to absorb calcium from the GI tract, and they may excrete abnormally large amounts of calcium in the feces, thus reducing the blood level of calcium. *Hypocalcemia* may also occur during the diuretic phase of acute renal failure as calcium is excreted.

The *patient with a calcium deficiency* usually *first complains of numbness and tingling of the nose, ears, fingers, and toes.* If calcium is not given at that time, painful muscular spasms, especially of the feet and hands (carpopedal spasm), muscle twitching, and convulsions may follow (*tetany*). The causes and symptoms of hypocalcemia are summarized in Box 7-8. *The two tests used to elicit signs of calcium deficiency are as follows:*
  1. *Trousseau's sign*
     a. Constrict the circulation of the arm by grasping the wrist or inflating a blood pressure cuff
     b. Positive sign of serious calcium deficit—hand goes into a position of palmar flexion
  2. *Chvostek's sign*
     a. Tap the face lightly over the facial nerve (just below the temple)
     b. Positive sign of calcium deficit—facial muscle twitching

The specific treatment for a low blood level of calcium is the administration of calcium gluconate or calcium chloride orally or intravenously.

Calcium excess (hypercalcemia)

A serum calcium level above 5.8 mEq/L is called hypercalcemia. It may be caused by calcium leaving the bone and concentrating in the ECF (as seen in bone diseases such as cancer or with prolonged immobilization) or by increased intake and absorption of calcium.

Normal retention of calcium in the bones is believed to be caused by the pressure exerted on bones by active movement or exercise. When a large amount of calcium accumulates in the extracellular fluid and passes through the kidneys, calcium can precipitate and form stones (calculi), a not infrequent complication of immobilization. Calcium precipitates more readily in alkaline solution. This can be a problem in a urinary tract infection, which increases the alkalinity of the urine. See Box 7-9 for a summary of causes and symptoms of hypercalcemia.

Treatment for hypercalcemia is removal of the cause. Intravenous saline and a diuretic (furosemide) may be given to promote renal excretion of the calcium. Oral or intravenous phosphate may also be given because calcium is excreted when phosphorus serum levels are increased. Mithramycin (Mithracin), a potent antitumor drug, has been used successfully to reduce serum calcium. If the hypercalcemia is caused by multiple myeloma or other cancers, glucocorticoids may be effective in reducing hypercalcemia, either because they decrease the size of the tumor or because the effect of the tumor on bone is reduced.

Because persons with marked hypercalcemia often are losing calcium from their bones or have malignant involvement of bone, special care should be taken to prevent pathologic fractures. Even the pressure used in giving a back rub must sometimes be avoided.

Careful *attention* must be *directed* to the *prevention of calcium stone formation in the kidneys.* Acid-ash fruit juices, cranberry and prune juice, or ascorbic acid can be given to promote urinary acidification and discourage stone formation. Urinary tract infections must be avoided. Good perineal care and meticulous technique in caring for Foley catheters are mandatory.

Unless they are contraindicated, persons with *hypercalce-*

7-10	Causes and symptoms of hypomagnesemia

Causes

Decreased intake
  Prolonged malnutrition
  Starvation
Impaired absorption from GI tract
  Alcoholism
  Hypercalcemia
  Diarrhea
  Draining intestinal fistulas
Conditions causing large losses of urine

Symptoms

Mental changes
  Agitation, depression, confusion
Paresthesias
Tremors
Ataxia
Cramps, spasticity, tetany
Tachycardia
Hypotension
Dysrhythmias

7-11	Causes and symptoms of hypermagnesemia

Causes

Renal failure
Diabetic ketoacidosis with severe water loss

Symptoms

Hypotension
Vasodilation
  Heat
  Thirst
  Nausea/Vomiting
Loss of deep tendon reflexes
Respiratory depression
Prolonged severe excess
  Coma
  Cardiac arrest

mia are *encouraged to drink 3000 to 4000 ml of fluids per day* to reduce the possibility of renal calculi and to overcome the thirst that accompanies hypercalcemia.

Magnesium

The normal serum magnesium level is within the range of 1.5 to 2.5 mEq/L. About 50% of magnesium is located in bones, 5% in ECF, and the remaining 45% within the cells. It functions in the activation of enzymatic reactions, especially in carbohydrate metabolism. Magnesium has a sedative effect on the CNS similar to that of calcium. High serum levels result in vasodilation and lowering of blood pressure; this is a rare occurrence except with kidney failure.

Metabolically, magnesium is closely interrelated with both calcium and potassium. In the presence of a large amount of calcium in the GI tract, calcium is absorbed in preference to magnesium, and the magnesium is excreted. Conversely, low calcium levels increase magnesium absorption. The kidneys effectively conserve magnesium when intake is low.

Magnesium deficit (hypomagnesemia)

Hypomagnesemia is a serum magnesium level below 1.5 mEq/L. It may be caused by impaired absorption from the GI tract, excess loss through the kidneys, or prolonged malnutrition.

A low serum magnesium level leads to increased neuromuscular irritability. Hypomagnesemia is usually manifested by behavioral and neurologic symptoms such as confusion, hallucination, convulsions, increased reflexes, muscle spasms, and paresthesias (see Box 7-10).

Nursing responsibilities for the person with hypomagnesemia include the following:

1. Encouraging foods high in magnesium (fruits, green vegetables, whole grain cereals, milk, meats, and nuts)
2. Careful observation and supervision of the patient who is confused or hallucinating
3. Providing for patient safety if convulsions occur

Magnesium excess (hypermagnesemia)

Hypermagnesemia is a serum magnesium level greater than 2.5 mEq/L. The action of magnesium is on the myoneural junction where a high magnesium level blocks acetylcholine release, decreasing the excitability of the muscle cells. Hypermagnesemia rarely develops unless there is renal failure, although it has been identified in diabetic ketoacidosis where there is severe water loss. In persons with renal failure, frequent use of magnesium-containing antacids or cathartics can cause toxicity. The vasodilating effect of magnesium is accentuated in hypermagnesemia and can lead to hypotension. There may be loss of deep tendon reflexes, respiratory depression, and cardiac arrest (see Box 7-11).

Correction of the underlying cause corrects magnesium excess. If renal failure is present, dialysis is necessary. Intravenous calcium gluconate may be a useful temporary treatment, because calcium has an antagonistic effect on magnesium.

ASSESSMENT OF FLUID AND ELECTROLYTE BALANCE

Patient Data

The nurse should be familiar with signs and symptoms of fluid and electrolyte disturbances. Because these *symptoms are frequently subtle,* it is necessary to have a high degree of sensitivity to the possibility of occurrence in certain persons, as in the following:

1. Has an illness of a type that usually disrupts fluid and electrolyte balance
2. Has medical or surgical treatments that result in imbalances

Table 7-9 Data supporting fluid and electrolyte imbalances

	Signs and symptoms	Imbalance
Change in mental status	Irritable, restless	Sodium or potassium excess
	Confusion, lethargy	Sodium or calcium excess or deficit
		Hyposmolar fluid excess
		Isosmolar fluid deficit
Head/neck	Dry, sticky mucous membranes	Sodium excess
	Facial puffiness (edema)	Isosmolar fluid excess
	Distended neck veins	Isosmolar fluid excess
	Thirst, dry mucous membranes, longitudinal furrows on tongue	Isosmolar fluid deficit
	Flat neck veins in supine position	Isosmolar fluid deficit
Temperature	Increase	Water loss, sodium excess
	Decrease	Fluid excess
GI	Absent bowel sounds (ileus)	Potassium deficit
	Anorexia, nausea, vomiting	Fluid excess or deficit
		Potassium excess or deficit
		Calcium excess
Circulation	Increased blood pressure	Increased circulatory volume
		Magnesium deficit
	Decreased blood pressure	Decreased circulatory volume
		Magnesium excess
	Increased pulse, slow vein filling	Potassium excess or deficit
		Isosmolar fluid deficit
	Bounding pulse	Increased circulating volume
		Potassium excess or deficit
		Sodium excess
	Weak, irregular pulse	Potassium excess or deficit
	Cardiac dysrhythmias	Potassium excess or deficit
Respiration	Dyspnea, orthopnea, moist breath sounds	Isosmolar fluid excess
	Decreased rate	Magnesium excess
Skin	Pale, cool extremities (without edema)	Decreased circulating volume
	Pitting edema	Isosmolar fluid excess
	Poor turgor (test over sternum)	Fluid deficit, sodium excess
	Dryness in groin, axillae	Isosmolar fluid deficit
	Flushed dry skin	Sodium excess
Neuromuscular	Numbness, tingling around mouth, fingers, toes	Calcium deficit
	Increased irritability, muscle spasms	Calcium deficit
	Muscle weakness, paralysis	Potassium deficit
	Decreased muscle tone, decreased deep tendon reflexes	Magnesium deficit
	Abdominal cramps	Potassium excess

3. Has considerable limitation of food and fluid intake
4. Sustains significant loss of body fluids

By knowing of conditions that put an individual at risk and making careful ongoing assessments, the nurse can prevent or detect imbalances before they become severe.

Subjective data include *thirst, headache, pain, nausea, dyspnea,* and *orthopnea.* The time of origin and a description of symptoms are noted. *Objective data,* as noted in Table 7-9, *can be compared to the baseline assessment* obtained at the time of the patient's initial contact with health care providers.

Laboratory Values

Laboratory determinations of serum levels of the specific electrolytes help in making decisions concerning electrolyte excesses or deficits. When electrolyte disturbances develop slowly, symptoms may not be pronounced, and the problem may be detected only by a determination of the electrolyte concentration in the patient's blood. When there is *excess water, hemodilution occurs* and the *hemoglobin* and *hematocrit levels decrease.* With excessive fluid loss, there is hemoconcentration and the hematocrit and BUN levels increase.

Additional Data

Important data to be considered in assessing fluid balances are comparison of fluid intake to output and changes in patient weight. Acutely ill medical patients and patients undergoing major surgery need to have their fluid intake and output and daily weight closely monitored. The practice of totaling the fluid intake and output every shift or every 24 hours provides additional data for determining whether or not the patient has a fluid imbalance.

Table 7-10   GI output

Type of fluid	Consistency	Color	Odor
Gastric	Watery	Pale yellow-green	Sour
			Fruity odor with metabolic acidosis
Biliary	Thicker than gastric	Bright yellow to dark green	Acrid odor and bitter taste
Intestinal	Thick	Dark green to brown	Fecal

Fluid intake

The intake record should show the type and amount of all fluids the patient has received and the route by which these were administered. This includes fluids given orally, parenterally, rectally, or fluids administered by tubes and retained by the patient. Foods that are eaten in a semisolid state but are basically liquid, such as gelatin or ice cream, are recorded as fluids. To record the fluid intake of ice chips, the amount of ice chips is divided by two (60 ml of ice chips equals 30 ml water). Patients may receive considerable amounts of fluid through the frequent sucking of ice chips.

Fluid output

Urinary output

Urinary output is recorded as to time and amount of each voiding to help evaluate renal function. If renal function is a major concern, such as in the patient with shock, an indwelling catheter is used so the amount of urine can be recorded every hour and fluid intake regulated accordingly.

Wound drainage

Any drainage from a catheter draining a wound is measured and the amount and character of the drainage is recorded. If there is excessive drainage on dressings, it may be necessary to weigh the dressings. Fluid loss equals the difference between the wet weight and dry weight of the dressing.

GI drainage

Electrolytes are lost in large amounts with vomiting, diarrhea, and gastric and intestinal drainage. The amount and kind vary according to the type of GI fluid lost. For determination of the amount and type of fluid replacement, vomitus, GI drainage, and liquid stools are measured as accurately as possible and are described as to consistency, color, and odor (Table 7-10). Fluid used to irrigate nasogastric tubes is subtracted from total drainage before the amount of drainage is recorded.

Other output

Fluid aspirated from any body cavity, such as the abdomen or pleural spaces, must be measured. This fluid contains not only electrolytes but also proteins.

Diaphoresis is difficult to measure. If the clothing and linen become saturated, there may be as much as 1000 ml of fluid lost in perspiration. Dry and wet weights may be taken to get a more accurate measure of the amount of fluid loss.

Daily weight

The *daily weight record* is *the best way to determine the onset of dehydration or the accumulation of fluid* either as generalized edema or as "hidden" fluid in body cavities. *An increase of 1 kg in weight is equal to the retention of 1 L of fluid.* If the weight record is to be useful, the *patient must be weighed* on the *same scale* and at the *same hour* each day and must be *wearing the same amount of clothing.* Usually weights are taken in the early morning before the patient has eaten or defecated but after voiding.

Urine specific gravity

The specific gravity of urine is a measure of the density (amount of solutes) in a sample of urine compared with the density of pure water (which is 1.000). Normal range for urine specific gravity is approximately 1.003 to 1.030. A person with renal impairment excretes a small amount of dilute urine (low specific gravity) because of the inability of the kidneys to concentrate solutes in the urine. The relationship between specific gravity and fluid deficit or excess is summarized as follows:

Fluid deficit: small urine volume with *high specific gravity*
Fluid excess: large urine volume with *low specific gravity*

INTERVENTIONS FOR PATIENTS WITH FLUID AND ELECTROLYTE IMBALANCE

Important nursing functions include prevention of fluid and electrolyte imbalance, assessment of patients to recognize and report early signs of imbalance, planning and carrying out actions related to therapy to correct the condition, and relief of symptoms.

Prevention of Fluid and Electrolyte Imbalance

Unless preventive measures are employed, many medical-surgical conditions and therapies may lead to fluid and electrolyte imbalance. In some frequently encountered situations, attention to preventive aspects may lessen the possibility of the development of serious fluid and electrolyte imbalance.

Prevention of inadequate fluid intake

Any patient who is unable to ask for fluids, to identify a need for fluid, or to swallow easily may develop a fluid deficit. The fluid intake of these patients is monitored, and specific plans are made to offer fluids at regular intervals. Some conditions placing persons at risk for fluid deficit are as follows: aphasia, catatonia, confusion, disorientation, dysphagia, weakness, and tube feedings.

Assessment

Obtain careful medication history: diuretics and laxatives (frequently taken by elderly) may promote dehydration.

Monitor fluid intake and output. Confusion or apathy may lead to decreased fluid intake.

Monitor dietary intake; decreased intake leads to decreased fluids (found in foods) and decreased electrolyte intake that can affect electrolyte balance. Decreased food intake may result from lack of teeth, poorly fitting dentures, decreased taste sensation from loss of tooth buds, or inability to purchase or cook foods at home.

Assess for signs of **dehydration** because of decreased ability to concentrate urine. Dehydration may occur more frequently and more rapidly in elderly than in younger adults.

Monitor urine specific gravity; this is usually lower in the elderly (1.026).

Watch for symptoms of dehydration that may include mental status changes, such as apathy, dulled mentation, confusion, irritability, and weakness.

Monitor for signs of volume depletion such as brown furry tongue, dry mucous membranes, decreased saliva pool under tongue; skin turgor is *not* a good indicator of dehydration in the elderly because of loss of skin elasticity with age.

BUN is normally increased in elderly (21 mg/dl).

Monitor carefully IV fluid rate and assess patient for signs of pulmonary edema (coughing, dyspnea, moist breath sounds). **Fluid overload** may occur more readily because of decreased cardiac reserves, decreased vasomotor response, or decreased urinary function.

Interventions

Facilitate fluid intake of at least 1500 ml/day. Smaller more frequent amounts of fluid are better tolerated.

Extra free water is essential when giving tube feedings to promote excretion of high-solute loads (up to 1000 ml daily).

Use measures to encourage a balanced dietary intake (within prescribed restrictions); small frequent meals may be better tolerated than 3 large meals per day.

Report and record early signs of dehydration (especially mental changes) or of IV fluid overload.

Teach patient the need for adequate hydration, control of sodium (as pertinent), and foods high in potassium (if taking diuretics).

Common disorders in elderly

Dehydration
IV fluid overload
Sodium excess
Potassium excess

Prevention of imbalances from GI fluid loss
Vomiting and diarrhea

Vomiting and diarrhea are common symptoms of many illnesses. Sodium and some potassium are lost in vomiting and diarrhea, whereas chloride is lost only from vomitus. As soon as fluids are tolerated, the patient may be served salty broth and tea or another fluid high in potassium to replace the losses. Dry salty crackers often are tolerated when fluids are not and can be used to replace sodium. These measures often keep the patient from feeling weak and exhausted.

Draining fistulas

A patient with a *draining fistula* from any portion of the GI tract loses *sodium, calcium,* and some *potassium,* and dietary supplements are needed. Extra milk can replace all the losses if tolerated by the patient. The vitamin D in the milk enables the body to use the calcium in the milk. Patients with a permanent fistulous opening, such as an ileostomy, need to be especially careful to supplement their sodium and potassium intake when vomiting, diarrhea, or fever adds to the already unusually large loss of electrolytes.

Nasogastric drainage

Routine *intravenous replacement usually is adequate to compensate* for *losses through nasogastric drainage, unless* the *patient* has *been sucking many ice chips or the tube has been irrigated frequently with water.* Both of these practices, although they seem to be harmless because the fluid is removed immediately through the aspiration apparatus, stimulate the secretion of gastric juices. Aspiration of gastric juices of the stomach at rest may lead to loss of electrolytes and fluid. If irrigation of the tube is necessary, normal saline is used.

Enemas

Repeated enemas may result in water intoxication and potassium loss. If there is an order for enemas until the returns are clear, it is best not to give more than three enemas at one time without consulting the physician. If an elderly person living at home complains of pronounced weakness without apparent cause, the person is asked whether cathartics or enemas are being taken. If so, stopping this practice, eating foods with high potassium content, and increasing fluid intake may relieve the symptoms. Methods to combat constipation without taking laxatives or frequent enemas are then taught.

Prevention of excessive fluid loss from skin, lungs, kidneys
Diaphoresis

Diaphoresis may result from heat, strenuous exercise, or fever. Even the healthy person who is perspiring profusely needs extra salt in the diet and should drink extra fluids. Some salty fluids are needed by the patient with a fever. Patients on salt-restricted diets and those with draining fistulas are especially likely to suffer from sodium depletion and should increase their salt intake slightly when perspiring profusely.

Diuretics

Diuretics are administered to encourage excretion of sodium and water in excess of body needs. However, potassium, which may not be in excess, is also lost with the increased urinary output. The patient receiving diuretics is encouraged to eat foods that are *high in potassium but low in sodium.* Good sources are bananas and other fresh fruits (see Box 7-6, p. 123).

Diuretics such as the thiazides may eventually cause sodium depletion; therefore the person receiving extensive diuretic treatment is taught to observe for symptoms indicating sodium depletion (p. 121) and to report these symptoms to the physician. Table 7-7 lists some commonly used diuretics.

Renal or circulatory impairments

Any patient with renal or circulatory impairment, as may occur in *shock, cardiac failure, renal insufficiency,* or *constriction of blood vessels* because of disease, *may develop a fluid and electrolyte imbalance.* Common imbalances include the following:

1. Edema from sodium and water retention
2. Hyperkalemia
3. Hyponatremia
4. Acidosis from inadequate tissue oxygenation
5. Overhydration

Patients with the above conditions are instructed to avoid taking too much food containing sodium, potassium, or bicarbonate. They should not drink carbonated beverages. The nurse must be especially aware of overhydration whenever intravenous fluids are being given to persons with renal or circulatory impairment.

Respiratory impairments

Patients with diseases such as emphysema that limit lung excursion and therefore limit exchange of O_2 and CO_2 should *not take carbonated beverages or bicarbonate of soda.* These substances tend to make the blood more alkaline than normal, and respiration is depressed in an effort to correct this imbalance. Depression of respiration is highly undesirable for patients with obstructive lung diseases. Early recognition and treatment of these lung diseases may help prevent acid-base imbalances.

Replacement Therapy

Fluids may be replaced by various routes as follows: orally (preferred route), by intravenous infusion, or by tube feedings (see Chapter 5).

Spacing of fluids

Fluids given by any route should be spaced throughout a 24-hour period. Not only does this practice help to maintain normal body fluid levels, but it also provides for better regulation of the electrolyte balance by the kidneys and prevents the end products of metabolism and toxic materials from being excreted in concentrated form. In this way the danger of renal damage, formation of calculi, and irradiation of the lower urinary tract are reduced. In addition, fluid spacing prevents overloading of the circulation.

Concentration of fluids

Infusing *concentrated solutions* rapidly and in *large amounts into the alimentary tract causes the blood volume to drop because large amounts of fluid are needed to dilute the substance. If the circulating volume becomes considerably depleted, irreversible shock can result.* The "dumping syndrome," which sometimes occurs after gastric resection, is caused by this abnormal shift of fluid. Concentrated solutions sometimes are given intentionally to reduce cerebral edema.

Concentrated intravenous solutions of sugar or protein should also be given slowly in small amounts because they require fluid for dilution. *Hypertonic saline solution may cause fluid to diffuse from the tissues to equalize the concentration of salt in the intravascular compartment.* The superior vena cava is the preferred site for infusions of hypertonic solutions, such as parenteral hyperalimentation, because of the rapid dilution by the larger amount of blood at this site. *If any of these concentrated solutions flows too rapidly into the vascular system, pulmonary edema can develop.*

Oral intake

Adults who have no circulatory or renal malfunction usually need between 1500 and 3000 ml/day of fluid, depending on the amount of food consumed. Patients who have anorexia and are not eating well require more fluid to maintain a fluid balance. Medical prescriptions for fluid restriction are usually given for patients who have fluid excess (edema or water intoxication) or whose kidneys are not functioning well.

A medical prescription may be given to the patient to "force fluids" or the nurse may make the decision that a large intake of fluids is desirable, such as for prevention of urinary stasis with its subsequent complications. No standard amount can be stated because the amount required depends on the following:

1. Size of the patient
2. Patient's circulatory and renal status
3. Amount of food intake
4. Amount of fluid loss (if appropriate)

It must be remembered that people with small or inelastic vascular systems become overhydrated easily. If the person has had a large portion of the body such as a limb removed either by surgery or trauma, the person's size is thereby decreased. If there is a question concerning the amount of fluids a patient should be encouraged to drink, the physician is consulted.

Parenteral fluids
Type of fluid

The nurse needs to know the common solutions used parenterally (Table 7-11). Some of the reasons for giving the more common intravenous solutions are listed in Box 7-12. Potassium chloride may be added to maintain normal intake of potassium and to replace losses. Ascorbic acid and vitamin B (Solu-B) may be added for nutritional purposes.

Whole blood, plasma, concentrated albumin, or plasma volume expanders can be given to substitute for blood protein loss and are used to establish normal blood volume

Table 7-11 Solutions for intravenous use

Type of solution	Cations (mEq/L)					Anions (mEq/L)			Glucose (g/L)
	Na$^+$	K$^+$	Ca^{++}	Mg^{++}	NH$_4^+$	Cl$^-$	HCO$_3^-$ lactate	PO$_4^-$	
5% Dextrose in water									50
10% Dextrose in water									100
Normal saline (0.9%)	154					154			
3% Saline	513					513			
Ringer's solution	147	4	4			155			
5% Dextrose in Ringer's lactate	130	4	3			109	28		50
Ringer's lactate	130	4	3			109	28		
Ammonium chloride (0.9%)					170	170			
Sodium lactate ⅙ molar	167						167		
5% Dextrose in 0.2% saline	34					34			50
5% Dextrose in 0.45% saline	77					77			50

7-12

Uses of common intravenous solutions

Solution	Use
Dextrose	
5% in water	Maintenance therapy when sodium not desirable
5% in saline (0.9%, 0.45%, 0.2%)	Maintenance therapy depending on desired amount of sodium
Sodium chloride (0.9%)	For large losses of sodium, as in loss of GI fluids, burns
One-sixth molar lactate	Replacement of sodium but not chloride
Ringer's lactate	Balanced solution containing Na$^+$, K$^+$, Ca^{++}, Cl$^-$

and prevent shock. *Dextran is* the most *generally accepted plasma volume expander.* It increases the oncotic pressure of the blood, thus increasing the reabsorption of fluid from interstitial spaces. This creates an increase in plasma volume. *Low-molecular dextran* decreases the viscosity of the blood, allowing greater blood flow through the capillaries; thus it is useful in treating cardiogenic, hemorrhagic, or septic shock. It may cause prolonged bleeding time and should not be used if renal disease with severe oliguria or anuria is present. The patient is monitored for signs of anaphylactic reaction (apprehension, dyspnea, wheezing, respirations, tightness of chest, itching, hypotension) when dextran is being given.

Intravenous fluids containing electrolytes should be run slowly to allow the body to regulate their use. The patient is monitored for signs of intoxication (excess of fluids or electrolytes) and satisfactory urinary output. *Increased serum potassium (hyperkalemia) can be particularly dangerous, because it may cause cardiac arrest.* Renal failure and untreated adrenal insufficiency are contraindications for the use of potassium. Many physicians do not start intravenous therapy until chemical analyses of the blood have been reported for the day.

Amount and rate of administration

The administration rate of fluids usually is ordered by the physician and depends on the patient's illness, the kind of fluid given, and the patient's size and age. Approximately 30 ml/kg body weight is needed to meet daily fluid requirements. Fever increases water needs by about 15% for each 1 degree Centigrade rise in a patient's body temperature.[11] If there has been an acute illness resulting in a significant fluid deficit, fluid is replaced at the rate of 1000 ml/kg loss in weight. The physician calculates water needs based on the amount needed to replace losses and the amount required to meet daily needs.

The usual rate for replacement of fluid loss is 3 ml/min; it is rarely run at a rate faster than 4 ml/min. If fluids are given continuously or if they are given when there is impaired renal or cardiac function, they are rarely run faster than 2 ml/min. Intravenous infusions that are run at too rapid a rate (sometimes seen when an infusion is "speeded up" to complete the treatment at a specified time) may result in overloading of the circulatory system and pulmonary edema. At the first signs of increased blood volume (p. 119) in any patient receiving an intravenous infusion, the rate of flow is reduced and the physician notified.

Relief of Thirst

Thirst, the first and most insistent sign of dehydration, sometimes causes the patient more misery than surgery or the symptoms of a disease. It may develop even when fluids have been withheld only for a number of hours. If fluid is being withheld intentionally, thirst often is made more bearable by explaining to patients why fluid is withheld and when they can expect to receive some.

Thirst usually is relieved rather readily by taking fluids. If fluids cannot be taken orally, the administration of fluids parenterally usually gives relief. It is often helpful to explain to the patient who is receiving an infusion that the procedure will soon provide some relief from thirst.

Mouth care allays some of the discomfort from thirst and may need to be repeated every hour. If patients can be trusted not to swallow, they may be given ice chips, which are held in the mouth and then spit out. Hard candies often give relief, even though they also must be expelled. The chewing of gum may help to relieve dry mouth.

Pronounced and continued thirst, despite the administration of fluids, is not normal and is reported. In the patient recently returned from surgery, *this kind of thirst may indicate internal hemorrhage, elevation of temperature, or some other untoward development. Thirst may also be an indication of hypercalcemia or the onset of diabetes mellitus.*

SUMMARY

1. Losses of fluid and electrolytes occur through the skin by diaphoresis and oozing from severe wounds or burns; from GI drainage and enemas; from the kidneys because of diuretic use and polyuria; from hemorrhage; and through the trapping of fluids by wound swelling, edema, ascites, and intestinal obstruction.
2. A low sodium level in the blood can indicate either a deficit of sodium or an excess of water.
3. Muscle weakness, anorexia, nausea or vomiting, diminished deep tendon reflexes, lethargy, cardiac arrhythmias, and ECG changes are symptoms of hypokalemia.
4. Nursing responsibilities for the person with hypercalcemia include active exercises for immobilized persons, increased fluid intake, prevention of urinary tract infections, and gentle handling to prevent pathologic fractures.
5. Monitoring fluid and electrolyte balance is particularly important in persons with an illness of the type that disrupts fluid and electrolyte balance, with medical-surgical treatments that result in imbalances, with considerable limitation of food and fluid intake, and in persons who have sustained significant loss of body fluids.
6. Assessment of fluid and electrolyte balance includes the monitoring of laboratory values, fluid intake, fluid output (urinary output, wound drainage, GI drainage, fluid from any body cavity, diaphoresis), daily weight, and urine specific gravity.

STUDY QUESTIONS

- What would you recommend to young women to prevent osteoporosis?
- How would you explain a low potassium diet to an elderly patient with a hearing deficit?
- Explain the relationship between vitamin D, parathyroid hormone, and calcium absorption.
- Why are the elderly at particular risk for dehydration?
- What is the best method to administer water, electrolytes, and nutrients? Why?

REFERENCES AND SELECTED READINGS

1. Ashby D: Balancing fluids and electrolytes in the PACU, *J Post Anesth Nurs* 2(2):114-116, 1987.
2.* Barta M: Correcting electrolyte imbalances, *RN* 50(2):30-34, 1987.
3.* Bowman M, et al: Effect of tube-feeding osmolality on serum sodium levels, *Crit Care Nurse* 9(1):22-28, 1989.
4. Brocklehurst JC, Allen S: *Geriatric medicine for students,* ed 3, New York, 1987, Churchill Livingstone.
5.* Calloway C: When the problem involves magnesium, calcium, or phosphate, *RN* 50(5):30-36, 1987.
6.* Felver L, Pendarvis J: Electrolyte imbalances: intraoperative risk factors, *AORN J* 49(4):992-1008, 1989.
7.* Gasparis L, Murray EB, Ursomanno P: IV solutions: which one is right for your patient? *Nurs 89* 19(4):62-64, 1989.
8.* Gershan JA, et al: Fluid volume deficit: validating the indicators, *Heart Lung* 19(2):152-156, 1990.
9. Goldberger E: *A primer of water, electrolyte, and acid-base syndromes,* ed 7, Philadelphia, 1986, Lea & Febiger.
10. Groer M, Shekelton ME: *Basic pathophysiology: a conceptual approach,* St. Louis, 1989, Mosby–Year Book.
11. Guyton A: *Textbook of medical physiology,* ed 7, Philadelphia, 1986, WB Saunders.
12. Innerarity SA: Electrolyte emergencies in the critically ill renal patient, *Crit Care Nurs Clin North Am* 2(1):89-99, 1990.
13.* Kee JL: *Fluid and electrolytes with clinical applications (programmed approach),* ed 4, New York, 1986, John Wiley & Sons.
14.* Mathewson M: Intravenous therapy, *Crit Care Nurs* 9(2):21-23, 26-28, 30-36, 1989.
15. Methany NM: *Fluid and electrolyte balance: nursing considerations,* ed 3, Philadelphia, 1987, Lippincott.
16. Miller L, Holloway N: Water intoxication: psychogenic hyperdipsia, *Crit Care Nurse* 9(7):74-78, 1989.
17. Plumer AL: *Principles and practice of intravenous therapy,* ed 4, Boston, 1987, Little, Brown.
18.* Rinardi G: Water intoxication, *Am J Nurs* 89(12):1635-1638, 1989.
19. Sabiston DC (editor): *Textbook of surgery,* ed 13, Philadelphia, 1986, WB Saunders.
20. Smith LH, Wyngaarden JB: *Cecil review of general internal medicine,* ed 4, Philadelphia, 1989, WB Saunders.
21.* Sommers M: Rapid fluid resuscitation: how to correct dangerous deficits, *Nurs 90* 20(1):52-59, 1990.
22.* Symposium on fluid, electrolytes, and acid-base balance, *Nurs Clin North Am* 22(4):749-872, 1987.
23.* Valle G, Lemberg L: Electrolyte imbalances in cardiovascular disease: the forgotten factor, *Heart Lung* 17(3):324-329, 1988.
24. Vander AJ, Luciano DS: *Human physiology: mechanisms of body functioning,* ed 5, New York, 1989, McGraw-Hill Book Co.
25.* Weldy NJ: *Body fluids and electrolytes (programmed presentation),* ed 6, St. Louis, 1991, Mosby–Year Book.
26. Woodward W, Woodward T: Management of dehydrating diarrhea, *Hosp Pract* 21(3):60, 63, 67-68, 1986.
27.* Yarnell RP, Craig MP: Detecting hypomagnesia: the most overlooked electrolyte imbalance, *Nurs 91* 54(7):55-57, 1991.
28.* Young M, Flynn K: Third spacing: when the body conceals fluid loss, *RN* 51:46-48, 1988.

*Recommended for student reading.

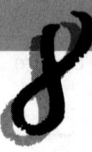

Acid-Base Imbalances

Mary Kay Lehman

After studying this chapter, the learner should be able to:

- Describe the mechanisms that maintain acid-base balance.
- Differentiate between metabolic and respiratory acidosis and alkalosis.
- Describe the causes and effects of metabolic and respiratory acidosis and alkalosis.
- Identify data indicating acid-base imbalances.
- Develop a nursing care plan for a patient with an acid-base imbalance.

This chapter reviews the regulation of normal acid-base balance. Mechanisms that regulate acid-base balance, including chemical buffer systems, the respiratory system, and the kidneys, are explored. Causes, effects, and interventions for acid-base imbalances are discussed.

Although the prescription of medical therapy to prevent and treat imbalances is the responsibility of the physician, nurses must carry out the following vital functions:

1. Recognizing situations likely to cause imbalances
2. Intervening to prevent imbalances
3. Carrying out preventive and therapeutic measures prescribed by the physician and monitoring patients' responses to these measures
4. Recognizing signs and symptoms of acid-base disturbances
5. Monitoring patients to prevent imbalances related to their specific conditions or treatments
6. Alleviating the effects of disturbances on the comfort and safety of patients

ACID-BASE BALANCE AND IMBALANCE

Regulation of Acid-Base Balance

Cells are sensitive to changes in the pH (hydrogen ion concentration) of body fluids. The maintenance of a stable pH of body fluids is essential to life. Normal body fluid is slightly alkaline (pH 7.35 to 7.45). A pH reading less than 7.35 is present in acidosis, and a reading greater than 7.45 is present in alkalosis. Limits of pH compatible with life are 7.0 to 7.8. The pH is kept relatively constant by the buffer systems in the body. Mechanisms that regulate acid-base balance include chemical buffer systems, the respiratory system, and the kidneys (Table 8-1).

Buffer system

A *buffer is a substance that can act as a chemical sponge,* either soaking up or releasing hydrogen ions so that the pH remains relatively stable. The main buffer systems of the body are the carbonic acid–bicarbonate system, the phosphate system, and protein. The carbonic acid–bicarbonate system is the most important clinically. If this buffer system is stable, the other buffer systems are stable.

Two types of carbonate are present in body fluids—carbonic acid (H_2CO_3) and bicarbonate (HCO_3^-). The ability of the body to keep the pH of body fluids within normal limits relies essentially on maintenance of the normal ratio of *one part of carbonic acid to 20 parts of bicarbonate* (Fig. 8-1).

Carbonic acid concentration is controlled by the lungs, because if carbon dioxide is retained in large amounts, more is available to combine with water to form carbonic acid in the following chemical reaction:

$$CO_2 + H_2O \rightleftarrows H_2CO_3$$

The amount of carbon dioxide expelled is varied by the rate and depth of respiration.

Bicarbonate concentration is controlled by the *kidneys,* which selectively retain or excrete bicarbonate, depending on body needs.

Respiratory control of pH

The respiratory control center in the brain responds to increases of carbon dioxide and hydrogen ions in body fluids. Rate and depth of respiration are in turn controlled by the respiratory control of pH as follows: (1) when pH decreases (more acid), respiratory rate and depth are increased, and there is greater excretion of carbon dioxide through the lungs; thus less carbon dioxide is present to produce carbonic acid by the reaction: $CO_2 + H_2O \rightleftarrows H_2CO_3$, and the pH increases toward alkalinity; and (2) when pH rises above the normal range (more alkaline), the respiratory center is depressed, rate and depth of respiration decrease, carbon dioxide is retained, and more carbonic acid is formed, moving the pH toward acidity.

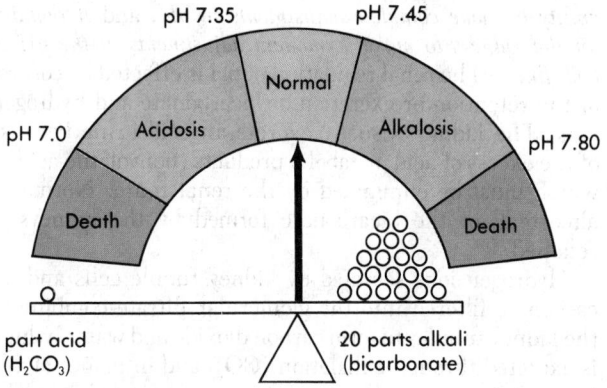

Fig. 8-1 Note that the relationship of 1 part carbonic acid to 20 parts bicarbonate maintains hydrogen ion concentration (pH) within normal limits. Increase in H_2CO_3 or decrease in HCO_3^- causes acidosis; similarly, decrease in H_2CO_3 or increase in HCO_3^- causes alkalosis. (Redrawn from Abbott Laboratories: *Fluid and electrolytes,* North Chicago, 1970, Abbott Laboratories.)

Table 8-1 Mechanisms regulating acid-base balance

	Action time	Effect
Chemical buffers in cells and body	Instantaneous	Combine with acids or bases added to the system to prevent marked changes in pH
Respiratory system	Minutes to hours	Controls CO_2 concentration in ECF by changes in rate and depth of respiration
Kidneys	Hours to days	Increases or decreases quantity of $NaHCO_3$ in ECF
		Combines HCO_3^- or H^+ with other substances and excretes them in urine

Table 8-2 Serum levels of pH, Pco₂, HCO₃⁻ seen in acidosis and alkalosis

| | Metabolic levels | | Respiratory levels | |
	Acidosis	Alkalosis	Acidosis	Alkalosis
Serum pH	Below 7.35	Above 7.45	Below 7.35	Above 7.45
Pco₂	Normal	Normal	Increases above 40 mm Hg (because of excessive retention of carbon dioxide)	Decreases below 40 mm Hg (result of excessive loss of carbon dioxide)
	Begins to decrease to less than 40 mm Hg to compensate	Begins to increase to more than 40 mm Hg to compensate		
HCO₃⁻	Decreases below 27 mEq/L	Increases above 27 mEq/L	Normal	Normal
			Increases to more than 27 mEq/L to compensate	Decreases to less than 27 mEq/L to compensate
Urine pH	Less than 6.0	More than 7.0	Less than 6.0	More than 7.0

Because carbon dioxide is constantly being formed as a product of metabolism, the concentration of carbon dioxide in the body must be continuously balanced between the rate of metabolism and the rate of pulmonary excretion. *The buffering capacity of the respiratory system is more than double that of all the chemical buffers combined.*

Renal regulation of pH

Both chemical buffers and respiratory regulation have limited ability to make complete adjustments in pH, and it remains for the kidneys to make permanent adjustments in the pH of body fluids. The renal regulation of pH is effected by control of the retention or excretion of bicarbonate and hydrogen ions. The kidneys usually excrete an acid urine because of the excess of acid metabolic products (nonvolatile acids), which must be eliminated by the renal route. Normally, almost all of the bicarbonate formed by the kidneys is retained.

Hydrogen ions secreted by kidney tubule cells and bicarbonate filtered into the glomerular filtrate combine in the kidney tubules to form carbon dioxide and water, which is excreted through exhalation (CO_2) and in urine (H_2O). In acidosis, excess hydrogen ions are secreted into the kidney tubules, where they combine with buffers and are excreted in the urine. In alkalosis, bicarbonate ions enter the tubules, where there is a lack of the hydrogen ions with which they normally combine to form carbonic acid; the bicarbonate ions combine instead with sodium or other cations and are excreted in the urine. Hydrogen ions can be exchanged for sodium and potassium ions in the kidney tubules; therefore excretion or conservation of hydrogen ions can result in imbalances of sodium and potassium.

Compensation

Carbonic acid (H_2CO_3) excess or deficit is referred to as *respiratory* acidosis or alkalosis, whereas base bicarbonate change is called *metabolic* acidosis or alkalosis. Changes in laboratory values are illustrated in Table 8-2.

Maintenance of the 1:20 ratio of carbonic acid to bicarbonate is crucial to keeping serum pH within the normal range. Actual amounts of both bicarbonate and carbonic acid may vary, but the pH remains normal as long as the 1:20 ratio exists. For example, if the Pco₂ indicator of carbonic acid rises, the bicarbonate rises to keep the normal

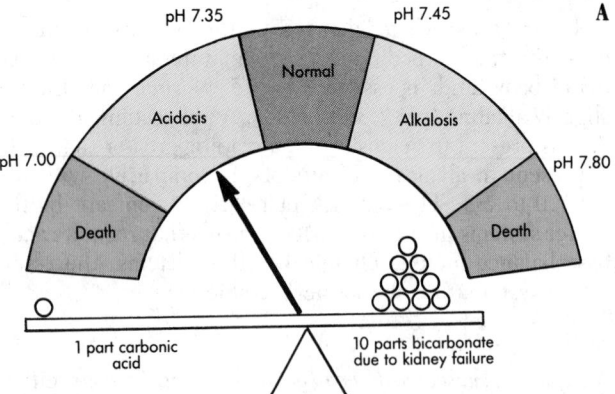

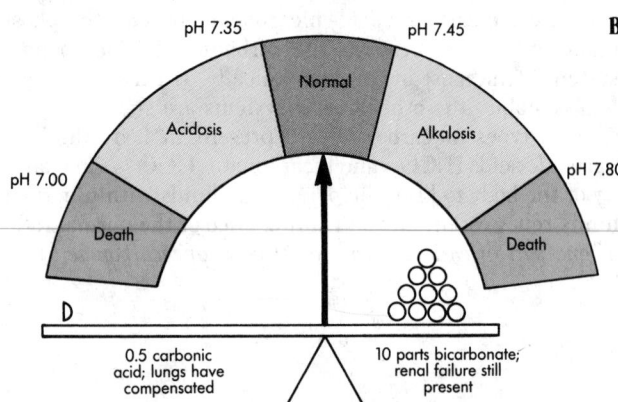

Fig. 8-2 A, Example of metabolic acidosis. Bicarbonate decreased because of renal failure. Carbonic acid to bicarbonate ratio is 10:1; acidosis is present. **B,** Example of compensation. Note that bicarbonate is still decreased, but now carbonic acid is also decreased. Ratio returned to 20:1; pH is normal.

Table 8-3   Types of acid-base disturbances and compensatory mechanisms

Disturbance	Physiologic causes	Method of compensation
Respiratory acidosis	Carbonic acid excess: lungs not removing sufficient CO_2 (hypoventilation)	Bicarbonate production by kidneys increased; bicarbonate retained and chloride excreted instead by kidneys; secretion and excretion of hydrogen ions in urine increased
Respiratory alkalosis	Carbonic acid deficit: lungs removing too much CO_2 (hyperventilation)	Kidneys increase excretion of bicarbonate ions
Metabolic acidosis	Bicarbonate deficit: retention of acid metabolites, diabetic ketoacidosis, excess acid intake (salicylate poisoning), loss of bicarbonate, hyperkalemia	Increased rate and depth of respiration cause increased excretion of CO_2 by lungs; formation of bicarbonate ions in the kidneys increased
Metabolic alkalosis	Bicarbonate excess: excess intake (sodium bicarbonate, carbonated drinks) or retention of bicarbonate Potassium depletion Loss of acid	Rate and depth of respiration decreased; lungs retain more CO_2; kidneys excrete bicarbonate

Table 8-4   Laboratory values in uncompensated and partially compensated acid-base disturbances

	pH	P_{CO_2}	HCO
Respiratory acidosis			
Uncompensated	Below 7.35	↑	Normal
Partially compensated	Move toward normal, but still ↓	↑	↑
Respiratory alkalosis			
Uncompensated	Above 7.45	↓	Normal
Partially compensated	Move toward normal, but still ↑	↓	↓
Metabolic acidosis			
Uncompensated	Below 7.35	Normal	↓
Partially compensated	Move toward normal, but still ↓	↓	↓
Metabolic alkalosis			
Uncompensated	Above 7.45	Normal	↑
Partially compensated	Move toward normal, but still ↑	↑	↑

ratio between these two substances intact. This effort of the body to maintain normal pH when acidosis or alkalosis occurs is known as *compensation.*

In compensation, the kidneys attempt to compensate for changes in blood CO_2 by making a corresponding change in blood *bicarbonate,* and the lungs attempt to compensate for abnormal changes in blood bicarbonate by making corresponding changes in blood CO_2. Compensation is an effort to maintain the normal 1:20 ratio. Figure 8-2 illustrates what happens in metabolic acidosis and how compensation of acid-base imbalance can occur.

Another compensatory mechanism that can be used by the body in the presence of acid-base problems is *shifting of hydrogen ions from the extracellular to the intracellular compartment or vice versa.* When there is an increased level of hydrogen ions (metabolic acidosis), these ions can be shifted into the intracellular compartment in exchange for *potassium.* This shift alone increases the pH in the blood. In addition, because the hydrogen ion concentration is now higher in the renal tubule cells, hydrogen will be excreted in exchange for the reabsorbed sodium. In *metabolic alkalosis,* hydrogen ions will be pulled from the intracellular compartment, and potassium ions will be shifted into the

intracellular compartment. Again, this shift alone will help to lower the pH. Also, because potassium ion concentration is now higher in the renal tubule cells, potassium will be excreted for the conserved sodium, and hydrogen ions will also be conserved. These *compensatory mechanisms can lead to hyperkalemia when metabolic acidosis is present* and *hypokalemia when metabolic alkalosis is present.*

It must be remembered that the buffer systems and the compensatory mechanisms provide for only temporary adjustment, and the underlying cause of the disturbance must be identified and corrected. However, the kidney can make permanent adjustments as seen in persons who have respiratory acidosis as a result of chronic obstructive pulmonary disease (see Chapter 24).

Types of Acid-Base Disturbances

There are two types of acidosis (respiratory and metabolic) and two types of alkalosis (respiratory and metabolic). Table 8-3 shows the four types that occur and their compensatory mechanisms. The *major effect of acidosis is depression of the CNS* as evidenced by *disorientation* followed by *coma* (Table 8-4). *Alkalosis is characterized* by *overexcitability of the nervous system,* and *the muscles may go into a state of tetany and*

8-1

Causes and effects of respiratory acidosis

Causes

Damage to respiratory center in medulla
Depression of respiratory center by drugs (narcotics)
Obstruction of respiratory passages: pneumonia, chronic bronchitis
Loss of lung surface for ventilation
  Atelectasis
  Pneumothorax
  Emphysema
  Pulmonary fibrosis
Weakness of respiratory muscles
  Poliomyelitis
  Hypokalemia

Effects

Rapid breathing
Visual disturbances
Behavioral changes
Confusion
Drowsiness
Headache
Coma

8-2

Causes and effects of respiratory alkalosis

Causes

Hyperventilation syndrome (caused by anxiety, hysteria)
Hyperventilation caused by:
  Fever
  Hypoxia
Pulmonary disorders
Lesions affecting the respiratory center in the medulla
  Brain tumor
  Encephalitis
Excess assisted ventilation
Hyperthyroidism

Effects

Lightheadedness
Paresthesias: numbness and tingling around mouth and in extremities
Inability to concentrate
Blurred vision
Dry mouth
Coma

---

convulsions. Acid-base imbalances always produce an imbalance of the body's electrolytes as well; therefore symptoms of these imbalances also occur.

Laboratory tests

Information about a patient's acid-base status is obtained by testing a sample of arterial blood (arterial blood gas) for the following values:

1. pH (normal 7.35-7.45): measure of hydrogen ion concentration.
2. P_{CO_2} (normal 40 mm Hg): partial pressure of carbon dioxide.
3. Bicarbonate (normal 27 mEq/L): sometimes reported as carbon dioxide content, which is a measure of all carbon dioxide dissolved in the blood as carbonic acid and bicarbonate. The approximate bicarbonate can be determined by subtracting 1 mEq/L from the carbon dioxide content.

The P_{O_2}, partial pressure of oxygen, is also measured and indicates how well the patient is obtaining oxygen, but does not indicate the acid-base status.

Table 8-4 shows whether laboratory values characteristic of the four types of acid-base disturbances are increased or decreased and the results of the body's compensatory efforts.

Carbonic acid excess (respiratory acidosis)

Any condition that decreases the rate of pulmonary ventilation increases the concentration of dissolved carbon dioxide and hydrogen ions and results in a build-up of carbonic acid known as respiratory acidosis. The *excess of carbon dioxide (hypercapnia) can cause carbon dioxide narcosis.* In this condition *carbon dioxide levels are so high* that *they no longer stimulate the respiratory center* (medulla) *but depress*

it. Associated with the decreased respiratory rate are lack of oxygen and hypoxia. *During respiratory acidosis, potassium moves out of the cells,* producing *hyperkalemia. Ventricular fibrillation may occur if the blood potassium level is greatly increased.* Box 8-1 contains a summary of the causes and effects of respiratory acidosis.

Treatment is aimed at increasing the alveolar ventilation rate to improve the exchange of carbon dioxide and oxygen. This objective is accomplished with bronchodilators, postural drainage, and chest clapping in patients with obstruction of respiratory passages. Because the respiratory center is narcotized by increased amounts of carbon dioxide, the lowered oxygen tension of the blood maintains respiration. If a patient whose respiratory drive is dependent on a low P_{O_2} is given large amounts of oxygen, the stimulus for breathing is removed, and respirations will cease. For this reason, oxygen is never given to patients with carbon dioxide narcosis. Low-flow oxygen (1 to 3 L/min) is given to a patient with chronic obstructive pulmonary disease who maintains a chronically high P_{CO_2}. Respiratory treatments are usually given using compressed air or room air instead of oxygen in these situations.

The major nursing responsibility is to recognize patients who have the potential for developing respiratory acidosis because of conditions that interfere with normal respiratory gas exchange. A patient whose airway is compromised by the presence of secretions must be encouraged to cough frequently or may need to have nasopharyngeal or tracheal suctioning.

Carbonic acid deficit (respiratory alkalosis)

Excessive pulmonary ventilation decreases hydrogen ion concentration and the formation of carbonic acid, leading to respiratory alkalosis. A common cause of respiratory alkalosis is *hyperventilation.* A person who hyperventilates blows off large amounts of carbon dioxide.

8-3

Causes and effects of metabolic acidosis

Causes
Increased acid production
  Ketoacidosis (uncontrolled diabetes mellitus, starvation)
  Uremic acidosis (kidney failure)
  Lactic acidosis (shock, respiratory or cardiac arrest)
Increased acid ingestion
  Salicylates, ethanol, ethylene glycol
Loss of bicarbonate
  Severe diarrhea
  Intestinal fistulas

Effects
Hyperventilation
  Weakness
  Hyperkalemia
  Disorientation
  Coma

8-4

Causes and effects of metabolic alkalosis

Causes
Loss of stomach acid
  Gastric suctioning
  Persistent vomiting
Excess alkali intake
Loss of potassium
Intestinal fistulas

Effects
Depressed respirations
Mental confusion
Dizziness
Numbness and tingling in extremities
Muscle twitching
Tetany
Convulsions

Respiratory alkalosis can be prevented in a person who is hyperventilating by administering a few whiffs of carbon dioxide or by having the person breathe into a paper bag and then rebreathe the exhaled carbon dioxide. Care should be taken in adjusting mechanical respirators so that the patient is not being forced to breathe too deeply or too rapidly.

The *patient may complain of lightheadedness and numbness or tingling of the fingers and toes.* If the *alkalosis becomes more severe, tetany and convulsions may be present.* Serum potassium levels will decrease because potassium moves into the cells as hydrogen ions move out in an attempt to correct the alkalosis. The causes and effects of respiratory alkalosis are shown in Box 8-2.

Treating the underlying condition usually effectively resolves respiratory alkalosis. Respiratory alkalosis becomes especially dangerous when it leads to cardiac dysrhythmias caused partly by a decreased serum potassium level. If a patient who is receiving assisted ventilation complains of dizziness or shows any signs of muscle irritability, it is likely that the depth of respiration is too great, and the respiratory rate of the machine should be decreased. If tetany is present, calcium gluconate is given intravenously. Renal function must be maintained to promote renal compensation of the alkalosis.

Bicarbonate deficit (metabolic acidosis)

When acid production or addition of acid by ingestion exceeds acid loss, bicarbonates attempt to buffer the acid load; however, the *bicarbonate supply* soon *becomes depleted* and a *bicarbonate deficit, metabolic acidosis, results* (see Table 8-3). Bicarbonate may also become depleted by losses of large amounts of alkaline secretions, such as intestinal secretions.

Increased acid production occurs during the development of ketoacidosis, uremic acidosis, or lactic acidosis. In *ketoacidosis,* glucose either cannot be used or is not available for oxidation. The body compensates for this by using body fat for energy, thus producing abnormal amounts of ketone bodies, which are fatty acids. Ketoacidosis also develops in anyone who does not eat sufficient food to meet daily needs and in whom body fat must be burned for energy. It is the reason why extremely low-carbohydrate or high-protein—zero-carbohydrate reduction diets are criticized by nutrition experts.

Lactic acidosis results when lactic acid is produced in large quantities such as in prolonged strenuous muscle exercise or when oxidation takes place in cells without adequate oxygen such as occurs in heart failure and shock. Uremic acidosis results from the *inability of the failing kidney to excrete the acid end products of metabolism.*

Hyperkalemia may result during metabolic acidosis; as the hydrogen ion concentration of the extracellular fluid increases, hydrogen moves into the cell and potassium moves out into the bloodstream.

The *patient in acidosis becomes hyperpneic* and *has deep, periodic breathing. Hyperventilation* represents an attempt to blow off carbon dioxide and to lower the P_{CO_2}, thus compensating for the acidosis. If the *condition is untreated, disorientation, stupor, coma, and death occur.* Box 8-3 shows the causes and effects of metabolic acidosis.

Metabolic acidosis is controlled by giving an intravenous solution of sodium bicarbonate or sodium lactate. Sodium bicarbonate sometimes is given orally if it can be retained. Treatment of the condition precipitating the acidosis is then instituted.

Bicarbonate excess (metabolic alkalosis)

When acid loss is greater than acid production, hydrogen ions are lost from body fluids and bicarbonate excess (metabolic alkalosis) exists. An excess may also occur with an excessive intake of sodium bicarbonate or other alkaline salt, especially if renal function is impaired.

Loss of potassium can also *lead to metabolic alkalosis.* When potassium is lost from the body, hydrogen ions move into the cells to replace the lost potassium, leaving a decreased hydrogen ion concentration in the extracellular fluid, that is, metabolic alkalosis (see Table 8-3).

In *metabolic alkalosis, breathing becomes depressed in an effort to conserve carbon dioxide for combination with hydrogen ions in the blood to raise the blood level of carbonic acid* (see Table 8-3). Box 8-4 lists the causes and effects of metabolic alkalosis.

Treatment consists of administration of sodium chloride or ammonium chloride. If the condition is associated with a loss of sodium chloride, potassium must be restored because it is lost with the sodium.

The nurse assists in maintenance of good respiratory function so that compensation can take place through this mechanism. *Careful monitoring of the patient for adequate renal function and safety precautions are important in the nursing care of patients with metabolic alkalosis.* Because convulsions may occur, precautions are taken for the patient's protection.

Persons must be cautioned against the excessive use of sodium bicarbonate to alleviate indigestion. Controlling the conditions that can cause metabolic alkalosis can prevent this imbalance from developing. If drug therapy is causing the alkalosis, these drugs should be discontinued, and others substituted where possible.

SUMMARY

1. Mechanisms that regulate acid-base balance include chemical buffer systems, the respiratory system, and the kidneys.
2. The respiratory control center in the medulla oblongata responds to increases of carbon dioxide and hydrogen ions in body fluids by changing the rate and depth of respiration.
3. The renal regulation of pH is effected by control of the retention or excretion of bicarbonate and hydrogen ions.
4. The major effect of acidosis is depression of the central nervous system as evidenced by disorientation followed by coma.
5. Alkalosis is characterized by overexcitability of the nervous system, and the muscles may go into a state of tetany and convulsions.
6. Any factor that decreases the rate of pulmonary ventilation increases the concentration of dissolved carbon dioxide, carbonic acid, and hydrogen ions and results in respiratory acidosis.
7. Excess pulmonary ventilation will decrease hydrogen ion concentration and thus cause respiratory alkalosis.
8. When excess organic acids are added to the body fluids or when bicarbonate is lost, a metabolic acidosis results.
9. When excessive amounts of organic acid substance and hydrogen ions are lost from the body, or when large amounts of bicarbonate or lactate are added, the result is an imbalance in which there is an excess of base elements, resulting in metabolic alkalosis.

STUDY QUESTIONS

- Why is low-flow oxygen (1 to 3 L/min) given to patients with obstructive pulmonary disease?
- Explain one common method of preventing respiratory alkalosis.
- Which acid-base imbalance occurs frequently in persons with diabetes mellitus? Why?
- What is the role of potassium in acid-base balance?
- Kussmaul's respirations are an indication of which acid-base imbalance? What does this breathing pattern indicate?

REFERENCES AND SELECTED READINGS

1.* Brenner M, Welliver J: Pulmonary and acid-base assessment, *Nurs Clin North Am* 25:761-770, 1990.
2. Goldberger E: *A primer of water, electrolyte, and acid-base syndromes*, ed 7, Philadelphia, 1986, Lea & Febiger.
3. Guyton A: *Textbook of medical physiology*, ed 7, Philadelphia, 1986, WB Saunders.
4.* Janusek LW: Metabolic alkalosis: pathophysiology and the resulting signs and symptoms, *Nurs 90* 20(6):52-53, 1990.
5.* Janusek LW: Metabolic acidosis: pathophysiology and the resulting signs and symptoms, *Nurs 90* 20(7):52-53, 1990.
6.* Lindell KO, Wesmiller SW: Using arterial blood gases to interpret acid-base balance, *Orthop Nurs* 8(3):31-34, 1989.
7.* Mathewson M, Mathewson R: Establishing acid-base balance, *Crit Care Nurs* 7(5):77-86, 1987.
8.* Mims BC: Interpreting ABGs, *RN* 54(3):41-47, 1991.
9.* Middaugh R, Middaugh D, Menk E: Current considerations in respiratory and acid-base management during cardiopulmonary resuscitation, *Crit Care Nurs Q* 10(4):25-33, 1988.
10. Shapiro BA, et al: *Clinical application of blood gases*, ed 4, St. Louis, 1988, Mosby–Year Book.
11.* Symposium on fluid, electrolyte, and acid-base balance, *Nurs Clin North Am* 22:749-872, 1987.
12. Taylor DL: Respiratory alkalosis: pathophysiology, signs, and symptoms, *Nurs 90* 20(8):60-61, 1990.
13.* Taylor DL: Respiratory acidosis: pathophysiology, signs, and symptoms, *Nurs 90* 20(9):52-53, 1990.
14. York K, Moddeman G: Arterial blood gases as easy as ABG, *AORN J* 49:1308-1329, 1989.

Classic

15.* Metabolic acid-base disorders. I. Chemistry and physiology (programmed instruction), *Am J Nurs* 77:1619-1950, 1977.
16.* Metabolic acid-base disorders. II. Physiology abnormalities and nursing actions (programmed instruction), *Am J Nurs* 78:87-108, 1978.
17.* Metabolic acid-base disorders. III. Clinical and laboratory findings (programmed instruction), *Am J Nurs* 78:443-460, 1978.

*Recommended for student reading.

9

Shock

Martha L. Allen
Gail Osterfield

After studying this chapter, the learner should be able to:

- Contrast three major types of shock.
- Describe early and late pathophysiologic changes that occur with shock.
- Describe organ damage that may occur with shock.
- Describe different methods of monitoring for shock.
- Describe methods of fluid replacement during shock.
- Identify effects of pharmacologic agents used to treat shock and nursing measures for patients receiving drug therapy.
- Describe therapeutic measures for shock other than fluids and drug therapy.

9-1	**Types of shock**	
	Hypovolemic	From loss of fluid from vascular system (through blood loss or fluid loss)
	Cardiogenic	From inability of heart to pump blood to tissues (decreased cardiac output)
	Vasogenic	From massive vasodilation (from interference with sympathetic nervous system or effects of histamine or toxins)

Shock is a syndrome characterized by hypoperfusion of body tissues. Any condition that prevents cells from receiving an adequate blood supply can interfere with their metabolism and produce shock.

Blood flow depends on pressure changes within the vascular compartment. Blood flows from areas of greater pressure to areas of lesser pressure. In the systemic circulation, the mean pressure is highest in the aorta, where the blood leaves the left ventricle, and lowest in the right atrium. In order for the necessary pressure gradients to exist so that blood can flow, the following three factors are necessary:

1. An adequate amount of blood for the heart to pump around the body
2. Ability of the heart to pump blood
3. Blood vessels with good tone, able to constrict and dilate to maintain normal pressure

Shock results from the disruption of one or more of these factors.

ETIOLOGY/EPIDEMIOLOGY

Shock may be classified as hypovolemic, cardiogenic, or vasogenic (see Box 9-1).

Hypovolemic Shock

Hypovolemic shock is the most common type of shock. *Any condition that reduces the volume within the vascular compartment by 15% to 25% can result in hypovolemic shock.* Common causes include the following:

1. Excessive blood loss: trauma (most common cause), gastrointestinal bleeding, coagulation disorders, surgery
2. Loss of body fluids other than blood: excessive diuresis (diabetic ketoacidosis or other hyperosmolar states), plasma loss from burns, fluid loss from excessive vomiting or diarrhea
3. Movement of fluid into another body space (third space), for example, bowel obstruction (up to 5 or 10 L may collect in bowel) or peritonitis (4 to 6 L may collect in peritoneal cavity within 24 hours)

Characteristically, the signs and symptoms of hypovolemic shock progress in direct proportion to the percent of blood loss (see Table 9-1).

Cardiogenic Shock

Cardiogenic shock results from the inability of the heart to pump blood sufficiently to perfuse the cells of the body. When stroke volume falls initially, cardiac output may be maintained by an increase in heart rate (Chapter 25); however, an increase in the heart rate may further damage the heart. As the heart rate increases, the period of diastole shortens and the period of systole remains relatively constant. Because the coronary arteries fill during diastole, their filling time is reduced. The heart works for longer periods and requires more oxygen and nutrients. Thus tachycardia can both increase the oxygen need of the heart and decrease its oxygen supply.

Although cardiogenic shock may be caused by various cardiac conditions including cardiac tamponade, restrictive pericarditis, pulmonary embolism, severe valvular disease, or dysrhythmias, the most common cause by far is myocardial infarction. Studies have shown that in most patients who die from cardiogenic shock, at least 40% of the left ventricle was damaged by a recent infarction or by a recent infarction plus a previous scar. In spite of improvements in managing cardiogenic shock, the mortality still remains above 80%. (Additional information on cardiogenic shock is given in Chapter 25.)

Vasogenic Shock

Vasogenic shock is caused by massive dilation of the blood vessels, resulting in disproportion between the size of the vascular space and the amount of blood contained. As arterial blood pressure falls, the difference between arterial and venous pressures decreases. Because blood flow depends on pressure differences, blood flow decreases. Blood pools in the blood vessels, resulting in decreased venous return to the heart. Cardiac output falls, and blood pressure decreases even further.

Initially in vasogenic shock, the extremities are warm because of vasodilation. However, as cardiac output decreases and tissue perfusion is reduced, *compensatory vasoconstriction occurs.*

Loss of vascular tone may result from a number of conditions. *Neurogenic shock results from interference with the sympathetic nervous system, which helps maintain vasomotor tone.* Spinal cord injury, spinal anesthesia, and rarely, brain damage are among the causes. *Anaphylactic shock occurs when there is massive dilation of the blood vessels from the direct effect on the vessels of a substance such as histamine.* Histamine, released by mast cells and basophils, has a powerful dilating effect on blood vessels, particularly capillaries. The endothelial cells that line the capillaries separate and expose the basement membrane, which is permeable to fluid and plasma proteins, resulting in hypovolemia.[11]

Septic shock, another form of vasogenic shock, may result from various infections, including those caused by both gram-positive and gram-negative bacteria, viruses, and fungi, although it most commonly results from gram-negative bacterial infections. The primary sites of infection are usually the urinary tract, respiratory tract, or blood. Organisms that ordinarily dwell in the gastrointestinal tract may cause sepsis and shock if they enter the bloodstream.

Septic shock is commonly seen in hospitals. Approxi-

Table 9-1 Clinical manifestations of hypovolemic shock

Parameter (for a 70 kg male)	Class I early	Class II moderate	Class III major or progressive	Class IV severe or profound
Approximate blood volume loss (ml)	Up to 750	750-1500	1500-2000	2000 or more
% of blood volume	Up to 15%	15-30%	30-40%	40% or more
Neurological/behavioral status	Slightly anxious	Mildly anxious, restless; muscle fatigue and weakness evident	Agitated, confused; progressive decrease in activity; progressive thirst evident	Stuporous, lethargic, unconscious; dilated pupils may be evident
Heart rate	<100	>100 Mild tachycardia	>120 Tachycardia	140 or higher Irregular pulse, decreased pulse amplitude
Blood pressure	Normal	Normal	Decreased	Severe hypotension
Pulse pressure (mm Hg)	Normal or increased	Decreased	Decreased	Decreased
Respirations	14-20, normal	20-30, normal	30-40, hyperpnea	>35, shallow, irregular
Urine output (ml/hr)	30 or more	20-30	5-15	Negligible
Capillary blanch test	Normal	Slight delay	Defined delay	No refilling observed
Skin	Pale pink, slightly cool	Slightly cold, pale	Cold and moist	Cold and cyanotic, mottled

From McQuillian KA and Wiles CE: Initial management of traumatic shock. In Cardona DV and others: *Trauma nursing from resuscitation through rehabilitation.* Philadelphia, 1988, WB Saunders.

mately one in every 100 patients in hospitals will develop sepsis, and of these 40 will develop septic shock.[40] Conditions that predispose to septic shock include the following:

1. Age, both the very young and the very elderly
2. Malnutrition
3. General debilitation
4. Immunosuppressive and steroid therapy
5. Chronic disease of the immune system (for example, AIDS)
6. Any surgery (for example, urologic or gastrointestinal surgery)
7. All forms of instrumentation (for example, intravenous lines, indwelling catheters, and diagnostic procedures)

Elderly men are particularly susceptible to septic shock because of the high incidence of prostatic hypertrophy in this group. They are more likely to develop urinary tract infections and to have urologic surgical procedures.

The mechanism by which septic shock occurs is not completely understood. Some believe that early in sepsis, fluid leaks out of the vascular system, and the resultant shock is simply a form of hypovolemic shock.[29] Others see the primary cause as faulty cellular metabolism from the direct effect of the toxin.[50] *Although the early pathophysiology of septic shock is not completely understood, it is known that when some organisms enter the bloodstream, they are destroyed by the immune system and a toxin is released.* This toxin, in some way, causes the characteristic symptoms of early septic shock (increased cardiac output, peripheral vasodilation, skin flushing, hyperthermia, increased renal output, and respiratory alkalosis).[40] As septic shock progresses and cardiac output decreases, it resembles other types of shock, with low urinary output, vasoconstriction, and cool moist skin.

PATHOPHYSIOLOGY
Early Stage

In the early stage of shock the body responds to hypoperfusion as it would to any other stressor. Many of the changes that occur are mediated through the sympathetic nervous system. *Stimulation of the sympathetic nervous system results in secretion of epinephrine and norepinephrine by the adrenal medulla.* Both alpha- and beta-adrenergic receptors are stimulated throughout the body. *Alpha receptors respond by causing vasoconstriction,* and *beta receptors respond by causing vasodilation (beta 1)* and *increased rate and strength of contraction of the heart (beta 2).* The skin and the abdominal organs, which are rich in alpha receptors, receive a decreased blood supply because of vasoconstriction. The heart and skeletal muscles, which are rich in beta receptors, receive an increased blood supply because of vasodilation. The heart beats more rapidly and more forcefully and the respiratory rate increases in response to beta stimulation, thereby increasing oxygen delivery to the tissues. All of the compensatory responses that are mediated through the sympathetic nervous system occur rapidly.

Another compensatory response, mediated through the renin-angiotensin system, occurs more slowly. As cardiac output decreases, the blood supply to the kidneys also decreases. The juxtaglomerular cells respond by secreting *renin,* which *acts upon a plasma protein, converting it* to *angiotensin I.* This is converted to *angiotensin II,* which has *two major effects:* it causes *vasoconstriction* and it causes the *adrenal cortex to secrete aldosterone. Aldosterone* causes the kidneys to *retain sodium and water,* and *secrete potassium, resulting in an increased blood volume.* The secretion of potassium may result in *hypokalemia* during this stage of shock. *Decreased cardiac output* results in *decreased hydrostatic pressure in the capillaries,* causing *fluid to shift from the interstitial space into the capillaries*. This also improves blood volume.

For a short period of time the compensatory mechanisms have a beneficial effect. The most vital organs, the heart and the brain, receive an adequate blood supply at the expense of the less vital organs, such as the kidneys and other abdominal organs. This allows time for the underlying cause of shock to be corrected. However, if the underlying problem is not or cannot be corrected, the compensatory mechanisms will not be able to continue to supply sufficient blood to vital organs and the compensatory mechanisms themselves will have a deleterious effect on the body. Shock will then progress to a later stage.

Late Stage

As shock progresses, blood flow to all body tissues becomes impaired. Cells in vasoconstricted organs receive *insufficient oxygen*, and aerobic metabolism is replaced by *anaerobic metabolism.* Energy, in the form of adenosine triphosphate (ATP), is produced very inefficiently. *Lactic acid cannot be metabolized* in the *absence of oxygen*, so it accumulates in the body, resulting in *metabolic acidosis. With insufficient ATP, the sodium-potassium pump fails; potassium leaves the cells and sodium and water enter them.* Organelles within the cells are damaged. Rupture of the cell wall of the lysosomes is particularly dangerous. They normally have an important role in phagocytosis and contain digestive enzymes. When their cell walls are destroyed, the digestive enzymes are released into the cell and autodigestion of the cell occurs.[21] This process can spread from cell to cell, resulting in organ death.

Acid metabolites cause dilation at the arteriole end of the capillaries (precapillary sphincter) and constriction at the venule end of the capillary (postcapillary sphincter), increasing *intracapillary hydrostatic pressure.* This results in *a fluid shift out of the capillary, further decreasing blood* volume. Increased capillary permeability may occur, particularly in septic shock, as large amounts of *histamine* and *serotonin* are *released in response to gram-negative toxins.* As proteins leak out of the capillaries, fluid follows and the blood volume is even further reduced. As the *blood supply to the kidneys is decreased, oliguria* or *anuria* occurs. The *blood urea nitrogen* (BUN) and *serum creatinine* levels rise. *Cellular damage releases potassium* into the blood, and the impaired kidneys are unable to excrete it. *Hyperkalemia*, which results, *depresses the contractility and conduction in the heart.*

Vasoconstriction of the splanchnic vessels in response to sympathetic stimulation *causes ischemia of the abdominal organs.* Of *particular importance* is the *pancreas.* In response to hypoxemia the pancreas produces and secretes a substance called myocardial depressant factor (MDF), which depresses contractility of the heart. As compensatory mechanisms fail, blood supply to the heart decreases and electrical and mechanical activity are impaired.

Box 9-2 summarizes the pathophysiologic changes in early and late shock.

9-2

Major pathophysiologic changes in shock

Change	Effect
Early stage (compensatory stage)	
Increased epinephrine and norepinephrine	Increased cardiac output to send more blood to tissues
Alpha and beta receptors stimulated	
Alpha effects	
Skin	Vasoconstriction and decreased blood supply
Beta effects	
Heart and skeletal muscles	Vasodilitation and increased blood supply and heart rate
Renin-angiotensin response	Vasoconstriction and secretion of aldosterone; sodium and water retention and potassium loss
Increased glucocorticoids and mineralocorticoids	Sodium and fluid retention to increase intravascular volume
	Potassium loss
Hypoxemia ($\downarrow$ Pa$_{O_2}$)	Hyperventilation; provides more oxygen to tissues; may cause respiratory alkalosis
Decreased hydrostatic fluid pressure	Fluid shifts from interstitial space to capillaries to increase vascular volume
Late stage (noncompensatory stage)	
Decreased blood flow to heart	Impaired cardiac pumping ability (decreased cardiac output); blood pressure decreases
Anaerobic metabolism	Acidosis; decreased adenosine triphosphate (ATP); failure of cellular N$^+$-K$^+$ pump (K$^+$ leaves cell, Na$^+$ and water enter cell); cellular damage
Arteriolar dilation and venule constriction	Fluid shift from intravascular to interstitial space
Decreased blood flow to kidney	Decreased kidney function (oliguria or anuria, retention of nitrogenous waste products)
Decreased blood flow to pancreas	Production of myocardial depressant factor (MDF)

Shock is a dynamic process with shock itself causing shock[15] as is depicted in Fig. 9-1. At some point a cycle begins that cannot be interrupted, and an *irreversible stage of shock* ensues. *Even if the primary problem that caused the shock is corrected and good supportive care is given, the patient will die.* However, the exact point at which shock becomes irreversible cannot be determined. Regardless of the patient's symptoms, all efforts should be made to reverse the progression of shock.

ORGAN DAMAGE
Kidneys

The kidneys contain about 2,400,000 nephrons, each of which is capable of forming urine. Each nephron is composed of a glomerulus, made up of capillaries and the collecting tubules (Chapter 33). Under normal conditions the pressure within the glomerulus is sufficiently high to force fluid out of the capillaries into the collecting chamber. *When the systolic pressure falls below 70 mm Hg, glomerular filtration ceases and the body is unable to rid itself of fluid and nitrogenous wastes.*

The tubules, which are perfused by the peritubular capillaries, suffer from the lack of oxygen and nutrients. *Acute tubular necrosis* develops. The tubular epithelial cells slough and block the tubules, causing loss of function of the nephron and resulting in *acute* renal failure.

The kidneys often are affected in the early stage of shock, even before systolic blood pressure falls, because the renal vessels respond to sympathetic stimulation by constricting. *A decrease in urinary output is often an early sign of shock.*

Brain

The brain is not affected early in shock. Because it does not contain alpha-adrenergic receptors, its vessels do not constrict in response to the increased levels of epinephrine and norepinephrine, and blood is shunted to the brain (and heart) at the expense of the other organs. As shock progresses and compensatory mechanisms fail, the brain does suffer inadequate perfusion. As *cerebral hypoxia* occurs, *restlessness and anxiety, followed by lethargy and coma, may be seen. Cerebral function may* also be *altered* by the *increasing acidosis* and the *accumulation of toxic substances.*

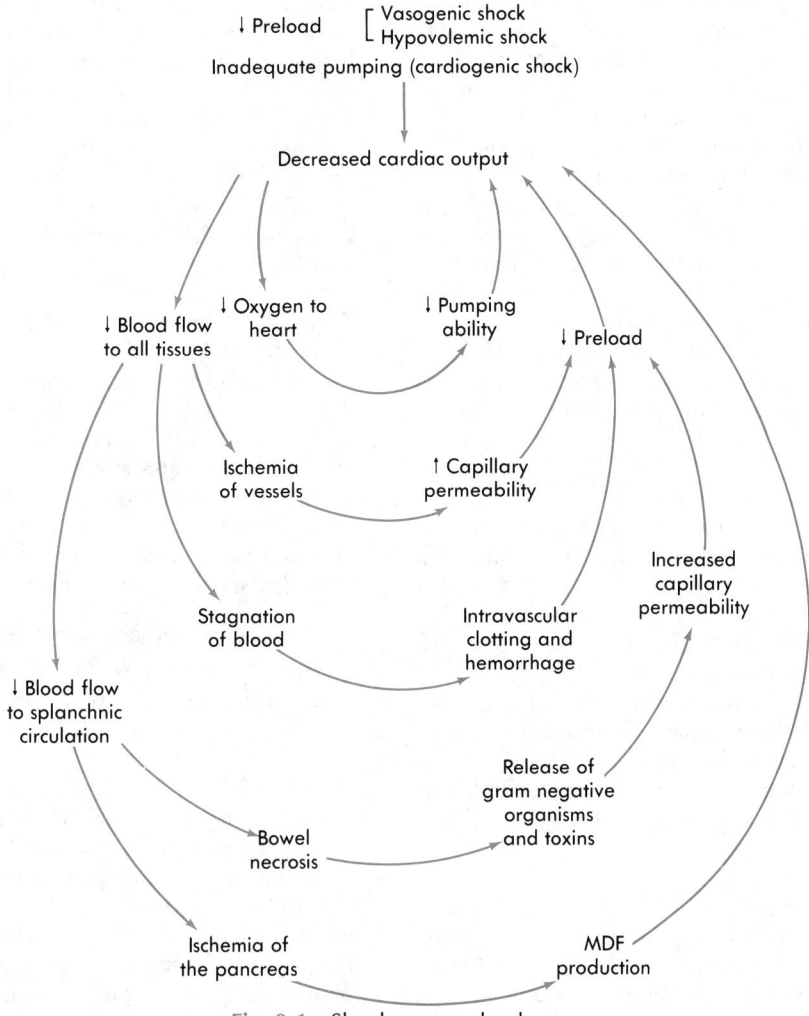

Fig. 9-1 Shock causes shock.

Heart

Although deterioration of cardiac function is a primary problem only in cardiogenic shock, the heart eventually is affected in all types of shock. As cited earlier, in the early stage of shock the heart is spared. *As shock increases, the pumping ability of the heart is affected and cardiac output decreases* (p. 141). As the heart muscle becomes increasingly hypoxic, it begins to show *disturbances of electrical activity.* Most *dysrhythmias have a detrimental effect on cardiac output*, and *some may be fatal.* In the *later stages* of shock, *deterioration of myocardial function* is probably the *most important factor* in the *further progression of shock.*[15]

Lungs

The effect of shock on the lungs has only been recently determined. During the Vietnam War, many victims of traumatic shock survived the early complications because of the use of massive blood transfusions and renal dialysis. The effect of shock on the lungs surfaced as a later complication. The pulmonary condition that results from hypoperfusion of the lungs has been known by a number of names, including shock-lung, white lung, and Da Nang lung. It is now known as adult respiratory distress syndrome (ARDS) (Chapter 24).

ARDS can result from any condition that causes hypoperfusion of the lungs, but is seen most commonly with traumatic or septic shock.[36] It is characterized by *increased permeability of the pulmonary capillaries* to *proteins* and *water*, resulting in *noncardiac pulmonary edema. Type 2 pneumocytes are destroyed, impairing* the *production* of *surfactant* that normally prevents collapse of the alveoli. *Alveoli either become filled with fluid or collapse*, and lungs *become stiff.*

In the early stages, *hypoxemia* results from impaired gas exchange and *hyperventilation* occurs, resulting in *hypocapnea* and *respiratory alkalosis.* Platelet aggregation in the pulmonary capillaries further damages the lungs. Hypoxemia persists despite administration of increasing amounts of oxygen. *As shock progresses, ventilation is impaired and carbon dioxide is retained. Respiratory acidosis* results. As hypoxemia increases, platelet aggregation increases, and a destructive cycle is initiated.

Gastrointestinal Tract

Sympathetic stimulation, which occurs early in shock, causes vasoconstriction and thus decreased blood supply to the organs of the gastrointestinal tract. Bowel function decreases, and *paralytic ileus* may result. If the *blood supply is severely impaired for a length of time, necrosis of the intestinal mucosa may occur. Microorganisms* normally *found in the bowel lyse* and release *endotoxins* when they are attacked by the leukocytes in the blood. *Shock*, from whatever cause, will now also have a septic component. The *gastric mucosa commonly ulcerates* when it *becomes ischemic*, which *may result in occult bleeding or massive hemorrhage.*

Liver

Sympathetic stimulation causes vasoconstriction in the liver. In the early stages of shock this can be beneficial. Normally the liver is capable of storing large amounts of blood in its veins. With *vasoconstriction* it can *release* up to *350 ml blood into the general circulation*, resulting in *improved cardiac output.*

With *continued sympathetic stimulation* and *decreased blood flow*, liver tissue is affected. In *septic shock* there is an *increase in oxygen uptake* and a *decrease in energy production* in the liver. All types of *shock affect the metabolic functions of the liver* including the *excretion of bile and cholesterol, gluconeogenesis, detoxification, and protein synthesis.*[23]

The sinusoids of the liver are lined with Kupffer cells, which are part of the reticuloendothelial system (RES). These cells are very powerful phagocytes and destroy the many bacteria from the colon that reach the liver by way of the portal system. *Normally, very few bacteria get past the RES. With the destruction of the RES, bacteria enter the general circulation and produce toxins*, which under normal circumstances would be detoxified by the liver. The liver can no longer perform this function, and *overwhelming infection and toxicity result.*

Blood

Disseminated intravascular coagulation (DIC) (Chapter 27) can be a cause or a result of shock. It is characterized by *intravascular clotting*, resulting in the *formation of microthrombi in the capillaries.* Some of the *factors that* activate *clotting factors in the blood* are *acidosis, stagnation*, and *procoagulant substances* such as *bacterial toxins.*[40] *Acidosis* and *stagnation of blood are present in all types of shock*, and bacterial toxins are found in septic shock. As clotting occurs in the capillaries, clotting factors in the rest of the body become depleted. Hemorrhage may then occur from incisions, punctures, the gastrointestinal tract, and other sites. A vicious circle ensues. Intravascular clotting results in even further decrease in tissue perfusion and acidosis. The *hemorrhage caused by DIC decreases* the *cardiac output even further* and *worsens tissue perfusion.* The mortality in patients with DIC in association with infection and shock is very high.

Nursing Process
Assessment

The signs and symptoms of shock are summarized in Table 9-2. There are few observable signs in the early stage; the patient may be restless and complain of feeling weak. Pulse and respiratory rates may be increased. Cool, clammy skin, decreased blood pressure, and lethargy or unconsciousness are signs of the later stage. The status of patients in shock is monitored by various methods. The parameters used in assessing shock appear in Box 9-3.

Hemodynamic assessment

Hemodynamic alterations are often the first sign of the onset of shock. The patient's hemodynamic status can be assessed at various levels (Fig. 9-2).

Vital signs

Objective data that are always indicators of physiological change are the vital signs. Any incremental change (e.g., 10 points or more in blood pressure or pulse) should be a clue to increase the frequency of monitoring of these clinical parameters. As shock progresses, the pulse becomes quite rapid and in the latter stages of shock becomes difficult to palpate. Irregularities in the pulse may develop as cardiac dysrhythmias occur.

Table 9-2   Comparison of signs and symptoms in early and late shock by body system

Body system	Early shock	Late shock
Respiratory system	Hyperventilation; $\uparrow$ minute volume; $\downarrow$ P_{CO_2}; normal P_{O_2}	Respirations shallow; breath sounds may suggest congestion; $\uparrow$ P_{CO_2}; $\downarrow$ P_{O_2}
Cardiovascular system	Blood pressure normal to slightly lowered; $\uparrow$ diastolic pressure; $\downarrow$ pulse pressure; cardiac output normal; tachycardia; mild vasoconstriction in hypovolemic and cardiogenic shock	$\downarrow$ Blood pressure; $\downarrow$ cardiac output; tachycardia continues; vasoconstriction worsens in hypovolemic, cardiogenic, and septic shock
Renal system	Normal to slightly depressed urine output; $\uparrow$ urine osmolality; $\downarrow$ urine sodium concentration Hypokalemia	Oliguria or complete renal shutdown; buildup of waste products Hyperglycemia
Acid-base balance	Respiratory alkalosis	Metabolic acidosis; respiratory acidosis
Vascular compartment	Fluids shift from interstitial space to vascular compartment; thirst	Fluids shift from vascular space to interstitial and intracellular space, causing edema
Skin	Minimal to no changes in hypovolemic and cardiogenic shock; warm, flushed skin in vasogenic shock	Cool, clammy skin in hypovolemic, cardiogenic, and septic shock; cool and mottled skin in other types of shock
Hematologic system	Release of red blood cells from bone marrow to increase vascular volume; platelet aggregation	Disseminated intravascular coagulation
Mental-neurologic system	Restlessness; alertness; confusion	Lethargy; unconsciousness
Gastrointestinal-hepatic system	No obvious changes	Perfusion decreases and bowel sounds may be diminished MDF production by hypoxic pancreas Liver dysfunction Possible bowel necrosis

---

9-3

Parameters for assessing status of patient in shock

Hemodynamic monitoring
Blood pressure (cuff and/or intraarterial)
Pulse
Central venous pressure
Pulmonary artery pressure
Pulmonary wedge pressure
Cardiac output
Electrocardiogram
Mixed venous O_2 saturation

Respiratory monitoring
Respiratory rate, depth
Breath sounds
Blood gases
  pH
  P_{O_2}
  P_{CO_2}
Percent O_2 saturation
Pulse oximetry

Fluid and electrolyte monitoring
Serum electrolytes
Blood lactate and pyruvate levels
Intake
  By mouth
  Intravenous
  Nasogastric
  Irrigation solutions
  Solution in medications
Output
  Urinary
  Gastrointestinal tract
  Sweating
  Dressings
Weight
Serum creatinine level
Blood urea nitrogen level
Serum and urinary osmolality
Urinary specific gravity

Neurologic monitoring
Alertness
Orientation
Mental acuity

Hematologic monitoring
Erythrocytes
Hematocrit and hemoglobin levels
Leukocytes
Platelets
Prothrombin and partial thromboplastin times
Clotting time
Fibrin degradation products

Other monitoring
Bowel sounds
Skin temperature

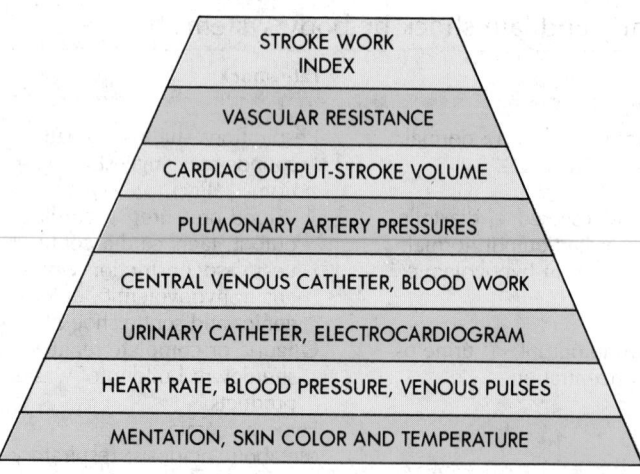

Fig. 9-2   Levels of hemodynamic monitoring. (From Ellerbe S: *Fluid and blood component therapy in the critically ill and injured,* New York, 1981, Churchill Livingstone.)

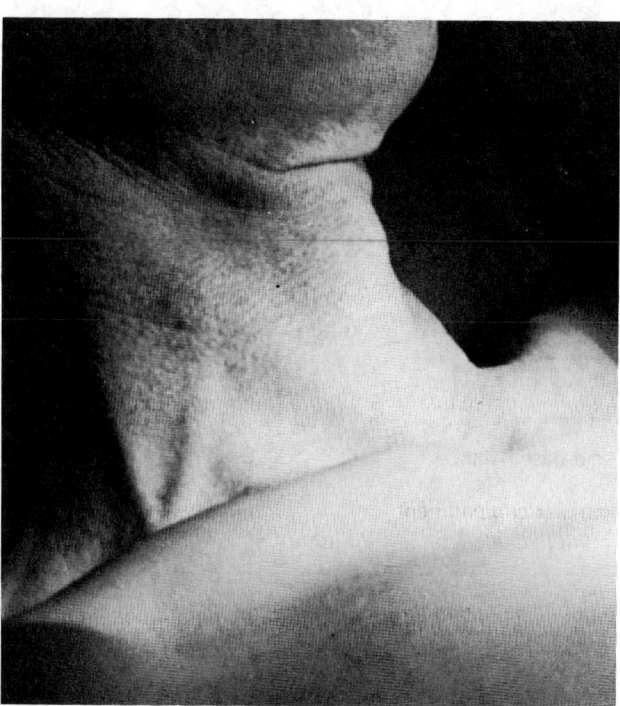

Fig. 9-3   Distended external jugular neck vein of a patient with right-sided heart failure. (From Daily EK, Schroeder J: *Techniques in bedside hemodynamic monitoring,* ed 4, St Louis, 1989, Mosby—Year Book.)

Early in shock the blood pressure may be normal or elevated because of compensatory vasoconstriction. Blood pressure can be heard without difficulty at this early stage. However, when blood pressure starts decreasing as the pulse rate is increasing, a heightened concern for clinical instability suggestive of *progressive shock* should be considered. The monitoring of vital signs at this point could be as frequent as every half hour to hour depending on the speed and magnitude of the changes being assessed. As shock progresses, the blood pressure may be difficult to auscultate, but it may be possible to obtain the systolic pressure by palpation. If intraarterial pressure monitoring is not instituted, Doppler ultrasound (Chapter 26) may be helpful in obtaining the blood pressure.

Venous pulsation in the neck is noted. Both the external and internal jugular veins should be examined. Generally, the external jugular vein is easier to see, but in some patients with heart disease the external jugular veins are occluded by fibrosis or are absent. Because of these potential problems, venous pulsation in the internal jugular vein may be a more reliable area to assess for signs of venous pulsation and right atrial pressure. Normally, *venous pulsations* are visible when the patient is lying flat but not when the head is elevated to 45 degrees (Fig. 9-3). Flat neck veins, when the patient is in a horizontal position, often indicate *hypovolemia,* common in most types of shock.

Central venous pressure

Central venous pressure (CVP) is a more accurate means of determining the fluid status of a patient in shock. CVP measures right ventricular filling pressure, which reflects venous return to the heart. CVP monitoring is most valuable in assessing status in patients with absolute or relative hypovolemia, including those with vasogenic, neurogenic, and hypovolemic shock. It is *less valuable* in *assessment in patients with cardiogenic shock, who may have intravascular fluid excess.*

To obtain an accurate CVP reading, a catheter is inserted into a major vein and threaded through the superior vena cava into the right atrium. The catheter is attached by a three-way stopcock to an intravenous infusion and a water manometer (Fig. 9-4). The intravenous solution (usually 5% glucose in water) is allowed to drip slowly into the vein to keep the vein open. When a reading is to be taken, the stopcock is opened to the manometer and the manometer is filled with the intravenous solution. The stopcock is then turned to the venous opening (the patient). The fluid level in the manometer should fluctuate with each respiration. The fluid is allowed to stabilize before a reading is taken, and the highest level of the fluid fluctuating in the column is used for the CVP reading. As soon as the reading is taken, the stopcock is turned to the solution position, and the infusion is continued.

For the CVP reading to be accurate, the patient must be relaxed, and the zero point of the manometer must always be at the level of the right atrium, which in most people is level with the midaxillary line. If the patient cannot be flat in bed, the zero point on the manometer is adjusted to the level of the right atrium in a sitting position. Any change in the patient's position requires that the zero point be reset. *The initial CVP reading and the position that the patient was in when it was taken should be recorded, because these will serve as a baseline for comparison with subsequent readings.* The patient should be placed in the same position for each reading, since even a slight change in position alters the CVP.

The normal values for CVP will vary with the use of different equipment; however, a range of 5 cm to 15 cm water is acceptable. It is important to note that a change

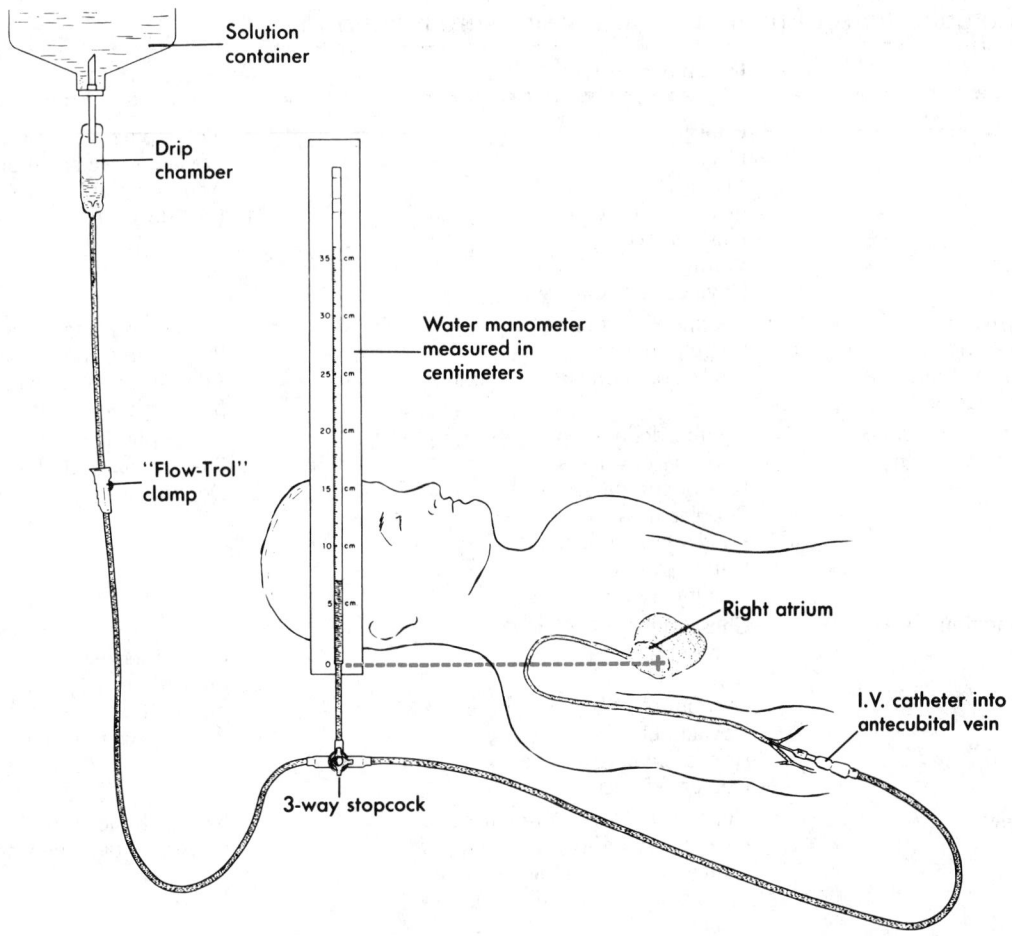

Fig. 9-4   Measurement of central venous pressure (CVP) using water manometer. Zero point on manometer is at level of midright atrium, and CVP reading is 7 cm of water.

or a trend in the CVP is more important than the actual numeric value.

Central venous catheters can also be used to obtain blood samples, to assess venous oxygen saturation determinations, and to administer fluids. The catheter insertion site should be kept scrupulously clean to minimize the possibility of phlebitis. Patient movement is not restricted as long as the catheter and tubing are secured adequately and intravenous flow is maintained.

Pulmonary artery pressures

The status of the left side of the heart can best be evaluated by the measurement of pulmonary artery pressure (PAP) *and pulmonary capillary wedge resection* (PCWP). A mean PAP of less than 10 mm Hg may indicate decreased blood volume resulting in decreased preload in the left ventricle. A mean PAP of more than 20 mm Hg may indicate poor myocardial contractility and left ventricular overload. These pressures are measured with a special triple-lumen balloon-tipped (Swan-Ganz) catheter (Fig. 9-5). The catheter is inserted into a vein, usually the *subclavian,* and advanced to the *right atrium.* The balloon is inflated and carried to the right ventricle and then to the pulmonary artery by the blood flow. The balloon is then deflated and the tip of the catheter

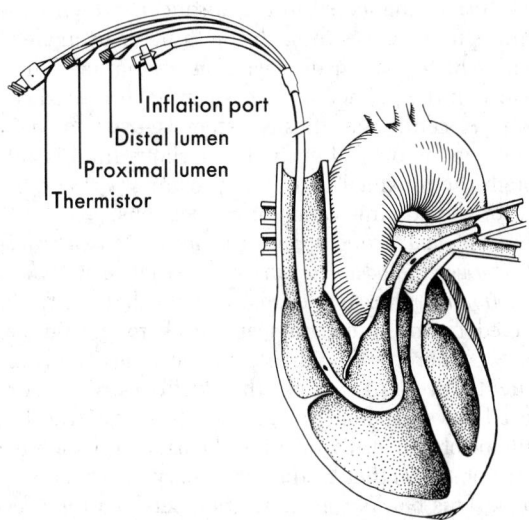

Fig. 9-5   Placement of Swan-Ganz catheter.

Table 9-3   Complications of pulmonary artery pressure monitoring

Complication	Indications	Interventions
Infection	Chills Headache Malaise Generalized aching Flushed face Warm skin Elevated temperature	1. Notify physician immediately. 2. Prepare for removal of catheter. 3. Administer antibiotics as ordered. 4. Provide symptomatic relief.
Ventricular arrhythmias: premature ventricular contractions, or short runs of ventricular tachycardia	"Skipped heart beats" Irregular pulse PVC's noted on cardiac monitor	1. Notify physician immediately. 2. Prepare for repositioning of catheter. 3. Administer antiarrhythmic drugs if problem persists after repositioning.
Sustained ventricular tachycardia, or ventricular fibrillation	Lightheadedness, progressing to loss of consciousness Loss of consciousness Pulselessness Dysrhythmia noted on cardiac monitor Respiratory arrest	1. Notify physician immediately. 2. Prepare for repositioning of catheter. 3. Defibrillate.
Pulmonary infarction	Chest pain Hemoptysis Fever Friction rub Elevated LDH Area of opacity on chest x-ray film Decreased PaO$_2$	1. Notify physician immediately. 2. Administer oxygen. 3. Prepare for repositioning or removal of catheter. 4. Provide symptomatic relief.
Valvular damage	Depends on extent of damage Patient may be asymptomatic, or may develop symptoms of congestive heart failure or new murmur	1. Notify physician of development of new murmur or new symptoms.

Modified from Asheervath J and Blevins D: *Handbook of clinical nursing practice,* Norwalk, Conn, 1986, Appleton-Century-Crofts.

is left in the *pulmonary artery.* The opening at the tip of the catheter communicates with the distal port. The lumen from the proximal port opens into the right atrium. The distal port is connected to a transducer, which converts the pressure it senses through the catheter to an electrical signal, which is then displayed on a monitor. Thus the pressure in the pulmonary artery can be measured continuously. A continuous flush system is used to maintain patency of the distal lumen. Intravenous fluid is infused through the proximal port. The proximal port can also be used for the administration of medications.

In individuals without lung or pulmonary vascular disease, *PAP is a good indicator of how well the left side of the heart is functioning.* Pressure changes in the left ventricle are reflected in the left atrium and back to the pulmonary artery. If there is any disease in the lungs, however, as frequently occurs in shock, the PAP does not accurately reflect left ventricular pressure. In this case, the PCWP should be obtained. By inflating the balloon, which is near the tip of the catheter, the pulmonary artery can be occluded. This blocks communication between the pressure in the pulmonary artery and the lumen of the catheter, allowing for pressure that is ahead of the occluded artery to be transmitted through the catheter. The PCWP is identical to the left atrial pressure.

The nurse caring for the patient with pulmonary artery pressure monitoring must be aware of the common complications that can occur with this type of invasive monitoring (Table 9-3). The appearance of either a *right ventricular* or *PCWP waveform* on the monitor can have serious consequences for the patient. Dislodgement of the tip of the catheter from the pulmonary artery into the right ventricle can result in the occurrence of *premature ventricular beats* or even *ventricular tachycardia.* Progression of the catheter into a small vessel in the pulmonary vasculature can occlude the vessel and result in *pulmonary infarction.* Prolonged inflation of the balloon can have the same effect. The nurse must be able to distinguish the normal PAP waveform from both right ventricular and PCWP waveforms (Fig. 9-6). It is essential that sterile technique be maintained during the insertion of the PAP catheter and during dressing changes.

Intraarterial assessment

Intraarterial monitoring is usually instituted along with pulmonary artery pressure monitoring. A catheter is inserted into a radial, brachial, or femoral artery and attached to a transducer in much the same way as the pulmonary artery catheter (Fig. 9-7). Because this is a high-pressure system, hemorrhage is a possible complication, and the

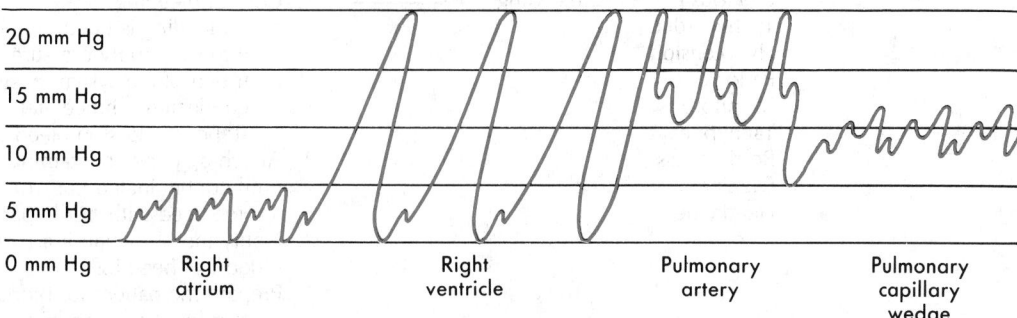

Fig. 9-6 Characteristic waveforms of pulmonary artery pressure monitoring. (From Asheervath J, Blevins D: *Handbook of clinical nursing practice,* 1986, Norwalk, Ct, Appleton-Century-Crofts.)

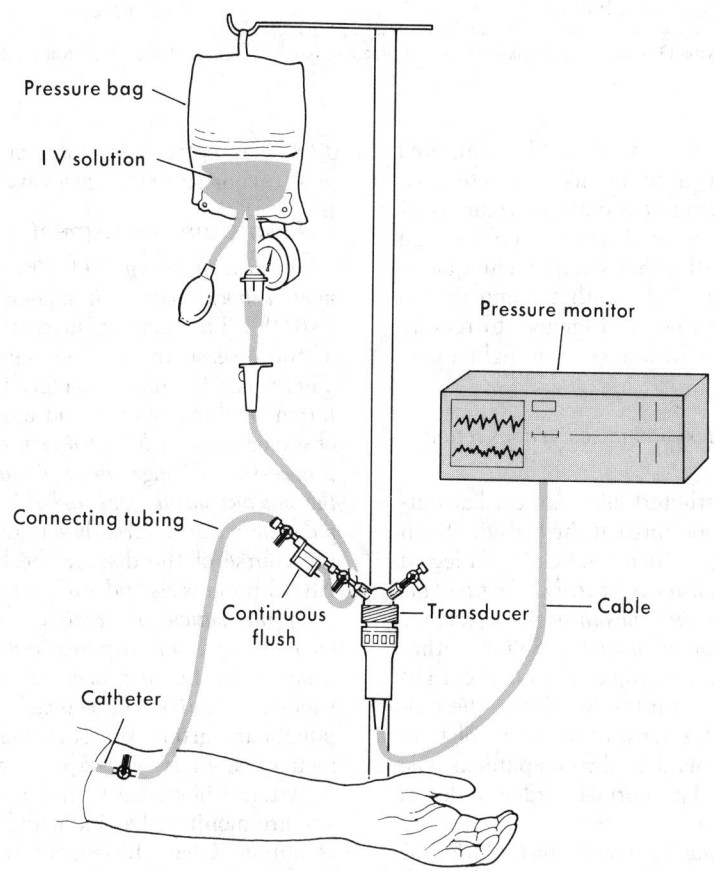

Fig. 9-7 Connections between intraarterial catheter, transducer, monitor, and fluid. (From Daily EK, Schroeder J: *Techniques in bedside hemodynamic monitoring,* ed 4, St Louis, 1989, Mosby–Year Book.)

Table 9-4   Complications of intraarterial pressure monitoring

Complication	Indications	Intervention

Hemorrhage	Obvious excessive bleeding
	Tachycardia
	Hypotension
	Pallor
	Diaphoresis
	Tachypnea
	Restlessness
	Dizziness
	Headache
		1. Control bleeding
		  a. If bleeding is occurring at the puncture site, apply pressure.
		  b. If part of the system has become disconnected, immediately turn the stopcocks to stop bleeding.
		2. Attach a syringe containing sterile saline until contaminated parts of the system are replaced with sterile parts.
		3. Notify the physician if a large amount of blood has been lost.
		4. Prepare the patient for blood replacement if loss has been large.

Thrombus or embolus	Pallor, loss of pulse, and coolness of skin distal to the site of the thrombus Pain	1. Notify the physician immediately. 2. Instruct patient to lie quietly. 3. Prepare to administer O_2.
Infection of catheter site	Redness and warmth at the site Possible fever	1. Notify the physician. 2. Prepare for removal of the catheter. 3. Send the catheter tip for culture.
Bacteremia	High fever Chills	1. Notify the physician. 2. Prepare for removal of the catheter.

Modified from Asheervath J and Blevins D: *Handbook of clinical nursing practice,* Norwalk, Conn, 1986, Appleton-Century-Crofts.

insertion and connections in the system must be monitored frequently. The extremity distal to the insertion site must be monitored for signs of arterial occlusion (color, temperature, movement, presence or absence of pulses, and pain) (Table 9-4). It is essential that sterile technique be maintained during insertion of the catheter and during dressing changes. A patient who is ill enough to require hemodynamic monitoring has little reserve to fight infection.

Cardiac output, cardiac index, and mixed venous return assessment

Some pulmonary artery catheters allow for cardiac output and cardiac index to be monitored at the bedside. Such catheters have a port through which fluid can be injected into the right atrium. *A thermistor is located at the tip of the catheter and attached to a wire that runs through the catheter and is attached to a cardiac output computer.* Saline, either iced or at room temperature, is injected into the right atrium. The solution travels with the blood into the pulmonary artery. The thermistor senses the extent of temperature change, and from this data the computer is able to calculate cardiac output. The normal cardiac index is 2.5 to 3.5 L/min/m².

Another version of the pulmonary artery catheter called the fiberoptic flow directed pulmonary artery catheter allows for continuous evaluation of the balance between supply of oxygen to the tissues and consumption of oxygen by the tissues. Values that reflect a normal balance between supply of oxygen and oxygen consumption are 0.68 to 0.77. High values (greater than 0.77) are associated with conditions of reduced oxygen consumption in the tissues (e.g., septic shock, hypothermia, deep coma). Low values (less than 0.68) may be seen in states of high oxygen consumption (e.g., major surgery, aggressive exercise).

Respiratory assessment

As cited earlier (p. 144), hypoperfusion of the lungs, common in shock, may result in adult respiratory distress syndrome (ARDS). This may be suspected very early in the course of the disease from changes in the patient's mentation. There may be minor changes in orientation, unusual interpersonal exchanges, and mood changes. The patient is observed for *cough* and *dyspnea,* which develop as ARDS progresses. *Changes in respiratory rate* and in the *color of the mucous membranes and skin are important indicators of pulmonary status.* Breath sounds are auscultated. Early in the course of the disease the lungs may be clear, but as ARDS progresses, *rales and rhonchi may be heard.*

If the patient is receiving mechanical ventilation, the amount of pressure required to deliver a specific tidal volume is noted. As the *lungs* become *increasingly* stiff, the *pressure required to deliver the volume increases.* With ARDS, the pulmonary artery pressure may rise, although the pulmonary capillary wedge pressure remains normal.[36]

Arterial blood gases may provide valuable information and are monitored as indicated depending on the patient's condition. Characteristically with ARDS, the PaO_2 falls, in spite of ventilation with increasing amounts of oxygen, because of *physiologic shunting* of blood through the lungs to the left side of the heart. Shunting occurs because many alveoli are either collapsed or filled with fluid, and diffusion cannot occur. In the earlier stages of ARDS, when a sufficient number of alveoli are functioning, the $PaCO_2$ is usually normal or more likely low because of the rapid diffusion of CO_2 and of hyperventilation that results from hypoxia. However, as the number of functioning alveoli decreases, the $PaCO_2$ increases.

Arterial blood gas determinations are also used to assess the *acid-base balance* of the patient in shock. In the early stages of shock, mild *respiratory alkalosis* is common from *hyperventilation* that is part of the stress response. As shock progresses and tissues become progressively hypoxemic, *anaerobic metabolism* takes place and *metabolic acidosis* occurs. In the *advanced stages of shock,* when *respirations decrease* and ARDS *becomes progressively worse, respiratory acidosis* may also *develop.*

Fluid and electrolyte assessment

The urinary output and the CVP most accurately reflect fluid status. An indwelling urinary catheter is usually inserted, and the urine output is measured hourly. Other output, such as gastrointestinal drainage, wound drainage, or perspiration, is measured or estimated as accurately as possible. *Body weight* often gives a more accurate assessment of fluid changes than the measurement of intake and output; however, this can be an inaccurate determinant of intravascular volume when "third spacing" of fluid occurs. *Noting* the presence of *edema, auscultating* the *chest* for the *presence of fluid,* and *measuring* the *abdominal girth* for the development of *ascites are means of assessing fluid collection in the third spaces.*

In the early stages of shock, the serum potassium concentration may be abnormally low as a result of increased levels of aldosterone in response to stress. However, as shock progresses, the serum K^+ level may become abnormally high as damaged cells release K^+. As urinary output falls, the body is unable to eliminate the excess amounts of K^+ that are accumulating in the serum. If K^+ is administered in the early stage of shock, it is extremely important that the urinary output and serum electrolytes be monitored frequently so that *hyperkalemia* can be *prevented* or *treated early* should it occur.

The concentration of other serum electrolytes may be abnormal as a result of acid-base abnormalities, altered renal function, or fluid therapy. Serum enzymes may be elevated because of ischemia and damage to the heart, liver, and pancreas.

Neurologic assessment

In shock, the brain may be adversely affected by hypoxia, acid-base imbalance, or toxins. Often, *subtle changes in mentation are the earliest signs of cerebral hypoxia.* The patient is observed for *increasing restlessness.* Sedation should not be given until the patient's status has been assessed further and it has been determined that the restlessness does not have an organic cause. In the *late stages, when perfusion of the brain is severely impaired, loss of consciousness* occurs. Vital signs and arterial blood gas determinations can aid in assessing the cause of subtle neurologic changes.

Hematologic assessment

The *hemoglobin* and *hematocrit* levels are valuable tools for assessing blood loss in *hypovolemic shock secondary to hemorrhage.* It must be remembered, however, that the *hemoglobin and hematocrit levels do not drop immediately with loss of an excessive amount of blood,* because *plasma is lost*

along with the blood cells. The *blood* that remains *in the intravascular compartment initially* will *have a normal concentration of RBCs in less plasma* and *the hematocrit will be increased.* Because the kidneys retain water in response to blood loss, the blood becomes more dilute and there is a decrease in the hemoglobin and hematocrit concentrations.

Patients in shock are assessed for the development of DIC. The nurse may be the first to observe that the patient is bleeding for an excessively long time after a venipuncture or that blood is oozing from an incision. If DIC is suspected, laboratory studies are initiated, then clotting factors (including fibrinogen and platelet counts) are decreased, prothrombin time and partial thromboplastin time (aPTT) are prolonged, and fibrin degradation products are increased.

Other assessment

Abdominal assessment is important in the patient in shock. Decreased blood flow to the intestines may result in decreased peristalsis or paralytic ileus (Chapter 31). *Decreased or absent bowel sounds are noted. Gastric drainage and stools are assessed for occult blood* because of the *high incidence* of *gastrointestinal tract bleeding* with *shock.*

Data analysis: nursing diagnoses

Nursing diagnoses are determined from analysis of patient data. Possible nursing diagnoses for the person with shock include, but are not limited to, the following:

Diagnostic title	Possible etiologies
Cardiac output, decreased	Myocardial hypoxia, myocardial depressant factor
Fluid volume deficit	Blood loss, increased capillary permeability, vasodilation
Gas exchange, impaired	Decreased lung compliance, interstitial edema
Tissue perfusion, altered cardiopulmonary	Hypovolemia, decreased cardiac output, redistribution of blood
Breathing pattern, ineffective	Inadequate perfusion of respiratory muscles
Airway clearance, ineffective	Decreased energy, endotracheal intubation
Anxiety	Threat of death
Oral mucous membrane, altered	Endotracheal intubation
Infection, high risk for	Invasive monitoring, Foley catheterization, decreased immune response
Sleep pattern disturbance	Intensity of nursing care
Activity intolerance	Imbalance between oxygen supply and demand

Planning: expected patient outcomes

Expected patient outcomes for the person with shock may include, but are not limited to, the following:

1. Cardiac output determination using thermodilution techniques confirms that the cardiac output is normal.
2. Intravascular volume (hemoglobin and hematocrit) returns to normal; urinary output and specific gravity are within normal limits.
3. Arterial blood gases (PO_2 and PCO_2) are within normal limits.

4. Vital signs (blood pressure, pulse) indicate normal tissue perfusion.
5. Respiratory rate and tidal volume are within normal limits.
6. Airway remains free from secretions.
7. Patient and significant others remain free of avoidable anxiety.
8. Oral mucous membrane remains moist and intact.
9. Patient is free from infection.
10. Patient sleeps for undisturbed periods of time.
11. Patient tolerates activity involved in care without an increase in pulse rate of more than 20 per minute.

Implementation
Assisting with achievement of therapeutic goals

Treatment of shock will vary to some extent, depending on the cause of the shock, the organ systems affected, and the preexisting condition of the patient. *In the early, acute phase of shock, the major role of the nurse is continuous assessment of the patient's clinical status and assisting with administration of therapies necessary to stabilize the patient's condition.*

Fundamentally, the same priorities that exist for treating any life-threatening emergency hold true for shock. The priorities for shock management are as follows:

1. Airway: A patent airway must be maintained to maximize oxygen uptake and carbon dioxide removal. To accomplish this, a nasal or oral airway may be inserted. When respiratory failure is a high potential, the airway is secured with an endotracheal tube.
2. Breathing: Oxygen is administered immediately at the level ordered. This may include preparations to ventilate the patient by mechanical ventilation. These measures support breathing and enhance ventilation and gas exchange between the airways and the circulation.
3. Circulation: The pump (the heart) is supported by the administration of fluids including blood to increase blood volume, improve cardiac output, and maximize oxygen transport to the cells. Vasoactive and cardiogenic drugs may also be prescribed to enhance cardiovascular functioning and oxygen transport to the cells.
4. Diagnosis: Shock can be treated most effectively if the underlying cause can be determined and treated. For example, if the cause of shock is hypovolemia secondary to massive bleeding, efforts will be made to find the site of the bleeding and stop it, if possible. Blood and fluids will be used to improve intervascular volume and cardiac output. This will then improve exchange of oxygen and carbon dioxide at the cellular level. If the cause of shock is sepsis, antibiotics will be administered intravenously, and if the cause is anaphylaxis, epinephrine is given.

Assisting with fluid replacement

The need to administer fluids to the patient with hypovolemic shock is obvious. At times, fluid replacement is the only therapy needed in this type of shock. Vasogenic and septic shock are accompanied by hypovolemia because fluid is leaking out of the capillaries. Fluid therapy is always a part of treatment in shock. In cardiogenic shock it is especially important to insert a pulmonary artery catheter to determine how much fluid of any type can safely be given.[41] For example, when the pulmonary capillary wedge pressure (PCWP) that reflects pressure and functioning of the left ventricle is low, fluid therapy may be beneficial in improving heart function.

What is less obvious is that fluid therapy rather than fluid restriction or removal of fluid is occasionally required in *cardiogenic shock.* Current therapies are focusing on *improving oxygen delivery to vital organs during shock to the point that the supply of oxygen will exceed the demand. Two ways this can be accomplished* are by *increasing the hemoglobin levels* (giving red blood cells) and by *increasing the cardiac output* from *the left side of the heart* (increased cardiac index through increasing volume in the left ventricle at the time the heart contracts). Because even patients with cardiogenic shock can have a problem with low circulating blood volume, "fluid challenges" or limited, quick intravenous infusions of crystalloids or colloids (e.g., packed red blood cells) may be given to improve oxygen delivery. Such fluid challenges tend to be no greater than 200 ml and are rarely given without exact monitoring of cardiac functioning using a pulmonary artery catheter.[2,41]

See Table 9-5 for fluids that are used in treating shock. The kind and amount of fluid are determined by the type of shock.

Various fluids may be given to the patient in shock. It is generally agreed that *the patient who has sustained a large blood loss will require blood replacement.* In preparation for giving fluids, it is customary to insert two IV lines attached to large bore needles in any patient in hypovolemic shock. The lines are kept open with normal saline until a decision is made about administering blood or other fluids. There is a great deal of disagreement concerning what other types of fluids should be used to treat shock. There are both advantages and disadvantages to all types of resuscitative fluids, including blood.

Administration of whole blood. The administration of whole blood has the obvious advantage of increasing the oxygen-carrying capacity of the blood. It also has many disadvantages (transmission of diseases, transfusion reactions, cost) (Chapter 41). If massive transfusions are given, additional problems may result. Because *blood for transfusion contains an anticoagulant* to prevent it from clotting while it is being stored, the *patient who receives large amounts of blood may develop clotting defects. Stored blood is also deficient in platelets and other clotting factors. Massive transfusions of cold blood* can result in *hypothermia,* which can cause cardiac arrhythmias.

Stored blood also contains some debris resulting from the aggregation of platelets, leukocytes, and fibrin. It is believed that some of this debris is able to pass through standard blood filters and is eventually filtered out of the blood by the pulmonary capillaries. This probably causes little difficulty in the patient who receives only a few units of blood, but is likely to cause a problem for the patient who receives massive transfusions. It is recommended by some that microfilters be used when large quantities of blood are transfused.[31]

The pH in stored blood is lower than in normal blood. The added anticoagulant makes the blood more acid. Also, because blood is stored in an airtight bag, the metabolism that continues is anaerobic, and the end products are *lactic* and *pyruvic acid*. With all of its disadvantages, until a blood substitute is available for general use, blood must be given to maintain relatively normal hemoglobin and hematocrit levels.[19]

Some patients who are losing large amounts of blood may be given transfusions with their own blood, collected from the bleeding site with special equipment. Autotransfusion has been used in patients bleeding massively from an uncontaminated wound as well as in patients who bleed excessively during surgery. Collecting the blood and keeping it from becoming contaminated are usually only possible in controlled settings, such as the operating room and

Table 9-5   Resuscitative fluids used in shock

Type	Uses/indications	Advantages	Disadvantages	Special considerations
Blood and blood products				
Whole blood	Replace blood volume and maintain hemoglobin (Hgb) at 12-14 g/100 ml	Provides intravascular volume Increases oxygen-carrying capacity of the blood	Potential associated risks of hepatitis and allergic reactions Delayed administration because of necessary typing and crossmatching Possibility of type and crossmatch errors	Whole blood should be stored at 0°-10° C (32°-50° F), but warmed at least 20-30 min before administration (never infuse cold blood) Use *fresh* whole blood whenever possible to avoid adverse metabolic changes related to stored blood
RBCs (packed, concentrate), fresh, frozen (also called leukocyte-poor)	Increase hematocrit to a minimum level of 30% Correct RBC deficiency and improve the oxygen-carrying capacity of the blood	Concentrated form helps to prevent excess fluid administration in patients with cardiogenic shock (increases oxygen-carrying capacity with less volume loading) Associated with fewer risks of metabolic complications when compared to stored whole blood (decreased amount of transfused antibodies, electrolytes, etc.) Provides economic use of blood as a resource; frees other blood components such as platelets and clotting factors to be concentrated and stored	Slow infusion rate because of increased viscosity Decreased content of plasma proteins and coagulation factors when compared with whole blood Inadequate (alone) for volume replacement and correction of hypovolemia Altered blood clotting with administration of more than 20 units; for every 4 units of RBCs over 20, 1 unit of fresh frozen plasma should be administered to replenish clotting factors High cost of frozen (thawed) RBCs	Administer via Y-connector tubing with normal saline to increase infusion flow rate Washed RBCs (resuspended in saline) can be given in shock to decrease red cell adhesiveness (washing decreases the cell's fibrinogen coating)
Human plasma (fresh, frozen, or dried)	Restore plasma volume in hypovolemic shock without increasing the hematocrit Restore clotting factors (except platelets)	Effective for rapid volume replacement Contains clotting factors	Expensive Deficient in RBCs	Human plasma carries the risk of viral hepatitis and allergic reactions Administer fresh frozen plasma promptly after thawing to prevent deterioration of clotting factors V and VIII

From Rice V: Shock: a clinical syndrome, the clinical continuum septic shock, *Shock management*, Secaucus, NJ, 1985, Critical Care Nurse/Hospitals Publications.

Continued.

Table 9-5 **Resuscitative fluids used in shock—cont'd**

Type	Uses/indications	Advantages	Disadvantages	Special considerations
Colloid solutions				
Plasma protein fraction (e.g., plasmanate, plasmaplex)	Expand plasma volume in hypovolemic shock (while cross-matching is being completed) Increase the serum colloid osmotic pressure	Can be used interchangeably with 5% human serum albumin Osmotically equivalent to plasma Associated with low risk of hepatitis	Expensive Deficient in clotting factors Associated with larger number of side effects such as hypotension and hypersensitivity than those reported with 5% albumin (because of presence of globulins) Hypotension induced by rapid intravenous administration (greater than 10 ml/min)	Plasma protein fraction is prepared from pooled plasma heated to 60° C (140° F) for 10 hr This procedure reduces the risk of transmission of hepatitis viruses Rapid administration of large dosages can alter blood coagulation This solution should be used cautiously in patients with congestive heart failure (caused by added fluid and rapid plasma volume expansion) and in patients with renal failure (caused by added proteins)
Albumin 5% 25% (salt-poor)	Increase the plasma colloid osmotic pressure Rapidly expand the plasma volume	Rare allergic reactions (less than 0.01% in all albumin solutions combined) Rare transmission of hepatitis virus	Potential leakage from capillaries in shock states associated with increased capillary permeability Possible precipitation of congestive heart failure after rapid infusion in patients with circulatory overload and compromised cardiovascular function	Albumin does not contain preservatives; therefore each opened bottle should be used at once Rate of administration of 5% albumin should not exceed 2-4 ml/min 25% albumin is reserved for use in patients with pulmonary or peripheral edema and hypoproteinemia Administer with a diuretic to ensure diuresis
Plasma expanders				
Dextran Low-molecular-weight dextran (LMWD) (Dextran 40) (Reomacrodex) (Gentran 40) High-molecular-weight dextran (HMWD) (Dextran 70) (Gentran 70-75) (Macrodex)	Rapidly expand plasma volume	All dextrans: associated with low incidence of anaphylactic reactions; less expensive than protein solutions LMWD: associated with fewer allergic reactions than HMWD; facilitates blood flow by decreasing RBC adhesiveness HMWD: leaks from the capillaries less readily than LMWD; can effectively increase plasma volume for up to 24 hr	LMWD: 70% excreted unchanged in urine, so urine osmolality and specific gravity are altered; potential osmotic-nephorisis and renal tubular shut-down; possible bleeding from raw surfaces caused by decreased platelet adhesiveness; side effects include decreased hemoglobin, hematocrit, fibrinogen, and clotting factors V, VIII, and IX	Avoid use of dextran in patients with active hemorrhage, hemorrhagic shock, coagulation disorders, and thrombocytopenia Bleeding times can be prolonged when the correct dose of dextran 70 (1.2 g/kg/day) or dextran 40 (2 g/kg/day) are exceeded Administer dextran in dextrose solutions to patients with sodium restriction

Table 9-5   Resuscitative fluids used in shock—cont'd

Type	Uses/indications	Advantages	Disadvantages	Special considerations
Plasma expanders—cont'd				
			HMWD: 50% excreted unchanged in the urine, so the urine osmolality and specific gravity are altered; higher incidence of allergic reactions when compared to LMWD; increases blood viscosity and platelet adhesiveness	
Hetastarch (Hespan) (Volex)	Expand plasma volume	Same volume expansion characteristics of albumin but with a longer duration of action (up to 36 hr) Associated with low risk of allergic and anaphylactic reactions (0.085%) Cost of hetastarch is about one half that of plasma protein fraction and albumin Nonantigenic No danger of transmission of hepatitis virus	Potential dilution of plasma proteins and decreased plasma colloid osmotic pressure Potential dilution of clotting factors with resultant coagulation changes Potential circulatory overload in patients with severe congestive heart failure and compromised renal function Increased serum amylase level (>200 mg/100 ml), peaking within 1 hour of intravenous administration of hetastarch and persisting for 3 to 4 days (caused by action of amylase in hetastarch degradation)	Do not use if the solution is cloudy or deep brown or if it contains crystals Monitor clotting studies and platelet counts, observe for prolonged prothrombin and partial thromboplastin times and thrombocytopenia Safety and compatibility of additives with hetastarch have not been established; the manufacturer recommends infusing hetastarch through a separate line, when possible, or piggybacking the second drug Maximum infusion rate in acute hemorrhagic shock is 20 ml/kg/hr Monitor serum albumin; if it falls below 2 g/100 ml, consider substituting albumin for hetastarch
Mannitol (Osmitrol)	Raise intravascular volume Reduce interstitial and intracellular edema Promote osmotic diuresis	Reduces intracellular swelling Increases urinary output	Potential circulatory overload in patients with congestive heart failure, pulmonary congestion, and renal dysfunction	
Crystalloid solutions (isotonic)				
Normal saline	Raise plasma volume when RBC mass is adequate Replace body fluid	Considered by some to be the single most important salt for maintaining and replacing ECF Increases plasma volume without altering normal sodium concentration or serum osmolality	Potential fluid retention and circulatory overload caused by sodium content	

Continued.

Table 9-5   Resuscitative fluids used in shock—cont'd

Type	Uses/indications	Advantages	Disadvantages	Special considerations
Lactated Ringer's solution (Hartman's solution)	Replace body fluid Buffer acidosis	Lactate is converted to bicarbonate (in the liver), which buffers acidosis Lactate replaces bicarbonate, preventing precipitation of calcium bicarbonate and calcium carbonate Lactate is more stable than bicarbonate and more compatible with ions present in the solution	Increased lactic acidosis in shock caused by lactate Fluid retention and circulatory overload caused by sodium content	Lactate conversion requires aerobic metabolism; therefore, it should be used cautiously in shock and other hypoperfusion states
Ringer's solution	Replace body fluid Provide additional potassium and calcium	Does not contain lactate, so can be given to patients with hypoperfusion	Potential hyperchloremic metabolic acidosis caused by high chloride concentration Potential fluid retention and circulatory overload caused by sodium content	
Crystalloid solutions (hypotonic)				
½ Normal saline	Raise total fluid volume		Potential interstitial and intracellular edema caused by rapid movement of this fluid from the vascular space Dilution of plasma proteins and electrolytes	
5% dextrose in water (D₅W)	Raise total fluid volume Provide calories for energy (200 cal/1000 ml)	Distributed evenly in every body compartment (acts like free water) Reverse dehydration Prevents hyperosmolar state Maintains adequate renal tubular flow (facilitates water excretion)	Dilution of plasma proteins and electrolytes caused by rapid metabolism of glucose and resultant free water	

selected intensive care units. While it does eliminate transfusion reactions and hepatitis associated with blood transfusions, it is not without risks. The most common complication of autotransfusion is *hemolysis* resulting in renal failure, coagulopathy, embolization of debris, and sepsis.[33] Its main use is in patients who are bleeding so rapidly that the supply of stored blood is becoming depleted.

Other types of fluid therapy. Other fluids given are classified either as crystalloid or colloid solutions (see Table 9-5). Controversy exists concerning which should be used. Those who favor the use of crystalloid solutions believe these are better able to restore and maintain urinary output.

In theory, colloids would seem to be superior because they should have the ability to hold fluid within the vascular compartment. However, when shock results in increased capillary permeability, the colloidal particle may leak into the interstitium and be followed by water. Another important consideration is cost. Colloids are generally much more expensive than crystalloids and therefore should be used only if their effect can be shown to be clearly superior to that of crystalloids.[12,50]

Regardless of the type of fluid that the patient receives, the nurse must carefully monitor the rate at which it is administered. The patient is assessed frequently for signs of hypovolemia, fluid overload, or adverse reactions to the type of fluid being administered (Chapter 7). Neck veins

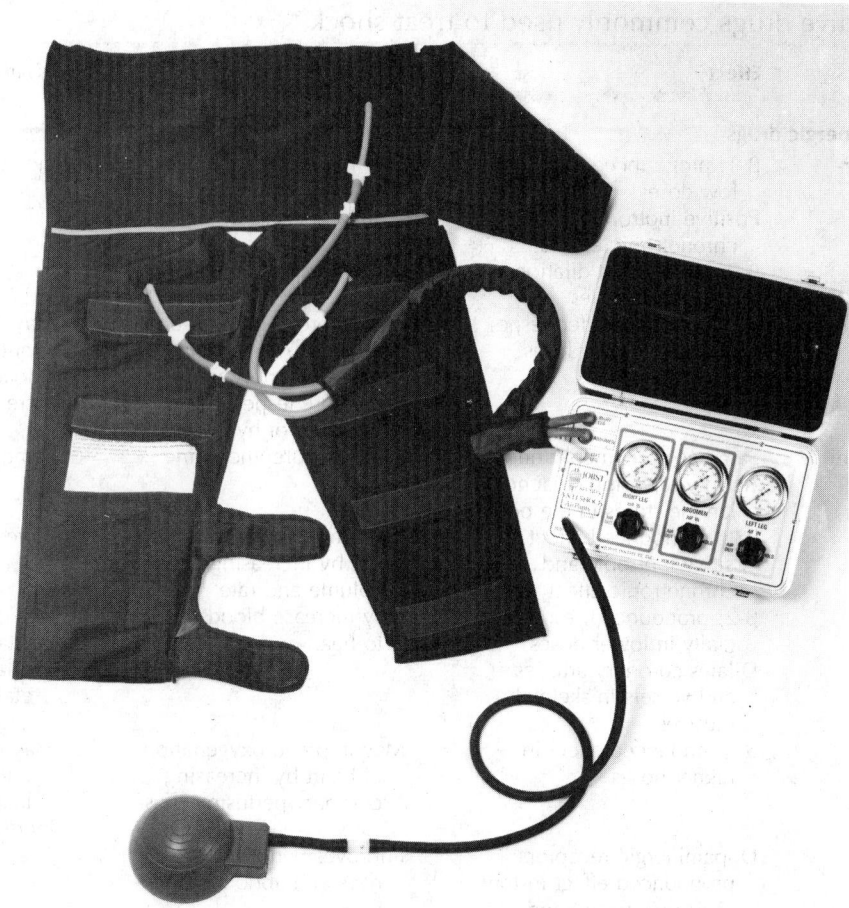

Fig. 9-8   Military antishock trousers (MAST) with inflation device and manometers. (Courtesy The Jobst Institute, Inc, Toledo, Oh. From Burrell LO, Burrell AL: *Critical care*, St Louis, 1982, Mosby—Year Book.)

are observed for distention, and lungs are auscultated for signs of fluid (rales, rhonchi).

Fluid redistribution. Another way in which fluid resuscitation may be accomplished is by the use of the MAST suit (Military Anti-Shock Trousers). The suit consists of three inflatable parts, one for each leg and one for the abdomen (Fig. 9-8). When inflated, the trousers "autotransfuse" the upper circulation with up to 2 L blood from the lower extremities, increasing blood to the heart, lungs, and brain.[32] The trousers also increase peripheral resistance, which helps compensate for decreased blood volume. If there is bleeding in the lower extremities, the MAST suit helps to control bleeding by tamponade (counterpressure). The suit is used as an emergency measure until adequate fluid can be administered. When the suit is to be removed, it must be deflated gradually to prevent a sudden fall in peripheral resistance and a return of shock.

Assisting with drug therapy

If fluid therapy alone is not sufficient to reverse the shock state, vasoactive drugs may be given (Table 9-6). Most vasoactive drugs are *catecholamines*, which stimulate *alpha* or *beta receptors* in the body. Generally, *stimulation of*

alpha receptors causes *vasoconstriction*, and *stimulation* of *beta receptors* causes *vasodilation*. *Stimulation* of *beta receptors* also causes the *heart* to *increase its rate* (*chronotropic* effect) and *strength of contraction* (*inotropic* effect). The abdominal viscera, skin, and muscles respond primarily to the alpha effects of the catecholamines.

Mixed alpha- and beta-adrenergic drugs are used most commonly. In the past, drugs that caused vasoconstriction were used because they enhanced the body's normal compensatory mechanisms. However, it was determined that vasoconstrictors were not helpful because they have an adverse effect on several organs: (1) as blood is shunted away from the kidneys to perfuse the heart and brain, renal perfusion decreases and renal failure severe enough to require dialysis may result, (2) bowel necrosis may develop, (3) the ischemic pancreas may begin to produce myocardial depressant factor, and (4) the ischemic liver can no longer perform its important functions.

Vasodilator drugs have been used to counteract the adverse effects of the body's compensatory mechanisms. They decrease the amount of pressure against which the heart has to pump, and thereby have the effect of increasing cardiac output without increasing the work load and oxygen need of the heart. *Fluid therapy must be given along with vasodilator*

Table 9-6   Vasoactive drugs commonly used to treat shock

Drug	Effect	Advantages	Disadvantages
Mixed α- and β-adrenergic drugs			
Norepinephrine (levar-terenol)	β-1: pronounced effect in low doses Positive inotropic and chronotropic effects	May improve cardiac output by increasing rate and stroke volume	Increases O_2 need of heart
	β-2: weak effect dilation of coronary arteries	May improve blood flow to heart	
	α: pronounced effect especially in higher doses Vasoconstriction	May improve oxygenation of heart by increasing coronary artery perfusion pressure (especially in presence of hypotension)	May decrease cardiac output by increasing afterload Increases O_2 need of heart
Metaraminol (Aramine)	Same as norepinephrine Acts by releasing catacholamine stores in the body	Same as norepinephrine	Same as norepinephrine
Epinephrine	β-1: pronounced effect Positive inotropic and chronotropic effect	May improve cardiac output by increasing stroke volume and rate	Increases O_2 need of heart
	β-2: pronounced, especially in lower doses Dilates coronary arteries and vessels in skeletal muscles	May increase blood supply to heart	May shunt blood away from vital organs because of dilation of vessels in skeletal muscles
	α: pronounced effect in higher doses	May improve oxygenation of heart by increasing coronary perfusion pressure	May decrease cardiac output by increasing afterload Increases O_2 need of heart
Dopamine	Dopaminergic receptors: pronounced effect in low (2-5 μg/kg/min) and moderate doses (5-10 μg/kg/min); α effect in high doses (greater than 10 μg/kg/min)	Improves perfusion of kidneys and abdominal viscera	
	β-1: pronounced effect in moderate dose range—positive inotropic and chronotropic effect	Improves cardiac output	Increases O_2 need of heart
	β-2: moderate effect Dilates coronary arteries	Increases blood supply to heart	
	α: pronounced in high doses Offsets dopaminergic and beta effects	May improve oxygenation of heart by increasing coronary perfusion pressure	May decrease cardiac output by increasing afterload Increases O_2 need of heart
Dobutamine	β-1: pronounced effect Positive inotropic effect	Improves the cardiac output by increasing stroke volume	Increases O_2 need of heart
	Minimal chronotropic effect	Lack of rate increase allows more coronary filling time than other inotropic drugs	
	β-2: weak effect Some dilation of coronary arteries α: minimal effect	May improve coronary artery blood flow	

Table 9-6   Vasoactive drugs commonly used to treat shock—cont'd

Drug	Effect	Advantages	Disadvantages
β-Adrenergic drugs			
Isoproterenol	β-1: very pronounced strong positive inotropic and chronotropic effects β-2: very pronounced Dilates coronary arteries and vessels in skeletal muscles Lowers peripheral resistance	Increases cardiac output by increasing stroke volume and rate May increase blood supply to heart May improve cardiac output by decreasing afterload	Pronounced increase in O_2 need of heart Cardiac dysrhythmias Decreased blood pressure may decrease coronary artery perfusion pressure
Vasodilators			
Nitroprusside	Acts directly on smooth muscle, dilating both veins and arterioles	Decreases O_2 need of heart by decreasing both preload and afterload Decreases pulmonary congestion by decreasing preload Increases cardiac output by decreasing afterload	Decreases in peripheral resistance can decrease coronary artery perfusion pressure
Nitroglycerine	Acts directly on smooth muscle Effect on veins: pronounced Effect on arterioles: weak	Decreases O_2 need of heart by decreasing preload and, to a lesser extent, afterload	Decrease in preload can decrease cardiac output and coronary artery perfusion pressure

drugs, or *the decrease in peripheral resistance can cause a decrease in venous return, thereby decreasing cardiac output. Cardiac output must be maintained when vasodilators are given, or the heart and brain may be poorly perfused.* The drug selected will depend to some extent on the cause of shock and how far shock has progressed.

Combinations of drugs may be given. Dopamine and nitroprusside may be given together to increase cardiac output by combining the inotropic effect of dopamine with the decreased peripheral resistance effected by nitroprusside. For these two drugs to work together effectively, adequate fluid must be administered.[45] Low-dose dopamine may be given for its effect on renal and mesenteric perfusion along with dobutamine for its inotropic effect.

Patients receiving vasoactive drugs require very careful monitoring (Box 9-4). Ideally, *intraarterial and pulmonary pressure monitoring should be instituted.* If the blood pressure is being measured by both cuff and intraarterial line, the two readings may vary. It is imperative that everyone working with the patient use the same measurements in adjusting the rate of drug infusion.

Steroids are often administered to patients in shock; however, their use is controversial. Many benefits from their use have been suggested, the most important of which is stabilization of lysosomal membranes, thereby preventing the leak of destructive enzymes. However, there is significant debate among physicians about whether steroids enhance survival chances with shock. For example, studies have consistently failed to show any increase in survival of patients after use of steroids in the treatment of septic shock.[40,43] Other drugs are being used experimentally at present and may become accepted therapeutic agents in

---

Box 9-4

Guidelines for care of the patient receiving vasoactive drugs

1. Monitor blood pressure every 5 to 15 minutes at the beginning of the infusion and every 15 minutes thereafter to maintain a *mean* blood pressure at prescribed level (usually 80 mm Hg).
2. Drug must be diluted in a compatible solution and administered slowly by intravenous pump (for control).
3. Observe peripheral site of infusion (if used) frequently for signs of infiltration (necrosis and sloughing of tissues may occur with infiltration).
4. If infiltration occurs, infiltrate area around site with norepinephrine blocker (Regitine) as prescribed.
5. Monitor urinary output.
6. When discontinuing drug infusion, taper infusion slowly while continuing to monitor blood pressure every 15 minutes.

---

the future; these include calcium channel blockers, Naloxone (a beta endorphin antagonist), monoclonal antibodies to endotoxins, receptor antagonists to other mediators that accelerate the septic shock process, and prostaglandins, which, among other things, may block the cardiovascular responses to shock.[5,14,27,45]

Assisting with cardiac support

When the left ventricle becomes severely impaired, as in cardiogenic shock, its function may be augmented by the use of the *intraaortic balloon pump* (Chapter 25). A balloon-tipped catheter is inserted into the aorta by way of the femoral artery. The catheter is attached to a machine that inflates and deflates the balloon in synchrony with the patient's cardiac cycle. During systole the balloon is deflated as the heart pumps blood into the aorta. During diastole the balloon inflates, enhancing blood flow to the heart, which is perfused during diastole, and to the rest of the body. During the next period of systole, the balloon deflates again, leaving a space in the aorta that must be filled. This causes a reduction in resistance, which allows the heart to eject a large quantity of blood with less effort than would normally be required.

Complications are not uncommon with use of the balloon pump. The most common complication is vascular insufficiency of the extremity distal to the insertion site. Frequent assessments are made of the pulses, color, temperature, movement, and sensation of the extremity, and any abnormality is reported immediately. Infection may occur with this procedure, as with any invasive procedure; therefore the patient's temperature is also monitored.

The use of the intraaortic balloon is a temporary measure used to enhance cardiac output only until the heart is able to function adequately on its own.

Assisting with respiratory support

Most patients in shock have some degree of *hypoxemia. Oxygen* is usually *administered* because *tissues* are already *suffering* from *oxygen deprivation* from *poor blood flow.* Because the energy system of the body is impaired, the muscles used in ventilation may not function adequately and breathing may have to be assisted. If symptoms of ARDS develop, positive end expiratory pressure (PEEP) may have to be used. Positive pressure at the end of expiration prevents surfactant-deficient alveoli from collapsing, resulting in atelectasis (see Chapter 24). Coughing and deep breathing are important, if the patient is able. If the patient is too weak to cough or if an endotracheal tube is in place, suctioning is necessary to keep the airway free of excessive secretions. Meticulous mouth care is necessary while the endotracheal tube is in place, because the mouth remains open and swallowing may be difficult. Turning the patient at least every 2 hours is important to aid in the mobilization of secretions.

Interventions to achieve patient outcomes
Preventing injuries

In the early stages of shock, the patient may exhibit *restlessness,* which may then progress to *confusion.* During this time, *injury is likely to occur if preventive measures are not taken. If the patient attempts to remove or disconnect life-saving equipment, soft restraints may have to be applied.*

Infections are very common in patients who are in shock, because of the many invasive procedures that are performed. Some *potential sources of infection are indwelling catheters, arterial lines, pulmonary artery catheters, intravenous lines, endotracheal tubes, surgical incisions, and traumatic wounds.* Meticulous sterile technique must be used with endotracheal suctioning, dressing changes, tubing changes, and urinary catheter care. *Patients who are receiving steroids or who have experienced excessive blood loss are at increased risk for developing infection.*

Complications of immobility must be prevented. It is not uncommon for the patient in shock to remain in one position for an extended period because of the constant activity that is occurring at the patient's bedside. This *immobility can predispose* the patient *to thrombi, pneumonia, and decubitus ulcers. Frequent turning and maintaining cleanliness of the skin will aid in the prevention of decubitus ulcers. If immobility is prolonged,* the use of special mattresses may be considered.

Maintaining comfort and rest

The patient should be kept as comfortable as possible. In the past, patients in shock were kept in the *Trendelenberg position* (head down), but this *is no longer recommended.* It is usually suggested that the *patient remain flat, with the legs elevated if necessary.* If a patient in shock has difficulty breathing, a small pillow may be used to elevate the head slightly.

Rest is important. All nonessential activities should be eliminated because *activity increases the body's need for oxygen and nutrients,* substances already deficient in the cells of the patient in shock.

Ambient temperature should be kept at a comfortable level. *Excessive warmth increases the metabolic rate of the tissues, thereby increasing* their *oxygen need.* Excessive coolness may cause the blood to flow even more sluggishly through the microcirculation, enhancing the formation of microthrombi. Patients with an endotracheal tube in place or who are very lethargic may not be able to express how they feel. Covers should be used according to the room temperature.

Both the *conscious patient and the family will probably experience considerable anxiety.* The *nurse should remain calm* and *explain all interventions whenever possible.* It may be necessary to repeat explanations frequently to both patient and family, because anxiety can interfere with their ability to comprehend and to remember.

Evaluation

Evaluation is based on expected patient outcomes, and questions used to measure them include the following:

1. Patient will be able to tolerate activity involved in care. Did pulse increase no more than 10 beats per minute? Did skin remain warm and dry? Did respiratory rate remain the same?
2. Patient's airway will remain free from secretions. Are lung sounds clear? Can suction catheter be inserted into airway easily?
3. Patient and significant others will remain free of avoidable anxiety. Are they able to verbalize fears? Are they free of signs of anxiety?
4. Patient will have a respiratory rate and tidal volume within normal limits. Are respirations regular? Is the respiratory rate between 16 and 22 per minute? Is the tidal volume normal for the patient's size?
5. Cardiac output will be within normal limits. Is the mean arterial blood pressure greater than 80 mm

Hg? Is the pulse rate between 60 and 100 beats per minute? Is the cardiac index 2.5 to 3.5 $L/min/m^2$? Is the PCWP between 10 and 20 mm Hg?

6. Patient will make his or her needs understood by verbal or alternate means of communication. Is the patient able to make his or her needs known? Is the patient free from anxiety when trying to communicate?

7. Intravascular volume will return to normal. Is the CVP between 6 and 15 cm water? Is the pulse volume normal? Is the pulse rate between 60 and 100 per minute?

8. Blood gases will be within normal limits. Are the blood gases within the following range? PO_2 80 to 100 mm Hg; PCO_2 35 to 45 mm Hg; HCO_3 22 to 26 mEq/L; pH 7.35 to 7.45.

9. Patient will be free from infection. Is the patient's temperature within normal range? Is the leukocyte count between 4500 and 11,000/mm? Are the catheter insertion sites free from redness, swelling, and drainage?

10. Oral mucous membrane will remain moist and intact. Is mucous membrane pink and moist? Are lips free from cracks? Is mouth free of excess mucus?

11. Patient will have adequate rest. Does patient appear rested? Has care been planned to allow for periods of undisturbed sleep?

12. Patient will have normal tissue perfusion. Is the urinary output greater than 30 ml/hr? Is the BUN between 8 and 25 mg/dl? Is the serum creatinine between 0.6 and 1.2 mg/dl? Is the lactic acid level less than 1.9 mEq/L? Is the serum potassium level between 3.8 and 5.0 mEq/L? Is the serum sodium level between 136 and 142 mEq/L? Is the patient's skin warm, dry, and pink? Is capillary refill less than 3 seconds? Is the patient's mental status the same as before the onset of shock?

13. Patient will remain free of injury. Is the patient free from nosocomial infections? Is the patient free of abrasions? Is the patient free of complications of immobility?

SUMMARY

1. Shock is a syndrome characterized by hypoperfusion of body tissues.
2. The major classifications of shock are hypovolemic, cardiogenic, and vasogenic shock.
3. Shock results in a derangement of cellular metabolism, and if not treated in the early stages, it can affect all body systems.
4. The early stage of shock is characterized by a stress response.
5. At some point in the progress of untreated shock, the process becomes irreversible and no treatment can save the patient.
6. The management of shock includes the following:
   a. Fluid therapy
      Blood and blood products
      Colloid solutions
      Plasma extenders
      Crystalloid solutions (isotonic)
      Crystalloid solutions (hypotonic)
   b. Drug therapy
      Mixed alpha and beta adrenergic drugs
      Beta adrenergic drugs
      Vasodilators
   c. Supportive care
      Support cardiac function
      Support respiratory function
      Prevent injury

STUDY QUESTIONS

- How would you define shock?
- What are the differences between the neurogenic form and the septic form of vasogenic shock?
- Metabolic acidosis and respiratory acidosis are typically signs of what stage of shock?
- Is fluid volume deficit a potential nursing diagnosis in all types of shock?
- When patients are receiving vasoactive drugs, how frequently should vital signs be taken?

REFERENCES AND SELECTED READINGS

1. Asheervath J, Blevins D: *Handbook of clinical nursing practice*, Norwalk, Conn, 1986, Appleton-Century-Crofts.
2. Barone JE: Treatment strategies in shock: use of oxygen transport measurements, *Heart Lung* 20(1):81-86, 1991.
3. Biharri DJ, Tinker J: The therapeutic value of vasodilator prostaglandins in multiple organ failure associated with sepsis, *Intens Care* 15(1):2-7, 1988.
4. Bonato J: Blood transfusions: are they safe? *Crit Care Nurse* 9(7):40-46, 1989.
5. Bone RC: A critical evaluation of new agents for the treatment of sepsis, *JAMA* 266(12):1686-1691, 1991.
6. Brandsetter RD: The adult respiratory distress syndrome-11986, *Heart Lung* 15(2):155-164, 1986.
7. Bulle TM, Rogers WJ: Cardiogenic shock. In Hardway RM: *Shock: the reversible stage of dying*, Littleton, Mass, 1986, PSG Publishing.
8. Calandra T, et al: Treatment of gram-negative shock with human IgF antibody to Escherichia coli J5: a prospective, double blind, randomized trial, *J Infect Dis* 58(2):312-319, 1988.
9. Clowes GHA Jr: *Trauma sepsis and shock: the physiological basis of therapy*, New York, 1988, Marcel Dekker.
10. Danner RL, Parrillo JF: The role of endotoxins in human septic shock: therapeutic potential of lipid A analogs, *Prog Clin Biol Res* 286:183-200, 1989, Alan R Liss, Inc.
11. Dickerson M: Anaphylaxis and anaphylactic shock, *Crit Care Nurs Q* 11(1):674-678, 1988.
12. Dislet L, et al: Cardiogenic shock in evolving myocardial infarction, *Heart Lung* 16:649-651, 1987.
13. Dunham CM, Cowley RA: *Shock trauma/critical care handbook*, Rockville, Md, 1986, Aspen Systems.
13a. Goldberg RJ et al: Cardiogenic shock after acute myocardial infarction, *N Engl J Med* 325(16):1117-1122, 1991.
14. Gorelick K, et al: Randomized placebo-controlled study of E5 monoclonal antiendotoxin antibody. In Larrick J, Borrebaeck C, eds: *Therapeutic monoclonal antibodies*, New York, 1990, Stockton Press.

*Recommended for student reading.

15. Guyton AC: *Textbook of medical physiology,* ed 7, Philadelphia, 1986, WB Saunders.
16. Halfman-Franey M: Current trends in hemodynamic monitoring of patients in shock, *Crit Care Nurs Q* 11(1):9-18, 1988.
17. Hammerschmidt DE, Vercellotti GM: Granulocytes of mediators of tissue injury in shock: therapeutic implications, *Prog Clin Biol Res* 236A:19-32, 1987, Alan R. Liss.
18.* Hancock BG, Eberhard NK: The pharmacological management of shock, *Crit Care Nurs Q* 11(1):19-29, 1988.
19. Hardway RM: *Shock: the reversible stage of dying,* Littleton, Mass, 1986, PSG Publishing.
20. Hesselvik JF, Brodin B: Low dose norepinephrine in patients with septic shock and oliguria: effects on afterload, urine flow, and oxygen transport, *Crit Care Med* 17(2):179-180, 1989.
21.* Houston MC: Pathophysiology of shock, *Crit Care Nurs Clin North Am* 2(2):143-149, 1990.
22. Jefferies PR, Whelan SK: Cardiogenic shock: current management, *Crit Care Nurs Q* 11(1):48-56, 1988.
23. Jurkovich GJ, Moore EE, Eisman B: The liver in shock. In Hardaway RM: *Shock: the reversible stage of dying,* Littleton, Mass, 1986, PSG Publishing.
24.* Lancaster LE, Rice V: Nursing care: planning overview and application to the patient in shock, *Crit Care Nurs Clin North Am* 2(2):279-286, 1990.
25. Lefer AM, Hock CE: Vascular mediators in circulatory shock. In Hardaway RM: *Shock: the reversible stage of dying,* Littleton, Mass, 1986, PSG Publishing.
26. Littleton MT: Pathophysiology and assessment of sepsis and septic shock, *Crit Care Nurs Q* 11(1):30-47, 1988.
27. Littleton MT: Prostaglandins and leukotrienes as mediators of shock and trauma, *Crit Care Nurs Q* 11(2):11-20, 1988.
28. MacLean LD: Shock, *Br Med Bull* 44(2):437-452, 1988.
29. Martin E, et al: Autotransfusion systems, *Crit Care Nurs* 9(7):65-72, 1989.
30.* McMorrow ME, Daniello MC: When to suspect septic shock, *RN* 54(10):32-37, October 1991.
31.* McQuillan KA, Wiles CE: Initial management of traumatic shock. In Cardona DV, et al: *Trauma nursing from resuscitation through rehabilitation,* Philadelphia, 1988, WB Saunders.
32. McSwam NE: Pneumatic anti-shock garment: state of the art, 1988, *Ann Emerg Med* 17(5):506-526, 1988.
33. Millar S: *AACN procedure manual for critical care,* Philadelphia, 1985, WB Saunders.
34. Nagy S: Cardiodepressant and cardiostimulant factors in shock, *Prog Clin Biol Res* 236A:599-610, 1987, Alan R Liss.
35. Parrillo JE: The cardiovascular pathophysiology of sepsis, *Ann Rev Med* 49:469-485, 1989.
36. Perry AG: Shock complications: recognition and management, *Crit Care Nurs Q* 11(1):1-8, 1988.
37. Rackow RC, Astiz ME: Pathophysiology and treatment of septic shock, *JAMA* 266(4):548-554, 1991.
38. Rackow RC, Astiz ME, Weil MH: Cellular oxygen metabolism during sepsis and shock, *JAMA* 259(13):1989-1993, 1988.
39. Rice V: *Shock: a clinical syndrome, the clinical continuum of septic shock, shock management,* Secaucus, NJ, 1985, Critical Care Nurse/Hospital Publications.
40.* Rice V: Shock, a clinical syndrome: an update. Part 1, an overview of shock, *Crit Care Nurs* 11(4):20-27, 1991.
41. Rice V: Shock, a clinical syndrome: an update. Part 3, therapeutic management, *Crit Care Nurs* 11(6):41-43, 1991.
42. Schedel I: New aspects in the treatment of gram-negative bacteremia and septic shock, *Infection* 16(1):4-7, 1988.
43. Schumer W: Corticosteroids in the treatment of shock, *Prog Clin Biol Res* 236B:249-259, 1987, Alan R Liss.
44. Shoemaker WC, et al: Therapy of shock based on pathophysiology, monitoring and outcome prediction, *Crit Care Med* 18(1):19-25, 1990.
45. Soulioti AM: Naloxone for septic shock, *Lancet* 2(8620):1133-1134, 1988.
46. Strange JM, editor: *Shock trauma care plans,* Springhouse, Penn, 1987, Springhouse.
47. Stroud M, Swindell B, Bernard GR: Cellular humoral mediators of sepsis syndrome, *Nurs Clin North Am* 2(2):150-160, 1990.
48. Summers G: The clinical and hemodynamic presentation of the shock patient, *Nurs Clin North Am* 2(2):161-166, 1990.
49. Tilkian SM, Conover MB, Tilkian AG: *Clinical implications of laboratory tests,* ed 4, St Louis, 1987, Mosby–Year Book.
50. Weil MH, Rackow EC: Colloidal osmotic pressure and its implication for the fluid management of patients in shock. In Hardway RM: *Shock: the reversible stage of dying,* Littleton, Mass, 1986, PGS Publishing.

Classics

51. Flower NO: Examination of the heart: inspection and palpation of venous and arterial pulses, New York, 1978, American Heart Association.
52. Perry AG, Potter PA: Shock: comprehensive nursing management, St Louis, 1983, Mosby–Year Book.

10

Pain

Judith H. Watt-Watson
Barbara C. Long

After studying this chapter, the learner should be able to:

- Describe some common misbeliefs about pain management.
- Describe the physiology of pain and related theories of pain transmission.
- Compare factors that influence perception and response to pain.
- Differentiate between acute and chronic pain assessment.
- Describe some assessment tools to use in clinical practice.
- Describe pharmacologic and nonpharmacologic approaches for pain management.
- Identify nursing implications for pain management.
- Explain the purpose and methods of the team approach for chronic pain management.

Pain is experienced by every person to some degree. It is, however, a very individualized experience and is difficult to define or understand. It is an unpleasant feeling, entirely subjective, that only the person experiencing it can describe or evaluate. It can be evoked by a multiplicity of stimuli, but the reaction to it cannot be measured objectively. Pain is a learned experience that is influenced by the entire life situation of each person.

Pain accompanies many disorders, as well as some therapies. It is a sensation that is frequently feared by persons undergoing surgery. Although many persons with cancer do *not* experience it, pain is one of the major concerns people have about cancer.

Relief of pain and discomfort is a major nursing intervention and one that requires skill in both the art and science of nursing. It requires knowledge about concepts related to pain, data collection, and useful therapies. It also requires sensitivity and empathy—an effort on the part of the nurse to understand what the patient is experiencing and to communicate understanding and caring. It requires that the nurse use a systematic approach (nursing process) with the patient in pain. Too often when a patient states that he or she has pain, medication is given without valid assessment and evaluation, resulting in undermedication, overmedication, or medication when other interventions would be more effective.

PHYSIOLOGY OF PAIN

Pain Receptors and Stimuli

Pain receptors, called *nociceptors*, are free nerve endings of unmyelinated or lightly myelinated afferent neurons. Nociceptors are located extensively in the skin and mucosa and less frequently in selected deeper structures, such as viscera, joints, arterial walls, and bile ducts. Nociceptors respond to harmful or potentially harmful stimuli that may be chemical, thermal, or mechanical.[12] Chemical stimuli for pain include histamines, bradykinin, prostaglandins, and acids, some of which are released by damaged tissues. Anoxic tissue also releases chemicals that lead to pain. Tissue swelling may cause pain by creating pressure (mechanical stimulation) on nociceptors in adjoining tissues.

After tissue injury and in some pathologic conditions, pain receptors do not adapt to repeated stimulation and may become more sensitive.[10] As a result, pain sensitivity to a normally painful stimulus may be increased (*hyperalgesia*) or a normally nonpainful stimulus, such as touch, may be painful (*allodynia*).

Pain Transmission

Pain impulses are transmitted to the spinal cord by two types of fibers: thinly myelinated faster-conducting A-delta fibers and slower-conducting unmyelinated C fibers. Pain that may be described as "sharp" or "pricking" and that can be easily localized results from impulses transmitted by the *A-delta fibers*. An example of this type of pain is that felt by a needle prick. Pain that may be described as "burning," "dull," or "aching" and that is more diffuse results from impulses transmitted by the *C fibers*. Impulses transmitted on the larger diameter myelinated A-beta and A-alpha fibers have an inhibitory effect on those transmitted over A-delta and C fibers.

The afferent nerve fibers enter the spinal cord through the dorsal root and synapse in the *dorsal horn* (Fig. 10-1). The dorsal horn consists of several layers (laminae) with interconnections. Lamina II comprises an area called *substantia gelatinosa* (SG). Substance P is released at synapses in the SG and is thought to be a major neurotransmitter of the pain impulses.

The pain impulses cross the spinal cord over interneurons and connect with *ascending spinal pathways*. The most important ascending pathways for nociceptive impulses located in the ventral half of the spinal cord are the spinothalamic tract (STT) and the spinoreticular tract (SRT). The STT is a discriminative system and conveys information about the nature and location of the stimulus to the thalamus and then to the cortex for interpretation. Impulses transmitted over the SRT (which goes to the brainstem and part of the thalamus) activate the autonomic and limbic (motivational-affective) responses.

Pain Modulation

Discovery of receptors in the brain to which opiate compounds bind led to the discovery of two naturally occurring endogenous morphinelike pentapeptides (5-amino acid compounds), met-enkephalin and leu-enkephalin. These enkephalins are classified as *endorphins* (from the terms endogenous and morphine). Other endorphins, such as beta-endorphin, have also been identified. The endorphins are thought to suppress pain by (1) acting presynaptically to *inhibit release* of the neurotransmitter substance P or (2) acting postsynaptically to *inhibit conduction* of pain impulses.[14] The endorphins are found in high concentration in the basal ganglia of the brain, thalamus, midbrain, and dorsal horn of the spinal cord.

Descending spinal pathways, from the thalamus through the midbrain and medulla to the dorsal horns of the spinal cord, conduct nociceptive *inhibitory* impulses. Serotonin is one neurotransmitter that supports these inhibitory impulses. The endogenous descending pain suppressive system is more effectively activated by nociceptive stimuli transmitted by A-delta fibers. Electrical stimulation by means of transcutaneous electrical nerve stimulation (TENS, p. 174) using low frequency and high intensity activates opiate analgesia. Acupuncture is also thought to use the opiate pathways.[14,52]

Theories of Pain Transmission

Various theories of pain transmission have been proposed[53] (Table 10-1). The affect specificity and pattern theories were early theories that led to the development of the gate control theory. Although the *gate control theory* does not fully explain pain transmission, it serves as a basis for understanding pain transmission.

The gate control theory was proposed by Melzack and Wall[58] in 1965. The theory proposes that the substantia gelatinosa (SG) in the spinal cord acts as a gating mechanism to permit or inhibit passage of pain impulses. The "gate" can be "closed" (so that the contact is not made, thus interrupting the pain impulse) by nerve impulses from the large non-nociceptive A-beta and A-alpha fibers or from the descending pathways. Impulses conducted over large fibers not only close the gate but also are sent immediately

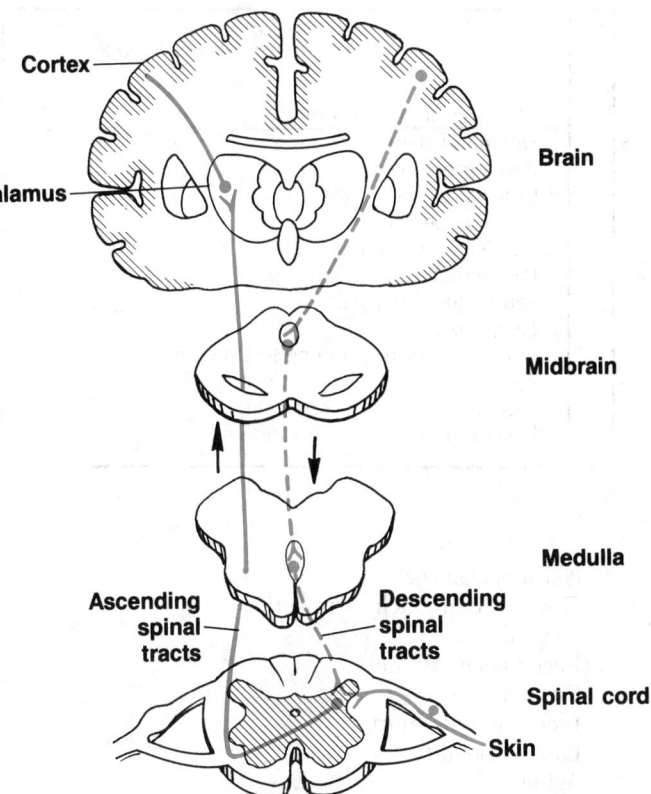

Fig. 10-1 Pathways of pain transmission to and from cortex.

Table 10-1 Theories of pain transmission

Theory	Description
Affect theory	Pain is an emotion and its intensity depends on the meaning of the part involved; does not include physiologic aspects.
Specificity theory	Specific pain receptors project impulses over neural pain pathways to the brain; does not account for psychologic aspects of pain perception and variability of response.
Pattern theory	Pain results from combined effects of stimulus intensity and summations of impulses in the dorsal horn of the spinal cord; does not account for psychologic aspects.
Gate control theory	Pain impulses can be controlled by a gating mechanism in the dorsal horn of the spinal cord to permit or inhibit transmission. Gating factors include effect of impulses transmitted over fast or slow conducting nerve fibers and effects of descending impulses from the brainstem and cortex.

Table 10-2 Factors affecting pain transmission based on the gate control theory

Site	Close gate (block transmission)	Open gate (permit transmission)
Fibers	Impulses transmitted by large fast myelinated A-beta and A-alpha fibers	Impulses transmitted by slow small A-delta and C fibers
	Stimulation of unaffected skin areas (for example, massage)	Stimulation of affected skin areas (for example, sunburned skin)
Brainstem (descending pathway)	Endorphin effect	No endorphin effect
	Sufficient or maximum sensory input (for example, distraction)	Insufficient sensory input (for example, monotony)
Cortex	Past experiences	Past experiences
	Feelings of pain control	Anxiety

to the cortex for rapid identification, evaluation, and modification of the sensory inputs.[59] Impulses sent to the brainstem, the center for motivational-affective and sensory-discriminative actions, can influence cognition or evaluation in the cortex. Impulses are then sent from the cortex back to the SG via corticospinal pathways to inhibit or permit passage of pain impulses. Note in Table 10-2 the various factors that can open or close the gate.

PAIN EXPERIENCE

The pain experience of every individual includes the perception of the pain sensation and the response to this perception. Tolerance to the noxious stimulus will influence both of these components.

Pain Perception

Perception of pain takes place in the cortex (cognitive-evaluative function) as a result of the stimuli transmitted up the spinothalamic and thalamic-cortical tracts. This thinking-feeling component of pain is subjective, highly complex, and individual; it is influenced by factors affecting stimulation of the nociceptors and transmission of the nociceptive impulse, as well as by cortical receptivity and interpretation:

1. Stimulation of nociceptors
   a. Increased number of stimuli
   b. Increased duration of the stimulus
2. Alteration of transmission
   a. Damage to nerve endings
   b. Inflammation, tumors, or injuries to spinal cord

10-1

Factors that influence pain tolerance

Increase tolerance	Decrease tolerance
Alcohol	Fatigue
Drugs	Anger
Hypnosis	Boredom
Warmth	Anxiety
Rubbing	Persistent pain
Distraction	
Faith	
Strong beliefs	

10-2

Factors that influence reaction to pain

Meaning of pain to individual
Degree of pain perception
Past experience
Cultural values
Social expectations
Physical and mental health
Parental attitudes toward pain
Setting in which pain occurs
Fear, anxiety
Usual way of responding to stressors
Age
Preparation for pain context
Health professionals' responses

---

3. Receptivity of cortex
   a. Inflammation, degenerative changes of brain
   b. Depression of brain function
   c. Anesthesia
4. Interpretation in cerebral cortex
   a. Childhood training
   b. Past experience with pain
   c. Cultural values
   d. Religious beliefs
   e. Physical and mental health
   f. Knowledge and understanding
   g. Attention and distraction
   h. Fear, anxiety, tension
   i. Fatigue
   j. State of consciousness

Pain perception, therefore, can be altered by usual activities, such as reading or socialization, as well as by abnormal conditions. Damaged nerve endings may not transmit pain sensation, such as from a severe burn, and the patient may not perceive a usually painful stimuli as such.

The intensity at which the noxious stimulus is subjectively judged as painful is called the *pain detection threshold*.[12] This sensory discrimination is relatively consistent within an individual and between different individuals, relative to the location and type of stimulus.

In contrast, *pain tolerance*, which is the maximum degree of pain intensity a person is willing to experience, is highly variable.[12] Numerous factors can increase or decrease pain tolerance (Box 10-1). Tolerance can vary between different individuals in the same situation and in the same individual in differing situations. For example, a woman with a tender breast lump may complain of more pain if her mother died of breast cancer. Individuals can respond in many ways to any level of pain intensity, and pain tolerance is influenced by the meaning of the pain to the individual. It is important to remember that there is no right or wrong way to experience pain and pain is whatever and whenever the patient says it is.[26]

Meaning of Pain

Pain has different meanings for each person, which may differ for the same person at different times. In general, most persons view pain as a negative experience, although it may also have some positive aspects. Some examples of the meanings of pain include the following:

Harm or damage
Complication, such as infection
New illness
Recurrence of illness
Fatal disease
Increasing disability
Loss of mobility
Aging
Healing
Necessary for cure
Punishment for sins
Challenge
Appreciation for suffering of others
Something to be tolerated
Release from unwanted responsibilities

Numerous factors influence the meaning of pain for an individual, including age, sex, sociocultural background, environment, and past or present experiences. For example, two women may be experiencing pain from a fractured leg. To the 75-year-old woman living alone with few social contacts, pain may be interpreted on the basis of fear of aging and inability to maintain her independent living status. The 28-year-old lawyer might interpret the pain as an expected nuisance, with the realization that healing will occur and she can get back to work soon.

Response to Pain

People respond to pain in different ways depending on their perception of the pain, including what it means to them. Some may be fearful, apprehensive, and anxious, whereas others are tolerant and optimistic. Some weep, moan, scream, beg for relief or help, threaten to destroy themselves, thrash about in bed, or move about aimlessly when in severe pain; others lie quietly in bed and may only close their eyes, grit their teeth, bite their lips, clench their hands, or perspire profusely when experiencing pain.

Some people, based on their cultural beliefs, are taught to endure severe pain without reacting outwardly, while others are very expressive about experiencing any degree of pain. People whose health beliefs and education emphasize prevention, tend to accept pain as a warning to seek help, and expect that the cause of pain will be found and cured.

Table 10-3 **Comparison of acute and chronic pain**

Characteristic	Acute pain	Chronic pain
Onset	Usually sudden	May be sudden or develop insidiously
Duration	Transient (up to 3 months)	Prolonged (months to years)
Pain localization	Pain vs. nonpain areas generally well identified	Pain vs. nonpain areas less easily differentiated; intensity becomes more difficult to evaluate (change in sensations)
Clinical signs	Signs of sympathetic overactivity (such as increased blood pressure)	Usually lacks changes in vital signs (adaptation)
Purpose	Warning that something is wrong	Meaningless; no purpose
Pattern	Self-limiting or readily corrected	Continuous or intermittent; intensity may vary or remain constant
Prognosis	Likelihood of eventual complete relief	Complete relief usually not possible

Numerous factors influence response to pain (Box 10-2). One cannot predict how any given person will respond, and value judgments should not be made concerning how a patient responds. It is very important for health professionals to recognize misbeliefs about expected pain response that prevent effective pain management (p. 171).

TYPES OF PAIN
General Types of Pain

There are two types of pain syndromes: acute and chronic. Unfortunately, a number of health care professionals provide care for the person experiencing chronic pain as though it were acute pain. There are many differences between acute and chronic pain (Table 10-3), and the approaches to pain relief are usually different, although some of the same techniques may be used.

Acute pain

Acute pain lasts no longer than 3 months. It is essentially a transient episode and informs the person that something is wrong. There is usually sudden onset from a perceived cause, and the painful areas can generally be well identified.

Sudden severe pain activates the autonomic nervous system, which may produce signs of sympathetic overactivity. These signs include tachycardia, increased blood pressure, pupillary dilation, diaphoresis, and stimulation of adrenal medullary secretion. In some situations, such as with severe visceral pain of sudden onset, vasodilation may occur with a subsequent fall in blood pressure and shock. Continuous painful stimulation can produce a steadily maintained reflex contraction of adjacent or distant muscles, such as abdominal rigidity, in people with intraabdominal pain.

Acute pain is commonly accompanied by increased muscle tension and anxiety, both of which may contribute to increased perception of pain (Fig. 10-2). If the pain is moderate or severe, overt physiologic and behavioral signs facilitate assessment of the pain. The person usually seeks pain relief.

Chronic pain

Pain that persists longer than 3 months is usually classified as chronic pain. Either the source of pain is unknown or

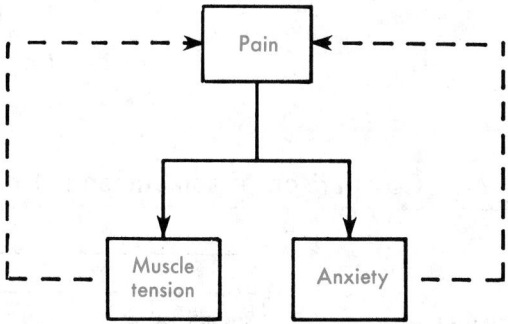

Fig. 10-2 Acute pain.

the pain cannot be eliminated. The pain sensation often becomes more diffuse, so that it is difficult for the person to identify a specific pain site. The pain may have originally been acute pain but persisted (for example, third-degree burns), or the onset may be so insidious that the person cannot state specifically when it was first experienced.

There are different types of chronic pain. *Intermittent* chronic pain occurs only at specific periods; at other times the person is pain free (migraine headaches). *Persistent* pain is always present, although there may be periods when pain is more or less intense (as seen with low back pain). One form of persistent pain may increase in frequency because of the pathologic condition (pain from incurable cancer). (Cancer pain is discussed in Chapter 11).

Chronic pain is characterized by irritability (often compounded by insomnia), which leads to decreasing interests and isolation from friends and family. Added to that is the centering of the person's life on the pain experience, with increasing feelings of helplessness and hopelessness as the pain persists. Ultimately the person withdraws from social interactions (Fig. 10-3).

The patient's world centers on ways to modify the pain experience. These patients experience tremendous disruptions in many aspects of their usual activities, including work, family roles, socialization, sleep, and leisure.[45] Some patients go from one physician to another seeking pain relief, which takes time, effort, and money. Even as they seek relief, they often lose faith in the ability of anyone to help them. The lack of continuity of care augments the

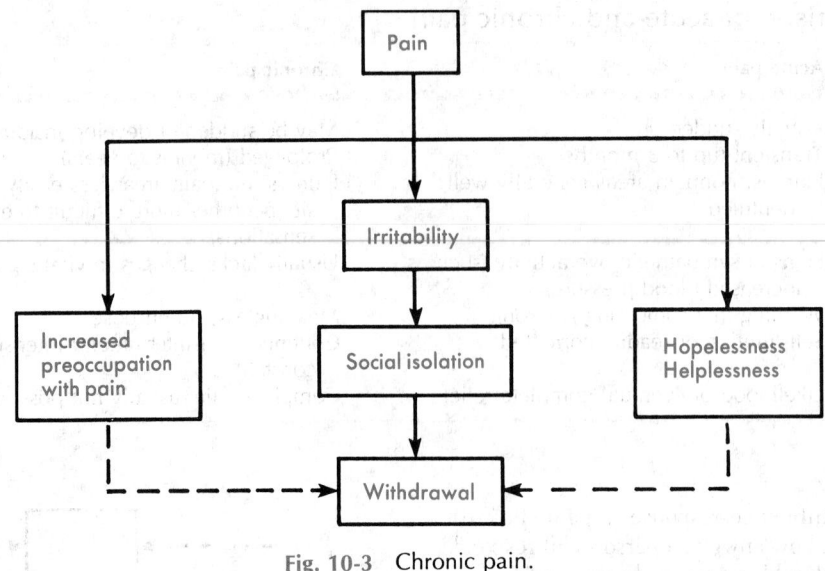

Fig. 10-3 Chronic pain.

Table 10-4 Comparison of somatic and visceral pain

| | Type of pain | | |
| | Somatic | | |
Characteristic	Superficial	Deep	Visceral
Quality	Sharp, pricking, burning	Sharp or dull and aching	Sharp, dull and aching, cramping
Localization	Good	Poor	Poor
Referred pain	No	No	Yes
Provoking stimuli	Cut, abrasion, excessive heat or cold, chemicals	Cut, pressure, heat, ischemia, displacement (bone)	Distention, ischemia, spasms, chemical irritants (no cutting)
Autonomic reactions	No	Yes	Yes
Reflex muscle contractions	No	Yes	Yes

problems. Physicians themselves may feel helpless when the patient continues to complain of pain. The development of pain clinics and inpatient teams has led to successful control of chronic pain for some (but not all) persons with chronic pain.

As a means of differentiating the acute and chronic types of pain, Crue has developed a taxonomy of pain, beginning with acute pain of short duration and ending with continuous intractable pain (unrelieved by therapeutic measures)[49]:

1. *Acute:* lasts a few days, is caused by tissue injury, and can be expected to end when source is removed
2. *Subacute:* similar to acute but persists days to weeks
3. *Recurrent acute pain:* exacerbations of chronic pain
4. *Ongoing cancer pain:* caused by progressive pathology
5. *Intractable benign pain* (adequate coping): pain is continuous but persons are able to live productive lives
6. *Intractable benign pain* (inadequate coping): person is completely disabled by the continuous pain

Specific Types of Pain
Somatic versus visceral pain

Pain may originate in the skin and subcutaneous tissue, (superficial), in the muscles and bones (deep somatic pain), or in the body organs (visceral pain). Somatic and visceral pain differ in their characteristics, particularly in the quality of pain, localization, causes, and accompanying symptoms (Table 10-4).

Referred pain

Referred pain is felt in areas other than those stimulated. It may occur when stimulation is not perceived in the primary areas. For example, the person having a heart attack may complain only of pain radiating down the left arm when in fact the tissue damage is occurring in the myocardium.

Referred pain occurs most often with damage or injury to visceral organs, and the pain is referred to cutaneous surfaces (Fig. 10-4). The origin of referred pain is complex

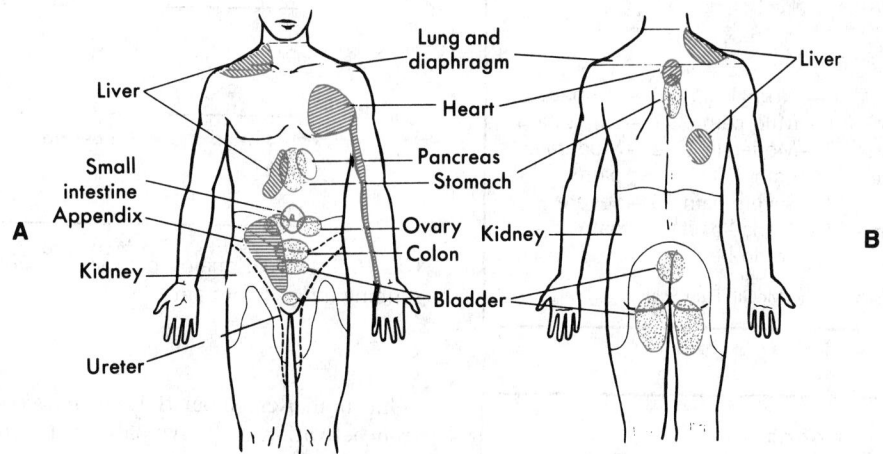

Fig. 10-4 Referred pain. **A,** Front. **B,** Back.

and not clearly understood and may relate to one or more of the following[14]:

1. Referred pain usually occurs in structures that developed from the same embryonic dermatome.
2. Visceral and somatic nerves enter the nervous system at the same spinal level and share the same spinothalamic tracts.
3. Somatic pain is more common and the person has "learned" to interpret signals conducted on certain pathways as being somatic in origin.

The cutaneous pattern of various referred pains is fairly constant and frequently seen in practice. The nurse should be able to recognize the possibility of visceral organ disease in patients who have appropriate complaints of cutaneous pain.

Psychogenic pain

The term "psychogenic" has been used to describe pain where no physical pathology has been found or where the pain appears to have a greater psychologic basis than a physical one.[39] A caution here is that diagnostic tests are not definitive measures and may not be sophisticated enough to detect pathophysiologic changes. Distinguishing between physical and emotional components of pain is difficult and it is important to remember that *all pain is real*.

Neurologic pain

Pain in the neurologic system occurs in different forms. *Neuralgia* is sharp, spasmlike pain along the course of one or more nerves. Two common areas of neuralgia are the trigeminal nerve in the face and the sciatic nerve in the lower trunk. *Causalgia,* a form of neuralgia, is severe burning pain associated with injury to a peripheral nerve in the extremities. The patient may go to great lengths to protect against irritating stimuli (which may be something as simple as the noise of a plane overhead).

Phantom limb pain is pain or discomfort perceived by the individual to be occurring in an extremity that has been amputated. It is more likely to develop in persons who had pain before amputation and may persist long after healing has occurred. The phenomenon of phantom limb pain is

poorly understood, and therefore, treatment is not very effective.

Nursing Process
Assessment
Acute pain

When a patient reports having pain or asks for pain medication, it is important to make a rapid assessment, collecting both subjective and objective data before taking any actions. Omission of assessment may lead to inadequate pain relief. For example, a young woman after pelvic surgery was crying loudly and demanding pain medication, which was given to her without assessment of the pain. No relief was obtained from the medication. When an assessment was finally made, it was discovered that she had a full bladder of which she was unaware. After she voided, the pain disappeared. Unfortunately, many patients continue to have pain postoperatively,[8] and many will not ask for help.[33] Use a rating scale to validate with patients the pain they are experiencing. This patient rating of pain intensity is assessed and recorded both before and 1 hour after giving any analgesic. If the pain intensity does not decrease after the analgesic, assess the adequacy and timing of the dose and necessity of change.

Subjective data

Data that are useful to obtain *before* pain is anticipated are the patient's expectations for pain relief from health care providers. Many persons are unaware of their expected role in speaking out when they have pain or discomfort. Some patients think they will be considered "complainers" or "bad patients" if they state that they are experiencing discomfort. In this situation, an explanation is given of the subjective nature of pain and the need for patient input to facilitate selection of effective pain relief measures.

The best assessment of pain is the patient's own evaluation. Data need to be gathered about the nature of the acute pain, that is, the location, intensity, quality, timing (onset, duration, frequency, cause), and provoking and palliative

<table>
<tr><td>10-3</td><td>**Pain scales**</td></tr>
</table>

10-3

Pain scales

0—No pain*	0—No pain	0—No pain
1—Mild pain	1—Mild pain	1—Slight pain
2—Discomfort	2—Moderate	2—Moderate
3—Distressing	pain	pain
4—Horrible	3—Severe pain	3—Severe
5—Excruciating	4—As bad as it	pain
	could be	

*NOTE: The first scale is the McGill Pain Scale.

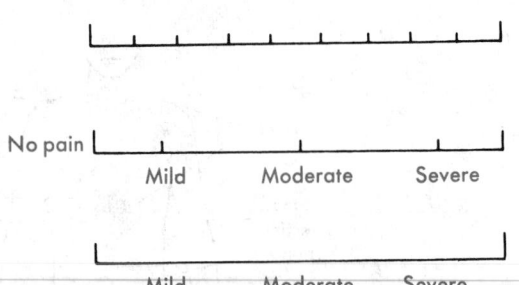

Fig. 10-5 Visual analog pain scales. Person marks line describing intensity of pain.

10-4

Objective signs of pain

Physiologic signs	Behavioral signs
Pulse: increased rate	Rigid body position
Respirations: increased	Restlessness
depth and frequency	Frowning
Blood pressure: increased	Clenched teeth
systolic and diastolic	Clenched fists
Diaphoresis, pallor	Crying
Dilated pupils	Moaning
Muscle tension (face, body)	
Nausea and vomiting (if	
pain is severe)	

factors. One approach for evaluating these characteristics is the use of the mnemonic PQRST[38]:

P Provoking factors: what makes the pain worse or relieves it
Q Quality: dull, sharp, crushing
R Region or radiation: site and radiation to other areas
S Severity or intensity
T Time: onset, duration, frequency, cause

Pain *intensity* can be determined by various means. One way is to ask the patient to describe the pain or discomfort, including a numerical rating between 0 (no pain) and 10 (worst pain possible). Other scales to assess pain intensity are outlined in Box 10-3. The obtained data is recorded. The pain scale score can also be recorded on a flow chart to provide ongoing assessment of progression of the pain. A third approach is to ask the patient to mark an X on a visual analog scale (Figure 10-5). Pain intensity should be assessed *at least once a shift* or more often if the patient is receiving interventions for pain (such as analgesics, relaxation exercises, or TENS). When acute pain has subsided, further data can be collected about the *meaning* of pain for the person.

Objective data

Objective data assist the nurse in identifying possible pain or discomfort in a person who has not reported pain and in helping to clarify the subjective response.

Objective signs of pain are of two types: physiologic and

behavioral. Remember that *physiologic* signs of pain result from activation of the sympathetic nervous system (see Box 10-4). With very severe acute pain, neurogenic shock may result from the stressful insult to the system. The *behavioral* signs are not specific to pain; therefore, if the observable data suggest that pain may be present, subjective data must be elicited to validate the assumption.

Specific objective data to be collected, therefore, include the following:

1. Appearance
2. Motor behavior
3. Affective and verbal responses
4. Vital signs
5. Skin: moisture, color
6. Inspection and gentle palpation of painful area; identify trigger points that initiate pain, if present

Sometimes the patient's subjective response differs from the objective signs. For example, the patient may request an analgesic, a back rub, or other measure to relieve pain, but when the nurse arrives to carry out the request, the patient is found to be asleep. The patient may be exhausted from the pain and thus falls asleep. The patient who is sleeping or quiet is not necessarily pain-free. It is important to reiterate that pain is what the patient says it is, and although objective data may assist in confirming the existence of pain, the diagnosis must include both subjective and objective data.

Chronic pain

Subjective data

Long-term pain requires a much more in-depth assessment of the pain syndrome. Hospitals or pain clinics that use a team approach in providing care to the person with chronic pain often develop their own pain history form or questionnaire (see references 26, 43, and 57 for examples). This history may be collected by one or more health team members. Types of data collected may include the following:

1. Demographic data
2. Sociocultural data
3. History of the pain pattern from time of onset
4. Factors perceived to increase or decrease the pain
5. Effects of the pain on the person's lifestyle
6. Meaning of the pain for the person
7. Effects of the patient's pain on other family members or friends
8. Measures used in the past and present for relief of pain

Objective data

Physiologic signs of pain may be absent in the person with chronic pain because of the body's compensatory mechanisms. Although there is adaptation to the pain stimuli, the pain persists. The absence of physiologic signs, therefore, does not indicate absence of pain. Prolonged pain, however, may create changes in the person's appearance over time, perhaps as a result of decreased appetite or lack of interest in appearance because of fatigue or depression.

Behavioral responses to chronic pain are varied and unique to the individual. Here, also, there may be few overt signs to indicate the presence of pain. Changes usually occur in daily patterns related to sleeping, eating, socialization, and libido. If the person is extremely depressed because of the ongoing pain, withdrawal behaviors may be noted.

Data analysis: nursing diagnoses

If pain is present for which specific nursing interventions may be effective, a nursing diagnosis is made of *Pain* (specify location). Possible etiologies may include but are not limited to: physiologic (specify), trauma, diagnostic tests, immobility, improper positioning, overactivity, or pressure points.

Pain may also be an etiologic factor for other nursing diagnoses, such as the following:

Anxiety related to increasing or threatened pain

Ineffective breathing pattern: related to pain in chest or abdomen

Impaired physical mobility: related to pain

Self-care deficit (describe) related to pain

Sexual dysfunction related to pain

Sleep pattern disturbance related to pain

Planning: expected patient outcomes

Expected patient outcomes for the person experiencing pain may include, but are not limited to, the following:

1. Patient states pain is relieved or reduced to a mild level.
2. Pain-related behaviors or signs (specify) are decreased or absent.
3. If pain is present when patient is discharged, patient or signifcant other can
   a. Describe general measures for pain relief (such as exercises, heat, ice)
   b. Explain prescribed medications (actions, dosages, frequency, side effects)
   c. Describe when to seek medical assistance if pain is not relieved as expected
4. Person with chronic pain can
   a. State plans to participate in ongoing therapies
   b. State plans for increasing independence in activities of daily living
   c. Identify supports for encouragement and help

The need to assess the person with pain is ongoing, yet the nurse must begin to plan an approach with the person in pain. Family members should be included when possible. The nurse is able to function independently with many interventions, but careful planning with other members of the health care team should ensure that all have the same patient outcomes or goals in mind.

One aspect of the treatment plan that is often forgotten or omitted is the incorporation of measures the patient thinks may help relieve the pain, even if these measures are different from those usually carried out in that institution. Without encouragement, the patient may hesitate to mention these possible remedies, for example, nonprescription liniments, special applications of heat and cold, unusual positioning, or favorite homemade foods or drinks. If there are no contraindications to the remedy the patient wishes to try, the health care team may consider using it before trying other relief measures.

The patient should be involved in planning the use of pain relief measures. For example, the patient may wish to receive parenteral analgesics at bedtime to improve sleep and to receive a less potent medication that causes less drowsiness before family members visit.

Planning for the same health care team members to care for the patient regularly should result in a more consistent approach and plan of care. Between the small group of health care team members and the patient, a plan of care can be developed in which the patient's decisions are honored, and a daily routine can be devised that will reduce anxiety and frustration about constant changes. This plan should include, if appropriate, such items as specified hours for analgesic administration before uncomfortable procedures, specified blocks of time for rest or napping, and coordination between various departments, such as physical therapy and occupational therapy. For some patients fatigue is a great problem, so regular visits to off-unit departments should be interspersed with rest periods; for other patients the most beneficial plan includes ensuring that they go directly from one department to the next so that time is not wasted getting in and out of bed or performing other painful maneuvers.

Implementation
Misbeliefs about pain and their effect on management

Ineffective pain management of both adults and children in a variety of settings has, unfortunately, been clearly documented.[9,33,37] There are some commonly held misbeliefs or incorrect beliefs that guide our practice and that may contribute to this ineffective pain management.[42]

Minimal or no pain should be the goal of pain management. A hospital admission should not automatically mean a pain experience for *any* patient, including elders, children, and infants. Patterns of pain intensity vary, and the diagnosis and/or type of surgery is *not* an effective primary basis for determining the amount of pain the person is experiencing or the analgesic required. Although not all pain can be removed, the use of multiple modalities can usually decrease it to at least the minimal range.

All pain tends to be assessed as acute pain. However, chronic pain differs from acute pain and needs to be assessed using different parameters (p. 170). It is important to believe that all pain is real and that malingerers (people who deliberately lie about their pain) are rare. Patients in pain will not necessarily ask for help until they are in severe pain,[33] and they may use words such as "pressure" or "soreness" instead of "pain."

Pain is a complex experience, and multiple strategies rather than only one approach are likely to be more suc-

Table 10-5   Equianalgesic* doses of commonly used opioids for moderate or severe pain

Generic name	Trade name	IM/SC dose (mg)	Oral dose (mg)	Duration of action (hours)
Morphine		10	20-30†	4
	MS Contin (slow release)	—	20-30	8-12
Hydromorphone	Dilaudid	2	4	4
Meperidine	Demerol	80-100	300	2-3
Codeine		120	200	3-4
Levorphanol	Levo-Dro-moran	2	4	4-6
Methadone	Dolophine	8-10	20	3-5
Oxycodone		15	30	3-4

*When given parenterally or orally, the drug produces approximately the same analgesic effect as 10 mg morphine (IM/SC).

†Oral to parenteral ratio for MS differs: 1:6, single dose for acute pain; 1:2 or 1:3, repeated doses for chronic pain. (Adapted from Tuttle CB: Drug management of pain in cancer patients, *Can Med Assoc J* 12:121-134, 1985.)

cessful. Incorrect beliefs about analgesic adminstration, particularly opioids, result in undermedication for patients.[48] Analgesics need to be given around the clock and titrated (regulated) so the pain levels are zero to mild. The fear of addiction should not prevent effective opioid doses as addiction rarely occurs.

It is difficult to understand and recognize another person's pain. Therefore it is crucial to gain as much information about the patient as possible instead of making assumptions about what may be happening. Recognizing misbeliefs (incorrect beliefs) is an important step to more effective pain management.

Pharmacologic approaches to pain management
Analgesics

Two groups of analgesics as well as adjuvant medications are important components of effective pain management. Opioid analgesics (also called narcotics), such as morphine, act mainly on the central nervous system to alter the perception of pain. Nonopioids, such as aspirin, block impulses mainly in the periphery and decrease inflammatory-related pain by inhibiting the synthesis of prostaglandins. For some types of pain, such as with bone cancer, analgesics from both groups are necessary. Adjuvant medications relieve pain, such as muscle spasms, or decrease the side effects associated with some analgesics, particularly opioids.

Nurses need to know the equianalgesic doses for both opioid and nonopioid analgesics. This means knowing the dose of any opioid that has the same strength (potency) as parenteral morphine 10 mg (Table 10-5).

Opioid analgesics. Opioids are the most effective analgesics for relief of moderate to severe pain. They must be given around the clock to reach and maintain the steady blood levels necessary for pain relief. Side effects of opioids vary with the physiologic state of the patient. Constipation is the most common side effect, and laxatives should be given to any patient receiving opioids on a regular basis. Nausea and vomiting are experienced by some; these patients usually respond well to antiemetics. Sedation and drowsiness may occur for the first 48 to 72 hours, but one needs to consider that the patient may be catching up on sleep lost because of pain. Respiratory depression is rarely a problem with standardized doses and careful titration (slowly increasing the dose). Narcan will reverse any depressive effect.

The oral route is preferred unless the patient is vomiting, unable or not permitted to swallow, or is in acute pain. Routes other than intramuscular or subcutaneous injection are rectal, intravenous, transdermal, or epidural (see Chapter 22).[17,34] Slow release preparations, such as MS Contin, are given every 8 to 12 hours, allowing less focus on the pain and better control with fewer side effects.

Concern for addiction. Persons receiving opioids for pain relief very rarely develop addiction. The incidence of opioid addiction in hospitalized patients is less than 1%.[61] Patients are taking opioids for pain relief and not for the psychologic effect. Unfortunately, health professionals are overly concerned about addiction, and opioids are underprescribed by physicians and underadministered by nurses.[48]

It is important to differentiate tolerance, dependence, and addiction, as summarized below:

Tolerance	Larger doses are needed to produce desired effects
Dependence	Need to continue use of drug to prevent symptoms
Addiction	Behavioral pattern of compulsive drug use; drug used for psychologic effect

Drug tolerance occurs with some patients and with some conditions, usually when the patient's pain is first being controlled and/or when the pain increases. This is a physiologic response and requires increasing the dose until pain relief is reached. There is no ceiling or maximum amount of opioid that can be given. *Physical dependency,* appearance of physiologic withdrawal symptoms, *rarely happens* because as pain decreases the dosage is gradually tapered, and no symptoms are experienced. Physical dependency and drug tolerance are involuntary behaviors.

Patient-controlled analgesia. One method of providing more adequate pain control with opioids is the system of patient-controlled analgesia (PCA). The system consists of a syringe-type infusion pump that is filled with the prescribed opioid and is piggybacked into an intravenous injection port. PCA is activated when the patient pushes a button to release a set amount of opioid by bolus. A refractory time prevents delivery of another bolus before a preset time interval. The device also records the patient's attempts to receive the opioid in a given time period. The physician determines the opioid dosage and the refractory time interval.

Experience has demonstrated that persons using PCA tend to take less than those receiving the standard method

Table 10-6   NSAIDs commonly used for mild to moderate pain

Generic name	Trade name	Dosage range
Fenoprofen	Nalfon	200 mg q 4-6 hr prn
Ibuprofen	Advil, Motrin	400 mg q 4-6 hr prn
Mefenamic acid	Ponstel	500 mg initially then 250 mg q 6 hr prn (not to exceed 7 days)
Naproxen	Anaprox, Naprosyn	550 mg initially, then 275 mg q 6-8 hr prn
Zomepirac	Zomax	50 to 100 mg q 4-6 hr prn

of intramuscular injections.[21,63] PCA has been used for postoperative pain, for other types of acute pain such as sickle cell crisis, and for cancer pain.[20,36] Nursing activities related to PCA include maintaining the system, recording the number of times the patient activates the system, and monitoring the patient's pain. The patient should be the only person who activates the PCA (presses the button); this serves as a safeguard to prevent oversedation.

Nonopioid analgesics. Mild to moderate pain can generally be controlled by nonopioid analgesics, most commonly nonsteroidal antiinflammatory agents (NSAIDs), such as aspirin, and by acetaminophen.

Acetaminophen (Tylenol, Datril) is comparable to aspirin for analgesic effects but is not antiinflammatory. It causes less alteration in prothrombin level and has fewer side effects but can cause severe liver damage. It is useful for persons who are allergic to aspirin and for whom aspirin is contraindicated.

Nonsteroidal antiinflammatory drugs. The nonsteroidal antiinflammatory drugs (NSAIDs) act primarily by inhibition of prostaglandin synthesis. In lower doses, these drugs have analgesic properties; in higher doses there is antiinflammatory action in addition to analgesia. The principal uses of NSAIDs are control of moderate pain of dysmenorrhea, arthritis and other musculoskeletal disorders, postoperative pain, and migraine. NSAIDs commonly used pain are listed in Table 10-6.

NSAIDs inhibit platelet aggregation with resulting increased bleeding time. Common side effects include gastrointestinal disturbances, dizziness, tinnitus, and headache. Persons who are hypersensitive to aspirin may also be hypersensitive to NSAIDs. Concurrent use of an NSAID with aspirin may lead to increased side effects.

Phenylbutazone (Butazolidin) is an NSAID with potent antiinflammatory properties given for short-term therapy for moderately severe arthritis, gout, or bursitis. Although the drug has analgesic activity, it is not used as a general analgesic for moderate pain because it is poorly tolerated by many persons and has numerous side effects, including hematologic changes, gastric irritation, and fluid and electrolyte disturbances.

Aspirin. Acetylsalicylic acid (aspirin) is the most widely used analgesic for mild to moderate pain. Salicylates produce analgesia by blocking pain impulses peripherally or centrally, possibly in the hypothalamus, and by inhibiting synthesis of prostaglandins. Aspirin is therefore also an

antiinflammatory agent. Aspirin has an onset of 15 to 20 minutes, peak of 1 to 2 hours, and duration of 3 to 4 hours.

Aspirin is a platelet aggregation inhibitor and a weak vitamin K antagonist. It produces an increased bleeding time and prolonged prothrombin time when given in large doses. Therefore, it is contraindicated for persons receiving anticoagulant drugs.

Irritation of the gastric mucosa is a common side effect of aspirin; therefore it should not be taken on an empty stomach. Aspirin is best taken after meals or with a snack such as a glass of milk. Persons with a history of peptic ulcer should avoid taking aspirin. Aspirin should also be avoided by persons taking phenylbutazone and spironolactone because of drug interaction and by adolescents and young adults because of risk of Reye's syndrome.

Other drugs for pain relief. *Smooth muscle relaxants* may be given for pain from muscle spasms and include propantheline bromide (Pro-Banthine) and drugs of the belladonna group, such as atropine. For example, belladonna and opium (B&O) suppositories are effective in relieving bladder spasms after prostatectomy.

Sedatives and antianxiety agents are sometimes prescribed for persons with pain. These drugs do *not* have analgesic effect but may permit relaxation and decrease anxiety and thus prevent potentiation of pain. The drugs may permit the person to sleep and thus be better able to cope with the pain. In some persons sedatives and antianxiety agents may lead to disorientation and agitation, which can increase the pain and decrease the person's ability to cope. Treating pain with analgesics is the more effective and preferred method.

Tricyclic antidepressants, such as amitriptyline (Elavil) produce analgesia at doses lower than those used for depression. These drugs are useful in nerve injury pain, such as with postherpetic neuralgia (shingles).

Counterirritants are over-the-counter (OTC) drugs that relieve local pain by producing counterirritation (stimulation of the large A-beta fibers). Examples of counterirritants include ointments containing methyl salicylate (oil of wintergreen) or ethyl aminobenzoate and oil of cloves (for toothaches).

Nonpharmacologic approaches to pain management

Nonpharmacologic approaches should be considered along with analgesics for effective pain management. This type of intervention can alter pain transmission, modify the response to pain, and modify the pain stimulus.

10-5

Methods of electrical stimulation for pain control	
Transcutaneous electrical nerve stimulator (TENS)	Manually controlled stimulation of specific pain areas through externally placed electrodes
Percutaneous implanted spinal cord epidural stimulator (PISCES)	Stimulation by an external transistorized receiver through leads inserted percutaneously in epidural space of spinal column
Dorsal column stimulator	Stimulation by a transistorized receiver, implanted surgically in an infraclavicular or abdominal skin pouch, through electrodes surgically implanted on dorsum of spinal cord

Alter pain transmission

Electrical stimulators. The purpose of electrical stimulators is to modify the pain stimulus by blocking or changing the painful stimulus with stimulation perceived as less painful. The success of this approach is thought to be explained by the gate control theory of pain transmission, that is, blockage of pain stimulus by stimulation of the large sensory fibers. Selected forms of electrical stimulation may activate the opiate or nonopiate descending pathways (see Box 10-5).

Transcutaneous electrical nerve stimulator. The transcutaneous electrical nerve stimulator (TENS) is a battery-powered stimulator worn externally. It is a convenient, nonintrusive, nonaddictive type of pain therapy that can be learned easily by the patient. Success is variable, and it is usually used along with other pain therapies.

A number of TENS devices are on the market; all consist of a battery-powered portable pulse generator about the size of a pocket paging device. Control knobs on the generator permit adjustment of the impulse. The generator is connected by a pair of cables to electrically conductive tape electrodes placed at appropriate sites on the skin. The TENS delivers a balanced biphasic potential in a waveform.

TENS appears to be more useful for postoperative pain, posttraumatic pain, phantom limb pain, peripheral neuralgias, low back pain, and muscle and bone pain. It is less effective with cancer pain, inflammatory arthritis, trigeminal neuralgia, or with anxious or depressed persons.[67]

TENS electrodes should not be placed over hair, irritated skin, sutures, carotid sinus (may produce bradycardia), laryngeal or pharyngeal muscles (may trigger spasms), or a pregnant uterus.[11] A cardiac pacemaker may interfere with TENS effects. Suggested electrode placement may include (1) directly over the painful area, (2) at trigger points along the nerve pathways, or (3) at trigger points in the same dermatome as the pain.[62]

Routine skin care at the electrode sites includes the following:

1. Remove and clean electrodes at least once a day.
2. Wash skin with soap and water.
3. Allow skin to air dry.
4. Wipe skin with a prep pad before reapplying conductor pad.

If the skin becomes irritated, it may be cleaned with milk of magnesia, rinsed well, then air dried.[62]

Spinal cord stimulators. Spinal cord stimulators are similar to the TENS except that they are intrusive procedures. Instead of electrode placement on the skin, the electrodes are placed on or near the spinal cord. This is done either surgically over the ventral surface of the spinal cord or percutaneously through the back into the epidural space. Because percutaneous placement of electrodes (PISCES) can be performed under local anesthesia, it is preferred over surgical placement of the dorsal column stimulator electrodes. Postoperative care after dorsal column stimulator implantation includes the same care that follows laminectomy, with monitoring for infection and leakage of cerebrospinal fluid (Chapter 37).

Neurosurgical procedures. Constant relentless chronic pain that cannot be controlled by analgesics (*intractable pain*) may be reduced or eliminated by one of various neurosurgical procedures (Table 10-7 and Fig. 10-6). Other forms of pain control are usually attempted before neurosurgical procedures.

Neurosurgical procedures do not play a major role in management of chronic pain. Major limitations include short duration of relief, occurrence of dysesthesia (pain induced by gentle touch of the skin), central pain syndrome (burning sensations in skin areas lacking sensation from surgical afferent interruptions), and possible further neurologic dysfunction.[64]

Neurectomy has limitations in that peripheral nerves may regenerate. Both rhizotomy and anterolateral cordotomy require laminectomy. A more commonly used procedure is percutaneous cordotomy, a closed stereotactic procedure in which the lesion is first located by using three-dimensional coordinates. The anterospinothalamic tracts are destroyed by electrodes inserted percutaneously. The patient is awake to provide feedback, thus providing more accurate site location and better pain relief. The effect usually lasts 18 to 24 months.[64]

Rhizotomy interferes with the ability to perceive heat and cold; therefore, protection from extremes in temperatures is important for prevention of injury. The advantages of cordotomy include a wide sense of analgesia below the surgical site while preserving other sensory and motor functions. After surgery there may be temporary leg weakness and loss of bowel and bladder control from edema of the spinal cord; these usually disappear within 2 weeks. If quadriceps setting exercises are begun in the early postoperative period, walking will be less difficult.

Table 10-7 Neurosurgical procedures for pain control

Procedure	Method	Use
Neurectomy	Severing of nerve fibers from the cell body	Trigeminal neuralgia (fifth nerve resection); incapacitating dysmenorrhea (presascral neurectomy)
Rhizotomy	Resection of posterior nerve root before it enters spinal cord	Severe pain in upper trunk (for example, lung cancer)
Cordotomy	Severing of ascending anterolateral pain-conducting pathways of spinal cord	Severe pain of lower body (for example, pelvic cancer)
Sympathectomy	Excision or destruction of one or more sympathetic ganglia or nerves	Pain secondary to vascular insufficiency of extremities (for example, Raynaud's disease)

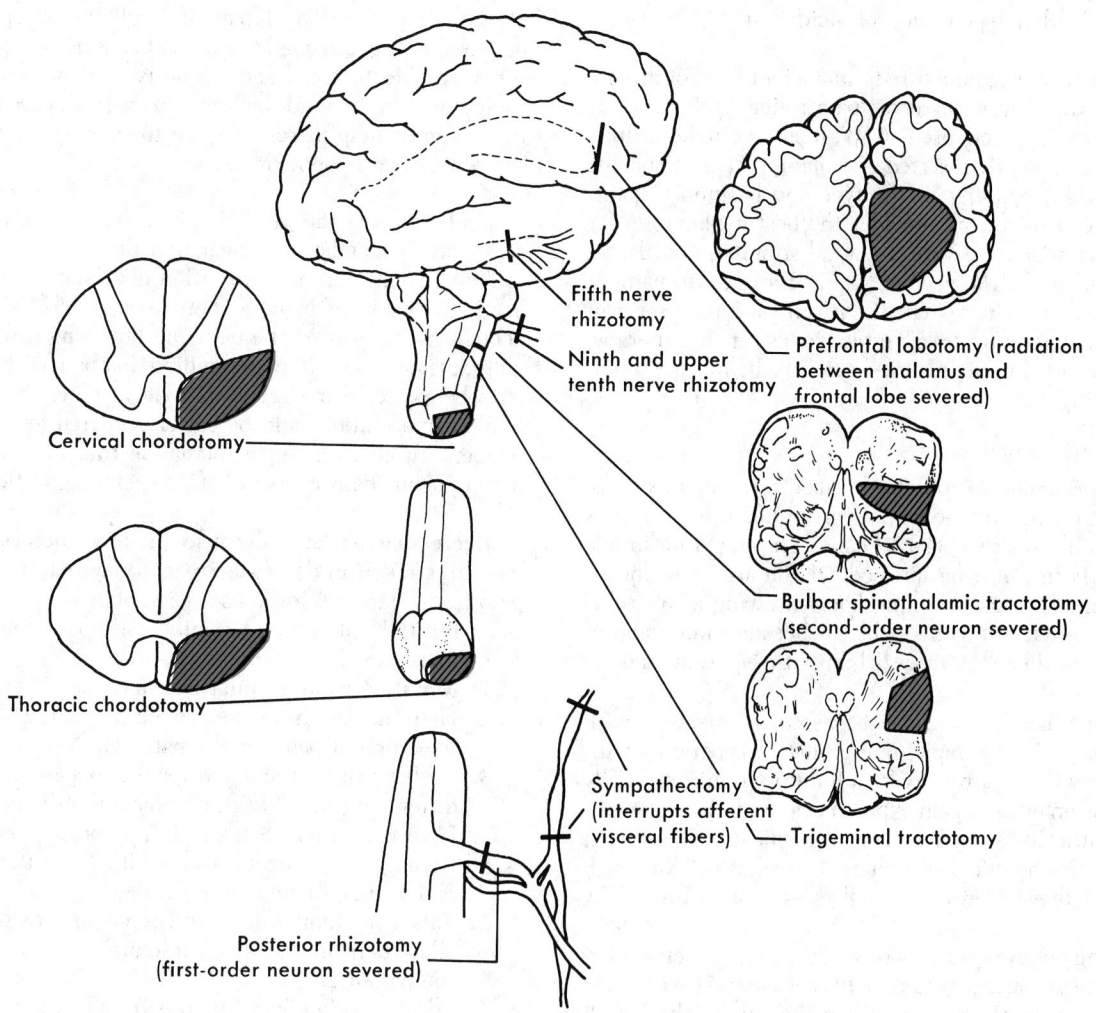

Fig. 10-6 Neurosurgical procedures for pain relief. (From Conway-Rutkowski BL: *Carini and Owens' neurological and neurosurgical nursing*, ed 8, St Louis, 1984, Mosby—Year Book.)

Pain pathways in the brain may also be interrupted by stereotactic techniques (tractotomy, thalamotomy, lobotomy). These surgical procedures are usually reserved as a final solution for patients with intractable pain, usually from malignant invasion of cranial or facial structures. Lobotomy usually results in a change in personality.

Nerve block. A nerve block involves the injection of substances such as local anesthetics or neurolytic agents (for example, alcohol or phenol) close to nerves to block the conduction of impulses over the nerves. Nerve blocks are frequently used for the symptomatic relief of pain. They are used to treat chronic pain associated with peripheral vascular disease, trigeminal neuralgia, causalgia, and cancer.

A nerve block may be unsuccessful because of difficulty in locating the correct nerve fiber or because of the complexity of the pain. Because the nerve fibers, ganglia, and roots contain fibers other than those for pain, and because some of the injected agents may leak out of the injection site and affect other nerves, the nerve block usually produces some other type of neurologic deficit.

Acupuncture. Acupuncture is an ancient form of disease treatment that can be used for pain relief. Only recently has the method been used in Western countries. Small needles are skillfully inserted and manipulated at specific body points, depending on the type and location of pain. The gate control theory provides the best explanation for the success of acupuncture: the local stimulation of large-diameter fibers by the needles "closes the gate" to pain. It is not known to what extent the psyche and the power of suggestion contribute to the effectiveness of this therapy. Nursing intervention includes careful client assessment and teaching.

Modify pain response

Behavior modification. Behavior modification consists of a planned change in the way a person behaves by means of rewarding desired behavior and ignoring undesirable behavior. Forms of behavior modification are used unconsciously all the time: a young boy "throwing a tantrum" may be ignored, but as his behavior becomes more appropriate his mother may reward him with her time and attention.

Behavior modification may be useful for persons with chronic pain. For example, one protocol for patients with chronic low back pain is to set a limit of 10 minutes daily for discussion of their pain experiences (with the exception of data-gathering interviews). Pain medications are given on a regular schedule to dissociate the feelings of pain with inappropriate use (reward) of analgesics or other unhealthy behaviors.

In using behavioral methods to alter pain-associated behavior or to encourage patient activities, success will occur only with a consistent approach on the part of the health care team. Although patients should always be praised for their efforts to comply or assist with treatment regimens, a true behavior modification program requires careful analysis of patient behavior and the development of a specific and comprehensive treatment plan.

Biofeedback and autogenic training. Some persons are able to alter their body functions through mental concentration. In biofeedback training a machine that monitors brain wave activity (electroencephalograph [EEG]) is used. The individual concentrates on slowing his or her brain wave activity to rates at which pain and distress are unlikely to cause discomfort (that is, complete relaxation). It may take many months of regular practice to achieve the desired level of control. The nurse should encourage and praise the person's efforts.

In autogenic training the same type of self-regulation is used to alter various autonomic nervous system functions, such as pulse, blood pressure, and muscle tension. Practiced use of transcendental meditation and other methods of concentration and self-control may achieve the same degree of autoregulation without the use of sophisticated physiologic monitoring equipment.

Hypnosis. Hypnosis may be used in the treatment of various conditions, particularly when these conditions are aggravated by tension and stress. Individuals are helped to alter their perception of pain through the acceptance of positive suggestions made to the subconscious. Many persons are able to learn self-hypnosis. Individuals vary in their suggestibility and readiness to try this approach. The nurse's most helpful role may be to support the patient's desire to make hypnotism work.

Explanation of the problem. As a result of nursing assessment, it may become clear that the patient's response to pain is really the manifestation of a lack of knowledge about the cause of pain. Sometimes a simple explanation about what is causing the pain and how long it will last is all that is necessary. Understanding that pain or discomfort is to be expected may relieve anxiety or help the patient to alter expectations and be better prepared for what will happen. In all cases, an explanation that includes information about pain is given before each diagnostic test.

Decreasing anxiety. Because anxiety increases pain, measures taken to decrease anxiety may help to decrease pain (see Chapter 6 for a discussion of anxiety). Interventions for the patient and family with pain include the following:
1. Maintain a calm, quiet manner.
2. Help the patient explore concerns related to the pain (meaning of pain for the patient).
3. Respect the patient's response to pain, even if it differs considerably from what the nurse expects.
4. Hold the patient's hand, if appropriate.
5. Arrange for someone to be with the patient if the patient fears being alone.
6. Talk with family or close friends and help them to allay their anxieties so these are not transmitted to the patient.
7. Teach the family and close friends ways in which they can help the patient, such as massage, encouraging the patient to use distraction or relaxation techniques, or supporting painful parts when moving. People often feel helpless when observing a loved one in pain and may need help themselves to cope.

Modify the pain stimulus

Cutaneous stimulation. Cutaneous stimulation innervates the large A-delta fibers to block the pain stimuli across the small C fibers. Methods of cutaneous stimulation include the following:
1. Lightly rubbing the affected area
2. Back rub
3. Application of heat or cold
4. Whirlpool massage

Reducing additional physical stimuli. Although in many instances pain cannot be prevented, it is often possible to avoid additional pain when pain is already present. For example, when moving the body or an extremity, supporting the trunk or extremity will prevent increasing the pain by unilateral pulling on muscles, joints, and ligaments. Interventions include the following list:
1. Use a turning sheet for patients with severe neck, back, or general trunk pain
2. Place a pillow under a painful joint when helping a patient change position
3. Support limbs at the joints rather than the muscle bellies when handling an extremity
4. Use special beds (Stryker frame, Foster bed, CircOlectric bed) for patients with severe general or trunk pain
5. Avoid bumping or moving the bed suddenly

Reducing auditory and visual stimuli. The patient may experience sensory overload with subsequent potentiation of pain sitmuli. If nurses could stand still for 5 minutes in the patient's environment and watch and listen, they might understand that some patients are simply bombarded with noise and visual stimulation. If these are problems, it may be possible to change the environment. Changes include the following:
1. Move the patient to a quieter room away from the center of activity.
2. Dim any bright lights; pull shades if sunlight is intense.
3. Keep verbal interactions at a minimum when pain is severe.
4. Keep television or radio at a resonable level but not loud.
5. Control the number of persons entering the patient's room according to patient's wishes.

Reducing social isolation. When external stimuli are decreased too much, the patient may lack distraction from the pain stimuli; thus pain perception is increased. Social isolation may occur for a variety of reasons: The serious nature of a patient's disease may necessitate being in a private room for an extended period; hospitalization far away from home may mean few family members and friends can visit; extended periods of hospitalization may result in friends losing interest in visiting; or the patient may complain so much that no one cares to visit to hear the monologue repeated.

Each of these causes of isolation may have a different solution. In any event, careful assessment may indicate that social isolation is a problem for the patient. Before determining the plan for addressing this problem, the patient should be consulted about the desire and need to alter the present situation. Possible nursing interventions include the following:
1. Place the patient with a compatible roommate
2. Plan frequent contacts with health team members
3. Facilitate visits by family and friends
4. Help patient to be as comfortable as possible during visits by family or friends

Therapeutic touch. A less traditional therapy, that of therapeutic touch, may be helpful to patients in pain. The rationale for the success of therapeutic touch is not clearly understood. The nurse undergoes a brief period of meditation before coming in contact with the patient. During this period the nurse quiets his or her internal energy levels and then touches the patient and transmits the healing energies. Few nurses are trained in the use of therapeutic touch as described. It does seem to be helpful for some patients and some kinds of pain.

Distraction and relaxation exercises. Patients can be taught to modify their sensory input to control pain by activities that promote distraction or relaxation.

Distraction. Distraction interferes with the pain stimulus, thereby modifying the awareness of the pain. Mild or moderate pain can be modified by focusing on activity in the environment. A very quiet environment providing little or no sensory input can actually intensify the pain experience because the individual has nothing to focus on but the painful stimulus.

Severe pain requires more active participation by the individual in an effort to block out the painful stimulus. This can be enhanced by involving two or more sensory modalities, such as vision, hearing, touch, or movement. The distractors must be powerful enough to involve the individual's total interest without resulting in fatigue. Pain of long duration requires a variety of meaningful distracters. Methods of distraction include the following:
1. Playing games, watching television
2. Talking with someone
3. Listening to favorite music
4. Rhythmic breathing
5. Focusing on an object

Waking-imagined analgesia. Waking-imagined analgesia is defined as imagining a pleasant situation when a noxious stimulus is applied. This intervention is similar to distraction except that the person concentrates on trying to relive the sensations that occurred during a previous pleasant experience rather than on enumerating the events that took place. Only a small percentage of the population in pain can use this method of analgesia; more can derive benefit from distraction alone.

Relaxation. Full relaxation decreases muscle tension and fatigue that usually accompanies pain. It also helps to decrease anxiety, thereby preventing augmentation of the pain stimulus. Carrying out relaxation techniques also serves as a form of distraction.

Not all persons with severe pain are able to achieve sufficient relaxation to have an effect on decreasing the pain sensation. Relaxation exercises may be especially beneficial for persons with chronic pain to help reduce stress that exacerbates the pain and to help the person achieve a sense of control, of being better able to cope with the pain. There are numerous forms of relaxation techniques (see Chapter 6). Success with a relaxation technique requires practice and encouragement.

Specific nursing implications for pain control

Specific nursing interventions for pain relief include those related to preventing pain, modifying the stimulus, and modifying the response to pain as previously described. General guidelines for pain relief are listed here.

Guidelines for pain relief measures

1. *Preparation for painful experiences*
   Prepare patients for what to expect in terms of discomfort and measures of pain control *before* pain occurs, whenever possible (such as before painful tests or treatments). Intensity and duration of pain are decreased because of decreased anxiety and the patient's sense of control.
2. *Preventive approach*
   Use pain relief measures *before* pain becomes moderate or severe. The more severe the pain the less the possibility of relief.
3. *Placebo response*
   Use methods that employ a placebo response, that is, some relief from discomfort not related specifically to the applied pain relief method. If the person expects relief from the pain, anxiety and muscle tension will decrease, and decreased pain is experienced. This can be accomplished by suggestion ("This should help you feel better") or by using methods the patient believes will work.
4. *Patient's ability or will to participate*
   Consider the patient's ability or will to be active or passive in using pain relief measures. Decreased ability results from severe pain, fatigue, sedation, or unconsciousness. Decreased will occurs with some persons with chronic pain who have experienced numerous failures in pain relief.
5. *Varying pain relief measures*
   Use more than one type of pain relief measure when appropriate. For example, give an analgesic, rub the patient's back, and then offer some distraction, or combine an analgesic with relaxation response.
6. *Introducing new pain relief measures*
   Introduce a new method in combination with known effective methods. Some measures, such as distraction or relaxation, require practice; do not discard the new method until after several tries.
7. *Giving analgesics*
   a. Assess and record the effectiveness of analgesics given.
   b. Ask the patient for a pain rating (0 to 10) on each shift, before, and 1 hour after each analgesic given.
   c. Give analgesics to prevent or minimize pain.
   d. Give opioids on a regular basis rather than as needed when acute pain is anticipated, such as after some general surgical procedures.
   e. If the medications will be given "as needed," instruct patient to report the presence of developing or recurrent pain, and ask regularly for pain ratings.
   f. Determine which patients are at high risk for developing pain and assess them frequently for presence of increasing pain.
   g. Use the oral route, when possible, where patient is not in acute pain, can swallow, and is not nauseated.
   h. Use the parenteral route in acute intermittent pain to provide immediate, short-term relief.

Team approach for chronic pain control

In recent years knowledge of the nature of chronic pain and the need for coordinated efforts of different health care professionals have resulted in the establishment of pain clinics and inpatient pain teams for control of chronic pain.

Pain clinics. Most pain clinics use a team approach that includes physicians (internists, dolorologists [pain specialists], surgeons, psychiatrists), nurses, physical and occupational therapists, social workers, psychologists, vocational rehabilitation counselors, and appropriate others. Each pain clinic is organized differently and places greater emphasis on different aspects of pain relief. Usual approaches to pain relief include the following:
1. Behavior modification (with patient's approval)
2. Medications: opioids, NSAIDs, laxatives, tricyclics
3. Exercise and activity prescriptions
4. Family training to support planned goals/activities.

The responsibility of the nurse varies depending on the available team members and may include patient assessment, documentation of observations, creating and maintaining a therapeutic milieu, providing emotional support for patient and family, and patient teaching. Nurses who work in pain clinics must be skilled in nurse-client interactions, be knowledgeable about the mechanisms of pain and the effectiveness of various treatment modalities, and possess patience and understanding as they assist patients in reaching their goals.

Inpatient chronic pain teams. Persons with chronic persistent pain are sometimes admitted to a hospital for evaluation or initiation of treatment by a multidisciplinary health team similar to that in a pain clinic. One example is a team for evaluation and treatment of chronic back pain. Each team member participates in the evaluation individually and collectively and in team conferences to develop a specific treatment plan. The culmination of the hospitalization is a discharge conference with the patient and family members in which future treatment plans and recommendations are presented and discussed.

Protocols are developed for the approach to be used in control of the chronic pain; all persons providing patient care during the hospitalization need to become familiar with the protocols so that a consistent approach is used for pain control. For example, protocols for control of chronic back pain in one large medical center include an initial immobilization phase in which patients are placed in pelvic traction and instructed to move as little as possible (for example, eat in side-lying position). This phase is followed by a mobilization phase in which the patients are encouraged to be active (for example, walk to physical therapy and to the cafeteria for meals and make their own beds). The type of nursing care is therefore different depending on which phase is being implemented.

Nursing responsibilities include patient assessment, documenting observations, carrying out phase-related activities, carrying out designated behavior modification modalities, and patient teaching.

Evaluation

Evaluation is an important component that is often forgotten in the care of the patient with pain. Evaluation is vital so that the effectiveness of the interventions continues, or that the interventions be modified, replaced with another intervention, or discontinued. The essential questions to consider in regard to *acute* pain are as follows.

Does the patient still have pain?

If so, how does it compare with the pain experienced before the intervention?

If it is better but still present, should the same intervention(s) be continued unchanged or modified?

Should new interventions be added?

If it is not better, were sufficient data obtained in the initial assessment to determine the cause of pain?

Are there new data to indicate a different diagnosis?

What are the patient's thoughts about the continuing pain and the modes of intervention?

The essential questions to consider in regard to *chronic* pain are as follows:

To what extent is the patient participating in the planned therapeutic program?

What is the patient's assessment of present pain?

Pain teams often have special evaluation guidelines specific to their patient population and treatment goals.

SUMMARY

1. Pain is a complex universal, yet individualized, experience.
2. Nociceptors are pain receptors that respond to chemical, thermal, electrical, or mechanical stimuli. Chemical stimuli released by damaged tissues include histamines, bradykinins, prostaglandins, and acids.
3. Pain impulses are transmitted over faster-conducting A-delta and slower-conducting C fibers to the substantia gelatinosa (SG) of the dorsal horn of the spinal cord. Ascending spinal pathways in the ventral spinal cord carry impulses to the thalamus and cortex.
4. Some descending spinal pathways carry pain inhibitory impulses back to the SG. Pain impulses transmitted over A-beta fibers also have a suppressive effect on impulses over the A-delta and C fibers.
5. Substance P is a neurotransmitter of pain impulses. Endorphins and serotonin are neurotransmitters of pain-inhibitory impulses.
6. The gate control theory proposes that the SG is a gating mechanism that may modify the pain experience by "opening" or "closing" the gate to pain impulse transmission. The gating mechanism is influenced by impulses from A-delta and C fibers and from descending pathways from the brainstem and cortex.
7. The pain experience is influenced by the individual's pain perception and response.
8. Pain perception is subjective, highly complex, and individual. It is influenced by characteristics of the pain stimuli and transmission and by receptivity and interpretation in the cerebral cortex.
9. Pain detection threshold is the intensity of the stimulus necessary for the person to perceive pain.
10. Pain tolerance is the maximum degree of pain intensity that the person is willing to endure before seeking relief. Pain tolerance may be increased by drugs, warmth, counterirritation, distraction, and strong beliefs; it may be decreased by fatigue, anxiety, boredom, continuous pain, or illness.
11. Pain response is influenced by the degree of pain perception, past experiences, sociocultural values, health status, anxiety, and age.
12. Acute pain is a sudden short-term event, usually with a known source and self-limiting or readily corrected. The typical clinical signs are usually present and pain areas generally well identified. It leads to action to relieve pain with likelihood of eventual relief. Acute pain is characterized by anxiety and muscle tension.
13. Chronic pain is a prolonged situation, often with no purpose. Pain areas are less easily defined. Pain may be continuous or intermittent and with few typical clinical signs. It leads to actions to modify the pain experience. Chronic pain is characterized by increased preoccupation with pain, hopelessness, and irritability, all leading to withdrawal.
14. Superficial somatic pain is sharp and pricking, well localized, and usually not accompanied by autonomic reactions. Deep somatic and visceral pains are sharp or dull and aching, poorly localized, and usually accompanied by autonomic reactions.
15. Referred pain is felt in areas other than those stimulated; it is usually visceral in origin.
16. Phantom limb pain is perceived to be occurring in a limb that has been amputated.
17. Pain intensity can be determined by the use of pain scales or visual analog scales in addition to asking the person to describe the pain.
18. Subjective data for pain include the location, intensity, quality, timing (onset, duration, frequency, cause), and provoking or palliative factors.
19. Objective data include appearance, motor behavior, affective and verbal response, vital signs, skin color and moisture, and inspection and palpation of painful areas.
20. Opioids provide relief of moderate to severe pain. Persons with severe pain rarely develop opioid addiction. Smaller, more frequent dosages of opioids are more effective for severe acute pain, whereas larger, less frequent dosages are more effective for severe cancer pain.

21. Patient-controlled analgesia is a system of self-administration by an intravenous set-up whereby a prescribed preset bolus of opioid may be taken but not repeated until a prescribed refractory time has occurred.
22. Acetaminophen and NSAIDs (such as aspirin) provide relief of mild to moderate pain.
23. Electrical stimulators include TENS and spinal cord stimulators. TENS is a nonintrusive system, easily learned by the patient and useful for postoperative, posttraumatic, peripheral neuralgia, and muscle and bone pain.
24. Approaches to modify the person's pain response include behavior modification, biofeedback and autogenic training, hypnosis, careful explanations, and anxiety reduction.
25. General nursing interventions for pain relief include preparing patients for painful experiences, using pain relief measures before pain becomes severe, using the placebo response, varying pain relief measures, trying new approaches, and giving analgesics as effectively as possible.
26. Nursing interventions to modify the pain stimulus include preventing pain when possible; modifying the pain stimulus by cutaneous stimulation, reduction of noise and visual stimuli, decreasing social isolation, therapeutic touch, distraction, and relaxation exercises; and modifying the pain response by careful explanations and measures to decrease anxiety.

STUDY QUESTIONS

* How does the assessment of acute pain differ from that of chronic pain? Think about two patients for whom you have provided care, one with acute pain and one with chronic pain. In what ways did their responses to pain differ, and how did these responses influence different management approaches?
* What misbeliefs are most prevalent in your areas of practice, and how have you tried to change them in relation to your practice and others?
* What are the equianalgesic doses and the duration of action for the most frequently administered analgesics?
* How do the following terms differ: *Pain tolerance* and *pain threshold*? *Pain tolerance* and *drug tolerance*? *Drug dependence* and *drug addiction*?
* Interview three or four patients who are using a non-pharmacologic pain intervention. Compare and contrast the method, frequency of use, patient satisfaction, and effectiveness for pain relief. Were several modalities used (including drugs), and was the combination of approaches successful?

REFERENCES AND SELECTED READINGS

1.* Amadio P, Cummings D, Amadio P: Pain in the elderly: management techniques, *Pain Manag* 6(12):33-41, 1987.
2.* Baquire ML: What matters most in chronic pain management, *RN* 52(3):46-50, 1989.
3. Barkas G, Duafala ME: Advances in cancer pain management: a review of patient controlled analgesia, *J Pain Sympt Manag* 3(3):150-160, 1988.
4.* Bast C, Hayes P: PCA, a new way to spell pain relief: patient controlled analgesia, *RN* 49(8):18-20, 1986.
5.* Copp LA, editor: *Recent advances in nursing, perspectives* and pain, New York, 1985, Churchill Livingstone.
6.* Coyle N: Analgesics and pain, *Nurs Clin North Am* 22(3):727-741, 1987.
7.* Dernham P: Phantom limb pain, *Geriatr Nurs* 7:34-37, 1986.
8.* Donovan M: Acute pain relief, *Nurs Clin North Am* 25(4):851-861, 1990.
9. Donovan M, Dillon P, McGuire L: The incidence and characteristics of pain in a sample of medical-surgical inpatients, *Pain* 30:69-78, 1987.
10. Dostrovsky J: Pathways of pain: update, *Persp Pain Manag* 1(1):4-8, 1991.
11. Driscoll CE: Pain management, *Prim Care* 14(2):337-352, 1987.
12.* Fields H: *Pain,* Toronto, 1987, McGraw-Hill Book Co.
13.* Fordham M: Psychophysiologic pain theories, *Nursing* (London) 3:360-364, 1986.
14. Ganong WF: *Review of medical physiology,* ed 15, Norwalk, Conn, 1991, Appleton & Lange.
15. Gorman ES, Warfield CA: The use of opioids in the management of pain, *Hosp Pract* 21(6):48A-48H, 1986.
16.* Grainger S: No cause, no cure—but he's still in pain, *RN* 50(2):43-45, 1987.
17. Haight K: What you should know about epidural analgesia, *Nurs 87* 17(9):58-59, 1987.
18.* Harrison M, Contanch PH: Pain: advances and issues in critical care, *Nurs Clin North Am* 22(3):691-697, 1987.
19.* Jacobs MK: Patient-controlled analgesia: who really benefits? *J Post Anesth Nurs* 3:404-407, 1988.
20. Kane N, et al: Use of patient-controlled analgesia in surgical oncology patients, *Oncol Nurs Forum* 15:29-32, 1988.
21.* Kleiman RL, et al: PCA vs regular IM injections for severe postop pain, *Am J Nurs* 87:1491-1492, 1987.
22. Lamb S, Barbaro NM: Neurosurgical approaches to the management of chronic pain syndromes, *Orthop Nurs* 6(1):23-29, 1987.
23. Lasagna L: Pain and its management, *Hosp Pract* 21(10):92C-92Y, 1986.
24.* Lisson EL: Ethical issues related to pain control, *Nurs Clin North Am* 22(3):649-659, 1987.
25.* McCaffery M: Giving meperidine for pain: should it be so mechanical? *Nurs 87* 17(4):61-64, 1987.
26.* McCaffery M, Beebe A: *Pain: clinical manual for nursing practice,* St Louis, 1988, Mosby—Year Book.
27.* McCaffery M, Ferrell B: Do you know a narcotic when you see one? *Nurs 90* 20(6):62-63, 1990.
28. McGuire DB, editor: Cancer pain seminar. *Semin Oncol Nurs* 1:81-150, 1987.
29.* McGuire L: Administering analgesics: which drugs are right for your patient? *Nurs 90* 20(4):34-41, 1990.
30.* McGuire L: The power of non-narcotic pain relievers, *RN* 53(4):28-35, 1990.
31.* Oberle K: Pain, anxiety and analgesics: a comparative study of elderly and younger surgical patients, *Can J Aging* 9(1):13-22, 1990.
32.* Olsson G, Parker G: A model approach to pain assessment, *Nurs 87* 17(5):52-57, 1987.
33.* Owen H, McMillan V, Rogowski D: Postoperative pain therapy: a survey of patients' expectations and their experiences, *Pain* 41(3):303-308, 1990.
34.* Paice JA: New delivery systems in pain management, *Nurs Clin North Am* 22(3):715-725, 1987.
35. Pearson BD: Pain control: an experiment in imagery, *Geriatr Nurs* 8:28-30, 1987.

*Recommended for student reading.

36. Royburn W, et al: Patient-controlled analgesia for postcesarean section pain, *Obstet Gynecol* 72:136-139, 1988.
37. Schecter M, Allen D, Hanson K: The status of pediatric pain control: comparison of hospital analgesic usages in children and adults, Pediatrics 77:11-15, 1986.
38. Sheehy SB, Barber J: *Emergency nursing: principles and practice*, ed 2, St Louis, 1985, Mosby–Year Book.
39. Sternbach RA: *The psychology of pain*, ed 2, New York, 1986, Raven Press.
40. Tuttle CB: Drug management of pain in cancer patients, *Can Med Assoc J* 12:121-134, 1985.
41.* Walker M, Wong DL: A battle plan for patients in pain, *Am J Nurs* 91(6):33-36, 1991.
42.* Watt-Watson J: Misbeliefs about pain. In Watt-Watson J, Donovan M, editors: *Pain management: nursing perspective*, St Louis, 1992, Mosby–Year Book.
43. Watt-Watson J: Neurological patient with chronic pain. In Baumann A, Dewis M, editors: *Decision making in neuroscience nursing*, St Louis, 1992, Mosby–Year Book.
44.* Watt-Watson J: Nurses' knowledge of pain issues: a survey, *J Pain Sympt Manag* 2(4):207-211, 1987.
45. Watt-Watson J, Evans R, Watson CP: Relationships among coping responses and perceptions of pain intensity, depression and family functioning, *Clin J Pain* 4(2):101-106, 1988.
45a. Wild L, Coyne C: Epidural analgesia: the basics and beyond, *Am J Nurs* 92(4):26-36, 1992.
46. Wright S: The use of therapeutic touch in the management of pain, *Nurse Clin North Am* 22(3):705-714, 1987.

Classic

47. Alberico JB: Breaking the chronic pain cycle, *Am J Nurs* 84:1222-1225, 1984.
48. Angell M: The quality of mercy, *N Engl J Med* 306(2):98-99, 1982.
49. Crue BL: The neurophysiology and taxonomy of pain. In Brena SF, Chapman SL (editors): *Management of patients with chronic pain*, New York, 1983, SP Medical and Scientific Books.
50.* Donovan MI: Relaxation with guided imagery: a useful technique, *Cancer Nurs* 3:27-32, 1980.
51.* Friedman FB: PRN analgesics: controlling the pain or controlling the patient? *RN* 46(3):67, 1983.
52. Huhman M: Endogenous opiates and pain, *ANS* 4(4):62-71, 1982.
53.* Kim S: Pain: theory, research and nursing practice, *ANS* 2:43-59, 1980.
54.* McCaffery M: When your patient's still in pain, don't just do something, sit there, *Nurs 81* 11(6):58-61, 1981.
55.* McCaffery M: Should you administer placebos for pain? *Nurs 82* 12(2):80-85, 1982.
56.* McGuire L, Wright A: Continuous narcotic infusion, *Nurs 84* 14(12):52-57, 1982.
57.* Meissner JE: McGill-Melzak pain questionnaire, *Nurs 80* 10(1):50-51, 1980.
58.* Melzack R, Wall PD: Pain mechanisms: new theory, *Science* 150:971-979, 1965.
59. Melzack R, Wall PD: The challenge of pain, New York, 1983, Basic Books.
60.* Moore DE, Blacker HM: How effective is TENS for chronic pain? *Am J Nurs* 83:1175-1177, 1983.
61. Porter J, Jick H: Addiction rare in patients treated with narcotics, *N Engl J Med* 303(2):123, 1980.
62. Rudy EF: Advanced neurological and neurosurgical nursing, St Louis, 1984, Mosby–Year Book.
63. Tamsen A, et al: Patient-controlled analgesic therapy: clinical experience, *Acta Anaesth Scand* 74(Suppl):157-160, 1982.
64. Warfield CA, Stein JM: Pain relief by electrical stimulation, *Hosp Pract* 18:207-218, 1983.

11

Cancer

Susan Moeller Schneider
Rosemarie M. Hogan

After studying this chapter, the learner should be able to:

- Discuss the epidemiologic variables related to cancer and the nurse's role in cancer epidemiology.
- List several factors that contribute to carcinogenesis.
- Outline the pathophysiology of malignant tumors, focusing on the concepts of tumor growth and metastasis.
- Describe the nurse's role in cancer prevention and health education.
- Conduct a holistic assessment of the oncology patient.
- Identify appropriate nursing diagnoses.
- Discuss the rationale for four categories of cancer therapy and nursing interventions for patients receiving those therapies.
- Formulate a plan of care for the patient with advanced cancer.

Cancer was recognized in ancient times by skilled observers who gave it its name (from the Latin *cancri,* crab) because it stretched out in many directions like the legs of a crab. It would be preferable if the image of the crab, suggested by Hippocrates for superficial cancer in the advanced stages, could be dropped, because it maintains a legend of incurability. Forms of cancer are found in plants and in humans and other animals. The term is somewhat general and is used interchangeably with *maglignant tumor* and *malignant neoplasm.*[27]

One of the least understood facts about cancer is that the name designates more than 200 diseases that have in common the production of abnormal cells that do not obey the laws of normal tissue growth.[41] Therefore cancer should never be looked on as a disease entity but only as a traditional term that describes a neoplastic process.

DEFINITION OF TERMS

The term *neoplasm* comes from the Greek word meaning "new growth" or "new formation." Normally, cell division is an orderly process with the distinct purpose of organism development or replacement of destroyed or injured cells. When cells divide without such a distinct purpose, they form neoplasms, sometimes referred to as *tumors.* Strictly speaking, a tumor is a swelling caused by any number of conditions, for example, inflammation or trauma. However, the terms *neoplasm* and *tumor* often are used interchangeably.

Oncology, a term used in association with the treatment and study of cancer, is the study of tumors (from the Greek *onkos,* mass). Neoplasms are classified broadly by distinguishing between those that are "benign" and those that are "malignant." A *malignant* neoplasm (that is, a cancer) will cause death if it is not controlled. A *benign* neoplasm usually will not cause death unless its location interferes with vital functions.[27]

ATTITUDES TOWARD CANCER

Cancer has become one of the more curable chronic diseases. Progress is evidenced by people's knowledge about the disease and the means to prevent it, more sophisticated diagnostic techniques revealing more cancers in the early curable stages, and improved methods of treatment, particularly with radiotherapy and chemotherapy.

More effective management of the side effects of therapy has improved survival rates. Advances in antimicrobial treatments and transfusion technology have helped to combat the life-threatening complications of sepsis and hemorrhage. Despite this progress, few diseases cause greater feelings of anxiety and apprehension. A diagnosis of cancer still may carry wtih it a social stigma. The myths surrounding malignant disease, often focusing on incurability, help foster feelings of hopelessness and dread.

Nurses may also have the same negative attitudes that exist in society. For this reason it is extremely important that all nurses examine their own feelings about cancer and try to work them through, both by increasing their knowledge of the diseases and treatments and by discussing feelings openly with members of the health team. Nurses who have worked through their feelings are more able to be of assistance to patients and their families than nurses who have not done so.

The nurse's role in helping cancer patients is broad in scope and area of influence. The nurse must have correct knowledge of prevention, control, and treatment of cancer and be able to apply this information in a variety of settings. Teaching about cancer is not limited to the hospital or clinic setting but takes place in industry, at PTA meetings, and at other public forums. In addition to teaching about prevention, the nurse has an active role in treatment and control programs in all settings in which clients are found. Clients and their families look to the nurse for assistance and guidance in all phases of illness from primary prevention to terminal care.

To be effective as a helping person, the nurse must be aware of the emotional impact that the diagnosis of cancer has on the patient and family, because this emotional response affects every aspect of nursing care. Cancer nursing is a challenge to the creativity, skill, and commitment of the nurse.

EPIDEMIOLOGY

Cancer is a disease that is universal in scope. It has existed since the beginning of history and affects humans wherever they live and whatever their race, color, level of culture, and material progress.[4]

Cancer ranks second to heart disease as the cause of death in the United States, but significant progress has been made in prevention and treatment. In the early 1900s few cancer patients had any hope of long-term survival. By the 1960s, 1 in 3 was alive at least 5 years after treatment. Today about 1 out of 2 cancer patients in the United States will be saved.[5] This success can be attributed to the following:

1. Diagnosis of more cancers in the early, localized stage
2. Treatment of more patients within 4 months of diagnosis
3. Development of new diagnostic and treatment modalities, especially chemotherapy

Despite these advances, it was estimated that about 510,000 persons would probably die in 1991 who might have been saved by earlier diagnosis and prompt treatment. There has been a steady rise in the age-adjusted national death rate for cancer, from 143:100,000 population in 1930 to 170:100,000 since 1984.[1] ("Age-adjusted" denotes a method used to make valid statistical comparisons by assuming the same age distribution among different groups being compared.) The major cause of the increased death rate has been cancers of the lung and breast. Death rates for other major sites are leveling off or declining (for example, stomach, uterine, and colon cancers).[5]

Epidemiologic Variables for Cancer

Although in general cancer shows no respect for economic or social status, there are some variations with regard to sex, site, age, race, and geographic location.

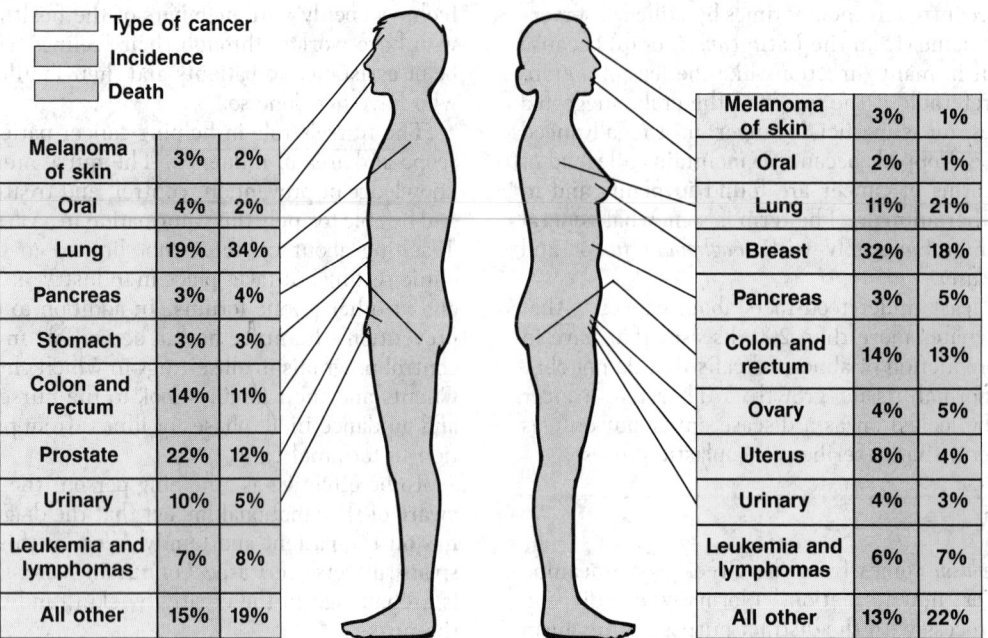

	Type of cancer	Incidence	Death
Melanoma of skin	3%	2%	
Oral	4%	2%	
Lung	19%	34%	
Pancreas	3%	4%	
Stomach	3%	3%	
Colon and rectum	14%	11%	
Prostate	22%	12%	
Urinary	10%	5%	
Leukemia and lymphomas	7%	8%	
All other	15%	19%	

	Incidence	Death
Melanoma of skin	3%	1%
Oral	2%	1%
Lung	11%	21%
Breast	32%	18%
Pancreas	3%	5%
Colon and rectum	14%	13%
Ovary	4%	5%
Uterus	8%	4%
Urinary	4%	3%
Leukemia and lymphomas	6%	7%
All other	13%	22%

Fig. 11-1 Comparison of cancer incidence and deaths by site and sex (1991 estimates). (From American Cancer Society: *Cancer Facts and Figures 1991*, New York, 1991, The Society.)

Sex and site

The average incidence of cancer is similar in both sexes. Overall survival rates (proportion of people alive 5 years after diagnosis) for some cancers have increased, such as those for cervical cancer. Rates for most other cancers have leveled off in the past 25 years. The average cancer mortality in developed countries is higher for men than for women.

Trends in age-adjusted cancer death rates per 100,000 population (1930 to 1991) indicated the following:
1. For both sexes
   a. Steady decrease in cancer of the liver and stomach
   b. Steady increase in cancer of the lung caused by cigarette smoking
   c. Steady increase, then leveling off, in cancer of the pancreas
2. For males
   a. Slight increase, then leveling off in prostate and colorectal cancer
3. For females
   a. Steady decrease in cancer of the uterus and breast
   b. Noticeable decrease in colorectal cancer[1]
   c. Constant rate for breast cancer.[5]

Fig. 11-1 compares cancer incidence and deaths by site and sex.

Age

Although more than three quarters of the deaths from cancer occur in persons over 55 years of age[12], cancer is the leading cause of death in women between 30 and 54 years of age, and more children aged 1 to 14 years die of cancer than of any other disease. However, mortality among children with cancer has declined.[5]

Race

Cancer incidence and mortality are higher for blacks than for whites. Statistics indicate that blacks have significantly lower survival rates for cancer of the breast, colorectum, and prostate.[4,5] Esophageal cancer has declined in whites but has risen rapidly in blacks of both sexes. Although incidence of invasive cervical cancer has declined in women of both races, the survival rate for white women is significantly higher than for black women.

Most differences in the cancer rates of black and white populations are attributed to environmental and social factors rather than to inherent biologic characteristics. One study showed that urban blacks tend to be less knowledgeable about warning signals and are less likely to seek medical care if symptoms do occur. These blacks also tended to underestimate the prevalence of cancer and the choices of cure.[25] Increased risk of exposure to industrial carcinogens and limited educational opportunities among those in the lower socioeconomic group may also be contributing factors, because a higher percentage of blacks are in the lower socioeconomic group.[4]

Geographic factors

Differences occur in the geographic distribution of cancer. For example, stomach cancer is common in Japan, Latin America, and Eastern Europe but uncommon in Australia, New Zealand, and the United States. Breast cancer is more common in Western countries but is rare in Japan. Cancer of the liver occurs frequently in parts of Africa and Asia but rarely in the United States.

Genetic differences between populations may contribute to international variations. However, observations of what happens to cancer incidence when people migrate from one country to another show that environmental (for

Table 11-1   Risk and epidemiology for six major cancer sites

Site	Estimated new cases 1991*	Estimated deaths 1991*	Risk factors	Comments
Breast	175,900	44,600	Over age 50, personal or family history of breast cancer, never had children, first child after age 30	Leading cause of death from cancer in women
Colorectum	157,500	60,500	Personal or family history of colon and rectum cancer, personal or family history of polyps in colon or rectum, ulcerative colitis, diet high in beef and/or deficient in fiber content	Considered a highly curable disease when digital and proctoscopic examinations are included in routine check-ups
Lung	161,000	143,000	Heavy cigarette smoking, history of smoking 20 or more years, exposure to certain industrial substances such as asbestos, particularly for those who smoke	Leading cause of cancer among men, and rising mortality among women
Oral	30,800	8,150	Heavy smoking and drinking, use of chewing tobacco	Many more lives could be saved, because the mouth is easily accessible to visual examination by physicians and dentists
Skin (melanoma)	32,000†	6,500	Excessive exposure to the sun, fair complexion, occupational exposure to coal tar, pitch, creosote, arsenic compounds and radium	Readily detected by observation and diagnosed by simple biopsy
Uterus	46,000†	10,000	Cervical cancer: early age at first intercourse, multiple sex partners. Endometrial cancer: history of infertility, failure of ovulation, prolonged estrogen therapy, late menopause, combination of diabetes, high blood pressure, and obesity	Cervical cancer mortality has declined 70% during past 40 years with wider use of Pap test Endometrial cancer has declined 50%

*American Cancer Society: 1991 *Cancer facts and figures,* New York, 1991, The Society.
†Does not include nonmelanoma skin cancer or carcinoma in situ.

example, air pollution) and clinical (for example, diet) factors play a more important role than genetic differences in the rate changes that occur.[7]

Nurse's Role in Cancer Epidemiology

Cancer is not only a threat to life, but its cost in loss of income and disruption of the lives of families cannot be estimated. Nurses must be in the forefront of the thousands of health professionals who are working to eradicate the disease. Cancer epidemiologic research has contributed to cancer prevention and control by identifying epidemiologic trends that can be used to determine individuals and groups at high risk for cancer. Nurses can play a vital role in cancer prevention by assessing people's cancer risks and teaching them about environmental and personal carcinogenic risk factors, including recommendations for prevention and early detection. Table 11-1 summarizes important epidemiologic aspects and risk factors for the six major cancer sites.

ETIOLOGY: CARCINOGENESIS

The factors that contribute to the development of cancer are many and at present are not fully understood; however, certain health practices are known to decrease the possibility that cancer may occur. Because cancer is not a single disease entity, it is not likely that there is a single cause. Cancer probably occurs as the result of the interaction of many risk factors or because of long-term exposure to a single carcinogenic agent. Factors involved in carcinogenesis include host susceptibility, environmental carcinogens, habits and customs, and viruses (Box 11-1).

Host Susceptibility
Genetic factors

Studies of genetic factors have focused on specific cancer sites and the disease in general. Chromosomes have been studied to find evidence of the genetic origin of cancer. Chromosomal abnormalities associated with neoplasia may consist of extra or missing chromosomes or the presence of abnormal chromosomes. The question is whether these changes are the cause or the effect of cancer.[16]

A second indication of genetic origin is that cancer cells are a population of cells descendant from a single cell of origin (clones). Future generations of cancer cells are always malignant; they inherit and pass on the trait. Finally, there is a possibility that cancer arises from an innate genetic inability, possibly a defect in mitotic regulation.

Some carcinogenic factors

Host susceptibility

Genetic factors
  Cancer family syndrome (CFS)
  Familial polyposis of colon
  Multiple endocrine adenomatosis (MEA)
  Retinoblastoma
Hormonal factors
  Estrogens
Precancerous lesions
  Polyps of colon and rectum
  Pigmented moles
  Cervical dysplasia
  Paget's bone disease
  Senile keratosis
  Xeroderma pigmentosum
Chronic irritation
  Coal tars and products in industry
  Sunlight overexposure
  Restrictive clothing
  Chronic use of laxatives
Immunologic factors
  Early childhood and old age
  Immunodeficiency disease
  Immunosuppressive therapy

Viruses

Herpesvirus hominis (HSV-2)—cervical cancer
Epstein-Barr virus—Burkitt's lymphoma

Psychosocial factors

Stressful life changes
Depression
Low social support and high need

Environmental factors

Ionizing radiation
  Radiographs
  Radioisotopes
Chemical pollutants
  Polycyclic hydrocarbons (soot, tar, pitch, mineral
    oils)
  Arsenic compounds
  Asbestos
  Aromatic amines
  Chromium compounds
  Benzol
  Nitrosamines (meat preservatives)
  Nitrates (food additives)
  Aflatoxin 13 (mold on nuts and grains)
  Vinyl chloride
  Diethylstilbestrol (DES)
  Red dyes (food coloring)
  Sweeteners (cyclamates and saccharin)

Health practices

Smoking
Nutrition
  Diets high in refined foods and low in roughage
    (colon cancer)
  Smoked foods ingestion
  High caloric intake
Alcohol
Sexual practices
  First coitus at an early age
  Multiple sex partners
  Uncircumcised sex partners

Familial polyposis of the colon, a precursor of cancer, is indisputably hereditary. There is also a high incidence of breast cancer in a vertical line of descent, such as from mother to daughter.[6] Risk of breast cancer in the first-degree relative of a patient is five times that of the general population. Heredity in some way seems to be connected with bronchogenic cancer. It seems to interact with cigarette smoking to cause a synergistic effect.[4]

In general, inherited cancers are a direct expression of an inherited defect, but these syndromes are rare and account for only a small percentage of familial cancer.[4] Studies have shown that the pattern of inheritance is not usually that of single mendelian gene, and it is still not known whether the incidences of many specific cancers are a result of a combination of genetic and environmental factors.[6]

Hormonal factors

Hormones do not appear to be primary carcinogens, but rather they seem to influence carcinogenesis in the following three ways:

1. By a preparative action on the target tissues, making them susceptible to the carcinogenic agent
2. By a "permissive" influence of carcinogenesis allowing the process to progress
3. By a conditioning effect on the tumor

Hormones are capable of restraining or enhancing the growth of tumors that have developed. Hormone therapy (p. 186) and some surgical therapies (hypophysectomy and oophorectomy) are based on this fact.

Evidence exists that tissues that are endocrine responsive (for example, breasts, endometrium, and prostate) do not develop cancer unless they are stimulated by their growth-promoting hormones. Estrogens have been associated with cancers such as adenocarcinoma of the vagina, hepatic tumors, breast tumors, and uterine cancer.

In addition to tissue stimulation by the hormone, carcinogenesis may be determined by the length of time of the hormonal effect. The longer the preparative influence of the hormone, the greater the chance of cancer development.

Precancerous lesions

Certain benign lesions and tumors have a tendency toward malignant change. These cancers are preventable if minor precursor conditions are treated carefully. Precancerous lesions are a large and heterogenous group. In some cancer is inevitable, whereas in others the risk is so low that medical management disregards the cancer risk. Some examples of precancerous lesions include actinic keratoses, which appear as rough, scaly, erythematous areas on skin that has usually been exposed to sun, and leukoplakia, which are white patches of the mucous membranes[12] (see Chapter 43).

Chronic irritation

It is also known that cancer may follow chronic irritation of any part of the body. There are many ways to prevent irritation that may lead to cancer. Effort is being made in industry to protect workers from coal-tar products known to contain carcinogens. Masks and gloves are recommended in some instances, and workers are urged to wash their hands and arms thoroughly to remove all irritating substances at the end of the day's work. Occupational health nurses participate in intensive educational programs to help workers understand the need for carrying out company rules that may help prevent cancer.

Prolonged exposure to wind, dirt, and sun may also lead to skin cancer.[6] Skin cancer of the face and hands is particularly common among outdoor workers who have fair complexions and who do not protect themselves from exposure. The incidence of skin cancer and melanoma is much higher in the "Sun Belt" region of the United States.[2]

Any kind of chronic irritation to the skin should be avoided, and moles that are in locations where they may be irritated by clothing should be removed. Shoelaces, shoetops, girdles, brassieres, and shirt collars are examples of clothing that may be a source of chronic irritation. Glasses, earrings, dental plates, and pipes that are in repeated contact with skin and mucous membrane may contribute to cancer. Cancer of the mouth is sometimes associated with rough jagged teeth and the constant irritation of tobacco smoke or alcohol. Indiscriminate use of laxatives is believed to have possible carcinogenic effects on the large bowel.

Immunologic factors

It may be possible that failure of the normal immune mechanism may predispose to certain cancers. The change from normal to malignant cells is relatively common. These new cells are antigenically different and are recognized as such by the body's immune system. If the immune response is initiated, the malignant cell will be destroyed. That a kind of immune surveillance system may exist is suggested by the following evidence:

1. The two peaks of high incidence of tumors in humans are in early childhood and old age.[12]
2. Individuals with rare immunodeficiency disease in which there is a defect in cellular immunity have increased evidence of tumor development.
3. Individuals receiving immunosuppressive drugs to prevent organ transplant rejection have an increased evidence of neoplasia.[6]

Cancer itself appears to suppress the immune response early in the disease, as well as late in its progression. It has not been definitely established that cancer develops because of failure in immune surveillance, and at present there is not enough data to make a strong case. (The role of the immune systems and cancer therapy is discussed later in this chapter and in Chapter 16).

Environmental Factors

It has been estimated that 70% to 90% of human cancers result from environmental factors and that we have the knowledge to prevent 30% to 40% of cancers in the United States. Occupational exposure causes 1% to 5% of human cancer, and the Environmental Protection Agency indicates that as many as 50,000 chemical substances, *excluding* pharmaceutical and food additives in common use, are carcinogenic.[42]

There are several types of chemical and physical carcinogens (cancer-producing substances). Various carcinogens may have an additive or enhancing effect on one another, and even small amounts of these substances may constitute a hazard. Carcinogens act on different organs depending on the portal of entry and the distribution in the body.[7]

Ionizing radiation

Radiographs and radium may cure cancer, but in other cases they cause it. Ionizing radiation consists of electromagnetic waves or material particles that have sufficient energy to ionize atoms or molecules (that is, remove electrons from them) and thereby alter their chemical behavior. In adequate amounts, it destroys the cells.[4]

Every living thing from the beginning of time has been exposed to small amounts of radiation from the sun and from certain natural elements in the earth, such as uranium, that emit gamma rays (γ-rays) in the process of their decay. This is called *natural background radiation*. No problem regarding radiation existed until after 1895, when the Roentgen ray (x-ray) machine was developed and became widely used in diagnosis of disease. The development of this machine was followed by the discovery of radium and the use of both radium and radiographs for treatment of disease such as cancer. With developments in the field of nuclear energy, it has been possible to produce radioactive isotopes of a number of the elements, although only a few of them, such as gold, iodine, cobalt, and phosphorus, have medical application at the present time.

The problem of overexposure and possible harm to patients and to personnel caring for them has increased greatly with the increased use of radiographs in diagnosis and treatment and the more recent use of radioisotopes in diagnosis and treatment. Also, radiation-producing substances are being used to greater extents in the work and home environments. High-dose exposures of ionizing radiation, such as those which occurred following the explosions of the atomic bomb in Hiroshima and Nagasaki, as well as the nuclear power accident in Chernobyl, have resulted in carcinogenesis. Survivors have an increased incidence of marrow suppression disorders such as leukemia, and also a higher risk of breast, thyroid, lung, and digestive cancers.[6]

No one really knows how much exposure to radiation is safe for persons working with patients and for patients having repeated radiographs taken for various purposes. Relatively small amounts of exposure have produced serious damage in experimental animals, but humans have not lived through enough generations of relatively high exposure for conclusive evidence of safe levels to be obtained. It is reasonable to assume that the less exposure one has the better. This does not mean that a patient receiving radiation treatment should not receive adequate nursing care. There are ways to protect persons from exposure, and hospitals are required to have protective procedures and guidelines for persons who care for patients receiving radiation therapy. Nurses should be familiar with the procedures used in the institution in which they are employed.

The ionizing effect of radiation on the body cells remains, so that exposure is cumulative throughout life.[6] Exposure of the entire body enormously increases the amount of radiation received. For this reason all of the body except the part being treated is protected from exposure when relatively high doses are given for therapeutic purposes.

The amount of exposure the patient receives from a series of radiographs taken for diagnostic purposes depends on the machine used and the technical skill involved. Usually, the fluoroscopic examination entails more exposure than radiography. To prevent excessive exposure with fluoroscopy, physicians allow time for their eyes to accommodate to the darkened room so that the patient can be observed with a lower intensity of the machine. The exposure of the average nurse working in a hospital and occasionally assisting a patient while a radiograph is taken is almost negligible.

Badges are worn by persons whose daily work exposes them to radiation. The badge, which contains photographic film capable of absorbing radiation, is developed each month. A darkening or blackening of the film indicates excessive exposure. Personnel who are becoming overexposed are removed, at least temporarily, from direct contact with radiation.

Because of the possible danger to the fetus, particularly between the second and sixth weeks of life, radiographs are seldom taken of pregnant women. Also, pregnant women usually are not employed in radiology departments or in caring for patients who are receiving radioactive materials internally.[6]

It should be noted that the energy of microwave radiation is too low to cause damage to DNA and that it is not likely to cause cancer.[4]

Chemical pollutants

Air pollution has been blamed for the rising cancer incidence in the twentieth century. Ten polycyclic aromatic hydrocarbons have been recognized as carcinogenic. Tar and pitch and their derivatives and mineral oils containing aromatic hydrocarbons were discovered to be carcinogenic many years ago. Bladder cancer from aromatic amines is an occupational disease of workers in the rubber industry.[2] The risk of contracting lung cancer is 15 to 30 times greater among those exposed to chromium compounds. Other common occupational cancers are respiratory cancers from asbestos and leukemia resulting from long-term inhalation of benzine.

A liver carcinogen, aflatoxin 13, has been isolated from a common mold that grows on peanuts, soybeans, fruit, some meats, and mild and cheddar cheese. A rare form of vaginal cancer in young women has been linked to the ingestion by their mothers of diethylstilbestrol (DES) prescribed to prevent spontaneous abortion.

In 1969 cyclamates, which were widely used as sugar substitutes, were banned when experimental studies revealed that in high doses they could produce cancer of the bladder in mice. Saccharin has also been identified as being carcinogenic in a study of rats, and the Food and Drug Administration has recommended that it not be used as an artificial sweetener. The use of some hair dyes has also been implicated in cancer.

Chemotherapeutic agents used to treat cancer are also considered carcinogens. Because these agents alter the ability of cells to replicate, they are capable of affecting healthy cells as well as tumor cells. Although data are inconclusive regarding how much risk is involved with handling antineoplastic agents, many groups recommend using protective gowns, gloves, and masks.[31] These medications should be prepared under a vertical laminar air flow hood. Nurses should be familiar with the policies and procedures of the institution where they are employed.[26]

Health Practices
Tobacco use

There is now no question that the rate of lung cancer during the past 70 years can be attributed to the use of cigarettes. The American Cancer Society estimates that cigarette smoking is responsible for 83% of lung cancer cases among men and 43% among women—more than 75% overall. Those who smoke two or more packs of cigarettes a day have lung cancer motality 15 to 25 times greater than nonsmokers.[2] In the past, more men than women smoked, and men smoked more heavily; however, the gap has been narrowing. The rise in the number of women smokers has captured the attention of cigarette manufacturers, who have increased their advertising efforts in this direction, to the point of designing cigarettes expressly for women.

Tobacco use accounts for about 30% of all deaths from cancers (some examples are mouth, pharynx, larynx, esophagus, pancreas, and bladder) and is also linked to heart disease, gastric ulcers, chronic bronchitis, and emphysema.[2] If smoking is discontinued, even after a habit of 30 years, there is a decrease in the evidence of lung cancer. Not smoking for 10 years reduces the risk of cancer to equal that of a person who has never smoked.[11]

The Cancer Prevention Study II by the American Cancer Society recently reported a steady decline in the proportion of adult smokers in the United States. The percentage of men smokers in the population had dropped from 50.2% in 1965 to 31.7% in 1987. The percentage of women smokers also decreased from 31.9% to 26.8% over the same time period. A corresponding decrease in lung cancer has occurred.[13] There are more than 33 million ex-smokers now living in the U.S. Of these, 95% quit on their own, without the aid of any organized program. However, for smokers who need more intensive assistance and group support, smoking cessation clinics are available in most communities.[1]

After the release of the Surgeon General's Report on Smoking and Health in 1964, the National Interagency Council on Smoking and Health was formed. This group, composed of 27 public and private health, educational, and youth organizations, has as its major objective combating smoking as a health hazard. Several of these participating organizations have produced films and other educational materials that are available to schools, organizations, and individuals. Assistance in securing films and other materials can be obtained from the Library, National Clearinghouse for Smoking and Health, Public Health Service.* One of the main concerns of the Interagency Council is how to convince young people not to start smoking. Educational and smoking control programs have been effective in college graduates, in whom smoking prevalence has decreased by 50%. Smoking rates of individuals with less than a high school education have not changed significantly since 1965.[13]

Smokeless tobacco has also been identified as a carcinogen and has been shown to cause cancer of the oral cavity. The trend among adolescents of using smokeless tobacco as snuff or chew has been linked to the rise in cancer of the mouth. The cancer occurs in the mucous membranes along areas where the tobacco is placed.[2] In recent years the scope of antismoking campaigns in the schools has broadened to include education regarding the hazards of smokeless tobacco. Antitobacco education in schools is conducted through school courses, assemblies, and exhibits.

Many smokers have switched to brands of cigarettes with filters that reduce the tar and nicotine (T/N) exposure. Although low T/N smokers may find it easier to quit smoking and the lung cancer mortality is reduced somewhat, many people only smoke *more* filtered cigarettes, resulting in no reduced lung cancer risk. In addition, certain filtered brands have been found to deliver more carbon monoxide than those without filters.[13]

Switching from a cigarette to a pipe or cigar also may reduce the risk of lung cancer but not the risk of cancer of the lips, pharynx, and esophagus. The smoke from pipes and cigars contains the same amount of tar and nicotine as cigarettes. It simply is not inhaled.[2]

The question of hazards for nonsmokers who breathe the smoke of others' cigarettes is not resolved, but recent studies have aroused concern. Two studies have shown increased risk of lung cancer among wives of cigarette smokers; however, another study found little, if any, risk for "passive smokers."[1]

Nurses have a responsibility, both as well-informed citizens and as professional persons, to be aware of the most recent antismoking programs and to interpret them to the public. One of the best ways for nurses to do this would be to stop smoking themselves. According to the American Cancer Society, approximately 24% of female nurses smoke and 41% of male nurses smoke.[14]

Nutrition

Nutritional habits are increasingly being investigated and implicated in the etiology of cancer. A high incidence of cancer of the colon occurs in populations whose diet is high in refined food and low in nonabsorbable cellulose "roughage" or fiber. Evidence indicates that the incidence of colonic carcinoma is low among persons who eat a largely vegetarian diet that has relatively few animal products[4] and is especially low in fats. Breast cancer appears to be associated with a diet high in animal fat, but the precise relationship has not been identified.[2]

Other factors in the daily diet may be responsible for

cancer. These are not only specific carcinogenic agents but also certain nutritional deficiencies. Ingestion of smoked foods, which contain benzopyrene, has been correlated with an increased incidence of stomach cancer. Some epidemiologic and experimental evidence suggests that high caloric intake may lead to cancer and calorie deprivation may prevent it. Obesity may increase the risk of breast, colon, gallbladder, prostate, and uterine cancer.[6]

Some foods may protect against cancer. The food additives butylated hydroxyanisole (BHA) and butylated hydroxytoluene (BHT) seem to inhibit cancer. Although reports are conflicting, some investigators believe vitamins A, B, C, and E actually have anticancer effects.[2] High-fiber foods such as fruits, vegetables, and whole grain cereals may decrease the incidence of cancer.[6]

Many food substances contain additives, contaminants, and naturally appearing substances such as aflatoxin, which may be carcinogenic. Food additives being studied include food dyes, flavoring agents, and antimicrobial preservatives such as sodium and potassium nitrite and nitrate. Although some potential carcinogens are present in the diet, the time trends do not indicate that additives now in use are significant in the etiology of cancer. The present government policy is to keep the levels of potential carcinogenic agents in food as low as feasible, recognizing that it is almost impossible to state with absolute certainty that any ingested chemical is safe.

The Delaney clause to the food additive amendment to the Federal Food, Drug and Cosmetic Act requires that no substance producing tumors in experimental animals should be permitted in food for human beings. The problem is that effects from ingesting carcinogenic agents may not be seen for decades because of the long latency periods. Childhood exposure, particularly, may provide the time for cancer to appear.

Alcohol

There is a significant association between alcohol intake and cancer of the mouth, pharynx, larynx, and esophagus.[6] However, alcoholism is often associated with smoking and with vitamin and dietary deficiencies, whose roles in the etiology of cancer are not known. It is speculated that alcohol and nutritional deficiencies enhance carcinogenesis by increasing the metabolic activities of specific tobacco carcinogens.[2] Tumors of the involved sites occur with greater frequency in men, blacks, lower socioeconomic groups, increasingly urbanized societies, and the elderly.[7]

Sexual practices

Carcinoma of the uterine cervix is less common in virgins than in married women. It is higher in those who have first coitus at an early age, who have an early first marriage, and who have had multiple sex partners. Cervical cancer is more frequent in women who have had multiple pregnancies, but this factor decreases in importance when the groups of women compared started their sex life at the same age. The development of cancer seems to be connected with coitus rather than pregnancy.[6]

Carcinoma of the penis is virtually unknown among circumcised men. The means by which circumcision provides protection is not clear, but it is probably related to better hygiene. There is also a lower incidence of cancer

---

*5401 Westbord Ave, Bethesda, MD 20016

of the uterine cervix in women whose sexual partner has been circumcised and in cultures in which the men, even though not circumcised, have a high standard of genital hygiene. Increased risk of testicular cancer is associated with undescended testicles.[6]

The correlation with sexual experience and breast cancer is the reverse of that for the uterine cervix. Breast cancer patients have usually been married and become pregnant later in life.[6] Lactation may provide some protection against breast cancer, since women who have breast-fed their infants show a lower incidence of breast malignancy. Cancer of the breast is reported to be unknown among Eskimo women and to be relatively rare among Japanese women; both cultures practice breast-feeding.

Viruses

There is strong evidence from animal studies that viruses play an important role in carcinogenesis, but evidence for viral etiology of human cancers is much less convincing. The strongest evidence of a causal relationship to cancer in humans is from studies of the DNA Epstein-Barr virus (EBV), a human virus known to be the etiologic agent of infectious mononucleosis and suspected in Burkitt's lymphoma and nasopharyngeal cancer.[6] However, a positive serum test for EBV antibody (indicating past exposure) has been found in healthy adults, suggesting that other factors need to be involved for cancer to develop.[36,41]

Cervical cancer may result from a virus introduced into the cervix during sexual intercourse. This virus may be a member of the herpes group, *herpesvirus hominis* (HSV-2). Carriers of HSV-2 in the population are generally uncircumcised males with poor personal hygiene.[2]

Even if the evidence of viral etiology were more conclusive, consideration needs to be given to the question of whether the virus is transmitted horizontally, from host to host, or vertically, from generation to generation via the viral chromosome. In addition, successful immunization against a virus would require the following:

1. Suppression of the genetic expression of the virus
2. Sufficiently high incidence of the type of cancer to justify the cost of immunization
3. Consideration of previous natural exposure to the virus
4. Consideration of the effects of the immunization on any other etiologic factors that may be linked to the occurrence of the cancer[36]

The viruses found in animal tumors indicate that viruses may act individually or as co-carcinogens in causing malignancy in humans. The question is no longer, however, whether viruses have a role in the cause of cancer but when they will be definitely implicated and whether one or many will be involved.

Psychosocial Factors

Stressors such as life changes, loss of a significant other, and personality variables have been suggested as etiologic factors in the development of cancer. Some researchers believe that stress alters the body's immune system, making a person more susceptible to cancer. Depression has also been linked to cancer deaths by causing changes in immune mechanisms.

Social support in the form of institutions, family, and friends may also be an important variable. The individual with low social support and high need may be at a higher risk for developing cancer. In addition, lack of social support may adversely affect coping responses to therapy and to the illness. At the present time, however, how one defines the nature of social support and the degree to which it is present or lacking is unclear.[16]

Conclusions

Carcinogenesis is a dynamic process that is influenced by many independent and poorly defined variables. The initial molecular changes are irreversible, but they may not be expressed when cooperative conditions are absent. Changes in these conditions may alter the carcinogenic process, resulting in either acceleration, inhibition, or even reversal of the process. Etiologic agents may be co-carcinogens. A genetic predisposition for a "weak" immune system along with a viral infection may lead to cancer, or oncogenic viruses may act as suppressants of the immune system. Chemical carcinogens may activate latent viral genes or inhibit the immune system's effectiveness in destroying cancer cells.

Nurses have a vital role to play in communicating to the public the factors involved in carcinogenesis. They can clarify misconceptions as well as do health teaching so that known carcinogenic practices may be eliminated. They can also set an example of good health practices for the general public, perhaps a more difficult role. As knowledgeable and concerned citizens, nurses must be initiators and supporters of efforts to have carcinogens removed from the environment.

PATHOPHYSIOLOGY

Characteristics of Malignant Cells

Normal tissue is composed of mature cells of uniform size and shape. Within each cell is a nucleus, which contains the chromosomes, a specific number for every species, and within each chromosome is deoxyribonucleic acid (DNA). DNA is a giant molecule whose chemical composition controls the characteristics of ribonucleic acid (RNA), which is found both in the nucleoli of cells and in the cytoplasm of the cell itself and which regulates cell growth and function. When ovum and sperm unite, the DNA and RNA within the chromosomes of each will govern the differentiation and future course of the trillions of cells that finally develop to form the adult organism. In the development of various organs and parts of the body, cells undergo differentiation in size, appearance, and arrangement; thus the histologist or the pathologist can look at a piece of prepared tissue through a microscope and know the portion of the body from which it came.

There are two categories of alterations in cell growth: benign and malignant. Benign neoplasms involve cellular proliferation of adult or mature cells growing slowly in an orderly manner in a capsule. These tumors do not invade surrounding tissue but may cause harm through pressure on vital structures. Benign tumors remain localized, do not metastasize (spread), and do not recur after they are completely removed (see Table 11-2).

Table 11-2   Characteristics of benign and malignant neoplasms

Characteristics	Benign	Malignant
Cell characteristics	Cells resemble normal cells of the tissue from which the tumor originated	Cells often bear little resemblance to the normal cells of the tissue from which they arose; there is both anaplasia and pleomorphism (assumption of two or more different forms)
Mode of growth	Tumor grows by expansion and does not infiltrate the surrounding tissues; encapsulated	Grows at the periphery and sends out processes that infiltrate and destroy the surrounding tissues
Rate of growth	Rate of growth is usually slow	Rate of growth is usually relatively rapid and is dependent upon level of differentiation; the more anaplastic the tumor the more rapid the rate of growth
Metastasis	Does not spread by metastasis	Gains access to the blood and lymph channels and metastasizes to other areas of the body
Recurrence	Does not recur when removed	Tends to recur when removed
General effects	Is usually a localized phenomenon that does not cause generalized effects unless by location it interferes with vital functions	Often causes generalized effects such as anemia, weakness, and weight loss
Destruction of tissue	Does not usually cause tissue damage unless location interferes with blood flow	Often causes extensive tissue damage as the tumor outgrows its blood supply or encroaches on blood flow to the area; may also produce substances that cause cell damage
Ability to cause death	Does not usually cause death unless its location interferes with vital functions	Will usually cause death unless growth can be controlled

From Porth C: *Pathophysiology: concepts of altered health states,* ed 3, Philadelphia, 1990, JB Lippincott.

A malignant cell is one in which the basic structure and activity have become deranged in a manner that is abnormal; the cause or causes are still poorly understood. It is believed, however, that the basic process involves a disturbance in the regulatory functions of DNA. It is known that the DNA molecule is affected by radiation in certain instances, and it is speculated that it may be affected by other factors as well.

In the neoplastic cell, normal restraints on growth are defective. It is believed that malignant neoplasms occur as the result of faulty mechanisms inside the cell nucleus.[27]

DNA, the permanent genetic material in nuclear chromosomes, contains information necessary for cell replication, the chemical code for cell growth and development. To convey this information, RNA serves as a messenger. Any small change in DNA (mutation) causes a distortion of biologic information, which may result in the affected cells running wild. The result is a malignant neoplasm.[2] The malignant cells lose the normal specialized function of the normal cell or may take on new characteristics and functions.

A characteristic of malignant cells that can be observed through a microscope is *loss of differentiation,* or loss of likeness to the original cell (parent tissue) from which the tumor growth originated.[15] This loss of differentiation is called *anaplasia,* and its extent is a determining factor in the degree of malignancy of the tumor.

Anaplasia is characterized by alterations in intracellular macromolecular synthesis and intercellular relationships and associations. Two types of anaplasia have been identified. In positional or organizational anaplasia, the usual distinct histologic patterns in tissues are altered. In cy-

11-2	**Characteristics of malignant cells**
	Nuclei are larger and irregular in shape. DNA is coarsely distributed and tends to appear near nuclear membrane. Nucleoli are large, usually increased in number, and contain more chromatin than usual. Mitosis is increased and atypical in appearance. Abnormal multipolar mitoses and multinucleated cells may appear. Cytoplasm is comparatively scanty and stains more deeply than normal cytoplasm (greater RNA concentration). Cells vary in size from normal cells. Surface characteristics of cells related to the cell membrane are altered: loss of contact inhibition, failure to form intracellular junctions, and impaired cell-to-cell communication.

tologic anaplasia, there is increased or altered nucleic acid synthesis in growing tissues.[7] Anaplasia is one of the most reliable indicators of malignancy. It is seen only in cancers and does not appear in benign neoplasms.

Other characteristics of malignant cells that can be seen through a microscope are the presence of nuclei of various sizes, many of which contain unusually large amounts of chromatin, and the presence of mitotic figures (cells in the process of division), which denotes rapid and disorderly division of cells. The proportion of cells actively proliferating in malignant tumors is generally greater than that of normal cells.

Malignant tumors have no enclosing capsule; thus they invade adjacent or surrounding tissue, including lymph and blood vessels, through which they may spread to distant parts of the body to set up new tumors (*metastases*). Unless completely removed or destroyed, they tend to recur after treatment, and their continued presence causes death by replacing normal cells and by other means not fully understood. Characteristics of malignant cells are summarized in Box 11-2.

Growth of malignant neoplasms

The term *neoplasm* has been defined as a relatively autonomous growth of tissues, the term *autonomy* meaning that a malignant tumor is not subject to the "rules and regulations" that govern cells and cell interaction of the healthy individual. This autonomy is relative in that the tumor is not completely independent of the tissue from which it arose.

There are considerable differences in the rate of growth of malignant tumors. The growth rate is often referred to in terms of tumor *doubling time*. Different types of tumors often have varying doubling times.[23] For example, lymphomas generally have a faster doubling time than cancers of the bone. It is also possible for tumors of the same tissue type to have different doubling times. A breast cancer may spread rapidly in one individual, whereas the growth in another individual could be extremely slow for a period of time and then could later accelerate. In general, it is has been calculated that a tumor mass will double in size 30 times before it is 1 cm in size, when there is a chance for it to be clinically detected[7] (Fig. 11-2). Occasionally, a tumor grows so slowly that it can be removed completely after a long period of time. This characteristic probably accounts for the good results obtained in a few circumstances even when treatment has been delayed. No physician, however, ever relies on this possibility to justify delay in treatment. Occasionally, a malignant tumor grows slowly for a long time and then undergoes change, and the rate of growth increases enormously.

Spread of cancer

The rate of growth of a malignant neoplasm determines its capacity to spread. Cancer may spread by direct extension, by gravitational metastasis, or by metastatic spread (Fig. 11-3).

Direct extension or invasion

Direct extension or invasion of neighboring tissue produces the typical local effects of ulcerating, bulky, hemorrhagic masses or indurative, fibrosing lesions with tissue fixation, distortion of the structure, and the pitting of the skin seen in some breast cancer. Infection may accompany this local infiltration. Because of local spread, any cancer excision must include a margin of surrounding tissues to ensure removal of all malignant cells.

Gravitational metastasis and seeding

Gravitational metastasis involves the erosion of cancer cells into body cavities and their dropping onto the serous membrane lining the cavity. The pathway is determined by gravity or movements of the body.[16] A tumor may penetrate the wall of the stomach and its cells implant on the surface of the peritoneal cavity. In the peritoneal cavity, cells tend to gravitate to the pelvis. Cells from neoplasm of the pleura of the thoracic cavity may "drop" to the diaphragm. Cancer cells can also be implanted by the surgeon into the operative area, causing metastatic lesions (mechanical transplantation).

Metastatic spread

Metastatic spread occurs when cancer cells invade vascular or lymphatic channels and travel to distant parts of the body where implantation occurs. Lymph node metastasis is present in approximately half of all fatal cancers. In *lymph vessels,* cells may detach and become emboli, which lodge in the regional lymph nodes that receive their drainage from the tumor site. Spread continues to the next group of nodes and into the other organs. Cells also may gain access to the bloodstream by way of the thoracic duct.[16]

Vascular embolism of malignant cells may occur through the veins or arteries to various parts of the body depending on the vascular drainage of the organs involved. The liver is a common metastatic site for cancers originating in the gastrointestinal tract, pancreas, and spleen because of routing through the portal vein before entering the general circulation. Because venous blood travels through the lungs, this is another common site for secondary growth via the venous system. Cancer cells in the arterial system frequently form secondary neoplasms in the bone and the brain, especially if the primary site is in the lungs, where cancer cells can gain direct access to the left heart and systemic circulation.

In metastatic spread, there is almost always a high degree of histologic, cytologic, and functional similarity between the primary cancer and these metastases. Consequently, the type of cell and the probable site of the primary tumor can be identified from the morphology of the metastasis. In addition, metastases usually mimic the primary tumor in the formation of cell products and secretions.

Naming and Classifying Neoplasms

Tumors derive their names from the parent tissue or the tissue type from which the growth originated (Table 11-3). This is often called the tissue of origin. In general, the names of benign tumors carry the suffix *-oma* following the name of the parent tissue, for example, *neuroma* or *fibroma*. Malignant tumors generally are of two types, those of epithelial and those of mesenchymal (connective tissue) origin. The term *carcinoma* denotes a malignant tumor of epithelial cells, and the term *sarcoma* denotes a malignant tumor of connective tissue cells.[16] Hematopoietic or blood-forming tissues are involved in malignant processes that are disseminated from the beginning, in contrast to solid tumors that initially are confined to a specific tissue or organ.

Tumors containing embryonic elements of all three primary germ layers, such as hair, teeth, and so on, are called *teratomas*. These are usually benign and often are found in the ovaries.

Some malignant tumors are known by the names of the

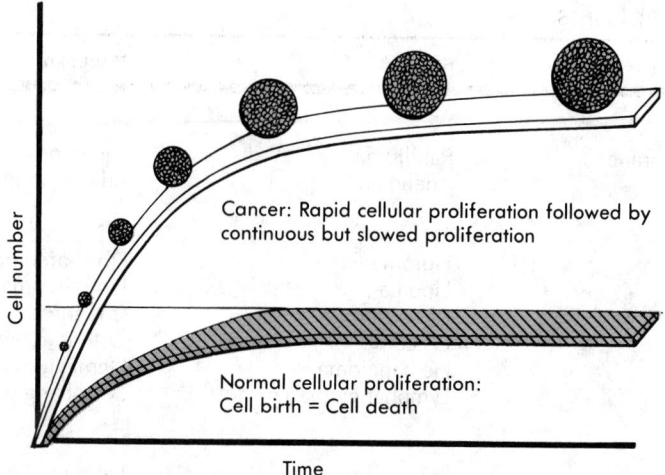

Fig. 11-2   Gompertzian function. (From Cancer: *chemotherapy and care*, Pt 1, Bristol Laboratories, Division of Bristol-Myers Co.)

CANCER SPREADS IN MANY WAYS:

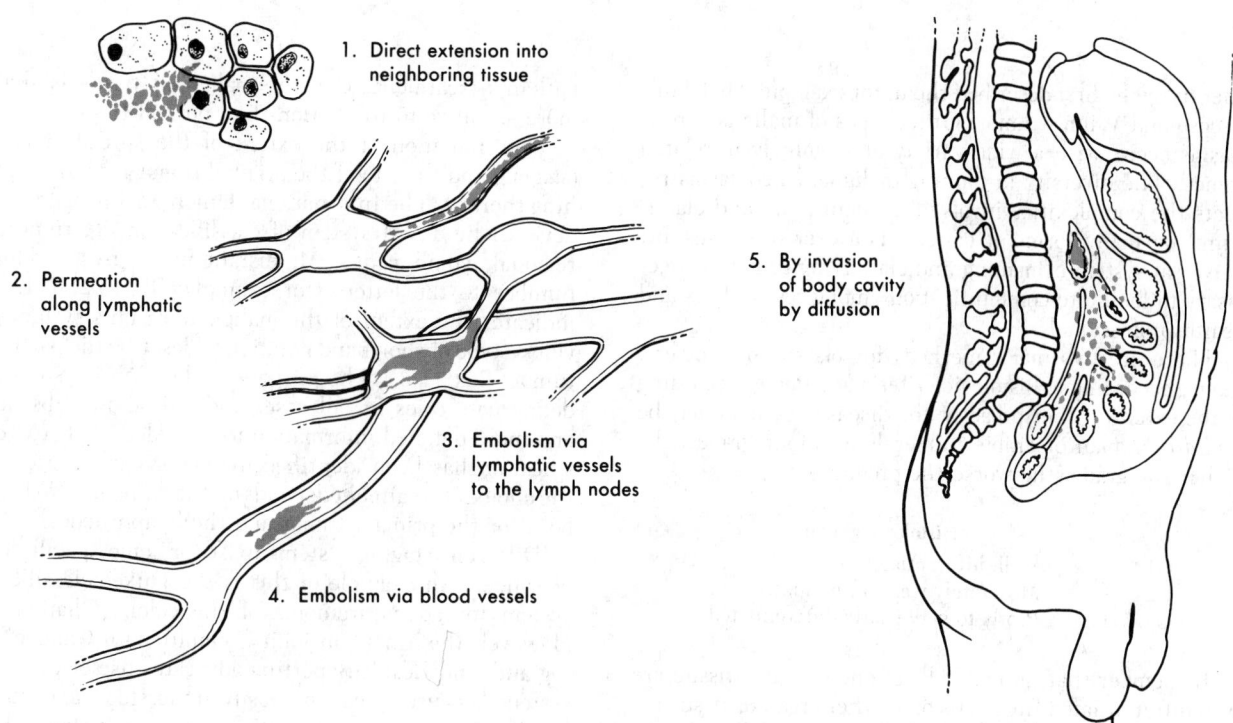

Fig. 11-3   Modes of dissemination of cancer.

Table 11-3 Names of neoplasms

Tissue type	Benign	Malignant
Epithelium		
Skin and mucous membrane	Papilloma	Squamous cell carcinoma
Glands	Adenoma	Adenocarcinoma
Connective tissue		
Fibrous	Fibroma	Fibrosarcoma
Adipose	Lipoma	Liposarcoma
Cartilage	Chondroma	Chondrosarcoma
Bone	Osteoma	Osteosarcoma
Blood vessels	Hemangioma	Hemangiosarcoma
Lymph vessels	Lymphangioma	Lymphangiosarcoma
Muscle tissue		
Smooth muscle	Leiomyoma	Leiomyosarcoma
Striated muscle	Rhabdomyoma	Rhabdomyosarcoma
Nerve tissue		
Nerve fiber end sheath	Neuroma	Neurogenic sarcoma
Ganglion cells	Ganglioneuroma	Neuroblastoma
Glia cells	Astrocytoma	Glioblastoma multiforme
Hematopoietic tissue		
Plasma cells		Multiple myeloma
Lymphoid		Lymphatic leukemia
Miscellaneous		
Placenta	Hydatiform mole	Chorioepithelioma (choriocarcinoma)

scientists who first described them, for example, Hodgkin's disease and Wilm's tumor. Other types of malignant neoplasms occur with a wide variety of seemingly unrelated names. The diversity in naming malignant neoplasms reflects the complexities involved in identifying and classifying the many forms of cancer. However, a consistent, universal system of naming and classifying tumors is necessary to facilitate communication among researchers and health professionals.

There are two major methods for classifying cancers: *grading* according to histologic criteria and *staging* according to the extent of the spread of the disease. Tumors may be *graded* by roman or arabic numerals into four grades; the higher the grade, the worse the prognosis.[15]

Histologic grading

G1	Well-differentiated
G2	Moderately well-differentiated
G3, G4	Poorly to very poorly differentiated

Remember that normal cells of one organ or tissue are well differentiated from cells of another organ or tissue (p. 191). Thus, a grade 1 tumor is the most differentiated (more like the parent tissue) and, therefore, the least malignant; grade 4 is the least differentiated (more unlike the parent tissue) and has a high degree of malignancy. These classifications are useful to the physician in knowing whether the tumor may be expected to respond to radiation treatment as well as in planning all other aspects of the patient's treatment. Usually, malignant tissue is slightly more sensitive to irradiation than normal tissue.

Determination of the extent of the spread of cancer (*staging*) and the site of the original tumor is vital for planning therapy. The International Union Against Cancer has devised the TNM system of classification: T, tumor; N, regional lymph nodes; M, distant metastases. Adding a number to the letters (for example, T1, T2, N1, N2) indicates the extent of the malignancy. This system provides a type of shorthand notation to describe the particular tumor (Box 11-3). The purpose of the TNM system is to define categories for all cases and also allow subsequent and more detailed information to be added. A TNM classification has been identified for major cancer sites, and the choice of treatment depends on the clinical TNM stage, both for the primary tumor and the lymph nodes.[2]

Different staging systems exist for some specific types of cancer. An example of this is the Dukes classification system for adenocarcinoma of the colon (Chapter 31). However, the American Joint Committee for Cancer Staging and End-Result Reporting advocates use of the TNM system because it can be easily understood and applied to all tumor types. The consistent terminology of the TNM system facilitates communication among health care providers.[15]

Physiologic Changes with Aging

The incidence of cancer is higher in the elderly population than in any other age group, and the chances of developing

11-3

TNM staging classification system

Tumor

T0	No evidence of primary tumor
TIS	Carcinoma in situ
T1, T2, T3, T4	Ascending degrees of tumor size and involvement

Nodes

N0	No regional nodes demonstrably abnormal
N1a, N2a	Demonstrate regional lymph nodes, metastasis not suspected
N1b, N2b, N3	Demonstrable regional lymph nodes; metastasis suspected
Nx	Regional nodes cannot be assessed clinically

Metastasis

M0	No evidence of distant metastasis
M1, M2, M3	Ascending degrees of metastatic involvement of the host including distant nodes

11-4

Dietary guidelines for cancer prevention[2]

Reduce the intake of saturated and unsaturated fats to 30% of total calories.

Increase intake of high fiber foods; include fruits, vegetables, and whole grain cereals. Eat fruits that are high in vitamin C, cruciferous vegetables (such as broccoli, cabbage, cauliflower), and vegetables that contain carotene (dark green and dark yellow-orange).

Avoid high doses of dietary supplements.

Minimize consumption of cured, pickled, and smoked foods, and alcohol.

cancer increase with each decade after an individual reaches the age of 60. While a variety of physiologic changes occur with the aging process that makes the host more vulnerable to malignant growth (see later chapters for specific changes), perhaps the most significant change is the exhaustion of the immune system. Antibody functioning becomes impaired and normal cells are subject to attack when the immune system falsely identifies them as foreign substances. The compromised immune system leaves the host more vulnerable to the development of malignancies and less capable of combating those malignancies when they do occur.[39]

Another theory regarding the increase of cancer incidence in the elderly is that a lifetime of exposure to carcinogens eventually leads to the development of cancer. The physiologic changes of aging do not naturally result in tumor formation, but it is the result of prolonged exposure to cancer-causing agents. Regardless of the cause of cancer in the elderly population, nurses need to remember to assess the patient thoroughly for the signs and symptoms of cancer.[4]

Because many older adults have chronic illnesses, early warning symptoms of malignancy are often attributed to other health conditions or are overlooked as part of the aging process.[39] As a result, many elderly patients are seen initially with advanced malignancies that are less amenable to treatment.

PREVENTION AND HEALTH EDUCATION

Primary Prevention

The American public is more widely read and informed about health problems than ever before. Health-seeking behavior and a desire to be more knowledgeable about

health problems are indicated by the frequency of articles on topics such as cancer in the lay press. The topic of cancer is also discussed more openly than ever before. Nurses have a major responsibility in the prevention of cancer. Because of their knowledge about the disease and their opportunity for contact with the public in the inpatient and outpatient setting, nurses have the opportunity to teach about cancer and to help motivate patients to seek treatment.

Self-care practices for primary prevention of cancer include (1) limiting sun exposure, (2) maintaining a healthy weight, (3) limiting alcohol consumption, (4) avoiding cigarettes and cigarette smoke, and (5) good hygiene. The nurse can be involved in primary prevention by educating individuals about the importance of these self-care practices, informing the public about the importance of screening examinations, and promoting the creation of a safe environment in which there is minimal exposure to carcinogens.[35]

Dietary modifications can also prevent the development of cancer. The National Cancer Institute recommends a prudent diet that limits the intake of fats, alcohol, and processed foods. Foods high in fiber are encouraged (Box 11-4).

Secondary Prevention

The approach to early detection of cancer is worldwide. General criteria for cancer screening and testing programs have been drawn up by the epidemiology section of the American Public Health Association, and these criteria have been adapted by the World Health Organization. Multiphasic screening and a periodic health examination are being accepted by the public. In some cases diagnosis can be made months before the development of symptoms causes the person to seek care.

Cancer detection is expensive. Education of the public often includes convincing them that a periodic health examination is a sound investment. Some cities have cancer detection centers where a complete physical examination including chest radiograph, Papanicolaou smear, breast examination, proctoscopy, urinalysis, and blood count are performed for a moderate fee. Nurses should be aware of clinics in their area where persons needing such resources may be referred.

Table 11-4 Guidelines for cancer related checkups*

Test or examination	Sex	Age (yr)	Recommendation
Papanicolaou test	Female	Over 18; under 18 if sexually active	After 3 consecutive years normal annual exams, Pap test at physician discretion
Pelvic examination	Female	Over 18	Yearly
Endometrial tissue sample	Female	At menopause if high risk	High risk: history of infertility, obesity, failure of ovulation, abnormal uterine bleeding, prolonged estrogen therapy
Breast self-examination	Female	Over 20	Monthly
Breast physical examination	Female	20-40	Every 3 years
		Over 40	Yearly
Mammogram	Female	35-40	One baseline mammogram
		40-50	Every 1-2 years
		Over 50	Yearly
Stool guaiac slide test	Male and female	Over 50	Yearly
Digital rectal examination	Male and female	Over 40	Yearly
Sigmoidoscopic examination	Male and female	Over 50	Every 3-5 years after two initial negative examinations 1 year apart

*American Cancer Society recommendations, 1991.

11-5

Cancer's seven warning signals

Change in bowel or bladder habits
A sore that does not heal
Unusual bleeding or discharge
Thickening or lump in breast or elsewhere
Indigestion or difficulty in swallowing
Obvious change in wart or mole
Nagging cough or hoarseness

11-6

Cancer's seven safeguards

Lung: Don't smoke cigarettes.
Colorectum: Have a proctoscopic exam as part of a regular checkup after age 40.
Breast: Practice monthly breast self-examination.
Uterus: Have a Pap test as part of a regular checkup.
Skin: Avoid overexposure to the sun.
Oral: Have a regular mouth examination by physician or dentist.
Complete body: Have an overall physical checkup annually or at 3-year intervals, depending on age.

The American Cancer Society has revised its guidelines for cancer-related checkups to provide essentially the same benefits with greatly reduced cost, risk, and inconvenience. Protocols for the early detection of cancer in asymptomatic persons are listed in Table 11-4. In general, persons over 20 years of age should have a cancer-related checkup every 3 years, and those over 40 should have one every year. These checkups should also involve health counseling including information about personal cancer risk factors.[2] Women should request that the Pap test (Papanicolaou stain) be done if it was inadvertently overlooked by the health care provider. The Pap test still is one of the best means of preventing death from cervical cancer.

Early detection of cancer can decrease mortality. The guidelines of the American Cancer Society have been developed for people *without* symptoms; however, those who have any signs or symptoms suggestive of cancer should report them immediately to a physician. The nurse must know and be able to explain the significance of the American Cancer Society's seven warning signals (Box 11-5) and seven safeguards (Box 11-6). Any of these signs should be investigated medically, but their occurrence does not necessarily mean that the person has cancer.

All persons should know the most common sites of cancer. In women these are the breast, uterus (cervix), lung, and colorectum (Fig. 11-1). Women should be taught to examine their breasts each month immediately after the menstrual period or, for postmenopausal women, on a designated day each month. Such self-examination is a much better method of detecting early breast cancer than an annual physical examination (see Chapter 36). Women of all ages should know the importance of reporting abnormal vaginal bleeding or other discharge between menstrual periods or after menopause. (Further information about cancer of specific organs can be found in appropriate chapters of this text.)

Testicular cancer accounts for only 1% of all male cancer, but it is the commonest carcinoma in the 15- to 35-year old age group.[5] Men, especially those in this young population, should be taught testicular self-examination (see Chapter 35). Testicular cancer, if diagnosed early, has an excellent chance for cure if treated with surgery and/or radiation therapy.

Two common misconceptions that lead the person to ignore symptoms should be corrected. The first is a belief that a disease as serious as cancer must be accompanied by weight loss. Weight loss is usually a late symptom of cancer, yet the person often remarks, "I wasn't losing weight so I thought nothing serious could be wrong." Another reason for neglect of cancer is that it may not cause pain, and again the person believes the absence of pain means that the indisposition is minor. It must be repeatedly emphasized to the public that pain is not an early sign of cancer and that cancer often is far advanced before pain occurs.

Nurses also have a role in prevention and early detection of genetic cancer. They systematically obtain family cancer histories, teach about health maintenance, and do genetic counseling.[35] They may be involved in centralized familial cancer registries analogous to the monitoring of communicable diseases by health departments. Familial cancer registries would be helpful in pooling data on suspected cancer-prone families, as well as in disseminating current methods of surveillance and management of the conditions.

In addition to being knowledgeable about measures for prevention and early detection of cancer, nurses must be aware of current therapeutic modalities and their rationales. Because of lack of information, misinformation, or fear of the effects of treatment, persons may put off seeking help. Clearly presented information about therapy will help to allay anxiety and confusion.

Tertiary Prevention

It is estimated that approximately half of the individuals diagnosed with cancer will survive at least 5 years or be cured.[5] As more and more individuals are cured or are living with cancer as a chronic illness, one of the major focuses in cancer care has become tertiary prevention. Many cancer centers offer nurse-coordinated support groups for cancer survivors. These groups discuss nutrition, insurance, reentry into the work force, body image, and various other issues that cancer survivors face.

Organizations that can help meet the needs of cancer survivors are listed on p. 199. Reach to Recovery and the United Ostomy Association are programs that help individuals cope with body image changes and the return to a healthy state of physical functioning following cancer surgery. The National Coalition for Cancer Survivorship is an organization that assists survivors with information on insurance, reemployment, and how to combat cancer-related discrimination. Even though patients are cured of cancer, they may still have many psychosocial and physical problems.

Factors that Interfere with Health-Seeking Behaviors

Even though there is more widespread knowledge of cancer, a more positive attitude toward the disease is essential if individuals are to follow good health practices and seek help when warning signs of cancer are noted. The public underestimates the incidence of cancer although they are aware of and concerned about it. This suggests that defense mechanisms are at work. The public does not view the conventional type of therapy as optimal, although they have a high level of awareness of cancer's warning signals. Less-educated people and men in general are less likely to have physical examinations.[40] These are all factors that may interfere with health-seeking behaviors.

Unfortunately, anxiety and fear may immobilize the individual. Despite all the public announcements that have been made in the last few decades, there are still people who think of cancer as a disgraceful disease that must be hidden from others. Cancer is talked about in whispers by some people who look on it as a punishment for past sins, a shameful disease, or a disgrace to the family. This attitude stems partly from the fact that cancer in its terminal stages may be a painful and demoralizing disease that is sometimes accompanied by body odor and other signs of physical debility that are deeply etched on the consciousness of friends and relatives. Actually, there is no characteristic odor of cancer, although diseased tissue that breaks down and becomes infected with odor-producing organisms will be as unpleasant as any other infected wound. The essential point—so often missed by the public—is that this tragic situation is an unusual one.

Some people fear cancer and shun persons who have the disease because they believe it is contagious. Scientific speculation on the possibility that a virus may be the cause has added to this fear. At this time, there is no conclusive evidence that cancer can be spread among humans in a way similar to the spread of infectious diseases, and absolute proof of the specific role of viruses in human malignancy is still not available.

The positive aspects of cancer care should be emphasized. It is estimated that approximately one half of the persons for whom a diagnosis is made are cured by medical treatment. Many more could perhaps be cured by medical treatment if the cancer is diagnosed early enough. Only a third have cancer occurring in locations in which the disease is advanced beyond permanent medical aid before sufficient signs appear to warn the patient of trouble. In spite of these facts, some persons think it is useless to report symptoms early, since they believe that if they do have cancer they cannot be cured. It can only be hoped that the recent publicity given to well-known persons who have been treated for cancer will help overcome some of these beliefs. If nothing else, the open discussion of the diagnosis and treatment in all types of media should result in a better informed public than ever before.

Unproven Methods of Cancer Management

Fatal delay in seeking medical care may occur because of the patient's reliance on a "quick, painless cure." Despite public education and efforts of the medical profession to control the extravagant claims of a few unethical practitioners, cancer quackery still exists, feeding on the ignorance and fear of the cancer patient and family.[18]

Quacks rely on testimonials of people they have "cured." Books and testimonials in magazines may be so appealingly written that the reader gets the impression that the content is factual and accurate. Electronic gadgets, dietary regimens, and various drugs and enzymes have all been purported to cure cancer.

Perhaps the most well-known drug in this category is Laetrile, a substance derived from apricot kernels. Use of

Unproven methods of cancer management

Antineoplastons
Chaparral tea
Contreras methods
Dimethyl sulfoxide (DSMO)
Electronic devices
Fresh cell therapy
Gerson method of treatment for cancer
Greek cancer cure
Hoxsey method (Hoxsey chemotherapy)
Immuno-augmentative therapy (Bahamas)
Issels combination therapy
Kelly malignancy index and ecology therapy
Koch antitoxins
Laetrile
PPLO vaccine and test
Macrobiotic diets
Metabolic cancer therapy
Revici cancer control

Modified from Unproven methods of cancer treatment (pamphlet), Amercian Cancer Society Area Office, 1010 Dixie Highway, Suite 404, Chicago Heights, IL 60411.

Laetrile for cancer therapy has been outlawed by the FDA, whose regulations prohibit the transportation of Laetrile across state lines. In response to active lobbying by various groups, however, 11 states in 1977 passed legislation legalizing use of Laetrile within their borders. The American Cancer Society and The American Medical Association do not recommend use of Laetrile because the drug has not been scientifically demonstrated to result in objective benefit to the person or to show evidence that metastatic growth has been controlled.

In 1979 the National Cancer Institute (NCI) announced that it would sponsor human testing of Laetrile. In 1981 investigators reported that the drug was a failure as a cancer treatment based on a study of 156 patients at four medical centers. These patients had advanced cancer, usually of the lung, breast, colon, and rectum, that could not be treated by standard methods. In addition to intravenous and oral administration of the drug, the patients received the metabolic program prescribed: vitamins, pancreatic enzymes, and a diet containing fresh fruits, vegetables, and whole grains. Within 1 month cancer had progressed in 50% of the patients and cancer had progressed in 3 months in 90%. Only one fifth were alive after 8 months, findings comparable to no therapy at all.

Laetrile advocates state that the drug was not pure Laetrile and charge that the study was designed to discredit Laetrile. However, NCI stated that the drug was structurally the same as that used in Mexico's Laetrile clinics. The tragedy in the use of these drugs is the false security the treatment gives to patients. The security results in delay in seeking medical care until it is too late.[18]

Federal legislation is aimed at controlling quackery, and the FDA has published a booklet, *The Big Quack Attack: Medical Devices*, that describes various methods of quackery and directs consumers where to report complaints regarding practitioners of these methods.*

In 1988, the American Cancer Society published a pamphlet listing unproven methods of cancer management (see Box 11-7).

Organizations Involved in Cancer Education, Detection, and Rehabilitation

Federal organizations

Federal recognition of the need to give intensive assistance to educational programs in cancer began in 1926 when Congress proclaimed April of each year as National Cancer Control Month. In 1937 the National Cancer Institute was created within the National Institutes of Health. This institute, with generous support from the federal government, conducts an extensive program of research in the field of cancer.

Cancer patients may also obtain help from both Medicare and Medicaid. The Community Services Administration provides services through state agencies such as Welfare and Aging or direct grants. The Rehabilitation Services Administration will arrange and pay for services that help the cancer patient return to productive living.[2] With the passage of the National Cancer Act of 1971, impetus was given for the development of Cancer Clinical Research Centers. The goal was to translate research results into medical practice so that no one would be denied professional advice and care because of lack of facilities and knowledge. These centers combine research capability, demonstration of recent techniques and therapy, and community outreach programs.

Nurses can be articulate speakers for the cause of cancer care and cure because they are intimately aware of the effects of cancer in threat to life and cost in dollars, disrupted lives, and human suffering. Nurses must assertively express to their representatives in government the importance of a combined effort to eradicate cancer.

National and regional organizations

The nurse should know of other sources of information and help for persons who have cancer. Organizations and programs offering services to the cancer patient and the family are listed in Box 11-8.

Nursing Process
Assessment
Subjective data

The physician obtains a careful medical history inquiring into family history to determine those with a familial tendency for cancer, social history, marital and sex history, habits, occupation, and past medical history, since all may provide valuable clues to the presence of cancer.

It is especially important that the nurse obtain baseline data in relation to the cancer patient's health and health habits, since the treatment of cancer often involves complex changes in the patient's ability to meet psychologic, physiologic, and sociologic health care. By careful collection of data the nurse can plan and carry out the complex nursing care that may be needed by the patient with cancer.

*FDA Office of Public Affairs, Rockville, Md 20857.

11-8

Organizations and programs offering services to the cancer patient and the family

Organization	General description
National organizations and affiliates	
American Cancer Society 1599 Clifton Rd. NE Atlanta, GA 30329	Voluntary organization offering programs of cancer research, education, and patient service and rehabilitation
CanSurmount	Composed of patient, family member, trained volunteer (also a cancer patient), health professional. Volunteers visit hospitals and homes.
I Can Cope	Addresses the education and psychologic needs of people with cancer.
International Association of Laryngectomees	Voluntary umbrella organization of 225 local clubs (varying names) that promote and support total rehabilitation program. Volunteers visit hospitals.
Reach to Recovery (Breast Cancer)	Provides rehabilitation support for women who have had mastectomies. Volunteers visit hospitals.
Cancer Information Service National Cancer Institute 1-800-4-CANCER	Telephone information and referral service supplemented by printed materials.
The Candelighters Childhood Cancer Foundation 7910 Woodmont Ave., Ste. 460 Bethesda, MD 20814	An international organization of self-help groups for parents of children/adolescents with cancer. Parent and youth newsletter.
The Concern for Dying 250 W. 57th St. New York, NY 10019	Nonprofit educational organization distributes the living will, a document that records patient wishes concerning treatment.
Leukemia Society of America 600 Third Ave. New York, NY 10016	Offers financial assistance and consultation services for referrals to other means of local support to cancer patients with leukemia and allied disorders.
Make Today Count P.O. Box 6063 Kansas City, KS 66106	More than 200 chapters comprising patients and family members, with the general goal of living each day as fully and completely as possible.
National Coalition for Cancer Survivorship 1010 Wayne Ave., Ste. 300 Silver Springs, MD 20910	A national communication network serving cancer survivors. Provides information and advocates against cancer-based discrimination.
The National Hospice Organization 1901 N. Moore St. Suite 901 Arlington, VA 22209	Membership organization consisting of groups providing or preparing to provide hospice care and institutions concerned with care of the terminally ill and their families.
United Ostomy Association 36 Executive Park, Ste. 120 Irvine, Calif. 92714	Nonprofit organization with more than 500 chapters in United States and Canada. General goal is to provide ostomy patients with mutual aid, moral support, and education. Members visit hospitals.

Knowledge of diagnosis

Some initial data are needed to plan care. The first important question to be answered is *whether the patient knows the diagnosis*. This information should be recorded on the nursing care plan and discussed with other health team members. This will ensure that the person does not receive different answers to the same questions from the health care providers. Some hospitals have partially overcome this problem by having regular meetings of all the members of the professional staff at which the information given to each patient is reviewed. If meetings of this type are not being held, nurses should take the initiative in planning such a meeting.

The nurse should also elicit from both the patient and the physician *what the patient has been told*. Because of anxiety and the need for denial to protect the ego, the patient may have only heard part of the information given by the physician or have misinterpreted the information. The nurse can identify any discrepancies to plan care on the basis of the patient's perceptions of the illness.

Members of the medical profession differ in their opinions regarding whether the patient with cancer should be told the diagnosis. The decision is usually made by the physician after consultation with the patient's family. The present trend is toward telling patients they have cancer. When patients are not informed, the reasons seem to be related much more to the physician's own attitudes and emotional reactions than to concern about patient's reactions. The nurse may help by discussing with the physician the reactions of the patient and the feelings expressed. It is the nurse's responsibility and sometimes a challenge to work effectively for the ultimate benefit of the patient within the seeming limitation it may impose.

Many spiritual advisors recommend telling the truth. Some persons, however, may not want to know the diagnosis and may ask and then answer their own questions negatively. Some do not ask for the diagnosis because they do not wish to have confirmed what they already suspect. Some insist on knowing the diagnosis and are preoccupied with every detail of their progress and treatment in a detached but completely abnormal fashion. Finally, there are some who wish to know the facts and who can accept them in a realistic way when given an opportunity to discuss their feelings with others. Some physicians prepare the patient over a period of time and tell the complete truth when they feel the patient is ready to accept it.

It is also important to determine *how long the patient has known the diagnosis*. The patient who has just been told may be going through the initial grief reactions. The person who has known for many years may have made a realistic adaptation and may see cancer as a chronic disease and not as a death sentence. The nurse should ascertain from the physician whether the cancer has already metastasized and, if so, whether the patient is aware of this fact. Responses of the patient with metastatic cancer will be different from those of the patient who can be more hopeful of a cure.

Coping skills

Coping skills should be identified, because the diagnosis of cancer is an enormous test of the person's inner resources, as well as those of friends and family. Some persons cope by directly verbalizing fears and seeking support from others, whereas other persons are less direct. Some deal with problems with a problem-solving approach; others try to avoid dealing with the problem.

The patient's and family's interpersonal, physical, and financial resources must be determined. What kind of support can be expected from the family? The financial burden the patient anticipates because of the therapy may affect the reaction to the disease.

Psychologic response to cancer

Once the diagnosis of cancer has been made, the patient and family may be overwhelmed and immobilized. As one patient stated, "I cried all day Saturday, Sunday, and Monday. My daughter and my husband wanted to help but they didn't know what to do or say. I know my daughter was scared that she'd get cancer, too." Not all patients can openly express their feelings. Consequently, the nurse may have difficulty gathering data in order to assess and plan intervention. Some individuals are stoic, feeling it is a sign of weakness to display their psychologic devastation in public. The nurse must be alert for subtle cues that may indicate that intervention is needed.

Grief. The general psychologic response to a diagnosis of cancer are those accompanying the grieving process (see Chapter 15). The patient and family may go through a period of denial, during which there may be a delay in beginning therapy. Anxiety, depression, regressive behavior, and anger may all be manifested (see Chapter 6).

To many the diagnosis of cancer signifies the end of life itself, the ultimate loss. Nurses must be careful that they do not communicate any negative reactions to cancer. Beginning practitioners must look at their own attitudes toward the disease.

Guilt. Guilt is also a frequent psychologic response. Cancer patients may feel that the disease is punishment for actions of their life. They may also feel guilty if they have delayed seeking treatment.

Sense of isolation. Perhaps one of the most prevalent reactions described by patients with cancer is a sense of isolation, of being cut off from those persons and things that are important to them. Patients with cancer may report that there is a gradual break in relationships. In some cases the isolation is patient initiated, in others it may result from actions of significant others because of their negative attitude toward the disease. Perhaps the most profound isolation is psychologic isolation, an inability to relate to and derive comfort from others, the feeling of being alone in a crowd.

Sexual disequilibrium. Nurses must be comfortable with their own sexuality and sensitive to the patients' responses, which may indicate that sexual tension is present.

Cancer is particularly destructive to the sexual relationship. It may so occupy the patient's life that all energy is directed to the illness. Sexual roles change. There may be fear that sexual activity may either cause the cancer to spread or that the well partner may "catch" it. Treatment modalities that affect the genital organs may cause sexual dysfunction, and the psychologic responses of anxiety, anger, depression, and body image changes may disrupt the sexual relationship[17] (see Chapter 34).

Fantasies of death and dying. Some patients report that they are overwhelmed with fantasies of death and dying. Most patients are more concerned about the process of dying, fearing pain, mutilation, and deterioration in both their physiologic and psychologic status, than with death itself. Patients may be open about their fantasizing, but they are more apt to communicate this in less obvious ways. Patients may focus their attention and discussion on the suffering and pain of others. They may express concern about the future of their families and may speculate on what will happen to their loved ones. The nurse must be alert to these signs that patients need to talk about their view of their future.

Objective data
Local effects

Benign tumors cause serious problems if they obstruct the lumen of tubular structures such as the ureter, trachea, or intestinal tract. Intraspinal and intracranial tumors cause problems because of the pressure they exert in a closed space. Tumors may also degenerate or by the pressure they exert cause atrophy and ulceration of overlying epithelium.

Malignant tumors may produce the same problems as benign tumors. In addition, because of their size and ability to infiltrate and destroy surrounding tissue, there is danger of obstruction, hemorrhage, ulceration, and secondary infection.

Systemic effects

The term *paraneoplastic syndrome* is used to describe the systemic effects of cancer. These can be divided into the following categories: (1) hematologic, immunologic, and vascular abnormalities; (2) hormonal and endocrine effects; (3) neuromyopathies; (4) skin and connective tissue disorders; (5) gastrointestinal disorders; and (6) general and metabolic disorders.[4]

Anemia, leukopenia, and platelet deficiency may result from replacement of bone marrow by cancer cells. Patients with cancer of the gastrointestinal tract often develop anemia secondary to chronic blood loss and malabsorption. Tumors of the endocrine glands usually cause an increase in secretion from the glands, resulting in various syndromes such as Cushing's disease or hyperthyroidism. In addition, some malignant tumors of the lung secrete trophic hormones, which can result in conditions resembling Cushing's syndrome.[8]

When there is a metastatic implant in the peritoneal or pleural cavity, this causes an increased production of serous fluid, and the patient develops either pleural effusion or ascites (peritoneal).

Degenerative changes can occur in the central nervous system of patients with advanced cancer, even in the absence of metastases to the area. The patient may show signs of cerebellar disease and peripheral neuritis.[4] There may be severe muscle weakness or dermatomyositis, and hemorrhage may occur if blood vessels are eroded by the growing tumor.

There is destruction of muscle protein, impaired cellular respiration (often a complication of anemia), and neuromyopathies followed by failure of important muscle masses, such as intercostal and abdominal muscle. This results in poor pulmonary ventilation, stasis of secretions, and pneumonia. Smooth muscle failure in the urinary bladder wall and the intestinal tract results in urinary tract infection or constipation.

Cachexia is almost universal at some point in the development of malignant disease and is usually a sign of advanced cancer. It is characterized by anorexia, hypermetabolism, excess of energy consumption over nutritional supply, and wasting as a result of negative protein and fat balance in the body. Weight loss may be gradual or rapid.

The following five factors are involved in the etiology of cachexia[3]:

1. It is possibly caused by inhibition of the hypothalamic appetite center. Appetite may fail to increase in the face of the increased nutrient needs of the tumor.
2. There is altered gastrointestinal function, malabsorption of nutrients, especially in the small intestine, and exudation of protein and electrolytes.
3. There is increased use of nutrients by some tumors that require more amino acids and vitamins than do normal tissues. There may also be insufficient use of available nutrients.
4. There is increased secretion of nutrients such as urinary excretion of electrolytes and metabolic products.
5. The disease process, and often the chemotherapy or radiation treatment, alter the patient's sense of taste and smell. Food is no longer appetizing.

In addition, other factors that may be implicated include immobilization, drugs, and reactive depression that may accompany metastatic cancer. Along with this may be insomnia and a feeling of hopelessness, which also may contribute to anorexia and cachexia. There is an increased susceptibility to infection. Therapy for the cachectic state is rarely successful unless the underlying cancer is treated.

Pain does not always occur with cancer; when it does occur, it is usually a late sign. Cancer pain is described later in this chapter (p. 221).

The paraneoplastic syndrome often results in devastating effects on the individual host; many of these effects are similar to the side effects of antineoplastic therapy. A common myth held by some general health care consumers is that the treatment for cancer is worse than the disease itself. It is important to remember that cancer, if left untreated, will eventually result in death. All health care professionals have an obligation to inform the public about the importance of early detection and treatment.

Diagnostic studies

The nurse needs to be able to give a simple description of various diagnostic procedures to patients and families. The tests may involve the use of complex equipment as well as the injection or ingestion of various substances.

The patient's anxiety may be high, and the nurse's ability to give factual information often will help to decrease this anxiety. Specific procedures before, during, and after diagnostic testing may vary slightly from institution to institution, requiring that the nurse be knowledgeable about the common as well as the possible unique characteristics of a diagnostic test. Table 11-5 lists and describes briefly the most common diagnostic procedures when the patient presents with signs and symptoms suggestive of malignancy.

Nursing intervention during assessment phase

The emotional climate produced during the period of diagnostic examination and initial treatment is very important in determining whether patients will continue diagnostic examination, treatment, or repeated follow-up care after discharge. The care they receive in the hospital may shape their attitudes toward the disease and may determine whether they can return home and either care for themselves or be cared for by the family. An important nursing function in the care of patients with cancer is

Table 11-5 Cancer diagnostic tests

Diagnostic test	Description
Physical examination	External and internal physical assessment to evaluate clinical signs and symptoms related to local or distant effects of cancer growth and development; internal assessment done through pelvic exam and/or rectal examination
Biopsy	Histologic testing (frozen or permanent section) to confirm malignancy and to determine type of cancerous cell and degree of cellular aplasia/differentiation (that is, grading)
Incisional biopsy	Surgical removal of section of neoplasm
Excisional biopsy	Removal of entire growth if tumor is small
Aspiration needle biopsy	Removal of small plug of tumor by use of needle and syringe
Cytology	Collection and slide preparation of exfoliated cells without the tissue framework provided in a biopsy; the Pap smear to determine abnormal or cancerous cells in the cervix is the most familiar example
Clinical laboratory tests	Include routine blood and urine studies as well as other biochemical and chromosomal analyses (for example, measurement of the enzyme acid phosphatase for cancer of the prostate)
Body imaging X-ray examinations	Provide good visualization of chest and bone (contrast to surrounding tissue); mammography (to detect breast cancer) differs from ordinary chest x-ray examination in that it uses very slow, nonpenetrating radiation and very sensitive film
Xerography	Uses a specially charged plate of selenium-coated metal, resulting in a detailed picture of soft tissue
Computed tomography (CT scan)	Uses an x-ray beam in conjunction with a computer permitting detailed study of small parts deep in the body without the necessity of invasive procedures
Magnetic Resonance Imaging (MRI)	Uses a very strong magnet combined with radio frequency waves and a computer to produce x-ray-like images of body chemistry in heart, brain, and other organs; no radiation is present
Contrast examination	Addition of contrast material for x-ray examination via swallowing of a liquid (for example, barium for gastrointestinal visualization) or injection of a dye into blood or lymph vessels (for example, lymphangiography)
Nuclear scans (radioactive isotopes)	Introduction of radioactive substance into body to detect primary or metastatic cancer; the isotopes concentrate in the tumor (hot spot) or in the normal tissue surrounding the tumor (cold spot) and create an image on a scintillation detector or on photographic film
Ultrasound (echography)	An electronic instrument detects and records echoes of sound when they are reflected at junction of tissues with different densities; not useful, at present, for lungs or stomach
Endoscopy	Uses a telescope-like optical instrument to look at the internal organs; x-ray examination or biopsy may be done simultaneously; instruments are named for the organs they visualize: • Bronchoscope: lungs • Laparoscope: abdomen • Cystoscope: bladder • Gastroscope: stomach • Sigmoidoscope: lower colon • Proctoscope: rectum

building up faith in the physician and in the clinic or the medical center where care is received. The patient needs to feel certain that everything possible is being done and that new measures will be tried if there is any promise whatsoever of their being helpful.

Many patients must undergo extensive diagnostic examinations and surgery in large medical centers a long distance from their homes. Some patients have reported that, although they were confident that they were in "good medical hands," such confidence did not make up for the feelings that they were not always known as individuals. They needed desperately to feel that at least one person knew and understood them. Some patients experience near panic at the thought of their loved ones coming to visit and being unable to locate them. In most instances it is best for the patient to be accompanied by a relative or a close friend. It should also be recognized that even a patient in familiar surroundings may feel very much alone when awaiting diagnostic tests or surgical treatment for known or suspected cancer.

Both patient and family need something to help pass the time during the period of diagnostic tests and treatment and between steps of treatment such as surgery or x-ray therapy. Psychologic relief may sometimes come from keeping occupied with usual daily activities. Anxious relatives also receive satisfaction from doing things that the patient would do, if possible, thus preserving parts of cherished routines.

Members of the family often need direction in their activity when they have just learned that a loved one has cancer. They may need to talk over immediate and long-term plans with someone not close to the family situation. The nurse can sometimes be this listening person. At other times the family can best be served by a social caseworker, who will help them talk through and think through a course of action.

Data analysis and planning

A sound personal philosophy and an objective, positive attitude toward the disease based on knowledge will help the nurse who is caring for the patient with cancer. The nurse should be able to give support and hope to the patient and family or friends.

Following an assessment that includes subjective and objective data, the nurse analyzes the information and formulates nursing diagnoses. Because cancer is a chronic illness that often involves numerous body systems, the list of pertinent nursing diagnoses can be extensive. It is often a challenge for the nurse to identify all of the pertinent diagnoses that will require nursing interventions for a specific person.

The following four principles should be considered by the nurse when planning nursing interventions that are patient centered:

1. Persons have a right to be part of the treatment team.
2. Persons have the right to choose the desired degree of privacy or communication.
3. The nurse must respect the coping mechanisms of patients who are trying to maintain themselves through a difficult illness.
4. The nurse must remember not to give the appearance of hurrying, thus blocking communications.

The plan of care that a nurse develops for a patient with cancer needs to be individualized to reflect problems unique to a particular disease, treatment regimen, or the personality and life situation of the patient. Table 11-6 provides guidelines for data analysis and planning by listing common problem areas, nursing diagnoses, and expected outcomes for the patient and family. The section that follows will detail the nursing interventions for the patient experiencing one or more of the four treatment modalities and for the patient with chronic pain and cancer that is terminal.

Table 11-6   Guidelines for data analysis and planning for patients with cancer

Problem area and possible nursing diagnoses*	Possible etiologies†	Expected patient outcomes*

Coping
  Anxiety
  Ineffective individual coping
  Ineffective family coping: compromised
  Altered family processes
  Fear (specify)
  Grieving (specify)
    Anticipatory
    Dysfunctional
  Powerlessness
  Body image disturbance
  Altered role performance
  Self-esteem disturbance
  Personal identity disturbance
  Social isolation
  Spiritual distress
	Threat to self-concept, threat of death, personal vulnerability, maladaptive coping styles, ambivalent family relationships, potential for loss of physiologic functioning, lack of ability to perform role, inadequate or impaired support systems, perceived helplessness, change in lifestyle, separation from religious/cultural ties, long-term illness	Within a level consistent with physical, psychosocial, and spiritual capacities and their value system, the person and family:
		1. Use appropriate resources for support in coping
		2. Communicate feelings about living with cancer
		3. Participate in care and ongoing decision making
		4. Identify alternative resources when present coping strategies do not provide support
		5. State accomplishable goals

*From Oncology Nursing Society and American Nurses Association Division on Medical-Surgical Nursing Practice: Outcome standards for cancer nursing practice, Kansas City, Mo, 1987, American Nurses Association.
†Based on suggested etiologies for nursing diagnoses from the North American Nursing Diagnosis Association, 1990.   *Continued.*

Table 11-6 Guidelines for data analysis and planning for patients with cancer—cont'd

Problem area and possible nursing diagnoses*	Possible etiologies†	Expected patient outcomes*
Comfort Pain Sleep pattern disturbance	Chronic physical disability, tumor necrosis, metastatic lesions, obstruction, pressure, ischemia, distention, environmental changes, anxiety	The person and family: 1. Report alterations in comfort level 2. Identify measures to modify psychosocial, environmental, and physical factors that influence comfort and enhance the continuance of valued activities and relationships 3. State the source of pain, the treatment, and the expected outcome of proposed intervention 4. Describe appropriate interventions for potential or predictable problems of pain and sleep management program
Nutrition Altered nutrition: less than body requirements	Chewing or swallowing difficulties, anorexia, nausea, emesis, impaired taste sensations, fatigue	1. Identify foods that are tolerated and those that cause discomfort or aversion 2. State measures that enhance food intake and retention 3. Select appropriate dietary alternative to provide sufficient nutrients when usual foods are not tolerated 4. State methods of modifying consistency, flavor, or amounts of nutrients to ensure adequate nutrient intake 5. State dietary modifications compatible with cultural, social, and ethnic practices 6. State foods and fluids that provide optimal comfort during the terminal stage of illness
Protective mechanisms (immune, hematopoietic, integumentary, and sensorimotor systems) Fluid volume deficit High risk for injury (specify) Knowledge deficit Altered oral mucous membrane Impaired skin integrity, high risk for altered protection	Neutropenia, thrombocytopenia, radiation, dehydration, ineffective oral hygiene, malnutrition, immobility, chemotherapy, cognitive limitation, lack of interest in learning, unfamiliarity with information resources	1. List measures to prevent skin breakdown, mucosal trauma, infection, and bleeding 2. Identify signs and symptoms of infection, bleeding, and sensorimotor dysfunction 3. Contact an appropriate health team member when initial signs and symptoms of infection, bleeding, or sensorimotor dysfunction occur 4. State measures to manage infection, bleeding, or sensorimotor dysfunction
Mobility Impaired physical mobility	Intolerance to activity, decreased strength and endurance, pain/discomfort, musculoskeletal impairment, depression	1. State the cause of the immobility, the treatment, and the outcome of treatment 2. Describe an appropriate management plan to optimally integrate the alteration in mobility into lifestyle 3. Describe optimal levels of activities of daily living in keeping with disease state and treatment 4. Identify health services and community resources available for managing changes in mobility 5. Use measures to aid or improve mobility 6. Demonstrate measures to prevent complications of decreased mobility

Table 11-6 Guidelines for data analysis and planning for patients with cancer—cont'd

Problem area and possible nursing diagnoses	Possible etiologies†	Expected patient outcomes

Elimination
  Constipation
  Diarrhea
  Altered patterns of urinary elimination
	Immobility, inadequate nutrition, inadequate fluid intake, chemotherapy, medications, radiation, alterations in peristalsis	1. State appropriate actions if changes in elimination patterns occur
		2. Describe the relationship between adequate elimination and physiologic integrity
		3. Identify and manage factors that may affect elimination, such as diet, stress, physical activity, and neurogenic conditions
		4. Develop a plan for managing an altered elimination route within personal life-style

Sexuality Sexual dysfunction	Change in body image, altered body structure, lack of knowledge, lack of privacy, psychologic stress, chemotherapy, radiation, fatigue	1. Client and partner identify potential or actual alterations in perception of sexuality or sexual function 2. Client and partner identify alternate methods of expressing sexuality

Ventilation
  Respiratory function, altered
    Ineffective airway clearance
    Ineffective breathing patterns
    Impaired gas exchange
	Infection, tumor, obstruction of airways, chemotherapy, radiation, fatigue, pain, anxiety, anemia	1. State plans for daily activity that demonstrate maximum conservation of energy
		2. List measures to reduce or modify pulmonary irritants from the environment, such as smoke, dry air, powders, and aerosols
		3. Describe the effect of environmental extremes on ventilatory function and oxygen use
		4. State effective measures to maintain a patent airway
		5. Identify reasons for altered ventilation, such as decreased hemoglobin, infection, anxiety, effusion, and obstructed airway
		6. Identify an appropriate plan of action should altered ventilation occur
		7. Develop a plan for managing an altered airway

Implementation

Often several physicians are involved in determining the appropriate treatment for cancer. The medical team decides on the choice of treatment on the basis of the biologic characteristic of the tumor, its clinical stage (p. 194), and the condition of the patient. The histologic type of the tumor is particularly important in determining the treatment to be used.

Therapy may be curative (removal of all traces of the disease from the body) or palliative (directed only toward relieving symptoms). At the present time there are four major forms of treatment: surgery, radiotherapy, chemotherapy, and immunotherapy. The latter is the newest form of treatment for cancer. Combinations of the four treatment modalities are often employed to achieve the best result for each patient.

Surgery

Surgery, the oldest method of treating cancer, may be either curative or palliative. The best treatment for cancer at present is complete surgical removal of all malignant tissues before metastasis occurs. Surgery must often be extensive and may require adjustments beyond those needed in many other conditions. There may not be time to accustom oneself gradually to the idea of surgery and the effect it can have on one's body and life-style. The individual often faces the prospect of mutilating surgery with only the hope that it will cure the cancer and be lifesaving. Concern about what will happen to the family may be utmost in the patient's mind. Obviously, the patient and family need empathy and understanding as they attempt to accept the recommendation for immediate surgery.

The operative procedures used to treat various types of cancer are discussed in the appropriate chapters of this book.

Radiotherapy

Radiotherapy, or the use of radiation in the treatment of disease, has been used in the treatment of cancer for about 90 years. It is estimated that approximately 60% of all cancer patients will receive radiation therapy.[4] The principal radiation agents are: (1) x-ray which consists of electromagnetic radiation produced by waves of electrical energy traveling at a very high speed; (2) radium, which is a radioactive isotope occurring freely in nature; and (3) the artificially induced radioactive isotopes produced by bombarding the isotopes of elements with highly energized particles in a cyclotron. The most common sources of radiation for external beam therapy are the linear accelerator (Fig. 11-4), and the cobalt-60 teletherapy machines. These machines produce radiation of varying types of energy, which control the depth of penetration of the x-rays into tissues.

Radiotherapy is effective in curing cancer in some instances; in other instances it controls the growth of cancer cells for a time. Because it may deter the growth of cancer cells, it may relieve pain even when extension of the disease is such that cure is impossible.

Principles underlying radiotherapy

Radiotherapy is based on the fact that rapidly reproducing malignant cells are more sensitive to radiation than are normal cells. Therapeutic doses of radiotherapy are calculated to destroy or delay the growth of malignant cells without destroying normal tissue. Rotation of either the target site in the patient or the radiation beam makes it possible to deliver a high total dose to the tumor while at the same time only part of the dose reaches the noncancerous tissue surrounding it.

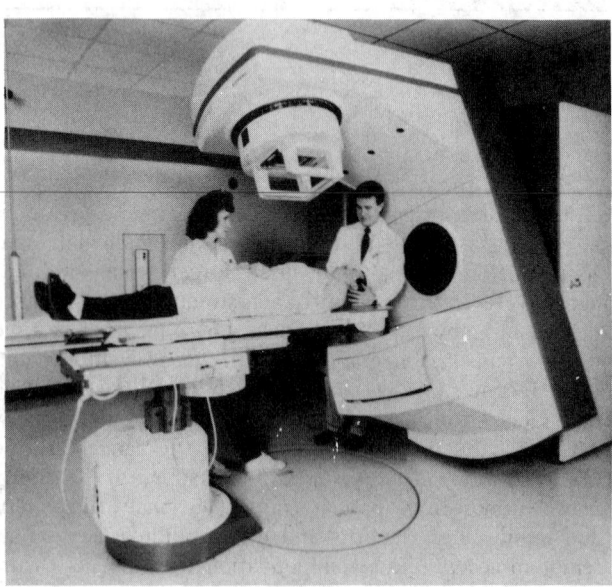

Fig. 11-4 Linear accelerator.

The radiation used medically consists of alpha- (α-), beta- (β-), and gamma- (γ-) rays (Fig. 11-5); α- and β- rays cannot pass through the skin. γ-rays, however, have been found to penetrate several inches of lead, although lead shielding offers a considerable degree of protection. X-rays, which are similar to γ-rays, require lead protection.

Teletherapy is the delivery of radiation to the patient *externally* by exposure to rays, such as from an x-ray machine or linear accelerator. Internal radiation is called *brachytherapy* and is administered by placing radioactive material such as radium within the tissues or body cavity (sealed internal radiation) or by administering the materials intravenously or orally so that they are distributed throughout the body (unsealed internal radiation).

Protection of health workers from radiation hazards

Radiation delivered externally (including x-rays) can do harm to persons working with the patient *only during* the time that the patient is being treated. This is true also of the radiation from some radioactive substances used for other methods of treatment. Patients with internal radiation who emit γ-rays, however, may expose other persons to radiation for varying periods of time, and the time one can be exposed safely to the patient is important in planning care. The time interval required for the radioactive substance to be half dissipated is called its *half-life* (Table 11-7). This period varies extremely widely, but as the end of the half-life is reached, danger from exposure decreases.

Exposure to radiation can be controlled three ways: *time, distance,* and *shielding.* All emanations are subject to the physical law of inverse-square. For example, a person who stands 2 meters away from the source of radiation receives only one fourth as much exposure as when standing only 1 meter away. At 4 meters, only one sixteenth of the exposure will be received. Therefore, increasing the distance from the emanations decreases the exposure (Fig. 11-6). When a patient such as an infant must be held for x-ray treatment, the nurse or person who holds the patient must be careful to keep at arm's length or as far away as possible and to avoid having any body part in the direct path of the rays. *Lead-lined gloves and a lead apron, which act as a shield to reduce exposure, should be worn by anyone who attends patients during x-ray treatment or during examination by fluoroscopy.*

When the nurse knows the kind of substance used, the kind and amount of rays it emits, its half-life, and its exact location in the patient and considers these facts in relation to control of exposure, safe and adequate care for the patient can be planned.

Nurses wishing to know about radioactive substances can obtain information from the Division of Radiological Health of the Public Health Service or from their state health department. Several drug companies also publish pamphlets that contain helpful information. In cities with large medical facilities a radiation physicist may be consulted.

Teletherapy

Preparation of patient. Teaching the patient and family is an important aspect of care. Orientation programs, information booklets, and weekly group sessions for patients

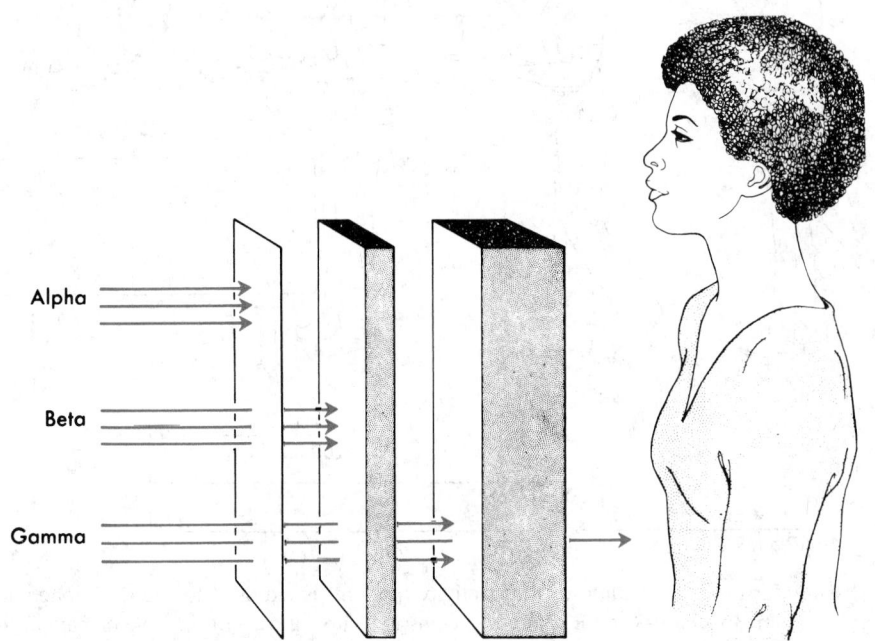

Fig. 11-5 Relative penetrating power of three types of radiation. (From Bouchard-Kurtz R, Speese-Owens N: *Nursing care of the cancer patient,* ed 4, St Louis, 1981, Mosby–Year Book.)

Table 11-7 Characteristics and uses of some commonly used radioactive agents

Radiation source	Half-life (where applicable)	Rays emitted	Appearance or form	Method of administration
X-ray	—	γ	Invisible rays	X-ray machine
Radium	1600 yrs	α β γ	In needles, plaques, molds	Interstitial (needles) Intracavitary (plaques, mold)
Radon	4 days	α β γ (low intensity)	In seeds, needles	Interstitial (seeds, needles)
Cesium (^{137}Cs)	33 yrs	β γ	In needles, capsules	Interstitial (needles) Intracavitary (capsules)
Cobalt (^{60}Co)	5 yr	β γ	External (cobalt unit) Internal (needles, seeds, molds)	Machine (teletherapy) Interstitial (needles, seeds)
Iodine (^{131}I)	8 days	β γ (low intensity)	Clear liquid	By mouth
Phosphorus (^{32}P)	14 days	β	Clear liquid	By mouth, intracavitary, intravenous
Gold (^{198}Au)	3 days	β γ	Purple liquid	Intracavitary
Iridium (^{192}Ir)	74 days	β γ (low intensity)	In needles, wires, seeds	Interstitial
Yttrium (^{90}Y)	3 days	β	Beads, needles	Interstitial

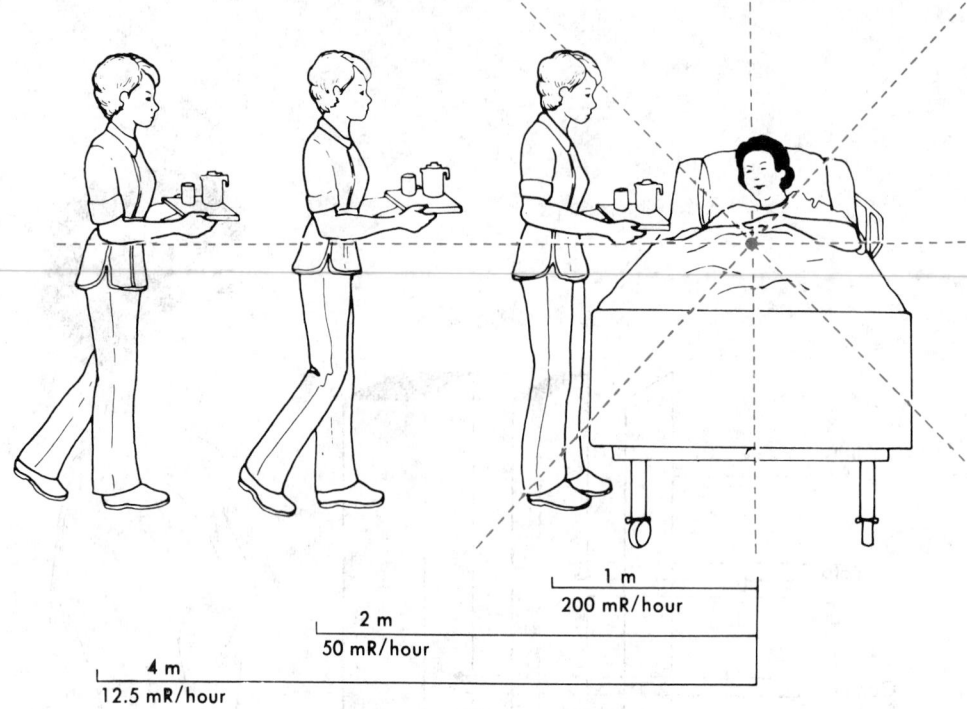

1 m
200 mR/hour

2 m
50 mR/hour

4 m
12.5 mR/hour

Fig. 11-6 Nurse nearest source of radioactivity (patient) is exposed to more radioactivity. (Modified from Bouchard-Kurtz R, Speese-Owens N: *Nursing care of the cancer patient,* ed 4, St Louis, 1981, Mosby–Year Book.)

and families are useful methods of communicating information. In group meetings, topics such as scheduling, whom to see for assistance with special problems, or care of the skin are discussed. There is an opportunity to discuss fears and misconceptions about radiation and cancer. Both inpatients and outpatients can attend.

Patients who are to receive radiation therapy should know that they will be attended by radiotherapists who will be stationed outside the treatment room and who will observe the treatment and be in communication at all times. The patient must often lie absolutely still for a period of time, a very tiring experience. There is no pain associated with radiation therapy.

Procedure. In giving treatment, rays can be directed at the tumor from several different angles so that normal tissue receives a minimum of exposure. The areas through which rays pass are known as *ports.* Different ports may be used on different days, or the position may be changed at intervals during a daily treatment so that only a certain amount is given through each of several ports. The patient may be placed on a rotating device such as a rotating chair so that although the tumor mass receives the full dose of radiation, skin areas receive less exposure.

In medical centers where hyperbaric oxygen chambers are available, patients may receive radiation therapy while receiving hyperbaric oxygen. The rationale for this combined therapy is that malignant cells, in which the oxygen tension is increased, are more susceptible to the effects of radiation. At the same time, the sensitivity of normal cells to the radiation effects is not increased.[4]

Early reaction. When radiation therapy is used, some degree of radiation reaction may occur. Early reactions include blanching or erythema of the skin and mucous membranes, possibly progressing to dry or moist desquamation. If the mucosa of the mouth, pharynx, bladder, or rectum is affected, there may be pain, inhibition of the normal secretions, and impairment of functions.[32]

When treatment is directed toward abdominal organs or any deep tissues there is almost always some skin reaction. There may be itching, tingling, burning, oozing, or sloughing of the skin. The term *burn* should never be used in referring to this reaction, since it implies incorrect dosage. Reddening may occur on or about the tenth day, and the skin may turn a dark plum color after about 3 weeks. The skin may also become dry and inelastic and may crack easily.

Gastrointestinal reactions to radiation therapy are more common when treatment includes some part of the gastrointestinal tract or when the ports lie over this system. The patient may have nausea, vomiting, anorexia, malaise, and diarrhea. Gastric emptying is slowed during the treatment phase, but usually returns to normal levels. Gastric reactions are extremely common, and almost all patients who receive moderate or large doses of radiation have these symptoms in varying degrees.

Radiation therapy also causes depression of the hematopoietic system and in turn a low white blood cell count, predisposing the patient to infection. Sloughing of tissue and subsequent hemorrhages are complications that must be considered when radiation is used in any form. Ambulatory patients are told that they should call the physician at once should any sloughing of tissue occur.

Late reaction. Effects of radiation may be apparent months or years after therapy. Genital tissue, muscles, and kidneys may be affected, resulting in painful radionecrosis. Radiation causes destruction of fine vasculature, and the skin may show signs of atrophy (thinning and blanching), pigmentation, and telangiectasis. If there is severe vascular damage or if there are other complications that require further surgery, the irradiated tissues may fail to heal.[32]

Nursing care of patients receiving external radiation. Nursing care is directed toward preventing skin breakdown, decreasing gastrointestinal upset, and preventing infection (Box 11-9). The area to be treated is usually outlined by the radiologist at the time of the first treatment. Occasionally, a small tattoo mark is used instead of the conspicuous skin markings when treatment is given to exposed parts of the body. Marks must not be washed off until the treatment is completed because they are important guides to the radiologist. Medicated substances that may contain heavy metals such as zinc are not permitted on the skin until the series of treatments is completed, because such substances may increase the radiation dosage.

If the radiation dosage has been high and blanching or discoloration of the skin has resulted, the patient may be advised to avoid exposure to temperature changes for several years. The patient may have to take much cooler baths or showers than formerly and may have to avoid sunbathing or any other extreme of temperature. Corn starch can be applied to dry, irritated skin.[32] If x-ray treatments have been given to a woman's face, she must be cautioned regarding the use of cosmetics to cover discolored skin. They may contain heavy, irritating oils and should not be used until consultation with the physician.

When treatment must be given to any part of the head, patients may ask about the possibility of loss of hair. Whether hair will return after falling out depends on the amount of radiation received. Attractive scarves and wigs are useful for patients with alopecia or when returning hair is too thin.

Brachytherapy

Internal radiation may be delivered by sealed or unsealed methods. In either type special precautions may be necessary, depending on the amount of radioactive material used, its location, and the kind of rays being emitted (Table 11-7). Special precautions may be taken if more than a tracer diagnostic dose has been given. Hospitals in which therapeutic doses of radioactive isotopes are administered are required to have a radiation safety officer. Quite often this person is a physicist. The radiation safety officer determines the precautions to be observed in each situation. Most hospitals have printed instruction sheets stating the precautions to be followed for each substance used. Personnel should be fully acquainted with all precautions and should be supervised in carrying them out. Generally, the patient will be placed in a single room or in a double room with another patient who is also receiving radiation ther-

---

11-9 | **Guidelines for Care**

Patients receiving external radiation

1. *Preventing skin breakdown*
   Skin preparation: cleansing.
   Care must be taken *not* to remove skin markings used to guide radiologist.
   Vegetable fat or oil may be ordered to protect the affected skin.
   Medicated solutions, ointments, or powders that may contain heavy metals such as zinc are *not* permitted on the skin.
   Consult radiologist about skin care for local radiation reactions; do *not* remove crusts.
   Keep dressings loose; use nonirritating tape and avoid pulling on affected skin.
   Teach patient to avoid constricting clothing or friction of any kind on exposed skin.
   Teach patient to avoid excesses of heat and cold to affected skin surfaces.
   Teach patient not to expose treatment area to the sun (sunburn).
2. *Decreasing gastrointestinal upset*
   Advise resting before and after meals to control nausea and vomiting.
   Breakfast is usually the best tolerated meal of the day.
   Suggest frequent small meals during the day.
   Sour beverages and effervescent liquids may relieve nausea.
   Suggest high-protein, high-carbohydrate, fat-free, low-residue diet to prevent nausea and vomiting; low-roughage diet for diarrhea.
   Administer palliative medications, as ordered.
3. *Preventing infection*
   Teach patient to avoid persons with upper respiratory infections.
   Use protective isolation if white blood count is low.
   Administer antibiotic drugs, as ordered.

---

apy. A radiation precaution sign should be placed on the door to the patient's room, and visitors should be restricted.

Sealed internal radiotherapy. Brachytherapy is used to deliver a concentrated dose of radiation directly to the malignant lesion or tumor area. Usually this involves insertion of radioactive substances within hollow cavities or within tissues. The radioactive isotopes commonly used are cobalt 60, iridium 192, iodine 125, phosphorus 32, cesium 137, gold 198, and radium 226[4] (Table 11-8). These radioactive substances may be used in the form of molds, plaques, needles, wires, special applicators, or ribbons that are carefully placed and left in position for a specified length of time (Fig. 11-7). Emanations from the radioactive substances may also be sealed in tiny gold tubes (seeds) and left indefinitely within the tissues into which they are inserted (Fig. 11-8). The half-life of the seeds is much less than that of the substances from which their emanations come.

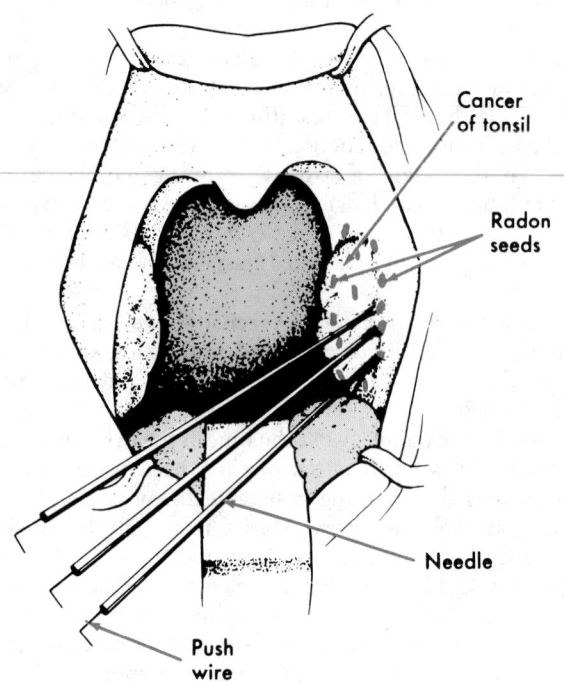

Fig. 11-8 Radium emanations may be sealed in tiny gold tubes (radon seeds) and left indefinitely within tissue into which they are inserted. Schema shows insertion into tonsil.

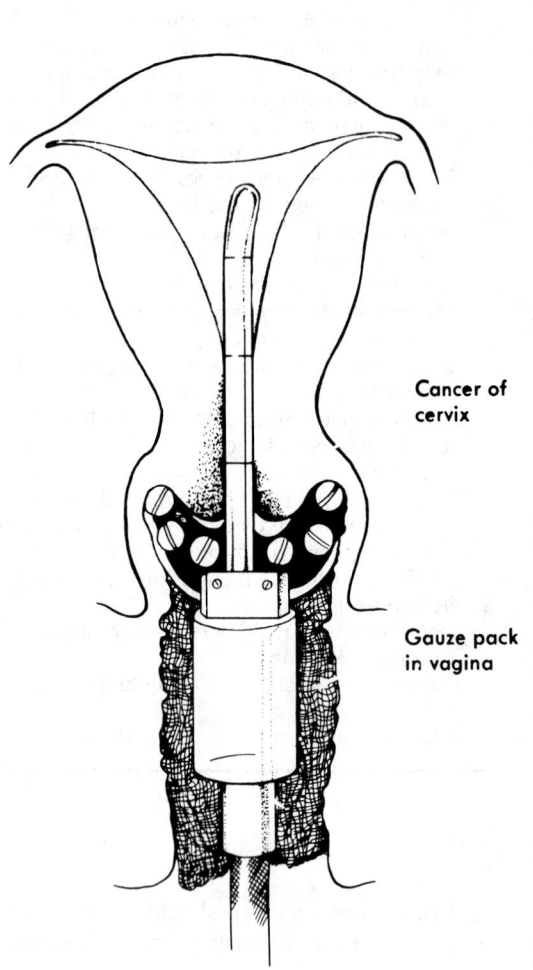

Fig. 11-7 Ernst applicator in place for treatment of cancer of cervix. Note gauze packing in vagina to help maintain applicator in position.

Table 11-8 Applications of brachytherapy

Type of application	Disease	Radioisotopes used
Sealed sources		
Intracavitary	Cervical cancer	Radium-^{226}Ra, cesium-^{137}Cs
	Uterine cancer	Radium-^{226}Ra, cesium-^{137}Cs
Interstitial	Breast cancer	Iridium-^{192}Ir
	Prostate cancer	Iodine-^{125}Ir, gold-^{198}Au
	Head and neck cancer	Iridium-^{192}Ir, cesium-^{137}Cs
Surface	Choroid cancer	Iodine-^{125}I
	Pterygium	Strontium-^{90}Sr
Unsealed sources		
Oral	Hyperthyroidism	Iodine-^{131}I
Intravenous	Polycythemia vera	Phosphorus-^{32}P
Intrapleural	Mesothelioma	Phosphorus-^{32}P
	Malignant pleural effusion	Gold-^{198}Au
Intraperitoneal	Ovarian cancer	Phosphorus-^{32}P

From Baird SB, McCorkle R, Grant M: Cancer nursing: a comprehensive textbook, Philadelphia, 1991, WB Saunders.

Table 11-9   Special precautions for unsealed internal radiotherapy

Substance or object	Radioactive element	Precautions
Urine	Iodine (^{131}I)	Urine emptied directly into lead-lined container. *All* urine must be collected (amount of radioactivity determines when patient may be removed from isolation). Urine in lead-lined container is stored in radioisotope laboratory until it can be safely disposed of.
Linen	Iodine (^{131}I)	Monitor with Geiger counter for contamination; if contaminated, place in special
Equipment	Phosphorus (^{32}P) Gold (^{198}Au)	container marked "Radioactive" and send to radioisotope laboratory.
Vomitus	Phosphorus (^{32}P)	Place vomitus in lead-lined container and send to radioisotope laboratory.
Wound drainage	Phosphorus (^{32}P) Gold (^{198}Au)	Place dressings in lead-lined container and send to radioisotope laboratory.

A fairly common site for the implantation of seeds is the mouth. Plaques and molds also are used for lesions in the mouth. Sealed internal radiation also is used widely in treatment of cancer of the cervix.

Prevention of radiation hazards. Safe practice for the nurse caring for a patient receiving sealed internal radiotherapy depends on the principles of time, distance, and shielding (p. 206). Radioactive materials for sealed internal therapy usually are kept in a lead-lined container in the radiology department and are inserted into the patient in the operating room. They should never be touched with bare hands. A pair of forceps should be kept in the patient's room for handling in case the radioactive implant becomes dislodged.

Sealed radioactive material is often reused. On removal from a patient the radioactive material should be cleansed using the precautions just described and returned to the radiology department in a lead-lined container at once so that it may be safe from accidental handling or loss. Even if it is not to be reused, it is returned in a lead-lined container. To prevent accidental loss in cleansing, radioactive material is cleansed in a basin of water instead of in an open sink. If a brush must be used, it must be grasped with forceps so that close contact with the material is avoided.

Exposure is sometimes termed *external* in that it can occur only by direct exposure to the encased radioactive substance. It cannot result from contact with linen, vomitus, or urine or from touching the patient. Knowing where the radioactive material is implanted helps the nurse to plan activities of care. If, for example, the substance is in the patient's mouth, there is less exposure if one stands toward the foot of the bed. If it is in the uterus or bladder, standing at the head of the bed is safer.

Unsealed internal radiotherapy. Unsealed internal radiation is delivered to the patient by mouth as an "atomic cocktail" or as a liquid instilled into a body cavity. Exposure for persons caring for the patient can result from direct contact with emanations from the substance in the patient (external exposure) or from contact with the patient's discharges that contain the radioactive substances (internal exposure). It may be inhaled, ingested, or absorbed through

the skin. The exposure varies with each of the substances used, and safety for the nurse and others caring for the patient depends on a thorough knowledge of the substance used and its action within the body. If only tracer doses (very small amounts) of radioactive substances are used, as for diagnostic purposes, no precautions are necessary.

Prevention of radiation hazards. Special precautions that need to be taken when using radioactive iodine, phosphorus, or gold are listed in Table 11-9. With radioactive iodine, small amounts will be present in sputum, vomitus, perspiration, feces, and urine. Protective gloves should be worn when giving direct patient care or handling body fluids.[4] The nurse should know the approved hospital procedure to safely dispose of any contaminated fluids that may be spilled.

No linen or equipment is removed from the room until it is monitored with a Geiger-Muller counter for contamination. Paper dishes are usually used and then burned. If the nurse's skin should become contaminated, it should be washed thoroughly with soap and water and then monitored. If contamination remains, washing should be continued until monitoring shows that additional cleansing is not necessary.

When the patient is removed from isolation, all equipment is monitored and carefully scrubbed by attendants who have been instructed in safe methods by persons who are in charge of the administration of the radioactive substances. It is then remonitored. The room is aired until monitoring shows that radioactivity is negligible and that the room is safe for any other patient. Airing takes at least 24 hours.

Nursing care of patients receiving internal radiotherapy. Nursing interventions consist of the following:
1. Teach routine and reasons for precautions
2. Decrease isolation by providing radio or television for outside contact and encouraging permissible interaction with nursing staff
3. Plan trips into room to include several tasks
4. Promote comfort: complete bath before treatment, clean bed linens, turn sheet, position pillow

The patient should know that isolation is temporary, that the restrictions will be removed on a certain day, and that members of the nursing staff will be available but that they will work quickly and will remain in the room only long enough to carry out essential activities. The patient can assist in notifying family and friends about the restriction on visitors and how long it will last. The patient should also know how the radioactive substance is eliminated to lessen worry about being a danger to others, particularly after therapy is concluded.

Trips made in haste into the patient's room are disturbing psychologically, because they imply that the patient is not acceptable to others. The nurse who plans thoughtfully might deliver a letter, fresh water, and the newspaper and make pertinent observations in less time than the one who plans less well and must make several trips into the patient's room.

Chemotherapy

Advances in knowledge of cancer growth and chemotherapeutic agents have led to concomitant advances in cancer treatment. Improvement in overall survival and longer disease-free intervals can be directly ascribed to the use of chemotherapeutic agents, particularly in combination chemotherapy regimens and as adjuvant therapy.

Benefits of chemotherapy

Chemotherapy is potentially curative in gestational choriocarcinoma, acute lymphocytic leukemia (ALL), Ewing's sarcoma, advanced Hodgkin's disease, diffuse histiocytic lymphoma, Burkitt's lymphoma, testicular cancer, and ovarian cancer. Prolonged disease-free or controlled intervals may be achieved by chemotherapy in the treatment of several non-Hodgkin's lymphomas, multiple myeloma, breast cancer, and oat cell carcinoma of the lung. In other advanced malignancies, such as colorectal carcinoma, chemotherapy rarely produces a complete response and only a few such patients experience an increased survival time. In the treatment of chronic myelogenous leukemia (CML) and chronic lymphocytic leukemia (CLL), although the duration of life may not be prolonged, the quality of life may be enhanced by chemotherapy because of control of symptoms. Patients and families may be told that incurable does not mean untreatable or uncontrollable.

In the care of an individual patient with cancer, the expected benefit of chemotherapy (cure, control, or palliation) should be known by the physician, nurse, and patient. This allows for realistic goal setting by the care givers, patients, and family. Such background also provides a perspective from which to view side effects. The potential for cure, prolonged disease-free survival, or reduction of symptoms is a benefit that most often outweighs the risk and discomfort of short-term toxicity and side effects. Conditions in which risk may outweigh benefits include overt or occult infections, bleeding dyscrasias, bone marrow depression, severe metabolic disturbances, renal or liver dysfunction, and pregnancy.

Adjuvant chemotherapy refers to chemotherapy administered after surgical removal of all known cancer present in the body. It is aimed at the destruction of micrometastases thought likely to be present but too small to be detected by current diagnostic techniques. Left untreated, the micrometastases have a high potential for tumor growth and cancer recurrence. With the use of chemotherapy at a time when the malignant cell population is small and likely to be susceptible, complete tumor cell eradication is possible. The goal is cure.

Adjuvant chemotherapy is now generally considered to be indicated after mastectomy in all women with involved axillary lymph nodes at the time of surgery and it has demonstrated a significant decrease in recurrence rates and prolonged disease-free intervals. Adjuvant chemotherapy also appears to be beneficial in osteogenic sarcoma and Wilms' tumor. Evidence is currently equivocal regarding its benefit in other malignancies, such as colon cancer and malignant melanoma. The precise role of adjuvant chemotherapy will be more clearly delineated during the next decade, but it is already established as one of the major developments in health care.

A feeling of well-being and knowledge that all diagnostic tests are negative for cancer understandably may cause the patient to question the need for adjuvant therapy. This is emphasized when side effects are experienced. A sensitivity to these feelings, coupled with the knowledge of the expected benefit of therapy, is the basis for both patient teaching and the supportive encouragement often needed for continued therapy.

Despite an intellectual understanding of the benefits of chemotherapy, it is sometimes difficult for a nurse to maintain an appropriately optimistic and realistic outlook if all one sees are those patients who did not respond to or are no longer responsive to therapy, manifest severe toxicity, or are dying. The practitioner must take into account the setting in which patients are seen. Hospital-based nurses tend to see patients at the time of diagnosis, when they are critically ill, or during the final days of life. The public health nurse may see the patient at comparable points of illness while providing nursing care in the home. Discussion between the nurse and primary physician, contact with the outpatient clinic, and readmission to the same nursing unit are useful ways of acquiring a more complete picture of an individual's response to treatment. Such positive experiences are a means of nurturing one's own faith in therapy so that a realistic and at times very optimistic approach to caring for, supporting, and teaching the chemotherapy patient exists.

Pathophysiologic principles of chemotherapy

Normal and malignant cells progress through various phases in the cell cycle as they replicate. Cancer chemotherapy is based on the action of certain drugs that create changes in the cell cycle phases and interrupt cell growth and replication. They specifically do this by disrupting production of essential enzymes, damaging structural proteins, and inhibiting DNA, RNA, and protein synthesis or direct interaction with DNA.

Some drugs are termed *cell cycle specific* because they are effective during a particular point of the cell cycle (Fig. 11-9). Antimetabolites interfere with DNA synthesis and affect the S phase of the cell cycle, whereas Vinca alkaloids, often called *mitotic inhibitors*, interfere with cell replication during the M phase. Drugs that are active throughout the cell cycle (*cell cycle nonspecific*) include the alkylating agents, antibiotics, and steroid hormones. Com-

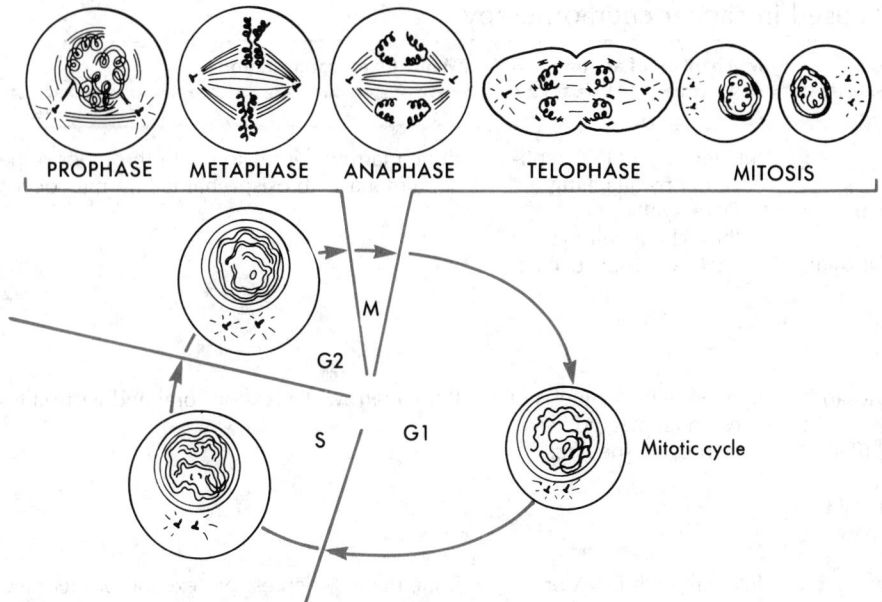

Fig. 11-9 Cell cycle. *G1*, RNA/protein synthesis; *S*, DNA synthesis; *G2*, RNA/protein synthesis and interphase; and *M*, mitosis. (Modified from Krakoff I: *Cancer chemotherapeutic agents*, American Cancer Society professional education publication, New York, 1977, The Society.)

binations of cycle-specific and cycle-nonspecific drugs have proved useful in planning treatment regimens. The goal is to use a combination of drugs that will destroy cancer cells at various stages of the replication process.

One major factor that influences the response of a cancer to chemotherapy is the fraction of tumor cells in replication at a given time, a percentage that varies among different tumors, individual patients, and at different times in the same patient. Malignancies with high growth fractions (proportion of cells in active cycle) and short cell cycle time (for example, leukemia) are most vulnerable to chemotherapy.[37]

Cell population growth. The concept of cell population growth recognizes the fact that the population of both normal cells and cancer cells contain more dividing cells when the overall cell population is small and fewer dividing cells when the overall cell population is large.[8] This relates to chemotherapy in that the choice of drug differs for large, slow-growing tumors as opposed to small tumors whose cell population is likely to be more rapidly proliferating. The latter, because of their sensitivity to interference with DNA, are susceptible to phase-specific drugs, whereas the large, slow-growing tumor is more likely to respond to phase-nonspecific drugs.[8]

Log cell kill hypothesis. The log cell kill hypothesis states that any dose of a chemotherapy drug will destroy only a fraction of the malignant cells.[8] Treatment must be repeated multiple times to eradicate the cancer. Moreover, clinical symptoms disappear before all malignant cells are destroyed, so treatment must often be continued even when all apparent evidence of disease has disappeared.

Chemotherapeutic agents

Drugs may be classified as alkylating agents, antimetabolites, plant (*Vinca*) alkaloids, antibiotics, and hormones (Table 11-10).

Alkylating agents. The alkylating agents are cell cycle nonspecific and act against already formed nucleic acids by cross-linking DNA strands, thereby preventing DNA replication and the transcription of RNA.

Antimetabolites. The antimetabolites act by interfering with the synthesis of chromosomal nucleic acid. Antimetabolites are analogs of normal metabolites and block the enzyme necessary for synthesis of essential factors or are incorporated into the DNA or RNA and thus prevent replication. Most antimetabolites are pyrimidine analogs, purine analogs, or folic acid antagonists and are, in general, cycle specific.

Vinca alkaloids. Vincristine sulfate and vinblastine sulfate are plant alkaloids that act as mitotic inhibitors. These agents exert their cytotoxic effect by binding to proteins within the cells. The *Vinca* alkaloids are cell cycle specific. Although these two agents are similar in composition, mechanism of action, and metabolism, their antitumor spectrum, dose, and clinical toxicity differ.

Antibiotics. Those antibiotics that demonstrate antitumor activity appear to affect either the function or synthesis of the nucleic acids. In addition, antimitotic and cell surface effects may be caused by these agents. The cytotoxic antibiotics are cell cycle nonspecific agents.

Table 11-10   Agents used in cancer chemotherapy

Agent	Mechanism of action[27]	Major toxic manifestations
Alkylating		
Busulfan (Myleran) Carmustine (BCNU) Chlorambucil (Leukeran) Cisplatin (Platinol) Cyclophosphamide (Cytoxan) Lomustine (CCNU) Melphalan (Alkeran)	Interfere with DNA replication by attacking DNA synthesis throughout cell cycle (cell cycle nonspecific)	Bone marrow depression with thrombocytopenia and bleeding; pulmonary fibrosis; renal failure may occur
Antimetabolites		
Cytarabine/ARA-C (Cytosar) 5-Fluorouracil (5-FU) Mercaptopurine/6-MP (Purinethol) Methotrexate/MTX (Mexate)	Interfere with synthesis of essential metabolites (cell cycle specific)	Bone marrow depression; oral and gastrointestinal ulceration
Antibiotics		
Bleomycin (Bienoxane) Dactinomycin (Cosmegan) Daunorubicin (Cerubidine) Doxorubicin (Adriamycin) Mitomycin (Mutamycin) Plicamycin (Mithracin)	Interfere with DNA or RNA synthesis, varying with the drug (cell cycle nonspecific)	Bone marrow depression (except for bleomycin); pulmonary fibrosis with bleomycin or mitomycin; renal failure with mitomycin; cardiac toxicity with doxorubicin
Plant alkaloids		
Vinblastine (Velban) Vincristine (Oncovin)	Interfere with mitosis	Bone marrow depression; areflexia Neurotoxicity with ataxia and impaired fine motor skills, paralytic ileus
Steroid hormones		
Adrenocorticosteroids (Prednisone) Androgens (testosterone proprionate) Antiestrogens, tamoxifen citrate (Nolvadex) Estrogens (DES) Progestins (Depoprovera)	Alter the host environment for cell growth (cell cycle nonspecific)	Specific for the actions of the hormone

Steroids. The corticosteroids are produced by the adrenal cortex and include mineralocorticoids and glucocorticoids. It is the glucocorticoids that, in addition to their use in numerous nonmalignant diseases, are effective in the treatment of many neoplastic disorders. In some malignancies (for example, lymphomas, breast cancer, multiple myeloma, acute lymphocytic leukemia, and chronic lymphocytic leukemia) steroids exert a direct antitumor effect by altering the environment. Steroids are also able to reduce edema and inflammation around a tumor and, therefore, are useful for symptom relief. Many side effects are associated with long-term steroid use, most notably a compromised immunologic response to infection, osteoporosis, and a cushingoid syndrome. Steroids in cancer treatment regimens are often given intermittently and for short periods of time and are not often associated with the debilitating side effects associated with chronic, long-term use. Patients often describe an improved sense of well-being and an increased appetite while receiving prednisone. With completion of a prescribed course of therapy, a brief period of fatigue, malaise, and emotional lability may be experienced.

Hormones. Hormonal alteration may be a desired therapeutic goal when tumor growth is directly influenced by certain hormones. The mechanism whereby the steroid hormones stimulate or inhibit cellular growth is not clear; an important mechanism may be interference or alteration at the cell membrane.

Estrogen receptor assays are now routinely done at the time of mastectomy for breast cancer. This technique has made it possible to evaluate the ability of a breast tumor to bind estrogen and thus project the probable sensitivity of the tumor to hormonal therapy.

Combination chemotherapy

Increased knowledge of how specific cytotoxic drugs exert their effect and of the potential for the emergence of tumor cells resistant to a specific therapy, similar to antibiotic resistance, has led to the use of combination chemotherapy. Combination chemotherapy demonstrates a therapeutic effect superior to single-agent therapy for many cancers. Drugs considered for combination chemotherapy are those that (1) are active when used alone, (2) have different mechanisms of action, (3) have a biochemical basis for possible synergism, (4) do not produce toxicity in the same organs, and (5) produce toxicity at different times after administration.[27] Repeated brief courses of drug therapy are given to reduce immunosuppressive effects.

Dose calculations

The dosage range for a particular drug is determined at the time of clinical trial and regimen development. Given these guidelines, the dosage for a specific individual must be calculated before starting therapy. Although some regimens may still prescribe milligrams per kilogram, drug doses are usually stated in terms of body surface area, and therefore, the doses are given in milligrams per square meter (m^2). An individual's height and weight are used to determine body surface; therefore, it is very important that height and weight be measured *accurately*.[26]

Methods of administration of chemotherapeutic agents

The route of administration is based on the metabolism and absorption of a given drug. The route of choice is that which will deliver the optimal amount of drug to the tumor. Chemotherapeutic agents are given orally, intravenously, intramuscularly, intraarterially, and by local instillation (that is; intrapleurally or intrathecally). If tumor cells are in an area that drugs cannot reach, cancer cells will survive with a consequent increase in disease recurrence. An example is the sanctuary effect afforded leukemic cells by the meninges in patients with acute lymphocytic leukemia. For this reason, local instillation of chemotherapy via an Ommaya cerebrospinal reservoir or intrathecally (directly into the spinal fluid by lumbar puncture) is used to treat tumor cells present in the CNS.

Before administering a cytotoxic drug, the clinician consults a reference for usual dosage, acceptable routes of administration, and any precautions that should be taken for that particular drug.[26] Since protocols may deviate from drug manufacturers' guidelines, discussion with the prescribing physician may also be indicated.

Oral administration. Many cytotoxic drugs are given in pill form. Since these may be prescribed on a daily basis to be taken at home, careful instructions need to be given to patients. Areas to be discussed include the importance of taking the drug as prescribed, the relationship to meals, fluid intake, and the use of an antiemetic.

Intravenous administration. The clinician must know specific properties for each drug to be administered. Of particular importance is the identification of those drugs that are vesicant (produce blisters). If infiltration and extravasation of a vesicant occur, extensive tissue damage and necrosis may result. Nitrogen mustard, doxorubicin (Adriamycin), vincristine, and vinblastine are the principal vesicant drugs. The intravenous site is evaluated before the administration of these drugs. If *any* suspicion of an infiltration or leak exists, the site is changed. Most often, vesicant drugs are given via the side arm of a running IV. If extravasation occurs, immediate action is taken to minimize damage.[30] Guidelines for treating extravasation vary and nurses should be aware of the policies that exist for the agency in which they are employed. Refer to Table 11-11 for suggestions.

For patients with poor venous access, either an in-dwelling Hickman catheter (Fig. 11-10) or an implantable infusion port (Fig. 11-11) may be used for chemotherapy administration. Nursing care considerations for these two types of venous access devices are described in Boxes 11-10 and 11-11. The skin around the catheter insertion site or implanted infusion port is inspected for redness, swelling, or drainage. Showering and bathing are permitted.[38]

Table 11-11   Treatment recommendations for vesicant extravasation

Antineoplastic agent	Local antidote	Application of heat or cold
Nitrogen mustard	Isotonic sodium thiosulfate	Cold
Doxorubicin	Hydrocortisone or dexamethasone and/or sodium bicarbonate	Cold
Vinblastine	Hyaluronidase	Warm

From Oncology Nursing Society: Cancer chemotherapy guidelines for nursing education and practice, Pittsburgh, 1988, The Society.

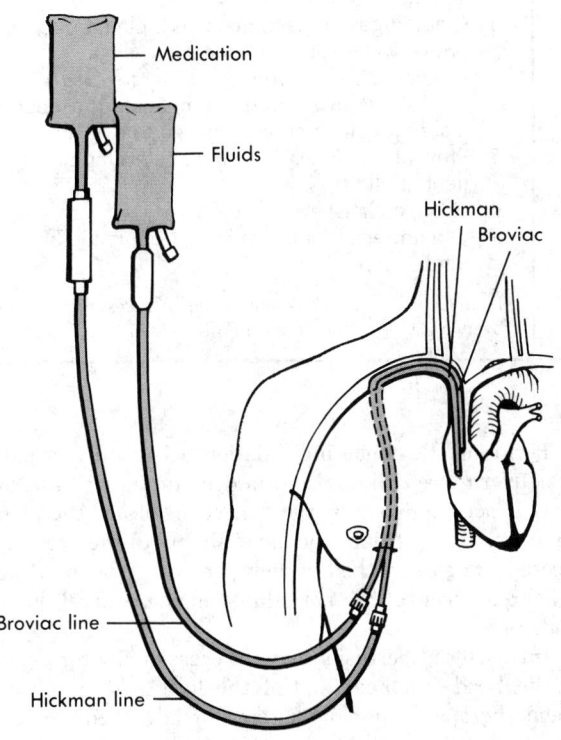

Fig. 11-10   Double lumen Hickman/Broviac catheter.

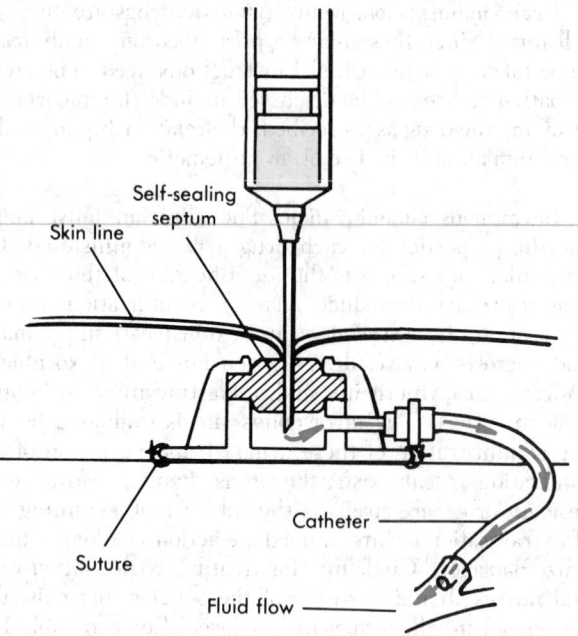

Fig. 11-11 Implantable infusion port. Drugs are administered through self-sealing port.

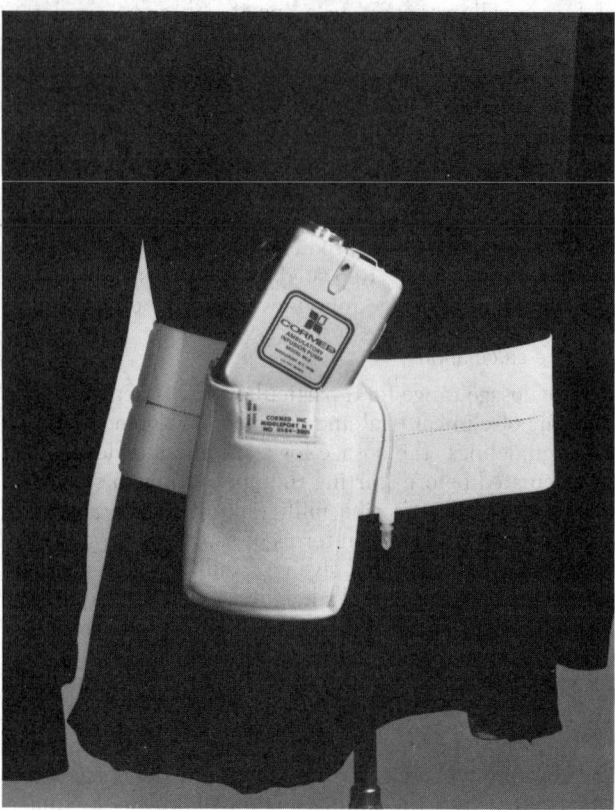

Fig. 11-12 Lightweight, battery-operated infusion pump for ambulatory patient. Flow rate is adjustable. (Courtesy CORMED, Inc, Middleport, NY.)

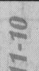

Routine care of Hickman/Broviac catheters

1. Irrigate catheter daily with 3 ml heparin-saline solution (10 U heparin/ml) to prevent clotting.
2. Irrigate briskly—may help prevent outflow obstruction.
3. Clamping is *not* recommended; clamp over protective covering if necessary.
4. Change dressing every other day for 2 to 3 weeks after insertion using meticulous aseptic technique, then apply bandage to exit site.
5. Prevent undue tension on catheter; tape to patient at all times.
6. Change cap(s) every 7 days.
7. Obtain repair kit for catheter from manufacturer.

From Goodman SG, Wickham R: Venous access devices: an overview, *Oncol Nurs Forum* 11(5):16–23, 1984.

Maintenance of implantable infusion port

1. Puncture with Huber point needle only.
2. Irrigate every 4 weeks with 3 to 5 ml heparin-saline solution (100 U heparin/ml).
3. Use 20 ml normal saline flush after blood drawing.
4. Irrigate arterial ports once a week with 3 to 5 ml heparin/saline solution (100 U heparin/ml).
5. Flush catheter after each use.
6. No restriction on patient because port is implanted.

From Goodman SG, Wickham R: Venous access devices: an overview, *Oncol Nurs Forum* 11(5):16-23, 1984.

Perfusion. Regional and isolation perfusion is a means of delivering a high dosage of a drug directly to a tumor. This is accomplished by the placement of a catheter into an artery that provides the blood supply to the area being treated. By this method, a high percentage of the drug is delivered because it is not diluted in the general circulation.

Intraarterial perfusion is used occasionally for cancers of the head and neck and of the liver and as adjuvant chemotherapy with radiotherapy for advanced cancer of the cervix. Because infusions may be continuous for long periods of time (several hours to days), the patient may be restricted in activity. However, intraarterial perfusion can be accomplished in ambulatory patients by means of a portable infusion pump (Fig. 11-12). Aspects of nursing care include assessment of the catheter insertion site, care of the line to maintain placement and prevent infection, and observation for bleeding. Outpatients need careful and detailed instruction so that these criteria can be maintained in the home. Hospital nurses involved in the discharge planning of such patients need to ensure that the community-based nurse also be informed of these detailed instructions.

11-12

Guidelines for Care

Patients receiving chemotherapy

Bone marrow suppression or infection

Check blood counts

Assess infection-prone areas daily to identify early
  signs of infection

Maintain medical asepsis through careful handwashing

Maintain intact skin and mucous membranes
  Teach avoidance of bumping and breaking skin
  Maintain aseptic technique during IV infusion and
    dressing changes
  Keep fingernails short
  Teach good perineal hygiene
  Teach avoidance of excessive friction and impor-
    tance of vaginal lubrication
  Teach avoidance of anal intercourse
  No enemas, rectal medications, or rectal ther-
    mometers
  Encourage fastidious orgal hygiene with a soft
    toothbrush
  Inspect mouth daily for ulcers and white patches
  Use lubricants to prevent drying and cracking of
    lips

Maintain optimal respiratory function
  Assess for early signs of respiratory infection
  Auscultate lung sounds
  Instruct family/friends not to visit if they have
    colds

Maintain reverse isolation if ordered

Gastrointestinal effects: stomatitis, nausea, vomiting

Administer oral nystatin, as ordered

Use a rinse and lidocaine before meals to lubricate
  and provide an analgesic effect

Use a cleansing rinse of plain water or normal saline
  after meals

Administer antiemetic as ordered

Determine from patient best time for food and fluid
  intake in relation to treatment

Teach relaxation techniques and imagery, if appropriate

Alopecia

Explain that drug-induced alopecia is not permanent

Allow expression of feelings about hair loss

Scalp tourniquets or scalp hypothermia via ice pack
  may be ordered for patients with solid tumors to
  minimize hair loss with some agents (for example,
  vincristine, adriamycin)

Encourage use of wigs, hats, and scarves

Effects on skin

Inspect administration site for signs of infiltration or
  extravasation

Organ toxicities

Assess signs and symptoms of liver dysfunction (see
  Chapter 30)

Monitor cardiac status (dysrhythmias, congestive
  heart failure) (see Chapter 25)

Assess signs and symptoms of pulmonary toxicity
  (see Chapter 24)

Urinary effects: hemorrhagic cystitis, renal toxicity

Maintain hydration by encouraging drinking of large
  amounts of fluid (if receiving cyclophosphamide)

Monitor renal function: check serum creatinine or
  creatinine clearance (with cisplatin or streptozotocin)

Sterility

Assess knowledge of known and possible effects on
  fertility

Provide birth control and reproductive counseling, as
  appropriate

Side effects and nursing intervention

Some degree of injury to normal cells often occurs with treatment by chemotherapeutic agents. The basis for normal cells being affected is their rate of proliferation. Many normal tissues have a high proliferation capacity, in some instances exceeding that of malignant disease. It is these rapidly proliferating tissues (the bone marrow, gastrointestinal epithelium, and hair follicles) that bear the brunt of the toxic effects of many of the cytotoxic drugs. Nursing care of patients receiving chemotherapy is summarized in Box 11-12.

Bone marrow suppression. Recognition of the bone marrow suppressive (myelosuppressive) potential of the chemotherapeutic agents is critical to the care of patients receiving chemotherapy. It is the major life-threatening toxicity associated with chemotherapy. Frequent blood counts are done to monitor this toxicity, and astute attention must be given to the results of the white blood count, platelet count, and hemoglobin, with appropriate modification of drug dosage. Patients who have received previous chemotherapy or radiation therapy, particularly to areas of bone marrow reserve (sternum, hips, or pelvis) may have an increased sensitivity to myelosuppression. Blood counts are done before the administration of chemotherapy and at regular intervals to assess the predictable lowest point, which varies with the drugs used. Nursing care of patients with neutropenia, thrombocytopenia, and anemia are discussed in Chapter 27.

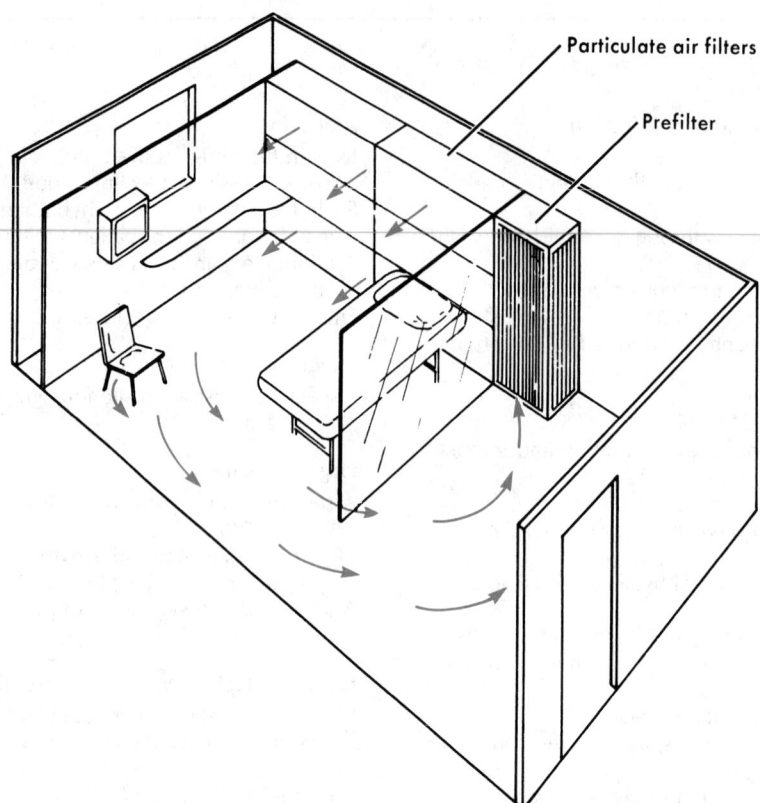

Particulate air filters

Prefilter

Fig. 11-13   In laminar airflow units, constant flow of purified air flows across width and breadth of room. (From American Cancer Society: *Proceedings of the National Conference on Cancer Nursing*, New York, 1973, The Society.)

Infection. The prevention of infection is of utmost importance in the care and teaching of the cancer patient. Body areas with high potential for infection should be inspected daily. The *skin and mucous membranes,* especially the mouth, axillae, and perineal areas, are infection prone. Assessment of the *respiratory tract* is also important to identify early signs of respiratory infection. Patients are susceptible to middle-ear infections, sinusitis, and pharyngitis. Pneumonia is especially prevalent in patients with leukemia and in elderly persons. Families of patients are instructed not to visit if they have colds.

Injections are usually avoided. Aseptic techniques must be scrupulously maintained during intravenous infusions and dressing changes. In preventing all types of infection, good medical asepsis and especially careful handwashing by the medical and nursing staff are important.

Use of patient isolation. If the white blood count is low, reverse isolation may be ordered to prevent infection and may include the use of private rooms with special air filtration systems. *Laminar airflow units* are rooms that have a constant flow of purified air across the width and breadth of the room (Fig. 11-13). Depending on the patient population and institutional policy, nurses may need to wear masks, gowns, and caps when caring for patients in isolation. Regardless of the specific isolation techniques, the most effective method for preventing infection is thorough

handwashing; this is essential for all individuals who enter the patient's room.

One problem with any type of isolation is that the patient may experience sensory deprivation and social isolation. In addition, when reverse isolation is terminated, the patient may feel unsafe, vulnerable, and angry because of removal from the protected environment.

Gastrointestinal effects. Changes in bowel habits commonly occur but usually do not require intervention. If diarrhea becomes marked or persists, an antidiarrheal medication such as diphenoxylate with atropine (Lomotil) may be prescribed. Metamucil is also recommended to increase bulk. Persons receiving vincristine are assessed for signs of paralytic ileus and are instructed to report constipation.

Stomatitis, an inflammation of the mucous membranes of the oral cavity, may range from an erythema of the oral mucosa to mild or severe ulceration. Methotrexate, 5-fluorouracil, doxorubicin, dactinomycin, and bleomycin are the chemotherapeutic drugs that most frequently cause stomatitis. Patients may also develop a superimposed *Candida* infection of the mouth and esophagus, and oral nystatin is usually prescribed. Good mouth care is important.

Nausea and vomiting. Nausea and vomiting are among the most uncomfortable and distressing side effects of chemotherapy. For the ambulatory patient, nausea may interfere with the ability to continue daily work. Persistent vomiting may result in fluid and electrolyte imbalance, general weakness, and weight loss. Decline of nutritional status renders the patient more susceptible to infection and perhaps less able to tolerate therapy. Such physiologic symptoms can accompany or precipitate psychologic responses that might include depression and withdrawal. Every effort must be made to minimize chemotherapy-induced nausea and vomiting. The onset and duration vary greatly among patients and with the drug given.

Antiemetics vary in success. Tetrahydrocannabinol (THC) taken in pill form produces an antiemetic effect in some patients who have not benefited from the commonly prescribed prochlorperazine (Compazine). Metoclopramide hydrochloride (Reglan) or onclansetron (Zofran) may be helpful for persons receiving cisplatin, and lorazepam (Ativan) is often effective in producing a relaxed state during which an individual is less sensitive to stimuli that can induce feelings of nausea. Timing of food and fluid intake in relation to treatment is often ascertained by the patient, as are the types of foods that are best tolerated. Relaxation techniques are useful for some patients.

Alopecia. Alopecia (loss of hair) may occur by two mechanisms. If the hair roots are atrophied, alopecia occurs readily. The hair either falls out spontaneously or by hair combing, often in large clumps. If the hair shaft is constricted because of atrophy or necrosis, the hair will break off very near the scalp. The root remains in the scalp and a patchy, thinning pattern of hair loss occurs. Hair loss may occur on other parts of the body in addition to the scalp. Loss of leg, arm, pubic, axillary, and facial hair is seen less often, although loss of eyebrows and eyelashes may occur.

The pattern and extent of hair loss cannot be accurately predicted for a given patient. When the treatment is given with a drug known to cause alopecia (Table 11-12), the patient needs to be told that severe hair loss can begin within a few days or weeks of treatment and that partial or complete baldness can quickly ensue. *Drug-induced alopecia is never permanent.* The patient may experience a change in hair color or texture when regrowth occurs.[37] Occasionally, hair growth may return while chemotherapy treatment continues. Given this perspective, coupled with the goal of disease control or cure, most patients tolerate the hair loss with minimal distress, although it is common and normal that some feelings are expressed about the hair loss.

Effects on skin. Vesicant drugs may cause severe tissue necrosis if infiltration should occur. Other skin reactions that might occur are hyperpigmentation, nail changes, and an increased sensitivity to the sun (photosensitivity).

Organ toxicities. *Liver* toxicity is uncommon but may occur. There may be a transient increase in liver enzymes. Alteration in liver function has been associated with Ara-C, methotrexate, and 6-mercaptopurine. *Cardiac* status is carefully monitored in patients receiving doxorubicin. A baseline echocardiogram is usually done before beginning treatment and at regular intervals while therapy continues.

Table 11-12 Alopecia as a side effect of chemotherapeutic drugs

Type of agent	Alopecia	No alopecia
Aklylating	Busulfan	Carmustine
	Cisplatin	Chlorambucil
	Cyclophosphamide	Lomustine
	Melphalan	
Antimetabolites	5-Fluorouracil	Cytabarine
	Methotrexate	Mercaptopurine
Antibiotics	Bleomycin	Plicamycin
	Dactinomycin	
	Daunorubicin	
	Doxorubicin	
	Mitomycin	
Plant alkaloids	Vinblastine	
	Vincristine	
Steroid hormones		All hormones

Two forms of cardiac damage may occur: dysrhythmias, most commonly associated with a preexisting cardiac disease, and a delayed moderate to severe congestive heart failure. Other drugs associated with some potential for cardiac toxicity are daunorubicin (Daunomycin) and high-dose cyclophosphamide (Cytoxan). *Pulmonary* toxicity may occur with methotrexate and some of the alkylating agents. The most common cause of chemotherapy-induced pulmonary toxicity is bleomycin. Pulmonary fibrosis can occur and may be irreversible. Each time bleomycin is administered, the pulmonary status of the patient is assessed by auscultation and questioning regarding the presence of cough or shortness of breath.

Urinary effects. Hemorrhagic cystitis occurs in about 10% of patients being treated with cyclophosphamide but rarely occur with other agents.[24] Patients receiving cyclophosphamide are encouraged to drink a large amount of fluid to minimize this effect. Taking the cyclophosphamide early in the day may also be of some benefit.[37] Renal toxicity is associated with several drugs, but most notably with cisplatin and streptozotocin. Before the administration of each dose of these drugs renal function is evaluated by either a serum creatinine or a 24-hour urine collection for creatinine clearance.

Sterility. Cancer chemotherapy reaches the reproductive organs at dose levels similar to those achieved at the site of the target tumor. The potential exists for a disruptive effect on genetic and fetal development. It is recognized that chemotherapy, particularly some of the alkylating agents, may cause transient or permanent sterility. Patients on chemotherapy need to be informed of the known and possible effects on fertility. Birth control and reproductive counseling need to be factors included in patient teaching.[3] If a nurse does not feel comfortable or qualified to discuss the topic, resources useful to the patient and spouse should be identified. Sperm banking before the initiation of therapy offers male patients the option of future conception.

Following completion of chemotherapy, conception and the birth of normal, healthy children are possibilities for couples. It is customary to recommend that procreation be avoided until at least 18 months after completion of treatment.

Biologic response modifier therapy (immunotherapy)
Pathophysiology

The role of biologic response modifier (BRM) therapy in the prevention and treatment of cancer is being studied. The term *BRM* actually applies to the broad category of biologic agents that have the potential to control the growth and metastasis of neoplasms. Immunotherapy is a subcategory of BRM therapies.[33]

Many scientists believe cancer occurs in the body more frequently than once in a lifetime; however, in most cases clinical evidence of the disease is not apparent. It is postulated that there is a natural immunity against the development of the disease and that cancer cells are destroyed almost as quickly as they develop.[16] Studies of cancer show that when the normal cell becomes malignant, it often undergoes biochemical changes resulting in formation of new cellular antigens that cause an immune response. Clinical malignancy may occur as a result of failure in the immunologic surveillance system of the body.

The immune response has two major components. The first, or *cellular immune response* (see Chapter 16), produces lymphocytes capable of destroying tumor cells on contact. These lymphocytes (T cells) undergo division and are released into the bloodstream when stimulated by an antigen. In addition to destroying cancer cells on contact, T cells may release cytotoxins, which cause holes in the cell membrane, eventually resulting in lysis or death of the malignant cell.

The second component of the immune response is *antibody production* resulting from activation of lymphocytes (B cells). When stimulated by antigens, B cells proliferate and differentiate into plasma cells, which are the major source of antibody production.

At the present time, the immune response can handle only a limited number of tumor cells, up to 10 million. After a growth to 100 million cells, the immune response is not capable of preventing further growth. Once the cancer is large, it cannot be totally controlled by the immune system, so immunotherapy cannot be the primary mode of cancer therapy at the present time. It is used after surgery, radiotherapy, and chemotherapy have removed the bulk of the tumor.

Much is yet to be learned about the immunology of cancers. The number of cancers once thought to be immunogenic and responsive to immunotherapy is less than originally supposed. If cancer vaccines are developed, they will be effective in tumors caused by viruses, and these are probably limited in number. Even if a cancer-carrying virus is isolated, it must be attenuated so it can be given safely.

Approaches used in BRM

Biologic response modifiers can be described as therapeutic agents that alter the interaction between tumor and host by influencing the host's biologic response to cancer cells. The two major categories of BRM therapies are distinguished by their mode of action. The first group consists of agents that *stimulate the general immune capacity* of the host. This group consists primarily of immunomodulators, including chemicals and synthetic compounds, that promote host resistance. The second group consists of effector cells, antibodies, and cytokines that have the ability to directly *destroy the tumor cells* or to indirectly *suppress the growth and metastasis of tumor cells.*[33] A discussion of several specific BRM therapies follows.

Cytokines

The term *cytokine* is a general one referring to the soluble products of cells. There are two major groups of cytokines: *monokines* derived from mononuclear phagocytes and *lymphokines* derived from lymphocytes. Interferon, tumor necrosis factor, and colony-stimulating factors are monokines; interleukin-2 is classified as a lymphokine.[4]

Interferons. Interferons are a family of secretory glycoproteins produced by leukocytes in response to viral infections or to other stimuli. Interferons induce cellular resistance to a broad spectrum of viruses and are a first line of defense against viral infections (see Fig. 16-5). In addition, they may protect against intracellular parasites, neoplastic changes in cells, and the tumor growth itself. They appear to have an inhibitory effect on DNA synthesis and cell growth and may suppress the tumor directly. Interferon's antitumor effect develops from its ability to augment natural killer (NK) cells (Chapter 16) and to stimulate the expression of antigens on the surface of lymphocytes and macrophages.[33]

When exposed to a virus, all nucleated cells are capable of interferon production. Three cell types produce interferon: leukocytes produce alpha interferon, fibroblasts produce beta interferon, and lymphocytes produce gamma interferon. Each type of interferon is distinctive in its ability to alter immunologic and biologic responses. Synthetic interferon has been manufactured by gene-cloning techniques.

Although interferon is not the cure for cancer that had been hoped initially, current research reports that interferon has antitumor activity against several cancers, including leukemia, lymphoma, and selected solid tumors. The FDA has approved interferon for use in treatment of hairy cell leukemia.[33]

Nursing intervention for persons receiving interferon therapy includes monitoring for side effects: fever, local discomfort at the injection site, and minimal nausea and vomiting. Acetaminophen (Tylenol) is given for discomfort and antiemetics are given for nausea and vomiting. If therapy is to be continued in the home setting, nurses may need to teach patients to give their own intravenous or intramuscular injections. Nurses must be careful not to raise false hopes in patients who may view interferon as a last-resort therapy.

Interleukin-2. Interleukin-2 (IL-2) stimulates formation of T cells and natural killer cells. Preliminary indications from clinical trials suggest that IL-2 may be useful as a curative agent for some malignancies and be beneficial in combination with other treatment modalities. It is administered by intravenous bolus or continuous infusion, by subcutaneous injection, and by peritoneal infusion. Identified side effects include confusion, psychosis, pulmonary edema, impaired renal functioning, dysrhythmias, and hypotension.[19] For some protocols, severe side effects, including capillary leak syndrome, require patients to be monitored in an ICU.

Tumor necrosis factor. Tumor necrosis factor (TNF) is a monokine capable of causing necrosis in existing tumors by selectively killing neoplastic cells. TNF alters the vascular endothelium, resulting in a hemorrhagic tumor necrosis. This biologic agent has been used with some success in patients with sarcoma; clinical trials are currently being conducted on various tumor types. Common side effects include chills, fever, headache, fatigue, and hypotension.[4] TNF is administered as an intravenous bolus, via continuous intravenous infusion, intramuscular injection, or subcutaneous injection. Intravenous tubing should be primed with human serum albumin to prevent the adherence of TNF to the tubing.[16]

Colony-stimulating factors. Colony-stimulating factors (CSFs), also called *growth factors*, are administered to cancer patients in hopes of decreasing the severity of neutropenia associated with chemotherapy. These monokines stimulate the maturation and production of blood cells. CSFs do not exhibit antitumor activity.

There are four types of CSFs. *Granulocyte-macrophage CSF* (GM-CSF) influences the maturation of granulocytes, monocytes, and macrophages. *Granulocyte CSF* (G-CSF) stimulates the development of granulocytes. *Interleukin-3* has been found to target a variety of blood cells in their very early phases of maturation. *Erythropoietin* affects formation of erythrocytes. These growth factors probably have some overlapping effects on blood cell development.

Erythropoietin received FDA approval in 1989. Its major use has been to decrease RBC transfusion needs in kidney dialysis patients (see Chapter 33). GM-CSF (Sargramostim) and G-CSF (Filgrastim) received FDA approval in 1991. Numerous clinical trials are currently being conducted to determine the potential of these new agents fully. The major clinical applications include decreasing or preventing neutropenia, which occurs as a side effect of chemotherapy treatments, or conditioning regimens for bone marrow transplant therapy (see Chapter 27). Use of CSFs allows patients to tolerate more easily the doses of chemotherapy needed to eradicate their malignancies.[34]

CSFs are administered by subcutaneous injection or by a variety of intravenous infusions ranging from bolus injections to continuous infusions. Patients who receive CSFs on an outpatient basis need to be taught subcutaneous injection techniques and should keep a log of any side effects that may occur.

Monoclonal antibodies

Monoclonal antibodies are produced by first injecting a mouse with a specific tumor antigen. The mouse's spleen cells are then removed and fused with myeloma cells. This fusion promotes the survival of the cells in cultures where they are cloned. The clones are then injected into a mouse. The result is a monoclonal hybridoma that secretes monoclonal antibodies that can be harvested from mouse and administered to humans.

Numerous clinical trials with monoclonal antibodies are currently being conducted, against both hematopoetic malignancies and solid tumors. Some studies are investigating the use of monoclonal antibodies conjugated with toxic substances.[33] Radioactive isotopes and cytotoxic agents are attached to antibodies to deliver these substances directly to the neoplasm. Monoclonal antibodies are administered by slow intravenous infusion. Side effects include but are not limited to fever, chills, and localized tumor pain.

Thymic factors

The two most common factors produced by the thymus gland are thymosin fraction 5 (TF-5) and thymosin alpha 1 (Tα-1). TF-5 is an extract of calf thymus and appears to be capable of restoring immunologic functioning when the thymus gland is absent or repressed. Tα-1 is a derivative of TF-5 and can be synthetically produced. Phase I research has demonstrated that thymic factors have immunostimulating capacities in immunosuppressed cancer patients. Some immunorestorative capacity has also been suggested using Tα-1 in clinical trials.[33]

Nursing interventions for BRM therapy

Clinical trials of biologic response modifiers are currently being conducted in many health care centers, and nurses must be familiar with the research protocols being tested in their particular setting. Consent forms need to be obtained. Medications are often administered in rigid schedules and nurses are particularly involved in monitoring for side effects. In general, BRM therapies can cause fever, malaise, arthralgias and myalgias, as well as anaphylactic types of reactions. These treatments are relatively new, and the incidence and severity of side effects are still being established. Thorough documentation of adverse reactions and their response to symptom management is essential. Patient teaching should emphasize the need to report all side effects, regardless of how subtle they may be.

Management of cancer pain

Pain is one of the most feared effects of cancer although, contrary to popular belief, it is frequently the last symptom to appear. Even in terminal stages, 60% of persons with cancer will experience mild or no pain. The etiology of cancer pain is complex because it has physical, psychologic, social, and spiritual aspects.

Stages of cancer pain

Three stages of cancer pain have been described: early, intermediate, and late. Early pain usually occurs after initial surgery for diagnosis or treatment and usually subsides after the third day; thus, this pain is an acute episode, that is, it is short term and temporary.

Intermediate-stage pain results from postoperative contraction of scars and nerve entrapment or from cancer recurrence or metastasis. This pain may subside or may be controlled by palliative therapy such as radiation, chemotherapy, neurosurgery, and analgesics. Therapy itself may initiate the pain.

Late-stage pain occurs in terminal cancer when therapy no longer controls the disease. This pain is chronic, may slowly increase in intensity, and at times may be intractable. Severe chronic pain occurs in only about 25% of patients who die from cancer.[11]

Pathophysiology

Malignant neoplasms cause pain by five physiologic changes: bone destruction, obstruction of lumens (viscera or vessels), peripheral nerve involvement, pressure of growing tumors causing ischemia or distention, and inflammation, infection, or necrosis of the tissue.

Bone destruction with infraction (fractures without displacement) is the most frequent cause of pain, usually resulting from metastatic lesions. Bone destruction may cause increased sensitivity over the area or sharp, continuous pain.

Obstruction of a viscus, such as in the gastrointestinal or genitourinary tract, causes severe, colicky, crampy-type pain. Visceral pain is dull, diffuse, and poorly localized. Obstruction of an artery, vein, or lymphatic vessel may initiate arterial ischemia, venous engorgement, or edema. This pain is dull, diffuse, and aching.

Infiltration or compression of peripheral nerves or nerve plexuses causes continuous, sharp, or stabbing pain sometimes accompanied by hyperesthesia or paresthesia.

Infiltration or distention of the integument, fascia, or tissue initiates a severe localized pain that is dull and aching, increasing in intensity as tumor size increases. An example of this is the pain resulting from distention of the abdomen by ascites or the stretching of the skin by carcinoma of the neck.

Finally, inflammation, infection, and necrosis of the tissue itself may cause pain by producing either pressure or ischemia. Chemical mediators of pain are present during inflammation and necrosis.

Psychosocial aspects

The psychologic component of cancer pain is associated with the patient's perception of the threat and stress of cancer and varies from individual to individual. Three categories of stressors have been identified: injury or threat of injury as a result of the cancer, loss or threat of loss (body part or death), and frustration of drives as a result of disabilities from the cancer per se or from the effect of therapies. Patients may respond with depression, decreased self-esteem, hostility, and irritability.

The sociologic effects include decreased interaction and participation in activities of daily living. There is decreased productivity characterized by absenteeism from work, economic problems, and deterioration in family relationships. The spiritual effects of pain are evidenced by loss of hope and trust and an overwhelming feeling of despair, rejection, and sense of isolation.

Side effects of cancer pain include fatigue, sleeplessness, anorexia, and decreased movement followed by the complications of immobility, namely, muscle weakness, decubiti, contractures, and respiratory dysfunction.[31]

Intervention

Medical therapy in early-stage pain focuses on therapy directed at the cancer per se. Late-stage pain is treated symptomatically by analgesia, neurosurgery, and nerve blocks. Surgical procedures to relieve the pain include simple intercostal nerve block where feasible, surgical section of posterior sensory roots adjacent to the spinal cord, and spinothalamic tractotomy (interruption of pain- and temperature-conducting tracts). Dorsal column stimulators and transcutaneous electrical stimulators (see Chapter 10) may be helpful in selected cases.

Cancer pain, like other types of severe pain, may occupy the patient's entire attention and, unless treated vigorously, may demoralize the patient and interfere with eating, resting, or sleeping. Interventions are directed toward helping the patient live as normal a life as possible and cope with the pain. Pain tolerance is increased when the patient's energy is preserved for enjoyable activities. General comfort measures to promote rest and sleep, good body positioning, and nutrition may do much to increase the patient's pain tolerance. Teaching patients conscious muscle relaxation during which they systematically contract and relax muscle groups throughout the body may decrease pain resulting from muscle tenseness as well as anxiety associated with the pain (see Chapter 10).

Diversionary activities help decrease the patient's perception of the pain by distraction. These activities may be physical (work, walking, rocking, swimming), social, or mental (watching television, reading, crafts). Some patients find imagery (waking-imagined analgesia) helpful. Others may try to separate the pain from their bodies thereby "quieting the mind by letting the body drop away."[31]

Medications. Drugs may be the one significant method that alleviates the pain of cancer. Aspirin is the most effective single analgesic for mild to moderate pain.[11] There is an additive and perhaps synergistic effect between aspirin and codeine; therefore, combinations of these drugs are useful in moderate acute pain and in chronic aching pain.

In severe chronic cancer pain the narcotics, with the exception of codeine and oxycodone, are the most effective. Although there are no significant differences among the various drugs in potency or side effects, there are significant differences in the duration of action. Those with long duration of action are preferred for relief of chronic cancer pain.[10] Tolerance and dependence related to these drugs is not an issue. Repeated studies show that, in general, patients with chronic physiologic pain do not become addicted to narcotic analgesics.[11]

There are three important principles in the administration of narcotics. The first is that the optimal dose must be determined, and initial pain control may require seemingly large doses of the narcotics. The second principle is to start with a dose that is too high rather than one that is too low because the person may become anxious if there is no analgesia despite analgesic administration. This anxiety may exacerbate the pain. The third and most important principle is that the narcotic must be *administered regularly*, not prn. Each dose must be given before the previous dose loses effect. Prevention of pain recurrence usually requires less analgesia than treatment of pain after it has recurred (Box 11-13).

Oral administration is preferred. Parenteral therapy produces higher initial serum and tissue levels of the narcotic, but the oral doses are as effective as parenteral doses in maintaining drug levels in the body. Intramuscular and subcutaneous injections are more difficult to administer and are painful to patients with marked muscle wasting. In addition, parenteral administration may make the patient dependent on others for drug administration.[10]

Phenothiazines are the principal adjunct drug given to control severe chronic cancer pain. They are effective as antiemetics and also have an antianxiety effect.

Nurses provide the psychologic and social support necessary to help the cancer patient cope with severe pain. Administration of analgesics over the 24-hour period and explanations of the physiologic and pharmacologic effects of the drugs can be very helpful to patients and their families (see Chapter 10).

Psychologic support of patient and family

Cancer nursing demands not only caring *for* the patient but also caring *about* the patient, who may be angry, depressed, and perhaps physically unattractive because of the effects of the disease or its treatment. Communication is vital in meeting the needs of the cancer patient and the family. Validating assumptions and assisting patients in describing, clarifying, and identifying reasons for feelings are important to promote communications. In addition, the nurse must try to make explanations clear and uncomplicated. Getting feedback from the patient is one way to ensure that the message has been received.

Nursing interventions to help patient cope

Because the threat to life and the potential for other losses are great for patients with cancer, they need especially to have their existing coping mechanisms supported or to receive support if coping mechanisms are inadequate to meet their needs.

Each patient's reaction to cancer is unique, so there can be no easy formula for care. The nurse must be able to work with and accept patients' behavior and coping style. Avoidance of false reassurance and pat answers that block communication will contribute to patient comfort. Openness, honesty, and creativity of the nurse are essential. The nurse reinforces patients' hope but is careful to avoid giving false hope, which can be more devastating than none at all. At times patients may need to deny their illness, while at other times they may want to talk about it.

Trusting patients' resilience and their will to try and helping them live as fully as possible are all appropriate interventions. When patients complain, perhaps the best response is, "Tell me how you feel. Perhaps we can do something about it." Self-esteem is maintained by fostering patients' independence, even if this only involves taking part in decision making about the care to be given.

Persons working with these patients must have confidence in themselves and the ability to suspend their own concerns, needs, and desires to concentrate on patients' problems. To do this one must be able to tolerate a high

11-13

Nursing Research

Ferrell B et al: Effects of controlled-release morphine on quality of life for cancer pain, *Oncol Nurs Forum* 16(4):521-526, 1989.

As the title indicates, the purpose of this study was to determine the effects of controlled-release morphine on the overall quality of life for patients with cancer. Data was collected from 83 subjects in a repeated-measure design every 2 weeks for 6 weeks, using five instruments to assess quality of life, pain, and functional status. Findings indicated improved pain management with improved quality of life as measured in the study. The study concludes that nurses can greatly enhance quality of life for the patient with cancer by providing appropriate pain therapies.

level of anxiety and to look at problems on both a feeling (affective) and a thinking (cognitive) level.

Listening carefully and attentively to concerns of patients helps to calm fears. In addition, nurses who are knowledgeable about cancer, who can answer questions and clear up misconceptions, help to promote the patient's psychologic well-being.

Nursing interventions to help family cope

The interventions that help the patient cope are also important in helping the family cope. The nurse must get to know them and their reactions. They may feel guilty, helpless, and angry, just as the patient does. Letting them know that their feelings are normal may increase their comfort. Families should not be pushed into responsibilities that they cannot handle. Some want to participate in care, others are overwhelmed by the disease and are afraid to or may not want to help. Their feelings need to be respected.

Teaching the family is a major responsibility. They should be reminded not to cut the patient off from family activities and concerns. If possible, the patient should be included in family decision making and planning. In their desire to help their loved ones, families may unintentionally contribute to the patient's sense of isolation by shielding him or her from family concerns.[29]

Interdisciplinary approach to care

The skills of many members of the health team may be required to meet the needs of the cancer patient. Clear, concise communication of ideas about care and the planned interventions is essential for coordination, continuity, and integration of care. Team conferences help establish goals and promote the sharing of expertise. The social worker, occupational therapist, minister, and psychologist may all be needed to contribute to the patient's well-being. The nurse, who spends the most time with the patient, may be the first person to recognize that the patient and family could benefit from the services of health team members.

Rehabilitation of the cancer patient to an optimal level of functioning through the efforts of many health team members results in a more satisfying life for the patient and the family. Often the community health nurse is called on to give care, teach, counsel, and support the patient and family after discharge.

Supportive care of the patient with terminal cancer
Planning care

When all possible therapies have failed to control the spread of cancer, the patient and family have many special problems. They need encouragement and help in living as normally as possible, in planning for the late stages of the patient's illness, and in adjusting to death and its implications for the family.

Before nurses can help the patient and family, they must have developed a mature philosophy that allows acceptance of death as an eventual reality for everyone. This philosophy is not acquired overnight. The nurse needs the opportunity to discuss feelings about caring for the patient whose death is imminent because the nurse's attitude toward death and suffering will affect the ability to plan and give care to the patient with advanced cancer. (See Chapter 15 for a discussion of death and dying.)

No one can say with certainty when death will come. The patient may ask about the length of time remaining, but no absolute answer can be given. Physicians may have made a statement to the patient about life expectancy. The nursing staff should know what the patient has been told because the patient's willingness to participate in self-care and attitude toward the illness may be influenced by his or her perception of life expectancy.

Planning, doing, and achieving are the best way to prevent the hopelessness and despair that may overwhelm the patient. Every effort must be put forth to meet the patient's physiologic needs so that higher-order psychologic needs may be expressed. The patient who is in pain or feels "dirty" will probably have difficulty expressing concerns and fears.

Other factors to consider in planning care are the personality of the patient, feelings about death and illness, and the reactions of those significant others whose opinion the patient values. The goal of nursing care should be to relieve physical, mental, and spiritual distress. The most common nursing diagnoses for the patient with cancer that is terminal are listed in Box 11-14.

Planning home care. At least half of all deaths from cancer occur in the patients' homes. Planning for home care of the patient without completely disrupting the rest of the family takes the concerted efforts of many people. Patients must always be consulted, and their wishes should be respected in the early stages of the disease. In the final stages they may be too ill to be bothered or concerned with making decisions. The physician, the social worker, and the nurse must work together with the local community agencies, such as the American Cancer Society, to ensure continuity of care from the hospital to the home. The principles governing suitability for home care are similar to those for any patient receiving home care, although the patient with cancer may not live as long as many others with chronic long-term illnesses. Medical and nursing supervision must be available; it must be possible for required care to be given; both patient and family must want the patient home; and home facilities must be suitable. Rehabilitation teams may also be sent into the home to help the patient and family.

The growth of the *hospice* concept, a place where patients may come for short or long periods for nursing care and then return to their homes as their condition warrants, is exciting. The hospice tries to maintain a homelike setting while relieving the family of the emotional and physical burden of constant care. Hospice programs provide medical, social, and psychologic support for patients and their families so that dying can be truly dignified.

The hospice concept may also be implemented as home care for the patient with the inpatient facility as a backup for home care. If a family wishes to go away on a trip, for example, the patient may request to stay in the hospice. The ultimate goal of the hospice is for the family to develop its ability to give care; thus the relationship of the hospice to the family becomes primarily one of consultation and referral. The family is aided in remaining the patient's primary support system.

Hospice staff are multidisciplinary and are employed and evaluated based on their interests and abilities to care for the terminally ill person. The focus of activities is care rather than cure, with an emphasis on symptom control. Actions are identified to help the patient and family deal with their chief concerns.[29]

Nursing interventions during advanced cancer stages
Counseling and guidance
Avoiding false hope. Occasionally, there is a mistake in diagnosis or the disease is in some way arrested for a long time. If the patient assumes that one of these occurrences may take place, the nurse should not suggest facing probable reality. The nurse must, however, avoid encouraging false hope. Many patients accept their prognosis philosophically, with the hope that a cure for cancer will be found before their disease is far advanced. Some patients are better able to accept the situation if their religious faith can be strengthened. Some patients and their families find it helpful to live each day as fully as possible without looking too far ahead. Sometimes patients with cancer have few symptoms and are able to carry on quite well until shortly before death.

Nurses also must be careful that they do not experience

11-14

Nursing diagnoses for the patient with terminal cancer

Airway clearance, ineffective
Constipation
Family processes, altered
Fatigue
Fear (specify)
Grieving: anticipatory, dysfunctional
Nutrition, altered: less than body requirements
Oral mucous membrane, altered
Pain
Powerlessness
Self-care deficit, bathing/hygiene
Skin integrity, impaired: high risk for
Social isolation

false hope. The inability to fulfill the hope to sustain life may make it more difficult for nurses to accept the patient's death and they may see themselves as having failed.[29]

Encouraging social and vocational activities. Patients with advanced cancer should resume their regular work if they can possibly do so, for work makes them feel as though they are still an active part of their group and worthy of the approval of others. It was said many centuries ago that employment is a person's best physician, and this concept applies particularly to persons whose existence is seriously threatened by cancer. Social activities and all experiences associated with normal family life should be continued whenever possible. There is probably no greater service the nurse can give to patients with uncontrollable cancer than to help them continue their everyday lives in any way possible. Family members often need guidance in seeing the patient's need to live as normally as possible.

Decreasing fear of helplessness. Patients may be haunted by fear of brain involvement, loss of mental faculties, and the possibility that they may become completely helpless and dependent on others. By these fears they express a basic human wish: the wish to leave the world with as much dignity as possible. The nurse should urge the patient and family to discuss such fears with the physician. The patient may feel that the physician is too busy and that questions are too trivial to justify the use of the physician's time. Some questions, however, are not trivial at all, and a satisfactory answer to them adds tremendously to the patient's peace of mind. Metastasis to the brain in persons who have other metastases is somewhat rare, and some patients suffer more from fear of damage to the brain than is justified. The patient should know that good general hygiene, good nutrition, being up and about for part of each day, and doing deep-breathing exercises with attention to posture all help to prevent helplessness. A positive approach to all problems certainly shortens the time of helplessness and makes the patient more content.

Facilitating activities of daily living.
Promoting comfort. Giving good nursing care to the patient in an advanced stage of cancer is challenging. Promoting the patient's comfort should be high on the list of goals. Nursing measures that increase rest and sleep and reduce pain (p. 222) will help maintain the patient's physical and psychologic well-being.

Maintaining nutrition. Cachexia is a frequent problem. Anorexia may accompany therapy, and the increased protein needs of the body resulting from tumor growth may be difficult to meet. Mealtimes should be incorporated with family visiting, or patients can eat together if possible. A high-protein diet enhances the response from therapy, and an adequate intake of calories spares protein for cell building. Because chewing may be difficult, food should be cut in small pieces and creamed or combined with cooked vegetables, rice, or noodles. Meat may also be ground or used as a base for soups or stews. Fish, cottage cheese, and eggs are also good sources of protein.

Total parenteral nutrition (TPN) may be used as an adjunct to therapy. TPN has not been found to stimulate tumor growth and it may result in a return of immune system competence, a decrease in sepsis, wound healing, and an increase in response to chemotherapy.

Maintaining elimination. Diarrhea may be a problem, but constipation is more likely. If the patient is receiving narcotics, especially opium derivatives, peristalsis is decreased.[10] Patients receiving the plant alkaloid vincristine (Oncovin) may develop neurotoxicity, causing a high fecal impaction. Increasing the intake of roughage and fluids in the diet, maintaining activity, and using stool softeners may be helpful. Enemas and laxatives may be necessary.

Maintaining personal hygiene. Careful and meticulous hygiene is essential. Careful bathing and attention to skin, hair, and clothing will all promote self-esteem in the patient. Odors from body exudates, draining wounds, and incontinence may occur. Soiled dressings and bed linen are changed immediately. Judicious use of deodorizers is helpful, but deodorizers do not take the place of good hygiene.

Preventing effects of immobility. Pressure sores may be a severe problem. The combination of inactivity, poor nutrition, and incontinence seen in patients with advanced cancer predisposes them to skin breakdown. Maintaining the patient's activity by getting him or her out of bed as much as possible will prevent pressure and also promote the patient's joint mobility and muscle strength.

Teaching patient and family. The nurse is involved in teaching during most interactions with the patient and family. Careful explanations about care and sensitivity to what the patient thinks and feels about the disease contribute to the nurse's effectiveness in promoting change in the patient's behavior. When possible, self-care activities should be emphasized. Maintaining the patient's independence whenever possible should be the goal while recognizing that the time may come when dependence is necessary.

Evaluation
Because of the diversity and complexity of cancer, evaluation of care is especially dependent on the expected patient outcomes that have been identified. Care is based on the person's level of physical and psychosocial capacities and value systems. Questions to consider include the following:
1. Have identified learning needs been met with patient teaching?
2. Have the person and significant others had opportunities to express feelings and concerns?
3. Has the person participated in decision-making as desired?
4. Has hope been maintained, without giving false hope?
5. Is the person as comfortable as possible?
6. Are good ventilation, nutrition, and elimination being maintained?

7. Are usual activities of daily living being carried out, with assistance given as needed?
8. Is the person active within existing limits?
9. Have coping methods been supported and support services been identified?

SUMMARY

1. The term *cancer* refers to more than 200 diseases that have in common the production of abnormal cells that do not obey the laws of normal tissue growth.
2. Early diagnosis and new treatment advances have increased the survival rate so that today one out of every two persons with cancer can survive.
3. Malignant cells are characterized by larger irregular nuclei, increased rates of mitosis, atypical appearance, loss of contact inhibition, and increased concentration of RNA.
4. Cancer spread occurs by three routes: direct extension or invasion, gravitational metastasis or seeding, and metastasis via blood or lymph vessels.
5. The chances of developing cancer increases with each decade after an individual reaches age 60. This may result from an exhaustion of the immune system or from a lifelong exposure to environmental carcinogens.
6. Environmental factors, host susceptibility, health practices, and psychosocial factors all contribute to carcinogenesis.
7. The most common sites of cancer in women are the breast, colorectum, lung, and uterus (cervix).
8. The most common sites of cancer in males are the prostate, lung, and colorectum.
9. Psychologic responses to cancer can range from stoicism to extreme anger. Loneliness, depression, denial, anxiety, and guilt are common reactions.
10. The term *paraneoplastic syndrome* is used to describe the systemic effects of cancer.
11. Surgery is the oldest treatment for cancer and involves removal of the tumor for cure or palliation.
12. Radiotherapy uses radiation to destroy or delay the growth of the rapidly reproducing malignant cells.
13. Chemotherapeutic drugs bring about changes in the cell cycle phases and interrupt cell growth and replication.
14. Biologic response modifier therapies are therapeutic agents that alter the interaction between the tumor and the host by influencing the host's biologic response to cancer cells.
15. Malignant neoplasms cause pain by five physiologic changes: bone destruction, obstruction of lumens, peripheral nerve involvement, pressure of growing tumors, and inflammation, infection, and necrosis of tissue.
16. Even in terminal stages, 60% of persons with cancer will experience mild or no pain.

STUDY QUESTIONS

- Look at Fig. 11-1. What are the three most common cancers for men and for women? What preventive measures can be taken for each of the common cancers?
- The physician's report states that the patient's tumor is staged as T1, N1, M0. What does this mean? What nursing implications does this have?
- What organizations in your community provide services to patients with cancer?
- What are the benefits and disadvantages of the four treatment modalities for cancer? What is the nurse's role in each of these modalities?
- What nursing care services are provided by hospices?

REFERENCES AND SELECTED READINGS

1. American Cancer Society, *Cancer facts and figures 1991*, New York, 1991, The Society.
2. American Cancer Society: *Cancer manual*, ed 8, Boston, 1989, The Society.
3. Averette HE, Boike GM, Jarrell MA: Effects of cancer chemotherapy on gonadal function and reproductive capacity, CA 40(4):199-209, 1990.
4. Baird SB, McCorkle R, Grant M: *Cancer nursing: a comprehensive textbook*, Philadelphia, 1991, WB Saunders.
5. Boring CC, Squires TS, Tong T: Cancer statistics, CA 41(1):19-36, 1991.
6. Crowley MJ: *Risk factors*. In Ziegfeld CR, editor: *Core curriculum for oncology nursing*, Philadelphia, 1987, WB Saunders.
7.* D'Agostino NS: Managing nutrition problems in advanced cancer, *Am J Nurs* 89:50-56, 1989.
8. DeVita V Jr, Hellman S, Rosenberg SA: *Cancer principles and practice of oncology*, ed 3, Philadelphia, 1989, JB Lippincott.
8a.* Dudjak LA, Fleck AE: BRMs: new drug therapy comes of age, *RN* 54(10):42-47, 1991.
9.* Ferrell BR, Schneider C: Experience and management of cancer pain at home, *Cancer Nurs* 11:84-90, 1988.
10. Ferrell B et al: Effects of controlled-release morphine on quality of life for cancer pain, *Oncol Nurs Forum* 16(4):521-526, 1989.
11.* Foley KM: The treatment of pain in the patient with cancer, CA 36(4):195-215, 1987.
12. Frank-Strombert M: The role of the nurse in early detection of cancer: population sixty-six years of age and older, *Oncol Nurs Forum* 13(3):66-74, 1986.
13. Garfinkel L, Silverberg E: Lung cancer and smoking trends in the United States over the past 25 years, CA 41(3):137-145, 1991.
14. Garfinkel MA, Stellman SD: Cigarette smoking among physicians, dentists, and nurses, CA 36(1):2-8, 1986.
15. Gordon D: *Staging: a classification system for cancer*. In Ziegfeld CR, editor: *Core curriculum for oncology nursing*, Philadelphia, 1987, WB Saunders.
16. Groenwald SL: Cancer nursing: principles and practice, ed 2, Boston, 1990, Jones & Bartlett.
17. Hogan R: Human sexuality: a nursing perspective, ed 2, New York, 1985, Appleton-Century Crofts.
18.* Jarvis W: Helping your patients deal with questionable cancer treatments, CA 36(5):293-301, 1986.
19.* Jassak PF, Stricklin LA: Interleukin-2: an overview, *Oncol Nurs Forum* 13(6):17-22, 1986.
20. Kane NE et al: Use of patient-controlled analgesia in surgical oncology patients, *Oncol Nurs Forum* 15:29-37, 1988.
21.* Lewandowski W, Jones SL: The family with cancer: nursing interventions throughout the course of living with cancer, *Cancer Nurs* 11:313-321, 1988.
22.* Lewis F, Levita M: Understanding radiotherapy, *Cancer Nurs* 11:174-185, 1988.

*Recommended for student reading.

23. Lovejoy N: *Alterations in cell biology.* In Ziegfeld CR, editor: *Core curriculum for oncology nursing,* Philadelphia, 1987, WB Saunders.

23a. McVey L: A direct assault on abdominal cancer, *RN* 55(2):46-52, 1992.

24.* Melone L et al: A teaching booklet for patients receiving GM-CSF therapy, *Oncol Nurs Forum* 18(3):593-597, 1991.

25. Million-Underwood S, Sanders E: Factors contributing to health promotion behaviors among African-American men, *Oncol Nurs Forum* 17(5):707-712, 1990.

26. Oncology Nursing Society: *Cancer chemotherapy guidelines for nursing education and practice,* Pittsburgh, 1984, The Society.

27. Porth C: Pathophysiology: concepts of altered health states, ed 3, Philadelphia, 1990, JB Lippincott.

28. Rose MA: Health promotion and risk prevention: applications for cancer survivors, *Oncol Nurs Forum* 16:335-340, 1989.

29.* Scanlon C: Creating a vision of hope: the challenge of palliative care, *Oncol Nurs Forum* 16(4):527-541, 1989.

30.* Schneider SM, Distelhorst CW: Chemotherapy-induced emergencies, *Semin Oncol* 16(6):572-578, 1989.

31.* Sprass J: Cancer pain and suffering: clinical lessons from life, literature, and legend, *Oncol Nurs Forum* 12(14):23-31, 1985.

32.* Strohl RA: The nursing role in radiation oncology: symptom management of acute and chronic reactions, *Oncol Nurs Forum* 15(4):429-434, 1988.

33. Suppers VJ, McClamrock EA: Biologicals in cancer treatment: future effects on nursing practice, *Oncol Nurs Forum* 12(3):27-32, 1985.

34. Taylor KM et al: Recombinant human granulocyte colon-stimulating factor recovery after high-dose chemotherapy and autologous bone marrow transplantation in Hodgkin's disease, *J Clin Oncol* 7(12):1791-1799, 1989.

35. Valentine A: *Early detection measures.* In Ziegfeld CR: *Core curriculum for oncology nursing,* Philadelphia, 1987, WB Saunders.

36. Varricchio CG: Cultural and ethnic dimensions of cancer nursing care: introduction, *Oncol Nurs Forum* 14(3):57-58, 1987.

37.* Walters P: Chemotherapy: a nurse's guide to action, administration, and side effects, *RN* 53(2):52-68, 1990.

Classic

38.* Goodman SG, Wickham R: Venous access devices: an overview, *Oncol Nurs Forum* 11(5):16-23, 1984.

39.* McIntire SM, Cioppa AL: Cancer nursing: a developmental approach, New York, 1984, John Wiley & Sons.

40. American Cancer Society: *Public attitudes toward cancer and cancer tests,* New York, 1980, The Society.

41. Rosenbaum EH: Living with cancer, St Louis, 1982, Mosby–Year Book.

42. Schottenfeld D, Haas JF: Carcinogens in the workplace, *CA* 29:173-183, 1977.

12

Sleep Disorders

Diane Broadbent Friedman

After studying this chapter, the learner should be able to:

- Take a complete sleep history.
- Describe the nature, pathophysiology, therapy, and teaching needs of persons with insomnia, narcolepsy, and sleep apnea.
- Describe the relationship of sleep to chronobiology and the implications for nursing research.

We usually divide our lives into two parts, waking and sleeping. We also commonly believe that our important activity occurs while we are awake and that sleep is a passive state initiated by simply closing our eyes. This belief contains the two most basic *misunderstandings* about sleep: that sleep is not active or very important to life and that sleep is something that simply comes "naturally." These misunderstandings contribute to health professionals and their patients overlooking sleep problems and the role sleep plays in healing and health maintenance.

12-1	**External factors regulating sleep/wakefulness**
	Sunrise, sunset, and length of day Ambient temperature Physical activity and rest Timing and composition of meals Timing of social/environmental cues, such as increased morning traffic noise

INTRODUCTION TO SLEEP PROBLEMS

Aspects of Normal Sleep

Sleep is difficult to define because as yet it is incompletely understood by researchers. From the sleeper's point of view, sleep is experienced as (1) being the deliberate initiation of a change or reduction in consciousness lasting an average of 8 hours, (2) commencing about the same time each 24-hour period, and (3) usually resulting in a feeling of restored physical, emotional, and intellectual energy. This definition contains three important concepts about normal sleep: *changes in consciousness, deliberate initiation of sleep,* and *timing of sleep.*

Although the sleeping person or observers may believe the sleeper is unconscious, the sleeping brain alternates among several active states during sleep, producing a series of predictable 90-minute sleep cycles. Unlike the unconsciousness produced by anesthesia, the brain maintains all body systems during sleep, some of which are more active in sleep (such as secretion of growth hormone), and allows for restoration of alertness if required. Also, unlike animals, only humans can deliberately postpone the initiation of sleep. The record for sleep postponement is about 10 days.

Sleep commences about the same time each 24-hour period. Sleep research at the cellular level indicates that changes in the neuronal cell membrane and in the cell nucleus in several brain areas alter the cell's excitability in different stages of sleep. The study of biologic rhythms places the study of sleep into a larger context. The timing for sleep is regulated by many subtle external factors (see Box 12-1). Internal hormonal factors and neurologic activity maintain internal biologic clocks. These factors tend to occur at the same time every 24 hours; therefore they help to "anchor" the onset and termination of sleep.

Normal Sleep Function

Sleep usually is initiated in the late evening about 8 hours before arising for morning work or daily routine. Some people require more or less than 8 hours to feel refreshed. Some people are "larks," falling asleep within moments of lying down and awakening alert and ready to go, whereas others are "owls," taking up to 30 minutes to fall asleep and feeling their most alert in the afternoon or early evening.

Sleep usually is initiated within 30 minutes of lying down. Sleep cycles of 90 minutes occur, initiated by very light stage I/II, followed by deep stage III/IV, and ending with lighter rapid eye movement (REM)/dream sleep. If awakened from light stage I sleep, sleepers state that they were not asleep, whereas if awakened from other stages, they state that they were asleep or dreaming. Arousal can occur after each REM cycle. As the night progresses, the amount of time spent in stage III/IV shortens and the amount of REM lengthens. Thus more dreaming time occurs in the morning hours just before final awakening.

Nature of Sleep Problems

It is estimated that more than one half of all adults cite difficulties with sleeping at some time in their lives. These problems result in suffering; risk of accident; worry about loss of emotional, intellectual, or neurologic functioning; embarrassment; and exacerbation of other health problems. In 1983 the National Institutes of Mental Health (NIMH) determined that 35% of a nationally representative sample reported "trouble sleeping" in the previous year and that half this group reported this as a "serious" problem. This means that approximately one of every three patients a nurse encounters may describe a sleep problem. Sleep problems have been historically overlooked, however, especially in the hospitalized patient when other circumstances appear more compelling.

Nurses can have a primary impact on helping persons with sleep problems and preventing sleep problems from starting. The following instances of sleep problems highlight the need to detect sleep concerns or to prevent sleep problems from developing.

1. A 50-year-old woman describes a 25-year history of inability to stay asleep beyond 5 AM, dating from the birth of her first child.
2. A 65-year-old man comes to the emergency room for contusions following a minor traffic accident. He works the night shift, driving a newspaper delivery truck, and then stays awake during the day to care for his chronically ill wife.
3. A downcast young boy leaves the examining room after his mother describes how he must pass up summer camp because of bed-wetting.
4. An executive, whose head is immobilized in halo traction following a neck injury, describes sleeplessness at night, distorted conversations with physicians (probably related to medications), being awakened at night for procedures, and being disturbed by noises and vibrations amplified by the tongs.
5. A woman states that her husband falls asleep readily, even while sitting up in a chair, and that his skin color becomes bluish as he snorts and breathes irregularly.

Sleep problems can be categorized by the disruption in one or more of the aspects of normal sleep. Box 12-2 identifies different types of sleep problems. This chapter discusses only the most common types of sleep disorders:

parasomnias or *disorders of arousal* dysfunction associated with sleep, sleep stages, or arousal
insomnia inability to initiate or maintain sleep
narcolepsy sleep intrusion into wakefulness
sleep apnea sleep problems involving other body systems

The last section of this chapter discusses research into sleep and circadian rhythms and its impact on nurses, both as researchers and as caregivers who must remain awake and alert at night.

PARASOMNIAS OR DISORDERS OF AROUSAL

Various types of parasomnias or disorders of arousal may occur (Table 12-1), especially in children who often outgrow the dysfunction.

Sleepwalking

Sleepwalking (somnambulism) usually occurs in children, although it may also be seen in adults. Children usually outgrow sleepwalking. It is characterized by sitting up or walking about during sleep. The sleepwalker's eyes are wide open, but the person appears in a daze, has purposeless movements, and may speak in short phrases, with

---

12-2

Classification of sleep and arousal disorders*

Disorders of initiating and maintaining sleep (DIMS)

Psychophysiologic: transient and situational, persistent
Associated with:
 Psychiatric disorders: symptom and personality disorders, affective disorders, other functional psychoses
 Use of drugs and alcohol: tolerance to or withdrawal from central nervous system (CNS) depressants, sustained use of CNS stimulants, sustained use or withdrawal from other drugs, chronic alcoholism
 Sleep-induced respiratory impairment: sleep apnea DIMS syndrome, alveolar hypoventilation DIMS syndrome
 Sleep-related (nocturnal) myoclonus DIMS syndrome and/or "restless legs"
 Other medical, toxic, and environmental conditions
 Child-onset DIMS
 Other DIMS conditions: repeated REM interruptions, atypical polysomnographic features
 No DIMS abnormality: "short sleeper," subjective DIMS complaints without objective findings

Disorders of excessive somnolence (DOES)

Psychophysiologic: transient and situational, persistent
Associated with:
 Psychiatric disorders: symptom and personality disorders, affective disorders, other functional psychoses
 Use of drugs and alcohol: tolerance to or withdrawal from CNS stimulants, sustained use of CNS depressants
 Sleep-induced respiratory impairment: sleep apnea DOES syndrome, alveolar hypoventilation DOES syndrome
 Sleep-related (nocturnal) myoclonus DOES syndrome and/or "restless legs"

Other medical, toxic, and environmental conditions
Other DOES conditions
Intermittent DOES (periodic) syndromes: Kleine-Levin syndrome, menstrual-associated syndrome
Insufficient sleep
Sleep drunkenness
Narcolepsy
Idiopathic CNS hypersomnolence
No DOES abnormality: "short sleeper," subjective DOES complaints without objective findings

Disorders of the sleep-wake schedule

Transient: time-zone (jet lag) syndrome, work shift change in conventional sleep-wake schedule
Persistent: frequently changing sleep-wake schedule, delayed sleep phase syndrome, advanced sleep phase syndrome, non-24-hour sleep-wake syndrome, irregular sleep-wake pattern

Dysfunctions associated with sleep, sleep stages, or partial arousals—parasomnias or disorders of arousal

Sleepwalking (somnambulism)
Sleep terror (pavor nocturnus, incubus)
Sleep-related enuresis
Other dysfunctions
 Dream anxiety attacks (nightmares)
 Familial sleep paralysis
 Impaired sleep-related penile tumescence
 Sleep-related epileptic seizures, bruxism, head banging (jactatio capitis nocturna), painful erections, cluster headaches and chronic paroxysmal hemicrania, abnormal swallowing syndrome, asthma, cardiovascular symptoms, gastroesophageal reflux, hemolysis (paroxysmal nocturnal hemoglobinuria)
Asymptomatic polysomnographic findings

*Adapted from Association of Sleep Disorder Centers and the Association for the Psychophysiological Study of Sleep, the diagnostic classification of sleep and arousal disorders, *Sleep* 2(1):21, 1979.

no recollection of sleepwalking in the morning. Twenty percent of sonambulists have a sleepwalking parent, and 5% to 15% of the population has sleepwalked at some time. Sleepwalking usually occurs in the first third of the night in stage III/IV sleep. Up to one half of all sleepwalkers either experience injury or narrowly avoid it.

Lead sleepwalkers back to bed without awakening them. If the sleepwalker must be awakened, do not slap or shake the person or splash cold water on the face, but do say the person's name over and over. If the sleepwalker lies down to sleep on the floor, cover the person and let him or her stay there until awakening spontaneously.

Protect the sleepwalker from injury. Place a bell at the bedside that will ring if the bedside is moved, or use a two-way radio in a child's room to awaken the parent when the child stirs. A protective gate or screen door may be placed across the entrance to the bedroom, but note that this blocks escape if there is a fire. Lock windows and doors to balconies. Imipramine, a tricyclic antidepressant, is sometimes prescribed for adult sleepwalkers who walk frequently and have been injured.

Sleep Terror

Sleep terror (pavor nocturnus) usually occurs in children during the first part of the night in stage III/IV sleep. The child screams, arises from bed, wanders about in panic, and cannot be awakened or consoled. Autonomic changes (rapid pulse and respirations, sweating) can be noted. The child may be amnesic for the event. Sleep terror is often associated with sleepwalking.

Interventions include planning sleep on a regular schedule. Do not try to awaken the child because this may worsen the confusion. Usually the child will lie back on the pillow after several minutes, never having awakened. Benzodiazepines are sometimes given to patients with severe episodes, because they suppress stage III/IV sleep.

Familial Sleep Paralysis

The person with familial sleep paralysis appears asleep but maintains consciousness. Occasionally, frighteningly vivid hallucinations may occur. The eyes may be open and can be moved, although the person is unable to move any other muscles. Although this is part of the tetrad of symptoms of narcolepsy, many normal people experience this. Intervention includes teaching family members to awaken the person by touch each day or training a pet dog or cat to awaken the person through touch.

Penile Erections

Men experience erections during REM sleep regardless of sexual activity or dream content. If impairment of erections occurs during sleep, an underlying illness may be present, such as diabetes mellitus, or it may result from the effect of medications. *Painful erections* may occur during sleep, even though erections are not painful or difficult while awake. There may be a problem with the foreskin in uncircumcised men or a problem with the penile blood vessels. The man should be referred to a urologist for evaluation.

INSOMNIA

Etiology/Epidemiology

Insomnia is the difficulty with initiating or maintaining sleep. Epidemiologic studies estimate the number of Americans experiencing insomnia to be in the millions. Insomnia

---

Table 12-1 Parasomnias or disorders of arousal

Type of dysfunction	Comments/definitions
Sleepwalking	Walking while asleep
Sleep terror	Panic attack while asleep
Sleep-related enuresis	Bed-wetting; event begins in stage III/IV sleep, and enuresis occurs as sleep lightens
Dream anxiety attacks	Nightmares; REM phenomenon
Sleep-related epileptic seizures	Seizures occur most often during sleep; explains why sleep is encouraged during short routine electroencephalograms (EEGs)
Sleep-related bruxism	Teeth grinding; dental assistance may be needed to preserve teeth
Sleep-related head banging (jactatio capitis nocturna)	Rhythmic head rocking and banging common in young children under age 5 years; occurs in stage I/II sleep
Familial sleep paralysis	Inability to move muscles when first awakening
Sleep-related cluster headaches	Associated with REM and relieved by indomethacin
Sleep-related abnormal swallowing syndrome	Inadequate swallowing of saliva during sleep
Sleep-related asthma	Early morning increase in bronchoconstriction; 46% of asthmatic attacks occur during last third of night
Sleep-related cardiovascular symptoms	Include paroxysmal nocturnal dyspnea, myocardial infarction (peak incidence, 4 AM to 6 AM), nocturnal angina, and premature ventricular contractions (more common in REM sleep)
Sleep-related gastroesophageal reflux	Caused more by posture than sleep
Sleep-related hemolysis	Probably related to combination of respiratory acidosis, change in acid-base balance, and renal clearance of defective red blood cells
Morning headaches	May be related to sleeping longer on weekends and delaying usual morning dose of caffeine
Impairment in penile erections	Changes in normal incidence of erections; painful erections

is experienced by adults and children and affects males and females equally.

Insomnia can be caused by various factors:

1. Transient situations of emotional upset (such as loss of a job) or family needs (such as a child's illness)
2. Adoption of nonfunctional sleep habits
3. Psychiatric disorders, such as depression or psychoses
4. Use of drugs or alcohol
5. Respiratory impairment (see later section on sleep apnea)
6. Medical conditions associated with pain, anemia, fever, changes in nutritional status, or immobility
7. Attempting to sleep in nonconducive environmental conditions

It is important to remember that in many instances *persons experience altered sleep patterns* when the actual cause of the sleep changes may have been resolved long ago. For example, a woman may describe that she habitually arose at 5 AM to nurse her baby, and now several years later, she still awakens at that time and cannot go back to sleep. Another person may report persistent inability to sleep coinciding with great anxiety associated with a job loss even though the person has now been happily employed for several years.

Prevention

Prevention involves teaching persons and families about normal sleep and counseling them to be aware of events and activities that can enhance or detract from sleep. Often persons take steps to remedy a sleep problem, such as taking sleeping pills, taking naps, or drinking alcohol, *which only exacerbate sleeping problems.* Nurses must also teach persons that it *is never too late to begin dealing with a sleep problem.*

Pathophysiology

Sleep onset can be delayed and arousal prolonged by active thought and worry, physical discomfort, or poor oxygenation. Worry and poor habits, such as sleeping with lights or a TV/radio on, delay sleep onset and cause arousals during light stage I sleep. Staying in bed longer than 8 hours or napping during the day fragments sleep; the person still sleeps 8 hours, but the total sleep time lengthens to fill 10 hours spent in bed. The person then believes the sleep is "poor."

Normally there is a clear boundary between and regular timing of sleep time and awake time. Meals and social and physical activities occur at predictable times during awake hours, and sleep occurs at night in a dark, quiet, comfortable, secure place. *Biologic clocks* are anchored in time by the regular occurrence of these events. For the person with insomnia, the distinction between waking/sleeping time is blurred by spending a prolonged time in bed, by not initiating the day's activities at a prompt time, or by staying up too late at night. These events cause a distortion in sleep and lead to a continuing cycle of poor sleep at the wrong time.

Clinical Manifestations

The person may describe insomnia in many ways, depending on which aspect of sleeplessness is most troubling.

Typical comments include: "I cannot go to sleep," "I am awake all night," and "I awaken early and can't go back to sleep." Persons with insomnia often monitor sleep by watching the clock. They may turn on the TV, read, or eat while waiting to feel sleepy. They may try to go to sleep earlier, stay in bed longer, take naps, use sleeping pills or alcohol to initiate sleep, or use caffeine to increase alertness during the day. They may also change their pattern of daily activities to compensate for a distorted sleep pattern by declining or omitting activities from the daily routine, saying "I'm just too tired." Some persons may not recognize a sleep problem at first because they have adapted to a changed sleep schedule over many years.

Diagnostic tests

Routine blood work, such as a SMA 18 and complete blood count (CBC), is used to determine if any hematologic, metabolic, cardiac, or respiratory diseases are contributing to sleeplessness.

A *polysomnogram* (PSG) consists of an all-night sleep study conducted in a certified sleep laboratory. Sleep technicians monitor the following:

1. Sleep time and quality
2. Brain EEG activity to determine stages of sleep
3. Respiratory activity: intercostal muscle movement, air passage from nose and mouth, oxygen saturation using an ear lobe oxymeter
4. Electrocardiogram (ECG) for monitoring cardiac rate
5. Electromyogram (EMG) monitoring of eye and facial muscles to determine onset of REM sleep and leg muscles to determine existence of "restless legs."
6. Occurrence of nightmares.

The PSG is performed when the person complains of insomnia and the physician is unable to make the diagnosis from a history and physical examination.

The *multiple sleep latency test* (MSLT) is a sleep study that takes place in the sleep laboratory during the day to measure daytime sleepiness. At times it is needed to distinguish the sleepiness caused by poor nighttime sleep and sleepiness caused by *narcolepsy.*

Medical Management

If the person has used sleeping pills or alcohol to help with sleep, supervised weaning from these substances is required. A schedule of reducing the dose of sleeping pills over a month or more, or a course of chlordiazepoxide hydrochloride (Librium) to assist with alcohol withdrawal, may be prescribed.

Nursing Process
Assessment

A complete nursing assessment of sleep disorders is listed in Box 12-3. Never jump to a conclusion about a sleep problem without asking systematic questions about all sleep disorders, because one sleep problem can resemble another superficially. Keep in mind that many times insomnia begins as an understandable response to a stress, such as the loss of a spouse, illness of a family member, or after a difficult hospitalization. The person may come to terms with the stress or loss, but the new maladaptive sleep habits are now in place. The person may state that the sleep

Sleep interview

General data

Statement of the sleep problem by patient, bed partner, or family: obtain a quantifiable answer regarding sleep, such as never sleeps, dozes off for an hour several times a night, or has trouble sleeping five nights out of seven, every other night, or on weekends only

Initiation of sleep problem: when possible, elicit cause

Factors that make it worse or better

Previous occurrences of sleep problems in patient or other family member or friend

Modifications that needed to be made for daytime activities or travel

Occurrences of frightening or upsetting incidences during sleep, such as sudden illness or death of a loved one or damage from storm, fire, or robbery

Occurrences of accidents or "near misses" as a result of sleep problems *(very important)*

Insomnia data

(Remember that a complaint of insomnia may be caused by sleep apnea or other difficulties with sleep.)

Time person gets into bed and time person falls asleep

Number and times of awakenings at night

Interval before returning to sleep after each awakening

Time of final awakening, time of arising from bed, and what wakes the person up, such as noises, alarm clock, or treatment

Daytime naps: number, when, and how long

Dozing off briefly (same question as napping, but some persons answer this question differently)

Lying down to rest on couch or "resting eyes for a moment" (this counts as napping because person may be falling asleep)

Practices used to assist with sleep: type and regularity of use

Changes in sleep patterns because of sleep deficit

Places where sleep occurs more readily, such as somewhere else in the house or on vacation

Concerns that delay getting into bed or falling asleep

Amount of and recent changes in caffeine intake (coffee, tea, colas, other caffeinated beverages, caffeinated gum) and alcohol

Types of weekly exercise and recreational activities

Methods of coping with concerns

Recent illness or loss of relatives, friends, or pets

Activities of others in house or neighborhood that affect sleep, such as child who returns home late, spouse who leaves home early in morning, noise from a neighbor or dog, and noise from a nearby highway or airport

Sleep apnea data

Description or reenactment by bed partner of the person's breathing pattern, including sound and volume of snoring, length of time that no air passes, and how the person starts to breathe again

Description by bed partner of differences in patient's breathing while on back, each side, and stomach and of changes in patient's skin color while asleep

Presence of morning headaches

Difficulty in awakening for the day

Number of pillows used; preference for sleeping in a certain chair

Degree of sleepiness during day; falling asleep at a movie, during a conversation, or while driving

Narcolepsy-related data

Presence of sudden irresistible urges to sleep; falling asleep and then awakening a few minutes later feeling refreshed

Experiences of a sudden loss of muscle tone, leading to drooping of the head or slumping to the floor, that occur during episodes of strong emotions (surprise, laughter, anger)

Experiences on awakening of feeling paralyzed until touched by another person

Presence of visual, auditory, or tactile hallucinations at time of sleep initiation or awakening

Family history of unusual experiences in sleep

Sleep schedule data

Working hours

Experience of going to bed later each night

Daily scheduled activities, flexibility of schedule

Changes in sleep schedule as a result of changes in life schedule, such as retirement or hospitalization

Interruption of sleep because of family activities

Practice of sleeping through the day or staying up at night because of a specific purpose, such as fear that a calamity will befall during the night

Other sleep-related events

Uncomfortable feelings in legs when ready to fall asleep: location, type of sensations, duration, actions that make it better or worse, attempted remedies, and effect on sleep

Reports from bed partner of patient kicking or moving legs in sleep

Bed-wetting: frequency, time of occurrence, actions that make it better or worse, and reports of any nights of dryness

Dreams: upsetting recurring dreams, frightening nightmares, or sleep terrors

Sleepwalking: initiation, frequency, ability to be awakened easily or guided back to bed, experience of injury while sleepwalking, actions that make it better or worse, and steps taken to keep the person safe

Teeth grinding during sleep

Dysfunctions associated with sleep, such as chest pain, shortness of breath, heartburn/ulcer pain, morning headache, asthmatic attacks, frequent awakenings to urinate, hot flashes in menopausal woman, coughing, choking and gagging, and arthritic or other neuromuscular pain

pattern began 5 years ago and that nothing is bothering him or her now to prevent sleep. This makes sense when one views insomnia as a series of decisions that *perpetuate* a certain sleep pattern, unfortunately a pattern that distresses instead of refreshes. The following data are important to highlight for a person with insomnia.

Subjective data

Assess the patient for:
1. Beliefs about the sleep problems and ability to sleep restfully. Some people believe that they have inherited or developed a permanent mental change or disorder that will prevent regaining normal sleep.
2. Knowledge about normal sleep.
3. Sources of pleasure and difficulty in the person's life and how the sleep problem has been affected by these.
4. Potential resources for life changes. For example, if a retired person has nothing to wake up for, can that person find a means of transport to a senior citizens center, volunteer job, or activity group?

Objective data

Objective data include results from diagnostic tests and reports from a bed partner. A person may be asked to keep a sleep diary, recording times of sleep initiation, arousals, naps, and time of awakening in morning.

Data analysis: nursing diagnoses

Nursing diagnoses are determined from analysis of patient data. Possible nursing diagnoses for the person with insomnia may include, but are not limited to, the following:

Diagnostic title	Possible etiologies
Knowledge deficit about insomnia	Incorrect self-monitoring and self-assessment of sleep
Sleep pattern disturbance	Adoption of counterproductive sleep habits
Diversional activity deficit	Immobility, depressed feelings, perceived loss of usefulness or of need for activity
Coping, ineffective individual	Habit of seeking sleep to avoid facing problems or of reviewing problems at sleep initiation
Fatigue	Reduced total sleep time
Fear	Personal concern about impossibility of every sleeping well again
Injury, high risk for	Sleepiness during the day

Planning: expected patient outcomes

Expected patient outcomes for the person with insomnia may include, but are not limited to, the following:
1. Patient/bed partner/family describe the basic aspects of normal sleep, with emphasis on factors that contribute to the person's problem.
2. Sleep patterns improve as patient/family carry out measures to reduce the insomnia.
3. Identifies impediments to activity and develops and implements a plan for increasing diversional activity.

4. Participates in a plan to solve problems and cope with difficulties; patient does not think about problems at time of sleep.
5. Fatigue lessens as sleep improves.
6. Has realistic expectations about the quality of sleep.
7. Patient does not suffer an injury.

Implementation

Interventions to achieve patient outcomes
Promoting knowledge of normal sleep

Teach aspects of normal sleep to patient and family. Persons typically monitor their own sleep. This can contribute to the sleep problem because the person may mistake a normal phenomenon for something abnormal or for a sign that the new sleep habits are not working.

Promoting sleep hygiene

A person with insomnia will benefit most from a reordering of sleep habits so that sleep pattern disturbance improves. Develop a plan for sleep hygiene with the patient and inform the physician of the plan, as appropriate. Physician advice may be required if intake patterns of alcohol, other drugs, or caffeine need to be changed. Patients must recognize that they must adhere to the plan faithfully every day, no matter what occurs. They are resetting their sleepwake cycle, which takes several weeks to a month to accomplish. In developing the plan, choose from the elements listed here those that apply to the individual's sleep hygiene problem. Not all elements are appropriate for each person. *The plan has three important parts: (1) what the person does during the day (use of time, naps, eating and drinking, exercise, diversion), (2) what the person does to prepare for sleep, and (3) how the person interprets his or her sleep experience.*

The plan is to be followed faithfully for 1 month. If sleep is improved, adjustments can be made for one element at a time, such as resuming a reduced intake of alcohol or caffeine. Once the sleep pattern is established, however, only one element should be modified at a time. If the sleep pattern is weakened, the person can identify an element to which he or she is sensitive. Check with the person weekly to identify how the new plan is proceeding. Be generous with encouragement. Remember that a new way of sleeping is being taught to a person who is still partly convinced that he or she is one of the few persons in the world who never sleeps.

Time spent in bed, sleep, and wake-up hours

The person, in collaboration with the health professional, selects a sleep time and a wake-up time for a total time spent in bed of 7 to 8 hours, depending on how much sleep the patient thinks is needed. Ask what constraints the person has, such as time to get up for work or time arriving home from evening work, and what time the person likes to go to bed, based on time spent with family members or favorite late-night TV shows. The bed time and wake-up time should be followed faithfully, without alteration, for 1 month, so planning ahead for life-style preferences is important. This means the person will follow this schedule even if he or she is out late on Saturday nights or wants to sleep in on Sunday mornings. If the person does not sleep well one night, the schedule must be kept because it is an investment in a better night's sleep the next night.

As sleeping improves, fatigue also improves and the patient is less fearful about not obtaining a good night's sleep. Because the patient is less drowsy during the day the risk of injury is reduced.

Napping

No naps should be taken. This means not lying down during the day and not closing the eyes while sitting in the chair after dinner. If the person gets sleepy reading the paper, the paper should be read while standing up at the counter. If the person is tired an hour before the agreed-on sleep time, he or she should walk around, engage in an activity, or stand up while watching TV. This gives the body a firm message that all sleep will take place in bed during the nighttime hours only. Taking naps at other times fragments nighttime sleep. If, in following the schedule, the person does not sleep much the night before, taking a nap only hinders the possibility that sleep will come more easily the next night, which perpetuates the problem.

Caffeine and alcohol

The best and fastest change in sleep quality comes from the elimination of caffeine and alcohol from the diet during the start of this plan. However, persons who drink a lot of caffeine or even one alcoholic drink each day could experience withdrawal symptoms, so it is best to work with the physician on a safe plan for withdrawal. Also, the strength of this plan is to help the person experience improved sleep without experiencing uncomfortable symptoms that might lead the person to resume the previous, more comfortable patterns.

Nutrition

It is important to eat three meals a day comprised of balanced nutrition at about the same time each day. On awakening in the morning, the person should wash, dress, and have some breakfast to give the body yet another message that it is time for the day to start. Breakfast may be large or simply toast and juice; the point is to give a regular nutritional time cue.

Exercise

Increasing activity gives the body another biologic message that the day is here. Even if the person is confined to bed, exercises can be developed to enhance a feeling of well-being. For persons who experience tension, stress, or worry or who face difficult problems, exercise can bring a respite from troubling thoughts or can be time for thinking through problems instead of at bedtime. Any exercise, from active sports to walking to stationary exercise, is encouraged.

Diversion

It is important for the person to do something each day that brings enjoyment. It is equally important to have both something in life a person can look forward to and something that requires a person's special participation, a feeling of being needed. A person facing a continuing illness often experiences a curtailing of usual outlets for diversion and participation. Remember that what a person does with time during the day influences sleep time as well. An important part of a plan for better sleep is life-participating activity. Even if the person is confined to bed, a telephone is a link with others who could use the person's support and good will.

Sleep environment

Evening routines, such as checking door locks or letting the dog out, should be completed before the predetermined bedtime. By bedtime the person should be in night clothes and ready to get into bed. The bed covers should provide the proper comfort. Lights, TV, and radio should be off. The person should not read or eat in bed. Persons can be advised to turn the clock around so it cannot be checked during the night. The person needs to understand that awakening during the night is normal and sleep activity does not need to be monitored.

Relaxation

The final component of a sleep plan is the relearning of skills of relaxing when the person wants to go to sleep. A person can easily adopt the habit of postponing thoughts about troubling issues until in bed with the lights off. This is a habit and can be replaced by a more useful habit. A person cannot lie in bed "thinking about nothing" because the mind simply searches for something interesting to think about and usually selects some unfinished, compelling issues. Relaxation exercises can help persons regain and strengthen the ability to select something enjoyable to think about. If the person consciously selects something pleasant, the tendency to ruminate over troubles is weakened. Relaxation exercises must be practiced each night. If the person has difficulty mastering this task, referral to a behavioral therapist may be appropriate.

Promoting realistic expectations of sleep

Reinforce that it is not realistic for the person to expect every night of sleep to be free of awakenings or disturbing thoughts and to be totally refreshing. The goal of the plan is to increase the number of nights that are restful. If sleep patterns unravel sometime in the future, the person now has the tools to get back on track.

Evaluation

Questions to be asked about the patient with insomnia include the following:

1. Can the patient/bed partner/family describe the basic aspects of normal sleep and the factors that contribute to patient's sleep problem?
2. Is the patient carrying out the measures designed to reduce insomnia?
3. Is the patient planning for diversional activities in his or her daily or weekly schedule?
4. Is the patient following the plan developed to assist with problem solving and coping?
5. Does the patient state that fatigue is lessened?
6. Does the patient express realistic expectations about the quality of sleep?
7. Has the patient been free of injury?

NARCOLEPSY

Narcolepsy is a neurologic condition characterized by short, irresistible episodes of sleep intruding into wakefulness and recurring at frequent intervals. *Five abnormal sleep features* may be present: (1) *irresistible sleep attacks with excessive daytime sleepiness,* (2) *hypnogogic hallucinations,* (3) *cataplexy,* (4) *sleep-onset REM periods,* and (5) *sleep paralysis.* Any combination of the five features can be seen in narcolepsy, but at least two must be present to make a diagnosis.

Epidemiology

Narcolepsy is not a rare condition. Its prevalence has been estimated at 0.05% to 0.06%, which indicates that about one of every 2500 people have this disorder. Males are somewhat more affected than females. The age of onset varies from childhood to the 50s, with a peak incidence in the second decade of life, usually after puberty. Unrecognized and untreated, these irresistible, unwanted sleep attacks can be totally disabling. They interfere with the concentration required in school or at work and can result in accidents, leading to injury and death.

Etiology

Two new research findings are fueling greater understanding of narcolepsy. First, several researchers have found a genetic link among persons with narcolepsy in which mild forms tend to cluster in some families, whereas more severe forms cluster in other families.[5] Some aspects of narcolepsy (cataplexy, excessive daytime sleepiness) are genetically transmitted in some breeds of dogs. Second, a genetic link has recently been discovered between narcolepsy and a class II antigen of the major histocompatibility complex known as DR2. Scientists theorize that narcolepsy may be a disease that links the involvement of the immune system and its response to severe psychologic stress with the development of disease in susceptible individuals.[5] This may help to explain the finding that in about one half of persons with narcolepsy, an abrupt change in the sleep/wake schedule and/or a major psychologic stress precede the first symptom.

Prevention

As yet, no clear evidence exists concerning the prevention of narcolepsy. More effort is being directed toward the early recognition of the disorder, particularly in relatives of affected family members. If a parent has narcolepsy, there is a 1 in 50 chance that each child will have it.

Characteristics of the Episodes

Occasionally a person with normal sleep patterns may experience any one aspect of narcolepsy. The combination of symptoms, however, experienced consistently, sets narcolepsy apart.

Irresistible sleep attacks and excessive daytime sleepiness

The sleep attacks, unpredictable and lasting a few moments to an hour, occur not only during monotonous sed-entary activity, but also during mental or physical stimulation. The person may also feel unpleasantly drowsy throughout the day, resulting in poor performance of tasks.

Sleep-onset REM periods

The normal sleeper passes through several stages of sleep and experiences REM sleep near the end of the 90-minute sleep cycle. In narcolepsy, when sleep occurs during the day in naps or during sleep attacks, the person goes into REM sleep within 5 minutes of going to sleep.

Cataplexy

Cataplexy is an abrupt, reversible loss of muscle tone usually brought on by strong emotions such as fright, laughter, anger, or sudden increased stress. Cataplexy can be experienced variously from a feeling of slight weakness to a loss of strength in skeletal muscles to a complete loss of posture. Typically, the jaw sags, the head nods, the arms droop, and the legs buckle. Because attacks can be precipitated by listening to a funny joke or reexperiencing in memory a strongly unpleasant experience, persons suffering from cataplexy often try to restrict their emotional responses to gain some control. *This atonia is similar to the atonia seen during REM sleep.*

Hypnogogic hallucinations

This is the experience of vivid, troubling hallucinations, usually on awakening. The hypnogogic hallucinations are usually visual but can be auditory or tactile.

Sleep paralysis

This frightening experience occurs just before falling asleep or on awakening. Sleepers find that, although they are completely awake, they cannot move the extremities, cannot speak, and may not even be able to breathe deeply. Sleep paralysis terminates spontaneously within several minutes but can be interrupted by being touched by someone. (One person who was plagued by sleep paralysis trained her dog to come and lick her hand each morning.) Often sleep paralysis is accompanied by hypnogogic hallucinations.

Pathophysiology
Loss of ability to suppress sleep

Normally the thalamus and cortical gray matter are highly active in wakefulness, resulting in general enhanced excitability of neurons as well as selective inhibition of input. In drowsiness, reduction of synaptic transmissions occurs in the thalamus, despite an unchanged level of sensory input. It is unknown exactly what neurotransmitters and synaptic receptors relate to maintenance of alertness and initiation of sleep. Interestingly, the activity of the gray matter and thalamus in REM sleep closely resembles waking activity.

It is also unknown what neuronal changes occur with narcolepsy. Because this condition responds to stimulant drugs such as amphetamine, pemoline, and methylphenidate, however, it is hypothesized that some ratio of adrenergic/cholinergic neuronal activity is disrupted in sleep attacks and restored by these drugs.

Episodic atonia

Normally, muscle tone is maintained during wakefulness and during all sleep stages *except REM* by activity in the cerebellum. In REM sleep, centers in the pons activate, producing active inhibition of muscle tone in all muscle groups except those of the eye, respiration, and penis. Usually this atonia is briefly interrupted or overcome by powerful excitatory inputs to muscle groups, resulting in the muscle twitches and jerks seen in REM sleep.

In cataplexy, sudden time-limited atonia is experienced, although no change occurs in consciousness. *Because this disorder responds to monoamine oxidase (MAO) inhibitors and other tricyclic antidepressants, it is theorized that cataplectic attacks* (as well as sleep paralysis and hypnogogic hallucinations) *result from some malfunction of norepinephrine, dopamine, and serotonin neurotransmitters or receptors in the brainstem.*

Aspects of dreaming intruding into wakefulness

Dreaming usually occurs in REM sleep. REM sleep occurs at the end of each 90-minute sleep cycle, and longer periods of REM sleep occur at the end of the night. On awakening, all features of REM sleep (atonia and resulting paralysis of all muscle groups except those for breathing and sight; dreaming) terminate. Less is known about the mechanisms of dreaming intruding into wakefulness. As just noted, however, because the person with narcolepsy responds to tricyclic antidepressants and MAO inhibitors, a disorder of neurotransmitters or receptors may exist somewhere in the brain.

Clinical Manifestations

The person with narcolepsy feels chronically drowsy, exhibits memory lapses and poor work performance, and may experience microsleeps, sleep periods of a few seconds that may appear as daydreaming. Night sleep can be frequently interrupted by frightening dreams and awakenings. Cataplexy may develop as long as 20 years after the more common symptom of sleep attacks and excessive daytime drowsiness. The paralysis may last from a few seconds to a few minutes. No known measures can terminate an attack, except to remove the emotional trigger so that another attack will not immediately follow recovery from the first.

Diagnostic tests

The PSG and MSLT (see p. 232) are the essential tests to distinguish narcolepsy from daytime sleepiness experienced by someone who simply sleeps poorly at night. The night sleep test (PSG) documents the night aspects of sleep. The MSLT, performed the following day, documents how readily the person falls asleep during a half-hour nap (four naps are observed during the next 8 hours after awakening from the PSG) and how quickly REM sleep occurs with each nap. A *normal* person may have one sleep-onset REM episode out of four naps and may not be able to fall asleep for all the nap periods. A *sleepy* person may be able to fall asleep each time but does not have more than one sleep-onset REM period. A *narcoleptic* person falls asleep readily during each nap period and has more than one sleep-onset REM period. The physician may try to record a cataplectic

attack if the patient reports a history of this with particular stressors.

Medical Management

The person who has sleep attacks and excessive daytime sleepiness is given CNS stimulants such as amphetamine, pemoline (Cylert), or methylphenidate (Ritalin). Some side effects, such as irritability, tachycardia, and nocturnal sleep disturbances, as well as tolerance and drug dependence, may occur. Persons experiencing cataplexy, sleep paralysis, or hypnogogic hallucinations receive a tricyclic antidepressant. Doses are usually adjusted to achieve the best balance between improved daytime alertness and unwanted side effects. An experimental drug, gamma-hydroxybutyrate, shows some promise.

Daytime naps may also be prescribed to assist with daytime alertness. Three 15- to 20-minute naps spaced evenly throughout the day often help restore a feeling of alertness.

Nursing Process
Assessment

A complete sleep history (see p. 232) is obtained from the person suspected of having narcolepsy. Data of particular importance include the following:

1. Understanding of narcolepsy and factors that increase or decrease symptoms
2. Experience with antinarcoleptic drugs and side effects (Are the drugs taken on holidays? Are doses self-adjusted?)
3. Safety practices and accident history, especially if the person drives
4. Family understanding and support
5. Problems and adjustments in employment or school performance

Data analysis: nursing diagnoses

Nursing diagnoses are determined from analysis of patient data. Possible nursing diagnoses for the person with narcolepsy may include, but are not limited to, the following:

Diagnostic title	Possible etiologies
Knowledge deficit about narcolepsy	Lack of information
Fatigue	Excessive daytime sleepiness
	Difficulty with treatment regimen, misunderstanding by family and employer or teacher
Injury, high risk for	Sleep attacks, cataplexy
Coping, ineffective individual	Purposeful emotional restriction and day-to-day difficulties

Planning: expected patient outcomes

Expected patient outcomes for the person with narcolepsy may include, but are not limited to, the following:

1. Describes the disorder and medication regimen and reports success with explaining narcolepsy to family or employer (or enlists the assistance of a person knowledgeable about narcolepsy).
2. Reports feeling less fatigue.
3. Reports improved job or school performance.
4. Demonstrates effective strategies for reducing ex-

posure to risk factors in the environment; avoidable accidents and injuries do not occur.

5. Describes a level of participation that satisfies family and work responsibilities.
6. Identifies purposeful avoidance of strong emotions to cope with cataleptic attacks.

Implementation

Interventions to achieve patient outcomes
Promoting understanding of narcolepsy

The major nursing strategies for the person with narcolepsy are teaching and support with effective ways of coping with the disorder. As control of sleepiness and cataleptic attacks is achieved, fatigue and job or school performance should improve and the potential for injury will decrease.

Teach aspects of narcolepsy and rationale for the treatment plan. It is important that the person maintain close contact with the physician and nurse to monitor effectiveness of medications and treatment. Telephone follow-up may be used to maintain contact and support. Encourage the person and family to contact the American Narcolepsy Association,* which can provide information on local support networks. The association's newsletter contains up-to-date information on recent research findings and provides a forum for sharing ideas.

Assess and support the person's efforts to teach others about narcolepsy. Remind the person that it may take some practice before he or she is at ease in teaching others.

Promoting safety and personal risk assessment

Teach the patient to consider carefully the risks of injury at home and at school or work. Rather than engage in denial or wishful thinking, the patient should consider problems caused by sleep attacks and cataleptic attacks. Some suggestions include the following:

1. Do not drive unless sleep attacks and cataleptic attacks are completely under control; avoid long-distance driving.
2. Do food preparation or self-grooming activities (handling knives, curling, or clothes iron; cooking on stove) during quiet times (such as before others in the house awaken) to avoid times of surprise or emotion that can trigger an attack.
3. Learn to use the microwave oven for cooking to avoid burns from the stove.
4. If possible, live in a dwelling that has either no stairs or an enclosed staircase to minimize injury during falls.
5. Ask family members/co-workers to use a gentle aural signal before approaching to prevent triggering a sleep attack.

Promoting participation in family life and work

Encourage the person to meet with other persons with narcolepsy for mutual support or with the nurse in times

of frustration as well as success. Suggest that family members join a local narcolepsy support group to help deal with their own concerns. Narcolepsy can be a very difficult disorder to live with, but personal isolation and withdrawal will only make life more difficult.

Evaluation

Questions to be asked about the patient with narcolepsy include the following:

1. Is the patient able to describe the disorder and medication regimen and can he or she explain narcolepsy to others?
2. Does the patient report less fatigue?
3. Does the patient report that work or school performance is improved?
4. Has the patient demonstrated strategies that are effective in reducing risk factors and in helping avoid accidents and injuries?
5. Is the patient able to participate in family and work responsibilities?
6. Has the patient been able to avoid strong emotions to cope with epileptic attacks?

SLEEP APNEA

Sleep apnea is a sleep problem involving other body systems. A mutual relationship exists between sleep and other body systems; the sleep state affects the functioning of all body systems to some extent. In addition, the functioning of any body system affects the states of sleep. Many disease processes affect sleep or are affected by sleep, including asthma, gastroesophageal reflux, epilepsy, headache, fibrositis, myocardial instability, and chronic pain. This section focuses on sleep apnea and the mutual relationship between body systems and sleep.

Etiology

The gradual development of sleep apnea and its sequelae is not completely understood. Although such factors as obesity and oropharyngeal architecture have been associated with this disorder, other neurologic and genetic factors may play a role even before any symptoms develop. Some researchers hypothesize that sleep apnea is a progressive illness resulting as a systemic response to years of decreased airway patency, reduced airflow, reduced ventilation,[5] and disruption of reflexes required to maintain breathing during sleep. This produces a maladaptive response that results in a feedback loop of greater impairment.

Many unanswered questions remain concerning sleep apnea, including the following:

1. How much time does it take for sleep apnea syndrome to develop or for cardiac rhythm changes and hypertension to become severe?
2. How many sleepers who snore quietly and sporadically early in life will subsequently develop sleep apnea?
3. How can one predict who will develop milder or more severe forms of sleep apnea?
4. What role does normal aging play in sleep and breathing?

*425 California St., Suite 201, San Francisco, CA 94104

Prevention

Because sleep apnea is not yet fully understood, steps to prevent its development are not completely known. In addition to encouraging normal weight and good pulmonary habits, it is advisable not to overlook or discount any reported symptoms of sleep apnea.

Pathophysiology

While reading the following discussion of normal and abnormal breathing during sleep, remember the following major points:

1. The understanding of breathing during sleep centers on the complex interrelationships and feedback loops between the neurologic and respiratory systems. These interrelationships have significant impact on the cardiovascular system and on sleep itself.
2. The two primary results of severely impaired breathing during sleep are (a) cardiac dysrhythmia, which can result in increased risk of cardiac fibrillation and death, and (b) excessive daytime sleepiness or reduction of daytime alertness, which can result in increased risk of accident, such as falling asleep while driving.

Control of breathing

Breathing is initiated by the respiratory center in the medulla. Breathing responds to body requirements through input from three sources: chemoreceptors in the carotid body, stretch/mechanical receptors located in the lung and chest wall, and input from other brain centers (see Chapter 24). In wakefulness, breathing is modified by conscious effort. *In sleep, breathing patterns show clear differences between stage I, deeper, and REM (dreaming) sleep, indicating that brain centers controlling sleep have a direct impact on breathing centers as well.* In persons with sleep apnea, chemoreceptor responsiveness is reduced, possibly as a result of years of decreased oxygen saturation and increased carbon dioxide levels during sleep. It is not known if ventilatory compensation for resistive loading (stretch receptor responsiveness) is maintained in sleep. During sleep apnea, when many arousals occur in the night, the person becomes sleepier, leading to decreased arousability and longer apneas.

Open passageway to lungs

The pharynx is the only nonrigid structure in the passageway to the lungs. Its diameter is maintained by toned muscle in pharyngeal walls, allowing for closure only during swallowing, regurgitation, and speech. In non-REM sleep, this muscle tone is reduced; in REM sleep, it is greatly reduced. Only intercostal, diaphragmatic, and ocular muscles maintain tone in REM sleep. Some sleep experts theorize that the evidence of diminished upper airway tone with maintenance of diaphragmatic and intercostal muscle tone suggests separate neural control of these respiratory muscle groups.[5] The oropharynx of persons with sleep apnea may be anatomically small or may contain enlarged structures, or it may once have been large enough but now has a reduced diameter because of fat deposition in tissues.

Response to internal/external stimuli

Breathing also depends on responsiveness to changed internal and external stimuli. In sleep, responsiveness to the following factors is reduced:

1. *Bronchial irritation.* Cough is reduced in REM and non-REM sleep and resumes only on arousal.
2. *Isocapnic hypoxia.* Partial oxygen pressure (Po_2) may fall as low as 70% of normal before sleepers are aroused. In REM sleep, arousal threshold is further reduced.
3. *Hypercapnia.* Most sleepers awaken before partial carbon dioxide pressure (Pco_2) rises by 15 mm Hg above wakefulness level. In REM sleep, arousal is further reduced.
4. *Alcohol and CNS depressants.* During sleep, these substances suppress upper airway tone as well as arousal by medulla and higher cortical centers.

Responsiveness to all these factors is depressed further in a person whose sleep has been so fragmented as to lead to further depressed arousal thresholds. *Moderate degrees of alcohol intoxication can decrease hypoxic and hypercapnic ventilatory responses to 50% of baseline values. Oxygen saturation less than 80% of normal is considered severe.*

Apneas/hypopneas

Different types of apneas occur (see Box 12-4 for definitions). Normal sleepers experience a few apneas/hypopneas each night; *the apneas may be obstructive, central, or*

12-4	Definitions of apnea/hypopnea	
	Apnea	Cessation of breathing for more than 10 seconds.
	Hypopnea	Reduction, rather than complete cessation, of breathing.
	Obstructive apnea	Breathing effort occurs with diaphragmatic and intercostal muscles, but no air passes through the mouth and nose. The pharynx collapses, producing obstruction.
	Central apnea	No breathing effort is expended by thoracic muscles (message to breathe not received by lungs from medulla).
	Mixed apnea	Begins as an absence of respiratory effort; when effort begins, however, obstruction results.
	Sleep apnea syndrome	More than five apneic events per hour of sleep.

mixed. These apneas are fewer and shorter in duration than those in sleep apnea syndrome. The normal sleeper has a transient drop in oxygen saturation, transient bradycardia or tachycardia, and a transient rise in blood pressure; all return to normal levels when the apnea episode is over. *The person with sleep apnea syndrome has decreased oxygen saturation (less than 80%) through the night that results in (1) maladaptive cardiovascular responses, (2) disrupted sleep, and (3) other difficulties, including morning headache, bed-wetting, and changes in mood, alertness, endurance, work performance, and intellectual and sexual functioning.* The most serious life-threatening results are hypertension, cardiac dysrhythmias (bradycardia, tachycardia, premature ventricular contractions, second-degree atrioventricular block, prolonged sinus pauses, atrial fibrillation), and accidents from falling asleep while driving or doing other monotonous tasks.

Clinical Manifestations

When sleep apnea is suspected, a sleeping partner is interviewed as well as the sleeper. The bed partner may report most or all of the following details:

> He falls asleep very easily in the chair or when he goes to bed for the night. Sometimes he is restless and dozes on and off for a while. He may begin snoring as soon as he falls asleep, or it may not start until later in the night. He used to snore only when he fell asleep on his back, but now he snores in any position. He snores very loudly, and you can hear him from other rooms in the house. Sometimes he stops breathing; after several moments, he snores loudly, shudders or kicks his legs, then takes a deep breath and goes back to sleep. He may answer me if I speak to him, but he doesn't recall it in the morning. He does this all night long, but I think it happens more often in the early morning. He may get up frequently to urinate in the night, and sometimes he perspires heavily from all the moving around in bed. I hate to admit it, but sometimes I have to sleep in another room because the noise and his restlessness keep me awake. Yet, I am worried that he needs me there to wake him up if he goes too long without breathing. I think I am developing a sleep problem.

Diagnostic tests

The PSG (see p. 232) is the primary test. It should be performed at night because apneic episodes may be more frequent during REM sleep, and a sleeper may not have any REM sleep during afternoon naps. The test may be repeated after the patient undergoes treatment for sleep apnea to determine the degree of response.

Almost routinely the patient is sent for a consulting examination with an otolaryngologist or maxillofacial specialist to determine the extent to which oropharyngeal architecture impacts on the obstructed airway. Pulmonary function tests may also be ordered to detect any underlying contributing factors. The physician may request that much of the pulmonary testing be performed with the patient in a supine position.

Medical Management

Medical management of the person with sleep apnea takes a graded approach to match the severity of the problem. *For mild sleep apnea syndrome, the patient is advised to sleep on a side and to lose weight if obese. In addition, the patient should avoid all sleeping medication, CNS depressants, and alcohol.* If these approaches do not provide improvement, drug therapy may be instituted. Medroxyprogesterone may be prescribed for those who also hypoventilate while awake. A trial of protriptyline is initiated for obese persons. Patients need to be followed closely because the side effects of the drugs may work against the patient taking them faithfully.

For moderate sleep apnea syndrome, an oral surgeon or ear, nose, and throat (ENT) specialist may suggest removal of tonsils or realignment of the bite, either through jaw surgery or use of an appliance during sleep, if specific upper airway obstruction is found. In the absence of obstruction, a nasal *continuous positive airway pressure* (CPAP) system may be recommended. A CPAP system consists of an air pump connected to a mask worn over the nose during sleep. *This air pump (to which supplemental oxygen may be added) delivers air to the oropharynx at a pressure sufficient to prevent collapse of the pharynx during sleep.* For the first several nights, the CPAP system is worn while the patient sleeps in the laboratory, where sleep technicians adjust the air pressure in the mask to the amount required. When the CPAP system reduces apneic events, the sleeper will experience deeper and longer periods of sleep for the next several nights; arousal to breathe is unnecessary. Because increased REM sleep also means increased time during which the sleeper does not arouse as easily, the person needs to be observed for any difficulties. Wearing the mask takes some personal adjustment; however, most patients experience quick relief from their problems of daytime sleepiness and nighttime symptoms.

When a patient demonstrates pronounced oxygen desaturation or frequent cardiac dysrhythmias (severe sleep apnea syndrome), more extreme therapy is recommended. A *uvulopalatopharyngoplasty* (UPPP) may be performed by an ENT surgeon experienced with the treatment of sleep apnea patients. This procedure removes almost all the soft tissue at the back of the mouth to widen the pharynx. The patient must be cautioned, however, that in some people snoring will disappear but apnea can still be present. In addition, during the first 3 days postoperatively, regional edema can occlude the airway. A tracheostomy may be required to prevent sudden death and a tracheostomy set is kept at the bedside. It may take a week to 10 days for the patient to swallow comfortably again. Special attention must be given to the obese person so that the airway will not occlude with supine sleeping postures.[6]

Nursing Process
Assessment
Subjective data

The following subjective data should be collected:
1. The patient's and family's understanding of the cause of the sleep apnea and the possible risks to health and life
2. Understanding of how the cardiac and respiratory systems work
3. Awareness of how excess weight and alcohol intake contribute to sleep apnea
4. Sleep history, including use of sleeping pills; use of stimulants; and work, hobby, and accident history
5. Understanding of possible courses of action

6. Assessment of any emotional, social, or economic factors that may contribute to reluctance of patient and family to take part in treatment

Objective data

The following data should be assessed:

1. Blood pressure, respiratory assessment (including breath sounds, chest movement, presence of any thoracic deformities), degree of obesity, oropharyngeal assessment, level of awareness, skin color
2. Results of CBC, pulmonary, cardiac, and sleep studies
3. Presence of any other health problems

Data analysis: nursing diagnoses

Nursing diagnoses are determined from analysis of patient data. Possible nursing diagnoses for the person with sleep apnea include, but are not limited to, the following:

Diagnostic title	Possible etiologies
Breathing pattern, ineffective	Airway obstruction or episodic loss of neurologic stimulus to breathe at night
Fatigue	Altered sleep pattern; oxygen desaturation and frequent arousals at night
Injury, high risk for	Increased daytime sleepiness, fatigue, reduced vigilance and response time
Knowledge deficit about sleep problem	Lack of information

Planning: expected patient outcomes

Expected patient outcomes for the person with sleep apnea may include, but are not limited to, the following:

1. Breathes easily at night.
2. Injuries do not occur as a result of daytime sleepiness, fatigue, or decreased awareness.
3. Patient/bed partner/family can describe the effects of sleep apnea.
4. Patient/family carry out a plan to remedy sleep apnea and will describe measures to take if sleep apnea does not respond to treatment.

Implementation

Interventions to achieve patient outcomes
Facilitating learning

Nursing intervention consists primarily of patient/family teaching, counseling, and support. As sleep apnea decreases with treatment, the breathing pattern improves and fatigue and potential for injuries are decreased.

It is important that both patient and bed partner/family understand normal breathing in sleep, the effects of sleep apnea, measures to take to prevent injury, and treatment regimen. Teaching includes the following:

1. Relationship between the pulmonary and cardiac systems
2. How sleep affects breathing
3. How uninterrupted sleep contributes to daytime functioning
4. How sleep apnea contributes to cardiac problems and leads to increased accident risk

5. Restrictions on operating machinery, including appliances and equipment at home, until risk of fatigue-related accident subsides
6. Drug therapy regimen, side effects, expected time to determine efficacy, and who to contact if difficulties occur

The nurse may anticipate that the patient or someone in the family may minimize the seriousness of sleep apnea and may not be totally supportive of the means required to respond to the problem. It takes teaching and support to help a family come to the understanding that "plain old snoring" can indicate a serious health problem. In some sleep laboratories the sleeper is videotaped throughout a night (with consent). If patients or family members doubt the seriousness of the problem, it can be instructive to let them see parts of the tape or sleep record to illustrate how long breathing does not occur or how often during the night the sleeper arouses.

In addition, a patient should be advised about the consequences of skipping a night of CPAP use. The patient may feel no ill effects and may be inclined to skip using it on succeeding nights. Sleep apnea symptoms will take several weeks to return, but they will. CPAP should not be discontinued except under direction of the physician.

Promoting effective team response

Successful treatment involves members of separate disciplines providing several modalities of therapy. A satisfactory therapeutic response from the family's point of view often hinges on one team member, such as the nurse, being willing to handle questions and concerns from family and other team members.

Obese patients need to lose weight. Successful participation in weight loss programs requires knowledgeable referral and supportive follow-up by a member of the treatment team. Surgical treatment requires input from many specialists, and patients and families benefit from someone who can handle questions and respond to concerns. A patient placed on CPAP will need information for the insurance company, as well as a 24-hour telephone number to call should problems with equipment occur in the middle of the night.

Evaluation

Questions to be asked about the patient with sleep apnea include the following:

1. Does the patient breathe more easily at night?
2. Is the patient free of injuries?
3. Can the patient/bed partner/family describe the effects of sleep apnea?
4. Has the patient been successful in carrying out a plan to remedy sleep apnea?
5. Can the patient state what to do if sleep apnea doesn't respond to treatment?

CLINICAL CHRONOBIOLOGY: THE DEVELOPMENT OF A NEW AREA OF SCIENCE

The study of normal sleep and sleep problems falls within the broader area of inquiry known as *chronobiology*, or the study of biologic activities as they vary or oscillate pre-

12-5

Nursing Research

Clapin-French E: Sleep patterns of aged persons in long-term care facilities, *J Adv Nurs* 11:57-66, 1986

In this study, 102 elderly residents of three long-term care facilities were interviewed to determine their current sleep patterns and problems and how they compared their current and preadmission patterns. In addition, the researchers compared this information with the quantity and quality of assessments documented by nursing staff at the three facilities. Residents reported that since their admission sleep was disturbed more by every factor except traffic noise. Many reported more napping, increased total sleep time, earlier bedtimes, and greater difficulty falling asleep. All these factors implied decreased satisfaction with sleep and were conceivably an explanation for increased sedative use after admission. The author cites the downward spiral of decreasing daytime alertness and vigor caused by patient's slower metabolism, a result of taking sedatives and hypnotics. This led to less active participation in daily activities and further sleep problems. Nursing assessment of sleep problems by all three staff groups was uneven. This study is a step toward a needed longitudinal study to determine what the nursing staff of a long-term facility can do to improve the sleep, rest, and daytime well-being of its residents.

dictably over time. Sleep is only one of many biologic events that occur at the same time every 24 hours. Other events that have predictable cyclic peaks and troughs every 24 hours include the following:

1. Core body temperature
2. Cell division
3. Production of red blood cells
4. Preferential migration of lymphocytes into spleen from the peripheral circulation
5. Production of hormones, such as cortisol and growth hormone
6. Muscle strength and alertness
7. Mental alertness[15]

Even more interestingly, some of these events are apparently controlled by the action of internal pacemakers that are somewhat insulated from the activity of the environment, whereas other biologic rhythms depend much more on and are driven by environmental cues. For example, some biologic events depend on the person turning out the lights and lapsing into sleep before they begin. Another compelling finding is that under circumstances of environmental change, such as changing time zones during airplane travel, working the night shift, or postponing sleep, some biologic rhythms are affected more than others and some take longer to readjust. Therefore, not only does an individual rhythm lose its pattern transiently, but all rhythms that act on this one rhythm can also become asynchronous.

These findings are pertinent at the clinical level because the biologic rhythms of both patients and caregivers are affected by the patient's hospitalization. Regarding the patient, the follow-

ing is only a partial list of factors at work when someone is hospitalized:

1. Pain, fatigue, uncertainty, and anxiety
2. Different bed and bedclothes in an unusual sleeping environment
3. Being awakened for procedures, monitoring of vital signs, or medications
4. Reduced opportunity for exercise
5. Nutrient timing changes or food withheld
6. Medications depressing or accelerating different biologic functions
7. Lights being turned on or off during the sleep time
8. Living in an environmental temperature (too hot or too cold) that is not under patient control

It is not yet known to what degree, if any, a change in environmental conditions affects healing, recovery time, feelings of well-being, or response to treatment. All these environmental factors and more are being studied as they impact sleep, response to treatment, and recovery time. What is most exciting for nursing research is that nurses make clinical decisions about many of these factors (see Box 12-5). Nursing research in the future will contribute to the determination of optimal timing for assessments and treatments and the creation of the chronobiologically most synchronous or most supportive environments for the patient.

Nurses must also remember that their own biologic rhythms are also responding to the environment. Ongoing research helps to determine optimal designs for shift hours and any effects on health or performance during the day, evening, or night shifts.[2,3]

Florence Nightingale is often pictured with a lamp as she watches over wounded and sick soldiers through the night. No more apt picture could illustrate the growing body of knowledge concerning the interrelationships among biologic rhythms, especially sleep, as they are challenged in illness, modified because of professional commitment, and highlighted by new nursing contributions to this developing research area.

SUMMARY

1. More than a half million adults have difficulty with sleeping at some time in their lives.
2. Sleep disorders can be categorized by the type of disruption they cause including the following:
   Parasomnia—disorders of arousal
   Insomnia—inability to initiate or maintain sleep
   Narcolepsy—sleep intrusion into wakefulness that can challenge the pattern of daily living
   Sleep apnea—sleep problems that involve other body systems and can be life-threatening
3. Persons with insomnia must be taught not to take naps, sleeping pills, caffeine, or alcohol because these may exacerbate insomnia.
4. Nurses need to understand the importance of a sleep schedule in treating sleep disorders.
5. Problems of initiating or maintaining sleep may continue over many years, even when the precipitating factor has been resolved.
6. Helping a patient master a problem with insomnia requires education about normal sleep and careful initi-

ation of new sleep practices.

7. Loud snoring and breathing disturbances in sleep are symptoms of sleep apnea.

STUDY QUESTIONS

- Taking into consideration the 90-minute sleep cycle, how could you best time the waking of a patient at night to take his or her vital signs?
- If a man with newly diagnosed sleep attacks caused by narcolepsy calls and states that his medication is not helping at all, what factors would you consider as you assess the situation?
- What might you expect as you assess a 70-year-old man whose spouse of 45 years has just mentioned that his snoring is a little louder than before, "but it's probably nothing"?
- What steps would you take to coordinate the care of a person having severe obstructive sleep apnea?

REFERENCES AND SELECTED READINGS

1.* Clapin-French E.: Sleep patterns of aged persons in long-term care facilities, *J Adv Nurs* 11:57-66, 1986.
2.* Czeisler CA et al: Exposure to bright light and darkness to treat physiologic maladaptation to night work, *N Eng J Med* 322:18, 253-259, 1990.
3.* Ferber R: *Solve your child's sleep problems*, New York. 1985, Simon and Schuster.

*Recommended for student reading.

4. Guilleminault E, editor: *Sleep and its disorders in children*, New York, 1987, Raven Press.
5. Kryger MH, Roth R, Dement WB: *Principles and practice of sleep medicine*, Philadelphia, 1989, WB Saunders.
6. Kuna ST, Sant'Ambrogio G: Pathophysiology of upper airway closure during sleep, *JAMA* 266(10)1384-1389, 1991.
7.* Metzler DJ, Finesilver CA: When to worry if your patient can't sleep, *RN* 53(3):52-57, 1990.
8.* Miles A, Philbrick DRS, Thompson C, editors: *Melatonin: clinical perspectives*, Oxford, 1988, Oxford University Press.
9. Parkes JD: *Sleep and its disorders*, London, 1985, WB Saunders Co.
10. Rogers AE, Rosenberg RS: Tests of memory in narcoleptics, *Sleep* 13(1):42-52, 1990.

Classic

11.* American Medical Association: *Straight talk no-nonsense guide to better sleep*, New York, 1984, Random House.
12.* Czeisler CA, Moore-Ede MC, Coleman RM: Rotating shift work cycles that disrupt sleep are improved by applying circadian principles, *Science* 217:460-463, 1982.
13. Guilleminault E, editor: *Sleeping and waking disorders: indications and techniques*, Menlo Park, Calif, 1982, Addison Wesley Publishing.
14. Kandel ER, Schwartz JH: *Principles and neural science*, New York, 1981, Elsevier Science Publishing.
15. Moore-Ede MC, Sultzman FM, Fuller CA: *The clocks that time us: physiology of the circadian timing system*, Cambridge, Mass, 1982, Harvard University Press.
16. Saunders NA, Sullivan CE: *Sleep and breathing*. In *Lung biology in health and disease*, vol 21, New York, 1981, Mattel Dekker.

13

Substance Abuse

Elizabeth Schenk

After studying this chapter, the learner should be able to:

- Name four negative compulsions that are considered addictions.
- Differentiate between tolerance (behavioral, pharmacologic, and cross tolerance) and dependence (physical, psychologic, and cross dependence).
- Name one legal effort and one educational effort to prevent alcoholism and chemical dependency.
- Define the terms *enabling* and *intervention*.
- Discuss two theories of the development of alcoholism.
- Name five disorders directly associated with alcoholism.
- Name three characteristics of the addicted person.
- Discuss alcohol withdrawal, including delirium tremens, and actions taken to prevent or reduce withdrawal.
- Define drug addiction.
- Name the six basic types of drugs, citing examples, how they are used, street names, effects and side effects, pathophysiology, and symptoms of overdose.
- Discuss why nurses are at increased risk for chemical dependency.
- Define the term co-dependency.

13-1

Terms used to describe responses to drugs/alcohol

Dependence (also called *habituation* or *compulsive use*)   Psychologic and/or physical need for a drug or alcohol
Psychologic dependence   Needing a substance in order to reach a maximum level of functioning or feeling of well-being
Physical dependence   Adaption of the body physiologically to chronic use of substance(s); symptoms of withdrawal occur when the substance is stopped or withdrawn
Tolerance   Need for higher and higher doses of a substance to achieve the same results
Cross tolerance   Development of tolerance to one drug of a class leads to tolerance to drugs of the same class
Withdrawal (abstinence syndrome)   Appearance of physiologic symptoms when a substance is stopped
Drug abuse   Use of mind-altering substances in a way that differs from generally approved medical or social practices
Metabolic tolerance   Substance is detoxified more quickly than normal
Pharmacologic tolerance   Tissue reaction to substance is diminished

---

The area of *substance abuse* is gaining increased attention as more and more nurses are working in this specialty. It is commonly accepted that substance abuse includes a complex set of behaviors that are covered under the term *addiction*. These addictions include *alcoholism, drug addiction, overeating, compulsive gambling,* and other negative compulsions. It is possible and likely that persons will have one or more of these addictions at the same time. An example is the alcoholic who is also a drug addict and a compulsive overeater. Only alcoholism and drug addiction will be discussed in this chapter.

Alcoholism and drug addiction are commonly referred to as *chemical dependency*. This is in recognition of the fact that alcohol is a drug and that the person addicted to alcohol is also at great risk for addiction to other drugs.

Dependency includes both *physical* and *psychologic dependency*. Terms used to describe responses to drugs and alcohol are listed in Box 13-1.

PREVENTION AND HEALTH EDUCATION

Problems that occur as a result of substance abuse can have devastating results. These results have an impact on almost every body system and produce changes that are *chronic* and *debilitating*.

Primary Prevention

The goal of primary, or early prevention is to stop involvement with drugs or alcohol before it ever occurs.[1] Although the cause of substance abuse is not clearly defined, efforts to prevent its occurrence have been made on several fronts. These include the following:
1. Legal
   a. Efforts to restrict sale of alcohol to minors
   b. Stringent legal consequences for use of drugs
   c. Strict DWI laws and serious consequences for driving while intoxicated
2. Education
   a. Teaching young children about the dangers of alcohol use and abuse

b. Working to increase self-esteem of children so that they can better withstand peer pressure
c. Educating family members and employers to assist the alcoholic or drug addict into treatment and to stop enabling behavior

Evaluations of programs where the focus of prevention has been mainly the presentation of facts has shown that increasing knowledge alone has no affect on subsequent abuse of substances.[33]

Alcoholics are usually surrounded by persons who *enable* them to use and abuse. *Enabling* is defined as a *set of behaviors that prevents the substance abuser from focusing on the abuse.* An example of this is the spouse who calls in to work for the sick mate and tells the employer that the mate is sick with the flu, when in reality the person has a hangover. Without this *enabling behavior,* the alcoholic is often forced to seek help sooner.

Secondary Prevention

The goal of secondary prevention is to identify the person in the early stages of substance abuse and to prevent negative consequences by convincing the person to stop the use through counseling or other treatment.[1]

Early diagnosis and treatment of substance abuse can be important in assisting abusers to once again become productive members of society and save themselves and others from expense, disability, and heartache.

Some still believe that it is only when the alcoholic desires and seeks help with his or her alcohol problem that treatment can be effective. Unfortunately, often by the time an alcoholic seeks help, many things have been lost. Recently the emphasis has been on the use of a process called *intervention* to assist the alcoholic in receiving help. This is sometimes called *raising the bottom.*

Interventions are *planned group confrontations* by individuals who care about the person. Rules for intervention include the following[20]:
1. Meaningful persons present facts or data. The employer of the person can often be a very meaningful participant.
2. The data presented is specific and descriptive of

events that have happened or conditions that exist.
3. The tone of the confrontation is nonjudgmental.
4. The chief evidence should be tied into alcohol or drug use.
5. The evidence of behaviors is presented in detail and should be explicit.
6. The goal of the intervention is to have the alcoholic see and accept reality so that the need for help is accepted.
7. The choices available for treatment should be offered. If possible, immediate help should be available.

It is often difficult to make the diagnosis of alcoholism or drug abuse without objective evidence. Some indications of problems include the following:
1. Frequent illnesses and related illnesses
2. Undue preoccupation with the intake of drugs or alcohol
3. Mood swings
4. Violent or acting-out behavior
5. Denial about the use of substances
6. Financial difficulties
7. Loss of control over use
8. Use of alcohol or drugs in such a way as to endanger physical health, interpersonal relationships, and/or economic functioning
9. Use of substances as the universal answer to all problems
10. Loss of ability to express feelings
11. Use of defense mechanisms, including a strong denial of the problem that drugs or alcohol is causing

Tertiary Prevention

The goal of tertiary prevention is to end the compulsive use of alcohol or other drugs or to minimize the negative effects of the use through treatment and rehabilitation. An example of tertiary prevention is the treatment of an alcoholic person in relapse with cirrhosis of the liver in a halfway house.[1]

It is important to consider *tertiary prevention*, or the prevention of complications, for the patient with substance abuse. These complications occur not only because of the effects of the substance itself, but also because of the nutritional deficits that usually accompany the problem. These problems include *infections, neuropathy,* and *myopathies.* Complications for persons with drug addictions often occur as a result of disease acquired from dirty needles or equipment. Many alcoholics and drug addicts continue to drink despite the development of life-threatening complications. This fact is often difficult for health professionals to understand.

Many patients with substance abuse will have to deal with these complications long after they have stopped the use of the substance.

ALCOHOLISM

Alcoholism is very common and may complicate the problems of a person with other health problems. It is recognized today as a treatable disease.

Alcoholism is the third most serious major health problem in the United States.[21] Conservative estimates are that at least 90 million persons use alcohol and that at least 10% of them are alcoholics or *"problem drinkers."* It is estimated that between 3% and 10% of Americans will at some time in their lives be problem drinkers. In addition, alcohol negatively affects the health or functioning of another 30 million persons. As many as one third of American families will be touched by alcoholism. It has been estimated that 70% of alcoholics are male, but the number of females who are alcoholic is increasing.[34] Women are more likely to hide their problem and are not as likely to be detected. Also, drinking has increased at an alarming rate among adolescents.

Alcohol is involved in nearly half of all deaths caused by motor vehicle accidents and fatal intentional injuries such as suicides and homicides. It has been found that victims are intoxicated in about one third of all homicides, drownings, and boating deaths.[33] Alcohol is involved in at least a quarter of all admissions to general hospitals. The costs of alcohol-related problems in the United States have been estimated to exceed $70 billion per year, with an additional $44 billion attributed to problems related to drug use.[37]

The use of alcohol predates recorded history. It has been used in rites of passage, to celebrate significant events, and to mourn the dead. Alcohol has also been used as magic, as a medicine, and as a part of worship services.

There have been changes in attitudes and laws about the use of alcoholic beverages in the United States. In 1642 Maryland made drunkenness punishable by a fine. In 1790 the U.S. government passed a law that gave every soldier a daily portion of hard liquor. In 1919 a law was passed that prohibited the production and sale of alcoholic beverages in the United States. This period of *prohibition* was repealed in 1933.[56] The average consumption of alcohol by persons aged 14 and older in 1987 was calculated as 2.54 gallons, down from a peak of 2.76 gallons per person over the age of 14 in 1981.[45] It is believed that the decreasing trend in alcohol consumption can be attributed to changing life-styles and heightened awareness of the health and safety risks of alcohol use. Another factor that may be significant is that all 50 states now have raised the legal age of drinking to 21.

Numerous theories have been suggested to explain the cause of alcoholism.[56] These theories have been divided into three categories that include the following:
1. Physiologic theories
   a. Genetotropic-etiologic: related to genetically determined biochemical defect
   b. Endocrine-etiologic: caused by dysfunction of endocrine system
   c. Genetic: alcoholism is part genetically determined (risk of sons of alcoholic men developing alcoholism over their lifetime is 30% to 50%). Identical twins of an alcoholic parent will be alcoholic in 60% of cases)[13]
2. Psychologic theories
   a. Oral fixation: resulting from lack of a warm, loving relationship with a mother figure as a child
   b. Behavioral learning theory: association of alcohol

13-2

Disorders associated with alcoholism	
Hepatic	Alcoholic hepatitis, Laennec's cirrhosis, fatty liver
Gastrointestinal	Gastritis, pancreatitis, duodenal ulcers, malabsorption syndromes, cancer of mouth and esophagus
Neurologic	Peripheral neuropathy, Wernicke-Korsakoff's syndrome, organic brain disease
Cardiovascular, hematologic	Cardiomyopathy, hypertension, familial type-IV hyperlipidemia, hypoglycemia, anemia, hyperuricemia, coronary artery disease, congestive heart failure
Musculoskeletal	Skeletal myopathies
Immunologic	Increased susceptibility to infections

ingestion with positive experience leads to alcoholism

3. Sociocultural or cultural-etiologic theories
   a. Cultural: relationship between various societal groups and incidence of alcoholism (Jews, Mormons, and Moslems have low rate; the French have high rate)
   b. Moral etiologic: alcoholism is a moral fault or sin of the alcoholic

Research is ongoing to determine the causes of alcoholism but, so far, no one theory can completely explain the syndrome. It is apparent, however, that alcoholics share common behavioral characteristics that usually include dependency, denial, rationalization, and projection.

Alcohol abusers continue compulsive use in the presence of consequences, focus on obtaining the drug or alcohol, and have relapses after treatment. Although alcoholism is not a personality disorder, there is evidence that two personality types are particularly susceptible to alcohol abuse—the antisocial personality, found chiefly in men, and the borderline personality, found chiefly in women.[13] Alcohol abuse can become a problem over a variable period of time. The abuse of alcohol is often so episodic that it is difficult to identify. Some persons can drink large amounts for years without becoming alcoholic, whereas other persons become alcoholic after just a short period of heavy drinking. Some alcoholics drink only on weekends. Many may not drink for months at a time. Some drink only episodically, but when they do, the drinking is in the form of a binge, with the person often drinking to the point of unconsciousness.

In alcoholics, however, there is evidence of progression. There is concern about the drinking or use. The alcoholic begins to develop an increasing physical dependence on and tolerance for alcohol. The drinking becomes uncontrollable and secretive. *Blackouts* (loss of memory from episodes of drinking) may start to occur. Feelings of guilt, shame, and remorse may occur, and the alcoholic drinks more to relieve these feelings. The person *drinks to live and lives to drink.*

Pathophysiology

Alcohol is a central nervous system (CNS) *depressant*. It affects the brain by suppressing the activity of the neurotransmitter gamma aminobutyric acid (GABA), an inhibitory neurotransmitter. The so-called stimulating effects of alcohol occur because the first areas affected by the suppression of GABA are the higher centers of the brain governing self-control and judgment, which are inhibitory functions. Slowing the release of GABA to those areas results in a seemingly "stimulating" effect. As alcohol continues to accumulate in the brain, areas of the limbic system and brainstem become inhibited. Unconsciousness may set in and the brain can become so overwhelmed by alcohol that it can stop functioning. Other organ systems are also affected. (See Box 13-2.)

The active ingredient in alcoholic beverages is *ethyl alcohol* or *ethanol*. Most American beers contain 3% to 6% alcohol, wine contains 2% to 21% alcohol, and hard liquors contain 40% to 50% alcohol. A 12-ounce bottle of beer, a 4-ounce glass of wine, and 1½ ounces of hard liquor contain similar amounts of alcohol.

Alcohol is absorbed in both the stomach and intestine. It does not require digestion. Absorption is hastened by increased alcohol concentrations and an empty stomach. After absorption, alcohol is distributed equally throughout the body, passing across cell membranes. Between 2% and 10% of the alcohol will be lost through the lungs through breathing. Some is also lost in the urine. About 90%, however, is broken down by a metabolic process that occurs primarily in the liver. This accounts for the high level of liver damage in persons who are alcoholic.

Cirrhosis of the liver, largely related to heavy alcohol consumption, is the ninth leading cause of death in the United States. Rates of death for nonwhites are almost 70% higher than rates for whites[45] and the rates for Native American males is triple that of white men.[36]

Alcohol has a diuretic effect, caused partly by the increased amounts of fluid ingested. Increased amounts of electrolytes, especially potassium, magnesium, and zinc, may be excreted in the urine of a heavy drinker. Also, continued use of alcohol has a toxic effect on the intestinal mucosa; this results in decreased absorption of thiamine, folic acid, and vitamin B_{12}.

Because alcohol is not converted to glycogen, it cannot be stored and provides 200 kcal per ounce but no minerals or vitamins. These *empty calories* can add weight to a person who, at the same time, is suffering from malnutrition (see Fig. 13-1). In addition, alcohol acts as an appetite suppressant in most people.

Alcohol ⟶ Acetaldehyde ⟶ Acetic acid ⟶ CO_2, calories, and energy
(toxic) (no food value)

Fig. 13-1 Metabolism of alcohol.

Table 13-1 Effects of blood alcohol levels on average-sized nontolerant adult

Blood alcohol levels (per dl of blood)	Effects
50-75 mg	Pleasant, relaxed state, mild sedation, loosening of inhibitions
100-200 mg	Overt signs of intoxication: loosening of tongue, clumsiness, beginning emotional changes
200-400 mg	Severe intoxication: difficulty speaking, stumbling, emotional lability
400-500 mg	Stupor, coma
Over 500 mg	Usually fatal

The amount of alcohol in the blood at any one time is called the *blood alcohol level*. This level depends on the amount ingested and the size of the individual. Most laws designate blood alcohol levels of 100 mg/100 ml (0.10%) as the legal limit for intoxication. There is currently a movement to allow a blood alcohol level of only .04% for drivers over the age of 21 and 0% for those under the age of 21. States that have adopted lower legal blood alcohol levels for those under 21 have shown a decreased number of fatalities in this age group.[45] As blood alcohol levels increase, the side effects become more serious (Table 13-1).

Fetal Alcohol Problems

Fetal alcohol problems occur in newborns whose mothers drank during pregnancy. The amount of alcohol that causes damage to the fetus is disputed at this time. According to one source, a woman who has six drinks a day will give birth to a child with a full-blown case of *fetal alcohol syndrome*.[13] Studies have shown that the effects of alcohol may be more serious when a given amount of alcohol is taken in large amounts rather than in small amounts. There is also evidence that the timing of the drinking may be important—a few binges early in pregnancy may be dangerous even if drinking stops after that.[13]

Also unknown is the amount of alcohol use that is safe. It has been found that as little as two drinks a day throughout pregnancy may cause decreased birth weight, increase the risk of miscarriage, abortion, or stillbirth, and result in a child with significant lags in mental and motor development.

Fetal alcohol syndrome occurs in about 1 in 500 to 1 in 1000 live births.[13] The syndrome can include the following:

1. Retarded growth
2. Physical defects and deformities (especially facial)
3. Mental retardation
4. Abnormalities of brain function and behavior (intellectual and emotional)[13]

Alcohol Withdrawal

With sustained drinking, a physiologic dependence on alcohol and increasing tolerance occurs. When the alcohol is unavailable, the person suffers *withdrawal*. Symptoms range from *mild tremors* to *severe agitation* and *hallucinations*. The type and severity of symptoms depends on several factors. Alcoholics at high risk include the following:

1. Older persons
2. Persons who have had previous delirium tremens (DTs) or seizures
3. Persons with coexisting acute illnesses
4. Persons with nutritional deficiencies

See Box 13-3 for symptoms of the alcohol withdrawal syndrome.

Tremors. The tremors associated with alcohol withdrawal usually are observed 6 to 48 hours after withdrawal from alcohol. They may persist from 3 to 5 days. The hands are involved first, but the tremors may become generalized with involvement of the extremities, tongue, and trunk.

Seizure disorders. Seizures usually occur from 12 to 24 hours after the last drink. Usually these are *grand mal* seizures and are not preceded by an aura. They are followed by a postictal period, however.

Delirium tremens. Delirium tremens, or DT, is an *acute complication* of alcohol withdrawal that is a serious medical concern. It is a pathologic state of consciousness that results from interference with brain metabolism. DTs that are treated have a 5% mortality rate, whereas untreated ones have a 15% mortality rate. Signs of impending alcohol withdrawal include *restlessness and irritability*, *headache*, *nausea*, *insomnia*, and *nightmares*. Before the onset of full-blown DTs, withdrawal signs may include *visual and tactile hallucinations* that are followed by *seizures*.

The onset of DTs is often sudden and dramatic. It usually occurs 3 to 4 days after the last drink. The condition lasts from 2 to 3 days to a week, but at times it can last 4 to 5 weeks. It may follow injury, infectious disease, anesthesia, or surgery and may develop in patients who have not told their physicians that they are heavy drinkers. Thus treatment of the DTs may be delayed.[13] See Box 13-4 for symptoms of DTs.

Wernicke-Korsakoff's Syndrome

At one time Wernicke-Korsakoff's syndrome was believed to be the result of the neurotoxic results of long-term alcohol use. It is now known, however, that nutritional deficiency is the causative factor. The specific nutritional deficiency in most of the cases is thiamine.

Symptoms present with this syndrome include ocular disturbances, which may include nystagmus and a paralysis of the lateral rectus muscle of the eye. Ataxia may be

13-3	**Symptoms of alcohol withdrawal syndrome**
	Diaphoresis, tachycardia, and elevated blood pressure Tremors Nausea or vomiting Anorexia Restlessness Hallucinations Convulsions Delirium tremens

13-4	**Symptoms of delirium tremens (DTs)**
	Increased psychomotor activity and tremulousness Confusion and disorientation Fearfulness Signs of vasomotor lability Tachycardia Temperature elevations (100° to 105° F) Delusions and hallucinations (visual and tactile, including terrifying animal images and crawling skin sensations)

present, along with symptoms of disturbed mental functioning. The latter can include symptoms of delirium tremens as well as apathy, listlessness, psychosis, and severe confusion. Other problems associated with Korsakoff's psychosis are often seen; these include a problem with memory and confusion.

With this syndrome, the patient may recover from the initial illness, but amnestic psychosis continues. The patient may very well be left with a serious residual mental illness that will require close supervision and intensive care.

Nursing Process
Assessment
Subjective data

1. Normal using or drinking patterns
2. Date and time of last drink or use
3. Substances used
4. Quantity used
5. Past history of blackouts, tremors, hallucinations, or DTs
6. Past periods of abstinence
7. Normal dietary patterns
8. Any legal problems
9. Any family problems
10. Any occupational problems
11. Family history of alcoholism
12. Other medications used

It is important to realize that the cardinal symptom of untreated alcoholism is *denial*. As a result, the information gathered from the patient may not always be accurate, and it is helpful to validate it with a family member of significant other.[13] Despite a variety of symptoms and the tendency of the alcoholic to be vague about the amount of alcohol used, diagnosis by clinical interview is usually accurate.[13]

Objective data

1. Abnormal response to preoperative medication, anesthetics, or sedatives
2. Presence of tremor (usually worse in the morning)
3. Morning nausea
4. Abnormal laboratory studies
5. Presence of pellagra—redness, dryness, scaling, and edema of skin

6. Body weight in relation to height
7. Mental functioning
8. Memory loss
9. General behavior
10. Vital signs (especially tachycardia or hypertension)
11. Presence of ascites
12. Positive blood alcohol or urine alcohol level
13. Petechiae
14. Presence of polyneuropathy

Criteria system

The National Council on Alcoholism divides alcoholism into a *major and minor criteria system* and outlines the development of alcoholism on two tracks as follows.[2]

Major criteria

Track I
Physiologic
1. Withdrawal syndrome
2. Tolerance
3. Blackout periods
Clinical
1. Alcoholic hepatitis
2. Laennec's cirrhosis
3. Wernicke-Korsakoff syndrome
Track II
Behavioral, psychologic, attitudinal
1. Drinking despite medical contraindications
2. Drinking despite social contraindications
3. Subjective complaint of loss of control

Minor criteria

Track I
Physiologic and clinical
1. Odor of alcohol on breath
2. Alcohol facies
3. Abnormal liver function test
4. Blood-alcohol level over 300 mg/100 ml at any time
Track II
Behavioral
1. Gulping drinks
2. Morning drinking
3. Missing work
4. Frequent automobile accidents

Psychologic and attitudinal
1. Frequent talk about drinking
2. Drinking to release stress
3. Spouse complains about drinking
4. Family disruption

Diagnostic tests

Routine blood tests will often reveal abnormalities that are directly related to alcoholism. These include elevated liver enzymes (serum glutamic-oxaloacetic transaminase [SGOT], serum glutamic pyruvic transaminase [SGPT], alkaline phosphatase, and bilirubin). Hypoglycemia may also be present if glycogen stores have been depleted. In addition, hypoalbuminemia and hyperglobulinemia are present in patients with cirrhosis of the liver. Magnesium is often decreased in persons who are alcoholic, usually because of poor dietary intake. It is not uncommon to find anemia and other indications of poor nutrition in alcoholic patients. Patients may have an increased mean corpuscle volume (MCV) because of the number of immature RBCs produced in response to the anemia. This and an elevated gamma glutamyl transferase (GGT) are strong indicators of a possible diagnosis of alcoholism.

Other diagnostic tests will demonstrate the concomitant diseases that usually accompany alcoholism.

Data analysis: nursing diagnoses

Nursing diagnoses are determined from analysis of patient data. Possible nursing diagnoses for the person with alcoholism may include, but are not limited to, the following:

Diagnostic title	Possible etiologies
Airway clearance, ineffective	Fatigue, infection, trauma, decreased consciousness
Activity intolerance	Generalized weakness
Adjustment, impaired	Disability requiring change in lifestyle
Anxiety	Change in health status/role functioning
Body temperature, altered	Environmental exposure, dehydration, sedation
Breathing pattern, ineffective	Cognitive impairment
Coping, ineffective family: compromised or disabling	Inadequate or incorrect information of understanding, prolonged disability of significant person
Coping, ineffective individual	Maturational crises
Denial	Alcoholism or drug abuse
Family processes, altered	Situational crisis of alcoholism or other drug abuse
Fluid volume deficit, actual or potential	Decreased fluid intake, abnormal fluid loss
Grieving, anticipatory	Loss of use of alcohol or other drugs
Hopelessness	Loss of beliefs
Infection, high risk for	Decreased nutrition, decreased immune response
Injury, high risk for	Sensory deficits, lack of awareness of environmental hazards
Knowledge deficit	Lack of exposure/recall, cognitive limitation
Mobility, impaired physical	Decreased strength and endurance, perceptual/cognitive impairment
Noncompliance	Alcoholic life patterns
Nutrition, altered, less than body requirements	Anorexia, inability to obtain food
Powerlessness	Inability to control alcoholism or drug addiction
Self-esteem disturbance	Inability to hold job, do necessary tasks; altered thought processes
Sleep pattern disturbance	Pain/discomfort related to withdrawal of substance being abused
Social isolation	Unacceptable social behaviors
Spiritual distress	Questioning of personal, spiritual values
Thought processes, altered	Alcohol- or drug-induced dementia

Planning: expected patient outcomes

Expected patient outcomes for the patient with alcoholism may include, but are not limited to, the following:
1. Maintains a patent airway.
2. Has minimal deficits in ADL.
3. States plans to stop drinking or using drugs.
4. Demonstrates the ability to maintain abstinence at home.
5. Demonstrates minimal anxiety.
6. Maintains a normal body temperature.
7. Patient and family demonstrate improved and effective coping mechanisms.
8. Admits he or she is alcoholic.
9. Patient and family verbalize plan to improve family processes.
10. Maintains adequate hydration.
11. Patient has begun to verbalize grief over not being able to drink.
12. Patient verbalizes sense of hope.
13. Remains free of infection.
14. Does not experience injury.
15. Patient and family verbalize knowledge of disease and treatment.
16. Patient has optimal mobility.
17. Does not demonstrate violent behavior.
18. Maintains optimal nutrition.
19. Verbalizes powerlessness over drugs or alcohol.
20. Verbalizes an improved self-concept.
21. Maintains normal sleep pattern.
22. Demonstrates improved social interactions.
23. Has decreased spiritual distress.
24. Maintains cerebral perfusion.

Implementation
Assisting with achievement of therapeutic goals
Management of acute withdrawal

Care for the alcoholic patient in the acute phase usually involves *detoxification efforts* to prevent acute *withdrawal*. Detoxification is undertaken in a controlled environment where the patient can be monitored and complications prevented, as possible.

Medications. Medication used in the initial period of detoxification include chlordiazepoxide (Librium) or another central nervous system depressant, usually a benzodiazepine. The drug is used in decreasing doses for its sedating and anticonvulsant effect during detoxification.

The dosage can be as great as 50 mg every 3 hours in the first 24 hours. Anticonvulsant therapy that includes phenytoin (Dilantin), as well as magnesium sulfate (2 ml of a 50% solution every 8 to 12 hours for several doses) are also used. Dilantin is likely to be continued past the initial period of detoxification if the patient has a history of seizures.

The drug Atenolol may be used to reduce tremors and lessen the danger of cardiovascular symptoms by lowering heart rate, blood pressure, and body temperature during alcoholic withdrawal. This drug suppresses the sympathetic nervous system. The use of Atenolol has also been found to speed withdrawal by a day or two. Antipsychotic drugs are used only for hallucinations. Antidepressants may be used if the person is found to be depressed.

Because of the nutritional problems common with the disease of alcoholism, multivitamin supplements are usually prescribed. These include thiamine in combination with other B-complex vitamins.

Specific medications may differ from setting to setting. Whatever the medication used, it is wise to remember that many alcoholics need to receive medication, sometimes in large doses, to safely withdraw from alcohol.[13] There is no reason for the alcoholic to suffer because health professionals believe that they deserve to feel some pain. Unfortunately, these beliefs sometimes still exist.

Delirium tremens

Treatment of delirium tremens (DTs) consists of the use of tranquilizing drugs such as chlordiazepoxide (Librium) or diazepam (Valium) and sedatives such as paradehyde given rectally, intramuscularly, or orally. High-calorie and high-vitamin diets may have to be given by nasogastric tube.

Wernicke-Korsakoff syndrome

Treatment of Wernicke-Korsakoff syndrome includes strict abstinence from alcohol and the administration of large doses of B-complex and C vitamins. A danger in treating patients with Wernicke-Korsakoff syndrome is the use of intravenous glucose solution. This solution may exhaust the patient's last reserve of B vitamins and cause rapid worsening of the disease. Because of this, B vitamins must be added when parenteral glucose is given.

When severe brain damage has occurred, long-term custodial care may be required. Family members who assume the care of the patient require much support and education.

Interventions to achieve patient outcomes
Promoting effective airway clearance

The patient withdrawing from alcohol is prone to aspiration because of nausea and a decreased mental status and level of consciousness. The head of the bed should be elevated at least 30 degrees and a suction machine should be readily available, either at the bedside or close by. Fluids should *not* be offered by mouth until the patient is fully alert.

Decreasing anxiety

Anxiety and depression are common in alcoholics. The patient is encouraged to share concerns and feelings and to learn to deal with anxious feelings. Generally, medications are not used to treat anxiety because of the risk of the person developing cross dependence on them. Relaxation exercises and techniques are taught and practiced. The patient is encouraged to keep a feeling log that may be helpful in learning to identify specific feelings and what triggers them. Anxiety usually decreases as long-term sobriety is attained. If not, psychiatric help may be necessary.

Maintaining normal body temperature

Alcoholics, especially homeless ones, are often victims of hypothermia. Alcohol ingestion makes the person unaware of temperature extremes and in winter some alcoholics have frozen to death while sleeping on the street.

If a patient experiencing *withdrawal* from alcohol also has *hypothermia*, his or her temperature should be monitored frequently. The extremities should be checked for *signs of frostbite* and *resulting ischemia*. Extra blankets should be used to assist in warming the patient.

Maintaining an effective breathing pattern

Because the *effects of alcohol* can cause *respiratory depression*, the patient should be assessed for *apnea* or other *breathing difficulties*. Medications that will further compromise respirations, such as morphine, are not given. If narcotic use is suspected, Narcan may be administered. The patient should also be encouraged to turn, cough, and breathe deeply at frequent intervals to prevent atelectasis.

Promoting activity and mobility

The person entering treatment may be weak because of poor nutrition as well as because of complications of the alcoholism. As the withdrawal from alcohol occurs, strength improves. Many alcoholics will not have a regular program of physical exercise, and for this reason most inpatient treatment programs include daily periods of physical conditioning. Patients recovering from alcoholism are urged to maintain a regular exercise program after discharge.

Facilitating adjustment and coping

It is often difficult for the alcoholic person to adjust to the diagnosis of alcoholism, especially if alcoholism is seen as morally wrong. Denial that alcohol is a problem may be part of the difficulty. Denial is discussed later in this chapter. The patient is encouraged to focus on one day at a time and to not consider having to stay sober forever. The patient is educated about the disease concept of alcoholism, which usually helps with adjustment. Attendance at *Alcoholics Anonymous (AA)* meetings is usually required as a part of both inpatient and outpatient treatment programs. Through daily assignments the person is helped to learn about himself or herself in relation to alcoholism.

Psychotherapy cannot help the patient who continues to drink. It can, however, be helpful as a part of the treatment program. Emotional problems that occur as part of the drinking do not automatically disappear when the person stops drinking. Some patients have problems that are unrelated to their drinking and need to gain insight about them. Therapy directed toward personal insight has been found to be effective only after the patient attains stable sobriety.

The goals of a successful treatment program are:

1. That the person emerges with a commitment to a life of total abstinence from alcohol and other mood-altering drugs.
2. That the person accepts the fact that alcoholism is a chronic, progressive, fatal disease and he or she gains understanding of the nature of the disease.
3. That some of the damage from the drinking starts to heal.
4. That the process of personal change necessary to continue sobriety has begun.[10]

Decreasing denial

One of the real challenges in working with the alcoholic patient is facilitating the *breaking down of denial*. The patient characteristically is not aware of the havoc that his or her alcohol abuse has caused. Group therapy is used to enable the person to see the relationship between the use of alcohol and the negative consequences it has on his or her life. When the alcoholic becomes sober, many of the problems that have occurred in his or her life can be seen clearly for the first time.

Nurses working with these patients need to assist in pointing out areas of concern and consequences that the person has suffered as a result of alcoholism.

Improving family processes

As the alcoholic becomes more involved in the destructive process of the disease, the family also suffers. As a result, when an alcoholic family receives help, the family processes are usually in a state of dysfunction. Divorce may have occurred, or is being discussed. Spouses, parents, and children have lost respect for and trust in the alcoholic. Other family members may also have become very enabling and codependent.

It is unrealistic to think that family processes can be changed in a short period of time. Treatment of the family along with the alcoholic is important, not only to help the alcoholic recover, but also to allow the family to work through feelings of fear, distrust, and anger. Adult family members should be referred to Al-Anon, a twelve step support group for persons whose lives are affected by someone who is alcoholic. Children may be referred to Ala-Teen.

The patient and family often need additional counseling to help them grow together and not apart. In spite of this, the divorce rate among couples where one member is an alcoholic is high, even after the alcoholic achieves sobriety.

Maintaining adequate fluid volume

In the *initial period of detoxification*, the alcoholic patient may require *intravenous fluids*. *Nausea and vomiting* may be a real problem. As the withdrawal from alcohol occurs, the patient will be more able to tolerate liquids. Most detoxification centers attempt to restrict the use of beverages containing caffeine.

Facilitating grieving

Many alcoholics will actually go through a *grieving process for the loss of the alcohol*. For the recovering person, the loss and sadness over what has been given up (alcohol) can be quite intense. Practically all persons start drinking or using drugs because it is socially acceptable and fun. No one plans to become addicted and trapped in the compulsion to drink. For some, giving up alcohol may also mean the necessity of giving up their drinking friends. The alcoholic may be angry about the changes required and the realization that drinking is out of the question. *Grieving is a natural part of recovery because it implies an emotional response to loss*. The nurse can facilitate this grieving by encouraging the patient to talk about feelings and expressing the grief or anger. Letting the alcoholic know that this grief is normal and expected is helpful.

Depression may occur as the alcoholic recognizes and accepts the illness. Although the decision to stay sober will bring relief and assurance in the long run, the alcoholic will have periods when the desire for a drink is very strong and he or she may become discouraged, even though they are able, with support, to resist the temptation to drink.

Decreasing hopelessness

Many alcoholics enter treatment with a great sense of hopelessness. They may have attempted treatment before without success. They may also feel that they will never be able to stop drinking, and that they will never achieve sobriety. In addition, many alcoholics drink in order to block their feelings of hopelessness, especially about the loss of family and friends and perhaps the loss of a job.

Instilling hope in the alcoholic patient *takes time*. Often, the most important treatment is the contact the person has with other recovering alcoholics. Listening to recovering persons "lead" a group meeting will help to instill a beginning sense of hope. Seeing other persons who were worse off than they are may help them to see the chance for recovery.

Preventing infection

As alcoholics continue to drink, their health deteriorates. They may suffer from a variety of infections, including tuberculosis. It is important to observe the patient for signs of infection and administer antibiotics as ordered. The patient experiencing detoxification should be encouraged to cough and breathe deeply to prevent atelectasis. The position of the patient who is unable to respond is changed frequently.

Homeless alcohol abusers are at substantially increased risk of contracting tuberculosis. The nurse should monitor the patient for night sweats or other symptoms of tuberculosis. (See Chapter 24).

Good nutrition and adequate hydration are essential. If skin infections are present, appropriate treatment is begun. The nurse should also be aware that some alcoholics, especially the homeless, may have lice or scabies.

Preventing injury

The alcoholic who is still drinking is at high risk for injury from trauma. The best way to prevent this injury is to encourage the beginning of sobriety and to help the patient see the correlation between injuries and the drinking.

In the *initial withdrawal period*, the alcoholic may be at risk for *seizure activity*. *Medication is given as ordered to* prevent *delirium tremens*. Side rails should be kept up and the patient observed closely for signs of impending problems. See Chapter 37 for a description of appropriate action to take when a patient has a seizure.

The nurse must also realize that the person experiencing delirium tremens may become violent and inflict injury on others. If the person becomes so agitated as to pose a risk of harm to self or others, it may be necessary to place the person in leather restraints.

Facilitating knowledge

Education about the disease of alcoholism is extremely important for the alcoholic and the family or significant others. See Box 13-5 for important topics that need to be covered. These persons also become sick in the midst of the alcoholic becoming sicker and need understanding and education to help themselves and the alcoholic to recover.

Many over-the-counter drugs contain alcohol. Two examples of these are cough medicines and mouthwashes. The alcoholic also needs to know that the use of any mood-altering chemical may lead to relapse.

Decreasing noncompliance

The object of all treatment for alcoholism is to assist patients in achieving sobriety. When they do stop drinking, they are taught that they can never take one drink without the danger of relapse. In fact, the *most complicated and frustrating part of treatment is to prevent relapse.*

Some have suggested that alcoholics may be taught to become "social drinkers," but this has not been substantiated. Alcoholics who are currently drinking are never considered cured, only recovering.

Behavior modification may be used to discourage drinking behaviors. The best-known aversive agent is disulfiram (Antabuse), which blocks the enzymatic action necessary to metabolize alcohol. If the person drinks, Antabuse will cause nausea, vomiting, palpitations, and general ill feeling with even a small sip of alcohol. This conditions the person to avoid alcohol. Disulfiram is usually used with other therapy and may help the alcoholic attain a period of sobriety so that other therapy may be effective.

Maintaining adequate nutrition

Many alcoholics enter treatment with a history of poor nutritional habits. They may have received as much as a third of their daily intake of calories from alcohol. They often may have been too intoxicated to eat or have had no appetite for normal food. Also, *alcohol is the most common cause of acute gastritis, which can result in severe vomiting, contributing to poor nutrition.* Often they have consumed many "empty calories" and are malnourished. In the initial detoxification period, diet is as tolerated, including liberal fluids. As the condition of the alcoholic improves, appetite usually improves also. Then the emphasis is on three well-balanced meals a day, with free access to snacks. Many patients find that they crave sugar during this initial period, and it is not discouraged because withdrawal from alcohol is the first priority.

Patients usually benefit from assessment by a nutritionist or dietitian. Education about the importance of improved nutrition is essential. If the patient has liver in-

---

13-5

Patient Teaching

The patient with alcoholism

Disease concept of alcoholism
Medical aspects of the disease, including complications
Need for continued abstinence
Importance of expressing feelings to stay sober
Defense mechanisms
Drugs to avoid
Products that contain alcohol (for example, mouthwash and cough medicine)
Importance of being honest with physician and dentist
Signs and symptoms of impending relapse
Importance of aftercare, including AA

---

volvement with cirrhosis, dietary medications are usually necessary. The reader is referred to the section on cirrhosis in Chapter 30 for further information.

Accepting powerlessness

The alcoholic person needs to accept that he or she is powerless over alcohol. This is the basis of almost all treatment approaches. It may be a difficult concept for the alcoholic to understand, that through becoming powerless they achieve the ability to stay sober. Attendance at Alcoholics Anonymous meetings, group therapy, and discussions with other alcoholics, all can help with this. The alcoholic needs to understand that taking even one drink of alcohol can start them on the process of active drinking again. *Inherent in accepting this powerlessness is the realization that they have no control over alcohol, but that it controls them.*

Increasing self-esteem

It is important for these patients to build positive self-esteem, enabling them to acknowledge that they are worthwhile. This is important because many alcoholics continue to drink to cover their feelings of inadequacy and lack of self-worth. Positive self-esteem is important for continued recovery.

An important part of treatment of alcoholism leading to positive self-worth is positive reinforcement. This usually occurs in the context of interpersonal relationships with nurses and other staff, as well as with other patients. Caring, emotional support, and encouragement are very important. This is demonstrated within the context of honesty and also by pointing out negative behaviors, defense mechanisms, and problems.

Encouraging normal sleep patterns

It is very common for the patient going through withdrawal to have insomnia. It may take several months for sleep to return to a normal pattern. Regular physical activity and establishment of a daily routine may help. What is most important is not to use sleeping medication, because the alcoholic is at risk of becoming dependent on the medication. Relaxation tapes and decreasing caffeine use may be helpful in inducing sleep.

Decreasing social isolation

The *social isolation* experienced by alcoholics can best be handled in a *support group*. The best-known group is Alcoholics Anonymous (AA), which is a group of self-acknowledged alcoholics whose aim is to stay sober and to help other alcoholics gain sobriety. AA was founded in the 1930s and now sponsors 60,000 groups in 112 countries. In the United States, it reaches 650,000 alcoholics a year.[13]

AA meets regularly in most communities. Meetings are of various types and include the following:

1. Open meetings—may be attended by anyone
2. Closed meetings—limited to persons who are alcoholic
3. Lead meetings—a recovering alcoholic tells his or her personal story of alcoholism
4. Discussion meetings—topic is discussed

There are meetings in most communities for women only, men only, young people, gay persons, and in larger communites, the deaf. There is no charge for attendance at the meetings, but a free-will offering is usually taken.

Local AA groups are sometimes listed in the telephone directory, and larger communities will publish and distribute directories of meetings. A phone call to AA (often called the central office) will bring help in the form of telephone conversation, or an AA member may visit the alcoholic who needs help.

In some communities some AA members are reluctant to have persons with other addictions attend AA meetings. This is partly because of a lack of information about the disease of chemical dependency; it is also based partly on fear. With improved methods of diagnosing drug abuse and alcoholism, especially among younger persons, many AA groups are faced with younger people who have not suffered the same number or kind of consequences that the older members may have.

The AA philosophy focuses on the opportunity for the alcoholic to share *personal experiences* of alcohol abuse and control. Participation in AA may or may not be accompanied by the participation of the patient in other types of treatment. The success of AA has led to the formation of other groups that share the same twelve-step spiritual approach (see Box 13-6). These groups include Al-Anon, Families Anonymous, Narcotics Anonymous, Overeaters Anonymous, Emotions Anonymous, Cocaine Anonymous, and Gamblers Anonymous.

The twelve steps assist the alcoholic in admitting his or her powerlessness over alcohol and other drugs. This is seen as essential for continued sobriety. Some persons may have a difficult time at first with the concept of a higher power or God. They are often encouraged to use the power of the group as a higher power, until they are able to recognize and accept a sense of *spirituality*. This sense of spirituality is not the same as a religion or church.[50]

Decreasing spiritual distress

Many alcoholics enter treatment spiritually bankrupt. Generally, they have been cut off from nurturing relationships with others, with self, and with a higher being. The person is forced, because of defense mechanisms, into a grandiose position of becoming a God of sorts. As the disease progresses, values decrease. Many persons may also see God as a punishing force who could never forgive the person for things done while he or she was drinking.

If the patient desires, the services of a chaplain should be offered. The patient should be educated about the difference in the spirituality talked about in AA and religion. As mentioned above, some persons may have difficulty with the concept of a higher power or God. They can be encouraged to use a power of the group as a higher power until they are able to accept a sense of spirituality.

Maintaining thought processes

The patient experiencing *alcohol withdrawal* or *delirium tremens* may have *altered thought processes*. It is important to reorient the patient as needed and to reassure family members that mentation usually clears as the symptoms of withdrawal end. If this does not occur, the patient will be evaluated for Wernicke-Korsakoff's Syndrome (see p. 248).

13-6

Twelve steps of Alcoholics Anonymous

1. We admitted we were powerless over alcohol—that our lives had become unmanageable.
2. Come to believe that a power greater than ourselves could restore us to sanity.
3. Made a decision to turn our will and our lives over to the care of God as we understood him.
4. Made a searching and fearless moral inventory of ourselves.
5. Admitted to God, to ourselves, and to another human being the exact nature of our wrongs.
6. Were entirely ready to have God remove all these defects of character.
7. Humbly asked him to remove our shortcomings.
8. Made a list of all persons we had harmed, and became willing to make amends to them all.
9. Made direct amends to such people whenever possible, except when to do so would injure them or others.
10. Continued to take personal inventory and when we were wrong promptly admitted it.
11. Sought through prayer and meditation to improve our conscious contact with God as we understood Him, praying only for knowledge of His will for us and the power to carry that out.
12. Have had a spiritual awakening as a result of these steps, we tried to carry this message to alcoholics, and to practice these principles in all our affairs.

Evaluation

Evaluation of the patient with chemical dependency involves input from the patient, as well as the family members or significant other. Questions to consider include the following:

1. Is the patient sober?
2. Is the patient able to hold a job?
3. Is the patient's medical problem under good control?
4. Is the patient attending aftercare, including AA?
5. Is the patient's skin intact?
6. Is the patient able to carry on home maintenance activities?
7. Is the patient able to carry on ADL with minimal difficulty?
8. Is the patient able to function with minimal anxiety?
9. Is the patient demonstrating positive coping mechanisms?
10. Does the patient have a stable support system?
11. Is the patient free of infection?
12. Is the patient free of traumatic injury?
13. Is the patient able to verbalize knowledge of the disease concept of alcoholism?
14. Is the patient able to verbalize knowledge of any prescribed medications?
15. Can the patient explain the importance of notifying his or her doctor or dentist about the history of alcoholism?
16. Is the patient able to state what medications and other products to avoid?
17. Is the patient free of violent behavior?
18. Is the patient's nutritional status improved?
19. Is the patient verbalizing powerlessness over alcohol and/or drugs?
20. Does the patient verbalize a more positive self-concept?
21. Is the patient sleeping normally?
22. Is the patient interacting with others in a more socially acceptable way?
23. Is the patient having less spiritual distress?

DRUG ABUSE

Because alcohol is in itself a drug, alcoholism and drug abuse are considered part of the disease of chemical dependency. There is an increasing tendency for persons who abuse substances to mix a variety of drugs and alcohol. Much of the information already covered in the section on alcoholism also pertains to drugs.

The history of nonmedical drug use is thousands of years old. As early as 5000 BC, the Sumèrians referred to a "joy plant." This is believed to be a reference to the opium poppy plant.[56] Since then drugs have played a significant role in almost every culture. Different drugs have assumed importance in different periods of history. For instance, today cocaine is more problematic than ever before, especially in the form of "crack." Another recent problem is the class of designer drugs, which were unheard of several years ago. Designer drugs result from attempts to produce synthetic narcotics in "home laboratories." The drugs that result can cause dangerous side effects such as severe and nonprogressive Parkinsonian syndrome characterized by a loss of spontaneous movements, rigidity, a coarse resting tremor of the hand, muteness, and loss of reflexes. In recent years the use of drugs has decreased, at least in some populations.[28] However, the toll exacted on society, health, and the economy is staggering. In the inner cities, the drug problem seems to be worse, with a corresponding increase in violent crime.[45]

Adolescents who use drugs (and alcohol) are much more likely than nonusing teens to experience serious problems such as failure in school, delinquency, early sexual activity, sexually transmitted diseases, and unwanted pregnancy.[36] Drug use among teens appears to develop in predictable

Table 13-2 Effects of mind-altering drugs

Drug	Tolerance	Physical dependence	Psychologic dependence
CNS depressants			
Narcotics	High	High	High
Barbiturates	Moderate	High	High
Glutethimide (Doriden)	Moderate	High	High
Methaqualone (Quaalude, Sopor)	Moderate	High	High
Tranquilizers	Moderate	Moderate	High
CNS stimulants			
Amphetamine	High	Low to moderate	High
Cocaine	Low	Low to moderate	High
Hallucinogens			
LSD	Moderate	None	Moderate
Mescaline	Low	None	Moderate
Phencyclidine (PCP, angel dust)	Low	None	Low
Cannabis			
Marijuana	Low	None	Moderate

ways, starting with gateway drugs (cigarettes, alcohol, or marijuana) and then progressing to other drugs.[36] It has been found that persons who begin smoking in childhood are more inclined to heavy smoking and drinking at an earlier age and are more likely to abuse other drugs. Teens are unlikely to develop drug and alcohol problems if the age of first use is delayed beyond adolescence.[39]

The term *addiction* has been used to define the nature and extent of drug use. *Drug addiction involves craving, psychologic dependence,* and *physical dependence.* It includes development of tolerance for increasing dosages of the drug and the appearance of withdrawal symptoms on cessation of the drug. *Drug dependence* is another term that may be used. This refers to a *psychologic* or *physical dependence* on a *drug that is taken regularly* (see Table 13-2).

According to the Controlled Substance Act of 1971, there are five basic kinds of drugs:

1. Stimulants
2. Depressants
3. Hallucinogens
4. Narcotics
5. Cannabis

To this list can be added solvents such as glue and paint thinner.

Another form of classification of drugs is that of the Drug Enforcement Agency (see Table 13-3).

Table 13-3 DEA drug schedules with examples

Schedule	Examples
I (high abuse, low usefulness)	Heroin Hallucinogens Marijuana Methaqualone (Quaalude)
II	Opium or morphine Codeine Synthetic opiates (Demerol) Barbiturates (Seconal) Amphetamines, methylphenidate (Ritalin) and phenmetrazine (Preludin) PCP
III	Aspirin with codeine Paregoric Methylprylon (Noludar) Glutethimide (Doriden)
IV	Chloral hydrate (Noctec) Ethchlorvynol (Placidyl) Flurazepam (Dalmane) Pentazocine (Talwin) Chlordiazepoxide (Librium) Propoxyphene (Darvon) Diethylpropion (Tenuate)
V (low abuse, high usefulness)	Narcotic-atropine mixtures (Lomotil) Codeine mixtures (<200 mg)

Adapted from Grinspoon L and Bakalar J: Alcohol abuse and dependence, *The Harvard Medical School Mental Health Review,* 1990.

Stimulants

Stimulants are natural and synthetic drugs that have a strong stimulating effect on the central nervous system. They are accompanied by a feeling of alertness and self-confidence.

Drugs included in this category are amphetamines, cocaine, caffeine, and nicotine.

Amphetamines

Amphetamines and amphetaminelike drugs are *synthetic psychoactive drugs* that are available legally by prescription. They are available in both capsule and tablet forms. A powdered or crystalline form of amphetamine is *methamphetamine,* which must be injected. It is no longer legally produced in injectable form.

Medical uses of amphetamines include the treatment of *narcolepsy, fatigue,* and *depression.* Ritalin, an amphetaminelike drug, is used to treat children who are hyperactive. Common brand names of amphetamines include dextroamphetamine (Dexedrine), metamphetamine (Methedrine), and amphetamine (Benzedrine). See Box 13-7 for common street names for amphetamines.[40]

Pathophysiology

Amphetamines are CNS *stimulants.* When swallowed or injected, they speed up the activity of the heart and brain. Other results include the following:

1. Dilation of the pupil of eye
2. Increase in pulse and blood pressure
3. Reduction of fatigue
4. Reduction of appetite
5. Increase in concentration
6. Sense of confidence and well-being

However, *when the feeling of alertness wears off, the person experiences fatigue* and *depression.*

Amphetamines have the potential to produce *tolerance* but usually not physical withdrawal. However, psychologic dependence is common.

Side effects of amphetamine usage include *restlessness, dizziness, insomnia, headaches, diarrhea, constipation,* and *lack of appetite.* Persons who ingest a large amount of amphetamines over a period of time may experience extreme agitation and anxiety. They may become paranoid and suffer from a temporary *paranoid psychosis* that is a psychiatric emergency. Death by overdose does not usually occur, but death may occur from *cerebral hemorrhage* or *heart attack.* Persons can also collapse from exhaustion because the use of amphetamines hides a sense of fatigue. Withdrawal from the drug can lead to profound depression and may lead to suicide.[57]

13-7	**Street names for amphetamines**	
	Pep pills	Speed
	Dexies	Crystal
	Bennies	Meth
	Ups	Whites

Cocaine

Cocaine is a psychoactive drug that comes from the leaves of the South American cocoa bush. It was first used by the members of early South American tribes. When the Spanish conquistadors discovered the Inca empire, they also found cocaine. They encouraged its use when they found that the natives worked longer and harder and needed less food when they used cocaine. The statistics for cocaine use are alarming. Twenty one million persons have tried cocaine and nearly three million use the drug on a regular basis.[15] Also alarming is the use of crack, which is even more addictive. Among those who used cocaine in the past year, over twice as many young persons reported smoking it as did their older peers.[29]

The active ingredient in cocaine was isolated in its pure form in the nineteenth century. During that time the drug was also used as an ingredient in many products, including *syrups, nasal sprays, cigarettes,* and *liquors.* At one time it was an ingredient in Coca-Cola and was also recommended as a treatment for alcoholism. In 1914 the nonmedical use of cocaine was prohibited by the Harrison Narcotic Act. During the past 15 years, cocaine has become increasingly popular as a recreational drug.[30]

Medical uses for cocaine include use as an *anesthetic of choice* for *certain procedures and surgery involving the nose, throat, larynx, and lower respiratory passages.* It may also be used as an ingredient in Brompton's mixture, which is used to relieve pain in terminal cancer patients.

Cocaine is used by *sniffing, smoking,* or *injecting.* When it is sniffed or snorted, the effect of the drug is realized when the cocaine is absorbed through the mucous membrane in the nose. Cocaine may be *free-based.* This is a process of heating the drug to separate it from whatever adulterants it may contain. It is then smoked.

A newer form of cocaine is called *crack.* It is a free-base form of cocaine hydrochloride, so called because the cocaine has been separated from its hydrochloride base. It is called crack because of the characteristic crackling sound that is made when the crystals are heated. Cocaine powder is not smoked because heat destroys its effects. Crack is heat resistant and reaches the brain faster and in higher concentrations, producing a more intense euphoria within about 6 seconds.[25] The high is also more intense because crack contains as much as 90% pure cocaine, whereas cocaine hydrochloride may contain only 15% to 25% of pure cocaine. The feeling of exhilaration lasts a much shorter time, however, 5 to 7 minutes in contrast with 30 minutes after using powdered cocaine.[25] Crack is less ex-

pensive than other forms of cocaine and is available in crystal form. Crack is considered to be even more addictive than other forms of cocaine.

See Box 13-8 for common street names for cocaine.

Pathophysiology

Cocaine acts as a CNS *stimulant.* It blocks the uptake or reabsorption mechanism of the neurotransmitters, thus prolonging the effects of norepinephrine and dopamine on the brain and peripheral nerves. It also breaks down neurotransmitters. The habitual use of cocaine eventually depletes the brain's supply of dopamine and norepinephrine.[25]

Because of the stimulation of the brain by cocaine, there is a surge in the systolic blood pressure with its use. This surge in blood pressure has been linked with sudden neurologic insults, including *subarachnoid hemorrhage. Cocaine use* in *high doses can precipitate fatal ventricular arrhythmias, as well as seizures.*

The use of cocaine during pregnancy causes constriction of the uterine blood vessels, leading to deprivation of oxygen and nutrients to the developing fetus. This increases the risk of spontaneous abortion during the first trimester, and can cause premature delivery and premature separation of the placenta. It can also slow fetal growth and cause congenital abnormalities. Use during the first trimester of pregnancy can interfere with the formation of neurologic pathways of the brain of the fetus.[15] Cocaine has also been found to lead to in-utero brain hemorrhage and stroke.[8]

Results of the use of cocaine include the following:
1. Stimulation of respiration and heart rate
2. Raising of blood pressure and blood sugar levels
3. Suppression of appetite
4. Dilation of the eyes
5. Constriction of certain blood vessels
6. Increase in levels of physical activity
7. Insomnia
8. Trembling
9. Sensations of extreme euphoria
10. Feelings of energy, power, confidence, and talkativeness

There is a letdown effect of cocaine crash that occurs when the effect of the drug wears off.

Chronic sniffing of cocaine can destroy the nasal tissues. Smoking it can cause lesions in the lungs. Tolerance and psychologic dependence can develop, and *an overdose can* cause *convulsions, respiratory paralysis,* and *death.* A cocaine psychosis has been reported that is characterized by a loss of pleasure, loss of orientation, hallucinations, insomnia, concern with minor details, stereotyped behavior, and an increased potential for violence. Abrupt withdrawal from cocaine does not lead to physical symptoms of withdrawal. However, symptoms that do occur include depression, fatigue, hyperphagia, and possible suicide ideation.

Caffeine

Caffeine is the most accepted and used psychoactive substance in the United States. Many beverages and other products contain caffeine. Because of its availability and widespread use, most people do not view caffeine as a drug.

The use of tea leaves in China dates back at least 4000 years. In the 1200s the Arabians used coffee. Caffeine was

---

13-8	**Street names for cocaine**	
	Blow	Snow
	Coke	Superblow
	Dust	Toot
	Flake	White
	Nose candy	White girl
	Rock	Crack

13-9	Caffeine content of products	
	Coffee (per cup)	
	Brewed	75 to 155 mg
	Instant	60 to 90 mg
	Decaffeinated	2 to 4 mg
	Carbonated sodas	
	(All colas, Dr Pepper, Mountain Dew, Sunkist Orange, unless they are labeled caffeine free)	30 to 70 mg
	Chocolate	
	Hot cocoa	30 to 70 mg
	Candy (1 ounce)	6 mg
	Over-the-counter drugs	
	Anacin, Excedrin, Vanquish, Doan's Pills	16 to 65 mg
	No-Doz, Vivarin	100 to 200 mg
	APC tablets	30 to 100 mg
	Diet aids	
	AYDS, Dexatrim, Prolamine	140 to 200 mg
	Tea (per cup)	25 to 75 mg

13-10	Nicotine withdrawal symptoms
	Decrease in heart rate
	Weight gain
	Impairment of psychomotor performance
	Nervousness and anxiety
	Headaches
	Fatigue
	Insomnia
	Constipation or diarrhea

first isolated from coffee in 1820. In its pure state, caffeine is a white powder or white needle-shaped crystals. It has been used as an additive in carbonated beverages since the early 1900s.

Medically, caffeine is present in many headache remedies, cold medications, diuretics, diet aids, and other prescriptions. See Box 13-9 for the amount of caffeine in commonly used beverages.

Pathophysiology

Caffeine *stimulates* the CNS, the digestive system, and the kidneys. Body metabolism is increased, and the blood pressure is raised. Urination is also increased, and the secretion of gastric acid is stimulated. Large doses of caffeine cause *tachycardia, headaches* and *nervousness, insomnia,* and *stomach distress.* Physical dependence occurs with a regular intake of 350 mg for an adult. The withdrawal symptoms include *severe headaches, irritability,* and *tiredness.*[40]

Caffeine makes most people feel energetic and alert. Too much caffeine can precipitate an *anxiety attack.* Long-term involvement can lead to depression, persistent anxiety, low-grade fever, nausea, ringing in the ears, and chronic insomnia. A fatal dose of caffeine is considered to be about 10 g or 10,000 mg. Some research has indicated that excessive use of caffeine may contribute to the development of heart disease and bladder cancer.

Nicotine

Over 50 million Americans smoke more than 600 billion cigarettes yearly. It is one of the most physically damaging and addictive habits that a large number of people engage in. Smoking has been linked to heart and blood vessel disease, chronic bronchitis and emphysema, and cancer of the lungs, larynx, mouth, esophagus, bladder, pancreas, and kidneys. It is far easier to become addicted to cigarettes than to alcohol or other drugs. Tobacco is used by *smoking, chewing,* or *inhaling.* Snuff is usually placed between the gums and the cheek.

The tobacco plant belongs to the genus *Nicotina,* a member of the *nightshade* family. Evidence has been found that cigarette use occurred as far back as 200 AD. When Columbus reached the New World, the sailors saw the natives smoking and soon picked up the habit. The cigarette-rolling machine was invented in the 1880s. This added greatly to the number of people who abused tobacco. In 1964 the surgeon general of the United States issued a report that linked smoking with several diseases. Cigarette packages are now so labeled. *Cigarette smoking is the chief preventable cause of death in present-day society.*[57]

Pathophysiology

The nicotine in tobacco acts as a *stimulant* to the CNS. Nicotine is present in the brain within a few seconds of the beginning of smoking. Smokers claim that smoking produces relaxation; however, smoking releases epinephrine, which may cause psychologic stress. Nicotine acts as an *appetite suppressant.* In large doses it produces *tremors, decreased urine output,* and a *rapid respiratory rate.*

Withdrawal symptoms occur with the stoppage of cigarette smoking. See Box 13-10 for symptoms of withdrawal. The craving for a cigarette often continues for an extended period of time.[57]

Depressants

Depressants are *synthetic* drugs that have a *depressant* action on the CNS. Drugs included in this category are the following:

1. Barbiturates
2. Nonbarbiturates
3. Benzodiazepines

Barbiturates

Barbiturates are *synthetic* drugs that are classified as *"sedative hypnotics."* They arise from barbituric acid. They are used medically to treat high blood pressure, epilepsy, and insomnia, and to sedate patients before and during surgery. Barbiturates are often available on the street.

Barbiturates are swallowed (capsule or elixir), used as a suppository, or injected. The drug was first synthesized in the early 1900s by two German scientists. Currently, about ten derivatives of barbituric acid are in use.

There are many common street names for barbiturates. They refer to the drug type, the drug effect, the drug name, or the color of the particular capsule. See Box 13-11 for common street names.[40]

Pathophysiology

Barbiturates cause *depression* of the CNS, including *slowing of physical and mental reflexes.* The continued use of these drugs can cause physical and psychologic dependence, as well as tolerance. Barbiturates produce a feeling of well-being, euphoria, and relief from anxiety. Some side effects of barbiturates include *difficulty in breathing, lethargy, allergic reactions, nausea,* and *dizziness.*

Alcohol and other CNS depressants tend to potentiate the effects of barbiturates. Accidental overdoses are common when taken with alcohol. Another feature of barbiturates that makes them especially dangerous is that although patient tolerance to them increases, the lethal dose remains the same. This increases the risk of a fatal overdose. A person who is physically dependent on barbiturates will experience various withdrawal symptoms on the stopping of the drug. Mild withdrawal includes *irritability, restlessness, anxiety,* and *sleep disturbances.* An extreme form of barbiturate withdrawal can be life threatening and includes symptoms of *convulsions* and *delirium.* Detoxification includes appropriate medication, which may include a long-acting barbiturate given in diminishing dosages.[40]

Nonbarbiturates

Almost all of the nonbarbiturates were introduced as drugs that were nonaddictive and safe substitutes for the barbiturates. They were developed synthetically to overcome some of the drawbacks of barbiturate hypnotics, such as the drug-induced sleep disturbances and the high risk of overdose. However, these drugs have been found to share the dangers of the barbiturates.

Nonbarbiturates include the following:
1. Methaqualone (Quaalude)
2. Ethchlorvynol (Placidyl)
3. Methprylon (Noludar)
4. Glutethimide (Doriden)
5. Chloral hydrate (Noctec)
6. Paraldehyde

Pathophysiology

Nonbarbiturate depressants slow the CNS and impair coordination, walking, and talking. The primary effect is drowsiness. If the user resists the sleep-inducing effects of the drug, he or she experiences a mellow sense of well-being.

The repeated use of these drugs produces tolerance, as well as physical and psychologic dependency. Withdrawal from these drugs produces headache, fatigue, dizziness, nausea, anxiety, skin problems, abdominal cramping, seizures, and vomiting if the withdrawal is not accomplished under medical supervision. Withdrawal requires the use of a medication such as diazepam or phenobarbital.

13-11

Common street names for barbiturates	
Yellow jacket (pentobarbital)	Barbs
	Downs or downers
Red devil (secobarbital)	Rainbows
Phennie (phenobarbital)	Blues
Blue heaven or blue devil (amobarbital)	Goof balls

Overdoses occur when the CNS-depressing effects of the drugs in this group slow the person's rate of breathing to the extent that unconsciousness occurs. Most overdoses occur when the drug is combined with other drugs such as alcohol that potentiate its action. Symptoms of overdose include delirium, coma, restlessness, convulsions, and vomiting.

Benzodiazepines

Minor tranquilizers are *psychoactive drugs* that are taken to reduce anxiety. They may also be used as *muscle relaxants. They are the most commonly prescribed drugs in the world today.* Tranquilizers are available in prescription form in capsule, tablet, and liquid forms. Illicitly, they are sometimes injected. Common types of tranquilizers are those found in the benzodiazepine family and include the following:
1. Chlordiazepoxide (Librium)
2. Diazepam (Valium)
3. Prazepam (Antrax or Vestram)
4. Oxazepam (Serax)
5. Lorazepam (Ativan)
6. Clorazepate (Tranzene)
7. Xanax

These drugs are relatively new; the first tranquilizer was developed in 1950. Diazepam was first marketed in 1963.[57]

A newer benzodiazepine, buspar (Buspirone) has been found in the first controlled studies to have no hypnotic effect, while decreasing anxiety.[33]

Pathophysiology

Minor tranquilizers *slow* the activities of the CNS. They also have *anticonvulsant* and *muscle-relaxant properties* and produce a sense of *well-being.* When the effects of the drug wears off, users frequently experience an *increased level of anxiety. Tranquilizers cause physical and psychologic dependence, and tolerance to them can develop.*

Side effects reported for these drugs include *skin rash, headache, nausea, impairment of sexual function, dizziness,* and *light-headedness.* Other CNS-depressing drugs potentiate the action of the tranquilizers. Signs of an overdose include *sleepiness, confusion, loss of consciousness,* and *diminished reflexes.*

Withdrawal symptoms from benzodiazepines occur from 48 hours after the last use of Xanax or 8 to 10 days for Valium. These symptoms include *anxiety, sweating, insomnia, vomiting, tremors, delirium,* and *seizures.* The patient must be detoxified with medications in a controlled environment.

13-12	**Common street names of hallucinogens**	
	LSD	Acid, barrels, blotter, domes, micro-dots, purple haze, windowpane
	Mescaline	Buttons, cactus, mesc, mescal buttons
	MDA	Love drug, mellow drug of Americ~
	Psilocybin	Magic mushroom, shroom

Hallucinogens

Hallucinogens are natural and synthetic drugs that affect the mind and produce *changes in perception* and *thinking*. One drug included in this category is phencyclidine (PCP), which will be discussed separately from the hallucinogens.

Hallucinogens include *lysergic acid diethylamide (LSD), mescaline, psilocybin,* and *3,4-methylenedioxyamphetamine (MDA), dimethytryptamine (DMT), diethyltriptamine (DET),* and *2,5-Dimethoxy-4-methylamphetamine (DOM or STP).* They are found on the streets in a wide range of forms, including powder, peyote buttons, mushrooms, capsules, and tablets. LSD may be found as tablets, pellets, blotter paper, chips, and sheets of paper containing tattoos or stamplike pictures of cartoon figures. Hallucinogens are taken orally, although MDA can be sniffed and injected. They may be put on sugar cubes or mixed in other food. See Box 13-12 for common street names of hallucinogens.[40] Other substances that may be considered in this class include catnip, locoweed, morning glory seeds, and nutmeg. These are used in a variety of ways, including smoking and eating.

Psilocybin and mescaline have been used in religious rites by cultures in the Western hemisphere for centuries. MDA was first synthesized in the 1930s and used as an appetite suppressant. LSD was first synthesized in 1938, and the first "trip" that was documented occurred in 1943 when the drug was accidentally ingested.

The use of LSD was prohibited in 1965. Before that time it had been used as a therapeutic treatment for neurotic and psychotic patients. Some medical experiments were conducted in the use of this drug with alcoholics and terminal cancer patients.

Pathophysiology

Most of the effects of hallucinogens are *psychologic,* although *nausea* and *vomiting* are not uncommon reactions. These drugs act as stimulants at first and produce *anxiety, depressed appetite, dilated pupils,* and *increases in body temperature, heart rate,* and *respirations.* With psilocybin, dizziness, numbness of the face, and shivering may also occur. Tolerance to these drugs occurs rather quickly (usually after 3 days of use), and there is cross tolerance among the four drugs.[40]

Hallucinogens also may have a profound psychologic effect on most people. The effect has been described as a process of *amplification,* with the drug acting as a *catalyst.* Hallucinogens amplify the users' experience of the environment and put them in touch with thoughts and feelings. In low doses, MDA produces a peaceful euphoria. With higher doses, it mimics LSD experiences minus the hallucinations.

All four drugs produce *altered sensory awareness.* The senses become more acute, and it is thought that colors can be heard and sounds seen. Fantasies and illusions occur, along with hallucination-like happenings, although the user is aware that they are not real. With LSD the mood changes can be rapid. Past and present experiences meld together, and some have described a feeling of "oneness, compassion, and love for all things."

The feelings brought on by MDA, mescaline, and psilocybin last from 6 to 8 hours, whereas those of LSD usually last from 8 to 12 hours. Toward the end of the "trip," the person will gradually reenter reality. A "bad trip" often is a reflection of the emotional state of the person or a contaminated drug.

Flashbacks may occur with the use of hallucinogens. In these the user reexperiences the effects of the drug without having taken it. *Bad trips are described as being characterized by tremendous confusion, unpleasant sensory images,* and *extreme panic.* Care during these situations includes getting the person into a nonstimulating environment and staying with the person until the effects of the trip wear off. Reassuring the person that he or she is experiencing a drug trip is helpful.

Although there have been no reports of deaths from LSD, there have been documented instances in which the person died as a result of trying to do something impossible while on a "trip." An example of this is trying to fly, that is, the person actually believes he or she will be able to fly, and may jump from a high place.

Phencyclidine

Phencyclidine (PCP) is a synthetic drug that is generally described as an *anesthetic-hallucinogen.* However, it is chemically unrelated to hallucinogens such as LSD or mescaline. It is water soluble and is stored in fatty tissue. As a result it has a long half-life.

PCP was first synthesized in 1957 and tested as a general anesthetic for humans. Testing stopped in the mid-1960s because of side effects of *agitation* and *delirium.* It presently is available as an anesthetic agent for use by veterinarians. In the 1960s and 1970s the drug became available as a street drug. It was banned from legal manufacture in 1978 but it is still produced illegally.

PCP, produced as a white or yellowish white powder, has a variety of forms, including tablets and capsules. As *angel dust* it is sprinkled on tobacco or marijuana and smoked. When it is combined with marijuana it is called *sheba.* PCP may also be injected or snorted. See Box 13-13 for common street names for PCP.[40]

13-13	**Common street names for PCP**	
	Angel dust	Embalming fluid
	Animal tranquilizer	KJ killer
	Crystal	Peace pill
	Dust	Synthetic marijuana
	Hog	

13-14	Physical effects of PCP	
	Dose	Effects
	5 mg	Physical sedation
		Numbness of extremities
		Loss of muscle coordination
		Dizziness
		Constricted pupils, blurred or double vision, and involuntary eye movement
		Flushing and profuse sweating
		Nausea and vomiting
		Increase in blood pressure, heart rate, and respiratory rate (breathing is shallow)
	5 to 10 mg	Marked drop in blood pressure, breathing, and heart rates
		Shivering, increased salivation, and watering of the eyes
		Loss of balance, dizziness, and rigidity of muscles
		In some cases, repetitive movements, such as rocking
		Analgesic and anesthetic properties apparent
	Over 10 mg	Extreme agitation followed by seizures or coma
		Symptoms similar to mental confusion and delusion similar to schizophrenia

From Scott L: *PCP* (pamphlet), Charlotte, NC, 1981, The Drug Center, Inc.

13-15	Psychologic effects of PCP	
	Low dose	Euphoria and sense of alcohol-like intoxication
		Changes in body image
		Mood swings from ecstasy to panic
		Hallucinations and confusion about time and space
		In final stage in some cases, a sense of despair and emotional isolation
		Feeling of paranoia
		Sense of impending death
	Moderate dose	Increase in effects felt at low dose
		Loss of sense of contact with environment
	High dose	Symptoms of mental and emotional confusion similar to schizophrenia

From Scott, L: PCP (pamphlet), Charlotte, NC, 1981, The Drug Center, Inc.

Pathophysiology

Different doses of PCP provide different physical effects. These can be found in Box 13-14.

Psychologic effects of PCP ingestion last from 1 to 6 hours, with 24 hours needed to return to baseline. Research seems to indicate that the bad trip rate of PCP is five times that of other drugs. Chronic users may have flashbacks. The dose of PCP may indicate the nature of the effects. These are found in Box 13-14. Toxic reactions to PCP are not only life threatening but tend to be the longest-acting of any reactions produced by a drug of abuse.

Although there is disagreement about whether PCP is physically addictive, there is wide agreement that it is psychologically habit forming. Abruptly stopping the use of PCP can result in feelings of fearfulness, tremors, and in some cases, facial twitching.

PCP overdoses are dangerous because the person may die as a result of *respiratory or cardiac arrest.* Symptoms of PCP intoxication include variable responses such as the following:

1. Violence or combativeness to near unconsciousness
2. Little or no response to pain
3. Inability to speak
4. Elevated blood pressure and pulse rate with slight fever
5. Comalike state

The person intoxicated by PCP becomes more agitated by noise, bright lights, and talking.[40]

PCP may result in psychosis that lasts from several days to 6 weeks. It is often mistaken for acute schizophrenia. Individuals may be actively suicidal and become depressed when the acute psychosis has passed.

During an acute reaction to PCP, the nurse protects the patient from injury as well as protecting others from being injured by the patient. The patient's behavior may be highly unpredictable and the event is treated as a psychiatric emergency. See Box 13-15 for psychologic effects of different doses of PCP.

Narcotics

Narcotics are drugs that are derived from the opium poppy or produced synthetically. The use of narcotics has been recorded far back in history. Synthetic production of narcotics has occurred in the past 30 to 50 years. In general, narcotics lower the perception of pain.

Heroin is one narcotic that is abused to a great extent. There is some evidence recently that as sources of cocaine are decreasing, use of heroin is increasing. The shift has been toward younger addicts of heroin. On the street, heroin is known as *H, horse, junk, hard stuff, smack,* or *scag.* The use of heroin is an expensive habit; addicts frequently resort to crime to support their habit.

There are several different forms of narcotics. See Table 13-4 for a listing of these drugs, their medical use, and route of administration.

Pathophysiology

Effects of the use of narcotics include *shallow breathing; reduced hunger, thirst,* and *sexual drive;* and *drowsiness.* The person may also experience *euphoria, lethargy, heaviness of limbs,* and *apathy.* The ability to concentrate is lost, along with judgment and self-control. Overdoses of narcotics can cause coma, convulsions, respiratory arrest, and death. As in the case of heroin, when the drug is injected, there are

Table 13-4   Narcotics

Name	Medical use	Route of administration
Heroin	None in the United States	By injection or sniffing
Morphine	Ease pain	By injection, smoking, or by mouth
Opium	Ease pain, treat diarrhea, and suppress cough	By mouth or smoking
Codeine	Suppress cough and reduce pain	By mouth or injection
Meperidine	Relieve pain	By mouth or injection
Methadone	Ease pain and help those dependent on heroin	By mouth or injection

From O'Brien, R, and Cohen, S: The encyclopedia of drug abuse, New York, 1984, Facts on File, Inc.

associated risks of hepatitis, acquired immune deficiency syndrome (AIDS), and other infections such as septicemia. Narcotic addicts develop both *tolerance* and *physical and psychologic addiction*. Withdrawal may be uncomfortable and should be under medical supervision. Clonidine (catepres) is often used for purposes of detoxification from narcotics.

The heavier the usage, the longer detoxification may take. Symptoms of withdrawal may include nausea, cramps, chills, sweating, watery eyes, running nose, and restlessness.[40]

Methadone may also be used to withdraw the narcotic abuser safely. However, much controversy exists about methadone clinics. Recent research has shown that buprenorphine may have positive benefits in the treatment of opiate addiction. It reduces the high from heroin or other narcotics, has a history of good compliance, and may reduce cocaine use in opiate addicts.[11]

Cannabis

Cannabis, or *marijuana*, comes from the Indian hemp plant. It can grow wild or is fairly easily cultivated. Marijuana is usually smoked as a cigarette (joint, reefer) or in a pipe. Other drug paraphernalia may be used, including "bongs." There are many slang terms for marijuana, including *dope, grass, herb, joint, pot, reefer, roach, smoke, snuff,* and *weed.*

Marijuana has been used both medically and nonmedically for more than 3000 years. It has been used since the 1850s in the United States. Its popularity as a street drug began in the twentieth century. It is still one of the most popular and commonly abused drugs, especially among young people.[57] In the 1988 household survey by the National Institute on Drug Abuse (NIDA), 21.1 million Americans reported use of marijuana in the past year, and 65.7 million reported having used marijuana at least once.[20]

Hashish, or *hash*, is a resinous extract of the leaves and flowering part of the marijuana plant. It is more concentrated than marijuana and has more intense effects.

Marijuana's role in reducing eye pressure in glaucoma patients and controlling side effects of cancer chemotherapy, especially nausea, is being evaluated in research studies.

Pathophysiology

Physical effects of marijuana include drying of the eyes and mouth, increase in appetite, reddening of the eyes, and impairment of short-term memory. It also impacts the way stress affects the heart and circulation, and it raises the heart rate and blood pressure. Lowered body temperature, loss of coordination, and possible confusion and distortion of reality may occur. In addition, research indicates that marijuana may affect chromosome segregation during cell division leading to birth defects. Because marijuana is a fat-soluble molecule, parts of it may be stored in the body for up to 30 days or more.[57]

Psychologic effects of marijuana include an *altering of perception* of sight, sound, touch, sense of time, and taste. The user usually has a feeling of well-being and intoxication, although depression and panic may occur. Psychologic addiction develops in users. Crisis situations may occur in the form of an anxiety reaction to the marijuana high. A calming and reassuring approach has been found to be helpful.

Deliriants

Deliriants are any chemicals that give off fumes or vapors, that, when inhaled, produce symptoms similar to intoxication. They may also be called *inhalants*. Vasodilators such as amyl and butyl nitrite are also considered inhalants.

The fumes or vapors from inhalants are sniffed through the nose, or the vapors are put into a bag or captured in a balloon to increase the concentration of the inhaled fumes.

The history of the use of inhalants is traced back to ancient Greece. Sniffing of glue and other commercial products and solvents was first documented in the 1950s. There is no medical use for commercially prepared inhalants. Of course, vasodilators and anesthetic agents have a legitimate medical purpose.

The deliriants or inhalants have a *psychoactive* or *mood-altering effect* when the vapors are inhaled or sniffed. Most fall into one of the three following categories.[57]

1. Solvents
2. Aerosol sprays
3. Anesthetics

Solvents include commercial products that are *not* commonly thought of as drugs. They are fat soluble and easily cross the blood-brain barrier to produce a change in the state of consciousness.

Some inhalants cause tolerance. Physical dependence is a possibility. Symptoms of withdrawal have included chills, hallucinations, headaches, stomach pains, cramps, and delirium tremens.

The psychologic effects of deliriants include a feeling of stimulation and energy. At higher doses, the user may feel intoxicated. Psychologic dependence is likely.

Use of large amounts of aerosols or solvents can cause death as a result of *cardiac arrest* following dysrhythmias. Death from inhalants is usually caused by *suffocation* because of the displacement of oxygen in the lungs. Sniffing inhalants from a bag or balloon increases the risk of suffocation. Misuse of commercial aerosol products used to chill food have been reported to cause death by freezing of the lungs of the user.

The CNS effect of inhalants are *potentiated* by other CNS depressants. This increases the chances of overdose.[57]

Nursing Process
Assessment
Subjective data

Subjective data of drug use include the same factors listed in the assessment section for alcoholism found on p. 249. Although the alcoholic may underestimate the use of alcohol, the drug abuser may deliberately overestimate the amount used in order to convince health professionals of the need to prescribe large amounts of drugs during the detoxification period.

Objective data

Objective data for drug abuse include the factors listed in the section on alcoholism. In addition, the individual may show the following symptoms:
1. Abrupt changes in behavior; mood swings
2. Loss of interest in school, work, sports, and social or other activities
3. Frequent talking and reading about drugs
4. Loss of appetite
5. Presence of "track marks"

Breaks in the skin are an objective sign that must be noted when assessing for drug addiction. If the person has been *mainlining* (that is, injecting the drug directly into the vein), needle marks, scars, or small scabs can be seen on the hands and forearms or the instep. However, many other veins are used as points of entry to conceal addiction, including the dorsal vein of the penis and the conjunctival artery of the eyelid.

Because of the expense involved, users often sell their belongings, steal, or become prostitutes to get money to supply their drug habit. Abuse of drugs costs the American economy millions of dollars each day.

Occasionally, patients must be given narcotics to control pain over a long period of time and nurses may worry about them becoming addicted. It is rare, however, for addiction to develop in those patients given narcotics for real pain, and nurses should not let the fear of the development of addiction keep them from administering prescribed narcotics to patients hospitalized and in pain. This is important because studies have indicated that many patients are *undermedicated* because nurses hesitate to give narcotics as prescribed.

Diagnostic tests

One diagnostic test used to test for drug abuse is urine or blood drug testing. Some employers demand "clean urines" as a condition of employment. Members of sports teams are asked to give samples at regular intervals. Jobs may be lost as a result of drugs in the urine.

The amount of time after use that drugs can be detected in the urine varies from a very short time for alcohol and cocaine to a long time for benzodiazepines and cannabis. In fact, cannabis may be found in the urine for as long as a *month* after the last use. It is possible to have a minimally positive drug test for cannabis because of a long period of "passive inhalation" from close contact with someone smoking and exhaling marijuana fumes.

Urine testing is usually not used to detect alcohol because it is metabolized very rapidly. Alcohol blood levels are much more accurate. The breathalyzer is used by law enforcement agencies to determine alcohol levels in the blood.

Although some persons are concerned that routine testing violates civil liberties, efforts will continue to develop an accurate objective method for determining whether a person is under the influence of drugs or alcohol.

Other diagnostic tests that may be used include testing for hepatitis and HIV. Blood cultures may show the presence of septicemia.

Data analysis: nursing diagnoses

See this section in the discussion of alcoholism in this chapter (p. 250).

Planning: expected patient outcomes

The reader is referred to this section in the part of this chapter dealing with alcoholism (p. 250). The nursing diagnoses and patient outcomes are the same whether the person is abusing alcohol or another drug.

Implementation

Table 13-5 lists the symptoms and treatment for acute intoxication and withdrawal. Rehabilitation follows the same guidelines discussed for the treatment of the alcoholic (p. 251). Today, most treatment centers treat alcoholics and drug addicts together because the majority of persons receiving treatment for chemical dependency have a history of abuse of both alcohol and drugs.

A real challenge for health professionals is how to handle the manipulation of the drug-addicted patient; they may be more intimidating and threatening to deal with than the alcoholic patient. Nurses caring for these persons need to set specific limits on behavior. They should be aware that some patients may attempt to obtain drugs even when hospitalized, including stealing drugs from the medication area.

Assisting with achievement of therapeutic goals
Methadone maintenance

One approach to the treatment of narcotic addiction is the *methadone maintenance program*. Methadone is a synthetic drug, and the average narcotic user's daily dose is much less expensive than that for heroin or morphine. The drug is given legally as a part of a rehabilitation program that should include group or individual therapy or both. Methadone reduces the severity of heroin withdrawal, and the user can maintain employment while undergoing treatment. Methadone itself is addictive and the use of it must be tapered off or the person may continue the habit for the rest of his or her life. Because methadone is easily

Table 13-5   Acute intoxication and withdrawal of mind-altering drugs

| Drug group | Acute intoxication | | Withdrawal symptoms |
	Symptoms	Treatment	
Narcotics	Respiratory depression, depressed respirations (12 or below) bradycardia, hypotension, cold clammy skin, decreased body temperature; deep sleep, stupor, or coma; pinpoint pupils	Maintain ventilation, provide oxygen Give narcotic antagonist: naloxone (Narcan) 0.4 mg IV Monitor vital signs every 15 to 30 min until patient is conscious Treat for shock	*Not life threatening* Early; restlessness, irritability, drug craving, yawning, lacrimation, diaphoresis, rhinorrhea; followed by "yen" sleep (intense desire to sleep; sleeps restlessly) Later: awakens with more severe symptoms, nausea, vomiting, anorexia, abdominal cramps, bone and muscle pain, tremors, piloerection ("gooseflesh")
Other CNS depressants	Same as narcotics (above)	Lavage if recent oral ingestion Maintain ventilation, provide oxygen Monitor vital signs every 15 to 30 min until patient is conscious Position patient side-lying or prone, not supine Treat for shock Hemodialysis for renal shutdown	*May be life threatening* Insomnia, restlessness, tremors, anorexia, followed by convulsions, and symptoms similar to delirium tremens (confusion, visual and auditory hallucinations), fever, dehydration
CNS stimulants	Labile cardiovascular symptoms (flushing or pallor, pulse and blood pressure changes, dysrhythmias), hyperpyrexia, mental disturbances (agitation, paranoia, hallucinations), convulsions, circulatory collapse	Give chlorpromazine, 25 to 50 mg IM Provide a quiet environment Orient patient to reality Monitor vital signs until stable	*Withdrawal is not severe* Somnolence, apathy, irritability, depression, fatigue
Hallucinogens	Physiologic toxicity low at doses that produce strong psychologic effects Acute panic reaction ("bad trip") may lead to suicide "Flashback" episodes Prolonged psychotic disorders (paranoia, depression) Phencyclidine: CNS depression or stimulation may lead to death	Provide quiet, supportive environment and constant attention Give diazepam (Valium), 2 to 10 mg IM for severe anxiety	No evidence of withdrawal symptoms
Cannabis	Adverse reactions infrequent Simple depression, paranoid ideation, confusion, disorientation, hallucinations	Provide support and reassurance Give tranquilizer for agitation	*Withdrawal symptoms rare* Insomnia, anorexia

available through legal channels and permits the person to work, some experts believe that using it is essentially the same as taking maintenance doses of other drugs such as insulin, steroids, or digoxin. *There are other experts, however, who believe that methadone treatment should be abolished because it promotes substance abuse.*

Treatment programs

Long-term residential programs were started in the 1970s and 1980s. Today they have been largely replaced by inpatient detoxification programs, drug and alcohol rehabilitation programs, and outpatient services. Much of the treatment of substance abusers is now taking place in day programs or outpatient settings. Relapse prevention programs have been instituted in many areas of the country.

Treatment helps the chemically dependent person focus on his or her use of drugs or alcohol. These programs attempt to help the person increase self-understanding and to change life-style. Group therapy is provided.

Halfway houses or three-quarter houses (which are less structured than halfway houses), are shorter-term residential settings that admit persons after they have completed residential treatment and assist them in reentry to the community. The usual length of stay in a halfway house is 3 to 6 months.

Risk of disease

Because many addicts inject drugs they are at risk for diseases such as hepatitis and AIDS. Often addicts share needles and equipment or reuse them without sterilizing them between periods of use. Addicts may also demonstrate resistance to more responsible use of drugs or equipment because of impulsivity and the need for the immediate relief provided by the drug.

Estimates of intravenous drug users who test positive for the AIDS virus are from 50% to 75% in some metropolitan areas such as New York City. Efforts to assist them in using clean or new equipment have not been very successful up to this point. Some have advocated supplying the addict with clean needles for no charge. This is not suggested to condone drug use, but as a means to prevent the spread of disease. The risk of AIDS for drug users is especially critical because they spread the disease to both men and women and to infants born to these women. Because of their mental condition while under the influence of drugs they may not remember the persons with whom they had sexual contact or shared drug equipment.

Interventions to achieve patient outcomes
Facilitating learning

The teaching for the patient with substance abuse is the same as that for the alcoholic patient (p. 253). It is especially important to teach about over-the-counter drugs that may be a hazard to the recovering person. These include the antihistamines, benadryl, which is included in some over-the-counter cold medications, and diet pills.

Evaluation

The evaluation of care of the patient who is a drug abuser is the same as that for the alcoholic patient (see p. 255).

Nursing Care Plan	**Person with substance abuse**

DATA: Mrs. T. is a 50-year-old secretary who was admitted to the emergency room after having been found lying in the snow. She was disoriented and had the smell of alcohol on her breath. Her blood alcohol level was 0.23. Her temperature was 97.4° and the respiratory rate was 10. Blood pressure was 90/56 and her pulse was 50. Physical examination showed an enlarged liver, as well as petechiae over parts of her body. She had dry skin in general. Laboratory studies showed low hemoglobin and hematocrit levels, a low RBC count, and elevated liver function test results. X-ray films showed two broken ribs. The urine screen was positive for Valium. Mrs. T. was started on Librium 25 to 50 mg q4h. She was admitted for observation and detoxification.

Because of her intoxicated state, it was difficult to obtain a nursing history. Her husband stated that she drank at least a pint of gin per day. In addition she was taking Valium that had been prescribed by her family doctor. Her husband stated that she hadn't been eating well for several months. He wasn't sure when the drinking started, but knew it had been going on for several years.

Collaborative nursing actions include those to prevent further complications caused by possible aspiration or alcohol withdrawal. Immediate reporting of signs and symptoms may prevent serious effects. Nursing actions include monitoring for the following:
1. Signs of respiratory difficulty caused by secretions or alcohol effects: slower, shallower breathing; inability to rouse; aspiration of vomitus.
2. Signs of alcohol withdrawal: diaphoresis, tachycardia, hypertension, tremors, nausea or vomiting, restlessness, or hallucinations
3. Seizures: presence of abnormal muscle movement without aura
4. Signs of delirium tremens: visual and tactile hallucinations, nightmares, insomnia, extreme restlessness or irritability

Continued.

Nursing Care Plan | Person with substance abuse—cont'd

Nursing diagnosis: Airway clearance, ineffective: related to fatigue and infection

Expected patient outcomes	Nursing interventions	Rationale
Mrs. T. will maintain patent airway	Keep head of bed at 30-degree angle	Position will help respiratory effort
	If LOC occurs	Turn on side to prevent aspiration
	Observe her carefully for aspiration	Aspiration may occur because of nausea and impaired mental status
	Have suction machine at bedside	Suction may be needed to clear airway

Nursing diagnosis: Breathing pattern, ineffective: related to cognitive impairment from effects of alcohol

Expected patient outcomes	Nursing interventions	Rationale
Mrs. T. will maintain adequate breathing pattern	Assess respiratory rate at regular intervals	Effects of alcohol can cause respiratory depression
	Give no medications that would further compromise respirations (such as morphine)	Some medications potentiate the effects of alcohol

Nursing diagnosis: Potential fluid volume deficit, high risk for related to decreased access to fluids and diuretic effect of alcohol

Expected patient outcomes	Nursing interventions	Rationale
Mrs. T.'s fluid volume will be maintained at optimal level	Weigh Mrs. T. daily	Comparing daily weights is most accurate way to determine fluid volume
	When Mrs. T. is more alert, offer fluids, including juices	Extra fluid will help correct fluid deficit
	Use intravenous fluids as ordered	IV feeding may be necessary in the presence of nausea or vomiting

Nursing diagnosis: Hypothermia: related to malnutrition and alcohol ingestion, as well as time spent in snow

Expected patient outcomes	Nursing interventions	Rationale
Mrs. T.'s temperature will be within normal limits	Monitor Mrs. T.'s temperature frequently	Temperature should increase gradually
	Check extremities for signs of frostbite	Decreased body temperature and time in snow may have caused decreased blood supply to the area
	Use extra blankets on bed to help Mrs. T. warm to normal temperature	Use of blankets should be adequate to assist in warming patient

Nursing diagnosis: Infection, high risk for: related to decreased nutrition and fractured ribs

Expected patient outcomes	Nursing interventions	Rationale
Mrs. T. will not develop atelectasis	Encourage coughing and deep breathing q4h	May be reluctant to breathe deeply because of fractured ribs
	Assist in changing position q2-3h	Changing position will assist with lung expansion

Nursing diagnosis: Injury, potential for: trauma, related to lack of awareness of environmental hazards

Expected patient outcomes	Nursing interventions	Rationale
Mrs. T. will be free of injury from withdrawal from alcohol	Give Librium as ordered to prevent withdrawal symptoms	Most alcoholic patients require medication
	Orient Mrs. T. frequently to place and time	She may be confused
	Keep bed side rails up	Used to prevent falling from bed
	Observe for signs of delirium tremens or seizures	She may need more aggressive medical treatment
	Give multivitamins, including B vitamins and thiamine as ordered	B vitamins and thiamine needed to prevent or decrease complications such as Wernicke-Korsakoff syndrome

Nursing diagnosis: Nutrition, altered: less than body requirements, due to anorexia and disinterest in eating

Expected patient outcomes	Nursing interventions	Rationale
Mrs. T.'s nutritional status is improved	Encourage snacks	Patient may not be able to tolerate large meals because of nausea or gastritis
	Encourage well-balanced meals	Good nutrition is important in preventing long term complicaitons from alcoholism
	Consult with dietician about need for special diet	Abnormal liver function studies may necessitate protein restriction

Mrs. T. is successfully detoxified from alcohol using Librium over the next 3 days. She is persuaded to accept treatment and is transferred to a nearby treatment facility. At this time additional nursing diagnoses are evident. These include those that follow:

Nursing diagnosis: Adjustment, impaired: related to disability requiring change in life-style and altered locus of control

Expected patient outcomes	Nursing interventions	Rationale
Mrs. T. will make positive adjustment to disease concept	Educate Mrs. T. about disease concept of alcoholism	Education will help with adjustment
	Encourage Mrs. T. to share experiences with other patients in group and informally	Peer support will assist with adjustment
	Encourage Mrs. T. to complete assignments directed at breaking down denial	Self-knowledge will assist in adjustment
	Have Mrs. T. attend AA meetings	Necessary for long-term adjustment

Nursing diagnosis: Anxiety: related to situational crisis

Expected patient outcomes	Nursing interventions	Rationale
Mrs. T. will demonstrate minimal anxiety	Encourage Mrs. T. to share feelings and concerns	Sharing feelings will ease anxiety
	Educate Mrs. T. about importance of not taking medications to ease anxiety	Mrs. T. will not be able to medicate feelings
	Teach Mrs. T. relaxation exercises	Will ease anxiety
	Have Mrs. T. keep feelings log	Will help Mrs. T. identify sources of anxiety
	Educate Mrs. T. on 12 steps of AA	Turning life and will over to higher power will lessen anxiety

Continued.

Nursing Care Plan — Person with substance abuse—cont'd

Nursing diagnosis: Family process, altered: related to situational crisis

Expected patient outcomes	Nursing interventions	Rationale
Mrs. T.'s family will demonstrate positive family processes	Encourage Mrs. T.'s family to attend family program	Knowledge of disease will assist family to recover
	Encourage Mrs. T. to keep in contact with family	Their support of patient is important to her recovery

Nursing diagnosis: Knowledge deficit (alcoholism) related to lack of exposure and lack of interest in learning

Expected patient outcomes	Nursing interventions	Rationale
Mrs. T. will verbalize understanding of alcoholism	Teach Mrs. T. about disease concept of alcoholism	Well-informed patient will be better able to stay sober
Mrs. T. will verbalize understanding of need to abstain from alcohol and mood-altering drugs	Teach Mrs. T. about drugs to avoid	See above
Mrs. T. will verbalize knowledge of complications of substance abuse	Teach Mrs. T. about complications	See above
Mrs. T. will verbalize knowledge of importance of good nutrition	Teach Mrs. T. about optimal nutrition	Good nutrition is important to prevent complications of alcoholism
Mrs. T. will verbalize knowledge of relaxation techniques	Teach Mrs. T. about ways to reduce stress	Mrs. T. will no longer be able to medicate stress
Mrs. T. will verbalize knowledge of importance of aftercare, including AA	Teach Mrs. T. about importance of aftercare	Aftercare has been found to be essential for continued sobriety

Nursing diagnosis: Powerlessness: related to alcoholism

Expected patient outcomes	Nursing interventions	Rationale
Mrs. T. will verbalize knowledge of powerlessness	Assist Mrs. T. in learning about and taking first step in AA	First step of AA involves admitting powerlessness
		Recognition of powerlessness is important for continued recovery

Nursing diagnosis: Self-esteem disturbance: related to change in life-style

Expected patient outcomes	Nursing interventions	Rationale
Mrs. T. will verbalize positive self-concept	Give Mrs. T. positive reinforcement of work and breakthroughs	Will assist in building self-esteem
	Demonstrate to Mrs. T. that she is not unique	Alcoholics tend to think they are unique
	Encourage Mrs. T. to share with other alcoholics	They will be support to her

Nursing diagnosis: Spiritual distress: related to personal/spiritual values

Expected patient outcomes	Nursing interventions	Rationale
Mrs. T. will verbalize less spiritual distress	Encourage Mrs. T. to learn about 12 steps of AA	12 steps of AA will assist patient in regaining sense of spirituality
	Ask chaplain to see Mrs. T. if she wishes	Source of support
	Encourage Mrs. T. to talk about prayers at AA meetings	This may surprise patients at first
	Encourage Mrs. T. to talk about difference between spirituality and religion	Many patients may be turned off by formal religion

IMPAIRED NURSES

Over the last several years many states have developed programs to assist nurses who are impaired by either alcohol or drugs. This has occurred for a number of reasons, one of the main ones being that the rate of chemical dependency among nurses and other health providers is *greater* than that of the general public. Part of the reason for this is that health care workers have greater access to mood-altering substances and many of them are in very stressful jobs. For instance, nurses may handle narcotics every day and may succumb to the temptation to use them. Before the inception of *Peer Assistance Programs*, through either state boards of nursing or state nursing associations, the nurse would often be fired and would be free to migrate to another facility, where the cycle of drug abuse would continue.

In March 1978 nurses from several states attended a meeting held in Manhattan to discuss the problems of the alcoholic nurse. By 1980 two organizations of nurses interested in alcoholism were active in encouraging help for impaired nurses. These were the Drug and Alcohol Nursing Association (DANA) and the National Nurses Society on Addiction (NNSA). In 1981 the American Nurses Association (ANA) created a Task Force on Addiction and Psychological Disturbance to formulate guidelines for state nursing associations to develop programs to help the impaired nurse. At the 1982 ANA convention, the American Nurses Association adopted a resolution that recognized the profession's responsibility to assist the nurse who is impaired.

In 1980 two states, Maryland and Ohio, had peer assistance programs in place. By April 1982 four state programs were in place and, as of fall 1983, 25 states either had programs in place or were planning to start one. As of 1991, only a few states do not have such a program.

Peer Assistance Programs have several goals: (1) to assist the nurse who is impaired to receive treatment; (2) to protect the public from the untreated nurse; (3) to help the recovering nurse reenter nursing in a systematic, planned, and safe way; and (4) to assist in monitoring the continued recovery of the nurse for a period of time, usually 2 years. The reentry of the nurse may include the restriction from handling narcotics for a period of time.

The basis of these programs is one nurse helping another nurse. Most volunteers in these programs are nurses who are recovering themselves or are working in the field of chemical dependency or psychiatric nursing. The program can work very effectively in states where the Peer Assistance Program, the state board of nursing, hospital administration, and law enforcement agencies all work together to assist the impaired nurse and safeguard the public.

CODEPENDENCY

The term *codependency* often has been used to describe a person who is emotionally involved with a chemically dependent person. The codependent is someone who develops an unhealthy pattern of coping as a reaction to someone else's drug or alcohol use. *Recently, however, the definition of codependency has been expanded. It is now seen as a disease entity with a definable onset, a set of physical and psychologic symptoms, and a predictable medical course.*

Definitions of codependency vary, but there is agreement that the person manifests dysfunctional responses to life and that he or she derive self-esteem from the ability to control themselves and others.

Characteristics of codependency include the following[11]:
1. Perfectionism
2. Denial
3. Poor communication
4. Caretaking
5. Inability to identify, express, and manage feelings
6. Difficulty forming and maintaining close relationships
7. Feeling responsible for others' behavior or feelings
8. Constantly seeking the approval of others
9. Feelings of powerlessness
10. Feeling morally superior
11. Difficulty in setting limits
12. Feeling "super-responsible" or "super-irresponsible"
13. Martyrdom
14. Need to control
15. Any addictive behavior
16. Stress-related illness

Many nurses suffer from the disease of codependency. It is thought to be a chief cause of "burn-out." Nurses who give too much of themselves to others become depleted.

Recovery from codependency starts with the person learning to care for himself or herself. The use of a journal to record feelings may be helpful. Breaking through the denial of the codependent is often difficult. The person also requires help to learn to set appropriate boundaries, grieve past losses, and acquire the skill of reparenting. Daily affirmations may be used to reinforce the self-worth of the person.[14]

FOCUS ON THE FUTURE
Goals for the Year 2000

The report to the Surgeon General on health goals for the year 2000 contained several recommendations regarding alcohol and other drugs. The goals include the following:
1. Reduce deaths caused by alcohol-related motor vehicle crashes to no more than 8.5 per 100,000 people from an age adjusted baseline of 9.8 per 100,000 in 1987. Special target populations for this goal are presented in Table 13-6.[45]

Table 13-6   Alcohol-related motor vehicle crash deaths per 100,000[45]

	1987 Baseline	2000 Target
American Indians/Alaskan men	52.2%	44.8%
People aged 15-24	21.5%	18.0%

Table 13-7   **Target goals for high school seniors who perceive social disapproval with use of drugs**[45]

Behavior	1989 Baseline	2000 Target
Heavy use of alcohol	56.4%	70%
Occasional use of marijuana	71.1%	85%
Trying cocaine once or twice	88.9%	95%

Table 13-8   **Target goals for high school seniors who associate physical or psychologic harm with use of drugs**[45]

Behavior	1989 Behavior	2000 Target
Heavy use of alcohol	44%	70%
Regular use of marijuana	71.5%	90%
Trying cocaine once or twice	54.9%	80%

2. Reduce cirrhosis deaths to no more than 6 per 100,000 people from an age-adjusted baseline of 9.1 per 100,000 in 1987.
3. Reduce drug-related deaths to no more than 3 per 100,000 people from an age-adjusted baseline of 3.8 in 1987.
4. Reduce drug abuse-related hospital emergency department visits by at least 20%. No baseline data was available at the time the report was published.

Risk reduction objectives related to alcohol and other drugs include the following:

1. Increase by at least 1 year the average age for first use of cigarettes, alcohol, and marijuana by adolescents aged 12 to 17. Baseline was age 11.6 for cigarettes, age 13.1 for alcohol, and age 13.4 for marijuana in 1988.
2. Reduce the proportion of high school seniors and college students engaging in heavy drinking of alcohol to no more than 28% of high school seniors and 32% of college students. Baseline was 33% of high school seniors and 41.7% of college students in 1989.
3. Reduce alcohol consumption by people aged 14 and older to an annual average of no more than 2 gallons of alcohol per person.
4. Increase the proportion of high school seniors who perceive social disapproval associated with the heavy use of alcohol, occasional use of marijuana, and experimentation with cocaine as follows (Table 13-7).
5. Increase the proportion of high school seniors who associate risk of physical or psychologic harm with heavy use of alcohol, regular use of marijuana, and experimentation with cocaine as shown in Table 13-8.

All 50 states are developing plans to meet these and other recommendations. It is evident that there is increased public awareness of the problems related to drug abuse. Organizations like Mothers Against Driving Drunk (MADD) and Students Against Driving Drunk (SADD) have been active in urging those who drink to designate as a driver someone who will abstain from drinking. They also have been effective in getting the drinking age raised to 21 in all 50 states and in lobbying for stronger laws against those who drive under the influence of alcohol or other drugs.

Nurses can play an important role in these goals being achieved through counseling and teaching of the public, especially of teenagers and young adults.

SUMMARY

1. Substance abuse includes a complex set of behaviors known as addictions.
2. Examples of addictions include alcoholism, drug addiction, compulsive overeating, and compulsive gambling.
3. Alcoholism and drug addiction are commonly referred to as chemical dependency.
4. Dependency includes both physical and psychologic dependency and is defined as the need to continue use of drugs/alcohol to prevent withdrawal symptoms.
5. With increased use of alcohol and drugs, the person develops tolerance, which is defined as a decreased susceptibility to the effects of the substance.
6. Efforts to prevent substance abuse have included legal and educational efforts.
7. Enabling behavior by spouses and employers allows a person to continue the use of drugs and alcohol.
8. Interventions are planned confrontations by individuals who care about the person and present meaningful data in a nonjudgmental way.
9. The goal of an intervention is to have the substance abuser recognize and accept reality so that the need for help is accepted.
10. Alcoholism is the third major health problem in the United States, affecting at least 9 million persons.
11. Theories concerning the cause of alcoholism include physiologic, psychologic, and sociocultural or cultural-etiologic theories.
12. Alcohol is a central nervous system depressant that affects the brain by suppressing the activity of the neurotransmitter gamma aminobutyric acid (GABA).
13. The so-called stimulating effects of alcohol occur because the first areas of the brain affected are the higher centers affecting self-control and judgment.
14. The active ingredient in alcoholic beverages is ethyl alcohol or ethanol.
15. Ninety percent of alcohol is metabolized in the liver.
16. Because alcohol is not converted to glycogen, it cannot be stored and provides 200 kcal but no minerals or vitamins.
17. The amount of alcohol in the blood at any one time is called the blood alcohol level.
18. Fetal alcohol syndrome occurs in children whose moth-

ers drank several times daily; it includes mental retardation, microcephaly, growth deficiencies, and malformations of skeletal and urogenital systems.

19. Alcohol withdrawal includes symptoms ranging from
mild tremors to severe agitation and hallucinations.

20. Delirium tremens (DT) is an acute complication of
alcohol withdrawal. It is a serious medical concern
that has a 5% to 15% mortality rate and requires
aggressive treatment.

21. Medication used in the initial period of detoxification
includes chlordiazepoxide (Librium), phenytoin (Dilantin), magnesium sulfate, and multivitamins.

22. Wernicke-Korsakoff's syndrome is a complication of
alcoholism that includes symptoms of pscyhosis, amnesia, and apathy.

23. Alcoholics Anonymous (AA) is a group of self-acknowledged alcoholics whose aim is to stay sober and to help
other alcoholics to gain sobriety.

24. Using the twelve steps of AA will assist the alcoholic
to accept his or her powerlessness over alcohol.

25. Alcohol is considered a drug.

26. Drug habituation is repeated use of a drug to a point
where there is psychologic dependence.

27. Drug addiction includes craving, psychologic dependency, and physical dependence.

28. The basic categories of drugs include stimulants, depressants, hallucinogens, narcotics, cannabis, and de-
lirants.

29. Caffeine is the most accepted and used psychoactive
substance in the United States and is found in many
beverages and health products.

30. Flashbacks may occur with the use of hallucinogens
and include reexperiencing the effects of the drug
without retaking the drug.

31. Drug addicts who inject drugs are at increased risk of
contracting AIDS and hepatitis.

32. Nurses are at increased risk for the development of
chemical dependency and codependency.

33. The goals for year 2000 place emphasis on reducing
the number of deaths caused by alcohol-related motor
vehicle crashes and increasing by at least 1 year the
age at which adolescents first use cigarettes, alcohol,
or marijuana.

34. The goals also include increasing the proportion of
high school seniors who associate risk of physical or
psychologic harm with heavy use of alcohol, regular
use of marijuana, and experimentation with cocaine.

STUDY QUESTIONS

- Why does psychotherapy prove ineffective for the alcoholic or drug abusing patient who is not sober?
- Are there differences between the person who abuses
drugs and the person who abuses alcohol?
- What knowlege is it important to teach the alcoholic or
drug-addicted patient who is newly sober and leaving
treatment?
- Why are nurses prone to the development of chemical
dependency?
- Why does codependency lead to burnout in nurses?

REFERENCES AND SELECTED READINGS

1. American Medical Association Board of Trustees Report:
Drug abuse in the United States: strategies in prevention,
JAMA 265(16):2102-2107, 1991.
2. American Psychiatric Association: *Diagnostic and statistical
manual of mental disorders,* ed 3, Washington DC, 1987,
American Psychiatric Association.
3. Beattie M: *Co-dependent no more: how to stop controlling others
and start caring for yourself,* Center City, Minn, 1987, Ha-
zelton Foundation.
4. Bluhm J: *When you face the chemically dependent patient: a
practical guide for nurses,* St Louis, 1987, Ishiyaku Euro-
America Inc.
5.* Captain C: Family recovery from alcoholism: mediating family factors, *Nurs Clin North Am* 24(1):55-68, 1989.
6. Caroselli-Karinja M: Drug abuse and the elderly, *J Psychosoc
Nurs Ment Health Serv* 23:25-30, 1985.
7. Christ M, Hohloch F: *Gerontologic nursing,* Springhouse,
Pennsylvania, 1988, Springhouse Publishing Co.
8. Dixon S, Bejar R: Brain lesions in cocaine and methamphetamine exposed neonates, *Pediatr Res* 23405A, 1988.
9.* Dubiel D: Action stat! Cocaine overdose, *Nurs '90* 20(3):33,
1990.
10. Fitzgerald L: *Alcoholism: the genetic inheritance,* New York,
1988, Doubleday.
11. Frances R: Substance abuse, *JAMA* 265(23):3171-3172,
1991.
12. Green P: The chemically dependent nurse, *Nurs Clin North
Am* 24(1):81-94, 1989.
13. Grinspoon L, Bakalar J: Alcohol abuse and dependence, The
Harvard Medical School Mental Health Review, 1990.
14.* Hall S, Wray L: Codependency: nurses who give too much,
Am J Nurs 89(11):1456-1461, 1989.
15. House M: Cocaine, *Am J Nurs* 90(4):40-45, 1990.
16. Hughes T: Models and perspectives of addiction: implications
for treatment, *Nurs Clin North Am* 24(1):1-12, 1989.
17. Jack L: Use of milieu as a problem-solving strategy in addiction treatment, *Nurs Clin North Am* 24(1):69-80, 1989.
18. Jacques J, Snyder N: Newborn victims of addiction, *RN*
54(4):47-51, 1991.
19. Johnson L: How to diagnose and treat chemical dependency
in the elderly, *J Gerontol Nurs* 15(12):22-26, 38-39, 1989.
20. Johnson V. *Intervention,* Minneapolis, 1987, Johnson Institute.
21. Joyce C: The woman alcoholic, *Am J Nurs* 89(10):1314-1318,
1989.
22. Kimball B: The alcoholic woman's mad, mad world of denial
and mind games, Center City, Minn, 1987, Hazeldon Foundation.
23. Kircus E, Brillhart B: Dealing with substance abuse among
people with disabilities, *Rehab Nurs* 15(5):250-253, 1989.
24. Kirk E, Bradford, L: Effects of alcoholism on the CNS:
implications for the neuroscience nurse, *J Neurosci Nurs*
19(6):326-335, 1987.
25.* Levy G, Hickey J: Fighting the battle against drugs, *RN*
54(4):44-47, 1991.
25a*. Lippman H: Addicted nurses: tolerated, tormented, or
treated? *RN* 55(4):36-41, 1992.
26. Milkman H, Shafferm H, editors: *The addictions: multidisciplinary perspectives and treatments,* Lexington, 1985, DC
Heath & Co.
27.* Miller H: Addiction in a coworker: getting past the denial,
Am J Nurs 90(5):72-75, 1990.

*Recommended for student reading.

28. National Institute on Drug Abuse: National household survey on drug abuse: main findings 1988, DHHS Pub No (ADM)89-1636, Washington, DC, 1989, US Department of Health and Human Services.

29. National Institute on Drug Abuse: National household survey on drug abuse: main findings 1988, DHHS Pub No (ADM)90-1682, Washington, DC, 1990, US Department of Health and Human Services.

30. Nuckols C, Greenson J: Cocaine addiction: assessment and intervention, *Nurs Clin North Am* 24(1):33-44, 1989.

31. Oswald L: Cocaine addiction: the hidden diagnosis, *Arch Psych Nurs* 3(3):134-141, 1989.

32. Parette H: Nursing attitudes toward the geriatric alcoholic, *J Gerontol Nurs* 16(1):26-31, 28-29, 1990.

33.* Perrine M et al: Epidemiological perspectives on drunk driving. In Surgeon General's workshop on drunk driving: background papers, Washington, DC, 1989, US Department of Health and Human Services.

34.* Pires M: Substance abuse: the silent saboteur in rehabilitation, *Nurs Clin North Am* 24(1):291-296, 1989.

35. Povenmire K: Recognizing the cocaine addict, *Nurs 90* 20(5):46-48, 1990.

36. Public Health Service, Health United States 1989 and prevention profile, Washington, DC, 1990, US Department of Health and Human Services.

37. Rice D et al: The economic costs of alcohol and drug abuse and mental illness, San Francisco, 1990, Institute for health and aging.

38.* Rich J: Action stat: acute alcohol intoxication, *Nurs 89* 19(9):33, 1989.

39. Robins L, Przybeck T: Age of onset of drug use as a factor in drug and other disorders. (NIDA research monograph No 56.) In Jones C, Battjes R, editors: *Etiology of drug abuse: implications for prevention*, Washington, DC, 1985, US Department of Health and Human Services.

40. Schuckit M: Drug and alcohol abuse: a clinician's guide to detoxification and treatment, New York, 1989, Plenum Medical Book Co.

41.* Sullivan E: A descriptive study of nurses recovering from chemical dependency, *Arch Psychiatr Nurs* 1(3):194-200, 1987.

42. Sullivan E: Nursing and health care: the supplement: chemical dependency in the nursing profession (pamphlet), NLN Pub No 41-2365, 1990.

43.* Sullivan E et al: *Chemical dependency in nursing*, Menlo Park, California, 1988, Addison Wesley Publishing Co.

44. Tweed S: Identifying the alcoholic client, *Nurs Clin North Am* 24(1):13-32, 1989.

45. United States Department of Health and Human Services: Healthy people 2000: National health promotion and disease prevention objectives, Washington, DC, 1990, US Government Printing Office.

46. Vandagaer F: Cocaine, the deadliest addiction, *Nurs 89* 19(2):72-74, 1989.

47. Watson M, Gold M: *Cocaine: a clinician's handbook*, New York, 1987, Guildford Press.

48. Williams E: Strategies for intervention, *Nurs Clin North Am* 24(1):95-108, 1989.

49. Zerwekh J, Michaels B: Co-dependency: assessment and recovery, *Nurs Clin North Am* 24(1):109-120, 1989.

Classic

50. *Alcoholics Anonymous*, ed 3, New York, 1976, Alcoholics Anonymous World Services Inc.

51. American Nurses Association: States start assistance programs for impaired nurses, *Am Nurse* 15:6, 1983.

52. Bissell L, Haberman P: *Alcoholism in the professions*, New York, 1984, Oxford University Press.

53. Bissell L, Jones R: The alcoholic nurse, *Nurs Outlook* 29:96-101, 1981.

54. Johnson V: I'll quit tomorrow, San Francisco, 1980, Harper & Row.

55. Kandel D: Reaching the hard to reach: illicit drug use among high school absentees, *Addictive Diseases* 1:465-480, 1975.

56. O'Brien R, Chafetz M: *The encyclopedia of alcoholism*, New York, 1982, Facts on File Inc.

57. O'Brien R, Cohen S: *The encyclopedia of drug abuse*, New York, 1984, Facts on File Inc.

58. Scott L: PCP (pamphlet), Charlotte, NC, 1981, Charlotte Drug Educational Center Inc.

59. Symposium on alcoholism and drug addiction, *Nurs Clin North Am* 19:77-87, 1984.

60. Valiant G: Natural history of alcoholism: causes, patterns, and paths to recovery, Cambridge, Mass, 1983, Harvard University Press.

61. Zimberg S: *The clinical management of alcoholism*, New York, 1982, Brunner Mazel, Inc.

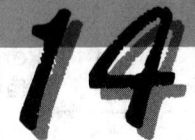

Chronic Illness

Wilma J. Phipps

After studying this chapter, the learner should be able to:

- Differentiate between acute and chronic illness.
- Describe factors that influence chronic illness.
- Identify areas of assessment for the chronically ill person.
- Describe physical and psychosocial interventions for the person with a chronic illness.
- Define rehabilitation and the roles of team members (especially the nurse) and of the patient.
- Describe different patterns and facilities for continuing care.
- Identify major health goals related to chronic health problems to be achieved by the year 2000.
- Describe provisions of the Americans with Disabilities Act.

Table 14-1 Persons with activity limitation, by selected chronic conditions and income, United States, 1980 and 1985 (figures in millions of persons affected)

| | 1980 | 1985 | Family income for 1985 only | | |
			Under $20,000	$20,000-$34,999	$35,000 and over
Age (years)					
All ages	31.4	32.7			
Under 45	10.2	11.6	16.6	7.1	4.7
45-64	10.4	10.4			
65 years and over	10.8	10.7			
Sex					
Male	15.5	15.3			
Female	15.9	17.4			

From US Department of Commerce, Bureau of the Census: Statistical Abstract of the United States 1990, Washington DC, 1990.

Prevention and control of chronic disease constitutes one of the major health problems in the United States today. In the past the impact of chronic diseases on individuals, families, and communities has been overlooked. Currently, there is increasing awareness in the United States of great pockets of unmet needs among people with long-term health problems. These individuals have needs that extend beyond the strictly medical. Their problems demand the use of multiple sources of help and care. In many cases the coping capacities of chronically ill individuals are reduced because of advancing age, serious functional impairment and disability, and limited personal, social, and financial resources.

Chronic disease is not an entity in itself but an umbrella term that encompasses long-lasting diseases, which are often associated with some degree of disability. Each chronic illness is unique and has a different impact on the individual, family, and community. Nevertheless, common problems and complications that accompany the various chronic health problems can be studied in general to help the nurse understand and care for individuals with specific long-term illnesses.

The incidence and prevalence of chronic diseases have increased since the beginning of the twentieth century. *Incidence* refers to the number of cases of illness that had their onset during a specified period of time. Commonly health statistics report the number of new cases for a calendar year. *Prevalence* refers to the total number of cases at a given point in time. Thus, prevalence rates are higher than incidence rates because they include all persons (cases) with a specified condition (old cases) and those who acquired the condition during a specified period of time (new cases).

The reason that both the incidence and prevalence are increased for *chronic diseases* is because fewer persons are dying from *acute diseases*. There is decreased mortality from infectious diseases such as whooping cough and chickenpox in children and tuberculosis and pneumonia in persons of all ages. Improved sanitation, the introduction of effective vaccines and mass immunizations, and the discovery of antibiotics have all contributed to this decrease in deaths from infectious diseases. Unfortunately measles immuni-

zation rates for children have declined recently and in 1991 several young children died from the consequences of measles. Most of these deaths were in children living under the poverty level with limited access to medical care. Also, several states stopped providing free immunization services because of budget restrictions at the Federal and state levels.

The latest available figures from the U.S. Bureau of the Census show that the number of persons with some limitation in activity increased from 1980 to 1985. Another finding of interest is that the number of persons with limited activity decreased as family income increased (See Table 14-1). This last finding seems to indicate that persons from higher income levels may be better educated about preventive health measures and they are able to afford better diet, better housing, and better medical care.

Disability refers to any long- or short-term *reduction of activity* as the result of an acute or chronic condition. *Limitation of activity* is used to describe a *long-term reduction* in a person's ability to perform the kind or amount of activity associated with a particular age group. *Restriction of activity* is generally used to refer to a relatively short-term reduction in a person's activity below his or her normal capacity.

Death rates from heart disease decreased so dramatically in persons 45 to 64 years of age from 1970 until the present that heart disease is no longer the leading cause of death. Cancer has replaced it as the leading cause of death in persons between 25 and 65 years of age. The other top causes of death are injury, stroke, suicide, liver disease, chronic lung disease, homicide, HIV infection, and diabetes (see Fig. 14-1). All the leading causes of death have risk factors associated with life-style and many of these diseases could be prevented by effective control of smoking, blood pressure, diet, and alcohol consumption.

While death rates from heart disease were decreasing dramatically, death rates from other conditions were increasing. The death rate from AIDS increased from 8.3 to 9.1 per 100,000 population from 1988 to 1990. This represented an increase in death rates of 9.6% in 1989 and 1990 alone. Deaths from homicides increased by 23% from 1987 to 1990. Most of this increase has been in young black males from 15 to 24 years of age. This black on black crime has been attributed to drugs, alcohol, and street gangs. Death rates also increased for diabetes with an increase of 23% from 1984 to 1990. The increase in deaths from diabetes was 15% from 1988 to 1990 alone, with the increase being in persons from 55 to 85 years of age.

At the same time, The National Health Survey of 1982 identified major disparities in the health of black Americans and other minorities in the United States when compared with the white population. As a result of these findings, the Secretary of the US Department of Health and Human Services (DHHS) established a Task Force on Black and Minority Health. The findings of the task force are discussed on p. 276.

According to the surgeon general's report, 80% of the over-65 population has one or more chronic diseases.

DEFINITION OF ACUTE AND CHRONIC ILLNESS

An *acute illness* is one caused by a disease that produces symptoms and signs soon after exposure to the cause, that runs a short course, and from which there is usually a full recovery or an abrupt termination in death. An acute illness may become chronic. For example, a common cold may develop into chronic sinusitis. A *chronic illness* is one caused by disease that produces symptoms and signs within a variable period of time, that runs a long course, and from which there is only partial recovery. The National Health Survey defines chronic conditions as follows: (1) the conditions were first noticed 3 months or more before the date of the interview, or (2) they belong to a group of conditions (including heart disease, diabetes, and others) that are considered chronic regardless of when they began.[41] This follows the pattern of the *Commission on Chronic Illness*, which in 1949 *defined chronic illness as any impairment or deviation from normal that has one or more of the following characteristics.*

1. The illness or impairment is permanent.
2. The illness or impairment leaves residual disability.
3. The illness or impairment is caused by nonreversible pathologic alteration.
4. The illness or impairment requires a long period of supervision, observation, or care.

This definition is still in use more than 40 years later.

The symptoms and general reactions caused by chronic disease may subside with proper treatment and care. The period during which the disease is controlled and symptoms are not obvious is known as *remission*. However, at a future time the disease may become active again with recurrence of pronounced symptoms. This is known as an *exacerbation* of the disease.

Exacerbations of chronic disease often cause the patient to seek medical attention and may lead to hospitalization. The needs of a patient who has an acute illness may be very different from those of the patient with an acute exacerbation of a chronic disease. For example, a young person may enter the hospital with complaints of fever, chest pain, shortness of breath, fatigue, and a productive cough. If the diagnosis is pneumonia, the patient usually can be assured of recovery after a period of rest and a

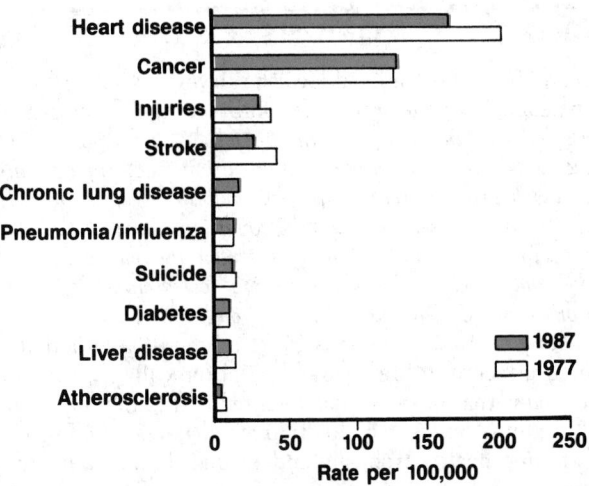

Fig. 14-1   Comparison of leading causes of death 1977 and 1987. (From US Dept of Health and Human Services: Healthy People 2000, *National health promotion and disease prevention objectives*, Washington, DC, 1990, US Government Printing Office.)

course of antibiotic treatment. However, if the diagnosis is rheumatic heart disease and if the patient is being admitted to the hospital for the third, fourth, or fifth time, the reassurance needed will not be so definite, clear-cut, or easy to give. In such a case it is necessary to begin planning care that will extend beyond the period of hospitalization, taking into consideration many aspects of the patient's total life situation. The concerns of the patient who has repeated attacks of illness will be very different from the concerns of the one who has a short-term illness.

Further, the needs of patients who are admitted to the hospital with an acute illness but who also have an underlying chronic condition must not be overlooked. For example, elderly patients who enter the hospital with pneumonia may receive treatment for the pneumonia and recover from their illness. However, they may still be hampered by the arteriosclerotic heart disease and arthritis that they have had for years. Also these two chronic conditions may have been aggravated by the acute infection, or the return to former activity may be hindered by joint stiffness resulting from bed rest and inactivity. Consideration of a patient's several diagnoses can help in preventing new problems associated with the chronic illness.

Strauss,[44] a well-known medical sociologist, has described the following problems experienced by persons with chronic illness:

1. Preventing and managing medical crises
2. Controlling symptoms
3. Following prescribed regimen
4. Maintaining normal interactions with others
5. Adjusting to recurrent patterns in the course of the disease
6. Arranging payment for treatment

The emotional, social, and economic implication of chronic illnesses are discussed later in this chapter.

IMPACT OF CHRONIC ILLNESS ON SOCIETY

According to the National Health Survey of 1989, 80 million people have one or more chronic conditions. *The survey classified chronic conditions in the following categories: (1) selected skin and musculoskeletal conditions, (2) impairments (visual, hearing, speech, paralysis, deformity, or orthopedic impairment), (3) selected digestive conditions, (4) selected conditions of the genitourinary, nervous, endocrine, metabolic, and blood and blood-forming systems, (5) selected circulatory conditions, and (6) selected respiratory conditions.*[42]

Many of these conditions cause a limitation of activity, which affects the life-style of the chronically ill. One of the trends that has been documented is that the impact of acute illness has seemed to diminish, whereas the burden of chronic health problems and related disability has increased. *Limitation of activity is a measure of long-term disability resulting from chronic health problems or impairment and is defined as the inability to carry on the major activity for one's age group, such as cooking, keeping house, going to school, or going to work.*

Approximately 15% of the population experience some limitations in their activities, whereas almost half of the persons over 65 years of age are limited in their activities by one or more chronic conditions. Some activity limitations are associated with mental disabilities, but most are the result of physical handicaps caused by heart conditions and arthritis. *Because chronic disability increases in direct proportion to age, persons over 65 years of age are most prone to severe chronic disability.*

As the population of the United States ages, the number of persons with chronic illness will continue to increase. The inability to work or to move about influences greatly the kind of medical treatment and health supervision needed by persons who have a chronic illness. Some persons only need periodic medical examination and perhaps continuing treatment with medications; others may require complete physical care. Some have a disease that progresses very slowly without remissions, whereas others may have episodes of acute illness and then seem comparatively well for a time. Each person requires a thorough assessment to determine the stage of the illness, the course the illness is likely to take, the type of care needed, and the method by which that care will be delivered if the individual is to be helped appropriately.

Factors That Influence Chronic Illness
Age

Different age groups have different kinds of experience with acute and chronic diseases. The young are more likely to experience short, intense, acute conditions that are quickly over. The elderly are more likely to have long, drawn-out chronic diseases; nevertheless, it is true that anyone can have either an acute or a chronic disease at any age. Chronic illness and disability may date from birth (for example, spina bifida with neurologic damage), or it may originate in childhood, adolescence, or early adult life (for example, multiple sclerosis, rheumatoid arthritis). *The major chronic illnesses among those 65 years and over identified in the National Health Survey were arthritis, diabetes, heart disease,* and *hypertension.*

Because of strides made in pediatric medicine, children who 30 years ago would have died from diseases such as cystic fibrosis are living longer. The reduction in death rates among the younger age groups has allowed a higher percentage of the population to reach the age of greatest risk from chronic diseases. Cancer develops far more frequently in older people. Because the average age of our population continues to rise, about 30% of people now alive will eventually contract cancer.[1]

Much remains to be learned about interactions of the normal, pathologic, and physiologic changes of aging with various diseases. A common question that is asked is "When does aging end and illness begin?" Differences found in age groups or changes found in individuals as they age represent normal aging; that is, a universal, intrinsic process of growth and development that is inevitable, irreversible, unpreventable, but ultimately detrimental. Even though aging, a normal process, is distinct from chronic disease, a pathologic process, *chronic illness often accompanies aging.* The problems of aging and chronic disease are influenced in major ways by each other; for example, the social problems confronting the aged are strongly influenced by the presence and severity of chronic disabilities. Remissions and exacerbations are possibilities with chronic illness; they are not with aging.

Healthy People 2000[28] makes the following comments about age and chronicity. People in the United States who reach the age of 65 can now expect to live into their 80s. However, it is not likely that all those years will be active and independent ones. Thus, improving the functional independence and not just the length of later life is an important element in promoting the health of this group.

One measure of health that considers quality as well as the length of life is the years of healthy life. Whereas people aged 65 and older have 16.4 years of life remaining on average, it is estimated that they have about 12 years of healthy life remaining. *Thus quality of life is determined by the individual's ability to perform activities of daily living so that he or she can be independent.*

Race and ethnicity

Race or ethnic group membership is a factor that influences chronic health problems. Race-specific rates measure the association between disease occurrence and race. Data on specific conditions indicate not only that some problems are more prevalent among nonwhites (blacks, American Indians, and Asians) but also that many nonwhites fail to receive necessary care. *For example, nonwhites are more than three times more likely to die of hypertension than whites of the same age group.*[41] *The findings of the Task Force on Black and Minority Health, which were released late in 1985, found that 60,000 excess deaths occur each year in minority populations.*[30]

The excess number of preventable deaths is derived by calculating the difference between the number of deaths in the black population and the number that would have been expected to occur by applying the average annual age-specific rates of the U.S. white population to the U.S. mid-period black population (as of 1983).[24] *This means that there would be no excess black deaths if the mortality rates of blacks and whites were the same.*

Table 14-2   Number of selected reported chronic conditions per 1000 persons by race and age: United States, 1989

Chronic conditions	White		Black	
	65-74	75 years and over	65-74	75 years and over
Arthritis	431.7	562.8	520.4	525.3
Diabetes	80.2	82.0	148.2	196.0
Heart disease	234.7	366.7	207.8	243.3
Hypertension	367.8	366.9	534.0	490.1

From National Center for Health Statistics, Division of Interview Health Statistics. Data from National Health Interview Survey, 1989.

Table 14-3   Comparison of life expectancy for the black and white populations from 1980 to 1989-1990

Population	Life expectancy in years	
	1980	1989-1990
Black males*	63.8	66
White males	70.7	72.6
Black females	72.5	74.5
White females	78.1	79.3

From National Center for Health Statistics, Division of Interview Health Statistics. Data from National Health Interview Survey, 1989.
*Increase in life expectancy for all except those 15-24 years of age in which the death rate increased each year since 1980.

Seven causes of death were identified that together account for more than 80% of the excess mortality. The health problems related to excess deaths are listed below in alphabetical order:

1. Cancer: 16% of excess mortality among black males under age 70 and 10% among black females.
2. Cardiovascular disease and stroke: 24% of excess mortality among black males and 41% among black females. Most of these deaths were due to hypertensive heart disease.
3. Chemical dependency (measured by deaths resulting from cirrhosis of the liver, associated with excessive use of alcohol): 13% of excess mortality among Native American males and 22% among Native American females under age 70 years of age.
4. Diabetes: 38% of excess deaths among Mexican-born Hispanic females.
5. Homicides and accidents (unintentioned injuries): 60% of excess mortality among Hispanics under age 65 years of age.
6. Unintentional injuries cause 44% of excess death among male and 30% among female Native Americans. Homicides and unintentioned injuries account for 19% of excess mortality among black males under age 70 and 38% among those under age 45. The figures for black females are 6% and 14%, respectively. A substantial portion of excess deaths in this category may be associated with excessive use of alcohol and other drugs.
7. Infant mortality: of excess deaths among black females up to age 45 years, deaths in the first year of life account for 35%.[20]

Table 14-2 compares the rates of four major chronic illnesses for white and black Americans.

The life expectancy for both black and white populations in the United States increased from 1980 to 1990 for all age categories except black males from 15 to 24 years of age (see Table 14-3).

Cultural values

Western culture tends to be cure oriented, therefore, health care for acute conditions is often more valued than is health care for the chronically ill. In contrast to the exciting aspects of sophisticated and mechanical technology, caring for chronically ill persons is often considered boring. The continued struggle to cope with day-to-day living soon becomes tedious for ill persons, their families, and health professionals. *The rewards of treating chronic illness cannot be measured by a cure but by the prevention of complications and by helping individuals function at their optimal level.*

The cultural context has many symbolic meanings, beliefs, and values that health professionals need to understand to meet individual's health needs. Some individuals may view their chronic disease as a form of punishment from God (see Chapter 3). Thus they may experience a sense of guilt. Individuals who view their chronic disease as a "leper phenomenon" may experience a sense of social rejection. Others may see their chronic illness as a destructive force without meaning or simply as a physical response of their body. Appreciation of the person's beliefs and behavior in the context of his or her cultural heritage rather than denial of the cultural influence increases understanding between the health professional and the chronically ill person. Differences need not imply deviance. It is possible to introduce health practices in a manner congruent with the individual's cultural values (see Chapter 3).

Cost of Disability

Chronically ill persons and their families are subjected to great personal and emotional losses that must be dealt with—loss of self-esteem, loss of status within the family, loss of independence, feelings of rejection, and feelings of helplessness are only a few. These can be more devastating than economic deprivation, which is a constant problem.

The economic cost to the patient and family is considerable. The cost of hospitalization rises yearly. Frequent or extended hospitalization and medical expenses can be ruinous if the patient is inadequately insured or if he or she cannot afford medical insurance or has been dropped by an insurance company because of the chronicity of their condition. In 1991 it was estimated that 30 million Americans had no medical insurance.

Many are forced to seek public assistance merely to survive. Placement in quality nursing homes, which commonly costs $3000 or more a month, is financially impossible for most patients or their families to manage. The cost of medications to control or maintain a patient's health status may require a major portion of the family budget. Additional expenses may include special diets and equipment, home modifications (for example, ramps or widening of doors for wheelchairs), transportation, and support services provided by homemakers, day or live-in attendants, or nurses.

The ability of the individual family to pay its own way is determined in part by which member of the family becomes disabled. Older studies showed that the family suffered less economic deprivation if the wife was disabled. In those studies, three fourths of the chronically ill persons unable to carry out their jobs were men. Today, however, more and more households are headed by women who are single parents and are the only wage earners for the family. Women who head households will need additional help and support and nurses should be sensitive to their needs.

Some financial assistance is provided by Medicare. This federally administered program provides hospital and medical insurance protection for individuals 65 years of age and over as well as for people under 65 who are disabled and eligible for Social Security benefits. Persons under age 65 who are medically indigent because of health problems may be eligible for assistance through the Medicaid program.

However, recent changes in federal funding have altered Medicare and Medicaid programs. Persons over age 65 receiving Social Security have a higher fee deducted from their monthly payments to pay for their Medicare premiums. Medicare Part A pays for hospitalization; Medicare Part B covers medical expenses and physician care. As of January 1, 1991, Medicare Part A pays all but $628 for the first 60 days of hospitalization and Medicare Part B covers physician bills, physical therapy treatments, rental of wheelchairs, and so on. Part B does not cover the cost of medicines, eye glasses, hearing aids, or dentures. Medicare reimbursement is commonly 80% of the amount billed. Most persons covered by Medicare purchase supplemental health insurance to cover the expenses not reimbursed by Medicare.

There have been severe cutbacks in Medicaid, which is administered by state governments. For example, persons seeking Medicaid assistance in Ohio are not eligible if they have assets (excluding their home) of more than $1500.

During 1991-1992 several governors proposed even more stringent eligibility standards for Medicaid because of large state budget deficits.

Thus persons with chronic illnesses may have considerable difficulty in paying for prescribed therapy. For example, antiinflammatory agents used to treat arthritis are very expensive. Many of these medications cost between $0.75 and $1.00 each and the usual dose is three times daily. It is not uncommon for the person with limited resources to weigh whether to purchase medications or food because there is not enough money to do both.

In considering the cost of disability to the community, it must be realized that most individuals who are unable to work must be supported by others, either from private or from public funds. There are 3 million adults between the ages of 18 and 64 years who are unable to work because of chronic disabilities. There are an additional 9.4 million who are partially limited in their ability to work.

CHRONICALLY ILL PERSONS AND THEIR FAMILIES

The effects of chronic illness on individuals and their families are numerous and varied. The first impact of the disability may nearly immobilize them. Time must be provided them to talk through their concerns and fears before they can be expected to begin coping with their new situation.

Marked changes often take place, and are often required to take place, in family living as a result of chronic illness. Some families may find themselves drawn closer together. Other families may drift apart, the individual members being incapable of helping one another. At times, chronic illness may threaten an individual's basic emotional stability, and the whole situation may be unbearable to others. Sometimes the individual's emotional needs may not have been apparent to the family early in the illness, but when such needs grow obvious, relatives feel inadequate to cope with the situation. *The length of illness, periodic hospitalizations, and increased financial, emotional, and social burdens are stressors that threaten the family's integrity.*

Many persons struggle on their own to assume the full financial burden of the illness and consequently expose other members of the family to lower standards of nutrition, housing, and care. Many times relatives move in with one another, arguments develop, and family ties are strained or broken. Public assistance may be acceptable to some families, whereas others find it impossible to accept.

Chronic illness imposes additional problems of learning how to cope with restrictions on activities of daily living, how to prevent or identify medical crises that occur, and how to carry out treatment regimens as delineated by the health care provider. Family members also need to learn about the restrictions, not only to be of assistance to the chronically ill person, but also because their own activity patterns may be disrupted by the person's activities.

Because chronic illness may have periods of exacerbation when symptoms become more acute and medical crises may occur, patients and family members need to know which symptoms must be reported to the health care provider as well as the time interval for reporting these symptoms. They also need to know how to contact the provider and what measures to take if a medical crisis occurs. For example, the person who has a history of myocardial infarction and that person's family members must know what to do if the person experiences severe chest pain. Should the person be taken immediately to a hospital emergency room or should the physician be contacted first? Patient and family should plan in advance the sequence of actions to take during a medical crisis, depending on the nature and extent of the presenting symptoms.

Compliance and Noncompliance

Persons with chronic illness are often labeled as "compliant" or "noncompliant" in carrying out regimens prescribed for them. There are many factors that influence the person's ability or motivation to carry out the prescribed regimen. If the person does not carry out the regimen

<table>
<tr><td>

14-1

Levels of prevention

Primary
Health promotion
Specific protection against diseases (vaccines)

Secondary
Early detection of disease
Prompt intervention to halt progression of disease

Tertiary
Rehabilitation (appropriate to the stage of disability)
Prevention of further complications
Restoration of optimal functioning to highest possible level

</td></tr>
</table>

(noncompliant), it does not necessarily mean that the individual is refusing to do so deliberately, although this may sometimes occur.

Before the nursing diagnosis of noncompliance is made, the nurse needs to assess the situation to determine the reasons that the patient is not complying with therapeutic recommendations. The etiology of noncompliance includes the patient's value system (health beliefs, cultural influence, spiritual values).[37] The following are some possible reasons for nonadherence to a prescribed therapy:

1. Failure to understand or internalize the reason for the recommendations
2. Procedures that are difficult to learn and carry out
3. Time required to carry out therapy
4. Inability to pay for prescribed therapy
5. Side effects of therapy (medications, exercises, etc.)
6. Being embarrassed when carrying out regimen in front of others
7. Social isolation and lack of support and positive reinforcement

Conflicts occur within the family structure when one family member recognizes the importance of carrying out the prescribed regimen but another does not. For example, a wife may see the need for continuing checkups and medication for her husband's hypertension, whereas he may perceive this as a needless expense because he feels well and has no symptoms. Persons vary from time to time in the extent of compliance. Individuals who are not hospitalized are their own health care agents and they (or their significant others) determine the actions that are taken.

Coping mechanisms that have been developed should not be tampered with unless, based on a thorough understanding of the situation, viable and more appropriate alternatives can be proposed. If the goal of maintaining the chronically ill person in the optimal state of health is being interfered with by the individual's or the family's attitudes or capacities, a change in those attitudes or capacities is necessary, but it must be a change that is mutually acceptable.

Prevention of Chronic Illness

Because chronic disease evolves over time and pathologic changes may become irreversible, the goal is to detect risk factors as early as possible.

Generally, prevention means inhibiting the development of a disease before it occurs. The term includes several levels of prevention to interrupt or slow the progression of disease (see Box 14-1).

Chronically ill persons and their families require long-term care. The nursing profession has been concerned with chronic health problems and the challenge involved in providing long-term nursing care to chronically ill individuals and their families.

The American Academy of Nursing has made the following statement regarding long-term care:

> Long-term care is the provision of that range of services—physical, psychological, spiritual, and social, including socio-economic—needed to help people attain, maintain, or regain their optimal level of functioning. It includes health maintenance throughout the life span as well as care during acute and protracted illness and disability. Such care is the legitimate province of nurses who now are making social contributions through health teaching and promotion, prevention of illness, and rehabilitation.[33]

In the past nursing has followed the general pattern of providing health services by placing the emphasis on acute and episodic care rather than on health promotion and health maintenance. However, there is an emerging consensus among the health community that the health strategy must be changed dramatically to emphasize the prevention of disease. In the same vein, the American Academy of Nursing has proposed that "nursing assume major responsibility for health promotion, maintenance, and teaching within the context of its definition of long-term care."[33]

Another way of looking at prevention has been identified by Albee. He has developed a "prevention equation" for preventing dysfunction:

$$\text{Incidence of dysfunction} = \frac{\text{Stress} + \text{Constitutional vulnerabilities}}{\text{Social supports} + \text{Coping skills} + \text{Competence}}$$

The two major strategies for preventing dysfunction are decreasing the values in the numerator (that is, decreasing stressors or constitutional vulnerabilities) and increasing the values in the denominator (that is, increasing social supports, coping skills, and competence). It is more difficult to have an impact on the numerator of the prevention equation because stressors in our lives cannot always be controlled; however, creative ways to decrease individual and societal stressors must continually be sought. It is easier to affect the denominator by strengthening social supports, coping skills, and competence. For more information see Chapter 6 for a discussion of stressors, stress, and stress management.

One valuable tool that has been developed to assist persons to identify their own risk factors and change their life-styles is the health hazard appraisal (HHA).[36] The HHA is a screening process that includes a comprehensive questionnaire and the taking of certain physical measurements. Based on probability tables, a risk assessment is then calculated from each person's profile along with goals that would result in risk reduction. Counseling and follow-up are provided to reinforce the data.

Nursing Process
Assessment of the person with a chronic illness

Before a plan of care can be devised for the chronically ill person, a thorough assessment of needs and capabilities must be carried out. Included in such an assessment are the individual's *physical, psychologic, social, and financial status.*

Physical status

Because medical diagnoses do not accurately reflect the physical status and functioning of the chronically ill person, the use of a profile system or assessment tool may be instituted as a guide for those working with the patient. One such tool[39] provides a guide for grading the patient in six different categories: (1) physical condition including cardiovascular, pulmonary, gastrointestinal (GI) genitourinary, endocrine, or cerebrovascular disorders; (2) upper extremities, structure and function, including the shoulder girdle and cervical and upper dorsal spine; (3) lower extremities, structure and function, including the pelvis and lower dorsal and lumbar sacral spine; (4) sensory components relating to speech, vision, and hearing; (5) excretory function, including the bowels and bladder; and (6) mental and emotional status. The ability of the person to carry out activities of daily living (for example, dressing, feeding, bathing, brushing teeth, combing hair, toileting, and moving from place to place) specifically need to be assessed. The completed assessment should indicate in what areas the patient has difficulty and the extent of that difficulty. Such a guide can be used in planning goals for care, both immediate and long term, and will be useful in assisting the individual and the family to make realistic plans for care. Because a chronic condition is not static, reassessment should be carried out at regular intervals whether there is improvement or regression.

The impact of chronic illness on the person's desire for or ability to participate in sexual activities should be assessed. Changes in body appearance, shortness of breath, and musculoskeletal or neurologic impairments may make it seem to the person that they can no longer be sexually active. In addition, the side effects of certain medications tend to decrease sexual desire or cause impotence. The nurse should determine if concern about sexual ability is a problem for the person, and if it is, appropriate action including referral can be taken. (See Chapter 34 for more information about sexuality in health and illness.)

Psychologic status

Assessment of the individual's psychologic needs and capabilities includes determining attitudes and stage of adaptation to the illness, feelings concerning how illness affects the family or significant others, and the person's own goals in regard to living with an illness. For example, individuals who are almost totally helpless as a result of an accidental spinal cord injury may seem to have no interest in learning ways to help themselves. Their families may react in the same manner and be of little help to them. Both the individuals and their families need interest and support from nurses and other professionals as they learn to cope with the change in their life situations.

Feelings of anxiety, frustration, irritability, bitterness, and guilt may be expressed by some chronically ill persons who face unending pain and loss of economic and social security. Some persons become obsessed with their health problems, and spend much of each day thinking about what will happen and what to do. Guilt may result from being unable to work and support oneself or from the belief, as a result of a search for some purpose or reason for the affliction, that one must deserve the suffering. *Depression is common among chronically ill persons, especially those who feel powerless. Powerlessness can be the result of feeling unable to control or overcome what has happened to one.*[17]

Social and financial status

Social and financial status must be considered because they relate specifically to the kind of support and resources available to the individuals in meeting their goals. It would be unrealistic, for example, to plan for a hydraulic bathtub chair if the patient could not afford it, family members were unavailable to help operate it, or the patient's apartment manager would not permit it to be installed. Alternative methods of helping the patient to take a tub bath would have to be explored.

The social assessment includes living arrangements, family roles, support of significant others, cultural and social group memberships, education, and vocational and avocational activities. The data collected through the performance of this kind of thorough assessment should make it possible to devise a *plan of care directed toward the accomplishment of attainable goals that are mutually acceptable to the patient, the family, and the caregivers.*

Data analysis: nursing diagnoses

Nursing diagnoses are determined from analysis of patient data. Possible nursing diagnoses for the person with a chronic illness may include, but are not limited to, the following:

Diagnostic title	Possible etiologies
Activity intolerance	Bed rest, immobility, generalized weakness, sedentary life-style
Adjustment, impaired	Disability requiring change in life-style; inadequate support systems; impaired cognition, sensory overload; altered locus of control; incomplete grieving
Anxiety	Threat to self-concept; threat of change in health status, socioeconomic status, and role functioning
Breathing pattern, ineffective	Neuromuscular impairment, pain, musculoskeletal impairment
Communication, impaired verbal	Aphasia, physical impairment
Constipation	Change in life-style, immobility, inadequate nutrition, inadequate fluid intake

Diagnostic title	Possible etiologies
Coping, ineffective family: compromised	Inadequate or incorrect information, temporary family disorganization and role changes, prolonged disability of significant person
Diversional activity deficit	Long-term hospitalization
Fear	Loss of body part, long-term illness, pain, life-style changes
Health maintenance, altered	Altered communication skills, decreased motor skills
Home maintenance management, impaired	Insufficient family resources, lack of knowledge/role modeling, inadequate support systems
Hopelessness	Prolonged activity restriction, failing physical condition, long-term stress
Incontinence, functional	Altered environment; sensory, cognitive, or mobility deficits
Incontinence, reflex	Neurologic impairment
Injury, high risk for	Sensory/motor deficits, lack of awareness of environmental hazards
Knowledge deficit	Lack of exposure/recall, cognitive limitation
Mobility, impaired physical	Intolerance to activity; decreased strength/endurance; pain/discomfort; cognitive, neuromuscular, or musculoskeletal impairment; depression; severe anxiety
Nutrition, altered: less than body requirements	Chewing or swallowing difficulties, inability to obtain food
Pain	Immobility, improper positioning, pressure points
Powerlessness	Health care environment, illness-related regimen, life-style of helplessness
Self-care deficit, bathing/hygiene, dressing/grooming, feeding/toileting	Intolerance to activity/fatigue, pain/discomfort, perceptional/cognitive impairment, musculoskeletal impairment, depression
Self-esteem disturbance	Severe trauma, change in body appearance, change in social involvement
Sexual dysfunction	Altered body structure, physiologic limitations
Skin integrity, impaired	Mechanical forces (pressure, shearing), immobility
Social interaction, impaired	Poor communication skills, self-concept disturbance, absence of supportive others, altered thought processes

Planning: expected patient outcomes

Because outcomes for specific chronic diseases are discussed in the chapters dealing with those diseases not all possible outcomes will be discussed here. However, in general it may be stated that on discharge from the hospital or other care facility, patients with chronic disease or their family members should be able to do the following:

1. Demonstrate or explain those measures that must be taken to avoid further preventable disability.
2. Demonstrate or explain those self-care activities of which they are capable.
3. Identify those activities for which help is needed.
4. Explain who will be available to help with those activities and on what basis that help will be available.
5. Recognize the effect that change in body appearance and social involvement have on self-esteem.
6. Recognize the need to work on coping skills of patient and family.
7. Explain what community resources are available and how to obtain them.
8. Discuss in reasonable detail their plans for follow-up care and reevaluation.

Implementation
Interventions to achieve patient outcomes
Limiting Disability

The first focus in intervention for the chronically ill person is on preventing and reducing disability and enabling the person to remain a socially functioning individual in every respect. Some disabilities among chronically ill persons might have been prevented if prompt, aggressive, suitable medical and nursing care had been available at the onset of the illness. *Many of the difficulties that limit these individuals may not have been caused by the disease itself but may have developed because of immobility during the acute phase of the illness.*

Keeping the person's body in good alignment, maintaining joint range and strength, and preventing decubitus ulcers are physical measures that must constantly be borne in mind. (For further information, see Chapter 43.) A careful plan of rest and activity helps preserve physical resources and makes the day purposeful. If assistance is needed, it should be given until the person can manage the activity by himself or herself or until an alternative method of management can be taught.

Promoting self-care

Asking the person to identify what is meaningful is a primary step toward helping develop self-care. Physical needs are of paramount importance for chronically ill persons. Meeting these physical needs provides a way to convey to such individuals an interest in their progress and welfare. For chronically ill persons who must be hospitalized, it is important that they be allowed to perform as much of their own care as possible. Persons who have been independent in self-care before hospitalization should not be allowed to regress in these abilities if at all possible. Helping them to take their own baths, attend to toilet needs, and groom themselves can give some sense of accomplishment and help them maintain their self-respect. Helping them to be dressed appropriately promotes a sense of wellness. Success in performing portions of their own self-care may be stimulating enough to strengthen ill persons' motivation; they and their families then may make amazing strides in thinking through and working out future problems themselves. For their planning to be realistic and ultimately functional, all health care personnel must teach chronically ill persons the total physiologic ramifications of their disability as well as methods of coping with those ramifications.

Persons who are in their homes or in substitute homes should be encouraged to dress in regular, comfortable street clothing rather than pajamas or gowns. Visitors to the home and family members who constantly see such individuals dressed in bedclothes think of them as sick and are reminded of their illness. Seeing them dressed as usual helps to maintain normal attitudes, relationships, and expectations.

Promoting self-esteem

The care of chronically ill persons requires alertness in feeling, seeing, and hearing. Continued warmth and interest are necessary to the self-esteem of any chronically ill person. Very often a relationship based on an understanding of these requirements promotes self-esteem and helps the individual to become highly motivated. It may be taxing to listen to the same questions and say the same things day after day, but the nature of chronic illness may require this attention, and the manner in which responses are given will convey warmth and interest. The world of chronically ill persons, whether they are in the hospital or elsewhere, becomes narrowed and circumscribed. They treasure and are interested in those things and those people who are close to them. Their conversations may be largely about themselves, their immediate environment, a few close objects, and the persons who are close to them. Although they may be confined to bed and to their room, others can keep them up-to-date on outside news. Depending on their level of adaptation to their illness, they may welcome hearing about outside events, or they may not be able to think beyond themselves. When they reach the stage of being able to look beyond themselves, newspapers, magazines, radio, television, or creating something with their own hands may help to keep up their interest in others and in outside events.

Supporting coping skills

Coping skills may be challenged by persistent, ongoing problems such as chronic pain, recurring medical expenses, or continuing difficulties in carrying out activities of daily living. Usual coping methods may become impossible; for example, a person who usually copes by *expending energy in physical activity* may become unable to do so. The person who *usually copes by discussing problems with family members* will need to find an alternative method if family communication patterns break down. The person can be helped to identify usual coping methods and to explore alternative approaches when necessary.

It is important to recognize that chronically ill persons or their families may suffer from unresolved sadness known as *chronic grief*. Chronic grief may be defined as accumulated or prolonged grief. It extends over long periods, with permanent characteristics developing in many persons, and carries with it a potential for decreased functioning. The causes are varied, and new waves of grief are constantly triggered. One example is grief caused by the losses associated with aging: youth, dreams, jobs, hair, friends, family, health, visual acuity, social role, money, body parts, and mobility. Each loss is accompanied by grief, which builds on previous grief like bricks in creating a wall. In chronic grief the person may be faced with repeated acute episodes. These episodes may coincide with exacerbation of the condition, facing a new limitation, or meeting new indignities. Each new episode requires a renewed struggle back and forth through the various stages of grief.[43]

The nurse can assist by listening and helping the person explore feelings and the content related to these feelings. Because the grief is ongoing, family members can also be helped to identify their feelings and strengthen the communication patterns within the family structure for mutual support of its members.

Clarifying nurse-patient values

Before nurses can work effectively with chronically ill persons they need to be able to distinguish between their own values, standards, and goals and those of the patient. In day-to-day contact with individuals who are making little or no progress, it is tempting to make plans for their future because of a sincere interest in helping them. This is particularly true when the patient's age is similar to one's own. There may be a feeling that something must be done to speed progress. One may become frustrated by the feeling of wanting to do something or wanting to see some marked change. However, the nurse must recognize that *management of chronically ill persons requires a slow-moving, persistent pace* with *possibly little or no change for a long time*. The person's physical and mental condition must be maintained at its present level or improved, and efforts must be made to progress and encourage the family's adaptation to the patient's condition. Eagerness and readiness to progress will be determining factors for the future. *The "doing" in the care of the chronically ill person is not always a physical action with the hands. Often the maintenance of a positive approach and attitude and a demonstration of real interest are the greatest help to the patient.* Teaching patients to perform activities related to their own care independently rather than performing those activities for them may also lead to progress.

Supporting the person with a progressive disability

Health care personnel must also be prepared to provide care for patients whose disease will follow a course of progressive disability, as in multiple sclerosis or rheumatoid arthritis. In these instances, goals of care must be modified to retard the downhill progression of disability rather than to achieve maintenance or improvement of physical status. Helping the patient and family cope with progressive deterioration and in some cases eventual death is a demanding task. Those who wish additional information relating to this aspect of care are referred to the literature on this subject.[45]

Persons with a disability, whether obvious to others or unrecognizable, should not be viewed from the standpoint of the disability alone but for their abilities as well. Usually the greatest need is for comprehensive health services and continuing care. Comprehensive care is provided to patients according to their needs in an appropriate, continuous, and dynamic pattern. Accommodating the plan of care to the needs and goals of individual patients rather than to those of the providers is the essence of comprehensive care.

Providing community resources

There has been an increasing interest in providing programs for chronically ill persons and in assisting them and disabled persons to assume a more active role in their communities. Volunteer workers may act as readers both in hospitals and in homes or may assist with other diversional activities (Fig. 14-2). Institutions receiving federal funds are required to make aids such as ramps available to individuals who are unable to climb stairs or who are in wheelchairs. See p. 292 for discussion of Americans with Disabilities Act. With the development of structural changes that facilitate mobility, some persons with physical limitations are more involved in local activities and associations. Nurses can assist by supporting the further development of these structural changes in all community buildings and by encouraging the participation of chronically ill persons in community activities of interest. Various information sources may be obtained from national organizations, involved with chronic illness and disability. Many of these agencies have services available in the community (see Box 14-2). Programs, facilities, and legislation of this nature reflect the public's increasing awareness of the difficulties faced by chronically ill and disabled persons.

Evaluation

Questions to be asked about the patient with a chronic illness include the following:

1. Can the patient or family demonstrate or explain the measures necessary to avoid further preventable disability?
2. Can the patient demonstrate or explain the self-care activities of which they are capable?
3. Can the patient identify the activities for which help is needed?
4. Can the patient explain who will be available to help with the above activities and on what basis they will be available?
5. Can the patient verbalize the effect that change in body appearance and social involvement has had on his or her self-esteem?
6. Do interactions between the patient and family members give evidence that they have been working to improve their coping skills?
7. Can the patient or family explain what community resources they are using and how they obtained them?
8. Can the patient discuss plans for follow-up care and reevaluation?

REHABILITATION

Rehabilitation is the process of assisting the individual with a handicap to realize his or her particular goals, physically, mentally, socially, and economically. As such, *rehabilitation*

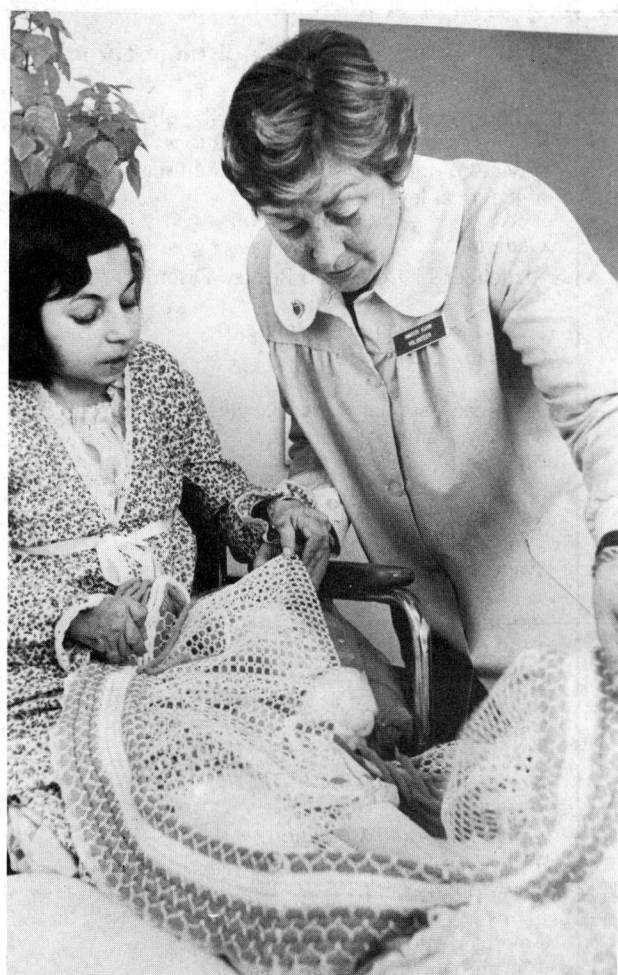

Fig. 14-2 Volunteer helping patient who has a chronic illness with some handwork.

is *an active concept* and *must be clearly differentiated from the concept of maintenance care.* Following a thorough assessment of patients' disabilities and capabilities, assumptions can be made regarding the potential for improving their conditions. If improvement can be made, patients are candidates for rehabilitation. If improvement cannot be made, care is directed toward maintaining the current condition, that is, preventing further disability. The process of rehabilitation can be viewed more appropriately as *patient education* rather than *patient care.* One must remember, however, that the rehabilitation of every patient will reach an end point, that is, a point at which no further progress is possible. At that time, the focus of care reverts to that of maintenance.

The purpose or extent of rehabilitation ranges from employment or reemployment for the handicapped person to the more limited achievement of developing self-care abilities. This latter accomplishment can be just as important to the individual as earning money and may represent that person's greatest life achievement. This might

14-2

Community resources involved in chronic health problems

Various types of information may be obtained by writing to these national organizations. In addition, services of the various agencies are usually available at the local level.

General

Alzheimer's Disease and Related Disorders Association
360 N. Michigan Ave., Suite 601
Chicago, IL 60641

American Association of Diabetes Education
3553 W. Peterson Ave.
Chicago, IL 60659

American Association of Retired Persons
1909 K St., N.W.
Washington, DC 20006

American Cancer Society
1599 Clifton Rd., N.E.
Atlanta, GA 30329

American Diabetes Association
1 W. 48th St.
New York, NY 10020

American Heart Association
44 E. 23rd St.
New York, NY 10010

American Lung Association
1740 Broadway
New York, NY 10019

American Parkinson Disease Association
147 E. 50th St.
New York, NY 10022

Arthritis Foundation
221 Park Ave. S.
New York, NY 10003

Easter Seal Society for Crippled Children and Adults
2023 W. Ogden Ave.
Chicago, IL 60612

Juvenile Diabetes Foundation
23 E. 26th St.
New York, NY 10010

Leukemia Society of America, Inc.
211 E. 43rd St.
New York, NY 10017

Mental Health Materials Center
419 Park Ave. S.
New York, NY 10016

Muscular Dystrophy Association, Inc.
810 7th Ave.
New York, NY 10019

National Aid to Retarded Citizens
   (formerly N.A.R. Children)
2709 E. St.
Arlington, TX 76011

National Association for Down's Syndrome
628 Ashland Ave.
River Forest, IL 60305

National Association for Mental Health, Inc.
1800 N. Kent St.
Rosslyn Station
Arlington, VA 22209

National Association for Sickle Cell Disease, Inc.
945 S. Western Ave., Suite 206
Los Angeles, CA 90006

National Association for Visually Handicapped
305 E. 24th St.
New York, NY 10010

National Asthma Center
875 Avenue of the Americas
New York, NY 10001

National Council on the Aging
1828 L. St. NW
Washington, DC 20036

National Cystic Fibrosis Research Foundation
3379 Peachtree Rd., N.E.
Atlanta, GA 30326

National Epilepsy League
6 N. Michigan Ave.
Chicago, IL 60602

---

be true, for example, for a person who was born with a severe physical handicap such as cerebral palsy.

Success in learning to adjust to living with a disability depends on the *person's premorbid personality, total life experience*, and *premorbid family relationships*, as well as the *person's current behavior and motivation*. Certainly, some rehabilitation can occur in any health agency; nevertheless, the greater the number of rehabilitation disciplines made available as needed to individuals, the greater is their chance of achieving their highest potential. The rehabilitative process, as with any form of education, is involved

as deeply in the motives and purposes of the teacher as in those of the learner.

Persons with disabilities, whether obvious to others or unrecognizable, should not be viewed from the standpoint of their disability alone. Usually the greatest need is for comprehensive health services and continuing care. *Comprehensive care is that which is provided to patients according to their needs in an appropriate, continuous, and dynamic pattern.* Accommodating the plan of care to the needs and goals of individual patients rather than to those of the providers of care is the essence of comprehensive care.

National Head Injury Foundation
333 Turnpike Rd.
Southborough, MA 01772

National Foundation—March of Dimes
1275 Mamaroneck Ave.
White Plains, NY 10605

National Genetics Foundation
250 W. 57th St.
New York, NY 10019

National Hemophilia Foundation
25 W. 39th St., Rm. 903
New York, NY 10018

National Kidney Foundation
116 E. 27th St.
New York, NY 10016

National Multiple Sclerosis Society
205 E. 42nd St.
New York, NY 10017

Nutrition Foundation, Inc.
489 5th Ave.
New York, NY 10017

Parents of Down's Syndrome Children
11507 Yates St.
Silver Spring, MD 20902

Shriners Hospital for Crippled Children
323 N. Michigan Ave.
Chicago, IL 60601

Stroke Clubs of America
805 12th St.
Galveston, TX 77550

United Cerebral Palsy Association, Inc.
66 E. 34th St.
New York, NY 10066

United Ostomy Association
1111 Wilshire Blvd.
Los Angeles, CA 90017

Rehabilitation

American Coalition of Citizens with Disabilities
1346 Connecticut Ave. N.W., Rm. 817
Washington, DC 20036

Architectural and Transportation Barriers Compliance
  Board
330 C St. W.W., Rm. 1010
Washington, DC 20201

Closer Look, National Information Center for the
  Handicapped
Box 1492
Washington, DC 20013

Mainstream, Inc.
1200 15th St., N.W., Rm. 403
Washington, DC 20005

National Center for a Barrier-free Environment
8401 Connecticut Ave.
Washington, DC 20015

National Center for Law and the Handicapped
1235 N. Eddy St.
South Bend, IN 46617

National Congress of Organizations of the Physically
  Handicapped
7611 Oakland Ave.
Minneapolis, MN 55432

National Paraplegia Foundation
333 N. Michigan Ave.
Chicago, IL 60601

Paralyzed Veterans of America
7315 Wisconsin Ave. N.W.
Washington, DC 20014

President's Commission on Employment of the
  Handicapped
111 20th St. N.W., Rm. 636
Washington, DC 20210

Interdisciplinary Approach

The number of professional people required to assist the patient and family with rehabilitation will vary. *Most often the patient, the family, the physician, and the nurse can work out a practical plan.* If a patient's problems are complex, other members may be added to the team. Typically, such a team consists of a physician, nurse, discharge coordinator, medical social worker, vocational counselor, psychologist, speech pathologist, occupational and physical therapists, and a caseworker from the patient's social agency. Fig. 14-3 shows members of an interdisciplinary team planning care for a patient. Teamwork requires that members of the team be able to use their special knowledge and skill and understand the value of their contribution to the patient's care. In addition, team members need some understanding of each other's professional functions and contributions. *One of the cooperative efforts of the involved team members is to meet regularly to evaluate patients and their abilities thoroughly. Based on this assessment, each patient and the team devise a plan to foster readjustment, compensation, and the learning of new ways to manage self-care and living.*

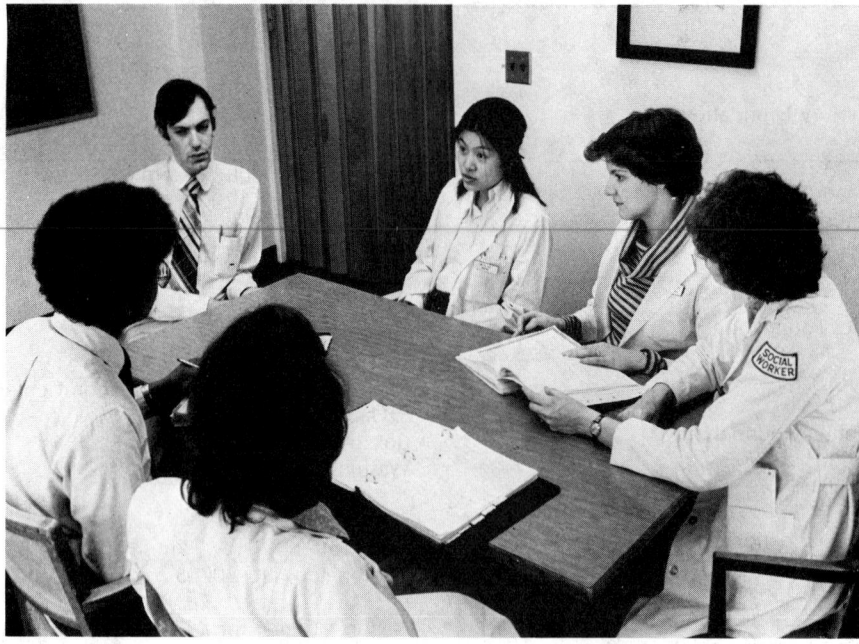

Fig. 14-3 The team approach to rehabilitation is essential. Here, physicians, nurse, physical therapist, and social worker review a patient's program and progress.

Rehabilitation Centers

Persons with very complex problems of rehabilitation may need to receive care at specialized centers for rehabilitation, or they may receive care at home combined with visits to day rehabilitation centers. The variety of specialized centers includes teaching and research centers (centers located in and operated by hospitals and medical schools), community centers with facilities for inpatients, community outpatient centers, insurance centers, skilled nursing homes with an active rehabilitation service and staff, including physical and occupational therapists, and vocational rehabilitation centers. In addition to centers that provide multiple services for the physically disabled, specialized centers provide rehabilitation for blind, deaf, mentally ill, and mentally retarded persons. Most centers offer a wide range of services that usually fall into the following three areas:

Physical area

Physical, nursing, and medical evaluation
Physical therapy
Occupational therapy
Speech therapy
Medical and nursing supervision of appropriate activities

Psychosocial area

Evaluation
Personal counseling
Social service
Psychometrics
Psychiatric service
Recreational therapy

Vocational area

Work evaluation
Vocational counseling
Prevocational experience
Industrial fitness of programs
Trial employment in sheltered workshops
Vocational training
Terminal employment in sheltered workshops
Placement

Several advantages exist for patients participating in organized programs for rehabilitation. They have an opportunity to see and be with others who have similar or more extensive disabilities. Often they progress more rapidly when they realize that others have similar difficulties and are overcoming them. Group therapy often arouses a competitive spirit, and a formerly reluctant person may become willing and diligent. On the other hand, all personnel need to be alert to those patients who have had the opposite reaction. Patients who see others advance in activity while they either do not improve or progress very slowly may become so discouraged that they give up trying. In some cases, the person becomes very depressed and may be suicidal. The nurse should be aware of changes in the person's behavior and be sensitive to any expression of suicidal ideas.

On a rehabilitation unit activities are scaled so that individuals can see their own progress in comparison with their beginning abilities. Patients may take an active interest in keeping their own scores. After a program of therapy has been planned and is scheduled as to time of day, patients can help to keep themselves on the schedule by having a copy of it at the bedside. Individuals can then be assisted to gradually assume more responsibility for readying themselves for scheduled activities. In addition, a master plan of activities for all patients on the unit can be a useful device for nurses, physicians, and therapists. The plan can be kept in a central place on the unit and should list name, activity, and time of activity for each patient. This type of plan is also helpful when a patient's progress is to be reevaluated.

A public program for vocational rehabilitation has been serving the United States since 1920. The program involves a partnership between the state and the federal governments. Services for disabled persons are provided by state divisions of vocational rehabilitation. The federal govern-

ment, through the Social and Rehabilitation Service (SRS), administers grants-in-aid and provides technical assistance and national leadership for the program. Opportunities and services are available in all 50 states, the District of Columbia, and Puerto Rico. All persons of working age with a substantial job handicap resulting from either physical or mental impairment are eligible for help or assistance. The purpose of this service is to *preserve, develop,* or *restore* the ability of disabled persons to earn their own livings. The individual services offered are medical care, counseling and guidance, training, and job finding. All 50 states have separate rehabilitation programs for blind persons. Application for such services can be made to the SRS or to the agency in the state for serving the blind.

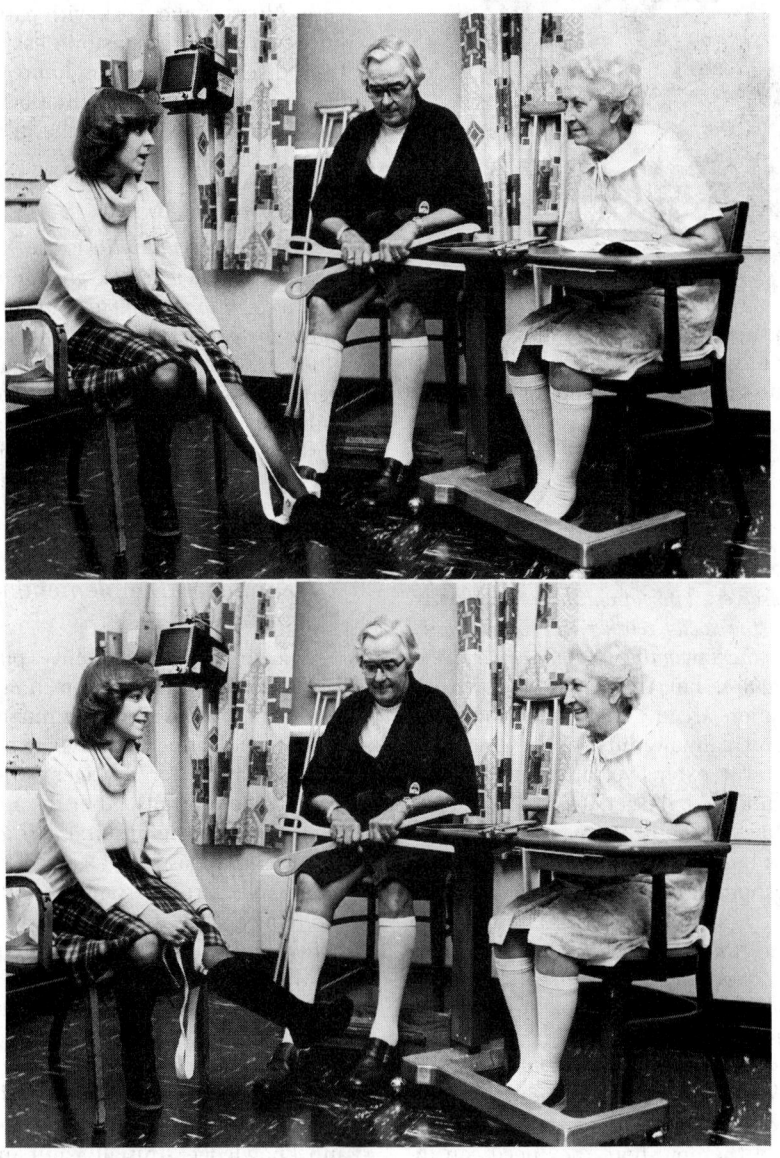

Fig. 14-4 The occupational therapist is concerned with helping patients make necessary adaptations in activities of daily living to permit independent functioning. Here the occupational therapist demonstrates the use of a stocking aid that to the delight of the patients really works.

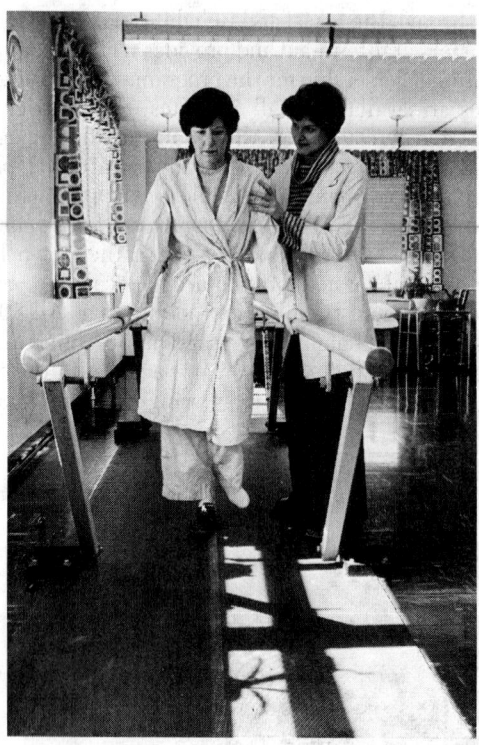

Fig. 14-5 A physical therapist begins a patient's ambulation training by teaching her to walk with the support of parallel bars. The patient wears no shoe on her left foot to remind her not to bear weight on it.

Role of the Patient in Rehabilitation

The most important contributions to patients' rehabilitation are made by the patients themselves. The patient, his or her family, the nurse, the physician, the social worker, the occupational therapist, and sometimes others planning together can arrive at the best plans for the future, but the patient's attitudes, acceptance, and motivation are the most important considerations. If the patient cannot adjust to the disability, whatever it is and however extensive, attempts at rehabilitation usually are hindered. Patients must make the decisions and they change at their own pace. If they are agreeable to suggestions but make little or no effort to try them, one should question if they really have accepted them.

Self-care is encouraged within existing limitations. The patient's behavior from day to day can be the first indication of the direction of positive motivation. For example, if the patient makes every effort to resume normal daily activities such as feeding, bathing, and dressing, one can be certain that the person has a sincere desire to be independent. As patients become ready for more advanced activities, such as ambulation and work in the occupational therapy shop, they need continuing genuine interest and support (Fig. 14-4 and 14-5). As obstacles arise, patients may be able to accept and eventually overcome them. Patients who are truly motivated toward helping themselves never seem to give up, finding ways of accomplishing activities that professional personnel might believe impossible. Each person working with the

chronically ill patient has seen that many times life has meaning for the individual even though it may not be readily apparent to others. Some patients, however, when faced with an added burden, cannot accept it and give up trying. Guidance and support for the families of such patients become tremendously important. Health care personnel who understand these attitudes and behaviors can help make life more satisfying for the chronically ill person and can positively influence the behaviors of the family, professional co-workers, and the public.

Role of the Nurse in Rehabilitation

The concepts of comprehensive nursing care and rehabilitation can be considered synonymous. Helping the patient and family to help themselves is an integral part of nursing care. Nurses who work with patients who have disabilities have two major responsibilities: (1) to ensure that disability from disease or disuse is limited as much as possible and (2) to see that a rehabilitation program is planned and implemented. Details of the nurse's role and responsibilities are listed in Box 14-3.

Limiting disability

Limitation of disability is the *nurse's first responsibility* and *requires attention to the prevention of complications, to the early recognition of symptoms of exacerbations or complications, and to the prevention of deformity.* For patients with chronic illnesses, the onset of exacerbations or complications is frequently subtle, marked by minute changes in functional ability or general performance or attitude. Nurses, working closely with such patients and understanding the pathophysiology of their diseases, are frequently the first to recognize initial signs of difficulty and make provision for appropriate intervention.

Planning and implementing a rehabilitation program

The second responsibility, planning and implementing a program of rehabilitation in *accordance with the patient's goals,* is a process in which nurses are intimately involved. Nursing personnel are likely to be in contact with a patient and the family for a longer period of time each day than are members of any other discipline on the rehabilitation team. Both in the hospital and in the home, nurses are in an excellent position to assist the patient in planning a reasonable care program, as well as to teach the patient, the family, and, if necessary, the employer, about the patient's limitations and rehabilitative expectations.

Much of the nursing activity in the rehabilitation process is no different from the nursing care given to all patients. Measures such as appropriate bowel and bladder programs, providing proper diet and fluid requirements, implementing new methods of bathing, and maintaining skin integrity fall within the domain of nursing concern and knowledge. Initially, nursing personnel may assume almost total responsibility for performing these activities for the patient. After assessing patient abilities in these areas, nurses formulate, implement, and evaluate a teaching plan in much the same way as do therapists from other disciplines. The assistance nurses can give the patient and family depends on nurses' ability to understand themselves,

14-3

The nurse's role and responsibilities in rehabilitation

I. Limit disability from disease as much as possible.
  A. Prevent complications.
    1. Ensure early recognition of symptoms indicating patient's condition is worsening.
      a. Review signs and symptoms and pathology of the chronic illness to recognize changes.
      b. Review signs and symptoms of complications frequently associated with the chronic illness, such as infection.
    2. Prevent deformities.
      a. Maintain proper body alignment.
      b. Position limbs to prevent contractures.
      c. Turn frequently; keep skin clean and dry to prevent skin breakdown.
      d. Provide adequate nutrition.
      e. Provide adequate fluid intake to maintain bladder and bowel program.
      f. Take precautions to prevent infection.
II. Plan and implement rehabilitation program appropriate to patient.
  A. Determine patient's own goals for rehabilitation.
  B. Plan appropriate nursing interventions based on mutually agreed-on goals.
    Early in rehabilitation nurse may have to assume total responsibility for assisting with activities of daily living (ADL), bathing, dressing, intake of food and fluids, bowel and bladder programs, maintaining skin integrity, turning patient, and so on.
  C. Plan nursing interventions that encourage patient to assume responsibility for own ADL as soon as possible.
    1. Set short-term goals with patient.
    2. Goals should be realistic and attainable.
    3. Reinforce patient's progress (no matter how small) with positive feedback.
    4. Work with other members of the rehabilitation team in providing a consistent, coordinated rehabilitation plan.
    5. Keep patient's significant others informed of patient's progress so they can give positive feedback to patient.
    6. Reassess goals periodically and set new goals as appropriate.
    7. Teach patient, family, and, if necessary, employer about patient's limitations and rehabilitative expectations.

personal feelings, and personal behavior as well as the behavior of the patient, family, and other professional team members.

One of the most important aspects of giving continuing care to a patient with a disability is the nurse's own attitude, perseverance, and expectations. Improvement may be slow, and patients may reach a plateau in their progress. Such a time can be critical for patients because they may become discouraged and not wish to continue with their program of care. *Realistic encouragement can often sustain patients so that they will not regress before some improvement is noted.*

Patients in a rehabilitaton program must often learn and practice special physical techniques to strengthen muscles and to improve mobility. Such measures as physical exercise to improve walking, activities to improve self-care abilities, and the use of prostheses require the special knowledge and skills of physical and occupational therapists. *To be effective in the rehabilitation process, nurses must have an understanding of the techniques used by the various therapists so that they can plan and work cooperatively with them in caring for the patient. This knowledge is also used to help the patient employ appropriate techniques in carrying out activities of daily living.*

CONTINUING CARE

Traditionally, health care professionals have assumed responsibility for the patient's well-being within the hospital and little to no responsibility for the patient and family in the home setting. This dichotomy between health care in the home and hospital facility made little sense. With chronically ill individuals the dichotomy interferes with a smooth transition from hospital to home. *The major portion of health care for persons with chronic illnesses occurs in the home; thus ongoing communications must exist between the patient and health professionals.* Strauss et al.[45] advocate that sick people participate more in their care within health facilities and that health care professionals play a greater role in aiding chronically sick people *and* their families to cope with their problems at home. Social forces such as shorter hospital stays have made it necessary for nurses to be more aware of home health care needs.

Self-Help Groups

Self-help groups are associated with self-care. These groups may or may not include the guidance of health care providers. They provide social support to their members through the creation of a caring community, and they increase members' coping skills through the sharing of information, experiences, and problem solutions. Examples of self-help groups include those for women who have had mastectomies and those for individuals who have colostomies, diabetes, or obesity. There are now self-help groups or clubs for patients with a variety of conditions. Nurses should learn what groups are available to patients in their community. A telephone call to a health agency such as the American Cancer Society, American Heart Association, or American Lung Association can elicit information about clubs available to patients who have the specific condition served by the agency.

In some hospitals and nursing homes nurses have been instrumental in setting up support groups for families of patients with chronic health problems such as Alzheimer's disease.

It can be expected that more support groups, both those for patients and those for families, will be developing in the near future. Some of the impetus for these groups can be traced to changes in health care reimbursement. With prospective reimbursement and the use of diagnosis related groups (DRGs) as a basis for reimbursement for patients whose care is being paid for with federal dollars (Medicare and Medicaid), the need for such groups has increased. Prospective reimbursement has resulted in shorter hospital stays for both acute and chronic illnesses. As a result, patients and their families need to be better prepared to care for the patient in the home because patients are sent home sooner than in the past and their needs for continuing care are greater.

Facilities for Continuing Care

It is impossible to include here all the facilities that provide continuing care. Each of the programs mentioned has its own criteria for acceptance of patients for the services it renders. *Before application for service is made and before the program is discussed with the patient and family, the individual patient's eligibility for that service should be determined.*

Ambulatory care

The term *ambulatory care* is used interchangeably with *outpatient care* and *refers to first-contact health care services as well as to continuing contact services in settings that do not require overnight stays.* The use of ambulatory care facilities has expanded because of the increase in chronic illness and the increase in cost of inpatient services. A good ambulatory care service constitutes one of the most important elements of the hospital's contribution to community health. There is a trend toward development of ambulatory care facilities in neighborhood health centers to assist disabled, aged, or disadvantaged persons to obtain needed health care. An ambulatory care center usually provides long-term follow-up care needed by the person with a chronic illness, in addition to preventive health care, diagnostic workups, and treatment of acute illnesses for which hospitalization is unnecessary.

Home care

Before World War II the home was the place where medical treatment was given. Well-to-do persons rarely went to a hospital; they received the services of a private physician in their own home, and the family or nurses employed by the family were responsible for the day-to-day care. Poor families were among the first persons to use hospitals. The philosophy of home care can be traced as far back as 1796, when the Boston Dispensary provided medical care to the sick poor in their homes.

One of the most obvious reasons for the development of home care programs was to provide care to patients with long-term illnesses who did not need the around-the-clock services of an institution and yet who were too ill to go to an outpatient center. Caring for patients at home is often desired by the individual and family, and it also releases hospital beds for use by acutely ill patients. See the section on home care of the adult in Chapter 47 for more information.

Today home care is being provided for acutely ill patients discharged from the hospital earlier than in the past. Prospective reimbursement for hospitals under diagnosis-related groups (DRGs) has meant that many patients are being discharged while they still need skilled nursing care. As a result, many hospitals have set up *home care programs* to supply nursing care and other services to their patients after discharge. Hospitals that have not set up their own programs are contracting with the Visiting Nurse Association and other nursing agencies to supply nursing care for their patients after discharge.

Frequently the issue arises as to who should pay for home health services and who should be reimbursed for health care provided. The American Nurses Association's position is that reimbursement systems should foster care of individuals in their homes based on the following premises[4]:

1. Home health care is humane and respectful of the individual's dignity and integrity.
2. Home care or care within the community can be less costly than institutional care.
3. Nursing care is the primary element in home care.
4. Payment systems for home care should recognize nurses as the major providers of home care, and nurses should be reimbursed on their own authority.

Home care may not be possible for all patients. For those living in smaller dwellings, adequate space for the patient, necessary equipment (oxygen, intravenous fluids, and so on) and for other members of the family may be at a premium. The choice of home care, independent living center, or institutional care depends not only on the desires of the patient and the family, but also on the ability to finance the care. Despite many inconveniences, some families wish to have the patient with them. The family's understanding of the patient and their ability to assist one another will make a great difference in choosing between home care or other living arrangements. Not only may space be inadequate, but many times it is impossible to have a family member in attendance with the patient during the day. Family members who work cannot afford to sacrifice jobs to stay with the patient. However, many families find it easier financially to have the patient at home and are able to make satisfactory arrangements even though the facilities are limited.

Many communities now provide portable meals (Meals-on-Wheels) for homebound persons. Most programs provide one hot meal daily and food that does not need to be heated for at least one other meal. The cost differs widely and depends on the services offered, such as special diets, and on the sponsorship of the plan. Volunteer groups frequently deliver the meals. This service alone often makes it possible for a chronically ill or aged person to remain at home.

Home health aide services

Home health aide services were increased when Medicare came into existence. The greater number of persons eligible for such services under Medicare spurred their growth. The early discharge of patients from hospitals has increased the need for these services even more. Home health aides provide physical care to the patient after a registered nurse evaluates the home situation and the patient's need for physical personal care. They are also responsible for keeping the patient's environment clean and for preparing the patient's meals. Ongoing supervision of the home health aide is the responsibility of the registered nurse assigned by the agency providing the home care.

Homemaker services

Homemaker services also have developed with the increased use of home care. These services are increasingly in demand in many communities and may be sponsored by a public or voluntary health or welfare agency or by a private agency that bills the family. Homemakers provide service to families with children and to the person who is convalescing, aged, or acutely or chronically ill. Homemakers are trained to assist in homes where the responsible family manager is temporarily unable to perform his or her usual responsibilities because of illness or absence.

Day care centers

In many communities some senior centers and nursing homes are expanding their facilities and services to include day care centers. Many chronically ill persons are able to live with their families but require 24-hour attendance. Often the caretaker in the family has to work. Homemaker or home health care aide services are generally not available for the time the caretaker is at work. Day care centers provide a place where the chronically ill person can be looked after on a daily basis. Nursing services, physical and occupational therapy, recreational therapy, meals, and, in some instances, transportation to and from the center are provided. This form of service may allow a person to remain at home with the family rather than having to resort to institutional care.

Respite care services

Some nursing homes maintain a specified number of beds for respite care. As the name implies, these beds are available on a short-term basis to provide respite for families who have a chronically ill person at home. The day-to-day care of the patient, often 24 hours a day, is a very trying experience for any family. To provide the family or primary caretaker with a period free of this responsibility, respite care may be the answer. Usually the cost of respite care is not reimbursable; however, it may be the only alternative if the primary caregiver cannot continue to care for the family member without a break.

Community health agenices, such as the Visiting Nurse Association, are providing respite services in some cities. They supply respite care in the patient's own home for part of a day, for 24 hours, or for extended periods depending on need. As mentioned, the cost of this service is usually not reimbursable.

Independent living centers

Some persons with chronic illnesses may be unable to cope with the demands of maintaining a home but wish to live as independently as possible. Various options are available in some communities; these range from living units where persons cook their meals but have the unit maintained, to assisted living units where persons can have their own physical living area but where one or more meals a day and other services are available. Living units are designed with such features as handrails for support in ambulation, wide doors to facilitate passage of wheelchairs, and emergency call systems.

Foster homes

Care in foster homes is a service that is now being widely used in many communities. Carefully selected families volunteer to take chronically ill persons into their own homes and provide the nonprofessional care needed. The family is paid either by the patient or the patient's family, from public funds, or by some social agency. The plan is primarily for those patients who have no family and cannot live alone, but who neither desire nor need institutional care.

Institutional care

Institutional care may be necessary when alternatives are not available, or the type of care needed by the patient requires close professional supervision. This includes chronic disease hospitals, skilled care facilities, convalescent homes, rest homes, homes for the aged, and nursing homes. Veteran's Administration hospitals provide services for men and women who have served in one of the U.S. Armed forces. The patient's potential for rehabilitation, need for maintenance care, or the level of physical disability are factors that determine eligibility for placement in any of these facilities. A large or limited selection of outside facilities may be available, depending on the community.

Role of the Nurse in Continuing Health Care

A nurse may be involved in continuing health care in several ways: (1) as an independent nurse practitioner assisting the person with chronic illness to cope with problems incurred by the illness; (2) as a public health nurse or visiting nurse involved in a primary rehabilitative program in the home; (3) as a supervisor of home health aides; or (4) as a nurse in a hospital concerned about the care patients will be receiving after they leave the hospital, particularly when the patient's rehabilitation program is not completed before discharge or when rehabilitation is not possible. Any of these nurses may also be involved in research pertaining to chronic illness. Some concepts that need further study in the area of chronic disease include social stigmatization, effects of isolation, and effects of chronic illness on the family, marriage, and domestic and occupational roles. Research will make a major contribution to clarification of these general concepts by identifying their relationship to chronic health problems.

Nurses must know the community resources available to patients to inform them and their families about what resources they might obtain, the types of service from which they may benefit, and what referrals they need for obtaining those services (see Box 14-2 for a list of community resources). The hospital nurse should clearly communicate to the continuing care agency the data pertinent to the patient's care so that continuity is ensured. Teamwork and continuity are the keys to successful rehabilitation and management services for patients, and they must be practiced at all stages of care if patients are to realize their fullest potential.

FOCUS ON THE FUTURE

Americans With Disabilities Act

In 1990 Congress passed the Americans with Disabilities Act (ADA), which some call the Civil Rights Act for the disabled. This law provides protection to the estimated 48 million Americans with disabilities. It has *four main components*, which *address employment*, *public services*, *public accommodations* and *services operated by private entities*, and

telecommunication services. The provisions under each of the components are listed in Box 14-4.

Implications for nursing

It is important for nurses to know about the provisions of the Disability Act so that they can inform the disabled about their rights under the law.

Nurses working in the rehabilitation settings will be able to employ nursing interventions that will assist the disabled person to function at his or her highest possible level. The role of the nurse in rehabilitation is discussed earlier in this chapter (see p. 288).

All nurses as citizens can be advocates for the disabled and help articulate their needs to the general public. Nurses can be active in their own communities to ensure that the public accommodations and public service provisions are carried out.[32]

A copy of the Americans with Disabilities Act, PL101-336, may be obtained free from the U.S. Government Documents Office in Washington, D.C. or from your congressional representative.

Center for Medical Rehabilitation Research

Another event that should have a favorable impact on persons with disabilities was the signing into law by President

---

14-4 **Provisions of Americans with disabilities employment act**

1. Employers may not discriminate against a qualified person with a disability in hiring or promotion.
2. Employers can ask about the person's ability to perform a job, but may not ask if someone has a disability or use tests that tend to screen out persons with disabilities.
3. Employers need to provide "reasonable accommodation" to individuals with disabilities including job restructuring and modification of equipment.
4. Employers do not need to provide accommodations that impose an "undue hardship" on business operations.
5. Employers with 25 or more employees must comply by July 26, 1992.
6. Employers with 15 to 24 employees must comply by July 26, 1994.

Transportation

1. New public transit buses ordered after August 26, 1990 must be accessible to persons with disabilities.
2. Transit authorities must provide comparable paratransit or other special transportation services to persons with disabilities who cannot use fixed route bus service, unless an undue burden would result.
3. Existing rail systems must have an accessible car per train by July 26, 1995.
4. New rail cars ordered after August 26, 1990 must be accessible.

5. New bus and train stations must be accessible.
6. Key stations in rapid, light, and commuter rail systems must be made accessible by July 26, 1993, with extensions up to 20 years for commuter rail (30 years for rapid and light rail).
7. All existing Amtrak stations must be accessible by July 26, 2010.

Public accommodations

1. Restaurants, hotels, and retail stores may not discriminate against persons with disabilities, effective January 26, 1992.
2. Auxiliary aids and services must be provided to individuals with hearing or vision impairments or other individuals with disabilities, unless an undue burden would result.
3. Physical barriers in existing facilities must be removed, if removal is readily achievable. If not, alternative methods of providing the service must be offered, if they are readily achievable.
4. All new construction and alterations of facilities must be accessible.

Telecommunications

Companies offering telephone service must offer telephone relay services to individuals who use telecommunication devices from the deaf (TTDs) or similar devices, effective July 26, 1993.

State and local governments

State and local governments may not discriminate against qualified individuals with disabilities.

Bush of a bill creating The Center for Medical Rehabilitation Research. The Center, which will be within the National Institutes of Child Health and Human Development, will be involved in basic, clinical, and applied rehabilitation research. It is expected to have a significant impact on the development of medical rehabilitation therapies and services.[11]

Health Care Goals for the Year 2000

In 1979, the surgeon general's Report established five goals concerned with major health problems in the United States.[47] The time frame for the achievement of those goals was to be 1990. By 1987, progress was made in reducing mortality in all the targeted age groups. Table 14-4 shows the progress made toward the 1990 goals.

As follow-up to the 1990 goals, work was begun in 1987 on developing health care goals for the year 2000. These goals are published in *Healthy People 2000: National Health Promotion and Disease.*[28]

The development of the year 2000 goals was a national effort that involved health professionals, citizens, private organizations, and public agencies from every part of the United States. Almost 300 national membership organizations and health departments from the 50 states were involved in the development. Nurses were represented by the American Nurses' Association, the National League for Nursing, and several speciality organizations.

Before discussing the goals for the year 2000, it is important to describe the changes in the U.S. population that are expected to occur between now and 2000.

Profile of the American people in the year 2000

Healthy People 2000[28] describes the demographic changes that will occur between 1990 and 2000.

1. By the year 2000, the population of the United States will have grown about 7% to approximately 270 million people. The slowest growth rate in the history of the country is projected to occur between 1995 and 2000. Average household size is expected to decline from 2.69 in 1985 to 2.48 in 2000, with husband-wife households decreasing from 58% to 53% of all households.
2. By the year 2000, the American population will be older with a median age of more than 36 years, compared to 29 years in 1975. The number of children under age 5 will decline from more than 18 million to fewer than 17 million between 1990 and 2000.

3. By the year 2000, 35 million people over age 65 will represent 13% of the population as compared to 8% in 1950. The "oldest old"—those over age 85—will increase to 30% to a total of 4.6 million by 2000.
4. By the year 2000, the racial and ethnic composition of the American population will change. Whites will decline from 76% to 72% of the population. Hispanics have been forecasted to increase from 8% to 11.3%, to more than 31 million Hispanic people by 2000. Blacks will increase from 12.4% to 13.1% Other racial groups, including American Indians and Alaska Natives, and Asians and Pacific Islanders will increase from 3.5% to 4.3% of the total population.
5. By the year 2000, reflecting changes in racial and ethnic populations, the entry rate of blacks, Hispanics, Asians and Pacific Islanders, and American Indians and Alaska Natives into the workforce will be higher than for Whites. Women of all racial and ethnic groups will be the major source of new entrants into the labor force. The women in the work force will comprise 47% of the total workforce as compared to 45% in 1988. White men will make up only 25% of the net growth of the labor force.
6. Occupations most likely to grow include service, professional, technical, sales, and executive and management positions.
7. By the year 2000, the American population may increase by up to 6 million people through immigration. This immigration will be to certain states and cities, with the greatest number settling on the east and west coasts.

According to *Healthy People 2000,*[28] the purpose of the report was to commit the nation to the attainment of three broad goals that will bring us a nation to our full potential. The three broad goals can be found in Box 14-5.

The goals to be achieved by the year 2000 are divided into 22 priority areas. The first 21 of these goals are grouped into three broad categories: *health promotion, health protection,* and *preventive services.* It seems clear that the achievement of the three broad goals would reduce the number of people in the United States with chronic health problems. These goals and the three approaches to them *require that individuals take more responsibility for their own health and in preventing chronic illnesses.* At the same time, health professionals are called upon not only to treat disease but to prevent disease and conditions that result in premature death and chronic disability.

The challenge spelled out in *Healthy People 2000* is for communities to translate these national objectives into state and local action.

Table 14-4   **Progress in meeting 1990 health goals**

Life stage	1990 goals	1987 status
Infants	35% lower death rate	28% lower
Children	20% lower death rate	21% lower
Adolescents/ young adults	20% lower death rate	13% lower
Adults	25% lower death rate	21% lower
Older adults	20% fewer days of restricted activity	17% lower

14-5   Three broad goals for the year 2000

1. Increase the span of healthy life for all Americans.
2. Reduce health disparities among Americans.
3. Achieve access to preventive services for all Americans.

Table 14-5 Target populations years of healthy life by year 2000

Populations	1980 baseline	2000 target
Blacks	56	60
Hispanics	62	65
People 65 and older—years of healthy life remaining	12	14

Table 14-6 Prevalence of disability in special population targets

Prevalence of disability	1989 baseline	2000 target
Low-income people (Annual family income: $10,000 in 1988)	18.9%	15%
American Indian/Alaskan natives	13.4%	11%
Blacks	11.2%	9%

Not all the goals for 2000 can be discussed in this chapter. Only those objectives related to chronic conditions will be presented. Other goals related to persons with specific health problems will be discussed in the appropriate chapters of this text.

Health status objectives related to chronic disabling conditions

Health status objectives related to chronic disabling conditions include the following:

1. Increase years of healthy life to at least 65 years from an estimated baseline of 62 years in 1980. Special target populations are listed in Table 14-5.
2. Reduce to no more than 8% (from a baseline of 9.4% in 1988) the proportion of people who experience a limitation in major activity due to a chronic condition. Special target populations for this objective are presented in Table 14-6.
3. Reduce to no more than 90 per 1000 people the proportion of all people aged 65 and older who have difficulty in performing two or more personal care activities (bathing, dressing, using the toilet, getting in and out of bed) thereby preserving independence. The baseline was 111 per 1000 population in 1984 to 1985. The special target population for this objective is people aged 85 years and older.
4. Reduce to no more than 10% the proportion of people with asthma who experience activity limitation as compared with a baseline of 19.4% in 1986 to 1988.
5. Reduce activitity limitation resulting from chronic back conditions to a prevalence of no more than 19 per 1000 by the year 2000 as compared with a baseline of 21.9 per 1000 in 1986 to 1988.
6. Reduce significant hearing impairment to a prevalence of no more than 82 per 1000 people by the year 2000, from a baseline of 88.9 per 1000 people during 1986 to 1988. Special target population is persons 45 years and older in whom a prevalence of hearing impairment would be no more than 180 per 1000 as compared with a baseline of 203 per 1000 in 1986 to 1988.
7. Reduce significant visual impairment to a prevalance of no more than 30 per 1000 people by the year 2000, from a baseline average of 34.5 per 1000 during 1986 to 1988. Special target population is people aged 65 and older in whom a prevalence of visual impairment would be 70 per 1000 as compared to 87.7 in 1986 to 1988.
8. There are several objectives related to diabetes. These are presented in Chapter 28.

Services and protection objectives

Services and protection objectives related to the health status objectives include:

1. Increase to at least 60% the proportion of providers of primary care for older adults who routinely evaluate people aged 65 and older for urinary incontinence; impairments of vision, hearing, and cognition; and functional status. Baseline data was not available.
2. Increase to at least 90% the proportion of premenopausal women who have been counseled about the benefits and risks of estrogen replacement therapy (combined with progestin, when appropriate) for prevention of osteoporosis. Baseline data was not available.
3. Increase to at least 75% the proportion of worksites with 50 or more employees that have a voluntarily established policy or program for hiring people with disabilities. The baseline was 37% of medium and large companies in 1986. This objective reflects the intentions of the Americans with Disabilities Act (see p. 292).
4. Increase to 50 the number of states that have service systems for children at risk of chronic conditions, as required by Public Law 101-239 (Americans with Disabilities Act (p. 292).

All nurses need to be aware of the goals spelled out in *Healthy People 2000*,[28] and the plans developed in the state in which they are residing for bringing these goals into fruition. The goals, if met, should assist all persons in the United States to have as healthy a life as possible.

Management System for Persons With Chronic Conditions

In looking at health care for the chronically ill in the United States, it seems obvious that some changes need to be made. One consultant to hospitals has suggested that hospitals need to look at their focus on acute care and give higher priority to care of the chronically ill.[14] He recommends that hospitals develop Chronic Disease Centers just as they have developed Ambulatory Surgery Centers. He points out that the present health care delivery system is oriented to intervening in the disease process and "fixing" the condition whereas persons with a chronic condition are trying to minimize their chronic condition and live as normal lives as possible.

He also suggests that Chronic Disease Centers could become the primary care provider for persons with chronic conditions. His suggestion will not be acceptable to all care providers including many nurses who believe that clinical nurse specialists and nurse practitioners are the ideal health care providers for these patients because much of their care involves teaching and counseling, which are central parts of the nursing role.

Burkhardt et al. describe the results of a research project using the Quality of Life Scale (QOLS) and point out what nurses might wish to keep in mind as they work with persons with chronic conditions.[2]

> There is no reason to believe persons with a stable chronic illness or condition cannot have as high a quality of life as those without chronic illness although care must be taken to see that the definition and measurement of *[quality of life]* be *[clearly subjective satisfaction]* and not be confounded with objective measure of health status.

SUMMARY

1. Chronic health problems are one of the major health problems in the United States.
2. The incidence and prevalence of chronic diseases have increased in this century and can be expected to increase even more as the population ages.
3. The Bureau of the Census estimates that approximately 110 million persons in the United States have one or more chronic illnesses.
4. There are major disparities in the health of black Americans and other minorities in the United States when compared with the white population.
5. The characteristics of chronic illnesses include one or more of the following: (1) illness or impairment that is permanent, (2) residual disability, and (3) nonreversible pathologic alteration, which requires a long period of care.
6. Chronic illnesses may be present from birth or develop during childhood, adolescence, early adult life, or old age.
7. Today some children with chronic illnesses such as cystic fibrosis live into early adulthood because of more effective treatment.
8. Major chronic illnesses of adults include arthritis, diabetes, heart disease, and hypertension. The rates for arthritis and hypertension are higher in blacks than in whites.
9. Cultural values determine how both nurses and patients view chronic illness.
10. The economic costs of chronic illness are considerable and many persons will require some type of financial assistance.
11. Failure to understand or internalize the reason for therapeutic recommendations, procedures that are difficult to learn and carry out, time necessary to carry out therapy, side effects of therapy, inability to pay for prescribed therapy, and social isolation and lack of support and positive reinforcement are possible reasons why a person may be noncompliant with therapeutic recommendations.
12. It is important that nurses be involved in prevention of chronic illness.
13. There are three levels of prevention: primary, secondary, and tertiary, and the nurse has an important role to play at each level.
14. Primary prevention involves health promotion and specific protection against disease (such as immunization against poliomyelitis).
15. Secondary prevention includes early detection of disease and prompt intervention to halt progression of disease.
16. Tertiary prevention includes rehabilitation appropriate to the stage of disability, prevention of further complications, and restoring optimal functioning to the highest possible level.
17. Depression is common among the chronically ill, especially those who feel powerless about controlling or overcoming what has happened to them.
18. Rehabilitation is best carried out in a setting where an intradisciplinary team of nurses, physicians, physical and occupational therapists, social workers and, when necessary, speech therapists are available to work together in planning the therapeutic regimen for the patient and in assisting and supporting the patient with the prescribed therapy.
19. The two major roles of the nurse working with persons with disabilities are (1) to limit disability from disease as much as possible and (2) to see that the rehabilitation program is planned and implemented.
20. The nurse should be familiar with the facilities for continuing care in his or her community and the eligibility requirements for each facility.
21. The Americans with Disabilities Act passed by Congress in 1990 provides protection for the disabled in terms of employment, public services, public accommodations, services operated by private entities, and telecommunication services.
22. *Healthy People 2000* is a publication prepared for the Surgeon General of the United States. It presents more than 300 objectives to improve the health of U.S. citizens by the year 2000.
23. Nurses need to be aware of the plans of the state in which they reside for meeting the goals for the year 2000.

STUDY QUESTIONS

- What types of patients do you think are most in need of rehabilitation? Outline the rehabilitation needs of a patient you are now caring for or have cared for in the past.
- What proportion of the patients on the hospital unit to which you are assigned has a chronic illness as either a primary or secondary diagnosis? What proportion has more than one chronic health problem? What age group is affected most by more than one chronic health problem?
- What resources are available in your community for the care of the chronically ill? Are the facilities adequate for the number of persons needing care? How are these facilities supported financially?
- From what you have learned in anatomy, outline in detail the physical movements necessary to rise from a sitting position in a chair to a standing position. Describe how you would assist a patient to stand while allowing him or her to be as independent as possible.

REFERENCES AND SELECTED READINGS

1. American Cancer Society: 1991 *Cancer facts and figures,* Atlanta, 1991, The Society.
2.* Burckhardt CS et al: Quality of life of adults with chronic illness: a psychometric study, *Res Nurs Health* 12:347-354, 1989.
3. Centers for Disease Control Report to the Secretary's task force on black and minority health, *MMWR* 35(8), 1986.
4.* Centers for Disease Control chronic disease reports, *MMWR* 38(S-1), 1989.
5.* Centers for Disease Control: Progress in chronic disease prevention, *MMWR* 38(8), 1989.
6.* Centers for Disease Control: Progress in chronic disease prevention, *MMWR* 38(12), 1989.
7.* Centers for Disease Control: Health objectives for the nation, *MMWR* 38(37), 1989.
8.* Centers for Disease Control: Chronic disease reports in the morbidity and mortality weekly report (MMWR) 38(S-1), 1989.
9. Council on Ethical and Judicial Affairs: Black-white disparities in health care, *JAMA* 263(17):2344-2346, 1990.
10. Council on Scientific Affairs: Home care in the 1990s, *JAMA* 263(8):1241-1244, 1990.
11. DeLisa JA, Jain SS: Physical medicine and rehabilitation, *JAMA* 265(23):358-359, 1991.
12. Dittmar S: *Rehabilitation nursing,* St Louis, 1989, Mosby–Year Book.
13.* Older Americans present a double challenge: preventing disability and providing care, *Am J Pub Health,* 81(3):287-288, March 1991 (editorial).
14. Henry WF: Chronic care needs to be a higher priority, *Hospitals* Feb 20: 68, 1991.
15. Kahn KL et al. Comparing outcomes of care before and after implementation of the DRG-based prospective payment system, *JAMA* 264(15):1984-1988, 1990.
16. Kemper P, Murtaugh CM: Lifetime use of nursing home care, *New Engl J Med* 324(9):595-600, 1991.
17.* Lambert VA, Lambert CE, editors: Adaptation to chronic illness, *Nurs Clin North Am* 22:527-644, 1987.
18.* Leidy NK: A structural model of stress, phychosocial resources, and symptomatic experiences in chronic physical illness, *Nurs Outlook* 34(4):230-236, 1990.
19. Lubkin IM: *Chronic illness: impact and interventions,* Boston, 1986, Jones & Bartlett Publishing.
20. National Center for Health Statistics: *Vital statistics of the United States, 1980,* vol 11, Mortality, part B, DHHS, Pub No (PHS) 85-1102, Washington, DC, 1985, US Government Printing Office.
21.* Pollock SE: Human response to chronic illness: physiologic and psychosocial adaptation, *Nurs Res* 35:90-95, 1986.
22. Primomo J, Yates BC, Woods NF: Social support for women during chronic illnesses: the relationship among sources and types to adjustment, *Res Nurs Health* 13:153-161, 1990.
23. Public Health Service: Vital and health statistics: current estimates from the National Health Interview Survey, 1989, US Department of Health, Education, and Welfare.
24.* Schwartz E, et al: Black/white comparisons of deaths preventable by medical intervention: United States and the District of Columbia 1980-1986, *Int J Epidemiol* 19(3):591-598, 1990.
25. Shaughnessy PW, Kramer AM: The increased needs of patients in nursing homes and patients receiving home health care, *New Engl J Med* 322(1):21-27, 1990.
26.* Stewart AI, et al: Functional status and well-being of patients with chronic conditions, *JAMA* 262(7):907-193, 1989.
27. US Bureau of the Census: *Statistical abstract of the United States, 1986,* annual ed 107, Washington, DC, 1987, US Government Printing Office.
28. US Department of Health and Human Services: *Healthy People 2000: national health promotion and disease prevention objectives,* Washington, DC, 1990, US Government Printing Office.
29. US Department of Health and Human Services: *Vital and health statistics: current estimates from the national health interview survey, 1989,* Washington, 1990, US Government Printing Office.
30. US Department of Health and Human Services, Secretary's task force on black and minority health, Washington, 1985, US Government Printing Office.
31.* Van Horne WA, Tonnesen TV, editors: *Ethnicity and health,* Madison, 1988, The University of Wisconsin System Institute on Race and Ethnicity.
32.* Watson PG: The Americans with Disabilities Act: More rights for people with disabilities, *Rehab Nurs* 15(6): 325-328, 1990.

Classic

33.* American Academy of Nursing: Long-term care: some issues for nursing, Kansas City, Mo, 1976, American Nurses' Association.
34.* American Nurses Association: A national policy for health care: principles and positions, Kansas City, Mo, 1977, The Association.
35. Expectation of life in the United States at a new high, *Stat Bull* 61(4):13-15, 1980.
36.* Johnson JH, editor: Rehabilitation nursing: *Nurs Clin North Am* 15:2, 1980.
37. Leslie PM: Nursing diagnosis: use in long-term care, *Am J Nurs* 81:1012-1014, 1981.
38. Morris R, editor: Allocating health resources for the aged and disabled, Lexington, Mass, 1981, Lexington Books.
39. Moskowitz E, McCann CB: Classification of disability in the chronically ill and aging, *J Chronic Dis* 5:342-346, 1957.
40.* Olson EV: The hazards of immobility, *Am J Nurs* 67:780-797, 1967.
41. Public Health Service: *Vital and health statistics: current estimates from the Health Interview Survey (1981),* series 10, No 141, Rockville, Md, Oct 1982, US Dept of Health, Education, and Welfare.
42. Public Health Service: *Vital and health statistics: health characteristics of persons with chronic activity limitations (1979),* series 10, No 137, Rockville, Md, Dec 1981, US Dept of Health and Human Services.
43. Ryan S, Wassenberg C, editors: Community health and home care nursing, *Nurs Clin North Am* 15:2, 1980.
44.* Sorensen K, Armis DB: Understanding the world of the chronically ill, *Am J Nurs* 67:811-817, 1967.
45.* Strauss AL et al: Chronic illness and the quality of life, ed 2, St Louis, 1984, Mosby–Year Book.
46. Thom A: Home health care agencies in the 1980s, *Home Health Care Serv Q* 3:5-24, 1982.
47.* US Dept of Health, Education, and Welfare: *Healthy people, Surgeon General's report on health promotion and disease prevention,* Washington, DC, 1979, US Government Printing Office.
48.* Wright BA: Value-laden beliefs and principles for rehabilitation, *Rehabil Lit* 12:266-269, 1981.

*Recommended for student reading.

15

Loss, Dying, and Death

Sally M. Featherstone

After studying this chapter, the learner should be able to:

- Describe losses to self, external losses, and factors influencing loss experiences.
- Describe the phases of life-threatening illness.
- Discuss the basis tasks of grief.
- Discuss the crisis model as an assessment tool for coping.
- Describe nursing interventions for patients/families coping with life-threatening events.
- Compare patient/family tasks associated with each phase of the dying process.
- Discuss the process and stress of nurses' grief and survival strategies when working with dying patients and bereaved families.

Nurses who work with the terminally ill and bereaved persons often develop a heightened empathy and identification with their patients. This occurs because the loss experience is so universal that everyone has experienced its impact. These losses can prepare us for the ultimate loss in death. Grief is the normal and universal response to loss.

Dying and death are not synonymous; they are distinct and separate events. Almost nothing can be known about death, at least on this side of parapsychology and faith. A great deal, however, can be known about dying. A pattern of dying is lived by each person in his or her lifetime. Life can be described as a migration through many little dyings, losses, and grieving for those losses. Growth, change, and maturing occur by adaptation to the losses occurring throughout one's lifetime. Nurses can learn about the "big" dying by understanding the "little" dyings.[38]

UNDERSTANDING LOSS

Basic Assumptions

When people do not do "grief work" following any significant loss, they are at risk for emotional, mental, and social problems. A review of the literature reveals many examples of increased morbidity, both physical and mental, following significant losses.[9,16,21,23,43] There is an increase in the breakup of marriages and other significant relationships following the loss of a child or when one partner suffers a loss of body part or function.[24]

Loss is defined as any change in a person's situation that reduces the probability of achieving goals or when a person is without something he/she formerly possessed. It can be anticipatory. A loss need not have occurred to stimulate a grief response. Loss is inevitable and inescapable—no one is exempt from loss. There are hardly any gains in life that have not grown out of or been accompanied by loss; for example, a person who receives a promotion gains in stature and income, but may simultaneously lose the support of his or her previous peer group. Losses accumulated without resolution lead to energy depletion and increased vulnerability to psychologic stress. Loss is a complex phenomenon.

Categories of Loss

Losses can be described as related to the self or as external to the self (Box 15-1). Self losses include the loss of the psychologic self, the sociocultural self, the physical self, and the spiritual self. The ultimate loss of self is the loss of self because of death. External losses include the loss of objects, possessions, loved ones, support, and environment.[25]

Self losses

Loss of the psychologic self includes loss of self-esteem and personal identity. Some examples are:

1. Mrs. Smith, who has been married for many years suddenly loses her husband. She not only loses her husband, but she also loses all that being Mrs. Smith meant.
2. John Jones has been a Professor of English for 30 years. He recently retired and no longer has the

responsibilities that go with being a teacher. He is no longer Professor Jones, just Mr. Jones.

Any loss that affects the way one perceives oneself as a competent and capable person impacts the psychologic self.

Loss of the sociocultural self includes the loss of language, associations, and the meanings of one's cultural heritage. Loss of the sociocultural self occurs when a person is suddenly thrust into an alien culture or has divided loyalties to different cultures. A nurse can belong to a religious group whose beliefs are in conflict with her work assignments, as in the case of a Catholic who is assigned to work in a family planning clinic. Society's demand for conformity places much pressure on people with different values and beliefs and often causes a person to be separated from familiar and comforting surroundings and people. The Native American culture is a good example of this. Native Americans have been forced to integrate into the Anglo-Saxon way of life. When confronted with life-threatening situations, they may well worry about possible discrimination and, fearful of giving expression to their needs, remain silent.[10] This can also be seen when patients are hospitalized. They no longer have control over their surroundings. They are expected to learn how to be "good" patients. People are shaped by the cultural values of the ethnic, religious, and social segment of the society in which they are reared. When access to that network is denied, the person suffers the loss of the sociocultural self.

Losses of the physical self are more obvious, but their impact is not necessarily so clear. The extent, duration, and visibility of the loss will influence how the individual responds to the loss. Loss of one leg could be less significant that the loss of both legs. A temporary loss of body function is much more easily adapted to than a permanent loss would be. Persons confined to wheelchairs often report being treated as incompetent persons. Beland relates the story of going shopping in a wheelchair—the store clerk asked Beland's companion what Beland wanted instead of speaking to Beland directly.[24] The meaning of the particular body part involved will also have an impact. It will make a significant difference if the persons losing the use of their legs are football players or accountants. The loss to the football player is central to his life goals and therefore is likely to have a much greater impact than the same loss

---

15-1 | **Categories of loss**

Self losses
    Loss of the psychologic self
    Loss of the sociocultural self
    Loss of the physical self
    Loss of the spiritual self
External losses
    Objects, possessions
    Loved ones
    Environment
    Support
Real or imagined losses
Present or anticipated losses

might have on an accountant whose legs are not critical to success as an accountant.

Loss of the spiritual self refers to the loss of hope, values, and beliefs. Many writers have identified the critical role that maintenance of hope plays for the person with a life-threatening illness. Without hope, despair sets in and the patient gives up.*

External losses

External losses includes the loss of objects, possessions, loved ones, environment, and support. These losses can be real or imagined, present or anticipated. The importance of the loss of objects or possessions is influenced by the value of the object, both monetary and sentimental, and the usefulness of the object. A lost loved one may be a family member, a friend, or an acquaintance. The loss can occur through separation, moving, promotion, or death. The loss of familiar surroundings or other supports can leave one feeling vulnerable and lonely. The impact of loss through the death of a loved one is discussed on p. 299.

Factors Influencing Loss

Loss is a complex phenomenon, influenced by many factors (Box 15-2). A review of these factors is helpful in understanding what a specific loss means to an individual. Generalizations about personal experiences and behavior are useful only when one is committed to understanding and accepting individual variations.

Childhood experiences can impact the way one perceives and reacts to a loss. How parents handle losses can influence a child's view of loss as a challenge or something to be avoided at all costs. If parents protect a child from experiencing the grief associated with loss, the child may think that loss is something bad. A child's first experience with death is often the death of a pet, such as when a pet goldfish dies. Parents can use this as an opportunity to discuss death or they can cover it up by replacing the dead fish before the child knows what has happened. A child who is punished for losing things, as in the nursery rhyme about the three little kittens who lost their mittens, may later experience guilt as the predominant emotion related to loss.

The significance assigned the loss can be related to the objective or subjective value of the object. An illustration of this is the story of a couple who is in the process of moving. The wife has a heavy old mantle clock that has been in the family for generations. The husband thinks the clock is ugly and it weighs a ton. The movers lift the clock out of the moving van and drop it. The clock shatters. The wife is horrified and bursts into tears. The husband can barely contain his glee. The objective value of the clock is the same, but its subjective value to each of the persons involved has a major impact on their response to the loss.

One's *physical and emotional status* at the time of a loss can have a significant influence on one's response. Nurse Nelly is getting ready for work. She woke up with a headache and she is running late; the alarm did not go off. She is anxious because her new supervisor starts today. Nelly

*References 1, 3, 7, 8, 12, 15.

15-2	**Factors influencing loss experiences**

Childhood experiences
Significance assigned to the loss
Physical and emotional state
Accumulated loss experience
View of loss as crisis
Visibility
Duration and timing
Abruptness or suddenness
Financial impact
Availability of resources
Cultural factors
Personal attributes
Relationship with the lost person
Death surround

---

can't find her car keys. She feels overwhelmed and dissolves into a sobbing heap on the floor. On a normal day she would have been slightly irritated and would have remembered that she has a spare set of keys and would only have lost a few minutes.

Accumulated losses can impact how a person responds to a current loss, especially if there are unresolved losses. A nurse was interviewing a family after the loss of a baby to Sudden Infant Death Syndrome. The grandparents were present. The grandmother began to sob uncontrollably. The nurse inquired about the grandmother's past experience with loss and found that she had recently lost a son in a car accident and had a history of miscarriages that she had never been able to talk about.

View of the loss as a crisis is an important factor. It can be helpful to understand how a person experiencing the loss perceives his or her ability to cope. A crisis is defined by the person experiencing the event. The balancing forces of crisis are: (1) The person's view of the situation; (2) the feelings experienced and expressed; (3) previous problem solving efforts made in this situation; and (4) the person's support system, both internal and external. If any of these balancing forces are absent or unavailable to persons coping with the loss, they will likely perceive themselves as being in crisis.

Visibility can have both a positive and negative effect on the loss. Visibility of the loss can increase the support offered, as in the example where a family loses its home in a fire and the neighborhood offers support through donations and assistance. Visibility can have a negative effect when it brings forth nonsupportive expressions, as in the situation of a person who has experienced a facially disfiguring accident that causes people to stare in horror. Other losses may fail to call forth support because they are invisible, as in the case of the loss of a baby before term.

Duration and timing can impact a loss depending on the degree of goal disruption that results from the time spent in resolving the loss. An athlete who suffers a broken leg may only be disrupted temporarily. However, if the break occurs before a key event, it may result in the athlete not getting an opportunity to go to the college of his or her choice. If the break is of short duration and timing is not

Table 15-1   **Children's responses to loss and death**

Age	Developmental stage/task	Concept of death	Grief response
2-4	Egocentric. Believes world centers around self. Narcissistic. No cognitive understanding. Preconceptual, unable to grasp concepts.	Seen as abandonment. Seen as reversible. "Did you know my daddy died—when will he be home?"	Intense, brief. Very present oriented. Most aware of altered pattern of care.
4-7	Gaining sense of autonomy. Exploring world outside of self. Gaining language. Fantasy. Initiative phase. Concerns of guilt.	Death still seen as reversible. Personification of death. Feels responsible, because of wishes, thoughts. "It's my fault. I was mad at her and wished she would die."	Verbalization. Great concern with process. How? Why? Repetitive questioning.
7-11	Concrete. Industry versus inferiority. Begins socialization. Developing of cognitive ability. Begins logical thinking.	Death as punishment. Fear of bodily harm, mutilation. Difficult transition period; still wants to see death as reversible, but beginning to see it as final.	Specific questions. Desire for details. Concern with how others respond. What is the right way? How should they respond? Begins to mourn.
11-18	Formal problem solving. Abstract thinking. Integration of own personality.	"Adult" Approach. Conceptualizes death. Works at making sense of teachings.	Depression. Denial. Repression. Willing to talk to people outside family. Traditional mourning.

Modified from Metzgar M: Little ears, big issues: children and loss, Seattle, 1990 (pamphlet).

an issue, the athlete may resume his or her career with little effect. However, an accident that results in permanent paralysis will have a major impact on the loss adjustment of the individual.

Abruptness or suddenness of the loss will influence how one copes with it. It is generally agreed that a sudden loss is more difficult to cope with than one that is expected and for which a person has had time to prepare.

Financial impact adds a secondary loss. The longer and more extensive the loss, the greater the expense usually involved. This is particularly significant when the primary loss results in the inability of the individual to return to work. Bereaved families have been known to express a great deal of anger and pain upon receiving a large hospital bill for a family member who died because it adds insult to injury.

Availability of resources, both internal and external, are important to the individual's ability to cope with the challenges resulting from the loss. Prior experience in successfully coping with loss can provide the internal support to deal with the current loss. However, if the loss is sufficiently different and catastrophic, such as a sudden violent death, previous coping is not likely to suffice to support the individual. External support from family, friends, acquaintances, and professional or community supports is essential.[9]

Culture is the dynamic system of values that informs and influences most loss situations. Culture is an integrated system of learned patterns of behavior, ideas, and products that are characteristic of a society. It affects the assessment of comfort needs of the dying and the kind of care provided. It influences the selection, perception, and evaluation of health care providers and their methods. It shapes beliefs about the cause of loss and death. It determines the disposition of the body and funeral and burial rites. It influences grief responses and bereavement roles.[47]

The nurse must not rely on stereotypes because there are variations within any group of people (see Chapter 3). Each patient and family's grief reactions will be a blend of culture, personal habits, and raw emotion.

Personal attributes that affect loss include age, sex, socioeconomic status, and education or occupation. The age at which a loss is experienced will impact the loss (Table 15-1). In their review of the literature, Stroebe and Stroebe[21] concluded that men and younger people were at greatest risk, with social support likely to be the moderating factor. Socioeconomic status and education affected the response to loss only in terms of the options for coping made available to the person experiencing the loss.

Relationship with the lost person will impact the loss according to the meaning and significance of the relationship to the survivor. It cannot be automatically assumed that one type of loss is more serious than another. It is not necessarily true that the loss of a parent will bring more grief than the loss of a grandparent. The griever may have had a more intimate relationship with the grandparent. The qualities of the relationship are more important than the relationship itself. For some persons the loss of a pet may be a more significant loss than the loss of a person. The psychologic nature of the relationship and the strength of the attachment will have a significant impact on the griever. For example, a relationship characterized by ambivalence is more difficult to resolve than one that is not conflicted. Those who are strongly dependent upon the lost person often have more problems than others.[47] It has been said that to lose your parents is to lose your past, to lose your child is to lose your future, and to lose your spouse is to lose your present.

The *death surround* refers to the immediate circumstance of the death or loss. It includes the location, type of loss or death, the reason for the loss, and the degree of preparation for the loss. Ideally the griever will feel that the

Beneficial ways in which death affects our perceptions of life

It helps us savor life.

It provides an opposite by which to judge being alive.

It gives us a sense of a real, individual existence.

It gives meaning to courage and integrity, allowing us to express our convictions effectively.

It provides us with the strength to make major decisions.

It reveals the importance of intimacy in our lives.

It helps us to ascribe meaning to our lives; this is especially useful to older people.

It shows us the importance of ego-transcending achievements.

It allows us to see our achievements as being significant.

From Rando TA: *Grief, dying, and death,* Champaign, Ill, 1984, Research Press.

Phases of life-threatening illness

Prediagnostic phase. Often precedes diagnosis. Here the client recognizes symptoms or risk factors of illness. The basic ongoing process is a health-seeking one in which the client recognizes some element of risk and selects strategies to cope with this perceived threat.

Acute phase. Centers around the crisis of diagnosis. The client is faced with a diagnosis of life-threatening illness and now must make a series of decisions—medical, psychologic, and interpersonal—on how, at least initially, to cope.

Chronic phase. The client is struggling with the disease and its treatment. Many clients may attempt, with varying degrees of success, to live a reasonably normal life within the confines of the disease. Often this period is punctuated by a series of illness-related crises.

Terminal phase. The disease has progressed to a point in which death is inevitable. Death is no longer merely possible, it is now likely.

Data from Doka K: *The Terrible Threat,* Book in preparation, 1992.

circumstances are appropriate. To the extent the "surround" can be accepted, the grief will be more amenable to resolution.[47]

DYING AND DEATH

Dying is an integral part of life. It is as natural and predictable as being born. Death is dreaded, whereas birth is often welcomed and celebrated. Death is an issue to be avoided. Throughout history, humanity has been concerned with death. Philosophy, religion, and science have all attempted to find answers to explain and control death. In spite of technologic advances, death continues to be inevitable, and this knowledge influences how we look at life.

Death affects our perceptions of life in beneficial ways, such as giving us an appreciation for living, helping us savor life, and giving us a sense of real existence (Box 15-3). It can however, also threaten us with the negation of ourselves and all that we value. We tend to be future-oriented and the thought of no future arouses anxiety. Attitudes toward death may range from complete denial to complete and existential acceptance. The particular attitude adopted influences our lives significantly.[19,47]

One person may choose to deny the reality of death, will avoid talking about it, will not attend wakes or funerals, may postpone making a will, or getting a physical examination. Another person will have faith in life after death and, through religion, can believe that this life is merely a prelude to the afterlife. It is critical to understand not only how our patients view death, but also our own personal feelings about death. We can have a variety of personal gut-level responses to death, but these responses do not prevent our being effective in working with the dying and the bereaved, if we are aware of them. It is normal and natural to have less-than-positive feelings about death.[37]

There is a "living-dying" interval between the time of diagnosis and death. Pattison offers a model of the dying process that emphasizes three phases: an acute phase that centers around the issue of diagnosis, a chronic phase that emphasizes living with disease, and the terminal phase when the impending death is both certain and paramount.[46] Doka[5] has adapted this model to a model of "life-threatening illness" (Box 15-4). It is clear that throughout each phase the patient and family will be coping with different loss issues. Dying or coping with illness is not an isolated process; rather it is part of the process of life. Models are valuable because they help organize information, but they are at best generalities. Models can be helpful when they contribute to our understanding of the individual experiences, but they are destructive when they impose that reality on the patient.

Kubler-Ross's model of the five stages of dying: denial, anger, bargaining, depression, and acceptance, has been misused when nurses tried to classify the many different responses of patients into one of the five stages or to move the patient from denial to acceptance.

GRIEF, MOURNING, AND BEREAVEMENT

The terms *grief, mourning,* and *bereavement* have been used interchangeably and have been assigned specific meaning. In this chapter they mean the following:

Grief is the process of psychologic, social, and somatic reactions to a perceived loss. It is manifested in all three areas and changes over time. It is a natural, often expected reaction, to many kinds of loss, not just death. Grief is based on the unique, individual perception of the loss by the griever.

Table 15-2 **Comparison of major theories of grief**

Kubler-Ross stages	Lindemann stages	Parkes/Bowlby phases	Engel
Denial and isolation	Shock/disbelief	Numbness	Shock/disbelief
Anger	Acute mourning	Yearning/searching	Developing awareness
Bargaining	Resolution of grief	Disorganization and despair	Restitution
Depression		Reorganization	Resolve the loss
Acceptance			Idealization
			Final outcome

Mourning includes a wide array of intrapsychic processes, conscious and unconscious, that are the result of loss. It is also a response to loss that is culturally and socially influenced. Grief may be conceptualized as a transitional phase in the overarching process of mourning.

Bereavement is the state of having suffered a loss.

Basic Tasks of Grief

An understanding of the grief process requires knowledge of the basic tasks of grief. Lindemann offered his conceptualization in 1944 and his theory has been incorporated into contemporary researchers' definitions of the grief process.[22,45,47] There are three basic tasks that constitute grief work:

1. Emancipation from the bondage of the lost object.
2. Readjustment to the environment in which the lost object is missing.
3. Formation of new relationships.

Emancipation from the lost object is the task of "untying the ties that bind" the griever to the lost person or object. This does not mean that what is lost is forgotten or not loved, but rather that the griever can invest the energy previously placed in the lost person in new relationships. The relationship with the lost person remains, but in altered form, in the mind and heart of the griever. What is changed is the ongoing investment in and attachment to the lost person as living. The energy that previously kept that relationship alive must now be channeled elsewhere, where it can be returned.

Readjustment to the environment is the task in which the griever accommodates to a world without the lost object or person. The griever experiences many distressing feelings while struggling to bear the pain of separation and becoming accustomed to the loved one's absence.

Formation of new relationships involves the reinvestment of the emotional energy that is withdrawn from the previous relationship in someone or something else. The time it takes before a griever can reinvest will depend on a host of factors, but at some point in time the griever should be able to take the energy that had been used to keep the previous relationship alive and redirect it towards establishing and maintaining rewarding investments in others.[47]

Lindemann's term "grief work" is accurate because grief requires the expenditure of both physical and emotional energy. The work of grieving involves grieving for the actual lost person or object and for all the hopes, dreams, fantasies, and unfulfilled expectations the griever had in terms of the relationship. The loss of a child not only involves the loss of the person, but all the dreams the parents had for the child and the parents' expectation that they would outlive their child. It does not seem to matter if the child was lost before birth or at a later age. From the moment that parents become aware of the child's conception, they begin to dream.

Another complicating factor in accomplishing the grief work is that loss resurrects old issues and conflicts in the griever. The feelings reawakened by these memories can be overwhelming. Conflicts around childhood dependency, ambivalence, parent-child relationships, and security can be stirred by the experience of loss and may make the work of grief more difficult.

Many theorists have described the grief process as having stages or phases (Table 15-2). The responses described include: (1) shock, disbelief, and numbness; (2) intense mourning, developing awareness and acceptance of the unwanted reality of the loss, accompanied by disorganization; and (3) reestablishment of homeostasis, recovery, restitution, and reorganization.

Engle[28] describes successful mourning as being evident in the ability to remember comfortably and realistically both the pleasures and disappointments of the lost relationship. Most theorists agree that mourning generally lasts a year or more. There is no one right way or one right time frame for grief.

More and more death educators and counselors are looking to task theories to assist in understanding the needs of grievers. Worden[22] described four tasks of grief and mourning:

1. To accept the reality of the loss.
2. To experience the pain of the grief.
3. To adjust to an environment in which the deceased is missing.
4. To withdraw emotional energy and reinvest it in another relationship.

In describing a model bereavement program, O'Toole[15] integrates the tasks of grieving into three phases of caring for the patient and family coping with a life-threatening illness: (1) living with illness phase, (2) active dying phase, and (3) follow-up bereavement phase. These are discussed in the section on nursing care of the patient/family coping with life-threatening illness and death (p. 304).

Complicated Mourning/Dysfunctional Grieving

There are four possible types of complicated outcomes of grief: (1) persevering, unusually intense or distorted occurrences of normal grief symptoms; (2) syndromes of expression (absence, inhibition, or delay), distortions

Symptoms and behaviors of unresolved grief[22,41,42]

Overactivity without a sense of loss.
Acquisition of symptoms belonging to the last illness of the deceased.
Development of psychosomatic illness.
Alteration in relationships with friends and relatives.
Furious hostility against specific persons somehow connected with the death.
Wooden and formal conduct masking hostile feelings.
Lasting loss of patterns of social interaction.
Actions detrimental to one's social and economic well-being; for example, giving away belongings.
Agitated depression with tension, agitation, insomnia, feelings of worthlessness, bitter self-accusation, obvious need for punishment, and even suicidal tendencies.
History of delayed or prolonged grief.
A feeling the death occurred yesterday, even though the loss took place months or years ago.
Unwillingness to move the possessions of the deceased after a reasonable amount of time.
Inability to discuss the deceased without crying, particularly over a year after the loss.
A relatively minor event triggering major grief reactions.
False euphoria subsequent to the death.
Overidentification with the deceased.
Phobias about illness or death.

15-6

Nursing Research

Lasker JN, LJ Toedter: Acute versus chronic grief: the case of pregnancy loss, *Am J Orthopsychiatry* 61(4):510-522, 1991.

This study considered some of the problems in measuring the extent of grief for any type of loss, but particularly "chronic" or "complicated" grief. A scale for measuring grief after pregnancy loss was tested on data from a longitudinal study of 138 women and 56 men who had experienced a perinatal loss. The results suggested that it is possible to distinguish between less severe (crying and sadness) and more severe dimensions of grief (withdrawal and despair). It was found that it may be possible to identify the long-term potential for chronic disturbed responses soon after the loss. Measures were taken at 2 months and 2 years. Scores on "Difficulty coping" and "Despair" are the best predictors, as represented by the level of one's mental health and social and marital support.

(rooted in anger, guilt, or lack of anticipation,) or problems ending (that is, chronic grief); (3) diagnosable mental or physical disorders; and (4) suicide.[19]

Six high risk factors make it more likely that such complications will occur: (1) sudden, unanticipated death, especially when it is traumatic, violent, mutilating, or random; (2) ambivalence or marked dependence or co-dependence in the relationship with the deceased; (3) perceived lack of social support, especially for disenfranchised grief; (4) liabilities of the mourner, including mental health problems; (5) loss of a child; and (6) perception of the death or the suffering as preventable (for example, cases in which persons take "too long" to die.)[19]

Various theorists have described behaviors indicative of unresolved grief (Box 15-5). There is disagreement whether these behaviors are indicative of "dysfunctional grieving" or complicating factors influencing the manifestation of grief. Whatever the case, it is important for the nurse to recognize and refer these patients for appropriate counseling and/or treatment (Box 15-6).

Nursing Process
Assessment of patient/family experiencing loss/dying/death

It is recognized that each loss experience is different. Generalizations are made for the sake of discussion. The focus of the nursing process discussion will be primarily on the

patient coping with a life-threatening illness, dying, and death. (The use of the term *family* throughout this chapter refers not only to legally defined family, but recognizes the nontraditional relationships or significant others as family).

Crisis assessment

The crisis model provides the nurse with an ongoing framework to help determine how much and what type of assistance is needed by the patient or family. A crisis is subjectively defined by the patient or family when they perceive the situation with which they are confronted as sufficiently different from previous experiences or so overwhelming that habitual problem-solving activities are not adequate to resolve the challenge.

There are four balancing forces to be assessed. First, the nurse needs to determine how realistic a view the patient and family have. Do they see the illness as fatal or are they able to see possible alternatives for the future? If their view of the situation is distorted, then the first challenge will be to provide them with accurate information; if it is clear that their misperception is caused by anxiety, then reducing the level of anxiety will be the necessary first step.

The second balancing force is the ability to identify and express feelings related to the situation. For example, after the loss of a child, fathers identify feeling the same emotions as mothers, but their modes of expression are often different. Fathers often chose activities for expressing feelings, whereas mothers will frequently cry and exhibit other overt expressions of sorrow. It is important not to assume that just because fathers are not showing their feelings they are not experiencing as much pain as mothers. Another example would be at the time of diagnosis of a life-threatening illness that has been described as a turning point, a time of crisis when the patient's whole orientation changes: one's worst fears may be realized and patients may recognize or perceive that they are now either in a struggle for life or an inexorable slide toward death. This confrontation with death can overwhelm the patient and family.[5]

The third balancing force is having successful problem-solving skills. Death is not as frequent an occurrence as it was in the past. It is an unfamiliar and frightening experience for many people. Confrontation with a life-threatening illness and possible death calls upon all the problem-solving skills a patient and family can muster. It would not be surprising that they would need assistance to cope with this event. The process of rendering a diagnosis is often very difficult; during this time patients undergo a multiplicity of tests and procedures and also experience a great deal of uncertainty. Despite the uncertainty of both diagnosis and prognosis, being diagnosed as having a life-threatening illness is an intense crisis filled with anxiety, affect, and a host of personal and interpersonal issues. Tensions and anxieties mount and individuals must either mobilize coping mechanisms or experience personal disorganization. Despite this crisis of uncertain nature, patients often have to make decisions that may radically affect the quality, nature, and even duration of life.[5]

The fourth balancing force is support. Coping with a life-threatening illness or loss due to a death is inevitably a family issue, for everyone's life is changed when one member of a family experiences illness or dies. The grief and emotional responses of each family member may be so intense that they are unable to provide each other the support they need.

Nursing assessment is an ongoing process throughout the illness and into the dying phase. A thorough assessment includes input from the patient and significant others (Box 15-7).

15-7

Nursing assessment: input from patient with life-threatening illness and significant others

General perception of each individual

Awareness of clinical diagnosis and prognosis
Philosophy of living and beliefs about dying
Expected physiologic and behavioral changes
Past experiences with major illness, loss, or crisis
Shared experiences with major illness or crises
Concurrent life crises or losses
Financial impact of illness, loss, or death
Degree of dependence or autonomy of family members

Perceived strengths, desires, and hopes

Personal abilities and coping techniques
Personal support systems
Availability of resources
Beliefs, religious convictions, and cultural views of dying, death, and bereavement
Past experiences with loss, dying, and death
Expectations about care, use of life supports, and advanced directives
Communication patterns

Tasks of the living-dying phase

The nurse assesses the tasks confronting the patient and family at each phase of the living-dying continuum. O'Toole has described these phases and their related tasks: (1) the living with illness phase, (2) the active dying phase, (3) the time of death and (4) the follow-up bereavement phase.[15]

The living with illness phase begins for the patient at the time when the illness is first diagnosed; for the nurse it begins with the initial assessment. The key tasks for the patient and family during this phase include:

1. The need to obtain and gain understanding and information regarding the illness process. This can include information about medical and nursing treatments, what to expect, and what patient and family need to do. It may also include having access to information regarding all treatment options available, both traditional and alternative methods. At this time it is appropriate to assess the patient and family's understanding of the grief process.

2. The need for assistance and information about limitations imposed by the illness and what resources are available to assist them.

3. A period of adjustment as family members develop new roles.

4. The patient and family's need to develop a trusting relationship with their caregivers.

5. The need for assistance in maintaining hope while dealing with the reality of the disease process and the implications of the threat to life.

6. The family's needs to develop strategies to meet the needs of the ill person that recognize the need of the ill person to retain as much control over his or her life as possible.

7. The patient and family's need to discover coping patterns that will assist in limiting their awareness of the impact of losses and conserve energy so that living can continue.

8. The need to maintain and/or restore relationships with significant persons; the need to tie up loose ends.

9. The time, to some degree, to recognize and to resolve unfinished business.

10. The caregivers' need to develop a system that permits them to care for themselves and continue living as fully as possible. The focus for the patient and family is on *living*.

It would be ideal, if in every case there could be sufficient time in the phases of illness and dying to allow the patient and family adequate time to complete all their tasks. All too often the living-dying period is too short, leaving the patient and family with unfinished business. That is why familiarity with the tasks confronting the patient and family, along with a careful assessment, completed as rapidly as possible, will provide the nurse with the data needed to plan optimal care.

Patient/family tasks of the active dying phase

The active dying phase is characterized by the period of physical and mental decline that indicates that death is near. Tasks of this phase are an integral part of the grief process of the survivors, just as the tasks of the earlier phase were a preparation for this phase. Completion of the tasks of this phase are significant in how the bereaved survivors will later remember the dying experience. This phase is often seen as part of the shock or numbing experience of grief when memories are recorded, stored, and frozen in vivid and graphic forms. Patient/family tasks of the active dying phase include the following:

1. If the patient is cared for at home the caregivers will need instruction on the care of the terminally ill.
2. The family caregiver needs to regulate emotions to attend to personal needs, the dying person's need, and the family system needs.
3. The patient and family will experience the pain of separation, as the patient may begin to withdraw.
4. The need to remain sufficiently engaged to provide care, comfort, and presence to the dying person and other family members.
5. The time for completion of significant issues of reconciliation and forgiveness.
6. As far as possible, the time to accept or recognize that earth life is ending.
7. The need for some form of acknowledgment of the bonds of the dying person to those who remain and some formalization of the creation of memories.
8. The dying person's needs for assurance that he or she will be remembered. Fears most often associated with dying are the fear of pain, disfigurement, abandonment, helplessness, loss of self-worth, and extinction.

Tasks at the time of death

1. Assessment of the need and wish of family to be present at the time of death.
2. The patient should not be left alone at the time of death.
3. Assessment of who the patient/family want present, such as clergy, other family members, or friends.
4. The family's needs for information about what to expect at the time of death.
5. The family's need for assistance in notifying the appropriate persons about the death, such as a funeral home.
6. The family's need for permission to remain alone with the patient's body after death.

Family tasks after death

1. If the patient died at home, the family needs assistance with preparing the body.
2. They may need assistance in arranging funeral/memorial rituals meaningful to them and the deceased.
3. They may want and need encouragement to use this period to reminisce about the "good days" prior to and during the illness.
4. They may need support in experiencing the tasks of grief, described earlier, and in expressing their grief, both individually and as a group.

Not all bereaved persons need or want formal intervention following the loss of a loved one. They will ultimately move through their grief work with or without intervention; however there is evidence that suggests people move faster through the grieving process when they receive formal support. The need for support is determined through careful crisis assessment and determination of possible dysfunctional grieving.

Data analysis: nursing diagnoses

Nursing diagnoses are determined from analysis of patient data. Possible nursing diagnoses for the person coping with loss, dying, or death may include, but are not limited to, the following:

Diagnostic title	Possible etiologies
Anxiety	Threat to self-concept, change in health status/socioeconomic status/role functioning/environment, crisis, and threat of death
Role performance, altered	Changes in social involvement due to life-threatening illness
Hopelessness	Failing physical condition, abandonment
Denial	Threat to life
Powerlessness	Health care environment, interpersonal interaction, illness-related regimen
Grieving, anticipatory	Potential loss of significant person/object/body part
Social interaction, impaired	Poor communication skills, self-concept disturbance, absence of supporting others, altered thought processes
Social isolation	Alteration in physical appearance, state of wellness or altered mental status, death of a significant other
Grieving, dysfunctional	Actual or perceived loss

Planning: expected patient outcomes

Planning patient and family care is a team effort including the patient, family, physician, nurse, social worker, and other health care providers, as appropriate. Successful planning incorporates the needs and goals of the family as well as the goals of the health care team.

Two major pieces of legislation impact the options patients must consider during this time, if not before. Most states now have legislation requiring hospitals to formulate policies and procedures for the identification and referral of potential organ or tissue donors to procurement agencies. More recently, states have also begun to mandate that hospitals provide patients with information about "Advanced Directives."

The National Task Force for Organ and Tissue Donation issued a report in 1986 that precipitated legislation requiring hospitals to offer patients and families the option to donate. The task force recommended that discussion be conducted in a sensitive and caring manner. The intent of the legislation was to ensure an adequate number of organs and tissues for those whose lives depend on transplantation of healthy organs or tissues. There remains an acute shortage of donated organs, eyes, and tissues. Over 16,000 people were listed on the national computer as awaiting transplants in December 1988. Another important benefit is that the option to donate may offer a sense of comfort to the grieving family of a dying loved one.[17]

Each hospital has implemented the program based on their own needs. The pastoral care department has been designated to make the requests in some hospitals, social work and nursing departments do so in others. It is incumbent on nurses to know the policy in the institution where they work, as well as being knowledgeable about the basic information regarding organ donation. It is often the nurse at the bedside who has the opportunity to discuss this issue with the patient or family.

The issue of advance directives has come to the forefront in many states within the last few years. Advance directives are signed and witnessed documents providing specific instructions for health care treatment in the event that a person is unable to make those decisions personally at the time they are needed. The legally recognized form varies from state to state. Documents may take the form of the standard Health Care Treatment Directive (see Box 15-8 for one example), additional specific written instructions, a Values History, a written statement that provides infor-

---

15-8

Health care treatment directive (This document is an expanded "Living Will")

I _____ make this Health Care Treatment Directive to exercise my
PRINT NAME
right to determine the course of my health care and to provide clear and convincing proof of my treatment decisions when I lack the capacity to make or communicate my decisions and there is no realistic hope that I will regain such capacity.

If my physician believes that a certain life prolonging procedure or other health care treatment may provide me with comfort, relieve pain or lead to a significant recovery, I direct my physician to try the treatment for a reasonable period of time. However, if such treatment proves to be ineffective, I direct treatment be withdrawn even if so doing may shorten my life.

I direct I be given health care treatment to relieve pain or to provide comfort even if such treatment might shorten my life, suppress my appetite or my breathing, or be habit-forming.

> I direct all life prolonging procedures be withheld or withdrawn when there is no hope of significant recovery, and I have:
> - a terminal condition; or
> - a condition, disease or injury without reasonable expectation that I will regain an acceptable quality of life; or
> - substantial brain damage or brain disease which cannot be significantly reversed.
>
> 1. When any of the above conditions exist, I DO NOT WANT the life prolonging procedures which I have initialed below. (You should assume any treatments not initialed may be administered to you.)
>   - surgery .... _____ initials
>   - heart-lung resuscitation (CPR) .... _____ initials
>   - antibiotics .... _____ initials
>   - dialysis .... _____ initials
>   - mechanical ventilator (respirator) .... _____ initials
>   - tube feedings (food and water delivered through a tube in the vein,
>   nose or stomach .... _____ initials
>   - other _____ .... _____ initials
> 2. I make other instructions as follows: (You may describe what a minimally acceptable quality of life is for you.)
>
> _____
> _____
> _____
> _____

> If you do not wish to name an agent as referred to on the reverse side, initial here _____, write "None" in the space provided for agent's name, sign document, and have notarized.

Discuss this document and your ideas about quality of life with your agent, physician(s), family members, friends and clergy and provide them with a signed copy (or photocopy thereof). You may revoke or change this document. Periodic review is recommended. If there are no changes after each review, initial and date in the margin.

(Courtesy the Kansas City Metropolitan Bar Association and its foundation, the Metropolitan Medical Society of Greater Kansas City, Midwest Bioethics Center and the Missouri Lawyer Trust Account Foundation.)

mation about the person's personal values as they relate to life and health care, and a Durable Power of Attorney for Health Care Decisions. It is important to know what the laws in your state are and your nursing responsibilities in seeing that they are not violated.

The advance directives are based on the person's right to self-determination. Every adult has the freedom to accept or refuse any recommended medical treatment. Every person who completes an advance directives should give a copy to his or her regular physician and to family or friends to ensure that it is available when necessary. Advance directives should be seen not only as legal protection for personal rights, but also as a guide to a person's health care providers.[6]

In states that recognize advance directives, the attending physician and hospital must comply with the provisions of the patient's Health Care Treatment Directive or transfer the patient to another physician, unless there is reason to doubt the validity of the Health Care Treatment Directive.

A person may revoke his or her Health Care Treatment Directive at any time and in any manner in which the person is able to communicate his or her intent.

Expected patient/family outcomes for the persons coping with loss, dying, or death may include, but are not limited to, the following:

1. Experience a reduced anxiety level as evidenced by: decreased tension, less apprehension, ability to discuss anxiety related to illness, the ability to identify stressors, and the ability to learn.
2. Demonstrate effective coping skills as evidenced by the ability to problem solve.
3. Engage in functional role performance as evidenced by being able to discuss role expectations and changes with each other and by using constructive strategies to cope with the changes related to the patient's deteriorating condition.
4. Hope is maintained as evidenced by the patient performing self-care activities as long as possible, by participating in diversional activities as long as possible, by participating in diversional activities and maintaining relationships. Patient and family will be able to express feelings, both verbally and nonverbally, as they choose. They will identify realistic goals.
5. Denial will be at a level that supports the patient's progress. They will express some reduction in concerns.
6. Participate during the living-with-illness phase in constructive anticipatory grief work as evidenced by: discussing thoughts and feelings related to anticipated losses, utilizing appropriate resources, meeting ongoing needs, and maintaining constructive relationships.
7. Demonstrate increased ability to cope with interpersonal encounters and social situations. They will express feelings in a constructive, socially acceptable manner.
8. The patient will experience a reduced level of social isolation and spend time daily with trusted persons.
9. Demonstrate normal grief work, acknowledging awareness of loss, verbalizing or in some comfortable manner expressing thoughts and feelings related to their losses. They will develop goals that are congruent with loss and that reflect individual values and choices.[8]

It is imperative that nurses include themselves in the assessment and planning phase. It is important to be aware of one's own loss experiences, unresolved griefs, beliefs about loss, dying, and death. Nurses who have not worked

---

15-9

The dying person's bill of rights

I have the right to be treated as a living human being until I die.

I have the right to maintain a sense of hopefulness however changing its focus may be.

I have the right to be cared for by those who can maintain a sense of hopefulness, however changing this might be.

I have the right to express my feelings and emotions about my approaching death in my own way.

I have the right to participate in decisions concerning my care.

I have the right to expect continuing medical and nursing attention even though "cure" goals must be changed to "comfort" goals.

I have the right not to die alone.

I have the right to be free from pain.

I have the right to have my questions answered honestly.

I have the right not to be deceived.

I have the right to have help from and for my family in accepting my death.

I have the right to die in peace and dignity.

I have the right to retain my individuality and not be judged for my decisions, which may be contrary to beliefs of others.

I have the right to discuss and enlarge my religious and/or spiritual experiences, whatever these may mean to others.

I have the right to expect that the sancity of the human body will be respected after death.

I have the right to be cared for by caring, sensitive, knowledgeable people who will attempt to understand my needs and will be able to gain some satisfaction in helping me face my death.

This Bill of Rights was created at a workshop on "The Terminally Ill Patient and the Helping Person," in Lansing, Mich, sponsored by the Southwestern Michigan Inservice Education Council and conducted by Amelia J. Barbus, Associate Professor of Nursing, Wayne State University, Detroit, 1975.

through their own grief issues are vulnerable when exposed to the loss of others. Unresolved griefs can be reactivated, preventing nurses from being able to respond to the needs of the patient or family. It colors their perceptions and ability to assess accurately and objectively. Rando[47] noted the following prerequisites for working with the dying:

1. A personal confrontation with death in the sense of having started to come to grips with one's own mortality. This can never be done completely, but the issue needs to have been addressed.
2. An understanding of the grief process and an appreciation for the total experience of the dying patient.
3. Effective listening skills and the ability to respond appropriately, nonverbally as well as verbally.
4. A commitment to giving part of oneself to the dying person and to working with families after death when appropriate.
5. A knowledge of one's own personal limits, knowing when there is a need to get away from death and how to avoid burnout.

Planning patient/family care must also take into consideration the "Dying Person's Bill of Rights" created at a workshop on "The Terminally Ill Patient and the Helping Person" in Lansing, Michigan in 1975 (Box 15-9).

Implementation
Living with illness phase

Many interventions are appropriate throughout the care period. The thrust of intervention with patients and families coping with life-threatening illness is the maintenance of hope, dignity, and quality of life.

Establishing a trusting relationship is key to all that follows. It is important that, as much as possible, the same nursing staff work with these patients and families. It is threatening to come into a foreign environment and undergo strange procedures that are often painful. Patients and families need someone they can rely on, who knows them and can assist them through this frightening and anxiety-producing experience. The nurse promotes the trusting relationship by first listening to the patient and family and hearing where they are in their coping process and what they say they need, not what they should need. E.J. Daniel[27] expressed it poignantly:

> This time
> those-in-white-in-colors
> seem on my side,
> caring about me
> but my friends don't,
> saying I'm manipulative
> and can be/do
> all that I'm supposed to be/do
> regardless of how I'm feeling.
> and I think I'll just run—
> find anyone
> who meets me where I am
> not where they say I should be—
> lovingly, gently helping
> me accept that point,
> so I can grow into
> a better me—
> somehow.

Be physically and emotionally present to offer security and support. When persons are feeling anxious or emotionally stressed they often respond positively to the gentle touch of a hand or the offer of a hug. However, be aware that some people are not comfortable with being touched or would not welcome it from a relative stranger. Be aware of nonverbal feedback and, if in doubt, ask permission before touching such persons.

The health care team can then move on to assisting the family in recognizing, accepting, and using their individual and collective coping styles to meet their needs. The family will need information and assistance in meeting the physical needs of the patient. In the hospital, the nursing staff provides most of the patient's care, including the family when appropriate and assuring them of their continued importance in the patient's care. Some families want to do as much as possible for their loved one; others are not able to participate. It is important to respect the choices of the patient and family in these matters. The patient and family should be included in decisions throughout the hospitalization and preparation for discharge. Encourage the person with the illness to retain as much control as possible.

The nurse can begin to explore with the family the impact of the illness and assist them in preparing for possible role changes. This can be especially important if the relationship involves dependency of the well partner. Encourage and assist the family to maintain as high a degree of normal living as possible. Recognize special events such as birthdays and anniversaries as a way to affirm that life is still valuable and in process and to encourage reminiscences. Normalize the experience, discussing common emotional responses and anticipatory grieving. Assist the patient and family in recognizing that they are grieving for themselves and for the other and of the naturalness of these reactions. Provide information on the grief process. As appropriate, encourage and provide opportunities for families to meet with each other to obtain information and clarification, to express feelings, to identify their needs for reconciliation, and to recognize and accept their various coping styles. Encourage patient/family support networks and assist in identifying resources, both personal and community.

When families choose to take the patient home for care, be sure that they are well prepared before discharge for what they will need to know. Teach them basic care, including feeding techniques when appropriate. Assist them in selecting foods that will be easy to chew and swallow and that are as palatable as possible. Have them assist in bathing, mouth care, and other hygiene measures so they will know how to perform these when they return home. Teach them simple transfer techniques to prevent injury to themselves and the patient. Discuss routines, including the need for rest periods. Arrange for the hospice services to assist the family if they are receptive; emphasize the importance of continuity of care and 24-hour availability for periods when the patient is experiencing an emotional or physical crisis and needs ongoing support.

Provide teaching, information, and encouragement in the use of creative outlets for expressing feelings and communicating with others. Encourage the use of taperecorded messages, drawings, writings, imagery, music, and poetry.

This also assists patients and families in creating memories that can be very comforting later. Teach the patient and family relaxation techniques.

The maintenance of hope can be difficult during this time. As the patient's condition deteriorates, the challenge becomes one of assisting the patient and family in translating their hope for a cure into realistic hopes that are focused on short-term achievable goals. This may be the hope for a comfortable and painfree life, or the desire to live long enough to participate in some important family event, like the wedding of a son. Hope can take many forms; the challenge for the nurse is to help the patient and family identify those hopes that are most important to them and that will help them cope.

Active dying phase

It is important to provide the family with realistic information about the course of the illness and the signs and symptoms of impending death. Hospices frequently give families both verbal and written information (Box 15-10) whereas in hospitals this is rarely discussed. Families have often expressed fear of what happens at the time of death and consequently may avoid being present, leaving the patient feeling alone and abandoned. When possible, encourage family members to have someone supportive be with them during this time. Ensure that they take adequate breaks and supplement their vigil if needed by people from the family support network, staff, or volunteers.

Continue to listen and to provide a supportive presence. Coach the family and model for them ways to interact with the dying patient. Speak to the patient, even if unresponsive and call him or her by name. Encourage family members to talk to the patient and assure him or her that he or she is significant to the family and will be remembered. Encourage the family to recognize that in terminal illness, dying is a process that often occurs over time and that the patient, although dying, is still alive.

It may be necessary to give the family permission to recognize that it is "okay" for them to continue to live even in the presence of death. Encourage them to bring food or beverages into the patient's room. Provide them with opportunities to express their sorrow and the pain of the loss. At the same time, demonstrate acceptance and support to family members who do not express their feelings.

When appropriate, model and coach the family in giving the patient "permission to die" and in saying "goodbye." If needed, give family members the permission to not be present during this stage; convey your acceptance of such a decision. Keep the family informed as the patient's condition changes. If the family chooses to be present, offer support, acceptance, and assurance, especially to those who fear the time of death or of being present at the time of death.

At time of death

Offer to call the clergy or other support persons identified by the patient and family. Allow the family time to be alone with the body of their loved one if they wish. Model acceptance of the body, by touching and calling the dead person by name. If the family was not present at the time of death, encourage them that this is a time when

15-10

Signs and symptoms of approaching death

The arms and legs may become cool to the touch and the underside of the body may become darker in color. These symptoms are the result of the blood circulation slowing down.

The patient will spend more and more time sleeping during the day and at times will be difficult to arouse. This results from slowing of the body's metabolism.

The patient may lose bladder or bowel control, resulting in incontinence.

Oral secretions may become more profuse and collect in the back of the throat, producing what is commonly referred to as the "death rattle." This is a result of decreased fluid intake and the patient's inability to cough up normal saliva.

The patient's vision and hearing decrease slightly, with hearing generally being the last sense to be lost.

The patient may become restless, pulling at bed linen and having visions of people or things. This is the result of decreased oxygen to the brain, as well as the decreased metabolism.

The patient will have a decreased need for food and drink.

The patient's breathing pattern will change during sleep to an irregular pace with 10- to 30-second periods of no breathing.

Signs of death include no breathing, no heartbeat, no response to shaking or shouting, loss of bladder and bowel control, eyelids slightly open with eyes fixed on one spot, and jaws relaxed and mouth slightly open.

Note: Not all these symptoms will appear at the same time and some may never appear.

they can still say anything that they will later regret not having said. Point out that we do not know how long the patient's life force is present and that there is still time to say "I love you" or whatever else they want to say. Give and model comfort and caring through shared tears, touch, listening, and acceptance. Provide a calm, reassuring, and caring presence.

Assist or prepare the body according to hospital protocol; in the home, assist the family prepare the body for removal to the funeral home. If requested or needed, support the family in arranging funeral or memorial rituals that are meaningful to them. If possible, attend the wake, funeral home visitation, or memorial service and let the family know of your presence and that you care. A special bond often forms between the family and the nurse because of having shared one of the most important events of their lives.

Care for nurse caregiver
Process and stress of nurse's grief

Because more patients die in hospitals than in homes, nurses have evolved in the role of "surrogate griever."

Nurses who work with the terminally ill and with bereaved persons develop a heightened empathy and identification with their patients. This occurs because the loss experience is so universal that we have all experienced its impact. Dying and bereaved individuals force us to confront death and loss. Nurses take emotional risks and form bonds that demand a grief response. When this is experienced intensely in a serial fashion without adequate processing, nurses can become subject to bereavement overload.[47]

Nurses are susceptible to all the emotions of grief: frustration, sadness, guilt, anxiety, depression, helplessness, and anger. They need to do for themselves what they do for their patients to help them with their grief work. There are however, roadblocks to nurses' grieving:

- Social negation of the loss and isolation from support: few hospitals provide opportunities for nurses to grieve lost patients formally. The nurses' families and friends often cannot understand how the death of a relative stranger can cause such intense grief. Hence the nurse is left to grieve alone or to go on as if nothing important has occurred.
- "Professionalism": Nurses are expected to be strong.
- Ambivalence and feelings of guilt toward the dead person can result when the nurse had mixed feelings about the patient. If the patient was a particularly difficult person to get along with or to care for, the nurse may even feel a sense of relief when death occurs. This can be incompatible with the idea that a nurse is "supposed to love everyone equally."
- Nurses often have a need to be in control, so they may not be able to show how they feel or may even suppress their feelings.
- Multiple losses can be overwhelming. It is not uncommon on some nursing units for several patients to die in a very short period of time, leaving little or no time for proper processing of the nurses' grief.
- Old, unresolved losses suffered by the nurse can be reawakened and can prevent the nurse from dealing with the current losses.

Nurses' responses to loss are subject to the same influences discussed earlier in this chapter. Other factors include: unique genetic and developmental history, prior loss history, stress management, professional training, values and beliefs, the particular developmental period in the nurse's life, the number and intensity of life changes at any given period of time, the nurse's personal motivation for working with the terminally ill, and the nurse's personal level of energy and rest requirements.

Strategies for survival

It is incumbent upon the hospital or other work group employing nurses in the care of the terminally ill to build into the organization a formalized process for recognizing and allowing the grieving process to take place. This can be done on the unit level or hospitalwide. Some hospitals have instituted regular memorial services that the staff can attend to share the losses they have experienced and to talk about patients who have recently died.

Nurses have the responsibility to take steps to care for themselves:

1. Take regular breaks or time-outs from the patient care area and consider rotating out of high-stress nursing areas.
2. Identify specific patients that are most difficult, so that they can be anticipated and counteracted. Trade off patients or ask for special assistance in working in these specific situations.
3. Acknowledge physical needs as key factors in stress reduction.
4. Integrate decompression routines into daily life. Before leaving the work area take a moment to review the day and set it aside before going home.
5. Engage in life-affirming activities, for example, spend time with lively healthy children.
6. View losses as an opportunity to reevaluate and grow.
7. Avoid the "rescuer" or "savior" complex; recognize limits.
8. Recognize the need for support and do not hesitate to ask for it.
9. Say "I choose" rather than "I should."
10. Develop the skills of setting limits and feeling okay about saying "no."
11. Laugh and play in the face of tragedy without guilt.
12. Seek consultation on a regular basis.

Evaluation: patient/family/nurse

A review of the projected outcomes provides the evaluation criteria:

1. Did the patient or family express a positive reduction in their initial level of anxiety and an increase in positive coping skills?
2. Were patient and family able to make the necessary role adjustments while preserving the patient's self-esteem and without overwhelming the family with the new responsibilities?
3. Did the patient and family find satisfactory expression of their feelings and grief?
4. Was hope redefined as the patient's condition changed?
5. Were patient and family able to maintain an appropriate level of denial, allowing them to adjust to the patient's deteriorating condition?
6. Did the patient and family maintain social interaction throughout the illness-dying process at a level satisfactory to them?
7. Did the nurse develop useful strategies for dealing with stress related to working with loss, dying, and death?

SUMMARY

1. Dying and death are distinct and separate events that are part of the continuum of life. Grief is the normal response to any loss. It is a lifelong normative process as each new loss experience is met. Grief is an active, not a passive process; it takes work and emotional energy. When people do not do "grief work" following any significant loss, they are at risk for emotional, mental, and social problems. The role of the nurse is to assist the patient and family in making choices related to their tasks of grieving.

2. Loss is inevitable and inescapable.
3. Losses can be described as self losses or external losses.
4. Self losses include the loss of the psychologic self, the sociocultural self, the physical self, and the spiritual self.
5. External losses include loss of objects, possessions, loved ones, environment, and support.
6. Losses can be real, imagined, present, or anticipated.
7. Many factors influence the way an individual responds to loss: childhood experiences, significance assigned the loss, the physical and emotional state of the individual, accumulated loss experiences, view of loss as crisis, visibility, duration and timing, abruptness or suddenness, financial drain, availability of resources, cultural factors, personal attributes, relationship with the lost person, and the death surround.
8. Dying is an integral part of life, as natural and predictable as birth.
9. Dying can help us to appreciate and understand life.
10. Models of dying and grief are useful in conceptualizing the processes, but should never be used prescriptively.
11. The terms *grief*, *mourning*, and *bereavement* are used to describe the process and state of having suffered a loss.
12. The tasks of grief help in understanding the needs of the griever.
13. Complicated or dysfunctional grief should be identified by the nurse and referred for appropriate intervention.
14. The crisis model provides a framework for assessing patient and family perspectives on loss as a possibly overwhelming event that needs professional intervention.
15. Nursing assessment includes a review of the tasks confronting patients and families during each phase of the living-dying continuum.
16. The nurse needs to be aware of the patient's wishes with regard to organ/tissue donation and advanced directives, as well as state and hospital regulations on these issues.
17. Nurses experience all the emotions of grief not only in response to their own losses but also in response to the deaths of their patients.
18. It is imperative that nurses care for themselves.
19. Patients and families properly supported through their early illness and final living-dying experiences will be able to make the necessary emotional adjustments to the changes in their lives so that growth and maturing are more likely to occur.

STUDY QUESTIONS

- Complete the following "Personal Loss" Inventory[39] and discuss your responses with a classmate:
- List the three most significant losses you have personally sustained in life to date. They do not need to be in any hierarchical order and can involve people, things, hopes, beliefs, or attitudes. Be brief and concrete.
- In which of these losses have you completed your grief work? How has this promoted self-affirmation, creative living, and growth? Be specific.

- In which of the three losses noted have you *not* completed your grieving? In what ways is this manifest in your living today?
- How would you explain the grieving process to a patient with a newly diagnosed life-threatening illness?
- Differentiate between the dying process and death.
- Select a patient you are currently working with and review the patient's loss history. What factors influencing loss are most pertinent in planning care?
- Share with a classmate the steps you take to manage the stress in your life.

REFERENCES AND SELECTED READINGS

1. Bruss CR: Nursing diagnosis of hopelessness, *J Psychosoc Nurs* 26(3):28-31, 1988.
2. Corr CA: A task-based approach to coping with dying. Paper presented at the ADEC conference, Duluth, Minn, April 1991.
3. DeSpelder LA, Strickland AL: *The last dance: encountering death and dying*, ed 2, Mountain View, Calif, 1987, Mayfield Publishing.
4.* Dobratz, MC: Hospice nursing: present perspective and future directives, *Cancer Nurs* 13(2):116-122, 1990.
5. Doka KJ: *The terrible threat*, Book in preparation, 1991.
6. Emanuel LL, Emanuel EJ: The medical directive, *JAMA*, 261(22):3288-3293, 1989.
7.* Grollman EA: *In sickness and in health: how to cope when your loved one is ill*, Boston, 1987, Beacon Press.
8. Kim MJ, McFarland GK, McLane AM: *Pocket guide to nursing diagnosis*, ed 3, St Louis, 1989, Mosby–Year Book.
9. Lasker JN, Toedter LJ: Acute versus chronic grief: the case of pregnancy loss, *Am J Orthopsychiatry* 61(4):510-522, 1991.
10.* Lawson LV: Culturally sensitive support for grieving parents, *MCN* 15:76-79, March/April 1990.
11. Leavitt PF, McDowell WA, Lewis SJ: *The patient who is dying*. In Lewis S et al, editors: *Manual of psychosocial nursing and interventions*, ed 3, Philadelphia, 1989, WB Saunders.
12. Longo DC, Williams RA, editors: *Clinical practice in psychosocial nursing: assessment and intervention*, ed 2, Norwalk, Conn, 1986, Appleton-Century-Crofts.
13. Metzgar M: *Little ears, big issues: children and loss*, Seattle, 1990.
14.* Mount BM: Dealing with our losses, *J Clin Oncol* 4(7):1127-1134, 1986.
15. O'Toole D: *Bridging the bereavement gap*, ed 2, LaPeer, Mich, 1985, The Bereavement Project.
16. Parkes CM: *Bereavement: studies of grief in adult life*, ed 2, Madison, Conn, 1987, International Universities Press.
17. Perryman JP: Providing the option to donate, *The Forum*: (Newsletter of the Association for Death Education and Counseling) 13:6, 1989.
18. Rando TA: *Loss and anticipatory grief*, Lexington, Mass, 1986, Lexington Books.
19. Rando TA: *Treatment of complicated mourning*, Book in preparation, 1992.
20. Redmond LM: *Surviving: when someone you love was murdered*, Clearwater, Fla, 1989, Psychological Consultation and Education Services.
21. Stroebe W, Stroebe MS: *Bereavement and health: the psychological and physical consequences of partner loss*, Cambridge, UK, 1987, Cambridge University Press.
22. Worden JW: *Grief counseling and grief therapy: a handbook for*

*Recommended for student reading.

the mental health practitioner, ed 2, New York, 1990, Springer Publishing.

23. Zisook S: *Biopsychosocial aspects of bereavement,* Washington, DC, 1987, American Psychiatric Press.

Classic

24. Beland-Werner JA, editor: *Grief responses to long-term illness and disability: manifestations and nursing interventions,* Reston, Va, 1980, Reston Publishing.
25. Bower F, editor: *Nursing and the concept of loss,* New York, 1980, Wiley Medical Publications.
26. Bowlby J: *Attachment and loss: loss, sadness, and depression,* vol 3, New York, 1980, Basic Books.
27. Daniel EJ: *Any other song: a plea for holistic communication,* Bowie, Md, 1980, Prentice-Hall.
28. Engel G: *Psychological development in health and disease,* Philadelphia, 1962, WB Saunders.
29. Feifel H: *New meanings of death,* New York, 1977, McGraw-Hill.
30.* Glaser BG, Strauss AL: The social loss of dying patients, *AJN* 63:119-121, 1964.
31.* Glaser GB, Strauss AL: *A time for dying,* Chicago, 1968, Aldine de Gruyter.
32. Glick IO, Weiss RS, Parkes CM: *The first year of bereavement,* New York, 1974, Wiley.
33. Harper GC: *Death: the coping mechanism of the health professional,* Greenville, SC, 1977, Southwestern University Press.
34. Jackson EN: *Understanding grief: its roots, dynamics, and treatment,* Nashville, 1957, Abingdon Press.
35. Kalish RA: *Death, grief, and caring relationships,* Monterey, Calif, 1981, Brooks/Cole.
36. Kastenbaum RJ: *Death, society and human experience,* St Louis, 1977, Mosby–Year Book.

37.* Kavanaugh R: *Facing death,* Baltimore, 1974, Penguin Books.
38.* Keleman S: *Living your dying,* New York, 1983, Bantam Books.
39. Knott JE, et al: *Thanatopics: a manual of structured learning experiences for death education,* Kingston, RI, 1982, SLE Publications.
40. Koestenbaum P: *Is there an answer to death?* Englewood Cliffs, NJ, 1976, Prentice-Hall.
41.* Kubler-Ross E: *On death and dying,* New York, 1969, Macmillan.
42. Lazare A: Unresolved grief. In Lazare A, editor: *Outpatient psychiatry: diagnosis and treatment,* Baltimore, 1979, Williams & Wilkins.
43. Lindemann E: Symptomatology and management of acute grief, *Am J Psychiatry* 101:141-148, 1944.
44. Maslach C: *Burnout—the cost of caring,* Englewood Cliffs, NJ, 1982, Prentice Hall.
45.* Parkes CM, Weiss RS: *Recovery from bereavement,* New York, 1983, Basic Books.
46. Pattison EM: The living-dying process. In Garfield CA, editor: *Psychosocial care of the dying patient,* New York, 1978, McGraw-Hill.
47. Rando TA: *Grief, dying, and death,* Champaign, Ill, 1984, Research Press.
48. Raphael B: *The anatomy of bereavement,* New York, 1983, Basic Books.
49. Simos BG: *A time to grieve: loss as a universal human experience,* New York, 1979, Family Service Association of America.
50. Vachon MLS: Motivation and stress experienced by staff working with the terminally ill, *Death Education,* 2:113-122, 1978.

Infection

Unit Four

16

Biologic Defense Mechanisms

E. Ronald Wright

After studying this chapter, the learner should be able to:

- Differentiate between the concepts of self and nonself.
- Identify the external and internal nonspecific biologic defense mechanisms.
- Relate the steps of the inflammatory process to the symptoms of inflammation.
- Describe the relationship between antigens and antibodies and the process of antigen-antibody interactions.
- Differentiate between B cells and T cells and their roles in the humoral and cell-mediated responses to antigens.
- Explain the immunologic bases for passive and active immunizations, cancer, and tissue transplatation.

CONCEPT AND SCOPE OF BIOLOGIC DEFENSE

The human body has developed a wide variety of mechanisms designed to protect itself from the encroachment of antagonistic agents in its environment. Those agents can be *exogenous* (from outside the body), for example, foreign animal cells, parasites, microorganisms, drugs, toxins, or inorganic substances; or they may be *endogenous* (from within the body), for example, damaged or worn out tissues and cells, obstructive agents, or neoplasms. Life as we know it could not exist without the ability to withstand and deal with these extrinsic and intrinsic onslaughts. In this chapter the interactive biologic mechanisms designed to provide this protection are described and the consequences of their failure or inappropriate functioning are briefly discussed.

The significance for medical-surgical nursing practice of an understanding of how these mechanisms function cannot be overemphasized. Much of preventive, compensatory, and restorative nursing practice is built on the maintenance and restoration of the systems and mechanisms of these biologic functions. Knowledge of these basic structures and mechanisms helps in the understanding of the following:

1. Resistance and immunity to infectious diseases
2. Diagnosis of diseases and physiologic functions
3. Rejection of tissue transplants and reactions to transfusions
4. Adaptations of the aging process
5. Development of allergic and hypersensitivity reactions
6. Immunization against infectious diseases
7. Expression of autoimmune diseases and immunodeficiences
8. Signs and symptoms of local and systemic inflammation
9. Development and treatment of neoplastic disease

Concept of Self Versus Nonself

Every human being can be regarded as a "one of a kind" collection of tissues, cells, and molecules that comprises a biologic unit of *self*. The exact nature of this unit is determined by a combination of genes inherited from one's parents, which encode for a unique array of structures and proteins that is not repeated exactly in any other individual. The only exception to this occurs in the case of identical twins. Therefore, every other individual or cell or biologic product can be considered to be *nonself*. It is the function of the biologic defense mechanism of the body to recognize and protect against encroachment by nonself agents while maintaining, monitoring, and supporting all that is self.

These defense mechanisms are composed of structural, chemical, cellular, special protein, and tissue elements that form an interrelated system of protection throughout the entire body (see Box 16-1). The mechanisms serve to protect self from both external and internal destructive agents by the following:

1. *Exclusion* of harmful agents from the body
2. *Recognition* of harmful agents within the body
3. *Response* designed to rid the body of the harmful agents that do gain access (Fig. 16-1)

The sources of these harmful nonself materials are generally external and include nonliving materials of the environment such as potentially harmful inorganic chemicals and compounds produced by other living organisms. The most serious external threats to biologic integrity, however, come from the living organisms that constantly surround the body. Some of these organisms pose no real threat because the mechanical, biochemical, and metabolic processes of the human body will not support them or offer them shelter. There are many living forms, on the other hand, for which the human body would be an ideal haven for growth and survival. Most of these organisms, if allowed to penetrate the body, would wreak havoc on the normal functioning of the body. The living forms that come to

16-1	Biologic defense mechanisms	
	Structural	Skin, mucous membranes
	Chemical	pH, blood proteins
	Cellular	White blood cells, phagocytes
	Special proteins	Interferon, immunoglobulins
	Tissue	Lymph nodes, thymus gland

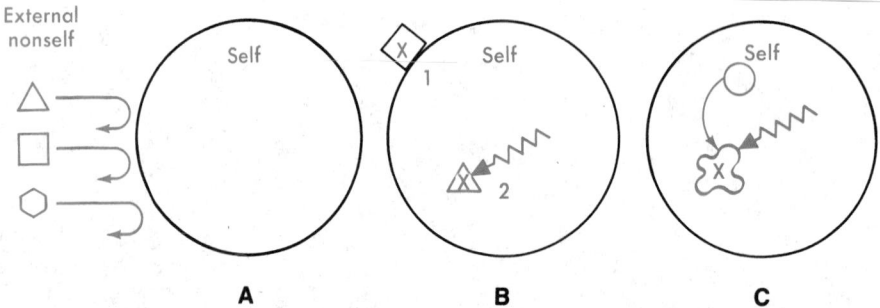

Fig. 16-1 Mechanisms of biologic defense in human body. **A,** Exclusion of external nonself. **B,** Destruction of external nonself by *(1)* nonspecific external mechanisms and *(2)* nonspecific internal mechanisms. **C,** Destruction of altered self. *X* indicates nonspecific mechanisms; indicates specific mechanisms.

mind in this regard are the organisms classified as pathogenic (disease causing). Although it is true that the progress of these organisms in the body can be altered by external agents such as antibiotics, the eradication of the offending organism from the body must be accomplished by the host's own adaptive mechanisms.

In addition to protection against external agents, the defense mechanisms also protect against the accumulation of damaged or dysfunctional self material. If it were not for these processes that carry out the systematic, specific removal of damaged or worn-out cellular material, the body would become clogged with debris. Still another general function of these systems is recognition of the alteration of self to a potentially dangerous state. When this defense function falters, cancer results.

The overall importance of this sytem has recently been illustrated by the problems that develop when one part of the defense mechanisms is compromised by the infection of the human body with human immunodeficiency virus (HIV). Infection with HIV leads to the progressive destruction of one group of cells of this system, the helper T cells (see p. 327). Without the protection afforded by these cells, the body becomes susceptible to the following: (1) infection by a variety of microorganisms that normally do not cause symptomatic infections (such as yeasts, herpes zoster, atypical mycobacteria); (2) infection by normally noninfective parasites (such as *Pneumocystis carinii, Toxoplasma, Cryptosporidium*); and (3) development and spread of cancers that are normally halted by the immune system (such as Kaposi's sarcoma, lymphomas).

On the other hand, if the immune response system incorrectly identifies self as nonself, it would bring to bear its destructive mechanisms against healthy cells or tissues. The result of such an inappropriate action against self produces cell and tissue damage referred to as *autoimmune disease* (see Chapter 41). Among the diseases caused by this failure in distinguishing self from nonself are rheumatoid arthritis, autoimmune thyroiditis, and systemic lupus erythematosis.

Recognition of Self From Nonself

It follows from the above discussion that a critical feature of the protective mechanisms of the immune response system of the human body is the ability to discriminate between self and nonself materials. This is accomplished by the presence of certain specific protein molecules that are embedded in the cell membrane of all human body cells (Fig. 16-2). The recognition process then occurs at the cell membrane surface. Immunoresponsive cells (lympho-

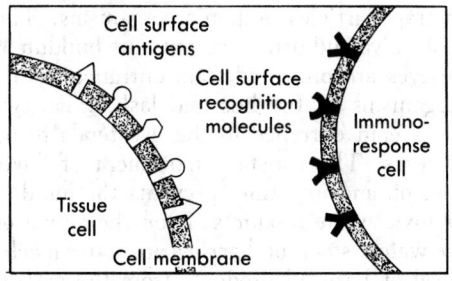

A. CELL SURFACE MARKERS

Cell surface antigens

Cell surface recognition molecules

Immuno-response cell

Tissue cell

Cell membrane

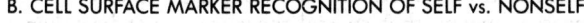

B. CELL SURFACE MARKER RECOGNITION OF SELF vs. NONSELF

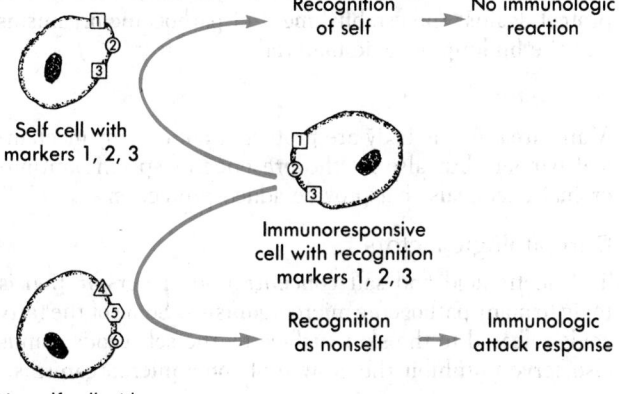

Recognition of self → No immunologic reaction

Self cell with markers 1, 2, 3

Immunoresponsive cell with recognition markers 1, 2, 3

Recognition as nonself → Immunologic attack response

Nonself cell with markers 4, 5, 6

Fig. 16-2   Cell surface markers for recognition of self versus nonself.

Table 16-1   ## Biologic defense mechanisms

Nonspecific mechanisms	Specific mechanisms
External	
Mechanical exclusion	Iummunoglobulin A
Physical structures	In mucosal secretions
Skin	In mucosal cells
Mucous membranes	
Specialized structures	
Physical actions	
Biochemical factors	
Body secretions	
pH	
Lysozyme	
Microbial antagonism	
Internal	
Reticuloendothelial system	Antigen processing by macrophage
Blood	Primary immune response
Cellular components	Humoral immune response
Fluid components	Synthesis of circulating immunoglobulins by B cells
Complement	
Acute-phase proteins	
Phagocytosis	Interaction of immunoglobulins with antigen
Inflammatory response	Cell-mediated immune response
Interferons	Activation of T cell response
	Lymphokines
	Combined immune response
	Secondary immune response

cytes) have specific protein molecules embedded in their membranes that recognize foreign (nonself) proteins. A person's own immunoresponsive cells recognize nonself proteins on cells that are genetically different, and this triggers a sequence of cellular reactions within the immune response system. This sequence of cellular reactions leads to the elaboration of materials and cells that attack the nonself materials. Contact with self proteins (markers) does not produce an immune attack. This explains why cells from different species or genetically dissimilar members of the same species cannot be transplanted from one host to another without triggering an immunologic attack and rejection of the tissue.

Scope of Defense Mechanisms

The array of defense mechanisms that have been adapted to protect the normal human body is formidable and complex. For the sake of orderly presentation they may be divided into *nonspecific* and *specific* mechanisms (Table 16-1). The specific and nonspecific mechanisms can be further divided on the basis of where the lines of defense are formed, that is, *external* for the mechanisms of mechanical exclusion, biochemical destruction, and microbial competition and *internal* for the physiologic reactions. The nonspecific mechanisms are nonselectively directed against *any* foreign substance. The specific mechanisms are specifically elicited by *unique* substances to which the body has *acquired* the ability to respond.

EXTERNAL NONSPECIFIC DEFENSE MECHANISMS

Anatomic Structures and Mechanical Actions

Skin and mucous membranes

The first line of defense against penetration by foreign materials, including pathogenic microorganisms, is the skin and mucous membranes. The intact skin is an extremely efficient physical barrier to harmful agents and environmental forces, such as heat, cold, and trauma. This protection is afforded by the keratinized surface cells, which provide a tough, dense, waterproof covering. Beneath this outermost layer is a dense layer of highly vascularized connective tissue (see Chapter 43, Fig. 43-1).

Even though some of the fatty acids derived from sebaceous gland secretions have antimicrobial activity, the environment provided by the skin does allow the growth of microorganisms on its upper layers and within hair follicles and sweat glands. For the most part these resident microorganisms are nonpathogenic; however, when these organisms gain entrance to the tissue of a host exhibiting reduced resistance, they may cause significant problems. Because even thorough scrubbing with soap and water removes only the surface organisms, the skin can never be considered sterile.

Any time the physical integrity of the skin is broken, such as in surgery, in-dwelling venous catheterization, or physical irritation or trauma, the risk of microorganisms gaining entrance to the body is very great. The skin must be kept relatively dry because the continued presence of moisture tends to cause maceration of the skin. Further, when essential oils are lost from the skin surface, they should be supplemented by lotions to maintain the resilience and unbroken texture of the surface cells. Adequate care of the skin of the hospitalized patient is not just a luxury but a necessity for the provision of an extremely important aspect of biologic defense.

Mucous membranes protect the eye and line all body tracts that have external openings. When intact, the mucous membranes, like the skin, are basically impervious to foreign materials and microorganisms. The surfaces are covered by a viscous secretion that tends to trap and inactivate microorganisms. The mucous membrane of the respiratory tract is further protected by the surface activity of the ciliated epithelial cells, which sweep foreign material upward and out of the tract. The mucous membranes are highly vascularized so that the internal defense mechanisms are readily available to attack any microorganisms that do gain access to the surface of these cells.

Also found in the mucosal secretions and in high concentration within the secretory mucosal cells of the respiratory and intestinal tracts are a specific class of immunoglobulins (antibodies) known as immunoglobulin A (IgA) (see p. 325). These specific antibodies are secreted from the mucosal cells and have antibacterial, antiviral, and antitoxic properties. These antibodies serve to prevent microbial adherence and colonization of these tracts by pathogens.

Specialized structures and mechanical functions

Other structures and functions of the human body that are generally taken for granted actually serve extremely important roles in defense. The filtration action of the nasal hairs serves to trap particles and microorganisms. The flushing action of saliva and urine prevents the buildup of organisms. The eyes are protected from entrance of dirt particles and organisms by the lids and lashes. Foreign material that does gain entrance to the eye tends to be washed out by tears. The constant movement of foods through the stomach and intestines prevents the buildup of organisms or toxic waste products. Even the action of vomiting and the watery stools of diarrhea are active mechanisms of removal of harmful products from the gastrointestinal tract. Dysfunction or blockage of any of these processes means that special measures must be taken to protect against the establishment of pathogenic organisms and the buildup of toxic materials.

Biochemical Factors

Many areas of the body are protected not only by mechanical barriers but also by the presence of specific antimicrobial chemicals that provide added protection.

Dermatologic factors

The acetic acid and salt concentration of perspiration is toxic to many pathogenic microorganisms. Some of the fatty acids released to the skin surface by the sebaceous glands also serve to inhibit the growth of some microorganisms.

Gastrointestinal factors

In the stomach the acidity (approximate pH 2) of the gastric juice kills many organisms and detoxifies certain potentially toxic substances. For this reason, when gastric acidity is

Table 16-2   Distribution of normal microbic flora

Region of body	Sterile areas	Nonsterile areas	Microorganisms
Skin	None	All skin	*Staphylococcus, Bacillus, Corynebacterium, Mycobacterium, Streptococcus,* transient environmental organisms
Respiratory tract	Larynx, trachea, bronchi, bronchioles, alveoli, sinuses	Nose, throat, mouth	*Staphylococcus, Candida, Streptococcus, Neisseria, Pneumococcus,* oral organisms
Gastrointestinal tract	Esophagus, stomach, upper small intestine	Esophagus and stomach (transiently), large intestine	Gram-negative rods, *Streptococcus, Bacteroides, Proteus, Clostridium, Lactobacillus*
Genitourinary tract	Cervix, uterus, fallopian tubes, ovaries, prostate gland, epididymis, testes, bladder, kidney	External genitalia, anterior urethra, vagina	Skin organisms, *Lactobacillus, Bacteroides*
Body fluids and cavities	Blood, pleural fluid, synovial fluid, spinal fluid, lymph, etc.	None	

low, special precautions must be taken to avoid introduction of organisms through the nose and mouth. Low gastric acidity is characteristic in neonates; therefore, special care should be taken in feeding and handling babies to prevent exposure to pathogens by the oral route. The upper intestine is generally freed of organisms by the action of bile and other proteolytic enzymes.

Vaginal factors

Vaginal secretions allow certain harmless acid-producing bacteria to colonize the vagina and create an acidic environment. This reduces the chance of the colonization of the vagina by pathogens. When either the amount or the acidity of the vaginal secretions is decreased, there is a much greater chance that a vaginal infection will develop. Because vaginal secretions are not present before puberty and are greatly decreased after menopause, young girls and older women are more prone to vaginitis. Birth control pills may cause a shift in the composition of pH of the vaginal secretions, which increases the possibility of colonization of the vagina, especially by the causative agent of gonorrhea. *Neisseria gonorrhoeae.*

Lysozyme

The most ubiquitous antimicrobial factor in the body is the enzyme lysozyme. It is capable of lysing (splitting) the bacterial cell wall of many gram-positive organisms, causing their destruction. Lysozyme is present in mucus, tears, saliva, and skin secretions and is also found in many of the internal fluids and cells of the body. Within the body it tends to work in combination with complement and other blood factors to destroy bacteria directly.

Microbial Antagonism

The skin and mucosal surfaces offer varying nutritional and environmental conditions for the growth and multiplication of certain microbial cells. Although the surfaces of the body are constantly exposed to temporary contamination by organisms from the environment, most of these organisms, known as *transient flora,* do not find conditions

suitable for the colonization of the body; however, many microorganisms, known as *normal microbic flora,* do colonize the skin and mucosal surfaces. Although this normal flora varies from site to site within the body and may vary in response to environmental, hygienic, and physiologic changes, it is capable of reestablishment and reflects a fairly predictable pattern. Table 16-2 provides an overview of the body areas normally colonized and shows which organisms most often make up the normal flora of the various areas.

The maintenance of this balanced microbic flora serves to make it difficult for pathogenic organisms to establish themselves on the body surfaces. Because the normal flora have a selective advantage in their environmental niche, they compete for nutrients and space. Some release antimicrobial substances to retard the growth of transient organisms seeking to occupy the same site. Such microbial interference is called *microbial antagonism.*

Most of the normal microbic flora are basically non-pathogenic; however, some overtly pathogenic organisms, such as *Staphylococcus aureus* and *Streptococcus pyogenes,* can be part of the normal flora. The individual who harbors such organisms without demonstrating any symptoms of disease is known as a *carrier.* This carrier state is of significance because the carrier may be unknowingly shedding organisms into the environment and infecting others.

The protective effects of the normal microbic flora become most apparent when something upsets the microbic balance within the body. The extended use of broad-spectrum antibiotics frequently creates such an effect. The imbalance may allow a segment of the normal flora to gain ascendency, causing adverse reactions. An example of this phenomenon is seen when certain orally administered antibiotics induce marked shifts in the normal intestinal flora, allowing organisms that are generally suppressed by the growth of competitors to thrive to an unusual degree. This imbalance may induce uncomfortable gastrointestinal tract problems or even allow gastroenteritis to develop. Oral or vaginal *Candida* (yeast) infections may also develop from extended antibiotic therapy and depression of normal flora.

INTERNAL NONSPECIFIC DEFENSE MECHANISMS

Once a foreign agent (living or nonliving) penetrates the external resistance barriers, it is met by an even more complex array of defense mechanisms, which provides for the recognition, capture, and disposal of the foreign material. The key to this process is the specific recognition and vigorous action taken against the foreign material while at the same time protecting the host tissues from extensive damage. The physiologic reactions that serve to contain and inactivate the foreign agent are carried out through interactions of cells and molecules of the blood, reticuloendothelial system, vascular system, and body tissues.

Reticuloendothelial System

The reticuloendothelial system (RES) is a widespread system of phagocytic (devouring) cells scattered throughout various body tissues (Fig. 16-3). The role of these cells is to ingest foreign particulate matter and damaged host tissues. *Some of the phagocytic cells are fixed in a variety of tissues, such as lymphoid tissue, liver, spleen, bone marrow, lungs, and blood vessels.* Within the different tissues these anchored cells have been given unique names (Table 16-3). It is the function of the fixed cells to capture and destroy foreign materials found in the fluids of their environment.

Other cells making up the reticuloendothelial network are not stationary and are called *wandering macrophages.* Depending on where they are found, they may be known as *monocytes* (in the bloodstream) or *histiocytes* (in loose connective tissues). *The wandering macrophages carry out the important role of final cleanup of a damaged site in preparation for repair.* The cells have the capacity to engulf and destroy virtually any type of foreign material or debris within the body. Macrophages also play an important role in the specific response mechanisms.

Blood

Blood is one of the primary sources of elements designed to provide protection against injurious agents. It transports these active factors to the site of an injury or intrusion and through specific vascular changes concentrates these materials at the site. Both the fluid and cellular constituents of blood contain these factors.

Cellular components

The cellular components of blood that are of importance in this nonspecific response include granulocytes, lymphocytes, monocytes, and thrombocytes (platelets). *The granulocytes, also referred to as polymorphonuclear leukocytes (PMNs), and the monocytes are the most important because of their phagocytic activity.*

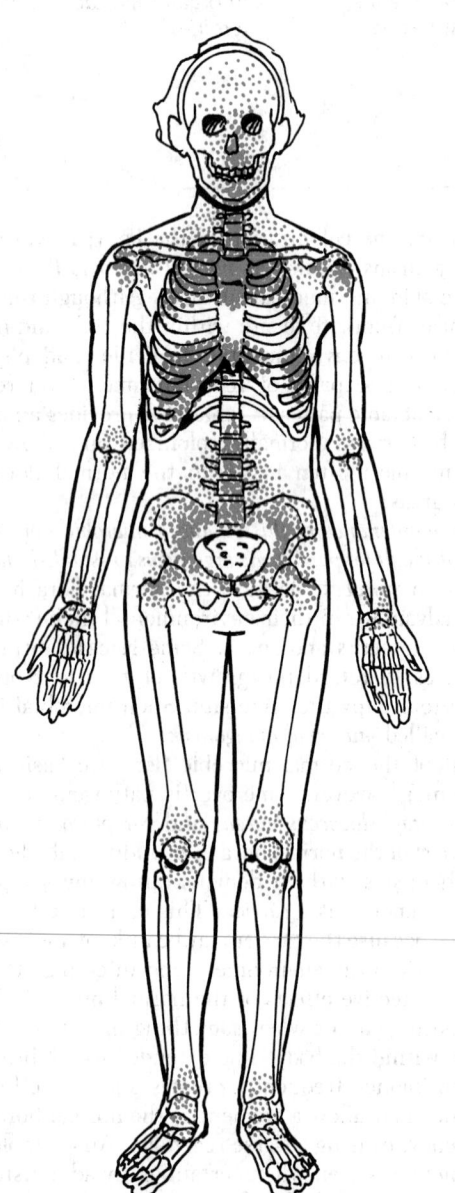

Fig. 16-3 Reticuloendothelial system. Note anatomic distribution of maximal activity in system, as indicated by darker areas. Note definition of liver, spleen, and active bone marrow in axial skeleton and proximal parts of long bones. (Redrawn from Smith AL: *Microbiology and pathology,* ed 12, 1980, St Louis, Mosby–Year Book.)

Distribution and names of macrophages in various tissue sites

Tissue	Macrophage
Peripheral blood	Monocytes
Loose connective tissue	Histiocytes
Liver	Kupffer's cells
Spleen and reticuloendothelial system	Wandering or fixed macrophages
Lung	Alveolar macrophages or dust cells
Granulomatous tissue	Epithelioid and giant cells
Peritoneal cavity, pleural cavity, and bone	Macrophages

One of the key methods of nonspecific defense is the ingestion of microorganisms and other particulate matter by the phagocytic white blood cells. The phagocytes carry out the process of *phagocytosis* in several discrete steps (Fig. 16-4). Most infecting microbes are quickly and efficiently destroyed by phagocytosis; however, some pathogens exhibit methods of escape from this destruction. Some bacteria, such as strains of the streptococci and staphylococci and *Bacillus anthracis* (anthrax), actually produce factors that will kill the phagocyte. Other organisms resist ingestion or digestion. Some organisms may survive within the phagocytes or reticuloendothelial cells and multiple there. This may lead to the transport of the organism to other sites in the body or serve as a chronic focus of continued infection.

Granulocytes can be divided on the basis of their structure and function into *neutrophils, eosinophils,* and *basophils.* The "granules" found within these cells represent discrete packets of degradative enzymes used to digest the ingested materials. The neutrophils are the most numerous in circulation and are the most efficient and responsive phagocytic cells involved in the inflammatory process. When there is adequate blood supply to a region, the phagocytes are constantly available to move from the blood vessels to the site of injury or infection. Neutrophils and monocytes are actually attracted to the scene by chemicals released during infection or injury. This *cellular response to chemical attraction is known* as *chemotaxis,* and the substances released are called *chemotactic substances.*

Fluid factors

The fluid portion of uncoagulated blood is called *plasma.* Some of the components of plasma provide important constituents for the internal defense mechanisms. *Plasma transports* the *circulating antibodies* produced in specific response to antigenic stimulation. These antibodies, when bound to their specific antigens, enhance the ability of white blood cells to engulf the clumped and sticky antigens. The antibodies of the blood that create this coating effect are known as *opsonins. Another plasma constituent, fibrin, may create a meshwork around the injured area, causing the sealing off of the area. Microorganisms may also become trapped within this meshwork, where they are more easily captured by phagocytic cells.*

One of the most important constituents of plasma is a complex series of 11 proteins known by the singular name of complement. The primary role of complement is to provide specific lysis (rupturing) of cell membranes. The initiation of the "complement cascade" is most often triggered by the binding of the first complement protein to complement-

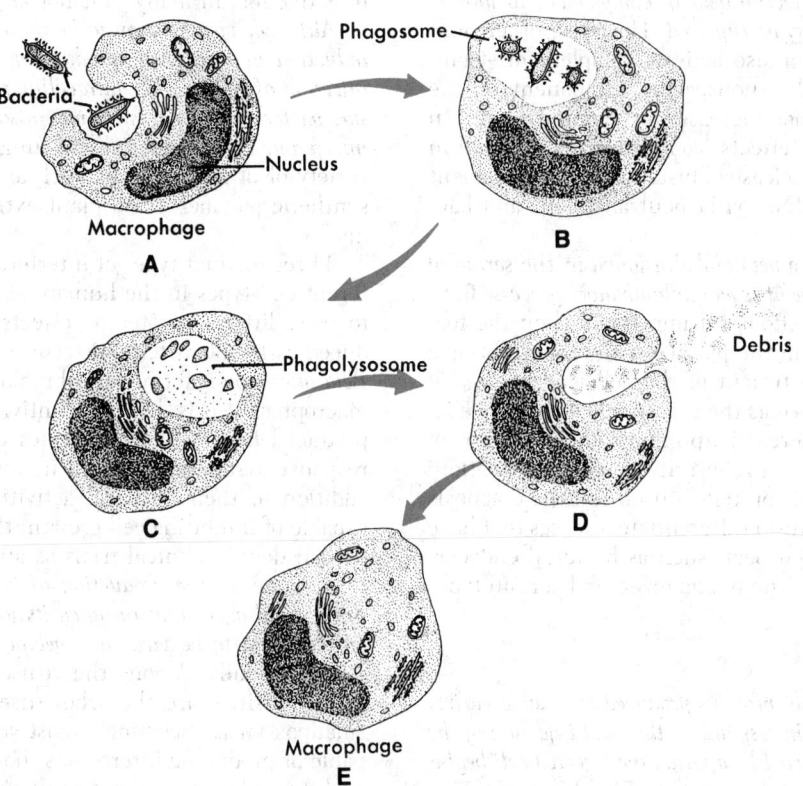

Fig. 16-4 Phagocytosis sketched in macrophage. **A,** Opsonized bacteria engulfed by phagocyte (macrophage). **B,** Phagosome formed. **C,** Phagosome becomes phagolysosome; bacteria digested. (To this point process of phagocytosis is comparable to either macrophage or neutrophil, not shown.) **D,** Debris is egested. (Neutrophil would succumb here.) **E,** Macrophage returns to resting state. (From Smith AL: *Microbiology and pathology,* ed 12, St Louis, 1980, Mosby—Year Book.)

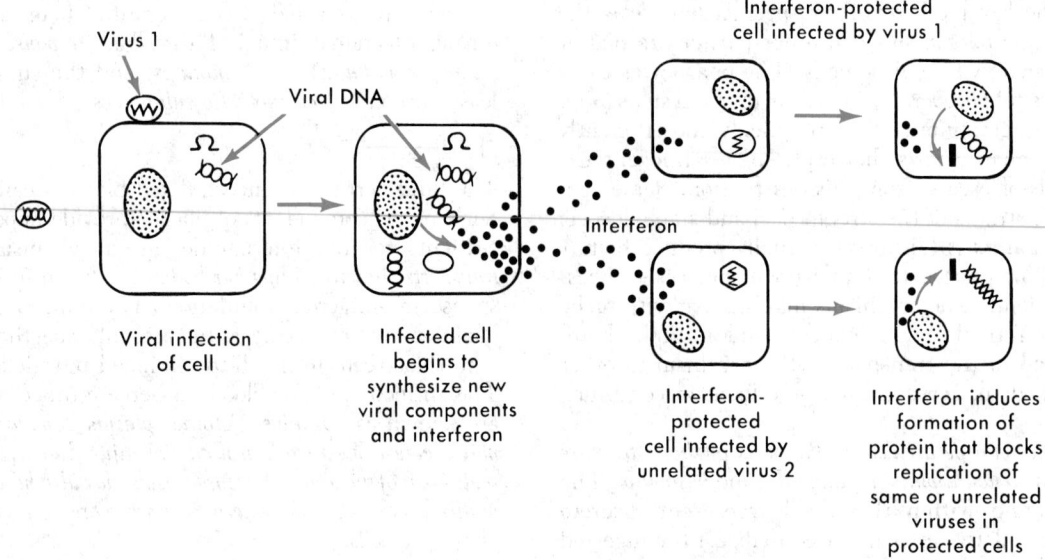

Virus 1

Viral DNA

Interferon-protected cell infected by virus 1

Interferon

Viral infection of cell

Infected cell begins to synthesize new viral components and interferon

Interferon-protected cell infected by unrelated virus 2

Interferon induces formation of protein that blocks replication of same or unrelated viruses in protected cells

Fig. 16-5 Mechanisms of interferon action.

binding antibodies that have already bound to their antigens. *Thus complement serves to accentuate or complete the action of an antibody. The antibody by itself cannot produce cell lysis, but with the recruitment of complement to join in the reaction, the cell may be ruptured.* However, other nonimmune substances can also activate complement. Complement is considered a nonspecific component of the plasma because it is not increased by immunization. In addition to its cytolytic effects, complement is involved in leukocyte chemotaxis, release of histamines, enhancement of phagocytosis by PMNs, viral neutralization, and bactericidal activity.

C-reactive protein is a beta globulin found in the serum of individuals with *any type of severe inflammatory process.* Both infectious and noninfectious inflammations elicit the formation of this protein in the plasma. The protein forms a precipitate with a constituent of the cell wall of *streptococcus pneumoniae* known as the C polysaccharide, hence its name. The amount of C-reactive protein found in the serum is roughly proportional to the severity of the inflammation; therefore, a test for this protein is useful in the diagnosis and management of hard-to-differentiate diseases that have a hidden inflammatory aspect, such as bacterial endocarditis, cryptic abscesses, rheumatic fever, and certain types of cancer.

Interferons

Interferons are a group of proteins produced by a wide variety of human cells, usually in response to the viral infection of the cell. When a cell is infected by a virus, the infected cell begins to make interferon almost immediately (Fig. 16-5). The interferon is released into its surrounding environment where it induces uninfected cells to produce alterations that protect those cells from viral multiplication. This antiviral action is exerted before the synthesis of immunoglobulins specific for the virus reaches protective levels.

The elaboration of interferons from virally infected cells continues for a few hours (up to about 24 hours) following infection, thereby playing a significant role in isolating the infective foci in many (but not all) viral infections.

Although viruses seem to be the most potent agents for the induction of interferon, production is not restricted to virus infection of cells. Other intracellular parasites such as rickettsia, bacteria, and parasites may also trigger the formation of interferon. Even bacterial and fungal extracts, as well as a variety of other materials such as double-stranded RNA, synthetic polymers, and plant extracts, may serve as signals.

Three distinct types of interferons are produced by different cell types in the human body, and each type seems to exert different protective effects. *Alpha interferon is produced by lymphocytes and seems to have antiviral activity. Beta interferon is formed by fibroblasts, epithelial cells, and macrophages; it is definitely antiviral. Gamma interferon is produced by T-cell lymphocytes of the specific immune response system and has an immunoregulatory effect.* In addition to their antiviral activities, the interferons are capable of inhibiting cell growth; therefore, they are being used widely in clinical trials as an *antitumor agent.*

In general, *the production of interferon occurs regardless of the viral agent that initiated its formation; therefore, interferon is said to be virus nonspecific.* It does not inhibit all viruses equally. Among the viruses that seem to be especially sensitive are the arboviruses, influenza virus, and smallpox virus. Seemingly most vertebrate species are capable of producing interferons: however, the interferon of each animal species is protective against viral infection only in that species. This means that bovine (cow) interferon has only limited protective value in the human and vice versa. The term *species specificity* is used to describe this quality. This characteristic limited early research into the effects of interferon, because it was difficult to obtain

Table 16-4   Steps of the inflammatory response

Steps	Mediators	Outcome
1. Injury	Physical, chemical, biologic, immunologic stimulus	Cell and tissue injury
2. Vascular response		
a. Vascular dilation	Histamine, plasmin, serotonin, kinins, prostaglandins released or activated by injury	Dilation of vessels causing stasis of blood and margination of leukocytes
b. Fibrin clot formation	Activation of clotting mechanism	Containment of irritants
3. Fluid exudation	Histamine, kinins, prostaglandins cause opening of venule–endothelial cell junction	Fluid exudation into tissues
4. Cellular exudation		
a. Leukocyte exudation	Chemotactic substances released by complement activation, clot formation, and injured cells	Passage of leukocytes from blood to site of injury and accumulation there
b. Attack and engulfment of foreign materials	Neutrophils and macrophages	Removal and digestion of bacteria, foreign particles, and damaged tissues
5. Healing	Fibroblasts produce collagen fibers and tissue regeneration	Resolution of inflammation and formation of scar tissue

enough human interferon to conduct clinical trials. Through the use of recombinant-DNA technology the human interferon gene has been introduced into bacterial cells. By growing such bacteria in culture, large amounts of specific types (alpha [α], beta [β], and gamma [γ]) of interferon can be harvested, purified, and used in clinical studies. The other benefit of this application of genetic engineering is to greatly reduce the cost of the purified interferon.

Inflammatory Response

When injury occurs in the body, all the nonspecific and, to some degree, the specific defense mechanisms are directed toward localizing the effects of the injury, protecting against microbial invasion at the site, and preparing the site for repair. This process is called *inflammation*. When inflammation occurs at a particular site in the body, the suffix *-itis* is added to the site designation to indicate the pathologic state; for example, an inflammatory response on the pericardium is termed *pericarditis*, and of the bladder, *cystitis*.

The inflammatory response can be initiated by any type of injury, for example, heat, cold, irradiation, chemicals, trauma, infection, immunologic injury, or neoplasm. Whatever the stimulus, the response of the body is the same, but the extent of the involvement of the various facets of the nonspecific response system depends on the extent and severity of the injury.

Inflammations can be classified as either acute or chronic. Acute inflammations are those characterized by a sudden onset and an increased fluid exudative response. Chronic inflammations have a slower, more insidious onset, and they are characterized by increased cellular exudation (see below).

Steps of the inflammatory response

Three major physiologic responses occur in the inflammatory process: vascular response, fluid exudation, and cellular exudation (Table 16-4). The inflammatory process occurs during the early part of wound healing (see Chapter 22).

Vascular response. The first response to cellular injury is a transitory vasoconstriction (stress response); however, this is followed immediately by *vasodilation* as a result of chemical substances such as histamine or kinins released at the site of injury or invasion. The amount of *blood flow* to the area is *thus increased (hyperemia), causing redness and heat.* Blood flow slows as the capillaries dilate. Permeability of the capillary walls is increased, facilitating fluid and cellular exudation to the injured tissue.

Fluid exudation. Fluid exudation from the capillaries into the interstitial spaces begins immediately and is most active during the first 24 hours after injury or invasion. Initially, the fluid exudate is primarily serous, but as the capillary wall becomes more permeable, protein (albumin) is lost into the interstitial spaces. Loss of large amounts of serum protein in major injuries, such as burns, leads to loss of plasma osmotic pressure (see Chapter 44). *Movement of protein into the interstitial spaces increases tissue osmotic pressure, which encourages more fluid exudation.* The *swelling from the fluid* in the *interstitial spaces is called edema* (see Chapter 7).

Cellular exudation. *Cellular exudation refers to the migration of white blood cells (leukocytes) through the capillary walls into the affected tissue.* An increased number of white blood cells is attracted to the vessels in the affected area as a result of chemotactic substances being released from the tissues by cell injury and complement activation. The white blood cells adhere to the capillary wall and then pass in ameboid fashion through the widened endothelial junctions of the capillary wall. Neutrophils (PMNs), which make up about 60% of the circulating white blood cells, are the first leukocytes to respond, usually within the first few hours. The neutrophils ingest the bacteria and dead tissue cells (*phagocytosis*) (see Fig. 16-4); then they die, releasing proteolytic enzymes that liquefy the dead neutrophils, dead bacteria, and other dead cells (pus). Monocytes and lymphocytes appear later. The macrophages continue the phagocytosis, and the lymphocytes play a role in the antigen-antibody response at the site.

<table>
<tr><td colspan="2">**16-2**
Causes of the cardinal symptoms of inflammation</td></tr>
<tr><td>Redness</td><td>Hyperemia from vasodilation</td></tr>
<tr><td>Heat</td><td>Vasodilation—blood vessels closer to skin surface</td></tr>
<tr><td>Swelling</td><td>Fluid exudation into tissue</td></tr>
<tr><td>Pain</td><td>Chemical (bradykinin) irritation of nerve endings and pressure of fluid in tissues</td></tr>
<tr><td>Loss of function</td><td>Tissue swelling and pain</td></tr>
</table>

<table>
<tr><td colspan="2">**16-3**
Some types of inflammations</td></tr>
<tr><td>**Cellulitis**</td><td>Inflammation involving cellular and connective tissue</td></tr>
<tr><td>**Lymphadenitis**</td><td>Inflammation of lymph nodes</td></tr>
<tr><td>**Lymphangitis**</td><td>Inflammation of lymphatic vessel</td></tr>
<tr><td>**Bacteremia**</td><td>Presence of bacteria in blood</td></tr>
<tr><td>**Septicemia**</td><td>Systemic disease associated with pathogenic microorganisms and their toxins in the blood</td></tr>
<tr><td>**Abscess**</td><td>Collection of pus localized by a zone of inflamed tissue</td></tr>
<tr><td>**Sinus**</td><td>Suppurating channel from an abscess to the surface of the body or into a body cavity</td></tr>
<tr><td>**Peritonitis**</td><td>Inflammation of the peritoneum</td></tr>
<tr><td>**Pleuritis**</td><td>Inflammation of the pleura</td></tr>
<tr><td>**Empyema**</td><td>Collection of pus in a body cavity, especially the pleural cavity</td></tr>
</table>

Effects of inflammation

Local effects of inflammation. The *five local cardinal symptoms of inflammation*, identified many centuries ago, are *redness (rubor)*, *heat (calor)*, *swelling (tumor)*, *pain (dolor)*, and *loss of function*. These symptoms result from vasodilation and fluid exudation as well as irritation from chemotactic substances (Box 16-2).

The inflammatory response serves to prepare the tissue for healing and to contain the spread of bacterial invasion. To prevent the spread of bacteria, fibroblasts are attracted to the area and secrete fibrin, a threadlike substance that encircles the affected area to wall it off from healthy tissue. If there is interference with this walling-off process, bacteria can spread into the surrounding tissue. This explains why an abscess should not be incised and drained until it has "come to a head," or until the walling-off process is completed.

No healing will occur until inflammation has subsided and pus and dead tissue have been removed. Pus is a local accumulation of dead phagocytes, dead bacteria, and dead tissue. The bacteria most commonly causing this reaction are the staphylococci, streptococci, *Neisseria*, and *P. aeruginosa (pyocyanea)*.

Lymph node involvement. *Bacteria may fail to be contained locally and may spread to other parts of the body by means of the lymph system* (lymphogenous) *or bloodstream* (hematogenous) (Box 16-3). If picked up by the lymph stream , the bacteria will be carried to the nearest lymph node. These nodes are located along the course of all lymph channels, and here too bacteria can be ingested and destroyed. If the bacteria are virulent enough to resist the action in the lymph nodes, leukocytes are brought in by the bloodstream to attack and engulf the bacteria in the node. The node then becomes swollen and tender because of the accumulation of phagocytes, bacteria, and destroyed lymphoid tissue. This is known as *lymphadenitis.* Swollen lymph nodes can be palpated primarily in the neck, axilla, and groin.

Systemic effects of inflammation. Moderate to severe inflammatory responses can produce generalized systemic effects. Products from the breakdown of bacteria and white blood cells can affect the temperature-regulating center in the hypothalamus and produce *fever.* A severe infection without accompanying fever may suggest a poor prognosis. *Loss of appetite* (anorexia) and *fatigue* may be caused by conservation of body energy needed to resist the infection. The body increases the production of white blood cells to help fight the infection, and *leukocytosis* (serum white blood cell levels $>10,000/mm^3$) may occur. With infection the *blood sedimentation rate* is also increased, that is, when an anticoagulant is added to the blood in the laboratory, the red blood cells settle to the bottom of a test tube more rapidly than normal. This increase in the sedimentation rate is believed to be caused by an increase in fibrinogen (a blood protein essential to the healing process). The sedimentation rate is elevated during the acute inflammatory stage of infection. An elevated sedimentation rate is considered to be a *non-specific* test because it indicates that inflammation is present, but not what is causing it. It also indicates that the body's defense mechanism for the repair of damaged tissue is operating. Because the sedimentation rate gradually returns to normal as tissues heal, it also is used to determine when physical activity can be safely resumed after an acute infection.

Resolution and healing

After the infected area is clean, new cells are produced to fill in the space left by the injury. They may be the normal structural cells, or they may be fibrotic tissue cells known as *scar tissue.* If they are fibrotic cells, they will not function as formerly but only serve to fill in the injured area. Some body cells readily regenerate; for instance, after the bowel has healed it is almost impossible to find the injured area. The respiratory tract also regenerates its tissues readily. Liver tissue has the capacity to regenerate, but over a longer priod of time. Some nerve cells are always replaced with fibrous tissue. If a large amount of tissue is destroyed, structural cells may not be replaced, regardless of the type of tissue. (See Chapter 22 for discussion of wound healing.)

SPECIFIC DEFENSE MECHANISMS
Concept of Specific Immunity

Nonspecific response mechanisms are often inadequate to cope with foreign agents. This is especially true when the agent is capable of multiplication and invasion of host tissues, as is the case with infectious disease microorganisms (viruses, bacteria, fungi). The body responds by activation of the specific immune response system.

The *fundamental nature* of the *specific immune response* is *characterized by diversity, specificity, recognition, memory,* and *action.* Among the most intriguing aspects of immune response is *the diversity of its ability to respond* while at the same time responding with *specificity of action.* Almost any conceivable organic molecular array on the surface of a molecule has been shown to be able to induce a series of cellular events culminating in the production of *antibodies.* These antibodies combine with the inducing *antigen* by virtue of combining sites on the antibody molecule, which exhibit an extremely narrow specificity. The remainder of the antibody molecule is chemically and structurally quite similar to all other antibody molecules with distinctly different combining site specificities. *Recognition* and *memory* are two other aspects of this system that make it unique. *The normal organism recognizes its own antigenic makeup and will not produce antibodies against its own antigens.* This is known as *recognition of self.* At the same time, this intricate system of self-recognition must be able to recognize extremely subtle changes in its own cells when tumors that differ only slightly in antigenic constitution are forming. Further, once the immune system has responded to an antigen, subsequent encounters with that antigen produces an even more vigorous and rapid response. This response includes a wide variety of mechanisms designed to take *action* against the offending agent. Many of these actions are among the most potent biochemical and cellular reactions that the body is capable of producing, yet they are focused so discretely that the foreign agent is rapidly destroyed with a minimum of damage to the host.

Basic Design of the System

The basic design of the specific immune response system is such that the body provides itself with cells and molecules distributed throughout the body that can respond to encroachment by "nonself" materials rapidly and efficiently and block the encroachment. The system has two major interactive divisions:

1. Humorally mediated system: specific blood proteins known as *antibodies* or *immunoglobulins.*
2. Cellularly mediated system: specific WBCs known as *activated lymphocytes* or *T cells.*

Both divisions are usually triggered to respond to encroachment; however, only one division may provide the majority of protection against certain types of encroachment.

The *humorally mediated system* provides our major immunity against the following organisms:

1. Bacteria that produce acute infection (such as *Staphylococcus, Streptococcus, Hemophilus*),
2. Bacterial exotoxins (diphtheria, botulinal, tetanus toxins),
3. Viruses that must enter the bloodstream to reach their target tissues (such as poliomyelitis, hepatitis virus)
4. Organisms that enter the body from the mucosal tissues (such as cold viruses, enteroviruses, influenza viruses)

Even though circulating antibodies may be produced against other organisms (such as tuberculosis, HIV, fungi), these antibodies do not protect the body from infection.

The *cell-mediated system* on the other hand offers protection from the following:

1. Chronic bacterial infections (such as syphilis, tuberculosis, leprosy)
2. Many viral infections (such as measles, herpes virus infections, chicken pox)
3. Fungal infections
4. Parasitic infections
5. Tissue transplants or transformed cells (such as cancer cells).

An individual can be immunodeficient (see Chapter 41) in one or both of these systems. When one system is not functioning properly, the individual becomes susceptible to infection or encroachment by the agents against which that system provided primary protection. If both systems are lost or compromised, the individual is fully susceptible to infectious agents and cannot survive in an unprotected, nonsterile environment.

Immune Response System
Antigens and antibodies
Antigens (immunogens)

An antigen is defined as a substance that, when introduced into an animal, elicits the formation of antibodies, or specifically sensitized cells. The antigen must be recognized as "nonself" or "foreign" material within the body. Although most antigens are naturally occurring proteins of at least 10,000 molecular weight, other substances such as polysaccharides, nucleoproteins, lipoproteins, and glycoproteins may also serve as antigens. The bulk of the antigen consists of subsurface molecular structures that do not elicit an immune response but do serve as carriers for the multiple *antigenic determinants* on the surface. Most antigens have multiple antigenic determinants and are termed *multivalent antigens;* however, some molecules may be monovalent.

Certain molecules, because of their small size, cannot by themselves induce the synthesis of antibodies; however, when they are coupled with a high-molecular-weight carrier, they can serve as antigenic determinants. These molecules are known as *incomplete antigens,* or *haptens.* These molecules take on special significance in the consideration of hypersensitivities (allergies to low-molecular-weight compounds such as certain drugs and antibiotics) (Chapter 41).

Antibodies (immunoglobulins)

The body's response to the introduction of an antigenic substance is the production of a specific, soluble *antibody* or a sensitized (antigen reactive) lymphocyte population. The type of antigen introduced will determine the immune response: antibody synthesis, antigen-reactive lymphocyte, or a combination of both.

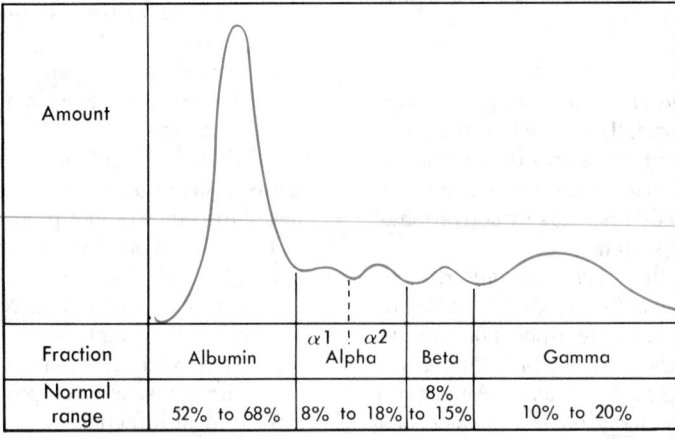

Fig. 16-6 Electrophoretic separation of major serum proteins. Majority of antibody activity lies within gamma globulin fraction. Gamma globulin fraction rises with active synthesis of antibodies in response to antigenic stimulation.

Table 16-5   Characteristics of immunoglobulin classes

Immunoglobulin class	Function	Body distribution	Activate complement	Cross placenta
IgA	Protects mucosal surfaces from bacteria, viruses, and toxins	Mucosal and exocrine secretions	No	No
IgD	Does not have antibody function but may play a role in signaling B cell differentiation	Membrane of circulating B cells	No	No
IgE	Protects against parasitic infections and responsible for Type I hypersensitivity	Membrane of mast cells and basophils	No	No
IgG	Protects against microorganisms and toxins in blood and body fluids	Major immunoglobulin in serum and other body fluids	Yes	Yes
IgM	Protects against microorganisms in blood	Confined to vascular system	Yes	No

The circulating antibodies represent modified (that is, antigen specific) globulin proteins found in blood serum. The serum contains several distinct protein fractions, which are separable on the basis of their net electrical charge, molecular size, and molecular conformation into several fractions: albumin, alpha globulins, beta globulins, and gamma globulins (Fig. 16-6). The antibody activity of the serum is characteristically associated with the gamma globulin fraction. Those gamma globulins with the ability to bind antigens are called *immunoglobulins*.

Five different classes of immunoglobulins are actually produced within the body. Each immunoglobulin class varies in structure, distribution in the body, and protective function. Some of these variations in function have significant clinical implications; for example, only one class of immunoglobulins, IgG, can cross the normal placenta; immunoglobulin E (IgE) binds to receptors on the membranes of mast cells and basophils to mediate one type of allergic reaction. Table 16-5 summarizes the characteristics of the different immunoglobulin classes.

Antigen-antibody interactions

When an immunoglobulin comes in contact with its specific antigen, a physical interaction occurs between the two, causing a reversible binding of the antibody to the antigen. The affinity that the antibody has for the antigen and the avidity, or tightness, of the binding depend on the location and spatial arrangement of the antigenic determinants on the surface of the antigen and how well the antigen-combining site on the antibody molecule "fits" the antigenic determinant. Because the antigen is usually multivalent and the antibody is generally at least bivalent, the antigen molecules may be cross bound and clumped (agglutinated, precipitated) by antibody molecules (Fig. 16-7).

Within the body the binding of antibody to the antigen can have direct beneficial effects, such as detoxification of toxins, inactivation of viruses, or, coupled with complement, the direct lysis of cells. However, in most cases the antigen-antibody combination initiates and facilitates the nonspecific defense mechanisms (phagocytosis, complement, inflammatory response, and so forth).

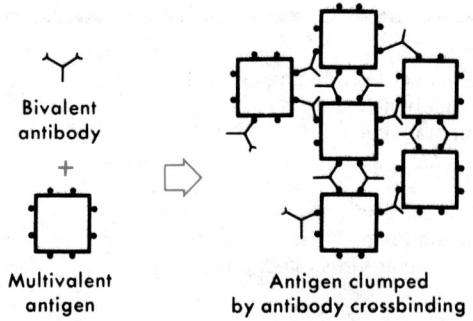

Fig. 16-7   Clumping of multivalent antigen by its specific antibody.

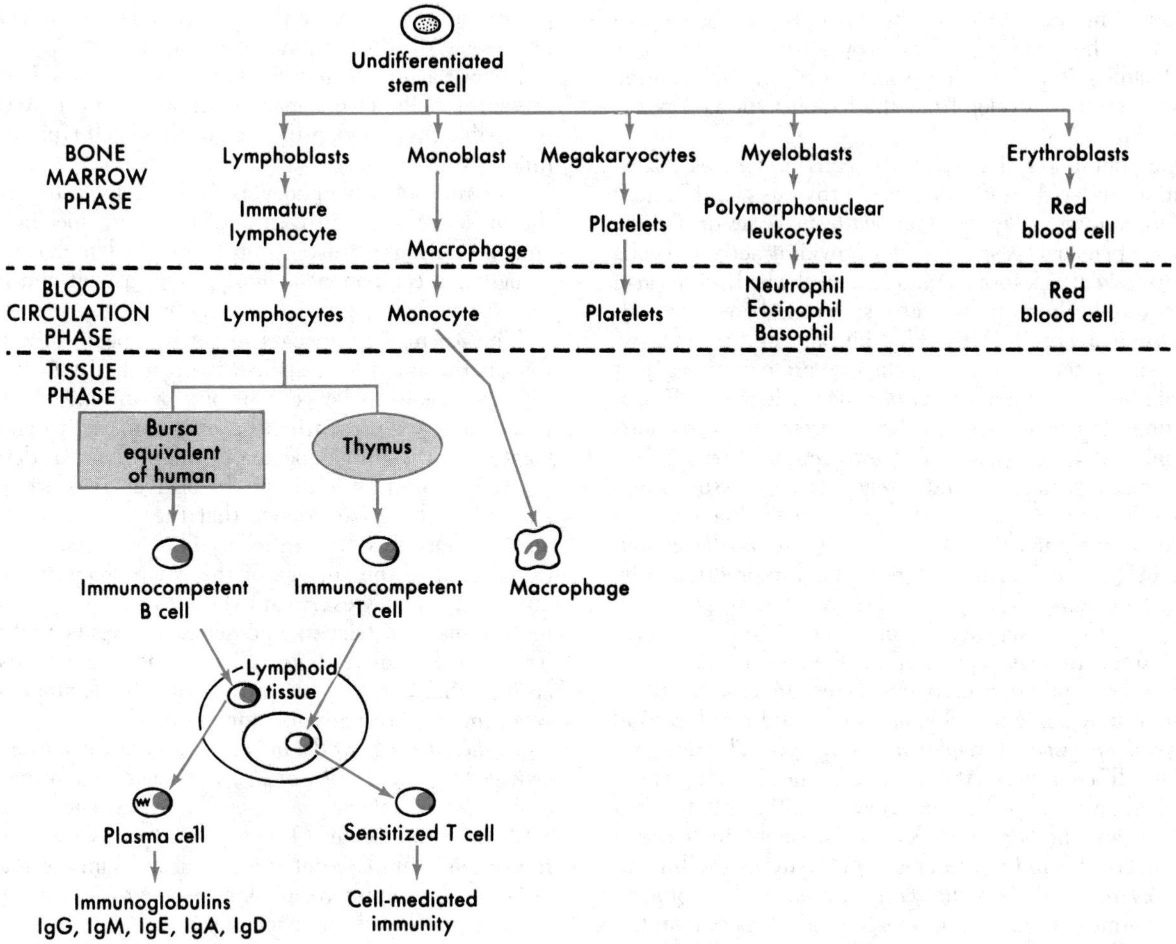

Fig. 16-8   Development of B and T cell lymphocytes.

Table 16-6 Protection provided by humorally mediated and cell-mediated immune response systems

Characteristic	Specific immune response system	
	Humorally mediated system	**Cell-mediated system**
Lymphocytes	B cells	T cells
Immunologically active effector	Plasma cells producing circulating immunoglobulins	Antigen-specific activated T cell producing lymphokines, cytotoxic T cells
Memory cells	B memory cells	T memory cells
Control cells	—	T helper cells (T_4) T suppressor cells (T_8)
Primary protection against	Acute bacterial infections Biologic toxins Extracellular virus infections	Chronic bacterial infections Fungal infections Protozoan infections Intracellular virus infections Foreign tissues

Cells involved

The cells in the specific immune response are all derived from the original undifferentiated stem cells of the bone marrow. The stem cell has the possibility of developing into any of the blood cells of the body depending on various signals and influences. The primary cells of the immune response system develop from the lymphocytic cell population (Fig. 16-8).

One population of lymphocytic cells undergoes differentiation under the influence of the thymus gland. These cells are known as *thymus-dependent lymphocytes* or *T cells.* They are primarily responsible for providing activated cells that directly attack foreign materials in the body. This arm of the specific immune response system is known as *cell-mediated immunity* (CMI). This division of the immune response system provides primary protection against chronic bacterial infection (tuberculosis, leprosy), fungal infections (thrush, athlete's foot), protozoan infections (pneumocystis, toxoplasmosis), intracellular virus infections (measles, herpes), and foreign tissues (tissue transplants) (Table 16-6). T cells also produce cells that exercise control of immunologic response. *T helper cells* (designated as T_H or T_4 cells) enhance immunoglobulin production by B cells and amplify cell-mediated immune response. *T suppressor cells* (designated T_S or T_8 cells) inhibit immunoglobulin synthesis and T cell cytotoxic activity.

Another population of lymphocytes undergoes differentiation independent of thymic control and is referred to as *thymus-independent lymphocytes* or *B cells.* The designation "B cell" comes from the fact that in the chicken, where these cells were first detected, they are differentiated in a single organ, the *bursa of Fabricius.* No such single organ site has been found in humans, so the site in the human is simply referred to as the *bursa-equivalent.* The process of commitment to the B-cell lineage probably occurs in the bone marrow during cell maturation. B cells produce immunoglobulins that appear in blood, lymph, mucus, and virtually all body fluids. This division of immune response provides the body's primary protection against acute bacterial infections (staphylococcal or streptococcal infections), biologic toxins (diphtheria or tetanus toxin), and certain viral infections (common cold, rabies, polio).

The proteins (markers) on the membranes of immune response cells vary according to the type of immune response cell it is. B-cell lymphocytes have immunoglobulins present on their surface that are missing from T-cell lymphocytes. All T cells have a marker called T_1; helper T cells have a unique marker known as T_4 (or CD4); suppressor T cells have a marker known as T_8 (or CD8). It is possible then to identify each of these cell types by their unique surface markers.

The role of the lymphocytes (B or T cells) is to recognize the presence of an antigen and to initiate specific mechanisms of disposal. Just as important, the lymphocyte must recognize a component of host tissues as self and protect that tissue from immunologic reactions.

The *macrophage* appears to act nonspecifically, but its role in the immune response is critical. First, the macrophage seems to be responsible for initially capturing, processing, and presenting the antigen to the lymphocytes. Capture of the antigen occurs by phagocytosis as described (p. 323). The processing of the antigen is poorly understood, but there is evidence that the macrophage digests and concentrates the antigen. This processed signal is transferred to the surface of the macrophage for presentation to lymphocytes. An antigen presented to lymphocytes in this manner triggers the series of events within the lymphocytes that leads to full immunologic response. An antigen that escapes this processing will stimulate only a weak immune response or none at all.

At the other end of the immune response the macrophage is activated to its maximum of phagocytic efficiency by the release of stimulatory, soluble substances, known as *lymphokines,* by activated lymphocytes (Table 16-7). In this way the macrophage is stimulated at the site of an immune reaction. Other of the soluble lymphokines serve to attract the macrophages to the site by chemotaxis.

Organs and tissues involved

The organs and tissues of the specific immune response system include the central organs (bone marrow and thymus) and the peripheral organs (lymph nodes, spleen, and lymphatic vessels). Within the central organs the immune response cells are synthesized and matured, whereas

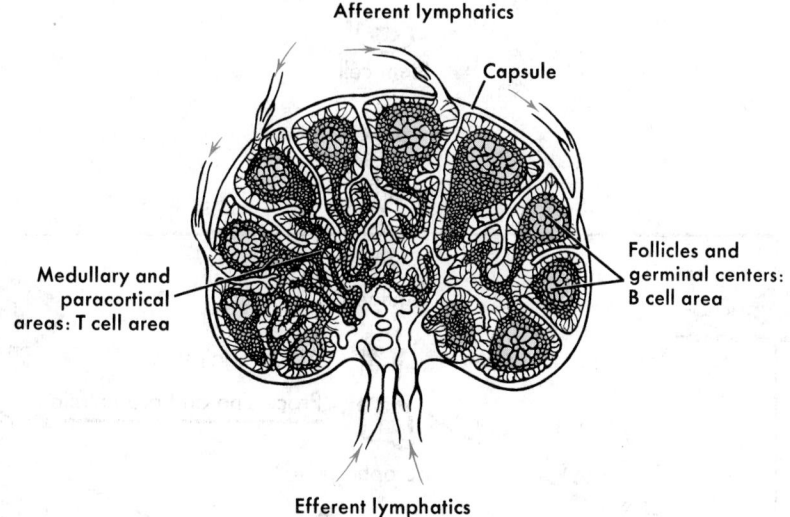

Fig. 16-9 B and T cell areas of lymph node.

Table 16-7 Lymphokines liberated by activated T cell lymphocytes

Lymphokine	Function
Lymphocyte-derived chemotactic factors	Chemotactic for macrophages
Lymphocytotoxins	Nonspecific lysis of cells
Macrophage inhibition-activation factors	Maintains macrophage at site and activates it
Interferon	Inhibits replication of viruses
Lymphocyte-activating factors (interleukins)	Activates nonsensitized lymphocytes

within the peripheral organs the mature cells are concentrated.

The *thymus serves as the control organ of the immune system.* It is the *site of differentiation of the T-cell lymphocytic* populations and through certain soluble thymic hormones *serves to regulate the overall immune system.* The activity of the thymus reaches its peak in childhood, and the organ begins to shrink in size after puberty. If the thymus is removed (thymectomy) very early in the life of an animal, a severe state of immunodeficiency is induced and T-cell—mediated immunity never develops. After thymectomy, a wasting disease develops, characterized by stunted growth, diarrhea, and death from massive infection by intestinal or respiratory tract normal flora. The B-cell function is also reduced, pointing to the cooperative effect between the two basic systems. In the adult animal the loss of the thymus creates less severe reactions, probably because of an already functional, long-lived population of T cells.

The *lymph nodes* and *the spleen serve as the primary sites of localization of the immune response cells.* The lymph node serves to filter the lymph drained from a region of tissue. The structure of the lymph node (Fig. 16-9) consists of an inner medullary and paracortical region primarily populated with T cells and an outer cortex composed of clusters or germinal centers of B cells known as follicles. The spleen is structured on somewhat the same pattern, with diffusely packed T-cell areas and germinal centers of

tightly packed B cells. In certain types of antigenic stimulation, either the T-cell areas or the B-cell areas will show tissue proliferation, whereas the other area remains quiescent. By the same principle, if there is a basic primary immunodeficiency of one system, the corresponding area of lymph nodes and spleen may not be populated by the normal cells (hypoplastic).

During the course of the immune response reaction, within the lymph nodes there is significant proliferation of specific cells or migration of phagocytic cells to the site, which may lead to lymph node enlargement. Enlargement of the lymph nodes in a region may be the result of infection, immune disease, intrinsic neoplasm of the lymph node, or metastatic spread of malignant cells to the node. The presence of an enlarged spleen or enlarged lymph nodes is virtually always an important clinical finding.

Primary immune response
Antigenic challenge

When an antigen is introduced into the body, it can trigger a wide or narrow spectrum of response mechanisms. The specific pattern of response depends on the amount of antigen introduced, the site of introduction, and the type of antigen introduced.

Small amounts of a noninvasive, large, particulate antigen introduced at a single body site are quickly and efficiently handled at a local site with little or no systemic

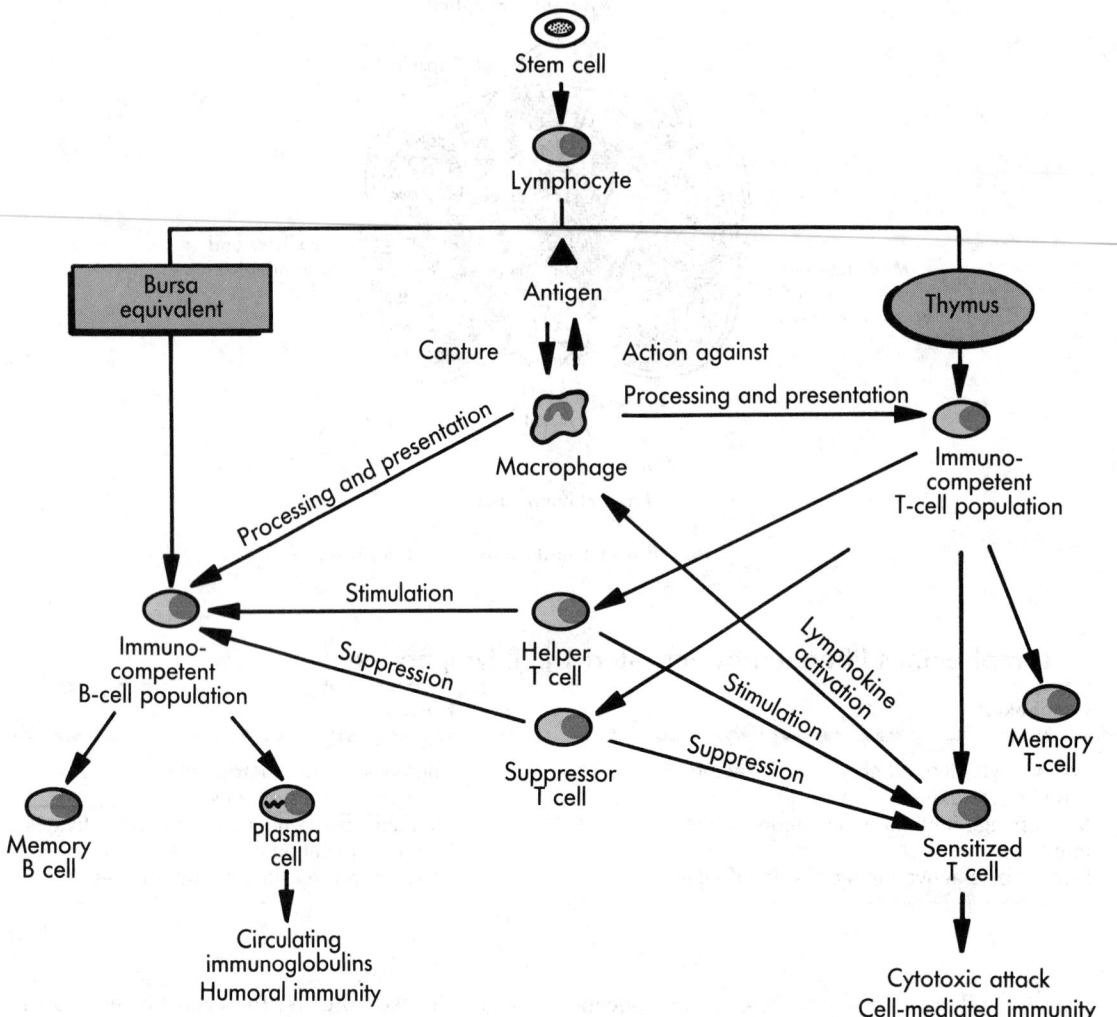

Fig. 16-10 Combined response of B and T cell systems.

involvement beyond the local lymph node. Because the inflammatory response and local lymph node can localize the spread of the antigen, the immune response may go completely unnoticed by the host organism. Larger, particulate antigens are readily cleared, but small, soluble antigens are more difficult to clear from the circulation.

Large amounts of an antigen may allow the antigen to escape from the local site by simply overwhelming the local defense mechanisms. Even though the lymph nodes and reticuloendothelial organs can clear 80% to 90% of an antigen on a single pass, if the amount of the antigen is extremely large, some antigen may escape the local site.

Highly invasive antigens (for example, bacteria such as Staphylococcus aureus or Streptococcus pyogenes) or those introduced directly into the bloodstream by blood transfusion, intravenous catheterization, or injection can immediately establish a systemic type of immune response. This is why extreme care must be exercised in the use of any type of medical procedure that could allow the introduction of organisms into the general circulation. The localization action of the immune response is critical to efficient functioning of the response.

Humoral response

When the antigen is introduced for the first time, one of three basic mechanisms of response will be elicited: (1) a response mediated primarily by B cells, (2) the humoral response; a response in which the T cells are primarily involved, the cell-mediated response; or (3) a combined type of response.

If the antigen is of the type that triggers a humoral response, the first time the body is exposed to the antigen the B cell system responds with the synthesis of circulating immunoglobulins (Fig. 16-10). The encroaching antigen is phagocytosed by a lymph node macrophage or tissue-active macrophage. The macrophage processes the antigen and presents the antigenic stimulus to a B cell that has been preprogrammed to respond to the introduced antigen. These antigen-specific B cells bear receptors on their surface, which allow them to recognize their antigenic stimulant. Only a few lymphocytes within a lymph node have the ability to respond to the antigen. The stimulated B cell then begins a process of proliferation (increase in number) and differentiation (change in structure and function). The progeny of the stimulated cell increase in number within the lymph node, forming *clones* of *specifically adapted lymphocytes*. With each generation of new cells within the clone, the lymphocytes become more differentiated toward a cell population ideally suited for the synthesis and release of immunoglobulin. These cells are known as *plasma cells*. With the development of this cell population in the lymph node (several days after the introduction of the antigen), antibodies can be detected in the lymph node. However, *it is not until about 1 to 2 weeks after the antigenic challenge that detectable levels of specific antibodies appear in the serum.* The plasma cell population of the lymph node and the levels of antibody in the blood continue to increase for another 2 to 3 weeks, and then both begin to retreat.

Two types of immunoglobulins are produced and released into the circulation, immunoglobulin M (IgM) and immunoglobulin G (IgG). *Immunoglobulin M (IgM or macroglobulin) is especially effective at attaching to particulate antigens such as bacterial cells and, with the activation of the complement system in the serum, causes the lysis of those cells.* Because IgM antibodies are so large, they cannot leave the blood vessels, so they are restricted to a role in the bloodstream.

Immunoglobulin G (IgG) makes up about 85% of the antibodies found in the serum. This immunoglobulin is smaller and can move from the blood and lymph into virtually all body fluids and can also cross the placenta from maternal circulation into fetal circulation. This class of immunoglobulin provides most of our protection against bacterial, viral, and toxic agents in the body. Usually when the term *antibody* is used, this is the type of immunoglobulin that is meant.

Some of the lymphocytes of the activated clone may become "memory cells," which are much more responsive, both in time of reaction and efficiency of antibody synthesis, to subsequent contact with the antigen.

The humoral response serves to protect the body from such agents as microbial toxins, bacteria within the extravascular spaces in the blood and on mucosal surfaces, and viruses that must pass through the circulatory system to reach their site of infection (for example, poliomyelitis virus).

Cell-mediated response

Certain antigens trigger a response mediated by T-cell proliferation and reaction. A T cell that has received its antigenic stimulus is referred to as a sensitized T cell lymphocyte (Fig. 16-10).

The initial steps of the cell-mediated response, those involving the antigen processing by the macrophage, seem to be the same as in the humoral response. Following presentation of the antigenic stimulus of lymph node T cells, there is proliferation in the T-cell domain. Circulatory *antibodies are not released; rather, activated lymphocytes are released into the circulation. These cells migrate to the site of the entrance of the antigen into the body, where the invading agent or residual antigen is found.* These activated lymphocytes, along with macrophages, *infiltrate the regions of the tissue* and *begin a direct attack* on the *antigen or tissue cells labeled with the antigen.* The T cells participating in this direct attack are known as *cytotoxic T cells.*

To amplify the site reaction further, the sensitized lymphocytes activate the nonspecific phagocytotic cells (mac-

rophages, PMNs, and noncommitted lymphocytes) in the region of the antigen. This is accomplished through the release of the soluble lymphokines (see Table 16-7), which recruit additional cells to attack the antigenic materials.

The cell-mediated response is especially effective in protection against diseases that grow and do their damage intracellularly where the circulating immunoglobulins cannot reach them. Diseases of this type include viral and rickettsial diseases and those produced by certain chronic types of infective agents, fungal pathogens and tubercle bacillus being the most outstanding examples. One other important function of this system is the provision of *cancer cell surveillance.*

Combined immune response

Most antigens do not cause a purely humoral or purely cell-mediated response; rather, both types of response are evoked. Likewise, our protection against most harmful antigens is the result of both of these specific response systems being brought to bear on the antigen involved. In the *combined type of response., an initial perturbation occurs within the T-cell areas of the lymph node.* This becomes obvious within about 2 days after the introduction of the antigen. About 3 to 5 days later, the B cell areas begin to proliferate.

To mount a maximal immune response, the cooperative action of the three central cell types is necessary. The macrophage serves to capture, process, and present the antigen to immunocompetent cells of both T- and B-cell ancestry. The T cells aid in the direct cell-mediated response, but a population of T cells also serves to interact with the B cell and a T-cell population controls the development of an effective immune response. A *helper T-cell* population cooperates with the B cells and T cells to enhance the activation and proliferation of the immunoglobulin synthesizing cells. The existence of the helper T cell explains the observation noted earlier in this chapter that the removal of the thymus from the neonate not only compromises the cell-mediated immune response but also significantly reduces the host's ability to mount a humoral immune response. T helper cells also mediate the normal expression of the cell-mediated immune response; therefore, the reduction or loss of this population of cells as occurs in acquired immunodeficiency syndrome (AIDS) would lead to progressive loss of immune response protection.

Another group of T cells also exerts an effect on the synthesis of circulating antibodies. *Cells known as suppressor T cells may provide a negative control function over B-cell clones and other T-cell clones, preventing the expression of an immunologic response.*

Secondary immune response

As emphasized at the outset of this section, one of the touchstone characteristics of the specific response system is the ability of the system to remember prior contact with an antigen and to provide a more rapid and efficient protective reaction on subsequent contact. The *first contact between the immune response system and an antigen leads to the primary response, the events of which have been laid out in the preceding paragraphs.* When antibody synthesis is measured in a primary response, there is a significant lag time

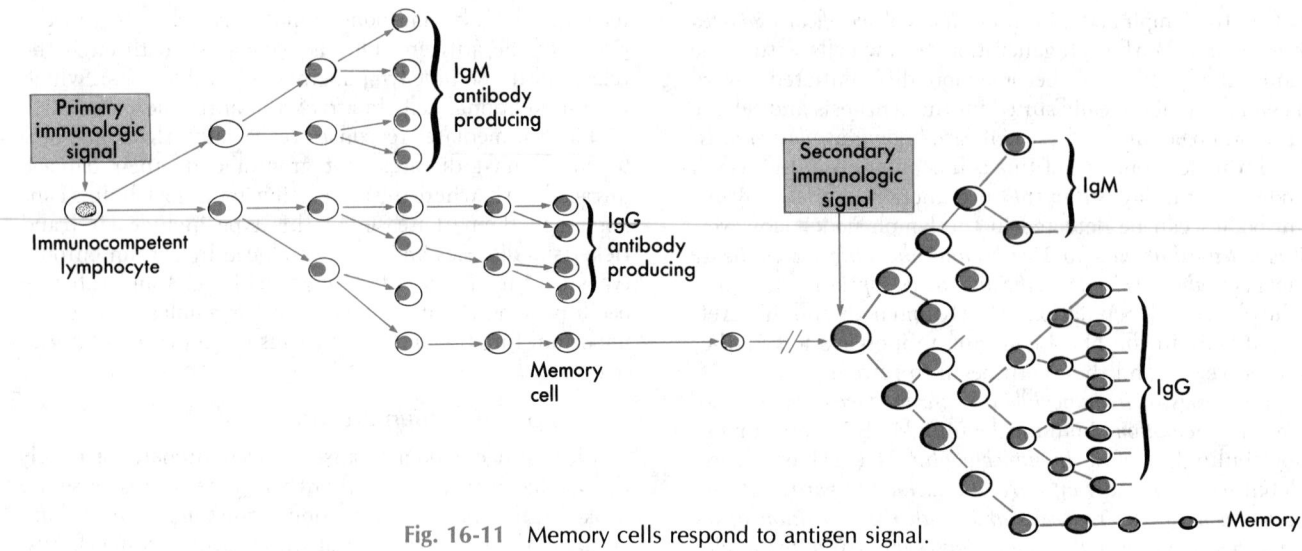

Fig. 16-11 Memory cells respond to antigen signal.

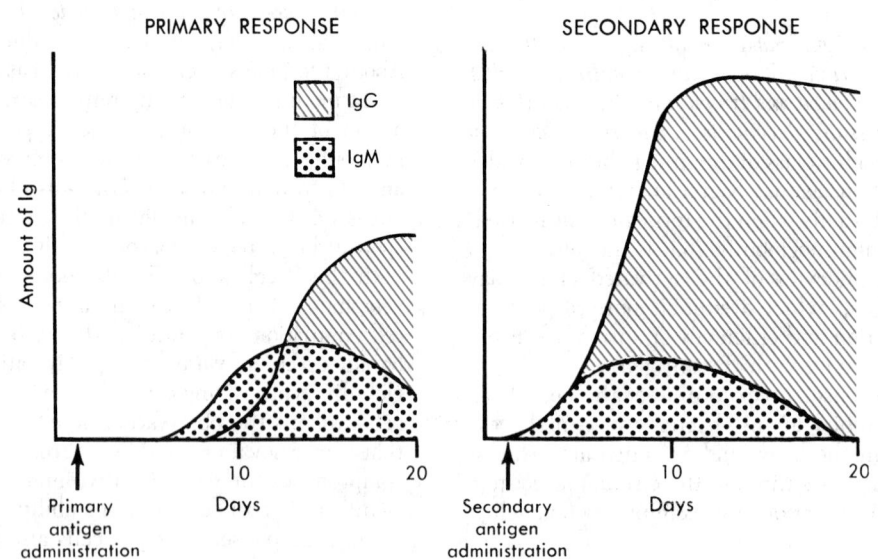

Fig. 16-12 Primary and secondary humoral responses.

to the appearance of antibodies in the circulation (Figs. 16-11 and 16-12). Immunoglobulins of the IgM class are the first to appear, but they maintain protective levels for only a short period. Specific IgG antibodies follow and reach protective levels within 12 to 14 days, but they too fall off fairly quickly with only this initial exposure.

When the "primed" immune response system encounters the antigen again, a *secondary response* ensues, which is more rapid, of greater intensity, and longer lasting than the primary response. This secondary response is also termed an *anamnestic response*. This "remembered" response is a characteristic of both the B- and T-cell systems. The prior contact with the antigen is stored in special memory cells of both cell lines. As illustrated in Fig. 16-11, the memory cells response immediately to the antigenic signal, so that the lag time between exposure to the antigen

and production of protective antibody levels is greatly reduced. This phenomenon provides the basis for active immunization and "booster" doses to maintain the protective levels of immunity. In an immunized individual the memory cells elicit the rapid response in time for the immune system to overwhelm the pathogen or toxin before it can produce its damage. These memory cells are very long-living lymphocytes that are able to respond for years following their development.

Developmental Aspects of the Immune Response

Lymphoid cells first appear in the fetus as stem cells in the fetal liver at about the end of the first trimester. The lymphoid tissues of the thymus also develop fairly early in the fetus. At birth, however, the lymph nodes and spleen are still underdeveloped, but T- and B-cell responsiveness

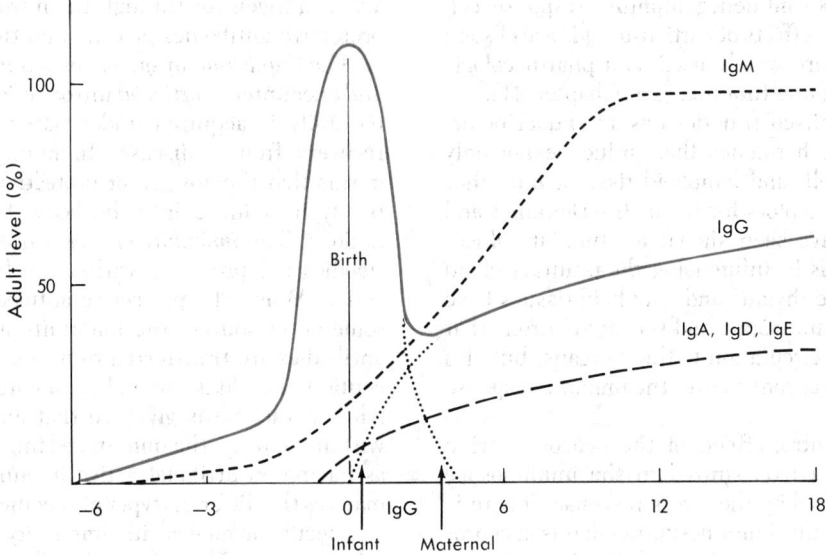

Fig. 16-13 Immunoglobulin levels in fetus and neonate.

is fully functional. The fetus is capable of some immune response if challenged by an in utero (within the uterus) infection, such as in the case of congenital syphilis or rubella. Unless the fetus has been exposed to a congenital infection, at birth the neonate-synthesized immunoglobulin levels are low (Fig. 16-13). The child does have high levels of transplacentally acquired maternal IgG antibodies. These maternal antibodies have a half-life of about 30 days in the child, and this coupled with the increase in blood volume in the growing infant leads to a drop in the IgG levels of the blood over the first 3 months. Thereafter the rate of the child's own synthesis of IgG provides for a steady increase in the immunoglobulin concentration within the serum. IgM levels reach adult concentrations by about the age of 9 months.

Numerous studies in both animals and humans have shown that during the aging process there is a progressive loss of immunologic vigor. *The prime immunologic age probably is achieved during the late teens, when virtually the full complement of immunities has been developed and the responsiveness of the system peaks.* The middle years are characterized by a plateau and slowly falling curve until the later years of life, when a sharp decline in both the cell-mediated and humoral response systems becomes evident. This *loss in immunologic sensitivity is associated with an increasingly less effective and more misdirected immune response.* There is an *increasing frequency of autoimmune disease, susceptibility to pathogenic and opportunistic microorganisms, and incidence of cancer.*

Development of Immune Tolerance

Immune tolerance is defined as the state of immunologic nonresponsiveness. By some mechanisms the body becomes tolerant to self while maintaining responsiveness to foreign materials. Evidence establishes that self-tolerance is acquired during embryonic development; however, the exact mechanisms by which it develops remain an issue. During fetal devel-

opment the immune system is presented with antigens from the developing tissues; these become identified as self-antigens, so that when exposed to these antigens postnatally the individual is tolerant of them.

One proposed mechanism by which this state could be induced is known as the *clonal selection theory.* This theory states that when potentially responsive clones of B or T cells come into contact with an antigen prenatally, the responsive cell line is killed, thus eliminating the responsiveness of that antigen from the body. This produces a state of *natural tolerance.* This theory is supported by experimental data that show that by exposing experimental animals to foreign antigens in utero a tolerance to that antigen is developed; however, some antigens introduced in this manner are found to be more *tolerogenic* (capable of inducing tolerance) than others. Further, the clonal selection theory does not explain how it is possible to break tolerance in adults, as indicated in certain experimental studies or as in the case of certain of the autoimmune diseases (see Chapter 41). In many cases tolerance is not the result of the total elimination of specifically reactive cells but of the blocking of expression or temporary inactivation of the responsive cells. The action of suppressor T cells or the failure of mobilization by helper T cells plays a significant role in maintaining the state of self-tolerance.

Neuroendocrine Factors Influencing Immune Response

The cells of the immune response system are influenced by and in turn influence the other regulatory communications in the body, that is, *the endocrine system* and *the neural system.* Immune response cells have receptors on their surface to receive modifying inputs from hormones. Glucocorticosteroids, testosterone, estrogen, and progesterone have been shown to depress immune function. Insulin, growth hormone, and thyroxine tend to improve immune function. Neurotransmitters and other hormones found in lower doses in the body also influence immune response cell function. The negative effects of corticosteroids are of such magnitude that they are widely used as a pharmacologic agent to suppress immune function (see Chapter 41).

The thymus gland itself functions as an endocrine organ, releasing thymic hormones that influence not only immune-responsive cells and lymphoid tissues, but other body cells that have receptors for them. Interleukin-1 and other lymphokines have been shown to stimulate glucocorticosteroid synthesis by influencing the pituitary gland to release ACTH. The thymus and lymphoid tissues have direct innervation by autonomic and sensory neurons that control not only blood circulation to these organs, but also seem to have more direct control over the immune response cells themselves.

The physiologic control effects of the neuroendocrine function have long been recognized in the immunosuppressive effects produced by the stress response. There is growing evidence that this immunosuppression is also produced indirectly through neural signals to the immunoresponsive tissues.

These *interconnections between the three major communication systems of the body have led to the concept that* although many aspects of each system can be considered to stand alone, *from a broader, more holistic perspective they can be seen as functioning as an interrelated complex.* The term *psychoimmunoendocrine system* has been developed to reflect this more inclusive concept. Psychotherapeutic methods and cognitive visualization has been increasingly used as adjunctive therapy in immune-related disease and cancer. However, because most of the connections between these systems are fairly indirect and because our understanding of the control functions of each is still uncertain, these therapies should never be relied on as a primary therapeutic approach. In fact, there is some potential danger in leading patients to believe that they can exercise direct cognitive control over their pathologic condition. When they are not successful, they become disillusioned and hopeless, which then removes whatever positive aspects might be derived. The emphasis should be on the indirect and broad improvement of their general immune state.

APPLICATIONS AND IMPLICATIONS OF IMMUNE RESPONSE

Concept of Immunity

The *objective of the biologic defense mechanisms is to provide the host with protection.* The ultimate protection would be total resistance to encroachment or damage by an organism or agent; this is usually termed *absolute immunity. Absence* of such *protective barriers* is called *susceptibility.* Although generally applied to immunity from infectious organisms, these terms can be used to describe the relative susceptibility to encroachment by any external agent. *Nonspecific immunity* (or *innate immunity*) is provided when the external and internal nonspecific defense mechanisms serve as the barrier excluding or destroying the invading agent. *Specific immunity* protects against a single unique agent through the development of specific antibodies or responsive cells in the body. It is *acquired* from prior contact with that

agent (antigen) or through the introduction of specifically protective antibodies or cells into the body.

The *acquisition of specific immunity* may result from *natural* encounter or *artificial* introduction. Immunity acquired naturally is acquired under natural conditions, such as recovery from a disease. Immunity acquired artificially means that the antigen or protective antibodies were purposely introduced into the body (for example, by vaccination). The *immunity may be active or passive.* When antibodies are produced within the body, the immunity is active. When the protective antibodies are received from some other source, the immunity is passive. Thus when antibodies are transferred from the mother across the placenta, the child is said to have a natural passive immunity; when a vaccine is given so that antibodies are produced within the body, the immunized individual is characterized as having an artificial active immunity. Table 16-8 summarizes the different types of specific acquired immunities.

Specific or nonspecific immunity to harmful agents is a relative state. The effects of different dosages of an infectious organism or the toxic products of such organisms in experimental studies clearly demonstrate that administration of sufficiently large numbers of an organism or high dosages of a toxin can overwhelm even the most highly immunized animal. Further, when the normal mechanisms of defense are breached, even in the highly resistant host, disease can result. Thus acquired immunity to infection is not always an absolute condition but depends on a large number of complex variables. These include not only the defense mechanisms and physical state (such as oxygenation, nutrition, or metabolic state) of the host, but also the dosage, route of contact, and virulence of the harmful agent.

Immunization

Long before the mechanisms of immune response were worked out, it was recognized that recovery from certain diseases conferred protection against subsequent exposure. From the days of Jenner's vaccination with cowpox exudate to protect against smallpox (1798), through the success of Pasteur with anthrax and rabies (1880s), to the present, the specific protective mechanisms of the immune system have been used against serious infectious diseases.

Passive immunization

Temporary protection, usually measured in days or at most weeks, is afforded by the acquisition of preformed antibody from another host. As the acquired antibodies are used up through binding with antigen or by being catabolized, the protection is lost.

Transplacental passive immunization occurs through the transfer of IgG antibodies from the maternal circulation across the placenta to the fetal blood. Some immunoglobulins are acquired through the colostrum of the mother's milk. There is a common misconception that infants acquire large amounts of circulating antibodies from breast milk that are added to their circulating antibodies. Most of the protective immunoglobulins that are passed in maternal milk are of the IgA class and serve to offer some degree of protection to the gastrointestinal tract of the infant. An

Table 16-8   Types of acquired specific immunity

Type of immunity	Acquisition of immunity	Development	Duration	Protection	Example
Active Antibodies synthesized by body in response to antigenic stimulation	*Natural* Natural contact with antigen through clinical or subclinical case	Develops slowly; protective levels reached in a few weeks	Long term; often lifetime	Specific to antigen contacted	Recovery from childhood diseases (for example, chickenpox, measles, mumps)
	Artificial Immunization with antigen	Develops slowly; protective levels reached in a few weeks	Several years; extended protection with "booster" doses	Specific to antigen immunized against	Immunization with live or killed vaccines; toxoid immunization
Passive Antibodies produced in one host (can be human or animal) are transferred to another	*Natural* Transplacental and colostral transfer from mother to child	Immediate	Temporary, up to several months	All antigens to which mother has immunity	Maternal immunoglobulins in neonate
	Artificial Injection of serum from immune human or animal	Immediate	Temporary, up to several weeks	All antigens to which source has immunity	Injection of pooled human gamma globulin; injection of animal hyperimmune sera

timicrobial factors other than immunoglobulins are also present in the milk and probably account for most cases of decreased incidence of infections observed in breast-fed versus bottle-fed infants.

Artificial passive immunization may be necessary if the individual to be immunized has suffered exposure to a serious infectious agent to which he or she has no immunity or if the individual's own immune system is impaired or deficient. The sources of these preformed antibodies are pooled human adult gamma globulin or heterologous (from another species) globulin fractions. *Pooled human gamma globulin has been used to modify the effects of measles,* particularly in premature infants, in children with primary immunodeficiencies, and in patients undergoing immunosuppressive therapies. Persons who have contact with persons with hepatitis and smallpox may also be protected by this method. It should be noted, however, that isolated *gamma globulin preparations* tend to form small protein aggregates, and these, *if injected intravenously, could lead to severe anaphylactic reactions. For this reason the material is always administered intramuscularly.*

The most commonly used heterologous antibody fractions are antitetanus and antidiphtheria antisera derived from horse globulins. Because these are foreign proteins, they can lead to the development of serum sickness (Chapter 41). Serum sickness is more likely to occur in individuals already primed by previous contact with horse globulin; thus multiple use of heterologous sera is to be avoided.

Active immunization

The *objective of active immunization* is to *provide effective long-term immunity by establishing within the individual's body* the capacity to produce effective levels of immune response and to establish a population of sensitive cells that can respond to a subsequent antigenic contact.

Immunizing agents ideally should be noninjurious to the individual being immunized. To accomplish this, the pathogenic effects must be modified while at the same time maintaining the antigenicity of the agent. Bacteria exotoxins such as those produced by the diphtheria and tetanus bacteria can be successfully detoxified by formaldehyde treatment without destroying the major antigenic determinants on the protein molecule. Such detoxified antigenic materials are called *toxoids.* The use of *killed vaccines of viruses and bacteria* can also *provide a safe antigen for immunization.* Killed vaccines include those for pertussis (whooping cough), typhoid, and cholera, and the Salk poliomyelitis vaccine. The protection conferred by these vaccines is generally inferior to that produced by live vaccines. A number of the most successful vaccines consist of living organisms that have been modified so that they are nonvirulent. The *attenuated live vaccines provide excellent protection, but* there is *some risk in their use* because of the slight risk of reversion to the virulent form of the organism or the possibility that the individual being immunized has some degree of immunodeficiency, in which case the attenuated organism might produce pathologic effects. Live vaccines that are of importance include those for measles, mumps, and tuberculosis (BCG), and the Sabin poliomyelitis vaccine.

The provision of protective levels of residual immunity depends on the inducement of the right type of response (that is, cell-mediated or humoral), in sufficient amounts, at the right place (that is, where the immune response can contact the antigen), and against the right antigenic determinants (that is, the antibodies formed produce an inactivating effect). Simply inducing an immune response is not sufficient to provide protection. For example, the early killed virus measles vaccines elicited a splendid production of circulating antibodies against the measles virus, but protection against measles is most effectively mediated by cellular immune responses. The humoral protection did not prevent infection.

Another problem of immunization for which provision must be made is the *interference that one antigen may have with another if the two are given simultaneously.* The live virus vaccines occasionally interfere with each other; they each interfere with the development of immunity by the other. This is probably the result of interferon production. Some live virus vaccines contain more than one strain of the virus, and these can cross-inhibit. In the case of the Sabin oral polio vaccine, three separate doses are required because there are three strains within the same vaccine. With the initial dose, immunity to only one strain may develop if the strain interferes with the other two.

Complications of immunization

Although *immunization is the most successful approach to the control of many infectious diseases, there are small but still real risks involved.* The development of postvaccination encephalitis or other neural autoimmune complications is a serious risk with vaccines such as those for smallpox or rabies. Children with immunodeficiencies may be overwhelmed by vaccination with live vaccine. With viral vaccines, which are produced in monkey kidney of human cell culture, there is a slight risk of the introduction of oncogenic (cancer-causing) viruses. A fetus may be significantly at risk if the mother receives a live virus vaccine during pregnancy. Vaccines such as live influenza should never be administered to a pregnant woman. It is still unclear whether the rubella virus harms the fetus, so it too should be avoided. Besides these rather serious risks, general discomfort is to be expected from some forms of immunization. The typhoid vaccine, for instance, is composed of large numbers of killed salmonella bacteria; because the endotoxic cell wall materials of these cells is a pyrogenic (fever-producing) substance, fever and malaise are not uncommon sequelae. The influenza vaccines often produce febrile reactions in children.

Cancer Immunology

One of the functions of the cell-mediated immune response system is the recognition and destruction of cancer cells within the body. It is postulated that, by the same mechanisms that are operative in an allograft rejection, the immune system continually protects against the establishment of certain types of tumor growths. The recognition of these cells as nonself is based on the appearance of "new" surface antigens that allow identification. A growing body of evidence supports the view that this is a vital function of the immune system. *Patients in whom the cellular immune system is impaired (immunosuppressed) or defective (immunodeficient) for significant periods are at especially high risk of certain neoplastic diseases.* To these data is coupled the observation that cancers are most prone to appear early in life before

the immune system is fully functional or in later life as the system becomes less effective.

Cancers may become established in the body by escaping the surveillance mechanisms or by growing so rapidly that they outdistance the immune system's ability to respond. Experimentally, if a few thousand tumor cells are transferred from a cancerous animal to a noncancerous animal, the latter is capable of responding and destroying the tumor; however, if the tumor cell load is increased to several billion cells, the tumor may become established. The humoral immune system may actually serve to protect the developing cancer by producing noncytotoxic antibodies *(enhancing antibodies)* that coat the tumor cell surfaces and mask the surface from recognition by sensitized lymphocytes. As a tumor grows, it is capable of both specific and nonspecific suppression of the immune system. This further reduces the effectiveness of a response.

Some of the new surface antigens, (known as *tumor-specific transplantation antigens* [TSTA]) *appearing on the cancerous cell are shed into the circulation and can be immunologically detected there.* Some of these antigens, such as carcinoembryonic antigen (CEA) and alpha feto-protein (α-FP), are present during fetal development but are not expressed in the adult. Their reappearance lends support to the theory that cancer represents a dedifferentiation to a more primitive cell caused by the introduction of oncogenes (Chapter 11). These antigens, termed *oncofetal antigens* (OFA), are of some significance in early detection, diagnostic confirmation, and determination of malignant disease progress.

Some very early progress has been made in stimulating, both specifically and nonspecifically, the body's immunologic response to cancers in the hope of preventing further growth of the tumors. With further knowledge of both the cancer process and the immune response mechanisms, the possibility of using immunotherapy, immunoprophylaxis, and immunodiagnosis as specific tools against malignancies seems quite realistic.

Immunologic Disorders

As expected in such an interrelated, complex system as is operative in the mechanisms providing biologic defense, there are *innumerable points at which the system may malfunction.* The immunologic disorders that have been characterized may result from the following:

1. Nonresponsiveness
2. Blocked responsiveness
3. Limited responsiveness
4. Misdirected responsiveness
5. Overresponsiveness

The underlying causes of the disorders may be attributed to developmental defect, infection, malignancy, trauma, metabolic state, or pharmacologic intervention. The severity of the disorders ranges from creation of a minor nuisance (for example, mild hayfever) to a life-threatening situation (for example, anaphylactic shock). The disorders may be classified into the following general categories:

1. *Immunodeficiencies:* deficiencies in the proper expression of the immune response system, parts of the system, or individual cell types within the system

2. *Gammopathies:* abnormal production of immunoglobulins
3. *Hypersensitivities:* exaggerated or inappropriate response to specific antigens
4. *Autoimmunities:* immunologic attack on self-antigens

Each of these immunologic disorders is discussed in Chapter 41.

Monoclonal Antibodies

A recent technologic breakthrough in tissue culture technique has made it possible to develop and isolate antibodies of great specificity for single antigenic determinants. Normally immunoglobulins that are produced in the body in response to antigenic challenge bind to various antigenic determinants introduced on the multivalent antigen. The antibodies themselves are produced by a variety of B cells responding to the antigen signal; thus 90% of the antibodies produced have little or no affinity for specific antigenic determinants. A single, highly specific antibody, large quantities of highly antigen-specific antibodies can be isolated by a technique for the production of immortal clones of *hybridoma* cells (made by the fusion of normal antibody-producing B cells with an appropriate B-cell tumor line) and selection of single clones of cells. These immunoglobulins are known as *monoclonal antibodies.*

The clinical and diagnostic implications for the use of monoclonal antibodies are enormous. It is now possible to identify individual cell types (such as T_H versus T_S lymphocytes, partially differentiated versus mature cells) with very specific cell markers, to diagnose malignant transformed cells, or to type tissue using monoclonal antibodies

for each HLA subtype. Therapeutically, it is possible to bind a toxic molecule or radioactive isotope to the monoclonal antibody and have it delivered specifically to a tumor cell bearing a specific tumor-cell marker, thus sparing all nontumor cells of the body. Monoclonal antibodies will dramatically alter our ability to identify, characterize, and treat many of the most significant pathologies.

Tissue Transplants

The transfer of healthy tissues and organs from one individual to replace damaged or diseased tissues in another has been surgically possible for many years. Early attempts failed because of the rejection of the foreign cells and tissues by the body. With the growing knowledge of the immune response, the mechanisms of this rejection process become more apparent, and it is now possible to make judgments and predictions concerning the likelihood of success of transplantation. It has become possible to control the course of the graft transfer process to favor the acceptance of the transplanted tissue.

The antigenic determinants of the tissues that lead to graft rejection are primarily found on the surface of the cells within the transplanted tissues. These antigens are known as *histocompatibility antigens* and are controlled by independently segregating genes within the chromosomal structure of the animal. They are also called *human leukocyte antigens (HLA).* Some of the histocompatibility antigens are more antigenic than are others; thus some antigens are referred to as *major* and others as *minor.* The major transplantation antigens are those of the ABO and Rh blood groups and the HLA antigens (Chapter 41).

Table 16-9   Effect of selected drugs on the immune system

Drug	Immune system impairment	Indications for immunosuppressive therapy
Corticosteroids	Impairment of T cell function Catabolism of immunoglobulins (decreased IgG) Lymphocytopenia Type 1 hypersensitivity: vasoconstriction, eosinopenia Type 3 hypersensitivity: decreased vascular permeability Type 4 hypersensitivity: decreased macrophage function	Diseases where immune disorder is unknown Tissue and organ transplantation Autoimmune diseases
Antimetabolites (azathioprine)	Interference with RNA, DNA, and protein synthesis Depression of bone marrow and antibody reproduction Decreased primary immune response	Autoimmune diseases Tissue transplantation Dermatologic diseases (pemphigus, psoriasis) Neoplasia
Alkylating agents (cyclophosphamide)	Interference with DNA, RNA, and protein synthesis Lymphocytolytic effect Suppression of primary immune response	Autoimmune diseases Tissue transplantation Inflammatory disease of unknown cause
Antilymphocytic serum (ALS, ALG)	Inhibition of lymphocyte stimulation by specific antigens Inhibition of lymphocyte mobility Agglutination and lysis of lymphocytes in the presence of complement	Renal transplantation Bone marrow transplantation Autoimmune diseases
Antibiotics (actinomycin D, chloramphenicol, tetracycline, cyclosporine)	Interference with DNA-directed RNA synthesis Suppression of primary immune response Inhibition of protein synthesis	None, except for cyclosporine (tissue transplantation)

Graft rejection can be minimized by the use of chemical (drug) or physical (radiation) agents that nonspecifically or specifically interfere with the development of an immune response reaction against the foreign tissue. Clinically, four types of chemical immunosuppressive agents are effective in providing the transitional protection needed to promote the graft establishment (Table 16-9).

Glucocorticoids, especially prednisone, are significantly antiinflammatory and impair lymphocyte (B- and T-cell) activation and function. Prednisone exerts a wide spectrum of activity against all immune response and inflammatory response mechanisms. Although it suppresses the cell-mediated system to a greater degree than the humoral system, the continued high dosage needed to maintain cell-mediated suppression creates significant risks because it reduces the responsiveness of the humoral system.

Antimetabolites and alkylating agents, such as azathioprine and cyclophosphamide, act nonspecifically against rapidly dividing cells within the body, and for this reason they are used for cancer chemotherapy. They interfere with DNA synthesis and with the B- and T-cell systems.

A more specific immunosuppression of the T-cell system is achieved with the use of *antilymphocytic serum* (ALS). ALS blocks the action of the sensitized cells in circulation while leaving the lymph node B-cell system only slightly suppressed. This leaves the host with protection against the humorally protected infectious agents while providing protection against the most active rejection system.

Cyclosporine is an antibiotic derived from fungi that exerts its action on the T lymphocytes. This drug has greatly improved the prognosis after transplantation (see Chapter 42).

SUMMARY

1. The concept of "self" refers to the collection of tissues, cells, and molecules that is unique to each human being. Every other individual, cell, or biologic product is therefore considered as "nonself." The body has mechanisms to recognize and protect against encroachment by nonself agents.

2. Biologic defense mechanisms may be structural (skin and mucous membranes), chemical (pH, blood proteins), cellular (WBC, phagocytes), special proteins (interferon, immunoglobulins), or tissue (lymph nodes, thymus gland). These mechanisms may be external or internal and specific or nonspecific.

3. External nonspecific biologic defense mechanisms include the skin and mucous membranes (first line of defense), nasal hairs, tears, peristalsis, antimicrobial chemicals (acidity, lysozyme), and the microbial antagonism of normal skin flora.

4. Internal nonspecific defense mechanisms are carried out by the phagocytes in the reticuloendothelial system and the blood, other blood components, interferon, and the inflammatory response.

5. Interferons enhance synthesis in uninfected cells of a protein that inhibits entry of any viral particles into the interferon-protected cell for about 24 hours.

6. The inflammatory response consists of an immediate vascular dilation to facilitate margination of leukocytes on the vessel walls before exudation. This is followed by exudation first of fluid to the injured area, then of phagocytes to remove and digest foreign substances.

7. The five cardinal symptoms of inflammation and their causes are redness and heat (vascular dilation), edema (fluid exudate), pain (pressure of the fluid exudate on nerve endings and chemical irritation of the nerve endings), and loss of function (swelling and pain).

8. Infection is contained by fibroblasts walling off the affected area: interference with this process may lead to spread of the infection.

9. The immune response is a biologic defense mechanism consisting of specific responses to specific antigens.

10. Antigens are substances that elicit the formation of antibodies when introduced into the body; there are five different types of immunoglobulins (antibodies), each with different structures and functions.

11. The two types of cells involved in the immune response are T cells that attack foreign material directly in the body (cell-mediated immunity) and B cells that produce immunoglobulins (humoral immunity). T helper cells enhance immunoglobulin synthesis and T-cell cytotoxic activity, whereas T suppressor cells inhibit these actions.

12. Lymphokines are soluble substances released by activated T cells; their functions include attracting and activating macrophages for phagocytosis, nonspecific lysis of cells, inhibiting replication of viruses (interferons), and activating nonsensitized lymphocytes (interleukins).

13. Three basic mechanisms of response may be elicited when an antigen is first introduced (primary immune response): humoral response (primarily B cells), cell-mediated response (primarily T cells), or combined B-cell—T-cell immune response.

14. An important characteristic of the specific response system is the ability of the system to remember prior contact with an antigen (during the primary immune response) and to provide a more complete protective reaction on subsequent contact (secondary immune response). The secondary response is more rapid, of greater intensity, and longer lasting than the primary response.

15. Immunity, or nonsusceptibility to specific antigens, may be natural or acquired artificially through immunization. Passive immunization is the receipt of antibodies either transplacentally (infant) or by injection (gamma globulin and antitetanus or antidiphtheria antisera). With active immunization, persons develop their own antibodies from injection of killed vaccines or toxoids. Passive immunization provides temporary protection, whereas active immunization provides long-term immunity.

16. Persons who are immunosuppressed or immunodeficient are at a higher risk for certain neoplastic diseases because the body does not recognize cancer cells as nonself. Tumors may also suppress specific and nonspecific immune responses, thus reducing effectiveness of the responses.

17. The body recognizes tissue transplants as foreign (nonself) and evokes the immune response to destroy the

new tissue; graft rejection can be minimized by suppression of the immune response with drugs or radiation.

STUDY QUESTIONS

- What would happen if the immune response system did not properly distinguish "self" cells and inappropriately labeled them as "nonself"?
- We have come to regard fever and leukocytosis as negative pathologic responses that call for intervention, such as antipyretic therapy. Why may this be inappropriate?
- Upon observing a finger wound, you note that there is pus in the wound and that the surrounding tissue is reddened, warm, and puffy. The person complains of pain and difficulty in moving the finger. How do these findings relate to the inflammatory process?
- What are the differences between B cells and T cells in terms of origin and function? How do they relate to each other?

REFERENCES AND SELECTED READINGS

1.* Ada GL, Nossal G: The clonal selection theory, *Sci Am* 257:52-69, 1987.
2. Alt FW et al: Development of primary antibody repertoire, *Science* 238:1079-1087, 1987.
3. Barrett JT: *Textbook of immunology,* ed 5, St Louis, 1987, Mosby–Yearbook.
4. Bartlett J: Current and future treatment of HIV infection, *Oncology* 4:19-26, 1990.
5. Berkelman RL, Curran JW: Epidemiology of HIV infection and AIDS, *Epidemiol Rev* 11:222-226, 1989.
6.* Besedovsky HO, DelRay AE, Sorkin E: What do the immune system and brain know about each other? *Immunology Today* 4:342-437, 1986.
7.* Cassileth B: Mind over body, *Cancer News* 6-20, Winter 1986.
8. Centers for Disease Control: Public Health Service statement of management of occupational exposure to HIV including consideration regarding AZT postexposure use, *MMWR* 39(suppl RR1):1-30, 1990.
9.* Cohen IR: The self, the world, and autoimmunity, *Sci Am* 258:52-60, 1988.
10.* Cohn ZA, editor: *Innate immunity: current opinion in immunology,* vol 1, London, 1988, Current Science Ltd.
11. Forrest BD: Women, HIV, and mucosal immunity, *Lancet* 337:835-840, 1991.
12. Graziano FM, Lemanske RF: *Clinical immunology,* Baltimore, 1989, Williams & Wilkins.

13.* Grey HM, Sette A, Baus S: How T cells see antigens, *Sci Am* 261:56-64, 1989.
14.* Griffin JP: Hematology and immunology: concepts for nursing, Norwalk, Conn, 1986, Appleton & Lange.
15.* Gurevich I: The competent internal immune system, *Nurs Clin North Am* 20(1):151-161, 1985.
16.* Hall NR, Goldstein AL: Thinking well: the chemical links between emotions and health, *Ann NY Acad Sci* 34:40-45. 1986.
17. Hallerstein MK, et al: Current approach to the treatment of HIV-associated weight loss, *Semin Oncol* 17:17-28, 1990.
18.* Hood LE: Interferon: getting in the way of viruses and tumors, *Am J Nurs* 87:459-455, 1987.
19. Hooper C: Eavesdropping on rare "silent" HIV-1 infection, *J NIH Research* 3:71-75, 1991.
20. Horoszewkz JS, et al: Interferon: a review of its development and potential clinical applications, *Hosp Formul* 22:776-779, 1987.
21. Law SKA, Reid KBM: *Complement,* Oxford, 1988, IRL Press.
22.* Lydyard DM, editor: *Immune response: current opinion in immunology,* vol II, London, 1988, Current Science Ltd.
23. Male D: *Immunology: an illustrated outline,* St Louis, 1985, Mosby–Year Book.
24. Marrack P, Kappler J: The T-cell receptor, *Science* 238:1073-1078, 1987.
25. Porth CM: *Pathophysiology,* ed 3, Philadelphia, 1990, JB Lippincott.
26.* Rennie J: The body against itself, *Sci Am* 263(6):106-115, 1990.
27. Richmond DO: Selection of AZT resistance variance of HIV by therapy, *J NIH Research* 3:83-86, 1991.
28. Roitt I: Essential immunology, ed 6, London, 1988, Blackwell Scientific Publications.
29. Roitt I, Brostoff J, Male D: *Immunology,* ed 2, St Louis, 1989, Mosby–Year Book.
30.* Rosenberg SA: Adoptive immunotherapy for cancer, *Sci Am* 262(5):62-69, 1990.
31. Rosenberg ZF, Fauci AS: Activation of latent HIV infection, *J NIH Research* 2:41-44, 1990.
32.* Seeley RR, Stephens TD, Tate P: *Lymphatic system and immunity: anatomy and physiology,* St Louis, 1991, Mosby–Year Book.
33.* Smith KA: Interleukin-2, *Sci Am* 262(3):50-57, 1990.
34. Stites DP, Terr AT: *Basic and clinical immunology,* ed 7, Norwalk, Conn, 1990, Appleton & Lange.
35. Truitt RL, Gale RT, Bortin MM, editors: *Cellular immunotherapy of cancer,* New York, 1987, Alan R. Liss.
36. Underdown BJ, Schiff JM: Immunoglobulin A, *Annu Rev Immunol* 4:389-417, 1986.
37. Vitetta ES, et al: Redesigning nature's poisons to create antitumor reagents, *Science* 238:1098-1104, 1987.
38. Widman FK: *An introduction to clinical immunology,* Philadelphia, 1988, FA Davis.

*Recommended for student reading.

17

Infection Control

Grace A. Rotter
Dora Rice
Elizabeth Cameron Eckstein

After studying this chapter, the learner should be able to:

- Describe the chain of infection.
- Identify high-risk factors for infection.
- Describe white blood cell response to infection.
- Identify community approaches to infection control and describe immunization programs.
- Define nosocomial infections and measures of prevention and control (bacteremia, and urinary, wound, and respiratory infections).
- Compare category-specific isolation precautions and body substance isolation, including major components of each.

HISTORICAL PERSPECTIVE

Infection control became a recognized discipline in 1970, but the principles governing it had been in existence for some time. In the middle of the nineteenth century Semmelweiss, an obstetrician in Vienna, demonstrated the significance of hand washing in combating the transmission of infection. He showed that when medical students and physicians were required to wash their hands and rinse them in a chlorinated lime solution before a delivery, the incidence of puerperal fever decreased markedly. The idea that hand washing alone could prevent the spread of disease met with much opposition by his colleagues. Better acceptance came after Pasteur, Lister, and Koch developed the germ theory of disease and related asepsis to the prevention of the spread of disease. At about the same time, Nightingale made significant contributions to sanitation and isolation practices. From this evolved an era in which medical asepsis was practiced more by ritual than with the true understanding of the scientific principles on which it was based.

A turning point came during World War II when the sulfonamides and penicillin were first used successfully to treat infections. As new antibiotics were developed, a false sense of security developed about infection control. It soon became apparent, however, that antibiotics were not the sole answer to infection control. Organisms, once well controlled by antibiotics, demonstrated the ability to develop resistant strains. In the late 1950s and the 1960s outbreaks of penicillin-resistant *Staphylococcus aureus* infections were common, and gram-negative organisms such as *Pseudomonas,* which were previously considered nonpathogenic (incapable of producing disease), were suddenly implicated as the cause of infections acquired in the hospital. Along with the emergence of drug-resistant strains and newly recognized pathogens came an increase in the number of persons at risk for secondary infections. An increase in life expectancy, the use of immunosuppressive agents, and an increase in the use of invasive procedures to diagnose and treat disease all increased the risk of infection in certain persons.

The rise in the number of hospital infections made apparent the need to examine preventive and control measures, including a reemphasis on aseptic techniques. Since 1970 an international conference to address the problem of hospital-acquired infections has been held every 10 years in Atlanta. As a result, the Centers for Disease Control (CDC) in Atlanta set forth guidelines for prevention and control of infections in hospitals. The CDC is constantly updating and revising its recommendations based on epidemiologic studies and research findings. The American Hospital Association (AHA) and the Joint Commission on Accreditation of Health Care Organizations (JCAHO), a major private accrediting agency, looked at the ethical and economic issues concerning hospital-acquired (nosocomial) infections and established standards for programs in infection control. The purpose of these programs was to decrease morbidity and mortality of infections, as well as to reduce the cost of infections that could have been prevented. Consumer awareness of the problem also contributed to the attention given the issue of infection control.

In the early 1970s only 10% of U.S. hospitals had infection surveillance and control programs; by the end of the decade nearly all had them.

The field of infection control is a challenging one, with the identification of new pathogens (for example, human immunodeficiency virus or HIV) and advances in research uncovering new information that may change current thinking and practices. Infection control practitioners (ICPs) serve as a valuable resource because they interact with virtually every department in a hospital as they survey for infections and teach staff how to prevent and control infection. The ICP is an important link between personnel from various hospital departments. When there is a question or problem regarding infection control, the ICP should be called on without hesitation.

The epidemiologic method used by infection control practitioners now serves as a model for the study of other adverse outcomes of hospitalization, for example, falls. Quality management departments of many hospitals consult infection control practitioners in the design and implementation of monitors and focused studies. Informing health care workers of rates of patient outcomes results in changes in practice, which ultimately improves patient outcomes.

The current epidemic of acquired immunodeficiency syndrome (AIDS), caused by the HIV, has presented infection control practitioners with the challenge of developing a system of isolation that would prevent transmission of this and other frequently undiagnosed infections in health care settings and the community. Body substance isolation (BSI) is a new system developed by ICP's Jackson and Lynch.[31] This system emphasizes universal precautions when in contact with the body fluids of all patients.

This chapter presents an overview of the role of the nurse in the prevention and control of infection. For further information regarding a specific infectious disease, the reader should consult the chapter in which the site of the disease is discussed, for example, Chapter 30 for hepatitis, Chapter 24 for tuberculosis, and so on.

THE INFECTIOUS DISEASE PROCESS

Definitions

A number of definitions are useful when describing certain conditions related to the infectious disease process. These are presented in Table 17-1.

The question of whether a person has an infection or colonization can be difficult to answer. What is important to realize is that persons who are colonized, as well as infected persons, can easily serve as a source of infection to themselves and to others who are at risk.

Chain of Infection

Essential to appropriate intervention in the prevention and control of infection is an understanding of the infectious disease process. All infectious diseases occur as a result of a sequence of events (Fig. 17-1). Often the reservoir for an agent responsible for an outbreak of an infection is not readily apparent and, in fact, may never be identified. If the process of infection is well understood, however, appropriate and effective control measures can be instituted

Table 17-1 **Selected definitions related to the infectious disease process**

Term	Definition
Pathogen	Microorganism or substance capable of producing disease
Pathogenicity	Capability of a pathogen to infect and produce disease; determined by ability to survive and multiply outside host, virulence, dose, host specificity, and resistance of host
Invasiveness	Injury to host as a result of presence and spread of pathogen through body tissues
Toxigenicity	Injury to host as a result of effects to host of toxins produced by pathogen
Incubation period	Period of time after pathogen enters host and before clinical symptoms of infection appear
Infection	Presence in the body of a pathogen that multiplies and produces effects injurious to the host
Apparent (symptomatic, clinical)	Clinical signs and symptoms present
Inapparent (asymptomatic, subclinical)	No perceivable signs or symptoms present
Acute	Rapid onset, immediate host response, severe symptoms, and usually short course
Chronic	Insidious onset, delayed host response, mild symptoms, and long course
Latent	Pathogen ever-present in host, symptoms present only intermittently, often in response to a stimulus; pathogen dormant at other times
Localized	Focal point of symptoms or injury
Generalized	Systemic, whole body involvement
Superinfection	New infection by a pathogen different from one that caused initial infection
Colonization	Presence of pathogenic microorganisms in or on a host that do not produce injury or incite an injurious body response
Normal flora	Presence of nonpathogenic microorganisms that normally reside in various body locations without invasion or harm (may become pathogenic if introduced into an area in which they do not normally reside)
Contamination	Presence of pathogenic micoorganisms on inanimate objects or in substances

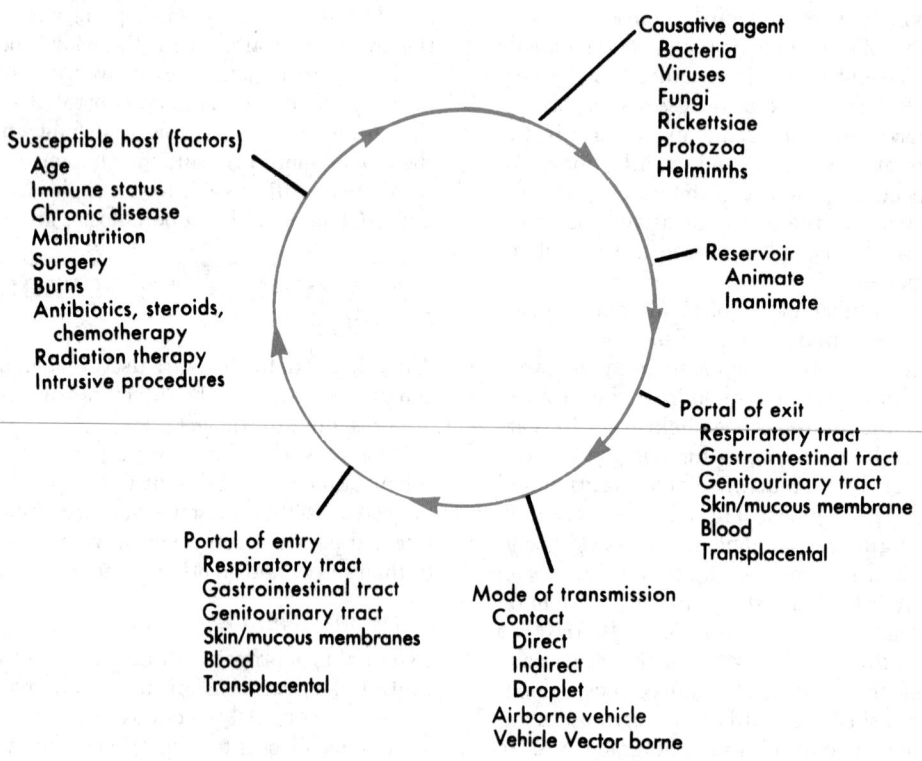

Fig. 17-1 The infectious disease process.

Examples of modes of transmission of infection

Mode	Example
I. Contact	HIV infection, gonorrhea, syphilis
Direct: (source to host)	
Indirect: by way of intermediate object	
Hands	*Staphylococcus aureus* wound infection
Fomites (e.g., hypodermic needle)	Hepatitic B, HIV infection
Surgical instruments	*Staphylococcus aureus* wound infection
Droplet (large particles)	Meningococcal meningitis, influenza
Host inhales droplets expelled from reservoir	
II. Airborne: host inhales droplet nuclei (1 to 5 micrometers) in air	Chickenpox (varicella), pulmonary tuberculosis
III. Vehicle: ingested or administered substance	
Food, water	Hepatitis A, salmonellosis
Blood products	Hepatitis B, HIV infection
IV fluids	Enterobacter bacteremia, fungemia
IV. Vector: animate intermediary (usually insect)	Malaria, Rocky Mountain spotted fever, yellow fever, Lyme disease

even though the original source of the causative agent is not known.

Once the agent has left the reservoir, it needs a *mode of transmission* to a host. Modes and examples of how infection is spread by each mode are explained in Box 17-1.

Entry of an infectious agent into a host does not mean that the agent will proliferate and cause infection. Infection depends on the dose and virulence of the agent and the *susceptibility of the host*. The healthy human body is extremely resistant to infection; however, when the basic biologic defense mechanisms of the body are compromised, an infectious organism has a much greater chance of causing an infection. Chapter 41 deals with many of the factors of biologic defense exhibited by the host to prevent infection and injury. Some of the factors that affect host susceptibility to infection are included in Box 17-2.

No one factor alone is responsible for an infection. Rather, there are a number of variables—the *agent*, the *environment*, and the *host*—that determine the outcome and toward which prevention and control measures are directed. To intervene effectively in the infectious disease process it is important that all of these concepts be understood.

Assessment

The establishment of an infection within the human body leads to a number of specific and generalized manifestations. The exact signs and symptoms elicited in the host depend on the agent responsible for the infection and the site of the infection. (For details on host response to specific infectious disease, see the particular chapter that discusses the disease site.) Early recognition of infection is a crucial step to initiating prompt treatment. There are some general subjective, objective, and diagnostic findings that can alert the nurse to suspect an infection, even if the causative agent is not known. These are summarized here.

The normal WBC count in blood is 5000 to 10,000

Factors affecting host susceptibility to infection

Age	Young and old—most susceptible
Impaired immune status	HIV infection, leukemia, immunosuppressive drugs, radiation therapy, steroids
Chronic diseases	Diabetes, cancer, COPD, end-stage renal disease
Poor nutritional status	
Invasive devices, surgery	Intravenous catheters, chest tubes, urinary catheters, artificial airways
Impaired skin integrity	Burns, decubitus
Altered body flora	Antibiotics, antacid therapy

WBC/mm³. With the presence of a serious infection the number of WBCs rises above 10,000/mm³ in response to the infectious inflammation. Leukocyte values between 10,000 and 20,000 are considered slightly elevated, 20,000 to 40,000 moderately elevated, and greater than 40,000 greatly elevated. In a few infectious diseases the number of WBCs in circulation actually drops, which is also a significant piece of diagnostic data.

Five types of mature WBCs are found in circulation: neutrophils, eosinophils, basophils, lymphocytes, and monocytes. Each type of WBC plays a more or less specific role in body defense (Chapter 41); therefore, different diseases produce different reactions among the white cell populations in the blood. These changes in patterns of distribution are detected not just by counting the total

Table 17-2 White blood cell response to infections

Leukocyte response	Associated infectious process
Increase in neutrophils (neutrophilia)	Acute local and systemic infections caused by bacteria (especially pyogenic bacteria), rickettsia, some viruses, and a few protozoa
Decrease in neutrophils (neutropenia)	Salmonellosis, brucellosis, whooping cough, overwhelming bacterial infections, influenza, infectious mononucleosis, infectious hepatitis, mumps, rubella, rubeola, and some rickettsial and protozoan diseases
Increase in eosinophils (eosinophilia)	Allergic reactions, chronic skin disease, helminthic infections, and scarlet fever
Increase in lymphocytes (lymphocytosis)	Chickenpox, mumps, measles, infectious mononucleosis, influenza, whooping cough, syphilis, tuberculosis, salmonellosis, viral hepatitis, and viral pneumonia; sometimes in convalescence from acute bacterial infection
Decrease in lymphocytes (lymphopenia)	AIDS/AIDS-related complex (ARC)
Increase in monocytes (monocytosis)	Tuberculosis, chickenpox, brucellosis, mumps, syphilis, and certain rickettsial diseases; may occur in certain viral and protozoan diseases and in convalescent phase of acute bacterial infections

number of WBCs in a stained blood smear but also by classifying them according to morphology and calculating the relative percentage of each cell type present. This type of a count is known as a differential count. For example, an increase in the number of immature neutrophils is commonly referred to as a "shift to the left" and may be indicative of an acute infection. The differential count may provide information that can be correlated with other clinical data to help diagnose a situation. Table 17-2 provides some general correlations between leukocyte response and infectious diseases.

None of the signs and symptoms present in localized or generalized infections are diagnostic in themselves. many can be demonstrated by other disease processes. They can, however, serve as helpful clues in the diagnosis of a suspected infectious process.

Diagnostic Tests

Diagnostic tests are important in the diagnosis of an infection. Some of the diagnostic tests used to obtain data are the following:

    Bacterial, viral, and fungal cultures, gram stain
    Antigen/antibody detection
    Blood counts
    Skin tests
    Radiologic tests
    Gallium scans
    Ultrasound examinations
    CT scan
    MRI examinations

Specimens for microbiologic testing are perhaps the most frequently ordered when an infection is suspected.

Proper collection and handling of laboratory specimens are essential to ensure accurate laboratory results. Inappropriate collection or handling of specimens may lead to unnecessary delays in test results or to inaccurate results, thus affecting the therapy given to the patient. When an infection is suspected, cultures are taken of the suspected site. If the patient has a fever and the site of infection is unknown, cultures are commonly taken of the blood, urine, sputum, and any other possible sites of infection. This may

---

17-3

General guidelines for specimen collection

Objective

To obtain specimen containing infecting pathogen that is free of contamination

Method

1. Wash hands.
2. Prepare site aseptically.
3. Collect specimen using aseptic technique; wear gloves if appropriate; avoid coughing, sneezing, or talking.
4. Obtain adequate amount of specimen.
5. Collect and transport in sterile container appropriate for type of specimen.
6. Label requisition with patient's name, location, date and time of collection, type of specimen, how obtained (for example, clean void or catheter urine), test requested, and current antibiotic therapy.
7. Store properly and transport promptly to laboratory.
8. Keep record of test.

---

include spinal fluid cultures, aspirates of body fluid, or intravenous catheter tips. *It is imperative that these cultures be obtained before the initiation of antibiotic therapy whenever possible because antibiotics can suppress any bacteria that are present and give inaccurate or false-negative culture results.* Cultures should be obtained in a manner that avoids contamination. Aseptic preparation of the site to be cultured, observance of aseptic technique, and placing specimens in an appropriate container are crucial factors to be observed in ensuring the best sample. Once obtained, the specimen must be properly stored and transported promptly to the laboratory. Each institution should have guidelines for the proper method for collecting and handling specimens for the laboratory (Box 17-3).

Interpretation of laboratory results is sometimes difficult. Certain body sites have bacteria known as normal flora, which reside there in a commensalistic (intimate) relationship with the host. These bacteria do not cause infection in the normal host. The skin, upper respiratory tract, vagina, urethra, and bowel are examples of body sites in which normal bacterial flora can be found. The bacteria found vary from site to site, and knowing the normal flora is helpful in discerning the significance of laboratory culture results. A *Clinician's Dictionary of Bacteria and Fungi*[15] is an excellent publication that lists in detail the normal flora of various sites. It must be emphasized that laboratory results alone cannot be used to make diagnostic and therapeutic decisions. Rather, they are used in conjunction with the clinical status of the patient to make appropriate diagnostic and therapeutic decisions.

Knowledge about the infectious disease process and about how to recognize or suspect an infectious process is vital to the prevention and control of infectious diseases in both community and hospital settings.

INFECTION CONTROL IN THE COMMUNITY

An infectious disease is termed a communicable disease when it is highly transmissable to other persons. Smallpox is an example of a communicable disease that, through cooperative efforts worldwide, has been successfully eradicated. The methods used to eradicate smallpox throughout the world can serve as a model of how to eliminate other communicable diseases. The eradication of smallpox also demonstrates the importance of accurate reporting of communicable diseases to the proper authorities so that prevention and control measures can be instituted.

The community health nurse plays a vital role in the collection of data, surveillance activities, immunization programs, education, and other control measures. Physicians and health care facilities have a responsibility to report communicable diseases promptly to the health department. Health agencies in the community can use the reported data to determine potential or real problems, to identify the causative agent and its source (if possible), and to identify the population at risk. A method to control the problem, care for the exposed, and protect the population at risk can then be devised and implemented.

The HIV epidemic has posed the greatest communicable disease threat in recent years. Since first identified as a communicable disease in 1981, much has been learned through epidemiologic research. AIDS was first described in homosexual males and then in intravenous drug users and hemophiliacs. This discovery helped to identify the routes of transmission as sexual contact, contaminated needles, and blood transfusions. In 1983 the virus was first isolated. In the United States the virus was named human *T lymphotrophic virus III (HTLV III)*. The French named the same virus *lymphadenopathy virus (LAV)*. Later the virus was renamed *human immunodeficiency virus (HIV)*. Since first recognized as a communicable disease, no new routes of transmission have been identified.

In April 1985 the screening of all blood and blood products for HIV antibody was begun in the United States. This has almost eliminated blood transfusions as a source of HIV infection. Today, those most at risk for HIV infection are persons who engage in high-risk behaviors: having multiple sexual partners, sharing intravenous needles, or being a sexual partner of a person who engages in high-risk behaviors. In addition, HIV infection may be transmitted from an infected mother to fetus in utero from maternal circulation or during labor and delivery. Casual contact has not been identified as a means of transmission. Nonsexual cohabitants of HIV-infected persons have not become infected. The risk of transmission of HIV to a health care worker from an infected patient via needlestick has been calculated as 1:250.[21] Improved technology to decrease exposure of health care workers to needles and other sharps is needed. In 1991, the first case of transmission of HIV from health care worker to patient during an invasive procedure was reported.

Until a cure or vaccine is available, the only effective control measure is education. Educational programs emphasize the routes of transmission, identify high-risk behaviors, and instruct in safer sexual practices. Nurses participate in AIDS education programs in schools, in the media, community centers, and churches. Nurses are also engaged in HIV counseling. It is essential that the nurse be well informed and provide accurate information in a sensitive and nonjudgmental manner.

AIDS is discussed in detail in Chapter 19.

Prevention and Control Measures

One method of prevention and control of disease in the community involves environmental control measures such as sanitation techniques that ensure a pure water supply and proper disposal of sewage and other potentially infectious materials. These measures have been legislated into building codes, state laws, and federal regulations. Similarly, there are regulations regarding health practices in institutions that handle, package, and prepare foods. Another example of an environmental control measure is the spraying of a designated area to kill mosquitos, which are implicated in the spread of viral encephalitis. Spraying usually is done only after an outbreak has been identified.

Depending on the communicable disease, care of exposed persons and protection of the population at risk for contracting the disease may entail prophylaxis, immunization, or only careful monitoring of new cases. Often, simple adherence to basic principles of hygiene is sufficient. Determination of additional required measures should be made by the local or state health department. Attempts are made to reach those at risk and inform them of the preventive measures. Education of the public is a key component of these efforts.

In the United States there has been a significant reduction in recent years in the incidence of infectious diseases, such as measles, whooping cough, and poliomyelitis, which can be prevented by immunization. Concern is being expressed, however, about the decrease in the number of children presently being immunized, despite the fact that these immunizations can often be obtained free of cost. Additionally, concern is being expressed that federal monies used to support local immunization efforts has been reduced to such a level that free immunizations are no longer equally available in all 50 states. Infections formerly

Artificial immunization

Active

Produce own antibodies after being inoculated with vaccine made from attenuated, killed organisms, or modified toxins (toxoids).
Examples: Smallpox, diphtheria, tetanus, pertussis, rubella, mumps, rubeola, polio (OPV), pneumococcal, hepatitis B, influenza, typhoid, *Haemophilus* polysaccharide conjugated vaccine.

Passive

Injected with antibodies produced by other persons or animals. This protection is temporary, lasting a few weeks without stimulating antibody production in the recipient.
Examples: immune human serum globulin, hepatitis B immune globulin (HBIG), mumps hyperimmune gamma globulin, rabies human immune globulin, tetanus immune globulin, varicella zoster–immune globulin.

Persons for whom hepatitis B vaccine is recommended

Health care and public safety workers having blood contact
Clients and staff of institutions for developmentally disabled
Hemodialysis patients
Sexually active homosexual men
Users of illicit injectable drugs
Recipients of certain blood products
Household and sexual contacts of hepatitis B carriers
Prison inmates
Heterosexuals with multiple partners

From *MMWR* 39(RR-2): 14-16, 1990.

seen only in children are now being seen more frequently in young adults because of the failure of the population to develop acquired immunity during early childhood.

A more recent concern because of air travel is the elimination of the barriers of time and distance and the possibility of a person with an infectious disease being brought from a remote area of the world to a major population center where the disease can be readily spread to a susceptible public.

The dramatic control of several infectious diseases has been caused by the development and use of a variety of *inactivated vaccines* and *live attenuated antigens*. The potential for eradication of common infectious diseases brings with it major responsibilities for public health agencies, physicians, and nurses. Ways must be found not only to carry out planned programs of immunization, but also to educate the public to the hazards of apathy and failure to maintain proper levels of immunization. Progress in control and eradication requires that all aspects of these programs be continually evaluated.

Immunization Programs

Immunization programs have played and continue to play a primary role in the control of infectious disease throughout the world. The body can be stimulated to produce antibodies against some specific diseases without actually having the disease (*active artificial immunity*). Temporary protection sometimes can be provided by injecting antibodies produced by other persons or animals into the bloodstream of a human being (*passive artificial immunity*).

Recommendations concerning current immunization schedules are found in the *Red Book* published by the Committee on Infectious Diseases of The American Academy of Pediatrics and in *Morbidity and Mortality Weekly Reports*, which present recommendations of the United States Public Health Service's Advisory Committee on Im-

munization Practices (ACIP). The reader should refer to these resources when there are questions about proper immunization practices, prophylaxis, interruption in immunization schedules, or adverse reactions and side effects. A summary of active and passive immunization appears in Box 17-4.

Active immunization

If 90% of the population is protected against organisms that required continued passage through human beings to reproduce and live, the disease caused by the organism can be virtually eliminated because there are too few susceptible hosts for organism spread. Smallpox has been eliminated from the world in this way. This type of protection of a group is called *herd immunity*. It is ineffectual, however, against organisms such as tetanus bacilli that can exist indefinitely (in the soil), and in this instance each person must be immunized to be protected. If the disease is one not prevalent in the environment, such as diphtheria in the United States, or is not spread from person to person by direct contact, such as tetanus, the inoculation must be repeated at regular intervals to maintain protection. This inoculation is called a *booster dose*, and usually one tenth of the original inoculating dose is sufficient.

An inoculation often causes a local tissue response. Symptoms of inflammation (redness, tenderness, swelling, sometimes ulceration) appear at the site of the injection, and generalized symptoms of widespread tissue involvement (slight febrile reactions, general malaise, muscle aching) for 1 or 2 days are common.

Active artificial immunization against many bacilli and viruses is now available. All persons should be encouraged to avail themselves of the protection advised by health officials in their local area. They also should be advised to keep a permanent record of the date of each immunization.

Primary immunization schedules

In the United States, the ACIP recommends that all children be immunized against diphtheria, pertussis, (whooping cough), tetanus (DPT); measles, mumps, and rubella (MMR); and poliomyelitis (OPV). *Haemophilus* b polysaccharide conjugated vaccine (HbCV) is also recommended

Table 17-3   Recommended schedule for active immunization of normal infants and children (see individual ACIP recommendations for details)

Recommended age	Vaccine(s)*	Comments
2 months	DTP #1, OPV #1	Can be given earlier in endemic areas
4 months	DTP #2, OPV #2	Six-week to 2-month interval desired between OPV doses
6 months	DTP #3	Additional dose of OPV at this time optional in areas with high risk of polio exposure
15 months	MMR, DTP #4, OPV #3	Completion of primary series
18 months	HbCV	Conjugate preferred over polysaccharide vaccine (HbPV)
4 to 6 years	DTP #5, OPV #4	At or before school entry
14 to 16 years	Td†	Repeat every 10 years throughout life

From Centers for Disease Control: Recommendations of the ACIP: general recommendations on immunization. *MMWR* 38(13):210, 1989.
*DTP, Diptheria, tetanus, pertussis; OPV, oral poliovirus vaccine; MMR, measles, mumps, rubella; HbCV, vaccine composed of *Haemophilus* b polysaccharide antigen conjugated to protein carrier.
†Tetanus and diptheria toxoids, adsorbed (for use in persons age 7 years and older); contains same amount of tetanus toxoid as DTP but reduced dose of diphtheria toxoid.

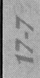

17-6

Persons for whom yearly influenza vaccine is recommended

Adults 65 or older
Person 6 months or older with chronic pulmonary, cardiovascular, metabolic, renal, or immune deficiency disease
Children age 6 months to 18 years receiving long-term aspirin therapy (danger of developing Reye syndrome after influenza)
Residents of nursing homes and other long-term care facilities
Note: Health care workers are also encouraged to be immunized yearly to reduce exposure of high-risk patients

From *MMWR* 40(RR-6): 4-5, 1991.

17-7

Persons for whom pneumococcal polysaccharide vaccine is recommended

Adults 65 or older with chronic illness or after splenectomy
Immunocompromised adults with Hodgkin's disease, renal disease, lymphoma, or multiple myeloma
Persons with HIV infection
Children 2 or older with chronic illness associated with increased risk of complications from pneumonia

From *MMWR* 38(5): 64-76, 1989.

---

for all children attending day care centers (Table 17-3). Children who have not been immunized as infants can be immunized at any age. All susceptible children, adolescents, and adults should be immunized unless contraindicated.

Routine vaccination against smallpox is no longer recommended by the CDC because the side effects and complications of the vaccine are greater than the danger of acquiring the disease. The vaccine is indicated only for laboratory workers who are directly involved with smallpox or closely related orthopox viruses. However, the U.S. armed forces require smallpox vaccination for recruits.

At the present time, immunization against typhoid fever is recommended only when there is exposure to a typhoid carrier in the household, when there is an outbreak of typhoid in a community, or for travelers to countries where typhoid is endemic (always present).

Immunization to protect against other diseases is given on a selective basis; that is, groups at a high risk are immunized. Hepatitis B vaccine is an excellent example of a vaccine that is only recommended for persons at high risk of acquiring the virus (see Box 17-5).

Because of the prevalence of *influenza* (flu) and its po-

tential for causing death, the ACIP recommends immunization against influenza for all individuals at increased risk of adverse consequences from infection of the lower respiratory tract (see Box 17-6).

A vaccine is currently available that protects against 23 types of Streptococcal pneumonia (88% of the strains seen in the United States). See Box 17-7.

Passive immunization

Passive immunization usually is reserved for situations in which the disease would be detrimental to the person. For example, it is rarely given to prevent a disease such as chickenpox or mumps in children because they are at an optimal age for the body to respond immunologically with minimal inflammatory response. On the other hand, an adult exposed to the same diseases often would be given antibodies because adults may have a severe pathologic response. *Immunization is given to all age groups exposed to pathogens that cause serious diseases such as hepatitis, poliomyelitis, diphtheria, tetanus, or rabies.* Antivenims, which are given to people bitten by poisonous snakes or black widow spiders, are other examples of passive immunologic products.

Products used for passive immunization may be specific to the disease. Antitoxins and immune animal and human sera are examples. These materials contain elevated levels of immune globulins, which can specifically detoxify the toxin, neutralize the virus, or inactivate the bacterium. The whole blood of a patient who has recently recovered from a disease against which antibodies are produced also may be used. Antitoxins are available for diphtheria, tetanus, botulism, gas gangrene, and the venom of snakes. *Human immune serum* is available for mumps, measles, pertussis, rabies, poliomyelitis, and tetanus.

Immune serum globulin (ISG), or gamma globulin (γ-globulin), is an antibody-rich fraction of pooled plasma from normal donors. The rationale for pooling plasma is that someone among the donors will have had the diseases and will have developed antibodies against them. The *globulin fraction* of the plasma carries the antibodies, and because it is known not to transmit the virus of hepatitis, it is considered safe to use. Because of occasional side effects, it is now recommended that the use of immune serum globulin be limited to those disorders in which its efficacy has been definitely established. These are measles pro-

phylaxis or modification, viral hepatitis type A prophylaxis or modification, and immune deficiency diseases.

Special human immune serum globulins are derived from the sera of persons previously immunized or convalescing from specific diseases. Tetanus immune globulin (human) is of value in prophylaxis and treatment of tetanus in persons who have not received prior immunization. Pertussis immune globulin (human) and mumps immune globulin (human) are of uncertain or unproved value in the prevention and treatment of pertussis and mumps, respectively. Hepatitis B immune globulin (human) is available for prophylaxis after exposure to hepatitis B. Zoster immune globulin (human) is available for restricted use for prophylaxis against chickenpox.

Nursing responsibilities
Teaching

The greatest responsibility of the nurse in immunization programs is to teach the public the advantages of immunization and encourage widespread participation in programs recommended by the local public health officer.

Table 17-4 Description of selected vaccines

Vaccine	Description	Comments
DPT		
Diphtheria	Toxoid Inactivated Diphtheria toxin	Booster dose every 10 years
Tetanus	Inactivated Tetanus toxoid	Booster dose very 10 years For contaminated wound management, additional booster given if more than 5 years since last booster dose
Pertussis	Killed whole *Bordetella pertussis*	Not recommended for individuals over 7 years of age because risk of pertussis low and reaction possibly severe
Measles	Live attenuated virus vaccine	Contraindications: pregnancy, immunocompromised state, history of anaphylactic reaction to eggs
Mumps	Live attenuated virus vaccine	Contraindications: pregnancy, immunocompromised state, history of anaphylactic reaction to eggs
Rubella	Live attenuated rubella virus grown in human diploid cells	Contraindications: pregnancy, immunocompromised state
Polio		
OPV	Live attenuated oral poliovirus vaccine	Contraindications: pregnancy, immunocompromised state
IPV	Inactivated poliovirus vaccine	Administered by subcutaneous injection, contraindicated in pregnancy
Influenza	Inactivated whole or disrupted (split) influenza viruses	Antigenic content annually changed to reflect influenza A and B virus strains in circulation; admininstered annually; contraindication: history of anaphylactic hypersensitivity to eggs
Pneumococcal	Purified preparation of 23 different types of pneumococcal capsular polysaccharide	Should be given only once to adults because of possible adverse reactions; data are not currently available regarding revaccination of children; should be given only to children 2 years and older who have chronic illnesses specifically associated with increased risk for pneumococcal disease
Hepatitis B		
Recombinant deoxyribonucleic acid (DNA)	Purified surface antigen of virus produced by recombinant yeast cells	Given in series of three injections; first followed by other two 1 and 6 months later; indicated for persons who have routine or frequent contact with blood and body fluids; contraindicated for persons allergic to yeast
Human serum	Purified, inactivated surface antigen of virus from plasma of human carriers	Administration schedule same as for recombinant DNA form; recommended for hemodialysis patients
Haemophilius influenzae b (HbCV)	Bacterial polysaccharide conjugated to protein	Administered at age 18 months to 5 years, up to sixth birthday

In teaching it is advisable to provide the public with the following information: (1) *against what disease protection is being given,* (2) *why immunization is desirable,* and (3) *when booster doses should be obtained.* The relative safety of the immunization and the advantages of immunization early in life should be stressed.

The nurse is responsible for assessing persons before immunization because there are some contraindications to receiving certain immunizing substances. Those that are prepared in chicken or duck embryos may cause an allergic reaction in persons who are allergic to eggs. Many people are allergic to horse serum, and substances containing horse serum, such as tetanus antitoxin, should never be given unless a small amount of the substance has been injected intradermally (a sensitivity test) and after 20 minutes produces no "hive" reaction about the injection site. *Active immunologic products should not be given while a person has a cold or other infection because the inflammatory reaction from the immunization will be greater than usual* (Table 17-4).

Live attenuated virus vaccines should *not be given* to *persons* with *alterations in their immune status* because virus replication after administration may be unchecked in these individuals. OPV viruses are excreted by the recipient of the vaccine and are communicable to other persons, so individuals who live with an immunocompromised person should not receive OPV. See Box 17-8 for additional considerations about vaccines.

Before leaving the clinic, the person or family members should be instructed about the expected effects of an inoculation and told to contact the physician or to report to a hospital emergency room if any other symptoms develop. The person is cautioned not to scratch any lesion produced by an inoculation. If a severe local reaction with redness, swelling, and tenderness occurs, the physician may order the application of hot, wet dressings. If the lesion is open, these dressings should be sterile.

When antitoxins, antisera, or antivenims are given, the patient is kept under observation for 20 to 30 minutes. Symp- *toms of severe allergic response usually will appear within that period of time.* The responsibility of the nurse working in employee health programs is to educate personnel to achieve and maintain immune status and participate in screening programs, for example, tuberculosis, varicella, and rubella.

Yearly chest x-ray examinations are no longer recommended for the routine management of persons with positive tuberculin skin tests. Health care workers with negative tuberculin tests should be tested yearly. If a worker who has had a negative test turns positive, he or she should be offered prophylactic isoniazed (INH). Additionally the source of the infection should be identified if possible. (For more information see Chapter 24.) After the initial chest x-ray examination following a skin test conversion, yearly chest x-ray examinations have not been shown to be of significant clinical value and are not cost effective in monitoring persons for early disease. Health care and public safety workers who have contact with blood should maintain their immune status against hepatitis B.

Home care

Persons with communicable diseases are frequently cared for at home. The community health nurse is often asked to teach family members how to care for the patient and how to protect family members, friends, and neighbors. The same principles apply in the home as in the hospital.

Regardless of the disease, good hand washing technique should be practiced and gloves should be worn for contact with any body substance. A smock or apron can be worn to protect the clothes from soiling. A mask, if indicated, can be improvised from any closely woven absorbable material, or disposable ones can be purchased at a pharmacy. All liquid wastes can be flushed down a toilet. Garbage and other wastes containing body substances can be wrapped in newspaper and placed in a plastic bag before being discarded in a rubbish container. Dishes should be washed in hot, soapy water. Separate dishes are not required. Laundry should be washed in a washing machine with a detergent. Chlorine bleach or a disinfectant should be added if linen is soiled with body substances. The local health department should be consulted for full information regarding specific communicable diseases.

The special problems the nurse encounters in controlling *hospital-acquired infections* will be the focus of the remainder of this chapter.

INFECTION CONTROL IN THE HOSPITAL
Scope of the Problem

A *nosocomial* infection is one that is not present or incubating at the time a person is admitted to the hospital but develops after admission. A *community-acquired* infection is one that is present or incubating at the time of admission to the hospital. The nurse should be aware of the problem of nosocomial infections, their effects on patient morbidity, mortality, and increased hospital costs, as well as the legal aspects concerning them. The nurse also should be knowledgeable about the types of infections seen most often, the common pathogens and how they are transmitted, factors that predispose a patient to a nosocomial infection, how to

---

17-8

Additional considerations for vaccine administration

In general, inactivated vaccines and live vaccines (except cholera and yellow fever) can be administered simultaneously at separate sites.

Whenever possible, live vaccines should be administered on the same day or at least 30 days apart.

PPD (purified protein derivative) testing for tuberculosis can be done on the same day as live virus vaccines or 4 to 6 weeks later.

Live attenuated vaccines should not be given at the same time as passive immunization because passively acquired antibodies can interfere with the response to live attenuated virus vaccines.

Pregnant women should not receive live attenuated vaccines because of the theoretic risk to the fetus.

If a person has a febrile illness, it is usually best to wait until recovery before vaccination.

Table 17-5   Infection rates per 1000 discharges by site and hospital category, 1984

	UTI	SWI	LRI	BACT	CUT	OTH	All sites
Nonteaching hospital	9.9	3.6	4.2	1.3	1.1	2.0	22.2
Small teaching hospital	13.9	6.0	5.4	1.9	1.8	4.7	33.8
Large teaching hospital	14.2	6.6	7.7	3.9	2.6	6.4	41.4

From Centers for Disease Control: CDC Surveillance Summaries, 1986; 35 (No. 1SS).
UTI, Urinary tract infection; *SWI,* Surgical wound infection; *LRI,* Lower respiratory tract infection; *Bact,* Primary bacteremia; *CUT,* Cutaneous infection; *OTH,* Other.

recognize persons at risk of infection, and the prevention and control measures necessary to decrease the incidence of nosocomial infections.

It is estimated that 3% to 5% of all patients discharged from U.S. hospitals each year develop nosocomial infections.[25] In addition to the considerable morbidity and mortality caused by these infections, their diagnoses and treatment (including additional days of hospitalization) cost more than $1 billion per year. The JCAHO requires that those institutions seeking accreditation have a program of infection control centered around monitoring (1) patients with infections, (2) patient care practices, (3) antibiotic usage, (4) health of personnel, and (5) the environment of the institution. The AHA and the CDC have developed guidelines for the prevention and control of infectious diseases for use in patient care centers. Because of these external forces, as well as to provide the best possible care for their patients, hospitals are recognizing the need to increase infection surveillance and to upgrade programs to prevent nosocomial infections.

As seen in Table 17-5, the incidence of nosocomial infections varies with the type of hospital, and this can be attributed to differences in the size of hospitals, the severity of illness in the patient population, the susceptibility of the patient population, and the number of personnel who have hands-on contact with the patients. The patient with the greatest risk of developing a nosocomial infection is one with a chronic illness, a prolonged hospital stay, and the most direct contact with various hospital personnel (that is, physicians, students, nurses, or therapists). These factors hold true not only for variations of infection rates from institution to institution, but also for variations in infection rates within an institution. Certain patient care areas are considered to be *high-risk areas* for developing nosocomial infections. These areas understandably are those that care for patients who have decreased host defenses, are immuno-compromised, or in whom invasive procedures and devices are common. Areas generally considered to be high risk are (1) intensive care units (including neonatal units), (2) burn units, (3) dialysis units, and (4) oncology units. The infection rate in these areas may be well over 20%.

According to the Surgeon General's report, although ICU patients account for only 15% of hospital admissions, they account for 50% or more of nosocomial infections.[26] The report has set the following goal to be met by the year 2000: reduce by at least 10% the incidence of surgical wound infections and nosocomial infections in intensive-care patients.[26]

Persons at Risk

The nurse needs to be able to recognize those patients who are at the greatest risk of a nosocomial infection. Some of the factors that predispose a person to infection are mentioned on p. 343. Probably the single most important factor predisposing a patient to a nosocomial infection is the severity of the patient's underlying disease.

A patient admitted to the hospital with an infection may develop during the hospitalization a *superinfection* with another organism. Often this superinfection is with a more virulent or drug-resistant organism. For example, a patient admitted with a leg ulcer infected with *Staphylococcus aureus* may develop further infection (not colonization) with *Pseudomonas aeruginosa.* Furthermore, if this infection progresses to involve the bloodstream, then a *secondary bacteremia* has occurred. Infection can occur secondary to (1) an existing infection, (2) an underlying disease process, or (3) an anatomic defect that may be causing obstruction. An example of this is the man who has benign prostate hypertrophy (BPH) and who develops a urinary tract infection secondary to the obstruction caused by the BPH.

The most common site for a nosocomial infection is the urinary tract; 75% of these infections are related to instrumentation, including in-dwelling urinary catheters, catheterizations, and urologic procedures. Infected surgical wounds, followed by lower respiratory tract infections, and then bloodstream infections (some associated with the use of intravascular lines) are the next most frequently encountered types of nosocomial infections. Together these sites account for about 80% of all nosocomial infections.

Pathogens Causing Nosocomial Infections

The pathogens commonly responsible for nosocomial infections and their common sources are listed in Table 17-6. Changes in the etiologic agents of nosocomial infections have occurred in the 1980s. Organisms causing these infections are increasingly likely to be resistant to most antibiotics, which leaves fewer options for treatment.

According to National Nosocomial Infections Surveillance System (NNIS) data from 1986 to 1989, *Escherichia coli* continues to be the most common pathogen responsible for hospital-acquired infection. Other pathogens responsible for 10% or more of the total number of infections include enterococci, *Pseudomonas aeruginosa,* and *Staphylococcus aureus.* Coagulase negative staphylococcus, once considered an insignificant source of nosocomial infection, is now responsible for close to 10% of all hospital-acquired infections. These infections are primarily seen in patients

Table 17-6 Modes of transmission of some common pathogens

Pathogen	Source
Gram-positive cocci	
Staphylococcus aureus	Contaminated objects, hands, and nasal tracts of health care workers, air, self
Coagulase-negative staphyloccus	Self, hands of health care workers, invasive devices
Group A *Streptococcus* organisms	Direct contact, air, hands, rarely objects
Enterococcus organisms	Self, hands of health care workers, contaminated environmental sufaces
Gram-negative rods	
Escherichia, Klebsiella, Enterobacter	Self, hands of health care workers, contaminated solutions
Proteus, Salmonella, Providencia, Serratia, Citrobacter	Contaminated food and water, hands of health care workers, self
Pseudomonas	Contaminated environment, hands, self
Anaerobic bacteria	
Clostridium, Bacteroides	Self, contaminated environment, hands
Fungal organisms	
Yeasts	Self, hands of health care workers
Fungi	Air, contaminated environment
Viruses	
Varicella	Air, direct contact
Herpes	Self, direct contact, air
Rubella	Direct contact, air
Hepatitis B	Contaminated instruments or injectables, direct contact

with intravascular devices and are caused by the ability of the organism to adhere to the walls of the device.

Serratia marcescens is a gram-negative organism responsible for 2% of nosocomial infections. Its ability to rapidly develop resistance to antibiotics has made it a potential source of nosocomial infection outbreaks, especially in intensive care units. Because the mode of transmission is direct or indirect contact on the hands of personnel or on contaminated articles, *good hand-washing* and *aseptic techniques are the most effective measures to prevent outbreaks.*

Candida albicans is a yeastlike fungus that can *cause infection, especially in immunocompromised patients* or in *patients receiving antibiotics.* These patients have a decrease in their normal flora, which provides a niche for *Candida* organisms to settle in and proliferate. *Candida vaginitis and oral thrush are common complications of antibiotic therapy.* Antibiotics suppress bacterial growth but do not affect fungal growth; special antifungal agents are necessary to control these infections unless the normal flora returns following discontinuance of the antibiotics.

Methicillin-resistant *Staphylococcus aureus* (MRSA) is a pathogen causing increasing concern among health care workers. Methicillin is one of the penicillins specifically developed to treat *S. aureus* infections. Because *S. aureus* is a common surgical wound pathogen, the concern is that MRSA infections will be more difficult and expensive to treat. Currently the antibiotic of choice for treating MRSA infection is vancomycin, which must be given intravenously and may be ototoxic and nephrotoxic. It is considerably more expensive than the methicillin-group antibiotics. Once introduced into an institution, MRSA becomes endemic, and eradication measures have been largely unsuccessful. The hands of health care givers have been associated with cross-infections. Patients colonized with MRSA should not be transferred to another health care institution because institutions are afraid of the spread of this pathogen.

Prevention and Control Measures

In the hospital there are many potential sources of infection, including patients, personnel, visitors, equipment, and linen. The patient may become infected with organisms from either the external environment (*exogenous*) or, as is often seen in the severely immunocompromised host, from their own internal organisms (*endogenous*). Virtually any microorganism can be a potential pathogen to the immunocompromised patient. Most of the causative organisms are present in the external environment of the patient and are introduced into the body through direct contact or by contact with contaminated materials. In many instances nosocomial infections could be prevented by strict aseptic technique when giving care to the patient and by greater restraint in the use of invasive procedures and antibiotics. A summary of some of the prevention and control measures is presented in Box 17-9. The reader is referred to Reference 39 for greater detail.

Prevention of urinary tract infections

As mentioned previously, *urinary tract infections* (UTIs) are the *most common nosocomial infections* seen in the hospital. The majority of these infections are associated with catheterization and instrumentation of the urinary tract. Urinary catheters should be used only when absolutely necessary. If a catheter must be used, it should be discontinued as soon as medically feasible because the longer the catheter is in place, the greater the risk of developing an infection. As small a catheter as possible should be used to minimize urethral trauma.

Intermittent catheterization should be considered for patients requiring long-term urinary catheterization because this technique has been shown to reduce the infection risk. External urinary drainage devices such as condom catheters, however, have not been shown to significantly reduce the risk of urinary tract infection.

Strict aseptic technique is necessary when inserting the catheter to prevent transmission of bacteria into the bladder. Bacteria that are present around the catheter meatal junction can also be transmitted on the tip of the catheter into the bladder along the thin layer of mucus that surrounds the catheter in the urethra. For this reason, the catheter should be securely anchored to prevent it from

Prevention of and control measures for nosocomial infections

Control of external environment (exogenous sources of infection)
Health care providers
1. In good health—do not care for patients when ill
2. Keep immunizations current
3. Practice effective hand washing between each patient
   If skin dry, rough, or broken, seek appropriate attention
   If active herpes simplex infection of hand (herpetic whitlow), do not give direct patient care until lesion healed
4. Wear gloves when contact with any body substance is anticipated

Housekeeping and sanitation
1. Bed linens not shaken in air or thrown on floor
2. Proper disposal of wastes—solid and liquid
3. Proper cleaning and sterilization of contaminated articles
4. Proper ventilation for adequate air exchanges
   Modern hospitals—patients' rooms under negative pressure
   Negative pressure keeps air from patients' rooms from moving into hallways
5. Proper mopping and damp dusting to remove dust and other environmental reservoirs of infection

Control of internal environment (endogenous sources of infection)
1. Preventive measures aimed at increasing patient's defense mechanisms and thus reducing risk of infection
   Teach patient about good nutrition
   Teach patient about personal hygiene, especially hand washing
2. Be aware that normal flora of patient can be disrupted when patient is receiving antibiotics or chemotherapy and colonization may occur
   Give antibiotics on time as scheduled
   Teach patient about appropriate use of antibiotics and dangers of taking them when not prescribed by physician

moving in and out of the urethra. Movement of the catheter can track bacteria into the urethra and up into the bladder along the mucous sheath. Furthermore, *the catheter-meatal junction should be kept clean;* the patient incontinent of stool can pose a problem in this regard. *Good hand-washing techniques by personnel, cleansing of the patient's meatal area with soap and water, and proper anchoring of the catheter are considered to be effective ways to reduce the incidence of UTIs in patients with in-dwelling catheters.*

Another portal of entry for bacteria is through the distal catheter–proximal drainage tube junction. Every time the system is disconnected there is an increased risk of introducing bacteria into the system. For this reason a sterile closed drainage system should be maintained. The tubing should be fastened to the bedsheet so that there are no kinks that could lead to an obstruction. Bladder irrigations should not be a routine practice. If irrigation is necessary, a sterile disposable syringe and sterile solution should be used, and the catheter-tubing junction should be disinfected before disconnection. If frequent irrigations are necessary, as in patients who have had a transurethral prostatectomy (TURP) in which blood clots are common, a three-way catheter drainage system with continuous bladder irrigation is recommended. In this way a closed system is maintained. Urine specimens should be obtained from the rubber portal on the drainage tubing. The portal should be cleansed with an antiseptic before insertion of the sterile needle into the portal.

Another portal of entry of bacteria into the system is *through the collection bag. The bag should be kept below the bladder level at all times to prevent reflux of urine into the bladder.* It also should be kept off the floor and the emptying spout should be cleansed with an antiseptic before and after the urine is emptied from the bag. The container used to collect the urine from the bag must be used for only one patient; it should not be shared between patients. Catheters should not be changed on a routine basis. Rather, they should be replaced only when they become obstructed, or when concretions are detected in the tubing, which can lead to obstructed flow. A final control measure in preventing nosocomial UTIs is to place patients with urinary catheters in separate rooms. This is helpful in preventing cross-infection between patients.

Prevention of surgical wound infections

Surgical wound infection is primarily related to the degree of contamination, endogenous or exogenous, during the surgical procedure and to specific host factors (underlying illnesses and the presence of a remote untreated infection at the time of surgery). The degree of contamination is related to the anatomic wound site, the wound classification, and the duration of surgery. Operations involving the abdominal cavity, as well as wounds classified as contaminated or dirty, increase the patient's risk of surgical wound infection. Surgical procedures lasting longer than 2 hours also increase the risk of postoperative infection. The duration of the surgical procedure is often considered a function of the surgeon's skill and experience. The surgical wound infection rate is rarely affected by postoperative nursing care because the closed wound serves as a barrier to further contamination from exogenous organisms. However, aseptic technique during dressing changes and when emptying closed wound drainage systems is important for all personnel having contact with the surgical wound. Studies have shown that the most effective approach to reducing surgical wound infection in both high- and low-risk patients involves two components. The first consists of an ongoing surgical wound infection surveillance program with routine reporting of surgical wound infection rates back to the surgeons. The second component is the use of a hospital epidemiologist with specific training in hospital infection control who is an active member of the Hospital Infection Control Committee. Findings from the Project Study on the Efficacy of Nosocomial Infection Control demonstrated that hospitals in which programs featured both components had a 35% reduction in high-risk and 41% reduction in low-risk surgical wound infection rates.[25] Keeping the surgeons and operating room nurses informed about specific infection rates results in a heightened awareness of the importance of aseptic technique and efficiency during surgery. Other measures that minimize the risk of infection include the appropriate use of prophylactic antibiotics, limiting the period of preoperative hospital stay, preoperative bathing with antiseptics, hair removal (preferably by depilatory or clipping) in the period immediately before the surgery, and traffic control in the operating room.

A summary of the ways in which surgical wounds are classified can be found in Box 17-10.

Prevention of respiratory tract infections

Nosocomial pneumonia is associated with the highest mortality rate of all nosocomial infections. Respiratory intubation is a major risk factor because endotracheal, nasotracheal, and tracheostomy tubes bypass the patient's defense mechanisms of the upper respiratory tract. The importance of proper maintenance and decontamination of respiratory therapy equipment in preventing nosocomial pneumonias is well established. Hand washing is essential before and after contact with patients and respiratory assistive devices because these devices contain moisture, making them ideal reservoirs for gram-negative organisms such as *Pseudomonas* and *Serratia* species. In addition, *gloves should be worn for handling all respiratory secretions and devices. Suctioning is a sterile procedure* necessitating the use of sterile equipment and irrigants (Chapter 23). Surgical procedures that lead to impaired coughing are also a risk factor. Preoperative teaching stressing the importance and proper technique of coughing and deep breathing is essential to the success of postoperative pulmonary toilet. Inappropriate use of antibiotics should be avoided to minimize oropharyngeal colonization with gram-negative organisms, which, if aspirated, may lead to a more serious pneumonia. Debilitated patients should be protected from the hazards of aspiration when eating or being fed.

Prevention of bacteremias

Many blood infections (bacteremias) occur secondary to infections at another site; thus prevention may depend a great deal on control of the underlying infection. Some bacteremias are the result of the use of intravascular devices and systems. The sources of infection in these instances are the hands of personnel, the patient's skin, or infusions that are contaminated either from mishandling by hospital personnel or, less commonly, at the time of manufacture. Intravenous and intraarterial catheters should be inserted under aseptic conditions, and catheter insertion sites should be cared for aseptically. A sterile dressing should cover the insertion site. The insertion site is inspected frequently for any sign of infection, such as redness, swelling, exudate, purulence, or warmth. The patient may also complain of pain at the site. Peripheral catheters should be changed every 72 hours or more often if there is a complication such as infiltration or phlebitis. The catheter is secured to prevent in-and-out movement and tracking

17-10	**Surgical wound classification**

Wound classification	Description and example
Clean	Wounds in which the GI or respiratory tract is not entered; no inflammation or break in aseptic technique. Cholecystectomy, hysterectomy
Clean contaminated	Clean operation in which the GI or respiratory tract is entered. Colon resection
Contaminated	Nonpurulent inflammation, gross spillage from GI tract, fresh traumatic wounds, or major breaks in sterile technique. Gunshot wound
Dirty or infected	Old traumatic with dead tissue, pus encountered, or perforated viscus found. Ruptured abscess

of bacteria into the cannula site. Aseptic technique should be followed when mixing and adding drugs, changing the infusion, or manipulating connections or stopcocks. It is recommended that the tubing be changed every 72 hours (24 to 48 hours for hyperalimentation). Before hanging a solution, the nurse should check it for turbidity and particulate matter and for leaks in the system. Solutions should be discarded after 24 hours. Hyperalimentation solutions require special adherence to these practices because they are composed of nutrients that are an excellent culture media for organisms. *Candida infections are commonly seen in patients who are receiving hyperalimentation, particularly among those who are immunocompromised.*

Protection by isolation

The purpose of isolation is to protect both the health care giver from exposure to infectious agents and the patient from cross-infection. In 1983 the Centers for Disease Control (CDC) published revised guidelines for isolation precautions in hospitals. Two systems were offered for use. One was based on categories of isolation, and the other listed disease-specific isolation precautions. Hospitals were advised to choose the system most appropriate for their needs. There were seven major categories of isolation: strict, contact, respiratory, tuberculosis (AFB), enteric, drainage/secretion, and blood/body fluid. Protective isolation was eliminated as a category because it has not been shown to reduce the risk of infection in the immunocompromised patient.

The current HIV epidemic has emphasized the need for health care givers to consider the blood and body fluids of all patients as potentially infectious. Although it has been shown that the risk of HIV transmission to health care givers is low, other pathogens such as hepatitis A virus, hepatitis B virus, hepatitis virus C, cytomegalovirus, herpes simplex virus, Epstein-Barr virus, and *Staphylococcus aureus* are more easily transmitted in health care settings. Infections with these agents are frequently undiagnosed before initial contact with the patient. Therefore, taking precautions with the body fluids of all patients will both protect the health care giver and reduce nosocomial transmission of pathogens. In August 1987 the CDC published new recommendations for the prevention of HIV transmission in health care settings. These guidelines recommend the elimination of a separate blood/body fluid category, because these precautions are to be taken with all patients. Many hospitals have eliminated all the old isolation categories and implemented a system called *body substance isolation* (BSI). BSI protects both the health care worker and patients because it is not dependent on a diagnosis to initiate precautions. Following are explanations of (1) category-specific isolation and universal blood/body fluid precautions (Box 17-11) and (2) BSI (Box 17-12).

General principles of isolation

Some general principles apply regardless of the type of isolation. Gowns, gloves, and masks should be used only once and then discarded in an appropriate receptacle before leaving the patient's room. Supplies should be available convenient to each patient's room. Hands must be washed before and after patient contact, even when gloves are a required part of the isolation procedure. Masks become ineffective when they are moist and therefore should never be reused. They should be worn over the nose and mouth and should not hang around the neck and then be reused. Disposable used articles and other waste should be placed in an impervious bag and the bag should be securely closed before it is discarded. Mattresses and pillows should be covered with impervious plastic.

The reader can see the similarity between the CDC's universal blood/body fluid precautions and BSI. The difference is that BSI does not require the other categories except for airborne transmitted diseases because the BSI technique prevents the transmission of the diseases in the other categories. There is redundancy in the CDC's category-specific and universal blood/body fluid precaution system.

(Text continued on p. 358.)

17-11

Category-specific isolation precautions

Strict isolation

Strict isolation is designed to prevent transmission of highly contagious or virulent infections that may be spread by both air and contact.

Specifications for strict isolation

1. Private room is indicated; door should be kept closed. In general, patients infected with the same organism may share a room.
2. Masks are indicated for all persons entering the room.
3. Gowns are indicated for all persons entering the room.
4. Gloves are indicated for all persons entering the room.
5. Hands must be washed after touching the patient or potentially contaminated articles and before taking care of another patient.
6. Articles contaminated with infective material should be discarded or bagged and labeled before being sent for decontamination and reprocessing.

Diseases requiring strict isolation

Diphtheria, pharyngeal
Lassa fever and other viral hemorrhagic fevers, such as Marburg virus disease*
Plague, pneumonic
Smallpox*
Varicella (chickenpox)
Zoster, localized in immunocompromised patient or disseminated

Contact isolation

Contact isolation is designed to prevent transmission of highly transmissible or epidemiologically important infections (or colonization) that do not warrant strict isolation. All diseases or conditions included in this category are spread primarily by close or direct contact. Thus masks, gowns, and gloves are recommended for anyone in close or direct contact with any patient who has an infection (or colonization) included in this category. For individual diseases or conditions, however, one or more of these three barriers may not be indicated. For example, masks and gloves are not generally indicated for care of infants and young children with acute viral respiratory infections, gowns are not generally indicated for gonococcal conjunctivitis in newborns, and masks are not generally indicated for care of patients infected with multiple resistant microorganisms, except those with pneumonia. Therefore, some degree of "overisolation" may occur in this category.

From Garner JS, Simmons BP: Guidelines for isolation precautions in hospitals, *Infect Control* 4:245-325, 1983.
*A private room with special ventilation is indicated.

Specifications for contact isolation

1. Private room is indicated. In general, patients infected with the same organism may share a room. During outbreaks, infants and young children with the same respiratory clinical syndrome may share a room.
2. Masks are indicated for those who come close to the patient.
3. Gowns are indicated if soiling is likely.
4. Gloves are indicated for touching infective material.
5. Hands must be washed after touching the patient or potentially contaminated articles and before taking care of another patient.
6. Articles contaminated with infective material should be discarded or bagged and labeled before being sent for decontamination and reprocessing.

Diseases or conditions requiring contact isolation

Acute respiratory infections in infants and young children, including croup, colds, bronchitis, and bronchiolitis caused by respiratory syncytial virus, adenovirus, coronavirus, influenza viruses, parainfluenza viruses, and rhinovirus
Conjunctivitis, gonococcal, in newborns
Diphtheria, cutaneous
Endometritis, group A *Streptococcus*
Furunculosis, staphylococcal, in newborns
Herpes simplex, disseminated, severe primary or neonatal
Impetigo
Influenza, in infants and young children
Multiply resistant bacteria, infection of colonization (any site) with any of the following:
1. Gram-negative bacilli resistant to all aminoglycosides that are tested (in general, such organisms should be resistant to gentamicin, tobramycin, and amikacin for these special precautions to be indicated)
2. *Staphylococcus aureus* resistant to methicillin (or nafcillin or oxacillin if they are used instead of methicillin for testing)
3. *Pneumococcus* resistant to penicillin
4. *Haemophilus influenzae* resistant to ampicillin (beta lactamase positive) and chloramphenicol
5. Other resistant bacteria may be included if they are judged by the infection control team to be of special clinical and epidemiologic significance.
Pediculosis
Pharyngitis, infectious, in infants and young children
Pneumonia, viral in infants and young children

Pneumonia, *Staphylococcus aureus* or group A *Streptococcus*
Rabies
Rubella, congenital and other
Scabies
Scalded skin syndrome, staphylococcal (Ritter's disease)
Skin, wound, or burn infection, major (draining and not covered by dressing or dressing does not adequately contain the purulent material) including those infected with *Staphylococcus aureus* or group A *Streptococcus*
Vaccinia (generalized and progressive eczema vaccinatum)

Respiratory isolation

Respiratory isolation is designed to prevent transmission of infectious diseases primarily over short distances through the air (droplet transmission). Direct and indirect contact transmission occurs with some infections in this isolation category but is infrequent.

Specifications for respiratory isolation

1. Private room is indicated. In general, patients infected with the same organism may share a room.
2. Masks are indicated for those who come close to the patient.
3. Gowns are not indicated.
4. Gloves are not indicated.
5. Hands must be washed after touching the patient or potentially contaminated articles and before taking care of another patient.
6. Articles contaminated with infective material should be discarded or bagged and labeled before being sent for decontamination and reprocessing.

Diseases requiring respiratory isolation

Epiglottitis, *Haemophilus influenzae*
Erythema infectiosum
Measles
Meningitis
   Haemophilus influenzae, known or suspected
   Meningococcal, known or suspected
Meningococcal pneumonia
Meningococcemia
Mumps
Pertussis (whooping cough)
Pneumonia, *Haemophilus influenzae*, in children (any age)

Continued.

Category-specific isolation precautions—cont'd

Tuberculosis isolation (AFB isolation)

Tuberculosis isolation (AFB isolation) is an isolation category for patients with pulmonary tuberculosis who have a positive sputum smear or a chest x-ray film that strongly suggests current (active) tuberculosis. Laryngeal tuberculosis is also included in this isolation category. In general, infants and young children with pulmonary tuberculosis do not require isolation precautions because they rarely cough, and their bronchial secretions contain few AFB, compared with adults with pulmonary tuberculosis. On the instruction card, this category is called AFB isolation to protect the patient's privacy.

Specifications for tuberculosis isolation (AFB isolation)

1. Private room with special ventilation is indicated; door should be kept closed. In general, patients infected with the same organism may share a room.
2. Masks are indicated only if the patient is coughing and does not reliably cover mouth.
3. Gowns are indicated only if needed to prevent gross contamination of clothing.
4. Gloves are not indicated.
5. Hands must be washed after touching the patient or potentially contaminated articles and before taking care of another patient.
6. Articles are rarely involved in transmission of tuberculosis. However, articles should be thoroughly cleaned and disinfected, or discarded.

Enteric precautions

Enteric precautions are designed to prevent infections that are transmitted by direct or indirect contact with feces. Hepatitis A is included in this category because it is spread through feces, although the disease is much less likely to be transmitted after the onset of jaundice. Most infections in this category primarily cause gastrointestinal symptoms, but some do not. For example, feces from patients infected with "poliovirus" and coxsackieviruses are infective, but these infections do not usually cause prominent gastrointestinal symptoms.

Specifications for enteric precautions

1. Private room is indicated if patient hygiene is poor. A patient with poor hygiene does not wash hands after touching infective material, contaminates the environment with infective material, or shares contaminated articles with other patients. In general, patients infected with the same organism may share a room.
2. Masks are not indicated.
3. Gowns are indicated if soiling is likely.
4. Gloves are indicated when touching infective material.
5. Hands must be washed after touching the patient or potentially contaminated articles and before taking care of another patient.
6. Articles contaminated with infective material should be discarded or bagged and labeled before being sent for decontamination and reprocessing.

Diseases requiring enteric precautions

Amebic dysentery
Cholera
Coxsackievirus disease
Diarrhea, acute illness with suspected infectious etiology
Echovirus disease
Encephalitis (unless known not to be caused by enteroviruses)
Enterocolitis caused by *Clostridium difficile* or *Straphylococcus aureus*
Enteroviral infection
Gastroenteritis caused by
  Campylobacter species
  Cryptosporidium species
  Dientamoeba fragilis
  Escherichia coli (enterotoxic, enteropathogenic, or enteroinvasive)
  Giardia lamblia
  Salmonella species
  Shigella species
  Vibrio parahaemolyticus
  Viruses—including Norwalk agent and rotavirus
  Yersinia enterocolitica
  Unknown etiology but presumed to be an infectious agent
Hand, foot, and mouth disease
Hepatitis, viral, type A
Herpangina
Meningitis, viral (unless known not to be caused by enteroviruses)
Necrotizing enterocolitis
Pleurodynia
Poliomyelitis
Typhoid fever (*Salmonella typhi*)
Viral pericarditis, myocarditis, or meningitis (unless known not to be caused by enteroviruses)

Drainage/secretion precautions

Drainage/secretion precautions are designed to prevent infections that are transmitted by direct or indirect contact with purulent material or drainage from an infected body site. This newly created isolation category includes many infections formerly included in wound and skin precautions and discharge (lesion), and secretion (oral) precautions, which have been discontinued. Infectious diseases included in this category are those that result in the production of infective purulent material, drainage, or secretions, unless the disease is included in another isolation category that requires more rigorous precautions. For example, minor or limited skin, wound, or burn infections are included in this category, but major skin, wound, or burn infections are included in contact isolation.

Specifications for drainage/secretion precautions

1. Private room is not indicated.
2. Masks are not indicated.
3. Gowns are indicated if soiling is likely.
4. Gloves are indicated for touching infective material.
5. Hands must be washed after touching the patient or potentially contaminated articles and before taking care of another patient.
6. Articles contaminated with infective material should be discarded or bagged and labeled before being sent for decontamination and reprocessing.

Diseases requiring drainage/secretion precautions

Abscess, minor or limited
Burn infection, minor or limited
Conjunctivitis
Decubitus ulcer, infected, minor or limited
Skin infection, minor or limited
Wound infection, minor or limited
These infections are included in this category provided they are *not* (1) caused by multiple resistant microorganisms, (2) major (draining and not covered by a dressing or dressing does not adequately contain the drainage) skin, wound, or burn infections, including those caused by *Staphylococcus aureus* or group A *Streptococcus,* or (3) gonococcal eye infections in newborns. See contact isolation if the infection is one of these three.

Universal blood/body fluid precautions

Because medical history and examination cannot reliably identify all patients infected with HIV or other blood-borne pathogens, blood and body fluid precautions should be consistently used for all patients.

Specifications for universal blood/body fluid precautions

1. Gloves are worn for touching blood and body fluids, mucous membranes, or nonintact skin of all patients, for handling items or surfaces soiled with blood or body fluids, and for performing venipuncture and other vascular access procedures. Gloves should be changed after contact with each patient.
2. Masks and protective eyewear or face shields should be worn during procedures that are likely to generate droplets of blood or other body fluids to prevent exposure of mucous membranes of the mouth, nose, and eyes.
3. Gowns or aprons should be worn during procedures that are likely to generate splashes of blood or other body fluids.
4. Hands and other skin surfaces should be washed immediately and thoroughly if contaminated with blood or other body fluids. Hands should be washed immediately after gloves are removed.
5. Disposable articles contaminated with body substances should be bagged and discarded according to local and state regulations.
6. Care should be taken to avoid needle stick injuries. Used needles should not be recapped or bent; they should be placed in a designated puncture-resistant container as close to point of use as possible.
7. Blood spills should be cleaned up promptly with a solution of 5.25% sodium hypochlorite diluted 1:10 with water or an approved "hospital disinfectant" that is also tuberculocidal.

Universal blood and body fluid precautions protect the caregiver from blood-borne communicable diseases. Diseases recognized as being transmitted by blood include:

Acquired immunodeficiency syndrome (AIDS)
Arthropod-borne viral fevers (for example, dengue, yellow fever, and Colorado tick fever)
Babesiosis
Creutzfeldt-Jakob disease
Hepatitis B (including HBsAg carrier)
Hepatitis C
Leptospirosis
Malaria
Rat-bite fever
Relapsing fever
Syphilis, primary and secondary (skin and mucous membrane lesions)

17-12

Body substance isolation

All body substances are potentially infectious. Feces, sputum, and wound drainage always contain infectious organisms, whereas blood, urine, and other body fluids sometimes contain infectious organisms. The colonized, subclinical, and diagnosed infections are all communicable. However, category-specific or disease-specific isolation only protects against the diagnosed communicable infection. Therefore, protection against communicable disease transmission (health care worker and patient) can be achieved only by taking precautions with the body substances of all patients. Precautions should be determined by the anticipated interaction with a patient's body substances. Under this system, labeling patients with diagnosed infections would serve as a hindrance and support a double standard of practice. For example, a double standard exists when caregivers wear gloves when handling the urine of a patient with diagnosed *Serratia* urinary tract infection but not when handling the urine of other patients. Under BSI, the caregiver would be instructed to wear gloves for handling the urine of all patients.

Specifications for body substance isolation

1. Gloves for contact with mucous membranes, nonintact skin, and moist body substances. Gloves are changed after each patient contact.
2. Gown or plastic apron if soiling of clothing is likely.
3. Mask and eye protection if splashing of moist body substances is likely.
4. A private room is indicated if personal hygiene is poor or if body substances contaminate the environment.
5. Trash and linen bagged securely to prevent leakage.
6. Needles are disposed of uncapped and unbent at the point of use in a puncture-resistant container. Safe recapping using a one-handed or device-assisted technique is used when necessary.
7. Blood spills of all persons should be cleaned by a gloved person using a solution of 5.25% sodium hypochlorite (household bleach) diluted 1:10 in water or a hospital disinfectant that is tuberculocidal.
8. A sign explaining BSI technique is placed in each patient's room.
9. Patients with airborne transmitted diseases require a private room with a sign to alert persons to check with the nurse before entering the room. Special ventilation is indicated. A mask is required to enter the room of a patient with pulmonary tuberculosis or meningococcal disease. Only immune persons should enter the room of a patient with chickenpox.

From Lynch P, Jackson M: Isolation practices: How much is too much or not enough? *Asepsis: The Infection Control Forum* 8(4):2-5, 1986.

SUMMARY

1. Infection control programs originated to decrease morbidity, mortality, and cost of nosocomial infections.
2. The sequence of events in the chain of infection involve (1) a causative agent, (2) a reservoir, (3) a portal of exit, (4) a mode of transmission, (5) a portal of entry, and (6) a susceptible host.
3. Modes of transmission are (1) contact (direct, indirect, and droplet), (2) airborne, (3) vehicle, and (4) vector.
4. In a serious infection, the WBC count usually rises above $10,000/mm^3$.
5. Whenever possible, appropriate cultures should be obtained before the initiation of antibiotic therapy.
6. In the United States, the ACIP recommends that children be immunized against diphtheria, pertussis, and tetanus (DPT); measles, mumps, and rubella (MMR); *Haemophilus influenzae* b (HbCV) and poliomyelitis (OPV).
7. Health care givers who have frequent contact with blood and blood products should be immunized against hepatitis B virus.
8. Passive immunity is temporary, lasting a few weeks without stimulating antibody production in the recipient.
9. A nosocomial infection is one that is not present or incubating at the time a person is admitted to the hospital and develops after admission.
10. A community-acquired infection is one that is present or is incubating at the time of admission to the hospital.
11. Hand washing is the single most important measure in preventing cross-infections.
12. Urinary catheterization is associated with increased risk for nosocomial urinary tract infection.
13. Aseptic technique is an important factor in preventing nosocomial infection.
14. Two systems of isolation are (1) CDC category-specific isolation with universal blood/body fluid precautions and (2) body substance isolation (BSI).
15. Adherence to currently recommended isolation practices is the best protection that health care workers have from occupationally acquired infection.
16. Health care workers should direct problems concerning any aspect of infection control to the infection control nurse, the hospital epidemiologist, or the infection control committee in their institution.

REFERENCES AND SELECTED READINGS

1. American Hospital Association: AIDS/HIV infection policy: ensuring a safe hospital environment, *AHA Report*, pp 1-27, 1987.
2. American Public Health Association: *Control of communicable disease in man*, ed 15, New York, 1990, The Association.
3. Bennett JV, Brachman PS, editors: *Hospital infections*, Boston, 1986, Little, Brown & Co.
4. Bowell B: Assessing infection risk, *Nursing (London)* 4(12):12-23, 1990.
5. Centers for Disease Control: Nosocomial infection surveillance, 1984, *MMWR* 35(1SS):17-29, 1986.

6.* Centers for Disease Control: Recommendations for prevention of HIV transmission in health-care settings, *MMWR* 36(2S):3-17, 1987.

7.* Centers for Disease Control: Perspectives in disease prevention and health promotion: Public Health Services Guidelines for counseling and antibody testing to prevent HIV infection and AIDS, *MMWR* 36(31):509-515, 1987.

8. Centers for Disease Control: Recommendations of the Immunization Practices Committee (ACIP): Pneumococcal polysaccharide vaccine, *MMWR* 38(5):64-76, 1989.

9. Centers for Disease Control: Recommendations of the Immunization Practices Advisory Committee (ACIP): General recommendations on immunization, *MMWR* 38(13):206-227, 1989.

10.* Centers for Disease Control: Recommendations of the Immunization Practices Advisory Committee (ACIP): Protection against viral hepatitis, *MMWR* 39(RR-2):1-26, 1990.

11. Centers for Disease Control: Recommendations of the Immunization Practices Committee (ACIP): Prevention and control of influenza, *MMWR* 39(RR-7):1-15, 1990.

12. Centers for Disease Control: Guidelines for preventing the transmission of tuberculosis in health-care settings with special focus on HIV-related issues, *MMWR* 39(RR-17):1-28, 1990.

13. Centers for Disease Control: Update: Transmission of HIV infection during an invasive dental procedure—Florida, *MMWR* 40(2):21-27, 1991.

14. Centers for Disease Control: Recommendations of the Immunization Practices Advisory Committee (ACIP): Diptheria, tetanus, and pertussis: recommendations for vaccine use and other preventive measures, *MMWR* 40(RR-10):1-28, 1991.

15. *A clinician's dictionary of bacteria and fungi,* Indianapolis, 1986, Eli Lilly.

16.* Cooper D: Optimizing wound healing, *Nurs Clin North Am* 25(1):165-180, 1990.

17. Craven DE, Steger KA, Barber TW: Preventing nosocomial pneumonia: state of the art and perspectives for the 1990s, *Am J Med* 91(suppl 3B):44-53, 1991.

18. Friedland GH, Klein RS: Transmission of human immunodeficiency virus, *N Engl J Med* 317(18):1125-1135, 1987.

19. Garner JS, et al: CDC definitions for nosocomial infections, *Am J Infect Control* 16:128-140, 1988.

20. Gaynes RP: The NNIS system: plans for the 1990s and beyond, *Am J Med* 91(suppl 3B):116-120, 1991.

21.* Gerberding JL: Reducing occupational risk of HIV infection, *Hosp Prac* June 15, 1991, pp 103-117.

22. Gerberding JL, Henderson DK: Design of rational infection control policies for human immunodeficiency viral infection, *J Infect Dis* 156(6):861-864, 1987.

23. Haley RW: The nationwide nosocomial infection rate: a new need for vital statistics, *Am J Epidemiol* 121(2):159-166, 1985.

24. Haley RW: Measuring the costs of nosocomial infections: methods for estimating economic burden on the hospital, *Am J Med* 91(suppl 3B):32-38, 1991.

25. Haley RW, et al: The efficacy of infection surveillance and control programs in preventing nosocomial infections in US hospitals, *Am J Epidemiol* 121(2):206-215, 1985.

26. Healthy people 2000: National health promotion and disease prevention objectives, US Department of Health and Human Services, Washington, DC, 1990.

27. Infection control in critical care units, *Crit Care Nurs Quart* 11(4), 1989.

28.* Jagger J, Pearson RD: Universal precautions: still missing the point on needlesticks, *Infect Control Hosp Epidemiol* 12(4):211-213, 1991.

29. Kunin C: *Detection, prevention, and management of urinary tract infections,* ed 4, Philadelphia, 1987, Lea & Febiger.

30. Larson E: Infection control, *Ann Rev Nurs Res* 7:95-113, 1989.

31. Lynch P, Jackson M: Isolation practices: how much is too much or not enough? Asepsis: the Infection Control Forum 8(4):2-5, 1986.

32.* Lynch P, et al: Why not treat all body substances as infectious? *Am J Nurs* 15(3):1137-1139, 1987.

33.* Mooney BR, Armington LC: Infection control—how to prevent nosocomial infections, *RN* 50(9):21-23, 1987.

34. Nafziger DA, Wenzel RP: Catheter-related infections: reducing the risk and the consequences, *J Crit Illness* 5(8):857-865, 1990.

35. Nichols RL: Surgical wound infection, *Am J Med* 91(suppl 3B):54-64, 1991.

36. Norwood S, et al: Catheter-related infections and associated septicemia, *Chest* 99(4)968-75, 1991.

36a. Shovein J, Young MS: MRSA: Pandora's box for hospitals, *Amer J Nurs* 92(2):48-52.

37. Stamm WE: Catheter-associated urinary tract infections: epidemiology, pathogenesis, and prevention, *Am J Med* 91(suppl 3B):65-75, 1991.

38.* Wysocki AB: Surgical wound healing, *AORN* 49(2):502-524, 1989.

Classic

39. Garner JS, Simmons BP: Guideline for isolation precautions in hospitals, *Infect Control* 4(4):245-325, 1983.

40. Larson E: Clinical microbiology and infection control, 1984, Cambridge, Mass, Blackwell Scientific Publications.

*Recommended for student reading.

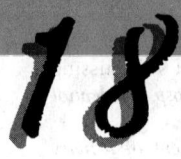

18

Sexually Transmitted Diseases

Wilma J. Phipps

After studying this chapter, the learner should be able to:

- Define sexually transmitted diseases (STDs).
- Describe the transmission, prevention, and control of STDs.
- List the causative agent, incubation period, signs and symptoms, medical therapy, and long-term effects of gonorrhea, syphilis, herpes genitalis, and chlamydia infection.
- Describe the subjective and objective data to be collected from a person suspected of having an STD.
- Write a teaching plan for a unit on the prevention of STDs for a sex education course for adolescents.

ETIOLOGY/EPIDEMIOLOGY

Sexually transmitted diseases (STDs) are diseases that usually are or can be transmitted from one person to another with heterosexual or homosexual intercourse or intimate contact with the genitalia, mouth, or rectum. Until the 1980s, only five veneral diseases (syphilia, gonorrhea, chancroid, lymphogranuloma venereum, and granuloma inguinale) were regularly monitored. In the 1980s several diseases were added to the list of STDs. These include *Chlamydia trachomatis,* genital herpes, human papillomavirus, genital mycoplasmas, cytomegalovirus, hepatitis B, vaginitis, enteric infections, and ectoparasitic disease.[14]

Early in the 1980s the human immunodeficiency virus (HIV) was identified and AIDS emerged as a major sexually transmitted disease. Because of its profound affect on the immune system Chapter 19 is devoted to the discussion of AIDS.

The diseases classified as STDs and their causative organisms are listed in Box 18-1. Because of improved laboratory and epidemiologic methods, the prevalence, modes of transmission, and clinical consequences of these newer STDs are better understood than in earlier decades. In addition, many of the newly recognized STDs have become epidemic or hyperendemic as a consequence of changing sexual behavioral patterns. Not only has the incidence of many STDs increased, but for agents with multiple modes of transmission (for example, hepatitis B virus, enteric pathogens), the proportion of infections that are transmitted sexually has also increased. In addition to the immediate consequences of STDs there are the recognized effects on maternal and infant morbidity as well as on human reproduction and fertility.

All states require that each case of syphilis and gonorrhea be reported to the state or local health officer. Most states also require the reporting of chancroid, granuloma inguinale, and lymphogranuloma venereum. Herpes genitalis, trichomoniasis, and candidiasis do not need to be reported in any state. The true incidence of STDs is not known because of variable reporting requirements and also because many cases are not reported by the clinicians who treat them.

In the United States almost 12 million cases of STDs occur yearly, 86% of them in persons aged 15 to 29 years. By the age of 21, approximately one out of every five young persons has undergone treatment for a sexually transmitted disease. Because only some teenagers are sexually active, this amounts to an effective rate of at least 25% among those who are sexually active.[14]

In addition, to the immediate consequences of STDs there are serious complications, most of which have the greatest impact on women and children. The most serious complications are pelvic inflammatory disease (PID), sterility, ectopic pregnancy, blindness, cancer associated with the human papillomavirus, fetal and infant deaths, birth defects, and mental retardation. The proportion of the population most affected are the medically underserved, the poor and racial and ethnic minorities.[14] The total societal costs of STDs exceeds $315 billion annually, with the cost of PID and PID-associated ectopic pregnancy and infertility alone exceeding $2.6 billion.

In explaining the trends of reported cases of STDs in the United States, *three changes* occurring since the 1960s are often referred to in the literature. The *first* of these concerns the use of antibiotics and changes in the antibiotic susceptibility of pathogenic organisms. The widespread, perhaps indiscriminate, use of penicillin and other antibiotics between the late 1940s and early 1950s parrallels the decline in both syphilis and gonorrhea. It is said that the organisms developed a greater resistance to antibiotics over time and that antibiotics have therefore become less effective than previously. There is no firm evidence to indicate a decrease in effectiveness of penicillin against syphilis. However, the gonococcus tends to develop resistance to antibiotics and this has been increasing.

A *second* explanation for the rise in incidence of STDs is that they are more likely to occur if a social system is permissive. During times of war and other catastrophes, it is easier for agencies to control interpersonal behavior, whereas in times of peace and absence of national crisis, civil liberties tend to flourish. The incidence curve of syphilis and gonorrhea after the years of World War II seems to support this thesis.

The *third* explanation centers around sexual behavior patterns and includes permissiveness. Concern has been expressed particularly about the prevalence of gonorrhea among adolescents and young adults who are considered to be promiscuous. In fact, rates for gonorrhea show young adults of 20 to 24 years of age accounted for 40% of reported cases of gonorrhea, while persons 15 to 19 years of age accounted for 25% of cases. The highest morbidity for males was in the 20- to 24-year age group; for females it was in the 15- to 19-year age group.

The above discussion makes an assumption of sexual promiscuity, and in doing so, requires acknowledgement of advances in contraceptive technology, especially "the pill." These social changes are often termed the three Ps (permissiveness, promiscuity, and the pill).[49] The underlying idea is that, with the advent of antibiotics and the pill, people began to lose fear of untreated venereal disease and pregnancy and that sexual promiscuity increased significantly, leading to increased exposure to infection.

If the definition of promiscuity is that sexual relations are not restricted to one partner, studies show that patients diagnosed in clinics as having STD are not promiscuous.

	Sexually transmitted diseases	
Type of organism	**Disease**	
Bacteria	Gonorrhea, chancroid, granuloma inguinale, *Gardnerella vaginalis*	
Spirochete	Syphilis	
Chlamydia	Nongonococcal urethritis, epididymitis, cervicitis, PID, lymphogranuloma venereum	
Virus	Herpes genitalis, hepatitis B, cytomegalovirus, AIDS, genital warts	
Protozoa	Trichomoniasis	
Yeast	Candidiasis	
Parasites	Pediculosis pubis, scabies	

18-1

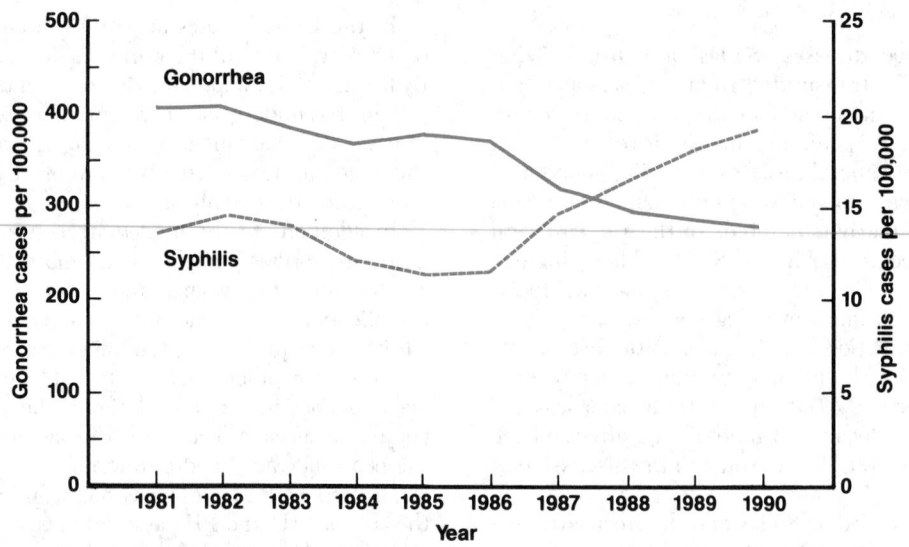

Fig. 18-1 Trend in the incidence of gonorrhea and primary and secondary syphilis, 1981 to 1990. (From Centers for Disease Control: Summary of notifiable diseases 1990, *MMWR* 39(53):1990.)

In one study 66.4% of patients having an STD named only one sexual contact. It must be realized, however, that persons may hesitate to admit to having more than one sex partner for any number of reasons.

In the past, prostitution has been considered a major force in the transmission of STDs. Before World War II it was estimated that approximately 75% of all STDs could be traced to prostitutes and that at least 10% of all prostitutes had contracted an STD at least once. Today less than 5% of patients with syphilis can be classed as prostitutes. Also, most persons with gonorrhea are single and under 25 years of age, and most clients of prostitutes are usually older, married men. *Chlamydia trachomatis* and herpes are two STDs that are very common in middle-class America.

Before 1960, homosexuals were rarely mentioned in the literature as carriers of STDs. Since the early 1970s much more attention has been given to the risk of STDs among homosexual and bisexual men. Homosexual men carry pathogens in the rectum and colon, including gonococcus, *Giardia,* ameba, *Shigella,* and *Camphylobacter.* Although lesbians are at low risk for contracting STDs and gay males are at higher risk, it is important to note that sexual orientation does not prescribe individual forms of sexual behavior.

The condom was the main method of contraception used before the advent of antibiotics and oral contraceptives. The use of the condom may have prevented the spread of the STDs by providing a mechanical barrier to the organisms. The pill revolutionized contraception practices, and it is known that neutralization of the vaginal and cervical environment by estrogenic substances predisposes to infection.

Several events during the 1980s bear mentioning. They are:

1. The designation of AIDS as a sexually transmitted disease put other STDs in competition with it for attention and resources.[7]

2. Studies of the sociodemographic and geographic distribution of gonorrhea clearly indicate that the transmission of gonorrhea is predicated on the existence of small groups of persons who share common sociodemographic, behavioral, and geographic characteristics of a so-called "core group." This concept was verified empirically in such diverse locations as New York state; Colorado Springs, Colorado; Dade County Florida; and Liverpool, England. With the understanding of a core group pattern comes the opportunity to design intervention programs tailored to the group at risk.

3. During the 1980s there was a substantial decline in the occurrence of gonorrhea. However, this decline was accompanied by an increase in penicillin-resistant organisms and further concentration of the disease in young minority populations.

4. While the incidence of gonorrhea decreased, the incidence of syphilis increased dramatically (Fig. 18-1). In 1990, the 50,223 reported cases of primary and secondary syphilis were the single largest yearly total since 1948. This epidemic is occurring primarily among young, heterosexual, minority populations and may be related to cocaine use and exchange of sex for drugs, especially crack cocaine.[7]

SEXUAL TRANSMISSION

The STDs are contagious diseases spread almost exclusively by contact during sexual intercourse; that is, when mucous membrane surfaces come in contact during genital, oral, or anal sexual activity. Because the causative organisms survive only very briefly outside a warm, moist environment, there is almost no way to contract STDs from toilet seats, towels, or bed linens. Although STDs are not usually transmitted in public restrooms, conditions caused by fungi, bacteria, and lice can be transmitted from water in unclean toilet bowls. Women using a conventional toilet expose the vaginal and anal area to pathogens that can be introduced by the back splash of contaminated toilet water.

There are some notable exceptions to sexual transmission. During pregnancy the fetus may become infected in utero by placental transmission, and the infant may acquire congenital syphilis or be stillborn. Infants of mothers with gonorrhea may contract infections of the eyes (ophthalmia neonatorum) during birth, and unless treated, this can lead to permanent blindness.

Prevention and Health Education

Prevention and control measures for STDs include three levels of prevention. *Primary prevention* is directed at preventing the disease. This includes educating uninfected persons so that they can take responsibility for their own health and not expose themselves to an infected person; identification and treatment of exposed persons who are asymptomatic; interviewing persons with infection for identification of contacts; examination and preventive treatment of contacts; educational programs for the public; and active involvement of professionals in programs of control. The goal of these efforts includes eradication of the reservoir of disease in the population. *Secondary prevention* is directed toward prevention of complications. *Tertiary prevention* focuses on the following: (1) prevention of complications, (2) supporting and counseling infected persons to receive treatment, and (3) asking infected persons to notify their sexual partners so that they can be examined and treated if infected.

Partner notification (contact investigation)

In the prevention and control of STDs, especially gonorrhea, emphasis was once placed on interviewing for information regarding sexual contacts. The named contacts were sought out for examination and treatment. Lay people knowledgeable about the required reporting to the local health department of some of the diseases were very hesitant to name their sexual contacts. Young people often feared that their parents and the parents of the sexual partner would find out about their infection. Minors need to know that they can probably obtain treatment without parental consent. Presently most states permit physicians to treat minors for STDs without obtaining parental consent, and several states are proposing changes in existing legislation restricting treatment of minors. People also may perceive reporting of STDs as a threat from an official agency and may hesitate to name their contacts out of a sense of protection if they do not know that no punishment is involved.

Interviewing the patient for contacts is done at the time of the initial visit in the event that the patient does not return for follow up. It is probably best that this interview takes place after the patient is examined, the type of infection is determined, and the treatment is prescribed. If assessment is accompanied by information giving, the person should be better informed about STDs and how they are treated, and be more willing and able to give information about sexual contacts.

Interviewing for contacts involves two aspects. The patient is first asked to name sexual contacts. Second, the patient is interviewed for "cluster suspects," who are friends or acquaintances who may have been exposed to the same contacts, or who have symptoms of an STD.

Because one focus of STD control is increasing self-referrals, the patient is asked to inform known contacts (partner notification) and cluster suspects to come in for examination and treatment. Confidentiality is stressed. There is reason to believe that patients do not name all their contacts at the time of the first interview and that a reinterview will usually result in additional names of contacts. Because of the understandable reluctance of many people to name their sexual contacts, the patient may be given the responsibility of informing the contacts and advising them of their need for treatment. (The contacts are not named, but instead cards that permit both examination and treatment without identification are given to the contacts by the patient.) Local health departments cooperate in locating, examining, and treating these contacts as necessary.

Whenever possible, the contacts of the infected person are located and advised to have an examination and tests as soon as possible. If the sexual partner(s) does not have symptoms of infection at the time of the first examination, treatment is instituted to abort infection. Giving preventive treatment to named contacts who have no clinical evidence of infection has gained popularity and acceptance in the United States, and there are indications that this same approach is being used more often in management of patients having the "minor" STDs.

CURRENT NEEDS

In its Annual Report for 1990, the Division of STD/HIV Prevention of the Centers for Disease Control defined the problem as follows:

> Sexually transmitted diseases continue as one of the nation's most serious public health problems. Not only is HIV infection the most devastating public health problem of this century, but also infectious syphilis has continued an unprecedented increase since the advent of penicillin therapy; resistant gonococcal infection is steadily increasing; chlamydial infections account for twice as many cases as gonorrhea; studies of human papillomavirus associate it with the development of cervical dysplasia; and trichomoniasis and other vaginal infections are being recognized as potently major contributors to premature birth.

In addition the CDC lists estimates that threaten the health of Americans, primarily adolescents and young adults (Box 18-2).

18-2

Estimated STD threats

1.4 million cases of gonorrhea
130,000 cases of syphilis
4 million cases of chlamydia
500,000-1,000,000 cases of human papillomavirus
200-500,000 cases of genital herpes
3 million cases of trichomoniasis
270,000-300,000 cases of hepatitis B
1.2 million cases of urethritis (non GC, non-CT)
1 million cases of mucopurulent cervicitis (non-C, not CT)

GOALS FOR THE FUTURE

Healthy People 2000 established several goals to be attained by year 2000.[14] These are listed below.

1. Reduce gonorrhea to an incidence of no more than 225 cases per 100,000 people as compared with a baseline of 300 per 100,000 in 1989.
2. Reduce *Chlamydia trachomatis* infections, as measured by a decrease in the incidence of nongonoccal urethritis, to no more than 170 cases per 100,000 people compared with a baseline of 215 cases per 100,000 cases in 1988.
3. Reduce primary and secondary syphilis to an incidence of no more than 10 cases per 100,000 people, as compared with a baseline of 18.1 per 100,000 in 1989.
4. Reduce congenital syphilis to an incidence of no more than 50 cases per 100,000 live births from a baseline of 100 per 100,000 live births in 1989.
5. Reduce herpes and genital warts, as measured by a reduction to 142,000 and 385,000 respectively, in the annual number of first-time consultations with a physician for these conditions. The baseline for 1988 was 167,000 and 451,000 cases per 100,000 persons respectively.
6. Reduce the incidence of pelvic inflammatory disease, as measured by a reduction in hospitalizations for pelvic inflammatory disease to no more than 250 per 100,000 women aged 15 to 44. The baseline was 311 per 100,000 in 1988.
7. Reduce sexually transmitted hepatitis B infection to no more than 30,500 cases from a baseline of 58,300 cases in 1988.

Risk reduction objectives to assist in achieving the above goals include the following:[14]

1. Reduce the proportion of adolescents who have engaged in sexual intercourse to no more than 15% by age 15 and no more than 40% by age 17. The baseline was 27% of girls and 33% of boys by age 15; 50% of girls and 66% of boys by age 17, as reported in 1988.
2. Increase to at least 50% the proportion of sexually active, unmarried people who used a condom at last sexual intercourse. The baseline was 19% of sexually active, unmarried women aged 15 to 44 who reported that their partners used a condom at last intercourse in 1988.

The special target population targets for this objective appear in Table 18-1.

To achieve these very important goals, changes need to occur in agencies that deliver primary care such as family planning clinics, maternal and child health clinics, drug treatment centers, and primary care clinics that screen, diagnose, treat, counsel, and provide (or refer for) partner notification services for HIV infection and bacterially sexual transmitted disease (gonorrhea, syphilis, and chlamydia). The CDC wants the goals to occur in at least 50% of the health care providers as compared with 40% of family planning clinics for 1989.

Another need to achieve the objectives relates to education of the young. The CDC recommends that instruction in STD prevention be included in the curricula of all middle and secondary schools, preferably as part of quality school health education.

In addition, to increase to at least 90% the proportion of primary care providers treating patients with STDs who correctly managed cases, as measured by their use of appropriate types and amounts of therapy. The baseline was 70% in 1988. The success of this objective will be monitored by the number of women treated for gonorrhea and pelvic inflammatory disease. For example, one study found that only 10% of primary care providers assessed the sexual behavior of their patients. Also, a large proportion of providers did not prescribe combination antibiotics to treat polymicrobial PID.

Another need to achieve the goals relates to counseling services. It is recommended that at least 75% of primary care and mental health care providers provide age-appropriate counseling on the prevention of HIV and other STDs. As mentioned above, baseline figures for 1987 indicate that only 10% of physicians reported that they regularly assessed the sexual behaviors of their patients in 1987.[14]

The goals for year 2000 also recommend an increase to at least 50% for the proportion of all patients with bacterial sexually transmitted diseases (gonorrhea, syphilis, and chlamydia) who are offered provider referral services. The baseline was 20% of those treated in STD clinics in 1988.

Provider referral services (previously called *contact tracing*) is the process by which health department personnel notify the sexual partners of infected individuals that they have been exposed to an infectious disease. The goal of provider referral is to find other persons who may be infected and to get them under treatment so that they can be adequately treated and the transmission of the STD is stopped within the community. Proper treatment also helps prevent complications among those already infected.[14]

Table 18-1 Special population targets for condom use

Use of condoms	1988 baseline	2000 target
Sexually active young women aged 15-19 (by their partners)	25%	60%
Sexually active young men aged 15-19	57%	75%
Intravenous drug abusers	—	60%

Table 18-2   Selected sexually transmitted diseases

Disease	Incubation period	Signs and symptoms	Medical therapy
Gonorrhea	Men: 3 to 30 days Women: 3 days to an indefinite period	Men: purulent urethral discharge, dysuria, epididymitis, prostatitis Women: asymptomatic in early stages; cervicitis with purulent discharge, bartholinitis, salpingitis	Ceftriaxone 250 mg IM once plus doxycycline 10 mg PO twice a day for 7 days
Syphilis	3 weeks (9 days to 3 months)	Positive serologic tests, chancre in stage I	Benzathine penicillin G 2.4 million units IM
Herpes genitalis	3 to 14 days	Vesicles that rupture and form ulcerations, pain, inguinal lymph node enlargement, dysuria, flulike symptoms	Symptomatic; topical acyclovir
Chlamydia	5 to 10 days or longer	Women: painful or difficult urination, abnormal vaginal discharge or bleeding, pain or bleeding with coitus, irregular menses. One third are asymptomatic. Men: testicular pain, nonspecific urethritis or epididymitis	Doxycycline 100 mg PO twice a day for 7 days or tetracycline 500 mg PO 4 times a day for 7 days
Condylomata acuminata (genital warts)	1 to 6 months	Horny papules on vulva, vagina, cervix, perineum, anal canal, urethra, glans penis	Cryotherapy

Even though the provider may be involved in the notification process, it is crucial that infected persons be supported and coached so that they can do partner notification themselves. This is especially so because provider referral is labor intensive and current resources (budget constraints) may not allow health departments to notify all persons named by infected persons. Partner notification should help the infected person internalize the need to assume more responsibility for his or her health and for the well-being of their sexual partners.[14]

SIGNS AND SYMPTOMS

Vaginitis, cervicitis, lower abdominal pain, urethritis, epididymitis, pharyngitis, proctitis, and skin or mucous membrane lesions are common in persons with STDs (see Table 18-2). Some people may be asymptomatic.

MEDICAL THERAPY

Treatment depends on the causative organisms identified through the history, physical examination, and laboratory tests and is discussed in detail in the following pages. It is not unusual for an individual to harbor two or more organisms simultaneously.

Nursing Process
Assessment
Subjective data

The following information is collected from the person suspected of having an STD:
1. Exposure to STD contact including HIV
2. Prior STD history, treatment
3. Sexual orientation: "Have you been having sex with men, women, or both?"
4. Timing of last sexual activity
5. Number of sexual partners in the past 2 months
6. Women are questioned about:
   a. Vaginal discharge
   b. Vulvar itching
   c. Dysuria
   d. Urinary urgency
   e. Lower abdominal pain
   f. Rectal symptoms
   g. Sore throat
   h. Genital lesions
   i. Skin rashes or itching
   j. Menstrual periods
7. Heterosexual men are questioned about:
   a. Urethral discharge
   b. Dysuria
   c. Genital lesions
   d. Skin rashes
   e. Itching
   f. Testicular pain
   g. Sore throat

8. Gay or bisexual men are asked the same questions as heterosexual men plus the following:
   a. Rectal symptoms such as pain, bleeding, discharge, and diarrhea
9. If hepatitis is also suspected, the person is questioned about:
   a. Dark-colored urine
   b. Clay-colored stools
   c. Fatigue
   d. Jaundice

Objective data

Objective data include the following:
1. Inspection and palpation of the integumentary system, reproductive system, and anorectal area.
2. Examination for women includes the following:
   a. Inspection of skin of lower abdomen, inguinal area, hands, palms, and forearms
   b. Inspection of pubic hair for lice and mites
   c. Inspection and palpation of external genitalia, including perineum and anus
   d. Speculum examination of vagina and cervix
   e. Bimanual pelvic examination
   f. Palpation for inguinal and femoral lymphadenopathy
   g. Inspection of mouth and throat, including tonsils
3. Examination of heterosexual men includes the following:
   a. Inspection of the skin and pubic hair
   b. Inspection of the penis, including the meatus, with retraction of the foreskin and "milking" of the urethra
   c. Palpation of the scrotum
4. Examination of homosexual or bisexual men is the same as for heterosexual men plus the following:
   a. Inspection of the mouth, throat including the tonsils, and anorectal area
   b. Anoscopic examination if there are rectal symptoms

Diagnostic tests

Specific diagnostic tests are used to establish the diagnosis of each of these diseases. Diagnostic tests will be discussed under the specific disease later in this chapter.

Data analysis: nursing diagnoses

Nursing diagnoses are determined from analysis of patient data. Possible nursing diagnoses for the person with a sexually transmitted disease, may include but are not limited to, the following:

Diagnostic title	Possible etiologies
Knowledge deficit	Lack of exposure/recall, information misinterpretation, lack of familiarity with information sources about STDs
Health maintenance, altered	Lack of knowledge, cultural practices, lack of material resources

Planning: expected patient outcomes

Expected patient outcomes for the person with a sexually transmitted disease may include, but are not limited to, the following:
1. Person and/or partner can explain the etiology and factors contributing to the STD.
2. Person and/or partner can state the name, dosage, and schedule of administration of drug therapy, as well as its possible side effects.
3. Person and/or partner can explain the need for adherence to the entire treatment regimen.
4. Person and/or partner can state the reasons for abstaining from sexual activity during the infectious stages of the STD.
5. Person and/or partner can state effects of the STD on the reproductive system of oneself and one's partner.
6. Person and/or partner can state indications for seeking immediate health care if signs and symptoms reappear.
7. Person and/or partner can explain necessity for treatment of sexual partner or partners.
8. Person and/or partner can accept the occurrence of the STD.
9. Person and/or partner can explain how to prevent the transmission of STDs by using safer sex practices including the type of condom to use, when and how to apply it, and how to remove it. Recommendations on the proper use of condoms to prevent transmission of STDs can be found in Box 18-3.

Implementation
Assisting with achievement of therapeutic goals

Medical therapy for each STD will be discussed under the specific diseases.

Interventions to achieve patient outcomes
Facilitating learning

The nurse's first responsibility in STD control is to educate patients who have a sexually transmitted infection or may develop one. Nurses must be knowledgeable about the diseases most prevalent, the signs and symptoms, methods used in diagnosis, treatments used, and where individuals can obtain help and information. They also can influence the knowledge and attitudes of their colleagues and peers toward STD and its control. Nurses can exert influence in the community by taking an active role in programs of education. Perhaps the best way to reduce the risk of STD is for persons who are sexually active to know their sexual partners. Sexual activity with different partners increases the risk of infection.

Preventive measures such as washing or showering with soap and water and using a condom are recommended but are no guarantee against STD. Good laundry and personal hygiene practices also may help reduce risk.

Before nurses can be effective in working with patients who have STDs, they must confront their own feelings and attitudes about STDs. The patient is often young, fearful of pain, and unaccustomed to surroundings in a clinic or physician's office. Young patients especially fear that their families and friends may learn they have an STD.

18-3

Recommendations from the CDC for the use of condoms

The following recommendations for proper use of condoms to reduce the transmission of STD are based on current information:

1. Latex condoms should be used because they offer greater protection against viral STD than natural membrane condoms.
2. Condoms should be stored in a cool, dry place out of direct sunlight.
3. Condoms in damaged packages or those that show obvious signs of age (for example, those that are brittle, sticky, or discolored) should not be used. They cannot be relied upon to prevent infection.
4. Condoms should be handled with care to prevent puncture.
5. The condom should be put on before any genital contact to prevent exposure to fluids that may contain infectious agents. Hold the tip of the condom and unroll it onto the erect penis, leaving space at the tip to collect semen, yet ensuring that no air is trapped in the tip of the condom.
6. Adequate lubrication should be used. If exogenous lubrication is needed, only water-based lubricants should be used. Petroleum- or oil-based lubricants (such as petroleum jelly, cooking oils, shortening, and lotions) should not be used because they weaken the latex.
7. Use of condoms containing spermicides may provide some additional protection against STD. However, vaginal use of *spermicides* along with condoms is likely to provide greater protection.
8. If a condom breaks, it should be replaced immediately. If ejaculation occurs after condom breakage, the immediate use of spermicide has been suggested. However, the protective value of postejaculation application of spermicide in reducing the risk of STD transmission is unknown.
9. After ejaculation, care should be taken so that the condom does not slip off the penis before withdrawal; the base of the condom should be held while withdrawaling. The penis should be withdrawn while still erect.
10. Condoms should never be reused.

From US Department of Health and Human Service, Public Health Services; Condoms for the prevention of sexually transmitted disease, MMWR 37(9):133-137, 1988.

Once the diagnosis, tentative or conclusive, is made, focus should first be placed on obtaining a cure and preventing complications and reinfection. Many lay people know that the treatment for syphilis and gonorrhea is penicillin, but they may not be fully informed about this and other aspects of treatment. Because some of the diseases respond to penicillin or other antibiotics, many people believe that all genital infections can be cured easily, and this is not so. Some people believe that antibiotics not only cure an infection but that they produce immunity against

reinfection well. Persons receiving an antibiotic or other medications for STDs must be informed of the action of the drug, its duration of effectiveness, side effects, chances of cure, and the need for follow-up. They need to be advised that treatment failures do occur and that reinfection rates are high. Return visits should be encouraged whenever possible, because adequacy of treatment of all of the STDs is evaluated best by laboratory analysis for the specific organism.

Providing social and emotional support

Many patients focus on how the diseases are spread rather than on the consequences of having an infection. For single persons, contracting an STD and securing help means they must admit to sexual activity, and some of them may feel guilty. Their self-esteem may be threatened by what has happened to them. Patients with an STD have not only a physical but a social, emotional, and perhaps economic problem as well. They need constructive and comprehensive help. The nurse who is successful in working with persons having an STD is one who can create an atmosphere of trust in which the person feels free to discuss all aspects of the problem.

Persons who seek help recognize they have a problem; they want to get better and stay well. Because of this they are highly motivated to do what is necessary, receptive to information and advice, and attentive when advice is given. Nurses can take advantage of the patient's readiness to learn and motivation to improve and maintain health.

Promoting self-care

Persons treated for sexually transmitted infections need information about self-care. To understand their therapy and to responsibly engage in self-care, they must be informed about the sexual nature of the infection, how it is transmitted, and the *possibility of reinfection and infection of their sexual partner or partners*. The patient needs to know that it is important for sexual partners to be checked for signs of infection, to be advised of what the signs are, and have a culture for asymptomatic infection. Patients should be advised to abstain from intercourse until cured. *It also should be stressed that condoms should be used to prevent infection or reinfection, if persons persist in engaging in intercourse even when advised not to.*

Teaching about hygiene and personal health practices is beneficial in reducing the chances of secondary infection, recurrence, and infections of various types in the future. Frequent bathing and hand washing are indicated. It is known that many of the organisms causing STDs are destroyed by soap and water. *For women, douching is contraindicated unless it is prescribed for the purpose of applying heat or applying medication.* All women should be informed that, for personal cleanliness, frequent douching at any time is *not* advisable, because this may disturb the vaginal and cervical environments and predispose the woman to infection. If douching is prescribed by the physician, the patient should be instructed in the procedure.

If the lesions are present on body surfaces, the patient should be instructed in their care. Unless contraindicated, a hot bath is taken two to three times a day; and lesions are kept as dry as possible between baths. Both men and women should be advised to wear cotton underwear, and women should be advised to avoid wearing pantyhose, because they tend to trap moisture and prevent circulation of air to the genitalia. Unless they are specifically prescribed as local medications, the patient should not apply any lotion, cream, or ointment to any of the lesions associated with an STD.

Self-examination is important for sexually active people, especially those with more than one partner. Inspecting skin, mouth, genitals, and perianal areas for lesions and discharges is recommended. In addition, people can learn to casually inspect their partners during the initial period of lovemaking to identify any signs of STDs. Urinating after sexual activity can be helpful in cleansing the urethra of organisms.

Promoting healthy sexual attitudes

Opportunities for promoting healthy attitudes about sexual activity and STDs frequently arise. These topics are approached tactfully and with consideration of the patient's feelings. Adolescents especially require an approach that indicates understanding balanced with the ability to help them set limits. They need to understand that they are responsible for their own bodies and they do not have to give in to sexual pressures. It is well documented, however, that the strongest influence on teenagers comes from their peer group. For this reason, discussion with groups of teenagers about their sexual responsibilities may be helpful. In the climate of the 1990s there should be no doubt that abstinence is the only absolute way to prevent STD. If a teen elects to be sexually active he or she needs to understand that the consequences of unprotected sex may include unwanted pregnancy and STD. Monogamous relationships and the proper use of condoms should be stressed for those who are sexually active.

Evaluation

Evaluation is based on the expected patient outcomes. Questions to be asked include the person's and/or partner's ability to do the following:

1. State the factors that contributed to the present infection with STD (multiple sexual partners; not using a condom).
2. State the drug therapy to be followed including name of drug, dosage, schedule of administration, and side effects.
3. Explain why the therapy must be taken without interruption (to prevent resistant strains of organisms from developing).
4. State why he or she should not engage in sexual activity while the STD is infectious.
5. State effects of STDs that may develop in the reproductive system of either partner.
6. State signs and symptoms (fever, pain, discharge) that indicate need for immediate health care.
7. Verbalize understanding of the necessity of treatment for his or her sexual partner or partners.
8. Verbalize that she or he has an STD and identify ways to prevent further STD infections.
9. Explain what is meant by practicing "safer sex" including what type of condom to use, when and how to apply it, and how to remove it.

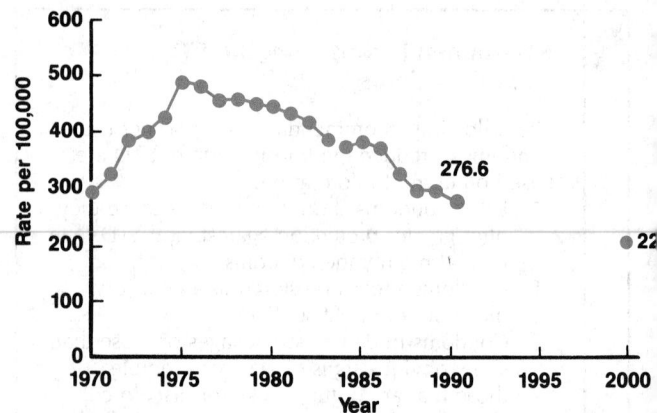

Fig. 18-2 Incidence of gonorrhea in the United States from 1970 to 1990. The rates are per 100,000 population. The number 225 is the goal for year 2000. (From US Dept of Health and Human Services: *Healthy people 2000: national health promotion and disease prevention objectives,* Washington, DC, 1990, US Government Printing Office.)

GONORRHEA

Etiology, Epidemiology, and Pathophysiology

There is no clinical difference in the infections caused by resistant strains of *N. gonorrhoeae* and those caused by sensitive strains. When there are a high number of resistant strains in a community, there is more likely to be an increase in sequelae of acute gonococcal infections such as pelvic inflammatory disease (PID), gonococcal ophthalmia, and disseminated gonococcal infection (DGI).[38]

The costs of patient management in communities with a high rate of resistant strains of *N. gonorrhoeae* are increased because of (1) additional laboratory tests, (2) added drug costs, (3) extra clinic visits, and (4) more extensive disease intervention.

Not all laboratories are prepared to test for all three forms of resistant strains. Therefore, emphasis is placed on identification of plasma-mediated resistance to penicillin by having all isolates of *N. gonorrhoeae* tested for beta-lactamase production.[38]

The incidence of gonorrhea in the United States decreased dramatically in the 1980s (Fig. 18-2). Since 1981, cases of gonorrhea decreased 29% in males and 24% in females. There is concern, however, that the rates will not continue to decrease because of an increase in the number of cases caused by antibiotic-resistant organisms. Despite these decreases the CDC estimated that there would be 1.4 million cases of gonorrhea in 1991. The proportion of antibiotic-resistant gonococcal organisms increased from 0.8% in 1985 to 7% in 1989 (Fig. 18-3). The incidence of gonorrhea is accepted to be much higher than shown because it is known that the cases of many patients treated by private physicians are never reported to public health authorities and therefore are not reflected in the statistics. It is generally accepted that only 25% to 50% of cases treated by private physicians are reported. In addition, women have few, if any, signs or symptoms of gonorrhea

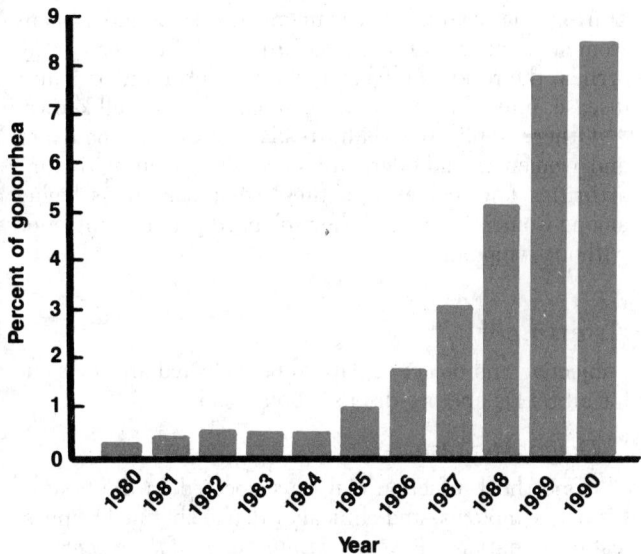

Fig. 18-3 Percentage of antibiotic resistant strains of gonorrhea in the United States 1980 to 1990. (From Centers for Disease Control: Summary of notifiable diseases 1990, *MMWR* 39(53):1990.)

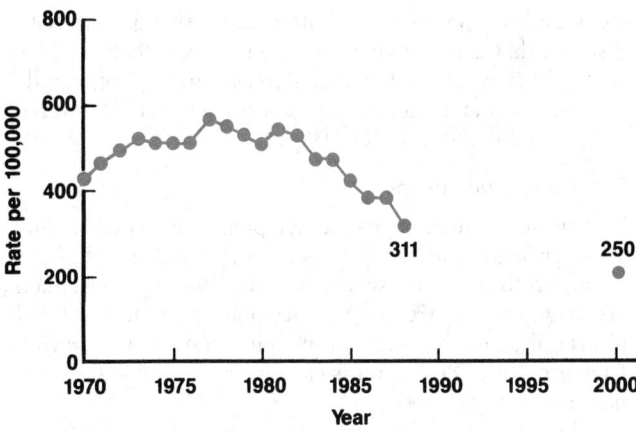

Fig. 18-4 Cases of pelvic inflammatory disease per 100,000 women. The number 250 per 100,000 is the goal for the year 2000. (From US Department of Health and Human Services: *Healthy people 2000: national health promotion and disease prevention objectives*, Washington, DC, 1990, US Government Printing Office.)

and thus are often not diagnosed. For this reason, it is commonly believed that the actual number of cases per year in the United States is probably more than 2 million.

Compounding the problem is the rapid increase of cases of gonorrhea caused by resistant strains of *N. gonorrhoeae.* Clinically significant resistance to the three widely used classes of drugs—the penicillins, the tetracyclines, and the aminoglycosides—has been reported.[38] Plasma-mediated resistance to penicillin (penicillinase-producing *N. gonorrhoeae*) first emerged in 1976.

Resistant strains of the gonococcus can be *plasma-mediated, chromosomally mediated,* or *both* and many varieties have been identified. The three most important in terms of public health are (1) plasma-mediated resistance to penicillin (PPNG); (2) chromosomally mediated resistance to penicillin (CMRNG); and (3) plasma-mediated, high-level tetracycline resistance (TRNG).[38]

Young adults 20 to 24 years of age are at highest risk of acquiring gonorrhea, with the next highest rates found among teenagers 15 to 19 years of age. In fact, 1 of every 30 teenagers in this age group will acquire gonorrhea each year.

It is estimated that the total cost of gonorrhea in the United States is several billion dollars yearly. Women and their offspring suffer the major physical, emotional, and economic burden. Pelvic inflammatory disease occurs in 10% to 20% of women with gonorrhea; and even when treated, these women are likely to suffer from recurrent salpingitis, ectopic pregnancy, infertility, and menstrual abnormalities and may face surgical removal of the pelvic organs, as well as fetal loss.

More than 1 million cases of PID are diagnosed and treated yearly. According to one report the cost of pelvic inflammatory disease and associated ectopic pregnancy and infertility exceeded 2.6 billion dollars yearly. Fig. 18-4

shows the number of cases of PID in the United States.

Asymptomatic persons or those with few symptoms are an important reservoir for infection, because they usually remain untreated. As many as 10% to 40% of gonorrheal infections in men are asymptomatic, and in women as many as 80% of infections are asymptomatic. Homosexual men can harbor reservoirs of anorectal and pharyngeal infections.

Gonorrhea, often referred to as *GC* or *the clap* by lay people, is caused by *N. gonorrhoeae.* Gonorrhea is of great concern because persons with it often have another STD such as chlamydia or HIV. They also have a high reinfection rate and serious residual effects. The incubation period is 3 to 30 days in men and 3 days to an indefinite period in women.

Prevention and Health Education

Prevention of gonorrhea and its complications can be achieved in three stages. The *first* and most crucial *stage, primary prevention,* is prevention of the disease. The *second stage, secondary prevention,* involves prevention of complications of the disease such as pelvic inflammatory disease. The *third stage, tertiary prevention,* is reversal of the damage caused by the disease, such as by tubal reconstruction.

Early treatment of infected persons is the most effective method to prevent new infection of sexual partners. Mechanical barrier methods such as condoms used with spermacides may reduce, but not prevent gonorrhea.[33] Education to acquaint people with the symptoms of gonorrhea, the efficacy of condoms, and the availability of diagnostic and treatment resources is also important. Early detection through partner notification and screening can reduce the serious complications of gonorrhea. There is no effective vaccine for gonorrhea, although clinical trials have been attempted.[33]

Some physicians believe that all persons with gonorrhea should be treated for chlamydia even though there are no signs and symptoms of it. There is no therapy for both diseases that is effective when given in a single dose. This will be discussed further under treatment. It is generally accepted that all patients with gonorrhea should be offered testing and counseling for HIV.

Signs and Symptoms

The most common signs and symptoms are listed in Box 18-4. In men, the gonococcus is introduced into the anterior urethra during sexual activity. Because most men are diagnosed and treated early, complications and residual effects of gonorrhea are uncommon among men. Sterility from orchitis or epididymitis can occur as a residual effect, but this is rare.

The incidence of *asymptomatic gonorrhea* in men is believed to be low; however, there is an increasing awareness of the importance of men with asymptomatic infection in the transmission of gonorrhea. Some men have been found to have no symptoms of infection despite positive tests for gonorrhea 2 weeks after exposure.

Gonorrhea in women most often begins as asymptomatic cervicitis, and the infection can be present for extended periods without causing noticeable signs. Hence there are a high number of infected, asymptomatic women. These women do not receive treatment unless gonorrhea is diagnosed through screening or unless the woman is identified by the sexual partner and presents herself for treatment. Frequently, complications are the first indicators of gonorrhea in women. *Salpingitis is the most common complication, with 10% to 20% of women presenting themselves with symptoms of salpingitis as the first sign of gonorrhea.*

During the course of treatment for salpingitis, many women are surgically sterilized. In cases of untreated gonorrhea, the residual effects of chronic pelvic inflammatory disease, infertility, and ectopic pregnancy are well known.

Other complications of untreated gonorrhea in both men and women include dermatitis, carditis, meningitis, and arthritis. The incidence of these complications is higher among women because of the prolonged period of infection without symptoms.

Nursing Process
Assessment

Subjective and objective data to be collected are the same for all STDs and are discussed on p. 365.

Diagnostic tests

Gonorrheal infection may be suspected on the basis of history, symptoms, and clinical evidence obtained by physical examination. However, *identification of the organism is necessary to confirm the diagnosis* and to rule out other problems. In men the diagnosis is confirmed by gram-stained smear of the discharge from the penis. Culture of the discharge from the penis is usually reserved for those whose smears are negative in the presence of strong clinical evidence.

Gram-stained cervical smears are inadequate for diagnosing gonorrhea in women. These smears are negative in about 50% of women having gonorrhea and are falsely positive in some cases. Therefore, cultures from the cervix, urethra, throat, and anus are usually taken. Because of the great length of time required to obtain reports of cultures for gonorrhea, treatment is usually begun on a presumptive basis.

Data analysis: nursing diagnoses

The nursing diagnoses are the same for all STDs and are discussed on p. 366.

Planning: expected patient outcomes

See p. 366 for a discussion of the patient outcomes for any of the STDs.

Implementation
Assisting with achievement of therapeutic goals
Medications

Therapy for gonorrhea presents a greater problem than for syphilis, because the gonococcus tends to develop resistance to antibiotics. It also is believed that *inadequate therapy is common in the United States.* Several drug regimens are in use. Emphasis is on single-dose treatment because it avoids the need for follow-up and patient cooperation.

The treatment regimen recommended by the CDC[40] is as follows:

1. Ceftriaxone (Rocephin) 250 mg IM in a single dose.
2. Alternative therapy includes Spectinomycin 2 g IM once, Ciproflaxin 500 mg PO once, or Narflaxacin 800 mg PO once.

Spectinomycin is recommended by the CDC for the treatment of persons with resistant strains of *N. gonorrheae.*

18-4

Signs and symptoms of gonorrhea

Heterosexual men

1. Urethritis—often first symptom
2. Severe dysuria—especially with first voiding in morning
3. Purulent discharge from urethra
4. Swelling of the penis and balanitis—rare symptoms

Homosexual and bisexual men

1. Rectal gonorrhea is common—usually asymptomatic and discovered by rectal culture
2. Pharyngeal gonorrhea—usually asymptomatic

Women

Women rarely have early, distressing symptoms such as men have. When symptoms are present, they include the following:
1. Slight purulent vaginal discharge
2. Vague feeling of fullness in pelvis
3. Discomfort or aching in abdomen
4. If bladder is involved—burning, frequency, and urgency, which usually cause the person to seek medical attention

The first three symptoms are so slight that they may be ignored by the person.

Because of the inconvenience of IM injections and concern about the possible needle-sticks associated with IM injections in persons who may also have HIV, a recent study using oral medication was undertaken. In this study Cefixime (400-800 mg) orally was found to be as effective as Ceftriaxone (250 mg IM) in treating uncomplicated gonorrhea.[12] Cefixime has excellent activity against *N. gonorrheae* with and without chromosomally medicated or plasmid-medicated antimicrobial resistance.[12] Further study of its use will probably be necessary before the CDC changes its recommendations for treatment of gonorrhea.[12] Nurses need to be alert to changes in CDC recommendations, which would be printed in the Morbidity and Mortality Weekly Report (MMWR).

Interventions to achieve patient outcomes

Facilitating learning, providing emotional and social support, promoting self-care, and promoting healthy sexual attitudes are important interventions. They are discussed earlier in the chapter (see p. 366).

Evaluation

The questions to be answered in evaluation are the same for all STDs (see p. 368).

SYPHILIS

Epidemiology, Etiology, and Pathophysiology

Syphilis is the third most frequently reported communicable disease in the United States, exceeded only by chickenpox and gonorrhea.[51]

Reported cases of syphilis reached an all-time high during World War II, with 575,593 cases being reported in 1943. The number of cases dropped sharply in the 1950s and began to rise again in the 1960s. There was a steady yearly increase in the number of cases until 1977, when the total number of cases leveled off until 1986 when the number of cases increased.

Recently there has been a dramatic increase in the number of cases of infectious syphilis (primary and secondary) reported to the CDC. The number of cases increased more than 55% between 1986 and 1989. In 1990 there were 50,223 reported cases of syphilis, which was the single largest yearly total since 1948[11] (Fig. 18-5).

As mentioned earlier in the chapter, the current syphilis epidemic is occurring primarily among young, heterosexual minority populations and is believed to be related to cocaine use and the exchange of sex for drugs. This same population is at risk for HIV infection and treatment of syphilis is more problematic in the presence of HIV infection.[11]

The incidence of syphilis went down among homosexual/bisexual men, especially white males. This decrease in incidence is believed to result from safer sexual practices by this population because of education about how to prevent HIV infection.

The cause of the increase in syphilis is unknown, but suggests a shift in epidemiology of the disease in the United States. Possible reasons for this increase identified by the CDC include the following:

1. Anecdotal reports from persons interviewing syphilis patients and their sexual partners indicate that prostitution that involves *nonintravenous* drugs (especially "crack" cocaine) may be partially responsible.
2. Routine use of spectinomycin to treat gonorrhea in areas where resistant strains of *N. gonorrhoeae* are common may have contributed to the increase in syphilis *because spectinomycin does not appear to cure incubating syphilis.* This is supported by data from New York City, Florida, and Los Angeles where spectinomycin was widely used to treat resistant strains of *N. gonorrhoeae.* However, it does not explain the nationwide increase in syphilis.
3. In some of the high-incidence areas there had been a decrease in the amount of money allocated to syphilis control programs and fewer interviewers were available in six of the high-incidence areas. However, the relationship between the number of interviewers and the increase in the incidence of syphilis was *not* statistically significant.

The increases in infectious syphilis among females and heterosexuals are causing concern for three reasons:

1. An increase in syphilis in females will probably be followed by increased incidence and deaths from congenital syphilis.
2. The marked increase in syphilis among inner-city, heterosexual minority groups indicates that *high-risk sexual activity is increasing despite the risk of HIV infection.* This is especially alarming because among these groups risks are already increased because of the high prevalence of intravenous drug abuse in their communities.
3. Studies in Africa and in the United States suggest that genital ulcer diseases such as primary syphilis increase the risk of HIV transmission.[43]

The trends for early congenital syphilis (CS) have paralleled the trends for primary and secondary syphilis among women. Factors thought to contribute to the sustained level of early CS are (1) an increase in the incidence of early infectious syphilis among pregnant women, (2) lack of

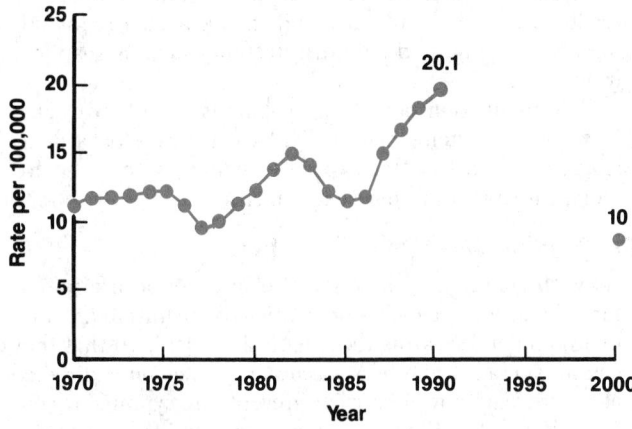

Fig. 18-5 Incidence of primary and secondary syphilis per 100,000 of the U.S. population from 1970 to 1990. The number 10 per 100,000 is the goal for the year 2000. (From US Department of Health and Human Services: *Healthy people 2000: national health promotion and disease prevention objectives,* Washington, DC, 1990, US Government Printing Office.)

Table 18-3 Stages of syphilis

	Primary	Secondary	Latent	Late
Duration	2-8 weeks	Appears 2-4 weeks after chancre appears; extends over 2-4 years	5-20 years	Terminal if not treated
Signs and symptoms	Hard sore or pimple on vulva or penis that breaks and forms painless, draining chancre; may be a single chancre or groups of more than one; may be present also on lips, tongue, hands, rectum, or nipples; chancre heals leaving almost invisible scar	Depends on site; low-grade fever, headache, anorexia, weight loss, anemia, sore throat, hoarseness, reddened and sore eyes, jaundice with or without hepatitis, aching of joints, muscles, long bones; sores on body or generalized fine rash; condylomata accuminata (venereal warts) on rectum or genitalia	No clinical signs	Tumorlike mass, (gumma), on any area of body; damage to heart valves and blood vessels; meningitis; paralysis; lack of coordination; paresis; insomnia; confusion; delusions; impaired judgment; slurred speech
Communicability	Exudates from lesions and chancre are highly contagious	Exudates from lesions highly contagious; blood contains organisms	Contagious for about 2 years; not contagious to others after that; blood contains organisms; may be transmitted placentally to fetus	Noncontagious; spinal fluid may contain organisms

available prenatal care, and (3) failure of the prenatal system to provide timely serologic testing and prompt follow-up.

In addition, it is believed that the greatest percentage of cases of syphilis go unreported and thus the incidence is much greater than the figures indicate.

Syphilis is caused by a spirochete, *Treponema pallidum*, that gains entry into the body through either the mucous membrane or skin during intercourse. The organism is readily destroyed by physical and chemical agents, including heat, drying, and mild disinfectants such as soap and water.

The incubation period for syphilis is usually 3 weeks. However, symptoms can appear as early as 9 days or as long as 3 months after exposure, which is the case for rectal infections in homosexual men.

Prevention and Health Education

As with gonorrhea, three levels of prevention are important. *Primary prevention* is prevention of the initial infection by finding and treating those with the disease so that they cannot spread it to others. *Secondary prevention* is directed at early treatment of cases to prevent late syphilis or congenital syphilis. Finally, as *tertiary prevention*, efforts can be made to treat the complications of syphilis when they occur. Contact investigation, which is necessary for all STDs, is discussed on p. 363.

Signs and Symptoms

The signs and symptoms of the four stages of syphilis are listed in Table 18-3. If syphilis is adequately diagnosed and treated during the primary stage, the other stages can be prevented.

Assessment

The subjective and objective data to be collected from a person suspected of having any STD are discussed on p. 365.

Diagnostic tests

Syphilis is most often diagnosed by standard serologic tests. Massive screening programs in the past made serologic diagnosis of syphilis very common. Mass screening with the VDRL test is no longer practiced except in high-risk populations, pregnant women, sexually active women, and couples who are applying for a marriage license. Dark-field microscopic examination of tissue scrapings from lesions or material obtained by aspiration of regional lymph nodes also reveals the presence of the spirochete, especially during the primary and secondary stages. A presumptive diagnosis is made on the basis of suspicious lesions, positive serologic tests, known exposure to infection, and involvement of regional lymph nodes. False-positive VDRL reactions are common among persons previously treated for syphilis, but fluorescent treponemal antibody (FTA) and absorption (ABS) tests are more specific (Table 18-4). Also, *once a VDRL test is positive, it remains so and is not useful for identifying reinfection.* Infectious mononucleosis, hepatitis, pregnancy, viral pneumonia, malaria, chickenpox, measles, and smallpox vaccination, narcotic addiction, and terminal malignancy have also been associated with false-positive VDRL results.

Table 18-4   Serologic tests for syphilis (STSs)

Type	Description	Examples	Comments
Flocculation	Antibody-antigen reaction produces a precipitation (flocculation)	VDRL RPR	Used primarily for screening; performed in standard laboratories
Complement fixation	Complement is used up in antigen-antibody reaction (fixed); hemolysis occurs	Reiter (Wasserman outdated)	Nonspecific; used less frequently; performed in standard laboratories
Fluorescent antibody	Antigen of killed *Treponema pallidum* is labeled with a fluorescent dye	FTA FTA-ABS	More specific than flocculation or complement-fixation test; differentiates false-positive from true syphilis positive results; performed in special laboratories
T. pallidum immobilization	Serum is mixed with live *T. pallidum*; presence of antibody decreases organism mobility	TPI	Most sensitive test; performed only at CDC laboratory in Atlanta

Implementation
Assisting with achievement of therapeutic goals
Medications

Syphilis can be successfully treated at any stage of the disease, although treatment may have to be more prolonged in latent and late syphilis. Even though syphilis can be cured in late stages, the damage to the body is much more difficult to manage.

Because penicillin continues to be effective in the treatment of syphilis, it remains the drug of choice. All types of penicillin are effective, but penicillin G benzathine is preferred because it is long-acting and can be given in a limited number of injections.

Patients with primary, secondary, and latent syphilis (and their sexual partners) are usually given 2.4 million units of penicillin intramuscularly in one dose. Patients with late syphilis are generally given 2.4 million units intramuscularly at 7-day intervals until a total of 7.2 to 9.6 million units has been given. When the use of penicillin is contraindicated because of drug sensitivity, doxycycline 100 mg orally twice a day for 2 weeks or tetracycline 500 mg orally four times a day for 2 weeks is given. For persons who cannot take tetracycline, erythromycin 500 mg four times a day for 2 weeks may be given. Compliance with any oral treatment regimen can be difficult, especially when the person is a chronic drug abuser and engages in other high-risk behaviors. The patient will need follow-up reminders to take the drug as prescribed.

If there is a question of whether or not the person is allergic to penicillin, penicillin skin tests and desensitization should be considered (see Chapter 41).[26]

Pregnant women with penicillin sensitivity pose problems for treatment. In the large dosage required to treat syphilis, tetracycline produces mottling and staining of fetal teeth and possible abnormal bone formation. If given the usual adult dose, inadequate placental transfer of tetracycline is likely, and congenital syphilis would probably develop. Erythromycin in a dose of 30 g over a period of 15 days seems to be the best alternative treatment for pregnant women with syphilis. Neurosyphilis is treated with intravenous penicillin. Sexual partners are treated with 2.4 million units of penicillin G benzathine.

Interventions to achieve patient outcomes

The nurse's role in the care of patients with syphilis is the same as for other STDs and includes facilitating learning, providing social and emotional support, promoting self-care, and promoting healthy sexual attitudes. All of these are discussed earlier in this chapter (p. 366).

Evaluation

The outcomes to be evaluated are the same as for any patient with STD (p. 368).

HERPES GENITALIS
Etiology, epidemiology, and pathophysiology

Herpes genitalis (genital herpes, HVH-2) is caused by infection with *Herpesvirus hominis* type 2 (HVH-2). Herpes genitalis was the most important STD of the 1970s. Its chronicity, frequent recurrences, and difficult treatment and prevention distinguish it from other STDs. It is estimated that about 400,000 to 600,000 new cases occur annually.[45] It is believed that at least one in six Americans now suffer from genital herpes and that because of poor control measures the number of cases is increasing dramatically. Its peak incidence parallels the young age groups affected by other STDs. Once acquired, herpes genitalis is a lifelong disease and carries with it not only intense and recurrent discomfort, but also anxieties about future childbearing, malignancy, and sexual and marital function. In early pregnancy women infected with herpes have an increased chance of miscarriage. Because genital herpetic lesions endanger the fetus during delivery, caesarean delivery is often necessary. Genital herpes has also been associated with cervical cancer. It is now generally accepted that HVH-2 is spread by sexual contact.

The incubation period is 3 to 7 days. The primary lesion appears as a vesicle on the external genitalia in men; often in the rectum in homosexual men; and on the vagina, cervix, or external genitalia in women. These lesions often ulcerate, especially when located on moist surfaces. Following primary herpes, the virus persists in a *latent* or *unrecognized* form in most patients. It is believed that latent infections are localized in the ganglia of sensory nerves to the genitalia. When the host factors favor it, the *latent infection* becomes clinically apparent as *recurrent herpes.*

Prevention and Health Education
Primary prevention

Primary prevention of herpes depends on limiting sexual contact between infected individuals and uninfected partners. There is preliminary evidence that the herpes virus may survive on towels for up to 20 minutes; therefore it is important to use separate linens. *Refraining from sexual intercourse while lesions are present and for 10 days after they heal is essential.* Sexually active young persons should be taught to examine themselves and prospective partners for such lesions. In some communities there are groups of individuals with herpes who have chosen to restrict themselves to sexual contact only with others who already have been exposed to herpes. Condoms may be helpful. Transmission to the fetus may be prevented by caesarean section. Infected neonates may develop subsequent mental retardation or die. If drug therapy for HVH-2 is effective, it will help limit new infections by eradicating at least some of the reservoir of infected individuals by preventing reactivation of HVH-2.

Secondary prevention

Secondary prevention is aimed at reducing or eliminating complications such as cervical cancer. A yearly Pap smear is recommended. Another important complication of herpes genitalis is its ability to create great psychologic pain and anxiety, to disrupt normal social and sexual relationships, and to stigmatize its victims. In the event that secondary prevention is not possible, efforts to detect and treat cervical cancer in its early stages are essential.

Assessment

The subjective and objective data to be collected from any person suspected of having a sexually transmitted disease is discussed on p. 365.

Signs and symptoms

The common signs and symptoms of primary herpetic infection are the following:
1. Local inflammation
2. Pain
3. Enlargement of inguinal lymph nodes
4. Generalized signs of infection
   a. Photophobia
   b. Headache
   c. Flulike symptoms

Although primary herpetic lesions begin as single or multiple reddish papules that then develop into clear, fluid-filled vesicles. Once they rupture they form ulcerations that may fuse with other lesions to form large ulcerated areas. The disease tends to be more extensive in women than in men. In some women cervical infection accompanies the external lesions, and in certain cases it may be the only infected site. Cervical involvement may be mild or severe with extensive ulceration and pus. Genital lesions often worsen during the first 10 to 15 days but usually heal within 3 to 4 weeks. These symptoms usually lead the individual to seek medical attention.

Vaginal discharge is common among women, and discharge from the urethra is usual in men having primary infections. Urinary tract involvement may occur and is reflected in symptoms of dysuria or urinary retention. The lesions can cause severe pain, requiring hospitalization for parenteral analgesia. Subclinical infections in which patients are unaware of any problem occur in only about 10% of the cases of genital herpes. Unfortunately, about 75% of all patients have at least one recurrence. Fortunately, recurrent infections are usually milder and of shorter duration than primary infections and usually produce local rather than systemic reaction. The patient experiencing a recurrent infection often has prodromal signs of paresthesia and burning at the site where the lesion will erupt. Factors known to predispose to recurrent infection include fever, emotional upsets, premenstrual states, and overexposure to heat and sunshine. Although the mode of recurrent infection is not clear, it has been theorized that during primary infection the virus ascends sensory nerve sheaths, localizing in corresponding nerve ganglia, and that when the environment becomes favorable, the virus is reactivated. Recurrent herpes usually begins with abnormal sensation or itching of a localized genital area. Lesions of recurrent infections usually occur at the site of the primary infection. Herpes encephalitis may also occur.

Diagnostic tests

Diagnosis of herpes genitalis is made by isolation of the virus from specimens obtained from lesions. Pap smears or fluid from the vesicles collected in transport medium demonstrates cellular characteristics of viruses.

Implementation
Assisting with achievement of therapeutic goals
Symptomatic therapy

Treatment for genital herpes has most often been symptomatic, because there is no known cure for the disease. Acyclovir appears capable of inhibiting the replication of herpetic viruses in vitro; in clinical trials with patients who had antibodies against herpes simplex viruses, acyclovir prevented active herpes infections. Acyclovir ointment, 5%, is recommended for genital herpes. The ointment is applied to cover all lesions every 3 hours, six times a day for 7 days. The acyclovir treatment reduces viral shedding and the duration of the disease in patients with primary initial infections who are treated within 6 days of the onset of symptoms. It does not prevent recurrences. There is no effective treatment to prevent recurrences or to shorten their duration.

Symptomatic treatment consists of using Burow's solution or hydrogen peroxide and soap and water to cleanse the lesions. The involved areas are blown dry with a hair dryer, and the skin is then dusted with cornstarch. Women are advised to use a mirror to examine the vulva, vagina, and cervix for hidden lesions.

Interventions to achieve patient outcomes
Facilitating learning

Persons with herpes should *abstain from sexual contact while the lesions are present and for 10 days after the lesions heal.* Risk of transmission during asymptomatic periods is unknown. Some experts advise using condoms to prevent transmission of the disease.

Providing social and emotional support

Because herpes genitalis is a recurrent disease with no cure, patients infected with the virus require considerable support. Some infected persons tend to withdraw from an active social life rather than face the possibility of making a commitment that will require them to share knowledge of their disease with another person. For this reason, in some communities support groups have been formed for persons who have herpes genitalis.

CHLAMYDIAL INFECTION

Etiology/Epidemiology

Chlamydia trachomatis is caused by the gram-negative obligate, *C. trachomatis*. It is recognized as the most prevalent of the STDs in the United States. Because it is not a reportable disease, the actual number of cases is unknown. It is estimated, however, that each year 3 to 4 million Americans suffer from epidemic chlamydial infections. In England and Wales, where nongonococcal urethritis (about half the cases of which are caused by *C. trachomatis*) is a reportable disease, the incidence has nearly doubled in the last decade.[49]

Chlamydial infections are responsible for about 20% to 30% of diagnosed pelvic inflammatory disease cases, and it is estimated that about 11,000 women each year become involuntarily sterilized and 36000 suffer ectopic pregnancies as a result of this organism.[50] Chlamydial infections can be transmitted to infants during delivery, causing conjunctivitis and pneumonia in many.

C. trachomitis is the leading cause of pneumonia in infants less than 6 months of age. The rate of infection with pneumonia is 3 to 10 per 1000 live births and may go as high as 50 to 60 per 1000 in areas where *C. trachomitis* is epidemic. The organism has superseded *N. gonorrheae* as a cause of neonatal conjunctivitis.[8]

Chlamydia is highest in young, promiscuous, indigent, unmarried women who live in the inner city and in those who have had a prior history of STD.

Pathophysiology

C. trachomatis is a parasite that has specific requirements for adenosine triphosphate (ATP) and amino acids. There are two stages in the life cycle of the organism. In *stage 1*, the *infective stage*, the *elementary body attaches* to the host cell and is ingested by phagocytosis. In *stage 2*, the *elementary body undergoes metamorphosis* to become a *reticulate or initial body*. This is the *metabolic phase* of the life cycle. The initial body duplicates by binary fission and changes into the elementary body. The host cell, which contains the elementary bodies, undergoes lysis, liberating infectious organisms that are capable of reinfecting new cells.[8]

Serotypes L1, L2, and L3 are responsible for lymphogranuloma venereum (LGV), which is common in South America and the far East.

Serotypes D through K cause chlamydial infections. It is estimated that between 20% and 40% of sexually active women have been exposed to the bacterium and have an-

Table 18-5   Chlamydia trachomatis infections

Males	Females	Infants
Transmission		
Males ⇄ Females → Infants		
Infections		
Urethritis	Cervicitis	Conjunctivitis
Postgonococcal urethritis	Urethritis	Pneumonia
Proctitis	Proctitis	Asymptomatic pharyngeal carriage
Conjunctivitis	Conjunctivitis	Asymptomatic gastrointestinal carriage
Pharyngitis	Pharyngitis	
Subclinical lymphogranuloma venereum	Subclinical lymphogranuloma venereum	
Complications		
Epididymitis	Salpingitis	
Prostatitis	Endometritis	
Reiter's syndrome	Perihepatitis	
Sterility	Ectopic pregnancy	
Rectal strictures*	Infertility	
	Vulvar/rectal carcinoma*	
	Rectal stricture*	

From Centers for Disease Control, Chlamydia Trachomatis Infections, Policy Guidelines for Prevention and Control, MMWR (suppl) 35:54, 1985.
*Associated with lymphogranuloma venereum.

tibody titers to *C. trachomatis*.[8] Table 18-5 shows how the infection can be transmitted between male and female sexual partners and from females to infants. It also lists the various ways the disease is manifested in males, females, and infants.

Prevention and Health Education

Primary prevention of chlamydial infections consists of limiting sexual contact with infected partners. *Secondary prevention* requires early diagnosis and treatment.

Risk assessment factors require special attention. Age, number of sex partners, socioeconomic status, and sexual preference are predictors of infection with C. trachomatis.[36] These factors include the following:

1. Age—Infection rates are 2 to 3 times higher in sexually active women under age 20 than in those over age 20. The rates for women between 20 and 29 years of age are considerably higher than for women over age 30. The rates of urethral infection are higher for teenage males than for adult men.

2. Number of sex partners—Persons with several sex partners are at higher risk of infection.

3. Socioeconomic status—Some studies have shown that persons of lower socioeconomic status are at increased risk for infection with C. *trachomatis*.

Clinical clues used to diagnose chlamydia in women

Purulent discharge
Endocervical mucous
Spotting after intercourse
Spotting between periods
Vague lower abdominal pain
Cervical atypia (not normal)
Infertility
C. trachomatis should be looked for when there is premature rupture of amniotic membranes

Data from Faro S: *Chlamydia trachomatis* infection. In Rakel RE, editor: *Conn's current therapy*, Philadelphia, 1991 WB Saunders.

Clinical cues to chlamydial infection

Presence of mucus in the endocervical canal
Microscopic examination
 Presence of WBCs
 Absence of bacteria on gram stain
 Decrease of 10 squamous eopithelial cells per high-powered field
Hypertrophy of columnar epithelium of endocervix
Pyuria but no bacteria on gram strain or culture of urine

From Faro S: *Chlamydia trachomatis* infection. In Rakel RE, editor: Conn's current therapy, 1991 Philadelphia, 1991, WB Saunders.

4. Sexual preference—The prevalence of urethral chlamydial infection among homosexual men is one-third that among heterosexual men. However, 4% to 8% of homosexual men seen in STD clinics have rectal chlamydia infection.

Assessment

Signs and symptoms

The clinical cues used to diagnose chlaymdia in women are presented in Box 18-5. Men usually have nonspecific urethritis or may seek treatment for epididymitis. However, up to 80% of women and 25% of men may be asymptomatic.

Box 18-6 lists the clinical findings in women with *C. trachomitis* infection.

Diagnostic tests

C. trachomatis infection may be diagnosed by traditional tissue culture or by one of the new rapid tests listed below.

1. Enzyme immunoassay (EIA) (chlamydiazime or test patch (Abbott)
2. Direct immunofluoresence—several of which are commercially available
3. If none of the above are available, a tentative diagnosis can be made by microscopic examination of an endocervical specimen.

Implementation

Assisting with achievement of therapeutic goals
Medications

1. Doxycycline 100 mg orally twice a day for 7 days or
2. Tetracycline 500 mg PO four times a day for 7 days
3. During pregnancy, erythromycin 500 mg orally four times a day for 7 days or
4. Erythromycin ethyl succinate 400 to 800 mg orally four times a day for 7 days.

Because neonatal infection rates of infants of untreated women approach 50%, all women diagnosed during pregnancy should receive treatment. Their sexual partners must be treated simultaneously, otherwise the women can be reinfected. The follow-up culture should be performed 7 to 14 days after treatment is completed.[8]

Patients with pelvic inflammatory disease being treated with cephalosporin must also be given an agent effective against chlamydia, such as doxycycline or erythromycin.

Interventions to achieve patient outcomes
Facilitating learning

It is important that the patient encourage their sexual partner(s) to seek care as soon as possible to avoid reinfection of the patient and complications in the partner.[20] Patients who are sexually active should be advised to wear condoms or use spermicides to reduce reinfection.

Providing social and emotional support

Social and emotional support of these patients is as important as it is with any person with an STD (p. 367).

LYMPHOGRANULOMA VENEREUM
Etiology/Epidemiology

Lymphogranuloma venereum (LGV) is a systemic, sexually transmitted disease caused by serotypes L_1, L_2, and L_3 of *C. trachomatis*. Other species of *Chlamydia* are the causative organisms of trachoma and psittacosis. The disease is contracted by vaginal, anal, or oral intercourse; primary inoculation with the organism may occur at any site involved in close contact. The incubation period is 7 to 12 days. Lymphadenitis of regional lymph nodes draining the site of primary infection occurs, and the disease spreads by way of the lymphatic system.

LGV is most prevalent in the tropics. In the United States it is found most often in the southern states, but epidemiologic studies are needed to determine its true incidence. Reports of the incidence of LGV indicate less than 500 cases annually. The symptoms of LGV resemble those of other sexually transmitted diseases, and its reported incidence may be influenced by this fact.

Pathophysiology

There are three clinical phases of infection in LGV: (1) inoculation and appearance of the primary lesions, (2) lymphatic spread and generalized symptoms, and (3) late complications. In individual cases any one of the phases may be absent or go unnoticed.

The primary lesion, which is transient, appears as a papule, small erosion, or vesicle. The most common sites of the primary lesion are the prepuce and glans in men and the vagina and cervix in women. Because it is painless, the primary lesion may go unnoticed, especially in women. Localized edema may be present. If the rectum is infected, there is a bloody discharge followed by a mucopurulent discharge, diarrhea, and cramping.

Involvement of the lymphatics occurs 1 to 4 weeks after the appearance of the primary lesion. If the primary lesion is on the penis, anal margin, clitoris, or upper vulva, the superficial inguinal lymph nodes are involved. Infection of the vagina or cervix as the primary site produces involvement of the deep iliac and anorectal lymph nodes. The large lymph nodes or *buboes* that appear are firm and lobular. The skin over the superficial nodes is bluish red and adheres to the nodes.

Assessment
Signs and symptoms

The first indication of infection in most patients is a feeling of stiffness and aching in the groin followed by swelling in the inguinal area. Symptoms of nongonococcal urethritis may be present. Constitutional symptoms of infection may or may not appear at this time. The involved lymph nodes may suppurate, causing extensive scarring. Obstruction of the lymphatics may result, leading to chronic edema and ulceration. Lymphatic spread of the infection is accompanied by generalized symptoms. Mild to severe fever, malaise, nausea, and vomiting may occur. Abdominal pain, symptoms of cystitis, and urinary retention are common when pelvic lymph nodes are involved. Acute proctocolitis is common in homosexual men.

Among the most severe complications of LGV are development of perianal abscesses, rectovaginal or rectovesical fistulas, and rectal strictures. In the last clinical phase, generalized infection is indicated by blood values showing anemia, leukocytosis, and an elevated sedimentation rate.

Diagnostic tests

LGV is isolated from aspirate from an affected lymph node. The LGV complement-fixation test (LGV-CFT) is a test for antibodies. A positive LGV-CFT test along with a careful history and physical examination affords the best chances for diagnosing LGV.

Implementation
Assisting with achievement of therapeutic goals
Medications

Early antibiotic therapy is essential for controlling and reducing morbidity from LGV, and it is generally agreed that treatment should not be delayed until diagnostic test results are obtained. Tetracycline in a dosage of 500 mg four times a day for 3 to 4 weeks or until all signs and symptoms are resolved is the treatment of choice. If drug sensitivity or pregnancy precludes use of tetracycline, erythromycin, 500 mg four times daily for 2 to 6 weeks, is used.

If cost is not a factor, doxycycline, 100 mg twice daily for 2 weeks, is preferred because it is better tolerated than tetracycline. Other drugs that are effective in treating LGV are chloramphenicol, minocycline, and rifampin. Sexual partners should receive the same therapy. If lymphadenopathy does not respond to therapy in 1 to 2 weeks, an alternate drug may be required. In some patients therapy must be continued for as long as 6 weeks. Sexual partners should also receive the therapy for the same period of time.

Other therapy

Fluctuant lymph nodes may be aspirated with a large-bore needle and syringe to prevent tissue breakdown and the formation of draining sinuses.[47] If rectal stricture supervenes, rectal dilation at 2-week intervals may be attempted. Development of fistulas is especially distressing and requires surgical repair. LGV is a disease characterized by remissions and exacerbations, and thorough surveillance is important. Antibiotic therapy should be reinstituted as soon as symptoms of reactivation occur. *Biopsy of lesions and lymph nodes is advised in chronic cases of LGV, because cancer may develop in the ulcerative lesions and may be overlooked as a result of similarity in appearance.*

Interventions to achieve patient outcomes

These patients may require much counseling and teaching as they deal with their disease. Because the fluctuant lymph nodes may be disturbing to the patient's self-image, social and emotional support is very important. See p. 367 for more discussions of these topics.

CHANCROID
Etiology/Epidemiology

Chancroid is a sexually transmitted disease caused by a gram-negative bacillus, *Haemophilus ducreyi.* Although chancroid is less common in the United States, there has been a tenfold increase per 100,000 population in the past decade.

Since the early 1980s epidemics associated with prostitutes have occurred in Boston, New York City, Dallas, Florida, and Orange County, California.

Although it is found worldwide, chancroid is most prevalent in tropical and semitropical areas in the Orient, the West Indies, and North Africa. The disease occurs more often in men than in women and more often among nonwhite than white people. It is possible that returning military personnel may have introduced the disease into areas where it did not previously exist. The incubation period varies from 1 to 14 days and averages 4 to 5 days.

Pathophysiology

The initial lesion(s) are acutely tender genital ulcers, lymphodenopathy, and tender buboes. The buboes may suppurate and lead to abscesses. Exudate from the ulcers or aspirate from the buboes are stained and may demonstrate a "school-of-fish" pattern on microscopic examination by someone experienced in interpretation.[32]

Assessment
Signs and symptoms

In women, the lesions of chancroid are most often found on the labia, anus, clitoris, vagina, and cervix. A few women do not have any lesions but may have signs of mild vaginitis. In men the lesions appear on the prepuce, glans, or shaft of the penis.

The ulcers found in chancroid are typically ragged and irregular. They are highly infectious and autoimmunity may occur, resulting in multiple lesions. The ulcers appear excavated, have a granulating, purulent surface, and are painful. Often, edema of the surrounding tissues is present. Involvement of the inguinal lymph nodes occurs in about 50% of all cases of chancroid within 2 weeks after appearance of the primary lesion. The buboes are most often unilateral, painful, and spherical in shape. The skin over the buboes is inflamed. The buboes tend to become softer as abscesses form. These abscesses in turn may suppurate and rupture, further spreading the infection. Generalized symptoms of infection usually appear when inguinal abscesses form.

Diagnostic tests

Diagnosis of chancroid depends on growth of the organism on special media. A specimen is collected by aspiration of a vesicle, pustule, or lymph node, or from the margin of an ulcer. Sensitivity testing has become more important because antibiotic resistance is increasing.

Implementation
Assisting with achievement of therapeutic goals
Medications

The treatment of choice is erythromycin, 500 mg orally four times daily for 7 days, or ceftriaxone 250 mg IM once. Other antimicrobial therapies are available but are not considered to be as effective. Plasma-mediated resistance to tetracycline has been documented in the United States and in other countries where chancroid is endemic.

Other therapy

Suppurative buboes are aspirated, preferably through normal skin. Warm saline compresses may be helpful for ulcerations.

Interventions to achieve patient outcomes
Facilitating learning

Patient follow-up is essential because treatment failure can occur. The patient is taught to report any signs or symptoms that persist or worsen during treatment. They also should be advised to abstain from sexual activity until all lesions are healed. Proper use of a condom should also be stressed (see Box 18-3, p. 367).

GRANULOMA INGUINALE (DONOVANOSIS)
Etiology/Epidemiology

Granuloma inguinale or granuloma venereum is believed to be most often transmitted by sexual contact, although nonsexual transmission has been reported. The infection is caused by a gram-negative bacillus, *Calymmatobacterium (Donovania) granulomatis*, widely referred to as *Donovan bacillus*. The organism is related to *Klebsiella*. The incubation period is uncertain but is about 8 to 12 weeks.

Donovanosis is common in tropical and subtropical areas and rarely occurs in the United States. It is very common in New Guinea, India, and the Caribbean. The disease is mildly contagious and probably requires repeated exposures

for spread of infection. Predisposing factors are poorly understood. The disease is more common in men than women and is especially common among homosexual men. The incubation period varies from several days to several months.

Assessment
Signs and symptoms

Lesions appear on the genitalia and in the perianal area. The most common sites of lesions are the prepuce and glans in men and the vagina and labia in women. The infection first appears with development of subcutaneous nodules. These elevated areas eventually ulcerate, producing sharply defined, painless lesions. The ulcers enlarge slowly and bleed on contact. With ulceration, the infection tends to spread along the pubic region. Involvement of the lymph nodes is uncommon but can occur and produce occlusion of the lymphatics, resulting in elephantiasis.

Diagnostic tests

Smears of exudates taken from the lesions do not always demonstrate the causative organism, even when donovanosis is present. Therefore, a sample of tissue is taken from the lesion, crushed between two slides, and stained with Wright's or Giesma stain. The specimen is examined for the presence of Donovan bodies, which represent the intracellular stage of the causative organism. Examination of a tissue sample also makes it possible to differentiate between donovanosis and cancer.

Implementation
Assisting with achievement of therapeutic goals
Medications

There is no standard treatment. Tetracycline 500 mg four times a day for 14 to 21 days is the treatment of choice. If tetracycline fails, streptomycin or gentamycin may be prescribed.

TRICHOMONIASIS
Etiology, Epidemiology, and Pathophysiology

A protozoan, *Trichomonas vaginalis*, is the causative organism of trichomoniasis. Evidence suggests that the incubation period ranges between 4 and 28 days.[23] Trichomoniasis may well be the most frequently acquired STD in the United States, with an estimated incidence of 3 million cases occurring annually. *T. vaginalis* organisms are found in 3% to 15% of women under the care of private physicians, 13% to 23% of women attending gynecologic clinics, and 50% of women who have gonorrhea. It is most often sexually transmitted. The parasite commonly exists in vaginal and cervical secretions and in seminal fluid. It is estimated that one of five females will have a trichomonal infection during her lifetime.

Trichomoniasis is frequently viewed as an innocuous infection, yet there are serious implications for health. During the postpartum period in women who have trichomoniasis, the rate of persistent fever, prolonged vaginal discharge, and endometritis is twice as high as in women who do not harbor the organism. About 90% of patients with trichomoniasis have cervical erosions and leukorrhea, and it has been suggested that chronic irritation may predispose to cervical cancer. Interpretation of cervical cytology, as in the Pap test, is unreliable in the presence of trichomoniasis, because the infection produces atypical cervical cells. Unless repeated cervical smears are taken, cancer of the cervix may be missed. Trichomoniasis results in urethritis; it also causes prostatitis in men 40% of the time; and, finally, reversible sterility can occur as a result of inhibition of sperm motility by toxins produced by the organism.

Assessment
Signs and symptoms

Only 25% of women harboring the organism are asymptomatic. Pruritus of the vulva and vagina is the predominant symptom among women. The itching may be so severe as to awaken the patient from sleep, and excoriation from scratching is common. Secondary infection of the broken skin may result.

Classically, the symptoms of trichomoniasis in women are a copious, frothy, green or greenish-yellow vaginal discharge, inflammation of the labia minora and lower vagina, and a red-speckled appearance of the vaginal canal and cervix known as "strawberry patches." Only a small number of patients present this classic picture that is usually described in texts.[23] Most patients have a vaginal discharge, but it is small in amount and white and watery, and there is some inflammation of the labia and vagina. Itching is almost universally present, however; and dyspareunia, dysuria, and urinary frequency may also occur.

In men, urethritis and its symptoms of purulent discharge, itching, burning, and inflammation are the signs of trichomoniasis most often seen. Prostatitis, epididymitis, and urethral stricture may occur as complications among men. However, these consequences of trichomoniasis have not been extensively studied and are not well documented.

Diagnostic tests

Diagnosis of trichomoniasis is most often made by preparing a hanging drop slide containing a specimen of the discharge and observing the motile organism under the microscope. Serologic and skin tests are currently being investigated but lack reliability so far. Because of the high incidence of coexisting gonorrhea, smears or cultures for gonococci should also be taken.

Implementation
Assisting with achievement of therapeutic goals
Medications

The recommended treatment is metronidazole (Flagyl) 2 g by mouth in a single dose. An alternative regimen would be metronidazole 250 mg orally three times daily for 5 to 7 days.

The CDC recommends that both partners should be treated simultaneously to prevent reinfection by the untreated partner at a later date. Vaginal inserts of metronidazole are less effective. The drug is known to cross the placental barrier. For this reason, it is not given to pregnant women until after the first trimester.

BACTERIAL VAGINOSIS (*GARDNERELLA VAGINALIS*)
Etiology

Bacterial vaginosis (BV) can be cultured from 23% to 96% of women with vaginitis and is recovered from up to 50% of asymptomatic women.

Assessment
Signs and symptoms

G. vaginalis infection is characterized by a small amount of homogeneous gray or grayish white discharge. The discharge usually has a disagreeable odor, and because it is less irritating than discharges caused by other organisms, pruritus is mild or absent. On inspection, the vaginal walls are slightly reddened, and the discharge appears to adhere to the mucosal lining. Some women are asymptomatic despite positive cultures.

Diagnostic tests

The diagnosis is confirmed by microscopic examination of a smear or culture of the vaginal discharge.

Implementation
Assisting with achievement of therapeutic goals
Medications

Treatment of *G. vaginalis* consists of oral metronidazole, 250 mg to 500 mg twice a day for 7 days. The CDC *does not* recommend treating the patient's sexual partner at the same time.

HUMAN PAPILLOMA VIRUS (GENITAL WARTS)
Etiology, Epidemiology, and Pathophysiology

Genital warts caused by the human papilloma virus (HPV) are important because of their possible role in the development of cervical cancer. There are between 500,000 and 1 million cases per year in the United States. Genital warts occur in or around the vulva, vagina, cervix, perineum, anal canal, urethra, and glans penis. They enlarge during pregnancy and may cause hemorrhage or obstruction during delivery. The disease is most common in adolescent girls and young women. The HPV can remain dormant for decades before recurrences appear.

Assessment
Diagnosis

Diagnosis is made by clinical appearance or histologic examination.

Implementation
Assisting with achievement of therapeutic goals
Cryotherapy

The Centers for Disease Control recommends cryotherapy as the treatment of choice. Podophyllum, which was previously recommended, is less effective and is toxic if applied to a wide area at one time. It still may be used in a 25% solution in benzoin to treat one or two lesions. Neither treatment cures the disease.

Interventions to achieve patient outcomes
Facilitating learning

Prevention of HPV should be stressed. It includes (1) avoiding sexual relationships with persons in known high-risk groups, (2) using latex condoms if having sexual intercourse, and (3) avoiding anal intercourse.

The CDC does not recommend a caesarean birth to prevent transmission of HPV to newborns. A C-section may be indicated for warts obstructing the pelvic outlet or if a vaginal birth would cause excessive bleeding of the warts.[23] Because genital warts sometimes undergo malignant change, the patient is advised to have an annual Pap smear. Malignant changes, especially in the cervix, may not be apparent for 5 to 40 years.

HEPATITIS B
Etiology/epidemiology

In the United States, hepatitis B is most frequently transmitted by sexual contact. Persons at high risk for sexual transmission of HBV include homosexual/bisexual men, heterosexual men and women with multiple sex partners, and sex partners of intravenous drug users.

Etiology is established by serologic testing. Most persons with acute viral hepatitis are asymptomatic. Because there is no specific treatment for HBV, emphasis is placed on prevention.

Prevention and Health Education
Primary prevention

The CDC recommends *vaccination* for all the persons identified above as being at high risk. In addition, residents of correctional or long-term care facilities, persons seeking treatment for STD, and prostitutes should be vaccinated. Vaccination is also recommended for health care workers because of the possibility of needle-sticks.

Secondary prevention

The CDC recommends that *postexposure prophylactic treatment* with hepatitis B immune globulin (HBIG) should be considered in the following situations: sexual contact with a person who has active hepatitis B or who contracts hepatitis B and sexual contact with a hepatitis B carrier (blood test positive for hepatitis B surface antigen). The prophylactic treatment should be given within 14 days of sexual contact.

Because pregnant women can transmit HBV to their infants at delivery, HBIG and hepatitis B vaccine is given to the infant after birth. All pregnant women should be screened during their first obstetric visit for the presence of HBsAg. If they are HBsAg positive, their newborns should be given HBIG as soon as possible after birth and subsequently immunized with hepatitis B vaccine. HBIG is also given to health care workers who suffer a needle-stick. For more information about hepatitis see Chapter 30.

OTHER SEXUALLY TRANSMITTED DISEASES

In addition to those diseases already discussed, pediculosis pubis and scabies are also considered to be STDs.

Pediculosis pubis, also known as "crabs," is caused by pubic lice. Although lice can be transmitted by bedding or clothing, they are often transmitted during sexual contact. They produce erythematous, itchy papules. The lice adhere to hair around the pubic area, anus, abdomen, and thighs. Diagnosis is made by observation of lice or microscopic observation of nits at the base of hair. Recommended treatment is 1% Kwell lotion or shampoo. One treatment per episode is necessary, but itching may persist.

Scabies, caused by mites known as *Sarcoptes scabiei*, is transmitted by close body contact, bedding, and clothing. Diagnosis is made from linear burrows, often characterized by a reddened papule containing the mite. Common sites are finger webs, wrists, elbows, ankles, and the penis. Nocturnal itching is common. A one-time use of 1% Kwell shampoo is recommended. Family, household, and sexual contacts should also be treated.

SUMMARY

1. The term *sexually transmitted diseases* refers to diseases that are usually transmitted by heterosexual or homosexual intercourse.
2. The five classic venereal diseases are gonorrhea, syphilis, chancroid, lymphogranuloma venereum, and granuloma inguinale.
3. In the 1980s chlamydia trachomatis, genital herpes, human papillomavirus, genital mycoplasmas, cytomegalovirus, hepatitis B vaginitis, enteric infections, and ectoparasitic disease were added to the list of STDs.
4. Three changes have affected the incidence of STDs in the United States since World War II: (1) antibiotics and antibiotic resistance, (2) social permissiveness, and (3) sexual behavior patterns.
5. The highest incidence of STDs is in young adults and adolescents. This is believed to be because of permissiveness, promiscuity, and "the pill."
6. Partner notification (formerly called *contact investigation*) is important to identifying persons who may have been exposed to an STD and in trying to identify the source of the infection.
7. Latex condoms are recommended to prevent the transmission of STDs. They are recommended because they provide greater protection against viral STDs than natural membrane condoms.
8. During the 1980s there was a decline in the incidence of gonorrhea. However, it remains an important risk for young minority populations who practice unprotected sex.
9. A major concern in the treatment of gonorrhea is the increased resistance of the organism to penicillin and other antibiotics.
10. Gonorrhea in women is often asymptomatic and is only diagnosed when complications such as salpingitis occur.
11. The incidence of syphilis increased dramatically in the late 1980s, and in 1990 the reported cases of primary and secondary syphilis were the highest they had been since 1948.
12. The increase in syphilis has been in young, hetero-

sexual, minority populations and may be related to cocaine use and the exchange of sex for crack cocaine.

13. The drug of choice in the treatment of syphilis is penicillin G benzathine (2.4 million units IM).

14. Herpes genitalis is a lifelong disease with no cure. It can be transmitted to the fetus during delivery and thus caesarean delivery is often recommended.

15. Treatment for herpes genitalis is symptomatic, and acyclovir ointment applied to the lesions reduces viral shedding and the duration of disease. It does not prevent recurrences.

16. *Chlamydia trachomatis* infections are recognized as the most prevalent STD in the United States.

17. *C. trachomatis* can be spread between sexual partners during intercourse and from mothers to infants.

18. Chlamydial infections are most common in women under the age of 20. They are also more common in persons who have several sex partners.

19. The treatment of choice for chlamydial infections is doxycycline, 500 mg twice daily for 7 days or tetracycline, 500 mg four times daily for 7 days.

20. Condylomata accuminata (genital warts) is caused by the papilloma virus; it is most common in adolescent girls and young women.

21. Genital warts are of particular concern because they can undergo malignant changes after a latent period of 5 to 40 years.

22. In the United States hepatitis B is most often transmitted by sexual contact.

23. The CDC recommends that all persons at high risk for hepatitis B be vaccinated. This includes health care workers because of the possibility of needlesticks.

STUDY QUESTIONS

- What is the incidence of STDs in your community?
- How does the incidence in your community compare with the incidence in other parts of the country?
- What services are available in your community for detection and treatment of STD?
- Are human sexuality and prevention of STDs taught in your local schools?
- Are similar teaching programs available for adults in the community in which you reside?
- Describe the nurse's role in working with persons with a newly diagnosed STD.

REFERENCES AND SELECTED READINGS

1. Bauer HM, et al: Genital human papillomavirus infection in female university students as determined by the PCR-based method, *JAMA* 265(4):472-477, 1991.
2. Brown ZA, et al: Effects on infants of a first episode of genital herpes during pregnancy, *N Engl J Med* 317:1246-1251, 1987.
3. DeBuono BA, et al: Sexual behavior of college women in 1975, 1986, and 1989, *N Engl J Med* 322(12):821-825, 1990.
4.* Dirubbo NE: The condom barrier, *Am J Nurs* 87:1306-1309, 1987.

5. Dodson MG, Faro S: The polymicrobial etiology of acute pelvic inflammatory disease and treatment regimens, *Rev Infect Dis* 4(suppl):5696-5702, 1985.
6. Sexually transmitted diseases in the 1990s (editorial) *N Engl J Med* 325(19):1368-1370, 1991.
7. Those other STDs (editorial), *Am J Public Health* 81(10):1250-1251, 1991.
8. Faro S: *Chlamydia trachomatis infection.* In Rakel RE: *Conn's current therapy 1991,* Philadelphia, 1991, WB Saunders, pp 1012-1014.
9. Feldblum PJ, Fortney JA: Condoms, spermicides, and the transmission of human immunodeficiency virus: a review of literature, *Am J Public Health* 78:52-54, 1988.
10. Fogel CL: Gonorrhea: not a new problem but a serious one, *Nurs Clin North Am* 23:885-897, 1988.
11. Gersham KA, Rolfs RT: Divergent gonorrhea and syphilis trends in the 1980s: are they real? *Am J Public Health* 81(10):1263-1267, 1991.
12. Handsfield HH: A comparison of single-dose cefixime with ceftriaxone as treatment for uncomplicated gonorrhea, *N Engl J Med* 325(19):1337-1341, 1991.
13. Hanssen PW, Kiviat NB, Holmes KK: Atypical pelvic inflammatory disease: subacute, chronic, or subclinical upper genital tract in women. In Holmes KK, et al: *Sexually transmitted diseases,* ed 2, New York, 1990, McGraw Hill.
14. *Healthy People 2000: National health promotion and disease prevention objectives,* U.S. Dept. of Health and Human Services, Public Health Service, Washington, DC, 1990.
15. Holmes KK, et al: *Sexually transmitted diseases,* ed 2, New York, 1990, McGraw-Hill.
15a. Hook EW, Marra CM: Acquired syphilis in adults, *New Eng J Med* 326(16):1060-1069, 1992.
16. Kahn JG, et al: Diagnosing pelvic inflammatory disease, *JAMA* 266(18):2594-2604, 1991.
17. Kaler SR: Epididymitis in the young adult male, *Nurs Pract* 15(5):10-16, 1990.
17a. Keller ML, Jadack RA, Mims LF: Perceived stressors and coping response in persons with recurrent genital herpes, *Res Nurs Health* 14:421-430, 1991.
18. Lafferty WE, et al: Recurrences after oral and genital herpes simplex virus infection, *N Engl J Med* 316:1444-1449, 1987.
19. Landrum S, et al: Racial trends in syphilis among men with same-sex partners in Atlanta, Georgia, *Am J Public Health* 78:66-67, 1988.
20.* Loucks A: Chlamydia: an unheralded epidemic, *Am J Nurs* 87:920-922, 1987.
21.* Lucas VA: Human papillomavirus infection: a potentially carcinogenic sexually transmitted disease, *Nurs Clin North Am* 23:917-935, 1988.
22.* Lutz R: Stopping the spread of sexually transmitted diseases, *Nurs 86* 16:47-50, March 1986.
23. Maberry MC: *Vulvovaginitis.* In Rakel RE: *Conn's current therapy: 1991,* Philadelphia, 1991, WB Saunders.
24.* McElhouse P: The "other" STDs as dangerous as ever, *RN* 52-58, June 1988.
25. Nettina SL, Kauffman FH: Diagnosis and management of sexually transmitted genital lesions, *Nurs Pract* 15(1):20-39, 1990.
26. Noble RC: *Syphilis.* In Rakel RE: *Conn's current therapy,* 1991, Philadelphia, 1991, WB Saunders Co, pp 685-688.
27. Peterson HB, et al: Pelvic inflammatory disease, *JAMA* 266:(18):2605-2612, 1991.
28. Ralel RE: *Conn's current therapy 1991,* Philadelphia, 1991, WB Saunders.
29.* Romanowski B, Harris J: Sexually transmitted diseases, *Clin Symp* 36(1):2-32, 1985.
30. Rotherberg RB, Potterfat JJ: *Strategies for management of sex*

*Recommended for student reading.

partners. In Holmes KK, et al: *Sexually transmitted diseases,* ed 2, New York, 1990, McGraw Hill.

31.* Secor RMC: Bacterial vaginosis: a comprehensive review, *Nurs Clin North Am* 23:865-875, 1988.

32. Sherertz EF: Chancroid. In Rakel RE: *Conn's current therapy 1991,* Philadelphia, 1991, WB Saunders.

33. Smith CE, McAllister CK: *Gonorrhea.* In Rakel RE: *Conn's current therapy 1991,* Philadelphia, 1991, WB Saunders.

34.* Smith LS: Ethnic differences in knowledge of sexually transmitted diseases in North American Black and Mexican-American migrant farmworkers, *Res Nurs Health* 11:51-58, 1988.

35. Strauss R, Glimp T: Sexually transmitted diseases, *Top Emerg Med* 7(2):73-84, 1985.

35a.* Touchstone DM, Davis DD: Consider chlamydia, *RN* 55(2):32-36, 1992.

36.* US Department of Health and Human Services, Public Health Services: Chlamydia trachomatis infections, policy guidelines for prevention and control, *MMWR* 34(3S):54S-73S, 1985.

37. US Department of Health and Human Services, Public Health Service: 1985 STD treatment guidelines, *MMWR (suppl)* 34(4S):76S-108S, 1985.

38. US Department of Health and Human Services, Public Health Service: Antibiotic-resistant strains of *Neisseria gonorrhoeae:* policy guidelines, *MMWR* 36(5S):1S-18S, 1987.

39.* US Department of Health and Human Services, Public Health Service: Progress toward achieving the 1990 objectives for sexual diseases, *MMWR* 36(12):173-176, 1987.

40. US Department of Health and Human Services, Public Health Service: Self-reported changes in sexual behaviors among homosexual and bisexual men from the San Francisco MMWR City Clinic Cohort, *MMWR* 36(12):187-189, 1987.

41. US Department of Health and Human Services, Public Health Service: Increases in primary and secondary syphilis—United States, *MMWR* 36(25):393-396, 1987.

42. US Department of Health and Human Services, Public Health Service: Sentinel surveillance system for antimicrobial resistance in clinical isolates of *Neisseria gonorrhoeae,* *MMWR* 36(35):585-593, 1987.

43. US Department of Health and Human Services, Public Health Service: Continuing increase in infectious syphilis—United States, *MMWR* 37(3):35-38, 1988.

44. US Department of Health and Human Services, Public Health Service: Condoms for the prevention of sexually transmitted diseases, *MMWR* 37(9):133-137, 1988.

45.* US Public Health Service, 1989 STD treatment guidelines, *MMWR* (suppl) 38(8):Sept 1, 1989.

46.* Whelan M: Nursing management of the patient with *Chlamydia trachomatis* infection, *Nurs Clin North Am* 23:877-883, 1988.

47. Wilms NA: Lymphogranuloma venereum. In Rakel RE: *Conn's current therapy,* 1991, Philadelphia, 1991, WB Saunders.

48. Zimmerman HL, et al: Epidemiologic differences between chlamydia and gonorrhea, *Am J Pub Health* 80(11):1338-1342, 1990.

Classic

49. Darrow WW: Changes in sexual behavior and venereal disease, *Clin Obstet Gynecol* 18:255-267, 1975.

50. Thompson SE, Washington AE: Epidemiology of sexually transmitted *Chlamydia trachomatis* infections, *Epidemiol Rev* 5:96-123, 1983.

51. US Department of Health and Human Services, Public Health Service: *STD fact sheet,* ed 35, HHS pub no (CDC) 81-8195, Atlanta, 1981, Centers for Disease Control.

52. US Department of Health and Human Services: Sexually transmitted diseases: treatment guidelines: morbidity and mortality, *MMWR* 31S-62S, 1982.

53. US Department of Health and Human Services, Public Health Service: *Annual Summary 1983, reported morbidity and mortality in the United States,* 32(54), Atlanta, 1984, Centers for Disease Control.

19

Management of Person with HIV Infection and AIDS

Denise M. Kresevic

After studying this chapter, the learner should be able to:

- Describe three common ways by which the HIV infection is spread.
- List the infection control measures to be used when caring for a person with AIDS.
- Identify three nursing problems and interventions for patients with HIV infection.
- Make a teaching plan on AIDS and its prevention for a high school class you have been asked to teach.
- Discuss the role of the nurse in addressing psychosocial, legal, and ethical issues related to the HIV epidemic.

Since the time of Florence Nightingale, nurses have provided care for individuals and families with communicable disease. One of the most dreaded communicable diseases of the twentieth century is AIDS (acquired immunodeficiency syndrome). AIDS is caused by the human immunodeficiency virus (HIV). Individuals infected with this virus suffer severe compromise of the body's ability to fight various infections and rare forms of cancer. The incidence of AIDS and HIV infection continues to increase steadily in the United States and worldwide. Therefore it is crucial that nurses have an understanding of (1) epidemiology, (2) disease prevention, (3) pathophysiology, and (4) nursing care of individuals infected with HIV.

EPIDEMIOLOGY AND PREVENTION

In 1981 the phenomenon of AIDS began to emerge. At that time the Centers for Disease Control (CDC) recognized that several previously nonlethal cases of *Pneumocystis carinii* pneumonia and a rare skin cancer called Kaposi's sarcoma were killing homosexual men at alarming rates in Los Angeles and New York City. By late 1986 more than 27,000 cases had been reported to the CDC, with over 15,000 fatalities. Epidemiologists and researchers studying these cases concluded that the cause of the fatal pneumonias and skin cancers was an underlying immune deficiency syndrome. Research efforts continued to isolate the causative immune deficiency virus. Before 1986 different researchers attributed various names to the virus: AIDS-related virus (ARV), lymphadenopathy-associated virus (LAV), and human T-lymphotropic virus type III (HTLV III). It was not until 1986 that the virus believed to cause AIDS was defined and named HIV.

By May 1991, 132,510 cases of AIDS had been reported in the United States (Table 19-1). It is estimated that another 1 to 1.5 million people are infected but asymptomatic. The World Health Organization (WHO) estimates that more than 600,000 persons are known to have AIDS worldwide; another 6 to 10 million in over 152 countries are infected but asymptomatic. The numbers of infected women and elderly continue to rise. It is also estimated that by the year 2000 from 12 to 18 million persons worldwide will be infected with HIV.

Virus Transmission and Risk Behaviors

A critical need exists to educate health care professionals, patients, and families about disease transmission and identified risk behaviors for HIV infection. The human immunodeficiency virus has been found in a variety of body fluids including blood, semen, cerebrospinal fluids (CSF), urine, stool, and saliva. Blood serum and CSF of infected individuals contain the highest concentrations of the virus and thus are the most likely means of transmission. Although HIV has also been found in varying concentrations in urine, stool, and saliva, no evidence exists that disease transmission has occurred via these body secretions.

There are *three major methods of HIV transmission:* (1) *intimate contact with body secretions,* including *semen* and *vaginal secretions* that occur *during sexual intercourse,* (2) *contact* with *infected blood* through *blood transfusions* or the *sharing of needles* during intravenous drug use, and (3) *maternal-infant transfer* via *placental exchange* or *breast milk.*

Although any member of the population may acquire AIDS, certain behaviors place individuals at increased risk for exposure to HIV based on disease transmission patterns. Populations at highest risk for exposure to HIV include homosexual and bisexual men, intravenous drug users, heterosexual partners of HIV-infected individuals, infants born to HIV-infected parents, and individuals who have received blood or blood products, especially before 1985 (Table 19-2).

The number of women with AIDS continues to increase with the greatest risk factor in 1990 being intravenous drug use. The incidence of AIDS in the elderly has been relatively low. Ten percent of all cases of AIDS have been reported in those aged 50 years and over. Of those cases, only 4% have occurred in those aged 70 years and older. Because of the latency period (up to 10 years) of this disease it is expected that the number of cases among the elderly will continue to increase.

More than 60% of the reported cases of HIV infection and AIDS have been in homosexual and bisexual men.[13] The greatest identified risk factors for HIV transmission in this group is anal intercourse. Such intercourse may be traumatic to fragile mucous membranes, resulting in microscopic tears and possible semen-blood transmission of the virus. The appropriate and consistent use of latex condoms, nonoxynyl-9 spermicide, and water-soluble lubricants may decrease the risk of trauma and disease transmission with anal intercourse in this risk group.[29]

Table 19-1 Distribution of AIDS cases in the United States as of May 1990*

Category	%	Category	%
Age		**Race ethnicity**	
<13	2	White	57
13-19	<1	Black	27
20-29	21	Hispanic	15
30-39	46	Other	1
40-49	21	Unknown	<1
49-70	6		
>70	4	**Sex**	
		Male	90
		Female	10
TOTAL CASES	132,510		

*Data from Centers for Disease Control, Atlanta.

Table 19-2 Number of AIDS cases in the United States by exposure category as of March 1992

Risk group	Number of cases
Homosexual and bisexual men	124,961
Heterosexual IV drug abusers	48,312
Homosexual and bisexual IV drug abusers	13,813
Heterosexual men and women	12,881
Recipients of blood products	457
Persons with hemophilia	1,812
Children of parents with/at risk for AIDS	3,133

Data from Centers for Disease Control, Atlanta.

Transmission of HIV by vaginal heterosexual intercourse is also possible. Associated risk factors for heterosexual transmission include anal intercourse, multiple sexual partners who may be infected and asymptomatic, and frequent sexual intercourse with multiple partners; these behaviors increase opportunities for exposure to infected body fluids. Studies on nonsexual household contacts, sharing of eating utensils and bathroom facilities, and close personal contact have *not* resulted in the transmission of HIV.[29,41]

Although the risk of HIV infection to health care workers is low, it remains a potential risk for those workers exposed to body secretions such as blood, urine, and stool. As of June 1990, 34 cases of occupational exposures had been reported to the Centers for Disease Control. Eighty percent of the exposures were attributed to needle-sticks. This represents a .05% risk of HIV seropositive conversion if stuck with a contaminated hollow-bore needle. To address this problem several syringe and needle manufactures have offered various anti-stick systems. These new products may offer additional protection from accidental needle-sticks to caregivers. *Several medical centers are studying the prophylactic use of AZT, an antiviral drug, for caregivers with accidental needle-sticks and mucous membrane exposures. Mucous membrane exposure* occurs *by blood splashing into the mouth, nose, or open cuts on the hands.*

Clearly the most important strategies for health care workers are good handwashing, avoidance of recapping needles, and the use of gloves whenever exposure to any patient's body secretions is likely to occur.[52]

For health care workers infected with HIV and desiring to continue to practice, the CDC recently issued guidelines. These guidelines recommend these health workers refrain from invasive procedures, such as surgery.[14a]

Infection Control Measures

In addition to health education strategies, infection control is one of the most important areas of concern for nurses caring for patients with HIV infection, whether in the hospital or home environment. Infection control procedures based on knowledge of disease transmission are essential to dispel the many emotional fears and myths surrounding the HIV infection. *Handwashing* remains the single most important principle of infection control for all diseases.[51] Handwashing is critical to protect immunocompromised patients and caregivers; it should be performed before and after contact with each patient and after removal of gloves. *Gloves* should be used whenever there will be *contact with body secretions: during care of lesions,* when *coming into contact with blood* (such as during dressing changes or starting intravenous lines), when *cleaning incontinent patients of urine or stool,* when *changing soiled linens,* and when *performing oral care.* In addition, caregivers should *keep fingernails cleaned* and well *trimmed to prevent punctures to gloves* and *possible transmission of the virus.*

Gloves are not necessary for casual contact such as bathing (without the presence of lesions), feeding, or ambulating patients.[52]

Soiled dressings, wet linens, and respiratory equipment should be discarded in heavy plastic bags. Puncture-resistant needle disposal containers should be in close proximity to all patient care areas. Needles should be disposed of promptly, *WITHOUT RECAPPING,* because recapping is the most frequent cause of accidental needle-sticks. Soap dispensers should be within close proximity of all patient care areas, and gloves should be worn for cleanup of urine, stool, or blood spills.

Standard household and institutional cleaning is important to protect all immunocompromised patients. Institutional cleaning agents used for floor and bathroom facilities are sufficient. A freshly mixed solution of bleach and water in a 1:10 parts mixture is used for home cleaning of floors, countertops, toilets, and spills. Standard laundering using bleach, and dishwashing using hot water and air drying are sufficient to protect caregivers and family members from HIV infection. However, *personal care items such as razors and toothbrushes should never be shared because of possible transmission* by *blood serum.* Pet excretion may pose a unique threat to immunocompromised patients. Patients with HIV infection who desire to keep their pets may require assistance in care, especially in cleaning bird cages, cat litter boxes, or fish tanks.[52]

The infection control guidelines previously mentioned are sufficient to protect pregnant women. Clearly, use of infection control measures is essential for all patients, regardless of known HIV infection, because this is the only way to ensure protection of caregivers. Patients' family members and all members of the health care team, including dietary workers and transport personnel, need basic education about HIV infection and infection control policies.

PATHOPHYSIOLOGY
Mechanism of HIV Infection

Infection with HIV renders the immune system severely compromised (see Chapters 16 and 41). The immune system, composed of organs and cells, protects the body from infections, cell mutations, and environmental toxins. The cells of the immune system are composed of lymphocytes, macrophages, and monocytes. Lymphocytes are further differentiated as T cells or B cells. HIV attacks T cells, which are responsible for all mediated immunity and protect the body from malignant cells, viruses, and parasites. The T cells are formed in the bone marrow and develop in the thymus. Two types of T cells produced by the body are T_4 inducer or helper cells, and T_8 cytotoxic or suppressor cells.

Table 19-3   Common laboratory abnormalities associated with HIV infection and AIDS

Disorder	Laboratory Findings
Anemia	Hematocrit <30%
Leukopenia	WBC <2500/cm³
Lymphopenia	Helper T cells 400/mm³
Decreased T_4/T_8 ratio	Ratio 1:2
Thrombocytopenia	Platelets <150,000

HIV has an affinity for invasion of the T₄ helper cells, but it may also invade other components of the immune system, including B cells, macrophages, and nerve cells, severely compromising cell-mediated immunity.

Individuals infected with HIV usually have almost twice as many T₈ suppressor cells as T₄ helper cells. This abnormal cell ratio renders HIV-infected persons immunocompromised and thus susceptible to a host of infections, malignancies, and abnormal laboratory results (Table 19-3).[18,26,40]

HIV is classified as a retrovirus. Retroviruses carry their genetic code in RNA rather than DNA material. In retroviruses an enzyme known as reverse transcriptase converts RNA to DNA, which is incorporated into the host cell's genetic material. Thus the virus invades the host cell, living within it and replicating itself (Fig. 19-1). Based on these cellular pathologies of the HIV infection, the CDC *defines AIDS as "a disease at least moderately predictive of a cell-mediated immunity occurring in persons with no known cause for diminished resistance to that disease."*[41]

HIV Infection Continuum and Clinical Manifestations

HIV infection may remain dormant for several years, producing no clinical symptoms.[18] This prolonged incubation period is of great concern because individuals may be asymptomatic but contagious. Others infected with the virus may experience transient acute symptoms of fever, muscle aches, rashes, diarrhea, and gastrointestinal cramping that occur 2 to 6 weeks after exposure and then resolve (Fig. 19-2 and Table 19-4). Others patients exposed to the virus and harboring HIV antibodies exhibit chronic symptoms of diffuse noncancerous lymph node enlargement, or *persistent generalized lymphadenopathy* (PGL), fever, chills, night sweats, and weight loss.

Patients exposed to the virus, who are *harboring HIV antibodies and who experience night sweats, fever, weight loss, fatigue, edema, and abnormal laboratory immune values including altered T₄ and T₈ cell ratios, but who have no infections or malignancies, are diagnosed as having AIDS-related complex* (ARC). ARC can be a very debilitating disease.[9] However, *Acquired immunodeficiency syndrome,* or AIDS, is the most severe HIV disease. Patients with AIDS continue to experience all the same symptoms, including fatigue, weight loss, fever, diarrhea, and edema.[6] In addition, *opportunistic infections may be life-threatening,* and rare forms of cancers also invade the body (Table 19-5). *Opportunistic infections* prey on compromised immune systems.

Patients with AIDS, similar to patients with cancer, patients with an organ-transplant, and those receiving immunosuppressive therapy to prevent rejection, become susceptible to infections that individuals with intact immune systems are able to fight.

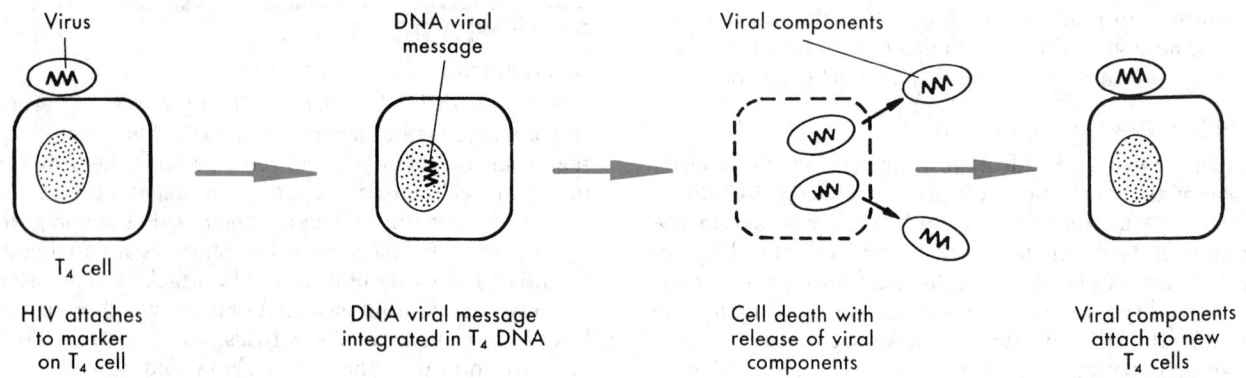

Fig. 19-1 Mechanism of HIV action.

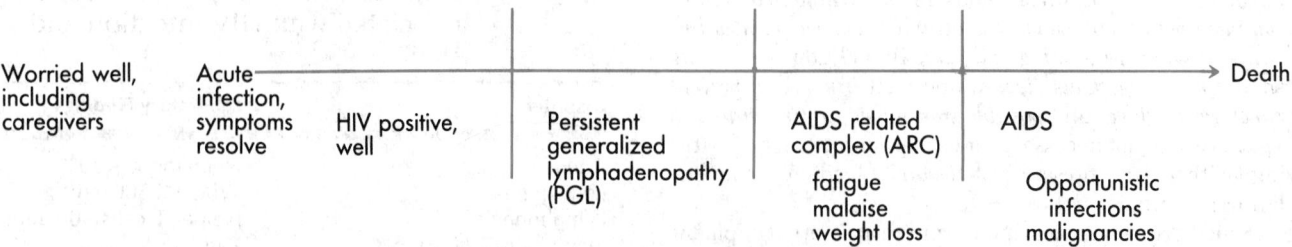

Fig. 19-2 Continuum of HIV infection; only some persons proceed from infection to AIDS and death.

Table 19-4   Progression of HIV infection[11]

Group	Type	Characteristics
I	Acute infection	Fever, malaise with seroconversion
II	Asymptomatic infection	Seroconversion; no symptoms
III	Persistent generalized lymphadenopathy (PGL)	Lymphadenopathy more than 3 months in absence of explainable illness
IV	Other HIV disease	(See subgroups)
IV-1	Constitutional disease (ARC)	Diarrhea or fever persisting more than 1 month; involuntary weight loss of greater than 10% of baseline
IV-2	Neurologic disease	HIV encephalopathy or dementia; peripheral neuropathy
IV-3	Secondary infectious diseases	*Pneumocystis carinii* pneumonia; candidiasis; extrapulmonary cryptococcosis; mycobacterial infection; CMV infection; herpes infections
IV-4	Secondary cancers	Kaposi's sarcoma, non-Hodgkin's lymphoma, primary lymphoma of the brain

Modified from Centers for Disease Control: Pneumocystis pneumonia: Los Angeles, *MMWR* 30:250-252, 1981.

Table 19-5   Opportunistic infections and neoplasms associated with HIV infection

Agent	Body system affected
Infection	
Protozoal	
Pneumocystis carinii	Respiratory
Toxoplasma gondii	Neurologic and disseminated
Cryptosporidium	Gastrointestinal
Bacterial	
Mycobacterium avium intracellulare	Disseminated
Mycobacterium tuberculosis	Respiratory, neurologic, or disseminated
Fungal	
Candida albicans	Gastrointestinal (mouth and or esophagus)
	Disseminated
Cryptococcus neoformans	Neurologic or disseminated
Viral	
Herpes simplex	Integumentary (mouth, genital, perianal)
Varicella-zoster	Integumentary
Cytomegalovirus	Neurologic (eyes) disseminated
Neoplastic diseases	
Kaposi's sarcoma (epidemic form)	Skin and mucous membranes
Burkitt's lymphoma	Lymph system
Non-Hodgkin's lymphomas	Lymph system
Hodgkin's disease	Lymph system
Chronic lymphocytic leukemia	White blood cells

19-1

Signs and symptoms of HIV infection

Chills and fever	Malaise
Night sweats	Fatigue
Dry productive cough	Oral lesions
Dyspnea	Skin rashes
Lethargy	Abdominal discomfort
Confusion	Diarrhea
Stiff neck	Weight loss
Seizures	Lymphadenopathy
Headache	Progressive generalized edema

Nursing Process
Assessment

Some patients may be asymptomatic; others may report nonspecific "flulike" symptoms of fever, chills, night sweats, or dry, nonproductive cough. The clinical diversity of the HIV infection (see Box 19-1) can make identification and assessment of infected patients difficult. Nurses may encounter patients experiencing various clinical symptoms including fatigue, fever, diarrhea, or confusion, depending on the continuum of illness. Patients identified at risk for HIV infection either by sexual history, drug history, or flulike symptoms should be further assessed for the presence of opportunistic infections, rashes, and neoplasms (see Table 19-5).

Identification of persons at risk

Health assessments of all patients should include an appraisal of potential risk factors for HIV infection. Obtaining a complete, accurate history of sexual behavior, including past and present sexual activities, will be necessary and requires skillful interviewing techniques and a professional relationship based on trust. Nurses need to be comfortable explaining the need for information on intimate sexual activities, and phrasing questions in appropriate but comprehensible terms. The sexual health history, in addition to identifying individuals at risk for possible HIV infection, may also be an opportunity for health education and disease prevention (see Box 19-2).

19-2

19-2 Sample sexual history

1. When did you first become sexually active? With whom? For how long? Type of sexual activity practiced:
   - Mutual masturbation
   - French kissing
   - Vaginal intercourse
   - Anal intercourse
   - Oral intercourse
   - Use of objects to enhance stimulation
   - Use of contraceptives
2. Are you currently sexually active? With whom? For how long? Type of sexual activity?
3. Do you currently have any concerns about your sexuality or sexual activity?
4. Do you suspect that any of your sexual partners have been infected with herpes, syphilis, gonorrhea, or AIDS? (Patients may need further explanations of specific types of infections and symptoms).

Information on the use of mood-affecting drugs such as alcohol, marijuana, heroin, cocaine, crack, barbiturates, tranquilizers, butyl nitrate, or amphetamines should also be obtained. Frequency and routes of administration including oral, smoking, sniffing, snorting, or injecting drugs should be explored. Needle exposure through the sharing of drug paraphernalia, tattoos, or acupuncture treatment should also be assessed.[39]

Individuals identified as being at risk for HIV infection should be counseled about the significance of testing and the necessity for follow-up. Patients with evidence of risk factors and any clinical symptoms should be referred for blood testing and medical evaluation of symptoms to diagnose exposure to the HIV infection.

AIDS and the elderly

Although much is still unknown about the immune function and aging, in general aging is associated with depressed cell-mediated immunity, impaired antibody production, and increased autoantibody production (see Chapter 41). These aging changes often result in decreased capacity to resist infections.

The majority of elderly persons with AIDS to date have been traced to blood transfusions associated with common surgical procedures such as coronary bypass and valve surgery and joint replacements. Given the long incubation period, the risk of contamination from blood transfusions, and the decreased capacity of the elderly to resist infections the incidence of HIV in this age group is projected to rise steadily.

Recognition of the HIV infection in the elderly may be difficult for several reasons. A diagnosis of AIDS may be missed in the elderly who frequently have symptoms such as pneumonia, dementia, shortness of breath, weakness, fatigue, poor nutritional intake, and weight loss. In addition, caregivers may fail to evaluate thoroughly such risk factors as intravenous drug use and homosexuality in this age group.

The elderly with compromised immune functions or chronic illnesses such as heart and respiratory disease often have little reserve to resist or fight the multiple infections that may accompany the HIV infection. In general, this age group exhibits more side effects from aggressive antibiotic therapy used to fight infections. Increasing numbers of acutely ill elders suffering from multiple infections associated with the HIV infection poses unique clinical challenges for nurses in all settings.

Diagnostic tests: HIV seropositivity

Individuals who have been exposed to HIV and have had sufficient time for increased antibody production can be tested for infection. Two tests may be used to diagnose infection. The most common test is the enzyme-linked immunosorbent assay (ELISA). This test was originally developed as a screening tool for potential blood donors. Because the ELISA is a sensitive screening test for HIV infection, *false positive* tests are possible. Individuals who are not infected with HIV but have had multiple blood transfusions or pregnancies may have false positive results. In addition, a *false negative* ELISA test may occur during the so-called "window period." The window period is that time between exposure to the virus and the development of sufficient antibodies. The window period for HIV may be a few weeks or up to 3 months.[40] An additional confirmatory test called the *Western Blot* is usually used as a means of accurately diagnosing HIV-infected persons. In general, the use of both the ELISA and Western Blot is able to provide over 99% accurate diagnosis of HIV infection.

A person with a positive test result is called HIV seropositive. This result indicates exposure to the HIV infection. Although it is not known at present how many seropositive individuals develop AIDS, it is believed that a majority die of AIDS complications.[40] Legal and ethical issues surrounding mandatory HIV testing for employment and insurance coverage continue to present an emotional challenge.

Data analysis: nursing diagnoses

Because of the different HIV infection categories on the HIV infection continuum and the great variety of symptoms, nursing care plans for persons with HIV infection or AIDS will show a variety of nursing diagnoses based on analysis of patient data. Some possible nursing diagnoses for the person with HIV infection include, but are not limited to, the following:

Diagnostic title	Possible etiologies
Knowledge deficit	Lack of exposure/recall, misinterpretation of information about HIV
Infection, high risk for	Decreased immune response
Body temperature, altered, high risk for	Infection, dehydration
Nutrition, altered: less than body requirements	Nausea, vomiting, diarrhea, alterations in oral mucous membranes, dysphagia
Coping, ineffective individual, family	Inadequate or incorrect information or understanding, crisis, prolonged disability of significant person, societal mores

Diagnostic title	Possible etiologies
Anxiety	Threat to self-concept, threat of death, threat to/change in health status/socioeconomic status
Injury, high risk for	Confusion, dementia, weakness
Skin integrity, impaired	Pressure sores, infected lesions
Self-care deficit	Activity intolerance, dyspnea, fatigue, depression, visual impairments, cognitive dysfunction
Social isolation	Societal biases, alteration in physical appearance or mental status, lack of knowledge about AIDS virus transmission
Grieving, anticipatory	Probable patient death

Planning: expected patient outcomes

Expected patient outcomes for the person with HIV infection or AIDS may include, but are not limited to, the following:

1. The patient and significant others verbalize an understanding of disease pathophysiology, transmission of the virus, basic infection control measures, diagnostic tests, and common treatment modalities.
2. Secondary infections do not occur or are identified early for treatment. HIV transmission to significant others and caregivers does not occur.
3. Body temperature decreases.
4. Weight loss, electrolyte imbalance, and discomfort are minimized. Patient ingests adequate fluids and a balanced diet daily.
5. Patient and significant others describe usual coping strategies and explore alternative strategies.
6. Patient demonstrates fewer signs of anxiety.
7. Patient will remain free from injuries such as falls.
8. Skin and mucous membranes are moist; skin turgor is good.
9. Patient participates in ADL at optimal level of functioning.
10. Patient has opportunities to interact with others on a social basis.
11. Patient and significant others engage in anticipatory grieving through communication that leads to sharing of feelings, decision making, and problem resolution, as pertinent.
12. The patient and family will be able to discuss perceptions related to the meaning of their life, their suffering, and wishes for continued treatment or withholding of treatment.

Implementation

Interventions to achieve patient outcomes
Facilitating learning for persons at risk

Nursing care needs vary along the illness continuum of HIV infection. Interventions are directed toward several groups of patients, including (1) "worried" well, (2) individuals with risk factors, (3) asymptomatic HIV-infected, (4) HIV-infected patients with clinical symptoms and their families; and (5) terminally ill HIV-infected individuals and their families. Nursing care of worried well individuals and family emphasizes education about HIV infection. Nurses will be required to serve as health resources for various community and institutional settings ranging from hospitals, churches, and schools to occupational settings. A majority of health education about HIV infection focuses on clarifying myths and helping individuals cope with their anxiety and emotional-laden fears surrounding this epidemic. The challenge for nurses providing health education about HIV infection is to impart accurate, concise information that addresses the fears of contagion and disease transmission. Inherent in such education is a multitude of complex educational issues, including human sexuality.

Educational strategies, whether directed toward the worried well or those infected with HIV, must emphasize accurate information about disease transmission and safer sex practices. Safe sex refers to abstinence or a mutually monogamous sexual relationship with a noninfected partner. Risky sexual practices include multiple sexual partners and anal sex. The use of water-soluble lubricants and latex condoms with the spermicide nonoxynol-9 may increase the safety of vaginal and anal intercourse.

Both the worried well and those identified as being at risk for HIV infection need education and referral for antibody tests. Before testing, individuals require extensive counseling on the significance of test results and follow-up care and treatment. It is *important to stress* in counseling *that a one-time negative antibody test is meaningless if exposure to risk factors continues.* Some patients practicing intravenous drug use need additional referral and treatment to eliminate the risk behavior. One of the most difficult issues in caring for patients at high risk of contracting and transmitting the HIV infection is the balance of patient confidentiality and the caregiver's responsibility to share information regarding potential risk to the patient's sexual partners and loved ones. Education and counseling may be accomplished through individual teaching, role modeling, informal group discussions, or lectures. However, teaching requires more than spoken words. Learning should be reinforced by allowing persons to express their concerns, an-

---

19-3

Guidelines for teaching patients with HIV and their significant others

Common risk factors for transmission of HIV infection include sharing of needles and other drug paraphernalia by IV drug abusers, anal intercourse, and blood transfusions.

Ways to prevent spread of HIV infection, including limiting sexual partners and using latex condoms with nonoxynol-9 spermicide, cleaning of needles by IV drug abusers and not sharing needles with others, and autologous blood donations before elective surgery.

Symptoms of AIDS—fevers, dry cough, and night sweats.

Diagnostic tests—ELISA and Western Blot.

Healthful living practices—good nutrition, exercise, and stress reduction.

Community resources available to persons with HIV infection including health clinics, support groups, homecare nurses, Legal Aid Society, and resources for AIDS education.

swering questions, and using printed resources for future reference; repetition is essential. See Box 19-3 for guidelines for teaching.

The Department of Health and Human Services report to the Surgeon General of the United States established health goals to decrease the spread of HIV infection by the year 2000. Some of these goals can be found in Box 19-4.

Patients and families along the HIV continuum, from the worried well to those terminally ill with the virus, require much health teaching and counseling. The goal of counseling is to impart accurate information that empowers patients and families to make informed decisions and mobilize adequate mechanisms of support and adaptation for coping with multiple stressors.

Patients with HIV infection have many questions and concerns about the disease and its transmission, prognosis, and treatment. Initially, most patients are in a state of shock and disbelief. Information should be given in small segments with opportunities for repetition. Many patients require assistance with the decision to share the fact of their illness with significant others. All sexual partners who are potentially at risk for contracting the disease have the right to know of their own potential risk of illness.

Additional information may be obtained from the following sources: PHS AIDS Hotline (800-342-AIDS, 800-342-2437; good source for statistics and clinical drug trials) and National Sexually Transmitted Disease Hotline, American Social Health Association (800-227-8922). Both lines are accessible 24 hours a day.

Preventing infections

Normal environments can be a source of lethal infections for the immunocompromised patient. Nursing care for persons with HIV infection or AIDS must stress meticulous personal hygiene, close observation of potential sources of infection, frequent handwashing, and avoidance of environmental microbes. Infection control measures (p. 385) are essential.

Patients with HIV infection are encouraged and assisted to bathe daily. Most patients will require a bed bath; tub baths should be avoided if the patient has a rash. Whenever possible, showers are recommended. Patients suffering from diarrhea require frequent cleaning with a gentle soap and liberal application of moisture barriers to prevent skin breakdown. Special attention to oral care to prevent infection and promote adequate nutrition and comfort is important. Soft toothbrushes and nonabrasive toothpaste and rinses will decrease the chances of trauma and secondary infections. Rinses with sodium bicarbonate, saline, or lemon and hydrogen peroxide are useful before meals and

---

19-4

Health status objective for HIV infection for year 2000

1. Confine annual incidence of diagnosed AIDS cases to no more than 98,000 from an estimated 44,000 to 50,000 diagnosed cases in 1989, with the following goals for special target populations:

Diagnosed AIDS cases	1989 baseline	Year 2000 target
Gay and bisexual men	26,000-28,000	48,000
Blacks	14,000-15,000	37,000
Hispanics	7000-8000	18,000

2. Confine the prevalence of HIV infection to no more than 800 per 100,000 people with the following goals for special target populations:

Population	1989 baseline per 100,000	Year 2000 target per 100,000
Homosexual men	2000-42,000	20,000
Intravenous drug abusers	30,000-40,000	40,000
Women giving birth to live infants	150	100

3. Reduce the incidence of sexual intercourse among adolescents.
4. Increase to at least 50% the proportion of sexually active unmarried people who use condoms.
5. Increase to at least 50% from an estimated 11% in 1989 the proportion of opiate abusers who are in treatment.
6. Increase to at least 50% from a baseline of 25% to 35% in 1989 the proportion of intravenous drug abusers not in treatment who use only uncontaminated drug paraphernalia.
7. Increase to at least 80% percent from an estimated 15% in 1989 the proportion of HIV-infected people who have been tested for HIV infection.
8. Increase to at least 95% the proportion of schools that have age-appropriate HIV education curricula for students in the fourth through twelfth grades.
9. Provide HIV education for students and staff at at least 90% of colleges and universities.
10. Extend to all facilities where workers are at risk for occupational transmission regulations to protect workers from exposure to bloodborne infections, including HIV infection.

From *Healthy people 2000: national health promotion and disease prevention objectives,* Department of Health & Human Services, Public Health Service, Washington, DC, 1991, Government Printing Office.

at bedtime. Oral care after meals helps prevent tooth decay and infections.

Pulmonary infection occurs frequently with HIV. Thus patients are taught and coached through deep-breathing and coughing exercises at least every 4 hours while awake to promote airway clearance and prevent atelectasis.

Meticulous skin care is necessary to minimize infections and promote comfort. Patients with decreased mobility may benefit from the use of air mattresses and frequent turning schedules to prevent decubiti. Turning sheets are used when necessary to prevent friction and injury. A high-protein diet will help prevent skin breakdown by providing essential amino acids for healing. Edematous limbs are elevated using pillows to promote circulation. Emollients can be used liberally to prevent skin drying and cracking. Skin lesions are washed separately using a clean washcloth and gloves to prevent contamination.

Biopsy sites and intravenous insertion sites can be sources of infection. Observe sites daily for redness, warmth, pain, or drainage. Sites that are suggestive of infection should have wound cultures to confirm or rule out infection. Avoid plastic occlusive dressings; they have been shown to increase the risk of infection in some immunocompromised patients. Change dressings at least every other day. Avoid sources of microbes, such as fresh plants and dietary servings of rare meat and fresh vegetables or fruits.

Attention must be paid to the patient's environment. The room should be dusted and mopped daily using damp cloths to prevent air distribution of microbes. Supplies should be neatly stocked. Dietary trays are removed after meals, and additional dietary supplements are stored outside the patient's room. In most cases, except with airborne infections such as tuberculosis, the patient's door may be kept open to minimize odors, promote adequate ventilation, and decrease feelings of isolation. Private rooms for patients with HIV infection are not usually necessary except with specific infections such as tuberculosis. Patients are not placed in a room with another patient who has an infection. The single most important factor that protects immunocompromised patients from infections is the practice of consistent good handwashing techniques by patients, caregivers, and visitors. Care of the person with HIV infection is summarized in Box 19-5.

Guidelines for Care   **19-5**

The patient with HIV infection/AIDS

Prevent infection.

1. Wash hands frequently and use emollient for patient and caregiver.
2. Use a gentle liquid soap (such as Castile); avoid bar soaps that may irritate skin.
3. Provide for daily showering or basin bath; avoid tub bath if rashes are present.
4. Use a separate washcloth for lesions.
5. Use soft toothbrushes, nonabrasive toothpaste; and mouth rinses with sodium bicarbonate, saline, or lemon and hydrogen peroxide before meals and at bedtime.
6. Use measures to prevent skin pressure, such as turning sheets, sheepskin, or eggcrate or air mattresses.
7. Elevate and support areas of edema.
8. Observe biopsy sites and IV insertion sites daily for signs of infection.
9. Change dressings at least every other day; avoid plastic occlusive dressings.
10. Avoid sources of microbes, such as fresh plants or ingestion of fresh fruits and vegetables.
11. Carry out measures to prevent spread of infection; use of gloves for contact with bodily secretions, double plastic bags to dispose of bodily secretions, use of bleach and water (1:10) for cleaning of contaminated areas.

Modify alterations in body temperature.

1. Administer prescribed antibiotics, IV fluids, or antipyretics.
2. Encourage fluid intake >2500 ml.
3. Maintain daily intake and output records.
4. Weigh daily.
5. Provide tepid sponge baths and linen changes as necessary.
6. Instruct patient in deep-breathing and coughing exercises to prevent atelectasis and additional fever.

Promote good nutrition.

1. Provide instruction for high-calorie, high-protein, high-potassium, low-residue diet.
2. Encourage high-calorie, high-potassium snacks.
3. Suggest foods that are easy to swallow (gelatin, yogurt, puddings) when dysphagia is present.
4. Avoid foods that are spicy or acidic, rare meats, and raw fruits and vegetables.
5. Provide oral care before patient eats.
6. Encourage patient to get out of bed and sit up for meals if possible.
7. Avoid odors by aerating room.
8. Make appropriate dietary consultations.

Promote self-care.

1. Assess realistic functional ability.
2. Plan, supervise, and assist with ADL as necessary.
3. Encourage patient to be as active and independent as possible.
4. Assist patient with range-of-motion exercise to prevent contractures.
5. Provide equipment such as assistive eating devices, walkers, and commodes to promote patient independence.
6. Pace activities and schedule rest periods to prevent fatigue.

Provide counseling.

1. Assess and support patient coping mechanisms.
2. Explore with patient and significant others normalcy of grief responses.
3. Assist patient and significant others in acknowledging and planning for anticipated losses.
4. Provide information as desired and necessary, depending on the ability to perceive.
5. Suggest appropriate religious support.
6. Facilitate participation in support groups or individual counseling as pertinent.

Modifying alterations in body temperature

Fever, a common result of HIV infection, may be caused by dehydration or multiple infections, including *P. carinii* pneumonia, cytomegalovirus, and *mycobacterium avium intracellulare*. Fevers may also be caused by infection from intravenous lines or biopsy sites.

All patients with HIV infection should be monitored for fever and adequate fluid intake. Temperatures of hospitalized patients are assessed every 4 hours, body temperatures greater than 37.5° C or 101.5° F are reported to the physician for medical follow-up. Diagnostic tests for fevers may include chest x-ray examinations or blood cultures for detection of specific pathogens. Patients with fevers may require several tepid sponge baths and linen changes to promote comfort. Fever and sweating may increase fluid loss and contribute to dehydration, therefore patients should ingest at least 2500 ml of fluid per day. Accurate daily intake and output are recorded and evaluated.

Daily monitoring of intravenous sites and other wounds for possible infection is also critical. Fevers are cautiously treated with antipyretics such as acetaminophen (contraindicated with use of the drug Retrovir). The use of aspirin is contraindicated with HIV infection because the infection itself may alter normal blood coagulation. Intravenous therapy may be necessary to provide adequate hydration. Despite meticulous personal hygiene and nursing care, some patients with HIV infection may continue to have persistent temperature elevation with no explained cause.

Promoting optimal nutrition

Patients with HIV infection are frequently plagued by alterations in gastrointestinal function, such as dysphagia, nausea, vomiting, and diarrhea. Infections such as *Candida* and *Cryptosporidiosis* also contribute to alterations in food and fluid intake and absorption, resulting in reduced nutrition. Depression may be manifested by changes in appetite.

Daily weight and food and fluid intake are monitored and recorded. Nutritional intake may be increased by attention to oral hygiene, positioning, socialization, and attention to individual preferences. Patients and caregivers are taught about nutritional factors that contribute to health despite the HIV infection.

Patients are encouraged to get out of bed and sit up for meals to aid digestion and decrease the possibility of aspiration. Odors should be minimized because they may contribute to nausea. Oral hygiene, including mouth rinses before meals, enhances the taste of food and stimulates digestive juices. Whenever possible, significant others can be encouraged to visit during meals and to bring home-prepared food. Patients may prefer frequent small meals or snacks spaced throughout the day to prevent indigestion and fatigue.

Adequate nutrition can be enhanced by the following:
1. Daily oral intake of 2500 ml to 3000 ml of fluids to prevent dehydration, especially with diarrhea; suggested fluids are water, fruit juices, soups, and gelatin.
2. Foods high in potassium (to replace that lost by diarrhea) include bananas, apricots, and orange juice.
3. Textured foods that are easy to swallow and tolerate include gelatin, yogurt, and pudding.
4. Foods high in protein that are easily tolerated include peanut butter, honey, and instant breakfast drinks.
5. Avoid foods with naturally occurring microbes (rare meat, raw fruits and vegetables) and foods that aggravate dysphagia (spicy, acidic, or raw fruits and vegetables).

Multiple medications may alter the normal taste of foods, and patients may need to be encouraged to try new or differently prepared foods. Collaboration with nutritionists may be useful. At times, dietary supplements may be needed to maintain adequate caloric intake. All supplements, especially those containing lactose, should be evaluated as potentially causing diarrhea. Dysphagia resulting from oral *Candida* may be treated with oral medications such as Nystatin or lidocaine to decrease discomfort and increase nutritional intake. Patients living alone in their own homes often require assistance with shopping and meal preparation.

Some severely malnourished patients may require oral nutritional supplements or parenteral hyperalimentation (Chapter 31).

Assisting with coping

Individuals who are exposed to HIV infection, but are without symptoms or complications of infections or cancers, live with a great deal of uncertainty and anxiety interspersed with denial and hopefulness. The role of the nurse in this stage of the disease process is to provide continued education about the disease of AIDS, as well as to assist in realistic goal setting. Patients are encouraged to participate in their own care and to maintain positive relationships.

As the HIV infection progresses with clinical complications of infections and cancers, patients experience multiple losses including loss of energy, self-care deficit requiring assistance with activities of daily living, and loss of independence, employment, finances, and hope. The reality of death emerges. Nursing care focuses on a philosophy of facing life a day at a time and living each day to the fullest extent possible by resolving multiple conflicts. This may be a time for strengthening personal and spiritual relationships.

Empathic listening and the ability to help patients find meaning in life become critical nursing interventions. Assisting families and significant others, including lovers, to provide support to the terminally ill patient despite their own anger and grief is a unique nursing challenge. Such care, although emotionally draining for the nurse, can provide tremendous positive feelings of professional accomplishment.

Box 19-6 presents the results of a research study of persons with HIV infection and AIDS.

The diagnosis of HIV infection, with its social stigma, poor prognosis, and lethal nature, is indeed a catastrophic event for patients and caregivers. Patients experience a variety of intense emotions that threaten self-esteem and predispose to depression and feelings of powerlessness. Anxiety is a response that pervades the entire HIV illness continuum. Anxiety and denial often accompany the initial diagnosis and intensify with physical decline and loss of independence, job, and finances. Anxiety may be incapacitating as death becomes a reality. Nursing interventions to promote effective coping focus on exploring and strengthening healthful coping strategies and maintaining sources of psychologic support.

Reducing anxiety

Individuals experiencing the anxiety of HIV infection are often in a state of crisis (see Chapter 6 for further information). Continued clarification and education about the HIV infection, complications, and treatment are critical. Every effort should be made to include the patient in planning medical and nursing care. An assessment of past coping styles and support systems should be made early and continually reevaluated. Healthful patterns of coping, such as talking or relaxation and meditation, are encouraged. Relationships with family, friends, and lovers should be maintained and may be strengthened through the HIV crisis. Conversely, past conflicts, especially among family members, may persist and intensify during the HIV crisis.

Occasionally anxiety, denial, depression, and even grief may persist for extended periods, interfering with daily functioning, productive communication and relationships, and even the ability to make decisions. The nurse must be able to assess normal periods of anxiety, depression, and grief, as well as refer patients and significant others for psychologic evaluation and counseling for ineffective coping patterns. Although reactions of anxiety and depression are normal, professional intervention is necessary whenever they preclude communication and daily functioning for an extended time (usually longer than 3 months). Patients with HIV infection and depression should be assessed for suicidal ideation because this phenomenon occasionally occurs in terminally ill patients who are experiencing anxiety and fear of further pain and physical decline. Early recognition of depression is critical because some cases of depression and anxiety may respond to medications and psychotherapy.

Individuals with diffuse anxiety often feel they have little control over their daily existence. A schedule of activities that patients develop with guidance from health care professionals may decrease anxiety and feelings of powerlessness. Opportunities for spiritual support and comfort should be explored. Significant others may also experience anxiety. Community support groups for patients and significant others may offer additional sources of support and contribute to healthful coping. Planned uninterrupted time with only the nurse, patient, and significant other may create a supportive environment that decreases anxiety and promotes healthful coping.

Preventing injury

Safety is a critical need for patients with HIV infection who are at increased risk for accidents and injury because of decreased physical and cognitive function. The patient's environment is assessed to ensure strategic placement of items such as call lights and urinals. Use of siderails and restraints may be necessary to prevent injury but should never be substituted for frequent observation. Both patients and significant others should be aware of safety needs

19-6   **Nursing Research**

Korniewicz DM, Obrien ME, Larson E: Coping with AIDS and HIV: psychosocial adaptation *J Psychosoc Nurs Men Health Serv* 28(3):14-21, 1990.

In this study four groups of patients were interviewed: those with HIV risk factors such as homosexuality but with unknown seropositive status, HIV-infected individuals with no symptoms, HIV-infected individuals with early symptoms of AIDS such as vomiting and weight loss, and those with late symptoms of AIDS including opportunistic infections. Through patient interviews and chart reviews these investigators found that individuals infected with the HIV virus but not yet exhibiting symptoms, experienced the greatest feelings of powerlessness. Based on these findings *the researchers recommend that nurses providing care to HIV-infected patients pay particular attention to newly diagnosed individuals rather than postpone psychosocial interventions until physical symptoms of AIDS are apparent.*

and the rationale for interventions to prevent injury. Referrals to occupational and physical therapy may be useful in developing a coordinated plan of care to maximize safe independent functioning.

Promoting skin integrity

As the patient becomes increasingly ill and is unable to meet self-care needs, the potential for skin breakdown is high. Nursing emphasis is on frequent turning and keeping the skin clean, dry, and well lubricated with moisturizers. Special mattresses or beds may be used to minimize pressure on bony prominences. Improving the patient's nutritional intake will also help prevent skin breakdown.

Promoting self-care and safety

Many persons infected with HIV suffer from fatigue, dyspnea, depression, or cognitive impairments requiring assistance with activities of daily living. Immunocompromised persons are particularly vulnerable to environmental pathogens and require meticulous daily hygiene. A daily schedule of activity that includes turning, positioning, sitting up for meals, bathing, and toileting will minimize the risks of secondary infections and contribute to feelings of positive self-esteem.

Patients are encouraged to remain as active and as independent as possible. The use of energy conservation and pacing of activities is very effective in maintaining independence and comfort. Adaptive equipment such as assistive eating devices, walkers, or bedside commodes may also promote independence and safety. Some patients may require assistance with range-of-motion exercises to prevent contractures.

Supporting interactions to minimize social isolation

The psychosocial aspects of AIDS are devastating. Because no cure presently exists for the HIV infection, the diagnosis of HIV infection, like a diagnosis of cancer, brings potential denial, fear, depression, and anger. The social stigma of AIDS, based on associations with homosexuality, intravenous drug abuse, and sexual transmission, cannot be minimized.[49] One of the earliest issues that HIV-infected individuals face is sharing the information with significant others. Tremendous fear of family anger, rejection, or abandonment is a real concern.

Often families and friends who are struggling with their own anxieties and fears abandon the patient. When this happens, the nurse should try to assist the patient to find other sources of social support. In some cities there are support groups for patients and separate groups for significant others. HIV-infected individuals who have been exposed by contaminated blood or unknowingly through heterosexual relationships may feel unique and intense anger and hostility. These patients are usually supported by their families and friends. They can be isolated by other persons who do not understand that HIV and AIDS are not spread by casual contact.

Assisting with grieving

Like patients with other terminal illnesses, patients diagnosed with the HIV infection may experience strong emotions of fear, anger, denial, or quiet depression. Some patients benefit from individual empathic listening and exploring feelings, fears, and treatment options. Other patients may benefit from support groups with patients experiencing similar feelings. Significant others, including family and lovers, experience their own feelings of fear, anger, and embarrassment. Individual counseling and support groups may be helpful for loved ones who will need to be a source of support for the patient. Practical issues such as employment disability, housing discrimination, insurance coverage, and preparation for death also need to be addressed. Referral to social workers and appropriate community agencies can alleviate many concerns that plague acutely and terminally ill patients. Continued participation in religious services and the support of fellow worshippers and clergy should not be overlooked as a source of healthy coping. Many members of the clergy are experienced in grief counseling and can be helpful to patients and significant others.

Evaluation

Evaluation is based on the expected patient outcomes. Questions to consider include the following:

1. Can the patient and significant others explain the disease pathophysiology, transmission of the virus, basic infection-control measures, diagnostic tests, and common treatment modalities?
2. Have secondary infections been avoided or identified early, and has HIV transmission to significant others and caregivers been avoided?
3. Has the patient's body temperature decreased?
4. Have weight loss, electrolyte imbalance, and discomfort been minimized, and is the patient ingesting adequate fluids and a balanced diet daily?
5. Can the patient and significant others describe usual coping strategies and have they developed alternative strategies?
6. Is the patient's anxiety reduced?
7. Has the patient remained free from injuries such as falls?
8. Are the patient's skin and mucous membranes moist, and is skin turgor good?
9. Does the patient participate in ADL at the optimal level of functioning?
10. Does the patient have opportunities to interact with others on a social basis?
11. Have the patient and significant others engaged in anticipatory grieving?
12. Can the patient and significant others discuss perceptions regarding the meaning of their lives, their suffering, and their wishes for the continuation or withholding of treatment?

HIV COMPLICATIONS: AIDS

The clinical presentation of AIDS can be attributed to secondary opportunistic infections and malignancies that occur with a compromised immune system. The following is a summary of these opportunistic infections and related patient care needs. See p. 399 for nursing care plan for a person with HIV complications.

PNEUMOCYSTIS CARINII PNEUMONIA

The most common opportunistic infection that occurs with HIV infection is *Pneumocystis carinii* pneumonia (PCP). This pneumonia is caused by a protozoa and is seen in 60% of all patients with HIV infection. PCP is not airborne and thus is not transmitted from person to person as are most other types of pneumonia. Clinical manifestations include malaise, fatigue, increased respiratory rate, dry cough, fever, night sweats, and shortness of breath. Chest x-ray examinations show diffuse interstitial infiltrates. Diagnosis of PCP can be made from patient history, bronchoscopy, sample of secretions obtained from sputum specimens, and tissue from lung biopsies.[42]

The majority of patients with PCP are hospitalized. Some require mechanical ventilation as a supportive therapy. The usual medical treatments for PCP include intravenous antibiotics such as Bactrim or Septra (Table 19-6) and pentamidine given intravenously or as an aerosolized respiratory treatment. These two medications have many potentially toxic effects, and nurses must carefully monitor patients for progression of clinical symptoms, as well as for toxic effects of the drugs. In rare cases, pentamidine may be given as an intramuscular injection. Sterile abcesses at the injection sites are common with IM injections, which is why pentamidine is usually given orally. Patients are usually treated for about 3 weeks in the hospital and are discharged on a regimen of oral Bactrim or Septra. They may continue to receive aerosolized pentamidine at home or in the outpatient clinic as a means of prophylaxis.[42]

Nursing care of patients with PCP focuses on relieving symptoms and monitoring for complications. Patients with PCP suffer extreme fatigue, shortness of breath, cough, and fever. Many patients are treated with multiple antibiotics and are at risk for untoward side effects, such as nausea and vomiting, that threaten nutritional intake and further contribute to fatigue and weakness. The most important nursing care goal for patients with PCP is the maintenance of adequate ventilation and comfort.

Table 19-6 Pharmacologic treatment of HIV infections and malignancy

Trade name	Generic name	Infection/malignancy	Side effects
Adriamycin	Doxorubicin (systemic)	Kaposi's sarcoma	Leukopenia or infection (fever, chills, sore throat); stomatitis; esophagitis, flank, stomach, or joint pain; pain at injection site; peripheral edema; fast or irregular heartbeat; shortness of breath; gastrointestinal bleeding; thrombocytopenia (unusual bleeding or bruising); changes in skin color; diarrhea, nausea, vomiting; skin rash or itching; hair loss; reddish color to urine
Bactrim Septra	Sulfamethoxazole and trimethoprim (systemic)	*Pneumocystis carinii* pneumonia	Skin rash or itching; Stevens-Johnson syndrome (myalgia, arthralgia, redness, blistering, peeling or loosening of the skin); extreme fatigue, dysphagia, fever, leukopenia (sore throat); thrombocytopenia (unusual bleeding or bruising); hepatitis (dark urine, pale stools, yellow skin, and/or sclera); crystalluria, hematuria, diarrhea, dizziness, headache; anorexia, nausea, vomiting
Blenoxane	Bleomycin (systemic)	Kaposi's sarcoma	Cough, shortness of breath, pneumonitis, fever, chills, stomatis, confusion, syncope, diaphoresis, changes in skin color and texture, rashes, swelling of fingers, nausea, vomiting and anorexia, weight loss, hair loss
DHPG	9-(1.3-dihydroxy-2 propoxymethyl) guanine (systemic)	Cytomegalovirus (CMV) (CMV retinitis and CMV colitis)	Under investigation Leukopenia, bone marrow depression, elevation of serum liver enzymes, neutropenia, eosinophilia, decreased platelet count; edema, nausea, myalgias, headache, anorexia, disorientation, hallucinations, rash, phlebitis
Fluconazole	Diflucan	Candidiasis, Cryptococcal meningitis	Nausea, headache
Fungizone	Amphotericin B (systemic)	Cryptococcus	Anorexia, headache, fever, chills and rigors, convulsions, myalgia, pain at injection site, tinnitus, hypotension, atrial fibrillation, hypokalemia, decreased renal function, anaphylactic reactions
Ketoconazole	Nizoral	Candidiasis (oral and systemic) Histoplasmosis	Headache, dizziness Nausea, vomiting Itching, nervousness Gynecomastia Hepatotoxicity
Pentam	Pentamidine	*Pneumocystis carinii* pneumonia	*Parenteral*: anorexia, nausea and vomiting, leukopenia, thrombocytopenia, hypoglycemia, hypotension, pain at injection site, hepatotoxicity, decreased renal function *Aerosol*: bronchospasm, fatigue, dizziness, burning pain in back throat, bitter metabolic aftertaste, conjunctivitis, hemoptysis
Zovirax	Acyclovir	Herpes simplex Herpes zoster Varicella	*Oral*: change in menstrual period, skin rash, diarrhea, dizziness, headache, myalgia, nausea and vomiting, acne, anorexia, somnolence *Parenteral*: skin rashes or hives, hematuria, lightheadedness, headaches, hypotension, diaphoresis, confusion, tremors, abdominal pain, dyspnea, oliguria, unusual thirst, extreme fatigue
Dapasone (experimental)		Dermatitis herpetiformis	Nausea and vomiting, abdominal pains, vertigo, blurred vision, tinnitus, insomnia, fever, headache, psychosis, phototoxicity, tachycardia, albuminuria, nephrotic syndrome, hypoalbuminemia, male infertility

19-7

Nursing Research

Longo MB, Spross JA, Locke AM: Identifying major concerns of persons with acquired immunodeficiency syndrome: A replication. *Clin Nurs Spec* 4(1)21-26, 1990.

This exploratory study used semistructured interviews to elicit concerns of patients with AIDS. Areas of concern most often reported included uncertainty about the future, desire to maintain physical and psychologic health, social unacceptability, fatigue, and weight loss. Adaptive responses such as verbalizing feelings and energy conservation are discussed.

Patients suffering from PCP should have a detailed respiratory and cardiovascular assessment including observation of respiration, mucous membrane color, and activity and fatigue levels; auscultation of breath sounds and heart sounds; and measurement of pulse, blood pressure, and respiratory rate. The nursing care plan should focus on promoting independence in activities of daily living while preventing fatigue. Pacing of activities and scheduling of rest periods are important for energy conservation. Maintaining adequate hydration of 2½ to 3 liters of fluid, positioning in semi-Fowler's or high-Fowler's position while in bed, spending short periods in a chair or ambulating combined with deep-breathing exercises, and using an incentive spirometer will enhance the patient's airway clearance and help prevent respiratory complications. Some patients with PCP may require oxygen for adequate ventilation. Patients with severe forms of PCP may require intubation and mechanical ventilation and bronchotracheal suctioning to ensure adequate respiratory function (see Chapter 24).

Box 19-7 discusses findings of an exploratory study of persons with AIDS.

CANDIDA INFECTIONS

Candidiasis, a *fungal infection* caused by a yeast of the genus *Candida,* is *common in HIV-infected* and *immunocompromised individuals.* The most common candidiasis symptom is oral thrush, with creamy whitish-yellow patches in the mouth and throat, but it may also infect the entire gastrointestinal system. Some individuals may be affected with skin lesions.

Commonly used drugs in the treatment of candidiasis are nystatin (Mycostatin), ketoconazole (Nizoral), and clotrimazole (Lotrimin, Mycelex). Although side effects from Mycostatin and Lotrimin are uncommon, some individuals may experience abdominal cramps, nausea, vomiting, and diarrhea. Nizoral is useful in the treatment of candidial esophagitis. Toxic effects include nausea, diarrhea, chemical hepatitis, itching, skin rashes and drowsiness. Clotrimazole cream is used to treat cutaneous candidiasis rashes and lesions.[23]

Patients with candidiasis are at risk for dysphagia from a painful oral inflammation (stomatitis), diarrhea and skin irritation, and nutritional deficiency. Nursing care priorities include oral hygiene and adequate food and fluid intake. Because patients with HIV infection are also at risk for bleeding secondary to clotting disorders, oral hygiene must be accomplished without trauma (Chapter 27).

Patients with candidiasis should have oral mucous membranes inspected daily for lesions, integrity, and bleeding. Oral hygiene measures such as brushing teeth with nonabrasive paste, rinsing with saline and hydrogen peroxide, and applying ointment to chapped lips will provide comfort, enhance nutritional intake, and minimize further spread of infection. In addition to routine oral hygiene measures, medications such as Nystatin, Xylocaine, and Mycelex will also prevent infection spread. Daily monitoring of food and fluid intake, urine and stool output, weight, skin turgor, and serum albumin levels will alert the nurse to potential problems of nutritional intake (p. 392) are instituted.

For disseminated *Candida* lesions along the GI tract, the potent intravenous antibiotic amphotericin B may be given (see Table 19-6). Patients receiving amphotericin B must be tested with a small dose of the drug to rule out sensitivity. Even in patients without sensitivity to small test doses, reactions of hypotension and severe shaking, called *rigors,* may occur. Frequent observation of vital signs during amphotericin B administration is necessary. Some patients may receive premedications of Tylenol or Benadryl, or hydrocortisone may be added to amphotericin solutions to prevent reactions. Should patients suffer severe reactions such as rigors, it is important to stop the infusion and initiate medical intervention quickly. The medications listed above for premedication are also used to treat a reaction. In some cases rigors may be treated with meperidine injections.

CRYPTOSPORIDIOSIS

Cryptosporidiosis is a common protozoan infection found in patients with HIV infection. This organism causes malaise, nausea, abdominal cramping, and massive watery diarrhea leading to weight loss. Some patients with cryptosporidiosis may lose up to 15 L of fluid per day, resulting in severe dehydration, malnutrition, and electrolyte imbalance. There is currently no effective medical treatment for cryptosporidiosis.[45] Symptomatic treatment using antidiarrheal medication and intravenous fluid therapy may be helpful in preventing dehydration and electrolyte imbalance.

Nursing care priorities for patients suffering from cryptosporidiosis include providing adequate nutrition, maintaining skin integrity, minimizing fatigue and discomfort, and preventing dehydration. Diets low in residue, which exclude items such as nuts, fried foods, and grains, may be beneficial in decreasing episodes of diarrhea. Hydration with 3000 ml of oral fluids including water, juices, and caffeine-free, noncarbonated fluids should be planned over 24 hours.

Skin care for patients suffering from cryptosporidiosis and massive diarrhea includes pressure relief by frequent position changes, range-of-motion exercises, and devices such as air mattresses. Cleansing of skin after episodes of diarrhea involves gentle washing with mild soap and a soft cloth, followed by application of moisture barrier creams. Occlusive dressings such as Duoderm and Op-site are contraindicated in immunocompromised patients because some studies have demonstrated an increased risk of infection with their use.

HERPESVIRUS INFECTIONS

Cytomegalovirus Infection

A common infection in the herpesvirus family is *cytomegalovirus* or CMV. Over half of the general population has been exposed to CMV early in life and has built up antibodies. However, latent CMV may be a significant cause of disease in immunocompromised persons. The virus can cause damage to the lung, large intestines, and retina. The diagnosis of CMV infection can be confirmed from blood cultures or organ biopsies. At present no effective medical treatment of CMV is available. However, the experimental use of the drug DHPG (see Table 19-6) an Acyclovir derivative, is showing some promise.[25,45]

Patients with CMV often suffer from fever, fatigue, malaise, weight loss, and facial edema. The most devastating form of CMV is retinal CMV, leading to blindness.[47] All patients with HIV infection should be assessed routinely for visual changes, which must be promptly reported. Patients with CMV retinitis often suffer light sensitivity. Rooms should be dimly lit, and the use of sunglasses may minimize discomfort indoors and outdoors. Nursing care of patients with CMV retinitis centers on patient teaching related to visual changes and anticipatory grief, as well as planning for safe activities of daily living. Early referrals to community sight centers will provide adequate time for adaptation to decreasing vision, as well as an additional support network to facilitate healthy grieving.

Herpes Zoster

Another herpesvirus, varicella zoster, causes chickenpox in children and herpes zoster (shingles) in older immunocompromised patients (Chapter 43). Vesicular eruptions, which are accompanied by painful tingling and itching, will rupture and finally crust over, lasting about 3 weeks. Diagnosis is made by clinical evaluation of the lesions and occasionally confirmed by cultures of the lesions. The drug Acyclovir, administered orally or intravenously for an indefinite period, may be used to treat herpes varicella zoster in HIV-infected immunocompromised patients.[23]

Herpes Simplex

Oral and genital-rectal lesions caused by the herpes simplex virus are a fairly common occurrence with HIV infection and an immunocompromised host. Vesicular lesions vary in size; some become ulcerated, causing wound discharge, bleeding, and—at times—excruciating pain. Oral or intravenous Acyclovir may be useful in treating herpes simplex. In many cases medication therapy must be administered indefinitely to control the virus. Nursing care for individuals receiving Acyclovir should focus on the monitoring and timely reporting of all medication side effects (see Table 19-6).

Nursing care of patients with herpes lesions focuses on promoting comfort and minimizing the spread of infection to the patient and caregivers. Patients with HIV infection should be assessed daily for intact skin, rashes, or lesions. All rashes and lesions are promptly reported for medical follow-up. *Patients with herpes lesions should avoid tub baths and the use of bar soap that may cause dissemination of the lesions. A separate clean washcloth should be used to bathe areas with lesions. Patients and caregivers should wear gloves whenever cleaning or applying medications to lesions.*

MYCOBACTERIAL INFECTIONS

Mycobacterium avium intracellulare (MAI) is a bacteria commonly found in the environment. MAI rarely causes severe infection except in patients infected with HIV virus. Clinical symptoms caused by MAI include fever, diarrhea, abdominal pain, weight loss, *pancytopenia*, abnormal food absorption, and abnormal liver function test results. MAI may be cultured from blood, sputum, body organs, bone marrow, and lymph nodes.[23,42] Various drug therapies including rifampin, ethambutol, amikacin, ansamycin, and clofazimine have been used in attempts to treat MAI. These drugs, however, have shown little success.

Mycobacterium tuberculosis (MTB) is being found more frequently in HIV-infected patients and is one reason why TB rates have been on the increase (Chapter 24). MTB may be found in any organ system, the lymph system, meninges, bones, peritoneum, and pleura. Diagnosis is based on the clinical symptom of fever and associated infected organs and is confirmed by the presence of acid-fast bacillus. Similar to HIV-infected patients with PCP, patients with MAI and MTB require nursing care to minimize the effects of fever, weakness, nausea, vomiting, and dyspnea.

CENTRAL NERVOUS SYSTEM INFECTIONS

Toxoplasmosis, caused by the protozoon *Toxoplasma gondii*, often results in focal *encephalitis* in immunocompromised patients. Symptoms include fever, headache, lethargy, decreased cognitive ability, confusion including memory loss, personality changes, and seizures. The CSF in patients with *Toxoplasma gondii* contains increased protein and white blood cells. CT scans may reveal masses, but a brain biopsy may be required to establish a definitive diagnosis of toxoplasma trophozoite in brain tissue. Medical treatment includes the use of antibiotics such as clindamycin, trimethoprim-sulfamethoxazole, spriamycin, pyrimethamine, and sulfadiazine.

Meningitis, caused by the fungus *Cryptococcus neoformans,* causes fever, headache, nausea, vomiting, blurred vision, stiff neck, varying degrees of confusion, lethargy, and possibly seizures. A lumbar puncture is needed to confirm the diagnosis of cryptococcus; a positive result is CSF infiltration of white blood cells, protein, an increased cryptococcal antigen titer, and abnormally low glucose levels.[45]

The human immunodeficiency virus itself may invade the central nervous system, causing HIV *encephalopathy* or *dementia*. It is believed that about 60% of all HIV-infected individuals suffer HIV encephalopathy. Initially, encephalopathy may be manifested by progressive loss or decline in cognitive, motor, or behavioral function. Early signs of HIV encephalopathy are subtle and may be confused with normal grieving and depression. These signs include reduced concentration, slowness of speech, and impaired memory. As HIV encephalopathy progresses, dementia results with further decline in the individual's ability to walk, control body functions, perform self-care, and make decisions. HIV encephalopathy may progress to coma. Treatment is primarily palliative and supportive. AZT (azidothymidine) has been used with some improvement in neurologic function in the early stages of the disease.[45]

Nursing care of patients with toxoplasmosis or meningitis resulting in encephalitis and cognitive impairment is aimed at relieving symptoms such as headaches and lethargy, and promoting safety during seizures, delirium, and depression.

Although some patients with cognitive impairment may be acutely aware of their deficits and need for assistance with activities of daily living, others may have little insight into these needs (Chapter 37). A major focus of nursing care for patients with cognitive impairment is the support and education of caregivers. Caregivers require instruction and supervision in patient bathing, positioning, skin care, oral care, transferring, use of assistive devices, range-of-motion exercises, feeding and nutrition, bowel and bladder management, and environmental safety, including infection control measures. Patients who are aware of declining cognitive abilities and the terminal nature of their HIV infection are at high risk for suicide. Therefore all patients with a diagnosis of HIV infection should be assessed for depression and suicide ideation. Referral to mental health professionals for caregivers suffering extreme grief and care burdens, as well as for depressed patients can be useful in addressing quality-of-life issues despite terminal illness.

TUMORS

Malignant lymphomas of the *central nervous system* are common in patients with HIV infection and often indicate poor prognosis. These lymphomas include non-Hodgkins lymphoma and Burkitt's-like lymphomas (Chapter 11). Clinical symptoms include malaise, myalgias, lymphadenopathy, and abdominal discomforts associated with weight loss.[45]

Kaposi's sarcoma (KS) is by far *the most common neoplasm found in patients with HIV infection*. KS affects vascular epithelium and results in red-purplish cutaneous lesions (Chapter 43). Lesions may appear on the trunk, arms, legs, head, and neck. Extracutaneous lesions may also occur in mucous membranes, lymph nodes, lungs, and the gastrointestinal tract. Kaposi's sarcoma tumors can block lymphatic drainage, resulting in severe edema to the face or extremities. Pulmonary lesions may result in respiratory distress and even death. Although some patients have no clinical symptoms associated with KS, others complain of malaise, weight loss, swollen lymph nodes, generalized edema, and shortness of breath. Kaposi's sarcoma may be diagnosed by tissue biopsy. Radiation therapy may be used as a palliative measure in some progressive forms of KS lesions.

Symptoms of KS depend on involved body systems. KS may invade cutaneous tissue, causing edema and skin lesions; lung tissue, causing shortness of breath and a productive cough; gastrointestinal system, causing diarrhea; or the brain, causing cognitive changes and gait disturbances. Radiation therapy has been used in the treatment of KS lesions, although some patients may suffer additional complications of therapy, such as nausea and vomiting.[42]

Nursing care priorities for patients depend on the particular system affected by KS. Care considerations include skin care of lesions, promoting comfortable ventilation, and maintaining a safe environment. Prevention of the effects of edema may be a major nursing care strategy for patients with KS. Elevating the head of the bed or affected extremities may produce some relief. Facial edema may be alleviated by cool compresses. Maintaining skin integrity despite edema and radiation therapy is indeed challenging.

Gentle massages with creams and oils help promote drainage, reduce discomfort, and prevent skin breakdown. KS lesions that are dry may be left open to the air. For draining KS lesions, cleansing with mild soap and patting dry, applying normal saline wet dressings, or applying Bacitracin and Neomycin creams and covering with nonadhering dressings such as Telfa may provide some comfort and prevent the spread of lesions. Similar to patients with PCP, patients with pulmonary Kaposi's sarcoma will require nursing interventions to reduce dyspnea and promote comfortable effective airway clearance.

DRUG THERAPY

Because there is no cure for HIV infection at present, treatment has been aimed at slowing progression of the disease, managing symptoms, and providing palliative care. Multiple clinical trials of various drugs to slow progression of the HIV infection are now under way. In 1987 the first such drug, azidothymidine (AZT), also known as Zetrovir or Zidovudine, was released for treatment. AZT acts by inhibiting the replication of the human immunodeficiency virus. In some individuals, AZT has been effective in reducing the number of opportunistic infections and dementia symptoms.

AZT, however, has many side effects including malaise, headache, fever, nausea, vomiting, insomnia, and myalgia. Toxic effects occur in about 50% of patients. These include anemia, bone marrow suppression, reduced white blood count, and low platelet counts. Patients on AZT require weekly blood testing to monitor for toxic effects.[42] Some patients on AZT may require blood transfusions to counter the toxic effects of AZT.

AZT therapy has also been suggested as a preventive measure in the management of occupational exposure to HIV.[14] Lower doses of it are being prescribed prophylactically for health care workers who have had an occupational exposure.

In addition, two other oral agents—DDI (videx, didanosine) and DDC (didexoxycytidine, zalcitabine)—have shown promise in slowing virus progression. These agents, like AZT, inhibit the enzyme, reverse transcryptase, and prevent the HIV from multiplying. Patients on DDI are monitored for the following side-effects: diarrhea, insomnia, headache, peripheral neuropathy, and pancreatitis.

Nursing Care Plan

Person with HIV complications

DATA: Mr. C. is a 32-year-old computer programmer. He was born in a small town in the Midwest but has lived on the West coast for the past 10 years. He has had little contact with his family because of the painful situation when he left home; his family was "disgraced" by the fact that he was "gay." For the last 5 years he has been living with his lover, Mr. J. Mr. C. reveals that before moving in with Mr. J., he had multiple homosexual and heterosexual experiences. Mr. J. and Mr. C. have lived in a monogamous relationship for the last 3 years. Mr. C. describes Mr. J. as a "dependent" person who rarely "hangs onto a job for very long." Mr. C. is being admitted to the hospital for a medical evaluation of 4 months of fatigue not relieved with sleep. He has lost 20 pounds, and reports night sweats that frequently awaken him, a rectal rash, and a dry cough with fevers. Mr. C.'s illness has caused him to use all of his sick time from work and he is afraid he will lose his job. He also says he is terrified that he might be dying. Mr. J. also reports that his friend suffers from intermittent confusion.

The nursing history identified the following:

- Mr. C. has multiple risk factors for contracting the HIV infection, including multiple sexual partners, homosexual experiences, and anal intercourse
- Mr. C. has several persistent clinical symptoms or evidence of new clinical symptoms indicative of HIV infection: fatigue, weight loss, dry cough, fevers, and a rectal rash
- Mr. C. has multiple sources of stress, including his alienation from family members because of his sexual preference, possible loss of his job due to his persistent illness, and his concern over his lover's ability to cope with stress while Mr. C. is ill.

Collaborative nursing activities include:

- Assessment of Mr. C.'s understanding of HIV testing, AIDS, and treatment regimens
- Assessment of progression of clinical symptoms or evidence of new clinical symptoms indicating complications such as infections and altered cognitive function
- Referral to a social service agency for investigation of health disability insurance and unemployment benefits
- Assessment and possible referral for mental health counseling for Mr. C. and Mr. J.

Nursing activities include monitoring the following:

- Temperature, particularly fever
- Daily food and fluid intake and weight
- Cognitive ability and neurologic status
- Ability to care for self
- Spread of, or drainage from, rectal rash
- Lung sounds and sputum production
- Appetite, ability to sleep, ability to discuss concerns, and other clinical indicators of anxiety or depression
- Laboratory results of ELISA, Western Blot, T-cell ratios, WBCs, PT, PTT, and serum electrolytes
- Support systems

Nursing diagnosis: Anxiety (Mr. C. and Mr. J.) related to persistent debilitating illness, with an unknown etiology but with evidence of terminal illness; related to threatened loss of independence, job, and social relationships

Expected patient outcomes	Nursing interventions	Rationale
Mr. C. and Mr. J. will identify previous coping strategies for stress, verbalize sources of anxiety, identify possible coping strategies for present anxieties, and articulate decreased symptoms of anxiety such as anorexia and sleeplessness.	Acknowledge multiple sources of stress as evidenced from history. Explore with Mr. C. past life crises and strategies of coping, as well as sources of support. Spend time with Mr. C., explaining procedures and treatments Spend uninterrupted time with Mr. C. and Mr. J. individually to allow for empathic listening. Monitor for increasing anxiety and report to physician. Assess for depression and suicidal ideation.	Patterns of past successful coping are indicators of present resources and strengths. Empathy as a counseling therapy utilizes realistic description stressors, reflective listening, physical presence, and clarification. Anxiety may increase with procedures and terminal diagnosis.

Continued.

Nursing Care Plan

A person with HIV complications/AIDS—cont'd

Nursing diagnosis: Knowledge deficit (HIV risk factors, disease transmission, test significance, HIV pathophysiology) related to lack of exposure

Expected patient outcomes	Nursing interventions	Rationale
Mr. C. and Mr. J. describe rationale of diagnostic tests, HIV risk factors, and strategies for prevention of HIV transmission.	Using discussion with repetition and printed materials, review diagnostic tests such as ELISA, Western Blot, and T-cell ratios, risk factors and prevention strategies of HIV infection, clinical symptoms of HIV infection, immune system, function	Patients have a right to information related to health. This information will promote their ability to make decisions to prevent disease and to seek medical treatment to alleviate symptoms and complications. Anxiety decreases the ability to take in information and requires repetition and multiple learning strategies.

Nursing diagnosis: Nutrition, altered: less than body requirements, related to diarrhea as evidenced by undesired weight loss

Expected patient outcomes	Nursing interventions	Rationale
Mr. C. and Mr. J. describe a meal plan with adequate calories and hydration. Mr. C. ceases to lose weight. Mr. C.'s serum albumin, potassium, and sodium remain within normal limits.	Plan with Mr. C. and nutritionist a daily schedule of six small meals including 3000 ml of fluids and 3000 calories, excluding dairy products, and raw fruits and vegetables.	Small meals prevent gastric distention and nausea; 2500-3000 ml provides adequate hydration for febrile adult; 3000 calories will prevent weight loss and negative nitrogen balance. Lactose in dairy products may enhance diarrhea; raw foods contain naturally occurring microorganisms that may increase infection in immunocompromised hosts.
	Plan routine oral care and rinses before and after meals.	Oral care before meals enhances appetite and flow of digestive juices; oral care after meals helps to prevent oral lesions and infections.
	Assist Mr. C. to be out of bed or sitting up.	Upright positioning prevents aspiration and pneumonia.
	Weigh Mr. C. daily at same time on same scale, and record.	Weight is a clinical indicator of adequate nutrition.

Nursing diagnosis: Activity intolerance related to weight loss, sleeplessness, and fatigue

Expected patient outcomes	Nursing interventions	Rationale
Mr. C. sleeps 6-8 hours at night, is independent in ADLS, and states decreased feelings of fatigue.	Plan and teach Mr. C. about pacing activity and the use of energy conservation measures. Include in plan uninterrupted period for sleep. Review with Mr. C. relaxation techniques at bedtime such as deep breathing, tepid baths, use of a radio. Increase nutritional intake. Assist with ADL, encourage patient participation.	Pacing of activity and energy conservation conserves patient's energy balanced with activity. Relaxation promotes comfort and contributes to sleep. Provides calories for energy consumption, thereby decreasing some fatigue.

Nursing diagnosis: Skin integrity, impaired, related to genital herpes; skin integrity, impaired, high risk for, related to fatigue and immobility

Expected patient outcomes	Nurisng interventions	Rationale
Rectal rash will heal and Mr. C. will report increased comfort. Herpes infection will not spread on Mr. C.'s body or to caregivers. Further skin breakdown does not occur.	Assist Mr. C. to clean rectal area after each episode of diarrhea using a mild soap such as liquid Castile soap; use gloves and good handwashing after cleaning. Assist Mr. C. to turn in bed at least every 2 hours. Assist Mr. C. with daily bathing; encourage shower, avoid tub baths. For basin baths, use clean washcloth for rash area and do not reuse Apply gloves (self or Mr. C.) for cleansing or application of medications to rash.	Herpes rashes cause local irritation and discomfort; healing is promoted by gentle clenaing, allowing regeneration of epidermis. Decreased pressure promotes healing and comfort by increased circulation. Daily hygiene prevents secondary infections and spread of existing infections. Showers provide continued washing away of microorganisms. Herpes and other rashes may be spread to patient and caregiver by skin contact.

Nursing diagnosis: Thought processes, altered, secondary to clinical manifestations of opportunistic infections and lymphoma of the brain.

Expected patient outcomes	Nursing intervention	Rationale
Mr. C. will remain safe within his environment	Assess orientation. Reorient as needed. Assess environmental safety including nightlights and cues such as clocks, calendars, and newspapers. Be consistent in daily routines and care. Use short repetitive phrases. Provide verbal reassurance.	Infections may cause increased intracranial pressure, resulting in confusion or dementia.

SOCIAL, ETHICAL, AND LEGAL ISSUES

The HIV epidemic has brought with it not only a dismal prognosis, but also severe social stigmatization, public fear, and a growing number of legal and ethical issues. Nurses providing care in a variety of settings will face many of these issues that may jeopardize the quality of patient care. In addition, nurses caring for patients with the HIV infection will face many personal stresses including fear of personal contamination and disease transmission to family members, and burnout related to caring for terminally ill young patients with controversial life-styles. The professional commitment needed by nurses who provide care to HIV-infected patients requires clarification of personal values regarding the issues of homosexuality and drug use.

Inherent in nursing is a respect for life, dignity, and social justice. The American Nurses Association Code of Ethics clearly reaffirms that the profession of nursing provides services with respect for human dignity and the uniqueness of each client, unrestricted by social or economic status, personal attributes, or the nature of health problems.

The very nature of nurses' work constitutes a level of risk for various diseases that does not exist in other professions. In upholding the moral principle of justice, risks and withholding of care must be carefully balanced with potential benefits of care. In addition, individual nurses and institutions have a responsibility to take reasonable precautions to protect caregivers from harm while providing medical and nursing care to patients.

As long as the HIV infection remains a downhill continuum with multiple complications and eventual death, nurses caring for patients with progressive AIDS will be involved in decisions regarding the selective withholding of treatment while preserving the quality of life and human dignity. The role of nursing in the terminal phase of illness is a critical one. When no medical treatments can be offered to the patient, nursing has everything to offer, including providing physical care that makes the patient more comfortable, identifying values, exploring the meaning of life with the patient and significant others, supporting bonds between the patient and significant others, and providing comfort measures and support that will allow the patient to have a peaceful death.

Nurses must continually help the health care team, family, and significant others to focus on the patients' desires. This principle of autonomy, as endorsed by the American Nurses Association, is a valuable guide for many ethical decisions regarding terminally ill patients. Nurse caregivers providing such intense physical and psychologic care also need support. Peer support through informal sharing or a structured support group is an effective strategy that may alleviate feelings of helplessness.

Legal issues such as confidentiality, mandatory testing, employee screening, and school attendance of children infected with HIV remain controversial. Therefore it will be important for all nurses to keep themselves informed of policy developments and to influence, whenever possible,

such decisions based on the ethical principle of justice. (For further information about ethical issues, see Boxes 19-8 and 19-9.)

19-8 **Nursing Research**

Flaskerud JH, Lewis MA, Shin D: Changing nurses' AIDS-related knowledge and attitudes through continuing education, *J Cont Ed Nurs* 20(4):148-154, 1989.

The purpose of this study was to measure changes in nurses' knowledge and attitudes following attendance at a continuing education conference. The conference topics included epidemiology of AIDS, infection control, sexual history taking, counseling, and psychosocial and institutional support for health care workers. Using a pretest, posttest, and a 3-month follow-up structured questionnaire, the researchers found significant increases in knowledge and attitude scores.

19-9 **Nursing Research**

Martin DA: Effects of ethical dilemmas on stress felt by nurses providing care to AIDS patients, *Crit Care Nurs Quar* 12:53-62, 1990.

The purpose of this study was to examine the nature and prevalence of ethical dilemmas encountered by nurses who provide care to patients hospitalized with AIDS-related illnesses. Half of the nurses reported a high degree of emotional exhaustion. However, there was a correlation between overall years of nursing experience and ability to cope. *The most frequent dilemmas reported were related to issues of dying* and "do not resuscitate" orders. The *second category of dilemmas surrounded issues of pain and symptom management*. Coping strategies ranged from venting emotions to deciding to leave the nursing unit or institution.

SUMMARY

1. The three major methods of transmission of human immunodeficiency virus (HIV) are by intimate contact with semen or vaginal secretions through sexual contact, by infected blood through blood transfusions or sharing of IV drug needles, and by mother-to-infant transfer through placenta or breast milk.
2. Risk behaviors for HIV infection include anal intercourse, frequent sexual intercourse with multiple partners, and sharing IV drug needles.
3. Populations at highest risk include homosexual and bisexual men, IV drug users, heterosexual partners of HIV-infected individuals, infants born to HIV-infected parents, and individuals who received blood transfusions before 1985 and their sexual partners.
4. HIV infection is not spread by nonsexual household contacts.

5. Infection control measures include handwashing before and after patient contact and after removal of gloves; wearing gloves whenever there will be contact with body secretions; disposing of soiled dressings, wet linens, and respiratory equipment in heavy plastic bags; disposing of needles *without capping* in puncture-resistant needle disposal containers; environmental cleaning with institutional cleaning agents or a 1:10 dilution of bleach and water; and use of bleach when laundering.

6. The human immunodeficiency virus is a retrovirus that invades helper T cells, incorporates its DNA into the genetic material of the helper T cell, and replicates itself, destroying the helper T cell. The decreased number of helper T cells causes immunodeficiency.

7. Persons exposed to HIV may develop an acute infection (similar to mononucleosis) or may be asymptomatic, harboring the virus for several years. The asymptomatic person may unknowingly transmit the virus to others. Some persons develop a persistent generalized lymphadenopathy in the absence of explainable illness. Not all persons appear to progress to AIDS-related complex (ARC) or AIDS.

8. ARC is a debilitating syndrome of fever, diarrhea, weight loss greater than 10% of baseline, fatigue, edema, and abnormal laboratory immune values (altered T_4/T_8 ratio, leukopenia, lymphopenia, thrombocytopenia).

9. AIDS is the most severe HIV disease. In addition to the symptoms of ARC, the AIDS patient develops opportunistic infections and/or malignancies. Death eventually ensues.

10. Opportunistic infections may be protozoal, bacterial, viral, or fungal; the most common infection is *P. carinii* pneumonia. The most common malignancy is Kaposi's sarcoma.

11. The ELISA test, indicating the presence of HIV *antibodies,* is the most often used diagnostic test for HIV infection. If this test is positive, a Western Blot test is used to confirm the results.

12. Interventions for persons with HIV infection depend on the symptoms and presence of infections or malignancies. Nursing interventions include prevention of infection, modification of alterations in body temperature, promotion of self-care, safety, and good nutrition, counseling, assisting with coping; and patient teaching.

13. Treatment for persons with *P. carinii* pneumonia includes antibiotics (Bactrim or Septra, pentamidine), administered intravenously or by aerosol. Mechanical ventilation may be necessary. Nursing interventions include maintenance of adequate ventilation, promotion of comfort, conservation of energy, and promotion of adequate hydration and nutrition.

14. Treatment for candidiasis (fungal infection of GI tract, particularly the mouth) includes use of the antifungal drugs nystatin, ketoconazole, or clotrimazole. Nursing interventions include oral hygiene and promotion of adequate food and fluid intake.

15. Cryptosporidiosis is a protozoal infection affecting the GI tract with massive diarrhea leading to weight loss.

Treatment is symptomatic with antidiarrheal medication and fluid replacement. Nursing interventions include preventing dehydration, promoting nutrition, energy conservation, and comfort, and maintaining skin integrity.

16. Cytomegalovirus (CMV) infection is caused by a herpesvirus. It can affect the lung, large intestines, and especially the retina, leading to blindness. No effective medical treatment is available, although the experimental drug DHPG is being used. Persons with CMV retinitis must be prepared for eventual loss of sight.

17. Individuals with herpes simplex or herpes zoster may be prescribed Acyclovir, which in many cases must be administered indefinitely to control the virus. Nursing interventions include promoting comfort and minimizing spread of infection.

18. Mycobacterial infections include *M. avium intracellulare* (MAI) or *M. tuberculosis* (MTB). Nursing interventions include promotion of comfort and ventilation.

19. CNS infections include encephalitis, meningitis, encephalopathy or dementia, and coma. Nursing care is aimed at relief of symptoms and promotion of ADL and safety.

20. Lesions of Kaposi's sarcoma may affect the skin, mucous membranes, lymph nodes, lungs, and GI tract. Radiation may be used as a palliative measure. Nursing care depends on the location of lesions, but may include maintaining skin integrity, promoting ventilation, and maintaining safety.

21. To slow progression of HIV infection, azidothymidine (AZT) is now being used. AZT acts by inhibiting the replication of HIV. There are many toxic effects, and patients receiving AZT require weekly blood tests, and may require blood transfusions to treat toxic effects. Lower doses of AZT may be prescribed prophylactically for persons with occupational exposure. Two newer oral agents—didanosine (DDI) and didexoxycytidine (DDC), whose action is similar to AZT, are being tested in patients.

22. Numerous social, ethical, and legal issues need to be considered regarding care of persons with HIV infections.

STUDY QUESTIONS

• You have been assigned to care for your first HIV-infected patient. What things should you consider before providing care?

• The local school has asked you to give a presentation on AIDS. What areas of content will you include? What teaching strategies and media might be helpful?

• Several of your peers confide in you that they would never care for a patient with AIDS. What ethical principles can help you clarify your views on this issues?

• What strategies can nurse caregivers use to alleviate fear and stress while caring for terminally ill HIV-infected patients and their families?

• You are preparing a family to provide home care for their son with AIDS. What learning needs must you assess?

REFERENCES AND SELECTED READINGS

1. Ahluwalia IB: The epidemiology of AIDS. In Blanchet KD, editor: *AIDS: a health care management response,* Rockville, Md, 1988, Aspen.
2. American Nurses Association: *Code for nurses with interpretative statements,* Kansas City, Mo, 1985, The Association.
3. American Nurses Association: *Nursing and the human responses to AIDS/HIV infection,* Kansas City, Mo, 1988, The Association.
3a.* Anastasi JK: Why give corticosteroids for *Pneumocystitis carinii* pneumonia? *Am J Nurs* 92(2):30-32, 1992.
3b.* Anastasi JK and Riviera JL: AIDS drug update, DDI and DDC, *RN* 52(11):41-43, 1992.
3c.* Andrullis DP, et al: Comparisons of hospital care for patients with AIDS and other HIV-related conditions, *JAMA* 267(18):2482-2486, 1992.
4.* Barrick B: Light at the end of the tunnel, *Am J Nurs* 90(11):37-40, 1990.
5.* Beckham MM, Rudy EB: Acquired immunodeficiency syndrome: impact and implication for the neurological system, *Neurosci Nurs* 18:7-10, 1986.
6. Bennett J, Gee G: History and overview of HIV infection. In Gee G and Moran TA, editors: *AIDS: concepts in nursing practice,* Baltimore, 1988, Williams & Wilkins.
7. Blanchet KD: *AIDS: a health care management response,* Rockville, Md, 1988, Aspen.
8. Carey JT: The clinical spectrum of AIDS. In Blanchet KD: *AIDS: a health care management response,* Rockville, Md, 1988, Aspen.
9. Carpenito LJ: *Nursing diagnosis: application to clinical practice,* ed 2, Philadelphia, 1987, JB Lippincott.
10. Carr G: Medical treatment of persons with AIDS/ARC. In Lewis A, editor: *Nursing care of the person with AIDS/ARC,* Rockville, Md, 1988, Aspen.
11. Centers for Disease Control: Classification system for human T-lymphotropic virus III/lymphadenopathy-associated virus infections, *MMWR* 35:334-339, 1986.
12. Centers for Disease Control: Revision of the CDC surveillance case definition for acquired immunodeficiency syndrome, *MMWR* 36:3-16, 1987.
13. Centers for Disease Control: Update: universal precautions for prevention of transmission of human immunodeficiency virus, hepatitis B virus, and other bloodborne pathogens in health care settings, *MMWR* 37:24, 1988.
14. Centers for Disease Control: Public Health Service statement on management of occupational exposure to HIV, including considerations regarding zidovudine postexposure use, *MMWR* 39(RR-1):1-14, 1990.
14a. Centers for Disease Control: Recommendations for preventing transmission of human immunodeficiency virus and hepatitis B virus to patients during exposure-prone procedures, *MMWR* 40(RR):1-9, 1991.
14b. Centers for Disease Control: *HIV-AIDS surveillance report,* January 1992, 1-22.
15. Christ GH, Weiner LS: Psychosocial issues in AIDS. In DeVita VT Jr et al, editors: *AIDS: etiology, diagnosis, treatment, and prevention,* Philadelphia, 1985, JB Lippincott.
16. Cohen F: Immunologic impairment, infection and AIDS in the aging patient, *Crit Care Nurs Q* 12(1):38-44; 1989.
17.* Durham J, Cohen F: *The person with AIDS: nursing perspective,* New York, 1987, Springer.
18. Fauci AS, et al: The acquired immunodeficiency syndrome: an update, *Ann Intern Med* 102:800-813, 1985.

19.* Flaskerud JH: AIDS: the psychosocial dimension, *J Psychosoc Nurs* 25:4-36, 1987.
20. Flaskerud JH: Nurses call out for AIDS information, *Nurs Health Care* 8:557-562, 1987.
21.* Flaskerud JH: *AIDS/HIV infection: a reference guide for nursing professionals,* Orlando, Fla, 1989, WB Saunders.
22.* Fillit H, et al: AIDS in the elderly, *AIDS Patient Care* 4(1):8-12, 1990.
22a. Graham MH, et al: The effect on survival of early treatment of human immunodeficiency virus infection, *N Engl J Med* 326(16):1037-1041, 1992.
23. Hatfield S, Dunkel J: Understanding and working with the emotional reactions of staff. In Lewis A, editor: *Nursing care of the person with AIDS/ARC,* Rockville, Md, 1988, Aspen.
24. *Healthy people 2000: National health promotion and disease prevention objectives,* Department of Health & Human Services, Public Health Service, Washington, DC, Government Printing Office, 1990.
25. Hughes AM, et al: *AIDS home care and hospice manual,* San Francisco, 1987, AIDS Home Care and Hospice Program, UNA of San Francisco.
26. Justice AC, Feinstein AR, Wells CK: A new prognostic staging system for the acquired immunodeficiency syndrome, *New Engl J Med* 320(22):1388-1489, 1989.
27. Kaplan LD, Wofsy CB, Volberding PA: Treatment of patients with acquired immunodeficiency syndrome and associated manifestations, *JAMA* 257:1367-1374, 1987.
28.* Koenig BA: Ethical and legal issues in the AIDS epidemic. In Lewis A, editor: *Nursing care of the person with AIDS/ARC,* Rockville, Md, 1988, Aspen.
29. Koop CE: *Surgeon General's report on acquired immune deficiency syndrome,* Rockville, Md, 1986, US Dept of Health and Human Services.
30. Leads from MMWR: Acquired immune deficiency syndrome, *JAMA* 252:1298-1301, 1985.
31.* Lewis A: *Nursing care of the person with AIDS/ARC,* Rockville, Md, 1988, Aspen.
32. Masur H, et al: Infectious complications of AIDS. In DeVita VT Jr, et al, editors: *AIDS: etiology, diagnosis, treatment, and prevention,* Philadelphia, 1985, JB Lippincott.
33. Menke EM: *HIV and AIDS: an introduction for nurses,* Columbus, Ohio, 1989, East Central AIDS Education and Training Grant.
34.* Nelson WJ: Nursing care of the acutely ill person with AIDS. In Durham JD and Cohen FL, editors: *The person with AIDS: nursing perspective,* New York, 1987, Springer.
35. Pender NJH: *Health promotion in nursing practice,* Norwalk, Conn, 1987, Appleton & Lange.
36.* Scherer P: How AIDS attacks the brain, *Am J Nurs* 90(1):44-53, 1990.
37. Smith CL: Nursing management of aerosolized pentamidine administration, *AIDS Patient Care* 4(1):13-17, 1990.
38. Ulrich SP, Canale SW, Wendell SA: *Nursing care planning guides: a nursing diagnosis approach,* Philadelphia, 1986, WB Saunders.
39.* Ungarvski PJ: Learning to live with AIDS, *Nurs Mirror* 160:20-22, 1985.
40. Ungarvski PJ: *Living with AIDS: a caregivers guide,* New York, 1987, National Center for Homecare Education Research.
41. Volberding PA: The clinical spectrum of the acquired immunodeficiency syndrome: implications for comprehensive patient care, *Ann Intern Med* 103:729-733, 1985.
42. Volberding PA: Kaposi's sarcoma and the acquired immunodeficiency syndrome, *Med Clin North Am* 70:665-675, 1986.
43.* Weaver K: Reversible malnutrition in AIDS, *Am J Nurs* 91(9):34-31, 1991.

*Recommended for student reading.

44. White K: "Why weren't you just more careful?" *AIDS Patient Care* 4(3):13-16, 1990.
45. Wolfe P: Clinical manifestations and treatment. In Flaskerud JF, editor: *AIDS/HIV infection: a reference guide for nursing professionals*, Philadelphia, 1989, WB Saunders Co.

Classic

46. American Nurses Association: *Nursing: a social policy statement*, Kansas City, Mo, 1980, The Association.
47. Beauchamp T, Childress J: *Principles of biomedical ethics*, New York, 1979, Oxford University Press.
48. Centers for Disease Control: *Pneumocystis* pneumonia: Los Angeles, *MMWR* 30:250-252, 1981.
49. Fowler MDM: *Ethics and nursing, 1893-1984: the ideal of service, the reality of history*, Los Angeles, 1984, University of Southern California.
50. Jameton A: *Nursing practice: the ethical issues*, Englewood Cliffs, NJ, 1984, Prentice Hall.
51.* Ungvarski PJ: Acquired immune deficiency syndrome, *Nurs Mirror* 157:17-20, 1983.
52. Ungvarski PJ: Infection control in the patient with AIDS, *J Hosp Infect* 5(A):111-113, 1984.

Perioperative Nursing

20

Preoperative Intervention

Carole G. Phipps
Barbara C. Long

After studying this chapter, the learner should be able to:

- Differentiate among ways of admitting surgical patients.
- Describe different purposes of surgery.
- Identify psychologic and physiologic responses to surgery.
- Identify risk factors for surgery.
- Explain the nature of informed consent and related nursing responsibilities.
- Explain the rationale for collection of physiologic data for the preoperative patient.
- Explain the preoperative preparation of the patient (diet, bowel and skin preparation).
- Identify common learning needs of preoperative patients and methods for deep breathing and coughing and leg exercises.
- Identify final preparation of the patient for surgery.

Surgery is one of the major modes of medical therapy. It is a stressful experience because it involves a threat to body integrity and sometimes a threat to life itself. Pain frequently occurs. The nurse can assist the person to cope with the stressors, to seek relief from the pain, and to return to optimal functioning.

The surgical (perioperative) experience can be divided into three stages: preoperative, intraoperative, and postoperative. The next three chapters discuss knowledge basic to the care of the patient during each of the three stages. This chapter discusses admission for surgery; types, responses, and risk factors of surgery; informed consent for surgery; and the use of nursing process with preoperative patients.

ELECTIVE ADMISSION FOR SURGERY

Persons scheduled for elective surgery were formerly all admitted to the hospital 1 or more days before surgery for medical workup, laboratory testing, and patient teaching, the necessary elements of preoperative care. Increasingly in recent years, patients scheduled for many types of surgery are either admitted to the hospital as inpatients on the day of surgery (same-day surgery), or to an ambulatory surgical center (either hospital- or community-based). One major reason for these changes has been the emphasis on cost containment in health care services and the subsequent need to shorten hospital stays.

Ambulatory Surgery

Ambulatory patients are admitted to the ambulatory center on the morning of surgery, remain there for their immediate postoperative care, and are then discharged to their homes before the end of the day. The surgery itself is uncomplicated and does not require expert postoperative care.

Success in ambulatory surgery depends on several factors, including preoperative testing and teaching facilities, physical status of the patient, and home care support persons. Most ambulatory surgical patients are either healthy or may have a mild systemic disease, such as diet-controlled diabetes mellitus, moderate obesity, chronic bronchitis, old MI, or mild hypertension. In selected instances persons with a severe systemic disease but who are in a stable condition may be considered.[27] Persons who are poor risks for ambulatory surgery include those with brittle diabetes mellitus, morbid obesity, or a systemic disease that places them in constant threat, such as cardiac, pulmonary, renal, hepatic, or endocrine insufficiency.[27]

Age per se is not a limiting factor, and in fact, many elderly persons have increased benefits from ambulatory surgery versus inpatient surgery. Benefits for the elderly include decreased risk of complications such as pneumonia or infection, increased mental and physical functioning because the environment is less foreign, decreased cost, and maintenance of contacts with family and friends.[5] Additional care requirements may be needed for elderly persons, including providing time and attention needed for adjustment.

Same-Day Surgery

Surgical patients who are admitted to the hospital approximately 2 hours before surgery and who require inpatient postoperative care are classified as undergoing same-day surgery (also called *same-day admit*, AM *admission*, or *day-of-surgery admission*). Same-day surgery patients require their preoperative preparation before the day of surgery because of time constraints. The admission management involves the necessary medical workup and testing procedures, as well as comprehensive preoperative nursing assessment, patient education, and discharge planning.[21] The establishment of preadmission testing and teaching programs provides this comprehensive patient care *before* the day of surgery and admission.

Early Hospital Admission

Patients who are admitted 1 or more days before planned surgery are those whose medical condition warrants it (such as patients with brittle diabetes) or those who require parenteral antibiotics or hydration, or bowel preparation.

Whether persons are admitted to the hospital the day before surgery, a few hours before surgery (same-day surgery), or for ambulatory surgery, they all require the necessary *preoperative preparation* (Box 20-1). The management of patient care is based on a person's medical and nursing history. The nurse in the preoperative prehospital period is in a position to perform the required comprehensive assessment to plan and initiate interventions from admission to discharge. This is of utmost importance for the ambulatory surgical patients who must have a responsible person take them home and provide any necessary care.

20-1 | **Components of preoperative preparation**

Preoperative tests (see Table 20-6)
History and physical examination
Anesthesia consult
Nursing assessment
Preoperative education

TYPES OF SURGERY

Classification

Surgeries may be classified in several ways, such as by location, extent, or purpose of the surgery.

Location

Surgery may be performed externally or internally. In *external surgery* the skin or underlying tissues are readily accessible to the surgeon. External surgery has disadvantages; it may result in scarring or disfiguration that may be readily visible, leading to great concern and distress for some patients. *Plastic surgery* (Chapter 43) is an example of external surgery; it is directed toward reconstruction and repair of deformed tissues. *Internal surgery* involves penetration of the body. The scars of internal surgery may not be visible but may lead to complications such as adhesions. Surgery of major internal organs may lead to decreased function if sufficient tissue is removed.

Table 20-1 Purposes of surgery

Type of surgery	Reason performed	Examples
Diagnostic	Determine cause of symptoms	Biopsy, exploratory laparotomy
Curative	Removal of diseased part	Appendectomy
Restorative	Strengthen weakened areas	Herniorrhaphy
	Correct deformities	Mitral valve replacement
	Rejoin a separated area	Bone pinning
Palliative	Relieve symptoms without curing disease	Sympathectomy
Cosmetic	Improve appearance	Rhinoplasty

Surgery may also be classified by location of body parts or systems, such as cardiovascular surgery, chest surgery, neurologic surgery, and so on. Information specific to these types of surgery can be found elsewhere in the text.

Extent

Surgery may be classified as minor or major. *Minor surgery* is simple surgery that presents little risk to life. It may be performed in a surgeon's office, a clinic, or an outpatient or inpatient surgical suite. Many minor surgeries are performed with the patient under local anesthesia, but general anesthesia may also be used. Although the operation is termed "minor," it is frequently not viewed as a minor episode by the patient and may evoke some fears and concerns.

Major surgery is usually performed under general anesthesia or a spinal block in an inpatient surgical suite. It is more serious than minor surgery and may involve risk to life.

Purpose

There are several reasons for performing surgery (Table 20-1). The surgeon explains the method and purpose for the proposed surgery to the patient and family. Because the preoperative period is often a time of increased anxiety for the patient or family, they may not perceive or understand the reason for the surgery and may require further clarification, which the nurse can provide.

Surgical Procedures

Most surgical procedures are given names that describe the site of the surgery and the type of surgery performed. For example, a hysterectomy is the removal of (-ectomy) the uterus (hyster-).

Common surgical suffixes

-ectomy	Removal of an organ or gland
-rrhapy	Suturing or stitching
-ostomy	Providing an opening (stoma)
-otomy	Cutting into
-plasty	Plastic repair
-scopy	Looking into

Some surgeries, however, carry the name of the surgeon who developed the technique, such as the Heineke-Mikulicz procedure (widening of the pyloric opening of the stomach).

The most common method of performing surgery is cutting into the tissue and exposing the operative field. Tissues or organs are removed with a scalpel and bleeding vessels are tied with ligatures. In recent years the "scope" approach has been introduced for certain types of surgery, for example, arthroscopy (knee) or laparoscopy (removal of gallbladder). It is estimated that by the year 2000 a majority of elective surgery will be performed through a scope (see Fig. 35-10). In this method, a very small puncture incision is made to introduce the scope, which is attached to a video screen for visualization of the operative area. Two to three additional puncture incisions are made to introduce manipulating forceps and other instruments. Lasers can be used (with great caution) to cut away tissue, obliterate tissue, repair tissue, or stop bleeding. The advantage of the scope method of surgery is more rapid patient recovery, with less discomfort.

EFFECTS OF SURGERY ON THE PATIENT

Surgery is a potential or actual threat to a person's integrity and thus may produce both physiologic and psychologic stress reactions. The physiologic stress reaction is directly related to the extent of the surgery, that is, the more extensive the surgery, the greater the physiologic response. The psychologic response, however, is not directly related. A relatively minor surgical procedure, such as removal of a cyst from the face, may evoke a greater psychologic response than removal of an organ such as the spleen because of the former's potential for scarring. Removal of the uterus, however, may evoke a greater response than would removal of the spleen. This is because of the implications and values attached to the uterus.

Physiologic Responses

Major surgery is a stressor to the body and evokes a neuroendocrine response. The response, which consists of sympathetic nervous system and hormonal responses (Table 20-2), serves to protect the body from the threat of injury (Fig. 20-1). (Review Chapter 6 for the neuroendocrine response to stress). When the stress to the system is severe or if blood loss is excessive, the body's compensatory mechanisms are overwhelmed, and shock is the result. Certain types of anesthesia used may also contribute to shock formation.

Metabolic responses also occur. Carbohydrates and fats are metabolized to produce energy. Body proteins are broken down to provide a supply of the amino acids used to build new tissues. Those amino acids that are not used are

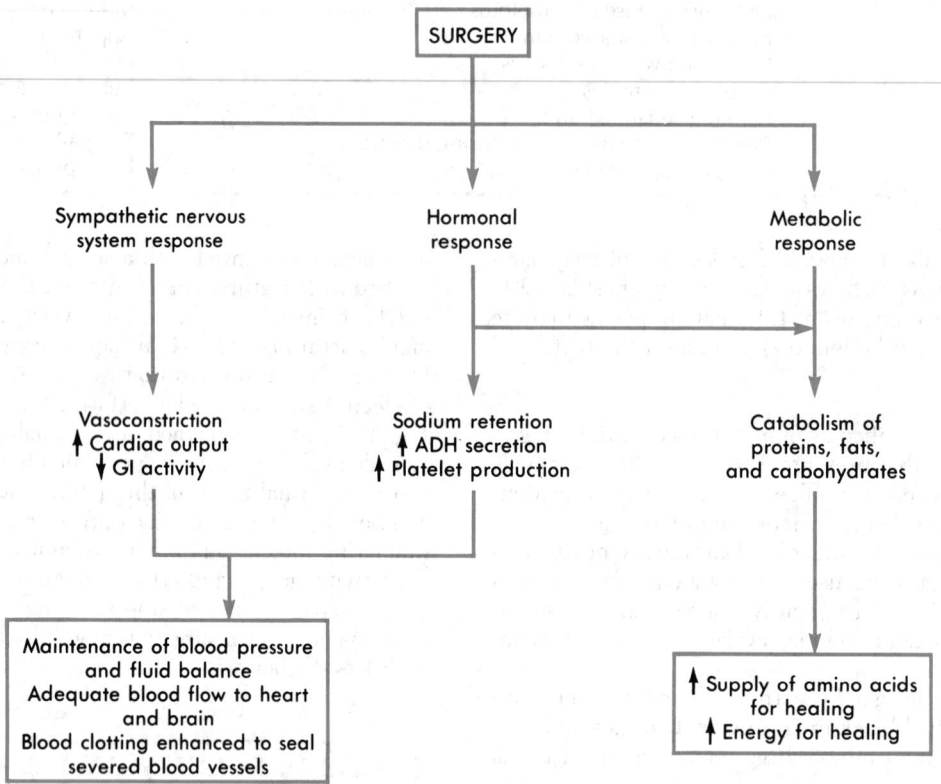

Fig. 20-1   Positive effects of the pathophysiologic response to surgery.

Table 20-2   Effects of physiologic responses to surgery

Response	Positive effect	Negative effect
Sympathetic nervous system		
Vasoconstriction	Maintain blood pressure, adequate blood flow to heart and brain	
Increased cardiac output	Maintain blood pressure	
Decreased GI activity		Anorexia, gas pains, constipation
Hormonal		
Increased glucocorticoid secretion (adrenal cortex)		
Sodium retention	Increased blood volume	Potassium loss
Protein and fat catabolism	Increased energy, amino acids available for healing	Weight loss
Increased platelet production	Prevent bleeding through clotting	Possible thrombus formation
Increased ADH secretion (posterior pituitary)	Increased blood volume	Possible fluid overload

Table 20-3   Potential postoperative complications in elderly persons

Dysfunction	Possible effects
Decreased circulation	Shock, wound infection, thrombophlebitis
Decreased kidney function	Prolonged response to anesthesia, fluid and electrolyte imbalances (especially overhydration)
Decreased respiratory function	Atelectasis, pneumonia
Decreased mobility	Atelectasis, pneumonia, thrombophlebitis, constipation, or fecal impaction

broken down to nitrogen end products, such as urea, and excreted. This leads to *a negative nitrogen balance;* that is, nitrogen loss exceeds nitrogen intake. All these factors lead to weight loss after major surgery. A high protein intake is necessary for restoration of needed proteins for healing and for restoration of optimal functioning.

Psychologic Responses

Persons differ in the way they perceive the meaning of surgery, and thus they respond in different ways. There are, however, some common fears and concerns. Some of the fears underlying preoperative anxiety are elusive, and the person may not be able to identify the cause. Others are more specific. Following is a list of these fears.

General	Specific
Fear of unknown	Diagnosis of malignancy
Loss of control	Anesthesia
Loss of love from significant others	Dying
	Pain
Threat of sexuality	Disfigurement
	Permanent limitation

Fear of the unknown is the most common. If the diagnosis is uncertain, fear of malignancy is frequent, regardless of the probability of occurrence. Fears concerning anesthesia are usually related to dying, "going to sleep and never waking up." Some persons are concerned about what they will say when they are awakening from anesthesia; if they do speak, their words often make little sense. Fears concerning pain, disfigurement, or permanent disability may be realistic or may be influenced by myths, lack of information, or lurid stories told by friends. The patient may also have other concerns related to hospitalization, such as job security, loss of income, and care of family.

Persons with anxiety so high that they cannot talk about and begin to cope with their anxiety before surgery frequently experience difficulty in the postoperative period. They are more apt to be angry, resentful, confused, or depressed. They are also more vulnerable to psychotic reactions than are persons with lower levels of anxiety.

Lack of any emotional response to surgery may indicate denial; this precludes dealing with and coping with the anxiety before surgery. Some anxiety enables the individual to identify and begin to cope with feelings. These persons usually have a smoother postoperative course.

Elderly Persons' Response to Surgery

The ability of the elderly patient to tolerate surgery depends on the extent of physiologic changes that have occurred with the aging process, the duration of the surgical procedure, and the presence of one or more chronic diseases.

Elderly persons vary greatly in the extent to which they incur physiologic changes. The changes that affect responses to surgery are cardiovascular, renal, pulmonary, and musculoskeletal (Table 20-3).

The greater the number of changes present, the greater the potential for the development of a postoperative complication. Heart rate changes in the elderly occur more slowly than in younger persons; therefore, the pulse rate *may not* be a good index in assessment of shock, and a longer period of time may be necessary to wait for pulse stabilization after activity.

The duration of the surgical experience can affect the response of elderly persons to surgery. Surgery of short duration is more easily tolerated. Presence of chronic diseases such as pulmonary, cardiac, or CNS disease limits the elderly person by prolonging recovery or be increasing the risk of mortality. Certain types of surgery present low or high risks for elderly persons:

Lower risk	Higher risk
Elective	Thoracic
Away from diaphragm	Radical head and neck
Not involving infections	Closure of wound dehiscence
Permitting early mobility	Perforated ulcer
Requiring minimal narcotics	Colostomy following obstruction

RISK FACTORS FOR SURGERY

A number of variables influence physiologic and psychologic responses throughout the surgical experience.

Age

Surgery can be performed on persons of any age, from newborns (and even on the fetus) to the very old. Persons at extremes of age are less able to tolerate stress such as tissue trauma (surgery) or infection. The specific factors influencing the surgery of the elderly are noted in the previous section.

Nutrition

Malnourished persons (nutritional deficits or excess) are poorer surgical risks than the well nourished and are more likely to develop postoperative complications. *Undernourished* persons already have diminished reserves of carbohydrates and fats. Body proteins will be used to provide the necessary energy requirement to maintain metabolic functioning of cells; thus nitrogen imbalances will be greater than normal and less protein will be available for healing. Wound healing becomes considerably delayed in undernourished persons because protein forms the collagenous matrix for wound closure, and wound separation and infection may occur. If surgery is not an emergency, it is delayed until the patient's nutritional status is improved. Conditions predisposing the person to preoperative malnutrition include chronic inflammatory disorders, liver and renal disease, gastrointestinal cancer, and congestive heart failure.

The *obese* person presents numerous risks during the surgical experience:

Respiratory complications
Vital signs fluctuations
Wound separation and infection
Incisional hernias
Thrombophlebitis

The organs are enlarged and excessive demands are placed on the cardiovascular system. Fatty tissue has reduced circulation so wounds heal more slowly. Obese persons have greater difficulty expanding their chests, moving in bed, and walking.

Neuroendocrine Response Ineffectiveness

The neuroendocrine response assists the person in coping with the stress of surgery. If this response is ineffective, postoperative complications such as shock and delayed wound healing may occur. In addition, anesthesia may be tolerated poorly, and fluid and electrolyte imbalances are more likely to occur because of insufficient adrenocortical activity. Persons with diseases of the adrenal gland or the sympathetic nervous system or those who are under a great deal of stress before surgery may do less well postoperatively because of inability to retain sodium. Infants and elderly also have diminished neuroendocrine responses.

Chronic Disease

The existence of one or more chronic diseases does not necessarily increase surgical risk. The nature and extent of the diseases and the degree to which they are under control are the important variables.

Pulmonary disease, such as chronic obstructive pulmonary disease (COPD), may affect the person's response to the anesthetic and ability to cope with respiratory problems after surgery (see Chapter 22). In persons with a history of recent respiratory infection, surgery will be delayed until optimal patient condition is achieved.

Cardiovascular disease can affect the individual's response to surgery because a heart that pumps effectively and blood vessels that constrict effectively are necessary for the prevention of shock and of fluid imbalances. To withstand blood loss and facilitate the inflammatory response to the trauma of surgery an adequate supply of red and white blood cells are required. Surgery is usually postponed if possible when the cardiovascular status of the patient is not at the optimal level of functioning.

Renal insufficiency can increase the risk of surgery because of difficulty in the removal of increased amounts of electrolytes, especially potassium, and waste products from catabolism. Persons with renal disease are prone to developing fluid overload from parenteral fluids if urine production is not adequate.

The patient with *diabetes mellitus* should have the disease well controlled before surgery. Glucocorticoid activity and potassium changes following surgery can influence insulin utilization (see Chapter 28).

Smoking

Smoke irritates the tracheobronchial tree, resulting in increased secretions that impinge on the airway and decrease ventilation. Therefore, smokers are at higher risk for developing postoperative pulmonary complications. Most surgeons and anesthesiologists prefer that persons who smoke stop smoking for a period of time before surgery.

INFORMED CONSENT

Written permission must be obtained from the patient for each operation performed and is usually obtained for major diagnostic procedures, such as thoracentesis, cystoscopy, or bronchoscopy, which involve entry into the body cavity. The consent implies that the patient has been provided with the knowledge necessary to understand (1) the nature of the procedure to be performed, (2) the available options, and (3) the risks associated with each option. Signed permission protects the patient from undergoing unauthorized surgery and protects the surgeon and hospital against claims of unauthorized surgery or that the patient was unaware of the risks involved.

Legal responsibility for obtaining informed consent from the patient resides with the physician. Oral consent is as binding as written consent.[32] Physicians will document that the necessary information has been provided the patient. Signing of the official consent form is primarily evidence that the *consent process* has occurred—that the patient is aware of the concept of informed consent. The signatures of the health care personnel (as required by specific states or hospitals) merely provide witness to the signature of the patient or family member. Thus the nurse's signature does not reflect the substance of the informed consent process.

What then is the role of the nurse in the decision-making process? In the role of patient advocate, the nurse

Table 20-4 Medications that can adversely affect anesthesia or surgery

Medication	Effect
Antibiotics	Potentiate muscle relaxants
Anticoagulants	Increase bleeding and hemorrhage
Antihypertensives	Affect anesthesia and compensatory ability (hypotension may occur)
Aspirin	↓ Platelet aggregation
	Potentiates effect of anticoagulants
Diuretics (thiazides)	Possible potassium imbalance
Steroids	↓ Neuroendocrine response
	Antiinflammatory effect, may delay wound healing
Tranquilizers	Potentiate effect of narcotics and barbiturates
	Hypotension

identifies that the patient has discussed with the physician the risks and benefits of the procedure and the alternatives. If this has not been done, the nurse consults with the physician. The professional nurse then uses skills of teaching and counseling to clarify any patient misconceptions and to facilitate the decision-making process by the patient. This process must occur before the patient receives any sedation. Patients may decide to refuse surgery, and it is their right to do so. Nurses have the responsibility to see that the decision is an *informed* decision.

If an adult is incapable of giving informed consent, consent must be obtained from the next of kin. The order of kin relationship for an adult, as determined from legal intestate succession, is usually spouse, adult child, parent, sibling.[26] A parent or legal guardian usually provides consent for a minor child. "Emancipated minors," that is, persons who are married or earning their own livelihood

and retaining the earnings, can sign their own permit. The signature of the husband or wife of a married minor is also acceptable.

In an emergency situation, the surgeon may operate without written permission of the patient or family, although every effort is made to contact a family member or guardian if time permits. Consent in the form of a telephone call is permissible in this situation.

Nursing Process
Assessment

Data are collected by the nurse in the preoperative period, often before admission, to identify the patient's (1) knowledge of events that will occur, (2) psychologic readiness for surgery, and (3) physiologic status before surgery. Specific data to be collected are listed in Box 20-2.

20-2   **Preoperative nursing assessment**

Subjective data
Knowledge and past experiences
   Understanding of proposed surgery
      Site
      Type of surgery to be done
      Information from surgeon regarding extent of
         hospitalization, postoperative limitations
      Preoperative routines
      Postoperative routines
      Preoperative tests
   Previous surgical experiences
      Type, nature, response
      Time interval
Psychologic readiness for surgery
   Concerns or fears about proposed surgery
   Usual coping methods
   Religion and its meanings for patient
   Living will or Advance Directives
   Cultural beliefs or practices related to surgery
      Refusal of treatment such as transfusion of blood
         or blood products
   Family and close friends
      Accessibility (distance)
      Perception of family and friends as source of
         support
      Present living situation
   Changes in sleep patterns
   Increased urinary frequency
Physiologic status
   Medications that may interfere with anesthesia or
      contribute to postoperative complications (Table
      20-4)
   Allergies: medications, soaps, adhesive tape, foods
      such as iodine-based salt
   Sensory: difficulties with vision, hearing, or speech
   Nutrition: adequacy of dietary intake (food, fluids),
      nausea, anorexia
   Elimination: problems with constipation, last
      bowel movement, problems with urination, last
      menstrual period

Motor: difficulties with ambulation, movement of
   arms and legs, arthritis, previous orthopedic surgery (joint replacement, spinal fusion), use of
   walking aids
Prosthetic devices: dentures, artificial eye or limb,
   contact lenses, pacemakers, broviac mediport
Comfort: ability to sleep, presence of pain or discomfort, expectations regarding relief of postoperative pain
Risk factors: smoking, alcohol, illicit drugs

Objective data
Speech patterns: repetition of themes, change of
   topic, avoidance of topics related to feelings (anxi-
   ety); ability to understand English
Degree of interaction with others (anxiety)
Behavior: excessive hand movements, restlessness,
   withdrawal, or excessive activity (anxiety)
Height and weight
Vital signs
Sensory: ability to see, hear, and speak
Skin: turgor, presence of lesions, rashes, or bruising
Mouth: dentures, condition of teeth and mucous
   membranes
Chest: breath sounds (presence, character), chest expansion, ability to do diaphragmatic breathing,
   heart sounds (baseline for postoperative compari-
   son)
Extremities: muscle strength (especially legs), character of peripheral pulses before vascular or limb
   surgery
Motor ability: any limitation to walking, sitting, or
   moving in bed, coordination with ambulation

Table 20-5 Five dimensions of preoperative education

Dimension	Description
Situational information	Description of activities; explanation of events, time sequence, and equipment
Sensational/discomfort information	Explanation of what patient may experience and interventions available for alleviation
Role information	Clarification of expected ways to participate in one's care to accomplish goals and assist in recovery
Psychosocial support	Identification of concerns and exploration of ways to decrease anxiety and enhance coping
Skills training	Explanation and demonstration of skills to aid in recovery

From Torrington KG, et al: Perioperative respiratory therapy (PORT): a program of preoperative risk assessment and individualized posterative care, *Chest* 93:946-951, 1988.

Patient knowledge

A major nursing strategy in the preoperative period is teaching the patient about forthcoming events and exercises that can be used in the postoperative period to decrease the potential for complications (Table 20-5). Before teaching can take place, it must be determined what the patient knows about the proposed surgery and the preoperative and postoperative routines. The nurse must be sensitive to the person's readiness to learn, and teach at the person's level of understanding.

Psychologic readiness for surgery

The degree of anxiety felt by the patient needs to be assessed. Patients may not be able to identify specific concerns, and further exploration may be necessary. If the nurse has identified clues from the patient's behavior that moderate to severe anxiety is present, these complications need to be validated with the patient. (Review Chapter 6 for further information about anxiety, if necessary.) If the collected data indicate that the patient is severely anxious or if the patient describes fear of dying while in surgery, report this information to the physician for further evaluation. Surgery may need to be postponed in these situations.

Knowledge of the meaning of religion for the patient can help the nurse identify a possible source of support. The effect of family members or significant others on the patient's level of anxiety needs to be determined. Some family members or friends increase the patient's anxiety by transmitting their own anxiety—hovering over the patient, displaying anxious behaviors, or offering false reassurances. Others are calm, and it is observed that the patient's anxiety is reduced when they are present.

Changes in sleep patterns or frequent urination also provide clues about increased anxiety. Major causes of insomnia are worry, fear, and concerns about the future.

Signs of anxiety in the preoperative patient are no different from those in other persons. Physical signs include an increased pulse rate and respiratory rate, moist palms, constant hand movements or motor-verbal activity, and restlessness.

Physiologic status

Data are collected in the preoperative period concerning the patient's physiologic status to obtain baseline data for comparison in the intraoperative and postoperative phases and to identify potential postoperative problems requiring preoperative intervention. Admission histories and physical examinations by the physician and nurse are good sources of pertinent data. The physician may order special tests (Table 20-6) to detect the presence of diseases that may affect the perioperative course. Patients often need explanations concerning the necessity for the sometimes numerous tests.

Ability to communicate

Data relating to the senses and language indicate the patient's ability to understand directions and to receive support during the perioperative experience. Deficits need to be communicated with the operating room staff.

Oxygenation

Respiratory data are especially important for determining the person's ability to expand the lungs, the risk for postoperative atelectasis or pneumonia, and the ability to carry out deep breathing exercises. Circulatory data are particularly important when the patient is elderly or is undergoing vascular or heart surgery. Persons with chronic lung, heart, or peripheral vascular disease may have more difficulties with tissue oxygenation in the postoperative period.

Nutrition

The height-to-weight ratio indicates whether the patient is overweight or underweight (see Chapter 5). Persons who are at risk for postoperative nutritional deficiency should be identified early. Inadequate dietary intake, nausea, anorexia, and poor conditions of the mouth and teeth will influence preoperative nutritional intake and may be factors to consider in the postoperative period.

Elimination

Decreased activity after surgery predisposes a patient to constipation. Persons with a history of chronic constipation have a higher probability for developing constipation or fecal impaction postoperatively.

Activity

Mobility and ambulation are important activities in the postoperative period for preventing postoperative complications. The patient's ability to move and walk preoperatively will determine actions that must be taken to enhance maximum mobility.

Table 20-6   Preoperative tests to establish baselines and detect presence of diseases that can affect patient responses in intraoperative or postoperative phases

System	Test	Disease or condition
Respiratory	Chest radiograph	Tuberculosis or other pulmonary disease
	Vital capacity	Tuberculosis, chronic obstructive lung disease, bronchitis, asthma
	Pulmonary function	
	Blood gas studies	
Circulatory	Electrocardiogram, echocardiogram	Cardiac dysrhythmias, myocardial damage
	Blood studies	
	WBC and differential	Chronic infection
	RBC, hemoglobin, hematocrit	Anemia
	Electrolytes	Electrolyte imbalances
	Platelet count, bleeding and clotting times, prothrombin	Liver disease, blood dyscrasias
	Typing and crossmatching	Compatibility for transfusion
	Blood volume	Heart disease
Renal	Urine studies	
	Bacteria	Urinary tract infection
	Albumin, specific gravity	Kidney disease
	Blood studies	
	Creatine, BUN, NPN, electrolytes	Kidney disease
Metabolic	Blood sugar, urine sugar, acetone	Diabetes mellitus
		Starvation

Comfort

Many persons are not aware of the hospital's routines or the nursing staff's expectations regarding the giving of medications for postoperative pain. The routines need to be clarified to the patient to prevent misunderstandings. The various modalities for pain management also need to be explained, depending on the anticipated management. Pain modalities may include patient-controlled analgesia (PCA) or the use of an epidural catheter (see Chapter 22). Because the epidural catheter is placed before general anesthesia is given, the anesthesiologist or surgeon discusses this with the patient preoperatively.

Data analysis: nursing diagnoses

Nursing diagnoses are determined from analysis of patient data. Possible preoperative nursing diagnoses may include, but are not limited to, the following:

Diagnostic title	Possible etiologies
Anxiety	Threat of death, threat to role functioning, threat of unmet needs, fear of the unknown
Fear	Anesthesia, surgery (type), loss of body part, anticipated pain, possible lifestyle changes
Knowledge deficit (events pertaining to surgery)	Lack of exposure/recall, information misinterpretation, cognitive impairment, severe anxiety
Infection, high risk for	Lack of knowledge, decreased nutrition
Injury, high risk for	Sensory/motor deficits, lack of awareness of environmental hazards

Planning: expected patient outcomes

Expected patient outcomes for the preoperative patient may include, but are not limited to, the following:

1. Demonstrates no more than moderate anxiety.
2. Describes (if conscious) the surgery to be performed and has signed the operative consent form.
3. Describes the sequence of events and physical activities expected in the early postoperative period (turning, effective deep breathing, and leg exercises).
4. Wears a legible identification band that has been checked and an allergy band (if pertinent).
5. Does not wear nail polish or acrylic nails, hairpins or wigs, dentures, or jewelry to the O.R. (articles have been stored for safekeeping).
6. Voids before going to O.R.
7. Receives preanesthetic medication as ordered, if informed consent is signed.

Implementation

Assisting with achievement of therapeutic goals
Medical interventions: correction of existing deficiencies

Postoperative complications can be minimized if existing medical conditions are treated or are under good control before surgery. Measures to treat wound infections are carried out before secondary closure or skin grafting. Dehydration from vomiting and diarrhea is treated with parenteral fluids to reestablish fluid and electrolyte balance.

Patients with chronic diseases should be at their optimal health level before surgery. The undernourished patient is placed on a high-protein, high-carbohydrate diet rich in vitamins B_1, C, and K. Supplementary vitamins may be ordered. If an oral diet is poorly tolerated or poorly absorbed, total parenteral nutrition (TPN) will be initiated. The obese patient is placed on a weight-reducing diet. Both the undernourished and the obese patient should understand the rationale for the diets. They may need considerable support and encouragement to maintain the diets.

Patients with low hematocrit levels from autologous blood donation (Chapter 41) are prescribed iron-rich diets and iron supplements.

Patients with chronic obstructive pulmonary disease are frequently placed on vigorous respiratory therapy to ensure maximal ventilation and to decrease postoperative respiratory complications. This therapy usually includes postural drainage, aerosol inhalations, and antibiotics. Smoking is restricted for all patients preoperatively and especially for patients with lung disease. Diabetes mellitus should be under good control.

Preoperative preparation

Diet. Except in bowel surgery for which patients may be placed on a low-residue or clear liquid diet, a regular diet is permitted on the day before surgery. However, nothing by mouth (no food or liquids) is permitted after midnight before the surgery. Presence of food or fluids in the stomach increases the possibility of aspiration of gastric contents should the patient vomit while under anesthesia. This can lead to aspiration pneumonia. If it should be discovered that the patient has consumed food or fluids when ordered "nothing by mouth" (NPO), the surgeon should be notified because this may necessitate rescheduling the surgical procedure. If a local or spinal anesthetic is planned, it is still common practice to keep the patient NPO.

Patients who are dehydrated will usually have parenteral fluids initiated before surgery. If it is anticipated that the patient may have decreased peristalsis after surgery (as a result of anesthesia or manipulation of the abdominal viscera), a nasogastric tube may be inserted during surgery.

Bowel preparation. Enemas are usually given preoperatively only for surgery of the GI tract or the pelvic, perineal, or perianal areas. If a preoperative enema is ineffective, it may be repeated. The purpose of the preoperative enema is to prevent injury to the colon, to provide better visualization of the surgical area, and to prevent constipation or fecal impaction postoperatively.

If enemas are to be given until the returns are clear, it is important to remember that fluid excess and potassium deficits can occur with repeated enemas. It is common practice to check with the physician if returns are not clear after the third enema. One method is to give up to three enemas on the evening before surgery, and then if the returns are still not clear, to repeat the enemas the following morning. Repeated enemas are very tiring for the patient and may irritate rectal and bowel mucosa. If antibiotic enemas are ordered for the purpose of decreasing intestinal bacteria before intestinal surgery, synthesis of vitamin K by the intestinal bacteria may be inhibited. Supplementary vitamin K may be given to prevent bleeding after surgery.

Patients may be given a glycerine suppository to use the night before surgery to clean out the lower bowel. This helps to prevent postoperative constipation when ambulation is delayed. Magnesium citrate or GoLYTLEY may also be prescribed for bowel cleansing.

Skin preparation. The purpose of preoperative skin preparation is to free the operative site of as many microorganisms as possible. In many instances showering well with hexachlorophene soap will suffice. In certain types of surgery, such as for placing orthopedic implants, infections can lead to dysfunction so several showers are prescribed. Same-day surgery patients are given Hibiclens and instructed to shower twice, the night before surgery and on the morning of admission. No soap, alcohol, or alcohol-based solutions should be used in conjunction with hexachlorophene solutions as these substances decrease the antiseptic properties of hexachlorophene.

Hair is removed from the surgical site because microorganisms cling to the hair. Shaving or clipping of the hair may be ordered either the night before or immediately before surgery (preferred approach). A sharp disposable razor is used with good lighting. Shaving must be *against the grain* of the hair shaft for a closer shave. The skin should not be scratched or nicked because microorganisms can harbor in broken skin surfaces. A depilatory may be used if the skin is not sensitive to the depilatory.

Shaving of hair on certain areas of the body may have a special meaning for some persons. These areas include the face, head, and pubic area. If the entire head is to be shaved, it is frequently carried out after the patient has been anesthetized. The eyebrows are not shaved. Pubic hair is shaved only when necessary; the regrowth of this hair is uncomfortable to many patients.

Some hospitals have specified procedures delineating the size of the area to be shaved. The surgeon usually specifies which of the areas is to be shaved. An area larger than the anticipated incision is shaved to permit flexibility in location and size of incision.

Interventions to achieve patient outcomes
Preparing patient psychologically for surgery

Both patient and family need opportunities to discuss their concerns and fears about the forthcoming surgery. The assessment of the patient's psychologic readiness for surgery provides the nurse with data about the patient's specific fears and concerns.

By providing time during the preadmission appointment for patients to talk with a supportive, knowledgeable individual helps them to begin to identify the reasons for their anxiety and to marshal coping responses. It is helpful for the nurse to provide for a quiet unhurried time to sit down with the person or family and give them an opportunity to ask questions and to talk about concerns. Touch is often a helpful form of communication, sending the message, "I care," and some persons will talk more readily while receiving a back rub. Knowing that a nurse is interested and cares helps to reduce anxiety. If the person knows also that anxiety is a normal reaction to the threat of surgery, it may help to remove the often self-imposed expectation, "I shouldn't be nervous."

Loss of control is one of the fears associated with surgery. It is important that a patient talk with the anesthesiologist preoperatively to understand the type of anesthesia recommended. Allowing persons to participate in decision making in regard to their own care, when feasible, helps

Table 20-7 Surgeries for which coughing is contraindicated or modified

Surgery site	Effect of coughing
Intracranial	Coughing increases intracranial pressure (ICP), leading to cerebral spinal fluid leak
Eye	Coughing increases ICP, which then increases intraocular pressure, causing pressure on suture line
Ear	Mouth must be kept open if coughing occurs to prevent pressure backup through eustachian tube to middle ear, causing pressure on suture line
Nose	Mouth must be kept open if coughing occurs to prevent dislodgement of clot with subsequent bleeding
Throat	Vigorous coughing may dislodge a clot with subsequent bleeding

---

20-3

Helpful information for preoperative patients and families

Preoperative tests—reason, preparation
Preoperative routines; sequence of events
Special equipment needed
Transfer to operating room (time, checking procedures)
Recovery room
    Place where patient will awaken
    Frequent monitoring of vital signs
    Return to room when vital signs stable
Probable postoperative therapies
    Need for increased mobility as soon as possible
    Need to keep respiratory passages clear
    Anticipated treatments (for example, I.V.)
    Pain medication routines (timing sequence, "as needed" [prn] status), and modalities of management

---

20-4

High-risk factors: pulmonary complications

Inhalant anesthesia	Tight abdominal
Thoracic surgery	binders
Upper abdominal	Body casts
surgery	Obesity
Smoking	Advanced age
Chronic lung disease	

---

them partially to meet the need for control. Identifying and carrying out measures to help the patient meet physical needs in the preoperative phase may help provide a feeling of security about having postoperative needs met and thus allay some anxiety.

Teaching (from preparation for surgery to home-going instructions) is an important nursing function in the preoperative phase, which may begin several days before admission. This teaching helps to allay anxiety when the patient knows what to expect. Also, if persons are to move toward self-care and independence, they need to know early the what, why, and how of activities that will help them regain an optimal level of functioning after surgery. They also need to know what to expect when they go home or go to a rehabilitation or extended-care facility. Waiting until the patient has sufficiently recovered from the insult of surgery before teaching is started means a considerable loss of time, and learning may be less effective. In addition, the patient may be discharged before teaching is completed. It is particularly useful to provide *written* instructions whenever possible, especially for activities the patient and family are to carry out.

Explaining events

Fear of the unknown can be decreased by an understanding of the events that will occur. The amount of information to give preoperatively depends on the background, interest, and stress level of the patient and the family. A good rule to follow is to ask patients what they would like to know about forthcoming surgery and to base responses on the types of questions asked. Simple explanations are indicated for persons under considerable stress or those with severe pain. A highly anxious person may not take in and remember information given. Information helpful for preoperative patients is listed in Box 20-3.

Facilitating teaching

Effective deep breathing exercises. Some persons are at high risk for developing postoperative pulmonary complications such as atelectasis or pneumonia (see Box 20-4).

These persons need to carry out deep breathing exercises in the early postoperative period.

Coughing is *contraindicated* in intracranial surgery and surgery of the eye, ear, nose, and throat, because it either increases pressure, causing tissue damage and dislodging of sutures, or dislodges a clot (Table 20-7). Waiting until after surgery to teach persons how to carry out the exercises decreases the effectiveness of the outcome, because anesthesia and pain will decrease the patient's ability to retain information.

The person needs to know how to perform diaphragmatic breathing, as this increases lung expansion by permitting the diaphragm to descend fully. Many males normally breathe diaphragmatically, whereas few females do. With diaphragmatic breathing, the abdomen *rises with inspiration* and *falls with expiration*. The nurse assesses the person's normal breathing pattern by placing a hand lightly on the person's abdomen and asking the person to take a deep breath. If diaphragmatic breathing does not occur naturally, the person can be taught to inspire deeply while pushing the abdomen up against the hand.

The method for effective deep breathing exercises is listed as follows:

1. Lie in semi-Fowler's or high Fowler's position with knees flexed to relax abdomen and allow full chest expansion.

2. Place a hand lightly on the abdomen.
3. Breathe in slowly through nose, letting chest expand and feeling abdomen rise against hand.
4. Hold breath for 5 seconds.
5. Exhale slowly through pursed lips (abdomen contracts).
6. Inhale and exhale 7 more times.

This exercise creates negative pressure and pulls air into the alveoli of the lung and stimulates the cough reflex if secretions are present. If a thoracic or high abdominal incision is present, the person can "splint" the incision with a pillow during coughing to relieve stress or pull on the incision. The use of an incentive spirometer (Chapter 22) or Respirex during pulmonary exercises helps to measure the depth of inhalation and breath hold.

Leg exercises. Venous stasis in the postoperative period may lead to thrombophlebitis (blood clot). Persons at high risk include those who (1) will have decreased mobility after surgery, (2) have a history of decreased peripheral circulation, or (3) undergo cardiovascular or pelvic surgery. These patients will need to carry out exercises postoperatively to prevent venous stasis in the legs. Tightening and relaxing leg muscles help to "pump" the blood along the veins. Valves in the veins prevent back flow of blood.

Persons at high risk may have sequential compression devices (SCD) (see Chapter 22) applied before, during, and after surgery to promote venous return. Antiembolic stockings, either thigh-high or knee-high, may also be used. Persons who will be restricted to bed rest for several days after surgery will need to exercise the legs to maintain muscle tone to facilitate ambulation at a later date. These persons need to learn to carry out ankle pumps, quadriceps sets, and gluteal tightening exercises (see Box 20-5).

20-5

Postoperative leg exercises

Ankle pumps
1. Move both ankles by pointing toes up, then down, then in circles
2. Repeat at least 10 times every hour
3. Do this while on back or when sitting and dangling feet over side of bed

Quad sets
1. Lie on back with both legs straight
2. Tighten thigh muscles so backs of knees press down on bed
3. Hold muscles tight for 5 seconds
4. Exhale slowly while holding muscles tight
5. Relax. Repeat at least five times every hour

Gluteal tightening
1. Lie on back
2. Tighten buttock muscles tightly as if to restrain a bowel movement
3. Hold muscles tight for 5 seconds
4. Exhale slowly while holding buttocks tight
5. Relax. Repeat at least five times every hour

Promoting mobility

Moving and turning in bed helps to prevent pulmonary and circulatory complications, prevent decubiti, stimulate peristalsis, and decrease pain. During the preoperative period, persons can be taught how to use the side rails effectively for turning. They can also be taught how to sit up on the side of the bed with the least amount of pull on the incision:

1. Move to edge of bed
2. Raise head of bed to high Fowler's position
3. Drop feet over side of bed
4. Push up to sitting position with hand closest to edge of bed

Carrying out final preparation for surgery

Preventing injury. Measures taken to protect the patient from errors of identification or injury include the following:

1. Check identification band for secureness and legibility and allergy band if allergies present.
2. Remove hair pins and wigs; protect hair with a cap.
3. Remove jewelry; wedding ring may be taped to patient's finger.
4. Remove nail polish and acrylic nails (for assessment of circulation during surgery).
5. Remove contact lenses and store in proper container.
6. Remove any prostheses (dentures, false eyes, and so on); store prostheses in a safe place.
7. Leave hearing aid in place if patient is unable to hear without the aid (inform operating room nurse).
8. Apply SCDs and/or antiembolic stockings if patient is at high risk for thromboembolism or shock (elderly, marked varicosities, pelvic surgery, time-consuming surgery).
9. Have patient empty bladder immediately before receiving preanesthetic medication.
10. Instruct patient to stay in bed until transported to the operating room.

Administering preanesthetic medication. If a patient is in the hospital the night before surgery, a sedative may be prescribed to ensure a full night's sleep. If additional sedation or medication for pain is given during the night, it must be given intramuscularly at least 4 hours before the preanesthetic medication (12 hours if taken by mouth) to prevent oversedation.

Preanesthetic medications, commonly referred to as *premedication,* are given when the patient is "on call" for the operating room (usually about 45 to 90 minutes before surgery is anticipated). Preanesthetic medications are given to decrease anxiety, to provide a smoother induction and maintenance of anesthesia, to diminish undesirable reflexes during emergence from anesthesia, to decrease salivary and respiratory secretions, and to block vagal impulses that produce bradycardia.

The effects of commonly used preanesthetic medications are listed in Table 20-8. Adults frequently receive a combination of drugs. Dosages may be decreased in the elderly.

Any delay in giving the medication is reported to the anesthesiologist. All preoperative routines are completed before the preanesthetic medication is given. The patient should remain in bed following administration of the medication to promote maximum effect and to prevent falls from dizziness. The side rails are raised, the bed is placed in low position, the call signal is placed within reach, and the patient is instructed not to get out of bed.

One major effect desired before surgery is decreased anxiety. It must be reemphasized that psychologic preparation of the patient for surgery is the most effective approach to help allay anxiety. The administration of preanesthetic medication without any attempt at psychologic preparation may render the patient drowsy, but it does not reduce anxiety. Occasionally, music or imagery is used to decrease anxiety. Advance preparation is needed for these approaches.

Some drugs other than preanesthetic agents, such as insulin, antihypertensive agents, and cardiac medications, may be prescribed for the day of surgery. Oral medications are given with only a small sip of water. Administration of these medications is recorded on the chart before patient transfer to surgery.

Recording. A check-off list that includes the final preparations is often used. A final nurse's note is written listing the times the patient voided, when the patient leaves for surgery, and any final pertinent remarks regarding the patient's condition and emotional response. Presence of any handicaps such as blindness or deafness should be noted for use by the surgical staff.

Table 20-8   **Commonly used preanesthetic medications**

Drug	Desired effect	Undesired effect
Benzodiazepines		
Midazolam (Versed)	Reduces anxiety, promotes sleep, causes amnesia	May cause respiratory depression, especially in debilitated or elderly persons
Diazepam (Valium)	Reduces anxiety, promotes relaxation	Orthostatic and general hypotension; drowsiness and decreased coordination
Lorazepam (Ativan)	Same as for midazolam	Respiratory depression
Narcotics		
Morphine sulfate	Reduces anxiety, promotes relaxation, decreases preoperative pain, decreases amount of anesthetic needed	Depresses respiration, circulation, and gastric motility; may cause nausea and vomiting
Meperidine hydrochloride (Demerol)	Same as for morphine sulfate	Same as for morphine sulfate
H₂ receptor antagonists		
Cimetidine (Tagament)	Decreases gastric acid and gastric volume	Rare; confusion may occur in elderly persons
Famotidine (Pepcid)	Decreases gastric acid	Same as for cimetidine
Ranitidine (Zantac)	Decreases gastric acid	Same as for cimetidine
Antacid, nonparticulate		
Sodium citrate (Bicitra)	Increases gastric pH; less pulmonary damage with aspiration	None
Antiemetics		
Metoclopramide (Reglan)	Enhances gastric emptying	Restlessness, confusion
Droperidol (Inapsine)	Decreases risk of nausea and vomiting, sedation	Restlessness, confusion, extrapyramidal reaction
Neuroleptanalgesic agent		
Fentanyl and droperidol (Innovar)	General quiescence, state of indifference, decreased motor activity, analgesia, antiemetic	Respiratory depression, muscle rigidity, hypotension
Anticholinergics		
Atropine sulfate	Decreased secretions, prevention of laryngospasms and bradycardia	Excessive dryness of mouth, tachycardia, confusion, restlessness
Scopolamine hydrochloride (Hyoscine)	Decreased secretions, amnesia, state of indifference, sedation	Excessive dryness of mouth; profound confusion and restlessness in the elderly
Glycopyrrolate (Robinul)	Same as atropine sulfate	Same as atropine sulfate

Nursing Care Plan	Preoperative patient

DATA: Mrs. G. is an active 76-year-old widowed homemaker with a history of osteoarthritis in her left hip. She has been experiencing difficulty ambulating and has had increased pain, especially at night. She denies any history of falls or trauma. She is scheduled for a total hip replacement.

1. Mrs. G. has been hospitalized only once before and has never had major surgery.
2. She lives alone in a two-story house with a bathroom on the second floor.
3. She states she is worried about being anesthetized and of the pain after surgery.
4. She expresses much anxiety about being a burden on her family and not going back to her home after surgery.
5. Mrs. G. has strong supportive family and friends.

Nursing diagnosis: Knowledge deficit related to lack of information regarding hip replacement surgery

Expected patient outcomes	Nursing interventions	Rationale
Mrs. G. describes the sequence of events that will occur on the morning of surgery	Review with Mrs. G. and family what to expect in terms of activities related to the day of surgery	Knowledge of expected events helps to decrease anxiety and facilitate coping
Mrs. G. repeats preoperative expectations	Provide rationale for preparation for surgery and give written instructions	Knowing why the preoperative activities are necessary and having notes to refer to will facilitate her carrying out the instructions
Mrs. G. demonstrates effective deep breathing exercises	Teach rationale and method of effective deep breathing exercises; have her give a return demonstration and suggest she practice at home	Mrs. G. will be less mobile after surgery; she is at high risk for pulmonary complications

Nursing diagnosis: Anxiety, related to surgery and threat of losing independence

Expected patient outcomes	Nursing interventions	Rationale
Mrs. G. is relaxed before surgery	Clarify her understanding of anesthesia, its administration and effects	Mrs. G. may have heard inaccurate stories about anesthesia or may be worried about waking up. Clarification will decrease anxiety
	Explain methods of postoperative pain relief and control she may have	Knowing that pain control is possible decreases anxiety

Nursing diagnosis: Home maintenance management, impaired related to inadequate living situation

Expected patient outcomes	Nursing interventions	Rationale
Mrs. G. states she is comfortable about her decision to go to an extended-care facility for 4 to 5 days before going home	Call social service to arrange for placement	Mrs. G. will be unable to go home until she can climb stairs with crutches or walker
	Arrange for transportation to extended-care facility	Mrs. G. will require transportation because of her limited mobility
	Order equipment and supplies for home care after surgery	Mrs. G. will require equipment for home care; advance ordering will facilitate her return home

Before the patient leaves for surgery the chart is checked for completeness as to the following:

1. Skin preparation done and checked by nurse
2. Vital signs (temperature, pulse, respiration, blood pressure) charted
3. Premedications charted
4. Regular medication charted
5. Weight and height recorded (for use by anesthesiologist)
6. Operative permit signed, witnessed, and attached to chart
7. All recent laboratory, radiographic, and ECG reports attached to chart
8. Previous hospital charts

Evaluation

Questions to ask may include the following:

1. Is the patient's anxiety level no more than moderate?
2. Does the patient understand the nature of the surgical procedure to be performed, and has the operative permit (consent form) been signed?
3. Has the patient been taught the physical activities to be performed in the early postoperative period, as pertinent (turning, effective deep breathing, and leg exercises)?
4. Is the patient wearing a legible identification band that has been checked?
5. Have all removable objects been stored for safekeeping?
6. Has nailpolish or acrylic nails been removed?
7. Did the patient void just before receiving premedication?
8. Has the premedication been given and charted?
9. Is the chart complete?

TRANSPORTATION TO OPERATING ROOM

Personnel transporting the patient bring the stretcher from the operating room and identify themselves to the nurse. The unit nurse assigned to prepare the patient for surgery checks the patient record, accompanies the transportation attendant to the patient's bedside, checks the patient's identification band, and signs the patient identification form. This form is usually then attached to the stretcher. Patients should be protected from drafts. Because the operating room is kept cool, cotton blankets are used to keep the patient warm.

The patient's family or close friends are provided with the following information:

1. Where to wait until patient returns to the unit
2. Availability of coffee shop, cafeteria, and so on
3. Expected time intervals
   a. Patient is sent to surgery 45 to 60 minutes before surgery actually commences
   b. Surgery may be delayed if the previous surgery took longer than anticipated
   c. Patient will be sent to a postanesthesia room (recovery room) after surgery for varying periods of time
4. Method of receiving information when surgery is completed

5. Visit by surgeon after surgery (if this is the policy)
6. What to expect when patient returns from surgery (condition, special equipment, and so on)

SUMMARY

1. Elective admission for surgery may be by way of ambulatory surgery, same-day surgery, or early hospital admission. All preoperative patients require the necessary preoperative preparation.
2. Surgery may be classified by location (external, internal, or body system) or by extent (major or minor).
3. The purpose of surgery may be diagnostic, curative, restorative, palliative, or cosmetic.
4. Surgery is a stressor; therefore, it evokes neuroendocrine and metabolic responses to stress. Neuroendocrine responses include vasoconstriction, increased cardiac output, decreased GI activity, increased glucocorticoid secretion, and increased ADH secretion. Metabolic responses include utilization of carbohydrates and fats for energy and protein catabolism.
5. Anxiety and fear are common responses to anticipated surgery. Persons with severe anxiety are poor candidates for surgery.
6. Risk factors for surgery include extremes of age, malnutrition, neuroendocrine response ineffectiveness, selected chronic diseases, and smoking.
7. Patients must know about the nature and risks of the proposed surgery and available options for care before signing a consent form (informed consent). The physician is responsible for obtaining informed consent; the nurse facilitates the process and ensures that the consent form has been signed before surgery.
8. Data are collected by the nurse in the preoperative period to identify the patient's knowledge about surgery and psychologic response (for planning of preoperative care); physiologic data are collected to establish a baseline for future comparison and to identify potential postoperative problems.
9. Preoperative medical care includes treatment of existing medical conditions, including nutritional status, to facilitate optimal health status (except in emergency surgery).
10. Dietary restrictions for adults having major surgery usually include nothing by mouth after midnight.
11. The skin is usually prepared by careful cleansing. Shaving is best done in the operating room immediately before surgery to prevent infection.
12. Psychologic preparation of the patient for surgery includes helping the person explore concerns or fear about surgery and providing desired information about the perioperative experience.
13. Teaching of necessary postoperative patient activities, such as effective deep breathing exercises, leg exercises, and turning in bed, is best done in the preoperative period.
14. Final preparations before the patient is transported to surgery include removing nonattached objects and nail polish, ensuring proper patient identification, providing a hair cap, and asking the patient to void.
15. Preanesthetic medications are given to decrease anx-

iety; facilitate induction, maintenance, and emergence from anesthesia; decrease secretions; and prevent bradycardia. The patient must remain in bed after premedication has been given to facilitate drug effects and to prevent falls from dizziness.

STUDY QUESTIONS

- What general reactions do you believe you would have if told you must have immediate major surgery? What questions would you want answered? Based on this, what would be important to include in your preoperative teaching?
- Using Fig. 20-1, explain in lay terms the positive effects of the pathophysiologic responses to surgery.
- Examine the informed consent form of your agency. What is your responsibility in this situation?
- Examine the charts of several patients who have had surgery. What preanesthetic medications were given? What were the purposes of these medications?

REFERENCES AND SELECTED READINGS

1. Anderson R, Zimbra C: Same day surgery: coordinating the admission process, *Nurs Manage* 17(12):23-25, 1986.
2. Association of Operating Room Nurses Inc: *AORN standards and recommended practices for perioperative nursing*, Denver, 1989, The Association.
3. * Blackwood S: Back to basics: the preop exam, *Am J Nurs* 86:39-44, 1986.
4. * Connoway CA, Blackledge D: Preoperative testing center: central location to evaluate and educate patients, *AORN J* 43:666-670, 1986.
5. * Crawford FJ: Ambulatory surgery: the elderly patient, *AORN J* 41:356-369, 1985.
6. Emery P: Ambulatory surgery. In Rothrock JC: *Perioperative nursing care planning*, St Louis, 1990, Mosby–Year Book.
7. Evaluating the usefulness of routine preoperative tests, *AORN J* 45:696, 1987.
8. Garibaldi RA, et al: The impact of preoperative skin disinfection on preventing wound contamination, *Infect Control Hosp Epidemiol* 9(3):109-115, 1988.
9. Hathaway D: Effect of preoperative instruction on postoperative outcome: a meta-analysis, *Nurs Res* 35:269-275, 1986.
10. * Hogue E: What you should know about informed consent, *Nursing 86* 16(6):47-48, 1986.
11. * Jackson MF: Implications of surgery in very elderly patients, *AORN J* 50:859-866, 1989.
12. Johnston M: Preoperative emotional states and postoperative recovery, *Adv Psychosom Med* 15:1-22, 1986.

13. Kaplan EB, et al: The usefulness of preoperative laboratory screening, *JAMA* 253:3576-3581, 1985.
14. Kneedler J, Dodge G: *Perioperative patient care*, ed 2, Boston, 1987, Blackwell.
15. Knight CG, Donnelly MK: Assessing the preoperative adult, *Nurs Pract* 13(1):6-17, 1988.
16. * Latz PA, Wyble SJ: Elderly patients: perioperative nursing implications, *AORN J* 46:238-253, 1987.
17. * Litwack K: Administering preoperative medications, *Nursing 91* 21(8):44-47, 1991.
18. Meeker MH, Rothrock JC: *Alexander's care of the patient in surgery*, ed 9, St Louis, 1990, Mosby–Year Book.
19. Mortensen M, McMullin C: Discharge score for surgical outpatients, *Am J Nurs* 86:1347-1349, 1986.
20. * Murphy EK: Informed consent, pt I, *AORN J* 47:1009-1016; pt II, 47:1295-1298, 1988.
21. Phipps C: Effectiveness of the clinical nurse specialist in preadmission testing, *Health Matrix* 5(4):23-27, 1988.
22. Rogers M, Reich P: Psychological intervention with surgical patients: evaluation outcomes, *Adv Psychsom Med* 15:23-50, 1986.
23. * Rothrock JC: Preoperative nursing research: preoperative psychoeducational interventions, *AORN J* 49:597-616, 1989.
24. Schoessler M: Perceptions of preoperative education in patients admitted the morning of surgery, *Patient Educ Counsel* 14(2):127-136, 1989.
25. Torrington KG, et al: Perioperative respiratory therapy (PORT): a program of preoperative risk assessment and individualized postoperative care, *Chest* 93:946-951, 1988.
26. Way LW: *Current surgical diagnosis and treatment*, ed 9, Norwalk, Conn, 1991, Appleton & Lange.
27. * Wetchler BV: Patient selection criteria for 1987: ambulatory surgery, *AORN J* 44:30-36, 1987.
28. * Williams D: Preoperative patient education: in the home or in the hospital? *Orthop Nurs* 5(1):37-41, 1986.
29. Worley B: Preadmission testing and teaching: more satisfaction at less cost . . . surgical admissions, *Nurs Manage* 17(12):32-33, 1986.

Classic

30. Alexander J, et al: The influence of hair removal methods on wound infections, *Arch Surg* 118:347-352, 1983.
31. American College of Surgeons' Committee on Pre- and Postoperative Care: *Manual of preoperative and postoperative care*, ed 3, Philadelphia, 1983, WB Saunders.
32. * Cushing M: Informed consent: an MD responsibility? *Am J Nurs* 84:437-440, 1984.
33. * Does preop medication promote stress? *Am J Nurs* 84:1202, 1984.
34. * Fraulini KE: Coping mechanisms and recovery from surgery, *AORN J* 37:1198-1208, 1983.
35. * Horsely J, Crane J: *Structured preoperative teaching*, New York, 1981, Grune & Stratton.

*Recommended for student reading.

21

Intraoperative Intervention

Mary Jo Boehnlein

After studying this chapter, the learner should be able to:

- Explain concepts basic to perioperative nursing.
- Relate the nursing process to each of the three phases of the patient's surgical experience.
- Explain the roles and responsibilities of each team member.
- Describe the principles of aseptic technique.
- Identify infection control practices used in the operating room.
- Identify practices that promote patient safety in the operating room.
- Describe basic intraoperative patient positions and the nursing care planning required for each patient.
- Identify common anesthetic agents and the methods used to anesthetize patients.
- Describe basic standards for intraoperative patient monitoring.
- Identify nursing interventions to ensure safe patient care at the completion of surgery.

Surgical intervention is a distinctive event for patients. Individuals face this particular event with their own values. Every patient not only has specific expectations of the surgical experience but also has distinct hopes for the outcome of the surgery.

The primary role of the perioperative nurse is that of a patient advocate. In order to fulfil this role the perioperative nurse must possess scientific and technical knowledge and also acquire a variety of technical skills. Incorporation of this knowledge with the nursing process enables the nurse to collaborate with other team members to provide effective, safe, and efficient care for the patient undergoing surgical intervention.

CONCEPTS BASIC TO PERIOPERATIVE NURSING

Perioperative Nursing

The practice of having registered nurses work in the surgical suite began in the mid 1890s. Initially nurses were brought to work in the operating room to provide technical service to the surgeon and his assistants. This highly technical role easily matched the description of the nurse as the physician's handmaiden. However, the role of the registered nurse in the operating room has been expanded, refined, and standardized through the efforts of the members of the operating room nurses' professional organization, the Association of Operating Room Nurses (AORN).

AORN has defined standards of patient care and recommended practices for perioperative nurses. The following statement of *Perioperative Nursing Practice* summarizes the role and responsibilities of the registered nurse working in the operating room:[1]

> The registered nurse in the operating room is responsible for providing nursing care to surgical patients. Perioperative is used as an encompassing term to incorporate the three phases of the surgical patient's experience. This includes the preoperative, intraoperative, and postoperative periods. Practice refers to expected behavior patterns reflecting professional activities, which include the range of clinical activities performed during the preoperative, intraoperative, and postoperative phases. Perioperative practice incorporates both technical and professional components of nursing practice. The perioperative nurse delivers care through the use of the nursing process as reflected in the *Standards of Perioperative Nursing Practice* in a manner that is cost effective without compromising quality of care.

The *preoperative* phase of the surgical experience begins when a patient elects to undergo a surgical procedure; it is completed when the individual is brought into the operating room and moved onto the surgical bed. It is throughout this period that the perioperative nurse compiles data and makes a nursing assessment of the patient's psychologic, physiologic, and sociologic needs (see Chapter 20). Once the assessment has been completed, the perioperative nurse formulates a plan of nursing care to meet the needs of the individual patient. The plan of care includes preparing the OR environment for the patient. Assembling special supplies and equipment and ensuring that the equipment is in working order are some of the activities the OR nurse performs to ensure an operating room that is ready to receive the patient.

Movement of the patient onto the OR bed begins the *intraoperative phase;* this period lasts until the patient is admitted to the postanesthesia care unit (PACU). During the entire intraoperative period, the perioperative nurse implements the nursing care plan while functioning as an active team member who is able to alter the plan of care quickly in response to emergency situations and/or changes in the patient's condition.

Evaluation of intraoperative care begins as the patient is being prepared for transfer to the PACU and continues into the postoperative period.

The *postoperative period* begins when the patient is admitted to the PACU. This period ends when there is a follow-up evaluation of the care the patient received. This evaluation can be completed in the PACU with a report to the PACU nurse, with a postoperative visit to the patient's room, or in the case of ambulatory surgery patients, with a telephone call to the patient's home. Examples of the perioperative nursing activities performed throughout the three phases of the patient's surgical experience can be found in Table 21-1.

When delivering patient care, the perioperative nurse uses knowledge and skills on a continuum. The continuum ranges from a level of basic competency to that of excellence or mastery (Fig. 21-1). At the basic competency level, the nurse applies fundamental nursing principles to patient care situations. In order to provide care that is excellent in quality, the perioperative nurse must constantly acquire and update knowledge and skills and use the new knowledge to deliver patient care.

Standards of Perioperative Nursing Practice

In 1975, the *Standards of Practice: Operating Room* were developed by a joint committee of the American Nurses' Association Division on Medical Surgical Nursing and AORN. These were reviewed and revised in 1981 and were published as the *Standards of Perioperative Nursing Practice.*

The standards are based on the nursing process. They are broad in scope and are meant to (1) guide the practice of perioperative nursing, (2) illustrate nursing's concerns for quality patient care, and (3) provide criteria to evaluate the competency of the nursing that individuals receive during surgical intervention throughout each of the four phases of the nursing process (Table 21-2).

The goal of perioperative nursing practice is to provide continuity of care throughout the preoperative, intraoperative, and postoperative phases. The *Standards of Perioperative Nursing Practice* and the *Patient Outcome Standards* are guides for nurses to provide care to individuals undergoing surgical intervention and also to provide a method for measuring the quality of care that the patient received.

INTRAOPERATIVE PATIENT CARE TEAM MEMBERS

Operating Team

The coordinated efforts of the surgical team are required to deliver safe and effective intraoperative care for the surgical patient. In order to achieve this goal, team members must work rapidly and efficiently as a coordinated unit. Each member of the surgical team must be familiar with the specific surgical procedure, adhere to policies and

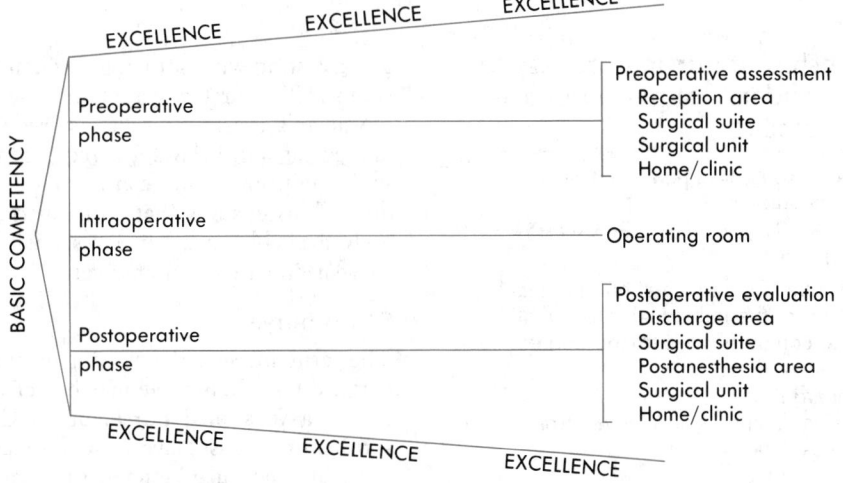

Fig. 21-1 Perioperative nursing practice: a continuum. (From AORN standards and recommended practices for perioperative nursing, Denver, 1991, AORN Inc.)

Table 21-1 Examples of nursing activities in perioperative nursing practice

Preoperative phase	Intraoperative phase	Postoperative phase

Preoperative assessment
Home/clinic
  1. Initiates initial preoperative assessment
  2. Plans teaching methods appropriate to patient's needs
  3. Involves family in interview
Surgical unit
  1. Completes preoperative assessment
  2. Coordinates patient teaching with other nursing staff
  3. Explains phases in perioperative period and expectations
  4. Develops a plan of care
Surgical suite
  1. Assesses patient's level of consciousness
  2. Reviews chart
  3. Identifies patient
  4. Verifies surgical site
 	
Planning
  1. Determines a plan of care
 	
Psychologic support
  1. Tells patient what is happening
  2. Determines psychologic status
  3. Gives prior warning of noxious stimuli
  4. Stands near/touches patient during procedures/induction
  5. Communicates patient's emotional status to other appropriate members of the health care team
	Maintenance of safety
	  1. Ensures that the sponge, needle, and instrument counts are correct
	  2. Positions the patient
	    a. Functional alignment
	    b. Exposure of surgical site
	    c. Maintenance of position throughout procedure
	  3. Applies grounding device to patient
	  4. Provides physical support
	
	Physiologic monitoring
	  1. Calculates effects on patient of excessive fluid loss
	  2. Distinguishes normal from abnormal cardiopulmonary data
	  3. Reports changes in patient's pulse, respirations, temperature, and blood pressure
	
	Psychologic monitoring (prior to induction and if patient is conscious)
	  1. Provides emotional support to patient
	  2. Continues to assess patient's emotional status
	  3. Communicates patient's emotional status to other appropriate members of the health care team
	
	Nursing management
	  1. Provides physical safety for the patient
	  2. Maintains aseptic, controlled environment
	  3. Effectively manages human resources
		Communication of intraoperative information
		  1. Gives patient's name
		  2. States type of surgery performed
		  3. Provides contributing intraoperative factors, that is, drain, catheters
		  4. States physical limitations
		  5. States impairments resulting from surgery
		  6. Reports patient's preoperative level of consciousness
		  7. Communicates necessary equipment needs
		
		Postoperative evaluation
		Recovery area
		  1. Determines patient's immediate response to surgical intervention
		Surgical unit
		  1. Evaluates effectiveness of nursing care in the operating room
		  2. Determines patient's level of satisfaction with care given during perioperative period
		  3. Evaluates products used on patient in the operating room
		  4. Determines patient's psychologic status
		  5. Assists with discharge planning
		Home/clinic
		  1. Seeks patient's perception of surgery in terms of the effects of anesthetic agents, impact on body image, distortion, immobilization
		  2. Determines family's perceptions of surgery

Table 21-2   Relationship of nursing process to AORN standards of perioperative nursing practice

Principles of nursing process	AORN standards of perioperative nursing practice
Assessment	Standard I The collection of data about the health status of the individual is systematic and communicated to appropriate persons. Standard II Nursing diagnoses are derived from health status data.
Planning	Standard III The plan of nursing care includes goals derived from the nursing diagnoses. Standard IV The plan for nursing care prescribes nursing actions to achieve the goals.
Implementation	Standard V The plan for nursing care is implemented.
Evaluation	Standard VI The plan for nursing care is evaluated. Standard VII Reassessment of the individual, reconsideration of nursing diagnoses, resetting of goals, and modification and implementation of the nursing care plan are continuous.

procedures, and be able to adjust quickly to alterations in the surgical procedure.

The OR team is divided into categories based on the duties of its members. Members of the *scrubbed* sterile team scrub their hands and arms, put on sterile gowns and gloves, and work in the sterile field. Members of this team consist of:

1. Primary surgeon
2. Assistants to the surgeon
3. Scrub nurse

Members of the *nonscrubbed* nonsterile surgical team function outside the sterile field. The team members are responsible for maintaining sterile technique, handling nonsterile supplies and equipment, and providing items for the sterile team. Members of the nonsterile team consist of:

1. Circulating nurse
2. Anesthesiologists and anesthetists
3. Others

Primary surgeon and assistants

The primary or operating surgeon has the knowledge, skill, and expertise to perform the identified surgical procedure successfully. The surgeon is responsible for the preoperative diagnosis, the choice and execution of the surgical procedure, and the postoperative management of the patient's care.

Under the direction of the operating surgeon, the surgeon's assistant is responsible for exposing the surgical site, suctioning blood to prevent it from obscuring the anatomy,

and assisting with suturing throughout the operative procedure. The first assistant may be a surgeon, resident, physician's assistant, or a registered nurse. In the majority of medical staff bylaws it is required that a physician work with the primary surgeon during a major surgical procedure. This ensures that a qualified individual is immediately available to assume responsibility for the primary surgeon in case of an emergency.[16]

Scrub nurse

The scrub nurse is the nursing team member of the sterile surgical team. This role may be performed by a registered nurse, a vocational nurse, or an OR technologist. The scrub nurse must have an understanding of the specific surgical procedure along with a knowledge of the basic anatomy and physiology involved in the procedure. Some of the responsibilities of the scrub nurse are:

1. Preparing the supplies and equipment on the sterile field
2. Maintaining the safety and integrity of the sterile field throughout the surgical procedure
3. Observing the scrubbed team members for breaks in sterile technique
4. Providing appropriate sterile instrumentation, sutures, and supplies to the operating surgeon
5. Watching the sterile field and anticipating and responding to the surgeon's needs
6. Adhering to established policies and procedures for sponge, instrument, and sharp counts.

In order to perform this role effectively, the scrub nurse must possess manual skills and dexterity, strictly adhere to the principles of aseptic technique, and consistently perform all duties with precision and accuracy to ensure the safety and welfare of the surgical patient.

Circulating nurse

The circulating nurse is a registered nurse whose responsibility is to serve as the patient advocate while coordinating the course of events before, during, and following the surgical procedure. Whereas the surgeon is responsible for the activities at the operating field, the circulating nurse is responsible for managing the activities outside the sterile field and providing nursing care for the patient.

Before and during administration of the anesthetic, the circulating nurse provides emotional support to the patient and assists the anesthesia team during the induction period. Throughout the surgical procedure, the circulating nurse obtains supplies and equipment for the sterile team members, enforces policies and procedures, and takes measures to ensure patient safety. The circulating nurse is also responsible for documenting intraoperative nursing care and ensuring that surgical specimens are identified and placed in the appropriate medium. Other responsibilities include but are not limited to:

1. Using the nursing process to ensure patient care needs are met
2. Developing and maintaining a safe environment for the patient
3. Ensuring that there are no breaks in aseptic technique
4. Recognizing and taking action to resolve possible en-

Table 21-3 Traffic control zones

Zone	Dress code	Areas
Unrestricted	Street clothes	Lounge, dressing rooms, scheduling office, patient holding area
Semirestricted	Scrub attire and caps	Storage for clean and sterile supplies, work areas for processing supplies and equipment, corridors to restricted zones
Restricted	Scrub attire, caps, and masks	Operating rooms, scrub room, substerile rooms

vironmental hazards that involve the patient or surgical team members

5. Ensuring that sponge, instrument, and sharp counts are completed and appropriately documented
6. Documenting intraoperative patient care
7. Communicating relevant information to individuals outside the operating room such as family members and other health care workers.

Anesthesiologist and anesthetist

An anesthesiologist is a physician who specializes in the art and science of administering anesthetic agents. An anesthetist is an individual, most commonly a certified registered nurse, who administers anesthetics under the direct supervision of an anesthesiologist or surgeon.

In the preoperative period, the anesthesiologist and anesthetist evaluate the patient and determine the appropriate anesthetic to be administered. Intraoperative responsibilities include anesthetizing the patient, providing appropriate levels of pain relief for the patient, and providing the best operative conditions for the surgeon. In the immediate postoperative period, the anesthesiologist assumes responsibility for the supervision of the recovery room management of the patient.

Other Personnel

Radiology technicians, perfusionists, pathologists, laboratory technicians, environmental services personnel, patient transporters, central service employees, and clerical staff are just a few of the many individuals whose skills and expertise are needed to provide assistance to the surgical team.

DESIGN OF THE SURGICAL SUITE

A surgical suite is designed to meet the requirements of the expected type and number of surgical procedures to be performed. The design of the suite addresses issues of traffic patterns, infection control, safety, efficiency, potential for expansion, and accessibility to other departments.

Traffic Control

Traffic control patterns are designed to address activity and movement into and out of the surgical suite as well as within the suite. The three-zone concept was developed to define areas within the surgical suite by the types of activities that occur within each area. The three zones are known as the *unrestricted area*, the *semirestricted area*, and

the *restricted area*. Table 21-3 provides further information on these areas.

Infection Control

The design of the operating room and the materials used within it are chosen to address issues of infection control and safety. Some infection control and safety control issues that are addressed in the design of the operating room include:

1. Ceilings and walls that are nonporous, fire resistant, smooth, and easy to clean
2. Ceiling-mounted versus track-mounted operating room lights. (Track mounted lights are not recommended because they are not easily accessible for cleaning and can produce fallout of dust each time they are moved.)
3. Recessed storage cabinets and view boxes
4. Sliding doors versus swinging doors. (The movement of swinging doors increases air turbulence. Fire regulations dictate that it should be possible to swing open sliding doors if necessary.)
5. Presence of an effective ventilation system to exchange air on a frequent basis. (This is necessary to decrease potential bacterial contamination at the operative site.)
6. Floor coverings that are easy to clean and highly wear resistant. (Slip-proof surfaces are used for the floors where scrub sinks are located.)

Environmental Conditions

Temperature and humidity are environmental conditions that need to be controlled to reduce the incidence of surgical infections. To decrease the surgical patient's metabolic demands, temperature within an operating room is maintained between 20° C and 27° C (68° F 80° F). Humidity in the operating room is maintained at a minimum level of 50%. This level of humidity diminishes bacterial growth and restricts static electricity.

Communication System

A reliable communication system is essential in the surgical suite. It is needed to call for assistance or to communicate with other members of the health care team. Telephones and intra- and interdepartmental intercom systems are used to make instant consultation by means of direct communication possible. In addition to intercom systems, a call light system can be used to call for assistance from the anesthesia department, pathology department, and environmental services department.

ASEPTIC TECHNIQUE AND INFECTION CONTROL

The antiseptic era and the modern age of surgery began in the mid 1800s with the work of Louis Pasteur and Joseph Lister. Lister recognized the relationship between Pasteur's germ theory and the process of infection and began promoting the use of carbolic sprays for hands, wounds, instruments, dressings, and the operating room itself. The advent of Lister's antiseptic practices resulted in a decrease in surgical mortality rates from 45% to 15% and led to the development of the modern principles of surgical asepsis. As a result of his work, Joseph Lister is known as the Father of Antiseptic Surgery.[19]

Asepsis is defined as the absence of microorganisms that cause disease.[2] *Surgical asepsis* promotes tissue healing by deterring pathogens from coming into contact with the surgical wound. Practices that suppress, reduce, and inhibit infectious processes are known as *aseptic technique*.

Infection control policies and procedures guide the practice of aseptic technique in the operating room. The policies and procedures are based on principles of microbiology and bacteriology. Infection control protocols include procedures for housekeeping activities, cleansing of skin, sterilization of supplies and equipment, cleanliness of the air in the surgical suite, and apparel of operating room personnel.

All members of the operating room team are responsible for strict adherence to aseptic technique. It is essential that OR nurses acquire a surgical conscience. A *surgical conscience* means vigilant adherence to aseptic technique throughout the entire perioperative period. This involves constant examination and observation of the patient, OR environment, and personnel. A surgical conscience is completely developed when the nurse automatically attends to sterile technique. To develop a surgical conscience the nurse must:

1. Understand the principles of aseptic technique
2. Acquire self-discipline in managing hygiene, dress, and nursing practice with special attention given to breaks in technique
3. Anticipate supply and equipment needs for the surgical team and the patient
4. Develop good communication and assertiveness skills to identify patient needs and communicate breaks in sterile technique
5. Demonstrate the ability to overcome personal prejudices in order to provide optimum patient care in spite of the specific surgical procedure or the patient's circumstances.

Basic Rules of Surgical Asepsis

The Association of Operating Room Nurses (AORN) has developed five recommended practices for aseptic technique. These were designed to establish guidelines for creating and maintaining a sterile field. Strict adherence to the following principles minimizes the chances of contamination and the potential for infection:

1. Gloves and gowns used by scrubbed personnel are sterile
   a. The gown of a scrubbed team member is considered sterile in front from the chest to the level of the

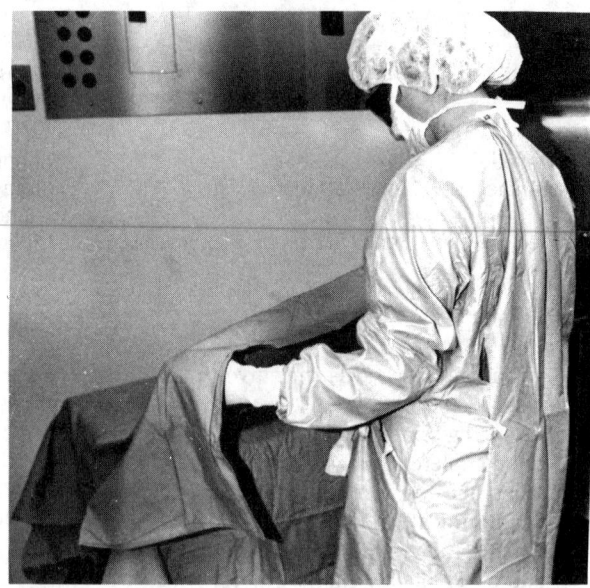

Fig. 21-2 Scrub nurse protects gloves with cuff of drape when opening inner wrapper of pack, which will serve as sterile table cover. (From Meeker MH, Rothrock JC: *Alexander's care of the patient in surgery*, ed 9, St Louis, 1991, Mosby–Year Book.)

sterile field, the sleeves are sterile from 2 inches above the elbow to the stockinette cuff
   b. The stockinette cuff portion of the gown is unsterile and needs to be completely covered by sterile gloves
   c. The unsterile areas of the surgical gown include the neckline, shoulders, axillary region, and the back
   d. Articles dropped below the waist or table level are contaminated
2. Sterile drapes are used to create a sterile field
   a. Draped tables are sterile only at the table level; items extending over the table edge are contaminated
   b. Sterile drapes are placed on the patient, equipment, and furniture used within the sterile field
   c. Handling of drapes should be kept to a minimum
   d. When placing drapes, gloved hands are protected by a cuff or the drape (Fig. 21-2)
3. All items used in the sterile field are sterile. If there is a question about the sterility of an item, it must be considered unsterile. Packages must be checked for moisture, seal integrity, tears, pinholes, and the presence of a sterilization indicator
4. Supplies introduced into the sterile field are delivered in a manner that ensures the sterility of the item and maintains the integrity of the sterile field
   a. A sterile package is opened from the far side first and the near side last; wrapper tails are held when the item is presented to the sterile field (Fig. 21-3)
   b. Solutions are poured so as to prevent splashing of liquids onto the field (Fig. 21-4)
   c. Once a bottle of sterile solution is opened the entire contents must be presented to the sterile field or discarded. (The edges of a bottle cap are considered

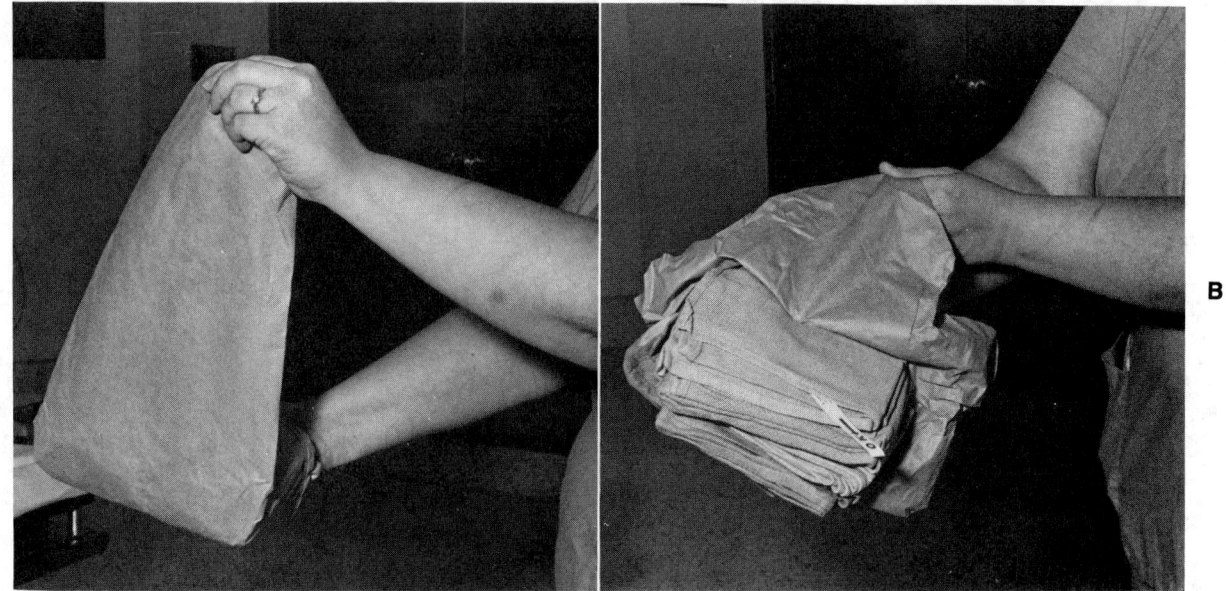

Fig. 21-3   A, Sterile wrap is opened farthest flap first. **B,** Wrapper flap ends are held back when placing item on sterile field.

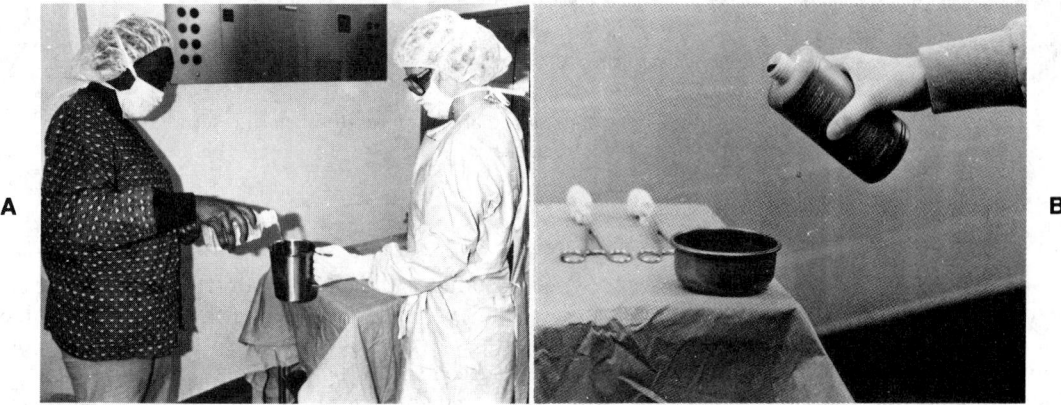

Fig. 21-4   A, Scrub nurse stands well back from solutions being poured into sterile receptacle to avoid contamination. **B,** Receptacle receiving fluid is placed near edge of table to permit circulating nurse to pour without reaching over sterile field. (From Meeker MH, Rothrock JC: Alexander's care of the patient in surgery, ed 9, St Louis, 1991, Mosby–Year Book.)

nonsterile once the cap is removed. If the cap is replaced, the sterility of the bottle contents cannot be assured, therefore the remaining contents must be discarded.)
5. The sterile field must be constantly monitored
   a. The sterile field should be established as close to the scheduled time of use as possible
   b. Unattended sterile fields are considered contaminated
   c. The integrity of the sterile field must be maintained by individuals moving within or around the sterile field
     (1) Scrubbed personnel only touch and reach over sterile areas

     (2) Unscrubbed personnel only touch and reach over nonsterile areas
     (3) Sterile persons remain close to the sterile field and never turn their back to the field
     (4) Sterile individuals change positions by passing back to back or face to face (Fig. 21-5)
     (5) Unscrubbed team members must not walk between sterile fields and must approach sterile fields by facing them
   d. The sterile dressing is applied before the surgical drapes are removed so as to prevent contamination of the incision.[1]

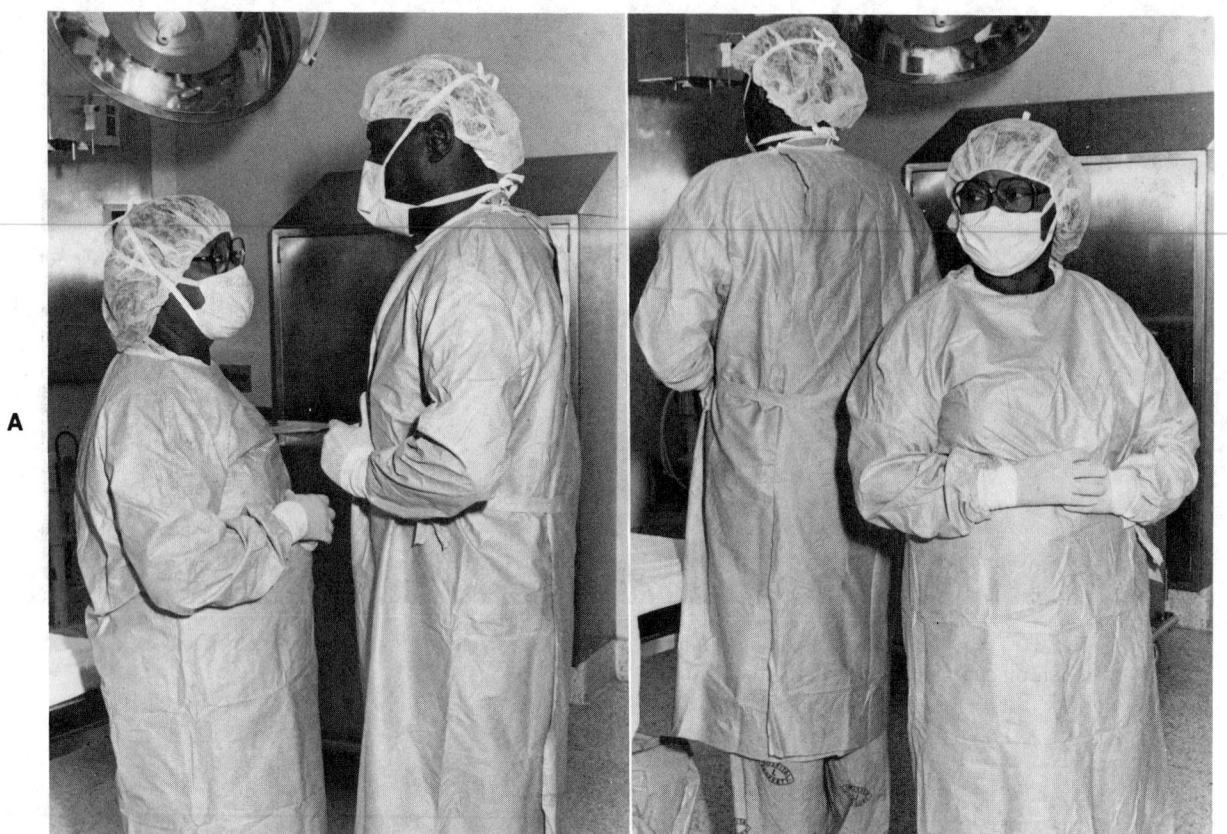

Fig. 21-5 Maintaining principle of sterile-to-sterile and unsterile-to-unsterile, scrubbed team members pass **A,** face to face, or **B,** back to back.

Infection Control Practices for Operating Room Personnel

All individuals working in the operating room serve as a major source of microbial contamination to the environment because of the large quantities of bacteria that are present in the respiratory tract, on the skin, hair, and attire of all persons. To reduce the risks of OR personnel serving as sources of infection for the patient, it is necessary for everyone to adhere strictly to OR dress code policies.

Daily personal hygiene is another important factor affecting the numbers of pathogens individuals bring into the OR environment. Hair, which is a fertile source of bacteria, may shed bioparticulate matter into an open surgical wound. Individuals with draining wounds or other types of infection should not work in the operating room. Institutional polices should identify circumstances that prohibit working in the operating room.

Operating room attire

Street attire cannot be worn in the semirestricted or restricted areas of the OR suite. The surgical suite should be designed so that dressing areas are provided for personnel to change into clean OR attire and directly enter the semirestricted areas of the surgical suite without going through unrestricted areas.

Dressing in OR attire proceeds from head to toe. The *surgical cap* is put on first to prevent contamination of scrub clothes with hair or dandruff. The cap must be clean, free of lint, and completely cover all head and facial hair. If the cap does not provide sufficient coverage of facial hair, a hood should be worn.

Surgical suits are put on after the hair is covered. The suits, which are laundered daily, should be made of materials that meet the requirements of the National Fire Protection Agency and should be closely woven to minimize bacterial shedding.

Scrub shirts are either tied at the waist or tucked into the scrub pants. This is done to decrease bacterial shedding and to prevent contamination of the sterile field by a loose shirt.

The legs of *scrub pants* should not be dragged on the floor when they are put on. Scrub pants should have some type of ankle closure to reduce bacterial dispersion (Fig. 21-6).

Unscrubbed personnel should wear *warm-up* jackets with stockinette cuffs to prevent possible shedding of microorganisms from bare arms. The jacket should remain closed to prevent the possibility of brushing against the sterile field.

Footwear should be comfortable. In the interest of safety, clogs, open-toe, and cloth athletic shoes are not recommended. Either OR-restricted shoes or shoe covers should be worn. Data show that unprotected street shoes

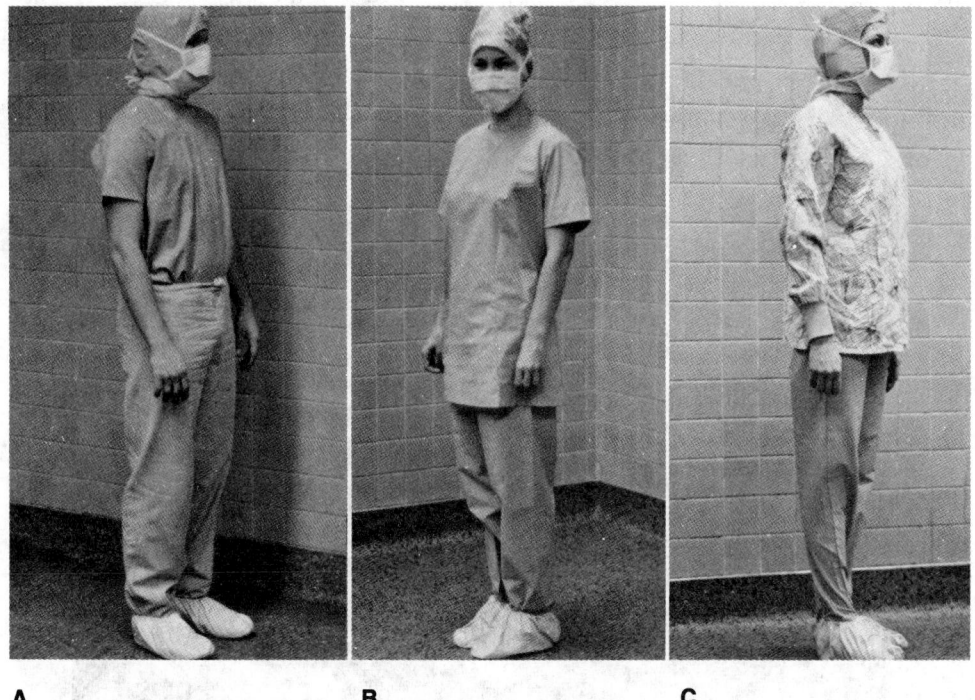

A   **B**   **C**

Fig. 21-6 Proper operating room attire. **A,** The scrub top should be tucked into pants. **B,** Tunic top that fits close to body may be worn outside of pants. **C,** Nonscrubbed personnel should wear long-sleeved jacket that is buttoned or snapped closed. (From Meeker MH, Rothrock JC: Alexander's care of the patient in surgery, ed 9, St Louis, 1991, Mosby—Year Book.)

carry a significant number of bacteria into the operating room. The practice of wearing OR-restricted shoes or shoe covers significantly decreases the number of bacteria transferred onto the OR floor.[6]

Wear OR-restricted shoes and shoe covers only in the semirestricted and restricted areas of the surgical suite. Shoe covers should completely cover the shoe and be changed when torn, soiled, or wet. Remove them when leaving the semirestricted area and put clean ones on when returning to the area. This practice is necessary to prevent cross-contamination to and from other areas of the institution.

Masks are necessary to prevent contamination of the surgical environment by respiratory droplets. Masks are worn at all times in the restricted areas of the surgical suite. Disposable masks of high microbial efficiency of 95% or greater are used; cloth or gauze masks are unsuitable because of their inefficient filtration.

Masks must totally cover the nose and mouth and must be secured to prevent ventilation from the sides of the face. They are either on or off. They should not be saved by being hung around the neck, placed on the forehead, or in a pocket. Masks should be changed between procedures. To avoid contamination of the hands, care must be taken to avoid touching the filter portion of the mask. It should be removed only by touching its strings (Fig. 21-7). Once it is removed, the mask should immediately be discarded. Following disposal, the individual should thoroughly wash and dry the hands.

If *jewelry* is worn in the operating room, it must be completely confined within scrub clothes or cap. Complete confinement of jewelry decreases the possibility of it falling into the surgical wound.

Wearing *fingernail polish* is forbidden in the operating room because it may crack, chip, and peel, which would then provide a medium to harbor bacteria. Artificial or *acrylic nails* are also not to be worn in the surgical suite. Studies have reported that fungal growth frequently occurs under and around these nails, which creates a possible source of contamination in the operating room.[4]

Ideally, OR attire should never be worn outside the surgical suite; however, this is not always possible. If a scrub suit is worn outside the operating room it must be covered. The preferred method is to use a clean cover gown that closes in the back. If a lab coat is worn, it must be completely buttoned to protect the front of the scrub suit. Upon return to the department, clean scrub attire should be put on in the appropriate order.

Universal precautions

The risk of patient-to-caregiver transmission of viruses and bacteria is a great concern to individuals working in the OR environment. Hepatitis B is a major infectious occupational health hazard, but OR personnel are also at risk for acquiring other bloodborne pathogens.[17]

The Centers for Disease Control (CDC) has recommended that all health care workers strictly adhere to blood and body fluid precautions for all patients regardless of the

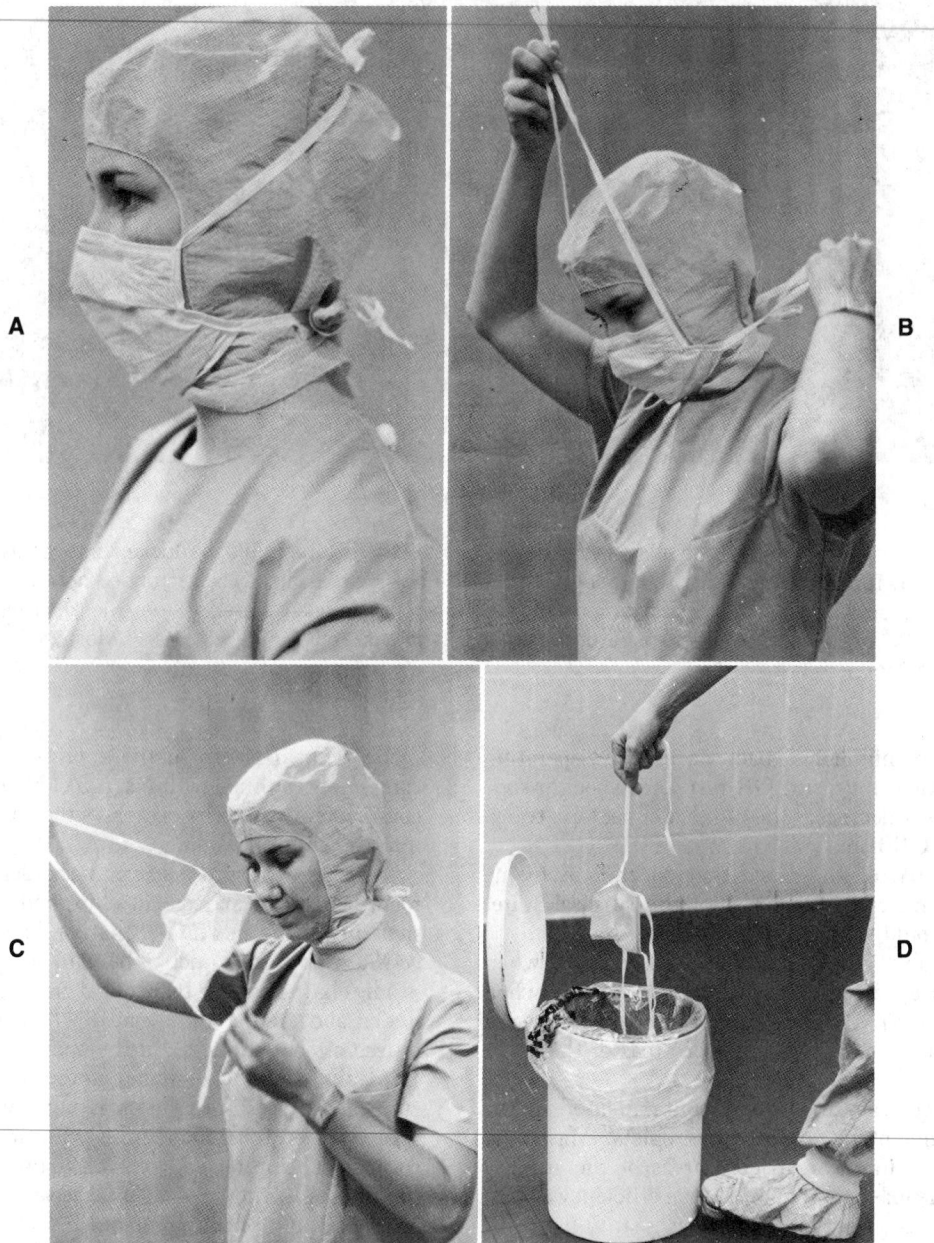

Fig. 21-7 Proper handling of mask. **A,** Edges of properly worn mask conform to facial contours when mask is applied and tied correctly. **B** and **C,** Avoid touching filter portion of mask when removing it. **D,** Discard mask upon removal. (From Meeker MH, Rothrock, JC: Alexander's care of the patient in surgery, ed 9, St Louis, 1991, Mosby–Year Book.)

Table 21-4   Intraoperative applications of universal precautions

Nursing action	Potential contaminant	Precautions
Changing the blood-filled suction liner at the end of the procedure	Blood splashing out of suction liner	Goggles or face shield, gloves
Transferring an actively bleeding trauma patient to the OR bed	Direct contact with blood	Goggles or face shield, gloves, fluid-resistant apron or gown
Organizing blood-filled sponges for the sponge count	Direct contact with blood-contaminated items	Goggles or face shield, gloves
Removing or changing the surgical knife blade	Cuts and direct contact with blood	Instrument or surgical clamp to disassemble knife blade and handle

patient's known or suspected bloodborne infection status. These recommendations, which are known as *universal precautions*, were developed because of the difficulty in identifying patients with the human immunodeficiency virus (HIV).

The universal precautions state that the blood and body fluids of all patients are potentially infectious for HIV, hepatitis B, and other bloodborne pathogens. The CDC has recommended that whenever an invasive or surgical procedure is performed, OR personnel should follow the universal blood and body fluid precautions combined with the following recommendations to prevent skin and mucous membrane contact with the blood and body fluids of all patients.[6]

1. Gloves and masks must be worn by all individuals who come in direct contact with blood, body fluids, and mucous membranes of any patient.
2. Gloves should be worn when touching items or surfaces that have been soiled with blood or body fluids.
3. Gloves should be changed following contact with each patient.
4. Gloves that are torn or contaminated by a needle or instrument should be removed as soon as possible. The needle or instrument must be removed from the sterile field.
5. Protective eyewear or a face shield should be worn for procedures that produce splashing of blood or irrigations, or the formation of bone chips.
6. Protective fluid-impervious gowns or aprons should be worn when there is exposure to gross contaminants such as blood or other body fluids.

The proper handling and disposition of needles, knife blades, and sharp instruments, along with strict compliance with the CDC practices of universal precautions, protects OR staff members. Adherence to these practices along with strict adherence to aseptic technique minimizes the chance of cross-contamination of pathogens between patients and personnel. Table 21-4 gives some examples of how OR nurses can apply these principles.

Scrubbing, gowning, and gloving

The purpose of a surgical scrub is to remove dirt and microorganisms from the hands, fingernails, and forearms; decrease the resident microbial count to minimum levels; and retard the regrowth of microorganisms. This is accomplished by a mechanical washing of the fingernails, hands, and arms with an antimicrobial soap.

The microbial flora of the skin is classified as transient and resident bacteria. *Transient flora* are acquired by contact, and loosely adhere to the skin. The majority of transient microorganisms are removed by chemical and mechanical methods.

Resident flora are found deep in the skin in hair follicles and sebaceous glands. These microorganisms are emitted from the body with the movement of old cells from the dermal to the epidermal layer of the skin with perspiration and other skin secretions. Because of these actions, the resident flora area is a potential source of contamination. Resident bacteria are decreased but are not completely removed during the surgical scrub.

The skin can never be sterilized; however, it can be made surgically clean. Obtaining surgically clean skin involves a mechanical process that removes transient flora with friction along with a chemical process that decreases the number of flora on the dermis with the use of an antimicrobial detergent.

Various antimicrobial detergents meet the criteria for effectiveness. The effective agent must be a broad-spectrum antimicrobial, fast-acting in decreasing the microbial count, able to leave a residue on the skin to reduce regrowth of bacteria, and nonirritating and nonsensitizing. The most commonly used agents are povidone-iodine and hexaclorophenes.

The actual procedure and types of materials used for the surgical scrub varies from one institution to another. Every institution should have written policies and procedures to standardize the scrub procedure for all personnel. Regardless of the specific policies and procedures, there are certain criteria that must be met by all personnel before beginning the surgical scrub.

Only individuals who are free of skin problems and upper respiratory infections should scrub. Skin cuts and abrasions can discharge serum, which is an environment for microbial growth and therefore increases the potential for infection. Fingernails must be short, clean, and free of polish to prevent harboring of microorganisms. Proper scrub attire is worn to decrease contamination that may pass from OR personnel to the surgical patient.

There are two accepted methods for performing a surgical hand scrub; the timed scrub procedure, and the brush-stroke-count procedure. Both are effective and follow an anatomic pattern of scrub, beginning at the fingertips and ending with the elbows.

Table 21-5   **Surgical scrub guidelines**

Action	Comments
1. Put on surgical attire making sure all hair and jewelry is covered and mask is properly secured.	Surgical attire decreases possible contamination from the operating room to the patient.
2. Remove all jewelry from hands and arms.	Jewelry harbors microorganisms that may not be removed with handwashing.
3. Moisten hands and arms and wash to 2 inches above the elbows with an antiseptic agent.	A pre-scrub loosens surface debris.
4. Clean nails and subungual areas with nail cleaner under running water.	Improperly cleaned fingernails and subungual areas can harbor microorganisms.
5. Rinse hands and arms. Allow water to flow from fingertips to elbows, taking care not to splash surgical attire.	Elevating hands higher than the elbows facilitates water flowing from the cleanest area down the arm. Moisture on scrub attire contaminates the sterile gown.
6. Moisten scrub brush, create a lather, and begin the surgical scrub at the fingertips, progress to the digits, palm, and back of the hand.	The scrubbing is done vigorously with the scrub brush held perpendicularly to the digit. All sides of the digit and web spaces are scrubbed. Depending on institutional policy, this step initiates either the timed scrub or the scrub-count process.
7. Scrub forearms to 2 inches above the elbow.	Each side of the arm is scrubbed in a circular motion to 2 inches above the elbow.
8. Discard the scrub brush into the appropriate container. Rinse hands and arms thoroughly. Keep hands elevated and proceed into the operating room.	Same comments as for No. 5.

The *timed scrub* takes a minimum of 5 minutes to complete. A 10-minute scrub versus a 5-minute scrub provides no appreciable reduction of microorganisms. In the timed scrub each anatomic area of the hands and forearms is scrubbed for an identified length of time with special attention given to the fingers and hands. At the conclusion of the timed scrub, the hands and arms are rinsed.

The *brush-stroke-count scrub* also takes approximately 5 minutes to perform. This method differs from the timed scrub method only in that there is a defined number of brush strokes used for each area of the fingers, hands, and arms. Methods of rinsing and entering the operating room are the same as for the time scrub process. See Table 21-5 for surgical scrub guidelines.

Once inside the operating room, the individual must dry the hands and arms with a sterile towel before putting on the sterile gown. Dry hands and arms facilitate gowning and putting on sterile gloves. More importantly, dry arms prevent contamination from the strike-through of moisture to the sleeves of the sterile gown.

The type of *sterile gown* used (disposable versus nondisposable) is determined by institutional policy. The method of donning the surgical gown and gloves is dependent on the type of gown used and whether or not the gowning and gloving is done by another sterile team member. Once the sterile gown is on, sterile gloves are put on.

Sterile gloves may be put on by one of two methods, either the closed glove method or the open glove technique. Both approaches are acceptable, although the closed method has the advantage of preventing the bare hands from coming in contact with the outside of the sterile glove. A more detailed explanation of the gowning and gloving process can be found in reference 19.

Patient Skin Preparation

The purpose of skin preparation, also known as the *prep*, is to make the surgical incision site as free as possible from transient and resident microorganisms. It is the first step in the prevention of a surgical wound infection.

The skin preparation, which may include hair removal, can be performed before the anesthetic induction. If the prep is done when the patient is awake, the circulating nurse needs to explain the purpose of the procedure, attend to the patient's privacy by avoiding unnecessary exposure, and provide for the patient's comfort and safety.

Removal of hair from the surgical site is done only as necessary. Methods for hair removal include wet shaving, use of clippers, and use of a depilatory. It has been shown that there is a greater incidence of wound infection in patients who are shaved preoperatively than for patients who have no shave prep, who have a smaller amount of hair clipped, or on whom a depilatory is used.[1]

Data also support the fact that the amount of time between the shave and the operation has a relationship to the wound infection rate. If a wet shave is ordered by the physician it should be performed immediately before the surgery in a well-lit area that provides privacy. The shave should be performed by an individual who has demonstrated skill in the shave procedure. When performing a shave prep, care should be taken to prevent knicks, scratches, or cuts because any breaks in the skin surface provide a medium for the growth of microorganisms and a resultant infection.

Once the shave prep has been completed the patient's skin is cleaned with an antiseptic agent. The choice of agents depends on the surgeon's preference and institutional policy. Other considerations used in the selection of the appropriate agent are:

1. Patient sensitivity and skin condition
2. Spectrum of activity (the agent must have a broad spectrum of antimicrobial action)
3. Toxicity of the agent (some agents can be absorbed from the skin and be neurotoxic)[1]
4. Length of antimicrobial action.

Necessary supplies for the skin prep include sponges, gloves, towels, drapes, and solutions. These are all arranged on a separate table. The prep begins with a mechanical scrubbing at the incision site and is extended in a circular fashion away from the site to the periphery. At the periphery the prep sponge is considered contaminated and is discarded. The soiled sponge is never brought back over the area previously scrubbed. Each time the area is scrubbed a new sponge is used.

The area of skin that is prepped needs to be large enough to avoid wound contamination by movement of the surgical drapes, to accommodate any necessary extensions of the incision, and to include all drain sites.

When it is necessary to prep an area that includes an open draining wound or a body orifice, the practice of cleansing from the incision site to the periphery is modified. The alterations of the prep are based on the principle that cleaning proceeds from clean to dirty areas. The most contaminated area is scrubbed last even if it is the site of the surgical incision.

Sterile Draping

Covering the patient, tables, and equipment with sterile sheets and towels creates an area that is known as the sterile field. Only sterile items are used within the sterile field. This practice prevents the transmission of microorganisms to the surgical wound.

The drapes used in creating the sterile field establish a barrier that eliminates the passage of microorganisms between sterile and nonsterile areas. Drapes may be disposable or reusable. Effective draping materials meet the following criteria:

1. Meet the standards of the National Fire Protection Agency
2. Are lint free
3. Resist moisture strike-through
4. Resist bacterial penetration
5. Are drapeable.

Components of a draping system include plain or whole sheets to cover instrument tables and body regions, towels to drape the operative site, fenestrated sheets to drape the patient and expose the operative site, and plastic incisional drapes.

Plastic incisional drapes used along with other draping materials are applied directly to the skin. Use of plastic incisional drapes eliminates the need for skin clips, holds other drapes in place, prevents skin excretions and bacteria from entering the wound, and isolates surrounding contaminated areas such as stomas.

Identifying the area to be draped and the type of drape to be used is the surgeon's responsibility. Maintaining an awareness of the limits of the sterile field and maintaining asepsis throughout the surgical procedure is the responsibility of the entire surgical team.

SAFETY AND PROTECTION OF THE PATIENT
Admission of Patient to Operating Room

The process for admitting a patient to the surgical suite should be defined by institutional policy. In some circumstances patients are admitted to a holding room before being transferred to the operating room.

The *holding room* is a separate area within the surgical suite where patients wait until the operating room is ready. It is in this area that patient identification and planned surgical procedure are confirmed by the holding room nurse. Intravenous lines are started, preoperative medications may be given, and, if necessary, a preoperative shave prep may be performed.

Some institutions do not have any holding rooms. In those institutions the patient arrives in the surgical suite and waits in a hallway until the operating room is ready.

While waiting in the holding room or other areas of the surgical suite the patient is separated from family members and is faced with the upcoming surgery. As a result the patient may experience feelings of fear, anxiety, and helplessness.

Regardless of where the patient is waiting, the nurse's first responsibility is to establish rapport with the patient. The nurse can then provide emotional support to the patient and help decrease anxiety by permitting expression of feelings, answering questions, and informing the patient of delays. Other nursing activities performed by either the holding room or circulating nurse include the following:

1. Identification of the patient with a verbal confirmation of name by the patient or significant other and a visual check of the identification bracelet. The visual check includes a comparison of the patient's name and the medical record number on the identification bracelet with the information on the chart.
2. Verification of the patient's adherence to dietary and fluid restrictions. NPO status is essential to prevent aspiration of gastric contents during anesthesia induction.
3. Verification of allergies.
4. Review of the operative consent and special consent form for:
   a. Clear precise description of the proposed surgical procedure
   b. Identification of the operating surgeon
   c. Patient signature
   d. Signature of the individual who witnessed the patient's signature.
5. Verification of the operative site and procedure with the patient.
6. Review of the chart for:
   a. Medical history and results of physical examination
   b. Laboratory examination results; any abnormal results are reported to the surgeon and anesthesiologist
   c. Radiology reports
   d. Other studies and examinations as required by institutional policy. A preoperative checklist is often used to ensure that all appropriate studies have been completed and the results have been documented.
7. Examination of the patient for the presence of personal belongings such as jewelry, wigs, dentures, and hearing aids. The nurse is responsible for the safe and proper disposition of the item(s).
8. Documentation of medications, fluids, or blood administered in the immediate preoperative period.

Transferring and Positioning Patient for Surgery
Transfer to operating room bed

When all sterile supplies have been opened onto the sterile field and the sponge, sharp, and instrument counts have been completed, the operating room is ready. The circulating nurse is responsible for planning for the patient's safety throughout the surgical procedure. Implementation of the plan includes the following safety precautions when transferring the patient to the OR bed:

1. Both the OR bed and gurney are securely locked during patient transfer to the OR bed.
2. All tubings such as intravenous lines, chest tubes, and in-dwelling catheters are appropriately secured and protected.
3. The anesthesiologist supports the patient's head during movement.
4. The surgeon is responsible for movement and protection of unsplinted fractures.
5. Geriatric, handicapped, and heavily medicated patients are moved slowly and smoothly to permit the circulatory system to adjust and to prevent shearing forces to the skin.

Once the patient is on the OR bed the circulating nurse places a restraint snugly across the patient's knees and ensures that there is no pressure on any bony prominences or nerves. The circulating nurse pads muscles, nerves, and bony prominences to prevent injury. The patient's legs and ankles must not be crossed as this will cause pressure on the nerves and legs and thereby compromise circulation. Once the patient has been draped, it is the responsibility of the nursing team to make sure all sterile tables are placed in a manner to prevent pressure on the patient's body and to remind sterile team members not to lean on any part of the patient.

Patient positioning

Proper patient positioning is a crucial element in the execution of a safe efficient surgical procedure. All members of the surgical team are responsible for safeguarding the patient from any harmful effects of the surgical position.

Intraoperative patient position is dictated by the surgical procedure and surgeon preference. Proper patient positioning provides optimum anatomic exposure and access to the surgical site; maintains proper body alignment, circulatory, and respiratory functions; allows patient accessibility for anesthesia personnel to monitor the airway, administer anesthetics, medications, and intravenous fluids; protects the patient from nerve and skin injury; and provides patient privacy and comfort.

The circulating nurse needs to be aware of the anatomic and physiologic changes that occur as a result of the surgical procedure, patient position, and anesthetic agents. Changes in the patient's position affect the circulatory, respiratory, nervous, and musculoskeletal systems.

In the preoperative assessment, the circulating nurse assesses the patient's physical limitations, height, weight, nutritional status, skin condition, and the presence of any preexisting medical problems. This information is used to determine any potential problems the patient may experience in coping with the surgical position.

Intraoperative nursing care is planned to meet the goal of preventing postoperative complications relating to the patient's position. This goal is achieved by ensuring the presence of positioning devices in the operating room that are clean and in working order; communicating special patient needs to anesthesia and surgical personnel; and ensuring the presence of personnel to assist in positioning the patient.

The circulating nurse takes an active role in positioning the patient. During the positioning process the nurse helps to maintain the patient's body alignment and ensures that all bony prominences and skin pressure areas are protected and padded. Once the patient has been positioned, the nurse reassesses body alignment and tissue integrity.

Types of positions

Surgical procedures are performed with the patient lying on his or her back, side, or abdomen. The three basic positions, dorsal, lateral, and prone can be modified in a variety of ways for specialized surgical procedures.

Dorsal or supine

The dorsal or supine position is the most neutral position for the body at rest and is used most frequently. In this position the patient is flat on the OR bed with arms at the side or on armboards with the palms down (Fig. 21-8, A). The head is positioned so that the cervical, thoracic, and lumbar spine are in a straight line. Small pillows may be placed under the head and lumbar curvature to maintain alignment and prevent muscle strain. The legs are in line with the spine. The feet are slightly separated, uncrossed, and supported by a padded foot extension to prevent foot drop. Heels are protected from pressure with a pillow, ankle roll, or foam heel protectors.

Trendelenburg

The Trendelenburg position is one modification of the supine position. In this position the table is tilted downward at a 45-degree angle at the head. The knees are flexed at the break of the bed to prevent pressure on the peroneal nerves or phlebitis (Fig. 21-8, B). Padded shoulder braces may be used to prevent the patient from slipping and to maintain the proper body position.

The Trendelenburg position is used for surgical procedures in the pelvis or lower abdomen. In this position the abdominal viscera are tilted away from the pelvic area to obtain a better surgical exposure. Although this position improves surgical exposure, the pressure of the organs against the diaphragm decrease lung volume. Blood pools in the upper torso resulting in an elevated blood pressure. When the patient is returned to a supine position hypotension may occur; therefore, movement from this position must be gradual to allow the heart time to accommodate to changes in the blood volume.

Reverse Trendelenburg

The reverse Trendelenburg position is used for procedures performed on the head, neck, and upper abdomen. In the reverse Trendelenburg position the OR bed is tilted so that the patient's head is higher than the feet (Fig. 21-8, C). A padded footboard and pillows under the knees and lumbar curve help support the patient in this position.

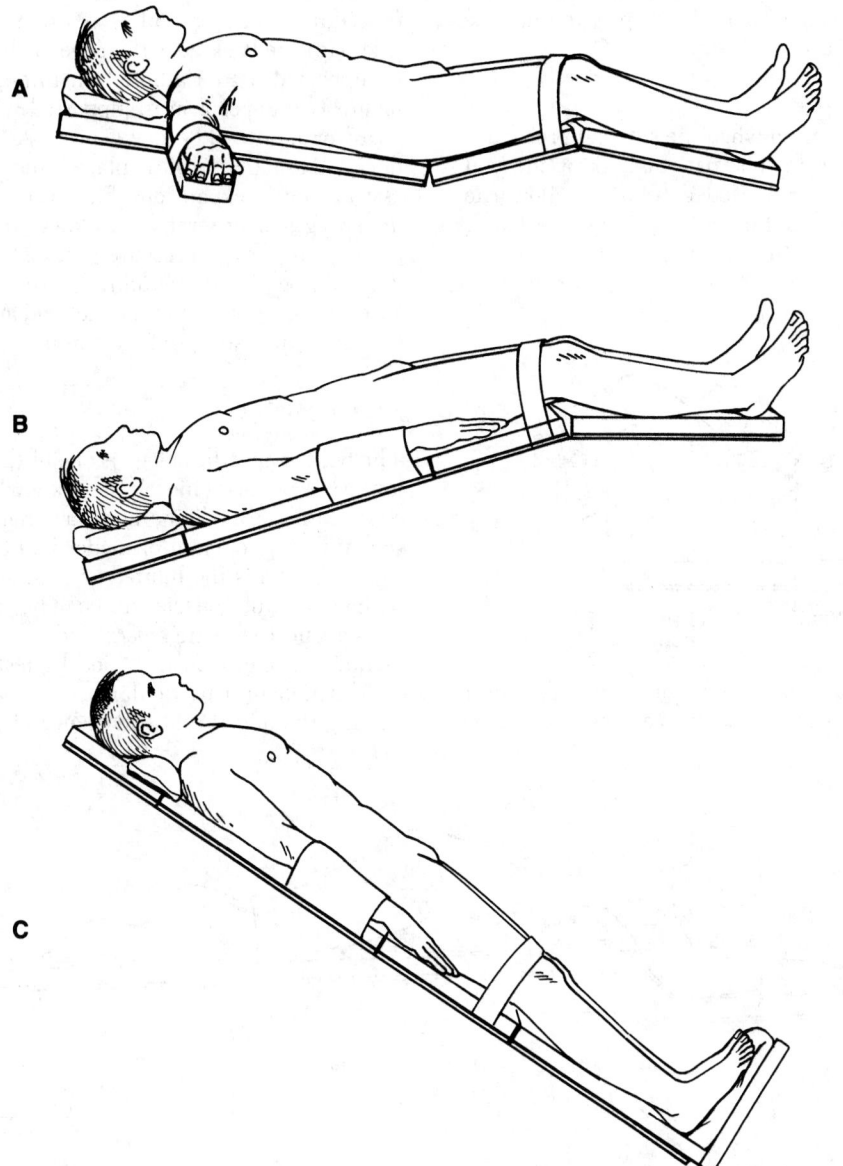

Fig. 21-8   **A,** Dorsal or supine position. **B,** Trendelenburg position. **C,** Reverse Trendelenburg position.

Lithotomy

The lithotomy position is the most extreme variation of the supine position. It is used for vaginal and some rectal procedures. With the patient in a supine position the legs are raised and abducted and placed in stirrups to expose the perineal area (Fig. 21-9). Appropriate placement, adjustment, and padding of the stirrups prevent damage to superficial nerves and veins on the lateral and medial aspects of the legs and thighs. In this position the sacrum supports most of the body weight. Extra padding may be required to avoid pressure on this area.

Prone

The prone position is used when the surgical procedure requires a dorsal approach. The patient is positioned on the abdomen with rolls or a padded frame to allow the diaphragm to move freely and permit the lungs to expand. The arms are positioned either at the patient's side or on

padded armboards with the arms extended outward and upward, and with the elbows flexed and palms down (Fig. 21-10). The feet are raised off the bed and supported with a bolster or pillow to prevent pressure on the toes and plantar flexion. Other padding may be necessary to protect the shoulders, elbows, anterior iliac spine, and knees.

Lateral

The lateral position is used for hip, kidney, or chest procedures. The patient is positioned on the unaffected side with the back near the edge of the OR bed. The head is supported with a pillow to maintain proper body alignment. The upper arm is supported with an elevated armboard or pillow. The down arm is slightly or completely flexed. An axillary roll is placed under the lower axilla to assist in chest expansion. The lower leg is flexed and the upper leg is kept straight. Pillows are positioned between the legs to prevent pressure (Fig. 21-11). Additional padding may be placed around the lower knee to prevent pressure on the peroneal nerve. Feet and ankles are also padded to prevent pressure and foot drop.

ANESTHESIA

The field of anesthesiology is one of the most rapidly growing areas of medicine. It is acknowledged as the major contributor to medicine and has enabled the growth and scientific development of modern surgery.[9]

Anesthesia is the limited or total loss of feeling with or without loss of consciousness. The two broad classifications of anesthesia are *general* and *local*. General anesthesia produces unconsciousness; local anesthesia creates a loss of sensation in a particular area. The method of administering the anesthesia and choice of anesthetic agent for

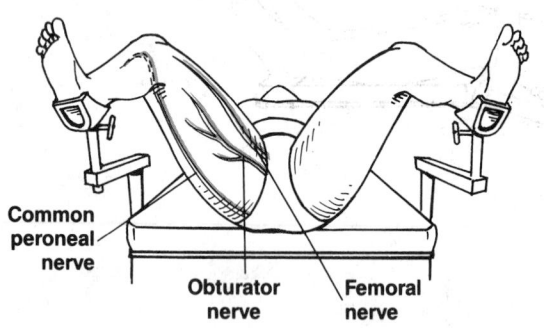

Fig. 21-9 Lithotomy position. The location of the nerves must be known to prevent pressure on the groin and popliteal area.

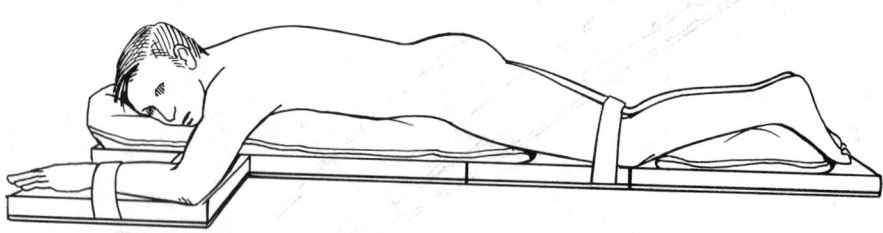

Fig. 21-10 Prone position.

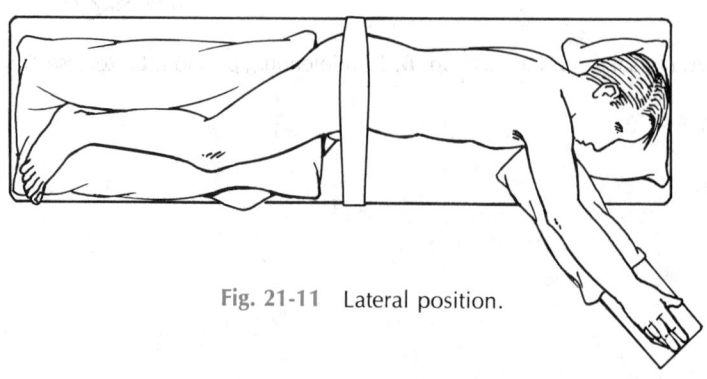

Fig. 21-11 Lateral position.

a particular patient is made by the anesthesiologist. Factors that influence the decision include:

1. Patient preference
2. Age of patient
3. Patient's physical and emotional status
4. Presence of coexisting disease
5. Type and length of surgical procedure
6. Position of patient during the surgical procedure
7. Surgeon's preference

Operating room nurses do not administer anesthetic agents but they must have an understanding of the various anesthetics used in surgery, the methods of administration, and the potential side effects and complications (Table 21-6). This knowledge enables the nurse to plan intraoperative nursing care and to assist the anesthesia team.

Table 21-6   Commonly used anesthetic agents

Agents	Common usage	Advantages	Disadvantages
Inhalational agents			
Nitrous oxide (N₂O)	Maintenance; sometimes for induction	Rapid induction and emergence; additive effects to other anesthetics	Poor muscle relaxation; can depress myocardium
Halothane (Fluothane)	Maintenance; sometimes for induction	Rapid induction and emergence; pleasant, nonirritating odor	Sensitizes myocardium to epinephrine; decreases heart rate and arterial blood pressure; poor muscle relaxation
Enflurane (Ethrane)	Maintenance; sometimes for induction	Good relaxation; permits larger amounts of epinephrine to be used than with halothane	Can cause increased heart rate and decreased blood pressure; slightly irritating odor
Isoflurane (Forane)	Maintenance; sometimes for induction	Good relaxation; smooth rapid induction and emergence	Increases heart rate; slightly irritating odor
Intravenous anesthetics			
Thiopental sodium (Pentothal)	Induction	Fast, smooth induction and emergence	Large doses may cause respiratory and cardiovascular depression
Ketamine (Ketalar)	Induction, occasional maintenance (IV or IM)	Short acting; patient maintains airway	Large doses may cause emergency delirium and respiratory depression
Diazepam (Valium)	Amnesia; hypnotic; preoperative medication; used for IV conscious sedation	Good sedation	Prolonged duration
Midazolam (Versed)	Hypnotic; used for IV conscious sedation	Excellent amnesia; water soluble (no pain with IV injection); short acting	Slower induction than thiopental
Depolarizing muscle relaxants			
Succinylcholine (Anectine)	Intubation; short cases	Rpaid onset; short duration	May cause muscle fasciculations, postoperative arrhythmias
Nondepolarizing muscle relaxants (longer onset and duration)			
d-Tubocurare (Curare, tubocurine)	Maintenance		May cause histamine release
Pancuronium (Pavulon)	Maintenance		May cause increased heart rate and elevated blood pressure
Local anesthetics			
Bupivacaine (Marcaine, Sensorcaine)	Epidural, spinal, or local infiltration	Good relaxation; long acting	Overdose can cause cardiac arrest
Chloroprocaine (Nesacaine)	Epidural anesthesia	Extremely short acting; good relaxation	Can lead to neurotoxicity if injected directly into CSF
Lidocaine (Xylocaine)	Epidural, spinal, peripheral, IV blocks, and local infiltration	Short acting; good relaxation; low toxicity	Overdose can lead to convulsions
Tetracaine (Pontacaine)	Spinal anesthesia	Long acting; good relaxation	

Patient Preparation

Patients experience numerous fears and stresses when they undergo surgical intervention. Preoperative medication is ordered to sedate the patient and decrease anxiety. The medication is usually given 60 to 90 minutes before the surgical procedure; however, there are times when it is administered intravenously in the surgical suite. Ambulatory surgery patients usually do not receive preoperative medications because the effects of the drugs can remain after the patient has been discharged.

Fear of anesthesia cause high levels of anxiety for patients. Some of the common concerns are:

1. Fear of death
2. Fear of the unknown
3. Loss of control
4. Fear of pain
5. Fear of waking up before conclusion of the surgical procedure
6. Fear of having the mask over the face during induction.

In the preoperative interview the circulating nurse assesses the patient's level of apprehension and plans interventions to decrease the patient's anxiety. Some nursing interventions include answering questions the patient has about the anesthesia; assuring the patient that there is continuous monitoring of the levels of anesthesia throughout the surgical procedure; explaining that patients generally do not speak during induction and if they do, the speech in unintelligible; and relaying the patient's fears and concerns to the anesthesia team and the surgeon. During the administration of anesthesia the circulating nurse is at the patient's side to provide emotional support and assist anesthesia personnel as necessary. Holding the patient's hand during induction can be one of the most effective nursing actions to provide comfort to the patient.

General Anesthesia

General anesthesia is the depression of the central nervous system with the administration of drugs or inhalation agents. The exact methods with which general anesthetic agents produce unconsciousness, analgesia, and muscle relaxation are unknown. It is believed that each anesthetic affects the central nervous system and musculoskeletal system in unique ways and works with various areas and systems to create these effects.[19]

In order for anesthesia to be safe, the anesthesiologist must monitor its depth or level. Guidelines to estimate the depth of anesthesia used to be based on clearly delineated physiologic changes that were seen with the administration of ether (Box 21-1). Because of the variety of anesthetic agents and anesthetic techniques used there are no consistent physiologic responses for estimating the exact depth of anesthesia. Determination of the depth of anesthesia is achieved by monitoring physiologic changes in the patient's heart rate, blood pressure, temperature, respiratory rate, oxygen saturation, and airway CO_2 tension.

Phases of general anesthesia

There are three phases of general anesthesia: the induction phase, the maintenance phase, and the emergence phase. *Induction* begins with the administration of intravenous

---

> **21-1**
>
> ### Stages of anesthesia
>
> **Stage I** begins with the administration of anesthetic agents and ends with the loss of consciousness. This is also known as the *relaxation stage.*
>
> **Stage II** begins with the loss of consciousness and ends with the onset of regular breathing and loss of eyelid reflexes. This stage is referred to as the *excitement* or *delirium phase* because it is often accompanied by involuntary motor activity. It is important that the patient receives no auditory or physical stimulation during this period.
>
> **Stage III** begins with the onset of regular breathing and ends with the cessation of respirations. This stage is known as the *operative* or *surgical phase.*
>
> **Stage IV** begins with cessation of respiration and leads to death.

---

agents or with the inhalation of a combination of anesthetic gases and oxygen. Endotracheal intubation is performed during this phase. The period is completed when the patient is ready for positioning, skin preparation, or the incision.

Once it is safe for any one of these activities to commence, the patient has entered the *maintenance phase* of anesthesia. During this phase the anesthesiologist maintains the appropriate levels of anesthesia with inhalation agents and/or intravenous medications. The anesthesiologist pays close attention to the surgical field and anticipates the surgeon's actions in order to alter the depth of anesthesia whenever necessary.

The *emergence period* begins when the anesthesiologist decreases the anesthetic agents and the patient begins to awaken. This period is completed when the patient is ready to leave the operating room. Extubation occurs during this period.

Inhalation anesthesia

Inhalation anesthesia is produced by administering anesthetic gases, which are mixed with oxygen, directly to the lungs. The gases are passed into pulmonary circulation and are delivered to the brain and other body tissues. These agent are administered to the patient by a face mask or directly into the lungs through an endotracheal tube. The inhalation agents are readily eliminated through the respiratory system.

Nitrous oxide, which is the most commonly used inhalation agent, is not potent by itself. It is used to supplement other drugs such as analgesics and sedatives and it is combined with stronger anesthetics to provide a more satisfactory intraoperative and postoperative course. The combined use of nitrous oxide with more potent agents helps decrease excessive depths of anesthesia, and decreases circulatory and respiratory depression; the initial recovery is rapid.

Halothane (Fluothane) is a potent, nonflammable, volatile liquid. It decomposes when exposed to light and can harm rubber, plastic, and some metals. Halothane provides a rapid, smooth induction and emergence with minimum excitement. It produces poor muscle relaxation and therefore requires the use of additional muscle relaxants. Halothane decreases arterial blood pressure and heart rate; it can also sensitize the myocardium to epinephrine. It is useful in the management of patients with airway difficulties because it is a potent bronchodilator and it also suppresses airway reflexes.

Enflurane (Ethrane) is a stable, nonflammable, volatile liquid. It produces a rapid induction, satisfactory maintenance, and a rapid recovery. Ventilatory and cardiovascular depression and muscle relaxation are dosage related.

Isoflurane (Forane) is a stable, nonexplosive, nonflammable, clear liquid. It has clinical properties similar to halothane and enflurane. Isoflurane provides a rapid induction and emergence. It is a good muscle relaxant and does not significantly alter cardiovascular output.

Intravenous anesthesia

Intravenous drugs are also given to cause a safe reversible state of anesthesia. These drugs can be used alone as anesthetics or as supplements to inhalation agents. Unlike the inhalation agents that are reversed by turning the agent off and ventilating the lungs with 100% oxygen, intravenous drugs must be metabolized in the liver and excreted by the kidneys. These agents are not quickly reversed.

Patients usually prefer an intravenous induction because it is rapid and generally pleasant. Because of patient satisfaction, it has become a routine practice to induce general anesthesia with intravenous agents regardless of the agent used for maintenance.

Barbiturates are the most commonly used intravenous induction agents. Thiopental (Pentothal) and methoxitral (Brevital) are the most commonly used barbiturates.

Barbiturates have a rapid onset of action and are short acting. Unconsciousness occurs approximately 10 to 20 seconds after an initial intravenous dose. The depth of anesthesia can increase for 40 seconds, but then it rapidly decreases.[33] By themselves, barbiturates are not usually sufficient for most surgical procedures although they can be used with nitrous oxide for short procedures that do not require muscle relaxation. Depending on the dosage and rate of administration, barbiturates can cause cardiovascular and respiratory depression. Because of these factors, resuscitative equipment must always be available.

Phenocyclidine

Ketamine, a phenocyclidine drug, is widely used to produce a state of dissociative anesthesia. Dissociative anesthesia produces unconsciousness, analgesia, and amnesia. Patients who receive Ketamine appear to be awake because the eyes remain open and move, but patients lack awareness and are anesthetized to pain. In the immediate postoperative period patients have been known to experience unpleasant dreams and hallucinations, a condition that is known as *emergence delirium*. Valium or droperidol can be given to minimize these effects as well as having the patient recover in an area where there is minimum sensory stimulation.

Ketamine can be used as the sole agent for minor surgical procedures that do not require muscle relaxation, or it can be used as an induction agent. Ketamine increases the heart rate and blood pressure and therefore is contraindicated in patients with coronary artery disease or angina.

Benzodiazepines

Many benzodiazepines are available for use. Diazepam (Valium), lorazepam (Ativan), and midazolam (Versed) are most commonly used as adjuncts for intravenous anesthesia induction. These drugs all produce sedation, amnesia, muscle relaxation, and anxiety relief. These effects, along with cardiovascular and respiratory depression, are patient specific and dosage dependent.

Neuromuscular blocking agents

Neuromuscular blocking agents are used as adjuncts to anesthetic agents. They are used to facilitate the passage of endotracheal tubes, prevent laryngospasms, control muscle tone throughout the surgical procedure, and decrease the amount of general anesthesia used. Muscle relaxation can be controlled with neuromuscular blocking agents. These agents interfere with the transfer of impulses from the motor nerves to the voluntary muscle cells. There are two categories of neuromuscular blocking agents, the depolarizing and nondepolarizing agents. Depolarizing agents react with receptors at the end plate region of the muscle and begin depolarization of the muscle membrane, which causes muscle contraction.[9] The muscle contraction is uncoordinated and is known as muscle fasciculation. Postoperatively patients may complain of muscle stiffness and soreness, which is caused by muscle fasciculation. Succinylcholine is a depolarizing agent. This drug causes muscle relaxation within 1 minute of intravenous administration. Because of its rapid action it is most frequently used for endotracheal intubation.

Flaxedil (gallamine), Pavulon (pancuronium bromide), Curare (d-tubocurarine), and Norcuron (vecuronium) are all nondepolarizing agents. Nondepolarizing agents cause paralysis of the voluntary muscles, are slower acting, and have a longer duration than depolarizing agents.

The major action of neuromuscular blocking agents is the relaxation of voluntary muscles. Nondepolarizing agents can interact with other drugs such as antibiotics and lead to a prolonged muscle relaxation. This occurs more frequently with intravenous administration of antibiotics or when the peritoneal cavity is irrigated with antibiotic solutions.

Balanced anesthesia

Balanced anesthesia is one of the most frequently used methods of administering anesthesia. This term is used to describe the practice of combining various agents to produce hypnosis, analgesia, and muscle relaxation, with a minimum of physiologic disturbances. Each agent is administered for a specific purpose. Intravenous barbiturates are used for induction, regional anesthetics are used for muscle relaxation and analgesia, and inhalation agents are used for maintenance. Variations of this technique are used depending on the patient's status and the requirements of the surgical procedure.

Malignant Hyperthermia

Malignant hyperthermia is the most serious and potentially fatal complication of anesthesia. Even though this disease occurs most frequently during induction or during the surgical procedure, it can occur in the PACU or on the nursing unit.

Malignant hyperthermia is a genetically transmitted disease of the musculoskeletal system that is caused by a disorder of muscle metabolism. It is triggered by certain anesthetic agents (Box 21-2), and extreme physiologic and emotional stress. There is believed to be a defect in the muscle cell membrane, which permits anesthetic agents to trigger a sudden increase of calcium ions within the muscle cells. The rapid increase of calcium starts a series of biochemical reactions that elevate the metabolic rate, causing heat and muscle rigidity.

The earliest most consistent clinical sign of malignant hyperthermia is unexplained *tachycardia*. Other clinical symptoms include:

1. Tachypnea
2. Cyanosis
3. Dysrhythmias
4. Skin mottling
5. Rigidity
6. Metabolic and respiratory acidosis
7. Unstable blood pressure
8. Increased body temperature along with profuse sweating (Body temperature can rise 1° to 2° C within 5 minutes and can reach as high as 46° C (114.8°F).[18]

21-2

Anesthetic agents triggering malignant hyperthermia

Halothane	Enflurane
Isoflurane	Succinylcholine
d-Tubocurarine	Gallamine

Treatment of the patient in a malignant hyperthermia episode includes stopping immediately the inhalation agent and/or muscle relaxants; administrating 100% oxygen; cooling with ice packs or cooling blankets; lavaging body cavities with iced saline; restoration of acid-base balance; and rapid intravenous infusion of dantrolene. Dantrolene provides skeletal muscle relaxation and retards the biochemical actions that cause muscle contractions. The dosage is 1 mg/kg of body weight (10 mg/kg is the recommended maximum dose).

Malignant hyperthermia presents a rare crisis situation in the operating room. It is a life-threatening event and it is necessary for all members of the surgical team to be familiar with the disease and know the protocols for treatment. The coordinated efforts of all members of the surgical team are necessary to provide life-saving patient care.

Regional Anesthesia

Regional anesthesia causes a temporary loss of sensation in a particular portion of the body from the action of local anesthetics. Local anesthetics (Table 21-6) temporarily prevent generation and conduction of nerve impulses, and

Table 21-7 Advantages and disadvantages of regional anesthesia

Advantages	Disadvantages
Simplicity Reasonable costs Easily induced Minimum equipment required Decreased postoperative care requirements	Lack of patient acceptance Patient's fear of being awake during the surgical procedure
Avoidance of adverse effects of general anesthesia Decreased nausea and vomiting	Impracticality of anesthetizing certain areas of the body
Can be used for a variety of patients in circumstances where general anesthesia is contraindicated Patient who recently ingested food or liquids	Insufficient duration of anesthesia Patients fear anesthetic will wear off prematurely
	Rapid absorption of agent into bloodstream Can lead to cardiac arrest

may or may not affect motor functions. Local anesthetics do not cause unconsiousness.

Regional anesthetics are used on patients in whom general anesthesia is contraindicated. The advantages and disadvantages of its use are outlined in Table 21-7. The types of regional anesthesia include spinal, epidural, nerve blocks, and intravenous regional anesthesia.

Spinal anesthesia

Spinal anesthesia is usually administered for surgical procedures performed on the lower abdomen, inguinal region, perineum, or lower extremities.

With the patient lying on one side curled into a fetal position or in a sitting position, a local anesthetic agent is injected into the cerebrospinal fluid in the subarachnoid spaces (Fig. 21-12). After the local anesthetic is injected there is an almost immediate onset of anesthesia at the site. Withdrawal of neural functions generally occurs in the following sequence with the disappearance of:

1. Autonomic activity
2. Superficial pain
3. Temperature sensitivity
4. Vibratory and position sense
5. Motor power
6. Touch

Nerve function returns in the reverse order of onset.[9]

The duration and level of spinal anesthesia is determined by the site and speed of injection, body height or length of the vertebral column, the specific gravity of the anesthetic agent, intraabdominal pressure, and the position of the patient immediately following injection. Patient position is extremely important when using hyperbaric agents (agents with a specific gravity heavier than that of spinal fluid), because gravity moves the anesthetic agents to the lowest point of the vertebral column.

One of the most common postoperative complaints of patients who have spinal anesthesia is that of headache.

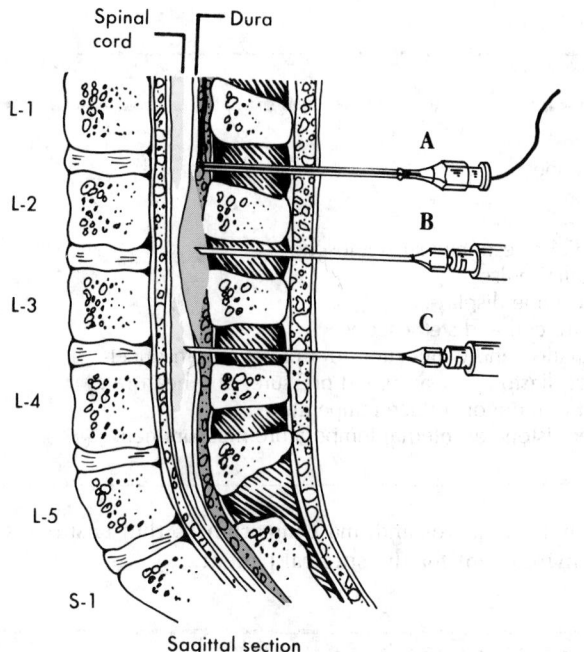

Spinal
cord ┐ ┌ Dura

L-1

L-2

L-3

L-4

L-5

S-1

Sagittal section

Fig. 21-12   Location of needles and injected anesthetic relative to the dura. **A,** Epidural catheter. **B,** Single injection epidural. **C,** Spinal anesthesia. (From Meeker MH, Rothrock JC: Alexander's care of the patient in surgery, ed 9, St Louis, 1991, Mosby–Year Book.)

The headache occurs because cerebral spinal fluid leaks out of the dura from the opening made by the spinal needle. This causes a decreased pressure in the spinal cord, which causes the headache when the patient assumes an upright position. Some treatment modalities include strict bedrest for 24 to 48 hours, hydration, and application of an abdominal binder to increase pressure.

Epidural anesthesia

Epidural anesthesia is achieved when a local anesthetic agent is injected into the space surrounding the dura matter in the spinal column (Fig. 21-12). This type of anesthesia is used in abdominal procedures and orthopedic procedures. A distinct advantage of epidural over spinal anesthesia is the absence of postoperative headaches.

Nerve block

A nerve block is achieved with the injection of a local anesthetic into or around a nerve or group of nerves that enervates the operative site. Nerve blocks are frequently used for surgical procedures performed on the upper extremities.

Intravenous regional anesthesia

Intravenous regional anesthesia is achieved by administering local anesthetic agents into the venous system of an exsanguinated extremity. A tourniquet is used to prevent the agent from entering the systemic circulation. Advantages of this technique are that the onset of anesthesia is quick and recovery time is short. The major disadvantage of this technique is that the tourniquet can only be inflated for 2 hours before causing tissue damage.

Intravenous Conscious Sedation

The practice of using intravenous conscious sedation along with the use of local anesthesia is becoming increasingly popular for outpatient use and for short surgical or diagnostic procedures that require sedation and amnesia. Intravenous conscious sedation is a state in which the patient maintains the ability to independently and continuously maintain an airway and appropriately respond to physical stimulation and verbal commands.

The primary objective of intravenous conscious sedation is to allay the patient's fear and anxiety. Other objectives include:

1. Maintenance of consciousness and protective reflexes
2. Patient cooperation
3. Elevation of pain threshold
4. Some degree of amnesia.[31]

Benzodiazepines are the most commonly used agents for intravenous conscious sedation. They are used because of their effects on the central nervous system and because they have the ability to be administered in combination with narcotic agents.

Midazolan (Versed) and diazepam (Valium) are the two most frequently used medications to produce conscious sedation. Table 21-8 shows a comparison of their actions.

Narcotics such as fentanyl, meperidine, and morphine are also used for analgesia and sedation. These agents are frequently used in combination with benzodiazepines. When narcotics and benzodiazepines are used together, the doses of each agent can be decreased by 30% to 50%.

Monitoring the Patient

During any surgical procedure the patient is subjected to many stresses. Potent anesthetic agents, tissue trauma, blood loss, and positioning are all stresses that can interfere and alter the patient's respiratory and cardiovascular sta-

Table 21-8   Comparison of midazolan and diazepam

	Midazolan	**Diazepam**
Onset of action	3-4 minutes	Somewhat longer
Duration of action	Short; elimination half-life from 1-4 hours	Longer; elimination half-life from 1-2 days
Water solubility	Soluble; causes less pain on injection and less venous irritation	Poor; causes pain on injection
Recovery time	Usually less than 2 hours	Usually longer than 2 hours
Amnesia effect	Anterograde	Retrograde

Table 21-9   Monitoring during anesthesia

Parameter	Method
Respiratory status	Direct observation of chest movements
	Auscultation of the chest with a stethoscope
Arterial oxygenation	Pulse oximetry
Circulatory status	Palpation of superficial artery
	Auscultation of the heart with a precordial or esophageal stethoscope
	Doppler monitoring probe applied to radial pulse
	Electrocardiogram with continual oscilloscope display
Arterial blood pressure	Auscultation method using blood pressure cuff and stethoscope
	Direct measurement with arterial cannulation and connection to a pressure transducer
	Automatic device that measures systolic, diastolic, mean blood pressure, and heart rate
Body temperature	Temperature sensor applied to forehead to monitor surface temperature
	Esophageal thermometer containing thermistors for internal temperature measurement
Urinary output	Indwelling urinary catheter

tus. Continuous monitoring and assessment is necessary to detect changes in the patient's physiologic status and initiate any necessary treatment in a timely manner.

Basic intraoperative monitoring standards have been developed by the American Society of Anesthesiologists to be followed by anesthesia personnel. The Association of Operating Room Nurses has also developed recommended practices to provide guidelines for nurses who monitor patients receiving local anesthetics. Both organizations have determined that the basic standards include performing ECGs, monitoring blood pressure, heart rate, and temperature, and continuous monitoring of ventilation and circulation. There are various methods for monitoring the patient and there are also automatic devices that assist in the monitoring process (Table 21-9). It is imperative that the anesthesiologist and nurse be familiar with the functions and uses of the specialized equipment and ensure that it is in proper working order. Even with the availability of automatic monitoring equipment it is necessary for the anesthesiologist, or in the case of local anesthesia, the nurse, to remain in close contact with the patient to observe any significant physiologic changes immediately.

Electrical Hazards

The operating room has a multitude of electrical equipment, all of which poses a potential threat to patient safety. Faulty electrical equipment can cause current leakage, which can result in fire or explosion. A current leakage can also include the patient in completing an electrical circuit; enough current may flow through the patient to cause burns, muscular contractions, or ventricular fibrillation.

In order to ensure patient safety, it is imperative that all members of the surgical team are aware of the electrical dangers in the operating room. Everyone should know the purpose of the electrical equipment that is used and the necessary precautions for preventing accidents. Federal agencies regulate the type of electrical equipment used in operating rooms and the Joint Commission for Accreditation of Healthcare Organizations (JCAHO) has specific standards addressing issues of electrical safety. Institutions have policies and procedures outlining the process for routine electrical maintenance checks on equipment. These routines keep the institution in compliance with federal safety standards and, most importantly, they ensure a safe environment for the surgical patient.

COMPLETION OF SURGERY

Near the end of the intraoperative period the circulating nurse must coordinate several activities to prepare the patient for admission to the appropriate area for recovery. These activities include assisting with the application of dressings, assisting anesthesia personnel during extubation, reporting to the nurses in the PACU, and documenting intraoperative care.

Dressings and Drains

Following the surgical procedure a dressing is usually applied to the incision site. Dressings are applied to absorb drainage, protect the wound from gross contamination, support the incisional area, and aid in hemostasis.

The primary dressing is applied directly over the wound by a scrubbed team member. Cotton or synthetic gauze is used for dressing material because it absorbs drainage and prevents adherence to the wound. The secondary dressings, which are used to absorb excess drainage, are applied over the primary dressing. The secondary dressing may or may not be applied by a sterile team member.

Dressings are usually secured with tape. The type depends on the size of the incision, the patient's sensitivity to the tape, and the amount of elasticity required. Montgomery straps can be used instead of tape when numerous dressing changes are expected. Soft padding, splints, and casts are used as a secondary dressing when it is necessary to immobilize an area.

Sometimes there are no dressings applied to the surgical site so as to expose the wound to air to promote healing. This also permits easy observation of the wound, prevents tape reactions, and increases patient comfort.

Drains are inserted at the time of surgery through a separate incision. There are many types available; the selection depends on the surgeon's preference and the intended use. Drains are used to provide a means for body fluids such as serum and blood to be removed from the surgical site. They may also be used to prevent deep-wound infections.

The type of drain used and its location must be documented in the intraoperative nursing notes. This information is important for nurses who care for the patient in the PACU and on the nursing units.

Documentation

Intraoperative care must be recorded to inform other health care team members of the care the patient received during the intraoperative period and the outcome of the care. Documentation provides a method to improve communication to personnel caring for the patient in the postoperative period; it also provides a method for ensuring continuity of care.

In the *Recommended Practices for Documentation of Perioperative Nursing Care,*[1] AORN recommends that the intraoperative patient care record should include but not be limited to documenting:

1. Evidence of patient assessment upon arrival in the operating room. The assessment should include the patient's level of consciousness, emotional status, and skin condition.
2. The presence and disposition of prosthetic devices the patient brought to the surgical suite.
3. The intraoperative patient position, including positioning devices and the types of supports used.
4. The placement of monitoring electrodes, temperature probes, and dispersive electrodes.
5. Placement of the tourniquet cuff, the inflation and deflation times, and the pressure settings.
6. Any medications administered by the registered nurse.
7. The presence of drains, packings, dressings, and catheters.
8. The size and types of prosthetic devices implanted.
9. The results of the sponge, sharp, and instrument counts.
10. The time of discharge and the disposition of the patient's condition and method of transfer should also be included.

Evaluation

Evaluation of the care the patient received during the perioperative period is the final phase of the nursing process. The Patient Outcome Standards for Perioperative Nursing provide a guide for the nurse to evaluate the individual patient's observable physiologic and psychologic responses to the surgical intervention. To evaluate if desired observable patient outcomes have been achieved, questions to consider include the following:

1. Is patient able to verbalize an understanding of the events during the perioperative period?
2. Is patient able to cope with preoperative anxiety?
3. Has the patient received emotional support from all health care team members until the anesthetic has taken effect?
4. Have complications resulting from intraoperative positioning, foreign objects left in the wound, or improperly functioning equipment been avoided?
5. Has skin integrity not been altered during the intraoperative period?
6. Is patient free from infection?

TRANSFER OF PATIENT TO POSTANESTHESIA CARE UNIT

Following the application of the wound dressings, the circulating nurse prepares the patient for transfer to the PACU. The patient's skin is cleaned, monitoring devices are removed, and a new gown and blanket are applied. The circulating nurse also ensures that all intravenous tubes and drains are unobstructed before transferring the patient to the recovery room bed.

The coordinated efforts of at least four people are required to move the patient from the operating room bed to the recovery room bed. One individual remains at the patient's head, one person is at the feet, and one person is on each side of the patient. During the transfer, the anesthesiologist maintains the airway and protects the patient's head. The individuals on either side grasp the lift sheet while the individual at the foot of the bed holds the patient's feet. The anesthesiologist gives the command to move the patient onto the recovery bed. The transfer is slow and smooth to prevent circulatory depression. The patient is positioned on the recovery room bed in a comfortable position that is conducive to respiration and circulation. Once the patient is positioned, the circulating nurse ensures that all intravenous lines and drainage systems are appropriately connected. In some institutions the circulating nurse and the anesthesiologist accompany the patient to the PACU. This provides continuity of care and permits the circulating nurse to inform the PACU nurse of the events that transpired during the preoperative and intraoperative periods.

SUMMARY

1. Perioperative nursing activities in the preoperative, intraoperative, and postoperative phases are performed by the registered nurse.
2. Members of the sterile scrub team include the primary surgeon, surgeon's assistants, and the scrub nurse.
3. Members of the nonsterile surgical team include the circulating nurse, the anesthesiologist and/or the anesthetist, and other personnel such as radiologists, perfusionists, and laboratory technicians.
4. The circulating nurse is a registered nurse who serves as the patient's advocate and coordinates activities in the operating room.
5. Strict adherence to principles of aseptic technique is essential to prevent patient infection.
6. Adherence to infection control practices and universal precautions minimizes the chance of cross-contamination of pathogens between patients and OR personnel.
7. Patient safety is a primary concern for all surgical team members. Policies and procedures address issues of patient identification and admission to the operating room; pre- and postoperative patient transfer; and electrical safety.
8. Intraoperative patient position is dictated by the surgical procedure and surgeon preference. There are three basic positions, which can be modified for spe-

cific surgical procedures. Extreme care must be taken to prevent injury from intraoperative positioning.

9. *General* and *local* are the two broad classifications of anesthesia. General anesthesia produces unconsciousness and local anesthesia creates a loss of sensation in a specific region.

10. There are three phases of general anesthesia: the induction, maintenance, and emergence phases. The depth of anesthesia is determined by the patient's physiologic response to the various agents.

11. Malignant hyperthermia is a life-threatening, genetically transmitted disease that is triggered by certain anesthetic agents, emotion and physical stresses.

12. Intravenous conscious sedation is used for many diagnostic and outpatient procedures. The primary objective of intravenous conscious sedation is to decrease the patient's fear and anxiety level.

13. Basic intraoperative monitoring parameters include monitoring of blood pressure, heart rate, body temperature, electrocardiogram, and respiratory and circulatory status.

14. Nursing care responsibilities near the end of the intraoperative period include application of dressings, assisting anesthesia personnel during extubation, transferring the patient to the recovery room bed, reporting to the PACU nurses, and documenting intraoperative nursing care.

STUDY QUESTIONS

• What nursing actions are taken to ensure the patient's safety in the preoperative and postoperative periods of surgical intervention?

• What are some actions that are taken in the operating room to minimize the risks of patient infection?

• What are some common concerns patients have when undergoing general anesthesia? What concerns do patients have regarding regional anesthesia? What nursing actions can be implemented to address these patient concerns?

REFERENCES AND SELECTED READINGS

1. Association of Operating Room Nurses: Standards and recommended practices for perioperative nursing, Denver, 1991, The Association.

2. Atkinson LJ, Kohn ML: *Berry and Kohn's introduction to operating room technique,* ed 6, New York, 1986, McGraw-Hill.

3.* Bland DS: Pulse oximetry monitoring arterial hemoglobin oxygen saturation, *AORN J* 45(4):964-967, 1987.

4. Burns S: A multiple evaluation study on artificial nails, *J Nurs Qual Assur* 2:77-79, 1988.

5.* Caldwell LM: Surgical outpatient concerns: what every perioperative nurse should know, *AORN J* 53(3):761-767, 1991.

6. Centers for Disease Control: Recommendations for prevention of HIV transmission in health-care settings, *MMWR* 36:2S, 1987.

7. Centers for Disease Control: Update: universal precautions for prevention of transmission of human immunodeficiency virus, hepatitis B virus, and other bloodborne pathogens in health-care settings, *MMWR* 37(24):377-388, 1988.

8. Copp G, et al: Footwear practices and operating room contamination, *Nurs Res* 36(61):366-369, 1987.

9. Dripps RD, Eckenhoff JE, Vandam LD: *Introduction to anesthesia: principles of safe practice,* ed 7, Philadelphia, 1988, WB Saunders.

10. Eubanks JR: Midazolam: saint or sinner? *AORN J* 50(1):155-156, 1989.

11.* Gerberding JL: Reducing occupational risk of HIV infection, *Hosp Pract* 26(6):103-118, 1991.

12.* Gillette MK, Caruso CC: Intraoperative tissue injury: major causes and preventive measures, *AORN J* 50(1):66-78, 1989.

13. Groah LK: *Operating room nursing: the perioperative role,* Norwalk, Conn, 1990, Appleton & Lange.

14. Hildebrand RD: Muscle relaxants: a review, *J Post Anesth Nurs* 3(3):165-167, 1988.

15. Ivey DF: Local anesthesia: implications for the perioperative nurse, *AORN J* 45(3):682-689, 1987.

16. Kneedler JA, Dodge GH: *Perioperative patient care,* ed 2, Boston, 1987, Blackwell Scientific Publications.

17. Kneedler JA, Purcell SK: Perioperative nursing research. Part III: Potential intraoperative biological hazards to personnel, *AORN J* 49(4):1066-1082, 1989.

18. Larew EB: Malignant hyperthermia: quick recognition and treatment to avoid death, *Postgrad Med* 89(8):117-120, 1989.

19. Meeker MH, Rothrock JC: *Alexander's care of the patient in surgery,* ed 9, St Louis, 1991, Mosby–Year Book.

20.* Miner D: Patient positioning: applying the nursing process, *AORN J* 45(5):1117-1118, 1987.

21. Moylan JA, Fitzpatrick KT, Davenport KE: Reducing wound infections, improved gown and drape barrier performance, *Arch Surg* 122:152-157, 1987.

22. Newberry JE: Malignant hyperthermia in the postanesthesia care unit: a review of current etiology, diagnosis, and treatment, *J Post Anesth Nurs* 5(1):25-28, 1990.

23. Pottinger J, Burns S, Manske J: Bacterial carriage of artificial versus natural nails, *Am J Infect Control* 17:340-344, 1989.

24.* Rathburn AM, Holland L, Geelhoed G: Preoperative skin decontamination: a study on efficiency and effect, *AORN J* 44(1):62-65, 1986.

25.* Richards ML: Perioperative nursing research. Part IV: Postoperative phase, *AORN J* 50(1):120-137, 1989.

26. Rothrock JC: *The RN first assistant: an expanded perioperative nursing role,* Philadelphia, 1987, JB Lippincott.

27. Rothrock JC: Perioperative nursing research. Part I: Preoperative psychoeducational interventions, *AORN J* 49(2):597-616, 1989.

28.* Sinkovitch DD, Mitch-Resignalo AE: Malignant hyperthermia, *Orthop Nurs* 10(1):39-43, 1991.

29. Slone LA, Burkholder A, Campion N: Nursing care documentation: creating a perioperative nursing record, *AORN J* 49(3):808-813, 1989.

30. Watson DS: Pharmacist's corner: safe administration of midazolam, *AORN J* 53(1):162-165, 1991.

31.* Watson DS, James DS: Intravenous conscious sedation: implications of monitoring patient receiving local anesthesia, *AORN J* 51(6):1512-1522, 1991.

32. Watson DS, Kaempf G: *Monitoring the patient receiving local anesthesia,* ed 2, Denver, 1991, Association of Operating Room Nurses.

33. Waugaman WR et al: *Principles and practice of nurse anesthesia,* Norwalk, Conn, 1988, Appleton & Lange.

34. Wlody GS: Malignant hyperthermia: Potential crisis in patient care, *AORN J* 50(2):286-289, 1989.

35.* Wolcott K, McDonnell A: Malignant hyperthermia: nursing implications, *Crit Care Nurse* 10(3):8-85, 1990.

Classic

36. Le Maitre G, Finnegan JA: *The patient in surgery,* ed 4, Philadelphia, 1980, WB Saunders.

*Recommended for student reading.

22

Postoperative Intervention

Barbara C. Long

After studying this chapter, the learner should be able to:

- Identify nursing interventions to meet patient needs in the postanesthetic period.
- Discuss the rationale for collection of data necessary to plan nursing care when the patient returns to the clinical unit.
- Describe the types and process of wound healing and interventions that promote wound healing.
- Explain wound dehiscence and evisceration and appropriate nursing interventions.
- Identify postoperative respiratory and circulatory problems, assessment parameters, and preventive measures.
- Describe possible postoperative problems with fluid and electrolyte balance, nutrition, elimination, and inactivity, and the assessment parameters and preventive measures.
- Describe measures to promote patients' physical and psychologic comfort in the postoperative period.

The postoperative period begins as soon as the operation is completed. If a general anesthetic has been given, the patient is usually taken to a postanesthesia care unit (PACU) for the postanesthetic phase.

POSTANESTHETIC PHASE

The immediate postanesthetic period is critical. The patient must be observed diligently and must receive intensive physical and psychologic support until the major effects of the anesthetic have worn off and the overall condition stabilizes. The nurse is largely responsible for the care of the patient at this time.

The patient is accompanied to the PACU by the anesthesiologist and another member of the operating room professional staff. The recovery room nurse assesses the patient's status, obtains report, and begins recording the recovery room notes.

Much of the ongoing nursing care provided in the immediate postanesthetic period depends on the surgical procedure performed and type of anesthetic given, and is discussed elsewhere in this text (see specific surgical care for each body system). Some outcomes, however, are the same for all patients: pulmonary ventilation, circulation, and fluid and electrolyte balance are maintained, injury is prevented, and comfort is promoted.

Nursing Process
Assessment

The initial patient assessment may be done by the PACU nurse or jointly with a member of the OR team. Data are primarily objective because the patient is often partly asleep. Data are collected pertaining to airway patency, vital signs, pressure readings, level of consciousness, patient position, tissue oxygenation, and dressings, or suture line, fluids lines, and tubes (Box 22-1). Many PACUs use a rating scale (PACU score card) to evaluate postanesthesia recovery. Ongoing data is collected on these same parameters and recorded on flow sheets or nurses notes to show changes in the patient's status.

Data analysis: nursing diagnoses

Nursing diagnoses are determined from analysis of patient data. Possible nursing diagnoses for the postanesthesia patient may include, but are not limited to, the following:

Diagnostic title	Possible causes
Airway clearance, ineffective	Inability to remove secretions, relaxed tongue blocking airway
Gas exchange, impaired	Anesthetic, narcotics, incisional pain
Cardiac output, decreased	Anesthetic, blood loss
Hypothermia	Anesthetic, body exposure in cold operating room
Fluid deficit	Blood loss, fluid loss
Fluid excess	Fluid replacement in excess of body's ability to remove fluids
Injury, high risk for	Anesthetic, immobility
Pain	Incision
Anxiety	Knowledge deficit, fear of results of surgery

22-1

Postanesthesia assessment

Airway	Patency, presence/adequacy of artificial airway
Vital signs	Respiratory rate, depth, character
	Heart rate (pulse, pulse oximeter, or cardiac monitor)
	Blood pressure (cuff or arterial line)
	Temperature
Pressure readings (as indicated)	Pulmonary artery wedge pressure (Chapter 9), central venous pressure (Chapter 9), intracranial (Chapter 37)
Level of consciousness	
Patient position	Position to facilitate breathing, to prevent pressure on body parts or invasive lines, and to promote comfort
Tissue oxygenation	Skin: color, temperature, moisture
	Nail beds: color, capillary refill
	Lips/oral mucosa: color
	Pulse oximetry
	Peripheral pulses: presence, strength (as indicated)
Dressing/suture line	Dressings: dry or minimal drainage
	Suture line (if visible): color, approximation of wound edges
Fluid lines/tubes	Intravenous fluids: rate, amount in bag, infusion site
	Other lines: patency, connection
	Drainage tubes: patency, connection, character and amount of drainage

Planning: expected patient outcomes

Expected patient outcomes for the postanesthesia patient may include, but are not limited to, the following:

1. Breath sounds are clear.
2. Respiratory rate is 12 to 20 breaths per minute and regular.
3. Oxygen saturation levels are within normal levels.
4. Blood pressure returns to patient's usual level.
5. Temperature returns to patient's usual level.
6. Skin is warm and dry, pulse is regular, urinary output usually slightly less than fluid intake.
7. Pulmonary edema does not occur.
8. Sleep is quiet and face is relaxed.

Implementation
Maintaining pulmonary ventilation

In the immediate postanesthetic period, two of the most common causes of inadequate pulmonary exchange are airway obstruction and hypoventilation.

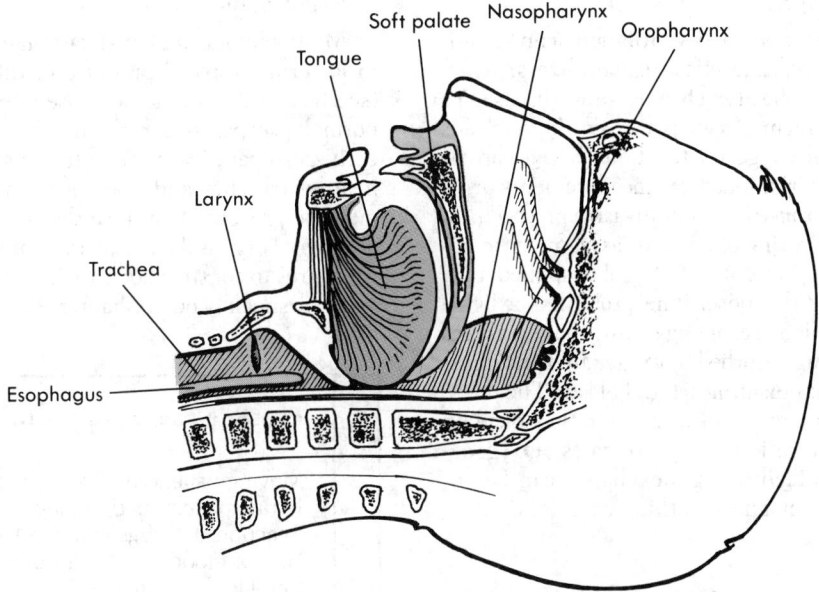

Fig. 22-1   Obstruction of airway by tongue blocking oropharynx in unconscious person lying in supine position.

Airway patency

Airway obstruction most frequently occurs as a result of the tongue, which is relaxed against the pharynx (Fig. 22-1), or of secretions or other fluids collecting in the pharynx, trachea, or bronchial tree. This can be prevented by proper positioning, use of an artificial airway, or removal of secretions.

Positioning. Until protective reflexes have returned, the best position for the majority of patients is a *side-lying* or *semiprone* position with the head tilted back and the jaw supported forward. It is important to remember that aspiration can occur unless the *whole body* is turned. Turning the patient's head while the chest and shoulders remain in the back-lying position is useless.

Artificial airway. Some patients are admitted to the PACU with an *endotracheal tube* in place; however, the endotracheal tube is usually removed in the operating room. (Care of the patient with an endotracheal tube is described in Chapter 24.)

An oropharyngeal or nasopharyngeal airway is often left in place after administration of a general anesthetic to keep the passage open and the tongue forward until pharyngeal reflexes have returned (Fig. 22-2). These artificial airways are made of rubber, plastic, or metal. They are removed as soon as the patient begins to awaken and has regained coughing and swallowing reflexes. After this time their presence can be irritating and can stimulate vomiting or laryngospasm. The pharyngeal reflex can be tested by touching the posterior pharynx with a tongue blade to produce gagging.

Removal of secretions. If the patient cannot cough up and expectorate secretions, they must be removed by suctioning. Pharyngeal suctioning is usually all that is necessary, although intratracheal suctioning may be indicated.

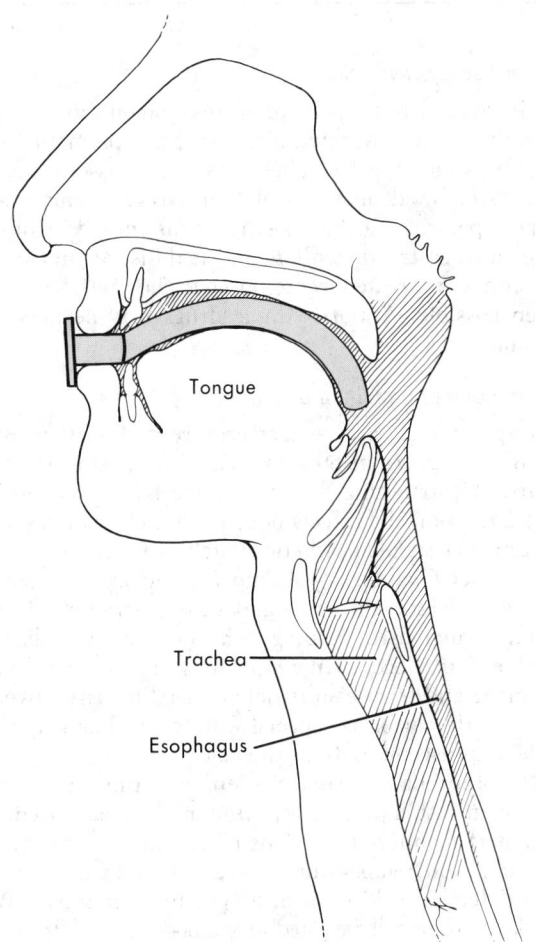

Fig. 22-2   Airway in place to prevent tongue from falling back against pharynx and blocking airway.

Adequate ventilation

Immediate postoperative hypoventilation can result from drugs (anesthetics, narcotics, tranquilizers, sedatives), incisional pain, obesity, chronic lung disease, or pressure on the diaphragm. Inadequate ventilation leads to hypoxemia. Arterial oxygen saturation (SaO_2) can be monitored either by arterial blood gas measurements or by pulse oximetry. *Pulse oximetry* is a noninvasive method providing continuous monitoring of SaO_2 for assessment of gas exchange. The system consists of a probe applied to a finger, toe, earlobe, or the nose. The probe has a light-emitting sensor, and a light-receiving sensor that measures the amount of light being absorbed by oxygenated and deoxygenated hemoglobin in pulsating arterial blood. The probe is connected to a computer with a monitor that displays hemoglobin oxygen saturation and pulse rates. Oxygenation and ventilation to facilitate gas exchange can be enhanced by oxygen therapy and breathing exercises.

Oxygen therapy

Oxygen is usually given postoperatively because after anesthesia almost all patients have decreased pulmonary expansion and areas of atelectasis, both of which result in hypoxemia. Oxygen is administered by nasal cannula, disposable face mask or shield, or endotracheal or tracheostomy tube if one is in place. Patients with thoracic or upper abdominal incisions or with preexisting pulmonary disease may be given oxygen for several hours or even into the next day.

Breathing exercises

Deep-breathing exercises are started as soon as the patient is conscious and able to follow directions. Considerable encouragement and repetition of directions are needed because of amnesia related to the anesthetic. If the patient is unconscious or will not breathe deeply when stimulated, the nurse can hyperventilate the lungs passively by using a breathing bag and mask.

Maintaining circulation

Hypotension and cardiac dysrhythmias are the most common cardiovascular complications in the immediate postanesthetic period. Early recognition and management of these complications before they become serious enough to diminish cardiac output depend on frequent assessment of the patient's vital signs.

Blood pressure, pulse, and respirations are usually taken as follows: (1) every 15 minutes until stable, (2) every half hour for 2 hours, then (3) every 4 hours until ordered otherwise. More frequent monitoring may be indicated. In many hospitals, the monitoring of vital signs every 15 minutes is continued for as long as the patient is in the PACU and for at least 1 hour after leaving the PACU. The pulse rate, volume, and rhythm, and the respiratory rate and character are carefully noted and recorded. Preoperative vital signs are used as a baseline for comparison.

Cardiac output may be monitored by the thermistor of a pulmonary artery catheter if one is in place. Cardiac dysrhythmias can be noted on a cardiac monitor. Auscultation of heart and lung provide additional data.

Hypotension

Many factors can cause circulatory changes that result in lowering of blood pressure in the postoperative patient (see Box 22-2). A mild decrease in blood pressure from the normal preoperative range is not uncommon during the early postoperative period. It is usually well tolerated in healthy patients and does not require treatment. Shock must be prevented because the brain, heart, kidneys, and other vital organs do not tolerate long periods of hypoxemia. Measures to control shock are immediately instituted when signs of shock occur (Chapter 9).

22-2

Possible causes of postoperative shock

Moving patient from operating table to bed
Jarring patient (bed) during transport
Reactions to drugs and anesthesia
Loss of blood and other body fluids
Cardiac dysrhythmias
Cardiac failure
Inadequate ventilation
Pain
Residual sympathectomy from conductive anesthesia

Cardiac dysrhythmias

Hypoxemia and hypercapnia are common causes of postoperative cardiac dysrhythmias, especially premature beats and sinus tachycardia. These dysrhythmias often can be suppressed by adequate ventilation. Other common causes of postoperative cardiac dysrhythmias include pain, hypovolemia, gastric distention, and acidosis. Significant dysrhythmias are treated by attending to the underlying cause when possible. Antiarrhythmic drugs may be prescribed (Chapter 25).

Promoting normal temperature

Hypothermia, a core temperature of less than 36° C (96.8° F), occurs in 60% to 80% of all postoperative patients.[2] Contributing factors include body exposure in a cold OR room, the effects of cold solutions, and as a consequence of some anesthetics (such as halothane and enflurane; see Chapter 21). Compensating body responses to the cold include shivering and vasoconstriction. Cardiac output is increased, leading to hypertension; cardiac dysrhythmias may occur. Increased oxygen consumption from shivering and from caloric deficits lead to tissue hypoxia. The elderly person is especially affected. The patient experiences discomfort from the cold.

Hypothermia increases the length of time spent by the patient in PACU unless warming methods are used. The patient is monitored for signs of continued hypothermia: persistent low temperature, shivering, and patient reports of still feeling cold even after warming methods. Warm blankets are usually applied to the body, especially around the feet, and adding warmth around the head is also helpful. Other methods include radiant heaters, and heated mattresses and solutions. A newer method is convective warming therapy in which a disposable cover inflated with warm air from a heating unit is placed over the patient; warm air passes out through the underside, providing constantly moving warm air.[2]

Maintaining fluid balance

Fluid deficit may result from inadequate replacement of body fluids lost during surgery or from continued fluid losses. *Fluid excess* may occur from large volumes of fluids replaced by intravenous fluids when kidney function is inadequate (as evidenced by oliguria). Most patients admitted to the PACU receive intravenous fluids as a means of maintaining fluid balance. Careful monitoring of intravenous fluids and urinary output is essential to ensure adequacy of replacement and prevention of fluid overload (Chapter 7).

Preventing injury

To prevent falls after anesthesia, side rails on the stretcher or bed are raised and left so until the patient is fully awake. The patient is turned frequently and placed in good body alignment to prevent nerve damage from pressure and muscle and joint strain from lying in one position for a long time. Patients who have nausea and vomiting are positioned in a side-lying position to prevent aspiration.

Relieving pain

Postoperative pain management in the PACU is now usually under the direction of the anesthesiologist.[56] Narcotics, especially morphine, are the drugs of choice. Narcotics may be given intramuscularly, intravenously, by patient-controlled analgesia (PCA), by continuous epidural infusion, or intrathecally. The anesthesiologist determines the method of administration on the basis of the type of surgery and patient factors. Intravenous dosages are titrated based on pain level and vital signs. *PCA* is now commonly used because it affords better control of postoperative pain and requires smaller dosages of narcotics as compared to narcotics given on demand.[56]

Good postoperative pain control is also achieved by narcotics (morphine, fentanyl, sufentanil, meperidine) given by continuous drip or by PCA in the *epidural* space. This method reduces respiratory, sympathetic, motor, and sensory disturbances as compared to parenteral administration. The epidural catheter is usually inserted preoperatively and an infusion is started. Patients may be placed on this system for 1 to 4 days following intraabdominal, thoracic, or joint replacement surgeries. Epidural analgesia blocks innervation of the bladder, leading to an inability to void; therefore an in-dwelling catheter is necessary during therapy. Other side effects may include pruritus and nausea. Side effects can be relieved by intravenous naloxone (Narcan); this does not reverse the analgesia.

Transcutaneous electrical nerve stimulation (TENS) may also be used for pain control. Other forms of pain management are also important, such as providing information to decrease anxiety (which intensifies the pain experience), and encouraging methods to promote relaxation (Chapter 10).

Promoting psychologic comfort

The immediate postanesthetic period is often frightening for the patient. Psychologic support is imperative for physical as well as emotional well-being. While awakening from anesthesia, the patient needs frequent orientation to place and reassurance of not being alone. The patient also needs to know that the operation is over and that recovery from anesthesia is satisfactory. Careful explanations of procedures being carried out are given even when it appears that the patient is not alert. The need for privacy is considered at all times. Patients who receive this type of support frequently recover from anesthesia faster, with fewer complications and less incisional pain.

Evaluation

Evaluation is based on the identified expected patient outcomes. Questions to consider include the following:

1. Are breath sounds clear?
2. Is respiratory rate 12-20/min and regular?
3. Are oxygen saturation levels within normal levels?
4. Is blood pressure at patient's usual level?
5. Is temperature at patient's usual level?
6. Is skin warm and dry, pulse regular, and urinary output slightly less than fluid intake?
7. Has pulmonary edema been avoided?
8. Is patient's sleep quiet and face relaxed?

Discharge from PACU

Patients are discharged from the PACU when the following criteria have been met:

1. Vital signs are stable and indicate adequate respiratory and circulatory function.
2. Patient is awake or easily aroused and can call for assistance if needed.
3. Postsurgical complications have been thoroughly evaluated and are under control.
4. After regional anesthesia, motor and partial sensory functions have returned to all anesthetized areas.

Acutely ill patients who require further close supervision are transferred to an intensive care unit. Most patients are transferred to a clinical unit. The unit is notified to expect the patient, and all pertinent information concerning the patient's status is communicated to the nurse who will continue to provide postoperative nursing care. The recovery room nurse writes a discharge summary note before the patient leaves the PACU.

ADMISSION OF PATIENT TO CLINICAL UNIT
Preparation on Clinical Unit

The patient's room is prepared to facilitate patient transfer and monitoring (see Box 22-3). The family is notified of the patient's expected return.

Most surgeons discuss the results of the operation with the family immediately after surgery and also visit the patient to describe briefly what was found and to provide reassurance. The family is frequently highly anxious concerning the patient's condition and may not perceive or understand all that the surgeon tells them. Patients frequently experience periods of amnesia during the hours

Preparing room for patient's return from surgery

1. Make an open surgical bed to facilitate easy transfer of patient.
2. Provide sufficient covers (patient may feel cold).
3. Clear a passageway to the bed.
4. Provide necessary equipment
   a. Intravenous pole
   b. Sphygmomanometer
   c. Any special equipment as designated by recovery room nurse.

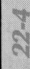

Patient assessment on return from recovery room

Respiratory status
Patency of airway
Respirations: depth, rate, character
Breath sounds: presence, character

Circulatory status
Pulse, blood pressure, temperature
Skin color, temperature
Capillary filling

Neurologic status
Level of consciousness, ability to move extremities

Dressing
Presence of drainage
Presence of tubes to be connected to drainage systems

Comfort
Presence of pain, nausea, vomiting
Patient positioned for comfort and to facilitate ventilation

Safety
Necessity for side rails
Call cord within reach

Equipment
Monitors connected and functioning
Intravenous fluids: rate, amount in bag, patency of tubing
Drainage systems (for example, nasogastric, chest, urinary): type, patency of tubing, connection of appropriate container, character and amount of drainage

when they first regain consciousness and may not remember what they have been told. The nurse needs to know what information was given to the patient and family to be able to answer their questions. The family also needs to know what to expect when the patient returns to the unit.

Safety

Bed siderails are kept raised until the patient is fully awake and responding or to prevent the heavily medicated patient from falling. The patient is instructed early regarding permissibility of ambulation and the need to call for assistance for initial attempts. The call cord should be easily accessible to the patient.

Family members

If family members are present in the room when the patient returns, they may be asked to step outside until the patient has been transferred and assessed. Before leaving the patient, the nurse invites the family to return, explains equipment, and describes the patient's state of awareness and comfort. Family members who understand what is occurring can offer support to the patient. Explanations should be simple but concrete and accurate.

Nursing Process
Assessment
Initial assessment

As soon as the patient is positioned on the bed in the clinical unit, the nurse makes a rapid assessment of the patient's condition. Parameters to assess include respiratory, circulatory, neurologic status, dressing, patient comfort and safety, and functioning of equipment (see Box 22-4). (See also Postoperative nursing care of elderly on p. 456 for special considerations of elderly persons.)

Subjective data

The patient is asked for symptoms of discomfort after having been transferred to the bed and positioned in supportive body alignment. This gives the nurse a quick indication of the level of alertness and symptoms of discomfort. An indirect question such as, "How do you feel?" will elicit data concerning nausea or pain without focusing on a specific area where there may be no discomfort. Pain perception is frequently increased at this time because of the movement from stretcher to bed. It is important to find

out location, onset, and change in pain intensity and not to assume that the pain is incisional.

Nausea occurs less frequently postoperatively with the use of newer anesthetics. There is greater possibility of nausea when the stomach has been manipulated extensively during the surgical procedure or if considerable amounts of narcotics have been administered. The emesis basin should be easily available but not in sight if vomiting is a possibility.

Objective data
Respiratory status

Respirations may be increased or decreased (see Table 22-1). If hypoventilation is present, oxygen may be given if a nasal cannula is in place.

Very noisy respirations may be heard without the aid of a stethoscope. Noisy respirations may be caused by airway obstruction from the tongue falling back against the pharynx or from secretions. The patient with noisy respirations is assisted in coughing and then positioned side-lying if possible. Suctioning may be indicated if coughing does not clear the airway.

Table 22-1   Some causes of vital sign changes in early postoperative phase

Vital sign	Increase	Decrease
Temperature	Stress reaction (low-grade fever)	Cold operating room and recovery room
Pulse rate	Jarring during transfer	Digitalis overdose
	Shock, hemorrhage	Cardiac dysrhythmias
	Hypoventilation	
	Acute gastric dilation	
	Pain	
	Anxiety	
	Cardiac dysrhythmias	
Respiratory rate	Hypoventilation: poor positioning, tight chest or upper abdominal dressing, obesity, gastric dilation	Drugs: anesthetics, narcotics, sedatives
Blood pressure	Anxiety ($\uparrow$ systolic)	Jarring during transfer
	Pain	Severe pain
	Distended urinary bladder	Cardiac dysrhythmias
		Shock: fluid loss, hemorrhage, acute gastric dilation

Postoperative Nursing Care of Elderly

Assessment

Assess breath sounds because thorax stiffening may impair ability to breathe deeply; use pulse oximetry to measure oxygen saturation.

Monitor pulse rate and characteristics. Be aware that heart changes may lead to decreased pulse rate stabilization after insult in the elderly.

Monitor blood pressure and assess for shock; a decrease from the elderly person's *usual* blood pressure may be a sign of shock even if the reading is within general normal limits.

Monitor awakening in PACU; delayed awakening may result from decreased drug clearance from decreased glomerular filtration rate (GFR) and nephron activity or from decreased hepatic function.

Assess patient orientation following surgery; confusion may result from decreased cardiac output, decreased vasomotor contol, or prolonged effects of anesthetic agents.

Assess fluid and electrolyte balance.
Fluid overload may occur from decreased vasomotor control.
Edema may be a sign of heart failure.
Dehydration and sodium retention may result from decreased ability to concentrate urine.
Acid-base imbalance may result from decreased urinary ammonia formation or increased carbon dioxide retention from decreased respiratory function.

Monitor wound healing; malnutrition or decreased circulation may impair healing.

Monitor bowel elimination; constipation may occur more readily because of decreased gastrointestinal muscle tone or loss of elasticity of abdominal muscles.

Monitor for thrombophlebitis from decreased peripheral circulation or increased peripheral resistance.

Intervention

Encourage frequent deep breathing and provide pain relief to encourage effective deep breathing.

Assist patient to change position slowly when getting up to prevent orthostatic hypotension; give the elderly person time to respond to vasomotor changes.

Monitor rate of intravenous fluids carefully; keep patient hydrated.

Orient patient to surroundings as necessary and explain nursing activities. Protect patient from environment.

Use good sterile technique when changing dressings because the elderly are more susceptible to infection from a decreased immune response. Report and record early signs of infection. Be aware that fever is not a good indicator of infection in the elderly person.

Provide support stockings and encourage patient activity in and out of bed to prevent thrombophlebitis.

Use measures to encourage normal bowel activity.

Clarify with patient the availability of home support persons for assistance when patient returns home.

Common complications in elderly

Hypoxia leading to atelectasis and pneumonia
Hypotension and shock
Heart failure with pulmonary edema; dysrhythmias
Fluid and electrolyte imbalances
Drug overdose (anesthetic or other drugs)
Wound complications
Thrombophlebitis
Constipation

If respirations are not noisy, the lungs are auscultated to establish a baseline for future comparison and to identify adventitious sounds. Absent breath sounds indicate hypoventilation of the lobe (Table 22-1). Coarse rales (crackles) indicate secretions in air passages. Presence of adventitious sounds indicates the need for energetic ventilatory exercises. Deep-breathing and coughing measures are instituted immediately in all patients who have had general anesthesia (Chapter 20).

Circulatory status

The pulse, blood pressure, skin color and temperature, and capillary filling are assessed (Table 22-1). Signs of shock or hemorrhage are reported immediately to the surgeon. Hypotensive changes may be related to shock, although other signs of shock usually occur before changes in blood pressure. The skin often feels cool to the touch after surgery as a result of coolness of the surgical suites, hypovolemia from blood loss, or vasoconstriction from stress. Restlessness is an early sign of shock.

After surgery of the extremities, local circulation is assessed by the presence and strength of peripheral pulses *distal* to the operative site or plaster cast. If the dressing is too tight, it should be loosened, if permissible, or reported at once to the physician.

Level of consciousness

Level of consciousness can be ascertained by asking the patient to respond to simple questions or commands. Variations in consciousness level from alertness to drowsiness will be observed. If the patient is not easily aroused, these data are compared with the patient's consciousness status at the time of discharge from the recovery room. A decrease in consciousness level may indicate shock (from jarring motions during the transfer) and should be reported to the surgeon at once along with any other pertinent data.

Dressing

The entire dressing is inspected with the covers pulled back or the patient turned as necessary. A dressing applied to the side, such as after kidney surgery, may appear dry on the top visible area if the patient is supine but may have excess drainage on the lower portion as a result of gravity. Excess drainage is reported immediately.

Whenever it is anticipated that fluid may collect in a body area postoperatively, leading to delay in healing, the surgeon usually inserts a tube or drain to permit escape of the fluid. One end of the tube or drain is placed in or near the organ or cavity to be drained, and the other end is passed through the body wall, usually through a separate stab wound.

After most types of surgery, the surgeon usually changes the dressing for the first time. If small amounts of unexpected drainage are observed, especially bright red drainage, the area can be outlined with a pen on the dressing so that the rate of drainage can be easily determined. Dressings that *cannot* be changed by the nurse are reinforced with dry dressings if drainage penetrates the outer layer; this prevents bacterial contamination by capillary action through the wet dressings. If these additional dressings become wet, they are removed and replaced with new dressings, leaving the original dressing intact. Dressings that *can* be changed by the nurse are changed as often as necessary to prevent maceration of the skin and to promote patient comfort.

Body position

The patient is placed in a position of comfort that aids good ventilation. Except after spinal anesthesia or in certain types of eye surgery or neurosurgery when the bed must remain flat, most patients prefer the head of the bed slightly elevated. The patient who is not very alert needs to be placed in a position of good alignment. There should be no strain on the area surrounding the incision. Pillows should *not* exert pressure on the popliteal area (behind the knee), because this leads to venous obstruction and potential thrombophlebitis.

Assessment of fluid lines

Fluids may be ordered to be given intravenously or instilled in body cavities for irrigation, such as in the bladder (see Chapter 33). The contents of the fluid containers, the patency of the tubing, and the rate of fluid administration are checked. Fluids are usually given intravenously at rates ranging from minimal (to keep the line open, K/O) to 3 ml/min (180 ml/hr). If the rate is greater than 3 ml/min, and if the physician's order sheet is not available in the patient's room, the rate should be slowed, the order checked immediately, and the rate adjusted appropriately. Rate of administration varies with the amount of fluid lost, size and age of the patient, and the underlying illness (Chapter 7). The patient and family should be instructed early concerning permissibility of fluids taken orally.

Drainage from tubes can be accomplished by either gravity or suction (Table 22-2). Each tube is connected to a separate drainage receptacle. All tubing is connected to the drainage receptacle and checked for patency. The amount of fluid in each receptacle is marked on the receptacle and recorded as baseline for future comparison. Color and consistency of drainage are noted.

Data from patient's chart

After the patient has been assessed and positioned comfortably and safely, the nurse gathers additional data from the patient's chart (Table 22-3) before planning and initiating general postoperative care.

Table 22-2   **Drainage systems**

Tube	System
Nasogastric tube	
Levine tube	Intermittent low electric suction
Sump tube	Constant low electric suction
Urinary catheter	Gravity urinary drainage system
Chest tube	Waterseal drainage system (gravity or suction)
Incisional tubes	Low negative pressure: Hemovac (Fig. 22-3), Jackson-Pratt (Fig. 22-4), or low constant electric suction

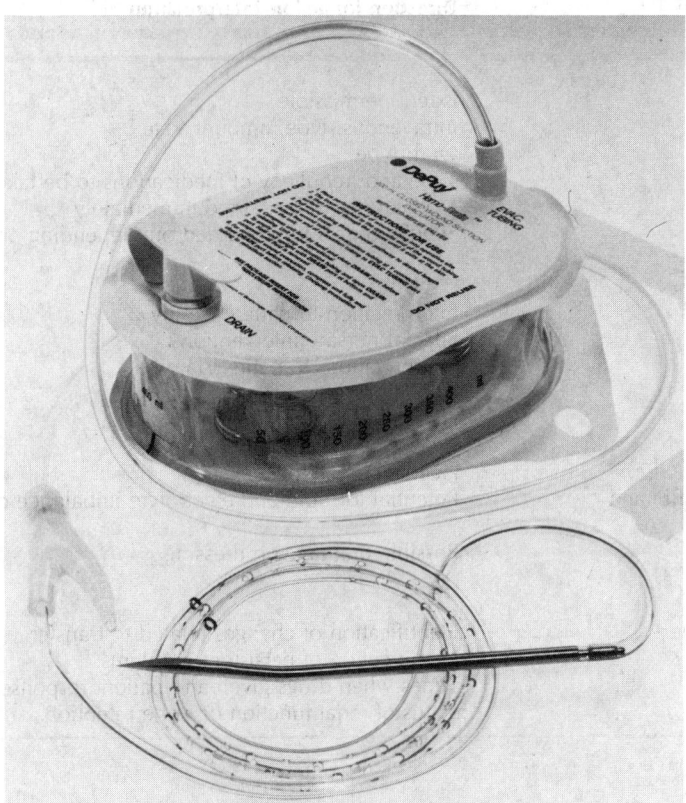

Fig. 22-3   Hemo-drain for low-suction wound drainage. Unit is compressed, then drain cap closed. Inner spring expands slowly creating suction through tube. (Courtesy DePuy, Warsaw, Ind.)

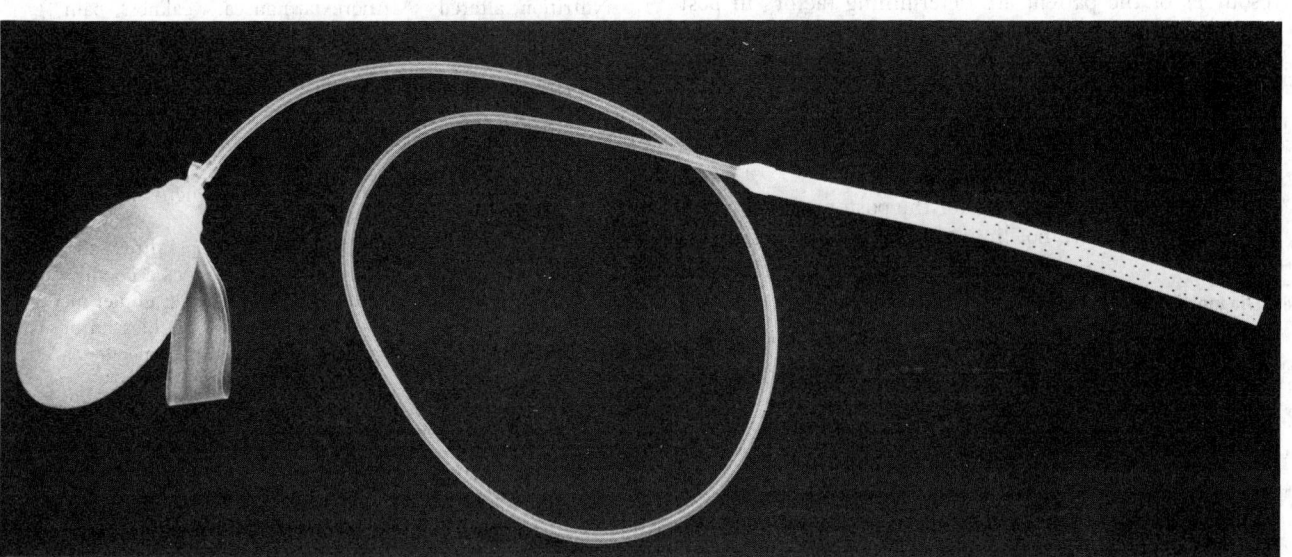

Fig. 22-4   Jackson-Pratt wound suction apparatus. After emptying through spout, reservoir bulb is kept compressed until spout is closed. Slow expansion of bulb creates low-pressure suction.

Table 22-3   Chart data useful in planning postoperative care

Data	Direction for action/interpretation
Surgeon's orders	
Activity	Extent permissible
Fluids, food	Intravenous: type, amount, rate
	Oral: type
Medications	Type and frequency of medications to be taken as needed
	Medications to be started immediately
Other orders	Special orders to be carried out depending on type of surgery
Surgical notes	
Postoperative diagnosis	Interpretation to patient/family
Type of surgery	Special nursing interventions
	Interpretations to patient/family
Anesthetic	
Inhalant	Need for deep-breathing measures
Muscle relaxants	Assessment of respiratory distress
Spinal	Headache may occur
Estimated blood loss (EBL) and fluid replacement	Potential for fluid and electrolyte imbalance or transfusion reactions
Drains	Possible drainage on dressing
Recovery room notes	
Vital signs before transfer	Identification of changes related to transfer
Patient progress	Identification of persistent problems
Medications given	Times when drugs given and patient response
Urinary output	Status of renal function or urine retention

Data analysis: nursing diagnoses

The collected data are recorded in the nursing admission notes and used to identify the specific needs of the patient in the postoperative period. The preoperative condition of the patient, type of surgery performed, and strengths and resources of the patient are determining factors in postoperative discomfort or complications. In planning the patient's care, the nurse uses previously collected data, present data, knowledge of factors related to specific types of surgery (as illustrated in succeeding chapters of this text), and specific postoperative needs and possible postoperative complications.

Possible nursing diagnoses for the postoperative patient may include, but are not limited to, the following:

Diagnostic title	Possible etiologies
Injury, high risk for: wound dehiscence	Excessive coughing, distention, dehydration, obesity
Infection, high risk for (wound)	Poor aseptic technique, malnutrition
Breathing pattern, ineffective	Increased respiratory secretions, dry sticky secretions, decreased thorax expansion, pain, tight bandages or casts, abdominal distention, medications
Tissue integrity, impaired, high risk for	Inactivity, shock, obesity, pressure on popliteal area, tight dressings or cast
Fluid volume excess	Age (elderly), large fluid volume intake

Diagnostic title	Possible etiologies
Comfort, altered, nausea	Anesthetic, narcotic, electrolyte imbalance
Pain	Incisional pain, sore throat from endotracheal tube, tissue anoxia from tight dressings/cast, abdominal distention
Nutrition, altered: less than body requirements	Anorexia, nausea, weakness, pain
Urinary retention	Position for voiding, anesthetic, narcotic, pelvic surgery
Constipation	Anesthetic, narcotic, inactivity, inadequate nutrition, stress
Mobility, impaired physical	Pain, decreased strength and endurance, multiple tubes
Anxiety	Threat to self-concept; threat or change in health status, socioeconomic status, role functioning; unmet meets
Knowledge deficit	Lack of exposure or recall: routines, preventive measures, specific care requirements

Planning: expected patient outcomes

Expected patient outcomes for the postoperative patient may include, but are not limited to:

1. Incision heals well without separation or infection.
2. Breath sounds are clear; atelectasis or pneumonia do not occur.
3. No pain or redness of calf/thigh occur (thrombophlebitis).
4. Fluid intake is more than fluid output for first 24 to 48 hours, then becomes essentially equal (no overhydration or urinary retention).

5. States feeling comfortable; lies quietly when at rest with no outward signs of discomfort.
6. Eats well from prescribed diet; weight loss is minimal or stabilized.
7. Stools return to usual pattern within 3 to 4 days after major surgery (earlier with minor surgery; longer after GI surgery)
8. Carries out activities of daily living at an optimal level, although fatigue may still be present; ambulates at prescribed levels.
9. Shows no outward signs of anxiety; identifies concerns, including sexual concerns, as pertinent.
10. Can explain at discharge:
    a. Home treatments, if pertinent
    b. Home medications (name, dosage, frequency, side effects)
    c. Dietary changes required by surgery
    d. Activity limitations incurred by surgery and any exercise programs to be carried out at home
    e. When and where to go for follow-up care by surgeon

Implementation
Promoting wound healing
Pathophysiology of wound healing

Understanding the pathophysiology of wound healing and the factors that influence wound healing provides the basis for some of the postoperative nursing care, particularly wound care, dietary requirements, and need for physical activity.

Result of wound healing. Wounds may heal by *regeneration* of the tissue or by *scar* formation. Injured cells that have the capacity to regenerate (Fig. 22-5) will do so if the underlying structure has not been destroyed. Muscle and nerve cells rarely undergo mitotic division and are usually unable to regenerate. When muscle cells are injured, satisfactory performance may result by hypertrophy of marginal cells. Nerve cells in the central nervous system do not regenerate. In the peripheral nervous system there is no regeneration if the cell body is destroyed; however, if the axon is injured, there is partial degeneration of the axon, followed by regeneration.

In a typical surgical incision, muscle tissue is cut into. Although the epithelial cells regenerate over the scar tissue, the epithelial layer is so thin that the scar tissue is visible.

Types of wound healing. Tissue may heal by primary, secondary, or tertiary intention (Fig. 22-6). Healing by *primary intention* occurs with surgical wounds; all layers of the wound are closely approximated by suturing. If not infected, the wound heals quickly with minimum scarring. Healing by *secondary intention* occurs when a wound, such as an ulcer with edges that cannot be sutured, heals by filling in the area from the bottom. The wound is open, with increased chance of infection, and heals slowly with considerable scarring. With healing by *tertiary intention,* the wound is sutured several days after wounding. This may occur if the wound was very dirty and had to be cleaned out before suturing could be done, or if a surgical wound breaks open after several days. The wound is more contaminated than with primary intention so scarring is greater, but less than with secondary intention.

Process of wound healing. Regardless of the type of wound healing, the process is the same. The difference is in the length of time for each phase of healing and the extent of granulation tissue formed. When tissue is injured, two major responses occur initially, the *stress response* (Chapter 6) and the *inflammatory response* (Chapter 16). The inflammatory response serves to prepare the tissue so

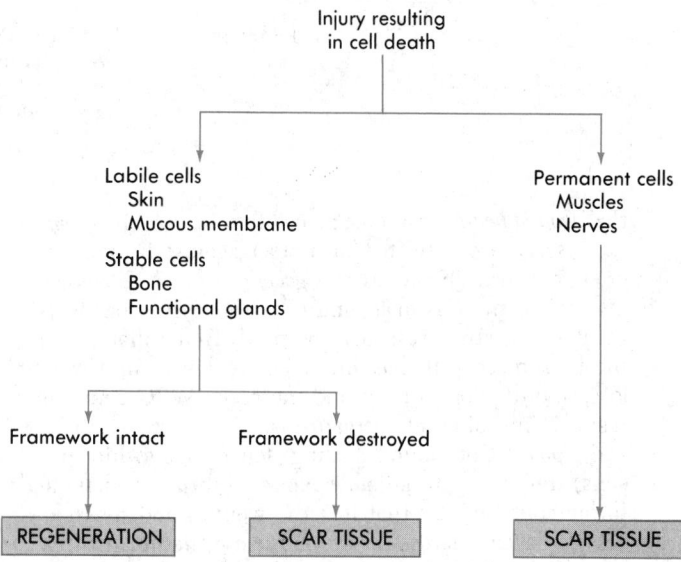

Fig. 22-5 End results of wound healing.

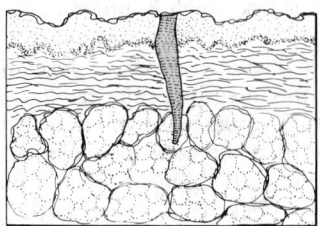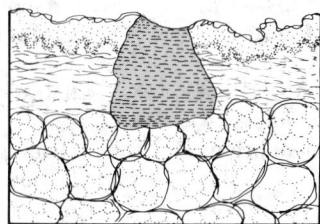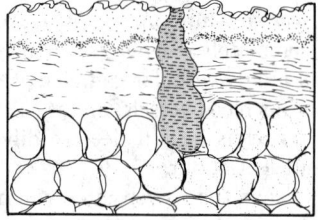

Fig. 22-6 Types of wound healing: primary, secondary, and tertiary intention.

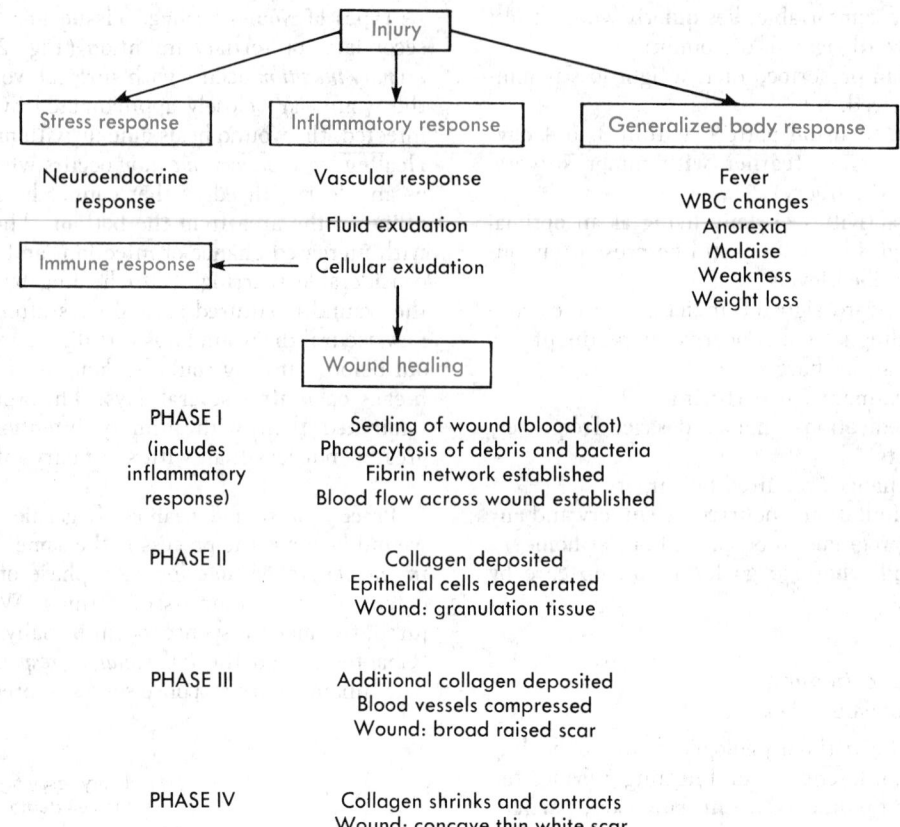

Fig. 22-7   Response of body to injury.

that *wound healing* can take place (Fig. 22-7). The *immune response* is also activated to protect against invading microorganisms (Chapter 16). A *generalized body response* occurs when there is major injury to the tissue, partly as a result of the stress response and partly from inflammation; the person feels ill, has anorexia, weakness, and weight loss, and develops a fever and increased WBC count as a result of invading microorganisms.

In *phase I* of wound healing, leukocytes (white blood cells) ingest bacteria and debris. Fibrin is deposited throughout the clot that fills the wound, and new blood vessels develop across the wound using the fibrin threads as a framework. A thin layer of epithelial cells migrate across the wound and help to seal the wound. The wound strength is low but sutured wounds will hold together if sutured correctly. After major surgery the patient looks and feels ill during this first phase, which lasts 3 days.

Phase II lasts from 3 to 14 days after surgery. The leukocytes start disappearing and the space begins to fill with *collagen*, a white protein fiber. All layers of epithelial cells are completely regenerated in about 1 week. The new tissue is a highly vascular connective tissue, reddish from the numerous blood vessels, and is called *granulation tissue.* If scraped, this tissue will bleed readily. The patient begins to look and feel better.

The collagen that is deposited will provide good support for the wound in 6 to 7 days. Thus sutures are often removed about this time, depending on the site and extent

of surgery. Skin sutures that are commonly used include black silk, fine wire, metal skin clips, and metal staples.

During *phase III,* collagen continues to be deposited. This compresses the new blood vessels, and blood flow decreases. The wound now looks like a broad pinkish raised scar. During this phase, which lasts from about the second to the sixth week after surgery, the patient should avoid heavy use of the affected muscles.

The final phase, *phase IV,* lasts for several months after surgery. The patient may complain of itching around the wound. Although collagen continues to be deposited during this time, the wound shrinks and contracts. If the wound is near a joint, contractures may occur. Because of the shrinkage the wound becomes a concave thin white line. Scar tissue is acellular, avascular collagen tissue. It will not tan with sunlight nor sweat nor produce hair.

Interventions to promote healing

1. Promote intake of foods high in protein and vitamin C. Protein is needed for the formation of collagen. Vitamin C also facilitates collagen formation and helps maintain the integrity of the capillary walls.
2. Carry out measures to increase circulation (p. 464). Healing requires that the necessary cells to fight infection and nutrients be brought to the wound and that the debris and dead cells be removed.
3. Avoid antiinflammatory drugs (such as steroids) when healing is desired; inflammation is a desired part of the healing process.

Table 22-4 Surgical tubes and drains

Type	Purpose	Examples	Comments
Tubes	Prevent blockage of drainage Drain an area by suction	T-tube (Fig. 22-8) Abramson all-purpose tube (Fig. 22-9) Saratoga sump tube (Fig. 22-9)	Connect to drainage system as ordered
Drains	Drain an area by gravity	Penrose drain (Fig. 22-10) Cigarette drain (Fig. 22-10)	Use a safety pin to prevent drain from sliding back into abdomen Encase outer end of drain in a dressing

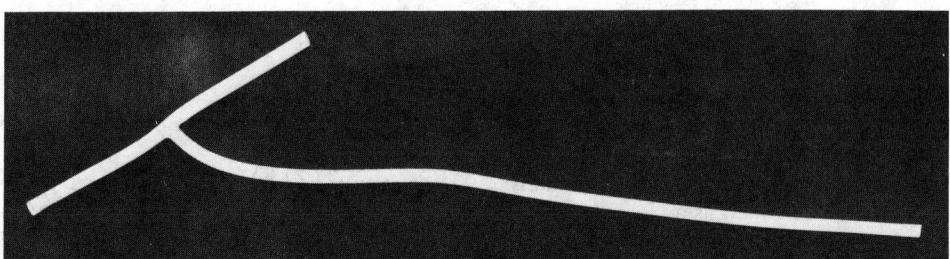

Fig. 22-8 T tube for draining common bile duct.

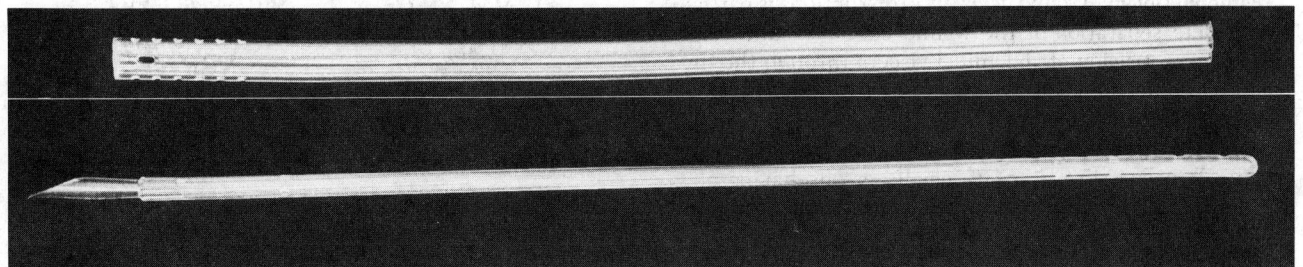

Fig. 22-9 Surgical drain tubes. *Top,* Abramson all-purpose drain has three lumens: for aspiration, irrigation, and instillation. *Bottom,* Saratoga sump drain has a tube within a tube for low-pressure suction.

4. Prevent infection that delays healing:
   a. Change soiled wet dressings immediately.
   b. Use strict aseptic technique when changing dressings.
   c. Cover moist dressings with a dry sterile cover.
5. Irrigate contaminated wounds well to remove foreign substances that create an excessive inflammatory reaction and infection, which delay healing.
6. Maintain suction of wound catheters. Fluid remaining in a wound space delays healing.

Care of the surgical wound

Surgical wounds, because they are aseptically created, generally heal well and quickly. For psychologic reasons and to prevent trauma until epithelialization occurs, the wound is usually covered initially by a dressing.

Incisional coverings may be gauze, semiocclusive, or occlusive dressings. Gauze dressings permit air to reach the wound; semiocclusive dressings permit oxygen but not air to pass; occlusive dressings permit neither air nor oxygen to pass. Occlusive and semiocclusive dressings are thought to promote healing by keeping wounds moist (yet sterile) so epithelial cells can slide more easily over the surface of the wound during epithelialization.[42] Dressings over closed wounds are usually removed by the third or fourth day.

Tubes and drains (Table 22-4) are used to prevent or remove accumulation of fluid from the surgical site. Because the drain provides a passage out of tissues or body cavities, microorganisms can also travel into these areas. Aseptic technique is therefore essential in caring for tubes and drains; they are removed by the surgeon as soon as unnecessary. Tubes and drains are usually brought out of a separate incision (stab wound) to prevent infection of the operative wound. Soft drains, such as a Penrose drain (Fig. 22-10) are either stitched to the skin or have a large safety pin fastened at the distal end to prevent slippage back into the body. If an open drainage system is present, the open

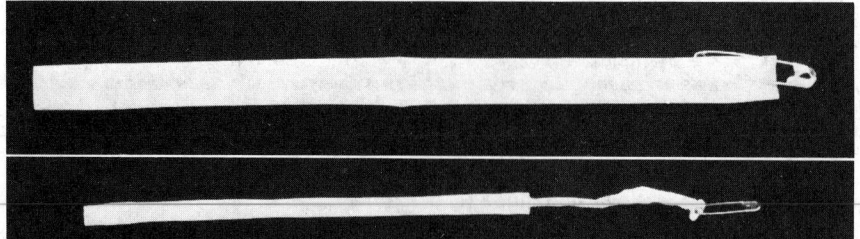

Fig. 22-10 Wound drains. *Top,* Penrose drain. *Bottom,* Cigarette drain.

end of the drain should be encased in an absorbable sterile dressing to protect the skin; this dressing is changed frequently. Fewer open drainage systems are being used, however, in preference to closed drainage systems that diminish the possibility of infection. A firm catheter is used in place of a soft drain for closed drainage. The catheter is usually attached to low-pressure suction such as a Hemovac (Fig. 22-3, p. 452) or a suction machine with low pressure. A sump drain (Fig. 22-9) has an airflow system that facilitates fluid removal; it must be connected to constant suction.

Wound dehiscence and evisceration

Pathophysiology. Wound *dehiscence* (disruption) is partial to complete separation of the wound edges. Wound *evisceration* is protrusion of abdominal viscera through the incision and onto the abdominal wall (Fig. 22-11).

Wound dehiscence is rare in persons under 30 but occurs in 5% of persons over age 60 who are having laparotomy. It occurs in 1% to 3% of all persons having abdominal surgery.[56] Thoracic wounds are less apt to dehisce than abdominal wounds.

Wound separation that occurs during the first 3 postoperative days (phase I of wound healing) are usually a result of inadequate surgical closure. During the next 10 days, wound separation is usually associated with postoperative complications, such as excessive coughing or vomiting, distention, dehydration, or infection. Many of these complications can be prevented by careful assessment and continued monitoring and by the institution of vigorous preventive measures (ventilatory exercises, ambulation, adequate fluid intake, aseptic technique) on the part of the nurse. Wound separation during phase III (after 2 weeks) is usually associated with metabolic factors such as cachexia, obesity, hypoproteinemia or avitaminosis, increased age, decreased resistance to infection, malignancy, multiple trauma, or hypothermia. These factors can also cause wound separation at an earlier time.

Assessment. The patient may complain of a "giving" sensation at the incision or a feeling of wetness with dehiscence. If evisceration has occurred and a loop of bowel is obstructed, the patient will complain of severe pain at the incision. On inspection the dressing will be found to be saturated with clear pink drainage. The wound edges may be partially or entirely separated, and loops of intestine may be lying on the abdominal wall. Signs of shock may be present.

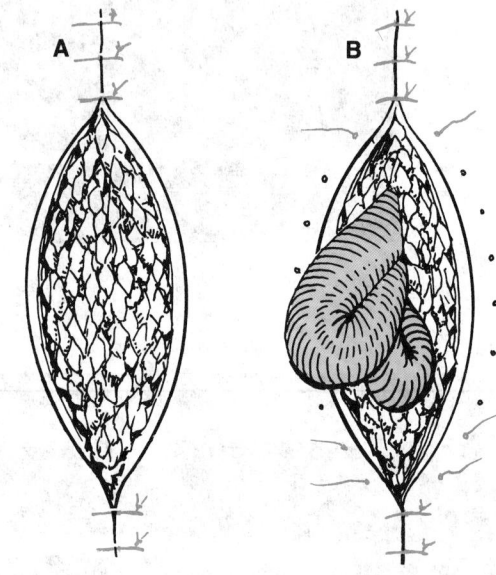

Fig. 22-11 **A,** Wound dehiscence. **B,** Wound evisceration.

Intervention

1. Put patient in bed in low Fowler's position to ease strain on the incision.
2. Tell patient to lie quietly and not cough, eat, or drink until seen by the physician.
3. Cover protruding viscera with a dressing moistened with warm sterile saline solution to prevent tissue dryness and necrosis.
4. Notify physician.
5. Remain with the patient until the physician arrives if evisceration is present; monitor vital signs for shock.

The treatment for wound dehiscence or evisceration is immediate closure of the wound under local or general anesthesia. If the patient is in shock, the preanesthetic medication may be omitted. Convalescence is usually prolonged, although the wound usually heals surprisingly well after secondary closure.

Promoting adequate respiration

Pathophysiology. Postoperative patients are at high risk for developing pulmonary complications (Table 22-5). The pulmonary complications are often preventable by nursing

Table 22-5   Risk factors in development of postoperative pulmonary complications

Risk factors	Effect
Increased respiratory secretions	
Smoking	Irritation of lining of tracheobronchial passages
Intubation	Decreased ciliary action to remove secretions
Inhalant anesthetics	Secretions will block bronchial passages or alveoli
Chronic lung disease	
Upper respiratory infection	
Dry sticky secretions	
Chronic lung disease	Difficult to cough up secretions
Dehydration	Secretions will block bronchial passages
Decreased thorax expansion	
Pain (chest, upper abdomen)	Lung does not expand fully, resulting in hypoventilation
Obesity	of alveoli
Age	
Tight binders or casts	
Skeletal abnormalities (for example, scoliosis)	
Decreased diaphragm mobility	
Abdominal distention	Decreased lung expansion, leading to hypoventilation
Surgery of chest or upper abdomen	
Muscle relaxants	
Neurologic deficit	
Depression of respiratory center	
Sedatives	Depressed respirations result in hypoventilation
Narcotics	
Acid-base imbalance	
Aspiration of gastric contents	
Vomiting	Causes aspiration pneumonia

management. The most common respiratory complications are atelectasis and hypostatic pneumonia.

In *atelectasis* a bronchiole becomes blocked by secretions and the distal alveoli collapse as the existing air is absorbed, producing hypoventilation (Fig. 22-12). A major bronchus or many small bronchioles may be involved. The latter situation is frequently undetected because there are few symptoms. The extent of atelectasis is determined by the site of the blockage; if the main stem bronchus to one lung is blocked, that *lung* will be atelectic. If a bronchus to a lobe is blocked, that *lobe* will atelectic.

Hypostatic pneumonia is inflammation of the lung from stasis of secretions. Both atelectasis and hypostatic pneumonia decrease oxygenation, prolong recovery, and add to the patient's discomfort.

Assessment. The patient is assessed frequently during the first 24 to 48 hours after an inhalant anesthetic, depending on the number of risk factors present. A person at high risk may need to be assessed as often as every hour. Assessment includes monitoring respirations and chest expansion, auscultating the lungs, evaluating the productiveness of the cough, and observing for signs of atelectasis and pneumonia (see Box 22-5).

Intervention. After general anesthesia most patients will need to ventilate their lungs well *at least* every 1 to 2 hours

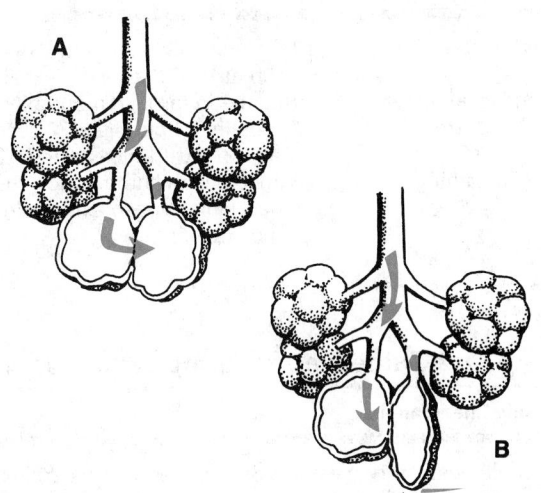

Fig. 22-12   Mucous plug blocking alveolar duct in obstructive atelectasis. **A,** Aeration of blocked alveolus through interalveolar duct with deep inspiration. **B,** Collapse of blocked alveolus with shallow inspiration.

during the first postoperative day, and then every 3 to 4 hours while awake for several days if not active. The decision for the type and frequency of preventive respiratory measures is based on each patient's risk factors and hour-by-hour and day-by-day response. Measures effective in increasing ventilation in one patient may be less effective in another patient.

Ventilatory measures. A number of ventilatory measures (Table 22-6) can be used in the postoperative period to prevent atelectasis by inflating the alveoli as fully as pos-

sible. Once the alveoli are fully inflated, they will remain open for at least 1 hour. The two most effective ventilatory maneuvers that lead to maximum alveolar inflation are the yawn and the incentive spirometer (Fig. 22-13). Guidelines for using ventilatory measures are described in Table 22-7.

Positioning and turning. If the patient lies in one position with continuous pressure from body weight against the chest wall, proper ventilation and drainage of secretions on that side of the chest are not possible and atelectasis can develop (Fig. 22-14). Turning and changing of position frequently (at least every 2 to 3 hours) provide for better ventilation of the lungs. Encourage the patient to help in the turning; the activity will increase the depth of respirations. Alternating the height of the bed is useful: high Fowler's position facilitates diaphragm movement; low Fowler's or a flat position facilitates drainage and expectoration of respiratory secretions.

Maintaining circulation

Pathophysiology. Thrombophlebitis, which results from venous stasis, is a preventable postoperative complication in many situations. Platelets adhere to the venous wall, with resultant thrombus formation (Fig. 22-15). Venous stasis occurs postoperatively for a number of reasons (see Box 22-6).

Assessment. If a patient complains of any discomfort in a leg, examine the leg (with gentle palpation) for redness and tenderness along the course of a vein if a superficial vein is involved or for tenderness and edema if a deep vein

22-5	Signs of postoperative pulmonary dysfunction	
	Hypoventilation	Rapid shallow respirations Absent or diminished breath sounds in lower lobes Decreased chest expansion
	Increased secretions in airways	Rales heard on auscultation Nonproductive cough
	Atelectasis	Signs may be absent Fever, increased pulse and respirations; dyspnea, cyanosis, and shock if a large bronchus is blocked
	Hypostatic pneumonia	Fever, dyspnea, chest pain, cough productive of mucopurulent sputum

Table 22-6 Common postoperative ventilatory maneuvers

Manuever	Method	Comments
Yawn	Inhale deeply with mouth open (yawn), hold breath for 3 seconds, exhale	Easy to do; good deep breath when yawn occurs
Incentive spirometer	Breathe in through mouthpiece as deeply as possible, hold breath 3 seconds, exhale; work toward increasing inspiratory effort	Promotes sustained maximal inspiration; requires minimal instruction; avoid using at mealtimes (may cause nausea)
Deep breathing	Inhale deeply through nose using diaphragm (abdomen rises), exhale slowly through pursed lips	Effectiveness depends on depth of respirations; patients with chest or abdominal incisions tend to limit depth; patients need encouragement

Table 22-7 Guidelines for using ventilatory measures in postoperative patients

Nursing interventions	Rationale
Schedule ventilatory measures 30 minutes after narcotic is given, if possible	Facilitates patient cooperation
Place patient in high Fowler's position, if permitted	Facilitates diaphragm and chest expansion
Auscultate lungs	Baseline assessment
Suggest patient take three to five normal breaths between each deep inspiration	Prevents dizziness from hyperventilation
Splint chest or abdominal incision with towel, small pillow, or hand before cough, if necessary	Prevents additional pain and muscle strain; provides support to incision to encourage deep cough
Auscultate lung	Comparison with baseline for evaluation of effectiveness

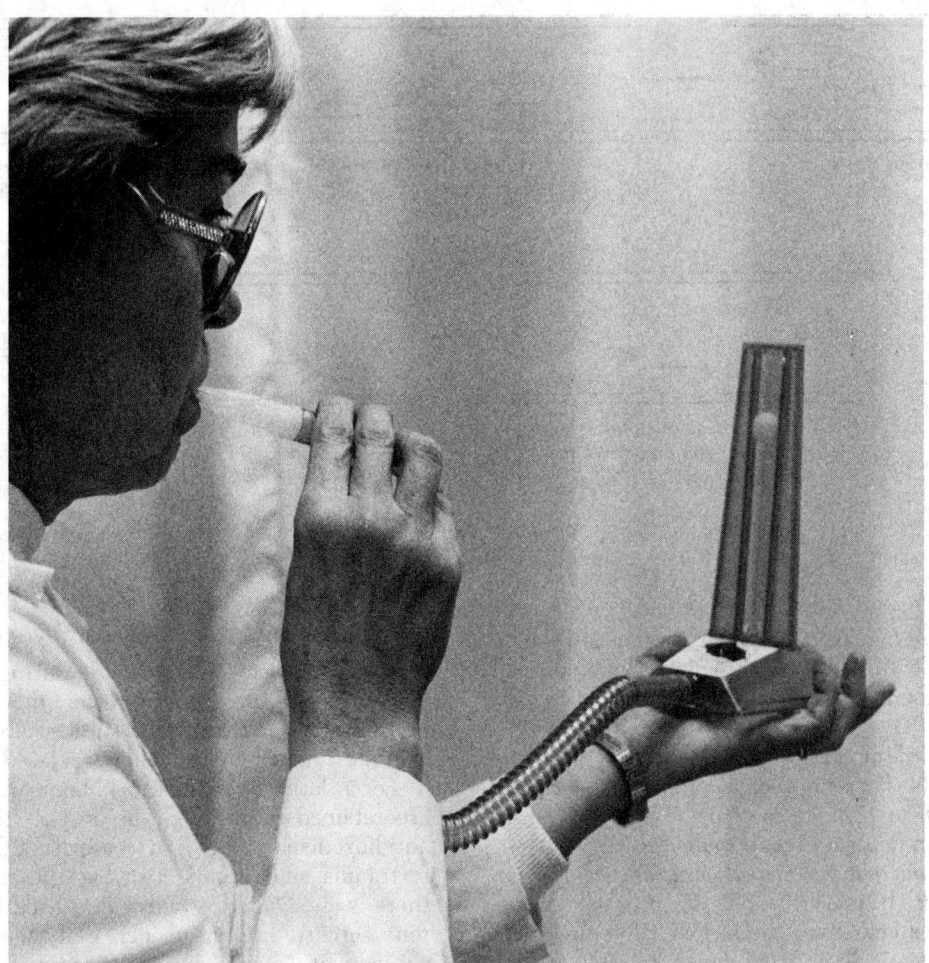

Fig. 22-13   Incentive spirometer. Ball rising with inspiration is a visual cue of deep breathing for patient.

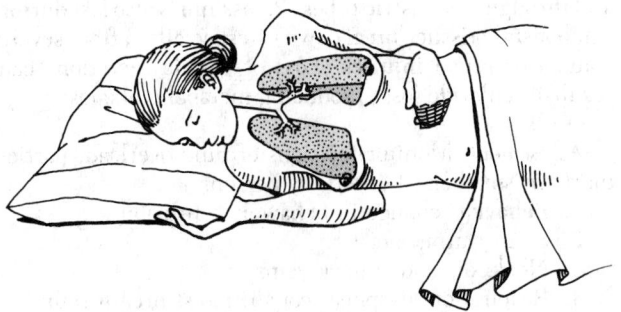

Fig. 22-14   Schematic of lungs illustrating pooling of secretions in dependent alveoli.

22-6	Risk factors for postoperative thrombophlebitis	
	Intrinsic factors	Older age, obesity, malnutrition, contraceptive use
	Pathologic condition	Malignancy, congestive heart failure, history of previous deep-vein thrombosis, polycythemia
	Types of surgery	Pelvic, abdominal, thoracic; fracture of hip or lower extremity
	Effects of surgery	Anesthesia, shock, decreased mobility
		Prolonged sitting with legs crossed
		Pressure on popliteal area
		Tight dressings or cast on lower extremities

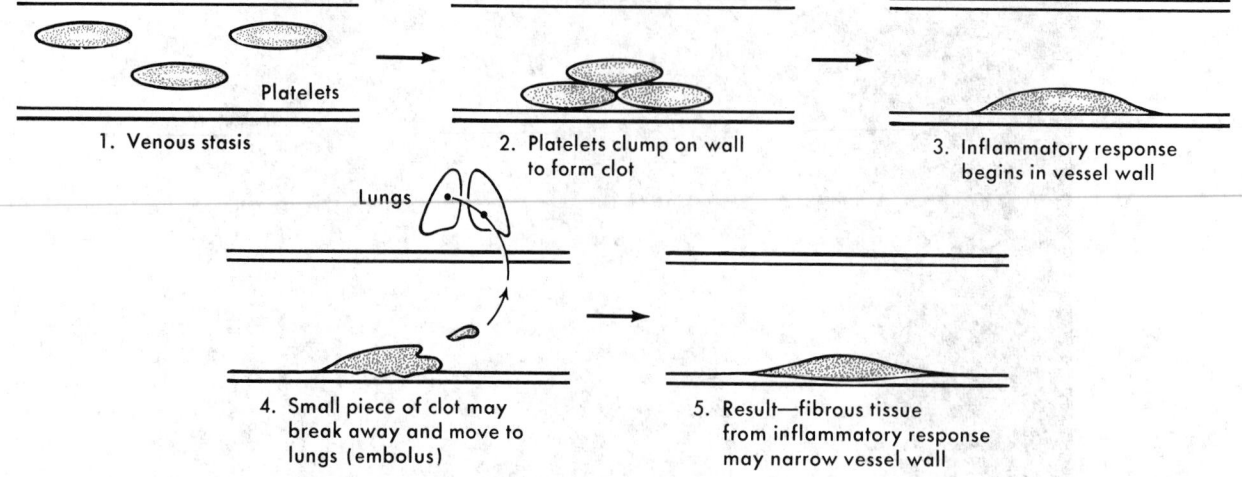

Fig. 22-15 Diagram illustrating formation of thrombus on wall of vein following venous stasis resulting in narrowing of blood vessel.

is involved. There may be pain on dorsiflexion of the foot (Homan's signs) with deep vein thrombosis, but this sign is not always present.

Prevention. *Medical* preventive measures in high-risk patients include (1) heparin prophylaxis given 2 hours preoperatively and 8 to 12 hours postoperatively, (2) aspirin in instances when heparin is contraindicated, (3) dextran, or (4) warfarin. *Intermittent external pneumatic compression* to the legs may also be prescribed. This consists of a pneumatic cuff that extends from the feet to below the knee. The cuff is automatically inflated rapidly to 40 to 50 mm Hg pressure, held for 10 to 12 seconds, and then deflated for 45 seconds. This procedure is not uncomfortable and has demonstrated marked effectiveness in high-risk patients.

Nursing preventive measures include the following:
1. Use elastic stockings, both in and out of bed, on patients at high risk to promote venous return by counter-pressure on leg muscles.
2. Teach patient to avoid sitting for long periods (pressure on popliteal area) and to elevate feet on a stool when sitting to promote venous return.
3. Avoid any pressure on popliteal area (for example, pillow under knee or elevating knee-gatch of bed) that can impede venous return.
4. Avoid leg massage postoperatively; massage may loosen a newly formed clot, causing an embolus.
5. Teach and encourage leg exercises (Chapter 20) for the inactive patient.
6. Encourage early ambulation to facilitate venous return and thus prevent venous stasis.

Intervention. The care of the patient with thrombophlebitis is discussed in Chapter 26. At the first sign of possible thrombophlebitis, ask the patient to return to bed and notify the physician. Rest, heat, elastic bandages, and anticoagulant therapy are usually prescribed. Monitor the patient for signs of pulmonary embolus (chest pain, dyspnea).

Maintaining fluid and electrolyte balance

Pathophysiology. Fluid is lost during surgery through blood loss and increased insensible fluid loss through the lungs and skin. During the surgical procedure the blood loss is estimated and fluids are replaced intravenously.

For at least the first 24 to 48 hours after surgery, fluids are retained by the body because of the stimulation of antidiuretic hormone (ADH), as part of the stress response to trauma and the effect of anesthesia. During surgery there is also renal vasoconstriction and increased aldosterone activity, leading to increased sodium retention and subsequent water retention. *Overhydration* can occur with vigorous fluid replacement, especially in very small or elderly persons. Both water intoxication and pulmonary edema can occur, depending on the type and amount of fluids given. (For further information on fluid overload, see Chapter 7).

Sodium and potassium depletion can occur in the postoperative patient from the loss of blood or body fluids during surgery or the loss of gastrointestinal secretions by vomiting and through nasogastric tubes. Potassium is also lost during catabolism (tissue breakdown), especially after severe trauma or crush injuries. Loss of gastric secretions can result in chloride loss, producing metabolic alkalosis.

Assessment. Monitor for signs of fluid overload, particularly in small sized or elderly persons:
1. Behavior: change in behavior, confusion
2. Skin: warm, moist
3. Neck: distended neck veins
4. Respiration: dyspnea, cough, moist breath sounds
5. Anorexia, nausea, vomiting
6. Fatigue
7. Weight gain (weigh high-risk patients)

Intervention. Intravenous administration of fluids is monitored carefully so that fluids are given evenly over the entire 24 hours. Usually 2000 to 2500 ml of 5% dextrose in normal saline or Ringer's lactate is given daily. (For further information on intravenous fluids, see Chapter 7).

If signs of fluid overload appear, slow the intravenous fluid to a keep-open rate and notify physician.

Fluids are started orally as soon as peristalsis is present. Sips of water are offered first to see if fluids can be tolerated. Some persons better tolerate sucking on ice chips. Ice chips must be recorded as fluid intake (two parts ice equal one part water). As soon as the patient can tolerate drinking fluids, the physician discontinues the intravenous fluid administrations.

Promoting comfort

The major discomforts after surgery are nausea and vomiting, abdominal distention and gas pains, and incisional pain. *Sore throat* may also occur from irritation of the endotracheal tube used during anesthesia. Throat lozenges may ease the discomfort. Notify the anesthesiologist if hoarseness persists longer than 24 hours, signifying possible injury to a laryngeal nerve.

Nausea and vomiting

Nausea and vomiting, which occur less frequently with the newer anesthetic agents, may be related to a number of factors (Box 22-7). Nausea resulting from anesthesia is self-limiting, and usually lasts only 24 to 48 hours. Reassure the patient and provide general nursing measures for nausea.

22-7
Causes of postoperative vomiting
Anesthetic agent Narcotic Abdominal distention (fluid, gas) Pain Electrolyte imbalances Drug idiosyncrasies

Persistent postoperative vomiting is usually a symptom of pyloric obstruction, intestinal obstruction, or peritonitis. Vomiting tires the patient, puts strain on the incision, and causes excessive loss of fluids and electrolytes. Choking while vomiting may lead to aspiration pneumonia.

Interventions for the person who is experiencing vomiting include the following:
1. Side-lying position to prevent aspiration
2. No food or fluids until vomiting subsides
3. Sips of fluid (ice chips, ginger ale, hot tea) or dry solid food (crackers) after vomiting subsides
4. Frequent oral care
5. Prescribed antiemetics given parenterally

Abdominal distention and gas pains

Pathophysiology. Postoperative *distention* results from accumulation of nonabsorbable gas in the intestines caused by decreased intestinal activity from handling of the bowel during surgery, by swallowing of air during recovery from anesthesia or attempts to overcome nausea, and by movement of gases from the bloodstream to the atonic portion of the bowel. Narcotics also decrease intestinal activity. Distention will persist until the tone of the bowel returns to normal and peristalsis resumes. Distention is experienced to some degree by most patients after abdominal and renal surgery. *Gas pains* are caused by contractions of the unaffected portions of the bowel in an attempt to move the accumulated gas through the intestinal tract.

Assessment. If the patient complains of diffuse or cramping abdominal pain, monitor the following:
1. Measurement of abdominal girth with tape measure to determine degree of distention
2. Percussion of distended abdomen for drumlike (tympanic) sounds
3. Presence of signs of shock from acute gastric dilation

Intervention. If the stomach is distended, the fluid and gas can be aspirated with a nasogastric tube. General distention or gas pains from sluggish intestinal peristalsis can be relieved by passage of flatus.

There are a number of interventions that may be helpful in moving the gas along the colon and facilitating passage:
1. Ambulation: most effective method to stimulate peristalsis and get the gas moving so it can be expelled
2. Avoidance of very hot or cold liquids that tend to cause gas buildup: sucking ice chips does not have the same effect because the water warms before it reaches the stomach
3. Exercise to stimulate movement of the gas from right to left and prevent buildup:[44]
   a. Lie on back with legs extended and a pillow under knees.
   b. Bend right knee, moving it toward abdomen.
   c. Put hands on knee and pull down toward abdomen.
   d. Hold position for count of 10.
   e. Lower leg slowly.
   f. Take 2 to 3 slow deep breaths.
   g. Repeat action with left leg.
   h. Repeat steps *a* through *g* 3 to 4 times.
4. Pelvic rock to stimulate peristalsis[25]:
   a. Lie on back.
   b. Exhale slowly while contracting abdominal muscles, simultaneously pressing small of back to bed.
   c. Relax and then repeat actions several times.
5. Abdominal massage to help push gas along colon[44]:
   a. Make a fist with both hands.
   b. Place one fist on lower right abdomen, rolling knuckles upward.
   c. Keeping first fist in place, put second fist above it and roll upward.
   d. Work hand over hand up to lower edge of ribs, across abdomen, then down left side (following course of the colon).
6. Rectal tube for 20 minutes every 4 hours as necessary: tube stimulates lower colonic peristalsis and permits easy passage of the gas past the anal sphincters
7. Heat to the abdomen (heating pad or hot water bottle): heat expands the gas, stimulating peristalsis; this method is most effective combined with a rectal tube
8. Prescribed enema to stimulate peristalsis

Pain

Pathophysiology. Pain is common after nearly all types of surgical procedures in which there has been cutting, pulling, or manipulation of tissues and organs. It may result from stimulation of nerve endings by chemical substances released at the time of surgery or from tissue ischemia caused by interference of blood supply to the part, such as by pressure, muscle spasm, or edema. After surgery other factors can add to the sensation of pain, such as infections, distention, muscle spasms surrounding the incisional area, and tight dressings or casts (see Box 22-8).

22-8

Common postoperative pain syndromes

Pain with fever
Pain with vomiting and abdominal distention
Suprapubic discomfort
Pain with coldness or numbness to part
Wound infection
Gas collecting in intestinal tract
Full bladder
Decreased circulation from tight dressing or cast
  or from venous stasis

Postoperative pain usually lasts 24 to 48 hours but may continue longer depending on the extent of the surgery, the pain threshold of the patient, and response to pain (Chapter 10). The presence of pain can prolong convalescence because it may interfere with return to activity.

Assessment. When the patient complains of pain in the postoperative period, do not assume that the pain is incisional. It is important to try to ascertain the possible cause of the pain. Subjective data include origin, area involved, nature of the pain, and possible cause from the patient's point of view. Objective data include observation of facial expressions, body position, activity, muscle rigidity, and pulse rate. If the patient is having severe pain, the assessment should be made gently and quickly but thoroughly.

Intervention. It is often impossible to prevent postoperative pain, but it can be minimized so that the patient is relatively comfortable. Patients with adequate preoperative instructions and confidence in the surgeon, the nurse, and the outcome of the surgery usually have less postoperative pain than apprehensive patients, because they have less tension. Measures to reduce anxiety and apprehension will also help reduce pain. Relief of pain may encourage the patient to move and breathe more deeply, thus preventing postoperative complications, which cause more pain.

If the cause of pain is determined to be other than incisional, measures are taken to relieve the cause. Emptying a full bladder can relieve what was thought to be pain from a lower abdominal incision. Elevation of a part may relieve venous stasis. Loosening of a tight bandage, if permissible, will relieve ischemic pain.

Incisional pain can be relieved by nursing measures and by analgesics.

1. Encourage patient to move in bed or to ambulate, to decrease pain from muscle tension and increase circulation to the part.
2. Move the injured part as a whole; for example, move trunk as one unit.
3. Support an injured limb during a move (a pillow is a useful support).
4. Teach patient to use siderails in moving to decrease incisional pull.
5. Teach relaxation and distraction techniques, if suitable (Chapter 6).
6. Give PRN medications according to the guidelines for acute pain (Chapter 10).
   a. Narcotics are usually required on a regular basis for 12 to 48 hours after major surgery. Do not hesitate to use full narcotic dosages as prescribed; narcotic addiction is unlikely with postoperative pain. Pain is not fully relieved with inadequate dosage.
   b. Assess the patient for pain frequently during this period. Tell patient to request medication *before* the pain becomes severe. Analgesia is less effective when pain is severe.
   c. Monitor patient receiving meperidine (Demerol) for signs of orthostatic hypotension (dizziness, fainting, rapid pulse) during ambulation.
   d. Nonnarcotics may provide relief after 48 to 72 hours following major surgery.

Epidural analgesia is now commonly used following major surgery; it improves pain relief with less sedation and facilitates postoperative mobility. The anesthesiologist inserts a small-lumen epidural catheter that can be fitted with an injection cap or can be attached by tubing to a continuous infusion pump. When injecting a bolus dose through the cap, aspirate to verify catheter location in the epidural space before giving the drug. If more than 0.5 ml is aspirated (indicating probable misplacement of catheter in the subarachnoid space), do not inject the aspirate or drug and notify the physician responsible for the epidural anesthesia.[57] Morphine sulfate is the primary analgesic of choice, although fentanyl and preservative-free meperidine or hydromorphone may also be used. Bolus doses of 2 mg to 5 mg of morphine q6-12h are commonly given following surgery (lower doses for elderly). Pain relief begins in 30 to 60 minutes and lasts 6 to 12 hours.[57] Better pain relief results with a regular dose schedule than PRN. No other narcotics or CNS depressants should be given concurrently unless prescribed by the responsible clinician. Keep an ampule of naloxone (0.4 mg) at the bedside (to counteract an opioid overdose).[57] Monitor the patient for decreasing level of consciousness and shallow respirations (indicating altered respiratory function from opioid overdose); intake and output (to distinguish between hypovolemia and urinary retention resulting from opioid action); and signs of epidural catheter leakage, infection, or bleeding.[57]

Patient-controlled analgesia (PCA) is also commonly used for control of severe pain following major surgery. PCA is a method by which the patient can self-administer the narcotic by pressing a button to deliver (intravenously or by epidural catheter) a predetermined dose of morphine (usually 1 mg to 3 mg).[56] Controls are built into the system to prevent overdosage (see Chapter 10). Because pain is a powerful respiratory stimulant, narcotics rarely produce respiratory depression when given for postoperative pain. Patients using PCA usually have better relief of postoperative pain and use smaller dosages than narcotics given on demand (PRN).[56]

Transcutaneous electrical nerve stimulation (TENS) is an additional method for postoperative pain relief (see Chapter 10). The conductive tape electrodes are usually applied to the skin on either side of the incision. The electrodes are then connected to a battery-powered portable pulse generator about the size of a pocket paging device. The stimulation is patient-controlled.

For relief of postoperative pain, a *high-frequency* (80 to 100 Hz) *low-intensity* (12 to 20 mamp) impulse appears to be the most effective. The intensity is determined preoperatively on a trial-and-error basis by the patient who locates a point just below the threshold of discomfort. A tingling sensation may be experienced. The patient can vary the intensity according to the pain level. The best results are obtained when the TENS is used at periodic intervals, such as for a 60-minute period, rather than continuously. It may be helpful to provide stimulation for about 30 minutes before painful activities, such as ambulation.

Maintaining adequate nutrition

Pathophysiology. Convalescence can be shortened if protein deficiency does not develop. The best way to supply essential foods is orally. Weight loss usually occurs after surgery as a result of catabolism, nutrients used for healing, and inadequate caloric intake while receiving fluids intravenously. A gradual loss of about 0.15 to 0.25 kg (⅓ to ½ lb) per day indicates tissue loss. Rapid weight loss indicates *fluid* loss: rapid weight gain indicates fluid retention.

Two food substances of special importance in wound healing are protein and vitamin C (p. 460). During catabolism in the early postoperative period, a negative nitrogen balance occurs; more nitrogen is lost than is taken in. Nitrogen is an essential constituent of amino acids, the building blocks of proteins. Protein intake is necessary to restore nitrogen balance and to provide the necessary amino acids for anabolism. Vitamin C is stored only in small amounts in the tissues, so must be supplied daily from an external source.

Peristalsis decreases temporarily after *abdominal and pelvic* surgeries because of handling of the gastrointestinal organs during surgery. Peristalsis then returns gradually in 24 to 48 hours (72 hours after colon surgery). Peristalsis is not affected in other types of surgeries.

Assessment

1. Monitor bowel sounds until heard regularly, or patient passes flatus, indicating return of peristalsis.
2. Weigh the patient for whom weight loss may present a problem, that is, the person who is severely undernourished or receiving feedings intravenously for 1 week or longer.
3. Monitor meal trays to identify those persons who are not eating foods high in protein and vitamin C.

Intervention. After abdominal or pelvic surgery, the patient usually receives intravenous fluids until bowel sounds are heard (indicating gastrointestinal movement). Poorly nourished patients may require total parenteral nutrition (TPN). When peristalsis has been identified, clear liquids (water, tea, coffee, broth, juice) are permitted until they are well tolerated. Full liquids (milk products, cream soups, high-protein drinks, ice cream) are then introduced. Soft foods are then permitted, and finally, a regular diet is permitted, as tolerated by the patient. The goal is to move the patient to a full nourishing diet as soon as possible. Persons having other than abdominal or pelvic surgery are usually encouraged to take fluids and food as tolerated.

Other nursing interventions include the following:

1. Encourage and teach postoperative patients to eat foods high in protein and vitamin C.
2. Do not force food if patient is anorexic. Instead, offer frequent small amounts of food or high-protein, high-calorie liquids (such as milkshakes or eggnogs).
3. Encourage activity to improve desire to eat.
4. Discuss with underweight persons their plans for obtaining the desired nutrients after discharge.

Maintaining elimination
Urine elimination

Pathophysiology. A patient who is well hydrated usually voids within 6 to 8 hours after surgery. Although 2000 to 3000 ml solution usually is given intravenously on the day of surgery, the first voiding may be 200 ml or less, and the total urinary output for the day may be less than 1500 ml. The small amount of urinary output results from the loss of body fluid during surgery, increased insensible fluid loss, vomiting, and increased secretion of antidiuretic hormone. As body functions stabilize, fluid and electrolyte balance returns to normal in about 48 hours.

Urinary retention, or the inability to void, may occur in the early postoperative period for several reasons (see Box 22-9). A full bladder may increase pressure on an abdominal or pelvic incision, causing bleeding and pain. *Urinary tract infections* may occur in patients who must have prolonged bed rest after surgery, have a history of urinary tract infections, have had pelvic surgery, or have in-dwelling catheters.

Assessment

1. Monitor urinary output until output equals fluid intake.

22-9	**Causes of postoperative urinary retention**

Recumbent position
Nervous tension
Anesthetic; decreased bladder sensation and ability to void
Narcotic: decreased bladder sensation
Pelvic surgery: interference with innervation of bladder muscles, local edema

2. If patient does not void sufficiently, especially within 6 to 8 hours after surgery, assess for urinary retention (suprapubic distention, sensation of full bladder, suprapubic discomfort).
3. If patient complains of frequency of urination with burning, check body temperature, send a clean voided urine specimen to laboratory for culture and sensitivity (if protocols permit), and notify physician.

Intervention. If urinary retention is present, carry out measures to facilitate voiding (Chapter 33). Catheterization may be delayed longer than the usual 8 hours postoperatively for patients other than those having lower abdominal or pelvic surgery, in the hope that the patient will void normally. Bethanechol chloride (Urecholine) may be ordered by the physician for acute postoperative urine retention; it may be given orally or subcutaneously but not by intramuscular injection because this may induce circulatory collapse.

If the bladder must be catheterized repeatedly after surgery, an in-dwelling catheter may be inserted. Fluids are then encouraged up to 3000 ml, unless contraindicated, to prevent urinary stasis that leads to infection. Prophylactic antibiotics may be prescribed.

Bowel elimination

Pathophysiology. Peristalsis will be decreased for at least 24 hours after abdominal or pelvic surgery and for several days after surgery of the gastrointestinal tract. No bowel movement can occur when peristalsis is absent or significantly decreased. *Constipation* occurs frequently after major surgery for several reasons (see Box 22-10). A bowel movement may be intentionally delayed after burns of the buttocks or extensive rectal surgery (by administration of paregoric orally) to prevent additional trauma.

22-10	**Causes of postoperative constipation**
	Neuroendocrine response to stress (decreased gastrointestinal motility)
	Anesthetic agents
	Narcotics
	Inactivity
	Decreased intake of high-fiber foods

Assessment
1. Monitor daily for bowel movement. If absent, ask if patient is passing flatus.
2. After abdominal surgery, assess and record signs of returning peristalsis (bowel sounds, passing flatus).
3. Examine stool for amount and consistency; small dry, hard stool indicates constipation.

4. Assess for potential constipation:
   a. Narcotics given frequently or in high doses
   b. Inactivity
   c. Fluid intake less than 1200 ml/day
   d. Previous history of constipation

Intervention
1. Institute measures to *prevent* constipation for the first 2 or 3 days after major surgery:
   a. Facilitate fluid intake of 2000 to 3000 ml/day
   b. Encourage maximal activity within prescribed limits
   c. Provide bathroom privileges as early as possible
2. If no bowel movement within 3 or 4 days after surgery:
   a. Give prune juice, if permissible and desirable
   b. Consult physician about a laxative order. A hypertonic (Fleet) enema or small soapsuds enema may be necessary if laxative is ineffective
   c. Encourage intake of foods high in fiber, if permissible

Maintaining activity

Pathophysiology. Early ambulation has been a significant factor in hastening postoperative recovery and preventing postoperative complications. Numerous benefits are derived from the exercise of getting in and out of bed and walking during the early postoperative period (see Box 22-11 and Fig. 22-16). Ambulation is usually contraindicated when there is a severe infection or thrombophlebitis.

22-11	**Effects of early postoperative ambulation**
	Increased rate and depth of breathing
	Prevention of atelectasis and hypostatic pneumonia
	Increased mental alertness from increased oxygenation to brain
	Increased circulation
	Nutrients required for healing are more available to wound
	Prevention of thrombophlebitis
	Increased kidney function
	Increased micturition
	Decreased pain
	Increased metabolism
	Prevention of urinary retention
	Prevention of loss of muscle tone
	Restoration of nitrogen balance
	Increased peristalsis
	Promotion of expulsion of flatus
	Prevention of abdominal distention and gas pains
	Prevention of constipation
	Prevention of paralytic ileus

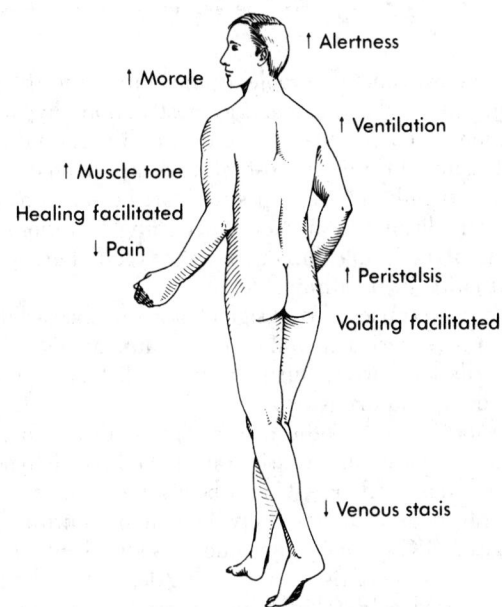

↑ Alertness

↑ Morale

↑ Ventilation

↑ Muscle tone

Healing facilitated

↓ Pain

↑ Peristalsis

Voiding facilitated

↓ Venous stasis

Fig. 22-16   Benefits from early postoperative ambulation.

Assessment. Before helping the patient to ambulate for the first few times after major surgery, an assessment is made of the patient's level of alertness to follow directions, cardiovascular status, and motor status:

1. Level of alertness: ask patient simple questions or to follow simple commands
2. Cardiovascular status
   a. Assess pulse and respiratory rate and depth while supine, then after sitting
   b. Observe skin color for pallor while sitting
   c. Note complaints of dizziness when sitting
3. Motor status
   a. Assess muscle strength of legs
   b. Assess sitting ability:
      (1) Assist patient to sitting position on side of bed
      (2) Ask patient to maintain an erect position while being gently pushed sideways.

It is also important to know of any limitations to ambulation present preoperatively. The patient with arthritis or arteriosclerosis may take longer to move and to adjust to standing and walking. The patient who used a walker preoperatively will need assistance for a longer time before progressing to using the walker again.

Intervention

1. Encourage muscle-strengthening exercises before ambulation:
   a. Bend knees, lower knees, press back of knees hard against bed.
   b. Alternately contract and relax calf and thigh muscles 10 times using the following cycle: contract, relax, rest.

2. Have patient sit on side of bed (legs dangling) to become accustomed to upright position before ambulating the first time. Be sure *pulse has stabilized* (returned to baseline) before ambulation is attempted:
   a. Clamp off nasogastric tube until patient has ambulated, then reconnect.
   b. Keep urinary tube connected to drainage bag; carry bag or pin bag to inside of robe.
   c. Attach intravenous bag to a movable pole.
4. Use two people to assist a weak patient receiving intravenous fluids to ambulate.
5. Encourage patient to walk farther at each ambulation.

The word *ambulate* means to move from place to place, to walk. Sitting in a chair is not considered ambulation. After ambulating, the patient may sit in a chair if permitted, but should be advised to stand and walk at intervals and to elevate the legs while sitting to prevent venous pooling in the extremities. Sitting in a chair for long periods is to be avoided.

Helping meet psychologic needs

Psychologic factors. Some of the concerns that were present preoperatively may continue into the postoperative period. These concerns fall into essentially three categories: concerns specific to the surgery performed, concerns over loss of a body part, and concerns about the future. Future concerns include those related to changes in sexuality, economic status, prognosis, or permanent effects. Sexuality may be threatened by enforced absence from home or by a specific surgical procedure. Sexual concerns may center around the effect of the surgery on the spouse relationship or on sexual performance itself.

Assessment. Anxieties will be expressed in many different ways. It must be remembered that expressions such as anger, resentfulness, crying, excessive joking, inappropriate laughter, or withdrawal may all be signs of anxiety and are often seen in the postoperative period. Some of these feelings may be projected against the surgeon, nurse, housekeeping aide, food, and such.

Intervention. Sitting down and talking with surgical patients about their concerns is as important a nursing action in many instances as any of the physical activities. Time must be planned for this. If a specific concern is expected, such as sexual functioning after a perineal prostatectomy, the topic may have to be introduced by the nurse who has established rapport with the patient in order to let the patient know that it is permissible to talk about it.

Evaluation

Evaluation is based on the identified outcomes, which vary greatly, depending on the type of surgery performed and the patient response to surgery. Questions to consider include the following:

1. Have postoperative complications or injury been avoided?

2. Is the incision healing well?
3. Are breath sounds clear and have atelectasis and pnuemonia been avoided?
4. Has thrombophlebitis been avoided?
5. Has overhydration been avoided?
6. Does the person state feeling comfortable?
7. Has weight been stabilized?
8. Have usual elimination patterns been reestablished?
9. Does the person carry out ADL at an optimal level and ambulate at prescribed levels?
10. Has the person had an opportunity to explore concerns related to surgery?
11. Does the person know the medication therapy, treatments, dietary restrictions, or activity prescription to be carried out at home and when to report for follow-up care?

DISCHARGE PLANNING

During hospitalization the patient and family should be prepared for any care that must be given at home, and any necessary arrangements for convalescent care should be completed before discharge. Because patients are discharged earlier than in the past, discharge planning must begin as soon as possible. Patients are helped to become as self-sufficient as possible before being discharged so they do not have to depend any more than necessary on the assistance of relatives and friends.

If dressings are needed, the patient may be given a 48-hour supply to take home unless a family member has already obtained them. The patient and family must know where in the community they can get dressings and other needed materials. A community health nurse is a useful resource person when treatment of almost any kind is to be provided at home.

On discharge the patient is given an appointment for a follow-up examination in the surgeon's office or clinic. This appointment is usually for 1 to 2 weeks after discharge. The patient should understand the importance of returning for the medical examination, (which is usually included in the surgeon's operating fee).

With modern surgical techniques the wound usually heals well within 1 week. Therefore, the convalescent period usually is relatively short, and most patients may return to their usual activities and occupation within 2 to 4 weeks. Normal activities should be resumed gradually. Driving is usually permitted 2 weeks after major surgery, but the patient should avoid any heavy lifting, pushing, or pulling for at least 6 weeks following surgery.

SUMMARY

1. The most common problems encountered in the postanesthetic phase are airway obstruction, hypoventilation, hypotension, cardiac dysrhythmias, and pain.
2. Measures to prevent postanesthesia pulmonary problems include side-lying position, artificial airway until patient begins to awaken, suctioning secretions that patient is unable to cough up, oxygen therapy, and initiation of breathing exercises.
3. Common causes of vital sign changes in the early postoperative period include shock, pain, anxiety, hypoventilation, jarring during transfer, distended urinary bladder, and drugs.
4. Postoperative hypothermia may cause discomfort, hypertension, cardiac dysrhythmias, and tissue hypoxia.
5. Narcotics in the PACU may be given intramuscularly, intravenously, intrathecally, by patient-controlled analgesia (PCA), or by continuous epidural infusion.
6. Regeneration of tissue or scarring depend on the types of injured cells (skin, mucous membrane, muscles, nerves) and intactness of the underlying structure.
7. Healing by primary or tertiary intention involves suturing the incision, immediate or delayed; healing by secondary intention consists of filling the area in from the bottom.
8. Responses that occur following tissue injury include stress, inflammatory, immune, and generalized body responses followed by wound healing.
9. Phase I of wound healing includes the inflammatory response, reestablishment of blood flow across the wound, and initiation of epithelialization.
10. Phase II of wound healing consists mainly of filling in the spaces with collagen and completing epithelialization.
11. During the phases III and IV of wound healing, further collagen is deposited, compressing the new blood vessels, then shrinking and contracting.
12. Interventions to promote wound healing include intake of protein and vitamin C, avoidance of antiinflammatory drugs, and prevention of wound infection and of fluid build-up in wound spaces.
13. Wound dehiscence (separation of wound edges) and wound evisceration (protrusion of viscera through incision) may be prevented during phase II of wound healing by early institution of ventilatory exercises, ambulation, adequate fluid intake, and aseptic technique during dressing changes.
14. Persons at high risk for postoperative pulmonary complications are those with increased or dry respiratory secretions, decreased thorax expansion, decreased diaphragm mobility, depression of respiratory center by drugs, or aspirated gastric contents.
15. Measures to prevent postoperative thrombophlebitis include providing elastic stockings for persons at high risk, avoiding pressure on popliteal area or leg massage, and encouraging leg exercises and early ambulation.
16. Water intoxication or pulmonary edema are more likely to occur postoperatively in elderly persons receiving intravenous fluids.

17. Incisional pain can be relieved or modified by medication in combination with encouraging the person to move in bed and ambulate, teaching relaxation and distraction techniques, and supporting injured parts.
18. Gas pains may be relieved by ambulation, avoidance of very hot or cold liquids, specific exercises or massage, rectal tubes, heat to the abdomen, and enemas.
19. Causes of weight loss after surgery include catabolism and inadequate nutrient intake plus additional nutrient usage for healing. This leads to loss of stored nutrients.
20. The patient is monitored in the early postoperative period for urinary retention; measures are taken to encourage voiding.
21. Constipation may be prevented postoperatively by encouraging maximal fluids and ambulation, as permitted, and by providing bathroom privileges as early as possible.
22. Early ambulation increases alertness, ventilation, muscle tone, and peristalsis; decreases pain and venous stasis; facilitates healing and voiding; and promotes increased morale.

STUDY QUESTIONS

* After the same type of major surgery, in what ways should the general postoperative care differ between a male athlete aged 25 and a man aged 75 with arthritis of hands and hips? Explain the rationale for your answer.
* Examine the charts of two or three postoperative patients.
  * What changes in vital signs occurred during the early postoperative period as compared to the preoperative baseline? What were the possible reasons for these changes?
  * What types of preventive respiratory measures were used and what was the effect? What other nursing actions could have been taken?
  * Did any postoperative complications occur? If so, what risk factors were present? How could the complication have been prevented?
  * How did the patients compare in their response to postoperative ambulation? Did some need more encouragement than others? What positive effects would ambulation have for each patient?

REFERENCES AND SELECTED READINGS

1. Atsberger DB, et al: Postoperative pain management in the PACU: nurse's challenge, *J Post Anesth Nurs* 3:399-403, 1988.
2. Augustine SD: Hypothermia therapy in the postanesthesia care unit: a review, *J Post Anesth Nurs* 5:254-265, 1990.
3. Blansett MT: The effects of rewarming hypothermic postanesthesia patients using thermadrape covering, heat lamps, and warmed cotton blankets, *J Post Anesth Nurs* 5:80-84, 1990.
4. Bragg CL: Practical aspects of epidural and intrathecal narcotic analgesia in the intensive care setting, *Heart Lung* 18:599-608, 1989.
5.* Bray CA: Postoperative pain: altering the patient's experience through education, *AORN J* 43:672-683, 1986.
6.* Brozenec S: Caring for the postoperative patient with an abdominal drain, *Nursing 85* 15(4):55-57, 1985.
7.* Burge S, et al: How painful are postop incisions? *Am J Nurs* 86:1263-1265, 1986.
8.* Carroll PF: Artificial airways: real risks, *Nursing 86* 16(8):56-59, 1986.
9.* Cerrato PL: What diet does for wound healing, *RN* 51(6):73-77, 1988.
10.* Closs SJ: An exploratory analysis of nurses' provision of postoperative analgesic drugs, *J Adv Nurs* 15:42-49, 1990.
11. Coleman DL: Control of postoperative pain: nonnarcotic and narcotic alternatives and their effect on pulmonary functioning, *Chest* 92:520-528, 1987.
12.* Crocker DG: Acute postoperative pain: cause and control, *Orthop Nurs* 5(2):11-15, 1986.
13. David JA: *Wound management,* Springhouse, Penn, 1988, Springhouse.
14.* Deters GE: Managing complications after abdominal surgery, *RN* 50(3):27-32, 1987.
15. Drain CB, Christoph SS: *The recovery room: a critical care approach to postanesthesia nursing,* ed 2, Philadelphia, 1987, WB Saunders.
16. Ehrenwerth J, Donielson D: Pulse oximetry in the postanesthesia care unit, *J Post Anesth Nurs* 2: 9-11, 1987.
17.* Erhardt BS: Pulse oximetry: an easy way to check oxygen saturation, *Nursing 90* 20(3):50-54, 1990.
18.* Fay MF: Drainage systems: their role in wound healing, *AORN J* 46:442-455, 1987.
19. Fraulini KE, Borchardt AC: Guide to solving postanesthesia problems, *Nursing 88* 18(5):66-86, 1988.
20. Fulk C, Hadley JC: Something for pain: new trends in epidural analgesia, *J Post Anesth Nurs* 5:247-253, 1990.
21.* Gilbert HC: Pain relief methods in the postanesthesia care unit, *J Post Anesth Nurs* 5:6-15, 1990.
22. Hargreaves A, Lander J: Use of transcutaneous electrical nerve stimulation for postoperative pain, *Nurs Res* 38(3):159-161, 1989.
23. Heffline MS: Exploring nursing intervention for acute pain in the postanesthesia care unit, *J Post Anesth Nurs* 5:321-328, 1990.
24. Jackson MF: Implications of surgery in very elderly patients, *AORN J* 50:859-866, 1989.
25.* Kearns PC: Exercises to ease pain after abdominal surgery, *RN* 49(7):45-48, 1986.
26. Kennedy-Caldwell C: The morbidly obese surgical patient, *Crit Care Nurse* 7(5):87-89, 1987.
27. Kneedler J, Dodge G: *Perioperative patient care,* ed 2, Boston, 1987, Blackwell Scientific Publications.
28.* Kresl JS: Patient-controlled analgesia, *AORN J* 48:481-487, 1988.
29.* Latz PA, Wyble SJ: Elderly patients: perioperative nursing implications, *AORN J* 46:238-253, 1987.
30.* Leeson IL: Pain and the postoperative patient, *Nursing (Oxford)* 2:1289-1290, 1985.
31. Lemmink JA: Infection control: when a surgical wound becomes infected, *RN* 50(9):24-27, 1987.
32.* Litwack K, Lubenow T: Practical points in the management of continuous epidural infusions, *J Post Anesth Nurs* 5:327-330, 1989.
33.* Litwack K, Parnass S: Practical points in the management of postoperative nausea and vomiting, *J Post Anesth Nurs* 3:275-277, 1988.
34.* McCaffery M: Narcotic analgesia for the elderly, *Am J Nurs* 85:296-298, 1985.
35. Meeker MH, Rothrock JC: *Alexander's care of the patient in surgery,* ed 9, St Louis, 1990, Mosby–Year Book.

*Recommended for student reading.

36.* Miller KM: Deep breathing relaxation: a pain management technique, *AORN J* 45:484-488, 1987.

37.* Miracle VA: How to perform basic airway management, *Nursing 90* 20(4):55-60, 1990.

38.* Montanari J: Wound dehiscence, *Nursing 86* 16(20):33, 1986.

39. Morttenson M, McMullin C: Discharge score for surgical outpatients, *Am J Nurs* 86:1347-1348, 1986.

40. Murray SE: Patient assessment in the postanesthesia care unit: a critical care approach, *J Post Anesth Nurs* 4:232-238, 1989.

41. Musgrave SF: Acute postoperative pain: the cause and the care, *J Post Anesth Nurs* 5:329-337, 1990.

42.* Neuberger GB: Wound care: what's clear, what's not, *Nursing 87* 17(20):34-37, 1987.

43.* Neuberger GB, Richling JB: A new look at wound care, *Nursing 85* 15(2):34-41, 1985.

44.* Nichols RR: Simple remedies for postoperative gas pain, *RN* 49(2):42-44, 1986.

45.* Powell AH, Bethbova M: How do you give continuous epidural fentanyl? *Am J Nurs* 89:1197-1198, 1989.

46. Roth RA, Verbridge N: Surgical wound surveillance, *AORN J* 47:722-729, 1988.

47. Rothrock JC: *Perioperative nursing care planning*, St Louis, 1990, Mosby–Year Book.

48.* Rowland MA: Myths and facts about postop discomfort, *Am J Nurs* (5):61-64, 1990.

49. Short LM, et al: Medicating the postoperative elderly: how do nurses make their decisions? *J Gerontol Nurs* 16(7):12-17, 1990.

50.* Smith CE: *Detecting abdominal distention: what to look for, what to do.* In *The Nursing Institute's CE test handbook*, vol 3, Hicksville, NY, 1988, Springhouse.

51.* Spyr J, Preach MA: Pulse oximetry: understanding the concept, knowing the limits, *RN* 53:38-43, 1990.

52. Stone HH: Infection in postoperative patients, *Am J Med* 81(1A):39-44, 1986.

53. Torrington DG: Perioperative respiratory therapy (PORT): a program of preoperative risk assessment and individualized postoperative care, *Chest* 93:946-951, 1988.

54. Villamiel LM: Help! This postanesthesia care unit patient is hypothermic, *J Post Anesth Nurs* 5:75-79, 1990.

55. Warfield CA: Management of postoperative pain, *Hosp Pract* 24(5A):53-59, 1989.

56. Way LW: *Current surgical diagnosis and treatment*, ed 9, Los Altos, Calif, 1991, Appleton & Lange.

57. Wild L, Coyne C: Epidural analgesia: the basics and beyond, *Am J Nurs* 92(4):26-36, 1992.

58. Williams SR: *Essentials of nutrition and diet therapy*, ed 5, St Louis, 1990, Mosby–Year Book.

59.* Wound management: Update 88, *Nursing 88* 18(6):33-37, 1988.

60.* Wysocki AB: Surgical wound healing, *AORN J* 49:502-518, 1989.

Gas Transport Problems

23

The Patient
with
Nose and Throat
Problems

Wilma J. Phipps

After studying this chapter, the learner should be able to:

- Describe pathophysiologic bases of upper respiratory infections and therapeutic modalities.
- Discuss the nursing care of persons having nose and sinus surgery and tonsillectomy.
- Describe etiology and symptoms of cancer of the larynx and postoperative care following surgery.
- Write a nursing care plan for a person having a radical neck dissection.

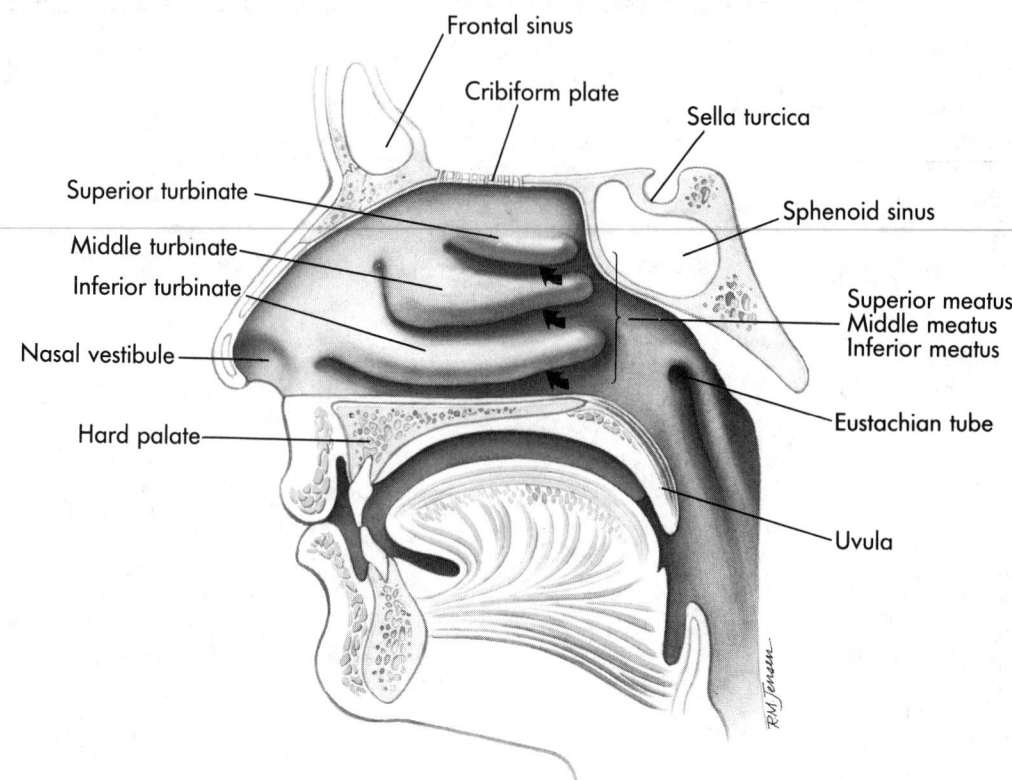

Fig. 23-1 Lateral wall of nose, showing superior, middle, and inferior turbinates. (From DeWeese DD, et al: *Otolaryngology—head and neck surgery,* ed 7, St Louis, 1988, Mosby–Year Book.)

Disorders of the nose and throat are very common, and nurses in particular are often asked to give advice about these problems. To be effective, nurses need a basic understanding of the structure and function of the organs of the upper airway, as well as knowledge of the medical and nursing regimens for problems affecting the upper airway.

ANATOMY AND PHYSIOLOGY

Nose and Sinuses

The nose is supported by the nasal bones, the nasal processes of the maxillary bones, the cartilaginous and bony parts of the septum, and the upper and lower nasal cartilages. The septum, which divides the nares, is rarely straight in adults because at some time it has been injured.

The nasal cavities are located between the roof of the mouth and the frontal, ethmoid, and sphenoid bones. Three projections, which are lined with mucous membrane and called the *turbinate bones,* are located on the lateral walls of each nasal cavity (Fig. 23-1). Their purpose is to increase the mucous membrane surface over which air passes as it travels to the nasopharynx, thus allowing for precipitation of inhaled particles and warming and moistening the inhaled air.

The mucous membrane posterior to the vestibule (anterior part) of the nose contains cilia that beat in a constant wavelike motion to carry mucus into the nasopharynx.

Trapped in the mucus are bacteria, dust, and other foreign matter entering the nose. The olfactory epithelium is located in a small area superiorly and provides the end organ of smell.

There are four sets of paranasal sinuses located on either side of the head (Fig. 23-2). These sinuses are air-filled spaces in the skull that drain into the nasal cavities through openings behind the turbinates. The maxillary sinuses are the largest and most accessible. The sinuses are lined with mucous membrane continuous with that of the nose.

Upper Throat: Pharynx and Tonsils

The pharynx is the space behind the oral and nasal cavities that extends from the base of the skull to the larynx. The pharynx can be considered in three parts: the nasopharynx, the oropharynx, and the laryngopharynx (Fig. 23-3). It is lined with mucous membrane.

The opening of the eustachian tubes and the adenoids are located in the nasopharynx, the palatine tonsils anterior to the oropharynx, and the lingual tonsils in the hypopharynx. The adenoids and tonsils are lymphoid tissue that help to filter the circulating lymph of bacteria or other foreign matter that penetrate the body, especially by way of the nose or mouth.

The oral pharynx serves both the respiratory and digestive systems. In the lower regions of the laryngopharynx the *larynx* and *esophagus* form separate passageways for air and food.

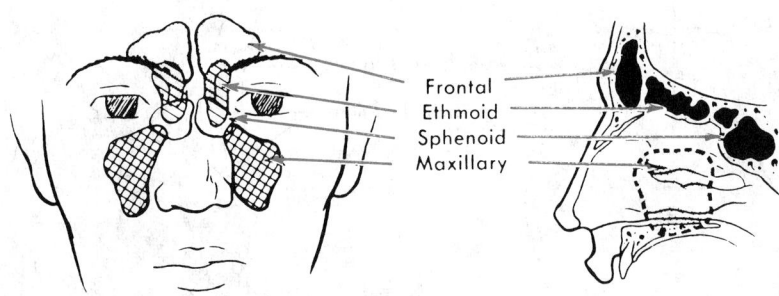

Fig. 23-2   Location of sinuses.

Frontal
Ethmoid
Sphenoid
Maxillary

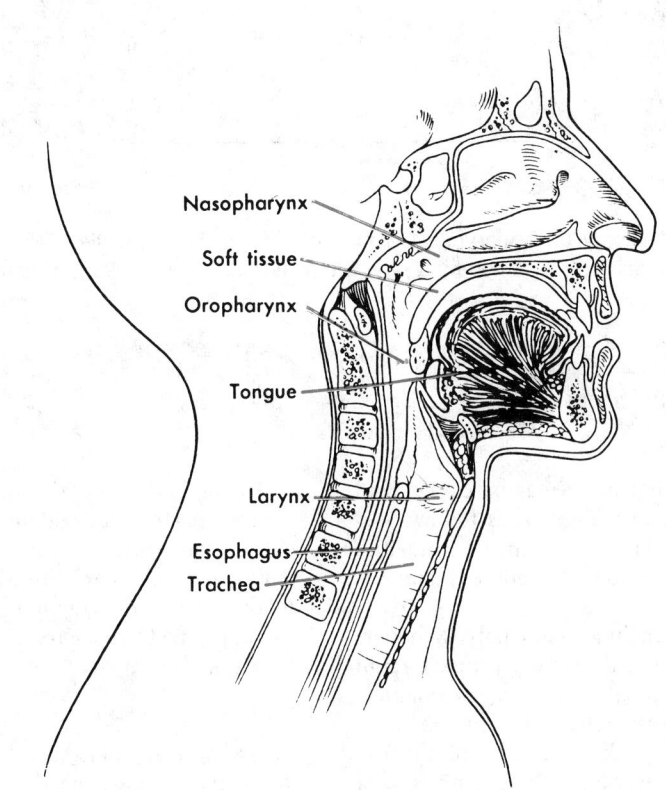

Nasopharynx
Soft tissue
Oropharynx
Tongue
Larynx
Esophagus
Trachea

Fig. 23-3   Sagittal section of head showing pharynx and larynx.

Lower Throat: Larynx and Laryngopharynx

The larynx ("voice box") forms the upper extremity of the trachea. The framework of the larynx is made up of several cartilages held together by muscle and ligaments (Fig. 23-4). The cartilaginous framework protects the vocal cords and affords a stiffness that permits an airway. The thyroid cartilage, the "Adam's apple," is the largest cartilaginous element in the larynx and protects the inner structures. The hyoid bone forms an attachment for the larynx and tongue. The larynx is lined with mucosa continuous with that of the laryngopharynx and trachea. The vagus nerve innervates the larynx.

The chief function of the larynx is to serve as an airway between the pharynx and trachea. A leaf-shaped lid of fibrocartilage (epiglottis) protects the glottis by covering the entrance to the larynx during swallowing to prevent aspiration of food or fluids. The closing of the glottis also allows for an increase of intrathoracic pressure, which is needed, for example, in coughing or lifting. This increased pressure increases the use of the muscles of the shoulder and thorax.

In addition, a most important function of the larynx is phonation. The larynx creates sounds as a result of vocal cord vibrations that are formed into speech patterns by the movement of the pharynx, palate, tongue, teeth, and lips.

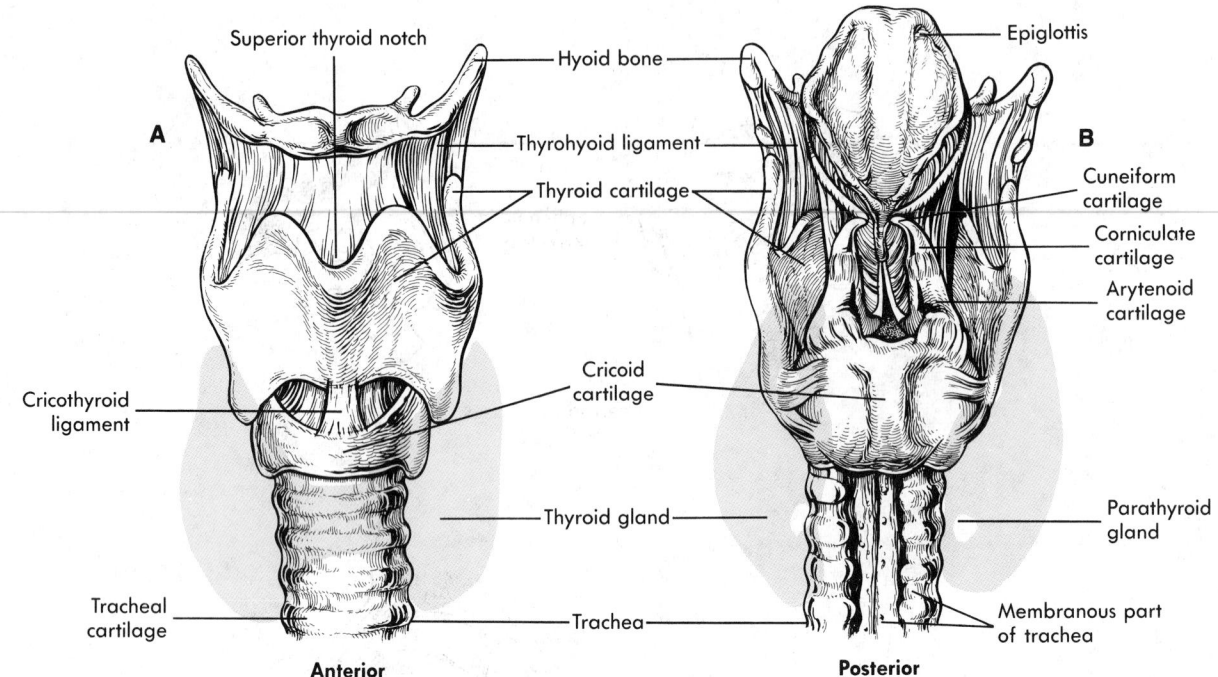

Fig. 23-4 Anatomy of the larynx. **A,** Anterior view. **B,** Posterior view. (From Seeley RR, Stephens TD, and Tate P: *Anatomy & physiology,* ed. 2, St Louis, 1992, Mosby–Year Book.)

MAJOR HEALTH PROBLEMS OF THE NOSE AND THROAT

Most disorders of the nose and throat may be categorized as inflammatory, obstructive, or malignant as follows:

1. Inflammatory disorders include rhinitis, sinusitis, pharyngitis, tonsillitis, peritonsillar abscess, and laryngitis.
2. Obstructive disorders include nasal polyps, hypertrophy of the turbinates, a deviated septum, foreign bodies, and fractures (nasal, maxillary, zygomatic). Airway obstruction is discussed in Chapter 24.
3. Malignant disorders include carcinoma of the nasopharynx, of the maxillary and ethmoid sinuses, of the tonsil, and of the larynx.

INFLAMMATIONS OF THE NOSE AND SINUSES

Inflammations may develop in the nose and sinuses (Table 23-1). A more detailed discussion of these conditions follows.

Etiology

Inflammations of the upper airway structures may result from numerous viruses and bacteria. Many filtrable viruses (such as the more than 100 identified rhinoviruses, adenovirus, echovirus, influenza and parainfluenza viruses, and coxsackievirus) may serve as etiologic agents of inflammations. Bacteria include primarily streptococci, staphylococci, and pneumococci.

Inflammations of the nose and sinuses, are often an allergic reaction to pollens of grasses and flowers, dust, animal dander, wool, and certain foods. Maxillary sinusitis may also occur as an extension of infection from abscessed teeth and tooth extraction, because the apices of many of the upper teeth roots are in close contact with the mucosal lining of the sinus.

Pathophysiology

Signs and symptoms seen with inflammations of the nose and throat result from the inflammatory process. Redness and edema of the mucous membrane occur early. Discharge from the nose and sinuses include fluid exudate from the inflammatory process (which may be serous or purulent if infection is present), as well as mucous secretions. General malaise and fever are part of the systemic response to inflammation.

INFECTIONS OF THE NOSE AND SINUSES

The skin around the external nose is easily irritated during acute attacks of rhinitis or sinusitis. Furunculosis and cellulitis occasionally develop. Infections around the nose are extremely dangerous because the venous blood supply from this area drains directly into the cerebral venous sinuses. Septicemia, therefore, can occur easily, and for this reason no pimple or lesion in the area should ever be

Table 23-1   Infections of the nose and sinuses

Disorder	Signs and symptoms	Medical therapy
Acute rhinitis (coryza, common cold)	Initial: dryness of mucous membranes, chills, general malaise 12-24 hrs: profuse watery discharge, sneezing, tearing of eyes	Rest, fluids, moist inhalations, antihistamines and decongestants
Allergic rhinitis (hay fever)	Sneezing, nasal obstruction, watery nasal discharge, frontal headache, itching of eyes and nose	Separation of person from sensitizing allergens, desensitization, antihistamines; topical nasal steroids
Chronic rhinitis	Stuffiness and pressure in the nose; nasal discharge, which may be serous, mucopurulent or purulent; polyp formation; frontal headache; vertigo; sneezing	Antibiotics, avoidance of the offending allergens, antihistamines, polypectomy may be necessary
Sinusitis		
Acute	Constant severe headache, pain over sinuses, orbital edema, nasal discharge, fever	Rest, analgesics, oral nasal decongestants, systemic antibiotics, local heat, topical nasal decongestants
Chronic	Chronic purulent nasal discharge, dull sinus headache, loss of ability to smell	Surgery; sinus irrigations

squeezed or "picked." Hot packs may be used. If any infection in or around the nose persists or shows even a slight tendency to spread or increase in severity, a physician should be consulted.

RHINITIS
Etiology/Epidemiology

Rhinitis refers to inflammation of the mucous membrane of the nose. It may be acute or chronic.

Acute rhinitis (coryza, common cold) is an inflammatory condition of the mucous membranes of the nose and accessory sinuses caused by a filtrable virus. It affects almost everyone at some time and occurs most often in the winter, with additional high incidence in early fall and spring. Some of the known causes of the common cold are more than 100 seratypes of rhinoviruses, adenoviruses, echoviruses, influenza and parainfluenza viruses, and coxsackievirus. The common cold is spread by droplet nuclei from sneezing, and the condition is contagious for the first 2 to 3 days.

Most persons with colds contaminate their hands when coughing or sneezing, contaminating everything they touch. Others can become infected when touching the telephone, computer, or anything else that has been touched by the person with the cold. Also, many colds are believed to be spread when shaking hands with the person who has a cold.

Secondary invasion by bacteria may complicate the cold, possibly causing pneumonia, bronchitis, sinusitis, and otitis media.

Allergic rhinitis (hay fever) can be acute and seasonal when caused by the pollens of grasses and flowers, or it may be chronic and perennial when associated with numerous allergens, such as house dust, animal dander, wool, and certain foods.

Chronic rhinitis is a chronic inflammation of the mucous membrane caused by repeated acute infections, by an al-

---

23-1

Correct administration of nose drops

1. Wash hands.
2. Assume a position that facilitates flow of medication.
   a. Sit in chair and tip head well backward, or
   b. Lie down with head extended over edge of bed, or
   c. Lie down with pillow under shoulders and head tipped backward
3. Turn head to side that receives the drops.
4. Place no more than 3 drops of solution into each nostril at one time (unless otherwise prescribed).
5. Remain in position with head tilted backward for 5 minutes to permit solution to reach posterior nares.
6. If marked congestion is still present 10 minutes after nose drop insertion, another drop or two of solution may be administered (nasal constriction of swollen mucosa from first insertion may facilitate additional drops reaching posterior nares).

---

lergy, or by vasomotor rhinitis. The cause of vasomotor rhinitis is unclear, but this condition may result from an instability of the autonomic nervous system caused by stress, tension, or some endocrine disorder. Often it is mistaken for nasal allergy, but the allergen cannot be identified. Formation of nasal mucus is increased, leading to a runny nose. Rhinitis can also be caused by the overuse of nose drops (*rhinitis medicamentosa*); a rebound phenomenon occurs after the immediate effect of the nose drops with the return to congestion. Discontinuing use of the nose drops usually clears up this condition within a week or two. The correct administration of nose drops is listed in Box 23-1.

Table 23-2   Signs and symptoms of rhinitis

	Acute rhinitis	Allergic rhinitis	Chronic rhinitis
Nasal discharge	Initially watery, then mucoid	Thin, watery	Serous, mucopurulent, or purulent
Eyes	Tearing during early phase	Tearing, itching	No tearing
Turbinates	Edematous	Pale, edematous, mucoid	Enlarged
Nasal polyps	No	Yes	Yes
Headache	Generalized	Frontal	Frontal

In all forms of rhinitis sneezing, nasal discharge with nasal obstruction, and headache are present, but the form of these symptoms varies with the type of rhinitis (Table 23-2). Acute rhinitis also includes signs of acute inflammation (early chilliness followed by "feverishness" and malaise). A painful throat is not always associated with a cold. However, the pharynx may feel sore because of early dryness followed by irritation from postnasal drainage. If uncomplicated, the cold is usually self-limiting and lasts for about 1 week.

In chronic rhinitis acute symptoms are absent. The chief complaint is nasal obstruction accompanied by a feeling of stuffiness and pressure in the nose. Polyp formation (p. 491) may occur and vertigo may be present.

Interventions

No specific treatment is available for the common cold. Over-the-counter cold remedies usually contain one or more drugs, including antihistamines, sympathomimetics, and analgesics. Differences of opinion exist concerning the effectiveness of antihistamines in relieving cold symptoms. If taken during the onset of the cold, the allergic manifestations (sneezing, tearing, watery discharge) may be relieved; use during the latter stages may only cause drowsiness. Sympathomimetic drugs (such as phenylephrine [Neosynephrine] and phenyl-propanolamine) are nasal decongestants and help to relieve the nasal stuffiness. Vitamin C has no significant protective or inhibitory effect on colds.[10] Antibiotics are used only for complicating secondary infections. Nursing management of the person with a cold centers around teaching (Box 23-2). Also see the Nursing Process section under Sinusitis (p. 485).

Nose drops are sometimes recommended for infrequent use (every 4 hours for a few days) if there is some nasal obstruction. Many otolaryngologists now believe that the frequent use of nose drops results in rhinitis medicamentosa, an "addiction" of the nasal mucosa to their use.[10] Some physicians believe that the obstruction of the nose may be a protective device that prevents the spread of infection to other parts of the body.

For allergic rhinitis, the treatment consists of maintaining an allergen-free environment (see Chapter 41). Hyposensitization or desensitization (administering the allergen in gradually increasing doses to establish an "immunity") may be helpful. Antihistamines give relief to most persons, but their effectiveness often decreases as the "hay fever season" continues.

For chronic rhinitis, antihistamines may give relief. When nasal obstruction persists, surgery may be necessary

Patient Teaching

23-2

The patient with rhinitis

Get additional rest
Drink at least 2 to 3 L fluid per day
Medications
    Antihistamines
        Effective only during initial period of cold
        Be cautious about their sedative effects when driving or working with heavy machinery
    Nose drops: use correct procedure (see Box 23-1)
Prevention of further infection
    Blow nose with both nostrils open to prevent infected matter from being forced into eustachian tube
    Cover mouth with disposable tissues when coughing and sneezing to prevent droplet nuclei from entering the air
    Dispose of used tissues carefully
    Avoid exposure when possible (that is, avoid crowds, people with colds, specific allergens). Elderly persons and those with chronic lung disease are particularly vulnerable
Wash hands frequently and especially after coughing, sneezing, and so on. Evidence suggests that many colds are transmitted from person to person by hand contact and from touching objects handled by person with a cold.
Seek medical attention if the following are present:
High fever, severe chest pain, earache
Symptoms lasting longer than 2 weeks
Recurrent colds

to remove polyps (polypectomy) or to remove tissue obstruction (septoplasty).

Nasal irrigations are now seldom used in the treatment of chronic rhinitis. Details of the procedure are described in texts on fundamentals of nursing or otolaryngology. Care should be taken to ensure that both nostrils are open and that the pressure in the nostrils is not excessive (the irrigating container should not be higher than 12 to 15 in above the level of the nose). Excess pressure may force infected material into the sinuses or the middle ear.

SINUSITIS

Etiology/Epidemiology

The sinuses are air-filled cavities lined with mucous membrane. Any inflammation of the mucous membranes of the

Table 23-3   Sinusitis: signs and symptoms and treatment

Type	Signs and symptoms	Medical therapy
Acute suppurative sinusitis	Stuffy nose, slowly developing pressure over involved sinus. General malaise, toxicity, headache, slightly elevated or normal temperature	Antibiotics for 14 days. Cefaclor, cefuroxime axetil, penicillin V, and erythromycin are effective against the three most common pathogens. Bed rest, humidity, hydration, decongestations, and expectorants. *Antihistamines should be avoided.* Relief of pain may require codeine or meperidine. Wet hot packs over affected sinus continuously or for 1-2 hr, four times a day
Subacute suppurative sinusitis present in about 10% of patients	Persistent purulent nasal discharge that lasts longer than 2 weeks but less than 4 weeks	Vasoconstrictors, heat, and irrigation of involved sinus
Chronic suppurative sinusitis	Purulent nasal discharge, persistent nasal congestion, postnasal drip, halitosis, anosomia, and sometimes sinus headache. Persistent headache requires surgical consult	A small percentage of patients may be cured by repeated irrigation, antihistamines, and antibiotics. Most patients require surgery: Caldwell-Luc surgery most common surgical procedure

sinuses is called *sinusitis*. This is still a frequent disorder, although it is less common since the advent of antibiotics. Often patients who complain of sinusitis do not have a sinus infection but some other disorder. When an otolaryngologist refers to sinusitis, *a bacterial invasion of the mucous membrane is implied.* Only about 10% of the patients who consult an otolaryngologist because of "sinus trouble" are diagnosed as having sinusitis.

Sinusitis is classified as follows:

- Acute suppurative
- Subacute suppurative
- Chronic suppurative
- Allergic
- Hyperplastic

The most common cause of *acute suppurative sinusitis* is the obstruction of the paranasal sinuses that blocks the egress of secretions from the sinuses. These secretions become infected, giving rise to acute suppurative sinusitis. The organisms most often responsible are *Streptococcous pneumoniae*, beta-hemolytic *Streptococcus*, *Haemophilus influenzae*, coagulase-positive *Staphylococcus aureus*, and *Klebsiella pneumoniae*. More than 50% of maxillary sinus infections are caused by *S. pneumoniae* and *H. influenzae*. Another 30% are caused by anerobic bacteria, which are often dental in origin. *Cultures are not helpful* because multiple organisms are usually found.

Acute Suppurative Sinusitis

The signs and symptoms of acute suppurative sinusitis are listed in Table 23-3. Symptoms worsen over 48 to 72 hours until there is severe localized pain and tenderness over the involved sinus (see Box 23-3). The patient often believes

---

23-3

Location of pain with sinusitis

Sinus	Pain location
Maxillary	Over cheek and upper teeth (Fig. 23-5)
Frontal	Above the eyebrow (Fig. 23-5)
Ethmoid	Medial and deep in the eye. (Fig. 23-5)
Sphenoid	Deep behind the eye, over the occiput, or top of head

---

that the pain is due to an infected tooth. Pain is localized and may be referred to another site (Fig. 23-5).

In acute frontal and maxillary sinusitis, pain usually does not appear until 1 to 2 hours after awakening. It increases for 3 to 4 hours and then becomes less severe in the afternoon and evening.

There may be bloody or blood-tinged discharge from the nose in the first 24 to 48 hours. The discharge rapidly becomes purulent and copious, blocking the nose. The throat may become inflamed and sore on one side because of the purulent discharge.

On examination, the involved nasal mucosa is hyperemic and edematous, and the turbinates are enlarged. X-ray films show that the involved sinus is clouded, and a fluid level is visible (Fig. 23-6). Usually the diagnosis is established without radiographs. If there are recurrent episodes of acute sinusitis, radiographs or CT scan are indicated to rule out underlying pathology.

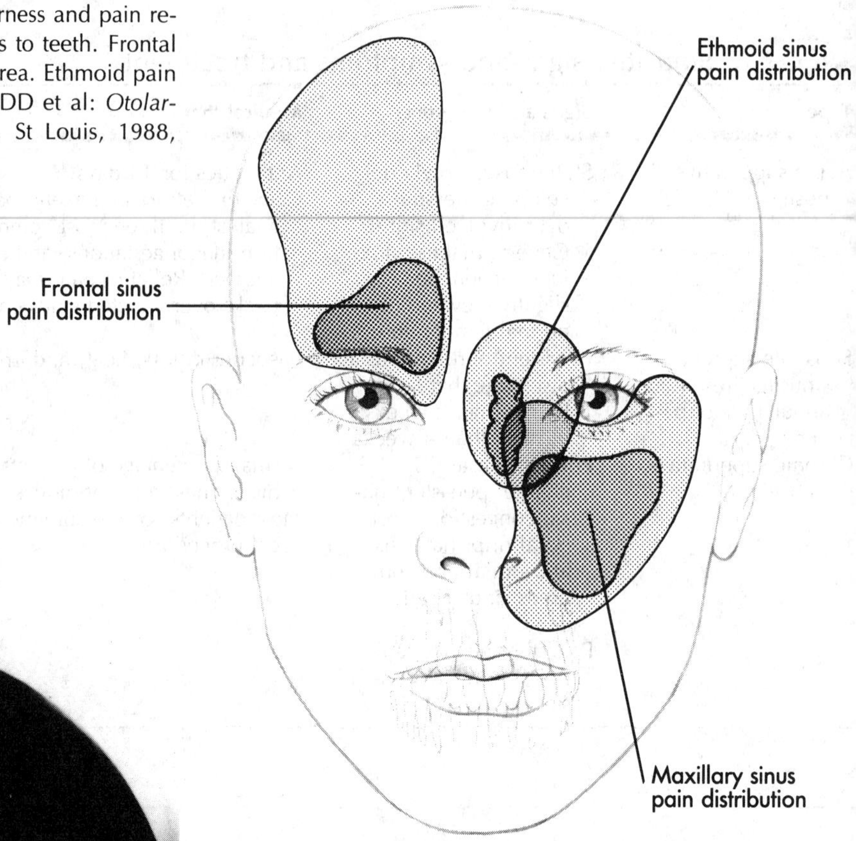

Fig. 23-5 Sinus pain—area of local tenderness and pain referral. Maxillary sinus pain frequently refers to teeth. Frontal pain is generally localized to supraorbital area. Ethmoid pain is generally deep to eye. (From DeWeese DD et al: *Otolaryngology—head and neck surgery*, ed 7, St Louis, 1988, Mosby–Year Book.)

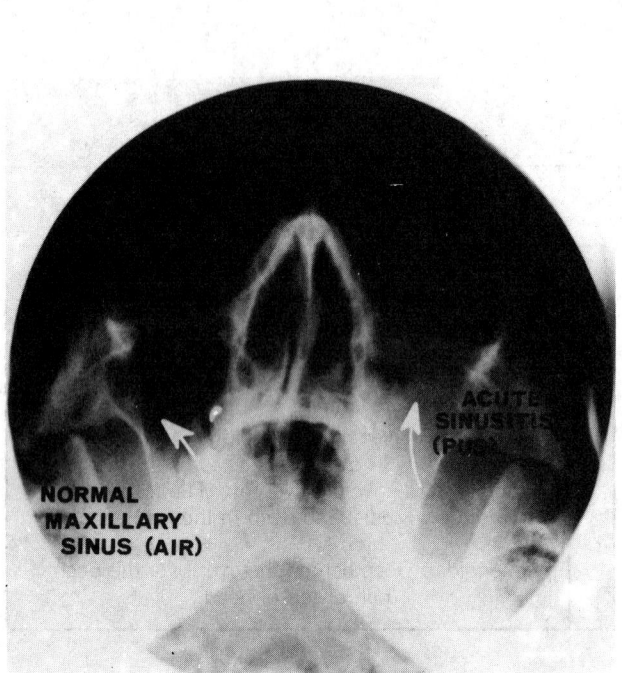

Ethmoid sinus pain distribution

Frontal sinus pain distribution

Maxillary sinus pain distribution

Fig. 23-6 Roentgenogram of maxillary sinus showing normal sinus on left and acute sinusitis on right. (From Saunders, WH, et al: *Nursing care in eye, ear, nose, and throat disorders*, ed 4, St Louis, 1979, Mosby–Year Book.)

Subacute Suppurative Sinusitis

The measures described in Table 23-3 under Medical Therapy cure more than 90% of patients with acute suppurative sinusitis. A subacute infection persists in the remaining 10%. Persistent purulent discharge is the only constant symptom. A radiograph or CT scan is indicated to determine whether one or more sinuses are involved. Because it is uncommon for acute sinusitis to persist, the causative organism may be unusual.[10] Special culture techniques may be necessary, and antibiotics sensitivity studies are essential. The most commonly isolated organisms are *H. influenzae*, *H. pneumoniae* and *Branhamella catarrhalis*. *B. catarrhalis* is not sensitive to penicillin or amoxicillin,

and treatment requires systemic sulfonamide therapy or erythromycin with a sulfonamide. Pain is not severe and requires no medication. Treatment consists of vasoconstriction of nasal mucosa, heat, and irrigation of the involved sinus (Table 23-3).

Antral irrigation, in which the anterior wall of the maxillary sinus is punctured, is the preferred treatment for subacute sinusitis. Anesthesia is obtained with an injection of 2 to 3 ml of 1% lidocaine (Xylocaine) with 1:100,000 epinephrine under the upper lip. A 16-gauge needle (with stylet in place) is rotated through the soft tissue and bone (Figs. 23-7 and 23-8). When proper placement of the needle is assured, saline solution is instilled to wash out the sinus. Antibiotic solutions may be used, but mechanical cleansing is more important than the solution used.[10]

It is not possible to irrigate the ethmoid sinuses directly, and *ethmoiditis* is treated with systemic antibiotics. The antibiotics should be continued for 10 to 14 days.[10] Proper treatment of subacute sinusitis is the best means of preventing *chronic suppurative sinusitis*.

Chronic Suppurative Sinusitis

When suppurative sinusitis is not treated or is inadequately treated during the acute or subacute phase, or when the mucosa is damaged from recurrent attacks, permanent change may occur. Bacteria can invade the tissue of the sinuses, become walled off, and produce chronic inflammation. With prolonged infection of soft tissue, pathologic change may become irreversible and the patient has *chronic suppurative sinusitis*.[10]

The most common and sometimes only symptom is purulent nasal discharge. In a small percentage of patients,

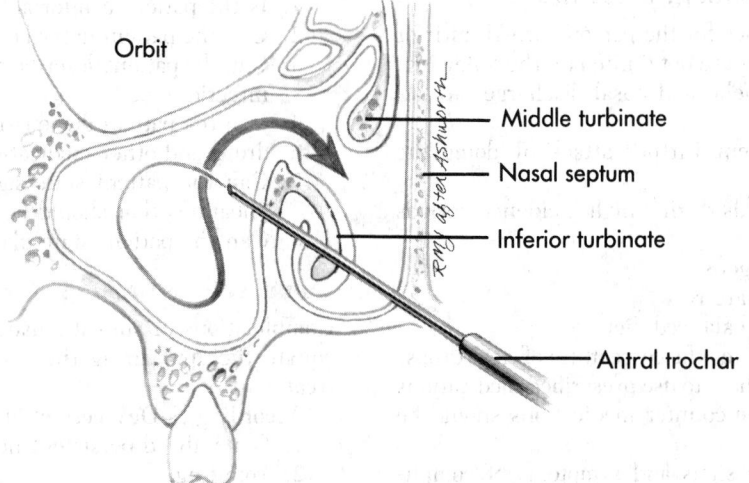

Orbit

Middle turbinate

Nasal septum

Inferior turbinate

Antral trochar

Fig. 23-7   Trochar inserted under the inferior turbinate (through the medial wall of the antrum). Contents of the sinus are washed into the nose through the natural ostium. (From DeWeese DD, et al: *Otolaryngology—head and neck surgery*, ed 7, St Louis, 1988, Mosby—Year Book.)

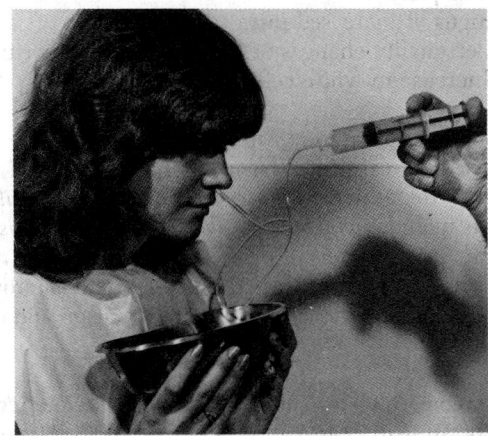

Fig. 23-8   Irrigation of the maxillary sinus. With the head tipped forward, solution returns via the natural ostium and out the anterior nose for examination and/or culture. (From DeWeese DD, et al: *Otolaryngology—head and neck surgery*, ed 7, St Louis, 1988, Mosby—Year Book.)

repeated irrigation, antihistamines, and antibiotics may cure the disease. However, most patients must be treated surgically. Surgical treatment is discussed on p. 486. *Anosomia* (loss of smell) or *parasomia* (a perverted sense of smell) may result from nasal blockage.

Nursing Process
Assessment
Subjective data
1. Obstruction of nares
   a. History of mouth breathing—time of day or night when it occurs, duration and frequency
   b. History of nasal surgery or injury to nose
   c. Use of nasal drops or spray—type, amount, frequency, and duration of use
2. Nasal discharge
   a. Color, amount, and consistency of discharge
   b. Prevalence of discharge—early AM, constant flow, and so on
   c. Nasal bleeding (epistaxis)—one or both nares
   d. Presence of nasal crusting or pain
3. History of sinusitis
   a. Headaches—location and severity
   b. Relationship of sinusitis to certain seasons or types of weather
4. Other general symptoms such as malaise

Objective data
1. Fever and drainage (serous, mucopurulent, purulent) in laryngopharynx
2. Polyps (pale, soft, edematous out-pouching of nasal mucosa)—may be present and are usually bilateral in inflammations of the nose and sinuses
3. Redness and edema of mucous membrane

Diagnostic tests
1. Culture of nose or throat for causative organism
2. Radiographs of sinuses are used to determine the presence and extent of the disease and whether there is involvement of the bony walls (Fig. 23-6). When an infection is present, the film appears cloudy. In persons with chronic sinusitis the sinus radiographs demonstrate thickening of the mucous membrane and diffuse cloudiness.

Data analysis: nursing diagnoses
Nursing diagnoses are determined from analysis of patient data. Possible nursing diagnoses for the person with rhinitis or sinusitis may include, but are not limited to, the following:

Diagnostic title	Possible etiologies
Pain: headache, throat, sinus	Inflammation in nose or sinuses
Knowledge deficit	Lack of exposure to information or misinterpretation of information

Planning: expected patient outcomes

Expected patient outcomes for the person with rhinitis or sinusitis may include, but are not limited to, the following:

1. Symptoms (headache and nasal discharge) are alleviated.
2. Patient can prevent further attack by doing the following:
   a. Avoiding crowds during high-incidence periods of infection
   b. Avoiding allergens
   c. Getting adequate rest
   d. Eating a well-balanced diet
3. Patient demonstrates the correct use of nose drops.
4. Patient can state how to use prescribed medications and what over-the-counter medications should be avoided.
5. Patient can state signs and symptoms of complications (bleeding, increased temperature, increase in drainage, change in color of drainage) that should be reported to the physician.
6. Patient states plans for follow-up care.

Implementation

Assisting with achievement of therapeutic goals
Medications

1. Give medications as prescribed (antihistamines, decongestants, antibiotics).
2. Provide an allergen-free environment. (See Chapter 41.)

Interventions to achieve patient outcomes
Assisting with comfort and ADL

1. Apply local heat as prescribed.
2. Provide moist inhalations as prescribed.

Facilitating learning

1. Avoid factors that contribute to the sinusitis.
   a. Avoid chilling and cold, damp atmospheres.
   b. Avoid air conditioning when outside air is warm and moist if this precipitates sinus irritation.
   c. Avoid smoking (further irritates damaged mucous membranes).
   d. Avoid fatigue.
   e. Try to avoid upper respiratory tract infections.
   f. Protect nose during swimming; avoid diving.
   g. Inform dentist of chronic sinus condition before tooth extraction.
2. If allergens are a contributing factor, prepare an environmentally controlled bedroom (Chapter 41).
3. Use acetaminophen rather than aspirin for pain relief; apply moist heat over sinus.
4. During an acute sinus infection, get additional rest and drink 2 to 3 L fluids per day.
5. Take antibiotic for prescribed time period, even if symptoms abate.
6. Keep room temperature constant (changes in room temperature aggravate sinusitis).

Evaluation

Evaluation is based on the expected outcomes for patients with rhinitis or sinusitis. Questions to consider may include the following:

1. Is the patient comfortable?
2. Can the patient describe the required care at home?
3. Can the patient describe measures to prevent further infection?
4. Can the patient demonstrate the correct use of nose drops and other medications?
5. Can the patient state signs and symptoms of complications that should be reported to physician?
6. Can the patient state plans for follow-up care?

Complications of Sinusitis

Complications of sinusitis usually are the result of inadequate therapy during the acute stage or by a delay in treatment.

According to DeWeese et al.[10] complications include:
1. Generalized persistent headache
2. Vomiting
3. Convulsions
4. Chills or high fever
5. Edema or increasing swelling of the forehead or eyelids
6. Blurring of vision, diplopia, or persistent retroocular pain
7. Signs of increased intracranial pressure
8. Personality changes or dulling of the sensorium
9. Increase in white cell count above 20,000

Orbital complications. Most orbital infections (75%) are caused by extension from paranasal sinusitis. Most frequently the ethmoid sinuses are involved. *Orbital complications* include *inflammatory edema, orbital cellulitis, subperiosteal abscess, orbital abscess,* and *cavernous sinus thrombosis.* Complications are treated vigorously with appropriate antibiotics and, in the case of abscess, incision and drainage.

Cavernous sinus thrombosis. This very serious complication of sinusitis can cause death in 48 to 72 hours if untreated. More than 25% of patients who develop this complication will die even when adequately treated. The primary treatment is with intravenous antibiotics.

Cavernous sinus thrombosis occurs when there is extension of infection through the venous pathways (usually the angular vein) to the cavernous sinus. The patient is very ill, with chills and a temperature as high as 41° C (106° F). Pain is deep behind the eye and the patient becomes toxic and may become semicomatose.

Surgery of the Sinuses

Treatment of *chronic suppurative sinusitis* involves surgery to remove all diseased soft tissue and bone, adequate postoperative drainage, and obliteration of the sinus cavity where possible. The goal of surgery is to eradicate infection and leave contiguous structures normal. Preoperative teaching is outlined in Box 23-4.

Caldwell-Luc surgery

The Caldwell-Luc procedure is the generally accepted operative procedure for chronic maxillary sinusitis. It is also called a *radical antrum* operation. Local or general anesthesia may be used.

Preoperative teaching for sinus surgery

Determine what patient understands about the surgical procedure. Clarify misconceptions and answer patient's questions. Explain that he or she:

- Will have nothing to eat or drink 6 to 8 hours preoperatively.
- Will receive sedative medication before surgery.
- Will feel pressure, not pain, during surgery.
- Will have a nasal pack for 24 to 48 hours postoperatively.
- Will have a mustache dressing postoperatively.
- Will have some ecchymosis and swelling around the nose and eyes for 1 to 2 weeks postoperatively.

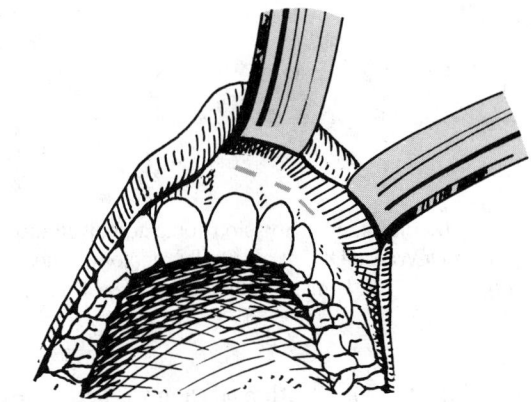

Fig. 23-9   The incision into the maxillary sinus (Caldwell-Luc surgery) is made under the upper lip.

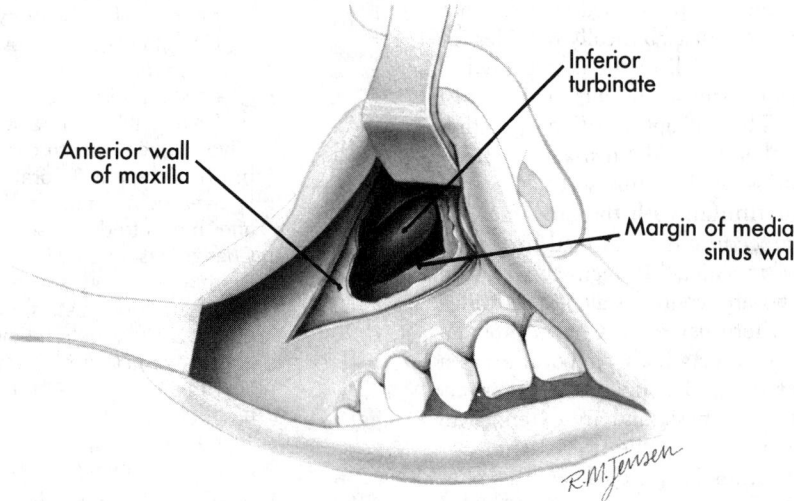

Fig. 23-10   After removal of the sinus mucosa or polypoid tissue, a window is made into the nose along its floor, allowing dependent drainage from the maxillary sinus. Incision is closed with absorbable sutures. (From DeWeese DD, et al: *Otolaryngology—head and neck surgery,* ed 7, St Louis, 1988, Mosby–Year Book.)

The procedure is performed through an incision under the upper lip (Fig. 23-9). Part of the anterior bony wall of the antrum is removed, producing a permanent window (Fig. 23-10). All of the diseased mucosa and periosteum is removed through the window. The bone of the lateral wall of the nose in the inferior meatus, which divides the nose from the antrum, is removed.[10] The mucous membrane and periosteum of the lateral wall of the nose are preserved, and fashioned into a hinged flap.

The antrum may be packed to prevent bleeding. Packing is removed through the nose 24 to 48 hours postoperatively. As the maxillary sinus heals, the exposed bone is covered by mucosa. Numbness of the upper lip and upper teeth may be present for several months after a Caldwell-Luc operation because some nerves to these structures pass through the site of the incision. Interference with eating occurs initially. Only liquids are given for at least 24 hours, followed by a soft diet for several days.

In addition to general care of the patient following sinus surgery, patient teaching specific to Caldwell-Luc surgery includes the following:

1. Do not chew on affected side until incision heals.
2. Use caution with oral hygiene to avoid injury to the incision.
3. Avoid wearing dentures for about 10 days.
4. Avoid blowing nose for about 2 weeks after packing has been removed.

Ethmoidotomy and ethmoidectomy

The external approach is preferred for ethmoid surgery because it allows better visualization and reduces the risks of complications such as damage to the optic nerve and central spinal fluid leak. Ethmoidotomy is an opening made for drainage, whereas an ethmoidectomy entails removal of ethmoid tissue (Table 23-3). The incision is made in the inner half of the eyebrow downward along the side of

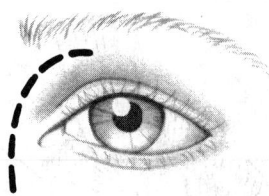

Fig. 23-11 Medial canthal incision for external ethmoidectomy. (From DeWeese DD, et al: *Otolaryngology—head and neck surgery,* ed 7, St Louis, 1988, Mosby—Year Book.)

the nose (Fig. 23-11).[22,31] Ethmoidectomy is performed for correction of nasal polyps and for ethmoiditis because nasal polyps frequently originate in the ethmoid cells.

Osteoplastic flap surgery

The advent of the osteoplastic flap operation makes frontal sinus surgery different from that performed on the other sinuses. Surgery of the other sinuses basically provides for an open, well-drained cavity, which in the past proved to be inadequate for the frontal sinuses because recurrence of disease was common. The osteoplastic flap operation allows for complete removal of diseased mucosa of the frontal sinus and for obliteration of the sinus so that it is no longer functional or in continuum with the inner nose.

The osteoplastic flap procedure is performed through a "gull-wing" or "cross-bow" incision.[53] In men, the incision extends along the eyebrows and connects along the bridge of the nose. In women, where baldness is not a problem in later life, the incision connects both temporal areas a few centimeters posterior to the hairline. Both incisions give excellent postoperative cosmesis and are extended to the periosteum of the bone overlying the frontal sinus.

The skin overlying the sinus is reflected, and a radiograph of the frontal sinus (obtained preoperatively) is used as a template for sawing the lateral and superior borders of the anterior frontal bone. The anterior bone is then reflected inferiorly, thus exposing the entire contents of the frontal sinus. The mucosa is removed under direct vision, and an operating microscope is used to ensure that all fragments of mucosa are removed. An incision is then made in the left-lower abdominal quadrant and subcutaneous fat obtained for placement into the frontal sinus cavity. The bony flap and skin are then repositioned. Nasal packs are not required.

Postoperatively, pain in the frontal area is not significant after 24 hours. Pain in the abdominal area, however, often lasts several days and serous drainage from this area is common after the drain is removed. Sutures are removed about the fifth postoperative day. *Because nasal packs are not used, special oral hygiene care is not needed.*

Postoperative care for sinus surgery

Care of the patient following sinus surgery is described in Box 23-5. Gauze packing is usually inserted into the nares and removed after 48 hours. The patient thus breaths through the mouth, with subsequent dryness of mouth and lips. Mouth care is required, and warm or cool vapor inhalations often are prescribed. If there is an oral incision,

---

23-5

Guidelines for Care

Postoperative care of the patient following surgery of sinuses

1. After general anesthesia, position patient well onto the side to prevent swelling or aspiration of bloody drainage.
2. When the patient is awake, remind him or her to expectorate secretions and not swallow them.
3. Encourage mid-Fowler's position when fully awake to promote drainage and decrease edema.
4. Apply ice compresses over nose (or ice bag over maxillary or frontal sinuses) in the early postoperative period.
5. Monitor the patient for:
    a. Excessive bleeding from nose (may be evidenced by repeated swallowing).
    b. Decreased visual acuity, especially *diplopia*, indicating damage to optic nerve or muscles of globe of eye.
    c. Complaints of pain over the involved sinus, which may indicate infection or inadequate drainage.
    d. Fever—take temperature rectally.
6. Give frequent mouth care using a soft toothbrush. If there is an oral incision, mouth care is given before meals to improve appetite and after meals to decrease danger of infection.
7. Change nasal pad when it is soiled.
8. Apply ice compresses to ecchymotic areas to constrict blood vessels, decrease oozing and edema, and to help relieve pain.
9. Encourage liberal fluid intake. Patient may be very thirsty because of dry mouth from mouth breathing.
10. Teach patient to:
    a. Avoid blowing nose for at least 48 hours after packing is removed to prevent bleeding.
    b. Report signs of infection (fever, purulent discharge) to surgeon.
    c. Expect tarry stools from swallowed blood for a few days.
    d. Avoid constipation (Valsalva maneuver can cause bleeding).
    e. Expect that ecchymosis of nose and eyes will begin to change color over next 1 to 2 weeks.
    f. Take prophylactic antibiotics as prescribed. Do not stop until all medication is taken.

---

mouth care is given before meals to improve appetite and after meals to decrease danger of infection. Antibiotics may be prescribed prophylactically. For 1 or 2 weeks swelling or ecchymosis may be present around the nose and eyes. Ice compresses will constrict blood vessels, decreasing oozing and edema, and help relieve pain.

REVIEW

Table 23-4   Infections of the pharynx and larynx

Disorder	Signs and symptoms	Medical therapy
Pharyngitis Acute	Redness and soreness of throat, difficulty in swallowing, fever Hacking cough	Warm saline gargles, ice collar, aspirin, moist inhalations, antibiotics, anesthetic lozenges may be given
Tonsillitis Acute follicular	Sudden onset of sore throat, dysphagia, fever, chills, malaise	Rest, fluids, warm saline gargles, ice collar, antibiotics, analgesics; tonsillectomy may be necessary when recurrent infections do not respond to antibiotics
Laryngitis Acute	From slight huskiness to total voice loss, sore throat, dry harsh cough	Symptomatic treatment, voice rest; steam inhalations; avoidance of smoking and being near those who are smoking

INFECTIONS OF THE PHARYNX AND LARYNX

ACUTE PHARYNGITIS

Etiology/Epidemiology

Acute pharyngitis is the most common throat inflammation. It may be caused by hemolytic streptococci, staphylococci, or other bacteria or viruses. There is an increased incidence of gonococcal pharyngitis caused by the gram-negative diplococcus *Neisseria gonorrhoeae*. The disease is increasingly found in both men and women who engage in oral-genital sex. When gonorrhea is suspected, a throat culture should be obtained.

A severe form of acute pharyngitis often is referred to as *strep throat* because of the frequency of streptococci as the causative organisms.

Symptoms usually precede or occur simultaneously with the onset of acute rhinitis or acute sinusitis. Pharyngitis can occur after the tonsils have been removed because the remaining mucous membrane can become infected. Pharyngitis is also a common manifestation of infectious mononucleosis.

Pathophysiology

Table 23-4 summarizes the signs and symptoms and therapy for infections of the pharynx and larynx. Nursing care includes the points listed in Box 23-6 and in the following discussion:

1. Give medications as prescribed. Penicillin or erythromycin may be prescribed prophylactically to prevent superimposed infections, especially in persons with a history of rheumatic fever or bacterial endocarditis.
2. If the diagnosis is gonococcal pharyngitis, the patient will need instruction in how to avoid reinfection (see Chapter 18).
3. Provide moist inhalations and ice collar if ordered.
4. Provide a liquid diet with at least 2-3 L of fluids.
5. Bedrest if temperature is elevated; otherwise, extra rest.

23-6

Patient Teaching

Teaching for the patient with an infection of the nose or throat

1. Get additional rest (hastens recovery)
2. Drink at least 2 to 3 L of fluid every day
3. Medications
   a. Antihistamines are effective primarily during the initial period only; care should be taken when driving or working with heavy machinery when taking antihistamines
   b. Take prescribed antibiotics for bacterial infections for the prescribed period of time
   c. If using nose drops:
      (1) Place no more than 3 drops of solution in each nostril at one time (unless otherwise prescribed)
      (2) Keep head tilted back for about 5 minutes to permit solution to reach posterior nares
      (3) Insert 1 to 2 additional drops after 10 minutes if marked congestion is still present
   d. If using atomizer:
      (1) Occlude opposite nostril with finger pressure to prevent entrance of air
      (2) Administer no more than 3 sprays of solution in each nostril at one time
4. Promote throat comfort through use of the following:
   a. Warm saline gargles
   b. Ice collar
   c. Throat lozenges
   d. Moist inhalations
5. Avoid further upper respiratory infections
   a. Avoid direct exposure to others with respiratory infections, if possible
   b. Teach all persons to cover nose and mouth with tissue when coughing or sneezing
   c. Wash hands after disposing of tissues
6. Explain rationale for prophylactic antibiotics for persons with a history of rheumatic fever or bacterial endocarditis
7. Medical attention is required for recurring symptoms (fever, excessive pain, dysphagia, expectoration of pus)

ACUTE FOLLICULAR TONSILLITIS
Etiology/Epidemiology

Acute follicular tonsillitis is an acute inflammation of the tonsils and their crypts. It is usually caused by the *Streptococcus* organism. It is more likely to occur when the person's resistance is low and is very common in children. (See Table 23-4 for summary of signs and symptoms and medical therapy.)

Complications of untreated tonsillitis include heart and kidney damage, chorea, and pneumonia. Incidence of these complications is decreasing with the widespread use of penicillin and early diagnosis.

Interventions

Most physicians believe that persons who have recurrent attacks of tonsillitis should have a tonsillectomy. This procedure is usually performed from 4 to 6 weeks after an acute attack has subsided.

23-7

Guidelines for Care

Postoperative care of the patient following tonsillectomy

1. Side-lying position until awake, then mid-Fowler's
2. Monitor for signs of hemorrhage
   a. Repeated swallowing
   b. Vomiting of bright red blood
   c. Increased pulse rate while sleeping
3. Diet
   a. Offer fluids when vomiting has ceased
   b. Encourage patient to take large swallows (more comfortable than small sips)
   c. Avoid using a straw (suction may cause bleeding)
   d. Ice-cold fluids better tolerated
   e. Offer bland nourishment:
      Ice cream, cold custards, cream soups, and bland juices (for example, pear) offered initially
      Refined cereal and soft-cooked egg usually better tolerated morning after surgery
      Avoid citrus juices, hot fluids, rough or highly seasoned foods for 1 week
4. Relieve throat discomfort:
   a. Apply ice collar as desired
   b. Give prescribed analgesic (avoid aspirin, which can increase bleeding)
5. Teach patient about the following:
   a. Avoid vigorous exercise, coughing, sneezing, clearing throat, and vigorous nose blowing for 1 to 2 weeks
   b. Report signs of bleeding immediately to physician
   c. Drink fluids (2 to 3 L/day) until mouth odor disappears
   d. Stools may be tarry for several days from swallowed blood
   e. Throat discomfort may increase slightly between fourth and eighth postoperative day (membrane separation)

Because the person with acute tonsillitis is usually cared for at home, the nurse should help in teaching the general public the care that is needed (Box 23-6 outlines teaching priorities). The office nurse, the clinic nurse, the nurse in industry, the school nurse, and the community health nurse have many opportunities to do this teaching.

Tonsillectomy

Tonsillectomy for the adult may be performed under local or general anesthesia. Hemorrhage may occur postoperatively. The physician may be able to control minor postoperative bleeding by applying a sponge soaked in a solution of epinephrine to the site. The person who is bleeding excessively often is returned to the operating room for ligation or cauterization of the bleeding vessel. If sutures must be used, the person has more pain and discomfort than following a simple tonsillectomy. The patient may not be able to take solid food for several days. Some surgeons no longer prescribe aspirin for pain after tonsillectomy, as it increases the tendency to bleed. Acetaminophen or another aspirin substitute is usually ordered.

A tough, yellow, fibrous membrane that forms over the operative site begins to break away between the fourth and eighth postoperative days, and hemorrhage may occur. The separation of the membrane accounts for the throat being more painful at this time. Pink granulation tissue soon becomes apparent, and by the end of the third postoperative week, the area is covered with mucous membrane of normal appearance.

Postoperative care is outlined in Box 23-7.

LARYNGITIS
Simple Acute Laryngitis

Simple acute laryngitis is an inflammation of the mucous membrane lining the larynx and is accompanied by edema of the vocal cords. It may be caused by a cold, by sudden changes in temperature, by irritating fumes, by excessive use of the voice, or excessive smoking. Symptoms vary from a slight huskiness to complete loss of voice. The throat may be painful and feel scratchy, and a cough may be present. (See Table 23-4 for signs and symptoms and therapy.)

Chronic Laryngitis

Some people who use their voices excessively, who smoke a great deal, or who work continuously where there are irritating fumes develop a chronic laryngitis. Hoarseness usually is worse in the early morning and in the evening. There may be a dry, harsh cough and a persistent need to clear the throat.

Treatment may consist of removal of irritants, voice rest, correction of faulty voice habits, steam inhalations, and cough medications. The physician may order spraying of the throat with an astringent antiseptic solution such as hexylresorcinol (S. T. 37). To carry out this procedure properly the patient must use a spray tip that turns down at the end so that the medication reaches the vocal cords and is not dissipated in the posterior pharynx. The spray

REVIEW

Table 23-5 Obstructions of the nose

Disorder	Signs and symptoms	Medical therapy
Nasal polyps	May cause anosmia, obstruction of breathing, blockage of sinus drainage	Aerosol sprays or polypectomy
Hypertrophy of turbinates	Nasal obstruction	Aerosols containing corticosteroids; cryosurgery or electric fulguration may be used
Deviated septum	Noisy, difficult breathing; postnasal drip; dry mucosa and crusts	Septoplasty or submucous resection
Foreign bodies	Nasal obstruction, discharge, bleeding	Topical vasoconstrictors; extraction of foreign body

tip is placed in the back of the throat with the bent portion behind the tongue. The patient should then take one or two deep breaths and spray the medication on inhalation. This procedure may cause temporary coughing and gagging. Many medications used as throat sprays are now sold in plastic squeeze bottles with tube and spray tip attached.

OBSTRUCTIVE DISORDERS OF THE NOSE

Trauma or polyps in the nose, nasal bones, turbinates, maxillary bones, and zygomatic bones may cause obstruction (Table 23-5). Many persons with obstructions of the nose may be diagnosed and treated on an ambulatory basis.

Etiology

Obstruction may be caused by a deviated septum, either congenital or, more commonly, as a result of trauma. Allergy and chronic sinusitis may lead to the development of nasal polyps, grape-like growths of mucous membrane and loose connective tissue in the sinus mucosa. Fractures of the nasal, maxillary, and zygomatic bones may result from falls, motor vehicle accidents, and fights. Displaced fragments from the fracture obstruct passage of air. Malignant growths may also cause obstruction.

Nosebleeds may result from a number of causes (see Box 23-8). When the bleeding stops, some nasal obstruction may occur from the blood clot until the mucosa heals. In adulthood, nosebleeds are more common in men than in women.

NASAL POLYPS
Pathophysiology

Nasal polyps are grapelike growths of mucous membrane and loose connective tissue. They are usually bilateral and are usually caused by allergic rhinitis. Polyps cause *anosmia* by preventing air from reaching the olfactory mucosa high in the nose.

23-8 **Common causes of nosebleeds**

Local irritation of superficial blood vessel
Trauma
Chronic infection
Lack of humidity in air breathed
Violent sneezing or noseblowing
Nose picking (most common cause)

Systemic causes
Hypertension
Blood dyscrasias (for example, leukemia)
Deficiency in vitamin K

Interventions

Because they may obstruct breathing or block sinus drainage, nasal polyps are removed surgically if they do not respond to treatment with aerosol sprays containing corticosteroids. Even when they do respond to corticosteroid sprays, polyps reappear when the steroids are discontinued.

HYPERTROPHY OF THE TURBINATES

Enlarged inferior turbinates sometimes cause considerable nasal obstruction. They may be medically treated by the use of aerosols containing corticosteroids such as dexamethosone (Decadron, Turbinaire). These aerosols are used for their antiinflammatory response and have proven effective for allergic and inflammatory nasal conditions as well as for treatment of nasal polyps.

Although not used as often since the advent of the corticosteroid aerosols, local surgery of the turbinates, such as cryosurgery or electric fulguration, may still be used to restore the airway. Resection of the hypertrophied mucosa may be necessary.

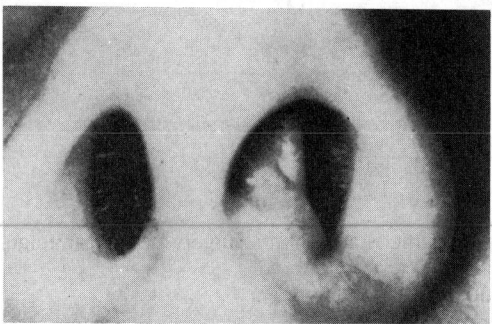

Fig. 23-12   Septal deviation. Anterior end of septal cartilage is dislocated and projects into nasal vestibule. (From Saunders, WH, et al: *Nursing care in eye, ear, nose, and throat disorders,* ed 4, St Louis, 1979, Mosby—Year Book.)

FRACTURES OF NASAL BONES AND SEPTUM

Fractures of the nasal bones and septum commonly occur from relatively minor injuries, such as falls, or from more severe injuries, such as automobile accidents or fights. If there is no displacement of the bone, no obstruction to the airway, and no cosmetic deformity, treatment is not needed. When airway obstruction or bone displacement occurs (Fig. 23-13), simple reduction is performed. Most simple nasal fractures can be reduced by applying firm pressure on the convex side of the nose. Nasal fractures should be reduced within the first 24 hours if at all possible. Local anesthesia is used. After 24 hours reduction becomes more difficult and may require general anesthesia.

FRACTURES OF MAXILLARY AND ZYGOMATIC BONES

Fractures of the maxillary and zygomatic bones are seen after automobile accidents and fights.[10] These fractures are generally reduced under anesthesia. Patients may also require wiring of the teeth with all the attendant problems of that procedure.

Nursing Process
Assessment
Subjective data

Symptoms of nasal obstructions include the following:
1. Noisy, difficult breathing
2. Dry mucosa
3. Postnasal drip
4. Nasal discharge
5. Anosmia
6. Bleeding from nose

If nasal trauma is present, additional symptoms include displacement of the bones, cosmetic deformity, pain, and ecchymosis around the eyes or jaw.

Objective data

1. Inspection for deformity or asymmetry
2. Some septal deviation is common in adults (Fig. 23-12) and is asymptomatic
3. Check for abnormal findings in nose.

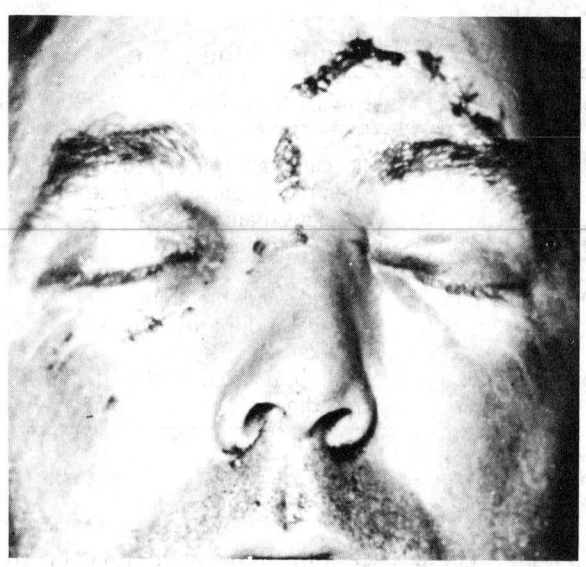

Fig. 23-13   Laterally displaced fracture of nose secondary to trauma. Pressure on convex side will restore alignment. (From Saunders WH, et al: *Nursing care in eye, ear, nose, and throat disorders,* ed 4, St Louis, 1979, Mosby—Year Book.)

a. Excessive redness
b. Edema
c. Exudate
d. Bleeding

Data analysis: nursing diagnoses

Nursing diagnoses are determined from an analysis of patient data. Possible nursing diagnoses for the person with obstruction of the nose may include, but are not limited to, the following:

Diagnostic title	Possible etiologies
Body image disturbance	Severe trauma/disfiguring surgery
Pain	Trauma/obstruction
Knowledge deficit	Lack of exposure to information, misinterpretation of information
Sensory/perceptual alterations: olfactory	Trauma/surgery

Planning: expected patient outcomes

Expected patient outcomes for the person with an obstruction of the nose may include, but are not limited to, the following:
1. Patient maintains positive body image.
2. Patient states he or she is comfortable.
3. Patient can state care required after surgery and discharge from hospital.
4. Patient knows how to prevent nosebleeds or to treat them if they occur.
5. Patient can state signs and symptoms of complications (bleeding, drainage, and fever) that need to be reported to the surgeon.
6. Patient can breathe more easily.

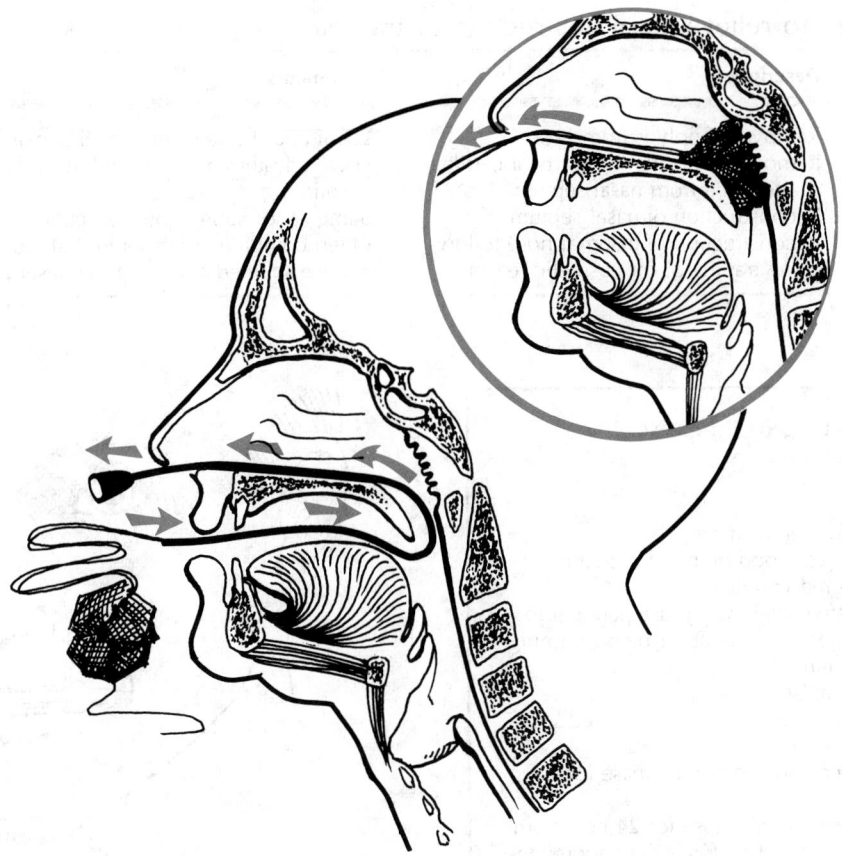

Fig. 23-14   Postnasal packing. Pack is attached to catheter then pulled through mouth to posterior nasopharynx.

Implementation
Assisting with achievement of therapeutic goals
Controlling nasal bleeding

Nosebleeds from the tiny blood vessels in the anterior part of the septum are usually controllable by compressing the soft tissue of the nose against the septum with a finger. Firm pressure should be maintained for at least 5 to 10 minutes, and it may be necessary for as long as 30 minutes. The person should breathe through the mouth during this time. Ice compresses may be applied over the nose; however, the primary benefit of the application of ice is that it requires the patient to remain still.

Bleeding may also be controlled by placing a cotton ball soaked in a topical vasoconstrictor such as phenylephrine (Neo-Synephrine) in the nose and applying pressure. Other first-aid measures include having the person sit quietly with the head up and inclined slightly forward to prevent blood from entering the pharynx and causing gagging or swallowing of blood. The person is instructed not to blow the nose for several hours after a nosebleed.

If these measures do not control bleeding, the help of a physician should be sought. After identifying the site of bleeding, the physician may cauterize the bleeding vessel with a silver nitrate stick or electrode cautery.

Bleeding from the posterior part of the nasal septum is more common in elderly persons and is more likely to be severe. If the bleeding point cannot be seen and cauterized,

a postnasal pack may be inserted (Fig. 23-14). Because this procedure is extremely painful and sometimes causes faintness, patients may be admitted to the hospital. Pain medication, antibiotic therapy, and sedation may also be ordered for a person with posterior packing. Sedation may be ordered, because bleeding tends to be increased by apprehension and restlessness. The pack is left in place for 2 to 5 days and then gently removed.

Severe bleeding results in a drop in blood pressure, which may cause the bleeding to stop; therefore, exsanguination from the usual nosebleed is rare. To prevent recurrent hemorrhage, the person is warned not to blow the nose vigorously and to avoid dryness of the nose. This can be accomplished by using saline or nasal lubricants.

Persistent or recurrent profuse epistaxis, especially posterior epistaxis, may require surgical ligation of the external carotid artery, the ethmoid artery, or the internal maxillary artery, all of which supply blood to the nose.

Nasal surgery

When there is obstruction of the nasal passages, surgery is usually necessary. The most common surgeries are presented in Table 23-6.

Polypectomy is usually performed under local anesthesia. Polyps are removed with a small snare or biting forcep, and the nostrils are packed for 24 hours. Because polyps tend to recur, especially if allergy is the underlying cause,

Table 23-6   Surgeries to relieve nasal obstruction or trauma

Procedure	Description	Comments
Nasal polypectomy	Removal of polyps from nose	Local anesthesia given; nasal packing for 24 hours
Submucous resection	Removal of obstructive parts of cartilage and bone from nasal septum	Local anesthesia given; both nostrils packed to provide splinting
Nasoseptoplasty	Reconstruction of nasal septum	Same as for submucous resection
Rhinoplasty	Reconstruction of external nose following trauma or for cosmetic reasons	Often combined with septoplasty following nasal trauma; nose splinted after surgery; nasal packing

---

Guidelines for Care   23-9

Postoperative care of the patient following nasal surgery

1. Assessment
   a. Monitor for hemorrhage
      (1) Excessive blood on nasal dressing
      (2) Bright red vomitus
      (3) Repeated swallowing (use penlight to check back of throat for blood running down throat)
      (4) Rapid pulse
   b. Monitor for infection: fever, elevated WBC
2. Discomfort
   a. Mid-Fowler's position to decrease local edema
   b. Ice compresses over nose for 24 hours prn
   c. Support and sedation for patient apprehension because of difficulty in breathing caused by blockage of nasal passages
   d. Frequent oral care
   e. Change dressing under nose prn
3. Nutrition
   a. Food as tolerated
   b. Encourage increased fluid intake
4. Patient teaching
   a. Avoid blowing nose for 48 hours after packing removed
   b. Avoid constipation (Valsalva maneuver) and vigorous coughing until healing occurs (can initiate bleeding)
   c. Expect stools to be tarry for several days
   d. Expect face to be discolored around eyes and nose for several days
   e. Cosmetic effect from nasal surgery cannot be judged for 6 to 12 months (time for tissue to return to normal and for scar resolution)
   f. Signs and symptoms of complications (bleeding, drainage, fever) that should be reported to the surgeon.

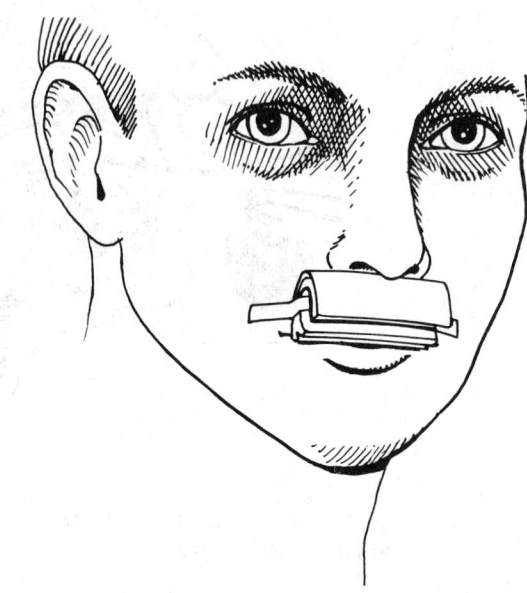

Fig. 23-15   Dressing placed under nose for nasal drainage.

usually performed under local anesthesia. With rhinoplasty, the nasal bones or cartilaginous framework of the nose are altered. The nose is usually protected with a plaster-of-Paris splint, adhesive tape dressing, or plastic mold following a plastic procedure on the nasal bones. Firm healing develops on about the tenth day. Usually only the surgeon changes a rhinoplasty dressing.

Monitoring after surgery

Following nasal surgery, the patient is placed in mid-Fowler's position to decrease local edema, and ice compresses are usually applied to the nose to lessen the discoloration, bleeding, and discomfort. Patients can usually apply their own ice compresses.

The patient is monitored for signs of hemorrhage (Box 23-9). Some oozing on the dressing below the nose (Fig. 23-15) is expected and this dressing may be changed as necessary. If bleeding becomes pronounced, the surgeon is notified and material for repacking the nose is prepared. This material consists of a hemostatic tray containing gauze packing, umbilical tape for posterior packing, a few small gauze sponges, small catheter (used for inserting a postnasal plug), packing forceps, tongue blades, and scissors. The surgeon may require a head mirror, good light, epi-

further surgery is often necessary. Ethmoidectomy and sphenoidectomy and even a Caldwell-Luc procedure (p. 486) may be necessary.

Nasoseptoplasty involves reconstruction of the septum and is replacing submucous resection as the operation of choice for deviated nasal septum. Reconstruction of the external nose *(rhinoplasty)*, often used for cosmetic reasons (Chapter 43), is often combined with septoplasty. It is

Table 23-7   Malignant disorders of nose and throat

Disorder	Description	Signs and symptoms	Medical therapy
Nasopharyngeal carcinomas	Carcinomas that obstruct nose first on one side then the other	Nasal obstruction, early metastasis to neck, bleeding	Surgery; radiation therapy
Carcinoma of maxillary and ethmoid sinuses	Relatively uncommon	Loosening of upper teeth; nasal obstruction, nosebleeds, displacement of eye, anosmia, tearing and diplopia	Chemotherapy; radiation; surgery that removes entire upper jaw (maxillectomy) and one eye (orbital exenteration)
Cancer of tonsil	May be carcinoma, lymphoepithelioma, or lymphosarcoma	Local ulceration, enlarged tonsil, pain	Surgery; radiation
Carcinoma of larynx	Squamous cell carcinoma of vocal cords and surrounding tissue	Progressive hoarseness that lasts longer than 2 weeks	Partial or total laryngectomy; radiation therapy before or after surgery

nephrine 1:1000 or other vasoconstrictor, 4% topical lidocaine (Xylocaine) or 4% cocaine solution, applicators, nasal speculum, and suction.

Because packing blocks the passage of air through the nose, a partial vacuum is created during swallowing, and the person may complain of a sucking action when attempting to drink. Postnasal drainage, the presence of old blood in the mouth, dryness of the mouth from mouth breathing, and loss of the ability to smell often lead to anorexia. Antihistamines may be prescribed to reduce nasal secretions, and frequent mouth care is important. Postoperative care is described in Box 23-9.

Interventions to achieve patient outcomes
Facilitating learning

Persons with trauma to the nose should be encouraged to seek medical attention, even if obstruction is not present, because a broken nose can lead to chronic problems (for example, chronic sinusitis) if not treated.

Teaching the person who has had nasal surgery is described in Box 23-9. If deformities are present, the person may be disturbed about body image because of the high visibility of the face. These persons need an opportunity to talk about their feelings and are encouraged to talk to the physician about possible long-term positive changes through plastic surgery (see Chapter 43).

Evaluation

Evaluation is based on expected patient outcomes. Questions to consider may include the following:
1. Does the patient exhibit a positive body image?
2. Is the patient comfortable?
3. Can the patient describe care required at home following surgery?
4. Can the patient describe ways to prevent nosebleeds?
5. Can the patient describe the expected time frame for positive cosmetic effects following rhinoplasty?
6. Can the patient list the signs and symptoms of complications (bleeding, drainage, and fever) that should be reported to the surgeon?
7. Is the patient able to breathe more easily?

MALIGNANCIES OF THE NOSE AND THROAT

Malignancies may develop in the nasopharynx, sinuses, tonsils, and larynx.

Pathophysiology

Nasopharyngeal carcinomas obstruct the nose; they metastasize early to the neck. Carcinomas of the maxillary and ethmoid sinuses may erode the adjacent nasal walls and bleed easily. Carcinoma of the maxillary sinus causes dental problems initially; other effects may include nasal obstruction, nosebleeds, and displacement of the eye. Carcinoma of the ethmoid sinus causes outward displacement of the eye, disturbance of the sense of smell, and nosebleeds. The prognosis is grave. The signs and symptoms and medical therapy of these disorders are listed in Table 23-7.

MALIGNANCY OF SINUSES

The most frequent malignancy of the nasal cavity and the paranasal sinuses is squamous cell carcinoma. The lesion is most common in the maxillary sinus. Unfortunately, there are no early symptoms to warn the patient.[10]

The diagnosis is confirmed by biopsy and CT scan, which are used to differentiate between benign and malignant lesions and to determine how far the tumor has extended.

Treatment consists of irradiation and surgery. Some surgeons prefer to irradiate the involved area before surgery, whereas other surgeons use irradiation after surgery.

Chemotherapeutic agents may also be prescribed in addition to surgery and radiation therapy.[10]

Maxillectomy and Orbital Exenteration

Surgery for malignancies of the sinuses consists of removal of the entire upper jaw (maxillectomy) and one eye (orbital exenteration). Split-thickness skin grafts (see Chapter 43) are usually applied to the operative area. Postoperatively, the deformity of the jaw is managed with a dental prosthesis, which closes off the defect in the mouth. Several prostheses may be needed because of shrinking of the cavity as healing progresses. Radical surgery is required because of the danger of recurrence.

Postoperative care includes the following:
1. Monitor for signs of meningitis (fever, headache, neck rigidity).
2. Provide care related to nasogastric intubation (see Chapter 31).
3. Provide mouth care.
   a. Use a gentle spray or oral irrigation.
   b. Use saline with hydrogen peroxide, weak sodium bicarbonate, or prescribed antibiotic solution.
   c. Aspiration of drainage may be necessary (care is taken to prevent trauma from suction tip).
4. Provide pain medication as needed.
5. Give prescribed prophylactic antibiotics.
6. Encourage early ambulation.
7. Provide emotional support.

Persons who undergo radical surgery of this type have a number of emotional adjustments to make.[25,26] The alteration in their physical appearance is readily visible; the person feels conspicuous and different. In addition to disfigurement, the person has all the normal fears of surgery and of cancer. Fear, anger, and grief are normal reactions to the situation. Fear is focused on concerns about the future, the ability to live normally, and also of being rejected. Anger and grief are common responses to the loss and the helplessness to control the loss. Oral communication also may be a problem immediately following surgery, and every effort is made to allow the person to express needs and feelings by writing if necessary. Conveying compassion and concern to the person is important.

MALIGNANCY OF TONSILS

Etiology/Epidemiology

Malignancy of the tonsils can be one of three types: *carcinoma, lymphoepithelioma,* or *lymphosarcoma.* Carcinomas are more common in men, possibly related to the longer smoking history of some men. The carcinomas spread upward into the soft palate and usually metastasize early to the neck.

Pathophysiology

Local ulceration and otalgia (earache) are early symptoms. Lymphoepithelioma often remain small and do not ulcerate, but neck metastasis occurs early. Lymphosarcomas produce large tonsils, usually without ulceration or pain, and metastasize early to the neck.

Medical Treatment

Medical interventions for tonsillar malignancies may include radiation in conjunction with an extensive surgical procedure to remove all the malignant tissue. Chemotherapy may be used also, but it is still being tested for effectiveness. The cure rate has improved using this combined technique.[10] Recurrence often occurs locally or with distant metastasis.

MALIGNANCY OF LARYNX

Etiology/Epidemiology

Squamous cell carcinoma of the larynx is increasing in frequency. It is estimated that in the United States there are over 12,500 new cases and over 3650 deaths every year.[1]

Cancer of the larynx is five times more common in men than in women, and it occurs most often in persons over 60 years of age. There appears to be some relationship between cancer of the larynx and heavy smoking, alcohol use, chronic laryngitis, vocal abuse, and family predisposition to cancer. Because of the number of women who continue to be heavy smokers, the incidence of carcinoma of the larynx has increased in women. According to the American Cancer Society the percentage of deaths from laryngeal cancer in women increased 150 percent when figures from 1955 to 57 and 1985 to 87 are compared.[1]

Pathophysiology

Cancer of the larynx that is limited to the true vocal cords grows slowly because of the lymphatic supply. Elsewhere in the larynx (epiglottis, false vocal cords, and pyriform sinuses) lymphatic vessels are abundant, and cancer of these tissues often spreads rapidly and metastasizes early to the deep lymph nodes of the neck.

Any smoker who becomes progressively hoarse or is hoarse for longer than 2 weeks should be urged to seek medical attention at once. Hoarseness is an early symptom of cancer of the vocal cords. If treatment is given when hoarseness appears (caused by the tumor's preventing the complete approximation of the vocal cords), a cure usually is possible. Signs of metastases of cancer to other parts of the larynx include a sensation of a lump in the throat, pain in the Adam's apple that radiates to the ear, dyspnea, dysphagia, enlarged cervical nodes, and cough). The diagnosis of cancer of the larynx is made from the patient's history, from visual examination of the larynx with indirect laryngoscopy, and from a biopsy and microscopic study of the lesion.

Diagnostic tests

A laryngeal mirror is used to visualize the larynx.

Direct laryngoscopy

When there are suspicious lesions of the larynx, a direct laryngoscopy is performed. It is usually performed with the patient under local anesthesia with 10% cocaine or under general anesthesia. A sedative (for example, secobarbital, meperidine, or other narcotic) and atropine sulfate (to decrease secretions) are given 1 hour before the examination. The person is placed in a reclining position

Table 23-8   Laryngectomy surgery for cancer

Type	Description	Voice result
Partial laryngectomy		
Hemilaryngectomy	Opening into larynx through thyroid cartilage with removal of diseased false cord, arytenoid, and one side of thyroid cartilage	Hoarse voice
Supraglottic partial laryngectomy	Horizontal incision passes above true cords (left intact) with removal of epiglottis and diseased tissue	Normal voice
Total laryngectomy	Removal of epiglottis, thyroid cartilage, and 3 or 4 tracheal rings; closure of pharynx with trachea; permanent tracheostomy	No voice

with the head in a head holder or with the head extended over the edge of the table and manually supported by a physician or nurse. The laryngoscope is inserted through the mouth and laryngopharynx, making the interior of the larynx easily visible. Minor surgical procedures, such as a biopsy, may be performed through the laryngoscope.

If local anesthesia has been given, the patient should not eat or drink anything until the gag reflex returns, usually within 2 hours. The gag reflex can be tested by touching the back of the throat with a tongue blade or applicator. After the gag reflex returns, the patient should first try to drink water because it is the fluid least likely to cause aspiration pneumonia if it is accidentally aspirated into the trachea or lungs.

Surgery of the larynx

Treatment of carcinoma of the true vocal cord depends on the extent of the tumor involvement. If the tumor is limited to the true cord without limitation of cord movement, then radiation therapy is the best course of treatment, with cure rates of 80% to 90%. Surgical intervention is considered when extension of the tumor fixes one of the cords or extends upward or downward from the larynx. Surgery may include a partial or total laryngectomy, or radical neck dissection. Table 23-8 lists the types of laryngectomy surgery.

Partial laryngectomy

Hemilaryngectomy. In this procedure, which is also called a *vertical partial laryngectomy*, one half or more of the larynx is removed. Persons suitable for this procedure have malignancies involving one true vocal cord or one true vocal cord and a portion of the other. This procedure is usually well tolerated, and difficulty in swallowing is minimal. Although the quality of the voice is altered, it is adequate for communication.[10]

Supraglottic laryngectomy. When the supraglottis is invaded by cancer, a *supraglottic laryngectomy* (horizontal partial laryngectomy) is performed. The procedure usually involves the removal of endolaryngeal structures from the tip of the epiglottis down to and including the laryngeal vertical. Because the true vocal cords are preserved, the patient's voice quality is excellent. The major postoperative problem is the danger of aspiration because of difficulty in

swallowing. Aspiration may occur because the major reflex arc that causes closure of the larynx is initiated by sensory receptors in the supraglottic larynx, which has been removed. These patients will need special swallowing training postoperatively. Although patients take variable amounts of time to learn to swallow safely, most will be able to take feedings by mouth.

After partial laryngectomy, a temporary tracheostomy tube is inserted and removed when edema in the surrounding tissues subsides. The person is not permitted to use the voice until the surgeon gives specific approval (usually 3 days postoperatively). In the past whispering was allowed, but it is now believed that whispering can further damage the voice. This problem is currently under study. The person usually adjusts quite readily to relatively minor limitations of speech. The main problems encountered by persons undergoing partial laryngectomy are those of swallowing and aspiration.

Total laryngectomy. When cancer of the larynx is advanced, a total laryngectomy may be performed. This includes removal of the epiglottis, thyroid cartilage, hyoid bone, cricoid cartilage, and three or four rings of the trachea. The pharyngeal opening to the trachea is closed, the anterior wall of the laryngopharynx (hypopharynx) is closed, and the remaining trachea is brought out to the neck wound and sutured to the skin. It forms an opening (permanent tracheostomy) through which the patient breathes (Fig. 23-16). The presence of a tracheal stoma affects the sense of smell because breathing through the nose is impossible; therefore, the person does not receive olfactory sensations. The person has no voice because of removal of the larynx. The nursing care of the patient with a laryngectomy is outlined in Box 23-10.

Radical neck dissection. A radical neck dissection may be performed along with a laryngectomy in patients whose risk of metastases to the neck from carcinoma of the larynx is high. This includes *primary tumors whose size and location are known to result in metastasis and palpable cervical lymph nodes at time of surgery.* In a radial neck dissection the submandibular salivary gland, sternocleidomastoid muscle, internal jugular vein, and spinal accessory nerve are removed to assure complete removal of nodal-bearing tissue.[10] In some patients a modification of a radical neck dissection

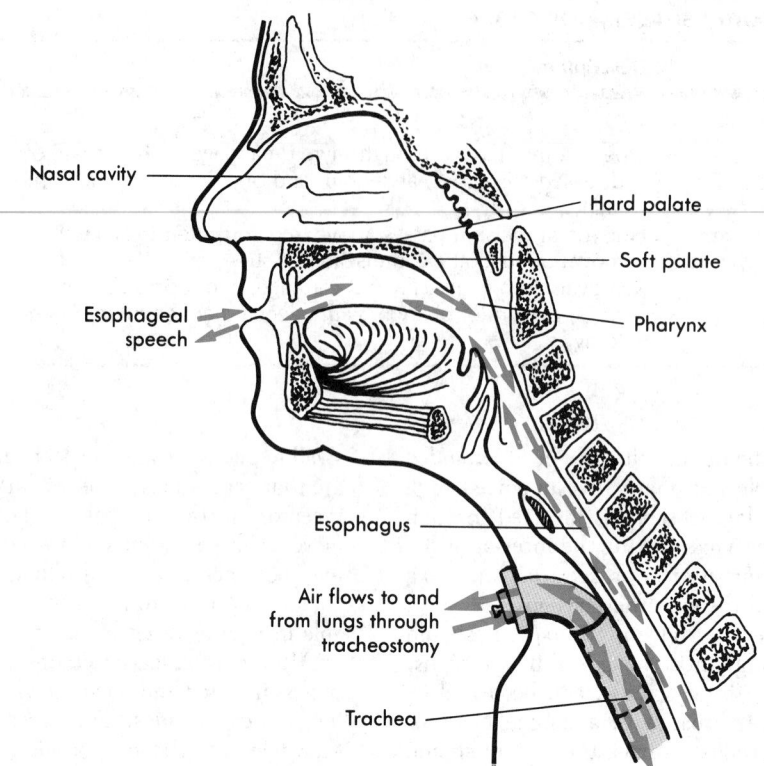

Fig. 23-16 Permanent tracheostomy: no connection exists between trachea and esophagus.

is performed. These are referred to as a *modified, conservation,* or *functional* neck dissections and are used when the nodal metastatic disease is not far advanced. These procedures cause atrophy of the trapezius muscle, and the shoulder droops on the side of surgery.

Patients can be taught to do exercises with other muscles that gradually replace the function of the lost muscles. Most patients have difficulty lifting their heads. They can be taught to place both hands behind their necks with fingers interlocked when lifting the head from the pillow. The patient is more comfortable and can breathe better when placed in mid-Fowler's position. Pressure dressings are best avoided in radical neck dissection because they compromise the blood supply to the skin flaps protecting the vital neck structures.

The Hemovac (Fig. 23-17) is one device available to keep constant drainage from the neck wound without pressure on the flaps. The Hemovac must be checked to see that it is working properly and that there is no edema, which might indicate hematoma. The tubing is milked every 1-2 hours for the first 24 hours postoperatively and then every 4 hours and prn. Changes in the amount or color of drainage should be reported to the surgeon.

Some alteration of appearance is readily visible, which may cause the person to feel somewhat conspicuous. Anger, grief, or denial may be part of the normal response to the change in body image. (For further information on psychologic support, refer to Chapter 11.)

Radical neck dissection can be performed without laryngectomy for persons whose primary malignant lesion is in the tongue, tonsil, lip, nasopharynx, or thyroid. Often

the procedure accompanies other procedures and is termed a *composite resection.* Composite resections may include either radical neck dissection in addition to the removal of the mandible; removal of the mandible and resection of the floor of the mouth; or removal of the mandible, floor of the mouth, and the tongue. The nursing care for these patients is outlined in Box 23-11. Emotional reactions to this type of radical surgery may be profound. Disfigurement is readily visible, and reactions to the change in body image are marked. In addition to the usual fears of surgery and cancer, the patient having a composite resection may have fears of rejection and fears concerning the future.

Preoperative care. The person who is to have a laryngectomy is told by the physician that breathing will occur through a special opening made in the neck and that normal speech will not be possible. This is often depressing to the patient because it may threaten economic status, as well as life. In some instances, it is helpful to receive a visit from another person who has made a good recovery from laryngectomy and who has undergone rehabilitation successfully. In other instances, this visit may depress the patient further. Careful assessment must be made to determine if the person will benefit from such a visit and whether the visit should be made preoperatively, immediately after surgery, or later in the recovery period.

Often no one else can give a person reassurance that speech can be regained as well as a fellow patient. Many large cities have a Lost Chord Club or a New Voice Club, and the members are willing to visit hospitalized patients. Information regarding these clubs may be obtained by writ-

Postoperative care of the patient following a laryngectomy

Elevate head of bed 45 degrees
Encourage coughing, deep breathing every 4 hours. Maintain oxygen to trach collar.
Incentive spirometry if ordered
Assess airway patency every shift and prn
　Vital signs
　Quality and rate of respiration
　Skin color (pallor, cyanosis)
　Auscultation of lungs every shift and prn
Monitor hydration and ensure adequate fluid intake to maintain healthy oral mucosa; provide mouth care at least three times a day
　Record intake and output every shift
　Weigh daily at the same time and in same amount of clothing
Provide stoma and stoma vent care every shift and prn
Ambulate tid and prn
Begin teaching laryngectomy care
Assess anxiety level and provide emotional support
Assist patient in communicating
　Provide patient with Magic Slate
　Use questions that can be answered yes or no
　Reinforce use of artificial speech device and encourage its use
Assess suture line and stoma site every 4 hours. Report erythema, purulent drainage, hematoma
Care for suture line and stoma site as ordered by surgeon
Monitor drain function and output
　Maintain suction to drain at level ordered
　Milk tubing every 1-2 hours for 24 hours; and then every 4 hours and prn
　Report changes in amount and color of drainage
Administer enteral feedings per order
　Assess patient's tolerance of feedings
　Assess bowel sounds every shift and prn
　Report intolerance to feedings (nausea, fullness, inability to tolerate prescribed amount of feedings)
　Record amount, consistency, and frequency of stools
　Assess swallowing ability and provide support when oral diet resumes
Monitor patient's reaction to change in body image
　Be sensitive to patient's reactions to changes in appearance
　Provide time to listen to patient
　Enourage use of Lost Chord Club
Prepare patient for discharge
　Monitor ability of patient or significant other to perform airway management care
　Provide patient with list of supplies necessary for home care
　Review written instructions in home-going booklet

Postoperative care of the patient following a total neck dissection

Elevate head of bed 30 degrees
Maintain oxygen mist therapy if ordered
Encourage coughing and deep breathing and use of incentive spirometer
Assess airway for signs and symptoms of increasing airway obstruction (stridor, dyspnea, increased pulse and respiratory rate)
Keep tracheostomy set at bedside
Monitor vital signs every 4 hours
Assess for early signs and symptoms of bleeding (potential for carotid hemorrhage)
　Ensure blood availability with blood bank
　Maintain venous access with large bore needle
　If hemorrhage occurs: STAT page physician, apply direct pressure, suction airway, reassure patient
Care for suture line as ordered
Maintain drainage function and output
　Maintain suction to drain
　Milk tubing every 1-2 hours for 24 hours; and then every q4h prn
　Assess output and document every shift
Assess for signs and symptoms of infection of suture line (erythema, pus, elevated temperature)
Assess skin flap every shift for signs and symptoms of poor drain patency or infection
Monitor intake and output and record every shift
Monitor for evidence of chylous fistula (lymphatic leak from thoracic duct into neck wound)
　Opaque or milky drainage from wound
　Observe color and amount of drainage and report any change to physician
　Place on lactose-free diet
Monitor shoulder droop secondary to loss of nerve supply to trapezius muscle
　Inability to raise hand over head
　Reinforce need to do shoulder strenthening exercise tid
　Consult physical therapist with concerns about patient's exercises
Monitor patient's ability to ingest optimal caloric intake
　Observe swallowing attempts and assess for aspiration
　Report inability to comply with recommended intake for physician and dietitian
　Provide emotional support during eating
Monitor depression which is not uncommon following disfiguring surgery
　Identify patient support system and involve them and patient in planning and giving care
　Plan for specific time to provide emotional support
　Help patient verbalize feelings about having cancer, changes in body image, and lifestyle
Encourage adequate caloric intake
　May have difficulty in swallowing related to postoperative swelling and radiation preoperatively
　Weigh daily at same time and with same amount of clothing
　Monitor attempts to swallow and check for aspiration
　Consult with dietitian and physician if desired caloric intake can not be met
　Teach patient about role of diet in wound healing

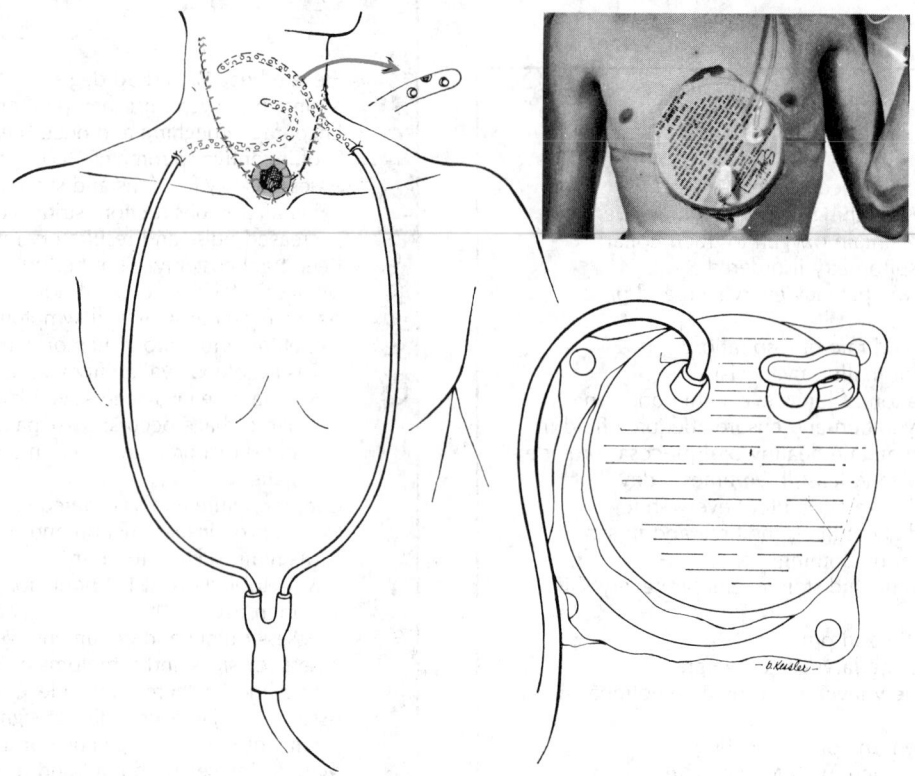

Fig. 23-17 Hemovac apparatus for constant closed suction. In this system of wound drainage, suction is maintained by plastic container with spring inside that tries to force apart lids and thereby produces suction that is transmitted through plastic tubing. Neck skin is pulled down tight, and no external dressing is required. Container serves as both suction source and receptacle for blood. It is emptied as required, and drainage tubes are left in neck for 3 days. (From DeWeese DD, Saunders WH: *Textbook of otolaryngology,* ed 6, St. Louis, 1982, Mosby—Year Book.)

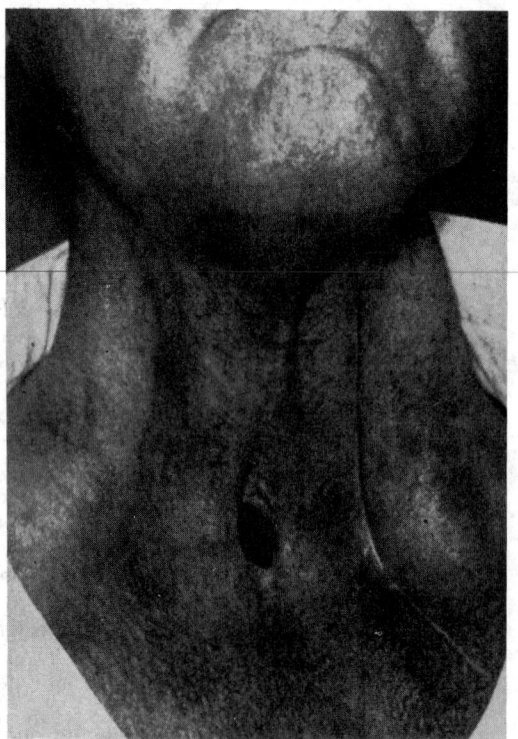

Fig. 23-18 After laryngectomy. Note scars of bilateral radical neck dissections. (From DeWeese DD, Saunders WH: *Textbook of otolaryngology,* ed 6, St. Louis, 1982, Mosby—Year Book.)

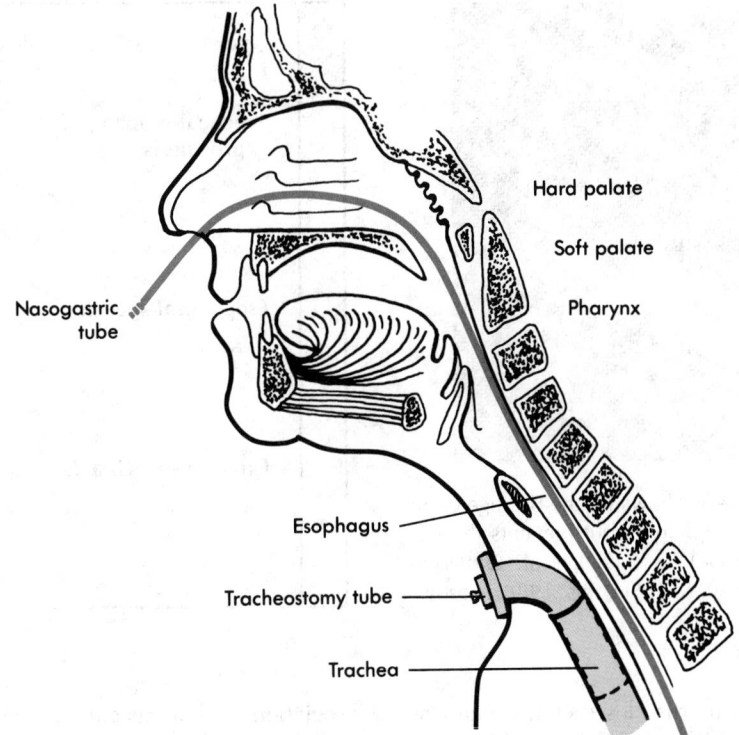

Fig. 23-19   Position of tracheostomy tube and nasogastric tube following total laryngectomy.

ing to the International Association of Laryngectomees.[*]
Local speech rehabilitation centers may supply instructive
films and other resources. The local chapter of the American Cancer Society and the local health department also
have information available. If possible, the family also
should learn about the method of esophageal speech that
the person will learn to use.

Postoperative care. Postoperative care of the person is
essentially the same as that described for tracheostomy
(Chapter 24) except that these persons will have a *laryngectomy tube* in place, a tube that is shorter and wider in
diameter than a tracheostomy tube. Some patients may not
have a tube in the stoma after the operation because the
stoma is a permanent one kept open initially by the sutures
and because their surgeon believes that there is less tissue
reaction and a better stoma if no tube is used. If a laryngectomy tube is used, it remains until the wound is
healed and a permanent fistula has formed, usually in 2
to 3 weeks (Fig. 23-18). Frequent suctioning is necessary
in the early postoperative period to keep the trachea free
of secretions.

A *nasogastric tube* is usually inserted during the surgical
procedure for the instillation of food and fluids at regular
intervals postoperatively for about 10 days (Fig. 23-19).
The use of the tube to give food is thought to minimize
contamination of the pharyngeal and esophageal suture
lines and to prevent fluid from leaking through the wound
into the trachea before healing occurs. The nasogastric

tube is removed as soon as the person can safely swallow.
The person then needs careful attention in the first attempts to swallow. There may be the sensation of choking
and severe coughing, which is frightening and painful.
Aspiration cannot occur because the trachea no longer
communicates with the esophagus.

The sense of smell is affected after laryngectomy because breathing through the nose is impossible, therefore,
the patient does not receive olfactory sensations.

Speech rehabilitation. Until recently, *esophageal speech*
was the primary speech method after laryngectomy. Although this method of speech was successful for many
laryngectomees, others could never learn to use it. In addition, the increased use of radiation therapy after laryngectomy causes fibrous tissue to form, making *esophageal
speech* less possible.

For a number of years, surgeons had been working to
develop other forms of speech after laryngectomy. In 1980
the first successful procedure using surgical-prosthetic
voice restoration was introduced. In this procedure, a *tracheoesophageal puncture* (TEP) is made to create a tracheoesophageal fistula large enough to permit the insertion of
a valve prosthesis. The TE fistula is created after the
larynx has been resected and a frozen section indicates
that all of the carcinoma has been removed. A red rubber
catheter is pulled through the fistula into the esophagus
and sutured in place. The end of the catheter is occluded
with an umbilical clamp. The patient is discharged with
the catheter in place.[43] The prosthesis is a hollow tube
open at the tracheal end and closed with a horizontal slit
at the laryngopharyngeal end (Fig. 23-20). When the pa-

[*]American Cancer Society, Inc, 1599 Clifton Road NE, Atlanta, GA
30329.

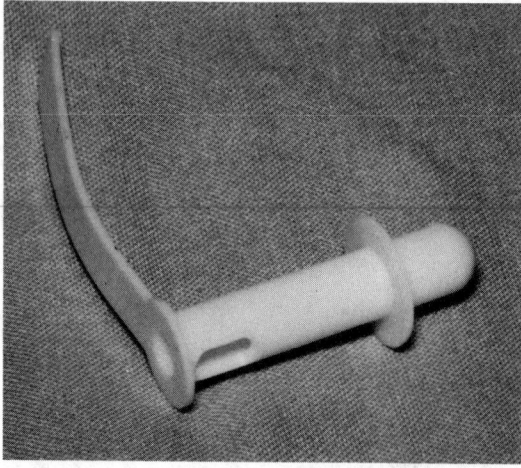

Fig. 23-20   This vocal prosthesis allows for the passage of air from the trachea into the hypopharynx but prevents the opposite flow of saliva. (From DeWeese DD, et al: *Otolaryngology—head and neck surgery*, ed 7, St Louis, 1988, Mosby–Year Book.)

23-12	Speech methods following total laryngectomy	
	Tracheal-esophageal prosthesis	Formation of a tracheal-esophageal fistula with insertion of a silicone prosthesis that produces a sound in the esophagus (Fig. 23-20)
	Esophageal speech	Speech produced by expelling swallowed air (burping) across constricted tissue in the pharyngoesophageal segment
	External speech aids	Mechanical devices, such as a vibrator or electronic artificial larynx, used externally (Fig. 23-21)

tient talks, air pressure opens the closed end, permitting air to enter the laryngopharynx. When the patient stops talking, the laryngopharyngeal end closes preventing saliva from draining into the trachea. Because air is diverted from the trachea into the esophagus, this form of speech is referred to as *tracheoesophageal speech.*

The stoma must be occluded during speech, either by placing a finger over the opening or by using a special tracheostomal valve inserted after the patient has learned to use the prosthesis. The patient or family must be taught to remove, clean, and reinsert the voice prosthesis rapidly so that stenosis of the fistula does not occur. Not all patients and families are comfortable with removing and cleaning the prosthesis, and considerable support by the speech pathologist may be necessary. Ideally, the patient should be able to use the prosthesis for speaking and be able to clean and reinsert it before discharge from the hospital.

Early evidence indicates that there are several advantages of *tracheoesophageal speech.* These include more rapid restoration of voice, speech that is closer to normal in rate and phrasing, and speech that is more pleasing than speech with an electrolarynx. Disadvantages include reliance on a prosthesis and the rapidity with which the tracheoesophageal fistula may undergo stenosis.[10] For this reason, all three methods of speaking are still in use, and none are mutually exclusive. In fact, some patients find it useful to use more than one of the methods (Box 23-12).

Information about devices used to produce electronic speech can be obtained from the American Cancer Society or from the local telephone company. Information about esophageal speech can be obtained from the American Speech and Hearing Association,* the International As-

sociation of Laryngectomies, and the American Cancer Society.

Teaching the patient to use *esophageal* speech is started as soon as the esophageal suture line is healed. To learn esophageal speech, the patient must first practice burping. This provides the moving column of air needed for sound, while folds of tissue at the opening of the esophagus act as the vibrating surface. The patients must learn to coordinate articulation with esophageal vocalization made possible by aspirating air into the esophagus. The new voice sounds are natural, although somewhat hoarse. The qualities of speech provided by the use of the nasopharynx are still present. The patient may have digestive difficulty while learning to speak; this is caused by swallowing air during practice, by unusual strain on abdominal muscles, and by nervous tension. Digestive difficulties usually abate with proficiency in speaking.

Most patients learn esophageal speech best at a special clinic. Although some individuals may need to go to a nearby city for this instruction, they usually must remain away from home for only 1 or 2 weeks. Motivation and persistent effort are essential in learning this kind of speech; encouragement and support from the professional staff and the patient's significant others are important to the patient's morale. About 75% of all patients who have their larynx removed master some sort of speech, and the average person can return to work 1 or 2 months after leaving the hospital. Information on esophageal speech can be obtained from the American Speech and Hearing Association, the International Association of Laryngectomees, and the American Cancer Society.

If a person is unable to learn esophageal speech in 60 to 90 days after surgery, a *speech aid* such as a vibrator or an electronic artificial larynx (Fig. 23-21) may be prescribed. Various mechanical devices are available, and the new ones permit a natural type of speech, providing pitch inflections and volume control. The local chapter of the

*American Speech and Hearing Association, 10801 Rockville Pike, Rockville, MD 20852.

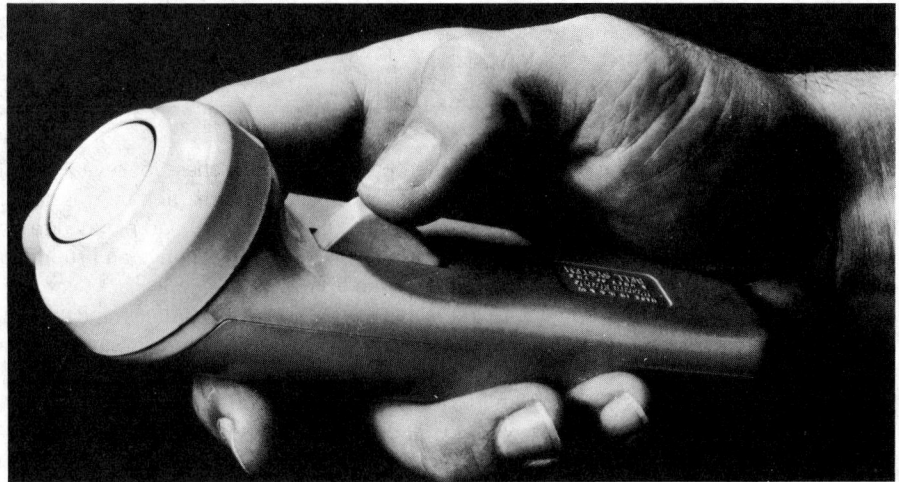

Fig. 23-21   Battery-powered electronic artificial larynx for patient who has total laryngectomy and cannot learn esophageal speech. (Courtesy Illinois Bell Telephone Co.)

American Cancer Society or the local telephone company can provide information about the purchase of these devices.

Reconstructive surgery. Because of the extensive surgery required to treat malignancies of the head and neck, reconstructive surgery may be necessary. In the past, skin grafts and pedicle or rotation skin flaps were used for reconstruction. Today the *myocutaneous flap* is the major reconstructive flap used after radical neck dissection and traumatic defects of the head and neck.

Myocutaneous flaps use the axial blood supply that supplies muscle mass, as well as cutaneous and subcutaneous tissue. The inclusion of muscle with its blood supply when transferring the skin allows for a much greater range of rotation of the flap. The *pectoralis major*, the *latissimus dorsi*, the *trapezius*, and the *sternocleidomastoid muscles* can be used for *myocutaneous flaps*.

The care of these patients is complex, and there are many nursing requirements both preoperatively and postoperatively. For further information, references 29 and 38 are two excellent articles on the nursing care of these patients.

Discharge teaching. Persons with laryngectomies must take special precautions because of the permanent tracheostomy (Box 23-13). Usually by the time of discharge, patients with laryngectomies do not need suctioning of the tracheostomy but can cough up secretions. If suctioning is deemed necessary, patients or their families need to be told where to secure the necessary suction equipment and how to care for themselves. Suction equipment can be rented for home use or obtained in many communities through the local chapter of the American Cancer Society.

Nursing Process
Assessment
Subjective data

Persons with carcinomas of the larynx can have a variety of symptoms, which include the following:

23-13

Patient following total laryngectomy

1. Wear a scarf or shirt with closed collar of porous material (to warm and screen air over stoma).
2. Use caution while taking a bath or shower (to prevent aspiration of water in stoma).
3. Check with surgeon concerning swimming or boating; if swimming is permitted, use a special snorkle device designed for tracheostomees.
4. Use available community resources for support and speech rehabilitation as necessary (for example, laryngectomee clubs, American Cancer Society).
5. Seek immediate medical attention for respiratory tract infection or signs of stomal bleeding.
6. Continue medical follow-up per physician instructions.

---

1. Persistent hoarseness (2 weeks or longer)
2. Sore throat
3. Odynophagia (pain when swallowing).

Objective data

1. Hoarseness is obvious when speaking.
2. Patient appears restless and anxious and has many questions about impending surgery.

Data analysis: nursing diagnoses

Nursing diagnoses are determined from an analysis of patient data. Possible nursing diagnoses for the person undergoing total laryngectomy may include, but are not limited to, the following:

Diagnostic title	Possible etiologies
Airway clearance, ineffective	Presence of laryngectomy tube, increased tranchobronchial secretions

Nursing Care Plan	**Person with laryngectomy**

DATA: Mr. K., a 68-year-old man, had noted progressive hoarseness for several months. Indirect laryngoscopy and biopsy confirmed cancer of the larynx, and he was admitted for a total laryngectomy. His wife accompanied him to the hospital and planned to be with him as much as possible during his hospitalization. She was attentive and supportive.

The following pertinent data were identified on admission:

1. He was visibly apprehensive (pacing the floor, restless, asking repeated questions).
2. His major concerns centered on the extent of the cancer and on communication problems following the surgery.
3. His height is 175 cm (5 ft 10 in), weight 68 kg (150 lb).
4. He wears glasses; near vision is poor without glasses.

Before surgery, Mr. K.'s primary nurse spent time with him, encouraging him to express his concerns and providing information about what to expect in the postoperative period and care that would be provided. Following the interaction, Mr. K.'s restlessness decreased and he was observed talking quietly with his wife and watching TV.

The larynx was removed during surgery; a permanent tracheostomy was performed, with insertion of a temporary laryngectomy tube. A tracheal esophageal catheter was in place. The end of the catheter was occluded with an umbilical clamp to prevent drainage of gastric contents into the surgical wound. A nasogastric tube was inserted, to be removed after Mr. K. was swallowing well. During the first postoperative day, Mr. K. again appeared apprehensive (restlessness, pointing frequently to the tracheostomy, pulling on his wife's hand, and pointing to call cord to call the nurse). Breath sounds in the upper lobes were clear but were absent in the lower lobes. Codeine and acetaminophen were prescribed for pain.

Nursing diagnosis: Anxiety, related to breathing difficulties and inability to communicate

Expected patient outcomes	Nursing interventions	Rationale
Mr. K. rests quietly and does not call frequently for suctioning	Explain suctioning procedure and carry out regular suctioning of tracheostomy	If Mr. K. knows tube will be suctioned frequently, fear of possible asphyxiation should decrease
	Develop a means of communication (such as cards, with needs printed clearly, a magic slate, or paper for writing); be sure Mr. K. wears his glasses	If Mr. K. can communicate needs, anxiety should decrease; his glasses are needed for visual communication
	After initial period and if wife is willing and able, teach her to help with suctioning tracheostomy	Participating in husband's care may assist wife in feeling she is helping, thus decreasing her anxiety (anxiety can be transmitted to patient)
	Encourage Mr. K. to care for own tracheostomy when feasible	Self-care enhances feeling of control of situation

Nursing diagnosis: Airway clearance, ineffective: related to secretions in upper airway and laryngectomy tube

Expected patient outcomes	Nursing interventions	Rationale
Respirations are effortless, quiet, and at baseline rate	Place Mr. K. in semi-Fowler's position	Position uses gravity to help expand thorax and decrease pressure on lower lobes
Breath sounds are clear at all lobes	Suction laryngectomy tube as often as needed as evidenced by noisy respirations, increased pulse and respiratory rate, and restlessness (may be as often as every 5 min initially)	Air blowing through secretions produces noisy respirations; pulse and respirations are increased when oxygen intake is decreased; restlessness may indicate decreased oxygen
	Provide tracheostomy care, including suctioning as needed	Keeping tube patent will facilitate air interchange
	Provide air humidification	Humidity will help keep secretions liquid for easier removal
	Encourage deep breathing and coughing	Deep breathing will help aerate lower lobes; coughing will help expel secretions

Nursing diagnosis: Nutrition, altered: less than body requirements related to difficulty in swallowing

Expected patient outcomes	Nursing interventions	Rationale
Weight is not more than 5 lb from baseline	Give prescribed tube feedings via N/G tube until patient can swallow well (usually 7 days)	Tube feedings provide more nutrients than IV fluids; swallowing is impaired initially from postoperative edema of lower pharynx
	When N/G tube is removed, give fluids only until Mr. K. is swallowing well	Fluids are easier to swallow than solid food until edema subsides
	Explain anatomic changes to Mr. K (no connection between esophagus and tracheostomy)	May help to decrease Mr. K's concern about choking
	Stay with Mr. K. during initial eating of semisolid and solid foods	Mr. K. may fear choking and not be willing to swallow initially; encouragement by nurse with assurance of suctioning if necessary may inspire more confidence
	Use measures to encourage eating as necessary (tray for wife so they can eat together, selection of desired foods, and a pleasant atmosphere)	Return to usual eating patterns may encourage Mr. K. to eat
	Encourage Mr. K. to monitor weight 2 to 3 times a week until baseline weight is regained	Participating in monitoring own weight may motivate Mr. K. to eat

Nursing diagnosis: Pain: related to surgery

Expected patient outcomes	Nursing interventions	Rationale
Mr. K. is relaxed and signals feeling comfortable	Give prescribed analgesic for pain	Analgesics will decrease transmission and interpretation of pain stimuli
	Encourage other pain-relieving measures such as relaxation exercises or distraction	Help to minimize pain perception
	Provide nose and mouth care while N/G tube is in place	Tube may irritate nose; mouth becomes dry an uncomfortable from open mouth breathing and decreased lubrication (unable to swallow fluids)

Continued.

Nursing Care Plan	**Person with laryngectomy—cont'd**

Nursing diagnosis: Knowledge deficit: related to need to care for self after discharge

Expected patient outcomes	Nursing interventions	Rationale
Mr. K. describes self-care	Teach Mr. K. description of anatomic changes Provide written instructions for all aspects listed below Teach Mr. K. care of stoma including self-suctioning Teach Mr. K. methods to protect stoma	Providing own care will give Mr. K. self-confidence; care is needed to keep the tracheostomy open for air exchange
	Advise Mr. K. of availability of community resources and provide written list	Mr. K. may be interested in the Lost Chord Club for sharing of experiences
	Teach Mr. K. how to reinsert TE tube and to go to hospital if cannot reinsert	Need to maintain TE fistula so tracheoesophageal speech can be achieved

Nursing diagnosis: Communication, impaired verbal related to laryngectomy

Expected patient outcomes	Nursing interventions	Rationale
Mr. K. communicates with others	Encourage Mr. K. to communicate using system devised with him preoperatively (hand signals, writing)	Absence of larynx makes speech impossible
Mr. K. understands need to retain tracheoesophageal catheter in fistula	Reinforce with Mr. K. peroperative teaching about tracheoesophageal speech and purpose of a catheter	Catheter in fistula prevents aspiration and maintains patency of TE fistula
Mr. K. understands options available to assist with speech	Review instructions about esophageal and electroesophageal speech	TE prosthesis will be fitted at first postoperative visit Electronic devices are available to assist him to speak as necessary
Mr. K. understands need for follow-up care after discharge	Reinforce need for regular followup with speech pathologist and surgeon after discharge	For best speech results he will be followed at least 1 year by surgeon and speech pathologist

Diagnostic title	Possible etiologies
Anxiety	Threat to self-concept, inability to speak, threat to socioeconomic status
Aspiration, potential for	Presence of laryngectomy tube
Body image disturbance	Disfiguring surgery
Infection, potential for	Surgical incision
Nutrition, altered; less than body requirement	Swallowing difficulty
Oral mucous membrane, altered	Surgery
Pain, postoperative	Surgery
Communication, impaired verbal	Laryngectomy

Planning: expected patient outcomes

Expected patient outcomes for the person undergoing total laryngectomy may include, but are not limited to, the following:

1. Patient maintains respiratory rate of 12-18 breaths/minute.
2. Respirations are quiet: breath sounds are clear in all lobes.
3. Patient does not exhibit signs of anxiety (restlessness, increased pulse and respiration).
4. Patient is able to swallow without aspirating.
5. Patient verbalizes acceptance of laryngectomy and begins to acknowledge feelings about change in body image.
6. Patient does not develop an infection in the suture line.
7. Patient's weight at time of discharge from hospital is not less than 5 lbs from baseline weight.
8. Patient's oral mucous membrane is moist and pink.
9. Patient signals that he or she is feeling comfortable.
10. Patient communicates using hand signals or Magic Slate.
11. Patient is willing participant in speech rehabilitation.

Implementation

Assisting with the achievement of therapeutic goals

Nursing interventions can be found in the Nursing Care Plan on p. 505 and Box 23-10.

Evaluation

Evaluation is based on expected patient outcome. Questions to consider about a patient having a laryngectomy and TEP may include the following:

1. Does patient maintain respiratory rate of 12-18 breaths/minute?
2. Are respirations quiet and breath sounds clear in all lobes?
3. Does patient exhibit minimal signs of anxiety?
4. Is the patient able to swallow without aspirating?
5. Does the patient verbalize acceptance of laryngectomy?
6. Is the patient beginning to acknowledge how he or she feels about the change in body image?
7. Is the patient free of infection in the suture line?
8. Is the patient's weight within 5 pounds from baseline at discharge?
9. Is patient comfortable?
10. Is the patient able to communicate using hand signals or in writing?
11. Is the patient a willing participant in speech rehabilitation?

SUMMARY

1. The major infections of the nose and sinuses are rhinitis (common cold), allergic rhinitis (hay fever), chronic rhinitis secondary to repeated infections or allergy, and sinusitis caused by a bacteria or virus.
2. Persons with allergic rhinitis (hay fever) are usually sensitive to pollen of grasses such as ragweed (see Chapter 41).
3. It is important for persons who are allergic to know which allergens they are allergic to and to avoid these allergens if at all possible. For this reason, they need to know how to prepare an environmentally controlled bedroom (see Chapter 41).
4. Persons with acute sinusitis usually have a severe headache and pain over the infected area. Fever is common and is related to the amount of sinus obstruction. If the sinus is abscessed, fever may be as high as 40° C (104° F).
5. Subjective assessment of the person with a nose or sinus problem includes a careful history of previous infections, how they were treated and self-treatment by the person including the use of over-the-counter medications.
6. Acetaminophen is recommended instead of aspirin in persons with nasal problems because aspirin may be associated with nasal polyposis.
7. There are five surgical procedures that may be used to treat chronic sinusitis: Caldwell-Luc procedure, ethmoidotomy, sphenoidotomy, ethmoidectomy, and osteopathic flap.

8. Postoperative care for persons having sinus surgery includes the following:
   a. Place patient in side-lying position until reacted from anesthesia and then mid-Fowler's position.
   b. Place ice compresses over nose or ice bag over maxillary or frontal sinuses.
   c. Monitor for bleeding and for decreased visual acuity such as diplopia, which indicates damage to the optic nerve.
   d. Provide frequent mouth care.
   e. Change nasal pad when soiled.
   f. *Teach patient not to blow nose for at least 48 hours after packing is removed.*
   g. Instruct patient to avoid constipation because Valsalva maneuver can cause bleeding.
9. The most common throat inflammation is acute pharyngitis. Hemolytic streptococci, staphlyococci, and other bacteria and viruses may be the source of infection. Pharyngitis caused by *Neisseria gonorrhoeae* is being seen more commonly in both men and women.
10. To obtain material for culture and sensitivity, a throat culture is taken to identify the organism and determine appropriate antibiotic therapy.
11. Prophylactic antibiotics are often prescribed for persons with pharyngitis who have a history of rheumatic fever or bacterial endocarditis.
12. Obstructions of the nose, such as a deviated septum, are often treated surgically by septoplasty or submucous resect ion (SMR). SMR is being used less frequently than in the past.
13. Postoperative care following nasal surgery includes the following:
   a. Monitor for hemorrhage.
   b. Place patient in mid-Fowler's position to decrease local edema.
   c. Place ice compresses over the nose for 24 hours and as needed.
   d. Provide food and fluids as tolerated.
   e. Provide frequent oral care.
   f. Change dressing under nose as needed.
   g. Teach patient to avoid blowing nose for 48 hours after packing is removed to prevent bleeding.
   h. Teach patient to avoid constipation and vigorous coughing until healing occurs because coughing and Valsalva maneuver may initiate bleeding.
   i. Explain that stools may be tarry for several days.
14. Progressive or persistent hoarseness that lasts longer than two weeks requires medical evaluation for cancer of the larynx.
15. Carcinoma of the larynx is treated with a partial or total laryngectomy.
16. Partial laryngectomy may be achieved by a hemilaryngectomy, or supraglottic partial laryngectomy after which the person will be able to speak.
17. Total laryngectomy is necessary when cancer of the larynx is far advanced. Persons with total laryngectomy are unable to speak normally, but will be able to have some form of speech.
18. There are three major forms of speech following laryngectomy: esophageal, tracheoesophageal, and external speech aide.

19. Tracheoesophageal speech requires the formation of a fistula after all the carcinoma has been removed. This procedure is called a trachealesophageal puncture (TEP).
20. A radical neck dissection is commonly performed along with total laryngectomy because of the possible metastasis to the neck.
   a. Postoperatively the person will have a laryngectomy tube and a nasogastric tube in place.
   b. Communication is impaired because of the loss of ability to speak and the person will require speech rehabilitation.

REFERENCES AND SELECTED READINGS

1. American Cancer Society: *19 Cancer facts and figures*, Atlanta, 1991, The Society.
2. Baker, KH, Feldman JE: Cancers of the head and neck, *Cancer Nurs*, 10(6):293-299, 1987.
3. Brown PE, Coleman JJ: The role of radiotherapy and musculocutaneous flaps in oropharyngocutaneous fistulas, *Am J Surg* 156 and 256-260, 1988.
4. Burke RH: A simplified nasal packing, *J Oral Maxillofac Surg* 43:555, 1985.
5. Calhoun KH: Otolaryngology—head and neck surgery, *JAMA* 265(230):3152-3154, 1991.
6. Carroll PF: Laryngospasm, *Nurs 86* 16(5):33, 1986.
7. Causes of stuffy nose: external nasal deformity, *Hosp Med* 21(5):194-198, 1985.
8.* Chisholm S, et al: Duck-bill prosthesis: words of hope for the laryngectomy patient, *Nurs 86* 16(3):29-31, 1986.
9. Clark KM: *Hoarseness and laryngitis*. In Rakel RE, editors: *Conn's current therapy 1990*, Philadelphia, 1990, WB Saunders.
10. DeWeese DD, Saunders WH: *Otolaryngology, head and neck surgery*, ed 7, St Louis, 1987, Mosby–Year Book.
11. Dropkin MJ: Coping with disfigurement and dysfunction after head and neck cancer surgery: a conceptual framework, *Semin Oncol Nurs* 5(3):213-219, 1989.
12. Ebersole P, Hess P: *Toward healthy aging*, ed 3, St. Louis, 1990, Mosby–Year Book.
13. Eichel B: Ethmoiditis: pathophysiology and medical management, *Otolaryngol Clin North Am* 18(1):43-53, 1985.
14.* Feinstein D: What to teach the patient who's had a total laryngectomy, *RN* 59(4):53-57, 1987.
15. Fosso BA: Sore throat, antibiotics and rheumatic fever, *Fam Pract* 2:101-107, 1985.
16. Gantz NM: *Streptococcal pharyngitis*. In Rakel RE, editor: *Conn's current therapy 1990*, Philadelphia, 1990, WB Saunders.
17.* Grant M, Rhimer J, Padilla GV: Nutritional management in head and neck cancer patient, *Semin Oncol Nurs* 5(3):195-204, 1989.
18.* Griffin CW, et al: Learning to swallow again, *Am J Nurs* 87:314-315, 1987.
19. Harold ML: Rehabilitation of the dysphagic client following ablative surgery for laryngeal cancer, *J Soc Otorhinolaryngol Head Neck Nurses* 5(2);16-18, 1987.
20.* Harris LL, Kraege J: After T-E puncture: relearning to speak, *Am J Nurs* 86(1):55-58, 1986.
21.* Harris LL, Smith S: Chemotherapy in head and neck cancer, *Semin Oncol Nurs* 5(3):174-181, 1989.
22. Hendrickson FR: Radiation therapy treatment of larynx cancers, *Cancer* 55:2058-2061, 1985.
23. Innes AJ, Gates N: ENT surgery and disorders, with notes on nursing care and clinical management, London, 1985, Faber & Faber.
24. Jafek BW: Intranasal ethmoidectomy, *Otolaryngol Clin North Am* 18(1):61-67, 1985.
25.* Kennedy DW, et al: Endoscopic sinus surgery: ambulatory surgery, *AORN J* 42:932-936, 1985.
26. Kennedy DW, Shikhani AH: *Sinusitis*. In Rakel RE, editor: *Conn's current therapy 1990*. Philadelphia, 1990, WB Saunders.
27. Knegt PP, et al: Carcinoma of the paranasal sinuses: results of a prospective pilot study, *Cancer* 56:57-62, 1985.
28. Konda M, et al: Prognostic factors influencing relapse of squamous cell carcinoma of the maxillary sinus, *Cancer* 55:190-196, 1985.
29.* Mahon SM: Nursing interventions for the patient with a myocutaneous flap, *Cancer Nurs* 10(1):21-31, 1987.
30. Mandel JH: Pharyngeal infections: causes, findings, and management, *Postgrad Med* 77;187-193, 1985.
31. Martin LK: Management of the altered airway in the head and neck cancer patient, *Semin Oncol Nurs* 5(3):182-190, 1989.
32. Mathieson CM, Stam JH, Scott JP: Psychosocial adjustment after laryngectomy: a review of the literature, *J Otolaryngol* 19(5):331-336, 1990.
33. Minx SM, et al: Carcinoma of the parasinus: perioperative nursing responsibilities, *AORN J* 42:671-681, 1985.
34. Neal GD: External ethmoidectomy, *Otolaryngol Clin North Am* 18:55-60, 1985.
35. Panje WR: *Sinusitis*. In Rakel RE, editor: *Conn's current therapy 1991*, Philadelphia, 1991, WB Saunders.
36. Parsons JT, et al: Neck dissection after twice-a-day radiotherapy: morbidity and recurrence rates, *Head Neck* 11(5):400-404, 1989.
37.* Patry-Lahey R: Doing it better: helping a laryngectomy patient go home, *Nurs 85* 15(3):63-64, 1985.
38.* Rodzwic D, Donnard J: The use of myocutaneous flaps in reconstructive surgery for head and neck cancer, *Oncol Nurs Forum* 13(3):29-34, 1986.
39. Romm S: Cancer of the larynx: current concepts of diagnosis and treatment, *Surg Clin North Am* 66:109-118, 1986.
40.* Rook IL, Rook M: Head and neck cancer, *J Postanesth Nurs*, 4(6):363-372, 1989.
41.* Sawyer DL, Bruya MA: Care of the patient having radical neck surgery or permanent laryngostomy: a nursing diagnostic approach, *Focus Crit Care* 17(2):166-173, 1990.
42. Schleper JR: Prevention, detection, and diagnosis of head and neck cancers, *Semin Oncol Nurs* 5(3):139-149, 1989.
43. Schwartz SS, Yuska CM: Common patient care issues following surgery for head and neck cancer, *Semin Oncol Nurs* 5(3):191-194, 1989.
44. Sigler BA: Nursing care of patients with laryngeal carcinoma, *Semin Oncol Nurs* 5(3):160-165, 1989.
45. Strohl RA: Radiation therapy for head and neck cancers, *Semin Oncol Nurs* 5(3):166-173, 1989.
46.* Trudeau MD, Schuller DE: *Mechanism for vocal communication following total laryngectomy*. In Jacobs C, editor: *Carcinomas of the head and neck: evaluation and management*, Boston, 1990, Kluwer Academic Publishers.
47.* Ulbricht GF: Laryngectomy rehabilitation: A woman's viewpoint, *Women Health* 11:131-136, 1986.
48. Wetmore SJ, et al: Long-term results of the Blom-Singer speech rehabilitation procedure, *Arch Otolaryngol* 111:106-109, 1985.
49. Williams L, Stieg F: Clinical practice: neck masses, *Plast Surg Nurs* 10(3):131-135, 1990.

*Recommended for student reading.

Classic

50. Annvas AA, et al: Groningen prosthesis for voice rehabilitation after laryngectomy, *Clin Otolaryngol* 9:51-54, 1984.
51. Estelle R, Simons R, Simons KJ: Pharmacologic treatment of rhinitis, *Clin Rev Allergy* 2:237-253, 1984.
52.* Gannon EP: Giving your patient meticulous mouth care, *Nurs 80* 10(3):70-75, 1980.
53. Hassard AD, Holness RO: The "crossbow" incision and nasal flap: its blood supply and clinical application, *Head Neck Surg* 7;135-138, 1984.
54. Holt JE: Orbital blowout fractures, *Ear Nose Throat J* 62:346-351, 1983.
55.* Hutton B, Hutton J: Living with facial prosthesis: a guide to patient care, *Am J Nurs* 84:50-52, 1984.
56. Johnson JT, Neman RK, Olson JE: Persistent hoarseness: an aggressive approach for early detection of laryngeal cancer, *Postgrad Med* 67:122-126, 1980.
57.* Kane KK: Carotid artery rupture in advanced head and neck cancer patients, *Oncol Nurs Forum* 10(1):14-18, 1983.
58.* Key G: Stopping nosebleeds in the elderly: pressure, cautery, or packing? *Geriatrics* 36:74-80, 1981.
59. Konrad HR: Carcinoma of the larynx, *Hosp Med* 20(8):165-179, 1984.

60.* Larson GL: Rehabilitation for the patient with head and neck cancer, *Am J Nurs* 82:119-120, 1982.
61.* Lyons RJ: Surgical implants: voice prosthesis, *AORN J* 37;1369-1373, 1983.
62.* Lyons RJ: The head and neck patient, *AORN J* 40:751-760, 1984.
63. Mack RM: Lessons from living with cancer, *N Engl J Med* 311-1640-1644, 1984.
64. McCormick GP, et al: Artificial speech devices, *Am J Nurs* 82:121-122, 1982.
65. Norris JL: Fiberoptic endoscopy: where to go from here, laryngoscopy, *AANA J* 52:611-613, 1984.
66. Segal C, et al: Adenotonsillectomies on a surgical day-clinic basis, *Laryngoscope* 93:1205-1208, 1983.
67. Singer MI, Blom ED, Hamaker RC: Voice rehabilitation after total laryngectomy, *J Otolaryngol* 12:329-334, 1983.
68.* Stephens DJ: An information guide for patients receiving head and neck irradiation, *Oncol Nurs Forum* 11(5):75-80, 1984.
69. Yarington CT: The Caldwell-Luc operation revisited, *Ann Otol Rhinol Laryngol* 93:380-384, 1984.

24

The Patient with Pulmonary Problems

Wilma J. Phipps

After studying this chapter, the learner should be able to:

- Differentiate between restrictive and obstructive pulmonary disorders.
- Describe the nature of viral respiratory infections and methods of assisting effective coughing.
- Compare classic, atypical, aspiration, and hematogenous pneumonia.
- Describe measures to promote oxygenation, facilitate breathing, and provide ventilation and hydration.
- Describe incidence, preventive measures, and therapeutic approaches to tuberculosis.
- Compare fungal infections of the respiratory tract.
- Explain the pathophysiology of adult respiratory distress syndrome (ARDS).
- Describe incidence, prevention, and therapy for lung cancer.
- Describe types of chest surgery and the care of the patient undergoing chest surgery (including patients with chest tubes).
- Describe the pathophysiologic conditions of chest trauma (for instance, fractured ribs, penetrating wounds, and pneumothorax).
- Explain the pathophysiologic conditions and interventions for chronic obstructive pulmonary disease.
- Describe the nature of respiratory insufficiency and the care of the patient with an artificial airway or mechanical ventilation.

ANATOMY AND PHYSIOLOGY OF THE RESPIRATORY TRACT

The main purpose of respiration is to provide oxygen to body cells and to remove excess carbon dioxide from them. For respiration to take place there must be a way to deliver oxygen (O_2) to the body and a circulatory system to carry it to the cells and to remove carbon dioxide (CO_2) from them. The transport of O_2 is accomplished through the upper and lower airway.

Upper Airway

The upper airway consists of the nose and sinuses, the pharynx and tonsils, and the larynx and laryngopharynx.

Nose and sinuses

The nose is supported by the nasal bones, the nasal processes of the maxillary bones, the cartilaginous and bony parts of the septum, and the upper and lower nasal cartilages. Air enters the nose through the two nostrils (nares), which are separated by the septum. The septum, which is usually straight and thin in the child, is rarely straight in adults because in many cases, it has been injured.

The nasal cavities are located between the roof of the mouth and the frontal, ethmoid, and sphenoid bones. Three projections, lined with mucous membrane and called the turbinate bones, are located on the lateral walls of each nasal cavity. The turbinates provide a large surface area with a rich blood supply that warms and humidifies ambient air as it passes through this area. Large particles are filtered out of inhaled air by precipitation or by stim-

511

ulation of mechanical receptors located in the nasopharynx, which results in the sneeze reflex.

The vestibule of the nose is the anterior part of the nose. The vestibule extends posteriorly a short distance to a point at which its lining changes from skin to mucous membrane. This mucous membrane posterior to the vestibule contains cilia that beat in a constant wavelike motion to carry mucus into the nasopharynx. Trapped in the mucus are bacteria, dust, and other foreign matter entering the nose. The olfactory epithelium is located in a small area superiorly and provides the end-organ of smell. The lateral walls of the nose contain the opening for the paranasal sinuses and the nasolacrimal ducts. These openings provide a means of aeration of and mucus drainage from the sinuses. The blood supply to the nose comes from both the external and internal carotid systems.

Four sets of paranasal sinuses are located on either side of the head. These sinuses are air-filled spaces in the skull that serve to lighten the head. They drain into the nasal cavities through the openings behind the turbinates. The maxillary sinuses are the largest and most accessible. The sinuses are lined with mucous membrane that is continuous with that of the nose. *The functions of the nose and nasal sinus are to warm, moisten, and filter air in preparation for the lungs; to house receptors for olfaction; and to promote vocal resonance.*

Upper throat: pharynx and tonsils

The pharynx is the space behind the oral cavity that extends from the base of the skull to the larynx. The pharynx can be considered in three parts: the *nasopharynx*, the *oropharynx*, and the *laryngopharynx*. It is lined with mucous membrane.

The *adenoids* are located in the *nasopharynx*, the *palatine tonsils anterior to the oropharynx*, and *the lingual tonsils in the laryngopharynx*. The adenoids and tonsils are made up of lymphoid tissue that helps to filter the circulating lymph of bacteria or other foreign matter that penetrate the body, especially by way of the nose and mouth.

Lower throat: larynx and laryngopharynx

The larynx forms the upper extremity of the trachea. The framework of the larynx is made up of several cartilages held together by muscle and ligaments. The cartilaginous framework of the larynx protects the vocal cords and affords a stiffness that permits an airway.

The chief function of the larynx is to serve as an airway between the pharynx and trachea. A leaf-shaped lid of fibrocartilage (epiglottis) protects the glottis by covering the entrance to the larynx during swallowing to prevent aspiration of food or fluids. *The closing of the glottis also allows for an increase of intrathoracic pressure, which is needed, for example, in coughing or lifting. The cough reflex, like the sneeze reflex, helps remove inhaled particles from the respiratory tract.*

This increased pressure gives added advantage to the use of the muscles of the shoulder and thorax. In addition to these, a most important function of the larynx is *phonation*. The larynx creates sounds as a result of vocal cord vibrations that are formed into speech patterns by the movement of the pharynx, palate, tongue, teeth, and lips.

Structure and function of the respiratory tract

The *conducting airways* (trachea, right and left mainstem bronchi, and bronchioles), which terminate into *respiratory units* (respiratory bronchioles, alveolar ducts, and alveoli), make up the lower airways (Figs. 24-1 and 24-2).

In addition to providing a passageway for air, the *conducting airways serve three functions: filtering, warming, and humidifying air.* Air inspired through an intact respiratory tree is cleansed of all particles larger than 2 μm in diameter before reaching the alveolus. The removal of particulate matter such as dust and bacteria preserves the sterility of the alveolus. The removal of particulate matter, such as dust and bacteria, is accomplished by the *mucociliary system, one of the lung's primary defense mechanisms.* The mucociliary system consists of *cilia*, which line the respiratory tract from the laryngopharynx through the terminal bronchioles, and a dual-layered *fluid lining* secreted by *goblet cells* and *subendothelial glands*. The fluid lining that lies on top of the cilia consists of a lower serous and an upper mucopolysaccharide (mucous) layer. Inhaled particles are trapped in the mucous layer and are propelled upward toward the pharynx by the continuous rapid beating of the cilia. After reaching the pharynx, mucus and particles are removed from the airways by swallowing, coughing, or sneezing. The process of particle removal by the mucociliary system is often referred to as the *mucociliary escalator*.

The warming and humidifying functions are made possible by the rich capillary blood supply in the submucosal layer of the airways. During inspiration, air is heated to body temperature, and up to 1000 ml/day of water is used to raise the humidity of the inspired air to at least 80%. On expiration, some of this water is reabsorbed, thus conserving fluid; an average of 300 ml/day is lost in normal respiration.

Within the respiratory unit, respiration occurs only in the alveoli. Alveoli, which number 300 million in adults, are minute sacs that arise from the walls of the respiratory bronchioles and alveolar ducts. *The alveolus itself is composed of a single layer of squamous epithelium and an elastic basement membrane. These two layers, together with the interstitum and the endothelial and basement layers of the adjacent capillary, form the alveolar-capillary membrane or interface.* It is across this membrane, a distance less than 1 μm, that *diffusion of carbon dioxide and oxygen occurs* (Fig. 24-3). The spherical interconnected structure of the millions of alveoli provides a large (50 to 100 m) surface area for gaseous diffusion to occur.

In addition to their respiratory function, the alveoli prevent lung collapse by producing surfactant, a phospholipid that decreases surface tension and prevents interstitial fluid from traversing into the lung space. Any foreign matter that deposits in healthy alveoli is engulfed by macrophages and disposed of through the circulatory system.

Lungs and thoracic cavity

The lungs themselves are subdivided into lobes. The *right lung has three lobes: upper, middle, and lower. The left lung has only two lobes: upper and lower.* Air is conducted to each lobe through lobar bronchi that branch off the main-stem bronchus. An important difference between the right and left lungs is the size of the airways leading to

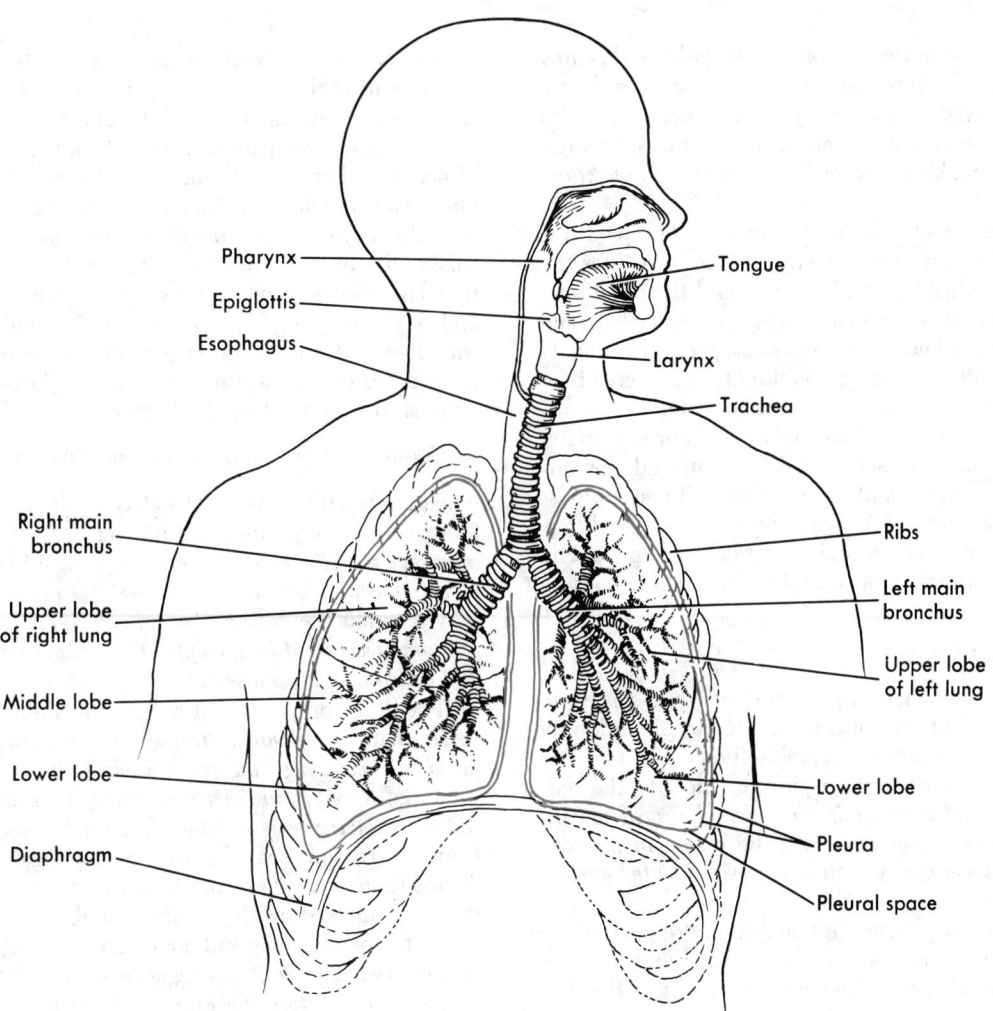

Fig. 24-1   Anatomy of the thorax and lungs.

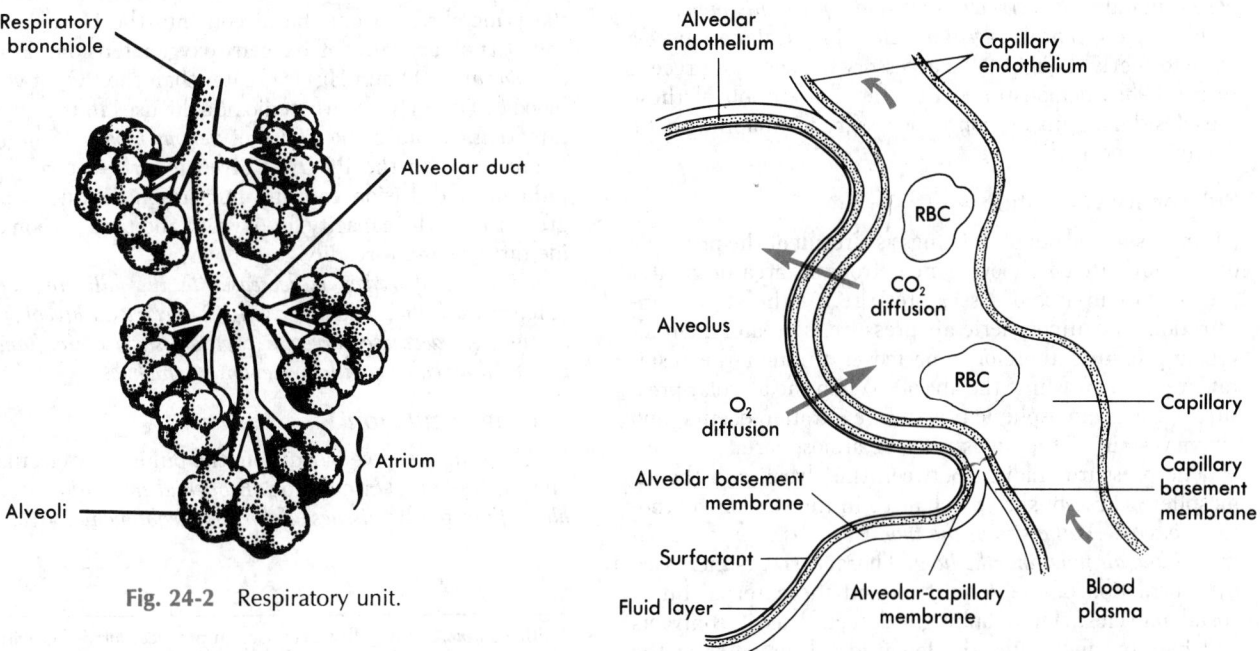

Fig. 24-2   Respiratory unit.

Fig. 24-3   Alveolar-capillary membrane.

them. *The right bronchus is significantly wider and shorter and extends at a straighter angle from the trachea, making it the more likely lodging point of aspirated material.* The *left bronchus* is narrower and extends at more of a right angle off the trachea, making it *more difficult to suction secretions from the left lung.*

The thoracic cavity is lined with pleura. The pleura is a continuous *serous* membrane; one surface of it lines the inside of the rib cage (parietal pleura), and the other surface (visceral pleura) covers the lungs. The space between the two surfaces is known as a *potential space.* It normally contains a few milliliters of serous fluid that prevents friction rub when the two surfaces come together.

The lungs lie in and are protected by the thoracic cavity. This bony cage is composed of the sternum and ribs anteriorly and the ribs, scapulae, and vertebral column posteriorly. On the anterior surface, the apices of the lungs lie just above the clavicles and posteriorly extend to the eleventh or twelfth rib. Figure 24-1 illustrates the borders of each lobe.

Respiratory muscles

The major function of the respiratory muscles is to pump air in and out of the lungs, thereby maintaining arterial blood gases within acceptable limits.[112]

The primary muscles of inspiration include the *diaphragm, the external intercostals, the internal parasternal intercostals, and the scalene muscles.* The major inspiratory muscle is the *diaphragm,* which is *innervated by the phrenic nerves.*

Although normal quiet expiration does not require active muscle contraction, relaxation of the abdominal muscles at the end of inspiration allows passive ascent of the diaphragm during expiration. When expiration is active, for example as a result of exercise, the *internal intercostal and abdominal muscles contract to assist expiration of air out of the lungs.*

Accessory muscles that are used when breathing is labored include the *sternocleidomastoids, pectoralis major and minor, trapezii, and laryngeal muscles.* The scalene muscles were formerly thought to be accessory muscles, but recent research has demonstrated that the contraction of these muscles during inspiration is necessary for diaphragmatic descent to occur.[112]

Pulmonary ventilation

Air moves in and out of the lungs as a result of the principle of gas flow; that is, movement is from an area of greater pressure to an area of lesser pressure. At the start of inspiration, the atmospheric air pressure is greater than alveolar pressure; therefore, air moves through the respiratory passageway into the alveoli. When the alveolar pressure exceeds atmospheric pressure, expiration occurs, and air moves out of the lungs into the atmosphere.

The pressure gradient between the alveoli and the atmosphere is established by changes in the size of the thoracic cavity. *As the size of the thorax increases, pressure decreases and air flows into the lung.* Thoracic size is increased by contraction of the diaphragm and the external intercostal muscles. The diaphragm descends as it contracts and flattens, increasing the longitudinal diameter of the thorax. The external intercostals, parasternal internal in-

tercostals, and the scalene muscles pull the ribs up and out, elevating the sternum and increasing both anteroposterior and lateral diameter of the chest.

As the thorax expands, it pulls the lungs with it because of cohesion between the moist surfaces of the lungs and chest wall. *Expiration is normally a passive process that results from the elastic recoil of the lungs and thoracic muscles.* It is this ability of the lungs to stretch and recoil that is evaluated by *pulmonary function testing* (see Table 24-6, *B*). The ability of the lungs to stretch is measured in terms of compliance. Compliance is the volume increase in lungs for every unit increase in intraalveolar pressure. This relationship is defined by the formula:

Compliance = Change in volume/Change in pressure

Thus lungs with increased (high) compliance have a larger increase in volume for each unit of pressure. *Lungs with increased compliance characterize a group of pulmonary disorders known as obstructive diseases.* Lungs with decreased (low) compliance *have a diminished volume for each unit of pressure. Decreased lung compliance characterizes lung disorders called restrictive diseases.*

The other property that affects the ability of the lungs to ventilate is *pulmonary resistance.* This property is *evaluated by measuring lung volume and airflow over time* (see Table 24-6, *C*). *Pulmonary resistance is made up of tissue resistance and airway resistance.* Tissue resistance results from the friction created as tissues move against each other during lung expansion. Airway resistance results from friction encountered by air passing through the airways. The major factor affecting pulmonary resistance is the radius of the airways. *The following factors alter airway radius:* (1) *bronchial innervation (for example: bronchospasm);* (2) *external compression (for example: thoracic tumor);* and (3) *internal obstruction (for example: mucus).*

Gas exchange (diffusion)

In the alveoli, oxygen diffuses across the alveolar-capillary membrane from the alveoli into the blood because the partial pressure of oxygen (oxygen tension, PO_2) of *alveolar air* (100 mm Hg) is greater than the PO_2 of venous blood (40 mm Hg). Carbon dioxide diffuses in the opposite direction, because the PCO_2 of *venous blood* (46 mm Hg) is greater than the PCO_2 of alveolar air (40 torr*). The pulmonary diffusion capacity for carbon dioxide is much greater than the capacity for oxygen, and thus carbon dioxide diffuses more readily.

Diffusion of oxygen is decreased by the following factors: (1) *decreased atmospheric oxygen,* (2) *decreased alveolar ventilation,* (3) *decreased alveolar-capillary surface area,* and (4) *increased alveolar-capillary membrane thickness.*

Lung circulation

The lungs receive blood from the pulmonary circulation and the bronchial circulation. *Bronchial circulation provides blood flow* to the *tissues of the tracheobronchial tree.* Pul-

---

*Although *mm Hg* is still widely used in practice, *torr* is becoming the accepted unit of pressure measurement in the scientific literature; 1 torr = 1 mm Hg.

monary circulation is made up of the entire blood volume received from the right ventricle of the heart. The deoxygenated blood from the right ventricle is carried through the main pulmonary artery to successively branching vessels that follow the bronchi to the respiratory units. *Within the alveolar walls, the branching capillaries form a dense network that has been described as a sheet of blood.* Thus the circulatory system matches the vast surface created by the alveoli to provide for the rapid efficient exchange of oxygen and carbon dioxide. Newly oxygenated blood then travels via the four pulmonary veins back to the left atrium where it is circulated throughout the body via the aorta.

Ventilation-perfusion relationships

As discussed above, exchange of oxygen and carbon dioxide between alveolar air and pulmonary capillary blood occurs by gaseous *diffusion*. It is imperative that lung *ventilation (airflow) and perfusion (bloodflow)* are relatively evenly matched so that adequate oxygen and carbon dioxide exchange can occur. Both airflow to the alveoli and blood flow to the pulmonary capillaries have volumes of 4 to 6 L/min. *A normal ratio between ventilation and perfusion ranges from 0.8 to 1.2.* A low ventilation-to-perfusion ratio exists when alveoli cannot receive ambient air. Blood flowing through the capillaries in contact with the occluded alveoli would have low oxygen and high carbon dioxide levels. A clinical situation that can cause *low ventilation-to-perfusion ratios is when secretions block* bronchioles leading to alveoli (Fig. 24-12). A *high ventilation-to-perfusion ratio exists when a pulmonary capillary is blocked.* In this situation, oxygen and carbon dioxide levels in the alveoli remain the same as ambient air (Fig. 24-12). A clinical situation that can cause high ventilation-to-perfusion ratios is pulmonary emboli.

Control of respiration

Breathing is an automatic process, but it may also be controlled voluntarily; that is, although humans do not have to think about breathing, they can breathe slower or faster at will. Voluntary control of respiration is centered in the cerebral cortex, from which impulses are sent to innervate the muscles of respiration.

Automatic control of respiration is centered in the medulla and pons. The pons is responsible for maintaining rhythmicity of respirations. The respiratory center that is located in the medulla is controlled primarily by *central chemoreceptors* that are sensitive to carbon dioxide tension (PCO_2), oxygen tension (PO_2), and acidity (pH) of arterial blood.

Peripheral chemoreceptors, located in the carotid body and aortic arch, respond to low arterial blood oxygen levels. The peripheral sensor mechanism is believed to be a built-in backup mechanism, and it does not function under normal physiologic conditions.

When the central chemoreceptor is not functioning because of elevated carbon dioxide levels of more than a few days' duration CO_2 narcosis results. When this occurs it is only the person's peripheral chemoreceptor response to a decreased oxygen level that maintains respiration. Elevating the oxygen level without simultaneous lowering of the carbon dioxide level will result in apnea and death.

Factors necessary for oxygen–carbon dioxide exchange

For breathing to take place normally, several factors are necessary: (1) an adequate supply of oxygen in the environment, (2) a patent airway, (3) a normally functioning bellows motion of the chest wall and diaphragm, (4) an adequate number of functioning alveoli and capillaries that together form a terminal respiratory unit (TRU), (5) an adequate amount of hemoglobin to carry oxygen to the cells, (6) an intact circulatory system and an effective heart pump, and (7) a functioning respiratory center. Problems in one or more of these can result in inadequate exchange of oxygen and carbon dioxide and, if severe enough, can cause death. Table 24-1 lists some of the conditions that can lead to inadequate oxygen-carbon dioxide exchange. Each of these factors is discussed here.

Maintaining an adequate supply of oxygen in the environment

High altitudes do not change the composition of the air, but the oxygen pressure (PO_2) decreases.[122] Persons exposed to high altitudes, such as pilots, astronauts, mountain climbers, and those moving to high altitudes, have various reactions depending on the rate at which hypoxia develops, the degree of oxygen requirements as determined by physical exertion, and the duration of exposure.[122]

The initial reaction to high altitudes results in the same signs and symptoms seen in anyone experiencing oxygen lack. *Headache, dizziness, breathlessness, weakness, nausea, sweating, palpitation, dimness of vision, partial deafness, and sleeplessness occur with moderate hypoxia.*[122] With exertion, dyspnea and other symptoms worsen. These signs and symptoms have been referred to as *mountain sickness* because they are evident as persons drive or take a train through altitudes higher than those to which they have been accustomed.

These symptoms gradually disappear over days or weeks depending on the altitude, and the person is eventually able to carry out more activities without becoming short of breath. This is known as *acclimatization* and is caused in part by an increased capacity for supplying oxygen to the tissues and in part by overcoming the consequences of hypocapnia produced by excessive breathing.[122]

The *factors involved in acclimatization include:* (1) *a sustained increase in alveolar ventilation,* (2) *adjustment in the acid-base composition of the blood and other body fluids,* (3) *an increase in oxygen-carrying capacity,* and (4) *an increase in cardiac output.*[122]

Persons moving to higher altitudes, such as mountain climbers, are advised to allow time for their bodies to adjust to changes in various altitudes. Trained climbers, especially those ascending to very high altitudes, allow themselves weeks or even months at base camps at various altitudes in preparation for their ascent.[122]

Maintaining a patent airway

Several measures may be used to ensure a patent airway. The most basic measure involves simply positioning the person in such a way as to prevent obstruction of the airway. This is most relevant in resuscitation or in caring for an unconscious person. The position of choice is supine or side-lying with the neck hyperextended. Persons who

Table 24-1   Factors interfering with oxygenation and normal oxygen–carbon dioxide exchange

Necessary component	Interference
Adequate supply of oxygen	Inhalation of air containing oxygen at subnormal pressure caused by: Smoke inhalation Carbon monoxide poisoning High altitudes
	Dilution of inspired air with inert gases (nitrogen, helium, hydrogen, methane, or anesthetic gases such as nitrous oxide)
Patent airway	Interference with the passage of oxygen from air through tracheobronchial tree to alveolar-capillary membrane caused by mechanical obstruction such as drowning or foreign bodies in tracheobronchial tree: Children (aspiration of objects such as pennies, pins, or jacks) Unconscious adults (tongue obstructing airway, aspirated vomitus, or loose dentures) Mucus plug resulting in atelectasis
	Allergic reactions resulting in bronchoconstriction, increased mucus secretions, and increased capillary permeability
Normally functioning bellows	Trauma to chest wall with possible sequelae of paradoxical breathing, pneumothorax, and mediastinal shift
	Muscle or nerve trauma or impairment (quadriplegia, paraplegia, poliomyelitis, myasthenia gravis, Guillain-Barré syndrome, Landry's ascending paralysis, and muscular dystrophy)
Adequate functioning alveoli and capillaries (TRU)	Pulmonary edema Adult respiratory disease syndrome (interstitial edema) Physiologic shunts Damage to alveolar-capillary membrane secondary to conditions such as pulmonary emphysema
Adequate amount of hemoglobin	Severe anemia Carbon monoxide poisoning Methemoglobinemia
Intact circulatory system and pump	Congestive heart failure Hemorrhage
Functioning respiratory center	Depression of respiratory center by drugs (heroin, morphine, barbiturates, alcohol, or a combination of alcohol with a tranquilizer or barbiturates) Increased intracranial pressure (head injury or disease such as meningitis)

are unconscious or very lethargic may suffer airway obstruction if the tongue should fall back and cover the glottis; the side-lying position prevents this from happening.

When a person has a mechanical obstruction of the airway and is expected to be unconscious for some time, it may be necessary to use an artificial airway (p. 616).

Maintaining bellows function of the chest wall and diaphragm

Whenever there is interference with the bellows function of the chest wall, there are changes in breathing pattern. The major cause of disruption of the bellows function is trauma to the chest involving fractures of the ribs or penetrating chest wounds. These conditions and their sequelae of paradoxical breathing and pneumothorax are discussed on p. 577.

Maintaining an adequate number of terminal respiratory units

The individual with pulmonary disease may have impaired ability to aerate alveoli. The impairment may be related to several factors. These include (1) inability to move adequate amounts of air in and out of the lungs, (2) interference with alveolar expansion secondary to an accumulation of secretions resulting in collapse of portions of the lungs (*atelectasis*), and (3) restriction of lung expan-

sion by mechanical factors such as air in the pleural space (*pneumothorax*) or fluid or blood in the pleural space (*pleural effusion* or *hemothorax*). An increase in respiratory rate and pulse rate indicates that the body is trying to compensate for hypoxia. Patients who must make a conscious effort to breathe become very fatigued. They also become anxious because of shortness of breath and hypoxia.

Maintaining transportation of oxygen and adequate oxygenation of tissues

For oxygen to be supplied to the cells there must be (1) *an adequate amount of hemoglobin available to transport oxygen* and (2) *an effective heart pump and circulatory system to deliver the oxygen to the tissues.* The amount of oxygen delivered to body tissues each minute equals the cardiac output in liters per minute times the number of milliliters of oxygen contained in 1 L of arterial blood. In the resting state this is about 5×200, or 1000 ml O_2/min. About one fourth of this is used by the tissues, and three fourths returns to the heart in mixed venous blood. During exercise the amount of oxygen contained in 1 L of arterial blood does not increase, but the cardiac output does increase. With a cardiac output of 24 L/min, the oxygen delivered would be 24×200, or 4800 ml/min. The tissues would use three fourths of this amount, and only one fourth would be returned to the heart in mixed venous blood.[99]

An *inadequate amount of hemoglobin* (such as occurs in anemia), *an inadequate heart pump*, or *a problem with the circulatory system can all have a deleterious effect on the delivery of oxygen*. In these situations the basic problem is treated in an attempt to increase the amount of available hemoglobin, to strengthen the heart pump and thus increase the cardiac output, or to improve the circulatory system. As can be seen in Table 24-1, *severe anemia, carbon monoxide poisoning, methemoglobinemia, congestive heart failure*, and *hemorrhage are possible interferences that must be corrected before an optimal amount of oxygen is available to the tissues*.

If *hypotension is present secondary to hemorrhage* or a *failing heart pump*, there may be *several sequelae*. These include (1) *anginal pain, because the coronary vessels that normally extract almost the maximal amount of oxygen* are not receiving sufficient oxygen to supply the myocardium and (2) *changes in sensorium and behavior secondary to cerebral anoxia*. If this situation continues and there is inadequate oxygenation of tissues, respiratory or cardiac arrest may result. If an arrest occurs, cardiopulmonary resuscitation (CPR) must be instituted. CPR is discussed in detail in Chapter 25, and the reader is referred there for details.

Maintaining a functioning respiratory center

Hypoventilation or apnea can occur if there is *depression of the respiratory center by general anesthesia*, or by drugs such as morphine, heroin, barbiturates, or alcohol. Diseases of the central nervous system, such as bulbar poliomyelitis or meningitis, also depress the respiratory center, as does an increase in intracranial pressure. In these situations the patient's respirations must be assisted until the patient is able to maintain his or her own breathing. Intubation with an endotracheal tube, supplemental oxygen, and artificial respiration with a ventilator may all be required. The conditions causing depression of the respiratory center need to be identified and treated while the person's ventilation is being maintained by a ventilator. Details of management of patients in respiratory failure are discussed on p. 615.

Physiologic Changes With Aging

Several changes occur in the lungs and other parts of the respiratory tract with aging.

Structural alterations in the thorax may limit lung expansion. Ribs do not move as freely because of cartilage calcification and partial contraction of respiratory muscles. Kyphosis (hunchback) secondary to osteoporosis decreases the transverse measurement of the thorax. The lungs become more rigid and less elastic. *There is a decrease in both residual volume and a decrease in vital capacity* (see Table 24-6) *secondary to a decrease in the strength of the inspiratory and expiratory muscles*. The result is incomplete lung expansion and basilar lung collapse. These changes may *not* cause an obvious decrease in lung performance unless there is an increase in activity or stress when dyspnea and other symptoms occur.

As a result of these changes older people are very vulnerable to respiratory problems if they develop a pulmonary infection or other illness that places stress on their already compromised respiratory system. For instance, changes in the thorax and altered muscle strength cause a decreased ability to clear the airway and cough effectively.

PHYSICAL EXAMINATION OF THE CHEST

Physical examination of the chest provides objective data that, along with information obtained during the interview, forms the database necessary to formulate nursing diagnoses appropriate to the individual. The pulmonary examination should be conducted with the person sitting upright on the edge of the bed, if possible. Adequate lighting and a relaxed, quiet environment are essential to obtain maximum information.

Detailed instruction in the techniques for performing the chest examination is beyond the scope of this book. The reader is referred to a textbook of physical assessment for in-depth information on the techniques of pulmonary physical assessment. Three of the steps in the physical examination of the chest are *inspection, palpation,* and *percussion*.

Inspection

The patient is observed for general appearance, respiratory rate and pattern, and thoracic configuration (Figs. 24-4, A and B). It is important to take adequate time to thor-

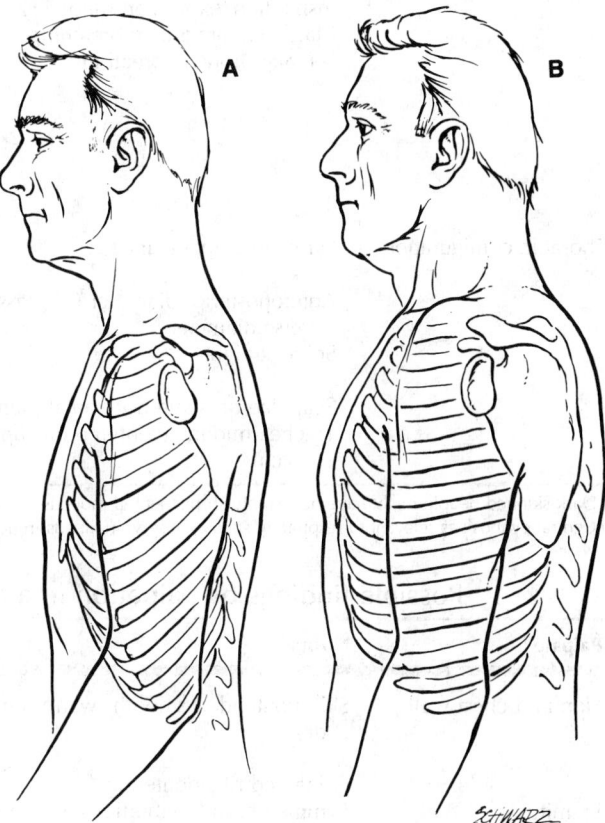

Fig. 24-4 A, Normal thorax configuration. **B,** Increased anteroposterior diameter. Note contrasts in the angle of the slope of the ribs and the development of the accessory muscle of respiration in the neck. (From Malasanos L, Barkauskas V, Stoltenberg-Allen K: *Health assessment,* ed 4, St Louis, 1990, Mosby–Year Book.)

Table 24-2 Possible findings by inspection in a pulmonary examination

Observe	Normal	Abnormal
General appearance	Quiet respiration Sitting or reclining without difficulty Skin translucent, appears dry Nailbeds pink	Lips puckered when exhaling Restless and apprehensive Leans forward with hands or elbows on knees Skin: diaphoretic, dull pale, or ruddy
	Mucous membranes pink and moist* Cyanosis or pallor assessed by establishing an early individual baseline	Cyanosis: Skin or mucous membrane has bluish cast Central cyanosis: results from decreased oxygenation of blood† Peripheral cyanosis: result of local vasoconstriction or decreased output Nail clubbing: painless enlargement of terminal phalanges related to chronic tissue hypoxia (see Fig. 24-42)
Trachea	Midline in neck	Tracheal deviation; displacement either lateral, anterior, or posterior Jugular venous distension (see Chapter 25) Cough: strong or weak, dry or wet, productive or nonproductive Sputum production: amount, color, odor, consistency
Rate	Eupnea: 12 to 20	Tachypnea: rate >20 breaths/min Bradypnea: rate <10 breaths/min
Breathing pattern	Minimal effort with inspiration: passive, quiet expiration Inspiration/expiration ratio: 1:2 Male: diaphragmatic breathing Female: thoracic breathing	Hypernea: increased breathing rate Accessory muscle breathing Apnea: total absence of breathing Biots: irregular rhythm with periods of apnea Cheyne-Stokes: cyclical deeper and shallower breaths followed by periods of apnea Kussmaul's: deep, rapid, and regular breathing Paradoxical: portion of chest wall moves in during inhalation and out during exhalation Stridorous: audible, loud, low-pitched sound with inhalation and exhalation
Thoracic configuration	Symmetric appearance Anteroposterior diameter (AP) less than transverse diameter Spine straight Scapulae on same horizontal plane Trachea midline (centered on suprasternal notch)	Chest expands unevenly Muscular development asymmetric Barrel chest: AP diameter increased in relation to transverse diameter (see Fig. 24-4) Kyphosis: increased thoracic curvature Scoliosis: increased lateral curvature Scapular placement *asymmetric* Trachea right or left of midline

*Dark-skinned people might have normal bluish pigmented mucous membranes.
†Central cyanosis is relevant to respiratory status. Observe nailbeds, mucous membrane, and lips.

Table 24-3 Possible findings by palpation in a pulmonary examination

Palpate	Normal	Abnormal
Skin and chest wall	Skin nontender, smooth, warm, and dry Spine and ribs nontender	Skin moist or exceedingly dry Crepitation—"crackling" when skin palpated—due to air leak from lung into subcutaneous tissue Localized tenderness
Fremitus*	Symmetric, mild vibrations felt on chest wall during vocalization	Increased fremitus—a result of vibrations through more solid medium such as lung tumors Decreased fremitus—a result of vibration through increased space in the chest such as pneumothorax or obesity. Asymmetric fremitus is always abnormal
Lateral chest expansion	Symmetric 3 to 8 cm expansion†	Expansion less than 3 cm, painful or assymetric†

*Normal fremitus varies from person to person. An individual's baseline must be established.
†Reduced expansion can result from either an overexpanded chest (barrel chest) or from a restricted chest.

Table 24-4   Possible findings by percussion in a pulmonary examination

Percussion	Normal	Abnormal
Lung fields	Resonant low-pitched, hollow, easily heard sounds; equal quality bilaterally	Hyperresonant: heard with air trapping or pneumothorax Dull or flat: results from decreased air in lungs (tumor, fluid)
Diaphragm position and movement	Resting diaphragm at 10th thoracic vertebrae Each hemidiaphragm moves 3-6 cm (Fig. 24-5)	High position—stomach distension or phrenic nerve damage Decreased or no movement in either hemidiaphragm*

*Decreased excursion can result from hyperinflated lungs pushing down on diaphragm, diaphragmatic disorders, or loss of diaphragmatic innervation.

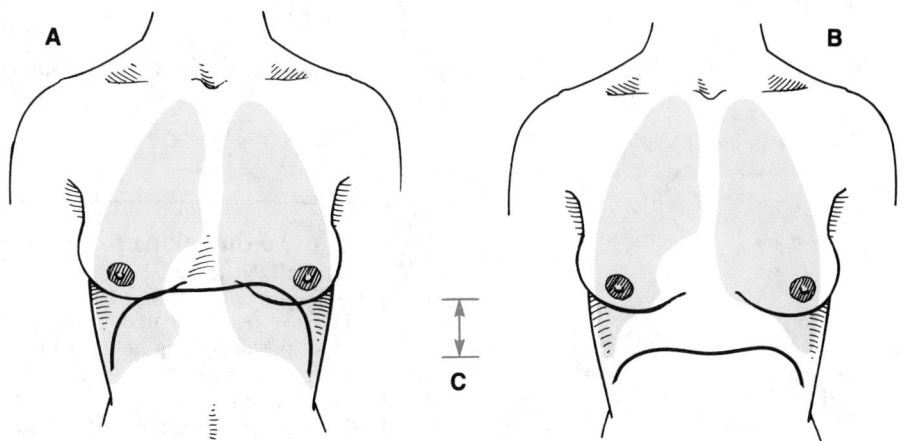

Fig. 24-5   Diaphragmatic excursion. **A,** Full-end expiration. **B,** Full-end inspiration. **C,** Range of diaphragmatic movement—distance from A to B.

oughly observe the patient before moving to the "hands on" component of the examination. By observing general appearance, respiratory rate and pattern, the presence and character of the person's cough, and sputum production, the nurse can determine which components of the pulmonary examination are appropriate for assessing the patient's current respiratory status. Table 24-2 indicates the normal and abnormal findings for each component of inspection.

Palpation

The chest is palpated to evaluate skin and chest wall status. Palpation of the chest and spinal column is a general screening technique to identify the presence of underlying abnormalities such as inflammation. The chest is also palpated for *fremitus, which are vibrations felt on the chest surface when sound passes through underlying tissue and air- or fluid-filled space.* Fremitus can be caused by secretions in the large airways, a pleural friction rub, or lung consolidation. Vocal (tactile) fremitus is normally present; thus it is necessary to determine whether fremitus is increased or decreased. The chest is also palpated for symmetry and degree of lateral chest expansion from maximal exhalation to maximal inhalation. Possible normal and abnormal findings are presented in Table 24-3.

Percussion

Percussion is used to assess the lung fields and the position and movement of the diaphragm (excursion). *Percussion notes are produced from vibration created by tapping the chest wall.* The quality of the percussion note depends on the density of underlying tissue and the amount of air through which the vibration passes. Table 24-4 identifies common normal and abnormal percussion findings.

Pulmonary Auscultation

Auscultation of the lungs enables a nurse to establish baseline data for identifying current and potential lung problems that require nursing interventions, such as determining the frequency for breathing exercises or the need for or effectiveness of suctioning. Landmarks for pulmonary auscultation are illustrated in Fig. 24-6.

Breath sounds

Breath sounds result from the movement of air through the lungs and air passages. The sounds are thought to occur as a result of two elements, the vesicular and bronchial elements. The vesicular element occurs when the walls of the alveoli are separated by air entering the alveoli from inspiration. The bronchial element is a hisslike sound re-

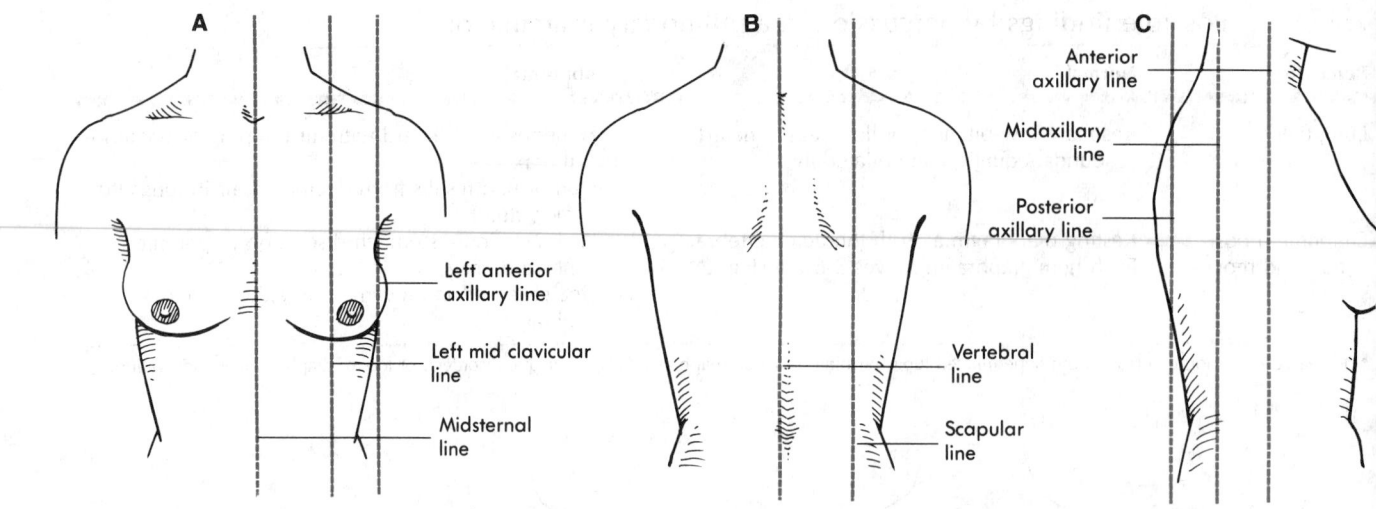

Fig. 24-6 Topographical landmarks. **A,** Anterior thorax. **B,** Posterior thorax. **C,** Lateral thorax.

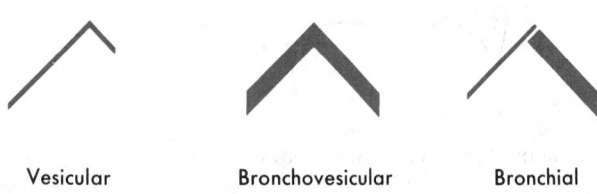

Vesicular   Bronchovesicular   Bronchial

Fig. 24-7 Schematic representation of the three types of breath sounds.

sulting from air flowing past the bronchi and across the vocal chords.

The three types of breath sounds that can be heard are vesicular, bronchovesicular, and bronchial (Fig. 24-7). *Vesicular breath sounds are heard over most of the lungs because of the prominence of the alveoli.* The sounds are of a low pitch and have a soft rustling or swishing quality. The sound of the inspiratory phase is longer and higher in pitch than that of the expiratory phase, which is a soft, short, low-pitched, almost inaudible sound. The relative loudness of inspiration may differ among listening sites; the sounds are usually softer at the bases of the lungs.

Bronchovesicular breath sounds are heard as one auscultates toward the main bronchi. Inspiration and expiration are loud and nearly equal in duration and intensity because of auscultating closer to the vocal chords.

Bronchial breath sounds normally are not heard over any area of lung tissue and their presence indicates consolidation such as occurs in pneumonia, or compression of lung tissue or a pleural effusion. These breath sounds are high pitched and loud; during the expiratory phase they increase in duration, pitch, and intensity.

General directions for pulmonary auscultation

1. Have person seated if possible for auscultation of posterior lung fields. The female patient may be easier to auscultate anteriorly if she is lying down.
2. Use the diaphragm of the stethoscope. Press firmly to produce a blanched ring when the diaphragm is removed. Hold the diaphragm in such a way as to decrease extraneous sounds (fingers not touching skin and diaphragm, or tubing of stethoscope not touching clothing or other objects).
3. Provide counter support for the person with your free hand.
4. Tell person to (a) turn head away, (b) breathe *slightly* deeper but *not* faster, and (c) breathe through the mouth.
5. Listen in a consistent, systematic manner.
6. At each listening site (Figs. 24-8 to 24-10), listen for one full breath and identify:
   • Type of breath sound
   • Intensity of breath sound
   • Presence of adventitious sounds

Adventitious abnormal lung sounds

Adventitious lung sounds are abnormal sounds superimposed on breath sounds. There are essentially two kinds of abnormal sounds: (1) *crackles* or *rales* (rhymes with *pals*) caused by air flowing through moisture in the air passages and (2) *wheezes* or *rhonchi* caused by air flowing through narrowed air passages (Table 24-5). A third type of sound occurs outside the lung; a *pleural friction rub* results from the rubbing of inflamed pleura between the lung and chest wall. Box 24-1 lists the steps of pulmonary auscultation.

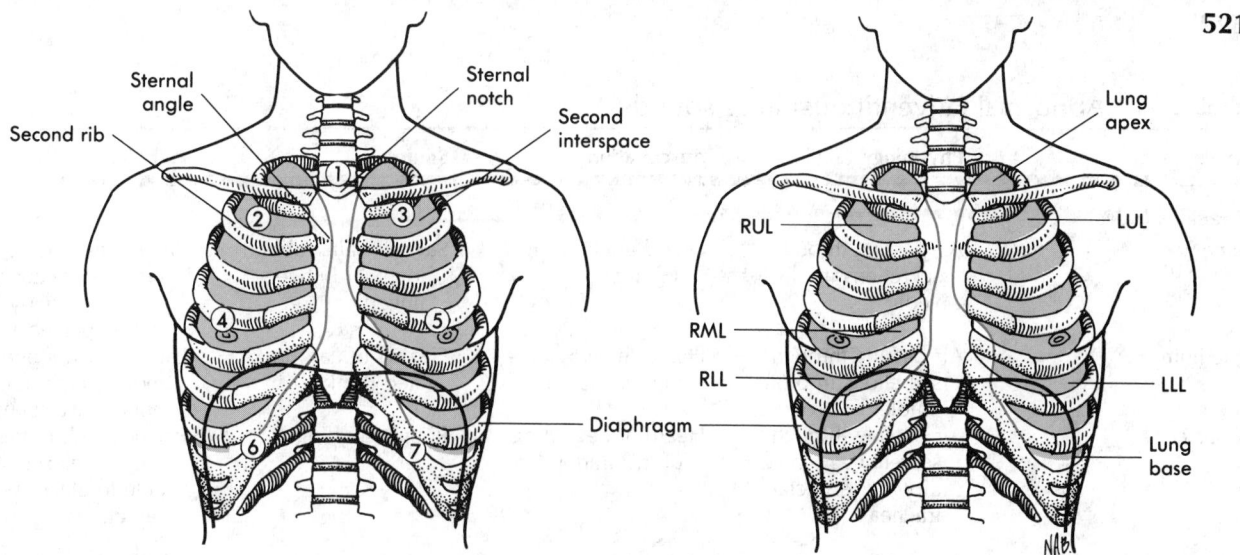

Fig. 24-8 Anterior thorax showing placement of stethoscope when listening to breath sounds and position of lobes of lungs.

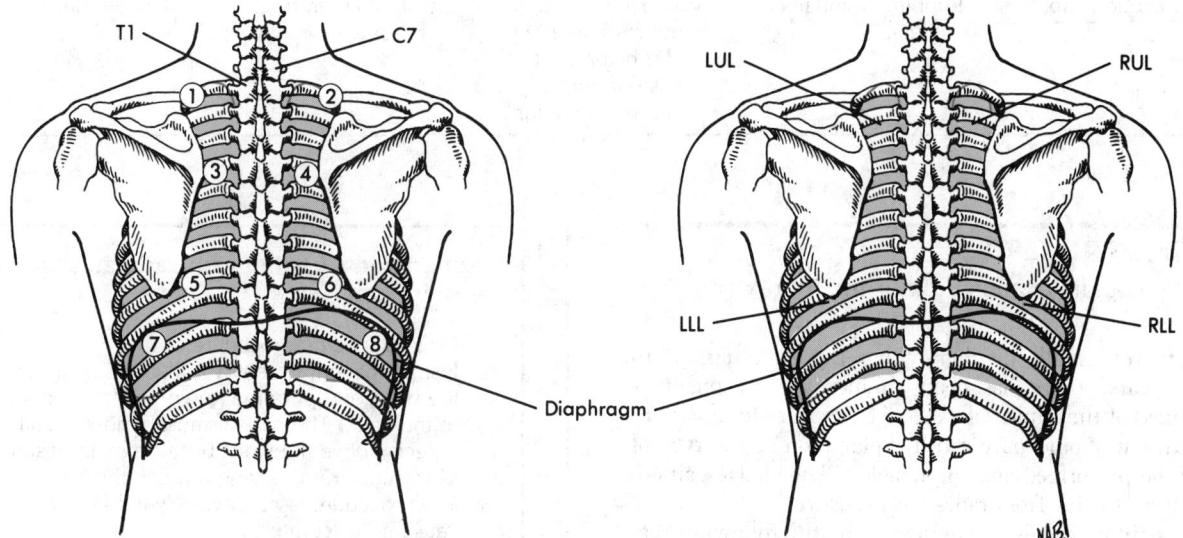

Fig. 24-9 Posterior thorax showing placement of stethoscope when listening to breath sounds and position of lobes of lungs.

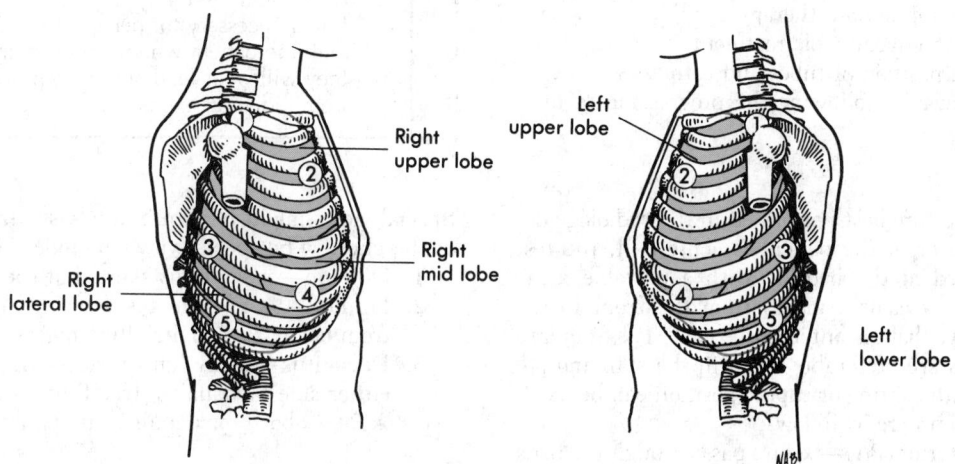

Fig. 24-10 Lateral thorax showing placement of stethoscope when listening to breath sounds and position of lobes of lungs.

Table 24-5 Abnormal (adventitious) lung sounds

Type	Physiology	Auscultation	Sound	Pathology
Crackles (rales)				
Fine	Air passing through secretions in alveoli	Heard at end of inspiration	Several hairs rubbed together between fingertips	Pneumonia, heart failure (may occur normally in elderly bedridden persons)
Medium	Air passing through secretions in bronchioles or bronchi	Heard midway during inspiration	Fizzing of carbonated drink	Later stages of pneumonia, heart failure, pulmonary edema
Coarse	Air passing through secretions in large airways, especially trachea	Heard at beginning of inspiration	Rough gurgling	Persons with repressed cough reflexes, unable to clear own secretions
Wheezes (rhonchi)	Air passing through narrow passages	Heard mostly during expiration, but may also occur with inspiration	Loud musical gurgling	Obstructive lung disease
Pleural friction rub	Rubbing of inflamed pleura	May occur throughout respiratory cycle, heard best at base of lung at end of expiration	Scratching, grating, rubbing	Inflamed pleura

DIAGNOSTIC TESTS

Roentgenologic examination of the thorax and lungs

Patients are usually familiar with x-ray examination. In recent years, there has been an increase in consumer awareness of the danger of excessive exposure to radiation. The patient should have a full explanation of the type of test to be performed and the benefits (knowledge gained) in relation to risk from radiation exposure.

Chest film studies are indicated for the following reasons:

1. Detect alterations of the lung caused by pathologic processes such as tumors, inflammation, fractures, fluid or air accumulation
2. Determine appropriate therapy
3. Evaluate effectiveness of treatment
4. Determine position of tubes and catheters
5. Provide a way of following the progression of lung disease

Chest films

Chest film studies are best performed in the radiology department. However, if the patient is acutely ill, the test can be completed at the bedside with a portable x-ray camera. The x-ray camera moves from the front to the back of the body; that is, anteroposterior (AP). Standard chest x-ray films are preferably taken in the standing position, although the sitting or supine position can be used. The standard views are as follows:

1. Posteroanterior (PA)—x-rays pass through the back to the front of the body
2. Lateral—x-rays pass through the side of the body (usually left side)

24-2

Preparation of patient for radiographic examination

1. Explain specific procedure.
2. Instruct patient to remove all clothing above the waist and put on a gown with an opening in the back. The patient must remove metal objects above the waist because metal restricts x-ray films from passing through the body.
3. The procedure is noninvasive and should cause no discomfort.
4. Patient will probably be alone in the room, but someone is nearby and always has voice contact.
5. Patient will probably be asked to take a deep breath and hold it.
6. If it is necessary for persons to be in the room with the patient while x-ray is being taken, they will wear lead aprons to protect them from radiation exposure.

Special views might be required to visualize specific parts of the chest. The special views include the following:

1. Oblique—x-ray films slanted at specific angles
2. Lordotic—x-ray films slanted at 45-degree angle from below to visualize lung apices
3. Decubitus—x-ray films taken with patient lying on either side to visualize free fluid in chest

See Box 24-2 above for details of preparation procedure.

Tomography

Tomography is a special technique that permits better visualization of a single layer or plane of the lungs. It is used to study cavities, neoplasms, and lung densities. The patient is required to lie still while an x-ray tube is rapidly moved over the lung at approximately 1-cm intervals. The procedure takes approximately 15 minutes.

Computed tomography

Computed tomography (CT) is rapidly replacing standard tomographic examination. Conventional tomography resulted in a blurred film, except for the one plane being observed. CT scanning uses computer programming to enhance and process the x-ray film "slices" to produce a clear picture of the chest cavity structures.

Fluoroscopic examination

When dynamic information about the chest such as diaphragmatic movement, lung expansion and contraction, or cardiac action is required, fluoroscopy is the preferred examination.

Ultrasound (echogram)

In an ultrasound examination, a harmless, high-frequency sound wave is emitted and penetrates the thorax. These sound waves bounce back and are converted by a transducer to a pictorial image of the area being studied. Ultrasound of the thorax can provide information about pleural effusion or opacities in the lung.

Bronchography

A bronchogram enables the physician to visualize the bronchial tree by x-ray film after the introduction of an iodized radiopaque liquid, which coats the bronchial mucosa. The pharynx, larynx, and major bronchi are anesthetized with a topical anesthetic before introduction of a metal cannula into the trachea. The radiopaque substance is then introduced, and the patient is tilted in various positions to distribute the dye to the bronchi and bronchioles. A series of x-ray films are then taken. See Box 24-3 for details.

Preparation of patient for a bronchogram

Prebronchogram
1. Patient is instructed to do complete mouth care night and morning before procedure.
2. Patient does not eat or drink for 8 hours before procedure.
3. Dentures are removed. Document any loose teeth on preoperative sheet.
4. Shortly before the examination, patient receives a short-acting sedative and an antispasmodic.

Postbronchogram
1. Postural drainage is initiated unless contraindicated to assist in the removal of radiopaque substance.
2. Food and fluid are withheld until gag reflex returns.
3. Deep breathing, coughing, and moving about are encouraged to maintain a clear airway.

Preparation for lung scan or pulmonary angiography

Radiopaque iodine is the radionucleotide usually used for both pulmonary angiography and lung scan. Always carry out the following activities.
1. Check patient for iodine allergy.
2. Obtain an order (often a standing order) to administer 10 drops of Lugol's solution several hours before the test to block thyroid uptake of radioactive iodine.

Roentgenologic Examination of Ventilation and Perfusion

Lung scan (pulmonary scintiphotography)

Lung scan procedures involve the use of a scanning device that records the pattern of pulmonary radioactivity after the inhalation or intravenous injection of gamma ray—emitting radionucleotides, thus providing a visual image of the distribution of ventilation or blood flow in the lungs. These studies provide valuable information about ventilation-perfusion patterns and aid in the diagnosis of parenchymal lung disease and vascular disorders such as pulmonary embolism. See Box 24-4 for preparation procedures.

In a *perfusion scan, radiopaque iodine is injected intravenously.* The lungs are then scanned, and the pattern of particle distribution in the lung vasculature is recorded. Areas of poor radionucleotide uptake are suggestive of pulmonary vascular disorders. In a *ventilation scan, the radioactive gas is inhaled, and the lungs are scanned to detect abnormal diffusion of the gas throughout the lungs.*

Pulmonary angiography

Pulmonary angiography is used to detect pulmonary emboli and a variety of congenital and acquired lesions of the pulmonary vessels. A radiopaque material is injected via a catheter into a systemic vein, the right chambers of the heart, or the pulmonary artery; and the distribution of this material is recorded on film.

Positron emission tomography (PET)

PET uses the capability of computerization to study regional pulmonary perfusion and ventilation-perfusion relationships. A radioisotope that releases positrons (positively charged particles with the same mass as an electron) is inhaled by or injected into the individual. As the short-lived radioisotope decays, it releases gamma rays that are recorded by the computerized scanner.

Examination of Sputum

Sputum analysis

Examinations of sputum are usually required when chest disease is suspected. The mucous membrane of the respiratory tract responds to inflammation by an increased flow of secretions that often contain causative organisms. The volume, consistency, color, and odor of the sputum are observed and recorded (see Box 24-5).

24-5

Sputum color analysis

1. Colorless or clear mucoid: noninfectious process
2. Creamy yellow: staphylococcal pneumonia
3. Green: *Pseudomonas* pneumonia
4. "Currant jelly": *Klebsiella* pneumonia
5. Rusty: pneumococcal pneumonia
6. Pink frothy: pulmonary edema

Sputum examination includes the following tests:

1. *Gram stain* usually gives enough information about organisms and cells present to give a presumptive diagnosis.
2. *Culture* identifies specific organisms to enable making a definitive diagnosis. It should be collected before initiation of antibiotic therapy and thereafter to monitor effectiveness of antibiotic therapy.
3. *Sensitivity* serves as a guide to antimicrobial therapy by identifying antibiotics that prevent growth of the organism present in the sputum. It is collected before initiation of antibiotic therapy. Culture and sensitivity (C & S) are usually ordered together.
4. *Acid-fast bacilli* (AFB) determines the presence of mycobacterium tuberculosis which, after taking up a dye, is not decolorized by acid alcohol.
5. *Cytology* assists in identification of lung carcinoma. Sputum contains coughed cells from tracheobronchial tree; thus malignant cells might be present. Although the presence of malignant cells indicates carcinoma, the absence of cells might indicate that either there is no tumor or that the tumor is not shedding cells.
6. *Quantitative test* is the collection of sputum over a period of 24 to 72 hours.

Sputum collection

Tests to be performed on sputum are explained to the patient so that a suitable specimen will be obtained. The patient is instructed to collect only sputum that has come from deep in the lungs. When not instructed adequately, patients often expectorate saliva rather than sputum. They are likely to exhaust themselves unnecessarily by shallow, frequent coughing that yields no sputum suitable for study and that affords them little relief from discomfort. *The first sputum raised in the morning is usually the most productive of organisms.* During the night, secretions accumulate in the bronchi, and just a few deep coughs will bring them to the back of the throat. If patients do not know this fact, on awakening they may almost unconsciously cough, clear their throats, and swallow or expectorate before attempting to produce the specimen.

The patient should be supplied with a wide-mouthed container and instructed to expectorate directly into it. Because the sight of sputum is often objectionable to the patient and to others, the outside of a glass container is covered with paper or other suitable covering. Usually 4 ml of sputum is sufficient for laboratory tests and examinations. Nursing implications for sputum collection include the following:

1. Patients who have difficulty producing sputum or who have very tenacious sputum might be dehydrated. Encourage fluid intake.
2. Collect specimen before meals to avoid possible emesis from coughing after eating.
3. Instruct patient to rinse mouth with water before collecting specimen to decrease contamination.
4. Instruct patient to notify staff as soon as specimen is collected so that it can be sent to the laboratory as soon as possible.

Occasionally patients have difficulty producing sputum for examination. Inhalation of a hypertonic solution such as 10% saline in distilled water is used to temporarily stimulate sputum collection. Other methods to collect sputum include the following: (1) endotracheal aspiration with a suction catheter and special sputum collection container, (2) transtracheal aspiration (insertion of a needle with a catheter through the cricothyroid cartilage), and (3) fiberoptic bronchoscopy (p. 528).

Gastric washings

Gastric aspiration is occasionally used to collect gastric contents, which may contain swallowed sputum. It is usually performed when the diagnosis or suspected diagnosis is tuberculosis. Because most patients swallow sputum when coughing in the morning and during sleep, an examination of gastric contents can reveal causative organisms.

The procedure requires the following steps:

1. Breakfast is withheld before aspiration.
2. A nasogastric tube is passed into the stomach.
3. A large syringe is connected to the nasogastric tube, and a specimen of stomach contents is gently withdrawn.
4. The specimen is placed in a covered container.
5. The nasogastric tube is withdrawn.

Skin testing

For various pulmonary disorders, the skin is tested for an antigen-antibody reaction to the proteins of the infectious agent. This cell-mediated or delayed hypersensitivity reaction is manifested by induration caused by cellular infiltration at the site of the injection in persons who have been sensitized to the proteins of the infectious agent. Skin testing for *Mycobacterium* tuberculosis with either tuberculin purified protein derivative (PPD) or old tuberculin (OT) is the most common type of test. However, skin testing also can be conducted for *atypical tubercule bacilli* and for *fungal infections* resulting from *coccidioidin, histoplasmin,* and *blastomycin.* The primary purpose of skin testing is to detect individuals who are infected with the suspect organism but who do not have the disease. In this capacity, skin testing is primarily a screening device. Skin antigens can also be used for presumptive diagnosis; however, a positive skin test reaction must be substantiated with other diagnostic evidence before active disease can be confirmed. Skin testing can produce false-positive and false-negative results (usually in immunosuppressed, older, or newly infected people).

24-6

Administration technique for the mantoux test

1. Draw up 0.1 ml of PPD, OT, atypical (tuberculin), or fungal antigen, using a tuberculin syringe and ½ inch 24- to 26-gauge needle.
2. Cleanse the site (dorsal surface of forearm).
3. Keeping skin slightly taut, insert the needle bevel upward just beneath the skin surface.
4. Inject the solution, creating a 6 to 10 mm wheal.
5. Read the test site with a millimeter ruler 48 to 72 hours after injection. The site should be lightly palpated to determine the presence or absence of induration. The largest diameter of induration should be measured and recorded in millimeters. Any erythema at the site should also be noted.
6. Interpretation of induration:
   a. 10 mm or more = highly significant for past or present infection.
   b. 5 mm through 9 mm = doubtful reaction except in persons with HIV infection.
   c. 0 through 4 mm = little or no sensitivity, however if patient's history indicates exposure, the test should be repeated.

Skin test administration

Skin tests can be administered by intracutaneous injection (Mantoux method), jet gun or multiple puncture tests (tine, mono-vacc, and heaf-type). The *Mantoux test is the only method used for diagnosis.* The jet gun or multiple puncture methods are used *only* for screening tests. (See Box 24-6 for details of administration.)

Pulmonary Function Tests

Pulmonary function testing is a noninvasive method of assessing the functional capacity of the lungs. These tests cannot be used by themselves to diagnose specific diseases, but they are an integral part of the diagnostic process. Pulmonary function tests (PFTs) are used for the following purposes:
1. Screening for the presence of pulmonary disease
2. Preoperative evaluation
3. Evaluating the patient's condition for weaning from a ventilator
4. Researching pulmonary physiology
5. Documenting the progression of pulmonary disease or effects of therapy
6. Studying the effects of exercise on respiratory physiology

Assessment of lung properties

The functional ability of the lungs is assessed by measuring properties that affect ventilation and respiration.

1. Ventilation
   a. Static properties focus on lung distensibility; that is, on the bellows action of the thorax and lungs. Static properties are assessed through measurement of lung volumes and functional capacities (Table 24-6, *A* and *B*).

b. Dynamic properties are those aspects of lung mechanics that affect the resistance within the airways. These properties are assessed by pulmonary function tests that measure volume/time relationships (Table 24-6, *C*).
2. Respiration
   a. Diffusion properties are those aspects of lung function that affect the ability of gas to move across the alveolar-capillary membrane (Table 31-8, *D*).
   b. Perfusion properties affect the supply of blood to the lungs (Table 24-6, *D*).

Normal values for pulmonary function tests are calculated by taking into consideration the following variables for each individual being evaluated: (1) age, (2) sex, (3) height and weight, and (4) individual effort in performing each test.

Measurement of ventilation

Ventilatory studies are performed by having the patient breathe through a mouthpiece connected to a spirometer that measures the air moving through the apparatus. The spirometer is connected to a recording device that documents air volume, usually in liter measurements. Some measurements such as the residual volume cannot be measured directly and are calculated mathematically. The interrelationship of lung volumes and capacities that measure *static properties* is shown in Fig. 24-11. The volumes and capacities are defined, and clinical implications of each measurement are given in Table 24-6.

Spirometric measurement of lung *dynamic properties* are of particular clinical significance because they relate the volume of air expired to the time required for expiration. One meaningful clinical measurement is the forced expiratory volume (FEV). The FEV measures the amount of air in liters forcefully expired over 1, 2, or 3 seconds after a full inspiration. *The FEV is an accurate indicator for obstructive diseases because airway obstruction becomes worse on expiration and particularly when expiration is forceful and rapid. The FEV at 1 sec is the most clinically accurate of the three measurements and is particularly* useful when expressed as a percentage of the forced vital capacity (FVC). An FEV_1/FVC of 80% or greater is considered normal.

Measurement of respiration

It is best to measure efficiency of respiration by both PFTs and other parameters such as arterial blood gas measurements. Two variables affecting respiration that PFTs can measure are the ability of gas to diffuse across the alveolar-capillary membrane and the ratio of ventilated alveoli to perfused capillaries.

Alveolar-capillary diffusion

The ability of gas to diffuse across the alveolar-capillary membrane is measured by a test called *diffusing capacity* (D_x). The patient breathes a measured amount of carbon monoxide from a closed system. The rate of carbon monoxide removal from the closed system indicates the status of the alveolar-capillary membrane.

Ventilation-perfusion relationship

In order for the lung to perform gas exchange efficiently, the ventilation-perfusion ratio (V/Q ratio) must be balanced. That is, areas that receive ventilation should be

Table 24-6   Definitions and implications of pulmonary function tests

Definitions		Clinical implications	
		Obstructive diseases	**Restrictive diseases**
A. Lung volume (nonoverlapping measures)			
Tidal volume (TV)	Volume of gas inspired and expired with a normal breath	General measure of ventilatory ability	
Inspiratory reserve volume (IRV)	Maximal volume that can be inspired from the end of a normal inspiration	↓	↓
Expiratory reserve volume (ERV)	Maximal volume than can be exhaled by forced expiration after a normal expiration	Clinically useful when combined with RV-FRC	
Residual volume (RV)	Volume of gas left in lung after maximal expiration	↑	↓
B. Lung capacities (combinations of various volumes)			
Inspiratory capacity (IC)	Maximal amount of air that can be inspired after a normal expiration (TV + IRV)	↓	↓
Functional residual capacity (FRC)	Amount of air left in lungs after a normal expiration (ERV + RV)	↑	↓
Vital capacity (VC)	Maximal amount of air that can be expired after a maximal inspiration (TV + IRV + ERV)	↓	↓
Forced vital capacity (FVC)	Maximal amount of air that can be expelled with a maximal effort after a maximal inspiration	↓	↓
Total lung capacity (TLC)	Total amount of air in lungs after maximal inspiration (TV + IRV + ERV + RV)	↑	↓
C. Volume/time relationships			
Minute volume (MV)	Volume inspired and expired in 1 min of normal breathing	↑	↓
Forced expiratory volume in 1 sec (FEV_1)	Amount of air expelled in the first second of the forced vital capacity maneuver	↓	—
FEV_1/VC ratio	Amount of air forcefully expelled in 1 sec compared to total amount forcefully expelled	↓	—
Maximal voluntary ventilation (MVV), also termed maximal breathing capacity (MBC)	Amount of air exchanged per minute with maximal rate and depth of respiration	↓	—
D. Diffusion/perfusion measurements			
Diffusing capacity (D_x)	Assesses ability of gas molecules to cross alveolar-capillary membrane	↓	↓
Nitrogen washout (N_2)	Measurement of amount of nitrogen in lungs at end expiration; indicates uniformity of gaseous distribution in lungs	↓	↓

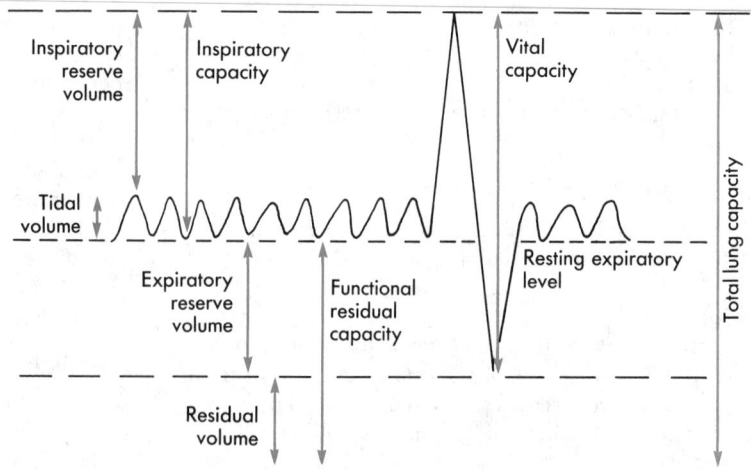

Fig. 24-11   Lung volumes and capacities illustrated by spirography tracing. (Modified from Wade JF: *Respiratory nursing care*, ed 2, St Louis, 1977, Mosby–Year Book.)

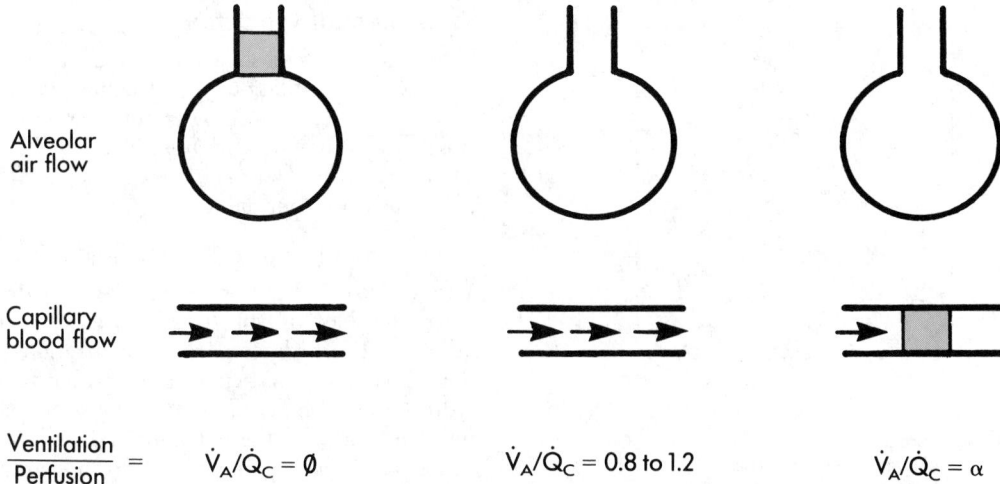

Fig. 24-12 Ventilation/perfusion relationships are as follows: *left,* bronchus blocked with secretions equals decreased ventilation, and normal perfusion equals zero gas exchange; *center,* normal ventilation and normal perfusion is Va/Q_c of 0.8 to 1.2; *right,* normal ventilation and decreased perfusion from blocked capillary as found in pulmonary emboli equals zero gas exchange. (Modified from West JB: *Ventilation, blood flow and gas exchange,* ed 3, Oxford 1977, Blackwell.)

well perfused with blood, and areas that receive blood flow should be capable of ventilation (Fig. 24-12). Although in the normal lung with its many millions of gas exchange units some imbalance in ventilation and perfusion exists, this has little effect on overall gas exchange function. In fact, adaptive mechanisms appear to exist that divert blood flow to the best ventilated regions of the lungs or redirect ventilation away from nonperfused areas in order to maintain a normal ratio in the range of 0.8 to 1.2. Alteration in ventilation-perfusion relationships (either overall or in circumscribed areas of lung tissue) is largely responsible for the *hypoxemia* or *hypercapnia* seen in patients. The nitrogen washout test measures ventilation/perfusion relationships. Ambient air, and thus air in the lungs, is known to contain 80% nitrogen. The nitrogen washout test requires the patient to breathe 100% oxygen to wash out all the nitrogen from the lungs. After a measured period of time, the patient's expired air is measured for nitrogen content. Unevenly ventilated alveoli that receive less of the inspired oxygen will take longer to wash out lung nitrogen.

For pulmonary function testing, patients are required to breathe into a mouthpiece while wearing a noseclip; thus they often fear smothering or having a dyspneic episode. Thorough preparation for the test includes an explanation of the procedure to decrease the patient's apprehension.

Arterial Blood Gas Analysis

Arterial blood gas analysis provides objective determination of the following: (1) arterial blood oxygenation, (2) gas exchange, (3) alveolar ventilation, and (4) acid-base balance. The arterial blood gas parameters that assess function of the respiratory system are shown in Table 24-7. A blood sample is obtained from a radial, brachial, or femoral artery with a preheparinized syringe to prevent clotting.

Table 24-7 **Arterial blood gases**

Respiratory function	Measurements	Normal value
Acid-base balance	pH-hydrogen ion concentration	7.35-7.45
Oxygenation	PaO_2:partial pressure of dissolved O_2 in blood	80-100 mm Hg
	SaO_2:percentage of O_2 bound to hemoglobin	95%-98%
Ventilation	$PaCO_2$:partial pressure of CO_2 dissolved in blood	38-45 mm Hg

The syringe is capped after obtaining the blood sample to prevent contact with air and is placed in an ice-water container until analyzed. Pressure is maintained over the puncture site for at least 5 minutes after needle withdrawal to prevent bleeding.

Patients with blood-clotting abnormalities may require that pressure be applied to the sample site for longer than 5 minutes. Nursing implications include assessing the site periodically and applying pressure for as long as necessary to prevent hematoma formation or bruising.

Measurement of oxygenation

Both PaO_2 and SaO_2 are used to determine the adequacy of arterial blood oxygenation. The PaO_2 measures oxygen dissolved in the blood; however, the amount of oxygen

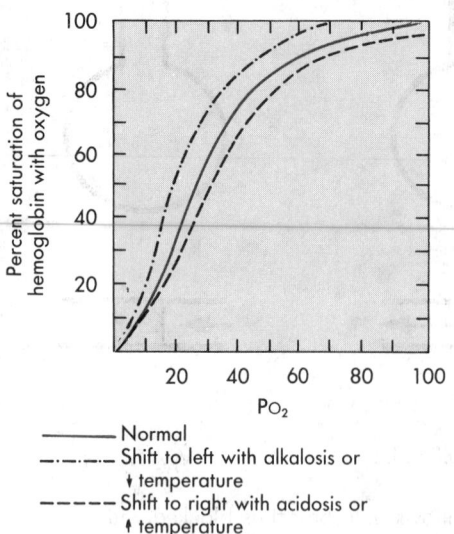

Fig. 24-13 Oxyhemoglobin dissociation curve. (From Comroe JH Jr: *Physiology of respiration*, ed 2, St Louis, 1974, Mosby–Year Book.)

carried in the blood in this form is small. Most oxygen is transported in chemical combination with hemoglobin. The SaO_2 measures the oxyhemoglobin saturation or that percentage of the hemoglobin that is combined with oxygen. More than 90% of the oxygen-carrying capacity of blood is accounted for by oxyhemoglobin, with the partial pressure of oxygen acting as the driving force for this chemical combination.

The relationship of PaO_2 to SaO_2 is demonstrated in the oxyhemoglobin dissociation curve. This relationship is not directly linear; many factors affect the affinity of the heme molecule for oxygen. The sigmoid curve represents the saturation percentages that occur at various PaO_2 levels. As can be seen in the oxyhemoglobin dissociation curve (Fig. 24-13), in the upper portion of the curve, hemoglobin has an increased affinity for oxygen, so that large changes in PO_2 levels can be tolerated without significantly changing the saturation. For example, at a PO_2 of 100 mm Hg, hemoglobin saturation is almost total, 97%; even if the PO_2 should fall to 70 mm Hg, the saturation would only decrease to 94%. This serves as a protective mechanism that ensures adequate tissue oxygenation even when there is mild hypoxemia. It should be noted, however, that once the PO_2 level falls below 60 mm Hg, saturation begins to decrease sharply, thus reducing the ability of the hemoglobin to transport oxygen.

The oxygen affinity of hemoglobin is influenced by various factors. Those factors that cause the curve to shift to the left (that is, hypothermia, alkalosis, and hypocapnia) increase the affinity of oxygen but diminish the release of oxygen to the tissues. Factors that cause a shift to the right are fever, acidosis, and hypercapnia. The primary impact of a shift to the right is reduced affinity of hemoglobin for oxygen.

The PaO_2 and SaO_2 must be evaluated in relation to the amount of hemoglobin. Because SaO_2 measures saturation of hemoglobin, an anemic person can have a normal saturation but still be inadequately oxygenated.

Assessment of ventilation

The $PaCO_2$ is used as a measurement to determine the adequacy of ventilation and depends on the amount of carbon dioxide produced by the body and the ability of the lungs to eliminate it. *Hypoventilation* is shown by an elevated $PaCO_2$ and *hyperventilation* is indicated by a decrease in $PaCO_2$ below normal levels.

Measurement of acid-base balance

Arterial blood pH is a measurement of hydrogen ion concentration. Because pH is expressed as a negative logarithm, as the hydrogen ion concentration increases and blood becomes more acid, the pH value falls. When the hydrogen ion concentration decreases, the blood becomes more alkaline, and the pH value rises.

The lungs play an important part in maintaining normal body pH (7.35 to 7.45) by regulating $PaCO_2$ through ventilation. The $PaCO_2$ is related to the pH by the chemical reaction of carbon dioxide and water in the blood, which results in the formation of carbonic acid. Carbonic acid, in turn, dissociates to form hydrogen and bicarbonate ions, as illustrated in the following equation:

$$CO_2 + H_2O \rightleftarrows H_2CO_3 \rightleftarrows HCO_3^- + H^+$$

The maintenance of a normal pH depends on a ratio of 20 bicarbonate ions to 1 hydrogen ion. It can be seen from the equation that the presence of an elevated $PaCO_2$ shifts the equilibrium equation to the right and will result in an excess of H^+ ions. When this occurs, the pH falls, and the patient is said to be in *respiratory acidosis*. Conversely, when $PaCO_2$ is decreased, the equation shifts to the left, resulting in an increased pH and *respiratory alkalosis*.

Endoscopic Examination
Bronchoscopy

A bronchoscopic examination is performed by passing a bronchoscope into the trachea and bronchi (Fig. 24-14). By use of either a rigid bronchoscope or a flexible fiberoptic bronchoscope, the larynx, trachea, and bronchi can be visualized. Diagnostic bronchoscopic examination includes observation of the tracheobronchial tree for abnormalities, tissue biopsy, and aspiration of sputum for testing. Therapeutic bronchoscopic examination can be performed to remove an aspirated foreign body, to facilitate free air passage by removal of mucus plugs with suction, or to control bleeding.

Preparation for a bronchoscopy is similar to that for bronchography, except that postural drainage is less often ordered. If the patient is very apprehensive or if a sponge biopsy (abrasion of a lesion with a sponge) is to be performed or a tissue biopsy specimen is to be obtained, intravenous anesthesia can be used.

Nursing care for patients after bronchoscopy is as follows:
1. Patient is NPO until gag reflex returns.
2. Patient is positioned in semi-Fowler's position or on either side to facilitate removal of secretions, unless physician specifies position.
3. All sputum is saved for culture and cytologic studies. *Note:* If bronchograms were performed, sputum cannot be used for cytologic examination, because the dye impedes cell fixation.

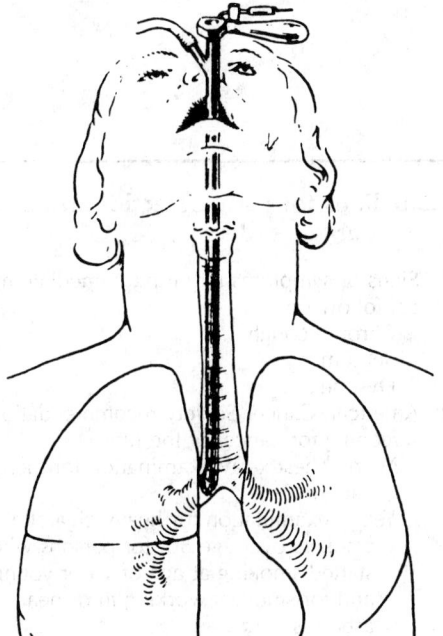

Fig. 24-14   Bronchoscope inserted through trachea into bronchus. (From DeWeese DD, Saunders WH: *Textbook of otolaryngology,* ed 7, St Louis, 1987, Mosby–Year Book.)

4. Patient is monitored for signs of laryngeal edema or laryngospasms such as stridor or increasing shortness of breath.
5. If lung tissue biopsy is taken, sputum is monitored for signs of hemorrhage. *Note:* Blood-streaked sputum can be expected for a few days after biopsy.

Mediastinoscopy

In mediastinoscopy a *mediastinoscope,* which is an instrument much like a bronchoscope, is inserted through a small incision in the suprasternal notch and advanced into the mediastinum where inspection and biopsy of the lymph nodes can then be carried out. Because these lymph nodes receive lymphatic drainage from the lungs, they are of diagnostic value for carcinoma, and granulomatous infections such as sarcoidosis. This procedure is performed in the operating room, and the patient usually receives a general anesthetic.

Thoracentesis

Thoracentesis involves the insertion of a needle into the pleural space. Indications for a thoracentesis include the following:
1. Removal of pleural fluid for diagnostic purposes
   a. The pleural fluid can be examined for specific gravity, white blood cell count, differential cell count, red blood cell count, protein, glucose, and amylase concentrations.
   b. The fluid can be cultured and checked for the presence of abnormal or malignant cells.
   c. The gross appearance of the fluid, the quantity obtained, and the location of the site of the thoracentesis should be recorded.
2. Biopsy of the pleura
3. Removal of pleural fluid when it is a threat to patient safety or comfort

---

24-7 | *Guidelines for Care*

The patient undergoing thoracentesis

Explain procedure. Emphasize the importance of not moving, breathing quietly, and not coughing during the procedure to avoid damage to the pleura. Although a local anesthetic is used, discomfort may be felt when the needle enters the pleura.

Patient's respiratory status and vital signs are assessed before the procedure to collect baseline data.

If possible, the patient sits on the side of the bed with feet supported in a chair. With the use of an elevated overbed table, the patient is helped to maintain a position with the head resting upon folded arms. Patients who are unable to sit up should be turned onto the unaffected side with the head of the bed elevated 30 degrees.

Reassure and provide physical support, such as holding patient's hand.

Monitor vital signs, general appearance, and respiratory status throughout the procedure. No more than 1500 ml of pleural fluid should be removed within a 30-minute period because of the risk of intravascular fluid shift with resultant pulmonary edema.

After the needle is withdrawn, a sterile occlusive dressing and pressure is applied to the site.

After thoracentesis, the patient is positioned on the unaffected side with the insertion site up.

Monitor respiratory status, vital signs, and puncture site. Observe for signs of the following complications:

Intravascular shift: hypotension, a rapid thready pulse, and increasing shortness of breath.

Lung trauma: coughing paroxysms, bloody sputum, or tracheal deviation.

---

4. Installation of medications into the pleural space. Box 24-7 lists the nursing care for a patient having a thoracentesis.

PREVENTION AND HEALTH EDUCATION

Disorders of the respiratory tract are probably the most common health problems for most persons in the Western world.

The objectives of health education in relation to pulmonary diseases are the same as for other diseases. *Prevention, early diagnosis, prompt and often continued treatment, limitation of disability, and rehabilitation should be emphasized for all persons.* Early symptoms of respiratory diseases are probably those most often ignored by the general population. Perhaps this is because, with the exception of influenza and some types of pneumonia, respiratory diseases often develop slowly and progress without the individual's awareness.

Because of the deleterious effects of cigarette smoking on the cardiopulmonary systems, a concerted effort is indicated to teach persons about the hazards of smoking. In recent years many organizations, most notably the American Lung Association (ALA), the American Cancer So-

24-8 Prevention of respiratory infections

Preventing spread of infection
1. Isolate the infected person.
2. Teach the infected person to cover nose and mouth with tissue when coughing or sneezing so that droplet nuclei are not released into the air.
3. Wash hands after coughing or sneezing.

Maintaining resistance to infection
1. Eat a balanced diet.
2. Get adequate rest and sleep.
3. Avoid crowds during periods of prevalent respiratory infections.
4. Receive annual influenza immunization and pneumonia vaccine every 3 to 5 years if over age 65 or if younger with chronic heart, lung, or renal disease.

24-9 Guidelines for early detection of major pulmonary disorders

1. Signs or symptoms requiring immediate medical follow-up
   Chronic cough
   Sputum
   Dyspnea
2. American Cancer Society recommendations for screening for cancer of the lung
   Yearly chest x-ray examination for men over age 40
   Yearly examination for heavy cigarette smokers over age 50, for persons who started smoking at age of 15 or younger, and for smokers working in or near asbestos

ciety (ACS), the American Heart Association (AHA), and the federal government, have launched campaigns to reduce cigarette smoking in the United States. These campaigns have been somewhat successful, and it is now estimated that only 28% of the adult population in the United States smokes. However, the number of women smokers has increased, and this is reflected in the ever-rising increase in morbidity and mortality from lung disease, especially cancer of the lung and chronic obstructive pulmonary diseases, among women. A major emphasis has been on preventing children and teenagers from beginning to smoke. Unfortunately, smoking among teenagers remains a problem.

Primary Prevention: Prevention of Disease

Because the cause of many respiratory disorders is known, prevention is possible. The major emphasis is on avoiding respiratory infections and educating the public about the risks of cigarette smoking. Health practices helpful in preventing infection are outlined in Box 24-8.

Secondary Prevention: Early Detection

Medical attention should be sought for respiratory symptoms that do not subside within 2 weeks. Guidelines for early detection are listed in Box 24-9.

MAJOR HEALTH PROBLEMS OF THE RESPIRATORY SYSTEM

There are several ways to classify disorders affecting the lung and respiration, but one of the most useful and commonly used is to divide them into restrictive and obstructive diseases.

In *restrictive lung disease, there is a restriction in lung volume and a reduction in lung compliance.* As a result there is a reduction in total lung capacity (TLC) and a decrease in vital capacity (VC) to less than the predicted norm.

In contrast, *in obstructive lung disease, there is an increase in airway resistance resulting in prolonged exhalation.* This results in an increase in residual volume (RV) while TLC may be normal or increased. Thus pulmonary function tests are necessary to establish the diagnosis. A comparison of the characteristic changes in pulmonary function tests for restrictive and obstructive disease is shown Table 24-8.

Table 24-8 Comparison of pulmonary function test results in restrictive and obstructive disease

Test	Restrictive	Obstructive
FVC	Decreased	Decreased or normal
RV	Decreased	Increased
TLC	Decreased	Normal or increased
RV/TLC	Normal or increased	Significantly increased
$FEV_{1.0}$/FVC	Normal or increased	Decreased
$FEV_{3.0}$/FVC	Normal or increased	Decreased

From Morrissey W: *Respiratory diseases.* In Kaye D, Rose LF, editors: *Fundamentals of internal medicine,* St Louis, 1983, Mosby–Year Book.

Table 24-9   Restrictive pulmonary disease

Alteration	Disease example
Parenchymal inflammation	Pneumonia, adult respiratory distress syndrome
Space-occupying lesions	Tumors, malignancies
Diffuse pulmonary disease	Silicosis, fibrosis
Pleural disease	Pleural effusion
Lung collapse	Pneumothorax, atelectasis
Resectional surgery	Pneumonectomy
Neuromuscular disorders	Poliomyelitis, Guillain-Barré syndrome, myasthenia gravis
CNS depression	Narcotics, cerebral edema
Limitation of thoracic mobility	Abdominal tumors, ascites, paralytic ileus
Changes in bony thorax	Kyphoscoliosis

There are several conditions that can cause restrictive pulmonary disease and examples of these can be found in Table 24-9. It is impossible to discuss all of these conditions in this chapter. Atelectasis, which is the most frequent postoperative complication, is discussed in Chapter 22, Postoperative Intervention.

Conditions that result in restrictive or obstructive pulmonary disease that are discussed in this chapter are the following.

1. Restrictive pulmonary disorders
   a. Infectious diseases of the pulmonary tract
      (1) Viral: acute bronchitis
      (2) Bacterial: pneumonia, tuberculosis
      (3) Fungal: histoplasmosis, coccidiomycosis, blastomycosis
   b. Occupational lung disease
      (1) Inhalation of inorganic dust: silicosis
      (2) Inhalation of organic dust: allergic alveolitis (farmer's lung)
   c. Adult respiratory distress syndrome (ARDS)
   d. Carcinoma of the lung
2. Obstructive pulmonary disorders
   a. Chronic bronchitis
   b. Pulmonary emphysema
   c. Asthma
   d. Cystic fibrosis

INFECTIOUS DISEASES: VIRAL DISEASES OF THE RESPIRATORY TRACT

For a viral infection of the lung to occur, pathogens must be able to enter the lower respiratory tract. This means that the defense mechanisms of the lung must be overcome in some manner. There are many lung defense mechanisms, including upper airway defenses, lower respiratory tract clearance mechanisms, and intrapulmonary detoxification mechanisms. These mechanisms are outlined in Box 24-10.

Many respiratory diseases are probably caused by viral infections. Presently, more than 30 diseases have been found to be directly related to viral infections, and there are probably many more. Some diseases may be caused by one virus; different viruses may cause the same symptoms.

If specific signs are not evident, the clinical illness is termed a common cold, viral infection, fever of unknown origin (FUO), or acute respiratory illness. The most common specific respiratory diseases caused by the various viruses are epidemic pleurodynia (Bornholm's disease), acute laryngotracheobronchitis, viral pneumonia, and influenza. Most adults have developed antibodies for the more common viruses, and most viral infections are relatively mild. However, they are frequently complicated by secondary bacterial infections. When new strains of the influenza virus develop, severe epidemics may ensue, and many people may die from secondary infections such as pneumonia.

ACUTE BRONCHITIS
Etiology/Epidemiology
Bronchitis can be acute or chronic (chronic bronchitis will be discussed later in this chapter). Acute bronchitis is an inflammation of the bronchi and sometimes the trachea (tracheobronchitis). Although it occurs most often in persons with chronic lung disease, it also occurs as an extension of an upper respiratory infection in persons without underlying lung disease and is therefore communicable. It also may be caused by physical or chemical agents such as dust, smoke, or volatile fumes. As air pollution increases, the incidence of acute bronchitis increases. *Acute bronchitis is typically viral in origin, but bacterial pathogens such as Streptococcus pneumoniae and Haemophilus influenzae may also caused bronchitis, either as a primary or secondary infection.*

Nursing Process
Assessment
Subjective data

1. Onset and duration of symptoms (see Table 24-10)
2. Medications taken for cough and their effectiveness

Objective data

1. Vital signs—temperature may be elevated; tachypnea frequent with severe bronchitis
2. Rasping cough with mucoid sputum
3. Chest percussion—normal
4. Auscultation—vesicular breath sounds, vocal fremitus normal, adventitious sounds—localized rales and sibilant rhonchi

Data Analysis: Nursing Diagnoses
Nursing diagnoses are determined from analysis of patient data. Possible nursing diagnoses for the person with acute bronchitis may include, but are not limited to, the following:

Diagnostic title	Possible etiologies
Airway clearance, ineffective	Tracheobronchial infection, obstruction, or secretion
Breathing pattern, ineffective	Decreased energy, fatigue
Pain	Rib or muscle trauma from coughing; inflammation of tracheobronchial tree
Knowledge deficit	Lack of exposure to information

24-10

Lung defense mechanisms

I. Upper airway defenses against pulmonary infection

Removing particulate matter from inspired air

Particles greater than 20 μm settle back on surfaces

Particles 5-10 μm deposited in nose

Particles 0.1-10 μm remain suspended in air for long periods and are then inhaled

Particles 1-5 μm deposited in tracheobronchial tree

Droplet nuclei 2-4 μm (dried particles from sneezing, coughing, talking)

May contain viruses or bacteria

Spread organisms from person to person

Minimizing the microbial population on membranes of upper respiratory tract

Mucocillary transport

Posterior two thirds of nasal cavity, sinuses, and nasopharynx lined by *ciliated epithelium* covered with thin layer of mucus

Dense concentration of small blood vessels present beneath ciliated epithelium and mucous layers

Mucus and fluid produced = 1000 ml/24 hr in normal persons

Mucus and fluid carried at rate of 5-10 mm/min back into hypopharynx by beating action of cilia

Substances in secretions inhibit microbial growth and prevent organisms from sticking to mucous membranes

Immunoglobulins (secretory IgA)

Lysozyme

Complement

Minimizing possibility of aspiration

Motor function of upper airway

Laryngeal mechanism—closes glottis when swallowing to protect larynx

Gag reflex also closes glottis

Clearing throat, spitting, clear upper airway

Contamination of lower respiratory tract

Impaired clearance of particles in upper airway = spread of bacteria

Accumulation of debris and microbes → penetration of tissues = sinusitis, otitis media

Accumulation of debris and microbes → aspiration into trachea; lung abscess caused by anaerobic bacteria secondary to severe gingival disease

Intoxication or distraction → aspiration

Normal sleep → minor aspiration

Aspiration of pharyngeal contents → lung → bacterial pneumonia

II. Lower respiratory tract clearance mechanisms

Pulmonary reflex

Cough—an involuntary reflex elicited by stimulation of irritant receptors in subepithelium of hypopharynx, larynx, and tracheobronchial tree: mediated by vagus nerve

Facilitator of mucociliary clearance

Aids in dealing with gross contamination from above larynx

Bronchoconstriction—reflex response to airway irritants

Decreased size of bronchus and forced expiration and cough propel debris toward mouth

Excessive bronchoconstriction (asthma) = decreased expiratory airflow, air trapped in lung, effective cough difficult

Mucociliary clearance

Mucus secreted by epithelial goblet cells from submucosal glands; 0.10-100 ml passes up trachea into hypopharynx and is swallowed; amount and nature of mucus secreted are controlled, in part, by parasympathetic nervous system affected by neurohumoral stimulation (adrenergic or cholinergic) and by direct mucosal irritation

Cilia (200 cilia/each cell surface) beat rhythmically 1200 beats/min mouthward beginning at terminal bronchioles → larynx; beating of cilia → overlying mucous layer → mouthward at rate of 0.5 mm/min in small airways to about 10 mm/min in major bronchi

Clearance increased by:

Bronchodilator drugs

Beta-adrenergic agents (ephedrine) stimulate transport of water and salt into mucus = ↓ viscosity of mucus

Methylxanthines (aminophylline) → ↑ mucus production and ciliary activity

Adapted from Light B: *Respiratory infections.* In Kryger MH, editor: *Pathophysiology of respiration,* New York, 1981, John Wiley.

Ciliary function depressed by:
  Chronic exposure to airway irritants—cigarette smoke and other irritants
  Pharmacologic agents—100% O_2, anticholinergic agents, alcohol
  Infection such as viral bronchitis
Mucous production increased by:
  Chronic irritation of respiratory tract → increase in number of mucus-secreting goblet cells = ↑ mucus
  Inflammatory response to irritation → ↑ numbers of phagocytic cells and amount of cellular debris in mucus (especially DNA) = ↑ viscosity of mucus, which is less readily moved along by ciliary action
  Immotile cilia—congenital impairment
    Kartagener's syndrome—sinusitis, recurrent lung infection and sinus inversus
    Cystic fibrosis—infection, chronic inflammatory increases in respiratory mucus volume and viscosity = impaired lung clearance and progressive lung damage
III. Intrapulmonary detoxification mechanism
  Phagocytes
    Alveolar macrophage
      Phagocytosis of particles—inhaled particulate debris, bacteria, or cell constituents
      Kills most microbes
    Polymorphonuclear neutrophil present in blood (normally only small number in lung)
    Avid phagocyte—kills microbes
    Defends against established infectious processes
    Infection—products of inflammation attract neutrophils to site of infection (chemotaxis)
  Factors interfering with phagocytosis
    Inhibition of alveolar macrophage function
      Cigarette smoke
      Other inhaled pollutants—ozone, nitrogen dioxide, oxygen
      Drugs—corticosteroids, antineoplastic and antiinflammatory cytoxic agents, and ethanol (alcohol)

Metabolic derangements—uremia, hyperglycemia of diabetes mellitus
Acquired granulocytopenia—bone marrow depression from cytoxic drugs
Immunoglobulins
  IgG and IgA—most important for lung defense; present in secretions of respiratory tract as well as in blood
    IgA antibodies—specific for viral antigens; neutralize viruses and prevent infection
    IgG predominates in terminal lung units; antigen-specific IgG contributes to local defense against bacterial infections (important in neutralizing highly pathogenic encapsulated bacteria [especially *Streptococcus pneumoniae* and *Hemophilus influenzae*], which are resistant to phagocytosis)
Cell-mediated immunity (CMI)
  One half of lymphocytes in and around airways are thymus-derived lymphocytes, or *T-cells*
    Found in lymphoid aggregates adjacent to bronchi (bronchus-associated lymphoid tissues, or BALT)
    T cells important in:
      Resistance to some viral infections
      Resistance to most fungal infections
      Infections by organisms that survive and multiply inside host cells: *Mycobacterium tuberculosis*, *Brucella*, *Listeria monocytogenes*, and *Pneumocystis carinii*
  Impaired CMI = ↑ susceptibility to infection
    Deficient T-cell function (anergy) associated with:
      Neoplasms—lymphoma
      Cytotoxic or corticosteroid therapy
      Systemic diseases—sarcoidosis, malnutrition
    Some lung infections occur almost exclusively with severely impaired CMI—pneumonia caused by cytomegalovirus, herpes zoster, aspergillus species, or *Pneumocystis carinii*

Table 24-10 Signs and symptoms and medical therapy for acute bronchitis

Symptoms	Signs	Medical Therapy
Cough	Sputum production: Viral-clear to mucopurulent: bacterial-purulent	No specific therapy for viral infection, therapy directed to relief of symptoms, i.e., cough medicine, vaporizer; fluid intake 3-4 L/day
		Bland diet
Chest pain	Tachypnea	Antibiotics for bacterial infection (elevation in temperature and mucopurulent sputum)
	Diffuse rhonchi/wheezes	
	Chest x-ray—clear, differentiates bronchitis from pneumonia	Rest
		Avoiding exposure to further infection

Planning: Expected Patient Outcomes

Expected patient outcomes for the person with acute bronchitis may include, but are not limited to, the following:

1. Patient demonstrates effective cough with adequate sputum production.
   a. Both cough and sputum production decrease within 72 hours of treatment initiation.
   b. For persons with chronic lung disease, sputum becomes clear and thin (return to prebronchitis status).
2. Patient demonstrates effective breathing patterns.
3. Patient demonstrates prebronchitis vital signs.
4. Patient reports that chest pain is decreased or absent.
5. Patient describes the cause and factors contributing to the occurrence of acute bronchitis and names common symptoms of it.

Implementation

Assisting with achievement of therapeutic goals
Medications for bacterial primary or secondary infection

Therapy for bacterial primary or secondary infections is as follows:

1. Antibiotic therapy
   a. Ampicillin, 250 mg, four times a day to 500 mg every 6 hours, or
   b. Tetracycline, 250 mg, four times a day or every 6 hours
2. Bronchodilator
   a. Aminophylline, 200 mg, four times a day

Interventions to achieve patient outcomes
Assisting with coughing

Assist the patient to cough effectively. Coughing is normally a mechanism that aids in the removal of inhaled foreign materials. When an infection is present the throat becomes dry and irritated and there is an increase in mucus production as part of the lung defense mechanisms.

Receptors for the cough reflex are located in the tracheal and bronchial mucosa with the largest concentration of them being found in the larynx, carina, and bifurcations of the large- and medium-sized bronchi. When these receptors are stimulated, impulses are transmitted primarily via the afferent nervous pathways (vagus, phrenic, and spinal motor nerves) to expiratory musculature (larynx, tracheobronchial tree, diaphragm, and the abdominal wall).

To produce an effective cough there must be a deep inspiration followed by maximum expiratory effort against a closed glottis. This results in a tremendous increase in

Table 24-11 Medications used to treat cough

Desired effect	Medications prescribed
↑ Secretions	Expectorants
	Ammonium chloride
	Ammonium carbonate
	Sodium iodide
	Potassium iodide (saturated solution-SSKI)
	Terpin hydrate
↓ Secretions	Anticholinergic agents
	Atropine
Thin secretions	Mucolytic agents
	Acetylcysteine (Mucomyst)
	Desoxyribonuclease (Dornavac)
Depress cough reflex	Antitussives
	Narcotic
	Codeine
	Nonnarcotic agents
	Benzonatate (Tessalon)
	Noscapine (Nectadon)
	Dextromethorphan hydrobramide (Romilar)
	Carbetapentane citrate (Toclase)
	Levopropoxyphene napsylate (Novrod)
	Chlophedianol hydrochloride (Ulo)

intrathoracic pressure. As the glottis opens, mucus and inhaled particles are forced out of the airways at a high velocity.

Persistent coughing can be very annoying and tiring to the patient and those around him or her. Complications of persistent coughing include insomnia, exhaustion, vomiting, urinary incontinence, rib or muscle trauma, pneumothorax, or fainting. If cough is present, give prescribed medication. Table 24-11 lists commonly used medications and their desired effects.

Assist with coughing as necessary by supporting chest (front and back) as patient coughs. Teach patient to cough effectively to maintain a clear airway and collect required specimens. Tell patient to take a deep breath, force the air out down to residual volume, contract the diaphragm, exhale forcefully and then cough. Successful airway clearance and an effective breathing pattern should help return vital signs to prebronchitis levels.

Additional assistance in achieving therapeutic goals includes the following:

1. Provide for good drainage of tracheobronchial secretions.

2. If antibiotics are prescribed, give on time to maintain therapeutic blood levels.
3. If steam vaporization is prescribed, administer it using precautions described on p. 540.

Assisting with comfort and ADL

1. Place patient in position of comfort; semi-Fowler's or high-Fowler's position should improve the patient's ability to breathe.
2. Assist with ADL as necessary during acute phase of illness.

Facilitating learning

The patient should be taught to avoid persons with upper respiratory infections. If respiratory infection does occur, the patient should seek medical attention.

If the patient smokes cigarettes, he or she should be encouraged to quit smoking. Group programs are helpful to some persons and the local branches of the American Lung Association, American Cancer Society, or American Heart Association can supply the names of local programs to assist persons to stop smoking.

Evaluation

Evaluation is based on patient outcomes. Questions to be asked include the following:

1. Have the patient's cough and sputum production decreased?
2. Is the patient breathing effectively?
3. Have the patient's vital signs returned to prebronchitis level?
4. Has the patient's chest pain decreased?
5. Can the patient list common symptoms and describe the cause of and factors contributing to acute bronchitis?

INFECTIOUS DISEASES: BACTERIAL DISEASES OF THE RESPIRATORY TRACT

As mentioned under viral infections, the protective mechanisms of the respiratory tract must be compromised before an infection can take hold.

PNEUMONIA

Etiology/Epidemiology

Acute pneumonias are responsible for 10% of hospital admissions in the United States. Pneumonia can occur in any season but is most common during winter and early spring. Persons of any age are susceptible, but pneumonia is more common among infants and the elderly. Pneumonia is often caused by aspiration of infected materials into the distal bronchioles and alveoli. *Certain individuals are especially susceptible*, including *persons whose normal respiratory defense mechanisms are damaged or altered (those with chronic obstructive pulmonary disease, influenza,* and *tracheostomy,* and *those who have recently had anesthesia); persons who have a disease affecting antibody response (those with multiple myeloma, hypogammaglobulinemia, and so on);* and *alcoholics in*

24-11

Organisms causing infectious pneumonia in adults

Typical or classic pneumonia syndrome
Bacterial pneumonia
  Common
    Streptococcus pneumoniae empyema, met
  Uncommon
    Haemophilus influenzae, Staphylococcus aureus

Atypical pneumonia syndrome
Common
    Mycoplasma pneumoniae
    Viral pathogens
Uncommon
    Legionella pneumophila
    Pneumocystis carinii

Aspiration pneumonia syndrome
Hospitalized, debilitated, or antibiotic-treated patients
    Mixed anaerobic/aerobic pharyngeal flora
    Staphylococcus aureus
    Klebsiella pneumoniae
    Pseudomonas aeruginosa
    Serratia marcescens
    Acinetobacter species
    Enteric gram-negative aerobes (*Escherichia coli* and *Enterobacter* and *Proteus* organisms)
Outpatients with normal pharyngeal flora
    Mixed anaerobic/aerobic pharyngeal flora

Hematogenous pneumonia syndromes
Staphylococcus aureus
Escherichia coli
Enteric/pelvic anaerobes

Adapted from Frame PT: *Basics RD* 10:1-8, 1982.

---

whom there is increased danger of aspiration and persons with delayed white blood cell response to infection. Increasingly, nosocomial pneumonia (acquired in the hospital) is a cause of morbidity and mortality. This is the direct result of an increase in the number of patients with impaired defenses resulting from certain types of therapy and of an increase in the number of patients whose lives are being prolonged with life-support therapy.

Pneumonia is a communicable disease; the mode of transmission is dependent on the infecting organism. Pneumonia is classified according to the offending organism rather than the anatomic location (lobar or bronchial) as was the practice in the past. A classification of pneumonia and its causative organisms in adults is presented in Box 24-11.

Pathophysiology

Pneumonia is an inflammatory process in which there is consolidation in the lung *caused by exudate filling the alveolar spaces. Gas exchange cannot take place in consolidated areas, and blood is shunted around the nonfunctioning alveoli. Hypoxemia* may occur depending on how much lung tissue is involved. About 60% of patients with pneumococcal pneu-

Table 24-12 Signs and symptoms and drug therapy of pneumonia

Pneumonia	Risk factors	Signs and symptoms	Drug therapy
Typical syndrome			
S. pneumoniae, uncomplicated; Streptococcus p., complicated (empyema, metastatic infection)	Sickle cell disease Hypogammaglobulinemia Multiple myeloma	Sudden onset with shaking, chill Fever (39° to 40° C), pleuritic chest pain, productive cough Sputum—green and purulent and may be blood tinged; "rusty" Respirations—rapid and shallow with "grunting" at end of each breath Nasal flaring, intercostal rib retraction, use of accessory muscles, and cyanosis may be present	*Drugs of choice* Penicillin G procaine, IM Aqueous crystalline penicillin G, IV Penicillin V *Other effective drugs* Erythromycin, clindamycin, cephalosporins, other penicillins, trimethoprim with sulfamethoxazole
H. influenzae, S. aureas	Advanced age COPD Alcoholism Recent influenza		Penicillin G Ampicillin *Other effective drugs* Chloramphenicol, cefamandole, trimethoprim with sulfamethoxazole, nafcillin *Other effective drugs* Methicillin, oxacillin, cefazolin, cephalothin, vancomycin, clindamycin Vancomycin, IV Cafazolin, IV, plus gentamicin or tobramycin
Atypical syndrome			
Common causes: mycoplasma pneumoniae, viral pathogens	Childhood, young adults	Onset gradual over 3 to 5 days Malaise, headache, sore throat, dry cough May have chest wall soreness from coughing	*Drug of choice:* Erythromycin *Other effective drugs:* Tetracycline None
Uncommon causes: Legionella pneumophilia	Recent URI; influenza	Above plus abdominal pain and diarrhea Temperature 40° C or greater Shaking chills Respiratory distress Renal failure, hyponatremia, hypophosphatemia, elevated creatine phosphokinase	*Drug of choice:* Erythromycin *Other effective drugs* Rifampin, gentamicin
Pneumocystic carinii	Immunologic deficiency Renal transplantation Autoimmune disease Debilitation	Gradual onset with increasing dyspnea, dry cough, tachypnea, hypoxemia X-ray film—diffuse interstitial involvement	Trimethoprim Pentamidine
Aspiration			
Gram-negative bacilli; Klebsiella, Pseudomonus, Serratia, Enterobacter, Escherichia, Proteus, gram-positive bacilli	Alcoholism Debilitation Hospitalization (that is, nosocomial infection)	Mixed anerobic: At first gradual onset Low-grade fever, cough Sputum—increased production, foul smelling Chest x-ray film—interstitial involvement in dependent portion of lung	Antibiotic therapy dependent on pathogen causing infection
S. aureus, gastric acid aspiration	Altered consciousness Aspiration of inert substances: water, barium, nutritional supplements	Gram-negative or positive infection: may present same clinical picture as classic pneumonia Sudden onset of respiratory distress, severe dyspnea, cyanosis, coughing, hypoxemia, followed by signs and symptoms of secondary infection	
Hematogenous Staphalococcus, E. coli, enteric anerobes	Infected intravascular catheter Endocarditis, IV drug abuse Intraabdominal abscess Pyonephrosis Empyema of gallbladder	Pulmonary symptoms minimal compared with the symptoms of septicemia Nonproductive cough and pleuritic pain similar to that seen in pulmonary embolism are most common complaints	*Drugs of choice* Nafcillin IV; ampicillin IV; plus gentamicin or tobramycin Clindamycin IV; plus gentamicin or tobramycin

monia have some degree of pleural effusion. Empyema may also occur in some patients with pneumonia.[116]

Typical or Classic Pneumonia

Typical or classic pneumonia occurs in both males and females of any age. It is found both in persons without underlying disease and in those with diminished defense mechanisms. *Commonly, there is a history of alcoholism, recent respiratory tract infection, or viral influenza* (Table 24-12).

Atypical Pneumonia
Etiology/epidemiology

The most common form of atypical pneumonia in adults is caused by *Mycoplasma pneumoniae*. *Legionella pneumophila* is an uncommon cause of atypical pneumonia. It occurs more commonly in older adults and in persons who smoke or have abnormal pulmonary defenses.[117] *Legionella pneumophila* is the agent causing Legionnaires' disease (legionellosis). It is three times more common in men than in women. *A number of conditions are believed to predispose one to legionellosis. These include chronic renal disease, chronic bronchitis or emphysema, diabetes, cancer, immunosuppressive medications, and smoking.* It is estimated that about 25,000 cases of Legionnaires' disease occur each year.

Both epidemics and sporadic cases of Legionnaires' disease occur. Epidemics have been associated with common source exposures such as air conditioning, water-cooling towers, and excavation sites. *Legionella pneumophila* has been isolated from soil and fresh water and from shower heads in hospitals.

Fine inspiratory rales may be present, but there is no evidence of consolidation. A roentgenogram of the chest shows patchy segmental infiltrates, which may progress from unilateral to bilateral. Pleural effusion is uncommon. Patients with legionellosis may have renal failure, hyponatremia, hypophosphatemia, and an elevation of creatine phosphokinase.

Medical therapy

The usual treatment for both *Mycoplasma pneumoniae* and *Legionella pneumophila* pneumonia is erythromycin (see Table 24-12). If a patient is seriously ill with Legionnaires' disease, rifampin may be added to the treatment with erythromycin. Rifampin should never be used alone because of the great likelihood of resistant organisms developing during monotherapy. *Because relapses have occurred within 1 to 2 weeks of therapy, it is recommended that treatment for Legionnaires' disease be continued for 3 weeks.*

The overall mortality of Legionnaires' disease is almost 15%. Most of this is attributed to respiratory failure.

When *Mycoplasma* pneumonia is untreated, the fever and malaise generally resolve in 1 to 2 weeks. Serious systemic complications are quite rare, although hemolytic anemia, disseminated intravascular coagulation (DIC), thrombocytopenic purpura and renal failure, myocarditis and pericarditis, meningoencephalitis and other neurologic syndromes, arthritis, and hepatitis have been reported.[117] The mortality for *Mycoplasma* pneumonia is less than 1%.[117]

24-12

Types of aspiration pneumonia

Noninfectious aspiration pneumonia
1. Aspiration of gastric acid
   a. Only a small quantity of aspirated gastric acid causes severe respiratory distress within a few seconds.
   b. Bacterial superinfection, if it does occur, does not become evident for 48 to 72 hours.
2. Aspiration of large quantities of inert substances
   a. Common substances include water, barium, tube-feeding liquids, and nonacid gastric contents.
   b. Aspirated substances obstruct airways, causing respiratory distress.
   c. Secondary bacterial infection may occur in lung segments that have obstructed airways.
3. Noninfectious aspiration syndrome is witnessed or identified from suctioning of foreign material from lungs.

Bacterial aspiration pneumonia
1. High-risk persons
   a. Persons with disorders of consciousness (for example, anesthesia, coma, seizures, or alcoholism).[117]
   b. Persons with poor cough mechanisms (for example, laryngeal dysfunction or respiratory muscle paralysis).
2. Mixed anaerobic and aerobic flora of the upper respiratory tract is most common cause.

Pneumocystis carinii

For approximately 40 years, *Pneumocystis carinii* has been recognized as a cause of pneumonia in immunosuppressed patients. *Pneumocystis carinii* is the most common life-threatening infection to persons with acquired immunodeficiency syndrome (AIDS). Malaise, fever, nonproductive cough, and dyspnea are the usual symptoms. A roentgenogram of the chest shows diffuse bilateral pulmonary infiltrates, although the infiltrates may be found only in upper or lower lobes.

Medical treatment includes the intravenous administration of trimethoprim-sulfamethoxazole. Pentamidine isethionate may be used in place of trimethoprim-sulfamethoxazole in persons intolerant to it. The relapse rate of *Pneumocystis carinii* in persons with AIDS is estimated to be approximately 20% to 30%. Failure to respond to therapy, the necessity of mechanical ventilation, and repeated episodes of *Pneumocystis carinii* are all associated with a poor prognosis. (See Chapter 19 for further discussion of AIDS.)

Aspiration Pneumonia

The common factor in all forms of aspiration pneumonia is the aspiration of material into the airways. Aspiration pneumonia can occur while the patient is in the hospital, but diligent nursing care may prevent it. The types of aspiration pneumonia are listed in Box 24-12.

Hematogenous Pneumonia

Bacterial infections of the lung can also occur when pathogenic organisms are spread to the lungs through the bloodstream. See Table 24-12 for signs and symptoms and medical therapy of this type of pneumonia.

Nursing Process
Assessment

Subjective data

1. Onset and duration of:
   a. Cough
   b. Fever
   c. Shaking chills
   d. Chest pain
   e. Sputum production (amount, color, and consistency; see Box 24-5, p. 524)
2. Self-care modalities used to treat symptoms
3. History of exposure to:
   a. Persons with infection
   b. Pulmonary irritants

Objective data

1. Observe for signs of other chronic disease and general debilitation
2. Monitor vital signs
   a. Elevated temperature (39° C to 40° C; 102.2° to 104° F) or low-grade temperature elevation
      Tachycardia
      Tachypnea
3. Pulmonary examination
   a. Inspection
      (1) Accessory muscle retraction
      (2) Central cyanosis
      (3) Respiratory grunting on expiration
      (4) Guarding and restricted chest movement on affected side
   b. Palpation
      (1) Decreased expansion on affected side of chest
      (2) Increased tactile fremitus
   c. Percussion
      (1) Dullness on percussion
   d. Auscultation
      (1) Bronchial breath sounds
      (2) Inspiratory crackles (rales)
      (3) Decreased vocal fremitus (pleural effusion)
      (4) Egophony (consolidation)
4. Assess laboratory findings
   a. Chest x-ray
      Diffuse involvement—atypical pneumonia
      Lobar involvement—typical pneumonia
   b. Hematology
      (1) WBC—elevated 15,000 to 25,000/mm³
      (2) Cold agglutins—complement fixation/viral or *Mycoplasma pneumoniae*
   c. Arterial blood gas studies
      (1) Hypoxemia/respiratory alkalosis
      (2) If underlying chronic pulmonary disease, respiratory acidosis

Data analysis: nursing diagnoses

Nursing diagnoses are determined from analysis of patient data. Possible nursing diagnoses for the person with pneumonia may include but are not limited to:

Diagnostic title	Possible etiologies
Airway clearance, ineffective	Decreased energy, fatigue, tracheobronchial inflammation
Gas exchange, impaired	Alveolar-capillary membrane changes, altered oxygen delivery
Pain	Pleural inflammation, coughing paroxysms
Infection, high risk	Compromised lung defense system
Knowledge deficit: conditions and its treatment	Lack of exposure to or unfamiliarity with information
Nutrition, altered: less than body requirements	Increased metabolic needs Anorexia due to infectious process, sputum production

Planning: expected patient outcomes

Expected patient outcomes for the person with pneumonia may include, but are not limited to, the following:

1. Patient demonstrates effective cough with adequate sputum production. (Both cough and sputum production decrease within 72 hours of treatment initiation. Patient with chronic lung disease returns to prepneumonia status.)
2. Patient demonstrates improved ventilation and adequate oxygenation of tissues
   a. pH returns within normal limits.
   b. PO_2 during active disease—60 to 80 mm Hg; after resolution of disease, PaO_2 within normal limits.
3. Patient reports absence of chest pain.
4. Patient does not develop a superinfection.
5. Patient states when influenza and pneumonia vaccines should be taken.
6. Patient can state the signs and symptoms that should be reported to the physician.
7. Patient describes the cause and factors contributing to the occurrence of pneumonia and names common symptoms indicating pneumonia.
8. Patient maintains prepneumonia body weight.
9. Patient's appetite improves and weight gain returns weight to near preillness level.

Implementation

Assisting with achievement of therapeutic goals
Medications

1. Before beginning administration of prescribed antibiotic, sputum is collected for culture. If blood culture is ordered, blood is also drawn before therapy is begun.
2. Antibiotic blood levels are monitored by giving antibiotics at scheduled times. (Table 24-11 lists the antibiotic therapy currently employed in treating pneumonia.)
3. Give medication prescribed to relieve pain. Codeine may be prescribed because it is less likely to inhibit the cough reflex than more potent narcotics.

Oxygen therapy

Oxygen by mask or cannula (Figs. 24-15 and 24-16) is usually ordered when PO_2 is less than 60 mm Hg.[117] When supplemental oxygen is necessary it may be administered by nasal prongs or by mask. The method used depends on the patient's condition and the concentration of oxygen required. The nurse should be familiar with the various devices used to administer oxygen, and when oxygen is in use the nurse should check the equipment frequently to be sure that it is working properly.

When the patient is having difficulty exchanging oxygen and carbon dioxide, such as occurs in pulmonary edema, oxygen may be given under positive pressure. In some situations, such as chronic obstructive pulmonary disease, low-flow rates of oxygen are indicated. The use of low-flow oxygen is discussed on p. 615. *In all situations, the nurse should remember that a patient suffering from hypoxemia may not be breathless or cyanotic because cyanosis does not occur until there is 5 g or more of deoxygenated hemoglobin.* In persons with anemia, all the available heme is completely saturated with oxygen and thus they are never cyanotic even though they may be hypoxemic. *For this reason an increase in the pulse rate may be the first indication that the patient is experiencing hypoxemia.* Patients receiving oxygen therapy are monitored by arterial blood gas studies. These studies are explained on p. 527.

Interventions to achieve patient outcomes
Facilitating breathing

Assist the patient to breathe deeply and expand the chest to increase ventilation.

1. Place patient in position to facilitate breathing—usually upright or semi-upright position (Fig. 24-17).

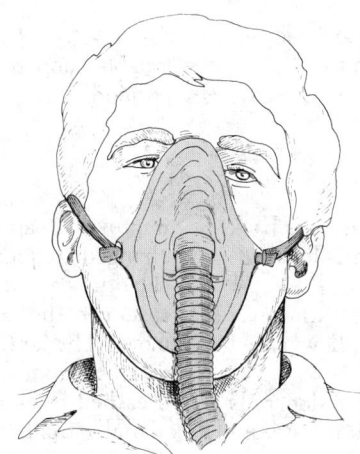

Fig. 24-15   Simple face mask. (From Abels LF: *Mosby's manual of critical care,* St Louis, 1979, Mosby–Year Book.)

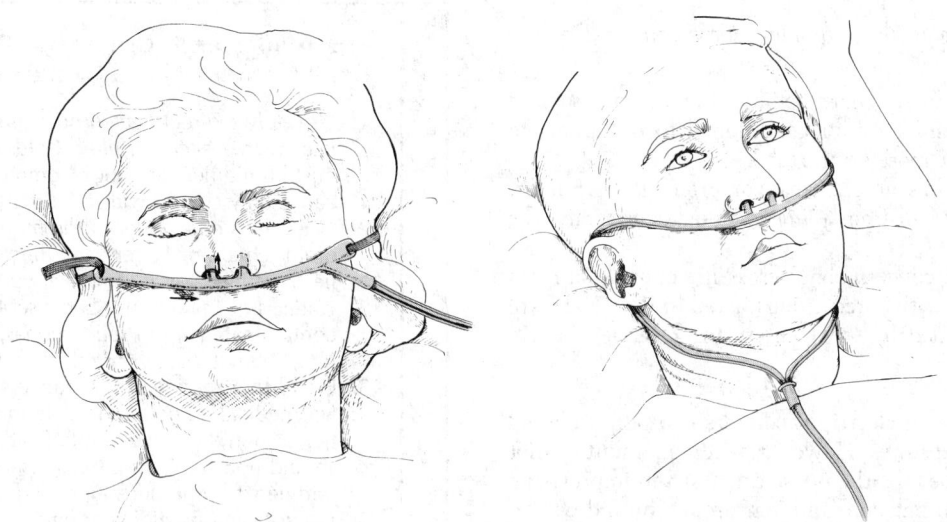

Fig. 24-16   Two types of nasal cannulas. (From Abels LF: *Mosby's manual of critical care,* St Louis, 1979, Mosby–Year Book.)

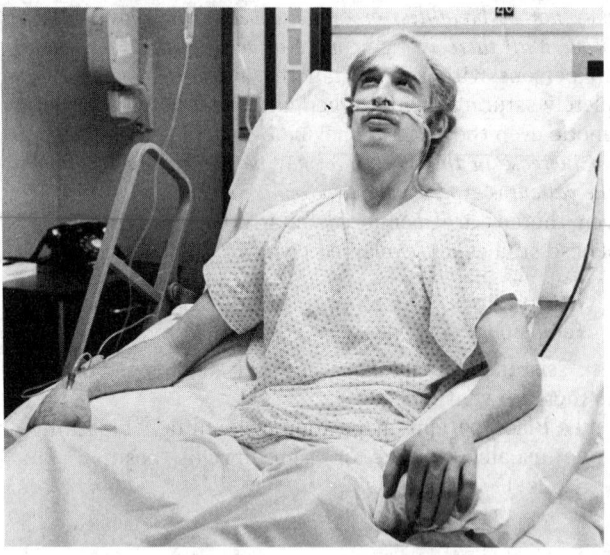

Fig. 24-17 Patient sitting upright with pillows under head and each arm to promote chest expansion and comfort.

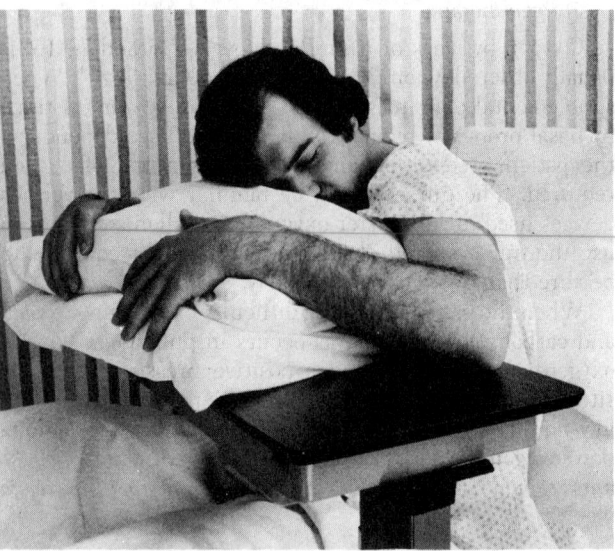

Fig. 24-18 Pillows placed on over-bed table provide comfortable support for the patient who must sleep in a sitting position.

2. A pillow may be placed lengthwise at patient's back to provide support and thrust thorax slightly forward, allowing freer use of the diaphragm.
3. The patient who must be upright to breathe may find it restful to rest head and arms on a pillow placed on an overbed table (Fig. 24-18).
4. For the patient with severe hypoxemia, side rails should be in place. Patient can use them to assist in moving about in bed.
5. Some patients may breathe best when sitting up in a large armchair while leaning on a smaller chair placed in front of them. This chair is blocked to prevent it from slipping.

Maintaining ventilation, humidity, and a comfortable temperature

1. Most patients are most comfortable if air is cool and not too humid. An air-conditioned room may make the patient more comfortable.
2. If patient has nose, throat, or bronchial irritation, warm moist air from a *humidifier* or *vaporizer* may be helpful.
3. Because of concern about cross-infection from room humidifiers, the precautions listed in Box 24-13 are recommended by the Centers for Disease Control (CDC).

Vaporizers. Small electric vaporizers can be purchased at most local drugstores. However, when a patient cannot afford to purchase one, the nurse can assist in improvising equipment for inhalation and for proper humidity. An empty coffee can or a shallow pie tin can be filled with sterile water and placed on an electric plate in the person's room to increase humidity. If the inhalation is to be directed, an ordinary steam kettle or a tea kettle with a longer improvised paper spout may be used. The paper should be changed frequently. A few drops of menthol or oil of eucalyptus can be put into the water. Benzoin causes corrosion in the kettle, which is exceedingly difficult to remove. The kettle and electric plate should be placed a safe distance from the face so that the medicated steam can be breathed freely but the person cannot be burned by accidentally tipping the kettle or by touching the hot plate. After the 25- to 30-minute treatment, equipment should be removed from the bedside.

24-13

Precautions from Centers for Disease Control when using a humidifier

1. *Use only a direct heated humidifier or nebulizer with a bacterial filter.* Cold vapor or cool mist humidifiers are not recommended because they cannot withstand daily sterilization.
2. *Use only sterile water in the humidifier* and drain remaining water each time the humidifier is refilled, or at least every 24 hours. Tap water is not safe to use because it is frequently contaminated with *Pseudomonas, Flavobacterium, Actinetobacter,* or other oganisms.
3. Establish a routine maintenance schedule.
4. Set medical guidelines to determine which patients should receive humidification and which should not. It may not be advisable to use humidifiers for immunosuppressed patients.
5. *Do not send humidifying unit home with patients because of the concern about transporting highly resistant hospital organisms into the community.*

Hydration. Dehydration results in thick, tenacious secretions. *The best liquefying agent is water, and it is preferable to adequately hydrate the patient rather than attempt to loosen secretions with mist therapy.* If the patient does not have cardiovascular disease requiring fluid restriction, a fluid intake of 3 to 4 L/day should be provided.

Assisting with comfort and ADL

1. Place patient in position of comfort—patients are usually most comfortable with head of bed elevated 45 to 90 degrees.
2. Support the patient's chest during coughing.

Preventing spread of infection

1. When universal precautions are used, respiratory isolation is unnecessary.
2. Hand washing is the most important way to prevent spread of pneumonia from one patient to another via the hands of hospital personnel.

Facilitating learning

The major emphasis is on prevention.

1. Two vaccines are now available to prevent respiratory infections: influenza vaccine and pneumococcal vaccine.
2. Persons at high risk for developing complication of influenza (pneumonia) should be immunized unless they are allergic to eggs or egg products or have had a previous reaction to vaccine.
   a. Influenza vaccine is given yearly.
   b. *Pneumonia polysaccharide* vaccine is given only every 3 to 5 years.[117]
3. Attention needs to be paid to reducing the likelihood of gram-negative colonization of patients. For this reason many hospitals have instituted tighter control policies on the use of antibiotics except in situations where a review panel of physicians approves their use. A reduction in use of antibiotics also reduces the incidence of antibiotic-resistant hospital flora, which are the source of many nosocomial infections. (See Chapter 17.)

Complications of pneumonia

With the advent of antibiotics and better diagnostic measures such as x-ray procedures, complications during or following pneumonia are rare in otherwise healthy persons. *Atelectasis, delayed resolution, lung abscess, pleural effusion, empyema, pericarditis, meningitis, and relapse are complications that were common in the past.* The fact that pneumonia and influenza rank fifth as a cause of death in the United States is an impressive reason for strict adherence to the prescribed medical treatment. Careful and accurate observation as well as sufficient time for convalescence also helps to ensure that the average patient has a smooth recovery. Elderly persons and those with a chronic illness are likely to have a relatively long course of convalescence from pneumonia, and there is a greater possibility of their developing complications. *There has been an increase in the incidence of staphylococcal pneumonia subsequent to influenza. Consolidation of lung tissue, pleural effusion, and empyema frequently occur soon after onset of this type of pneumonia and may cause death.*

The Elderly with Pulmonary Problems

Assessment

Assess lung sounds; diminished lung sounds are common in the elderly because of thickened alveoli and decreased rib cage expansion (thorax stiffening).

Assess respiratory status with activity; dyspnea with exertion may occur from decreased pulmonary oxygen diffusion.

Monitor effects of drugs that may interfere with breathing, such as narcotics and hypnotics. Elderly persons may have decreased drug clearance from decreased glomerular filtration rate (GFR) and nephron activity or from decreased hepatic function.

Monitor for signs of pneumonia, to which older persons are highly susceptible. Elderly patients may present with symptoms of mental confusion, tachycardia, or dyspnea rather than the customary signs of cough, fever, and rales (crackles).

Intervention

Encourage as much activity as the person can tolerate to promote ventilation, such as paced walking.

Suggest patient sit upright for meals and for 20 to 30 minutes after meals, to prevent pulmonary aspiration during eating.

Encourage pneumococcal and influenza vaccine prophylaxis.

Teach patient the importance of oral care to help prevent pneumonia.

For the elderly patient with pneumonia, maintain good hydration (with close monitoring to prevent fluid imbalances) and assist with respiratory therapy and position changes.

Common disorders in elderly

Pneumonia
Lung cancer
COPD

Evaluation

Evaluation is based on patient outcomes. Questions to be asked include the following:

1. Have the patient's cough and sputum production improved?
2. Have the patient's PaO_2 and pH returned to normal limits?
3. Does patient state that chest pain is absent?
4. Is the patient free of a superinfection?
5. Can the patient state the cause of and factors contributing to pneumonia?
6. Can the patient state the common symptoms of pneumonia?
7. Can the patient state when influenza or pneumonia vaccines should be taken?
8. Can the patient state the signs and symptoms that should be reported to the physician?
9. Is the patient's appetite improved and weight returning to prepneumonia levels?

TUBERCULOSIS

Etiology/Epidemiology

In 1900 tuberculosis was the leading cause of death in the United States. It remained a major cause of death until the introduction of antituberculosis drug therapy in the late 1940s and early 1950s. The most effective of these agents is isoniazid, which first became available clinically in 1952. The use of isoniazid in combination with two agents introduced earlier, streptomycin and paraaminosalicylic acid, resulted in a striking decrease in tuberculosis mortality rates. It also made it possible for patients with tuberculosis to be treated on an outpatient basis. However, some patients still have to be hospitalized during their illness, and most nurses will care for a patient with tuberculosis at some time in their careers.

Although tuberculosis is considered a preventable and curable disease, it is a disease that demands constant public health surveillance. The case rates for tuberculosis in the United States declined steadily from 1953, when there were 84,304 reported cases, to 1984, when there were 22,225 reported cases. Beginning in 1986, when the number of cases increased by 3%, the rates have continued to increase yearly. There was a 5% increase in 1989 and a 6% increase in 1990[12] (Fig. 24-19).

These new cases were not evenly distributed throughout the population, however, and some differences bear mentioning. The highest number of cases were in the 25- to 44-year age group. This is a change from the 1970s and early 1980s, where the highest cases rates were in white males aged 65 years and older.

In addition, the highest case rates between 1985 and 1990 were found in Miami, Atlanta, San Francisco, Newark, Tampa, and New York City.[12a] These states have the highest number of HIV-positive persons, especially among drug abusers. These states also have a large number of immigrants, many of whom come from countries in which tuberculosis is endemic. Of particular concern has been an increase in the cases of tuberculosis among children under the age of 15. It is assumed that most of these

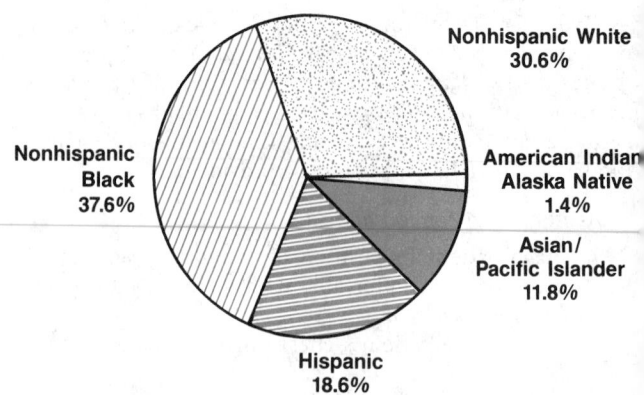

Fig. 24-20 Tuberculosis case rates by race and ethnicity, United States 1990. (From Centers for Disease Control: Tuberculosis morbidity in the United States: final data, 1990, *MMWR* 40 (SS3):23-28, 1992.)

children were infected by persons in the 25- to 44-year age group in which the incidence of tuberculosis is highest. Also of concern is that many persons with HIV infection have organisms resistant to most of the chemotherapeutic agents used to treat tuberculosis. When this is true, the infected person passes his or her resistant organisms to those they infect, making treatment of the newly infected particularly difficult. In all age groups, cases *increased* among non-Hispanic blacks, Hispanics, and Asian/Pacific Islanders but *decreased* among non-Hispanic whites and American Indians/Alaskan natives (Fig. 24-20). Increases in cases occurred among both males and females. In 1990 there were 17,814 reported cases (69.3%) in persons of racial/ethnic minorities and 7,836 cases (30.5%) among non-Hispanic whites.[12a] The increases in these racial/ethnic groups primarily reflects the increase in tuberculosis in persons infected with the human immunodeficiency virus (HIV).[24]

Because HIV infection is an important risk factor for developing clinically apparent tuberculosis among persons already infected with the tubercule bacillus, the CDC recommends that all HIV-infected persons be screened for tuberculosis and latent tuberculous infection and, if infected, placed on appropriate therapy. Also, persons with tuberculosis and known tuberculin-positive persons should be evaluated for HIV infection so that appropriate counseling and treatment can be given.

Tuberculosis is caused by the bacillus, *mycobacterium tuberculosis,* or tubercle bacillus, a gram-positive and acidfast organism. If microscopic study of a slide prepared from the sputum of an individual reveals tubercle bacilli, the individual is said to have positive sputum; and this confirms the diagnosis of tuberculosis. However, most persons with tuberculosis will not have positive sputum on smear, and a *positive sputum culture* will be necessary to confirm the diagnosis. Patients who have a positive culture and negative smear are less infectious than are those with both a positive smear and culture.

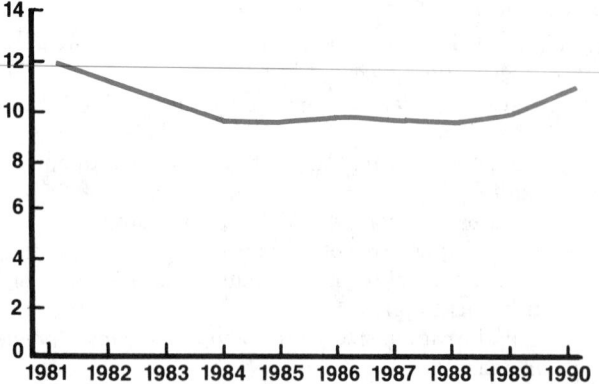

Fig. 24-19 Tuberculosis case rates 1981-1990. (From Centers for Disease Control: Tuberculosis Morbidity in the United States: Final Data, 1990, *MMWR* 40 (SS3):23-28, 1992.)

When a person with tuberculosis speaks, coughs, sneezes, or sings, minute droplets fall to the ground; the smaller ones evaporate, leaving *droplet nuclei* that remain suspended indefinitely in the air and are carried on air currents. Droplet nuclei are 1 to 10 μm in size and are small enough to be inhaled into the alveoli. Thus tuberculosis is transmitted by inhalation of tubercle-laden droplet nuclei.

Pathophysiology

When an individual with no previous exposure to tuberculosis (negative tuberculin reactor) inhales a sufficient number of tubercle bacilli into the alveoli, tuberculosis *infection* occurs. The body's reaction to the tubercle bacilli depends on the *susceptibility of the individual, the size of the dose, and the virulence of the organisms*. Inflammation occurs within the alveoli (parenchyma) of the lungs, and natural body defenses attempt to counteract the infection.

Macrophages ingest the organisms and present the mycobacterial antigens to the T cells. CD4 cells secrete lymphokines that enhance the capacity of the macrophages to ingest and kill bacteria. Lymph nodes in the hilar region of the lung become enlarged as they filter drainage from the infected site. The inflammatory process and cellular reaction produce a small, firm, white nodule called the *primary tubercle*.[2] The center of the nodule contains tubercle bacilli. Cells gather around the center, and usually the outer portion becomes fibrosed. Thus blood vessels are compressed, nutrition of the tubercle is interfered with, and *necrosis* occurs at the center. The area becomes walled off by fibrotic tissue around the outside, and the center gradually becomes soft and cheesy in consistency. This latter process is known as *caseation necrosis*. This material may become calcified (calcium deposits), or it may liquefy and is known as *liquefaction necrosis*. The liquefied material may be coughed up, leaving a *cavity* or hole in the parenchyma of the lung. The cavity or cavities are visible on chest x-ray films and result in the diagnosis of *cavitary disease*. Most individuals who are exposed to tuberculosis and develop a tuberculosis infection (confirmed by a positive tuberculin test) do not develop an active case of tuberculosis. The only x-ray evidence of their tuberculosis infection is a calcified nodule known as the *Ghon tubercle*. The evidence on x-ray film of enlarged hilar lymph nodes and a Ghon tubercle is referred to as the *primary complex*.

Persons who have the *primary complex* have become sensitized to the tubercle bacillus, and an antigen-antibody reaction results. When the person receives the antigen in the form of a purified protein derivative (PPD) or old tuberculin (OT) in a tuberculin test the reaction results in a positive tuberculin test. This sensitization, once developed usually remains throughout life unless something interferes with the immune response. Evidence suggests that most tuberculin reactors who take isoniazid prophylactically for 6 months convert back to negative test results. This protection is believed to last for life. A *positive tuberculin test does not mean that one has tuberculosis, however, and nurses should explain this fact to persons undergoing the test.*

Tuberculosis infection is unlike other infections. Usually, other infections disappear completely when overcome by the body's defenses and leave no living organisms and generally no signs of infection. However, a person who has been infected with tubercle bacilli harbors the organism for the remainder of his or her life unless they have received prophylactic isoniazid. Tubercle bacilli remain in the lungs in a dormant, walled-off, or so-called resting state. When a person is under physical or emotional stress, these bacilli may become active and begin to multiply. If body defenses are low, active tuberculosis may develop. Most persons who have active tuberculosis developed it in this manner. However, it is generally accepted that only 1 out of 10 persons with a positive tuberculin test will ever develop active tuberculosis, and the incidence is expected to be much lower among those who receive preventive therapy with isoniazid.

When tuberculosis occurs several years after the primary infection, it is known as *reactivation tuberculosis*. The development of active tuberculosis is believed to be caused by defects in T-cell or macrophage functions or both.[2]

Tuberculosis is more likely to occur in persons with HIV infection because in HIV infection there are progressive depletion and dysfunction of CD4 cells, along with defects in macrophage and monocyte function. Epidemiologic evidence suggests that because of these changes, persons with HIV infection and a positive tuberculin test (primary infection) are at risk for *reactivation tuberculosis*. At the same time persons with HIV infection who have negative tuberculin tests are at risk of going right from a primary infection to active tuberculosis when exposed to someone with tuberculosis. Also, extrapulmonary tuberculosis is more common in persons with HIV infection and when it is diagnosed in them it becomes an AIDS-defining condition. This means that tuberculosis is a more opportunistic infection than is *P. carinii* and other infections that indicate that a person has gone from HIV infection to AIDS.[2]

Two mycobacterial organisms are found in persons diagnosed as having AIDS. In developed countries, the *Mycobacterium avium* intracellular complex (MAC) is the organism found in middle-class AIDS patients who have no history of intravenous drug use. Pulmonary tuberculosis caused by *M. tuberculosis* is more common in AIDS patients from *developing countries* and *in persons from inner-city minority populations who have a history of intravenous drug use.*[35]

Classification of Tuberculosis

The classification used by states and territories of the United States when reporting tuberculosis cases to the CDC of the Public Health Service is outlined in Table 24-13. The six basic classifications cover the total child and adult population, those unexposed to tuberculosis, those uninfected even though exposed, those with evidence of tuberculosis infection without disease, those with current disease, those with evidence of tuberculosis without current disease, and those in whom tuberculosis is suspected (diagnosis pending).

REVIEW

Table 24-13   Classification of tuberculosis

Class	Description	Medical therapy
0	No TB exposure, not infected	None
1	TB exposure, no evidence of infection	Preventive chemotherapy may be given for persons converting their tuberculin test from negative to positive
2	TB infection, no disease	Isoniazid (INH) for 1 year (preventive chemotherapy) for *positive reactors* under age 35
3	TB: current disease (persons with completed diagnostic evidence of TB: both a significant reaction to tuberculin skin test and clinical and/or x-ray evidence of TB)	Antituberculosis drugs: at least 2 of the first-line drugs (INH, ethambutol, rifampin, streptomycin)
4	TB: no current disease (persons with previous history of TB or with abnormal x-ray films but no significant tuberculin skin test reaction or clinical evidence)	No new therapy (persons may still be receiving chemotherapy)
5	TB: suspect (diagnosis pending); used during diagnostic testing of suspect persons, for no longer than a 3-month period	Preventive chemotherapy may be instituted

---

24-14

Priorities for preventive therapy among TB-infected persons

1. Persons with HIV infection
2. Recent contacts of persons with infectious TB
3. Persons with recent skin test conversions
4. Persons with recent TB disease who have been inadequately treated
5. Persons with negative sputum cultures and stable fibrotic lesions on chest radiographs consistent with inactive TB
6. Persons with medical conditions that increase the risk of TB
   - Leukemia or lymphoma
   - Silicosis
   - Diabetes mellitus
   - Gastrectomy
   - End-stage renal disease
   - Antibodies to human immunodeficiency virus (HIV)

Primary and Secondary Prevention

To eliminate tuberculosis, the organism must be prevented from being transmitted from one person to another. Preventive measures are directed toward the latest recommendations from the Advisory Council for the Elimination of Tuberculosis (ACET). These recommendations can be found in Box 24-14.

Persons over 35 years of age without the risk factors listed here are not given preventive chemotherapy because of the risk of isoniazid-associated hepatitis. Although the risk is small, it is age related and increases from less than 0.2% in those under age 20 to up to 2.3% in those 50 to 64 years of age.

If isoniazid-associated hepatitis occurs, the symptoms are mild, nonspecific, and resemble those of any viral illness. (See Chapter 30 for a discussion of viral hepatitis.)

Contraindications to the use of isoniazid preventive therapy are (1) previous isoniazid-associated liver disease; (2) severe adverse reactions to isoniazid, including fever, chills, rash, and arthritis; and (3) *acute* liver disease of any cause.

Persons receiving isoniazid preventive chemotherapy should be seen monthly by a health care provider for the purpose of reinforcing the necessity of taking the chemotherapy regularly and to monitor the patient for any serious side effects. Because most cases of tuberculosis in patients with HIV infection occur in those with a history of a positive tuberculin test, all persons with HIV infection should be considered for preventive therapy with isoniazid. Groups that should receive particular attention are intravenous drug users, prison inmates, and the homeless, because they have an extraordinarily high incidence of HIV and tuberculosis infection.[2]

Because of the difficulty in preventing tuberculosis among homeless persons special recommendations have been made for the group[12a]:

1. The highest priority should be given to 1) detection, evaluation, and reporting of homeless persons who have current symptoms of active TB and 2) completion of an appropriate course of treatment by those diagnosed with active TB.
2. The second priority should be screening and preventive therapy for homeless persons who have, or are suspected of having, human immunodeficiency virus (HIV) infection.
3. The third priority should be the examination and appropriate treatment of persons with recent TB that has been inadequately treated.
4. The fourth priority should be screening and appropriate treatment of persons exposed to an infectious (sputum-positive) case of TB. Because contacts are difficult to define in a shelter population, it is usually necessary to screen all residents of a shelter when an infectious case is identified.
5. The fifth priority should be screening and preventive

therapy for homeless persons with known medical conditions that increase the risk of TB, for example, diabetes mellitus and other conditions listed in Box 24-14, Number 6.

Preventive chemotherapy in the United States is isoniazid daily for 6 months. The usual adult dose is 300 mg in a single dose daily. If the person has antibodies to the human immunodeficiency virus (HIV), isoniazid is given daily for 1 year.

In 1989, the CDC's Advisory Committee for the Elimination of Tuberculosis (ACET) published *A Strategic Plan for Elimination of Tuberculosis in the United States*. The committee recommended that a goal be established to eliminate tuberculosis by the year 2010. To achieve the goal, a case rate of 0.1 per 100,000 persons was set for the year 2010, with an interim goal of a case rate of 3.5 per 100,000 population by the year 2000. This goal may not be easy to accomplish, in view of the 1990 case rate of 10.0 per 100,000.[22]

Vaccination

Efforts continue in search of a more satisfactory tuberculosis vaccine. Presently, bacillus Calmette-Guérin (BCG) vaccine is used worldwide except in the United States and the Netherlands. The vaccine contains attenuated tubercle bacilli that have lost their ability to produce disease. It is administered only to persons who have a negative reaction to the tuberculin test. It is not widely used in the United States because of disagreements among physicians as to its safety and effectiveness. Also, vaccination with BCG induces hypersensitivity to tuberculin (positive tuberculin reaction) in vaccinated persons.

Most persons who have received BCG will have a skin test reaction of less than 10 mm. If a larger reaction occurs to purified protein derivative (PPD), it can be assumed that the person has a TB infection.

The vaccine should be given only by persons who have had careful instruction in the proper technique. A multiple-puncture disk is used. When there is a positive reaction to skin testing with tuberculin, when acute infectious disease is present, or when there is any skin disease, BCG vaccine is not given. Possible complications following vaccination are local ulcers, which occur in a relatively high percentage of persons vaccinated, and abscesses or suppuration of lymph nodes, which occur in a small percentage.

In countries where living conditions are such that transmission of tuberculosis is to be expected, BCG vaccine is given at birth and then repeated after 12 to 15 years. The intradermal method is used to administer the vaccine so that a uniform controlled dose can be given. BCG vaccine, as mentioned above is not widely used in the United States, although some highly susceptible groups such as migrant workers may be vaccinated.

Diagnostic Tests

Each of the tests used to diagnose tuberculosis are described earlier in this chapter. The tests and the pages on which the tests are discussed are listed below.

1. Tuberculin skin testing (p. 523).
2. Chest x-ray (p. 522).
3. Sputum smear and culture (p. 524).

Additional information about each of the tests in the diagnosis of tuberculosis is next.

Tuberculin skin testing

Tuberculin skin testing provides evidence of whether the individual tested has been infected by tubercle bacilli. It is based on the fact that a hypersensitivity reaction develops to certain products of *Mycobacterium tuberculosis*. This cell-mediated or delayed hypersensitivity reaction is manifested by induration caused by cellular infiltration at the site of the injection in persons who have been sensitized to the tubercle bacillus. Such persons are called *reactors*. In the past the terms *negative* and *positive* were used to describe the results of tuberculin testing. In 1981 the American Thoracic Society (ATS), the medical section of the American Lung Association, suggested that the terms positive and negative are not the most accurate way to describe the results of tuberculin skin testing. They recommend that the number of millimeters of induration be recorded and then interpreted appropriately, with persons being classified as reactors or non-reactors.

A tuberculin reaction may begin after 12 to 24 hours with an area of redness and a central area of induration, but it reaches its peak in 48 hours. *The area of induration* (not the erythema) *indicates how positive (reactive) the test is.* Induration should be examined in a good light and palpated gently. Tuberculin reactions should always be measured and recorded in millimeters at the largest diameter of the induration. When successive dilutions are being used, it is advisable to have tests read by the same person so that individual variation in interpretation can be prevented. If the response to the test is non-reactive (negative), there may be no visible reaction or there may be only slight redness with no induration.

One of the most important steps in tuberculin testing is the accurate measurement of reaction. A reaction is considered to be significant when it is 10 mm or more in diameter. Reactions between 5 and 9 mm are considered to be doubtful reactions and are more likely to indicate infection with atypical acid-fast bacilli than with *Mycobacterium tuberculosis*, except in persons who are suspects or close contacts of persons with tuberculosis. In this instance a reaction of 5 mm or more is considered significant.

Roentgenographic examinations

Persons with positive tuberculin tests undergo chest x-ray examinations to determine if there is evidence of active tuberculosis. Standard posteroanterior and lateral chest films are usually ordered. Body-section roentgenograms (tomography) also may be ordered (see p. 522). These views are helpful in defining nodules, cavities, cysts, calcification, and vascular details in the parenchyma of the lung.

Tuberculosis lesions usually occur in the apical and posterior segments of the upper lobe or in the superior segment of the lower lobe.

Pleural effusion may be the only x-ray finding evident with pleural tuberculosis.

Sputum examination

For the diagnosis of tuberculosis to be made there must be microscopic identification of *M. tuberculosis* (acid-fast bacillus).

24-15	**Guidelines for sputum specimen collection**

1. Patients who have difficulty producing sputum or who have very tenacious sputum may be dehydrated. Encourage fluid intake.
2. Collect specimens before meals to avoid possible emesis from coughing.
3. Instruct patient to rinse mouth with water before expectorating into sterile specimen bottle to decrease sputum contamination.
4. Notify staff as soon as a specimen is collected so it can be sent to the laboratory without delay.

Tests performed on sputum are explained to the patient so that a suitable specimen is obtained. See p. 524 for more information. Box 24-15 lists guidelines for sputum collection.

Establishing the diagnosis of tuberculosis

Results of roentgenograms and sputum examinations will either rule out the possibility or confirm a diagnosis of tuberculosis. Bacteriologic confirmation of the presence of *M. tuberculosis* is necessary to establish the diagnosis of tuberculosis. Because it is impossible to differentiate between typical and atypical acid-fast bacilli by a sputum smear, cultures are obtained on all persons. Cultures are also used for antimicrobial susceptibility (sensitivity) studies. *Despite the introduction of improved culture media, the tubercle bacillus grows slowly on artificial media, and culture reports are not available for 3 to 6 weeks.*

Blood-streaked sputum in the absence of pronounced coughing may be the first indication to the person that something is wrong. Pathologic changes may have occurred in the lungs, but sputum examination may not show tubercle bacilli. However, if the nodules produced in the parenchyma of the lung become soft in the center and then caseated and liquefied, the liquefied material may break through and empty into the bronchi and be raised as sputum. Cavities in the lung may appear on x-ray film and may be present in more than one lobe of the lung.

Nursing Process
Assessment
Subjective data

Early in the course of tuberculosis, the person may be *asymptomatic. Later symptoms include cough with sputum production, afternoon temperature elevation, and night sweats.* Blood-streaked sputum in the absence of pronounced coughing may be *the first indication to the person that something* is wrong. It is important to determine whether the patient was exposed to a person with tuberculosis. *Often the source of the infection is unknown and may never be determined.* At the same time, close contacts of the patient need to be identified so that they may undergo follow-up to determine if they are infected and *have active disease or* have a tuberculosis infection (tuberculin reactor with negative sputum tests).

Objective data

1. Productive cough
2. Afternoon temperature elevation
3. Tuberculin skin test reaction of 10 mm induration or more
4. X-ray film showing a pulmonary infiltrate

Data analysis: nursing diagnoses

Nursing diagnoses are determined from analysis of patient data. Possible nursing diagnoses for the person with tuberculosis may include, but are not limited to:

Diagnostic title	Possible etiologies
Knowledge deficit about tuberculosis—spread and treatment	Lack of exposure to information
Airway clearance, ineffective	Increased sputum, decreased energy/fatigue
Fear	Long-term illness requiring long-term chemotherapy, lifestyle changes until no longer infectious

Planning: expected patient outcomes

Expected patient outcomes for the person with tuberculosis may include, but are not limited to, the following:

1. Patient can explain how tuberculosis is spread and those measures necessary to prevent spread of tuberculosis (remain on chemotherapy, cover mouth and nose when coughing or sneezing)
2. Patient can explain basic food groups and how a nutritionally adequate diet will be achieved
3. Patient can state name, dose, actions, and side effects of prescribed medications
4. Patient can state why two or three chemotherapy agents must be taken together
   a. Can explain drug-resistant organisms and relate this to the need to take chemotherapy as directed
   b. Can explain why the health care provider should be notified immediately if for any reason (for example, side effects) chemotherapy cannot be taken
5. Patient can state where to receive new supply of chemotherapy and date it is to be obtained
6. Patient can state plans for follow-up care
   a. Can list signs and symptoms that indicate need for immediate medical care (increased cough, hemoptysis, unexplained weight loss, fever, night sweats)
   b. Can state when next sputum test or x-ray film is to be taken and where
   c. Can state plans for ongoing follow-up care
7. Patient is able to maintain a clear airway as chemotherapy decreases the amount of sputum.
8. Patient states that he or she is less fearful about the future.

Implementation
Assisting with achievement of therapeutic goals
Medications

Medical treatment is with antituberculosis drug therapy. The drugs used to treat tuberculosis, their classification, side effects, and tests for side effects can be found in Table 24-14.

Table 24-14 Drugs used to treat tuberculosis

Drug	Classification	Common side effects	Tests	Remarks
Isoniazid (INH)	Bactericidal; penetrates all body tissues and fluids, including CSF	Peripheral neuritis hepatitis, rash, fever	SGOT, SGPT (not as routine)	Daily alcohol intake interferes with metabolism of isoniazid and increases risk of hepatitis; antacids containing aluminum interfere with absorption of INH.
Rimfampin (RIF)	Bactericidal; penetrates all body tissues including CSF	Hepatitis, febrile reactions, thrombocytopenia (rare), hepatotoxicity increases when given with INH	SGOT, SGPT, platelet count (not as routine)	Urine, sweat, tears may turn orange temporarily; decrease effectiveness of oral contraceptives, anticoagulants, corticosteroids, barbiturates, hypoglycemics, and digitalis
Ethambutol (EMB)	Bacteriostatic; does not penetrate CSF; penetrates other body fluids	Optic neuritis (reversible with discontinuation of drug; very rare at 15 mg/kg; skin rash)	Visual acuity; red-green color discrimination; GI irritation	No significant reaction with other drugs. Check vision monthly; give with food
Pyrazinamide (PZA)	Bacteriostatic or bactericidal depending on susceptibility of myocobacterium	Hyperuricemia, hepatitis, arthralgia, GI irritation	Uric acid, SGOT, SGPT	Obtain baseline liver function tests and repeat regularly. Give with food; Drink 2 L of fluid daily.
Streptomycin (SM)	Bactericidal, aminoglycoside; disrupts protein synthesis; poor penetration into body tissues and CSF	Eighth cranial nerve damage (vestibular portion); often damage is irreversible; nephrotoxicity	Vestibular function; audiograms; renal function; creatinine level determined before therapy started	Monitor kidney function monthly, monitor vestibular function with caloric stimulation test monthly. Monitor hearing with audiograms monthly. Meningitis treated with intrathecal or subarachnoid instillation of SM

At least two drugs are given together to prevent the development of resistant strains of the tubercle bacillus. A commonly used treatment schedule uses three drugs in combination: isoniazid, 300 mg/day: rifampin, 600 mg/day for 6 months: and P2A, 15 to 30 mg/kg/day, up to 3 g maximum during the first 2 months of treatment. Ethambutol may also be added for two months, especially in the homeless.

When drug resistance develops, other drugs to which the patient's organisms are sensitive are prescribed.

Some persons are infected with resistant strains of the tubercle bacillus. Resistance is most common to isoniazid and streptomycin. There are race/ethnic differences in rates for primary drug resistance. Asians and Hispanics have the highest rates, followed by blacks, whites, and American Indians.[12] Primary drug resistance rates vary widely in the United States and Canada, and nurses need to know the local resistance rates for areas where they are working. It can be assumed that resistance rates are highest in those areas where large numbers of persons with HIV infection live and among drug abusers and the homeless.

Interventions to achieve patient outcomes
Preventing contamination of air with droplet nuclei

Preventing contamination of air with tubercle bacilli is accomplished by: (1) treating the patient with antituberculosis drugs and (2) preventing contamination of air with tubercle bacilli.

24-16

Patient Teaching

Preventing the transmission of tuberculosis

Patient must take antituberculosis drugs as prescribed.

Drugs are always taken as combination of two or three drugs.

Drugs must be taken uninterruptedly.

Both of the above are necessary to prevent development of resistant strains of *M. tuberculosis.*

Preventing contamination of air with *M. tuberculosis.*

Cover nose and mouth with disposable tissues when coughing, sneezing, or laughing.

Place used tissues in paper bag, which should be burned.

Facilitating learning

The most effective way to achieve the prevention of the transmission of tuberculosis is by patient teaching (Box 24-16).

Evaluation

Evaluation is based on patient outcomes. Questions to be asked include the following:

1. Does patient cover nose and mouth when coughing, sneezing, or laughing?

2. Are the patient's sputum cultures negative, indicating that antituberculosis drugs are effective and are being taken as prescribed?
3. Can the patient state name, dosage, and side effects of prescribed antituberculosis drug therapy?
4. Can the patient explain why two or more drugs are prescribed and why they must be taken without interruption?
5. Can the patient state the signs and symtptoms that indicate a need for immediate medical care?
6. Can the patient state the dates of the next sputum and x-ray examinations and the importance of keeping these appointments?
7. Can the patient state the date of the next medical appointment and the importance of keep the appointment?
8. Is the patient less fearful about his or her future?

Extrapulmonary tuberculosis

Tuberculosis may affect other parts of the body besides the lungs, such as the larynx, gastrointestinal tract, lymph nodes, skin, skeletal system, nervous system, urinary system, and reproductive system. Tuberculosis is spread to other parts of the body hematogenously or lymphogenously.

Extrapulmonary tuberculosis has taken on increased importance because of its extremely high frequency, usually with concomitant pulmonary tuberculosis in persons with HIV infection. The most frequent site of extrapulmonary tuberculosis in persons with HIV infection are the lymph nodes; miliary disease, in which the chest x-ray looks like millet seeds spread throughout both lungs, is also common. Involvement also occurs in bone marrow, genitourinary tract, and central nervous system.

Because persons with HIV infection and tuberculosis infection usually have bacteremia, blood cultures are recommended when the diagnosis is suspected.

Infection with atypical acid-fast bacilli

Pulmonary disease that is indistinguishable from tuberculosis can be produced by a number of species of mycobacteria other than *M. tuberculosis*. These organisms are strongly acid fast but differ from *M. tuberculosis* on culture. Four groups have been classified by Runyon: group I, *M. kansasii* (photochromogens); group II, scotochromogens, which are commonly found in soil and water; group III, Battey bacilli (nonchromogens), which are found mainly in Georgia; and group IV, *M. fortuitum* (rapid growers). These atypical organisms are found in various geographic locations. *Group I is the most widely distributed, and many organisms have been identified in the Midwest.* Group III is found more in the southeastern portion of the United States. The pulmonary disease caused by atypical bacilli closely resembles tuberculosis. The disease often causes lung cavities, responds poorly to antituberculosis drugs, and often requires surgery. It occurs most commonly in persons in high socioeconomic groups—especially those residing in suburban areas of large cities. Infection with atypical acid-fast bacilli is three to four times more common in men than in women. Most of those infected are middle-aged or older, and men with emphysema seem to be particularly susceptible. Atypical bacilli are not believed to be airborne; thus isolation is not required. Because of the

seriousness of the pulmonary disease caused by these organisms, patients are usually given multidrug chemotherapy for at least 2 years and should have careful medical follow-up examinations after discharge from the hospital. It is possible for persons to be infected with both *M. tuberculosis* and atypical bacilli at the same time.

INFECTIOUS DISEASES: FUNGAL INFECTIONS OF THE RESPIRATORY TRACT

There are three major fungal infections of the lungs: *histoplasmosis, coccidioidomycosis,* and *blastomycosis.* They are classified as deep mycoses because there is involvement by the parasite of deeper tissues and internal organs. The incidence and prevention of these fungal (mycotic) infections are discussed in Table 24-15.

HISTOPLASMOSIS
Etiology

Inhalation of spares of *Histoplasma capsulatum* is the cause of histoplasmosis.

Pathophysiology

The inhaled spores are phagocytized by alveolar macrophages within which they germinate. They form yeast cells and multiply by budding. In persons previously uninfected there is a primary or initial infection that resembles the infection in primary tuberculosis with involvement of regional lymphatics and early dissemination via lymphatics and blood to other organs. Yeast cells spread hematogenously and are phagocytized by reticuloendothelial cells in the liver, spleen, and bone marrow. The process in the lung is similar to that seen in tuberculosis with necrosis and healing by fibrosis encapsulation. Eventually, the areas show calcification in the original parenchymal foci in the lung and in the hilar lymph nodes. Usually the initial infection is self-limiting and does not require antifungal chemotherapy. However, some persons, such as infants and adults with immunologic imcompetence (lymphoma), may develop a rapidly progressive primary infection that can be fatal without antifungal therapy.

Reinfection histoplasmosis and *progressive histoplasmosis* can also occur. Reinfection with histoplasma causes an illness resembling the initial infection. Because some degree of immunity to histoplasmosis is conferred by the initial infection, the extent of disease is modified by the degree of fungal immunity.[105] Heavy inoculation may cause *pneumonitis,* which is usually self-limiting over days to weeks. *The onset is acute with nonproductive cough, fever, malaise, and dyspnea.* Some persons who are fully immune may develop a hypersensitivity-like pneumonitis with small, discrete granulomatous foci that may give a *miliary* appearance on x-ray examination. This means that the infection is spread throughout the lung, giving the appearance of the presence of small millet seeds throughout the lung.

Progressive histoplasmosis is usually chronic; chronic pulmonary histoplasmosis is the most frequently encountered

Table 24-15   Incidence and prevention of fungal infections

Type of infection and source	Incidence	Prevention
Histoplasmosis		
Soil contaminated with fowl excreta. Bats may be infected and areas they inhabit (caves, attics, hollow trees) can be extremely infectious.	Quite high in United States. Endemic areas in Missouri, Kentucky, Tennessee, southern Illinois, Indiana, and Ohio.	Locate areas where soil is infected with fowl excreta. Teach public to avoid inhalation of dust from infected soil. Infants and the elderly are especially susceptible.
Coccidioidomycosis		
Soil contaminated with spores. Heavy rainfall in the desert enhances growth of the fungus—sunlight inhibits it. Liberation of dust in the spring disperses anthrospores, which are inhaled.	Endemic to well-defined areas in southwestern United States, Mexico, and South America. In United States, endemic in San Joaquin Valley, southern Arizona, New Mexico, and southwestern Texas.	Persons working in desert dust, archeologists, and construction workers should wear masks.
Blastomycosis		
Soil contaminated with spores that are carried on air currents and inhaled by humans and animals. Dogs can acquire the disease. Not believed to be spread from animals to man; believed that both humans and animals are infected by inhaling spores.	Most prevalent in the United States and Canadian valley areas surrounding the Mississippi, Missouri, Ohio, and St. Lawrence rivers. Also present in Africa, South America, and Mexico.	Avoid inhalation of spores in areas where cases have been identified.

symptomatic form of the disease. It develops almost exclusively in middle-aged white men who have chronic obstructive pulmonary disease. There are recurrent episodes of necrotizing segmental or lobar granulomatous pneumonitis, which have a tendency to cavity formation, contraction, fibrosis, and compensatory emphysema.

Progressive disseminated histoplasmosis usually occurs as a consequence of the initial infection in persons with very low resistance to the infection (for instance, infants and persons with immunologic incompetence). Rarely, it can occur in adults of both sexes and all ages with no known immune disorder. These persons have fever, weakness, weight loss, hepatosplenomegaly, leukopenia, and mucous membrane ulceration involving the oropharynx, tongue, or larynx. Adrenal insufficiency occurs in about 50% of these persons.[105]

COCCIDIOIDOMYCOSIS

Etiology

Inhalation of the spores of *Coccidioidoides immitis* is the cause of coccidioidomycosis.

Pathophysiology

The process following inhalation of spores is believed to be very similar to that described under histoplasmosis. The arthrospores reach the alveoli, where they are phagocytized. If the disease becomes disseminated, there is marked hilar adenopathy, and fungi can be isolated from lymph nodes. A pneumonic disease with necrosis and cavitation may occur after development of delayed hypersensitivity.[104] The disease process is controlled and resolved in most persons as the result of cell immunity to infection. *Thus progressive disseminated coccidioidomycosis or progressive pulmonary disease is found only in those persons whose ability to*

resist infection or develop immunity has been compromised in some way. Susceptibility to infection is in part genetically determined. Coccidioidomycosis is 50 times more common in Filipino men and 10 times more common in black men than it is in white men.[104] This increased susceptibility to progressive disease in these groups of men parallels their susceptibility to tuberculosis. The increased susceptibility of some races to diseases such as coccidioidomycosis and tuberculosis is believed to be the result of a genetically determined impairment of their capacity to develop cellular immunity to infection.[104]

Skin testing with coccidioidin, 1:10 or 1:100 is available to test for the disease. The test is read in 48 hours. It takes 3 to 6 weeks after exposure for the test to become positive. In severe disseminated disease the test may be negative, indicating that the patient's immune system is no longer able to respond to the antigen, coccidioidin.

Roentgenograms of the chest may exhibit pneumonic infiltrate, hilar adenopathy, pleural effusion, or a cavitary lesion. About 5% of persons with primary pulmonary involvement have residual lung lesions such as cavities or nodules. Only about 0.5% of infected individuals go on to develop a severe, progressive mycosis.

Extrapulmonary dissemination of coccidioidomycosis can occur. One of the most frequent sites of dissemination is the meningeal surfaces of the brain. If there is any indication of involvement of the central nervous system, a lumbar puncture is performed. A positive complement fixation titer in the spinal fluid is diagnostic of meningitis.

Dissemination can also occur to skin, soft tissue, and bones, and the patient is monitored by physical examination of the skin, gallium scanning of soft tissues, and bone scans. A bone scan should be performed before starting amphotericin B therapy.

Surgical intervention for localized lesions may involve either excision or drainage to facilitate healing.

BLASTOMYCOSIS

Etiology

Blastomycosis is believed to be caused by the inhalation of *Blastomyces dermatitidis*.

Pathophysiology

Although skin lesions are the first evidence of blastomycosis, it is believed that the initial site of infection is in the lung. It is assumed that spores are inhaled and phagocytized in the alveoli as part of the primary infection. Thus the pathogenesis of blastomycosis is similar to that of tuberculosis, histoplasmosis, and coccidioidomycosis. The infection is spread by the lymphatics throughout the body. The skin lesions represent metastatic infection from the primary pulmonary disease.[104]

Acute pulmonary blastomycosis in the form of a self-limited pneumonia can occur. Otherwise, blastomycosis is a chronic progressive disease with a mortality of about 90% when untreated. For this reason it is recommended that every person in whom the diagnosis is established be treated.

Nursing Process
Assessment
Subjective data

1. Onset and duration of signs and symptoms. (See Table 24-16 for common signs and symptoms.)
2. History of exposure to soil contaminated with spores

Objective data

1. Palpation of chest to check for limited expansion
2. Percussion of chest to check for dull to flat sounds
3. Auscultation to check for type of breath sounds or adventitious sounds

Diagnostic tests for fungal infections

1. Direct demonstration of intracellular yeasts in smears of bone marrow and biopsy of lymph nodes, liver, and spleen; cultures of bone marrow, blood, or sputum.
2. Serologic tests. Agglutination, precipitation, and complement-fixation tests are used to help establish diagnosis of histoplasmosis and coccidioidomycosis. Serologic tests become positive about 1 month after the primary infection. Titers of serial tests are used to determine activity of the infection.
3. Skin testing. Skin test for histoplasmosis is only used for screening purposes. In endemic areas, between 90% and 95% of young adults have positive test results. The person should be tested with histoplasmin, tuberculin, blastomycin, and coccidioidin because of the likelihood of cross-reaction. The strongest reaction indicates the likely cause of the infection.
4. In histoplasmosis and coccidioidomycosis, chest x-ray films demonstrate a nodular infiltrate similar in appearance to tuberculosis. In blastomycosis, chest x-ray films may be nonspecific.
5. White blood cell count is usually normal but in acute causes may increase to 13,000/mm².
6. Leukopenia and anemia may be present in persons with disseminated disease.

Data analysis: nursing diagnoses

Nursing diagnoses are determined from analysis of patient data. Possible nursing diagnoses for the person with *severe* mycotic infection may include, but are not limited to, the following:

Diagnostic title	Possible etiologies
Airway clearance, ineffective	Tracheobronchial infection and increased tracheobronchial secretions
Breathing pattern, ineffective	Musculoskeletal impairment, fatigue
Pain	Rib or muscle trauma
Gas exchange, impaired	Ventilation and perfusion impairment
Knowledge deficit	Lack of exposure to information

Planning: expected patient outcomes

Expected patient outcomes for the person with *severe* mycotic infection may include, but are not limited to, the following:

1. Patient demonstrates cough with adequate sputum production.
2. Patient states that chest pain is reduced.
3. Patient demonstrates improved ventilation and oxygenation of tissues. Arterial blood gases are improved.
4. Temperature returns to normal.
5. Amphotericin insertion site is free of complications such as local phlebitis.
6. Patient knows source of infection and can teach others to avoid infected areas (Table 24-16).
7. Patient states plans for follow-up care.

Implementation
Assisting with achievement of therapeutic goals
Medications

1. Administer medications as prescribed and monitor patient for side effects.
   a. Amphotericin B (Fungizone Intravenous) is the standard therapy for mycotic infections. The dose and length of therapy are determined by the difficulty in eradicating the infection and the likelihood of relapse.[105] The therapy may last 2 to 3 weeks or 2 to 3 months.
   b. Amphotericin B must be given intravenously and has many toxic side effects, including local phlebitis at insertion site, systemic reactions, renal toxicity, hypokalemia, and anemia. In rare instances anaphylaxis, bone marrow suppression, and cardiovascular and hepatic toxicity develop.
   c. Systemic toxicity (chills, fever, aching, nausea, and vomiting) can be lessened by premedication with 600 mg of aspirin along with 25 to 50 mg of diphenhydramine (Benadryl) or promethazine (Phenergan) or 10 mg of prochlorperazine (Compazine) orally.[105] Heparin and hydrocortisone succinate (Solu-Cortef) are sometimes added to the infusion to minimize phlebitis.
   d. A reversible azotemia occurs regularly when amphotericin B is administered. The level of azotemia is monitored by biweekly BUN and serum creatinine determinations. A BUN of greater than 40 or a creatinine nearing 3 indicates a need to

Table 24-16   Signs and symptoms and medical therapy for fungal infections

Type of infections	Signs and symptoms	Medical therapy
Histoplasmosis	*Severe infections* Acute onset with fever, chest pain, dyspnea, prostration, weight loss, widespread pulmonary infiltrates, hepatomegaly, and splenomegaly. Some persons show no symptoms; others have benign acute pneumonitis	*Drug(s) of choice* Amphotericin B or Ketoconazole orally
Coccidioidomycosis (Valley fever, San Joaquin Valley fever)	Asymptomatic upper respiratory tract infection in about 60% of those who inhaled spores; 40% have symptoms ranging from flu-like illness to frank pneumonia	Amphotericin B IV severe cases Ketoconazole—less severe cases Therapy required for only 10% of those with symptoms, remainder have spontaneous remission
Blastomycosis	Skin lesions that appear as small papular or pustular lesions on exposed parts of the body such as hands and face Lesions develop peripherally, may become raised and do *not* itch	Amphotericin B IV

temporarily reduce or stop the drug. Therapy is not continued until the azotemia is improved.[105] Serum potassium levels are checked biweekly, and hypokalemia is treated with oral potassium. Anemia is common, and the hematocrit level usually stabilizes at 25% to 35%.[105]

   e. Ketoconazole (Nizoral) is a newer drug, administered orally, and is effective in the treatment of systemic mycotic infections. It is given daily for a minimum of 6 months. Toxicity appears to be minimal; pruritus, minor gastrointestinal intolerance, and liver function abnormalities have been reported. It is not known whether late relapses of histoplasmosis will occur in persons treated with ketoconazole because the drug has been in use for only a short time.

   f. Resectional pulmonary surgery is seldom required, and it is reserved for patients with adequate pulmonary reserve and residual cavities who are not able to tolerate amphotericin B.

2. Effectiveness of drug therapy should improve breathing pattern and gas exchange.

Interventions to achieve patient outcomes
Assisting with comfort and ADL

1. Place patient in position to facilitate breathing
2. Take measures to reduce fever (if present) by cool sponge baths, and so on.
3. Maintain room temperature desired by patient.

Facilitating learning

1. Review precautions for preventing reinfection (avoid infected areas).
2. Assist patient with plans for recuperation after leaving hospital.

Evaluation

Evaluation is based on patient outcomes. Questions to consider may include the following:

1. Is the patient raising adequate sputum?
2. Is the patient's breathing pattern effective?
3. Is the patient comfortable?
4. Have the patient's arterial blood gas findings improved?
5. Is the patient's temperature normal?
6. Is the amphotericin insertion site free of complications?
7. Can the patient identify the source of his or her infection and teach others to avoid infected areas?
8. Can the patient state plans for follow-up care?

OCCUPATIONAL LUNG DISEASES

Etiology/Epidemiology

Many pulmonary diseases are believed to be caused by substances inhaled in the work place. They are more common (1) in blue-collar workers than in white-collar workers, (2) in industrialized areas than in rural areas, and (3) in small and medium-sized businesses than in larger industrial plants.

In some instances it is debatable whether a person's lung disease is clearly occupation specific. This is especially so in cases of bronchitis, asthma, emphysema, or cancer because all of these conditions can be caused or aggravated by several factors found in many different occupations and by nonoccupational factors such as smoking and pollution of the atmosphere.[109]

Millions of Americans are believed to be suffering from job-related diseases. Because these diseases are not reportable, exact statistics do not exist. The Department of Health and Human Services has estimated that 400,000 persons develop job-related diseases each year. They also estimate that there are 100,000 deaths each year from occupational diseases. The National Heart, Lung, and Blood Institute report that lung diseases cause more than half of these deaths.[109] Several billion dollars a year are paid out in workers' compensation for job-related illnesses and injuries.

Table 24-17   Major occupation-related lung disease

Type	Etiologic and epidemiologic factors	Pathophysiologic conditions	Signs and symptoms
Pneumoconioses*	1 million people in United States run risk of developing silicosis		
Chronic silicosis	Inhaled silica dust; commonest form seen in miners, foundry workers, and others who inhaled relatively low concentrations of dust for 10-20 yr	Dust accumulated in tissue → tissue reaction with whorl-shaped nodules throughout lungs	Breathlessness with exercise
Coal worker's pneumoconiosis (CWP; black lung disease)	150,000 coal miners in the United States at risk; amount, size, and nature of dust in air vary according to type of coal, machinery, and technique used, efficiency of ventilation, and other dust control measures; 10%-30% of all coal miners develop simple form of the disease; more prevalent in miners of anthracite, or hard coal; other minerals found in miner's lung (silica, kaolin, mica, beryllium, copper, cobalt, and others); unknown whether these minerals contribute to development or progression of CWP	Simple CWP: dust accumulation in lungs visible on x-ray film; over years piles up and respiratory bronchioles are dilated (called *focal emphysema*)	Simple CWP: no symptoms, no respiratory difficulty
Complicated CWP or progressive massive fibrosis (PMF)	3% of persons with simple CWP develop complicated form; more often occurs in miners with heavy deposits of coal dust in lungs; may appear suddenly years after miner has left the mines; can stop suddenly for no discernible reason; smoking seems to have no affect on development of CWP, but smoking has adverse effect on miners' health; miners who smoke have 5-6 times more lung obstruction than nonsmoking miners; cigarette smoking causes chronic bronchitis and emphysema as in nonminers	Fibrosis develops in some dust-laden areas; fibrosis spreads and fibrotic areas coalesce, eventually most of lung is stiffened and useless; silica plays some role in fibrosis but despite international research, role of silica in CWP is not understood	PMF shortens life span; may die from respiratory failure, cor pulmonale, or superimposed infection Prevention: dust control; reduced levels of coal dust can lower simple CWP and reduce number of miners who develop complicated CWP

From American Lung Association: *Occupational lung diseases: an introduction,* New York, 1979, The Association.
*Also known as "dust in the lungs."

Table 24-17   Major occupation-related lung diseases—cont'd

Type	Etiologic and epidemiologic factors	Pathophysiologic conditions	Signs and symptoms
Asbestos-related lung disease†	Asbestos is one of the most dangerous occupational hazards; can cause both fibrosis and cancer in asbestos workers; also a general environmental hazard because of its extensive use before health hazards were recognized; most dangerous to those who mine the ores and process the crude material into pure form; no asbestos mines in United States, but it is processed and used in United States; federal agencies and state governments moving to tighten controls on use of asbestos; lung cancer associated with all types of asbestos; 20%-25% of deaths of workers with heavy exposure are from lung cancer; cancer is related to degree of asbestosis and to cigarette smoking, which enhances carcinogenic properties of asbestos; asbestos worker who smokes is 90 times as likely to get lung cancer as smoker who never worked with asbestos	Asbestos occurs in several different forms or ores; commercially important ores are chrysolite, crocidolite, and amosite; most hazardous medically are crocidolite and amosite; fibrosis caused by asbestos is called *asbestosis*; asbestos fibers accumulate around terminal bronchioles; body surrounds fibers with iron-rich tissue = asbestos body with characteristic picture on x-ray film; more asbestos bodies as more fibers are inhaled; after 20-30 yr of exposure, fibrosis begins in lungs; if heavy exposure, fibrosis appears in 4-5 yr	After fibrosis begins, cough, sputum, weight loss, increasing breathlessness; most die within 15 yr of first symptoms
	Mesothelioma (cancer of the pleura) accounts for 7%-10% of deaths of asbestos workers; inoperable and always fatal; can occur after very little exposure to crocidolite; has been reported in wives of asbestos workers and in persons living near asbestos plants; cigarette smoking not a contributing factor; only a few fine, straight crocidolite fibers are necessary; asbestos workers have a higher incidence of other cancers (esophagus, stomach, and intestines); swallowing of asbestos-contaminated sputum responsible for these cancers	Occurs in persons exposed to crocidolite fibers of a certain size; a few cases involve amosite fibers; needlelike shape of crocidolite fibers enables them to pass through lung tissue to pleura	Prevention: number of asbestos-related diseases has been increasing despite recognition of hazards and dust-control measures; much tighter controls are needed; some countries have taken such steps; there is need for massive efforts to educate general public of danger of asbestos

†Asbestos is a fire-proofing and insulating agent.

Continued.

Table 24-17   Major occupation-related lung diseases—cont'd

Type	Etiologic and epidemiologic factors	Pathophysiologic conditions	Signs and symptoms
Hypersensitivity diseases	Hypersensitivity diseases fall into occupational category when antigen is found primarily in work place; lung hypersensitivity can occur in bronchi; bronchioles, or alveoli; coarse dust causes bronchial reactions; fine dust provokes small airway and alveolar reactions		
Occupation-related asthma	More common in the 10% of the population who are atopic (genetic tendency to develop an allergy); nonatopic persons can also become sensitized; substances with antigenic properties include detergent enzymes, platinum salts, cereals and grains, certain wood dusts, isocyanate chemicals used in polyurethane paints and other products, and agents used in printing and some pesticides	Hypersensitivity reaction mediated by histamine → bronchoconstriction and ↑ mucus production; repeated attacks if cause unrecognized and asthma is untreated may lead to permanent obstructive lung disease; asthmatic response that is well established can be provoked by other factors (house dust, cigarette smoke) and by fatigue, breathing cold air, and coughing	Wheezing is major symptom Prevention: total elimination of antigen, desensitization not successful
Allergic alveolitis (farmer's lung)	Hypersensitivity disease caused by fine organic dust inhaled into smallest airways: cause of farmer's lung is moldy hay; other dusts can cause allergic alveolitis: these include moldy sugar cane and barley, maple bark, cork, animal hair, bird feathers and droppings, mushroom compost, coffee beans, and paprika; often disease is named for cause (mushroom worker's lung, etc.); fungus spores growing in the apparent antigen are thought in many cases to be real cause of the disease	Alveoli are inflamed, inundated by WBCs, sometimes filled with fluid; if exposure is infrequent or level of dust low, symptoms are mild; if treatment not sought, chronic form develops over time; eventually, fibrosis occurs, and fibrosis may be so well established that it cannot be arrested	Symptoms begin some hours after exposure to offending dust and include fatigue, shortness of breath, dry cough, fever, and chills; symptoms may be severe enough to require emergency treatment and hospitalization; acute attacks treated with steroids; recovery may take 6 wk and patient may suffer residual lung damage; real cure is permanent separation of patient and antigen Prevention: properly dried and stored farm products (hay, straw, sugar cane) do not cause allergic alveolitis; presumably fungi only grow in moist conditions
Byssinosis (brown lung)	Occupation-related disease occurring in textile workers; mainly in cotton workers but also afflicts workers in flax and hemp industries; cause is found in bales of raw cotton that contain not only cotton fibers but fragments of cotton plant; something in plant matter, rather than pure cotton, is cause	Chronic bronchitis and emphysema develop in time; constriction of bronchioles in response to something in crude cotton; symptoms of asthma and allergy persist as long as there is exposure to cotton antigen	Tightness in chest on returning to work after a weekend away (Monday fever); strong relationship between amount of dust inhaled and symptoms; persistent productive tight chest with chronic bronchitis and emphysema; person leaves industry as respiratory cripple Prevention: dust control measures; pretreating bales of cotton by washing with steam and other agents may inactivate causative agent; try to detect persons who are likely to become sensitized to cotton dust and keep them out of high-risk areas

Prevention

Occupational lung diseases are preventable. However, there must be a concerted effort by the public, governmental agencies, and industry if these diseases are to be prevented.

Governmental action has been slow and has only occurred, in some instances, in response to environmental and health agencies, such as the American Lung Association, that have lobbied for stricter regulation of harmful substances. But countervailing political pressures have sometimes prevented laws from being passed, have resulted in less strict laws because of the costs involved in meeting the strict standards required to control certain hazards, or have resulted in less strict enforcement of existing laws.

The year 2000 national health goal for occupational lung diseases is to establish in the 50 states exposure standards to prevent the major occupational lung diseases to which their worker populations are exposed (byssinosis, asbestosis, coal workers' pneumoconiosis, and silicosis). Because these diseases are not reportable, no baseline data were available. The reader is urged to contact his or her state's Department of Health to see what progress has been made in establishing exposure standards for these diseases.

The American Lung Association believes that several things need to be done to reduce the incidence of occupation-related diseases: (1) education of the public about the relationship between polluted air in the work place and lung diseases; (2) general commitment to reducing, eliminating, or avoiding air pollution of the work place; and (3) elimination of the most prevalent and notorious lung hazard, cigarette smoke. (The reader is referred to reference 109 for more information.)

Education of the public includes not only employers and employees but also engineers and planners who design operations; buyers and purchasers who select ingredients, cleaning agents, and equipment; and physicians who see persons with occupation-related diseases. Many times, workers who are instructed about the hazards involved in certain occupations and work places are helpful in deciding what preventive measures need to be taken to combat or minimize the effects of hazards. The commitment to reduce, eliminate, or avoid pollution of work place air requires full consideration of possible health effects whenever operations are planned, and improvement of conditions whenever possible.

It is well documented that smokers get occupation related lung diseases more often than nonsmokers and that smokers' lungs are more vulnerable to the effects of these diseases than are nonsmokers' lungs. The combined effects of cigarette smoke and industrial pollutants are very great. *The risk of developing chronic bronchitis, emphysema, lung cancer, and heart disease is much increased when a worker smokes.*[109] Some of these risks, such as lung cancer in asbestos workers who also smoke, are becoming more commonly known.

Occupation-related lung diseases can be divided into several categories. The major ones are (1) *the pneumoconioses, including silicosis and coal miner's pneumoconiosis (black lung disease)*; (2) *asbestos-related lung disease*; and (3) *hypersensitivity diseases, including occupation-related asthma, allergic alveolitis (farmer's lung), and byssinosis (brown lung disease)*. The etiology, pathophysiologic conditions, signs and symptoms, and prevention of these diseases are listed in Table 24-17.

The medical therapy and nursing care of these patients is dependent on the patient's signs and symptoms and complications. The reader is referred to other sections of this chapter for discussion of these topics.

The major role of nurses is to be knowledgeable about the cause and prevention of these diseases so that appropriate information and teaching can be presented to the public.

ADULT RESPIRATORY DISTRESS SYNDROME

Etiology/Epidemiology

Adult respiratory distress syndrome (ARDS) is the name given to a syndrome of acute hypoxemic respiratory failure without hypercapnia. The syndrome was first described by T.J. Petty in 1967. ARDS is often fatal and is characterized by severe dyspnea, hypoxemia, and diffuse bilateral pulmonary infiltrations after lung injury in previously healthy persons. Recently, the term *hyperpermeability pulmonary edema* (HPPE) has been used to describe the condition that affects between 150,000 and 200,000 critical care patients yearly.[85] Causes of ARDS are presented Box 24-17.

24-17

Clinical conditions associated with ARDS/HPPE

Shock
  Septic
  Hemorrhagic
  Cardiogenic
  Anaphylactic
Trauma
  Pulmonary contusion
  Nonpulmonary, multisystem
Infection
  Pneumonia
    Viral
    Bacterial (staphylococcal or streptococcal)
    Legionellosis
  Miliary tuberculosis
Disseminated intravascular coagulation (DIC)
Fat emboli
Near-drowning
Aspiration: highly acid gastric contents (pH <2.5)
Inhaled toxic agents
  Smoke
  Phosgene
  Oxides of nitrogen
Pancreatitis
Oxygen toxicity
Narcotic drug abuse
  Heroin
  Methadone
  Propoxyphene (Darvon)
Radiation pneumonitis
Drugs
  Ethchlorvynol
  Salicylates

Adapted from Petty TL: *Adult respiratory distress syndrome.* In Kryger M: *Pathophysiology of respiration,* New York, 1981, John Wiley.

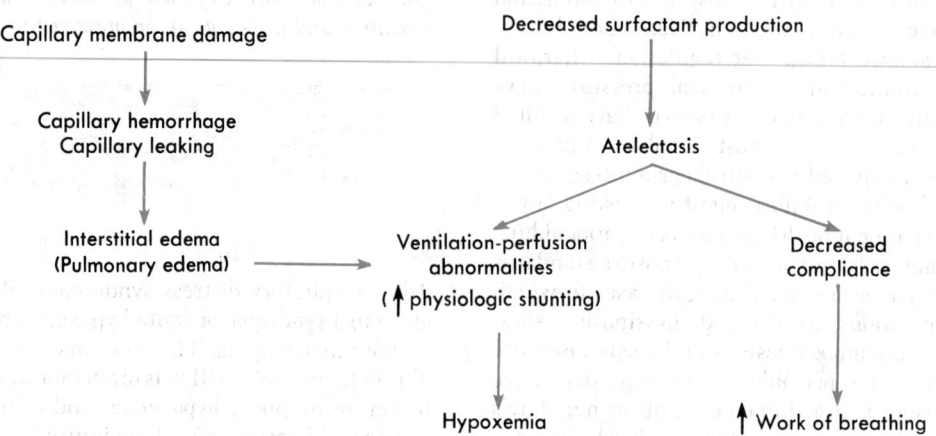

Fig. 24-21 Pathophysiologic events in adult respiratory distress syndrome.

Prevention

Prompt treatment of the underlying cause of ARDS is the major focus of preventive care. Additionally, judicious use of the mechanical ventilator and oxygen therapy is required to avoid inducing ARDS as an untoward complication of these treatments.

Pathophysiology

The pathophysiologic alterations that result in ARDS are typically initiated by a major trauma to the body, often a physical insult to a body system other than the pulmonary system (see Fig. 24-21). The following physiologic alterations result in the clinical syndrome identified as ARDS:

1. As a consequence of the precipitating insult, the complement cascade is activated, which in turn increases capillary wall permeability.
2. Fluid, granular leukocytes, red blood cells, macrophages, cell debris, and protein leak into the interstitial spaces between the capillaries and alveoli, and ultimately into the alveolar spaces.
3. Because of the fluid and debris in the interstitium and alveoli, the surface area for oxygen and carbon dioxide exchange is decreased, resulting in low ventilation/perfusion ratios and hypoxemia.
4. Compensatory hyperventilation of functional alveoli occurs, resulting in hypocapnia and respiratory alkalosis.
5. Cells that normally line the alveoli are destroyed and replaced by cells that do not produce surfactant, thus increasing alveolar surface tension and resulting in atelectasis and increased alveolar opening pressures.

The normal function, pathophysiology, and clinical picture of a person with ARDS/HPPE is presented in Table 24-18.

Clinical Manifestations

ARDS usually occurs in a person who has had a recent physical trauma, although it can appear in persons who appeared to be healthy immediately before onset (for example, someone with sudden onset of an acute infection). There is usually a latent period of 18 to 24 hours from the time of lung injury to the development of symptoms. The syndrome runs a variable course from a few days to several weeks' duration. Patients who appear to be recovering from ARDS may suddenly relapse into acute pulmonary disease from a secondary insult such as pneumothorax or an overwhelming infection. Signs and symptoms of ARDS include the following:

1. Acute respiratory distress: tachypnea, dyspnea, accessory muscle breathing, and central cyanosis
2. Dry cough and fever that develop over a few hours or days
3. Fine crackles throughout both lung fields
4. Altered sensorium ranging from confusion and agitation to coma

Radiologic and laboratory findings include the following:

1. Chest x-rays—diffuse, bilateral, and usually symmetric interstitial and alveolar infiltrations
2. Arterial blood gases
   Hypoxemia PO_2 less than 50 mm Hg
   Hypocapnia
   Respiratory alkalosis
3. End-stage: hypercapnia and respiratory acidosis

Table 24-18   Normal function, pathophysiology, and clinical picture of a person with ARDS/HPPE

Normal function	Pathophysiology	Clinical picture
Alveolar capillary membrane Oxygen and carbon dioxide exchange between alveolar air and pulmonary capillaries	Increased capillary wall permeability blood plasma contents infiltrate interstitial and alveolar spaces, resulting in hypoxemia, alveolar hyperventilation, and respiratory acidosis	PaO_2 ↓ $PaCO_2$ ↓ pH ↑ Fine crackles auscultated throughout lungs
Lung parenchyma Lung tissue that makes up the alveoli	Destruction of normal lung tissue, in particular, alveolar septal walls, normal cells replaced by nonsurfactant producing cells, and presence of edema and debris result in decreased lung compliance (stiff lung). Fibrosis may also develop.	Functional residual capacity, need to use high pressures to ventilate patient Dyspnea at rest

Medical Management

Patients with ARDS are critically ill and are best managed in an intensive care unit. Medical management focuses on the following aspects of care:

1. Oxygenation
   a. Initially may need to administer highest concentration of oxygen available (100%—using nonrebreathing face mask). However, oxygen delivered at levels greater than 50% are associated with oxygen toxicity that worsens already existing ARDS pathology. Oxygen concentrations can usually be lowered below 50%, by using positive-end expiratory pressure (PEEP) to open closed alveoli for increased ventilation.
   b. Goal is PaO_2 = 50 to 60 mm Hg.
   c. Gradually reduce FiO_2 while maintaining adequate arterial oxygen levels.
2. Ventilatory support
   a. If oxygen therapy alone is unsuccessful in providing adequate arterial oxygenation, the patient is intubated and placed on a mechanical ventilator.
      (1) A volume-limited ventilator is preferred.
      (2) Ventilator is set to provide tidal volume equal to 10 to 12 ml/kg body weight, respiratory rate equal to 10 to 14/min FiO_2 = 50%, PEEP used.
      (3) If individual's spontaneous respiration is adequate, intermittent mandatory ventilation (IMV) mode or continuous positive-airway pressure (CPAP) is used. When spontaneous ventilatory patern interferes with providing adequate ventilation, the patient is sedated or paralyzed with Pavulon. The control mode is then used. See p. 623 for more information on care of the patient on a ventilator.
3. Fluid volume
   a. Insert balloon-tipped pulmonary artery catheter to measure pulmonary capillary pressure.
   b. Diuretics, fluid volume expanders, and hypotensive medications are administered as indicated to maintain optimal fluid volume.
4. Treat underlying cause of ARDS.

Nursing Process
Assessment

Nursing assessment of the patient with ARDS must be tailored to maximize information obtained without increasing respiratory distress.

Subjective data

Background information and history of present illness can be obtained from family members because the patient is usually too ill to give details.

Objective data

The process of gathering objective data is the same as that described for respiratory failure (see p. 615).

Data analysis: nursing diagnoses

Nursing diagnoses are determined from analysis of patient data. Possible nursing diagnoses for the person with ARDS may include, but are not limited to, the following:

Diagnostic title	Possible etiologies
Gas exchange, impaired	Ventilation/perfusion inequality
Tissue perfusion, altered (cardiopulmonary)	Fluid mobilization to (and from) third space (interstitium and alveolar space)
Nutrition, altered: less than body requirements	Unable to take in adequate nutrition to meet increased metabolic workload from increased work of breathing
Anxiety	Threat of death Physiologic factors (arterial blood gas derangements)

Planning: expected patient outcomes

Expected patient outcomes for the person with ARDS/HPPE may include, but are not limited to:

1. Improved ventilation and oxygenation
   a. PaO_2 is maintained at 50 to 60 mm Hg during acute phase of illness.
   b. Upon resolution of ARDS PaO_2, pH, and PCO_2 return to acceptable baseline limits.
   c. Sensorium returns to preillness level.

d. During acute phase of illness, patient is able to tolerate mechanical ventilatory assistance.
e. Inspiratory to expiratory ratio is 5:10 seconds.
f. Respiratory rate and tidal volume are within normal limits.
g. Patient does not complain of dyspnea.
2. Adequate tissue perfusion
   a. Pulmonary capillary wedge pressure (measure of pulmonary capillary pressure) below 18 mm Hg
   b. Urinary output of at least 30 ml/hr
   c. Peripheral pulses present and extremities warm to touch
3. Increased physiologic and psychologic comfort
   a. Tolerates ventilator and artificial airway
   b. Acknowledges and expresses fears
   c. Communicates personal needs effectively with staff and family
   d. Cooperates and assists with care
4. Stable body weight within 5 pounds of preillness weight
5. Patient and family anxiety is decreased

Implementation

Patients with ARDS are critically ill and are usually cared for in an intensive care unit. Caring for these patients focuses on the following measures.

Assisting with achievement of therapeutic goals
Maintaining adequate gas exchange

Oxygenation
1. Maintain oxygen therapy as ordered.
2. Monitor for signs of hypoxemia (p. 615).

Ventilatory support. Provide ventilatory support as follows:
1. Maintain a patent airway.
2. If artificial airway present (endotracheal tube or tracheostomy) provide necessary care.
   a. Secure tube to avoid movement either in or out of established position.
   b. Position patient for optimal oxygenation (see p. 540).
   c. Auscultate lungs hourly to assess placement of endotracheal tube (may slip into right mainstem bronchus).
3. Suction endotracheal tube as needed.
4. Administer bronchodilators as ordered.
5. Check ventilator settings frequently.

Interventions to achieve patient outcomes
Maintaining adequate tissue perfusion

The maintenance of adequate tissue perfusion is a nursing responsibility.
1. Monitor pulmonary capillary wedge pressure.
   a. Notify physician if pressure is above or below established range.
   b. If pressure is below established range, plasma volume expanders or hypotensive medications are given as ordered.
   c. If pressure is high, administer diuretics or vasodilators as ordered.

2. Assess urine output, vital signs, and pulses in extremities hourly.

Maintaining adequate nutrition

Nutritional interventions for patients are the same as those for the patient with COPD (see nursing care plan for person on mechanical ventilation with PEEP on p. 559).

Decreasing patient and family anxiety

1. Ensure proper ventilator function to deliver adequate tidal volume and oxygen concentration: If patient appears to be in respiratory distress although ventilator is functioning properly, assess arterial blood gas levels
2. Identify a way for patient to be able to communicate concerns and express feelings (if unable to verbalize because intubated, try alternative ways of communication)
3. Provide simple explanations about procedures to patient and family, orient patient to surroundings, and repeat explanations regularly.
4. Offer explanations of care routines and environment to family. Encourage family to approach, talk, and touch patient as they desire.

Evaluation

Evaluation is based on patients' outcomes. Questions to consider may include the following:
1. Is the patient able to maintain own airway so that ventilation/perfusion are equal?
2. Are the arterial blood gases within normal limits?
3. Is the patient's weight within 5 pounds of preillness weight?
4. Do the patient and family appear to be calm and free of anxiety?

CANCER OF THE LUNG

Etiology/Epidemiology

During the past 50 years there has been a startling increase in the incidence of cancer of the lung.

The ACS estimates 161,000 new cases in 1991 and 143,000 deaths. In 1986, cancer of the lung surpassed breast cancer to become the number one cancer killer of women. Thus lung cancer is now the leading cause of death from cancer in both men and women.

The increase in death rates for both men and women is directly related to cigarette smoking. A history of smoking, especially for 20 years or more, is considered to be a prime risk factor. Other risk factors include exposure to certain industrial substances such as asbestos particularly in those who smoke (p. 561).

It is estimated that asbestos workers who smoke have six to ten times more lung cancer than the general population at large. There also is some evidence of a genetic predispostion to lung cancer.[30]

In the United States the age-adjusted death rate from cancer has been steadily increasing. Most of the increase

DATA: Mr. R. is a 28-year-old married male admitted to the Surgical Intensive Care Unit after a motor vehicle accident. Injuries sustained include a ruptured spleen and liver laceration resulting in hypovolemic shock. Mr. R. was taken to the operating room where his injuries were repaired and blood losses replaced. His early postoperative course was unremarkable. On Mr. R.'s third postoperative day, he began to experience some respiratory difficulties with a deterioration in his arterial blood gases. Because of severe hypoxemia, Mr. R. was intubated. His chest x-ray revealed diffuse interstitial and alveolar infiltrates. He had developed ARDS and eventually required 16 cm H_2O of PEEP.

Mr. R.'s wife visited her husband daily and often attempted to communicate with him. She would reassure and calm him when he became anxious and resisted the ventilator. Mrs. R. would ask the nurse many questions about her husband's status.

The nursing history identified the following:
- Mr. and Mrs. R. have been married 5 years; they have no children.
- Mr. R. has full hospitalization and medical coverage through insurance at work.
- Mr. and Mrs. R. come from large families that appear supportive.
- Mr. R. is a nonsmoker.

Collaborative nursing actions include those to assist in improving oxygenation through evaluating FiO_2 and levels of PEEP as well as techniques used to wean AR from the ventilator.

Nursing actions include:
- Supporting oxygenation and ventilation to maintain PaO_2 over 60 mm Hg and to maximize functional residual capacity
- Weaning from FiO_2 and levels of PEEP gradually while monitoring arterial blood gases.
- Monitoring patient for signs of hypoxia.

Nursing diagnosis: Gas exchange, impaired, related to ARDS

Expected patient outcomes	Nursing intervention	Rationale
Mr. R. will remain adequately oxygenated as evidence by: 1. PaO_2 on arterial blood gas >75 mm Hg 2. Adequate color 3. Adequate peripheral circulation	Monitor arterial blood gases to determine PaO_2 Suction only when necessary to prevent loss of PEEP secondary to disconnection from ventilator Monitor required levels of PEEP and FiO_2 Assess peripheral circulation for pulses, color of extremities, and warmth Monitor mixed venous blood oxygen levels	ARDS is an acute lung injury that results in increased capillary permeability, which permits proteins and fluids to leak out into alveoli and interstitial spaces, thus preventing normal gas exchange to occur.

Nursing diagnosis: Cardiac output, decreased, related to decreased venous return

Expected patient outcomes	Nursing interventions	Rationale
Mr. R. will not experience hemodynamic compromise related to PEEP	Monitor vital signs every hour and as needed Monitor hemodynamic parameters for signs of decreased cardiac output, hypotension, elevated CVP, and oliguria Monitor intake and output Check peripheral circulation every 2 to 4 hr and PRN Elevate foot of bed 10 to 20 degrees to encourage venous return Perform passive range of motion exercises every 4 to 6 hr to encourage venous return Administer adrenergic agents as ordered to improve cardiac output Notify physician of hemodynamic complications	PEEP may cause decreased cardiac output by increasing intraalveolar pressures, thereby decreasing venous return to the heart

Continued.

Nursing Care Plan	Person on mechanical ventilation with PEEP—cont'd

Nursing diagnosis: Breathing pattern, ineffective, related to altered lung/thoracic pressure relationship

Expected patient outcomes	Nursing interventions	Rationale
Mr. R. will not experience pulmonary complications secondary to PEEP 1. Atelectasis 2. Pneumothorax 3. Pneumomediastinum 4. Subcutaneous emphysema	Monitor respirations every hour and as needed Assess breath sounds for adventitious findings Administer pulmonary toilet every 2 hr and as needed 1. Frequent turning 2. Chest physiotherapy Monitor for signs of pulmonary complications and respiratory distress 1. Asymmetric chest excursion 2. Sudden sharp pain 3. Cyanosis 4. Anxiety Assess for subcutaneous emphysema Keep chest tube set up at bedside Monitor arterial blood gases as needed Notify physician of respiratory complications	When walls of alveoli cannot withstand the positive pressure from PEEP, perforation may occur. As a result, air leaks into the pleural space, mediastinum and/or its subcutaneous space. The result is a pneumothorax, pneumomediastinum or subcutaneous emphysema, respectively

Nursing diagnosis: Nutrition, altered: less than body requirements, related to intubation

Expected patient outcomes	Nursing interventions	Rationale
Mr. R. will receive adequate nutritional intake while intubated	Administer hyperalimentation or arterial feedings as prescribed Intake and output Daily weights Administer albumin or volume expanders as prescribed Monitor serum albumin level	Nutritional status must be maintained to assist in weaning process; proteins and volume expanders will increase serum colloidal osmotic pressure, thus maintaining fluid in the intravascular compartment

Nursing diagnosis: Anxiety, related to ARDS, intubation, and discomfort from PEEP

Expected patient outcomes	Nursing interventions	Rationale
Mr. and Mrs. R. will exhibit behavioral signs of decreased stress and anxiety	Assess for signs of anxiety Explain ARDS to Mrs. R., including rationale for mechanical ventilation and PEEP Allow Mr. and Mrs. R. to express concerns and fears Explain procedures before performing them Provide comfort measures Provide for a means of communication between Mr. R. and his wife Attempt to anticipate their needs Administer light sedation/antianxiety medications if necessary, as ordered Attempt to calm and reassure Mr. R. if he begins to "buck" or resist the ventilator Provide Mr. R. and his wife distraction from the ICU environment • soft music, TV • breaks from the ICU for Mrs. R.	The intensive care unit, mechanical ventilation, the inability to communicate, and fear of the unknown all contribute to feelings of stress and anxiety for the patient in the ICU and his or her significant others Positive-pressure exhalation is often uncomfortable for the patient who may respond by resisting ventilator

is directly related to rise in lung cancer death rates. Age-adjusted rates for other cancer sites have been leveling off and, in some cases, declining. There has been a decline in cancer death rates for all age groups, sexes, and blacks and whites, except in people 55 years old and older, in whom the cancer death rate has been increasing.[30]

Because of the relationship between cigarette smoking and the incidence of lung cancer, emphasis is continuing to be placed on reducing smoking. The relationship between smoking and lung cancer is shown in Table 24-19.

The mortality of persons with lung cancer depends primarily on the specific type of cancer and the size of the tumor when detected. *Squamous cell carcinoma is the most common, followed by adenocarcinoma; undifferentiated small cell (oat cell) carcinoma is the least common.* Most people who develop the disease are over 50 years of age. Some of the factors believed to be involved in the increased incidence of cancer of the lung include an increase in smoking among women, more accurate diagnoses, and a tendency to name the lung as the primary site.

Only 13% of lung cancer patients live 5 years or more after diagnosis. The survival rate is 37% for cases detected in a localized stage; only 20% of lung cancers are discovered that early. Survival rates have improved only slightly over the past 10 years.[1]

Cancer of the lung may be either metastatic or primary. *Metastatic tumors may follow malignancy anywhere in the body. Metastasis from the colon and kidney is common.* Metastasis to the lung may be discovered before the primary lesion is known, and sometimes the location of the primary lesions is not determined during the person's life.

Prevention

The cause of cancer of the lung is closely related to cigarette smoking. Table 24-19 shows the extreme increase in mortality from lung cancer in those persons who smoke. Prevention is the best protection against cancer of the lung because early detection of the disease is difficult. The cancer death rates for male cigarette smokers is more than double that for nonsmokers, and the rate for female smokers is 67% higher than that for nonsmokers.[7]

Because there is no effective treatment for lung cancer, emphasis is placed on prevention. *Nearly 90% of persons with lung cancer die within 5 years of diagnosis.* This figure could be lowered with early diagnosis and treatment. Unfortunately, about one third of the cases of lung cancer are inoperable when first seen by a physician. Another one third are found to be inoperable when an exploratory thoracotomy is performed.

The goal set for year 2000 in *Healthy People 2000* is to *slow the rise* in lung cancer deaths to no more than 42 per 100,000 people as compared with an age-adjusted baseline of 37.9 per 100,000 in 1987. Thus the only hope is to slow the number of deaths because *decreasing* the number of deaths appears to be impossible at this time.[30]

From available research data it seems evident that curtailing smoking is a primary preventive measure. The nurse should be active in teaching the dangers of smoking and should set a positive health example in this regard. It is especially important that teenagers be given specific facts

Table 24-19   Deaths caused by lung cancer, according to smoking habits*

	Deaths per 100,000 population
Nonsmokers	3.4
10-20 cigarettes per day	54.3
20-40 (1-2 packs) per day	143.9
More than 40 (2 packs) per day	217.3

*From American Cancer Society: *Cancer facts and figures.* New York, 1976. The Society.

about the dangers of cigarette smoking because they are not likely to be habitual smokers at that age. *Recent studies indicate that the incidence of smoking among teenagers is increasing.* People who are already habitual smokers should also be urged to stop smoking, although it may be difficult for them to do so. Various types of programs are available to assist persons to stop smoking. Because air pollution affects the lungs and may predispose to the development of cancer, nurses should encourage and actively support community programs to decrease the amount of air pollution.

Pathophysiology and Clinical Manifestations

Because most new growths in the lungs arise from the bronchi, the term *bronchogenic carcinoma* is widely used. The signs and symptoms that a patient has depend on several factors including the location of the lesion.

Signs and symptoms of a *lesion in the bronchus* and lung include the following:

1. Ten percent of patients are asymptomatic and the disease is picked up on routine chest x-ray.
2. Seventy-five percent will have a cough.
3. Fifty percent will have hemoptysis.
4. Shortness of breath and a unilateral wheeze are common.

If peripheral pulmonary lesions perforate into the pleural space, there will be extrapulmonary intrathoracic signs and symptoms. These include:

1. Pain on inspiration
2. Friction rub
3. Pleural effusion
4. If the superior vena cava is involved, edema of face and neck
5. Fatigue
6. Clubbing of fingers (Fig. 24-38)

Diagnostic tests include:

1. Chest x-ray (p. 522)
2. Sputum cytology test (p. 524)
3. Fiberoptic brochoscopy (see p. 528) (sometimes biopsy taken)

In the later stage of the disease, *weight loss and debility usually indicate metastases, especially to the liver.* Cancer of the lung may metastasize to nearby structures such as the prescalene lymph nodes, the walls of the esophagus, and the pericardium of the heart, or distant areas such as the brain, liver, or skeleton.

24-19

Histologic subtypes of cancer of the lung and the therapy of each type

Type	Classification and percentage of cases	Therapy
Small cell carcinoma	Small cell lung cancer (SCLC); 25% of cases	Combination chemotherapy such as (1) cyclophosphamide, doxorubicin, and vincristine, or (2) cyclophosphamide, doxorubicin, and etoposide, or (3) cisplatin plus etoposide
Squamous cell carcinoma Adenocarcinoma Large cell carcinoma	All three classified as non-small cell lung cancer (NSCLC); 75% of cases	Pulmonary resection—only one third are operable; one third unoperable because of advanced lung cancer; one third unoperable because of distant metastases

24-20

International TNM staging for lung cancer*

Tumor size (T)

TX = Occult carcinoma (cytologically positive; bronchoscopically and radiographically nondetectable)

T1 = Tumor 3 cm or less surrounded by lung or visceral pleura

T2 = Tumor more than 3 cm

T3 = Tumor of any size with direct extension into chest wall, or with 2 cm of the carina, or associated with atelectasis or obstructive pneumonia of the enitre lung

T4 = Tumor of any size invading the mediastinal structures or vertebral body, or presence of malignant pleural effusion

Nodal status (N)

N0 = No hilar or mediastinal nodal involvement

N1 = Ipsilateral hilar nodal involvement

N2 = Ipsilateral mediastinal nodal or subcarinal nodal involvement

N3 = Contralateral hilar or mediastinal nodal involvement, supraclavicular nodal involvement (ipsilateral or contralateral)

Metastases (M)

M0 = No distant metastases

M1 = Distant visceral metastases present

Stage

Occult carcinoma	TX, N0, M0
Stage I	T1-2, N0, M0
Stage II	T1-2, N1, M0
Stage IIIA	T3, N0-1, M0
	T1-3, N2, M0
Stage IIIB	T-4, N1-3, M0
	T1-3, N3, M0
Stage IV	Any T, any N, M1

*Adapted from Mountain CF: A new international staging system for lung cancer, Chest 89(suppl):2255, 1986.

24-21

Five-year disease-free survival rates for surgical resection in patients with non-small cell lung cancer

Stage		5 yr Disease-free (%)
I	T1, N0, M0	70-85
	T2, N0, M0	55-65
II	T1, N1, M0	30-50
	T1, N2, M0	25-30
IIIA	T3, N0, M0	25-35
	T3, N1, M0	15-20
	T1-2N2, M0	9-24
	T3, N2	0-5

From Bonomi P: *Primary lung cancer.* In Rakel RE, editor: *Conn's current therapy,* 1990, Philadelphia, 1990, WB Saunders.

Medical Management

The treatment of lung cancer depends on the type and stage of the disease. *Histologically, lung cancer is divided into four major subgroups: small cell carcinoma, squamous cell carcinoma, adenocarcinoma,* and *large cell carcinoma.* Box 24-19 lists the types, percentage of cases in the subtypes, and recommended therapy. As with other types of cancer, lung cancer is staged (see Chapter 11 for more details about staging). The international Tumor, Node, Metastasis (TNM) Staging for Lung Cancer is presented in Box 24-20.

Because patients with early lung cancer have no symptoms, they are often inoperable by the time they are seen. Some patients with cancers of the lung are first diagnosed after chest x-ray as part of a routine physical examination. Other patients are not diagnosed until they seek medical treatment for symptoms related to metastases.

Survival rates of patients with non-small cell lung cancer (NSCLC) obviously depend on the size of the tumor, nodal status, and degree of metastases. Box 24-21 gives the 5-year survival rates for patients with non-small cell cancers.

Some patients who undergo surgical resection (pneumonectomy or lobectomy) may also receive radiation therapy or chemotherapy. These adjuvants are mainly used to treat metastases and to relieve some of the patient's symptoms. Both of these therapies are discussed in detail in Chapter 11. Because surgery is the treatment of choice, it is discussed next.

Thoracic Surgery

Intelligent nursing care of patients undergoing thoracic surgery depends on knowledge of the anatomy and physiology of the chest, of the surgery performed, and of procedures and practices that assist the patient to recover from the operation. When endotracheal anesthesia became possible, surgery of the chest was given a great impetus.

Principles of resectional surgery. Principles of resectional surgery are as follows:
1. Endotracheal anesthesia is used for surgery involving the lung in which the pleural space is entered.
2. With endotracheal anesthesia it is possible to keep the uninvolved ("good") lung expanded and functioning when the chest is opened and atmospheric pressure enters the pleural space.
3. To understand resectional surgery and the purpose of chest tubes and water-seal drainage, an understanding of the following is necessary.
   a. *Physiology of breathing*
      (1) The pressure in the pleural space (the space between the visceral and parietal pleura) is subatmospheric (less than 760 mm Hg) and is referred to as *negative*.
      (2) The pressure in the pleural space is usually 756 mm Hg and goes down to 751 mm Hg before inspiration. This change in pressure allows air (atmospheric pressure) to enter the lungs.
      (3) When the pleura is entered surgically, atmospheric pressure enters the pleural space, and the lung collapses.
   b. *Purpose of chest tubes and water-seal drainage*
      (1) After resectional surgery of the lung (except pneumonectomy), one or two drainage tubes are inserted into the pleural space. Each tube is connected to a water-seal drainage bottle containing 1 to 2 cm of sterile water (see Fig. 24-23) or to another negative pressure suction system (Fig. 24-22).
      (2) The glass rod connected to the chest tube is under water. This "seals" the chest tube, allowing air and fluid to drain from the pleural space into the water-seal bottle, and preventing air or fluid from entering the pleural space.
      (3) In all resectional surgery (except pneumonectomy), the remaining portions of the lung must overexpand and fill the space left by the resected portion.
      (4) The removal of air and fluid from the pleural space accomplishes two basic purposes. These are to (1) *aid in the expansion of the remaining portion of the lung as air (positive pressure) and fluid escapes through the drainage tubes*, and (2) *to reestablish negative pressure in the pleural space*.

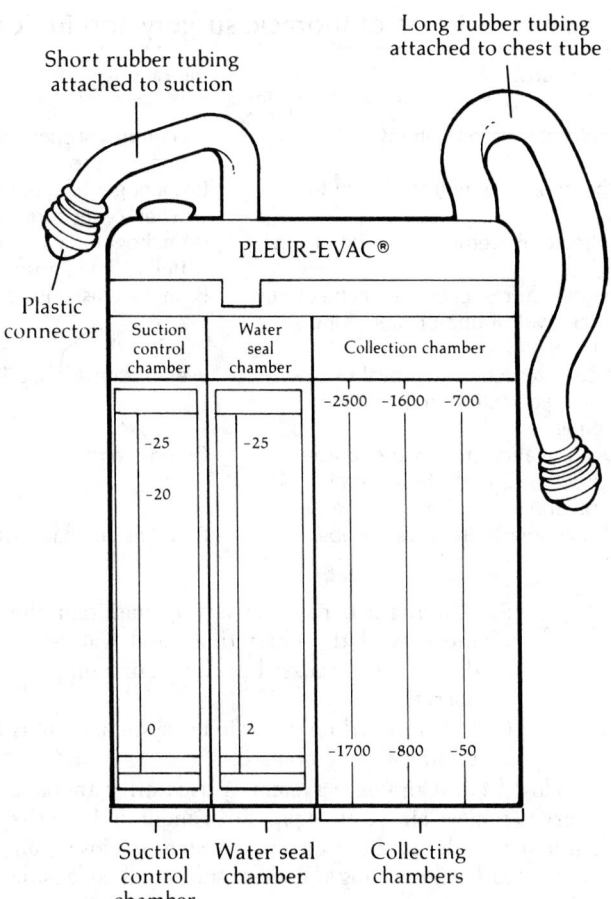

Fig. 24-22 Pleurevac—one of several available brands of chest drainage systems. The system functions like a three-bottle system in that the unit collects drainage, maintains a seal to prevent air from entering pleural cavity, and prevents excessive build-up of negative pressure. (From Thompson JM, et al: *Mosby's manual of clinical nursing*, ed 2, St Louis, 1989, Mosby–Year Book.)

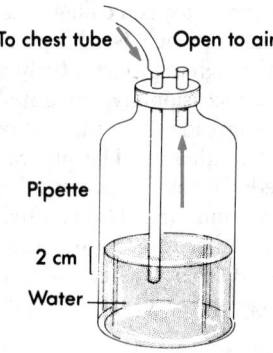

Fig. 24-23 Water-sealed closed chest drainage showing type of tube under water. (From Abels LF: *Mosby's manual of critical care*, St Louis, 1979, Mosby–Year Book.)

Table 24-20   Types of thoracic surgery and indications for their use

Procedure	Indications
Exploratory thoracotomy	To confirm suspected diagnosis of lung or chest disease, especially carcinoma; to obtain a biopsy
Pneumonectomy (removal of lung)	Bronchogenic carcinoma when lobectomy will not remove all of lesion; tuberculosis when other surgery will not remove all of diseased lung
Lobectomy (removal of lobe of lung)	Bronchogenic carcinoma confined to a lobe, bronchiectasis, emphysematous blebs or bullae; lung abscess, fungal infections, benign tumors; tuberculosis
Segmental resection (segmentectomy removal of one or more lung segments)	Bronchiectasis; lung abscess or cyst; metastatic carcinoma
Wedge resection (removal of pie-shaped section from surface of lung)	Well-circumscribed benign tumors, metastic tumors, or localized inflammatory disease
Decortication (removal of a fibrinous peel from the visceral pleura)	Chronic empyema
Thoracoplasty (removal of ribs)	Residual air space after surgery; chronic empyema space

(5) Nursing actions necessary to maintain the integrity of the chest tubes and water-seal drainage is discussed in the section on postoperative care.

(6) Other closed chest drainage system such as Pleurevac may be used.

A closed chest drainage system is used after thoracic surgery to remove air (positive pressure) and fluid from the pleural space. Because the drainage system is closed, air is prevented from entering the chest tubes and collapsing the lung.

Today closed chest drainage system such as the Pleurevac (Fig. 24-22) are commonly used. However, the general principles underlying this type of drainage are best understood if an older (but still used) system of water-sealed drainage bottles is explained first. Once the principles of water-sealed drainage are understood, this knowledge can be used to understand other types of closed drainage systems.

Type of resectional surgery. Table 24-20 presents the types of resectional surgery and the indications for the use of each type. A brief discussion of each type of resectional surgery follows.

Exploratory thoracotomy. An exploratory thoracotomy is performed to confirm a suspected diagnosis of lung or chest disease. The usual approach is by a posterolateral parascapular incision through the fourth, fifth, sixth, or seventh intercostal space. Occasionally, an anterior approach is used. The ribs are spread to give the best possible exposure of the lung and hemithorax. The pleura is entered, and the lung examined; a biopsy usually is taken; and the chest is closed. This procedure may also be used to detect bleeding in the chest or other injury after trauma to the chest. Because the pleural space was entered, a chest tube and water-seal drainage are necessary (Fig. 24-23).

Pneumonectomy. A pneumonectomy, the removal of an entire lung, is most commonly performed to treat bronchogenic carcinoma (Fig. 24-24, *B*). It may also be used

to treat tuberculosis. However, a pneumonectomy is only performed in those instances when a lobectomy or segmental resection will not remove all the diseased tissue. A thoracotomy is made in either the posterior or anterior chest using the method described under exploratory thoracotomy. Before the lung can be removed, the pulmonary artery and vein are ligated and then cut. The main-stem bronchus leading to the lung is clamped, divided, and sutured, usually with black silk. To ensure an airtight closure of the bronchus, a pleural flap is placed over it and sutured into place. The phrenic nerve on the operative side is crushed, causing the diaphragm on that side to rise and reduce the size of the remaining space. Because there is no lung left to reexpand, drainage tubes are not used. Ideally, the pressure in the closed chest is slightly negative. The fluid left in the space will consolidate in time, preventing the remaining lung and heart from shifting toward the operative side (mediastinal shift).

Lobectomy. In a lobectomy one lobe of the lung is removed (Fig. 24-24, *C*). It is used to treat bronchiectasis, bronchogenic carcinoma, emphysematous blebs or bullae, lung abscess, benign tumors, fungal infections, and tuberculosis. For a lobectomy to be successful, the disease must be confined to one lobe, and the remaining lung tissue must be capable of overexpanding to fill the space of the resected lobe. One or two chest tubes are connected to water-seal bottles for postoperative drainage.

Segmental resection (segmentectomy). In a segmental resection, one or more segments of the lung are removed. This operation is used in an attempt to preserve as much functioning lung tissue as possible. It is a very taxing operation for the surgeon because the dissection between segments must be performed very carefully and slowly, and the identification of the segmental pulmonary artery and vein and bronchus is more difficult than when a lobe is involved. Because there are ten segments in the right lung and eight in the left lung, only a portion of a lobe or lobes may need to be removed. The most common indication for segmentectomy is bronchiectasis. It is also used to treat the other conditions listed in Table 24-20. Chest tube(s)

Table 24-21   **Long-term complications of resectional surgery**

Complications	Signs and symptoms	Treatment
Empyema Pus in the pleural space is a dreaded complication of thoracic surgery. Pus may drain from chest tube(s) or if chest tubes are already removed can be obtained on thoracentesis (insertion of a needle attached to a syringe with a threeway stopcock used to remove fluid, blood, or pus from pleural space).	Unexplained elevation in temperature Evidence of pleural exudate on x-ray film	*Dependent drainage* by thoracentesis, intercostal chest tube, or open drainage with rib resection. Chest tube may be connected to water-seal bottle or cut off and allowed to drain into chest dressings. Water-seal no longer necessary if empyema space has a thick wall and there is no danger of lung collapse. Over time as empyema drains out of tube, the space becomes smaller and fills in with granulation tissue. If space persists, a *thoracoplasty* will be necessary. (p. 567).
Bronchopleural fistula Opening in the sutured bronchus that permits communication between bronchus and pleural space. Space usually becomes infected and empyema develops.	Persistent cough (usually nonproductive), fever, leukocytosis, anorexia, expectoration of purulent sputum, and evidence of pleural exudate on x-ray film	Chest tube connected to water-seal, as there is a direct communication between bronchus (positive pressure being inspired) and the pleural space. A persistent bronchopleural fistula is treated by thoracoplasty and a muscle implant to seal off the bronchus.

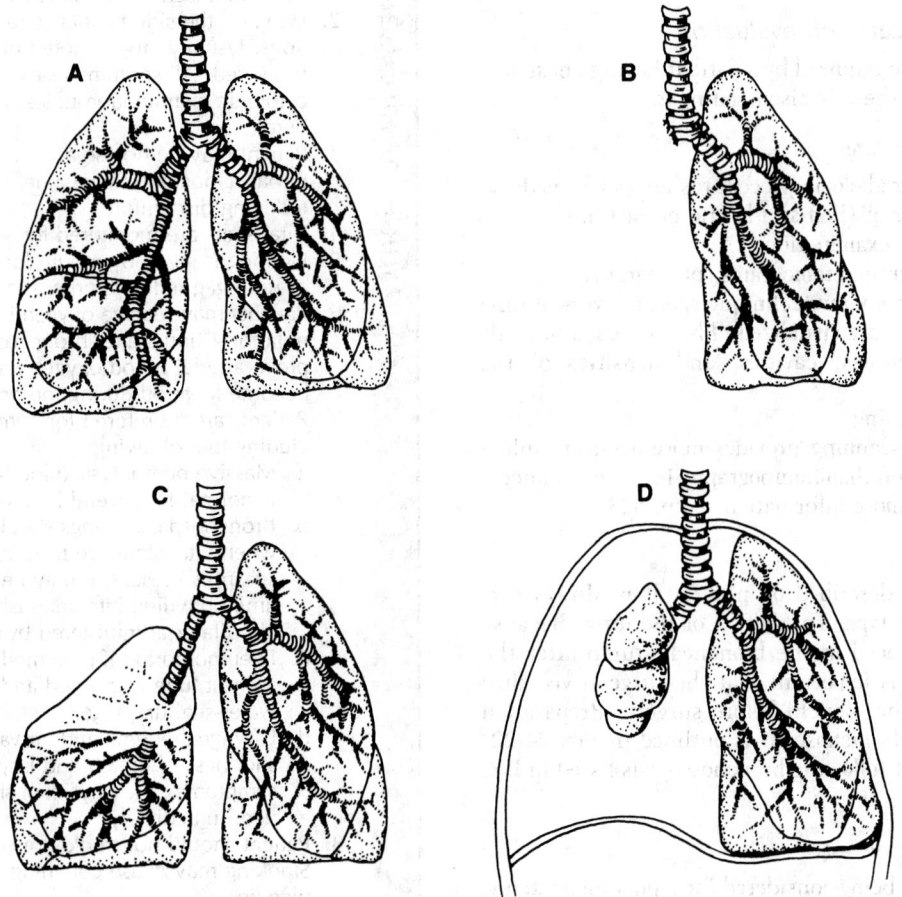

Fig. 24-24   A, Normal lungs. **B,** Surgical absence of right lung after a pneumonectomy. **C,** Surgical absence of the right upper lobe after a lobectomy. **D,** Complete collapse of right lung as a result of air in the pleural cavity (pneumothorax).

and water-seal drainage are necessary postoperatively. Because of air leaks from the segmental surface, the remaining lung tissue may take longer to reexpand.

Wedge resection. In a wedge resection, a well-circumscribed diseased portion is removed without regard to the segmental planes. The area to be removed is clamped, dissected, and sutured. Chest tube(s) and water-sealed drainage are used postoperatively.

Decortication. In a decortication a fibrinous peel is removed from the visceral pleura, allowing the encased lung to reexpand and obliterate the pleural space. This procedure is discussed further under the treatment of empyema (Table 24-21). Chest tube(s) and chest suction are used to facilitate the reexpansion of the lung. If the lung has been encased for a long time, it may be incapable of reexpanding after decortication. In this situation thoracoplasty may be necessary.

A newer procedure that makes it possible to preserve more lung tissue is a *bronchoplastic* or *sleeve resection.* In this procedure one lobar bronchus and part of the right or left bronchus are excised. The distal bronchus is anastomosed to the proximal bronchus or the trachea. This procedure is used to treat bronchogenic carcinoma.

Preoperative care and evaluation

Special tests are required by a patient having chest surgery, and each of these is discussed next.

Radiologic procedures

The following radiologic procedures are performed:
1. Posteroanterior (PA) and lateral chest films
2. Other x-ray examinations
   a. Laminograms (tomograms, planograms)
      (1) In this x-ray technique special layers of lung tissue are visualized. They are used to study neoplasms, cavities, and densities of the lung.
   b. CT scanning
      (1) CT scanning provides more accurate information than laminography in some instances. For more information see p. 523.

Bronchoscopy

Brochoscopy is described on p. 528. It is always performed before any type of resection of the lung. Because sutures will be placed in the broncheal stump after the lung resection, it is important that the surgeon visualize the condition of the bronchi before surgery. Preparation of the patient for bronchoscopy is outlined in Box 24-22. Care of the patient following bronchoscopy is listed in Box 24-23.

Pulmonary function tests

For the patient being considered for a pneumonectomy, the preoperative evaluation is even more precise because whether the uninvolved lung will be able sustain the patient's respiration after surgery needs to be determined.

24-22

Preparation of patient for bronchoscopy

1. Physician should explain procedure to patient and obtain patient signature on informed consent form.
2. Patients are advised not to smoke for at least 24 hours.
3. Dentures are removed. Loose teeth are noted and called to physician's attention.
4. Preanesthetic medications are administered 30 to 60 minutes before procedure. Commonly prescribed are the following:
   a. Morphine sulfate, 5 to 15 mg IM, to suppress cough and relieve pain and anxiety. Demerol 50 to 100 mg IM is used in persons who have asthma or bronchospasm.
   b. Diazepam (Valium), 5 to 10 mg IM, for sedation and to protect against convulsive reactions to local anesthetic agents.
   c. Atropine sulfate, 0.4 to 1 mg IM, to reduce vasovagal reflex and decrease oral secretions.

24-23

Guidelines for Care

The patient following bronchoscopy under local anesthesia

1. Patient lies flat or is placed in semi-Fowler's position based on physician's preference.
2. Lying on the side facilitates removal of secretions. Usually large amount of secretions are produced. All sputum is saved for culture and cytologic examination unless otherwise ordered.
3. Patient may be hoarse and complain of sore throat. Lidocaine (Xylocaine) is often helpful in reducing discomfort.
4. Vital signs are monitored for several hours.
5. Nothing is given by mouth for at least 2 hours or until gag reflex returns.
6. Patients may receive oxygen by mask or cannula for 4 hours after bronchoscopy to improve arterial blood oxygen levels, which may become lowered during the procedure.
7. Patients are monitored for complications including the following:
   a. Massive hemoptysis (blood-tinged sputum is normal for several hours after procedure)
   b. Bronchospasm: lungs should be auscultated when vital signs are taken. If bronchospasm is present, it may be treated with aminophylline intravenously or by bronchodilator administered by aerosol.
   c. Pneumothorax: if pneumothorax is present, a chest tube is inserted and connected to water-seal drainage.
   d. Laryngeal edema and airway obstruction: shortness of breath and laryngeal stridor are symptoms. The physician should be notified immediately.
8. Patient should not smoke for several hours. Smoking may cause coughing and initiate bleeding.
9. Sputum may be blood streaked for a few days. Pronounced bleeding should be reported at once.

Pulmonary function tests are usually used to determine the patient's ability to withstand pneumonectomy. In one center, patients who are being considered for pneumonectomy are evaluated on the basis of their forced expiratory volume in the first second (FEV_1) as follows:

1. If the FEV_1 is greater than 70% of the predicted normal level (approximately 2.5 L of flow), the patient's lung function is essentially normal, and the patient should be able to tolerate a pneumonectomy as long as cardiac status and arterial blood gas levels are acceptable.
2. If the FEV_1 is less than 35% of the predicted normal level (less than 1.1 L of flow), there is severe ventilatory impairment, and *surgical resection is not feasible.*
3. If the FEV_1 is between 35% and 70% of the predicted normal level (1.2 to 2.4 L of flow) there is mild-to-moderate ventilatory impairment, and further studies will be necessary to determine the maximal tolerable resection.

The nurse should be sure that the patient understands what tests are to be performed and the preparation for them. The person's significant others also are kept informed. Pulmonary function tests are described on p. 525.

Preoperative teaching

The proposed surgery is discussed with both patient and family. The goal of teaching is to prepare the patient for what he or she is expected to do postoperatively. In some hospitals nurses from the operating room, recovery room, or intensive care unit do the preoperative teaching. Even when this is so, the nurse caring for the patient is responsible for determining what the patient understands about the impending surgery and to be sure that preoperative teaching is completed.

Points to be discussed in teaching include:
1. Patient's knowledge of procedure
2. Explanation of procedure as necessary, including intubation for anesthesia, site and length of incision, and chest tube(s) and drainage system
3. Where patient will go immediately following surgery
   a. To recovery room—for how long
   b. To intensive care unit—for how long
4. Oxygen
5. Intravenous fluid and/or blood administration
6. Pain medication
7. What patient will be asked to do
   a. Coughing and deep breathing
   b. Arm exercises
   c. Ambulation

Postoperative care

The care of the patient after thoracic surgery centers on promoting ventilation and reexpansion of the lung by maintaining a clear airway, promoting comfort by pain relief, promoting reexpansion of the lung by proper maintenance of the water-seal drainage system, promoting arm exercises to maintain full use of the patient's arm on the operated side, promoting hydration and nutrition, and monitoring the incision for bleeding and subcutaneous emphysema. These will be discussed in the Implementation section on p. 569.

In most hospitals the patient will go from the recovery room to the intensive care unit. The immediate postoperative nursing care is outlined here.

Care after pneumonectomy

The postoperative care discussed in the box applies to all patients with resectional surgery except those having a pneumonectomy. The special care required after pneumonectomy is outlined in Box 24-24.

Complications of resectional surgery

In the immediate postoperative period (24 to 48 hours) hypotension, cardiac dysrhythmia, pulmonary edema, and subcutaneous emphysema may occur. Long-term complications include a residual air space, which results from failure of the remaining portions of the lung to reexpand and fill the space. If this space is small, no treatment is indicated. Two major complications of chest surgery tend to occur later in the postoperative period and require treatment: empyema and bronchopleural fistula. The patient may have empyema alone or empyema and a bronchopleural fistula. The signs and symptoms and treatment of these two complications are outlined in Table 24-21.

Thoracoplasty

A thoracoplasty is an extrapleural procedure involving the removal of ribs to reduce the size of the chest cavity. Before the widespread use of resectional surgery, thoracoplasty was the basic surgical treatment for tuberculosis. Today *thoracoplasty is used infrequently and then only to prevent or treat the complications of resectional surgery.* When it is thought that a patient's lung may not be able to expand sufficiently after a resection to fill the space, a thoracoplasty is performed 2 to 3 weeks before the resection. It also may be performed before pneumonectomy. This will reduce the size of the cavity on the operative side and decrease the chance of mediastinal shift toward that side. This type of thoracoplasty is often called a *preresection* or *tailoring* thoracoplasty, that is, the chest wall is tailored to reduce its size.

If the remaining portions of the lung fail to reexpand sufficiently after resection or if another complication such as empyema occurs, a thoracoplasty is performed. *In general, it is used when there is a space in the chest that cannot be obliterated by other means.* Usually no more than three ribs are removed; therefore, paradoxical motion after thoracoplasty is seldom seen anymore. Paradoxical motion is discussed under chest injuries (p. 577).

Nursing Process
Assessment
Subjective data
1. Onset and duration of signs and symptoms
2. What the patient understands about why he or she is hospitalized
   a. For diagnostic tests
   b. For chest surgery or radiation or chemotherapy
3. Whether the patient states that carcinoma of the lung is present or suspected
4. Smoking history
5. Occupational history of exposure to asbestos or other carcinogenic agents

24-24

Special care following pneumonectomy

1. Chest tubes are not necessary because there is no lung left to reexpand on the operative side.
2. Patient may lie on back or *operated side only*. Patient is not allowed to lie with operative side uppermost because of fear that the sutured bronchial stump may open, allowing fluid to drain into the unoperated side and drown the patient.
3. Pressure in the operative side will be checked in the operating room after the chest is closed. A pneumothorax apparatus (which can instill or remove air) will be used to check the pressure in the operative space, and air will be removed or intilled as necessary to bring the pressure to slightly negative (slightly less than 760 mm Hg).
4. The surgeon will palpate the patient's trachea at least daily to determine if it is in midline. Deviation of the trachea toward either the operated or unoperated side is a sign of *mediastinal shift*. If pressure builds up in the operated side, the trachea will deviate toward the unoperated side. The treatment is to remove air (positive pressure) with a pneumothorax apparatus. Mediastinal shift toward the "good" lung can seriously compromise ventilation and needs to be treated promptly. Deviation of the trachea toward the operated side indicates that more pressure (air) needs to be instilled into the empty space so that the mediastinum will shift back to its normal position.
5. The patient's trachea should be palpated to be sure it is in midline and the position should be recorded. If there is a change in the position of the trachea, it should be reported immediately.
6. The patient with a mediastinal shift resembles the patient in congestive heart failure. Neck veins are distended, the trachea is displaced to one side, pulse and respirations are increased, and dyspnea is present.
7. Serous drainage will collect in the operated space and over time will congeal to the consistency of axle grease. This is often sufficient to keep the mediastinum from shifting toward the operative side. Persistent mediastinal shift toward the operative side may have to be treated with *thoracoplasty* (removal of ribs) to reduce the size of the remaining space and assist in maintaining the mediastinum in midline. Thoracoplasty is described on p. 567.
8. It usually takes 2 to 4 days for the remaining lung to adjust to the increase in blood flow. For this reason the amount of fluids and blood given intravenously is monitored closely to prevent fluid overload. CVP monitoring is common. Rales are commonly heard over the base of the remaining lung, and vascular markings will be more prominent on x-ray films. Any increase in rales, in pulse or blood pressure, and in dyspnea may indicate circulatory overload and should be reported immediately. Treatment may include diuretics and/or digitalization along with discontinuing intravenous fluids.
9. Deep breathing, coughing, and arm exercises are described (p. 574).
10. Patients who have had a lung removed may have a lowered vital capacity, and excercise, and activity should be limited to that which can be performed without dyspnea. Because the body must be given time to adjust to having only one lung, the patient's return to work may be delayed.
11. If the diagnosis is cancer, radiation therapy is usually given, and it may be started before the patient leaves the hospital. (See Chapter 11 for further discussion of nursing care for patients receiving radiation therapy.)
12. The patient who has had a pneumonectomy for cancer is urged to report to the physician at once if hoarseness, dyspnea, pain on swallowing, or localized chest pain develop because these symptoms may be signs of complications.

Objective data

1. Presence of cough and whether or not productive of sputum
2. If sputum is present, whether blood-tinged
3. Hemoptysis
4. Shortness of breath when talking or on exertion
5. Unilateral wheezing on auscultation

Data analysis: nursing diagnoses

Nursing diagnoses are determined from analysis of patient data. Possible nursing diagnoses for the person with bronchogenic carcinoma having resectioned surgery may include, but are not limited to, the following:

Diagnostic title	Possible etiologies
Anxiety	Threat of death
	Threat/change in health status/scocioeconomic status/role functioning environment
Gas exchange, impaired	Ventilation/perfusion impairment
Pain	Pleuritic chest pain (if pleura involved)
Knowledge deficit: about the disease and its treatment	Lack of exposure/unfamiliarity with information sources
Airway clearance, ineffective	Decreased energy/fatigue
Disuse syndrome, high risk for	Surgical incision involving trapezius muscle
Tissue integrity, impaired	Surgical incision

Planning: expected patient outcomes

Expected patient outcomes for the person undergoing resectional surgery may include, but are not limited to, the following:

1. Patient is coping effectively with anxiety.
2. Patient's gas exchange is within normal levels as evidenced by arterial blood gone.
3. Patient's postoperative pain is controlled by medication.
4. Patient is maintaining a patent airway.
5. Patient is able to put operative arm through normal range of motion.
6. Patient's incision is healing well.
7. Patient can explain regimen to follow after discharge including the following:
   a. Explain recommended changes in ADL
      (1) Which usual activities to limit and for how long
      (2) Exercise program
   b. Explain any changes required in life-style (reason and plans for changes in occupation and habits such as smoking, activity level, and so on).
   c. State name, dose, action, and side effects of medications ordered
      (1) How and when to use PRN medications
      (2) Schedule for other medications and how to take them
   d. Describe professional and community resources necessary for structuring an environment compatible with convalescence
      (1) Plans for obtaining assistance of agencies such as Visiting Nurses Association
      (2) Plans for necessary modifications of home
   e. Describe plans for follow-up care.
      (1) Signs or symptoms requiring immediate medical assistance
      (2) State plans for ongoing medical care

Implementation
Assisting with achievement of therapeutic goals
Maintaining chest tube(s) and drainage

All patients who have resectional surgery of the lung, except those having a pneumonectomy, will require drainage of the pleural space by one or two chest tubes connected to closed drainage. The tubes are inserted immediately after the operative incision is closed. Usually two tubes are used, although some surgeons may prefer only one tube. When two tubes are used, one catheter is inserted through a stab wound in the anterior chest wall above the resected area. This is referred to as the *anterior* or *upper tube*. It is used to remove air from the pleural space. The second tube is inserted through a stab wound in the posterior chest and is referred to as the *posterior* or *lower tube*. It is primarily for the drainage of *serosanguineous* fluid that accumulates as the result of the operative procedure. The lower tube may be of a larger diameter than the upper tube to prevent it from becoming plugged with clots. Fig. 24-25 shows the placement of tubes within the pleural space. When only one chest tube is used, it is usually placed anteriorly above the resected area of the lung.

When initiating chest tube drainage, a 2 L clear glass bottle is usually used for each chest tube, although other commercial devices, such as the Pleurevac system (Fig. 24-22) are available. Approximately 300 ml of sterile water, or enough to fill the bottles 1 to 2 cm from the bottom, is then added. If considerable drainage accumulates in the bottle, the amount of subatmospheric (negative) pressure in the system will increase, and it will be more difficult for the patient to expel air and fluid from the pleural space.

Fig. 24-25   A, Drainage tube being inserted into pleural space. **B,** Note that upper and lower tubes are placed well into pleural space. (From Johnson J, MacVaugh H III, Waldhausen JA: *Surgery of the chest, a handbook of operative surgery,* ed 4, Chicago, 1970, Mosby–Year Book.)

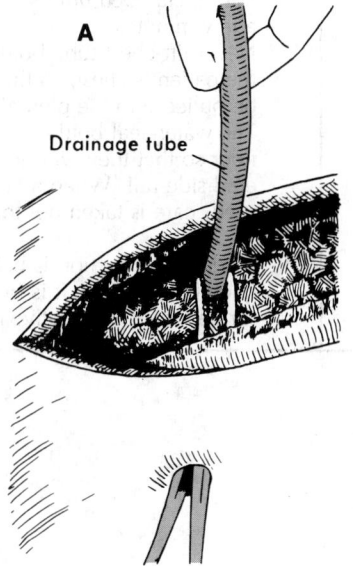

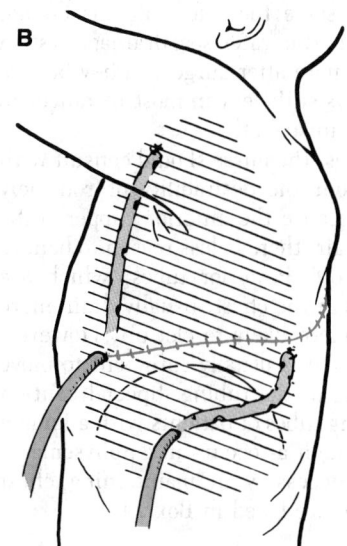

In this instance, the glass rod may be pulled up so that less of it is under water, or the surgeon may order that the drainage bottle be changed. In this case a sterile setup is prepared. When the sterile bottle with sterile water and the tubing are ready, the chest tube is clamped as close to the patient's chest as possible. The chest tube is then disconnected from the drainage tubing, the sterile setup is connected, and the chest tube is unclamped. The amount of drainage in the bottle should be measured and usually is sent to the laboratory for examination.

As the patient breathes, there will be movement of fluid in the glass tube that is under water. This is known as *fluctuation* or *oscillation*, and *the column will move up when the patient inhales or coughs, and it will fall when the patient is exhaling.*

Some thoracic surgeons wish to have the chest tubes "milked" or "stripped" to prevent formation of clots that could plug the tubes; *the practice of routinely stripping chest tube(s) is becoming less common, however, because it increases the negative pressure exerted on the pleural space.* A study by two clinical nurse specialists revealed the following: (1) The pressure generated by stripping was considerably higher than the suction pressures of -15 to -20 cm of water commonly applied to chest drainage systems; (2) the amount of pressure was directly related to the length of the tubing stripped; and (3) even stripping only a few centimeters produced pressures near -100 cm of water, stripping the entire tube produced pressures exceeding -400 cm of water.[113] They also found that higher negative pressures resulted when a roller was used to strip the tubes rather than the hands.[113]

Undesirable side effects of increased levels of negative pressure reported in the literature include (1) lung entrapment in the thoracic tube eyelets and focal tissue infarction and (2) persistent pneumothorax.[126] The persistent pneumothorax occurs when the pleural surface of lung, which normally has air leaks at the close of the operative procedure, does not "seal off." Usually fibrin will seal the air leaks; however, the presence of an increased amount of negative pressure may prevent the air leaks from sealing off and may even increase the size of the air leaks. This is the reason why some thoracic surgeons do not attach additional suction to the water-seal drainage system for the first 24 hours or more after surgery. They believe that this amount of time is sufficient in most instances to allow the pleural surface to seal off.

In view of these findings, the nurse should consult with the thoracic surgeon about the desirability of routinely stripping chest tubes. Because the anterior (upper) tube usually evacuates mainly air, there is less reason to believe that this tube will clot off. Posterior tubes, which are commonly inserted lower in the chest, usually drain more fluid and blood and are more likely to clot off. However, gentle squeezing of the tube is usually sufficient to move the bloody drainage along in the tubing. Special caution should be used in stripping tubes of patients with a known history of fragile tissue, such as occurs in emphysema.[119] The nursing measures necessary in maintaining chest tubes and closed drainage are listed in Box 24-25.

24-25

Maintaining chest tubes and closed chest drainage bottles

1. Mark water level in bottle with strip of adhesive tape so that amount of drainage can easily be determined. Write date and hour on tape.
2. Fasten tubing to the bed so that there are no dependent loops between the bottles and the bed (see Fig. 24-26). Dependent loops allow fluid to collect in tubing and impede removal of air and fluid from pleural space.
3. Be sure that tip of chest tube is 1 to 2 cm under water so that if the bottle accidentally tips over, the tube will remain under water.
4. Check the glass rod in the bottle for fluctuation frequently. If the column of water is not fluctuating:
   a. Be sure patient is not lying on tubes.
   b. Check connections to be sure chest tube system is intact.
   c. Ask patient to cough or change position to see if fluctuation is restored.
   d. Fluctuation will stop when lung is reexpanded. Call the surgeon if the tubes are not patent (column of fluid not fluctuating).
5. Keep two hemostats at the bedside so that the chest tube can be clamped if a bottle is accidentally broken. When a bottle is broken, the chest catheter should be clamped and then reconnected to a sterile setup as soon as possible. Sterile water should be used in the bottle. As soon as the system is reconnected with the tip of the tube under water, the clamp should be removed. *Except in case of an emergency such as a broken bottle, most thoracic surgeons prefer that tubes not be clamped, and a specific order is written if clamping is desired.*
6. Never clamp chest tubes unless a bottle breaks (a rare occurrence) or without a written order. When chest tubes are clamped, air (positive pressure) may be trapped in the pleural space and further collapse the lung. If a patient is being transported from one place to another, such as to the x-ray department, tubes should not be clamped unless it is necessary for only a few minutes.
7. Never lift chest tube bottles above the level of the patient's chest, as this would allow fluid to be pulled into the pleural space.
8. The water-seal bottles should be placed on the floor so that they will not be broken by a lowered side-rail. When a Hi-Lo bed is being used, care is taken not to lower the bed onto the bottles.
9. If additional suction is being used, check frequently to be sure it is functioning at the prescribed level of negative pressure.

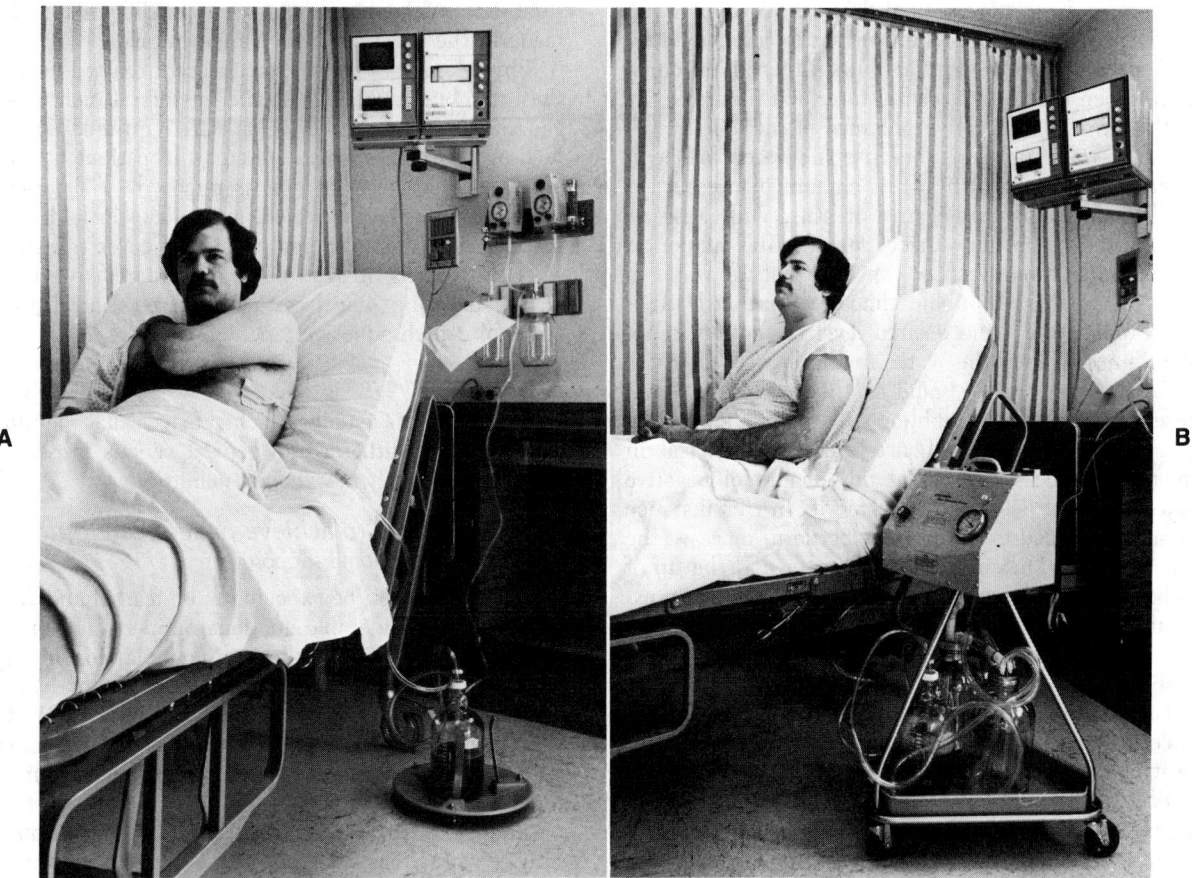

Fig. 24-26 Chest tube with water-seal suction. **A,** Wall outlet provides source of suction. Note holder used to secure bottle in upright position. **B,** Emerson suction machine as source of vacuum.

Additional suction. Suction is usually used to speed reexpansion of the lung after surgery, using either wall suction (Fig. 24-26, *A*) or an Emerson suction machine (Fig. 24-26, *B*). Most often −30 cm of suction is applied, but this amount varies according to the surgeon's preference. When it is particularly important to regulate the exact amount of suction used, a "breaker" bottle may be added to the system between the suction source and the patient's drainage bottle. The use of a breaker bottle provides for control of the amount of suction that is applied to the water-sealed bottle and thus to the patient's pleural space. The stopper in the control bottle has three openings. One is connected to the water-sealed bottle, one is connected to the suction source, and the third contains a glass rod that is under water and open to the outside (Fig. 24-30). The amount of suction produced will be determined by the distance between the surface of the water and the tip of this tube.

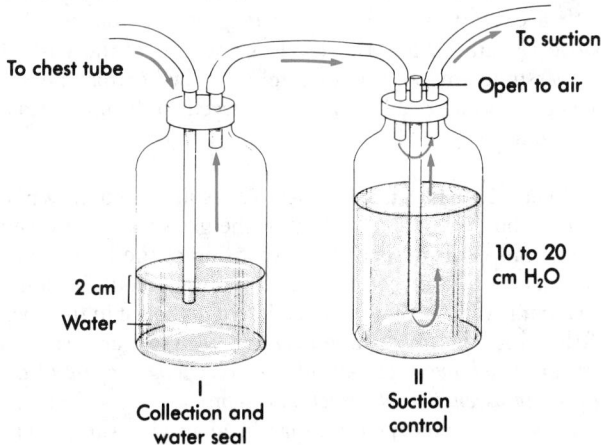

Fig. 24-27 Water-sealed closed drainage system with suction control bottle. (From Abels LF: *Mosby's manual of critical care,* St Louis, 1979, Mosby—Year Book.)

When the suction source is turned on, the level of water in the open tube will sink in proportion to the amount of negative pressure in the system. Thus if there is 15 cm of water between the surface of the water and the tip of the tube, the amount of negative pressure in the system will be 15 cm of water pressure. Because the water will be at the bottom of the tube when this amount of pressure is reached, any increase in negative pressure will cause air to be drawn in from the outside, *breaking* the suction at this level. Therefore, it can be expected that the water in the breaker bottle will bubble almost continuously. If it fails to bubble at all, the desired level of suction is not being attained. When the water in the breaker bottle is not bubbling, the tubing should be checked for air leaks. If there are no leaks and bubbling still does not occur, the surgeon should be notified at once because the air leak in the pleura may be so great that the amount of negative pressure is not sufficient to overcome it. In this instance water may be added to the breaker bottle to increase the distance between the surface of the water and the tip of the tube, thereby increasing the amount of negative pressure being exerted on the pleural space.

The distance the tube is placed under water in the breaker bottle is determined by the surgeon. A breaker bottle and suction may be attached to one or both tubes. Most commonly it is attached to the upper tube because this is where air is most likely to be leaking from the pleural surface. A small empty trap bottle is usually attached by tubing between the breaker bottle and the suction source. The purpose of this bottle is to protect the suction motor from becoming wet should the breaker bottle overflow. See the box on p. 570 for a summary of actions to maintain chest tubes.

Ambulation. There is no contraindication to ambulating with a chest tube in place. As long as the water-sealed bottle remains below the level of the chest, the patient may assume any position of comfort in bed or may be out of bed in a chair. The patient is urged to be up at least 2×'s day.

Removal of chest tubes. Chest tubes are removed when there is no fluctuation of fluid in the glass rod, and when x-ray films confirm the full reexpansion of the lung. Most patients have their chest tube(s) removed about 72 hours postoperatively. If there is a persistent air space in the apex of the lung, the upper tube may be left in longer. *Surgeons are concerned about leaving tubes in very long because of the risk of an ascending tube track infection.*

A well-accepted practice has been to give the patient pain medication 30 minutes before removal of chest tube(s). However, a recent study of sensations experienced by patients during chest tube removal raises questions about this practice. In this study, burning was the most frequently reported sensation, followed by pain, pulling, and pressure. The authors of the article recommend that preparing patients to experience a brief sensation of burning or pain may be the only preparation necessary. They also question the influence that the nurse's manner may have on the patient's reaction to the procedure.[48] For this reason, we recommend the nurses review this study with their surgeon colleagues to see if modification might be made in the practice in their institutions.

Physicians vary in the exact procedure used to removed the tube, but generally a sterile scissors, 4 inch × 4 inch gauze squares, and adhesive tape are required. The suture holding the tube in place is cut, the patient is asked to exhale deeply, and the tube is removed. If a pursestring suture was used, it is retied, and a dry sterile dressing is placed over the site. Some physicians cover the site with a Telfa dressing instead of gauze squares to ensure an airtight dressing. The dressing is covered securely by three strips of 2-inch adhesive tape.

Hemodynamic monitoring

The patient is usually attached to a cardiac monitor and a Swan-Ganz catheter and central venous pressure line may be used for hemodynamic monitoring.

Interventions to achieve patient care outcomes
Providing emotional support

All patients can be expected to be fearful and anxious, and require considerable emotional support. The nurse and physician should discuss the treatment plan for the patient, so that all information given to the patient and family is carefully coordinated. In addition, the patient and family should be encouraged to verbalize their fears and concerns. The nurse should be supportive without giving unrealistic reassurance.

Because of the very poor survival rate in persons with lung cancer, a major role of the nurse is to teach the public how lung cancer can be prevented or at least diagnosed as early as possible. Points to be emphasized in teaching are listed in Box 24-26.

24-26

Prevention and early detection of lung cancer

1. Smoking control programs
   a. Encourage young persons not to start smoking.
   b. Educate public about hazards of smoking.
   c. Provide self-help materials to assist persons to quit smoking.
   d. Refer to stop-smoking programs sponsored by organizations such as the ACS, ALA, and American Heart Association.
   e. Stress that there is no such thing as a "safe cigarette," but that persons who smoke cigarettes lower in tar and nicotine find it easier to quit smoking.[1]
   f. Support nonsmoking areas in public places such as restaurants and meeting places.
   g. Support legislation to establish nonsmoking areas in public meeting places.
2. Urge all individuals over 40 years of age to have a chest x-ray periodically in addition to a yearly physical examination.
3. Know the cancer detection centers in your community or other resources to which persons can be referred for evaluation.

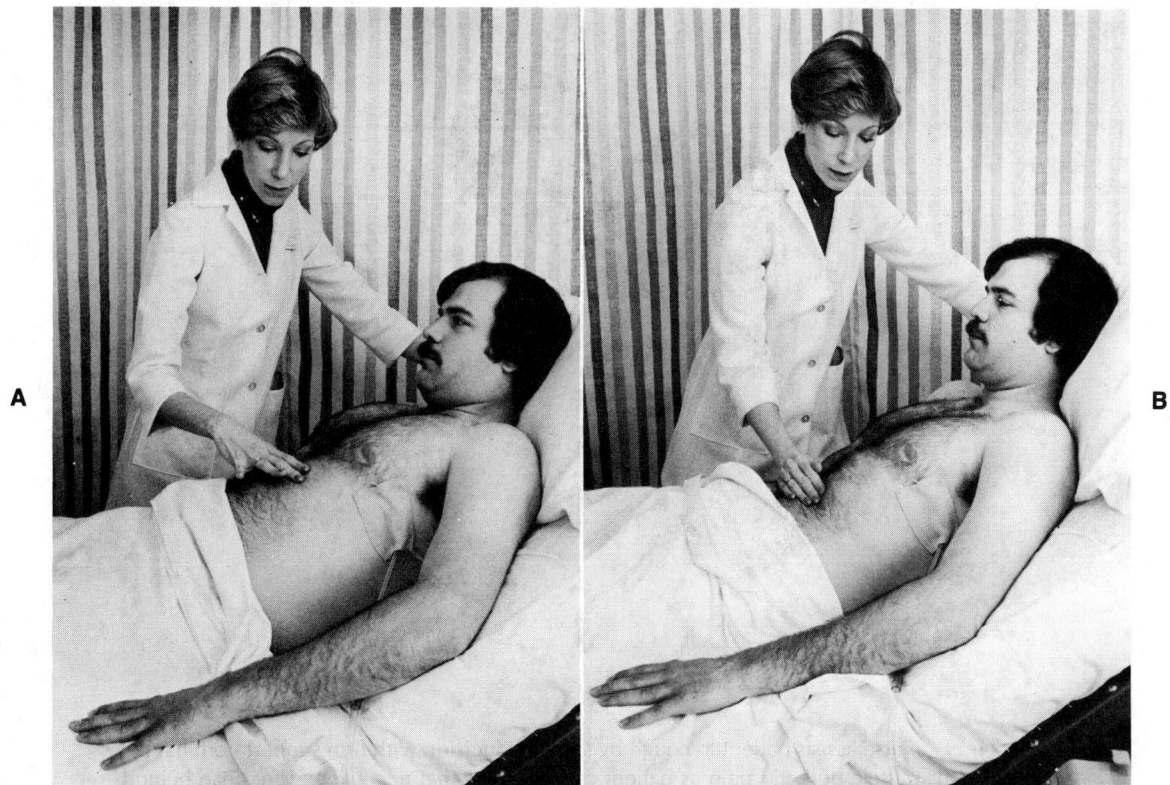

Fig. 24-28   A, Physical therapist assists patient in learning augmented abdominal breathing. Patient is instructed to inhale through nose, using abdominal muscles and concentrate on moving lower ribs under therapists hand. This exercise improves ventilation of bases of lungs. **B,** Physical therapist places hand on upper abdomen in assisting patient to exhale fully.

Maintaining oxygen therapy

Oxygen is attached to the endotracheal tube. After extubation, oxygen is given by cannula, usually at 6 L/min. An oxygen mask is not used because of a need to have the patient cough and raise secretions frequently.

Promoting gas exchange by positioning of patient

The patient is kept flat in bed or with head elevated slightly (20 degrees) until blood pressure is stabilized to preoperative levels. Once blood pressure is stabilized, the patient can usually breathe best in semi-Fowler's position with a pillow under the head and neck but not under the shoulder and back because of the subscapular incision.

Promoting abdominal breathing

Abdominal breathing exercises are a valuable adjunct to the care of the patient with chest surgery because they improve ventilation without increasing pain and assist in coughing more effectively (Fig. 24-28). The exercises should be taught *preoperatively* so that the patient has time to practice them before surgery. The patient can cough most effectively 20 to 30 minutes after receiving pain medication, and this should be capitalized on by the nursing staff.

Monitoring vital signs

Vital signs are taken every 15 minutes until the patient is well recovered from anesthesia and then every hour until condition has stabilized. It is not unusual for blood pressure to fluctuate during the first 24 to 36 hours, and close monitoring of the patient is essential. A persistently low blood pressure is reported to the surgeon.

Promoting comfort by pain relief

Morphine or meperidine hydrochloride is usually ordered for pain. Medication for pain should be given as needed and may be required as often as every 3 to 4 hours during the first 48 to 72 hours. The patient is extremely uncomfortable and will not be able to cough or turn unless there is relief from pain. In some instances the dose of the narcotic is decreased so that it may be given more frequently and yet not depress respirations. The tubes in the chest cause pain, and the patient may attempt rapid, shallow breathing to splint the lower chest and avoid motion of the catheters. This impairs ventilation, makes coughing ineffective, and causes secretions to be retained. Thus it is a nursing responsibility to make the patient comfortable, because this facilitates deep breathing and coughing. *Pain medication should never be withheld without first consulting with the surgeon because undermedication is counterproductive.*

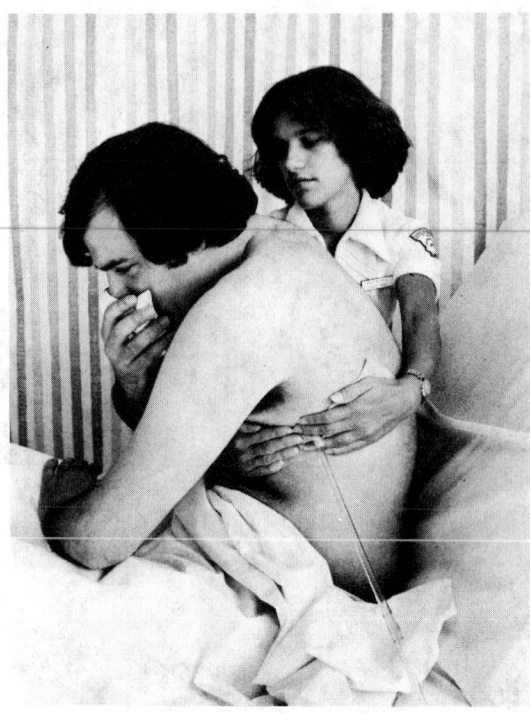

Fig. 24-29   Nurse assists patient to cough by splinting incision with firm support from hands. This lessens muscle pull and pain as patient coughs. Note that nurse keeps her head behind patient while he coughs, and patient uses tissue to cover mouth.

If, despite all efforts the patient's discomfort is interfering with adequate chest excursion, an intercostal nerve block may be performed.

Initiating coughing and deep breathing exercises

The patient should be assisted to cough as soon as conscious. If the blood pressure is stable, the patient is assisted to a sitting position, and the incision is supported anteriorly and posteriorly by the nurse's hands. Firm, even pressure over the incision with the open palm of the hand is a most effective method. The nurse's head should be behind the patient when the patient is coughing (Fig. 24-29). The patient is encouraged to breathe deeply, exhale, and then cough. Sips of fluids, especially of warm ones such as tea or coffee, often facilitate coughing. Mist therapy may be used to loosen secretions. Coughing *keeps the airway patent, prevents atelectasis, and facilitates reexpansion of the lung*. The patient should be assisted to cough every hour for the first 24 hours, and then every 2 to 4 hours. The patient should cough until the chest sounds clear. Otherwise, secretions will accumulate in the tracheobronchial tree.

When a patient is unable to cough effectively, tracheobronchial suctioning is performed. If suctioning fails to clear the airway, bronchoscopy may be necessary because it is crucial that the airway is kept clear. In these situations, *bronchoscopy* is performed at the bedside with a *fiberoptic bronchoscope* (Fig. 24-30).

Promoting hydration and nutrition

The patient is encouraged to take fluids postoperatively and to progress to a general diet as soon as it is tolerated. Forcing fluids helps to liquefy secretions and makes them easier to expectorate. A diet adequate in protein and vitamins (especially vitamin C) facilitates wound healing.

Promoting arm exercises

Passive arm exercises are usually started on the evening of surgery. The purpose in putting the patient's arm through range of motion is to prevent restriction of function from disuse. Most patients are reluctant to move the arm on the operative side, but with proper preoperative instruction and postoperative follow through they do so readily. *It is important for both the patient and nurse to understand that the longer the arm is unexercised, the stiffer it will become. The patient should put both arms through active range of motion two or three times a day within a few days.* The recommended exercises are similar to those done after mastectomy (see Chapter 36). The exercises are best performed when the patient is upright or lying on the abdomen. Exercises such as elevating the scapula and clavicle, "hunching the shoul-

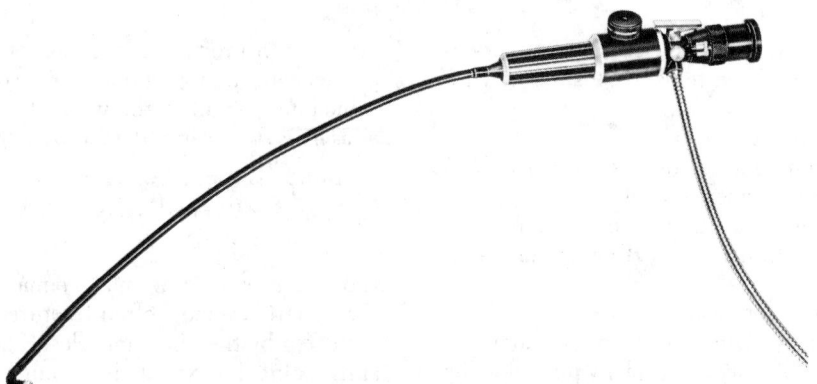

Fig. 24-30   Fiberoptic bronchoscope. Because of its flexibility it allows better visualization of bronchi. (Courtesy American Cystoscope Makers, Inc, Pelham, NY.)

ders," bringing the scapulae as close together as possible, and hyperextending the arm can only be performed in these positions. Because lying on the abdomen may not be possible at first, these exercises are performed with the patient sitting on the edge of the bed or standing.

Monitoring the incision for bleeding or subcutaneous emphysema

The outer dressings are checked periodically for evidence of bleeding. *Blood on the dressings is unusual and should be reported to the surgeon at once.* The time and amount of blood is recorded in the patient's record. The surgeon may reinforce the dressing, and, in the rare instance when bleeding persists, the patient may be taken back to surgery. The chest will be reopened and the source of bleeding located and ligated.

Subcutaneous emphysema is not unusual after chest surgery. In subcutaneous emphysema, *air leaks from the pleural space through the thoracotomy incision or around the chest tubes into the soft tissues.* When palpating the chest, the presence of air under the skin is readily detected and has been described as feeling like "tissue paper" or "Rice Krispies" under the skin. Subcutaneous emphysema is most notable in the neck and chest, and, if considerable air is leaking, the patient's face and neck will become considerably enlarged. Small amounts of air will reabsorb over time and cause no problem, but if subcutaneous emphysema is worsening, the chest tube may be changed by the surgeon and a larger one inserted, because air is leaking into the tissues faster than it is being removed by the tube. Additional suction may also be applied to the chest tube(s) in an attempt to remove air more rapidly. Rarely a patient will need to return to surgery for closure of air leaks.

The patient with a pneumonectomy should have only a small amount (if any) of subcutaneous emphysema. *Progressive subcutaneous emphysema after pneumonectomy is very serious, and should be reported to the surgeon immediately because it could indicate a major leak in the bronchial stump.* This also is a rare occurrence, requiring immediate return to surgery for reclosure of the bronchial stump.

Facilitating learning

For the patient whose cancer is successfully removed at surgery and who will be discharged home, the following points need to be emphasized.

Because of early discharge, the patient will need to make some changes in ADL. This may include taking frequent rest periods or at least a nap in the morning and afternoon for a week or two. The patient's activities are guided by fatigue. When the patient begins to get tired, he or she should stop and rest.

Exercising of the arm on the operative side should continue with the arm being put through range of motion at least twice daily. It is important that the patient understands that if the exercises are discontinued, the arm will become stiff and restricted motion will result. This is referred to by some as a *frozen shoulder.*

If the patient has not already stopped smoking, he or she will need support to do so. The patient can be referred to a support program for those wishing to stop smoking. These programs are frequently offered by the American Lung Association or the American Cancer Society.

The patient needs to understand the purpose, dosage, and so on of any prescribed drugs. Following successful surgery, the only medication prescribed may be an oral analgesic.

Although the patient may not appear to need the assistance of community resources at discharge, he or she should be informed of what is available. For example, a person living alone may wish to use a service such as Meals on Wheels until he or she feels more like cooking.

The patient should be able to describe plans for follow-up care including signs and symptoms such as blood in sputum, chest pain, or unexplained fever, which should be reported to the surgeon.

The patient should know the time and date of the next appointment with the surgeon. If a patient is not able to put the operative arm through full range of motion, a follow-up appointment with the physical therapist would also be scheduled.

Evaluation

Evaluation for the patient having resectional surgery is based on patient outcomes. Questions to consider may include the following:

1. Is patient's anxiety reduced?
2. Is patient maintaining adequate gas exchange?
3. Is the patient's pain under control?
4. Is the patient able to maintain a clear airway?
5. Is the patient able to move arm through full range of motion?
6. Is the patient's incision healing well?
7. Can patient explain regimen to follow at home including changes in lifestyle and plans for follow-up care with surgeon?

CHEST TRAUMA

Etiology/Epidemiology

Trauma to the chest is a major problem most often seen first in the emergency department. *Injury to the chest may affect the bony chest cage, pleurae and lungs, diaphragm, or mediastinal contents. Injuries to the chest are broadly classified into two groups—blunt and penetrating. Blunt, or nonpenetrating, injuries damage the structures within the chest cavity without disrupting chest wall integrity. Penetrating injuries disrupt chest wall integrity and result in alteration in intrathoracic pressures.*

The leading cause of blunt chest injuries in the United States is motor vehicle steering wheel impaction in the person not wearing a seat belt. Blows to the chest with blunt objects or as a result of a fall also cause nonpenetrating chest injury. Penetrating wounds usually result from gunshot or stabbing injuries.

Both penetrating and blunt chest injuries can be fatal. The common chest injuries and their sequelae are classified as primarily penetrating or nonpenetrating chest wounds in Table 24-22.

Table 24-22 Types of penetrating and nonpenetrating (blunt) chest injuries

Penetrating	Blunt
Open pneumothorax (sucking chest wound)	**Closed pneumothorax**
Hemothorax	Tension pneumothorax
Tracheobronchial injury	Tracheobronchial injury
Pulmonary contusion	Flail chest
Diaphragm rupture	Diaphragm rupture
Mediastinal injury	Mediastinal injury
	Fractured ribs

Prevention

Nurses can promote prevention of chest trauma through public education programs focused on safe practices in vehicle usage and in the work place. *The major preventive measure is the use of seat belts when operating a motor vehicle.*

CHEST CAGE INJURIES: RIB FRACTURES

Pathophysiology

Rib fractures are the most common chest injury. Ribs 3 through 10 are most often fractured because they are less protected by the chest muscles. The ribs usually fracture at the point of maximal impact but may fracture at a distant site from impact. Fractures of the ribs are caused by blows, crushing injuries, or strain caused by severe coughing or sneezing spells. If the rib is splintered or the fracture displaced, sharp fragments may penetrate the pleura and the lung, resulting in a hemothorax or pneumothorax.

Common signs and symptoms of rib fracture include the following:

1. Pain at the site of injury, increasing on inspiration
2. Localized tenderness and crepitus on palpation
3. Splinting of the chest and taking shallow breaths

Medical Management

Treatment is individualized, based on the patient's age, whether there is a history of preexisting chronic pulmonary disease, and the number and location of ribs fractured. Medical treatment includes the following:

1. Stabilization of the fracture site with a rib belt or Ace bandage
2. Analgesics as needed
3. For severe pain, performance of a regional nerve block

Nursing Process

Assessment

Subjective data

Subjective data include the nature of the injury and when it occurred. If patient is unable to answer questions, data are obtained from those with the patient.

Objective data

1. Pain at site of injury that increases on inspiration
2. Area tender to the touch
3. Patient splints chest and takes shallow breaths

Diagnostic tests

Fractures are confirmed by chest x-ray findings.

Data analysis: nursing diagnoses

Nursing diagnoses are determined from analysis of patient data. Possible nursing diagnoses for the person with rib fracture may include, but are not limited to, the following:

Diagnostic title	Possible etiologies
Pain	Trauma to the rib cage
Airway clearance, ineffective	Pain/trauma to rib cage

Diagnostic title	Possible etiologies
Anxiety	Threat to change in health status
Breathing pattern, ineffective	Pain, musculoskeletal impairment
Knowledge deficit	Lack of exposure to information or misinterpretation of information

Planning: expected patient outcomes

Expected patient outcomes for the person with fractured ribs may include, but are not limited to, the following:
1. Pain is improved.
2. Patient maintains a patent airway.
3. Patient is less anxious.
4. Patient is breathing effectively.
5. Patient understands follow-up therapy.
6. Patient understands that physician is to be notified if shortness of breath, hemoptysis, or temperature elevation occur.

Implementation
Assisting with achievement of therapeutic goals
Initial care for fractured ribs

If ribs are fractured and the rib has not penetrated the pleura, the chest is strapped with adhesive tape or an Ace bandage or chest binder is applied.
1. Check strapping to be sure it is secure.
2. Give analgesics as ordered.

Interventions to achieve patient outcomes
Assisting with comfort and ADL

1. Place patient in position of comfort. May be able to breathe easier in Fowler's or semi-Fowler's position.
2. Give prescribed analgesics.
3. If pain persists despite analgesics, notify the physician, who may infiltrate the intercostal spaces above and below the fractured rib(s) with 1% procaine.

Assisting with airway clearance

1. Assist patient to deep breathe and cough to clear airway.
2. If cough is ineffective, suction airway.

Providing emotional support

1. Monitor level of anxiety.
2. Check on patient frequently to reassure him or her that they are in a safe environment and their needs will be met.
3. Provide time to listen to patients' concerns and provide realistic reassurance.

Facilitating learning

1. Teach patient symptoms (increase in pain, shortness of breath) to report immediately.

Evaluation

Evaluation is based on patient outcomes. Questions to consider may include the following:
1. Is the patient's pain improved?

2. Is the patient able to breathe effectively?
3. Is the patient less anxious?
4. Can the patient state plans for follow-up care?
5. Can the patient state the signs and symptoms (shortness of breath, hemoptysis, or elevated temperature) that require immediate medical attention?

FLAIL CHEST
Pathophysiology

When multiple ribs or the sternum are fractured in more than one place, a portion of the chest wall becomes separated from the chest cage, resulting in a *flail chest*. That is, the chest wall no longer provides the rigid bony support that is necessary to maintain the bellows function required for normal ventilation. This causes *paradoxical respiratory* movement. On inspiration the dislocated segment is pulled inward by the subatmospheric intrapleural pressure. During expiration the dislocated segment bulges outward as intrapleural pressure becomes less negative (Fig. 24-31, *C* and *D*).

Flair chest usually causes localized atelectasis secondary to decreased ventilation, resulting in hypoxemia. Because of the increased work of breathing, the individual may also develop hypercapnia and respiratory acidosis.

Assessment
Subjective data

Data to be collected includes the nature of the injury and when it occurred. Often the patient is too badly injured to answer questions, and data are obtained from those accompanying the patient.

Objective data

1. Pain is severe and increases with each respiratory movement.
2. Mediastinum oscillates, or "flutters," with each respiration.
3. Breath sounds are decreased on auscultation.
4. If there is severe interference with cardiac function, neck veins will be distended.
5. Vital signs: increased pulse and respiratory rate. Blood pressure will fall if paradoxical motion is not relieved.

Diagnostic tests

1. Chest x-ray examination to determine extent of trauma.
2. Arterial blood gasses to determine PaO_2 and $PaCO_2$.

Medical Management

Treatment includes the following:
1. Stabilize the flail segment. After initial stabilization the individual is usually intubated and placed on a *volume-controlled ventilator*. Postive-pressure mechanical ventilation provides internal stabilization of the chest, decreases the work of breathing, and initiates the bellows function normally provided by the

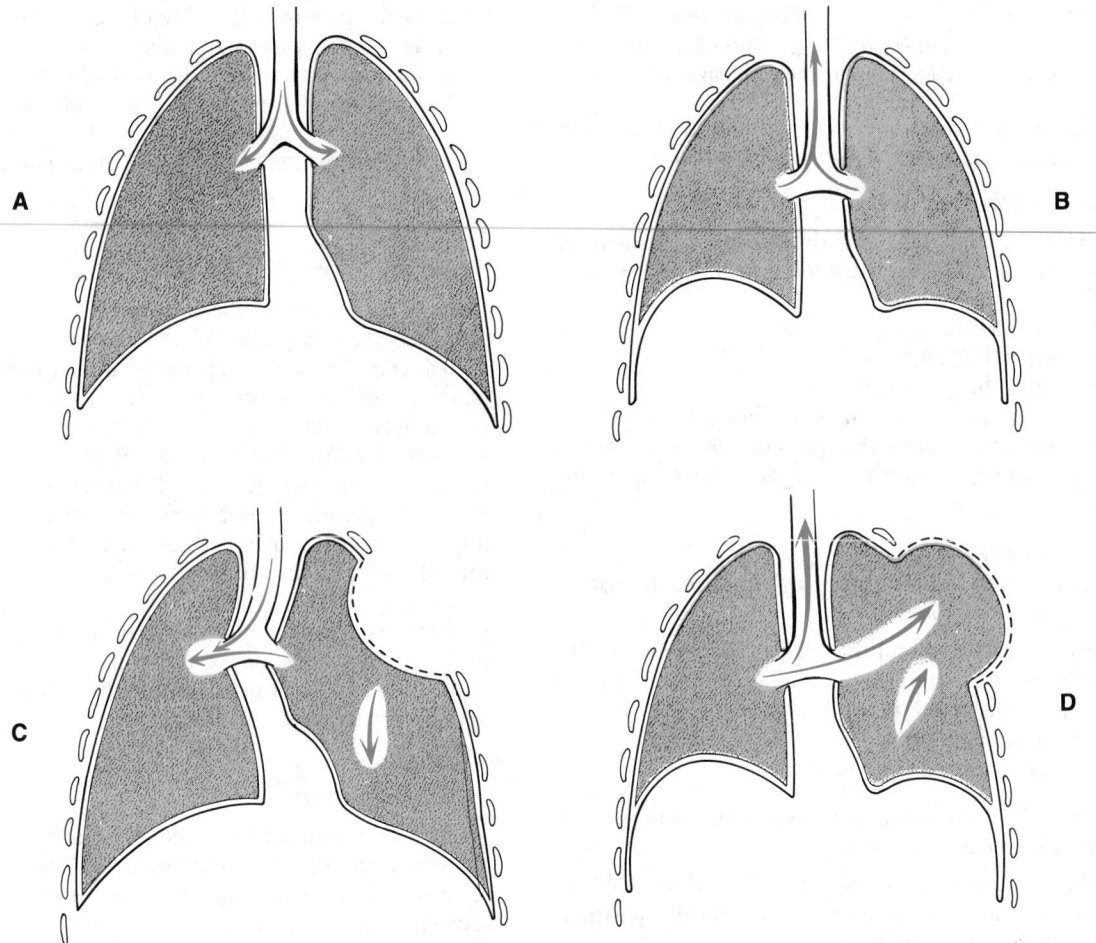

Fig. 24-31 Normal respiration. **A,** Inspiration; **B,** Expiration. *Paradoxical motion:* **C,** Inspiration, area of lung underlying unstable chest wall sucks in on inspiration. **D,** Same area balloons out on expiration. Note movement of mediastinum toward opposite lung on inspiration.

intact bony chest cage. If prolonged ventilatory support is required, a tracheostomy is performed.

2. Provide supplemental oxygen.
3. Correct acid-base imbalance. Mechanical ventilation is used to correct respiratory acid-base imbalance.
4. Provide analgesics for pain control.

PENETRATING CHEST WOUNDS

Pathophysiology

When a knife, bullet, or other flying missile enters the chest, a penetrating wound occurs. The major problem in penetrating injury is not injury to the chest wall but injury to the structures within the chest cavity. Penetration of the lung is associated with leakage of air from the lung into the pleural cavity (pneumothorax) (Fig. 24-32, *B*). Blood may also leak into the pleural cavity (hemothorax). As the air or fluid accumulates in the pleural cavity, it builds up positive pressure, which causes the lung to collapse and may cause a mediastinal shift toward the unaffected lung. This compresses the opposite lung and inter-

feres with cardiac action. The person then has serious difficulty in breathing and may go into shock.

Assessment
Subjective data

Subjective data to collect include the nature of the injury and when it occurred. If the patient is too badly injured to answer questions, data is obtained from those accompanying the patient.

Objective data

1. Signs of shock—weak and thready pulse, falling blood pressure, and cold and clammy skin
2. Severe shortness of breath
3. Check for mediastinal shift—trachea deviated from midline

Diagnostic tests

1. Chest x-ray examination to determine extent of injury
2. Arterial blood gases to determine PaO_2 and $PaCO_2$

Medical Management

If an open sucking wound of the chest has been sustained, it should be covered immediately to prevent air from entering the pleural cavity and causing a pneumothorax. Several thicknesses of nonporous material such as plastic food wrap may be used, and these are anchored with wide adhesive tape, or the wound edges may be taped tightly together. If an object such as a knife is still in the wound, it is *not* removed until a physician arrives. Its presence may prevent the entry of air into the pleural cavity, and its removal may cause further damage. *The person who sustained a penetrating wound of the chest should be placed in an upright position and taken to the nearest emergency room.*

Emergency treatment is directed toward *sustaining oxygen exchange and correcting circulatory failure.* Usually the patient is intubated with an endotracheal tube and then is checked for air or blood in the pleural cavity. An emergency thoracentesis is performed, and air and fluid are removed by syringe. Usually a catheter is inserted into the pleural space and connected to water-seal drainage (p. 563). If the lung fails to reexpand with this treatment or there is evidence of internal bleeding, surgical exploration may be necessary and will be performed as soon as shock and other complications are under control.

To monitor the patient for hypovolemia, a central venous pressure (CVP) line is inserted. This line can also be used to administer intravenous fluids and blood as necessary. The CVP is a very effective way to monitor for cardiac tamponade. A pressure above 15 cm of water or a rising CVP in a patient in shock with penetrating trauma in the region of the heart often indicates cardiac tamponade.[124] If it is suspected that cardiac injury and tamponade may be present, a *pericardiocentesis* will be done.

PNEUMOTHORAX
Pathophysiology

In pneumothorax air enters the pleural space between the lung and the chest wall. It can occur spontaneously or as a result of penetrating or nonpenetrating injuries.

A *closed pneumothorax* is caused by a blunt injury resulting in fractured ribs piercing the pleural membranes or by a sudden compression of the rib cage. Air enters the pleural space, increasing intrapleural pressure, which collapses the lung (Fig. 24-32, *B*). A variant of a closed pneumothorax is a *spontaneous pneumothorax* that can result from the rupture of an emphysematous bleb on the lung surface or that may follow severe bouts of coughing in persons with a chronic pulmonary disease such as asthma. Frequently, it occurs as a single or recurrent episode in an otherwise healthy young person. If large enough and left untreated, a closed pneumothorax can become a tension pneumothorax.

A *tension pneumothorax* occurs when air leaking into the intrapleural space cannot escape during expiration. *Although usually a result of a closed pneumothorax, a tension pneumothorax can be caused by a penetrating chest injury.* The accumulating air builds up positive pressure in the chest cavity, resulting in (1) lung collapse on the affected side, (2) mediastinal shift toward the unaffected side, and (3)

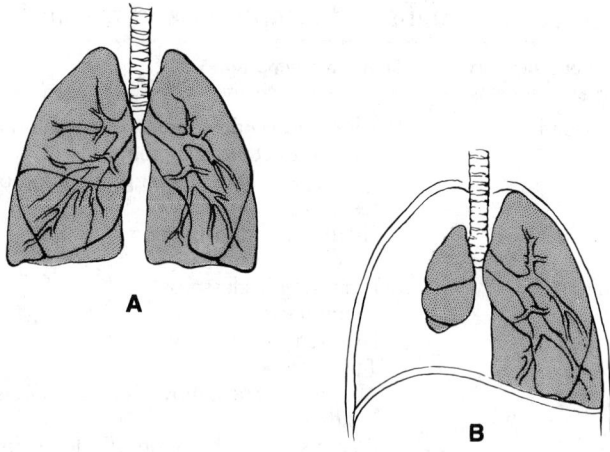

Fig. 24-32   A, Normal expanded lungs. **B,** Complete collapse of right lung caused by air in pleural cavity (pneumothorax).

compression of mediastinal contents (heart and great vessels), resulting in decreased cardiac output and decreased venous return.

An *open pneumothorax* occurs when a penetrating chest wound opens the intrapleural space to atmospheric pressure. Each time the patient inspires, air is sucked into the intrapleural space, increasing intrapleural pressure. An open pneumothorax is also called a sucking chest wound because the wound makes a sucking sound on inspiration and expiration. Blood also may leak into the pleural cavity creating a *hemothorax.*

The signs and symptoms and medical management of the various types of pneumothorax are presented in Table 24-23.

Nursing Process
Assessment
Subjective data

1. The nature of the injury
2. When injury occurred
3. Sudden, sharp pain in chest

Objective data

1. Dyspnea, anxiety, diaphoresis, weak and rapid pulse
2. Cessation of normal chest movements on affected side
3. Trachea deviated toward unaffected side
4. Hyperresonance on percussion
5. Breath sounds decreased or absent
6. Vocal fremitus depressed or absent
7. No adventitious sounds

Diagnostic tests

1. Chest x-ray examination
2. Arterial blood gas determinations of PaO_2, $PaCO_2$, and pH.

Data analysis: nursing diagnoses

Nursing diagnoses are determined from analysis of patient data. Possible nursing diagnoses for the person with a

Table 24-23 Signs and symptoms and medical therapy for pneumothorax

Pneumothorax	Signs and symptoms	Medical management
Closed	Small or slowly developing pneumothorax may produce no symptoms Larger or rapidly developing pneumothorax results in: Sharp pain on inspiration Increasing dyspnea Increasing restlessness Diaphoresis Hypotension Tachycardia Absence of chest movement on affected side Breath sounds absent on affected side Hyperresonance on affected side	Observation on an outpatient basis Supplemental oxygen Needle aspiration of air from pleural space Insertion of chest catheter connected to water-sealed drainage system
Spontaneous	Sudden, unexplained shortness of breath	If there are frequent recurrences, silver nitrate is instilled into the pleural space to cause adhesions between the pleurae; if this procedure fails, lung portion with defect is resected and parietal pleura is abraded
Tension	Severe dyspnea Agitation Trachea deviated from midline toward unaffected side Jugular venous distension Absence of chest movement on affected side Hypotension, tachycardia Breath sounds absent on affected side Hyperresonance on affected side Diminished heart sounds	Same as open pneumothorax
Open	Sucking sounds at wound site with respiration Tracheal deviation (trachea moves toward unaffected side during inspiration and returns toward midline with expiration)	Occlude open wound Same as closed pneumothorax

pneumothorax may include, but are not limited to, those listed in Table 24-24 and the following:

Planning: expected patient outcomes

Expected patient outcomes for the person with a pneumothorax may include, but are not limited to, the following:
1. Patient is able to clear airway without difficulty.
2. Lung is reexpanded and cardiac output is normal.
3. Patient has arterial blood gases within normal limits.
4. Patient states plans for follow-up care.

Implementation

Assisting with achievement of therapeutic goals
Initial care for spontaneous pneumothorax

When a spontaneous pneumothorax is suspected, a physician should be summoned immediately. The patient should not be left alone, should be reassured, and should be urged to remain still and not move about. Oxygen and equipment for a thoracentesis should be prepared. Air is immediately aspirated from the affected pleural space, and the intrapleural pressure is brought to normal if possible. If air continues to flow into the pleural space, a chest tube is inserted and connected to water-seal drainage (p. 571). Medication is given for pain.

Vital signs are monitored every 15 minutes until stabilized and then every hour for the first 24 hours (see Table 24-24 for other nursing interventions).

Interventions to achieve patient outcomes
Follow-up care for spontaneous pneumothorax

When air no longer is expelled from the pleural space through the underwater drainage system and a roentgenogram reveals that the lung has completely reexpanded, the chest tube is removed and the person is allowed out of bed. Strenuous exertion, which increases the rate and depth of respirations, should be avoided, but relatively normal activity may be resumed rather quickly. If there are frequent recurring episodes, some physicians instill silver nitrate into the pleural space to cause adhesions to form between the visceral and parietal pleurae. If this procedure is unsuccessful, the portion of the lung containing the defect may be resected and the parietal pleura abraded so that it adheres to the visceral pleura and obliterates the pleural space.

Assisting with breathing and ADL

1. Place patient in upright position to facilitate breathing and comfort.

Table 24-24   Nursing diagnoses and interventions for pneumothorax

Pneumothorax type	Nursing diagnoses	Nursing interventions
Closed (spontaneous)	Knowledge deficit	For the outpatient or patient who has had chest tube removal, instruct patient to: 1. Report any increased dyspnea to physician 2. Avoid strenuous exercise or activity that increases rate and depth of breathing 3. Avoid holding breath 4. Follow physician's instructions about resuming normal activity
	Gas exchange, impaired	1. Place in a semi-Fowler's position 2. Administer oxygen 3. Monitor vital signs 4. Obtain a thoracentesis tray and water-sealed drainage equipment. See p. 570 for care of the patient with chest tubes.
Tension	Knowledge deficit	Same instructions as for patient with closed pneumothorax.
	Gas exchange, impaired	A tension pneumothorax is a life-threatening event. It is imperative that interventions be carried out immediately to relieve the increased intrapleural pressure. Interventions are the same as those listed for closed pneumothorax.
	Cardiac output, decreased	1. Monitor vital signs frequently. 2. Observe for cardiac dysrhythmias. 3. Palpate for subcutaneous emphysema in upper chest and neck. 4. When pressure in pleural space returns to normal, cardiac output will also return to normal.
Open	Knowledge deficit	Same instructions as for closed pneumothorax.
	Gas exchange, impaired	1. Occlude wound with nonporous covering. 2. Same interventions as for closed pneumothorax. 3. Monitor arterial blood gases to determine effectiveness of treatment. Goal is to have PO_2 and PCO_2 within normal limits.

2. Assist patient to keep physical activity at minimum for 24 hours.
   a. Place call light and other necessary objects within easy reach of patient.
   b. Caution patient not to stretch, reach, or move suddenly.
3. Give analgesics as necessary to relieve pain.

Monitoring gas exchange and cardiac output
See Table 24-24 for interventions.

Evaluation

Evaluation is based on patient outcomes. Questions to consider may include the following:
1. Is patient able to clear airway without difficulty?
2. Has the patient's lung reexpanded?
3. Has the patient's cardiac output returned to normal?
4. Are the patient's blood gases within normal limits?
5. Can the patient state plans for follow-up care?

CHRONIC OBSTRUCTIVE PULMONARY DISEASE

Etiology/Epidemiology

As mentioned on p. 531, *chronic obstructive pulmonary disease (COPD)* refers to diseases that produce obstruction of airflow and includes *chronic bronchitis, pulmonary emphysema,* and *asthma*. The disease spectrum associated with this diagnosis ranges from pure obstructive airway disease with the presence of bronchitis but no emphysema, through various combinations, to severe emphysema without bronchitis. The pathophysiologic processes that cause

Table 24-25 **Possible variants of COPD***

Predominant disease entity	Associated obstructive disease		
	Asthma	Chronic bronchitis	Emphysema
Chronic bronchitis	Chronic bronchitis with asthma	Pure chronic bronchitis	Chronic bronchitis with emphysema
Emphysema	Emphysema with asthma	Emphysema with chronic bronchitis	Pure emphysema
Asthma	Pure asthma	Asthma with bronchitis	Asthma with emphysema

*In addition to the nine variants above, the individual may have a combination of asthma, bronchitis, and emphysema.

these changes are neither static nor are they necessarily progressive. Thus all stages are possible, from reversible abnormalities to relentlessly progressive cardiopulmonary insufficiency. There has been much confusion concerning the clinical use of the terms *chronic bronchitis, emphysema,* and *asthma;* therefore the term *chronic obstructive pulmonary disease* is now used rather than a designation of the specific disease. Frequently by the time the patient seeks medical attention, pathologic changes have occurred and symptoms are often moderately severe.

In 1988, nearly 13 million persons in the United States reported that they had chronic bronchitis or emphysema. When persons with asthma are included in this statistic the total number of persons affected by COPD totals 17 million. Persons with chronic bronchitis or emphysema had 169 million days of restricted activity per year, or nearly 2 months of restricted activity yearly for each person. For employed persons with these diseases frequent absences from work are likely to threaten their jobs.[30]

Both the prevalence of COPD and the death rates attributed to it have reached epidemic proportions. In 1989, COPD was the fifth cause of death in the United States, following heart disease, cancer, strokes, and accidents. According to the Centers for Disease Control, the death rate increased 32.9% from 1979 to 1989. For this reason there is no hope of reducing the death rate by the year 2000. The goal set for that year is to slow the rise in deaths from COPD to no more than 25 per 100,000 people. The age-adjusted baseline was 18.7 deaths per 100,000 in 1987. If the 1987 trend continues, the CDC estimates that the death rate for COPD will reach 26 to 28 deaths per 100,000 in the year 2000. Given the difference between 18.7 deaths per 100,000 and 26 deaths per 100,000, considerable change will have to occur if the year 2000 goal is to be achieved.

The increase in the death rate from COPD is believed to be related to (1) the growing tendency of physicians to list it as a primary cause of death, (2) the greater use of pulmonary function testing, and (3) more emphasis in medical literature on the importance of this syndrome. Despite these facts, it is believed that the mortality is even higher than reported because many persons who were reported to have died from pneumonia, asthma, or congestive heart failure probably had COPD. The major factors in this increase in mortality, in addition to improved reporting and the increased aging of the population, is a history of cigarette smoking. These diseases are more prevalent among men than women, but death rates are now showing a higher percentage rate of increase in women than in men. This is directly related to the increase in smoking among women.

Although asthma, chronic bronchitis, and emphysema are classified under the common category, it is clinically important to identify the predominant type of pulmonary disease that is the basis for the individual's COPD. Therefore, in the following presentation, COPD is divided into three major obstructive diseases: chronic bronchitis, emphysema, and asthma. Because the clinical management of chronic bronchitis and emphysema is similar, the care for patients with either of these diseases is presented together. (See nursing care plan for person with COPD on p. 600.)

CHRONIC BRONCHITIS

Chronic bronchitis is defined *clinically* by hypersecretion of mucus and recurrent or chronic productive cough for a minimum of 3 months per year for at least 2 consecutive years in patients in whom other causes have been excluded. It is characterized *physiologically* by hypertrophy and hypersecretion of the bronchial mucus glands and structural alterations of the bronchi and bronchioles.

Etiology/Epidemiology

As indicated in Table 24-26, chronic bronchitis is caused by the inhalation of physical or chemical irritants or by viral or bacterial infections. The most common inhaled irritant is cigarette smoke, and heavy cigarette smoking is believed to be the major cause of the disease. Occupations in which dust or other irritants are inhaled may cause bronchitis, but the evidence for this is not conclusive. However, in Great Britain it has been recognized for years that the highest incidence of bronchitis occurs in large industrial cities with high levels of air pollution.

Prevention

The overall focus for prevention of chronic bronchitis is to alleviate whatever irritant appears to be causing the associated symptoms in the individual. Of all the known risk factors, the most clearly implicated is smoking. The continued inhalation of tobacco smoke leads to worsening of bronchial inflammation and hypersecretion. Thus smoking cessation is an essential step for the prevention of chronic bronchitis. Additionally, such preventive measures as avoidance of repeated infections and prompt treatment of upper and lower respiratory infections are important steps to avoid disease progression. National standards for

Table 24-26   Factors in development of COPD*

Chronic bronchitis	Emphysema	Asthma
Cigarette smoking	Cigarette smoking	Allergy
Atmospheric contaminants	Atmospheric contaminants	Hypersensitivity
Infection	Antienzyme and enzyme deficiencies (alpha, alpha$_1$, and alpha$_2$)	Infection
Chronic irritation	Advanced pulmonary fibrosis	Environment
Gastroesophageal dysfunction	Destruction of lung parenchyma (necrosis, ischemia)	Drugs
		Emotions
		Social conditions
		Exercise

From Tomashefski JF, editor: Chronic obstructive pulmonary disease: a perplexing and challenging spectrum: core curriculum symposium (pulmonary disease), *Postgrad Med* 62:87-151, 1977.

air quality and governmental actions related to improving the quality of the air we breathe should be of concern to everyone.

Progress in the prevention of chronic bronchitis has been impeded by the slow and insidious onset of the disease. Recent advances in pulmonary function testing have allowed identification of abnormalities in the small airways of the lungs. It is believed that peripheral airway changes occur early in the development of obstructive lung disease. Research has indicated that some of the abnormalities associated with small airway changes may be reversible. Thus if high-risk populations could be identified and a feasible screening test developed, preventive measures could be instituted before permanent lung damage and chronic disease occur.

Pathophysiology

The two pathologic changes that typify chronic bronchitis are hypertrophy of mucus-secreting glands and chronic inflammatory changes in the small airways. First, there is glandular hypertrophy. *Mucous gland hypertrophy* and *hyperplasia* from chronic irritation cause excessive mucus production. The excessive mucus and impaired ciliary movement associated with chronic bronchitis increase susceptibility to infection. Bacteria proliferate in the mucous secretions in the lumen of the bronchi. The most common infectious agents are *S. pneumoniae* and *H. influenzae*. As bacteria multiply, they exert a neutrophilic chemotaxis, and pus cells migrate from between bronchial epithelial cells to produce a mucopurulent exudate in the lumen, or the disease may progress to ulceration and destruction of the bronchial wall. The presence of granulation tissue and peribronchial fibrosis result in stenosis and airway obstruction. Small airways may be completely obliterated, and others may become dilated. This chain of events further traps secretions and promotes multiplication of bacteria. There is some evidence that the pathologic changes occur initially in small airways and move to larger bronchi.[107]

Second, persons with chronic bronchitis develop increased airway resistance as a result of bronchial wall tissue changes, mucosal edema, and excessive mucus production. Excess mucus in the airways not only obstructs airflow but also often causes bronchospasm, which further increases airway resistance.

Third, there is altered oxygen-carbon dioxide exchange.

Airway obstruction resulting from all the pathophysiologic changes that increase airway resistance may impair the ability of the lungs to exchange oxygen and carbon dioxide. Obstructed airways cause ventilation-perfusion mismatching at the alveolar-capillary membrane by decreasing the amount of oxygenated air that reaches the alveoli. Additionally, the obstructed airways may lead to atelectasis, which further diminishes the surface area available for respiration. The result of these pathophysiologic alterations is hypercapnea, hypoxemia, and respiratory acidosis (see discussion of arterial blood gases; see p. 527).

Fourth, right ventricular decompensation (cor pulmonale) may result. The hypercapnia and hypoxemia commonly associated with chronic bronchitis cause pulmonary vascular vasoconstriction. The increased pulmonary vascular resistance results in pulmonary vessel hypertension that in turn increases vascular pressure in the right ventricle of the heart.

Clinical Manifestations

Signs and symptoms of chronic bronchitis are manifestations of the underlying physiologic abnormalities that have occurred. Table 24-27 relates normal function, primary pathophysiology, and the clinical picture observed in chronic bronchitis.

The earliest symptom of chronic bronchitis is a productive cough, especially on awakening. This symptom is often ignored by cigarette smokers who become so accustomed to an early morning cough that they take it for granted; some of them even refer to it as their "cigarette cough."

Persons with chronic bronchitis often unconsciously adapt their activity level to accommodate their respiratory symptoms in their daily lives. Thus they do not seek medical help until they experience a severe exacerbation of their symptoms, usually precipitated by a respiratory infection.

Pulmonary function testing reveals a limitation to airflow on expiration as evidenced by a diminished FEV_1. Vital capacity is also reduced, indicating diminished air movement both in and out of the lungs. Lung volumes are usually within normal limits until later in the course of the disease, when the lung volumes may be increased. There usually is no loss of diffusing capacity.

Early in the course of chronic bronchitis, the symptoms

Table 24-27   Normal function, primary pathophysiology, and the clinical picture in chronic bronchitis, emphysema, and asthma

Normal function/ pathophysiology	Clinical picture		
	Chronic bronchitis	**Emphysema**	**Asthma**
Bronchial mucus-secreting glands produce mucus to trap foreign particles and transport them out of lungs	Productive chronic cough, grayish-white sputum; when infected sputum is yellow, inspiratory; crackles (rales)		Inflammation, hypersecretion; eosinophils in sputum
Bronchi and bronchioles			
Carry oxygenated air to alveoli and carry deoxygenated air out of lungs	Inspiratory, expiratory rhonchi; dyspnea: episodic or continual; ↓ FEV, ↓ VC with small response to bronchodilators*	Early-onset dyspnea on exertion, which progresses to continuous dyspnea. Rhonchi, crackles, accessory muscle breathing ↓ FEV, ↓ VC with no response to bronchodilators	Episodic dyspnea, accessory muscle breathing; inspiratory/expiratory wheezing. ↓ FEV, ↓ VC with good response to bronchodilators. ↑ Work of breathing, pulsus paradoxus
Alveolar-capillary membrane			
Semipermeable membrane where oxygen diffuses from alveoli to blood and carbon dioxide diffuses from blood to alveoli	Respiratory acidosis, hypoxemia, polycythemia, tachycardia, cyanosis	Early stage: normal or mild hypoxemia, respiratory alkalosis; late stage: hypoxemia, respiratory acidosis, ↓ diffusing capacity	Respiratory alkalosis with mild hypoxemia Status asthmaticus: respiratory acidosis with hypoxemia
Right side of heart			
Carries deoxygenated blood to pulmonary vasculature for oxygen/carbon dioxide exchange	Jugular vein distention, hepatomegaly, peripheral edema	Right ventricular decompensation	
Lung and chest wall compliance			
The relationship between lung and chest wall ability to expand and contract during inhalation and exhalation		↑ A-P diameter, ↓ lateral expansion, ↓ diaphragmatic excursion, ↓ breath, heart, and voice sounds, ↑ RV, ↑ FRC, ↑ TLC₃, hyperresonance, complaint of episgastric fullness	↓ Fremitus, ↓ lateral expansion, hyperresonance, ↓ breath sounds, ↓ diaphragmatic excursion

*FEV, forced expiratory volume; VC, vital capacity.

tend to be episodic in nature. As the disease progresses in severity, the patient's symptoms are constantly present to some degree. The patient appears increasingly dyspneic, using accessory muscles to breathe. *Chronic hypoxemia resulting in polycythemia causes the patient to appear to be cyanotic.* Increased pulmonary vascular resistance caused by respiratory acidosis and hypoxemia increases pressure on the right side of the heart, ultimately resulting in right heart failure (cor pulmonale). The person with late-stage chronic bronchitis and cor pulmonale appears stout or overweight from edema. Because of the edema and dusky skin color these people are often referred to clinically as "blue bloaters." The person with preceding characteristic appearance is classified by some as a person with type B COPD.

Patients with chronic bronchitis complicated by cor pulmonale often have chronic respiratory failure (gradual onset of PaO_2 <50 and a $PaCO_2$ >50). They are also prone to developing acute respiratory failure (sudden onset of a $PaCO_2$ <50 and a $PaCO_2$ >50) as a complication of a respiratory infection superimposed on their already-diseased lung.

Medical Management

The process of medical diagnosis of chronic bronchitis may include any of the following:
1. Patient history
2. Physical examination
3. Diagnostic studies
   a. Chest x-ray: typical findings with chronic bronchitis increased bronchovascular markings
   b. Sputum studies for culture and sensitivity: neutrophils and bronchial epithelial cells usually present in chronic bronchitis

REVIEW

Table 24-28 Signs and symptoms of and medical therapy for chronic bronchitis and pulmonary emphysema

Chronic bronchitis	Pulmonary emphysema
Signs and symptoms	
Early symptoms	
Productive cough on awakening; often ignored by cigarette smokers who refer to it as their "cigarette cough"	Dyspnea on exertion indicating acute respiratory distress Using accessory muscles to breathe; ruddy color Thin with a "barrel chest" Usually able to maintain resting Pao_2 Cyanosis uncommon Sometimes referred to as "pink puffer"
Later symptoms	
Significant physical incapacity; breathlessness even when walking on a flat surface; noticeable shortness of breath (SOB) and use of accessory muscles to breathe. Cyanosis is common. Ankle edema, bloated appearance, distended neck veins; sometimes referred to as "blue bloater"	
Late in disease	*Late in disease*
Cor pulmonale (right ventricular hypertrophy), right-sided heart failure, and respiratory failure are frequent complications	$Paco_2$ ↑ Cor pulmonale and respiratory failure possible complications
Pulmonary function test findings	
↓ Expiratory flow rates ↓ Vital capacity ↑ Residual volume Total lung capacity usually within normal limits	↓ Expiratory flow rates, especially forced expiratory volume and maximal midexpiratory flow ↑ Total lung capacity ↑ Residual volume Vital capacity may be normal or slightly reduced until late stages of disease. Change in FEV_1/VC ratio
Arterial blood gas findings	
Low resting Pao_2 Elevated $Paco_2$ (if obstruction severe) During exercise $Paco_2$ ↑ and Pao_2 may also ↑	Pao_2 normal or slightly reduced at *rest;* falls during exercise Normal $Paco_2$ Late in disease, elevated $Paco_2$

Medical therapy

Medical therapy for chronic bronchitis and pulmonary emphysema is similar and dependent on symptoms, pulmonary function test results, and blood gas findings. Therapy may include all or some of the modalities outlined here.

Supportive measures

Education of patient and family about:
  Avoidance of cigarette smoke
  Avoidance of other inhaled irritants
  Avoidance of persons with upper respiratory infections
  Control of environmental temperature and humidity
  Proper nutrition
  Adequate hydration

Specific therapy

Medications

Bronchodilators (Table 24-29)
  Antimicrobials
    Tetracycline or ampicillin usually prescribed to treat respiratory tract infections
  Corticosteroids
    May be prescribed to alleviate acute symptoms. Inhaled steroids being used more frequently. Oral prednisone also prescribed.
  Digitalis
    May be prescribed to treat left ventricular failure.

Respiratory therapy

Aerosol therapy

Used to deliver bronchodilators through metered cartridge devices or hand-held nebulizers

Oxygen therapy

  Required for patients who are unable to maintain a Pao_2 of 50 mm Hg or more at rest or who cannot carry out ADL without becoming short of breath; 1 to 2 L of O_2 given by nasal prongs (p. 539)

Continued.

Table 24-28   Signs and symptoms of and medical therapy for chronic bronchitis and pulmonary emphysema—cont'd

Chronic bronchitis/Pulmonary emphysema

Physical conditioning

Relaxation exercises
  Progressive relaxation exercises are encouraged. Best practiced before meals or 2 hours or more after eating because digestion seems to interfere with ability to relax (p. 599)
Meditation
  Meditation more widely used to assist patients to relax (p. 599)
Breathing retraining
  Pursed-lip breathing (Fig. 24-33)
  Leaning forward position for exhalation (Fig. 24-35)
  Abdominal breathing (p. 593)
  Inhalation-exhalation exercises (p. 595)
  Exhalation with exertion (p. 595)
Rehabilitation
  Muscle reconditioning programs specific for the patient

---

  c. Arterial blood gas studies: see discussion under clinical manifestations
  d. Hematology studies: CBC
  e. Pulmonary function testing: see discussion under clinical manifestations
Effective health care management programs for persons who have chronic bronchitis or any of the variant combinations of pulmonary diseases that make up COPD requires a multidisciplinary approach. The multidisciplinary approach to the management of COPD is included in the discussion of implementation of care for patients with COPD later in this chapter.

Medical management of a person with chronic bronchitis is included in Table 24-28, which summarizes a typical multidisciplinary program for a person with COPD.

Nursing Process
Assessment
Subjective data
  1. History of character of onset and duration of:
     a. Cough
     b. Sputum production (amount, color, and consistency)
     c. Dyspnea
     d. Pain in right upper quadrant (hepatomegaly)
  2. Smoking history
  3. Disease history
     a. Influenza
     b. Pneumonia
     c. Repeated respiratory tract infections
     d. Chronic sinusitis
  4. Past or present exposure to environmental irritants at home or at work
  5. Self-care used to treat symptoms
  6. Medications taken and their effectiveness in relieving symptoms

Objective data
  1. Assess general appearance
     a. Patient may appear overweight or bloated.

  b. Check for dependent edema and jugular vein distention
  c. Abdominal assessment may indicate hepatomegaly
  2. Assess vital signs
     a. Elevated temperature
     b. Tachycardia
     c. Tachypnea
  3. Pulmonary examination
     a. Inspection
        (1) Accessory muscle breathing
        (2) Forward leaning posture
        (3) Central cyanosis
        (4) Clubbing of fingers
        (5) Altered sensorium (restlessness or lethargy)
     b. Palpation
        (1) Increased tactile fremitus
     c. Percussion—normal
     d. Auscultation
        (1) Inspiratory crackles (rales)
        (2) Inspiratory and expiratory rhonchi
  4. Assess laboratory findings
     a. Arterial blood gases
        (1) Respiratory acidosis
        (2) Hypoxemia
     b. Hematology
        (1) Elevated hemoglobin and hematocrit
        (2) Elevated WBC
     c. Pulmonary function tests
        (1) Decreased FEV_1
        (2) Normal diffusing capacity
        (3) Normal lung volumes (in end-stage chronic bronchitis lung volumes may appear similar to those found with emphysema)

Planning: expected patient outcomes
Nursing diagnoses and expected outcomes for patients with COPD are similar, regardless of the underlying obstructive airway disease. Thus outcomes for patients with chronic bronchitis are included later in this chapter under the outcomes for patients with COPD (p. 589).

Implementation

See Implementation section for COPD on p. 590.

Evaluation

See Evaluation section for COPD on p. 602.

EMPHYSEMA

Emphysema is defined *pathologically* by destructive changes in alveolar walls and enlargement of air spaces distal to the terminal nonrespiratory bronchioles. It is characterized *physiologically* by increased lung compliance, decreased diffusing capacity, and increased airway resistance.

Etiology/Epidemiology

Although it is not known when emphysema actually begins, there appear to be many years between the initial pathophysiologic changes and the onset of overt symptoms. Symptoms associated with emphysema usually appear in the fourth decade, and disability from disease usually occurs in the fifth or sixth decade of life. The typical individual with emphysema is a male about 55 years of age with a history of tobacco smoking.

The cause of emphysema is not known; however, recent evidence suggests that proteases released by polymorphonuclear leukocytes or alveolar macrophages are involved in the destruction of the connective tissue of the lungs. Connective tissue in the lungs is primarily composed of elastin, collagen, and proteoglycan, which can be damaged and destroyed by enzymes such as proteases and elastase. It has been demonstrated that elastase (produced by alveolar macrophages) can destroy or damage the elastin in the connective tissue of the parenchyma of the lung. Normally, inhibitors found in human serum, lung tissue, peripheral airways, and bronchial mucus protect the lung from the proteolytic enzymes. It is believed that some change in the enzyme-inhibitor balance occurs, which allows the proteolytic enzymes to attack lung tissue.

It has been known since 1965 that some persons have a deficiency of alpha$_1$-antitrypsin and that these persons develop severe, disabling emphysema, usually of the bullous type, early in life. Recent studies indicate that cigarette smoke increases the amount of elastase secreted by the alveolar macrophages and neutrophils and that it impairs the inhibitor functions of alpha$_1$-antitrypsin.

It is estimated that *1% of persons with COPD have a congenital alpha$_1$-antitrypsin (AAT) deficiency.* The mean age for onset of dyspnea related to COPD was 40 to 45 years in persons with AAT. Their mean life expectancy was 50 to 65 years of age with smokers dying about 10 years earlier than nonsmokers.[55]

Patients with AAT can be treated with human alpha$_1$ proteinase inhibitor (Prolastin), which has been approved by the Food and Drug Administration. The cost of Prolastin, which is given intravenously once a week, is estimated to be about $30,000 a year.[55] A recent study indicates that treating patients with AAT would be cost effective because it would decrease complications in those with AAT and increase their life span. Because AAT cannot be prevented, it is important that persons who have it not smoke.[55]

It is not known why some smokers develop bronchitis and others develop emphysema. Differences in susceptibility and the predominant type of disease are believed to be influenced by hereditary or environmental factors or those related to the patient's history.[106] It is established, however, that there is familial tendency to alpha$_1$-antitrypsin deficiency and that relatives of persons with this type of emphysema should be screened and provided with counseling as discussed next.

Primary Prevention

The cornerstone of prevention of emphysema is education. Public education must focus on the pulmonary health risks associated with inhaled irritants, regardless of their source. Increased public awareness of the vital role clean air plays in pulmonary health is essential for the success of any legislative actions promoting air quality standards. Individuals must also be educated to understand the importance of personal responsibility to decrease their own health risk through smoking cessation.

Persons with a family history of emphysema should be screened for alpha-$_1$antitrypsin deficiency. It is imperative that persons with this enzyme deficiency take active measures to prevent additive lung damage from smoking, air pollution, and infection. Persons identified as being at high risk for emphysema may require vocational counseling if their current work environment is known to have inhaled irritants. These individuals also should be counseled to receive the influenza vaccine yearly, and the pneumococcal vaccine once.

Pathophysiology

The type of emphysema can be determined only by descriptive morphology. There are two principal types of emphysema morphologically—*centrilobular* emphysema (CLE) and *panlobular* emphysema (PLE). In CLE, there is distention and damage of the respiratory bronchioles selectively. Openings develop in the walls of the bronchioles; they become enlarged and confluent and tend to form a single space as the walls enlarge. The disease tends to be unevenly distributed throughout the lung but usually is more severe in the upper portions.

In PLE, there is a more uniform enlargement and destruction of the alveoli in the pulmonary acinus. PLE is usually more diffuse and is more severe in the lower lung. It is found in elderly persons who have no evidence of chronic bronchitis or impairment of lung function.[106] It occurs just as commonly in women as in men, but PLE is less common than CLE. PLE is a characteristic finding in persons with homozygous alpha$_1$-antitrypsin deficiency.[106]

The clinical diagnosis of emphysema is inferred from signs and symptoms that are manifestations of known pathophysiologic changes associated with the disease. Physiologic abnormalities characteristic of emphysema include the following alterations:

1. Increased lung compliance. Loss of elastic recoil resulting from destruction of elastin in lung parenchyma causes the lungs to become permanently overdistended. Thus, compared to normal lungs, emphysematous lungs have a larger increase in volume relative to the pressure change that occurs during inhalation.

2. Increased airway resistance. Destruction of elastic lung tissue causes the small airway to either collapse or narrow, particularly during expiration. Thus air becomes trapped in the distal airspaces, contributing to the lungs' overdistended state. The overdistended lungs press against the diaphragm, diminishing its ventilatory effectiveness. Accessory muscles are used to breathe as the body attempts to compensate and force the trapped air out of the lungs. This causes an increase in intrapleural pressure that increases airway collapse.

3. Altered oxygen-carbon dioxide exhange. Destruction of alveolar and respiratory bronchiole walls decreases the alveolar-capillary membrane surface area, which in turn may diminish gaseous diffusion. Persons with emphysema are able to compensate for these destructive changes by increasing their respiratory rate. Thus arterial blood gases remain relatively normal, although mild hypoxemia may be present. Late in the course of the disease, extensive surface area loss coupled with ventilation-perfusion inequalities usually cause respiratory acidosis and hypoxemia.

Normal function, pathophysiology, and clinical picture of emphysema is presented in Table 24-27.

Clinical Manifestations

Typically, the first symptoms heralding the onset of emphysema is dyspnea on exertion (DOE), which progresses to continual dyspnea. Sputum production tends to be scant or absent. Persons with emphysema usually appear thin and manifest a "barrel chest" with an increased anteroposterior (AP) diameter from hyperinflation. The characteristic breathing pattern of the emphysematous individual includes accessory muscle breathing, an increased respiratory rate, and a prolonged expiratory phase resulting from airway narrowing or collapse on expiration. These individuals will spontaneously exhibit pursed-lip breathing (Fig. 24-33), which facilitates effective air exhalation. (Pursed-lip breathing elevates end-expiratory pressures, which inhibits airway collapse during expiration.)

Pulmonary function studies demonstrate an increased residual volume, functional residual capacity, and total lung volume. Diffusing capacity is significantly reduced because of lung tissue destruction. Diminished respiratory air flow is demonstrated by a decreased forced expiratory volume (FEV) and maximal midexpiratory flow rate (MMFR). The vital capacity (VC) may be normal or only slightly reduced until late in the disease; thus the FEV_1/VC ratio is decreased. The degree of respiratory impairment may be estimated on the basis of the ratio of FEV to FVC (see Box 24-27). A significant finding that differentiates emphysema from the other obstructive airway disorders is the failure to show improvement in pulmonary function tests in response to bronchodilators.

Arterial blood gases are often near normal because of the individual's ability to compensate through increased respiratory rate and tidal volume. Indeed, many people with emphysema overcompensate and develop a mild respiratory alkalosis from hyperventilation. Because resting hypoxemia is absent and ventilation is high, these individuals maintain a normal PCO_2 despite abnormal gas ex-

---

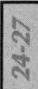

24-27	**Estimate of pulmonary dysfunction based on FEV/VC ratio**
	Normal lung function—greater than 80% predicted values
	Mild impairment—65% to 85% of predicted values
	Moderate impairment—50% to 64% of predicted values
	Severe impairment—49% or less of predicted values

---

change and are described as "pink puffers." A person exhibiting these symptoms of pure emphysema is classified as having type A COPD. Late in the course of the disease the PCO_2 is elevated, which leads to cor pulmonale and respiratory failure.

The terms "blue bloater" and "pink puffer" represent the two extremes seen in persons with chronic airway obstruction. Recently, it has been suggested that the underlying disease alone does not determine whether the person is "blue" or "pink," but rather the interaction between the lung disease and the person's drive to breathe. For example, the pink puffer may just fight harder to maintain a normal PCO_2, whereas the blue bloater settles for less work and allows the PCO_2 to rise.

Medical Management

The medical diagnosis of emphysema may include any of the following:

1. Patient history
2. Diagnostic studies
   a. Chest x-ray: positive finding = increased radiolucency of lungs with diaphragm in a low flat position
   b. Arterial blood gas studies
   c. Pulmonary function testing
   d. Hematology
      (1) alpha₁-antitrypsin assay
      (2) CBC; usually normal
   e. Sputum for culture and sensitivity

Medical management of emphysema includes the same modalities as those used in the treatment of chronic bronchitis. Table 24-28 presents the components of medical therapy used in the treatment of both chronic bronchitis and emphysema.

Nursing Process
Assessment
Subjective data

1. History of and onset of the following:
   a. Dyspnea—(important to investigate if patient correlates the occurrence of dyspnea with any specific illness or other life event; establish how the patient's dyspnea affects ADL)
   b. Cough—usually mild or may be absent
   c. Sputum production—usually scant white sputum
2. Smoking history

3. Family history of emphysema
4. Past or present exposure to environmental irritants at home or at work
5. Self-care modalities
6. Medications or other prescribed therapies and their effectiveness in relieving symptoms

Objective data

1. Assess general appearance
   a. Patient usually appears thin with a large chest. (Note: this is a normal variant in the elderly; thus it does not always signify pulmonary disease.)
2. Assess vital signs for:
   a. Tachycardia
   b. Tachypnea
3. Pulmonary examination
   a. Inspection
      (1) Accessory muscle breathing
      (2) Forward-leaning posture
      (3) Pursed-lip breathing
      (4) Prolonged expiration
      (5) Barrel chest, increased A-P diameter
   b. Palpation
      (1) Decreased lateral expansion
      (2) Decreased fremitus
   c. Percussion
      (1) Hyperresonance
      (2) Low diaphragm
      (3) Decreased diaphragmatic excursion
   d. Auscultation
      (1) Decreased breath and heart sounds
      (2) Late inspiratory crackles
      (3) Rhonchi (Note: adventitious sounds are often not present with emphysema.)
4. Assess laboratory findings
   a. Aterial blood gases
      (1) Early stage emphysema-respiratory alkalosis with mild hypoxemia
      (2) Late stage emphysema-respiratory acidosis with hypoxemia
   b. Hematology
      (1) Positive alpha$_1$-antitrypsin assay
   c. Pulmonary function
      (1) Decreased FEV_1, VC, and diffusing capacity (D_L)
      (2) Increased total lung capacity, functional residual capacity (FRC), residual volume (RV)

Data analysis: nursing diagnoses

Nursing diagnoses for patients with COPD are similar regardless of the underlying obstructive airway disease..

Nursing diagnoses are determined from analysis of patient data. Possible nursing diagnoses for the person with COPD include, but are not limited to, the following:

Diagnostic title	Possible etiologies
Gas exchange, impaired	Low ventilation/perfusion ratio
Breathing pattern, ineffective	Decreased energy/fatigue, airway changes

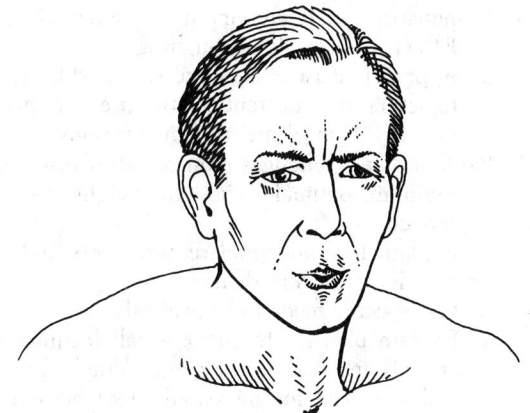

Fig. 24-33   Pursed-lip breathing.

Diagnostic title	Possible etiologies
Airway clearance, ineffective	Hypersecretion, tracheobronchial infection, decreased energy/fatigue
Nutrition altered: less than body requirements	Dyspnea, anorexia, sputum production, medication side effects, fatigue
Infection, high risk for	Decreased lung defenses
*Fluid volume excess	Pulmonary hypertension with resultant increased cardiac workload
Activity intolerance	Imbalance between oxygen demand and requirement
Sleep pattern disturbance	Dyspnea
Fear	Long-term illness and disability, change in role functioning
Knowledge deficit: condition and its treatment	Lack of exposure/recall, cognitive limitation, unfamiliarity with information source

Planning: expected patient outcomes

The following expected patient outcomes and implementation sections apply to patients with chronic bronchitis, emphysema, or any combination of these two obstructive airway diseases.

The patient will:
1. Demonstrate improved ventilation and oxygenation
   a. Arterial blood pH and P_{CO_2} that returns or stays within acceptable baseline limits
   b. PaO_2 at optimal level for individual
   c. Explains how and when to use oxygen therapy
2. Demonstrate an effective breathing pattern
   a. Inspiratory to expiratory ratio = 5:10 seconds
   b. Pursed-lip breathing (Fig. 24-33)
   c. Appropriate use of leaning forward postures
   d. Diaphragmatic breathing (abdominal muscle breathing)
   e. Exhales with activity
   f. Respiratory rate within near normal limits, moderate tidal volume

---

* More common with bronchitis

3. Demonstrate adequate airway clearance
   a. Effective methods of coughing
   b. Appropriate use of nebulizers, humidifiers, mistometers, intermittent positive pressure breathing (IPPB) machine, and medications
4. Explain dietary changes required after discharge
   a. Maintain optimal weight for height, age, and gender
   b. Explain food and fluid requirements and daily plan for achieving them
   c. List specific foods to be avoided
   d. Explain plan for frequent, small feedings that are soft and that do not require much chewing, and the need for increased time required for eating if indicated
5. Remain infection free
   a. Temperature remains normal
   b. Sputum does not change in color, amount, or consistency
   c. If the above occur, health care provider should be informed
6. Achieve a normal fluid balance
   a. Daily weight remains stable
   b. Electrolyte levels remain within expected levels
   c. Diuretics and digitalis, if prescribed, are taken as ordered
   d. If signs of edema (weight gain, increase in dyspnea) occur, health care provider is notified
7. Maintain or work toward an optimal activity level
   a. Pacing activities
   b. Planning for simplification of activities
   c. Participating in planned muscle conditioning program
8. Demonstrate activities to control stress response to symptoms
   a. Muscle relaxation
   b. Meditation
   c. Participation in support group
9. Use effective measures to promote sleep
   a. Determine best position in bed (number of pillows) to minimize dyspnea
   b. Practice methods that promote sleep (relaxation exercises, meditation, guided imagery, or soft music)
10. List common signs and symptoms that require reporting to the health care provider
    a. Change in sputum color, amount, and consistency
    b. Increased coughing
    c. Change in behavior
    d. Increased fatigue
    e. Increased dyspnea
    f. Weight gain or loss
    g. Peripheral edema
    h. Elevated temperature
11. Demonstrate how to carry out the specific exercise program to be followed at home including:
    a. Specific exercises to be completed
    b. Frequency of each exercise
    c. Criteria for monitoring physical response to exercises such as heart rate increase or perceived fatigue

12. Demonstrate comprehension of self-care activities
    a. Explain health maintenance or therapeutic follow-up program
    b. Describe any home medication or treatment program
    c. Explain exercise program to be followed at home
    d. Describe how to obtain professional and community resources necessary to structure a satisfactory environment at home
    e. State plans for ongoing follow-up care
13. Explain the following aspects of home medication or treatment regimens:
    a. State name, dose, action, and side effects of each medication to be used at home
    b. How and when to use medications ordered on an as needed basis (for example, bronchodilators, antibiotics, steroids, antacids)
    c. Techniques necessary for follow-up care (for example, segmental postural drainage, clapping and vibrating, inhalation therapy treatments)
    d. How to obtain and maintain any needed equipment or supplies such as oxygen, nebulizers, humidifiers, mistometers, IPPB machine, syringes, and medications
14. List names and telephone numbers of appropriate community support services such as the Visiting Nurse Association and a home medical equipment supplier

Implementation

COPD and all of its actual or potential impact on the individual's life are most effectively managed by a multidisciplinary team. Pulmonary health care teams consisting of physicians, nurses, respiratory therapists, occupational therapists, physical therapists, dieticians, social workers, and psychologists or psychiatrists provide a comprehensive approach to assist patients to attain or maintain their optimal level of function within the constraints of their pulmonary disability.

A typical multidisciplinary program incorporates the areas listed in Box 24-28.

Although it is difficult to measure the physiologic effects of these programs, hospitalization of patients who have participated in them is less frequent, and most people state that they feel better.

Although the complex multidisciplinary rehabilitation team is the ideal, the nurse functioning in a small community hospital or community health agency can provide effective rehabilitation activities for the person with COPD.

Nursing interventions for persons with chronic bronchitis and pulmonary emphysema are the same and center around the following.

Assisting with the achievement of therapeutic goals
Medications

The types of medications that may be prescribed for persons with COPD include bronchodilators, expectorants, antimicrobials, corticosteroids, digitalis, diuretics, and psychopharmacologic agents.

Table 24-29   Bronchodilators commonly used to treat COPD

Name	Mode of action
Methylxanthines	
Aminophylline	Block action of phosphodiesterase and interfere with degradation of cyclic AMP, resulting
Theophylline	in bronchodilation
Dyphylline	
Sympathomimetics*	
Beta$_1$-receptor sites	Activate adenylcyclase leading to increased production of cyclic AMP, resulting in relaxa-
Epinephrine (adrenaline HCl)	tion of smooth muscle of airway; increase in cyclic AMP also inhibits release of chemi-
Isoproterenol (Isuprel)	cal mediators that cause bronchospasm (histamine and SRS-A)
Beta$_2$-receptor sites	
Terbutaline (Brethine)	
Metaproterenol (Alupent)	
Isoetharine (Bronkosol)	

*Beta-adrenergic drugs.

24-28

Multidisciplinary programs for patients with COPD[57]

Patient Teaching

Patient and family education
  Pharmacotherapy
  Conditioning exercises
    Cardiopulmonary conditioning
    General muscle conditioning
  Pulmonary hygiene modalities
  Relaxation training
  Counseling
    Psychosocial counseling
    Vocational counseling

24-29

Using an inhaler with a spacer

Patient Teaching

1. Exhale fully.
2. Position nebulizer in mouth without sealing lips around it.
3. Take a deep breath while releasing a puff of medication into spacer.
4. Hold breath for 3 to 4 seconds at full inspiration.
5. Exhale slowly through pursed lips.
6. Usually one or two puffs are prescribed.
7. Several breaths may be necessary to receive the entire dose from the spacer.
8. The mouth should be rinsed after completing treatment.
9. The inhaler and spacer are washed with warm soapy water, rinsed, and dried thoroughly.

24-30

Using a hand-held nebulizer

Patient Teaching

1. Exhale fully.
2. Position nebulizer in mouth *without* sealing lips around it.
3. Take a deep breath through mouth while squeezing the bulb of the nebulizer *once*.
4. Hold breath for 3 to 4 seconds at full inspiration.
5. Exhale slowly through pursed lips.
6. Usually one inhalation is sufficient. Several inhalations of a bronchodilator may cause medication overdosage and result in side effects (for instance, tachycardia, palpitation, and nervousness).

Bronchodilators. There are two basic categories of *bronchodilators*—sympathomimetic (adrenergic) agents and xanthine compounds. These bronchodilators act at different sites and appear to work synergistically when used together.[57] Table 24-29 lists the commonly used bronchodilators and their mode of action. Adrenergic agents that work at beta$_2$ sites located in smooth muscles of the airways have fewer cardiac side effects than do beta$_1$ agents whose receptor sites are in the myocardium. For this reason, isoetharine, metaproterenol sulfate, and terbutaline sulfate may be prescribed for patients with hypertension and those who have excessive palpitations or tachycardia from beta$_1$-agents.

Aerosol therapy. Aerosol therapy is one of the most effective ways to deliver bronchodilators and corticosteroids. The most commonly used ways to deliver an aerosol include a freon-propelled metered dose cartridge inhaler (MDI), hand-held nebulizer, or IPPB machine. IPPB is used less frequently and is reserved for persons who cannot inhale repetitively enough to near total lung capacity (TLC) or who are unable to use a hand-held nebulizer or MDI because of lack of coordination or fatigue. Box 24-29 gives directions for using an inhaler with a spacer, and Box 24-30 gives directions for teaching patients to use a hand-held nebulizer. When administering bronchodilators, the solution should be diluted with either water or saline. Some experts recommend that the diluent be water because saline solutions already contain a solute (NaCl) in water. All bronchodilator solutions are high-molecular weight concentrated solutions and have a high solute content. When

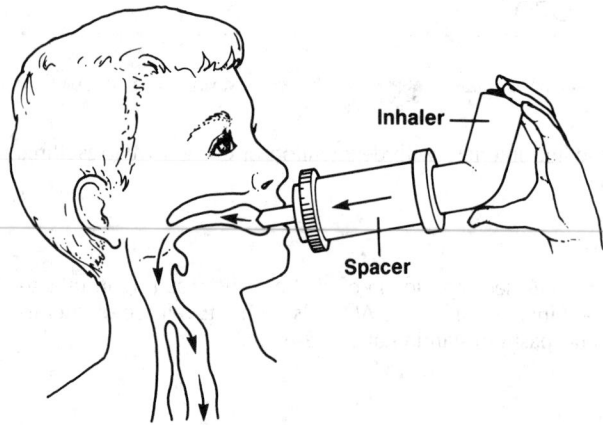

Fig. 24-34   Patient using inhaler with spacer attached to allow for better dispersal of medication.

they are diluted with water, there is a maximal decrease in solute concentration; thus smaller particle size and deeper deposition of the aerosol in the smaller airways results.

Aerosol devices are excellent sites for bacterial growth, and patients using such equipment at home should be advised on how to clean them appropriately.

When a spacer (Fig. 24-34), a molded plastic chamber, is fitted on an inhaler, medication can be delivered more safely and effectively for the following reasons. (1) Large droplets of the aerosol, which would tend to settle in the mouth and on the vocal cords, land on the walls of the spacer instead; (2) the finer droplets in the aerosol disperse more fully within the spacer and can be carried farther into the airways; (3) it is not necessary to coordinate breathing as carefully as it is with the standard inhaler and thus patients are medicated more effectively; and (4) spacers can reduce the number and volume of puffs required, thereby reducing the cost of medication because each dose is used more efficiently.[54]

After the medication is in the spacer, the patient can take several breaths, inhaling each time from the spacer, to receive the entire dose. Inhalers with spacers can be used to deliver steroids, beta$_2$ drugs, and cromolyn.

Expectorants. Although expectorants are sometimes prescribed, some experts believe they do more harm than good.[57] Water is still considered to be the best expectorant, and adequate hydration without fluid overload should be encouraged. Usually 3 to 4 L of fluids daily are recommended unless the patient has *cor pulmonale* and is on fluid restriction.

Antimicrobials. Antimicrobials are prescribed to treat respiratory tract infections in persons with COPD. The most commonly used ones are *tetracycline* and *ampicillin*, 1 to 2 g/day for 7 to 10 days. Some patients have a prescription on hand and self-administer the antimicrobial after telephone consultation with their physician. Antimicrobials should be started within 24 hours of the first sign of a respiratory infection (increased sputum production and

purulence). In patients who are febrile or have other signs and symptoms of infection that do not respond to the prescribed therapy, a sputum specimen should be sent for a Gram stain and culture and sensitivity studies. When antibiotics are used inappropriately, especially in patients who are not adequately clearing their lungs of secretions, superinfection with bacteria or fungi may occur.

Corticosteroids. Corticosteroids may be prescribed for patients with intermittent bronchial obstruction and blood or sputum eosinophilia whose condition is not controlled by bronchodilators. They can be administered orally or by inhaler with the latter becoming the most common method. Usually a short course of corticosteroids is prescribed to alleviate acute symptoms. Prednisone is often prescribed for a total of 7 to 10 days. In some patients with asthma, a longer course of prednisone may be prescribed and some patients are on low-maintenance doses (5 to 10 mg/day) for several months or even years. Long-term corticosteroid therapy is usually not recommended for patients with chronic bronchitis or emphysema unless their disease is rapidly progressing.[57]

Persons who are on long-term steroid therapy should have a tuberculin test before initiation of therapy. Those with tuberculin reaction of 10 mm induration or more are candidates for isoniazid therapy (p. 544). The purpose of isoniazid therapy is to prevent reactivation of tuberculosis, which is likely to occur, in persons receiving prolonged steroid therapy.

Digitalis. Digitalis may be prescribed for patients with COPD and left ventricular failure. The patient receiving a digitalis preparation should be carefully monitored for side effects (Chapter 25).

Patients with increased dyspnea secondary to pulmonary edema, or with right ventricular failure, or corticosteroid-induced fluid retention may benefit from *diuretics*. When diuretics are given, the patient should be carefully monitored for side effects. Those on thiazide diuretics need to be told to eat foods high in potassium such as bananas, oranges, prunes, and raisins.

Psychopharmacologic agents. Psychopharmacologic agents may need to be prescribed for some patients with severe emotional disturbances. The type of agent and size of dose are individually determined, but in general, the older the patient, the smaller the dose. When these agents are prescribed, a pharmacology book should be referred to for information about the side effects and precautions to be used in administering these agents.

Oxygen therapy

Oxygen therapy is required for patients with COPD who are unable to maintain Po$_2$ of greater than 55 mm Hg or an Sao$_2$ of greater than 85% or more at rest and for those who cannot carry out ADL (breathing, eating, dressing, toileting) without becoming very short of breath. In these instances, 1 to 2 L of oxygen is usually given via nasal prongs to relieve hypoxemia and decrease pulmonary hypertension, which in turn, decreases the load on the right side of the heart. It has been demonstrated that

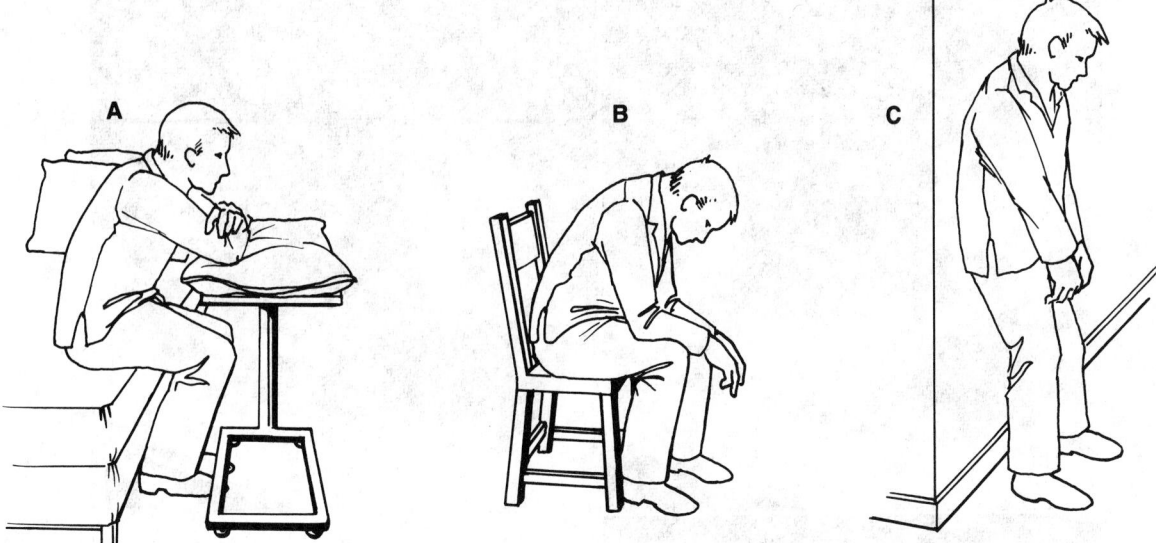

Fig. 24-35 Forward leaning position. **A,** Patient sits on edge of bed with arms folded on pillow placed on elevated bedside table. **B,** Patient in three-point position. Patient sits in chair with feet approximately 1 foot apart and leans forward with elbows on knees. **C,** Patient leans against wall with feet spread apart allowing shoulders to sag forward with arms relaxed.

patients receive the most benefit from oxygen therapy if the oxygen is used continuously. A common misunderstanding expressed by patients requiring ongoing oxygen therapy is that they should only use their oxygen when they are symptomatic (that is, short of breath) in order to avoid becoming habituated to the oxygen and thus requiring higher levels of oxygen. It is imperative that the nurse clarify that habituation does *not* occur and that it is important to use oxygen continuously in order to receive maximal benefits of oxygen therapy.

Interventions to achieve patient outcomes
Improving gas exchange

Arterial blood gases are monitored for indications of hypoxemia, respiratory acidosis, and respiratory alkalosis.

Hypoxemia and hypercapnia often occur simultaneously, and the signs and symptoms of each are similar. These include headache, irritability, confusion, increasing somnolence, asterixis (flapping tremors of extremities), cardiac dysrhythmias, and tachycardia.

If hypocapnia is developing, tachypnea, vertigo, tingling of the extremities, muscular weakness, and spasm are commonly present. It is important to remember that the presence of signs and symptoms associated with altered levels of O_2 and CO_2 depend more on the *rate of change* than on the *degree of change. Rapidly changing signs usually indicate a rapid worsening of the patient's condition.* At the same time, patients with long-standing hypoxemia and hypercapnia may be relatively asymptomatic because they have physiologically accommodated to increased levels of CO_2 and decreased levels of O_2.

Improving efficiency of breathing pattern

1. Teach patient to slow respiratory frequency and to breathe slowly and rhythmically.

2. Discourage patient from taking big gulps of air.
3. Teach patient to increase inspiratory to expiratory ratio so that expiration takes twice as long as inhalation.
   a. Teach patient to count in seconds and to concentrate on increasing time taken to exhale.
   b. Count to 5 on inhalation and to 10 on exhalation.

Teach pursed-lip breathing if the patient is not already using it (Fig. 24-33). Teach the forward-leaning position for exhalation. Using a forward-leaning position of 30 to 40 degrees with the head tilted at a 16- to 18-degree angle is a very effective way to improve exhalation (Fig. 24-35). As mentioned earlier, patients with emphysema have increased TLC and residual volume (RV) with the diaphragm in a fixed flattened position. For this reason, the diaphragm cannot assit in exhalation as it does normally. Leaning forward allows more air to be removed from the lungs on exhalation. The leaning-forward position can be achieved in either a sitting or standing position. For example, (1) the patient can sit on the edge of the bed or a chair and lean forward on two or three pillows placed on a table or overbed stand; (2) the patient can sit in a chair with the legs spread apart shoulder width (or wider, if obese) with the elbows on the knees and the arms and hands relaxed; or (3) the patient can stand with the back and hips against the wall with the feet spread apart and about 12 inches (30 cm) from the wall. The patient then relaxes and leans forward. In these positions the patient cannot use the accessory muscles of respiration, and the upward action of the diaphragm is improved.

Abdominal breathing and exercises. Teach abdominal breathing, leg raising exercises, inhalation-exhalation exercises, and muscle reconditioning exercises.

Abdominal breathing improves the breathing efficiency

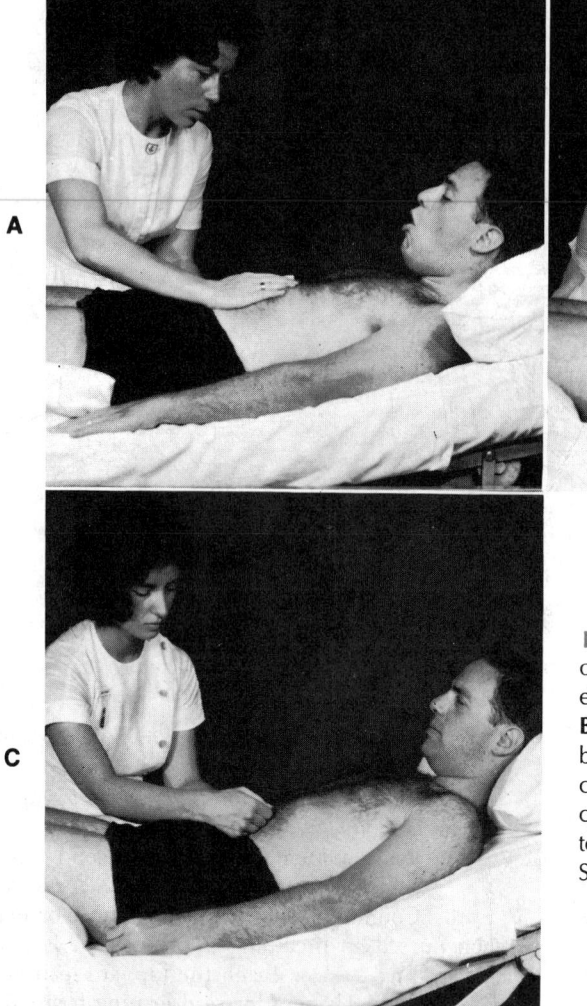

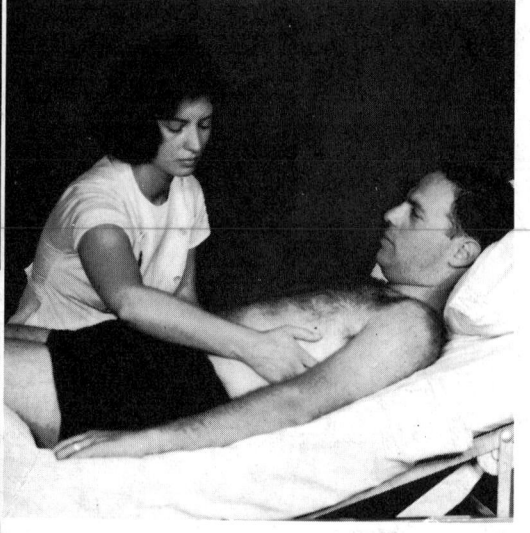

Fig. 24-36 A, When made to breathe against the resistance offered by the therapist's hands, the patient is made aware of every phase of his respiration and use of muscle groups. **B,** The patient learns how to fully expand his lower lobes by breathing against counterpressure applied to the side of the chest during inspiration. **C,** The patient is taught diaphragmatic control by breathing against a resistance applied in the costophrenic angle. (From Bendixen HH, et al: *Respiratory care,* St Louis, 1965, Mosby—Year Book.)

of persons with COPD because it assists the patient to elevate the diaphragm. Abdominal breathing can be taught in the sitting or lying position. In the sitting position, the patient sits on the side of the bed or in a chair and holds a small pillow or a book against the abdomen. The patient then exhales slowly while leaning forward and pressing the pillow or book against the abdomen. In the lying position, a small pillow or a book is placed on the abdomen and the patient is asked to "puff out" the abdomen and raise the pillow or book as high as possible. The patient then exhales slowly through pursed lips while pulling in on the abdominal muscles. Manual pressure on the upper abdomen during expiration facilitates this maneuver (Fig. 24-36). In addition to abdominal breathing, exercises to strengthen the abdominal muscles assist patients to use their abdominal muscles more effectively in emptying their lungs.

This "controlled" breathing pattern is to be used while performing various activities of daily living—from sitting, standing, walking, and climbing stairs to more complex activities. As this pattern becomes natural, it will be used automatically during periods of increased shortness of breath. Persons who do not know how to use controlled breathing tend to increase their respiratory rate and their

work of breathing when they are short of breath. As a result, physiologic obstruction increases, oxygen requirements increase, and effective ventilation decreases. Changing a person's respiratory pattern requires a great deal of effort by both the individual and those providing care.

This same method of teaching augmented abdominal (diaphragmatic) breathing can be used to teach the patient to cough. The difference is that expiration is forced down to residual volume. This maneuver often stimulates the cough reflex. If it does not, the person is taught to actively cough at the end of full expiration. Physiologically, forced expiration simulates the effects of a cough and is, therefore, more effective than telling the patient to take a deep breath and then cough.

Leg-raising exercises, with each leg being raised alternately as the patient exhales, is one way to strengthen abdominal muscles. Another way is to have the patient raise the head and shoulders from the bed while he or she exhales. Not all patients can do all exercises, but most can do some of them on a daily or twice-daily basis. With practice and encouragement the patient can do the exercises 10 times each morning and evening after clearing the lungs as completely as possible of secretions.

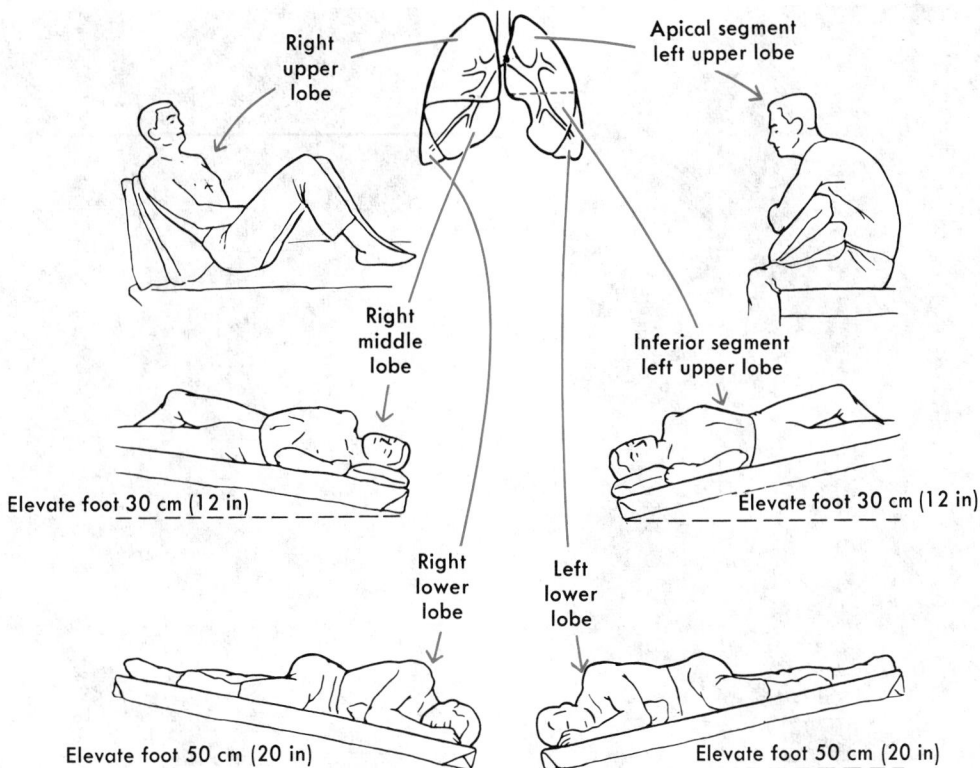

Right upper lobe

Apical segment left upper lobe

Right middle lobe

Inferior segment left upper lobe

Elevate foot 30 cm (12 in)

Elevate foot 30 cm (12 in)

Right lower lobe

Left lower lobe

Elevate foot 50 cm (20 in)

Elevate foot 50 cm (20 in)

Fig. 24-37   Postural drainage requires that the patient assume various positions to facilitate the flow of secretions from various portions of the lung into the bronchi, trachea, and throat so that they can be raised and expectorated more easily. Drawing shows the correct position to drain various portions of the lung.

Inhalation-exhalation exercises emphasize the need to prolong exhalation about four to five times longer than inhalation. Patients who walk can be taught to count in seconds and to concentrate on exhaling slowly and fully. While learning to *exhale with exertion,* the patient exhales during an activity such as bending over or sitting down.

Muscle reconditioning refers to a variety of exercises that tone muscles. For patients who are able to be out of bed, walking, using a treadmill, or riding a stationary bicycle is helpful. The exercise period is started slowly with 10 minutes twice daily three times a week, increasing to 20 minutes twice daily three times a week. The patient needs to be assessed for his or her ability to carry out such an exercise program, and a staff member should be present during the exercise period.

Pulmonary physiotherapy.   The person who has difficulty breathing may be taught how to increase the efficiency of his or her breathing pattern. Breathing exercises are usually a part of pulmonary physiotherapy, which may also include *segmental postural drainage, clapping,* and *vibrating.* Although pulmonary physiotherapy activities may be performed by a physical therapist, they are often part of a nurse's responsibility. Regardless of where the primary responsibility lies, nurses must be familiar with the techniques so that they can demonstrate and reinforce them and ensure that the individual is doing them correctly. Also, the need for pulmonary physiotherapy may occur at a time when the physical therapist is not available to the patient.

Segmental postural drainage.   Segmental postural drainage with clapping and vibration is a technique used to combine the force of gravity with the natural ciliary activity of the small bronchial airways to move secretions upward toward the main bronchi and the trachea. From this point the patient can cough secretions up, or they can be suctioned. In the treatment of chronic obstructive pulmonary disease, drainage of all segments is usually accomplished by placing patients in various postural drainage positions (Fig. 24-37). Treatment may also be directed at draining specific areas of the lung. While the patient is in each position, *clapping* with a cupped hand is performed over the area being drained. This maneuver helps to loosen secretions and stimulate coughing (Fig. 24-38). After clapping the area for approximately 1 minute, the patient is instructed to breathe deeply. *Vibrating* (pressure applied with a vibrating movement of the hand on the chest) is performed during expiratory phase of the deep breath (Fig. 24-39). This assists the patient to exhale more fully. The procedure is repeated as necessary. When the patient cannot tolerate a head-down position, a modified position is used.

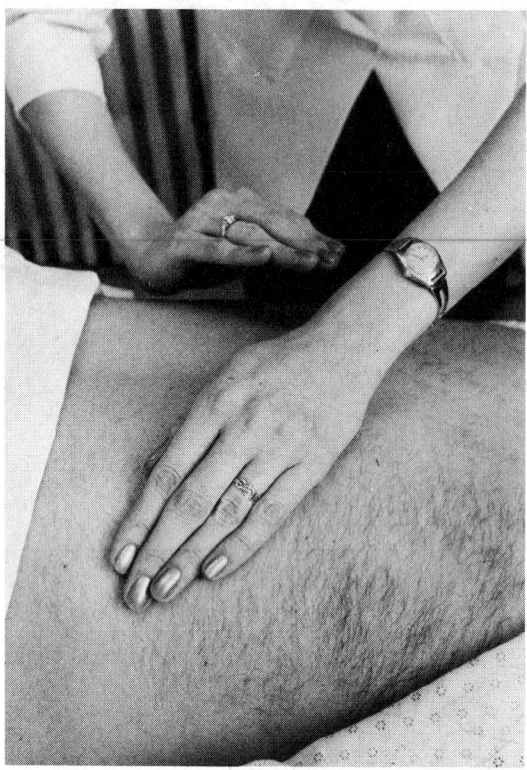

Fig. 24-38 Position of the hands for clapping the chest to loosen secretions.

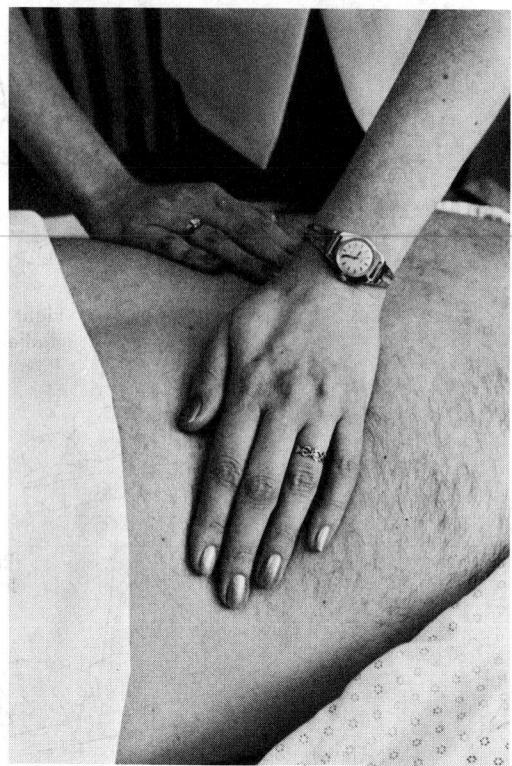

Fig. 24-39 Position of the hands for vibrating the chest at the end of prolonged expiration. Upper hand is cupped in preparation for clapping. Lower hand at end of clapping motion.

Positions that provide gravity drainage of the lungs can be achieved in several ways, and the procedure selected usually depends on the age and general condition of the person as well as the lobe or lobes of the lungs where secretions have accumulated. A young person usually can tolerate greater lowering of the head than an elderly person whose vascular system adapts less rapidly to change of position. A severely debilitated patient may only be able to tolerate slight changes in position.

Postural drainage can be accomplished in several ways. Electric hospital beds can be tilted into a head-down position with little difficulty. If an electric bed is not available (for example, in the home), blocks can be placed under the casters at the foot of the bed or a hydraulic lift can be used under the foot of the bed. If these are not available, the foot of the bed can be supported on the seat of a firm chair to provide a position in which the head is lowered.

The nurse needs to know the part of the lung that is affected and how to position the patient to drain that portion of the lung. For example, if the right middle lobe of the lung is affected, drainage will be accomplished best by way of the right middle bronchus. The patient should lie supine with the body turned at approximately a 45-degree angle. The angle can be maintained by pillow supports placed under the right side from the shoulders to the hips. The foot of the bed is raised about 30 cm (12 inches). This position can be maintained fairly comfortably by most patients for half an hour at a time. On the other hand, if the lower posterior area of the lung is affected, the foot of the bed can be raised 45 to 50 cm (18 to 20 inches) with

the patient assuming a prone position for drainage. A summary of the positions for segmental postural drainage is given in Table 24-30.

Postural drainage and percussion should be planned so as to achieve maximal benefit. The best time is generally in the morning soon after arising and at night before retiring. Frequency of treatments depends on each person's needs, but care should be taken to avoid exhaustion, which results in shallow ventilation and negates the positive effects of the treatment.

Patients having postural drainage of any kind are encouraged to breathe deeply and to cough forcefully to help dislodge thick sputum and exudate that is pooled in distended bronchioles, particularly after inactivity. Humidity, bronchodilators, or liquefying agents often are given 15 to 20 minutes before postural drainage is started, because they facilitate the removal of secretions. The patient may find that sputum can best be raised on resuming an upright position even though no drainage appeared while lying down with the head and chest lowered.

Because some patients complain of dizziness when assuming positions for postural drainage, the nurse stays with the patient during the first few times and reports any persistent dizziness or unusual discomfort to the physician.

Postural drainage may be contraindicated in some persons because of *heart disease, hypertension, increased intracranial pressure, extreme dyspnea,* or *advanced age.* However, most people can be taught to assume the positions for postural drainage and can proceed without help after being supervised once or twice.

Table 24-30   Positions for segmental postural drainage, clapping, and vibrating

Area of lung	Position of patient	Area to be clapped or vibrated
Upper lobe		
Apical bronchus	Semi-Fowler's position, leaning to right, then left, then forward	Over area of shoulder blades with fingers extending over clavicles
Posterior bronchus	Upright at 45-degree angle, rolled forward against a pillow at 45 degrees on left and then right side	Over shoulder blade on each side
Anterior bronchus	Supine with pillow under knees	Over anterior chest just below clavicles
Middle lobe (lateral and medial bronchus)	Trendelenburg's position at 30-degree angle or with foot of bed elevated 35-40 cm (14-16 inches), turned slightly to left	Anterior and lateral right chest from axillary fold to midanterior chest
Lingula (superior and inferior bronchus)	Trendelenburg's position at 30-degree angle or with foot of bed elevated 35-40 cm (14-16 inches), turned slightly to right	Left axillary fold to midanterior chest
Apical bronchus	Prone with pillow under hips	Lower third of posterior rib cage on both sides
Medial bronchus	Trendelenburg's position at 45-degree angle or with foot of bed raised 45-50 cm (18-20 inches) on right side	Lower third of left posterior rib cage
Lateral bronchus	Trendelenburg's position at 45-degree angle or with foot of bed raised 45-50 cm (18-20 inches) on left side	Lower third of right posterior rib cage
Posterior bronchus	Prone Trendelenburg's position at 45-degree angle with pillow under hips	Lower third of posterior rib cage on both sides

Chest percussion (clapping) is *contraindicated in patients with pulmonary emboli, hemorrhage, exacerbation of bronchospasms,* or *severe pain* and *over areas of resectable carcinoma.* Often patients with a chronic pulmonary problem need to be taught to perform postural drainage independently so that they can continue it at home. The position usually is maintained for 10 minutes at first, and the period of time is gradually lengthened to 15 to 30 minutes as the patient becomes accustomed to the position. At first, elderly persons usually are able to tolerate these positions only for a few minutes. They need more assistance than other patients during the procedure and immediately thereafter. They should be assisted to a normal position in bed and required to lie flat for a few minutes before sitting up or getting out of bed. This helps to prevent dizziness and reduces the danger of accidents from orthostatic hypotension.

The patient may feel nauseated because of the odor and taste of sputum. Therefore, the procedure should be timed so that it comes at least 1 hour before meals. A short rest period following the treatment often improves postural drainage. Aromatic mouth washes should be available for frequent use by any patient who is expectorating sputum freely.

Improving nutritional intake

Persons with COPD often demonstrate excessive weight loss. Some of the factors that may contribute to weight loss are:

1. A feeling of satiety with small amounts of food because of compression of abdominal contents by the flattened diaphragm
2. Dyspnea interfering with eating
3. Increased dyspnea when eating caused by stomach pushing up against the diaphragm
4. Decreased appetite secondary to chronic sputum production
5. Gastric irritation associated with bronchodilators and steroids
6. Increased work of breathing requiring increased caloric intake to maintain weight; makes it imperative that the patient with COPD maintain adequate nutritional levels because:
   a. A diminished total weight is correlated with a dramatic decrease in respiratory muscle (especially the diaphragm) size and strength[101]
   b. Inadequate nutritional status and in particular deficiencies in vitamins A and C decrease resistance to infection
   c. Protein insufficiency decreases colloid osmotic pressure, which increases the risk of pulmonary edema

Nursing actions focused on assisting the patient with COPD to maintain adequate nutrition include the following:

1. Explore usual dietary habits (collect a 24-hour diet history).
2. Counsel patient to select foods that provide a high-protein, high-caloric diet (see Box 24-31).
3. Encourage vitamin supplementation. It is important to counsel the patient to select foods that provide higher calorie levels through higher fat content rather than by high carbohydrate levels. Persons with advanced chronic bronchitis or emphysema are unable to breathe off the excess carbon dioxide that is a natural end product of carbohydrate metabolism. Therefore, calories obtained from high carbohydrate foods may elevate arterial carbon dioxide levels in persons with COPD.

24-31

Foods to increase protein and caloric intake*
Offer frequent small feedings of foods high in protein and calories such as the following: Milk shakes Flavored gelatin or pudding with whipped cream Cream soups made with half-and-half Peanut butter spread on crackers, bananas, pears, or apples Crackers and cheese, nuts, dried fruits, and ice creams readily available for snacks
*Excellent sources for suggestions to increase protein and calorie intake are McCauley K and Weaver R: Cardiac and pulmonary diseases-nutritional implications. *Nurs Clin North Am* 18:81-95, 1983; and Spector N: Nutritional support of the ventilator-dependent patient. *Nurs Clin North Am* 24:407-414, 1989; and Cerrato PL: The special nutritional needs of a COPD patient, *RN* 11:75-76, 1987.

4. Prepackaged food supplements such as milk shakes or snack bars taken between meals provide an excellent source of protein and calories.
5. Smaller, more frequent meals are often tolerated better than three larger meals.
6. Consider financial and ethnic background when planning for meals.

Preventing infection

The *most common complication of COPD* and cause of most hospital readmissions, is *respiratory infection*. Pulmonary system response to the infectious process includes increased respiratory rate, mucosal irritation, and increased mucus production. Because of these localized responses, patients may present with bronchospasm and a change in their pattern of sputum production (see list of signs and symptoms on p. 585). If the infection remains untreated, the end result is an overall increased work of breathing with eventual respiratory failure. Thus for the person with COPD, it is imperative that respiratory infections be avoided. The patient should be counseled to take the following steps to *decrease* the chance of contracting a pulmonary infection.

1. Avoid large crowds, especially during known influenza seasons.
   a. Avoid contact with people who have an upper respiratory infection.
   b. Get influenza and pneumonia immunizations
2. Contact health care provider if the following common signs and symptoms occur:
   a. Change in sputum color, amount, and consistency
   b. Increased cough
   c. Change in behavior (for example, more argumentive than usual) that indicates an increase in PCO_2
   d. Increased fatigue
   e. Increased dyspnea
   f. Weight gain
   g. Peripheral edema
   h. Elevated temperature

Antimicrobial agents are prescribed to treat respiratory tract infections in persons with COPD. The most commonly used antimicrobials are tetracycline or ampicillin, 1 to 2 g/day for 7 to 10 days. Some patients have a prescription on hand and self-administer the antimicrobial agent after telephone consultation with their physician. Antimicrobials should be started within 24 hours of the first signs of a respiratory infection. Patients who have a fever or who have other signs and symptoms of infection that do not respond to the prescribed therapy should have a sputum specimen sent for a gram stain and culture and sensitivity studies. When antibiotics are used inappropriately, especially in patients who are not adequately clearing their lungs of secretions, superinfection with bacteria or fungi may occur. Although these regimens of prophylactic treatment do not appear to decrease the incidence of infection, they do decrease the severity and duration of the infection.[25]

Preventing fluid volume excess

Low arterial blood oxygen is a potent pulmonary vasoconstrictor. Pulmonary vasoconstriction increases pulmonary arterial pressure. If pulmonary hypertension exists for a prolonged period of time, the increased workload on the heart's right ventricle will ultimately result in *right ventricular failure* and what is known as pulmonary heart disease or *cor pulmonale*. Depending on its severity and duration, cor pulmonale may be characterized by neck vein distention, hepatomegaly, dependent peripheral edema, and, as oncotic pressure is exceeded, ascites and pleural effusions. Nursing interventions for fluid volume excess resulting from cor pulmonale are based on the understanding that the disease is treated by intervening with the underlying cause of the pulmonary hypertension. Therefore, nursing interventions focus on promoting adequate ventilation for optimal oxygen/carbon dioxide exchange and relieving symptoms that result from the fluid volume excess. Thus a nursing plan of care for the person with COPD that promotes optimal ventilation also intervenes with fluid volume excess resulting from cor pulmonale. Additionally, interventions focused on the symptoms of fluid volume excess include:

1. Weigh daily in the same amount of clothing and at the same time of day on the same scale.
2. Monitor intake and output accurately. (Note: Although it is unknown if fluid restriction is effective in the actual treatment of cor pulmonale, excess fluid intake may overwhelm an already compromised cardiac system.)
3. Encourage moderate exercise or change patient's position frequently to promote adequate perfusion in lung.
4. Measure abdominal girth at regular intervals to assess the possible presence or progression of ascites.
5. Administer diuretics as ordered. When diuretics are given, the patient should be carefully monitored for side effects. Those on thiazide diuretics will need to be taught about eating foods high in potassium such as bananas, oranges, prunes, and raisins.
6. Administer digitalis as ordered. (Note: Digitalis is of questionable usefulness in pure right-sided heart failure.) Persons receiving digitalis should be carefully monitored for side effects.

24-32

Progressive relaxation exercises[84]

1. Contract each muscle to a count of 10 and then relax it.
2. Do exercises in quiet room while sitting or lying in a comfortable position.
3. Do exercises to relaxing music, if desired.
4. Have another person serve as a "coach" by giving command to contract muscle, count to 10, and relax muscle.
5. The following are examples of exercises helpful to some persons with COPD.
   a. Raise shoulders, shrug them, and relax for 5 seconds; then relax them completely.
   b. Make a fist of both hands, squeeze them tightly for 5 seconds, and then relax them completely.

24-33

Meditation exercises

1. Sit or lie quietly with eyes closed and attempt to relax all muscles, beginning with feet and moving upward (see relaxation techniques at left).
2. Breathe in through the nose slowly (may help to count slowly to four on inhalation), exhale slowly through pursed lips (mentally count to six) with a natural rhythm, relaxed and peaceful (this can be coached or done privately).
3. Survey the body for points of tension. Consciously relax the tense areas. The body is peaceful and relaxed.
4. Continue breathing as above, aware of the feeling of well-being throughout your body. This can be continued for 10 to 20 mintues, or after 5 minutes go to step 5.
5. Listen for (or visualize) a special relaxing sound (or image) such as relaxing sound or picture. Listen to it closely (or visualize) all the while breathing as above.
6. At this point positive suggestion can be used; for example, "I am in control of my body. When I find myself getting tense I can take a moment to stop and breathe in all the air that I need and let the tension flow away."
7. After mental suggestion continue breathing easily and slowly come back to normal alert mental state.
8. Meditation can be used at any time to induce a relaxed state of mind (for example, to promote sleep).

Assisting with breathing and rest

1. Place patient in position of comfort, usually Fowler's or high Fowler's.
2. Assist patient with progressive relaxation exercises and meditation (see Boxes 24-32 and 24-33).

Assisting with control of environment

Abrupt changes in weather or hot or cold environments can increase sputum production and bronchial obstruction.

Temperature and humidity

1. Humidity of 30% to 50% is ideal. This can be achieved by a humidifier as necessary.
2. An air conditioner may reduce dyspnea by controlling temperature and preventing pollutants from outside air from entering. The cost of an air conditioner is a medically deductible expense for persons with COPD.
3. Wearing a scarf over the nose and mouth in cold weather helps to warm the air and prevent bronchospasm. Masks for this purpose are also available.
4. Moving to another climate is usually not advised unless there is some other medical indication for doing so. Persons living at high altitudes may be advised to move to a lower altitude or use supplemental oxygen continuously.
5. Travel by airplane is possible. The airline needs to be informed in advance of the need for supplemental oxygen during the flight.

Avoiding inhaled irritants

Air pollution is a common problem in modern civilization and is a real threat to persons with COPD who should observe the following:

1. Heed announcements on radio and television regarding pollution alerts and avoid being outdoors when an alert is in effect.
2. Use an air conditioner or high-efficiency particulate air filter or electrostatic filter to remove particulate matter from air.

   a. Keep filters clean.
   b. Follow manufacturer's directions for use.
3. Use an activated charcoal filter if offending odors or gas pollutants are a problem.
4. Avoid second-hand smoke.

Improving activity tolerance

1. Allow ample time for activities; do not rush patient.
2. Provide oxygen as needed before and during activities.
3. Encourage gradual increase in activities such as walking.
4. Provide positive feedback on progress and encourage new endeavors when patient is ready.

Assisting with sleep pattern disturbance

Persons with COPD usually only sleep for short periods of time. Most are most comfortable sleeping in an upright position in bed or in a lounge chair with foot rest.

1. Assist with relaxation exercises at bedtime.
2. Give backrub at bedtime and encourage family member to do so at home.
3. Provide relaxing music at bedtime and encourage same at home.
4. Ascertain preferred position for sleep, usually high Fowler's.

Nursing Care Plan

Person with COPD

DATA: Mrs. D. is a 54-year-old housewife with a past medical history of severe chronic obstructive pulmonary disese with cor pulmonale. She has a 75-pack-a-year history of cigarette smoking and stopped smoking 2 years ago (husband still smokes). Patient states: "I am unable to walk back from the bathroom to the living room without a 30- to 60-minute rest." Lung sounds are diminished throughout. Chest x-ray indicates overinflation of the lungs. Pulmonary function tests show severe obstructive ventilatory dysfunction with hyperinflation. Arterial blood gases are: pH = 7.34, $PaCO_2$ = 48, PaO_2 = 69, oxygen saturation = 94%. Current medications include metaproterenol inhaler, Theo-Dur, terbutaline, hydrochlorothiazide, K-Lyte, and nitroglycerin sublingual tablets as needed for chest pain. She is seeking outpatient rehabilitation, including muscle reconditioning and education.

The nursing history identified the following:
- Mrs. D. continues to be exposed to cigarette smoke because of her husband's continued cigarette smoking. Patient stated, "He's never without a cigarette in the house."
- Mrs. D. indicated that her husband's smoking makes it hard for her not to smoke. Patient indicated that she occasionally had a cigarette.
- Mrs. D. is fearful of becoming a "bedridden invalid like my mother." Patient's mother had COPD and in her last years had a cerebrovascular accident, which left her totally dependent on her daughter for care until her death 5 years ago.

Collaborative nursing activities include those to assess (1) Mrs. D.'s current pulmonary function status, (2) establish individualized rehabilitation, and (3) evaluate current theophylline levels. Nursing actions include the following:
- Prepare patient for pulmonary function testing. Explain her role in the testing procedure and describe what she might expect to feel during testing.
- Participate in rehabilitation team meetings for planning Mrs. D.'s program. Encourage Mrs. D. to actively participate in the planning process to establish realistic individualized program goals. Elicit feedback to assess her understanding of the program activities and goals.
- Assess theophylline blood levels and presence of any medication side effects.

Nursing diagnosis: Activity intolerance, related to tissue hypoxia associated with impaired gas exchange/fatigue

Expected Patient Outcome	Nursing Intervention	Rationale
Mrs. D. demonstrates increased tolerance for activity.	Provide frequent rest periods. Instruct patient in energy-saving techniques. Reinforce use of pursed lip breathing. Gradually increase activity.	Improve activity tolerance.

5. Establish regular bedtime to meet patient's usual schedule.
6. Give bedtime snack, if desired.

Assisting with anxiety reduction

Persons who are short of breath are very anxious and frightened.
1. Encourage patient to talk about anxiety and fears with nurse and family members.

2. Take measures already discussed to improve airway clearance and breathing.
3. Do not leave patient alone during periods of breathlessness.
4. Explain to family reason for not leaving patient at home alone for long periods; assist them with securing community resources to assist as necessary (for instance, Homemakers, Visiting Nurses Association, and so on).

Nursing diagnosis: Gas exchange, impaired, related to decrease in effective lung surface for diffusion

Expected patient outcomes	Nursing interventions	Rationale
Mrs. D.'s dyspnea is decreased	Assess respiratory status	Obtain baseline information
	Provide low-flow oxygen as prescribed	Many persons with COPD depend on hypoxemia as stimulus to breathe
	Provide breathing retraining	Decreased work of breathing
	Provide rest periods	Improve tolerance

Nursing diagnosis: Infection, high risk for, related to increased secretions, decreased motility in lungs

Expected patient outcomes	Nursing interventions	Rationale
Mrs. D.'s infections are minimized	Restrict persons with upper respiratory infections	Decrease exposure
	Teach Mrs. D. measures to prevent infections	
	Encourage Mrs. D. to get annual influenza immunization	

Nursing diagnosis: Self-esteem disturbance, related to changes in life-style, dependence on others

Expected patient outcomes	Nursing interventions	Rationale
Mrs. D. participates in necessary activities	Give Mrs. D. opportunities to express concerns about limitations.	Allow for communication
	Provide rationale for necessary activities.	Maintain sense of control.
	Discuss with family and friends the need for patient to maintain role relationships	Increase self-esteem
	Assist patient to identify personal strengths	
	Provide information about community resources.	

Nursing diagnosis: Knowledge deficit, related to lack of exposure/lack of recall.

Expected patient outcomes	Nursing interventions	Rationale
Mrs. D. describes therapeutic regimen and health maintenance	Teach Mrs. D.	Increase self-care abilities and self-esteem
	1. Nature of COPD and need to follow prescribed therapy and activities	
	2. Home medication and treatment plans	
	3. Home exercise plan	
	4. Avoidance of respiratory irritants and infections	
	5. Signs requiring medical attention	
	6. Professional and community resources	

Facilitating learning

Persons with COPD play a major role in monitoring their own condition and in maintaining their physical and psychologic functioning at the maximum possible level.

For these reasons, it is imperative that the nurse thoroughly assess the patient's knowledge about COPD, including its cause and treatment. Individualized teaching plans based on the patient's knowledge level can then be developed. Areas that may be included in the teaching program are listed in Box 24-34.

According to the Centers for Disease control, only 30% of persons at high risk for influenza-related complications, such as persons with COPD, are vaccinated.[16] A Year 2000 national health objective is to achieve influenza vaccination levels of at least 60% in noninstitutionalized high-risk persons. Unless more persons who are at high risk can be convinced to receive influenza vaccine, it is obvious that this goal will not be reached by the year 2000.[30]

Patient Teaching

The patient with COPD

The following areas should be addressed in a typical teaching program for persons with chronic bronchitis or emphysema:

I. Patients should be able to explain, in lay terms, the basic function and pathology of their lungs. The ALA offers several excellent booklets for the lay population. (Your local branch of the ALA can provide you with a complete listing of their various publications).

II. The avoidance of respiratory irritants and maintenance of a proper environment should be emphasized to people with COPD. As discussed earlier, inhaled irritants (especially cigarette smoke) pose a serious threat to these persons. Steps the patient can take to reduce or avoid exposure to these irritants are listed below.

  a. Stop smoking. There are many community agencies, including the ALA, American Heart Association, and American Cancer Society that offer programs for persons who want to stop smoking. The nurse should be familiar with community programs and give a list of them to the patient.

  b. Ask other persons not to smoke in the immediate environment. Inhalation of secondary smoke can exacerbate symptoms.

  c. Pay heed to announcements on radio and television warning of pollution alerts. Do not go outside during an alert.

  d. Use an air conditioner or high-efficiency particulate air filter or electrostatic filter to remove particulate matter from air.
    1. Keep filters clean.
    2. Follow manufacturer's directions for use.

  e. Use an activated charcoal filter if offending odors or gas pollutants are a problem.

  f. Avoid abrupt environmental temperature or humidity changes because they can increase sputum production and cause bronchospasm.

1. Use an air conditioner in hot weather.
2. Use a face mask when going out in cold weather.
3. Use a dehumidifier or humidifier as appropriate to maintain a humidity of 30% to 50%.

  g. If air travel is requird, check with physician about the need for supplemental oxygen.

  h. Avoid large crowds, especially during known influenza seasons.
    1. Avoid contact with people who have an upper respiratory infection.
    2. Get influenza and pneumonia immunizations.

III. The patient should be able to explain the following aspects of the home medication or treatment regimen.

  a. State name, dose, action, and side effects of each medication.

  b. Explain how and when to use medications ordered on an as needed basis (for example, bronchodilators, antibiotics, steroids, antacids).

  c. Demonstrate techniques necessary for follow-up care (for example, postural drainage, clapping and vibrating, aerosol therapy).

  d. Describe how to obtain and maintain any needed equipment or supplies such as oxygen, nebulizers, humidifiers, aerosols, IPPB machines, syringes, and medications.

4. The patient should demonstrate how to carry out the specific home exercise program.
  a. Specific exercises to be completed
  b. Frequency of each exercise
  c. Criteria for monitoring physical response to exercises such as heart rate increase or perceived fatigue

5. The patient should be able to list the names and telephone numbers of appropriate community support services such as the visiting nurse association and a home medical equipment supplier.

Evaluation

Evaluation is based on patient outcomes. Questions to consider may include, but are not limited to, the following:

1. Are patient's arterial blood gases within acceptable baseline limits?

2. Is patient using an effective breathing pattern? Inspiratory-expiratory ratio of 5:10 seconds? Pursed-lip breathing? Using leaning forward position to empty lungs? Exhaling with activity?

3. Is patient using appropriate means to clear airway? Coughing effectively? Using MDI with spacer correctly?

4. Is patient able to explain the dietary plan to be followed after discharge?

5. Is the patient free of a superinfection?

6. Is the patient able to achieve a normal fluid balance?

7. Is patient able to maintain an optimal activity level? Pacing activities? Doing muscle conditioning exercises?

8. Is patient able to demonstrate activities to control stress response to symptoms (muscle relaxation, meditation)?

9. Is the patient successful in using measures to promote sleep?

10. Is patient able to list sign and symptoms (change in sputum, amount of coughing, fatigue, dyspnea, elevated temperature, weight gain, peripheral edema, or change in behavior) that should be reported to health care provider?

11. Is patient able to demonstrate specific exercise program to be followed at home?
12. Is the patient able to discuss how self-care activities will be accomplished after discharge?
13. Is patient able to explain home medications (name, dose, action, side effects) and how to take prescribed medications?
14. Is patient able to demonstrate how to do postural drainage and other treatments and where to obtain necessary equipment?
15. Does patient have a list of names and telephone numbers of community services?

ASTHMA

Asthma is discussed separately from bronchitis and emphysema because it results in intermittent rather than continuous, irreversible airway obstruction. Its onset is sudden as opposed to the slow insidious progression of symptoms seen in bronchitis and emphysema. Asthma is characterized by increased responsiveness of the trachea and bronchi to various stimuli that cause narrowing of the airways and difficulty in breathing.

Etiology/Epidemiology

Asthma is known to affect nearly 10 million persons in the United States, two thirds of whom are adults. Both hospitalizations for treatment of asthma and deaths from it have been increasing. In 1978, there were just under 2000 deaths from asthma. This number more than doubled in the 1980s and was 4800 in 1988. Although no firm figures are available as yet for the 1990s, both morbidity and mortality are believed to be increasing. The reasons for these increases are not well understood. The figures available show that the death rate for blacks is higher than that for whites. Some experts have suggested that the reason is that more blacks are among the medically underserved. Women have higher death rates than men, but the highest death rates are among the elderly (age 65 and over). Deaths in the elderly show increases during December through February, suggesting that a concomitant respiratory infection (influenza, pneumonia) contributed to the severity of asthma, the need for hospitalization, and the number of deaths.

Table 24-31 lists the traditional classification and general causative factors associated with asthma. In any type of asthma, the airway is in a state of easy provocation, and attacks may be precipitated by a variety of factors. Although the classification listed in Table 24-31 is still the most commonly used way of differentiating types of asthma, there is a move away from using this classification system. Clinically, most people with asthma fall into the mixed classification of asthma types; thus the traditional asthma classification is of limited usefulness in establishing individual treatment programs. Experts in asthma treatment are recommending that asthma be grouped as *syndromes* and *classified according to precipitating factors* and *individual response patterns to precipitating factors.*[55] Table 24-32 presents some of the common syndromes of asthma using the currently recommended classification.

Prevention

Prevention of immunologic (atopic) asthma is focused on identification of the allergens to which the person is sensitive. In nonimmunologic or mixed asthma, factors precipitating the exacerbation of symptoms may be obscure. However, identification of causative or aggravating factors is still imperative in order to avoid or decrease the incidence of asthma attacks.

There is perhaps no disease in which knowing the patient well is more important than in asthma. Because sensitivity tests can be performed with only a very small frac-

Table 24-32   Asthma syndromes classified by precipitating factor and response pattern

Asthma syndromes	Characteristics
Atopic asthma	Childhood onset, allergic rhinitis, allergic dermopathy, identifiable environmental precipitating events
Exercise-induced asthma	Airway contriction after exercise
Aspirin-hypersensitivity triad	Presence of nasal polyps, urticaria, and asthma after aspirin ingestion
Bronchospasm associated with nonbacterial upper respiratory tract infections	As described by patient
Industrial asthma	Bronchoconstriction associated with certain industrial precipitating factors

Table 24-31   Traditional asthma classification

Type	Immunologic (allergic, extrinsic)	Nonimmunologic (nonallergic, intrinsic)	Mixed (combined immunologic, nonimmunologic)
Onset	Usually in childhood	Usually after age 35	Any age
Causative agent/precipitating	Any extrinsic protein (antigen)	Nonspecific stimulus	Allergen or nonspecific stimulus
Associated factors	Other allergic-based disorders (that is, eczema) Elevated IgE (see Chapter 41)	Respiratory infections, influenza	Nonspecific

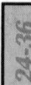

Identifying factors precipitating asthma

1. Be alert for casual comments about daily activities the patient might consider insignificant.
2. Encourage patient to keep a symptom diary. Ask patient to perform the following tasks.
   a. Use a small notebook that can be carried at all times.
   b. Record everything that occurred and was present during 24 hours before and during the onset of the attack.
      When the attack began: What were you doing? Where were you? Who or what else was present? What was the weather like?
   c. Note the time and date that the attack occurred.
3. Write down what you think caused the symptoms to occur, even if it is a guess.
4. Observe patient's interaction with others and reaction to stressors that might aggravate and/or precipitate an attack.

Common factors triggering an asthmatic attack

Environmental factors
   Change in temperature, especially cold air
   Change in humidity—dry air
Atmospheric pollutants
   Cigarette and industrial smoke, ozone, sulfur dioxide, formaldehyde
Strong odors—perfume
Allergens
   Feathers, animal dander, dust mites, molds, allergens; foods treated with sulfites (beer, wine, fruit juices, snack foods, salads, potatoes, shellfish, and fresh and dried fruits)
Exercise
Stress or emotional upset
Medications
   Aspirin and nonsteroidal antiinflammatory drugs (NSAIDs), beta-blockers (including eye drops), cholinergic drugs (to promote bladder contraction and as eyedrops for glaucoma)
Enzymes—including those in laundry detergents
Chemicals—toluene and others used in solvents, paints, rubber, and plastics

---

tion of the substances with which the patient is in contact, the physician usually makes the diagnosis on the basis of a careful history. Knowing about the person's life-style such as the type of work, leisure-time activities, and even food preferences may give useful clues as to what precipitates the asthmatic attack. Nursing strategies for identifying causes are included in Box 24-35.

It is imperative to understand that even though psychologic factors may precipitate an attack, the response to it is physiologic and requires the same treatment as that prescribed for an attack precipitated by an allergen or any other factor.

Pathophysiology

An asthmatic attack results from several physiologic alterations, including altered immunologic response, increased airway resistance, increased lung compliance, impaired mucociliary function, and altered oxygen-carbon dioxide exchange. Each of these alterations is discussed below.

Altered immunologic response

No matter what the precipitating factors are, the basis of asthma appears to be genetic or immunologic factors. The basis of nonimmunologic asthma is less well understood than is immunologic asthma.

Immunologic asthma is the result of an antigen-antibody reaction in which chemical mediators are released. The chemical mediators, which include histamine, slow-releasing substance of anaphylaxis (SRS-A), eosinophilic chemotactic factor of anaphylaxis (ECF-A), and perhaps others, cause three main reactions: (1) constriction of smooth muscles of both the large and small airways, resulting in bronchospasm; (2) increased capillary permeability that results in mucosal edema and further narrows the airways; and (3) increased mucous gland secretion and increased mucus production. As a result, the person with an asthmatic attack struggles to breathe through a narrowed airway that is in spasm. Because breathing is labored, the person breathes through the mouth, which dries the mucus and further occludes the airway.

Common factors triggering an asthmatic attack are presented in Box 24-36. Although allergic mechanisms are important in the pathogenesis of asthma, the many nonimmunologic precipitating factors indicate that other pathophysiologic processes, such as parasympathetic and sympathetic nervous system reactivity, are active in the onset of asthma. *Hypoxemia, hypercapnia,* and *overuse of bronchodilators may lead to an acute asthma attack.*

Increased airway resistance

Increased airway resistance results from bronchial smooth muscle spasm, mucosal inflammation, and hypersecretion of mucus. These airway changes cause obstruction to airflow both in and out of the lungs.

Increased lung compliance

The lungs become hyperinflated during an acute asthmatic attack as a result of air that becomes trapped in the distal airspaces. During the acute attack the person with asthma demonstrates the same symptoms of increased lung compliance that are observed in the patient with emphysema.

Impaired mucociliary function

Hypertrophy of mucus-secreting glands, thickened mucus, and slowed ciliary movement are common findings in persons with asthma. During an asthma attack, increased mucus production combined with slowed clearance of mucus due to decreased ciliary movement results in *increased water loss from mucus.* Thus, the *mucus becomes increasingly viscous* and *can ultimately result in the development of mucous plugs, which may block airways.*

Altered oxygen-carbon dioxide exchange

Increased airway resistance and hyperinflation cause the respiratory muscles to work harder, resulting in muscle fatigue and ultimately exhaustion. In mild or short-term asthmatic attacks, the individual compensates with an increased respiratory rate, which results in respiratory alkalosis. Mild hypoxemia from altered ventilation-perfusion ratios usually accompanies the alkalosis.

In a severe or prolonged attack, if the increased work of breathing cannot be relieved, respiratory muscle exhaustion will result in hypoventilation, which in turn causes respiratory acidosis and severe hypoxemia. If the process cannot be reversed, the person may die.

Clinical Manifestations

The signs and symptoms associated with asthma are correlated with normal lung functions, and underlying pathophysiologic origins (see Table 24-27). *The character of asthmatic attacks can vary on a continuum from chronic or acute mild intermittent attacks to life-threatening status asthmaticus.*

With chronic mild asthma, symptoms are not noticeable when the person is at rest. However, *after exertion such as laughing, singing, vigorous exercise, or emotional excitement, dyspnea and wheezing develop rapidly.* These attacks are controlled with medications, and patients usually can continue their mode of living with a few modifications and no serious lung changes. They are not hospitalized, but they sometimes come to outpatient clinics for medical supervision.

Acute asthmatic attacks often occur at night. The person awakens with a sensation of choking caused by the mucosal inflammation and hypersecretion of mucous. Bronchospasm, with resultant increased airway resistance, causes audible *expiratory* and *inspiratory wheezing. During the acute attack patients appear to be in acute respiratory distress and typically demonstrate tachypnea, accessory muscle breathing, and nasal flaring. They appear to be apprehensive and diaphoretic, and their attention is totally focused on their breathing.* If the treatment is successful, the attack usually ends with the coughing up of large quantities of thick, tenacious sputum. Most attacks subside in 30 minutes to 1 hour, although repeated asthmatic attacks associated with infection may continue for days or weeks. The person is usually exhausted and should rest quietly after the attack.

Persons who are severely affected by asthma and who have attacks that are difficult to control with the usual medications may develop *status asthmaticus.* In this case, the symptoms of an acute attack continue *despite measures to relieve them. Air trapping in the distal airspaces ultimately leads to respiratory muscle exhaustion and severe ventilation-perfusion abnormalities with resultant respiratory failure and hypoxemia.*

Patients with *status asthmaticus* often demonstrate respiratory distress so severe that they are unable to talk. They may be moving minimal air in and out of the lungs; thus audible wheezing and adventitious lung sounds may *not* be present. *During this phase of the attack the patient will appear cyanotic and may demonstrate both pulsus paradoxis and sensorium changes.* This is a medical emergency and the patient requires immediate therapy. Most patients arrive in the emergency room where treatment is begun. The patient remains in the emergency room until his or her condition is stablized. Most patients are then admitted to the hospital for ongoing therapy and observation.

Repeated attacks of status asthmaticus may cause irreversible emphysema, resulting in a permanent decrease in total breathing capacity.

Pulmonary function studies characteristic of asthma show reduction in FEV_1 to less than 25% of predicted. The FEV is usually markedly reduced in proportion to the FVC, although the FVC may also be decreased. Improved flow rates after administration of bronchodilators indicating reversible bronchospasm is a characteristic finding with asthma.

The results of arterial blood gas studies can vary from respiratory alkalosis with mild hypoxemia to severe respiratory acidosis with profound hypoxemia, depending on the severity and duration of the asthmatic attack.

Medical Management

The objectives of medical management of asthma are to promote normal functioning of the individual, to prevent recurrent symptoms, prevent severe attacks, and prevent side effects from medication. The chief aim of various medications is to afford the patient immediate, progressive, ongoing bronchial relaxation. One approach is presented in Table 24-33.

Maintenance Therapy

Concern has been raised recently that many patients may be undertreated and that this may have contributed to the increase in death rates.[54]

As a result, more consideration is being given to the role of inflammation as the fundamental process in asthma. Thus, inhaled steroids along with inhaled beta$_2$-adrenergic agents are being ordered more frequently. The use of inhaled steroids ensures that the drugs reach deeper into the lung and do not cause the side effects associated with oral steroids.[54]

It is recommended that the inhaled beta$_2$-agonist must be given first to open the airway and then the inhaled steroid will be more beneficial.

In one study, patients were given peak-flow meters and taught how to use them. If their peak expiratory flow-rate (PEFR) was below 70% of normal, inhaled medication was increased; if below 50%, oral steroids were added; below 30%, emergency measures were called for and the patient called the physician and went to the emergency room for treatment with oxygen and additional drug therapy.

In Great Britain the use of peak-flow meter regimen was compared with a program based on symptoms alone. Patients were taught what to do if their breathing felt tighter, if they awoke at night with wheezing, if the inhaled bronchodilator lasted less than 2 hours or if relief lasted only 30 minutes, or if they had difficult talking. The study found that the daily use of peak-flow meters made no significant contribution. The important thing was that patients had a systematic way to evaluate their symptoms and knew what to do when they occurred.

Table 24-33 Treatment of an acute asthmatic attack[68]

Therapy	Effects and precautions
Inhaled beta-agonist such as albuterol sulfate (Proventil, Ventalin) or metaproterenol sulfate (Alupent, Metaprel) in normal saline	Stimulates beta$_2$ receptors in bronchial smooth muscle = relaxation. Starts to act in 10 min, effects last 4-6 hours. Monitor vital signs, lung sounds, and peak expiration flow rate (PEFR) before and after each treatment
If above is not successful Methylprednisolone (Solu-Medrol) intravenously. Loading dose 2 mg/kg or about 125 mg every 6 hr then 60-125 mg every 6 hr for 48 hr total or until patient stable. When patient is *stabilized*, change IV to 60 mg prednisone daily or every other day. Nebulized atropine sulfate may be tried or aminophylline may be given intravenously—a pump is used for better control of infusion. Loading dose of aminophylline 4 to 6 mg/kg over 15 to 30 min and then continuous infusion of 0.45 to 0.70 mg/kg/hr. Patients who have been on aminophylline at home will be placed on continuous IV therapy. Rate of infusion is determined by theophylline blood level. Desired level is 10 to 20 µg/ml.	Reduces inflammation and edema of airway and decreases hyperactivity of airway. Benefit seen within 6 hours—full effect in 6-8 hours. Oral prednisone should be tapered off by 7-10 days. Taper 60 mg × 2 days, 40 mg × 2 days, 30 mg × 2 days, and 10 mg × 2 days. Relax bronchial smooth muscle. *Too rapid an infusion may cause severe hypotension, premature ventricular contractions, and cardiac arrest.* Monitor heart rate and rhythm closely and report any changes immediately. Theophylline metabolized by the liver. For persons with liver disease, smaller doses are used. Patients taking Tagamet, erythromycin, or ciprofloxacin require smaller doses. Smokers and those taking Dilantin require larger doses to maintain blood levels.

Nursing Process

Assessment

Subjective data

1. History of asthma onset and duration
2. Precipitating factors
3. Current medications
4. Medications used to relieve asthma symptoms
5. Any recent changes in medication regimen
6. Self-care methods used to relieve symptoms

Objective data

1. Assess general appearance.
   a. Does patient appear apprehensive?
   b. Is there any evidence of altered sensorium?
2. Assess vital signs.
   a. Tachycardia
   b. Pulsus paradoxus (diminished pulse with inspiration, confirmed by a 6 to 8 mm Hg drop in systolic blood pressure during inspiration)
   c. Tachypnea
3. Pulmonary examination
   a. Inspection
      (1) Accessory muscle breathing
      (2) Forward leaning posture
      (3) Dyspnea
      (4) Prolonged expiration
      (5) Cyanosis
   b. Palpation
      (1) Decreased lateral expansion
      (2) Decreased fremitus
   c. Percussion
      (1) Hyperresonance
      (2) Decreased diaphragmatic excursion
   d. Auscultation (Note: as *patient approaches exhaustion from increased work of breathing, breath sounds and adventitious sounds may be absent or faint*)
      (1) Inspiratory and expiratory wheezing
      (2) Rhonchi
4. Assess laboratory findings
   a. Arterial blood gases
      (1) Short-term or moderate attack—respiratory alkalosis with mild hypoxemia.
      (2) Prolonged or severe attack—respiratory acidosis with severe hypoxemia.
   b. Sputum—for eosinophilia.
   c. Pulmonary function testing—decreased FEV and VC.

Data analysis: nursing diagnoses

Nursing diagnoses are determined from analysis of patient data. Possible nursing diagnoses for the person with asthma may include, but are not limited to, the following:

Diagnostic title	Possible etiologies
Airway clearance, ineffective	Ineffective technique, decreased energy/fatigue, impaired mucociliary clearance mechanism, inadequate fluid intake
Anxiety	Threat of unknown or death
Breathing pattern, ineffective	Bronchoconstriction, underuse of bronchodilator medications
Gas exchange, impaired	Mucous plugs, ventilation/perfusion imbalance
Knowledge deficit of predisposing factors and prevention/treatment	Lack of exposure to information, unreceptiveness to information, unfamiliarity with information sources

Planning: expected patient outcomes

Expected outcomes for the person with asthma may include, but are not limited to, the following:

The patient will:

1. Demonstrate effective airway clearance
   a. Effective methods of coughing
   b. Appropriate use of medication and equipment
2. Demonstrate activities to control anxiety response to symptoms
   a. Muscle relaxation
   b. Meditation
   c. Appropriate use of medications
3. Demonstrate effective breathing patterns
   a. Inspiratory to expiratory ratio = 5 seconds: 10 seconds
   b. Respiratory rate within near-normal limits
4. Demonstrate improved ventilation and oxygenation
   a. Arterial blood pH and $PaCO_2$ that returns or stays within acceptable limits
   b. PaO_2 at optimal level for individual
5. Patient or significant other can state the factors most likely to precipitate an asthmatic attack (for example, stress, allergens, and infections).
6. Patient or significant other can state the importance of keeping a diary of symptoms and medications (time and dose) during an asthmatic attack.
7. If the cause is allergic, state how to prepare an environmentally controlled bedroom (Chapter 41).
8. Patient or significant other can explain any home medication program.
   a. Give name, dose, action, and side effects of each medication.
   b. State conditions under which medications might be increased (for example, infection—start or increase antibiotics; increased stress or worsening of symptoms—increase corticosteroids).
9. Patient or significant other can demonstrate how to take inhaled medications (p. 591).
10. Patient or significant other can describe what to do when an acute attack occurs (for example, take medication and be quiet).
11. Patient or significant other can state signs and symptoms that indicate need for immediate medical attention (for example, asthmatic attack unrelieved by usual treatment).
12. If receiving corticosteroid therapy, patient can show card to be carried at all times giving data about the drug, dose, and name of physician; alternative is to wear Medic-Alert bracelet.
13. Patient can state plans for ongoing follow-up care including plans for desensitization if appropriate.

Implementation
Assisting with achievement of therapeutic goals
Medications

1. Given medications as ordered. Monitor IV rates closely.
2. Monitor patient closely for side effects of medications (Table 24-34).

Interventions to achieve patient outcomes
Improving airway clearance

During an asthmatic attack secretions tend to become sticky and can plug airways, causing increased airway obstruction. By mobilizing secretions, the need for intubation and artificial ventilation can often be prevented.

1. Ensure adequate systemic fluid intake (Note: Research findings suggest that overhydration may not increase secretion clearance above levels obtained by normal hydration levels)
2. Provide adequate nutritional levels
3. Provide extra humidity
4. Medicate with bronchodilators
5. Teach effective cough maneuver (see p. 594)
6. If cough ineffective to produce sputum, administer chest physiotherapy (see p. 595).

Providing emotional support and preventing anxiety

1. Do not leave patient alone during an attack
2. Encourage relaxation techniques
3. Guide/assist patient with respiratory maneuvers
4. Assess for possible medication overuse or underuse

Improving breathing patterns

The nursing role in improving breathing patterns and gas exchange is as follows:

1. Place patient in high Fowler's position
2. Encourage slow rhythmic breathing
3. Encourage patient to breathe through nose and exhale through pursed lips
4. Administer bronchodilator and an antiinflammatory medication (corticosteroid) as ordered. Monitor patient for both therapeutic response and side effects to medications. Table 24-34 lists medications, dosage, action, and side effects of medications commonly used to treat asthma.

Improving gas exchange

Arterial blood gas results should be monitored as follows:

1. If respiratory alkalosis is present, encourage slower breathing
2. If respiratory acidosis and hypoxemia are present
   a. Administer O_2 as prescribed
   b. If O_2 does not relieve the attack, intubation and ventilatory assistance may be required

Facilitating learning

After the patient has recovered from an acute attack, the patient's knowledge about asthma is assessed, and the following points are stressed.

1. Keep a symptom diary (p. 604) to help identify:
   a. Possible precipitating factors
   b. Symptom pattens
   c. Efficacy of self-treatment modalities (include time and dose of any medications self-administered)
2. Signs and symptoms
   a. Tightness in chest
   b. Restlessness or vague feeling of uneasiness
   c. Dyspnea
   d. Increased wheezing
   e. Productive cough

Table 24-34   Medications used in treatment of asthma

Medications	Dosage	Action	Side effects
Epinephrine 1:1000	0.3 to 0.5 ml subcutaneously, may need to repeat 2-3 times at 20-30 min intervals	Short-acting bronchodilator	Tachycardia Palpitations Elevated blood pressure
Ephedrine	25-50 mg PO q 4-6 hr	Long-acting bronchodilator	Cerebral agitation (often given with phenobarbital)
Terbutaline	2.5 mg PO	Bronchodilator	Tachycardia Tremors Headache Spasms in extremities
Isoproterenol .25% (Isuprel)	1-2 inhalations, q 3 hr (max. 8 day)	Bronchodilator	Headache Tremors
Metaproterenol (Alupent, Metaprel)	20 mg PO tid or 1-2 inhalations	Bronchodilator	Tachycardia Tremors Nausea
Cromolyn sodium (Intal)	20 mg qid inhaled	Antiasthmatic mast cell stabilizer used as prophylactic against asthma attacks	Nasal congestion Nausea Bronchospasm
Corticosteroids Hydrocortisone	200-400 mg IV (up to 1 g first 24 hr) PO or IV	Antiinflammatory	Corticosteroid withdrawal syndrome, sodium retention, GI disturbance
Dexamethasone	Varies with individual response and disease severity		
Beclomethasone	Inhaled: 100 μg 3-4 times/day		
Theophylline	Dosage to maintain serum concentrations between 10-20 μg/ml	Bronchodilator	Nausea and vomiting CNS irritability Tachycardia Hypotension

3. Self-treatment of signs and symptoms
   a. Take bronchodilator as ordered.
   b. Take epinephrine if prescribed by physician.
   c. State conditions under which medication might be increased (infection-start or increase antibiotics; increased stress or worsening of symptoms increase inhaled corticosteroid)
   d. If another person is not present, call someone so patient will not be alone.
   e. Try to remain calm and breathe slowly; use relaxation techniques at first sign of attack
   f. If symptoms are not relieved, call physician or go to nearest emergency facility.
4. Know how to use special equipment (metered dose inhaler [Box 24-37], inhaler with spacer [Box 24-29], nebulizer [Box 24-30], and peak flow meter if one is prescribed).

Evaluation

Evaluation is based on patient outcomes. Questions to consider may include the following:
1. Can the patient demonstrate ways to maintain a clear airway?
2. Can the patient demonstrate muscle relaxation and meditation exercises used to control anxiety?
3. Does the patient demonstrate a respiratory rate that is within near-normal limits?

Correct way to use a metered-dose inhaler

1. Inhale through nose, then slowly breathe out completely.
2. Place mouthpiece in mouth.
3. Press down on inhaler, while simultaneously inhaling one puff deeply. Breathe in air from around the mouthpiece while inhaling.
4. Hold breath for a few seconds, then exhale.
5. Repeat second puff if one is ordered.
Caution: Some persons with asthma may experience bronchoconstriction after using a metered-dose inhaler. Patients who complain of chest tightness after using a metered-dose inhaler may be reacting to the propellant gases used to deliver metaproterenol.

4. Are the patient's arterial blood gas findings at acceptable levels?
5. Can the patient state factors that need to be avoided to prevent an asthmatic attack?
6. Does the patient have a symptom diary so that he or she can track time of regular medications and the onset of symptoms?

7. Can the patient discuss what he or she has done to prepare an environmentally controlled bedroom?
8. Can the patient state the purpose, dosage, and side effects of each prescribed medication?
9. Can the patient state conditions under which medication might be increased or changed? Infection—start or increase antibiotics; increased stress—increase dose of inhaled corticosteroid.
10. Can the patient state what to do if usual therapy does not improve symptoms (call physician or go to an emergency facility, preferably one where the patient and his or her history and treatment are known).
11. Does the patient carry a card stating drugs, doses, and name of physician or does the patient wear a Medic-Alert bracelet?
12. Can the patient state time of next medical appointment?

CYSTIC FIBROSIS

Etiology/ Epidemiology

Cystic fibrosis (CF) continues to be the most common lethal genetic disease among whites. It is an autosomal recessive disease, and one of every 22 individuals carries the CF gene. When both parents are carriers (heterozygotes), there is a one in four chance with each pregnancy that their child will have CF (Fig. 24-40).

Approximately 25,000 individuals with CF live in the United States. Of that population, 6500 individuals are adults according to the Cystic Fibrosis Foundation Patient Care Registry. More important, the number of adults with CF continues to increase steadily because of increased life expectancy and diagnostic advances. (Fig. 24-41).

Inheritance possibilities

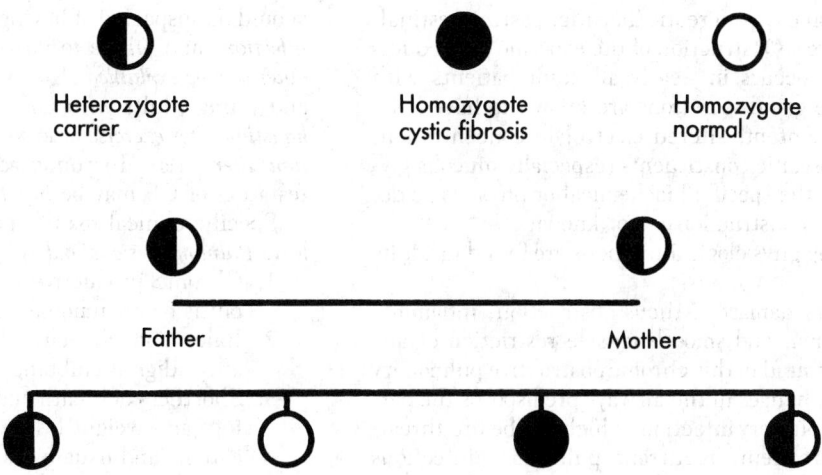

Inheritance ratio equally distributed among sexes (boys and girls)

Fig. 24-40   Inheritance of cystic fibrosis when both mother and father are carriers of cystic fibrosis gene (Modified from CF Foundation Fact Sheet, 1980, Bethesda, Maryland).

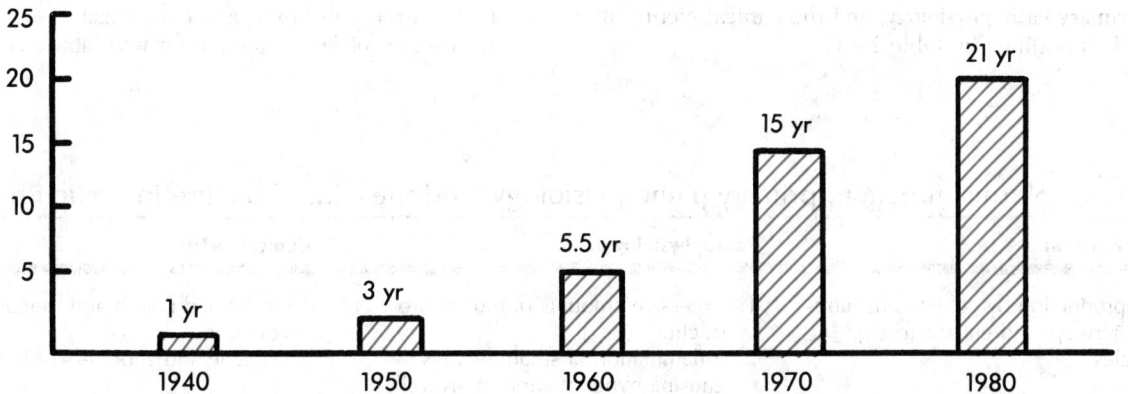

Fig. 24-41   Life expectancy of children born with cystic fibrosis. The number of children surviving to adulthood continues to increase (Modified from CF Foundation Fact Sheet, 1988, Bethesda, Maryland).

Two groups make up this adult CF population: Infants and children and adolescents and adults. Recent statistics indicate that approximately 20% of the adult CF population is diagnosed after age 15.[111]

Reaching adulthood is now a realistic expectation for infants and children with CF. The average life expectancy is 24 years with a maximum survival of 30 to 40 years. The major contributing factors to this increased life expectancy include diagnostic advances and therapeutic interventions.

Prevention

Because CF is a genetically inherited disease, identification of carriers who may pass on the defect and disease to offspring remains the most important preventive strategy. Early identification of carriers combined with genetic counseling minimizes the chance of offspring inheriting this lethal genetic disease. Family histories of possible incidences of CF should be followed up by genetic testing.

Pathophysiology

Cystic fibrosis is an exocrine gland disease involving various systems (pulmonary, pancreatic/hepatic, gastrointestinal, and reproductive). Obstruction of the exocrine gland ducts or passageways occurs in nearly all adult patients with CF.[128] Exocrine gland secretions are known to have a decreased water content, altered electrolyte concentration, and abnormal organic constituents (especially mucous glycoproteins); yet the specific biochemical or physiologic defect that leads to obstruction is not known.

The following physiologic alterations are found in adults with CF.

1. Pulmonary damage. Mucus obstruction, inflammation, edema, and smooth muscle restriction of airways are found in this chronic obstructive pulmonary disease. Changes in the airways predisposes the person to respiratory infection, which can be life-threatening. Frequent, recurrent pulmonary infections erode blood vessels. Brachial arteries branching from the aorta and the lung at high pressures are most at risk for bleeding (hemoptysis).

   Other complications of damage to the airways include *pneumothorax, respiratory insufficiency*, and *cor pulmonale*. These complications account for 95% of the deaths in adults with CF. The normal function, primary pathophysiology, and the clinical picture in CF is outlined in Table 24-35.

2. Gastrointestinal and pancreatic involvement. Intestinal obstruction occurs in 20% of adult patients with CF. Generally, pancreatic insufficiency predisposes to intestinal obstruction. Cramps and abdominal pain in adults with CF should arouse suspicion of intestinal obstruction. Pancreatic insufficiency is reported in 80% to 90% of adults with CF. The pathologic lesions in the pancreas decrease pancreatic enzyme production and lead to malabsorption of fat.

3. Glucose intolerance. About 40% of adults with CF have glucose intolerance caused by obstruction of islets of Langerhans by pancreatic fibrosis.[128]

Clinical Manifestations

Three major clinical symptoms are associated with CF: *recurrent respiratory infections, malnutrition*, and *excessive salt losses*. Early identification of CF often rests on the presence of several otherwise unexplained clinical symptoms. In infants, clinical symptoms of CF may include meconium ileus and failure to thrive. Excessive salt losses in infants may first be detected by the infant's mother who reports that the child tastes salty when kissed. Older children should be suspected of having CF when *recurrent respiratory infections* and *failure to thrive despite large appetites cannot otherwise be explained. Excessive salt losses* in older children and young adults with CF may be manifested by *heat exhaustion after exercise or exposure to hot weather*, or *dehydration after fevers*. In young adults, the *only* clinical manifestation of CF may be *infertility*.

Specific clinical manifestation by system are listed below. *Pulmonary signs and symptoms of CF include:*

1. Chronic productive cough and/or recurrent bronchitis or pneumonia
2. Rales and rhonchi, decreased pulmonary compliance, digital clubbing (Fig. 24-42).
3. Shortness of breath and dyspnea on exertion, wheezing, and weight loss occur with respiratory complications and usually indicate need for vigorous therapy

Gastrointestinal signs and symptoms include:

1. Frequent, bulky, greasy stools
2. Weight loss
3. Cramps and abdominal pain—should make one suspect an obstruction is present

Glucose intolerance signs and symptoms include:

1. Polyuria, polydipsia, and polyphagia
2. Absence of ketoacidosis even with above signs

Table 24-35   Normal function, primary pathophysiology, and the clinical picture in cystic fibrosis

Normal function	Pathophysiology	Clinical picture
Mucus production by goblet cells lubricates airways and entraps foreign particles	1. Excessive amounts of mucus production 2. Inflammation of small airways, causing hyperinflation of alveoli 3. Chronic bacterial infections 4. Eroding of a major blood vessel secondary to infection	1. Increased cough and mucus production 2. Fatigue and shortness of breath 3. Fever, fatigue, shortness of breath 4. Hemoptysis

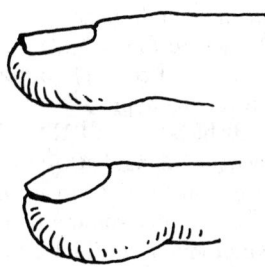

Fig. 24-42 Comparison of normal nail *(top)* and digital clubbing *(bottom)*.

Diagnostic Tests

The diagnosis of CF is confirmed by the presence of *at least two* of the *following:*
1. A positive sweat test with a chloride level greater than 60 mEq/L
2. COPD
3. Exocrine pancreatic insufficiency
4. A positive family history of CF

Medical Management

The goals of medical management of CF are to *minimize bronchial plugging and to inhibit bacterial colonization.*[111]

Measures to minimize bronchial plugging include:
1. Chest physiotherapy with chest percussion and postural drainage for 20 minutes two to three times daily and sometimes much more frequently.
2. Mucolytic agents may be ordered to thin secretions, although ensuring that the patient is well hydrated may be sufficient to thin secretions.
3. Humidification of air is controversial because it has been associated with bronchospasm and bacterial colonization. It may be helpful for some patients, however, and some physicians may prescribe it.

To minimize bacterial colonization during acute phases of the disease, sputum should be cultured and tested for sensitivity. Antibiotics are prescribed based on the results of these tests. Combination therapy with two or three antibiotics is recommended to prevent bacterial resistance and is usually prescribed for 14 days. *Shorter courses of antibiotic therapy are associated with reexacerbation of symptoms.* Oral antibiotics may be prescribed for long-term therapy to inhibit bacterial colonization, although there is little scientific basis for this practice. *Inhaled antibiotics are given in very high doses because only about 10% of the inhaled drug is absorbed.*

Complications and their Management
Pulmonary infections

Pulmonary infections compromise respiratory status and usually result in the patient being hospitalized for routine pulmonary physiotherapy or "clean out." This includes:
1. Vigorous postural drainage and clapping. Some patients will spend up to 8 hours a day consumed by clapping, vibrating, and postural drainage (see p. 595). Mechanical vibrators may be purchased by the patient with CF when physical therapists, nurses, respiratory therapists, or family members are not able to provide the necessary therapy. The majority of patients must have postural drainage with clapping every 4 hours. Respiratory personnel and nurses share the treatments.
2. Room humidification if ordered.
3. Aerosols with a bronchodilator such as Brokosol R or antibiotics may be administered before postural drainage and clapping.

Hemoptysis

Hemoptysis occurs when a blood vessel is eroded as a result of pulmonary disease. The patient may expectorate as much as 300 to 500 ml of blood in 24 hours. When a patient with a pulmonary disease such as CF has an uncontrollable urge to cough, this usually indicates blood in the airways from hemoptysis. The patient will be very anxious and should not be left alone.

Nursing and medical care during hemoptysis includes the following:
1. Elevate head of bed 45 to 90 degrees.
2. Turn patient's head to left side.
3. Have emesis basin and tissues ready for expectoration of blood.
4. Provide clean basin frequently so that patient is not made more anxious by amount of blood.
5. Measure amount of hemoptysis and record time and amount.
6. *Postural drainage and clapping are withheld during acute episodes of bleeding, usually for at least 24 hours.*
7. Vitamin K_1, (Mephyton) by mouth or subcutaneously is ordered sometimes to control bleeding.
8. Stay with patient until bleeding has subsided and patient is made comfortable and is less fearful.
9. Hemoptysis usually subsides without surgical intervention. If hemoptysis become life threatening, surgical intervention, such as removal of the bronchiectatic lobe, may be necessary. Unfortunately, in most patients, the pulmonary disease is too extensive to permit surgery.[111]
10. Bronchoscopy with endobronchial tamponade may be successful in stopping bleeding in patients with minimal bleeding.

Pneumothorax

Pneumothorax occurs when apical cysts rupture, allowing air from the lung to enter the pleural space. *Sudden sharp chest pain in adults with CF should suggest spontaneous pneumothorax.* Pneumothorax occurs in 20% of adult CF patients and has a recurrence rate of 50%. Symptomatic pneumothoraces (increasing shortness of breath, mediastinal shift) are treated with intercostal drainage as follows:
1. Stab wound is made between ribs and chest tube is inserted.
2. Chest tube is connected to a closed drainage system (p. 563).
3. After lung is reexpanded, pleural sclerosis with tetracycline or guinacrine may be used. This procedure causes the visceral pleura to adhere to parietal pleura, obliterating the pleural space.
4. If there is a persistent air leak or pleural sclerosis fails, a partial pleurectomy should be performed.[111] In a partial pleurectomy, the portion of pleura overlying the cysts that ruptured is removed.

Cor pulmonale

As the airways become progressively plugged, *atelectasis* and *air trapping* occur. The result is a progressive ventilation/perfusion mismatch, resulting in progressive *hypoxemia*. Cor pulmonale can be expected to develop in patients with cystic fibrosis and advanced lung disease. A resting PaO_2 of less than 50 mm Hg, and a $PaCO_2$ greater than 45 mm Hg usually indicate cor pulmonale. Treatment of cor pulmonale includes the following:

1. Supplemental O_2 to help reverse pulmonary vasoconstriction caused by the hypoxemia and to improve myocardial performance. Oxygen therapy via cannula during sleep is commonly prescribed for patients with a daytime resting PaO_2 less than 60 mm Hg. Continuous O_2 is prescribed for patients with daytime resting PaO_2 less than 50 mm Hg.
2. Long-term diuretic therapy and fluid restriction may be effective therapy. The patient is monitored closely for electrolyte imbalances.
3. Digoxin is of questionable value in patients with right ventricular failure. However, many patients with CF have both right and left ventricular failure, and digoxin may be of therapeutic value. Patients are monitored closely for hypoxemia and hypokalemia, both of which increase the risk of digitalis toxicity.

Gastrointestinal complications

Gastrointestinal complications are common and are treated as follows:

1. Supplemental fat-soluble vitamins are used to aid digestion and improve weight.
2. Most patients take multivitamins and Vitamin E.
3. Pancreatic enzyme supplement doses are individualized and titrated by patients to control fatty stools to less than three per day.
4. When a patient is NPO, minimal doses of pancreatic supplements are necessary.
5. If adequate intake cannot be maintained orally, intravenous feedings or gastrostomy may be necessary.

Nursing Process
Assessment

Assessment data need to be collected in three areas—pulmonary, nutritional/gastrointestinal, and psychosocial. Data to be collected in each of these areas are listed below.

Pulmonary
Subjective data

1. Onset and description of symptoms such as shortness of breath, dyspnea on exertion, fatigue, and wheezing
2. Patient's understanding of CF pathophysiology and treatment regimens, including postural drainage and clapping, antibiotics, aerosol therapy, and nutritional supplements such as pancreatic enzymes and vitamins

Objective data

1. Auscultation for adventitious breath sounds
2. Chest pain on inspiration
3. Cyanotic mucous membranes
4. Digital clubbing (see Fig. 24-42)
5. Productive cough and color of sputum
6. Presence of fever, tachypnea
7. Review arterial blood gases (ABGs) for indications of falling PaO_2 or rising $PaCO_2$; review results of pulmonary function tests (decrease in tidal volume, FEV_1 (forced expiratory volume in 1 minute)
8. Signs and symptoms of antibiotic toxicity that may cause renal toxicity.
9. Side effects of aerosols (bronchodilators) that may cause tachycardia

Nutritional-Gastrointestinal
Subjective data

1. Description of color, consistency, and frequency of stools
2. Description of color, smell, and frequency of urination
3. Description of appetite and ability to swallow food
4. Description of daily eating pattern
5. Medications taken at home and their effectiveness in decreasing stool frequency
6. Onset and duration of abdominal discomfort
7. Signs or symptoms of gastric reflux
8. Weight loss; when began

Objective data

1. Color, consistency, and frequency of stools
2. Weight loss
3. Presence of polyuria, polydipsia, or polyphagia
4. Dietary intake
5. Intensity, frequency, and location of abdominal pain
6. Absence of bowel sounds

Psychosocial
Subjective data

1. Description of daily routines as it relates to work or school, pulmonary regimen, medications, and leisure activities
2. Description of current coping strategies and support network
3. Concerns about sexuality or fertility
4. Method of financial support (job, family, other forms of assistance)
5. Patient and family's understanding of CF

Objective data

1. Identify stage of grieving: symptoms that would infer that patient is grieving: anxiety, sleeplessness, hallucinations
2. Identify patient and family strengths
3. Identify patient support structure
4. Identify normal adult developmental needs (see Chapter 4)
5. Identify need for genetic counseling, career counseling, social services

Data analysis: nursing diagnoses

Nursing diagnoses are determined from analysis of patient data. Possible nursing diagnoses for the adult with CF may include, but are not limited to:

Diagnostic title	Possible etiologies
Airway clearance, ineffective	Obstruction/thick secretions, tracheo-bronchial infection, hemoptysis
Fatigue	Decreased oxygenation, inadequate nutrition, inadequate rest
Gas exchange, impaired	Ventilation/perfusion imbalance
Grieving, dysfunctional	Loss of fertility/loss of independence/loss of job or role/loss of control of one's life; unhealthy grief work/withdrawal, preoccupation, sleeplessness
Infection, high risk for	Increased mucus in airway, decreased nutrition
Nutrition, altered: less than body requirements	Pancreatic insufficiency resulting in malabsorption, glucose intolerance/weight loss; shortness of breath makes eating difficult

Planning: expected patient outcomes

Expected patient outcomes for the person with CF may include, but are not limited to, the following:
1. Patient will have improved airway clearance
   a. Decreased mucus production
   b. Clear breath sounds
   c. Decreased fatigue and shortness of breath
   d. Absence of fever
   e. Absence of hemoptysis
2. Patient's fatigue will be improved
   a. Oxygenation will be improved and patient will have less shortness of breath
   b. Will be able to sleep better
3. Patient's gas exchange will be improved
   a. PaO_2 will be above 50 mmHg
   b. $PaCO_2$ will be less than 45 mmHg
4. Patient's grieving skills will be improved
   a. Verbalizes actual and potential losses
   b. Identifies own strengths and personal goals
   c. Identifies support persons to assist with coping and achievement of goals
5. Patient's potential for infection is decreased
   a. Decreased mucus in airway
   b. Environment free of pathogenic bacteria
   c. Nutrition is improved
6. Patient demonstrates improved nutrition
   a. Maintains weight within 20% of ideal weight.
   b. Maintains normal blood glucose
   c. Is able to eat small frequent feedings that permit eating when less fatigued and short of breath

Implementation

Because the adult with CF is most commonly admitted to the hospital when the airway is compromised, considerable nursing care will be necessary. The care of the adult with CF centers around the following measures.

Interventions to achieve patient outcomes
Improving airway clearance

1. Provide with postural drainage with clapping every 2 to 4 hours, depending on the severity of the infection
2. Assist to cough effectively
3. Assess breath sounds before and after each treatment

4. Encourage patient to increase fluid intake to 3 to 4 L every 24 hours unless contraindicated
5. Monitor food intake; provide frequent snacks when energy level is improved
6. Provide quiet environment with frequent monitoring and reassurance
7. Maintain cool room with temperature below 70° F.

Monitoring fatigue

The nurse is responsible for monitoring the patient's fatigue and instituting methods to decrease as prevent it.
1. Assess fatigue frequently
2. Provide rest periods between activities
3. Provide frequent small feedings, which will increase energy stores
4. Visitors may need to be limited

Improving gas exchange

The nursing role is as follows:
1. Place patient in high Fowler's position.
2. Encourage slow rhythmic breathing.
3. Encourage patient to breathe through nose and exhale through pursed lips.
4. Monitor ABGs findings.

Assisting the patient to cope with grief

The nurse can play a major role in assisting the patient to work through the grieving process.
1. Identify stage of grieving.
2. Allow time for patient to verbalize feelings, hopes, and fears.
3. Support expressions of hope but avoid false reassurance.
4. Support patient and family through grief work. Recommend CF support groups as indicated.
5. Refer as appropriate for genetic counseling, career counseling, or social service.
6. Intervene for pathologic symptoms of grief such as anxiety, sleeplessness, and hallucinations.
7. Be aware of your own feelings of grief and share these with peers or a support group for nurses and other health care providers.

Monitoring for infection

Because the adult with CF is very vulnerable to infection or superinfection, the nurse needs to be aware of providing an environment that is as free of pathogens as possible.
1. Monitor patient's temperature frequently.
2. Monitor color, volume, and consistency of sputum.
3. Collect sputum specimens correctly and send for culture and sensitivity as indicated.
4. Give antibiotics as prescribed and on time to maintain adequate blood level.
5. Keep all persons with upper respiratory infections away from patient.
6. Wash own hands frequently and encourage visitors to wash hands before touching the patient.
7. Provide frequent mouth care, especially after postural drainage.
8. Assist patient to wash hands after coughing.

Promoting adequate nutrition

Because the patient with CF often has difficulty in maintaining nutrition, the nurse may need to be ingenious in promoting nutrition.

1. Perform baseline and periodic assessment of nutrition including food history, recording of daily intake, output, and daily weight.
2. Monitor blood glucose levels so that insulin can be given as prescribed according to blood glucose findings.
3. Provide small, frequent feedings.
4. Work with dietitian and patient to provide feedings that appeal to patient.
5. Administer pancreatic enzymes and vitamins as ordered.

Facilitating learning

Because the adult patient has had CF for several years, teaching is more in the form of review and reinforcement. In addition to the teaching guidelines for patients with COPD in Box 24-34, the following areas should be addressed with the patient with CF:

1. Review daily nutrition requirements, vitamins, and the need to check weight daily.
2. Review daily pulmonary exercises and treatments.
   a. Postural drainage and clapping
   b. Aerosol bronchodilators before postural drainage
3. Review medications in terms of usual dose, expected effects, and side effects. In some sections of the United States, medications can be obtained at substantial discount through the local Cystic Fibrosis Foundation.
4. Review clinical symptoms that indicate that the health care provider should be notified.
   a. Signs of an acute respiratory infection such as fever, increased fatigue, shortness of breath, increased production of sputum, or change in color of sputum.
   b. Hemoptysis
   c. Sudden sharp chest pain

5. Assess patient's knowledge and understanding of fertility, genetic testing, and contraceptive methods
6. Assess patient and family knowledge of community and social resources for assistance with health care reimbursement programs, disability insurance, and finding an appropriate support group.

Evaluation

Evaluation is based on patient outcomes. Questions to consider may include the following:

1. Can the patient maintain a clear airway?
2. Is the patient able to pace self so that fatigue is avoided as much as possible?
3. Is the patient's PaO_2 above 55 mm Hg and $PaCO_2$ less than 45 mm Hg?
4. Is the patient able to discuss feelings about having CF and the restriction it places on his or her life?
5. Is the patient free of a superinfection?
6. Is patient able to maintain weight within 20% of ideal?

Respiratory Failure

Patients with CF eventually succumb to progressive respiratory and cardiac failure. Because these patients have a fatal disease they usually have "do not resuscitate" (DNR) orders and are not intubated or placed on mechanical ventilation. The patient and family have to be involved in the DNR decision, and nurses play an important role in supporting the patient and family in their decision. The median age of death of adults with CF is 22 for women and 28 for men.

Research

There is considerable ongoing research on CF. Table 24-36 summarizes research projects, findings, and future goals. The indentification of the CF gene, in 1989, was a major breakthrough and has raised hopes for future progress in preventing and treating CF.

Table 24-36 Research in the prevention and treatment of cystic fibrosis

Subject	Topic	Findings	Future goals
Prevention	CF gene	Gene identified in 1989—location, size mutations, and defective protein	To define protein structure and function To treat or alter defective protein To identify and change sodium and chloride ion movement in CF cell To identify causes of CF
	Vaccinations		To develop vaccines to prevent lung infections
	Genetic counseling	Phosphatase and pancreatic trypsin for neonatal diagnosis	To identify CF carriers—prenatal and neonatal diagnosis
Treatment	Antibiotics	Prophylactic use Early use Aerosolized antibiotic Oral route effectiveness	To treat lung infections effectively To decrease side effects of frequent treatment To decrease hospitalizations
	Lung transplantation		To replace damaged lungs

RESPIRATORY INSUFFICIENCY AND RESPIRATORY FAILURE

Etiology/Epidemiology

The term *respiratory insufficiency* is usually used to indicate that the exchange of oxygen and carbon dioxide is not adequate to meet the needs of the body during normal activities. *Respiratory failure* is said to occur when ventilation is not sufficient to achieve adequate gas exchange even at rest. Many disorders can lead to or are associated with both respiratory insufficiency and failure; these are listed in Table 24-37.

The diagnosis of respiratory insufficiency or failure is based on arterial blood gas studies, pulmonary function testing, and the clinical status of the patient. The criteria listed in Box 24-38 are generally used in defining a state of failure. However, it cannot be overemphasized that these parameters are only *guidelines* and must be applied in light of the individual's history, age, and overall condition.

Pathophysiology and Clinical Picture

Regardless of the underlying condition, the resultant events or processes that occur in respiratory failure are the same. With inadequate ventilation, the arterial P_{O_2} falls and tissues cells become hypoxic. The P_{CO_2} increases, leading to a fall in pH, and the patient becomes acidotic. The nurse must keep in mind while working with the patient with COPD who has developed respiratory failure that this patient normally exists in a compensated state with decreased Pa_{O_2} levels and elevated Pa_{CO_2} levels. Thus the parameters in Box 24-38 are not applicable; the pH level, however, is a useful guide in assessing the degree of insufficiency. When the pH begins to fall below 7.3, it is an indication that the patient is no longer able to compensate for the elevated Pa_{CO_2} level.

Respiratory insufficiency and failure can result from a worsening in the condition of the patient with any of the disorders already mentioned.

24-38	Criteria for diagnosis of respiratory failure
	Pa_{O_2} <60 mm Hg when breathing room air
	Pa_{CO_2} >50 mm Hg
	Vital capacity <15 ml/kg
	Respiratory rate >30/min or below 8/min

Interventions

Intervention for the patient who has respiratory insufficiency or failure always begins with a recognition of the underlying disease state or cause of the disturbance in ventilation. Therapy is first directed at improving the underlying condition, such as sepsis, or by removing the cause, such as fluid overload.

The goals of intervention are to improve oxygenation and ventilation to restore the person's Pa_{O_2} and Pa_{CO_2} to their previous levels. The initial medical management can often be conservative if the diagnosis is made early enough.

Oxygen

Particular care is needed in working with the patient who has chronic lung disease. As mentioned earlier, *individuals with COPD normally are CO_2 retainers and exist with elevated Pa_{CO_2} levels and have lost the usual respiratory drive, carbon dioxide stimulation.* They no longer respond to increased carbon dioxide levels by increasing their rate and depth of respiration; rather, the elevated Pa_{CO_2} depresses the respiratory center. Their respiratory drive is now derived from their low Pa_{O_2} levels; therefore, even though these persons lack oxygen, it is extremely dangerous to raise their Pa_{O_2} to normal levels. If the arterial P_{O_2} is normal and there is retention of carbon dioxide (*hypercapnia*), the person will have no respiratory drive. Hypoventilation becomes more severe and Pa_{CO_2} continues to rise. This situation results in *carbon dioxide narcosis*, a markedly elevated carbon dioxide level that causes coma or semicoma. Persons with COPD are, therefore, treated with low-flow or controlled-

Table 24-37   Disorders associated with respiratory insufficiency and failure

Pulmonary disorders	Nonpulmonary disorders
Severe infection	CNS disturbance secondary to drug overdose, anesthesia, head injury
Pulmonary edema	Neuromuscular disorders (for example, Guillain-Barré syndrome, myasthenia
Pulmonary embolus	gravis, multiple sclerosis, poliomyelitis, muscular dystrophy, spinal cord in-
COPD	jury)
Adult respiratory distress syndrome (ARDS)	Postoperative reduction in ventilation following thoracic or abdominal surgery
Cancer	Prolonged mechanical ventilation
Chest trauma	
Severe atelectasis	
Airway compromise secondary to trauma, infection, or surgery	

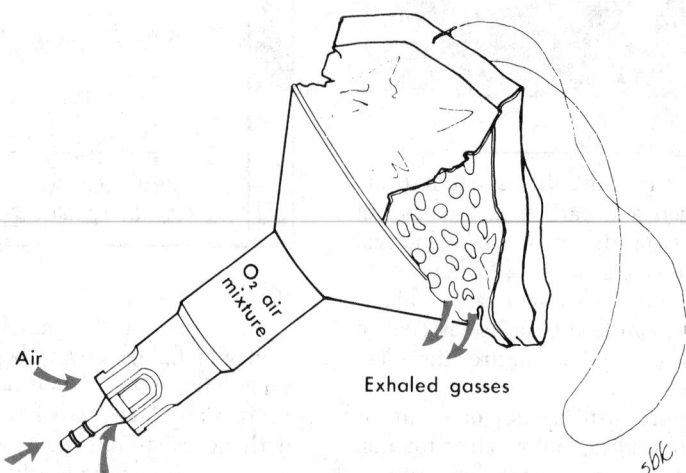

Fig. 24-43 Ventimask allows air to be mixed with oxygen to provide diluted oxygen to patient. (From Wade JF: *Comprehensive respiratory care*, ed 3, St Louis, 1982, Mosby—Year Book.)

flow oxygen; that is, inspired oxygen concentrations of 24% to 30%. These concentrations can easily be obtained by using a Ventimask (Fig. 24-43) or a two-pronged nasal cannula with a 1 to 2 L oxygen flow. This amount of oxygen can significantly increase the amount of oxygen carried by hemoglobin without a significant increase in arterial PO_2; therefore, the patient's blood carries much more oxygen even though hypoxemia is still present. The person continues to have respiratory drive, and the $PaCO_2$ does not rise.

By the use of low-flow oxygen, the amount of oxygen carried in the patient's blood can often be increased enough to maintain basic body functions without further reduction of ventilation. Persons who do not have COPD, who have a normal $PaCO_2$, but who are hypoxic are usually able to tolerate high flow rates of oxygen (5 to 10 L/min). Oxygen is an integral part of the therapy of patients with respiratory insufficiency and failure; however, some hazards are associated with prolonged use.

Oxygen toxicity is the term used to describe the damage to lung tissue that results from prolonged exposure to high concentrations of oxygen. Although the exact effects of oxygen in any one individual may depend on the person's underlying pathologic condition, it is believed that exposure to greater than 60% oxygen for a period of more than 36 hours, or exposure to 100% oxygen for a period of more than 6 hours, results in atelectasis and alveolar collapse. Breathing very high concentrations of oxygen (80% to 100%) for prolonged periods (24 hours or more) is often associated with the development of ARDS (p. 555). Thus it is a firm general principle that the lowest amount of oxygen that will achieve an acceptable PO_2 is the amount that should be given.

Airway management

In addition to providing supplemental oxygen, care of the person with respiratory insufficiency usually includes aggressive airway management and attempts to improve ven-

tilation. Suctioning, IPPB, ultrasonic mist therapy, and postural drainage with clapping and vibrating are all employed in an attempt to halt the progression of insufficiency. When the patient develops respiratory failure and can no longer maintain his or her own respirations, an artificial airway is necessary.

Types of artificial airways

An endotracheal tube is usually chosen initially as a means of providing an airway; tracheostomy is only performed if airway maintenance is necessary for a prolonged period of time or if trauma to the airway prevents the use of an endotracheal tube. Although a tracheostomy has the *disadvantage* of a higher risk of infection, it is often elected for long-term airway management because it is *much more comfortable than an endotracheal tube and allows the person to eat.*

In endotracheal intubation a tube is passed through either the nose or mouth into the trachea; in a tracheostomy an artificial opening is made in the trachea into which a tube is inserted (Fig. 24-44). These procedures are used (1) to establish and maintain a patent airway, (2) to prevent aspiration by sealing off the trachea from the digestive tract in the unconscious or paralyzed person, (3) to permit removal of tracheobronchial secretions in the person who cannot cough adequately, and (4) to treat the patient who requires positive pressure ventilation that cannot be given effectively by mask. Whether an intubation or a tracheostomy is performed initially depends on the facilities available and the preference of the physician. Most physicians now consider it safer to do an emergency endotracheal intubation and then perform a tracheostomy as a nonemergency procedure in the operating room if prolonged support of the airway is needed. In this instance the endotracheal tube is not removed until after the tracheostomy opening is made.

A tracheostomy is necessary when an endotracheal tube cannot be inserted or when it is contraindicated, as in

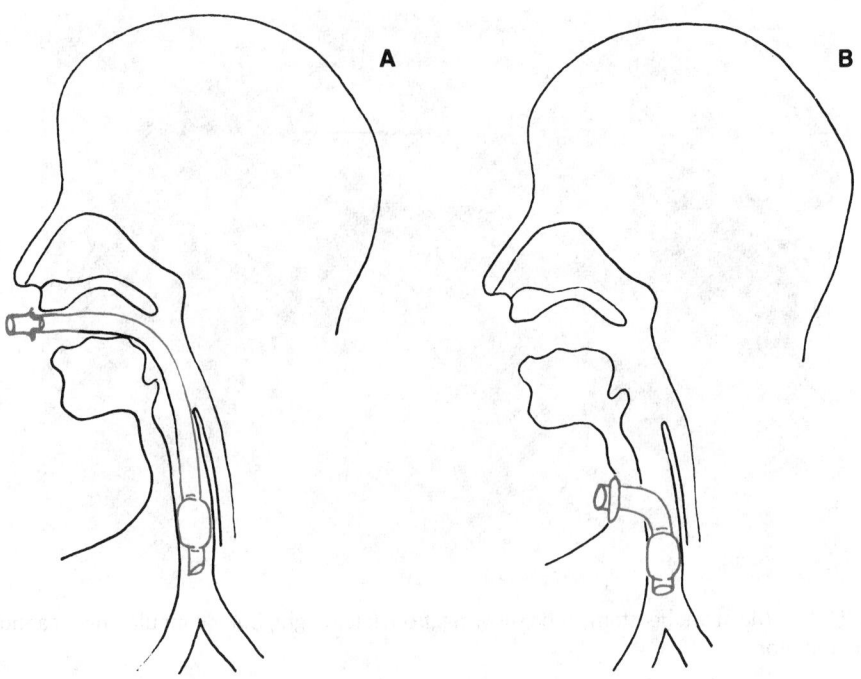

Fig. 24-44 **A,** Position of endotracheal tube. **B,** Position of tracheostomy tube.

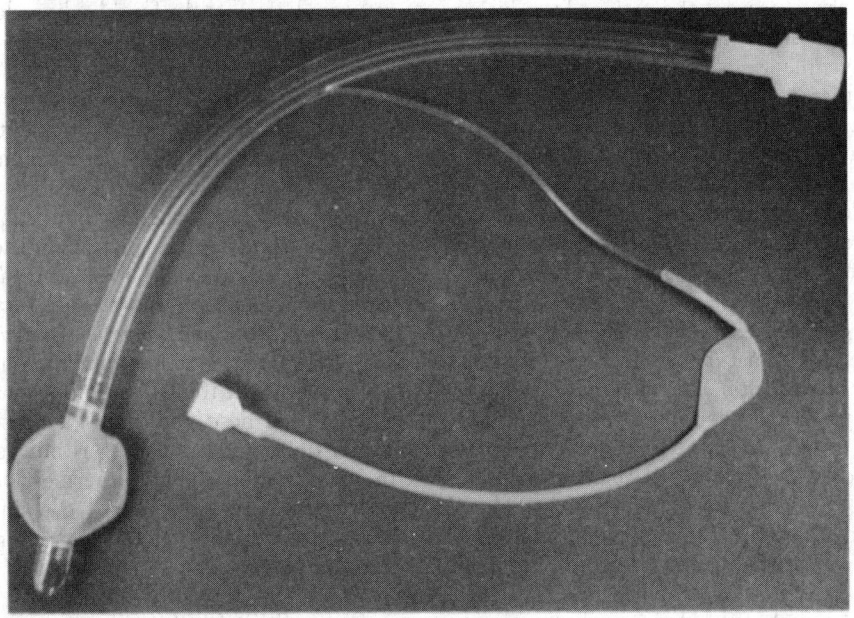

Fig. 24-45   Forregar high-volume, low-pressure cuffed endotracheal tube. Cuff shown here is not inflated. Low-pressure cuff is preferred because it is less likely to cause tracheal damage.

severe burns or laryngeal obstruction caused by tumor, infection, or vocal cord paralysis. Tracheostomy may also be required when a patient is conscious and cannot tolerate an endotracheal tube. Once the airway is secured either by intubation or by tracheostomy, secretions are aspirated and well-humidified oxygen is usually given. If the patient is unable to sustain respiration, a mechanical ventilator (for example, a Bennet or a Bird ventilator) is attached to the endotracheal tube or the tracheostomy tube. When

mechanical ventilation is required, a cuffed tube is used. Usually an endotracheal tube is not left in place longer than 10 to 14 days. If the patient is unable to maintain an open airway after this period of time, a tracheostomy is performed.

The endotracheal tube is made of plastic, with an inflatable cuff so that a closed system with the ventilator may be maintained (Fig. 24-45). The tube is inserted via the mouth or nose through the larynx into the trachea. If

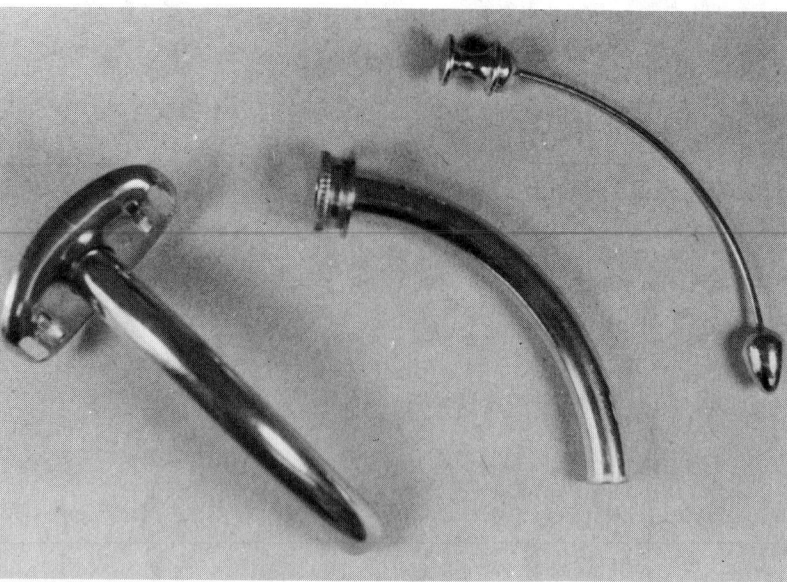

Fig. 24-46 Metal tracheostomy tube showing, from left to right, outer cannula, inner cannula, and obturator.

an oral endotracheal tube is used, a rubber airway or bite block is often necessary to prevent the patient from biting down on the tube and obstructing the airway.

The tracheostomy tube is usually made of plastic or metal. It may be either a single-lumen or double-lumen (Jackson) type (Fig. 24-46). Both types of tubes may be cuffed, and the newer plastic tubes come with high-volume, low-pressure cuffs that are less likely to cause damage to the trachea. Single-lumen tubes must be changed about every 72 hours, because they are more difficult to clean and more likely to become plugged than are double-lumen tubes.

Metal tubes are commonly available in sizes 00 to 8 (No. 00 is used for the premature or newborn infant; a No. 6 or 7 is used for most adults). The metal tracheostomy tube consists of two parts, an inner and an outer cannula. The outer cannula is removed only by the physician, whereas the inner cannula is removed regularly by the nurse for cleaning. The metal tracheostomy tube has a lock that must be turned to remove the inner cannula. The lock should be secured when the inner cannula is reinserted after cleaning. Twill tapes attached to either side of the tube are tied securely behind the neck to prevent the tube from becoming dislodged when the patient coughs or moves about.

Should the tube be coughed out, the opening may close, and the patient will be unable to breathe. Therefore, a tracheal dilator or curved hemostat is always kept at the bedside so that the opening can be held open if the tube is dislodged. Some surgeons prefer to place a retention suture on each side of the tracheostomy opening and tape the end of the suture to the skin. If the opening shows signs of closing, tension can be placed on the sutures to widen the opening.

The operative wound may be sealed with a plastic spray, or a small dressing may be placed around the tracheostomy tube. Although drainage should be minimal, the wound is inspected frequently for bleeding during the immediate postoperative period. The dressings are changed as they become soiled with mucus drainage.

Depending on the patient's condition, a tracheostomy can be either temporary or permanent; the person who has a laryngectomy will have a permanent tracheostomy. Any patient who has had a tracheostomy is apprehensive and is often fearful of choking. Thus when feasible, the procedure is thoroughly explained to the patient before surgery. Both patient and family need to understand that the *patient will be unable to speak* and that *constant attendance will be provided until the patient can give self-care safely.*

A fenestrated tracheostomy tube has an opening on the upper surface of the outer cannula that allows air inspired through the nose and mouth to pass through the tube. When the external opening is plugged, air can pass over the vocal cords, allowing the individual to talk. If ventilatory assistance is required, the inner cannula can be inserted so that the patient can be connected to a ventilator.

General care of the person with an endotracheal or tracheostomy tube

An endotracheal or tracheostomy tube provides a direct route for introduction of pathogens into the lower airway, increasing the risk of infection. It is essential that the following preventive nursing interventions be consistently implemented.

1. Minimize infection risk
   a. Endotracheal tubes irritate the trachea, resulting in increased mucus production. Assess the patient regularly for excess secretions, and suction as often as necessary to maintain a patent airway. See Box 24-42 for sterile suctioning procedure.
   b. Provide constant airway humidification. Endotracheal airways bypass the upper airway that

normally humidifies and warms inspired air. An external source of warmed, humidified air must be provided to avoid thickening and crusting of bronchial secretions.

c. All respiratory therapy equipment should be changed every 24 hours. In addition:
   (1) Replace any equipment that touches the floor.
   (2) Remove water that condenses in equipment tubing. Do not poor condensed water back into humidifier reservoir.

d. Provide frequent mouth care. Secretions tend to pool in the mouth and in the pharynx, particularly if the cuff of the tube is inflated. There is an increased risk of ulceration or abrasion of the lips and oropharynx when an endotracheal tube or oral airway is present.
   (1) Gently suction oropharynx as needed.
   (2) Inspect the lips, tongue, and oral cavity regularly.
   (3) Clean the oral cavity with swabs soaked in saline.
   (4) Apply moisturizing agent to cracked lips.

e. Maintain adequate nutritional levels.
   (1) The person with an endotracheal tube is allowed nothing by mouth. Nourishment will be given parenterally or by gastrointestinal feedings. Gastrointestinal supplemental feedings pose less infection risk and are more economical. See Box 24-39 for guidelines for administering gastrointestinal feedings to the intubated patient.
   (2) The patient with a tracheostomy tube is usually able to swallow and have a normal oral intake. Some experts prefer that the cuff on the tracheostomy tube be inflated while the patient is eating to prevent aspiration. Others believe that the inflated cuff bulges into the esophagus and makes swallowing more difficult, and they therefore prefer that the cuff be deflated. Nursing assessment will determine which technique to use. Methylene blue dye can be swallowed before each feeding or mixed with the tube feeding. If the dye does not appear in tracheal secretions, it is safe to proceed with the meal.

2. Ensure adequate ventilation and oxygenation.
   a. Assess lung sounds regularly. Unless the individual's underlying lung pathology alters lung ventilation, breath sounds should be heard bilaterally, and chest expansion should be symmetric. If a cuffed tube is inserted too far, it will slip into one of the main-stem bronchi (usually the right) and occlude the opposite bronchus and lung, resulting in atelectasis on the obstructed side. Even if the tube is still in the trachea, airway obstruction will result if the end of the tube is located on the carina (area at lower end of trachea at point of bifurcation of main-stem bronchi). This will result in dry secretions that obstruct both bronchi. Although these compli-

Care of the intubated patient receiving gastrointestinal feedings

1. Assess for the presence of bowel sounds.
2. Elevate the head of the bed at least 30 degrees.
3. Inflate the tube cuff.
4. Administer the gastrointestinal feeding to which methylene blue dye has been added.
5. Assess at regular intervals for aspiration. The presence of methylene blue in secretions indicates aspiration.
6. Regularly assess for tube placement and residual stomach contents.

cations are more common with the use of an endotracheal tube, they can occur with a tracheostomy tube, especially in a small person with a short neck. In either case the tube is pulled back until it is positioned below the larynx and above the carina. The tube is then fastened securely in place with adhesive tape or twill ties.

b. Turn and reposition the patient every 2 hours for maximum ventilation and lung perfusion.

c. Assess respiratory frequency, tidal volume, and vital capacity.

d. Perform postural drainage, cupping (clapping), and vibrating as appropriate (p. 595).

3. Provide safety and comfort.
   a. Most endotracheal and tracheostomy tubes have cuffs for the following reasons:
      (1) To provide a sealed airway for positive–pressure ventilation
      (2) To prevent aspiration in the unconscious person, during meals or during tube feedings
      (3) To exert pressure on bleeding sites following throat or neck surgery
   b. Assess tube placement at regular intervals.
      (1) The tube is secured around neck with tape or specially designed ties.
      (2) The endotracheal tube is marked to establish a landmark for position comparison and to measure and document the length of tube that extends beyond the patient's lips
   c. Change tapes or ties whenever soiled to decrease skin irritation.
   d. Always keep a spare tube at the bedside.
   e. Minimize sensory deprivation.
      (1) Patients with endotracheal tubes or tracheostomy tubes with the cuff inflated cannot talk. Therefore an acceptable communication mode must be established.
         (a) Organize questions so that the patient can use a simple "yes" or "no" response, nodding head or using hand signals.
         (b) The patient may be able to use an erasable board (Magic Slate) or note pad to communicate.
         (c) Always talk to the patient and explain all procedures.

24-40

Inflating an endotracheal or tracheostomy cuff

The cuff should be inflated to a volume that provides adequate occlusion around the tube without increasing the risk of tracheomalacia, tracheal stenosis, tracheoesophageal fistula, or erosion through a major blood vessel. Many experts recommend the "minimal leak technique," which is described below.

1. Using a 10- or 20-ml syringe, slowly inject air into cuff.
2. As air is introduced, assess for air leak around tube. This is determined (1) by ability of patient to talk or make sounds, and (2) being able to feel air coming from patient's nose or mouth.
3. When the airway is sealed and no passage of air around the tube can be detected, remove 0.5 ml of air. This creates a "minimal leak" and ensures that the lowest possible pressure is being exerted on the tracheal wall.
4. Auscultate over the trachea while ventilating the patient with either an Ambu bag or mechanical ventilator. A small amount of air should be heard gurgling past the cuff.
5. If an adequate seal cannot be obtained with 25 ml of air, notify the physician.

24-41

Routine tracheostomy care

Materials: Suction catheter, cleansing solutions (usually hydrogen peroxide and saline), tracheostomy care kit or two sterile basins, sterile applicators, sterile gloves, tracheostomy dressing (must be a nonshredding material), twill tape, disposable bag, and antibiotic ointment.

1. Wash hands and apply nonsterile gloves.
2. Explain procedure.
3. Suction mouth or orophayrnx if needed.
4. Prepare sterile work field.
5. Remove soiled tracheostomy dressing and discard in disposable bag.
6. Put on *sterile gloves.* If tracheostomy has an inner cannula, remove and clean it in hydrogen peroxide solution. Rinse with saline solution.
7. Inspect inner cannula lumen for patency before reinserting it.
8. Replace tracheostomy ties if soiled. Always hold tracheostomy in place with one hand while ties are being changed. If possible, a second nurse can assist to ensure that tube is not accidentally dislodged.
9. Tie end of twill tapes in a square knot on one side of neck.
10. Using sterile technique, clean tracheostomy incision. Apply antibiotic ointment.
11. Apply sterile tracheostomy dressing.

(d) Reorient the patient frequently.
(e) Encourage family and frieds to talk to the patient.
(f) Keep call light (or tap bell) within patient's reach.
(g) Reinforce that the ability to speak will return when the tube is removed.

4. Observe special considerations during immediate extubation period.
   a. Monitor for signs such as increased respiratory distress, increased hoarseness, and laryngeal stridor, indicating upper airway obstruction secondary to laryngeal edema.
   b. Assess for adequacy of cough and gag reflex.
   c. After removal of a tracheostomy tube there is a temporary air leak at the incision site.
   d. The stoma can be suctioned. However, frequent use of the stoma for suctioning can delay closure and healing of the tracheostomy incision.

Although the low-pressure cuffs used today reduce the risk of tracheal wall damage, it is important to inflate the cuff with the correct amount of air (Box 24-40).

Care of the patient with a tracheostomy

Although nursing care of patients with endotracheal and tracheostomy tubes is similar, patients with tracheostomies have additional nursing care needs. Analgesics and sedatives are given judiciously so as not to depress the respiratory center. The patient is suctioned as often as necessary, possibly every 5 minutes during the first few postoperative hours. The need for suctioning can be determined by the sound of the air coming from the tracheostomy tube, especially after the patient takes a deep breath. *When respirations are noisy and pulse and respiratory rates are increased, the patient needs to be suctioned.* Patients who are conscious can usually indicate when they need to be suctioned. With any sign of respiratory distress, the tube should be suctioned. If mucus is blocking the inner cannula of a metal tube and cannot be removed by suction, the inner cannula is removed to open the airway. When the mucus is thick, the inner cannula should be cleaned and replaced at once because the outer tube may also become blocked. If, despite these measures, the patient becomes cyanotic, the physician should be summoned at once. A patient who is able to cough up secretions probably will require suctioning less frequently. The amount of mucus subsides gradually, and the patient eventually may go for several hours without being suctioned. However, even when secretions are minimal, the patient is apprehensive and needs constant attendance. Box 24-41 describes routine tracheostomy care.

See p. 621, Box 24-42, for the details of suctioning an endotracheal or tracheostomy tube.

Care of the patient discharged with a tracheostomy

Patients to be discharged with a tube in place are taught to care for and change the tube while in the hospital (Fig. 24-47). A mirror will be necessary to perform this procedure, which may be begun a few days after surgery.

Suctioning a patient with an endotracheal or tracheostomy tube

1. All patients with tubes require suctioning and should be suctioned as often as necessary. The frequency of suctioning is determined by auscultation. Much of the ability to produce an effective cough is lost because it is impossible for the person who is intubated to build up the pressure needed to create an expulsive cough.

2. The mouth and oropharynx above the cuff are suctioned first. This catheter is discarded, and a *sterile catheter* and sterile technique are used to suction the trachea.

   It is not necessary to deflate the cuff each time the patient is suctioned. The nurse may wish to deflate the cuff once per shift to remove secretions pooled on top of the cuff and to ensure that it is properly sealed. Deflation should be performed when the nurse is ready to suction the trachea.

3. Suction as deeply as possible. In an adult, a catheter can be introduced through an endotracheal tube approximately 45 to 55 cm (18 to 22 inches). The recommended depth through the tracheostomy tube is 20 to 30 cm (8 to 12 inches). The catheter should be approximately one-half the diameter of the tube.

4. A fenestrated catheter with a whistle tip is attached to the suction outlet. The catheter is always inserted without suction being applied. Once the catheter is in place, suction is applied by placing the thumb over the fenestration in the catheter.

5. Before suctioning, the patient is hyperoxygenated with 100% oxygen. An Ambu, anesthesia, or Laerdal bag is used to deliver 6 to 10 breaths of 100% oxygen. Preoxygenation with 100% oxygen is necessary because oxygen will be removed during suctioning.

6. The suction catheter is lubricated with sterile water or a water-soluble lubricant. In the person with a tracheostomy, suctioning usually stimulates coughing. If the patient coughs, the catheter is removed because its presence obstructs the trachea and the patient must exert extra pressure to cough around it. As coughing occurs, the nurse or the patient should have tissues ready to receive mucus, which may be ejected with force.

7. If mucus is thick, sticky, and difficult to remove, sterile saline solution may be instilled into the tube just before suctioning. From 5 to 15 ml is commonly used.

8. Although some clinicians recommend that the patient's head and shoulders be turned to the right when suctioning the left bronchus and vice versa, there is no objective evidence that this technique improves suctioning the desired bronchus. In most people the right main-stem bronchus is easier to enter anatomically and thus is suctioned more often than the left bronchus. The catheter is rotated as it is withdrawn with the suction on.

9. To prevent hypoxia, the patient must **not** be suctioned longer than 10 to 15 seconds at a time and should rest 1 to 3 minutes between aspirations, and 100% oxygen should be administered between suctioning. If secretions are interfering with breathing, suctioning may have to be more frequent.

10. The patient is monitored for signs of hypoxia such as tachycardia, bradycardia, or ectopic beats.

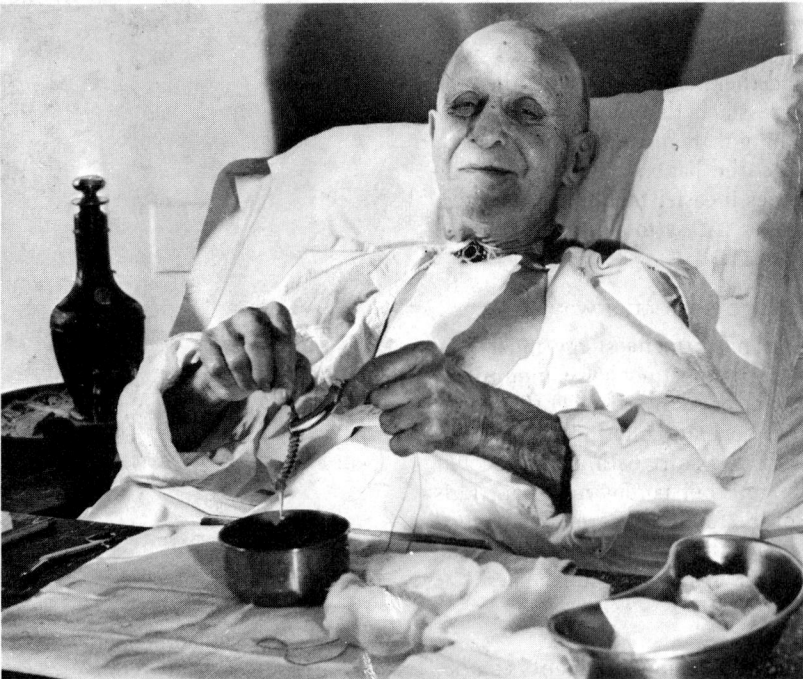

Fig. 24-47 This 82-year-old man cares for his own tracheostomy tube. He is about to clean inner tube with small tube brush. (From Anderson HC: *Newton's geriatric nursing,* ed 5, St Louis, 1971. Mosby–Year Book.)

Patients who go home with the tracheostomy tube in place must be provided with necessary supplies or with instructions as to where to secure them and with knowledge of how to care for themselves. They should have suction equipment, which can be rented for home use or obtained in many communities through the local chapter of the American Cancer Society. Suction can be provided by attaching a suction base to a faucet. Many hardware stores carry the necessary equipment. The amount of suction is controlled by the stream of water.

Maintaining air humidification

Because the insertion of the endotracheal or tracheostomy tube bypasses the upper airway, the patient's ability to humidify and warm inspired air is lost. Therefore, whether the patient is on or off the respirator, the inspired air should be heated and humidified to prevent mucosal irritation and drying of secretions. *Large-bone* tubing is needed to provide this mist because water particles condense in *small-bore* tubing. A noticeable difference in the viscosity of secretions is evident in patients who do not receive mist for even as short a period as 30 minutes. Other important nursing care measures and observations vary with the route of intubation—via the larynx or from below the larynx. The patient who has an endotracheal tube in place usually has an increased volume of oropharyngeal secretions because of irritation from the tube. The patient also has great difficulty in swallowing (especially if an oral tube is used), necessitating frequent oropharyngeal suctioning.

Providing nourishment

The patient with an endotracheal tube is allowed nothing by mouth. Nourishment is given intravenously or by nasogastric tube feedings. The patient with a tracheostomy tube in place is usually able to swallow and have a normal oral intake. As mentioned earlier, some experts prefer that the cuff on the tracheostomy tube be inflated while the patient is eating to prevent aspiration. Others believe that the inflated cuff bulges into the esophagus and makes swallowing more difficult, and therefore, they prefer the cuff to be deflated. Nursing assessment determines which technique to use. In determining if the patient aspirates food, it is often helpful to feed the patient red gelatin. The consistency of gelatin makes it easier to swallow than water, and the red color makes it easy to detect if aspirated into the lower airway.

Maintaining precautions to protect airway

Persons who have a permanent tracheostomy must take some special precautions. They must not go swimming and must be careful while bathing or taking a shower that water is not aspirated through the opening into the lungs. They are advised to wear a scarf or a shirt with a closed collar that covers the opening, yet is of porous material. This material performs some of the functions normally assumed by the nasal passages, such as the warming of air and the screening out of dust and other irritating substances.

Providing adequate rest

The patient who is subjected to many treatments can become excessively fatigued, further compromising ventilatory capacity. Frequent rest periods must be interspersed with treatments, and it is the nurse's responsibility to see that the patient has a quiet environment and is not disturbed by unnecessary interruptions at rest times. Unfortunately, persons who have severe respiratory insufficiency must have frequent treatments and interventions; it is *not appropriate, although the person may be quite tired, to allow the patient to sleep through the night and to omit treatments.* This inevitably leads to a worsened status.

Although persons with respiratory insufficiency are often anxious and frightened, sedation is contraindicated because it depresses respirations. Therefore, it is especially important that the nurse be supportive of the patient and be skillful in assisting the patient to breathe effectively. The patient can be extremely demanding, and the nurse must understand the fear and anxiety that is often the basis for the patient's behavior.

Monitoring ventilation

Aggressive, constant nursing care is essential for these patients. The nurse must be continually alert to clinical changes that represent changes in the patient's ventilation. Increasing confusion and behavioral changes often indicate an elevated $PaCO_2$. The behavioral changes may range from pugnacious, combative behavior to lethargy. Other clinical signs of *hypercapnia* are flushed skin caused by reflex vasodilation, muscle twitching, and headache. Signs commonly seen in hypoxemia include tachycardia, increased pulse rate, cyanosis, changes in blood pressure, and changes in behavior. In *early* stages of hypoxemia the blood pressure is elevated as a result of vasoconstriction and

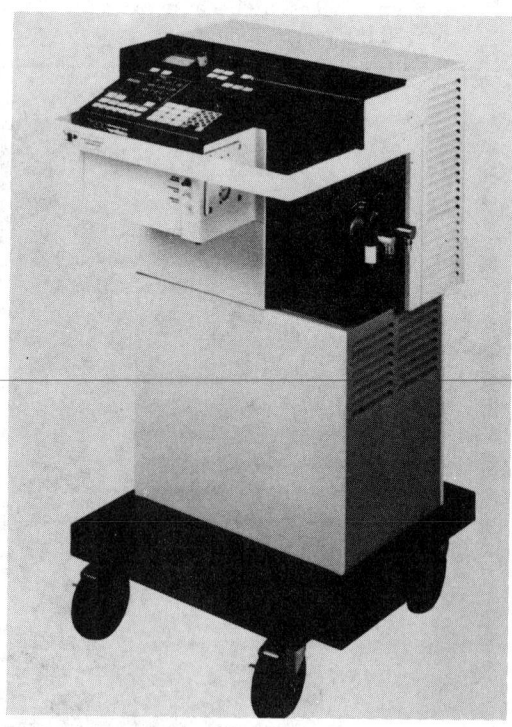

Fig. 24-48 Puritan-Bennett 7200 ventilator shown with optional pedestal and compressor. (Courtesy Puritan-Bennett Corp, Kansas City, Mo.)

increased peripheral resistance. In *later* stages, the blood pressure falls to hypotensive levels and circulatory arrest can occur. It is important to point out that cyanosis is not an early sign of hypoxia because it does not occur until arterial oxygen saturation is less than 85%; thus the nurse needs to be alert to the earlier signs of hypoxemia mentioned earlier.

Mechanical ventilation

If the patient is unable to maintain ventilation (as indicated by a rising arterial P_{CO_2}), mechanical ventilation is necessary. The ventilator will be attached either to an endotracheal or to a tracheostomy tube (p. 616).

The goal of mechanical ventilation is to deliver a minute ventilation (respiratory rate × tidal volume) with an enriched concentration of oxygen sufficient for adequate tissue oxygenation.[96] The usual tidal volume delivered by a ventilator is in the range of 10 to 15 ml/kg, compared with a spontaneous tidal volume of 5 ml/kg.

Because of the complexity of mechanical ventilation, the ideal place for these patients is in the intensive care unit where experienced nursing staff can care for them. Additionally, ventilators are constantly being improved and new models are introduced periodically. For this reason, an ongoing staff development program is mandatory. The general principles for care of patients on ventilators follow. However, it must be stressed that a nurse can only become proficient in working with the patient after repeated experience under the preceptorship of more experienced nurses.

Many different kinds of ventilators are available. In general, there are two types: pressure-cycled and volume-limited. The Bird and Bennett (PR series) are pressure-limited ventilators. They are mainly used for IPPB treatments. Volume-cycled ventilators include the Air Shields, Bennett MA series, Bennett 7200 (Figs. 24-48 and 24-49), BEAR 2 (Fig. 24-50), Emerson, Engstrom, Ohio 560, and Siemens-Servo. Table 24-38 lists the types of ventilators and their mode of function.

Volume-cycled ventilators are currently the most commonly used. They provide a wide range of flexibility to meet individual requirements for adequate oxygen and carbon dioxide exchange. The functions that can be adjusted on the volume-cycled ventilator are listed in Box 24-43.

With a *volume-cycled* machine a *constant volume* of air is delivered with each breath. The volume is preset and is delivered to the patient at whatever pressure is necessary to attain that volume. A volume-cycled machine should have a pressure cutoff valve. Such a mechanism allows a pressure limit to be set. If the pressure required to deliver the set volume exceeds the pressure limit, the machine will turn off before the entire volume is delivered. *The pressure limit on a volume-cycled machine usually has an audible alarm. The nurse can set the limit slightly above (approximately 5 cm of water) the pressure required to ventilate the patient. The alarm will then go off if the patient coughs, accumulates secretion, or starts to resist the machine.*

Regardless of which type of ventilator is used, mechanisms for various regulations are necessary if the machine

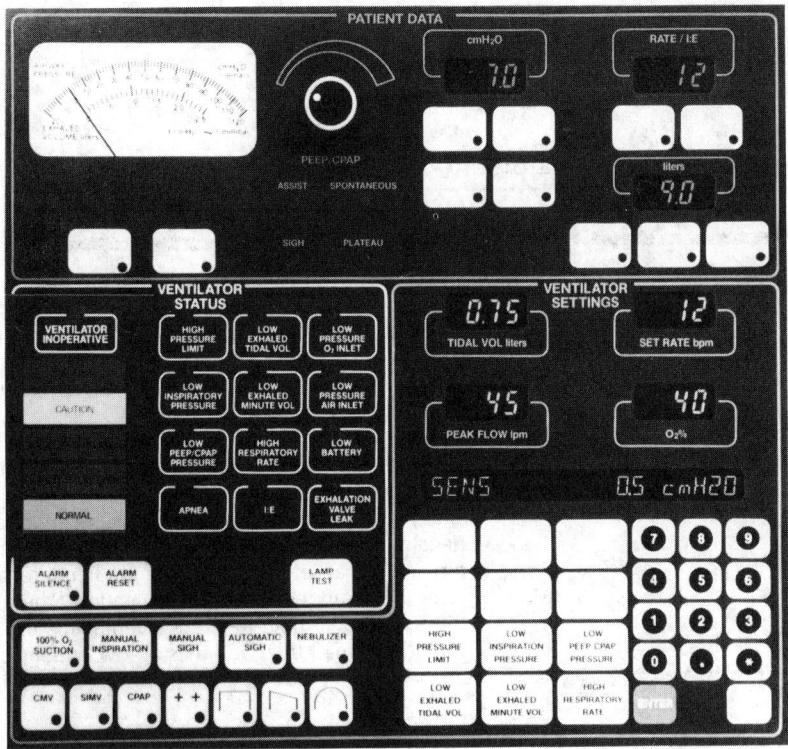

Fig. 24-49   Control panel of Puritan-Bennett 7200 microprocessor ventilator. (Courtesy Puritan-Bennett Corp, Kansas City, Mo.)

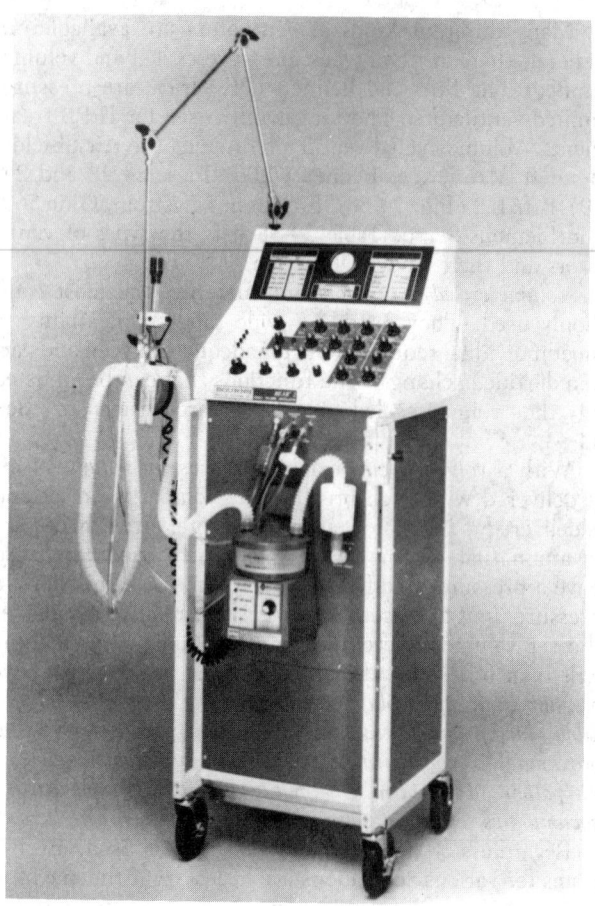

Fig. 24-50 BEAR 2 adult volume ventilator. (Courtesy BEAR Medical Systems, Inc, Riverside, Calif.)

24-43

Functions that can be adjusted with volume-cycled ventilators

Tidal volume—volume of air in a normal breath
Sigh—periodic deep breath; used to prevent microatelectasis and decreased lung compliance; decreased need for sigh function because ventilating with larger tidal volumes
FiO_2—oxygenation concentration delivered through the ventilator
Alarm systems—vary from machine to machine; basic alarms usually present are:
  1. High-pressure alarm—increased resistance somewhere in system from lungs to machine
  2. Low-pressure alarm—system not reaching minimal pressure required for ventilation
  3. Low-volume alarm—when volume of ventilation does not equal the amount set
Control modes—Degree of ventilation that is controlled by the ventilator; can vary from complete ventilator control to almost total patient control (see Table 24-38)

Table 24-38 Types of mechanical ventilators

Types		Basic function mode
Positive-pressure ventilator		Types of positive-pressure ventilators are based on how inspiratory phase is ended.
Pressure-cycled ventilator	(require intubation)	Inspiration ends at a preset pressure limit; time and volume are variable.
Time-cycled ventilator		Inspiration is preset for a given time interval; volume and pressure are variable.
Volume-cycled ventilator		Preset volume of air is delivered. Time and pressure are variable. However, volume-cycled ventilators often have pressure- and time-cycled capacities.
Negative-pressure ventilator (intubation not required)		Thorax, at least, is encapsulated. When ventilator expands, it creates negative pressure by pulling the thorax outward. Air rushes into the airways because of the pressure gradient created.
High-frequency ventilation (requires intubation)		System is still under clinical investigation. There are several variants of this system. All high-frequency ventilators use high respiratory rates to deliver small tidal volumes at low pressures.

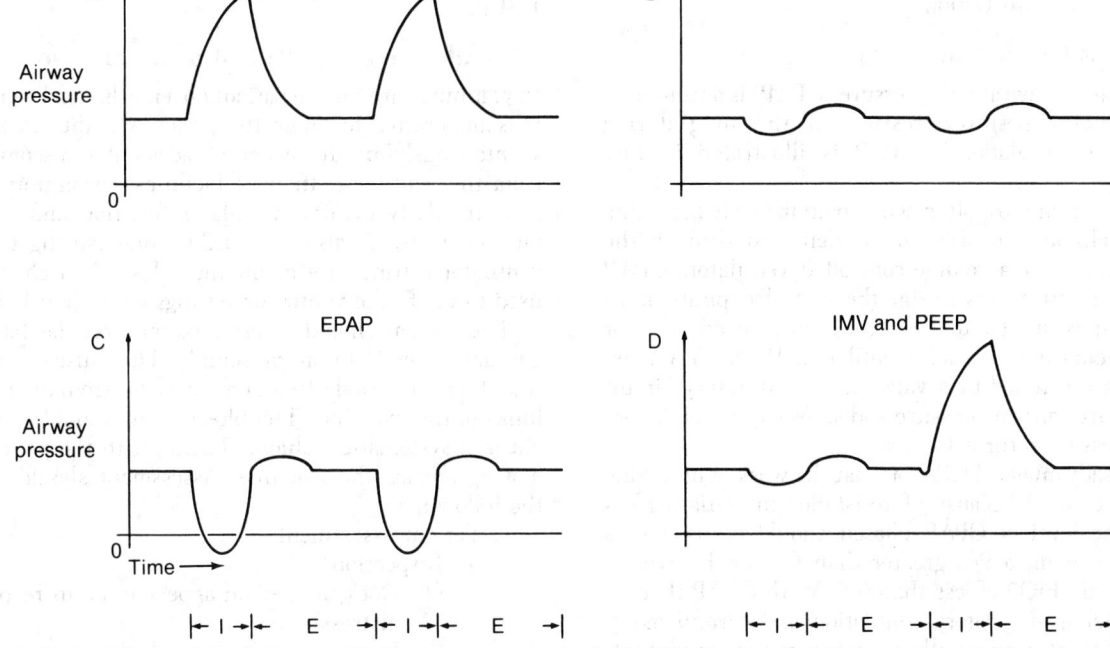

Fig. 24-51   Three forms of positive expiratory pressure. (From Dupuis YG: *Ventilators: theory and clinical applications,* ed 2, St Louis, 1992, Mosby–Year Book.)

is to be adjusted to each patient. It is preferable to have a respirator that can be used to assist or control the patient's breathing. *"Assist" means that the patient's own inspiratory effort triggers (turns on) the machine.* Most respirators have a *sensitivity control knob* that can be adjusted to respond to weak inspiratory efforts. *"Control" implies the use of automatic cycling.* The patient may be apneic and the machine set at the desired rate; the patient's own respiratory rate may be too slow, and the automatic cycling can be used to force an increase in the rate; or the patient's own respiratory efforts can be ignored and an automatic rate used to ventilate the patient. (Some machines with automatic cycling do not allow for the latter adjustment). It is also helpful to be able to regulate the flow rates at which the gas is delivered to the patient. For example, patients breathing at rapid rates and high volumes need faster flow rates than those breathing slowly and at moderate volumes. A final necessity is the ability to regulate the inspired concentration of oxygen from 20% (room air) to 100%.

All mechanical ventilators must do the following:

1. Provide for the heating and humidification of inspired air
2. Provide a means for measurement of expired volumes
3. Be dependable for long periods of use
4. Be easily cleaned

Any patient on continuous mechanical ventilation should be "sighed" (given a deep breath) several times an hour. Some ventilators automatically "sigh" the patient, while with others the patient is "sighed" manually using a self-inflating (Ambu) or anesthesia bag. This periodic deep breathing is necessary to prevent alveolar collapse and resultant atelectasis.

Positive End-Expiratory Pressure

Positive end-expiratory pressure (PEEP) is a ventilator mode that has been shown to increase the effectiveness of mechanical ventilation in certain patients. PEEP involves the maintenance of positive pressure, at the end of expiration, rather than allowing airway pressure to return to normal (atmospheric) as usually occurs (Fig. 24-51, A). By maintaining positive pressure, alveoli that would otherwise collapse on expiration are held open, thus increasing the opportunity for gas exchange across the alveolar-capillary membrane. This is accomplished by the increase in functional residual capacity. The result is a decrease in physiologic shunting and the ability to achieve a higher level of PaO_2 with lower concentrations of delivered oxygen (FiO_2). PEEP has its greatest use in the treatment of adult respiratory distress syndrome (ARDS), but is also used in treating any patient who would otherwise require unacceptably high concentrations of oxygen.

The hazards of PEEP are related to the increase in intrathoracic pressure. Most serious of the dangers related to this technique is the increased incidence of pneumothorax, particularly in those with friable lung tissue, as seen in persons with emphysema or lung cancer. *The sudden disappearance of breath sounds on one side, in conjunction with signs of respiratory distress, in the patient being ventilated with PEEP must be taken as an indication of a pneumothorax.* This can develop into a life-threatening episode if the pneumothorax is large, and the physician must be called immediately. Another *less serious consequence* of PEEP may be a *reduction in venous return, which is impeded by the increased intrathoracic pressure, and a subsequent fall in cardiac output.* This effect seems to be particularly common in patients who are relatively dehydrated and can sometimes be avoided by careful fluid administration.

Continuous Positive Airway Pressure

Continuous positive airway pressure (CPAP) is a technique that maintains positive pressure in the lung during spontaneous ventilation.[36] CPAP is illustrated in Fig. 24-51, B.

CPAP is used most often with spontaneously breathing patients, although it also can be delivered through the tubing circuits of a volume-controlled ventilator. CPAP maintains positive pressure at the end of expiration. In this way it is similar to PEEP, which is used only for patients being mechanically ventilated. With CPAP, expiration is controlled by a valve in the expiratory circuit that measures airway pressure and stops expiration before airway pressure returns to zero.

One disadvantage of CPAP is that the work of breathing may be increased because of resistance in initiating gas flow.[96] The level of CPAP chosen should be as low as possible to obtain a PO_2 greater than 60 mm Hg with a relatively safe FiO2 of less than 0.6. With CPAP there is lack of backup mandatory ventilation and careful monitoring of O_2 saturation with oximeters is very important. Respiratory rates, level of agitation, and blood gases must be monitored to prevent unrecognized hypercapnia.[96]

Pressure Support Ventilation

Pressure support ventilation (PSV) is another mode of ventilation. It relies on patient effort to determine tidal volume and frequency. This mode differs from CPAP in that the patient's inspiratory efforts trigger ventilator air flow until a preset airway pressure is reached. Air flow continues as long as the patient is making sufficient inspiratory effort to keep airway pressure below the preset limit. The advantages of pressure support ventilation may include overcoming the circuit-resistance breathing associated with spontaneous breathing through a ventilator. By decreasing the level of "pressure support" over time, this mode of ventilation can be an effective weaning technique.[96]

Biphasic Airway Pressure

A recent addition to the ventilator mode is biphasic airway pressure (BiPAP), which delivers pressure support ventilation (PSV) for inspiration and CPAP on expiration. It is used primarily to assist breathing during sleep for patients with neuromuscular disorders such as muscular dystrophy and central sleep apnea. To deliver BiPAP, a small mask is fitted over the nose. The use of BiPAP during sleep allows the patient to obtain a restful night's sleep and to awake feeling more refreshed.

Suctioning the Patient

When the patient on a ventilator needs suctioning, a closed system is preferred. In closed system endotracheal suctioning, an adaptor is inserted at the endotracheal tube–ventilatory circuitry interface. This allows patients to be suctioned without disconnecting them from the ventilator. The potential benefits of this form of suctioning are (1) the maintenance of positive-pressure ventilation, (2) the

continuation of oxygen supply, and (3) the stability of PEEP.

General Care of the Patient on a Ventilator

In planning care for the patient on a mechanical ventilator, it is imperative to know the patient's ability to breathe spontaneously in the event of accidental disconnection from the ventilator. In most facilities, respiratory therapists regularly monitor ventilator function and settings, but the nurse is also responsible for ensuring that the ventilator settings are maintained. Usually a checklist is used to verify the ventilator settings on an hourly basis.

The patient should be assessed on a regular basis and any time a ventilator alarm sounds. The cause of an alarm sounding can be a dysfunction anywhere from the person's lungs to the machine. Trouble-shooting should be carried out in a systematic fashion, starting with the patient and moving toward the machine. Assessment should include the following:

1. Patient assessment
   a. Inspection
      (1) Does the person appear to be in respiratory distress?
      (2) Is the person's chest moving with machine-cycled inspiration?
      (3) Is the chest moving bilaterally?
   b. Auscultation
      (1) Are breath sounds present?
      (2) Are adventitious sounds present?
      (3) Are breath sounds coordinated with ventilator inspiration?
2. Tubing to machine assessment
   a. Inspection
      (1) Is there an air leak around the endotracheal cuff?
      (2) Is there excess condensation in the tubing? (Always remove water from tubing system. Do not empty back into humidifier reservoir). Note: Not all ventilators have humidifiers.
      (3) Check all ventilator settings and readouts.

If the alarm continues to sound and the cause cannot be determined or the patient is in respiratory distress, the patient is disconnected from the machine and manually ventilated with an Ambu bag with oxygenated air until the problem can be resolved.

Weaning From the Ventilator

The decision to wean a person from the ventilator is based on clinical evidence of improved physical status. Weaning is most successful when performed by a nurse who has developed a trusting relationship with the patient. The underlying condition that compromised the patient's respiratory status must be stabilized. Weaning is initiated when the patient meets certain physiologic criteria, such as:

1. Acceptable arterial blood gases
2. Tidal volume greater than 10 ml/kg
3. Vital capacity greater than 15 ml/kg
4. FiO_2 less than 0.5
5. Maximal inspiratory pressure greater than 20 cm of water

The patient should be able to breathe on his or her own through the endotracheal tube for at least 30 minutes.

The weaning process is individualized to meet the patient's needs. The three most common forms of weaning are as follows:

1. T-piece weaning with or without CPAP.
   a. Place patient in upright sitting position.
   b. Deflate endotracheal or tracheostomy cuff.
   c. Disconnect patient from ventilator.
   d. Connect a T-piece (Fig. 24-52) to endotracheal tube cuff to provide oxygenated humidified air.
2. Intermittent mandatory ventilation (IMV) weaning (particularly useful for the person who is difficult to wean from the ventilator). Fig. 24-51, *C*, illustrates IMV and PEEP. In comparing *B* and *C* of Fig. 24-51, it can be seen that IMV and PEEP is a combination of PEEP and CPAP.
   a. Patient remains connected to the ventilator. The number of mandatory breaths delivered by the machine is gradually reduced, allowing the patient to take an increasing number of breaths independently.
   b. Patient is disconnected from the ventilator when predetermined physiologic criteria are maintained.
3. Pressure-support ventilation (PSV) as described on p. 626. It is a newer method and less widely used than IMV or T-piece weaning.

A recent article on weaning divides the process into three phases: *preweaning, weaning,* and *extubation.*[66]

During the *preweaning stage* special attention is given to ensuring that the patient will have *normal electrolytes* including *phosphate, calcium,* and *magnesium.* Malnutrition is to be avoided, but the patient should not be overfed. *Overfeeding with carbohydrates (CHO) and extra calories may result in increased CO_2 production and increased ventilatory demand.* The recommended 24-hour caloric intake is 1500 to 2500 calories, which should ensure adequate calories for energy expenditure. Protein intake is important and 1 to 1.5 mg/kg has been suggested. Tube feedings containing these requirements are given to prepare the patient for weaning. Nursing interventions during the weaning process include the following:

1. Before initiating weaning, prepare the patient. Teach effective breathing techniques. Inform the patient that weaning may take several attempts.
2. Obtain baseline vital signs, tidal volume, and vital capacity.
3. Stay with the patient during the initial weaning process.
4. Coach the patient as needed to breathe slower and deeper.
5. Suction as needed.
6. Monitor for the clinical signs of hypoxemia and hypercapnia (tachycardia, dysrhythmias, increased blood pressure, agitation, diaphoresis, or increased somnolence).
7. If patient is unable to breathe on own, reconnect to ventilator.
8. Weaning may require several attempts for increasingly longer periods of time before the ventilator can be disconnected.

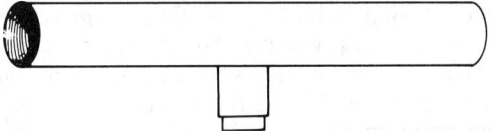

Fig. 24-52   T-piece used for weaning from ventilator. (From Abels LF: *Mosby's manual of critical care.* St Louis, 1979. Mosby–Year Book.)

Care of the Patient Discharged on a Ventilator

It is becoming more common for patients who cannot be weaned from the ventilator to be sent home on the ventilator. Before discharge, careful planning is required to assure that the home can accommodate the patient and the necessary equipment. Home care of patients such as these are discussed in detail in Chapter 47.

SUMMARY

1. In restrictive lung disease, there is a restriction in lung volume and a reduction in lung compliance. In obstructive lung disease, there is an increase in airway resistance resulting in prolonged exhalation.
2. Acute bronchitis, pneumonia, tuberculosis, fungal infections, occupational-related lung diseases, adult respiratory distress syndrome, and cancer of the lung are examples of restrictive lung diseases.
3. Chronic obstructive lung disease refers to diseases that produce obstruction of airflow and includes asthma, chronic bronchitis, pulmonary emphysema, and cystic fibrosis.
4. Primary prevention of respiratory infections includes prevention of the spread of infection by teaching the infected person to cover nose and mouth with a tissue when coughing or sneezing so that *droplet nuclei* are not released into the air.
5. Histoplasmosis, coccidioidomycosis, and blastomycosis are three major fungal infections of the lungs. Amphotericin B is the standard therapy for mycotic infection.
6. Adult respiratory distress syndrome is often fatal and is characterized by severe dyspnea, hypoxemia, and diffuse bilateral pulmonary infiltrations following lung injury in previously healthy persons.
7. The cause of cancer of the lung is closely related to cigarette smoking. From available research data, it seems evident that curtailing smoking is a primary preventive measure.
8. Efforts to detect malignant lesions of the lungs early, while curative treatment may be possible, are critical. The nurse should encourage all persons over the age of 40 to have an x-ray examination of the chest periodically in addition to a yearly physical examination.
9. Postoperative care of the patient after thoracic surgery centers on promoting ventilation and reexpansion of the lung by maintaining a clear airway; promoting

comfort by pain relief; promoting reexpansion of the lung by proper maintenance of the water-seal drainage system; promoting arm exercises to maintain range of motion; and monitoring the incision for bleeding and subcutaneous emphysema.

10. If an open sucking wound of the chest has been sustained, the wound should be covered immediately to prevent air from entering the pleural cavity and causing a pneumothorax.

11. Persons with chronic bronchitis are sometimes referred to as "blue bloaters." Persons with pulmonary emphysema are sometimes referred to as "pink puffers."

12. Cystic fibrosis is an inherited disease that causes airway obstruction. It usually develops in childhood.

13. Because of better treatment, more patients with CF are living into their twenties.

14. Asthma results in intermittent rather than continuous airway obstruction.

15. Respiratory failure is said to occur when ventilation is not sufficient to achieve gas exchange even at rest.

16. Patients in respiratory failure require intubation and mechanical ventilation.

STUDY QUESTIONS

• What is the quality of air in the community in which you reside? If air pollution is a problem, what are the major contributing factors (industries, automobile exhaust, and so on)? Are there community groups working to improve the problem? If so, what activities are they involved in and how might a nurse be helpful to their efforts?

• Where is the branch of the American Cancer Society and the American Lung Association nearest your community? What services do they provide for health professionals and for patients?

• What is the tuberculosis case rate in the area in which you live? Is this higher or lower than the national rate of 10.9/100,000 population? List the factors that contribute to a higher or lower case rate in your community.

• List the services available in your community to assist persons who wish to stop smoking and to which you could refer patients or friends.

• Design a teaching plan or project that you believe would help convince teenagers they should not smoke. Would you use a different approach for females than for males?

• Plan a 3000-calorie, high-protein diet for a 60-year-old man with pulmonary emphysema who is very short of breath and finds eating to be a chore.

REFERENCES AND SELECTED READINGS

1. American Cancer Society: *Cancer facts and figures 1991*, Atlanta, Ga, 1992, The Society.
2. Barnes P et al: Tuberculosis in patients with human immunodeficiency virus infection, *New Engl J Med*, 324(23):1644-1649, 1991.
3.* Barry MA et al: Tuberculosis infection in urban adolescents: results of a school-based testing program, *Am J Pub Health* 80:439-441, 1990.
4. Bates D: *Respiratory function in disease*, ed 3, Philadelphia, 1989, WB Saunders.
5. Bonomi P: *Primary lung cancer*. In Rakel RE, editor: *Conn's current therapy 1990*, Philadelphia, 1990, WB Saunders.
6. Bradley RB: Adult respiratory distress syndrome, *Focus on Critical Care* 14:48-59, 1987.
7. Brisette S, Zinman R, Reidy M: Nursing care plans for lessons in young adults with advanced cystic fibrosis, Issues in contemporary pediatric nursing 10(2):87-97, 1987.
8. Callahan M: A prudent pulmonary rehabilitation program, *Am J Nurs* 85:1368-1369, 1985.
8a.* Carroll PL: What's new in chest-tube management, *RN* 54(5):34-40, 1991.
8b. Carroll P: Nursing the thoractomy patient, *RN* 55(6):34-42, 1992.
9.* Carroll PL: Cyanosis: the sign you can count on, *Nurs 88* 18(3):50, 1088.
10.* Carroll PL: Lowering the risks of endotracheal suctioning, *Nurs 88* 18(5):46-50, 1988.
11.* Caruthers DD: Infectious pneumonia in the elderly, *Am J Nurs* 90(2):56-60, 1990.
12. Centers for Disease Control: CDC Surveillance Summaries, Dec 1991, Tuberculosis morbidity in the United States: final data, 1990, *MMWR* 40 (no. SS3):23-28, 1992.
12a.* Centers for Disease Control: Prevention and control of tuberculosis among homeless persons. Recommendations of the Advisory Council for the Elimination of Tuberculosis, *MMWR* 41(no. RR5):1-23, 1992.
13. Centers for Disease Control: Nosocomial transmission of multi-drug resistant tuberculosis among HIV-infected persons—Florida and New York, 1988-1991, *MMWR* 40(34)585-591, Aug 20, 1991.
14. Centers for Disease Control: State tobacco prevention and control activities: results of 1989-1990 association of state and territorial health officials (ASTHO) survey—final report, *MMWR* 40(RR-11):1-41, Aug 16, 1991.
15. Centers for Disease Control: Purified protein derivative (PPD)—tuberculin anergy and HIV infection, *MMWR* 40 (no. RR-5); 27-33, April 28, 1991.
16. Centers for Disease Control: Influenza activity-world-wide, 1990-1991, *MMWR* 40(41):709-712, 1991.
17. Centers for Disease Control: Prevention and control of influenza, *MMWR* 40 (no. RR-6):1-15, May 24, 1991.
18. Centers for Disease Control: Summary of notifiable diseases, United States, 1990, *MMWR* 39 (53):1-62, Oct 4, 1991.
19. Centers for Disease Control: Tuberculosis among foreign-born persons entering the United States, *MMWR* 39 (RR-18), Dec 28, 1990.
20. Centers for Disease Control: The surgeon general's 1990 report on the health benefits of smoking cessation—executive summary, *MMWR* 39 (no RR-12):1-12, Oct 5, 1990.
21. Centers for Disease Control: Screening for tuberculosis and tuberculosis infection in high-risk populations and the use of preventive therapy for tuberculosis infection in the United States, *MMWR*, 29 (no RR-8):1-12, May 18, 1990.
22. Centers for Disease Control, Morbidity and Mortality Weekly Report: update: tuberculosis elimination—United States, *MMWR* 39 (10):153-156, 1990.
23. Centers for Disease Control, Morbidity and Mortality Report: Cigarette smoking—behavioral risk factor surveilliance system, *MMWR* 38(49):845-848, 1989.
24. Centers for Disease Control, Morbidity and Mortality Weekly Report—Summary of notifiable disease United States 1988, *MMWR* 37(54):41-43, 1988.

*Suggested for student reading.

25. Cherniack RM: Current therapy of respiratory disease—two, Toronto, 1986, BC Dekker.

26.* Chulay M, Graeber GM: Efficacy of a hyperinflation and hyperoxygenation suctioning intervention, *Heart Lung* 17:1:15-22, 1988.

27. Cobb N, Etzel RA: Unintentional carbon monoxide related deaths in the United States, 1979 through 1988, *JAMA* 266(5):659-663, 1991.

28.* Cornell C: Tuberculosis in hospital employees, *Am J Nurs* 88(4):484-486, 1988.

29. Davis PB: Pathophysiology of pulmonary disease in cystic fibrosis, *Semin Resp Med* 6(4):261-269, 1985.

30. Dept of Health and Human Services: *Healthy people 2000: national health promotion and disease prevention objectives*, Washington, DC, 1990, US Govt Printing Office.

31. DeVito AJ: Rehabilitation of patients with chronic obstructive pulmonary disease, *Rehab Nurs* 10:12-15, 1985.

32.* Dooley SW et al: Guidelines for preventing the transmission of tuberculosis in health care settings, with special focus on HIV-related issues, *MMWR* 39 (RR-17):1-26, 1990.

33.* Dougherty S: The malnourished respiratory patient. *Crit Care Nurs* 8:13-15, 18-22, 1988.

34.* Douglas RG: Prophylaxis and treatment of influenza, *N Engl J Med* 322(7):443-449, 1990.

35. Dowling PT: Return of tuberculosis: screening and preventive therapy, *AFP* 43(2):457-467, 1991.

36. Dupuis YG: Ventilators theory and clinical application, ed 2, St Louis, 1991, Mosby—Year Book.

37.* Durham E, Frost-Hartzer P: Relaxation therapy works, *RN* 54(8):40-42, Aug 1991.

38.* Engelking C: CE lung cancer therapy, *Am J Nurs* 87:1438-1439, 1987.

39.* Engelking C: Teaching, counseling, and caring, *Am J Nurs* 87:1439-1440, 1987.

40.* Engelking C: CE lung cancer: the language of staging, *Am J Nurs* 87:1434-1437, 1987.

41. Ferland PA: Are you ready for ventilator patients? *Nurs 91*, 21(1):42-47, Jan 1991.

42.* Finesilver C: Perfecting the art of respiratory assessment, *RN* 55(2):22-30, Feb 1992.

43. Forouzesh M, Price JH, Taylor C: Pulmonary disease, *Nurs Care* 15:19-22, 1992.

44. Fraser RG et al: *Diagnosis of disease of the chest*, vol 3, ed 3, Philadelphia, 1990, WB Saunders.

45.* Freedberg PD et al: Effect of progressive muscle relaxation on the objective symptoms and subjective responses associated with asthma, *Heart Lung* 16:24-30, 1987.

46.* Fuchs Carroll P: Caring for ventilator patients, *Nursing* 86 16(6):34-39, 1986.

47.* George MR: CF not just a pediatric problem anymore, *RN* 53(9):60-65, Sept 1990.

48. Gift AG, Bolgiano CS, Cunningham J: Sensations during chest tube removal, *Heart Lung* 20(2):131-137, 1991.

49. Hahn DL, Dodge RW, Golubjatnikov R: Association of *Chlamydia pneumoniae* (strain TWAR) infection with wheezing, asthmatic bronchitis, and adult-onset asthma, *JAMA* 266 (2):225-230, 1991.

50. Handwerger S et al: Tuberculosis and the acquired immunodeficiency syndrome at a New York city hospital, *Chest* 91(2):176-180, 1987.

51. Hanley MV, Tyler ML: Ineffective airway clearance related to airway infection, *Nurs Clin North Am* 22(1):135-149, 1987.

52. Hartman B et al: *Pneumocystis carinii* pneumonia in the acquired immunodeficiency syndrome (AIDS)—diagnosis with bronchial brushings, biopsy, and bronchoalveolar lavage, *Chest* 87:603-607, 1985.

53. Harvard Medical Health Letter: *Asthma*, part 1, Harvard Medical School, 16(7):5-7, May 1991.

54. Harvard Medical Health Letter: *Asthma*, part 2, Harvard Medical School, 16(8):1-4, June 1991.

55. Hay JW, Robin ED: Cost-effectiveness of alpha₁ antitrypsin replacement therapy in treatment of congenital chronic obstructive pulmonary disease, *Am J Pub Health* 81(4):427-433, 1991.

56.* Hefts D: Chest trauma, *RN* 54(5):28-32, 1991.

57. Hodgkin JE, Petty RL: *Chronic obstructive pulmonary disease: current concepts*, Philadelphia, 1987, WB Saunders.

58.* Hoffman LA: Airway management for the critically ill patient, *Am J Nurs* 87(1):39-43, 1987.

59.* Hoffman LA, Maskiewicz RC: The specifics of suctioning, *Am J Nurs* 87(1):44-53, 1987.

60.* Irwin M, Openbrier D: A delicate balance—strategies for feeding ventilated COPD patients, *Am J Nurs* 3:274-280, 1985.

61. Janson-Bjerklie S, Shnell S: Effect of peak flow information on patterns of self-care in adult asthma, *Heart Lung* 17:543-549, 1988.

62. Johnson A: The elderly and COPD, *J Gerontol Nurs* 14:20-24, 1988.

63.* Jordan K: Chest trauma, *Nursing* 90(9):34-42, 1990.

64.* Kersten LD: *Comprehensive respiratory therapy*, Philadelphia, 1989, WB Saunders.

65. Klinger JR, Nichols NS: Right ventricular dysfunction in chronic obstructive pulmonary disease, *Chest* 90(3):715-723, 1991.

66.* Knebel AR: Complications in critical care weaning from mechanical ventilation: current controversies, *Heart Lung*, 20(4):321-331, 1991.

67.* Krokosky NJ: Black lung and silicosis, *Am J Nurs* 85:883-886, 1985.

68. Larson EB, Ramsey PG, editors: *Medical therapeutics*, Philadelphia, 1989, WB Saunders.

69. Lewis MI, Belman MJ: Nutrition and respiratory muscles, *Clin Chest Med* 9:337-348, 1988.

70. Lordi GM, Reichman LB: Tuberculosis and other mycobacterial disease. In Rakel RE, editor: *Conn't current therapy 1990*, Philadelphia, 1990, WB Saunders.

71.* Madsen LA: Tuberculosis today, *RN* 53 (3):44-50, 1990.

72. Mapp CS: Trach care—are you aware of the danger? *Nurs* 88 18(7):34-42, 1988.

73. Marx JL: The cystic fibrosis gene is found, *Science* 245:923-925, 1989.

74.* Mathews PJ, Mathews LM, Mitchell RR: Artificial airways resuscitation guidelines you can follow, *Nurs 92*, 22(1):53-59, Jan 1992.

75.* McNaull FH: CE lung cancer: tobacconism in America, *Am J Nurs* 87:1430-1432, 1987.

76.* McNaull FW: CE lung cancer: What are the odds? *Am J Nurs* 87:1428-1429, 1987.

77. Norton LC et al: Common problems and state of the art in nursing care of the mechanically ventilated patient, *Crit Care Nurs* 6:23-37, 1986.

78.* Openbrier DR, Hoffman LA, Weismiller SA: Home oxygen evaluation, *Am J Nurs* 88(2):192-197, 1988.

79.* Openbrier DR, Fuoss C, Mall CC: What patients on home oxygen therapy want to know, *Am J Nurs* 88(2):198-202, 1988.

80. Orsi AJ: Asthma—the danger is real, *RN* 54(4):58-62, April 1991.

81.* Preucser BA et al: Effects of two methods of preoxygenations on mean arterial pressure, cardiac output, peak airway pressure, and past suctioning hypoxemia, *Heart Lung* 17(3):290-298, 1988.

82. Ramsdell JW: *Bronchodilator drugs*. In Bordow RA, Moser KM: *Manual of clinical problems in pulmonary medicine*, Boston, 1988, Little Brown.

83. Ray JW, Robin ED: Cost-effectiveness of alpha-₁ antitrypsin replacement therapy in treatment of congenital chronic obstructive pulmonary disease, *Am J Pub Health*, 81(4):427-433, 1991.

84.* Renfroe KL: Effect of progressive relaxation on dyspnea and state anxiety in patients with chronic obstructive pulmonary disease, *Heart Lung* 17:408-413, 1988.

85. Roberts SL: High-permeability pulmonary edema: nursing assessment, diagnosis and interventions, *Heart Lung* 19(3):287-299, 1990.

86. Rogge JA et al: Effectiveness of oxygen concentrations of less than 100% before and after endotracheal suction in patients with chronic obstructive pulmonary disease, *Heart Lung* 18:64-71, 1989.

87. Schmidt GA, Hall JB: Acute and chronic respiratory failure assessment and management of patients with COPD in the emergent setting, *Concepts Emerg Crit Care* 261:3444-3453, 1989.

88. Schumann L, Parsons GH: Tracheal suctioning and ventilator tubing changes in adult respiratory distress syndrome: use of a positive end-expiratory pressure valve, *Heart Lung* 14, 362-367, 1985.

89. Shapiro BA, Harrison RA, Trout CA: *Clinical application of respiratory care*, ed 3, Bowie, Md, 1985, The Charles Press.

90. Shekelton ME: Coping with chronic respiratory difficulty, *Nurs Clin North Am* 22(3):569-581, 1987.

91.* Slonim NB, Hamilton LH: *Respiratory physiology*, ed 5, St Louis, 1987, Mosby–Year Book.

92.* Sonnesso G: Are you ready to use pulse oximetry? *Nurs 91* 21(8):60-64, August 1991.

93. Spector N: Nutritional support of the ventilator-dependent patient, *Nurs Clin North Am* 24:407-414, 1989.

94.* Stevens SA, Becher KL: Respiratory assessment, *Nurs 88* 18(1):57-63, 1988.

95.* Stiesmeyer JK: What triggers a ventilator alarm? *Am J Nurs* 91(10):61-64, 1991.

96. Struve SW, Dean NC: *Acute respiratory failure*. In Rakel RE, editor: *Conn's current therapy*, Philadelphia, 1991, WB Saunders.

97. Taggart JA, Dorinsky NL, Sheahan JS: Airway pressure during closed suctioning, *Heart Lung* 17(5):536-542, 1988.

98. Tiep BL et al: Pursed-lip breathing training using ear oximetry, *Chest* 90:218-221, 1986.

99. Traver G, Mitchell JT, Flodquist Prestley G: *Respiratory care: a clinical approach*, Gaithersburg, Md, 1991, Aspen.

100.* Walsh LM, Johnson CC: Update on microbial agents, *Nurs Clin North Am* 26(2):341-360, June 1991.

101. West JB: *Pulmonary pathophysiology—the essentials*, ed 3, Baltimore, 1987, Williams & Wilkins.

102. Whitney E: Chronic bronchitis and emphysema, *Nurs 92*, 22(3):34-42, 1992.

103. Yeaw EMJ: Good lung down? *Am J Nurs* 92(3):27-32, 1992.

104. Youmans GP, Patterson PY, Sommers HM: *The biologic and clinical basis of infectious diseases*, ed 3, Philadelphia, 1986, WB Saunders.

Classics

105. Alford RH: Histoplasmosis. In Conn HF: *Current therapy 1982*, Philadelphia, 1982, WB Saunders.

106.* American Lung Association: *Chronic obstructive pulmonary disease*, New York, 1981, The Association.

107. American Lung Association: *Diagnostic standards and classification of tuberculosis*, New York, 1981, The Association.

108. American Lung Association: *The asthma handbook*, New York, 1984, The Association.

109. American Lung Association: *Occupational lung disease: an introduction*, New York, 1979, The Association.

110. Centers for Disease Control: *Humidifiers: tips given on trimming hazards*, Atlanta, 1979, The Centers for Disease Control.

111. Davis PB, diSant' AP: Diagnosis and treatment of cystic fibrosis—an update, *Chest* 85(6):802-808, 1984.

112. DeTrayer A, Estenne M: Coordination between rib cage muscles and diaphragm during quiet breathing in humans, *J Appl Physiol* 57:899, 1984.

113.* Duncan C, Erickson R: Pressures associated with chest tube stripping, *Heart Lung* 11-166-171, 1982.

114.* Erickson R: Solving chest tube problems, *Nursing 81* 11(6):62-68, 1981.

115.* Erickson R: Chest tubes: they're really not that complicated, *Nursing 81* 11(5):34-43, 1981.

116. Fletcher CM, Pride NB: Definition of emphysema, chronic bronchitis, asthma, and airflow obstruction: 25 years from the CIBA symposium, *Thorax* 39:81-85, 1984 (editorial).

117.* Frame PT: Acute infectious pneumonia in the adult, *Basics RD* 10:3, 1982.

118. Godfrey S: *Exercise-induced asthma*. In Clark TJH, Godfrey S, editors: *Asthma*, ed 2, London, 1983, Chapman and Hall.

119.* Gold W: Restrictive lung disease, *Phys Ther* 48(5):455-466, 1982.

120. Hagarty E: Weaning your COPD patient from the ventilator, *RN* 47(7):36-40, 1984.

121. Harris B, Hyman RB: Clean vs sterile tracheostomy care and level of pulmonary infection, *Nurs Res* 33:80-85, 1984.

122. Kryger M, editor: *Pathophysiology and respiration*, New York, 1981, John Wiley.

123. Langston HT, Barker WS: *The adult thoracic surgical patient*. In Neville WE, editor: *Intensive care of the cardiopulmonary patient*, ed 2, Chicago, 1983, Yearbook.

124. Leininger BJ: *Thoracic trauma*. In Neville WE: *Intensive care of the surgical cardiopulmonary patient*, Chicago, 1983, Yearbook.

125.* Matthews LW, Drotar DD: Cystic fibrosis—a challenging long-term chronic disease, *Pediatr Clin North Am* 31(1):133-152, 1984.

126. Stahley TL, and Trench WD: Lung entrapment and infarction by chest tube suction, *Radiology* 122:307, 1977.

127. Treoloar D, Stechmiller J: Pulmonary aspiration in tube-fed patients with artificial airways, *Heart Lung* 13:667-671, 1984.

128. Wood RF, Boot TF, Doershuk CF: Cystic fibrosis: state of the art, *Am Rev Resp Dis* 113:833-877, 1976.

25

The Patient with Cardiovascular Problems

Terri Abraham
Mary A. (Sandy) Wyper

After studying this chapter, the learner should be able to:

- Differentiate between data obtained from a 12-lead ECG and data obtained from a cardiac monitor.
- Explain the differences between dysrhythmias that are a result of arrhythmogenic mechanisms.
- Identify life-threatening dysrhythmias.
- Describe treatment modalities for cardiac dysrhythmias.
- Identify risk factors for CAD.
- Explain the pathophysiologic basis, therapeutic modalities, and nursing interventions for angina pectoris, myocardial infarction, and congestive heart failure.
- Plan teaching needs of patients with angina, myocardial infarction, and congestive heart failure, and patients undergoing cardiac surgery.
- Describe the pathophysiologic bases for pulmonary edema and cardiogenic shock and the relation of the therapeutic modalities for these conditions to those for congestive heart failure.
- Explain the pathophysiologic bases for disorders of the various layers of cardiac tissue (pericardium, myocardium, epicardium), the cardiac valves, and the aorta.
- Describe surgical intervention for repair of cardiac valves and aortic aneurysms and the pre/postoperative nursing care required.

Cardiovascular disorders are a major health problem in the United States, although deaths from myocardial ischemia and its complications have decreased significantly since the 1970s. Key factors contributing to this decline include (1) advances in medical and surgical treatment of coronary disease, (2) reduction in cigarette smoking, (3) improved screening and treatment of hypertension, and (4) an overall increase in health awareness, notably increased interest in exercise or fitness and improved nutritional habits.

In 1991 approximately 1.5 million people in the United States will sustain myocardial infarction (heart attack), of which 500,000 (33%) will not survive. More than 300,000 people a year die before reaching the hospital.[3] These statistics strongly support the need for public education about the early recognition of cardiac emergencies and basic cardiac life support measures. It is hoped that effective application of the increased knowledge of cardiovascular disease and its risk factors will enable health care professionals to assist persons more effectively in achieving and maintaining optimal health.

ANATOMY AND PHYSIOLOGY
Basic Structure of the Heart

The heart is a small organ (about the size of a fist) located in the middle and slightly to the left of the mediastinum, where it is partially overlapped by the lungs. The heart is wider at the top (base) than at the bottom (apex) and is positioned in the chest so that the blunt tip of the apex projects forward and to the left. The lower border of the heart rests on the diaphragm.

The heart is enclosed by the *pericardium,* which consists of two layers: the inner layer (visceral pericardium) and the outer layer (parietal pericardium). The two pericardial surfaces are separated by a pericardial space that normally contains approximately 10 to 20 ml of thin, clear pericardial fluid. This lubricating fluid moistens the contacting surfaces of the pericardial layers and reduces the friction produced by the pumping action of the heart. If too much fluid collects in the pericardial space (pericardial effusion), pressure is exerted on the heart muscle, leading to decreased pumping efficiency.

There are three layers of cardiac tissue:

Epicardium: Outer layer of the heart
   Same structure as the visceral pericardium
Myocardium: Middle layer of the heart
   Composed of striated muscle fibers
   Responsible for the heart's contractile force
Endocardium: Inner layer of the heart
   Consists of endothelial tissue
   Lines the inside of the chambers and covers the heart valves

Chambers

The heart is divided into two halves by a muscular wall (septum) (Fig. 25-1). Each half has an upper collecting chamber (atrium) and a lower pumping chamber (ventricle), for a total of four chambers. Oxygen-poor venous blood enters the right atrium, flows from the right atrium to the right ventricle (mainly by gravity) when the tricuspid valve is opened, and is pumped to the lungs through the pul-

monary artery. Oxygen-rich blood returns from the lungs to the left atrium, enters the left ventricle when the mitral valve is opened, and is ejected into the aorta for distribution to the peripheral tissues.

The *right atrium* is a thin-walled structure that serves as a reservoir for venous blood returning to the heart via the superior and inferior vena cava and the coronary sinus. The right atrium stores this blood during right ventricular systole (contraction). The *right ventricle* receives venous blood from the right atrium during ventricular diastole (relaxation) and then propels this blood through the pulmonic valve into the pulmonary artery and then to the lungs. The overall workload of the right ventricle is less than that of the left ventricle because the pulmonary system is a low-pressure system.

The thin-walled *left atrium* receives oxygenated blood from the four pulmonary veins and serves as a reservoir during left ventricular systole. Blood flows by gravity from the left atrium into the *left ventricle* through the opened mitral valve during ventricular diastole. Blood is then ejected from the left ventricle through the opened aortic valve into the systemic arterial circulation during ventricular systole. The left ventricle has thick walls because it must contract against a high-pressure systemic circulation to deliver blood to the peripheral tissue.

Valves

The four cardiac valves are flaplike structures that function to maintain unidirectional (forward) blood flow through the heart chambers. These valves open and close in response to pressure and volume changes within the cardiac chambers. The cardiac valves can be classified into two types: the atrioventricular (AV) valves, which separate the atria from the ventricles, and the semilunar valves, which separate the pulmonary artery and the aorta from their respective ventricles.

Atrioventricular valves

The AV valves are the *tricuspid* valve, located between the right atrium and the right ventricle, and the *mitral* (bicuspid) valve, located between the left atrium and left ventricle. The tricuspid valve contains three leaflets held in place by fibrous cords called the *chordae tendineae,* which in turn are anchored to the ventricular wall by the papillary muscles. The mitral valve on the left side of the heart has two valve cusps or leaflets (Fig. 25-2). It is attached in the same manner as the tricuspid valve. The chordae tendineae are important because they support the AV valves during ventricular systole to prevent valvular prolapse into the atrium. A degree of leaflet overlapping during closure of the AV valves helps prevent the backward flow of blood. Damage to the chordae tendineae or to the papillary muscles would permit blood to regurgitate (flow backward) into the atrium during ventricular systole. The AV valves are *closed during ventricular systole (contraction) and open during diastole (relaxation).*

Semilunar valves

The semilunar valves include the *aortic* and *pulmonic* valves. The structural design of the semilunar valves is quite different from that of the AV valves; each consists

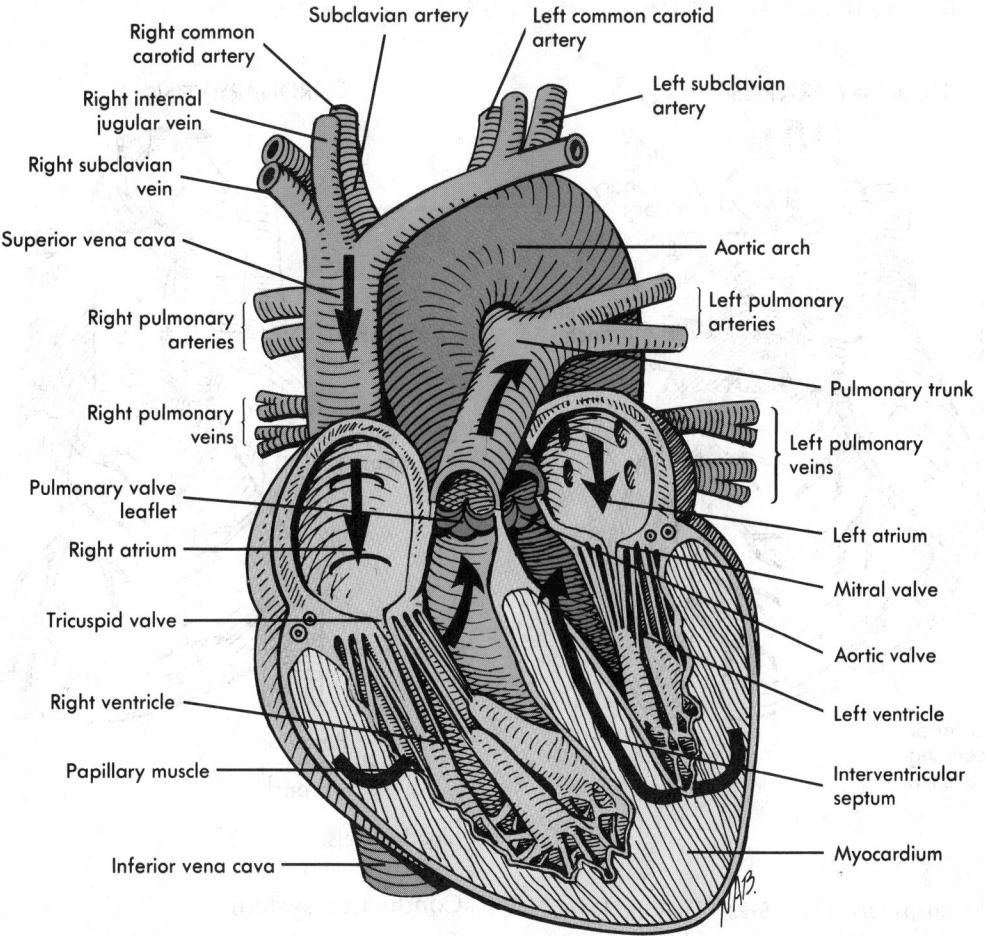

Right common
carotid artery

Right internal
jugular vein

Right subclavian
vein

Superior vena cava

Right pulmonary
arteries

Right pulmonary
veins

Pulmonary valve
leaflet

Right atrium

Tricuspid valve

Right ventricle

Papillary muscle

Inferior vena cava

Subclavian artery

Left common carotid
artery

Left subclavian
artery

Aortic arch

Left pulmonary
arteries

Pulmonary trunk

Left pulmonary
veins

Left atrium

Mitral valve

Aortic valve

Left ventricle

Interventricular
septum

Myocardium

Fig. 25-1   Heart in frontal section: course of blood through the chambers.

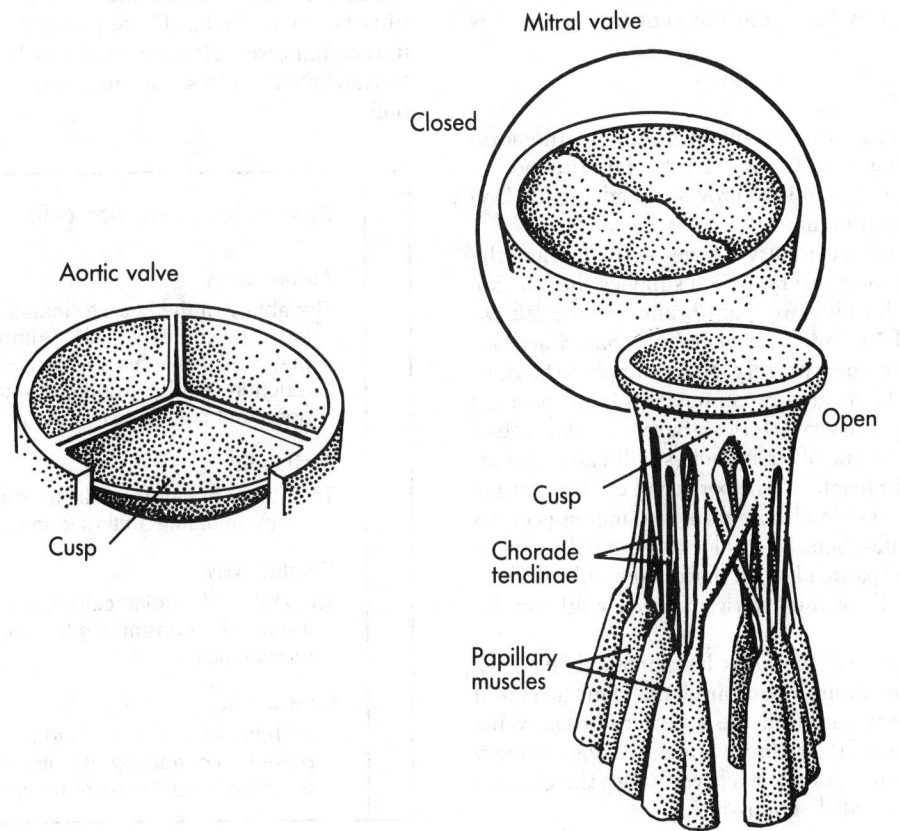

Mitral valve

Closed

Aortic valve

Open

Cusp

Cusp

Chorade
tendinae

Papillary
muscles

Fig. 25-2   Mitral and aortic valves.

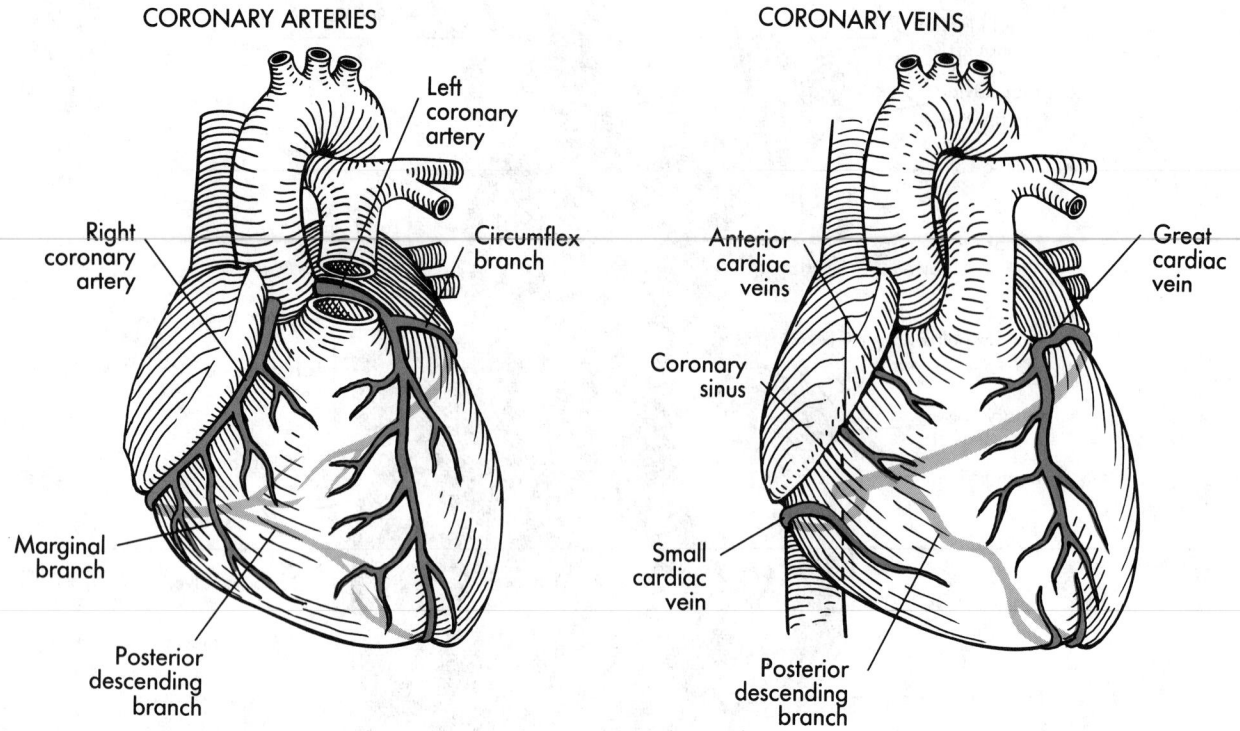

Fig. 25-3 Coronary blood vessels.

of three cuplike cusps (see Fig. 25-2). They lie between each ventricle and the great vessel into which it empties. These valves are *open during ventricular systole* to permit blood flow into the aorta and pulmonary arteries and *closed during diastole* to prevent retrograde flow from the aorta and pulmonary artery back into the ventricle when it is relaxed.

Coronary arteries

The coronary arteries arise at the beginning of the aorta right behind the aortic valve (Fig. 25-3). The function of the coronary artery system is to provide an adequate blood supply to the myocardium.

There are two main coronary arteries—the left and the right. The left coronary artery, which supplies the left side of the heart, divides into two main branches, the *left anterior descending* (LAD) and the *circumflex coronary* arteries (CCA). The right coronary artery (RCA) supplies the right side of the heart. There are few connections (anastomoses) between the main coronary arteries; therefore, blockage of a coronary artery or one of its branches will cause diminished blood flow (ischemia) to the portion of cardiac muscle supplied by that vessel and may result in angina pectoris or a myocardial infarction. Such blockages may be caused by coronary artery spasm, clots or, more commonly, by fatty deposits in the walls of the arteries (coronary atherosclerosis).

The venous system of the heart has three subdivisions: the thebesian veins drain a portion of the right atria and right ventricular myocardium; the anterior cardiac veins drain a large portion of the right ventricle; and the coronary sinus and its branches drain the left ventricle (the greatest portion of the myocardial venous return).

Conduction system

The mechanical contraction of the heart is the product of a stimulus-response process. Properties that are integral components of the electromechanical events in the heart are automaticity, excitability, conductivity, and contractility (see Box 25-1). These properties allow the heart to initiate impulses (either spontaneously or from a stimulus), to transmit impulses, and to respond by muscle contraction.

25-1

Properties of cardiac cells

Automaticity

The ability of the heart to initiate impulses regularly and spontaneously. (Although most cardiac cells have this ability, it is the primary function of the SA node, designating it the dominant pacemaker in the normal heart.)

Excitability

The ability of cardiac cells to respond to a stimulus by initiating a cardiac impulse.

Conductivity

The ability of cardiac cells to respond to a cardiac impulse by transmitting the impulse along cell membranes.

Contractility

The ability of cardiac cells to respond to an impulse by contracting. (Contractile cells comprise the largest mass of the myocardium.)

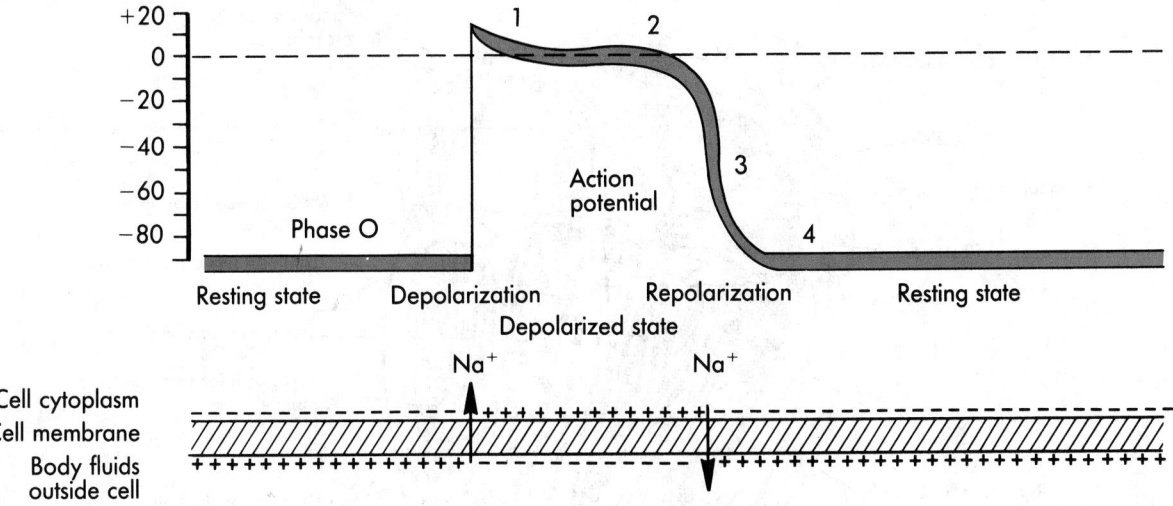

Fig. 25-4   Phases of the action potential of cardiac muscle.

Action potential

The resting myocardial cell has a membrane potential (that is, an electrical charge) as a result of the relative distribution of extracellular and intracellular sodium and potassium ions. Whenever the cell is stimulated, the membrane potential changes. A graphic record of this change forms the basis for an electrocardiogram (ECG). The change in electrical potential in response to a stimulus is known as the action potential. The two components of the action potential are *depolarization* (generation of the impulse) and *repolarization* (return of cell to resting state.) The electrical current stimulates the release of calcium ions, which catalyze the reaction of myocardial contraction.

Resting membrane potential

In the resting state, the inside of the cell is negative with respect to the outside (Fig. 25-4). Initiation and conduction of cardiac impulses depend on the cell's ability to maintain an electrical potential gradient when the cell is at rest. The main factor that contributes to the -90 mV resting membrane potential (see Fig. 25-4) is the cell's permeability to potassium and nonpermeability to sodium. Because more sodium is pumped out of the cell via the sodium-potassium exchange pump than potassium is moved in, a net outward current of positive ions further enhances the cell's negativity during the resting phase.

Depolarization

The initiation of a cardiac impulse begins with the process of depolarization, which indicates the rapid reversal of the resting membrane potential. Depolarization results from increased cell membrane permeability to sodium and subsequent rapid intracellular sodium influx as well as potassium movement out of the cell. This movement of ions across the membrane creates an electrical current. When the amount of sodium entering the cell reaches a critical level, an electrical impulse is generated. The impulse may spread as a wave of depolarization to adjacent cells.

Repolarization

Repolarization is the process by which the cell returns to the resting state. The following sequence occurs: (1) cell membrane permeability to sodium decreases, and (2) sodium leaves the cell while potassium returns through an active ion transport system.

Sequence of cardiac activation

The primary structures of the conduction system are listed in Box 25-2 and illustrated in Fig. 25-5. The sequence of cardiac activation is as follows:

1. Depolarization is initiated by an impulse from the SA node.

25-2

Structure of the conduction system of the heart

Sinoatrial (SA) node
Pacemaker node located in right atrium near opening of superior vena cava

Bachmann's bundle
Facilitates spread of impulse to left atrium

Internodal tracts
Connect SA and AV nodes

Atrioventricular node (AV)
Located on right side of interatrial septum

Bundle of His
Thick cable of fibers starting at the AV node, bifurcating into left and right bundle branches (LBB and RBB) down the two sides of the interventricular septum; the LBB bifurcates into anterior and posterior divisions

Purkinje fibers
Network of fibers at end of bundle of His that transmits impulse to both ventricular walls

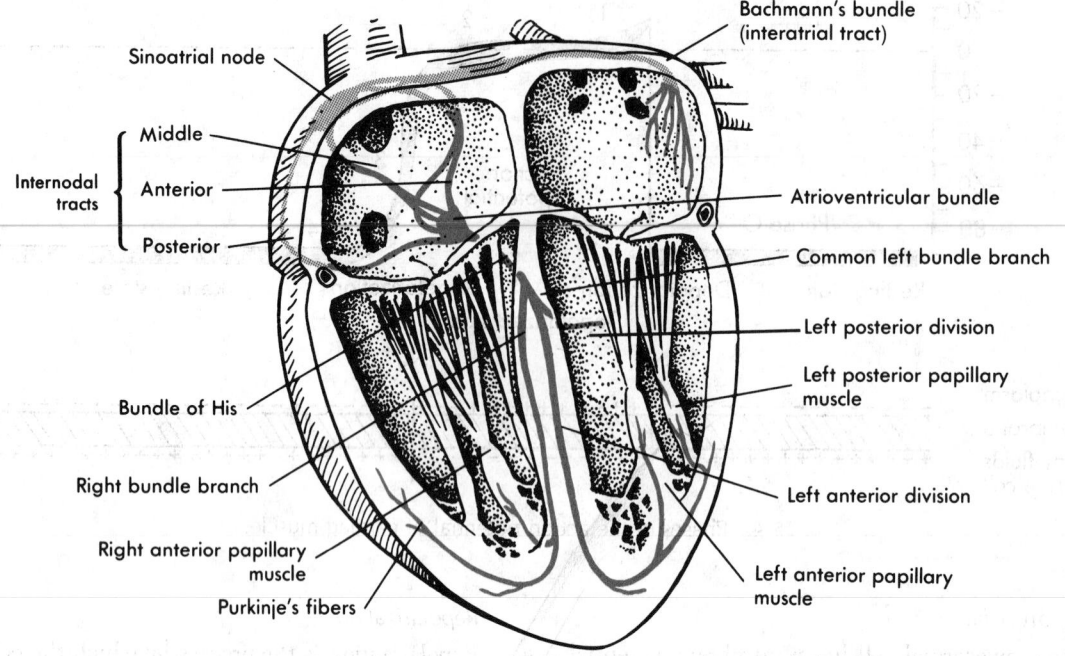

Fig. 25-5 Schematic diagram of heart illustrating the conduction system.

2. The impulse spreads through both atria.
3. The impulse reaches the AV node, which delays the impulse about 0.1 second.
4. The impulse is transmitted along the branches of the bundle of His to the Purkinje fibers, activating both ventricles almost simultaneously.
5. Activation of ventricular muscle proceeds from apex toward base of heart.

Cardiac Cycle

The cardiac cycle has two phases—diastole and systole. Relaxation and filling of the chambers take place during diastole. Contraction and emptying occur during systole.

Diastole

It is useful to envision the cardiac cycle starting at a point immediately after ventricular systole. At this time the AV valves are closed, and the atria are rapidly filling with blood (atrial diastole) (Fig. 25-6). Ventricular diastole is conceptualized in the following phases:

1. *Isovolumetric ventricular relaxation*: ventricular muscle relaxed but not yet filling
2. *Rapid ventricular filling*: passive gravity flow of blood from atria to ventricles; starts when atrial pressure exceeds ventricular pressure and AV valves open
3. *Slow ventricular filling*: occurs as increasing blood volume causes ventricular pressure to rise, which slows further filling

4. *Atrial systole*: atrial musculature contracts, propelling an additional 20% to 30% of blood into the ventricle before ventricular contraction. Atrial contraction occurs following electrical depolarization of the atria.

Systole

Electrical activation (depolarization) precedes mechanical contraction of both atria and ventricles. The ventricular systolic phase is comprised of the following:

1. *Isovolumetric ventricular contraction*: increase in myocardial tension and intraventricular pressure without change in blood volume; AV valves closed.
2. *Maximal ventricular ejection*: greater pressure in ventricles than in aorta or pulmonary artery forces open semilunar valves, and blood is pumped into pulmonary and systemic circulation
3. *Reduced ventricular ejection*: ventricles remain contracted and a small quantity of blood is ejected from momentum built up by contraction; higher pressure in the aorta and pulmonary artery than in ventricles causes closure of semilunar valves—the end of ventricular systole

The familiar "lub-dub" heard when listening to the heart corresponds with the closure of the valves. The first sound results from closure of the atrioventricular valves at the beginning of ventricular systole. The second sound results from closing of the semilunar valves at the end of ventricular systole.

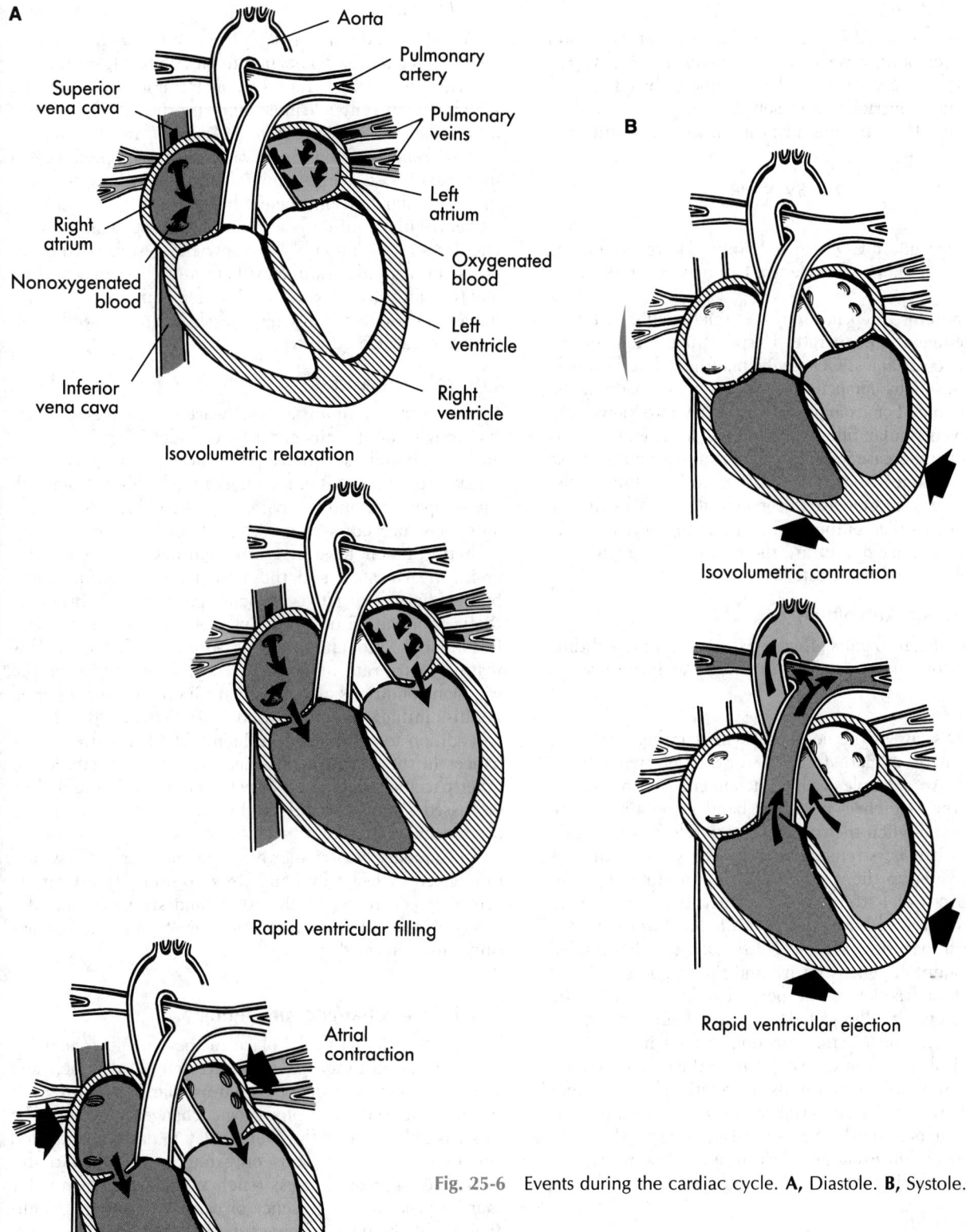

Fig. 25-6 Events during the cardiac cycle. **A,** Diastole. **B,** Systole.

Cardiac Output

The amount of blood ejected from the left ventricle into the aorta per minute is called *cardiac output* (CO). CO is equivalent to *stroke volume* (SV) (volume of blood ejected from the left ventricle with each contraction) multiplied by *heart rate* (HR) (number of heart beats per minute):

$$CO = SV \times HR$$

The average adult CO is 5.6 L/min. However, during periods of strenuous exercise the CO may reach 20 to 25 L/min.

CO therefore depends on the relationship between stroke volume and heart rate. Despite fluctuations in one of these two variables, CO can be maintained at relatively constant levels by compensatory adjustments made in the other variable. For example, if the heart rate slows, the time for ventricular filling (diastole) is lengthened. This allows for an increase in preload and a subsequent increase in stroke volume. Conversely, if the stroke volume falls, the heart rate can increase to compensate temporarily and to maintain cardiac output. Therefore, the actual determinants of cardiac output are the mechanisms regulating stroke volume and heart rate.

Control of stroke volume

Three significant factors affecting stroke volume and thus cardiac output are preload, contractility, and afterload.

Preload

Starling's law of the heart states that myocardial fiber responds with a more forceful contraction when it is stretched. An example of this phenomenon is that of increasing the stretch of a rubber band to obtain a more forceful recoil when the rubber band is released. Myocardial fibers can be stretched by increasing the volume of blood delivered to the ventricles during diastole. The degree of myocardial stretch before contraction is expressed in terms of preload. *Preload is related to the volume of blood distending the ventricles at the end of diastole.* It is determined by the amount of venous return and the ejection fraction. The ejection fraction is the portion of the end-diastolic volume that is actually ejected (normally about two thirds). A decrease in the ejection fraction results in a greater amount of blood left in the ventricle at the end of systole.

Since Starling's length-tension relationship is functional only within certain physiologic limits, it is important to note that prolonged, excessive stretching of the myocardial fibers will eventually lead to a *decrease* in cardiac output by reducing the stroke volume.

Contractility

Contractility refers to a change in the inotropic state (force of contraction) of the muscle without a change in myocardial fiber length or preload. Contractility can be increased by sympathetic stimulation or by the administration of substances such as calcium or epinephrine. Increased contractility improves ventricular emptying during systole, thereby increasing the stroke volume.

Afterload

Afterload is defined as *the amount of tension the ventricle must develop during contraction* to eject blood from the left ventricle into the aorta. The major impedance against which the left ventricle must pump is primarily determined by *peripheral vascular resistance.* Increase in pressure resulting from hypertension or vasoconstriction produces an increased resistance to pumping and requires an increase in ventricular tension to eject blood.

Ventricular tension is also directly proportional to ventricular size. Dilation of the ventricles resulting from increased ventricular volume will elevate ventricular tension and thus afterload. Excessive elevation of the afterload may impair ventricular emptying, thereby reducing stroke volume and cardiac output.

Control of heart rate

Under normal circumstances, heart rate is regulated by the activity of the sinoatrial (SA) node. The number of electrical impulses initiated per minute by this pacemaker is primarily the result of its innervation by fibers from both the sympathetic and the parasympathetic branches of the autonomic nervous system (ANS). Impulses from the sympathetic branch have a positive chronotropic effect (increase heart rate), and those from the parasympathetic branch have a negative chronotropic effect. Parasympathetic innervation occurs by way of the vagus nerve and is commonly thought to act as a "brake" that maintains resting heart rate at 65 to 75 beats/min. Some of the common conditions associated with increased or decreased impulse initiation by the SA node are listed in (Box 25-3). In addition to factors that influence the SA node, disturbances in the heart's conduction system and excitation of other pacemaker cells can affect heart rate. These will be discussed in more detail in the next section on cardiac dysrhythmias (p. 646).

In summary, ventricular function and therefore CO are influenced by heart rate and stroke volume. Heart rate is primarily controlled by the ANS, and stroke volume depends on the three distinct variables of preload, contractility, and afterload.

Physiologic Changes with Aging

Age-related changes take place in the chemical composition, cells, and tissues of the heart and blood vessels and influence many aspects of cardiovascular functioning.[21,33] However, despite the physiologic changes of aging, the heart is able to meet the average day-to-day demands and function adequately. It is only under unusual circumstances or increased stress (such as sudden demands for more oxygen or the presence of cardiac pathologic conditions) that the deteriorating function of the heart is most apparent. For instance, *asymptomatic ischemia* may cause significant functional impairment. Not only is coronary atherosclerosis more prevalent in the elderly, but it frequently manifests as an occult (hidden) disease. It is crucial to detect the occult form of this disease to determine necessary interventions, such as pharmacotherapy and alterations in life-style.

With advancing age, life-styles often change with regard to eating, drinking, smoking, and physical activity. A sedentary life-style versus habitual exercise can produce a significant difference in cardiac output.

A number of physiologic factors reduce the efficiency of the heart as a pump as evidenced by a 30% reduction in cardiac output by age 65. Atrophy of muscle cells may lead to decreased muscle mass. Increased amounts of connective tissue add to myocardial stiffness and decrease cardiac compliance. The aorta and the major arteries also become less elastic, which compounds problems in filling and emptying the ventricles. The amount of subendocardial fat may increase, and the endocardium undergoes fibrosis, thickening, and sclerosis. In addition, delays may occur in the ability of myocardial cells to recover following electrical stimulation. The efficiency of the cardiac pump is also diminished because of decreased production of enzymes that influence the force and speed of ventricular contractions.

The aorta and its branches and the major pulmonary arteries and their branches undergo progressive dilation and elongation with age. Because the enlargement is transverse and longitudinal, the aorta tends to become tortuous. These alterations are caused by fragmentation, degeneration, and reduction in the amount of elastic tissue, as well as by increased collagen deposits and structural changes. Because of decreased vascular distensibility, arterial pulse pressure increases secondarily to increased systolic pressure (with less change in diastolic pressure).

Increased amounts of connective tissue in the SA node, internodal tracts, AV node, and bundle branches may cause conduction defects and a less effective heart rate response to exercise. The heart rate tends to return to normal more slowly following any type of exertion. In addition, the elderly may be more prone to dysrhythmias because of increased sensitivity to stimulation of the carotid sinus and an overall reduction in coronary blood flow.

The cardiac valves are also affected by the aging process. The mitral and aortic valves seem particularly vulnerable to fibrosis and calcification and can become somewhat rigid. Distortion of the aortic valve cusps can occur and may actually interfere with blood flow to the coronary arteries. These rigid valves can lead to audible systolic murmurs, usually of an ejection nature.

Confusion or decreased mental alertness may be early signs of a significant decrease in cardiac output in the elderly. These findings may mask other pertinent symptoms of decreased cardiac functioning, such as pain, fatigue, or dyspnea. Therefore, thorough evaluation of cardiovascular functioning should always be included in the assessment of changes in mental status.

Age-related changes in the cardiovascular system are significantly more pronounced in response to *exercise*. The overall increase in heart rate during vigorous exercise is less in elderly persons. Older people without significant coronary artery disease may demonstrate increases in stroke volume greater than those in younger individuals. These increases compensate for the lesser increases in heart rate. Left ventricular ejection fraction has been shown to decrease, or fail to increase, with more exercise in persons with coronary artery disease.

25-3

Factors affecting sinus node

Increase heart rate
Emotions (fear, anger)
Pain
Decreased blood pressure
Increased body temperature
Exercise
Epinephrine

Decrease heart rate
Stimulation of baroreceptors in carotid sinus or aortic arch
Decreased body temperature
Increased intracranial pressure
Digitalis excess
Beta blockers

CARDIAC AUSCULTATION

Auscultation of *heart sounds* enables a nurse to establish baseline data for identifying current and potential cardiac problems that require nursing intervention. Cardiac auscultation also assists the nurse in evaluating a patient's progress (for example, effect of activity on heart rate) or in monitoring responses to medications (for example, quinidine or digitalis preparations).

First and Second Heart Sounds

The familiar "lub-dub" heard when taking an apical pulse are the first and second heart sounds (S_1 and S_2) and mark the beginning and end of each ventricular contraction; hence rate, when obtained by auscultation, is determined by counting each set of "lub-dubs" as one beat. Whether these sounds occur regularly or irregularly determines the assessment of cardiac rhythm.

The *first heart sound* (S_1) is the result of the closure of the *mitral* and *tricuspid* atrioventricular valves (Fig. 25-7). This sound is heard best at the apex of the heart (normally the fifth left intercostal space at the midclavicular line) (Fig. 25-8). The valves do not close at precisely the same time. However, the fact that the time difference between their closure is measured in terms of hundredths of a second and that a greater volume of sound is produced by the mitral valve generally results in only one detectable noise. Occasionally the tricuspid component may be heard along the lower left sternal border.

The *second heart sound* (S_2) is the result of the closure of the semilunar valves (*aortic* and *pulmonic*). This sound is usually heard best at the base of the heart in the aortic area (second right intercostal space). The aortic valve closes slightly ahead of the pulmonic valve but produces a louder sound, so S_2 is also often detected as only one sound. When auscultating in the pulmonic area (second left intercostal space) one may hear the pulmonic component of

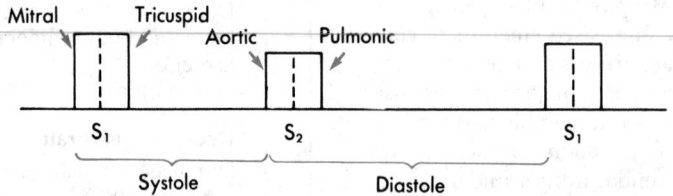

Fig. 25-7 Heart sound S_1 is the closure of mitral and tricuspid valves; S_2 is the closure of aortic and pulmonic valves. Systole is the time interval between S_1 and the start of S_2. Diastole is S_2 to the start of S_1. Diastole is longer than systole.

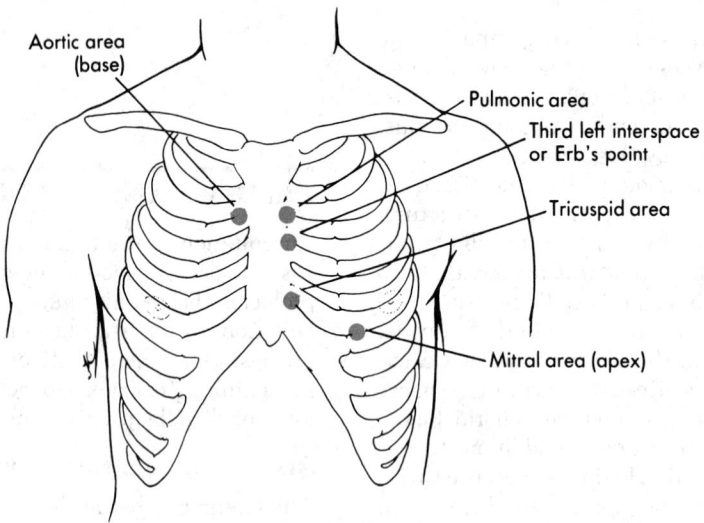

Fig. 25-8 Topographic areas for cardiac auscultation.

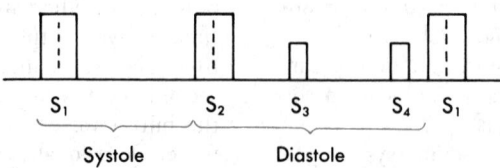

Fig. 25-9 Location of extra heart sounds during cardiac cycle.

S_2 (producing what is then referred to as a *split sound*) in a phasic manner, that is, the splitting is heard for a few beats and then is absent for a few beats. This phasic appearance of a split S_2 is the result of alterations in right ventricular volume (and therefore contraction time) related to the respiratory cycle. Under normal circumstances the split S_2, if heard at all, is detected during inspiration.

Extra heart sounds

With some exceptions, the occurrence of any additional heart sounds would be considered an abnormal finding. Abnormal cardiac sounds include gallops (S_3 and S_4), murmurs, opening snaps, and clicks.

Ventricular diastolic gallop (S_3) is a faint, low-pitched sound produced by rapid ventricular filling in early diastole (Fig. 25-9). Ventricular "gallop" describes the canter of a horse, which is frequently mimicked at heart rates greater than 100 beats per minute. When this sound is present in healthy children and young adults, it is almost always a normal condition and is referred to as a physiologic S_3. An S_3 heard in an older person is usually a pathologic sign and is frequently one of the first signs of serious heart disease or cardiac decompensation as seen in congestive heart failure.

Atrial diastolic gallop (S_4) is a low-pitched sound that occurs late in diastole when atrial contractions eject blood into a noncompliant ventricle. It may be heard in such states as hypertensive cardiovascular disease, coronary artery disease (especially during an attack of angina pectoris), and aortic stenosis.

Murmurs are audible vibrations of the heart and great vessels that occur because of turbulent blood flow. They may occur either during systole or diastole or through both phases. The intensity may be faint or loud; the pitch may be high (sharp) or low (dull), and the quality is described as harsh, blowing, rumbling, or musical. Murmurs may be organic (structural cardiovascular abnormalities), functional (increased blood flow through normal structures), or physiologic.

Other sounds that may be heard include a high-pitched clicking sound heard during systole (ejection sounds) or a high-pitched snapping sound heard in early diastole (opening snap of stenosed mitral valve).

General directions for cardiac auscultation

1. Locate the landmarks for auscultation: the second and fifth intercostal spaces.
2. Start at either the mitral or aortic areas.
3. Move the stethoscope at very short intervals (inching method) along the fifth interspace to sternum, then along the left sternal border to the second left interspace, then across the sternum to the right second interspace (or vice versa) (see Fig. 25-8).
4. Go through the listening sequence at least two times, first with the diaphragm for high-pitched sounds, then with the bell for low-pitched sounds. It is easier to follow the sequence three times (twice with the diaphragm listening first for normal sounds S_1 and S_2; second, for extra high-pitched sounds; and third, with the bell for extra low-pitched sounds).
5. Press firmly when using the diaphragm, but rest the bell only lightly on the skin.
6. When listening to normal heart sounds, note intensity of sounds and presence of splitting. Splitting of S_1 can be heard best at the tricuspid area and splitting of S_2 at the pulmonic area. The carotid pulse can be used to verify S_1 if needed. If splitting of S_2 is heard, note timing in relation to respiratory cycle.
7. Describe any extra sounds in terms of timing (systolic or diastolic), intensity, pitch character, and location where heard on thorax. For example, a sound might be described as "a high-pitched, blowing, systolic murmur of medium intensity, best heard along the left sternal border."

CARDIAC DYSRHYTHMIA

Persons with heart disease or with conditions that can affect heart function may experience cardiac dysrhythmias, which in certain situations may lead to cardiac arrest. Although the term dysrhythmia is preferred to denote a disturbance or variation from normal heart rhythm, the term *arrhythmia* can be used interchangeably with dysrhythmia.

The discussion of dysrhythmias is intended as a brief introduction to the more common dysrhythmias. Nurses who are responsible for dysrhythmia interpretation must undertake an in-depth study of electrophysiology and electrocardiography.

The hemodynamic consequences of dysrhythmias are extremely variable. Some cause no significant alteration in CO, although they may produce annoying symptoms such as a "fluttering" feeling in the chest or the sensation that the heart has "flipped over." Other dysrhythmias cause reductions in CO that result in symptoms of decreased perfusion. This is particularly likely if the dysrhythmia is associated with a very fast or very slow heart rate. Two dysrhythmias, ventricular fibrillation and ventricular stand-still, cause death if not promptly treated, because they result in *no* CO. There are many causes of dysrhythmias, some of which are not primarily related to a cardiovascular disease.

Accurate assessment of heart rate and rhythm and comparison of findings with baseline data will allow the nurse to detect some changes in the heart's electrical activity, but not all dysrhythmias are easily noted by physical assessment. A visual display of cardiac electrical activity on the oscilloscope of a cardiac monitor or a graphic record such as an ECG is always required for definitive identification of cardiac dysrhythmias.

Detection of Cardiac Rhythms
Electrocardiogram (ECG)

An ECG is a graphic record of the electrical activity of the heart muscle. The recording is made at a standard speed on a grid that allows measurement of both the intensity of electrical events (voltage) and their duration. Intensity is measured on the vertical axis in millivolts (mV), and time is measured on the horizontal axis in seconds. Each small square on the grid is equivalent to a known unit of time (0.04 sec) and voltage (0.1 mV), which allows rapid calculation of both these parameters (Fig. 25-10).

The ECG may be recorded by a special technician by health care professionals who have been trained in

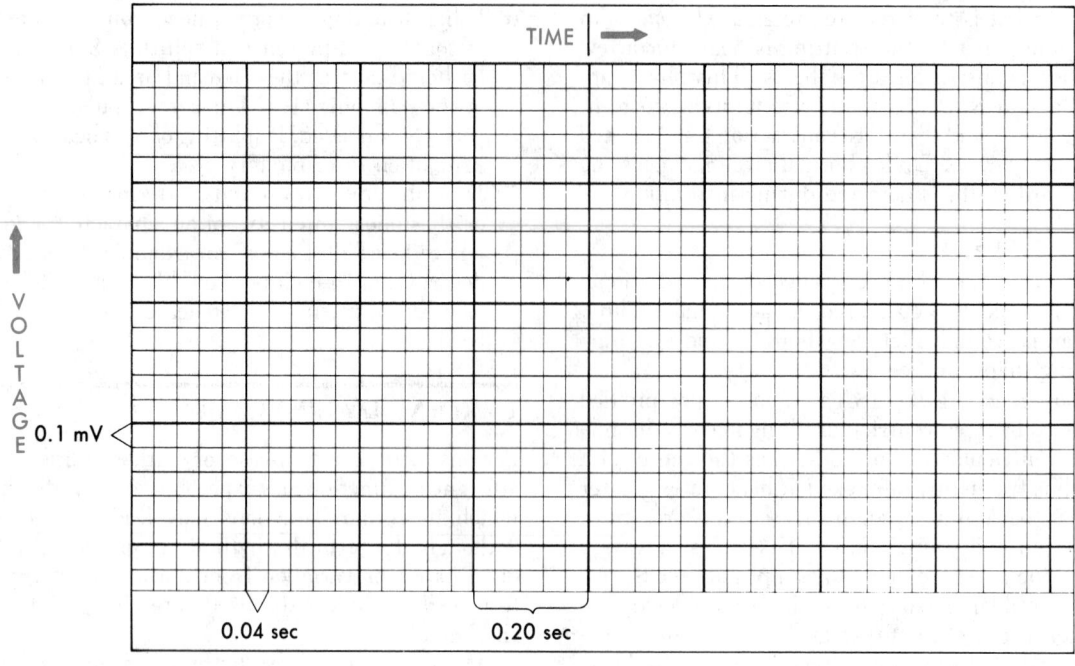

Fig. 25-10 Components of ECG paper.

Components of the 12-lead electrocardiogram

Standard (bipolar) limb leads	Lead I, II, III
Augmented (unipolar) limb leads	aVR, aVL, aVF
Chest leads	V₁ through V₆

Standard (bipolar) limb leads — Lead I, II, III

Augmented (unipolar) limb leads — aVR, aVL, aVF

Chest leads — V_1 through V_6

procedure. It is essential that the patient be relaxed and cooperative, so the nurse must be able to explain both the purpose of this test and the procedure itself. It is important to emphasize that the ECG machine is merely *recording* electrical energy produced by the body and is not delivering any electrical current to the body. The patient's comfort and safety are maintained by preventing unnecessary exposure and by ensuring adequate grounding of the ECG machine.

In brief, recording electrodes are placed on the patient's four extremities and on the anterior thorax. A conductive substance (jelly, paste, or a specially prepared disposable pad) is placed between the skin and the electrodes to facilitate high-quality recording. The patient must lie still during the procedure, which is not painful and takes less than 5 minutes. The operator controls the ECG machine, which is designed to record electrical activity in several planes.

Typically, 12 different views are recorded, hence the term *12-lead* ECG (Fig. 25-11). The 12 typical views of the heart's electrical activity actually represent three methods of recording and provide information about activation

Table 25-1 Normal cardiac electrical activity and resultant electrocardiographic findings

Cardiac electrical event	Electrocardiographic finding
Firing of SA node	Not recorded
Spread of impulse through the atria (atrial depolarization)	P wave
AV node delay	Isoelectric baseline between P and QRS
Atrial repolarization	Not recorded
Spread of impulse through the ventricles (ventricular depolarization)	QRS complex
Ventricular repolarization	T wave

on both the frontal (vertical) and horizontal planes. The subdivisions of the 12-lead ECG and the names of the leads are described in Box 25-4.

Normal cardiac electrical activity as described earlier in the chapter and the resultant electrocardiographic findings are found in Table 25-1. When cardiac electrical activity occurs in a normal manner, a *cardiac complex* such as the one schematically depicted in Fig. 25-12 is produced. The voltage and major deflection (above or below the isoelectric baseline) of each component of the cardiac complex vary with the specific lead being recorded. A chest lead is compared with one of the standard leads shown in Fig. 25-13.

The nature of cardiac dysrhythmias can be inferred by observing the presence, rate, and regularity of the various

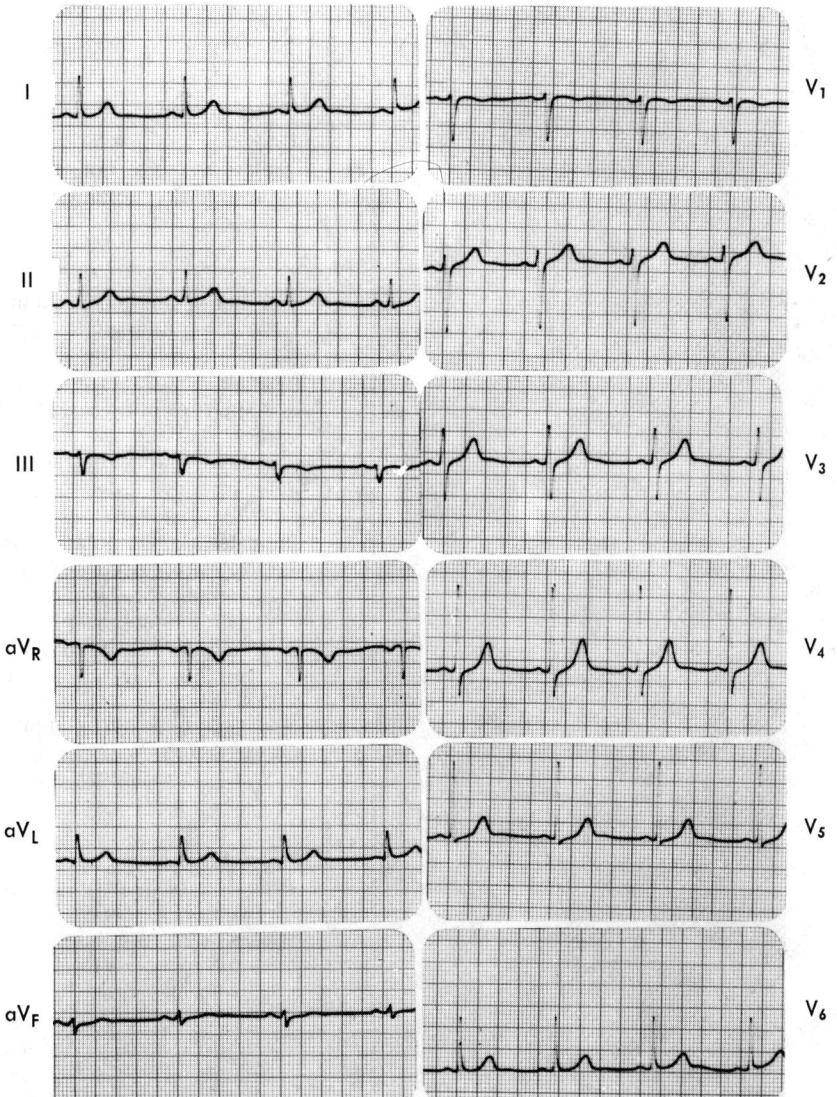

Fig. 25-11   Twelve-lead ECG showing normal sinus rhythm. (From Anderoli KG et al: *Comprehensive cardiac care,* ed 6, St Louis, 1987, Mosby—Year Book.)

"QRS"

R

P

q   s

T

Fig. 25-12   Normal cardiac complex as seen in lead II.

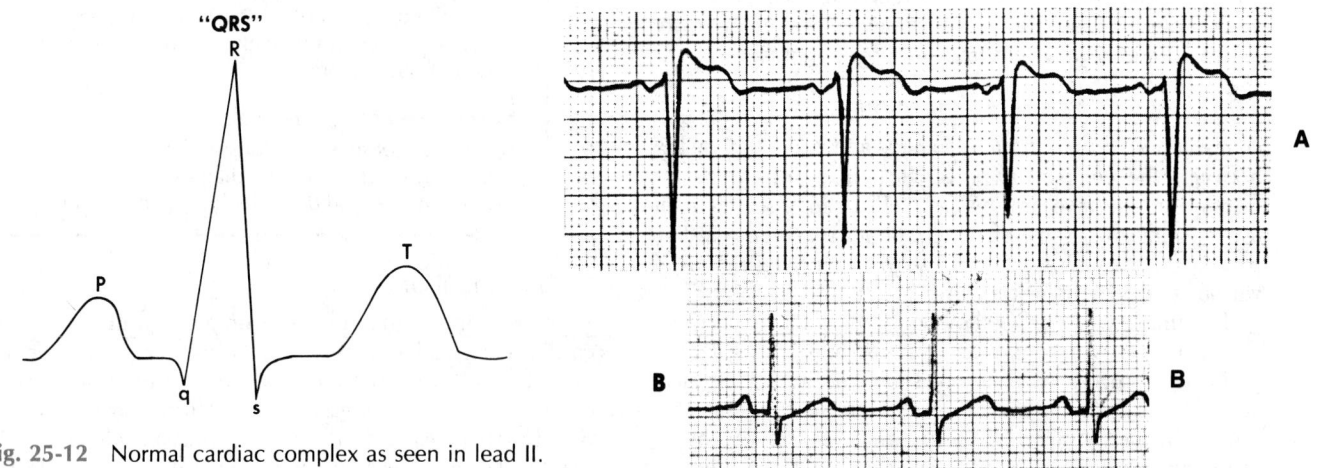

Fig. 25-13   **A,** Normal ECG in lead V_1. **B,** Normal ECG in lead II.

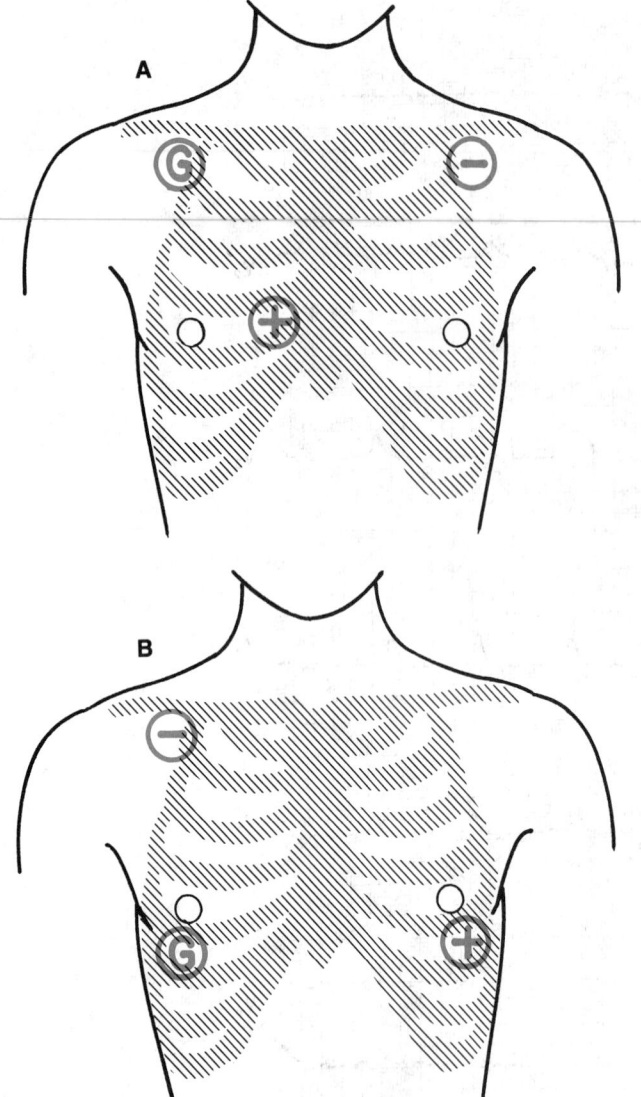

Fig. 25-14   Placement of ECG electrodes on anterior chest wall. **A,** Lead V$_1$: grounding electrode is on upper right chest, negative electrode on upper left chest, and positive electrode on right lower chest along sternal border. **B,** Lead II: grounding electrode is on lower right chest, positive electrode on lower left chest, and negative electrode on upper right chest.

Rhythm strip analysis

Heart rhythm

Does this produce a pulse that is regular or irregular? Assess by noting whether the distance between QRS complexes (RR) interval is consistent.

Heart rate

Number of ventricular contractions/min. Calculate by counting QRS complexes in 6 seconds and multiplying by 10 or by dividing number of small squares between two consecutive QRS complexes into 1500 (1500 × 0.04 sec = 60 sec). The latter method can be employed only if the rhythm is regular.

Presence of P wave

Indicates atrial depolarization.
   Do P waves occur regularly? The sinus node normally fires in a rhythmic fashion. Assess by noting whether PP interval is consistent.
   Atrial rate: number of atrial contractions per minute. Calculate as with heart rate but use P waves.
   Is each wave followed by a QRS complex? If so, this verifies conduction of impulse from atria into ventricles; if not, a conduction defect is present.

P-R interval

Time from onset of atrial depolarization to onset of ventricular depolarization. It includes passage of impulse through the AV node.
   Length of PR interval. Measure from beginning of P to beginning of QRS. Normal duration is 0.12 to 0.20 second. Longer than 0.20 second indicates a conduction delay in AV node.
   Is length of PR interval consistent? If not, it may indicate lack of association between P and QRS.

QRS duration

Time needed for ventricular depolarization. Normal duration is 0.06 to 0.10 second. Longer than 0.10 second indicates abnormal ventricular depolarization.

ST segment and QT interval

Assessment of these portions of the cardiac complex provides additional diagnostic information but is not required for rhythm interpretation.

---

components of the cardiac complex and the relationship between the component parts. Ischemia, injury, or infarction of the myocardium, as well as an assortment of other conditions (some of which do *not* represent cardiac pathology), may alter the size, shape, or configuration of various components of the cardiac complex.

   In summary, the ECG shows only the electrical activity of the heart, which may or may not be disturbed by a pathologic process. It does not show the actual physical state of the heart or indicate its ability to function as a pump. Its most important diagnostic uses are the interpretation of abnormal cardiac rhythms and the identification of ischemia or pathology resulting from coronary atherosclerotic heart disease.

Cardiac monitors

It is common practice to assess on a continuing basis the cardiac electrical activity of persons who are known or suspected to have dysrhythmias or who are prone to develop dysrhythmias. This assessment is performed with a cardiac monitor that displays information from *one* electrocardiographic lead on an oscilloscope. The lead chosen for display varies with the condition of the patient, but standard lead II or MCL$_1$ (a close facsimile of V$_1$) is frequently used (Fig. 25-14).

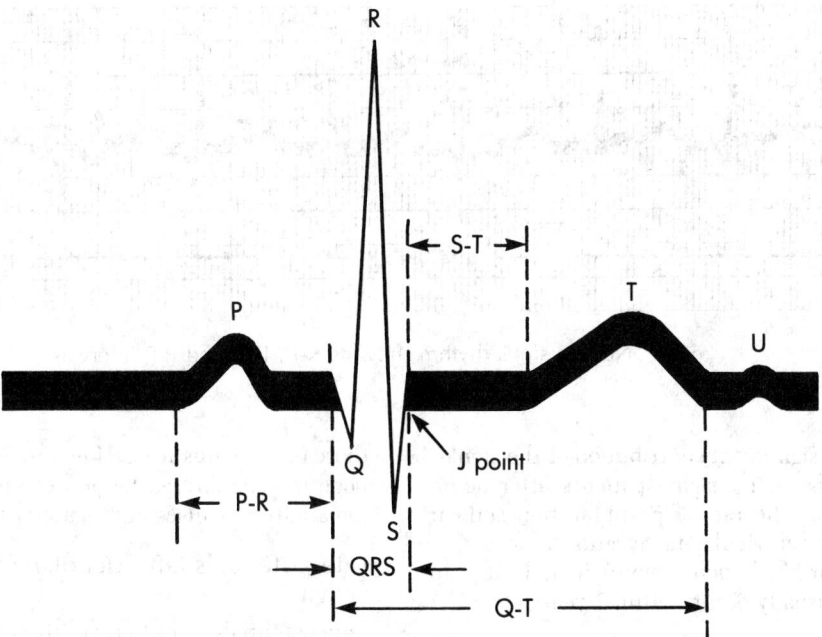

Fig. 25-15   Schematic drawing of ECG waves produced by the cardiac cycle.

Most monitors provide a visual display of cardiac electrical activity and the current heart rate. Preset alarms warn of heart rates that exceed or drop below limits considered acceptable for each patient. More sophisticated monitors are designed to detect and tentatively interpret dysrhythmias and their frequency with a computer.

Acutely ill persons are monitored in intensive care settings, but the increased use of battery-powered ECG transmitters that do not require direct connection of the patient to the oscilloscope (*telemetry monitoring equipment*) has expanded the use of such equipment to other patients as well. This development has resulted in the need for nurses working on general medical-surgical units to become familiar with monitoring equipment and to acquire some basic skills in rhythm interpretation.

Attachment to a cardiac monitor does not significantly alter a person's need for nursing care. Placement of the monitoring electrodes on the anterior thorax rather than the extremities leaves the patient relatively free to carry on usual activities. Special attention should be paid to the electrode sites to ensure a constant tight seal between the electrode and the skin and to note the development of any skin irritation. If a rash appears, the electrodes must be switched to alternate sites. Instructions supplied by individual electrode manufacturers guide the nurse in the application procedure and in necessary routine maintenance. Periodic checking of the monitoring system to ensure proper grounding and secure connection of all component parts is another general nursing responsibility.

Format for rhythm interpretation

A permanent graphic record of the heart's electrical activity can be obtained by a standard ECG machine or a "write-out" component of a cardiac monitor. The monitor write-out is usually activated automatically when the monitor alarm sounds and can also be activated manually whenever a written record is desired for analysis. The record produced is commonly called a *rhythm strip* and should be at least 6 seconds long for proper interpretation. A long strip may be required if the heart rhythm is irregular.

Interpretation of a rhythm strip involves knowledge of normal electrophysiology and a measure of deductive reasoning. Systematic collection and analysis of the data listed in Box 25-5 are required. (The important segments and intervals of a single cardiac complex are schematically depicted in Fig. 25-15).

Electrographic signal averaging

Signal averaging of the surface QRS complex is now being used to detect low-amplitude, high-frequency signals in the terminal portion of the QRS complex or in the early ST segment. It is a new, noninvasive, computerized method of analyzing standard ECGs that identifies patients at risk for lethal ventricular dysrhythmias.

Electrocardiographic signal averaging involves amplification of electrical heart signals that have a voltage too small to be recorded by a standard ECG. Ischemia and infarction can cause the extreme slowing of conduction that results in this delayed activity. Typically, approximately 200 identical QRS complexes are grouped and averaged, resulting in a waveform that appears smooth and continuous.

Equipment necessary to perform signal averaging includes ECG leads, an amplifier, an analog-digital converter, and a personal computer with software to average the QRS waveforms and store data. Patient interface with the electrodes is of primary importance to obtain and analyze data. Cleansing and mildly abrading the skin must precede electrode attachment.

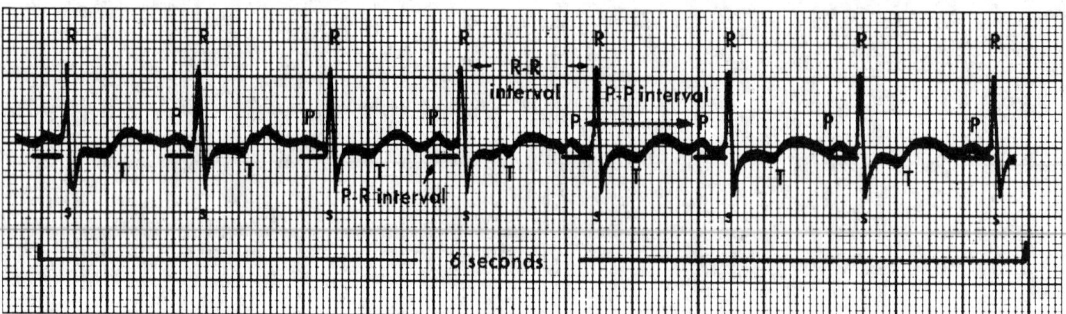

Fig. 25-16   Normal sinus rhythm showing R-R, P-P, and P-R intervals.

Probably the most significant contribution of the signal-averaged ECG will be in managing patients after acute myocardial infarction. The rate of postinfarction sudden death precipitated by ventricular tachycardia that degenerates into ventricular fibrillation is approximately 10% to 15%. These deaths usually occur within 2 years after the myocardial infarction.

Normal Sinus Rhythm

The term *normal sinus rhythm* (NSR) implies that cardiac electrical activity is within normal limits as indicated by the following criteria (Fig. 25-16).
1. P waves present and regular. If the SA node is initiating electrical activity in a rhythmic manner, atrial depolarization should occur in a rhythmic manner.
2. Atrial rate (P waves) between 60 and 100 beats/min. This represents the range of normal rates for SA node.
3. Each P wave is followed by a QRS complex. This verifies conduction of the impulse initiated by the SA node into the ventricles and implies that the heart rhythm is regular and the heart rate is also between 60 and 100 beats/min.
4. In addition, normal P/R interval and QRS duration indicate normal functioning of all components of the conduction system.

Arrhythmogenic Mechanisms

Most dysrhythmias are believed to be caused by (1) abnormalities in impulse formation because of altered automaticity (enhanced or abnormal automaticity) or late potentials (afterdepolarizations or triggered activity), (2) abnormalities of conduction caused by a block or reentry, or (3) a combination of these. The following is a brief discussion of these mechanisms.

Altered automaticity

Remember that cardiac cells are able to maintain an electrical potential across their cell membranes. When an impulse of sufficient magnitude that exceeds their threshold potential arrives, these cells depolarize. Some cardiac cells have the additional property of automaticity (ability to depolarize spontaneously without external stimulation). Control of the cardiac conduction system belongs to the cells with the most rapid spontaneous depolarization, normally

those of the sinus node. The rate of discharge of the sinus node may be altered by any condition that enhances automaticity or causes automaticity to be abnormal.

Late potentials (afterdepolarizations or triggered activity)

Late potentials refer to repetitive ectopic (nonsinus) firing, which is the result of afterdepolarizations. These afterdepolarizations occur during or after repolarization. Triggered activity results only when the afterdepolarization achieves threshold potential. The afterdepolarizations may reach threshold because of a shortened cycle length or an increased level of catecholamines.

Reentry

Reentry occurs when an impulse is delayed long enough within a pathway of slow conduction to be still viable when the remaining myocardium repolarizes (Fig. 25-17). The impulse then reenters surrounding tissue and produces another impulse. The initiating impulse may be normal sinus or ectopic. One-way conduction is necessary because without it the impulse would cancel itself out within the area of slow conduction. Any condition that decreases the amplitude of the action potential, such as ischemia, hypercalcemia, or calcification of the conducting fibers, can cause cardiac conduction disturbance. This results in heart block or a reentry rhythm.

Types of Dysrhythmias

The many types of dysrhythmias are grouped in the following discussion according to anatomic origins. These dysrhythmias are summarized in Table 25-2.

Dysrhythmias originating in the sinus node
Sinus dysrhythmia

Sinus dysrhythmia is the most frequently noted dysrhythmia. It is typically found in young adults and the elderly. The P waves are of sinus origin and have a constant morphology. There are two forms of sinus dysrhythmia—respiratory and nonphasic. In the respiratory form, the cyclic pattern of changing P/P or R/R intervals correlates with the patterns of inspiration and expiration. During inspiration, the intervals shorten as the heart rate increases. Conversely, the intervals lengthen during expiration. These phenomena result from a reflex inhibition of vagal tone, an enhancement of sympathetic tone, or both.

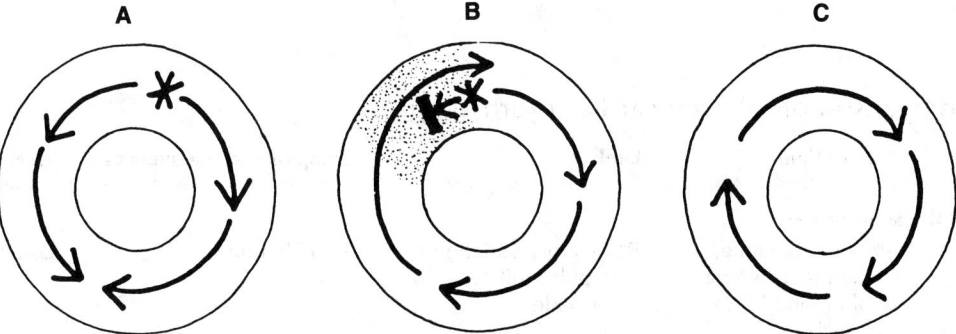

A   **B**   **C**

Fig. 25-17   Mechanisms of reentry. In **(A)** the impulses travel from the stimulus in opposite directions around the ring to meet and cancel each other out. In **(B)** pressure has been applied at the shaded area in the ring, at which point the impulse is blocked and travels only in the opposite direction. Pressure is then removed, and the impulse continues around and around **(C)** on its one-way journey as long as refractory tissue is not encountered. (From Marriott HJL, Conover MB: *Advanced concepts in arrhythmias,* ed 2, St Louis, 1989, Mosby–Year Book.)

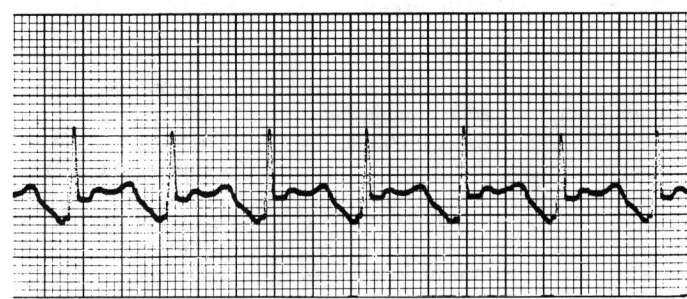

Fig. 25-18   Sinus tachycardia. Lead II showing heart rate of 115 beats/min, regular rhythm, normal PR interval, and normal QRS duration.

The nonphasic form has no correlation to respiration. It may be caused by vagal stimulation from other vagally innervated organs.

Sinus dysrhythmia is a benign rhythm that usually requires no treatment. With slow heart rates, some persons may experience palpitations or dizziness. In such cases, exercises or medications that increase the heart rate will abolish the dysrhythmia.

Sinus tachycardia

Sinus tachycardia is the result of the SA node firing at a faster than normal rate (that is, greater than 100 beats/min). Any condition that increases the body's demand for oxygen may cause this dysrhythmia, which is a normal response to exercise, excitement, and fever. Sinus tachycardia may also be a compensatory response to anemia, heart failure, and hemorrhage. The ECG appearance (Fig. 25-18) is the same as with normal sinus rhythm except for the faster atrial and ventricular rates (usually 100 to 150 beats/min). The general result of sinus tachycardia is an increased CO, although a prolonged episode may precipitate ventricular failure caused by decreased ventricular filling time and therefore decreased cardiac output. When the underlying cause has been treated, the SA node returns to a normal rate.

Sinus bradycardia

Sinus bradycardia is the result of the SA node firing at a slower than normal rate (that is, less than 60 beats/min). This dysrhythmia may be a normal finding in athletes or others whose heart muscles contract at peak efficiency. It may also be the result of stimulation of the parasympathetic nervous system, increased intracranial pressure, myocardial infarction, or lack of blood and oxygen in the SA node. The ECG appearance (Fig. 25-19, p. 650) is the same as for normal sinus rhythm except for the slower atrial and ventricular rates (usually 40 to 60 beats/min).

Generally, sinus bradycardia is a benign rhythm. Often in association with myocardial infarction, it is a compensatory rhythm because it reduces myocardial oxygen demand. If the heart rate is too slow to maintain adequate cardiac output, the person may be predisposed to syncope and congestive heart failure. Administration of atropine or isoproterenol is usually effective in increasing the heart rate. The person with refractory bradycardia who is symptomatic may require a permanent implantable pacemaker.

Sick sinus syndrome

Sick sinus syndrome (SSS) is a term describing several clinical disorders of SA node function. The tachycardia-

Table 25-2   Comparison of selected cardiac dysrhythmias

Dysrhythmia	Description	Etiology	Symptoms/consequences	Treatment
Dysrhythmias of the sinus node				
Sinus dysrhythmia	Phasic shortening, then lengthening of PP and RR interval	Respiratory variation in impulse initiation by SA node	Usually none	Usually none
Sinus tachycardia	P waves present followed by QRS Rhythm regular Heart rate 100-150	Increased metabolic demands Decreased oxygen delivery, congestive heart failure, shock, hemorrhage, anemia	May produce palpitations Prolonged episodes may lead to decreased cardiac output	Treat underlying cause Occasionally sedatives
Sinus bradycardia	P waves present Rhythm regular Heart rate < 60	Physical fitness Parasympathetic stimulation (sleep) Brain lesions Sinus dysfunction Digitalis excess	Very low rates may cause decreased cardiac output; lightheadedness, faintness, chest pain	Atropine if cardiac output is decreased Pacemaker Treat underlying cause if necessary
Atrial dysrhythmias				
Premature atrial beats	Early P wave QRS may or may not be normal Rhythm irregular	Stress, ischemia, atrial enlargement, caffeine, nicotine	May produce palpitations Frequent episodes may decrease cardiac output Is sign of chamber irritability	Sedation Quinidine May require no treatment
Atrial tachycardia	P wave present (may merge into previous T wave), QRS usually normal, rapid heart rate usually >150/min	Sympathetic stimulation, chemical stimuli (caffeine, nicotine), drug toxicity	Palpitations Possible anxiety	Usually none Prolonged episodes may require carotid sinus pressure, vagal stimulation, or verapamil, digitalis, or beta blockers
Atrial fibrillation	Rapid, irregular waves (over 350/min) Ventricular rhythm irregularly irregular Ventricular rate varies, may increase to 120-150/min if untreated	Rheumatic heart disease Mitral stenosis Atrial infarction Coronary atherosclerotic heart disease Hypertensive heart disease Thyrotoxicosis	Pulse deficit Decreased cardiac output if rate is rapid Promotes thrombus formation in atria	Digitalis Quinidine Cardioversion
Ventricular dysrhythmias				
Premature ventricular beats	Early wide bizarre QRS, not associated with a P wave Rhythm irregular	Stress, acidosis, ventricular enlargement Electrolyte imbalance Myocardial infarction Digitalis toxicity Hypoxemia, hypercapnia	Same as for premature atrial beats	Procainamide Quinidine Disopyramide (Norpace) Lidocaine Oxygen Sodium bicarbonate Potassium Treat congestive heart failure

Table 25-2   Comparison of selected cardiac dysrhythmias—cont'd

Dysrhythmia	Description	Etiology	Symptoms/consequences	Treatment
Ventricular tachy-cardia	No P wave before QRS; QRS wide and bizarre; ventricular rate >100, usually 140-240	PVB striking during vulnerable period; hypoxemia; drug toxicity; electrolyte imbalance; bradycardia	Decreased cardiac output, hypotension, loss of consciousness, respiratory arrest	Lidocaine Procainamide Bretylium Cardioversion
Ventricular fibrillation	Chaotic electrical activity No recognizable QRS complex	Myocardial infarction Electrocution Freshwater drowning Drug toxicity	No cardiac output Absent pulse or respiration Cardiac arrest	Defibrillation Epinephrine Sodium bicarbonate Bretylium CPR
Ventricular stand-still	Can be distinguished from ventricular fibrillation only by ECG P waves *may* be present No QRS "Straight line"	Myocardial infarction Chronic diseases of conducting system	Same as for ventricular fibrillation	CPR Pacemaker Intracardiac epinephrine Isoproterenol
Impulse conduction deficits				
First-degree atrio-ventricular block	PR interval prolonged >0.20 sec	Rheumatic fever Digitalis toxicity Degenerative changes of coronary atherosclerotic heart disease Infections ↓ oxygen in AV node	Warns of impaired conduction	Usually none as long as it occurs as an isolated deficit
Bundle branch block	Same as NSR except QRS duration >0.10	Hypoxia, acute myocardial infarction, congestive heart failure, coronary atherosclerotic heart disease, pulmonary embolus, hypertension	Same as first-degree block	Usually none unless severe blockage of left posterior division (see text)
Second-degree blocks	P waves usually occur regularly at rates consistant with SA node initiation; Not all P waves followed by QRS; PR interval may lengthen before nonconducted P wave or may be consistent; QRS may be widened	Acute myocardial infarction	Serious dysrhythmia which may lead to ↓ heart rate and ↓ cardiac output	May require temporary pacemaker
Complete third-degree atrio-ventricular block	Atria and ventricles beat independently P waves have no relation to QRS Ventricular rate may be as low as 20-40/min	Digitalis toxicity Infectious disease Coronary artery disease Myocardial infarction	Very low rates may cause decreased cardiac output: lightheadedness, faintness, chest pain	Pacemaker Isoproterenol to increase heart rate Epinephrine if isoproterenol is ineffective

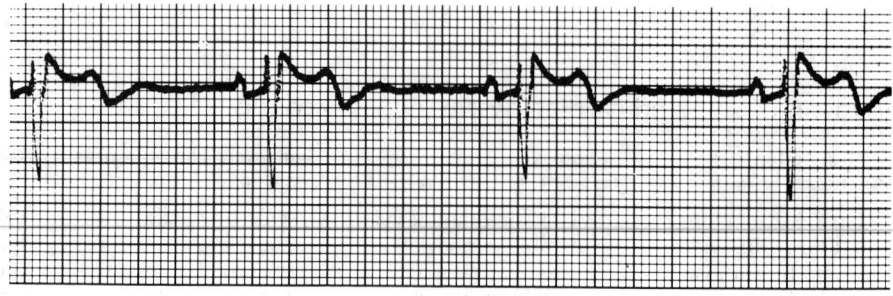

Fig. 25-19 Sinus bradycardia (lead V₁). P waves are present and regular. Atrial and ventricular rates are 44 beats/min. Each P is followed by a QRS.

V₁

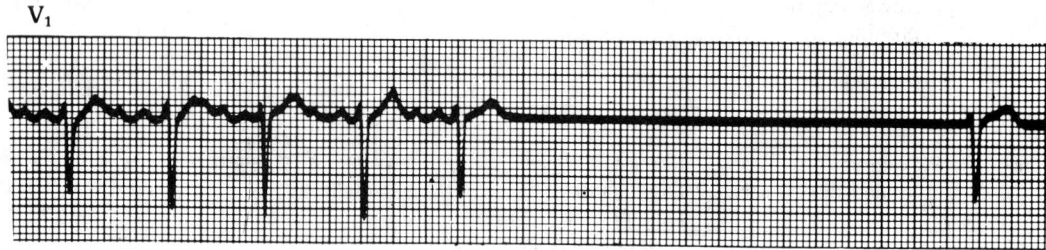

Fig. 25-20 Sick sinus syndrome caused by bradycardia-tachycardia. (From Marriott HJL, Conover M: *Advanced concepts in arrhythmias,* ed 2, St Louis, 1989, Mosby–Year Book.)

A

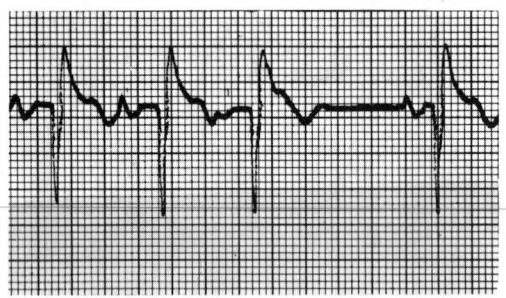

Fig. 25-21 A, Premature atrial beat (lead V₁). Third beat is premature atrial beat with abnormal early P wave followed by normal QRS complex. **B,** Premature ventricular beats (lead II). Fourth and tenth beats are premature with no P wave and wide, bizarre QRS. Different shapes of PVBs indicate two different ectopic sites in ventricles.

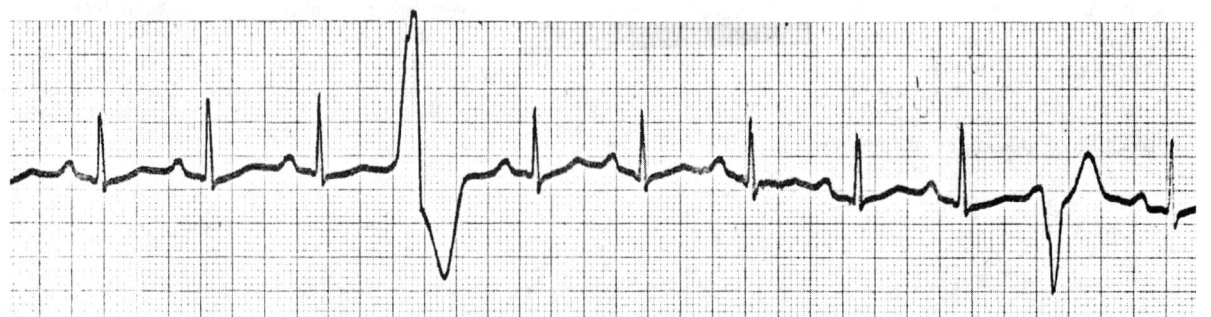

B

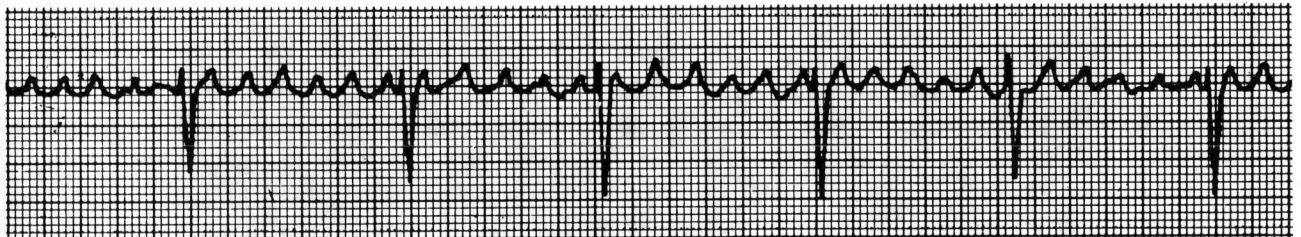

Fig. 25-22   Atrial flutter (V₁). Rate of atrial flutter waves is 300/minute. Ventricular rate is 50 to 75/minute.

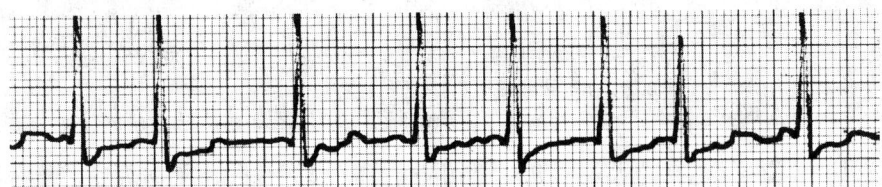

Fig. 25-23   Atrial fibrillation (lead II). Atrial rate is rapid with varying conduction to ventricles, rhythm is irregular, QRS complex is normal, and no definite P waves are visible.

bradycardia syndrome is the most common type of SSS. It is characterized by the presence of a sinus bradycardia with intermittent episodes of atrial tachydysrhythmias (Fig. 25-20). Complications of this inefficient rhythm include congestive heart failure and cerebrovascular accidents resulting from thromboembolisms. Some individuals may remain asymptomatic or complain only of palpitations. For the severely symptomatic person, the heart rhythm should be stabilized by a permanent implantable pacemaker.

Dysrhythmias originating in the atria
Premature atrial beat

The premature atrial beat (PAB) is initiated by an ectopic focus (outside the SA node) in the atria (Fig. 25-21). It is characterized by a premature P wave with a contour different from that of a sinus P wave. The QRS complex may or may not be normal, and the PAB is followed by a pause approximately equal to the sinus cycle (measured R to R). The atrial impulse may be nonconducted (blocked) because of refractoriness of the ventricles at the time the impulse arrives. The nonconducted atrial beat (blocked PAB) is the most common cause of irregularities in the heart rhythm.

In the absence of organic disease, such as ischemia, no treatment is required. Often the omission of caffeine and tobacco will suppress the atrial focus. If symptoms are present or organic disease is known, PABs may be suppressed by digitalis, quinidine, or procainamide.

Atrial tachycardia

In atrial tachycardia, the atrial rate is approximately 150 to 250 beats per minute. The QRS complex is generally normal, and the ventricular rate is regular.

When atrial tachycardia occurs suddenly, it is called paroxysmal atrial tachycardia (PAT). Transient episodes of PAT may occur in children and young adults in the absence of heart disease. When underlying disease is present, it is usually rheumatic heart disease. The person may complain of palpitations and experience anxiety during a tachycardic episode. Short, infrequent episodes require no treatment. Lengthy occurrences may require carotid sinus pressure, vagal stimulation, or intravenous administration of digitalis, verapamil, or beta blockers to restore sinus rhythm.

Atrial flutter

The characteristic feature of atrial flutter is the presence of a sawtooth pattern of rapid atrial activity (Fig. 25-22). The atria depolarize at a rate of 250 to 350 beats/min. These atrial depolarizations produce flutter (F) waves that give the baseline a sawtooth appearance. The QRS configurations are normal. Physiologically, the AV node usually prevents conduction of each atrial impulse to the ventricles. Despite this protective mechanism, ventricular rates of greater than 150/min can occur. There is no true PR interval, and it is impossible to discern which atrial impulse is actually conducted to the ventricles.

The potentially rapid ventricular rate of atrial flutter may decrease cardiac output. Control of the ventricular rate or conversion to sinus rhythm is the major treatment goal. Direct-current cardioversion is the treatment of choice in the patient with an acute myocardial infarction to protect an already compromised myocardium from the metabolic demands of a rapid ventricular rate.

Atrial fibrillation

Atrial fibrillation (Fig. 25-23) is the most rapid of atrial dysrhythmias. The atria beat chaotically at rates of 350 to 600 beats/min. The baseline is characteristically composed of irregular undulations without definable P waves. The QRS complex is usually normal, but the ventricular rhythm is irregularly irregular. If untreated, the ventricular rate will generally be 100 to 180 beats/min. Atrial

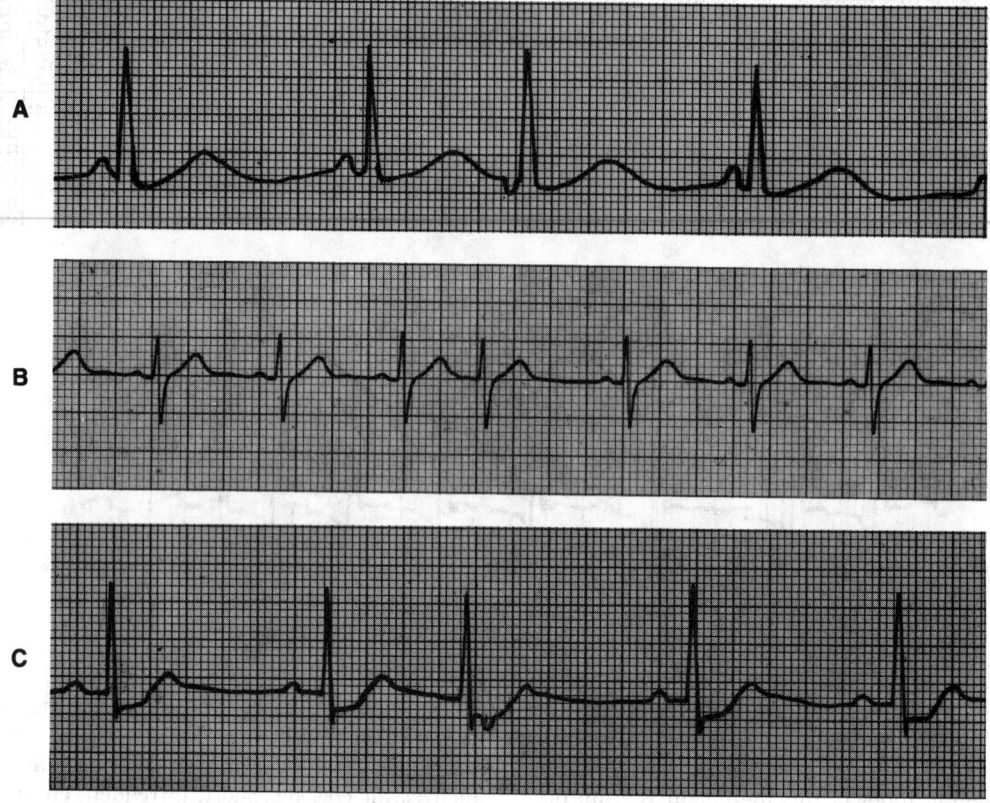

Fig. 25-24 Premature junctional beats (PJBs). **A,** Inverted P wave (third QRS complex). **B,** P wave hidden in fourth QRS complex. **C,** P wave follows third QRS complex. (From Conover MB: *Understanding electrocardiography: arrhythmias and the 12-lead ECG,* ed 6, St Louis, 1992, Mosby–Year Book.)

fibrillation may be paroxysmal and transient, or it may be chronic. The latter generally indicates underlying heart disease.

Because of ventricular rhythm irregularity and the loss of synchronous atrial contractions (atrial kick), cardiac output is decreased and a pulse deficit often exists. In the presence of mitral stenosis, thrombi may form in the atria and cause embolisms affecting the lungs or periphery. The goal of therapy is to prevent these complications by controlling the ventricular rate and giving anticoagulants to certain patients.

Dysrhythmias originating in atrioventricular junction
Premature junctional beats

The premature junctional beat (PJB) arises from an ectopic focus near the junction of the AV node and the bundle of His. PJBs may occur in the normal heart; they are also associated with digitalis toxicity, congestive heart failure, ischemia, and hypokalemia. The P waves may occur before, during, or after the QRS. The QRS is normal, and the ventricular rhythm is regular (Fig. 25-24).

When the automaticity of a junctional pacemaker increases to a rate greater than 60/min, it may override the SA node as the pacemaker of the heart. This rhythm is called *accelerated junctional rhythm* if it occurs at 60 to 100

beats/min. A *junctional tachycardia* exists when the rate exceeds 100 beats/min.

Treatment should correct the underlying cause. Quinidine, propranolol, and procainamide may suppress PJBs. Phenytoin (Dilantin) is particularly effective in suppressing PJBs secondary to digitalis toxicity.

Dysrhythmias originating in the ventricles
Premature ventricular beats

The premature ventricular beat (PVB) arises from an ectopic focus in the ventricles. The characteristic wide, bizarre QRS complex (usually greater than 0.12 second) makes the PVB readily recognizable on the ECG tracing (Fig. 25-25). No associated P wave precedes the QRS complex, and the T wave is in the opposite direction from the main QRS deflection. Frequently PVBs are followed by a compensatory pause so that the interval from the beat preceding to the beat following the PVB is equal to two sinus cycles.

Even in the absence of heart disease, PVBs occur often and increase in number with a person's age. The incidence and frequency of occurrence are higher, however, for the population with heart disease. Clinically, PVBs are associated with myocardial infarction, congestive heart failure, digitalis toxicity, drug therapy, and electrolyte imbalances. Pharmacologic suppression of PVBs is most often accomplished with lidocaine, procainamide, and quinidine.

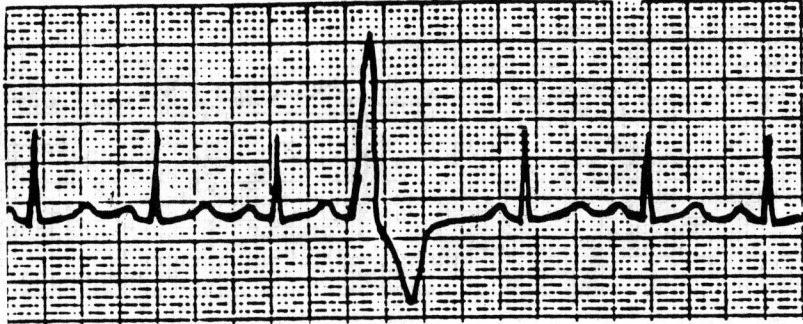

Fig. 25-25   Premature ventricular beat. Lead II showing fourth beat is a PVB with wide early QRS complex; no P wave associated with beat.

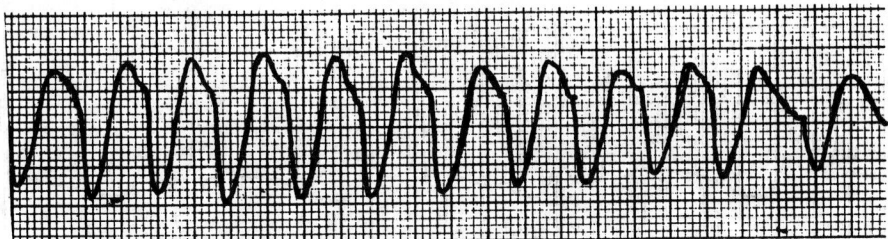

Fig. 25-26   Ventricular tachycardia at a rate of approximately 150/minute; rhythm is slightly irregular.

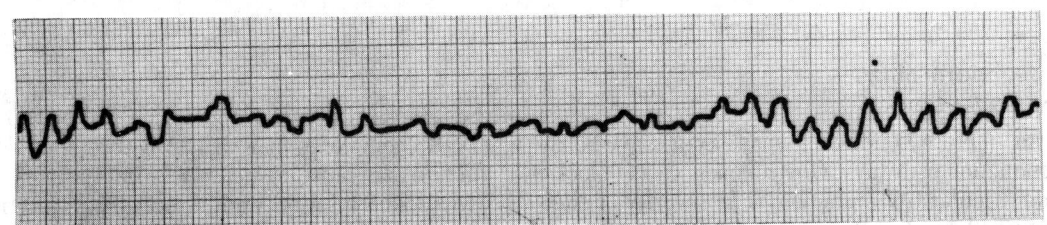

Fig. 25-27   Ventricular fibrillation (lead II). Tracing shows electrical chaos in myocardium. There are no QRS complexes and no definite P waves visible.

Ventricular rhythms and tachycardia

If the SA node and AV junction fail to initiate impulses, a ventricular pacemaking cell will automatically begin to initiate impulses at an inherent rate of 20 to 40 beats/min. This is known as *idioventricular rhythm*. If the ventricle-initiated rhythm increases to 40 to 100/min, it is known as *accelerated idioventricular rhythm*. It may be seen in digitalis toxicity or as a complication of an acute myocardial infarction. Generally, neither of these rhythms is treated except to correct underlying abnormalities.

By definition, three or more successive PVBs constitute *ventricular tachycardia* (Fig. 25-26). The ventricular rate is usually 150 to 250 beats/min. Although P waves may be present, they are not associated with the QRS complexes. Ventricular tachycardia may complicate any form of heart disease. If the patient remains stable, treatment may include intravenous lidocaine, procainamide, or bretylium. If pharmacologic measures are unsuccessful, the alternative is cardioversion.

Ventricular fibrillation and standstill

In *ventricular fibrillation,* the ventricles twitch chaotically, much as they do in atrial fibrillation. Individual muscle fibers are depolarizing but in a disorganized fashion. Thus, they fail to produce a proper ventricular contraction. Common causes for this lethal dysrhythmia include ischemia in the ventricles, electrocution, drowning, electrolyte imbalances, and toxic doses of digitalis or quinidine. The ECG tracing consists of a bumpy line of unidentifiable waves (Fig. 25-27).

In *ventricular standstill* (asystole), the ECG tracing is a flat line. No electrical activity is noted; all pacemaking cells have failed. Clinically, ventricular fibrillation and standstill cannot be differentiated without an ECG. Both are fatal dysrhythmias requiring immediate measures. The patient has no blood pressure, pulse or audible heartbeat, or respirations and quickly loses consciousness. CPR must be instituted immediately and defibrillation performed within 1 minute to prevent biochemical derangements that further compromise the patient.

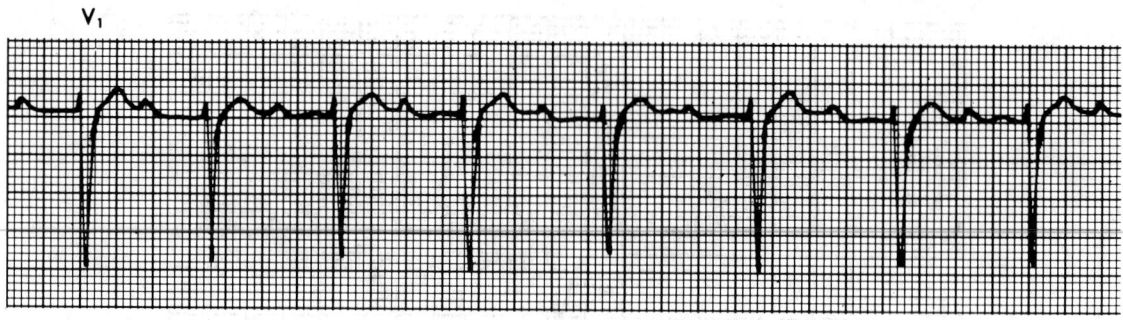

Fig. 25-28 First-degree AV block; the PR interval is 0.33 second (too long). (From Conover MB: *Cardiac arrhythmias,* ed 2, St Louis, 1978, Mosby–Year Book.)

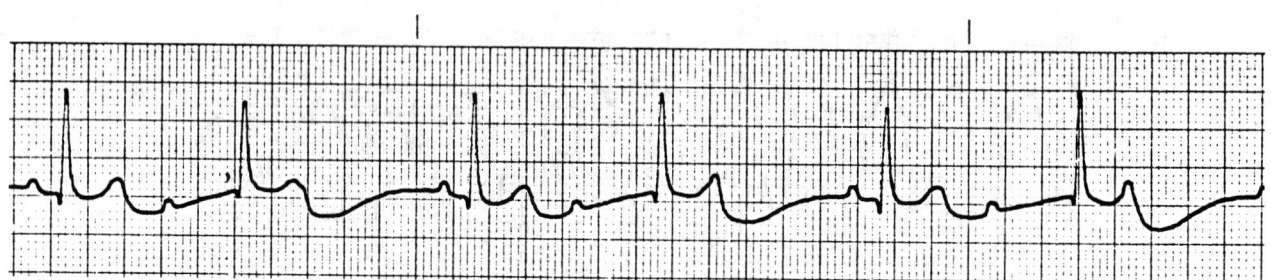

Fig. 25-29 Second-degree AV block, type I (Wenckebach). Every third P wave is hidden in preceding T wave; conduction is 3:2. Note progressive lengthening of PR interval before dropped QRS.

Conduction abnormalities
Atrioventricular block

A block to impulse conduction may occur anywhere along the conduction pathways. One common area of block is the atrioventricular (AV) junction. The severity of the block is identified by degrees: first-, second-, or third-degree AV block.

First-degree atrioventricular block

First-degree AV block is present when the PR interval is prolonged to greater than 0.20 second, indicating a conduction delay in the AV node (Fig. 25-28). The clinical implications of a prolonged PR interval depend upon the level of the lesion. It may be associated with acute myocardial infarction (usually inferior). When a first-degree AV block occurs as an isolated defect, no treatment is necessary.

Second-degree atrioventricular block

In second-degree AV block, some of the atrial impulses are not conducted to the ventricles. There are two types of second-degree AV block: type I (Wenckebach or Mobitz I), when pathology is in the AV node, or type II (Mobitz II), when the lesion is within or below the bundle of His. Each type has different clinical implications, treatment, and prognosis.

Type I second-degree AV block is characterized by a PR interval that progressively lengthens until a P wave is not followed by a QRS complex (Fig. 25-29). The nonconducted beat is the result of the arrival of the impulse during the refractory period of the AV node. The ratio of P waves to QRS complexes may vary. Any drug that slows AV conduction may cause a type I block. It often occurs in patients with acute inferior wall myocardial infarction. Type I blocks are often transient and reversible and generally require no treatment unless the patient becomes symptomatic.

Type II second-degree AV block is less common but more serious than type I. A type II block is characterized by nonconducted sinus impulses despite constant PR intervals (Fig. 25-30). Usually the QRS complexes are widened because of a bundle branch block. The dropped beat represents a form of intermittent blockage of both bundle branches. Type II blocks are most often seen with acute anterior wall myocardial infarction and may progress to third-degree or complete heart block. A temporary pacemaker is often used prophylactically until the condition stabilizes.

Third-degree atrioventricular block

In third-degree AV block (complete heart block), all the sinus or atrial impulses are blocked, and the atria and ventricles are forced to beat independently. The ventricles are driven by a junctional or ventricular pacemaker cell. The rate and dependability of the ventricular rhythm are related to the level of the lesion. If a junctional pacemaker drives the ventricles, ventricular rate will be at least 40 to 60 beats/min (Fig. 25-31). Atropine may be useful in restoring conduction.

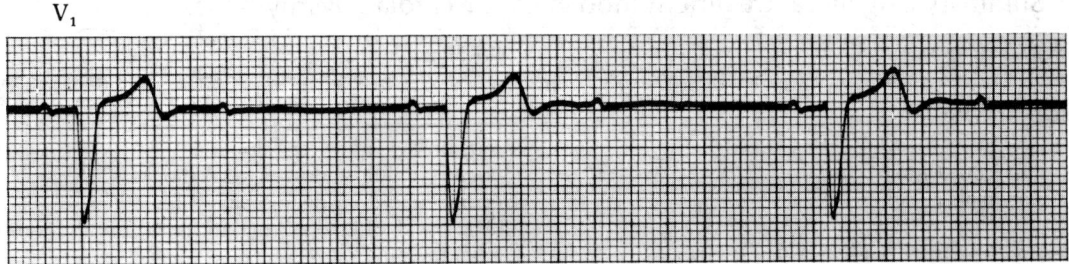

Fig. 25-30 Second-degree AV block, type II with 2:1 conduction. (From Conover MB: *Understanding electrocardiography: arrhythmias and the 12-lead ECG*, ed 6, St Louis, 1992, Mosby–Year Book.)

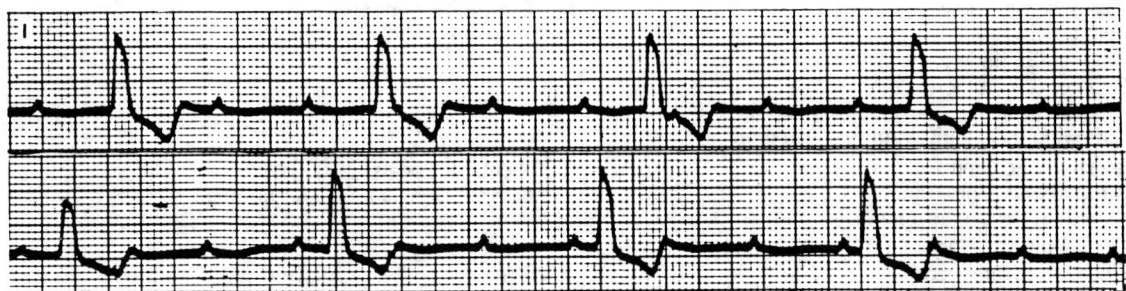

Fig. 25-31 Complete (third-degree) AV block. The strips are continuous. In the presence of sinus tachycardia (rate 108/minute), an independent idioventricular rhythm occurs (rate 36/minute). Note that the ventricular rhythm is absolutely regular, whereas the P-R relationship is constantly changing. (From Marriott HJL, Conover MB: *Advanced concepts in arrhythmias*, ed 2, St Louis, 1989, Mosby–Year Book.)

If a ventricular pacemaker controls the ventricles, the rate will be 20 to 40 beats/min, and the patient may experience syncope, congestive heart failure, altered mentation, or angina. Generally the patient will require a permanent artificial pacemaker. Intravenous epinephrine or isoproterenol may increase the ventricular rate temporarily until artificial pacing can be instituted.

Bundle branch block

A bundle branch block (BBB) occurs as a transient block or permanent defect secondary to tachydysrhythmias, congestive heart failure, acute myocardial infarction, pulmonary embolus, hypoxia, or metabolic derangement. The electrical impulse spreads from one ventricle to the other by abnormal pathways producing distinct ECG tracings and widened QRS complexes.

Bundle branch block may occur in the right bundle branch, the more delicate structure of the two bundles. In the younger person, right bundle branch block (RBBB) often results from right ventricular hypertrophy, whereas coronary artery heart disease is usually the cause in the older person. In the absence of other conduction defects, no intervention is necessary.

The left bundle branch has a main trunk that bifurcates into the left anterior and left posterior divisions. A block may occur in the main trunk or in either of the two divisions. A block in the main trunk produces a complete left bundle branch block (LBBB). LBBB is associated with severe coronary atherosclerotic heart disease, valvular disease, hypertensive disease, cardiomegaly, and acute ante-

---

25-6

Therapies to relieve underlying cause of dysrhythmias

Oxygen to relieve hypoxia
Provision of depleted serum electrolytes (especially potassium)
Treatment of heart failure
Relief of anxiety
Removal of noxious stimuli (for example, caffeine)

---

rior wall myocardial infarction. For in-depth discussion on this topic, see specific cardiology texts.

Treatment Modalities

Three major treatment modalities are employed for cardiac dysrhythmias:

1. Therapy aimed at relieving the underlying cause of the dysrhythmia (see Box 25-6)
2. Drug therapy aimed at suppressing impulse formation by ectopic sites or enhancing impulse formation by the SA node
3. The use of electrical stimuli to suppress ectopic impulse formation or to initiate impulse formation in a regulated manner

Antiarrhythmic agents

The list of *antiarrhythmic drugs* in current use appears to grow almost daily. The development of drugs that are ef-

Table 25-3   Summary of general treatment modalties for cardiac dysrhythmias

Therapeutic aim/treatment	Indications for use
Increase heart rate	
Atropine	Sinus bradycardia (very slow rates)
Epinephrine, isoproterenol	Second- and third-degree heart blocks
Artificial pacemaker	Second- and third-degree heart blocks
	"Overdrive" of ectopic rhythms refractory to more usual therapy
Decrease heart rate	
Reduction of metabolic demands	Sinus tachycardia
Treatment of underlying cause of decreased stroke volume	Sinus tachycardia
	Ectopic tachycardias
Antiarrhythmic agents	Ectopic tachycardias
Verapamil	
Propranalol (Inderal)	
Esmolol (Brevibloc)	
Suppression of ectopic impulse formation	
Antiarrhythmic agents	Premature beats
Amiodarone (Cordarone)	Ectopic tachycardias and fibrillation
Bretylium tosylate (Bretylol)	
Disopyramide (Norpace)	
Flecainide (Tambocor)	
Lidocaine (Xylocaine)	
Mexiletine (Mexitil)	
Procainamide (Pronestyl)	
Propafenone (Rhythmol)	
Quinidine	
Tocainide (Tonocard)	
Verapamil (Calan, Isoptin)	
Cardioversion	Ectopic tachycardias and atrial fibrillation
Defibrillation	Ventricular fibrillation

fective and free of dangerous or annoying side effects has been a challenge to the pharmaceutical industry. The more common drugs are listed in Table 25-3; see pharmacology texts for specific information regarding antiarrhythmic agents.

Pacemakers

The use of various forms of electrical stimuli in the treatment of cardiac dysrhythmias has a number of nursing implications; therefore, these modalities will be discussed in detail.

An artificial pacemaker is a mechanical device that electronically stimulates impulse initiation within the heart. The pacemaker system is composed of a battery-powered energy source (technically called a *pulse generator* but more commonly called a *pacemaker*) and a wire or catheter that delivers the electronic stimulus to a point of contact in the atrial or ventricular myocardium or both. The purpose of artificial pacing is control of heart rate.

Pacemakers are primarily used to treat conduction defects, in which case the catheter is placed in the atria, ventricle, or both to ensure adequate depolarization beyond the site of impulse blockage (Fig. 25-32, A). These devices are also employed to remedy inadequate impulse initiation by the SA node and to suppress myocardial irritability that does not respond to antiarrhythmic therapy. In these in-

stances the catheter may be placed in the atrium, since the underlying problem does not involve failure of the conduction system (Fig. 25-32, B). Ventricular pacing is "nonphysiologic," since it does not result in coordination between atrial and ventricular mechanical activity. The CO thus achieved, however, is adequate for most persons requiring pacemakers.

Pulse generators

The pulse generator has a number of controls that can be easily manipulated in a temporary system (Fig. 25-33). These are more easily manipulated than those in permanent systems because of improvements in technology. These controls include energy output, heart rate, and pacing mode (asynchronous or demand).

Energy output refers to the intensity of the electronic stimulus delivered to the myocardium. Output is measured in milliamperes (mA), and relatively low levels of energy (approximately 1.5 mA) are usually sufficient to cause depolarization if the catheter is in proper contact with the myocardium. Energy output is set by the physician at the time of pacemaker insertion after determination of the "threshold level" of stimulation, that is, the lowest output that will achieve depolarization. Because of continuous minor fluctuations in the threshold, energy output is usually set at twice the initial level.

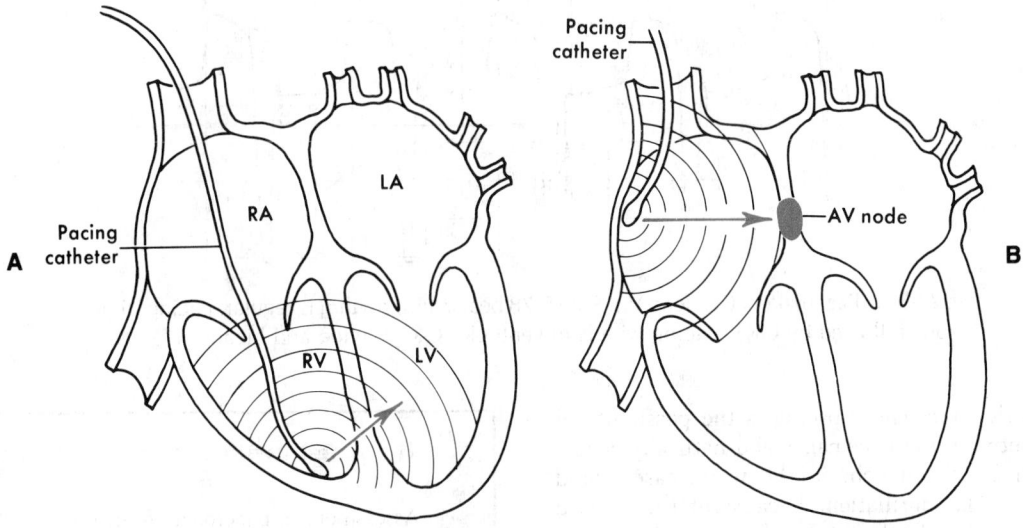

Fig. 25-32   A, Ventricular pacing: impulses are initiated in ventricle. **B,** Atrial pacing: impulses are initiated in atrium and travel to ventricles by normal conduction system.

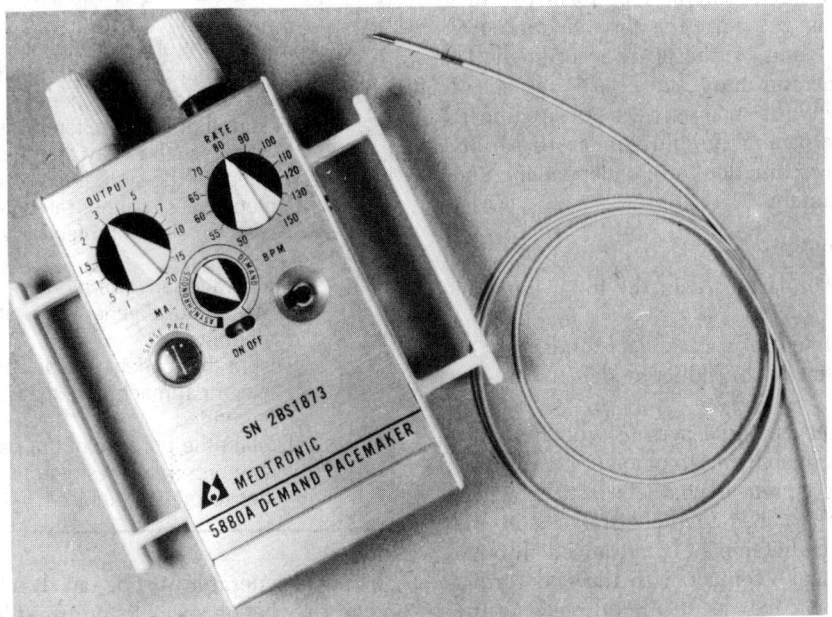

Fig. 25-33   Temporary (external) pacemaker. Pulse generator is battery powered. Electrode is passed into heart before being attached to pulse generator.

Heart rate is set according to the clinical condition of the patient and the desired therapeutic aim. With rare exceptions, the rate is set between 70 and 80 beats/min when the aim is simple maintenance of adequate cardiac output. If the purpose of pacing is the suppression of myocardial irritability, the rate is set higher, often as high as 100 to 120. The heart rate setting reflects the *lowest* anticipated heart rate in a properly functioning pacemaker system.

There has been a considerable evolution in *pacing modes* since the original introduction of artificial pacemakers. The pacemaker may function in the atria, the ventricles, or both cardiac chambers. The mode may be asynchronous (stimulation at a preset fixed rate) or demand (stimulation only in the *absence* of specified electrical activity such as a P wave or a QRS complex). The combination of chamber, mode, type of programmability, and function during tachydysrhythmias has become so complex that the Inter-Society Commission for Heart Disease (ICHD) has developed a code that allows easy identification of pacemaker function in a shorthand type of notation.[65]

An in-depth discussion of available multiple pacing modes is beyond the scope of this text. The reader is referred to specialized texts for more information. In general,

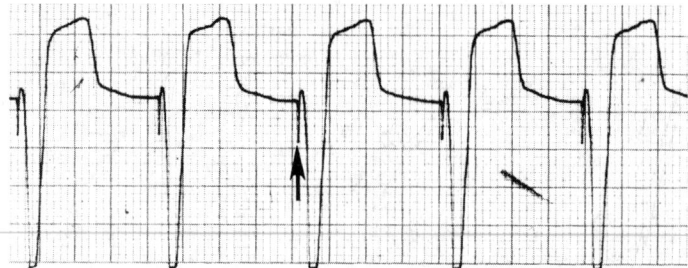

Fig. 25-34   Pacemaker ECG (lead V_1). Rate is 78 beats/min, rhythm is regular. Pacing stimulus *(arrow)* followed by QRS. Pacing wire is in ventricle. QRS is wide and bizarre.

the danger with *asynchronous* pacing is the possibility of competition between the pacemaker and naturally occurring electrical activity which, in the worst case, could result in ventricular fibrillation. Because of this hazard and the development of safer approaches to pacing, asynchronous pacing is rarely used today.

Demand pacing is the most frequently used mode and is characterized by stimulation of the myocardium *only* when the person's natural heart rate falls below the preset limit. This requires that the pulse generator perform two different functions. It must recognize the absence of natural electrical activity and stimulate the heart accordingly. In addition, the pulse generator must "sense" the presence of natural electrical activity that maintains the desired heart rate and withhold the pacing stimulus under those circumstances. These two functions are independent and must be assessed separately.

Temporary pacemakers

Temporary pacemakers are used in the following situations:

1. Emergency treatment of ventricular standstill
2. Short-term treatment of conduction defects causing decreased CO
2. Prophylactic management of persons who are prone to the sudden development of complete heart block

A temporary pacing system is characterized by an *external* pulse generator attached to the distal end of the pacing catheter. The catheter may be advanced through the venous system to make contact with the endocardial surface of the heart, or it may be sutured directly to the epicardial surface. The transvenous approach can be employed at the bedside under ECG guidance or in a special procedure room under fluoroscopy. Direct suturing of the catheter to the epicardium is performed during cardiac or thoracic surgery.

If the patient is connected to a cardiac monitor, the presence of the pacing stimulus (a small vertical spike that indicates that the pulse generator has sent a stimulus to the heart) and evidence that the stimulus actually causes depolarization (either a P wave or a QRS complex immediately following the stimulus, depending on where the catheter has been placed) will be noted (Fig. 25-34).

The pulse generator may be secured to an arm if the antecubital fossa is the insertion site of the pacing catheter. If a subclavian site is used (an approach that has become more common because it leads to greater catheter stability),

---

25-7 — **Guidelines for Care**

The patient with a temporary pacemaker

Assessment of pacemaker function
Assess heart rate to verify that it has not fallen below the preset level; if it has, notify physician
If patient is connected to cardiac monitor, monitor presence of pacing stimulus and that a P wave or a QRS complex immediately follows the stimulus

Maintenance of system integrity
Ensure that catheter terminals are securely connected to pulse generator
Ensure that pulse generator is attached to person in such a way that accidental dislodgement of the system does not occur

Maintenance of patient safety and comfort
Assess for signs of infection at catheter insertion site
Encourage range of motion in extremity to which pulse generator is attached, as permitted
Ensure that patient avoids contact with any electrical machinery that is not properly grounded
Explain the purpose of the pacing system and any prescribed restrictions on physical activities to prevent anxiety

---

the pulse generator may be taped to the chest or placed in a chest pocket on specially prepared hospital gowns. Nursing care of patients with temporary pacemakers is summarized in Box 25-7.

Permanent pacemakers

Permanent pacemakers are used in the long-term treatment of persistent dysrhythmias that are amenable to this type of therapy. The pacing system is totally implanted, with the pulse generator generally placed in a subcutaneous "pocket" beneath the clavicle (Fig. 25-35). As with temporary pacing systems, the catheter may be placed in contact with the heart by the transvenous or epicardial approach.

Permanent pacemakers (Fig. 25-36) are inserted in the operating room or in a special procedure room. The transvenous approach to insertion does not require general anesthesia, a fact that decreases the risk of this procedure.

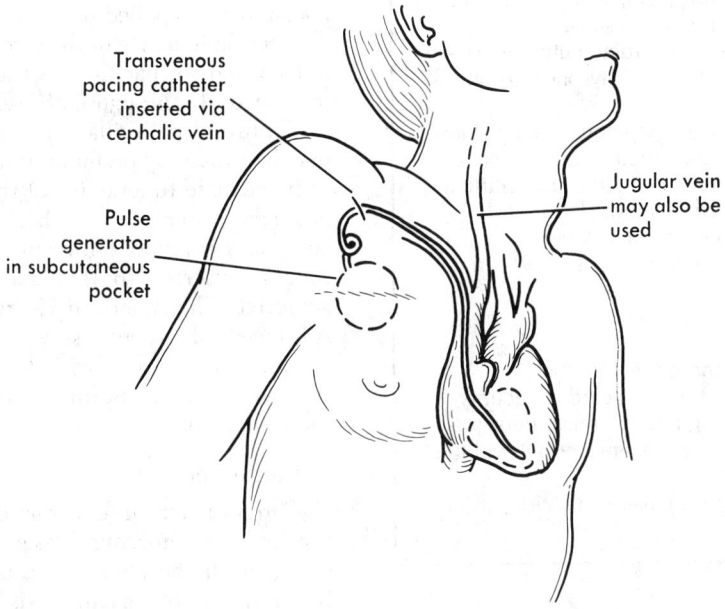

Fig. 25-35 Thoracic placement of a permanent pulse generator (pacemaker) and transvenous pacing catheter.

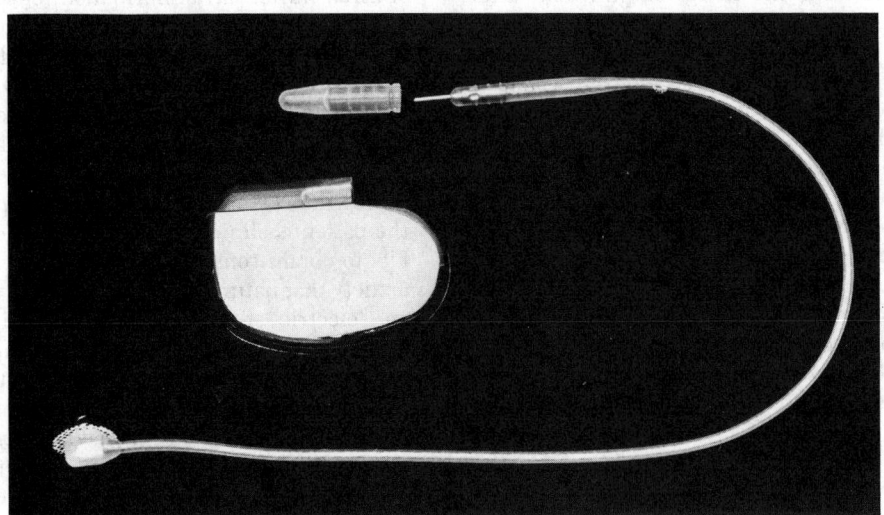

Fig. 25-36 One type of implantable pacemaker (pulse generator) usually implanted subcutaneously in right anterior chest below clavicle.

The patient with a permanent pacemaker

Count pulse daily for 1 full minute; report rate significantly above or below programmed rate to physician.

Report signs of infection (pain, redness, or drainage over incision site) to physician.

Report signs of decreased cardiac output (dizziness, fatigue, "palpitations," dyspnea) to physician.

Avoid holding electrical equipment (such as blow dryers, battery-operated toothbrushes) next to pacemaker (may cause interference, placing the pacemaker in a fixed mode or shut it off[65]).

Carry an identification card that states:
   Pacemaker's manufacturer, model, and serial number
   Implant date
   Programmed rates
   Physician's name and phone number

Show pacemaker identification card to security guards before passing through metal detectors (detector will not affect pacemaker but will trigger the alarm).

Report regularly for pacemaker evaluation, as instructed.

The generator is powered by a battery that has an expected life of 4 to 10 years.

Manipulation of heart rate and energy output has been difficult at best once the permanent unit was implanted; however, recent technologic advances have resulted in programmable pulse generators that allow variation in both the present heart rate and the energy output. The latter manipulation has proved useful in reducing battery drain.

Immediate postinsertion care of a person with a permanent pacemaker includes relief of incisional discomfort, monitoring for infection, and assessment of the system's functioning. Attaching the person to a cardiac monitor for 24 to 48 hours following insertion is the usual practice. Long-term follow-up of these persons is essential and is especially important within the last year of anticipated battery life. Pacemaker clinics have been established to facilitate follow-up, and in some instances, telecommunications systems allow telephone assessment of functioning. Literature published by pacemaker manufacturers and by the American Heart Association can be incorporated into teaching plans (see Box 25-8) for persons with permanent pacemakers.

Defibrillation and cardioversion
Defibrillation

Defibrillation operates on two electrophysiologic principles. The first is that electricity is a stimulus that can initiate depolarization. The second is that premature discharge of a normal pacemaker or an ectopic focus can upset its rhythmicity and momentarily suppress its activity. The application of electrical energy (200 to 360 joules) to the chest wall of a person in ventricular fibrillation allows enough current to reach the heart to cause depolarization of a critical cell mass. This suppresses the ectopic focus and, it is hoped, allows the SA node to regain control of cardiac electrical activity.

Defibrillation is achieved by placing the paddles from the defibrillator at the third intercostal space to the right of the sternum and the fifth intercostal space on the left midaxillary line. Either conducting gel or saline-soaked pads must be applied between the paddles and the skin to ensure conductance of the electrical energy. The machine is triggered so that the electrical energy is discharged simultaneously through both paddles.

Failure of defibrillation to achieve the desired results may be caused by profound myocardial ischemia, acidosis, or inadequate functioning of the SA node. Usual practice is to administer a second shock immediately and then proceed with adjunctive therapy if needed. An endotracheal tube is inserted so that adequate oxygenation can be achieved. The American Heart Association Standards for Advanced Life Support serve as a guide for training health professionals to deal with life-threatening dysrhythmias such as ventricular fibrillation and as criteria for evaluating their performance.

Cardioversion

Cardioversion differs from defibrillation in that it is a synchronized procedure designed to deliver the electrical energy to the heart at a set time during the cardiac cycle. In brief, once the machine has been discharged, the shock is withheld until the next QRS complex occurs. The purpose of synchronization is to prevent ventricular fibrillation from occurring as the result of an improperly timed electrical stimulus. It is clear that cardioversion is *never* used to terminate ventricular fibrillation, because there are no QRS complexes to trigger the release of electrical energy.

When cardioversion is elective (for example, conversion of atrial flutter, atrial fibrillation, or PAT), the procedure differs slightly. The patient receives nothing by mouth for 8 hours before the cardioversion. The daily digitalis is usually withheld on the procedure day (or for several days previously). Anticoagulant therapy is continued. In many instances, oral antiarrhythmic drugs are given in advance.

Cardioversion is largely an elective procedure that requires the person's consent. Exceptions would be made if the patient's clinical condition were deteriorating too rapidly to obtain consent. Premedication is given to allay the anxiety that naturally accompanies the thought of enduring an "electric shock." Diazepam (Valium) or midazolam (Versed) is frequently administered intravenously for this purpose because of its muscle relaxant and amnesic properties. An oral airway, oxygen, and emergency drugs should be available during this procedure. For most elective procedures, the amount of watt-seconds or joules required for cardioversion is lower than that required for defibrillation. The patient is monitored after cardioversion until vital signs are stable and the gag reflex has returned.

Automatic implantable cardioverter defibrillator

A sudden death occurring within 24 hours of the onset of symptoms account for more than half the deaths from coronary disease in the United States. Sudden cardiac death is due to a derangement in the heart's electrical stability, which most often deteriorates into ventricular fibrillation.

After several years of research and development, Mirowski and others implanted the first permanent *automatic* defibrillator in 1980.[70] This device automatically senses ventricular fibrillation and, within approximately 15 to 20 seconds, delivers an electrical countershock. It is also capable of identifying and correcting ventricular tachycardia with cardioversion. Defibrillatory energy requirements are considerably less because the shock is being applied directly within the heart.

The automatic implantable cardioverter defibrillator (AICD) consists of a pulse generator and two lead or sensing systems. The device is implanted surgically through a median sternotomy or lateral thoracotomy approach. This device has been approved by the Food and Drug Administration (FDA) for two categories of patients: (1) those who have experienced recurrent life-threatening ventricular dysrhythmias, inducible into sustained hypotensive ventricular tachycardia or ventricular fibrillation despite conventional antiarrhythmic drug therapy, and (2) those who have survived one or more episodes of sudden cardiac death resulting from ventricular tachycardia or ventricular fibrillation not associated with acute myocardial infarction.

MAJOR HEALTH PROBLEMS OF THE HEART

Alterations in cardiovascular structure or function affect circulation and may therefore be life threatening. Disease of the heart and major blood vessels may be classified in a variety of ways such as congenital versus acquired, identification of the structure involved (valvular heart disease, myocarditis, endocarditis), etiology of the disease (inadequate coronary artery blood flow, hypertensive cardiovascular disease, rheumatic heart disease), disruption of cardiac physiology (dysrhythmias), and disruption of cardiac function (heart failure, cardiogenic shock). The following common cardiac and aortic disorders are discussed in this chapter.

1. Interference with coronary blood flow: coronary artery disease (angina pectoris, myocardial infarction)
2. Failure of the heart as a pump: congestive heart failure, cardiogenic shock
3. Diseases of specific portions of the cardiac tissue: pericarditis, myocarditis, endocarditis
4. Diseases that are secondary to other diseases or conditions: cardiovascular syphilis, alcoholic cardiomyopathy, rheumatic heart disease, cocaine abuse
5. Inadequate valvular functioning: stenosis or insufficiency
6. Weakening of aortic wall: aortic aneurysms

CORONARY ARTERY DISEASE

Pathophysiology

Coronary artery disease (CAD) refers to a variety of pathologic conditions that obstruct blood flow through the arteries that supply the heart (see Box 25-9). Atherosclerosis is the most common etiologic factor leading to coronary atherosclerotic heart disease (CAHD).

25-9	Conditions that obstruct coronary blood supply
	Atherosclerosis
	Arteriosclerosis
	Arteritis
	Coronary artery spasms
	Coronary thrombosis
	Embolism

Atherosclerosis, the predominant type of arteriosclerosis in humans, is characterized by the accumulation of fatty materials (lipids) and fibrous tissue within the arterial walls. As these atherosclerotic changes progress, the lumen of the vessel becomes narrowed, and blood flow is obstructed to those areas of the myocardium supplied by the artery. Since this is a form of arteriosclerosis, the arterial wall also loses its elasticity and becomes less responsive to changes in blood volume and pressure.

Although several theories have been postulated to explain the pathogenesis of atherosclerosis, the etiology of this condition remains unclear. Atherosclerotic lesions usually develop near the origin and bifurcation of the main coronary arteries (see Fig. 25-2). The left coronary artery is more often affected than the right coronary artery. The disease process is initially localized but then becomes diffuse with advancing coronary atherosclerosis.

The first lesion to form within the coronary arterial wall is called a fatty streak (Fig. 25-37). This lesion begins to appear in coronary vessels as early as 15 years of age. Lipid-

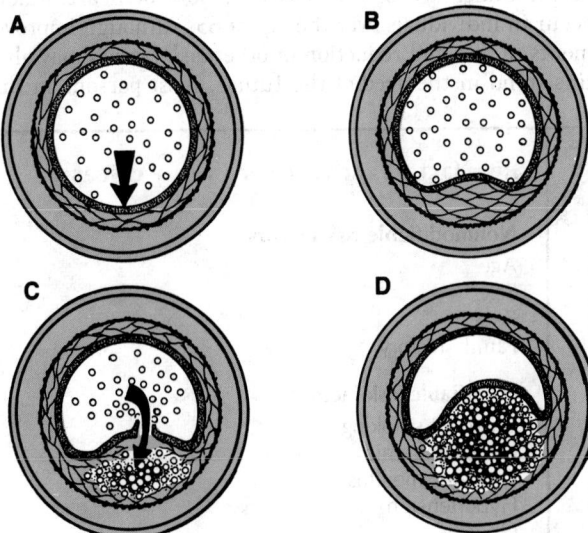

Fig. 25-37 Progressive development of coronary atherosclerosis. **A,** Injury to intimal wall. **B,** Lipoprotein invasion of smooth muscle cells. **C,** Development of fatty streak and fibrous plaque. **D,** Development of complicated lesion.

filled cells, or "foam cells," invade the intimal wall and produce a fatty streak. As the disease progresses, raised thick fibrous plaques form and with increasing size limit the luminal capacity of the vessel. These lesions are typically characteristic of advancing atherosclerosis.

An even more advanced stage of atherosclerosis is represented by a calcified fibrous plaque or complicated lesion. This calcified deposit can rupture and hence greatly increase the risk of spasm, thrombus formation, and embolization. It is this final type of atherosclerotic lesion that gives rise to the symptoms of CAHD. The arterial lumen becomes so narrowed that a great imbalance exists between myocardial oxygen supply and myocardial oxygen demand. Manifestations of myocardial ischemia do not usually occur until the artery is about 75% occluded. They include the following:

1. Angina pectoris
2. Myocardial infarction
3. Sudden death

Risk Factors

Extensive clinical research has identified several contributing factors that place an individual at risk for the development of coronary artery disease. The cumulative effect of these risk factors accelerates the atherosclerotic process. Risk factors are grouped into two basic categories: those that cannot be altered by the individual (nonmodifiable) and those that the individual has the capacity to change (modifiable) (Box 25-10).

Nonmodifiable risk factors
Age

Both morbidity and mortality of coronary artery disease increase with age. Clinical symptomatology may be seen as early as the second decade of life, but the incidence of CAHD steadily rises in the 30- to 50-year age group. As reported by the Framingham Heart Study, 5% of all heart attacks occur in people under age 40, and 45% occur in people under age 65.[3] In essence, 50% of heart attacks occur in individuals over the age of 65. Although improvements in diet and reduction of other risk factors may alter this trend in the aged of the future, most persons in this risk category today are a reflection of yesterday's poor health practices.[21]

Sex

Men are at a greater risk for the development of CAHD. Women are usually not affected by this disease until after menopause. The postmenopausal increase has been attributed to decreased levels of estorgens and rising blood lipids. The incidence of CAHD in women has been rising, and it is now a leading cause of death in women as well as men.

Race

Black Americans have a higher risk for CAHD than do whites. One possible explanation for this finding is their increased incidence of hypertension (33% higher than in the white population).[3]

Family history

A familial tendency toward the development of CAHD has been demonstrated. The presence of coronary atherosclerosis in a parent or sibling under 50 years old is associated with the same finding in another family member. The extent to which genetic and environmental factors contribute to this disorder, however, is still not known.

Modifiable risk factors
Cigarette smoking

Cigarette smoking is a major contributing factor of CAHD. Cigarette smokers have a two to three times greater risk of death from CAHD than nonsmokers. This risk is related to the number of cigarettes smoked per day; the more cigarettes smoked, the greater the risk. Individuals who quit smoking are at less risk than smokers.

Although the exact relationship between cigarette smoking and coronary atherosclerosis is unclear, it is thought to be associated with the effects of nicotine and the higher content of carbon monoxide produced by the smoker. Nicotine increases myocardial workload and subsequent oxygen demand. Carbon monoxide interferes with oxygen transport. The combination of these two factors may place an inordinate demand on a diseased heart.

Hyperlipidemia

Hyperlipidemia refers to the elevation of cholesterol and triglyceride levels within the blood. Cholesterol can be obtained directly from animal dietary sources (see Chapter 5) or manufactured by the liver and intestine. Triglycerides are derived from fatty acids found in adipose tissue or the diet. Cholesterol and triglycerides are involved in the transportation, digestion, and absorption of fats.

Individuals with cholesterol levels in excess of 300 ml/dl have four times the risk of CAHD of those with levels less than 200 mg/dl. There is also clinical evidence that high levels of a specific type of lipid-protein complex, the *low-density lipoproteins,* are indicative of CAHD. These lipoproteins transport plasma lipids and contain approximately 50% cholesterol. In contrast, the high-density lipoproteins are thought to have an antiatherogenic effect.

A diet high in saturated fat, cholesterol, and calories is thought to be a major factor in the development of hyper-

---

25-10

Risk factors for coronary artery disease

Nonmodifiable risk factors
Age
Sex
Race
Family history

Modifiable risk factors
Cigarette smoking
Hyperlipidemia
Diabetes mellitus
Hypertension
Obesity
Lack of exercise
Stress
Oral contraceptives

lipidemia. Dietary management, therefore, is an essential component in the prevention of this risk factor. Changes in long-established dietary patterns do not come easily, however. Awareness of the link between diet and the development of CAHD is frequently not sufficient motivation for modifications in diet that require a great deal of determination and creativity.

Diabetes mellitus

Individuals with diabetes mellitus are at much greater risk for CAHD. Coronary atherosclerosis has been found to be two to three times more prevalent in persons with diabetes, regardless of blood lipid levels. The mechanisms by which impaired glucose tolerance increases the risk for CAHD is unclear. A predisposition to vascular degeneration has been noted in diabetics, and abnormal lipid metabolism may also play a role in the development of atheromas.[45] Adherence to a prescribed medical regimen for glucose regulation may diminish the effect of this risk factor and is within the realm of individual responsibility.

Hypertension

The relationship between high blood pressure and CAHD has been attributed to acceleration of the process that results in coronary atherosclerosis. In addition, increased peripheral vascular resistance associated with hypertension increases afterload and the demand on the left ventricle. The result is an increased demand for myocardial oxygen in the face of a diminished supply. The effects of hypertension are potentially modifiable through adherence to a medical regimen for control of systolic and diastolic blood pressure.

Obesity

Obesity or excess body weight in relation to height increases the workload and hence the oxygen demand of the heart. Its effect as a risk factor is questionable, although obesity highly correlates with hypertension, hyperlipidemia, and diabetes. Specifically, obesity tends to be associated with increased caloric intake and elevated levels of low-density lipoproteins.

Lack of exercise

The lack of exercise has not been clearly linked to CAHD. It has been demonstrated, however, that exercise can improve the efficiency of the heart by the reduction of heart rate and blood pressure. Other physiologic effects of regular exercise, such as decreased levels of low-density lipoproteins, lowered blood glucose levels, and improved cardiac output, have been associated with a lesser chance of CAHD. The psychologic benefits of exercise, reduced anxiety and depression, may also be of significance.

Stress

The effect of stress on the pathogenesis of CAHD is controversial. Stress stimulates the cardiovascular system by the release of catecholamines, which in turn increase the heart rate and produce vasoconstriction. Stress also plays a major role in those individuals with type A behavior. Behaviors including ambitiousness, aggressiveness, competitiveness, impatience, muscle tenseness, vigorous speech, and rapid pace in all activities are indicative of the type A behavior pattern.[68] In early studies, people with type A personality characteristics were found to have twice the risk of developing CAHD compared with the type B personality, which has totally opposite characteristics. However, several recent prospective studies fail to confirm these earlier findings. In fact, it now appears that not only is the global type A behavior pattern not a reliable indicator of subsequent development of CAHD, but some aspects of this behavior pattern may even represent a positive and healthy coping pattern.[26]

Oral contraceptives

The use of oral contraceptives or birth control pills has been associated with an increased risk of CAHD. The nature of the association is not clearly understood. It is possible that this risk factor acts synergistically with others.

ANGINA PECTORIS

Etiology

Although angina pectoris is usually caused by atherosclerosis of the coronary vessels, the incidence is high in persons with hypertension, diabetes mellitus, thromboangiitis obliterans, aortic regurgitation caused by rheumatic heart disease or syphilis, periarteritis nodosa, and polycythemia vera. Other causes of anginal pain include aortic insufficiency, severe anemia, and coronary arterial spasm. Typically, angina is triggered by cold, exercise, or anything that increases cardiac workload and myocardial oxygen consumption.

Pathophysiology

Angina pectoris or chest pain is a clinical syndrome produced by insufficient coronary blood flow. An imbalance exists between myocardial oxygen supply and myocardial oxygen demand, which creates transient myocardial ischemia. The underlying mechanism to account for the experience of pain is probably related to the change from aerobic to anaerobic metabolism. By-products from anaerobic metabolism, specifically lactic acid, may initiate sensory receptors and cause pain. The release of other substances from the ischemic cells may also produce pain in this manner. Since the basic problem in angina is an imbalance between oxygen supply and demand, the primary goals of therapy are directed to the restoration of this balance (Table 25-4).

Two subcategories of angina should be distinguished from the classic condition. These are unstable angina and variant angina. A brief description of these forms of angina is presented here. For further information, consult a cardiology text.

Unstable angina

Unstable angina is also referred to as preinfarction angina, crescendo angina, or intermittent coronary syndrome. This type of angina is characterized by an increase in the severity, frequency, or duration of symptoms without infarction.

Table 25-4   Coronary artery disorders

Disorder	Signs and symptoms	Medical therapy
Angina pectoris	Chest pain (substernal, retrosternal), may radiate to neck, jaw, arm, back; usually brought on by exertion, emotional upsets; relieved by rest, nitroglycerin	Avoidance of precipitating factors Reduction of modifiable risk factors Medications: nitrates, beta-adrenergic blocking agents, calcium channel blockers Oxygen therapy ECG monitoring
Myocardial infarction	Severe, crushing chest pain; may radiate as with angina; not relieved with rest, nitroglycerin May be associated with dyspnea, diaphoresis, apprehension, nausea	Relief of pain (O_2, morphine, other analgesics) ECG monitoring Reduction of O_2 demand (rest) Prevention of complications (stool softeners, anticoagulants) Treatment of complications (dysrhythmias, CHF)

Variant angina

Variant angina, or Prinzmetal's angina, is thought to develop from intermittent coronary artery spasm with or without atherosclerotic heart disease. This type of anginal pain can occur during normal activities and is not necessarily precipitated by exercise or stress. Anginal pain in this condition often develops at the same time of day or night, demonstrating a cyclic pattern. Some persons with variant angina may also have typical exertional angina.

Nursing Process
Assessment
Subjective data

Collect data concerning the person's knowledge about the disorder, presence of risk factors, and perception of the anginal pain. Specific data related to pain include the following:

1. Location and radiation to other sites: the pain is most often substernal or retrosternal. Pain may radiate to other sites (Fig. 25-38) or may occur *only* in one of those sites.
2. Quality of the pain: the pain is frequently described as a tightness or heaviness in the chest. Pressure, or a squeezing sensation, may also be part of the description. The person may complain only of a vague discomfort that is sometimes misinterpreted as indigestion. Angina is *not* usually described as a "sharp" pain.
3. Onset and duration of the pain: usually of brief duration.
4. Precipitating factors: often identified as exertion, exposure to extreme hot or cold, stress or emotional upset, or a heavy meal. *No* precipitating factor may be identified with variant angina.
5. Associated symptoms: apprehension, nausea, diaphoresis may be noted but are not common.
6. Relieving factors: angina is usually relieved by rest and/or nitroglycerin.

The nurse should be especially alert to reports of *change* in the frequency, severity, precipitating factors, or duration of anginal attacks, as these may be warnings of worsening ischemia.

Objective data

1. Patient behavior: note presence of diaphoresis, apprehension. Persons with angina are sometimes seen pressing a fist against the sternum during an attack.
2. Changes in vital signs: increases in pulse rate, blood pressure, and respiratory rate may be noted.
3. Changes in cardiac rhythm.
4. Pattern of anginal attacks with particular attention to changes.

Diagnostic tests

The diagnosis of ischemic heart disease is frequently made on the basis of the patient's history. Diagnosis of angina may also be facilitated by electrocardiogram (ECG) (p. 641), Holter monitor, coronary angiography, and stress testing.

Electrocardiogram

Characteristic findings of ischemia, ST segment depression, and T wave inversion may be seen during chest pain. The absence of ECG changes does not exclude the diagnosis of ischemia.

Holter monitor

A Holter monitor is a small portable ECG monitor about the size of a large transistor radio. In nonacute situations, a patient can be connected to this monitor to evaluate chest pain during performance of daily activities. Two wires are attached to the patient's chest and connected to the monitor. The patient wears the monitor for 24 hours, during which time the ECG tracing is recorded on tape and the patient maintains a log of daily activities, medications, and unusual sensations. Compare the log with the corresponding segment of the ECG tracing.

Coronary angiography

Selective coronary angiography may be carried out as part of a catheterization of the left side of the heart. Injection of contrast medium into the coronary arteries is followed by cineangiographic films to monitor the progression of the "dye." The contrast medium outlines the entire

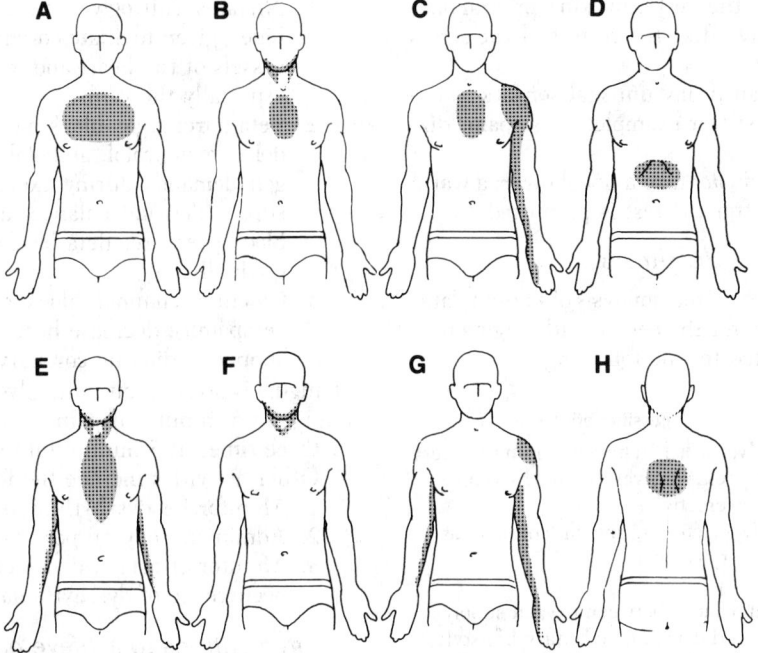

Fig. 25-38   Sites where ischemic myocardial pain may be referred. **A,** Upper chest. **B,** Beneath sternum radiating to neck and jaw. **C,** Beneath sternum radiating down left arm. **D,** Epigastric. **E,** Epigastric radiating to neck, jaw, and arms. **F,** Neck and jaw. **G,** Left shoulder, inner aspect of both arms. **H,** Intrascapular.

25-11	**Indications for stress testing**
	Evaluate symptoms of CAHD.
	Determine physical work capacity and aerobic capacity.
	Determine functional capacity following a myocardial infarction.
	Determine limitations for exercise programming.
	Evaluate dysrythmias that develop during exercise.
	Screen patients over age 40 and at risk for CAHD.
	Evaluate effect of pharmacologic agents on dysrhythmias and angina.

25-12	**Conditions requiring termination of stress testing**
	Ventricular tachycardia
	Marked decrease in peak systolic blood pressure
	Marked decrease in heart rate
	Vertigo
	Frequent premature ventricular beats
	Anginal pain
	Severe dyspnea
	Severe anxiety
	Diagnostic ST segment depression on ECG

coronary circulation and enables the examiner to evaluate the anatomy of the coronary arteries, as well as note the location and nature of any lesions (that is, areas in which the arteries are narrowed or obstructed) and the presence of collateral circulation.

Stress testing

Stress testing or exercise electrocardiography is a non-invasive test used to evaluate cardiovascular response to controlled physical work loads. The indications for performing a stress test are identified in Box 25-11.

During stress testing, the patient pedals a stationary bicycle or walks on a treadmill. Throughout the testing, the patient's blood pressure and ECG are recorded. Conditions that require termination of the testing are listed in

Box 25-12. The risk of developing a myocardial infarction is less than 1 in 500; the risk of death is less than 1 in 10,000.[8]

Adequate patient preparation is extremely important. The patient should do the following:

1. Get adequate rest the night before the test
2. Avoid coffee, tea, and alcohol the day of the test
3. Avoid smoking and taking nitroglycerin during the 2-hour period immediately before the test
4. Eat a light breakfast or lunch at least 2 hours before the test
5. Wear comfortable, loose-fitting clothes; women need to wear a bra for support
6. Wear sturdy, comfortable walking shoes
7. Consult with the physician regarding the taking of

medications before the test (digoxin, propranolol, and vasodilators may affect the results of the stress test)
8. Inform the physician if any unusual sensations develop during the test (for example, chest pain, dizziness)
9. Rest after the test; do *not* take a hot shower; a warm bath 1 or 2 hours after the test is permitted

Data analysis: nursing diagnoses

Determine nursing diagnoses from analysis of patient data. Possible nursing diagnoses for the person with angina may include, but are not limited to, the following:

Diagnostic title	Possible etiologies
Pain	Myocardial ischemia, coronary artery occlusion, vasospasm, hypoxia, overactivity
Tissue perfusion, altered: cardiovascular	Hypertension, angina, coronary artery occlusion
Activity intolerance	Imbalance between oxygen supply and demand, sedentary life-style, immobility, pain, fatigue, generalized weakness
Anxiety	Threat or actual change in health status, diagnosis of pathology involving a major organ, threat to self-concept, threat of death
Knowledge deficit	Lack of exposure/recall, information misinterpretation, unfamiliarity with information resources, cognitive limitation, lack of interest

Planning: expected patient outcomes

Expected patient outcomes for the person with angina may include, but are not limited to, the following:
1. States feeling more comfortable.
2. Demonstrates cardiac tolerance to increased activity (stable pulse and blood pressure).
3. Identifies factors that reduce activity tolerance and progresses to highest level of mobility possible.
4. Uses effective coping mechanisms in managing anxiety.
5. Identifies factors that increase cardiac workload.
6. Describes the following:
   a. Disease process, causes, variables contributing to symptoms, and interventions for disease or symptom control
   b. Events that may precipitate anginal attacks
   c. Medical regimen
   d. Plans to participate in a regular exercise program
   e. Rationale for and type of surgery to be performed, if surgery is indicated
   f. Plans for medical follow-up

Implementation
Assisting with achievement of therapeutic goals

The major medical therapy is pharmacologic. Medications are prescribed to dilate coronary arteries and decrease the workload on the heart. The drugs include the following:

1. Nitrates (nitroglycerin, amyl nitrate, and isosorbide): given to dilate coronary arteries and collateral vessels of the heart and to dilate peripheral vessels, especially the veins.
2. Beta-adrenergic blocking agents (propranolol, nadolol, metoprolol, atenolol, and esmolol): lower oxygen demands during exercise, improve the oxygen supply/demand balance, and lower heart rate and blood pressure. Beta blockers should be withdrawn gradually.
3. Calcium channel blockers (nifedipine, diltiazem, verapamil): decrease heart rate and improve oxygen supply by dilating coronary arteries.

If angina is present, give nitroglycerin sublingually. Repeat dosage in 5 minutes if pain does not subside. Repeat two or three times at 5-minute intervals.

Other activities include the following:
1. Monitor for dysrhythmias.
2. Administer oxygen per nasal cannula as prescribed.
3. Monitor effects of daily activities on cardiac status, occurrence of dysrhythmias, and need for oxygen.

Interventions to achieve patient outcomes
Promoting comfort

Reduce or remove any known factors (physiologic or psychologic) that are contributing to increased pain. Assess for causes of decreased pain tolerance, such as anxiety, fatigue, or lack of knowledge. Fatigue from increased oxygen demands with a decreased oxygen supply increases pain perception. Therefore take measures to reduce fatigue, such as providing rest periods if fatigue is present during physical activities. Provide a calm environment to decrease stress and anxiety that can increase the pain experience. Give nitroglycerin if angina is present.

Promoting tissue perfusion

Instruct patient to avoid becoming overly fatigued and to stop activity immediately in the presence of chest pain, dyspnea, faintness, or light-headedness, which indicate low tissue perfusion. Decreased tissue perfusion causes cellular hypoxia with subsequent ischemia, cellular swelling, and cellular death.

Promoting activity and rest

Enhance the patient's activity tolerance by encouraging slower activity or shorter periods of activity with more rest periods. Pulse increases of 50/min occur with strenuous activity; this rate is safe provided it returns to the resting pulse within 3 minutes. Most persons with angina pectoris can tolerate mild exercise such as walking and playing golf, but exertion such as running or climbing stairs rapidly causes pain. Anginal pain occurs more easily in cold weather. Some persons may have to take nitroglycerin prophylactically before they engage in exercise or sexual activity, but the key to healthful activity is to avoid overexertion.

Promoting relief of anxiety and feeling of well-being

Help the patient reduce the level of anxiety. Because excessive emotional strain also causes vasoconstriction by releasing epinephrine into circulation, the patient should minimize emotional outbursts, worry, and tension. Persons with angina may need continuing help in accepting situations as they find them. See Chapter 6 for approaches to assist persons cope with stress and anxiety.

Teaching patient/family

Delay teaching until the individual is ready. The patient needs to be relatively free of pain and excessive anxiety in order to learn. Promote a positive attitude and active participation of patient and family to encourage compliance. The teaching plan includes information about medications, approaches to minimize precipitating events, effects of exercise on reduction of myocardial oxygen needs, and the need for regular medical follow-up (Box 25-13).

Evaluation

Evaluation will be based on expected patient outcomes. Questions to ask may include the following:
1. Is patient able to control pain by use of prescribed medication?
2. Can patient describe ways to minimize events that may precipitate anginal pain?
3. Is patient engaged or planning to engage in a regular exercise program?
4. Does the patient use effective coping mechanisms to manage anxiety?
5. Does the patient know action, usage, and side effects of prescribed medications?
6. Does the patient know CAHD risk factors that can be modified?

MYOCARDIAL INFARCTION
Etiology

Acute myocardial infarction (AMI) is caused by sudden blockage of one of the branches of a coronary artery. It may be extensive enough to interfere with cardiac function and cause immediate death, or it may cause necrosis of a portion of the myocardium with subsequent healing by scar formation or fibrosis. Coronary occlusion is a general term for blockage of a coronary artery. The blockage may be caused by formation of a thrombus in the coronary artery (coronary thrombosis), sudden progression of atherosclerotic changes, or prolonged constriction of the arteries.

Pathophysiology

Prolonged ischemia lasting more than 35 to 45 minutes produces irreversible cellular damage and necrosis. The contractile properties of cardiac muscle within the necrotic areas become permanently impaired (Fig. 25-39). The final extent of the infarct depends on the ability of the surrounding ischemic tissues to recruit collateral circulation. Collateral circulation is the development of new vessels within the heart to compensate for the damaged artery.

The clinical features of a myocardial infarct are determined by the site and extent of the disease process. An occlusion in the *left anterior descending* coronary artery (LAD) typically results in an *anterior wall infarction*. Depending on the exact site of the occlusion, the area involved

---

Patient Teaching **25-13**

The patient with angina pectoris

Use of nitrate medications
  Use nitroglycerin prophylactically to avoid pain known to occur with certain activities
  Burning sensation on tongue indicates nitroglycerin is activated
  Throbbing sensation in head and flushing may occur
  Sit and stand slowly after taking nitroglycerin
  Place nitroglycerin tablets under the tongue at the onset of anginal pain; second tablet can be taken after 5 minutes and third tablet after another 5 minutes if pain is unrelieved
  Call physician if pain does not subside after third nitroglycerin tablet; go to nearest emergency department; do not drive yourself
  Always carry nitroglycerin
  Store nitroglycerin in dark bottle and keep in dry place
  Replenish nitroglycerin supply every 6 months or before expiration date
  Remove all old nitrate ointment just before application of new cream
Ways to minimize precipitating events
  Avoid overexertion
  Try to reduce stress and anxiety, which cause blood vessels to constrict
  Avoid overeating, as it places an increased work load on the heart
  Avoid cold weather (constricts coronary vessels to conserve body heat, hence anginal pain can develop more easily)
  Dress warmly in cold weather
  Avoid hot, humid conditions (increases work load of heart)
  Walk downhill and with wind since walking uphill and against wind increase work load of heart
Effects of exercise program in reduction of myocardial oxygen needs
  Engage in regular exercise program
  Exercise conditions heart muscle and can decrease oxygen demand during exercise
  Space exercise period with rest periods
  Take nitroglycerin before exertion
Need for regular medical follow-up

---

may be limited or massive. Substantial loss of left ventricular muscle mass is associated with severe hemodynamic consequences.

An occlusion in the *right* coronary artery (RCA) may result in an *inferior* or *posterior* wall infarction. Although the loss of muscle mass may not be as extensive as in anterior infarctions, the person with an inferior infarction may be predisposed to dysrhythmias and conduction defects because of the proximity of the RCA to the conduction system. A lateral wall infarction is usually caused by an occlusion of the *left circumflex* coronary artery. The signs and symptoms and medical therapies to curtail the complications of myocardial infarction are outlined in Table 25-4 (p. 664).

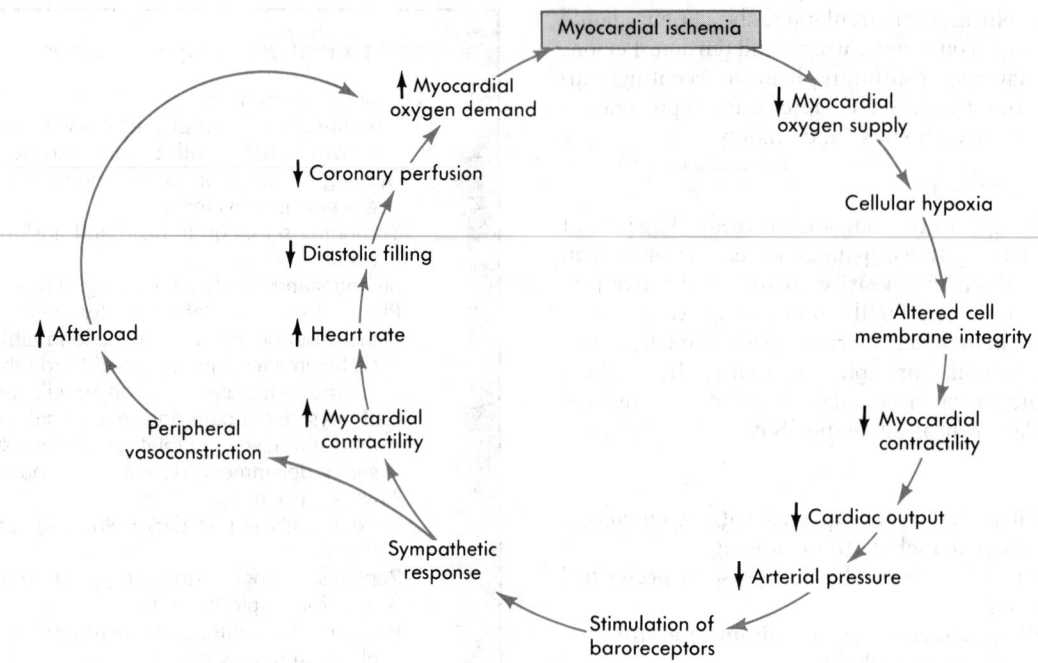

Fig. 25-39 Effects of prolonged myocardial ischemia.

Nursing Process

Assessment

Subjective data

Myocardial infarction (MI) can be equated with irreversible myocardial ischemia; hence many of the associated signs and symptoms are similar to those found with angina. Typically the symptoms are more severe and of longer duration than the person's usual angina attacks, although they may occur in a person who has never previously complained of angina. Symptoms are absent or unreported in about 15% of all myocardial infarctions. Data to be collected include the following:

1. Patient's perception of the pain
   a. Location and radiation to other sites (see Fig. 25-38)
   b. Quality of the pain: often described as crushing or viselike; often more severe than angina
   c. Onset and duration of pain: may be of sudden onset or may build up over a period of a few minutes; duration is longer than angina—may be several minutes to several hours
   d. Precipitating factors: often occurs with intense emotion or exertion but may also occur at rest
   e. Relieving factors: not relieved by rest, nitroglycerin, changes in body position.
2. Associated symptoms: may include nausea, dyspnea, dizziness, weakness, and a sense of impending doom

Ojective data

1. Behavior: often very apprehensive
2. Changes in vital signs: pulse rate may increase in response to pain or diminished cardiac output; may decrease if conduction defects develop; blood pressure may decrease if the extent of myocardial damage is significant; vital sign changes in elderly persons are noted in the box entitled "The elderly with cardiovascular problems."
3. Associated signs: may include diaphoresis, vomiting, pallor, cold clammy skin, cardiac dysrhythmias, labored respirations
4. Breath sounds: no change may be noted, but if pulmonary edema develops, rales will be present
5. Presence of risk factors

Diagnostic tests

Although the clinical picture of severe crushing chest pain, pallor, diaphoresis, and apprehension or a sense of impending doom is the classic description of a person having a myocardial infarction, it by no means describes *all* infarction patients. About 15% of myocardial infarctions occur without the characteristic signs and symptoms (called "silent infarctions"), and individual variation in the symptoms is to be expected. A variety of diagnostic tests are used, therefore, to verify the diagnosis. These tests include blood tests that detect both nonspecific and specific changes caused by the infarction, ECG, radiologic tests, and scintigraphic studies.

Blood tests

A nonspecific reaction to myocardial injury is an elevation in white blood cell count (12,000 to 15,000/mm³). This increase begins a few hours after the onset of pain and lasts for 3 to 7 days. In general, high white blood cell counts are associated with larger infarcts. Also, the erythrocyte sedimentation rate (ESR) rises during the first week after the infarction and remains elevated for several weeks.

Serum enzymes. As infarcted cardiac muscle cells die, cellular components are released into the vascular system.

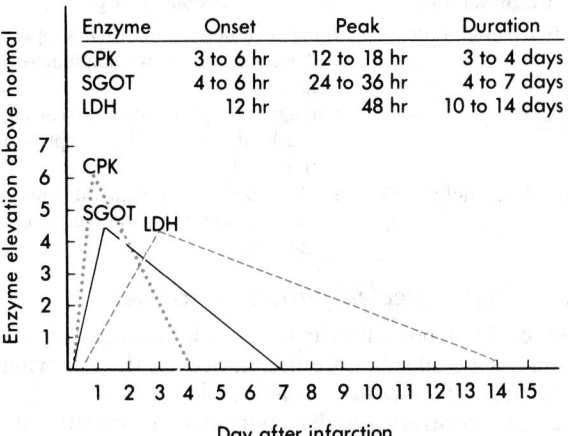

Enzyme	Onset	Peak	Duration
CPK	3 to 6 hr	12 to 18 hr	3 to 4 days
SGOT	4 to 6 hr	24 to 36 hr	4 to 7 days
LDH	12 hr	48 hr	10 to 14 days

Fig. 25-40   Patterns of serum enzyme levels following myocardial infarction.

Some of these components are enzymes that can be evaluated by blood levels. Creatine phosphokinase (CPK), serum glutamic-oxaloacetic transaminase (SGOT) (also termed serum aspartate amino-transferase [AST]) and lactic dehydrogenase (LDH) are found to be elevated at varying times following a myocardial infarction (Fig. 25-40).

Since these enzymes are not exclusively found in the heart, measurements of enzyme fractions or *isoenzymes* are more diagnostic of myocardial insult. Isoenzymes levels of CPK are the most reliable indicators of cardiac damage. The CPK isoenzyme that contains the MB subunits, CPK $(MB)_1$, is elevated for 48 hours after a transmural infarction. LDH can be fractionated into five distinct isoenzymes. Of these, LDH_1 and LDH_2 are most important. LDH_2 is found more abundantly in serum, whereas heart muscle is rich in LDH_1. An elevation in serum LDH_1, therefore, is confirmation of a myocardial infarction.

Electrocardiogram

Characteristic findings of infarction include ST segment elevation in leads overlying the infarcted area (an early finding) and the development of pathologic Q waves (a later finding). As the infarction "evolves," the ST segments return to baseline and the T waves become inverted. The electrocardiogram is considered to be one of the most reliable tools for diagnosing a myocardial infarction, but occasionally the "typical" changes do not develop, and serum enzymes must be relied upon to a greater extent.

Radiologic tests

An *x-ray film* of the chest may be taken to determine overall size and configuration of the heart as well as individual cardiac chamber size. Most abnormalities of heart size can be detected with a standard posteroanterior and lateral view of the chest. Calcifications in the large blood vessels, heart muscle, valves, and pericardium can also be visualized.

Cardiac fluoroscopy facilitates observation of the heart from varying views while the heart is in motion. Fluoroscopy can be used to detect ventricular aneurysms, which appear as a paradoxical bulging during systole.

The Elderly with Cardiovascular Problems

Assessment

Count the pulse for a full minute at rest and after exertion. The pulse is often slower and may be irregular because elderly are more prone to decreased cardiac output and dysrhythmias.

Monitor changes in blood pressure:

Systolic blood pressure in elderly may normally be as high as 160 mm Hg (as compared with 140 mm Hg in younger adults). A widened pulse pressure may also be observed.

Check blood pressure in a lying, sitting, and standing position to detect postural hypotension because vasomotor control is decreased in the elderly.

When assessing the heart, the apical impulse may be harder to locate. Murmurs are common from thickening and calcification of the valves.

Monitor for signs of mental confusion, lethargy, indigestion, and weakness in the elderly person; these may be early signs or cardiac disease. Angina is commonly noted with ischemic heart disease.

Assess elderly patient with myocardial infarction for signs of congestive heart failure, a common complication.

Intervention

Prevent falls in elderly that may be associated with bradycardia, postural hypotension, or myocardial infarction.

Teach the elderly to move and stand slowly to prevent falling because of hypotension (drop attacks).

Teach the patient who is taking diuretics or antihypertensives to move slowly and cautiously.

Teach the elderly to avoid standing for long periods (blood pooling), especially over a hot stove or in the shower (heat causes vasodilation thus lowering blood pressure).

Teach foot pumping exercises, which are performed before rising from bed or chair, to increase venous return.

Teach patient and significant others to seek early medical attention for unexplained illness, unrelieved indigestion, or sudden changes in behavior.

Common disorders in elderly

Congestive heart failure
Angina pectoris
Myocardial infarction
Dysrhythmias

Scintigraphic studies

Myocardial imaging. Myocardial imaging is a noninvasive procedure that aids in evaluating the myocardium and coronary arteries. The two most commonly used techniques are pyrophosphate scanning and thallium scanning. Even though these scans involve radioactive materials, they are safe for both patients and hospital personnel.

Pyrophosphate scanning. A radionuclide, technetium 99m pyrophosphate, is injected intravenously. The patient is scanned after 2 to 3 hours. This radionuclide is actively taken up by damaged myocardial tissue, producing a "hot spot" image. The scan takes 15 minutes to complete and is not painful. The scan will be negative during the first 12 hours after an infarction. Peak activity is evidenced at 36 hours.

Thallium scanning. Thallium 201 is an intracellular ion that is actively transported into normal cells. If the cell is ischemic or infarcted, the thallium will not be picked up, and a "cold spot" image is produced. This radioisotope is injected intravenously with the patient at rest or during stress testing.

MUGA scanning. Another way of imaging myocardial function is with a *dynamic* scan to assess cardiac wall motion and global left and right ventricular function. Multiple-gated acquisition cardiac blood pool imaging (MUGA scanning) can demonstrate cardiac wall motion, which permits assessment of injury as well as capacity of cardiac function.

A small amount of technetium 99m (attached to human serum albumin or to autologous RBCs) is injected intravenously. MUGA scanning reflects mild injury of the cardiac wall as hypokinesia versus a more severe disturbance producing akinesia or dyskinesia. It also reveals other important events, such as right ventricular infarction and aneurysm formation. In addition, it permits evaluation of the effects of pharmacotherapeutics (for example, nitroglycerin, vasodilators) on ventricular function.

Positron emission tomography. Positron emission tomography is a radionuclide-based imaging technique that uses short-lived radionuclides as tracers to report perfusion and metabolic events. These tracers are generally given by intravenous injection or inhalation and only occasionally by intraarterial injection. The trace elements readily pass through the tissues. Under normal circumstances, the well-perfused, aerobically metabolizing myocardium prefers free fatty acids for energy production from oxidative metabolism. When ischemia is present, more glucose and less fatty acid tends to be utilized.

Data analysis: nursing diagnoses

Nursing diagnoses are determined from analysis of patient data. Possible nursing diagnoses for the person with myocardial infarction may include, but are not limited to, the following:

Diagnostic title	Possible etiologies
Pain: chest	Persistent myocardial ischemia, hypoxia, immobility, overactivity, diagnostic tests, improper positioning
Tissue perfusion, altered: cardiovascular	Decreased cardiac output, pulmonary edema, CHF, angina, vasospasm or vasoconstriction
Cardiac output, decreased	Reduced stroke volume, cardiogenic shock, bradycardia, tachycardia
Constipation	Immobility in postinfarction period, opiate pain medication

Diagnostic title	Possible etiologies
Activity intolerance	Imbalance between oxygen supply and demand, immobility, angina, sedentary life-style
Anxiety	Change in health status, threat of death, threat to self-concept, situational crisis
Knowledge deficit	Lack of exposure/recall, information misinterpretation, ineffective coping patterns

Planning: expected patient outcomes

Expected outcomes for the person with myocardial infarction may include, but are not limited to, the following:
1. States feeling more comfortable.
2. Demonstrates cardiac tolerance to activity (stable pulse and blood pressure).
3. Identifies factors that increase cardiac workload.
4. States breathing is easier and fatigue is decreased.
5. Stools are soft and formed.
6. Identifies factors that reduce activity tolerance in a program of progressive activity.
7. Participates in a program of progressive activity.
8. Uses effective coping mechanisms in managing anxiety
9. Describes the following:
   a. Nature of MI and how the healing process relates to the treatment regimen
   b. Variables contributing to symptoms and interventions for disease or symptom control
   c. Risk factors that can be modified and plans to alter life-style
   d. Plans to participate in a regular exercise program
   e. Rationale for and type of surgery, if indicated
   f. Any dietary restrictions
   g. Plans for ongoing medical care

Implementation
Assisting with achievement of therapeutic goals

Medical interventions include promoting oxygenation of the tissues, relieving pain, preventing further tissue damage, promoting improved coronary circulation, and preventing complications. Analgesic drugs, such as morphine sulfate, can be administered for the relief of pain. Myocardial tissue oxygenation can be improved with supplemental oxygen. When relaxation occurs with pain relief and with improved tissue oxygenation, cardiac workload is reduced. Cardiac monitoring is used to detect the occurrence of dysrhythmias.

When complications are inevitable, the therapeutic aims are early detection and control. Healing of the myocardium is a natural process that is promoted by rest and reduction of myocardial oxygen demands. The trend toward early ambulation under carefully monitored conditions has reduced the incidence of complications, such as thromboembolic phenomena and psychologic manifestations of depression and hopelessness, which were largely related to a prolonged period of immobility.

In recent years, considerable attention has been directed toward therapies that limit the size of the infarcted area and prevent further tissue injury. One approach to this goal is reperfusion of the occluded coronary artery. To be effective, reperfusion must be attained within 3 to 5 hours following the onset of symptoms. Administration of fibrinolytic agents either systemically or directly into the coronary arteries activates mechanisms that lyse existing blood clots. Streptokinase, eminase, urokinase, and tissue plasminogen activator are currently used in reperfusion therapy. The use of laser angioplasty may also promote reperfusion and has the advantage of acting locally rather than initiating a more widespread fibrinolytic response.[45,49,52] Beta-adrenergic blocking agents reestablish the balance between myocardial oxygen supply and demand.

Nursing interventions include the following:

1. Administer medications as prescribed:
   a. Intravenous lidocaine is usually given prophylactically to prevent ventricular fibrillation
   b. Anticoagulants (heparin or coumadin) may be prescribed to decrease incidence of thrombophlebitis and pulmonary embolism
   c. *Avoid giving intramuscular injections* because these alter serum enzyme levels
2. Monitor for signs of complications of myocardial infarction (See relevant sections in this chapter for an expanded discussion of these conditions.):
   a. Congestive heart failure (crackles, tachycardia and tachypnea, dyspnea and increased respiratory effort, S_3 heart sound, weight gain, oliguria)
   b. Thromboembolic phenomena (pain in chest or legs)
   c. Pericarditis
   d. Mitral insufficiency
   e. Cardiogenic shock (decreased blood pressure, tachycardia, cold clammy skin, mental confusion, severe oliguria)
3. Maintain patient on prescribed low-cholesterol, low-salt diet without caffeine-containing beverages

Interventions to achieve patient outcomes

Promoting comfort

Perception of pain and discomfort by an individual is highly variable. After vascular access is established, morphine sulfate may be administered for relief of pain and apprehension and to produce vasodilation. Continued episodes of chest pain may be related to infarct size, insufficient collateral circulation, and increased myocardial consumption. Provisions for comfort and rest are essential to reduce sympathetic stimulation and subsequent myocardial oxygen demand.

Promoting tissue perfusion

Decreased tissue perfusion causes cellular hypoxia with subsequent ischemia, cellular swelling, and cellular death. Instruct the patient to avoid excessive fatigue and to stop activity immediately in the presence of chest pain, dyspnea, light-headedness, or faintness. Administer oxygen for 24 to 48 hours and longer if persistent pain, hypotension, dyspnea, or dysrhythmias occur.

Promoting adequate cardiac output

1. Monitor the patient for the following parameters:
   a. Dysrhythmias on ECG tracings
   b. Vital signs
   c. Effects of daily activities on cardiac status, as evidenced by occurrence of dysrhythmias and need for oxygen
   d. Signs of fluid overload and electrolyte imbalance
2. Document rate and rhythm of pulse.
3. Administer pharmacotherapy, as prescribed.
4. Plan nursing strategies to promote rest and minimize unnecessary disturbances.

Promoting elimination

Constipation is common from the effects of narcotics and decreased activity; a stool softener is usually prescribed. Avoid using bedpans and straining at stool because Valsalva's maneuver causes changes in blood pressure and heart rate, which may trigger ischemia, dysrhythmias, pulmonary embolus, or cardiac arrest.

Providing rest

The patient is usually placed on bed rest with commode privileges for 24 to 48 hours. Assist with activities of daily living during this period. Sedation with diazepam (Valium) or an equivalent may be prescribed to relieve anxiety and restlessness and to promote sleep.

Promoting activity

After the first 24 to 48 hours, patients are usually encouraged to increase their activity gradually, depending on the extent of the infarction. During this period, the person is continually monitored for signs of dysrhythmias, presence of cardiac pain, and changes in vital signs.

Promoting relief of anxiety and feeling of well-being

During hospitalization, many patients experience denial, depression, and anxiety. Depression may occur several days later and may continue after the patient is discharged. Generally, patients tend to become more anxious on the second day of hospitalization after the immediate threat of death from infarction has passed. Anxiety varies in intensity contingent on the severity of the threat as perceived by the individual, as well as the person's success in coping. Most persons who have a myocardial infarction, however, adjust extremely well. Over 85% of all patients with uncomplicated myocardial infarctions are able to return to work. This, along with resuming normal sexual functioning, aids tremendously in the adjustment process. Provide the patient and family with opportunities to explore their concerns and to explore alternative methods of coping, if appropriate.

Promoting patient/family learning

Education of the patient and family enables them to assume a more active role in the patient's health care. A great deal of anxiety and apprehension can be allayed by providing information about the cardiac condition and its management. Major points for teaching are outlined in Box 25-14.

The patients and their partners may need teaching and reassurance regarding resuming *sexual activities*. Many feel that their sex life is over after a myocardial infarction. Education should aim at supplying information and dispelling misinformation. Once patients with an uncompli-

25-14

Patient Teaching

The patient with a myocardial infarction

Effect of myocardial infarction, the healing process, and treatment regimen

Effect of medications in the treatment of myocardial infarction

Association between risk factors and coronary artery disease

Identify nonmodifiable risk factors

Identify modifiable risk factors (especially cigarette smoking)

Effect of dietary restrictions on CAHD: low salt, low cholesterol, no caffeine, fluid restrictions

Effect of activity on heart and need to participate in a progressive activity plan

Resumption of sexual activity (if appropriate)

Abstention of sexual intercourse as directed, usually for 4 to 6 weeks (sexual closeness, for example, cuddling, may be started earlier as desired)

Reporting to physician the following symptoms occurring during or following intercourse

Dyspnea or increased heart rate continuing for more than 15 minutes after intercourse

Extreme fatigue

Chest pain during intercourse

Palpitations for more than 15 minutes after intercourse

Insomnia after intercourse

---

cated myocardial infarction are capable of walking two flights of stairs without difficulty, they are generally able to perform sexual intercourse safely. Approximately 80% of all postcoronary patients will be able to resume sexual activity without serious risk. The other 20% need not totally abstain, but their sexual activity should be limited according to their cardiac capacity.

Evaluation

Evaluation will be based on the expected patient outcomes. Questions to consider include the following:

1. Was chest pain decreased?
2. Was need for additional oxygen decreased?
3. Are stools soft and formed?
4. Is activity tolerance increasing as evidenced by absence of fatigue, dyspnea, or discomfort with increasing activity?
5. Does the patient use effective coping mechanisms to manage anxiety?
6. Does the patient know the nature of the disorder, ways to decrease possibility of further ischemic attacks, activity prescription?
7. Has the patient made plans for follow-up medical care?

CARDIAC SURGERY FOR MYOCARDIAL ISCHEMIA

Surgical intervention is often necessary for patients with severe myocardial ischemia that is uncontrolled by medical

therapy. Recommendation for surgery is based on the assessment of the expected benefits of the procedure and the inherent surgical risks. Patients with cardiomegaly, severe congestive heart failure, recent myocardial infarction, high left ventricular end-diastolic pressure, and an inadequate ejection fraction are at higher risk.

Coronary Artery Bypass Graft

Surgical correction of myocardial ischemia is usually done through a bypass procedure in which a graft is sutured above and below the area of blockage in the coronary artery. Any number of bypasses can be performed, depending on the location and extent of the blockages. Blood flow to the ischemic areas of the heart is then conducted through the new grafts, thus "bypassing" the obstruction.

Bypass grafts are obtained from sections of the saphenous vein or the internal mammary artery. The saphenous vein is harvested from the inner thigh and sectioned. Removal of this vein does not compromise circulation in the leg, since there are numerous other vessels to assist in this function.

The heart is exposed through a median sternotomy or anterolateral thoracotomy; retractors are used to spread the chest wall. Saphenous vein sections are grafted from the aorta to the point beyond the blockage. The internal mammary artery remains attached proximally to the subclavian artery. The distal portion is grafted to the coronary artery beyond the occlusion (Fig. 25-41). Cardiopulmonary bypass is often used during cardiac surgery to allow the surgeon easier access to the operative site while maintaining perfusion of vital organs.

Cardiopulmonary bypass

Most heart surgeries require partial or total cardiopulmonary bypass. In *partial* bypass, pulmonary circulation is not interrupted. Oxygenated blood is drained from the left side of the heart, passed through a pulsatile pump, and returned through the descending aorta or common femoral artery (Fig. 25-42). *Total* cardiopulmonary bypass involves both circulation and oxygenation of the extracted blood. Cannulas are placed in the right atrium to drain venous blood. The machine oxygenates this blood and pumps it back into the ascending aorta or femoral artery.

Besides the capability of the heart-lung machine to provide extracorporeal circulation, it also serves as a direct route for medication administration and systemic hypothermia. Cooling of the machine solutions and subsequent body cooling lowers oxygen consumption by decreasing cellular metabolism.

Types of equipment

Many types of equipment are used during cardiac surgery. Some of these and their uses are described in the following list:

1. Endotracheal tube, ventilator: to maintain open airway, ventilation, and access to secretions
2. Cardiac monitor: to identify dysrhythmias
3. Intravenous line: to replace fluids, monitor central venous pressure, administer medications
4. Arterial line: to monitor blood pressure, obtain arterial blood samples

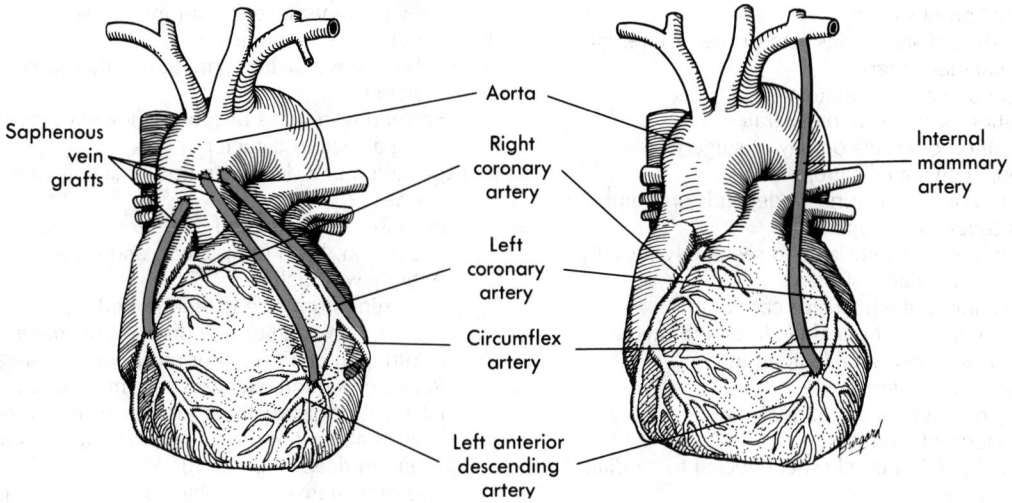

Aorta

Right coronary artery

Saphenous vein grafts

Left coronary artery

Circumflex artery

Left anterior descending artery

Internal mammary artery

Fig. 25-41   Coronary artery bypass grafts.

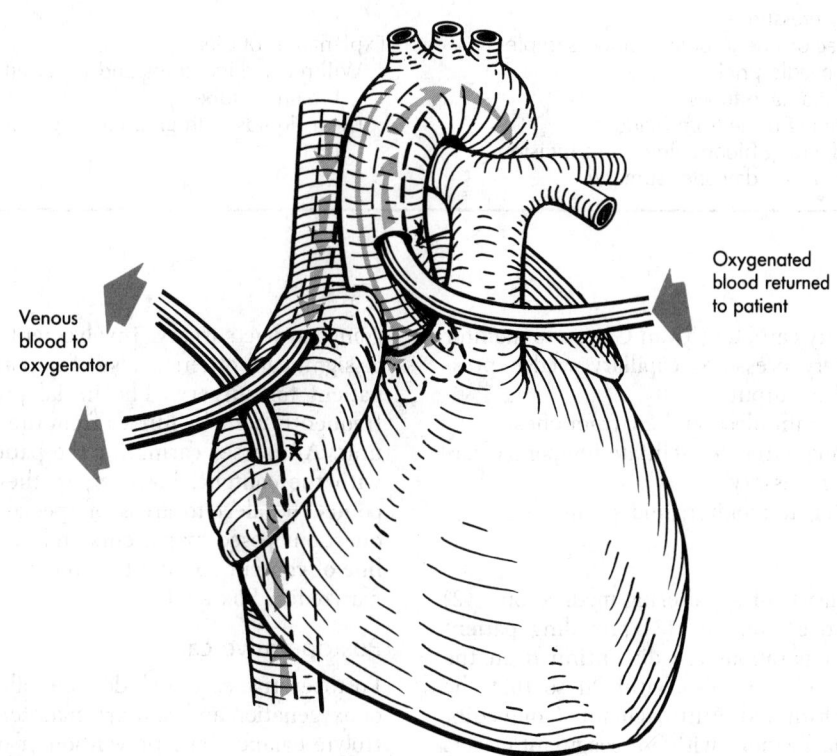

Venous blood to oxygenator

Oxygenated blood returned to patient

Fig. 25-42   Cardiopulmonary bypass.

The patient undergoing coronary artery bypass surgery

Simple explanation of anatomy of heart, function of coronary arteries, and effect of CAHD (use of heart drawings and models is helpful)
Explanation of surgery
  Removal of saphenous vein or use of internal mammary artery
  Effect on cardiac function
Definition of terms: *bypass, graft*
Explanation of events on day of surgery
  Preoperative medications
  Length of time in surgery (depends on number of arteries to be bypassed)
  Length of time until able to see family (usually 1½ to 2 hours after surgery)
Explanation of the intensive care unit
  Description of physical facilities and layout
  Nurse will be available at all times
  Visiting hours for family
  Length of stay in unit (2 to 3 days)
Explanation of monitors
  Round patches on chest connected to cardiac monitor
  Beeping sounds from monitors may be heard
Explanation of lines
  Intravenous routes for fluid and medications
  Central venous line in chest or groin to monitor fluid status
  Pulmonary artery line in chest or neck to measure pulmonary pressure
  Plastic connector line to obtain blood samples without a needle prick
Explanation of drainage tubes
  Catheter draining urine from bladder
  Chest tube draining bloody fluid from incision (usually removed day after surgery)

Explanation of breathing tube
  Tube in windpipe connected to machine called ventilator
  Tube prevents speech (can mouth words or write notes to communicate)
  Tube removed when patient is fully awake and stable
  Secretions in lungs or tube removed by nurse using a suction catheter
Explanation and demonstration of activity and exercises
  Purpose of activity and exercises is to promote circulation, keep lungs clear, and prevent infection
  Activity will include:
    Turning from side to side in bed
    Sitting on edge of bed on night of surgery
    Sitting in chair night or morning after surgery
  Range of motion exercises to arms and legs
  Effective deep breathing (use of sustained maximal inspiration, holding breath for 3 to 5 seconds at end of deep inspiration)
  Use of incentive spirometer (similar technique used to take deep breath)
Relief of pain
  Pain will be present at chest incision and leg incision
  Frequent pain medication will be given, but patient should always tell nurse when pain is present
Explanation of diet
  Will receive ice chips and water after removal of breathing tube
  Clear liquids with gradual progression to regular diet

---

5. Pulmonary artery catheter (Swan Ganz): to monitor pulmonary artery pressure, capillary wedge pressure, and cardiac output
6. Chest tube: to drain blood and air from chest
7. Epicardial pacing wires: to facilitate temporary cardiac pacing, if necessary
8. Urinary catheter: to monitor fluid status

Preoperative care

Preoperative care consists of (1) altering medications, (2) preparing the operative site, and (3) providing patient teaching. Digitalis preparations are discontinued on the day of surgery. Diuretics are also withheld so that the patient is adequately hydrated. Anticoagulants (coumadin, heparin) and other medications with anticoagulant effects (aspirin) are discontinued 48 hours before surgery.

In preparing the operative site, the patient showers with a special antimicrobial soap on the night before surgery. The chest and abdomen are shaved from neck to groin and from the left to the right midaxillary lines. If saphenous veins are needed for grafting, the inner aspects of the legs are also shaved.

Preoperative teaching is essential for a patient under-

going cardiac surgery. Involvement of the patient's family or significant others is also of importance in preparing the patient for surgery. The initial preoperative teaching is frequently done by nurses from the surgical intensive care unit. All nurses caring for the patient should be familiar with the content, however, so they may reinforce major points, be alert to areas of special concern, and answer questions posed by patients and family members. An outline of content specific to coronary bypass surgery is summarized in Box 25-15.

Postoperative care

Postoperative care includes the following goals: promotion of oxygenation and comfort, maintenance of fluid and electrolyte balance, and prevention or early detection of complications (thrombophlebitis, pulmonary embolus, cardiac tamponade, cardiac dysrhythmias, and cardiac failure).

Promoting oxygenation

1. Ventilate with supplemental oxygen
2. Turn from side to side
3. Keep head of bed elevated at least 10 to 20 degrees
4. Assess quality of breath sounds

5. Monitor arterial blood gases
6. Encourage performance of range of motion exercises
7. Encourage progressive activity level
8. Daily chest x-ray films will be obtained
9. Monitor patency and drainage from chest tube
10. Assist with deep breathing, coughing, and use of incentive spirometer

Maintaining fluid and electrolyte balance

Give crystalloid fluids intravenously to maintain adequate circulating blood volume. Administration of colloids (whole blood, packed cells, plasma, or plasma expanders) depends on the hemoglobin and total protein concentrations. Potassium is frequently required after heart surgery, and the patient is monitored for signs of hypokalemia. Nursing activities include the following:

1. Maintain prescribed flow rate of parenteral fluids
2. Maintain patency of chest tube and urinary catheter
3. Record amount of drainage accurately
4. Assess for signs of fluid loss (dry skin, dry mucous membranes, decreased skin turgor) and fluid overload (peripheral edema, neck vein distention, moist respirations)
5. Monitor central venous pressure (CVP) readings
6. Monitor daily weight
7. Assess serum electrolytes (especially potassium) and hematocrit
8. Monitor pulmonary artery parameters: pulmonary artery pressure, pulmonary capillary wedge pressure

Promoting comfort

1. Administer narcotic analgesics (morphine sulfate or meperidine) every 3 hours during first 24 hours, then as needed
2. Provide frequent mouth care until patient is taking fluids regularly
3. Eliminate unnecessary environmental stimuli (noise, lights) that impair ability to rest/sleep
4. Provide backrub for backache
5. Change linens if profuse nights sweats occur; assure patient that this commonly occurs
6. Group daily activities to allow for periods of uninterrupted rest/sleep
7. Encourage use of splinting devices (pillow, blanket) during coughing
8. Provide explanations for activities, as necessary
9. Monitor patient for changes in behavior and encourage patient to express concerns

Preventing/detecting complications

1. Thrombophlebitis/pulmonary embolism
   a. Encourage leg exercises until patient is ambulatory
   b. Encourage use of elastic stockings
   c. Encourage ambulation when permitted
2. Tamponade (compression of heart from accumulation of blood or fluid under pericardium)
   a. Monitor color and amount of chest tube drainage (change in color to bright red, sustained bleeding, or sudden cessation of drainage)

   b. Assess for increase in bleeding from midsternal incision
   c. Assess for other signs (restlessness, diaphoresis, hypotension, increased CVP, decreased urinary output)
3. Cardiac dysrhythmias
   a. Maintain continuous ECG monitoring
   b. Assess cardiac rhythm
   c. Monitor daily electrolyte values (especially potassium)
   d. Medicate with antiarrhythmic drugs as prescribed
   e. Assist in treatment of other underlying causes of dysrhythmias (decreased oxygenation)
4. Cardiac failure
   a. Monitor for signs of low cardiac output (hypotension, increased heart rate, restlessness, lethargy)
   b. Monitor CVP readings
   c. Monitor hourly urine output during initial period
   d. Monitor pulmonary artery
   e. Administer blood products and volume expanders as prescribed

Discharge planning

The usual hospital stay is 7 to 10 days after surgery, barring any complications. Before discharge, the patient and family need specific guidelines for physical activity level. Encourage activities at a slow progressive pace unless overexertion occurs. Daily walking and gradually increasing weekly distance are highly recommended. Caution patients to avoid heavy lifting (greater than 30 pounds) and activities that require repetitive arm movements, such as vacuuming and playing golf. Instruct patients not to drive a car or perform heavy labor until permitted by the physician.

Sexual intercourse can be resumed within the third or fourth postoperative week. Caution couples to avoid sexual positions in which the patient would be supporting weight. Patients should avoid large meals or the consumption of alcohol before sexual activity.

In summary, the following patient outcomes are expected:

1. Describe extent of permissible activity
   a. Describe plans for progressive return to physical activity as recommended by physician
   b. State awareness of when sexual activity may be resumed
   c. Describe criteria to use as a guide in determining if overexertion occurs (fatigue, dyspnea, pain)
   d. Describe plans to return to work if employed
2. Plan meals incorporating a balanced diet with any prescribed modifications
3. Describe any medication regimen
4. Describe plans for follow-up care
   a. Explain basis of any symptoms that may persist (dyspnea, pain, night sweats)
   b. Describe signs or symptoms requiring immediate medical attention (fever, increasing dyspnea, chest pain with minimal exertion)
   c. State plans for ongoing medical care

Percutaneous Transluminal Coronary Angioplasty

An alternative approach to coronary bypass surgery for selected patients with myocardial ischemia is percutaneous transluminal coronary angioplasty (PTCA). This procedure consists of dilating the coronary vessel wall by mechanical compression of the atheromatous plaque. PTCA is attractive because of a short recovery period, discharge within 3 days barring complications, and a shorter return-to-work time than with bypass surgery.[33]

Selection criteria for PTCA include persistent angina despite medical treatment and a lesion that is single, noncalcific, and located in a portion of a proximal vessel that does not involve a point of bifurcation. PTCA is not usually considered for lesions in the left main coronary artery. PTCA may also be used following thrombolytic therapy for myocardial infarction (see p. 671) and to dilate areas of stenosis in bypass grafts.

During PTCA, a pacemaker catheter is inserted as a precautionary measure through the femoral vein, and a specially designed catheter in the femoral artery. The catheter is advanced under fluoroscopy (similar to cardiac catheterization) to the site of the coronary obstruction. Once the catheter is in position, a balloon on the catheter is inflated to provide compression and rupture the atheromatous plaque. Heparin is infused during the procedure. Anticoagulation may be continued for several months after the procedure.

Following PTCA the patient may return to the general medical unit or may be admitted to an intensive care unit. In either case, nursing care includes immobilizing the legs for 6 to 12 hours, monitoring for bleeding at the catheter insertion sites, monitoring pedal pulses for indications of femoral artery thrombosis, and monitoring for chest pain that could be caused by an abrupt occlusion of the coronary vessel, restenosis of a dilated artery, coronary artery spasm, or pulmonary embolism. In the case of pulmonary embolus, the site of thrombus formation is usually the femoral vein puncture site. Chest pain requires an immediate ECG and the use of nitrates or calcium channel blockers as prescribed. ECG results may indicate the need for repeat PTCA or emergency coronary bypass surgery.

About 5% to 10% of patients who undergo PTCA have a major complication such as a myocardial infarction, the need for emergency coronary bypass surgery, or in-hospital death.[33] Minor complications include prolonged angina, bradycardia or transient ventricular dysrhythmias, and excessive blood loss. Over the long term, restenosis of the vessel is a significant complication and occurs in about 25% to 30% of patients, usually within the first 8 months following the procedure.

Intravascular Stenting

Restenosis persists as the single greatest limitation of PTCA. Stenosis recurs in 30% to 60% of patients, depending on the dilation location within the graft. A recent approach to solving the problem of restenosis has been to seek ways of "stenting," or maintaining the cylindrical lumen produced by the balloon. Two techniques are being investigated. The first is to produce a "biologic stent" during balloon dilatation through coagulation of collagen, elastin, and other tissues in the vessel wall by laser photocoagulation or radiofrequency-induced heat. The second method consists of prosthetic intravascular cylindrical stents capable of maintaining a cylindrical lumen after balloon deflation and withdrawal.

Laser Therapy for Cardiovascular Disease

Light is a form of electromagnetic energy that lasers use under controlled conditions. As laser light interacts with tissues, it is transmitted, scattered, reflected, or absorbed. A thermal reaction occurs when target tissue absorbs the laser light. This thermal reaction produces necrosis, hemostasis, coagulation, evaporation of tissue, cutting, or vaporization, depending on the time of application, power density, and focusing of spot size.

Nursing care after laser angioplasty is similar to postcatheterization care. Cardiac rehabilitation after laser therapy is important to heighten patients' awareness of the value of risk-factor reduction to prevent the advance of coronary artery disease.

CONGESTIVE HEART FAILURE

Heart failure (also known as cardiac insufficiency) is a state in which the heart is no longer able to pump an adequate supply of blood to meet the demands of the body. *Congestive heart failure* refers to a state of circulatory congestion resulting from heart failure and its compensatory mechanisms.[45] Heart failure may develop rapidly after a specific insult to the myocardium (such as an acute myocardial infarction) or may develop more gradually in response to a prolonged stress (such as hypertension). In the latter case, the person may initially seek medical attention with milder symptoms because the circulatory system has had more time to adjust to the heart's decreased performance and the resultant compensatory responses.

Etiology

The causes of heart failure can be categorized to correspond to the three determinants of stroke volume: myocardial contractility, preload, and afterload (see p. 638). Heart failure can also be the result of conditions that reduce ventricular filling. Examples of specific etiologies of heart failure are summarized in Box 25-16.

25-16

Causes of heart failure

Direct damage to the heart (reduction in contractile ability)
　Myocardial infarction, myocarditis, myocardial fibrosis, ventricular aneurysm
Ventricular overload
　Volume overload (increased preload): aortic regurgitation, ventricular septal defect
　Pressure overload (increased afterload): aortic or pulmonic stenosis, systemic hypertension, pulmonary hypertension
Restriction to ventricular diastolic filling
　Constrictive pericarditis or cardiomyopathy, rapid rate dysrhythmias, cardiac tamponade, mitral stenosis

From Spann JF, Hurst JW: *The recognition and management of heart failure.* In Hurst JW: *The heart, arteries and veins,* ed 6, New York, 1986, McGraw-Hill.

25-17	Compensatory responses to inadequate cardiac output	
	Response	**Initial effect**
	Stimulation of sympathetic nervous system	Increased rate and force of myocardial contraction
		Peripheral vasoconstriction—shunting of blood to vital organs, increased venous return, increased blood pressure
	Activation of renin-angiotensin system	Increased reabsorption of sodium and water—increased blood volume; peripheral vasoconstriction
	Ventricular hypertrophy	Increased myocardial contractility

Pathophysiology

Compensatory responses to inadequate cardiac output

Inadequate cardiac output triggers a number of compensatory responses that are geared toward maintaining adequate perfusion to vital body organs (see Box 25-17). The initial response is stimulation of the sympathetic nervous system, which has two main effects: (1) increased rate and force of myocardial contraction and (2) peripheral vasoconstriction. Peripheral vasoconstriction shunts arterial blood away from less vital organs such as the skin and kidneys and toward more vital organs such as the brain. Constriction of the veins increases venous return to the heart, which increases cardiac volume and dilates the ventricles. The increased stretch of myocardial muscle fibers enhances contractility.

Initially these responses may result in improvements in cardiac output, but, in the long run, afterload and myocardial oxygen demands are also increased, and stretch of myocardial fibers moves beyond a point where contraction is enhanced. Unless the person was in a state of fluid depletion to start with, the increased ventricular volume aggravates preload and compounds the failure.

A second type of compensatory response involves activation of the renin-angiotensin system (Chapter 33). A decrease in renal blood flow and, subsequently, of glomerular filtration rate triggers the release of renin, which interacts with angiotensinogen to form angiotensin I. Conversion of angiotensin I to angiotensin II results in further peripheral vasoconstriction and increased reabsorption of sodium and water by the kidneys. These events increase fluid volume and maintain blood pressure in the short term but increase both preload and afterload in the long term.

A third type of compensatory mechanism involves changes in the structure of the myocardium itself. Over time, the ventricular myocardium thickens or hypertophies to improve contraction, but this too results in increased myocardial oxygen demands.

Initially, one side of the heart fails. Since the left ventricle is most often affected by coronary atherosclerosis and hypertension, heart failure usually begins there. However, since both ventricles are part of the same system, the right ventricle often becomes impaired as well. The symptoms of heart failure are the result of decreased cardiac output and congestion that involves the venous system or the pulmonary system or both. The symptoms are summarized in Box 25-18. In general, the symptoms of heart failure are considered relative to the amount of associated physical exertion. A classification scheme developed by the New

25-18	Signs and symptoms of congestive heart failure

Signs and symptoms caused by decreased cardiac output to systemic tissues

Fatigue	Oliguria
Angina	Decreased GI motility
Anxiety	Skin cool, pale
S₃ heart sound	

Signs and symptoms caused by congestion backward from left ventricle

Dyspnea	Pulmonary rales (crackles)
Cough	
Orthopnea	X-ray evidence of pulmonary congestion

Signs and symptoms caused by congestion backward from right ventricle

Peripheral edema	Liver engorgement
Distended neck veins	Elevated central venous pressure

York Heart Association ranges from "asymptomatic with ordinary physical exertion" (Class I) to "symptomatic at rest" (Class IV).[45]

Left ventricular failure

Failure of the left ventricle to pump adequate amounts of oxygenated blood to meet the demands of the body results in two major consequences: (1) signs and symptoms of decreased cardiac output (see general symptoms of heart failure) and (2) pulmonary congestion (sometimes called backward failure). The reduced ejection fraction leads to increased end-diastolic volume (preload) and increased left ventricular end-diastolic pressure (LVEDP). This increased pressure is reflected backward into the pulmonary circulation, which is normally a low pressure, high capacitance circuit. Ultimately, increased pressure in the pulmonary circulation causes fluid to be forced into the alveoli and interstitial tissue. In severe cases, fluid may reach the bronchioles or the pleural space. The symptoms may range from mild dyspnea to those of frank pulmonary edema (p. 684) or pleural effusion.

Dyspnea

Dyspnea, or labored breathing, is an early symptom of left ventricular failure. It is caused by interference with gas exchange as a result of the fluid in the alveoli. It may occur or become worse only on physical exertion, such as climbing stairs, walking up an incline, or walking against the wind, since these activities require increased amounts of oxygen.

Orthopnea

Difficulty in breathing when lying flat may be present, and persons often must sleep propped up in bed or in a chair. When the person is lying flat, ventilation is decreased and the blood volume in the pulmonary vessels is increased. Orthopnea is often described by the number of pillows required for the patient to rest comfortably when in bed, for example, "three-pillow orthopnea."

Although orthopnea may occur immediately after lying down, it often does not occur for several hours. At that time, it causes the person to wake with severe dyspnea and coughing. This condition is known as *paroxysmal nocturnal dyspnea* and results from the accumulation of fluid in the lungs as the person is lying in bed. The patient usually has a feeling of suffocation and often awakens in panic.

Apnea and hyperpnea (Cheyne-Stokes)

The patient with heart failure may have alternating periods of apnea and hyperpnea called Cheyne-Stokes respirations. Pulmonary congestion results in decreased oxygenation of the blood, and altered cardiac function may cause an abnormally long circulation time between the lungs and respiratory control centers in the brain. Periods of hyperpnea cause carbon dioxide levels to fall to such an extent that the respiratory center is not stimulated. A period of apnea results that may last as long as 30 seconds. During this time the carbon dioxide levels build up again until respirations resume and another period of hyperpnea begins. This phenomena often begins as the patient goes to sleep and decreases as sleep deepens and ventilation decreases.

Cough

A persistent hacking cough is often a symptom of left-sided heart failure. It results from congestion of trapped fluid, which is irritating to the mucosal lining of the lungs and bronchi. The cough is usually productive of large quantities of frothy sputum, which is occasionally blood tinged. On auscultation *rales* (crackles) may be heard. Rales are the moist popping and crackling sounds heard most often at the end of inspiration.

Right ventricular failure

Right ventricular failure occurs when this chamber is unable to pump effectively against increased pressure in the pulmonary circulation. Most often the increased pressure is the result of blood backing up from a failing left ventricle, but right ventricular failure can also be a consequence of chronic pulmonary disease and pulmonary hypertension.

Inability of the right ventricle to pump blood forward into the lungs results in congestion that is reflected backward into the systemic circulation. Increased venous volume and pressure forces fluid out of the vasculature into interstitial tissue (*peripheral edema*). This edema is first likely to appear in dependent areas of the body such as the feet, ankles, and sacrum. It is usually nontender and may become pitting (easily depressed by the pressure of an examiner's thumb). As right ventricular failure worsens, edema progresses up the legs into the thighs, external genitalia, and lower trunk. Extremely engorged tissue causes the skin to crack, and fluid may "weep" from the tissues.

The *liver* may also become engorged with intravascular fluid, resulting in enlargement and tenderness in the right upper abdominal quadrant. As venous stasis increases, pressure within the portal system becomes so great that fluid is forced through the blood vessels into the abdominal cavity (ascites). The ascitic fluid can reach volumes of more than 10L, displacing the diaphragm and resulting in severe respiratory distress. A paracentesis (see Chapter 30) may be required to relieve the pressure on the diaphragm. *Distended neck veins* are a result of the increased systemic venous pressure and are usually observed when the patient is in a sitting position (see Fig. 9-3).

General symptoms of heart failure
Fatigue

Persons with heart failure commonly note fatigue following activities that ordinarily are not tiring. The fatigue results from impaired blood circulation to tissues as a result of the decreased CO. The reduction in tissue oxygen decreases the production of adenosine triphosphate (ATP), the immediate energy source for muscle contractions. In addition, the impaired circulation causes a decrease in the removal of metabolic waste products; the result of this is further decreased muscle function.

Anginal pain

Cardiac pain is *not* a typical symptom of heart failure; however, angina pectoris can occur from the decrease in CO. It is most likely to occur in patients with CAHD, which increases the patient's sensitivity to a deficiency in the oxygen content in the circulating blood. As heart failure develops, the blood is less effectively oxygenated and angina occurs. As the fluid overload state is corrected, the chest pain resolves.

Anxiety

Most persons are aware of the importance of an effectively functioning heart. Awareness that one has signs and symptoms of heart failure may therefore be anxiety producing, especially if the symptoms have occurred suddenly or are clearly getting worse. The frequent association of dyspnea with heart failure is another reason why anxiety is a common finding. Perceived difficulty with breathing can be a stressful experience, and anxiety may make the dyspnea worse. In extreme cases, anxiety may also increase oxygen demands on an already compromised heart.

Nursing Process
Assessment
Subjective data

Collect data concerning the occurrence of signs and symptoms that may indicate the presence of heart failure, the person's ability to cope with the physical limitations, knowledge of the condition and treatment regimen, and ability to adhere to the treatment regimen. Also elicit patient concerns and anxieties. Specific areas for assessment include the following:

1. Respiratory status—dyspnea, orthopnea (precipitating factors, severity, relieving factors)
2. Signs of fluid retention—recent weight gain, pedal edema (shoes too tight), skin feels tight
3. Ability to perform daily activities—fatigue, lack of endurance (precipitating factors, extent)
4. Comfort—anginal or abdominal pain
5. Knowledge of condition and treatment regimen
6. Ability to adhere to any prescribed treatment regimen; factors that make adherence difficult
7. Measures taken to compensate for physical limitations
8. Usual coping skills
9. Specific concerns related to condition

Objective data

1. Neck vein distention: presence, degree (Fig. 25-43)
2. Edema: site, degree of pitting
3. Abdominal distention
4. Daily weights: weigh on litter scale if severe heart failure present; weigh at same time of day (usually in morning after emptying bladder, before breakfast) and with same amount of clothing
5. Adventitious breath sounds
6. Gallop rhythm of heart on auscultation
7. Level of consciousness
8. Pulse changes and respiratory effort with activity

Diagnostic tests

Heart failure is typically diagnosed based on the clinical signs and symptoms and the presence of a precipitating cause. An electrocardiogram is usually done to determine the presence or absence of an acute myocardial infarction, to assess for dysrhythmias, and to identify compensatory responses such as ventricular hypertrophy. Chest x-ray films are done to assess pulmonary congestion and cardiac enlargement. Actual cardiac output may be determined by a variety of techniques, but this assessment is usually reserved for the more critically ill patient. A number of other tests have been devised to provide data about cardiac functioning and are discussed briefly below. They include echocardiograms, gated pool imaging, and pulmonary artery catheterization.

Echocardiogram

Information about the shape, size, and movement of the cardiac muscle and valves can be obtained through the use of ultrasonic sound waves directed to the heart. These waves are reflected by cardiac structures and can be visualized as an electronic wave form on an oscilloscope. The use of this noninvasive test to detect valvular abnormalities is discussed more fully on p. 695.

Gated pool imaging

Gated pool imaging involves the intravenous injection of technetium 99m. Three and 5 minutes after injecting the technetium, the patient is placed in a supine position, and computer outlines of the left side of the heart during all cardiac cycles are obtained. This procedure is used to evaluate left ventricular function and specifically to calculate the ejection fraction.

Pulmonary artery catheterization

The development of a balloon-tipped, flow-directed pulmonary artery catheter (commonly called a Swan-Ganz catheter in recognition of the physicians who developed it) has made possible significant advances in the diagnosis and treatment of cardiac failure. Specifically, its uses include the assessment of right and left ventricular function and evaluation of the effect of various cardiovascular drugs and other treatment modalities such as increasing or restricting intravenous fluids.

A flexible multilumen catheter (Fig. 25-44) is inserted into a major vein by means of a cutdown. The catheter is threaded through the superior vena cava, the right atrium, right ventricle, pulmonary artery, and into a small branch of this artery (pulmonary wedge position) (Fig. 25-45).

Representative waveforms are viewed on an oscilloscope and pressure readings can be obtained from various cardiac chambers (see normal pressures on p. 696). Pulmonary wedge pressure reflects left ventricular pressure and allows

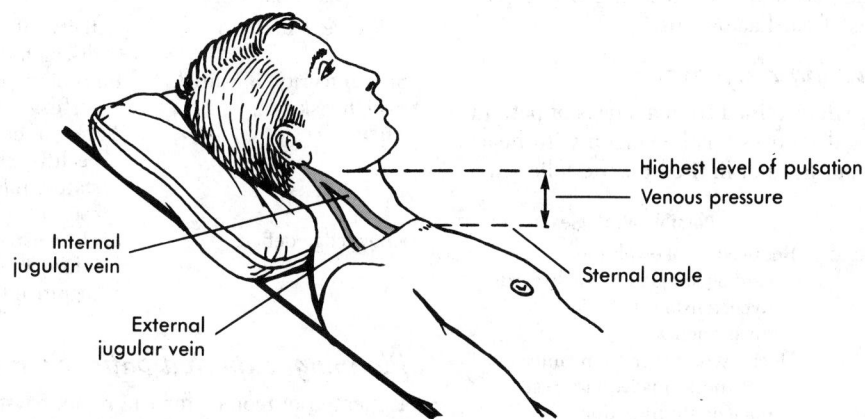

Fig. 25-43   Measurement of neck vein distention. Place person with head elevated at angle of 45 degrees. Measure highest level of neck vein pulsation above sternal angle.

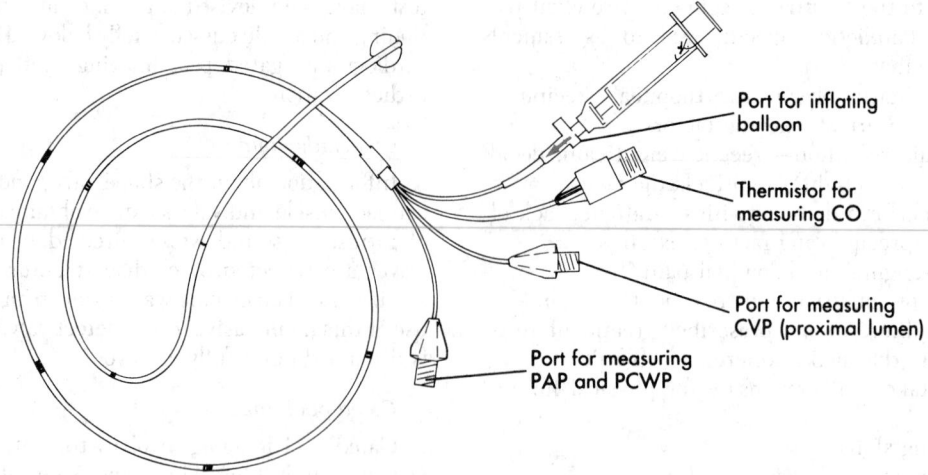

Fig. 25-44 Four-lumen thermodilution pulmonary artery catheter for measuring cardiac output *(CO)*, central venous pressure *(CVP)*, pulmonary artery pressure *(PAP)*, and pulmonary capillary wedge pressure *(PCWP)*.

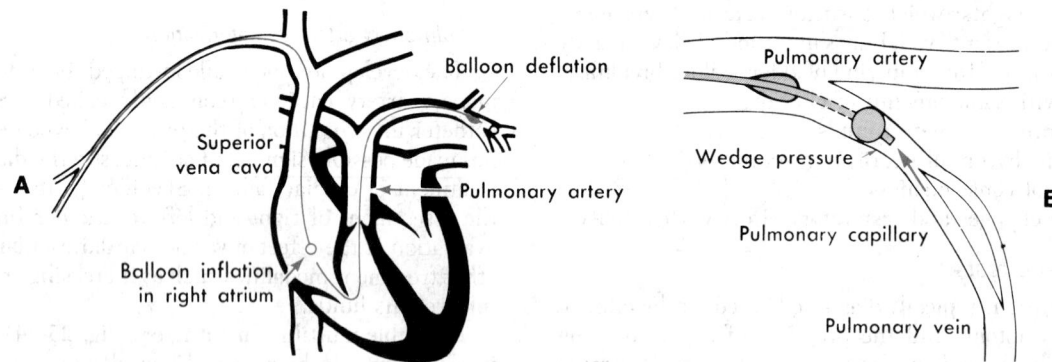

Fig. 25-45 **A,** Flow-directed pulmonary artery (PA) catheter showing inflation of balloon in right atrium and consequent "floating" of catheter through right ventricle and out to distal PA branch. Balloon is deflated, advanced slightly, and reinflated slightly to obtain PCW pressure. **B,** Initial placement of balloon in PA and again when advanced to take PCWP. (From Daily EK, Schroeder JS: *Techniques in bedside hemodynamic monitoring*, ed 4, St Louis, 1989, Mosby–Year Book.)

monitoring of preload. In addition, the thermistor port allows determinations of cardiac output.

Data analysis: nursing diagnoses

Nursing diagnoses are determined from analysis of patient data. Possible nursing diagnoses for the person with heart failure may include, but are not limited to, the following:

Diagnostic title	Possible etiologies
Cardiac output, decreased	Reduced stroke volume, cardiogenic shock, tachycardia, hypertension, valvular insufficiency
Fatigue	Decreased oxygenation, muscle weakness, inadequate rest, inadequate nutrition
Gas exchange, impaired	Ventilation/perfusion imbalance
Nutrition, altered: less than body requirements	Edema, dyspnea, fatigue, drug therapy

Diagnostic title	Possible etiologies
Self-care deficit	Activity intolerance/fatigue, pain/discomfort, anxiety
Skin integrity, impaired, high risk for	Immobility, decreased tissue perfusion to skin, edema
Anxiety	Threat of death; threat/change in health status, socioeconomic status, role; threat to self-concept
Knowledge deficit	Lack of exposure/recall, information misinterpretation, cognitive limitation

Planning: expected patient outcomes

Expected outcomes for the patient with heart failure may include, but are not limited to, the following:
1. Identifies factors that increase cardiac workload.
2. Performs ADL without undue fatigue.

3. Achieves normal respiratory rate without use of supplemental oxygen; states breathing is easier; confusion is decreased.
4. Demonstrates cardiac tolerance to increased activity (pulse and blood pressure are stable).
5. Eats prescribed diet.
6. Performs ADL within symptom limitations.
7. Skin remains intact.
8. Uses effective coping mechanisms in managing anxiety.
9. Describes the following:
   a. A modified plan for activity that avoids fatigue or dyspnea
   b. Plans for a diet in accordance with prescribed sodium or fluid restrictions
   c. Medication therapy, including adverse side effects
   d. Usage and precaution of supplemental oxygen therapy, if prescribed for home use
   e. Plans for follow-up health care

Implementation
Assisting with achievement of therapeutic goals

Treatment of congestive heart failure has the overall aim of restoring a supply of blood and oxygen that is equal to the demands of bodily tissues. Approaches to treatment therefore may focus on increasing oxygen supply, decreasing oxygen demand, or both (see Box 25-19). A second aim of treatment is reducing pulmonary and/or systemic congestion and the associated symptoms. Identification and treatment of the underlying etiology and factors that may have precipitated a particular episode of heart failure (that is, caused excessive demands on the heart) are important therapeutic goals.

At many acute care hospitals, patients with acute congestive heart failure are admitted to medical or cardiac intensive care units. Occasionally, the physician may elect to place the patient in the usual room accommodations, where the environment is less stressful and where family members can visit more routinely.

Medications

Digitalis therapy. Digitalis and its derivatives (cardiac glycosides) usually are effective in improving myocardial function in persons with congestive heart failure. The positive inotropic action of digitalis preparations enhances mechanical performance by strengthening the force of myocardial contractions. This leads to increased cardiac output and increased blood flow to the kidneys. Digitalis preparations also decrease heart rate (automaticity) and cardiac conduction velocity, which permits the ventricles to relax more and allow for better filling of the ventricles with blood.

When acute congestive heart failure occurs, the physician usually orders an *optimal therapeutic dose* of a digitalis preparation to slow the ventricular rate and decrease symptoms. This larger dose given over a short period of time, usually 24 to 48 hours, is called a *loading* or *digitalizing* dose. In some instances the dose may approach the toxic level, and the patient then requires careful observation for signs and symptoms of toxicity (see Box 25-20). After the

> **Medical therapy for congestive heart failure**
>
> Reduction of oxygen requirements
>   Treatment of precipitating causes
>   Rest
> Improvement of oxygen supply/reduction of congestion
>   Oxygen therapy
>   Positioning of patient to facilitate breathing
>   Increase myocardial contractility (positive inotropic drugs)
>   Reduce preload (sodium restriction, diuretics, venous dilating drugs)
>   Reduce afterload (arterial dilating drugs, mixed arterial/venous dilating drugs, ACE inhibitors)

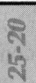

> **Signs and symptoms of digitalis toxicity**
>
> **Cardiovascular effects**
> Bradycardia
> Tachycardia
> Bigeminy (double beats)
> Ectopic beats
> Pulse deficit (difference between apical and radial pulse)
>
> **Gastrointestinal effects**
> Anorexia
> Nausea and vomiting
> Abdominal pain
> Diarrhea
>
> **Neurologic effects**
> Headache
> Double, blurred, or colored vision
> Drowsiness, confusion
> Restlessness, irritability
> Muscle weakness

optimal therapeutic dose has been determined, give the patient a daily maintenance dose of digitalis.

Numerous types of digitalis preparations may be used. Digoxin or digitoxin is most commonly used for maintenance drug therapy. Digoxin has a more rapid effect than digitoxin yet has sufficient duration for adequate maintenance therapy. If digoxin is given intramuscularly, inject it deeply and massage the area after injection because the drug is a tissue irritant.

Before giving a digitalis preparation, take the apical pulse rate. If this rate is below 60, withhold the medication until the physician has been consulted. Also evaluate the pulse for changes in rhythm. Always take the pulse rate of persons with irregular rhythm for a full minute for accuracy. Evaluate the response to digitalis on the basis of relief of symptoms, that is, decreased edema, loss of weight, fluid output greater than fluid intake, and no dyspnea or cyanosis.

Table 25-5 Diuretics used in treatment of heart failure

Type	Example	Side effects
Thiazide	Hydrochlorothiazide (Esidrix, Hydrodiuril) Chlorothiazide (Diuril)	Gastrointestinal upsets (can be minimized by taking medication with meals); hypokalemia; hyperglycemia
Loop	Furosemide (Lasix) Bumetanide (Bumex)	Similar to thiazide diuretics; also ototoxicity and blood dyscrasias
Potassium-sparing	Spironolactone (Aldactone) Triamterene (Dyrenium)	Gastrointestinal irritation; hyperkalemia

Diuretic therapy. Diuretic therapy is the most effective approach for symptomatic relief to patients with moderate to severe congestive heart failure.[55] The purpose of diuretic therapy is to decrease cardiac workload by reducing circulating volume and thus reduce preload.

Essential to proper initiation of diuretic therapy is determining how much fluid should be removed from the patient by establishing a "dry weight." This can be accomplished by gradually removing fluid with diuretics and assessing the patient's blood pressure. When the patient becomes hypotensive, particularly orthostatic, this signals the physician that too much fluid has been removed. The patient is then permitted to reaccumulate a small amount of fluid until hypotension no longer occurs. The weight at which this occurs is then considered the patient's dry weight.

Currently, thiazides (Table 25-5) are the diuretics of choice in the treatment of heart failure. The major complication is hypokalemia, which can be prevented by the intake of foods high in potassium or by potassium supplements. The most potent diuretics available are the loop diuretics (furosemide, bumetanide). These medications are reserved for severe congestive heart failure or when other forms of treatment are ineffective in relieving symptoms. These agents also increase renal blood flow and therefore may prove effective in treating heart failure when renal function is also impaired.

Other drugs. Vasodilators may be used to decrease afterload by decreasing resistance to ventricular emptying. Commonly used agents include nitroprusside (Nipride), hydralazine (Apresoline), and prozosin (Minipres). Nifedipine, a calcium channel blocker, also has vasodilator effects. Captopril (Capoten), an ACE inhibitor with hypotensive properties, is also a vasodilator and blocks sodium retention by suppressing aldosterone. Vasodilators are more effective in the treatment of acute rather than chronic heart failure.

Sodium-restricted diet

Edema is often effectively controlled in patients with heart failure by restricting sodium intake. The degree of restriction depends on the severity of the failure and the extent of diuretic therapy. The severely restricted sodium diet is rarely prescribed because this diet is unpalatable and expensive, which results in poor patient compliance.

The amount of sodium in the normal diet is 3 to 10 g/day. Sodium restriction in persons receiving diuretics may not be dropped below 3 to 5 g/day because of the dangers of hyponatremia. In mild cardiac failure, sodium may be restricted to 1 to 2 g/day; this is known as a no-added-salt (NAS) diet. It is essentially a normal diet, except that no extra salt is added to prepared foods and, obviously, salted foods such as potato chips are omitted. For moderate or severe heart failure, the amount of sodium permitted is specifically prescribed.

Low-sodium diets can be made more appealing by adding salt substitutes to food in place of table salt. Since many salt substitutes contain potassium, the patient's need for potassium must be assessed. Often the increased potassium is beneficial when the patient is on diuretic therapy. The use of herbs often makes the food more appetizing.

Fluid restriction is less commonly instituted than in the past as long as the person is on a sodium-controlled diet and is receiving diuretics or digitalis. If fluids are restricted, the amount of fluid permitted is prescribed by the physician and a plan is made, in conjunction with the patient if possible, to space the fluids over the day.

Interventions to achieve patient outcomes

Guidelines for nursing interventions for the person with congestive heart failure are summarized in Box 25-21.

Promoting rest and activity

Reducing the requirement for oxygen can best be effected by providing the patient with the degree of activity that does not compromise myocardial function, as demonstrated by the presence of symptoms. For mild heart failure, the patient may be treated on an ambulatory basis with only a regimen of less strenuous activity and more rest than usual.

For severe heart failure, a program of bed rest or limited activity may be necessary until symptoms abate. Permissible activity will be based on symptoms such as dyspnea and fatigue. A careful assessment must be made each day to determine the amount of rest required. If the patient has difficulty relaxing because of apprehension or anxiety, a tranquilizer may be prescribed.

Ambulation is started slowly to avoid overloading the heart. The regimen varies with individual patient response. When a patient has been on restricted bed rest, activities progress slowly from dangling, to sitting, to walking increased distances under close supervision. If signs of dyspnea, fatigue, or increased pulse rate that does not stabilize readily occur, the patient returns to bed. Oxygen is given for dyspnea, and the physician is notified.

The plan for increased activity is explained to the patient and family. They should understand that if activity tires the person excessively, it may be curtailed. Overactivity can produce physical and mental setbacks that delay ultimate recovery.

Rest to the heart is also promoted by preventing constipation, since straining at defecation places an extra burden on the heart. During straining against a closed glottis (Valsalva maneuver), venous return to the heart is decreased as a result of increased intrathoracic pressure. When this pressure is released after straining, a large amount of venous return creates an increased work load on the heart. The feces can be kept soft by stool softeners or bulk-forming laxatives. If an enema is necessary, it should be of low volume.

Providing oxygenation

In heart failure, the oxygen content of the bloodstream may be markedly reduced because of the less effective oxygenation of the blood as it passes through the congested lungs. The patient may be more comfortable and better able to rest when receiving oxygen, since it helps in reducing dyspnea and fatigue. Oxygen is usually administered by nasal cannula at 2 to 6 L/min. Obtain baseline arterial blood gases when oxygen therapy begins and intermittently during therapy to assess effectiveness of the treatment.

Breathing is often made easier by maintaining the patient in semi-Fowler's or high Fowler's position. These positions maximize oxygenation by permitting greater lung expansion. The patient is often orthopneic and tends to breathe more easily sitting than lying in bed. If the patient is sitting in a chair, elevate the feet to reduce pooling of fluid in the dependent limbs. When the patient is in high Fowler's position in bed, place a pillow lengthwise behind the shoulders and back so that full expansion of the rib cage is possible. The arms may be supported on pillows to reduce the pull on the shoulder muscles. An over-the-bed table may be placed close to the patient to allow resting of the head and arms.

Promoting nutrition

During the acute stage of congestive heart failure, the diet should be bland, low-calorie, low-residue with vitamin supplement (in addition to any sodium restrictions [p. 682]). Anorexia is often present because of edema in the gastrointestinal tract, dyspnea, fatigue, and the effect of medications. Frequent small feedings minimize exertion and reduce gastrointestinal blood requirements, which can tax the failing heart. Care must be taken to provide a diet that meets the metabolic demands of the body so that body wasting does not occur.

Although careful records of intake and output are kept on most patients with cardiac failure, the best method to estimate progress and response to prescribed diet, medications, and other forms of treatment is *daily monitoring of the patient's weight*. Weight gain indicates fluid retention. Carefully record the weight on admission and then daily while the patient is hospitalized. Weight loss in the patient stabilized at dry weight indicates inadequate nutrient intake.

Guidelines for Care 25-21

The patient with congestive heart failure

Provide oxygenation
  Administer oxygen by nasal cannula at 2-6 L/min as prescribed
  Give oxygen as needed for dyspnea
  Patient should be well supported in semi-Fowler's or high Fowler's position
Provide rest and activity
  Reinforce importance of conservation of energy and planning for activities that avoid fatigue
  Encourage activity within prescribed restrictions; monitor for intolerance to activity (dyspnea, fatigue, increased pulse rate that does not stabilize)
  Assist with ADL as necessary; encourage independence within patient's limitations
  Provide diversional activity that will assist in conservation of energy
Monitor for signs of fluid and potassium imbalance; record daily weights
Provide skin care, particularly over edematous areas; use prophylactic measures to prevent skin breakdown
Assist in maintaining an adequate nutritional intake while observing prescribed dietary modifications (sodium restrictions)
Monitor for constipation; give prescribed stool softeners
Give prescribed medications
  Digitalis (take apical pulse before administration)
  Diuretics (assess for hypokalemia)
  Vasodilators
  Drugs to reduce anxiety and promote sleep
Provide patient/family opportunities to discuss their concerns
Teach patient about the disorder and self-care (see Box 25-22)

Facilitating self-care and skin integrity

Careful daily assessments determine the extent to which the person can perform ADL such as eating and bathing. Most patients prefer to maximize their independence, and this is encouraged within the limitations of their symptoms.

Edematous skin is poorly nourished and very susceptible to breakdown. Edema of the sacrum is prevalent in patients with heart failure who are restricted to bed rest, and decubiti can develop quickly. Institute measures to prevent skin breakdown early.

Facilitating coping with anxiety

Because anxiety increases the symptoms of heart failure, take measures to help the person decrease anxiety. These measures include the following:

1. Identifying the feelings and the content related to these feelings
2. Identifying strengths that can be used for coping
3. Learning what can be done to decrease the anxiety, (for example, learning about measures to control heart failure and measures to reduce stress; see Chapter 7)

Working with family members in the same manner is also helpful to decrease their anxiety so they can be of greater support to the patient.

Facilitating patient/family learning

Patients who will be receiving oxygen therapy at home need to know how to manage the therapy. Instructions include the following:

1. Indication for initiating oxygen therapy
2. Method of initiating oxygen therapy
3. Precautions necessary when oxygen therapy is being used

Start teaching patients their dietary restrictions early during hospitalization to permit time for learning and asking questions. The patient may need frequent interactions with the dietitian and nurse before being able to follow a prescribed diet. Additional teaching includes the signs and symptoms that indicate recurring congestion, avoidance of fatigue and need for rest periods at home, and the medication regimen (see Box 25-22).

Evaluation

Evaluation will be based on the expected patient outcomes. Questions to ask may include the following:

1. Is the patient breathing more easily?
2. Is the patient more comfortable?
3. Is the patient less fatigued?
4. Does the patient know how to plan activities to prevent fatigue and dyspnea?
5. Is peripheral edema decreased?
6. Is the patient using effective coping mechanisms to manage anxiety?
7. Can the patient describe components of the treatment regimen?
8. Can the patient explain the rationale for the treatment regimen?
9. Can the patient state plans for follow-up care?

Pulmonary Edema

Acute pulmonary edema is the rapid effusion of serous fluid from plasma into the pulmonary interstitial tissue and alveoli. It is a medical emergency that requires immediate care. The causes of pulmonary edema include the following:

1. Severe left ventricular failure
2. Inhalation of irritating gases
3. Rapid administration of intravenous fluids (whole blood, plasma, crystalloid fluids)
4. Barbiturate or opiate overdose

Pathophysiology

In pulmonary edema caused by heart failure, cardiac output decreases, resulting in increased left atrial pressure. This increases pulmonary vein and capillary pressure. As the pulmonary capillary pressure exceeds the intravascular osmotic pressure, serous fluid is rapidly forced into the alveoli. Fluid rapidly reaches the bronchioles and bronchi, and patients literally begin to drown in their own secretions. As oxygenation decreases, the person shows signs of respiratory distress (see Box 25-23). The sputum is frothy

---

Patient Teaching

25-22

The patient with congestive heart failure

Monitor for signs and symptoms of recurring congestive heart failure and report these signs and symptoms to the physician or clinic:
Weight gain of 1-1.5 kg (2-3 lb) over a short period of time (about 2 days).
Loss of appetite.
Shortness of breath.
Orthopnea.
Swelling of ankles, feet, or abdomen.
Persistent cough.
Frequent nighttime urination.
Avoid fatigue and plan activity to allow for rest periods.
Plan and eat meals within prescribed sodium restrictions.
Avoid salty foods.
Avoid drugs with high sodium content (for example, some laxatives and antacids, Alka-Seltzer)—read the labels.
Eat several small meals rather than three large meals per day.
Take prescribed medications.
If several medications are prescribed, develop a method to facilitate accurate administration.
Digitalis: check own pulse rate daily; report a rate of less than 60/min to physician.
Diuretics
Weigh self daily at same time of day.
Report weight gain to physician.
Eat foods high in potassium and low in sodium (such as oranges, bananas).
Vasodilators
Report signs of hypotension (light-headedness, rapid pulse, syncope) to physician.
Avoid alcohol when taking vasodilators.
Report to physician for follow-up as directed.

25-23

Signs and symptoms of pulmonary edema

Restlessness
Vague uneasiness
Dyspnea
Tachycardia
Pallor or cyanosis
Cough productive of large quantities of blood-tinged frothy sputum
Audible wheezing

---

from air mixing with the fluid in the alveoli and blood-tinged from blood cells that have exuded into the alveoli.[44]

Medical therapy

Treatment for acute pulmonary edema involves a number of simultaneous interventions to promote oxygenation, improve cardiac output, and reduce pulmonary congestion.[59] Whenever possible, identify the underlying cause. The

Nursing Care Plan — Person with congestive heart failure

DATA: Mr. G. is a 59-year-old factory worker with a long history of hypertension. He has taken his antihypertensive medications only sporadically and frequently fails to keep follow-up appointments at the hypertension clinic. His blood pressure has never been under good control, and readings have typically been 160-190/96-100. Mr. G. has felt fatigued for several weeks and has noticed increasing difficulty with breathing, particularly when moving heavy equipment at work. At times he awakens during the night and feels like he is suffocating. He came to the clinic to get something to help him sleep better and was admitted to the hospital for evaluation. Tests revealed that he has hypertensive cardiovascular disease and congestive heart failure. Following loading doses of digoxin, he is being maintained on 0.25 mg PO qd. He is also on a low-sodium diet and hydrochlorothiazide 50 mg PO bid. His activity has been restricted to "up in room as tolerated."

The nursing history identified the following:
1. He and his wife have little understanding of the low-sodium diet that was prescribed years ago. He remembers the diet instructions as "not adding too much salt at the table." He frequently eats sandwiches of luncheon meat and cheese at work or has canned soup from the vending machine.
2. The episodes of nocturnal dyspnea have been very frightening to both Mr. G. and his wife. They have tried various preventive measures such as more fresh air, but nothing seems to work. Mrs. G. states that she is almost afraid to go to bed anymore.
3. He sees little need to take "medicine" if he doesn't feel sick. Now the doctor has prescribed more medicine for his heart when the trouble is his breathing.
4. He is reluctant to tell his boss about the dyspnea he encounters at work because he doesn't want to be labeled a "cry baby"—"It's better to just tough things out."

Collaborative nursing activites include those to assess (1) Mr. G.'s response to the therapeutic regimen and (2) the presence of any complications associated with the regimen. Nursing actions include monitoring the following:
1. Response to exertion—especially heart rate and respiratory effort
2. Breath sounds—location and extent of adventitious sounds such as rales (crackles)
3. Daily weights and intake/output
4. Blood pressure
4. Heart rate and rhythm; abnormal cardiac sounds such as an S_3 gallop
6. Serum electrolytes—especially potassium

Nursing diagnosis: Cardiac output, decreased, related to reduced stroke volume, resulting in a compromised state.

Expected patient outcomes	Nursing interventions	Rationale
Mr. G.'s pulse and respirations are within normal limits.	Organize care to provide scheduled periods for rest and to minimize unnecessary disturbances.	Exercise and physical activity increase cardiac output, heart rate, and blood pressure
Mr. G. identifies factors that increase cardiac workload.	Explain and encourage increases in activity and ambulation to prevent a sudden increase in cardiac workload.	Regular exercise makes the heart more efficient, so stroke volume increases and is not appreciably altered.
	Monitor respirations q4h for increased effort, pulse for tachycardia.	
	Monitor heart sounds q4h for presence of gallop rhythm.	
	Teach Mr. G. to avoid Valsalva's maneuver.	Surge of blood to heart after intrathoracic pressure decreases causes increase in cardiac workload.

Continued.

Nursing Care Plan

Person with congestive heart failure—cont'd

Nursing diagnosis: Tissue perfusion, altered, related to decreased blood flow to tissues and edema

Expected patient outcomes	Nursing interventions	Rationale
Mr. G. demonstrates improved circulation (decreased neck vein distention, decreased peripheral edema, decreased weight).	Assess neck vein distention, edema of extremities, and coolness of skin q4h; weigh daily.	Provides information on fluid retention from decreased circulation.
	Encourage movement and activity as tolerated.	Movement promotes circulation to tissues.
Skin breakdown does not occur.	Eliminate or reduce pressure points by changing position frequently, use of pressure mattress, etc. Give diuretics and sodium-restricted diet as prescribed.	Edema interferes with diffusion of O_2 to cells. Cellular nutrition depends on adequate blood flow.

Nursing diagnosis: Activity intolerance related to imbalance between oxygen supply and demand

Expected patient outcomes	Nursing interventions	Rationale
Mr. G. complains of less dyspnea on exertion.	Plan activities to conserve energy; allow for rest periods; provide assistance with aspects of physical care that are tiring; discuss ways to conserve energy at home and at work.	Pacing of activities will lessen myocardial oxygen demand. Any factor that compromises cardiovascular function reduces tolerance to activity

Nursing diagnosis: Anxiety (Mr. G. and his wife) related to perceived change in health status (onset of frightening symptoms) and uncertainty regarding cause or measures to control

Expected patient outcomes	Nursing interventions	Rationale
Mr. G. and wife express less anxiety about paroxysmal nocturnal dyspnea (PND) episodes.	Explain basis for symptoms and expectations of therapeutic regimen; suggest sleeping with head of bed slightly elevated.	Providing structure in a situation of uncertainty allows persons to gain control and feel less anxious.

Nursing diagnosis: Knowledge deficit (low-sodium diet, pathophysiology of heart failure, rationale for therapeutic regimen) related to lack of recall and lack of exposure

Expected patient outcomes	Nursing interventions	Rationale
Mr. G. and wife can describe CHF and explain the basis for symptoms.	Teach about the heart as a pump and effect of hypertension; select an appropriate analogy from Mr. G.'s home or work life regarding pumps and pressure.	Learning is easier when content can be related to something familiar.
Mr. G. can explain rationale for low-sodium diet, diuretic, digoxin.	Teach relationship between sodium, fluid retention, and hypertension; explain effect of digoxin on heart.	Understanding of the rationale for therapeutic regimen may improve compliance.
Mr. G. and/or wife can describe basic elements of a low-sodium diet.	Provide and discuss information on foods to avoid and foods that may be eaten liberally on this diet.	Providing information on activities that are allowed, as well as those that must be avoided, gives persons resources for coping with restrictions.

Nursing diagnosis: Noncompliance (previously) with therapeutic regimen possibly related to absence of physical symptoms or inability to cope with taking on any aspect of the "sick role"

Expected patient outcomes	Nursing interventions	Rationale
Mr. G. adheres to therapeutic regimen.	Explore previous noncompliance to determine reasons from Mr. G.'s perspective; identify difficulties foreseen with new regimen; help Mr. G. explore acceptable alternatives.	Data are insufficient to guide specific plan; Mr. G.'s perceptions of difficulties with therapeutic regimen provide avenues for intervention by nurse.

25-24

Medical therapy for acute pulmonary edema

Intervention	Rationale
Patient in high Fowler's position or over side of bed with arms supported on bedside table	Promotes expansion of lungs; legs in dependent position causes venous pooling and reduction in venous return (preload)
Morphine sulfate, 4 to 8 mg, intravenously	Decreases anxiety; slows respirations; reduces venous return
Oxygen at 40% to 70% by face mask; intubation as needed	Promotes oxygenation; increased tidal volume also promotes removal of secretions from alveoli
Rapid digitalization if patient not previously taking digitalis	Improves contractility; increases CO and reduces heart rate; converts rapid rate dysrhythmias such as atrial fibrillation
Aminophylline, 250 mg, given intravenously over approximately 30 min	Relieves bronchospasm and wheezing; acts as diuretic

Causes of cardiogenic shock

Myocardial infarction
Critical aortic stenosis
Intractable dysrhythmias
Ruptured aortic aneurysm
Severe congestive heart failure
Massive pulmonary embolism
Cardiac tamponade

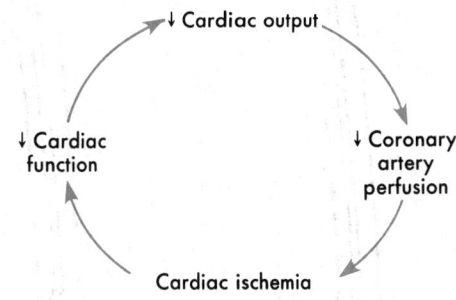

Fig. 25-46   Sequence of events in cardiogenic shock.

components of treatment are similar to those discussed for congestive heart failure but are applied more vigorously. Common interventions include patient positioning, morphine sulfate IV, oxygen, rapid digitalization, and aminophylline IV (see Box 25-24). Other measures to reduce circulating blood volume may include administering diuretics such as furosemide and ethacrynic acid, rotating tourniquets on three extremities, and performing a phlebotomy.

Cardiogenic Shock

Cardiogenic shock is a shock state of primary cardiac origin. It is most frequently caused by myocardial infarction but also may result from other cardiac disorders that lead to low cardiac output (see Box 25-25).

Pathophysiology

Cardiogenic shock occurs when cardiac function is severely impaired and cardiac output is low. As the shock progresses, coronary artery perfusion decreases, leading to cardiac muscle ischemia that leads to further decreased function (Fig. 25-46). The mortality rate is high. (See Chapter 9 for further discussion on shock.)

Medical therapy

Cardiogenic shock is a medical emergency that requires immediate intervention and constant attention to prevent irreversible cell damage and death. Therapy is aimed at correcting factors that contribute to decreased tissue perfu-

sion, such as cardiac dysrhythmias, hypoxemia, and pain.

Invasive monitoring lines that are usually placed include catheters in the pulmonary artery, systemic artery, and urinary bladder. The left ventricular end-diastolic pressure (LVEDP) is reflected in the pulmonary capillary wedge pressure, which is used as a guide to fluid therapy.

The following therapy may be initiated:

1. Vasopressors and cardiotonic agents (for example, dopamine, norepinephrine) to raise systemic arterial pressure without increasing cardiac work load; vasopressors are titrated to maintain systolic pressure, preferably above 90 mm Hg.
2. Hyperventilation and buffering agents (for example, sodium bicarbonate) to counteract lactic acidosis
3. Intravenous fluids if hypovolemia is present: care must be taken to prevent fluid overload with resulting pulmonary edema
4. Use of intraaortic balloon counterpulsation, if necessary (see discussion below)

General care of the patient in shock is described in Chapter 9.

Intraaortic balloon counterpulsation

A counterpulsation device facilitates blood circulation by decreasing aortic pressure during systole and increasing it during diastole. The overall effects include the following:

1. Increase in coronary artery perfusion
2. Decrease in preload (degree to which the myocardium is stretched before contracting)

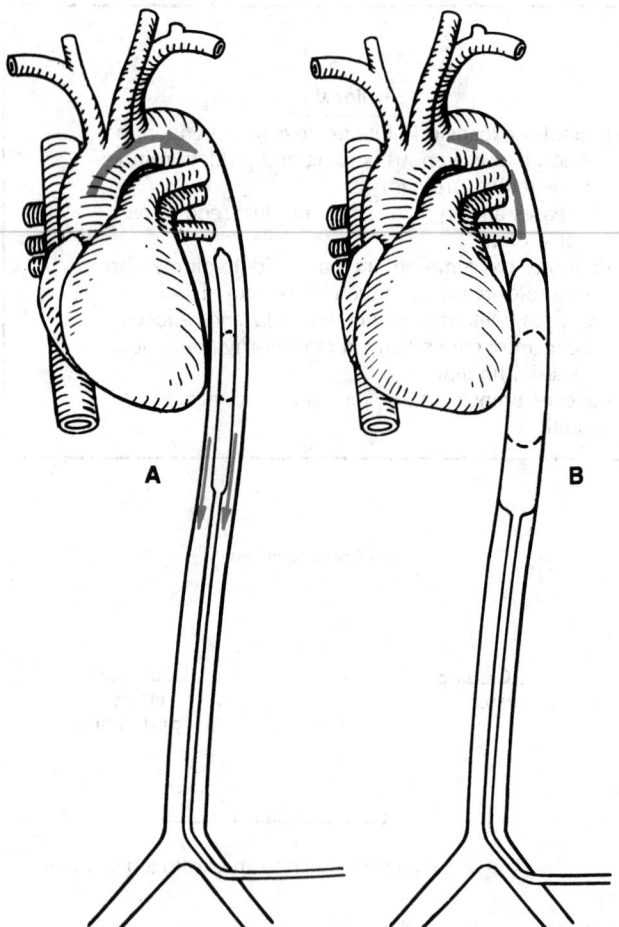

Fig. 25-47 Representation of intraaortic balloon positioned just distal to left subclavian artery. **A,** Balloon is deflated allowing forward blood flow during systole. **B,** Balloon is inflated to increase coronary perfusion during diastole.

3. Decrease in afterload (resistance against which blood is expelled).

In addition to being used in the situations producing cardiogenic shock, the intraaortic balloon pump may be used in unstable patients with cardiac disease before and during open heart surgery and in assistance when removing these patients from cardiopulmonary bypass following surgery.

Technique

The intraaortic balloon is inserted percutaneously or by cutdown into the right or left femoral artery. It is advanced into the thoracic aorta and sutured into place at the insertion site after the balloon tip has been correctly positioned just distal to the left subclavian artery (Fig. 25-47). The end of the balloon catheter is attached to a pump console, which alternately inflates and deflates the balloon using helium or carbon dioxide gas.

The timing of the inflation-deflation sequence is of the utmost importance in obtaining maximal counterpulsation effect. Using the ECG to trigger the pumping mechanism

and the arterial waveform to determine the effectiveness of the counterpulsation, the balloon is timed to inflate just at the beginning of ventricular diastole, immediately after closure of the aortic valve and thus enhances coronary artery filling. The balloon remains inflated during diastole and is then timed to deflate immediately before the next ventricular systolic ejection or just before the aortic valve reopens, thereby reducing afterload and secondarily decreasing preload. Improper timing of the balloon not only defeats the purpose of counterpulsation, but also could directly damage the myocardium. This is particularly true in early inflation or late deflation, in which the heart would be ejecting blood against a partially inflated balloon.

Nursing management

1. Monitor vital signs and indices of cardiac function at frequent intervals as specified
2. Position patient:
   a. Head of bed elevated no more than 30 degrees to prevent balloon migration upward in aorta
   b. Reposition patient every 2 hours on alternate sides to prevent skin breakdown and other consequences of immobility
   c. Avoid hip flexion on catheterized side; restrain leg if necessary.
3. Monitor circulation of both legs before catheter insertion and hourly thereafter until balloon is removed
4. Keep dressing on balloon insertion site clean and dry; change every 24 to 48 hours using sterile technique
5. Administer prescribed heparin or low-molecular-weight dextran to prevent blood clotting or emboli

Considerable psychologic support is necessary for the patient and family during such critical therapy. Not only is the physical size and noise of the pump console very intimidating, but its presence only reinforces everyone's awareness of the frailty of the patient's heart and uncertainty about the future. Careful but simple explanations of the pump's action are necessary for patients who are alert enough to understand; it is important that they not get the mistaken idea that the pump is working instead of their heart. Some patients with this type of misunderstanding fear that they will die if the pump stops even momentarily. Such terrific fear makes them anxious and restless and further increases the body's demand for oxygen. Continuous reassurance and repeated simple explanations are essential. Some patients may benefit from mild sedation.

INFLAMMATORY HEART DISORDERS

This section will discuss a group of cardiac conditions that are generally the result of inflammation. All cardiac tissues are susceptible to inflammation, and heart failure can be a serious and rapid result of the inflammatory process. The specific pathologic mechanisms for each disorder are discussed below, and in Table 25-6, signs and symptoms and medical therapy are summarized.

REVIEW

Table 25-6   Inflammatory heart disorders

Disorder	Signs and symptoms	Medical therapy
Pericarditis	*Acute:* Severe precordial chest pain referred to neck, shoulder, left arm; intensified when lying supine, coughing or breathing deeply or swallowing Pericardial friction rub Fever, leukocytosis, ECG changes Cardiac tamponade *Chronic:* Dyspnea, fatigue, congestive heart failure	*Acute:* Treatment of underlying condition Supportive care: salicylates, indomethacin, corticosteroids Pericardiocentesis for injection of antibiotic or sclerosing agent Pericardial fenestration *Chronic:* Digitalization, diuretics Low-sodium diet Pericardiectomy for severe cases
Myocarditis	May be asymptomatic Nonspecific complaints of dyspnea on exertion, palpitations, precordial chest pain, fever, tachycardia	Antibiotics Corticosteroids for severe cases Antiarrhythmic drugs for dysrhythmias
Endocarditis	Gradual onset: malaise, achiness, fever Splenomegaly, clubbing of fingers, Osler's nodes on fingers, petechiae in conjunctiva and mouth, cardiac murmur, anemia	Bed rest Antibiotics (IV) Prolonged antibiotic therapy Incision and drainage of abscesses Valve replacement
Rheumatic fever/rheumatic heart disease	Symptoms follow pharyngeal infection in 1 to 4 weeks Joint pain—recurrent Heart murmur, friction rub, cardiac arrhythmias, congestive heart failure	Antibiotics Antiinflammatory drugs (salicylates, corticosteroids) Early ambulation
Cardiovascular syphilis	Signs of aortic aneurysms, aortitis, aortic valve insufficiency, congestive heart failure	Penicillin Surgery for aneurysm or aortic valve insufficiency, if feasible Treatment of congestive heart failure, if it develops

PERICARDITIS

Pericarditis may result from bacterial, viral, or fungal infection. In addition, it may occur as a complication of a systemic disease, such as rheumatoid arthritis, systemic lupus erythematosus, scleroderma, uremia, or myocardial infarction or may result from trauma or neoplasm.

Pericarditis is an inflammatory process of the visceral or parietal pericardium or both. It may be acute or chronic, and infection may spread from or to the myocardium. *Acute pericarditis* is further classified as fibrinous or exudative. The exudate may be serous, purulent, or hemorrhagic. When fluid accumulates in the pericardial sac, *cardiac tamponade* (compression of heart from blood or fluid) causes decreased venous return to the heart and decreased ventricular emptying. Symptoms result from interference with ventricular functioning (see Box 25-26).

A known etiologic disease process is treated specifically, such as with antibiotic therapy, if indicated. Salicylates or indomethacin (Indocin) may be used to decrease inflammation. If the accumulation of pericardial fluid or effusion is large, the physician may remove the fluid by *percardiocentesis.* A *pericardial fenestration* (pericardial window) may be performed to provide continuous drainage of pericardial fluid.

Chronic pericarditis is referred to as chronic constrictive or adhesive pericarditis. It is three times more prevalent

Symptoms of cardiac tamponade

Diminished or absent point of maximal impulse (PMI)
Diminished peripheral pulses
Distended neck veins (secondary to increased CVP)
Decreased blood pressure (secondary to ineffective pumping action)
Narrowing pulse pressure (difference between systolic and diastolic blood pressure)
Paradoxical pulse (decrease in pulse strength during inspiration)
Diminished heart sounds

in men than women. It may result from fibrosing of the pericardial sac secondary to trauma or neoplastic disease. In the majority of cases, no specific pathogen can be identified as the causative agent. Chronic pericarditis is often associated with other disease processes (see Box 25-27). If the pericardium becomes a constrictive band surrounding the heart, it will prevent adequate filling and emptying of the ventricles, thus decreasing CO and ultimately producing cardiac failure.

Removal of the pericardium (*pericardiectomy*) may be

necessary to restore cardiac function. Postoperative care is similar to that of other surgery. Other measures to restore more efficient pumping include digitalization, diuretic therapy, and a low-sodium diet.

MYOCARDITIS

Myocarditis is an inflammatory disease of the myocardium that causes an infiltrate in the myocardial interstitium and injury to adjacent myocardial cells that is atypical of infarction. Myocarditis may be primary, with an unknown etiology, or secondary, from an identifiable cause such as drug hypersensitivity or toxicity and infection. In North America, infection is most often caused by a virus, including coxsackievirus, echovirus, viral encephalitis, rabies, and herpes simplex.

Myocarditis is difficult to study in human beings, because it frequently remains undiagnosed until chronic cardiac dysfunction and congestive heart failure become clinically obvious. Very often this inflammatory process develops secondary to acute endocarditis or pericarditis. Myocarditis may be classified as acute (benign or fulminant) or chronic.

Patients with myocarditis are often treated with bedrest and digitalis to prevent heart failure and cardiogenic shock. Immunosuppression may be beneficial in reducing myocardial inflammation.

ENDOCARDITIS

Endocarditis is an infection of the endocardium and most often of the heart valves. The more recent method of classification of infective endocarditis is on the basis of the causative organism, for example, enterococcal endocarditis or streptococcal endocarditis. It may occur in acute or subacute forms. Acute endocarditis occurs rapidly, often on normal heart valves, and if untreated may cause death within days or weeks. The subacute form develops more gradually, usually on previously damaged heart valves, and responds well to treatment.

Major causes of underlying cardiac pathologic conditions include rheumatic valvular disease, congenital heart disease, and degenerative heart disease. Endocarditis may also be preceded by intrusive procedures, such as gynecologic examinations or minor surgery. Other persons at high risk are IV drug abusers because of the possibility of bacteremia from contaminated needles and syringes.

The infecting organisms are carried by a turbulent blood flow and deposited on the heart valves or elsewhere on the endocardium. The turbulent blood flow occurs in areas of myocardial anomalies, such as prolapsed mitral valves or ventricular septal defects. The organisms bombard the heart valves, become embedded in the valve matrix, and result in vegetative growths that may scar and perforate the leaflets. Further risk results if the vegetative growths break free of the valves, enter the bloodstream, and cause emboli. If the vegetative emboli enter organs such as the spleen or kidney, abscesses may form.

Prevention of infective endocarditis includes correction of any underlying cardiac defect, as well as measures to prevent bacteremia. For persons with underlying cardiac disease, early and vigorous treatment of infections, good oral hygiene, and prophylactic antibiotic therapy when undergoing dental care or a surgical procedure are important. When infective endocarditis occurs, prolonged antibiotic therapy may be required after the organism is identified. Abscesses may require surgical drainage.

RHEUMATIC HEART DISEASE

Rheumatic fever is an acute inflammatory reaction. It is important in the discussion of inflammatory heart disease, as it has tremendous potential for causing chronic heart problems. In the United States today approximately 1,750,000 adults and 100,000 children have rheumatic heart disease.[3] Symptoms of cardiac involvement usually follow a group A beta-hemolytic streptococcus pharyngeal infection. Ninety percent of the victims are between the age of 5 and 15.

Rheumatic fever may progress with mild symptoms and go undiagnosed, or the disease may be subclinical with no symptoms. The patient develops cardiac manifestations years later. On careful history taking, a recollection of a childhood illness confirming the likelihood of rheumatic fever is usually found.

The pathophysiology of rheumatic heart disease remains unclear. The pericardium, myocardium, or endocardium can be involved. The affected tissue develops small areas of necrosis (*Aschoff bodies*), which heal, leaving scar tissue. Myocardial changes are usually reversible. In the pericardium and endocardium, however, the disease process is usually not reversible and produces the disabling effects of rheumatic heart disease. The valves are typically most affected and become fibrous and incompetent. The leaflets of a valve may fuse during the healing phase (p. 691).

CARDIOVASCULAR SYPHILIS

Cardiovascular syphilis usually occurs from 10 to 30 years after the primary syphilitic infection. Since the highest incidence of primary syphilis is among persons in their early twenties, persons with symptoms of cardiovascular syphilis are usually over 30 years of age.

Cardiovascular syphilis is an extremely dangerous complication of primary syphilis. The spirochetes attack the aorta, the aortic valve, and the myocardium. The ascending aorta is often affected. The wall of the aorta becomes weakened and an *aneurysm* (p. 698) develops. As the aneurysm grows, it may press on neighboring structures, such as the intercostal nerves, resulting in chest pain. An aneurysm may be present without symptoms. It may rupture as it increases in size. Because of this, the patient is encouraged to avoid strenuous activities that might suddenly increase blood pressure.

Spirochetes may also attack the aorta more diffusely, causing *aortitis*. The aorta becomes dilated, and calcium plaques are laid down. The junction of the aorta with the coronary arteries become constricted, resulting in angina (p. 663). Thrombi may also develop in the aorta, leading to the development of emboli and resulting in myocardial infarction or cerebral emboli.

Spirochetes may also attack the aortic valve, resulting in scarring. Aortic insufficiency may develop. This is often complicated by heart failure.

TOXIC HEART DISORDERS

Two common toxins that can affect the heart are alcohol and cocaine. The effects of alcohol are long term, whereas the effects of cocaine are immediate.

ALCOHOLIC CARDIOMYOPATHY

When any form of ethanol (the chief substance in alcoholic beverages) is consumed in large quantities over a period greater than 5 years, it has a direct toxic effect on cardiac tissue. Additives in alcoholic beverages may also create their own toxic effects. Persons with alcoholic cardiomyopathy are usually well-nourished individuals; only 15% of these patients have thiamin deficiency as is seen in many alcoholics.

Alcohol cannot function as an adequate source of calories. The oxidation rate of alcohol cannot be accelerated to meet demands for increases in energy. In chronic alcoholism, these metabolic disturbances result in visceral fatty degeneration of heart tissue. In the early stages, the disease process may be totally reversed by abstinence from alcohol. An enlarged heart is treated with vasodilators and bed rest. Heart failure is treated with the usual methods (p. 681).

CARDIOVASCULAR EFFECTS OF COCAINE ABUSE

Despite the widespread use of cocaine, medical investigation of its systemic effects in humans is sparse and frequently controversial. Cocaine is classified as a local anesthetic and a sympathomimetic drug. It is a tropane alkaloid of the evergreen shrub, *Erythroxylon coca*. Crack cocaine is a heat-stable, freebase form of cocaine that is suitable for smoking and that causes an almost immediate, often intense, response.

Cocaine toxicity is characterized by generalized stimulation including hyperthermia, acute agitation, tachycardia, hypertension, diaphoresis, and acidosis. Fatal pulmonary edema, myocardial ischemia and infarction, and respiratory arrest have been associated with cocaine intoxication. Treatment options include beta blockers for ventricular dysrhythmias, nitrates and calcium channel blockers if coronary pathogenesis is suspected, and aspirin or other thrombolytic agents for acute ischemic events.

VALVULAR HEART DISEASE

Pathophysiology

Valvular heart disease is a general term that refers to any one of a variety of conditions that affect the valves within the heart. Normal valves function to maintain a unidirectional flow of blood through the cardiac chambers by passively opening and closing in response to variant pressure gradients. The mitral and tricuspid valves (atrioventricular valves) prevent the backflow of blood from the ventricles into the atria during systole. Movement of the atrioventricular valves is facilitated by the chordae tendinae and papillary muscles (see Figs. 25-1 and 25-2). Similarly, the aortic and pulmonic valves (semilunar valves) prevent the backflow of blood from the aorta and pulmonary artery into their respective ventricles during diastole.

The two basic problems that compromise the normal function of the valves are stenosis and insufficiency. *Stenosis* is a thickening of the valvular tissue, which causes a narrowing of the valvular orifice. *Insufficiency* refers to the inability of the valve to close completely. An insufficient or incompetent valve allows blood to flow in a retrograde or regurgitant manner.

The predominant etiologic factor in the development of a stenosed or insufficient valve is rheumatic fever. Throughout the course of this disease, large hemorrhagic and fibrinous lesions vegetate along the inflamed edges of the valves.[29] These lesions frequently develop on adjacent valve leaflets so that the edges adhere together. As the disease process progresses, the leaflets become so scarred there is permanent leaflet fusion and limited valvular movement of the normally free-flapping edges.

Since these underlying pathologic changes occur over a period of time, the clinical signs and symptoms of a stenosed or insufficient valve do not usually show up until 10 to 40 years after the onset of rheumatic fever. Furthermore, the extent of valvular damage is largely dependent on its normal degree of motion. Since the pressures and consequent valvular movement on the left side of the heart are greater than those on the right, the mitral and aortic valves are more susceptible. The tricuspid and pulmonic valves are much less frequently affected by rheumatic fever.

The signs and symptoms and medical therapy of valvular heart disorders are outlined in Table 25-7 for each type of disorder. Additional information about specific valvular disorders is provided in the sections that follow.

Mitral stenosis

Mitral stenosis is more often found in women than men. As rheumatic fever is the primary factor in its development, the progressive destruction of the valve occurs over a 20-year period. Mitral commissures (junctions between adjacent cusps) fuse, and the valvular leaflets or cusps thicken and calcify. The chordae tendinae also become short and thick. These underlying changes result in a

Table 25-7   **Valvular heart disorders**

	Signs and symptoms	Medical therapy
Mitral insufficiency	Excessive fatigue, weakness, exhaustion Weight loss Exertional dyspnea, orthopnea, paroxysmal nocturnal dyspnea, rales Late stages: pulmonary edema, right-sided heart failure *Auscultation:* Palpable thrill at apex S₁ absent, soft, or buried in murmur Murmur: high pitched, blowing, swishing, throughout systole (at apex) S₃ low pitched	Activity limitations Sodium-restricted diet Diuretics Digoxin Treatment of atrial dysrhythmias Surgery: valvuloplasty, valvular replacement, annuloplasty
Mitral stenosis	Excessive fatigue, weakness Dyspnea, exertional dyspnea, orthopnea, paroxysmal nocturnal dyspnea Dry cough, bronchitis, rales Pulmonary edema Recurrent pulmonary emboli Hemoptysis Right-sided heart failure *Auscultation:* Palpable thrill at apex S₁ snapping, increased, loud Murmur: soft, low pitched, rumbling, diastolic (at apex)	Sodium-restricted diet Diuretics Activity limitations Oxygen therapy Anticoagulant therapy Surgery: valvulotomy, valve replacement
Aortic insufficiency	Palpitations, sinus tachycardia Exertional dyspnea, orthopnea, paroxysmal nocturnal dyspnea Excessive diaphoresis Angina Late stages: left- and right-sided heart failure *Auscultation:* Murmur: high pitched, blowing, diastolic (third intercostal space) Systolic ejection murmur at base	Digoxin Sodium-restricted diet Diuretics Nitroglycerin (angina) Penicillin therapy (if syphilis a cause) Surgery: valve replacement, valvuloplasty
Aortic stenosis	Angina Syncope Fatigue, weakness Exertional dyspnea, orthopnea, paroxysmal nocturnal dyspnea Pulmonary edema, rales Late stages: right-sided heart failure *Auscultation:* Murmur: low pitched, rough, rasping, systolic (at base or carotids) Systolic thrill at base of heart	Activity limitations Sodium-restricted diet Diuretics Digoxin Nitroglycerin (angina) Surgery: valve replacement
Tricuspid stenosis	Pulmonary congestion, dyspnea Right-sided heart failure Decreased CO: weakness, fatigue, weight loss, hypotension Late stages: cirrhosis, jaundice, malnutrition	Sodium-restricted diet Digoxin Diuretics Surgery: valvuloplasty, valve replacement
Tricuspid insufficiency	Right-sided heart failure Decreased CO: weakness, fatigue, weight loss, hypotension *Auscultation:* Murmur: blowing, throughout systole (left sternal border, increases with inspiration)	Sodium-restricted diet Digoxin Diuretics Surgery: narrowing of annulus, valve replacement

narrow mitral valve that impedes the normal blood flow. Nonrheumatic causes include atrial myxomas, bacterial vegetation, thrombus formation, or calcification of the mitral annulus.

To accommodate the increased work load required to move blood through this narrowed orifice, the left atrium hypertrophies. The resultant left atrial pressure exerts further pressure onto the pulmonary vasculature, causing pulmonary hypertension and pulmonary congestion. Eventually these conditions result in right ventricular failure and right-sided heart failure.

Another common complication of mitral stenosis is atrial fibrillation. Structural changes in the atrial wall from the increased pressure predispose to this dysrhythmia. The coupling of atrial fibrillation and pooling of blood in the atria increases the likelihood of thrombus formation and arterial embolization.

Mitral insufficiency

In contrast to mitral stenosis, mitral insufficiency is more commonly seen in men than women. Although the same pathologic processes occur as a result of rheumatic fever, several other acquired and congenital conditions, such as papillary muscle dysfunction, ruptured chordae tendinae, prolapsed mitral valve, bacterial endocarditis, and congenital abnormalities, can contribute to its development. The result is that the mitral valve leaflets fail to close fully. Consequently, a variable amount of blood leaks back through the valve from the left ventricle into the atrium.

The left atrium dilates and hypertrophies to compensate for the increase volume and pressure. The left ventricle also hypertrophies in response to the increased preload (blood that was regurgitated into the atrium during systole is returned to the ventricle during diastole). In other words, the ejection fraction is reduced and the end-diastolic volume is increased.

Aortic stenosis

Aortic stenosis constitutes 25% of all valvular heart diseases. Diseases of the aortic valve do not usually occur as a single entity; most often there is also involvement of the mitral valve. Aortic stenosis develops as a congenital or acquired condition (rheumatic fever, arteriosclerosis). Clinical symptoms of aortic stenosis are not manifested until the size of the opening in the valve has been reduced to approximately one third of normal. This situation may not occur until many years after the inception of the disease process. The asymptomatic nature of this disease is largely caused by the tremendous compensatory abilities of the left ventricle.

The left ventricle must generate an abnormally high pressure to eject blood through the narrowed aortic orifice. This added pressure requirement results in ventricular hypertrophy with a concomitant increase in myocardial oxygen demand. The oxygen demand may exceed the supply because of reduced cardiac output and inadequate coronary artery perfuson. Classic symptoms of angina may result.

The progressive stenosis accompanied by ventricular hypertrophy in the presence of mitral valve disease causes a decrease in CO. Symptoms of pulmonary congestion and eventually right-sided heart failure ensue.

Aortic insufficiency

Rheumatic fever accounts for approximately 80% of all cases of aortic insufficiency. In this instance the valve fails to close completely, and this results in a retrograde blood flow from the aorta into the left ventricle during diastole. The ventricle hypertrophies to hold all the regurgitant blood. Over time, the left ventricle cannot withstand the added work load, leading to the development of decreased CO, left ventricular failure, and right-sided heart failure. Other causes of aortic insufficiency include Marfan's syndrome, congenital anomalies, syphilis, severe hypertension, bacterial endocarditis, traumatic valve rupture, and dissecting aortic aneurysm.

Tricuspid stenosis

Tricuspid stenosis is a relatively uncommon valvular lesion that usually coexists with stenosis of the mitral or aortic valves. The major cause of this disease is rheumatic fever. The leaflets become thick and fuse together, and the chordae tendinae also become short and thick. Hence during diastole blood flow is reduced through the compromised valve. This blockage further causes a backflow of blood in the systemic circulation. Engorgement of the superior and inferior vena cava precede the development of right-sided heart failure.

Tricuspid insufficiency

Tricuspid insufficiency is a rare disorder that is more prevalent in children than adults. The disease usually develops secondary to marked dilation of the right ventricle and tricuspid valve ring.[8] The valve itself widens and the leaflets are unable to close properly. Therefore, there is regurgitant blood flow to the right atrium during systole. The right atrium hypertrophies to accommodate the increased volume, but invariably the CO decreases with the concomitant decreased blood flow to the left side of the heart. Eventually the excess volume in the atrium causes right-sided heart failure.

Pulmonic valve disease

Lesions of the pulmonic valve are extremely rare in adults. This valve is less likely to be affected by rheumatic fever and bacterial endocarditis. For a more detailed discussion of congenital pulmonic stenosis, refer to a standard pediatric text.

Nursing Process
Assessment

Assessment data that the nurse obtains are essentially the same for any patient with valvular heart disease. Many of the symptoms are related to decreased CO.

Subjective data

1. Ability to carry out ADL and other desired activities: changes in endurance, fatigue, weakness
   These symptoms result from inadequate CO with subsequent impairment in cellular oxygenation
2. Shortness of breath: occurrence, type
   The patient may have dyspnea on exertion (DOE), orthopnea, or paroxysmal nocturnal dyspnea (PND) (p. 678), depending on the degree of heart failure

3. Pain in chest (angina): occurrence, measures used to relieve pain
4. Palpitations: occurrence
   Palpitations are a sensation in the chest described as a bounding or pounding of the heart
5. Syncope: occurrence
   A patient may verbalize feelings of light-headedness, dizzy spells, or fainting; these symptoms can be associated with a decrease in CO
6. Peripheral edema: site, extent, time of day
   Swelling of legs during the day with decreased swelling at night when legs are elevated is usually reported
7. Body weight: perceived pattern of weight gain
8. Diet and medications: ability to carry out therapeutic regimen

Objective data
1. History of rheumatic fever
2. Observation/inspection
   a. Position and comfort level of patient
   b. Character and rate of breathing
   c. Use of supplemental oxygen
   d. Skin color and temperature
   e. Nailbed color and blanching (capillary filling)
   f. Diaphoresis
3. Auscultation
   a. Cardiac rate and rhythm
   b. Presence or change in heart sounds (murmurs, S_3, S_4, friction rub)
   c. Character of heart sounds at all auscultatory sites (aortic, pulmonic, tricuspid, mitral)
   d. Character and distribution of breath sounds

Table 25-8 **Findings in valvular heart disorders**

Disorder	Chest radiograph	ECG	Echocardiogram	Cardiac catheterization
Mitral stenosis	Left atrial enlargement Mitral valve calcification Right ventricular enlargement Prominence of pulmonary artery	Left atrial hypertrophy Right ventricular hypertrophy Atrial fibrillation	Thickened mitral valve Left atrial enlargement	Increased pressure gradient across valve Increased left atrial pressure Increased PCWP Increased right heart pressures Decreased CO
Mitral insufficiency	Left atrial enlargement Left ventricular enlargement	Left atrial hypertrophy Left ventricular hypertrophy Atrial fibrillation Sinus tachycardia	Abnormal mitral valve movement Left atrial enlargement	Mitral regurgitation Increased atrial pressure Increased LVEDP Increased PCWP Decreased cardiac output
Aortic stenosis	Left ventricular enlargement Aortic valve calcification May have enlargement of left atrium, pulmonary artery, right ventricle, right atrium	Left ventricular hypertrophy	Thickened aortic valve Thickened ventricular wall Abnormal movement of aortic leaflets	Increased pressure gradient across valve Increased LVEDP
Aortic insufficiency	Left ventricular enlargement	Left ventricular hypertrophy Tall R waves Sinus tachycardia	Left ventricular enlargement Abnormal mitral valve movement Increased movement of ventricular wall	Aortic regurgitation Increased LVEDP Decreased arterial diastolic pressure
Tricuspid stenosis	Right atrial enlargement Prominence of superior vena cava	Right atrial hypertrophy Tall peaked P waves Atrial fibrillation	Abnormal valvular leaflets Right atrial enlargement	Increased pressure gradient across valve Increased right atrial pressure Decreased CO
Tricuspid insufficiency	Right atrial enlargement Right ventricular enlargement	Right ventricular hypertrophy Atrial fibrillation	Prolapse of tricuspid valve Right atrial enlargement	Increased atrial pressure Tricuspid regurgitation Decreased CO

LVEDP, Left ventricular end-diastolic pressure; *PCWP*, pulmonary capillary wedge pressure.

e. Presence of adventitious breath sounds (rales, rhonchi)
   4. Palpation
      a. Warmth of extremities
      b. Equality of symmetry of pulses
      c. Presence of edema, pitting or nonpitting
      d. Signs of phlebitis (increased calf diameter, positive Homans' sign)
      e. Pulse rate and rhythm
   5. Change in body weight

Diagnostic tests

Four major diagnostic tests are used to determine the presence of valvular heart disease: chest radiograph, ECG, echocardiogram, and cardiac catheterization. Table 25-8 summarizes the findings that are indicative of each specific type of valvular disease.

Chest radiograph

A chest radiograph demonstrates the overall size and configuration of the heart and its chambers. Calcification in the pericardium, myocardium, valves, or large blood vessels is also evident on the film. Most cardiac abnormalities that are discernable on a chest radiograph can be detected with standard anterioposterior and lateral views of the chest.

Electrocardiogram

An ECG (p. 641) is helpful in the diagnosis of valvular heart disease. Hypertrophy of either chamber, as well as specific dysrhythmias, can be detected.

Echocardiography

Echocardiography is most useful in the detection of abnormalities in the mitral and aortic valves. It is some benefit in the diagnosis of tricuspid valve disease.

Echocardiography is a noninvasive technique that uses ultrasound to assess both the structures and motions within the heart. A small transducer is placed on the patient's anterior left chest and moved in various directions to visualize specific cardiac areas. This small transducer functions as a transmitter and receiver. It transmits high-frequency sound waves to the heart and then receives the reflected or echoed ultrasonic beams from the patient's heart. The ultrasonic beam is converted into electrical energy so that lines and spaces are displayed on the oscilloscope. These lines and spaces represent bone, cardiac chambers, valves, the septum, and muscle. A representative copy of the echocardiogram is obtained on paper to become a permanent record of the findings.

Since echocardiography is a noninvasive procedure, it is safer than cardiac catheterization. Hence, whenever possible, it precedes the cardiac catheterization. No special preparation is required for the test. The patient can eat and take medications as usual. Most importantly, the patient should be told about the purpose and procedure of this test. The patient must be aware of the importance of lying still for approximately 30 to 60 minutes. After the test the patient may resume normal activities, since there are no adverse effects from this test.

Cardiac catheterization

Cardiac catheterization is an extremely valuable diagnostic procedure that provides information about the structure and the function of the cardiac chambers, valves, and vessels. Since this is an invasive procedure, it is usually performed after several other diagnostic tests. A catheterization is performed on either the right or left side of the heart depending on the suspected valvular dysfunction. The purpose and procedure of each type are outlined in Box 25-28.

Normal pressure readings and oxygen concentrations for the chambers and great vessels are listed in Fig. 25-48. The right side of the heart is a low-pressure system with less oxygen saturation, since the blood there is going to the lungs. In contrast, the left side of the heart is a relatively high-pressure system with full oxygen saturation, as the blood there is returning from the lungs. Any changes

---

25-28

Cardiac catheterization

Right side	Left side
Purpose	
Confirm suspected valvular heart disease—congenital or acquired	Evaluate pressures on left side of heart
	Assess competency of valves
	Assess left ventricular function
Procedure	
Cutdown made in large vein in patient's arm	Cutdown made in large artery in patient's arm or groin
Catheter threaded via fluoroscopy through superior vena cava, right atrium, right ventricle, pulmonary artery and pulmonary capillaries	Catheter threaded via fluoroscopy through descending aorta, aortic arch, ascending aorta, aortic valve, and left ventricle
Blood sample obtained to determine oxygen content and saturation	Blood sample obtained to determine oxygen content and saturation
Pressures recorded for each chamber/vessel	Pressures recorded for each chamber/vessel
	Pressure gradient measurement across valves obtained

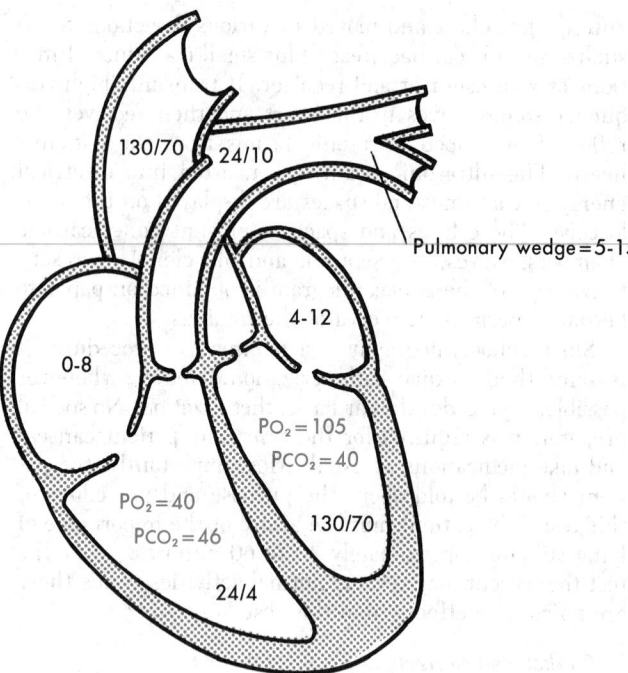

Fig. 25-48 Pressure readings and blood gases in millimeters of mercury (mm Hg) in chambers of heart and major blood vessels.

in normal pressures and oxygen saturation are significant. Abnormalities in pressure gradients across valve are also indicative of valvular heart disease.

Data analysis: nursing diagnoses

Nursing diagnoses are determined from analysis of patient data. Possible nursing diagnoses for the person with valvular disease may include, but are not limited to, the following:

Diagnostic title	Possible etiologies
Activity intolerance	Imbalance between oxygen supply and demand, weakness
Breathing pattern, ineffective	Decreased cardiac output, fatigue
Pain	Angina, organ congestion
Fluid volume, excess	Decreased cardiac output
Knowledge deficit	Lack of exposure/recall

Planning: expected patient outcomes

Expected therapeutic outcomes for the patient with valvular heart disease center around relief of symptoms and adequate cardiac functioning. Signs of pulmonary congestion and systemic venous congestion should be decreased, and improvement in cardiac output should be noted. The extent to which these outcomes are realized depends on the severity of the underlying problem, the presence or absence of other medical conditions, and the response of the patient to the treatment regimen. Outcomes related to the possible nursing diagnoses may include, but are not limited to, the following:

1. Rests between activities.
2. States that breathing is easier and fatigue occurs less frequently with activity.
3. States feeling more comfortable.
4. Coughs less frequently; pitting edema decreases.
5. Describes the following:
   a. Nature of valvular disease
   b. Medication regimen
   c. Prescribed dietary sodium modifications
   d. Work, rest, and activity program to conserve energy and decrease exertional dyspnea
   e. Rationale for and type of surgery to be performed, if indicated
   f. Plans for continued medical therapy.

Implementation
Assisting with achievement of therapeutic goals

1. Administration of medications, as prescribed (diuretics, digoxin, antiarrhythmics)
2. Continued monitoring for signs of decreased CO
   a. Daily intake and output
   b. Daily weights
   c. Respiratory rate and rhythm
   d. Auscultation of breath sounds and heart sounds
   e. Condition of skin and mucous membranes
   f. Capillary perfusion
   g. Equality and strength of peripheral pulses
   h. Presence and extent of edema.
   i. Blood pressure
3. Sodium restricted diet for fluid control of pulmonary or systemic venous congestion

Interventions to achieve patient outcomes
Assisting with comfort and ADL

1. Identify those activities of daily living which are fatiguing and for which patient may need some assistance
2. Design with patient a plan that will allow for completion of daily activities
3. Incorporate rest periods between activities
4. Maintain use of supportive oxygen therapy during activities, as necessary

Facilitating patient/family teaching

1. Effect of a sodium-restricted or fluid-restricted diet on cardiac function, as appropriate
2. Effects of medications: diuretics, cardiac glycosides, anticoagulants
3. Prophylactic use of antibiotics before and after dental work
4. How to check for buildup of fluid in legs
5. Purpose of procedure for diagnostic tests (echocardiogram, cardiac catheterization)
6. Purpose and nature of surgical intervention, if appropriate.

Evaluation

Evaluation will be based on expected patient outcomes. Questions to consider to include the following:

1. Is patient able to describe a work, rest, and activity program to conserve energy?
2. Can patient describe the nature of the valvular disorder?
3. Is patient able to explain any required dietary changes?

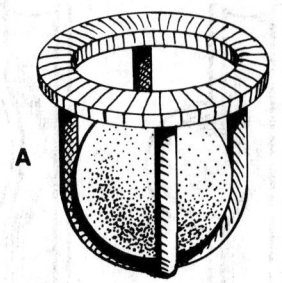 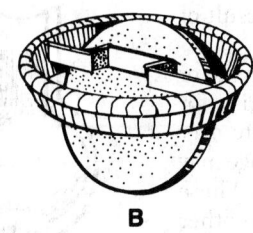 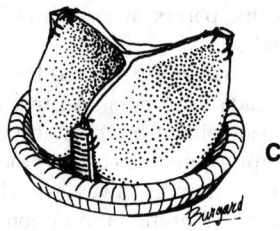

Fig. 25-49   Heart valve replacements. **A,** Caged-ball valve. **B,** Tilting-disk valve. **C,** Biological valve.

25-29

Types of valve repair

Valvuloplasty

Repair of valve, suturing of torn leaflets

Annuloplasty

Repair of ring or annulus of incompetent valve, tightening and suturing of annulus

Valvulotomy/commissurotomy

Repair of a leaflet or commisure, fibrous band, or ring

---

4. Can patient explain medication regimen?
5. Has patient made plans for continued medical follow-up?

Surgical Intervention

Surgical intervention is indicated for a patient whose lifestyle is severely compromised by valvular heart disease. If a patient has hemodynamically debilitating symptoms that are unsuccessfully managed by conventional medical therapies, surgery is then the recommended treatment modality. There are two basic surgical procedures: repair of the valve problem or replacement of the valve.

Repair of valve

Several terms are used to describe the specific anatomical structure undergoing repair (see Box 25-29). Valvulotomy or commisurotomy can be done as a closed or open procedure. A closed approach involves removing a rib with a small incision into the left atrium. A dilator is then used to widen the narrowed valve and free the stenosed leaflet. The atrium is also palpated for thrombi. In the open technique, used also for valvuloplasty and annuloplasty, the thorax is incised and the heart completely exposed.

Replacement of valve

Many types of valves can be used for replacement. A valve is selected on the basis of location of the incompetent valve, the underlying pathologic changes, and the age of the patient. The size of the prosthetic valve is of major importance. Valves are grouped according to their design and function: caged-ball, caged-disk, tilting-disk, and biologic valves (Fig. 25-49).

Caged-ball valves are the most durable. Their use, how-

25-30

Guidelines for Care

The patient undergoing valvular surgery

Preoperative care

Give medications as ordered

Digitalis preparations and diuretics are often discontinued before surgery to avoid dysrhythmias associated with digitalis toxicity that may be precipitated by cardiopulmonary bypass

If the patient has been receiving anticoagulants, vitamin K may be administered before surgery to return prothrombin time to normal

Antibiotics may be given to decrease incidence of postoperative endocarditis

Prepare patient for surgery by providing explanation of procedure and usual postoperative routines, addressing specific concerns of patient and family

Postoperative care

Administer anticoagulant therapy as prescribed

Assess apical heartbeat: a "click" sound is usually heard; reassure patient that this sound is normal; assess for development of murmur

Explain medication regimen to patient

Need for antibiotics for approximately 1 month following valve replacement

Need for cardiac glycosides to improve cardiac function and control dysrhythmias for prescribed time (usually 3 to 6 months after surgery)

---

ever, is restricted to patients with a large enough annulus and chamber to accommodate the cage itself. It is never used for tricuspid valve replacement because of the limited capacity of the right ventricle.

Caged-disk valves occupy less space in the ventricles than other valves and require less force to move the occluding disk. This type of valve creates more obstruction to blood flow than other types of valves. If the disk "sticks" in the cage, causing total obstruction of blood flow, hemodynamics are seriously compromised.

Tilting-disk valves have occluders that tilt or pivot within a ring rather than balls or disks that pop back and forth in a cage (Fig. 25-49, *B*). This type of valve produces nearly central blood flow through its orifice, providing more normal blood flow. However, the valve may develop areas under the pivoting points, where thrombi can form as a result of the blood stasis.

Biologic valves are derived from animal cardiac tissue or human cadaver donors. Animal valves carry less risk for thromboembolism; however, they tend to degenerate over time. Improvements in organ procurement and storage may make more human valves available in the future. These valves are less prone to infection and rejection than other replacements.

Preoperative and postoperative nursing care

Nursing care for the patient undergoing valvular heart surgery is essentially the same as that for patients undergoing coronary bypass surgery (p. 674). Specific nursing care related to valvular surgery is listed in Box 25-30.

ANEURYSMS

Pathophysiology

An aneurysm is a local or diffuse dilation of an artery. It occurs secondary to a variety of disease processes such as infections, hypertension, or syphilis, although arteriosclerosis is the predominant etiologic factor. Regardless of the pathogenesis, the musculoelastic middle (media) layer of the artery becomes weakened, and it produces stretching of the inner (intima) and outer (adventitia) layers. Blood pressure within the vessel continues to weaken its walls and to enlarge the aneurysm.

The extent of arterial damage and clinical symptomatology vary greatly according to the type, size, and location of the aneurysm. An aneurysm is classified on the basis of its shape and subsequent damage to the affected artery (Fig. 25-50). The *fusiform aneurysm,* the most common type, assumes a spindle shape around the entire circumference of the vessel. In contrast, a *saccular aneurysm* affects only a part of the arterial circumference. This type of aneurysm appears as a unilateral sac or outpouching on the side of the artery. Also, a saccular aneurysm is more likely to rupture. A *dissecting aneurysm* develops from a split or tear in the intimal wall overlying a diseased media. This relatively uncommon occurrence leads to the accumulation of blood in a newly formed cavity between the vessel layers.

Although these types of aneurysms can develop in any artery, the major site for aneurysm formation is the aorta. Since the aorta has such a large diameter and is subject to great pressures, it is often the location for underlying disease processes. Aortic aneurysms are found in the thoracic segment and, more commonly, in the abdominal portions (Fig. 25-51). Since there is some difference between aneurysms in these locations, they are discussed as separate entities.

Thoracic aortic aneurysms

Aneurysms within the thoracic area can develop in the descending, ascending, or transverse section of the aorta. Hypertensive men between 50 and 70 years of age are typically subject to this disease.

Aneurysms in the *descending aorta* are usually fusiform and originate just distal to the left subclavian artery. A

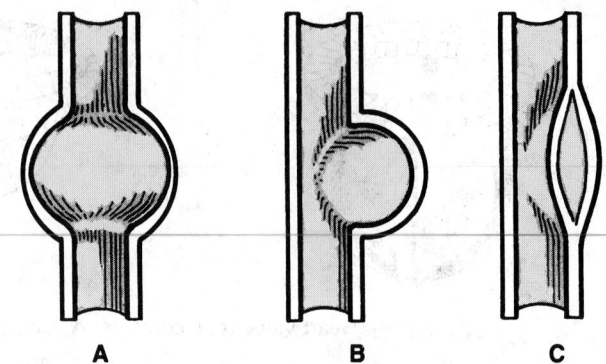

Fig. 25-50 Types of aneurysms. **A,** Fusiform. **B,** Saccular. **C,** Dissecting.

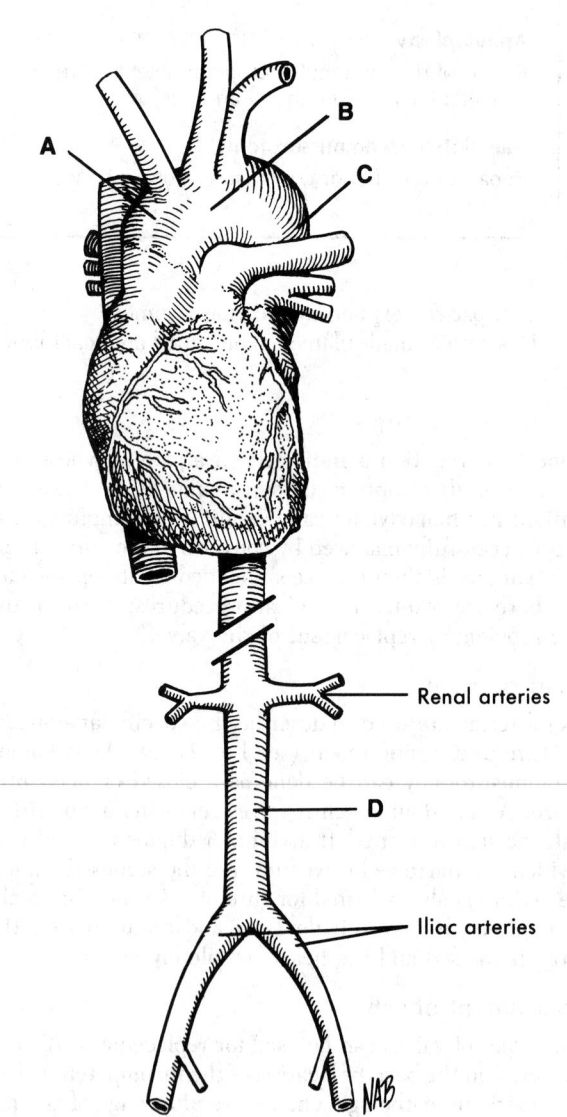

Renal arteries

Iliac arteries

Fig. 25-51 Common sites of aortic aneurysms. **A,** Ascending aorta. **B,** Transverse aorta. **C,** Descending aorta. **D,** Abdominal aorta.

Table 25-9   Aneurysms

Type	Signs and symptoms	Medical therapy
Abdominal aortic	Pulsating mass in mid-upper abdomen Systolic bruit over aorta Pain in mid-upper abdomen or in lower back or groin Long-standing cramps in buttocks, thighs, calves	Antihypertensive medications Pain medications Inotropic agents (for example, propranolol [Inderal]) Surgery: resection of aneurysm with graft replacement
Thoracic aortic	*Ascending aorta:* Chest pain: deep, diffuse, aching *Transverse aorta:* Dyspnea, cough, hoarseness *Dissecting aneurysm:* Tearing sensation in chest, pain radiating to neck, shoulders, lower back, abdomen	Antihypertensive medications Negative inotropic agents (for example, propranolol [Inderal]) Surgery: Resection of aneurysm with graft replacement Aortic valve replacement (if aortic insufficiency)

patient with this form of aneurysm is asymptomatic. Symptoms of chest pain are associated with aneurysms of the *ascending aorta* (Table 25-9). Less frequent are aneurysms of the *transverse aorta* or aortic arch. Symptoms of this type directly relate to the aneurysm's compression on surrounding structures, such as the lungs, trachea, and larynx. Operative mortality is highest in those persons who have an acute onset of symptoms and in whom a dissecting aneurysm begins in the ascending aortic arch and causes insufficiency of the aortic valve.

Abdominal aortic aneurysms

Aneurysms of the abdominal aorta are more prevalent in hypertensive men over 60 years of age. The vast majority of these aneurysms develop just below the renal arteries but above the iliac bifurcation. An abdominal aneurysm grows slowly, hence the patient is usually asymptomatic. At other times the person may have pain or tenderness in the mid or upper abdomen. The aneurysm can leak into the retroperitoneal or pelvic cavity, or dissect into the duodenum. As the aorta exceeds its normal 3 to 4 cm diameter at this point, there is an increased probability of rupture.

The prognosis for a patient with an abdominal aortic aneurysm depends not only on the size of the defect but, more importantly, on the extent of arteriosclerotic heart disease. The aneurysm may extend to impinge on the renal, iliac, or mesenteric arteries. The stasis of blood favors thrombus formation along the wall of the vessel, and if the aneurysm is large, the most feared complication is aneurysmal rupture. More than half of those with untreated abdominal aneurysm die within 2 years of diagnosis; over 85% die within 5 years.

Diagnostic Tests
Radiography

An aneurysm is most often detected accidentally by routine chest or abdominal radiograms, since symptoms are rarely manifested. Radiographic findings show widening of the aorta with a ring of calcification outlining the aneurysm and displacement of surrounding structures.

Angiography

An aortogram reveals the size and location of an aneurysm. This test determines whether an aneurysm is leaking, expanding, or dissecting. An aortogram is performed by insertion of a catheter into the femoral, brachial, or axillary artery. The patient may feel a burning sensation when the contrast dye is injected. Following injection of the contrast material, a series of radiograms are taken at intervals to determine an accurate flow study.

After the procedure, the patient must remain resting in bed for 6 to 12 hours with only minimal flexion of the cannulated joint. Monitor vital signs every 15 minutes for 2 hours. Assessment of pulses, skin color, temperature, movement, and numbness distal to the site is also important. Inspect the injection site whenever vital signs are taken for the presence of bleeding, swelling, or hematoma.

Sonography

Ultrasound is also helpful in determining the shape and location of the aneurysm. Special conducting gel is applied to the skin, and the Doppler probe head is placed over the gel to intensify sounds of pulse vibration. This procedure detects blood flow and presence of bruit. Since this is a noninvasive procedure, there are no special precautions or posttest care.

Surgery

Surgery is the treatment of choice for patients with large or dissecting aneurysms or with those aneurysms that produce symptoms with a significant risk of rupture. Elective resection at the time of the first symptoms is often advised, since emergency surgery increases surgical risks. Complications of surgery include massive hemorrhage, injury to adjacent structures (duodenum, ureters, kidneys), myocardial infarction, renal failure, stroke, or graft infection.

Procedures
Thoracic aorta

Surgical intervention for the patient with an aneurysm of the thoracic aorta is comparable to open heart surgery.

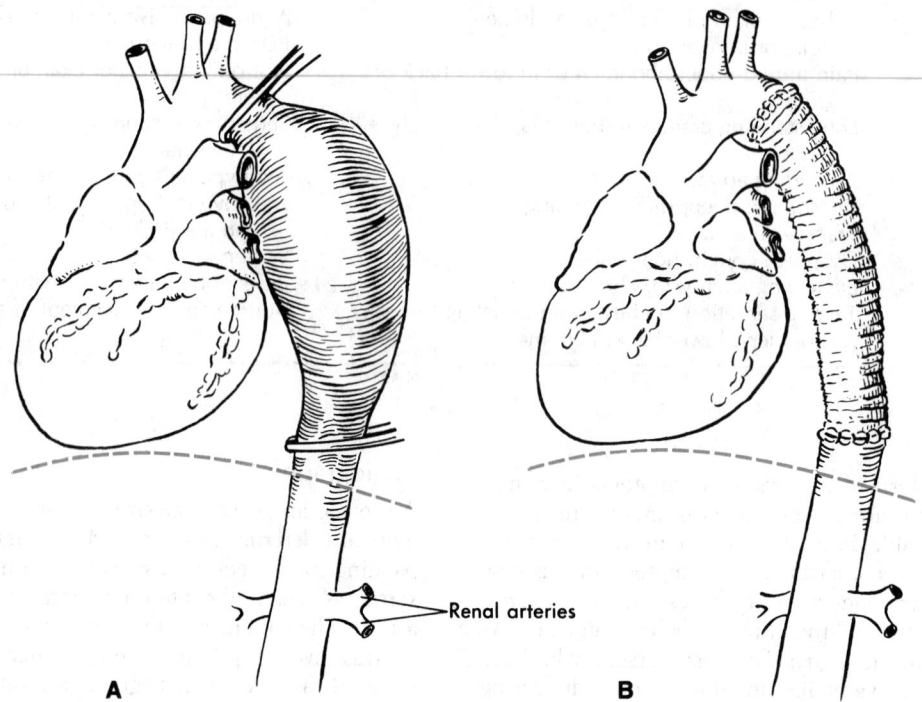

Fig. 25-52 Aneurysm of descending thoracic artery. **A,** Resection of throacic aorta with cardiovascular clamps in place. **B,** Permanent replacement graft after resection of aneurysm.

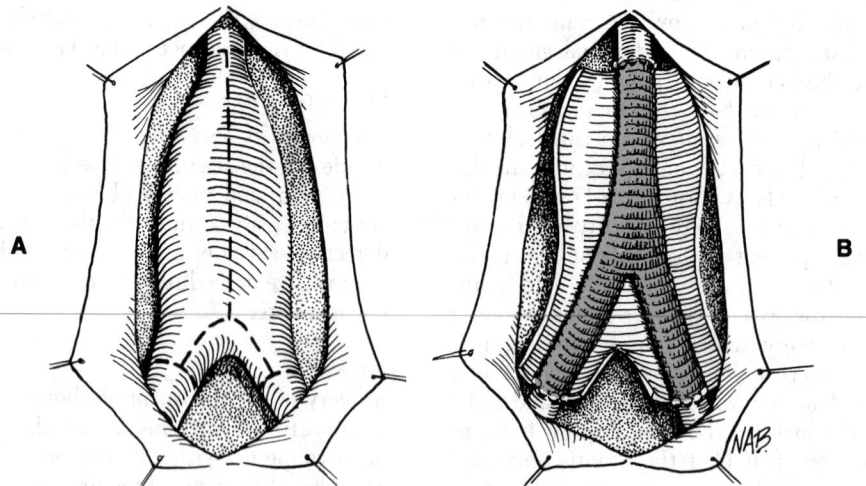

Fig. 25-53 **A,** Abdominal aneurysm of aorta and iliac arteries. **B,** Bifurcation graft used to replace excised aneurysm.

A midline thoracic incision is made, and the aneurysm is exposed. Cardiopulmonary bypass (p. 672) maintains tissue oxygenation during clamping of the aorta. Hypothermia may also be indicated to decrease the metabolic requirements of the tissues. While the aneurysm itself is being resected, cross-clamps are placed above and below the aorta to prevent blood flow into the operative area (Fig. 25-52). An artificial patch or tube (Teflon or Dacron) is grafted on the area.

Abdominal aorta

Surgical intervention for the removal of an abdominal aortic aneurysm is performed without use of heart and lung bypass, since arterial blood flow to lower extremities can be interrupted safely during the operative procedure. An abdominal incision is made, the aneurysm is opened, and any clots and debris are removed. A synthetic graft in the form of a patch or tube is sutured onto the tissues. Once the graft is replaced, the remaining arterial wall is sutured over the graft (Fig. 25-53).

Preoperative preparation

The physician explains the surgical risks when obtaining informed consent for the surgery. The nurse provides support for the patient during the decision-making process, since the surgery is associated with some mortality and morbidity.

The preparation and postoperative care for resection of a thoracic aortic aneurysm are similar to that for cardiac surgery (p. 674). Resection of an abdominal aortic aneurysm is similar to other abdominal surgery. Some surgeons additionally require a bowel preparation for optimal preparation, should bowel surgery be necessary. Heparin is usually given during surgery, before clamping of the artery.

Postoperative care (abdominal aortic aneurysm)

1. Monitor the following parameters:
   a. Vital signs until stable
   b. Central venous pressure (CVP), pulmonary artery pressure (PAP), pulmonary capillary wedge pressure (PCWP); observe for decrease indicating hypovolemia
   c. Dysrhythmias
   d. Hourly circulation checks with assessment of all pulses distal to graft site
      (1) Absent pulses more than 6 to 12 hours indicate arterial occlusion
      (2) Poor peripheral perfusion: marked decrease in blood pressure, weak thready pulses, cool skin temperature, diaphoresis
      (3) Advanced occlusion: pain, cramping, numbness in extremities; legs may be white or blue and cool to cold
   e. Neurologic: check level of consciousness and ability to move lower extremities every 1 to 2 hours
   f. Blood loss: monitor chest tube output every hour; report drainage of >100 ml/hr × 3 hr
   g. Electrolytes: hypokalemia, hypocalcemia; supplement when necessary
   h. Postoperative ileus or distention: NG output, bowel sounds, abdominal pain or discomfort
   i. Renal function (since aorta was clamped during surgery, preventing blood flow to kidneys)
      (1) Hourly urine flow greater than 25 to 30 ml through indwelling catheter
      (2) Urine color (hematuria may occur with renal damage)
      (3) Daily blood urea nitrogen (BUN)
2. Keep patient flat in bed without sharp flexion of hip and of knee to avoid pressure on femoral and popliteal arteries; turn patient gently side to side
3. Give medication for pain
4. Institute pulmonary ventilatory measures (deep breathing and coughing, and so on); use firm abdominal support to incision during coughing
5. Prevent postoperative thrombophlebitis
   a. Check for pain or cramps in calf, tenderness in specific areas of leg, redness along course of vein
   b. Encourage dorsiflexion and plantar flexion of feet
   c. Use elastic stockings
6. Encourage ambulation, when permitted

SUMMARY

1. Cardiac output is a function of heart rate and stroke volume.
2. Heart rate is generally under the control of the autonomic nervous system.
3. Stroke volume is determined by preload, contractility, and afterload.
4. Physiologic changes in cardiac functioning related to aging are most apparent in situations of increased stress on the cardiovascular system or in the presence of underlying cardiac pathologic conditions.
5. A less effective heart rate response to exercise and prolongation of the time required for the heart rate to return to normal following exercise are two common physiologic changes associated with aging.
6. An ECG is a graphic record of the electrical activity of the heart muscle. It is recorded on a grid that allows measurement of time and voltage.
7. A 12-lead ECG provides 12 different views of cardiac electrical activity; a cardiac monitor typically displays one view at a time.
8. A normal cardiac complex consists of a P wave, a QRS complex, and a T wave. The exact configuration of each component will vary according to the view or lead that is being recorded.
9. Normal sinus rhythm is characterized by a rhythm that is regular, a rate between 60 and 100 beats/min, and a cardiac complex that is within established criteria for configuration and duration of the components and intervals.
10. Components of the action potential include resting membrane potential, depolarization, repolarization, and atrial systole.
11. The three electrophysiologic mechanisms responsible for disorders of cardiac rhythm include reentry (or

circus movement), altered automaticity (enhanced or abnormal), and late potentials (afterdepolarizations or triggered activity).

12. Signal averaging of the surface QRS complex can be used to detect low-amplitude, high-frequency signals in the terminal portion of the QRS complex or in the early ST segment.

13. Dysrhythmias may originate in the sinus node, atria, atrioventricular junction, or ventricles. Conduction abnormalities include atrioventricular blocks and bundle branch block.

14. Treatment for cardiac dysrhythmias involves identification and elimination of the cause (if possible), drugs or electrical suppression of ectopic impulse initiation, and modalities to regulate heart rate (drugs, regulation of oxygen demand, and artificial pacemakers).

15. Two life-threatening dysrhythmias are ventricular fibrillation and ventricular standstill. CPR must be initiated and maintained until definitive treatment is effective.

16. Components of a teaching plan for patients with permanent pacemakers include the rationale for insertion, activities to avoid, the method for monitoring the function of their particular pacemaker, and symptoms to report to their physicians.

17. Atherosclerosis is the most common etiology of coronary artery disease.

18. Nonmodifiable risk factors for CAHD include advancing age, being of the male sex or black race, and a positive family history of CAHD.

19. Major modifiable risk factors for CAHD include cigarette smoking, hyperlipidemia, diabetes mellitus, and hypertension. A diet high in cholesterol and saturated fats contributes to the risk factors.

20. Angina pectoris is chest pain caused by reversible myocardial ischemia. Treatment involves increasing myocardial blood and oxygen supply (either with medication or surgical intervention) and reducing myocardial oxygen demands.

21. Teaching plans for patients with angina should include CAHD risk factor identification and reduction, interventions to use when chest pain occurs, methods of reducing myocardial oxygen demands, and symptoms to report to the physician.

22. The most commonly used drugs for reduction or control of angina are nitrates, beta blocking agents, and calcium channel blockers.

23. A myocardial infarction is the result of prolonged myocardial ischemia that causes irreversible cellular damage and necrosis.

24. The clinical consequences of a myocardial infarction depend on the location of the coronary artery occlusion and the extent of necrosis.

25. Diagnosis of myocardial infarction is based on the clinical picture, ECG findings, elevation of serum enzyme levels, and other procedures that allow direct visualization of the area of myocardial damage.

26. Medical therapy for myocardial infarction includes measures to reduce the size of the infarcted area, to reduce myocardial oxygen demands, and to prevent or treat complications.

27. Possible nursing diagnoses for the patient with myocardial infarction include activity intolerance, decreased cardiac output, chest pain, anxiety, knowledge deficit, and diagnoses related to psychosocial adjustment of the patient and the family.

28. The two most common complications of myocardial infarction are cardiac dysrhythmias and left ventricular failure.

29. Teaching plans for patients with myocardial infarction should include content on the pathophysiology of myocardial infarction, the healing process, the treatment regimen, risk factors for coronary artery disease, the relationship between the treatment regimen and risk factor reduction, and resumption of activities (including sexual activity) following the acute phase of illness.

30. Coronary artery bypass graft (CABG) is one type of surgical intervention to improve coronary blood flow. This procedure involves grafting a blood vessel such as a portion of the saphenous vein from the aorta to a point beyond the occlusion in a coronary artery.

31. Percutaneous transluminal coronary angioplasty (PTCA) is a newer procedure for improving coronary blood flow. This procedure involves insertion of a balloon-equipped catheter into a coronary artery and compressing or destroying an atherosclerotic plaque.

32. Intravascular stenting is an intervention designed to prevent restenosis by maintaining the cylindrical lumen produced by the balloon in angioplasty.

33. Heart failure is a state in which the heart is no longer able to pump an adequate supply blood to meet the demands of the body.

34. Congestive heart failure (CHF) refers to a state of circulatory congestion resulting from heart failure and its compensatory mechanisms. Symptoms of congestion may involve the pulmonary circulation, the systemic venous circulation, or both.

35. Signs and symptoms associated with CHF include those resulting from decreased cardiac output (forward failure) and those resulting from the subsequent congestion (backward failure).

36. Treatment for CHF involves improving oxygen supply to the tissues, decreasing oxygen demands on the myocardium, and relieving the symptoms of congestion. Common elements of treatment include oxygen, rest, positioning to facilitate optimal respiration, positive inotropic drugs, diuretics, sodium-restricted diet, and arterial/venous dilating drugs.

37. Teaching plans for patients with congestive heart failure include content on the pathophysiology of the condition, approaches to regulating and monitoring the effect of activity, avoidance of precipitating factors, rationale for the treatment regimen, approaches to implementing the treatment regimen, and signs and symptoms to report to the physician.

38. Pulmonary edema represents the most severe form of congestion resulting from left ventricular failure, and cardiogenic shock represents the most severe form of decreased cardiac output. Both conditions are medical emergencies and require immediate, intensive medical and nursing intervention.

39. Inflammation of the pericardium, myocardium, or en-

docardium may be a consequence of infectious diseases, neoplasms, and other metabolic disorders. Patients with these conditions have the usual signs and symptoms associated with the inflammatory process and may also develop heart failure. Measures to prevent further episodes are important aspects of the treatment regimen.

40. The two basic problems that compromise the normal functioning of the cardiac valves are stenosis and insufficiency. Stenosis causes a narrowing of the valvular orifice and impedes the forward flow of blood. Insufficiency causes incomplete closure of the valve and allows blood to flow backward.

41. Cardiac murmurs are a common physical finding in patients with valvular heart disease. Depending on the severity of the disease, the patient may or may not develop clinical symptoms such as those associated with heart failure.

42. Diagnosis of the nature and extent of valvular heart disease is frequently based on the findings obtained from a cardiac catheterization. Pressure gradients between relevant cardiac chambers and O_2 content of the blood are two parameters that are measured with this procedure.

43. Treatment for cardiac valvular disease involves management of the clinical symptoms. Surgical repair of the valve or replacement of the valve with an artificial prosthesis may be necessary.

44. An aneurysm is a local or diffuse dilation of an artery. Atherosclerosis is a common cause of this problem. Aneurysms may be fusiform, saccular, or dissecting and may form in the thoracic or abdominal aorta.

45. Depending on the location and size of the aneurysm, surgical resection may be necessary. An artificial tube is grafted onto the resected area.

STUDY QUESTIONS

• Using Box 25-5 (Rhythm strip analysis) as your guide, analyze Fig. 25-18 (Sinus tachycardia). How do your findings compare with those in the legend?

• Review the process of wound healing in Chapter 22. How can this process be applied to a myocardial infarction?

• What is being done in your community to increase the public's awareness of risk factors for CAHD? How would you go about teaching the lay public about this health problem?

• Examine the chart of a patient who has had a myocardial infarction. What ECG changes did you note? What changes occurred in the serum enzymes? How do the changes you noted compare to the usual pattern for MI? What significance do these changes have for nursing interventions?

• Mr. N. is scheduled for CABG surgery. He has never had surgery before and is very apprehensive. He lives out of town; his wife is staying at a nearby motel. What should be included in a preoperative teaching plan for Mr. N.?

• Examine the chart of a patient who has congestive failure. How do the patient's symptoms compare with the

usual symptoms for CHF? Did the patient have left- or right-sided failure or both? What was the etiology of CHF in this patient? What data would indicate an improvement in the pumping capabilities of this patient's heart? What nursing diagnoses did you identify for the patient? Could other diagnoses have been appropriate?

REFERENCES AND SELECTED READINGS

1.* Alpert JS: The pharmacologic management of coronary artery disease, *Heart Lung* 15:558-561, 1986.
2. Alpert JS, Rippe, JM: *Manual of cardiovascular diagnosis and therapy*, ed 3, Boston, 1988, Little, Brown.
3. American Heart Association: *Heart facts*, Dallas, 1991, The Association.
4. Ayres SM: The prevention and treatment of shock in acute myocardial infarction, *Chest* 93:17S-21S, 1988.
5.* Baggs JG, Karch AM: Sexual counseling of women with coronary heart disease, *Heart Lung* 16:154-159, 1987.
5a.* Bavin TK, Self MA: Weaning from intra-aortic balloon pump support, *Am J Nurs* 91(10):54-59, 1991.
6. Berne RM, Levy MN: Cardiovascular physiology, ed 6, St Louis, 1991, Mosby–Year Book.
7.* Borders CR: When the bypass patient returns home: problems your bypass patients face after discharge, *Patient Care* 19(13):65-76, 1985.
8. Braunwald E, et al: *Harrison's Principles of internal medicine*, ed 12, New York, 1991, McGraw-Hill.
9. Breithardt G, Borggrefe M: Recent advances in the identification of patients at risk of ventricular tachyarrhythmias: role of ventricular late potentials, *Circulation* 75:1091-1096, 1987.
10.* Burgess AW, Hartman CR: Patients' perceptions of the cardiac crisis, *Am J Nurs* 86:568-571, 1986.
11.* Carpenito LJ: Nursing diagnosis: application to clinical practice, ed 4, Philadelphia, 1991, JB Lippincott.
12. Cohn LH: Surgical treatment of acute myocardial infarction, *Chest* 93:13S-16S, 1988.
13. Conner WE, Bristow JD: Coronary heart disease: prevention, complications, and treatment, Philadelphia, 1985, JB Lippincott.
14.* Conover MB: *Understanding electrocardiography*, ed 6, St Louis, 1991, Mosby–Year Book.
15.* Conti CR: Advances and controversies: laser therapy for cardiovascular disease, *Heart Lung* 16:465-473, 1987.
16. Cosgrove D, et al: Results of mitral valve reconstruction, *Circulation* 74(suppl 1):182-187, 1986.
17.* Darovic GO: *Hemodynamic monitoring: invasive and noninvasive clinical application*, Philadelphia, 1987, WB Saunders.
18.* Deans K, Hartshorn J: Use of antithrombotic agents in valvular heart disease, *J Cardiovasc Nurs* 1(3):65-69, 1987.
19. Duncan C, et al: Effect of chest tube management on drainage after cardiac surgery, *Heart Lung* 16:1-9, 1987.
20. Dunn DL, Gregory JJ: Noninvasive temporary pacing: experience in a community hospital, *Heart Lung* 18:23-28, 1989.
21. Ebersole P, Hess P: Toward healthy aging: human needs and nursing response, ed 3, St Louis, 1990, Mosby–Year Book.
22.* Finesilver C, Metzle DJ: Right ventricular infarction: the critically different MI, *Am J Nurs* 91(4):32-36, 1991.
23. Gardin JM, et al: Effects of aging on peak systolic left ventricular wall stress in normal subjects, *Am J Cardiol* 63:998-999, 1989.
23a.* Gawlinski A, Jensen G: The complications of cardiovascular aging, *Am J Nurs* 91(11):26-30, 1991.

*Recommended for student reading.

24. Gold HK: Thrombolysis in acute myocardial infarction, *Chest* 93:10S-12S, 1988.
25. Gottleib SV: Ischemia as an indicator of future adverse events in patients with coronary artery disease, *J Myocard Ischemia* 1:20-28, 1989.
26. Groer MW, Shekleton ME: Basic pathophysiology: a holistic approach, ed 3, St Louis, 1989, Mosby–Year Book.
27. Guyton AC, et al: *Textbook of medical physiology*, ed 8, Philadelphia, 1991, WB Saunders.
28.* Hall LT: Cardiovascular lasers: a look into the future, *Am J Nurs* 90(7):27-30, 1990.
29. Hurst JW: *The heart, arteries, and veins*, ed 6, New York, 1986, McGraw-Hill.
30. Izor-Povenmire K, House AA: Acute crack cocaine intoxication: a case study, *Focus Crit Care* 16:112-119, 1989.
31.* Joseph DL, Bates S: Intraaortic balloon pumping: how to stay on course, *Am J Nurs* 90(9):42-47, 1990.
32. Kerber RE, et al: Energy, current, and success in defibrillation and cardioversion, *Circulation* 77:1038-1046, 1988.
33. Kinney MR, et al: *Comprehensive cardiac care*, ed 7, St Louis, 1991, Mosby–Year Book.
34.* Kleinhenz TJ: The inside story on preload and afterload, *Nurs 85* 15(5):50-55, 1985.
35. Krone R: Valvular heart disease. In Ahumadr G: *Cardiovascular pathophysiology*, New York, 1988, Oxford University Press.
36. Lakatta EG, et al: Human aging: changes in structure and function, *J Am Coll Cardiol* 10(2):42A-47A, 1987.
37.* Loan T: Nursing interaction with patients undergoing coronary angioplasty, *Heart Lung* 15:368-375, 1986.
37a.* Lothian CL: Laser angioplasty: vaporizing coronary artery plaque, *Nurs 92* 22(1):63-64, 1992.
38. Loveys VJ: Physiologic effects of cocaine with particular reference to the cardiovascular system, *Heart Lung* 16:175-182, 1987.
39.* Marrie TJ: Infective endocarditis: a serious and changing disease, *Crit Care Nurs* 7(2):31-46, 1987.
40. McGill HC Jr: The cardiovascular pathology of smoking, *Am Heart J* 115:250-257, 1988.
41.* Mickus D, Monahan KJ, Brown, C: Exciting external pacemakers, *Am J Nurs* 86:403-405, 1986.
42.* Misenski M: Pathophysiology of acute myocardial infarction: a rationale for thrombolytic therapy, *Heart Lung* 17:743-750, 1988.
43.* Norsen LH, Fox GB: Understanding cardiac output and the drugs that affect it, *Nurs 86* 16(5):43-45, 1986.
44. Porth CM: *Pathophysiology: concepts of altered health status*, ed 3, Philadelphia, 1990, JB Lippincott.
45. Price SA, Wilson LM: Pathophysiology: clinical concepts of disease processes, ed 3, New York, 1986, McGraw-Hill.
46.* Purcell JA, Burrows SG: A pacemaker primer, *Am J Nurs* 85:553-568, 1985.
47. Purdy RE, Boucek RJ: *Handbook of cardiac drugs*, Boston, 1988, Little, Brown.

48. Roberts WC: The aging heart, *Mayo Clin Proc* 63:205-206, 1988.
49.* Rodriguez SW, Reed, RL: Thrombolytic therapy for MI, *Am J Nurs* 87:632-640, 1987.
50. Roubin GS: Intracoronary stenting, percutaneous placement of intracoronary prosthesis: new solutions and new problems, *J Invasive Cardiol* 1(1):1-6, 1988.
51.* Runions J: A program for psychological and social enhancement during rehabilitation after myocardial infarction, *Heart Lung* 14:117-125, 1985.
52.* Sakallaris BR: Advances and controversies: laser therapy for cardiovascular disease, *Heart Lung* 16:464-473, 1987.
53. Saul L: Arrhythmia mimics. I. *Am J Nurs* 91(3):41-43, 1991.
54. Saul L: Arrhythmia mimics. II. *Am J Nurs* 91(5):41-45, 1991.
55. Schroeder SA, et al: *Current medical diagnosis and treatment*, ed 30, Norwalk, Conn, 1991, Appleton & Lange.
56.* Scordo KA: Hemodynamic monitoring: learning to read the waves, *Nurs 85* 15(7):40-42, 1985.
57. Sokolow M, McIlroy MB, Cheitlin MD: *Clinical cardiology*, ed 5, Norwalk, Conn, 1990, Appleton & Lange.
58.* Solomon J: Managing a failing heart, *RN* 54(8):46-50, 1991.
59. Spann JF, Hurst JW: The recognition and management of heart failure. In Hurst JW: *The heart, arteries, and veins*, ed 6, New York, 1986, McGraw-Hill.
60.* Summer SM, Grau PA: Guidelines for running a 12-lead ECG, *Nurs 85* 15(12):30-33, 1985.
61. Urban P, et al: Intravascular stenting for stenosis of aortocoronary venous bypass grafts, *JACC* 13:1085-1091, 1989.
62. Vatterott RJ, et al: Signal-averaged electrocardiography: a new noninvasive test to identify patients at risk for ventricular arrhythmias, *Mayo Clin Proc* 63:931-942, 1988.
63.* Weller S, Noone J: Mechanisms of arrhythmias: enhanced automaticity and reentry, *Crit Care Nurse* 9(5):42-66, 1989.
64. Wilhelmsen L: Coronary heart disease: epidemiology of smoking and studies of smoking, *Am Heart J* 115:242-249, 1988.
65.* Witherell CL: Questions nurses ask about pacemakers, *Am J Nurs* 90(12):20-26, 1990.
66. Yusuf S: The use of adrenergic blocking agents, IV nitrates and calcium channel blocking agents following acute myocardial infarction, *Chest* 93:25S-28S, 1988.
67. Zipes DP: Cardiovascular electrophysiology: promises and contributions, *J Am Coll Cardiol* 13:1329-1352, 1989.

Classic

68.* Chesney MA, Rosenman RH: Type A behavior: observations on the past decade, *Heart Lung* 11:12-18, 1982.
69. DeBakey M, et al: Surgical management of dissecting aneurysm of the aorta, *J Cardiovasc Surg* 49:130-149, 1965.
70. Mirowski M, et al: Termination of malignant ventricular arrhythmias with an implanted automatic defibrillator in human beings, *N Engl J Med* 303:322-324, 1980.

The Patient
with
Peripheral
Vascular
Problems

Eileen Walsh

After studying this chapter, the learner should be able to:

- Identify risk factors associated with the development of peripheral vascular disorders.
- Compare pathophysiology, nursing diagnoses, expected outcomes, and interventions for patients with arterial and venous disorders.
- Describe nursing interventions for patients having surgery for arterial and venous disorders.
- Describe the pathophysiology and nursing interventions for patients with leg ulcers and lymph disorders.
- Identify nursing diagnoses and nursing interventions to prevent and control hypertension.

Problems of the peripheral vascular system refer to a number of disorders that disrupt blood flow through the blood vessels. This classification generally excludes those conditions that affect the aorta and coronary arteries, which have a more direct relationship to the heart (see Chapter 25) and the cerebral vessels (Chapter 37). Specific alterations in arterial and venous blood flow in the lower and upper extremities are discussed in this chapter. Lymphedema is included because the lymphatic system complements the function of the vascular system. In addition, a section on hypertension is included because it is a major contributing factor to peripheral vascular problems.

ANATOMY AND PHYSIOLOGY

All the cells of the body depend on an intact and functioning vascular system. This vascular system is a closed circuit consisting of the systemic and pulmonary circulations. Blood circulates from the left side of the heart to the tissues and back to the right side of the heart. It then flows through the lungs and back to the left side of the heart. The main components of the vascular system are the arteries, capillaries, and veins. The vascular system is aided by the lymphatic system, which contains lymph vessels and nodes.

Arteries

Arteries are thick-walled vessels that transport oxygenated blood via the aorta away from the heart and to the tissues. As the arteries approach the tissues, they branch into smaller vessels called arterioles (Fig. 26-1). All arteries are composed of the following three basic tissue layers:

1. Inner layer of endothelium (intima)
2. Middle layer of connective tissue, smooth muscle, or elastic fibers (media)
3. Outer layer of connective tissue (adventitia)

The media comprises the major part of the vessel wall. In the large arteries the media is primarily composed of elastic and connective tissue, which enables the artery to respond to alterations of blood volume while maintaining a constant flow. Arterial constrictions (decreased arterial diameter) increases resistance to blood flow. There is much less elastic fiber in the smaller arteries and arterioles; these vessels have smooth muscle that contracts and relaxes through nervous, chemical, and hormonal factors.

Capillaries

The capillaries are minute, thin-walled vessels located in the tissues and are composed of a single layer of cells. The capillaries connect the arterioles to the smallest veins and venules, allowing for the exchange of essential cellular products. Nutrients, oxygen, and regulatory substances move into the cells, whereas waste products, carbon dioxide, and cellular secretions move from the cells into the blood.

Veins

Veins are thin-walled vessels that transport deoxygenated blood from the capillaries back to the right side of the heart. They are composed of three layers: intima, media, and adventitia. Unlike the arterial walls, there is little

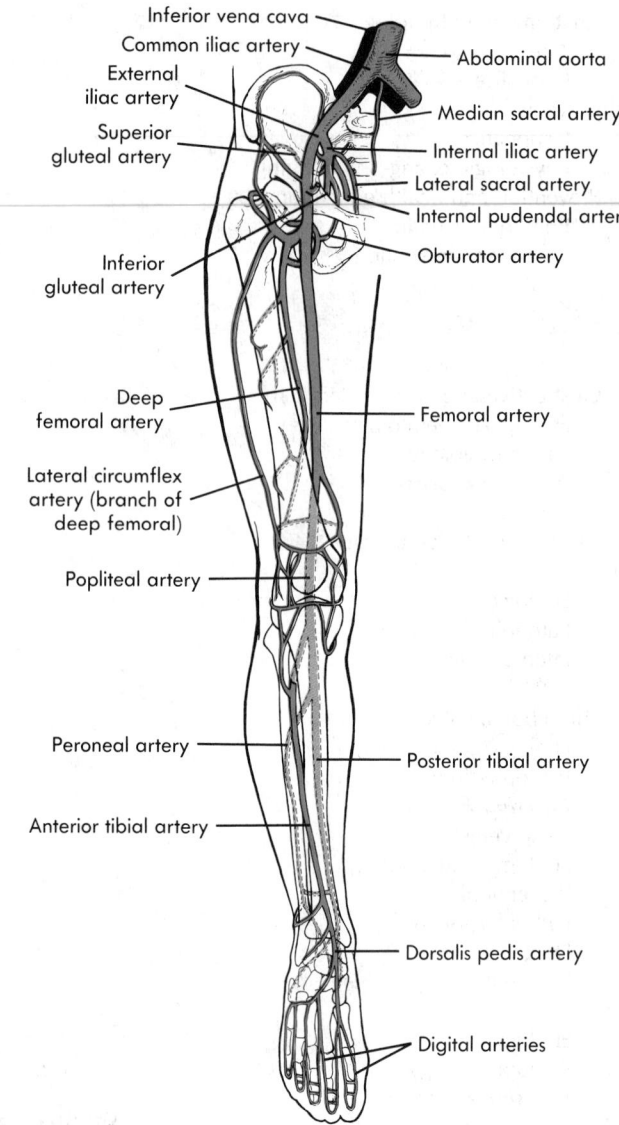

Fig. 26-1 Major arteries of lower limb. (From Seeley RR, Stephens TD, and Tate P: *Anatomy & physiology*, ed 2, St. Louis, 1992, Mosby–Year Book.)

smooth muscle and connective tissue. This make the veins distensible, enabling larger volumes of blood to accumulate. The sympathetic nervous system innervates the veins, causing vasoconstriction, decreased venous volume, and increased circulating blood volume. Major veins, particularly those in the lower extremities (Fig. 26-2) have one-way valves that allow blood to flow against gravity.

Lymphatics

The lymphatic vessels carry lymph from the tissues back into the venous circulation. This system is made up of small thin vessels located throughout the body in close proximity to the veins (Fig. 26-3). The lymphatics begin as capillaries that drain the tissues of lymph (a fluid similar to plasma) and tissue fluid containing cells, cellular debris,

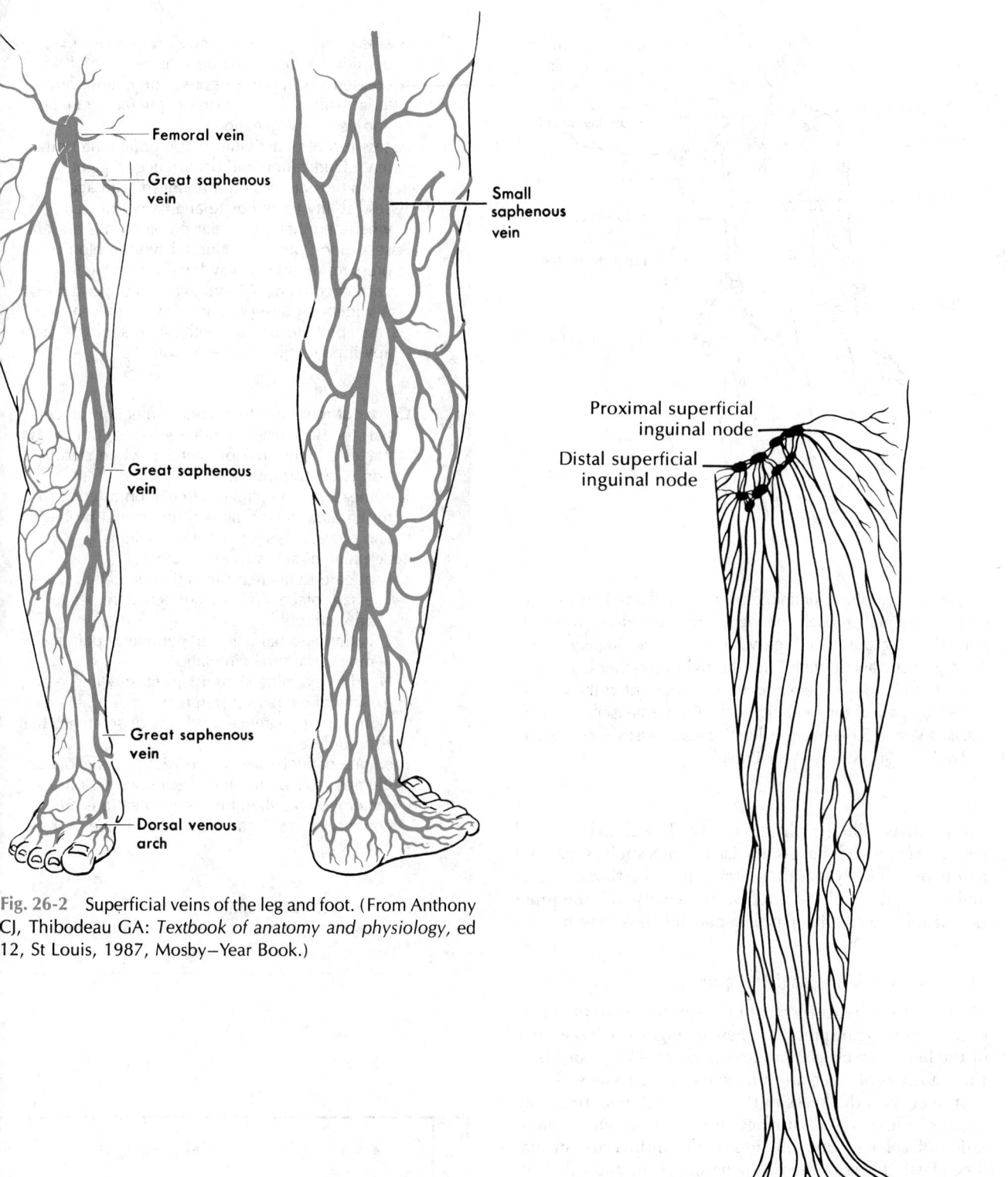

Fig. 26-2   Superficial veins of the leg and foot. (From Anthony CJ, Thibodeau GA: *Textbook of anatomy and physiology,* ed 12, St Louis, 1987, Mosby—Year Book.)

Fig. 26-3   Superficial lymphatics of medial aspect of lower extremity (after Sappey). (From Francis CC, Martin AH: *Introduction to human anatomy,* ed 7, St Louis, 1975, Mosby—Year Book.)

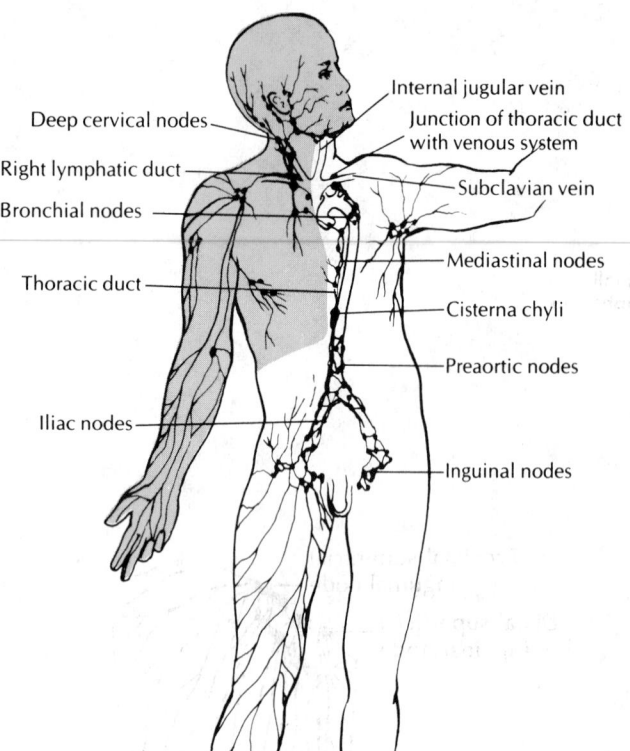

Fig. 26-4   Lymphatic drainage pathways. Shaded area of the body is drained through the right lymphatic duct, which is formed by the union of three vessels: the right jugular trunk, the right subclavian trunk, and the right bronchomediastinal trunk. Lymph from the remainder of the body enters the venous system by way of the thoracic duct. (From Malasanos L, Barkauskas V, and Stoltenberg-Allen K: *Health assessment,* ed. 4, St Louis, 1990, Mosby–Year Book.)

and proteins. The lymph flows through oval bodies called *lymph nodes,* which remove noxious agents such as bacteria and toxins. The lymph then drains into the thoracic duct and the right lymphatic duct, which empty into the junction of the internal jugular vein and subclavian vein (Fig. 26-4).

Physiologic Changes with Aging

Degenerative changes occur in the vascular system as part of the normal aging process. These changes affect the walls of the blood vessels and predispose persons to problems in the transport of blood and nutrients to the tissues. There is an increased thickness in the intima wall resulting from fibrosis. Further wall stiffness is caused by an accumulation of collagen and calcium in the intima and media. The elastic fibers of the media become thin and calcified. These changes markedly decrease the elasticity and flexibility of the vessels and hence increase peripheral vascular resistance, causing a rise in blood pressure. There is less blood flow through the vessels, leading to a decreased supply of oxygen and nutrients coupled with the accumulation of cellular secretions, waste products, and carbon dioxide. Gerontologic considerations for care are described in the box entitled "The elderly with peripheral vascular problems."

The Elderly with Peripheral Vascular Problems

Assessment

Assess peripheral pulses and skin of lower extremities of all elderly persons because of decreased vasomotor response and changes in arterial walls that decrease peripheral circulation and tissue oxygenation.

Assess extent of activities that produce intermittent claudication and occurrence at night; symptoms are more pronounced with age.

Assess ability to ambulate and carry out ADL when peripheral vascular problems are present.

Assess blood pressure. Normal systolic blood pressure in elderly may be 160 mm Hg (as compared with 140 mm Hg in younger adults). A widened pulse pressure may be present.

Assess ability to comply with pharmacologic therapy if patient has hypertension.

Intervention

Carry out measures to decrease infection potential; the decreased immune response of elderly places a higher risk of infection when circulation is compromised.

Use measures to increase circulation to compromised area: lower the legs for arterial problems and elevate legs for venous problems.

Teach patient and significant other:

Foot care to decrease infection potential; if necessary place lamb's wool between toes to prevent rubbing.

Location and palpation of peripheral pulses to monitor arterial circulation.

Need to examine skin of legs closely and report signs of decreased skin temperature, changes in skin appearance, and cuts or scratches that do not heal.

Facilitate patient compliance with pharmacologic therapy of hypertension. Decreased vision and remembering when to take medications are common factors that affect compliance of the elderly.

Common disorders in elderly

Arteriosclerosis obliterans
Leg ulcers from chronic deep vein insufficiency
Hypertension

26-1

Risk factors for peripheral vascular disorders

Cigarette smoking
Hypertension
Hyperlipidemia
Obesity
Physical inactivity
Emotional stress
Diabetes mellitus
Family history of atherosclerosis

PREVENTION AND HEALTH EDUCATION
Primary Prevention

Primary prevention is the most important means for reducing the incidence of peripheral vascular disorders. Nurses in all clinical settings can provide health education about the risk factors that affect development of peripheral vascular disorders. Because these disorders normally develop with advancing age, all individuals can benefit from this information, particularly those in the elderly age groups.

The risk factors associated with the development of peripheral vascular disorders are listed in Box 26-1. These factors are similar to those of other forms of cardiovascular diseases (Chapter 25). Specific health teaching is discussed on p. 713.

Cigarette smoking

Smoking is one of the major contributory factors in the development of peripheral vascular problems. Nicotine causes vasoconstriction and spasms of the arteries, thus reducing circulation to the extremities. The carbon monoxide inhaled in cigarette smoke reduces oxygen transport to the tissues.

Hypertension

Hypertension causes the elastic tissue in the arteries to be replaced by fibrous collagen tissue. This makes the arterial wall less distensible and increases the resistance to blood flow (p. 734).

Hyperlipidemia

Hyperlipidemia refers to the elevation of lipids, such as cholesterol and triglycerides, within the blood. Cholesterol and triglycerides contribute to the development of atherosclerotic plaques in the vessels (see Chapter 25).

Obesity

Obesity, or excess body weight in relation to height, places an added burden on the heart and blood vessels. Excess fat compromises blood vessels and contributes to increased venous congestion. Obese individuals are also more prone to physical inactivity, diabetes, hypertension, and hyperlipidemia.

Physical inactivity

Physical activity promotes muscle contraction and relaxation. It improves the return of venous blood to the heart by the pumping of muscle on the veins and aids in the development of collateral circulation, which is useful for venous return when veins are blocked.

Emotional stress

Emotional stress stimulates the sympathetic nervous system and causes peripheral vasoconstriction. Stress can also cause increased cholesterol and platelet levels, decreased clotting time, and sustained high blood pressure.

Diabetes mellitus

The exact mechanism by which diabetes contributes to the development of peripheral vascular disorders is unknown. The changes in glucose and fat metabolism are thought to affect the atherosclerotic processes.

Secondary Prevention

Secondary prevention is important because peripheral vascular disorders can become chronic and potentially disabling diseases. Persons with peripheral vascular disorders are subject to periods of exacerbation and complications such as infection, injury, thrombosis, and amputation. Persons with early symptoms are encouraged to seek medical care. Increasing the person's knowledge of the specific disorder and prevention of future occurrences is essential.

MAJOR HEALTH PROBLEMS OF THE PERIPHERAL VASCULAR SYSTEM

Changes in the peripheral vascular system may cause local arterial or venous disorders or may result in a systemic effect (for example, hypertension). Major peripheral vascular disorders that are discussed in this chapter include the following:

1. Arterial disorders
   a. Atherosclerosis
   b. Arteriosclerosis obliterans
   c. Thromboangiitis obliterans (Buerger's disease)
   d. Arterial embolism
   e. Aneurysm of lower extremity
   f. Raynaud's disease
2. Arteriovenous fistula
3. Venous disorders
   a. Thrombophlebitis
   b. Varicose veins
4. Leg ulcers
5. Lymphedema
6. Hypertension

ARTERIAL DISORDERS

Any disturbance in the structure of the arteries interferes with transport of blood from the heart to the tissues. The result is diminished blood and decreased oxygen and nutrients to the tissues. The symptoms of arterial disease are not caused by the degree of obstruction or narrowing but by the degree to which the involved body part is deprived of circulation. This in turn is affected by such factors as blood pressure and presence or absence of collateral circulation.

Signs and symptoms, and medical therapy for the various types of arterial disorders are listed in Table 26-1.

Table 26-1 Arterial disorders

Disease	Signs and symptoms	Medical therapy
Arteriosclerosis obliterans	Early: intermittent claudication, low skin temperature, diminished or absent arterial pulses distal to the obstruction, audible bruits	Cessation of cigarette smoking Regular exercise program Drug therapy with vasodilators (controversial)
	Late: burning pain at rest, pallor or cyanosis, persistent reddish-blue discoloration, dry shiny skin, loss of hair on legs, deformed toenails, numbness and tingling, ulceration and gangrene of toes and foot	Weight reduction Low-fat and low-cholesterol diets, antilipemic medications Control of hypertension and diabetes Surgery: removal of occlusion, bypass of occlusion Percutaneous transluminal angioplasty
Thromboangiitis obliterans	Pain in digits at rest, sensitivity to cold, intermittent claudication in arm or hand, reduced or absent distal pulses, digits pale or persistently red, numbness and tingling, ulceration and gangrene of digits	Cessation of smoking Keep body warm Prevent injury to feet and hands Drug therapy with vasodilators (controversial) Surgery: sympathectomy to decrease arterial spasms, amputation of areas of ulceration and gangrene
Arterial embolism	Sudden onset of pain, coldness, and numbness Burning or aching pain distal to occlusion Muscular weakness Diminished or absent pulses distal to occlusion Skin pallor or cyanosis Signs and symptoms of shock	Bed rest Drug therapy: anticoagulants, fibrinolytics (streptokinase) Treatment of shock Surgery: embolectomy
Aneurysm of the extremity	May be asymptomatic Large pulsatile mass in area of artery Audible bruit Pain, coldness, and numbness distal to aneurysm	Drug therapy to control hypertension Surgery: removal of aneurysm
Raynaud's disease	Chronically cold hands and feet Vasospastic attack in digits: pallor, cyanosis, coldness, numbness, occasional pain After attack: intense redness, tingling, or throbbing Symptoms intensify with cold and emotional stress Ulcerations of fingertips in advanced cases	Protection against exposure to cold Cessation of cigarette smoking Drug therapy: calcium antagonists, vascular smooth muscle relaxants, vasodilators Biofeedback Surgery: sympathectomy, amputation of areas of ulceration and gangrene

OBSTRUCTIVE ARTERIAL DISORDERS

Arterial disorders that may lead to arterial obstruction include arteriosclerosis obliterans, thromboangiitis obliterans, arterial embolism, and aneurysm of lower extremity.

Etiology/Epidemiology
Arteriosclerosis obliterans

Arteriosclerosis obliterans is a disorder in which there is segmented arteriosclerotic narrowing or obstruction of the intima and media of vessel walls. It results from advanced atherosclerotic plaque formation, and the risk factors are similar to those for atherosclerosis. Arteriosclerosis obliterans is the most common cause of arterial obstructive disease in the extremities of persons over age 30. It affects men more than women, with clinical symptoms evident in persons between ages 50 and 70. In the person with diabetes, the disease becomes more progressive, affecting the smaller arteries, primarily below the knee.

Thromboangiitis obliterans

This disorder, also called Buerger's disease, is an episodic and segmental obstructive and inflammatory disorder of the arteries and veins. It typically occurs in men between ages 20 and 40 and has been reported in all races. Although the cause is unknown, it almost always occurs in men who smoke.

Arterial embolism

Arterial emboli are blood clots floating in arterial blood. These clots most commonly originate in the heart as a result of atrial fibrillation, myocardial infarction, or congestive heart failure. The clots may also be associated with immobility, anemia, and dehydration.

Aneurysms of lower extremity

An aneurysm is an enlarged, dilated portion of an artery. Although it may follow trauma, such as an automobile accident, it is most commonly associated with atherosclerosis. Aneurysms of the lower extremity, particularly in the popliteal area (Fig. 26-5), are more common in persons over age 60 who have pronounced arteriosclerosis.

Pathophysiology
Atherosclerosis

Atherosclerosis is generally viewed as a type of arteriosclerosis or as a part of the aging process. This disease involves the development of lesions in the intimal wall.

Three types of lesions have been identified: (1) fatty streaks, which consist of smooth-muscle cells and lipid deposits that are present in all individuals, although they do not necessarily progress to produce disease; (2) fibrous plaques, which involve a thickening of the intima and are surrounded by lipids, collagen, smooth muscle cells, and plasma components; and (3) the complicated lesion that is a large mass consisting of calcified fibrous plaques.

The result of atherosclerosis is narrowing of the artery, which progresses to obstruction, thrombosis, aneurysm development, and rupture. In addition, nutrients and oxygen to the tissues can be reduced, resulting in ischemic necrosis of the tissue cells. (For further information on atherosclerosis, see Chapter 25.)

Arteriosclerosis obliterans

The primary lesion of arteriosclerosis obliterans is plaque formation on the intimal wall that causes partial or complete occlusion. In addition, there is calcification of the media and the gradual loss of elasticity that further weakens the arterial wall and predisposes the patient to aneurysmal dilation or thrombus formation. As a result, the artery is unable to transport an adequate blood volume to the tissues during exercise or at rest. Symptoms appear when the blood vessels can no longer supply the tissue with required nutrients and remove wastes.

The most common symptom of arterial insufficiency, *intermittent claudication*, occurs with exercise and consists of pain that develops during exercise in a muscle that has an inadequate blood supply. It is described as a cramp that disappears within 1 to 2 minutes of cessation of exercise. The pain is usually bilateral but may be unilateral. The muscles of the calf are more frequently affected because the femoral artery is often involved.

A gnawing or burning pain occurring at rest, especially at night, is indicative of severe disease. Feelings of coldness, numbness, and tingling may also occur concurrently with pain. In advanced disease, the ischemia may lead to necrosis, ulceration, and gangrene (particularly of the toes and distal foot) because of the decreased circulation.

Thromboangiitis obliterans (Buerger's disease)

In contrast to arteriosclerosis obliterans, this disorder develops in the small arteries and veins, primarily in the feet and hands, although the wrists and lower leg may also be involved. Symptoms are most always a result of occlusion of the arteries, leading to ischemia, complicated in later stages by infection. The main characteristic is inflammatory infiltration of vessel walls. Different segments of arteries may be involved. The process is intermittent, and arteries may recannulize during quiescent periods.

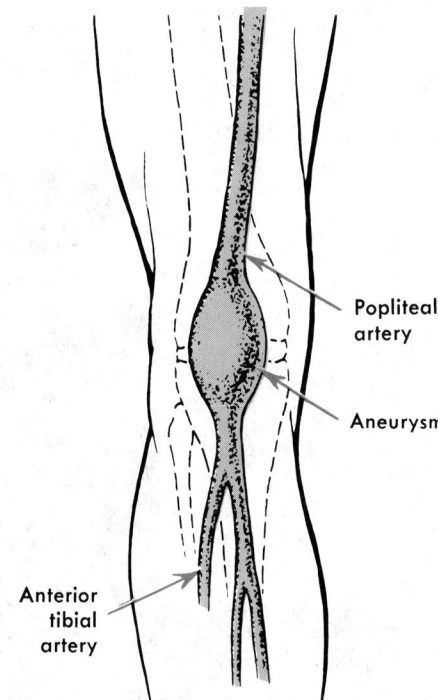

Fig. 26-5   Posterior view of the knee with an aneurysm of the popliteal artery. (From Anderson HC: *Newton's geriatric nursing*, ed 5, St Louis, 1971, Mosby—Year Book.)

The most common symptom is pain with exercise in the arch of the foot or instep claudication. With involvement of the hands, the pain is usually bilaterally symmetric. Pain at rest is frequent and persistent, particularly in the person with atherosclerosis. Changes in skin color or temperature, sensitivity to cold, and ulcers or gangrene of the digits may be present. Superficial thrombophlebitis is a common early sign.

Arterial embolism

A blood clot may become detached from the site of origin and travel through the arterial circulation. The embolus is frequently a fragment of arteriosclerotic plaque loosened from the aorta. Emboli tend to lodge in the bifurcation of arteries, especially in the femoral or popliteal arteries causing obstruction. Blood flow to sites distal to the lodged embolus is impaired, and ischemia occurs. Signs and symptoms depend on the size of the embolus, the presence of collateral circulation, and the proximity to a major organ. Abrupt cessation of blood flow causes severe pain. Distal pulses are absent, and the extremity becomes cold, numb, and pale. Shock may develop if an embolus blocks a large artery.

Aneurysm of lower extremity

Destruction of the medial layer of an artery leads to weakening of the arterial wall and to the eventual formation of an aneurysm. Thrombi form at the site of the aneurysm and break off, forming emboli that may travel and obstruct more distal portions of the artery. Symptoms of an aneu-

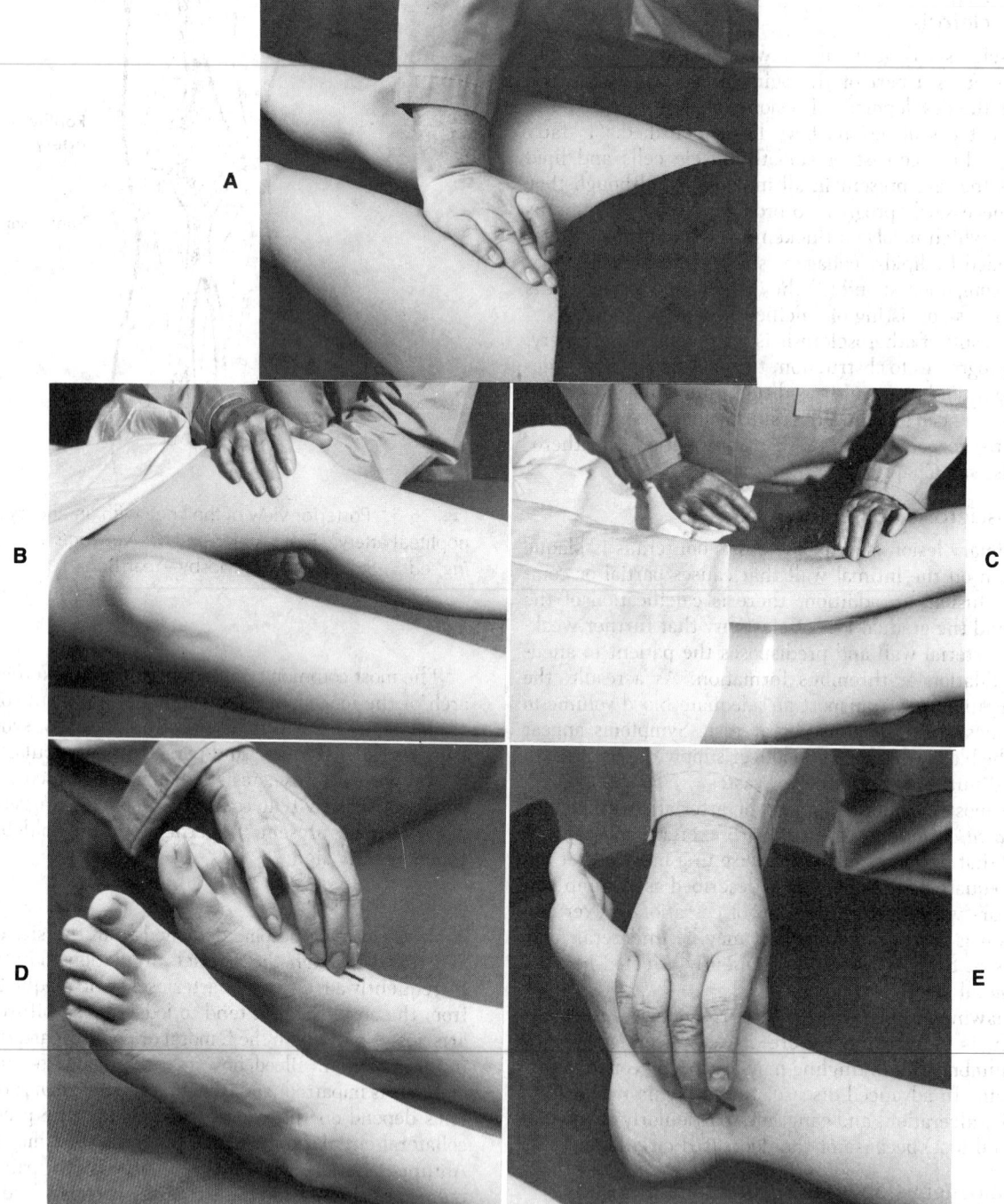

Fig. 26-6   Palpation of peripheral pulses. **A,** Femoral pulse. **B,** Popliteal pulse (recumbent position). **C,** Popliteal pulse (prone position). **D,** Dorsal pedal pulse. **E,** Posterior tibial pulse. (From Malasanos L, et al: *Health assessment,* ed 3, St Louis, 1985, Mosby–Year Book.)

rysm may be absent. A large pulsating mass may be palpated at the site of the aneurysm.

Nursing Process
Assessment

Data collection for the person with arterial insufficiency focuses on noted changes in the circulation of the extremities and possible causative factors.

Subjective data

1. Onset of symptoms: slow and progressive or sudden
2. Changes noted in skin color and temperature of extremities
3. Discomfort or pain in extremities: onset, location, quality, and occurrence with exercise or at rest
4. Effect on extremities of cold temperatures, cigarette smoking, or emotional stress
5. Effectiveness of measures used to relieve discomfort or pain
6. Presence of risk factors: cigarette smoking; physical inactivity; obesity; emotional stress; history of hypertension, hyperlipidemia, or diabetes; family history of atherosclerosis

Objective data

1. Skin changes indicating tissue anoxia:
   a. Appearance: shiny, taut, absence of hair on extremities (indicates lack of tissue oxygen)
   b. Color: pallor, redness, cyanosis
   c. Temperature: coldness
   d. Presence of ulcerations or gangrene
2. Condition of nail beds: opaque, thickened, capillary refill >3 seconds
3. Peripheral pulses (Fig. 26-6): presence and quality (*Note:* compare bilaterally)
4. Presence of audible bruit or palpable thrill over artery indicating turbulent flow through a narrowed vessel
5. Symmetry of extremities
6. Sensation in extremities: numbness, tingling
7. Muscle tone: weakness, loss of tone
8. Effectiveness of prescribed medications

Diagnostic tests

Several tests may be used in the diagnosis of arterial disorders. Noninvasive diagnostic tests such as segmental limb pressure and pulse volume recordings are often used. These diagnostic tests are outlined in Table 26-2.

Data analysis: nursing diagnoses

Nursing diagnoses are determined from analysis of patient data. Possible nursing diagnoses for the person with an obstructed arterial disorder may include, but are not limited to, the following:

Diagnostic title	Possible etiologies
Activity intolerance	Imbalance between oxygen supply and demand; immobility
Infection, high risk for	Lack of knowledge
Injury, high risk for	Sensorimotor deficits
Knowledge deficit	Lack of exposure, recall
Skin integrity, impaired, high risk for	Immobility, tissue anoxia
Tissue perfusion, altered peripheral	Decreased arterial blood flow

Planning: expected patient outcomes

Expected patient outcomes for the person with an obstructed arterial disorder may include, but are not limited to, the following:

1. Performs measures to increase peripheral perfusion.
2. Participates in activity, with a balance between activity and rest.
3. Describes ways to prevent skin lesions, infection, and injury.
4. Describes risk factors that may compromise arterial circulation and plans to avoid these factors, follows prescribed medication regimen, and plans for ongoing care.

Implementation
Assisting with achievement of therapeutic goals
Medications

The most frequently used medications to treat obstructive arterial disorders include anticoagulants, fibrinolytics, and vasodilators. *Anticoagulants* are used to prolong clotting time, thus preventing extension of a clot and inhibiting further clot formation. Heparin and warfarin sodium (Table 26-3) are the most commonly administered anticoagulants. *Fibrinolytics,* or thrombolytics, are useful in dissolving existing thrombi when rapid dissolution of the clot is required to preserve organ and limb function. Streptokinase and urokinase (Table 26-4) impair hemostasis by increasing fibrinolytic activity. After infusion of fibrinolytics, the patient is started on heparin or oral anticoagulants to prevent clot extension or formation. Guidelines for the care of the patient receiving anticoagulant or fibrinolytic therapy is described in Box 26-2. The use of *vasodilators* is controversial; most studies indicate that these drugs are not effective.

Interventions to achieve patient outcomes
Promoting tissue perfusion

Nursing interventions are directed toward activities that promote tissue oxygenation and include the following:

1. Maintain a warm environmental temperature of about 21° C. (70° F.).
2. Place legs in *slight dependency* (uses gravity to enhance tissue perfusion) and avoid elevating legs (impedes arterial flow).
3. Avoid pressure on affected extremity; use padding for severe ischemia.
4. Avoid vigorous massage of extremities (may promote embolus formation).
5. Teach patients to carry out above activities in addition to the following:
   a. Avoid chilling (causes vasoconstriction) and exposure to cold; layer clothing in cold weather.
   b. Avoid constrictive clothing that impedes circulation: rolled garters, socks with tight banding, girdles, tight waistbands, and tight shoelaces.
   c. Avoid crossing legs at knees (places pressure on arteries of legs).
   d. Quit smoking (nicotine causes vasoconstriction

Table 26-2   Diagnostic tests for arterial disorders

Test	Purpose	Procedure	Comments
Doppler ultraso-nography	Evaluate vascular network (arteries, veins) Measure blood flow through vessels Monitor status of bypass grafts	High-frequency sound waves directed to artery or veins through hand-held transducer moved evenly across skin surface; audible tone produced proportional to blood velocity	No discomfort experienced Noninvasive Explain to patient that noise will be heard
Segmental limb pressure	Evaluate arterial occlusion	Systolic pressure readings from each limb segment obtained by pneumatic pressure cuffs and Doppler probe; readings compared	Noninvasive
Pulse volume recordings	Substantiate diagnosis of arterial stenosis and occlusion	Pneumatic pressure cuffs attached to extremities; pressure changes recorded by pressure transducer as wave forms during cuff inflation and deflation	Useful to assess areas such as foot and toes, not easily evaluated by segmental limb pressure
Exercise testing	Determine amount of exercise that precipitates ischemia and claudication	Ankle pressure, pulse volume, and blood pressure measured while person walks on treadmill at specific speed for about 5 min or until onset of leg pain	Exercise should be stopped at onset of pain
Radionuclide scan	Visualize vascular system and detect changes in blood vessels Assess arterial blood flow; determine perfusion pressure Identify arterial obstruction or vascular abnormality Determine patency of bypass graft	Injection of radionuclide followed by scanning of area at predetermined intervals to determine accumulation of radionuclide	Explain to patient that radiation dose is usually less than that received from diagnostic x-rays Check for allergy to iodine, shellfish
Arteriography (angiography)	Visualize arterial system and detect vascular changes Assess arterial blood flow Identify arterial obstruction, vascular abnormality, or aneurysm	Dye injected through catheter inserted into femoral or brachial artery, followed by x-ray films	Transient flushing and burning sensation felt when dye is injected Posttest assessment includes the following: 1. Injection site for bleeding, hematoma, and swelling, especially thigh 2. Peripheral pulses distal to site qh for 4-8h 3. Allergic reation to dye (dyspnea, flushing, hives, nausea, vomiting) 4. Sensation distal to site Encourage patient to drink fluids to facilitate excretion of dye
Digital subtraction angiography	Visualize vascular system Determine presence and extent of occlusion	Dye injected through catheter inserted into blood vessel; x-ray signals are digitized	Same as for arteriography
Transcutaneous oxymetry	Evaluate severity of limb ischemia Assess healing of ulcers Determine level of amputation	Sensors placed on skin to measure oxygen diffusion gradient between electrode and capillaries	Explain to patient that measurements may be taken in several positions
Magnetic resonance imaging (MRI)	Evaluate vascular network (arteries, veins) Measure blood flow velocities Assess stages of vascular disease	Radiofrequency pulses excite protons, which give a signal creating an image	Explain to patient that the space is very tight Noise level may be high; ear plugs provided

Table 26-3   Anticoagulants used in treatment of vascular disorders

Drug	Action	Dosage	Side effects
Heparin	Forms complex with antithrombin III which inhibits thrombin action Intravenous route produces immediate action; duration is 2 h Subcutaneous route used for maintenance and prophylaxis	Intravenous: Loading dose 5000 U Continuous drip: 20,000-30,000 U/day at 0.5 U/kg/min in 5% dextrose or NS Intermittent: initial loading dose, then 5000-10,000 U q4h Subcutaneous: 5000 U 2 h before surgery and every 8-12 h thereafter Other: 10,000-12,000 U q8h 14,000-20,000 U q12h NOTE: dosage adjusted to maintain APTT at 2-2.5 times laboratory control Normal APTT = 33-45 sec Prolonged APTT = 60-100 sec	Hemorrhage, spontaneous bleeding, epistaxis, bleeding gums, hematoma, GI bleeding with black tarry stools
Warfarin sodium (Coumadin, Panwarfin)	Inhibits vitamin K dependent clotting factor synthesis (factors II, VII, IX and X) Depresses prothrombin activity Peaks in 36-72 h Duration is 2-5 days	Oral 10 to 15 mg/day until prothrombin time within therapeutic range Then 2 to 10 mg/day NOTE: dosage adjusted to maintain prothrombin time (PT) at 1.2 to 1.5 times laboratory control Normal PT = 11-12 sec Prolonged PT = 17-19 sec	Same as for heparin

Table 26-4   Fibrinolytics used in treatment of vascular disorders

Drug	Action	Dosage	Side effects
Streptokinase (Streptase, Kabikinase)	Synthetic protein derived from streptococcal bacteria Activates plasminogen by forming streptokinase-plasminogen complex	IV: Loading dose 250,000 IU over 30 min Then 100,000 IU/h for 24-72 h (arterial thrombosis) or 72 h (deep vein thrombosis)	Bleeding, bronchospasm, rash, urticaria
Urokinase (Abbokinase, Breokinase, Win-Kinase)	Human proteolytic enzyme derived from cultured kidney cells and urine Directly converts circulating plasminogen to plasmin	IV: Loading dose 4100 IU/kg over 10 min Then 4400 IU/kg/h for 12-24 h	Same as for streptokinase

The patient on anticoagulant or fibrinolytic therapy

Monitor the infusion accurately; maintain desired therapeutic rate of units per minute or hour.

Assess skin for signs of bleeding: bleeding gums, nosebleeds, petechiae (pinpoint red areas on skin), ecchymosis (bruising), hematoma formation, and venipuncture sites.

Monitor urine, stool, emesis, and gastric secretions for blood.

Avoid administration of medications by intramuscular route to prevent bleeding.

Avoid unnecessary bleeding.

Use a soft toothbrush and brush teeth gently.

Use an electric razor rather than razor blade for shaving.

Avoid use of rectal thermometers (may cause mucosal bleeding).

Special care with *anticoagulant therapy*

Give heparin by deep subcutaneous injection; use a fine gauge needle at a 90 degree angle; do not aspirate nor massage site after injection (can result in bleeding); rotate sites on a regular basis.

Administer protamine sulfate, if necessary, as a heparin antagonist to reverse anticoagulant effects.

Hold pressure for 3 to 5 minutes on venipuncture sites.

Monitor results of blood work: a partial thromboplastin time should be 2 times normal level (normal APTT is 33 to 45 seconds); a prothrombin time (PT) should be 1.2 to 1.5 times normal level (normal PT is 11 to 12 seconds).

Avoid use of aspirin; aspirin inhibits platelet adhesion, thus having an anticoagulant effect.

Special care with *fibrinolytic therapy*

Assess patient for signs of intracranial bleeding: headache, vomiting, disorientation, mental confusion.

Assess patient for signs of retroperitoneal bleeding: low back pain, muscle weakness, or numbness in lower extremity.

Avoid insertion of unnecessary venous and arterial lines; insert before initiation of therapy if necessary.

Hold pressure on all venipuncture or other bleeding sites for 20 to 30 minutes to promote blood clotting.

Give antiulcer medication, if prescribed, as a prophylactic measure.

General exercises

1. Engage in a regular aerobic exercise program that includes activities such as walking, swimming, jogging, or bicycling (see Chapter 5).
2. Do 30 to 45 minutes of activity with warm-up and cool-down activities on 3 alternate days.
3. Walk at a slow pace on a daily basis.

Special exercises

1. Perform the following Buerger-Allen exercises on a daily basis
   a. Lie flat with legs elevated above heart level for 2 to 3 minutes.
   b. Sit for 2 to 3 minutes with legs relaxed and slightly dependent.
   c. Flex, extend, invert, and evert feet for 30 seconds in each position.
   d. End by lying flat with legs at heart level and cover with warm blanket for 5 minutes.
2. Perform other exercises such as ankle rotations, ankle pumps, and knee extension on a daily basis.

Maintaining skin integrity and preventing infection

Because of decreased tissue oxygenation from decreased circulation, the skin is at high risk for breaking down and becoming infected. Nursing activities include examining the skin on a daily basis when the patient is hospitalized and encouraging the patient to be as mobile as possible. If redness or other signs of infection are noted, notify the physician. Teach the patient to monitor and protect the skin:

1. Assess skin on a daily basis for intactness, dryness, redness, and lesions; use mirror to inspect areas that are difficult to see, such as heels and plantar surface of toes.
2. Take a daily bath in tepid water (three times per week if skin is very dry).
   a. Use a neutral pH soap to prevent skin irritation.
   b. Wash gently; avoid scratching and vigorous rubbing.
   c. Dry skin gently.
   d. Lubricate skin with moisturizing agent; avoid using alcohol (dries skin).
3. Take meticulous care of feet.
   a. Bathe each toe and dry well.
   b. Use only prescribed foot powders.
   c. Wear clean cotton socks and change daily (synthetic fibers can cause irritation and do not absorb moisture).
4. Avoid wearing shoes that do not "breathe," such as those made of synthetic materials (prevents evaporation and contributes to fungal infections).
5. Avoid application of direct heat such as hot water.
6. Contact health care professional at onset of skin breakdown such as abrasions, lesions, or ulcerations.

Preventing injury

With decreased circulation to the extremities, sensation may decrease. Injuries may include cuts or abrasions, burns, and excessive pressure (leading to further ischemia). Teach the patient to carry out the following activities:

and vasospasms; inhaled carbon dioxide reduces oxygen-carrying capacity of blood).

Promoting activity

Activity improves circulation through muscle contraction and relaxation. Exercise also stimulates collateral circulation that increases blood flow to the ischemic area. Teach the patient to carry out general and specific exercises and to allow adequate time for rest between vigorous activities. Exercises include the following:

1. Wear comfortable protective shoes at all times (do not go barefoot); alternate shoes on a daily basis to allow for airing.
2. Trim nails carefully: Cut at regular intervals, soak in warm water to soften nails, use straight nail clippers, and avoid using scissors to prevent cutting skin.
3. Avoid scratching and rubbing feet to prevent abrasions.
4. Check water temperature carefully (ability to sense temperature may be decreased).
5. Seek medical advice for thickened or deformed nails, blisters, corns, calluses, and ulcerations (self-treatment may cause infection).

Facilitating patient learning

The patient is taught how to promote tissue perfusion, maintain skin integrity, and prevent infection and injury as described previously. In addition, teach the patient the medication regimen and importance of taking the prescribed medications. Special instructions for the patient receiving oral anticoagulant therapy at home are listed in Box 26-3. The patient also needs to know that arterial disorders are usually chronic disorders and that medical follow-up is important to help prevent advanced disease with necrosis and ulcerations.

Evaluation

Questions to consider may include the following:
1. Does the patient perform measures to increase peripheral perfusion?
2. Is the patient able to tolerate activity and balance activity with rest?
3. Is the skin intact?
4. Have infection and injury been prevented?
5. Can the patient describe:
   a. Daily physical activity to be carried out?
   b. Risk factors to be avoided?
   c. Medication regimen?
   d. Plans for continued medical follow-up?

Surgery

Surgery is indicated for patients who have advanced arterial disease in which ischemic changes are present or for patients with severe pain that impairs their activities. These surgical procedures include arterial bypass surgery, embolectomy, percutaneous transluminal angioplasty, removal of aneurysm and closure of a fistula, sympathectomy, and amputation.

Arterial bypass surgery and reconstruction

If *arteriosclerosis obliterans* is rapidly progressing and intermittent claudication has become gravely disabling, surgery to correct the obstruction is indicated. The most common procedure is a bypass of the obstructed arterial segment, using prosthetic material such as Teflon or Dacron or autogenous (the patient's own) artery or vein, such as the saphenous vein (Fig. 26-7). The bypass may involve the aorta itself, as with an aortofemoral bypass, or more distal vessels, such as the femoral-popliteal bypass. Procedures that are performed either in conjunction with a bypass or by themselves include *patch grafting* (replacing a

---

Patient Teaching · **26-3**

The patient receiving oral anticoagulant therapy

Know general action and side effects of prescribed drug; avoid taking medications containing aspirin, which also has an anticoagulant effect.

Take the anticoagulant at the same time every day; do not stop taking it until advised by physician.

Check for signs of bleeding (gum bleeding, nosebleeds, bruising, cuts that do not stop bleeding with direct pressure, blood in urine or stool); report these signs promptly to health care professional.

Wear a Medic-Alert bracelet or carry an identification card containing the drug name, drug dosage, and physician's name in case of emergency.

Report for prescribed blood tests (APTT, PT) used to adjust drug dosage.

Do not add dark green and yellow vegetables to diet (contain vitamin K, which counteracts the anticoagulant drug effect).

Restrict alcohol intake (increases anticoagulant effect).

Guidelines for Care · **26-4**

The patient following arterial surgery of limbs

Monitor skin color and temperature distal to the graft site every hour.

Assess sensation and movement in the distal limb.

Assess peripheral pulses in the involved limb.
   Sudden absence of pulse may indicate thrombosis.
   Mark location of peripheral pulse with a pen to facilitate frequent assessment.
   Use a Doppler if pulses are difficult to palpate.
   Compare pulses of involved limb with pulses of noninvolved limb.

Monitor extremity for edema.

Check incision for redness, swelling, and drainage.

Monitor and immediately report signs of complication, such as increasing pain, fever, changes in drainage, absent or weakening pulse, change in skin color, limitation of movement, or paresthesia.

Promote circulation.
   Reposition patient every 2 hours.
   Tell patient not to cross legs.
   Use a footboard and overbed cradle to keep linens off extremity.
   Encourage progressive activity when permitted.

Avoid sharp flexion in the area of the graft.

Monitor for signs of bleeding secondary to anticoagulation therapy.

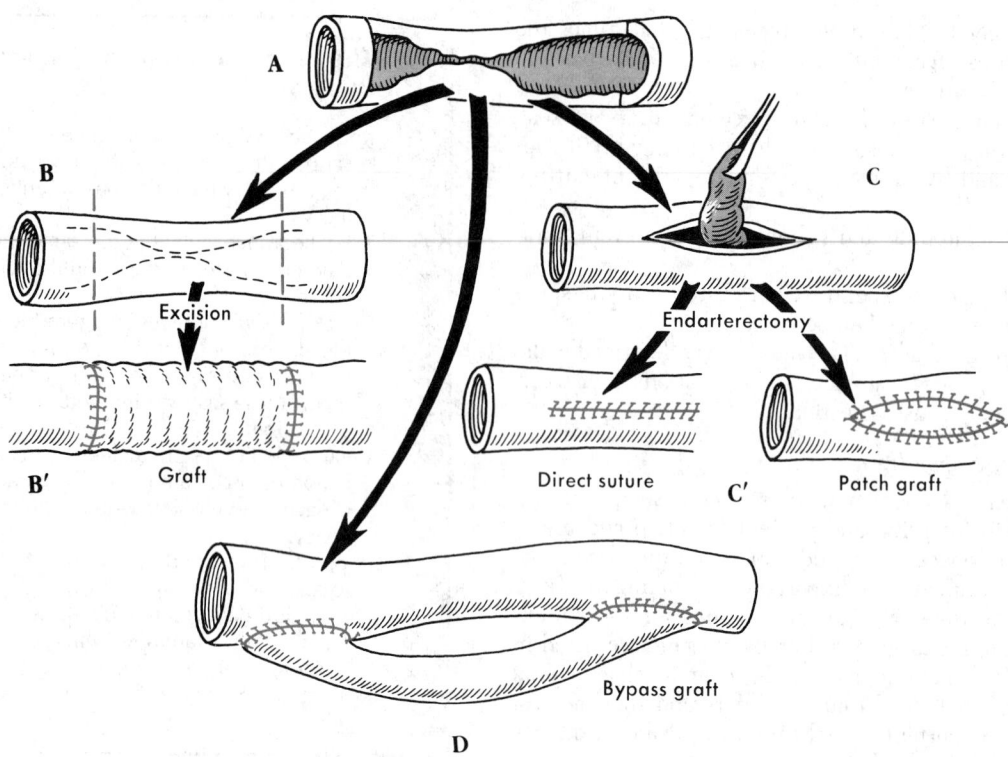

Fig. 26-7   **A,** Obstructed artery. Methods of restoring arterial blood flow include: **B** and **B'**, excision followed by grafting; **C** and **C'**, endarterectomy followed by either direct suture or patch graft; and **D,** bypass graft. (Redrawn from Juergens JL, et al: *Peripheral vascular disease,* Philadelphia, 1980, WB Saunders. By permission of Mayo Foundation.)

damaged segment of the arterial wall with a vein patch) and *endarterectomy* (stripping arteriosclerotic plaques from the intima and inner media using balloon catheters or other instruments). Care of the person with an aortic bypass graft is discussed under abdominal aneurysms in Chapter 25. Care following femoral-popliteal bypass is the same as for other arterial surgery (Box 26-4).

Embolectomy

An embolectomy is the surgical removal of a blood clot and is most often used when large arteries are obstructed. Success of the surgery depends on the length of time the extremity was ischemic; surgery must be performed within 6 to 10 hours to prevent muscle necrosis and loss of the extremity. Nursing care after embolectomy is described in Box 26-4. An endarterectomy, to remove the blood clot and strip the atherosclerotic plaque from the inner arterial wall, may also be performed.

Percutaneous transluminal angioplasty

Percutaneous transluminal angioplasty (PTA) may be used as surgical treatment for atherosclerotic obliterans or in the removal of a stenotic arterial graft. A specially designed catheter is inserted under fluoroscopy and advanced to the site of the obstruction. The balloon tip of the catheter is inflated to provide compression and rupture the atherosclerotic plaque. Thrombosis may occur after treatment; therefore, anticoagulants are usually prescribed. Care following PTA is similar to that following arterial surgery (Box 26-4).

Removal of aneurysm and closure of fistula

The blood vessel may be ligated unless the procedure is incompatible with the life of tissues distal to the lesion. Homografts or Teflon or Dacron grafts may be used in larger blood vessels of the extremities, either to replace the portion of the artery that contains the aneurysm or to bypass the abnormality. Fig. 26-8 illustrates the excision of an aneurysm and its replacement with a synthetic graft. Popliteal function is better at the flexion crease when the patient's own vein is used. Perioperative care is similar to that for the patient undergoing an embolectomy.

Amputation

Although a partial or complete amputation of an extremity may be necessary as a result of sarcoma or trauma, most amputations are indicated for patients with advanced atherosclerosis and gangrene of the extremities. The majority of amputations are of the lower extremity; the toes are the most amputated part of the body. An amputation may also be offered as an option to improve functional ability with a prosthesis.

The surgical goal is to remove the least amount of tissue possible and to create a stump adequate for the fitting of a prosthesis. The specific level of amputation is determined by the extent of the disease process. Below-knee (BK) amputations maintain knee function and allow for greater stability with a prosthesis. A BK amputation is usually done in the lower third of the leg, leaving a 12 to 18 cm stump. An above-knee (AK) amputation may be made at

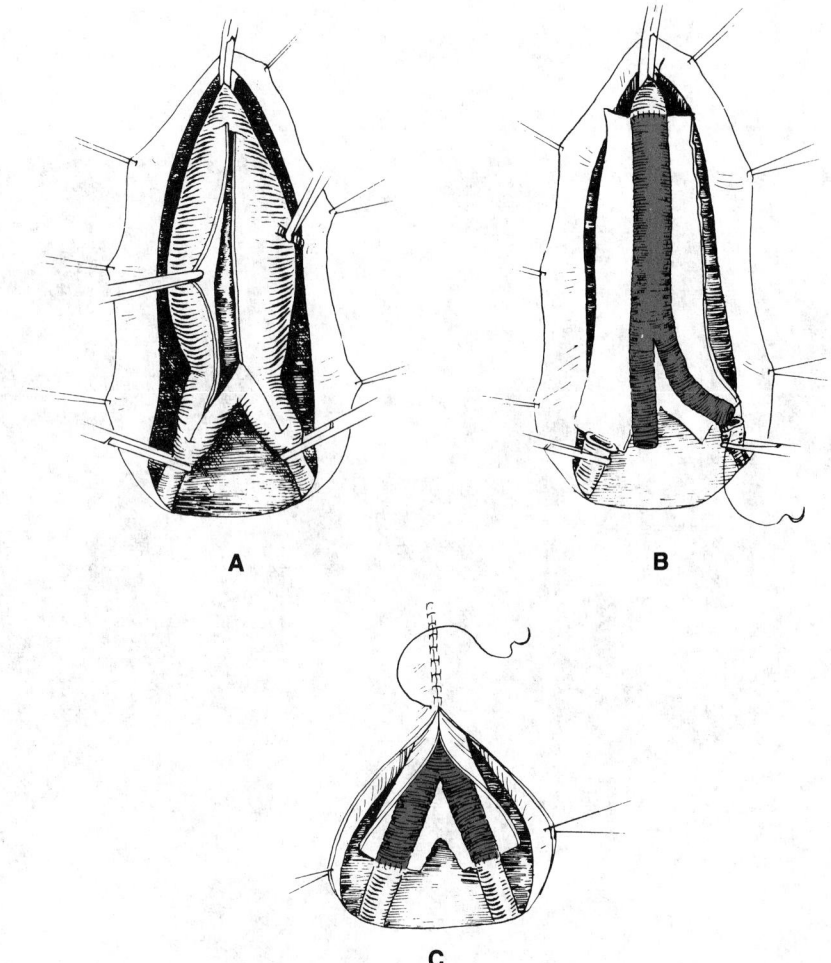

Fig. 26-8   Abdominal aneurysm. **A,** Aneurysm of aorta and iliac arteries. **B,** Bifurcation graft used to replace the excised aneurysm. **C,** Closure of the posterior peritoneum over the graft and suture line. (Redrawn from Crawford ES, et al: *Surg Clin North Am* 46:963-978, 1966.)

any level, although it is frequently below the middle of the thigh to preserve an adequate stump for satisfactory use of a prosthesis. AK amputations are often performed after unsuccessful BK amputations.

Amputation involves loss of a body part; therefore, feelings of grief related to loss are usually experienced. (For further discussion on loss and grief see Chapter 15). Before and after surgery the patient should exercise to strengthen arm and leg muscles to promote movement and ambulation and to prevent knee and hip contractures.

After surgery, most persons experience phantom sensations, or feelings related to the removed limb. About 10% of patients experience uncomfortable sensations (*phantom limb pain*) similar to the pain experienced before amputation or the sensation of a cramped or uncomfortable position. In most instances, this discomfort disappears with time, but the pain may become chronic for some persons. Even though the limb is removed, the pain is a real sensation and should not be dismissed as illusionary.

A *prosthesis* may be used immediately after or within 5 weeks of surgery. A cast may also be applied over the dressing to allow for attachment of a metal pylon prosthesis (Fig. 26-9). A permanent prosthesis is made 6 months after surgery to allow for stump shrinkage and molding.

Preoperative care includes the following:

1. Assist patient to express feelings, concerns, and fears; accept patient reaction of anger, discouragement, and grief.
2. Discuss postoperative regimen with patient and family.
   a. Frequent positioning to promote circulation
   b. Exercises to strengthen arm muscles for the use of crutches: push-ups and weight lifting
   c. Exercises to strengthen leg muscles to prevent knee and hip contractures and to promote ambulation: ankle rotations, ankle pumps, and quadriceps sets
3. Teach crutch walking if appropriate (usually done by physical therapist).

Text continued on p. 724.

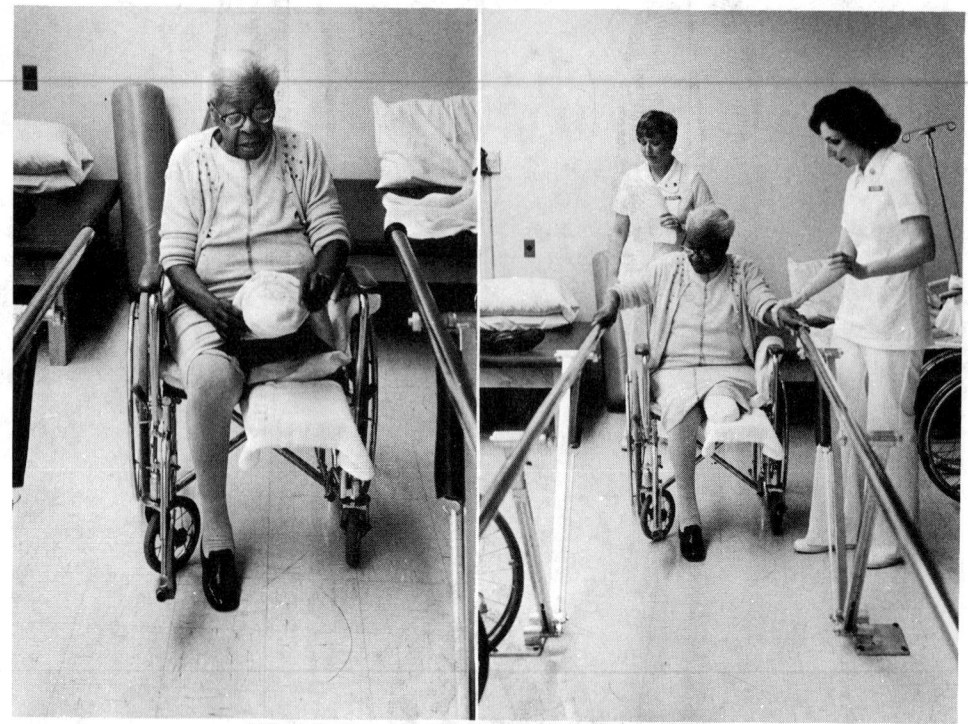

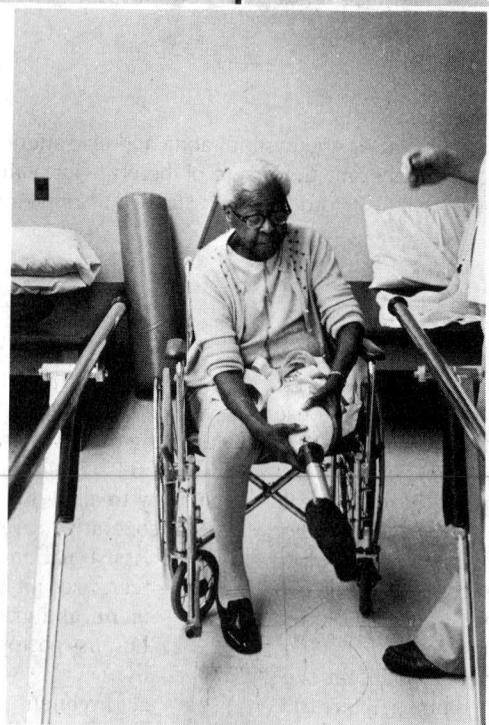

Fig. 26-9 Patient with cast on stump with metal pylon attached for weight bearing.

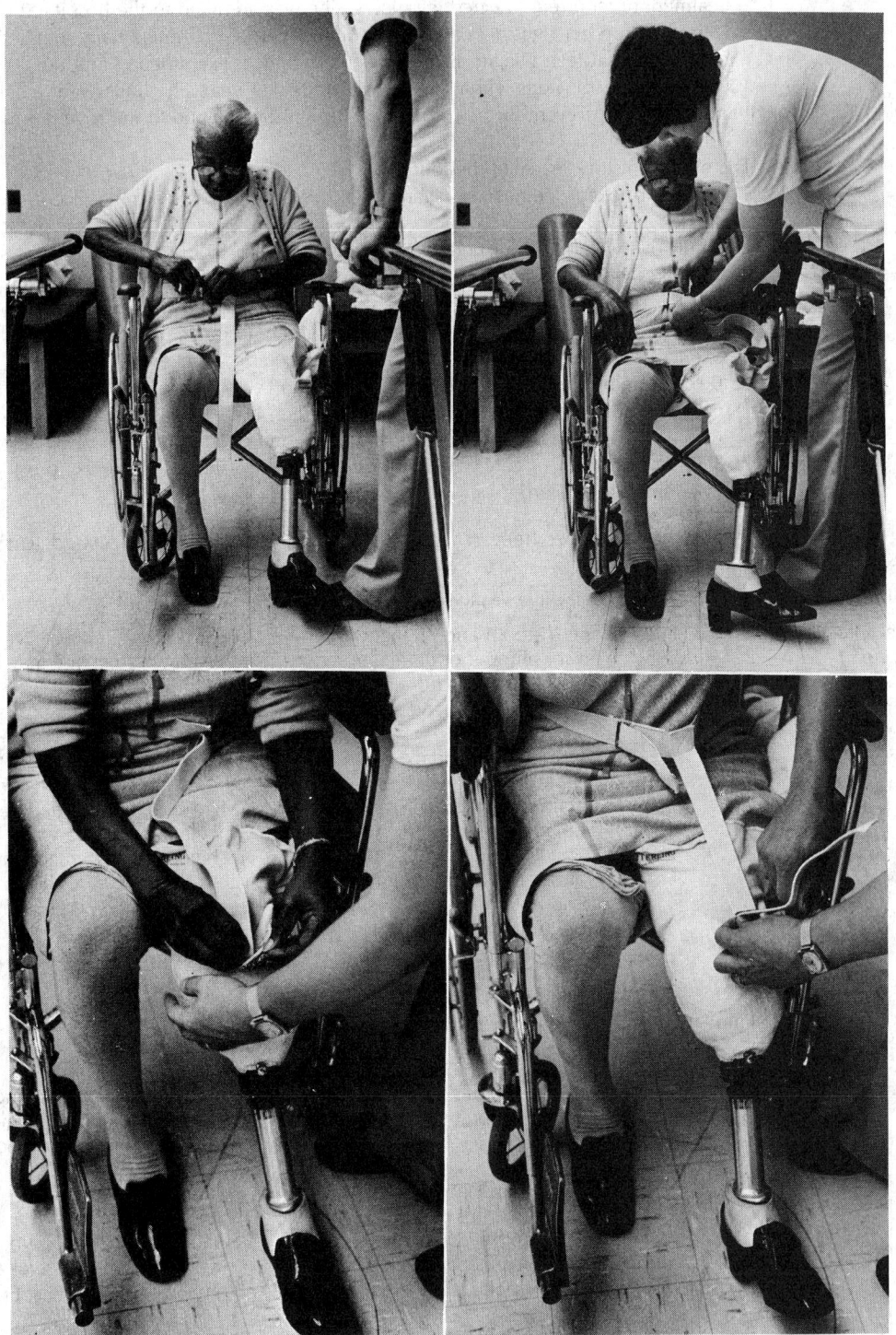

Fig. 26-9, cont'd.   Patient with cast on stump with metal pylon attached for weight bearing.

DATA: Mrs. R. is a 65-year-old widowed, retired sales clerk with a history of diabetes and peripheral vascular disease. During the past 3 years she has been in and out of the hospital for treatment of recurrent infected leg ulcers. She was admitted to the hospital 2 days ago with ulcers on her right heel and toes, complaining of cramplike pain with activity and a burning pain at rest. Diagnostic findings from clinical examination and tests revealed severe arterial occlusions within her bypass grafts of 1 year. She underwent a below-knee amputation to prevent further progression of her disease and to improve her functional ability.

The nursing history revealed the following:

1. She has smoked one pack of cigarettes per day for 40 years despite recent efforts to quit smoking.
2. She is overweight for her height: 5 feet 4 inches and 155 pounds.
3. She takes 24U NPH insulin every day to control her diabetes of 10 years duration.
4. She has not been able to prepare meals, clean house, or visit friends because of pain and discomfort in her legs and a decreased ability to move around.
5. She has been unsuccessful in establishing a regular daily exercise program.
6. Before surgery she said that she was resigned to be a "gimpy" for life; she had been expecting that she would eventually lose her leg, but she was concerned about how she would manage at home with meals, cleaning, and other chores.
7. She returned from surgery with a below-knee stump; she will receive a prosthesis after the stump has healed.

Nursing diagnosis: Injury, high risk for: hemorrhage, infection, and contractures related to surgery (BK amputation)

Expected patient outcomes	Nursing interventions	Rationale
Hemorrhage, infection, contractures do not occur	Monitor stump and drainage catheter for amount of drainage; report signs of increased drainage	Bleeding may occur from surgery; purulent drainage may be noted with infection
	Monitor vital signs and signs of shock	Severe bleeding may cause shock
	Apply pressure bandage over stump dressing	Pressure decreases bleeding and prevents fluid collection
	Maintain aseptic technique when changing dressing	Mrs. R. is diabetic and has poor circulation; therefore, she is at higher risk for infection
	Elevate stump on pillow, avoiding flexion of knee; place a support along outer side	Elevation decreases edema (from the trauma of surgery); contractures from constant knee flexion and outward rotation of leg interfere with use of prosthesis

Nursing diagnosis: Pain: in stump related to removal of lower leg

Expected patient outcomes	Nursing interventions	Rationale
Mrs. R. states she is feeling better	Provide analgesics as needed during early postoperative period	Analgesics may relieve incisional pain. Phantom limb pain is real pain and needs to be accepted as such
	Reinforce explanation of phantom limb pain if this occurs	
	Use other forms of pain management (such as backrubs, distraction, and relaxation exercises)	Nonmedicinal forms of pain management can be useful adjuncts to analgesics in reducing pain

Nursing diagnosis: Body image disturbance: related to loss of leg and change in body appearance

Expected patient outcomes	Nursing interventions	Rationale
Mrs. R. expresses feelings about loss of leg	Be aware that initial reaction after surgery may include shock and denial	Mrs. R. needs to begin to work through grieving process; an expression of feelings and obtaining support from family, friends, and nurse are helpful in working through this process
	Be accepting of Mrs. R.'s expression of frustration or anger	

Nursing diagnosis: Body image disturbance: related to loss of leg and change in body appearance—cont'd

Expected patient outcomes	Nursing interventions	Rationale
	Continue to provide Mrs. R. with opportunities to express feelings about the lost leg	
	Explain grief reactions if appropriate	
	Encourage supportive visits from family and friends	
	Encourage Mrs. R. to look at stump when ready	Looking at stump is the first step toward incorporating lost leg into new body image
Mrs. R. carries out ADL	Encourage Mrs. R. to move toward independence in ADL	Providing care to self and making decisions assist in regaining previous level of independent function and thus helps Mrs. R. feel better about self
Mrs. R. expresses confidence in self	Give Mrs. R. opportunity to make decisions about care when appropriate	

Nursing diagnosis: Impaired physical mobility: related to decreased strength and endurance, pain, loss of leg

Expected patient outcomes	Nursing interventions	Rationale
Mrs. R. performs preparatory exercises	Encourage Mrs. R. to do ROM of unaffected leg, biceps, triceps, and gluteal exercises	Active ROM exercises increase muscle strength and prevent contractures
Mrs. R. ambulates with crutches	Encourage Mrs. R. to ambulate using correct crutch-walking technique	Exercises and early ambulation promote circulation and wound healing; ambulating helps Mrs. R. begin to get a new sense of balance preparatory to using a prosthesis

Nursing diagnosis: Constipation: related to immobility and opiates

Expected patient outcomes	Nursing interventions	Rationale
Stools are soft, formed, and at Mrs. R.'s normal frequency	Monitor stools for constipation	Immobility and opiates are high risk factors for constipation
	Encourage fluids and high-fiber diet	Fluids and fiber promote bowel motility
	Encourage maximum activity and ambulation	Activity promotes bowel motility

Nursing diagnosis: Impaired home maintenance management: related to impaired mobility

Expected patient outcomes	Nursing interventions	Rationale
Home is clean and balanced meals are available	Explore with Mrs. R. ways in which housekeeping needs can be met	Involving Mrs. R. in planning helps ensure results
	Enlist help of social worker in plans for use of community resources	Social workers have access to community resources

Nursing diagnosis: Knowledge deficit: related to lack of exposure or recall

Expected patient outcomes	Nursing interventions	Rationale
Mrs. R. demonstrates proper crutch walking	Reinforce teaching of crutch walking	Reinforcement of earlier teaching helps promote retention
Mrs. R. demonstrates stump care	Teach stump care and how to get supplies for care in the community	Mrs. R. needs to care for stump at home
Mrs. R. describes plans to stop smoking and to lose weight	Review effect of smoking, obesity, and uncontrolled diabetes on circulation	Mrs. R. is at high risk for arterial insufficiency in other leg
	Discuss previous efforts to discontinue smoking and to lose weight; explore additional ways, especially group programs	Programs that include group support are often more successful than individual efforts

Postoperative care is described in Box 26-5. A sample nursing care plan is shown on p. 722.

VASOMOTOR ARTERIAL DISEASE— RAYNAUD'S PHENOMENON/DISEASE

Etiology/Epidemiology

Raynaud's *phenomenon* is characterized by episodic arterial spasms of the extremities, predominantly of the hands. It occurs secondary to other disorders, such as occlusive arterial diseases, connective tissue diseases, or neurogenic lesions. Raynaud's phenomenon develops more frequently in women between ages 20 and 40, and is more common during winter months. Raynaud's *disease* has no known cause, although immunologic factors, alterations in sympathetic innervation, emotional stress, and a hypersensitivity to cold have been suggested.

Pathophysiology

Symptoms of Raynaud's phenomenon or disease result from the episodic arterial spasms, usually in the fingers. Few pathologic changes occur in the early stages; with advancing stages, the intimal wall thickens and there is hypertrophy of the medial wall. The person typically complains of chronically cold hands and feet. During arterial spasms, sluggish blood flow causes pallor, coldness, numbness, cutaneous cyanosis, and pain. After the spasms, the involved area becomes reddened with tingling and throbbing sensations. With advanced disease, ulcerations can develop on the fingertips and toes.

Assessment

Subjective data include the following information:
1. Feelings in hands and feet: coldness, numbness, tingling
2. Measures used to relieve symptoms: effect of warmth
3. Presence of associated factors: emotional stress, cigarette smoking, exposure to cold

Objective data include observations of the hands and feet: temperature, skin color changes (white, blue, red), and presence of ulcerations on fingertips and toes.

A *diagnostic test* used for Raynaud's disease is the cold stimulation test. Skin temperature changes are recorded by a thermistor attached to each finger. The patient's hand is submerged in an ice-water bath for 20 seconds and ongoing temperatures are recorded. A comparison is made for baseline data.

Interventions

Medical therapy for the person with Raynaud's disease is primarily preventive. Drug therapy with calcium antagonists, vascular smooth muscle relaxants, and vasodilators may be prescribed to promote circulation and reduce pain. Biofeedback techniques to increase skin temperature and thereby prevent spasms have been beneficial in some cases. A *sympathectomy* may be indicated to relieve symptoms in the early stage of advanced ischemia. Sympathectomy involves removal of the sympathetic ganglia or a division of their branches. If the disease is advanced with ulcerations and gangrene, the involved area may have to be amputated.

Nursing interventions are similar to those for other arterial disorders in terms of preventing injury and promoting tissue perfusion (p. 713). Teaching the patient includes the following:

1. Effects of smoking on arterial flow (nicotine causes vasoconstriction); recommend techniques to quit smoking, such as behavior modification, stimulus control, biofeedback, nicotine gum, and hypnosis.
2. Ways of avoiding exposure to cold:
   a. Wear adequate clothing to promote warmth.
   b. Layer clothes as needed (several layers provide more warmth than one heavy layer).
   c. Wear gloves and warm socks during winter months.
   d. Use caution when cleaning refrigerator and freezer.
   e. Wear gloves when handling frozen foods.
   f. Avoid occupations that require constant exposure to cold.

26-5

Guidelines for Care

The patient after an amputation

Assess stump and monitor catheter drainage for color and amount; report signs of increased drainage.

Position patient with no flexion at hip or knee to avoid contractures; encourage prone position

Maintain patient in low-Fowler's or flat position after AK amputation.

Support stump with pillow for first 24 hours (according to physician preference and avoiding flexion); place rolled bath blanket along outer aspect to prevent outward rotation.

Encourage exercises to prevent thromboembolism.
  Active ROM of unaffected leg, ankle rotations and pumps
  Use of overhead trapeze when moving in bed
  Push-ups from sitting position and bed
  Quadriceps sets (Chapter 40)
  Lifting stump and buttocks off bed while lying flat on back to strengthen abdominal muscles

Teach care of stump.
  Inspect for redness, blister, and abrasions.
  Wash stump with mild soap, rinse with water, and pat dry.
  Avoid use of alcohol, oils, and creams.
  Remove stump bandage or stump sock and reapply as needed; use firm smooth figure-eight ace wrapping (Fig. 26-10) to reduce swelling and shape stump (if rigid dressing not used).

Encourage patient to ambulate using correct crutch-walking technique.
  Keep elbows extended; limit elbow flexion to 30° or less.
  Avoid pressure on axilla.
  Bear weight on palms of hands, not on axilla.
  Maintain upright posture (head up, chest up, abdomen in, pelvis in, foot straight)

Monitor patient's ability to use a prosthesis (Fig. 26-11)

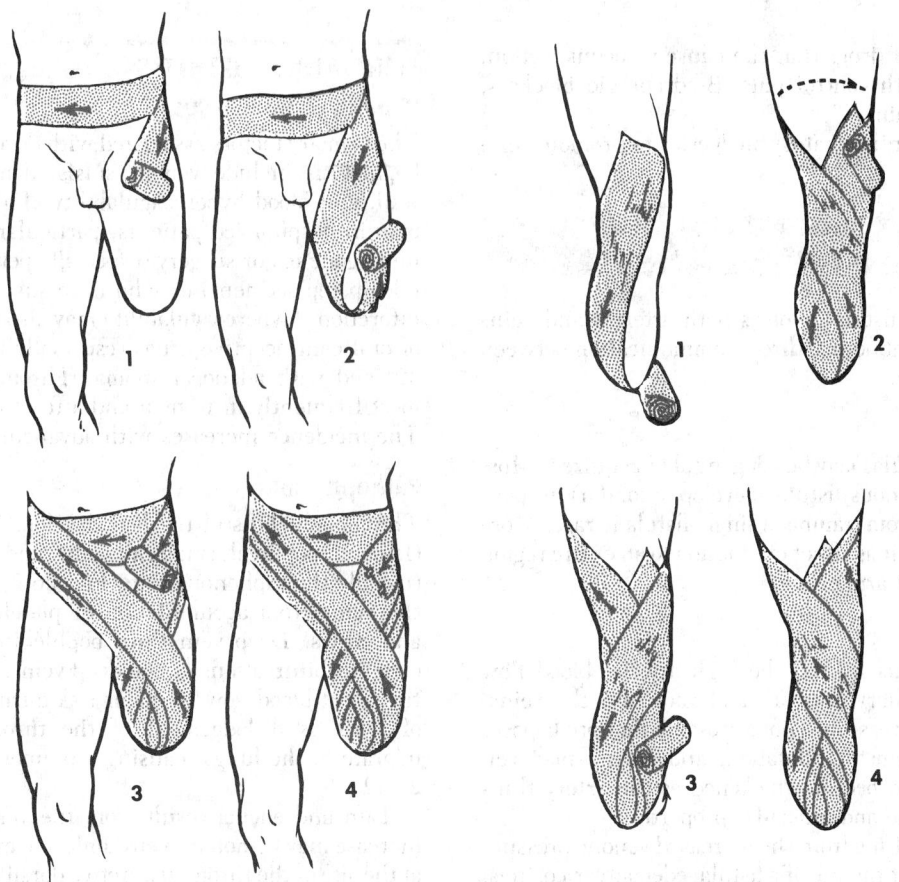

Fig. 26-10 *Left,* correct method of bandaging midthigh amputation stump. Note that the bandage must be anchored around patient's waist. *Right,* correct method for bandaging midcalf amputation stump. Note that bandage need not be anchored about waist.

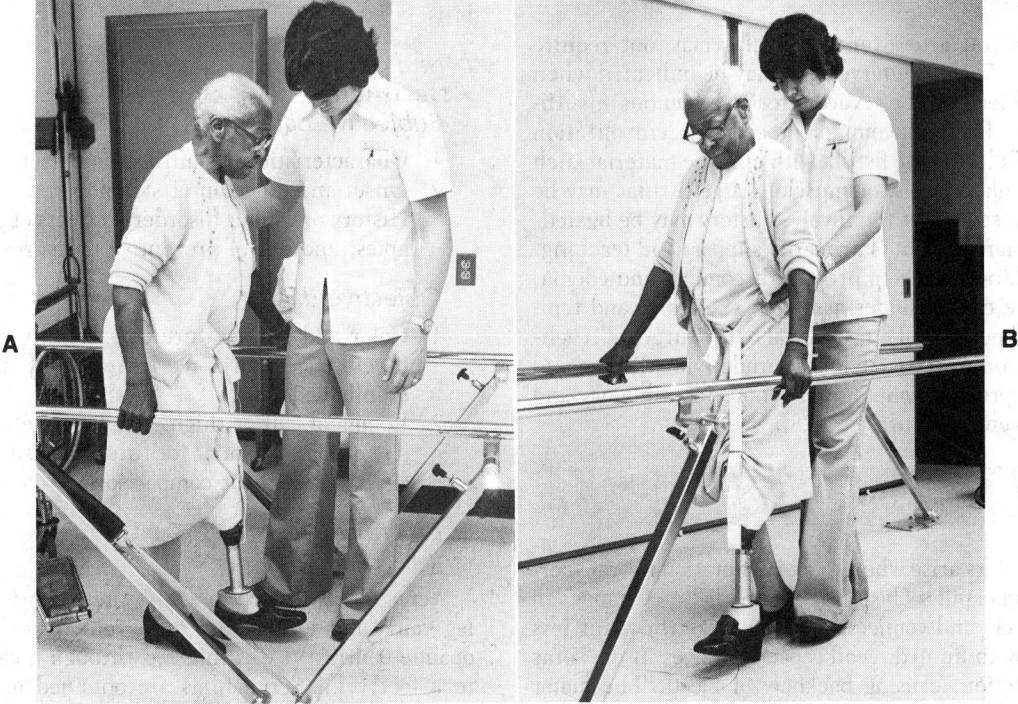

Fig. 26-11   A, Patient steps forward on the prosthesis while using the bars for stability. **B,** Walking behind the patient enables the therapist to assess the patient's gait.

3. Avoidance of drugs that can cause vasoconstriction, such as birth control pills, β-adrenergic blockers, and ergotamines.
4. Use of antiinflammatory analgesics to promote comfort.

ARTERIOVENOUS FISTULA

An arteriovenous fistula involves both arteries and veins and consists of an abnormal direct communication between an artery and vein.

Etiology

Arteriovenous fistulas may be congenital or acquired. Most acquired arteriovenous fistulas develop secondary to penetrating injuries from trauma; a single fistula is rare. More often, multiple fistulas affect circulation to an entire region or area such as an arm or leg.

Pathophysiology

In an arteriovenous fistula, the high arterial blood flow bypasses the capillary network and goes into the veins. This causes an increase in venous pressure that predisposes to venous engorgement, dilatation, and aneurysm development. The veins become thickened as the artery thins and loses its elastic and muscular properties.

Symptoms resulting from the increased venous pressure may include pain at the site of a fistula; edema, varicosities, and asymmetry of an extremity; tortuous, dilated superficial veins; and venous pulsations. Venous bruit and thrill may be heard from the turbulent blood flow. Testing includes arteriography and Doppler ultrasonography.

Interventions

Small peripheral arteriovenous fistulas may not require intervention. *Surgical* intervention may be indicated when ulceration, bleeding, or severe arterial or venous insufficiency occur. The most common procedure is embolization consisting of closing the fistula with embolic material such as Gelfoam, glass beads, or muscle. Large fistulas may be repaired or resected, or the involved artery may be ligated.

Nursing management is primarily support and teaching. Elastic stockings can help prevent discomfort and edema. Postoperative care includes assessing skin color and temperature and peripheral pulses distal to the surgery. Teaching includes information about the underlying disease and measures to prevent symptoms of venous insufficiency and to promote venous return (p. 728).

VENOUS DISORDERS

Venous disorders arise when there is alteration in transport of blood from capillary beds back to the heart. Changes in smooth muscle and connective tissue make the veins less distensible with limited recoil capacity. Valves in the veins may malfunction, causing backflow of blood. The major venous disorders are thrombophlebitis and varicose veins (Table 26-5).

THROMBOPHLEBITIS

Etiology/Epidemiology

The primary factors associated with development of thrombophlebitis include venous stasis, damage to the vessel wall, and blood hypercoagulability. This disorder is common in hospitalized patients, particularly those who have undergone major surgery (especially pelvic surgery and total hip replacement) or who have sustained a myocardial infarction. Hypercoagulability may also occur with the use of oral contraceptive drugs (especially in women over age 30) and with adenocarcinoma. Thrombophlebitis occurs most frequently in women and affects people of all races. The incidence increases with advancing age.

Pathophysiology

Thrombophlebitis of the legs develops in both deep veins (femoral, popliteal, small calf veins) and in superficial veins (usually the saphenous vein, Fig. 26-2). Thrombi form in the veins from accumulation of platelets, fibrin, WBCs and RBCs. Deep vein thrombophlebitis (DVT) tends to occur at bifurcations of the deep veins, which are sites of turbulent blood flow. A major risk during the acute phase of DVT is dislodgement of the thrombus, which can migrate to the lungs, causing a pulmonary embolus (Fig. 26-12).

Pain and edema result from the vein obstruction. An increase may be noted in circumference of the calf or thigh at the site of the thrombus. Active dorsiflexion may produce calf pain (Homan's sign); however, this action should be avoided because of increased risk of embolization. Because superficial veins are closer to the surface, signs of inflammation (redness, warmth, tenderness along the course of the vein) may be noted with superficial thrombophlebitis.

Nursing Process
Assessment
Subjective data

1. Characteristics of pain in the extremity
2. Onset and duration of symptoms
3. History of venous disorders, effects of previous therapies, and use of preventive measures

Objective data

1. Color and temperature of extremity (pale and cold if vein is occluded; red and warm if superficial vein is inflamed)
2. Edema of calf or thigh: Use tape measure and mark site of measurement for future measurements; measure both legs for comparison

Diagnostic tests
Venography

Venography is used to assess the condition of the deep leg veins and to diagnose deep vein thrombosis. A radiopaque contrast dye is injected through a catheter placed in a foot vein. Serial films are obtained to detect filling defects. Injection of the dye can cause a brief inflammatory response or allergic reaction.

Table 26-5   Venous disorders

Disease	Signs and symptoms	Therapy
Thrombophlebitis	Entire limb may be pale and cold Area along vein may be reddened and feel warm to touch Homan's sign: pain in calf on dorsiflexion Superficial veins feel hard and thready and are sensitive to pressure Difference in circumference of extremities	Bed rest during acute phase Warm moist heat to reduce discomfort and pain Elevation of extremity Elastic bandage Heparin and Coumadin Vasodilator to combat arterial spasms and improve circulation Fibrinolytics to resolve the thrombus Exercise program after acute phase

Varicose veins	Veins appear as darkened, tortuous, raised blood vessels; more pronounced on prolonged standing
	Feeling of heaviness in legs
	Fatigue
	Pain and muscle cramps
	Edema
		Conservative treatment:
		   Elevate legs at least every 2 to 3 hours
		   Wear elastic stocking
		   Avoid standing for long periods of time
		   Weight reduction if obese
		Surgery: venous ligation and stripping

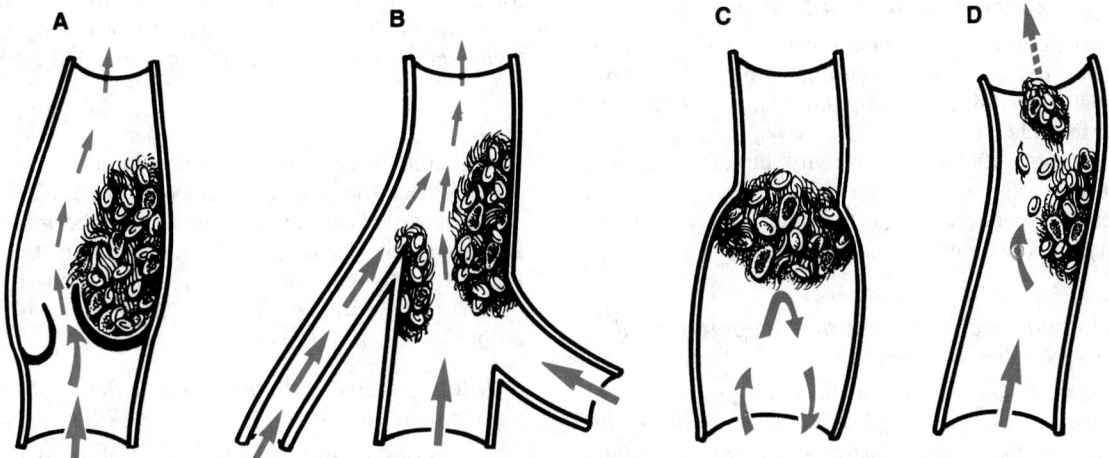

Fig. 26-12   Development of thromboemboli with arrows indicating direction of blood flow. **A,** Thrombus in a valve pocket of a deep vein with blood flowing beside thrombus. **B,** Thrombi tend to form at bifurcations of deep veins with some slowing of blood flow. **C,** Complete occlusion of vein by thrombus, forcing back flow of blood. **D,** Embolus, which has broken off from thrombus and is floating in blood stream, could migrate to lungs and cause pulmonary embolus.

Doppler ultrasonography

Doppler ultrasonography is used to measure flow through vessels. A probe or electronic stethoscope is placed over the patient's femoral and popliteal veins. The flow probe directs an ultrasound beam at the involved areas; the beam is reflected back off the red cells that circulate through the blood vessels. The reflection varies according to the rate of flow in the vessel. This change in the frequency of reflected sound according to velocity of the flow is referred to as a Doppler effect (Fig. 26-13). Both extremities are compared for diminished or absent readings over the veins.

Impedance plethysmography

Impedance plethysmography is used to measure changes in venous volumes and to detect deep vein thrombosis. A pressure cuff is applied to the thigh and electrodes are attached to the patient's leg. Venous volume tracings during inflation and deflation of the cuff are compared.

Data analysis: nursing diagnoses

Nursing diagnoses are determined from analysis of patient data. Possible nursing diagnoses for the person with thrombophlebitis may include, but are not limited to, the following:

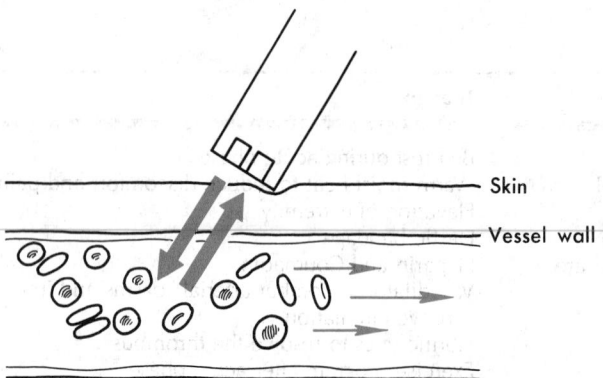

Fig. 26-13 Doppler effect showing red blood cells reflecting sound.

Diagnostic title	Possible etiologies
Knowledge deficit	Lack of exposure/recall
Pain, leg	Inflammation, edema, venous stasis

Planning: expected patient outcomes

Expected patient outcomes for the person with thrombophlebitis may include, but are not limited to, the following:

1. Shows signs of decreased pain; states feeling more comfortable.
2. Describes rationale for activity limitation during acute phase.
3. Describes pharmacologic therapy, signs of pulmonary embolus, and preventive measures.

Implementation

Assisting with achievement of therapeutic goals
Acute care for thrombophlebitis

Bed rest is prescribed during the acute phase for *deep vein thrombosis* to prevent embolus. The affected extremity is elevated periodically above heart level to prevent venous stasis and to reduce edema. Specific activity orders depend on physician preferences. When the patient begins to ambulate, elastic stockings or an elastic bandage is used to compress the superficial veins, increase blood flow through the deep veins, and prevent venous stasis. Anticoagulants are routinely given (p. 715), and vasodilators or fibrinolytics may also be prescribed.

Superficial thrombophlebitis is usually treated by rest; however, physicians differ in regard to the amount. Some physicians believe that complete immobilization is necessary to prevent emboli formation; others believe that clots are sufficiently adherent to vein walls and that mobility improves general circulation and prevents further venous stasis. Antiinflammatory drugs may be prescribed.

Surgery

Surgical intervention for venous thrombosis is indicated only when other conservative measures are unsuccessful. If the thrombosis is recurrent and extensive or if the patient is at high risk for pulmonary embolism, surgery may be necessary. A thrombectomy or a vena caval interruption may be performed. Vena caval interruption consists of

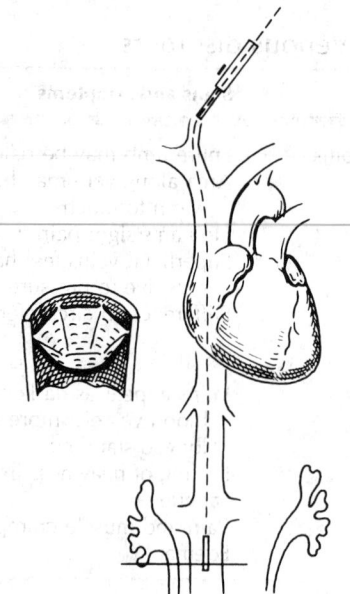

Fig. 26-14 Transvenous method of vena cava interruption using caval prosthesis of umbrella design. Inset illustrates open umbrella. (Redrawn from Fairbairn JF, Jurgens JL, Spittell JA: *Peripheral vascular disease,* Philadelphia, 1972, WB Saunders.)

transvenous placement of a grid or umbrella in the vena cava to block the passage of emboli (Fig. 26-14).

Preoperative care includes monitoring peripheral pulses and signs of bleeding from anticoagulant therapy and pulmonary emboli (for instance, sudden chest pain and cough). Postoperative nursing care is described in Box 26-6.

Interventions to achieve patient outcomes
Promoting comfort

Analgesics reduce pain and discomfort in the person with acute thrombophlebitis. Antiinflammatory medication decreases the inflammation, thereby contributing to increased comfort. Warm moist heat, heating pads, or ice packs may be prescribed to enhance resolution of the inflammation.

Teaching the patient

The major emphasis of nursing interventions for the person with a chronic venous disorder is patient teaching. Important topics for teaching are measures to increase tissue perfusion by preventing venous stasis (and thereby preventing pain) and measures to prevent recurrences.

1. Prevention of venous stasis
   a. Avoid prolonged sitting or standing.
   b. Elevate legs when sitting.
   c. Avoid crossing the legs at the knee.
   d. Wear elastic stockings (see Box 26-7).
   e. Avoid constriction on leg veins by tight bands (socks and garters).
   f. Carry out daily exercises and physical activity (promotion of blood flow by contraction of leg muscles).

(1) Practice dorsiflexion of both feet while sitting or lying down.
(2) Walk daily; increase distance as tolerated.
(3) Swim several times weekly if possible.
(4) Use stationary bicycle.
2. Prevent recurrence
   a. Maintain desired weight for height.
   b. Modify lifestyle (both at work and at home) as necessary to prevent long periods of standing or sitting.
   c. Follow activity program as described above.
   d. Take special precautions if pregnant (because of increased pressure on veins) or for any surgical procedure (especially pelvic surgery).

Evaluation

Evaluation is based on expected patient outcomes. Questions to consider may include:
1. Does patient state that leg pain is decreased?
2. Did patient remain inactive during acute phase?
3. Can patient describe the medication regimen, preventive measures, and signs to report to physician?

VARICOSE VEINS
Etiology/Epidemiology

Varicose veins can develop from the congenital absence of a valve or acquired valve incompetence. They often occur as a result of external pressure on the veins from pregnancy, ascites, or abdominal tumors. Other associated factors are prolonged standing, constricting clothing, and marked obesity. They may also occur from sustained elevations in venous pressure from heart disease or cirrhosis. From 10% to 20% of the world's population is affected. The highest incidence is in women aged 40 to 60.

Prevention

Persons with varicosities, especially if there is a family history of varicosities, should wear elastic stockings during activities that require prolonged standing or when pregnant. Moderate exercise and elevation of the legs when sitting help to prevent venous congestion. No continual pressure should be applied to the legs.

Pathophysiology

Varicose veins are abnormally dilated veins with incompetent valves occurring most often in the legs and lower trunk. The great and small saphenous veins are most often involved (Fig. 26-15). The precipitating factor is weakness of the vessel wall. The weakened area dilates, stretching the valves, which then become incompetent. This results in inability to support a column of blood, and venous pooling results.

Varicose veins may be primary or secondary. *Primary* varicosities have a gradual onset and affect superficial veins. Often there are no symptoms except the appearance of darkened tortuous veins. Symptoms include dull aches, muscle cramps, heaviness, or fatigue arising from decreased blood flow to the tissues. *Secondary* varicosities affect the deep veins and result from chronic venous insufficiency or venous thrombosis. Symptoms of edema, pain, changes in skin color, and ulceration may occur from venous stasis.

Diagnostic Tests

Trendelenburg's test is a simple noninvasive diagnostic tool to assess the competency of the venous valves through measurement of venous filling time. The patient lies down with the affected leg raised to allow for venous emptying. A tourniquet is then applied above the knee, and the patient stands. The direction and filling time of the veins are recorded both before and after the tourniquet is removed. Incompetent valves are evident when the veins fill rapidly from backward blood flow.

Interventions

Sclerotherapy consists of injection of a sclerosing solution at the sites of the varicosities. It produces permanent obliteration of the collapsed veins. Elastic bandages are applied for continuous pressure for 1 to 2 weeks. The procedure is performed as ambulatory surgery and offers good cosmetic results.

Surgical intervention is indicated for edema, recurrent leg ulcers, pain, or cosmetic reasons. Surgery consists of vein ligation and stripping. The great saphenous vein is ligated (tied) close to the femoral junction, if possible. The great and small saphenous veins are then stripped out

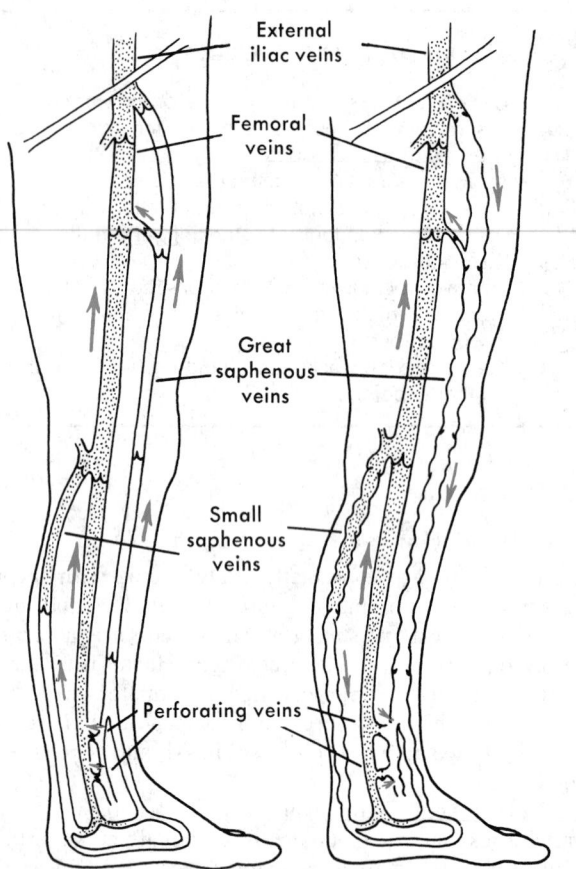

Fig. 26-15 *Left,* venous flow in normal veins. *Right,* venous flow in varicose veins. (Redrawn from Fairbairn JF, Jurgens JL, Spittell JA: *Peripheral vascular disease,* Philadelphia, 1972, WB Saunders.)

through small incisions at the groin, above and below the knee, and at the ankle (Fig. 26-16). An elastic bandage is applied firmly.

Postoperative nursing care includes the following:
1. Monitor for signs of bleeding; if bleeding occurs, elevate leg, apply pressure on wound, and notify surgeon.
2. Keep patient flat in bed for first 4 hours; elevate leg to promote venous return when lying or sitting.
3. Medicate 30 minutes before ambulation.
4. Keep elastic bandage snug and wrinkle free; do not remove bandage for daily care.

Because varicosities are chronic conditions, the person must know how to prevent venous stasis and encourage venous return. Preventive measures are listed on p. 728.

LEG ULCERS

Etiology

Most leg ulcers occur from chronic deep vein insufficiency or severe varicose veins, and less frequently from arterial obstruction. Other causes include burns, leg trauma, and neurogenic disorders. Persons with diabetes mellitus are

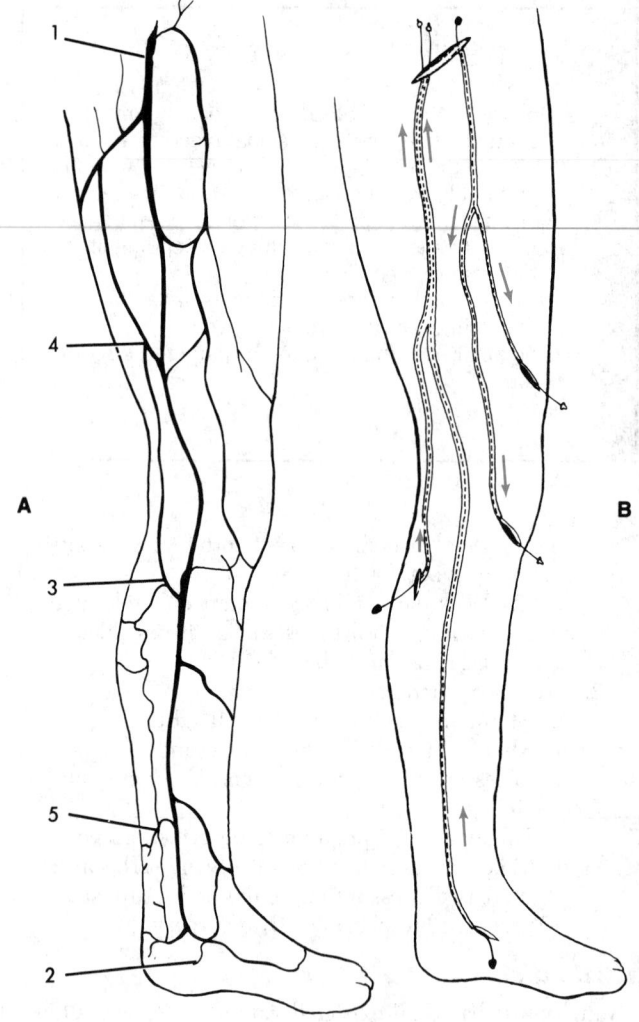

Fig. 26-16 **A,** Outline of incompetent great saphenous system with numerals indicating main tributaries. **B,** Passing of strippers in preparation of removal of incompetent veins.

at high risk for development of leg ulcers because of vascular insufficiency.

Pathophysiology

A leg ulcer is an open necrotic lesion that results from inadequate exchange of oxygen and other nutrients to the tissues because of decreased circulation. The same underlying pathophysiologic changes that contribute to chronic venous or arterial insufficiency are involved. Secondary bacterial infection occurs because of the decreased circulation that limits the body's response to infection. The infection, in turn, delays healing.

Clinical signs vary, depending on the underlying problem. A *venous ulcer* (stasis ulcer) is usually moderately painful and located on the medial aspect of the ankle. Edema and pigmentation are common around the ulcer because of venous stasis. Most venous ulcers heal with therapy. An *arterial ulcer* (ischemic ulcer) causes more pain and has a more necrotic, pale gray base because of lack of oxygen to the tissues. Pale or mottled skin is common around the ulcer base. Edema is infrequent. Peripheral pulses are diminished or absent. Arterial ulcers frequently develop on the heel, lateral malleolus, toes, and dorsum of the foot.

Nursing Process
Assessment
Subjective data

1. Onset and duration of symptoms
2. Extent and characteristics of pain
3. Limitations in mobility and activity
4. History of deep vein thrombosis, varicose veins, arterial insufficiency, or diabetes

Objective data

1. Appearance and temperature of the skin
2. Location and appearance of the ulcer
3. Presence and quality of all peripheral pulses
4. Presence of edema

Data analysis: nursing diagnoses

Nursing diagnoses are determined from analysis of patient data. Possible nursing diagnoses for the person with leg ulcers may include, but are not limited to, the following:

Diagnostic title	Possible etiologies
Tissue perfusion, altered peripheral	Decreased blood flow (arterial or venous)
Pain, ulcer	Inflammation, necrosis
Knowledge deficit	Lack of exposure/recall

Planning: expected patient outcomes

Expected patient outcomes for the person with leg ulcers may include, but are not limited to, the following:

1. Ulcer shows signs of healing and absence of further breakdown.
2. Patient participates in ADLs without discomfort or pain.
3. Patient describes measures to prevent infection and increase tissue perfusion, and care of the ulcer.

Implementation
Assisting with achievement of therapeutic goals

The primary goal in treating leg ulcers is to promote wound healing and prevent infection. Necrotic tissue is debrided by mechanical, chemical, or surgical means. A wet-to-dry dressing may be applied to debride the wound *mechanically.* The dressing is applied damp; when dry, it is removed, pulling off the debris that has adhered to the

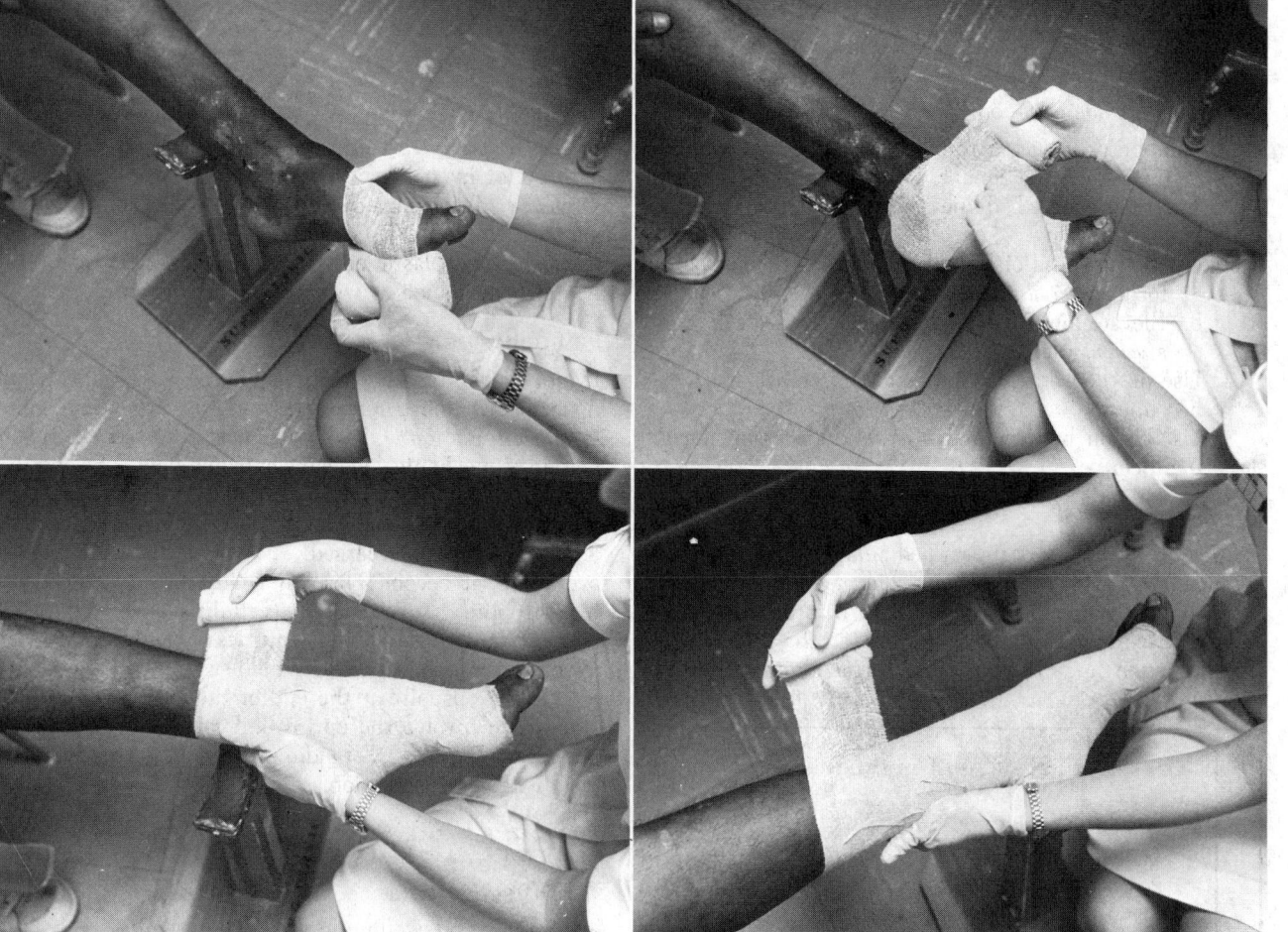

Fig. 26-17   Nurse applying Unna paste boot using specially impregnated gauze. Note ulcers on inferior aspect of patient's foot.

dressing. *Chemical* beads, such as Debrisan, and enzyme ointments, such as fibrinolysins (Elase), may be placed over the ulcer (avoiding healthy tissue) to break down the debris. Necrotic tissue can also be cut away with the aid of *surgical* instruments, usually a scalpel.

Topical and systemic *antibiotics* may be prescribed to prevent infection. Systemic antibiotic therapy is the most effective route in the treatment of leg ulcers. Periodic culture of wound drainage may be ordered to monitor the effectiveness of the antibiotics.

A *boot* may be applied to cover small, newly formed ulcers in ambulatory persons (Fig. 26-17). This boot protects the ulcer and provides constant and even support to the area. The boot is made from a special type of impregnated gauze (Unna paste) that hardens after it is wrapped around the patient's leg. The Unna boot is generally left on for 1 to 2 weeks, although it may be changed more often if there is copious drainage. Elastic bandages are applied to the leg after the ulcer has healed.

Surgery

Recurrent venous ulcers and nonhealing arterial ulcers may require surgical intervention. Ligation of incompetent veins may be necessary. Arterial bypass and reconstruction can be used to revascularize the artery and restore circulation (p. 717). Amputation may be required if less aggressive means are unsuccessful.

Interventions to achieve patient outcomes
Promoting tissue perfusion

Circulation of tissue surrounding the ulcer is encouraged by the following actions:
1. Maintain proper body positioning to improve circulation by gravity:
   a. Elevate head of bed on 3-inch to 6-inch blocks for an *arterial* ulcer.
   b. Elevate lower extremities to decrease edema for a *venous* ulcer.
2. Use overbed cradle to protect leg from pressure of bed linens.
3. Use cotton between toes to prevent pressure on a toe ulcer.

Promoting comfort

Encourage the use of prescribed analgesics and antiinflammatory medication to reduce pain and inflammation. Medicate for pain 30 to 45 minutes before a dressing change. Use aseptic technique in dressing changes to prevent infection and further discomfort. Administer pre-

scribed antibiotics on time to maintain blood levels for effective prevention or control of infection, thus relieving discomfort.

Teaching the patient

Teaching includes prevention of infection, maintenance of skin integrity, and measures to increase peripheral tissue perfusion (see pp 713 and 728). Teach the patient the correct method of dressing changes and discuss resources in the community for obtaining necessary supplies. Many of the patients with leg ulcers are elderly; therefore, ascertain if the patient is able to obtain supplies and carry out the dressing changes. If not, other persons in the home must be included in the teaching. If the person lives alone, other approaches must be explored.

Evaluation
Questions to ask may include the following:
1. Does the ulcer show signs of healing?
2. Is the patient able to participate in ADLs without pain?
3. Can the patient describe measures to prevent infection, increase tissue perfusion, and make necessary dressing changes?

LYMPHEDEMA

Etiology

Lymphedema is an abnormal collection of lymph in tissues. It may be *primary*, congenital or developing at puberty as a result of hypoplastic development of lymph vessels; or *secondary*, developing from obstruction, inflammation, or parasitic infection (see Box 26-8). The most common causes are neoplastic obstruction and surgical removal of lymph nodes, such as with radical mastectomy.

Pathophysiology

Lymphedema results when lymphatic vessels or lymph nodes become obstructed and cannot return tissue lymph to the circulation. Obstruction may result from inflammation or mechanical blocking of lymph flow. The obstruction may lead to incompetence of valves in the lymph vessels with resulting stasis of lymph flow and eventual fibrosis. The limb becomes enlarged. *Edema* is initially pitting; but over time, it becomes brawny (nonpitting) as the tissue hypertrophies. Inflammation (cellulitis or lymphangitis) may occur with minor limb injuries. Lymphedema of the lower extremities begins with mild swelling on the dorsum of the foot, usually at the end of the day, and gradually extends to involve the entire limb. The condition is aggravated by prolonged standing, pregnancy, obesity, warm weather, or menstruation.

Nursing Process
Assessment
Subjective data
1. Onset of swelling in affected extremity
2. History of secondary cause of lymphedema (Box 26-8)
3. Effectiveness of current therapy to reduce edema

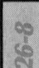

26-8	**Causes of secondary lymphedema**

Obstruction
 Malignant tumors
 Postsurgical removal of lymph nodes
 Mechanical trauma
 Postirradiation
Inflammation
Infection (parasitic)

Objective data

1. Observation of extremities for edema: unilateral, pitting or nonpitting
2. Comparison in size of extremities
3. Quality of peripheral pulses

Diagnostic tests

Lymphangiography consists of injection of a radiopaque dye directly into the lymphatic vessels. An x-ray examination is made after injection and 24 hours later. The lymph nodes can also be visualized. Periodic x-ray examinations can be made for up to 6 months because the dye remains in the lymph system.

Data analysis: nursing diagnoses

Nursing diagnoses are determined from analysis of patient data. Possible nursing diagnoses for the person with lymphedema may include, but are not limited to, the following:

Diagnostic title	Possible etiologies
Body image disturbance	Change in body appearance
Knowledge deficit	Lack of exposure/recall

Planning: expected patient outcomes

Expected patient outcomes for the person with lymphedema may include, but are not limited to, the following:

1. Expresses confidence in self, despite change in appearance of extremity.
2. Describes measures to decrease infection, maintain intact skin, and improve lymph drainage.

Implementation
Assisting with achievement of therapeutic goals

Therapy for lymphedema is conservative. The goal is to reduce edema and to maintain skin integrity. Therapy includes the following:

1. Passive and active exercises
2. Elevation of affected extremity
3. Elastic stocking to reduce edema of leg
4. Restriction of dietary sodium to reduce fluid retention and thereby decrease edema
5. Diuretic therapy to temporarily decrease limb size by decreasing total body fluid
6. Long-term antibiotic therapy to control recurrent cellulitis and infection

Most patients respond to conservative medical therapy and do not require surgical intervention. If indicated, surgery consists of removal of the edematous lymph tissues or reconstruction of the lymphatic drainage channels.

Interventions to achieve patient outcomes
Promoting positive body image

Lymphedema may cause a limb to become excessively large, which greatly alters the patient's appearance. Although the limb can be covered by clothing, the size cannot be hidden (except with a long skirt for women). The change in appearance can lead to a poor self-concept. The patient should be given opportunities to express feelings and encouragement to follow through on measures to decrease some of the edema. Positive attributes are emphasized.

Teaching the patient

Patient teaching includes measures to prevent infection and improve lymph drainage:

1. Take antibiotics for as long as prescribed to prevent infection.
2. Take measures to promote skin integrity and thus prevent infection:
   a. Monitor skin for intactness, swelling, redness, and lesions
   b. Seek medical assistance if skin changes occur
   c. Carry out special foot care (for leg edema) to prevent minor infection
3. Take measures to improve lymph drainage and decrease edema:
   a. Elevate affected extremity above heart level at frequent intervals
   b. Avoid prolonged standing
   c. Sleep with foot of bed elevated 4 to 8 inches
   d. Wear elastic stockings from arising until retiring at night
   e. Avoid constrictive clothing
   f. Exercise on a regular basis
   g. Take diuretics as prescribed
   h. Follow prescribed sodium-restricted diet
4. Carry out instructions for continued medical follow-up.

Evaluation

Questions to ask may include the following:

1. Is patient able to discuss feelings about altered appearance of the extremity?
2. Is patient taking measures to facilitate control of edema and thereby promote a more positive body image?
3. Can the patient describe ways to prevent infection and to improve lymph drainage?
4. Is the patient making plans for follow-up care?

HYPERTENSION

Hypertension can be considered with peripheral vascular disorders because they both involve problems of peripheral circulation and are affected by similar factors. Hypertension itself is a risk factor in atherosclerosis, the major cause of peripheral vascular disease.

Etiology/Epidemiology

Hypertension (HTN) is defined as a consistent systolic blood pressure >140 mm Hg and/or a consistent diastolic blood pressure >90 mm Hg. A more complete classification of blood pressure which was developed by a national task force to assist in establishing a more universal diagnosis of HTN, is listed in Table 26-6. It must be emphasized that the categorical classification is based on the average of two or more blood pressure readings, not a single elevated reading.

More than 59 million Americans have been diagnosed with elevated blood pressure or are taking antihypertensive medications. Additionally, it is estimated that another 50% of adults in the United States are undiagnosed hyperten-

Table 26-6 Classification of blood pressure* (age 18 and older)

Range (mm Hg)	Classification
Diastolic	
<85	Normal blood pressure
85-89	High normal blood pressuret
90-104	Mild hypertension
105-114	Moderate hypertension
≥115	Severe hypertension
Systolic	
<140	Normal blood pressure
140-159	Borderline isolated systolic HTN‡
>160	Isolated systolic HTN‡

*Based on average of two or more readings on two or more occasions.
†High normal blood pressure takes precedence over normal (systolic) blood pressure when both occur in same person.
‡Borderline isolated systolic HTN or isolated systolic HTN take precedence over high normal blood pressure when both occur in same person.

sives. The exact number is unknown because most individuals are symptom-free and others avoid pursuing treatment.

The incidence of HTN increases with age and varies considerably among different groups. HTN occurs more often in men than in women and is nearly twice as prevalent among blacks than whites. HTN in blacks is usually more severe than it is in similar hypertensive whites. There is an increased incidence and severity of HTN in blacks living in the southeastern United States, compared with blacks residing in other areas.

There are two types of HTN, essential (primary, idiopathic) and secondary. *Essential* hypertension accounts for 90% to 95% of all types of HTN. Although there is no generally accepted cause of essential hypertension, several theories have been suggested, including arteriolar changes, alterations in sympathetic tone, hormonal influence, and genetic factors. *Secondary* hypertension develops as a consequence of an underlying disease or condition (Table 26-7). In most instances, the HTN will subside when the disease is treated or corrected.

Prevention
Primary prevention

Primary prevention is aimed at reducing risk factors associated with HTN (see Box 26-9). Health education programs include teaching about moderate sodium intake, a decreased saturated-fat diet, maintenance of optimal body weight for height, cessation of cigarette smoking, moderate consumption of alcohol, and the use of effective coping strategies to minimize stress.

Secondary prevention

Secondary prevention consists of identification and control of HTN in high-risk groups, such as blacks (especially males), obese persons, and blood relatives of known hypertensives. A major effort should be made to contact people who have limited access to health care because of geographic or economic constraints. Follow-ups should be

Table 26-7 Causes of secondary hypertension

Disorder/condition	Mechanism
Kidney	
Renal parenchymal disease (glomerulonephritis, renal failure)	Most often cause a renin or sodium dependent HTN; physiologic changes relate to type of disease and severity of renal insufficiency
Renovascular disease	Decrease in renal perfusion from atherosclerotic or fibrotic narrowing of renal arteries; causes marked increase in peripheral vascular resistance and cardiac output
Adrenal cortex	
Cushing's syndrome	Increase in blood volume
Primary aldosteronism	Increase in aldosterone, causing sodium and water retention that increase blood volume
Pheochromocytoma	Excess secretion of catecholamines (norepinephrine increases peripheral vascular resistance)
Coarctation of aorta	Causes marked elevated blood pressure in upper extremities with decreased perfusion in lower extremities
Head trauma or cranial tumor	Increased intracranial pressure reduces cerebral blood flow; resultant ischemia stimulates medullary vasomotor center to raise blood pressure
Pregnancy-induced HTN	Cause unknown; generalized vasospasm may be a contributing factor

made after initial blood pressure measurements depending on the range of initial findings (see Table 26-8). Mass blood pressure screenings are currently not recommended. Most often these screenings occur at large-scale gatherings where environmental conditions may cause inaccurate blood pressure readings. In addition, these sites tend to be frequented by the same people.

Pathophysiology

Blood pressure is the pressure exerted by the blood on the vessels through which it flows. Systolic pressure is the pressure exerted during ventricular contraction; diastolic pressure is pressure during ventricular relaxation. Blood pressure is regulated by two factors: blood flow and peripheral vascular resistance. Factors that determine *blood flow* are the volume of blood ejected from the left ventricle with each contraction (stroke volume) and the heart rate (see Chapter 25). *Peripheral vascular resistance* is affected primarily by the diameter of the blood vessel and, to a lesser degree, by the viscosity of the blood. Increased pe-

<table>
</table>

26-9	**Risk factors in essential hypertension**

Risk factors in essential hypertension

Age: advancing
Sex: male
Race: black
Family history: hypertension
Obesity: associated with increased intravascular volume
Atherosclerosis: narrowing of arteries increases blood pressure
Smoking: nicotine constricts blood vessels
High-salt diet: sodium causes water retention, increasing blood volume
Alcohol: increases plasma catecholamines
Emotional stress: stimulates sympathetic nervous system

Table 26-8 **Recommendations for follow-up of initial blood pressure measurements in adults (over age 18)**

Range (mm Hg)	Recommended follow-up*
Diastolic	
<85	Recheck within 2 yr
85-89	Recheck within 1 yr
90-104	Confirm within 2 months
105-114	Evaluate or refer to source of care within 2 wk
≥115	Evaluate or refer immediately to source of care
Systolic	
<140	Recheck within 2 yr
140-199	Confirm within 2 months
≥200	Evaluate or refer to source of care within 2 wk

*If recommendations for follow-up of diastolic and systolic blood pressure are different, the shorter recommended time for recheck should take precedence.

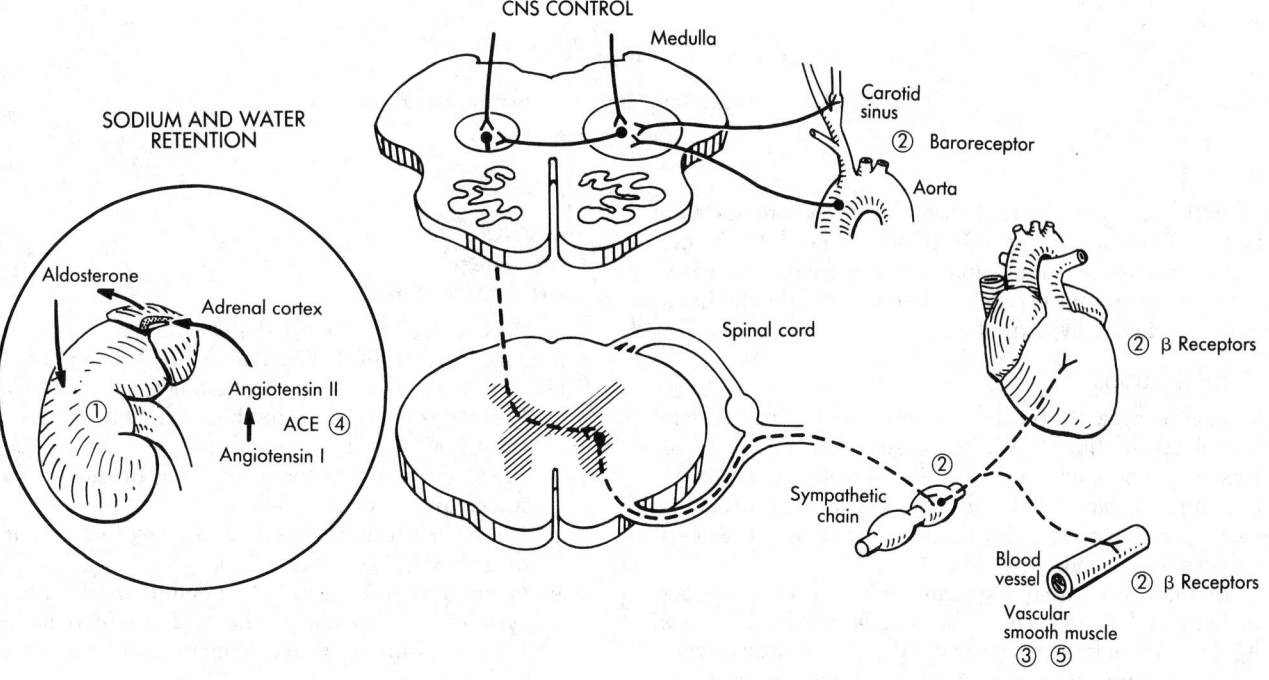

Fig. 26-18 Sites of blood pressure regulation and action of antihypertensive drugs. ① Diuretics. ② Adrenergic inhibitors. ③ Vasodilators. ④ ACE inhibitors. ⑤ Calcium antagonist.

ripheral vascular resistance as a result of narrowing of the arterioles is the most common characteristic in HTN.

Dilation and constriction of the peripheral arterioles are controlled by several mechanisms, primarily the sympathetic nervous system and the renin-angiotensin system. The vasomotor center in the medulla can be stimulated by the baroreceptors (Fig. 26-18) or by psychogenic stress. Impulses are then carried through the sympathetic nervous system, causing the release of catecholamines. Norepinephrine is released from the postganglionic fibers, causing blood vessel constriction and increased peripheral resistance. Epinephrine is secreted by the adrenal medulla and

causes vasoconstriction. Epinephrine also increases ventricular contraction force and cardiac output.

Renal regulation is an essential component of blood pressure control (Fig. 26-19). Activation of the renin-angiotensin system occurs when there is reduced blood flow to the kidneys. Renin leads to the formation of angiotensin, a potent vasoconstrictor. Angiotension stimulates the secretion of aldosterone, which promotes retention of sodium and water.

Hypertension is essentially a disease without symptoms. When symptoms do occur, they are usually indicative of advanced HTN. Signs and symptoms may include early

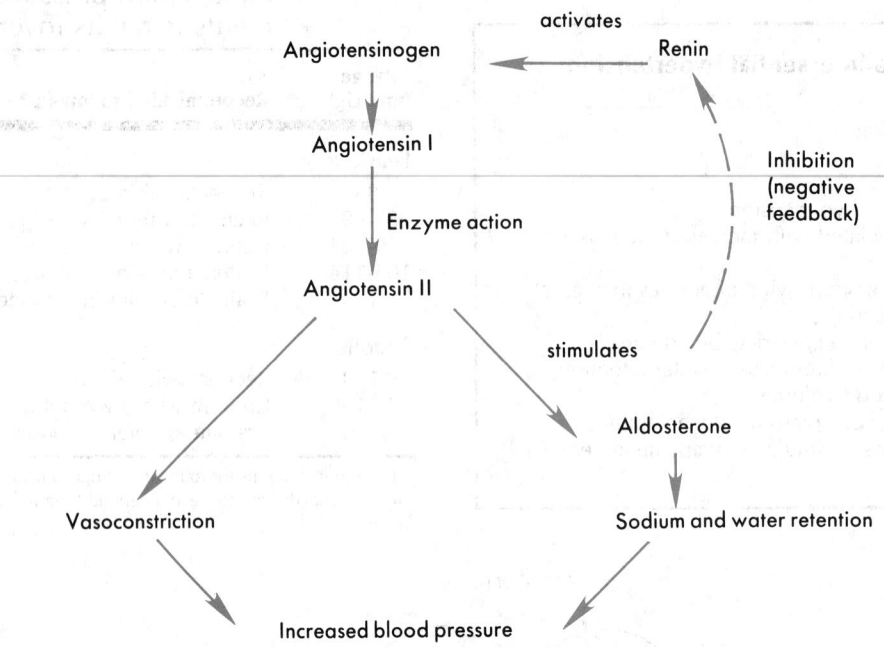

Fig. 26-19 Effect of renin-angiotensin system on blood pressure.

morning headache, blurred vision, and spontaneous nose-bleeds. Evidence of the effects of advanced HTN may include nausea, vomiting, and confusion (hypertensive encephalopathy), and exertional dyspnea and dysrhythmias (left ventricular hypertrophy).

Complications

With prolonged HTN, the elastic tissue in the arterioles is replaced by fibrous collagen tissue. The thickened arteriole wall becomes less distensible, creating even greater resistance to blood flow. This process leads to decreased tissue perfusion, especially in the target organs, the heart, kidneys, and brain.

In the cardiovascular system, decreased coronary perfusion may lead to *angina pectoris* or *myocardial infarction*. As the heart is forced to work against consistently elevated aortic pressure, left ventricular hypertrophy and *congestive heart failure* may result.

As the renal vessels thicken and perfusion diminishes, the glomerulus is deprived of its blood supply. Permanent kidney damage and *renal failure* may result. Cerebral ischemia and arteriosclerosis can result from the progressive effects of HTN; *stroke* or *cerebral hemorrhage* may occur.

Malignant hypertension is a severe, rapidly progressive elevation in blood pressure that causes damage to the small arterioles in major organ systems (heart, kidneys, brain, eyes). A primary distinguishing finding is inflammation of the arterioles (arteriolitis) in the eyes. Retinitis and papilledema occur in later stages. This type of HTN is most common in black males under age 40. Unless medical treatment is successful the course is rapidly fatal. The most common causes of death are myocardial infarction, congestive heart failure, stroke, or renal failure.

Nursing Process
Assessment
Subjective data

Subjective data are collected about the presence of any symptoms, history of HTN, and patient knowledge of HTN. These data may include the following:

1. Presence of early morning headache, blurred vision, confusion, exertional dyspnea
2. Presence of risk factors (Box 26-9) including stress in occupation or daily life
3. Course and compliance with therapy for previously diagnosed HTN
4. Current knowledge of HTN: definition, meaning of systolic and diastolic readings, and effects of high blood pressure on heart, kidneys, and brain.

Objective data

Two or more blood measurements are taken in both arms with the patient in both supine and sitting positions. Additional data include:

1. Height and weight (identification of obesity)
2. Examination of neck for carotid bruits and abdomen for abdominal bruits (sound of blood flow through narrowed passageways)
3. Auscultation of heart for abnormal heart sounds: S_3 and S_4, murmurs (evidence of left ventricular hypertrophy)
4. Palpation of peripheral pulses: rate, amplitude, bilateral symmetry (signs of peripheral vascular narrowing)
5. Funduscopic eye examination by trained clinician (presence of arteriolar narrowing or hemorrhage)

Diagnostic tests

Diagnostic tests used to determine the possible cause of HTN, to assess the effect of the disease on other organ systems, or to provide baseline information may include the following:

1. Serum levels of sodium, potassium, calcium, and creatinine as well as hemoglobin and hematocrit (severity and possible causes)
2. Urinalysis, BUN, and renal function tests (effect on kidneys and baseline for drug therapy)
3. ECG, chest x-ray, and possibly echocardiography (extent of left ventricular hypertrophy or aortic calcification)

Data analysis: nursing diagnoses

Nursing diagnoses are determined from analysis of patient data. Possible nursing diagnoses for the person with hypertension may include, but are not limited to, the following:

Diagnostic title	Possible etiologies
Knowledge deficit: nature of HTN, risk factors, drug therapy	Lack of exposure/recall, unfamiliarity with information resources
Noncompliance: drug regimen, ongoing care	Patient value system, treatment side effects
Sexual dysfunction	Lack of information of effects of medications

Planning: expected patient outcomes

Expected patient outcomes for the person with hypertension may include, but are not limited to, the following:

1. Explains nature of HTN and effects of HTN on heart, kidney, brain.
2. Demonstrates correct procedure for self-management and recording of blood pressure.

3. Maintains blood pressure within desirable range.
4. Describes therapeutic regimen.
5. Describes plan to participate in other measures to promote normal blood pressure (dietary changes, exercise, stress reduction).
6. Explains effects of prescribed antihypertensive medication on sexual function (as appropriate).
7. Takes antihypertensive medications as prescribed.

Implementation
Assisting with achievement of therapeutic goals

Medical therapy is directed at the control of HTN and the prevention of associated diseases. The primary goal is to maintain a systolic blood pressure of less than 140 mm Hg and a diastolic pressure of less than 90 mm Hg. The decision to treat HTN is based on degree of the blood pressure elevation, presence of risk factors, and extent of damage to associated organ systems. *Nonpharmacologic* means, such as dietary programs of weight control and reduction of sodium and saturated fats, as well as exercise programs, are prescribed. Most persons with HTN have difficulty maintaining the desired blood pressure with these measures alone; therefore drug therapy is usually prescribed.

Pharmacologic therapy

Antihypertensive medications have a protective effect against damage to the heart, kidneys, and brain in patients with mild HTN. Drug treatment has been shown to successfully lower a consistent diastolic blood pressure from higher than 94 mm Hg to less than 90 mm Hg. When a diastolic blood pressure is between 90 and 94 mm Hg, an individualized approach to drug therapy is used.

Commonly used hypertensive drugs are listed in Table 26-9. Drug selection is determined by use of a step-care

Table 26-9   Oral medications for treatment of hypertension

Drug	Action*	Side-effects*
Thiazide/thiazide-like diuretics		
Bendroflumethiazide (Naturetin) Benzthiazide (Aquatag, Exna) Chlorothiazide (Diuril) Chlorthalidone (Hygroton) Cyclothiazide (Fluidil) Hydrochlorothiazide (Esidrix, Hydrodiuril) Hydroflumethiazide (Saluron) Indapamide (Lozol) Methyclothiazide (Enduron) Metolazone (Zaroxolyn) Polythiazide (Renese) Quinethazone (Hydromox) Trichlormethiazide (Diurese, Metahydrin)	Block sodium reabsorption in cortical portion of ascending tubule; water excreted with sodium, producing decreased blood volume. NOTE: thiazides ineffective in renal failure	Increased BUN, uric acid, blood glucose, calcium, cholesterol, and triglycerides Decreased potassium Possible postural hypotension in summer from sodium loss GI upset, dry mouth, thirst, weakness, muscle aches, fatigue, tachycardia Sexual dysfunction May cause increased blood levels of lithium
Loop diuretics		
Bumetanide (Bumex) Ethacrynic acid (Edecrin) Furosemide (Lasix)	Block sodium and water reabsorption in medullary portion of ascending tubule; causes rapid volume depletion	Decreased potassium Thirst, skin rash, postural hypotension, nausea, vomiting

*Primary actions and most common side effects are included and are related to entire drug category; consult a drug reference or drug package insert for more specific information.

Continued.

Table 26-9   Oral medications for treatment of hypertension—cont'd

Drug	Action*	Side-effects*
Potassium-sparing diuretics		
Amiloride (Midamor)	Inhibit aldosterone; sodium excreted in exchange for potassium	Drowsiness, confusion
Spironolactone (Aldactone)		Increased potassium levels
Triamterene (Dyrenium)		Diarrhea
		Gynecomastia with Aldactone
Adrenergic inhibitors		
Beta-adrenergic blockers		
Acebutolol (Sectral)	Block beta-adrenergic receptors of sympathetic nervous system, decreasing heart rate and blood pressure	Bronchospasms
Atenolol (Tenormin)		Bradycardia, fatigue, insomnia
Metoprolol (Lopressor)		Sexual dysfunction
Nadolol (Corgard)		Peripheral vascular insufficiency
Pindolol (Visken)	NOTE: beta blockers should not be used in patients with asthma, COPD, CHF, and heart block; use with caution in diabetes and peripheral vascular disease	Increased triglycerides
Propranolol (Inderal)		
Timolol (Blocadren)		
Centrally acting alpha blockers		
Clonidine (Catapres)	Activate central receptors that suppress vasomotor and cardiac centers, causing a decrease in peripheral resistance. NOTE: rebound hypertension may occur with abrupt discontinuation of drug (except with Aldomet)	Drowsiness, sedation
Guanabenz (Wytensin)		Dry mouth
Guanfacine (Tenex)		Fatigue
Methyldopa (Aldomet)		Sexual dysfunction
		Orthostatic hypotension
		Positive Coomb's test with Aldomet
Peripheral-acting adrenergic antagonists		
Guanadrel (Hylorel)	Deplete catecholamines in peripheral sympathetic postganglionic fibers	Orthostatic hypotension
Guanethidine (Ismelin)		Lethargy, depression
Rauwolfia serpentina (Raudixin)	Block norepinephrine release from adrenergic nerve endings	Sexual dysfunction
Reserpine (Serpasil)		Nasal congestion (with Raudixin and Serpasil)
Alpha-1-adrenergic blockers		
Prazosin (Minipress)	Block synaptic receptors that regulate vasomotor tone; reduce peripheral resistance by dilating arterioles and venules	"First dose" syncope, orthostatic hypotension, weakness, palpitations, decreased low-density lipoproteins
Terazosin (Vasocard, Hytrin)		
Combined alpha- and beta-adrenergic blockers		
Labetalol (Normodyne, Trandate)	Same as for beta blockers	Bronchospasm, orthostatic hypotension, peripheral vascular insufficiency
Vasodilators		
Hydralazine (Apresoline)	Dilate peripheral blood vessels by directly relaxing vascular smooth muscle	Headache, dizziness
Minoxidil (Loniten)		Tachycardia, palpitations, fatigue, edema
	NOTE: usually used in combination with other antihypertensives as they increase sodium and fluid retention and can cause reflex cardiac stimulation	
ACE inhibitors		
Captopril (Capoten)	Inhibit conversion of angiotensin to angiotensin II thus blocking the release of aldosterone, thereby reducing sodium and water retension	"First dose" hypotension, headache, dizziness, fatigue
Enalapril maleate (Vasotec)		Increased potassium
Lisinopril (Prinivil)		Cough, skin reactions
Calcium antagonists		
Diltiazem (Cardizem)	Inhibit influx of calcium into muscle cells; act on vascular smooth muscles (primary arteries) to reduce spasms and promote vasodilation	Dizziness, fatigue, nausea, headache, edema
Felodipine (Plendil)		
Nifedipine (Procardia)		
Nitrendipine		
Verapamil (Calan, Isoptin)		
Verapamil SR		

Table 26-10   Medication for treatment of hypertensive emergencies

Drug	Action*	Side effects*
Vasodilators		
Sodium nitroprusside (Nipride, Nitropress) Nitroglycerine Diazoxide (Hyperstat) Hydralazine (Apresoline)	Dilate peripheral blood vessels by relaxing vascular smooth muscle	Headache, dizziness Tachycardia, palpitations, fatigue, nausea, edema NOTE: thiocyanate toxicity may occur with sodium nitroprusside
Adrenergic inhibitors		
Phentolamine (Regitine) Trimethaphan camsylate (Arfonad) Labetalol (Normodyne, Trandate) Methyldopa (Aldomet)	Block adrenergic receptors of sympathetic nervous system, thereby dilating peripheral blood vessels and reducing peripheral vascular resistance	Tachycardia, orthostatic hypotension

*Primary action and common side effects are included and are related to entire drug category; consult drug reference or drug package insert for more specific information.

approach. Therapy is started with a small dose of a less potent drug. Additions and substitutions of drugs, and dosage adjustments are based on the patient's response. The step-care approach is as follows:

Step 1: Use a diuretic, beta blocker, calcium antagonist, or angiotensin converting enzyme (ACE) inhibitor.

Step 2: If ineffective after 1 to 3 months, increase dosage of drug, add a second drug of a different class, or substitute another drug.

Step 3: Add a third drug of a different class or substitute a second drug.

Step 4: Add a fourth drug of a different class or substitute a third drug: evaluate further and refer to a specialist if ineffective.

After 1 year of satisfactory blood pressure control, a step-down approach may be effective in patients also adhering to nonpharmacologic measures.

Hypertensive crisis

Hypertensive emergency or crisis refers to a situation that requires immediate blood pressure lowering. Although such cases are relatively uncommon, prompt recognition and management are essential to prevent organ dysfunction. Clinical conditions that may precipitate a hypertensive crisis include hypertensive encephalopathy, intracranial hemorrhage, left ventricular heart failure, dissecting aortic aneurysm, severe hypertension of pregnancy, head trauma, extensive burns, unstable angina, or acute myocardial infarction. It may also occur in patients with poor hypertensive control and in those who abruptly discontinue their medications. Parenteral drug administration through IV and IM routes is used to quickly lower markedly elevated blood pressure. Intravenous medications are administered by drip and titrated according to the patient's response. Common drugs used in the treatment of hypertensive emergencies are listed in Table 26-10.

Interventions to achieve patient outcomes

The major nursing strategies in the care of the person with HTN are patient teaching and counseling. Teaching is directed toward increasing knowledge about HTN, risk factors, associated diseases, and the treatment regimen.

Counseling includes assisting the person in making behavioral changes to further reduce, control, or maintain blood pressure at acceptable levels, and in coping with sexual dysfunction.

Increasing knowledge of hypertension

The individual needs to understand the concepts of blood pressure and HTN. Use simple words to define systolic and diastolic blood pressure. Explain the effects of HTN on the heart, kidneys, and brain. Teach the person self-monitoring of blood pressure, as appropriate, and advise the person to purchase a reliable instrument; discourage use of coin-operated machines, which are often inaccurate. Have the person keep a written record of blood pressures, including date and any pertinent information if elevated or lowered.

Teaching about risk factors

Dietary modifications. Explain that excess salt intake will contribute to fluid retention; more fluid in the circulating blood will increase the blood pressure. Teaching should include the following:

1. Avoid adding salt to foods during preparation and at the table; substitute herbs for flavor.
2. Avoid highly salted foods, such as potato chips, pretzels, nuts, canned soups, and packaged luncheon meats.
3. Minimize eating in fast food restaurants (most of these foods have increased salt and fat content).
4. Reduce intake of saturated fats to maintain body weight and control atherosclerotic changes (see Chapter 5).
5. Use moderation in alcohol consumption: alcohol may potentiate certain antihypertensive medications in addition to raising blood pressure.

Other risk factors. Other behavioral changes to discuss include cessation of cigarette smoking, participating in exercise programs, and reducing stress.

1. Explain the effects of *nicotine* on blood vessels (p. 734); suggest use of behavior modification (Chapter 5), group therapy, or hypnosis as means of stopping smoking.

2. Discuss need to participate in a regular *aerobic* exercise program three times a week (Chapter 5), consisting of 20 to 45 minutes of activity with warm-up and cool-down periods.
3. Help patient identify sources of *stress*; demonstrate relaxation techniques such as deep breathing, progressive muscle relaxation, and imagery that can help lower blood pressure; suggest use of biofeedback techniques (Chapter 6).

Teaching about medications

Patients who are prescribed medications to control their blood pressure should know the name and type of drug, general action, dosage, and administration schedule. Common side effects include potassium depletion, orthostatic hypotension, and sexual dysfunction. *Potassium depletion*, seen mostly with use of diuretics, can be avoided by eating foods high in potassium (see Chapter 7) or by taking a multivitamin that contains potassium or a potassium supplement. *Orthostatic hypotension* is often worse in the mornings (when blood pressure is normally lower), after alcohol ingestion (vasodilator), and during immobility that follows exercise (pooling of blood in muscles). Orthostatic hypotension may be avoided by the following:

1. Rise slowly from a lying or sitting position to standing.
2. Sit down immediately if feeling faint; lower head.
3. Avoid long periods of standing (blood pools in legs, thereby temporarily causing hypovolemia)
4. Avoid very hot showers or baths (cause vasodilation, temporarily decreasing blood pressure)
5. Take medication at bedtime if drug can cause "first dose" hypotension or syncope.

Maintaining sexual function

Sexual dysfunction is a potential side effect of adrenergic inhibitors. In general, beta-adrenergic blockers and alpha blockers decrease ejaculation ability. Beta blockers also depress libido. Specific drugs, such as clonidine, interfere with erection. The patient needs to know about these effects. Do not make assumptions that the patient is not sexually active, despite marital status or age. Define terms of sexual dysfunction, such as libido, erection, and ejaculation, in simple language. Encourage the patient to report promptly any problems to a health care professional, and include the sexual partner in the teaching process, if possible (see Chapter 34). Suggest patient consult the physician concerning substituting an alternate medication.

Preventing noncompliance

Noncompliance with the therapeutic regimen is a major reason for inadequate HTN control. One reason is that symptoms are usually absent until advanced stages; hence the individual may not perceive a need to adhere to therapy. A second factor is the experience of unpleasant medication side effects and hesitancy to seek professional follow-up. If several medications are prescribed, it is sometimes difficult to remember to take the medications correctly. Well-controlled hypertensives have been found to have fewer HTN-related problems and lower blood pressures.

Measures to help increase compliance with therapy include the following:

1. Be sure that patient understands that absence of symptoms does not indicate control of blood pressure; remind patient that symptoms do not occur until advanced stages of the disease.
2. Advise patient against abrupt withdrawal of medication; rebound hypertension can occur.
3. Encourage patient to discuss unpleasant side effects of medication and other nonpharmacologic therapies with a health care professional.
4. If remembering to take medications is a problem, discuss alternate ways to remember, such as taking them with certain meals or placing medication in separate containers labeled with times of day.
5. Suggest patient participate in an exercise program with a friend (see Chapter 5) or pay for the program (more likely to participate "to get money's worth").
6. Include family and significant others in the teaching process to provide support and promote adherence to regimen.
7. Explain reason for regular health care follow-up (high blood pressure is a chronic disorder).
8. Contact patients who consistently cancel follow-up appointments.

Evaluation

Questions to ask may include the following:

1. Can patient explain the nature of HTN and effects on heart, kidney, and brain?
2. Can patient or significant other demonstrate correct procedure for self-measurement and recording of blood pressure?
3. Is blood pressure maintained within desirable range?
4. Can patient describe the drug regimen?
5. Is patient participating in dietary regimen, aerobic exercise program, and stress reduction activities?
6. Can patient explain effects of adrenergic inhibitors on sexual function, if indicated?
7. Is patient taking antihypertensive medication as prescribed?

SUMMARY

1. Risk factors associated with the development of peripheral vascular disorders include cigarette smoking, hyperlipidemia, hypertension, obesity, physical inactivity, emotional stress, diabetes mellitus, and a family history of atherosclerosis.
2. Primary prevention through health education about risk factors is the most important means to reduce the incidence of peripheral vascular disorders.
3. Arterial disorders occur when any disturbance in the structure of the arteries causes diminished blood flow and decreased oxygen and nutrients to the tissues.
4. The symptoms of arterial disorders are not caused by the degree of obstruction but by the extent to which the involved body part is deprived of circulation.
5. Medical therapy for patients with atherosclerosis include: smoking cessation; low-fat, low-cholesterol diet;

weight reduction; regular exercise; control of associated diseases (for example, diabetes and hypertension); and management.

6. Intermittent claudication is a symptom of arterial disorders. This term is used to describe a cramplike muscle pain that develops during exercise and is relieved after 1 to 2 minutes after stopping the exercise. It is usually unilateral and primarily affects the calf muscles.

7. Peripheral pulses may be absent or diminished in patients with arterial disorders.

8. Anticoagulants such as heparin and warfarin sodium (Coumadin) prolong clotting time, prevent extension of an existing clot, and inhibit further clot formation. Anticoagulants do not dissolve existing clots.

9. An important area to include in teaching a patient receiving Coumadin is the prevention of bleeding.

10. Protamine sulfate is a heparin antagonist, and vitamin K counteracts the effects of Coumadin.

11. Fibrinolytics such as streptokinase and urokinase dissolve existing thrombi.

12. Important nursing interventions for the patient undergoing arterial bypass surgery include: frequent assessment of peripheral pulses and the graft site, avoiding flexion in the area of the graft, and position changes to promote circulation.

13. Positioning a patient with an arterial disorder may include placement of the extremity flat in bed or in a slightly dependent (that is, 15 degree) position to promote circulation. Elevation is contraindicated in arterial disorders.

14. An important nursing intervention for the patient undergoing amputation surgery is to avoid flexion at the hip or knee to prevent contractures.

15. A teaching plan for a patient with arterial problems includes measures to prevent infection and injury, interventions to maintain skin integrity and to increase peripheral tissue perfusion, and methods to alter risk factors.

16. Thrombophlebitis can affect the superficial or deep veins. Thrombophlebitis in a deep vein can lead to a pulmonary embolus.

17. Deep vein thrombosis is treated by bed rest with periodic elevation of the affected extremity above heart level to prevent venous stasis and reduce edema.

18. Patients with chronic venous disorders such as varicose veins should be taught measures to increase perfusion. Measures to avoid include wearing restrictive clothing, crossing legs at the knee, and sitting or standing for long periods; measures to practice include elevating legs when sitting, wearing elastic stockings, and using good posture.

19. Leg ulcers can develop secondary to arterial or venous disorders. The primary goal in treating these ulcers is to promote wound healing and to prevent infection.

20. Wet-to-dry dressings and debriding chemicals remove necrotic tissue from leg ulcers. A special protective boot (Unna paste boot) may be applied over ulcers for ambulatory patients. Arterial bypass surgery or amputation may be necessary for nonhealing chronic ulcers.

21. Lymphedema results from interference with the drainage of interstitial fluid from the tissues; the affected part becomes greatly edematous.

22. Counseling and teaching the patient with lymphedema includes elevation of the affected extremity, wearing elastic stockings, taking diuretics as ordered, and avoiding an excess intake of foods high in sodium.

23. Hypertension is generally considered to be present when blood pressure levels persistently exceed 140/90. Most hypertension is idiopathic. It is a major cause of coronary artery disease, cardiac failure, strokes, and renal failure.

24. Drugs to control hypertension include diuretics (especially thiazides), peripheral and central acting adrenergics, beta blockers, and vasodilators. Medications are added in steps, as necessary, to control the blood pressure within normal limits.

25. Persons with hypertension should monitor their own blood pressure, continue prescribed medications, exercise, avoid salty foods, stop smoking, and continue with follow-up health care.

STUDY QUESTIONS

• What is the physiologic basis for the difference in leg positioning for arterial and venous disorders?

• What are the similarities and differences in patient teaching with arterial and venous disorders?

• Examine the chart of a patient with an arterial disorder. What diagnostic tests were done, and how would you explain these tests to a patient? What specific patient teaching is indicated? Is there notation of patient teaching on the chart?

• If you were directed to plan for hypertension screening in the community, which of the following sites would be most effective for identifying silent hypertension: malls, senior citizen centers, churches in black communities, blue collar workers in industrial centers? Give a rationale for your selection(s).

• Your 45-year-old neighbor tells you that she had her blood pressure taken by a friend and that it was 140/96. She says she's not worried because many of her family members also have high blood pressure. What actions would you take and why?

REFERENCES AND SELECTED READINGS

1.* Adelman EM: When the patient's blood pressure falls: what does it mean, what should you do? *Nurs 87* 17(10):66-73, 1987.

2.* Bartucci MR, et al: Factors associated with adherence in hypertensive patients, *ANNA J* 14:245-248, 1987.

3.* Beaver BM: Health education and the patient with peripheral vascular disease, *Nurs Clin North Am* 21:265-272, 1986.

4. Bergan JJ, Yao JT: *Venous disorders*, Philadelphia, 1991, WB Saunders.

5. Bernstein EF: *Noninvasive diagnostic techniques in vascular disease*, St Louis, 1990, Mosby–Year Book.

*Recommended for student reading.

6. Cotran RS, et al: *Robbin's pathologic basis of disease*, Philadelphia, 1989, WB Saunders.

7. Craeger MA: Preventing and treating deep vein thrombophlebitis, *Drug Ther* 15:16-25, 1985.

8. Crockett F: Varicose veins as a cause of venous ulceration, *Pract Cardiol* 11:191-199, 1985.

9.* Cunningham SG: Nonpharmacologic management of blood pressure, *J Cardiovasc Nurs* 23(4):18-22, 1987.

10.* Daeschner SA: Pulmonary embolism, *Nurs 88* 18(9):33, 1988.

11.* David JA: Wound management update, *Nurs 88* 18(6):33-37, 1988.

12.* Dixon MB, et al: Arterial reconstruction for atherosclerotic occlusive disease, *J Cardiovasc Nurs* 1(2):36-49, 1987.

13. Douglas MK, Shinn JA: *Advances in cardiovascular nursing*, Rockville, 1985, Aspen Systems.

14.* Doyle JE: Treatment modalities in peripheral vascular disease, *Nurs Clin North Am* 21:241-253, 1986.

15.* Ekers MA: Psychosocial considerations in peripheral vascular disease: cause or effect? *Nurs Clin North Am* 21:255-263, 1986.

16. Foreman MD: Arterial prosthetic graft injections: the pathophysiologic basis of nursing care, *Focus Crit Care* 12:23-28, 1985.

17. Ganong WF: *Review of medical physiology*, ed 15, Norwalk, Conn, 1991, Appleton & Lange.

18.* Gerdes L: Recognizing the multisystemic effects of embolism, *Nurs 87* 17(12):34-41, 1987.

19. Goldberg K, editor: *Vascular problems*, Springhouse, Penn, 1986, Springhouse.

20. Haimovici H, et al: *Vascular surgery: principles and techniques*, ed 3, Norwalk, Conn, 1989, Appleton & Lange.

21.* Henneman EA, Henneman PL: Intricacies of blood pressure measurement: reexamining the rituals, *Heart Lung* 18(3):263-271, 1989.

22.* Herman JA: Nursing assessment and nursing diagnosis in patients with peripheral vascular disease, *Nurs Clin North Am* 21:219-231, 1986.

23.* Hill MN, Cunningham SL: The latest words for high BP, *Am J Nurs* 89:504-509, 1989.

24.* Keller KB, Lemberg L: Vignettes in coronary care: hypertensive crisis, *Heart Lung* 20(4):421-424, 1991.

25.* Kleven MR: Comparison of thrombolytic agents: mechanisms of action, efficacy, and safety, *Heart Lung* 17(6):750-755, 1988.

26. Krakosky JN, Vanscoy GJ: Running an anticoagulation clinic, *Am J Nurs* 89:304-306, 1989.

27.* Massey JA: Diagnostic testing for peripheral vascular disease, *Nurs Clin North Am* 21:207-218, 1986.

28. McCarthy WJ, Williams LR: Femoral artery reconstruction, *Crit Care Q* 8:39-48, 1986.

29.* McMahan BE: Why deep vein thrombosis is so dangerous, *RN* 51:20-23, 1987.

30.* Miller RA, Evans WE: Immediate postop prosthesis, *Am J Nurs* 87:310-311, 1987.

31.* Moore LD, Pulliam CB: An on-the-spot guide to antihypertensive drugs, *Nurs 86* 16(1):54-57, 1986.

32. Moore WS: *Vascular surgery: a comprehensive review*, Philadelphia, 1991, WB Saunders.

33. Pender NJ: *Health promotion in nursing practice*, ed 2, Norwalk, Conn, 1987, Appleton & Lange.

34.* Ramsey R: Adjusting drug dosages for critically ill elderly patients, *Nurs 88* 18:47-49, 1988.

35. Report of the Joint National Committee on Detection, Evaluation, and Treatment of High Blood Pressure, US Department of Health and Human Services, Public Health Services, Bethesda, Md, 1988, National Institutes of Health.

36. Schmieder RE, Rockstroh JK, Messerli FH: Antihypertensive therapy: to stop or not to stop? *JAMA* 265(12):1566-1571, 1991.

37. Schroeder SA, et al: Current medical diagnosis and treatment, Norwalk, Conn, 1991, Appleton & Lange.

38. Schwartz SL, et al: *Principles of surgery*, ed 5, New York, 1989, McGraw-Hill.

39. Sobel BE: Fibrinolysis and activators of plasminogen, *Heart Lung* 17(6):775-779, 1987.

40.* Swithers CM: Tools for teaching about anticoagulants, *RN* 51(1):57-58, 1988.

41.* Turner JA: Nursing interventions in patients with peripheral vascular disease, *Nurs Clin North Am* 21:233-240, 1986.

42.* Vitello-Ciccio K: Thrombolytic therapy: urokinase, *J Cardiovasc Nurs* 1(2):59-62, 1987.

43.* Wagner MM: Pathophysiology related to peripheral vascular disease, *Nurs Clin North Am* 21:195-205, 1986.

44. Way LW: *Current surgical diagnosis and treatment*, ed 9, Norwalk, Conn, 1991, Appleton & Lange.

45. Wyngaarden JB, Smith LJ: *Cecil textbook of medicine*, ed 18, Philadelphia, 1988, WB Saunders.

46. Yee BH, Zorb SL: *Critical care nursing*, Boston, 1986, Little, Brown.

47. Young JR, et al: *Peripheral vascular disease*, St Louis, 1991, Mosby–Year Book.

27

The Patient with Hematologic Problems

Kathryn Sabo Thompson
Rosemarie M. Hogan

After studying this chapter, the learner should be able to:

- Differentiate among the functions of red blood cells, white blood cells, platelets, and the lymphatic system.
- Compare and contrast different types of anemia in terms of pathophysiology, assessment, and interventions.
- Contrast bone marrow aspiration and biopsy and the related care.
- Explain the genetic factors of sickle cell disease and describe sickle cell crisis.
- Compare and contrast disorders of coagulation (thrombocytopenia, hemophilia, DIC).
- Describe the four types of leukemia and their therapeutic modalities and nursing interventions.
- Differentiate between Hodgkin's disease and non-Hodgkin's lymphomas and related treatment modalities and nursing interventions.

Table 27-1 Normal adult values of cellular blood components

Type	Normal values	
Red blood cells	Male: 4.6-6.2 million/mm³	
	Female: 4.2-5.4 million/mm³	
White blood cells	4000-10,000/mm³	
Neutrophils	38%-70%	
Eosinophils	1%-5%	Differential blood count—
Basophils	0%-2%	totals 100%
Monocytes	1%-8%	
Lymphocytes	15%-45%	
Platelets	150,000-400,000/mm³	
Hematocrit	Male: 42%-53%	
	Female: 38%-46%	
Hemoglobin	Male: 13.4-17.6 g/100 ml	
	Female: 12-15.4 g/100 ml	
Mean corpuscular volume (MCV)	81-96 μm	
Mean corpuscular hemoglobin concentration (MCHC)	30%-36%	

Disorders related to the hematologic system are usually the result of problems in the normal production, development, and function of the components of blood or alterations in the rate of blood cell destruction. The illness can be chronic, acute, or a combination of both.

ANATOMY AND PHYSIOLOGY

The hematopoietic system includes blood and its components as well as the reticuloendothelial system (RES), which is located throughout the body. The RES's function is phagocytizing foreign materials and lysing (breaking down) red blood cells.

Components of the Hematopoietic System
Blood

Blood is a suspension of particulate materials in an aqueous colloid solution. The aqueous component of blood (plasma) is 91% to 92% water and 7% to 9% solids such as proteins, inorganic substances such as sodium, potassium, and calcium, and organic constituents such as urea, uric acid, and glucose.[26]

The cell components of blood include erythrocytes (or red blood cells [RBC]), leukocytes (or white blood cells [WBC]), and thrombocytes, or platelets (Table 27-1). All normal cells are derived from a single stem cell located throughout the bone marrow. The stem cell can divide into lymphoid and blood stem cells, which in turn become progenitor cells that divide along a specific single pathway (Fig. 27-1). This process is known as *hematopoiesis* and takes place in the bone marrow of the skull, vertebrae, pelvis, sternum, ribs, and proximal epiphysis of long bones. Production may take place in all the long bones during periods of increased demand, such as with hemorrhage or during blood cell destruction (hemolysis).

Red blood cells

An RBC is a nonnucleated biconcave disk that is soft and pliable. This property enables the RBC to change its shape during passage through the microcirculation. The RBC's major component is hemoglobin (Hb), a protein that transports oxygen and approximately 20% of carbon dioxide and maintains normal pH through a series of intracellular buffers (see Chapter 8). The Hb molecule contains globin (two pairs of polypeptide chains) and four heme groups. Each heme group contains an atom of ferrous iron. Oxygen is loosely and reversibly combined with hemoglobin to form oxyhemoglobin. Each molecule of hemoglobin can carry four bound molecules of oxygen, one oxygen molecule to each of the four heme groups. At the tissue site, the oxygen is released into the plasma and diffuses into the tissue cells to supply their needs.

Maturation of RBCs requires adequate amounts and use of vitamin B_{12}, folic acid, proteins, enzymes, and minerals such as iron or copper. *Erythropoietin*, a glycoprotein hormone believed to originate in the kidney, appears to stimulate RBC production (*erythropoiesis*). Tissue hypoxia resulting from changes in oxygen stimulates erythropoietin production. The stem cells involved in RBC production then initiate formation and maturation of the erythrocytes.

RBCs circulate for 120 days. Their cell membranes become fragile and rupture during passage through tight spots in the circulation. Many RBC fragments in the spleen are phagocytized and digested by RES cells. *Energy* in the form of ATP is required to maintain cell membrane integrity and the relatively low sodium and high potassium content of the red cell and for defense against oxidation and other environmental stressors.

White blood cells

WBCs may be classified into two groups: *granular leukocytes* (also called *polymorphonuclear* [PMN] *leukocytes*), consisting of neutrophils, eosinophils, and basophils; and *nongranular leukocytes*, consisting of monocytes and lymphocytes. The granulocytes contain enzymes that kill and digest bacteria upon degranulation of the cells.

Eosinophils have a weak phagocytic action and function in antigen-antibody reactions. Levels are elevated in asthmatic attacks, drug reactions, and certain parasitic infections. *Basophils* contain histamine and heparin; they release

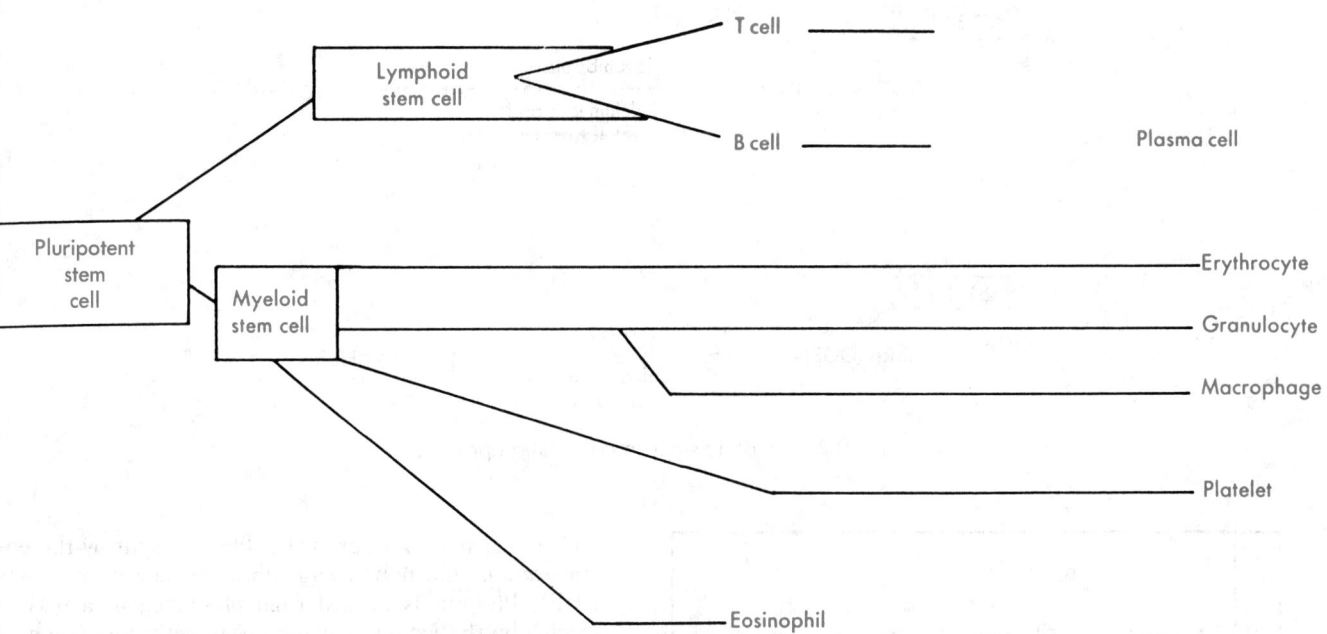

Fig. 27-1   Diagram of stem cell differentiation showing common progenitor cell for lymphoid cells, erythrocytes, granulocytes, and platelets. (Modified from Clinc M, Golde D: Blood 53:157-164, 1979.)

Table 27-2   Laboratory tests for hematologic assessment

Blood cell	Function	Diagnostic test
RBCs	Mediate the exchange of oxygen and carbon dioxide between lungs and tissue	RBC, hemoglobin, hematocrit, reticulocyte count Blood indices: Mean corpuscular hemoglobin concentration (MCHC), mean cell volume (MCV), mean corpuscular hemoglobin (MCH) Red cell fragility Morphologic description in stained smear
Platelets	Platelet plug; promotion of thrombin production	Platelet aggregation Platelet count Bleeding time
WBCs		WBC
Granulocytes		WBC with differential
Neutrophils	Phagocytosis	
Eosinophils	Parasitic infestation, allergic responses	
Basophils	Allergic (type I hypersensitivity) responses	
Lymphocytes	Immunlogic responses	
Monocytes	Phagocytosis	

histamine in allergic responses. Elevated basophil levels may be found in immunologic reactions and proliferative disorders of blood-forming cells.[26]

Neutrophils are present in the circulation or along the capillary walls (the margination pool). They move into the tissues and mucous membranes and serve as the body's primary defense against bacterial infection through the process of phagocytosis (see Chapter 16).

Monocytes are larger than neutrophils and have one large folded or indented nucleus. They leave the circulation and become tissue *macrophages*, which also have phagocytic ac-

tion, removing dead and injured cells, cell fragments, and microorganisms.

Lymphocytes are mononuclear with a round or oval nucleus. They originate primarily in lymphoid tissue (lymph nodes) but also in the bone marrow. There are two types of lymphocytes—T lymphocytes and B lymphocytes. T lymphocytes initiate the cellular immune response, while B lymphocytes (immunoglobulins) initiate the humoral immune response (see Chapter 16).

Laboratory tests have been developed to measure the amounts and functioning of all cellular components of the blood (Table 27-2).

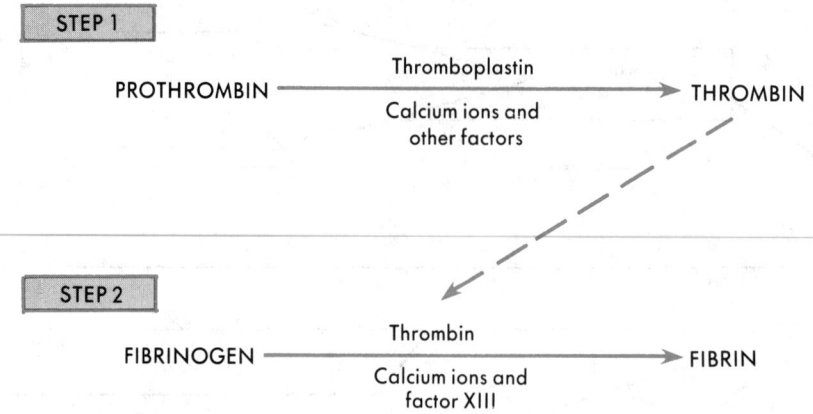

Fig. 27-2   Basic steps in coagulation process.

Coagulation factors

Factor I	Fibrinogen
Factor II	Prothrombin
Factor III	Thromboplastin, tissue thromboplastin
Factor IV	Calcium
Factor V	Proaccelerin, labile factor
Factor VI	Active form of factor *V*; no longer seen as separate factor
Factor VII	Serum prothrombin conversion accelerator (SPCA)
Factor VIII	Antihemophilic globulin (AHG) Antihemophilic factor (AHF)
Factor IX	Plasma thromboplastin component (PTC); Christmas factor
Factor X	Stuart factor
Factor XI	Plasma thromboplastin antecedent (PTA)
Factor XII	Hageman factor
Factor XIII	Fibrin-stabilizing factor, fibrinase

27-1

Platelets

Platelets (thrombocytes) are not cells but are granular disk-shaped, nonnucleated cell fragments. One third of the platelets are in the spleen as a reserve pool and the remainder in circulation. Platelets are derived from the stem cells that differentiate into the megakaryoblast, which in turn matures into megakaryocytes. These cells eventually break up into individual platelets that are essential to hemostasis and coagulation.

Hemostasis results from the adhesion and aggregation (clumping) capabilities of platelets to plug small breaks in blood vessels. Platelets also release *thromboplastin* (factor III), which, in the presence of calcium ions, converts prothrombin into thrombin in the first step of the coagulation mechanism (Fig. 27-2). In the second step of the coagulation mechanism, thrombin promotes the conversion of fibrinogen (a soluble plasma protein) into fibrin (an insoluble strand). Step one requires coagulation factors IV, V, VIII, IX, X, XI, and XII; whereas step two requires factors IV and XIII (Box 27-1).

Clot destruction occurs when fibrin is split by the enzyme *plasmin* (fibrinolysin) into fibrin degradation products (FDP). Plasmin is formed from plasminogen (a plasma protein) by the action of plasminogen activators (such as streptokinase, urokinase, tissue kinase, and factor XIIa). FDP interferes with thrombin activity, platelet functioning, and fibrin formation, thus dissolving the clot.

Reticuloendothelial system

The RES, also called the monocyte-phagocyte system or macrophage system, includes circulating monocytes and their precursor cells in the bone marrow. It also includes more or less fixed mononuclear phagocytic cells found in blood channels in the spleen and liver (Kupffer cells) and in the lymphatic system, serosal cavities of the body, lungs, general connective tissue, and bone marrow.

The important function of the RES is *phagocytosis*, that is, cleaning the blood, lymph, and intestinal spaces of foreign material, especially bacteria, that are removed in a few hours by macrophages (phagocytic cells) located throughout the body. This removal of foreign materials is the first step—essential in the chain of events leading to the immune response (Chapter 16).

In addition to phagocytosis, the RES removes the Hb of RBCs that have reached the end of their life span, splitting Hb into an iron-containing substance and bilirubin (see Chapter 30).

Physiologic Changes with Aging

The total number of leukocytes and differential counts show no variation through middle age and no gross changes in old age. In general the leukocyte count does not rise as high in response to infection, and studies suggest that the elderly have a diminished marrow granulocyte reserve.

The Hb level decreases after middle age, although the decrease in women seems to be relatively less than that in men. Unexplained anemia in the elderly has been noted, but iron absorption is not impaired. However, use of orally administered iron is reduced. This anemia does not appear to be related solely to age.[47] Serum iron and iron-binding capacity decrease in the elderly, and low serum vitamin B_{12} and folic acid levels occur in a significant proportion of elderly people but without anemia.

No age-related changes in platelets have been reported. RBC sedimentation rate increases significantly, but this rate is of limited value in detecting disease in the elderly. Some of the plasma coagulation factors have been reported to increase with age (factors I, V, VII, and IX). Partial thromboplastin time may be shortened.[18] Changes in lymphocyte (T cells and B cells) function are described in Chapter 41.

PREVENTION AND HEALTH EDUCATION
Primary Prevention

Health promotion for hematologic disorders includes health teaching to prevent the disorders, when possible. Exposure to certain chemicals and drugs places individuals at high risk, especially for aplastic anemia and the leukemias. Persons with inadequate dietary intake of iron and vitamins B_{12} or folic acid, alcoholics, and others with poor dietary habits because of inadequate knowledge or low income, are particularly susceptible to anemia. Women who have long-term blood loss because of heavy menstrual bleeding (menorrhagia) are also at risk for anemia, as are other persons with long-term slow blood loss, as with hemorrhoids.

Occupational health nurses provide information to workers about health risks in the environment and ways in which risk factors can be decreased. Nurses in all settings teach about dietary needs for iron and other vitamins. Persons with low incomes can be taught to identify inexpensive food sources of the vitamins and minerals necessary for hematologic health. Nurses can also become politically active to ensure that there is adequate government funding for food stamps and establishment or maintenance of other low-cost nutritional programs for those persons who have marginal incomes.

Secondary Prevention

Occupational health nurses are involved in identifying industrial chemicals or processes that place workers in danger and in screening employees as pertinent. Screening for anemias in any setting occurs during routine physical examinations with blood tests.

Diseases such as sickle cell anemia, the thalassemias, and hemophilia are hereditary; therefore, marriage between carriers of defective genes may result in children with the disease. One of the most difficult and sensitive roles for nurses is that of genetic counselor, communicating to individuals with hereditary problems the risk factors involved and possibility of having children with severe hematopoietic disease. Couples are allowed to make their own decisions after information has been shared with them. The decision to conceive a child, given the hereditary risk, is extremely difficult and can prove to be devastating to a couple.

MAJOR HEALTH PROBLEMS RELATED TO BLOOD AND LYMPH SYSTEMS

Disorders associated with the hematopoietic system are diverse in their underlying pathologic manifestations, disease course, and response to treatment. Most often, the symptoms are the result of interference with the normal development and function of the blood components and with altered hematopoiesis (blood cell production). Normally homeostasis is maintained through a balance between the rate of production of normal blood cells and the rate of destruction. Disorders of the blood are manifested when this hemostatic balance is lost. Disturbances in the coagulation mechanism also result in blood disorders.

In addition to primary hematologic disorders, secondary effects from disease of another body system may also manifest themselves in abnormal hematologic findings. For example, the anemia that is associated with azotemia is the consequence of disease existing outside of the hematopoietic system. Major health problems include the following:

1. RBC disorders
   a. Anemias
   b. Erythrocytosis: polycythemia
2. Coagulation disorders
   a. Platelet disorders: thrombocytopenia
   b. Hemophilia
   c. Disseminated intravascular coagulation (DIC)
3. WBC disorders: agranulocytosis, leukemia
4. Lymph system disorders: lymphadenopathy, lymphomas (Hodgkin's and non-Hodgkin's)
5. Plasma cell dyscrasias: multiple myeloma

DISORDERS ASSOCIATED WITH ERYTHROCYTES

Anemia (decreased RBCs) and erythrocytosis (increased RBCs) are the general categories of red cell disorders. Sickle cell anemia, a form of anemia, is discussed separately from the other types of anemia because of differences in nursing care.

ANEMIA

Anemia refers to a deficiency of RBCs as reflected in a decreased hemoglobin level, packed cell volume (hematocrit), and red cell count.

Etiology

Anemias may be divided into those that are the result of blood loss, impaired production of RBCs, increased destruction of RBCs, or nutritional deficiencies (Table 27-3).

Table 27-3   Disorders of red blood cells

Disorder	Signs and symptoms	Medical therapy
Anemias		
Secondary to blood loss Acute	Hypovolemic and hypoxemic symptoms (weakness, stupor, irritability, cool moist skin, hypotension, tachycardia, ↓ Hb and Hct, pallor)	Treat for shock: IV fluids, whole blood or packed cells; identify source of loss; administer iron
Chronic	Depends on degree of ↓ in Hb; if less than 8.0 g/dl: weakness, fatigue, ↑ pulse, pallor, exertional dyspnea	Packed cells, iron; identify source of loss
Aplastic anemia	As in chronic anemia plus those related to ↓ WBC and platelets (ecchymoses), petechiae, GI, GU, CNS bleeding, increased risk of infection)	Remove causative agent; supportive care until bone marrow is regenerated: transfusions; bone marrow transplantation, antithymocyte therapy
Hemolytic anemia Congenital Sickle cell anemia	↓ Hb; ↓ Hct; pain (bones, joints, back): generalized, localized or migratory; vomiting; fever; infections; chronic leg ulcers; cardiomegaly; murmurs; CHF; delay in growth and sexual maturation; swollen hands and feet (dactylitis); jaundice	No specific therapy; analgesics, oxygen, adequate hydration, treatment of infection, polyvalent pneumococcal vaccine to prevent pneumococcal infections, antisickling agents (experimental), therapeutic apheresis
	Thrombotic crisis: severe pain in abdomen and musculoskeletal system	Adequate hydration, exchange transfusions (replacing person's blood with packed red cells, unit for unit)
	Aplastic crisis: rapid ↑ in anemia	
Thalassemia	Thalassemia minor: mild anemia Thalassemia major: severe anemia	No therapy required; transfusions with severe symptoms or to maintain Hb near normal
Enzyme deficiency	Anemia when person exposed to oxidant drugs (aspirin, sulfonanmides, antimalarial)	Remove causative drug
Acquired hemolytic anemia	Same as with other anemias	Corticosteroids, splenectomy in those who do not respond to drug therapy
Nutritional anemia Iron deficiency anemia	Gradual development; may have few signs; fatigue, exertional dyspnea, severe anemia, brittle spoon-shaped (concave) nails with longitudinal ridges, atrophy of tongue papillae, smooth shiny tongue, cheilosis (cracks in corner of mouth); low serum iron, pallor, weakness	Determine and correct cause Oral iron administration (ferrous sulfate); parenteral iron if oral not tolerated or not absorbed via GI tract; adequate balanced diet
Megaloblastic anemia	Low serum B_{12} and folate levels, neurologic abnormalities (peripheral neuropathies, loss of balance), symptoms associated with underlying disease and anemia	Parenteral administration of vitamin B_{12}, usually once a month
Erythrocytosis		
Polycythemia vera (primary)	Absent in early stages; headache, tinnitus, blurred vision, reddened skin, nosebleeds, ecchymoses, GI bleeding caused by platelet dysfunction, thrombosis, hepatomegaly, splenomegaly, ↑ total RBC volume, ↑ or normal plasma volume	Periodic phlebotomy (removal of blood), radioactive phosphorus, chemotherapeutic agents such as busulfan
Secondary polycythemia	↑ RBC, ↑ Hct; symptoms may be similar to but less severe than those in polycythemia vera	Correct underlying condition
Pseudopolycythemia	As above; is self-limiting; symptoms are mild	Stress reduction

27-2	**Drugs that may cause aplastic anemia**
	Acetylsalicylic acid (aspirin) Lithium
	Benzene Mephenytoin
	Chloramphenicol D-Penicillamine
	Colchicine Phenobarbital
	Ibuprofen Sulfonamides
	Lead Trimethadione

27-3	**Pathophysiologic basis of symptoms of chronic anemia**
	Fatigue and weakness Decreased RBCs in superficial vessels.
	Tachycardia Increased cardiac pumping to deliver more oxygen to tissues with less Hb to carry oxygen.
	Exertional dyspnea Activity requires more oxygen, but the fewer RBCs cannot keep up with the increased demand for oxygen; the person becomes dyspneic trying to take in more oxygen.

Blood loss is a major cause of anemia. The anemia may be due to acute blood loss by hemorrhage or to blood loss over a period of time, as from slow bleeding from a peptic ulcer, GI tumor, bleeding hemorrhoids, or menorrhagia.

Impaired production of RBCs leads to *aplastic anemia*. Causes of aplastic anemia may be antineoplastic or cytotoxic agents, certain drugs (Box 27-2), and viral infections. At times no causative agent can be found (idiopathic aplastic anemia).

Anemias that result from destruction of RBCs are termed *hemolytic anemias*. Many are of *genetic* origin, including hereditary spherocytosis, and the hemoglobinopathies, including sickle cell anemia, thalassemia, and enzyme-deficiency anemia. *Acquired* hemolytic anemia may be caused by a drug (alpha methyldopa, penicillin) or an autoimmune response or may be idiopathic or secondary to lymphocytic lymphoma or chronic lymphocytic leukemias.

The final group of anemias are due to *nutritional deficiencies*. A major example of this type of anemia is *iron deficiency anemia*, which may result from chronic blood loss or from inadequate dietary intake. *Vitamin B$_{12}$ deficiency* anemia usually occurs from decreased absorption rather than decreased intake. *Folic acid deficiency anemia* results from inadequate dietary intake (often associated with alcoholism), malabsorption syndromes, and certain medications.

Pathophysiology
Anemia secondary to blood loss

Anemia associated with blood loss may be acute or chronic. *Acute anemia* is the direct result of the decrease in a large amount of circulating RBCs. An adult of average build can lose 500 ml of blood (out of a total of 6000 ml) without serious or lasting effects. Losses of 1000 ml or more can cause acute consequences. The severity of symptoms depends on the severity of blood loss and the resulting degree of hypoxia (inadequate tissue oxygenation); as the number of RBCs decreases, less oxygen is delivered to tissues. Sudden acute hemorrhage with loss of 30% or more of blood volume causes symptoms of diaphoresis, restlessness, tachycardia, tachypnea, shortness of breath and, without intervention, shock. The body's compensatory responses to hypoxia include the following[37]:

1. Increased cardiac output and respirations increasing oxygen delivery to the tissues
2. Increased release of oxygen by hemoglobin
3. Expanded plasma volume by pulling fluid from tissue spaces
4. Redistribution of blood to vital organs.

Compensatory vasoconstriction to shunt blood to vital organs is responsible for some of the signs and symptoms of anemia, such as pallor or cold or clammy extremities. Cerebral hypoxia causes symptoms of mental confusion, bizarre behavior and drowsiness, headache, dizziness and tinnitus (ringing of the ears).

Chronic anemia secondary to blood loss is the most common cause of iron-deficiency anemia (p. 750). The body has remarkable adaptive powers and may adjust fairly well to a marked reduction in RBCs and Hb, provided the condition develops gradually. An individual may remain asymptomatic even though the total RBC count may drop to almost half of its normal level or the Hb level to below 7 g/100 ml. When blood loss is continuous and moderate in amount, the bone marrow may be able to keep up with the losses by increasing RBC production. If the cause of chronic blood loss is not found and corrected, eventually the bone marrow will not be able to keep pace with the loss, and symptoms of anemia (Box 27-3) will appear. In addition, gastrointestinal symptoms (anorexia, nausea, constipation or diarrhea, stomatitis) may also occur as a result of chronic hypoxia.

Aplastic anemia

The word aplastic means no tendency to develop into new tissue. The defect leading to aplastic anemia is most likely injury or destruction of a common stem cell (see Fig. 27-1) that affects all subsequent cell populations. This produces a deficiency in blood cell production in bone marrow. Aplastic anemia is characterized not only by impaired RBC production but also by impairment of *all* blood-producing elements. A decrease in WBCs (leukopenia) and in platelets (thrombocytopenia) occurs. Loss of RBCs leads to symptoms of chronic anemia (see Box 27-3). Fewer WBCs increase the risk of infection, and decreased platelets may lead to bleeding in the tissue (ecchymoses), as well as GI, GU, and CNS bleeding.

Hemolytic anemias

Hemolytic anemia results when the RBCs are destroyed at such a rapid rate that the bone marrow is unable to compensate for the loss. The severity of the anemia is determined by the degree of lag between the rate of RBC destruction (hemolysis) and the rate of bone marrow production of red cells (erythropoiesis). *Hereditary sphero-*

27-4	**Descriptive cell characteristics in anemia**	
	Size	Macrocytic (large)
		Normocytic
		Microcytic (small)
	Hemoglobin	Normochromic
		Hypochromic (decreased)

cytosis, an inherited autosomal dominant trait, is characterized by a membrane abnormality leading to osmotic swelling of the red cell and susceptibility to destruction by the spleen. It is most commonly detected in childhood but may be noted initially in adulthood. Severe anemia (aplastic crisis, p. 755) may occur if bone marrow production is impaired, as by infection. Jaundice may result from the chronic RBC hemolysis in the spleen.

Hemoglobinopathies

Hemoglobinopathies are a group of hemolytic diseases in which one or more amino acids are substituted in the globin chain of the Hb molecule, leading to the formation of abnormal Hb (for example, hemoglobins S and C). The most common hemoglobinopathy is sickle cell anemia (p. 754).

Thalassemia, which is a hemoglobinopathy, is an inherited disorder characterized by a decreased synthesis of one of the globin chains of hemoglobin. The beta (β) chain is most often affected (β-thalassemia). As a result, hemoglobin synthesis decreases, although hemoglobin accumulates in the erythrocyte of the unaffected globin chain. These alterations result in decreased red cell production and a chronic hemolytic anemia. The red cells are characteristically hypochromic and microcytic (see Box 27-4). Hb electrophoresis is diagnostic.

There are two types of thalassemia: thalassemia minor, which is usually asymptomatic, and thalassemia major, which is characterized by severe anemia. Lifespan is significantly shorter, and frequent transfusion therapies may produce iron overload, a problem that can be ameliorated by an iron-chelating drug such as deferoxamine.

Another type of hemoglobinopathy is *enzyme deficiency*. Deficiency of enzymes in the pathways that metabolize glucose and generate ATP frequently leads to premature red cell destruction. The most common clinically significant enzyme abnormality is that of *glucose-6-phosphate dehydrogenase*. This disorder is common in a mild form among the black population in the United States and in the Mediterranean area and may cause chronic hemolytic anemia. When an oxidant drug puts the cells under stress, acute hemolysis results.

Acquired hemolytic anemia

Hemolytic anemia may be drug induced or may be caused by an autoimmune disorder. In the latter case an antibody develops that is directed against an antigen on the individual's own RBCs. The antibody-coated red cells are destroyed prematurely by reticuloendothelial cells, particularly in the spleen. Diagnosis is confirmed by demon-

strating the presence of the antibody on the red cells (antiglobin or Coombs' test).

Drugs produce hemolysis in a variety of ways. Alpha methyldopa (Aldomet) is associated with production of an autoantibody and a positive Coombs' test in approximately 20% of patients. More rarely, high-dose penicillin causes hemolysis by producing an antibody that requires the presence of penicillin on the red cell membrane for its effects to occur. This disorder is often fatal, in part because transfusion is often made difficult and dangerous by the fact that the autoantibody reacts not only with the patient's red cells but also with all donor cells.

Anemia secondary to nutritional deficiency

The nutritional anemias include iron-deficiency anemia and the megaloblastic anemias.

Iron deficiency anemia

Iron is a fundamental part of the Hb molecule, and its deficiency leads to production of red cells with a decreased amount of Hb and ultimately to a decreased number of red cells. The average adult body contains approximately 4 g of iron, 3 g of which are in Hb. Average daily loss of iron by the body is approximately 1.5 mg, which is compensated for by absorption from the diet of approximately that amount of iron daily. This tenuous balance may be compromised by chronic blood loss, which may be physiologic, as in menstruation, or pathologic, as in GI or other bleeding.

It is also common in menstruating women, pregnant women, and growing children. Aged individuals may eat an imbalanced diet because of limited income, mobility, and isolation from those people who might help with preparation or purchase of food.

The anemia is characteristically hypochromic and microcytic (see Box 27-4).

Megaloblastic anemia

Megaloblastic anemia is characterized by the presence of megaloblasts (immature progenitors of abnormal RBCs) in the bone marrow. The red cells are macrocytic. There is a deficit in the nucleus of the maturing red cell as a result of interference with DNA synthesis from a nutritional deficiency, primarily vitamin B_{12} or folic acid.

Vitamin B_{12} requires the presence of an intrinsic factor from gastric secretion for absorption in the ileum. Two interferences with absorption are lack of intrinsic factor or direct interference with the transport of vitamin B_{12} across the membrane in the ileum. Intrinsic factor may be absent as a result of genetic factors (*pernicious anemia*) or from surgical resection of the stomach. Malabsorption in the ileum may result from malabsorption syndromes, small bowel diverticuli, intestinal inflammations, or intestinal resection.

Because vitamin B_{12} can be stored in the body, deficiencies may not produce symptoms for many years. Diagnosis of pernicious anemia is confirmed by an abnormal Schilling test, which demonstrates the inability to absorb vitamin B_{12} unless intrinsic factor is administered.

Folic acid (folacin) is a vitamin of the B complex that is involved in the synthesis of amino acids and DNA and

Table 27-4   Clinical significance of abnormal blood counts

	Increased values	Decreased values
RBC	Polycythemia (erythrocytosis)	Leukopenia
WBC	Neutrophilia	Leukopenia
	Leukemias	Aplastic anemia
		Neutropenias
Platelets	Polycythemia	Aplastic anemia
		Thrombocytopenia
		Disseminated intravascular coagulation (DIC)
Hematocrit	Polycythemia	Anemias
		Hemorrhage
Hemoglobin	Polycythemia	Anemias
		Hemorrhage
Mean corpuscular volume (MCV)	Pernicious anemia	Iron deficiency anemia
	Folic acid deficiency	Chronic blood loss
Mean corpuscular hemoglobin concentration (MCHC)		Iron deficiency anemia
		Chronic blood loss

therefore in the maturation of RBCs. Certain medications inhibit the enzyme that is involved in normal absorption of folate through the intestinal wall. Vitamin B_{12} deficiency and folic acid deficiency often occur together.

Nursing Process
Assessment
Subjective data

Collect the following subjective data from patients with anemia:

1. Knowledge of cause of the anemia
2. Feelings of weakness or fatigue and ability to carry out ADL
3. Feelings of dyspnea and precipitating activities
4. Factors that appear to exacerbate symptoms
5. History of exposure to chemicals (insecticides, benzene products) or drugs that may cause aplastic anemia (see Box 27-2)
6. Family history of anemia

Objective data

Physical examination of the person with anemia usually shows normal findings. The skin and mucous membranes may appear pale and cool. If hemolytic anemia is present, the skin and eyeballs may appear yellowish from bile deposits. Labored breathing may be observed, especially with exertion. The pulse may be rapid. With severe anemia, monitor the patient's ability to respond to questions and for signs of confusion.

If blood loss has occurred or if the person has severe aplastic anemia, monitor and report signs of bleeding, external or internal (bleeding gums, melena). For aplastic anemia, monitor for signs of infection (from the leukopenia).

Diagnostic tests
Laboratory tests

Clinical significance of abnormal blood counts are noted in Table 27-4. RBCs are usually decreased but are not good indicators of anemia: hematocrit (Hct) and hemoglobin

(Hb) tests are better indicators. Normal values are listed in Table 27-1. The *hematocrit* (packed RBC volume) is the ratio of RBC volume to the whole blood volume. The Hct rarely falls below 25% in chronic anemia.[30] An Hb test measures the amount of Hb in circulation.

RBC indices provide a differential diagnosis of the type of anemia. The RBC indices include the *mean corpuscular volume* (MCV) and *mean corpuscular Hb concentration* (MCHC). The MCV estimates the average size of the RBC. The MCHC measures the content of Hb in RBCs. (The significance of changes in these indices are listed in Table 27-4.)

Peripheral blood smears provide information on the etiology of the anemia. Observe the size and shape of the RBC (Box 27-4), as well as extent of cell maturity and ratio of the various cell types to each other. WBCs can also be examined to provide information about adequate bone marrow production.

Bone marrow aspiration

Bone marrow aspiration is appropriate when the diagnosis is not clearly established by peripheral blood smears or when further information is needed. Aspiration is the most common procedure for obtaining a bone marrow sample. The procedure is possible because normal bone marrow is soft and semifluid and can therefore be removed by aspiration through a needle. Bone marrow aspiration is also used in the diagnosis of acute leukemia and thrombocytopenia.

The skin surrounding the puncture site (Fig. 27-3) is shaved, if necessary, and cleansed with an antiseptic such as povidine-iodine complex (Betadine). Sterile towels are placed around the site. The skin and periosteum are anesthetized to avoid pain. First, the most superficial layer of the skin is infiltrated with procaine. After a few seconds the needle is further advanced until bone is touched. Procaine is then injected to anesthetize the periosteum.

The marrow aspiration needle is inserted, and when the marrow cavity is entered, the marrow stylet is removed from the needle and a sterile syringe is attached. The

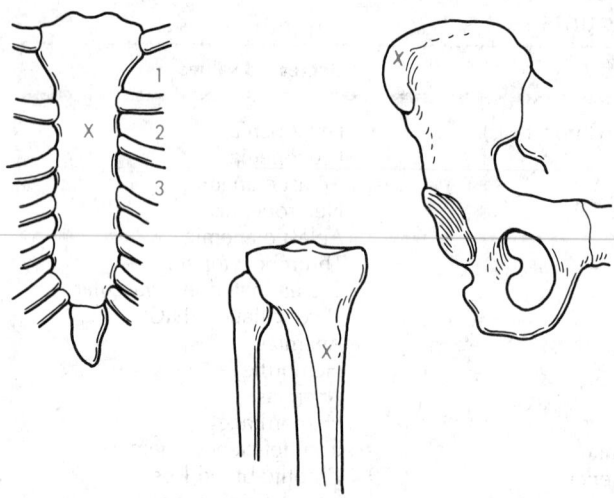

Fig. 27-3 Sites for bone marrow aspiration: sternum, iliac crest (most common) and tibia.

syringe plunger is drawn back until marrow appears in the syringe. As the plunger is drawn back the person will experience a brief, sharp pain, sometimes described as a burning sensation. The pain is caused by the suction exerted as the plunger is pulled back. Some persons may complain of tenderness at the aspiration site for a few days. Most often no pain or discomfort is experienced following the procedure.

Nursing care with bone marrow aspiration includes the following:

1. Explain procedure to patient, stating that there may be brief discomfort when the marrow is aspirated.
2. To prevent movement, place hands on patient's shoulders and instruct patient to remain still at the time of aspiration.
3. Apply pressure over aspiration site after needle is removed to prevent bleeding; apply pressure for 3 to 5 minutes if patient is thrombocytopenic.
4. Assess for bleeding from aspiration site.
5. Provide comfort measures to help patient relax.

Bone marrow biopsy

When a large sample of bone marrow is needed, a bone marrow biopsy may be performed. Persons most likely to undergo a bone marrow biopsy are those with pancytopenia (more than one altered cell type), metastatic tumor, lymphoma, and multiple myeloma.

The most common site for bone marrow biopsy is the posterosuperior iliac spine, although the sternum may also be used. The initial steps in the biopsy procedure are similar to those outlined for bone marrow aspiration. The use of a Jamshidi needle allows for a core of marrow to be collected (Fig. 27-4). Nursing care following a bone marrow biopsy is similar to that of bone marrow aspiration.

From microscopic examination of the bone marrow, iron stores can be determined, as can the morphology of the progenitor cell. Megaloblastic (RBC precursor) changes and the absence of cells may be observed. Infiltration with leukemic cells may also be determined.

Data analysis: nursing diagnoses

Nursing diagnoses are determined from analysis of patient data. Possible nursing diagnoses for the person with anemia may include, but are not limited to, the following:

Diagnostic title	Possible etiologies
Fatigue	Decreased tissue oxygenation, inadequate rest
Injury, high risk for falls, bleeding	Decreased cerebral oxygenation, decreased coagulation
Infection, high risk for	Decreased WBC, decreased immune response
Decisional conflict	Threat to health of future children
Knowledge deficit	Lack of exposure or recall

Planning: expected patient outcomes

Expected patient outcomes for the patient with anemia may include, but are not limited to, the following:

1. States feeling more rested and less fatigued.
2. No injuries have occurred from falls.
3. Bleeding is controlled.
4. No infection is present.
5. Makes decisions with spouse concerning conception based on knowledge of illness (hemolytic anemia).
6. Explains nature of anemia, measures to prevent injury and bleeding, replacement therapy, and follow-up care.

Implementation
Assisting with achievement of therapeutic goals

Transfusion therapy may be given for anemias from acute blood loss. With chronic blood loss, packed cells are more appropriate, if indicated, because the patient has had time to replace the plasma. Monitor the patient for signs of transfusion reactions (see Chapter 41).

Bone marrow transplantation is the treatment of choice for persons with severe aplastic anemia (aplastic crisis) who are under age 30 and who have HLA-matched siblings[30] (p. 768). Those over age 30 or without HLA-matched siblings are treated with immunosuppressive therapy such as antithymocyte globulin (see Chapter 41).

The medical treatment for nutritional anemias is primarily drug replacement (Table 27-3). Oral ferrous sulfate is the drug of choice for iron deficiency anemia or anemia from chronic blood loss. Parenteral iron may be given if GI disease is present or if blood loss continues. Iron therapy should be taken for 3 to 6 months after normal hematologic levels are restored to replenish iron stores.[30] Vitamin B_{12} replacement therapy must be given parenterally because of the decreased oral absorptive capabilities. Life-long therapy is necessary for persons with pernicious anemia. Folic acid replacement therapy is given orally.

Interventions to achieve patient outcomes
Promoting rest

Fatigue is a major problem for persons with anemia because of the decreased oxygenation to tissues from the decreased Hb. For the hospitalized patient, plan care so that there is a balance between activities and rest to prevent increased oxygen expenditure and hypoxemia. Persons at home need to plan ADL to allow rest periods.

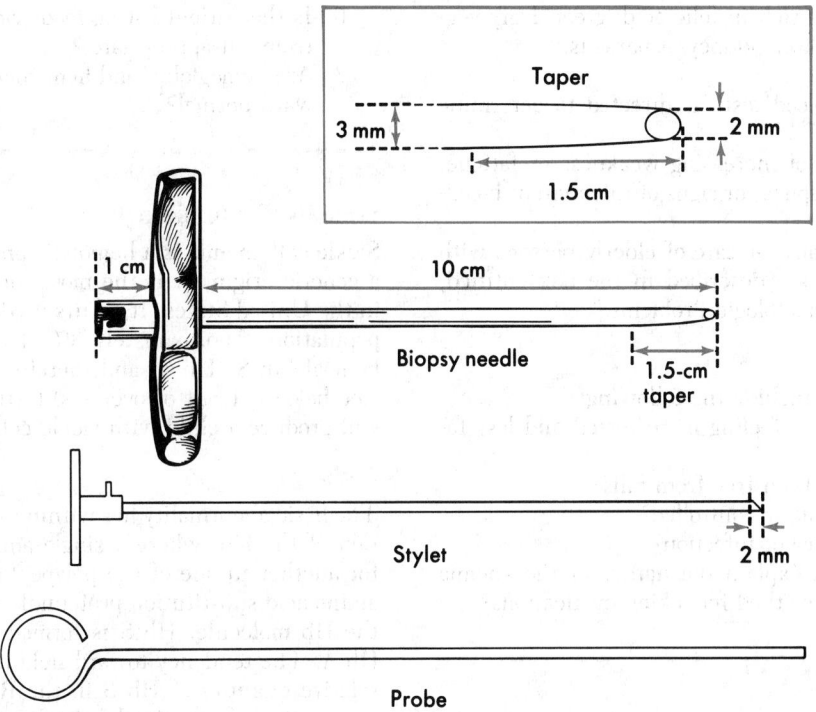

Fig. 27-4 Bone marrow biopsy needle showing shape and size.

Preventing injury

When muscle weakness or confusion is present with severe anemia (because of the decreased oxygenation to muscles and brain), supervise patient ambulation to prevent falls. Keep the room uncluttered. Encourage the patient to use handrails as necessary.

Remember that the patient with aplastic anemia is susceptible to bleeding because of decreased platelets. Apply direct pressure for 5 minutes after injection or if any external bleeding occurs. Encourage patient to use a soft toothbrush to prevent bleeding of the gums. Suggest that patient use an electric shaver to prevent skin breaks. Encourage fluids and dietary fiber to promote a soft stool, thus decreasing irritation of the rectum or hemorrhoids, which cause bleeding. Avoid drugs such as aspirin that have anticoagulant properties.

Preventing infection

Patients with severe aplastic or hemolytic anemia may be susceptible to infection because of decreased WBCs or decreased immune response. Persons with colds or other infections should avoid contact with the patient. Provide and teach good hygiene care. Avoid injections and other intrusive procedures, if possible.

Counseling patients

Persons who have a hereditary hemolytic anemia (hereditary spherocytosis, hemoglobinopathies, or enzyme deficiency) have the potential to transmit the trait to their children. It is therefore important for these persons to seek genetic counseling to assist them and their spouses in making decisions about bearing children. As cited in the discussion on prevention of hemotologic disorders (p. 747),

this is not an easy decision to make. The nurse can provide opportunities for the couple to explore their feelings and to help them use problem-solving techniques in coming to a conclusion. The decision is ultimately up to the couple.

Facilitating patient learning

Because anemia is often a chronic condition, patient teaching is an important part of nursing care and includes the following:

1. Knowledge about the cause of the anemia, preventive measures (if any), and therapeutic modalities.
2. Measures to prevent infection and bleeding (see above).
3. Replacement therapy when indicated for anemia from chronic blood loss or nutritional anemia.
    a. Iron
        (1) Take ferrous sulfate after meals to prevent GI irritation.
        (2) Stools will be black from digested iron.
        (3) Report signs of nausea or diarrhea to physician.
        (4) Eat iron-rich foods: organ meats (especially liver), seafood, whole or enriched grains, legumes, green leafy vegetables, and nuts.[36]
        (5) Take iron for 3 to 6 months after blood levels are restored, to build up iron stores.
    b. Vitamin B_{12}
        (1) Must be given parenterally because of decreased absorption.
        (2) Life-long therapy is necessary.
    c. Folic acid
        (1) Take prescribed oral folic acid.

(2) Eat foods rich in folic acid: green leafy vegetables, liver, kidney, asparagus.[36]

4. Follow-up care
   a. Report for blood tests as directed to determine progress.
   b. Report signs of increasing weakness or fatigue, increased dyspnea, or signs of infection or bleeding.

Special considerations for care of elderly persons with hematologic problems are described in the box entitled, "The Elderly with Hematologic Problems."

Evaluation

Questions to consider include the following:
1. Does patient state feeling more rested and less fatigued?
2. Has the patient been free from falls?
3. Is bleeding absent or controlled?
4. Is the patient free of infection?
5. Can the patient explain the nature of the anemia and the correct method for taking medications?

The Elderly with Hematologic Problems

Assessment

Assess adequacy of iron and folic acid intake.
Assess presence and extent of fatigue and ability to carry out ADL.

Intervention

Assist patient with nutritional deficiency anemia to plan diet that includes food rich in iron and folic acid, as appropriate.
Assist patient to plan for rest periods when fatigue is present.
Teach patient and significant others:
   Importance of prescribed replacement therapy and ways to facilitate compliance.
   Need to report signs of increasing fatigue to physician.
   Measures to prevent infection with leukemia. Elderly persons have the added risk factor of decreased immune response and are hightly susceptible to pneumonia.

Common disorders in elderly

Nutritional deficiency anemia
Leukemia (ANLL, CLL)
Lymphoma

---

6. Is the patient eating foods rich in the deficient nutrient (if appropriate)?
7. Are hemoglobin and hematocrit levels increasing toward normal?

SICKLE CELL ANEMIA

Etiology/Epidemiology

Sickle cell anemia is a hemolytic anemia (see p. 749) with a genetic origin. It is the most common genetic disorder in the United States. It occurs predominantly in the black population. Approximately 8% of American blacks carry hemoglobin S (Hb S) and therefore have sickle cell trait (see below); 1 out of over 400 births of American blacks will produce a child with sickle cell trait.[30]

Pathophysiology

The basic abnormality lies within the globin (protein) fraction of the Hb, where a single amino acid is substituted for another in one of the polypeptide chains. This single amino acid substitution profoundly alters the properties of the Hb molecule. Hb S is formed instead of the normal Hb A. The tendency toward sickling depends on both the relative quantity of Hb S in the RBCs and the levels of oxygen tension within the tissues of the body.

Different terminologies are used with sickle cell anemia: sickle cell trait, sickle cell disease, and sickle cell syndromes (Table 27-5). A person with sickle cell trait (Hb SA) has received an Hb S gene from one parent and an Hb A gene (normal) from the other.

The clinical manifestations of the disease result from the sickling phenomenon. Sickling occurs when red cells containing Hb S are deoxygenated; this is the result of the poor solubility of the Hb S, which crystallizes in the RBCs. The RBCs elongate and become rigid and crescent- or sickle-shaped (tactoid formation) (Fig. 27-5). Sickling is always present to some extent in the person with sickle cell anemia. Because of increased RBC destruction, patients are often jaundiced and may develop gallstones (cholelithiasis secondary to increased bilirubin).

Sickle cell crises

Basically, any event that increases the body's need for oxygen or that alters the transport of oxygen may lead to the exacerbation of symptoms called *crisis*. Symptoms may be exacerbated by pregnancy, infection, surgery, trauma, and dehydration. Sickle cell crises are primarily thrombotic or aplastic.

Table 27-5   Types of sickle cell disorders

Term	Characteristic	Hb Molecule
Sickle cell trait	Carrier of Hb S Persons are asymptomatic	Hb SA
Sickle cell disease	Presence of sickling with associated symptoms	Hb SS
Sickle cell syndromes	Diseases associated with presence of Hb S	Hb SC (sickle cell Hb C) Hb SD (sickle cell Hb D) Hb Sβ (sickle cell thalassemia)

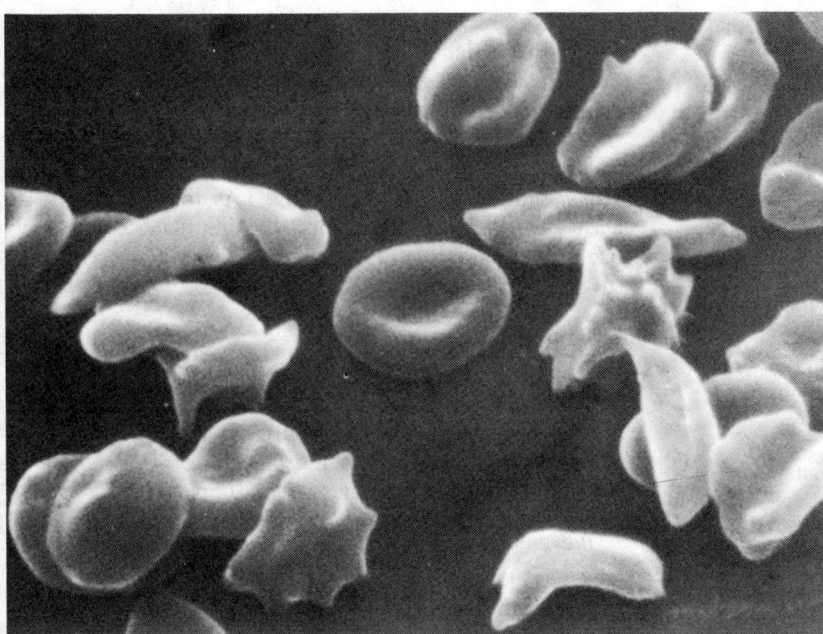

Fig. 27-5   Sickled red cells.

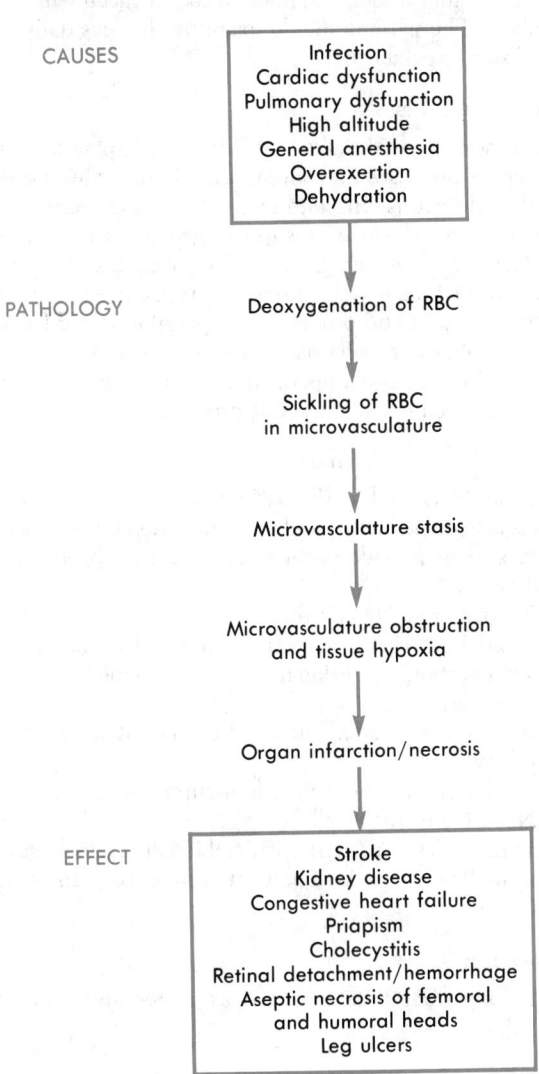

Fig. 27-6   Pathophysiology of sickle cell crisis.

Thrombotic crisis is the most common sickle cell crisis. Signs and symptoms occur as a result of occlusions in the microvasculature by sickled cells causing deoxygenation of tissues with pain and infarctions in organs such as the kidney, lung, bones, and central nervous system (Fig. 27-6). The sites most frequently affected in crises are the abdomen, back, chest, and joints.

Aplastic crisis, usually secondary to infection, involves cessation of bone marrow function and decrease in erythropoiesis and reticulocyte count. Signs of severe anemia are often present.

Megaloblastic crisis, the result of depletion of bone marrow stores of folic acid, is prevented or treated by folic acid administration. *Splenic sequestration crisis*, pooling of blood in the spleen, causes splenic enlargement and hypovolemia with signs of shock.

Nursing Process
Assessment
Subjective data

Data to be obtained from the patient with sickle cell disease include the following:
1. Knowledge of the disease and family history
2. Factors that precipitate crises or exacerbate symptoms
3. Presence of fatigue.
4. Presence of pain and measures taken for pain relief
5. Feelings of dyspnea and precipitating activities
6. Ability to carry out ADL

Objective data

Objective data collected by physical assessment and patient observation may include the following:
1. Skin: pale (anemia) or jaundiced (RBC destruction)
2. Legs: presence of infected ulcers on lower leg
3. Overt signs of pain

4. Temperature: elevation from infection (low-grade fever)
5. Pulse rapid (from decreased oxygenation)
6. Labored breathing, especially with activity

Data analysis: nursing diagnoses

Nursing diagnoses are determined from analysis of patient data. Possible nursing diagnoses for the patient with sickle cell disease may include, but are not limited to, the following:

Diagnostic title	Possible etiologies
Activity intolerance	Decreased oxygen transport
Tissue perfusion (peripheral, renal, pulmonary), altered	Dehydration, interruption of blood flow
Pain: joints, chest	Decreased tissue oxygenation, inadequate pain management techniques
Infection, high risk for	Anemia, tissue destruction, knowledge deficit
Anxiety	Threat to self-concept or life, situational crisis
Decisional conflict	Decision making regarding childbearing
Knowledge deficit	Lack of information or recall, poor motivation, anxiety

Planning: expected patient outcomes

Expected outcomes for the patient with sickle cell disease may include, but are not limited to, the following:
1. States feeling rested and that exertional dyspnea is lessened.
2. Drinks at least 4 L of fluid daily.
3. Demonstrates no signs of thrombosis.
4. States pain is modified or absent.
5. Signs of infection are absent.
6. Signs of anxiety are decreased.
7. Makes decisions with spouse concerning conception based on knowledge of illness.
8. Explains nature of sickle cell disease, factors that precipitate painful crises, fluid needs, counseling resources, and need for follow-up care.

Implementation
Assisting with achievement of therapeutic goals

Because there is no specific therapy for sickle cell disease, treatment is symptomatic. Transfusions may be given; the blood products generally used are packed RBCs. The goal of transfusion therapy depends on the specific condition: replacing RBCs for anemia; lowering the percentage of Hb S in an infarction; and increasing the amount of circulating Hb and thus oxygen in overwhelming infections, leg ulcers, pregnancy, and preoperatively. Exchange transfusions (replacement of patient's blood with normal blood) may be given for intractable crises, stroke, or as a preventive measure preoperatively.[30] Care of the patient receiving transfusions is discussed in Chapter 41.

Interventions to achieve patient outcomes
Promoting activity tolerance and tissue perfusion

Fatigue and dyspnea with activity result from decreased tissue oxygenation because of decreased oxygen-carrying capabilities of the hemoglobin. Assist and teach patient to maintain a balance between rest and exercise to prevent increased oxygen expenditure. Oxygen may be given during crises to increase oxygen blood saturation.

The vasoocclusive nature of painful episodes requires adequate *hydration* to decrease blood viscosity. During a crisis, the patient requires 6 to 8 L of fluids daily and at least 4 to 6 L at all other times. If IV fluids are necessary, use a small-bore (No. 23) needle and avoid multiple punctures and infiltration.[46]

Promoting comfort

Pain of sickle cell crisis is excruciating and involves all the principles of pain management (see Chapter 10). Pain medications (narcotics and nonnarcotics) must be given continuously—orally, intramuscularly, or intravenously. Evaluation of pain therapies is very important.

Preventing infection

The person with sickle cell disease is especially prone to respiratory infections and ulcers of the lower leg. Good hygiene is essential. The patient should avoid persons with upper respiratory infections; pneumococcal vaccine may be prescribed. The patient should examine the legs daily for signs of skin breakdown.

Counseling patients

Many persons with sickle cell disease display anxiety about recurring crises and the nature of their chronic illness. Provide counseling and suggest ongoing counseling (if needed) and the use of support groups. Information about local services can be obtained from the National Association of Sickle Cell Disease.* Assist the patient to be as independent and productive as possible in a difficult situation when sickle cell crises are frequent. *Genetic* counseling (p. 753) is also important to assist the couple in making informed decisions about procreation.

Facilitating patient learning

The family as well as the patient needs to know about the disease to dispel myths and misconceptions, to decrease anxiety, and to provide optimal care. Teaching includes the following:
1. Nature of sickle cell disease
2. Avoidance of situations that cause crisis (infection, overexertion, emotional stress, alcohol, cigarette smoking)[28]
3. Importance of adequate fluid intake (at least 4 to 6 L/day)
4. Availability of counseling and support services
5. Need for medical follow-up

Nursing care of the patient with sickle cell crisis is summarized in Box 27-5. A sample nursing care plan is described on p. 757.

Evaluation

1. Does patient state feeling more rested and comfortable?

---

*4221 Wilshire Blvd, Los Angeles, CA 90010.

DATA: Mr. S. is a 24-year-old, married, black mail carrier, who is father of one child. He was diagnosed at age 10 as having sickle cell disease but has been largely asymptomatic until 2 years before this admission. When he was first admitted with symptoms of sickle cell crisis, he had severe joint pain in upper and lower extremities, moderate fever (38.1° C), shortness of breath.

PHYSICAL EXAMINATION: Coarse rales in both lower lobes, cyanosis of lips and nailbeds, dry scaly skin on both legs, 2+ pitting edema with a small (2 cm) reddened area over each medial malleolus. No hair was visible on toes. His Hb was 9 g/dl.

PHYSICIAN ORDERS: Oxygen by nasal cannula, 4L/min, bed rest with bathroom privileges, morphine sulfate 15 mg IM q3-4h prn. Mr. S. was given two units of packed cells to be followed by IV fluids. Sickle cell crisis with congestive heart failure was diagnosed.

The nursing history identified the following:

1. Mr. S. is very "worried" about the outcome of the hospitalization and his ability to "catch his breath."
2. He expresses concern about his ability to support his family and be a "father" to his son and especially to take part in athletic events: "I'm hardly a man." His wife has assumed responsibility for some of the yard work, formerly his responsibility.
3. He continues to exercise and jogs several times a week. He smokes one pack of cigarettes per day and states he has never been "a big fluid drinker," although he does have a beer a day. He states that he does not know what brings on the crisis.
4. He is concerned about his sexual relationship with his wife because of his general fatigue. They had one child before he was aware of the genetic nature of the disease and expresses concern about having other children who might inherit the disease.

Collaborative nursing action includes those to maintain fluid and electrolyte balance and peripheral and pulmonary oxygen/carbon dioxide balance as well as to prevent further vascular occlusion.

Nursing actions include monitoring for the following:

1. Signs of infection: hyperthermia, abnormal fluid, positive blood and sputum cultures, tachycardia, tachypnea.
2. Signs of increased fluid/electrolyte imbalance, CHF and renal failure: hematocrit, electrolyte levels, intake and output, skin turgor; respiratory status (rate, depth of respiration, presence of crackles, skin color, level of consciousness), renal function: creatinine, blood urea nitrogen.

Nursing diagnosis: **Anxiety: related to threat to self-concept, health status and role functioning**

Expected patient outcomes	Nursing interventions	Rationale
Signs of anxiety are decreased	Give Mr. S. opportunities to explore concerns about the effects of the disorder. Assess his knowledge of sickle cell anemia and correct misunderstandings.	Making the unknown known may decrease anxiety.
	Teach relaxation measures.	Relaxation decreases the psychomotor responses to anxiety.

Nursing diagnosis: **Potential for infection: related to spleen dysfunction, inadequate primary defense (broken skin) and inadequate secondary defenses (decreased hemoglobin)**

Expected patient outcomes	Nursing interventions	Rationale
Infection does not occur.	Use good medical asepsis.	Aseptic technique decreases patient's contact with pathogenic organisms; infection is predicted on type and number of organisms to which individuals are exposed and patient resistance to infection.
	Restrict persons (staff/visitors) with any type of infection.	Restricting persons with infection decreases patient's contact with infectious agents.

Continued.

Nursing Care Plan	**Person with sickle cell crisis—cont'd**

Nursing diagnosis: Pain in joints and chest related to poor pain management techniques, lack of knowledge

Expected patient outcomes	Nursing interventions	Rationale
Mr. S. states feeling comfortable.	Give prescribed analgesics on a regular basis and evaluate effectiveness of medication: obtain orders for increased doses if necessary.	Pain of sickle cell crisis is excruciating: large doses of medication may be required.
	Identify measures Mr. S. has found helpful and include these measures in the care.	Patients often have the most accurate information for their pain control.
	Support joints gently when assisting patient to do ROM exercises.	Improper support increases stress on joints and increases pain.
	Use moist heat or massage, if helpful.	Heat dilates blood vessels and increases circulation to the area. Massage may increase circulation, relax tense muscles.
	Use other pain-relieving measures; person with frequent crises may benefit from learning special techniques such as biofeedback or self-hypnosis.	Biofeedback, self-hypnosis decrease the physiologic responses to pain (muscle spasm, increased pulse).

Nursing diagnosis: Activity intolerance related to decreased oxygen transport

Expected patient outcomes	Nursing interventions	Rationale
No dyspnea occurs with activity. Mr. S. states feeling rested.	Provide prescribed oxygen as needed.	High concentration of O_2 in alveoli increases diffusion across membranes.
	Limit activities and provide periods of rest.	Decreased activity decreases O_2 needs of body.
	Administer prescribed transfusion (packed red cells).	Packed cells increase the number of RBCs available to carry O_2 to tissue cells in the anemic person.

Nursing diagnosis: Potential sexual dysfunction: related to fatigue, pain, fear of pregnancy

Expected patient outcomes	Nursing interventions	Rationale
Mr. S. and wife state the sexual relationship is satisfying	Discuss coital positions that require less energy for the person who becomes tired easily.	Coitus requires energy and involves neuromuscular activity; sidelying or male-inferior position is less demanding for male patient.
	Suggest coitus at times of day when Mr. S. is less fatigued (morning, afternoon).	Fatigue increases with continued daily activities and demand on cardiovascular system.
	Discuss genetic counseling and contraceptive methods.	Knowledge of and use of reliable methods to prevent pregnancy reduce fear that may cause sexual dysfunction.

Nursing diagnosis: **Self-esteem disturbance: related to loss of body function, change in life-style and masculine role**

Expected patient outcomes	Nursing interventions	Rationale
Mr. S. states satisfaction with life and self.	Provide opportunities for Mr. S. to discuss feelings about inability to fulfill expected roles.	Verbalization of concerns decreases their impact and assists in problem solving.
	Assist Mr. S. to identify personal strengths.	Focusing on strengths and positive factors provides the baseline for personal growth.
	Assist Mr. S. to explore alternative ways to meet role expectations.	Concern over losses may immobilize patient; assistance in exploring alternatives is a therapeutic role of the nurse.
	Suggest joining a support group or obtaining counseling to minimize dependency behaviors.	Research shows that increased social support from family and groups increases recovery from disease and disability and facilitates rehabilitation.

Nursing diagnosis: **Knowledge deficit: related to lack of exposure/recall and unfamiliarity with information sources**

Expected patient outcomes	Nursing interventions	Rationale
Patient/family describe the nature of the disorder and care requirements.	Review with Mr. S. the basis of sickle cell disease and genetic effects.	Knowledge of causes of disease is *one* factor in ensuring patient compliance with medical regimen and adherence to preventative measures.
	Provide resources for family planning and genetic counseling.	Individuals and groups with indepth knowledge of family planning methods help patients identify a family planning method that conforms to the patient's cultural and religious values.
	Encourage Mr. S. to avoid situations that cause crises (see text).	(See first rationale and text).
	Encourage Mr. S. to drink 4 to 6 L fluid daily; explain rationale.	Dehydration is a primary cause of RBC sickling.

Guidelines for Care

Care of the patient with sickle cell anemia during crisis

Promoting adequate hydration
   Maintain intake of a least 4000 ml, unless contraindicated
   Maintain IV fluids as ordered
Maintaining tissue oxygenation
   Avoid overexertion by patient
   Maintain oxygen by mask or cannula as ordered
Preventing infection (sames as for leukemia, p. 768)
Providing comfort
   Give pain medication continuously during crisis
   Evaluate response to medication to determine if increased dosage is needed
   Do not discount severity of pain
Promoting psychologic comfort
   Encourage independence and productive life (refer to work classification clinic, if necessary)
   Be a good listener and give information to decrease anxiety

---

2. Is patient drinking at least 4 to 6 L/day?
3. Is patient free of thrombosis and infection?
4. Are signs of anxiety decreased and does patient state plans for counseling and support services as needed?
5. Have patient and spouse begun to deal with the problem of childbearing?
6. Can patient and family describe the nature of sickle cell disease, precipitating factors, and need for follow-up care?

ERYTHROCYTOSIS (POLYCYTHEMIA)

Etiology and Pathophysiology

Polycythemia, an abnormal increase in RBCs, may be primary or secondary. *Primary polycythemia (polycythemia vera)* is a proliferation disorder of unknown etiology. It is characterized by hyperplasia of the bone marrow; there is usually a simultaneous increase in WBCs and platelets.

Secondary polycythemia may result from cardiac, pulmonary, or renal disorders, or it may be stress related. Chronic hypoxia is a major cause of secondary polycythemia; it stimulates the production of the enzyme erythropoietin, which then stimulates the bone marrow to increase RBC production. More red cells are then available to carry oxygen.

The signs and symptoms of polycythemia (headache, dizziness, blurred vision, fatigue) are secondary to increased blood viscosity and total blood volume. Pruritus results from the increased number of basophils. Vasodilation occurs as a result of increased RBCs. There is also marked leukocytosis and thrombocytosis, which, along with the increased RBC count, predispose the person to thrombosis, tissue hypoxia, and bleeding (Table 27-3).

Nursing Process

Assessment

Subjective data and objective data

Subjective data include reports of headache, blurred vision, fatigue, and pruritus. Assess the person's knowledge about the nature of polycythemia. *Objective data* include observations for signs of bleeding, such as nosebleeds or areas of ecchymosis. Principal laboratory tests to determine the nature of the erythrocytosis consist of determination of the arterial oxygen concentration, red cell volume, and plasma volume.

Data analysis: nursing diagnoses

Nursing diagnoses are determined from analysis of patient data. Possible diagnoses for the person with polycythemia include, but are not limited to, the following:

Diagnostic title	Possible etiologies
Knowledge deficit	Lack of exposure to pertinent information

Planning: expected patient outcomes

Expected patient outcomes for the person with polycythemia may include, but are not limited to, the following:
1. Explains the nature of the disorder, importance of continued medical care, and reason for therapy.
2. Describes foods to avoid.
3. Describes signs of thrombosis.

Implementation

Patient teaching is the primary care for persons with polycythemia and includes the following:
1. Nature of the disorder
2. Importance of continued blood tests and medical care
3. Phlebotomy therapy
   a. Removal of 500 ml blood per week until hematocrit level reaches 45%
   b. Repeat phlebotomy when hematocrit level rises over 50% (usually every 2 to 3 months)
4. Avoidance of foods high in iron content (liver, oysters, legumes) because patient already has increased iron from increased RBCs
5. Signs of extremity thromboses (swelling, redness, pain) requiring medical attention

Evaluation

1. Can the person explain the nature of the disorder and rationale for therapy?
2. Does the person describe plans to avoid iron-rich foods?
3. Does the person know signs of thrombosis requiring medical intervention?

COAGULATION DISORDERS

Pathophysiology

Platelets are formed in the bone marrow. In the normal adult approximately 80% of the platelets are in free circulation and 20% are stored in the spleen. It is estimated

Table 27-6   Disorders of coagulation (platelets)

Disorder	Signs and symptoms	Medical therapy
Idiopathic thrombocytopenia purpura (ITP)	Petechiae, ecchymoses, easy bruising; platelet count below 10,000 mm³, prolonged bleeding time	Corticosteroids, splenectomy, therapeutic plasmapheresis
Secondary thrombocytopenia	Same as above	Correct underlying cause
Thrombocytosis	Bleeding (mucosal areas, especially GI tract); thrombosis (primarily venous, but may be arterial)	Cytotoxic drugs to decrease bone marrow activity; platelet pheresis, aspirin
Hemophilia	Life-long bleeding into any part of body, spontaneously or after trauma; may be into joints or retroperitoneal, intracranial areas; signs of blood loss	Replacement of deficient coagulation factor VIII or IX; topical coagulants (fibrin foam or thrombin); concentrated preparations of fibrinogen; plasma pheresis to remove antibody inhibitors against factor VIII
Disseminated intravascular coagulation (DIC)	Diffuse bleeding into mucous membranes and tissues, wound sites; renal failure; prolonged prothrombin time	Correct underlying problem, cardiovascular support, platelet packs, cryoprecipitate, fresh whole blood; hemodialysis for renal failure

Table 27-7   Common bleeding/coagulation blood tests

Test	Description	Normal value
Bleeding time	Evaluation of vascular and platelet factors—the time it takes for a small stab wound to stop bleeding	2 to 9 minutes
Clotting time	Time required for solid clot to form (less sensitive test than PTT)	5 to 10 minutes
Prothrombin time (PT)	Indicates rapidity of blood clotting (indicative of adequacy of extrinsic coagulation pathway; factors I, II, V, VII, X)	11 to 16 seconds; 100% as compared to control levels
Partial thromboplastin time (PTT)	More sensitive test than PT to evaluate adequacy of intrinsic coagulation pathway (fibrin clot formation)	60 to 90 seconds
Activated partial thromboplastin time (APTT)	Modified PTT; more sensitive; quicker to perform, frequently used to monitor heparin therapy and hemophilia	26 to 42 seconds

that the normal life span of platelets is approximately 10 days. Laboratory values for a normal adult platelet count range from 150,000 to 400,000/mm³.

Refer to p. 746, if necessary, for a discussion of the coagulation process. Remember that platelets release thromboplastin (factor III); therefore, changes in platelet *function* will interfere with coagulation. Platelets also plug small breaks in blood vessels by adhesion and clumping. Aspirin inhibits the release of intrinsic platelet ADP and produces a defect in platelet aggregation. The defect remains for the life of the platelet, and clot formation is inhibited.

Changes in circulating platelet *numbers* can also affect coagulation. *Thrombocytosis* (increase in number of circulating platelets) is usually seen in association with other diseases. The danger of thrombocytosis is that it may lead to thrombosis of abnormal bleeding (Table 27-6). Care of the patient is similar to that for persons receiving anticoagulation therapy. *Thrombocytopenia* (decrease in number of circulating platelets) leads to bleeding.

Coagulation disorders may be congenital or acquired.

The most common *congenital* coagulation disorders are the hemophilias. *Liver disease* is the most common *acquired* coagulation disorder. The liver produces most of the clotting factors: II, V, VII, IX, X, and fibrinogen. Liver disease may produce impaired production of these clotting factors and an elevated prothrombin time (Table 27-7). A deficiency in vitamin K can also affect clotting since vitamin K is a cofactor in the synthesis of clotting factors II, VII, IX, and X. Approximately 50% of required vitamin K is obtained from a normal diet, and the remainder is produced by intestinal bacteria. *Inactivation of intestinal bacteria* by intestinal antibiotics can lead to vitamin K deficiency. Disseminated intravascular coagulation (DIC) is also an acquired disorder of coagulation.

THROMBOCYTOPENIA
Etiology

Thrombocytopenia, a decrease in number of circulating platelets, can result from decreased platelet production or increased platelet destruction. Decreased production is

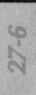

	Drugs with thrombocytopenic effects
	Alcohol
	Nonsteroidal antiinflammatory agents (azathioprine, D-penicillamine, phenylbutazone)
	Oral hypoglycemics
	Quinidine
	Salicylates
	Sulfonamides
	Thiazides

	The patient with thrombocytopenia
	Nature of the disorder
	Signs of decreased platelets (petechiae, ecchymoses, gingival bleeding, hematuria, menorrhagia)
	Name dosage, frequency, side effects of prescribed medications (corticosteroids) and importance of not stopping corticosteroid medications suddenly
	Measures to prevent injury/hemorrhage
	Use soft toothbrush or swab for mouth care
	Keep mouth clean and free of debris
	Avoid intrusions into rectum (for example, rectal medications, enemas)
	Use electric shaver
	Apply direct pressure for 5 to 10 minutes if any bleeding occurs
	Avoid contact sports, elective surgery, and tooth extraction
	Avoid picking or blowing nose forcefully
	Avoid trauma, falls, bumps, cuts; avoid contact sports
	Avoid use of aspirin or aspirin preparations
	Use adequate lubrication and gentleness during sexual intercourse
	Need for follow-up medical care

usually caused by drugs (Box 27-6) or bone marrow suppression from chemotherapy or radiotherapy.

Pathophysiology

The most common thrombocytopenia from increased platelet destruction is *idiopathic thrombocytopenia purpura* (ITP). It occurs most commonly in the second and third decades of life and is caused by production of an autoantibody (IgG), which is directed against a platelet antigen. It is manifested by excessive bleeding, which may be reflected in purpuric lesions on the skin or by visceral bleeding (Table 27-6).

Assessment
Subjective data and objective data

Subjective data include eliciting a history of recent viral infection, as this may produce transient thrombocytopenia. Also obtain a detailed history of drug and alcohol use.

Objective data include observing the patient for the presence of ecchymoses (bruises or black and blue marks caused by bleeding into the subcutaneous tissues and skin) and petechiae (1- to 4-mm flat, round, purple-red hemorrhagic bruises in the skin), bleeding gums, vaginal bleeding, GI bleeding, or hematuria.

Diagnostic tests

Diagnostic tests include laboratory studies (see Table 27-7) and bone marrow examination (p. 751). Commonly used tests for assessment of platelets include platelet count, peripheral blood smear, and bleeding time, which is usually prolonged. The bone marrow is examined for the presence of *megakaryocytes* (precursors of platelets in the bone marrow). Their presence suggests that the thrombocytopenia is caused by peripheral platelet destruction, and their absence or decrease suggests a failure of thrombopoiesis.

Implementation

The medical management of idiopathic thrombocytopenic purpura includes corticosteroid therapy, plasmapheresis, and splenectomy. Steroids appear to decrease the autoantibody that is directed against the platelet antigen. Splenectomy removes the organ primarily responsible for destruction of the antibody-coated platelets. Danazol, immunoglobulin, or immunosuppressive drugs also may be administered.

Nursing management is primarily teaching the patient with thrombocytopenia. Of primary concern is the bleeding tendency and measures taken to prevent hemorrhage and

injury (see Box 27-7). Bleeding associated with trauma is likely with a platelet count less than 60,000/mm³. The need for avoidance of trauma is obvious. Spontaneous hemorrhage looms as a life-threatening possibility in individuals with a platelet count of less than 20,000/mm³. Teaching also includes signs of decreased platelets (petechiae, ecchymosis, hematuria, menorrhagia) and the need for continuous follow-up medical care.

HEMOPHILIA
Etiology and Pathophysiology

Hemophilia is a hereditary coagulation disorder. Both hemophilia A (factor VIII deficiency) and hemophilia B, also called Christmas disease (factor IX deficiency), are inherited as sex-linked recessive disorders and are therefore almost exclusively limited to males. An example of the inheritance pattern of hemophilia is shown in Fig. 27-7.

The degree of bleeding is related to the amount of factor activity and the severity of injury. Spontaneous bleeding, joint bleeding (hemarthrosis), and deep tissue hemorrhage occur with factor levels less than 1%. Retroperitoneal and intracranial bleeding may also occur and may be life-threatening. Patients may experience bleeding after tooth extraction, minor trauma, or during surgical procedures. Any body system may be affected.

Assessment
Subjective data and objective data

Subjective data include the patient's and family's knowledge of the disorder, measures taken to prevent injury, and coping mechanisms. If pain or bleeding is present, explore

Table 27-8   Blood factor replacement therapy for hemophilia

Type	Clotting factors	Comments
Fresh frozen plasma	All	Thawed to 37° C before infusion; allergic reactions are common; fluid overload possible, especially in older persons
Cryoprecipitate	VIII, fibrinogen	Thawed at 37° C before infusion; occasional allergic reactions; low risk of hepatitis transmission, administer at 12-hour intervals
Lyophilized factor VIII concentrate	VIII	Stable at room temperature; possible hemolytic reactions for persons with blood types A, B, AB when given over prolonged period; allergic reactions rare
Vitamin K dependent complex	VII, IX, X, prothrombin	Keep refrigerated; higher risk of hepatitis transmission and thrombus formation (heparin usually given concurrently)

possible causes to ascertain if these could have been prevented (data useful for teaching future prevention). *Objective data* include presence of bleeding or swelling of joints (indicating joint bleeding).

Diagnostic tests

A diagnosis of hemophilia is made by specific assays for factors VIII and IX. The partial thromboplastin time (PTT) (Table 27-7) is prolonged in both types of hemophilia. The platelet count and prothrombin time are normal.

Implementation
Assisting with achievement of therapeutic goals

Bleeding disorders may require local treatment such as ice bags, manual pressure or dressings, immobilization, and elevation of a body part. Joint aspiration may be necessary. Muscle stretching exercises are begun after pain and bleeding have subsided (usually within 3 to 5 days). Active range of motion exercises are encouraged when swelling has subsided.

With major hemorrhages, careful monitoring is necessary to avoid fluid overload if large plasma volumes are given. Concentrates (Table 27-8) provide the deficient factors and prevent fluid overload and fewer side effects (such as urticarial or febrile reactions) in some patients. High cost and contamination with the virus of serum hepatitis are drawbacks, however, to the use of some of the concentrates. The heat treatment of factor VIII now reduces the likelihood of AIDS transmission.

Factor replacement therapy may be given on an outpatient basis, either in a clinic or in the home. Home infusion programs have gained interest and are seen as a way of controlling bleeding episodes more quickly, thereby decreasing the need for hospitalization and a long absence from school or work.

A synthetic drug that is effective against mild hemophilia and von Willebrand's disease (deficiencies in factor VIII and in platelet adhesion) is desmopressin (DDAVP). It is administered intravenously and can cause a threefold to sixfold increase in factor VIII activity.

The outlook for the person with hemophilia has been greatly improved by the availability of transfusion therapy. In the past many people with factor VIII deficiency died in the first 5 years of life. Today people with moderate or mild hemophilia may live normal, productive lives.

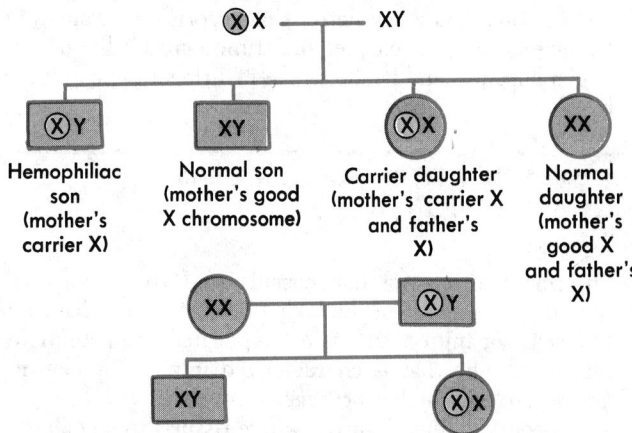

Fig. 27-7   Pattern of inheritance of hemophilia.

Counseling and teaching

Threat of spontaneous bleeding episodes and pain control are ongoing stressors the individual must confront. Important points for teaching are listed in Box 27-8. Those individuals who are able to meet the demands of their illness and adapt their life-styles accordingly are able to live productive lives as individuals, spouses, parents, and employees.

Genetic counseling, aimed at explaining the pattern of inheritance of hemophilia, may be of great value to adults contemplating parenthood. Such counseling can assist potential parents in evaluating realistically their ability to raise a child afflicted with hemophilia and to anticipate

27-8 The patient with hemophilia

Nature of disease: genetic basis
Prevention of hemorrhage
Possibility of bleeding after dental extraction
Avoidance of contact sports
Importance of carrying a card or wearing a
    Medic-Alert tag with name, blood type, physi-
    cian's name and phone number, and diagnosis
Community resources (National Hemophilia
    Foundation)
Family planning techniques if desired
Need for medical follow-up

27-9 The patient with DIC

Monitor continually for bleeding sites or changes
    in amount of bleeding (especially if heparin
    therapy is given)
Assess and record amount of drainage from chest
    and nasogastric tubes and oozing from incisions
Monitor fluid rates; be alert for signs of fluid over-
    load (increased pulse rate, distended jugular
    veins, and increased CVP)
Provide care for the critically ill patient (see
    Chapter 46)
Explain to family what is occurring and provide
    opportunities for expressions of feelings

ways to meet the demands placed on both of them and the child.[18]

The National Hemophilia Foundation* is an organization established for persons with hemophilia and their families. The basic function of the national organization is hemophilia research. In addition, it publishes literature, produces films, and promotes health care legislation in Washington. Local chapter services include special camps for children with hemophilia, counseling and group therapy sessions, and a newsletter that reports on advances in hemophilic care. A chapter may function as a liaison between hospitals and families with insurmountable bills for blood.

DISSEMINATED INTRAVASCULAR COAGULATION

Etiology

Disseminated intravascular coagulation (DIC) is a pathophysiologic response of the body's hemostatic mechanisms to disease or injury. DIC is a complicated and potentially fatal syndrome that is characterized initially by clotting and secondarily by hemorrhage.

It occurs in any condition where tissue thromboplastin is liberated subsequent to tissue destruction. One of the most common causes is abruptio placentae, or premature separation of the placenta. Tumor products, crushing trauma, burns, leukemia, vasculitis, sepsis and shock, as well as surgery (especially prostatic, orthopedic or open heart) may also initiate DIC.[26]

Pathophysiology

DIC is essentially an imbalance between the processes of coagulation and anticoagulation. The normal balance of clotting factors and fibrinolytic factors, which under normal conditions prevent bleeding while maintaining the fluidity of the blood, are altered.

The primary disease or injury initiates the clotting process. This response is generalized and occurs throughout the vascular system, creating a state of *hypercoagulability*.

*110 Green St., Rm 406, New York, NY 10012.

The fibrinolytic processes, which normally operate to limit clot extension and dissolve clots, are then stimulated (Fig. 27-8). As clotting factors are depleted and fibrinolysis continues, a state of *hypocoagulability* develops.

The most common sequela of DIC is hemorrhage. This paradox is caused by decreased platelets and the depletion of clotting factors, II, V, VIII, and fibrinogen and the production of fibrin degradation products (FDP) through fibrinolysis. FDP act as anticoagulants, which increase the hemorrhagic tendency (p. 746).

Assessment

The first signs and symptoms may be those of hemorrhage (oral, vaginal, rectal, after injection and venipuncture, petechiae, and ecchymosis). Pain may be present from joint bleeding.

Diagnostic tests

Laboratory findings, which may be the only indications of the syndrome in the early stages, may include the following:

1. Decreased circulating platelet count
2. Prolonged PT
3. Prolonged PTT
4. Decreased factors V and VIII
5. Decreased fibrinogen levels
6. Increased fibrin split products (fibrinolysis)
7. Abnormal RBCs on peripheral blood smear

Implementation

Medical management is aimed at correcting the underlying problem. Antibiotics, chemotherapeutic agents, and cardiovascular support may be used. Fresh-frozen plasma and packed RBCs may be administered to restore clotting factors and blood volume.

Nursing intervention in the care of the patient with DIC is extremely challenging (Box 27-9). The person is critically ill and frequently has numerous sites of bleeding before DIC becomes evident. Frequently the patient is comatose, and the presence of purpura, numerous intravenous lines, and drainage tubes makes the patient's ap-

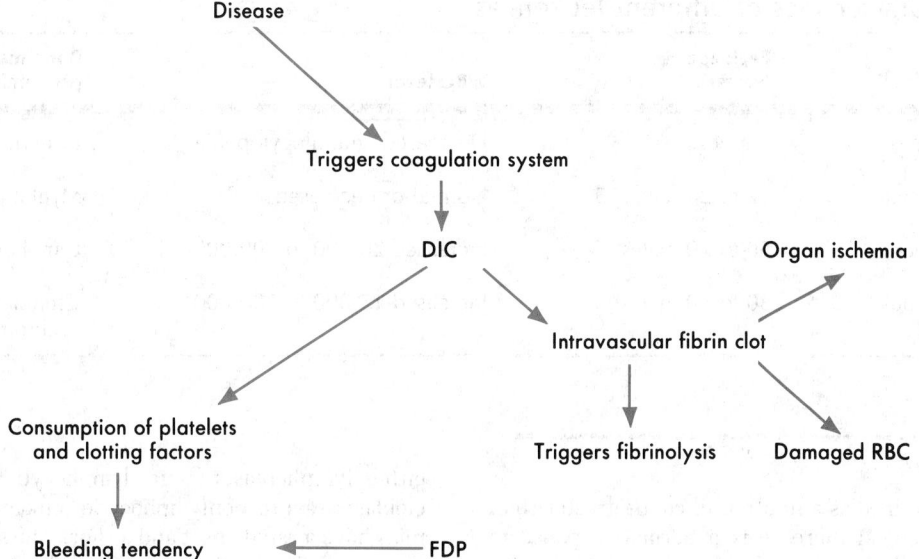

Fig. 27-8   Illustration of pathophysiology of disseminated intravascular coagulation, which may result in bleeding tendency, organ ischemia, and hemolytic anemia. (From Pagana KD, Pagana TJ: *Diagnostic testing & nursing implications: a case study approach*, ed 3, St Louis, 1990, Mosby—Year Book.)

pearance especially upsetting to the family. Most of the primary conditions associated with DIC are of a sudden nature, and the family requires help in understanding this catastrophic occurrence and support during the long period of treatment.

Interventions for thrombocytopenia (p. 762) are applicable to the patient with DIC. The patient requires careful monitoring of fluid replacement therapy, renal function and fluid output, and signs and symptoms of further bleeding.

DISORDERS ASSOCIATED WITH WHITE BLOOD CELLS

NEUTROPENIA (LEUKOPENIA)

Neutropenia is defined as a neutrophil count of less than 2000/mm³. It may occur as a primary hematologic disorder but is seen more often in association with other disorders, including malignant disease of the bone marrow, aplastic anemia, megaloblastic anemia, use of chemotherapeutic agents, starvation, and viral infections. Severe neutropenia can also occur as a reaction to drugs, particularly in the patient with aplastic anemia secondary to cytotoxic drugs. The degree of susceptibility to infection is in direct proportion to the degree of neutropenia. Individuals with marked neutropenia are at risk for contracting a life-threatening infection.

Agranulocytosis is an acute disease in which the number of WBCs suddenly decreases, usually as the result of chemicals or drugs (sulfonamides, propylthiouracil, chloramphenicol, and bone marrow depressant drugs such as che-

Patient Teaching   27-10

The patient with leukopenia: preventing infection

Use good handwashing technique.
Avoid contact with persons with infections.
Avoid sharing eating utensils and bath linens.
Take daily baths with meticulous perineal care.
Use good oral hygiene, avoiding gum injury.
Keep environment clean.
Monitor for signs of infection (if present) and report these to physician.
Avoid eating raw meats and fresh fruits and vegetables.

motherapeutic agents). Clinical signs include infection, malaise (discomfort, headache, lassitude, muscle aches), ulceration of mucous membranes, chills, and fever. A sepsis may develop, which may lead to death. Care is directed toward removing the causative agents and resolving infection. If bone marrow is not destroyed, the prognosis for recovery is good.

Granulocyte transfusions may be used for the patient with severe neutropenia. Nursing interventions focus on preventing infections (see Box 27-10) and careful monitoring for early signs of infection so that therapy can begin promptly. Because neutrophil count is low, some of the classic signs of infection and the inflammatory response (purulent drainage, abscess formation, sequestration of a local infection) may be absent (Chapter 16). Fever may also be absent because of a lack of the endogenous pyrogens that are produced by neutrophils in response to infection.

Table 27-9   Characteristics of different leukemias

Type	Peak age (years)	WBC level	Bone marrow cell predominance
Acute lymphocytic leukemia (ALL)	2 to 4	Decreased (granulocytopenia)	Lymphoblasts
Acute nonlymphocytic leukemia (ANLL)	12 to 20; after 55	Normal or decreased	Myeloblasts
Chronic lymphocytic leukemia (CLL)	50 to 70 males	Increased 20,000 to 100,000	Lymphocytes
Chronic myelogenous leukemia (CML)	30 to 50 males	Increased 15,000 to 500,000	Granulocytes, Philadelphia chromosome

NEUTROPHILIA

Neutrophilia is defined as a neutrophil count greater than $10,000/mm^3$. Such an increase is a normal response to infections, primarily bacterial. It may also increase with strenuous exercise. Prolonged elevation of the neutrophil count, especially in the absence of an apparent cause, is a reason for a diligent search for the underlying cause. Persistent elevated neutrophil counts are associated with leukemia, polycythemia vera, myeloid metaplasia, and a variety of systemic and inflammatory disorders. Treatment consists of therapy for the primary condition.

LEUKEMIA
Etiology

The cause of leukemia is unknown. An increased incidence of leukemia in siblings has led to hypotheses of genetic predispositions or viral origins. Radiation and chemicals (including benzene, arsenic, chloramphenicol, and antineoplastic drugs) have also been implicated.

Pathophysiology

Leukemias are malignant disorders of the hematopoietic system involving the bone marrow and lymph nodes; they are characterized by uncontrolled proliferation of leukocytes and their precursors. The large number of cells accumulate first at the site of origin (granulocytes in the bone marrow, lymphocytes in the lymph nodes), then spread to hematopoietic organs, leading to organ enlargement (splenomegaly, hepatomegaly). The proliferation of one type of cell often interferes with the normal production of other hematopoietic cells, leading to the development of immature cells and to cytopenias (decreased numbers). The immaturity of the white cells leads to decreased immunocompetence with increased susceptibility to infections.

Classification

The leukemias are classified as acute or chronic and further subdivided according to cell type or maturity of the cell (Table 27-9).

Acute leukemias

Acute leukemias involve immature cells and are classified according to the predominant cell in the bone marrow,

either lymphoblasts (acute lymphocytic leukemia) or myeloblasts (acute nonlymphocytic leukemia). Acute leukemias have a rapid onset and a short course, ending in death if untreated. The immaturity of the white cells leads to numerous infections, such as ulcerations of the mucous membranes, pneumonias, and septicemias. Early symptoms include fever, lymphadenopathy, pallor, and fatigue from anemia, and ecchymoses (Table 27-10). The WBC count may be normal or decreased.

Acute lymphocytic leukemia (ALL)

ALL arises from a single lymphoid stem cell (see Fig. 27-1) with impaired maturation and accumulation of the malignant cells in the bone marrow. It is common to find different stages of lymphoid development in the bone marrow from very immature to almost normal cells. The degree of immaturity is a guide to prognosis; the more immature the cells, the poorer the prognosis. Leukocytes in the bloodstream are predominantly in the blast form. The WBC count is often decreased, but a blood smear will show immature lymphoblasts. It is primarily a disease of children, but adults may develop it. Complete remissions are achieved in 70% to 90% of all newly diagnosed patients.

Acute nonlymphocytic leukemia (ANLL)

ANLL arises from a single myeloid stem cell (see Fig. 27-1) and is characterized by the development of immature myeloblasts in the bone marrow. The WBC count is usually in the low ranges of normal, and bone marrow aspiration reveals an increased number of myeloblasts. In the untreated patient or the person who is nonresponsive to therapy, the median survival time (MST) is approximately 2 to 3 months. Complete remission occurs in 50% to 75% of treated patients, and there is an MST of approximately 2 to 3 years. Approximately 20% of patients are in complete remission at 5 years and are capable of prolonged disease-free periods (remissions).

Chronic leukemias

Chronic leukemias are classified according to the predominant mature white cell, either lymphocytes (chronic lymphocytic anemia) or granulocytes (chronic myelogenous leukemia). Chronic leukemias have a more insidious onset and an MST of 4½ to 5½ years. Initially there are fewer infections than in acute leukemias because of the maturity

Table 27-10   Leukemias

Type	Signs and symptoms	Medical therapy
Acute lymphocytic leukemia (ALL)	Respiratory infections, anemia, bleeding of mucous membranes; proliferation of lymphoblasts in bone marrow, lymph nodes, spleen; hepatomegaly; splenomegaly; bone pain; CNS symptoms (headache, vomiting, seizures)	Combined chemotherapy, radiotherapy and immunotherapy; drugs: vincristine, prednisone, L-asparaginase
Acute nonlymphocytic leukemia (ANLL)	Same as above	Chemotherapy with daunorubicin, cytarabine, doxorubicin, 6-thioguanine
Chronic lymphocytic leukemia (CLL)	Painless and massive lymphadenopathy and splenomegaly; hepatomegaly with disease progression; anemia; thrombocytopenia; fatigue; weakness, pruritic vesicular lesions	Chemotherapy with alkylating agents (chlorambucil) and glucocorticoids (only when symptoms appear)
Chronic myelogenous leukemia (CML)	Fatigue, weakness, anorexia, weight loss; blastic (accelerated) phase: anemia, thrombocytopenia, fever, adenopathy, splenomegaly with sensation of abdominal fullness	Chemotherapy with agents used in AML; also vincristine, busulfan

of the white cells in the chronic disorder, but eventually infections of the skin and pneumonias result from decreased immunocompetence. Early signs of chronic leukemias include fatigue, weakness, anorexia, and weight loss characteristic of a hypermetabolic state. An enlarged spleen and liver can usually be palpated. The WBC count is usually elevated.

Chronic lymphocytic leukemia (CLL)

CLL is characterized by a proliferation of small, abnormal, mature B lymphocytes, leading to decreased synthesis of immunoglobulins and depressed antibody response. The accumulation of abnormal lymphocytes begins in the lymph nodes, then spreads to other lymphatic tissues. There is a marked increase in the number of leukocytes and mature lymphocytes. At the time of diagnosis the bone marrow is often filled by lymphatic infiltrations. The WBC count rises to a level between 20,000 and 100,000. Bone marrow biopsy shows infiltration of lymphocytes.

Chronic myelogenous leukemia (CML)

The primary defect in CML is an abnormal stem cell leading to an uncontrolled proliferation of the granulocytic cells. As a result of this proliferation, the number of circulating granulocytes increases markedly. In most cases, a characteristic chromosomal abnormality, the *Philadelphia chromosome*, is present. Diagnosis of CML is made on the basis of an elevated WBC count of 15,000 to 500,000, granulocytes on the peripheral blood smear that range in maturity from blast cells to mature neutrophils, granulocytic hyperplasia in the bone marrow, and the presence of the Philadelphia chromosome.

Nursing Process
Assessment
Subjective data and objective data

Subjective data include eliciting feelings of weakness and fatigue and a history of predisposition to infection. The person's knowledge of the nature of leukemia and concerns related to the disease are also obtained. The type of *objective data* depends on the type of leukemia and may include monitoring for lymphadenopathy, splenomegaly, fever, pallor, and bleeding. The mouth is examined for breaks in the mucous membranes. The person is also observed for behavioral signs of anxiety.

Diagnostic tests

Laboratory tests include bone marrow biopsy or aspiration, and WBC counts for differentiation of the type of leukemia (Table 27-9).

Data analysis: nursing diagnoses

Nursing diagnoses are determined from analysis of patient data. Possible nursing diagnoses for the person with leukemia may include, but are not limited to, the following:

Diagnostic title	Possible etiologies
Infection, high risk for	Decreased WBCs, chemotherapy, radiation
Injury, high risk for: hemorrhage	Disease process, trauma, chemotherapy
Anxiety	Threat of death, change in health status
Coping, ineffectual, individual/family	Situational crisis, prolonged disability, ineffective problem solving
Knowledge deficit	Lack of exposure or recall

Planning: expected patient outcomes

Expected patient outcomes for the person with leukemia may include, but are not limited to, the following:
1. Shows no signs of infection or excessive bleeding.
2. Shows evidence of problem solving and finding satisfying solutions.
3. Assumes activities of daily living.
4. Describes the nature of the disease, the therapeutic program, symptoms requiring follow-up, and available community resources.

Chemotherapeutic agents commonly used in leukemia therapy	
L-Asparaginase	Melphalan
Busulfan	6-Mercaptopurine
Chlorambucil	Methotrexate
Cyclophosphamide	Prednisone
Cytarabine	6-Thioguanine
Daunorubicin	Vincristine
Doxorubicin	

Implementation

Many of the interventions for the listed nursing diagnoses are discussed in the chapter on cancer (see Chapter 11).

Assisting with achievement of therapeutic goals

Leukemia, by its nature, is a diverse illness. The varied courses and response or lack of response to treatment also add to the diversity. Complete remission of the disease is the goal of medical therapy since cure is not possible at this time. Complete remission exists when all tests are normal, and all symptoms have disappeared. Partial remission occurs when symptoms have disappeared, but the disease remains in the bone marrow.

Chemotherapy

Chemotherapy is the primary treatment modality. The first phase of chemotherapy is termed *induction chemotherapy* and consists of combination chemotherapy (use of more than one chemotherapeutic agent, see Chapter 11). Commonly used agents in the treatment of leukemias are listed in Box 27-11. Bone marrow studies are conducted 2 and 3 weeks following initiation of therapy. A different drug regimen will be given if evidence of disease in the marrow is still present after 3 weeks.

During induction therapy, the patient is at high risk for hemorrhage or infection. Nursing care of the patient during this phase includes the following:
1. Monitor vital signs every 4 hours
2. Use bleeding precautions
   a. Use soft toothbrush or swabs for mouth
   b. No rectal temperatures, medications, or enemas
   c. Use electric razor
   d. Avoid aspirin
3. Monitor for signs of bleeding (observation of skin, testing urine with hemastix and stool for guaiac)
4. Give antibiotics on time to maintain blood levels if fever occurs
5. Monitor administration of whole blood or blood component therapy, if given
6. Assess intravenous site of chemotherapy for redness, swelling, tenderness, extravasation of drugs (Chapter 11)
7. Provide immediate care of extravasation of chemotherapeutic drugs (discontinue infusion, apply ice to area, infiltrate subcutaneous area with sodium bicarbonate or steroids)[39]

Maintenance therapy, the second phase of therapy, is usually required to maintain a complete remission. This therapy is often given on an outpatient basis. Appropriate duration of therapy in patients who continue free of disease varies, depending on the type of the disease and the patient's response to therapy. Chemotherapy is discussed in more detail in Chapter 11.

Bone marrow transplantation

Bone marrow transplantation, using HLA-identical bone marrow, has been used with increasing frequency and promises to have an increasing impact on the progress of ANLL. In addition to leukemia, bone marrow transplantation is being used for patients with lymphoma, aplastic anemia, thalassemia, and immunodeficiency disorders.

Pretransplant preparation is necessary for bone marrow transplantation. It has two goals: *immunosuppression* to allow acceptance of an immunologically nonidentical graft and *cytoreduction* to kill all tumor cells. This is accomplished by chemotherapy followed by total body irradiation.[15]

The procedure consists of taking 600 to 1000 to 2500 ml[30] of marrow cells by multiple needle aspiration from the posterior iliac crest of the donor under general or spinal anesthesia. After processing, the marrow is placed in a blood transfusion bag and administered intravenously through a Hickman catheter (see Chapter 11) at the same rate as RBC administration (about 4 hours).

Patients over 30 may develop severe acute graft-versus-host reaction (Chapter 41), which may be fatal. One approach being used to prevent graft-versus-host reaction is to treat the donor marrow with monoclonal antibodies before transplantation. This removes mature T cells, which cause the reaction, but leaves immature T cells to prevent infection (Chapter 11).

Another method to prevent graft-versus-host reaction is *autologous* bone marrow transplantation. Some of the *patient's* bone marrow is removed during a period of remission and is frozen. It is stored for transplantation when needed by the patient. Recombinant human granulocyte-macrophage stimulating factor (GM-CSF), produced by recombinant DNA technology, is being given to patients after undergoing autologous bone marrow transplantation to accelerate myeloid engraftment, decrease infectious episodes, and shorten hospital stay.

Nursing care is focused on preventing infection, providing emotional support and skin care, and maintaining fluid, electrolyte, and nutritional balance. Protective isolation (Chapter 11) may be used. Care of the patient with a transplant is discussed in Chapter 42.

Interventions to achieve patient outcomes
Preventing infection

Patients with leukemia are at high risk of infection as a consequence of leukopenia. They may suffer from recurrent perirectal abscesses, pneumonia, and septicemias. Measures to prevent infection include the following:
1. Place patient in a private room; avoid contact with visitors and staff who have infection.
2. Place patient in protective isolation (see Chapter 11).
3. Provide meticulous hygiene, including daily bath, careful oral hygiene, and perineal care; use antiseptic creams.

4. Avoid catheterizations.
5. Use povidone iodine skin cleansing for 1 minute before parenteral injections (or other preparations as prescribed).
6. Maintain a clean environment.
7. Provide emotional support for anxiety when infection occurs.

Preventing excessive bleeding

Patients with leukemia have fewer platelets, which causes bleeding, as evidenced by petechiae, ecchymosis (bleeding into the skin), epistaxis (nosebleeds), and GI and urinary tract hemorrhage. Measures to prevent excessive bleeding include the following:

1. Assess all sites for bleeding.
2. Test urine (Hemastix) and stool (guaiac) for blood.
3. Keep venipuncture and intramuscular injections to a minimum.
4. Apply pressure to venipuncture sites for 5 minutes, arterial sites for 10 minutes.
5. Use soft toothbrush or swab for mouth care.
6. Keep mouth clean and free of debris with normal saline rinse if bleeding occurs.
7. Avoid taking rectal temperatures, administering rectal medications, or giving enemas.
8. Avoid invasive procedures.

Counseling patient and family

Each person with leukemia responds in a different way. It cannot be predicted for certain whether an individual will respond to a prescribed treatment or how long a remission will last. Leukemia is a threat to life, a situational crisis. Both patient and family, therefore, can experience anxiety, especially when the diagnosis is first made and during acute phases. Even the patient in remission may experience periods of anxiety when other illnesses occur and be concerned that the acute phase has returned. Anxiety is also high during chemotherapy and bone marrow transplantation. Give patients and family members opportunities to talk, to share fear and concerns, to ask questions. Help them explore alternative methods of coping, if appropriate. Carefully explain therapies and planned activities. Include the family in all aspects of patient care.

Facilitating patient learning

How the individual incorporates the illness into life is also unique to each person. Nursing has the key role in patient education (Box 27-12). Of utmost importance in learning is the ability of the person to identify the body's signals that blood abnormalities exist. Bone pain, often severe, may signal blast crisis (acute proliferation of immature cells).

Individuals whose illness runs the course of several months to years often become very knowledgeable about their disease, blood components, related symptoms, and specific chemotherapeutic drugs. These persons sometimes discuss their progress in terms of changes in their blood counts. Over time many individuals become attuned to how such changes affect them. For example, they often can predict their count by how they feel. Many such persons respond well to being included in their plan of care during hospitalization and in preparation for discharge.

Evaluation

Questions to consider include the following:

1. Is the patient free of infection?
2. Is the patient assuming activities of daily living?
3. Is the patient free from anxiety?
4. Do the patient and family say they are coping with the illness?
5. Is the patient knowledgeable about the disease, its effects, and the treatment regimen?
6. Can the patient describe symptoms that require medical intervention?
7. Can the patient state importance of and schedule for chemotherapy and periodic blood tests?

DISORDERS ASSOCIATED WITH THE LYMPHATIC SYSTEM

LYMPHADENOPATHY

Lymph node enlargement (lymphadenopathy) may be caused by infection in the area drained by the lymph vessel containing the node or by systemic infection. Enlargement of the node, which in this situation is usually painful, is a positive sign indicating immune responsiveness to the invading microorganisms. Lymphadenopathy may also occur when the node is invaded by cells normally not present (leukemic cells, cancer cells) and is a pathophysiologic sign of lymphomas such as Hodgkin's disease. Some body areas where lymph nodes may be palpated are illustrated in Fig. 27-9.

Lymphangiography is a radiologic technique used for evaluation of lymph nodes to detect the presence of disease. This procedure is especially valuable in assessing those nodes that are anatomically too deep to allow for evaluation by palpation. For this procedure a small incision is made on the dorsal surface of each foot so that the small lymph glands are made accessible. A dye is slowly instilled over several hours, filling all lymph chains and nodes. Radiographs are usually done immediately after the dye is ab-

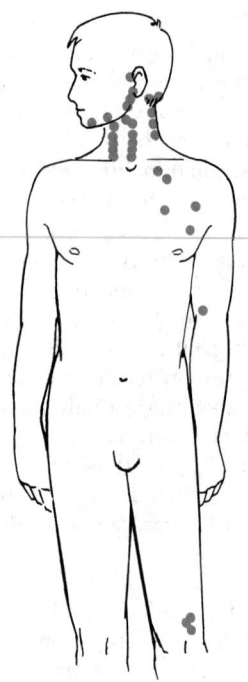

Fig. 27-9 Diagram of body areas where enlarged lymph nodes may be palpated.

Stage	Definition
I	Single abnormal lymph node
II	Two or more abnormal lymph nodes on the same side of the diaphragm
III	Abnormal lymph node regions on both sides of the diaphragm, which may also be accompanied by involvement of the spleen
IV	Diffuse or disseminated involvment of one or more extralymphatic organs or tissues with or without lymph node involvement

Staging of Hodgkin's disease

sorbed and again at intervals of 24 and 48 hours after the procedure. In addition, because the dye remains in the lymph nodes for as long as 6 months after the initial study, disease status and response to therapy can be periodically evaluated with routine abdominal x-ray films.

LYMPHOMAS

Lymphomas are malignant disorders of the lymph system. Hodgkin's disease is considered separate from other lymphomas (Table 27-11).

Etiology and Pathophysiology
Hodgkin's disease

Hodgkin's disease, which was considered fatal until fairly recently, is now potentially curable. Although the cause is unknown, it is thought that viruses may be implicated. The person has *defective cellular immunity (T cell disease)* and is therefore at high risk for infections. Four pathologic variants of Hodgkin's have been recognized: *lymphocyte predominant, nodular sclerosis, mixed cellularity,* and *lymphocyte depletion.* The lymphocyte predominant and nodular sclerosis types have the best prognosis, and lymphocyte depletion, the worst. Hodgkin's disease is usually characterized by the presence of the Reed-Sternberg cell, a large macrophage-derived cell.

The most important prognostic indicator is the stage of disease at the time of diagnosis. Accurate staging (see Box 27-13) is crucial to the subsequent treatment regimen. All stages are subclassified further, as follows:

A: No symptoms
B: Presence of weight loss, fever, profuse night sweats

Non-Hodgkin's lymphomas

Non-Hodgkin's lymphomas (NHL) include a broad spectrum of lymphoid malignancies with different histopathologies, disease courses, and responses to therapy. Accurate identification of the histopathology is crucial to the determination of the treatment plan. NHL can be categorized as *lymphocytic, histiocytic,* or *mixed cell types.* A lymphocytic cytology has the most favorable prognosis, and the histiocytic has the least favorable. Immature lymphocytes are produced, leading to impaired B-cell (humoral) immune response. These patients are therefore also at high risk for infections.

Nursing Process
Assessment
Subjective data and objective data

Subjective data include the following:
1. Knowledge of the disorder
2. Effect of fatigue on the ability to carry out ADL
3. Discomfort from night sweats or pruritus
4. Appetite and present nutritional status

Objective data include weight and condition of skin from scratching (for example, excoriations).

Diagnostic tests

Diagnostic tests for lymphomas may include a chest x-ray film to identify a mediastinal mass and lymphangiography to evaluate the retroperitoneal nodes. The liver and spleen are evaluated by radionuclide scanning or by computed tomography (CT scan). A staging laparotomy may be performed to obtain a biopsy specimen of retroperitoneal lymph nodes and of both lobes of the liver and to remove the spleen. The diagnostic workup is often arduous and difficult, and explanation of the diagnostic procedures helps provide the patient with the emotional support so often needed during this time.

Slides are often sent to major cancer centers for consultation regarding the classification of the disease. Once the diagnosis is made, the extent of the disease (staging) must be determined for planning the treatment regimen.

Data analysis: nursing diagnoses

Nursing diagnoses are determined from analysis of patient data. Possible nursing diagnoses for the person with

Table 27-11 Disorders of the lymphatic system

Disorder	Signs and symptoms	Medical therapy
Hodgkin's disease	Lymph node enlargement (firm, nontender, painless), fever, weight loss, night sweats, pruritus, fatigue	Radiation therapy for stages IA and IIA, radiation and chemotherapy for stage IIIA, combination chemotherapy for stages IIIB and IVB
Non-Hodgkin's lymphoma	Nontender "bulky" lymphadenopathy, moderate hepatomegaly and splenomegaly, fever, night sweats, weight loss	Initial localized radiotherapy; total nodal radiation and chemotherapy for multifocal lesions
Multiple myeloma	Severe disabling bone pain (especially in weight-bearing areas), hypercalcemia, renal failure, anorexia, CHF, bleeding tendency, coma	Radiation for bone pain, chemotherapy, hydration, ambulation, blood transfusions for anemia, analgesics

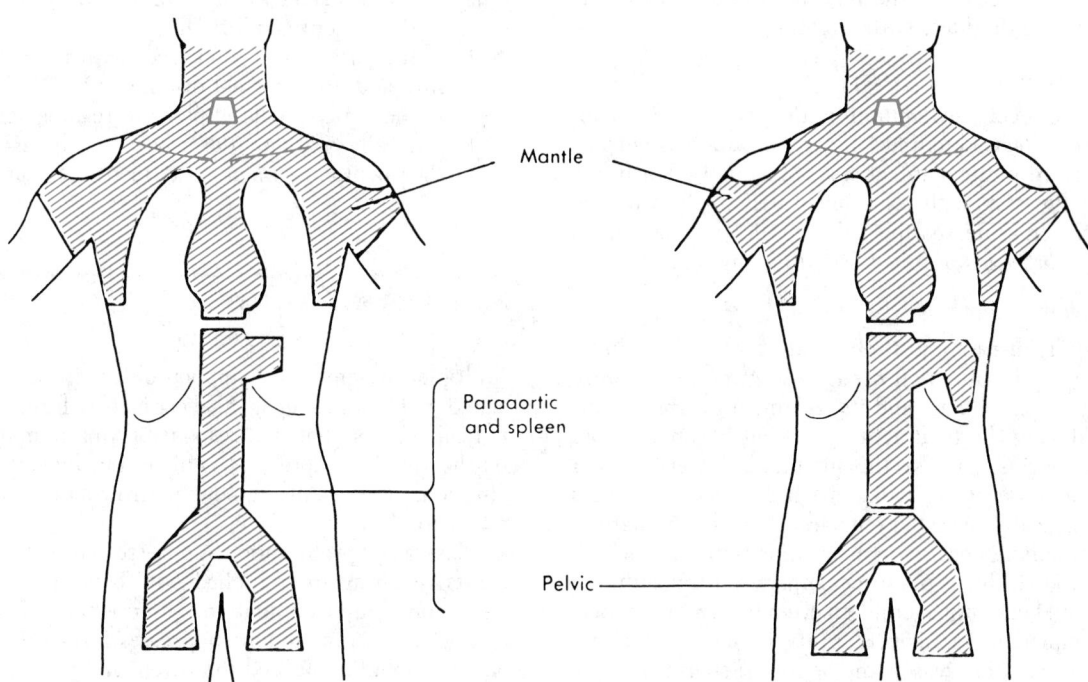

Mantle

Paraaortic and spleen

Pelvic

Fig. 27-10 Diagram of mantle and inverted Y fields used in total lymphoid radiotherapy of Hodgkin's disease. (From Rosenberg SA, Kaplan HS: *Calif Med* 113:23, 1970.)

lymphomas may include, but are not limited to, the following:

Diagnostic title	Possible etiologies
Comfort, altered: night sweats, pruritus	Hypermetabolism
Infection, high risk for	Defective immune response
Coping, ineffective individual	Situational crisis
Knowledge deficit	Lack of exposure or recall

Planning: expected patient outcomes

Expected patient outcomes for the person with lymphomas may include, but are not limited to, the following:

1. States feeling more comfortable without itching.
2. Is free from infection.
3. Discusses effects of illness on life's activities and methods of coping.
4. Describes the nature of the disorder, the therapeutic regimen, and community resources.

Implementation
Assisting with achievement of therapeutic goals

Chemotherapy and radiation therapy are the primary treatment modalities for the lymphomas (Table 27-11). For Hodgkin's disease, treatment yields a cure rate of approximately 90% for stage I and 80% for stage II. Combination chemotherapy is the treatment of choice for stages IIIb and IV. The most commonly used combination is the MOPP regimen (see Chapter 11). It is administered in a 2-week course each month with prednisone added during the first and fourth course. The drugs are administered for at least 6 months or for two or three courses following the attainment of complete remission. Complete remissions are achieved in approximately 80% of these patients, and long-term, disease-free remissions and probable cures occur in half of this group.

When nodal radiation is used, only those areas of the body to be irradiated are exposed; the other areas are protected by a mantle (Fig. 27-10).

Varying approaches are used for non-Hodgkin's lymphomas. Single alkylating agents, such as chlorambucil, or combination chemotherapy may be used. Local or total nodal radiation therapy may be given. Explanation of the treatment regimen is important to ensure patient understanding and compliance to achieve therapeutic goals.

Interventions to achieve patient outcomes
Promoting comfort

Fever, pruritus, and profuse night sweats may lead to general discomfort. Comfort measures for pruritus, such as baths and antipruritic medication (see Chapter 43), may be instituted. Frequent changes of night clothing or bed linens may be necessary, and high fluid intake is encouraged to replace fluid lost with sweating.

Preventing infection

Because of decreased immunity, the person with a lymphoma needs to avoid sources of infection, such as persons with upper respiratory infections. Thoroughly wash any breaks in the skin with soap and water, apply a topical antibiotic such as neosporin, and keep the area clean until healed. Report signs of infection to the physician.

Counseling patients

Hodgkin's disease most often affects young adults. Therefore special attention needs to be given to minimize the impact of the illness and its treatment on their lives, not only during the treatment period but beyond. Before treatment begins, discuss therapy-induced sterility. For young women receiving radiation therapy alone, ovaries may be surgically relocated outside the field of radiation. Sterility frequently occurs in association with chemotherapy. For women this is often temporary, and the ability to conceive and bear normal children often returns after therapy is completed. For men, sterility is more frequently permanent. For this reason the option of sperm banking should be discussed before beginning either radiation or chemotherapy.

To allow for work and career development, every effort should be made to schedule treatment at those times and days of the week that least interfere with work and other important events in the person's life. The nurse has a crucial role in assisting individuals to develop a realistic approach to the illness and in successfully meeting the demands and limitations imposed by the illness and its treatment.

Individuals with lymphomas may have periods of remission and recurrence. Such peaks and valleys are stressful and disruptive. Many patients describe subsequent courses of treatment following a recurrence as more stressful than the initial treatment. Comments include, "Is it worth it? I don't have the same faith." Other patients, realistically encouraged by the initial response to treatment, are able to express an optimistic outlook, "It worked the first time. It will work again." Recognition of the stress involved in therapy requires that support systems be available to the individual. The health care team can provide some of the needed support and guidance as the individual learns to incorporate the illness into daily life.

Facilitating patient learning

Teaching the patient includes the following:
1. Nature of the disorder
2. Importance of the extensive workup in identifying the treatment plan
3. Effects of therapy on sterility
4. Need for periodic blood counts
5. Side effects of radiation and chemotherapy and how to cope with them (see Chapter 11)
6. Need for continued medical follow-up
7. Community resources (American Cancer Society)

Evaluation

Questions to consider include the following:
1. Is the patient comfortable?
2. Is the patient infection free, with normal temperature and no abnormal discharges?
3. Is the patient making plans to resume activities?
4. Can the patient describe the disease process, therapeutic regimen, and identify community resources?

MULTIPLE MYELOMA
Etiology and Pathophysiology

Multiple myeloma is a lymphoproliferative disorder associated with plasma cells, the most mature form of activated B lymphocytes that are responsible for immunoglobulin synthesis (see Chapter 16). This is a malignant neoplastic disease that arises in the bone marrow and involves bones primarily.

Plasma cell proliferation suppresses normal marrow elements resulting in "punched out" bone lesions that are visible on x-ray examination. Functionally abnormal immunoglobulin production suppresses formation of normal immunoglobulins needed to prevent infections.[26]

Because of changes in the bone, patients develop severe disabling bone pain (especially in weight-bearing bones), pathologic fractures, neurologic symptoms from cord compression, hypercalcemia (because of bone destruction), with symptoms of renal failure, anorexia, confusion, and coma. Renal tubules may be damaged by myeloma proteins (Bence-Jones proteins).

Pneumonia, urinary tract infections, and bacteremia occur because of the decrease in normal immunoglobulins. Expanded plasma volume may lead to congestive heart failure. Increased plasma viscosity leads to visual problems, headache, immobility, and confusion. Hemorrhage may occur because the myeloma proteins interact with plasma coagulation factors and also coat platelets, decreasing their function.

Assessment
Subjective data and objective data

Subjective data include the presence of bone pain, anorexia, and neurologic symptoms such as numbness, tingling, and weakness. *Objective data* include skin color, urinary output, signs and symptoms of infection, level of consciousness, and signs of bleeding.

Diagnostic tests

Diagnostic tests include x-ray evaluation of bones, hematologic studies (serum protein electrophoresis and immunoelectrophoresis), Bence-Jones proteins, and calcium levels.

Implementation

There is no cure for multiple myeloma, and treatment is primarily palliative. The median survival is 5 to 6 years.[30] Combination chemotherapy is given for bone pain or other symptoms. Localized radiotherapy may also be used. During therapy, monitor renal and cardiac function.

Pain control includes analgesic administration and careful handling of extremities when mobilizing or turning the patient. Because immobility increases bone demineralization and osteoporosis, it is essential that the patient maintain mobility to prevent fractures. Use of splints, braces, and walkers may facilitate activity.

If the patient is prone to infection or bleeding, initiate interventions that prevent their occurrence (see p. 768). Counseling and teaching about these side-effects are essential, as well as providing psychologic support for an individual with a chronic debilitating disease.

SUMMARY

1. Major health problems of the hematopoietic system include RBC disorders (anemias, polycythemia), WBC disorders (leukemias), coagulation disorders (platelet disorders, hemophilia, DIC), lymphatic system disorders (Hodgkin's disease, non-Hodgkin's lymphoma), and plasma cell disorders (multiple myeloma).
2. Anemia may be caused by blood loss, impaired RBC production, increased RBC destruction, or nutritional deficiency.
3. Weakness and fatigue are major signs of anemia. They result from decreased oxygenation from lack of hemoglobin and increased energy needs required by increased RBC production.
4. Bone marrow samples may be obtained by aspiration or biopsy from the sternum, iliac crest, or tibia.
5. Sickle cell anemia is a hemolytic anemia with a genetic basis; a sickle cell crisis occurs when the RBCs become deoxygenated and sickle-shaped, thus causing stasis and obstruction of the microvasculature, leading to organ infarction and necrosis.
6. Ingestion of iron compounds is part of the therapy for iron-deficiency anemia or anemia from chronic blood loss only; it will not help the other types of anemias.
7. Thrombocytopenia is a decrease in the number of circulating platelets and leads to bleeding; persons with thrombocytopenia need to learn how to prevent injury and hemorrahge.
8. Hemophilia is a hereditary coagulation disorder; hemophilia A is a lack of coagulation factor VIII, and hemophilia B is a lack of factor IX; maintenance therapy consists of blood factor replacement therapy and prevention of injury.
9. Disseminated intravascular coagulation (DIC) is a coagulation disorder characterized initially by clotting and secondarily by hemorrhage. It results from an alteration in the balance between clotting factors and fibrinolytic factors; the person is usually critically ill.
10. Persons with alterations of WBCs are at high risk of infection, because leukocytes are a major factor in the body's defense against invading microorganisms.
11. The leukemias are malignant disorders characterized by uncontrolled proliferation of WBCs and their precursors; the cause is unknown.
12. Leukemias may be lymphocytic or myelogenous, and acute or chronic. Acute leukemias have a rapid onset and a short course, if untreated; chronic leukemias have a more insidious onset and longer course. The major therapies for leukemias are chemotherapy and bone marrow transplantation.
13. Lymphomas are malignant disorders of the lymphatic system. Persons with Hodgkin's disease have defective cellular immunity and are therefore at high risk for infection. Non-Hodgkin's lymphoma is a group of lymphoid malignancies. Chemotherapy and radiation are the primary treatment modalities for lymphomas.
14. Multiple myeloma is a lymphoproliferative disorder associated with plasma cells (B lymphocytes); it is a malignant disorder arising in the bone marrow and affects primarily bones. The person is at high risk for pathologic fractures.

STUDY QUESTIONS

- From your knowledge of physiology, explain why the patient who is anemic may have dyspnea, tachycardia, and fatigue.
- What is the difference between sickle cell anemia and nutritional deficiency anemia? How does treatment differ?
- Why does WBC count increase during infection? Why is a person with leukopenia more susceptible to infection?
- What are the differences in the four major forms of leukemia in terms of course and treatment?
- Why are patients with leukemia and multiple myeloma at high risk for infection, even though WBC counts may be elevated?

REFERENCES AND SELECTED READINGS

1.* Baker LS: *You and leukemia: a day at a time,* Philadelphia, 1988, WB Saunders.
2. Baum K, et al: The painful crisis of homozygous sickle cell disease, *Arch Intern Med* 147:1231-1234, 1987.
3.* Borley D: Oncology nursing: leukemia and bone marrow transplant. 3. *Nurs Mirror* 160(6):30-34, 1985.
4. Brain MC, Carbone PP: *Current therapy in hematology-oncology,* ed 4, St Louis, 1991, Mosby–Year Book.
5. Brannan D, Guthrie T: Idiopathic thrombocytopenia purpura in adults, *South Med J* 81(1):43-44, 1989.
6.* Cerrato PS: Could you spot the other anemia? *RN* 49(10):63-64, 1986.
7.* Coyle MK: Organic illness mimicking psychiatric episodes, *J Gerontol Nurs* 13(1):31-35, 1987.

*Recommended for student reading.

8. Dalton W, Miller T: Multidrug resistance, principles and practice of oncology, *Updates* 5(7):1-13, 1991.

9. DeVita V, Hellman S, Rosenberg S: *Cancer: principles and practice of oncology*, ed 3, Philadelphia, 1989, JB Lippincott.

10.* France-Dawson M: Sickle cell disease: implications for nursing care, *J Adv Nurs* 11(6):729-737, 1986.

11.* Fraser M, Tucker M: Second malignancies following cancer therapy, *Semin Oncol Nurs* 5(1):43-45, 1989.

12.* Freedman SL: An overview of bone marrow transplantation, *Sem Oncol Nurs* 4(1):3-8, 1988.

13.* Froberg J: The anemias: causes and courses of action, *RN* 52(1):24-29, 1989.

14.* Gallagher MT, Wyland N: Leukemia: when white cells run wild, *RN* 49(10):33-37, 1986.

15.* Gibson L: Bone marrow transplant: the process, *Nurs Times* 83(3):36-38, 1986.

16.* Goodman M: Managing the side effects of chemotherapy, *Semin Oncol Nurs* 5(2):29-52, 1989.

17. Haskell C: *Cancer treatment*, ed 3, Philadelphia, 1990, WB Saunders.

18.* Huckstadt A: Hemophilia: the person, family and nurse, *Rehab Nurs* 11(3):25-28, 1986.

19.* Lakhani AK: Current management of acute leukemias, *Nursing 88* (London) 3:755-758, 1987.

20. Lamb C: Managing sickle cell emergencies, *Patient Care* 19(1):92-95, 1985.

21. Mauer AM: Acute lymphoblastic leukemia in a young adult, *Hosp Pract* 22(9):145-156, 1987.

22.* McConnell EA: Leukocyte studies: what the counts can tell you, *Nursing 86* 16(3):42-43, 1986.

23.* Moeller KI: Suppressing the risks of bone marrow suppression, *Nursing 87* 17(3):52-54, 1987.

24. Pittiglio D, Sacher R: *Clinical hematology and fundamentals of hemostasis*, Philadelphia, 1987, FA Davis.

25. Post-White J: Glucocorticoid-induced suppression in the patient with leukemia or lymphoma, *CA Nurs* 9(1):15-22, 1986.

26. Price SA, Wilson LM: *Pathophysiology*, ed 3, New York, 1986, McGraw-Hill.

27. Ratnoff OD, Forbes CD: *Disorders of hemostasis*, ed 2, Philadelphia, 1991, WB Saunders.

28. Rifkind R, et al: *Fundamentals of hematology*, ed 3, Chicago, 1986, Year Book.

29.* Rooney A, Haviley C: Nursing management of disseminated intravascular coagulation, *Oncol Nurs Forum* 12(1):15-22, 1985.

30. Schroeder SA et al: *Current medical diagnosis and treatment*, Norwalk, Conn., 1991, Appleton & Lange.

31.* Simonson GM: Caring for patients with acute myelocytic leukemia, *Am J Nurs* 88:304-309, 1988.

32.* Smith D: Sexual rehabilitation of the cancer patient, *Cancer Nurs* 12(1):10-15, 1988.

33.* Terry BA: Hodgkin's disease and non-Hodgkin's lymphomas, *Nurs Clin North Am* 20(1):207-217, 1985.

34. Thomas ED: Bone marrow transplantation: present states and future expectations. In Isselbacker KJ et al: *Harrison's Principles of internal medicine*, ed 11, New York, 1987, McGraw-Hill.

35.* Trotta P: Nursing assessment of symptoms associated with hyperviscosity syndrome, *Oncol Nurs Forum* 14(1):21-27, 1987.

36. Williams SR: *Essentials of nutrition and diet therapy*, ed 5, St Louis, 1990, Mosby–Year Book.

37. Wyngaarden JB, Smith LH: *Cecil's Textbook of medicine*, ed 18, Philadelphia, 1988, WB Saunders.

Classic

38. Alcorn R, et al: Fluid therapy and exercise in the management of sickle cell anemia, *Phys Ther* 64:1520-1522, 1984.

39.* Campbell VB, Preston R, Smith KY: The leukemias: definition, treatment, and nursing care, *Nurs Clin North Am* 18(3):523-542, 1983.

40.* Gibbons PT: Transfusion therapy in sickle cell disease, *Nurs Clin North Am* 18(3):563-568, 1983.

41.* Hutchinson MM: Aplastic anemia: care of the bone marrow failure patient, *Nurs Clin North Am* 18(3):543-552, 1983.

42.* Hutchinson MM, King AH: A nursing perspective on bone marrow transplantation, *Nurs Clin North Am* 18(3):511-522, 1983.

43.* Lopez JA, Hausz M: Therapeutic apheresis, *Am J Nurs* 82:1572-1578, 1982.

44. Miller VG: The sickle cell anemia patient in surgery, *AORN J* 31:1080-1090, 1979.

45. Nausef WM, et al: A study of the value of simple protective isolation in patients with granulocytopenia, *N Engl J Med* 304:448-452, 1981.

46.* Rozell MS, Hijazi M, Pack B: The painful episode, *Nurs Clin North Am* 18(1):185-199, 1983.

47.* Williams I, Earles AN, Pack B: Psychological considerations in sickle cell disease, *Nurs Clin North Am* 18(1):216-230, 1983.

Metabolic and Endocrine Problems

Unit Seven

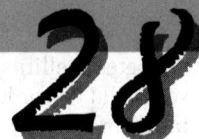

The Patient with Diabetes Mellitus

Dorothy Blevins
Virginia L. Cassmeyer

After studying this chapter, the learner should be able to:

- Differentiate between the two major types of diabetes mellitus (DM).
- Describe prevention and health education for DM.
- Explain the pathophysiologic bases for hyperglycemia, nonketotic coma, diabetic ketoacidosis, macrovascular and microvascular changes, neuropathy, and lower extremity changes.
- Identify assessment parameters of DM.
- Describe dietary recommendations and systems for learning dietary requirements.
- Explain the role of exercise in DM.
- Describe medication regimens for DM.
- Describe therapy for correcting acute metabolic crises.
- Explain the effect of surgery on the person with DM.
- Describe the 15 commandments of importance in teaching the patient with DM.

Diabetes mellitus (DM) is a complex chronic disease involving (1) disorders in carbohydrate, protein, and fat metabolism and (2) the development of macrovascular, microvascular, and neurologic complications. It is classified as an endocrine or hormonal disease because of its central feature of hyperglycemia, which results from a deficit in production or utilization of insulin.

ANATOMY AND PHYSIOLOGY

An insulin deficit hampers the metabolism of carbohydrates, proteins, and fats. The deficit may occur because the pancreatic beta cells do not secrete insulin properly or because hepatic or peripheral cell receptors are resistant to the binding of insulin or transfer of insulin across the cell membrane. Diabetes mellitus has been described as "cellular starvation in the midst of plenty"; cells are deprived of glucose while hyperglycemia exists. When glucose is not available for cellular function, cells use other fuels; these are derived from glycogen, amino acids, lactate, glycerol, and ketones. These energy substrates are stored chiefly in muscle, hepatic, and adipose cells.

Hormonal Regulation of Blood Glucose

The pancreatic hormone, *insulin,* has a major metabolic role during fed states; it promotes the use of available glucose and promotes the storage of fuels for later use. See Box 28-1 for the actions of insulin that are *hypoglycemic, antilipolytic, and anabolic.* Of the several hormones involved in the regulation of blood glucose levels, insulin is the only one that lowers blood glucose. In diabetes, an insulin deficit raises blood glucose above normal levels.

Glucagon, another hormone produced in the pancreas, maintains normal blood glucose levels during fasting states. Glucagon is called a counterregulatory hormone which acts "counter to insulin"; that is, it raises blood glucose. The major role for glucagon is during fasting states when it promotes the use of stored fuels by these processes: *glycogenolysis, gluconeogenesis, ketogenesis, and lipolysis.* The liver is a chief site for producing new glucose from glycogen and amino acids and releasing this into the blood. Free fatty acids are released from triglyceride stores and can be used as energy sources. In diabetes, excessive amounts of glucagon contribute to the hyperglycemia and other metabolic alterations of the disease.

Persons with normal metabolism are able to maintain blood glucose levels of 70 to 110 mg/dl (euglycemia) under markedly different conditions of food intake. In nondiabetic persons, blood glucose levels may rise to 120 to 140 mg/dl after eating (postprandial), but these then rapidly return to normal, as excess glucose is extracted from the blood and stored as glycogen in liver and muscle cells (glycogenesis).

Other counterregulatory hormones affect metabolism much as glucagon does. These include *growth hormone,* produced in the anterior pituitary gland, *epinephrine,* produced in the adrenal medulla, the *glucocorticoids,* produced in the adrenal cortex, and *thyroid hormone.* They also raise blood glucose and promote the use of stored fuels by one or more of the same processes listed above. The secretion of the counterregulatory hormones often increases during the stress response, thus providing glucose for increased energy needs. If there is sufficient insulin in stress states, blood glucose levels will stay within normal limits or be only slightly elevated for a short time. In diabetes, the insulin deficit is made worse by the effects of the counterregulatory hormone, and blood glucose levels can rise greatly during the stress response.

Anatomy

Insulin and glucagon are produced by the islet cells in the pancreas, which is both an exocrine and an endocrine gland. It lies retroperitoneally behind the stomach, with its head and neck in the curve of the duodenum, its body extending horizontally across the posterior abdominal wall, and its tail touching the spleen. More than 1 million islet cells are located throughout the organ. Three types of endocrine cells are alpha (α), which secrete glucagon, beta (β), which secrete insulin, and delta (Δ), which secrete gastrin and pancreatic somatostatin.

Physiology

Insulin is necessary for the transport of glucose, amino acids, potassium, and phosphate across cell membranes, especially those of adipose and resting muscle cells. Insulin is also needed to activate enzymes that promote intracellular metabolism. Insulin functions by a fixed receptor model; that is, it combines with a receptor on the plasma membrane of the cell and initiates a sequence of postreceptor cellular activities that are coordinated by a second messenger, most probably cyclic guanosine 3,5-monophosphate (CGMP). (See a physiology text for further detail on the action of insulin.)

It should be apparent that when there is a deficit of insulin, as in diabetes mellitus, *hyperglycemia, increased fat metabolism,* and *decreased protein synthesis* occur.

A small amount of insulin is secreted continually (basal secretion), and a bolus (surge) amount is secreted in response to intake of glucose and amino acids. Insulin is also secreted in response to a rise in hepatic glucose output (HGO), which is stimulated by glucagon and/or other counterregulatory hormones. This surge in HGO normally

28-1	**Actions of insulin**	
	Hypoglycemic	Decreases blood glucose level
		Increases uptake and utilization of glucose by adipose and muscle cell
		Increases phosphorylation of glucose by liver
		Increases glycogenesis
	Suppresses fat metabolism	Increases lipogenesis (antilipolytic)
	Promotes protein synthesis	Increases amino acid incorporation into protein (anabolic)

occurs at approximately 4 AM; it is reflected in rising blood glucose levels (*dawn phenomenon*).

Physiologic Changes with Aging

Diabetes mellitus affects about 15% to 20% of persons over the age of 65. The disease of diabetes in the elderly must be differentiated from the normal changes of aging that affect glucose tolerance.[42]

Carbohydrate tolerance gradually declines as people age. Glucose ingestion results in higher levels of blood glucose and longer durations of hyperglycemia in the elderly. After a loading dose of glucose, the 2-hour glucose blood level can be expected to increase approximately 10 to 15 mg/dl for each decade of life (Table 28-1). The change in fasting blood glucose levels related to age is less marked—only 2 mg/dl per decade.

This age-related carbohydrate intolerance has been variously attributed to reduced insulin release from beta cells, a delay in insulin release, and/or a decrease in peripheral sensitivity to insulin.

A second physiologic change associated with aging that is important in diabetes management is a rise in the renal threshold for glucose above the average of 160-180 mg/dl blood glucose.

Table 28-1   Glucose tolerance with aging (plasma glucose in mg/dl)

Age (yr)	Normal		
	Fasting	1 hr	2 hr
0-30	110	185	165
30-40	112	191	175
40-50	114	197	185
50-60	116	203	195
60-70	118	209	205
70-80	120	215	215

From Andres, R, adapted from Prout, TE: Diabetes mellitus, ed 4, New York, 1975, American Diabetes Association.

CLASSIFICATION OF DIABETES MELLITUS

This chapter focuses on insulin-dependent diabetes mellitus (IDDM, type 1) and non-insulin-dependent diabetes mellitus (NIDDM, type 2). These are two of eight diagnoses of glucose intolerance. Table 28-2 describes five of these, including IDDM and NIDDM and the criteria for their diagnoses. These are part of a classification system developed in 1979 by an international work group and adopted for use in United States and by the World Health Organization. This classification made labels previously used to categorize persons with diabetes (borderline, latent, juvenile, and adult onset) obsolete. The older terms were discontinued because they were not associated with

Table 28-2   Diagnoses of diabetes mellitus and other categories of glucose intolerance

Disorder	Description	Criteria for diagnosis
Diabetes mellitus Insulin dependent (IDDM), type 1	Insulin deficiency caused by islet cell loss; often associated with specific HLA types, predisposition to viral insulitis or autoimmune phenomena; *ketosis prone;* occurs at any age, common in youth	Unequivocal elevation of plasma glucose (≥200 mg/dl) and classic symptoms of diabetes (polydipsia, polyuria, polyphagia, weight loss), or Fasting plasma glucose (FPG) ≥140 mg/dl on two occasions, or FPG <140 mg/dl and 2 hr plasma glucose ≥200 mg/dl with one intervening value ≥200 mg/dl after a 75 g glucose load (OGTT)
Non-insulin-dependent (NIDDM), type 2	*Ketosis resistant;* more frequent in adults, but occurs at any age; majority of patients overweight; familial tendency; may require insulin for hyperglycemia during stress	Same as above
Diabetes associated with certain conditions or syndromes	Hyperglycemia occurring in relation to other disease states: pancreatic disease, drugs or chemicals, endocrinopathies, insulin receptor disorders, certain genetic syndromes	Same as above
Impaired glucose tolerance (IGT)	Abnormality in glucose levels intermediate between normal and overt diabetes; may progress to diabetes (25%), improve to normal, or remain unchanged	FPG <140 mg/dl and 2 hr plasma glucose ≥140 mg/dl and <200 mg/dl with one intervening value ≥200 mg/dl after a 75 g glucose load
Gestational diabetes (GDM)	Glucose intolerance with recognition of onset during pregnancy related to placental hormones antagonistic to insulin; 35% to 50% develop NIDDM within 8 years	Two or more of following plasma glucose concentrations met or exceeded using a 100 g glucose load: FPG 105 mg/dl; 1 hr, 190 mg/dl; 2 hr, 165 mg/dl; 3 hr, 145 mg/dl

Adapted from Shuman, CR, and Spratt, IL: Office guide to diagnosis and classification of diabetes mellitus and other categories of glucose intolerance, Diabetes Care 4(2):335, 1981. With permission from the American Diabetes Association, Inc.

Table 28-3   Comparison of insulin-dependent and non-insulin-dependent diabetes mellitus

	Insulin dependent DM (IDDM, type 1)	Non–insulin dependent DM (NIDDM, type 2)
Age of onset	More often in persons <40 years	More often in persons >40 years
Insulin	Absolute deficit	Relative deficit
Ketosis	Prone	Resistant
Serum insulin levels	Absent, low	Low, normal, or high
Insulin resistance	Occasional	Present
Complications	More often affects small blood vessels in eyes and kidneys	More often affects large blood vessels and nerves
Treatment	Insulin, diet, exercise	Diet and exercise; may be supplemented by oral hypoglycemic agents or insulin

clear diagnostic criteria. This classification specifies two other diagnoses of glucose intolerance:

1. Potential abnormality of glucose tolerance (in persons with known risk factors)
2. Previous abnormality of glucose tolerance (in persons who have had transient hyperglycemia)

The World Health Organization added an eighth type of glucose intolerance to the classification system. This is *malnutrition-related diabetes,* a disorder found in the tropics in young adults with a history of nutritional deficiency. In addition, there are subsets of these eight disorders of glucose intolerance. For example, MODY (mature onset of diabetes in youth) is characterized by mild hyperglycemia and has an autosomal-dominant mode of inheritance. Atypical diabetes is found predominantly in black children and is similar to IDDM at onset; however, after a period of insulin therapy, the insulin requirement decreases and the disease resembles NIDDM.[62]

Table 28-3 compares the essential features of the major two types of diabetes mellitus: insulin-dependent diabetes mellitus (IDDM) and non-insulin-dependent diabetes mellitus (NIDDM). In IDDM, little or no insulin is secreted by the beta cells, whereas in NIDDM, the beta cell defect and the amounts of insulin secreted are variable, depending on the course of the disease.

A major characteristic of IDDM is the therapeutic need for insulin for survival. This insulin deficiency is often termed absolute, in comparison with a relative deficit of insulin in NIDDM. Because of the complete dependency on exogenous insulin, persons with IDDM disease tend to have more severe and unstable glucose intolerance. In addition, they are prone to acute metabolic complications of ketosis and ketoacidosis (p. 786).

In NIDDM, hyperinsulinemia may be present, or normal or low amounts of insulin may occur in the blood. Although much is still unknown about NIDDM, it is understood that *insulin resistance plays a major role in NIDDM.* In this condition there are deficient numbers of effective insulin receptors, postreceptor defects or both. Early in NIDDM, insulin levels may be high as the pancreas responds to the failure of insulin and glucose to cross the cell membrane. Insulin secretion may be delayed in response to a glucose load; thus postprandially, blood glucose rises higher and stays higher than normal. The beta cell defect may worsen as the course of NIDDM progresses and result in low levels of insulin.[39]

Note that both forms of the disease may occur at any age; however, IDDM is more commonly associated with onset in childhood, adolescence, or young adulthood, whereas NIDDM is more commonly associated with onset after 40 years of age. Both forms of the disease are associated with vascular and neurologic complications; however, they differ in the organs most frequently affected.

Gestational diabetes mellitus (GDM) has its onset during pregnancy. If glucose tolerance remains impaired after the pregnancy, the disease is reclassified as IDDM or NIDDM. Pregnancy stresses glucose tolerance in all women, particularly in the latter half of pregnancy when placental hormones are secreted in increasing amounts. These hormones increase the supply of amino acids and glucose.

Pancreatectomy and chronic pancreatitis are obvious reasons why persons might develop hyperglycemia. So, too, are diseases or treatments that induce an excessive secretion of one or more counterregulatory hormones. Commonly used drugs that can induce hyperglycemia include furosemide (Lasix) and thiazide diuretics, glucocorticoids, epinephrine, phenytoin, and nicotinic acid.

PREVENTION AND HEALTH EDUCATION
Primary Prevention

It has been long known that three factors increase the risk of diabetes: a *family history* of the disease, *obesity,* and, for women, the *birth of a large-weight baby* (over 9 lb). Avoiding obesity and, if necessary, reducing weight under medical supervision are the major focuses in primary prevention of NIDDM (type 2).

The Surgeon General's Report, *Healthy People 2000,* established several goals in relation to diabetes.[25] One goal is to increase exercise in the general population, so that at least 30% of people aged six and older engage regularly, preferably daily, in light to moderate physical activity for at least 30 minutes per day. (Baseline: 22% of people aged 18 and older were active for at least 30 minutes five or more times per week and 12% were active seven or more times per week in 1985.) Note: Light to moderate physical activity requires sustained, rhythmic muscular move-

---

28-2

Recommended health behaviors for persons at risk for or with diabetes mellitus

Use dietary patterns to avoid hyperlipoprotein-
   emia, obesity
Develop pattern of consistent exercise
Seek detection and control of glucose intolerance,
   and hypertension
Avoid cigarette smoking

Table 28-4   **Special population targets**

Diabetes-related deaths	Baseline (per 100,000)	2000 Target (per 100,000)
Blacks	65	58
American Indians/ Alaska Natives	54	48

Note: Diabetes-related deaths refer to deaths from diabetes as a direct or contributing cause.

ments, is at least equivalent to sustained walking, and is performed at less than 60% of maximum heart rate for age. Maximum heart rate equals roughly 200 beats/min minus age. Examples include walking, swimming, cycling, dancing, gardening and yardwork, various domestic and occupational activities, and games and other childhood pursuits. This goal has relevance for the prevention of NIDDM because increased physical activity is being proposed as a primary prevention measure for NIDDM. Physical training is associated with lower plasma concentrations of glucose and increased peripheral sensitivity to insulin.[32] In a recent study, exercise was found to exert a preventive effect on the development of NIDDM in former college students who were studied for 15 years. There was an inverse relation between energy expenditure and the development of NIDDM. Because of the strong association of NIDDM with *hypertension, heart disease,* and *atherosclerosis,* health practices that diminish risk factors for these diseases are recommended for those identified at high risk for diabetes and for persons with diagnosed diabetes (Chapter 25).

Health behaviors recommended to modify the risk of diabetes mellitus or its complications are similar to those that modify the risk of cardiovascular disease (see Box 28-2).

Cardiovascular disease is the leading cause of death among persons with diabetes. It is estimated that the cardiovascular disease risk in diabetic persons could be decreased by more than one third if the following goal was achieved.

Reduce diabetes-related deaths to no more than 34 per 100,000 people. (Age-adjusted baseline: 38 per 100,000 in 1986.) The special target populations for this goal are listed in Table 28-4.

Genetic counseling is hindered by the current state of knowledge about modes of transmission. Persons with diabetes may be told that the rates of transmission from parent to child are low (2% to 5% for IDDM and 10% to 15% for NIDDM).[5] Current research is directed toward investigation of whether the expression of IDDM can be prevented in first-degree relatives of persons with diabetes. Previous research has demonstrated that insulin requirements can be minimized or delayed in persons with recent onset of IDDM by the use of immunosuppressants.[54] However, some subjects experienced nephrotoxicity. Long-term side effects may pose constraints on the widespread use of immunosuppressants.

Secondary Prevention: Detection of Diabetes Mellitus

The majority (90%) of persons with diabetes mellitus have NIDDM (type 2). It is estimated that more than 12.5 million persons in the United States have diabetes mellitus. Forty percent to 50% of these individuals have mild hyperglycemia and glucose intolerance and are relatively asymptomatic, and *the disease is undiagnosed.* However well they feel, they are at risk for developing more severe glucose intolerance and vascular and neurologic complications. NIDDM is a risk factor for heart disease, peripheral vascular disease, stroke, and hypertension. Although in some patients diabetes is diagnosed only when vascular or neurologic complications ensue, increasing evidence points to a relationship between the duration of the disease and metabolic control of blood glucose and the development of long-term complications of diabetes. Screening programs typically have an educational component to inform the public about the importance of the screening and the common signs and symptoms.

Screening programs

Screening programs are directed chiefly toward detection of NIDDM (type 2) for two reasons: (1) the incidence of NIDDM is greater, and (2) screening programs currently available are not effective in identifying IDDM before the actual onset, which is very sudden and severe. Many authorities believe screening of high-risk populations (elderly, poor, nonwhite, pregnant women) to be a better use of resources than screening entire populations.

A basic principle of screening programs is that adequate follow-up is available for persons with positive findings. Plans for screening for diabetes mellitus must take into consideration that the elderly, the poor, and nonwhite populations are medically underserved; therefore, community or neighborhood screening programs must involve the local health care providers in planning for adequate follow-up.

Educational and case finding programs can be carried out in health departments, neighborhood clinics, outpatient clinics, physicians' offices, local diabetes associations, industry, or in the community at health fairs or in mobile health units.

Screening methods

Community-wide screening programs may use tests to detect glycosuria or hyperglycemia. For screening purposes,

Table 28-5 Blood tests for diabetes mellitus*

Test	Procedure and preparation	Interpretation
Fasting plasma glucose (FPG) 70-110 mg/dl (venous plasma)	Fasting after midnight	Diagnostic criteria for DM: ≥ 140 mg/dl on at least two occasions or ≥ 200 mg/dl accompanied by classic symptoms of hyperglycemia; for IGT 115-140 mg/dl
2 hr postprandial blood glucose < 140 mg/dl	Blood glucose measured 2 hr after heavy meal or 2 hr after receiving loading of 100 g of sugar	Used for screening or evaluation of treatment; it is not diagnostic
Random blood glucose < 140 mg/dl		Used for screening; it is not diagnostic
Oral glucose tolerance test (OGTT) FPG < 115 mg/dl; ½ hr, 1 hr, 1½ hr: < 200 mg/dl; 2 hr < 140 mg/dl	Fasting after midnight, FPG obtained, 75 mg glucose load taken; blood (and urine) samples collected at ½, 1, and 2 hr; sometimes at 3, 4, and 5 hr	Diagnostic criteria for DM: FPG < 140 mg/dl but both 2 hr and one other value > 200 mg/dl on two occasions For IGT: FPG < 140 mg/dl; 2 hr value between 140 mg/dl and 200 mg/dl; and one other value ≥ 200 mg/dl OGTT should be performed only in patients who have been on unrestricted diet and physical activity 3 days before test; not recommended for (1) fasting hyperglycemia; (2) persons taking thiazides, phenytoin, propranolol, furosemide, thyroid, estrogens, birth control pills, glucocorticoid steroids; (3) hospitalized patients or acutely ill or inactive patients. The patient should remain seated and not smoke during the test.
Intravenous glucose tolerance test (IGTT)	Same as for OGTT	Performed when OGTT contraindicated (see OGTT) or in presence of gastrointestinal disorder that interferes with glucose absorption
Cortisone-glucose tolerance test	Performed similar to GTT except that cortisone is administered at start of test	Used when GTT results are inconclusive; cortisone causes an abnormal increase in blood glucose level and decreased peripheral utilization of glucose in persons predisposed to diabetes; blood glucose level of 140 mg/dl at end of 2 hr is considered positive result
Glycosated hemoglobin (hemoglobin Al$_c$) 3.8-6.4 mg/dl	Blood sample drawn	Useful in monitoring average blood glucose levels over previous 2- to 3-month period; hemoglobin is linked to glucose in proportion to circulating glucose
C-peptide 1-2 mg/ml (fasting) 5-6-fold increase after glucose load	12 hr fasting blood sample drawn before ingestion of glucose and at 1 hr (may be combined with serum insulin test)	Measures biologically inactive byproduct from conversion of proinsulin to insulin, thus can help determine insulin secretion
Serum insulin Fasting: 2-20 µU/ml Postglucose: up to 120 µU/ml	10-12 hr fasting blood sample drawn before ingestion of glucose and after 1 hr	Use is not clinically widespread; may be used in differential diagnosis of hypoglycemia or in diabetes research

*Values differ according to particular test used and whether measurement made on plasma or whole blood.

if screening for glycosuria is carried out, Tes-Tape and Diastix urine strips are more reliable than Clinitest because the former are specific for glucose, whereas Clinitest tablets show reactions to all sugars. Testing for hyperglycemia is a more reliable screening tool than testing for glycosuria; however, it is more costly. A random capillary blood test read by a meter is less costly and less reliable than a laboratory test of venous blood.

A fasting blood glucose (FBG) test is widely used to screen for diabetes in patients newly admitted to hospitals or ambulatory care centers and as a part of yearly screening in primary care.

A positive finding in a screening test is not sufficient for diagnosis. The physician usually chooses a FBG measurement for follow-up and may order a glucose tolerance

test (GTT). See Table 28-5 for a description of these tests and the values used to determine if diabetes is present. It should be clear from the table that if overt symptoms are present, one blood glucose finding over 200 mg/dl is sufficient for diagnosis; whereas, in other instances, the finding of two fasting blood glucose levels over 140 mg/dl is necessary to confirm the diagnosis.

Tertiary Prevention

Measures to prevent, detect early, and to treat acute and chronic complications of diabetes mellitus form a major portion of diabetes education for individuals and groups of patients and for health professionals. Table 28-6 shows a brief listing of measures used to detect early and to treat some of the long-term complications. These complications

Table 28-6   Prevention of long-term complications of diabetes mellitus[60]

Complication	Early detection	Early intervention
Eye problems	Ophthalmoscopic examination	Care by an ophthalmologist or retinal specialist Control of hyperglycemia Control of hypertension Laser photocoagulation Referral for low vision evaluation, optical aids, and rehabilitation
Kidney problems	Examination of urine for albumin and/or protein excretion Measurement of serum creatinine and creatinine clearance	Control of hyperglycemia Control of hypertension and other cardiovascular risk factors Consulation with a nephrologist Limiting protein intake Avoiding nephrotoxic agents Early treatment of urinary tract infections
Atherosclerosis	History for risk factors and symptoms Examination: ECG and serum lipids measurements, peripheral pulses	Control of hyperglycemia Control of hypertension Weight control Exercise Consultation with specialist: cardiologist, neurologist, vascular surgeon
Neuropathy	History of symptoms of pain, numbness and so forth Examination: orthostatic blood pressures, muscle strength, reflexes, and sensory function	Control of hyperglycemia Avoidance of neurotoxic agents Education about the importance of routine evaluation, foot care, and specific treatments of neuropathy
Foot problems	History of symptoms of numbness, infection and peripheral vascular insufficiency Complete foot examination	Control of hyperglycemia Control of atherogenic risk Education about the importance and methods of foot care Referral to a podiatrist and vascular surgeon Referral for special shoes, shoe inlays, assistive mobility devices and rehabilitation services

Table 28-7   Reduction of diabetic complications

Complications	1988 Baseline	2000 Target
End-stage renal disease	1.5/1000*	1.4/1000
Blindness	2.2/1000*	1.4/1000
Lower extremity amputation	8.2/1000*	4.9/1000
Perinatal mortality†	5%	2%
Major congenital malformations†	8%	4%

*1987 baseline
†Among infants of women with established diabetes

Table 28-8   Special population targets

	Baseline (per 1000)	2000 Target (per 1000)
ESRD from diabetes		
Blacks with diabetes	2.2*	2
American Indians/Alaska Natives with diabetes	2.1*	1.9
Lower extremity amputations from diabetes		
Blacks with diabetes	10.2†	6.1

*1983-1986.
†1984-1987.

are more completely described later in the chapter. Basic to the prevention of all complications is the control of hyperglycemia. Because long-term complications involve vascular and neurologic changes, it is not surprising to see that measures to decrease risk factors for cardiovascular and neurologic disease are given high priority.

The importance of patient education and the need to increase the availability of patient education to persons with diabetes led to one of the goals of *Healthy People 2000*,[25] which is to increase to at least 40% the proportion of people with chronic and disabling conditions who receive formal patient education, including information about community and self-help resources as an integral part of the management of their condition. The specific target for the year 2000 for patient education of people with diabetes is 75%; the 1983 to 1984 baseline is 32% (classes) and 68% (counseling).

Another goal of *Healthy People 2000* is to reduce complications of diabetes overall and in particular populations in which rates are extremely high.[25] The goal is to reduce the most severe complications of diabetes as shown in Table 28-7.

Table 28-8 lists specific target populations for end-stage renal disease and amputations.

ETIOLOGY/EPIDEMIOLOGY

Diabetes mellitus is not a single entity but a heterogenous group of diseases with diverse causes that are incompletely understood.[51] Both genetic and environmental factors have been implicated and are under study. A combination of factors is most likely responsible for both IDDM and

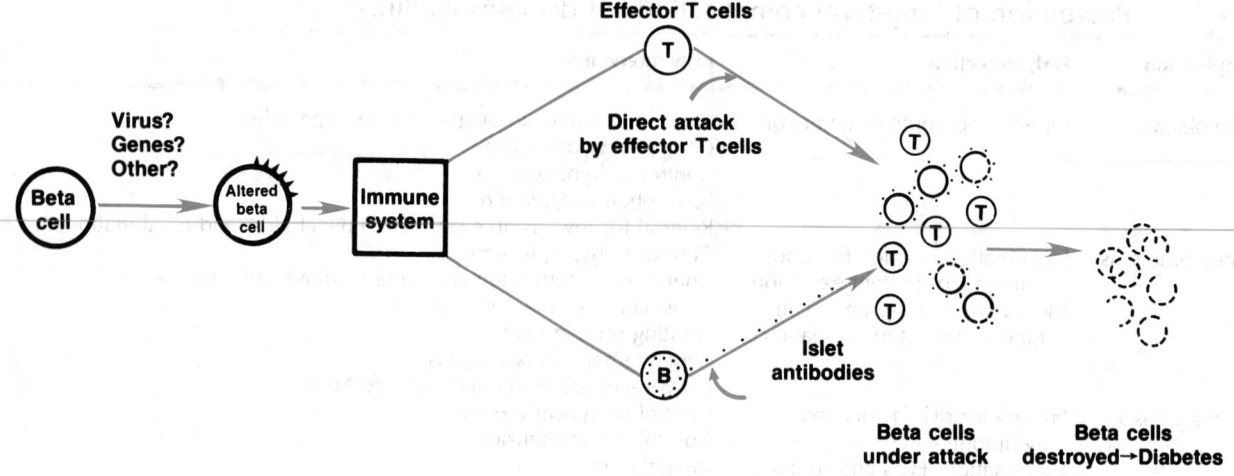

Fig. 28-1   Autoimmunity and diabetes.

Table 28-9   Heredity and diabetes mellitus

Evidence	IDDM	NIDDM
Concordance in monozygotic twins	Less than 50%	90%-100%
Autosomal dominant		Small subset of children with MODY (maturity-onset type of diabetes)
Presence of HLA antigens, DR3, DR4, DW3, DW4	Increase the risk four- to ten-fold	Present only in three populations: Pimas, Xhosas, and Fijans[51]
Prevalence rates in certain ethnic-cultural groups		American Indian tribes have rates of 1 in 3 compared to 1 in 20 for general population

NIDDM. Although the same etiologic factors relate to both NIDDM and IDDM, the relative importance of individual factors differ. A *family history of diabetes* is a risk factor for developing the disease; however, the relationship of genetic transmission to diabetes mellitus is not yet well understood. Table 28-9 shows that the evidence from studies of monozygotic twins indicates that genetic transmission is stronger in NIDDM than in IDDM. HLA typing has very low predictability in identifying persons at high risk for IDDM from the general population. The alleles associated with IDDM susceptibility are common in 30% to 40% of the general population, yet only 0.3% develop IDDM.[47] HLA alleles associated with IDDM are present in 95% of persons with IDDM. It is thought that there may be several genetic mechanisms involved in the transmission of diabetes; among these are HLA gene products, defects in insulin receptor genes, and insulin genes.[47]

IDDM is considered an *autoimmune disorder that destroys the beta cell.* Evidence for an autoimmune basis of the disease includes the immunogenetic association of IDDM with HLA haplotypes, lymphocytic infiltration of beta cells in persons with IDDM, the experimental reversal of IDDM by immunosuppressant therapy, and increased rate of other autoimmune diseases in patients with IDDM.[54] Three *immunologic markers* are *islet cell antibodies* (ICAs), *insulin autoantibodies* (IAAs), and *autoantibodies* to a 64,000M₁ islet protein.[47] These markers are present sev-

eral years before the onset of hyperglycemia, when most of the B cell functional reserve is lost.[47]

Multiple environmental agents have been proposed as important in the development of IDDM: viruses, diet, and toxins.[54]

An association between acute viral infections and the occurrence of IDDM in some communities has been noted. Certain viruses (coxsackie virus B, rubella, and mumps) have been implicated in particular cases. Fig. 28-1 shows a postulated interaction between viral agents and the beta cells.

The etiology of NIDDM is not well understood. Overweight adults, especially those with a family history of diabetes, are at high risk for NIDDM. About 25% of persons with impaired glucose tolerance (IGT) and 30% to 35% of women with gestational diabetes develop NIDDM. Controversy persists about whether a pancreatic islet cell disorder or insulin resistance at peripheral and hepatic cell membranes is the primary disorder.

Epidemiologic studies have *identified populations* of the *poor, the elderly,* and *the nonwhite* to be at *high risk for NIDDM.* The nonwhite populations also have higher incidence of diabetic complications and diabetes mortality rates that are double those of the white population. A goal of *Healthy People 2000*[25] specifies a reduction in the incidence of diabetes among the general population but emphasizes special populations. The goal is to reduce diabetes

Table 28-10   Prevalence of diabetes (per 1000)

	1982-1984 Baseline*	2000 Target
American Indians/ Alaska Natives	69†	62
Puerto Ricans	55	49
Mexican-Americans	54	45
Cuban-Americans	36	32
Blacks	36‡	32

*1982-1984 Baseline for people aged 20-72.
†1987 baseline for American Indians/Alaska Natives aged 15 and older.
‡1987 baseline for Blacks of all ages.

to an incidence of no more than 2.5 per 1000 people and a prevalence of no more than 25 per 1000 people (baseline: 2.9 per 1000 in 1987; 28 per 1000 in 1987). See Table 28-10 for prevalence rates in special target populations.

PATHOPHYSIOLOGY

To understand the complex changes that diabetes causes throughout the body, it is helpful to consider those that occur when insulin deficit induces hyperglycemia, those that occur when there is an acute metabolic crisis, and those that occur as a result of vascular and neurologic defects. Each is discussed below.

Hyperglycemia

Normally, when insulin is present, glucose intake (or glucose production) in excess of caloric needs is stored as glycogen in the cells of the liver and muscle or as fat. These processes of glycogenesis and lipogenesis prevent *hyperglycemia* (blood glucose concentration > 110 mg/dl). When *insulin deficit* is present, four metabolic derangements lead to hyperglycemia:

1. Transport of glucose across cell membranes diminishes.
2. Glycogenesis diminishes, and excess glucose remains in the blood.
3. Glycolysis increases; thus glycogen stores are reduced and "liver" glucose is added to the blood continually rather than when needed.
4. Gluconeogenesis increases, and more "liver" glucose is added to the blood from the breakdown (catabolism) of amino acids and glycerol from triglycerides.

The five classic signs of hyperglycemia are:

1. Polydipsia
2. Polyuria
3. Polyphagia
4. Weight loss
5. Fatigue

Associated with the hyperglycemia from the insulin deficit are abnormal levels of free fatty acids, cholesterol, and triglycerides in the blood.

Cellular Starvation

Blood glucose concentration is high in uncontrolled diabetes mellitus, yet cells are subjected to starvation conditions. Insulin deficiency impairs the uptake of glucose in insulin-dependent peripheral tissues (skeletal muscle and adipose tissue). If glucose is not available, muscle cells metabolize their own glycogen supply, and in prolonged fasting, they may use free fatty acids and ketones. Brain cells are not insulin-dependent and must have a constant supply of glucose; they can utilize ketones for part of their energy requirement.

Similarly, the uptake of amino acids is impaired. Instead of protein synthesis, *proteins are catabolized* and the amino acids are used to provide the substrate necessary for gluconeogenesis in the liver. Because of impaired metabolism, fatigue, loss of weight, and loss of strength may occur, with stunting of growth in children. Insulin deficiency can lead to the increased mobilization and metabolism of fats. Instead of lipogenesis, lipolysis occurs when insulin deficiency is severe, as in IDDM. Increased fatty acids, triglycerides, and glycerol circulate and provide the liver with substrates for ketogenesis and gluconeogenesis. There is a resultant production of ketones (highly acidic, intermediate metabolites of fat). *Ketosis* is the condition of ketone excess in the blood. If severe enough, ketosis can lead to a form of metabolic acidosis and coma, *diabetic ketoacidosis* (p. 786).

In NIDDM ketosis is usually absent. There seems to be enough effective insulin to suppress the breakdown of fats, but not enough or not enough effective insulin to control blood glucose at normal levels.

Insulin Resistance

Insulin can be present in the blood in normal and even in abnormally high amounts, yet be unable to effect cellular processes. In this condition, called *insulin resistance*, peripheral and hepatic cells are insensitive to insulin. Insulin resistance may be caused by any of several factors: decreased number of insulin receptors, decreased insulin binding, and/or postreceptor defects and hyperglycemia. *Insulin resistance is a major component of obesity and NIDDM.*

An exogenous source of animal insulin, particularly beef insulin, leads to the development of insulin antibodies. A rare *syndrome* of insulin resistance occurs in which insulin requirement exceeds 200 u/24 hr.

Hyperosmolality

A major pathophysiologic alteration associated with hyperglycemia is hyperosmolality. Blood glucose concentrations of 60 to 100 mg/dl correlate with normal blood osmolality values of 280 to 290 mosmol/kg. Hyperglycemia increases blood osmolality. Increases in blood glucose content and blood osmolality lead to *dehydration* by two mechanisms.

1. Glycosuria and osmotic diuresis ensue when blood glucose concentrations exceed the renal threshold. Large amounts of water and electrolytes may be lost, along with loss of calories.
2. Fluid shifts from the intracellular compartment to the more highly concentrated extracellular compartment, resulting in intracellular fluid deficit.

Osmotic diuresis increases urine volume (*polyuria*). Thirst is stimulated, and the patient drinks large amounts of fluid (*polydipsia*). Because of the calorie loss and cellular

Table 28-11 **Comparison of DKA and HHNC**

Factors	DKA	HHNC
Mortality rate	About 10%	About 50% in elderly
Blood glucose level	200-1000 mg/dl	600-2000 mg/dl
Ketonuria	Present	Absent
Metabolic acidosis	Present	Absent
pH	<7.2	
HCO₃	<15 mEq/L	
Kussmaul breathing	Present	
Flushed skin	Present	
Acetone odor to breath	Present	
Average fluid deficit	3-5 L	8-12 L
Abdominal pain	Frequent	Rare
Neurologic changes	Lethargy-coma	Lethargy-coma, but often accompanied by other neurologic deficits

---

28-3

Signs of dehydration

Dry mucous membranes
Loss of skin turgor (over sternum is most reliable site to assess)
Soft or sunken eyeballs
Red, parched lips and tongue
Tachycardia
Hypotension
Oliguria

28-4

Signs of hyperglycemic, hyperosmolar, nonketotic coma (HHNC)

Fluid deficit	Neurologic changes
Dehydration	Sensory deficits
Hypotension	Motor deficits
Anuria	Focal seizures
Circulatory collapse	Aphasia
Elevated body temperature	Coma

---

starvation, the appetite increases, and the person eats more (*polyphagia*). When combined with *loss of body weight* and *fatigue*, the "three p's" (polyuria, polydipsia, and polyphagia) are the classic signs of hyperglycemia. These symptoms are usually less severe in NIDDM, but the risks of dehydration are still present. The signs of dehydration are listed in Box 28-3.

Polydipsia is important in preventing hypovolemia because the resultant increase in fluid intake compensates for excess fluid losses caused by polyuria. As long as intravascular fluid volume is sufficient to maintain renal perfusion and glomerular filtration, the osmotic diuresis continues. When the fluid deficit is great enough to contract the intravascular fluid space and thus impair kidney function, *oliguria may signal a very severe fluid deficit.*

Hyperglycemic, Hyperosmolar, Nonketotic Coma (HHNC)

Table 28-11 compares the two major crises of diabetes mellitus that are acute and life threatening.

Blood glucose levels may exceed 1000 mg/dl, urinary glucose may be 5% to 10%, and serum osmolality may exceed 370 to 380 mosmol/kg in the absence of blood ketones. Coma in these circumstances is termed hyperglycemic, hyperosmolar, nonketotic coma (HHNC) and occurs in NIDDM. Most frequently, HHNC occurs in the elderly, debilitated, and those who have impairments of mobility or cognition. So long as persons with hyperglycemia and glycosuria can respond to thirst and replace fluids lost

by glycosuria and osmotic diuresis, the risk of HHNC is diminished.

If fluid intake is diminished and dehydration ensues, the risk becomes greater. Frequently an associated illness increases fluid losses (fever, diarrhea, vomiting) and insulin-antagonist hormones. Often, HHNC develops slowly over a period of days, and patients or caregivers may not identify the need for increased fluid intake. The elderly have less accurate thirst sensations, and they and persons who are acutely ill may not have access to fluids.

HHNC may also develop in nondiabetic persons receiving enteral or parenteral nutrition if hyperglycemia is induced. Adequate fluid intake and prompt recognition and treatment of hyperglycemia reduce the risk of HHNC in these persons. In some studies,[51] the mortality rate from HHNC is reported to be as high as 40% to 60%.

Blood hyperosmolality, marked dehydration, and resultant fluid shifts decrease intracellular fluid volume. Cerebral dysfunction reflects cell dehydration and is manifested by changes in neurologic parameters (see Box 28-4). Laboratory findings reflect the fluid deficit and hyperosmolar state: normal to high serum sodium and chloride concentrations, elevated glucose concentration, elevated hematocrit, and elevated blood urea nitrogen level.

Diabetic Ketoacidosis (DKA)

Diabetic ketoacidosis (DKA), a severe metabolic disorder, is characterized by hyperglycemia, hyperosmolality, and *metabolic acidosis*. The acidosis differentiates DKA from

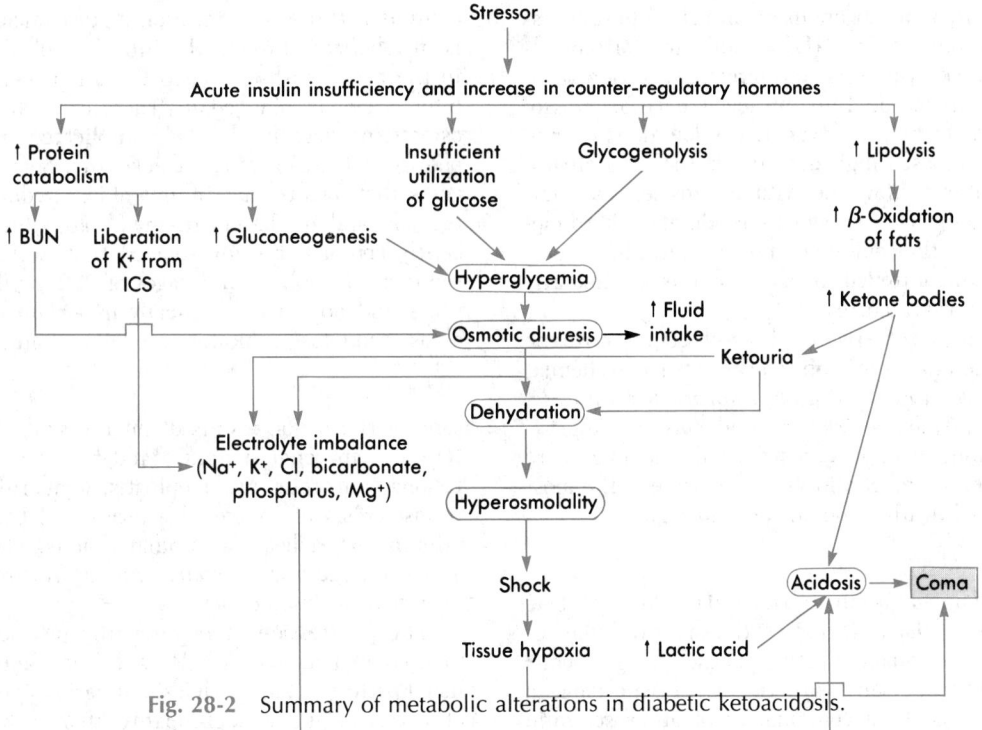

Fig. 28-2   Summary of metabolic alterations in diabetic ketoacidosis.

HHNC, as can be seen in Table 28-6. Six clinical signs are characteristic of DKA (see Box 28-5).

DKA is preventable and treatable. The mortality rate of 100% in the preinsulin era has steadily decreased. It is most frequently seen in persons with IDDM but can occur in NIDDM. It is usually precipitated in the known diabetic by stressors that increase insulin needs, although it may occur when diabetes is out of control because of noncompliance with prescribed therapy.

A frequent precipitating factor is an *infection,* such as those of the urinary or respiratory tracts. Other major stressors that can precipitate diabetic ketoacidosis are surgery, trauma, major illnesses, therapy with steroids, and emotional upset. Occasionally diabetic ketoacidosis is the initial symptom in adults with undiagnosed diabetes, and it is often the initial problem in children with diabetes.

Fig. 28-2 presents a schema of the major metabolic alterations of DKA. Increased lipolysis, oxidation of fats, and ketogenesis result in increased levels of organic acid (ketones) in body fluids. As ketones "use up" the body's alkali reserve for buffering, the pH of the blood decreases. Kussmaul breathing is stimulated to compensate for the metabolic acidosis. The *osmotic diuresis* is *made worse by* the *ketonemia* and from *protein catabolism,* which increases the nitrogen load to the kidney. *Ketones give the breath a fruity odor.* When the *extracellular fluid deficit is severe,* polyuria may decrease, and *anuria may be seen.* The detection of signs and symptoms of hyperglycemia, urinary ketones, sleepiness, "air hunger," nausea, and vomiting can alert diagnosed patients to seek medical help early so that prompt treatment can be given.

Signs of diabetic ketoacidosis

Dehydration
Lethargy leading to coma
Kussmaul breathing
Flushed face
Fruity breath odor
Nausea and vomiting

Macrovascular Changes

Atherosclerosis is a macrovascular disease. The vascular changes occur in the large arteries and are the same as those seen in nondiabetics. It is well known, however, that diabetics are prone to develop atherosclerosis at an earlier age, that the disease progresses faster, and that it is more severe and extensive in diabetics than in nondiabetics. In addition, the complications of atherosclerosis occur more frequently in diabetics than in nondiabetics. Coronary artery disease and cerebrovascular disease are three times more common, and peripheral disease is five times more common. Persons with NIDDM develop macrovascular changes more frequently than do persons with IDDM. Diabetes is associated with various atherogenic factors: abnormal lipid metabolism, changes in platelet adhesion, and hormonal changes (Chapter 25).

Insulin plays a major role in the metabolism of fats. *Lipid disorders* are frequently found in persons with diabetes mellitus. *Hyperinsulinism* also may be an atherosclerogenic factor.[34] In IDDM, peripheral hyperinsulinism may occur as a result of sufficient exogenous insulin given to suppress hepatic glucose output. In NIDDM, insulin resistance is often accompanied by excessive pancreatic secretion of insulin. Persistently elevated insulin levels have been associated with hypertension, elevated very low density lipid (VLDL) and decreased high density lipid (HDL) cholesterol concentrations, as well as with atherosclerosis.[34] *Hypertension* has long been known to accelerate atherosclerosis; in diabetes, the combination of uncontrolled hyperglycemia and uncontrolled hypertension is particularly damaging to the vasculature.

Decreased lumens of large blood vessels compromise the delivery of oxygen to tissues and can cause tissue ischemia, resulting in *cerebrovascular disease, coronary artery disease, renal artery stenosis,* and *peripheral vascular disease.* Approximately three fourths of all cerebrovascular accidents are related to diabetes; and cardiovascular disease is the most common cause of death among older diabetics.

Microvascular Changes

Microvascular changes occur in both IDDM and NIDDM and are unique to diabetes; that is, the microvascular lesions do not occur in nondiabetics. These changes occur most frequently in persons with IDDM. Tissue damage in organs is caused by a combination of atherosclerotic changes in large vessels and the defects in the microcirculation. *Changes in the microvasculature are particularly damaging to the retina, kidney, and nerves.* Two structural changes in the capillary are *thickening of the basement membrane* and *increased glycosylation of the collagenous* and *reticular fibers of the blood vessels.*[28] Increased rigidity of the vessel wall, decreased permeability of the vessel wall, capillary hypertension, and changes in blood flow through the capillary are some of the changes that interact to affect organ perfusion. Organ perfusion is increased early in the disease process, and the resultant hemodynamic changes may play a role in further structural damage. Later in the disease process, blood flow is impeded, and decreased organ perfusion results.

A *history of hyperglycemia* is *thought to play a major role in the development of microvascular lesions.* Studies have evaluated various factors, such as role of protein fractions, glycoproteins, lipids, and lipoproteins. One theory proposes that capillary damage may result from increased sorbital content within cells. Sorbitol, a sugar alcohol of glucose, is metabolized through the influence of aldose reductase in the polyol pathway when there is hyperglycemia. Sorbitol is slowly reduced to fructose. Sorbitol is a highly osmotic particle that has been implicated in microvascular changes such as capillary thickening. Some evidence suggests that agents that inhibit aldose reductase can slow retinal capillary basement membrane thickening. A recently completed study showed that Sorbinil, an aldose reductase inhibitor, in dosages of 250 mg daily for 2 to 3 years, did not have a clinically important effect.[59] Other aldose reductase inhibitors are being studied.

Nephropathy

One of the major results of microvascular changes is alterations in renal structure and function. Four types of lesions can occur: pyelonephritis, glomerular lesions, arteriosclerosis of the renal arteries and the afferent and efferent arterioles, and tubular lesions. *Diabetic nephropathy* is characterized by *albuminuria, hypertenson,* and *progressive renal insufficiency.*[28]

The progression of nephropathy has been well documented in persons with IDDM (see Table 28-12). The usual pattern begins with a silent period, with no clinically observable signs of nephropathy, that exists for about 15 years. However, researchers have demonstrated that microvascular changes occur soon after diagnosis. *Glomerular hypertrophy* related to mesangial capillary enlargement is often associated with increased kidney size.[41] An *increase in glomerular filtration rate* is typically found after the onset of hyperglycemia. There is early onset of *microalbuminemia,* defined as albuminuria of 30 to 300 mg/24 hr, that precedes by many years clinically detectable proteinuria (over 300 mg/24 hr).

Clinical period

Tests to detect *microalbuminemia* are not yet widely available,[45] whereas tests to measure larger amounts of albumin or protein are commonly used. The clinical onset of detectable *proteinuria* can thus be quite late in the course of nephropathy. As renal insufficiency develops, the *serum creatinine concentration* and *the blood urea nitrogen increase,* and other signs and symptoms of renal insufficiency and failure appear (Chapter 33).

Diabetes is present in approximately one fourth of all patients treated for end-stage renal disease in the United States at a cost of about $280 million.[60] The incidence is much higher in patients who develop diabetes before age 20 years. After a duration of 20 years, the chance of a diabetic person developing renal disease is estimated at 40% for those whose diabetes was diagnosed before age 20 years, and 2% to 4% in those diagnosed after age 20.[60] About equal numbers of persons with each type of diabetes develop ESRD each year. This occurs because of the greater number of persons with NIDDM (90%) than with IDDM (10%). Attention is directed toward control or prevention of factors known to increase the progression of renal disease in diabetic persons (see Box 28-6).

The *normalization of blood glucose levels* and the *control of hypertension* are high priorities. Recently, the use of a *lowered protein intake* (40 g/24 hr) and decreased use of

Table 28-12	Progression of diabetic nephropathy (IDDM) years after diagnosis[60]
Years	
Silent period	
0	Diagnosis of diabetes, development of microalbuminuria and hyperfiltration
Clinical period	
15	Onset of proteinuria and hypertension
19	Elevated creatine and blood urea nitrogen levels
23	*End-stage renal failure*

animal protein are being evaluated in research studies for their effectiveness in slowing the progression of microalbuminemia, hyperfiltration, and further renal damage.[28] *All nonpregnant adults with diabetes currently are encouraged to limit their daily protein intake to 0.8 g/kg of body weight.* This early intervention is an attempt to modify the hemodynamic changes occurring in the glomeruli by reducing the nitrogen load of the glomerular filtrate. ACE inhibitors have been shown to reduce microalbuminemia and are being evaluated for their effectiveness in decreasing the rate of development of nephropathy.[45] The value of controlling hyperglycemia in reversing some of the hemodynamic changes that occur within the glomerulus has been shown in animal and human volunteer studies; reversal of hyperfiltration and renal hypertrophy that were induced by amino acids in diabetic subjects occurred when hyperglycemia was corrected.[20]

The treatment and nursing care of renal insufficiency in persons with diabetes are similar to that in nondiabetics. It is important to remember that as renal insufficiency develops, the patient receiving insulin may require *less* insulin because it will be excreted more slowly. Renal transplantation is the treatment of choice, because diabetic complications progress rapidly in many patients who receive dialysis. If transplantation is not possible, dialysis is necessary to maintain life. Dialysis is often instituted earlier for those with diabetes and renal failure than for nondiabetics because renal failure causes progression of other complications such as neuropathy and retinopathy in the diabetic. There have been improved survival rates with dialysis for diabetic patients over the last decade. The improved rates may be due to beginning dialysis earlier, to improved control of hypertension, and to improved technical management of dialysis. Short-term survival rates at 5 years or less are now equivalent to those attained by transplantation.[41] Islet cell transplantation or pancreatic transplantation (Chapter 42) are being performed at the time of kidney transplantation in some medical centers.

Diabetic Retinopathy

Blindness in the diabetic person is most often a result of diabetic retinopathy and diabetic macular edema, the latter seen most frequently in those with NIDDM.[17] After 10 years, half of all patients with IDDM have diabetic retinopathy, whereas after 15 to 20 years, 1 in 10 patients with NIDDM will have retinopathy.[28]

Macular edema is characterized by retinal thickening, hard exudates, and/or areas of nonperfusion in the macular area. Destruction of the macular retina results in loss of central

vision. Diabetes is the leading cause of blindness in persons between the ages of 20 and 65 years. In addition to retinopathy, the diabetic person is also subject to increased *cataract* formation. *Cataracts may be caused by prolonged hyperglycemia that results in swelling of the lens and opacity formation.*

The early retinal lesion is a *microaneurysm* of the *retinal vessels. Microinfarction* and *exudate formation* follow. These early retinal changes may progress to a more serious stage, *proliferative retinopathy,* in which new blood vessels form in the retina (neovascularization). As these new vessels form, they shrink and cause traction in the retina. *Retinal detachment* and *hemorrhage* into the vitreous can result.

There are no symptoms of early retinal changes, and there may be no symptoms even when retinopathy is advanced. Early detection requires a complete ophthalmoloscopic examination. All patients with NIDDM should be referred at diagnosis to an ophthalmologist, and then seen yearly. (The disease of NIDDM usually has been present long before diagnosis.) All patients with IDDM should be referred to an opthalmologist for follow-up 5 years after diagnosis and yearly thereafter.

Animal studies demonstrate that early reversal of hyperglycemia (2 months after induction of diabetes) reduced the progression of retinopathy, whereas a longer period of hyperglycemia (3 months) was associated with retinopathy developing during the succeeding euglycemic period.[16] Although this study has not been replicated in humans, it has reinforced the evidence that *control of hyperglycemia soon after clinical onset can reduce the incidence and severity of diabetic eye disease.* There are no symptoms of early retinal damage. Laser-induced *photocoagulation,* when used at appropriate times, is effective in reducing the risk of blindness. This has been demonstrated in two significant studies. The Diabetic Retinopathy Study (DRS) resulted in recommendations that *scatter photocoagulation* be used for all eyes with *"high-risk" proliferative diabetic retinopathy.* The study used random assignment of one eye of a patient for treatment, and the other eye was assigned to follow-up without treatment. *Scatter photocoagulation reduced the risk of severe visual loss by more than 50%.*[17]

The second study, Early Treatment Diabetic Retinopathy Study (ETDRS), used a design similar to the DRS's to evaluate scatter or focal photocoagulation at an earlier point in the development of retinopathy. Recommendations from the ETDRS are: (1) while careful follow-up is recommended for patents with mild or moderate nonproliferative diabetic retinopathy, scatter photocoagulation is not recommended; (2) focal treatment should be considered for eyes with macular edema that involves or threatens the center of the macula; and (3) there are no ocular contraindications to aspirin treatment when it is required for cardiovascular disease or other reasons.[17] Photocoagulation uses thermal energy to seal capillary leaks, destroys new vessels, and causes adherence of the retina to the choroid. It is usually performed on an outpatient basis.

Vitrectomy, the removal of vitreous humor that has been infiltrated by hemorrhage, is another treatment for retinopathy. The removed vitreous humor is replaced by saline solution; unfortunately improved vision does not always result. Refer to Chapter 38 for a discussion of care, as-

---

28-6	**Factors accelerating renal disease in persons with diabetes**
	Uncontrolled hyperglycemia
	Hypertension
	Urinary tract infection
	Nephrotoxic drugs
	Radiologic contrast dyes

Table 28-13 Signs and symptoms of neuropathies

Type of neuropathy	Signs and symptoms
Symmetric polyneuropathies	
Acute painful neuropathy	Severe, burning pain; paresthesias
Small-fiber neuropathy	Varying degree of pain and sensory loss to temperature, pinprick, or pressure
Large-fiber neuropathy	Impaired distal vibration sensation and impaired distal position sense; reduced ankle reflexes, sensory ataxia, positive Romberg's sign
Focal neuropathy	Acute onset, asymmetric sensory or motor impairment of a nerve or group of nerves: e.g., cranial, truncal, radiculopathies
Autonomic neuropathy	
Gastric changes	Nausea, vomiting, weight loss, erratic glycemic control; e.g., episodes of hypoglycemia occurring at unusual times
Constipation or diarrhea	Diarrhea may be severe and watery and is often nocturnal; may alternate constipation with diarrhea
Incontinence	Loss of control of bowel or bladder function
Sexual dysfunction	Impotence in men, dyspareunia and decreased vaginal lubrication in women

sistive devices, and referral sources for rehabilitative services for the blind and for those with low vision. See page 806 for modifications useful in helping the visually impaired individual manage the diabetes regimen.

Neuropathy

Diabetes may affect peripheral sensory and motor nerves, the autonomic nervous system, or the central nervous system. Multiple and varied symptoms may result, depending on the neurons involved. The most common type of diabetic neuropathy is *symmetric peripheral polyneuropathy.*

Approximately 12% of patients display neuropathy on diagnosis of diabetes, and over 60% will have neuropathy after 25 years.[60] It is seen in both IDDM and NIDDM. As with all neuropathic syndromes, the pathology includes altered nerve conduction that is related to ischemia and/ or impaired neural metabolism. Usually the first symptom is *bilateral sensory loss in the distal lower extremities;* later, the upper extremities may be affected in a "stocking and glove" distribution. This sensory loss impairs the ability of the patient to detect pressure or pain. It is a major risk factor for amputation of the lower extremities. *The inability to detect pressure or pain in the feet often leads to neuropathic ulcers, infections, gangrene, and trauma. It is essential that patients with sensory loss be vigilant in performing foot care* (see page 792) and in protecting the feet from injury (for example, not walking barefoot).

Treatment includes *control of hyperglycemia.* When neuropathy is painful, treatment includes one or more psychotherapeutic agents such as amitriptyline, drugs usually used for anticonvulsant therapy (such as Tegretol or mexiletine), or capsaicin, a recently introduced local analgesic ointment.

See Table 28-13 for a listing of the neuropathic syndromes that may develop in the person with diabetes. All of these problems cause considerable distress to patients; on the whole, treatment is palliative. Safety issues become a major concern when patients develop orthostatic hypotension, hypoglycemic unawareness, or both.

Two *autonomic neuropathies* are of special concern in the management of hyperglycemia. *Delayed gastric emptying* slows the delivery of glucose to the blood from food intake. Insulin timing in relation to meals may need to be altered to prevent the occurrence of hypoglycemia. In addition, measures may include small, liquid, low-fiber, low-fat meals, and metoclopramide (Reglan). *Hypoglycemic unawareness* impairs the person's ability to detect and treat early hypoglycemia. It may necessitate maintaining an increased level of blood glucose as a therapeutic goal. It is essential that patients with these disorders, and their families, be well educated about the prevention and treatment of hypoglycemia.

Lower Extremity Changes

Macrovascular changes, microvascular changes, and neuropathies cause changes in the lower extremities. The interrelationships of vascular and nerve changes in diabetic foot lesions, which often result in amputation because of gangrene, are illustrated in Fig. 28-3.

Amputation occurs 15 times more frequently in diabetic persons than in nondiabetic persons; 5% to 15% of diabetic patients require a lower-leg amputation at some time.[46] Fifty percent of nontraumatic amputations in the United States occur in the diabetic population. Survival rates after amputation are very low (50% for the first 3 years; 40% after the first 5 years).[36]

The *three most common causes* of *amputation in diabetes* are *gangrene* (90%), *infection* (71%), and *nonhealing ulcer* (65%).[36] *Dry gangrene* occurs when tissue death is not associated with inflammatory changes; *autoamputation* (spontaneous detachment) is often the treatment of choice for toes affected by dry gangrene. The area is kept dry during the process with close monitoring of the integrity of proximal tissues. In contrast, *wet gangrene* is tissue death coupled with inflammation. Septicemia and septic shock may occur. Antibiotic therapy, debridement, and, often, amputation are treatment measures. Infections and nonhealing ulcers often lead to gangrene.

Infections of the lower extremity start in cracks in hypertrophied and dry skin, from ingrown toenails, under

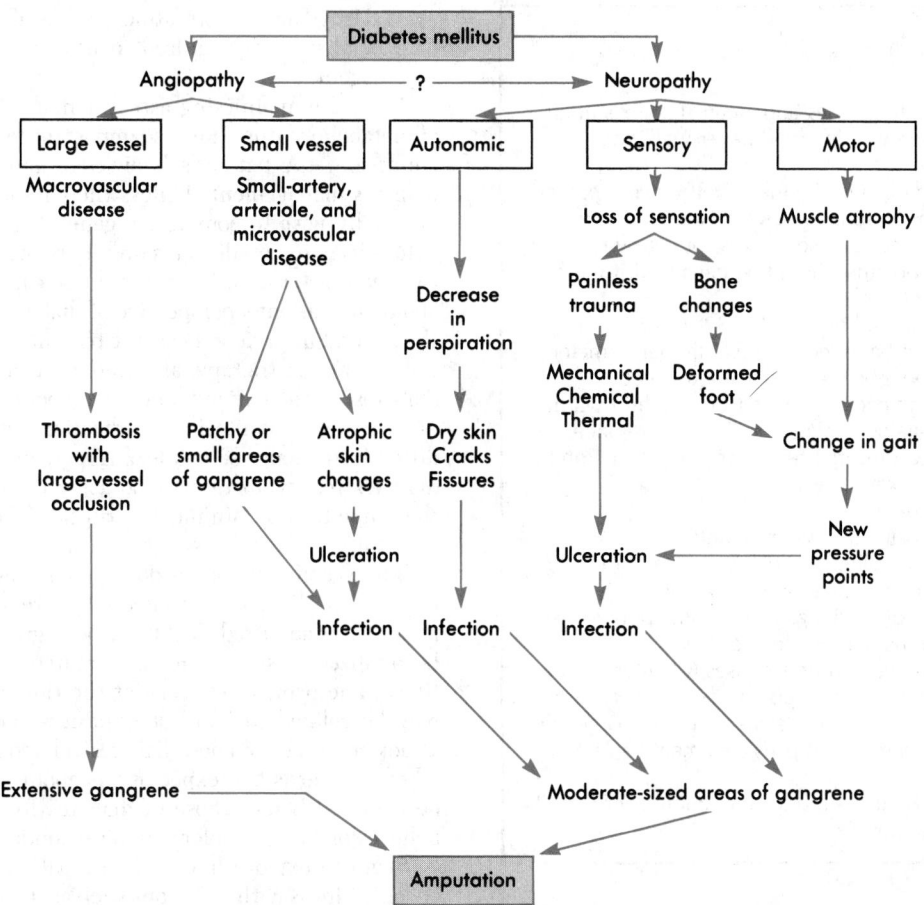

Fig. 28-3   How foot lesions from diabetes can lead to amputation. (Modified from Levin ME: *Pathophysiology, evaluation, and treatment.* In Levin ME, O'Neal LW, editors: *The diabetic foot,* ed 4, St Louis, 1988, Mosby–Year Book.)

corns and calluses, and in traumatized tissues. A *neurotropic ulcer* is one that develops under corns or calluses and is insensitive to pain. Fifteen percent of persons with diabetes have skin ulcers.[36] Infections in ulcers can appear superficial but be quite invasive. A recent clinical study found "clinically silent" osteomyelitis in 68% of ulcers; 64% of the ulcers had no associated signs of inflammation.[46]

Accurate diagnosis of osteomyelitis has been reported with the use of 24-hour leukocyte scanning with indium in 111 Oxyguinoline. This new noninvasive test has more sensitivity in identifying osteomyelitis than roentgenograms, bone scans, or 4-hour leukocytic scanning tests.[46]

In addition to antibiotics, *ulcer debridement* and *vascular reconstruction* are commonly used to facilitate wound repair in diabetic foot ulcers. Wound healing in diabetic ulcers may be enhanced by the application of PDWHF (platelet-derived wound healing formula [Procuren]), which contains at least five locally acting growth factors of importance in wound healing. Box 28-7 describes the results of one research trial with PDWHF.

Absence of weight-bearing is often necessary for healing of diabetic foot ulcers. Extra-depth shoes with custom-designed plastic insoles may help prevent recurrent ulcers.

Knighton DR et al: Stimulation of repair in chronic non-healing cutaneous ulcers. *Surg Gynecol Obstet* 170:56-60, 1990.

A double-blind, crossover, placebo-controlled trial was undertaken to test the independent effectiveness of PDWHF as a treatment measure for foot ulcers. Thirty-two patients were randomly assigned to a treatment or control group. About half of the patients had diabetes. Both groups were treated for a total of 8 weeks. Then the control group was crossed over to the positive (treatment) arm of the study and treated with PDWHF. For 13 patients finishing the positive arm of the study, 100% epithelization was achieved in 17 of 21 wounds in an average of 8.6 weeks. In the control group of 11 patients, 2 of 13 wounds healed during the initial 8 weeks of placebo treatment; while 11 of 13 wounds failed to heal in 8 weeks and were crossed over to the treatment group. One hundred percent epithelization was then achieved in an average of 7.1 weeks for these 11 wounds.

Diabetic foot care

Wear well-fitting shoes and clean stockings at all times when walking, and *never walk barefooted*.

Bathe feet daily and dry them well, paying particular attention to area between the toes.

Do not self-treat calluses, corns, or ingrown toenails; a podiatrist should be consulted if these are present.

Bath water should be 29.5° to 32° C (85° to 90° F) and should be tested with a bath thermometer or the elbow before immersing the feet.

Avoid heating pads, hot water bottles, and warming feet against radiator or close to fireplace.

Institute measures that help increase circulation to the lower extremities:

Avoid smoking.

Avoid crossing legs when sitting.

Protect extremities when exposed to cold.

Avoid immersing feet in cold water.

Use socks or stockings that do not apply pressure to the legs at specific sites.

Institute a regimen of exercises (Chapter 5).

Inspect feet daily and report any cuts, cracks, redness, blisters, or other signs of trauma to health care provider so that early treatment can be instituted.

If feet are dry, use a lubricating lotion or cream; if moist, use powder.

Foot care

Prevention of ulcers, trauma, and infections of the lower extremities is the key to prevention of amputation. The need for daily foot care, including inspection, cannot be overemphasized. The patient can use a mirror to examine soles of the feet. The nurse's effectiveness in teaching about foot care will be greater if the patient has previously included foot care as a part of daily care. Box 28-8 contains guidelines for instruction. Also teach patients to take shoes and stockings off at each medical visit and ask the physician to examine the feet. A podiatric evaluation is recommended for all diabetic patients; podiatric services are essential when there are vascular changes, neuropathy, or foot lesions such as calluses, corns, or bunions.

Nursing Process
Assessment
Subjective data

If the patient is acutely ill, the priority assessment is focused on the extent of metabolic imbalance and its effects on the patient's well-being. Does the patient complain of lethargy, air hunger, or the classic signs of hyperglycemia? Collect specific data about nausea, vomiting, abdominal pain, last food intake, and time and dosage of oral hypoglycemic agents, insulin, or both.

Take a thorough history to determine whether any conditions are present that affect blood glucose concentrations:

1. Food intake in excess of caloric requirements
2. Infection or other acute illness
3. Stress related to psychologic or social factors
4. Drugs or other treatments that affect blood glucose
5. Omission of required insulin or oral hypoglycemic agent

Do not limit nursing assessment to the determination of metabolic status. It is also important to assess, soon after admission, the patient's knowledge and coping ability in diabetes management. Unless the patient is acutely ill, it is usually wise to complete a general nursing assessment before focusing on diabetes and its related care. There are two reasons for this. First, the nurse can learn a great deal about the patient's perspective of diabetes self-care during the general interview. Does the patient specify the disease, the regimen of therapy, and state special needs relating to diabetes? Is the patient concerned about how the plans for diet, activity, monitoring, medications, and foot care will differ from home schedules? A person well educated in diabetes management will be assertive in planning with the nurse how to minimize disruption of care while in the hospital.

The second reason to do a general assessment before focusing on diabetes is related to the reason for which the patient was admitted. Most newly diagnosed adults are not hospitalized; instead, they are treated in ambulatory settings. The primary concern at the time of hospitalization may be related to fears of blindness, amputation, heart attack or stroke, or a non-diabetes-related medical problem. These concerns and expectations about treatment need to be explored before those of diabetes for the patient who believes diabetes problems to be secondary in importance.

Begin to explore how well the patient copes with this chronic illness with questions such as: How easy or difficult is it to stay on the diet? What is difficult or easy about diabetes or its treatment for you? Asking the patient to describe a typical day (meal intake and times, sleep and work schedules, social activities, exercise and monitoring schedules) will help the nurse understand how the therapeutic regimen is incorporated into the patient's life-style and help identify areas of conflict and strengths of the patient.

Assess for the presence of vascular and neuropathic complications: How is your vision? Do you have any problems with blood pressure, eyes, kidney, circulation, sensation? Ask these questions during the general nursing history. Most importantly, if the patient answers yes to any of these questions, what special care is needed?

In assessing learning needs, whenever possible observe actual self-care practices: insulin injection, urine or SBM testing, foot care, and so on.

Because education is an integral part of the treatment, assess the *learning needs* related to self-care of *all* patients who are diabetic. Do this assessment early in the hospitalization in order to increase the time available for teaching. Unfortunately, many patients who have had diabetes for a long time may have inadequate knowledge, skills, or attitudes to manage their diabetes at optimal levels. The development of vascular or neurologic complications may require learning modifications of self-care measures.

Objective data

Objective data to be collected include the following:

1. Level of consciousness
2. Blood and urinary glucose concentrations

3. Blood and urinary ketone concentrations
4. Blood urea nitrogen
5. Blood pressure, pulse, and respiratory pattern
6. Body temperature
7. Body weight
8. Urinary volume (per timed period)
9. Appearance of mucous membranes and skin
10. Presence of skin lesions
11. Skin turgor
12. Breath odor

When an acute metabolic crisis is suggested by the patient's clinical findings, further assessment is related to *metabolic acidosis* and *fluid imbalance* (p. 786). Table 28-11 is a comparison of signs and symptoms of the two metabolic crises: hyperglycemic, hyperosmolar, nonketotic coma (HHNC) and diabetic ketoacidosis (DKA).

Assessment of any adult patient with diabetes mellitus also includes data for identifying *abnormalities related to vascular or neurologic changes.* Measures directed toward prevention or treatment of these complications may be required. In addition, the patient often needs assistance with activities of daily living and modification of diabetes self-care activities. Assessment should always include attention to the *lower extremities, vision, cardiovascular-renal status,* and *neurologic status.*

Diagnostic tests

See Table 28-5 for laboratory tests used in the diagnosis and screening of diabetes mellitus and for the evaluation of therapy. *Fasting blood glucose* and *glucose tolerance* tests are most commonly used in diagnosis. Directions about timing and fasting requirements for a particular test must be explained to the patient. For the glucose tolerance test, give the patient specific, written directions because many variables interfere with the accuracy of this test. Table 28-5 summarizes the directions for patient preparation.

The table lists other tests that are used less commonly. Cortisone- and ACTH-stimulating tests are provocative tests that challenge the capacity to maintain normal blood glucose levels when a counterregulatory hormone is administered. The C-peptide test can be used to differentiate whether the source of circulating insulin is endogenous or exogenous, as well as to evaluate pancreatic secretion. C-peptide tests and serum insulin measurements are used more frequently in research than in clinical practice.

Monitoring glucose control

In the past, good to excellent control was defined by higher levels of blood glucose than is now thought to be ideal. Previously 5% to 10% of daily calorie loss through glycosuria was considered acceptable. Patients who received their diabetes education before 1980 may need reeducation about desired levels of control. Table 28-14 compares past and current criteria of blood glucose levels.

Once the diagnosis of diabetes mellitus is made, measurements of blood glucose are essential in evaluating the effectiveness of treatment measures. Tests that measure blood glucose levels may be ordered to be *fasting; postprandial* (1 hour, 2 hours or 3 hours after eating); and *preprandial* (½ to 1 hour before meals). All give useful information about control of blood glucose in relation to food, fasting, exercise, and the particular insulin or oral hypoglycemic agent being used.

Table 28-14   Criteria for strict control of blood glucose level

Past criteria (mg/dl)	Current criteria	
	Ideal (mg/dl)	Acceptable (mg/dl)
Fasting 60-130	60-90	60-130
Before meals	60-105	60-130
After meals (1 hr) <200	≤140	≤180
After meals (2 hr) <140	≤120	≤150

From Skyler J and others: Algorithms for adjustment of insulin dosage by patients who monitor blood glucose, Diabetes Care **4**:314, 1981. By permission of the American Diabetes Association, Inc.

Laboratory tests

For the hospitalized patient, a fasting blood glucose test often is ordered daily. Tests by the laboratory may be ordered at other times. In addition, capillary blood glucose obtained by fingerstick is often ordered before meals and at bedtime—more frequently for the person in acute metabolic crisis or if on sliding scale insulin.

When trying to correlate test results of laboratory and bedside meters, it is helpful to consider that normal values for glucose differ according to whether measurement is made using whole blood or plasma/serum, to the source of the whole blood, and to whether the patient was fasting or not. Laboratory tests of blood glucose are often performed on samples of plasma or serum, whereas capillary whole blood is tested in bedside meters. Plasma/serum glucose levels are usually 10% to 15% higher than simultaneously measured whole blood glucose levels. In addition, capillary whole blood in the fasting patient is normally 5 to 10 mg/dl higher than venous whole blood; capillary whole blood postprandially is normally 20 to 70 mg/dl higher than venous whole blood.[33]

Self-monitoring of blood glucose (SBM)

The technology now available for self blood glucose monitoring (SBM) has made it possible for persons with diabetes to manage their blood glucose at near physiologic levels.

Increasingly, persons with diabetes mellitus are using SBM to determine their metabolic status rather than testing urine for glucose. Various types of tests for home blood glucose monitoring correlate well with laboratory measurement of blood glucose level. A reflectance meter adds to the cost and inconvenience of monitoring but gives a precise numerical value (Fig. 28-4). Some test strips (Chemstrip bG, Visiden) do not require a meter and indicate only the *range* of blood glucose. For many patients, knowing the range is sufficient.

Self-monitoring has been found to facilitate glycemic control in all persons with diabetes. It is essential for patients who are pregnant, for those who use multiinjection insulin regimes or pump therapy, and for all those who want ideal glycemic control.

SBM is very helpful to the patient in making decisions

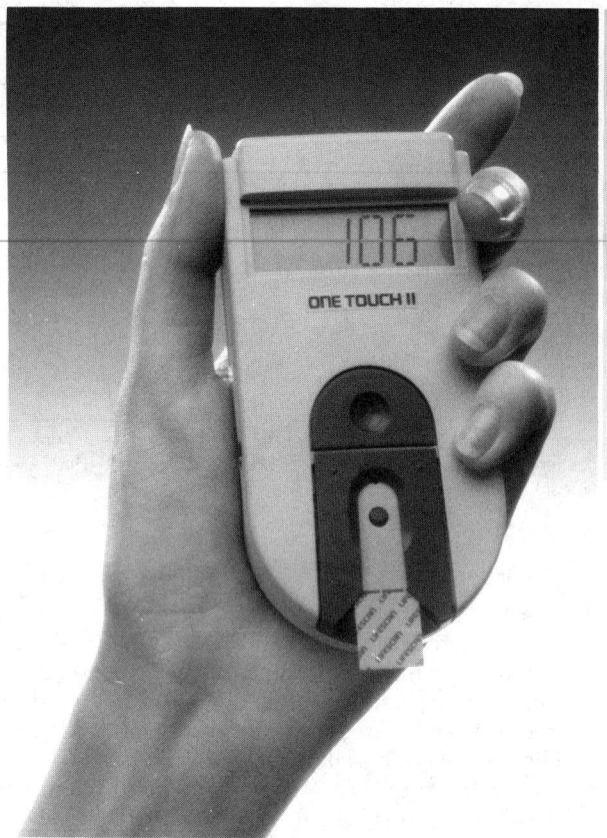

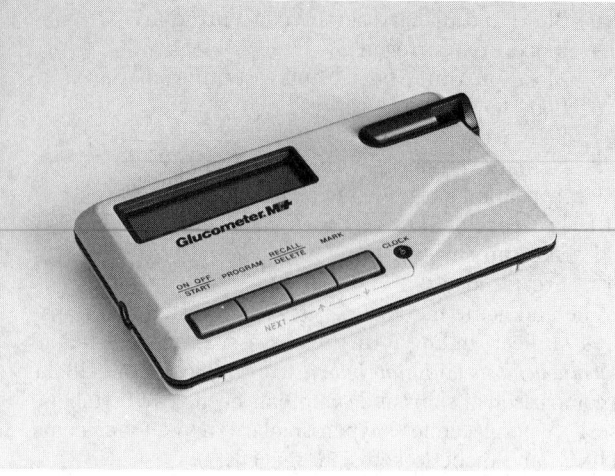

Fig. 28-4 Examples of reflectance meters used for self blood glucose monitoring (SBGN). **A,** One Touch II blood glucose monitor. **B,** Glucometer M+ blood glucose monitor. (**A,** courtesy Lifescan, Inc., Milpitas, California; **B,** courtesy Miles Diagnostics Division, Elkhart, Indiana.)

about exercise and food and in preventing hypoglycemia or severe hyperglycemia and metabolic crisis. Analysis of the patient's log of blood glucose levels, food intake, medication usage, and so on can uncover specific problems in blood glucose control. Patients can modify insulin timing or dosage, food intake, and or exercise. Some patients, after learning the use of insulin dosage algorithms, adjust insulin dosages according to a given protocol. See Table 28-15 for seven common problem patterns in controlling blood glucose and the necessary corrections.

Certain factors should be considered before recommending blood glucose monitoring to a particular patient. Those with neuropathy or vascular or inflammatory conditions of the fingers may be at risk for tissue injury from repeated pricking of the finger. Patients may not perceive the expense, discomfort, and inconvenience as barriers. Visual acuity must be adequate to "read" the color changes of the test strips or to read the digital display of the meter or a "talking" meter must be used. Those who believe that they have managed their diabetes well in the past with urine testing may have little incentive to do blood glucose monitoring. The most important factor, perhaps, is that the patient and the health care provider intend to use the information gained to achieve better blood glucose control than can be obtained with urine testing.

Physicians' recommendations for frequency of testing vary greatly. Some patients are advised to test before and after meals and at bedtime. For others who have established stable control, physicians may recommend testing frequently during one day of the week and whenever they feel ill.

To do the testing, the person sticks a finger and applies a drop of blood to a commercially prepared glucose oxidase stick. The timing for the reading and the preparation of the specimen are very important in obtaining accurate results. Self-monitoring of blood glucose is expensive, and not all insurance companies reimburse for this expense.

Monitoring of glycosylated proteins

Glycosylation results in the binding of glucose to proteins, and the amount of glycosylation of a particular protein correlates with blood glucose levels. Tests most frequently measure glycosylated hemoglobin A or $A1_C$ to monitor past blood glucose control.

Glycosylated hemoglobin accumulates during the lifespan of red blood cells and reflects the *average* glucose level over several weeks. In normal persons the level of Hb $A1_C$ is 3% to 6%. The goal of therapy is for the person with diabetes mellitus to be able to maintain Hb $A1_C$ within normal or at least no greater than one and one half times normal.

This test is the first measurement of how well patients have controlled blood glucose over a period of time. It is also used in research studies of blood glucose control and to differentiate noncompliance from an acute illness that results in an elevated level of blood glucose. Findings can be summarized as follows:

1. Any level of blood glucose with a high Hb $A1_C$ value suggests poor compliance over the previous 6 to 12 weeks
2. A high blood glucose level with a low Hb $A1_C$ value indicates recent onset of a hyperglycemic process,

Table 28-15   Common problem patterns found from blood glucose monitoring

	Potential cause*	Potential solutions
High fasting glucose	Insulin resistance,† insufficient insulin available overnight, rebound hyperglycemia overnight (Somogyi effect), dawn phenomenon	• Adjust p.m. intermediate- or long-acting insulin dose or time • Weight reduction to reduce insulin resistance
High glucose after breakfast	Inadequate insulin produced or injected to cover breakfast, peak insulin action not at anticipated time	• Adjust time or dose of short-acting a.m. insulin • Decrease size of breakfast or adjust amount of breakfast carbohydrate or divide breakfast into 2 smaller morning meals
Insulin reactions (hypoglycemia) before lunch	Insufficient breakfast for a.m. short-acting insulin or peak action later than anticipated time	• Adjust time or dose of a.m. short-acting insulin • Add morning snack or increase breakfast
Insulin reactions (hypoglycemia) in afternoon	Excessive a.m. intermediate-acting insulin, skipping or inadequate lunch	• Adjust time or dose of a.m. intermediate-acting insulin • Add afternoon snack • Adjust time or size of lunch
High glucose in afternoon	Inadequate insulin produced or intermediate-acting a.m. insulin is insufficient for need, or excessive snack or lunch	• Adjust dose of a.m. intermediate-acting insulin • Decrease or omit afternoon snack or decrease lunch
High glucose at night after evening meal	Inadequate insulin produced or insufficient insulin to cover dinner, or evening meal too large	• Adjust time or dose of p.m. insulin • Reduce size of meal or alter composition
Insulin reactions (hypoglycemia) at night	Excessive amount of insulin or insufficient dinner meal or evening snack	• Adjust time or dose of evening or bedtime insulin • Increase dinner and/or snack

*In addtion to food and insulin, other factors may affect blood glucose (e.g., exercise, sick days, infection).
†Insulin resistance associated with obesity is likely to result in high glucose levels throughout the day.
Reprinted with permission from Powers, *Diabetes Spectrum*, Vol. 4, No. 4, 1991. Copyright © 1991 by the American Diabetes Association.

Table 28-16   Urine tests for ketonuria

Test	Procedure	Interpretation
Acetest tablets	Use only whole tablets Place 1 drop of urine on tablet; read after 30 sec Lavender-purple	Differentiates level of ketones: small, moderate, large
Ketostix	Dip test strip quickly in and out of urine; hold in air for reading; read after 30 sec Lavender-purple	Differentiates level of ketones: 0, trace, small, moderate, large
Keto Diastix		Also tests for glucose (see Table 28-17)
Kyotest UGK	Dip test strip quickly in and out of urine; hold in air for reading; read after 50 sec Lavender-purple	Differentiates level of ketones: under ¼%, ¼%, ½%, 1% +. Also for glucose (see Table 28-17)

such as an infection or frequent episodes of hypoglycemia

The glycosylation of other proteins can also be measured. One test, fructosamine assay, indicates blood glucose control over the past 2 or 3 weeks. This assay is useful in pregnant women with IDDM or gestational diabetes and in puberty, when body changes are frequent and rapid.

Urine testing

Some patients monitor glucose levels by urine testing, even though the information obtained is imprecise and difficult to use in daily decision making about ways to achieve "strict" control. Nurses can help patients to understand that negative results of urine tests (in a patient with a renal threshold of ≥180 mg/dl) may mask significant hyperglycemia. In contrast, some patients, often children, have low renal thresholds and can control blood glucoses at optimal levels with urine tests alone. Some patients combine urine testing with blood glucose testing to monitor blood glucose in time periods between blood tests.

Urine testing for the presence of ketone bodies (Table 28-16) should be encouraged for the following persons:

Table 28-17 **Urine tests for glycosuria**

Test	Procedure	Interpretation
Clinitest tablets	Obtain freshly voided urine. Use only "fresh" whole tablets (off-white with blue specks) that completely dissolve. Use only the Clinitest dropper. Do not shake the tube during the reaction. Place required drops of urine (2 or 5) and *10* drops of *water* in a clean test tube. Drop 1 tablet into tube. Wait 15 sec after boiling has stopped to compare urine color with the proper color chart.	Clinitest is based on copper reduction of sugars, including glucose; thus false positive results can occur in the presence of other sugars. Other false-positive results can occur if patient takes large doses of vitamin C, more than 6 tablets of aspirin per day, and certain drugs (gantrisin, levodopa, probenecid, isonizid). Cephalosporins (for example, Keflex) may cause color reactions that make Clinitest results difficult to read.
2-drop method	Use *2* drops of urine and the 2-drop color chart. *Watch* the color reaction *during* the 15 sec waiting period.	Differentiates glucose content of 0.5%, 1%, 2%, 3%, and 5%. Large amounts of sugar may cause a "pass-through" reaction in which the color of the urine quickly changes from 5% to a lesser number.
5-drop method	Use *5* drops of urine and the 5-drop color chart.	Differentiates glucose content of 0.25%, 0.5%, 0.75%, 1%, and 2%.
Plastic, paper-impregnated strips, and paper tape	Dip the test strip or tape quickly in and out of urine; hold strips and tape in air for reading.	These strips and tapes show a reaction of urine and glucose oxidase, thus are specific for glucose. Inaccurate findings can occur if patients are taking ascorbic acid, pyridium, salicylates, or levodopa. More convenient and more costly than tablets.
Chemstrip uG	Read after 2 min: block 1, yellow to green; block 2, white to aqua.	Differentiates urine glucose content of $\frac{1}{10}$%, $\frac{1}{4}$%, $\frac{1}{2}$%, 1%, 2%, 3%, 5+%.
Chemstrip uGK		Also tests for ketones (Table 28-16).
Diastix	Read after 15 sec with proper color chart on container.	Differentiates urine glucose content of 0.1%, 0.25%, 0.5%, 1%, and 2%.
Keto Diastix		Also tests for ketones (Table 28-16).
Kyotest UGK	Read after 30 sec: shades of blue.	Differentiates urine glucose content of under $\frac{1}{4}$%, $\frac{1}{4}$%, $\frac{1}{2}$%, 1%+; also tests for ketones (Table 28-16).
Clinistix	Read in 10 sec with Clinistix color chart.	Estimates glucose presence as light, medium, and dark, thus most imprecise of all tests.
Tes-Tape	Tear 1½ inch from Tes-Tape roll; dip in urine and *read in air* after 1 or 2 min: 1 min, yellow-green, 0.25% 2 min, dark green, ≥0.5%; 2 min, green-black, ≤2%.	Differentiates urine glucose content as 0.1%, 0.25%, 0.5%, and 2%.

Table 28-18 Comparison of readings with various urine-sugar (glucose) tests

Product	Glucose concentration							
	$\frac{1}{10}$%	$\frac{1}{4}$%	$\frac{1}{2}$%	$\frac{3}{4}$%	1%	2%	3%	5%
Clinitest, 5-drop		Trace	+	+ +	+ + +	+ + + +		
Clinitest, 2-drop*			‡		‡	‡	‡	‡
Diastix	Trace	+	+ +		+ + +	+ + + +		
Clinistix†		Light (+)		Medium (+ +)		Dark (+ + +)		
Tes-Tape	+	+ +	+ + +			+ + + +		

*The 2-drop chart provides a "trace" color block without a percent value; a trace result only indicates less than ½%.
†Estimates relative presence of glucose, but cannot show percent amount.
‡Measures percent at these levels, but equivalent + signs not available.
NOTE: Blank spaces mean color blocks are absent for those concentrations.
From *Home urine testing for the diabetic*, Ames Company, Division of Miles Laboratories, 1976, Elkhart, Ind, p. 7.

1. All patients with IDDM (type I) with blood glucose over 250 mg/dl
2. All diabetics who feel ill

Often, a "double-voided" specimen is ordered as the sample to be obtained for urine testing of glycosuria. The patient is directed to empty the bladder one-half hour before the desired time of the specimen, drink water, and then void and test the freshly formed urine. See Table 28-17 for descriptions of urine tests for gycosuria.

Patients should record and report the extent of glycosuria by *percentage* rather than by plus signs (+, + +, + + +, + + + +); plus marks do not correlate with the same percentage of glycosuria on all urine tests. This can lead to errors in interpretation of the test results (Table 28-18).

The age of the individual, stability of disease, and renal threshold affect the physician's decision in advising the patient to use urine testing. The nurse can assist the person in interpreting the urine test results and in understanding the rationale for the specific regimen.

Data analysis: nursing diagnoses

Nursing diagnoses are determined from analysis of patient data. Possible nursing diagnoses for the person with diabetes mellitus may include, but are not limited to, the following:

Diagnostic title	Possible etiologies
Altered nutrition: more than body requirements	Excessive intake in relation to metabolic needs, established eating patterns, knowledge deficit, noncompliance
Self-care deficit in one or more activities	Perceptual impairment (visual, sensory), motor impairment
Impaired skin integrity or high risk for impaired skin integrity	Pressure from ill-fitting shoes, lack of podiatry services, knowledge deficit about foot care, visual or mobility impairment hampering inspection
Fluid volume deficit: actual or high risk for	Polyuria, other fluid losses, decreased fluid intake, insulin deficit
Knowledge deficit (diabetes managment)	Lack of exposure, poor recall, new diagnosis or new treatment, cognitive limitation
Noncompliance (with one or more aspects of diabetes regimen)	Cultural influences, established daily patterns of eating, activity, lack of resources

Planning: expected patient outcomes

Expected patient outcomes for the person with diabetes mellitus may include, but are not limited to, the following:

1. Blood glucose is at optimal level.
2. Ideal weight is maintained or achieved.
3. Is able to perform health care skills accurately, including insulin administration, test monitoring and interpretation of results, foot care, diet manipulation, and so forth.

4. Skin integrity is maintained; proper foot care is implemented.
5. Hydration is adequate.
6. Repeats accurate information about diabetes mellitus and measures for its control.
7. Can explain signs and symptoms of hypoglycemia and hyperglycemia and what to do when they occur.
8. Knows when to seek medical assistance.
9. Identifies one goal of improved health maintenance and states behavior necessary to achieve goal.

Implementation
Assisting with achievement of therapeutic goals
Promoting nutrition

Diet is considered to be the keystone of therapy in both IDDM and NIDDM with three nutritional goals[1]:

1. Control of blood glucose and blood lipid levels
2. Achievement and maintenance of desirable body weight
3. Provision of adequate nutrition and balanced diet

Dietary recommendations

1. Calories should be sufficient to promote normal growth and activity in the child and to maintain *ideal* weight and activity in the adult.
2. Calorie intake should be as follows:
   a. Protein, 12% to 20% (0.8 g/kg body weight)
   b. Carbohydrate, 55% to 60%
   c. Fat less than 30%
3. The amount of carbohydrate is individualized and depends on the impact of carbohydrate on blood glucose and lipid levels and individual eating patterns.
4. No more than 10% of calories from fat should be from saturated fats and the remainder from unsaturated fats. Cholesterol should be restricted to less than 300 mg daily.
5. Foods with unrefined carbohydrates and foods with fiber should be incorporated into the diet. The amount of highly refined carbohydrates low in fiber should be reduced; the diet should include 25 to 30 g of plant fiber/1000 Kcal.
6. Consistency in timing and the distribution of calories, carbohydrates, protein, and fat for each meal are most important in IDDM and in patients with NIDDM on insulin.
7. Weight control is more important in obese persons with NIDDM; balanced meals at consistent times aid in achieving this goal.
8. Sodium intake should be limited to 1000 mg/1000 Kcal of total intake, not to exceed 3000 mg/day.
9. A variety of nutritive and nonnutritive sweeteners should be encouraged.
10. Alcohol should be used in moderation, if at all. Alcohol has 7 Kcal/g when metabolized and must be included in calorie calculations. Patient should be aware of potential severe hypoglycemia from alcohol.

Some evidence indicates that *water-soluble fiber* helps to reduce blood glucose levels and blood lipids and to enhance bowel function. Fiber content should be increased grad-

28-9

Glycemic index

Food	
Glucose	100%
Rice, white	
Honey	70%
Potatoes	
Carrots	
Peanuts	
Lentils	<30%
Kidney beans	

From Franz, MJ: Evaluating the glycemic response to carbohydrates, Clin Diab 11:127-130, 1986.

ually to prevent abdominal discomfort. Additional fluids should be recommended when fiber intake is increased. Foods containing water-soluble fiber include the following:

1. Legumes
2. Oats
3. Barley
4. Fruit

Individualization of dietary recommendations for a particular patient has always been a principle of dietary therapy. This principle has been reinforced by recent knowledge about the many factors that influence the effect of specific starches on blood glucose levels. Beginning research indicates that some starches (complex carbohydrates) may raise blood glucose more than previously thought.

The term *glycemic index* is used to describe the change in blood glucose levels from ingestion of specific foods compared with that induced by a standard glucose load (see Box 28-9).

Many factors, including the preparation of foods and the combination of foods, influence the glycemic index. Too little is known at this time to make generalized recommendations using the glycemic index. However, individual patients may use blood glucose monitoring to assess the effect of particular food intake. A second benefit of the knowledge gained by research on the glycemic index is less reliance on *total* restriction of simple CHO. Small portions of foods containing sucrose can be eaten with meals, provided blood glucose levels are controlled.[19]

Patients may choose to include four "sweeteners" in their food. Aspartame (Nutrasweet) and saccharin are nonnutritive sweeteners; fructose and sorbital are nutritive sweeteners, with a caloric value of 4 cal/g. The Federal Drug Administration is reviewing two others, Sucralose and Alitame, and cyclomate, which may be reintroduced.[61]

Principles of dietary planning. Should a nutritional history reveal that the patient's food intake and patterns of eating incorporate the above recommendations, few changes would be recommended. It is often said that the diet needed by a diabetic person is that needed by all persons. However, most Americans find it necessary to change dietary habits to reduce hyperglycemia and maintain ideal weight. Recommendations need to be made with awareness

of the difficulty with which people change established eating habits. It is best to start with the patient's current diet and make as few modifications as necessary to achieve therapeutic goals.

Dietary planning should include considerations of the following factors:

1. The patient's personal, cultural, or religious food preferences
2. Life-style: working hours, family composition, financial resources
3. Activity: activity patterns; timing and level of exercise; periods of exercise, work, and sleep
4. Hypoglycemic drugs; onset, duration, and peak activity of insulin or oral hypoglycemic agents (p. 802)
5. Other modifications needed in consistency or nutrient content
6. Personal perceptions of ideal body weight

Systems for learning dietary requirements. There are several systems by which dietitians and nurses help patients learn dietary requirements.[69] The simplest system is providing patients with *sample diet plans* for each meal that can be used until they are able to learn and choose more options. For example, the plan for breakfast could be as follows:

4 oz orange juice
1 C cooked or dry cereal
1 slice toast with 1 tsp butter
1 C 2% milk
Coffee

A more complex system is *carbohydrate counting*, in which well-educated patients are taught to calculate carbohydrate intake in relation to regular insulin dosages taken at a mealtime by using a prescribed ratio of grams of carbohydrate to units of insulin.

The *food exchange system* has been widely used throughout the United States because of its ease in teaching. The exchange lists consist of six groups of food divided on the basis of similar amounts of *carbohydrates and fats*. Patients can learn to exchange foods within one list to obtain a variety of food intake. Some of the common foods in each of the food groups are listed in Table 28-19.

Information about the food exchange system is available from hospitals, clinics, and physicians' offices and in diabetic educational literature. Standardized diet plans have been developed for various levels of calorie intake and can serve as guides; however, these should not be used without attention to individual requirements. The dietitian translates the diet prescription into numbers of food exchanges and food distribution throughout the day that will meet the patient's nutritional requirements. Two sample meal plans for a day using a food exchange system appear in Table 28-20.

A dietary consultation should be initiated early in the educational program. The nurse and other health care professionals should not underestimate how difficult it is for persons to change food habits. There is no substitute for a careful dietary history and mutual planning by patient and dietitian (or nurse) about those changes necessary to control blood glucose levels or weight. The nurse can assist

Table 28-19   **Examples of food exchanges**

Food product	CHO (g)	Fat (g)	Equivalents
Milk and milk products			
Skim	12	Trace	1 C skim or nonfat milk
Lowfat (2%)	12	5	1 C yogurt
Whole	12	8	½ C evaporated milk
Vegetable			
Nonstarchy	5	2	½ C asparagus, carrots, eggplant, collards, tomatoes, and such
Fruit	15	—	1 Apple (2 inches across)
			½ C apple sauce
			½ banana
			½ grapefruit
Starch/bread	15	Trace	1 slice bread
			½ bagel
			1 tortilla (6 inches)
			½ hamburger bun
			3 graham crackers (2 × 2 sq)
			¾ C unsweetened cereal
Meat			
Lean	—	3	¼ C cottage cheese (dry)
			1 oz lean beef or fish
			¼ C tuna (water pack)
Medium fat	—	5	1 oz ground beef
			¼ C tuna (oil packed)
			½ C cottage cheese (creamed)
High fat	—	8	1 Tbsp peanut butter
			1 oz pork ribs or deviled ham
			1 oz cheddar cheese
			1 oz frankfurter
Fats	—	5	1 tsp margarine or butter
			1 strip crisp bacon
			2 tsp French dressing
Free food	—	—	Calorie-free beverages, unsweetened gelatin, and such: as desired

Adapted from American Diabetes Association, Inc: American Diabetes Association and National Institutes of Health, US Public Health Service exchange lists for meal planning, Chicago, 1986, The Association.

the patient in selecting foods in the hospital, in planning menus for home, and in reinforcing the dietary instruction (see p. 812).

Additional nursing activities related to dietary control include the following:

1. Helping the patient eat according to the diet plan
2. Monitoring and recording food intake
3. Obtaining substitutes for foods not desired or refused
4. Coordinating care so that patient's food is not delayed or omitted

The diabetic diet does not require the use of special or dietetic foods. Persons with diabetes must be warned about being misled by the word *dietetic.* Dietetic may refer to low sodium content rather than to low sugar content. Dietetic candies and foods labeled light (or Lite) also must be used with care. Dietetic foods are not necessarily low in calories and may have high fat content.

Some persons who develop diabetes are accustomed to having an alcoholic beverage daily. With approval of the physician, the diabetic may have small amounts of alcohol. Because alcohol is a high-calorie food, it must be exchanged for fat calories in the diet. The combination of alcohol and chlorpropamide should be avoided because of a severe Antabuse-like reaction.

Four strategies are useful in helping patients learn to manage blood glucose levels by diet:

1. Written instructions should accompany verbal discussion of the meal plan.
2. Weighing of meat and measuring of other foods acquaint patients with portion size.
3. Patients record of food intake can be correlated with records of blood or urine glucose tests, food intake, exercise, and medication.
4. Patients should be helped to apply dietary knowledge by doing exercises in which the person chooses foods from hospital and restaurant menus or from a variety of food items (models, pictures)

Participation in a behavior modification program for weight reduction and maintenance is highly recommended for obese persons with NIDDM. Teaching facts and principles about food intake and therapeutic requirements alone does not help the patient change eating behavior.

Promoting exercise

Exercise is the second treatment modality of diabetes mellitus. Glucose can enter *active* muscle cells without the action of insulin and can then be oxidized to carbon dioxide and water in most patients; thus *exercise has a hypoglycemic*

Table 28-20   Sample of two menu plans using the exchange list*

Exchanges	Menu 1	Menu 2
	Breakfast	**Breakfast**
1 Fruit	½ Glass orange juice	¼ Cantaloupe
1 Milk (skim)	1 Glass skim milk	1 Glass skim milk
1 Meat (medium fat)	1 Egg poached	1 Scrambled egg
3 Bread	2 Toast, ½ C oatmeal	1 English muffin, ½ C bran flakes
2 Fat	2 tsp margarine	2 tsp margarine
	Lunch	**Lunch**
1 Fruit	1 Peach	½ Banana
1 Milk (skim)	1 Glass skim milk	1 Glass skim milk
2 Meat (medium fat)	Tuna salad sandwich (¼ C tuna with celery, 2 slices	1 MacDonald's cheeseburger (2 bread, 2 meat)
2 Bread	bread, 3 tsp mayonnaise, and lettuce)	1 Lettuce salad with 2 Tbsp French dressing
3 Fat		
	Afternoon snack	**Afternoon snack**
1 Bread	6 Thin round crackers	¾ oz Pretzels
1 Fruit	1 Apple	15 Grapes
	Dinner	**Dinner**
1 Fruit	¾ C strawberries	¾ C pineapple
2 Vegetable	1 C green beans	Sliced tomatoes
4 Meat (lean)	4 oz round steak	4 oz chicken
1 Milk (skim)	1 Glass skim milk	1 Glass skim milk
2 Bread	1 Small baked potato	2 slices bread
	1 Roll	
3 Fat	1 Tbsp sour cream/2 tsp butter	1 tsp mayonnaise/2 tsp butter
	Evening snack	**Evening snack**
1 Bread	3 Rye wafers	6 Salt crackers
1 Meat	1 oz diet cheese	¼ C low-fat cottage cheese

Adapted from American Diabetes Association, Inc: American Diabetes Association and National Institutes of Health, US Public Health Service exchange lists for meal planning, Chicago, 1986, The Association.
*Diet distributed over three meals and two snacks. Diet based on 2000 calories with 45% CHO (225 g); 35% fats (78 g); and 20% proteins (100 g).

action. Exercise also decreases insulin resistance by increasing the number or activity of insulin receptors and promoting weight loss in the obese diabetic.

Persons with type 2 diabetes (NIDDM) benefit from regular exercise for 30 minutes three or four times a week. Results of exercise are improved glucose tolerance, insulin sensitivity, and weight loss. In addition, aerobic exercise improves cardiovascular function and lipid profiles.[22]

There are some cautions about exercise that patients must know. Exercise in the presence of hyperglycemia above 250 mg/100 ml can increase the hyperglycemia and even promote ketosis. Very intense exercise, even in persons with well-controlled blood glucose, can increase blood glucose levels.

Before an exercise program begins, the patient should have a complete cardiovascular examination, including a stress ECG if over age 35. Working capacity can be evaluated to determine the level of exercise that can be instituted safely. The person with diabetes mellitus should be evaluated for retinopathy, neuropathy, and hypertension because particular types of exercises should be avoided in these conditions.[22] Box 28-10 has information and guidelines for exercise in persons with diabetes mellitus.

Those persons receiving insulin or oral hypoglycemic agents should understand that diet and medications are planned around the usual activity level and pattern of exercise. Decisions about timing and duration of exercise are safer if the patient uses SBM. Optimal timing of exercise would be during periods of hyperglycemia (but with blood glucose levels below 250 mg/100 ml) and *not* during the peak action of insulin. Hypoglycemia is more likely to occur when exercise and peak action of insulin coincide. Encourage patients to use SBM one-half hour before beginning vigorous exercise and, if blood glucose is low (below 70 mg/100 ml), to eat a snack of complex carbohydrates and protein. Also encourage them to eat at 30-minute intervals during prolonged exercise. The increased sensitivity to insulin induced by exercise can last several hours and up to 3 days; inadequate food during this time can precipitate an episode of hypoglycemia. Changes in activity level require changes in diet or medication (Table 28-21).

Activity. In addition to stressing the importance of exercise, the nurse can assist the patient in planning how to incorporate regular exercise into the life-style after discharge. Previously sedentary adults should be encouraged to *gradually* increase activity and work up to 30 minutes of brisk walking, swimming, or low-impact aerobic exercises. Plans need to be reasonable and take into account previous activity level, cardiopulmonary status, mobility, and inter-

Guidelines for exercise program of the person with diabetes mellitus

Exercise type: aerobic, start with light level

Exercise session: Each session should include:
1. 5 to 10 minutes of warm-up stretching-limbering exercises
2. 20 to 30 minutes of aerobic exercise with heart rate in target zone (75% to 80% of maximum heart rate)
3. 15 to 20 minutes of light exercise and stretching to cool down

Exercise frequency: three to five times a week

Special precautions for diabetic who is being treated with hypoglycemic agent (insulin or oral)
1. Carry an ID card or wear bracelet identifying wearer as having diabetes mellitus and what to do if person is observed acting abnormally.
2. Monitor self during and after exercise for hypoglycemia (may include doing SBM at least at initiation of exercise program).
3. Carry a source of readily absorbable carbohydrate.
4. Avoid dehydration.
5. Consult professional (podiatrist) about footwear that is best for planned exercise.
6. Exercise when blood sugar is highest (1 to 3 hours after meals).
7. For regular, planned exercise, decrease insulin as prescribed.
8. Consume extra carbohydrate before, during, or after exercise; need is dictated by SBM, whether any reduction of insulin was instituted, length and level of exercise, presence of symptoms of hypoglycemia, and whether exercise was planned or spontaneous.

Precautions for selected persons
1. Persons with insensitive feet should avoid running and jogging and choose cycling or swimming.
2. Persons with proliferative retinopathy should avoid exercises associated with the Valsalva maneuver or that cause jarring and jolting of head and exercises associated with head in a lower position.
3. Persons with hypertension should avoid exercises associated with the Valsalva manuever and exercises involving intense exercise of the body and arms (exercises involving the lower extremities are preferred).

Modified from Rifkin H, editor: The physician's guide to type 2 diabetes (NIDDM): diagnosis and treatment, New York, 1984, American Diabetes Association.

Table 28-21   Effect of exercise on need for medication and food

	Increased exercise	Decreased exercise
Hypoglycemic agent	Decreased need	Increased need
Food	Increased need	Decreased need

ests. For example, an elderly hemiplegic patient could be encouraged to do range-of-motion and leg-raising exercises, and a younger person with no disabilities could be encouraged to develop interest in a specific exercise or sports program. Sports that are contraindicated for patients receiving insulin include those in which the dangers of hypoglycemia increase the hazard of the sport (for example, scuba diving or sky diving).

Medications
Insulin. Insulin is necessary for the survival of patients with IDDM. It is also used to treat NIDDM in some patients in whom other measures have not achieved a desired level of blood glucose control.

The current trend in treatment is to achieve the best control of blood glucose possible for each individual, that is, to achieve blood glucose levels near normal limits if this can be done without significant hypoglycemia.

Properties of insulin. Insulin preparations have four major properties that are incorporated into the prescription: (1) type of action, (2) strength, (3) species source, and (4) purity.

TYPE OF ACTION. All insulins are hypoglycemic, but they differ in the speed with which they begin to act *(onset)*, the period of time they have the strongest action *(peak)*, and how long they act *(duration)*. Insulins are classified as short, intermediate, and long acting. Table 28-22 gives the characteristics of seven standard insulin preparations. Nurses need to know the characteristics of each in order to coordinate food and activity with insulin action. This coordination is necessary so that (1) insulin is available for optimal metabolism when food is taken, and (2) food is available while insulin is acting to prevent hypoglycemic reactions.

Three principles are useful in coordinating food and hypoglycemic medications:
1. Food must be taken after insulin (or oral agent) within the time of onset; for example, with regular insulin, food must be taken within 1 hour after injection.
2. Intermediate- or long-acting insulins require that a supplemental feeding be given, timed to match the peak action of the insulin, for example, an afternoon feeding if NPH insulin given at 7 AM.
3. With intermediate- or long-acting insulin a bedtime feeding is required so that glucose is available through the night.

STRENGTH. Insulin preparations vary in the concen-

Table 28-22 Action of insulin preparations

Type of insulin	Time of onset (hr)	Peak of action (hr)	Duration of action (hr)	Insulin appearance
Rapid acting				
Regular	< 1	2-4	4-6	Clear
Semilente	< 1	4-7	12-16	Cloudy
Intermediate acting				
NPH	1-2	8-12	18-24	Cloudy
Lente	1-4	8-12	18-24	Cloudy
Long acting				
Ultralente	4-8	16-18	36 +	Cloudy

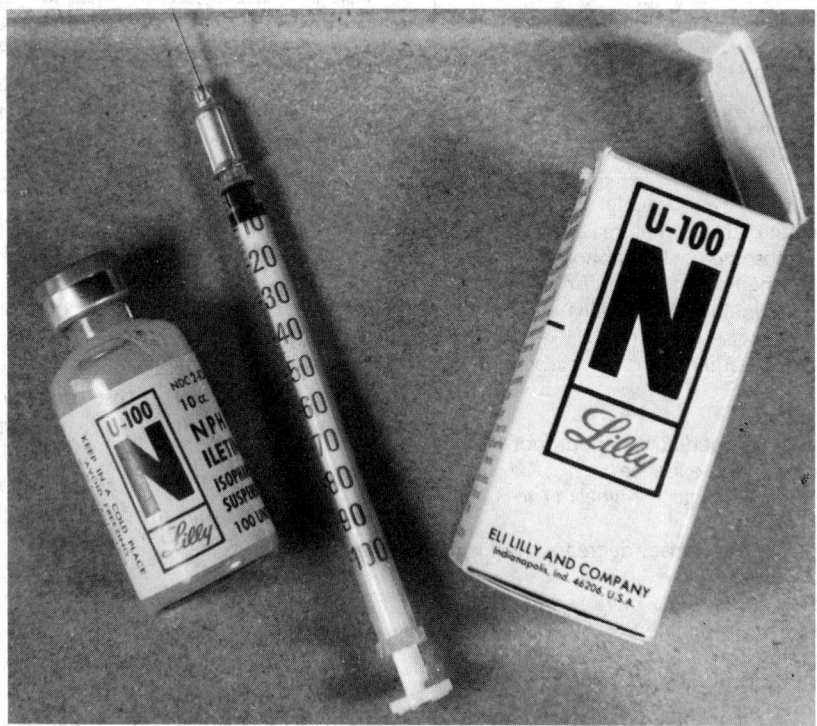

Fig. 28-5   U-100 insulin and disposable U-100 insulin syringe.

tration of insulin units in 1 ml volume. U-100 insulin, or 100 units/ml, is the strength most frequently used. A very concentrated preparation of insulin (U-500) may be used in implantable pump reservoirs or when daily insulin doses exceed 100 units. This large dosage may be necessary in a rare condition of insulin resistance.

It is very important that the insulin concentration and the insulin syringe calibration match in units per milliliter to prevent errors in dosing (Fig. 28-5).

SPECIES. In the past, most insulin was prepared from a combination of beef and pork pancreas. Single-species insulin (usually pork) could be obtained for patients with beef-insulin allergy or antibodies. (Pork insulin most closely resembles human insulin and is considered the least antigenic animal insulin.)

"Human" insulin is either porcine (pork insulin modified enzymatically to structurally resemble human insulin) or

bacterially produced by recombinant DNA techniques. It is increasingly prescribed in place of animal insulin, because it has less antigenicity than animal insulin, and it greatly expands the insulin resources of the world. As of December 1991, protamine zinc insulin was removed from the market. The insulins available in the United States today appear in Table 28-23.

PURITY. Over time, manufacturers have improved the purity of insulin preparations by reducing the amounts of proinsulinlike substances and other antigenic substances contained in the solution. All standard insulins now contain less than 50 ppm (parts per million) of these antigenic particles. Insulins labeled "highly purified" contain less than 10 ppm and may be prescribed in rare instances.

Because of the many changes being made in insulin preparations, the nurse must clarify the insulin prescription if the type, strength, purity, or species is unclear. A

Table 28-23   Insulins available in the United States as of December 1991

Duration/source	Product	Manufacturer	Strength
Short-acting			
Human	Humulin Regular	Lilly	U-100
	Humulin BR	Lilly	U-100
	Novolin R	Novo Nordisk	U-100
	Velosulin Human R	Novo Nordisk	U-100
Pork	Iletin II Regular	Lilly	U-100, U-500
	Regular	Novo Nordisk	U-100
	Purified Pork Regular	Novo Nordisk	U-100
	Velosulin	Novo Nordisk	U-100
Beef	Iletin II Regular	Lilly	U-100
	Semilente	Novo Nordisk	U-100
Beef/Pork	Iletin I Regular	Lilly	U-100
	Iletin I Semilente	Lilly	U-100
Intermediate-acting			
Human	Humulin L (Lente)	Lilly	U-100
	Humulin N (NPH)	Lilly	U-100
	Novulin L (Lente)	Novo Nordisk	U-100
	Novulin N (NPH)	Novo Nordisk	U-100
	Insulatard NPH Human	Novo Nordisk	U-100
Pork	Iletin II Lente	Lilly	U-100
	Iletin II NPH	Lilly	U-100
	Purified Pork Lente	Novo Nordisk	U-100
	Purified Pork NPH	Novo Nordisk	U-100
	Insulatard NPH	Novo Nordisk	U-100
Beef	Illetin II Lente	Lilly	U-100
	Iletin II NPH	Lilly	U-100
	Lente	Novo Nordisk	U-100
	NPH	Novo Nordisk	U-100
Beef/Pork	Iletin I NPH	Lilly	U-100
	Iletin I Lente	Lilly	U-100
Long-acting			
Human	Humulin U (Ultralente)	Lilly	U-100
Beef	Ultralente	Novo Nordisk	U-100
Beef/Pork	Iletin I Ultralente	Lilly	U-100
Fixed combinations (all are U-100, NPH/regular insulins)			
Human	Humulin 70/30	Lilly	70/30
	Novolin 70/30	Novo Nordisk	70/30
	Mixtard Human 70/30	Novo Nordisk	70/30
Pork	Mixtard	Novo Nordisk	70/30

From Campbell RK: *Practical diabetology,* 10(6):8-11, 1991.

change in any one of these properties may lead to significant differences in action. When the insulin prescription is changed, careful patient monitoring is necessary to identify the extent of clinical effect.

Insulin administration. Increasingly, physicians are attempting to simulate the normal bodily secretion of insulin that occurs in nondiabetics, that is, a continuous basal level of insulin that rapidly increases with food intake. In addition, they try to mimic the tendency for glucose to reach its lowest peak between 3 AM and 4 AM and a tendency for blood glucose and basal insulin secretion to rise between 5 AM and 8 AM before breakfast (dawn phenomenon). A description of various regiments is presented in Box 28-11; regimens 3 to 6 are designed to mimic the normal endogenous secretion pattern. These regimens are

termed *intensive therapy* and are aimed at "tight control" of blood glucose. Obviously the risk of hypoglycemia is increased with intensive therapy.

The insulin type and dosage are ordered in anticipation of food, activity, and other factors that balance or affect the insulin requirements. Regardless of the particular regimen, consider the following information before administering insulin:

1. Time of onset, peak, and duration of the insulin
2. Availability of food or adequate glucose at these times of action
3. Plans for treating hypoglycemia should it occur

Thus if a patient were ordered nothing by mouth for several hours, insulin should not be given until provision is made for an intravenous infusion of a dextrose solution.

ROTATION OF NEEDLE INSERTION SITES. The subcu-

28-11

Insulin therapy regimens

One injection of intermediate-acting insulin per day
  Most frequently used in persons with NIDDM who are not controlled with diet and/or oral hypoglycemic agents
  Does not mimic the normal endogenous pattern
  May be used with oral hypoglycemic agents
Two injections of intermediate-acting insulin per day
  Used mostly in persons with NIDDM
  Does not mimic the normal endogenous pattern
Split and mixed insulin regimen: injection of rapid-acting insulin and intermediate-acting insulin at breakfast and supper
  Used in many persons with IDDM
  Theorectically, the morning rapid-acting insulin covers breakfast and early morning, the morning intermediate-acting insulin covers lunch and afternoon, the evening rapid-acting insulin covers the evening meal, and the evening intermediate-acting insulin covers the bedtime snack and the *basal level needed* during the night
Split and mixed insulin regimens (similar to No. 3 above), except that the evening intermediate-acting insulin is given at bedtime instead of at supper time
  Used in persons with IDDM
  Theoretically provides better basal nighttime coverage and provides coverage for the natural prebreakfast elevation in glucose
Multidosage regimen: three injections of rapid-acting insulin, one before each meal; and one injection of intermediate insulin given at bedtime
  The rapid-acting insulin provides coverage for each meal
  The bedtime intermediate-acting insulin provides the nighttime basal level and coverage for the natural prebreakfast glucose elevation
Multidosage regimen: three injections of rapid-acting insulin, one before each meal; and an injection of long-acting insulin given at breakfast or at supper or split between breakfast and supper (provides the same coverage as No. 5 above)

---

taneous tissue of the upper arms, the anterior and lateral aspects of the thigh, most of the abdomen, and the buttocks may be used for insulin injections.[1a] It is very important that the site of injection of insulin be rotated to assure proper absorption of insulin and to prevent lipodystrophy.[1a] No injection site should be used more than once a month.

The older practice of randomly rotating sites between *anatomic areas such as the arms, thighs, buttocks, and abdomen* with each injection is no longer recommended. If possible *only one anatomic area is used throughout the patient's life* because the absorption rate of insulin varies among these sites.[1a] The rate of absorption of insulin from fastest to slowest is abdomen, arms, and legs. Some specialists are recommending that only the abdomen be used.[6,63] However, in a majority of instances it is not possible to use only one anatomic area.[13a] The abdomen or any other anatomic area might not provide a large enough surface area for multiple injections in a small person. Remember no one site should be used more than once a month and some persons will be on three to four injections a day, thus requiring 90 to 120 sites per month in one anatomic area. Some persons have an aversion to injecting themselves in the abdomen, and other persons find it difficult to use arms or legs.

The most commonly used recommendation is rotation of sites within one *anatomic area until no more sites are available,* and then movement to another anatomic area.[13a,23a,23c] For most persons, if this recommendation is followed a patient will use one anatomic area for 3 to 4 days up to several weeks. In some instances the person may use only two of the anatomic areas.[13a] That is, all sites in the arms will be used, then all sites in the abdomen will be used, and then the person will switch back to the arms.

Another variation in rotation being used with some persons is rotating within a geographic area for injections given at specific times of the day.[13a] That is, some specialists suggest that the abdomen and arms be used for AM insulin injections, when insulin resistance is the highest and the thighs and buttocks be used for PM (dinner and bedtime) insulin injections, to allow for longer absorption overnight. If this rotation schedule were used, a patient would be taught to give AM insulin in the abdomen until every available site has been used and then to switch to the arms and use every available site and then to switch back to the abdomen. PM insulin would be given in the thighs until every available site is used; then the person would switch to the buttocks and use every available site and then switch back to the thighs. This later type of rotation schedule is more complex and may not be started until the patient has mastered many of the other self-care skills. Important to remember is that the best, most effective plan for rotation of sites should be individualized for each person. The major areas for injection and the multiple sites within these areas are depicted in Fig. 28-6.

Two forms of *lipodystrophy* can occur: hypertrophy and atrophy. *Hypertrophy* is thickening of an injection site because fibrous scar tissue develops from repeated injections in the same site. A hypertrophic area is usually devoid of nerve endings, and the patient likes to reuse it because injections are painless. Absorption from this area is slow and erratic.

Atrophy is loss of subcutaneous fat. The cause is unknown. It is thought to result from repeated injections in the same site, faulty injection technique, or impurities in the insulin. Some researchers have successfully treated atrophy by injecting purified insulin into atrophic areas.

SELF-INJECTION OF INSULIN. Most persons are fearful of self-injection and would prefer to postpone learning this task; yet repeated practice is necessary if they are to safely administer an accurate dose using sterile technique. The nurse must teach this skill early and with attention to the patient's fear, whether that fear is or is not expressed.

One study supports the belief that adults can learn this skill most readily and cope best if the first self-injection is not delayed for practice with syringe, vials of medicine, or

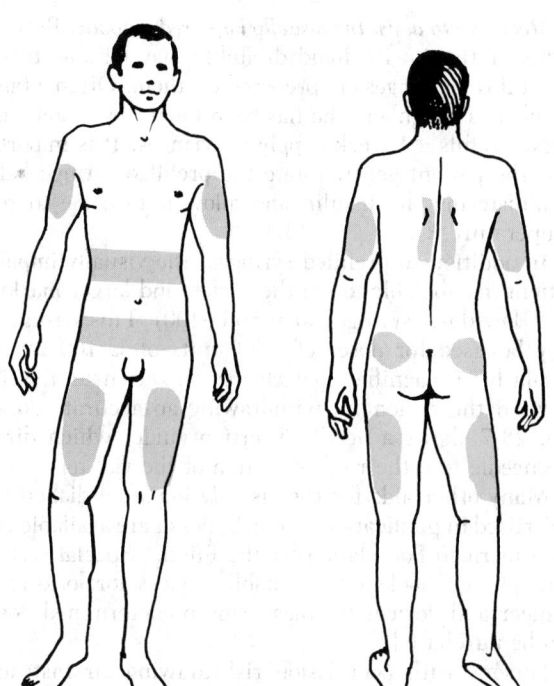

Fig. 28-6   Rotation of sites for insulin injection.

Guidelines for insulin administration

1. Always use an insulin syringe calibrated in the same units as the insulin.
2. Select insulin according to type, strength, species, purity, and brand name as specified by the prescription.
3. Rotate or gently roll or shake the bottle if it is other than regular insulin.
4. Do not inject cold insulin; allow it to come to room temperature if it is stored in the refrigerator before using.
5. Examine intermediate- and long-acting insulin vials for suspension of insulin (cloudy appearance); do not use if it is *not* cloudy. Examine human insulin for a frosty or clumping of precipitate—do not use if present.
6. Check for and remove any air bubbles after insulin is drawn into the syringe (do not use an air bubble to clear the needle after injection).
7. When mixing insulins, do not vary the sequence in which two insulins are drawn into the same syringe; inject air into both bottles—first into intermediate and then into regular; withdraw the insulin first from the regular vial and then from the longer-acting insulin vial. Commercially peremixed NPH and regular insulin may be prescribed, for example, Novalin 70/30, Mixtard Human 70/30, and Humulin 70/30. All contain 70% NPH and 30% regular insulin.
8. Insert the needle into fatty tissue closer to muscle than to skin; if there is little subcutaneous tissue, "pinch" up the skin and use a 45-degree angle and a ⅜ or ½ inch needle. Use a 90-degree angle when the fat pad is large.

any other equipment.[64] Traditionally, the patient has been given an orange to inject as practice before self-injection. Instead, the researcher suggests that the patient perform self-injection first.

The nurse should firmly encourage the patient to hold the syringe, cleanse and pierce the skin, and inject the ordered insulin (or an equivalent dosage of sterile saline) from the syringe previously prepared by the nurse. Verbal encouragement and a guiding hand may be necessary for the patient to self-inject successfully. After adults experience self-injection, they are better able to focus on preparation of the insulin syringe (see Box 28-12 for guidelines in insulin administration).

Help patients to determine the quantity of disposable syringes and needles and other supplies needed for at least a month. Cotton balls purchased in bulk and a bottle of 70% ethyl alcohol, as compared with individually wrapped alcohol pledgets, can reduce costs.

Set up typical trays for injection at home to use in demonstrations and for patient practice. Discuss boxes or trays that can be used at home to keep all equipment together. The equipment should be stored on a shelf or closet, out of reach of children and out of sight.

INSULIN PUMPS. Very close control of blood glucose can be achieved for some patients with IDDM with an insulin infusion pump. External insulin pumps, which are battery operated and portable, deliver regular insulin at a basal rate (continuously) and a bolus dose at meal times. The insulin is delivered from a reservoir through tubing to a needle placed in subcutaneous tissue. The external pump is only disconnected to change the needle (every 2 to 3 days), while bathing or swimming, and during sexual activity.

About the same size as a small calculator, the external pump can be worn on a belt at the waist or in a pocket.

The patient requires considerable education to ensure safe and effective insulin delivery. Complications include hypoglycemia, infection at the site of needle insertion, and rapid onset of ketoacidosis if the pump becomes disconnected. Pumps do not decrease the amount of attention the patient must give to diabetes management; pumps require the use of frequent SBM and decisions about food, exercise and insulin dosage. Thus the patient must be highly motivated. They do enable the patient to maintain blood glucose levels at near-normal ranges and to add flexibility to daily life.

Insulin pumps are expensive; however, insurance reimbursement of initial and maintenance costs is becoming more common. A policy statement by the American Diabetes Association cautions that the use of portable infusion devices be prescribed and managed by diabetologists trained and skilled in their use. Projected for the future is the closed-loop insulin delivery system, which will combine a pump, a blood glucose sensor, and a calculator to determine rate of delivery.

Insulin pumps now in use are open-loop systems. These pumps enable patients to avoid multiple insulin injections; however, patients must monitor blood glucose levels and manually set the insulin delivery rate.

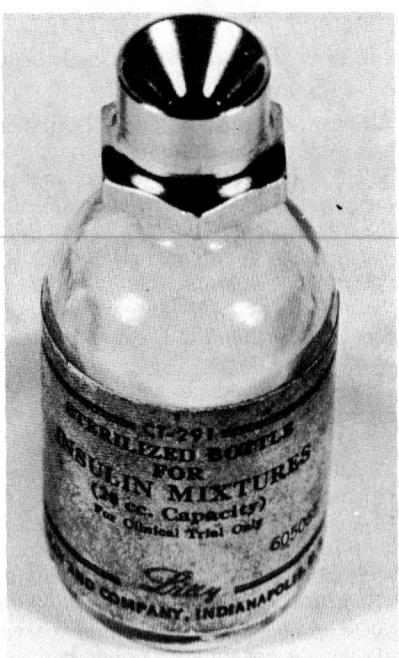

Fig. 28-7 Insulin needle guide that fits over top of insulin vial. Patient cleans stopper and guide with alcohol before placing guide on vial. Needle is laid in V of guide, and vial is pushed toward it. (Courtesy American Foundation for the Blind, Inc, New York.)

EXPERIMENTAL THERAPIES. Internal (implantable) pumps are now being used for some patients who are participating in clinical research trials. These devices are computerized and have a reservoir of insulin from which the programmed dose is injected into the peritoneal cavity. The patient transmits directions to the pump by radiotelemetry. Advantages of internal pumps are avoidance of peripheral hyperinsulinemia and suppression of hepatic glucose output. These devices use U-400 insulin. The reservoir is refilled every 40 to 60 days by transcutaneous injection.[55]

ALTERNATIVE DELIVERY SYSTEMS OF INSULIN. Over the years, there has been interest in developing systems to deliver insulin: by nasal spray, by skin patches, and by specially protected encapsulated forms for oral use.[7] To date, none of these have been satisfactorily developed for widespread clinical use.

Storage of insulin. Patients should be taught to give insulin at room temperature to decrease the risk of lipodystrophy and to decrease the antigenicity of the insulin. The current practice is to keep the currently used vial at room temperature if it can be used within 1 month, even though insulin vial labels direct the refrigeration of all insulin. It is known that regular insulin will remain stable for 12 months at 37° C (modified insulins for 24 months). Teach travelers to carry insulin with them rather than to pack it in baggage that might be subjected to extreme temperatures in car trunks or cargo compartments of planes or trains.

Refrigeration is recommended for additional vials and when prefilled syringes are used, to decrease the potential bacterial growth from contamination.

Measures to assist the visually impaired diabetic. Blind patients or those with hand disability may be able to self-inject if the syringes are prepared for them. Often a family member or neighbor who has been taught by a home-care nurse prefills a 1-week supply of syringes. It is important that the patient gently rotate the prefilled syringe before administering the insulin and allow it to come to room temperature.

In addition to prefilled syringes, the visually impaired patient may be able to see the darker and larger markings on a "low-dose" syringe (30 or 50 U-100). This syringe can only be used for doses of <50 units of U-100 insulin. Similarly, a magnifier that clamps on the insulin syringe may aid the patient in withdrawing an accurate dosage. Fig. 28-7 shows a needle insertion guide, which directs the needle into the rubber portion of the vial top.

Many other aids for the visually impaired diabetic are advertised in publications for diabetics or are available from the American Foundation for the Blind.* Special syringes with plunger locks or attachable devices for locking the plunger and devices for measuring predetermined dosage can be purchased.[27]

Persons with poor vision risk drawing air instead of insulin into the syringe. Caution them to invert the bottle completely and to insert the needle only a short distance. Often they are advised to use only about two thirds of the bottle of insulin and to have on hand another full bottle. Some persons have a community health nurse or a friend withdraw the last doses in a bottle of insulin for them or go to a clinic for the last few injections.

Carbohydrate blockers. A drug that inhibits the absorption of carbohydrates from the small intestine (acarbose) is reported to have beneficial effects on postprandial blood glucose levels in patients with NIDDM. Acarbose inhibits the degradation of starch, dextrins, maltose, and sucrose to absorbable monosaccharides. Further, acarbose had minimum side effects. Flatulence, which subsided, was reported in a double-blind, placebo-controlled study. Better glycemic control and a beneficial influence on triglyceride were reported.[24]

Oral hypoglycemic agents. Six orally administered agents are now available for controlling blood sugar levels in persons with diabetes mellitus; all are sulfonylurea compounds (Table 28-24). One drug from another class of oral hypoglycemic agents, biguanides, is being clinically tested at selected sites.[4a] Glypizide (Glucotrol) and glyburide (Micronase, Diabeta), are more potent than the first-generation compounds; thus doses are smaller. These drugs have fewer drug-drug interactions, because they are not so easily displaced (unbound) from albumin by other drugs.

The sulfonylurea compounds increase the ability of the islet cells of the pancreas to secrete insulin, although other methods of action are being studied. With long-term use they may increase the number of insulin receptors and correct defects in postreceptor insulin action.

Complications of oral hypoglycemic agents are infre-

---

*American Foundation for the Blind, Inc, 15 West 16th St, New York, NY 10011.

Table 28-24   Oral hypoglycemic agents

Agent	Proprietary name	Range of daily dose
Acetohexamide	Dymelor	250 mg to 1.5 g
Chlorpropamide	Diabinese	100 to 750 mg
Tolazamide	Tolinase	100 mg to 1 g
Tolbutamide	Orinase	250 mg to 3 g
Second generation		
Glyburide	Micronase, Diabeta, Euglucon	1.5 to 20 mg
Glipizide	Glucotrol	2.5 to 40 mg

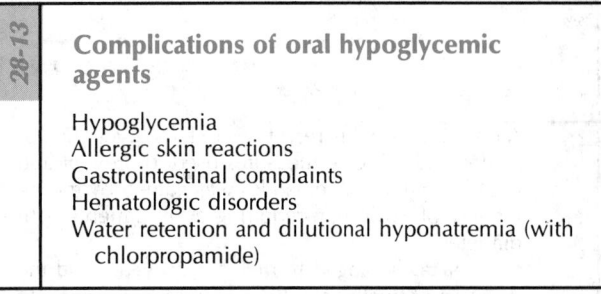

28-13

Complications of oral hypoglycemic agents

Hypoglycemia
Allergic skin reactions
Gastrointestinal complaints
Hematologic disorders
Water retention and dilutional hyponatremia (with chlorpropamide)

28-14

Signs and symptoms of hypoglycemia

Sympathetic nervous system activity

Pallor	*Perspiration
Piloerection	Hunger
Tachycardia	Palpitation
*Nervousness	Irritability
*Weakness	Trembling

Central nervous system activity

Headache	Blurred vision
Diplopia	Incoherent speech
Emotional changes	Fatigue
*Mental confusion	Numbness of lips,
Convulsions	tongue
	Coma

*Four signs most commonly reported by patients.

quent (see Box 28-13). Oral hypoglycemic agents differ in routes of excretion; the presence of liver or kidney dysfunction may increase the risk of complications. Chlorpropamide may prolong hypoglycemia because of its long half-life (36 hours) and duration of action (24 to 60 hours). See Table 28-24 for information about the hypoglycemic agents.

Chlorpropamide is usually given in one dose per day; Tolbutamide has the shortest duration of action (6 to 12 hr) and is ordered two to three times a day.

The drugs are not hormones, and it is inaccurate to refer to them as oral insulin.

Physicians vary in their use of these agents because of the controversial study conducted in the 1970s by the University Group Diabetes Program (UGDP). The FDA recommends that orally administered hypoglycemic agents be limited to persons with symptomatic adult-onset nonketotic diabetes mellitus that cannot be adequately controlled by diet or weight loss alone and in whom the administration of insulin is impractical or unacceptable. This recommendation was based on the report of the UGDP study that the death rate from cardiovascular disease was two and one half times higher in persons receiving tolbutamide as in those receiving a placebo. These results have been challenged by numerous groups.

These medications are not used to treat IDDM or in pregnant women. They are useless in the treatment of diabetic ketoacidosis. A few patients may be treated with a combination of insulin and oral agents.[8]

Persons taking oral hypoglycemia medications need to be as careful about taking the prescribed dosage, following the prescribed diet, maintaining the usual amount of exercise, testing by SBM, and taking general health precautions as do persons taking insulin.

Preventing, detecting, and treating hypoglycemia

Hypoglycemia (plasma glucose level <60 mg/dl) occurs in at least two circumstances in diabetes mellitus. It occurs by far more frequently in the patient receiving insulin or an oral hypoglycemic agent in whom there is an insulin excess relative to food intake or energy expenditure. Hypoglycemia in this situation occurs for the following reasons:

1. Too large a dosage taken in relation to the need for insulin
2. Too little food taken (meals delayed or omitted) or delayed gastric emptying
3. Exercise excessive in relation to food intake and hypoglycemic agent or insulin
4. Emotional stress
5. Vomiting, diarrhea, or decreased food absorption

A less common instance is hypoglycemia occurring in the early phase of NIDDM, when a sluggish release of insulin allows peak insulin activity to occur hours after food has been ingested.

The symptoms of *hypoglycemia* can occur when blood glucose level falls rapidly: that is, the blood glucose level may be >60 mg/dl, but the patient has the symptoms of hypoglycemia. Symptoms of hypoglycemic reaction can vary among patients and from time to time in one patient.

Symptoms of sympathetic nervous system (SNS) activity usually precede those of the CNS and are related to epinephrine action. Signs of cerebral dysfunction reflect hypoglycemia that interferes with the glucose supply of nerve cells (see Box 28-14). Prolonged attacks of severe hypoglycemia can cause brain damage.

For some patients, a disturbing development is a diminished ability to perceive hypoglycemic symptoms, particularly the early SNS symptoms. This dysfunction is associated with duration of disease, development of neuropathy, and use of certain drugs that affect the SNS (for example, beta blockers). Patients find this loss frightening because they no longer are able to intervene early in the

28-15

Nursing Research

Paulk LH. Hypoglycemic reactions: from the diabetic's perspective, unpublished master's thesis, Kent, Ohio, 1983, Kent State University.

A description of the responses to hypoglycemic episodes and self-care measures used to prevent and treat hypoglycemic episodes was gained by the interview of 30 insulin-requiring adult patients with diabetes.

Their ages ranged from 19 to 76 years and the duration of treatment with insulin ranged from 1 to 47 years.

Sixty percent of the sample reported the three most frequent symptoms of hypoglycemia to be: nervousness, weakness, and sweating (all early symptoms related to epinephrine activity).

Mental confusion was the most frequently reported symptom related to change in central nervous system activity. Sixty-two percent of the sample reported nocturnal reactions and severe reactions involving memory loss.

Thirty six percent of the subjects reported that they did nothing to prevent attacks and used the same substance (juice, candy) to treat all attacks. The recommendations of the researcher were that (1) the most frequently reported symptoms be used in initial teaching, (2) patients be taught to treat at the earliest symptom, (3) measures to prevent hypoglycemia be reinforced in patient teaching, and (4) patients learn to use more than one treatment substance. For the subset of patients with fear, hypoglycemic unawareness or severe reactions, an alternative plan for treatment must be developed with patient's significant others. Family members should be taught not to put food in mouth of the unconscious patient. A trained layperson can be taught to administer 1 mg glucagon (adult dose) into muscle or subcutaneous tissue.

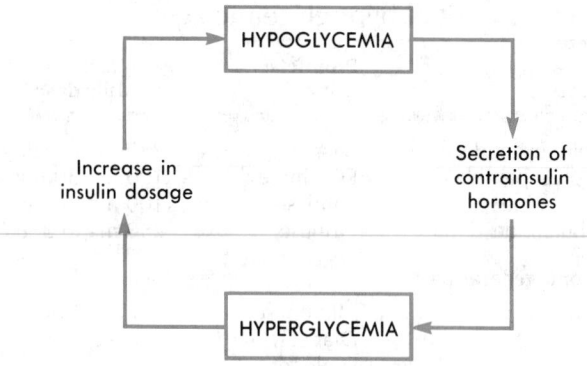

Fig. 28-8   Sequence of events in Somogyi phenomenon.

28-16

Carbohydrates (10 to 15 g) for relief of hypoglycemia

½ C fruit juice
½ C cola drink (not diet)
½ C gelatin dessert (not diet)
4 Cubes sugar
2 Packets sugar
2 Squares graham crackers

The nurse should not hesitate to treat the patient if symptoms of hypoglycemia occur. Hospital protocols should clearly describe prompt treatment of hypoglycemia in patients who cannot take anything by mouth.

To facilitate prompt treatment for unconsciousness, diabetic persons should carry identification cards with the insulin or hypoglycemic agent and dosage listed. Medic-Alert bracelets or necklaces can also alert others to the diabetic status.

Patients who are receiving insulin or orally administered hypoglycemic agents must know how to prevent, detect, and treat hypoglycemic reactions before discharge. The nurse provides and explains the following:
1. Written material describing symptoms and treatment
2. Written material describing exercise related to hypoglycemia
3. Diabetic identification card
4. Sample of quickly absorbed glucose to carry

Somogyi phenomenon. Some patients have great difficulty in stabilizing blood glucose levels. One cause of instability is the Somogyi phenomenon, a sequence of increasing peaks and valleys in blood glucose levels. It is often triggered by an insulin dosage in excess of true insulin requirements. The sequence of events is depicted in Fig. 28-8.

Very frequently the signs and symptoms of hypoglycemia are not obvious enough to be detected. In many instances the hypoglycemia occurs at night and is undetected. The hyperglycemia is not recognized until early morning, and it is assumed that the patient needs higher doses of insulin, but this treatment just makes the problem worse.

reaction, but only when signs of cerebral dysfunction alert others or themselves to a more severe hypoglycemic reaction. If a hypoglycemic reaction is suspected, obtain a blood glucose level if it can be done quickly. Encourage patients to use SBM and not to rely on subjective feelings alone. At the same time, encourage them to take action—to use SBM and ingest glucose when subjective feelings first occur. See Box 28-15 for a description of a research study of hypoglycemic reactions from the patient's perspective.

Hypoglycemia in a *conscious patient* is treated by administering a quickly absorbed sugar; 10 to 15 g carbohydrate should be given promptly (see Box 28-16). With this amount of food, the patient usually feels better within 5 to 15 minutes. Should symptoms not decrease, give another feeding after this time. With unconsciousness or severe hypoglycemia, give an intravenous bolus of 50% dextrose.

After recovery the patient should eat a snack consisting of complex carbohydrates and proteins (for example, milk and crackers) or eat the next meal if it is due. Ascertain the reason for hypoglycemia if possible, and monitor the patient more frequently, until duration of the action of the hypoglycemic agent is completed.

The signs and symptoms of the Somogyi phenomenon can be those normally seen with hypoglycemia, but frequently they consist only of nighttime sweats, nightmares, and a headache on arising. There may be weight gain in the presence of glycosuria, no glucose but ketone bodies in the urine (counterinsulin hormones stimulate lipolysis and beta-oxidation of fats), and wide fluctuations in blood and urine glucose levels unrelated to meals.

Monitoring the blood glucose once or twice during the night can help identify undetected hypoglycemia and help differentiate early morning hyperglycemia from the *dawn phenomenon* from elevated hyperglycemia from insulin-induced hypoglycemia (*Somogyi phenomenon*).

Treatment of Somogyi phenomenon consists of decreasing the insulin dosage. A primary nursing role is to document complaints of hypoglycemia, glucose intake, and laboratory results, and in particular to look for complaints of night sweats, nightmares, and early morning headaches. Correlating these complaints and laboratory results with the time of meals and insulin type and dosage will also help to identify the phenomenon.

Correcting acute metabolic crises

Diabetic ketoacidosis (DKA) and hyperosmolar nonketotic coma (HHNC) are medical emergencies that require intensive nursing care. Therapy is directed toward correction of hyperglycemia, dehydration, electrolyte imbalances, acidosis, and precipitating factors. All of these interventions should occur simultaneously. Intense monitoring is necessary to evaluate treatment effects. Review Table 28-11, on p. 786 for the differences in symptoms of DKA and HHNC.

Insulin. Insulin replacement is based on one or a combination of several indices of insulin deficit (see Box 28-17).

A low-dose insulin system of treatment is usually used for DKA. It includes the use of intravenous push and continuous intravenous infusion of regular insulin. *Regular insulin is the only insulin that may be given intravenously.* The low-dose regimen includes a bolus of 10 to 20 units of regular insulin given by intravenous push and then regular insulin infused continuously at a rate of 10 to 12 units/ hour. Most patients respond well to this regimen. Blood glucose levels should decrease by 50 to 100 mg/dl/hour. In a few patients, insulin resistance may be present, and the hyperglycemia and blood glucose levels do not decrease. This insulin resistance is treated with another bolus of regular insulin or by an increase in the infusion rate. If blood glucose decreases more rapidly than 100 mg/dl, the infused rate will be decreased or even stopped temporarily

and then restored at a lesser dosage. In the past, *high-dose* therapy consisting of an intravenous bolus of 50 to 150 units of regular insulin followed by repeated doses given either intravenously or subcutaneously was used. This form of therapy is not used frequently.

Patients with HHNC will usually be treated with the same low-dose insulin regimen. However, smaller doses of insulin are required.

As blood glucose level decreases and nears 200 to 300 mg/dl, close attention must be given to preventing and detecting the onset of hypoglycemic reactions. As hyperglycemia subsides, insulin resistance decreases and insulin sensitivity increases. For this reason the nurse should be more alert at this time for the symptoms of hypoglycemia and expect changes in insulin dosage that reflect the decreasing blood glucose levels.

Fluid and electrolyte replacement. The patient with HHNC may have a fluid deficit of 8 to 12 L, and the patient with DKA a deficit of 3 to 5 L. To correct the *dehydration and sodium deficit,* normal saline solution or 0.45% saline (half-strength normal saline) solution is given intravenously. Initially, the solution is infused rapidly and at a rate of 1 to 3 L/hr or more in adults without cardiac or renal failure. When the urine output is 1 to 2 ml/min and the blood pressure is stable, the rate is reduced to 1 L in 2 to 4 hours. When the blood glucose level falls to 300 mg/ dl, 5% glucose solutions are used. Monitor the patient very carefully for signs of fluid overload.

Potassium is not initially added to the intravenous fluids because the serum potassium level is usually *elevated* at the beginning of therapy in the patient with DKA, even though total body stores of potassium are depleted. With correction of the dehydration, acidosis, and insulin deficit, potassium moves back into cells and urinary excretion of potassium increases. *Hypokalemia* can develop rapidly. Serum potassium levels and ECG tracings are monitored to determine when potassium should be added.

The administration of fluids and insulin usually corrects the acidosis in DKA so that bicarbonate administration is seldom needed. Bicarbonate is not usually given unless serum bicarbonate is 5 mEq/L and blood pH is <7.

An additional electrolyte imbalance that may develop during ketoacidosis is *hypophosphatemia*. Without adequate phosphorus, decreased peripheral oxygen delivery and additional tissue anoxia may result. Phosphorus in the form of potassium phosphate may be given.

Nursing interventions planned for the patient depend on the severity of the clinical findings and the prescribed therapy. In all patients, careful and frequent monitoring of the following is necessary:
1. Vital signs
2. Level of consciousness
3. Intake and output
4. Resolution of other signs of dehydration and acidosis
5. Serum potassium levels and ECG changes
6. Signs and symptoms of fluid overload
7. Blood glucose and ketone bodies

The nurse must make sure that the specimens are collected as ordered and that the appropriate tests are done. It is important to document test results. The assessments made

---

28-17

Indices of insulin deficit

pH value <7.35
Blood glucose level
Degree of ketonemia
Clinical findings, including degree of coma

by the nurse and the results of laboratory tests will be used to make appropriate adjustments in therapy. A flow sheet with all pertinent laboratory and assessment data is instituted so that all changes in the patient's status are displayed in a readily comprehensible manner.

Treatment of precipitating condition. As therapy for acute metabolic imbalance begins (insulin, fluid and electrolyte replacement), attention is given to detecting and treating concurrent illness. Sometimes the precipitating factor is not determined until treatment is well under way and the patient is recovered from coma sufficiently to give a history of preceding events. Sometimes family members can give insight into possible etiology. A common cause of DKA and HHNC is infection. Antibiotic therapy should begin after specimens for culture and sensitivity of urine, sputum, wound drainage, or blood are obtained.

Should lack of knowledge or of compliance be implicated in DKA or HHNC, begin patient education or counseling as soon as the patient has recovered enough to be comfortable and is feeling well enough to learn or to explore causes of noncompliance.

Promoting safety and well-being. The patient with severe insulin deficit is critically ill and requires excellent nursing. Skilled care involves attending to the following:
1. Required monitoring (as discussed previously)
2. Prescribed therapeutic measures
3. Maintenance of airway in an unconscious patient
4. Frequent turning, mouth care, and skin care
5. Side rails and hand restraints, if necessary, to maintain intravenous lines and ensure patient safety
6. Attention to discomforts of abdominal pain, nausea, and vomiting usually present in the conscious patient
7. Maintenance of nutrition
   a. Fluids first when able to take something by mouth
   b. Solid foods as soon as possible to improve gastric tone
8. Maintenance of the flow sheet
9. Reassurance about care
10. Meeting psychologic needs of patient and family

Minimizing disruption of diabetes treatment

Disruption of blood glucose control often occurs when patients with diabetes are scheduled for surgery or diagnostic tests or when there is an intercurrent illness. This is particularly so when insulin or oral hypoglycemics are a part of the daily regimen. Medication, glucose intake, and frequency of monitoring are three measures that may need to be modified so that optimal metabolic balance can be achieved.

Effects of surgery on the person with diabetes. Surgery is a physical and psychologic stressor for anyone. For the person with diabetes mellitus there are additional risks. The stress of surgery can disrupt metabolic control. Persons with diabetes are at increased risk for the following:
1. Infection
2. Impaired wound healing

3. Age-related complications (many persons with NIDDM are elderly)
4. Postsurgical complications from macrovascular and microvascular changes

The person with diabetes mellitus is at risk for developing *hypoglycemia or hyperglycemia* during the perioperative period. During this period, patients usually are not given anything by mouth and are given fluid intravenously. This decreases total caloric intake and may also decrease insulin needs. However, the effects of surgery on counterregulatory hormones may increase the need for additional insulin. The stressors of surgery cause the release of ACTH, glucocorticoids, and catecholamines, all of which can elevate serum glucose levels.

Management of the diabetic person undergoing surgery. See Box 28-18 for modifications of therapy during the perioperative period. To minimize the disruption in metabolic control, the patient's metabolism should be thoroughly regulated before surgery. Maintain the normal food, fluid, and medication routine until the night before surgery. After surgery, perform blood glucose checks on an every 4 to 6 hour schedule; the results are used to determine the amount of insulin needed. Urine checks for ketones may also be done. To prevent starvation ketosis, all diabetic persons should receive 125 to 250 g carbohydrate/day until they resume a normal diet.

Care during surgery and diagnostic tests. When fasting is necessary, take care to avert hypoglycemia in the person who takes insulin or an oral hypoglycemic agent. Clarify orders as necessary to ensure that glucose is available while insulin is acting. Sometimes insulin administration is delayed until the patient finishes a specific test and can resume eating. When fasting must be prolonged for a diagnostic test or for surgery, provide caloric intake by intravenous infusion. The minimum intake recommended to prevent hypoglycemia and starvation ketosis and to provide basic energy requirements is 250 g/24 hr. An intravenous flow rate of a 5% glucose solution at a rate of 5 to 10 g of glucose per hour is commonly used. Frequent monitoring of blood glucose levels is very helpful in determining proper rates and concentrations of intravenous fluids containing glucose and the required dosages of insulin to maintain metabolic control.

It is routine to schedule diagnostic tests or surgery for diabetic patients early in the morning to minimize the amount of disruption in their regimen.

In general, surgery and anesthesia exert a diabetogenic effect as a result of the increased secretion of counterregulatory hormones (ACTH, glucagon, glucocorticoids, and catecholamines). Insulin resistance increases; in fact, insulin requirements may increase more in patients with NIDDM than in those with IDDM.[29] Decompensation of carbohydrate, fat, and protein metabolism is possible under the stressors of surgery and anesthesia, and the metabolic crises of DKA or HHNC may develop. Patients who have not needed insulin to control their NIDDM may require insulin during the perioperative period, and insulin-requiring patients often need additional dosages to maintain adequate control of hyperglycemia.

The person with diabetes during the perioperative period

Diabetics who receive insulin
  Preoperative
    Intravenous infusion of glucose on morning
      of surgery
    One-half usual insulin dose subcutaneously
  Intraoperative
    Monitoring of blood glucose levels if surgery
      is lengthy
    Additional insulin or glucose as needed
  Postoperative
    Intravenous infusion of glucose until food can
      be taken orally
    Insulin given subcutaneously in equally di-
      vided doses over 24 hours or added to in-
      travenous fluids
    Blood glucose and urine ketones monitored
      every 4 to 6 hours
    Additional insulin given if indicated from
      monitoring
Diabetics not normally given insulin
  Preoperative
    Intravenous infusion of glucose on morning
      of surgery
  Postoperative
    Blood glucose and urine ketone levels moni-
      tored every 4 to 6 hours
    Insulin given if indicated from monitoring
All diabetics
  125 to 250 g CHO/day until normal diet re-
    sumed
  Normal regimen reinsituted as soon as possible
  Continued monitoring of blood glucose and
    urine ketone levels even after usual diet re-
    sumed (increased insulin may be needed be-
    cause of catabolism from surgery)

There are additional risks for the patient with diabetes who has vascular or neurologic complications. Perform a thorough cardiovascular-renal-cerebral evaluation before surgery. The presence of any complication may necessitate additional evaluation and treatment before surgery, during surgery, and postoperatively. For example, the loss of neuroreflexes in patients with autonomic neuropathy may compromise cardiovascular and pulmonary function during anesthesia.[48] *"Silent" myocardial infarctions occur most often in diabetic patients.* Forty percent of diabetic patients have hypertension; a history of hypertension and antihypertensive drug therapy is taken into account in the selection of anesthesia and the management of hemodynamic changes during surgery.

Disruption of metabolic control places diabetic patients at higher risk for infection and for problems in wound healing. Compromised wound healing may occur because of impairments in cellular repair, phagocytosis, and fibroplastic proliferation.[58]

There are several protocols for perioperative management of insulin, fluids and electrolytes, and caloric intake in the patient with diabetes. Differences in management may occur because of the nature of the surgery (inpatient/outpatient, short/long, minor/major); the nature of anesthesia (type, length), and whether patients have used insulin or hypoglycemic agents before surgery. For example, the patient with well-controlled NIDDM, scheduled early in the day for outpatient tooth extraction, may not require any special modification of the diabetic regime except fasting after midnight, delay of insulin or oral hypoglycemic agent, and no food intake until after the surgery. (Intermediate-acting insulins are not acting during early morning; thus, the patient might be instructed to take the usual dose of NPH insulin and omit regular insulin before coming to the surgical center.)

In contrast, a patient with IDDM scheduled for cardiac bypass surgery requires significant modification of insulin and caloric intake throughout the perioperative period. Not only can extended length of surgery, anesthesia, and recovery be expected; but this type of surgery markedly increases requirements for insulin.[29]

Controversy exists about the best way to manage insulin regimens for patients undergoing major surgery. Still common is the practice of giving about 50% of the intermediate insulin dosage by subcutaneous injection before surgery and supplementing it with regular insulin during and after surgery as indicated by glucose monitoring. Increasingly recommended is intravenous administration of regular insulin only. The absorption of insulin from subcutaneous tissue becomes even more erratic when fluid shifts and hemodynamic changes occur as a result of anesthesia and surgery.[29]

Controversy also exists about the best way to administer insulin intravenously during the operative period and postoperatively. Physicians may order regular insulin to be given by bolus or by fixed-rate or variable-rate infusions. Better metabolic control has been reported with variable-rate infusions of glucose containing insulin and potassium.[29]

Three factors that affect the postoperative recommendations for management of insulin dosage are (1) postoperative dietary intake, (2) postoperative nausea and vomiting, and (3) the ability to use the results of capillary blood glucose monitoring. Although sliding scale insulin protocols are still in common use, the use of insulin logarithms, which better predict the doses of insulin required,[29] is increasing.

Care during concurrent illness. Concurrent illness may also disrupt diabetes control. All illnesses influence the status of diabetes control. In most instances the person with diabetes needs increased insulin in the presence of a concurrent illness, especially infection. Yet many mistakenly believe that if they cannot eat they do not need to take the prescribed insulin or oral hypoglycemic agent. *Failure of patients with IDDM to take insulin when ill is a frequent cause of ketoacidosis.* These persons should take their insulin and *carbohydrate* in some form.

"Sick days" is the name given to times when the person with diabetes feels ill and may have anorexia, nausea, and malaise and yet have no defined illness. For one or two sick days, teach the patient to maintain metabolic balance by the following guidelines:

1. Take prescribed dose of insulin.
2. Spread 50% of the daily CHO allowance over 24 hours.
3. Increase fluid intake.
4. Include food items with more simple sugars than regularly allowed, such as custard, nondiet soft drinks, nondiet gelatin.
5. Advance diet toward the normally prescribed diet as soon as possible.
6. Institute blood glucose and urine ketone monitoring on a more frequent basis.

The person must know when to call the primary health care provider. Each person will receive individual instructions, but in general the primary health care provider should be called if any of the following occur:

1. A full day's urine glucose test results are at maximum readings or blood glucose levels are consistently elevated beyond a specified level, often 200 mg/dl
2. Ketone bodies persist in the urine for 6 hours or more
3. The person is not able to take *any* food or fluids for longer than 4 hours
4. The person is febrile

Interventions to achieve patient outcomes
Preventing fluid deficit

Dehydration is a potentially dangerous sequella of hyperglycemia, and it is a corollary to the metabolic crises of diabetes: DKA and HHNC. An insulin deficit is the basic feature of both of these life-threatening states. The usual monitoring of fluid balance for any patient includes measuring weight, intake and output, and excessive losses from polyuria, vomitus, diarrhea, drainage, and so on. These measurements are as important in the diabetic patient as they are in any patient; however, in the diabetic patient, the monitoring of blood glucose and urinary ketones also is essential in order to detect, prevent and correct an insulin deficit. Report evidence of dehydration or hyperglycemia above 200 mg/dl to the physician and obtain directions for fluid replacement and insulin coverage.

Oral or intravenous fluids are necessary to compensate for excess losses that occur in the osmotic diuresis of glycosuria. When fluid intake is adequate, and when the renal threshold for glucose is normal, the patient can maintain a normal glomerular filtration rate (GFR) and is able to clear excess glucose and, to some extent, ketoacids from the extracellular fluids.[37] Decreases in GFR caused by volume depletion lead quickly to metabolic decompensation.

Patients who have age-related high renal thresholds for glucose or who have renal disease lack this "safety valve" of glycosuria and are at higher risk for developing hyperosmolar imbalance. Teach patients experiencing sick days to attempt to drink at least 8 ounces of fluids every hour they are awake.[37] Because they need to replenish electrolytes as well, these fluids should include soups, broths, colas, Gatorade, and so on, and not just water. It is essential to provide frail elderly or disabled persons with access to an adequate fluid intake, because they are at particular risk for HHNC.

28-19

Components of diabetes education

1. Definition of disease (general facts)
2. Nutrition
3. Activity (exercise)
4. Medication
5. Monitoring glucose control
6. Hypoglycemia
7. Illness
8. Psychologic adjustment
9. Hygiene and foot care
10. Follow-up
11. Community resources
12. Benefits and responsibilities of care
13. Relationship between nutrition, exercise, and medications
14. Complications
15. Use of health care systems.

Facilitating learning

An integral part of the treatment of diabetes mellitus is education of patients so they can assume responsibility for required self-care, including seeking medical advice or treatment when needed. Teaching should begin at the time of diagnosis and continue until the patient is competent in maintaining an optimal level of wellness. The American Association of Diabetes Educators has proposed 15 components for the educational program. (See Box 28-19)

Previous sections discussed the educational content of many of these components, particularly numbers 1 to 7 and number 14. The other components are discussed in this section along with suggested approaches to teaching.

The Association further proposes planning educational programs for diabetic persons in the following three phases:

1. *Initial management,* in which the knowledge and skills needed to survive are emphasized
2. *Home management,* in which patients learn to be self-sufficient in the daily management of the disease
3. *Improvement of life-style,* in which patients learn how to enrich their lives by gaining flexibility in management, insight, and self-determination

The three phases of diabetes education are illustrated in Table 28-25 for one component. Each phase is specified by objectives and the requisite knowledges, skills, and attitudes. The nurse should begin teaching about initial management before introducing more complex home management content. Evaluation of learning and reinforcement should be part of the plan.

It is important to set priorities in teaching and begin with the most basic information.

For example, when insulin is newly prescribed, teaching the patient how to administer insulin safely and accurately takes precedence over the other components, and related survival skills must be taught before more advanced content. The nurse would focus first on teaching the patient to:

1. Identify the prescribed insulin
2. Check the expiration date

Table 28-25   Phases of diabetes education

Initial management	Home management	Improvement of life-style
Survival knowledge and skills	Self-sufficiency in daily management of diabetes	Enrichment of life by flexibility in management, insight, and self-determination

Objectives for the component—definition of diabetes

Initial management	Home management	Improvement of life-style
States need for insulin in body Describes what happens in body when insulin is deficient States simple working definition of diabetes States role of food, activity, and medication in treatment of diabetes	Lists symptoms of diabetes Explains relationship of symptoms to insulin deficiency States how diagnosis of diabetes is made IDDM: States relationship of undernutrition to insulin deficiency NIDDM: States relationship between state of overnutrition, inactivity, and relative insulin deficiency	Identifies significance of hyperglycemia in relation to other metabolic problems and long-term complications States significance of hyperglycemia and glycosuria, or vice versa, relative to changes in renal threshold Lists main differences between insulin-dependent and non–insulin-dependent diabetes States current knowledge of hereditary aspects of diabetes Verbalizes concerns about diabetes in other family members

From A Joint Task Force for the American Diabetes Association and the American Association of Diabetes Educators, Spring 1979, American Diabetes Association.

3. Prepare and administer an accurate dose using sterile technique
4. Never change the insulin dosage, strength, type, species without the physician's direction
5. Plan the purchase, storage, and disposal of insulin and syringes and needles
6. Prevent, recognize, and treat hypoglycemia

It would be inappropriate when first introducing insulin therapy to teach about the various kinds of insulin or the different insulin regimes that are used.

It is also important to individualize the teaching plan according to the assessed needs for learning. All patients with diabetes need to be assessed for learning needs. It is important to understand that many patients who have had diabetes for years may not have adequate education or have not updated their knowledge and skills for some time. It is only through an individual assessment that the nurse can identify the specific knowledge, skills, and attitudes that require intervention.

There are usually assessment guides and teaching tools within a nursing department or agency that can facilitate teaching. Often, diabetes educators who can provide access to teaching materials and serve as consultants are available. If there is a centralized diabetes education program, promptly refer the patient and plan for collaborative efforts between staff nurses and the teaching team.

With short hospital stays, begin teaching as soon as the patient is judged ready to learn. Some interventions must be planned early by making appointments for specific times. These include:

1. Dietary consultation
2. Attendance at groups classes, if available
3. Involvement of family members in particular sessions

The teaching plan should clearly delineate when initial instruction and reinforcement is to take place for each of the components selected for teaching. If specific outcomes are clearly identified for the individual patient, evaluation

The Elderly with Diabetes Mellitus

Assessment

Assess for signs of diabetes mellitus; the elderly may have a history of recent weight loss, decreased vision, urinary tract infection, or mental changes rather than classic symptoms of diabetes mellitus.

Assess vision and ability to ambulate.

Monitor weight of elderly persons; Type 2 diabetes mellitus (NIDDM) is associated with obesity.

Monitor glucose levels; glucose levels may be tolerated at higher levels than in younger adults.

Intervention

Encourage regular exercise, such as paced walking, to decrease hyperglycemia and increase calorie expenditure.

Encourage a diet that promotes weight reduction if obesity is present.

Be aware that the elderly person with diabetes mellitus may have vision changes and plan care accordingly.

Teach patient to maintain hydration and eat prescribed diet (even when not hungry) to prevent hypoglycemic epsiodes (anorexia is common in the elderly).

Teach patient or significant other management of oral hypoglycemics (or insulin if used), diet, and blood sugar testing.

Teach importance of foot care to decrease potential of gangrene; the elderly person may have concurrent peripheral vascular problems.

Common complications in elderly

Vascular degeneration in kidneys, eyes, heart, and legs from lipidemia (causing atherosclerosis) and hyperglycemia

Infections and ulcers of the lower extremities

Cerebral vascular accidents

can be facilitated and needed modifications put in place as necessary.

Initial instruction for a hospitalized patient with newly diagnosed diabetes should encompass three factors:

1. Expected length of stay
2. Specific referrals for further teaching
3. Other concerns and teaching needs not related to diabetes self-care

Teaching sessions should include mutual planning and goal setting. Patients with diabetes often report that their education was "too much and too fast." Teaching approaches and methods need to be modified according to the learning style, motivation, and comfort level of the patient. Eliciting feedback from the patient during the instruction will help identify correct pace and depth and allow modifications to be made as needed.

Some teaching can focus on ongoing care activities: for example, plans should specify that foot care instruction be given along with foot care and that instruction related to blood glucose monitoring and medications be gradually introduced as these tasks are performed. Flow sheet information relating to status of diabetes and its treatment can be shared to illustrate the interactions of food, medication, illness, and so on. The patient can be helped to keep his or her own flow sheet at the bedside. This can serve as an introduction to the type of records to be kept after discharge.

Written materials should be selected carefully for accuracy and relevance to the individual's learning needs and reading level. For example, the patient with NIDDM need not be given materials that discuss the management of IDDM. Written materials should always be introduced to reinforce or amplify previous instruction. After the patient has read the materials, provide an opportunity to answer questions and clarify any misconceptions.

Follow-up. The many teaching needs of the person with diabetes mellitus have been discussed. Education is an integral part of therapy and must be planned over a period of time if the patient is to be capable of diabetes management. The knowledge and skills necessary for self-care are summarized in Box 28-20. Teaching usually begins at the time of diagnosis, but the nurse must be aware that everything cannot be learned during the first contact. Priorities need to be set: teach the person the skills necessary to meet immediate needs, and then refer to an ambulatory setting or home health care agency. Follow-up might take place in a clinic, physician's or nurse's office, or in a program sponsored by the local diabetes association or a local hospital.

In addition to securing follow-up education appointments, the nurse can do the following:

1. Reinforce the value and need of continued learning
2. Encourage family members to participate
3. Give the patient written instructions and educational literature
4. Ensure that the patient has a resource person to call if assistance is needed before the next appointment

Give the patient local sources of information, such as the public library and the local diabetes association, as well as specific appointment information.

28-20

Summary of knowledge and skills for adequate self-care of diabetes mellitus (survival level)

Basic understanding of diabetes mellitus and how metabolism is changed by it

Therapeutic regimen prescribed and how it works to keep the blood sugar level normal

Diet ordered (calories, CHO, and such), how to calculate diet requirements for each meal, ability to incorporate personal preferences

Exercise and its effect on caloric and insulin needs, and how to manage if exercise level is increased above usual

If receiving insulin:
   Type, amount, timing, method of administration
   Ability to give the insulin accurately
   Ability to care for equipment properly

If receiving oral hypoglycemic agents:
   Type, dosage, time schedule
   Potential side effects
   What to do if new or unexpected symptoms occur

Self-monitoring routine for glucose status (urine ketone and serum glucose monitoring):
   How to do the tests accurately
   What to do if results show hyperglycemia, ketonuria, or hypoglycemia
   How to care for equipment and supplies

Signs and symptoms of hypoglycemia, how to treat them, and what to do if they occur frequently

Signs and symptoms of hyperglycemia and what to do when they occur

How to manage diabetes mellitus on days when usual diet cannot be eaten because of illness

Measures to prevent lower extremity trauma or injury

Type of follow-up care necessary and whom to contact with questions

---

Promoting adherence to diabetic regime

The ability of the patient with diabetes mellitus to manage self-care at an optimal level on a daily basis is not only based on knowledge and skills, but on motivation, willingness, and ability to make behavioral changes. Many of these changes include those that are recommended for all people and are related to food intake, regular exercise, and participation in regular screening examinations. For the person with diabetes, however, failure to integrate the diabetes regimen into daily life leads to more frequent and more severe complications.

Adherence to the diabetes regimen may mean changing existing health behaviors for life. This change involves disruption of belief structures and organized patterns of living (eating, activity) and incorporation of new beliefs and patterns of behavior. For example, in IDDM, the requirement for insulin necessitates some loss in spontaneity and more attention to consistency in meal times and exercise. In the obese person with NIDDM, the requirement to lose weight and to maintain weight loss requires reordering caloric intake and caloric expenditure, both of which involve giving up some behaviors, changing some, and incorporating new ones into daily life patterns. Inability to make these changes independently and to maintain the changed behavior may be related to emotional responses, family conflicts, economic barriers, and perceived problems in communication with health care providers.

The emotional impact of the disease on the patient and the family can lead to nonadherence. Emotional responses to diabetes affect the patient's motivation and capacity to make changes. One researcher has described three phases of health and functioning in NIDDM[30]:

1. Up to 1 year post diagnosis. This phase involves a sense of helplessness, anxiety, and/or anger. During this time, increased feelings of vulnerability to illness, loss of function, amputation, and disabilities occur along with decreases in self-esteem. Depression may occur. Anxieties about work and marital roles and social functioning may persist. Patients who are over 40 may for the first time be confronted with a sense of their own mortality.
2. Middle phase of management. Characterized by relative well-being and functioning.
3. Final phase, for some. Adjustment to one or more permanent physical complications and physical impairments. Feelings of depression, anxiety, and helplessness coincide with the stressors associated with learning to adapt to the complication(s).

Patients and family members may receive some comfort by learning how adherence to blood glucose control can lead to benefits such as increased vigor and sense of well-being and a decrease in acute illness episodes. In addition, blood glucose control is the best means for preventing vascular and neurologic damage. Patients may be reassured by knowing that most people experience emotional distress on learning that they are diabetic, and that they may expect to feel more comfortable as they experience living with this chronic disease and becoming proficient in its management. Referral to a specialized counselor is helpful when severe or prolonged emotional responses interfere with quality of life or with carrying out the prescribed treatment measures.

Adherence is best promoted when the family and the patient work collaboratively on the tasks involved in managing this chronic illness. Integration of a diabetes regimen into one's life-style involves not only the person with diabetes, but also the family members. Sometimes compliance with the diabetic regime serves as a focal point for interpersonal conflicts. This is typically illustrated by the teenage patient's noncompliance being the focus for parent-teen conflicts about independence. Conflicts may be just as overt in the adult person and family; food often serves as an available forum for focusing interpersonal conflicts. Family members can be helped to assume supportive roles by involvement in educational programs and support groups. Specialized counseling can also be useful to patients and family members if dysfunctional behavior persists.

Adherence to diabetic regimes may be made more difficult when there are economic barriers. Restriction of access to health care, employment, and health insurance are problems for many patients with diabetes. Sometimes the problem can be ameliorated when the physician can document that the diabetes is under excellent control and that measures to prevent complication are being used. Encourage patients to consult their local diabetes association to obtain information about these issues and to seek guidance from their specific caregivers about certain cost-saving measures. For example, patients can split SBM testing strips, reuse syringes and needles, and decrease the frequency of SBM from that originally recommended.

Effective interpersonal communication is necessary between the patient and the health care provider in any chronic illness. A barrier to adherence exists if the patient perceives goals or recommendations as not achieveable yet is unable to share this perception with the health care provider. Help the patient to be assertive in asking questions, describing barriers, and seeking resources to improve their ability to maintain health.

There has been an increasing trend in diabetes treatment and education to use behavioral modification techniques and contracting, particularly in approaches to diet and exercise. Steps include selecting an achievable goal, selecting one or two behavioral changes, and using monitoring and positive reinforcement of the behavior.[32,49]

Persons can be referred to groups focused on weight loss, such as Weight Watchers, or support groups sponsored by local diabetes associations, where the focus arises out of the expressed needs of the group participants. These groups often include topics such as psychologic responses, socioeconomic strategies and handling of interpersonal conflicts, and information about current therapy. Formal programs in diabetes education may include follow-up group sessions for reinforcement of learning. At some agencies, recheck clinics are held at intervals and include laboratory testing, consultation, and planned instruction.

In addition to group activities, patients can be encouraged to subscribe to *Diabetes Forecast*,* a magazine published monthly by the American Diabetes Association for the lay public. This magazine gives current information about the disease and its treatment and focuses on the incorporation of diabetes self-care into daily life. It has an annual issue that compares various diabetic equipment and supplies, including costs.

Evaluation

Questions that guide the nurse's evaluation derive from an understanding of potential effects of diabetes mellitus on physical well-being, the importance of education for self-management of blood glucose control, and the psychologic impact of this chronic disease and its treatment.

Specific goals or objectives for each patient identify the intended outcomes of health care.

1. What level of blood glucose control has been achieved?
2. Has ideal weight been achieved or maintained?
3. Has the patient developed sufficient skill to be independent and safely carry out self-management of

---

*American Diabetes Association, 1660 Duke St. Alexandria, VA 22314.

Nursing Care Plan	**Person with diabetes mellitus**

DATA: Mrs. T. is an obese, 52-year-old married woman with NIDDM diagnosed 3 years ago. She was referred to a short-term ambulatory diabetes education program by her physician for instruction on insulin administration, since she had not achieved blood glucose control with dietary measures and oral agents.

The nursing history identified the following:

1. Mrs. T. saw referral as necessary but perceived it and the inability to control weight and blood glucose as a personal failure.
2. She maintained inconsistent sleep/activity schedule. (Worked as an LPN 8 PM to 8 AM Saturday and Sunday with 2 to 4 hours sleep during day; arose at 8 AM and retired at 11 PM on other days.)
3. She had accurate knowledge about dietary modifications and had participated successfully in several weight reduction programs with 20- to 40-pound weight loss each time.
4. She does not exercise consistently.
5. She has performed blood glucose monitoring on others and once or twice on self.
6. She states that work is important to her; she derives satisfactions from work group socialization and says it "keeps me busy."
7. She fears that her husband will die suddenly at home. Two years ago she performed CPR when he had a cardiac arrest at home. Realizes that she maintains work schedule "to keep me from worrying about my husband."

Objective data included blood glucose, 220 mg/dl; weight, 200 lb; height, 5'4"; BP 134/84; urine glucose 2% with no ketones present.

Collaborative nursing actions include teaching Mrs. T. those measures that would help her achieve control of blood glucose (insulin, diet, and exercise) and to detect, prevent, and treat hypoglycemic reactions. The nurse reported Mrs. T.'s work schedule to the physician and asked for insulin dosage alterations on weekends. The physician was unaware of her work schedule and stated that blood glucose control could not be optimum with this schedule.

Nursing diagnosis: **Knowledge deficit: self-injections, self–blood glucose monitoring related to lack of exposure**

Expected patient outcomes	Nursing interventions	Rationale
Mrs. T. will independently administer to self	Support Mrs. T. as necessary to self-inject insulin	Adults who perform this task have minimal discomfort and realize they are capable of giving own insulin
Mrs. T. will perform blood glucose monitoring (BGM) accurately	Observe patient's skill in BGM; correct as necessary	Evaluation of patient technique is necessary to ensure accuracy
Mrs. T. will use measurements obtained by BGM to achieve fasting blood glucose below 140 mg/dl	Review with Mrs. T. the effect of activity, dietary intake, and insulin on blood glucose. Instruct patient on frequency and timing of BGM	BGM gives immediate feedback about previous behaviors and reinforces value of therapeutic measures
Mrs. T. can detect and treat hypoglycemia	Review with Mrs. T. signs and symptoms and treatment measures	This knowledge assures that patient can safely give own insulin and decreases fear of a reaction
	Refer to dietician for modification of diet necessary with insulin, and for verification of diet knowledge	The dietician is the appropriate person to teach about diet

Nursing diagnosis: Altered health maintenance: related to ineffective coping skill

Expected patient outcomes	Nursing interventions	Rationale
Mrs. T. will state at least one change that will improve blood glucose control	Teach Mrs. T. effects of stress, lack of exercise, and activity pattern on blood glucose	If Mrs. T. understands how stress impairs health, likelihood of change is more likely
	Explore with Mrs. T. willingness and ability to change behaviors: sleep/activity, coping, and exercise	Goals are more likely to be achieved if Mrs. T. makes realistic choices after considering cost and benefits
	Engage Mrs. T. in mutual problem solving; refrain from prescribing	Increasing Mrs. T.'s sense of control can help with self-esteem and enhance attitudes toward change
	Explore sources for long-term support in learning more effective coping skills. Suggest support groups: 1. For spouses of patients with myocardial infarction 2. For weight loss *and maintenance* of weight loss 3. Available at work in health service program	Changing life-style, eating behaviors, and coping skills are very difficult; support over long periods of time is usually required
	Suggest to Mrs. T. that she seek a trial period on day shift on weekends	Trial period can help Mrs. T. make informed choices about work schedule in attaining goals

the disease in terms of administration of insulin injections or oral hypoglycemic agents, treatment of hypoglycemic reactions, and foot care?

4. Is proper foot care practiced? Is skin integrity present?
5. Has the patient maintained fluid balance?
6. Is the patient equipped with knowledge and skills to make decisions about food, exercise, medications, and when to seek medical advice?
7. Is the patient committed to prevention of short- and long-term complications (follow-up, self-management)?
8. Is the patient coping with diabetes self-care measures, fears and concerns, and life-style changes?

SUMMARY

1. Diabetes mellitus is a complex metabolic disorder and may be clinically expressed as non-insulin dependent diabetes mellitus (NIDDM) and as insulin-dependent diabetes mellitus (IDDM) in persons with onset generally before age 40.
2. Insulin deficit is a central feature of the disease; insulin deficit may be *absolute* when beta cells do not secrete insulin; or *relative*, when beta cell defect and peripheral resistance to insulin is present.
3. Glucagon excess and increase in other antagonists to insulin contribute to the hyperglycemia; these are increased during the stress response.
4. Measures to prevent and treat obesity are the focus of primary prevention of NIDDM; screening to detect persons who are undiagnosed (50%) is the focus of secondary prevention.
5. Insulin deficit and hyperglycemia lead to many immediate alterations in metabolism: hyperosmolarity and osmotic diuresis, glycosuria, cellular starvation, calorie loss, and increased fat metabolism and catabolism.
6. Diabetic ketoacidosis *(DKA)* and hyperglycemic, hyperosmolar, nonketotic coma *(HHNC)* are two life-threatening situations that occur in diabetes mellitus.
7. The duration of hyperglycemia seems a major predictor of the development of microvascular lesions (nephropathy, retinopathy), macrovascular lesions (atherosclerotic disease), and neuropathy.
8. Amputation in diabetes mellitus can result as a consequence of alterations in blood vessels and nerves, tissue trauma, and infection occurring in persons with inadequate skin integrity and insensitivity to pain or pressure. Proper foot care can reduce the risk of amputation.
9. Because patients must be capable in diabetes management, nursing assessment must address the knowledge and coping skills of a patient early in hospitalization so that appropriate education and counseling can proceed.
10. A well-educated person with diabetes will be assertive in describing special needs relating to patterns of food intake, exercise, monitoring, medications, and foot care.
11. Assessment of the person with diabetes includes collecting objective data about metabolic status, cardiovascular-renal status, vision, and nerve function. The lower extremities should be carefully examined.
12. Dietary recommendations in diabetes mellitus include the following: calorie distribution of CHO (55% to 60%), fat (20% to 30%) with restriction in saturated fat to 10%, and protein (20%); limitation of cholesterol, sodium, and refined simple CHO; and increased use of complex, unrefined CHO.
13. The three primary modalities of treatment of diabetes mellitus are diet, exercise, and hypoglycemic agents; education for self-management of these modalities is an integral part of treatment.
14. Exercise has a hypoglycemic action in most instances; but, it can increase hyperglycemia if blood glucose levels are very high or if exercise is intense. Exercise also aids in cardiovascular fitness and weight reduction and weight maintenance programs, and it decreases peripheral resistance.
15. Nurses and patients must be careful to use prescribed insulin: strength, species, length of action, purity.
16. The oral hypoglycemic agents used in NIDDM stimulate pancreatic beta cell secretion and decrease peripheral resistance. They may induce hypoglycemia.
17. Patients using insulin pump therapy or multiple injections always self-monitor blood glucose. These technologies make it possible to achieve normoglycemia in well-educated patients.
18. Hemoglobin Al_C measures the amount of glycosylation of normal hemoglobin A; it correlates with average blood glucose levels over the past 2 to 3 months.
19. The treatment of hypoglycemia must be prompt; give 10 to 15 g of simple CHO as soon as symptoms are detected. The first signs present are those of epinephrine excess; later signs are those of cerebral dysfunction.
20. Insulin or oral hypoglycemic agents should not be omitted when short illness occurs; about 50% of daily CHO intake should be distributed over 24 hours.
21. The impact of the diagnosis of diabetes mellitus and living with this chronic illness may be expressed by patients emotionally, in concerns about the future, in patient-family conflicts, and in noncompliance.
22. The treatment of DKA and HHNC requires replacement of insulin, fluids, and electrolytes; treatment of precipitating conditions; and monitoring and supportive nursing care of these acutely ill patients.
23. Patients fasting or undergoing surgery require modifications of insulin and food intake and increased monitoring of metabolic status.
24. Foot care includes daily inspection, measures to maintain integrity of skin, and prevention of injury. Referral to podiatric services is highly recommended.
25. Diabetes education must be individualized and planned over time. Initial instruction should be restricted to "survival skills" and beginning home management skills with referral for continued education.
26. An educational program for persons with diabetes mellitus has 15 components: these components include knowledge, skills, and attitudes for effective diabetes management (p. 812).

27. Evaluation of nursing interventions includes assessment of whether the metabolic balance is improved, whether the patient has the requisite knowledge and coping skills for self-management, and whether appropriate referrals were made.

STUDY QUESTIONS

- What are the major differences between insulin-dependent (IDDM) and non-insulin-dependent (NIDDM) diabetes mellitus?
- What information needs to be included on an assessment guide to elicit information about risks for metabolic crises, vascular and neurologic complications of diabetes mellitus, and nonadherence to prescribed regimen?
- What foods should be chosen for a day's diabetic diet to meet recommendations of the American Diabetes Association?
- What would be included in a teaching plan for a 22-year-old newly diagnosed person with IDDM and how would this differ for a 68-year-old person with NIDDM?
- What are the patient problems posed by "strict" versus "loose" control of blood glucose?

REFERENCES AND SELECTED READINGS

1. American Diabetes Association: Principles of nutrition and dietary recommendations for individuals with diabetes mellitus, *Diab Care* 10(1):126-132, 1987.
2. American Diabetes Association and American Dietetic Association: *Exchange lists for meal planning*, Alexandria, Va, 1986, The Association.
3. American Diabetes Association: A Position Statement: standards of medical care for patients with diabetes mellitus, *Diab Care* 12:365-368, 1989.
4. Andreoli FE, et al: *Cecil's essentials of medicine*, Philadelphia, 1986, WB Saunders.
5. Benson JW: In Metz R, Larson E (editors): *Blue book of endocrinology*, Philadelphia, 1986, WB Saunders.
6. Bantle JP: Injection site rotation: the downside, *Practical Diabetol* 9(5):1-3, 1990.
7. Beaser RS, Weir GC, Hill J: Diabetes research update, *Diabetes in the News* 10(1):7-1, 1991.
8. Bingham PR, Riddle MC: Combined insulin-sulfonylurea treatment of type II diabetes, *Diab Educator* 15:450-455, 1989.
9.* Brown S: Effects of educational interventions in diabetes care: a meta-analysis of findings, *Nurs Res* 37:223-230, 1988.
10.* Byrnes CA: What's new in the diabetic diet, *Nurs 87* 17(8):58-59, 1987.
11.* Callahan M, Bradley DJ: Why you should teach your diabetic patients to chart, *Nurs 88* 18(3):48-49, 1988.
11a. Christensen MH et al: How to care for the diabetic foot, *Am J Nog* 91(3):50-58, 1991.
12. Davidson MB: Aging: relation to diabetes and carbohydrate metabolism: conclusions, *Diab Spectrum* 2:190-192, 1989.
13. Davidson MB: How to get the most out of insulin therapy, *Clin Diab* 8:565-73, 1990.
14. DeAtkine D, Surwit R, Feinglos M: Stress and diabetes, *Practical Diabetol* 10(5):1-8, 1991.
15. DeFronzo RA: From research to practice: conclusions, *Diab Spectrum* 3:325-328, 1990.

16. Engerman RL, Kern TS: Progression of incipient diabetic retinopathy during good glycemic control, *Diabetes* 36:808-812, 1987.
17. Ferris FL, Early Treatment Diabetic Retinopathy Study Research Group: Photocoagulation for diabetic retinopathy, *JAMA* 266:1263-1265, 1991.
18.* Fondiller S: Meeting the growing challenge of diabetes, *Am J Nurs* 91(11):57-66, 1991.
19. Franz MJ: Evaluating the glycemic response to carbohydrates, *Clin Diab* 11:129-130, 1986.
20.* Gluck SL, Klahr S: Enlarging our view of the diabetic kidney, *N Engl J Med* 324:1662-1664, 1991.
21. Goetz FC, Moudry-Munns K, Sutherland DER: Whole-organ pancreas transplantation in the 1990's, *Clin Diab* 9:33-41, 1991.
22.* Graham C: Exercise in the elderly patient with diabetes, *Practical Diabetol* 10(5):8-11, 1991.
23.* Graham C, Lasko-McCarthey P: Exercise options for persons with diabetic complications, *Diab Educator* 16:212-219, 1990.
23a. Guthrie DW, Guthrie RA: *Nursing management of diabetes mellitus*, ed 3, New York, 1991, Springer.
23b. Guthrie RA: New approaches to improve diabetes control, *Am Family Physician* 43:570-578, 1991.
24. Hanefeld M et al: Therapeutic potentials of acarbose as first-line drug in NIDDM insufficiently treated with diet alone, *Diab Care* 14:732-737, 1991.
25. *Healthy People 2000: National Health Promotion and Disease Prevention Objectives*, US Dept of Health and Human Services, Public Health Service, Washington, DC, 1991.
26. Heins JM, Rosett JW, Davis SG: The new look in diabetic diets, *Am J Nurs* 87:196-199, 1987.
27.* Herget M, Williams A: New aids for low-vision diabetics, *Am J Nurs* 89:1319-1322, 1989.
28. Hernandes CG: The pathophysiology of diabetes mellitus; an update, *Diab Educator* 15:162-168, 1989.
29. Hirsch B, McGill B: Role of insulin in management of surgical patient with diabetes mellitus, *Diab Care* 11:980-991, 1990.
29a. Holmes CS, editor: *Neuropsychological and behavioral aspects of diabetes*, New York, 1990, Springer-Verlag.
30. Holmes DM: The person and diabetes in psychosocial context, *Diab Care* 9:194-206, 1986.
31. Jeweler D, Steinburg C: Finding more clues, *Diab Forecast* 43(9):31-38, 1990.
32. Horton ES: Exercise and decreased risk of NIDDM, *N Engl J Med* 325:196-198, 1991.
33.* Johnson CKH: Measuring blood glucose: does your meter agree with the lab, *Diab Forecast* 44(10):71-72, 1991.
34. Kaplan N: Hyperinsulinemia in diabetes and hypertension, *Clin Diab* 9(1):1-8, 1991.
35. Keegan DJ et al: Fighting diabetes: a global effort, *Diab Forecast* 44(9):35-40, 1991.
36.* Knighton DR et al: Treating diabetic foot ulcers, *Diab Spectrum* 3:51-56, 1990.
37.* Ley B, Goldman D: Sick-day management: preparing for the expected, *Diab Spectrum* 4:173-176, 1991.
38. Levin ME, O'Neal LW, editors: *The diabetic foot*, ed 4, St Louis, 1988, Mosby–Year Book.
39. Lorber DL: Commentary: what is type II diabetes . . . and what else is it, *Practical Diabetol* 9(5):9, 1990.
40. Lorber DL: Nonketotic osmolarity in diabetes, *Practical Diabetol* 10(1):5-9, 1991.
41. Matson MD, Kjellstrand CM: Long-term follow-up of 369 diabetic patients undergoing dialysis, *Arch Intern Med* 148:600-604, 1988.
42. Messana I, Beizer JL: Diabetes in the elderly, *Practical Diabetol* 10(1):1-4, 1991.

*Recommended for student reading.

43. National Institutes of Health: *The national long-range plan to combat diabetes*, DHHS Pub. No. PHS 87-1587, Bethesda, Md, US Dept of Health and Human Services, 1987.

44. Nelson RL: The OBTT: its practical use, *Diab Spectrum* 2:219-223, 1989.

45. Neuman RG, Cohen MP: Testing for microalbuminuria. *Diab Professional*, 90:1-4, 1989.

46.* Newman LG et al: Unsuspected osteomyelitis in diabetic foot ulcers, *JAMA* 266:1246-1251, 1991.

47. Palmer JP: From research to practice: commentary, *Diab Spectrum* 4:211-213, 1991.

47a. Peterson A, Drass J: Managing acute complications of diabetes, *Nursing 91* 21(2):34-40, 1991.

48.* Pfeifer M: Cardiovascular autonomic neuropathy, *Diab Spectrum* 3:18-19, 45-48, 1990.

49. Powers MA: Facilitating nutritional changes in difficult patients, *Diab Spectrum* 4(4):186-192, 1991.

50. Rickabaugh TE: Plan of attack is needed to scale exercise walls, *Diab in News* 10(4):50-51, 1991.

51. Rifkin H, Porte D, editors: *Ellenberg and Rifkin's diabetes mellitus, theory and practice*, ed 4, New York, 1990, Elsevier.

52. Rimoin DL, Rotter JI: Genetics and genetic counseling, *Diab Spectrum* 4:194, 1991.

53. Rost K: Research needs and strategies for the meantime. *Diab Dateline: Bull National Diab Information Clearing House* 9(2):1-2, 1988, US Depart of Health and Human Services, Public Health Service, NIH, Bethesda, Md, 1988.

54. Rossini AA, Mordes JP, Handler EW: A tumbler hypothesis: the autoimmunity of insulin-dependent diabetes mellitus, *Diab Spectrum* 2:195-200, 1989.

55. Saudek MD, Zacur HAA, Pitt HA: Implanted insulin pumps: a status report, *Practical Diabetol* 9(2):18-20, 1990.

56. Scharp DW, Lacy PE: The clinical feasibility of human islet transplantation, *Clin Diab* 9(4):42-45, 1991.

57.* Schwarts MJ et al: Unsuspected osteomyelitis in diabetic foot ulcers, *JAMA* 266:1246-1251, 1991.

58. Shuman CR: Controlling diabetes during surgery, *Diab Spectrum* 2:263-269, 1989.

59. Sorbinil Retinopathy Trial Research Group: A randomized trial of Sorbinil, an aldose reductase inhibitor, in diabetic retinopathy, *Diab Spectrum* 4:131-141, 1991.

59a. Tandan R et al: Topical capsaicin in painful diabetic neuropathy, *Diabetes Care* 15:8-14, 1992.

60. *The prevention and treatment of complications of diabetes: a guide for primary care practitioners*, Atlanta, 1990, 6-1 to 6-4, US Department of Health and Human Services, Centers for Disease Control.

61. Warshaw H: Sweet nothings; update on sugar substitutes, *Diab Self-Management* 8(2):34-37, 1991.

62.* Winter W: Atypical diabetes in blacks, *Clin Diab* 9(4):49-56, 1991.

63.* Zehrer MS, Hansen R, Bantle J: Reducing blood glucose variability by use of abdominal insulin injection sites, *Diab Educator* 16:474-477, 1990.

Classic

64. Carlyon PE: Diabetic self-injections: analysis or two teaching/learning approaches, unpublished masters thesis, Kent, Ohio, 1980, Kent State University.

65. Gabbay K, O'Sullivan J: The sorbitol pathway: enzyme localization and content in normal and diabetic nerve and cord, *Diabetes* 17:239-243, 1968.

66. Ganda OP, Soeldner SS: Genetic, acquired, and related factors in the etiology of diabetes mellitus, *Arch Intern Med* 137:461-469, 1977.

67. Gerich JE et al: Characterization of the glucagon response to hypoglycemia in man, *J Clin Endocrinol Metab* 1:77-82, 1974.

68. Indications for use of continuous insulin delivery systems and self-measurement of blood glucose: policy statement, American Diabetes Association, *Diab Care* 5(2):141-142, 1982.

69. Neville J: Management by nutrition. In Blevins D, editor: *The diabetic and nursing care*, New York, 1979, McGraw-Hill.

70. Office guide to diagnosis and classification of diabetes mellitus and other categories of glucose tolerance, *Diab Care* 4(2):335, 1981.

71. Paulk LH: Hypoglycemic reactions: from the diabetic's perspective, unpublished master's thesis, Kent, Ohio, 1983, Kent State University.

72. Skyler JS, Cahill G: Diabetes mellitus: progress and directions, *Am J Med* 70:101-104, 1981.

73. US Department of Health and Human Services: The treatment and control of diabetes: a national plan to reduce mortality and morbidity. A report of the National Advisory Board, NIH Publication No. 81-2284, Washington, DC, 1980, US Government Printing Office.

The Patient with Endocrine Problems

Virginia L. Cassmeyer
Dorothy Blevins

After studying this chapter, the learner should be able to:

- Describe the anatomy and physiology of the endocrine system.
- Describe the nature of hormonal imbalances in terms of hyposecretion and hypersecretion.
- Describe the pathophysiologic bases, signs, and symptoms of dysfunction of the endocrine glands.
- Develop a plan of care, including identification of appropriate nursing diagnoses, patient outcomes, and interventions for patients with selected endocrine problems.
- Explain the care of the patient undergoing surgery for problems of selected endocrine glands.
- Specify learning needs of patients receiving long-term hormonal replacement therapy.

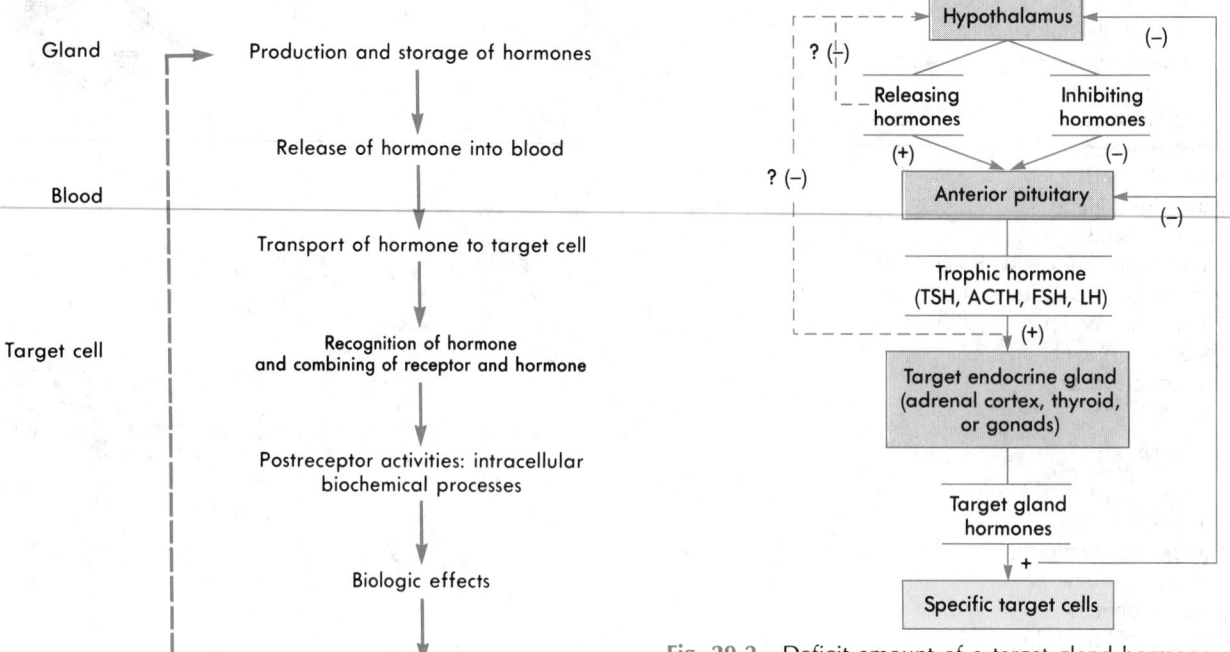

Fig. 29-1 Processes of endocrine system.

Fig. 29-2 Deficit amount of a target gland hormone allows development of more trophic hormone. This system controls the levels of some hormones secreted by the adrenal cortex (glucocorticoids), thyroid (T_3 and T_4), and the gonads. (Redrawn from Harvey, AM, et al: *The principles and practice of medicine,* ed 20, New York, 1980, Appleton-Century-Crofts.)

The endocrine system functions as the regulator of multiple body processes, primarily through the actions of hormones. Hormones are chemical compounds that are synthesized in glands under genetic control and then secreted into the blood. They affect specific target cells in the body and control diverse physiologic functions. Alterations in the function of the endocrine glands, hormones, or target cellular activities usually result in a wide variety of effects. Many endocrine diseases have a slow and subtle onset of signs and symptoms; yet, because many of the functions controlled by the endocrine system are vital, dysfunction can be serious and even fatal.

Research is advancing the knowledge of complex cellular activities that result from the presence of hormones. Fig. 29-1 illustrates a simple schema of the components of the endocrine system, that is, the series of processes that are now considered integral to the endocrine system. This chapter discusses the health problems related to the hormones of the anterior and posterior pituitary, adrenal cortex and medulla, thyroid, and parathyroid. The endocrine functions of the pineal and thymus glands are poorly understood. The gonads are discussed in Unit IX, the endocrine secretions of the gastrointestinal tract are discussed in Chapters 31 and 32, and pancreatic endocrine dysfunction is discussed in Chapter 28.

ANATOMY AND PHYSIOLOGY

Hormone levels are finely regulated in healthy persons. For hormones to initiate changes in cellular function the hormone must combine with a specific receptor located on the cell membrane or within the cell. Before the discussion of the anatomy and physiology of the specific endocrine glands, some information on hormonal regulation and receptor activity will be reviewed.

Hormonal Regulation

The amount of hormone available to receptors is critical for health. The amount is kept within definite limits by a number of factors. One factor, the closed-loop negative-feedback system, is shown in Fig. 29-2. It is an important regulating mechanism for hormones secreted by the hypothalamus, anterior pituitary, thyroid, adrenal cortex, and gonads. In this regulatory system, the hypothalamus stimulates gland A to produce trophic hormone X, which stimulates gland B to produce hormone Y; hormone Y then inhibits the secretion of hormone X by gland A and the hypothalamic hormone that started the stimulation. This regulating mechanism for cortisol secretion is called the hypothalamic-pituitary-adrenal cortex (HPA) axis.

A simpler and more direct feedback control is exhibited by other glands. For these glands feedback is exerted by the level of a particular substance in the blood on a particular hormone's production or secretion. For example, a lowered serum calcium concentration stimulates the secretion of parathyroid hormone (PTH) and a higher serum calcium level inhibits the secretion of PTH.

Other factors influencing secretion patterns of hormones include sleep-wake patterns, age, and growth and development. Hormones are not secreted at a uniform rate or steady flow but are released in bursts. Some hormones have cyclic rhythmic patterns of secretions, and thus rhythmic patterns of serum hormone levels can be noted;

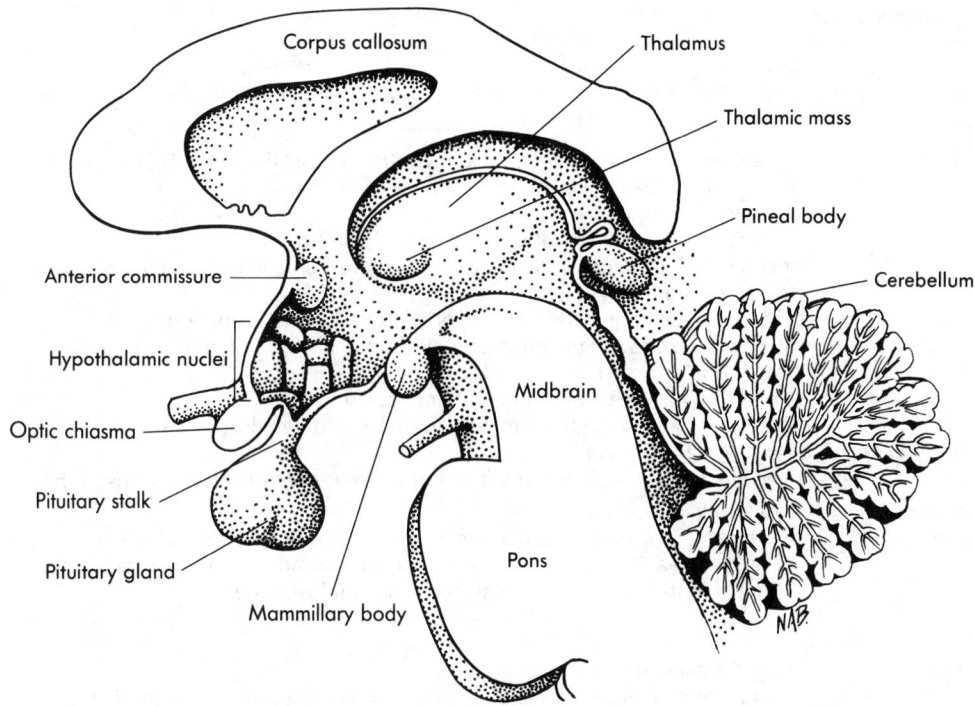

Corpus callosum
Thalamus
Thalamic mass
Pineal body
Cerebellum
Anterior commissure
Hypothalamic nuclei
Midbrain
Optic chiasma
Pituitary stalk
Pituitary gland
Pons
Mammillary body

Fig. 29-3   Sagittal section depicting the hypothalamus, pituitary gland, and related parts of the brain.

for example, cortisol has a diurnal pattern and estrogen has a monthly pattern.

The rate of excretion or metabolic inactivation also affects the levels of circulating hormones. Usually hormones have a very short activity period before they are degraded and excreted by the liver or kidneys. Diseases of these two organs can change hormone levels and activity.

Receptor Activity

It is hypothesized that hormones initiate cellular activity in one of two ways. In the *mobile receptor* model the hormones are thought to cross the plasma cell membrane and combine with receptors in the cytoplasm of the cell. The hormone-receptor complex then crosses the nuclear membrane and reacts with particular proteins in the chromatin of the nucleus or binds with deoxyribonucleic acid (DNA). In general, steroid hormones, such as adrenal cortical steroids, and androgen(s), estrogen, and progesterone act in this manner. Thyroid hormone may also act in the same way.

In the second model or the *fixed receptor* model, the hormone combines with a receptor on the plasma membrane of a cell and initiates a sequence of events coordinated by a second messenger causing the cell to initiate whatever activity it is equipped to do. Adrenocorticotropin hormone (ACTH), thyroid stimulating hormone (TSH), glucagon, insulin, PTH, and the catecholamines may initiate cellular activity in this manner.

Hypothalamus

The hypothalamus (see Fig. 29-3) is a very small area of the brain consisting of numerous poorly defined nuclei. It lies above the anterior and posterior pituitary. The hypothalamus receives input directly or indirectly from almost every part of the brain and is a major controller of both the anterior and posterior pituitary.

Pituitary Gland

The pituitary gland (hypophysis) (see Fig. 29-3) is approximately 1 cm in size and weighs 500 mg. It lies in the sella turcica of the sphenoid bone at the base of the skull and is separated from the oral cavity by the sphenoid bone. The sella turcica is close to the optic chiasma. The pituitary gland is actually two glands, the larger anterior pituitary or adenohypophysis and the posterior pituitary or neurohypophysis. The small size of the pituitary gland should not be misleading. The pituitary is often called the *master gland* because of its major influence on other glands and thus on the entire body. This influence is exerted by six hormones that are produced by different cells of the anterior pituitary gland and by two hormones released by the posterior pituitary gland. See Table 29-1 for the specific name and functions of each hormone.

Thyroid-stimulating hormone (TSH), adrenocorticotropic hormone (ACTH), and the gonadotropic hormones are called trophic hormones because the target cells for these hormones are other endocrine glands. As trophic hormones these hormones are necessary for the growth and maintenance of the size of the targeted endocrine glands, as well as functioning as major regulators of the synthesis and secretion of hormones from these targeted endocrine glands. The other pituitary hormones exert their influence directly on body cells.

Table 29-1   Pituitary hormones

Hormone	Function
Anterior pituitary	
Growth hormone (GH)	Target organ: whole body, possibly works on most tissue through action of somatomedin
	Concerned with growth of cells, bones, and soft tissues
	Increases mitosis
	Affects carbohydrate, protein, and fat metabolism
	Increases blood glucose by decreasing glucose utilization; insulin antagonist
	Increases protein synthesis
	Increases free fatty acid levels, lipolysis, and ketone formation
	Increases electrolyte retention and extracellular fluid volume
Prolactin (PRL)	Target organ: breast and gonads
	Necessary for breast development and lactation
	Regulator of reproductive function in males and females
Thyroid-stimulating hormone (TSH)	Target organ: thyroid
	Necessary for growth and functions of thyroid; controls all functions of thyroid
Adrenocorticotropin hormone (ACTH; corticotropin)	Target organ: adrenal cortex
	Necessary for growth and maintenance of size of adrenal cortex
	Controls release of glucocorticoids (cortisol) and adrenal androgens
	Minor role in release of mineralocorticoids (aldosterone)
Gonadotropins	
Follicle-stimulating hormone (FSH)	Target organs: gonads
	Stimulates gametogenesis and sex steroid production in males and females
Luteinizing hormone (LH)	
Posterior pituitary	
Antidiuretic hormone (ADH)	Target organ: kidney tubular cells
	Effects changes in kidney tubular membrane to increase water absorption; stimulates smooth muscle of intestines and blood vessels
Oxytocin	Target organs: breast, uterus
	Stimulates uterine contractions and breast milk ejection

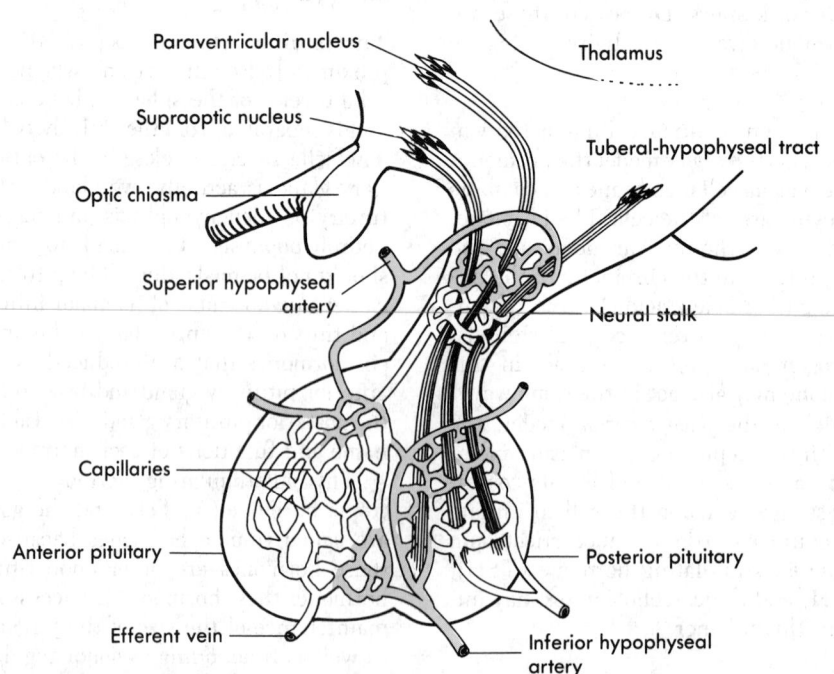

Fig. 29-4 Hypothalamic pituitary connections. The hypothalamus connects to the posterior pituitary gland by nerve tracts. The connection between the hypothalamus and the anterior pituitary gland is vascular.

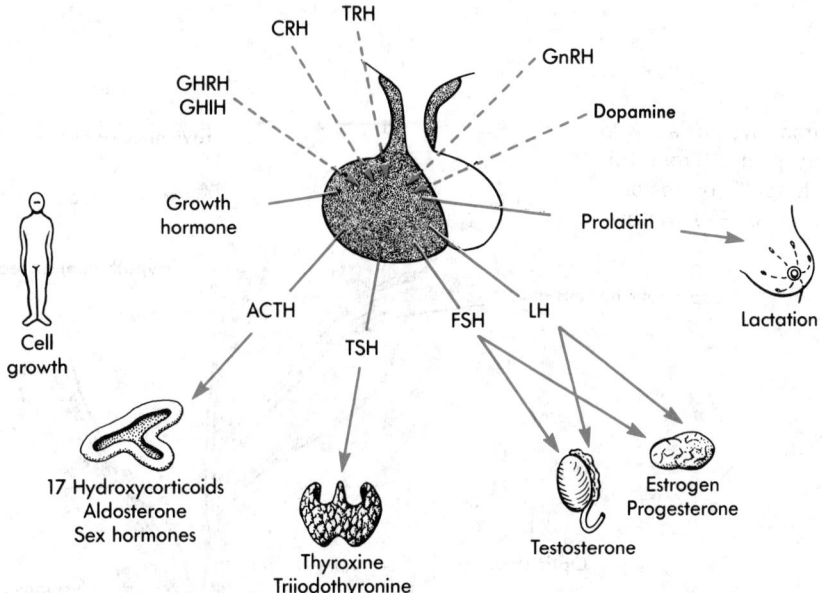

Fig. 29-5 Relationships between hormones of the hypothalamus, anterior pituitary gland, and target tissues are depicted. Six releasing or inhibiting hormones have been chemically identified: growth hormone–releasing hormone *(GHRH)*; growth hormone–inhibiting hormone *(GHIH,* somatostatin); thyrotropin-releasing hormone *(TRH)*; corticotropin–releasing hormone *(CRH)*; gonadotropin-releasing hormone *(GnRH)*; and dopamine, which acts as a prolactin inhibiting hormone *(PIH)*. Each anterior pituitary hormone is shown with its respective target tissues: body cells *(GH)*; adrenal cortex *(ACTH)*; thyroid *(TSH)*; testes and ovaries *(FSH and LH)*; and breasts (prolactin).

Relationship between hypothalamus and pituitary gland

The hypothalamus serves as a vital link between the neurologic and hormonal regulatory mechanisms. The hypothalamus and the anterior pituitary are connected by the hypothalamic-hypophyseal portal blood system, by which neurosecretory-releasing hormones and neurosecretory-inhibiting hormones are carried from the hypothalamus to the anterior pituitary (Fig. 29-4). The exact number of releasing and inhibiting hormones is not known. At present, six of these hypothalamic hormones have been identified. These hormones are depicted in Fig. 29-5. The interactions between the hypothalamus, anterior pituitary, and other endocrine glands or target organs are also summarized in the legend in Fig. 29-5.

The hypothalamus also exerts control over the posterior pituitary gland to which it is structurally connected. ADH and oxytocin are produced in the hypothalamus in the paraventricular and supraoptic nuclei and are carried down neurons by axonal transport to the terminal branches that are located in the posterior pituitary lobe (Fig. 29-6). There they are stored and then released.

Adrenal Gland

The two adrenal organs lie in the retroperitoneal area, each capping the upper pole of a kidney. There are two glands in each adrenal organ: the adrenal cortex, or outer layer, and the adrenal medulla, or central portion. The *adrenal cortex* secretes two groups of hormones that are necessary for life: the *glucocorticoids* of which cortisol is the principal hormone, and the *mineralocorticoids* of which

aldosterone is the principal hormone. The third group of hormones secreted by the cortex in both men and women is the androgens. Although these androgens do not have much intrinsic biological activity, they can be converted to testosterone or estrogen in the periphery. This source of androgens is an important consideration in certain pathologic conditions or when treatments require the absence of a particular sex hormone.

Table 29-2 lists the specific effects of each adrenal hormone. Although the glucocorticoids have other important functions, they have a major role in *nutrition* (cortisol has hyperglycemic, catabolic, and lipolytic effects) and in *biologic defenses* (cortisol has antiinflammatory and immunosuppressive effects).

The secretion of cortisol is regulated by ACTH (a pituitary hormone) under the influence of corticotropin-releasing hormone (CRH). Cortisol has a circadian diurnal pattern of release with peak levels occurring in the early morning following release of ACTH. This pattern of release follows sleep-wake cycles. Through a negative feedback system, serum levels of cortisol also are primary regulators for inhibition or stimulation of ACTH release. Low serum levels of cortisol stimulate the release of ACTH and then, as a result, the release of cortisol. High serum levels of cortisol inhibit the release of ACTH and thus its own release. However, during the stress response, hypothalamic stimulation (by CRH) of the pituitary results in increased ACTH secretion and stimulation of the adrenal glands that release cortisol. This stress response overrides the usual negative feedback system.

Mineralocorticoid secretion is increased during the

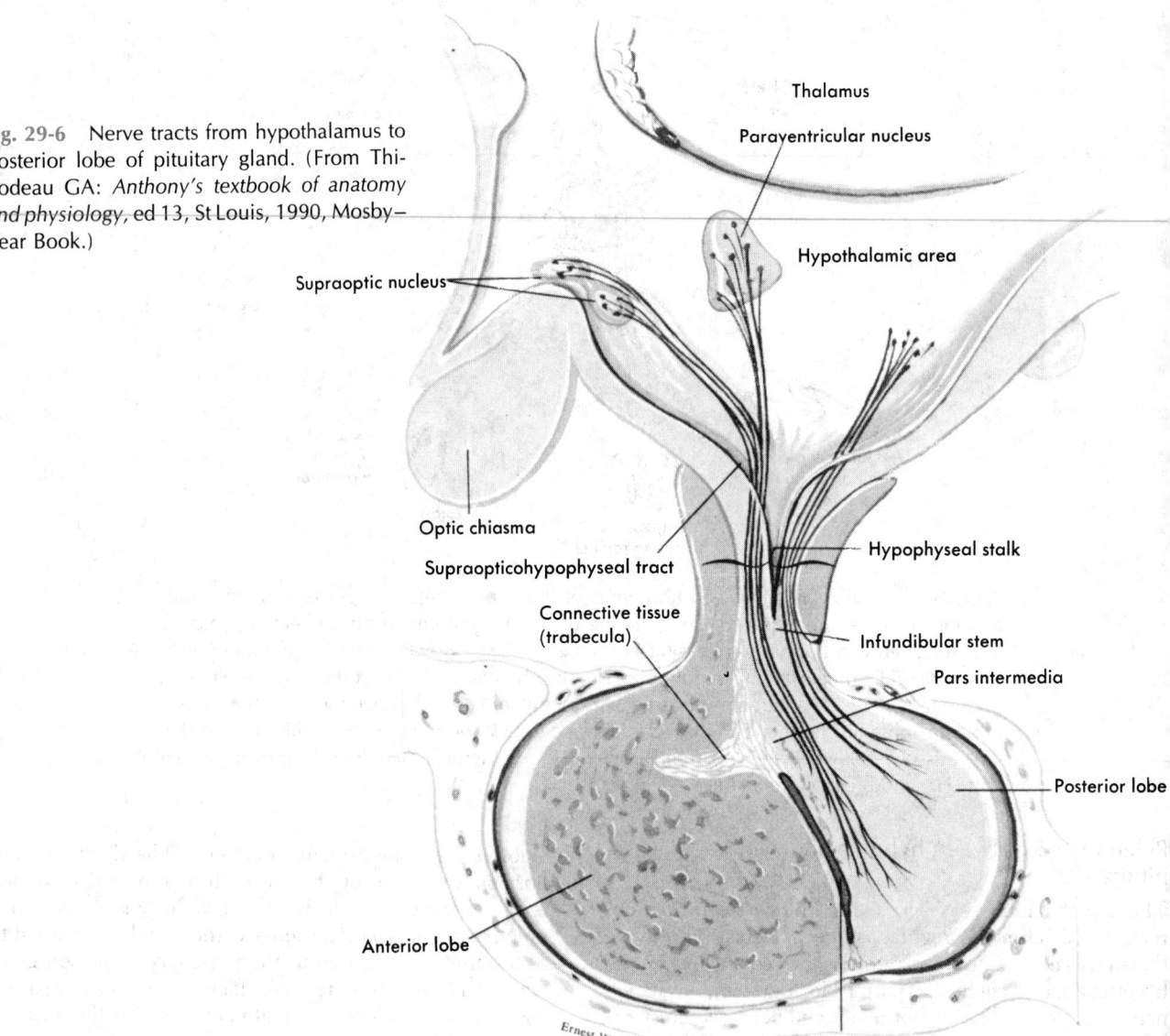

Fig. 29-6 Nerve tracts from hypothalamus to posterior lobe of pituitary gland. (From Thibodeau GA: *Anthony's textbook of anatomy and physiology*, ed 13, St Louis, 1990, Mosby–Year Book.)

Thalamus

Paraventricular nucleus

Hypothalamic area

Supraoptic nucleus

Optic chiasma

Supraopticohypophyseal tract

Connective tissue (trabecula)

Hypophyseal stalk

Infundibular stem

Pars intermedia

Posterior lobe

Anterior lobe

Cleft

Ernest W. Beck

stress response; however, the primary regulator at all times is the renin-angiotensin system (see Chapters 7 and 33). An increased serum potassium level also stimulates the adrenal cortex to increase its release of aldosterone. Mineralocorticoids are necessary for the maintenance of sodium, potassium, and water balance; they act on the kidneys to increase the retention of sodium and water and the excretion of potassium.

The *adrenal medulla* secretes epinephrine and norepinephrine, which augment the catecholamines produced by the sympathetic nervous system. These *catecholamines* secreted by the adrenal medulla are not necessary for life but, in excess, can be responsible for serious hypertension.

A small amount of the catecholamines is released at all times, but during the stress response, increased amounts are released as part of the *physiologic stress response*. Table 29-3 lists the multiple effects of increased adrenal-medullary stimulation. Different effects in the body are seen

as a result of stimulation of different receptors located on target organs. Receptors are classified as:

alpha (α)-adrenergic:

α_1-adrenergic receptors are on various target organs throughout the body and are excitatory.

α_2-adrenergic receptors are at presynaptic sites on nervous tissue and are inhibitory.

Beta (β)-adrenergic:

β_1-adrenergic receptors are located primarily in the heart.

β_2-adrenergic receptors are located elsewhere in the body.

Norepinephrine stimulates only alpha (α) receptors; epinephrine stimulates both beta (β) and α receptors.

Parathyroid Gland

The *parathyroid gland* consists of four minute glands that are variously located on the posterior aspect of each thyroid

Table 29-2 Functions of the adrenal hormones

Gland	Hormones	Functions
Adrenal cortex	Glucocorticoids (cortisol)	Overall effect is to maintain blood glucose level by increasing gluconeogenesis and decreasing rate of glucose use by cells Increases level of protein catabolism Promotes lipolysis Promotes sodium and water retention Antiinflammatory Degrades collagen Decreases T lymphocyte participation in cellular-mediated immunity by decreasing circulating level of T lymphocytes Increases serum level of neutrophils by increasing release and decreasing destruction but neutrophils are prevented from migrating to sites of injury Decreases new antibody release Decreases eosinophils, basophils, and monocytes Decreases scar tissue formation Increases RBC formation and possibly increases platelet formation Stimulates appetite Increases gastric acid and pepsin production Maintains emotional stability
	Mineralocorticoids (aldosterone)	Primary stimulus is the renin-angiotensin system Primarily responsible for maintenance of normovolemic state by increasing sodium and water retention in distal kidney tubules Causes potassium excretion Causes increased excretion of ammonium and magnesium ions
	Androgens	Same functions as gonadal sex hormones
Adrenal medulla	Epinephrine and norepinephrine	Necessary for maintenance of neuroendocrine integrating functions of body See Table 29-3 for a summary of the effects of these two catecholamines

Table 29-3 Effects of adrenal-medullary-sympathetic stimulation on body organs*

Organ	Effect	Organ	Effect
Heart	Increased conduction velocity, automaticity, contractility, rate, and stroke volume caused by β_1-stimulation	Gallbladder	Relaxation
		Kidney	Increased renin secretion caused by β_2-stimulation
Blood vessels		Urinary bladder	Relaxation of detrusor muscle and contraction of internal sphincter
Coronary vessels, brain, lungs	Dilation caused by β_2-stimulation and autoregulatory phenomena	Skin	Pilomotor muscle contraction and localized sweating
Skin, mucosa, abdominal viscera, renal and salivary gland vessels	Constriction caused by α-stimulation; renal vessels also have dopaminergic receptors	Liver	Glycogenolysis and gluconeogenesis caused by β_2-stimulation
Veins	Constriction caused by α-stimulation	Pancreas	Decreased secretion of acini cells; β_2-stimulation causes increased secretion of islet β-cells but α-stimulation causes decreased secretion of islet cells; α-effect predominates so insulin secretion decreased
Bronchial muscles	Relaxation caused by β_2-stimulation		
Gastrointestinal tract	Inhibition of production of gastrointestinal secretions; decreased motility and contraction of sphincters caused by β_2-stimulation	Fat cells	Lipolysis
		Brain	Increased alertness, restlessness
		Eyes	Dilation of pupils and relaxation of ciliary bodies

*These total effects would be seen in the physiologic response to stressors.

Table 29-4 Functions of parathyroid hormone (PTH)

Organ	Effects of PTH
Kidney tubule	Decreases urinary excretion of calcium
	Increases urinary excretion of phosphorus
	Inhibits H$^+$ ion secretion
	Decreases reabsorption of sodium and bicarbonate
	Increases renal threshold for glucose
Gut	Increases calcium and phosphorus absorption from intestinal tract (requires vitamin D)
Bone	Converts osteogenic osteocytes to osteolytic osteocytes
	Decreases the number of osteoblasts
	Decreases bone formation and increases bone breakdown

Table 29-5 Functions of thyroid hormone

Hormones	Functions
Thyroxine (T$_4$) Triiodothyronine (T$_3$)	Regulates protein, fat, and carbohydrate catabolism in all cells
	Regulates metabolic rate of all cells
	Regulates body heat production
	Insulin antagonist
	Maintains growth hormone secretion, skeletal maturation
	Affects CNS development and function
	Necessary for muscle tone and vigor
	Maintains cardiac rate, force, and output
	Maintains secretions of gastrointestinal tract
	Affects respiratory rate and oxygen utilization
	Maintains calcium mobilization
	Affects RBC production
	Stimulates lipid turnover, free fatty acid release, and cholesterol synthesis
Calcitonin	Lowers serum calcium and phosphorus levels
	Decreases calcium and phosphorus absorption in gastrointestinal tract
	Inhibits bone resorption

lobe. Occasionally extra glands are located on the thyroid, in the mediastinum, or behind the esophagus. Parathyroid hormone (PTH) regulates calcium and phosphorus metabolism by its effect on gastrointestinal absorption, kidney excretion, or bone resorption. A low serum calcium level stimulates the release of PTH. The specific functions of PTH are listed in Table 29-4.

Thyroid Gland

The thyroid gland is located in the anterior aspect of the neck and weighs about 20 g. It consists of two lobes connected by an isthmus and lies just below the larynx. The thyroid gland stores iodine and secretes the thyroid hormones and calcitonin. The two thyroid hormones are thyroxine (tetraiodothyronine, T$_4$) and triiodothyronine (T$_3$).

The production of the thyroid hormones is under the control of thyroid-releasing hormone (TRH) from the hypothalamus and thyroid-stimulating hormone (TSH) from the anterior pituitary. A primary regulator of T$_4$ and T$_3$ is the negative-feedback system depicted in Fig. 29-2. Calcitonin is primarily regulated by serum levels of calcium; elevated serum levels of calcium promote the release of calcitonin, and lowered serum levels of calcium inhibit calcitonin release.

The functions of the thyroid hormones and calcitonin are presented in Table 29-5. Overall, T$_3$ and T$_4$ regulate metabolic rate, growth and tissue differentiation. Calcitonin helps maintain serum calcium levels.

Physiologic Changes with Aging

Changes in the endocrine system are associated with normal aging. Endocrine dysfunction may result from cellular damage resulting from aging, wear and tear on the endocrine tissue from long-term use, or genetically programmed cellular changes. Endocrine changes may result in altered synthesis and secretion of hormones, altered metabolism of hormones, altered circulatory levels of hormones, altered biologic activity, altered target cell and target tissue responsiveness, or altered intrinsic rhythms. Although findings are not consistent, the following is a summary of the major alterations in endocrine function that are most frequently reported.*

1. The most commonly seen change is decreased ovarian functioning in females, resulting in increased gonadotropins and changes in reproductive and sexual functioning. No similar change in males has been reported.

2. Impaired secretion of hypothalamic hormones or impaired response to feedback may influence endocrine system responsiveness to alterations in the internal environment, and thus to stressors.

3. The anterior pituitary gland shows morphologic changes with increased fibrosis and microadenoma formation, a decrease in basal levels of prolactin in females and a decrease in growth hormone and somatomedins.

4. Antidiuretic hormone secretion in response to changes in serum osmolality is increased, resulting in increased levels of ADH. However, elderly persons also have alterations in renal function that decrease the ability to concentrate urine and can result in hyponatremia. Nocturia is commonly present.

5. Various changes in thyroid gland structure, including glandular atrophy, fibrosis, nodularity, and infiltrates have been found. The following changes in thyroid hormone levels have been reported:
   a. Decreased T$_4$ secretion and metabolism
   b. Decreased plasma T$_3$ levels
   c. Increased basal plasma TSH levels
   d. Decreased responsiveness in TSH secretion to TRH

---

*References 3, 4, 6, 8, 10, 34.

Hypothyroidism is very common in the elderly. Whether all these changes in thyroid structure, function, or disease can be attributed to the aging process is unclear. Some of the early clinical manifestations of hypothyroidism, such as skin and hair changes, neurologic changes, or gastrointestinal change can be seen in elderly persons for other reasons, leading health care professionals to ignore or potentially misdiagnose the changes.

6. Calcium homeostasis is altered in the older adult. Changes found include decreased intake of calcium, negative calcium balance, bone loss, decreased intestinal adaptation to varied calcium intake, hypercalciuria, and decreased vitamin D levels. Age-related alterations in PTH may explain some of the changes in calcium homeostasis, but more research is needed.

7. The adrenal cortex, which is small and contains fibrous tissue, responds to feedback mechanisms and maintains circadian patterns of cortisol secretion in response to circadian patterns of ACTH. However, the amount of cortisol secreted is decreased because of decreased metabolic clearance and decreased usage. Thus increased blood cortisol levels result in decreased secretion. The amount of androgens secreted by the adrenal cortex is decreased, and the renin-aldosterone response to postural changes and volume depletion is depressed.

If the endocrine changes described in the preceding section are ignored, the elderly may be misdiagnosed. That is, endocrine disease may not be diagnosed. Changes in serum sodium and potassium such as hyponatremia and hypokalemia must be carefully evaluated to differentiate changes related to endocrine changes with aging from those that might be due to drugs such as diuretics, other diseases such as congestive heart failure, or diet. The potential role of changes in PTH in development of metabolic bone disease contributing to osteoporosis needs more exploration. It is important to remember that the hypothalamic-pituitary-adrenal axis and the hypothalamic-pituitary-thyroid axis, which are important in daily living and response to stressors, are intact but may be slower to respond thus explaining in part the decreased ability to respond to physiological and psychological stressors.

Besides the changes listed above, changes in response to actual endocrine pathology have been reported. Some elderly persons with hyperthyroidism have subtle signs and symptoms that make diagnosis difficult. Elderly persons tolerate hypothyroidism better, and there may be a greater insufficiency of thyroid hormones when they are first diagnosed. Also, early signs and symptoms of hypothyroidism such as skin changes, change in hair, increased diastolic pressure, decreased memory and so forth may be overlooked because they are seen in many elderly persons even in the absence of thyroid pathology.

PREVENTION AND HEALTH EDUCATION
Primary Prevention

Few primary endocrine diseases can be prevented at this time. *Simple goiter,* a disease characterized by an enlargement of the thyroid gland, is an exception. This condition may occur because of a lack of ingested iodine. The nurse can participate in primary prevention by teaching the importance of eating foods that contain iodine, such as seafoods and leafy vegetables. In places where there is a known deficiency of iodine in the natural water (for example, the Great Lakes region), persons are encouraged to use iodized salt.

Diseases similar to endocrine hypersecretory states may be caused by inappropriate use of hormones for nonmedical purposes. This abuse of hormones is termed *factitious* and is often concealed from health care providers. Primary prevention education programs should focus on the use of gonadal steroids and growth hormones by athletes, glucocorticoids for mood elevating effects, and thyroid drugs by dieters.

Secondary Prevention

Malignant tumors of the endocrine gland are less prevalent than other forms of cancer. The thyroid gland can be easily palpated, and people should be encouraged to have yearly physical examinations to help in early detection of thyroid carcinoma. This cancer appears in all age-groups and especially in those with a history of irradiation to the neck structures. In recent years, there has been a concerted search in the United States for adults who received irradiation of the upper thorax, head, or neck for conditions such as thymus conditions, enlarged tonsils and adenoids, acne, disfunction of the eustachian tube and so forth during early childhood years. These individuals are urged to seek medical attention for detection of thyroid cancer.

Heart disease can be induced or aggravated by certain hormonal alterations. Thyroid and adrenocortical dysfunction are two disorders in which early detection and treatment can minimize cardiovascular disease. The nurse can assist in the early detection of these disorders by encouraging persons to seek medical attention for persistent vague complaints of decreased well-being that may include the following:

1. Fatigue
2. Altered nutritional intake
3. Changes in skin and hair appearance and condition
4. Changes in excretory patterns

Although endocrine diseases are not the only cause of these signs and symptoms, it is true that these are early signs and symptoms of many endocrinopathies.

Tertiary Prevention

A major contribution of the nurse to patients with diagnosed endocrinopathies is that of assisting them to learn self-management of their chronic diseases. The progression of many hormonal deficiency diseases can be halted or slowed by patients who are educated and motivated to follow prescribed regimens. Hormonal replacement, when necessary, is an important method of treatment that must be handled by the patient over a long period of time. It should be stressed that failure to maintain adequate hormonal replacement and other parts of the regimen can result in illness and death.

MAJOR HEALTH PROBLEMS OF THE ENDOCRINE SYSTEM

The classifications of hypersecretion and hyposecretion of hormones help organize the information in this chapter. Only those endocrine problems encountered most frequently are discussed; these are listed in Table 29-6. The most frequent endocrine disorder in the United States is diabetes mellitus, which is discussed in Chapter 28. The next most frequent disorder is thyroid dysfunction. All endocrine disorders can lead to significant health problems in individuals.

Regardless of the pathologic process involved, endocrine disorders are characterized by an alteration in *amount* of effective hormone, either an excess or a deficiency. Hormonal alterations *may result from* the following:

1. Change in the integrity of glandular tissue
2. Dysfunction of regulating mechanisms
3. Decrease in excretion or inactivation of hormones
4. Peripheral resistance to the action of the hormones

Etiologic factors of endocrine glandular disorders are classified as primary, secondary, or iatrogenic:

Primary: disorder of the gland

Secondary: disorder of a target gland because of disorder in the pituitary gland or the hypothalamus

Iatrogenic: hormonal disorders that occur because of treatment

Hyposecretory states may occur when there is absence of glandular tissue or when there is *hypoplasia* (decrease in number of functioning cells). *Atrophy* (decrease in gland size) and hypoplasia often occur together. Hypersecretory states may occur when there is *hyperplasia* (increase in number of active secreting cells) or a tumor. For example, pituitary hyperplasia might be a response to hypothalamic stimulation. *Hypertrophy* (increase in gland size) is not always accompanied by an increased secretion of hormone. One pathologic cause of hypersecretory states is the secretion of hormones by tissues in quantities not related to body needs. These tissues are not responsive to the regulating mechanisms, for example, to the negative feedback loops or to the trophic hormone stimulation or lack of stimulation. Affected endocrine glands are said to be *autonomous* when this escape from regulation occurs.

ANTERIOR PITUITARY DYSFUNCTION

Dysfunction of the anterior pituitary may involve increased or decreased secretion of one or more than one hormone. Important information related to hypersecretory and hyposecretory states is presented first followed by a discussion of the nursing process as it pertains to the most common situations affecting the anterior pituitary gland.

HYPERSECRETION

Hypersecretion of the anterior pituitary may involve one or more hormones.

Etiology/Epidemiology

The causes of hypersecretion of anterior pituitary hormones are multiple. Hypersecretion may be:

1. A primary problem (tumor or hyperplasia) in the anterior pituitary gland.
2. Secondary to hypothalamic dysfunction (increased secretion of releasing hormones or decreased secretion of inhibiting hormones.
3. Secondary to target gland dysfunction (lack of negative feedback).
4. Mimicked by excessive secretion of hormone by ectopic nonendocrine tissue.
5. Iatrogenic from drug therapy.

Pituitary adenomas are the most common cause of hyperpituitarism. Pituitary adenomas of the anterior pituitary gland account for 6% to 18% of all intracranial tumors.[42] In most patients the cause of the adenoma is unknown and no family history exists. Pituitary adenomas are almost always *secreting* or *functioning* tumors. These tumors are usually benign, but some can grow very aggressively. Classification usually is based on the specific hormone secreted, for example, prolactinoma, somatotroph tumors, corticotroph tumors, or gonadotroph adenomas. Tumors are also

Table 29-6   Health problems caused by imbalances in the endocrine system

Gland	Hyposecretion	Hypersecretion
Pituitary	Panhypopituitarism, hypopituitarism, dwarfism, pituitary adrenal insufficiency, thyroid deficiency secondary to pituitary deficiency, hypoprolactinemia, diabetes insipidus	Hyperpituitarism, acromegaly, gigantism, pituitary Cushing's syndrome, thyroid excess secondary to pituitary excess, hyperprolactinemia, syndrome of inappropriate ADH secretion (SIADH)
Thyroid	Hypothyroidism, cretinism, myxedema	Hyperthyroidism
Parathyroid	Hypoparathyroidism	Hyperparathyroidism
Adrenal cortex	Addison's disease	Adrenal Cushing's syndrome, hyperaldosteronism
Adrenal medulla		Pheochromocytoma
Pancreas (endocrine)	Diabetes mellitus (see Chapter 28)	Hypoglycemia (see Chapter 28)

classified by size (microadenomas and macroadenomas) and invasiveness of the sella turcica (enclosed or invasive).

Prolactin-secreting tumors[42] (prolactinomas) account for 60% to 80% of all pituitary tumors. The next most frequently occurring tumor secretes growth hormone (GH) (somatotroph tumor). Tumors that secrete adrenocorticotrophic hormone (ACTH) (corticotroph tumors) are the third most frequently occurring tumors. Gonadotroph adenomas, reported in the past to be rare, may be more common than initially thought.[32] It is possible that adenomas once classified as nonsecreting actually secrete gonadotropins or their subunits.[33] Thyroid-stimulating hormone (TSH)–secreting tumors are still considered to be rare. Pituitary adenomas can occur as part of multiple endocrine neoplasia, type 1 (MEN I). MEN I is a hereditary disorder that consists of primary hyperparathyroidism, pancreatic islet cell tumor, and pituitary adenoma. The pituitary adenoma in MEN I is secreting and usually secretes GH, but some secrete prolactin or ACTH.

Pituitary hyperfunctioning also can result from hyperplasia of pituitary tissue. The cause of hyperplasia is not always known, but one hypothesis is that altered feedback signals can cause hypersecretion.[42] Diminished feedback from target organ secretions can result in hyperplasia and hypersecretion.

Pathophysiology

Secreting pituitary tumors cause two clinical problems depending on the size, location, and *secreting capacity* of the tumor. These are (1) neurologic alterations resulting from pressure on surrounding nervous system structures and (2) hypersecretion of one or more anterior pituitary hormones (see Table 29-1, p. 824 for a review of functions of anterior pituitary hormones).

The major affects of hypersecretion of anterior pituitary hormones are presented in Table 29-7. The effects of growth hormone (GH) and prolactin excess are presented in more detail because these are the most common hypersecretory conditions seen in adults.

Growth hormone excess

An excess of GH is almost always caused by a secreting pituitary tumor, although occasionally there is no distinct tumor. Hypersecretion of GH that occurs in children before fusion of the epiphysis results in *gigantism*. Such children reach enormous proportions because of massive growth in

Table 29-7   Anterior pituitary dysfunction

Alteration in secretion	Signs and symptoms	Medical therapy
GH excess	Gigantism in children; acromegaly in adults: growth of soft tissues, cartilages, bones; enlargement and coarsening of facial features; enlarged tongue; visceral enlargement (liver, spleen, heart, kidneys); warm, moist, coarse skin; husky voice; prominent muscle development; insulin resistance	Removal of tumor: adenectomy, hypophysectomy; irradiation; medications that suppress GH: bromocriptine mesylate (Parlodel) or long-acting somatostatin analog (sandostatin, octreotide) (experimental)
GH deficiency	Dwarfism in children; sensitivity to insulin; fasting hypoglycemia	Growth hormone replacement in children
ACTH excess	Similar to Adrenal Cushing's syndrome (adrenocortical excess) (Table 29-11)	Pituitary ablation: adenectomy, hypophysectomy; radiation; surgical removal of ectopic source of ACTH
ACTH deficiency	Similar to Addison's disease (primary adrenocortical deficit) (Table 29-11); asthenia (weakness); nausea, vomiting; hypotension; hypoglycemia; hyponatremia; hyperkalemia	Glucocorticoid replacement
TSH excess	Same as primary hyperthyroidism (thyroid hormone excess) (Table 29-19)	Removal of tumor: adenectomy, hypophysectomy
TSH deficit	Same as primary hypothyroidism (thyroid hormone deficit) (Table 29-19)	Thyroid hormone replacement
Prolactin excess	Amenorrhea; galactorrhea; depressed libido; osteopenia, hirsutism and acne in women; impotence and oligospermia in men	Removal of tumor: adenectomy, hypophysectomy; irradiation; drugs to suppress prolactin: bromocriptine mesylate (Parlodel)
Prolactin deficit	Failure of postpartum lactation	
Gonadotropic hormone excess	Precocious sexual development in children; changes in secondary sex characteristics: hirsutism in women; gynecomastia in men	Removal of tumor: adenectomy, hypophysectomy
Gonadotropic hormone deficit	Delayed sexual development in children; in adults: female—amenorrhea, infertility; male—impotence; in both—changes in secondary sex characteristics	Replacement of gonadotropins in cyclic pattern

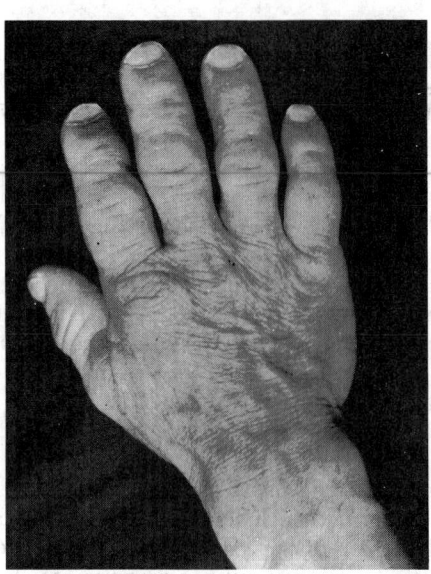

Fig. 29-7 Hand showing characteristics of acromegalic condition. (From Schottelius BA, Schottelius DD: *Textbook of physiology*, ed 18, St Louis, 1978, Mosby—Year Book.)

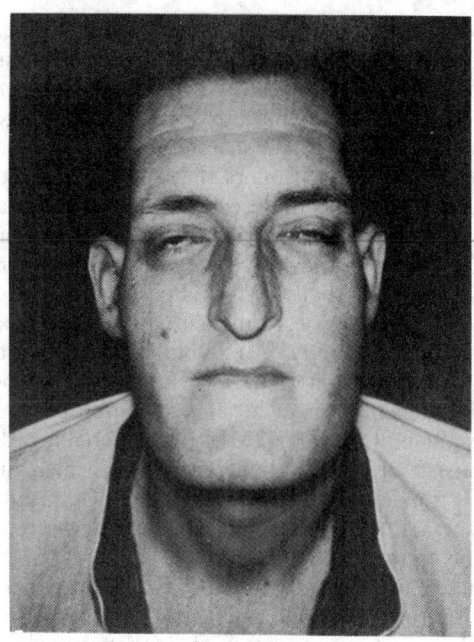

Fig. 29-8 Acromegaly. Note large head, exaggerated forward projection of jaw, and protrusion of frontal bone.

both the length and width of bones. Soft tissue enlarges along with the skeleton.

Hypersecretion of GH that occurs after the fusion of the epiphysis results in *acromegaly*. This disorder affects men and women equally and most frequently begins between the second and fourth decades of life. The changes are slow and progressive and frequently go unrecognized for some time. The adult with acromegaly may note an increase in ring, shoe, glove, and hat size. The hands become spadelike in appearance (Fig. 29-7). The enlargement of the mandible causes an under bite and increased spacing of the lower teeth. The forehead and orbital ridges become prominent (Fig. 29-8). Widening of spaces between joints occurs with increased cartilage growth. This leads to osteoarthritis with pain and limitation of joint motion. Changes in the spine may cause nerve root and cord compression.

The following systemic changes can result from excess in growth hormone:

1. Increased metabolic rate
2. Increased sweating and sebaceous gland activity
3. Glucose intolerance (50% of patients) and insulin resistance that can lead to diabetes mellitus
4. Hypertension (25% of patients) and cardiomegaly can lead to congestive heart failure (CHF)

Many patients with GH excess eventually develop neurologic alterations resulting from an expanding lesion. Frequently they do not seek help until neurological signs and symptoms occur. Common neurological alterations are described below.

Prolactin excess

Prolactin excess is usually caused by pituitary adenomas, usually microadenomas (tumors less than 1 cm in diameter), or hypothalamic dysfunction. Dopamine is the primary hypothalamic inhibitor of prolactin release; interruption of dopamine transmission to the pituitary can result in prolactin excess. Other causes are hypothyroidism, renal failure, and side effects of drugs. Levels of serum prolactin over 300 μg/ml suggest a prolactinoma.[20] Prolactin excess interferes with normal gonadal function by disturbing the hypothalamic-pituitary-gonadal axis. Persons usually seek help for gonadal dysfunction or changes in breast tissue before neurologic signs and symptoms from an intrapituitary mass are present. Women may complain of amenorrhea or galactorrhea. They often complain of depressed libido. Men may give a history of depressed libido, infertility, or impotence. Other signs and symptoms of hypogonadism, such as changes in secondary sex characteristics, may be present.

Neurologic alterations

Tumors larger than 1 cm in diameter (macroadenomas) cause compression of the pituitary and enlargement of the sella turcica; as they expand, they can invade or compress nearby tissue. The primary neurologic alteration is caused by pressure on the optic chiasma and optic nerves. Patients experience progressive loss of vision, and if untreated, permanent blindness results. Most adenomas cause midline pressure and damage the fibers subserving vision in the upper temporal fields. This causes loss of vision in one half of the visual field of both eyes (see Fig. 38-5).

Other symptoms include headaches that are characteristically bitemporal or bifrontal and result from pressure on the sella turcica. Confusion and impaired memory may occur but are rare. Symptoms of increased intracranial pressure may develop as lesions expand in size.

HYPOSECRETION

Hyposecretion of the anterior pituitary gland may involve one or more of the anterior pituitary hormones and is referred to as *hypopituitarism*. If all anterior pituitary hormones are deficit, as well as antidiuretic hormone from the posterior pituitary, the condition is called *panhypopituitarism*.

Etiology/Epidemiology

The cause of hypopituitarism or panhypopituitarism is most frequently the presence of a nonsecreting tumor of the pituitary that is compressing normal secretory tissue. Other causes of hyposecretion of anterior pituitary hormones include ischemia and necrosis after hemorrhage or trauma, infection, autoimmune problems, radiation, and developmental problems. Gonadotropin hormone deficits can result from severely malnourished states such as anorexia nervosa. In hypopituitarism or panhypopituitarism, unless due to removal of the pituitary or massive destruction of the pituitary, the hormone deficits of the anterior pituitary do not usually appear simultaneously. Deficits of GH and gonadotropins occur first, followed by deficits of TSH, and then ACTH.

Pathophysiology

The signs and symptoms associated with anterior pituitary deficiency vary widely depending on the hormones that are deficient and the cause of the deficiencies (see Table 29-1, p. 824 for a review of functions of anterior pituitary hormones). If a tumor is the cause of the problem, neurological alterations as described on page 832 can be present. Signs and symptoms associated with specific hormone deficiencies are summarized in Table 29-7.

Although growth hormone deficiency occurs first in hypopituitarism in the adult, it causes no striking effects except that it may aggravate hypoglycemia related to other problems. However, congenital deficiency of growth hormone in the child results in short stature (dwarfism). Pituitary dwarfism is a rare disorder and is characterized by short stature that is apparent at about 4 years of age (Fig. 29-9). The child typically appears immature and has increased truncal fat. Bone age and height age are usually approximate, and as the child matures, the body proportions approach those of an adult.

Deficiency of gonadotropins will result in various alterations in sexual and reproductive functioning. In adult women, amenorrhea and infertility occur. In adult males infertility and impotency occur. Changes in secondary sexual characteristics will also be present. Lack of TSH and ACTH results in signs and symptoms of primary hypothyroidism and primary adrenocortical insufficiency, which are discussed later in this chapter.

Nursing Process
Assessment

The application of the nursing process to patients with either *hypersecretion* or *hyposecretion* of the *anterior pituitary* focuses on patients with secreting pituitary tumors, pituitary surgery, and potential hormonal imbalances related to the surgery. Many of the descriptions of assessment,

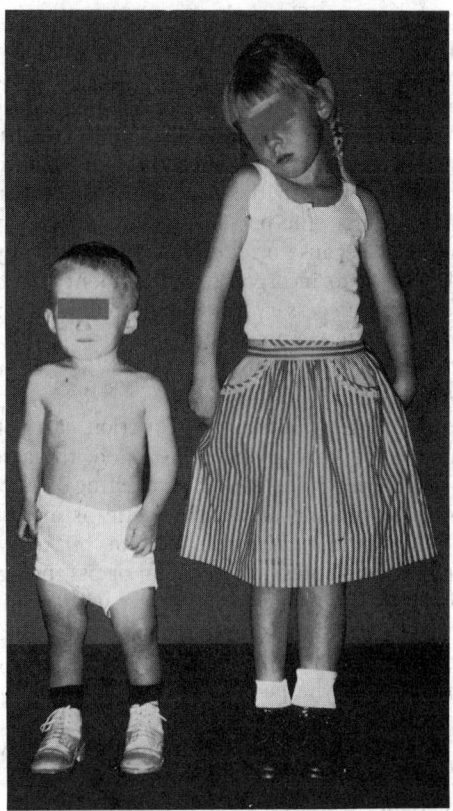

Fig. 29-9   Hypopituitary dwarfism in a 4-year-old boy whose height is 25 inches. Girl is also 4 years old and has a normal height of 39 inches. Dwarf has normal face, as well as head, trunk, and limbs of approximately normal proportions. (From Brashear HR, Raney RB: *Handbook of orthopaedic surgery*, ed 10, St Louis, 1986, Mosby–Year Book.)

data analysis, and planning discussed in this section can be applied to later sections in the chapter. The following are some common clinical problems seen in the various endocrine disorders discussed in this chapter:

1. Fatigue
2. Nutritional alterations
3. Fluid and electrolyte imbalances
4. Cardiovascular changes
5. Changed body characteristics
6. Intolerance to stressors
7. Emotional instability
8. Reproductive alterations

Nursing assessment should include the following:

1. Assessing for clinical signs and symptoms that indicate the extent of hormonal imbalances
2. Assessing for manifestations of potential complications of the endocrine disorder or its treatment
3. Eliciting the patient's and family's perceptions of health problems, their management, and the assistance needed
4. Determining the resources needed by the patient and family to cope with the disorder and to manage it in the hospital and after discharge

Assessment of psychologic and social factors is important

for several reasons. The endocrine diagnostic process can be lengthy, frightening, and costly. Stressors in the patient with pituitary hormonal imbalances should be avoided as much as possible, because the stress response places an additional burden on the impaired endocrine function. Body image changes and physical problems may influence the person's goals, activities of daily living, and relationships with others. The person's coping abilities may also be diminished because of energy depletion or physiologic crisis. Learning to incorporate a treatment regimen into daily life is often necessary for optimal treatment and sometimes necessary to maintain life.

Subjective data

Because anterior pituitary dysfunction can potentially affect almost every other endocrine gland, the assessment focuses on a variety of areas. The collecting of information regarding changes in body characteristics is important not only in defining the physiologic problem, but also in identifying potential or present emotional or psychologic problems. Some of the changes that occur with pituitary endocrine disorders are irreversible even when the physiologic problem is controlled. Body characteristics are part of the identity of the person, and the patient may have problems dealing with the changes.

The patient's or other's description of the following factors helps define the needs for assistance:

1. Fatigue, rest, and sleep patterns
2. Eating patterns (frequency of food intake)
3. Fluid intake and output patterns
4. Cardiovascular history
5. Special hygiene or grooming needs (hirsutism, perspiration, obesity)
6. Discomforts
7. Emotional response
8. Reproductive history
9. Medication usage
10. The endocrine disorder and its treatment

Objective data

Initially, inspection is used to assess the patient's body growth and developmental status and should include the following:

1. Height and weight
2. Body proportions
3. Amount and distribution of muscle mass
4. Fat distribution
5. Skin pigmentation
6. Hair distribution

A great variation exists in these characteristics in the general population, and often changes are not obvious. Inspection of family members for like characteristics provides information as to whether the characteristics seen in the patient are caused by heredity or pathophysiologic alterations. The patient's alertness and speech patterns can be assessed when the history is being collected. Physical assessment should be thorough in these patients because of the wide spectrum of bodily effects that occur with pituitary dysfunction.

The minimum baseline data should include the following:

Nutritional status: presence or absence of fat pads, truncal obesity, abnormal fat depositions; muscle mass, strength; serum levels of lymphocytes, albumin, glucose

Fluid and electrolyte status: vital signs, urine output, fluid intake; signs of fluid excess (edema, jugular vein distention [JVD], adventitious lung sounds) or deficit (orthostatic blood pressure, poor skin turgor, sunken eyeballs, dry mucous membranes); serum levels of electrolytes, BUN, creatinine

Cardiovascular status: blood pressure level including postural BP; pulses, skin color; signs of hypotension or cardiac failure; serum levels of electrolytes, triglycerides, cholesterol; ECG

Diagnostic tests

Usually target organ function is first studied to confirm the presence of a hormonal deficit or excess suggested by the patient's history and clinical findings. Thus measurement of cortisol, T_3 and T_4, and estrogen or testosterone are usually the first tests performed when pituitary disorders are suspected. These are followed by measurements of ACTH, TSH, and FSH and LH. The nontrophic hormones (GH and prolactin) will also be measured.

In comparing the results of these tests, the physician can often learn if the source of the endocrine problems is target gland or hypothalamic-pituitary dysfunction. For example, low levels of both trophic and target gland hormones indicate hypothalamic-pituitary hyposecretion, whereas a low level of target gland hormone and a high level of trophic hormone indicate target gland failure.

Further studies may be needed for exact diagnosis. Provocative tests involve the use of a stimulant or suppressant of the hormone and measurements of the effects on hormonal serum levels. Table 29-8 lists the most common tests of pituitary function. Provocative tests are not used in prolactin excess or deficit because serum levels give confirming data about pituitary function.

Skeletal and skull x-ray examinations are used to assess changes in bone structure and the size of the pituitary gland and sella turcica. Computed tomography (CT) scanning may be used to demonstrate the presence of intrasellar masses and to differentiate a pituitary tumor from an "empty" sella turcica. An enlarged sella turcica may be described as "empty," a condition resulting from herniation of the arachnoid and subarachnoid cistern into the pituitary fossa. The displacement of the pituitary gland is not always clinically significant.

Data analysis: nursing diagnoses

Nursing diagnoses are determined from the analysis of patient data. Possible nursing diagnoses for the person with anterior pituitary dysfunction (secreting pituitary tumors and/or postoperative pituitary surgery) may include, but are not limited to, the following:

Diagnostic title	Possible etiologies
Infection, high risk for	Leakage of spinal fluid through incisional site in dura
Fluid volume deficit	Compromised regulatory mechanism; inadequate conservation of sodium and/or water

Table 29-8   Tests of anterior pituitary function

Test	Procedure	Interpretation
Hormonal radioimmunoassay TSH, ACTH, prolactin, FSH, LH, GH	Blood sample, no special preparation in most cases Glucose may be administered before blood collection	Used to measure circulating hormonal levels; for hormones secreted in diurnal pattern (ACTH, GH), levels obtained in early AM and at intervals throughout day to determine cyclic pattern

Provocative tests
  TSH stimulation
    TRH
	All require basal rate established by pretest assay; stimulant is given and the hormonal levels repeatedly measured	Normal serum TSH begins to rise at 10 min and peaks at 45 min; subnormal values reflect decreased pituitary reserve

ACTH stimulation ACTH, insulin, metyrapone		Normal response of serum cortisol is doubling of normal baseline; subnormal values reflect pituitary or adrenal cortex deficiency
GH stimulation L-dopa, insulin, glucagon, exercise	IV glucose may be given before stimulant	Normal response is a peak in GH levels approximately 60 min after stimulation

Suppression tests
  ACTH suppression
    dexamethasone
	Basal rate established by pretest assay; suppressant is given and serum levels of cortisol are measured, as well as urinary excretion of cortisol and its metabolites
	Collection of 24-hr urine for 17-hydroxycorticosteroids (OHCS)
		Dexamethasone normally suppresses ACTH secretion and thus cortisol; less than normal suppression can reflect pituitary, adrenal cortex, or ectopic hypersecretion

GH suppression glucose	75-100 g glucose load Blood sample drawn every 30 minutes for 2 hours	Hyperglycemia normally suppresses GH secretion

Diagnostic title	Possible etiologies
Knowledge deficit: disorder, diagnostic or treatment measures, self-care measures	Lack of exposure, cognitive limitation
Impaired physical mobility	Intolerance to activity: decreased strength, pain
Body image disturbances	Change in body appearance or function
Sensory/perceptual alterations: visual	Altered sensory transmission

Planning: expected patient outcomes

Expected patient outcomes for the person with anterior pituitary imbalance may include, but are not limited to, the following:

1. Restoration of physiologic well-being, as evidenced by:
   a. Normal body temperature
   b. No evidence of CSF leakage
   c. Desired weight
   d. Balance of intake and output
   e. Stable blood pressure and pulse within optimal limits
   f. Prompt recovery from crisis
2. Explains planned diagnostic and therapeutic measures.
3. Explains rationale for medications and prescribed modification of food and fluid intake.
4. Demonstrates requisite knowledge, skill, and resources for self-management of treatment measures:
   a. Describes the hormonal imbalance and relates to signs and symptoms.
   b. Explains the planned treatment measures and effects of treatment.
   c. Explains the prescribed medication program.
      (1) Awareness of the need for lifelong replacement therapy
      (2) Drugs, dosage, and frequency of therapy
      (3) Desired effects and side effects of therapy
      (4) What to do when signs and symptoms of undertreatment or overtreatment occur
   d. Describes the times when extra hormonal therapy is necessary.
   e. Describes need to obtain MedicAlert symbol to wear.
   f. States plans for regular follow-up care.
5. Physical mobility increases. Receives needed assistance for activities unable to do because of decreased mobility.
6. Speaks of self in positive terms, listing strengths and ways to deal with deficits.
7. Explains to others the assistance needed because of visual defect or weakness.

Implementation
Assisting with achievement of therapeutic goals

Untreated GH-secreting tumors can result in major neurologic alterations as well as continual systemic changes if the hormone level is not returned to normal and if tumor growth is not inhibited. Treatment consists of surgery, radiation, or pharmacologic agents. The primary treatment is neurosurgery using a transsphenoidal approach. Radiation therapy may be used as an adjunct to surgery or as an alternative. Radiation lowers hormone levels much more slowly and is associated with a high incidence of hypopituitarism. Bromocriptine (Parlodel), a dopamine agonist, is effective in lowering GH levels but not always to the level needed, and therefore it is used mainly if surgery and radiation have not been effective.

A long-acting somatostatin analog (Octreotide, Sandostatin, SMS 201-995) is available and has been approved by the Food and Drug Administration (FDA) for use in treating carcinoid.[2] In experimental studies with persons with acromegaly, it has been found to be effective in reducing plasma GH levels as well as relieving some clinical manifestations of GH excess, such as headache, arthropathy, swelling of soft tissue, excess perspiration, sleep apnea, and neuropathy. Sandostatin must be given by subcutaneous injection three or four times daily. It also can be given by continuous subcutaneous infusion. Side effects include pain at injection site, diarrhea, steatorrhea, abdominal cramps, and flatulence. This drug has also been used preoperatively and appears to improve the success of surgery. The routine use of somatostatin analogs for persons with acromegaly will depend on future research.

For prolactin-secreting tumors, some authorities[40] have recommended no treatment for a microadenoma with no annoying symptoms and if the patient does not wish to become pregnant. Studies have shown that the incidence of microadenomas progressing to macroadenomas is very low.[21] However, the ovarian dysfunction and the low estrogen state that is associated with elevated prolactin levels may result in premature osteoporosis; thus other experts recommend that all prolactin-secreting tumors be treated.

When treatment is recommended, the dopamine agonist bromocriptine (Parlodel) is used for enclosed tumors. Drug therapy effectively returns hormone levels to normal, restores fertility, and decreases tumor size in most patients. Transsphenoidal adenectomy is still frequently used for invasive tumors and for some enclosed macroadenomas. Because the use of bromocriptine during gestation is very limited, patients who become pregnant after successful bromocriptine therapy are treated in various ways.[21] In persons with microadenomas, the drug may be stopped and the patient monitored for signs and symptoms of tumor enlargement. If signs and symptoms recur, the drug may be reinstituted. For larger tumors, pre-pregnancy surgery may be carried out. In some instances, bromocriptine may be continued throughout pregnancy. Visual testing is used to monitor for enlargement, and if enlargement is suspected, a CT scan or MRI is carried out. After delivery and if surgery was not carried out, bromocriptine is restarted.

Interventions to assist with patient outcomes
Preventing infection

The transsphenoidal approach is most frequently used to resect an adenoma. The sella turcica is entered through the sphenoid sinus, and the tumor is removed with the aid of a surgical microscope. The incision is made between the

---

29-1	**Activities that increase intracranial pressure**
	Coughing
	Sneezing
	Blowing the nose
	Bending over
	Straining
	Isometric exercises

---

gums and upper lip. This approach may also be used to implant [39]Y. The opening made in the dura mater on entering the sella turcica is frequently patched with a piece of fascia taken from the leg; thus the patient must be prepared for the leg incision. The patch is to prevent a cerebrospinal fluid (CSF) leak. Leaking of CSF may occur for a few days postoperatively but should then stop. The nose may be packed and a gauze sling placed under it to absorb drainage.

Monitoring for the presence of CSF leak is important. The following data should be noted:
1. Complaint of postnasal drip
2. Constant swallowing
3. Evidence on the nasal sling or gauze pads of a "halo ring" (clear CSF fluid marking around a darker center of serous fluid)
4. Presence of glucose in the nasal drainage
   CSF fluid contains glucose, whereas nasal drainage does not. If the glucose test is positive, a specimen should be sent to the laboratory for confirmation.

If a persistent leak occurs, bed rest with the patient's head elevated to decrease CSF pressure and place pressure against the patch is prescribed. Most often CSF leaks heal spontaneously, but occasionally surgical repair is necessary. Activities that increase intracranial pressure should be avoided (see Box 29-1).

Headache may be present and is treated with nonnarcotic analgesics or codeine. Persistent headache or nuchal rigidity (neck stiffness) may indicate the presence of meningitis and should be reported immediately. Because of the risk of infection, prophylactic antibiotics may be ordered preoperative or postoperatively.

Other nursing interventions for the patient with transsphenoidal surgery include the following:
1. Encourage oral fluids and a clear liquid diet as soon as the patient is alert and no longer nauseated from the anesthesia.
2. Increase the diet as tolerated (anorexia may result from a decreased sense of smell).
3. Reassure the patient that the loss of smell is temporary and should improve as soon as the nasal packing and sling is removed.
4. Provide oxygen and humidity as ordered to keep the nasal and oral mucous membranes moist.
5. Provide mouth care:
   a. Avoid toothbrushing to prevent disruption of the suture line.
   b. Use soft cotton swabs to cleanse the teeth.
   c. Offer mouth rinses frequently.

Signs and symptoms of adrenocortical insufficiency

Nausea, vomiting
Prolonged lethargy
More fatigue than expected
Slower recovery than expected
Mild hypotension

Signs of adrenal crisis

Hypotension
Dehydration
Hyponatremia
Hyperkalemia
Hypoglycemia

Monitoring of fluid, electrolyte, and hormonal status

The patient with panhypopituitarism after surgery or other intracerebral problems requires lifelong replacement of cortisol, thyroid, and in most instances, gonadotropins or sex hormones. The exception to replacement of gonadotropins or sex hormones is the patient with cancer whose pituitary was removed to eliminate gonadotropic stimulation of tumor growth, which is not being done very frequently.

ACTH deficiency and thus glucocorticoid deficiency occurs immediately if the total pituitary has been removed. Although it occurs rarely after transsphenoidal adenectomy, a temporary ACTH deficiency can result in adrenocortical insufficiency and even *adrenal crisis*. (See Boxes 29-2 and 29-3.) The patient is treated with replacement therapy as long as necessary. Plasma levels of cortisol will be assessed before discharge to make sure that the deficit has been corrected.

To detect adrenocortical deficiency and to determine adequacy of cortisol replacement, frequent monitoring of any patient with potential for adrenocortical insufficiency is necessary. Actions include the following:

1. Taking vital signs every hour and PRN after surgery until stable, then every 4 hours
2. Tabulating intake and output every 8 hours
3. Weighing patient daily

Electrolyte studies are ordered at least daily to monitor sodium and potassium levels. Signs of insufficient cortisol replacement are usually vague and nonspecific. Maintaining the patient's blood pressure at optimal levels is a major clinical guideline that determines the amount of cortisol replacement.

The signs and symptoms listed in Boxes 29-2 and 29-3 should be reported and carefully evaluated. Progression of symptoms can be rapid, and profound shock can develop. The treatment of adrenal crisis is discussed on p. 849. The critical treatment measure is the replacement of cortisol and administration of volume expanders.

The removal of the pituitary gland or edema of surrounding tissue can precipitate the sudden onset of *diabetes insipidus* from the lack of ADH. (Diabetes insipidus is described in more depth on p. 838). Disruption of the hypothalamic secretion of ADH can also result in ADH alterations. Diabetes insipidus is usually not permanent, even if all of the pituitary gland has been removed—ADH is produced in the hypothalamus and adequate amounts can be released from there.

Monitoring for patients who may develop diabetes insipidus includes the following:

1. Intake and output tabulated every 4 hours
2. Specific gravity determined on each urine specimen (continuously dilute urine with specific gravity of 1.000 to 1.005 is a sign of diabetes insipidus)

Polyuria makes it imperative that fluid intake be maintained to balance the urinary output. When diabetes insipidus occurs, thirst is a frequent complaint. It can usually be managed by providing ice chips and adequate water intake. If fluid deficit is severe, vasopressin (Pitressin) is administered.

Deficiency of TSH and of thyroid hormones usually does not occur on a temporary basis, and it is not seen immediately even after the total pituitary has been removed, because the thyroid stores enough hormone to last for several weeks. If the total pituitary has been removed, the patient will eventually require thyroid replacement.

Gonadotropin deficiency requires lifetime therapy to maintain normal sexual characteristics and reproductive ability. To maintain libido, secondary sexual characteristics, and well-being, men are given testosterone and women receive estrogen-progesterone preparations. If childbearing is desired, the gonadotropins (LH and FSH) must be replaced.

Facilitating learning

Nurses will be instituting various types of patient education interventions. First, patients will need to be prepared for laboratory tests (hormonal, chemical, and electrolyte studies) and x-ray procedures. Once the diagnosis is made, patients will need to be prepared for surgery or other therapy.

Nurses make an important contribution to patients with hypopituitarism resulting from the tumor or the surgery when they help them and their families understand the prescribed regimen for hormonal replacement. The serious nature of adrenocortical insufficiency should be stressed. Specific points to include in the teaching are listed in Box 29-4.

ADH deficiency following surgery is usually temporary. The patient does need to understand the replacement therapy and why signs and symptoms occur (thirst, polyuria). If other deficiencies (TSH or gonadotropins) occur, the patient will need to know how to manage replacement therapy.

Patients treated with bromocriptine alone or as adjunctive therapy must know how to self-administer the drug.

The patient who requires cortisol replacement

Never omit a dose of the drug.

Assist patient to develop a plan for replacement if a dose is missed.

Notify physician if a dose cannot be taken or retained.

Wear an identification bracelet.

Carry information concerning:

Name and dosage of drug to be given in case of an emergency.

Name and phone number of physician to be notified in an emergency.

Carry an emergency supply of a rapid-acting cortisone preparation with directions for use (for example, hydrocortisone 100 mg in a sterile syringe).

Report to physician any signs and symptoms of adrenocortical insufficiency.

Avoid stressors as much as possible.

Notify physician when illness, injury, or emotional crises occur.

Maintain regular medical follow-up.

For prolactin-secreting tumors, 2.5 to 15 mg of bromocriptine daily usually is effective. Higher doses may be necessary for growth-hormone–secreting tumors. The primary side effects are mild nausea, vomiting, and postural hypotension. Repeated hormonal analysis is carried out to monitor the effectiveness of therapy.

Assisting with adaptation to changes in body image and bodily functions

The changes in appearance that result from GH excess and sometimes the changes associated with other hormonal excesses or deficits are not always reversible with treatment. Additionally some of the losses in body function are not reversible. When dealing with changes in body image, nurses must help patients develop realistic images and maximize their ability to attain the desired images by strengthening the remaining functional abilities. Patients need to be shown that not all changes are negative and must be helped to see themselves in positive terms. Sometimes consultation with persons who specialize in make-up, clothing, and colors can be used to help accentuate the patient's best physical attributes.

Developing progressive activity plans with patients will assist them to regain some of the lost physical mobility and also will help to increase self-esteem. Increasing physical activity should be started as soon as possible. Referral to physical therapy may be helpful for some patients. Visual alterations, although usually not severe, require that first and foremost the patient is assessed to determine any special needs to maintain the patient's safety. Depending on the amount of loss, the patient may need care as described in Chapter 38 for the visually impaired.

Evaluation

Evaluation is based on the expected patient outcomes. Key questions to consider include the following:

1. Are a stable weight, blood pressure, intake and output, and temperature achieved?
2. Can the patient describe self-care needs?
3. Does the patient speak of self in positive terms?
4. Is the patient able to get around safely?

POSTERIOR PITUITARY DYSFUNCTION

The two hormones of the posterior pituitary are oxytocin and antidiuretic hormone (ADH). (See Table 29-1, p. 824 for a review of the functions of oxytocin and ADH). Refer to obstetrical nursing texts for further information about oxytocin. The two alterations of ADH secretion, ADH excess and deficit, are described in Table 29-9. The nursing process for the patient with either hyposecretion or hypersecretion of ADH starts on p. 839.

HYPOSECRETION OF ANTIDIURETIC HORMONE

Etiology

Pituitary diabetes insipidus (DI) results from a lack of sufficient ADH. The cause may be a brain or pituitary tumor, head trauma, encephalitis, meningitis, adenectomy or hypophysectomy, or other cranial surgery. The cause is often idiopathic, although a rare hereditary form of the disease occurs. Nephrogenic DI is a second form of the disorder and results from failure of the renal tubules to respond to ADH.

Pathophysiology

The secretion of ADH is an important and normal response to stressors or plasma hyperosmolality. ADH effects changes in the kidney tubular membrane to increase water absorption to dilute the hyperosmolality and to provide an adequate blood volume during the stress response. In the presence of ADH, the urine is concentrated. When ADH is absent, water is not reabsorbed in the tubules and a large amount (7 to 11 L/day) of dilute urine is produced.

When the posterior pituitary does not release ADH or the hypothalamus does not secrete ADH in response to a hyperosmolar state, diabetes insipidus results. The potential is great for severe dehydration and vascular collapse if the patient does not replenish fluids lost by the excessive urination. The three classic symptoms that should alert the nurse to diabetes insipidus are *polyuria, dilute urine,* and *polydipsia.*

Often the patient complains of insatiable thirst. Ice water is preferred, although the reason for this is unknown. Voiding may occur so often that there is interference with sleep and the patient complains of tiredness.

Table 29-9   Alterations in ADH (posterior pituitary) secretion

Alteration	Signs and symptoms	Medical therapy
ADH deficit: Diabetes insipidus	Polyuria, polydipsia, dilute urine (specific gravity 1.000 to 1.005); if fluid intake is insufficient: dehydration, vascular collapse; weakness, anorexia	Fluid intake to balance fluid output; vasopressin replacement: Pitressin, lypressin, (deamino-D-arginine vasopressin nasal spray or drops); surgical removal of tumor; drug therapy: thiazide diuretics, chlorpropamide
ADH excess: SIADH	*Dilutional hyponatremia:* Serum Na below 130 mEq/L; weakness; lethargy; confusion; convulsions; weight gain; edema	Surgical removal of ADH secreting tissue (pituitary or nonpituitary); water restriction of 800 to 1000 ml/day; hypertonic saline with diuretics (for critical levels of sodium); demeclocycline

HYPERSECRETION OF ANTIDIURETIC HORMONE

Etiology

The causes of syndrome of inappropriate antidiuretic hormone (SIADH) are many (see Box 29-5). This disorder is associated with various pathologic processes as well as with drug therapy.

Pathophysiology

In the syndrome of inappropriate antidiuretic hormone (SIADH), the patient is unable to excrete dilute urine and therefore retains water. Normally, ADH secretion is self-limiting; in SIADH, there is a continual release of ADH unrelated to plasma osmolality. Hemodilution results in depressed levels of solutes and electrolytes. CNS dysfunction occurs as a result of the hyposmolar state in which fluid shifts between intracerebral fluid compartments.

Nursing Process
Assessment

A history of polydipsia and polyuria should always be explored further. If the patient with *diabetes insipidus* (hyposecretion of ADH) is able to replenish lost fluids, few other symptoms will be noticed. There can be a severe and sudden onset of dehydration and hyperosmolar fluid imbalance in hyposecretion of ADH if oral intake is decreased.

29-5

Etiologic factors associated with SIADH

Pulmonary disorders: malignant neoplasms such as oat cell adenocarcinoma of the lung, tuberculosis, ventilator patients receiving positive pressure
Other malignancies: duodenum, pancreas, prostate lymphoma, sarcoma, leukemia
CNS disorders: tumors, infection, trauma
Endocrine disorders that result in hypovolemia and impaired free water excretion, particularly if associated with fluid replacement (adrenal insufficiency, anterior pituitary insufficiency)
Drugs such as colfibrate, chlorpropamide, thiazides, vincristine, cyclophosphamide, morphine
Stressors: fear, acute infections, pain, anxiety, trauma surgery

---

Most symptoms of ADH excess (see Table 29-9) are nonspecific. Mental status changes can occur with either hyperosmolar or hypo-osmolar fluid imbalances. The patient who is unconscious, such as after intracranial or pituitary surgery, cannot relate feelings of discomfort or thirst nor can the nurse assess mental changes. Careful documentation of patterns of fluid intake and output can help alert caregivers to fluid imbalances in these patients.

Subjective data

Subjective data can be obtained from the conscious patient. Data to collect include the following:
1. Fluid intake and output patterns
2. Use of Pitressin: frequency and side effects
3. Presence of thirst, weakness, and fatigue
4. Sleep patterns

Objective data

The following objective data center on fluid and electrolyte monitoring:
1. Mental status
2. Daily weight
3. Fluid intake and output every 8 hours or more frequently if risk of imbalance is high
4. Urine osmolality, specific gravity, and sodium content
5. Serum sodium and serum osmolality
6. Blood pressure

Diagnostic tests

Primary diabetes insipidus is rare, but secondary or iatrogenic diabetes insipidus is seen fairly often. Before diabetes insipidus is conclusively diagnosed, the patient must be shown to have a deficit of ADH, and the patient's kidneys must be able to respond to ADH to rule out nephropathy. (Table 29-10 lists tests of ADH function.)

Another diagnostic problem is the differentiation of ADH deficiency from neurogenic polydipsia (compulsive water drinking). A water deprivation test demonstrates ADH deficiency if urine output continues with no change in urine osmolality and sodium content when the patient is deprived of water. Close monitoring of vital signs is necessary to detect significant changes before vascular collapse occurs, which can occur with water deprivation in the presence of ADH deficiency. In neurogenic polydipsia, the water-deprived patient needs continual emotional support to endure the test and may exhibit extreme behavioral responses.

Table 29-10 Tests of ADH function

Test	Procedure	Interpretation
Radioimmunoassay of ADH	Blood sample	Clinical findings, sodium content and osmolality of blood and urine more commonly used
Water deprivation test	Water withheld until 2%-5% of body weight is lost; collect urine and serum samples for osmolality and sodium before test and at ordered intervals; measure intake and output every 1-2 hr, weigh every 8 hr	Normal response is an increase in osmolality and sodium content and decrease in urine volume; in diabetes insipidus, no changes occur
Vasopressor stimulation	Baseline urine osmolality obtained before and after administration of vasopressin	Urine osmolality rises after vasopressin; confirms renal responsiveness to vasopressin and rules out nephrogenic origin of polyuria

Usually laboratory studies of electrolytes and osmolality confirm the diagnosis of SIADH. A search for an extrapituitary source of ADH hypersecretion would include x-ray films, CT scans, or an MRI of the skull, chest, and abdomen.

Data analysis: nursing diagnoses

Nursing diagnoses are determined from the analysis of patient data. Possible nursing diagnoses for the person with imbalances of ADH may include, but are not limited to, the following:

Diagnostic title	Possible etiologies
For the patient with ADH hyposecretion:	
Fluid deficit, high risk for or actual	Compromised regulation of urinary excretion, inadequate fluid intake to balance loss, inadequate management, knowledge deficit
For the patient with ADH hypersecretion:	
Fluid excess, high risk for or actual	Compromised regulation of urinary excretion, improper management, knowledge deficit

See p. 835 for other nursing diagnoses, particularly *knowledge deficit*, applicable to patients with hormonal imbalance following surgery on the pituitary gland.

Planning: expected patient outcomes

Expected patient outcomes for the person with ADH dysfunction may include, but are not limited to, those for patients with hormonal imbalance listed on p. 835, particularly numbers 2 and 4. The following are specific expected outcomes:

1. Maintains weight appropriate for height and fluid status.
2. Urine volume is maintained between 800 and 2000 ml/24 hr. depending on intake; serum sodium is within normal limits.
3. Demonstrates correct use of ADH replacement agent or other drugs.
4. Complies with fluid restrictions.
5. Suffers no injury from mental status impairment associated with hypo-osmolality and hyponatremia.

Implementation

Assisting with achievement of therapeutic goals
Maintaining fluid balance

Frequent monitoring of these patients and early detection of problems assists in achieving fluid and electrolyte balance. High priority nursing actions that ensure adequate intake for patients with *diabetes insipidus* include the following:

1. Provide access to and assistance with oral fluid intake, as permitted.
2. Notify physician if fluid intake is inadequate, that is, intake not kept in balance with output.
3. Maintain ordered flow rates of intravenous infusions.

Water restriction is the key therapeutic measure for *SIADH-induced hyponatremia*. Fluids may be restricted to as little as 500 ml/24 hr. During changes in electrolyte levels and with the fluid restriction, thirst can be discomforting to the patient. The nurse can enhance the patient's comfort and assist in adherence to fluid restriction by the following:

1. Moistening the patient's mouth frequently by offering ice chips rather than water to allow more frequent intake
2. Offering mouth rinses to the patient
3. Planning with the patient and dietitian the most satisfactory fluid distribution

The use of hypertonic saline solution is usually reserved for patients who have severe hyponatremia ($Na^+ < 116$ mEq/L), disturbed sensorium, or convulsions. Appropriate safety measures must be provided for the patient at risk for mental confusion (place patient close to nursing station, provide frequent human contact and orientation, place on constant observation and so forth) until the serum sodium is returned to and maintained at 120 mEq/L or greater.

Diuretic therapy must be appropriately implemented in the patient with SIADH. The nurse needs to monitor the serum sodium very carefully because diuretics can worsen the hypo-osmolality and hyponatremia and precipitate changes in sensorium.

ADH replacement

The key therapeutic measure for diabetes insipidus is the administration of *antidiuretic hormone*. For immediate treatment of a crisis, aqueous vasopressin injection is used. Pitressin tannate in oil can provide longer-lasting duration of effect (over 3 days). It is only given intramuscularly; it is often painful, and swelling may occur. It is best to warm the vial and to shake it vigorously to disperse the active ingredient.

Most patients use nasal sprays of Pitressin (demopressin [DDAVP]) to maintain adequate ADH levels. They learn to determine the dosage in response to polyuria and thirst.

The patient is cautioned about overdosage and its symptoms. Usually 1 to 2 doses/24 hr are sufficient to maintain a urinary volume under 2000 ml. Overdosage of any Pitressin medication results in symptoms of ADH excess:

1. Weight gain
2. Hyponatremia and hypo-osmolality
3. Abdominal cramping
4. Neurological changes

Rhinopharyngitis may interfere with the absorption of nasal drops, sprays, or powders. For this reason, patients are taught to report this condition to the physician, as well as other medications that may be used in hyposecretion or hypersecretion of ADH listed in Table 29-9. The nurse will assist in administering these drugs and teaching the patient as appropriate.

Interventions to achieve patient outcomes

The nursing interventions for the nursing diagnoses related to fluid volume changes are largely collaborative, and these were discussed in the preceding section on assisting with the achievement of therapeutic goals.

Facilitating learning

A summary of the instructions required for the patient with diabetes insipidus is listed in Box 29-6. The patient

---

Patient Teaching 29-6

The patient with diabetes insipidus

Medication therapy
   Dosage and side effects of prescribed medication
   Correct use of prescribed Pitressin nasal spray
   Signs and symptoms (polyuria, polydipsia) that indicate the need to take prescribed medication
Signs of rhinopharyngitis (runny nose and red, painful mucous membranes) that need to be reported to the physician
Symptoms requiring immediate medical follow-up if not relieved by prescribed medications
An identification card or Medic Alert bracelet or necklace indicating the nature of the disorder needs to be carried at all times
Lifelong replacement therapy for diabetes insipidus probably will be necessary
Regular medical follow-up care that is needed

---

with chronic ADH excess will need teaching about how to manage required fluid restriction. Teaching should focus not only on the amount of the restriction, but also on helping the patient identify ways to deal with thirst.

Evaluation

Evaluation is based on the expected patient outcomes. Key questions to consider include the following:

1. Is weight maintained at normal level?
2. Is urine output equal to intake and within 800 to 2000 ml range?
3. Is serum sodium within normal limits?
4. Can patient manage self-care measures, that is, take ADH replacement correctly or maintain fluid restrictions as necessary?
5. Does the patient remain free of injuries?

ADRENAL GLAND DYSFUNCTION

Dysfunction of the adrenal gland can be manifested as an increased or decreased function of the cortex or an increased function of the medulla (Fig. 29-10). The three major hormones of the adrenal cortex are cortisol, aldosterone, and androgens. The adrenal medulla produces epinephrine and norepinephrine. The nursing process that starts on p. 845 applies to the various types of adrenal gland dysfunction that are discussed in this section.

HYPERSECRETION

Hypersecretion of the adrenal cortex can be of one hormone or all three. See Table 29-2, p. 827 for a review of functions of the hormones of the adrenal cortex. See Figure 29-2, p. 822 for a review of control mechanisms for glucocorticoids. Hypersection of adrenal medullary secretions can be epinephrine alone, norepinephrine alone, or both. See Table 29-3, p. 827 for a review of the effects of adrenal medullary stimulation.

Cortisol Excess
Etiology

Excessive production of cortisol, regardless of the cause, results in a group of signs and symptoms classified as *Cushing's syndrome*. The causes of Cushing's syndrome may be classified into four categories.

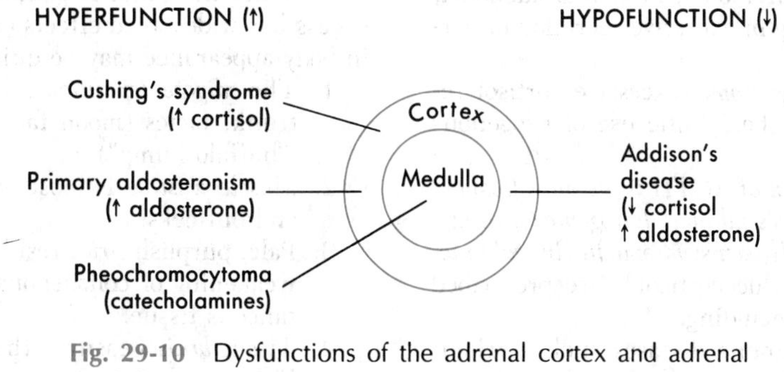

HYPERFUNCTION (↑)   HYPOFUNCTION (↓)

Fig. 29-10 Dysfunctions of the adrenal cortex and adrenal medulla.

Table 29-11 Adrenal gland dysfunction

Alteration in secretion	Signs and symptoms	Medical therapy
Adrenocortical excess	**Cortisol excess** Body appearance change Hyperglycemia, hypernatremia, hypokalemia Increased susceptibility to infections Emotional changes Hypertension, edema Weakness, fatigue	Surgery: adrenalectomy (unilateral, bilateral), excision of adrenal or pituitary tumor Irradiation of pituitary Drugs to suppress cortisol synthesis: mitotane, metyrapone, aminoglutethimide
	Aldosterone excess Hypertension Hypokalemia Hypernatremia Metabolic alkalosis Headache, edema Severe muscle weakness	Surgery: adrenalectomy, excision of tumor Spironolactone and antihypertensive agents
	Androgen excess Hirsutism, virilization, amenorrhea in females, precocious sexual development in young boys	Surgery: adrenalectomy, excision of tumor
Adrenocortical deficiency	**Cortisol lack** Weight loss, asthenia Hypoglycemia, hyponatremia, hyperkalimia Intolerance to stressors Hyperpigmentation GI complaints: nausea, vomiting, abdominal pain, diarrhea; Addisonian crisis: hypotension, vasomotor collapse, coma, hyperpyrexia	Replacement therapy: glucocorticoids (cortisone, hydrocortisone); mineralocorticoids (desoxycorticosterone, fludrocortisone) For addisonian crisis: hydrocortisone phosphate (IV), normal saline solution IV, rest
	Aldosterone lack Hypotension, hyponatremia, hyperkalemia	Replacement therapy: mineralocorticoids (desoxycorticosterone, fludrocortisone)
Adrenal medulla excess	Hypertension, episodic or sustained (usual) Occasional hypotension and tachycardia Headache, episodic Diaphoresis, pallor Palpitations Hyperglycemia during attacks Constipation or diarrhea	Surgery: excision of tumor Drugs to suppress catecholamine actions: Phenoxybenzamine (Dibenzyline), metyrosine, nitroprusside, propranolol (Indural) or metoprolol (Lopressor)

1. *Primary or adrenal Cushing's syndrome:* adrenal adenomas, adrenal hyperplasia, or adrenal carcinomas that produce excessive cortisol.
2. *Secondary or pituitary Cushing's syndrome* (also called Cushing's disease): excessive pituitary ACTH secretion resulting in excessive cortisol.
3. *Ectopic Cushing's syndrome* (also called secondary Cushing's syndrome): excessive secretion ACTH from nonpituitary sites, such as bronchogenic carcinoma, pancreatic carcinoma, bronchial adenoma, and so forth, resulting in excessive secretion of cortisol.
4. *Iatrogenic Cushing's syndrome:* excessive cortisol resulting from chronic therapeutic use of exogenous glucocorticoids.

Excessive pituitary secretion of ACTH is the most frequent pathological cause of Cushing's syndrome. Iatrogenic Cushing's syndrome is the most frequently seen syndrome in clinical practice. Therapeutic doses of glucocorticoids are prescribed for a variety of conditions including:

1. Treatment of autoimmune diseases such as rheumatoid arthritis and lupus

2. Prevention of rejection in organ transplantation
3. Prevention of excessive fibrosis (scarring) after certain surgeries or diseases particularly of the eye
4. Reduction of acute increased intracranial pressure or immediately after spinal cord injury
5. Treatment of inflammatory process associated with COPD, regional enteritis, and ulcerative colitis.

Pathophysiology

Whether the cause is pathologic or iatrogenic, cortisol excess has widespread effects (Table 29-11). The changes in body appearance may be quite striking:

1. The *adipose deposition* is classic in its distribution to trunk, facies (moon face), and intrascapular areas ("buffalo hump").
2. *Muscle wasting* is most obvious in the legs, thighs, and buttocks.
3. Pale, purplish *striae* result from thinning of skin and weakening of collagenous fibers that expose subcutaneous tissue.
4. Tissue *bruises* easily with ecchymosis formation from lack of collagen support of the blood vessels.

Conditions for which persons with cortisol excess are at high risk
Hypertension
Diabetes mellitus
Osteoporosis
Peptic ulcer
Psychoses
Infection

The affects of excessive cortisol place the patient at higher risk for many chronic illnesses (see Box 29-7). Increased gastric secretion and altered mucosal defense mechanisms increase the risk of peptic ulcers. In addition, the effects of cortisol excess on emotional stability are marked. Patients may report insomnia, nightmares, and mood swings. Frank psychoses can develop.

Many of the signs and symptoms of cortisol excess are related to its diabetogenic, catabolic, and ketogenic effects:

1. Loss of bone matrix and calcium from bones
2. Decreased glucose intolerance, decreased glucose use, and increased gluconeogenesis
3. Increased ketogenesis and fatty acid mobilization

Because cortisol has some mineralocorticoid-like activity, excessive sodium and water retention can occur.

Cortisol is immunosuppressive as a result of decreased lymphocyte production and cell-mediated immunity (Chapters 16 and 41). Although the number of neutrophils may be increased, the migration and thus activity of these cells are decreased and there are decreased fibrin deposits that limit localization of infections and allow systemic spread.

The potency of antiinflammatory action and mineralocorticoid activity vary among the many preparations (Table 29-12). The side effects of glucocorticoids place a limit on the dosage employed over time.

Beside the problems caused by corticosteroid therapy (cortisol excess), the patient is also at risk for an episode of *adrenocortical insufficiency* (cortisol deficit) should the medication be stopped suddenly or a severe stressor be encountered shortly after the medication is stopped (see section on adrenal corticoid insufficiency).

Aldosterone Excess
Etiology/epidemiology

The cause of excessive aldosterone secretion can be primary, resulting from an aldosterone secreting adrenal adenoma, or secondary. Secondary increases in aldosterone can follow increased renin production by the kidney and are associated with renal and hepatic disease and congestive heart failure. Primary aldosteronism is rare.

Pathophysiology

Three major effects of aldosterone excess are *hypertension, hypokalemia,* and *hypernatremia.* Hypertension results from the increased blood volume as a result of sodium reabsorption. As the sodium is retained, potassium is excreted and results in hypokalemia. Hypokalemia can result in the following:

1. Changes in excitability of muscle membrane, causing weakness, paresthesia, hypoactive bowel sounds, and hypoactive deep tendon reflexes
2. Cardiac arrhythmias, changes in ECG patterns (depressed or inverted T-wave is a major change), and increased sensitivity to digitalis preparations
3. Loss of the kidneys' concentrating ability: dilute urine, polyuria, and nocturia
4. Metabolic alkalosis

See Table 29-11 for a summary of signs and symptoms and medical therapy for aldosterone excess.

Androgen Excess
Etiology/epidemiology

Androgen excess can result from adrenal adenomas or carcinomas or adrenal hyperplasia. Androgen excess may occur in ovarian disease or as a side effect of some medications. Androgen excess often occurs in combination with cortisol excess in adrenal hyperplasia and with cortisol and aldosterone excess in adrenal carcinoma.

Table 29-12   Comparison of antiinflammatory and mineralocorticoid potency of derivatives of adrenocorticosteroids

Drug	Antiinflammatory potency*	Mineralocorticoid potency†
Hydrocortisone (Cortef)	1	0.03
Cortisone acetate (Cortone, Cortogen)	0.8	0.03
Prednisone (Deltasone, Meticorten)	4	0.04
Methylprednisolone (Medrol)	6	0.02
Triamcinolone (Aristocort, Kenacort)	5	None
Dexamethasone (Decadron)	30	None
Desoxycorticosterone (DOCA)	None	1
Fludrocortisone (Florinef)	10	4.2

*Potency relative to hydrocortisone, whose potency = 1.
†Potency relative to DOCA, whose potency = 1.

Pathophysiology

Androgen excess does not produce clinically significant signs in adult men. Two signs of androgen excess in women are *hirsutism* and *virilization.*

1. *Hirsutism:* an increase in coarse, dark hair on the face, abdomen, axillae, and pubes; increased sebaceous gland activity leading to oily skin and acne
2. *Virilization:* symptoms of amenorrhea or oligomenorrhea, clitoromegaly, frontal balding, deepening voice, and muscle hypertrophy

Catecholamine Excess

Etiology / epidemiology

Although rare, the most common cause of excess catecholamines in adults is *pheochromocytoma,* a catecholamine-producing tumor of the adrenal medulla. Approximately 10% of tumors of the medulla will be bilateral.[9a] These tumors arise from chromaffin cells which are derived from neural crest cells and thus similiar tumors can be found in the head, neck area, mediastinum, abdomen, bladder, testes, or anywhere along the sympathetic nervous system trunk. Ten percent or greater number of tumors are extra-adrenal.[9a] Pheochromocytomas can be benign or malignant. Approximately 10% are malignant and the malignancy rate increases in extra adrenal tumors and in children.[9a]

Pathophysiology

Although hypotension and tachycardia can be the major signs of an epinephrine secreting tumor, the *prominent sign of catecholamine excess is hypertension,* which may be labile, depending on blood levels of the catecholamines, or the blood pressure may stay persistently elevated. Most patients have an elevated blood pressure reading at least 50% of the time.[42] Headache is abrupt, severe, throbbing, and generalized; it usually is of short duration. The headache is often associated with sweating and palpitations. If hypertension is longstanding, the patient may develop hypertensive retinopathy. Other signs and symptoms along with the medical therapy are summarized in Table 29-11. An important point to remember is that a large percentage of patients remain hypertensive even after surgery.[9a]

Frequently the patient has a history of paroxysmal attacks that are precipitated by multiple factors. Postural changes (especially flexion or bending of the body), sneezing, abdominal pressure, sexual activity, eating, urination, Valsalva maneuvers, exercise, pain, and changes in environmental or body temperature are some of the major precipitating factors. In pheochromocytoma, the serum levels of catecholamines and their metabolites (metanephrines, vanillylmandelic acid [VMA]) in the urine are increased. The localization of the tumor is done with use of I-metaiodobenzylguanidine (^{131}I-MIBG) scintigraphy. CT scanning and MRI, which were once the major tools to localize tumors, are used to further delineate tumors.

HYPOSECRETION

The adrenal cortex is essential to life. Without its hormones, cortisol and aldosterone, the body's metabolic processes would respond inadequately to even minimal physical and emotional stressors, such as changes in temperature, exercise, or excitement. The normal functions of the adrenal cortex hormones are presented in Table 29-2, p. 827.

Adrenocortical Insufficiency

Etiology / epidemiology

The causes of adrenocortical insufficiency include the following:

1. Primary causes: adrenocortical destruction from infection, hemorrhage, or autoimmune processes; idiopathic atrophy; or congenital hypoplasia. Also called Addison's disease.
2. Secondary causes: adrenal hypoplasia resulting from lack of pituitary ACTH.
3. Iatrogenic: bilateral adrenalectomy, mitotane therapy, or sudden withdrawal of long-term glucocorticoid therapy.

Pathophysiology

Hypotension, hyponatremia, and hyperkalemia are characteristically seen in patients with primary adrenocortical insufficiency because of a lack of mineralocorticoids. These patients are subject to changes in cardiovascular status because of fluid and electrolyte alterations. A low circulating vascular volume and a decreased heart size develop. ECG changes (peaked T-wave is a major change) may occur with hyperkalemia.

Conversely, when there is hypoplasia secondary to decreased ACTH secretion, aldosterone secretion is not impaired. This occurs because ACTH has minimal influence on aldosterone secretion, which is under control of the renin-angiotensin system. However, there may be evidence of hyposecretion of other pituitary hormones.

Table 29-11 explains many of the signs and symptoms that occur with the lack of cortisol in primary, secondary, and iatrogenic insufficiency because of diminished protein, carbohydrate, and fat metabolism. These pathophysiological changes may lead to:

1. Hypoglycemia
2. Weight loss
3. Weakness, fatigue

Gastrointestinal symptoms (for example, anorexia, nausea and vomiting, or diarrhea) are often the reason that the person initially seeks help. Symptoms of adrenocortical insufficiency most often have a gradual onset and are vague. Asthenia (weakness) is a cardinal complaint, the intensity of which is out of proportion to other overt symptoms. It is usually more severe when stressors are present and eventually may force the patient to stay in bed.

The decreased cortisol level is often associated with mental and emotional changes: loss of vigor, depression, irritability, and loss of ability to concentrate. Apathy and generalized weakness contribute to decreased activity.

Hyperpigmentation with a bronzelike discoloration of skin and mucous membranes is a common sign in primary adrenal insufficiency. This is caused by increased levels of melanocyte-stimulating hormone (MSH) from the anterior pituitary. In normal persons, cortisol causes negative feedback inhibition of MSH, one of the precursors of ACTH. This lack of cortisol in adrenal insufficiency allows the

MSH level to increase along with the ACTH. Persons with secondary insufficiency do not usually have hyperpigmentation because their levels of MSH and ACTH are low (see Figure 29-2, p. 822 for a review of the negative feedback control of cortisol).

Iatrogenic adrenocortical insufficiency results from hypothalamic-pituitary-adrenal changes that are induced by corticosteroid therapy. An elevation of serum cortisol levels inhibits the secretion of ACTH and CRH; thus the responsiveness of the hypothalamic-pituitary-adrenal (HPA) axis and the stimulation of the cells of the adrenal cortex are decreased. This form of insufficiency shows up when the corticosteroid therapy is withdrawn. This suppression of the responsiveness of the HPA axis may persist for up to 1 year, if corticosteroid therapy is used in large doses or if therapy is prolonged. During the period of HPA axis suppression, stressors may precipitate acute adrenocortical insufficiency (adrenal crisis). Measures to reduce the suppression of the HPA axis include administering cortisol on alternate days in the morning or in a larger dose in the morning and a smaller dose in the early afternoon. Topical administration of corticosteroids causes less suppression than does systemic administration. Tapering with withdrawal is used to prevent reactivation or flare-up of the underlying disease and to determine the lowest adequate dosage.

Addisonian Crisis (Adrenal Crisis)

Adrenal crisis is a *severe* and *sudden* exacerbation of adrenal insufficiency. It can quickly lead to death unless it is treated promptly. It is usually precipitated by stressors. Adrenal crisis (*Addisonian crisis*) can occur in any person with adrenal insufficiency and is manifested by acute exaggeration of signs and symptoms and vascular collapse. (See Box 29-8.)

Nursing Process
Assessment
Subjective data

Common considerations in assessing patients with pituitary dysfunction (p. 833) are also pertinent for adrenal dysfunction because of the effect of the anterior pituitary on the adrenal glands. The nurse can gain insight into patient needs by considering the following data:

1. Extent of fatigue
2. Patient's perception of body image changes
3. Mood changes
4. Ability to tolerate stressors
5. Need for assistance with activities of daily living
6. Sleep patterns
7. Eating patterns
8. Knowledge of the adrenal dysfunction and its treatment
9. Medication regimen
10. Presence of discomforting symptoms

Objective data

Ongoing patient assessment should include the following:
1. Daily weight
2. Temperature and blood pressure every 4 hours and PRN

29-8	**Signs and symptoms of adrenal crisis**
	Hypotension
	Shock
	Fever
	Nausea and vomiting
	Confusion
	Electrolyte imbalances ($\downarrow$ sodium, $\uparrow$ potassium)
	Hypoglycemia

---

3. Intake and output every 4 hours
4. Skin integrity
5. Activity level
6. Food intake
7. Early signs of infection

The nurse should be alert for clinical findings that indicate excess or deficiency of adrenal hormones, including those of acute crises. Laboratory tests of serum glucose and electrolyte levels should be closely monitored.

Diagnostic tests

Diagnosis in adrenocortical dysfunction relies heavily on measurements of serum and urinary levels of hormones and metabolites (Tables 29-13 and 29-14). There is usually no special preparation needed for tests of blood hormonal values, unless provocative agents are used to test responses of the adrenal gland to a stimulant or depressant. Provocative agents could be medications, diet, or any stimulus that elicits a known response. For example, an upright position or sodium loading can be used to stimulate aldosterone secretion. When such tests are performed, special care must be taken to clarify any questions and avoid the need to reschedule that test. The measurement of VMA is influenced by the diet. Thus, before the test, dietary restrictions for approximately 3 days are necessary. Tests of adrenocortical function are described in Table 29-14. The presence of tumors of the adrenal cortex will require a CT scan or an MRI. Adrenal medullary tumors are confirmed by ^{131}I-MIBG scintigraphy.

Special care must be taken if provocative agents are used to test catecholamine secretion in suspected pheochromocytoma; histamine, which depletes catecholamines, may precipitate a hypertensive crisis. Regitine, an adrenergic-blocking agent, may induce severe hypotension. These agents are used infrequently today.

When urinary hormonal levels of metabolites are measured, timed specimens are collected. Important nursing actions include the following:
1. Start and stop the urine collection at the specified times; this is necessary if the pattern of diurnal secretion is to be analyzed correctly.
2. Obtain the specimen container and preservative required by the hospital laboratory; icing the specimen may be necessary.
3. Instruct the patient and involved staff in the procedure recommended by the laboratory.
4. Ensure that all urine voided in the time period is collected.

Table 29-13   Comparison of laboratory findings in hyposecretion and hypersecretion of adrenal gland

Substance	Hyposecretion	Hypersecretion
Adrenal cortex		
Plasma levels		
Cortisol	Low in all cases of adrenal cortex insufficiency	High in all cases of adrenal cortex hypersecretion
Aldosterone	Low in primary adrenal insufficiency	High in adrenal hyperplasia or aldosterone-secreting tumors
Androgen	Low in primary adrenal insufficiency	High in adrenal hyperplasia or androgen-secreting tumors
ACTH	Low in secondary and iatrogenic adrenal insufficiency	High in pituitary or ectopic hypersecretion of ACTH
	High in primary adrenal deficiency resulting from lack of feedback inhibition by cortisol	Low in primary adrenal hypersecretion because of inhibition by cortisol
MCH	High in primary adrenal insufficiency	Normal
Urinary excretion of cortisol metabolites	All usually are low in primary or secondary adrenocortical hyposecretion	All are high in primary adrenocortical hypersecretion
17-Ketogenic glucocorticoids (17-KGs) 5 to 23 mg/24 hr (male) 5 to 18 mg/24 hr (female)		
17-Hydroxycorticosteroids (17-OHCS) 3-10 mg/24 hr		
17-Ketosteroids (17-KS) (androgens) 5 to 18 mg/24 hr	17-KS may be normal with secondary adrenal insufficiency	17-KS may be high in androgen-secreting tumors or enzymatic deficiency
Aldosterone and 18-glucoronide 16 mg/24 hr	Aldosterone and 18-glucoronide may be normal with secondary adrenal insufficiency	Aldosterone elevated in hyperaldosteronism
Adrenal medulla		
Plasma levels		
Epinephrine		All are increased in pheochromocytoma
Norepinephrine		
Total catecholamines		
Urinary excretion		
Total catecholamines		All are increased in pheochromocytoma
Epinephrine		
Norepinephrine		
Metanephrine		Metanephrine is a urinary metabolite of epinephrine
Vanillylmandelic acid (VMA)		VMA is end product of catecholamine metabolism

a. Just before starting the collection, the patient should void and that urine is discarded.

b. The last urine collected should be of a voiding at the time the test ends.

Additional tests that the physician may order include the following:

1. Glucose tolerance test (Chapter 28)
2. Renal function tests (Chapter 33)
3. Roentgenograms of kidney or abdomen
4. Adrenal arteriograms

Data analysis: nursing diagnoses

Nursing diagnoses are determined from the analysis of patient data. Possible nursing diagnoses for the person with adrenal dysfunction may include those identified on p. 834 (with the exception of sensory/perceptual alterations) because anterior pituitary dysfunction may result in adrenal cortex dysfunction.

Other nursing diagnoses specific to adrenal hormonal imbalance include the following:

Diagnostic title	Possible etiologies
For the patient with Cushing's syndrome	
Infection, high risk for	Decreased immune response
Altered nutrition: more than body requirements	Excessive intake in relation to metabolic needs; lack of knowledge
Fluid volume excess	Compromised regulatory mechanism—inappropriate conservation of sodium and water
Fatigue	Muscle wasting and weakness, hypokalemia

Table 29-14   Tests of adrenocortical function

Function test	Procedure and preparation	Interpretation
ACTH stimulation test (various tests available)	Synthetic ACTH given in 500-1000 ml of normal saline at 2 units/24 hr; then 17-OHCS and plasma cortisol levels are measured; alternative is to infuse 25 units of ACTH over an 8 hr period on 2-3 days and measure 17-OCHS and plasma cortisol levels on these days	Normally 17-OHCS excretion increases to 25 mg/24 hr and plasma cortisol increases to 40 µg/100 ml or greater; in patients with secondary adrenal insufficiency, the 17-OHCS rate is 3-20 mg/24 hr and the cortisol level is 10-40 µg/dl
Screening ACTH stimulation test	ACTH, 25 units, is given IM and plasma cortisol level is measured before and at 30 and 60 min intervals	Normally plasma cortisol increases 7 µg/dl
Cortisol suppression test	Twenty-four-hour urine specimen for 17-OCHS is collected for baseline; dexamethasone, 0.5 mg, is given every 6 hr for 2 days; 24 hr urine is collected for 2 days	Dexamethasone normally suppresses pituitary secretion of ACTH and thus of steroids; normally by day 2 of dexamethasone, 24-hr urinary level of OHCS should drop more than 50% below baseline, patients with primary adrenocortical excess show decrease in 24-hr urine levels; patients with secondary adrenocortical excess have drop, but less than 50%
Screening cortisol suppression test	Dexamethasone, 1 mg, given at 12 PM; at 8 AM cortisol level is drawn	Normally cortisol should be less than 5 µg/dl
Mineralocorticoid suppression test (various tests are available)	IV infusion of saline 500 ml/hr for 4 hr	Normally saline infusion depresses plasma aldosterone to <8 µg/dl

Diagnostic title	Possible etiologies
Body image disturbance	Change in body appearance or function
Knowledge deficit: disorder, diagnostic test, self-care measures	Lack of exposure
For the patient with aldosterone excess	
Fluid volume excess—	Compromised regulary mechanism—severe retention of sodium and water
Knowledge deficit: disorder, diagnostic tests, self-care measures	Lack of exposure; new diagnosis
For the patient with adrenal androgen excess	
Body image disturbance	Compromised regulatory mechanism—occurrence of changes in sexual characteristics
For the patient with pheochromocytoma	
High risk for impaired tissue perfusion: cerebral	Impairment in blood perfusion associated with uncontrolled elevation in blood pressure
Fear	Paroxysmal attacks
Knowledge deficit: disorder, diagnostic tests, treatment, self-care needs	New diagnosis and no previous exposure to information
For the patient with adrenal insufficiency	
Decreased cardiac output	Reduced fluid and electrolyte intake; inadequate cortisol replacement, noncompliance, lack of knowledge
Fluid volume deficit	Compromised regulatory mechanisms—inadequate sodium and water conservation
Coping, ineffective individual	Impaired ability to mount stress response

Diagnostic title	Possible etiologies
Fatigue	Muscle weakness, hypoglycemia, hypokalemia
Knowledge deficit: disorder, diagnostic tests, therapy, self-care	New disease and no previous exposure to information

Planning: expected patient outcomes

Expected outcomes for the person with adrenal hormonal imbalances include those listed on p. 835. In addition, expected outcomes include, but are not limited to, the following:

1. Patient with Cushing's syndrome:
   a. Explains ways to avoid infections and describes what to do if infections occur.
   b. Describes dietary restrictions.
   c. Intake equals output, edema decreases, body weight decreases.
   d. Fatigue is decreased as rated by patient.
   e. States needs (if unable to meet by self because of fatigue) are met.
   f. Describes self in positive terms.
   g. Describes any therapeutic regimens prescribed for hypertension or diabetes mellitus, if appropriate.
2. Patient with aldosterone excess:
   a. Sodium and water balance return to normal.
   b. Blood pressure is within normal limits.
   c. Describes any therapeutic regimens prescribed for hypertension and hypokalemia.
3. Patient with androgen excess:
   a. Describes self in positive terms.

Table 29-15 **Comparison of clinical problems of Cushing's disease and Addison's disease**

Cushing's syndrome	Addison's disease
Hypertension	Hypotension
Hyperglycemia	Hypoglycemia
Hypervolemia	Hypovolemia
Hypokalemia	Hyperkalemia
Immunosuppression	Intolerance to stressors
Osteoporosis	

4. Patient with pheochromocytoma:
  a. Mental status and sensory and motor function remain normal.
  b. Describes what can and should do if attack occurs.
  c. Describes any diagnostic tests, planned therapy.
5. Patient with *adrenocortical insufficiency:*
  a. Blood pressure and pulse are returned to normal and are maintained; urine output is normal; skin warm and dry; mental status normal.
  b. Intake equals output and is within normal limits; body weight is returned to normal and maintained.
  c. Stressors are decreased until patient stable.
  d. Explains the effects of stressors on the need for medication.
  e. Identifies stressors in own life and ways to control them.
  f. States awareness of the need for additional medication in times of severe stress response.
  g. Describes any therapeutic plans and self-care needs.

Implementation

The interventions designed to assist in achievement of therapeutic goals and to achieve patient outcomes are presented together for each type of patient.

Certain nursing measures are appropriate regardless of the type of adrenal dysfunction. The *maintenance* of medication regimens is a high priority. Other measures include those that achieve the following:
1. Provision of adequate rest
2. Regulation of blood pressure levels within desired limits
3. Maintenance of fluid and electrolyte balance
4. Maintenance of adequate nutrition to maintain or achieve desired weight and to keep blood glucose levels within normal limits.
5. Provision of an environment that is as restful and as free of stressors as possible

The reasons for the above nursing measures are shown in Table 29-15.

The patient with Cushing's syndrome

Nurses can assist patients with specific therapy directed toward correcting the hormonal imbalance caused by dis-

ease. Measures may include one or more of the following:
1. Pituitary surgery or radiation
2. Unilateral or bilateral adrenalectomy
3. Drug therapy to suppress or block synthesis of cortisol (see Table 29-11)
4. Surgery to remove an ectopic source of ACTH

In iatrogenic Cushing's syndrome or when corrective treatment is not feasible, measures include those that control the side effects of the glucocorticoid therapy, that is, hypertension, hypokalemia, hyperglycemia, hypercalciuria, hypervolemia, infections, and osteoporosis.

Nurses can assist patients with the following:
1. Nutrition: calorie and sodium restrictions and potassium supplements to deal with the fluid volume excess, fatigue, and altered nutrition
2. Fluid and electrolyte balance: diuretics and potassium supplements; restriction of fluids to deal with fluid volume excess and fatigue
3. Blood glucose control: calorie restriction and insulin replacement to handle the altered nutrition and help with body image changes
4. Blood pressure control: antihypertensive agents and sodium restrictions to deal with the fluid volume excess
5. Ambulation to prevent osteoporosis and safety measures to prevent pathologic fractures when osteoporosis is present

Persons with Cushing's syndrome are at particular risk for *nosocomial infections* because of their immunosuppressed states. Immunosuppression combined with metabolic imbalance and obesity impairs wound healing. Careful handwashing and aseptic technique are essential. Patients must not be exposed to infection, and they should be separated from other patients with infections. Staff members who have *any* signs or symptoms of infection should not care for these patients.

Body image changes are numerous. They are reversible once the hypersecretion of glucocorticoids is controlled. However, for the patient with iatrogenic Cushing's syndrome counseling and care as described on page 838 is necessary.

The patient with pituitary, adrenal or ectopic Cushing's syndrome will need explanations about the disease, treatment, and expected outcomes. These patients are usually very ill and fatigue easily so teaching needs to be spaced at intervals. Adrenal surgery causes many problems the patient must be prepared for. Considerable hemodynamic and metabolic changes occur rapidly. A temporary cortisol deficit may occur after unilateral adrenalectomy or resection of an adenoma. The cortisol deficit results from the depressed responsiveness of the HPA axis and the atrophy of the normal adrenal gland, which is caused by HPA axis suppression by the previously high blood-cortisol levels. Bilateral adrenalectomy results in permanent cortisol deficit because surgery changes the hormonal imbalance from cortisol excess to cortisol deficit. After adrenal surgery the patient has iatrogenic adrenal insufficiency and is at risk for adrenal crisis. Hormonal replacement is essential for maintenance of life. After bilateral adrenalectomy, ACTH levels rise in the absence of the negative feedback control of cortisol-blood levels.

For the patient with iatrogenic Cushing's syndrome, the major focus of nursing care is patient teaching. The patient must be prepared for all potential side effects. They will need teaching about diet, fluid and electrolytes, blood glucose control, blood pressure control, ambulation, and avoidance of infection. Importantly, they must carry out the activities described in Box 29-4. Because the information and self care is so tremendous, several teaching sessions should be planned and written, verbal and audiovisual materials should be used.

The patient with primary aldosteronism

The fluid and sodium excess and hypertension associated with primary aldosteronism are usually treated with surgical resection of the adrenal adenoma or unilateral adrenalectomy. Bilateral hyperplasia is usually treated with sodium restriction, potassium replacement, and the aldosterone antagonist, spironolactone. These same measures may be used preoperatively.

After surgery a temporary suppression of renin-induced aldosterone production may be present and fluid deficit can occur. If the aldosterone deficit is severe, fludrocortisone may be necessary. If the deficit is mild, treatment of acidosis and hyperkalemia may be achieved with sodium bicarbonate and sodium polystyrene sulfonate (Kayexalate) after surgery. Usually aldosterone production returns to normal within 6 months. Surgery reverses hypertension in a majority of patients.

Patients will require teaching for the diagnostic test and for the adrenal surgery (see p. 850) or for life-long medications and dietary treatment. Written materials should be used to supplement verbal information.

The patient with androgen excess

Body image change is the major nursing diagnosis for the person with androgen excess. Nursing care will focus on helping patients manage and cope with these changes (see p. 838).

The patient with pheochromocytoma

The primary treatment of pheochromocytoma is surgical removal of the tumor. The priority of preoperative care is control of hypertension. Medication to control hypertension includes alpha and beta adrenergic blocking agents (see Table 29-11). During a hypertensive crisis, the patient should be admitted to an intensive care unit. Cardiac monitoring and frequent monitoring of vital signs are necessary. When the patient's blood pressure reaches the desired level, medication can be gradually decreased.

Maintaining blood pressure at a desired level is a major concern during anesthesia, surgery, and the postoperative period. The antihypertensive medication used preoperatively may influence the choice of anesthetic agent; manipulation of the tumor during surgery may release large bursts of hormones causing elevation of the blood pressure. When the tumor is removed sudden hypotension may occur. Hypotension is usually treated with plasma or a plasma substitute. Appropriately administered volume expanders (normal saline) usually control the hypotension, making vasopressors unnecessary.

On the first postoperative day, hypertensive episodes are common and caused by the response to pain and to hypervolemia caused by the treatment of hypotension after surgery. Currently, the most effective therapy for this hypertension is a rapidly acting diuretic such as furosemide (Lasix).

The patient will need careful preparation for diagnostic tests so that the tumor can be identified as quickly as possible. Preoperatively the blood pressure must be controlled for at least 1 week before surgery so patients will need to know self-care measures. Postoperatively, many patients remain hypertensive so the patient will need to know how to take any prescribed medications and the side effects to monitor for. The patient will be followed and reassessed for reoccurrence. The patient must understand the importance of this follow-up.

The patient with adrenal insufficiency

The primary nursing activities for a patient with severe adrenocortical insufficiency are directed towards improving and maintaining cardiac output and fluid volume and decreasing the number of stressors. Actions required include:

1. Hormonal replacement of glucocorticoids and mineralocorticoids
2. Administering sodium and fluids as ordered
3. Monitoring fluid status including intake and output, daily weights, urine specific gravity, blood pressure and pulse, mental status, and skin temperature and moisture
4. The number of stressors are decreased by using a private room, limiting disturbances, keeping temperature controlled, decreasing noise, and promoting physical and mental rest.

Fatigue will be partially relieved as cardiac output and fluid status are improved. The patient does need an adequate intake of carbohydrates and protein to meet glucose and protein needs.

The patient's adrenal insufficiency may be partial or complete, thus the doses of hormonal replacement will vary. In mild adrenocortical insufficiency, cortisol may be needed only during periods of stress, and mineralocorticoid insufficiency can be managed with high sodium intake. When cortisol and aldosterone deficit is absolute, as after bilateral adrenalectomy, the usual hormonal replacement is as follows:

1. Cortisone: 37.5 mg daily (25 mg in the early morning and 12.5 mg in the early evening)
2. Fludrocortisone: 0.1 to 0.2 mg daily

Synthetic preparations of cortisol may be used instead of cortisone.

Adrenal insufficiency after surgery of the pituitary gland or associated with other disease of the anterior pituitary gland was discussed on p. 837.

Once the patient is stable, patient education to promote self-care will be necessary. The patient will need all the information described in Box 29-4. Additionally the patient will have to institute monitoring to detect signs and symptoms of excess of glucocorticoids and mineralocorticoids because the needs vary from day to day (see page 842). Last the patient must be able to identify stressors, ways to minimize stressors, and how to change the medication at times of increased stressors.

The patient having adrenal surgery

Preoperative

Provide supportive care.

Assist patient with usual preoperative care.

Maintain nutritional status with a high-protein, prescribed calorie diet with adequate minerals and vitamins.

Assist with correction of fluid and electrolyte imbalance.

Assist with hormonal suppression as prescribed (see Table 29-11).

Assist with measures used to prevent or treat crises of adrenal hormonal excess or deficit.

Administer prescribed intravenous fluids and glucocorticoid before surgery.

Postoperative

Establish monitoring schedule to detect complications of surgery;
  Adrenal crisis
  Blood pressure alterations
  Blood glucose alterations
  Fluid and electrolyte imbalances

Pace postoperative activities with alternate periods of rest and gradual increase in self-care (because the patient may have unusual activity intolerance).

Provide measures to minimize effects of postural hypotension:
  Apply ace bandages or elastic stockings.
  Assess effects of posture on blood pressure.
  Change patient's positions slowly.
  Assist or accompany the patient during ambulation while blood pressure remains labile.

Provide measures to decrease risk of infection in the immunosuppressed patient (for instance, strict surgical asepsis, deep breathing, avoiding contact with persons with upper respiratory infections).

Administer cortisol replacement as prescribed:
  Intravenous route for the first 24 hours
  Intramuscular route the second day
  Oral route when patient is able to tolerate food by mouth

Administer mineralocorticosteroid (Fludrohydrocortisone) replacement, if prescribed.
  Typically prescribed when cortisol replacement is less than 40 to 50 mg/24 hr in the patient with bilateral adrenalectomy

Assist patient and family in learning about required hormonal replacement (see p. 838)
  Bilateral adrenalectomy: maintenance dose of cortisol and mineralocorticoids
  Unilateral adrenalectomy: doses of cortisol dependent on degree of suppression of HPA axis

Assist patient and family in learning about self-care needs:
  Monitoring for signs and symptoms of deficiency
  Monitoring for signs and symptoms of excess
  Dietary needs
  Ways to decrease stressors or to manage stressors
  How to manipulate steroids in relation to stressors

Inform patient of required follow-up

Surgery

The patient undergoing adrenal surgery usually has a preoperative state of hormonal excess (cortisol, aldosterone, or catecholamines) that is suddenly reversed by surgery. This rapid change is associated with instability in hemodynamic and metabolic functions and varies according to the hormones involved and the amount of functional adrenal tissue that remains. The patient must be given constant nursing attention until hormonal stability is regained or a maintenance regimen established.

When cortisol deficit is expected after surgery, glucocorticoid replacement is first given by intravenous drip throughout the perioperative period and then changed to oral doses. The dosage is adjusted by evaluating measurements of blood pressure, blood glucose, electrolyte, and serum cortisol levels. Monitoring for signs of adrenal insufficiency and adrenal crisis should be frequent. An increase in glucocorticoid medication is often required when blood pressure levels are less than adequate.

Along with hormonal, fluid, and electrolyte replacement, vasopressors may be necessary to maintain adequate blood pressure in the immediate postoperative period. Orthostatic hypotension is not unusual as the patient begins ambulation.

The patient is also observed carefully for signs of hypoglycemia (weakness, sweaty, nervous, tachycardia, skin moist, sluggish, increased appetite). This condition is most likely to occur if the patient had diabetes mellitus as a symptom, but it can occur in any patient who has adrenal gland surgery. Intravenous solutions containing glucose are usually ordered. If the patient is able to eat, the nurse should check to see that all food on the tray is consumed. A balanced diet of carbohydrates, proteins and fat is encouraged.

Teaching the patient about adrenocortical insufficiency and the importance of hormonal replacement was discussed previously for the patient having surgery on the pituitary. It is not unheard of for patients to be admitted to the hospital in adrenal crisis because they did not understand the need to take their medication as ordered. The nursing care for patients having adrenal surgery is summarized in Box 29-9.

Evaluation

Evaluation is based on the expected patient outcomes. Questions to consider may include the following:

1. For the patient with Cushing's syndrome:
   a. Were infections avoided?
   b. Were dietary restrictions maintained?
   c. Did intake and output stay in balance? And was an appropriate weight attained?
   d. Was fatigue controlled?
   e. Could patient accurately describe self-care?
2. For the patient with aldosterone excess:
   a. Was sodium and water balance restored and maintained?
   b. Was blood pressure kept within normal limits?
   c. Could the patient describe the self-care needs for elevated blood pressure and low potassium?
3. For the patient with androgen excess:
   a. Did patient describe self in positive terms?

4. For the patient with pheochromocytoma:
   a. Did mental status and sensory and motor function remain normal?
   b. If changes occurred, were they detected and reported immediately?
   c. Did the patient know what to do for paroxysmal attacks?
   d. Could the patient describe:
      (1) Purpose of diagnostic test?
      (2) Planned surgery and care associated with surgery?
      (3) Self care needs after discharge?
5. For the patient with adrenocorticoid insufficiency:
   a. Was blood pressure, pulse, urine output, intake and body weight returned to normal and maintained?
   b. Was fatigue decreased?
   c. Could the patient identify stressors and describe what to do when stressors increased?
   d. Could patient describe self care needs?

PARATHYROID DYSFUNCTION

Parathyroid hormone (PTH) is involved with maintenance of calcium and phosphorus levels (Table 29-4, p. 828 presents an overview of functions of the PTH). PTH and vitamin D are two major regulators of calcium metabolism. PTH excess results in increased blood calcium levels, whereas PTH deficit leads to hypocalcemic states. PTH excess leads to hypophosphatemia, whereas PTH deficit is associated with elevated serum levels of phosphorus.

PTH and vitamin D work together to promote absorption of calcium from the intestine. They both promote bone resorption of calcium. In hypoparathyroidism, PTH deficiency impairs the synthesis of vitamin D to its active form $(1,25[OH]_2D)$, and thus vitamin D deficiencies accompany PTH deficits. See Table 29-18 for information about vitamin D synthesis.

Calcitonin, a third regulator of calcium metabolism, has actions antagonistic to PTH and vitamin D. It is not involved in parathyroid disorders; however, it may be used for treatment of severe hypercalcemia. Calcitonin inhibits bone resorption. The signs, symptoms, and medical therapy for persons with various types of dysfunctions are summarized in Table 29-16. The nursing process for parathyroid dysfunction starts on p. 852.

PARATHYROID HORMONE (PTH) EXCESS
Etiology

Parathyroid hormone excess results from primary causes such as parathyroid gland adenomas and carcinomas and parathyroid hyperplasia. Secondary causes of parathyroid hormone excess include renal failure, rickets, PTH-resistant nephropathy, vitamin D intoxication, and ectopic secretion by parathyroid-like tumors. Parathyroid abnormalities in persons with renal failure are a common clinically seen cause of excess.

Pathophysiology

Normally, a low serum calcium level stimulates secretion of PTH, whereas a high serum level inhibits its secretion. In primary hyperparathyroidism, PTH does not become suppressed with the elevated serum calcium level (dysfunctional negative-feedback system), thus hypercalcemia results. In many instances elevated serum calcium is the only sign of parathyroid dysfunction and is detected on routine examination. Mild symptoms of weakness and easy fatigability may be present. In some patients severe effects of hypercalcemia (renal or bone disease) may be evident.

Most of the symptoms seen in PTH excess are a result of the hypercalcemia. The effect of increased calcium on the muscles leads to hypotonicity of gastrointestinal mus-

Table 29-16   **Parathyroid dysfunction**

Signs and symptoms	Medical therapy
PTH hormone excess	
Hypercalcemia and hypophosphatemia:	Hydration, normal saline infusion
Anorexia, nausea, vomiting, fatigue, depression, polyuria, polydipsia, dehydration; bone pain, muscle hypotonia and hyporeflexia; constipation	Furosemide (Lasix)
	Phosphate infusion or oral salts
	Calcitonin
	Mithramycin
	Dialysis
	Surgical excision of tumor or parathyroidectomy
	Antacids (phosphate-binders) for patients with renal failure
PTH hormone deficiency	
Hypocalcemia:	Calcium salts: give with food but not with dairy products; calcium gluconate, calcium chloride
Paresthesia, Chvostek's sign, Trousseau's sign, carpopedal spasm, marked anxiety, seizures, laryngeal stridor, dyspnea, cyanosis, arrhythmias	Vitamin D supplements: Hytakerol, calciferol
Hyperphosphatemia:	Dietary calcium and vitamin D
Soft tissue calcifications; nausea, vomiting, abdominal pain; dry scaling skin, brittle nails; patchy, thin hair	

cles, skeletal muscles, and tendon reflexes. Thus decreased bowel mobility, abdominal pain, nausea, vomiting, and anorexia are common and lead to weight loss and fatigue. Some patients have histories of peptic ulcer disease and GI bleeding. The fatigue associated with the weight loss is worsened by skeletal muscle weakness. Mental changes may vary from confusion to depression or psychosis. Relatively small elevations of calcium may cause major mental changes, especially in elderly persons.

The continued removal of calcium phosphate from the bones results in a variety of bone lesions. Bone pain may be severe, and bone fragility can predispose the patient to fractures. In primary hyperparathyroidism, hypophosphatemia occurs.

Secondary hyperparathyroidism develops from chronic hypocalcemic states, such as renal failure. Hyperplasia of the parathyroid glands develops with an increase in PTH. The hyperplasia and excessive production of PTH may be enough to keep the serum calcium normal, but this is at the expense of bone integrity. In some patients, the parathyroid glands become autonomous and lose their responsiveness to serum calcium levels (tertiary hyperparathyroidism). In renal failure the chronic hypocalcemia results from ↑ phosphorous, inability to activate vitamin D, and poor calcium intake and absorption.

Primary and most causes of secondary hyperparathyroidism result in *hypercalcemia* and *hypophosphatemia*. The patient has increased urinary excretion of both calcium and phosphorus with the following effects:

1. Inability of the kidney to concentrate urine
2. Polyuria
3. Increased risk of renal calculi with subsequent urinary obstruction or infection
4. Calcification of renal tubules

In hyperparathyroidism secondary to renal failure, the changes in urinary and kidney function as described in the preceding paragraph are not seen and hyperphosphatemia occurs.

When the serum calcium level rises above 16 to 18 mg/dl, acute hypercalcemic crisis occurs. Severe intractable vomiting leads to dehydration and electrolyte imbalances. Fever, severe mental changes, coma, and cardiac arrhythmias may result, ending in death if untreated.

PARATHYROID HORMONE (PTH) DEFICIENCY

Etiology

Parathyroid hormone deficiency results from autoimmune destruction of the gland, from idiopathic changes, or secondary to excision of the glands. Temporary hypoparathyroidism is a risk for every person undergoing thyroidectomy or surgical exploration of the neck.

Pathophysiology

With a diminished level of parathyroid hormone, there is decreased bone resorption, and the serum calcium level falls. Because parathyroid hormone is involved in the renal clearance of phosphate, serum phosphate levels increase. The decreased level of serum calcium results in neuromuscular irritability.

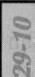

29-10

Signs of latent tetany

Paresthesia in fingertips and around mouth
Chvostek's sign (facial contraction on tapping facial nerve near jaw angle)
Trousseau's sign (carpal spasm after compression of upper arm with a cuff)
Carpopedal spasm (spasm of wrist and fingers and/or feet and toes)

Nerves show decreased thresholds of excitation, repeated responses to a single stimuli, and in severe cases, continuous activity. The neuromuscular irritability is manifested in both peripheral sensory and motor nerves and is responsible for the signs of latent tetany (see Box 29-10). Convulsions, laryngeal stridor and bronchospasm, and cardiac arrhythmias are possible if treatment is not instituted for the latent tetany.

Acute hypocalcemia (tetany) is life threatening, and the signs of latent tetany should always be promptly reported to the physician (see Box 29-10 and Table 29-16). Changes in electroencephalographic (EEG) patterns may be present, and a prolonged Q-T interval is frequently seen on the cardiac monitor.

It is important for the nurse to recognize that the clinical findings of hypocalcemia are more reliable than the total serum calcium level, which measures (1) the ionized (unbound) blood calcium, which is the active metabolic calcium, and (2) the nonionized (bound) calcium, which does not affect neuroactivity. A low serum albumin results in a decrease in nonionized (bound) calcium and total serum calcium. But because ionized calcium levels are normal, signs and symptoms of hypocalcemia do not occur.

The principal problem in acute hypoparathyroidism is hypocalcemia. In prolonged hypoparathyroidism, there may be other problems of calcium imbalance, such as cataracts, malabsorption, and decreased growth of skin and nails. Hyperphosphatemia is indicated by calcifications in blood vessels, nerves, and soft tissues.

Nursing Process
Assessment

The signs and symptoms of calcium excess and deficit are priority observations when patients are assessed for parathyroid dysfunction.

Subjective data

The following subjective data are obtained from the patient:

1. Presence of discomfort (bone pain), fatigue, or paresthesia
2. Elimination patterns (constipation, polyuria)
3. Gastrointestinal symptoms (anorexia, nausea, vomiting, abdominal pain, or history of constipation or ulcers)
4. Emotional changes (anxiety)
5. Medication usage

Table 29-17 Diagnostic tests for parathyroid function

Test	Procedure	Interpretation
Serum		
Total calcium 9.6-10.4 mg/100 ml	Blood sample No preparation	Measures both bound and ionized calcium; increased in primary hyperparathyroidism; decreased in hypoparathyroidism or with low albumin
Phosphorus 1.3-1.75 mEq/L	Blood sample	Decreased with hypercalcemia and elevated in hypocalcemia and in renal failure
Alkaline phosphatase 2-5 Bodansky units	Blood sample	Increased in bone demineralization, liver disease, and by certain drugs
Parathyroid hormone (PTH) by radioimmunoassay	Blood sample	Elevated in hyperparathyroidism and decreased in hypoparathyroidism
Urine		
Calcium	Collect single specimen	Decreased in hypoparathyroidism
Quantitative	24-hr collection	Elevated in hyperparathyroidism
Phosphorus	24-hr collection	Elevated in renal failure, hypocalcemic states, and PTH excess; decreased with PTH lack
Function tests		
Ellsworth-Howard excretion test (PTH infusion test)	Fasting required; 200 units of PTH extract administered IV; hourly urine collections	Normal response is 5-6 times increased urinary phosphate excretion; an increase of 10 times is found in hypoparathyroidism
Urinary cAMP	Urine sample	High levels of cyclic AMP found in hyperparathyroidism

6. Dietary history
7. Knowledge of condition

Objective data

Objective data include the following:
1. Mental status (signs of behavior changes)
2. Intake and output every 8 hours
3. Daily weight
4. Changes in reflexes (hypo- or hyper-reflexia)
5. Respiratory status
6. Muscle weakness or twitching
7. Electrolyte levels (calcium, phosphorus)
8. Condition of skin, hair, and nails

Diagnostic tests

Because the maintenance of normal calcium and phosphorus metabolism involves multiple systems besides the parathyroid (skeletal, gastrointestinal, and urinary), when parathyroid function is being assessed, the patient also undergoes diagnostic tests of these other systems. This is necessary to determine whether the problem with calcium and phosphorus metabolism is caused by parathyroid metabolism or other disease states. In addition, ECG, EEG, and sometimes nerve conduction studies may be performed in an effort to detect hypotonicity or neuromuscular irritability. Tests of parathyroid function are shown in Table 29-17.

Data analysis: nursing diagnoses

Nursing diagnoses are determined from the analysis of patient data. Possible nursing diagnoses for the person with parathyroid disorders include, but are not limited to the following:

Diagnostic title	Possible etiologies
For the patient with hyperparathyroidism and hypercalcemia:	
Impaired physical mobility	Pain, neuromuscular impairment
Nutrition, altered: less than body requirements	Anorexia, nausea, vomiting
Constipation	Decrease in GI motility
For the patient with hypoparathyroidism and hypocalcemia:	
Ineffective breathing	Neuromuscular impairment, obstruction of airway
Decreased cardiac output	Disturbed neurologic mechanisms: arrhythmias
For either patient:	
Injury, high risk for	Increased neuromuscular excitability; altered mental status leading to falls
Knowledge deficit: disease, diagnostic tests, treatment, side effects of treatment, follow-up, and self-care	New information; new problem

Planning: expected patient outcomes

Expected patient outcomes for the person with parathyroid disorders may include, but are not limited to the following:

The patient with *hyperparathyroidism* and *hypercalcemia* should be able to:
1. Maintain optimal mobility by pacing activities and scheduling analgesics.
2. Maintain adequate nutritional intake.
3. Maintain adequate bowel elimination.
4. Be up without falls or other injuries.
5. List signs and symptoms of calcium imbalance.
6. Describe symptoms requiring medical follow-up.
7. Explain planned medication regimen, if appropriate.
8. Describe plans for follow-up care.

The patient with *hypoparathyroidism* and *hypocalcemia* should be able to:

1. Maintain adequate air exchange, shown by adequate blood gases and absence of stridor and dyspnea.
2. Maintain adequate cardiac output as shown by blood pressure and perfusion to CNS, kidney, and periphery; experience no undetected cardiac arrhythmias.
3. Not experience any undetected increase in neuromuscular irritability and, if convulsions occur, not experience injury.
4. State plans for self-care:
   a. Explain the prescribed drug therapy (calcium, vitamin D)
   b. State reasons for lifelong calcium and vitamin D therapy, if total parathyroid function is lost.
   c. Plan a diet high in vitamin D.
   d. Describe symptoms for tetany or hypercalcemia that require immediate attention.
   e. State plans for ongoing follow-up care.

Implementation

The interventions to assist with achievement of therapeutic goals and achieve patient outcomes are discussed together for each specific pathological state.

Hyperparathyroidism

Correction of hypercalcemia and treatment of hyperparathyroidism

Definitive treatment of hyperparathyroidism requires surgical removal of the adenoma or of all but a part of one gland, if hyperplasia is the cause. Treatment varies depending on whether symptoms are present. In mild asymptomatic hypercalcemia when renal function, urinary calcium excretion, and skeletal system x-ray films are normal, surgery may be withheld until abnormalities occur. This type of patient should be evaluated every 6 to 12 months.

Medical treatment of hypercalcemia may be performed preoperatively and in some patients who are not suitable candidates for surgery. Normalization of electrolyte levels reduces the risk of surgery.

Hypercalcemia greater than 14 mg/dl requires immediate therapy if cardiac arrhythmias and coma are to be avoided.[20] Several measures can be used. The first step is diuresis; this involves hydration followed by a potent diuretic, such as furosemide (Lasix), for the excretion of several grams of calcium per day. This therapy can be used only in patients with adequate renal function. Intake and output must be monitored closely in all patients receiving this treatment. Replacement of electrolytes other than calcium may be necessary. This may include potassium, phosphorus, and magnesium. Drugs that inhibit bone resorption include salmon calcitonin (Calcimar), mithramycin, and phosphates (Neutra-Phos).

Calcimar may be given in acute hypercalcemia. It acts rapidly and causes an abrupt inhibition of bone resorption. Sensitivity skin testing may be performed with 1 MRC unit applied to the forearm. A rapid fall in the serum calcium level may occur after injection. Mithramycin is a cytotoxic antibiotic that has a potent effect on serum calcium levels; often only one dose is ordered. See Table 29-16 for other agents that are used as adjunctive therapy in selected instances of hypercalcemia.

Improving mobility and preventing injury

Activities that provide stress to long bones are known to increase bone formation, whereas immobilization fosters demineralization; thus ambulation should be promoted in these patients. A schedule of progressive activities should be planned with the patient, with attention to his or her level of weakness and pain. Activities should be spaced to lessen fatigue, and pain medication should be given before ambulation. Safety measures to prevent injury from falling are a high priority in these patients, who are weak, may have impaired cognitive function, and often have increased bone fragility.

Maintaining adequate nutritional intake and managing constipation

The hypercalcemia results in several problems that disrupt normal GI function, fluid and nutritional intake, and elimination. Nursing care to manage these needs includes:

1. Promoting urinary elimination by ensuring a fluid intake of 3 L/day unless contraindicated
2. Providing appetizing, small meals and liquids that the patient enjoys
3. Providing symptomatic relief and administering prescribed agents for bone pain or gastrointestinal distress
4. Preventing fecal impaction by careful attention to elimination patterns and use of dietary fiber, fluids, activity, and stool softeners, laxatives, or enemas
5. Monitoring for signs of renal calculi (Chapter 33)

Facilitating learning

This patient will first need explanations of the therapeutic interventions (fluids, medications) to elicit the patient's cooperation. The patient will then need information about the various diagnostic tests (blood, urine) that will be carried out. Lastly the patient will need information related to the surgery and the self-care after surgery. The information related to surgery is explained in the next section.

Parathyroid surgery

Partial parathyroidectomy is usually the treatment of choice in primary hyperparathyroidism. The usual surgery involves removing three glands totally and part of the fourth gland. An alternative approach involves removing all four glands and implanting some of the removed tissue into the muscle of the forearm. Implantation avoids vascular failure and death of residual parathyroid tissue left in the neck. If no glandular abnormality is found at the time of surgery, extensive exploration of the neck and surrounding areas for additional glands that could be the cause of the symptoms is necessary.

Postsurgical hypocalcemia. The serum calcium level decreases within 24 hours after successful surgery. The patient must be monitored carefully for signs of tetany. Parathyroid function usually returns to normal in 5 to 7 days after subtotal resection. By this time the remaining parathyroid tissue resumes normal secretion. If mild hypocalcemia occurs, oral calcium is given. If hypocalcemia is severe, calcium gluconate or calcium chloride is given intravenously. Calcium replacement is continued until the serum calcium level returns to normal, usually within a few days. If signs and symptoms of hypocalcemia continue to be present, calcium and/or vitamin D replacement therapy in the same amount as that used to treat hypoparathyroidism will be necessary. While patients are receiving replacement therapy, they must be monitored carefully for signs and symptoms of hypercalcemia.

If total parathyroidectomy is performed, hypoparathyroidism will develop, and the patient will need the same treatment as any other patient with hypoparathyroidism.

Hypoparathyroidism
Decreasing neuromuscular excitability and the resultant respiratory and cardiac problems and tetany that results in injury

When the patient has a known risk of tetany, nursing interventions include the following:
1. Prompt reporting to physician of any signs of hypocalcemia
2. Maintenance of emergency equipment (tracheostomy set and intravenous calcium) at bedside
3. Frequent assessment of signs of latent tetany (p. 852)
4. Administering ordered calcium and vitamin D replacement with aluminum-based antacids to patient with hyperphosphatemia
5. Maintaining a quiet, nonstressful environment

The symptoms of hypocalcemia are more severe in patients with alkalosis because alkalosis causes more of the dissolved calcium to bind to serum albumin. If more calcium is bound, less is ionized, and hypocalcemic symptoms occur more readily. Attention to acid-base balance includes the prevention and treatment of causes of alkalosis: hypokalemia and respiratory alkalosis (hyperventilation). Caution should be used with agents that promote alkalosis, such as certain drugs and gastrointestinal intubation.

Providing a nonstressful environment for the patient with hypoparathyroidism is a major nursing responsibility because stressors can promote hyperventilation, which can precipitate alkalosis and tetany and ineffective breathing. Actions might include the following:
1. Frequent contacts by nursing staff
2. Explanations of treatments geared to patient's level of understanding and concern
3. Plan visitations that are most calming for patient
4. Discussion with family members about avoiding disturbing discussions

If tetany develops, the nurse assists as needed in emergency treatment of airway obstruction, cardiac arrhythmia, and seizures.

After the patient has been stabilized and the risk of tetany is past, the patient will be started on long-term maintenance therapy to maintain serum calcium levels. Long-term maintenance of normal serum calcium levels can usually be achieved by daily calcium and vitamin D supplements. Replacement of PTH is not possible.

Large doses of vitamin D_2 or D_3 are required to overcome the effect of the lack of PTH on the synthesis of vitamin D. Use of one of the more potent vitamin D preparations such as Calderol or Rocaltrol (Table 29-18) necessitates frequent measurements of serum and urinary calcium.

Dietary intake of calcium may be limited by the neces-

Table 29-18   Vitamin D synthesis and synthetic preparations

Metabolic steps	Preparations
Vitamin D_2 (ergocalciferol) skin: photogenesis ingestion	Calciferol (Drisdol, Geltaps)
Vitamin D_3 (cholecalciferol)	Dihydrotachysterol (Hytakerol)
Liver synthesis of vitamin D metabolite, 25 (OH) D (hydroxycholecalciferol)	Calcifediol (Calderol)
Kidney synthesis of vitamin D metabolite, 1, 25 $(OH)_2D$ (dihydroxycholecalciferol) and vitamin 24, 25 $(OH)_2D$	Calcitriol (Rocaltrol)

sity for restricting phosphorus intake. When a low phosphorus intake is required, dairy products and egg yolks (good sources of phosphorus and vitamin D) are avoided. Phosphate-binders (such as aluminum-based antacids) may be prescribed to increase excretion of phosphorus. The amounts of elemental calcium contained in calcium preparations varies; for example, a 650 mg calcium lactate tablet contains 87 mg of elemental calcium, whereas an Os-Cal tablet contains 250 mg. Calcium salts may be given as lactate, gluconate, or carbonate; calcium phosphate is contraindicated.

Dosages of vitamin D and calcium are adjusted to maintain a normal serum calcium and to minimize urinary calcium excretion, to avoid the risk of renal calculi. The lack of PTH results in excessive urinary calcium levels. Thiazide diuretics and a restricted sodium intake are helpful in decreasing hypercalcinuria.

Medical follow-up with monitoring of laboratory tests of serum and urinary calcium levels is necessary to prevent hypercalcemia, renal colic, and metastatic calcifications. The patient must be well educated for self-management of the illness.

Facilitating learning
Vitamin D appears to be the principal regulator of the level of calcium ions in the body and therefore increases the absorption of calcium. The person with hypoparathyroidism needs a diet high in vitamin D. The amount of calcium and vitamin D is gradually adjusted until the serum calcium level is normal. Recognition of symptoms of hypocalcemia and hypercalcemia is important so that adjustment in dosage can be instituted. Other instructions for patient education are listed in Box 29-11.

Evaluation

Questions that the nurse can use to evaluate the nursing care of the patient with parathyroid dysfunction may include the following for the patient with hypercalcemia and hyperparathyroidism:
1. Was mobility maintained?
2. Was nutritional status maintained?
3. Was normal bowel elimination maintained?

29-11

Important information for the patient with hypoparathyroidism

Relationship of symptoms of hypocalcemia and hypercalcemia to
  Disease
  Medication usage
  Complications: tetany, hypercalcemia, renal stones
Importance of medical care at prescribed intervals and when untoward signs develop
Importance of taking prescribed medications daily
Importance of informing health care providers of the health problem
Consistent dietary inclusion of vitamin D and calcium-rich foods (excepting dairy foods that are high in phosphates)
Awareness that dietary intake alone is insufficient to maintain calcium levels in the absence of PTH
Need for lifelong management of calcium balance by replacement; the amount necessary is determined by serum calcium levels

---

4. Is patient prepared to manage treatment measures at home?
5. Is patient aware of need for lifelong replacement therapy, if indicated?

For the patient with hypocalcemia and hypoparathyroidism, evaluate on the following:

1. Were complications (tetany, impaired air exchange, decreased cardiac output) prevented by early detection and reporting of signs and symptoms?
2. Was the patient free of injuries?
3. Could the patient explain medications, diet, follow-up care, and signs and symptoms to report immediately?

THYROID DYSFUNCTION

Alterations in the thyroid gland may be associated with hyperthyroid, hypothyroid, or euthyroid metabolic states (Table 29-19). A review of the normal functions of the thyroid are presented in Table 29-5, p. 828.

A brief discussion of goiter and thyroiditis will be presented before an examination of the major problems of hypothyroidism and hyperthyroidism. This section concludes with the nursing process for patients with either hypersecretion or hyposecretion of the thyroid hormone or surgery of the thyroid gland.

Table 29-19 **Thyroid gland dysfunction**

Signs and symptoms	Medical therapy
Thyroid hormone deficit	Replacement therapy of thyroid hormones:
Hypothyroidism (early signs):	Thyroid
Weight gain; weakness, fatigue, lethargy; sluggishness; sleepiness; slowed mental process; slurred speech; intolerance to cold; constipation; dry skin; dry sparse hair; infertility; decreased libido; decreased body temperature; menorrhagia in young women	Levothyroxine sodium
(late):	Liothyronine sodium
Lethargy; periorbital puffiness; nonpitting edema of feet and hands; large tongue; dull facies; pale, cool, rough, "doughy" skin; coma	Thyroglobulin
Decreased urine flow and urine concentration; proteinuria (see text for cardiac, musculoskeletal, and gastrointestinal symptoms)	Liotrix
Thyroid hormone excess	Reduction of thyroid hormone
Hyperthyroidism	Antithyroid drugs; sodium iodide, propylthiouracil, methimazole
Loss of weight, fatigue, hyperthermia, change in fat metabolism	
Mental status: anxiety, poor concentration, restlessness, emotional lability, irritability, restlessness	Radioactive iodine
Nervous system: fine tremors, rapid tendon reflexes, decreased fine coordination	Surgery: subtotal or total thyroidectomy
Cardiovascular system: tachycardia, increased blood pressure, angina, arrhythmias, cardiac hypertrophy	
Respiratory system: decreased vital capacity and dyspnea	Thyroid crisis:
Gastrointestinal system: Increased frequency of stools, increased appetite, hepatic dysfunction	Antithyroid drugs; oxygen, hypothermia to reduce fever, IV fluids, steroids, sedatives, cardiac drugs as necessary
Muscle and bone changes: muscle weakness, atrophy, osteoporosis	
Skin changes: warm, moist skin, intolerance to heat, fine hair	
Dermopathy: pretibial myxedema, vitiligo, hyperpigmentation	
Sexual changes: amenorrhea, decreased libido	
Enlarged thyroid	

GOITER

Any enlargement of the thyroid gland is called a goiter. A goiter may be caused by various disorders that prevent the synthesis of normal quantities of thyroid hormones or when there is increased stimulation of the thyroid gland by thyroid stimulating hormone (TSH) or TSH-like substances. These disorders include the following:

1. Iodide deficiency
2. Congenital metabolic defects preventing synthesis of thyroid hormones
3. Blocking of hormone synthesis by chemical agents (e.g., substances in cabbage, turnips, soybeans)
4. Blocking of hormone synthesis by drugs (for example, thiocarbamides, sulfonylureas, and lithium)
5. Selected types of hyperthyroidism

Goiter occurs in the first four categories because of an impairment in hormonal synthesis associated with a reduction of the thyroid hormones T_3 and T_4. It is believed that this reduction prevents the normal feedback inhibition of TSH. The TSH level is increased, which in turn causes an increase in thyroid mass. This thyroid enlargement (Fig. 29-11) may be sufficient to allow for adequate hormonal synthesis. In the last category there is an increase in TSH or TSH-like substance from the disease with resultant thyroid enlargement and excessive production of T_3 and T_4.

Not all patients with goiter demonstrate an elevated level of TSH. Another hypothesis is that goiter results from the stimulation of the thyroid gland by thyroid growth immunoglobulins. Goiter may be diffuse or nodular; nodules are caused by an adenoma, a carcinoma, inflammatory processes, or a hemorrhage.

Simple goiter is the term used for thyroid enlargement that is not associated with hyperthyroidism, hypothyroidism, malignancy, or inflammation. It is frequently seen in females, appearing at puberty or during pregnancy.

THYROIDITIS

Inflammation of the thyroid gland may be acute, subacute, or chronic and is characterized by painful swelling of the thyroid gland. Acute thyroiditis following infections by a pyogenic organism and subacute thyroiditis that follows a viral infection are rare.

The most common form of thyroiditis is Hashimoto's thyroiditis, in which the thyroid is infiltrated with lymphocytes and plasma cells. Autoimmunity is considered to be the pathologic basis of this chronic thyroiditis. Early in the disease when functioning thyroid tissue is still present, excessive stored thyroid hormone may be released, resulting in signs and symptoms of transient hyperthyroidism. As the disease progresses, the thyroid gland may be destroyed, and signs and symptoms of hypothyroidism may develop. Antithyroid antibodies are present in the serum. Although TSH levels may be elevated in the early stages of the disease, serum T_4 and T_3 levels gradually decrease. There is diffuse enlargement of both lobes of the thyroid gland.

HYPOTHYROIDISM

Etiology

The causes of hypothyroidism may be primary, secondary, tertiary, or iatrogenic. Primary hypothyroidism can result from:

1. Congenital atrophy or congenital defect in enzyme production.
2. Idiopathic causes.
3. Iodine deficiency.
4. Chronic thyroiditis.

Secondary and tertiary causes of hypothyroidism include hypothalamic-pituitary dysfunction. Treatment with radioactive iodine, antithyroid drugs or surgery of the thyroid are iatrogenic causes of hypothyroidism.

Pathophysiology

Hypothyroidism is a hypometabolic state resulting from a deficiency of thyroid hormone that may occur at any age. Signs of infantile (congenital) hypothyroidism, or *cretinism*, are not usually seen until several months after birth; by then, mental and physical retardation are usually irreversible. Figure 29-12 shows an adult who had untreated infantile hypothyroidism.

In adults the most frequent causes of hypothyroidism are autoimmune thyroiditis, ablative therapy, and idiopathy. It may be secondary to pituitary failure and TSH lack or may result from hypothalamic disease that causes a deficiency of thyroid-releasing hormone. In hypothyroidism

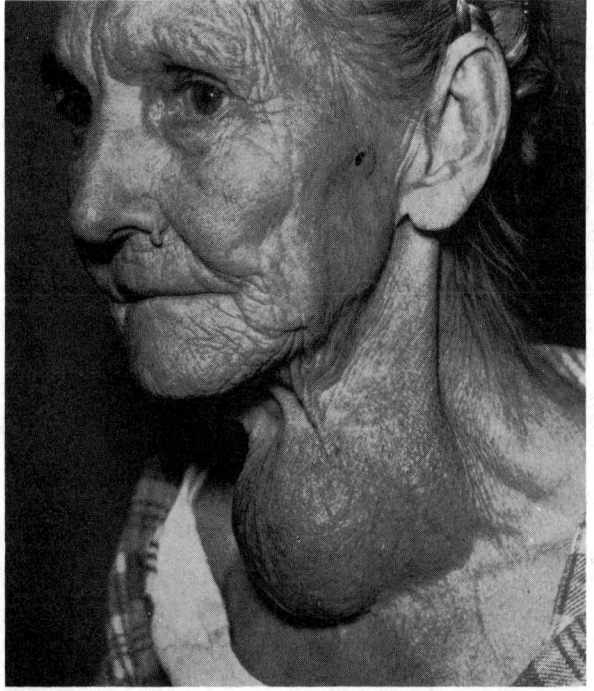

Fig. 29-11 Simple goiter. (From Prior JA, Silberstein JS, Stang JM: *Physical diagnosis: the history and examination of the patient*, ed 6, St Louis, 1981, Mosby–Year Book.)

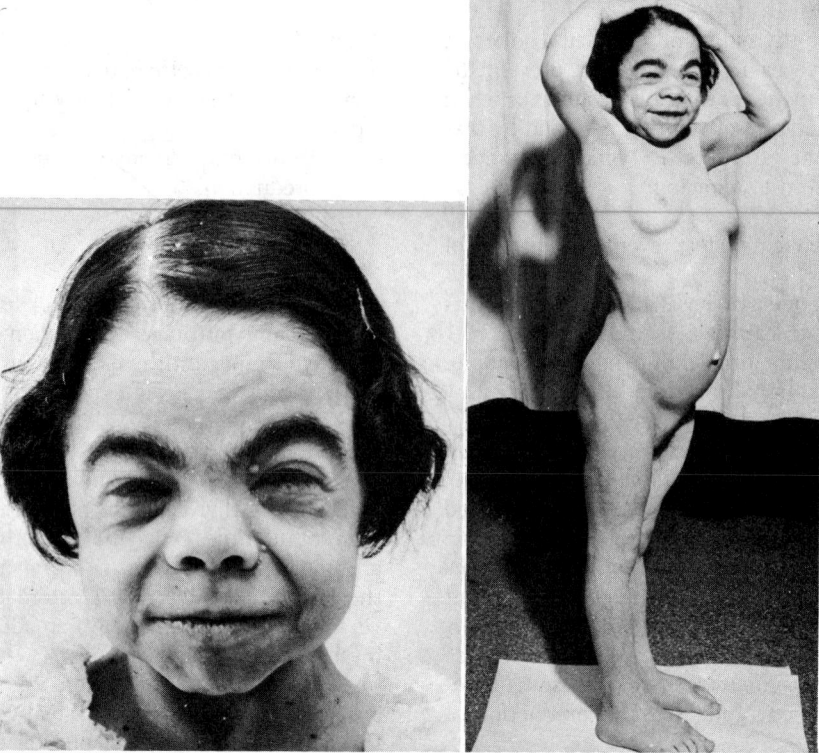

Fig. 29-12   Adult cretin (33 years old, untreated). Note characteristic cretinoid features, dwarfism (height of 44 inches), absent axillary and scant pubic hair, poorly developed breasts, potbelly, and small umbilical hernia. (From Schneeburg NG: *Essentials of clinical endocrinology,* St Louis, 1979, Mosby—Year Book.)

resulting from pituitary or hypothalamic problems, TSH is depressed and no hyperplasia occurs. In primary hypothyroidism, hyperplasia is present because a lack of T_4 and T_3 result in an increase in TSH.

The signs and symptoms of hypothyroidism result from a deficiency of T_3 and T_4, leading to a decrease in the normal metabolic functions that are under the control of these hormones. Usually the pathophysiologic changes develop slowly and early symptoms are vague (fatigue, weakness, lethary, and intolerance to cold). Table 29-19 lists some other early signs and symptoms of hypothyroidism.

The characteristics of hypothyroidism vary with the age of onset and the severity of the deficiency. There is an accumulation of hyaluronic acids and alteration of ground substances that result in mucinous edema. This development is responsible for the thickened tissues of hands, feet, and tongue and around the eyes and for effusions in the pleura, pericardium, and joints.

See Fig. 29-13 for an example of the facies characteristic of hypothyroidism. These patients often have course skin that bruises easily (because of increased capillary fragility) and is pale and yellow (because of anemia and hypercarotenemia). Hair becomes sparse, dry, and brittle. Mental processes slow, with loss of initiative, memory deficit, and slurred speech; somnolence, confusion, and even dementia may occur. Muscular and joint stiffness are common. Appetite decreases and decreased peristaltic activity lead to

constipation. Despite these marked changes, some individuals do not seem to be aware of the changes in their physical functioning, appearance, or behavior.

Cardiovascular dysfunction is a serious outcome of untreated hypothyroidism. Besides bradycardia, there may be elevation of diastolic blood pressure, cardiomegaly, and changes in cardiac output. Hypercholesteremia is often present. Angina or cardiac failure may occur. Diminished heart sounds may represent pericardial effusion. *Pleural effusion* and *ascites* can develop.

Myxedema coma occurs as the hypothyroidism worsens. The patient becomes less responsive and goes into a coma. An infection such as pneumonia, cellulitis, or pyelonephritis may precipitate the coma in a poorly treated patient.

HYPERTHYROIDISM
Etiology

The causes of hyperthyroidism include primary, secondary, tertiary, and iatrogenic causes. The primary causes include:

1. Toxic diffuse goiter (Graves' disease)
2. Toxic multinodular goiter
3. Toxic adenoma
4. T_3 thyrotoxicosis
5. Secreting thyroid cancer
6. Early stage of thyroiditis (temporary)

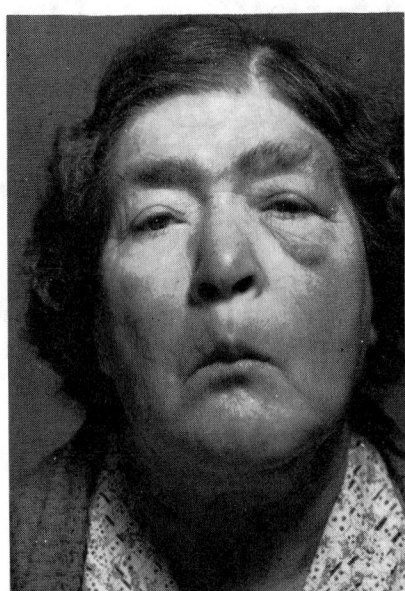

Fig. 29-13   Person with myxedema. (From Schottelius BA, Schottelius DA: *Textbook of physiology,* ed 18, St Louis, 1978, Mosby–Year Book.

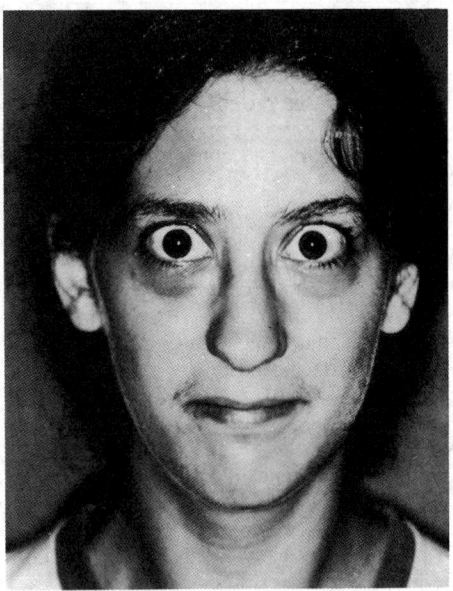

Fig. 29-14   Ophthalmopathy of Graves' disease. (From Kaye D, Rose LF: *Fundamentals of internal medicine,* St Louis, 1983, Mosby–Year Book.)

Secondary and tertiary causes of hyperthyroidism include hypothalamic-pituitary hyperfunction and some ovarian tumors. Factitious use of thyroid medication is an iatrogenic cause of hyperthyroidism.

Pathophysiology

Hyperthyroidism, a hypermetabolic state, is also called thyrotoxicosis. Hyperthyroidism results from excessive secretion of thyroxine (T_4) or triiodothyronine (T_3). The most common causes are toxic diffuse goiter (Graves' disease) and toxic nodular goiter. In both of these conditions, secretion of T_4 and T_3 becomes autonomous, and the thyroid gland is no longer regulated by TSH.

Hyperthyroidism is more common in women than in men, and there is a higher incidence between 20 and 40 years of age. It often appears after episodes of emotional trauma, infection, or increased stressors and occurs frequently in persons who have had other endocrine disturbances.

The cardiovascular system is seriously affected by hyperthyroidism because of the increased metabolic rate and the direct effects of thyroid hormones on the heart.

Sympathetic nervous stimulation is responsible for many of the symptoms of hyperthyroidism listed in Table 29-19. Atrial fibrillation and congestive heart failure may evolve in hyperthyroidism if not treated. Other symptoms are related to a chronic catabolic state or interactions with other hormones.

Because the pathophysiology of the two major causes of hyperthyroidism differ somewhat, each will be discussed individually.

Graves' disease (toxic diffuse goiter)

Graves' disease, which is characterized by a triad of symptoms—*goiter, hyperthyroidism,* and *exophthalmos* (abnormal protrusion of the eyes, Fig. 29-14)—is thought to be an autoimmune disease and is the result of thyroid-stimulating immunoglobulins (TSI), also called long-acting thyroid stimulator (LATS). The cause of the abnormal development of the immunoglobulins is unknown. Persons with specific haplotypes and monozygotic twins have a higher frequency of Graves' disease.

Retro-orbitally, there is edema with infiltration (fat, mucopolysaccharides, and lymphocytes) that results in proptosis. This process *is not closely correlated* with the severity of hormonal excess. The forward protrusion intensifies other signs related to the eye that result from increased sympathetic nervous sytem (for example, stare and lid lag). In severe *exophthalmos,* there may be an inability to close the eye and extraocular muscle weakness.

The amount of thyroid enlargement varies in Graves' disease, but it is diffuse and usually symmetric. An important sign of Graves' disease is a *bruit* heard over the thyroid; this sign reflects increased vascularity.

Toxic multinodular goiter

Milder hyperthyroidism and nodular disease are typical of toxic multinodular goiter. This condition usually occurs after age 50 and is most commonly seen in the elderly. Usually nontoxic nodular disease has been present for many years before health care is sought. In the elderly, signs of increased sympathetic activity (for example, tremors, hyperactivity, and heat intolerance) may not be as marked and can make diagnosis more difficult. Unexplained tachycardia or a decrease in mental status may lead to the diagnosis.

Thyroid storm

Thyroid storm (thyroid crisis) may occur in persons with uncontrolled hyperthyroidism. It is believed that in thyroid

Assessment

Assess for signs and symptoms of decreased alertness, decreased mobility, or increased susceptibility to cold, which may be signs and symptoms more typically noted with hypothyroidism in elderly.

Assess from signs of myxedema, seen with untreated hypothyroidism.

Assess for signs of drug toxicity because of decreased metabolic activity from diminished endocrine function.

Assess for signs of infection because thymic activity is decreased.

Intervention

Assist elderly patient to plan a way to remember taking replacment therapy; without a plan, the apathetic patient may forget to take the thyroid hormone replacement.

Teach patient and significant others the following:
Monitor for drug side effects.
Report signs of angina or congestive heart failure that may result from initial doses of thyroid hormone replacement.
Take precautions to avoid infections.
Take measures to prevent constipation, which often occurs with hypothyroidism, especially in the elderly.

Common disorders in elderly

Hypothyroidism
Infections

storm, increased amounts of hormones are released into the bloodstream and metabolism is markedly increased. It may be precipitated by infection, stressors, or thyroid surgery undertaken on a patient who was not adequately prepared with antithyroid drugs. The onset often occurs spontaneously. The patient's temperature may rise to 41°C (106°F) as the body becomes unable to release the heat formed with increased metabolism. The pulse will be rapid, and there is marked respiratory distress, apprehension, restlessness, irritability, and prostration. The patient may become delirious and finally comatose, with death resulting from heart failure.

Nursing Process
Assessment
Subjective data

Hypersecretion or hyposecretion of the thyroid gland has marked effects on the patient's ability to function, as well as on physiologic processes. The nurse collects data from the patient or a family member about the factors listed below. It is important to ask if there has been a change in any of these factors and when the change was first noted.

Energy level
Mood and mental ability
Ability to carry out activities of daily living
Ability to manage stressors
Intolerance to heat or cold
Food intake
Elimination patterns
Weight changes
Skin and hair changes
Changes in reproduction function

The interview should help the nurse determine the patient or family's understanding of the disease and its treatment and learn about the care needs of the patient.

Objective data

Initial physical examination should provide the following baseline information about the patient:

Mental status (ability to follow directions)
Nervous system status
Nutritional status
Cardiovascular status
Body characteristics
Skin appearance and texture
Hair quality and amount
Eye appearance and extraocular motion
Presence and location of edema
Neck appearance and range of motion
Abdominal girth
Muscle mass/strength

Diagnostic tests

Testing for thyroid function can be made at the hypothalamic, pituitary, thyroid, serum, or peripheral tissue levels. Table 29-20 presents the major test procedures and preparations and their interpretation. The most commonly used tests are serum T_4 and T_3 concentrations, and TSH levels. T_3 resin uptake is also frequently used. The T_3 resin uptake test evaluates changes in serum protein concentrations that can alter the binding of T_3 and T_4. Changes in thyroxine-binding globulins (TBG) and prealbumin may alter free T_4 concentrations and, to a lesser extent, T_3. The T_3 resin uptake along with the serum T_4 can be used to determine free T_4 levels.

An elevated T_4 level often confirms clinical findings of overt hyperthyroidism, whereas T_3 testing is more sensitive in discerning mild hyperthyroidism. TSH radioimmunoassay and stimulation testing can help differentiate primary and secondary hypothyroidism, hyperthyroidism, and the effectiveness of treatment. Investigation of thyroid nodules may require needle biopsy or surgical exploration.

Data analysis: nursing diagnoses

Nursing diagnoses are determined from the analysis of patient data. Possible nursing diagnoses for the person with thyroid hormone imbalance may include, but are not limited to the following:

Diagnostic title	Possible etiologies
Diagnoses specific for the patient with hypothyroidism:	
Self-care deficit	Intolerance to activity, cognitive impairment
Constipation	Immobility, inadequate fluid intake, inadequate bulk in diet
Potential decreased cardiac output	Impaired fat metabolism, muscle weakness, decreased sympathetic activity

Table 29-20   Diagnostic tests of thyroid function

Function test	Procedure and preparation	Interpretation
Tests related to serum levels of thyroid hormone		
Serum T_4 concentration	Blood sample, no special preparation	Measures circulating thyroxine that is bound and free; normal, 3-7 µg/100 ml; can be affected by pregnancy, estrogen, glucocorticoids, and hypoproteinemia.
Serum T_3 concentrations	Radioassay of blood sample, no special preparation	Measures circulating T_3 that is bound and free; normal values are 100-170 µg/100 ml
Thyroxine-binding globulin (TBG)	Blood sample, no special preparation	Measures levels of TBG; TBG can be elevated or depressed by other conditions and can alter free T_4 and T_3 concentrations
Triiodothyronine (T_3) resin uptake (T_3U)	Blood sample drawn; in laboratory, resin and radioactive T_3 are added to sample of blood; radioactive T_3 will first bind to unoccupied sites of thyroxine-binding globulin (TBG) and any extra radioactive T_3 will bind to resin; radioactive counts are performed on blood and resins to determine amount of T_3 (radioactive) bound to resin	Measures changes in thyroid-binding protein concentrations. Normally 25%-30% of radioactive T_3 will bind to resin. If binding sites of protein are saturated by high levels of T_4 then more radioactive T_3 will bind to the resin; higher T_3U levels may indicate hyperthyroidism; low levels may indicate hypothyroidism
Pituitary level test		
TSH radioimmunoassay	Blood sample, no special preparation	Directly measures TSH levels, measurement aids in differentiating primary and secondary hypothyroidism and in validating total T_4 and T_3 levels; values are elevated in primary hypothyroidism because of loss of negative feedback and low in hyperthyroidism
TSH stimulation test	Baseline level of TSH is measured, 500 ug of TRH is given; 30 min later, TSH again measured	Normally TRH causes a rise in TSH to 15-30 µg/ml; a flat response confirms hyperthyroidism; a marked response indicates primary hypothyroidism
Thyroid level test		
Radioactive iodine uptake (RAIU)	A tracer dose of radioactive iodine (^{131}I) is given by mouth. At 2, 6, and 24 hr after administration, scintillation detector is placed over neck in region of thyroid and amount of accumulated radioactive iodine is measured; excess iodine in any foods, cough medicines, x-ray media, other medications, and enriched iodine foods affect test by giving low readings. Fasting may be required.	Measures level of thyroid activity. Normal thyroid will take up 5%-35% of tracer dose; increased uptake occurs in hyperthyroidism; excess tracer dose is excreted in urine and can be measured; urine is collected for 24 hr; decreased amounts in urine indicate hypothyroid state
Thyroid scan	Dose of ^{131}I is given, and scintillation scan is done: a picture of distribution of radioactivity is recorded	Size, shape, and anatomic function of gland assessed; areas of increased or decreased uptake noted; iodine ingestion (in medicines and dyes) before test can modify results
Thyroid ultrasound	No preparation required	Ultrasonography used to find structural abnormalities; cysts, nodules, and other masses

Continued.

Table 29-20 Diagnostic tests of thyroid function—cont'd

Test	Procedure and preparation	Interpretation
Thyroid antibody test	Blood sample	Antibodies to thyroglobulin and microsomes are present in Hashimoto's thyroiditis
Thyroid-stimulating immunoglobulins (TSI)	Blood sample	If TSI antibodies are present, Graves' disease is confirmed
Tests related to peripheral effects of thyroid hormone		
Basal metabolic rate (BMR)	Patient at rest and fasted; amount of oxygen used while at rest is calculated; patient's oxygen use is compared with established norms for people of same sex, age, and size	Normal range is −15% to +15%; in hyperthyroidism patient's BMR will be greater than +15%; in hypothyroidism patient's BMR will be less than −15%; BMR is less accurate than other tests described above but may be used to evaluate therapy
Serum cholesterol level	Blood sample; patient placed on NPO night before	Normals vary from laboratory to laboratory; high levels found in hypothyroidism and low levels found in hyperthyroidism; data augment other tests

Diagnostic title	Possible etiologies
Diagnoses specific for the patient with hypothyroidism—cont'd:	
Knowledge deficit: disease, diagnostic tests and self care	Never exposed previously
Diagnoses specific for the patient with hyperthyroidism:	
Coping, ineffective individual or family	Inadequate information, temporary role change, crisis
Altered nutrition: less than body requirements	Increased metabolic demand; inability to digest sufficient amounts of foods
Sleep pattern disturbance	Anxiety, altered sensory state, environmental change
Potential decreased cardiac output	Muscle weakness, increased sympathetic activity
Knowledge deficit: disease, diagnostic tests, therapeutic management, and self care	New disease, never been exposed to information
Potential sensory perceptual alterations: visual	Impaired protective mechanisms of the eye

Planning: expected patient outcomes

Expected patient outcomes for the person with thyroid disorders may include, but are not limited to the following. Specifically, the patient with *hypothyroidism* should be able to perform the following:

1. Gradually increase independence in self-care abilities.
2. Employ measures to prevent constipation.
3. Blood pressure and cardiac output will be returned to normal and maintained within normal limits.
4. State plans for follow-up care:
   a. State symptoms of hypothyroidism requiring immediate follow-up.
   b. State plans for regular medical appointments.
   c. State need for daily replacement therapy.

The patient with *hyperthyroidism* should be able to perform the following:

1. Employ coping measures to decrease anxiety and interpersonal friction.

2. Describe ways to increase caloric and protein intake.
3. State ways to help improve sleep.
4. Cardiac output will be maintained.
5. State plans for follow-up care:
   a. State symptoms requiring immediate follow-up (signs of remission, thyroid crisis, hypothyroidism).
   b. State plans for regular medical appointments.
6. Describe eye care if exophthalmos is present.

Implementation
Assisting with achievement of therapeutic goals
Medications

Medications may be used to treat goiter, hyperthyroidism, or hypothyroidism.

The drugs used most commonly to treat *hypothyroidism* are listed in Box 29-12. It is important that dosages be increased gradually because a sudden increase in metabolic rate can cause cardiac failure.

Thyroid hormone replacement. The optimal dosage of levothyroxine is 1.5 to 1.7 μg/kg or about 100 to 125 μg/day.[41] Levothyroxine therapy is started with doses of 5 to 50 μg. Doses are then increased by increments of 25 to 50 μg every month until a normal metabolic rate is obtained.[41] The daily maintenance dose of thyroid hormones varies widely. The correct dose is determined by clinical status and assay of TSH levels. Diuresis with weight loss and regression of puffiness is an early response. Increased pulse rate, improvement of appetite, and relief of constipation are usually seen next. Most signs of hypothyroidism are eventually reversed.

Adults with hypothyroidism respond quickly to the administration of thyroid hormones. Changes in appearance and physical symptoms occur within 2 to 3 days. Treatment must be continued throughout life. Medication dosage may need periodic adjustments to avoid symptoms of hyperthyroidism or recurrence of hypothyroidism.

Table 29-21   Antithyroid drugs

Drug	Actions	Interventions

Iodide solutions
  Compound iodide solution
   (Lugol's solution)
  Saturated solution of po-
   tassium iodide (SSKI)
	Rapid action, block synthesis and release of thyroid hormone; less sustained action; reduce vascularity of the thyroid gland, thus often used in preparation for surgery; saturate(s) thyroid with iodide, thus radioactive iodine studies or treatment of thyroid cannot be carried out	Explain to patient that compliance with dosage schedule is necessary; give through a straw to avoid staining of teeth; give in milk or fruit juice; teach patient to report toxic symptoms: brassy taste, sore teeth and gums

Propylthiouracil
  (Propacil)
Methimazole
  (Tapazole)
	Blocks synthesis of thyroid hormone and the release of stored hormone
	Blocks synthesis of thyroid hormone, not the release of stored hormone
		Explain to patient that 2-4 weeks are necessary before improvement is noticed; teach patient to report toxic symptoms: fever, sore throat, skin eruptions; leukopenia or pancytopenia may occur

---

29-12

Replacement therapy for hypothyroidism

Levothyroxine sodium; L-thyroxine (synthetic T_4)
  Synthroid
  Levothroid
Liothyronine sodium; L-triiodothyronine (synthetic T_3)
  Cytomel
Liotrix (synthetic combination of T_4 and T_3)
  Euthroid
  Thyrolar
Thyroid extract (natural T_3 and T_4 preparation from animal thyroid); potency varies; rarely used today

---

Antithyroid drugs. Propylthiouracil or methimazole block thyroid hormone synthesis, thus they reduce the output of thyroid hormone in hyperthyroidism (see Table 29-21). Usually antithyroid drugs are used before ablation of thyroid tissue by radioactive iodine or surgery.

The patient usually is started on a relatively large dose of an antithyroid drug, and then the dosage is gradually reduced to a level sufficient to maintain the euthyroid state. When antithyroid drugs are used as the primary therapy, they commonly are continued for 6 to 18 months or longer. Some patients stay in remission without further therapy. Others require longer drug therapy, additional therapy, or lifelong therapy.

The patient should see the physician at regular intervals after drugs are discontinued so that early signs of recurrence are noticed. It is important to give the drugs at regularly spaced intervals, because the blood levels are reduced in about 8 hours. Some persons may not tolerate continued use of antithyroid drugs. Toxic side effects include agranulocytosis and cholestasis. Skin rashes, joint pains, and diarrhea may also occur.

Iodides. Lugol's solution or another iodide solution can rapidly reduce the patient's metabolic rate. It is given for short periods only. Its principal use is to decrease thyroid vascularity before surgery. Iodide administration saturates the thyroid gland with iodine and interferes with ablation of the thyroid by ^{131}I; therefore the administration of iodides is contraindicated before ^{131}I therapy. See Table 29-21 for important activities relevant to iodide administration.

Iodide may be used in concert with antithyroid therapy preoperatively; it is given *after* propylthiouracil has reduced the hyperthyroidism.

Radioactive iodine

Ablation of the thyroid gland may be achieved by radiation. The most commonly used isotope is ^{131}I. It is the treatment of choice for most persons with hyperthyroidism. A radioactive isotope of iodine, ^{131}I is given by mouth, is absorbed rapidly in the stomach, and becomes concentrated in the thyroid. Usually, a single dose is given in a radioactive "cocktail." It takes about 3 weeks for the symptoms of hyperthyroidism to subside, and more than 2 months for thyroid function to become normal. Occasionally, remission is not achieved with one dose, and the treatment is repeated after an interval of several months. Hypothyroidism frequently develops after ^{131}I therapy, and the onset can occur years after treatment.

Radioactive iodine is not used in pregnant women because iodine readily crosses the placenta and may affect the fetus. Some physicians do not prescribe ^{131}I for persons in the childbearing years because of the belief that there is a potential for damage to the gonads, although this belief is not supported by research.

Patients who receive radioactive iodine for hyperthyroidism need to have the treatment explained to them with special care, and they usually need repeated reassurance that the radioactive properties are quickly dissipated. Because persons with hyperthyroidism may be more emotional than other persons, they sometimes think they are experiencing reactions to the drug long after this is possible.

Surgery

Surgery of the thyroid is the procedure of choice for removal of goiters causing pressure, and for cancer of the thyroid. Part or all of the thyroid gland may be removed surgically. Total thyroidectomy (complete removal of the thyroid) may be performed for cancer of the thyroid, and the patient must then take thyroid hormone regularly for

Possible complications after thyroid surgery

Hemorrhage
Edema about vocal cords and larynx
Laryngeal nerve injury
Tetany

Guidelines for Care

The patient after thyroid surgery

Monitor for postoperative complications.
    Laryngeal damage: hoarseness, weak voice, stridor
    Hemorrhage or tissue swelling:
        Bleeding: check dressing and back by slipping hand gently behind neck and shoulders
        Choking sensation
        Difficulty in swallowing or coughing
        Sensation of dressing being too tight even after it is loosened
    Hypocalcemia (tetany):
        Parathesias
        Trousseau's and Chvostek's signs
        Carpopedal spasm
        Seizure activity
    Respiratory distress
Maintain equipment at bedside for treatment of laryngeal obstruction (tracheostomy set) and tetany (calcium gluconate).
For acute respiratory distress:
    Call for immediate medical assistance.
    If a physician is not readily available, remove clips and sutures as previously instructed.
Encourage high-carbohydrate fluids by mouth and a soft diet as tolerated.
Provide comfort.
    Use prescribed analgesics.
    Local agents (analgesic throat lozenges or gels) ease swallowing; give 30 minutes before meals.
    Avoid placing tension on suture line.
    After 5 to 7 days, gradual range of motion may be promoted.
Teach patient about required drugs (dosage, side effects) and importance of medical follow-up.

the remainder of his or her life. Hyperthyroidism may be treated surgically by removing approximately five sixths of the gland (subtotal thyroidectomy). In most cases this operation permanently alleviates symptoms, while the remaining thyroid tissue provides enough hormones for normal function. Hypothyroidism, if present, is treated with replacement doses of thyroid hormone. The remaining tissue can hypertrophy, however, and hyperthyroidism can recur.

Before thyroid surgery is undertaken, a normal (euthyroid) state must be produced by drug therapy. An ECG is made before surgery to detect evidence of heart damage.

Postoperative complications. The complications after thyroid surgery are extremely serious. Monitoring for these complications has the highest priority in postoperative care (see Box 29-13).

Hemorrhage can result in incisional bleeding or in compression of the trachea and surrounding tissue. Hemorrhage is most common in the first 12 to 24 hours after surgery.

Although slight hoarseness is normal, the patient is observed for any increase in hoarseness and accompanying respiratory difficulty. To reveal early symptoms of laryngeal nerve injury, patients are asked to speak as soon as they have emerged from anesthesia and at intervals of 30 to 60 minutes.

Respiratory obstruction can occur for many reasons. These include laryngeal nerve injury, compression of the trachea by hemorrhage, vocal cord edema or spasm, and tetany. Emergency measures for these complications are outlined in Box 29-14. Injury to the parathyroids is uncommon but may occur. Surgery or inflammation may block the normal release of parathyroid hormone, and symptoms of tetany caused by calcium deficiency may appear from 1 to 7 days after surgery. Serum calcium levels are usually monitored, and hypocalcemia is treated by replacement of calcium intravenously. Daily oral doses of calcium are then given until normal function returns.

Postoperative nursing interventions are summarized in Box 29-14.

Interventions to achieve patient outcomes

Interventions to assist in meeting the various outcomes are presented for each pathological state separately.

Hyperthyroidism. Since the advent of antithyroid drugs and ^{131}I therapy, most people with hyperthyroidism can be cared for at home. Although these persons usually are not particularly hyperactive, they are likely to be nervous and irritable. It is important that family and friends understand

that extreme sensitivity and irritability are part of the disease; otherwise, they may become upset with the individual and aggravate the situation. It may be necessary to assist these persons with activities requiring fine motor coordination and concentration, although they may appear physically able to perform the activities themselves. They will need an explanation about why they require such assistance.

The patient's cardiac status needs to be monitored closely. Rest periods need to be provided and encouraged. As activity is changed the patient's cardiac status needs to be reassessed.

Other interventions by nurses or caregivers at home indicated for the person with hyperthyroidism include:

1. Maintain a cool, quiet environment.
2. Assist person to obtain sufficient rest.
3. Encourage quiet activities that require gross motor movements (for example, weaving and reading), which the person can do without assistance.
4. Assist person with tasks requiring fine motor coordination (for example sewing and washing dishes).
5. Provide a high-calorie, high-protein diet; snacks be-

Nursing Care Plan	**Person with hyperthyroidism**

DATA: Mrs. T., a 28-year-old housewife, is admitted for diagnostic evaluation before a thyroidectomy, which is scheduled to be performed in 2 weeks. Graves' disease was diagnosed 2 days ago; hospitalization was delayed until child-care arrangements were made for her 6-year-old step-son. (The marriage occurred 3 months ago.) Initial therapy, started 2 days ago, is Tapazole and Lugol's solution. The ECG report is sinus tachycardia (rate 132).

The nursing history identified the following about the patient:

1. Mrs. T. feels overwhelmed, cries frequently, and fears losing control of temper.
2. She has lost 15 lb in 2 months and is always hungry, although she is eating large amounts of food.
3. She is bothered by heat, others' noisiness, and her own clumsiness.
4. She expects medicine to keep her feeling better and dreads surgery.

The physical examination revealed the following: BP: 140/90; T:38.0° C pulse: 136, R: 24. Staring gaze of eyes with proptosis (equal bilaterally); right eye slightly reddened. Skin warm and perspiration present. Increased muscle tone; quick muscle response to sudden noise; fine tremor of both hands. Diffuse enlargement of thyroid visible. *Bruit* present over thyroid.

Collaborative nursing actions include those to prevent further environmental stressors that could make the patient more uncomfortable and increase her signs and symptoms.

Nursing actions include monitoring for the following: temperature, pulse, respiration, blood pressure, weight, excessive hunger, and tremulousness.

Nursing diagnosis: Decreased cardiac output: related to environmental stimulation

Expected patient outcomes	Nursing interventions	Rationale
Pulse rate is less than 10 above baseline during first 72 h Pulse rate decreases gradually after 72 h Undetected cardiac arrhythmias do not occur	Assess vital signs, especially heart rate and rhythm at least q4h Instruct Mrs. T. to report palpitations, chest pain, and dizziness Assess daily weight, daily intake and output; assess for signs of edema, jugular vein distention and pulmonary congestion q8h Decrease known stressors; explain all interventions, and listen to Mrs. T. Balance periods of activity with rest Administer prescribed drugs and monitor therapeutic response	The early detection of cardiac changes such as atrial fibrillation or thyroid storm allows prompt treatment and prevents cardiovascular crisis

Nursing diagnosis: Coping ineffective individual: related to personal vulnerability to environmental stimuli

Expected patient outcomes	Nursing interventions	Rationale
Explains reason for change in behavior Emotional lability is minimized Identifies at least one coping mechanism that will help during periods of nervousness	Discuss reasons for emotional lability Maintain calm, relaxed environment Encourage visitors who are calm and will not upset her Provide privacy (such as a single room) Suggest that others avoid sharing distressing news with her Explain all interventions Avoid stimulants such as coffee, tea, caffeine, and alcohol Help her identify previous coping mechanisms or explore new ones	A supportive environment can reduce environmental stimuli and stressors and assist patient in coping

Continued.

Nursing Care Plan	**Person with hyperthyroidism—cont'd**

Nursing diagnosis: Altered nutrition: less than body requirements related to increased metabolic needs

Expected patient outcomes	Nursing interventions	Rationale
Normal weight is maintained Mrs. T. gains at least 0.5 kg/wk, if weight is below normal	Monitor weight qod to weekly Monitor serum albumin, hemoglobin, and lymphocyte levels Help her plan for high-calorie, high-protein, high-carbohydrate diet with selection from all food groups Suggest six meals per day or between-meal snacks	Increase nutrient intake to meet increased metabolic demand

Nursing diagnosis: Sensory/perceptual alterations: high risk for visual related to environmental agents

Expected patient outcomes	Nursing interventions	Rationale

Vision does not worsen
Explains measures to protect eyes
	Assess visual acuity, ability to close eyes, and photophobia
	Protect eyes from irritants:
	  Use patches or glasses when in high wind
	  Use artificial tears, if prescribed
	  Elevate head of bed at night
		These measures can prevent corneal injury and minimize risk of loss of vision

Nursing diagnosis: Hyperthermia: related to increased metabolic rate

Expected patient outcomes	Nursing interventions	Rationale
States that she feels more comfortable	Control environmental temperature for comfort (fans may be helpful) Suggest that she take frequent showers Encourage adequate fluid intake and monitor fluid losses	These measures keep her comfortable by increasing heat loss and preventing problems of increased fluid loss

Nursing diagnosis: Activity intolerance: related to generalized weakness and decreased cardiac reserve

Expected patient outcomes	Nursing interventions	Rationale
States fatigue is decreased	Assess activity schedule Suggest ways to modify fatiguing activities Identify activities than can be done by others until condition is controlled Schedule rest periods Encourage activities that promote sleep at night	Reduction of energy expenditure is necessary to reduce fatigue in persons with increased metabolism

Nursing diagnosis: Impaired home maintenance management: related to activity intolerance, fatigue, and emotional lability

Expected patient outcome	Nursing interventions	Rationale
States plan for home maintenance management	Assist her to identify home maintenance difficulties Assist her to identify persons who can provide temporary help Make referrals as needed, such as to social services Identify persons who can help monitor her compliance with medical regimen	These measures increase resources available to patient and reduce stress from inability to meet expectations of role

Nursing diagnosis: Knowledge deficit: therapeutic regimen related to lack of exposure to information

Expected patient outcomes	Nursing interventions	Rationale
Explains medical regimen and care needs	Explain how and when to take prescribed medications Describe symptoms of infection to be reported to physician, such as sore throat or fever Describe ways to plan prescribed dietary intake Provide required teaching about care needs (comfort, sleep, and rest)	These measures increase likelihood of compliance with therapy used to achieve euthyroid state and optimal physical status before surgery

tween meals may be necessary to maintain weight and meet energy requirements.

6. Discourage the use of caffeinated drinks.
7. If exophthalmos is present:
   a. Encourage use of dark glasses, which afford some protection from wind, sun, and dust.
   b. Administer soothing eye drops, such as methylcellulose, 0.5% to 1%, which may prevent drying of the eye and provide comfort.

The patient with hyperthyroidism requires education about the disease, diagnostic tests, treatment, and self-care needs (medications, eye care, diet). Educational sessions should be spaced, and written material should supplement verbal information.

Hypothyroidism. The patient's slowed mental and physical functioning requires understanding and patience on the part of caregivers. A thorough explanation of the cause of the changes in the patient's physical and mental responses also should be given to family or friends. As thyroid hormone levels return to normal, the patient's physical and mental state will return to normal and the patient will be able to take over own self-care.

Other nursing care includes the following:

1. Minimize environmental stressors, because the patient is less able to respond to them.
2. Administer replacement therapy and monitor patient for effectiveness of therapy and side effects.
3. Provide complete care at first and gradually increase patient's self-care.
4. Prevent constipation and fecal impaction by administering fluids, fiber, and stool softeners and by encouraging activity.
5. Monitor cardiac response to therapy and any increase in activity.

Patient education is an important part of the patient care. Because the patient has impaired cognitive functioning at the beginning of therapy, instructions need to be simple, concise, and repeated frequently. The patient needs to be taught about the need for life-long therapy and given suggestions on how to manage constipation. Other information on self-care must be discussed. The planned follow-up needs to be explained.

Evaluation

Evaluation is based on expected patient outcomes. Questions useful in evaluating nursing care of patients with thyroid dysfunction may include the following:

For the patient with hypothyroidism:

1. Were self-care needs met?
2. Was the patient able to maintain normal bowel elimination?
3. Was cardiac output returned to normal and maintained?
4. Is the patient prepared to manage self-care at home (diet, medications)?
5. Does the patient know plans for follow-up?

For the patient with hyperthyroidism:

1. Was the patient able to identify several coping measures to decrease anxiety?
2. Did the patient maintain adequate nutritional intake?

3. Did the patient attain adequate sleep/rest patterns?
4. Was cardiac output returned to normal and maintained?
5. Can the patient describe ways to meet self-care needs (handling medicines, eye care, rest/activity needs, diet)?
6. Does the patient know plans for follow-up care?

SUMMARY

1. Normal physiology depends on the proper amounts of hormones being available to act on cell receptors of target tissues.
2. Many factors influence secretory patterns and rates of secretion of hormones. Atrophy and hypoplasia of a gland result in hyposecretion, whereas hypertrophy and hyperplasia result in hypersecretion.
3. The hypothalamic-pituitary-target gland axis is a principal regulator of hormonal secretion of the adrenal, thyroid, and gonad glands.
4. Parathyroid hormone, vitamin D, and calcitonin are three regulators of calcium and phosphorus balance. The serum level of calcium is the principal regulator of parathyroid hormone secretion.
5. *Giantism* in children and *acromegaly* in adults are conditions resulting from growth hormone excess. Tumors or pituitary hyperplasia may be treated with surgery, irradiation, or growth hormone suppressants.
6. The most common pituitary tumor is a prolactinoma that may present with symptoms of galactorrhea or reproductive dysfunction.
7. Pituitary tumors may cause compression of normal tissue, resulting in hyposecretion of anterior pituitary hormones. They may also compress the optic chiasma and cause visual field defects.
8. Life-long replacement of cortisol is necessary to maintain life after a bilateral adrenalectomy or pituitary ablation or when disease or injury has destroyed the pituitary or adrenal cortex (for instance, in Addison's disease).
9. Administration of *therapeutic* doses of glucocorticoid medications produce iatrogenic Cushing's syndrome and place the patient at risk for adrenocortical insufficiency or crisis if abruptly stopped.
10. Diabetes insipidus results from ADH deficit and is characterized by polyuria and low specific gravity of urine. Overdosage of ADH replacement can induce weight gain and reduce urinary volume.
11. Cardiac problems may develop from several hormonal alterations: growth hormone, cortisol, thyroid hormone, and catecholamines. Cardiac arrhythmias may occur in hypoparathyroidism and hyperthyroidism.
12. Fluid and electrolyte imbalances are predominate features of disorders of the posterior pituitary and adrenal cortex.
13. Hypertension may result from adrenal medullary or adrenal cortical hypersecretion.
14. Nutritional problems are common with hormonal disorders. Excesses of growth hormone and cortisol can induce states of catabolism, ketogenesis, and hyperglycemia. Hyperthyroidism increases the amounts of

nutrients required. Hypothyroidism decreases the calories required.

15. Disorders of growth may be a reflection of hormonal alterations, for instance, in *pituitary dwarfism* and *congenital cretinism* (hypothyroidism). Skin, hair, and nails may be changed in appearance in several of the hormonal disturbances.

16. Skeletal abnormalities and loss of bone integrity is a hallmark of parathyroid dysfunction. *Osteoporosis* from excessive bone resorption of calcium may limit the amount of corticosteroid medications given in chronic inflammatory diseases. *Acromegaly* (growth hormone excess) induces bony growth, which alters the patient's appearance and may cause joint problems and compression syndrome.

17. Hypotension is of particular concern in deficits of ADH, glucocorticoids, and mineralocorticosteroids. Volume expanders may be required immediately after adrenal surgery or to treat Addison's crisis. Large doses of cortisol have mineralocorticoid effects.

18. Both vitamin D and calcium supplements are necessary to maintain serum calcium levels in *hypoparathyroidism* and to prevent *tetany*.

19. Neuromuscular irritability in hypocalcemia gives rise to the symptoms of latent tetany and to cardiac arrhythmias, laryngeal obstruction, and convulsions. *Trousseau's* sign, *Chvostek's* sign, *carpopedal spasm,* and *paresthesia* should be reported promptly.

20. The first priority in treatment of hyperparathyroidism is reducing severe hypercalcemia (that is, levels greater than 14 mg/dl); cardiac arrhythmias and coma can result if treatment is delayed.

21. Thyroid enlargement (goiter) may be detected by inspection and palpation and described as diffuse or nodular, and the qualities of symmetry and presence of pain or tenderness noted. *Simple goiter* is the term used to describe enlargement without thyroid hormone alteration.

22. *Hyperthyroidism* has many causes; excesses of T_3 and T_4 induce a hypermetabolic state and excessive sympathetic nervous system stimulation.

23. *Graves' disease* is characterized by hyperthyroidism, goiter, and exophthalmos. The presence of thyroid-stimulating antibodies confirms the diagnosis.

24. *Hypothyroidism* often has an insidious onset. A decrease in the metabolic functions under the control of T_4 and T_3 gives rise to multiple symptoms. Fluid retention results in weight gain, changes in appearance of skin, and effusions.

25. Hypothyroidism in the elderly may not be detected until severe changes in cardiac or mental status occur.

26. Thyroid hormone replacement reverses most signs of hypothyroidism in the adult; synthroid is a common drug used for maintenance therapy.

27. Treatment of Graves' disease, the most common disease associated with hyperthyroidism, may include medications, ^{131}I, or surgery.

28. Complications of thyroid surgery include hemorrhage, tetany, laryngeal nerve injury, and respiratory obstruction.

STUDY QUESTIONS

- What is the role of the adrenal gland in response to stressors?
- Giving a large amount of hormone such as cortisone to a person who is producing that hormone affects endogenous production in what way? Why does this change occur?
- How would you explain to a patient with hyperthyroidism that increased amounts of food are needed?
- Are there other patient situations where increased foods are needed for the same reason as occurs in hyperthyroidism?
- What potassium problems are caused by disorders of the adrenal cortex and anterior pituitary? Why do these problems occur?
- What nutritional guidelines should be taught to persons with hypersecretion and hyposecretion of the adrenal cortex or of the thyroid gland?

REFERENCES AND SELECTED READINGS

1. Bagdale JD: Endocrine emergencies, *Med Clin North Am* 70(5):1111-1128, 1986.
2. Barkan A: Acromegaly and gigantism. In The Endocrine Society: *41st post graduate annual assembly syllabus*, Bethesda, Md, 1989, The society.
3. Blackman M: Pituitary hormones and aging, *Endocrinol Metab Clin North Am* 16(4):981-994, 1987.
3a. Blondell RD: Hypopituitarism, *AFP* 43:2029-2036, 1991.
3b. Brunader RE, Moore DC: Education of the child with growth retardation, *AFP* 35:165-176, 1987.
4. Davis PJ, Davis FB: Endocrinology and aging. In Reichel W, editor: *Clinical aspects of aging*, Baltimore, 1985, Williams and Wilkins.
5. DeGroot L et al: *Endocrinology*, ed 2, New York, 1989, Grune and Stratton.
6.* Ebersole P, Hess D: *Toward healthy aging*, ed 3, St Louis, 1990, Mosby-Year Book.
7. Endocrine Society: *43rd post graduate assembly syllabus*, Bethesda, Md, 1991, The society.
8.* Feit H: Thyroid function in the elderly, *Clin Geriatr Med* 4:151-161, 1988.
9. Guyton AC: *Human physiology and mechanisms of disease*, ed 4, Philadelphia, 1987, WB Saunders.
9a. Hart JJ: Pheochromocytoma, *AFP* 42:163-169, 1990.
10. Ingbar SH: The effects of aging on the thyroid hormone economy in man, *Prog Clin Biol Res* 74:135-145, 1985.
11.* Lancaster LE: Renal and endocrine regulation of water and electrolyte balance, *Nurs Clin North Am* 22:761-772, 1987.
12. Lennquist S: The thyroid nodule: diagnoses and surgical treatment, *Surg Clin North Am* 67:213-232, 1987.
13.* Lockhart J: Actionstat, *Nurs 88* 18:33, 1988.
14. Loriauy DL: Cushing's syndrome. In the Endocrine Society: *41st Post graduate annual assembly syllabus*, Bethesda, Md, 1989, The society.
15. Marx SH: Familial multiple endocrine neoplasia type 1. In The Endocrine Society: *41st post graduate annual assembly syllabus*, Bethesda, Md, 1989, The society.
16.* Mathewson MK: Thyroid disorder, *Crit Care Nurse* 7(1):74-85, 1985.
17. Mazzaferri E et al: Solitary thyroid nodule: diagnoses and management, *Med Clin North Am* 72:1177-1211, 1988.

*Suggested for student reading.

18. McCance K, Huether SE: *Pathophysiology: the biologic basis for disease in adults and children,* St Louis, 1990, Mosby-Year Book.

19. Melmed S, Fagin JA: Acromegaly update—etiology, diagnoses, and management, *West J Med* 146:328-336, 1987.

20. Metz R, Larson EB: *Blue book of endocrinology,* Philadelphia, 1985, WB Saunders.

21. Molitch M: Lactation and prolactinomas. In The Endocrine Society: *41st post graduate annual assembly syllabus,* Bethesda, Md, 1989, The society.

22. Nabarro JD: Acromegaly, *Clin Endocrinol* 26:481-512, 1987.

23.* O'Neil J: Thyroid crisis, *Nurs 87* 17(11):335-338, 1987.

24. Robinson AG, Amico JA: Non-sweet diabetes of pregnancy, *N Engl J Med* 324:556-558, 1991.

25. Sakiyama R: Common thyroid disorders, *AFP* 38(1):227-238, 1988.

25a. Salman K, Miller JL, Rose LI: Selection of thyroid preparations, *AFP* 40:215-219, 1989.

26.* Sarsany S: Thyroid storm, *RN* 51(7):46-48, 1988.

27. Sawin CT: Hypothyroidism, *Med Clin North Am* 69:989-1003, 1988.

28.* Schira M: Steroid dependent states and adrenal insufficiency, *Nurs Clin North Am* 22:837-841, 1987.

28a. Shulman L, Miller JL, Rose LI: Growth hormone therapy, *AFP* 41:1541-1546, 1990.

29. Singer FR: Calcitonin: actions and therapeutic uses. In The Endocrine Society: *41st post graduate annual assembly syllabus,* Bethesda, Md, 1989, The society.

30. Sitges-Serra A, Caralps-Riera D: Hyperparathyroidism associated with renal disease, *Surg Clin North Am* 67:359-377, 1987.

31. Sivula A, Ronni-Sivula H: Natural history of treated primary hyperparathyroidism, *Surg Clin North Am* 67:329-341, 1987.

32. Snyder PJ: Gonadotroph cell adenomas of the pituitary, *Endocr Rev* 6:552-630, 1985.

33. Snyder PJ: The myth of the nonsecreting pituitary adenoma. In The Endocrine Society: *41st post graduate annual assembly syllabus,* Bethesda, Md, 1989, The society.

34. Spaulding S: Age and the thyroid, *Endocrinol Metab Clin North Am* 16(4):1013-1025, 1987.

35. Svee F: Steroid usage: too much of a good thing. In The Endocrine Society: *41st post graduate annual assembly syllabus,* Bethesda, Md, 1989, The society.

36. Thomas C, Groom RD: Current management of the patient with autonomously functioning nodular goiter, *Surg Clin North Am* 67:315-328, 1987.

37. Thompson N, Cheung P: Diagnoses and treatment of functioning and non-functioning adrenocortical neoplasms including incidentalomas, *Surg Clin North Am* 67:423-436, 1987.

38. Vance ML, Thorner MO: Prolactinomas, *Endocrinol Metab Clin* 16:731-753, 1987.

39. Verbalis JG: SIAD and other hyponatremic states. In The Endocrine Society: *41st post graduate annual assembly syllabus,* Bethesda, Md, 1989, The society.

40. Wilson JD, Foster DW, editors: *Williams' textbook of endocrinology,* ed 7, Philadelphia, 1985, WB Saunders.

41. Wolf PG, Meek JC: Practical approach to the treatment of hypothyroidism, *AFP* 45:722-731, 1992.

42. Wyngaarden JB, Smith LH, editors: *Cecil textbook of medicine,* ed 18, Philadelphia, 1988, WB Saunders.

Classic

43.* Camunas C: Pheochromocytoma, *Am J Nurs* 83:887-891, 1983.

44.* Evangelisti JT et al: Thyroid storm: a nursing crisis, *Heart Lung* 12:184-194, 1983.

45.* Gotch PM: Teaching patients about adrenal corticosteroids, *Am J Nurs* 81:78-85, 1981.

46.* Hoffman JT: Syndromes of ectopic hormone production in cancer, *Nurs Clin North Am* 15:499-509, 1980.

47. Hoffman JT, Newby TB: Hypercalcemia in primary hyperparathyroidism, *Nurs Clin North Am* 15:469-480, 1980.

48. Honigman RE: Deciphering diagnostic studies: thyroid function tests, *Nurs 82* 12(4):68-71, 1982.

49. Hurley JR: Thyroid disease in the elderly, *Med Clin North Am* 67(2):497-516, 1983.

50. Jones SG: Adrenal patient: proceed with caution, *RN* 45(2):69-72, 1982.

51.* Jones SG: Bilateral adrenalectomy: postop dangers to watch for, *RN* 34(2):66-69, 1982.

52.* Larson CA: The critical path of adrenocortical insufficiency, *Nurs 84* 14(10):66-69, 1984.

30

The Patient with Hepatic Problems

Virginia L. Cassmeyer
Dorothy R. Blevins

After studying this chapter, the learner should be able to:

- Describe the anatomy of the liver and the physiological functions of the hepatic system.
- Differentiate between diffuse and focal hepatocellular disorders.
- Differentiate between toxic and viral hepatitis, acute and chronic hepatitis, and among hepatitis A, B, C, D, and E.
- Explain the pathophysiologic basis for common manifestations of diffuse liver disorders and the signs and symptoms of cirrhosis.
- Describe preventive measures for hepatitis.
- Discuss the care of the patient with diffuse liver disorders such as cirrhosis or hepatitis or their sequelae.
- Describe the care of patients with liver abscesses, tumors, or trauma.

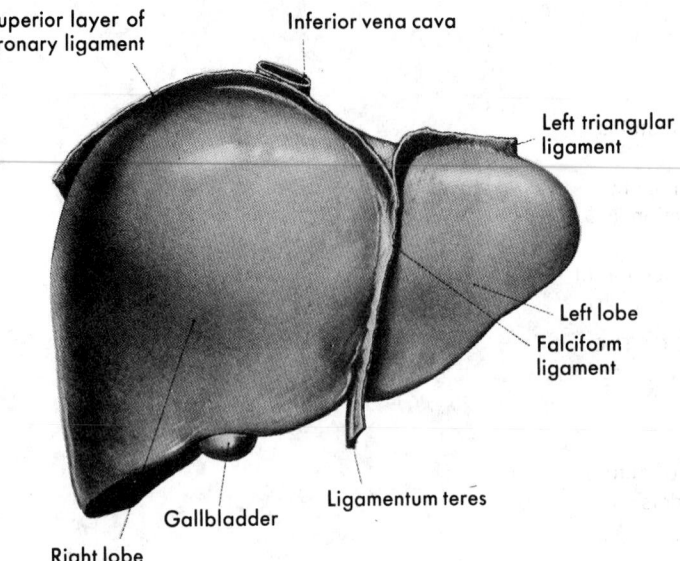

Fig. 30-1 Anterior view of liver. (From Hamilton WJ, editor: *Textbook of human anatomy*, ed 2, St Louis, 1976, Mosby—Year Book. By permission of Macmillan, London & Basingstoke.)

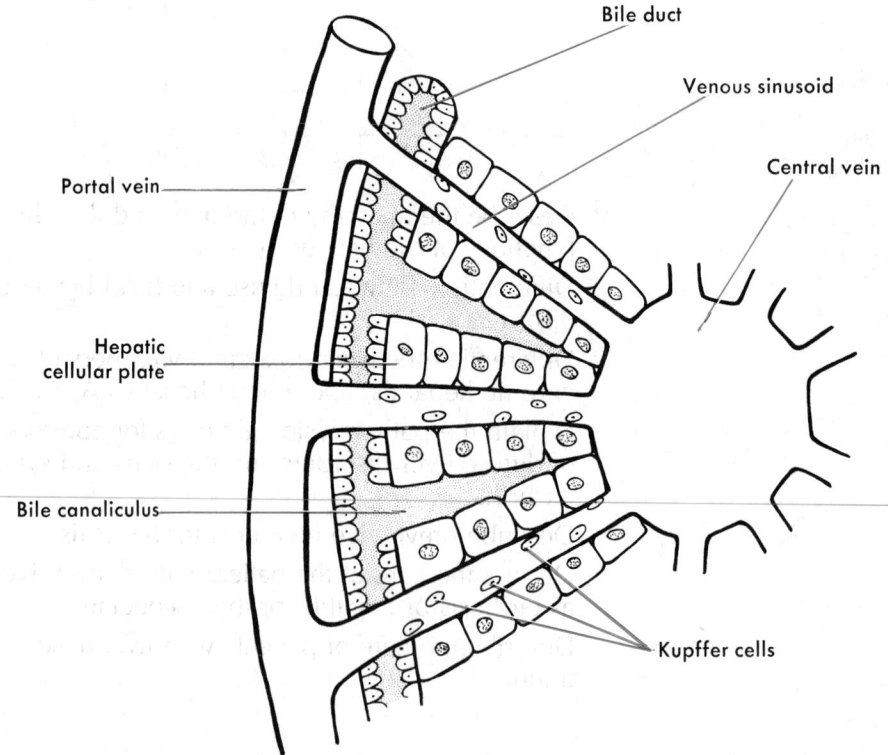

Fig. 30-2 Diagram of liver lobule. (Modified from Guyton A: *Textbook of medical physiology*, ed 4, Philadelphia, 1971, WB Saunders.)

The hepatic system is affected by a variety of pathologic processes that may severely affect normal metabolic processes. Many of the disorders of the hepatic system are chronic and require patients to make changes in their lifestyles, if optimal health is going to be maintained. These patients need nursing support to deal with their chronic health problems in the most effective ways.

ANATOMY AND PHYSIOLOGY

The hepatic system is a major system involved in regulation of body functions. The liver, which consists of two lobes, is one of the largest organs of the body and is located in the right upper quadrant of the abdomen under the diaphragm. It extends up under the ribs and is 4 to 8 cm in height in the midsternal line and 6 to 12 cm in height in the midclavicular line. It normally extends from the fifth intercostal space to just below the costal margin. The gallbladder lies under the inferior surface of the liver (Fig. 30-1).

The liver is made up of small liver lobules (Fig. 30-2) composed of hepatic cellular plates. Each hepatic cellular plate is usually two cells thick, and between these cells run biliary canaliculi. Venous sinusoids (also called hepatic sinusoids), which are capillaries of the liver that receive blood from both the portal vein and the hepatic artery, lie on the opposite sides of the hepatic cells. After flowing through the venous sinusoids, blood is emptied into the central vein and from there flows into the hepatic vein. The venous sinusoids are lined with Kupffer's cells, which are reticuloendothelial cells that phagocytize bacteria and other foreign products.

The liver is ideally structured to receive large supplies of blood to carry out its multiple functions, which are summarized in Box 30-1. Although only 25% of its blood supply is oxygenated, oxygen extraction by the liver is so efficient that there is little variation in oxygen consumption regardless of the rate of oxygen flow. The liver contains about 15% of the total blood volume and can quickly expel about half of this blood in situations of hemorrhage. The liver can also increase the percentage of blood volume it stores in the presence of vascular excess. Thus, the liver serves as a blood reservoir. (See Fig. 30-3 for diagram of the hepatic portal system.)

It is helpful to think of the liver as a metabolic factory and a waste disposal facility. The portal vein brings to the liver raw materials absorbed from the gastrointestinal tract, finished products are manufactured by the liver, and then the hepatic venules and biliary canaliculi act as the distributors of these products through blood and bile flow. Waste products that are produced through these metabolic processes are eliminated through bile flow or carried by blood to other parts of the body for elimination.

Carbohydrate, Protein, and Fat Metabolism

The liver has a major role in the metabolism of the major food nutrients. Through various enzymatic activities, the liver can oxidize carbohydrates, proteins, and fats for energy or use these nutrients to produce needed compounds, or to produce storage forms of these compounds for future use.

30-1

Summary of liver functions

Carbohydrate, protein, and fat metabolism
　Carbohydrate metabolism
　　Glycogen formation and storage
　　Glucose formation from glycogen (glycogenolysis) and from amino acids, lactic acids, and glycerol (gluconeogenesis)
　Protein metabolism
　　Protein catabolism
　　Protein synthesis
　　　Albumin
　　　Globulin
　　　Clotting factors
　　　C-reactive protein
　　　Transferrin
　　　Enzymes
　　　Ceruloplasmin, etc.
　　Formation of needed amino acids
　Fat metabolism
　　Oxidation of fatty acids for energy
　　Ketone formation
　　Synthesis of cholesterol and phospholipids
　　Formation of triglycerides from dietary fats and excessive dietary carbohydrates and proteins
　　Formation of lipoproteins
Production of bile salts
Bilirubin metabolism
Detoxification of endogenous and exogenous substances
　Ammonium
　Steroid hormones (aldosterone, estrogen, testosterone, etc.)
　Drugs
Storage of minerals and vitamins
Protection (Kupffer cells)

The liver helps maintain a normal blood glucose level. Immediately after meals, the liver cells extract glucose and other sugars from the sinusoidal blood and use them to form glycogen (glycogenesis). Between meals, or in longer fasting states, the liver provides glucose to the blood by breaking down glycogen (glycogenolysis) or by forming new glucose from amino acids, glycerol, and lactic acids (gluconeogenesis).

The liver provides needed amino acids through the process of transamination. In addition, it is the only source of albumin, which is necessary for the maintenance of osmotic pressure. The liver is the source of several clotting factors. It produces fibrinogen (factor I), prothrombin (factor II), proaccelerin (factor V), serum prothrombin conversion accelerator (factor VII), (Christmas factor) factor IX, Stuart-Prower factor (factor X), plasma thromboplastin antecedent (factor XI), Hageman factor (factor XII), and fibrin stabilizing factor (factor XIII). Although some of these may be produced elsewhere in the body, the levels decrease significantly with liver disease. The production of factors II, VII, IX, and X requires vitamin K. Because vitamin K is a fat-soluble vitamin, it requires adequate production and excretion of bile for its absorption. In addition to protein synthesis, the liver catabolizes proteins as necessary for energy.

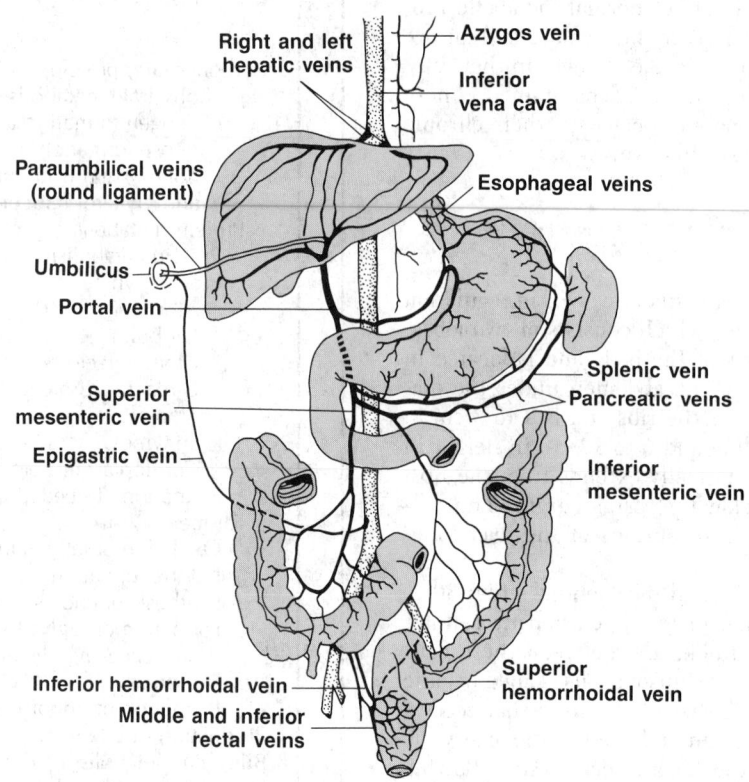

Fig. 30-3 Hepatic portal system. Blood is carried from the stomach, intestines, spleen, and pancreas into the venous sinusoids. Hepatic veins convey blood to the inferior vena cava. Clinically significant sites of anastomosis between the hepatic and systemic circulations are *(1)* the esophageal veins (portal tributary), which anastomose with the azygos veins (systemic tributary); *(2)* the paraumbilical veins in the round ligament originate in the left branch of the portal vein, which connect with the superficial veins of the anterior abdominal wall (systemic tributaries) in the area of the umbilicus; *(3)* the superior rectal or hemorrhoidal veins (portal tributary), which anastomose with the middle and inferior rectal veins (systemic tributaries); *(4)* the portal tributaries to the intestines, pancreas, and liver, which anastomose with the phrenic, renal, and lumbar veins (systemic tributaries not shown). In portal hypertension and chronic liver disease, blood may be backed up in these veins and be shunted around the liver through the points of anastomosis. (From Price SA, Wilson LM, eds: *Pathophysiology, clinical concepts of disease processes,* ed 4, St Louis, 1992, Mosby–Year Book.)

The liver is involved in multiple aspects of fat metabolism. Fatty acids that are metabolized by the liver are released from adipose tissue or derived from food. Triglycerides in the diet are absorbed in chylomicrons and metabolized to fatty acids. Fatty acids may be (1) oxidized, (2) metabolized to ketones, (3) converted to phospholipids, (4) used to form cholesterol esters, or (5) reesterified to triglycerides and combined with protein, cholesterol, and phospholipids to form lipoproteins.

Production of Bile Salts

Bile production is one of the major functions of the liver. Bile is a complex compound composed of cholesterol, phospholipids, bile salts, bile pigments (bilirubin), and a very small amount of proteins and electrolytes. Ninety-seven percent of bile is water. Metabolites of drugs and other substances that need to be excreted are also found in bile. Bile salts are necessary for the absorption of fats, cholesterol, and fat-soluble vitamins. Bile is released from the liver and concentrated and stored in the gallbladder. The liver secretes approximately 700 ml of bile daily. The bile salts released during each meal are reabsorbed into the enterohepatic circulation and recycled two or three times during a meal.

Bilirubin Metabolism

Bilirubin is a by-product of the heme portion of red blood cells and is released when red blood cells are destroyed. The bilirubin at this point is not water soluble *(unconjugated/indirect)* and is carried in the blood attached to protein. The liver is responsible for picking up this unconjugated bilirubin, for converting it a water-soluble form (*conjugated/direct*) and for secreting conjugated bilirubin into the bile. The bilirubin in bile is emptied into the duodenum and is broken down by bacteria into *urobilinogen*. Some of the urobilinogen is excreted with the feces, giving stool its brown color; some is eliminated in the urine; and the majority returns to the liver and is recycled. (See Fig. 30-4 for diagram of bilirubin metabolism.)

Detoxification

The liver has a prime role in detoxification of both exogenous and endogenous substances. Ammonia, from protein metabolism or from intestinal production, is one of the major toxic products handled by the liver. Because the liver extracts almost all the ammonia produced in the gut via the enterohepatic circulation and detoxifies this ammonia and the ammonia liberated in the liver itself, peripheral blood levels are kept very low. The ammonia is detoxified by conversion into urea, which is then excreted by the kidneys. The liver also has a major role in the detoxification of many drugs. All barbiturates (except phenobarbital and barbital) and many other sedatives are inactivated by the liver. The status of the liver plays an important role in the effectiveness of toxicity of these and other drugs. The liver also serves a function in metabolizing aldosterone, corticosterone, estrogen, and testosterone steroid hormones.

Storage of Minerals and Vitamins

The liver stores reserves of various minerals and vitamins. This storage prevents abnormal internal levels from occurring, although the intake may be very irregular. Vitamins A, D, and B_{12} are stored in sufficient quantities to prevent deficiencies for months. Vitamins E and K are also stored. Iron in the form of *ferritin* is stored and can be used to resupply iron for hemoglobin formation as needed; copper is stored as well.

Blood Reservoir

The liver, because of its tremendous vascular supply and sinusoidal system, can act as a reservoir for blood. When the venous vascular volume becomes greater than the right side of the heart can handle, blood will accumulate in the liver.

Protection

The Kupffer cells, which line the sinusoids of the liver, are phagocytic cells. These cells are very efficient in removing infective organisms and other foreign substances from the blood as blood flows through the liver. The phagocytic activity of the liver is very important in protecting the body from infections.

Physiologic Changes With Aging

Most of the functions of the liver do not seem to be affected by aging, even though the weight of the liver lessens and there are identifiable microscopic changes in liver cells. However, enzymes involved in the metabolism of drugs such as anticonvulsants, psychotropics, and oral anticoagulants are decreased.[44] Nurses need to be alert to signs and symptoms of excesses of these and other drugs metabolized by the liver.

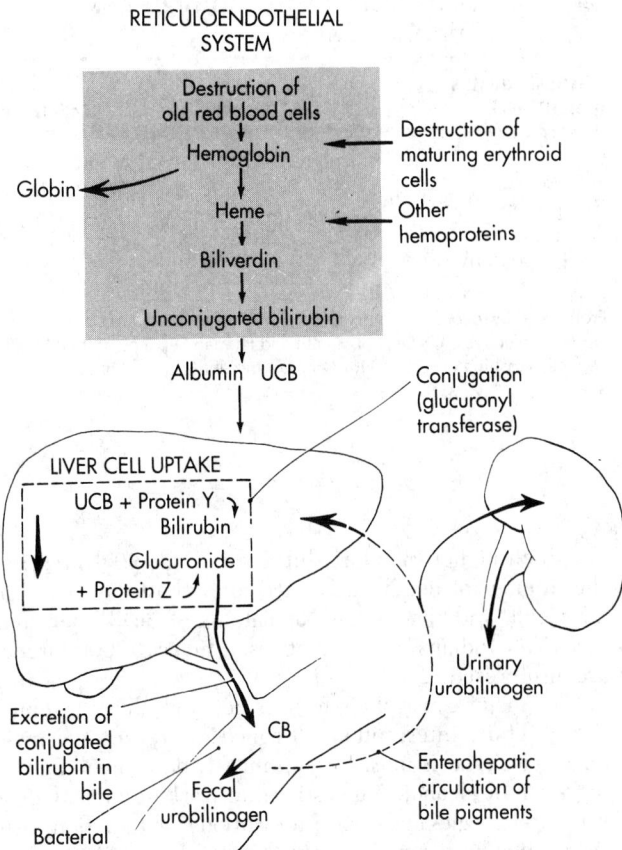

Fig. 30-4 Normal bilirubin metabolism. (From Price SA, Wilson LM, eds: *Pathophysiology, clinical concepts of disease processes*, ed 4, St Louis, 1992, Mosby–Year Book.)

PREVENTION AND HEALTH EDUCATION

Primary Prevention

Both hepatitis and cirrhosis, the two major diffuse hepatocellular problems, are preventable. *Healthy People 2000*,[14] which resulted from activities of the Public Health Services, lists several objectives relevant to nurses caring for persons with potential or acute hepatic problems. These goals are related to decreasing the incidence of and the death from cirrhosis and viral hepatitis. Every nurse has a responsibility to be involved in preventive care in whatever ways possible to promote appropriate health care that reduces the incidence of these diseases as well as others.

Cirrhosis

The term *cirrhosis* refers to several diseases that are characterized by diffuse inflammation and fibrosis resulting in major structural changes and functional loss. Although the incidence of deaths from cirrhosis has decreased for all persons, cirrhosis was still the ninth leading cause of death in 1985.[14] Importantly, the current death rates from cirrhosis for black men and American Indians/Alaska Natives

Table 30-1 Cirrhosis death and high-risk populations

Cirrhosis deaths (per 100,000)	1987 baseline	2000 target
All people	9.1	6
Black men	22	12
American/ Alaska Natives	25.9	13

From *Healthy people 2000: national health promotion and disease prevention objectives,* US Dept of Health and Human Services, Public Health Service, Washington DC, 1990, US Government Printing Office.

Table 30-2 Incidence of hepatitis and target populations for hepatitis B prevention

Incidence of viral hepatitis (per 100,000)	1987 baseline	2000 target
Hepatitis B	63.5	40
Hepatitis A	31	23
Hepatitis C	18.3	13.7

Special population targets for hepatitis B prevention	1987 baseline estimated	2000 target
Intravenous drug abusers	30,000	22,500
Heterosexually active people	33,000	22,000
Homosexual men	25,300	8,500
Children of Asians/Pacific Islanders	8,900	1,800
Occupationally exposed workers	6,200	1,250
Infants of hepatitis B carrier mothers	3,500	500 (new carriers)
Alaska Natives	15	1

From *Healthy people 2000: national health promotion and disease prevention objectives,* US Dept of Health and Human Services, Public Health Service, Washington DC, 1990, US Government Printing Office.

are much higher than for white men. Table 30-1 presents the number of deaths attributed to cirrhosis in 1987 for all people and the special populations of black men and American Indians/Alaska Natives. The year 2000 targets are also presented.

The major cause of cirrhosis is heavy alcohol consumption.[14] Thus, interventions designed to prevent the incidence of cirrhosis must focus primarily on controlling the ingestion of alcohol. Nurses need to work to identify preventive strategies and early interventions for addiction with special emphasis on getting this level of care to black men, American Indians, and Alaska Natives. (See Chapter 13 for a discussion of some interventions related to substance abuse.)

Hepatitis

Hepatitis refers to acute or chronic inflammation of the liver. It may be induced by toxins, including alcohol, viruses, or bacteria. Both toxic and viral hepatitis are preventable.

Toxic hepatitis

Toxic hepatitis may be induced by industrial toxins, household agents, alcohol, and prescription and nonprescription drugs. Toxic hepatitis due to alcohol is called *alcoholic hepatitis*. Nurses can assist in the prevention of toxic hepatitis by teaching the dangers of the injudicious use of materials that are known to be injurious to the liver and by emphasizing the need for a well-balanced diet with recommended dietary requirements of nutrients and minimal or *no alcohol*. Interventions designed to control ingestion of alcohol (Chapter 13) should be emphasized.

Because cleaning agents, solvents, and related substances sometimes contain products that are harmful to the liver, the public should read instructions on labels and follow them explicitly. Dry-cleaning fluids may contain carbon tetrachloride, which can cause liver injury if warnings to avoid inhalation of the fumes and to keep windows open are not heeded. If people must use these agents inside the home, a good practice is to open the windows wide, use the cleaning materials as quickly as possible, and then vacate the room, the apartment, or the house for several hours, leaving the windows open.

Many solvents used to remove paint and plastic material and to stain and finish woodwork contain injurious substances and should be used outdoors and not in the basement because dangerous fumes may spread throughout the house. Cleaning agents and finishes for cars should be applied outdoors or in the garage with the door open. Nurses in industry have a responsibility to teach the importance of observing regulations to avoid industrial hazards. Nitrobenzene, tetrachloroethane, carbon disulfide, and dinitrotoluoyl are examples of injurious compounds used in industry.

Some drugs that are known to cause mild liver damage must be used therapeutically. However, the nurse should warn the public about the use of preparations that are available without prescription that may be injurious (see Box 30-2, p. 884). Many drugs, prescription and nonprescription, reach the market before dangers resulting from their extensive use have been conclusively ruled out; for example, the prescription drug chlorpromazine, which was being widely used as a tranquilizer, has been found to cause stasis of bile in the canaliculi of the liver, which can lead to serious hepatic damage. A safe rule to follow is to avoid taking any medication except that specifically prescribed by a physician for a specific ailment. Other information related to toxic hepatitis is discussed on p. 884.

Viral hepatitis

The term *viral hepatitis* refers to five distinguishable forms of hepatitis: hepatitis A, B, C[7,9] (previously called *non-A, non-B* [parenteral form]), D, and E (previously called *non-A, non-B* [nonparenteral form]). Viral hepatitis is the most serious infection of the liver. It is a reportable disease in all states. Statistics from the Centers for Disease Control (CDC) indicate that viral hepatitis is one of the most frequently reported infectious diseases in the United States. It is well accepted that the figures for any given year may be grossly underestimated, because persons with subclinical manifestations are often not reported as having active disease.

The three major forms of hepatitis are hepatitis A, B, and C. These three forms of hepatitis are the focus of the Healthy 2000 goals. The goals related to reduction of the incidence of viral hepatitis are summarized in Table 30-2. For hepatitis B, the special targeted populations for interventions also are identified.

Prevention of viral hepatitis is related to knowledge about (1) the viral agents, (2) routes and modes of transmission, and (3) measures that are effective in controlling transmission. Preventive-care measures related to viral hepatitis can be categorized into three groups: general measures that help to prevent the spread of many infectious diseases, measures used with patients with known hepatitis, and prophylactic preventive measures for persons exposed to viral hepatitis or for persons at high risk for infection. Information about the viral agents and routes of transmission, along with information about measures to prevent hepatitis, is presented in detail in conjunction with other information about viral hepatitis (see pages 885 to 891).

Secondary Prevention: Detection of Disease

Most of the diseases of the hepatic system result in early signs and symptoms that are vague and nonspecific. Early detection of these signs and symptoms can result in more rapid initiation of effective nursing and medical interventions. Because of their holistic assessment nurses can identify persons with life-style patterns that would put them at high risk for hepatic dysfunction, and can encourage and refer persons who have vague signs and symptoms to seek additional evaluation as appropriate.

MAJOR HEALTH PROBLEMS OF THE HEPATIC SYSTEM

Disorders of the hepatic system that are encountered in clinical practice include not only those caused by infectious organisms and toxins, but also abnormalities from changes in structure and function. The more common disorders are discussed in this chapter and outlined below.

1. Diffuse hepatocellular disorders
   a. Cirrhosis of the liver
   b. Hepatitis
2. Focal hepatocellular disorders
   a. Liver abscess
   b. Trauma to the liver
   c. Tumors of the liver

The nursing process discussion that concludes this chapter applies to all the above disorders.

DIFFUSE HEPATOCELLULAR DISORDERS

Regardless of the specific pathologic condition, disorders secondary to diffuse parenchymal damage result in problems that are common to all these conditions. These problems will be discussed before the specific disorders of cirrhosis and hepatitis are discussed.

Common Manifestations of Diffuse Hepatocellular Disorders

Jaundice

Jaundice is a symptom complex caused by a disturbance of physiology of bilirubin metabolism and the excretion of bile and is present in many hepatic problems as well as in disorders of the pancreatic and biliary systems (See Fig. 30-4, p. 875.) Regardless of the course of jaundice, there is an *excess of bilirubin* in the blood that eventually is distributed to the skin, mucous membranes, and other body fluids and tissues, giving them a yellow discoloration. If bilirubin has been processed by the liver (extracted, conjugated, and secreted), it is water soluble and can be excreted in urine, which will be darker than usual. The presence of bilirubin in the skin causes *pruritis (itching)* in about 20% to 25% of the patients who have jaundice. Regardless of the type of jaundice, there will be an *increase in the total serum bilirubin* (normal: 0.1 to 1 mg/dl). Jaundice can usually be detected when bilirubin concentrations exceed 2.5 mg/dl. The changes in concentration of bilirubin and bilirubin metabolites in the serum, urine, or stool help in determining the type of jaundice. Serum bilirubin levels must be combined with other laboratory and diagnostic tests and interpreted in view of the history and clinical findings.

Jaundice can result from hemolysis and obstruction of extrahepatic and intrahepatic biliary ducts. Table 30-3 compares the different causes of jaundice. A common cause of *intrahepatic cholestasis* (stasis of bile within the small biliary canniculi of the liver) is drug reactions such as from phenothiazines. Clay-colored (grayish-white) stools indicate that bile is not reaching the intestine and suggest *extrahepatic obstruction* (obstruction of hepatic, gallbladder, or common bile duct). An absence of urobilinogen in the urine supports this inference because bile and bilirubin must reach the intestines for the normal formation of urobilinogen, some of which is usually excreted in the urine. Frequent causes of extrahepatic obstruction are gallstones lodged in the common bile duct, pancreatitis, and carci-

Table 30-3 Types of jaundice

Category	Pathology	Possible findings
Obstructive		
Intrahepatic	Suppression of bile flow in canaliculi or small biliary ductiles (cholestasis)	Direct* bilirubin elevated; alkaline phosphatase elevated; no enlargement of bile ducts seen on scan or ultrasound
Extrahepatic (biliary tract obstruction)	Obstruction of bile flow in large bile ducts	Direct* bilirubin elevated; alkaline phosphatase elevated; enlargement of bile ducts documented by scan, ultrasound; absence of urobilinogen in urine
Hepatocellular	Hepatocyte injury from toxins (toxic/alcoholic hepatitis), viruses (viral hepatitis) or as part of syndrome of cirrhosis	Transaminases (ALT, AST) elevated 10- to 15-fold; both direct* and indirect† bilirubin may be elevated (direct more than indirect); prolonged prothrombin time
Hemolytic	Excessive amounts of bilirubin are released from RBCs as would be seen in sickle-cell anemia; liver is unable to excrete bilirubin as rapidly as it forms	Usually mild elevation of total bilirubin (indirect more than direct)

*"Direct" measures conjugated bilirubin.
†"Indirect" measures unconjugated bilirubin.

noma of the head of the pancreas, all of which are discussed in Chapter 32.

In hepatocellular damage, there is interference with uptake, conjugation, and excretion of bilirubin into bile. Excretion is the most profoundly affected process and a predominantly *conjugated hyperbilirubinemia* is seen. *The level of jaundice does not correlate with the severity of hepatitis; however, in cirrhosis, jaundice suggests a poorer prognosis.*

Bleeding tendencies and anemia

Bleeding tendencies and anemia are common complications of hepatic disease. They may occur in persons with advanced cirrhosis or hepatitis. These tendencies are a result of deficiencies in the formation of clotting factors, thrombocytopenia, and a deficiency of erythrocytes. In patients with obstructive jaundice and hepatic disease, the synthesis of various clotting factors is impaired. If the patient's bile duct is obstructed, absorption of fat and vitamin K (fat soluble) is reduced. Even if vitamin K is absorbed, severely damaged liver cells may not synthesize adequate amounts of clotting factors, especially prothrombin. Other vitamin deficiencies (A, B complex, D) may also result from decreased absorption of fat-soluble vitamins or the inability to store the vitamins.

The patient with hepatic disease may also develop an enlarged spleen as a result of portal hypertension. This is believed to be a primary factor in thrombocytopenia and increased red blood cell destruction. In addition, alcohol has a direct toxic effect on bone marrow, which can cause thrombocytopenia and anemia.

Various other factors contribute to the anemia, including blood loss from gastrointestinal bleeding and decreased red blood cell production secondary to folic acid deficiency and poor protein intake.

Infection

The patient with diffuse hepatocellular disease is at risk for infection. Depressed protein synthesis, lymphatic obstruction of the splanchnic organs, impaired Kupffer cells, and depressed bone marrow all contribute to the increased risk. Leukopenia may be present.

Fluid and electrolyte alterations

Fluid volume deficit results when body losses exceed body gains and should be considered when the following symptoms are seen:

1. Vomiting
2. Anorexia with decreased intake
3. Hemorrhage
4. Diarrhea

It is important that nurses understand that patients with *hypoalbuminemia* (serum level below 4 g/dl) may have a contracted intravascular volume, *even in the presence of edema and ascites.* This phenomenon is seen most often in cirrhosis and results from the decreased production of albumin and the continued loss of this protein into the peritoneal cavity. As a result, the colloidal osmotic pressure of the blood is decreased (leading to increased fluid filtration through the capillary wall) while the return of fluid to the capillary is impaired. The patient is less able to maintain adequate perfusion of tissues should blood volume decrease further.

The several factors that lead to *ascites* (accumulation of serous fluid in the peritoneal cavity) are illustrated in Fig. 30-5. The sequence of these mechanisms and how they interact to intensify ascites is not well established. A vicious cycle is established as the albumin lost into the peritoneal cavity further decreases the patient's serum albumin levels, resulting in an increase in interstitial fluid. As a result, hydrothorax, and ankle and presacral edema may accompany the ascites. The patient with cirrhosis frequently is unable to excrete normal amounts of urinary sodium. *Hyponatremia* is frequent and reflects the disproportional retention of water in comparison to sodium.

Alterations in renal function may occur because of decreased blood volume, portal hypertension, and increased

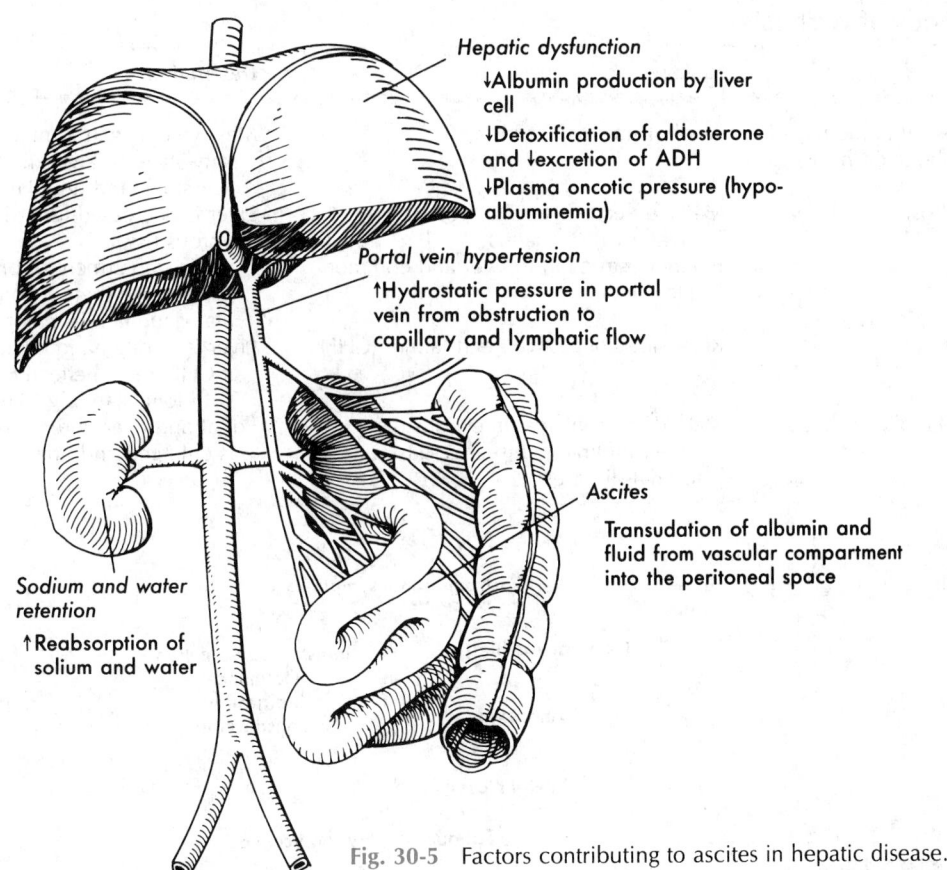

Hepatic dysfunction

↓Albumin production by liver cell

↓Detoxification of aldosterone and ↓excretion of ADH

↓Plasma oncotic pressure (hypo-albuminemia)

Portal vein hypertension

↑Hydrostatic pressure in portal vein from obstruction to capillary and lymphatic flow

Ascites

Transudation of albumin and fluid from vascular compartment into the peritoneal space

Sodium and water retention

↑Reabsorption of solium and water

Fig. 30-5   Factors contributing to ascites in hepatic disease.

circulating hormones. Decreased excretion of water, sodium, and metabolic wastes is common. Oliguria, azotemia (nitrogen wastes in the blood), and low urinary sodium (less than 10 mEq/L) may occur abruptly and signal hepatorenal syndrome. Although renal medullary blood flow is maintained in this condition, there is a marked decrease in renal cortical blood flow. Precipitants of hepatorenal syndrome, which has a mortality rate of nearly 90%, are the following:

1. Diuretic therapy
2. Paracentesis
3. Gastrointestinal hemorrhage

CIRRHOSIS OF THE LIVER

Cirrhosis of the liver is the term applied to chronic disease of the liver characterized by diffuse inflammation and fibrosis of the liver that result in drastic structural changes and significant loss of hepatic function. The basic processes leading to cirrhosis are liver cell death with scar tissue formation and regeneration of cell mass that causes distortion of the structure with a resultant change in circulation. Primary prevention of cirrhosis is discussed on p. 875.

Etiology/Epidemiology

The major types of cirrhosis are described in Table 30-4. Laënnec's cirrhosis is most frequently caused by chronic alcoholism. Malnutrition associated with other diseases

such as pancreatitis and ulcerative colitis may also cause Laënnec's cirrhosis. The major hepatotoxin leading to postnecrotic cirrhosis is viral hepatitis.

Postnecrotic cirrhosis is the most common type of cirrhosis on a worldwide basis. *Laënnec's cirrhosis is the most common type in North America.* More rare nonspecific types of cirrhosis account for about 10% of the deaths resulting from cirrhosis. Overall, cirrhosis is the ninth leading cause of death in the United States.[14]

Pathophysiology

Cirrhosis secondary to alcoholism and other causes is usually preceded by fatty infiltration of the liver, which is reversible if the causative factor is removed. The fatty infiltration is followed by acute inflammation (alcoholic hepatitis if due to alcohol) and finally cirrhosis, if the degenerative process continues. Fatty liver and alcoholic hepatitis are described on p. 884.

The end result of cirrhosis is loss of normal physiologic functions of the liver and obstruction of hepatic portal blood flow. Alterations in physiologic functioning are seen late in the disease because the liver has a large reserve capacity and remarkable powers of regeneration.

The fibrosis in the liver resulting from the continual destruction distorts the hepatic structures and obstructs splanchnic veins and portal blood flow. This vascular obstruction can worsen the fluid and electrolyte problems, bleeding, anemia, and other problems resulting from loss of normal physiologic function of the liver. Additionally,

Table 30-4 **Types of cirrhosis**

Type	Etiology	Description
Laënnec's cirrhosis (nutritional, portal, or alcoholic cirrhosis)	Alcoholism, malnutrition	Massive collagen formation; liver in early fatty stage is large and firm; in late stage it is small and nodular
Postnecrotic cirrhosis	Massive necrosis from hepatotoxins, usually viral hepatitis	Liver is decreased in size with nodules and fibrous tissue
Biliary cirrhosis	Biliary obstruction in liver and common bile duct	Chronic impairment of bile drainage; liver is first large then becomes firm and nodular; jaundice is major symptom
Cardiac cirrhosis	Right side congestive heart failure (CHF)	Liver is swollen and changes are reversible if CHF treated effectively; some fibrosis with long-standing CHF
Nonspecific, metabolic cirrhosis	Metabolic problems, infectious diseases, infiltrative diseases, gastrointestinal diseases	Portal and liver fibrosis may develop; liver is enlarged and firm

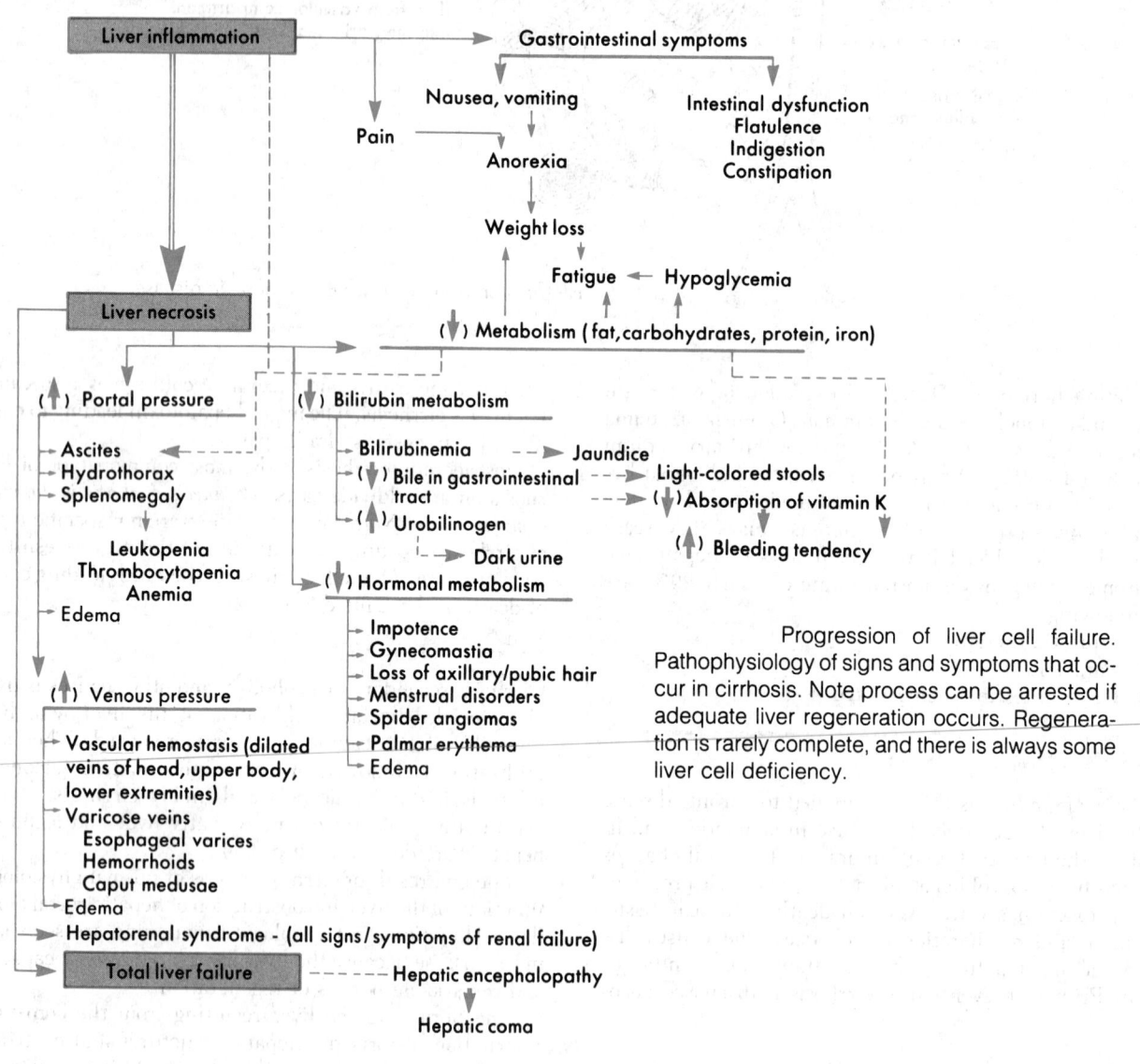

Progression of liver cell failure. Pathophysiology of signs and symptoms that occur in cirrhosis. Note process can be arrested if adequate liver regeneration occurs. Regeneration is rarely complete, and there is always some liver cell deficiency.

Fig. 30-6 Progression of liver cell failure. Pathophysiology of signs and symptoms that occur in cirrhosis. Note process can be arrested if adequate liver regeneration occurs. Regeneration is rarely complete, and there is always some liver cell deficiency.

this vascular obstruction can cause new problems. The portal hypertension associated with the obstruction of blood flow will cause vascular hemostasis, varicose veins, hemorrhoids, and esophageal varices.

A variety of signs and symptoms can be seen in persons with cirrhosis, regardless of the cause of cirrhosis. In Fig. 30-6 and Table 30-5 the multiple signs and symptoms associated with cirrhosis are presented and are related to the pathophysiologic changes. Any patient may exhibit any or all of the signs and symptoms. Frequently, the patient will have a long history of vague, nonspecific early symptoms

such as failing health, nausea, vomiting, anorexia, indigestion, flatulence, and constipation. Malnutrition and the resultant weight loss may not be obvious because of abnormal water retention or because of the calories obtained from alcohol. Abdominal pain may be present and is variable in character. It may be dull, mild, sharp, steady, or wavelike. It may be confined to the right upper quadrant by the liver or referred to the lower abdomen. Late signs and symptoms such as jaundice, ascites, and edema usually occur together.

Once cirrhosis is established it usually advances slowly

REVIEW

Table 30-5   Diffuse disorders of the liver

Disorder	Signs and symptoms	Medical therapy
Cirrhosis of the liver	Malaise	Rest
	Gastrointestinal symptoms: anorexia, indigestion, nausea, vomiting, flatulence, altered bowel function	Diet: high calorie, normal to high protein (unless ammonia toxicity is present), low fat, vitamin supplement (A, B, C, D)
	Malnutrition: muscle wasting, muscle weakness, possible loss of weight depending on fluid status	Bile salts Abstinence from alcohol
	Fluid retention: edema, ascites, abdominal distention, hydrothorax (often on right), weight gain	Sodium and water restriction Furosemide, spironolactone Albumin infusion (salt-poor) Peritoneal-jugular shunt (PJS)
	Jaundice: pruritus, hypoprothrombinemia, steatorrhea, light-colored stools, dark urine	Paracentesis Antihistamines
	Hepatomegaly, splenomegaly	
	Increased estrogen: palmar erythema, gynecomastia, spider angiomas, sparse body hair, testicular atrophy	
	Portal hypertension: caput medusae, hemorrhoids, esophageal varices, edema of lower extremities	Surgical procedures that shunt blood away from liver
	Gastrointestinal bleeding	Fresh blood transfusion, plasma expanders, normal saline (IV)
	Esophageal varices	Saline lavage Vasopressin or other pharmacologic therapy Injection of sclerosing agents Esophageal tamponade Other therapy as described in text
	Bleeding tendencies, purpura, hematuria, gingival bleeding, epistaxis, melena, hematemesis	Vitamin K Transfusions of whole blood, plasma, platelets
	Anemia: pallor, fatigue, and decreased RBC, hematocrit and hemoglobin	High protein diet with supplements of vitamins and folic acid Splenectomy
	Portal-systemic encephalophathy: Impaired attention span, impaired concentration, apathy, insomnia, slurred speech, yawning, asterixis, fetor hepaticus, coma, muscular rigidity, hyperreflexia, myoclonus seizures	Protein-free diet Enemas, cathartics Lactulose, neomycin Dialysis, exchange transfusion Corticosteroids Amino acid (arginine) or levodopa replacement
	Hepatorenal syndrome: Oliguria, azotemia, ↑ blood pressure, edema, hyponatremia, neurological changes, anorexia, fatigue, and weakness	Improve hepatic function Stop nephrotoxic drugs Maintain hemodynamic status Dialysis/ultrafiltration Liver transplantation

Continued.

Table 30-5   Diffuse disorders of the liver—cont'd

Disorder	Signs and symptoms	Medical therapy
Viral hepatitis	**Preicteric stage** Anorexia, nausea and vomiting, chills and fever, arthralgia, right upper quadrant tenderness, fatigue	Rest Diet: high calorie, high protein, low fat Avoidance of toxins
	Icteric stage Jaundice (yellow sclera and skin), dark urine, light colored stools	Vitamin K Diet as above Rest Avoidance of toxins
	Posticteric stage Fatigue	Rest Diet as above Avoidance of toxins

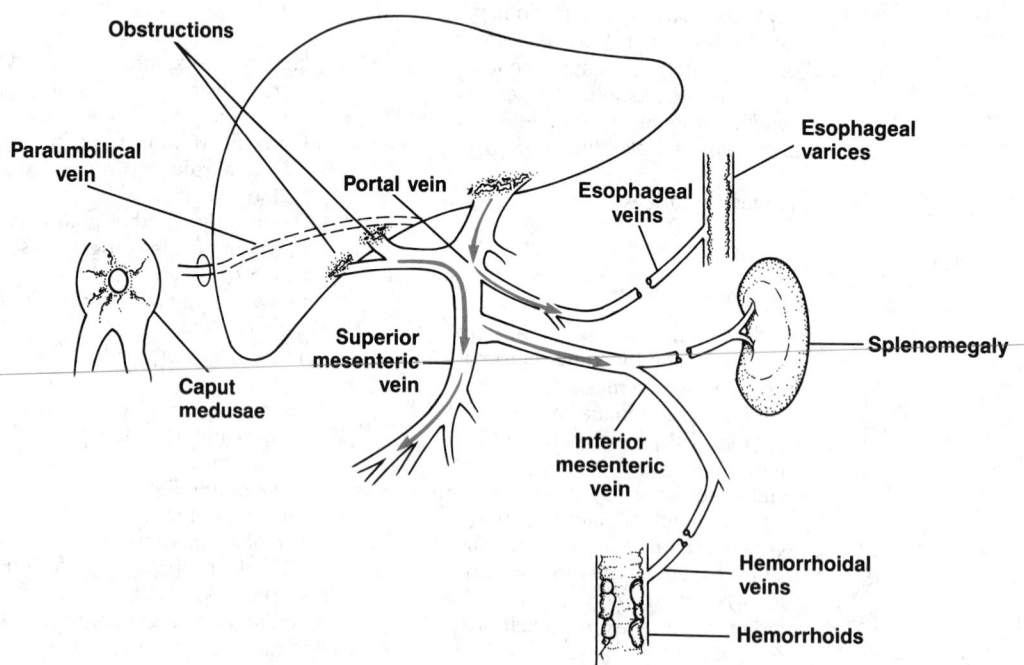

Fig. 30-7   Splanchnic veins. Venous drainage of splanchnic organs. When portal hypertension develops, other vessels can become engorged, leading to stasis and hypoxia of respective organs. The red lines indicate backflow when portal hypertension occurs, resulting in engorged veins and enlarged spleen.

to death. However, its progression can often be halted if prescribed therapeutic interventions are followed. Unfortunately, at times rapid deterioration occurs. Continued progression of the cirrhotic process will result in total liver failure, bleeding esophageal varices, portal-systemic encephalopathy, or renal failure.

Because of the severity of portal hypertension, esophageal varices, portal systemic encephalopathy, and hepatorenal syndrome, these four problems will be discussed in more detail.

Portal hypertension

As structural damage occurs and portal circulation is obstructed, portal hypertension occurs (Fig. 30-7). This hypertension results in a back flow of blood into the veins emptying into the portal veins. These veins in turn develop collateral channels of circulation. Collateral channels are most likely to occur in the paraumbilicus veins, the hemorrhoidal veins, and the veins at the cardia of the stomach that extend into the esophagus. These veins become distended and tortuous because they are not anatomically equipped to handle large volumes of blood. This results in hemorrhoids, esophageal varices, and a ring of varicosities surrounding the umbilicus (caput medusae). In addition, the spleen enlarges (splenomegaly) and sodium and water retention worsen, causing more edema. The increased pressure in the portal system results in transudation of albumin and fluid from the vascular compartment of the liver and other organs into the peritoneal cavity, worsening ascites. Lymphatic flow also is obstructed by the increased pressure, and this adds to the ascites.

Bleeding esophageal varices

Bleeding esophageal varices (Fig. 30-8) occur frequently in patients with cirrhosis of the liver and portal hypertension. The small vessels of the esophagus become tortuous and fragile and may be affected by mechanical trauma from ingestion of coarse foods and acid pepsin erosion, which may result in bleeding. Bleeding may also occur as a result of coughing, vomiting, sneezing, straining at stool (Valsalva's maneuver), or any physical exertion that increases abdominal venous pressure. Bleeding is frequently abrupt and without pain. Severe hematemesis and resultant shock may follow, requiring immediate emergency treatment. Treatment for this complication is summarized in Table 30-5.

Portal systemic encephalopathy

Portal systemic encephalopathy (PSE), formerly called *hepatic coma* or *ammonia toxicity*, is a metabolic encephalopathy associated with liver failure. This dysfunction of the central nervous system is thought to be related to several factors. Many patients with PSE have an increase in blood ammonia concentration. Normally, ammonia, which is formed in the intestines from the breakdown of protein by intestinal bacteria, is converted to urea in the liver. When liver failure occurs the detoxification ability of the liver may be decreased and thus ammonia is not converted into urea and ammonia concentration in the circulating blood is increased. Additionally, in liver failure, ammonia levels may be increased because blood is shunted past the liver.

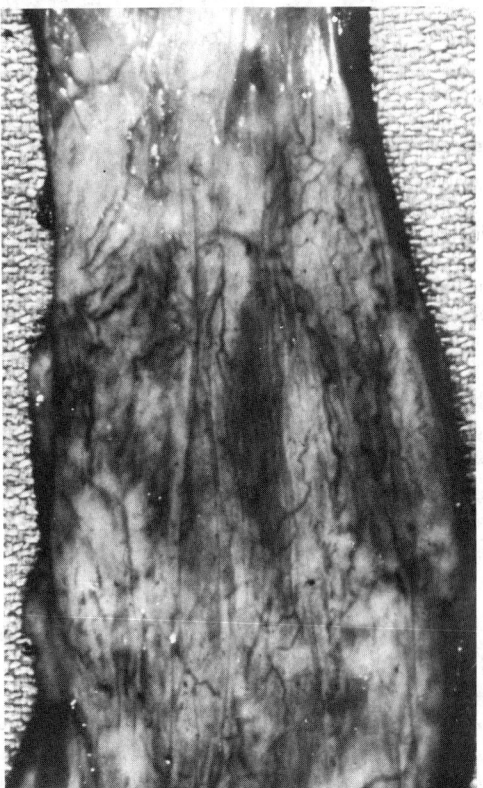

Fig. 30-8   Esophageal varices. Swollen varices and extensive collateral circulation are evident in segment of esophagus from patient with Laënnec's cirrhosis. (From Groer ME, Shekleton ME: *Basic pathophysiology: a conceptual approach,* ed 2, St Louis, 1983, Mosby–Year Book. Courtesy department of pathology, University of Tennessee, Knoxville.)

There are many factors that can increase blood ammonia levels (see p. 903).

It has been shown that patients with PSE have increased levels of aromatic or short-chain amino acids (SCAAs) and a decrease in branched-chain amino acids (BCAAs). Normally SCAAs are cleared by the liver. With liver failure they increase and cross the blood-brain barrier. These SCAAs such as phenylalanine, tryptophan, and tyrosine act as weak neurotransmitters and compete with regular neurotransmitters, resulting in an impairment of normal neurologic function.

Hypokalemia, alkalosis, sedation, and *gastrointestinal bleeding,* as well as other factors, are common precipitants of PSE. They induce PSE by the following mechanisms:

1. Hypokalemia results in a shift of potassium from the cells to the extracellular fluid in exchange for sodium and hydrogen. The shift of hydrogen (H) ion decreases the H ion concentration in the extracellular fluid and increases that within cells. The change in pH increase the formation of ammonia NH_3 in the extracellular fluids from ammonia NH_4. NH_3 is gaseous and crosses readily into cells where it exerts its toxic effects and where it may become trapped as nondiffusible NH_4.

Table 30-6 Stages of consciousness, intellectual behavior, and neurologic changes in portal-systemic encephalopathy

Stage 1 (prodromal)	Stage 2 (impending)	Stage 3 (stuporous)	Stage 4 (coma)
Change in sleep pattern	Lethargy	Confused, somnolent	Unconscious
Slow response	Disorientation to time	Stupor but arousable	No intellectual functioning
Shortened attention span	Impaired computation	Disorientation to place	Loss of deep tendon reflexes
Oppressed or euphoric	Decreased inhibition	Anger, rage, paranoia	If responsive, it is only to deep
Irritable	Anxiety or apathy	Increased reflexes	pain
Tremors	Inappropriate behavior	Clonus	
Some incoordination	Speech slurred	Babinski reflex	
Writing impaired	Decreased reflexes		
	Ataxia		

2. Alkalosis, from any cause, results in an increased formation of NH_3 in extracellular fluids, as described above.

3. In PSE, there is increased sensitivity to depressants, and any hypoxic insult or sedation may precipitate PSE.

4. Blood in the intestines increases the protein content, ammonia formation by bacteria, and ammonia absorption into the portal vein.

5. Constipation may increase the formation and absorption of ammonia from the gut or it may induce straining, precipitating esophageal bleeding.

6. Other factors such as exercise and infection may increase ammonia formation or change the blood flow to the liver and worsen hepatic function.

When one or more of these conditions exist, the nurse should institute intense monitoring for PSE. Treatment for PSE is started when the earliest signs are detected. Table 30-6 presents the stages of progression in impaired consciousness, intellectual behavior, and neurologic changes. The interventions for portal systemic encephalopathy is summarized in Table 30-5.

Hepatorenal syndrome

Hepatorenal syndrome is the sudden onset of renal failure from unknown causes in persons with progressive hepatic failure. A major factor is thought to be vasoconstriction of the renal vessels from an increase in renin, decrease in prostaglandins, release of endotoxins, or increase in sympathetic activity. The decreased renal blood flow can result in schemic damage and cell death. Oliguria, increased nitrogen waste products, and fluid and electrolyte imbalances occur. The patient will have the fatigue, anorexia, neurological changes, and weakness commonly seen in other causes of renal failure (see Chapter 33). The treatment for this problem is summarized in Table 30-5.

HEPATITIS

Hepatitis may be defined as an acute or chronic inflammatory disease of the liver. Although the term *hepatitis* is most commonly used in conjunction with viral hepatitis, the disease can be caused by toxic injury to the liver, including by alcohol, viruses, or bacteria.

Toxic hepatitis

The primary prevention of toxic hepatitis is discussed on p. 876. Box 30-2 lists some common hepatotoxins. Two types of chemical hepatotoxicity occur: direct toxic and idiosyncratic. In direct toxic hepatitis, the agent causes toxicity with predictable regularity and is dose dependent, such as with acetaminophen, tetracycline, alcohol, and carbon tetrachloride. The reactions in idiosyncratic toxic hepatitis are sporadic and not dose dependent, such as with isoniazid and chlorpromazine, which suggests idiosyncrasy in the host.

The pathologic changes in the liver will depend on the toxic agent. For example, necrosis and fatty infiltrates are present when the causative agent is carbon tetrachloride, whereas cholestasis with portal inflammation is seen when the toxic agent is chlorpromazine.

Fatty liver and alcoholic hepatitis

The leading cause of hepatic disease in the United States is alcohol. There are two reversible conditions for alcoholic liver damage: *fatty liver* and *alcoholic hepatitis*. In fatty liver, fatty deposits are seen within hepatocytes and the patient may complain of right quadrant tenderness. Hepatomegaly and elevated levels of transaminases are often present.

In alcoholic hepatitis, histologic examination reveals deposits of hyalin within hepatocytes, leukocytic infiltration and development of connective tissue surrounding hepatocytes and the central vein. The clinical presentation is varied; it can be asymptomatic or reflect liver failure. Anorexia, nausea, vomiting, weight loss, and abdominal pain are common.

30-2

Common hepatotoxins

Drugs: chlorpromazine, isoniazid, tetracycline, thiazides, thiouracil, acetaminophen
Organic solvents: carbon tetrachloride, methylenedianiline (MDA)
Phosphorus, heavy metals
Plant poisons
Alcohol

Alcohol has at least two toxic effects on fat metabolism that lead to fatty liver:

1. Increased NADPH generation, which promotes fatty acid synthesis and triglyceride formation
2. Inhibition of the release of triglycerides

In addition, acetaldehyde may be directly toxic to the hepatocytes. Factors that may enhance hepatotoxicity of alcohol include malnutrition, genetic susceptibility, and immune processes.

Viral Hepatitis

Viral hepatitis refers to several clinically similar but etiologically and epidemiologically distinct infections.

Etiology/epidemiology

There are currently five types of hepatitis: hepatitis A; hepatitis B; hepatitis C[7,9] (formerly called non-A, non-B hepatitis [parenterally transmitted form]); hepatitis D (formerly called delta hepatitis); and hepatitis E[7] (formerly called non-A, non-B hepatitis [nonparenterally transmitted form]). Some authorities suggest there is a sixth hepatitis virus.[34b] The vast majority of cases of hepatitis that are seen clinically are caused by hepatitis A or hepatitis B viruses. Most cases of all types of hepatitis occur in young adults. Factors such as viral agent, transmission, and high-risk groups vary for the types of hepatitis. Table 30-7 summarizes the difference between the types of hepatitis.

Table 30-7   Etiologic/epidemiologic/transmission characteristics of hepatitis

	Hepatitis A	Hepatitis B	Hepatitis C	Hepatitis D	Hepatitis E
Age group	Older children and young adults	Young adults because of life-style	All age groups but highest in adults because of more frequent blood transfusions	Same as for hepatitis B	Young to middle-aged
Transmission	Primarily person-to-person through fecal contamination; common source epidemics from contaminated food and water; rare transmission by blood; *not* transmitted by shared utensils and kissing	Percutaneous or permucosal routes through infected body substances introduced by contaminated needles and sexual contact; spread by personal contact in households and among children; rare transmission by blood transfusion, since screening of blood for presence of hepatitis B surface antigen (HB$_s$Ag); *not transmitted* fecal-oral route or by contaminated H$_2$O	Parenterally transmitted through infected blood and parenteral drug abuse; no clear evidence of transmission by surgery, dental work, acupuncture, or tattooing; no evidence of transmission by sexual and other personal contact or by contaminated secretions other than blood; perinatal transmission unclear. Importantly, many persons have no identifiable risk factor.	Routes same as those for hepatitis B	Enterically transmitted form of non-A, non-B spread by contaminated water and food
Incubation period	15-50 days; average 28-30 days	45-160 days, average 60-120 days	Variable—14-150 days; 50 days average	Unknown	6 weeks
Secretions that have been found to contain infective agent	Feces of infected persons	Highest in blood and serous fluids; also found in saliva, semen, urine, nasopharyngeal washings, feces, and pleural fluid	Blood	Blood	Feces
Greatest infectivity	2 weeks before onset of jaundice	—	—	Infections occur as either coinfection with hepatitis B or superinfection in hepatitis B carrier	—

Modified from Advisory Committee on Immunization Practices (ACIP): *MMWR* 39(52):1-26, 1990.

Continued.

	Hepatitis A	Hepatitis B	Hepatitis C	Hepatitis D	Hepatitis E
Clinical onset	Abrupt	Insidious	Insidious	Insidious	Insidious
Diagnostic serologic tests	Confirmed by presence of immunoglobin against hepatitis A virus (IgM-class anti-HAV) in serum (found during acute and early convalescent period)	Confirmed by HB$_s$Ag, hepatitis B$_e$ antigen (HB$_e$Ag), antibody against hepatitis B$_e$ antigen (anti-HB$_e$), antibody against core antigen (anti-HB$_c$)	Confirmed by antibody to hepatitis C virus (anti-HCV); Anti-HCV test does not differentiate acute and chronic forms of Hepatitis C. The Food and Drug Administration and the CDC recommend that all donated blood be screened for the presence of anti-HCV. Blood banks voluntarily began testing blood for anti-HCV in the United States in 1986 and 1987[31]	Delta antigen in serum during early infection; delta antibodies during or after infection (first test for antigen not available for routine use)	—
Indication of protective immunity	IgG-class anti-HAV appears during the convalescent period and indicates immunity	Antibody against hepatitis B, surface antigen (anti-HB$_s$) indicates immunity	No tests available; people have had repeated infections	No test available but can only occur if hepatitis B virus is present	—
Chronic carriers	None demonstrated	Frequent—6%-10% of adult persons with HBV become carriers; 90% of infected infants and 25%-50% of infected children become carriers	8% of persons with hepatitis C become carriers	80% of those persons who have superinfection with hepatitis D become carriers with superinfection	—
Mortality	Infrequent (<0.6%)	1%-2%	Unknown	Unknown	High mortality rate in pregnant women
Subsequent chronic disease	Virtually absent	About 10% develop chronic disease	High—20%-50% develop chronic disease	Frequent in persons who contact a superinfection of hepatitis D	—
High-risk groups	Staff and children at day-care centers where children in diapers are cared for; staff and persons in institutions for custodial care (prisons, institutions for developmentally disabled); international travelers to developing countries	Immigrants/refugees from endemic areas of HBV; clients and staff in institutions for developmentally disabled; users of illicit parenteral drugs; fetuses of infected mothers; homosexually active men; heterosexually active people; household and sexual partners of HBV carriers; patients on hemodialysis; male prisoners; health care workers with occupational exposure to body substances	Parenteral drug users; health care workers with occupational exposure to blood; hemodialysis patients; and recipients of whole blood, blood cellular components, or plasma	Same as for hepatitis B	Found in Southeast Asia, India, and North Africa; cases found in Western countries in travelers from these areas[34]

Prevention of incidence or transmission of hepatitis
General preventive measures

The major activity that can assist in the general prevention of viral hepatitis is thorough handwashing by all persons. All feces, urine, blood and other body fluids should be considered potentially infectious for a wide variety of organisms and disposed of properly. Nurses should be involved in the promotion of the development of adequate sewage disposal systems to prevent contamination of food and water supplies that may result in endemic forms of hepatitis A.

Because hepatitis B, hepatitis C, hepatitis D, and possibly hepatitis A, as well as carrier states of some types of hepatitis can be spread by contaminated needles and other equipment that comes in contact with infected blood and other body fluids, disposable and nondisposable needles, syringes, and other equipment used in patient care must be handled with great care. *All equipment should be treated as if it had been used on an infected person and handled using universal precautions or body substance precautions (an extension of universal precautions because it focuses on all body substances) no matter who the patient.*

Needles should *not* be recapped. They should be discarded in puncture resistant containers designed for this purpose. Other disposable equipment should also be discarded in appropriate containers; the containers are marked "Contaminated" to alert persons handling the rubbish.

Nondisposable equipment should be rinsed, packaged so sharp objects do not accidentally puncture someone, and sterilized by dry heat and steam under pressure (autoclaving), or by gas sterilization. If invasive reusable equipment is used in an environment in which autoclave sterilization is not available and boiling is the only available way to sterilize, the nurse should see that everything placed in the water sterilizer is covered completely and boiled for at least 30 minutes. The nurse should realize that the boiling time needed to destroy hepatitis virus is unknown and that water sterilization of invasive equipment, such as catheters, to be used for another patient is *not* an acceptable method for preventing the transmission of hepatitis.

Preventive measures used with persons with known hepatitis

Patients with known hepatitis A should be placed on *enteric precaution* (which is really an extension of universal precautions because it focuses on appropriate handling of contaminated gastrointestinal secretions). Children should be in private rooms, but responsible adults do not require one. Good handwashing after fecal and urine elimination is the major isolation measure. Anyone who must handle feces or potentially contaminated articles (bedpan, diapers, rectal thermometer) should wear gloves and gowns and wash hands thoroughly after completing care (see Box 30-3). Separate toilet facilities are sometimes used, but this is not necessary if fecal contamination, which might occur in a person who is confused, is not a problem. The toilet should be cleansed thoroughly daily. All disposable and nondisposable equipment and linens should be bagged properly and labeled correctly before being removed from the patient's room.

For patients with hepatitis B, C, and D, good hand washing and body substance precautions (an extension of universal precautions because it focuses on appropriate handling of *all* body substances) are used any time blood or other body fluids are handled. Gowns and gloves should be worn when the amount of potential contamination with blood or other body fluids is great (such as in the operating room or in intensive care). If splattering of contaminated blood and other body fluids is likely, goggles and a mask are worn. Care must be taken to avoid contact between the blood and other body fluids of an infected person and open cuts, the mucous membranes, or eyes of another

---

Nursing Research   30-3

Korniewicz DM., et al: Integrity of vinyl and latex procedures gloves, *Nurs Res* 38:144-146, 1989.

The use of protective gloves in the delivery of nursing care is a critical component in preventing the spread of hepatitis B virus (HBV) and human immunodeficiency virus (HIV). The risk of transmission of HBV exceeds that for HIV. The effectiveness of gloves in preventing transmission of HBV or HIV depends on the integrity of the gloves during use. This study was designed to determine the integrity of vinyl and latex procedure gloves under conditions that are present in clinical practice.

In this study, 645 latex and vinyl gloves from 28 lot numbers and five manufacturers were first tested for presence of visible defects when filled with water and allowed to hang vertically for 2 minutes. Next, 90 vinyl and 90 latex gloves with no visible defects were checked for permability to dye after being worn by one of 28 subjects during one of three levels of hand manipulation, some of which mimicked activities performed during routine patient care. The permeability of the gloves to *Serratia marcescens* also was tested using 50 of each type of glove.

Visible defects were present in 4.1% of the vinyl gloves and 2.7% of the latex gloves. Fifty-three percent of vinyl and 3% of the latex gloves showed dye penetration, and 20% of latex gloves and 34% of vinyl gloves that were water tight allowed for penetration of *S. marcescens*.

Glove standards set by the American Society of Testing and Materials (ASTM) allow for a failure rate of 1.5% for sterile surgical latex gloves and 2.5 for nonsterile latex gloves by the water-tight method. When the water-tight test was used in this study, the latex glove failure rate was equal to the standards established by ASTM, whereas the vinyl glove failure rate was much higher. When more sensitive tests were used to examine the gloves, both the latex and the vinyl gloves showed failure rates higher than the standard.

Latex gloves maintained better integrity when tested after in-use conditions than did vinyl gloves in all tests. Because all gloves showed leakage, this finding reemphasizes the need for excellent hand washing before and after all patient care activities, the importance of not reusing gloves, and the importance of not just washing the gloved hands between patients contacts. Additionally, in situations where high stress is placed on the gloves during patient care, gloves may need to be changed.

person. All invasive equipment such as needles, lancets, and dental drills should be disposed of properly or sterilized properly. All contaminated linens and other items should be bagged and labeled correctly. Persons who have had viral hepatitis should not be blood donors. The patient with acute hepatitis B, hepatitis C, and hepatitis D should not have intimate sexual contact during the period of infection. Protection of household and sexual contacts of persons who become hepatitis B carriers is discussed later in this chapter.

To prevent exposure of patients to hepatitis B virus from health care workers who are infected, the Centers for Disease Control has made several recommendations related to the care-giving practices of this group.[32] First, *it is important to remember that* the infected health care worker who maintains strict universal precautions and who is not performing invasive procedures poses no risk for the transmission of hepatitis B. There is a small risk for transmission when *invasive procedures* are performed by infected health care workers. To eliminate this risk, the CDC has developed recommendations that protect the patient, but do not limit unnecessarily the practice of the health care worker. The reader is encouraged to see the identified reference for the exact recommendations.[32]

Prophylaxis

Prophylaxis can be instituted either before exposure for persons at high risk and/or after exposure. The recommendations for prophylaxis vary for the different types of hepatitis and are reevaluated on a continual basis by the CDC.

Hepatitis A. For hepatitis A, the following recommendations have been made by CDC.[1]

Preexposure prophylaxis is recommended for travelers to developing countries who will be eating in settings of poor or uncertain sanitation or visiting extensively with local persons. The recommended therapy is immune globulin, 0.02 ml/kg, for persons traveling for less than 3 months, and 0.06 ml/kg every 5 months for those traveling for prolonged periods.

Postexposure prophylaxis is recommended for selected persons who have had contact with persons known to be positive for hepatitis A, if the prophylaxis is given *within 2 weeks* of exposure. Postexposure prophylaxis for the following people is recommended:

1. Close household and sexual contacts of persons with hepatitis A
2. *Staff* and *attendees* of day-care centers, if hepatitis A cases are recognized among attendees or employees or two or more households of center attendees have recognized cases; household members of families with children in diapers, if three or more families of attendees report cases
3. Residents and staff in institutions for custodial care who have close contact with person, with hepatitis A
4. Hospital staff who have close contacts with patients with hepatitis A (only if outbreaks occur)
5. Persons exposed to a common source of infection (infected food or water), if identified within 2 weeks of exposure

6. Food handlers working with another food handler diagnosed as having hepatitis A; patrons of food establishments only treated in rare instances

Hepatitis B. For hepatitis B, there is a vaccine available that provides active immunity (hepatitis B vaccine) and an immune globulin with high amounts of anti-HB_s (HBIG). The hepatitis B vaccine is used in both preexposure and postexposure prophylaxis. HBIG is used in only certain postexposure situations.

Hepatitis B vaccine is given as a series of three intramuscular injections (deltoid in adults and children; anterolateral thigh muscles in infants and neonates), with the second and third doses given 1 and 6 months after the first dose. The vaccine given in this manner has shown an efficacy of 90% to 95%. Some health care workers, hoping to decrease costs, have tried intradermal administration with smaller doses. This is not effective.[30] The effect of the vaccine on the developing fetus is not known. Because hepatitis B infection in pregnant women results in severe infection in the mother and chronic infection in the infant, and because the vaccine contains only noninfectious HB_sAg particles, pregnancy should not be considered a contraindication for its use if necessary.[1] Soreness at injection site is the most common side effect.[1] Hepatitis B vaccine causes *no adverse effects or benefits* in HBV carriers.

Preexposure vaccination is recommended for the following[1]:

1. Health care workers at high risk for exposure (medical technologists or staff, phlebotomists, most nurses in acute and critical care settings, surgeons, pathologists, oncology and dialysis unit staff, dentists, oral surgeons, dental hygienists, laboratory and blood bank technicians, emergency medical technicians, and morticians)
2. Clients and staff of institutions for the developmentally disabled
3. Hemodialysis patients
4. Sexually active homosexual men
5. Users of illicit injectable drugs
6. Recipients of frequent blood products, particularly patients with clotting disorders who receive frequent transfusions of clotting factors
7. Household and sexual contacts of HBV carriers
8. Some American populations, including infants, such as Alaska natives; native Pacific Islanders; immigrants and refugees and their infants from areas where hepatitis B is endemic, such as Eastern Asia; adoptees from countries of HBV endemicity and families of adoptee with positive HB_sAg tests
9. Long-term inmates of correctional facilities
10. Sexually active heterosexual persons with multiple sexual partners
11. International travelers who plan to reside for 6 months or longer in areas with a high incidence of hepatitis B

Postexposure prophylaxis for hepatitis B should be considered for the following[1]:

1. Infants born to HB_sAg-positive mothers
2. Persons who have percutaneous or permucosal exposure to HB_sAg-positive blood

3. Persons who have sexual contact with HB_sAg-positive persons
4. Infants <12 months of age exposed to primary care giver who has acute hepatitis B

Infants exposed perinatally are given HBIG at birth, and the hepatitis B vaccination series is started at the same time, if possible. Persons who have percutaneous or permucosal exposure and are unvaccinated are also treated with HBIG, and the hepatitis B vaccination series is started. If the exposed person has been vaccinated, he or she is checked for anti-HB_s and given HBIG immediately plus a booster dose of hepatitis B vaccine. The CDC also makes recommendations about prophylaxis after percutaneous or permucosal exposure from a source with unknown hepatitis B virus status.[1]

Booster immunization doses are recommended for previously vaccinated persons who experience percutaneous or needle exposure to HB_sAg-positive blood. In addition, it is recommended that patients on hemodialysis be assessed semiannually by antibody testing, and if their antibody level declines below 10 mlU/ml, they should be given a booster dose.[1] For persons with normal immune status, booster doses and routine serologic testing to assess antibody level are not necessary.[1]

Because the incidence of hepatitis B has not decreased in the manner it should have given that there is a vaccine available, in the Health Goals[14] for the year 2000 there are several goals related to decreasing the number of cases in selected groups of persons and increasing the number of high-risk persons who are immunized against hepatitis B. One high-risk group of concern is persons who are at risk of exposure because of their occupations. The goal related to this group of persons is to decrease the incidence of occupationally transmitted cases from the baseline of 6200 cases in 1987 to 1250 cases in the year 2000. This goal will be accomplished *in part* by enforcing work practices strictly. Importantly, this goal will require that more persons who are at high risk for hepatitis B from work exposure be immunized. The goal is to increase the level of hepatitis B immunization to 90% among occupationally exposed workers.[14] Hepatitis B is most frequently spread by sexual transmission. The persons who account for the most cases are intravenous drug abusers, sexual partners of infected heterosexuals, and homosexual men. Sexually transmitted hepatitis B has been decreasing among the homosexual population and increasing among heterosexuals.[14] The major ways to achieve a reduction in sexual transmission of hepatitis B is to continue to educate persons about its hazards and about the ways to avoid spread of the infection, and to increase the number of persons in these high-risk groups who are immunized. It remains a challenge to get these groups immunized because of a lack of awareness of the high-risk groups *by health care workers* and the difficulty in reaching these groups with the vaccination. Infants born of mothers who are hepatitis B surface antigen positive frequently become carriers of hepatitis B. This is another group targeted for immunization efforts by the year 2000.

To achieve the objectives related to immunization, the vaccine must be available. A year 2000 goal[14] related to this is to increase to at least 90% the proportion of public health departments that provide adult immunization for hepatitis B.

Hepatitis C and E. Prophylaxis for hepatitis C and E is not as effective as that for hepatitis B. For travelers to countries where hepatitis E occurs in endemic proportions, preventive health teaching is the best prophylactic measure. The value of immunoglobulin in this situation is unknown.[1] For postexposure prophylaxis in persons exposed through breaks in the skin to blood from a patient with hepatitis C, immunoglobulin may be given, but its value is uncertain.[1]

Hepatitis D. Hepatitis D requires the presence of hepatitis B virus; thus the preexposure and postexposure prophylaxes that are recommended for hepatitis B should suffice to prevent hepatitis D.[1] Currently there is no prophylaxis for preventing hepatitis D infection in HBV carriers except health teaching.

Pathophysiology

Viral hepatitis causes diffuse inflammatory infiltration of hepatic tissue. With typical acute viral hepatitis, there is no collapse of lobules, no loss of lobular architecture, and minimal or no fibrosis. Inflammation, degeneration, and regeneration may occur simultaneously, distorting the normal lobular pattern and possibly creating pressure about the portal vein. Laboratory findings include elevations in serum levels of transaminases (ALT and AST), prothrombin time, alkaline phosphatase, and bilirubin. Symptoms may vary in severity; many patients have very mild symptoms and do not have jaundice. Because the pathologic process is usually distributed evenly throughout the liver, biopsy in most cases is diagnostic for viral hepatitis.

In most instances of nonfatal viral hepatitis, regeneration begins almost with the onset of the disease. The damaged cells are removed by phagocytosis and enzymatic reaction, and the liver returns to normal.

The outcome of viral hepatitis may be affected by such factors as the following:

1. Virulence of the virus
2. Amount of hepatic damage sustained before exposure to the virus
3. Natural barriers to damage and disease of the liver
4. Supportive care the patient receives when symptoms appear

The majority of patients recover normal liver function, but the disease may take several courses; different terms describe each of these courses (Box 30-4).

30-4	**Atypical courses of hepatitis**	
	Submassive hepatic necrosis	Destruction of substantial group of adjacent cells but without destruction of the greater part of a lobule; most patients recover
	Massive hepatic necrosis	Destruction of whole lobule; most patients recover
	Fulminant viral hepatitis	Sudden and severe degeneration of the liver resulting in hepatic failure
	Subacute fatal viral hepatitis	Severe but slower degeneration of the liver

Table 30-8 **Serologic tests for hepatitis antigens and antibodies**

Test*	Definitions	Hepatitis A virus (HAV)	Hepatitis B virus (HBV)	Hepatitis C
HAV-Ab/IgM	Immunoglobulin (M class) against hepatitis A virus	Positive test, develops early in the disease, 4 weeks after infection	Not positive	Not positive
HB$_s$Ag	Hepatitis B surface antigen	Not positive	Positive test, develops about 3 weeks after infection; it is also positive in chronic infections with HBV and in carrier states	Not positive
HB$_e$Ag	Hepatitis B e antigen	Not positive	Develops about 3 weeks before onset of symptoms; usually clears in 1 month	Not positive
HB$_c$Ab	Antibody against hepatitis B core antigen	Not positive	Develops shortly after core antigens appear; positive in acute and chronic infections; indicated low infectivity	Not positive
HB$_e$Ab	Antibody against hepatitis B e antigen	Not positive	Develops about 4 weeks before onset of jaundice; may be persistently present in chronic infections	Not positive
HB$_s$Ab	Antibody against hepatitis B surface antigen	Not positive	Develops about 3-4 months after onset of symptoms; reflects clinical recovery and immunity	Not positive
Anti-HCV	Antibody against hepatitis C virus	Not positive	Not positive	Positive test develops about 18 weeks after exposure but sometimes not for 12 months

*Ab, antibodies; Ag, antigens; s, surface marker (viral coating); c, core viral material (Dane particle); e, envelope.

REVIEW

Table 30-9 **Focal disorders of the liver**

Disorder	Signs and symptoms	Therapy
Liver abscess	Fever, chills Vague abdominal discomfort, tenderness over liver, palpable liver Jaundice, leukocytosis ↑ Serum alkaline phosphatase ↑ ALT, AST	Surgical incision and drainage and broad-spectrum antimicrobial therapy for pyogenic abscess Amebic abscess: emetine hydrochloride, chloroquine, metronidazole (Flagyl)
Trauma to liver	Variable signs: pain, shock, abdominal rigidity Blood or bile with peritoneal tap	Drainage Suture and drainage Resection Blood volume management Antimicrobial therapy
Carcinoma of liver	Weight loss, weakness Jaundice, anemia Ascites, edema Upper right quadrant pain, hepatomegaly Unexplained fever Elevated liver enzymes (ALT, AST) Elevated sedimentation rate Elevated AFP	Surgical excision Chemotherapy: methotrexate, 5-fluorouracil, doxorubicin (Adriamycin), mitomycin C; often administered by hepatic artery perfusion Homotransplantation Decompression of biliary tract Palliative radiation

Signs and symptoms of the various types of viral hepatitis are not clinically distinctive from each other except that acute symptoms may be more severe in hepatitis A. Serologic tests are used to validate the type of viral hepatitis (see Tables 30-7 and 30-8). Symptoms appear before jaundice is apparent. Anorexia is one of the most frequent symptoms. This preicteric stage lasts for approximately 1 week and then subsides as hepatocellular jaundice occurs.

The icteric stage usually reaches its intensity in 2 weeks and may last from 4 to 6 weeks. The *posticteric* or convalescent stage begins with the disappearance of jaundice and may last from a few weeks to several months. Complete recovery is usually expected in 6 months. The disease may relapse during the posticteric stage, with recurrence of previous symptoms but to a milder degree. See Table 30-5 for a summary of the signs and symptoms of viral hepatitis and an overview of the medical therapy.

Chronic Hepatitis

If hepatitis lasts 6 months, it is classified as chronic hepatitis. Viral hepatitis is only one cause, but it is the most common etiology of chronic hepatitis (drugs, toxins, metabolic liver disease, and autoimmune processes are other causes).

Chronic viral hepatitis

Chronic viral hepatitis is not seen with hepatitis A. *Chronic active hepatitis* is the most serious form of chronic hepatitis. Twenty percent of cases follow HBV infection. There is extension of the necrosis with loss of normal structure and function. Very frequently the disease progresses to cirrhosis. If left untreated, most patients will die within 4 to 5 years; about 75% respond well to cortocosteroid treatment.

Chronic persistent hepatitis and *chronic lobular hepatitis* are characterized by abnormal liver function tests, fatigue, and hepatomegaly for greater than 6 months, but there is no necrosis and no increase in mortality.

FOCAL HEPATOCELLULAR DISORDERS

The three most common focal disorders of the liver, their etiologies, signs and symptoms, and medical therapies are listed in Table 30-9. Each disorder will be discussed briefly.

LIVER ABSCESS
Etiology/Epidemiology

Liver abscesses may result from a variety of organisms, including *Echerichia coli*, *Staphylococcus*, *Streptococcus*, *Pseudomonas*, *Proteus*, and *Klebsiella*. In patients with depressed immune functioning, such as those with neutropenia or leukemia, systemic candidiases with multiple hepatic abscesses have been found. Many persons with abscesses have multiple bacteria involved.[44] *Entamoeba histolytica* is an important worldwide cause of amebic liver abscess and dysentery. It most frequently is found in tropical and subtropical regions, but it is also found in temperate zones and in many parts of the United States.

Pathophysiology

Pyogenic abscesses can occur as either a singular large abscess or multiple small and/or microscopic abscesses. Amebic liver abscesses are typically large and singular.

Liver abscesses are usually a secondary site of infection. Pyogenic organisms originating in various areas of the body reach the liver through the biliary, vascular, or lymphatic systems. In addition, pyogenic organisms may be introduced by penetrating injuries to the liver or by direct contiguous extension. In amebic abscesses, the vegetative form of the organism moves from the gut to the small portal vessels and into the hepatic tissue, where it becomes activated and causes tissue destruction and abscess formation.

The abscess formation may disrupt hepatic function, but most of the altered physiologic functioning is caused by the presence of an acute infective process. If liver abscesses are not identified, they continue to increase in size and can perforate into the pleural cavity, the peritoneal cavity, or the pericardial cavity. The clinical manifestations of liver abscess are often nonspecific and are related to the infectious process. Patients present with tenderness of the right upper quadrant, hepatomegaly, and persistent fever; 20% to 40% show pleural involvement (effusion, pain on breathing, cough, crackles). The mortality rate for untreated liver abscess is 100%. Complications include sepsis, peritonitis from rupture of abscess, and respiratory complications (emboli, infection). See Table 30-9 for a summary of signs and symptoms of liver abscesses and the proposed medical therapy.

TRAUMA TO THE LIVER
Etiology/Epidemiology

Because of its location and size, the liver is frequently subjected to trauma, which may be either penetrating (gunshot wounds, stab wounds) or blunt (collision with steering wheel during automobile accidents, falls). If the injury is severe, rupture of the liver may occur with severe internal hemorrhage.

Pathophysiology

The pathophysiology seen varies with the types of injury. Liver injuries are graded on a scale of one to five.[37] In grade one there is laceration and capsular tear with minimal damage to the parenchyma. In grades two through five there is increasing parenchymal damage with fracture of the liver. In grade five, the damage extends into the retrohepatic vasculature. The liver is a highly vascular organ, and severe hemorrhage that results in hypovolemic shock may occur. Stab wounds often make a relatively superficial incision and may do no more damage than a needle biopsy of the liver. Gunshot wounds and blunt trauma often result in significant hemorrhage that results in hypotension or shock and leakage of bile from the biliary canaliculi. Hypovolemic shock may occur. If the peritoneal cavity has been contaminated by blood or bile, *peritonitis* (abdominal tenderness, rebound tenderness, muscle rigidity or spasm, decreased bowel sounds, increased white blood cell level, and fever) occurs. Less severe blunt trauma may result in subcapsular hematoma only.

Late complications of liver trauma may include the following:

1. Severe hemorrhage, resulting from disseminated intravascular coagulation that often accompanies shock during the total course of treatment
2. Degeneration and sloughing of segments of the liver that have had disruption in circulation with resultant hemorrhage.
3. Intrahepatic abscess formation
4. Traumatic hepatic cyst formation
5. Infections of other areas of the body following hepatic trauma
6. Subphrenic abscess formation
7. Biliary fistulas

The mortality rate for liver trauma has decreased over the years. The mortality rate depends on type of injury (highest for blunt trauma because of the larger portion of liver damaged and because of other associated injuries), severity of the injury (highest for those requiring resection of a large amount of liver), and the presence of associated injuries (increasing mortality with each additional injury to another organ). See Table 30-9 for an overview of signs and symptoms of and medical therapy for trauma of the liver.

TUMORS OF THE LIVER

Etiology/Epidemiology

Tumors of the liver may be either malignant or benign. Benign lesions include hemangiomas, cysts, and, rarely, adenomas. These benign tumors occasionally enlarge enough to become symptomatic and present problems in differentiation from a malignant tumor. Malignant tumors may be metastatic or primary. *Metastatic tumors* are common; they occur 20 times more frequently than primary tumors and rank second to cirrhosis as a cause of fatal liver disease.

Primary hepatic carcinomas may arise within the liver (hepatocellular) or the bile duct cell (cholangiocellular) or may be of mixed origin. Hepatocellular tumors are the most common, but primary liver cancer accounts for only 1% to 2% of malignant tumors found at death in the United States. They are more common in men and usually occur in the fifth and sixth decades of life.

Pathophysiology

The liver most commonly receives metastatic cells from tumors in the gastrointestinal tract, the lungs, the breast, the kidney, and melanomas of the skin. See Table 30-9 for common signs and symptoms of metastatic lesions of the liver. Metastatic carcinoma of the liver varies from a few small nodules to large nodes. Adjacent nodes may eventually grow together and compress the surrounding liver tissue. Usually different parts of the liver are uniformly involved so that liver biopsy may be a useful diagnostic aid.

Primary lesions may be multiple or singular, diffuse or nodular, and may spread to only a lobe or to the entire liver. The cancerous cells appear to compress the surrounding normal liver cells and to spread quickly by invading the portal vein branches. Spread may be by direct extension to surrounding tissue. Primary cancers also tend

to cause hemorrhage and necrosis. The most common site for metastasis of the primary liver lesion is the lung, but it may metastasize elsewhere. Primary lesions tend to grow rapidly, sometimes without signs or symptoms, and the patient may live only a short time after onset.

Jaundice and ascites are signs that the metastatic or primary process is quite far advanced. Extreme weakness is also usually an outstanding symptom. Ascites occurs secondary to compression of the portal vein. Gastrointestinal bleeding may also be present and may confuse the diagnosis. A special blood test that may be used to help diagnose primary liver carcinoma is a high serum concentration of alpha-fetoprotein (AFP). AFP in concentrations of 500 mg/ml is found in 70% of patients with hepatocellular cancer. (Lower levels may be found in patients with metastatic carcinoma or viral hepatitis.)

Nursing Process
Assessment
Subjective data

The patient's description of complaints or symptoms and course of illness yields useful data for the nurse who is planning care for the patient with hepatic disease. Among the potential symptoms, the following are explored:

1. Level of fatigue and amount of rest needed
2. Extent of pruritus and measures used to relieve it
3. Severity of anorexia; food intake patterns and likes and dislikes
4. Nausea or vomiting
5. History of edema or ascites
6. Changes noted in mood, alertness, and mental ability
7. Pain: onset, location, measures used to relieve it
8. Episodes of bleeding, lightheadedness, or syncope
9. Known allergies or toxic agents

When viral hepatitis is a potential medical diagnosis, the past history often contributes clues as to the time and type of contact (blood or sera, polluted water, food, shellfish, and so on). The past history is also vital in determining the injurious agent in toxic hepatitis. The patient's description of the course of illness in chronic hepatitis or cirrhosis can be helpful in giving the nurse insight into the patient's understanding of the disease, its prognosis, and whether the patient believes there is control over its progress.

When alcohol ingestion is a factor, data from the patient should include the patient's knowledge of the effect of the alcohol and the person's desire to abstain from drinking (see Chapter 13).

Objective data

A thorough physical assessment is required on admission to obtain data for baseline comparisons. There is a possibility that any of the manifestations listed in Box 30-5 will be present in a patient with a hepatic disease; in the patient with cirrhosis, these manifestations will be chronic in nature and subject to progressive worsening.

The patient with hepatic dysfunction can deteriorate rapidly, and many factors can depress hepatic function. It is helpful to have the same nurse responsible for the care of the patient and for documenting changes in mental functioning that can occur as hepatic dysfunction worsens (see Box 30-6).

30-5

Common manifestations of liver disease

Ascites and edema
Bleeding tendencies
Esophageal varices with gastrointestinal bleeding
Malnutrition
Jaundice
Portal-systemic encephalopathy (hepatic coma)

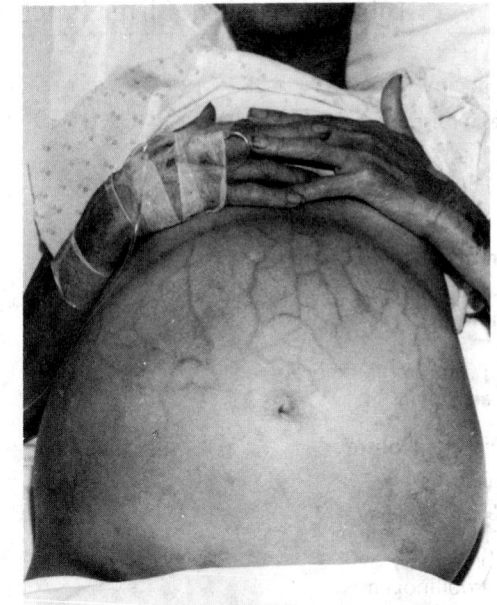

30-6

Parameters of mental functioning

Attention span
Ability to concentrate
Presence of irritability, apathy, or restlessness
Writing patterns
Speech patterns
Level of consciousness

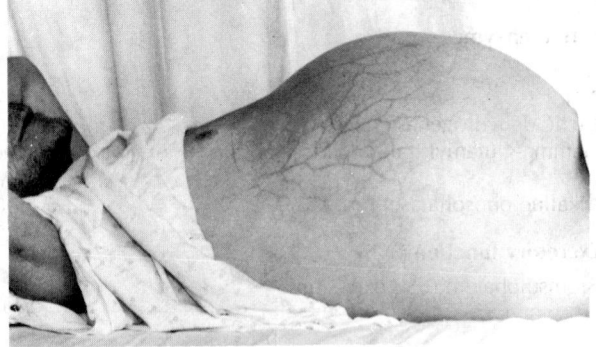

Fig. 30-9   Massive ascites. Note bulging flanks, dilated upper abdominal veins, and everted umbilicus. (From Prior JA, Silberstein JS, Stang JM: *Physical diagnosis: the history and examination of the patient,* ed 6, St Louis, 1981, Mosby–Year Book.)

Asterixis (liver flap) is a characteristic sign elicited by asking the patient to dorsiflex the wrist while the arm is extended. The patient's hand has a peculiar flapping tremor. *Fetor hepaticus* is a sweet but fetid breath odor. Asterixis, fetor hepaticus, and decreasing consciousness indicate progressing portal-systemic encephalopathy.

Ascites and peripheral edema are monitored by daily measurements of the abdomen and extremities. All patients with abdominal wounds or bleeding tendencies are monitored for signs of internal hemorrhage (shock). The liver may be examined while the abdomen is examined. The abdomen is first observed for the following signs:

1. Striae caused by stretching of skin with ascites
2. Engorged veins caused by obstruction of portal flow
3. Abdominal distention caused by ascites

Auscultation of the abdomen for bowel sounds is done before percussion or palpation. Percussion is used to assess the size of the liver as well as for ascites.

Percussion is used to check for the presence of *shifting dullness.* Ascites causes dullness and bulging of flanks when the patient is supine (Fig. 30-9); tympany may be found centrally. If the patient is turned to the side, the bulging and dullness is shifted to the dependent side.

While the patient is lying supine, the abdomen can be examined for presence of a *fluid wave.*

The liver may also be palpated by deep palpation. The liver edge, if palpable, presents a firm, sharp, regular ridge with a smooth surface. It is considered abnormal when felt more than 1 cm below the costal margin.

When caring for the patient with hepatic disease, the nurse should make ongoing observations about each of the following:

1. Body weight
2. Vital signs
3. Intake and output
4. General appearance: muscle mass, nutritional status, color of skin and sclera
5. Mental status
6. Breath sounds and respiratory effort
7. Abdomen, including abdominal girth
8. Skin: color, presence of spider angiomas, bleeding sites, excoriations, palmar erythema
9. Extremities: edema
10. Color of urine and stools

Diagnostic tests

Multiple tests may be necessary to determine the extent and seriousness of hepatic disease. Some of the laboratory

Table 30-10   Laboratory tests of liver function with possible changes seen in hepatocellular disease

Test	Normal	Hepatocellular disease
Fat metabolism		
Serum total cholesterol	150-200 mg/dl	Decreased
Cholesterol ester	70%	Decreased
Serum phospholipids	150-380 mg/dl	Decreased
Protein metabolism		
Total serum protein	6-8 g/dl	May be normal
Albumin	3.2-4.5 g/dl	Decreased
BUN	10-20 mg/dl	Varies
Serum prothrombin time	12-15 sec	Increased
Blood ammonia	< 75 µg/dl	Increased
Bilirubin metabolism		
Total bilirubin	0.1-1.0 mg/dl	Increased
Conjugated (direct)	0.1-0.3 mg/dl	Increased
Unconjugated (indirect)	0.2-0.8 mg/dl	Increased
Urine bilirubin	None	Increased
Urine urobilinogen	0.1-1.0 Ehrlich U/dl	Increased
Fecal urobilinogen	90-280 mg/day	Varies
Serum enzymes		
ALT	5-35 IU/L	Increased (nonspecific)
AST	5-40 IU/L	Increased
Lactic dehydrogenase (LDH)	90-200 IU/L	Increased (nonspecific)
Gamma-glutamyl transpeptidase (GGT)	Men: 10-38 IU/L	Increased
	Women: 5-25 IU/L	
Alkaline phosphatase	30-85 IU/L	Increased (slightly)
Excretory function		
Bromsulphalein (BSP excretion)	< 5% retained after 45 min	Increased

tests are listed in Tables 30-10 and 30-11. Additional studies may include abdominal films, barium swallow and enema, and endoscopic examinations. The diagnostic workup will frequently include one or several tests for examination of the biliary tract (see Chapter 32).

Liver biopsy

Biopsy of the liver presents the risk of hemorrhage because of the vascularity of the liver and the bleeding tendencies that often occur with liver disease. The procedure may be open or closed. The open procedure is done in the operating room, and the usual preoperative procedure is required.

The closed procedure is often done at the patient's bedside. This procedure is contraindicated if the patient has an infection of the right lower lobe of the lung, ascites, or a blood dyscrasia, or is unable to cooperate by holding a breath. The procedure consists of inserting a specially designed needle through the chest or abdominal wall into the liver and removing a small piece of tissue for study. Movement by the patient may tear the liver covering. Although no physical preparation is necessary for a closed procedure, written consent is usually required, a current hematologic and coagulation profile should be available, and food and fluids may be withheld after midnight the night before. Importantly, the patient needs teaching, time to have questions answered, and support. (see Box 30-7).

30-7

Liver biopsy

Preprocedure
Explain procedure to patient
Explain need to hold breath during the procedure; help patient practice holding breath and maintaining a sustained exhalation
Report inability of patient to hold breath on command
Give vitamin K as prescribed

Postprocedure
Maintain bed rest for prescribed period (8 to 24 hours)
Turn patient on *right* side for first few hours with pillow placed under the right side for pressure on liver
Monitor patient
First hour
    Observe site for hemorrhage every 15 minutes
    Monitor vital signs every 15 minutes
    Up to 24 hours, take vital signs hourly
Report signs of hemorrhage (increased pulse, decreased blood pressure, cold clammy skin) and peritonitis (increased temperature, pain in abdomen)
Provide analgesics as prescribed for mild right upper quadrant or right shoulder pain

Table 30-11   Diagnostic tests used in hepatic diseases

Procedure	Preparation	Interpretation
Ultrasonic hepatography (liver ultrasound)	Preparation includes enema and/or laxatives and sometimes dietary preparation to decrease intestinal gas (low carbohydrate, no carbonated beverages); barium studies should be done after ultrasonic exams or 48 hours before	Use of sound waves to bombard liver and surrounding areas; images caused by differences in sounds reflected by solid tissue, air-filled cavities, and fluid-filled cavities; can help in determining focal or diffuse liver disease
Computerized axial tomography (CAT scan)	No preparation needed; patient must lie still Sometimes dye studies of the biliary system are done at the same time; barium studies should be done after CT scan	Use of CAT scan provides radiographic visualization of liver and surrounding structures; a computer handles the complex calculations used to analyze the multiple images of serial sections of tissue
Radioisotope scanning ^{131}I rose bengal ^{99}Tc colloidal technetium ^{67}Ga gallium citrate Risa^{131} radioionated serum albumin ^{198}Au colloidal gold ^{99}TC-HIDA	Injection of radioisotope A scintillosope detects, amplifies, and records radiation No preparation necessary except for ^{67}Ga, for which enema and laxatives will be ordered to prevent absorption by GI tract	The liver will be outlined by radioisotope scanning techniques to help identify tumors, cysts and abscesses (Fig. 30-10); hepatocellular abscesses and carcinomas show as areas of heavy radioactivity with ^{67}Ga; decreased areas of radioactivity usually are those of nonfunctioning tissue
Angiography (catheterization of hepatic artery, portal venous system vein)	Preparation includes fasting and obtaining written consent; check for previous reactions to contrast media	The contrast medium provides visualization of the vascular supply of the liver and presence of masses, bleeding, and collateral circulation
Wedged hepatic vein pressure (WHVP) and portal vein pressure	This test may be done with angiography	The degree of portal hypertension can be determined
Percutaneous transhepatic cholangiography	Preparation includes fasting (up to 8 hours); written consent is required; explain that tilting of table will occur and patient must be securely fastened on table; check for previous reactions to contrast media	The contrast medium is directly inserted into biliary ducts and allows visualization of the biliary tree

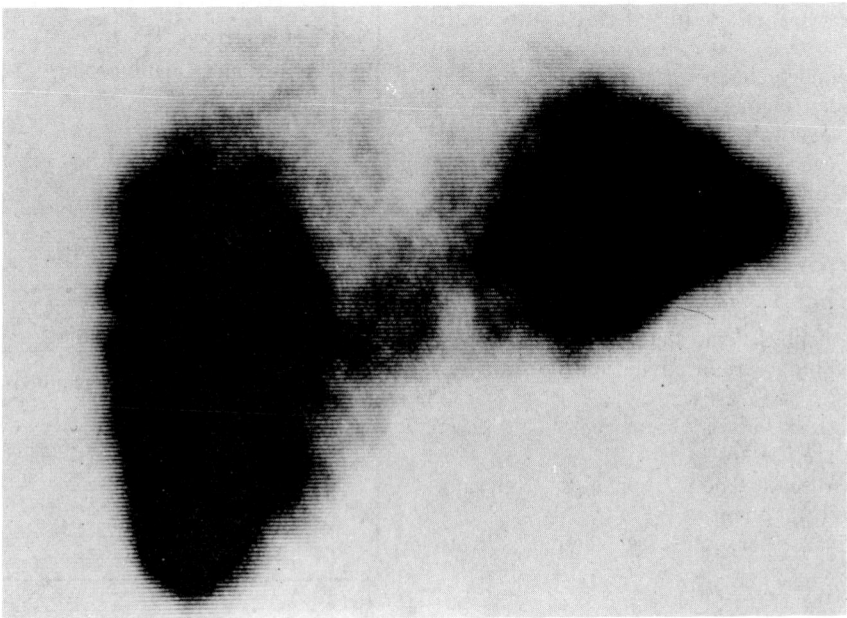

Fig. 30-10   Liver scan showing metastasis to liver (light area on right) of carcinoma of colon. (Courtesy Rejali AM, Department of Radiology, Case Western Reserve University, Cleveland.)

Data analysis: nursing diagnosis

Nursing diagnoses are determined from analysis of patient data. Possible nursing diagnoses for the person with diseases of the liver may include, but are not limited to, the following:

Diagnostic titles	Possible etiologies
Fatigue	Generalized weakness, imbalance between supply and demand of energy
Fluid volume excess or deficit	Compromised regulatory mechanisms, inappropriate fluid and sodium intake
Infection, high risk for	Decreased immune response, pruritus, skin lacerations, intrusive procedures, inadequate measures to prevent transmission of infection
Injury: high risk for: falls	Sensory/perceptual deficits, tremors, weakness, impaired cognition
Cardiac output, decreased (potential)	Potential for hemorrhage, potential for fluid deficit in response to diuretic therapy
Nutrition, altered: less than body requirements	Anorexia, inadequate intake, increased metabolic needs
Pain	Jaundice and pruritus, ascites
Breathing pattern, ineffective	Ascites, coma
Knowledge deficit: diagnostic tests, treatment, home care, follow-up care	Lack of exposure, potential cognitive limitations
Health maintenance, altered	Inability to make appropriate judgments because of alcoholism

Planning: expected patient outcomes

Expected patient outcomes for the person with hepatic dysfunction may include, but are not limited to, the following:

1. Demonstrates an increase in self-care ability each day.
2. Develops no undetected oliguria; does not exceed 1 kg loss of body weight per day.
3. Develops no new infections; temperature remains at a normal level.
4. Does not fall or suffer any injury.
5. Does not develop undetected bleeding and/or hypotension.
6. Eats diet high in calories and carbohydrates, with adequate vitamins, minerals, and protein as appropriate for pathophysiologic state.
7. States that itching is reduced and has no skin lacerations.
8. Normal breath sounds and a normal chest x-ray examination are present.
9. Explains the disorder and relationships to relevant symptoms and treatment.
10. Describes plans for self-care (activity, rest, sleep)
11. Gives detailed description about ways to manage diuretic therapy, water restriction, diet prescription, and avoidance of alcohol.
12. Describes signs and symptoms to report to physician.
13. If alcohol abuse is a problem, is able to make conscious decision about the use of services such as Alcoholics Anonymous.

Implementation

The patient with hepatic disease should be considered to have multisystem disorders and to be at risk for fluid and electrolyte imbalances, infection, alteration in mental status, and hemorrhage. Thus, regardless of the specific medical or nursing diagnoses or severity of distress, the nurse should institute a monitoring schedule that ensures early detection of at least those clinical findings listed in Box 30-8.

The frequency of monitoring depends on the current status of the patient, the medical and nursing diagnoses, and the estimation of risk. For example, the patient who is actively bleeding from liver trauma or esophageal varices requires continuous monitoring in an intensive care unit. In contrast, the patient who has bleeding tendencies because of a mild increase in prothrombin time may be monitored by routine vital signs, daily *guaiac* tests for occult blood in the stool, and daily prothrombin time, partial

---

30-8 | **Priorities in monitoring schedule**

Fluid and electrolyte problems
Ascites
Edema
Oliguria
Hypotension

Hemorrhage
Gastrointestinal bleeding
Hypotension
Tachycardia

Infection
Fever
Tachycardia
Abnormal breath sounds
Chills
Malaise
Cloudiness of body fluids

Portal-systemic encephalopathy
Mental status impairment
Change in sleep pattern, mood, behavior, perceptual ability
Lethargy
Slurred speech
Incoordination

thromboplastin time, and hematocrit. Institution of new therapeutic agents, a change in therapy (dosage of medication, amount of food, or fluid intake), or the onset of complications necessitates review of the monitoring plan to assess its adequacy.

Assisting with achievement of therapeutic goals

Rest, nutrition, and absence of toxin use are principal treatments for patients with hepatic disorders. Before the nurses' role in implementing these treatments is discussed, this section will discuss other treatments for specific hepatic lesions or dysfunctions.

Medications

The drugs to be described are antimicrobial and chemotherapeutic agents. Diuretics and drugs used to treat bleeding and PSE will be discussed later.

Antimicrobials. The nurse will be involved in the administration of antimicrobials to patients with bacterial infections of the liver (liver abscess, wound infections). The specific antibiotic therapy is based on culture and sensitivity studies of material obtained by percutaneous or surgical aspirations of the abscess or on studies of wound drainage. Blood cultures are usually done to determine if septicemia is present. Anaerobic organisms alone or in combination with aerobic organisms account for 50% of liver abscesses; common organisms are *Escherichia coli*, *Klebsiella*, and *Staphylococcus aureus*. Appropriate broad-spectrum antibiotics may be administered for 4 to 6 weeks to a patient with pyogenic liver abscess. Surgical drainage of the abscess is also frequently necessary. See Chapter 17 for details about administration of antibiotics.

Because patients with liver dysfunction may be immunosuppressed, they are subject to a variety of infections including superinfections and nosocomial infections. Therefore, the nurse may be involved in the administration of antibiotics to patients with liver disease who have infections of the urinary tract, pneumonia, peritonitis, or other infections. There is no antimicrobial therapy for hepatitis. The patient with amebic abscess is treated with amebicidal agents (see Table 30-9). Usually surgery is not done. Medication therapy must be prolonged; for example, metronidazole (Flagyl), 750 mg, might be ordered orally, three times a day for 5 to 10 days followed by diiochohydroxyquin (Diodoquin), 650 mg, three times a day for 20 days. Intravenous administration of metronidazole may also be used. Reconstituted vials of this medication should not be refrigerated and should be used within 96 hours. This drug may cause urine to have a reddish-brown color and gastrointestinal distress (nausea, diarrhea, abdominal cramps, and dizziness). A psychotic episode may be precipitated if metronidazole is combined with alcohol intake or disulfiram.

Chemotherapy. Chemotherapy is used to induce regression of primary and metastatic lesions of the liver; it also may be part of other therapy such as radiation or surgery.

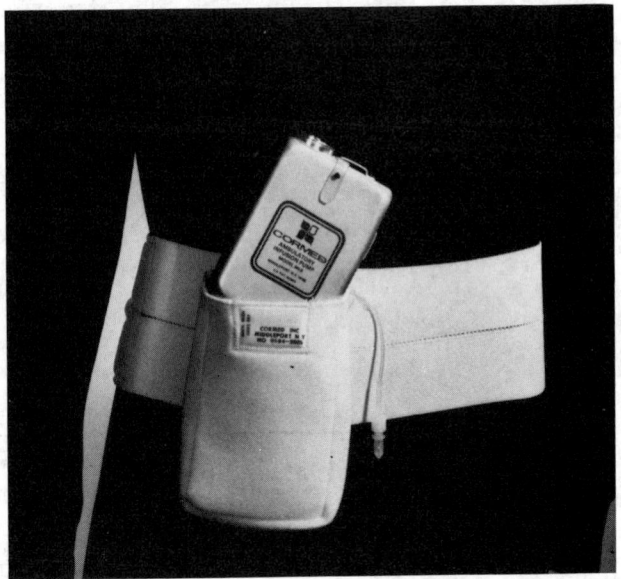

Fig. 30-11 Lightweight, battery-operated infusion pump for ambulatory patient. Flow rate is adjustable. Power pack operates for 7 days before needing recharging. (Courtesy CORMED, Inc, Middleport, NY.)

5-Fluorouracil (5-FU) and doxorubicin (Adriamycin) have been used as single-drug therapy. Combination chemotherapy with 5-FU and 1,3 bis-2 chloroethyl-1-nitrosurea (BCNU), methyl CCNU, or streptozotocin have also been tried. Chemotherapeutic agents have been given intravenously or by infusion into the hepatic artery.

Hepatic arterial infusion can be accomplished by one of two methods. In the first method, a percutaneous catheter is inserted into the hepatic artery using fluoroscopy. The catheter is attached to an external infusion pump (Fig. 30-11) that is filled with the appropriate chemotherapeutic agent and programmed to deliver the agent over a desired period of time. The catheter is removed after each drug treatment cycle. In the second method, a catheter is surgically inserted into the hepatic artery and connected to an implanted infusion pump (see Fig. 30-12). Characteristics of the infusaid pump (an internal pump) are described in Box 30-9.

The implanted pump can be filled with the correct amount of drug and programmed to deliver the chemotherapeutic agent over a desired time interval and at a desired dosage. In chemotherapy-free intervals the pump is filled with a heparin solution, so that patency of the hepatic artery catheter is maintained. Depending on flow rates and drug schedule, the chamber is refilled at various intervals that are scheduled so that the chamber never empties completely.

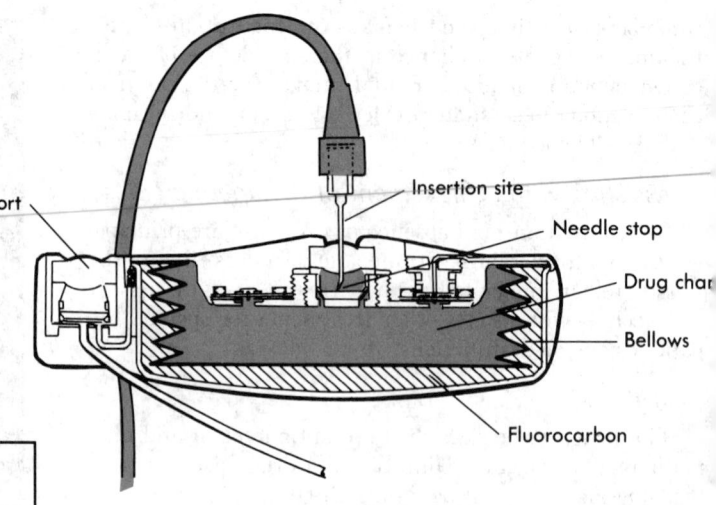

Fig. 30-12 Infusaid pump.

30-9

Characteristics of Infusaid pump

1. The pump has two chambers: one for the drug solution and one that contains a fluorocarbon.
2. The two chambers are separated by a flexible metal bellows.
3. The drug reservoir has a capacity of approximately 50 ml (model 400) and is refilled every 2 weeks by percutaneous injection into a special insertion site.
4. The fluorocarbon is temperature sensitive and converts from a liquid to vapor at body temperature.
5. The vapor exerts pressure on the bellows, forcing the drug solution from its reservoir into the catheter at a constant preset rate; typically 2 to 3 ml/day of solution is delivered.
6. *Drug dosage* is controlled by manipulating the concentration of the chemotherapeutic agent.
7. The fluorocarbon vapor is reliquefied as the drug chamber is refilled; vaporization again occurs, and the next dose is delivered.

Instructions regarding self-care for patients with implanted pumps

1. Avoid deep-sea diving or mountain climbing. These activities change atmospheric pressure and can change vaporization of the fluorocarbon and thus the delivery rate.
2. Monitor body temperature daily, and report elevations immediately.
3. Avoid long hot baths, saunas, and spas. These can change the flow rate.
4. Avoid contact sports because they can damage the pump.
5. Wear a Medic Alert bracelet or necklace that states that you have an implantable pump and give information such as physician's name.
6. Return for follow-up care as prescribed—usually every 2 weeks.
7. Contact nurse/physician/outpatient department any time questions arise.
8. Individualized instructions concerning side effects of the specific chemotherapeutic agents that need to be monitored for and reported need to be emphasized.

From Gullatte M, Foltz AT: Hepatic chemotherapy via implantable pump, *Am J Nurs* 83:1674-1678, 1983.

The implanted infusion pump allows the patient to be treated at home. The patient comes into an outpatient site at prescribed times for addition of drugs or heparin solution and a recheck of pump flow rate. The patient will need physical care before and after surgery similar to that of any patient having surgery (Chapters 20 to 22). Instructions regarding self-care and needs related to the chemotherapeutic agent being used (see Chapter 11 and a pharmacology text) are also needed. The nurse will also be involved in refilling the pump at the prescribed intervals.

Reduction of edema and ascites

Edema and ascites are typically found in patients with cirrhosis; however, they may occur in any patient whose hepatic dysfunction results in (1) hypoalbuminemia; (2) dilutional hyponatremia; and (3) portal hypertension. Under these circumstances, diuresis occurs slowly and is more difficult to accomplish than it would be in a patient with a normal serum colloidal osmotic pressure, a normal serum sodium-to-water ratio, and relatively similar hydrostatic pressures in portal and systemic venous circulations.

Sodium restriction and bed rest are usually the first approach to reducing edema. These measures and an adequate diet often result in a spontaneous diuresis that reflects improved hepatic function. The amount of sodium restriction may be based on 24-hour urinary excretion of sodium but is generally not less than 1 g daily. The lack of salt in food makes it less palatable, and the patient may not consume adequate protein and calories. Inadequate intake is reported to the physician and dietitian because adjustments may need to be made in sodium restriction. Salt substitutes may be permitted.

patient treated with spironolactone. The nurse should monitor the patient's potassium level and be alert for signs of potassium imbalance (see Chapter 7). Magnesium levels also need to be monitored carefully. Magnesium may be low because of a poor nutritional history, and diuretics will worsen the loss of magnesium. However, if hepatorenal failure is present, both potassium and magnesium may be high.

Infusions of salt-poor albumin in 25-g units may be given to increase the effectiveness of diuretic measures. These infusions expand the blood volume, thus increasing renal blood flow and serum osmotic pressure. They may also decrease the risk of oliguria, azotemia, and encephalopathy. The effects are short term and protein loss into the ascitic fluid continues. Albumin is very viscous and must be infused with a large-bore needle, such as a No. 18. It is often used to improve the patient status during acute crises or to prepare the patient for surgery. The administration of salt-poor albumin may expand the blood volume rapidly. During and following administration, the patient is monitored carefully for signs of pulmonary edema.

Paracentesis. A peritoneal tap may be done to obtain fluid for laboratory study but paracentesis places the patient at risk for complications such as shock, hypovolemia, azotemia, encephalopathy, and infection. Although once a standard mode of therapy, paracentesis is now used with caution and usually only as a last resort in patients with severe and chronic liver disease.

If the abdomen is taut with fluid and is producing dyspnea and anorexia, paracentesis may be necessary. In general, only enough fluid to relieve symptoms is removed; this decreases the risk of rapid fluid shifts and additional protein loss. One liter of ascitic fluid contains as much protein as 200 ml of whole blood. Salt-poor human albumin may be administered following this procedure to counteract the shift of fluid and protein into the peritoneal cavity. When paracentesis is done, the patient must be monitored for signs and symptoms of all complications. Monitoring would include blood pressure, pulse, temperature, skin color and temperature, urine output, mental status, and abdomen (for signs of peritonitis).

Peritoneal venous shunt. In chronic and resistant ascites caused by cirrhosis, a LeVeen or Denver peritoneal venous shunt may be used. The shunt allows for the continuous reinfusion of ascitic fluid back into the venous system through a silicone catheter with a one-way pressure sensitive valve. One end of the catheter is implanted in the peritoneal cavity, and the tube is channeled through subcutaneous tissue to the superior vena cava where the other end is implanted. The valve opens when there is a pressure differential greater than 3 mm of water between the abdominal cavity and the thoracic vein, allowing fluid to move from the peritoneal cavity into the superior vena cava.

Persons treated with a shunt may also receive furosemide therapy, and the two together have been successful in relieving ascites in some patients. Persons who have a shunt may still have severe problems, including disseminated intravascular coagulation, bleeding varices, and congestive failure.[5]

30-10

Assessment for patients with edema or ascites

Daily weights
Intake and output
Measurement of abdominal girth
Blood pressure
Mental status
Serum electrolytes

A second intervention that may be used, if hyponatremia is present, is fluid restriction. Fluids may be restricted to as little as 500 ml/day and will usually not exceed 1500 ml/day. The fluid restriction may affect the patient's food intake. The patient is encouraged to assist in planning the distribution of fluid intake. It is not unusual for fluid and sodium to be restricted and bed rest continued when diuretic therapy is ordered.

Nursing assessments to monitor fluid and electrolyte balance in patients with edema or ascites are listed in Box 30-10. These assessment measures enable the nurse to detect the onset of hypokalemia, oliguria, azotemia, and PSE (all of which are complications of diuresis in patients with hepatic dysfunction and are related to excessive fluid and potassium losses).

Ascites cannot be mobilized at rates greater than 900 ml/day (approximately 2 lb/day of weight loss).[36] Hypovolemia can occur if amounts greater than this are diuresed (unless peripheral edema is contributing the additional fluid). Azotemia and oliguria result from decreased renal perfusion in hypovolemic states. PSE may be precipitated by azotemia, hypovolemia, and hypokalemia.

Diuretic therapy. Furosemide (Lasix) alone or with spironolactone (Aldactone) is commonly used to promote diuresis in persons with hepatic dysfunction who do not respond to sodium restriction and bedrest. Spironolactone provides the benefit of retention of potassium along with the excretion of sodium.

Potassium supplements are often prescribed along with the furosemide and, at times, may be necessary for the

30-11

Assessment for bleeding

Check the following for blood:
  Urine, stool, vomitus, or gastrointestinal drainage
Assess the following for bleeding:
  Mouth
  Wounds
  Skin (for purpura, hematoma, or petechiae)
Monitor vital signs for the following:
  Hypotension
  Postural hypotension
  Tachycardia
Monitor results of the following:
  Prothrombin or partial thromboplastin times
  Platelet count
  Hematocrit level in concert with assessment of sodium and fluid status

30-12

Measures to minimize bleeding

1. Arrange with the laboratory to minimize number of venipunctures.
2. Start IV infusions when blood samples are drawn.
3. Apply pressure for 5 minutes to sites of venipunctures or injections, for 10 minutes to sites of arterial puncture.
4. Suggest patient use a soft toothbrush or cotton swab for brushing of teeth to prevent bleeding gums.
5. Serve the patient with esophageal varices only soft foods (for example, bread rather than toast).
6. Avoid taking temperatures rectally, and use gentle pressure and well-lubricated enema tips if hemorrhoids are present.
7. If injection must be given, use the smallest-gauge needle possible.
8. Instruct patient not to strain at stool and to avoid vigorous coughing or blowing of the nose.
9. Avoid clutter in patient's room and give adequate assistance in ambulating to prevent falls.

A modification of the original LeVeen peritoneal venous shunt, the Denver shunt, is sometimes used when ascites is marked and is the result of malignancy. Malignant ascites may contain a lot of particulate matter that can stop the flow of ascitic fluid through the tubing. The Denver shunt has a subcutaneous pump that can be compressed manually to irrigate the tubing. Increased comfort and improvement of renal and respiratory function have been reported.[48]

When shunts are first implanted and functioning, there can be dramatic changes such as hemodilution of intravascular fluid, decreased abdominal girth, and increased renal output. The rapid addition of ascitic fluid back to the vascular compartment can result in fluid overload with signs and symptoms of pulmonary edema. As peritoneal fluid is removed, less of a pressure gradient exists between the peritoneal fluid and the jugular vein. To force the valve open, deep breathing is encouraged at regular intervals with the patient in the supine position.

Control of bleeding

Bleeding tendencies or actual hemorrhage is common in patients with hepatic disorders. See p. 878 for the specific factors that may decrease coagulation ability in hepatocellular or biliary tract disease. Also, see p. 883 for the reason that dilated hemorrhoidal, gastric, and esophageal veins are frequent sites of bleeding when portal hypertension is present.

Gastrointestinal bleeding is not uncommon in patients with jaundice and/or portal hypertension. Patients with cirrhosis or recent alcohol intake may have bleeding from gastritis or peptic ulcers, as well as from hemorrhoidal or esophageal venous rupture.

Bleeding may also be prolonged in tissue injury and in surgical wounds. Assessment measures for bleeding and measures to minimize bleeding are presented in Boxes 30-11 and 30-12.

The nurse assists with specific medical therapies to improve the status of coagulation. A trial of vitamin K (usually daily for 3 days) may be ordered to determine whether the liver is able to manufacture prothrombin and other clotting factors when an adequate supply of vitamin K is given. Recall that shunting of blood around the liver or the absence of bile or bacteria in the intestine reduces the supply of vitamin K available to the liver. Vitamin K will not help if hepatic cell damage is the cause of reduced prothrombin formation. If this is the case, whole blood or plasma may be given to replace clotting factors at least temporarily. If the patient has a reduced platelet level, platelet transfusions may be given.

Table 30-5 lists some of the treatment measures used with bleeding esophageal varices. This hemorrhage is often massive and life-threatening; mortality rates are 30% to 60%.

Shunts and nonshunting operations

The first priority in the management of bleeding is to establish the source of bleeding. After diagnosis the goal is to control bleeding and to replace the blood volume. Bleeding may be controlled with:

1. Gastric lavage (see Chapter 31 for discussion of this procedure)
2. Pharmacologic therapy
3. Injection sclerotherapy
4. Balloon tamponade of varices
5. Endoscopic esophageal varix ligation (banding)
6. Surgery: shunts and nonshunting operations

Pharmacologic therapy. Vasopressin (Pitressin) is usually given intravenously (may be given into the mesenteric artery) at a dose of 0.2 μ to 0.8 μ/minute on an intermittent basis or as a continuous infusion. It lowers portal pressure by causing splanchnic vasoconstriction and thus can stop or control esophageal bleeding. Side effects, which the nurse will monitor for and report immediately, include hypertension, bradycardia, abdominal cramping and pallor

Fig. 30-13   Sengstaken-Blakemor tube with esophageal and gastric balloons inflated. (Redrawn from *Rubber appliances in surgery and therapeutics,* Providence RI, Davol, Inc.)

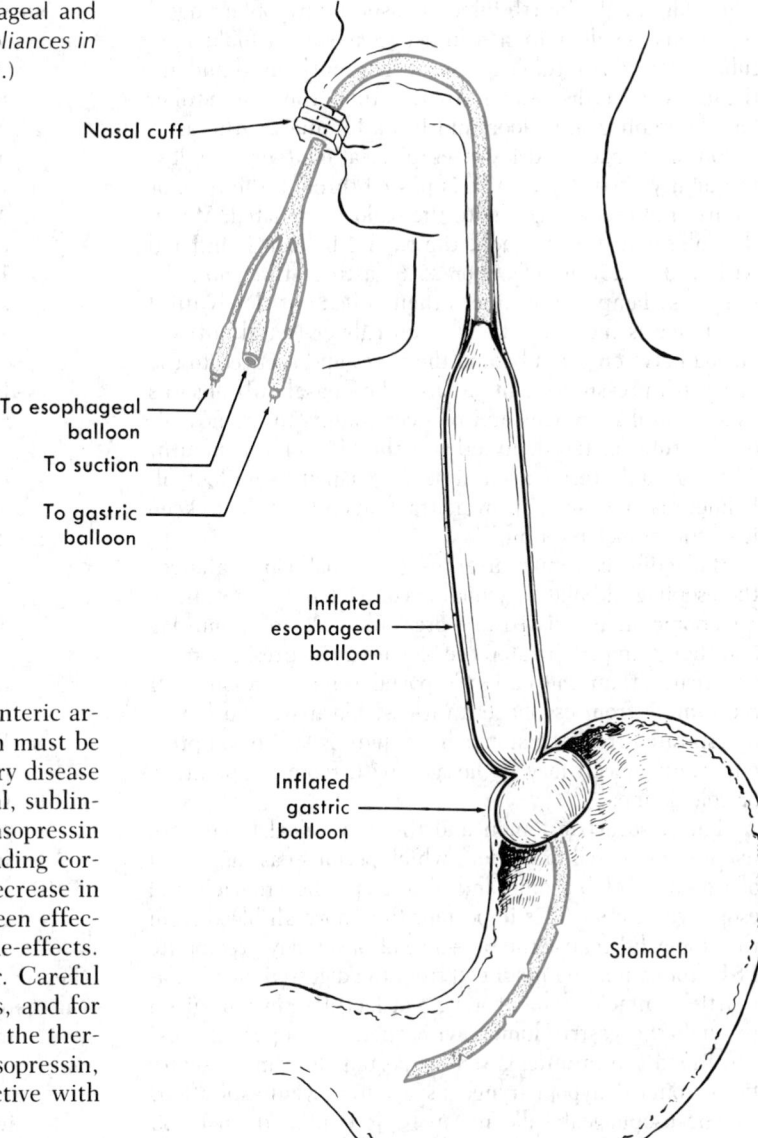

Coronary artery vasoconstriction as well as mesenteric artery vasoconstriction can occur; thus vasopressin must be used with caution in persons with coronary artery disease and in the elderly.[5,18] Nitroglycerine (transdermal, sublingual, or intravenous) has been combined with vasopressin to decrease the systemic vasoconstriction, including coronary vasoconstriction, while maintaining the decrease in portal pressure. The combination therapy has been effective in controlling bleeding while decreasing side-effects. With vasopressin water retention can also occur. Careful monitoring of blood pressure, pulse, fluid status, and for recurrence of bleeding must be carried out while the therapy is withdrawn. Glypressin, an analogue of vasopressin, given intravenously has been shown to be effective with fewer cardiac effects in preliminary studies.

Propranolol (Inderal), a beta-adrenergic blocking agent, has been shown to decrease esophageal bleeding in some patients, but not all studies support this finding.[5,18] Thus it is still used experimentally to treat variceal bleeding. Importantly, propanolol has been used to prevent the first episode of bleeding in persons with esophageal varices.[34a] Other drugs that have been used on limited numbers of patients include somatostatin, which reduces portal inflow and pressure, and other drugs (metoclopramide, clomperidone, and pentagastrin) that reduce blood flow in the azygos vessels and lowers varix pressure.

Injection sclerotherapy. For emergency treatment of varices and longer-term control or for control and prevention of rebleeding in patients who may not be candidates for surgery, injection sclerotherapy may be used. In this procedure a fiberoptic endoscope is introduced into the esophagus by the physician; and, once the bleeding site is identified, a sclerosing agent (sodium morrhuate, 5 ml) is injected into the varices. This agent causes thromboses and sclerosis of the vessel and should result in hemostasis in 3 to 5 minutes. If hemostasis does not occur, a second injection may be given. The procedure may be repeated as necessary and can be initiated while the patient is bleeding or as an elective procedure. Before the procedure the patient and significant others need an explanation of the procedure, and the patient should receive nothing by mouth for at least 6 hours. A mild sedative and a local anesthetic will be given. After the procedure the nurse will monitor the patient for complications (perforated esophagus, aspiration pneumonia, pleural effusion, and worsening of ascites). Respiratory support to ensure adequate air exchange must be provided. *Retrosternal pain* is often present and is treated with analgesics; fever is common for several days. The procedure has shown very favorable results in some patients.

Esophageal tamponade. The original Sengstaken-Blakemore tube is a three-lumen tube with two balloon attachments. One lumen serves as a nasogastric suction tube, the second is used to inflate the gastric balloon, and the third is used to inflate the esophageal balloon (Fig. 30-13).

The addition of a fourth lumen to aspirate hypopharyngeal secretions resulted in a 4-lumen Sengstaken-Blakemore tube.[6a] These two tubes are most frequently used and are the focus of this discussion. Another tube, the Linton tube, has no esophageal balloon and has a lumina for the aspiration of stomach and lower esophageal content; it is less frequently used.[6a] The tube is passed through the nose or mouth into the stomach with the balloons deflated. When the tube is in the stomach, the gastric balloon is inflated with 150 to 250 ml of air or 25% gastrograffin[6a] and the lumen is clamped; the tube is then pulled out slowly until resistance is met. A cube of foam rubber (nasal cuff) is placed between the tube and the nares and secured to the face with pressure-sensitive tape. The nasal cuff absorbs excess nasal secretions and reduces trauma to the nostril, or the tube is taped directly to the side of the mouth. Although only rarely used, a device shaped like a football helmet may be used to provide traction on the tube to keep it in the proper position.

If bleeding continues after the gastric balloon is inflated, the esophageal balloon, which is connected by a Y tube to a manometer, is inflated to a pressure of 30 to 40 mm Hg and then clamped. To stop the bleeding, the pressure must be greater than the patient's portal venous pressure. If bleeding is from esophageal varices, blood will no longer be aspirated from the stomach. If there is still blood present, the stomach may be lavaged with room temperature or cold saline.

The nasogastric lumen and the esophageal lumen are usually connected to suction, which permits easy appraisal of cessation of bleeding and also keeps the stomach and esophagus empty. It is important to remove all blood from the stomach because the presence of blood may precipitate PSE from ammonia produced from the digested blood. Cathartics, antacids, and neomycin or lactulose may be given through the gastric lumen with suction temporarily discontinued (20 minutes). It is important to remove secretions from the hypopharyngeal space to prevent aspiration.

The esophageal balloon can be left inflated up to 48 hours without tissue damage or severe discomfort. However, the esophageal balloon is usually deflated in approximately 12 hours to assess if bleeding has stopped. The fully inflated gastric balloon with or without traction exerted on it can compress the stomach wall between the balloon and the diaphragm causing ulceration of the gastric mucosa and severe discomfort. To offset the possibility of necrosis, the physician may release the traction and balloon pressures periodically.

The nurse must stay with the patient while balloons are deflated to secure the tube's position and to detect recurrence of bleeding. Intensive monitoring of the patency of the airway also is necessary when the balloons are inflated. *Asphyxiation* is a hazard if the inflated esophageal balloon moves into the upper airway. This can happen if the gastric balloon deflates or ruptures and the inflated esophageal balloon moves upward. If this happens, the esophageal balloon is deflated at once and the entire tube is removed. A scissors, which can be used to cut the tube and deflate balloons rapidly, must be at the bedside.

The nurse will be assisting with therapeutic measures aimed at restoration of blood volume and coagulation factors and the prevention and treatment of PSE.

Nursing care of the patient with esophageal tamponade includes the following:

1. Explain procedure and provide continued support to patient during the procedure.
2. Monitor vital signs every 15 minutes until stable and then hourly and PRN.
3. Ensure that patient does not pull at the tube.
4. Measure and record pressure of esophageal balloon every hour; maintain pressure at prescribed level.
5. Provide mouth and nares care every 1 to 2 hours.
   a. If the patient is alert, provide with tissues, and encourage spitting of saliva into a tissue or basin.
   b. If the patient is alert, have the patient rinse mouth well to remove any old blood; a Water Pik under low pressure may be used.
   c. Gently suction mouth and throat if patient is not alert, which is usually the case.
   d. Keep nostrils clean and lubricated with water soluble jelly.
6. Maintain transfusions and infusions at prescribed rate.
7. If cooled solutions are used, report patient chilling to the physician who may then order a warming blanket.
8. Record intake and output; test gastrointestinal output for occult blood (guaiac).
9. Consult physician concerning permissible patient movement; passive range of motion is usually allowed.
10. Provide comfort measures (for example, rub back, change patient's position).

The nurse will be assisting with the following additional therapeutic measures when hemorrhage from esophageal varices is present:

1. Administering prescribed fresh whole blood and intravenous infusions; fresh blood avoids the increased ammonia and citrate of stored blood and has relatively more coagulation factors
2. Administering saline cathartics as prescribed through the nasogastric lumen of the Sengstaken-Blakemore tube or through a nasogastric tube to hasten expulsion of blood from the gastrointestinal tract and to prevent an increase in production of ammonia. Enemas may also be ordered to decrease gut content and bacterial action on the blood
3. Administering lactulose or neomycin to decrease effect of bacteria on digested blood in the intestine (ammonia production) in an effort to prevent portal systemic encephalopathy

Endoscopic esophageal varix ligation

Endoscopic esophageal varix ligation (EVL),[40a] also called banding, is based on the principles employed for elastic band ligation of internal hemorrhoids. In this procedure, use of a special endoscope allows direct placement of a rubber band (elastic rubber "O" ring) around a targeted varix. This ligation of the varix results in necrosis, inflammation, shallow ulcer formation, and then healing with scar formation, which then obliterates the varix within 14 to 21 days. This procedure has been used at limited sites with good results.[40a] The procedure is done after bleeding is controlled. Repeat EVL sessions are necessary. Transient dysphagia was the only complication. Patients who completed the total series of sessions did not experience rebleeding. Continual study of this procedure is necessary.[40a]

Shunting and nonshunting operations

At this time endoscopic sclerotherapy is the therapy of choice to prevent rebleeding. However, there is still much disagreement over whether it is the definitive long-term therapy for esophageal varices. Both nonshunting operations, such as esophageal transection with or without esophagogastric devascularization, and shunting operations, such as splenorenal shunting, mesocaval shunting, and portacaval shunting, are still used in selected patients. All of these operative procedures are lengthy, highly invasive procedures requiring intensive care of the patient in the postoperative period. All are associated with the potential for major problems, including respiratory and cardiovascular complications, obstruction of the shunt, rebleeding, esophageal leaks, and PSE. Shunts are described in more detail on p. 904. The reader is referred to the identified references for more information on these procedures.[20a,20b,42a]

Treatment of portal-systemic encephalopathy

Treatment of PSE centers around finding and treating the precipitating cause (see pages 883 to 884), providing general supportive measures, and decreasing ammonia levels (Box 30-13).

Measures to decrease ammonia levels include the following:

1. Eliminate protein from the diet for several days.
2. Give carbohydrates by mouth or through nasogastric feedings to prevent protein catabolism. At least 200 g of carbohydrate should be given in 24 hours.
3. Administer intestinal antibiotics (for example, neomycin) that destroy or alter bacteria in the intestines and subsequently reduce the amount of ammonia absorbed into the blood.
4. Administer lactulose, which increases the excretion of ammonia via the gastrointestinal tract.

Neomycin (Mycitracin) may be prescribed orally or by rectal instillation. The adult dosage is 4 to 12 g/day. Lactulose is a synthetic disaccharide that is degraded in the lower intestine and acidifies the intestinal lumen. The lowered pH traps ammonia ions (as nondiffusible NH_4), which are then excreted into the stool. The dosage of lactulose syrup (Cephulac) is 30 to 45 ml initially, administered as often as hourly until the patient has a bowel movement. Then the dosage is usually lowered to 3 times a day. Lactulose causes a very irritating diarrhea. The skin should be cleansed promptly after each stool.

Many patients with PSE die of renal failure secondary to an inadequate circulating blood volume (hypovolemia) or hepatorenal syndrome. The treatment of PSE requires careful balancing of fluid administration to maintain adequate perfusion of the kidney without creating an excessive load on the cardiovascular system. Nursing activities include the following:

1. Monitoring desired intravenous flow rate very closely.

30-13	**Sources of ammonia**	
	Exogenous	**Endogenous**
	Dietary protein	Azotemia
	Whole blood transfusions	Blood in gastrointestinal tract
	Ammonium salts	Constipation
	Amino acids	Catabolism

2. Observing patient for signs of cardiovascular overload (dyspnea, moist respirations, coughing frothy sputum, distended neck veins, restlessness).
3. Monitoring urinary output from indwelling catheter.
4. Monitoring changes in CVP readings that are suggestive of either hypervolemia or hypovolemia.
5. Documenting all fluid losses including diarrhea.

The patient who has had definite or threatened PSE may be kept indefinitely on a low-protein diet. When protein is added to the diet, it is added gradually and often does not exceed 40 g/day (average intake in the United States is 70 to 80 g/day). In addition, the patient may receive neomycin or lactulose daily. Constipation must be avoided. Patients with chronic hepatic disease may go in and out of PSE; therefore, they are monitored for any change in behavior that would indicate early coma. The patient and family are taught to be alert to subtle changes in the patient's behavior and to seek medical assistance when changes occur.

Surgery

Focal liver disease. Treatment of liver abscess consists of incision and drainage of the abscess or abscesses and treatment with broad-spectrum antibiotics for pyogenic abscesses. Portal hypertension occurs in rare instances from scarring of the liver as part of the healing process. These patients require close follow-up after discharge from the hospital.

If trauma to the liver has occurred, blood volume replacement is usually required. Emergency surgery may be needed to repair the ruptured liver and local pressure may need to be applied to stop the bleeding. Removal of necrotic tissue may also be indicated, as well as drainage of any bile that may be leaking from the liver surface. The patient may require long-term follow-up to check for signs and symptoms of residual liver damage.

In most instances there is no corrective medical surgical treatment for metastatic or primary carcinoma of the liver because the disease is too far advanced when first diagnosed. Patients are usually alert at this time and will know the prognosis. The patient and family are assisted to live with the prognosis and to do the things they wish to do in the time remaining for the patient (see Chapter 11).

In a few patients with primary tumors, surgery may be possible. If the tumor is limited to a single lobe and there is no evidence of metastases elsewhere, a hepatic lobectomy may be done to remove metastatic as well as primary carcinoma. The remarkable regenerative capacity of the liver permits resection of 70% to 80% of the organ.

Homotransplantation of the liver has been performed in

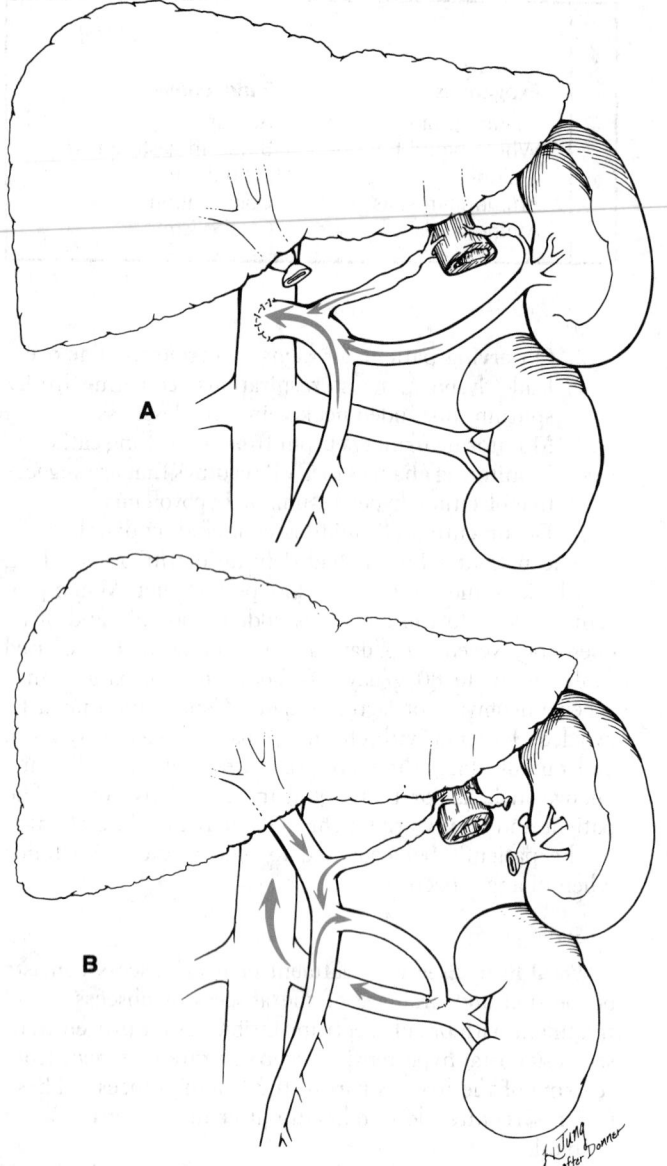

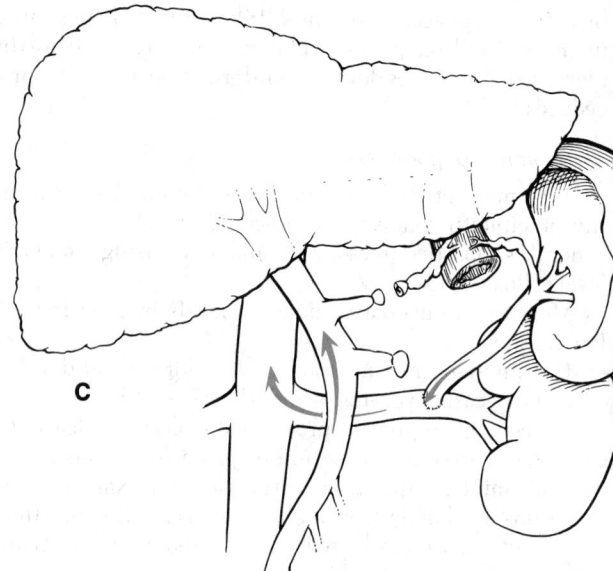

Fig. 30-14 Decompression operations for portal hypertension. **A,** End-to-side portacaval shunt. **B,** Splenorenal shunt. **C,** Distal splenorenal shunt.

a few medical centers. Rapid advances in technology and pharmacologic agents are occurring; however, availability of donor organs and high costs are major limitations.

Hepatic transplantation is done in selected cases of biliary atresia in children and chronic aggressive hepatitis, cirrhosis, and malignancy in adults. See Chapter 42 for a discussion of patient care associated with organ transplantation.

Portal-caval shunts. The only way to achieve permanent lowering of portal pressure is by surgical treatment to reduce blood flow through the portal system. Fig. 30-14, *A* and *B*, shows two different techniques to decompress the portal vein and one technique, *C*, to decompress the esophageal veins. It must be remembered that the patient with hepatic damage severe enough to cause bleeding esophageal varices is not a good operative risk.

The mortality rate when surgical shunts are used as immediate intervention for bleeding esophageal varices is 50%; it is 10% when performed in well-selected patients with portal hypertension who are not actively bleeding. It is generally believed that a prophylactic shunt is not justified. Shunts are recommended only when there has been at least one hemorrhage from esophageal varices and the patient does not respond to other therapy.

The shunts shown in Fig. 30-14, *A* and *B* create a connection between the high-pressure portal system and the low-pressure vena caval system, thereby decompressing the portal system. A major complication is PSE resulting from less venous blood passing through the liver. Nursing care of the patient having liver surgery is discussed in Box 30-14.

Interventions to achieve patient outcomes

The nursing care directed towards many of the nursing diagnoses such as fluid volume changes, high risk for infection, high risk for injury, decreased cardiac output, and ineffective breathing pattern are collaborative in nature

The patient undergoing liver surgery

Preoperative care

Assist patients and significant others to cope with anxiety and fear related to trauma or illness, surgery, and unknown outcomes.

Institute hemodynamic monitoring as required by severity of shock or hypotension, or risk of these complications (see Chapter 9).

Establish baseline data (neurologic, respiratory, renal), and monitor frequently for change in these and for peritonitis.

Assist in therapy to improve the patient's physiologic status and to protect the liver from further metabolic insult.

If the prothrombin level is low, vitamin K is given.

If the patient has upper respiratory disease or infection, vigorous respiratory therapy is given; because of the thoracoabdominal approach and postoperative splinting, postoperative atelectasis and pneumonia are frequent complications.

If malnourishment is present, protein hydrolysates are given by total parenteral nutrition (TPN), and blood transfusions and vitamins are given.

Salt-poor albumin may be given to increase blood colloidal osmotic pressure and vascular volume.

Administer antimicrobial (such as neomycin) to rid intestine of bacteria.

Avoid sedation and use judicious doses of CNS depressants if hepatic dysfunction is present; chlordiazepoxide (Librium), barbital, or phenobarbital are excreted by the kidney, and thus may be drugs of choice.

If the patient has a **pyogenic abscess**

Monitor for signs of rupture of the abscess, peritonitis.

Control pyrexia by cool sponge baths, antipyretics, and cooling blankets.

Administer broad-spectrum antibiotics as prescribed.

Provide comfort measures for chills, fever, and headache.

If the patient has **hepatic trauma**

Monitor intensively for change in hemodynamic, neurologic, and respiratory parameters, and peritonitis.

Assist with peritoneal tap, chest tube insertion, and measures used to maintain blood volume

For the patient who has a **portal-caval shunt**

Assist in measurement and treatment of edema, ascites, and hepatic dysfunction. When hepatic function is poor, coagulation problems, hypoglycemia, hypoalbuminemia, and ammonia excess are common.

Assist patients with comfort measures for pruritus and hemorrhoidal pain, and assist with positioning and self-care activities.

Postoperative care

Establish schedule for hemodynamic, neurologic, renal, and respiratory monitoring, and for detection of the following:

Hemorrhage, coagulation defects

Hypovolemia, oliguria

Postoperative care—cont'd

Hypoglycemia

Hypoalbuminemia

Infection: wound, subdiaphragmatic

Atelectasis or pneumonia

Fluid and electrolyte imbalance (dilutional hyponatremia, metabolic alkalosis, ascites, edema)

PSE

Give prescribed drugs for control of pain, observing the same precautions cited under preoperative care.

Assist with measures to improve or maintain respiratory function:

Have person breathe deeply.

Give respiratory treatments as prescribed.

Change position frequently.

Monitor chest drainage system.

Maintain patency and prescribed flow rates of intravenous fluids including blood, plasma, dextran, and parenteral nutrition substances.

Maintain patency of gastrointestinal tubes.

Nothing by mouth is usually maintained for several days. When food intake is begun, protein intake may be limited and advanced as the patient demonstrates ability to metabolize and excrete protein wastes (BUN, ammonia levels, mental status). Hypoglycemia may occur because of hepatic dysfunction or because of increased insulin capacity from parenteral nutrition.

Assist patient with ambulation. This may be slower than after other types of surgery depending on the patient's hemodynamic status. Carefully monitor pulse, blood pressure, and respiratory rate before, during, and after exertion.

Maintain asepsis in managing all wounds and insertion sites (cleansing, dressings, and drainage system).

Assist patient and family to cope with distress of postoperative period, prolonged and uncertain recovery, and issues related to chronicity, prognosis, and treatment options.

Assist with specific therapies, monitoring, and education related to the following:

Pyogenic abscess

Prolonged antimicrobial therapy, recurrence of infection

Hepatic trauma

Late complications: hemorrhage, cyst and abscess formation, biliary fistulas

Portal-caval shunts

Thrombosis at site of anastomoses: pain, distention, fever, nausea

Edema in lower extremities: sudden increase in blood flow into vena cava may cause venous congestion

Peritoneal venous shunt

Sudden change from shunting of ascitic fluid into venous system (hemodilution, increased renal output, decrease in abdominal girth)

Measures to increase shunt's effectiveness

Transplantation

Complications including rejection, infection, and need to continue immunosuppressive agents for life and were discussed in the preceding section. This section focuses on the other nursing diagnoses that are more independently cared for.

Promoting optimal balance between rest and activity and assisting with comfort

Hepatic repair and regeneration can be promoted by rest, nutrition, and avoidance of toxins and infection. The liver can best be allowed time for repair and regeneration by decreasing the metabolic demands of activity, of infection, of catabolism, and of the stress response.

The physician usually prescribes the desired amounts of rest and activity. In hepatitis, serum enzyme levels may indicate necrosis and may serve as a guide (the higher levels indicate a need for more rest and restricted activity). It is believed that activity and maintaining an upright position decrease hepatic blood flow, thus preventing optimal circulation to the already compromised liver. Relapses are frequently attributed to premature increases in activity.

Although the physician's prescriptions define whether complete bedrest or some ambulation is allowed, the nurse must use judgment in determining activity levels within these limits. The patient with hepatic dysfunction has overwhelming fatigue and benefits from a paced schedule, alternating self-care activities with rest. The schedule should include rest before meals and before family visits. The nurse can use the patient's rating of fatigue and the serum transaminase levels as guide to increases in activity. As patients recover and acute discomfort recedes, patients may need assistance in finding diversional activities that will dispel boredom, yet not be tiring. Boredom and social isolation are particularly difficult for patients who are placed in isolation. Recurrence of anorexia, enlargement or tenderness of the liver, or lack of progress as indicated by laboratory studies indicate a need to return to bed rest.

There are many sources of discomfort for patients with hepatic disorders. The nurse can promote rest by assisting patients to reduce discomfort by direct physical care measures:

1. Assist patients with ascites to shift position frequently. They often require a high Fowler's position for ease in breathing. Flotation or air mattresses and a trapeze may be helpful.
2. Provide assistance for acute symptoms of chills, fever, diaphoresis, nausea, vomiting, and diarrhea.
   a. Apply blankets to provide comfort during chills, yet not so many that temperature is increased.
   b. Use tepid sponge baths to lower temperature and apply cool cloths to the forehead.
   c. Change linens or dressings as frequently as necessary.
   d. Provide clean receptacles for emesis and diarrhea and remove them promptly.
   e. Provide quiet, cool, and pleasant environment.
3. Provide measures to decrease pruritus:
   a. Use cool, light, and nonrestrictive clothing and dry, soft bed linens.
   b. Avoid extremes of temperature in baths or compresses.
   c. Avoid stimulating perspiration.
   d. Maintain a cool environment.
   e. Administer prescribed antihistamines or cholostyramine (Cuemid, Questran).
   f. Use distraction to decrease patient's perception of pruritus.

Assisting with nutrition

Good nutritional intake is necessary for repair and regeneration of the liver. Rest and nutrition are key treatments for hepatitis, alcoholic lesions of the liver, cirrhosis, and during recovery from infections, surgery, or trauma of the liver. The patient with a malignant tumor of the liver also needs a focus on nutrition and rest. The liver's ability to excrete toxins and to carry on its many other functions may be seriously hampered by inadequate intake of protein and vitamin B complex. If hepatic damage has occurred, the organ's ability to store glycogen and vitamins A, B complex, C and D may also be decreased.

Although fat is a concentrated source of calories, most patients with diffuse hepatic disorders but not focal hepatic disorders have some fat intolerance. Oral bile salts may improve the digestion and absorption of fats and fat-soluble vitamins.

A diet high in calories, protein, and vitamins; fairly high in carbohydrates (unless weight reduction is desired); and with moderate amounts of fat is often ordered for patients with diffuse or focal hepatic disease.

However, a high-protein diet may not be possible if there is potential or actual PSE. In this case, protein restriction becomes necessary. If protein needs to be restricted for some time, the physician may prescribe an enteral or parenteral supplement that has selected BCAAs and a low content of SCAAs. (see p. 883).

Because alcohol is thought to interfere with hepatic conversion of folic acid to its active metabolites, many persons with cirrhosis have a folic acid deficiency anemia that usually responds well to treatment with oral doses of folic acid. Other nutritional anemias requiring nutritional supplements include vitamin B_{12} and iron deficiency anemias (see Chapter 27).

Anorexia and fatigue interfere with adequate food intake. Although large amounts of food may be prescribed, it is exceedingly difficult for patients to eat these amounts. The person with diffuse or focal liver disease is often anorexic, and it can become a challenge for the nurse to identify ways to encourage the person to eat the prescribed diet. It is important to remember that the nurse is the health team member who provides this direct assistance to the patient. The following are specific measures to promote nutritional intake:

1. Provide frequent oral hygiene.
2. Provide a pleasant atmosphere.
3. Incorporate patient's food preferences.
4. Serve small, frequent feedings.
5. Increase caloric content by adding calories to prepared foods (for example, powdered milk, sauces, butter).
6. Use calorie-rich juices and drinks as fluid allowance, particularly if fluids are restricted.
7. Request use of salt substitutes, herbs, and spices if sodium is restricted.

DATA: Mr. S. is a 55-year-old salesman with portal hypertension who is admitted to the hospital with upper gastrointestinal bleeding. Endoscopy revealed enlarged esophageal and upper gastric veins and a bleeding ulcer. Gastric lavage with iced saline controlled bleeding; 1 U of packed red blood cells was given. Treatment orders included protein (20 g/day) and sodium (1000 mg/day) restrictions, fluid (1000 ml/day) restriction, neomycin 1 g orally every 4 hours, thiamine 1 ml intramuscularly once a day for 3 days, vitamin K subcutaneously once a day for 3 days, and spironalactone 25 mg twice a day. A physical exam revealed slight jaundice of sclera and skin; ascites and peripheral edema; thin legs and arms with poor musculature; signs of increased estrogen; orientation to person, place, and time; and coherence; blood pressure of 116/60 mm Hg; pulse of 90 beats/min; and respiration rate of 32.

The nursing history identified the following:

- Mr. S. has participated in Alcoholics Anonymous (AA) for 1 year; he has not been drinking since then.
- Mr. S. has had infleunza-like symptoms the past 2 weeks but continued with his busy schedule. He complains of fatigue, anorexia, and itching.

Collaborative nursing actions include interventions to prevent further impairment of physical status from hemorrhage and ammonia toxicity and to assist in treatment of the gastric ulcer and fluid excess. Nursing actions include monitoring for the following:

- Signs of hemorrhage: hematemesis, decreased blood pressure, tachycardia, restlessness, stools testing positive for guaiac, and cool, moist skin
- Signs of portal systemic encephalopathy: change in mental status, asterixis, and change in handwriting or tremors

Nursing diagnosis: **Fatigue related to muscle wasting, blood loss, and potential anemia**

Expected patient outcomes	Nursing interventions	Rationale
Mr. S. will indicate on a weekly basis that he is less fatigued He will show improved rating of fatigue on a scale of one (no fatigue) to 10 (severe fatigue) Mr. S. will show a gradual increase in activities on a weekly basis	Ensure or maintain bed rest as prescribed during the acute phase After acute phase, encourage increasing activity interspersed with rest periods as tolerated; coordinate with patient Intervene if patient shows fatigue after or during visits by family or friends Make sure diet is well balanced nutritionally and that patient takes calories, protein, and sodium within proper restrictions	Graduated increase of activity is important so as not to overtax patient who has poor nutritional status and activity intolerance

Nursing diagnosis: **Nutrition, altered: less than body requirements related to anorexia and flu-like symptoms**

Expected patient outcomes	Nursing interventions	Ratioale
Mr. S. ingests required nutrients and adequate calories on a daily basis; signs of muscle wasting lessen	Assess knowledge of nutrient needs On a daily basis, plan and implement well-balanced, high-carbohydrate, low-protein diet with adequate vitamins Decrease roughage in diet Encourage use of salt substitute or alternative seasonings such as Mrs. Dash Give antiemetics as prescribed and extra mouth care if nausea is present Suggest small, frequent meals, 6 meals/day Use measures that encourage eating such as a clean environment and making sure patient is rested and comfortable Support continuation of AA activities while patient is hospitalized	Food intake within prescribed limitation can influence liver regeneration; nursing measures can influence amount of intake in anorectic patient. Low-roughage diet is necessary because of esophageal varices It is important that patient continue AA participation as he has for past year. AA representatives should be allowed to see patient as condition permits and patient desires

Nursing diagnosis: Fluid volume excess related to impaired metabolism of aldosterone and hypoalbuminemia

Expected patient outcomes	Nursing interventions	Rationale
Mr. S.'s weight and abdominal girth decrease daily Edema resolves Serum sodium and potassium levels remain within normal limits	Monitor weight daily, blood pressure q4h, assess edema every shift, and measure abdominal girth daily Monitor intake and output on every shift until excess fluid is excreted Teach patient the rationale for sodium restriction as the patient shows interest Provide bed rest for ascites Give the patient prescribed diuretics Restrict fluids; provide those that are best tolerated, and space the fluids througout 24 hours with greatest volume in daytime and least at night	Diuresis in cirrhosis is undertaken slowly using very conservative measures because of the contracted intravascular fluid volume. Diuresis in excess can jeopardize renal perfusion and precipitate portal-systemic encephalopathy, so careful monitoring is necessary

Nursing diagnosis: Breathing pattern, ineffective related to ascites and immobility and potential stasis of secretions

Expected patient outcomes	Nursing interventions	Rationale
Mr. S.'s dyspnea is decreased or does not worsen as indicated on a scale of 1 (no dyspnea) to 5 (severe dyspnea) Breath sounds are clear	Monitor respirations and breath sounds q4h Place in Fowler's position Encourage patient on bed rest to turn frequently, q2h Encourage deep breathing q2h	Nursing measures to encourage deep chest excursions are important when ascites and immobility are present. Fowler's position can relieve pressure on diaphragm, which can decrease chance of stasis of secretions

Nursing diagnosis: Skin integrity, impaired, high risk for, related to immobility, poor nutrition, edema, and jaundice

Expected patient outcomes	Nursing interventions	Rationale
Mr. S.'s skin remains intact	Assess patient's skin daily for signs of possible breakdown Use measures such as egg crate mattress and routine turning schedule to prevent skin breakdown Keep skin clean and moisturized. Clean and apply lotion every shift Keep nails short and clean Provide soft cloth to rub skin	Patient has poor nutrition, edema, immobility; all of these are risk factors for decubitus ulcers requiring preventive care. Jaundice could lead to scratching and requires preventive care

Nursing diagnosis: itching related to jaundice and environmental stimuli

Expected patient outcomes	Nursing interventions	Rationale
Mr. S. states that he feels more comfortable and that itching is decreased. Mr. S. is not observed scratching	Avoid heat and heavy clothing; provide a cool environment Apply antipruritic lotion as prescribed to skin as needed at least every shift Give prescribed antihistamines Use diversional activities such as music Keep patient's fingernails cut short and clean If patient must scratch, provide soft cloth to prevent excoriations Use tepid water for bathing	Nursing measures relieve or lessen the effects of environmental stimuli, reduce itching, and promote comfort

Nursing diagnosis: Infection, high risk for, related to immunosuppression

Expected patient outcomes	Nursing interventions	Rationale
Mr. S. develops no infections; temperature remains normal	Monitor patient for signs of infection every shift Use sterile technique for all invasive procedures Encourage pulmonary hygiene such as turning and deep breathing every 1 to 2 hr Restrict exposure to persons with infections	Infections in patient with cirrhosis can be life threatening because they can cause sepsis and can precipitate failure, which may result in portal systemic encephalopathy Measures to prevent infection are essential in persons whose immune systems are suppressed Early detection is important for early treatment

Nursing diagnosis: Coping, ineffective individual, related to health crisis

Expected patient outcomes	Nursing interventions	Rationale
Mr. S. will describe at least one coping mechanism to deal with health crisis	Assess patient's perception of health and present illness Identify and support patient's coping strategies such as prayer, music, conversation, etc Listen actively if patient expresses feeling of powerlessness, fears, or spiritual distress. Plan time daily for listening Assess and facilitate family support. Meet with family or significant other on a scheduled basis	Support of patient undergoing a health crisis can facilitate use of intrapersonal family resources. One can expect this patient to be discouraged and fearful. Ineffective coping may precipitate return to alcohol.

Nursing diagnosis: Injury, high risk for bleeding and falls related to decreased metabolic function of liver

Expected patient outcomes	Nursing interventions	Rationale
No undetected bleeding occurs Vital signs return to normal	Monitor the following for blood: urine, stool, skin, and mucous membranes Check patient's vital signs q4h and prothrombin and PTT levels and thrombocytes daily Avoid injections if possible; apply pressure at all puncture sites for 5 min Give prescribed vitamin K Teach patient to use soft toothbrush and to avoid straining or coughing	Patient's esophageal varices and cirrhosis make him a candidate for bleeding and falls; surveillance is the major nursing focus, as well as decreasing precipitating factors
No falls occur	Provide support when patient is ambulating to prevent falls Maintain safe environment	

Continued.

Nursing Care Plan   **Person with cirrhosis—cont'd**

Nursing diagnosis: Self-esteem disturbance related to inability to accept physical changes of increased abdominal girth, jaundice, and change in secondary sexual characteristics and potential changes in role

Expected patient outcomes	Nursing interventions	Rationale
Mr. S. describes self in realistic terms, which include positive characteristics	Encourage patient to participate in goal setting and decision making Help patient identify personal strengths and give positive feedback Assist family to understand patient's need for a positive self-concept and how they can help Assist patient to explore ways to diminish overt signs of jaundice and ascites and thus help body image	Poor self-esteem can lead to poor coping, causing the patient to resume alcohol consumption

Nursing diagnosis: Knowledge deficit: follow-up care and home care related to change in health status and previous inability to cope with information

Expected patient outcomes	Nursing interventions	Rationale
Mr. S. describes nature of cirrhosis and therapeutic regimen	Assess patient's knowledge and clarify the following, as necessary: basis of signs and symptoms and therapeutic regimen, dietary and fluid restrictions, medication therapy, avoidance of infection and bleeding, and signs (increased temperature, bleeding, worsening jaundice, change in mental status, etc) requiring immediate medical follow-up	Patient has had the medical problem for some time, so first assess his knowledge; he may not need teaching. The assessment will help identify other reasons for the delay in seeking help

Facilitating learning and promoting health maintenance

All patients need to be prepared for diagnostic tests, to understand their treatments, and to learn how to implement their therapeutic regimens at home. Patients with chronic hepatic dysfunction need to understand long-term care needs for changes in life-style, diet, fluid intake, and avoidance of toxins, including alcohol. Box 30-15 lists important points to consider for patients with various hepatic disorders. All patients should be taught how to prevent further hepatic damage from insults of inadequate food, toxins, including alcohol, and infections.

The patient with malignant tumors, whether primary or metastatic, needs help to deal with self-care needs and to deal with cancer (see Chapter 11). A major focus for many patients with cirrhosis is helping them to confront the effect of alcohol on their well-being. It requires willingness to engage in discussion about alcohol. Denial is a major part of alcoholism and "breaking through" denial is a part of treatment that occurs over time. Discussion of past alcohol intake and its effects on physical health, and social functioning (family, job, involvement with police, and accidents) is a necessary early part of improving health maintenance. Confrontation by family members, employ-ers, and friends may be part of intervention (see Chapter 13 for details and for other techniques and support systems to assist persons with alcohol problems).

The nurse can assist patients with alcoholism and cirrhosis due to alcoholism or other causes by giving them as much control as possible. This could include the following:
1. Involve the patient in goal setting and decision making.
2. Give positive feedback for accomplishments.
3. Support the patient in times of failure.
4. Help the patient recall past accomplishments.
5. Help significant others provide positive feedback.
6. Help the patient find ways to disguise jaundice or ascites.

A different set of issues is the focus of teaching and promotion of health maintenance in the patient with toxic or viral hepatitis. Often, patients with hepatitis are young adults who find that fatigue and slow recovery interfere with personal and career goals. The nurse can assist the patient and family to cope with these concerns by listening actively and supporting their coping mechanisms. Accurate information about rest requirements and infectiousness of viral hepatitis, as well as about measures that must be used

For patient with specific hepatic disorders

Tumors of the liver
  Balancing activity and rest
  Managing complications such as jaundice, ascites, and edema
  Managing symptoms due to metastasis to other sites such as respiratory distress
  (See Chapter 11 for care needs of cancer patient in general)
Hepatitis
  Activity restriction
  Food intake
  Measures to avoid transmission of disease and exposure to toxins
Liver abscess
  Long-term compliance with self-administered antimicrobial therapy
  Wound care
  Recurrence of infection; signs to watch for
Hepatic trauma and surgery
  Wound care
Peritoneal venous shunt
  Shunt care
  Self-monitoring of abdominal girth and weight
Transplantation
  (See Chapter 42)
Cirrhosis
  Self-monitoring of abdominal girth, edema, body weight, bleeding sites, jaundice
  Compliance and self-administration of diuretics: neomycin/lactulose; potassium replacements; fluid, and sodium restriction; avoidance of alcohol and other toxins; restriction of activity

at home to prevent transmission of viral hepatitis and further recovery should be provided. The patient and family need an opportunity to express their fears and concerns about care requirements, prognosis, and infectiousness.

Evaluation

Evaluation will be based on the identified patient outcomes. For the person with acute hepatic dysfunction, questions to consider may include the following:
1. Are signs and symptoms of fluid changes, infection, bleeding, or jaundice decreasing?
2. Have complications (infection, bleeding, respiratory dysfunction, skin breakdown) been avoided?
3. Have falls or other injuries been avoided?
4. Is the patient getting sufficient rest?

For persons with chronic hepatic dysfunction, do the patient and family know the following:
1. The nature of the disorder and need for continued medical follow-up?
2. Measures to prevent exacerbations and complications?
3. Signs and symptoms to be reported to the physician?
4. All information related to diet and medications?

SUMMARY

1. The anatomic structure of the liver has several specialized characteristics: the organization of cellular plates; the portal vein and hepatic arterial blood supply into the sinusoids; the biliary canaliculi emptying into the larger biliary ductules, ducts and common bile duct; and Kupffer's cells lining the blood vessels.
2. The liver is important for proper metabolism of fat, protein, and carbohydrate, for production of plasma proteins, for bilirubin metabolism and bile production, and for detoxification.
3. Physiologic changes that occur in aging may change the metabolism of drugs.
4. All types of jaundice are associated with increased serum levels of bilirubin; hemolytic jaundice is a problem of excessive red blood cell breakdown; obstructive jaundice is associated with an elevation of conjugated bilirubin (direct) and an absence of urinary urobilinogen, and hepatocellular jaundice is often associated with elevated serum transaminases.
5. An increased prothrombin time may be associated with a decrease in vitamin K or hepatocellular inability to form prothrombin even if vitamin K is adequate.
6. Increasingly severe histologic changes in liver cells are seen in alcoholic fatty liver, alcoholic hepatitis, and Laënnec's cirrhosis; the latter condition is not reversible.
7. In the United States, cirrhosis is most commonly a result of chronic alcoholism and is characterized by multiple changes in hepatic function. Portal hypertension, bleeding esophageal varices, and hepatorenal syndrome are three problems that threaten life.
8. The incidence of toxic hepatitis could be reduced by decreased use or proper use of toxins such as petroleum distillates; alcoholic hepatitis is the major type of toxic hepatitis in the United States.
9. There are five known types of viral hepatitis. Measures to control hepatitis A and hepatitis E are directed toward hand washing and interrupting the fecal-oral route of transmission. The other three types are spread through infected blood and other body fluids.
10. Anorexia and influenza-like symptoms are often more acute in hepatitis A but these symptoms occur in all types of hepatitis. They occur before icterus (jaundice) appears.
11. Most persons with viral hepatitis recover within 6 months and have no residual hepatic damage. Hepatitis B and C may lead to a carrier state, atypical course of illness, chronic hepatitis, or cirrhosis.
12. Preexposure and postexposure prophylaxis for hepatitis include immune globulin and HBIG (passive immunity) and hepatitis B vaccine (active immunity).
13. The CDC in Atlanta is the national authority for information about the prevention of infectious diseases.
14. There are many tests that use serologic markers (antigens, antibodies) for differentiating the type of hepatitis: HBsAg is one test for hepatitis B. Hepatitis A is detected by the presence of IgM-class anti-HAV, and hepatitis C is detected by anti-HCV.
15. The CDC considers hepatitis B to be the greatest

occupational hazard for health workers. Measures to decrease risk include hepatitis B vaccination, hand washing, and universal or body substance precautions used with all patients.

16. Common problems of diffuse hepatocellular disease are jaundice, bleeding tendencies, anemia, infection, and fluid and electrolyte imbalances.

17. Diuresis of ascitic fluid is slow and can induce complications: hypokalemia, magnesium deficit, oliguria, azotemia, and portal systemic encephalopathy. One kg of loss of body weight per day is the maximum safe amount of ascitic fluid loss.

18. Portal systemic encephalopathy (PSE) is associated with elevations of serum ammonia or other metabolic abnormalities. Central nervous system dysfunction is manifested in a sequential pattern leading to coma. Asterixis is an early sign.

19. Common precipitants of PSE are hypokalemia, alkalosis, sedation, and gastrointestinal bleeding.

20. Measures to control bleeding in esophageal varices include use of the Sengstaken-Blakemore tube, pitressin infusion and other drugs, injection sclerosis, esophageal variceal ligation, or surgery. Measures to prevent PSE are also started when there is gastrointestinal bleeding.

21. After esophageal hemorrhage unresponsive to other measures, elective surgical decompression of the portal vein may be done by creating a connection between portal and systemic venous circulation (liver bypass or shunting procedures); elective nonshunting procedures may also be done.

22. Portal-systemic encephalopathy may be treated by neomycin, lactulose, and no- or low-protein diet. These measures may be used as prophylaxis when there is gastrointestinal bleeding.

23. Liver abscesses may be pyogenic and treated with broad-spectrum antibiotics and surgery, or they may be amebic and treated with amebicidal drugs.

24. Metastatic tumors of the liver are 20 times more prevalent than primary tumors of the liver. Symptoms occur late; jaundice, ascites, and weakness are common.

25. Malignant lesions of the liver are treated by resection, palliative use of radiation, and chemotherapy by systemic routes or portal arterial infusion.

26. Assessment techniques of value in persons with hepatic diseases include percussion and palpation of the liver, and inspection, auscultation, and percussion of the abdomen. Palpating for fluid wave is helpful when ascites is present.

27. In liver biopsy, aseptic technique and assisting the patient to hold his or her breath during the procedure reduce risks of infection and hemorrhage.

28. Rest, nutrition, and abstinence from toxins are three major treatments of focal or diffuse hepatic disorders.

29. Patients with chronic diffuse hepatic disease will require extensive teaching to assist them to master self-care skills.

30. The patient with hepatic disease may need to make major changes in life-style (avoidance of alcohol or changes in sexual practices).

STUDY QUESTIONS

- Why does gastrointestinal bleeding, low serum potassium, or alkalosis increase the risk of portal-systemic encephalopathy?
- Why are persons with diffuse hepatic disease at greater risk for infection?
- What measures are needed to decrease incidence and transmission of hepatitis B?
- Why do persons in high-risk groups for hepatitis B not receive the correct primary preventive care?

REFERENCES

1.* Advisory Committee Immunization Practices (ACIP): Recommendation for protection against viral hepatitis, *MMWR* 39(S-2):1-26, 1990.

2.* Adinaro D: Liver failure and pancreatitis: fluid and electrolyte concerns, *Nurs Clin North Am* 22:843-852, 1987.

3. Alter MJ et al: The changing epidemiology of hepatitis B in the United States, *JAMA* 263:1218-1222, 1989.

4.* Anderson FP: Portal-systemic encephalopathy in the chronic alcoholic, *Crit Care Q*, 8(4):40-52, 1989.

5. Arora S, Kaplan MM: Cirrhosis. In Rakel RE, editor: *Conn's current therapy*, ed 28, Philadelphia, 1989, WB Saunders.

6. Berne R, Levy M, editors: *Physiology*, ed 2, St Louis, 1988, Mosby–Year Book.

6a. Blumgart LH, editor: *Surgery of the liver and biliary tract*, New York, 1988, Churchill Livingstone.

7. Bradley DW: Hepatitis non-A, non-B viruses become identified as hepatitis C and E viruses, *Prog Med Virol* 37:101-135, 1990.

8.* Brown M: Gastroesophageal varices, *Prim Care* 15:175-186, 1988.

9. Deinstag JL: Hepatitis non-A, non-B: C at last, *Gastroenterology* 99(4):1177-1180, 1990.

10.* Dobberstein K: The liver: to know it is to love it, *Am J Nurs* 87:74, 1987.

11. Franks AL et al: Hepatitis B virus infection among children born in the U.S. to Southeast Asian refugees, *New Engl J Med* 321:1301-1305, 1989.

12. Frey CF et al: Liver abscesses, *Surg Clin North Am* 69:259-271, 1989.

13.* Gillham MB, Southworth K, Dollahite J: Nutritional treatment for the alcoholic patient, *Crit Care Q* 8(4):20-28, 1986.

14.* Healthy People 2000: National Health Promotion and Disease Prevention Objectives, US Dept of Health and Human Services, Public Health Service, Washington, DC, 1990, US Government Printing Office.

14a. Heeg JM, Coleman DA: Hepatitis kills, *RN* 55(4):60-68, 1992.

15. Hoofnagle JH: Toward universal vaccination against hepatitis B virus, *New Engl J Med* 321:1333-1334, 1989.

16. Hoofnagle JH: Type D (Delta) hepatitis, *JAMA* 261:1321-1325, 1989.

17. Jensen DM: Portal-systemic encephalopathy and hepatic coma, *Med Clin North Am* 70:1081-1092, 1986.

18.* Keith JS: Hepatic failure: etiologies, manifestation, and management, *Crit Care Nurse* 5(1):60-86, 1985.

19. Korniewicz DM, Kirwin M, Larson E: Do your gloves fit the task? *Am J Nurs* 91(6):38-40, 1991.

20.* Korniewicz DM et al: Integrity of vinyl and latex procedure gloves, *Nurs Res* 38:144-146, 1989.

---

*Recommended for student reading.

20a. Levine BA, Sirinek KR: The portacaval shunt—is it still indicated? *Surg Clin North Am* 70:361-377, 1990.

20b. Lillemoe KD, Cameron JL: The interposition mesocaval shunt, *Surg Clin North Am* 70:379-393, 1990.

21. Ludwig J: Etiology of biliary cirrhosis: diagnositic features and a new classification, *Zentralbl Allg Pathol* 134:132-141, 1988.

22. Maddrey WC, Thiel DHV: Liver transplantation: an overview, *Hepatology* 8:948-959, 1988.

23.* Maloney JP: Surgical intervention in the alcoholic patient with portal hypertension, *Crit Care Q* 8(4):63-73, 1986.

24. Mattsson L, Weiland O, Glaumann H: Long-term follow-up of chronic posttransfusion non-A, non-B hepatitis: clinical and histological outcome, *Liver* 8:184-188, 1988.

25. Maxwell AJ, Mamtora H: Fungal liver abscesses in acute leukemia—a report of two cases, *Clin Radiol* 39:197-201, 1988.

26. Metzger U: Intraportal chemotherapy for colorectal hepatic metastases, *Antibiot Chemother* 40:51-60, 1988.

27. MMWR: Changing patterns of groups at high risk for hepatitis B in the United States, *MMWR* 37:429-437, 1988.

28.* MMWR: Hepatitis A among drug abusers, *MMWR* 37:297-305, 1988.

29.* MMWR: Hepatitis B among parenteral drug abusers—North Carolina, *MMWR* 35:481-483, 1986.

30. MMWR: Inadequate immune response among public safety workers receiving intradermal vaccination against hepatitis B—United States, 1990-1991 *MMWR* 40:569-571, 1991.

31. MMWR: Public Health Service inter-agency guidelines for screening donors of blood, plasma, organs, tissues, and semen for evidence of hepatitis B and hepatitis C, *MMWR* 40(RR-4):1-17, 1991.

32. MMWR: Recommendations for preventing transmission of human immunodeficiency virus and hepatitis B virus to patients during exposure-prone invasive procedures, *MMWR* 40(RR-8):1-9, 1991.

33. MMWR: Update on hepatitis B prevention, *MMWR* 36:353-366, 1987.

34. Price SA, Wilson LM: Pathophysiology: clinical concepts of disease processes, ed 4, St Louis, 1992, Mosby–Year Book.

34a. Rector WG, Jr: *Complications of chronic liver disease*, St Louis, 1992, Mosby–Year Book.

34b. Russell B: Score: hepatitis viruses 5, vaccines 1, *Amer Nurse* 24(8):2, 11, 1992.

35. Schreeder M: Viral hepatitis, *Prim Care* 15:157-173, 1988.

36. Schroeder SA, et al, editors: *Current medical diagnosis and treatment: 1990*, Norwalk, Conn, 1990, Appleton & Lange.

37.* Semonin-Holleran R: Critical nursing care for abdominal trauma, *Crit Care Nurse* 8(3):48-58, 1988.

38. Solomon J, Harrington D, Gogel HF: When the patient suffers from esophageal bleeding, *RN* 50(2):24-27, 1987.

39. Starzel TE, Iwatsuki S: Transplantation of the liver. In Schiff L, Schiff ER, editors: *Diseases of the liver*, ed 6, Philadelphia, 1987, JB Lippincott Co.

40. Steven CE et al: Epidemiology of hepatitis C Virus, *JAMA* 263:49-53, 1990.

40a. Stiegmann GV, Goff JS: Endoscopic esophageal varix ligation: preliminary clinical experience, *Gastrointestinal Endoscopy* 34:113-117, 1988.

41. Stone MD, Benotti PN: Liver resection: preoperative and postoperative care, *Surg Clin North Am* 69:383-391, 1989.

42. Vitale G, Heusen LS, Polk H: Malignant tumors of the liver, *Surg Clin North Am* 66:723-741, 1986.

42a. Wexler MJ, Stein BL: Nonshunting operations for hemorrhage, *Surg Clin North Am* 70:425-448, 1990.

43. Widmann F: *Goodall's Clinical interpretation of laboratory tests*, ed 10, Philadelphia, 1987, FA Davis.

44. Wyngaarden JB, Smith LH, Bennett JC, editors: *Cecil Textbook of medicine*, ed 19, Philadelphia, 1992, WB Saunders.

45. Zimmerman HJ, Maddrey WC: Toxic and drug-induced hepatitis. In Schiff L, Schiff ER, editors: *Diseases of the liver*, ed 6, Philadelphia, 1987, JB Lippincott.

Classic

46.* Freditti SL: When the liver fails, *Am J Nurs* 84:64-67, 1984.

47.* Gullate MM, Foltz AT: Hepatic chemotherapy via implantable pump, *Am J Nurs* 83:1674-1678, 1983.

48. Klopp A: Shunting malignant ascites, *Am J Nurs* 84:212-213, 1984.

Problems with Digestion or Elimination

31

The Patient with Gastrointestinal Problems

Barbara C. Long
Rebecca Roberts

After studying this chapter, the learner should be able to:

- Compare and contrast obesity and protein-calorie malnutrition and their nursing interventions.
- Compare and contrast the nature of common inflammatory disorders of the mouth, stomach, intestines, and appendix and nursing interventions for them.
- Describe the cause of dysphagia and heartburn and related therapeutic interventions.
- Differentiate gastric and duodenal ulcers and required medical and nursing care.
- Explain malabsorption syndrome and nursing interventions.
- Differentiate ulcerative colitis, Crohn's disease, and diverticular disease and the care required for each.
- Describe the nature and care of the patient with intestinal obstruction and with hernias.
- Differentiate preventive and therapeutic modalities for patients with cancer of the mouth, stomach, and bowel.
- Describe the care of persons with a stoma for fecal diversion.
- Differentiate types of surgery and nursing care for persons with anorectal lesions.

ANATOMY AND PHYSIOLOGY

Maintenance of adequate nutrition and elimination requires an intact and functioning gastrointestinal tract. Normally, food and fluids are placed in the mouth, chewed (if solid), pushed to the pharynx by the tongue, and swallowed by automatic reflex activity down the esophagus into the stomach. Digestion starts in the mouth and ends in the small intestine, although fluids continue to be reabsorbed in the colon. Fig. 31-1 shows the anatomic structures of the gastrointestinal tract. The gallbladder and pancreas, which are also involved with digestion, are discussed in Chapter 32.

Mouth and Esophagus
Salivation

The cortical thought of food initiates saliva production from the salivary glands. The salivary secretions consist of *serous secretion,* containing ptyalin for starch digestion, and *mucous* secretion for lubrication. These two secretions account for one half of the upper gastrointestinal tract secretions.

Mastication

The teeth initiate food breakdown; no other part of the gastrointestinal tract can perform this function if the teeth are missing. Enzymes can act only on the exposed surfaces of the food particles. Very fine particulation prevents excoriation of the lining of the tract, and the rate of digestion depends on the total surface area of food particle exposed. General health teaching for children and adults should stress the reason behind thorough mastication of all food substances that are ingested.

Swallowing

Swallowing must be accomplished without compromising respiration. The tongue forces the bolus of food into the pharynx, from which point the food moves to the upper esophagus and then down into the stomach. Food is prevented from passing into the trachea by the closing of the epiglottis over the trachea and the opening of the esophagus.

The esophagus is a hollow tube. The upper one third is composed of skeletal muscle and the remainder of smooth muscle. It is lined with mucous membrane, which secretes a mucoid substance for protection. The bolus of food arrives at the cardiac sphincter of the stomach usually within 5 to 10 seconds of ingestion.

The *cardiac sphincter* (at the junction of the esophagus with the stomach) prevents reflux of stomach contents into the lower esophagus. This area is heavily layered with mucoid glands. The secretions adhere to the food particles and prevent actual contact with the wall mucosa. The coated particles adhere to each other, forming a bolus for digestion. These secretions act as a protective mechanism for the sphincter zone, since they themselves are strongly resistant to digestion.

Stomach

The food bolus enters the stomach, the largest dilated portion of the tract. The stomach has relatively little muscular tone, which permits increased distention. *Peristalsis,* the alternate contraction and relaxation of the muscle fibers, propels the substance in a wavelike motion through the stomach and intestines.

The mucous membrane lining the stomach is arranged in thick folds known as *rugae* that provide an increased surface area for exposure and contain the openings of the gastric glands. The gastric secretions are clear and colorless and contain water, salts, enzymes, and hydrochloric acid. The amount of enzymes produced is in direct proportion to the amount needed, and the actual food substance stimulates the release of a particular enzyme. The gastric mucosa releases gastrin, which stimulates the production of *pepsinogen* (the precursor of pepsin), *rennin,* and *lipase.* Pepsin and rennin digest protein, and lipase splits fats. The production of hydrochloric acid (HCl) does not appear to depend on the presence of any particular food.

As the food moves toward the *pyloric sphincter* at the distal end of the stomach, peristaltic waves increase in force and intensity. The fluid bolus now becomes a substance known as *chyme.* Chyme is pumped through the pyloric sphincter into the duodenum. Two factors regulate emptying of stomach contents: consistency of the fluid chyme and receptiveness of the duodenum. The average length of time food remains in the stomach after a meal is 2 to 6 hours.

Intestines

The small intestine has three parts: the *duodenum,* which connects to the stomach, the *jejunum* or middle portion, and the *ileum.* The large intestine also has three parts: the *cecum,* which connects to the small intestine, the *colon,* and the *rectum.* The primary function of the intestines is to receive the chyme from the stomach and move the chyme forward to facilitate proper absorption of water, nutrients, electrolytes, and bile salts (Fig. 31-2). Secondary functions include secreting mucus and serving as a storage area before waste discharge.

Movement

Peristaltic movements that mix the intestinal contents propel the contents of the small intestine toward the anus. Chyme moves slowly and normally takes 3 to 10 hours to move from the stomach to the ileocecal valve (see Fig. 31-1). In the colon, the fecal contents are pushed forward by *mass movements* that occur only a few times each day. These mass movements are stimulated by gastrocolic reflexes initiated when food enters the duodenum from the stomach, especially after the first meal of the day. This is therefore the most frequent time of the day for defecation to occur.

The defecation reflex occurs when feces enter the rectum. Afferent impulses are transmitted to the sacral segments of the spinal cord, from which reflex impulses are transmitted back to the colon and rectum, initiating relaxation of the internal anal sphincter.

Secretion

Secretions of the small intestine, biliary, and pancreatic systems provide for the final digestion of food. As chyme enters the small intestine, gastric secretion of hydrochloric acid is slowed. Mucous secretion throughout the tract in-

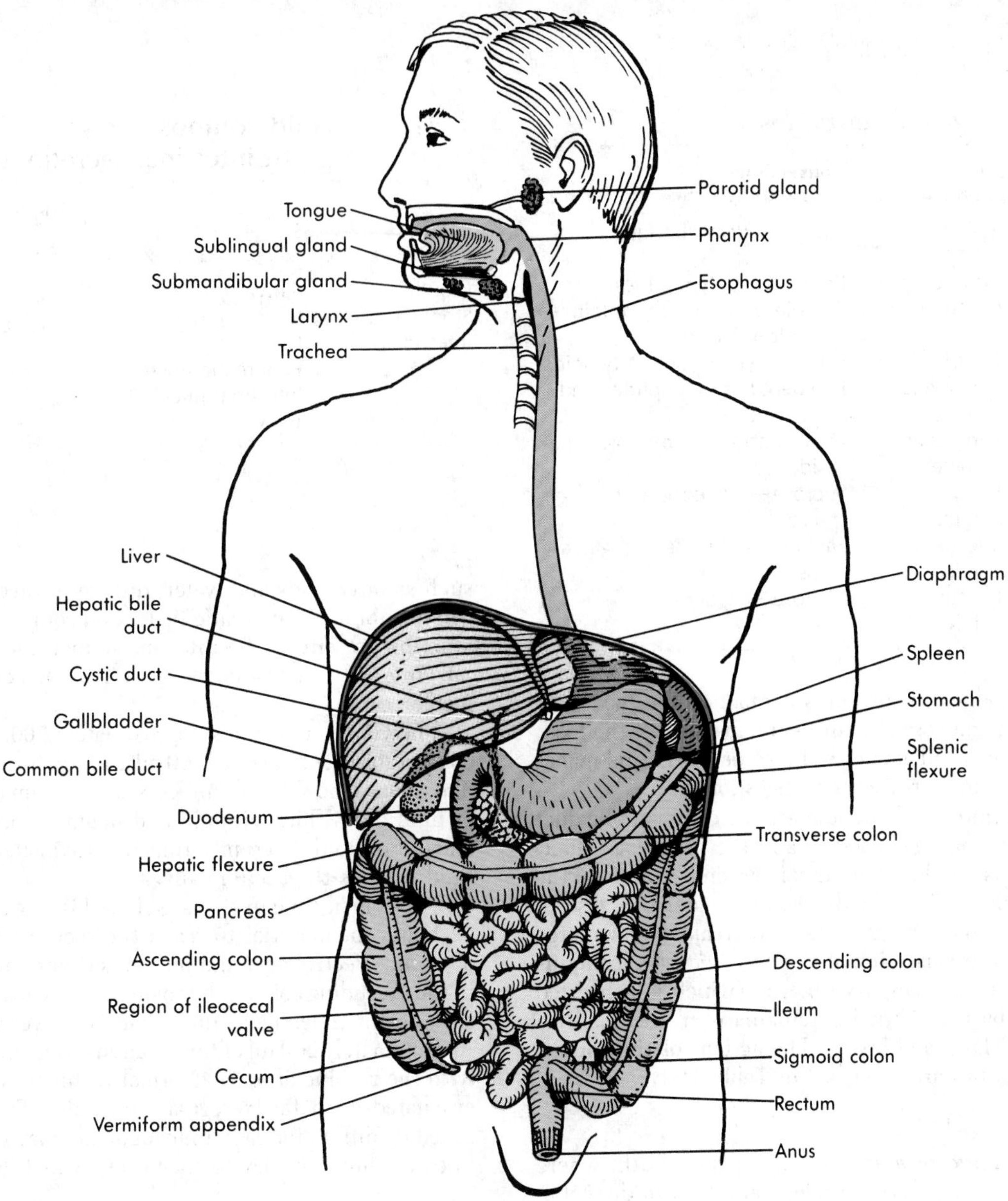

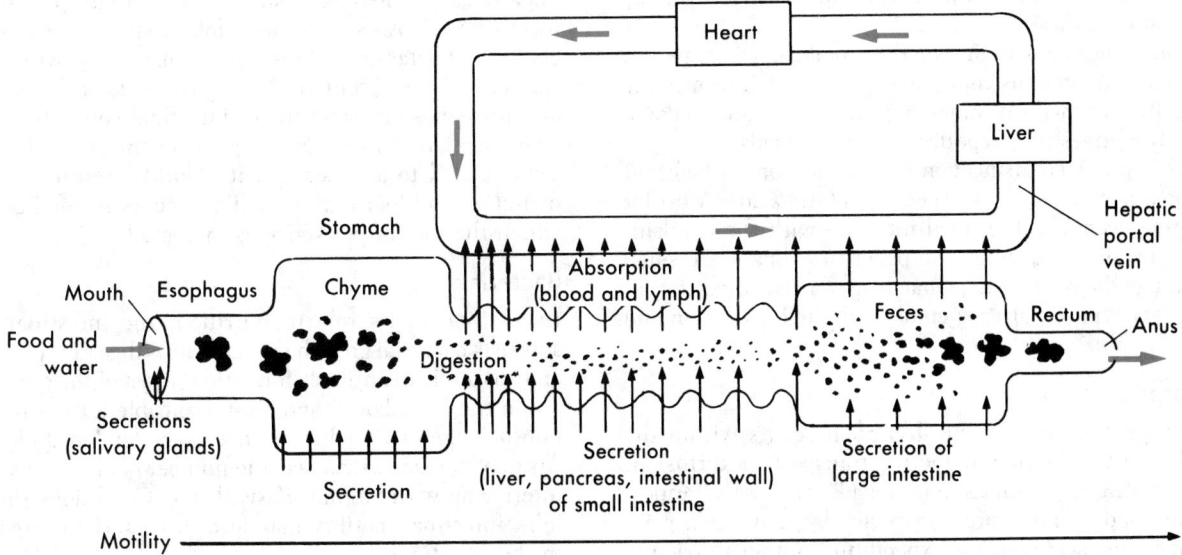

Fig. 31-1 Organs of digestive system and assorted structures.

Fig. 31-2 Summary of gastrointestinal activity involving motility, secretion, digestion, and absorption. (From Vander AJ, et al: *Human physiology*, ed 3, New York, 1980, McGraw-Hill. Used with the permission of McGraw-Hill.)

Table 31-1   Digestive enzymes

Enzyme	Location	Conversions
Amylase (ptyalin)	Saliva	Starch → disaccharides
Pepsin	Gastric juice	Protein → polypeptides
Renin	Gastric juice	Soluble milk casein (protein) → insoluble form
Lipase	Gastric juice	Fats → glycerol and fatty acids
Trypsin	Pancreatic juice	Polypeptides → peptides and amino acids
Amylase	Pancreatic juice	Disaccharides → monosaccharides
Sucrase	Intestinal juice	Sucrose → glucose and fructose
Lactase	Intestinal juice	Lactose → glucose and galactose
Maltase	Intestinal juice	Maltose → glucose

Table 31-2   Fluid composition of gastrointestinal secretions

Site	Secretion	Approximate amount (ml/day)
Mouth	Saliva	1500
Stomach	Gastric juice	2500
Intestines	Bile	500
	Pancreatic juice	1500
	Intestinal juice	1000
	TOTAL	7000

creases food adhesion, prevents contact of the food with the wall of the mucosa, enhances free passage of the food, neutralizes the small amounts of acid or alkali, and makes some particles more resistant to digestion.

Emptying into the duodenum are the common bile duct (from the liver and gallbladder) and the pancreatic duct. *Bile,* which is produced in the liver and stored in the gallbladder, drains into the duodenum to assist in absorption of fats by emulsifying the fat and breaking down large fat droplets into small droplets. *Pancreatic juice* contains three digestive enzymes, trypsinogen (which is converted into trypsin by the enzyme enterokinase in the small intestines), amylase, and lipase. The actions of the various digestive enzymes are described in Table 31-1.

Digestion

The digestion of *carbohydrate* begins in the mouth, where the breakdown of polysaccharides (starches) to disaccharides (sucrose, lactose, maltose) occurs by the action of amylase. The disaccharides are then broken down into monosaccharides (glucose, galactose, and fructose) by the action of the enzymes within the intestinal mucosa and by pancreatic amylase.

Protein digestion begins in the stomach, when pepsin breaks down proteins into polypeptides (an intermediate step). In the small intestine, trypsin further breaks down the polypeptides into peptides and amino acids.

Fat requires emulsification into small droplets before it can be broken down into glycerol and fatty acids. Most fat digestion occurs in the small intestine with the emulsification by bile and action of pancreatic lipase. A small amount of lipase in the stomach may begin digestion of some fats that are already emulsified, such as cream and butter.

Absorption

Ninety percent of nutrient absorption occurs within the small intestine, either by active transport or diffusion. Many nutrients, such as amino acids, monosaccharides, sodium, and calcium, are transported by active transport, requiring metabolic energy expenditure. Other nutrients,

such as fatty acids and water, diffuse passively across the cell membrane. Pancreatic lipase and conjugated bile salts must be present in the intestinal lumen for hydrolysis of fats into fatty acids to permit diffusion across the cell membrane.

The GI tract secretes approximately 7000 ml of fluids daily (Table 31-2); about 2000 ml are usually ingested daily. Therefore, the GI tract processes approximately 9000 ml of fluid daily. The jejunum and ileum absorb the largest amount of fluid (7500 ml); thus, approximately 1500 ml of fluid reaches the cecum daily.

The transit time in the large bowel is slow, taking about 12 hours for material to reach the rectum. Reabsorption of water, electrolytes, and bile salts occurs predominantly in the ascending colon. The colon has the capacity to absorb six to eight times more fluid than is delivered to it daily. Approximately 200 ml of fluid contents remains to be mixed with the residue of feces. Normally, this residue (feces) is evacuated on a fairly regular schedule. The evacuation schedule differs for each individual and may vary from one to three times per day to once every 3 to 4 days.

Fluid and electrolyte balance

Pathologic changes occur with the loss of particular segments of small or large bowel or when reabsorption is impaired. The loss of small bowel contents precipitates metabolic acidosis and hypokalemia from the loss of bicarbonate and potassium. This problem may occur with drainage of small bowel contents through a suction tube or fistula or with persistent vomiting of intestinal contents. Losses from the large intestine comprise mainly loss of water, sodium, and to a lesser extent chloride, resulting in dehydration and hyponatremia. This occurs in conditions in which the rate of peristalsis is increased.

Bacteria

In addition to its role in nutrition, the intestinal tract supports bacterial growth that enhances digestive processes and has a role in antibody formation. Most of the organisms are in the large bowel and are responsible for the production of vitamin K, which is necessary for blood clotting. Antibiotic enemas decrease the number of organisms, thus interfering with vitamin K synthesis. Conditions that inhibit intestinal motility may lead to bacterial overgrowth in the intestines.

Assessment

Assess for dry mouth (from decreased salivation), missing teeth, or poorly fitting dentures that may interfere with eating.

Assess mouth for early signs of periodontal disease (bleeding or receding gums, loose teeth) or oral cancer (white patches or red granular patches, especially on anterior side of tongue or floor of mouth).

Assess dietary intake for adequate fluid intake (at least 1500 ml daily), for adequate food intake, and for fiber-containing foods. Elderly persons, especially those living alone, often drink and eat less than adequate amounts; their diet may also be deficient in fiber, which is needed to maintain normal bowel elimination and help prevent colon cancer. Convenience foods are usually low-fiber.

Assess usual activity level; activity in the form of some type of exercise (based on the person's capabilities) facilitates normal bowel elimination.

Assess laxative use; if needed, bulk laxatives or stool softeners provide for normal stools without affecting bowel function.

Test stool for guaiac (occult blood), which may result from diverticular disease, GI cancer, or hemorrhoids, all commonly seen in elderly persons.

Intervention

Use measures that encourage eating when patient is anorexic (commonly seen in elderly persons).

Persons are more likely to eat types of food they usually eat (especially ethnic foods). Suggest family provide favorite foods.

If patient lives alone and is eligible, Meals on Wheels is available in some communities to provide a daily nourishing meal.

More spices, sugar, and salt (or substitute) may be needed in foods because elderly tend to lose their sense of smell and taste.

Assist elderly to complete hospital dinner menu, if necessary, because of poor vision or loss of fine motor control.

Suggest hospitalized patient sit in chair when possible to eat meals (usual pattern for eating).

Offer food supplements between the usual three times daily meal pattern; smaller more frequent meals are better tolerated. Offer substitutes for missed meals.

Following GI diagnostic procedures, provide oral fluids (if permitted) and opportunity to rest (these procedures are often lengthy and tiring). Monitor stools for barium excretion and constipation.

Promote normal bowel function with adequate fluid intake, dietary fiber, ambulation, and bulk laxatives or stool softeners.

If diarrhea is present, which may result in dehydration and hypokalemia in elderly persons, do the following:

Monitor I&O and serum potassium levels.

Report oliguria (less than 30 ml/hr for 2 to 3 hours) and serum potassium level greater than 3.0 mEq/L to physician.

Encourage fluid intake.

Monitor perianal skin for excoriations; keep the skin clean and apply a soothing ointment such as petrolatum (elderly skin is more fragile and susceptible to breakdown).

Teach patient:

Adequate fluid intake (use juices when possible for additional nutrient intake) and regular exercise to prevent constipation.

High-fiber diet to help prevent constipation, diverticulitis, and colon cancer. Omit fiber if symptomatic diverticulitis is present.

Avoid overuse of laxatives.

Common disorders in elderly

Hiatal hernia
Cancer of mouth, stomach, and colon
Constipation
Diverticulosis
Fecal incontinence

Physiologic Changes With Aging

Changes in the gastrointestinal tract structure and function may occur with aging but vary among individuals and may or may not cause altered functioning.

In the mouth, aging teeth become darker and may loosen from loss of supporting bone and gums. Teeth may become uneven or develop fractures, and circulation of the gums is reduced. Gum changes affect denture fit. Salivary gland output decreases, leading to increased dryness of mucous membranes and making them more susceptible to breakdown. Dryness of the mouth may also interfere with chewing.

Changes in the ability to digest and absorb foods are related to decreased secretion of most digestive enzymes and bile production. Absorption of fats and fat-soluble vitamins becomes impaired. The increased residue resulting from decreased digestion and absorption may lead to increased flatulence. Gas-forming foods may be less well tolerated than when the person was younger.

Decreased intestinal motility may result from decreased peristalsis, decreased muscular tone of the intestinal wall, and decreased abdominal muscle strength. Decreased anal sphincter tone may also be present. These changes contribute to the increased occurrence of constipation or loss of sphincter control in the older person. Considerations for the care of elderly persons with GI problems are listed in the special box.

PREVENTION AND HEALTH EDUCATION

Disorders of the digestive system are among the most commonly encountered health problems. Symptoms produced by digestive disorders are numerous and often lead to decreased employment productivity. Gastrointestinal symp-

Prevention of gastrointestinal problems

Oral hygiene

Brush teeth after meals with fluoridated toothpaste
to decrease caries.
Floss teeth to prevent plaque buildup.
Rinse mouth after eating sweets.
Have regular dental checkups.
Replace misfitting or broken dentures.

Nutrition

Plan meals based on basic four food groups
(Chapter 5).
Substitute high-vitamin fruits for sweets, especially
at end of meal (for example, apples, apricots,
peaches, pears).
Avoid *excessive* amounts of foods that are found
to irritate the oral mucosa (for example, raw tomatoes, hot peppers).
Avoid foods found to irritate one's stomach, such
as highly seasoned foods, large amounts of alcohol, or coffee.
Include high-fiber foods (vegetables, fruits, whole-
grain cereals) in the diet.
Avoid foods that may cause food poisoning: unrefrigerated mayonnaise; cream-filled foods; inadequately cooked eggs, poultry, or meat (especially pork); improperly canned foods.

Tobacco use

Avoid constant exposure of lips to hot pipe (to
prevent cancer of the lips).
Avoid chewing tobacco (to prevent cancer of the
mouth).
Discontinue cigarette smoking, if possible.

Stress

Identify and remove or minimize cause of stress,
if possible.
Use measures to reduce stress response when
stress occurs, for example, relaxation exercises
(see Chapter 6).
Get adequate sleep on a regular basis.

Early detection of major gastrointestinal disorders

Signs requiring immediate medical follow-up
Mouth

A sore that bleeds easily and does not heal
A lump or thickening
A persistent red or whitish patch
Difficulty chewing, swallowing, or moving
tongue or jaws

Abdomen

Persistent heartburn, indigestion
Abdominal pain, especially if accompanied by
nausea and vomiting

Elimination

Change in bowel habits
Blood in the stool

***American Cancer Society recommendations for
screening for cancer of colon and rectum***

Digital rectal examination by physician every
year after age 40
Stool guaiac test done by patient at home every
year after age 50
Sigmoidoscopic examination every 3 to 5 years
after age 50; following two initial negative
tests, 1 year apart.

toms, such as nausea and vomiting or diarrhea, often result
from disorders of other body systems. Interference with
functioning of the gastrointestinal system leads to temporary or long-term nutritional imbalances.

Primary Prevention: Prevention of Disease

Because the cause of many gastrointestinal disorders is
unknown, prevention may not be possible. Some health
practices that are either known to be or are thought to be
helpful in preventing disorders include good oral hygiene
and nutrition and avoidance of tobacco use and stress (see
Box 31-1).

Secondary Prevention: Early Detection

Early detection of major gastrointestinal health problems
can prevent serious complications such as a ruptured appendix with peritonitis. Persons at high risk for cancer of
the colon (p. 971) need careful screening to detect early
signs of cancer because the cancer may be in an advanced
stage before any symptoms occur. Guidelines for early detection are listed in Box 31-2.

MAJOR HEALTH PROBLEMS OF THE GASTROINTESTINAL SYSTEM

Nutritional excess (obesity) and deficit (protein-calorie malnutrition) are disorders that relate to ingestion of food. Gastrointestinal disorders may be classified according to their overall effect on gastrointestinal function or according to the function of specific areas.

CLASSIFICATION BY GENERAL FUNCTION

Disorders of the gastrointestinal (GI) tract may interfere with function in one of three ways: interference with motility and control, with digestion and absorption, and with mechanical passage of food, chyme, and feces.

Disorders of Motility

Interference with GI motility may occur in any part of the GI tract. Esophageal disorders interfere with swallowing and movement of food to the stomach. Vomiting is reverse peristalsis and may result from delayed gastric emptying. Surgical removal of part of the stomach leads to rapid emptying (dumping syndrome). Intestinal hypermotility produces diarrhea. Fecal incontinence results from loss of control. Decreased intestinal motility may lead to flatulence and constipation. Paralytic ileus is failure of intestinal peristalsis.

Disorders of Digestion and Absorption

Disorders that interfere with the digestion and absorption of food include inflammatory disorders, ulcerations, or malabsorptions. *Inflammatory* disorders may occur in any part of the GI tract (Fig. 31-3) and may be acute or chronic. Acute inflammations are painful and produce swelling of the mucosa that may interfere with absorption. Chronic inflammations create changes in the muscular walls, as well as in the mucosa. *Ulcerations* may also extend through the mucosa into the muscular wall and cause pain. *Malabsorption* disorders may alter digestion when nutrients are not broken down into a form that can be transported across cell membranes, or they may alter absorption of the nutrients across the cell membranes and into the lymphatic or circulatory system.

Obstructive Disorders

The GI tract may become obstructed at any point from the portal of entry (mouth) to the exit (rectum). Obstruction may occur from mechanical causes that physically impede passage of intestinal contents or from paralytic causes, in which the passageway is open but peristalsis ceases. Mechanical obstructive disorders include tumors, hernias, adhesions, twisting or telescoping of the intestines, and interferences with the vascular supply.

CLASSIFICATION BY SPECIFIC FUNCTION

GI disorders can also be grouped by functions of specific areas: ingestion via the mouth and esophagus, digestion in the stomach and duodenum, and elimination via the in-

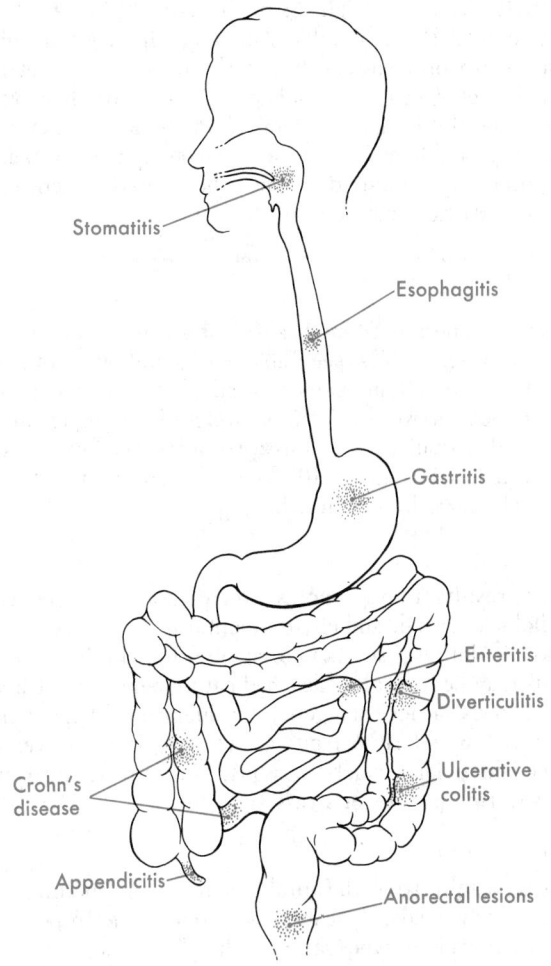

Fig. 31-3   Inflammatory disorders of gastrointestinal system.

testines. Common GI disorder classifications (as discussed in this chapter) are:
1. Ingestive disorders
   a. Inflammations of the mouth
   b. Esophageal disorders
   c. Cancer of the mouth and esophagus
2. Digestive disorders
   a. Gastritis
   b. Ulcerations of stomach and duodenum
   c. Cancer of the stomach
   d. Malabsorption syndromes
3. Elimination disorders
   a. Acute inflammatory intestinal disorders
   b. Chronic inflammatory intestinal disorders
   c. Ileus: paralytic, intestinal obstruction
   d. Hernias
   e. Anorectal lesions
   f. Colorectal cancer

NUTRITIONAL EXCESS AND DEFICIT

Ingesting more calories than are burned off by metabolism or activity leads to weight gain. Overweight (up to 20% above standard weight tables) does not in itself usually cause health problems, although the person is not at an optimal level of health (see Chapter 5). Obesity, however, does cause physiologic problems. Nutritional deficiencies also cause problems, the most common deficiency being protein-calorie malnutrition. Both obesity and protein-calorie malnutrition may require therapy.

OBESITY

Obesity is generally defined as weight greater than 20% of standard weight tables (see Table 5-1). One fourth of people in the United States can be classified as obese.[60] Persons who are 60% above the desirable weight have higher morbidity and mortality rates. *Massive* or *morbid obesity*, which is often defined as 45 kg (100 lb) over desirable weight, is extremely hazardous to health.

Etiology

Obesity results from a complex interrelationship of genetic, psychologic, social, and environmental factors (Box 31-3). Although "fatness" seems to occur in some families, much of this may be a result of learned eating behaviors of high caloric foods rather than genetic influence. Old age is not a factor; few elderly persons are obese. Mild overweight can be beneficial to elderly persons, as it provides nutrient stores during periods of stress and illness.

Pathophysiology

Obesity results from the intake of foods in amounts exceeding body needs; the excess is stored as fat. In persons of normal weight who gain weight, fat is deposited by *hypertrophy* of existing fat cells in adipose tissue. These people respond well to weight reduction regimens. Fat cells can also increase in number (*hyperplasia*). Excess food intake has been shown to stimulate hyperplasia. Hyperplasia is irreversible and conditions persons to be overweight throughout their lives.[31] Weight reduction in persons with hyperplastic obesity is difficult to achieve and to maintain.

Table 31-3 lists the physiologic effects of obesity. Increased fatty acid utilization, glucose, and body mass may contribute to the development of atherosclerosis, hypertension, emboli, gallstones, diabetes mellitus, osteoarthritis, angina and sudden death, and respiratory insufficiency.

Interventions

Nursing diagnoses, expected outcomes, and implementation of nursing actions to help the overweight person are described in Chapter 5. Persons with severe or massive obesity often have difficulty losing weight or maintaining weight loss by the usual dietary, behavior modification, and exercise approaches. These persons may require more drastic therapy.

Very low calorie diets

A variety of very low calorie diets (VLCD) have been used to treat obesity. VLCD consists of powdered formulas of egg and milk proteins that provide 400 to 800 kcal/day. Persons taking VLCD lose 2 to 4 lb/week over a 4- to 6-month program. Achievement of long-term weight loss requires a significant change in eating and exercise behaviors; therefore, the patient must follow behavior modification and exercise programs concurrently. Positive results of VLCD are rapid improvement in obesity-related diseases, but these benefits are offset by the potential for serious complications. Medical supervision is therefore essential. Side effects include hair loss, fatigue, cold intolerance, orthostatic hypotension, fluid and electrolyte disturbances,

---

Box 31-3

Factors influencing obesity

Genetic	Heavy bone structure, large muscle mass
Psychologic	Pleasure associated with eating Emotional problems (for example, grief, stress, or boredom) Interpersonal problems with family, friends, or coworkers
Sociologic	Learned behaviors of overeating or eating high caloric foods Reinforcement from others to eat large amounts of high caloric foods
Environmental	Easy availability of high caloric "junk" foods Availability of money to spend on high caloric foods

---

Table 31-3 Physiologic effects of obesity

Parameter	Metabolic effect	Associated disorder
Increased fatty acid utilization	Hypertriglyceridemia	Atherosclerosis, hypertension, emboli
	Increased cholesterol synthesis	Gallstones
Increased glucose	Hyperinsulinism leading to pancreatic β-cell failure	Diabetes mellitus
Increased body mass	Cumulative trauma to weight-bearing joints	Osteoarthritis
	Increased workload for heart	Angina, sudden death
	Decreased thorax expansion with decreased tidal volume	Respiratory insufficiency

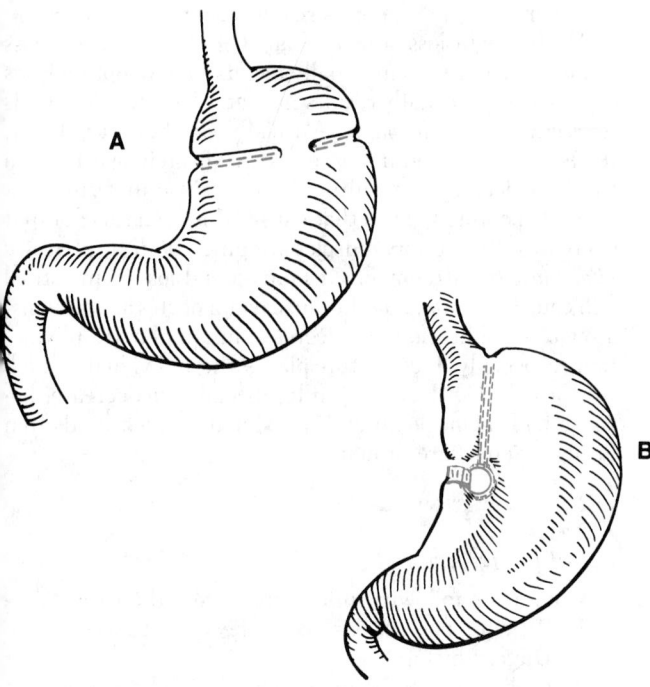

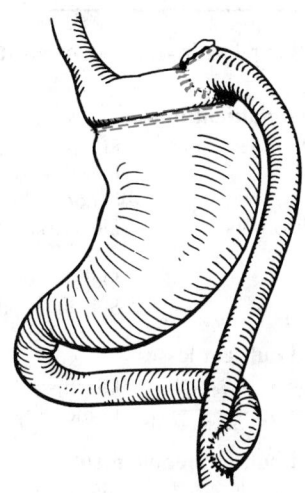

Fig. 31-5   Roux-en-Y retrocolic gastric bypass. Stomach is stapled completely horizontally; jejunum is resected from duodenum and connected to stomach entrance; distal duodenal stump is connected to jejunum to permit drainage of intestinal secretions.

Fig. 31-4   Gastric partitioning. **A,** Horizontal gastroplasty; **B,** vertical-banded gastroplasty.

and other signs of protein-calorie malnutrition. Long-term results are generally disappointing; the majority of these persons regain considerable weight.[16,60]

Surgery

When the person is morbidly obese and when other methods have been diligently tried and have failed, the physician may consider surgery. Criteria for surgery include morbid obesity for at least 5 years, no major illness, evidence of serious dietary efforts, and high motivation. Obese persons are a high surgical risk, however, and the surgery itself adds more risks.

The more common surgical approaches are *gastroplasty*, which reduces food intake (horizontal gastroplasty or vertical banding gastroplasty), and *gastric bypass* (see next discussion). The first type of surgery for massive obesity was an *intestinal bypass*, in which the jejunum was anastomosed to the ileum, thereby bypassing most of the small intestines. Serious metabolic complications have resulted from the intestinal bypass; therefore, this method is now rarely used.

Gastroplasty

This procedure makes the stomach smaller by placing sutures *horizontally* or *vertically* through the stomach walls (Fig. 31-4). A small pouch thus forms, which limits the amount of food the person can take without experiencing pain and vomiting. This type of surgery has fewer consequences than bypass surgery because the gastrointestinal tract is not opened and remains intact. The vertical banded gastroplasty is the preferred method.[68]

Postoperatively, if irrigation through the nasogastric

tube is necessary, only a small amount of fluid (30 ml) is used. The patient takes clear fluids on about the third day and, if they are tolerated, advances to a diet of pureed foods. The patient then follows a blenderized diet for 8 weeks, at which time small amounts of soft bland foods and vitamin supplements are introduced gradually. Solid foods are then introduced slowly. Foods to be avoided initially are meat and skin of poultry or fish, foods high in cellulose that are not easily digested, and high-calorie foods (such as milkshakes and alcohol). Upper abdominal pain radiating to the left shoulder following surgery may indicate perforation of the stomach by the staples. Occasional vomiting is commonly encountered.

Gastric bypass

A Roux-en-Y gastric bypass is illustrated in Fig. 31-5; the resected jejunum is attached to a closed-off pouch of the upper stomach created by complete horizontal stapling. This procedure involves intrusion of the gastrointestinal tract, and the care of the patient is similar to that for other gastric surgeries (p. 954). Foods are introduced as for postgastroplasty. Complications include dumping syndrome, uncontrolled vomiting, leaks in the suture lines, and pulmonary infections.

Gastric balloon

A different method to facilitate weight loss is the gastric balloon (Garren-Edward gastric bubble). This is a *temporary* method used in conjunction with dietary control, exercise, and behavior modification. The gastric balloon is a polyurethane balloon with a hollow central channel that is inserted by endoscopy into the stomach. The balloon is

<table>
<tr><td>31-4</td><td>

Causes of protein-calorie malnutrition

Decreased nutrient intake

Anorexia	Financial distress
Nausea	Inability to shop or
Dysphagia	cook
Mouth disorders	Decreased desire to
Pain	cook
	Depression
	Substance abuse

Increased nutrient losses

Vomiting	Diarrhea
Malabsorption	Immobility

Increased nutrient requirements

Surgery	Infection
Fever	Cancer

</td></tr>
</table>

then inflated with 200 to 220 ml of air through a catheter attached to a self-sealing valve. The balloon occupies about 25% of the stomach capacity and thus produces early satiety. Side effects include nausea, vomiting, crampy pain, and heartburn, especially during the first week. Some controlled studies, however, have not demonstrated significant increase in weight loss with the gastric balloon.[60]

PROTEIN-CALORIE MALNUTRITION

Etiology

Protein-calorie malnutrition is the most common form of nutritional deficiency in the United States. Causes include decreased nutrient intake, increased nutrient loss, and increased nutrient requirements (see Box 31-4). Approximately 20% of hospitalized patients have protein-calorie malnutrition. In developing countries, this disorder is a major health problem. It may occur in two forms, *Kwashiorkor* (protein deficiency when calorie intake is inadequate) and *marasmus* (deficiency of both proteins and calories). The typical child with kwashiorkor has thin extremities and ascites of the abdomen.

Pathophysiology

If diets contain sufficient carbohydrates and fats, the body will use these nutrients for energy needs. When the caloric intake is reduced, however, increased amounts of body proteins will be used for energy. The body will meet energy requirements at the expense of protein needs.

A deficiency of both calories and protein is characteristic of protein-calorie malnutrition in adults. Proteins are constantly being synthesized and broken down into amino acids in the body to be reformed into other proteins. Amino acids that are not used are excreted. The body can synthesize certain amino acids (nonessential) but depends on ingested proteins to supply the eight essential amino acids. When more nitrogen (the end product of amino acid breakdown) is excreted than is ingested in proteins, the body is said to be in *negative nitrogen balance*, and weight loss, decreased

muscle mass, and weakness result from tissue catabolism.

With weight loss of more than 10% of body weight, loss of physiologic function usually begins to develop, and loss of 35% to 40% usually results in death.[60] Protein loss leads to *decreased muscle mass*, especially in the liver, heart, lungs, GI tract, and immune system. Protein synthesis in the liver decreases, resulting in a decrease in serum proteins (hypoproteinemia) that cause *edema*. Cardiac output decreases. Respiratory muscles atrophy, leading to *decreased vital capacity*. Atrophy of GI mucosa and loss of intestinal villi cause *malabsorption*. Because lymphocytes are proteins, a major complication is a decrease in lymphocyte production, especially T cells; this places the individual at high *risk for infection*. Hemoglobin levels may also decrease, because both hemoglobin and transferrin (which binds iron in hemoglobin) are proteins.

Nursing Process

Assessment

Subjective data

Obtain the following information from the patient:
1. Patient's perceptions about the weight loss
2. Dietary history
3. Foods that can be tolerated; likes and dislikes
4. Ability and desire to eat
5. Facilities and ability for purchasing, storing, and preparing food
6. Financial resources, if appropriate

Objective data

Objective data include the following:
1. Weight and height
   Underweight is considered to be less than 90% of desirable weight (Chapter 5); severe weight loss is less than 75% of desirable weight
2. Signs of infection or skin breakdown

Diagnostic tests

1. Low hemoglobin levels in absence of blood loss
2. Plasma albumin level of less than 3.0 g/100 ml on two or more determinations, indicating decreased protein synthesis
3. Urinary creatinine of less than 20 mg/kg in 24 hours for males or less than 16 mg/kg in females, with a normal plasma creatinine level, indicating decreased muscle mass

Data analysis: nursing diagnoses

Nursing diagnoses are determined from analysis of patient data. Possible nursing diagnoses for the person with protein-calorie malnutrition may include, but are not limited to, the following:

Diagnostic title	Possible etiologies
Fatigue	Muscle weakness, inadequate nutrition
Infection, high risk for	Decreased nutrition, decreased immune response
Nutrition, altered: less than body requirements	Inadequate nutrient intake, increased nutrient losses, increased nutrient requirements

Planning: expected patient outcomes

If oral intake is permitted, the patient's fullest cooperation will be needed to increase the possibility of adequate nutritional intake. Patient participation in the planning is therefore a vital part of the care.

Expected patient outcomes for the person with protein-calorie malnutrition may include, but are not limited to, the following:

1. The patient includes rest periods in the day's activities.
2. Infection does not occur.
3. If eating is permitted, the patient:
   a. Participates in menu selection.
   b. Eats all food on tray, if hospitalized.
   c. Eats six small meals per day plus supplementary foods and vitamins, as planned, at home.
4. If tube feedings are given:
   a. Feedings are given at a slow, constant rate.
   b. Patient is hydrated.
   c. Patient states feeling comfortable.
   d. Complications do not occur or are quickly corrected.
5. If total parenteral nutrition (TPN) is given:
   a. Fluid and electrolyte balance is maintained.
   b. Hypoglycemia or hyperglycemia do not occur.
   c. Infection and air embolism do not occur.
   d. Patient states feeling comfortable.

Implementation
Assisting with achievement of therapeutic goals
Gastrostomy

Method. Gastrostomy is an alternative approach to nasogastric tube feedings when the person is unable to swallow for a long period. The procedure takes place under local or general anesthesia and involves the creation of an opening into the abdomen and insertion of the catheter through the stomach wall.

The *percutaneous endoscopic gastrostomy* (PEG) does not require incision into the abdominal cavity and is a safer and more rapid method. It is performed under local anesthesia; the patient is mildly sedated. A small incision is made on the skin of the abdomen, and a cannula is pushed through the adjacent abdominal and gastric walls while the site is observed through a gastroscope. A long silk suture is threaded through the cannula, grasped through the endoscope, and pulled up through the endoscope, which is then removed. The exit end of a specially prepared mushroom catheter is attached to the thread, and the catheter is then pulled in retrograde fashion through the esophagus and stomach and out the abdominal wall. Internal and external dams hold the catheter in place. A jejunostomy tube may be inserted by the same method.

Food and fluids. After gastrostomy tube insertion, the physician may order the tube to be attached to low intermittent suction for 24 hours, or fluids may begin the first day. The following method may be used for giving the initial feedings, as tolerated:[16]

Day 1: One half concentration of feeding solution at 25 ml/hr by continuous drip

Day 2: Full-strength feeding solution at 50 ml/hr by continuous drip

Day 3: Full-strength solution at 75 ml/hr by continuous drip

After day 3, as tolerated: change to bolus feeding of 500 ml every 4 to 6 hours for gastrostomies; jejunostomies require continuous infusions

Principles of administration are the same as for tube feedings. A dressing is not generally used to prevent the possibility of skin maceration, breakdown, or infection. Clean the skin with hydrogen peroxide solution to remove crusts and rinse with normal saline or water.

The psychologic trauma of not being able to eat normally is usually severe. The patient may become depressed and needs a great deal of encouragement. However, as most patients become proficient in feeding themselves, they gradually accept this method of obtaining nourishment as inevitable and adjust remarkably well.

Interventions to achieve patient outcomes
Preventing fatigue

The loss of muscle mass and the decreased utilization of nutrients lead to decreased energy production and fatigue. Rest periods are therefore essential to decrease energy expenditure. Dyspnea with exertion and pulse rates that take longer than 5 minutes to stabilize are signs that activities need to be modified.

Preventing infection

Maintenance of medical and surgical asepsis is particularly important for the person with protein-calorie malnutrition. These individuals should avoid any person with upper respiratory infections. If the patient is relatively immobile in chair or bed, good skin care is essential to prevent skin breakdown and subsequent infection. Surgical wounds may heal more slowly, and they require strict surgical asepsis.

Encouraging oral intake

Adequate nutrients to meet nutritional requirements can be taken by oral, enteral (tube feedings, gastrostomy), or TPN. The best way to receive nutrients is the oral route. Persons with inadequate nutrition stores need encouragement to eat, although forced feeding may lead to frustration or nausea and vomiting. Motivating a person with anorexia to eat can be a challenge. Interventions that can correct the cause will lead to improved appetite. Providing an environment conducive to eating and providing several small meals rather than three large meals per day may facilitate an adequate nutritional intake.

A high-calorie, high-protein diet is indicated if the patient can eat. The diet is essentially a normal one with added protein and supplementary high-calorie feedings. High-protein diets are contraindicated if there is liver disease.

Facilitating tube feedings

Nasoenteral tubes are used to provide nutrients when a person with normal intestinal function is unable to ingest sufficient nutrients by oral ingestion, has difficulty swal-

Table 31-4 Tube feedings

	Elemental	Supplemental	Liquid whole foods
Examples	Vivonex Flexical Pregestimil	Precision Vital	Ensure Sustacal Isocal
Content	Simple carbohydrates, amino acids	Complex carbohydrates, peptides	Complex carbohydrates, proteins
Osmolality	500-800 mOsm	450-600 mOsm	300-600 mOsm
Advantages	Given through small-bore tube Well tolerated for prolonged use	Can be given through small-bore tube More effective protein content than elemental	Lower osmolality Moderate price Acceptable flavor More nutritionally complete High fat content
Disadvantages	Unpalatable High osmolality Not well tolerated by bolus feeding Excellent culture media for bacteria Expensive Require monitoring of blood glucose and electrolytes	More expensive than liquid whole foods Tend to coagulate in tube Require monitoring of blood glucose and electrolytes	Tend to coagulate in tube May require a large-bore tube

lowing, or has mild to moderate malabsorption (short bowel syndrome). The tube is inserted through the nose and terminates in the stomach, duodenum, or jejunum.

Feeding tubes are soft polyurethane or silicone tubes with a narrow lumen (usually No. 5F to No. 8F), although in some instances a larger bore tube (No. 12F or No. 14F) may be necessary. Some tubes have a monofilament or stainless steel stylet for easy passage. A tube with a weighted end may be used to help pass the tube through the pylorus into the intestine, if desired.

Technique. Administration of tube feedings may be by bolus, gravity drip, or infusion pump. *Bolus* delivery consists of infusing 300 to 400 ml of formula over several minutes four to six times daily.[28] It is appropriate only for persons who can eat and are receiving supplemental tube feedings. The sudden influx of the feeding may cause nausea, cramping, diarrhea, or aspiration. The *gravity* method consists of placing the feeding in a feeding bag attached to the nasoenteral tube and allowing the fluid to run in by gravity. Disadvantages of this method include erratic fluid flow and greater potential of tube blockage. The gravity method may be used for intermittent or continuous administration. Most persons can tolerate 250 to 400 ml per feeding given over 20 to 30 minutes. The *infusion pump* is the preferred method for more constant administration rate and less probability of tube blockage or of diarrhea; however, it is more expensive. Pump accuracy must be checked routinely by comparing the actual drop count with the preestablished rate.

Solutions. Different types of fluids may be given by tube feedings (Table 31-4). Blenderized whole foods may be used; these are nutritious and less expensive, but they require large-bore tubes and are good culture media for bacteria. Elemental and semielemental feedings are more easily digested and can be given through small-bore tubes, but they are more expensive and less nutritionally complete than liquid whole foods.

Complications. Methods of preventing complications include the following:

1. Regurgitation with aspiration
   a. Keep head elevated to at least 30 degrees at all times.
   b. Monitor tube position every 4 hours.
2. Tube dislodgement: tape tube to nose.
3. Tube clogging
   a. Give fluid at a constant rate (by pump, if possible).
   b. Give water before and after intermittent feedings and medications, and q4h during continuous feedings.
   c. Give medications by *liquid* form; crushed tablets may clog tube.
4. Bacterial contamination
   a. Do not let feeding of freshly blended formulas (perishable) hang for more than 6 hours, ready-to-use formulas more than 24 hours, and all other formulas more than 12 hours.
   b. Use prefilled delivery sets if possible; if unavailable, use ready-to-use formulas that do not have to be diluted or reconstituted (the less the handling, the less the potential for contamination).
   c. Rinse delivery set before adding new formula.
5. Dehydration
   a. Give water as necessary; total fluid intake should equal urinary output.
   b. Iso-osmolality is 300 mOsm; the greater the osmolality of the feeding, the more water is needed.
   c. Give extra water if the need is increased, as with fever.
   d. Monitor for signs of dehydration: thirst, oliguria, decreased skin turgor, dry mucous membranes.
6. Diarrhea
   a. When starting tube feedings, initiate feedings slowly at half-strength, then increase concentration and rate gradually (at different times).

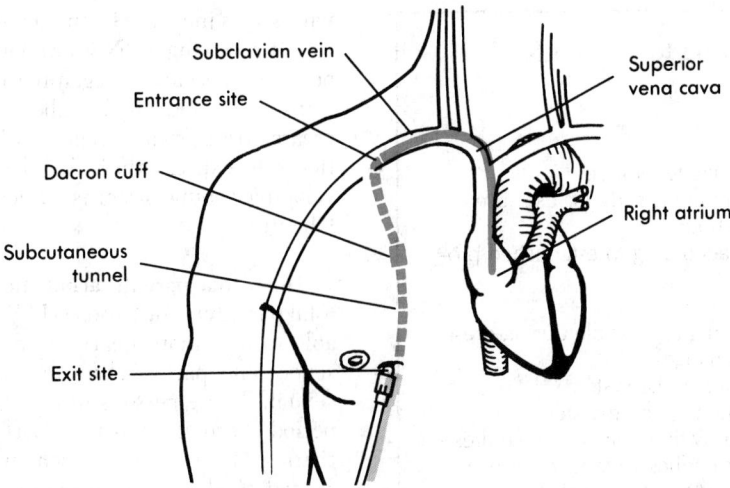

Fig. 31-6 Placement of Hickman catheter for administration of TPN solutions.

b. Dilute elixers and hypertonic oral suspensions before inserting through feeding tube.

d. If diarrhea occurs:
1. Check concurrent medications for those that may be causing the diarrhea; consult with physician.
2. If medication is not a cause, decrease rate of fluid flow.
3. Administer prescribed antidiarrheal medication through tube.

7. Hyperglycemia
a. Monitor urine for glucose and acetone every 4 to 6 hours until stable.
b. If urine tests positively, decrease rate of feeding flow and notify physician.

Home tube feedings. Patients can maintain home tube feedings after receiving instruction in insertion and care of the tube, in formula care and insertion, and in monitoring for complications. An enteral feeding pump may be rented or purchased. The person needs to know where in the community to purchase materials (tubes, administration sets, and formula bags).

Facilitating total parenteral nutrition

Total parenteral nutrition (TPN) is a method of giving concentrated solutions intravenously to maintain protein synthesis. Indications for this therapy are (1) major gastrointestinal diseases, fistulas, or inflammatory diseases; (2) extensive negative nitrogen balance, such as occurs with major body burns, extensive wounds, or cachexia; and (3) gastrointestinal side effects from radiation therapy.

Technique. Under strict aseptic conditions, a central venous catheter is inserted into the subclavian vein through the chest wall (Fig. 31-6) or into the basilic vein in the antecubital fossa and then threaded through to the superior vena cava. The large amount of blood in the superior vena cava helps to dilute the highly concentrated solution rapidly and thus prevent phlebitis or vein occlusion.

A Hickman catheter is commonly used in place of a standard intracatheter. This catheter is designed so that the end of the catheter can be capped between infusions. When infusion is complete, fill the catheter with heparinized saline solution to prevent clotting and cap it until the next infusion.

The catheter is secured with one suture and covered by an air-occlusive dressing. The dressing may be transparent (OpSite) or a gauze dressing covered entirely with adhesive tape. Start the infusion with a standard intravenous fluid (5% dextrose) until a radiograph confirms the location of the catheter tip in the superior vena cava.

Solutions. Solutions for TPN are good culture media and are prepared under strict aseptic conditions in the pharmacy under a laminar airflow hood. The physician orders the solution contents based on the person's nutritional needs. Keep the solutions refrigerated until ready for use and then warm them to room temperature before infusion. Use prepared formulas within 48 hours to prevent contamination.

TPN solutions usually consist of 25% to 35% dextrose, 3% to 5% amino acids, electrolytes, minerals, and vitamins. Fat emulsions (10% to 20%) may also be added through a separate peripheral IV over 4 to 12 hours or through a Y connector in the main line.[71] Dextrose and fat are given for caloric value to spare the proteins for anabolism. Fat provides twice the caloric value of glucose, exerts minimal osmotic pressure, and prevents fatty acid deficiency. Regular insulin may be added to the TPN solution or may be given by injection for glucose utilization.

Complications. Complications of TPN may be mechanical, infectious, or metabolic. *Mechanical* problems may include pneumothorax, hemothorax, air embolism, catheter misplacement, brachial plexus injury, and thromboembolism. These complications are rare with correct catheter insertion and maintenance. *Infection* is a serious complication but can be prevented by using conscientious aseptic technique during catheter insertion and subsequent care.

The major *metabolic* alterations are hyperglycemia or,

The patient receiving total parenteral nutrition

Prevent infection
Maintain strict aseptic technique
Keep solutions cold until ready for use; use within 24 to 36 hours
Change dressings according to established protocols
Prevent air embolism
Position patient as flat as possible during dressing and tubing changes
Tape all connections of the system
Clamp catheter when opening system
Cover insertion site with an air-occlusive dressing (covered with adhesive tape) or transparent polyurethane (Op-Site) dressing
Maintain fluid and electrolyte balance
Maintain a continuous uniform infusion rate
If rate is too *slow:*
Return rate to prescribed rate
If prescribed rate does not resume, ask person to change position
Monitor and report to physician signs of *hypoglycemia* (pallor, diaphoresis, tachycardia, hunger, trembling, behavioral changes)
If rate is too *fast:*
Slow infusion to prescribed rate
Monitor for signs of *overhydration* (neck vein distention, cough, weight gain)
Monitor for signs of *hyperglycemia* (sugar in urine, nausea, weakness, thirst, headache)
Monitor daily weights and intake and output
Monitor serum electrolyte, glucose, and blood urea nitrogen (BUN) levels
Encourage ambulation, activities of daily living
Promote comfort
Provide for good oral hygiene
Provide emotional support to enhance coping

more rarely, hypoglycemia. Other possible alterations include fluid imbalances; electrolyte imbalances in sodium, potassium, calcium, magnesium, and phosphates; and acid-base imbalances (primarily acidosis). Vitamin D deficiency and vitamin A excess may also occur. Monitor serum levels several times a week, and test urine for sugar and acetone. Weigh the patient daily for the first 2 weeks and three times a week thereafter. Early satiety may occur for several days after TPN is discontinued.

Patient care. Care of the patient receiving TPN consists of preventing infection and air embolism, maintaining fluid and electrolyte balance, encouraging ambulation and activities of daily living, and promoting comfort (see Box 31-5).

Patients may have many fears and concerns about being fed by intravenous fluids over a long period of time. They should understand what is occurring and the reason for the frequent dressing changes. Encourage them to sit at the dinner table to participate in the social interaction. If food is not permitted orally, persons may need aid in coping with stress incurred by the smell of food or watching others eat. If receiving TPN over a long period of time, they may be concerned about regaining taste or normal eating patterns. Being fed only by tube, even though temporary, may create stress from a change in body image. Encourage patients to express their feelings and support them in developing coping patterns to deal with these stresses (see Chapter 6).

Home total parenteral nutrition. Since the advent of home total parenteral nutrition (HTPN) many persons have been able to lead more nearly normal lives—going to work or school and participating in selected activities, including sexual. These persons infuse the solutions over a 12-hour period overnight and then participate in normal daily activities. Their lives are somewhat limited by being connected to the infusing equipment for the 12 hours, although there are vest systems that support the HTPN solution, tubing, and pump to provide increased mobility. There are also 24-hour battery packs to provide more freedom for the person who is connected to a pump that requires an electrical outlet.

Learning to mix, infuse, and disconnect the infusion and care for the equipment may be overwhelming at first for both patient and family. The hospital nurse begins teaching in the hospital well before the patient is discharged; the home health nurse continues the process at home. Teaching includes the following:

1. Principles of aseptic technique
2. Opening and setting up bags
3. Starting pump, stopping infusion, flushing tubing, clamping tube
4. Maintaining and troubleshooting equipment
5. Catheter care
6. Monitoring for signs of complications
7. Where to obtain supplies and need for storage space for supplies in the home

Companies that supply HTPN equipment and supplies often have a nutrition support nurse who can provide information as necessary and may have an instruction manual for patient use.[18]

HTPN teams are available to assist the person or family member to carry out TPN care at home. Before the patient is discharged, the home health nurse meets with other team members and the patient to facilitate the move home. The home health nurse then assists the person with HTPN at home until the person becomes self-sufficient and can manage independently. The patient maintains contact with the health team for assistance with changes that are needed and with problems that may arise. The person often requires changes in solution content depending on response to therapy.

Complications of HTPN are similar to those of TPN. However, risk of infection increases, mostly from *Staphylococcus aureus*. Catheter damage may occur from repeated cross-clamping; however, the catheter may be repaired with a catheter repair kit. An occluded catheter may be opened by instillation of urokinase or streptokinase into the catheter. Unusual metabolic deficiencies may occur with long-term therapy, such as deficiencies in chromium, selenium, molybdenum, and vitamins A and E.

HTPN is expensive, but the cost is considerably less than the similar care provided in a health care center. In addition, the person can remain at home and have continuity in activities of daily living.

Evaluation

Evaluation is based on expected patient outcomes. Questions to consider include the following:

1. Does the patient include rest periods in the day's activities?
2. Has infection been avoided?
3. If eating is permitted, does the patient participate in menu selection?
4. If tube feedings are given, is patient hydrated?
5. If TPN is given, have infection, air embolism, and other complications been avoided?

INGESTIVE DISORDERS

VOMITING

Although vomiting is a symptom rather than a disorder per se, it is a common disruption of motility of the upper GI tract and therefore is discussed here.

Pathophysiology

Vomiting is often preceded by nausea but may occur alone. It may be a symptom of a disease process (such as infection or uremia) or a response to drugs, visceral injury, pain, psychic trauma, radiation, or motion. Vomiting is initiated by the vomiting center in the brain. It is reverse peristalsis. Vomiting can be defined as forceful ejection of stomach contents. If the pyloric end of the stomach is obstructed, the vomitus will project away from the person (projectile vomiting).

Prolonged and severe vomiting will interfere with nutrition and cause fluid and electrolyte imbalance, specifically dehydration and metabolic alkalosis with loss of potassium, chloride, and hydrogen ions. The act of vomiting produces a strain on the abdominal muscles, and in some postoperative patients it may cause wound dehiscence or bleeding. Vomiting is especially dangerous for anesthetized patients, comatose persons, and infants because they are likely to aspirate the vomitus into the lungs. Aspiration may block oxygen intake (asphyxia) or lead to inflammation of the lung (atelectasis, pneumonitis), especially in an elderly person whose nasopharyngeal reflexes are less acute than those of a younger person.

Assessment

Subjective data: onset of vomiting, patient's perception of cause

Objective data: examination of vomitus

1. Greenish yellow: bile
2. Bright red: overt bleeding of recent origin
3. Brownish "coffee-ground": blood has been in the stomach for a period of time and is partly digested
4. Fecal odor: intestinal contents from an intestinal obstruction

Vomiting of blood is termed *hematemesis*. It is important to ascertain whether the content expelled from the mouth has been vomited from the stomach or coughed up from the lungs. Bloody sputum usually has a more frothy appearance than hematemesis. "Dry" emesis or retching may occur when the stomach is empty.

Implementation

1. Assisting with achievement of therapeutic goals
   a. If vomiting is anticipated (such as with radiation or motion), give prescribed antiemetic 30 minutes before the event.
   b. If vomiting is present, give prescribed antiemetic by suppository or *deep* intramuscular injection.
2. Assisting with comfort
   a. Provide a calm environment to decrease anxiety.
   b. Suggest deep breaths through the mouth if nausea or gagging occurs.
   c. Remove vomitus as soon as possible and provide oral hygiene.
   d. Provide fluids in small amounts after vomiting subsides; ginger ale and other effervescent drinks are usually well tolerated.
   e. Provide solid foods (after vomiting subsides) that are well tolerated, such as crackers, baked potato, or apple.

INFLAMMATORY DISORDERS OF THE MOUTH

Etiology

The mouth is an excellent barometer of general health, reflecting general disease and debility as well as good health. Specific diseases of the mouth most often occur when general nutrition and oral hygiene are poor, when people neglect their teeth, and when smoking is excessive.

In the mouth, inflammation may occur on the mucous membranes, gum, or tongue from viruses, bacteria, fungi, or irritants.

Pathophysiology

Several factors contribute to the development of oral inflammatory disorders: (1) poor oral hygiene, (2) stress, (3) nutritional deficiencies, (4) debilitating diseases, (5) heavy smoking, and (6) chemotherapy. Poor oral hygiene leads to mouth debris that can irritate the mucous membranes. Other irritants include smoke, broken teeth, and irritating foods. Stress, malnutrition, and chemotherapy interfere with the body's immune response, leading to breakdown of body defenses.

Inflammation of the mucous membranes (*stomatitis*) often results in small, painful ulcerations. Scarring rarely occurs, as only the mucous membrane is usually involved. Inflammation of the gums may cause teeth to loosen. Causative organisms include bacteria, viruses, or fungi.

Aphthous stomatitis (Table 31-5) occurs frequently, especially among young adults. The lesions are painful but usually heal in about 1 to 3 weeks. *Herpetic* stomatitis may occur only once or be recurrent. People receiving immunosuppressive drugs have increased susceptibility.

Thrush frequently occurs when antibiotics are given

Table 31-5 Inflammatory disorders of mouth

Disease	Signs and symptoms	Medical therapy
Aphthous stomatitis (canker sores)	Ulcer on mucous membranes becomes covered with opaque material; pain	Fluocinonide in emollient dental paste (Lidex in Orabase), hydrocortisone ointment
Herpetic stomatitis (cold sore, fever blister)	Painful vesicle formation on junction of lips to mucosa, lymphadenopathy, crusting, malaise	Symptomatic treatment: analgesics, bland mouth rinses; rest; avoidance of stress
Vincent's gingivitis (ulceromembranous stomatitis)	Malaise, acute painful bleeding gums, fetid breath, ulceration on margins of gums, dysphagia	Gentle debridement by dentist; mouthwashes with warm normal saline or 3% hydrogen peroxide; rest; antibiotics if severe
Candidiasis (thrush)	White patches (like milk curds) over inflamed membranes	Nystatin oral suspension Clotrimazole troches (Mycelex) Ketoconazole tablets (Nizoral)
Gingivitis (gums)	Red inflamed gums, bleeding with minimum injury, swelling of interdental spaces	Good oral hygiene and dental care
Periodontitis (loss of bone supporting teeth)	Same as for gingivitis, loose teeth, recession of gums, possible abscess formation	Dental care, dental surgery

over a period of time to control other infections. It is thought that the elimination of bacteria permits growth of the existing fungus, causing thrush. Persons at higher risk include denture wearers, persons with debilitating or acute illnesses, or those with impaired immune response.[60]

The parotid gland that drains into the mouth may also become inflamed (parotitis). Acute communicable parotitis (mumps) is caused by a virus that is transmitted by direct contact with the saliva. Noncommunicable parotitis occurs in debilitated persons whose oral hygiene is poor, whose mouths have been permitted to become dry, and who have not chewed solid foods regularly. Elderly persons are more susceptible than younger ones. Usually the *staphylococcus* organism is not present.

Nursing Process
Assessment

In patients at high risk of developing infections, assess the mouth daily for developing or healing inflammations.

Subjective data

Question the patient about the presence and extent of the following symptoms: (1) pain in the mouth, (2) loss of appetite, (3) nausea, (4) foul taste in the mouth, and (5) increase or decrease of salivation. The inflammatory response causes the pain, which restricts ability or desire to keep the teeth and mouth clean. This leads to the foul taste and loss of appetite. Swallowing of inflammatory debris may produce nausea.

Objective data

1. Mouth inspection
   a. Cleanliness
   b. Condition of teeth (caries, loose teeth, debris)
   c. Signs of inflammation (redness, edema, ulceration, or white curdlike patches of thrush)
   d. Bleeding of mucous membranes or gums
2. Ability of patient to carry out oral hygiene

   a. Mental status (decreased consciousness or confusion)
   b. Ability to open mouth (pain may limit mouth movement)
   c. Cleanliness of mouth after oral hygiene
3. Ability to ingest and swallow food

Data analysis: nursing diagnoses

Nursing diagnoses are determined from analysis of patient data. Possible nursing diagnoses for the person with a mouth infection may include, but are not limited, to the following:

Diagnostic title	Possible etiologies
Oral mucous membrane, altered	Poor oral hygiene, inflammation
Pain, mouth	Inflammation of mouth
Fluid volume deficit, high risk for	Foul taste, mouth discomfort
Nutrition, altered: less than body requirements	Difficulty chewing, foul taste, mouth discomfort
Knowledge deficit	Lack of exposure/recall

Planning: expected patient outcomes

Expected patient outcomes for the person with a mouth infection may include, but are not limited to, the following:
1. Mouth is clean; mucosa is pink and moist.
2. Says mouth feels comfortable.
3. Has a fluid intake greater than 1500 ml/day; skin turgor is good.
4. Eats a balanced diet; weight remains stable.
5. Describes risk factors to be avoided to prevent recurrence of oral inflammations.

Implementation
Assisting with achievement of therapeutic goals

If antibiotics are ordered, give them on time on a regular schedule to maintain blood levels. If the patient has dif ficulty swallowing tablets, crush the tablets, if possible, or give the antibiotics intramuscularly or intravenously. If nystatin is prescribed for oral thrush, the patient should hold the suspension and swish it through the mouth for as long as possible before swallowing it.

Interventions to achieve patient outcomes
Providing mouth care

Thorough and frequent mouth care is a must to remove the debris and to permit healing of the oral mucosa.
1. Frequency
   a. Mild stomatitis: at least every 4 hours
   b. Severe stomatitis: at least every 2 hours
2. Types of solutions
   a. Alkaline mouthwashes, such as sodium bicarbonate or sodium perborate
   b. Hydrogen peroxide diluted 1:4 with normal saline (mix just before use to prevent decomposition)
   c. Lidocaine rinses may be prescribed for stomatitis resulting from chemotherapeutic drugs
3. Removal of dentures if causing pain
4. Use foam-sponge toothbrushes, such as toothettes
5. If the toothbrush causes pain, gently wipe gum and teeth with moistened gauze wrapped around a tongue blade; rinse with solution followed by water

Promoting pain relief

Pain may be partially relieved by good oral hygiene. Smoking is contraindicated. Cold drinks or sucking on frozen Popsicles may be soothing. Analgesic drugs may be necessary, and lidocaine may be applied to provide topical anesthesia.

Facilitating eating and drinking

If the mouth is very sore and painful, eating may be difficult, and the patient may need considerable encouragement. Patients can best tolerate soft foods, including strained meats and fish, pureed vegetables and fruits (except citrus), cooked cereals, soups, flavored gelatin, and ice cream. Hot spicy foods are to be avoided; cold drinks may be soothing. High-protein, high-calorie drinks such as eggnog serve both nutritional and fluid needs.

Patient teaching

Persons at high risk for developing recurrent oral infections need to know about contributing factors that may be controlled, such as poor oral hygiene, poor nutrition, irritating foods, heavy smoking, and stress (see preventive measures, p. 922).

Evaluation

Evaluation is based on the expected patient outcomes. Interventions may have to be modified based on the severity of the oral infection. Assess mouth daily for cleanliness and extent of healing and comfort. Questions to consider include
1. Are mucous membranes clear and pink?
2. Does the patient state mouth feels comfortable?
3. Is the patient hydrated?
4. Has the patient's weight remained stable?
5. Can the patient describe ways to avoid recurrent infection?

CANCER OF THE MOUTH
Epidemiology

Cancer of the mouth (Table 31-6) accounts for about 3% of all cancers. Men are affected twice as often as women, and occurrences are more frequent after age 45; the average patient age is about 60.[60] An increasing number of teenagers are developing oral cancer from chewing tobacco or betel leaf. Although any part of the mouth may be affected, the lips and the anterior tongue and floor of the mouth are the most common sites.

Pathophysiology

Most oral cancers are squamous cell carcinomas; occasionally the tumor may be a basal cell carcinoma that starts on the skin and spreads to the lips. Risk factors include

Table 31-6   Cancer of mouth and esophagus

Place	Cases/year	Contributing factors	Signs and symptoms	Medical therapy
Mouth				
Lips	3600	Smoking, alcohol, sunlight	Fissure or painless indurated ulcer	Excision, jaw reconstruction if extensive
Anterior tongue and floor of mouth	17,800	Smoking, alcohol, chewing tobacco	Ulcer or growth	Local tissue perfusion with antimetabolites Partial or total excision of tongue Radical neck dissection if extensive Radiation therapy instead of or following surgery
Esophagus	9400	Alcohol, heavy smoking	Dysphagia, regurgitation, aspiration of fluids, foul breath odor	Upper and middle one third: esophagogastrostomy Lower one third: esophagogastrectomy

heavy tobacco and alcohol use; the combination causes an apparent breakdown in the immune system. Ultraviolet rays from the sun are a risk factor for cancer of the lips.

Oral cancers can be classified according to four stages. In stages I and II, there is no lymph node spread or metastasis; tumor size varies from less than 2 cm (I) up to 4 cm (II). In stage III, the tumor size is greater than 4 cm, and there may be a palpable node on one side. In stage IV, the tumor is invasive, and there may be metastasis to the liver or lungs. Surgery or radiation may be used to treat stage I cancers, and both therapies are used for stages II and III. Stage IV therapy is usually palliative.

Premalignant lesions (that may or may not become malignant) include *leukoplakia* (white patches), *erythroplasia* (red granular patches), and *erythroplakia* (white plaques within red patches). The red patches have a higher potential for malignancy than leukoplakia.[60]

The cure rate for cancer of the *lips* is high because the lesion is easily apparent to the patient and to others. Metastasis to regional lymph nodes has occurred in 10% of people when the case is diagnosed. In some instances a lesion may spread rapidly and involve the mandible and the floor of the mouth by direct extension.

Cancer of the *anterior tongue* and *floor of the mouth* may seem to occur together because their spread to adjacent tissues is so rapid. Metastasis to the neck has already occurred in more than 60% of people when the diagnosis is made because of the tongue's abundant vascular and lymphatic drainage. The mortality rate is high in stages III and IV. Lesions about the base of the tongue may go unnoticed by the patient and may be far advanced when treatment begins.

Prevention and Health Education

Primary prevention includes the following:
1. Avoid excess exposure to sun and wind on lips; use lip balm with sunscreen.
2. Eliminate smoking or chewing tobacco or betel leaf.
3. Maintain good oral hygiene and dental care.

Secondary prevention includes frequent dental examinations (the dentist may identify early lesions) and consulting the physician for a mouth lesion that does not heal within 2 to 3 weeks.

Nursing Process
Assessment
Subjective data

1. Eating patterns: changes may occur in the ability to eat certain foods, especially solids.
2. Discomfort in mouth (only seen with extensive lesions).
3. Concerns: the person's facial appearance will usually change, depending on the amount of tissue to be removed during surgery. Even with reconstructive surgery, noticeable changes will be present.

Objective data

Condition of mouth: persons with oral cancer frequently have poor dental hygiene; chemotherapy or radiation threatens intactness of mucous membranes; breath may be foul.

Data analysis: nursing diagnoses

Determine nursing diagnoses from analysis of patient data. Possible nursing diagnoses for the person receiving therapy for cancer of the mouth may include, but are not limited to, the following:

Diagnostic title	Possible etiologies
Oral mucous membranes, altered	Oral cavity radiation, decreased salivation
Nutrition, altered: less than body requirements	Chewing or swallowing difficulties, anorexia
Verbal communication, impaired	Resection of oral tissue
Body image disturbance	Actual/threat of facial/head disfigurement with therapy, foul breath

Planning: expected patient outcomes

Expected patient outcomes for the person receiving therapy for cancer of the mouth may include, but are not limited to, the following:
1. Incisions heal without infection.
2. Patient feeds self through appropriate means and consumes a nutritionally balanced fluid or soft diet.
3. Patient has a means of communication and is working to improve speech.
4. Patient interacts with others and states plans for gradual resumption of activities involving others.

Implementation
Assisting with achievement of therapeutic goals
Surgery

The tongue may be partially excised (hemiglossectomy) or totally excised (glossectomy). If the lymph nodes are involved, a radical neck dissection (Chapter 23) may be performed.

Antibiotics may be given *preoperatively* to decrease the number of bacteria present in the mouth. Prostheses of the palate and jaw may be designed to replace portions of tissue that have been resected. If a prosthesis is to be made, impressions will be taken during the preoperative period; the prosthesis will be fitted when healing has occurred postoperatively. If a composite resection including a radical neck dissection is to be performed, reconstructive surgery will be done, if possible, during the initial procedure; it may also be performed at a later date. *Postoperative* care of the patient is focused on promoting an adequate airway, mouth drainage, oral hygiene, comfort, nutrition, and speech (see Box 31-6).

Facilitating oral hygiene. Good mouth care is essential for comfort, prevention of infection, and promotion of healing. Teeth brushing is usually contraindicated because of discomfort and potential trauma. Use sterile equipment to prevent introduction of exogenous organisms, and encourage patients to assist in their oral hygiene as soon as possible.

Facilitating nutrition. Most patients can suction and feed themselves a few days after mouth surgery and are happier doing so. Chewing is difficult without the tongue, and the

The patient undergoing mouth surgery for cancer

Preoperative care

Clarify patient's knowledge of expected changes after surgery.

Explain expected postoperative measures (including suctioning, nasogastric tube).

Provide opportunities for patient and family to begin to express feelings about changes in body image.

Postoperative care

Monitoring

Assess facial movement for facial nerve damage (if parotid gland excised): ask patient to raise eyebrows, frown, smile, show teeth, pucker lips.

Assess degree and character of drainage.

Amount of drainage and presence of blood should be minimal.

Hemorrhage may occur with wide resection of tongue.

Maintaining adequate airway/promoting drainage

Have patient use side-lying position initially.

Have patient use Fowler's position when fully alert.

Suction mouth (except for lip surgery).

Gauze wick may be used to direct saliva into an emesis basin.

Maintain patency of drainage tubes, if used.

Promoting oral hygiene and comfort

Clean involved areas of mouth with cotton applicator moistened with hydrogen peroxide and saline.

Mouth irrigations

Use sterile equipment.

Use solution of sterile water, diluted hydrogen peroxide, normal saline, or sodium bicarbonate (avoid commercial mouthwashes).

Protect any dressings from getting wet.

A catheter may be inserted along the side of cheek and the solution injected with gentle pressure; a spray may also be used.

Give analgesics as indicated (pain is usually mild).

Promoting nutrition

Tube feedings will be used initially with hemiglossectomy.

Oral fluids: place in back of throat with Asepto syringe or feeding cup with attached tubing.

Eating soft foods

Encourage patient to feed self when possible.

Teach patient to follow all meals with clear water to cleanse mouth.

Avoid using fork, which may traumatize new tissue.

Foods

Avoid long-term use of commercial preparations such as instant breakfast drinks (may cause diarrhea or constipation).

Fruit-flavored yogurt preparations are less irritating than gelatin preparations and easier to swallow.

Avoid very hot or cold foods (hot foods irritate new tissue; cold foods may cause facial pain or paralyze oral functions).

Promoting speech

Limit patient responses initially to yes-no questions that can be answered by gestures.

Encourage patient when speech returns to speak slowly.

Listen carefully and validate communication before initiating action on requests.

Speak in a soft clear voice.

Refer patient to speech therapist if necessary.

Encourage socialization with others.

---

person has a problem getting the food to the posterior pharynx. Sensation in the mouth is decreased, and the patient has difficulty locating the position of the food in the oral cavity. One method of eating is for the person to use the forefinger to push the food to the posterior pharynx.

Facilitating communication. The patient commonly loses the ability to speak for short or long periods after surgery, but if the vocal chords are intact, speech will eventually return. A magic slate letter board or flash cards may be used for communication; however, some patients have difficulty using these methods because of visual impairments. Conversation can be carried out so that the patient's responses can be limited to affirmative or negative gestures. Loud noises are disturbing to the patient because the oral tissue loss may create a channel that amplifies sound; therefore address the patient in a soft, clear voice. Speech retraining may be necessary, and a tape recorder may be

useful for the patient to hear his or her own voice to work on improvements.

Radiation

Tumors of the mouth may be treated by radiation in various forms. Needles containing radium, radioactive cobalt, or other radioactive substances may be inserted and left in place for a prescribed time. Seeds containing emanations from radium or radioactive cobalt may be used and left in place indefinitely or else removed. External radiation treatment using x-rays or other radioactive substances may be prescribed.

Radiation therapy produces secondary effects in the mouth that include mucositis, dryness, dental decay, and tightening of the jaw muscle. Some of the changes may be permanent. The initial reaction is an inflammation of the mucous membrane. Sloughing of the tissues may occur and cause a fetid odor. Dentures are not tolerated for some

REVIEW

Table 31-7 **Esophageal disorders**

Disease	Signs and symptoms	Medical therapy
Achalasia (aperistalsis of esophagus)	Dysphagia for liquids and solids, weight loss, substernal chest pain	Forceful dilation of lower esophageal sphincter with pneumostatic or mechanical dilators
	Later: regurgitation	Cardiomyotony
Esophageal strictures	Dysphagia	Esophageal dilation, resection of stricture
Esophageal diverticulum (pouch in mucosa)	Dysphagia, fetid breath	Surgery for severe symptoms (excision of herniated sac)
Gastroesophageal reflux	Heartburn	Antacids; histamine-2 blockers (cimetidine [Tagamet], ranitidine [Zantac]); bethanechol chloride (Urecholine); metoclopramide (Reglan)
Hiatal hernia (diaphragmatic hernia)	50% asymptomatic, heartburn, dysphagia	No treatment if asymptomatic
Heartburn: high-protein, low-fat diet; antacids
Surgery for incarcerated hernias through thorax or abdomen

time thereafter because of the sensitivity of the tissues. Dryness of the mouth begins 1 to 2 weeks after radiation therapy begins and may persist throughout life. The dryness makes the mouth feel uncomfortable and gives an unpleasant taste.

Decreased salivary secretion and altered pH of the saliva contribute to rapid dental decay, especially at the gingival margins. The patient should begin an active dental control program before radiation therapy starts. Fluoride treatments to the teeth may be given and a conscientious toothbrushing regimen is instituted. Pilocarpine solution or bethanechol may be prescribed to enhance salivation.

The general care of the patient receiving radiation therapy is discussed in Chapter 11. Specific considerations for the patient receiving radiation of the mouth include the following:

1. Provide good oral hygiene.
2. Remove dentures at night; check dentures for fit.
3. Encourage fluid intake of at least 2500 ml/day unless contraindicated.
4. Encourage chewing sugar-free gum or lozenges to stimulate salivation.
5. Provide humidity in air for added moisture and comfort.
6. Avoid very hot or cold food, dry bulky foods, or smoking to decrease irritation of sensitive mucous membranes.

Palliative care

Tissue necrosis and severe pain occur in advanced cancer of the mouth, either from failure of treatment or from death of tissue as a result of radiation. The patient usually experiences difficulty in swallowing, fear of choking, and the constant accumulation of foul-smelling secretions. Good mouth care is extremely important. The danger of severe and even fatal hemorrhage must always be considered. It is very difficult to induce these patients to take sufficient nourishing fluids. A gastrostomy (p. 927) may be done to permit direct introduction of food into the stomach. Family members caring for the person at home need considerable support from hospice or other community health nurses.

Interventions to achieve patient outcomes
Counseling

The person with cancer of the mouth faces two threats: threat to life and possible disfigurement. Because the face and neck are readily visible to others, one of the major problems that the person will have to cope with and adapt to is the change in body image. The impact of the loss may be slightly minimized when the grieving process begins early. The full emotional impact of the loss, however, occurs after therapy.

Withdrawal because of not wanting to be viewed by others or because of foul breath odor is often observed in these patients. The patient needs to experience acceptance by health professionals. The family members may need help in understanding patient behavior and in coping with their own feelings concerning the patient's appearance. Patients are encouraged to identify their feelings and are provided with support and explanations as appropriate. Patients are encouraged to mingle with others as soon as clues indicating readiness are observed.

Evaluation

Evaluation is based on expected patient outcomes. Questions to consider include:

1. Have incisions healed without infection?
2. Can patient feed self, and is patient consuming a nutritionally balanced diet?
3. Does patient have a means of communication, and is patient working to improve speech?
4. Does patient interact with others and state plans for resumption of activities involving others?

COMMON ESOPHAGEAL DISORDERS

A number of esophageal disorders delay motility in the esophagus. Table 31-7 describes some of these disorders.

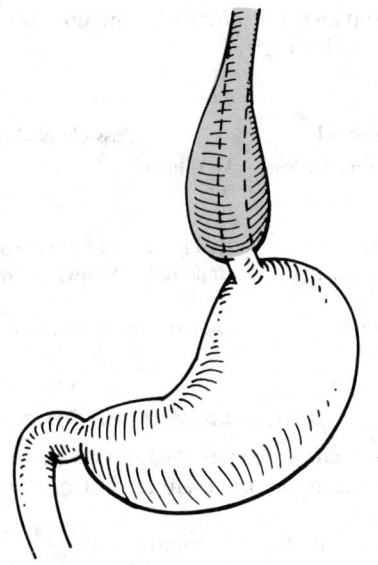

Fig. 31-7 Achalasia.

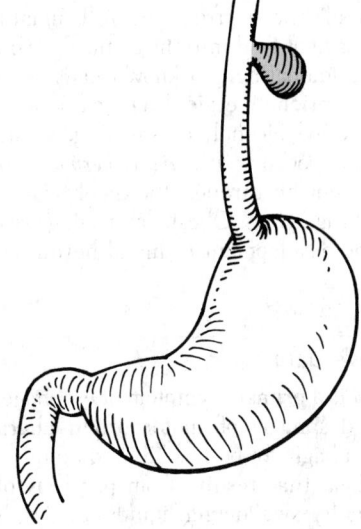

Fig. 31-8 Esophageal diverticulum.

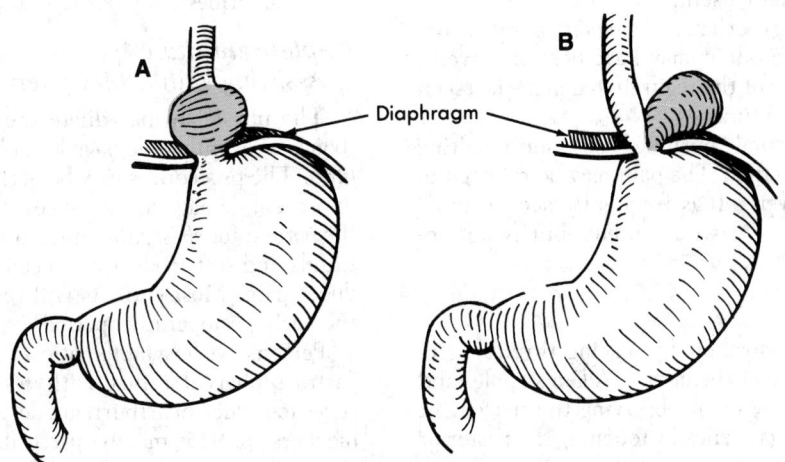

Fig. 31-9 Hiatal hernia. **A,** Sliding hernia. **B,** Paraesophageal hernia.

Etiology and Pathophysiology

Esophageal motility may be impaired by physiologic dysfunction or lack of peristalsis (achalasia), by a narrowed tract (stricture), by lack of structural integrity (diverticulum), or by irritation of the esophageal lining, particularly at the gastroesophageal junction (gastroesophageal reflux, hiatal hernia).

Various degrees of *achalasia* can exist; the cause is unknown. In addition to the absent peristalsis, the lower esophageal sphincter does not relax with swallowing. In severe conditions the portion of the esophagus above the achalasia dilates, and the person may have difficulty swallowing food and fluids past that point (Fig. 31-7). Chest pain results from esophageal spasms. Increased hydrostatic pressure (as with the Valsalva maneuver) helps to overcome the increased lower esophageal pressure.

Strictures may be corrosive or benign. Corrosive strictures occur from ingestion of a strong alkali (such as Drano) or strong acid (such as toilet bowel cleaner) that causes

severe esophageal burns. Benign strictures develop following inflammatory lesions (such as those occurring with gastroesophageal reflux), acute viral or bacterial diseases, or mucosal injury from prolonged presence of indwelling nasogastric tubes.[60] Narrowing of the esophagus makes swallowing difficult.

An *esophageal diverticulum* is a bulging of the esophageal mucosa and submucosa through a weakened portion of the esophageal muscle (Fig. 31-8). As food is ingested, some of it may collect in the pouch formed by the weakened area. After a sufficient amount of food has collected in the pouch, it overflows into the esophagus and is regurgitated. There is always danger that some of the regurgitated food may be aspirated in the trachea during sleep.

Gastroesophageal reflux occurs when the lower esophageal sphincter (LES), at the junction of the esophagus and stomach, becomes incompetent and permits reflux of gastric material into the esophagus. The acidity of the gastric juice irritates the esophageal mucosa, creating a muscle spasm. Chronic reflux may lead to stricture of the LES (as a result of fibrosis from the inflammatory process), delaying passage of food into the stomach. An incompetent LES may be idiopathic (no known cause) or may be exacerbated by anticholinergic drugs, caffeine, theobromine (chocolate), ethyl alcohol, or smoking. Gastroesophageal reflux may also occur with *hiatus hernia,* a protrusion of part of the stomach through the diaphragm into the thoracic cavity (Fig. 31-9). Obesity and aging are contributing factors to the development of hiatal hernias.

Nursing Process
Assessment
Subjective data

Dysphagia is a primary symptom of esophageal disorders. Esophageal dysphagia of motor origin characteristically produces dysphagia for both solids and liquids. This differs from dysphagia that results from paralysis of neurologic origin (difficulty swallowing liquids) or dysphagia caused by obstruction of the esophageal lumen (difficulty swallowing solids). If the patient has had dysphagia for a period of time, it is helpful to know what approaches to eating the person has found most useful.

Ask the patient who experiences *regurgitation* if it occurs at night (staining of the pillow may have been observed), and if there is a foul odor of the regurgitated material (seen with esophageal diverticulum).

Heartburn is a substernal "burning" sensation resulting from gastroesophageal reflux. The pain may be referred to the neck or back if severe. It is frequently accompanied by a sour regurgitation of gastric contents but is not accompanied by nausea.

Objective data

Assess the ability to swallow by placing three fingers over the thyroid cartilage of the larynx (Adam's apple) and ask the person to swallow or by observing the movement of the larynx. Elicit the gag reflex by touching the posterior tongue or pharynx lightly with a tongue blade. Do *not* check the gag reflex if there is no laryngeal movement. Persons who have difficulty swallowing may still have a gag reflex.[21] Make a further assessment, if necessary, by placing 4 to 5 ml of water in the oropharynx and asking the patient to swallow.

Diagnostic tests

The diagnosis of esophageal disorders is facilitated by x-ray films of the esophagus taken after barium swallow. The patient may be placed in Trendelenburg's position during the x-ray examination or fluoroscopy to identify gastroesophageal reflux.

A water siphon test is a fluoroscopic examination in which barium is swallowed followed by plain water. If the LES is incompetent, the barium will be seen to reflux into the esophagus. Overnight pH recordings measured from swallowed glass electrodes will demonstrate periods of increased gastric reflux.

Data analysis: nursing diagnoses

Nursing diagnoses are determined from analysis of patient data. Possible nursing diagnoses for the person with a common esophageal disorder may include, but are not limited to, the following:

Diagnostic title	Possible etiologies
Nutrition, altered: less than body requirements	Dysphagia
Pain: heartburn	Reflux of acid gastric contents
Aspiration, high risk for	Impaired swallowing, incompetent LES
Knowledge deficit	Lack of exposure/recall

Planning: expected patient outcomes

Expected patient outcomes for the person with a common esophageal disorder may include, but are not limited to, the following:
1. Eats a nutritionally balanced diet.
2. Describes any recommended dietary changes.
3. States feeling comfortable.
4. Does not aspirate.
5. Describes body-position and activity requirements.

Implementation
Assisting with achievement of therapeutic goals

The physician may dilate the esophagus with dilators (bougies) or inflatable bags for *achalasia* or *esophageal strictures.* The procedures may be performed under fluoroscopy to prevent damage to the mucosa. Postoperatively, monitor the patient for *chest pain,* indicating esophageal perforation. Fluids and soft foods are indicated when swallowing produces pain. Most patients will require pain medication in the early postoperative period.

Persons with symptomatic *hiatal hernias* usually have gastroesophageal reflux with resultant heartburn. Measures to reduce heartburn are described below. H_2 receptor blockers (p. 945) may be prescribed for hiatal hernias. If these measures are ineffective, surgery may be necessary. The fundus of the stomach is wrapped around the lower esophagus (Nissen fundoplication). Increases in intragastric pressure are thereby transmitted to the lower esophagus, facilitating closure of the esophageal sphincter.[68] Esophageal surgery is discussed on p. 939.

Interventions to achieve patient outcomes
Facilitating nutrition

People with esophageal disorders who experience *dysphagia* have difficulty swallowing both solids and liquids. Frequent small feedings may alleviate this difficulty. Some patients drink large amounts of fluid while swallowing solids to increase esophageal pressure, thus pushing the food into the stomach. The Valsalva maneuver can also be used to help push the food past the sphincter. Eating with the head elevated encourages movement of food through the esophagus by gravity. Regurgitation of food may occur several hours after eating, especially at night, when the body is horizontal (therefore eating is avoided for at least 2 hours before bedtime). Encourage people to sleep with the upper body elevated; wooden blocks may be used to raise the head of the bed.

Promoting comfort

The patient may decrease discomfort from heartburn by taking 30 ml of a liquid antacid 1 hour after meals, at bedtime, and whenever heartburn occurs. Gaviscon, which is a mixture of antacids with alginic acid, has been found to be effective in alleviating heartburn. Two to four tablets, when *chewed* thoroughly and then swallowed, produce a viscous antacid foam that coats the esophagus and floats on the gastric contents. If antacids are not effective, medications that increase LES contraction may be prescribed; these include bethanechol chloride (Urecholine) or metoclopramide (Reglan) to be taken 30 minutes before meals and at bedtime. Patients should avoid anticholinergic medications, because they decrease gastric emptying. Histamine-2 blockers (Tagamet, Zantac) suppress gastric secretions, thus preventing night reflux.

Preventing aspiration

Tell the patient to remain upright for at least 2 hours after eating to prevent regurgitation that may lead to aspiration. Also suggest that the patient sleep with the head elevated. The head of the bed can be raised on 15 cm blocks.

Facilitating patient learning

Prevention is the best approach to treatment of heartburn. Box 31-7 lists key points for patient teaching. Encourage a high-protein, low-fat diet. Protein stimulates gastrin release that increases LES pressure. Fats, however, stimulate release of the hormone cholecystokinin that decreases LES pressure. Other foods that decrease LES pressure include caffeine products, chocolate, peppermint and spearmint oils, and alcohol; therefore, these foods should be avoided.

Evaluation

Evaluation is based on expected patient outcomes. Questions to consider include:
1. Does the patient eat a nutritionally balanced diet?
2. Can the patient describe recommended dietary changes?
3. Does the patient state that he/she feels comfortable?
4. Has aspiration been avoided?
5. Can the patient state (1) body-position and activity requirements, (2) how to achieve comfort and an adequate diet when at home, (3) medication, dosage schedule and side effects, and (4) signs and symptoms that must be reported to the physician?

CANCER OF THE ESOPHAGUS
Epidemiology

Carcinoma is the most common condition causing obstruction of the esophagus and accounts for about 2% of all deaths from cancer in the United States. The incidence is more than twice as high in men as women but is increasing among women. Smokers, alcoholics, and persons with achalasia are at high risk.

The only possible hope for successful treatment lies in very early diagnosis and treatment. Any person who has difficulty in swallowing, no matter how trivial it may seem,

should be urged to seek medical advice at once. This applies particularly to people over 40 years of age because cancer of the esophagus occurs more often in middle and later life than at younger ages.

Pathophysiology

Cancer may develop in any portion of the esophagus but is most common in the middle and lower thirds. The tumor may be a squamous cell carcinoma originating in the esophagus or an adenocarcinoma that spreads upward from the stomach. The cancer may spread to adjoining areas by local invasion or by lymphatic spread. Symptoms depend on the area and extent of metastasis.

Implementation

The treatment for cancer of the esophagus is usually surgery, although radiation may be used. An *esophagogastrostomy* is a resection of a portion of the esophagus with anastomosis to the stomach. An *esophagogastrectomy* is resection of a lower esophageal section together with a proximal portion of the stomach, followed by anastomosis of the remaining portions of esophagus and stomach. Adjuvant chemotherapy enhances the prognosis.

Considerable psychologic support is usually required as the patient and family begin to cope with the diagnosis, prognosis, and physical debility of the patient. Encourage the patient to stop smoking, to avoid others with upper respiratory infections, and to seek medical help for even minor illnesses. Provide palliative and supportive care, as described in Chapter 11, as indicated.

ESOPHAGEAL SURGERY
Preoperative Care

The care of the person undergoing surgery of the esophagus is described in Box 31-8. Improving the nutritional status is particularly important before surgery because the person is usually malnourished because of dysphagia and anorexia from the foul taste. Total parenteral nutrition is often prescribed, although a temporary gastrostomy may be performed to supply food in the preoperative or early postoperative period.

The patient undergoing esophageal surgery

Preoperative care

Encourage improved nutritional status.
   Encourage high-protein, high-calorie diet if oral diet is possible.
   Total parenteral nutrition (TPN) may be necessary for severe dysphagia or obstruction.
Provide mouth care; vary the solution used.
Give preoperative preparation appropriate for thoracic surgery (Chapter 24).
Give prescribed antibiotics before esophageal resection or bypass.

Postoperative care

Promote good pulmonary ventilation.
Maintain chest drainage system as prescribed.
Maintain gastric drainage system.
Maintain nutrition.
   Start clear fluids at frequent intervals when oral intake is permitted.
   Introduce soft foods gradually with several small meals of bland foods.
   Have patient keep head elevated for 2 hours after eating and while sleeping if heartburn occurs.

Good mouth care is essential, especially when the patient is spitting up decomposed food, blood, or pus. Mouthwashes are useful in making the mouth feel fresher; offer them to the patient before meals. Vary the mouthwashes from time to time unless the patient has a preference, because sometimes the flavor of the solution may be identified with the unpleasant throat secretions and becomes almost as distasteful as the secretions.

Preoperative patient teaching includes the care of the patient experiencing chest surgery (Chapter 24) if this is appropriate. A nasogastric tube will be in place after surgery.

Postoperative Care

The immediate postoperative care centers on prevention of respiratory complications and maintenance of chest and gastric drainage systems. Postoperatively the nasogastric tube is usually left in place until complete healing of the esophageal anastomosis has occurred because esophageal tissue is very friable and because the anastomosis may be under tension. The nasogastric tube is not disturbed to prevent traction on the suture line. Small amounts of bright red blood may drain from the nasogastric tube for 6 to 12 hours after surgery. The color of the drainage then changes to greenish yellow.

When oral intake is permitted, give clear fluids first until well tolerated; then the diet progresses to soft foods. If part of the stomach has been pulled up into the thoracic cavity, the patient may complain of a feeling of fullness in the chest or difficulty in breathing after eating. Smaller, more frequent meals may alleviate this problem. Heartburn (p. 938) may result from gastric reflux if the esophageal sphincter has been removed or made incompetent.

DIGESTIVE DISORDERS

Most digestion takes place in the stomach, duodenum, and jejunum. Gastritis, peptic ulcer, cancer of the stomach, and malabsorption syndrome are the major digestive disorders (Table 31-8).

GASTRITIS

Etiology

Gastritis (inflammation of the stomach) is a common disorder characterized by anorexia, epigastric fullness and discomfort, and nausea and vomiting. The cause is often undetermined, but gastritis commonly results from stress, alcohol, or drugs (especially salicylates, antibiotics, indomethacin, sulfonamide, steroids). The disorder may also occur with bacterial or viral infections, from irritation by backflow of bile or pancreatic secretions, with radiation, or from corrosive substances.

Pathophysiology

Drugs, alcohol, bile salts, or pancreatic enzymes may damage the gastric mucosa (erosive gastritis), disrupting the gastric mucosal barrier and allowing a back-diffusion of acid and pepsin into the gastric tissue, causing inflammation. The gastric mucosa responds to most irritating agents by regeneration of the mucosa; therefore the disorders are often self-limiting. With continued irritation, the tissue becomes inflamed and bleeding may occur.

Ingestion of corrosive acids or alkalies can result in inflammation and necrosis of the stomach wall (corrosive gastritis). The necrosis may lead to perforation of the stomach wall with subsequent hemorrhage and peritonitis.

Chronic gastritis may be associated with atrophy of gastric glands and the appearance of patches of thin, gray, or greenish gray mucosa (atrophic gastritis). The loss of gastric mucosa will eventually reduce gastric secretion and lead to pernicious anemia. Atrophic gastritis may be a precursor to gastric carcinoma. Chronic gastritis may also be associated with peptic ulcer disease or may occur following gastrojejunostomy.[40]

Nursing Process

Assessment

Subjective data include presence of anorexia and nausea and the extent of abdominal discomfort. *Objective data* include (1) emesis (frequency, amount, presence of blood) and (2) signs of fluid and electrolyte imbalance (thirst, decreased skin turgor, dry mucous membranes, oliguria, muscle weakness).

Data analysis: nursing diagnoses

Nursing diagnoses are determined from analysis of patient data. Possible nursing diagnoses for the person with gastritis may include, but are not limited to, the following:

Diagnostic title	Possible etiologies
Pain: epigastric	Gastric irritation
Fluid volume deficit	Vomiting

REVIEW

Table 31-8   Digestive disorders

Disorder	Signs and symptoms	Medical therapy
Gastritis	Anorexia, epigastric fullness, nausea/vomiting, epigastric discomfort, hematemesis, or melena Shock and esophageal strictures	Mild: antacid, rest Severe: correction of fluid/electrolyte imbalances, sedatives, antacids, H_2 blockers
Peptic ulcer	Epigastric pain relieved by food or antacids	Antacids, H_2 blockers, sucralfate, surgery for intractable ulcers or complications
Gastric cancer	Few early symptoms: anorexia, weight loss, anemia Late symptom: palpable abdominal mass	Subtotal gastrectomy, chemotherapy, radiation
Malabsorption syndrome	Steatorrhea, flatulence, abdominal distention, anorexia, weight loss, signs of vitamin and protein deficiencies	Elimination of foods that cannot be tolerated; TPN when necessary; packed RBC for severe anemia

Table 31-9   Types of peptic ulcers

Type of ulcer	Location	Comment
Esophageal	Lower third of esophagus	Usually result from gastroesophageal reflux
Gastric	Usually on antrum or lesser curvature of stomach	Larger and deeper than duodenal ulcers; gastric malignancy must be ruled out
Duodenal	Usually in first part of duodenum	More common than gastric ulcers; not as well defined
Marginal	Jejunum near site of gastrojejunal anastomosis	Difficult to heal

Planning: expected patient outcomes

Expected patient outcomes for the person with gastritis may include, but are not limited to, the following:

1. States epigastric pain is minimized or relieved.

Implementation
Assisting with achievement of therapeutic goals

Mild gastritis is treated with antacids and rest. With severe gastritis, intravenous fluids and electrolytes are prescribed to maintain fluid balance until symptoms subside. Then give tea, broth, and ginger ale orally at frequent intervals. The patient can usually tolerate bland feedings of custard, gelatin, and cream soups after 12 to 24 hours, and then can tolerate other foods that are added gradually. People with chronic superficial gastritis will usually respond to a diet that avoids highly seasoned or greasy foods. Carbonated liquids are well tolerated.

Histamine H_2 blockers (p. 945) may be prescribed to inhibit gastric acid formation and thus decrease gastric irritation. Sucralfate (p. 945) may also be prescribed to protect the gastric mucosa by coating it to prevent back diffusion of acid and pepsin that causes irritation.

Interventions to achieve patient outcomes
Assisting with comfort

Antacids usually help to decrease epigastric discomfort. Good mouth care is indicated if vomiting is present. Rest and a calm environment help to decrease the effects of stress.

Evaluation

Evaluation is based on expected patient outcomes. Questions to consider include:

1. Does patient state that epigastric pain is minimized or relieved?
2. Is patient hydrated?

STRESS EROSIONS/STRESS ULCERS

Stress erosions or ulcers are a form of gastritis that may occur with stressful disorders such as shock, severe trauma, major surgery, sepsis, or severe burns. The lesions are usually superficial. The gastric mucosa becomes eroded or superficially ulcerated in multiple sites. Possible causative factors have been identified as mucosal ischemia or mucus deficiency. Stress erosions associated with the central nervous system, such as with brain tumors or injury or with cerebrovascular accidents, are termed *Cushing's ulcers* and are characterized by gastric hyperactivity. However, stress erosions from other causes do not demonstrate hyperacidity, and they may result from increased acid back-diffusion (similar to gastric ulcers).

Stress erosions can be prevented in high-risk persons, such as those in intensive care units, by administration of antacids and H_2 blockers or sucralfate. Stress erosions develop within 24 to 48 hours of the stressful episode. Note signs of upper GI bleeding (hematemesis, melena). Pain is not a prominent symptom. If bleeding is severe, the patient receives blood transfusions. Therapy consists of administration of antacids and H_2 blockers or sucralfate.

PEPTIC ULCER
Etiology/Epidemiology

A peptic ulcer is an acute or chronic ulcer that occurs in the area accessible to gastric secretions (lower esophagus, stomach, duodenum, jejunum) (Table 31-9). Peptic ulcers

---

31-9

Factors contributing to development of peptic ulcers

Smoking
Cigarette smokers have increased incidence of peptic ulcers and delayed healing of gastric ulcers.

Drugs
Prolonged aspirin intake may lead to peptic disease. Corticosteroids, salicylates, indomethacin, and phenylbutazone in massive doses may cause acute ulcers or exacerbate an already existing chronic peptic ulcer.

Emotional tension
No direct relationship has been demonstrated between personality and peptic ulcer, but emotional tension can alter gastric functioning. Stress may lead to a stress ulcer.

Genetic factors
A tendency for gastric or duodenal ulcers may be inherited.

Blood group
Duodenal ulcers occur more frequently in persons with type O blood.

31-10

Gastrointestinal series (upper GI x-rays)

Purpose
Visualization of the structure and motility of the stomach and intestinal tract by means of ingestion of radiopaque barium

Preparation of patient
1. Diet: No food or fluids 6 to 8 hours before examination (test is postponed if stomach is not empty)
2. Patient teaching
   Explain procedure.
   Time: approximately 45 minutes.
   Patient will need to drink all of fluid, which may taste chalky.

Procedure
1. Patient drinks approximately 250 ml (8 ounces) of barium while standing in front of a fluoroscopy tube.
2. Several successive radiographs will be taken.
3. The patient will be asked to assume different positions on the x-ray table to outline the stomach and small intestines.

After procedure
1. Provide food and fluids.
2. Administer laxative, if ordered, to speed elimination of the barium and prevent a fecal impaction.
3. Observe stool to determine complete elimination of barium; stool should be brown (barium is white) and of normal consistency.
4. Tell patient the reason for the change in stool color.

---

occur in the presence of gastric acid, but the cause of most peptic ulcers is unclear. The incidence of peptic ulcers in the United States has been declining, but they remain a common disorder.

A number of environmental, psychologic, and genetic factors may contribute to the development or delay of healing of peptic ulcers (see Box 31-9). A common belief is that persons exhibiting certain traits such as tenseness or a striving for perfection or success are more likely to develop peptic ulcers. Conclusive evidence to support this belief is lacking. Diet does not appear to be a predisposing factor, although caffeine-containing foods may exacerbate an ulcer. Cigarette smoking and regular use of aspirin are strongly associated with chronic peptic ulcers.

Ulcers in the duodenum occur more frequently than gastric ulcers and have a greater incidence in persons 20 to 45 years of age. Gastric ulcers occur more frequently in persons over age 40.

Pathophysiology

An *acute peptic ulcer* is usually superficial, involving only the mucosal layer. In most cases it heals within a relatively short time, but it may bleed, perforate, or become chronic. A *chronic peptic ulcer* is a deep crater with sharp edges and a "clean" base. It involves both the mucosa and the submucosa. If the ulcer penetrates the stomach wall and becomes adherent to an adjacent organ such as the pancreas, the organ may become the base of the ulcer.

Ulceration of the stomach and duodenum occur through different mechanisms. Persons with *gastric* ulcers have a normal gastric secretion and a normal emptying rate of the stomach but an increased diffusion of gastric acid *back* into the tissue (Fig. 31-10, *A*). Free acid that has been secreted into the stomach normally diffuses back slowly into the tissue. Rapid diffusion causes an inflammatory reaction in the tissue leading to tissue breakdown and bleeding. Gastric mucosa is normally protected from autodigestion by a thick layer of gastric mucus and by a gastric mucosal barrier.[55] Bile acids, alcohol, and salicylates can break down the natural barrier that slows the back diffusion. Cigarette smoking has been shown to increase bile reflux from the duodenum into the stomach.[72]

Persons with *duodenal* ulcers have a normal back diffusion of gastric acid but an increased gastric acid secretory rate and a markedly increased rate of gastric emptying (Fig. 31-10, *B*). Thus there is an increase in the amount of gastric acid in the gastric lumen, and if not buffered with a food such as protein or an antacid, the acid is propelled rapidly into the duodenum. The increased amount of acid in the duodenum irritates the duodenal mucosa, leading to tissue breakdown. Table 31-10 lists differences between duodenal and gastric ulcers.

Zollinger-Ellison syndrome refers to peptic ulceration as-

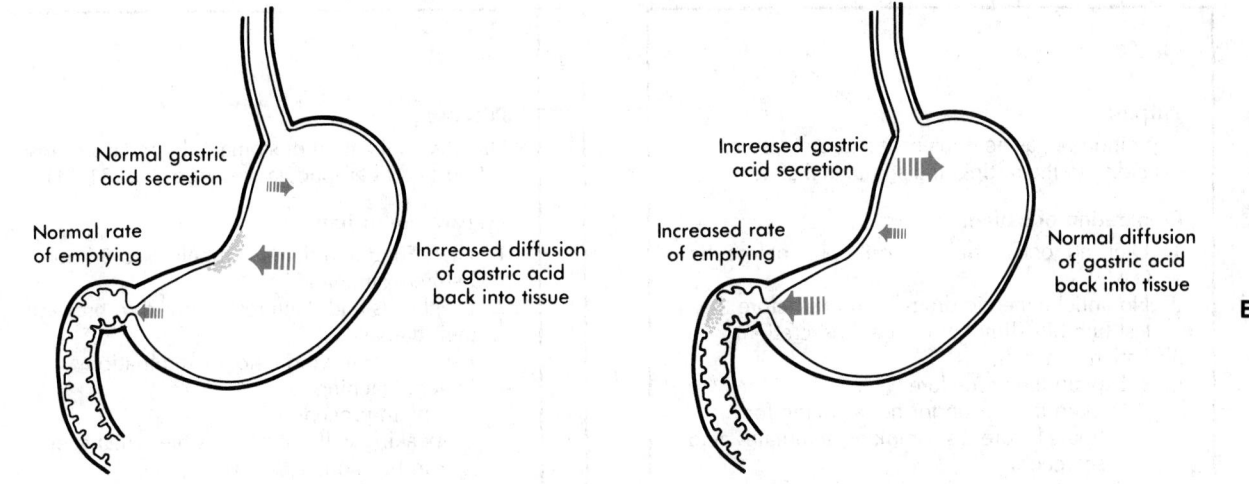

Fig. 31-10 Pathophysiology of peptic ulcer. **A,** Gastric. **B,** Duodenal. Note that with gastric ulcers the major alteration is increased back-diffusion of gastric acid whereas with duodenal ulcers gastric acid secretion and stomach emptying is increased.

Table 31-10 Comparison of duodenal and gastric ulcers

	Duodenal ulcer	Gastric ulcer
Pathophysiology	Normal back diffusion of gastric acid; increased gastric secretion and emptying rate	Increased back diffusion of gastric acid; normal gastric secretion and emptying rate
Epidemiology	2 to 5 times more common than gastric ulcers; most common in men 20 to 45 years of age	Less common than duodenal ulcers; most common in persons 40 to 60 years of age
Pain	Epigastric pain 45 to 60 minutes after eating and at night	Epigastric pain about 30 minutes after eating and on an empty stomach
Diagnostic studies	Upper GI series	Upper GI series; gastroscopy with biopsy to determine if ulcer is benign or malignant
Course	Can usually be controlled by medical therapy	More difficult to control medically; and recurs more frequently than duodenal ulcer

sociated with a non-insulin-producing islet cell tumor of the pancreas. The syndrome is characterized by one or more peptic ulcerations in the lower end of the esophagus, stomach, duodenum, and jejunum and by enormous gastric hypersecretion and acidity.

Nursing Process
Assessment
Subjective data

Pain, which is the major symptom of peptic ulcer, has the following characteristics:

1. Usually described as gnawing, aching, or burning
2. Usually confined to a small area of the upper abdomen near the midline
3. May radiate around the costal area to the back
4. Starts 1 to 2 hours after eating when the stomach begins to empty
5. May disappear with ingestion of food or an antacid
6. Frequently occurs at night when the stomach is empty

Assess the patient with a peptic ulcer for the presence, location, and character of pain as well as time of occurrence in relation to food and effectiveness of antacids. Some persons never experience pain, and the peptic ulcer may be discovered accidentally by x-ray or postmortem examination.

Objective data

Monitor the patient for signs of hemorrhage (hematemesis, tarry stools), perforation (severe abdominal pain, abdominal rigidity), or pyloric obstruction (weight loss, projectile vomiting).

Diagnostic tests

The diagnosis of peptic ulcer is made from the patient's history, a gastrointestinal series (Box 31-10), gastric analysis (Box 31-11), and stool examinations for occult (hidden) blood (p. 963). Direct visualization of the ulcer by gastroscopy (Box 31-12) differentiates gastric ulcer from gastric carcinoma.

Selective *angiography* is becoming useful in the diagnosis and evaluation of treatment of gastric hemorrhage when angiography is combined with endoscopy. With angiography a contrast medium is injected through an arterial cath-

31-11 Gastric analysis

Purpose
Aspiration of gastric contents to assess gastric acidity in the fasting and stimulated state

Preparation of patient
1. Diet: no food or fluids 6 to 8 hours before the test
2. No anticholinergic drugs 24 hours before the test (inhibits stimulation of acid secretion)
3. Patient teaching
   Explain the procedure
   Explain the reason for not smoking for 8 hours before test (smoking stimulates acid secretion)

Procedure
1. Nasogastric tube is inserted (p. 953).
2. Encourage patient to relax after tube is inserted.
3. Instruct patient to expectorate saliva rather than swallowing (saliva may act as a buffer).
4. Gastric contents are aspirated.
5. Betazole hydrochloride (Histalog) or histamine is given subcutaneously. (Histamine is *not* given to a person with a history of allergies.)
6. Monitor patient for side effects of medication.
   Take pulse and blood pressure immediately after giving medication (a slight increase in pulse and decrease in blood pressure may be noted).
   Side effects include flushing, feeling of warmth, slight headache, itching.
   Signs of adverse reaction include shock, intense headache, vomiting, diarrhea.
7. Have epinephrine available to counteract effect of histamine if sensitivity reaction occurs.
8. After giving histamine preparation, aspirate stomach contents every 10 to 20 minutes until desired number (usually three) of specimens obtained.
9. Tube is then clamped and withdrawn.

After procedure
1. Provide patient with tissues to wipe eyes and nose.
2. Offer mouth care.
3. Patient may resume food and fluids.
4. Benadryl may be prescribed for home use following a sensitivity reaction.

31-12 Gastroscopy

Purpose
Direct visualization of stomach by means of insertion of a fiberoptic gastroscope (Fig. 31-11)

Preparation of patient
1. Diet: Food and fluids withheld 6 to 8 hours before examination.
2. Eyeglasses and dentures removed to prevent their damage.
3. Ask patient to void before examination.
4. Patient teaching
   Explain procedure.
   Speaking will not be possible when scope is in position.
   Time: approximately 15 minutes.
   Sensation: feelings of pressure but no pain.
   Hoarseness and sore throat may be present for several days after examination.

Procedure
1. Topical anesthesia (spray or gargle) is applied to throat.
2. Valium or Versed is given parenterally to relax patient.
3. Gastroscope is inserted through mouth with patient sitting or lying down.
4. Air is insufflated through scope to visualize mucosa.
5. Biopsy may be obtained.
6. Scope is removed; patient is asked to sit up immediately and to deep breathe, cough, and expectorate.

After procedure
1. No food or fluids until gag reflex returns (2 to 4 hours).
2. Monitor vital signs every 30 minutes for 2 hours.
3. Monitor for dyspnea, dysphagia, abdominal pain, fever, bleeding.
4. Maintain safety precautions until effect of sedative wears off.
5. Tell patient sputum may be bloody (if biopsy performed).

Diagnostic title	Possible etiologies
Pain: epigastric	Ulceration of mucosa
Coping, ineffective individual	Situational stressors
Knowledge deficit	Lack of exposure/recall

eter for better visualization of bleeding areas and for differentiation between normal and tumor vessels. Following the procedure, observe the femoral insertion site for signs of bleeding, and take vital signs at frequent intervals.

Data analysis: nursing diagnoses
Nursing diagnoses are determined from analysis of patient data. Possible nursing diagnoses for the person with a peptic ulcer may include, but are not limited to, the following:

Planning: expected patient outcomes
Expected patient outcomes for the person with a peptic ulcer may include, but are not limited to, the following:
1. States pain is decreased, minimal, or absent.
2. Identifies life stressors and describes useful stress management techniques.
3. States plans to modify health-risking behaviors (smoking, alcohol ingestion) if pertinent.
4. Describes factors that contribute to healing, medication plan to be followed, and plans for follow-up care.

Table 31-11   Drug therapy for peptic ulcer

Drug	Action	Comments
Antacids	Neutralize gastric acid	Generally heal ulcers in 4 to 6 weeks Side effects limited to diarrhea or constipation Lack of adherence to regimen by many patients
Histamine H_2 receptor antagonists (cimetidine, ranitidine, famotidine, nizatidine)	Inhibit acid secretion	Generally heal ulcers in 4 to 6 weeks Side effects may interfere with administration
Sucralfate (Carafate)	Coats ulcer, prevents action of acid and pepsin on ulcer	Generally heals ulcers in 4 to 6 weeks Longer time span before recurrence Large capsule; may be difficult to swallow
Anticholinergics	Decrease gastric secretions, delay gastric emptying	Less effective than other drugs; now rarely used Side effects usually occur with therapeutic doses

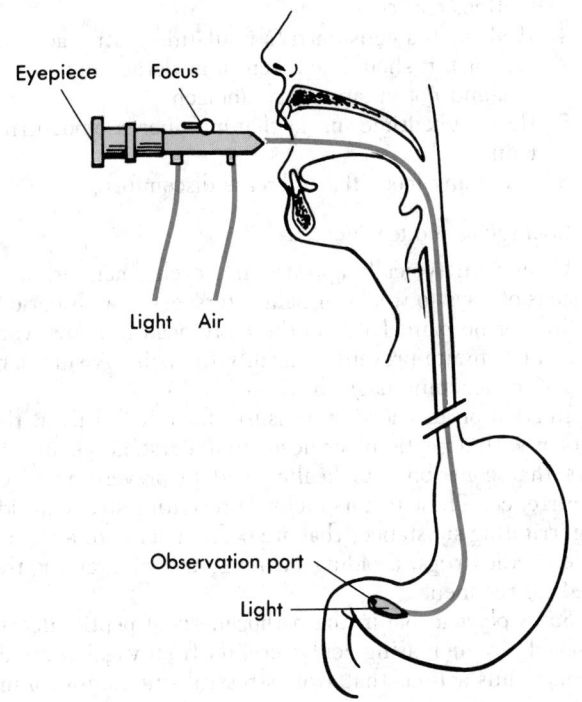

Fig. 31-11   Stomach may be visualized by means of a fiberscope.

Implementation
Assisting with achievement of therapeutic goals

The pain of peptic ulcer is directly related to periods of the day when gastric acidity is high, particularly several hours after meals and at bedtime, when acid secretion is high and the stomach is empty. Measures to decrease ulcer pain and promote healing include drug therapy (antacids, histamine H_2 blockers, sucralfate) (Table 31-11) and food to buffer the gastric acidity.

Antacids

Antacids are the most effective therapy for relieving peptic ulcer pain; they act by decreasing gastric acidity. Antacids of choice are the nonsystemic antacids (Table 31-

12), which are poorly absorbed from the stomach and therefore do not alter the pH of the blood or interfere with normal acid-base balance. Sodium bicarbonate is readily absorbed and therefore should be avoided as an antacid for relief of ulcer pain. Also, the reaction of sodium bicarbonate and hydrochloric acid forms carbon dioxide, which may cause distention.

Antacids may be administered frequently, and if symptoms are severe, it may be necessary to give them as often as every 30 to 60 minutes. When antacids are given to a person in a fasting state, the buffering power is usually transitory. For maximal effectiveness, antacids should be given 1 and 3 hours *after* meals; this produces a buffering effect that lasts approximately 3 to 4 hours. Aluminum hydroxide becomes less reactive over time and should not be given with anticholinergic drugs or with tetracycline because it interferes with absorption of these drugs. Liquids are more effective than tablets; if tablets are used, they are chewed slowly to permit complete pulverization.

Histamine H_2 receptor antagonists

One of the major stimulants of hydrochloric acid secretion in the stomach is histamine (in addition to gastrin and acetylcholine). In the body, histamine has two types of receptors, H_1 receptors, which mediate histamine action in the smooth muscle (and are blocked by antihistamines), and H_2 receptors, which mediate secretion of hydrochloric acid in the stomach. Histamine H_2 receptor antagonists, therefore, are drugs that block histamine's stimulation of gastric acid, either in the fasting state or the stimulated state.

Histamine H_2 receptor antagonists that are available for peptic ulcer therapy include cimetidine (Tagamet), ranitidine (Zantac), famotidine (Pepcid), and the newer drug nizatidine (Axid). The overall side effects are low but may include confusion, dizziness, and weakness (most common in elderly persons); diarrhea and abdominal cramps; bradycardia or tachycardia; impotence and gynecomastia; itching and rash; and thrombocytopenia. The patient needs to know about the possibility of a decreased libido and to monitor for signs of bleeding (from the thrombocytopenia). Cimetidine has increased toxicity when given concurrently with benzodiazepine, metoprolol, propanolol, phenytoin, theophyline, and tricyclic antidepressants.

Table 31-12   **Commonly used antacids**

Generic name	Trade name	Comments
Aluminum hydroxide	Amphojel ALternaGEL Alu-Cap Dialume	Slow buffering effect Constipating Decreased absorption of phosphates Contains sodium Edema of feet and legs with large doses
Aluminum carbonate	Basaljel	Same as for aluminum hydroxide
Aluminum and magnesium hydroxide	Maalox	A preferred antacid Good buffering effect Good taste Nonconstipating Low sodium content
Aluminum hydroxide and magnesium trisilicate	Gaviscon	Slower buffering effect Coats and protects ulcer Nonconstipating
Magaldrate	Riopan	A chemical combination of magnesium and aluminum hydroxide Intermediate buffering action Nonconstipating Low sodium content No acid rebound
Calcium carbonate	Alka-2	Rapid buffering effect Constipation may be severe May cause acid rebound May cause hypercalcemia Not suitable for long-term therapy
Magnesium and calcium carbonate	Marblen	Slow buffering effect Neutralizes more acid than other antacids Nonconstipating Low sodium content
Antacids with simethicone		
Aluminum and magnesium hydroxide, with simethicone	Mylanta Maalox Plus Gelusil	Same actions as aluminum and magnesium hydroxide alone Simethicone is non-gas-forming: lowers the surface tension of gas bubbles

Sucralfate

Sucralfate (Carafate) helps to heal ulcers and decrease pain by coating the ulcer, thus preventing irritation by gastric acid and pepsin (Table 31-11). Sucralfate decreases the absorption of tetracycline and phenytoin; therefore, administer these drugs at least 2 hours apart from sucralfate administration. Give antacids at least 30 minutes before or after sucralfate.

Interventions to achieve patient outcomes
Promoting comfort

Although modifying the diet has not been shown to accelerate healing of an uncomplicated ulcer, regulation of food may promote comfort. Food in the stomach, especially protein, buffers gastric acid; however, food also stimulates gastric acid secretion, which may irritate the ulcer and cause pain. Controversy exists concerning whether ulcer pain is better relieved by three regular meals or six small meals a day. The person with the pain can best judge which approach provides the maximum comfort. Suggest the following eating guidelines:

1. Eat meals slowly to prevent overdistention and gastric acid reflux.
2. Eat snacks if pain occurs between meals.
3. Restrict foods that stimulate gastric acid secretion (coffee, tea, cola).
4. If alcohol is consumed (stimulating gastric acid secretion), it should be taken in moderate amounts or less and not on an empty stomach.
5. Restrict bedtime snacks that may increase nocturnal pain.
6. Avoid any foods that increase discomfort.

Counseling and teaching

Ulcer pain typically appears in a cyclic manner, with periods of days to weeks of pain interspersed with periods of little or no pain. Patients therefore need to know what to do at home to prevent or modify the pain. A summary of patient teaching is given in Box 31-13.

In addition to knowing measures for relief of pain, the person with a peptic ulcer needs to understand about factors that contribute to healing and to preventing ulcer recurrence. These factors include preventing stress, avoiding irritating substances that are poorly tolerated, avoiding ulcerogenic drugs, avoiding smoking, and maintaining the medical regimen.

Stress plays a role in the pathogenesis of peptic ulcers, probably by increasing acid secretion from vagal stimulation.[55] Thus actions that avoid stressful situations or minimize the effect of stress can promote healing or prevent recurrence. If removal from stressful environmental influences is impossible, the person must learn to cope with the stressful situations without reactivating the ulcer. (Measures to decrease stress are described in Chapter 6.) Occasionally the person requires psychologic counseling to better understand the problems and develop more effective coping behaviors.

Since there seems to be a relationship between *smoking* and irritation of a peptic ulcer, most physicians believe that the person who has a peptic ulcer should give up smoking permanently. To do so is sometimes very difficult, since often the person's life and work situations as well as personality are such that a change of this sort is a major one. Encourage those few persons whose ulcers are reactivated when they attempt to give up smoking to at least moderate the habit.

If every consideration is given to adjusting the prescribed regimen to fit the appropriate physical, economic, and social pattern, the person with an ulcer will be better able to follow the medical treatment.

Table 31-13   Comparison of different types of vagotomy procedures for peptic ulcer

Type of surgery	Advantages	Disadvantages
Truncal vagotomy with pyloroplasty	Low operative mortality and morbidity	High recurrence rate
Selective vagotomy with pyloroplasty	Preservation of vagal innervation of viscus; fewer side effects than truncal vagotomy	More difficult to perform than truncal vagotomy
Proximal vagotomy	Preserves gastric emptying; low recurrence rate; fewer side effects; no intrusion of GI tract	Requires greater expertise
Vagotomy with antrectomy	Lower recurrence rate than for vagotomy with pyloroplasty	Higher operative mortality Greater side effects

---

Patient Teaching   31-13

The patient with a peptic ulcer

Medications

Know dosage, administration, action, and side effects.

Continue drug for prescribed time, even when symptoms abate.

Keep antacids available at all times.

Anticipate increased need for antacid during periods of stress.

Avoid self-medication with systemic antacids (bicarbonate of soda) that alter acid-base balance.

Avoid ulcerogenic drugs such as salicylates, ibuprofen, corticosteroids.

Use acetaminophen (Tylenol) or buffered aspirin (if tolerated) for relief of pain.

Smoking

Stop smoking if possible.

If stopping smoking increases discomfort from stress, try to decrease amount smoked.

Eating

Eat three balanced meals a day.

Eat between-meal snacks if this helps to relieve pain.

Avoid any foods that increase discomfort.

If alcohol is taken, drink in moderation and not on an empty stomach.

Avoid stress at mealtimes and plan for a quiet time after eating.

Relaxation and reduction of stress

Participate in recreation and hobbies that promote relaxation.

Provide for a good night's sleep on a regular basis.

Use relaxation techniques to decrease effects of stress.

Participate in a reasonable exercise program to promote well-being.

Structure home and work environment to keep stressors at a reasonable level.

Avoid factors found to increase symptoms, if possible.

Evaluation

Questions to consider for the person with a peptic ulcer include the following:

1. Has epigastric pain been relieved or minimized?
2. Does the person know measures to minimize the effects of stress in daily living?
3. Has the person made plans to avoid or modify activities that delay healing?
4. Can the person describe
   a. Correct administration of prescribed medications?
   b. Specific actions to take to promote healing of the ulcer and decrease recurrence?
   c. Plans for follow-up care?

Surgery for Peptic Ulcer

Emergency surgery is necessary when a peptic ulcer perforates and causes peritonitis or erodes a blood vessel, causing severe hemorrhage. Elective surgery may be performed if the ulcer does not respond to the medical regimen and continues to produce symptoms, if it causes pyloric obstruction, or if a chronic recurring gastric ulcer is thought to be premalignant. The basic surgical procedures for treatment of peptic ulcers are subtotal gastrectomy, vagotomy, and pyloroplasty. Subtotal gastrectomy is now rarely performed alone but is usually combined with a form of vagotomy. Pyloroplasty is also combined with a vagotomy. The several common surgical combinations are listed in Table 31-13.

Table 31-14 describes *subtotal gastrectomies*. The Billroth II (Fig. 31-12, *B*) is usually preferred for duodenal ulcers because of decreased duodenal recurrence. The duodenal stump is preserved to permit bile flow into the jejunum to mix with the food but may develop infection from stasis.

Part of the vagus nerve innervating the stomach is severed in a *vagotomy* for the purpose of decreasing gastric acidity. There are three types of vagotomies currently in use: truncal, selective, and proximal (Fig. 31-13). With both *truncal* and *selective* vagotomies, gastric emptying is inhibited; thus a pyloroplasty or antrectomy (removal of antrum or lower portion of stomach) must be performed to prevent gastric stasis by enlarging the pyloric opening. The *proximal* vagotomy severs only the branches of the gastric portion of the vagal nerve that innervate the upper two thirds of the stomach, thus maintaining effective gastric emptying. Because a pyloroplasty or antrectomy is unnecessary with a proximal vagotomy, there is no intrusion into the gastric lumen and side effects, especially diarrhea, are reduced.

Table 31-14   Comparison of subtotal gastrectomy procedures

	Gastroduodenostomy	Gastrojejunostomy
Common term	Billroth I	Billroth II
Procedure	Removal of lower part of stomach (antrectomy) with anastomosis to remaining segment of duodenum (Fig. 31-12, A)	Removal of lower part of stomach (antrectomy) with anastomosis to side of the proximal jejunum (Fig. 31-12, B)
Common use	Gastric ulcer	Duodenal ulcer
Side effects	Decreased gastric capacity, rapid emptying with decreased effect of pancreatic enzymes (malabsorption)	Same as Billroth I; stasis with subsequent infection in the blind duodenal loop

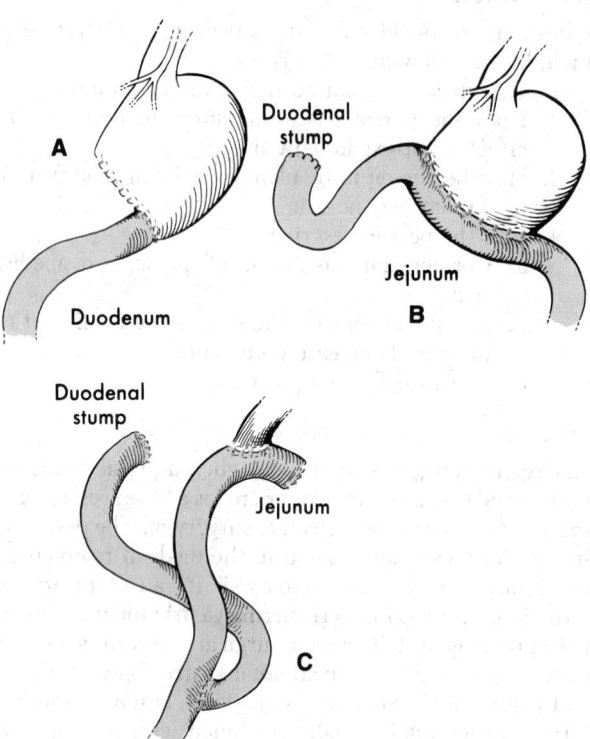

Fig. 31-12   Types of gastric resections with anastomoses. **A,** Billroth I. **B,** Billroth II. **C,** Total gastrectomy.

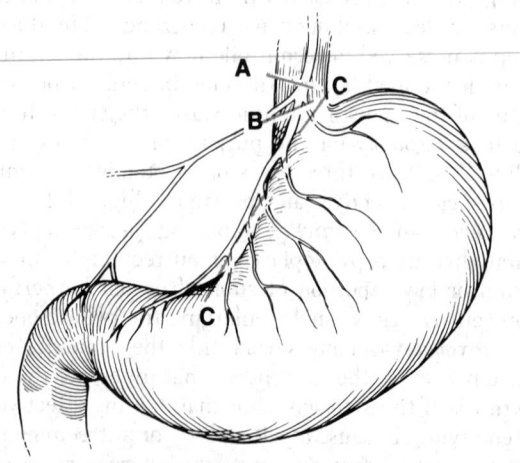

Fig. 31-13   Types of vagotomies: **A,** Truncal; **B,** Selective; **C,** Proximal or parietal cell.

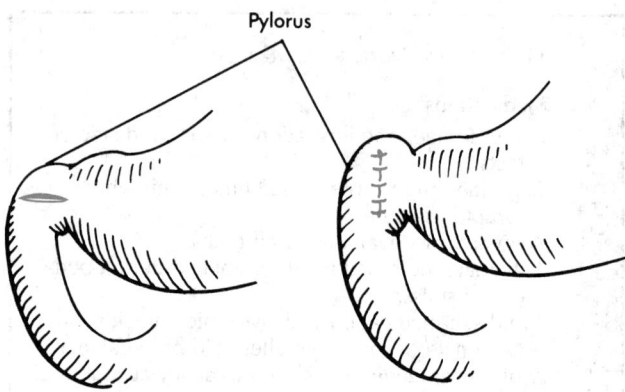

Fig. 31-14   Heineke-Mikulicz pyloroplasty. Longitudinal incision across pylorus is pulled apart and closed in transverse position to widen pyloric outlet.

A *pyloroplasty* or drainage procedure widens the pyloric outlet. It is performed with a truncal or selective vagotomy to prevent gastric stasis. One type of pyloroplasty is the Heineke-Mikulicz procedure (Fig. 31-14).

Care of the patient experiencing gastric surgery is described on p. 954.

Complications of Peptic Ulcer

A peptic ulcer may perforate a major blood vessel and cause hemorrhage, perforate the stomach or duodenal wall, or cause an obstruction at the pyloric end of the stomach.

Hemorrhage

Peptic ulcer is the most common cause of massive upper gastrointestinal bleeding. Duodenal ulcers have a higher incidence of bleeding than gastric ulcers. In some cases bleeding is slight, and the only symptoms are tarry stools and a developing iron deficiency. When a major blood vessel erodes, bleeding is massive.

The medical management of hemorrhage is summarized in Table 31-15. If endoscopy shows a bleeding ulcer, endoscopic hemostatic therapy (heater probe, electrocautery, or Nd:YAG laser) may be used.[68] Surgery is indicated for uncontrolled bleeding or for recurrence of hemorrhage. Vagotomy with pyloroplasty is preferred to gastrectomy. The drainage from the nasogastric tube is usually dark red for 6 to 12 hours after surgery but should turn greenish yellow within 24 hours. The patient may continue to pass tarry

Table 31-15   Complications of peptic ulcer

	Hemorrhage	Perforation	Pyloric obstruction
Occurrence with peptic ulcer	15% to 20%	10%	5% to 10%
Clinical picture	Hematemesis, tarry stools, shock	Sudden severe abdominal pain, usually several hours after eating; abdominal rigidity; decreased abdominal sounds; increased pulse and respiratory rate	Partial obstruction: epigastric fullness, anorexia, weight loss; complete obstruction: projectile vomiting of undigested food, dehydration
Diagnostic findings	Blood in vomitus and stool	Leukocytosis
X-ray film: air under diaphragm	Anemia, hypochloremia, hypokalemia, hyponatremia
X-ray film: large gastric fluid level
Medical treatment	Bed rest, sedation, blood transfusions, gastric lavage, treatment for shock, cimetidine
After bleeding stops: antacids hourly or by continuous drip	Gastric decompression, parenteral fluids, antibiotics, surgery	Gastric decompression, correction of metabolic alkalosis and dehydration
Antacids and liquids after 72 hours if obstruction decreased
Surgery if obstruction persists

stools for several days postoperatively, but this is usually because the blood from the hemorrhage before surgery has not yet completely passed through the gastrointestinal tract. Stools may be guaiac positive for several days after bleeding stops.

If gastric lavage is indicated, saline is usually used to minimize loss of electrolytes. No evidence supports the use of iced solutions.[56]

Nursing interventions during the phase of *severe gastric bleeding* include the following actions:
1. Assisting with achievement of therapeutic goals
   a. Monitor vital signs and urinary output for response to therapy for shock.
   b. Monitor nasogastric drainage, emesis, and stools for amount of blood loss (stools may be red or tarry depending on the length of time required for passage).
   c. Test stools daily for occult blood (guaiac) until bleeding has completely stopped.
   d. Assist with medical treatments (blood transfusions, saline gastric lavage) and monitor patient's response.
   e. Prepare patient for surgery if indicated.
2. Assisting with patient comfort
   a. Provide special mouth care after vomiting (a weak solution of hydrogen peroxide will help remove blood from the oral mucosa).
   b. Administer prescribed sedative/narcotic regularly to decrease apprehension.
   c. Remove all evidence of bleeding as quickly as possible.
   d. Tell patient rationale for blood transfusion.
   e. Tell patient that rest and quiet will help stop the bleeding.
   f. Maintain a calm approach.
   g. Restrict activities only to those deemed necessary until massive bleeding has slowed down or stopped.

Perforation

Perforation is an erosion of a peptic ulcer through the muscular wall, providing an opening from the gastrointestinal tract into the peritoneal cavity. Most perforated ulcers are located on the anterior duodenal wall. Immediately on perforation a chemical peritonitis results from contact with the gastrointestinal contents, and bacterial peritonitis results within 12 hours. Symptoms and medical management are listed in Table 31-15. Persons taking corticosteroids may develop a peptic ulcer and perforation without exhibiting any of the usual symptoms.

Some perforations are minor and close within a short time or wall themselves off. However, most perforations require surgery and should be closed surgically as soon as possible. Surgery may consist of simple laparotomy with closure (oversewing) of the perforation and aspiration from the peritoneum of all escaped GI fluid. Most people who have had a perforated ulcer, however, continue to have recurrences of ulcer symptoms. Therefore, most surgeons now perform definitive ulcer surgery, such as vagotomy with gastric resection or pyloroplasty, if the patient's condition permits. A pelvic abscess may require incision and drainage.

Nursing interventions for the person with a *perforated ulcer* include the following activities:
1. Assisting with achievement of therapeutic goals
   a. Connect the nasogastric tube initially to continuous suction until stomach is empty, then maintain at intermittent suction.
   b. Place patient in low Fowler's position to collect escaped fluids in pelvic cavity.
   c. Prepare patient for surgery, if indicated.
   d. Monitor postoperatively for continuing peritonitis and abscess formation (fever, respiratory distress, increased abdominal pain, distention, hyperactive or absent bowel sounds, inability to pass flatus or stool).

Nursing Care Plan

Person with peptic ulcer

DATA: Mr. J. is a 42-year-old single computer operator with a history of duodenal ulcer (diagnosed 4 years ago). He has had periods of epigastric distress for the past month with partial relief from Maalox. He was admitted 2 days ago with hematemesis, tarry stools, faintness, and a blood pressure of 96/54 (usual 124/84). Intravenous fluids were initiated. Endoscopy revealed a bleeding duodenal ulcer. A nasogastric tube was inserted and antacids prescribed hourly per tube. Cimetidine was started by intravenous push. His blood pressure is now stable and the nasogastric tube was removed early today. He is taking oral fluids and has been started on a soft diet. Current prescriptions include cimetidine 300 mg with meals and at bedtime and Maalox 30 ml 1 and 3 hours after meals.

The nursing history identified the following:
1. He is vague about the nature of peptic ulcer or possible complications.
2. He takes aspirin for headaches "from computer eyestrain."
3. He smokes 1½ packs per day; he has tried several times, unsuccessfully, to quit.
4. He spends two to three evenings a week at a local bar and "puts down quite a few beers."

Collaborative nursing actions include those to prevent further injury from hemorrhage or perforation. Immediate reporting of and treatment of early signs may prevent serious effects (loss of blood, peritonitis, or death). Nursing actions include *monitoring* for the following:
1. Signs of hemorrhage: hematemesis, decreased blood pressure, restlessness, cool moist skin, stools that test positive for guaiac
2. Signs of perforation: severe, sudden, sharp abdominal pain

Nursing diagnosis: **Pain: epigastric related to irritation of gastric acid on duodenal ulcer**

Expected patient outcomes	Nursing interventions	Rationale
Mr. J. states epigastric pain is decreased	Give prescribed cimetidine with meals and at bedtime (8 AM, 12 noon, 5 PM, and 9 PM)	Cimetidine encourages healing by decreasing gastric acid secretion; give with meals to inhibit food-stimulated HCl secretion
	Give prescribed antacid 1 and 3 hours after meals (9 AM, 11 AM, 1 PM, 3 PM, 6 PM, and 8 PM)	Antacids neutralize HCl; they interfere with absorption of cimetidine if given concurrently
	Teach relaxation measures as appropriate	Relaxation facilitates rest to promote healing

---

2. Assisting with patient comfort
   a. Give analgesic medications at regular intervals for pain control during acute phase.
   b. To decrease apprehension, explain what is being done.

Pyloric obstruction

Pyloric obstruction may be caused by edema of tissues around an ulcer or by scar tissue from a healed ulcer located near the pylorus. It may be only a partial obstruction and cause dilation of the stomach, or it may be complete. Obstruction caused by edema and spasm generally responds to medical management (Table 31-15).

At the end of a 72-hour period of gastric decompression, a *saline load test* is performed to assess the degree of gastric emptying: 700 ml of normal saline at room temperature is introduced through the nasogastric tube over a 3- to 5-minute period, and the tube is then clamped. After 30 minutes the stomach is aspirated. A residual volume of more than 350 ml indicates continued pyloric obstruction, and surgery consisting of either a vagotomy with pyloroplasty or gastrectomy is considered. If the saline load test demonstrates improved gastric emptying, oral liquids and antacids are introduced with continued assessment of gastric emptying for several days.

Nursing interventions for the person with a *pyloric obstruction* include the following activities:
1. Monitor for signs of increased severe abdominal pain and decreased abdominal sounds.
2. Assist with achievement of therapeutic goals.

Nursing diagnosis: Altered health maintenance: related to lack of knowledge

Expected patient outcomes	Nursing interventions	Rationale
Mr. J. states plans to decrease smoking and drinking and to avoid aspirin	Teach effects of aspirin, smoking, and alcohol on ulcer formation	Aspirin is ulcerogenic; smoking delays healing; alcohol stimulates HCl and may further irritate ulcer
	Discuss previous efforts at discontinuing smoking; explore additional ways, especially group programs, such as those provided by the American Cancer Society, American Lung Association, and American Heart Association	Programs that include group support are often more successful than trying to quit smoking by oneself
	Explore with Mr. J. reasons for frequent visits to bars, then explore other ways of meeting his needs (such as nonalcoholic drinks or substituting other social activities)	Assisting Mr. J. to think about reasons and alternate approaches will increase the potential for a behavioral change
	Suggest Mr. J. get his eyes examined (if appropriate); describe analgesics that do not contain aspirin (such as Tylenol and Anacin)	Headaches may be caused by strain from decreased vision; fewer headaches will decrease need for analgesics

Nursing diagnosis: Knowledge deficit: related to lack of recall or exposure

Expected patient outcomes	Nursing interventions	Rationale
Mr. J. describes nature of and therapy for peptic ulcer	Review nature of peptic ulcer and possible recurrence; review factors that contribute to healing (see Box 31-8); review methods of pain relief, including administration and side effects of cimetidine and antacids; review need to report symptoms of bleeding, perforation, or pyloric obstruction to physician immediately	Reinforcement of earlier teaching will help promote retention

a. Assist with gastric lavage and maintain gastric decompression.
b. Explain saline load test, when pertinent.
c. Prepare patient for surgery as necessary.

CANCER OF THE STOMACH
Etiology/Epidemiology

Almost all gastric tumors are malignant. The incidence of cancer of the stomach has decreased in recent years; nevertheless, gastric cancer is the seventh most common cause of cancer-related deaths.[4] It occurs more frequently in men than women. It rarely occurs in people under the age of 40 and is most frequent between the ages of 50 and 70. The cause is unknown, although the incidence is higher when gastric acid is low. Contributing factors, symptoms, and usual medical therapy are summarized in Table 31-8 (p. 941).

Pathophysiology

Cancer may develop in any part of the stomach but is found most often in the distal third. Most gastric cancers are adenocarcinomas and occur in polypoid, ulcerative, or infiltrative forms. The ulcerative form is the most common and may produce peptic ulcer–type symptoms that, unfortunately, tend to delay diagnosis and encourage self-treatment. Growths located at the entrance or exit of the stomach may lead to signs of esophageal or pyloric obstruction (heartburn or early satiety). In general, however, early signs of gastric cancer are absent.

Gastric cancer may spread directly through the stomach wall into adjacent tissues, to the lymphatics, to the regional lymph nodes of the stomach, to other abdominal organs, or through the bloodstream to the lungs or bones. Involvement of the regional lymph nodes occurs early, followed by involvement of the more distal nodes. There is a tendency toward intraperitoneal seeding, particularly to the peritoneal cul-de-sac. Prognosis depends on the depth of invasion and extent of metastasis.

Medical Therapy

Surgery is the primary therapy for gastric cancer. If the tumor has not spread beyond the stomach, a subtotal gastrectomy (gastroduodenostomy or gastrojejunostomy) is usually performed. Tumors high in the cardia of the stomach may require a total gastrectomy (esophagojejunostomy).[68] Palliative subtotal gastrectomy may be performed when hemorrhage or obstruction occurs.

Chemotherapy and radiotherapy may be given for metastatic disease to decrease symptoms and prolong survival. Only about 12% of persons with gastric cancer survive for 5 years.[68]

GASTROINTESTINAL INTUBATION

GI intubation consists of inserting a tube through the nose into the stomach (nasogastric) or beyond the stomach into the intestines (intestinal). Common uses of GI intubation include the following:

1. Nasogastric (N/G)
   a. Decompression of stomach
   b. Tube feedings, including medication administration (p. 927)
   c. Removal of gastric contents (gastric hemorrhage or perforation)
   d. After esophageal or gastric surgery to permit healing of suture line
   e. Gastric analysis (Box 31-11)
2. Intestinal: intestinal decompression

The following section discusses the use of GI intubation for decompression and drainage and the care of persons with a GI tube.

Types of Tubes

Different types of tubes are used depending on the purpose and site (Table 31-16). A *Levin* tube (Fig. 31-15) is used for gastric intubation; however, because it is a single-lumen tube, damage to the mucosa may result even with intermittent suction. A less traumatic approach, and a more commonly used N/G tube, is the double-lumen Salem *sump tube*. The larger lumen of the sump tube drains the area, while the smaller lumen provides a continuous flow of air at atmospheric pressure, thus maintaining the suction at a lower level and preventing adherence of the tube against the tissue wall. The air vent should never be clamped off or connected to suction.

Two tubes that may be used for intestinal decompression are the Miller-Abbott tube and the Cantor tube (Fig. 31-16). The length of these tubes permits their passage through the entire intestinal tract. A small balloon on the tip of each tube acts like a bolus of food when inflated with air or injected with water or mercury. This balloon stim-

Table 31-16   Nasogastric and intestinal tubes

Tube	Purpose	Characteristic	Use
Nasogastric			
Levin	Removes fluid and gas from stomach (decompression); may also be used to give tube feedings	Single lumen; easy to maintain; may cause trauma to stomach wall	Use intermittent suction at low pressure setting
Salem sump	Same purpose as Levin tube; more commonly used	Double lumen, one for drainage and one to provide an air vent to prevent tube adherence to stomach wall	Use low (30 mm Hg) *constant* suction; attach the larger lumen of tube only to suction
Entron	Tube feedings for gastric feedings only	No. 6 Fr (small bore); has a stylet for easier insertion but no weighted end	Clamp off when not in use; do not attach to suction (collapses)
Dobbhoff enteric	Tube feedings for gastric or intestinal feedings	No. 8 Fr (small bore); has a stylet for easier insertion and a weighted end to pass into intestines	Same as for the Entron tube
Intestinal			
Miller-Abbott	Removes fluid and gas from intestines (decompression)	Double lumen, one for balloon inflation and one for drainage	Use low pressure intermittent suction; clamp off balloon tube and attach drainage tube only to suction
Cantor	Same purposes as Miller-Abbott tube; (used less frequently)	Single lumen; mercury is injected into balloon with needle and syringe prior to insertion	Use low-pressure intermittent suction

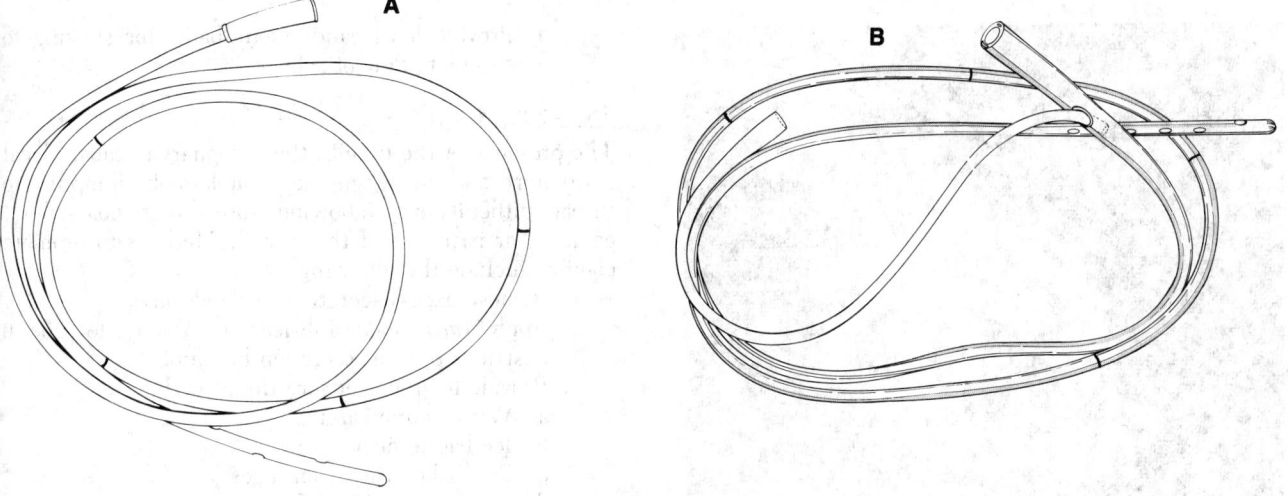

Fig. 31-15   Nasogastric tubes. **A,** Levin tube. **B,** Salem sump tube.

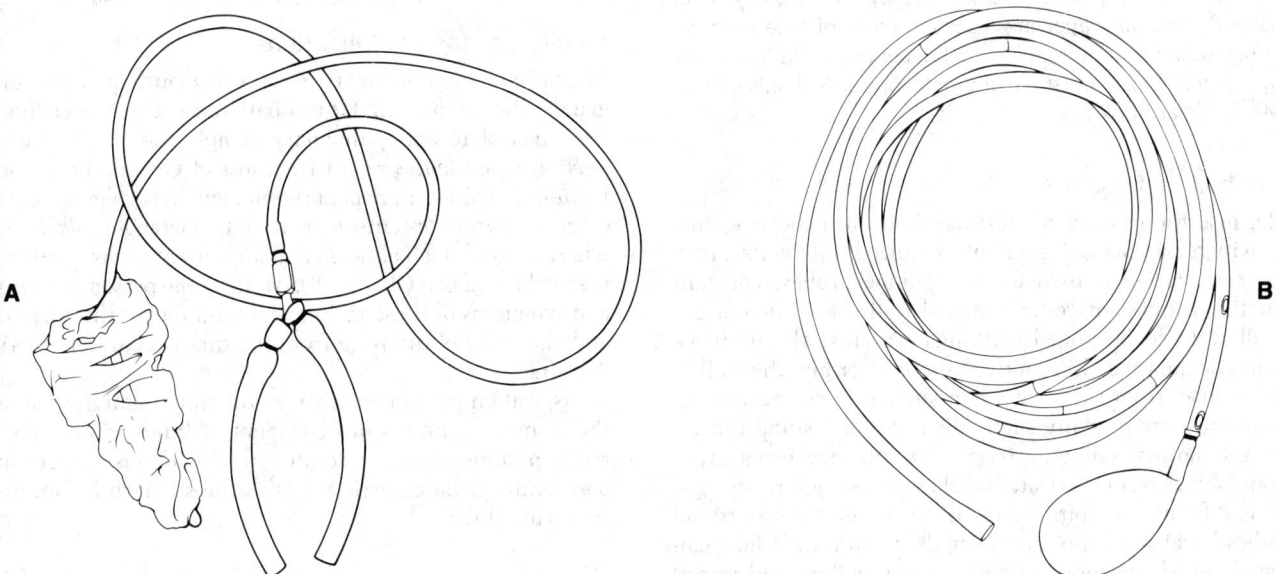

Fig. 31-16   Intestinal tubes. **A,** Miller-Abbott tube. **B,** Cantor tube.

ulates peristalsis, which advances the tube along the intestinal tract. If peristalsis is absent, the weight of the mercury in the balloon will usually carry it forward. When a Miller-Abbott tube is used, the mercury is inserted into the balloon of the tube after the tube is passed.

Insertion of Tubes

Nasogastric tubes may be inserted by the nurse or the physician. *Intestinal* tubes are more difficult to insert because of the addition of the balloon. The intestinal tube can be mechanically inserted only into the stomach. Its passage along the remainder of the GI tract depends on gravity and peristalsis. The weight of the mercury in the balloon helps propel the tube through the intestines.

The intestinal tube is passed in the same manner as the nasogastric tube. After the intestinal tube reaches the stomach its passage through the pylorus into the duodenum

is facilitated by positioning and activity.

1. Encourage the following patient positions;
   a. Right side for 2 hours, then
   b. Lying on back with head elevated for 2 hours, then
   c. Left side for 2 hours
2. Encourage patient ambulation following passage of tube into the pylorus (often assessed by x-ray film)
3. Advance the tube 2 to 10 cm (1 to 4 inches) at specified intervals to provide slack for peristaltic action
4. Secure tube to face *only* when desired point has been reached; coil extra tubing on bed or pin to clothing

The intestinal tube is usually monitored daily by x-ray film for signs of coiling or telescoping of the tube. Telescoping is movement of bowel along with the tube resulting in intussusception (p. 968), a serious complication.

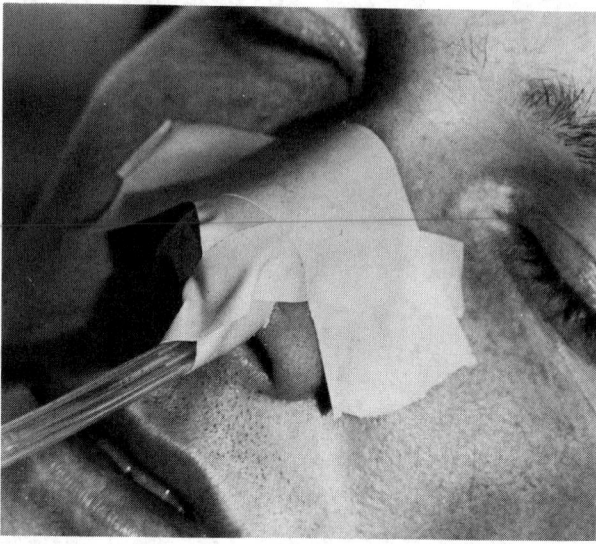

Fig. 31-17   Nasogastric tube secured by crossing tape over patient's nose and applying a second piece of tape over the bridge of the nose. (From Hirsch J, Hannock L, editors: *Mosby's manual of clinical nursing procedures,* St Louis, 1981, Mosby–Year Book.)

Facilitating Drainage

Because the gastric or intestinal fluid must move against gravity to be removed, suction is required. *Intermittent low-pressure suction* is used for single-lumen tubes; constant suction could damage the mucosal wall if a section of the wall were to be pulled continually against the drainage holes of the tube. Intermittent suction permits the wall to drop away from the tube when suction is not occurring. Constant low-pressure suction is used for a sump tube.

Use normal saline to irrigate the tube because a hypotonic solution such as water would increase electrolyte loss. It is difficult to aspirate irrigating solution from *intestinal* tubes because of the tubes' length. If no return flow can be obtained, use only a small amount of fluid and record the amount instilled.

Preventing Injury

Pressure of the tube against the nares may lead to irritation and tissue breakdown. The oropharyngeal mucosa or the parotid glands may become inflamed as a result of dry mucous membranes from oral breathing (nares plugged) or from GI bacteria that travels up the tube by capillary action. Discomfort at the jaw angle may indicate a parotitis. Methods to prevent injury from gastric intubation include the following:

1. Tape tube securely to nostril so that it does not press against nostril (Fig. 31-17)
2. Pin tube loosely to clothing to support weight of tube and permit free head movement
3. Prevent oral inflammations
   a. Keep oral mucous membranes moist
   b. Give frequent mouth care
   c. Use ice chips sparingly (ingestion of large amounts of hypotonic water from the melted ice may produce electrolyte loss through suction)

d. Provide hard candy (sour balls) for sucking to stimulate flow of saliva

Promoting Comfort

The presence of the tube in the nasopharynx causes local discomfort, and the person may complain of a lump in the throat, difficulty in swallowing, sore throat, hoarseness, earache, or irritation of the nostril. Methods to promote comfort include the following:

1. Remove excess secretions around nares.
2. Apply *water-soluble* lubricant (K-Y jelly) to tube at nostril to prevent secretion buildup.
3. Provide for relief of sore throat with:
   a. Warm saline gargles
   b. Ice bag to neck
   c. Prescribed throat lozenges
   d. Frequent position changes to relieve pressure of tube on throat
4. Use low- or mid-Fowler's position (unless contraindicated) to prevent esophageal reflux (heartburn).

Monitoring for Complications

In addition to inflammations of the mouth and parotid glands, the person with GI intubation may experience fluid and electrolyte and pulmonary complications. *Fluid and electrolyte imbalances* result from loss of GI secretions and include dehydration, hyponatremia, and hypokalemia. Loss of acid *gastric* contents may lead to metabolic *alkalosis,* whereas loss of alkaline *intestinal* contents may produce metabolic *acidosis* (Chapter 8). Monitor the person for signs and symptoms of these imbalances, and record the amount and character of drainage from the tubes accurately every 8 hours.

Aspiration pneumonia may result from regurgitation of the stomach contents or placement of fluids in an incorrectly positioned tube. Monitor breath sounds. Ascertain positioning of nasogastric tubes in the stomach before introducing fluids.

SURGERY OF THE STOMACH

A number of different surgical procedures may be performed on the stomach (Table 31-17). The suffix *-ostomy* means "an opening into," thus *gastrostomy* refers to an opening into the stomach. If only one prefix precedes the term *-ostomy,* then the surgical opening is made from the exterior, such as gastrostomy. When two prefixes precede *-ostomy,* the surgery consists of an opening made between two organs (*anastomosis*); for example, a gastroenterostomy is an anastomosis of a portion of the stomach (*gastro-*) with a portion of the small intestine (*entero-*). The surgical procedures more commonly used for cancer of the stomach are gastroduodenostomy (Billroth I) and gastrojejunostomy (Billroth II) (see Fig. 31-10).

Preoperative Care

If the nutritional status of the patient is poor, an attempt is made to improve nutrition preoperatively. Total parenteral nutrition (p. 929) or a temporary gastrostomy (p. 927) may be necessary. If the patient is to have surgery for an

Table 31-17   **Surgeries of the stomach**

Name	Description	Comments
Esophagogastrostomy	Anastomosis of esophagus and stomach	Usually involves removal of lower one third of esophagus; tissue graft may be used
Esophagojejunostomy	Removal of stomach (total gastrectomy) and anastomosis of esophagus to jejunum (Fig. 31-12, C)	Two portions of jejunum meeting esophagus are sometimes joined to form a reservoir for food
Gastrectomy	Removal of part (subtotal) or all (total) of stomach	Remaining portions are anastomosed to small intestine
Gastrostomy	Insertion of tube through abdominal wall into stomach	Permits esophageal bypass allowing for nutritional feedings into GI tract
Gastroduodenostomy	Formation of new opening between stomach and duodenum	In Billroth I surgery (Fig. 31-12, A) part of stomach is removed and remaining portion is anastomosed to duodenum
Gastrojejunostomy	Anastomosis of stomach with jejunum	In Billroth II surgery (Fig. 31-12, B) duodenal stump is closed after excision of lower part of stomach
Antrectomy	Removal of entire antrum (lower portion) of stomach	Usually followed by gastroduodenostomy
Pyloroplasty	Repair of pyloric opening of stomach	To enlarge opening and facilitate stomach emptying
Gastric partitioning	Stapling of stomach to reduce size	Staples applied in two rows partially across stomach for control of massive obesity (see Fig. 31-4)

Table 31-18   **Postgastrectomy complications**

Complications	Symptoms	Therapy
Bleeding at anastomotic suture line	Large quantity of blood in nasogastric tube drainage during day 1; may also occur on days 4 to 7	Treatment for upper GI hemorrhage (p. 949)
Duodenal stump leakage	Severe upper abdominal pain that may radiate to shoulder, fever, leukocytosis; usually occurs on days 3 to 6	Surgery
Gastric retention	Abdominal fullness, nausea, and vomiting after nasogastric tube is removed	Nasogastric suction for 48 hours then feedings resumed slowly; surgery if no improvement
Dumping syndrome	Weakness, faintness, tachycardia, diaphoresis during eating or from 5 to 30 minutes later	Small frequent feedings (low carbohydrate, high fat and protein); fluids only between meals
Blind loop syndrome (stasis in blind loop with bacterial proliferation)	Abdominal pain 15 to 30 minutes after eating; steatorrhea, diarrhea, weight loss	Antibiotics; surgery to change a Billroth II to a Billroth I may be necessary

ulcer, any special dietary prescriptions are continued through the preoperative period.

The major focus of preoperative nursing care is teaching the patient. Since the incision for gastric surgery is high in the abdomen, emphasize breathing exercises preoperatively (see Chapter 20). The patient should know that a nasogastric tube may be in place for several days postoperatively because of decreased peristalsis from manipulation of the gastrointestinal tract organs during surgery and to prevent trauma or pressure on suture lines.

Postoperative Care

The care of the patient after gastric surgery centers on promoting pulmonary ventilation, nutrition, and comfort and teaching the patient. Specific nursing care is listed in Box 31-14.

Promoting pulmonary ventilation

Patients with high abdominal incisions are at high risk of developing postoperative pulmonary complications because they are inclined to lie still and breathe shallowly to limit incisional pain. Measures to encourage movement and deep breathing take high priority.

Facilitating gastric drainage

Drainage from the nasogastric tube after surgery usually contains some blood for the first 6 to 12 hours, but bright red blood, large amounts of blood, or excessive bloody drainage is reported to the surgeon immediately (Table 31-18). *If the nasogastric tube stops draining, notify the surgeon,* since a buildup of gas or fluid can cause pressure on the suture line resulting in rupture or dislodgement of the sutures. Do not irrigate the N/G tube without physician

Guidelines for Care

The patient undergoing gastric surgery

Preoperative care

Teach breathing exercises and leg exercises.

Explain special postoperative measures: nasogastric tube and parenteral fluids until peristalsis returns.

Postoperative care

Promoting pulmonary ventilation

Encourage patient to turn and deep breathe at least every 2 hours or less until patient is ambulating well.

Give pain medication before activities to encourage active patient participation (thus increasing ventilation).

Position patient to promote chest expansion (mid- or high-Fowler's).

Promoting nutrition

Measure nasogastric tube drainage accurately for determination of fluid and electrolyte replacement.

Monitor patient for signs of leakage of the anastomosis (pain, fever) when oral fluids are initiated.

Add small amounts of bland food at frequent intervals until foods are well-tolerated.

Monitor patient for early satiety and regurgitation.

If regurgitation occurs:

Tell patient to eat less food at a slower pace.

Report persistent regurgitation to physician.

Report signs of dumping syndrome (weakness, faintness, palpitations of heart, diaphoresis, feeling of fullness, nausea, diarrhea) to physician.

Monitor weight.

Providing comfort

Provide special mouth care until oral fluids are resumed (p. 933).

Provide analgesic medications on a regular basis during first few days to prevent pain.

Splint incision before patient coughs.

Encourage ambulation.

Patient teaching

Gradually increase amount of food until able to eat three meals a day, if possible.

If discomfort occurs after eating, decrease size of meals and amount of fluids with meals and eat more slowly.

Avoid stress, if possible, during and immediately after meals; plan a rest period after eating.

Elevate head when lying down (if cardia of stomach removed) to prevent gastroesophageal reflux (heartburn).

Use measures to modify effects of stress (see Chapter 6).

Monitor weight regularly; report weight loss to physician.

Report signs of complications to physician (vomiting after meals, increasing feeling of abdominal fullness, increasing weakness, hematemesis, tarry stools, pain, persistent diarrhea).

---

approval. It is the *responsibility of the surgeon to adjust the placement of the nasogastric tube* so that inadvertent dislodgement of the sutures is prevented. Report signs of return of GI functioning (auscultation of bowel sounds, passage of flatus) to the surgeon.

Promoting nutrition

Until the nasogastric tube is removed and the patient is able to drink enough nutritious fluids, fluids are given parenterally. The average patient requires about 3500 ml of fluids intravenously each day (2500 ml for normal body needs plus enough to replace fluids lost through the gastric drainage and vomitus).

Fluids by mouth are restricted for about 12 to 24 hours after the nasogastric tube is removed. Fluids are then introduced slowly until well tolerated. Small amounts of bland food may be added until the patient is able to eat six small meals a day and to drink 120 ml of fluid every hour between meals. The dietary regimen must be adapted to the individual, since some persons tolerate increasing amounts of food and fluids better than others. Vitamins are usually prescribed until the patient is eating a full, well-balanced diet.

Early satiety and regurgitation after meals are common problems after gastric surgery. Eating less food more slowly and chewing thoroughly is usually effective. Persistent early satiety or regurgitation may be caused by edema of the suture line. A nasogastric tube may need to be reinserted until the edema subsides.

Dumping syndrome

After a gastric resection, the dumping syndrome occurs to some extent in most patients.[68] It may also occur in patients who had a vagotomy, antrectomy, or gastroenterostomy. The onset may occur during the meal or from 5 to 30 minutes after the meal. The attack may last 20 to 60 minutes. The patient complains of weakness, faintness, tachycardia, and diaphoresis. Other symptoms include a feeling of fullness, discomfort, nausea, and diarrhea.

The symptoms are thought to be caused by the entrance of hypertonic food directly into the jejunum without undergoing usual changes and dilution in the stomach. The food mixture, more hyperosmolar than the jejunal secretions, causes fluid to be drawn from the bloodstream to the jejunum. The reaction appears to be greater after the ingestion of sugar, since sugar is the most osmotically active food. The symptoms are also attributed to the sudden rise in blood sugar (hyperglycemia), with the entrance of glucose into the bloodstream, and the subsequent fall in the blood sugar level. The rapid gastric emptying and the propulsion of chyme into the small intestine are felt to initiate an intensive gastrocolic reflex and cause diarrhea and a feeling of fullness and discomfort.

Reactive hypoglycemia, sometimes called "dumping," has some of the same symptoms. It occurs 3 to 4 hours after eating.[68] Symptoms are relieved by ingestion of sugar.

Teaching for the patient who experiences dumping syndrome includes the following:

1. Eat a low-carbohydrate, moderate-fat, high-protein diet

2. Drink fluids only between meals

Table 31-19   Causes of intestinal malabsorption

Factors affecting absorption	Mechanism	Examples
Altered digestion (intraluminal phase)	Decreased gastric function	Subtotal gastrectomy
	Decreased pancreatic lipase	Pancreatic insufficiency: pancreatitis, cancer of pancreas, cystic fibrosis, Zollinger-Ellison syndrome
	Decreased conjugated bile salts	Liver disease, biliary tract obstruction, enteric fistulas
		Drugs that precipitate bile salts (neomycin, cholestyramine)
Altered mucosal cell transport (mucosal phase)	Genetic abnormalities	Lactase deficiency
	Small bowel disease	Crohn's disease, celiac disease, tropical sprue, Whipple's disease, infectious or allergic enteritis, parasitic infections, small bowel ischemia
	Inadequate surface	Intestinal resection or bypass
	Drugs	Para-aminosalicylic acid, colchicine, irritant laxatives, neomycin
	Radiation	Radiation enteritis
Altered lymph/blood transport (transit phase)	Lymphatic obstruction	Lymphoma
	Altered blood supply	Superior mesenteric thrombosis

3. Avoid eating large amounts of food at one time
4. Rest after meals (recumbent position for 30 minutes)
5. Take anticholinergic drugs before meals as prescribed

Total Gastrectomy

Total gastrectomies are now rarely performed. The nursing care of the patient who has had a total gastrectomy (esophagojejunostomy) differs in some ways from that of patients undergoing other types of gastric surgery. A thoracic approach is used, and the nursing care will be the same as that for the patient who has had chest surgery. Drains are usually inserted from the site of the anastomosis, and there may be serosanguineous drainage. There is little or no drainage from the nasogastric tube because there is no longer any reservoir in which secretions may collect, and there is no stomach mucosa left to secrete.

Following a total gastrectomy the maintenance of good nutrition is difficult because the patient can no longer eat regular meals and because the food that is taken is poorly digested and therefore poorly absorbed from the intestines. Since the patient also becomes anemic, ferrous sulfate, folate, and vitamin B_{12} are often prescribed. These patients rarely regain normal strength.

MALABSORPTION SYNDROME
Etiology

Malabsorption syndrome is a group of signs and symptoms resulting from inadequate absorption of fat in the small intestine. Because fat-soluble vitamins (A, D, E, and K) require fat for absorption, decreasing absorption of these vitamins usually accompanies fat malabsorption. In addition, fat malabsorption often is accompanied by decreased absorption of protein, carbohydrate, and minerals. Different signs and symptoms specific to various nutrients result from malabsorption of nutrients other than fat.

Adult lactase deficiency is a common disorder found among most populations of the world with the exception of northern European Caucasians and their descendants. In North America, Blacks, Jews, Orientals, American In-

dians, Eskimos, and Mexicans are frequently affected. Lactase deficiency is usually a congenital disorder, although symptoms may not occur immediately. It also occurs occasionally after a subtotal gastrectomy.

Some adults have an intolerance to gluten found in grains (wheat, rye, barley, oats). The disorder may be termed *adult celiac disease, celiac sprue,* or *gluten enteropathy*. These persons often have a history of childhood celiac disease or evidence of disease in relatives. Tropical sprue is different than celiac sprue and is endemic to the Caribbean, Southeast Asia, and India.

Pathophysiology

Malabsorption results when there are (1) alterations of digestion so that nutrients are not broken down into a form that can be transported across the cell membranes of the villi; (2) alterations in the transportation of nutrients across the cell membranes of the villi so that nutrients cannot be absorbed; and (3) alterations in the transport of nutrients, particularly fat, from the villi through the lymphatic or circulatory systems (Table 31-19).

Lactase deficiency results from a lack of the enzyme lactase, which hydrolyzes lactose (a disaccharide found in milk) into glucose and galactose for absorption. The undigested lactose acts as an osmotic agent drawing water into the intestinal lumen and a substrate for bacterial fermentation, producing abdominal distention and pain.

Intolerance to gluten found in grains leads to atrophy of the intestinal villi and microvilli. The proximal jejunum is the area most affected. This disorder is thought to be a hypersensitivity response. Tropical sprue has both a nutritional and infectious basis and responds to treatment with antibiotics, as well as to diet therapy.

Nursing Process
Assessment

The stool is assessed for presence of a light, greasy, bulky, mushy appearance and a foul odor. This is a sign of *steatorrhea* (excess fat in the stool). The stools float because of their low specific gravity and because of gas produced by action of intestinal bacteria on the undigested fat. Bowel movements may be limited to one bulky stool a day or may be frequent. If the malabsorption is caused by a lactase deficiency, the patient will have a watery, foul-smelling diarrhea. Malabsorption causes *flatulence* and abdominal distention. Decreased fat absorption leads to weight loss, weakness, fatigue, and anorexia.

If malabsorption is severe, the person will have signs of *vitamin deficiency* (bleeding, bone pain and fractures, hypocalcemia, anemia, inflammation of the tongue, muscle tenderness, peripheral neuritis, and dermatitis). *Protein deficiency* will be evidenced by edema, hypoalbuminemia and loss of muscle mass. The skin will be dry and scaly and may be hyperpigmented.

If acute generalized malabsorption is present, the patient is monitored for signs of *bleeding* (ecchymosis, hematuria), tetany, and skin breakdown.

Data analysis: nursing diagnoses

Determine nursing diagnoses from analysis of patient data. Possible nursing diagnoses for the person with a malabsorption syndrome may include, but are not limited to:

Diagnostic title	Possible etiologies
Nutrition, altered: less than body requirements	Malabsorption
Pain: abdominal, bone, muscle, dry mucous membranes	Malabsorption
Knowledge deficit	Lack of exposure/recall

Planning: expected patient outcomes

Expected patient outcomes for the person with a malabsorption syndrome may include, but are not limited to, the following:

1. Consumes nutrients that can be tolerated
2. States feeling comfortable
3. Describes diet to be followed and signs indicating need for dietary reevaluation

Implementation
Promoting nutrition

If intolerance to a specific substance is present, omit that substance from the diet. Thus, in adult *lactase deficiency*, all foods containing milk products or added lactose are avoided. Milk substitutes (such as Ensure Plus, Isocal) are available, and vegetable oils are used instead of butter. Some persons can tolerate some cheeses and yogurt. Calcium substitutes are required.

If *gluten intolerance* is present, exclude all cereal grains and their products (except for rice). This is a difficult diet to follow because many commercial foods, including some instant coffees, contain some wheat filler. Corn, soybean, and gluten-free flour are available for cooking.

If *generalized acute malabsorption* is present, the patient may require total parenteral nutrition or intravenous albumin, calcium, magnesium, and potassium. Packed red blood cells may be necessary if anemia is severe.

Providing comfort
Mouth care

Dry mucous membranes and enlarged tongue lead to oral discomfort. Good mouth care every 4 hours to maintain

---

31-15

Foods containing lactose or gluten

Foods containing lactose
Dairy products
Baked foods containing milk, butter, cheese
Commercial foods processed with lactose
Instant coffee
Chocolates
Cold cuts, hot dogs

Foods containing gluten
Foods containing wheat, rye, barley, oats
Commercial baked goods and pastas
Commercial salad dressings
Ice cream, candies
Beer, ale
Instant coffees using wheat flour as a filler

---

hydration will ease discomfort.

Bone and muscle pain

Analgesics may relieve bone or muscle pain. Aspirin may be contraindicated because of the bleeding tendency from vitamin deficiencies. Gentle handling of the extremities is indicated.

Anal care

The rectal area may become irritated with diarrhea. Provide for gentle personal hygiene after *each* loose stool.

Counseling and teaching

Because there is no "cure" for malabsorption syndrome, persons with these problems must learn to adjust their diets for life. Teaching the person includes the following:

1. Avoid all foods containing that which is not tolerated (Box 31-15).
2. Read carefully the labels of prepared foods.
3. Follow the appropriate diet (lactose-free or gluten-free) for life.
4. Reevaluate diet if symptoms reoccur.

Evaluation

Evaluation of the care of the person with malabsorption syndrome is based on the expected patient outcomes. Questions to consider are:

1. Is the patient consuming nutrients that can be tolerated?
2. Is the patient comfortable?
3. Does the patient know the types of food to be avoided?

FLATULENCE
Pathophysiology

Gas collects in the GI tract as a result of swallowed air, as gas formed by the action of intestinal bacteria, and as carbon dioxide formed by the action of bicarbonate with hydrochloric acid or fatty acids. Normally the gas is either reabsorbed or is expelled. When gastrointestinal motility is decreased, the gas collects in the stomach or intestines, causing abdominal distention and pain.

Assessment

"Gas pains" can cause severe abdominal discomfort. The abdomen is distended over the entire area (as differentiated from lower abdominal distention occurring from a full bladder). The abdomen has a drumlike sound if percussed.

Implementation

Some of the following interventions may help decrease the intestinal gas volume when a pathologic condition is not present:

1. Avoid activities that increase repetitive swallowing of air such as gum chewing.
2. Maintain an erect position after meals to facilitate gas rising to the fundus of the stomach and being expelled.
3. Eat a low-fat diet to decrease carbon dioxide production.
4. Take antacids containing hydroxide and simethicone (Maalox Plus, Mylanta) 1 hour after meals to neutralize acid and reduce flatus.
5. Avoid gas-forming carbohydrates that produce more discomfort (for example, selected vegetables, fruit, or bran).
6. Ambulate to increase peristalsis to move the gas through the intestinal tract, if discomfort is present.

ELIMINATION DISORDERS

The major disorders of the intestines are inflammatory disorders (acute and chronic) that may interfere with absorption and disorders that interfere with passage of the chyme and fecal matter (paralytic ileus, intestinal obstruction, hernias, and tumors). Anorectal lesions, which may be inflammatory or vascular (hemorrhoids), may interfere with passage of feces because of the discomfort produced.

ACUTE INFLAMMATORY INTESTINAL DISORDERS

Etiology

Inflammation of the intestines (enteritis) is a common occurrence and may occur alone or in combination with gastritis (p. 940). Gastroenteritis is often of viral origin. Some foods may irritate the intestinal mucosa, which leads to mild symptoms of belching, abdominal discomfort, and diarrhea.

Food poisoning occurs after the ingestion of food that is contaminated by bacteria containing toxins. Some examples of bacteria that cause food poisoning, along with the foods in which they are found or food preparation methods that produce the bacteria, are: (1) *Staphylococcus aureus*: enterotoxin in fish, meats, unrefrigerated mayonnaise or cream-filled foods; skin and respiratory tract of food handlers; (2) *Salmonella*: inadequately cooked pork, poultry, eggs; and (3) *Clostridium botulinum*: improperly canned or smoked foods. Bacteria and parasites may also cause intestinal inflammations (Table 31-20). The appendix may become inflamed (appendicitis); appendicitis is most common in males aged 10 to 30.

Pathophysiology
Enteritis

Acute enteritis can be caused by direct bacterial or viral infection or by the effect of neurotoxins produced by bacteria. This produces either an increased secretion of water and salt into the gut lumen or an increase in motility, causing large amounts of undigested food and fluid to be excreted. In the latter case, large amounts of gas and foul-smelling stool result. With profuse diarrhea, large amounts of fluid and electrolytes may be lost, leading to dehydration, hyponatremia, and hypokalemia (see Chapter 7).

REVIEW

Table 31-20

Disease	Signs and symptoms	Medical therapy
Gastroenteritis	Abdominal cramps, nausea and vomiting, diarrhea, headache	Nothing by mouth until nausea and vomiting subside, then fluids and bland diet; rest
Food poisoning	*Staphylococcus aureas:* Nausea and vomiting, abdominal pain, decreased temperature; diarrhea is variable	Bed rest, fluids
	Salmonella: Nausea and vomiting, abdominal pain, chills, fever, weakness	Bed rest, fluids
	Clostridium botulinum: Nausea and vomiting, double vision, flaccid paralysis of face and throat, dryness of skin and mucous membranes	Botulinum antitoxin, maintenance of ventilation and oxygen, parenteral fluids
Amebiasis	Early: abdominal cramps, intermittent diarrhea/constipation, flatulence	Amebicidal drugs
	Late: frequent liquid stools containing blood, mucus; fever, colicky abdominal pain	
Trichinosis	Edema of eyelids, muscle stiffness, weakness, fever, pain on eye motion, dyspnea	Symptomatic: bed rest, analgesics, steroids, thiabendazole
Appendicitis	Sudden onset, pain in midepigastrium becomes localized in right lower quadrant, nausea and vomiting, low grade fever, leukocytosis	Appendectomy when diagnosis confirmed

Parasitic infections

The most common parasitic infections are amebiasis and trichinosis (Table 31-20). *Amebiasis* is caused by the protozoan parasite that primarily invades the large intestine and secondarily the liver. The active motile form of the protozoa, the trophozoite, is not infectious and, if ingested, is easily destroyed by digestive enzymes. However, the inactive form (cyst) is highly resistant to extremes in temperature, most chemicals, and the digestive juices. When the cyst is swallowed in *fecally contaminated food or water*, it easily passes into the intestines, where the active trophozoite is released and enters the intestinal wall. Here it feeds on the mucosal cells, causing ulceration of the intestinal mucosa. Although the disease exists chiefly in tropical countries, it also prevails wherever sanitation is poor. The cyst can survive for long periods outside the body.

Trichinosis is caused by the larvae of a species of roundworm, which become encysted in the striated muscles of humans, hogs, and other animals (rodents) that eat infected pork in garbage. Trichinosis has a worldwide distribution with the highest incidence occurring in Europe and the United States. It occurs more often in hogs that have been fed garbage than in those fed on grain. The larvae do not form cysts in pork; therefore, they are not visible to the naked eye and cannot be seen by food inspectors.

Trichinosis is transmitted through inadequately cooked food. *Pork* is the most common source of infection. When infected food is eaten, live encysted larvae develop within the intestine of the host; they mate and produce eggs that hatch in the uterus of the female worm. The larvae are discharged in huge numbers into the lymphatics and lacteals of the host's small intestine at the rate of about two every hour for about 6 weeks. They pass to the muscles of the host, where they become encysted by the reaction of the host's body and may remain for many years.

The trichinosis parasite can be killed by cooking at the recommended temperature of 77° C (170° F) or by freezing at a temperature of −15° C (5° F) for 20 days.[60] They are not killed by smoking, pickling, or other methods of processing. Sausage and other infected pork products carelessly prepared are a source of infection in humans.

Appendicitis

Appendicitis is an inflammation of the vermiform appendix, located near the ileocecal valve. The inflammation may be initiated by obstruction from a fecalith (a stonelike mass formed from feces), infection from colon bacilli or streptococcus, or appendiceal kinking or occlusion. A small part of the appendix may be edematous or necrotic, or the entire appendix may be involved. Pressure within the appendix builds up rapidly, leading to early necrosis of the appendiceal walls with subsequent perforation. Heat and external pressure (such as that resulting from enemas) increase the appendiceal pressure, facilitating rupture of the appendix.

Although the typical symptoms of acute appendicitis (anorexia, nausea, and vomiting combined with abdominal pain that becomes located at McBurney's point halfway between the umbilicus and right ileal crest) are common

findings, many variations of these symptoms may occur. The pain may be located in other parts of the abdomen as a result of the stretching of the appendix or the location retrocecally or adjacent to the ureter. Low-grade fever and leukocytosis result from the inflammation.

Peritonitis

If peritonitis (inflammation of the peritoneum) results from a perforated appendix, adhesions form quickly in an attempt to wall off the infection, and the omentum helps to enclose areas of inflammation, forming an abscess. As healing occurs, fibrous adhesions may form, leading to intestinal obstruction at a later date. At other times the fibrous adhesions may disappear completely. Local inflammatory reactions of the peritoneum include redness, edema, and the production of large amounts of fluid containing electrolytes and proteins. Hypovolemia, electrolyte imbalance, dehydration, and finally shock develop from loss of circulating fluid if the infection is not contained. Intestinal peristalsis is halted by a severe peritoneal infection.

Nursing Process
Assessment

Subjective data to be collected from the person with an acute inflammatory disorder of the intestines include anorexia, nausea, and presence and extent of abdominal discomfort. If food poisoning is suspected, question the person about possible sources of food contamination. Abdominal pain is usually diffuse except if acute appendicitis is present. With appendicitis, there is often rebound tenderness over McBurney's point if pressure is applied lightly, then released suddenly.

Objective data to be collected include the following:
1. Emesis: frequency, amount, presence of blood
2. Stools: frequency, character, amount if liquid, presence of foul odor
3. Flatulence
4. Signs of fluid and electrolyte imbalance (thirst, dry mucous membranes, hemoconcentration, oliguria, muscle weakness)

Data analysis: nursing diagnoses

Nursing diagnoses are determined from analysis of patient data. Possible nursing diagnoses for the person with an acute inflammatory disorder of the intestines may include, but are not limited to, the following:

Diagnostic title	Possible etiologies
Fluid volume deficit	Diarrhea
Pain: abdominal	Intestinal inflammation
Infection: high risk for spread	Lack of knowledge

Planning: expected patient outcomes

Expected patient outcomes for the person with an acute inflammatory disorder of the intestines may include, but are not limited to, the following:
1. Patient is hydrated (moist skin and mucous membranes, good skin turgor).
2. Patient states feeling more comfortable.
3. Infection is not spread.

REVIEW

Table 31-21   Chronic inflammatory bowel disorders

Disease	Signs and symptoms	Medical therapy
Crohn's disease	Periods of exacerbation and remission Acute: colicky or steady right lower quadrant pain, malaise, moderate fever, mild diarrhea, mucus or pus in stool Chronic: weight loss, anemia, fistula formation, intestinal obstruction	Diet: high-calorie, high-protein, high-vitamin Sulfonamides, azathioprine (Imuran) Surgery for fistulas or intestinal obstruction (colectomy or colostomy)
Ulcerative colitis	Periods of exacerbation and remission Severe diarrhea (15 to 20 stools/day containing blood, mucus, pus); anorexia; weight loss; anemia; low grade fever Severe: weakness, debility, cachexia, dehydration, hypokalemia, hypoproteinemia	Diet: high-calorie, high-protein, high-vitamin (avoid milk) Sulfonamides, adrenocorticosteroids Surgery for refractory disease or complications (total colectomy with permanent ileostomy)
Diverticulitis of colon (inflamed mucosal pouches)	May be asymptomatic Intermittent lower left quadrant pain aggravated by emotional tension or eating Constipation alternating with diarrhea	Diet: high in vegetable fiber, unprocessed bran Bulk stool additives; analgesics (pentazocine [Talwin]), anticholinergics (dicyclomine [Bentyl], propantheline [Pro-Banthine]) Bed rest, sedation, and parenteral or oral fluids for severe episode Surgery for complications of perforation or obstruction (colectomy, temporary colostomy)

Implementation
Assisting with achievement of therapeutic goals

When *appendicitis* is suspected, the patient usually is hospitalized at once and placed on bed rest for observation and the necessary diagnostic procedures (serum WBC, urinalysis, flatplate abdominal x-ray film) that must be performed. Because an operation may be performed shortly after admission, do not give the patient anything by mouth until blood count reports are available. Parenteral fluids may be given during this time. Do not give narcotics until the cause of the pain has been determined because they would mask signs or symptoms. Sometimes an ice bag to the abdomen is ordered to help relieve pain. *Heat and enemas are contraindicated,* as they may cause the appendix to rupture. Explain to the patient that a rectal examination (given by the physician) is necessary to help establish the diagnoses. Surgery consists of an appendectomy (removal of the appendix).

Interventions to achieve patient outcomes
Promoting hydration

When nausea and vomiting are present, give the person nothing by mouth until symptoms subside. With severe vomiting, replace fluids and electrolytes intravenously. A sedative such as sodium phenobarbital or an antiemetic such as prochlorperazine (Compazine) or trimethobenzamide (Tigan) may be prescribed parenterally or by suppository. When vomiting subsides, give tea, broth, and ginger ale orally every hour. Bland feedings of custard, gelatin, and cream soups are usually tolerated after 2 to 24 hours. Carefully measure and record intake and output.

Assisting with comfort

Abdominal cramping from diarrhea may be relieved by constipating agents containing an opiate, such as paregoric,

diphenoxylate (Lomotil), which is chemically related to meperidine (Demerol), or loperamide (Imodium). Belching and defecation also often relieve the discomfort. If appendicitis is ruled out, heat to the abdomen may offer some relief.

Preventing spread of infection

Universal precautions help to control spread of infection in the hospital. Stress cleanliness, and advise patients that it is important to wash their hands well after bowel movements and before meals to prevent spread of infection.

Evaluation

Evaluation is based on expected patient outcomes. Questions to consider include:

1. Is patient hydrated, with moist skin and mucous membranes and good skin turgor?
2. Is the patient more comfortable?
3. Has the spread of infection been avoided?

CHRONIC INFLAMMATORY BOWEL DISEASE

Chronic inflammations of the bowel include two disorders, Crohn's disease and ulcerative colitis, that are fairly similar and are referred to as chronic inflammatory bowel disease (IBD). Another chronic inflammatory disorder is diverticulitis (inflammation of colon diverticula), but because it is a different entity, it is discussed separately. Table 31-21 lists signs and symptoms and usual medical therapies of these disorders.

Table 31-22   Comparison of Crohn's disease and ulcerative colitis

	Crohn's disease	Ulcerative colitis
General appearance	Usually normal	May feel and look ill
Age	Peak: 15 to 30 years	Bimodal: high peak 15 to 30 years, lower peak 50 to 70 years
Area affected	Mainly terminal ileum, cecum, and ascending colon (right side)	Colon only, primarily the descending colon (left side)
Extent of involvement	Segmental areas of involvement	Continuous, diffuse areas of involvement
Inflammation	Mostly submucosal	Mostly mucosal
Mucosal appearance	Cobblestone effect; granulomas	Ulcerations
Cancer potential	Normal incidence	Increased incidence
Character of stools	No blood; may have some fat; three to four semisoft per day	Blood present; no fat; frequent liquid stools
Reasons for surgery	Fistulas; intestinal obstruction	Poor response to medical therapy; hemorrhage; perforation
Complications	Fistulas; perianal disease; strictures; vitamin and iron deficiencies; fistulas to other organs	Pseudopolyps; hemorrhage; toxic megacolon; cachexia; perforation less often, causes peritonitis

Etiology/Epidemiology

Chronic inflammatory bowel disease occurs primarily in young adults ages 15 to 30 but may occur up to age 70. The cause is unknown, although both genetic and environmental factors have been implicated. There is a higher incidence of IBD in Western Europe and the United States. Ulcerative colitis occurs twice as often as Crohn's disease, but incidence of the latter is increasing.

Pathophysiology

Ulcerative colitis and *Crohn's disease* differ in terms of location and type of lesions (Table 31-22). Ulcerative colitis starts in the rectosigmoid colon and spreads upward. Crohn's disease can affect both the small and large intestines, and the areas of inflamed tissue are often separated by normal tissue. The lesions of ulcerative colitis are mucosal ulcerations that bleed easily. As the lesions advance, the bowel mucosa becomes edematous and thickened with scar formation. The colon may lose its elasticity and absorptive capability. The lesions of Crohn's disease are granulomatous ulcers that may involve deeper structures. The ulcers may perforate and form fistulas (Fig. 31-18). Scar tissue may lead to intestinal obstruction.

The loss of absorptive capability in both ulcerative colitis and Crohn's disease leads to anorexia, weight loss, malaise, and diarrhea. Severe diarrhea leads to dehydration from fluid loss, hypokalemia from loss of potassium-rich intestinal secretions, and hypoproteinemia from loss of protein through the damaged intestinal epithelium.[72]

Nursing Process
Assessment

Collect subjective and objective data about the patient's knowledge of the disorder, nutritional status, pattern of elimination, comfort, and ability to cope with stress.

Subjective data

1. Patient's understanding of the disorder
2. Patterns of bowel elimination: frequency, character, amount; presence of blood, fat, mucus, or pus
3. Pain: location, character, frequency, relief with passage of stools, relief measures taken
4. Nutritional status
   a. Intolerance to certain foods
   b. Intake of caffeinated drinks, alcohol
   c. Appetite, presence of nausea
   d. Usual weight, recent weight loss
   e. Weakness, fatigue
5. Sleep: interference because of diarrhea or pain
6. Stress
   a. Perceived sources of stress in daily life
   b. Occupation: nature, hours of work, job satisfaction
   c. Usual coping methods and present effectiveness
7. Social relationships
   a. Extent of social activities and interferences as a result of illness
   b. Availability and perceived support of significant others
8. Sexual: effect of illness on sexual relationships
9. Medications taken at home: type, dosage, effect

Objective data

1. Weight
2. Temperature
3. Observable eating patterns
4. Signs of dehydration with severe ulcerative colitis (decreased skin turgor, dry mucous membranes)
5. Stool: number, character, amount, presence of blood (overt, positive guaiac test), pus, mucus
6. Condition of perianal skin with severe diarrhea
7. Behavior: signs indicating stress or anxiety (for example, restlessness, pacing, twisting hands, verbal comments indicating concerns)

Information about the patient's understanding of the nature and precipitating factors is helpful in planning necessary teaching. Analyze the diet of the person with ulcerative colitis or Crohn's disease for nutritional adequacy. Compare the person's usual daily intake to the basic four food groups to determine quality of nutrient intake. Anorexia and intolerance to milk products are characteristic of ulcerative colitis. With severe ulcerative colitis or Crohn's disease, there is weakness from loss of weight because of the decreased nutrient intake and decreased absorption. Cachexia may result.

The pattern of bowel elimination for the person with chronic bowel inflammation may vary as follows:

Ulcerative colitis	Severe diarrhea (15 to 20 stools/day) stool may contain blood, pus, mucus
Crohn's disease	Mild diarrhea; stool may contain mucus, fat or pus; no blood
Diverticulitis	Constipation or constipation alternating with diarrhea; stool may contain blood

With ulcerative colitis, abdominal cramps may occur with or without bowel movements. The colicky right lower quadrant abdominal pain of Crohn's disease is often relieved by a bowel movement. The pain of diverticulitis may be aggravated by eating.

Symptoms of chronic inflammatory bowel disorders may be exacerbated by stress or tension. Knowledge of the patient's perception of the effect of stress on the onset of symptoms and of the patient's usual coping patterns is useful for planning measures to relieve or reduce effects of stress.

Diagnostic tests

Laboratory tests are conducted for the presence of anemia and for blood in the stools. IBD is diagnosed by means of radiographs, sigmoidoscopy, or colonoscopy. A biopsy of tissue may be taken during sigmoidoscopy or colonoscopy.

Stool examination for occult blood

Occult blood may be identified by one of three tests: guaiac (Hemoccult), benzidine, or orthotoluidine (Occultest). The *guaiac* test is the least sensitive but does not require special preparation. With the *benzidine* or *orthotoluidine* tests, false readings may be obtained if the patient ingests meat (false-positive) or vitamin C in quantities greater than 500 mg/day (false-negative). Ask patients about whether they have taken these substances before performing the benzidine or orthotoluidine tests.

Radiographs

The barium enema (Table 31-23), also called lower GI series, helps identify the lesions of IBD, as well as complications such as fistulas, strictures, polyps, and megacolon of perforation (Fig. 31-18).

Endoscopy

Sigmoidoscopy (Table 31-23) is a common procedure for visualizing the rectum and sigmoid colon just past the sigmoid flexure. Colonoscopy is a more exacting procedure and is usually performed only when clinically necessary.[72] Neither sigmoidoscopy nor colonoscopy is performed during acute episodes of IBD.

Data analysis: nursing diagnoses

Nursing diagnoses are determined from analysis of patient data. Possible nursing diagnoses for the person with

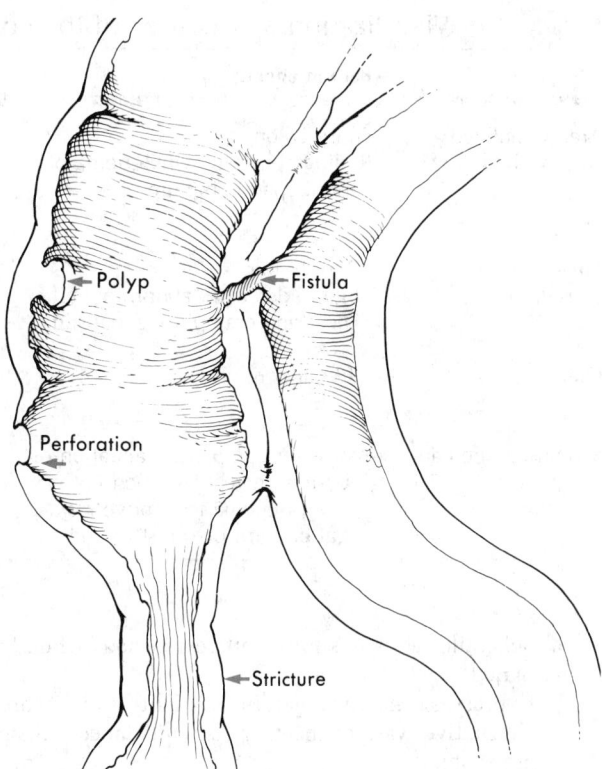

Fig. 31-18   Selected complications of chronic inflammatory bowel disease.

chronic inflammatory bowel disease may include, but are not limited to, the following:

Diagnostic title	Possible etiologies
Nutrition, altered: less than body requirements	Loss of nutrients in diarrhea, anorexia
Fluid volume deficit, high risk for	Diarrhea
Pain: abdominal, anus	Diarrhea, anal skin irritation
Skin integrity, impaired, high risk for	Malnutrition
Coping, ineffective individual, family	Chronicity of disorder, situational crises
Fatigue	Anemia, malnutrition, inflammatory response, stress
Sexual dysfunction	Malnutrition, diarrhea
Knowledge deficit	Lack of information or recall

Planning: expected patient outcomes

Expected patient outcomes for the person with a chronic inflammatory bowel disorder may include, but are not limited to, the following:

1. Eats a high-protein, high-calorie, high-vitamin, well-balanced diet.
2. Drinks 2500 ml/day; skin and mucous membranes are moist.
3. States feeling more comfortable.
4. Skin of elbows, sacrum, and rectal area is intact.
5. Describes alternative coping measures, if appropriate.

Table 31-23   Visualization procedures of the colon

	Barium enema	Colonoscopy	Sigmoidoscopy
Area visualized	Entire colon	Entire colon	Sigmoid colon
Approach	Radiographs following enema of radioopaque barium	Direct visualization through a colonic fiberscope (105 to 185 cm)	Direct visualization through a sigmoidoscope (30 to 65 cm)
Time	30 to 45 min	30 to 120 min	10 to 15 min
Sensation	Urge to defecate, abdominal fullness and cramping, exhausting	Uncomfortable; sedation given	Urge to defecate, minimal abdominal cramping
Diet	NPO after midnight	Clear liquids for 3 days or administration of GoLYTELY; NPO for 8 hr before procedure	Light breakfast
Postprocedure care	Assess for complete evacuation of barium; give prescribed laxative or enema to remove residual barium; plan rest period	Plan rest period; monitor vital signs q4-6h; monitor for signs of bowel perforation (abdominal pain, rise in body temperature, gross blood in stools)	No special care

6. Schedules activities to permit rest periods when fatigued.
7. Expresses concerns regarding sexuality and explores alternative ways of meeting sexuality needs, if appropriate.
8. Describes nature of illness and prescribed therapy, measures to promote relaxation and rest, symptoms requiring medical attention, and plans for regular follow-up care.
9. Family/friends describe:
   a. Approaches to promote patient independence and control of own daily activities.
   b. Approaches to cope with own feelings regarding patient's illness.

Implementation
Assisting with achievement of therapeutic goals

Therapy for IBD during exacerbations is primarily supportive and includes nutritional therapy and rest. Medications include the following:

1. Sulfasalazine: the most commonly prescribed drug. Patient instructions include drinking 2000 to 2500 ml/day to prevent crystallization in kidneys and avoiding sunlight or using sunscreen because of photosensitivity. Infertility may occur.
2. Mesalamine (5-ASA, the active ingredient of sulfasalazine): given by enema for ulcerative colitis; oral forms (mesalamine, mesalazine) are available in many countries[68]; has fewer side effects than sulfasalazine.
3. Corticosteroids: given in high dosages over a limited time for severe disease to suppress inflammation; dosages are decreased gradually before drug is discontinued.
4. Antibiotics: given to acutely ill patients with signs of peritoneal irritation or with a fistula.
5. Bulk hydrophilic agents such as psyllium (Metamucil) in preference to the antimotility drugs for diarrhea.
6. Vitamin supplements, particularly when anorexia

and nausea are present; replacement of vitamin B$_{12}$ when there is a marked loss of ileum.
7. Iron dextran (Imferon): given by Z-track for anemia (oral iron intake is ineffective because of intestinal ulceration).

Interventions to achieve patient outcomes
Promoting nutrition

A low-residue diet to promote bowel rest and to avoid irritation of the mucosal lining is recommended during exacerbations. The diet should be high in proteins and calories to replace lost nutrients. With IBD, large amount of proteins are lost through the intestinal wall by exudation or bleeding. Calories are needed for energy to spare the protein for healing. Fats are sometimes not well tolerated because of malabsorption. Some persons with ulcerative colitis have an intolerance to lactose, and these person should avoid milk products. In acute stages, give an elemental diet that is almost residue free (products that are generally used for tube feedings but are here given orally). Palatability may be a problem; serving fluids chilled and offering a variety of flavors increases patient acceptance. For severe exacerbations, total parenteral nutrition (TPN) is commonly used.

Promoting fluid balance

Profuse diarrhea leads to loss of fluids and electrolytes. Encourage fluids to 2500 ml/day for persons on oral diets. Keep the mouth moistened and apply lotion to the skin. Monitor weight for marked changes resulting from fluid losses or gains. Monitor fluid intake and output daily in the hospitalized patient.

Promoting comfort and skin integrity

Encourage patients to use the toilet or commode whenever possible, but a weak, acutely ill person usually want the bedpan accessible at all times. Empty and clean the bedpan as often as it is used, which may be frequently for patients with ulcerative colitis. Room deodorizers may be necessary. Patients who brace themselves on the bedpan by leaning on their elbows may develop pressure areas; these areas will need to be protected and massaged frequently.

The anal region often becomes excoriated from the frequent stools. Painful anal fissures and fistulas may also develop. Keep the anal area clean and dry. Medicated wipes (such as "Tucks") can provide greater comfort than toilet tissue. Frequent sitz baths also promote comfort and cleanliness. Ointments such as Desitin or zinc oxide may be used to protect the perianal skin.

Facilitating coping

Ulcerative colitis and Crohn's disease are lifelong illnesses with periods of exacerbation and remission that can disrupt the person's life. Emotions and stress have been noted to play a role in exacerbations. If the disease is of long duration, the patient is usually thin, nervous, and apprehensive and is inclined to be preoccupied with physical symptoms. Insecurity, dependency, and depressed or hostile behavior may be present. Family and friends may take over control of the person's life, adding to the person's feelings of loss of self-control.

The caregiver may also experience feelings of frustration and dissatisfaction. Empathic communication over time is usually needed to establish a helping relationship. It may be necessary to plan to spend time with the person and with the family on a regular basis.

Help the person with chronic inflammatory bowel disease to identify possible sources of life stressors and to examine ways to possibly reduce or modify the stress. Assess the person's usual coping mechanisms for effectiveness, and discuss alternate coping strategies as appropriate (see Chapter 6). Knowledge about the illness, diagnostic tests, and therapy may help to decrease anxiety. Patients need to be included in planning of activities to gain some control over their lives. During periods of remission, the person may need to be encouraged to participate in social activities.

Promoting rest

Fatigue is common because of increased energy demands from the inflammatory process and decreased energy supply from malnutrition and anemia. Include planned rest periods in the daily activities. When fatigue subsides, encourage progressive activity. During periods of remission, encourage the person to participate in social activities but not overextend to the point of fatigue.

Promoting sexuality

Sexual response may be decreased by chronic inflammatory bowel disease and may interfere with sexual relationships. Malnutrition and frequent diarrhea lead to decreased libido. Give the person an opportunity to discuss any sexual concerns, and assist the person to communicate these concerns with the involved party. Alternate ways of meeting sexuality needs can be explored (see Chapter 34).

Facilitating patient learning

Patient teaching is important on an ongoing basis to help the person learn effective self-care. Main points to be included in teaching are listed in Box 31-16. Pamphlets

---

Patient Teaching

31-16

The patient with a chronic inflammatory bowel disease

Diet
Eat a high-protein, high-calorie, high-vitamin diet (avoid milk products with ulcerative colitis).

Elimination
Take medications as prescribed.
Drink at least 8 glasses fluid daily.
Keep rectal area clean; use analgesic rectal ointment or take sitz bath for anal discomfort.

Promotion of rest
Use relaxation measures (such as breathing exercises) when emotional tension is present.
Identify sources for an ongoing supportive relationship.
Maintain a regular sleep schedule.
Schedule daily activities to avoid fatigue; rest as necessary.

Health maintenance program
List signs indicating possible exacerbation or complications (abdominal pain, increasing diarrhea or constipation, presence of blood or pus in the stool, fever, progressive weight loss).
Plan for regular follow-up care.

---

about inflammatory bowel disease to be used in patient teaching can be obtained from the National Foundation for Ileitis and Colitis.*

Evaluation

Evaluation is based on expected patient outcomes. Questions to ask may include the following:

1. Is the patient eating a well-balanced, high-protein, high-calorie diet and drinking 2000 to 2500 ml/day?
2. Does the patient feel comfortable and rested?
3. Is skin intact on elbows, sacrum, and rectal area?
4. Are patient and family coping with the changes caused by IBD?
5. Does the patient schedule activities to permit for rest periods?
6. Has the patient expressed concerns regarding sexuality and explored alternative ways of meeting sexual needs?
7. Can the patient describe the nature and therapy for IBD and need for medical follow-up?
8. Can family and friends describe their approaches to promote patient's independence?

Surgery

Ulcerative colitis can be treated by surgery. The trend is toward earlier surgical intervention for the acutely ill person and for persons experiencing frequent exacerbations. Surgery is clearly indicated when complications are pres-

---

*National Foundation for Ileitis and Colitis, 444 Park Ave, New York, NY 10016.

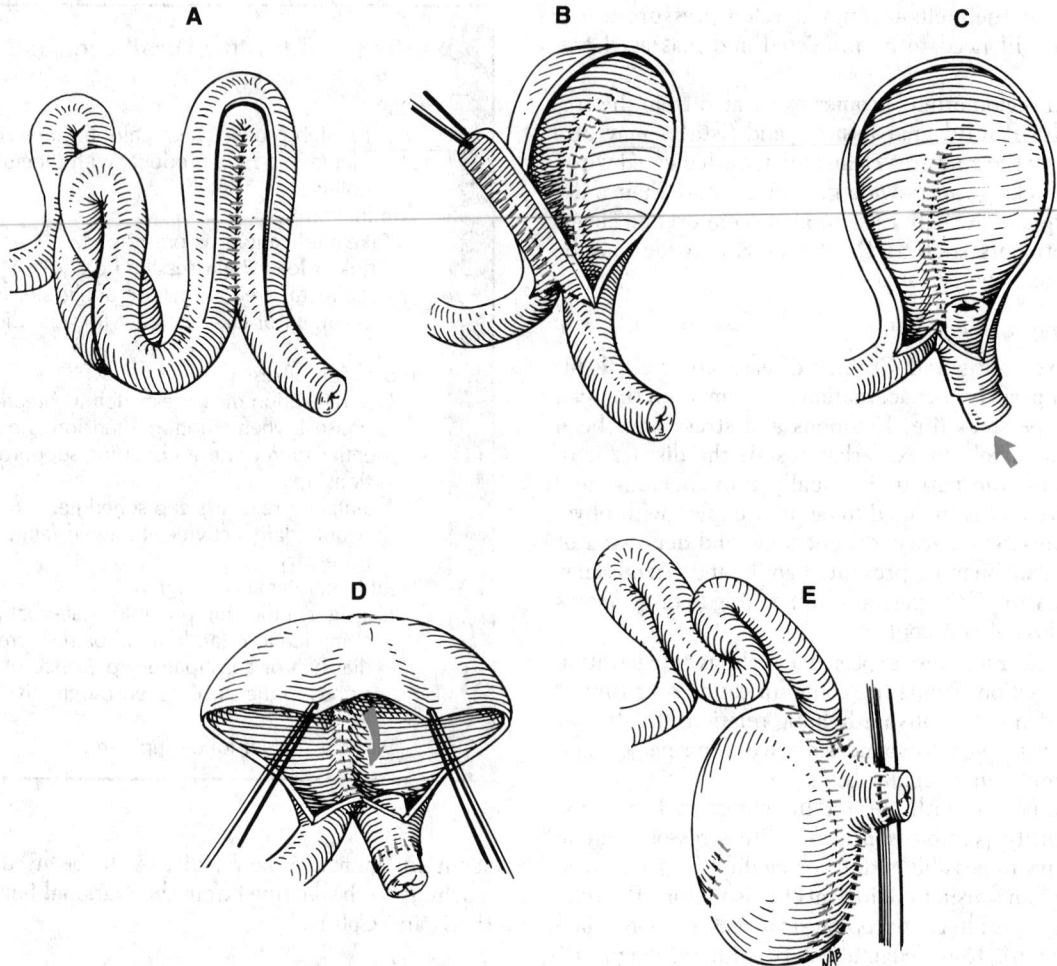

Fig. 31-19 Continent ileostomy (Kock pouch). **A,** Loop of bowel sewn together. **B,** Removal of anterior portion. **C,** Nipple valve made by pushing bowel back on itself. **D,** Pouch formation. **E,** End brought through stoma.

ent, including massive hemorrhage, perforation of the colon, strictures, and medically unresponsive toxic megacolon (dilation and hypertrophy of the colon).

Different types of surgery may be performed. A common procedure is removal of the diseased colon and rectum, with the end of the ileum being brought out through the abdominal wall (*ileostomy*). If the rectum is only mildly diseased, an ileorectal anastomosis may be performed with preservation of rectal function.

A different type of surgical approach is the *continent ileostomy* or *Kock's pouch* (Fig. 31-19). An intraabdominal reservoir with a nipple valve is formed from the distal ileum to provide continence. The capacity of the pouch increases slowly over months until it can hold approximately 500 ml. Contents of the pouch are removed several times a day by catheterization. Difficulties have occurred with valve failure and in keeping the ileal contents from becoming too thick and plugging up the stoma.

Total colectomy and mucosal proctectomy with *ileoanal anastomosis* (with or without a valveless pouch) consists of resection of the colon, removal of rectal mucosa leaving rectal muscle intact, and anastomosis of ileum with the

anal sphincter. A J-pouch (Fig. 31-20), an S-pouch, and a W-pouch are approaches that can be used. These methods are now used more frequently than the continent ileostomies. A 2-month temporary ileostomy is performed to permit healing of the anastomosis. Bowel incontinence may be a sequela.

Crohn's disease does not respond well to surgery and has a high recurrence rate. Surgery is indicated when complications occur (bowel obstruction, fistulas, abscesses). Types of surgery include (1) segmental *resection* of the diseased bowel with anastomosis (preferred method) or (2) bowel *bypass* by anastomosing the ileum to the disease-free colon, leaving the diseased bowel intact. A newer procedure is *strictureplasty*, in which blocked or narrowed bowel segments are widened, leaving the bowel intact.

Ileostomy care

The general care of the patient with an ileostomy is similar to that of the patient with a colostomy (p. 979).

Fecal drainage from the ileostomy stoma begins within 72 hours. It is liquid and may be constant. Within 10 to 15 days, the ileostomy output will be a soft, slightly formed

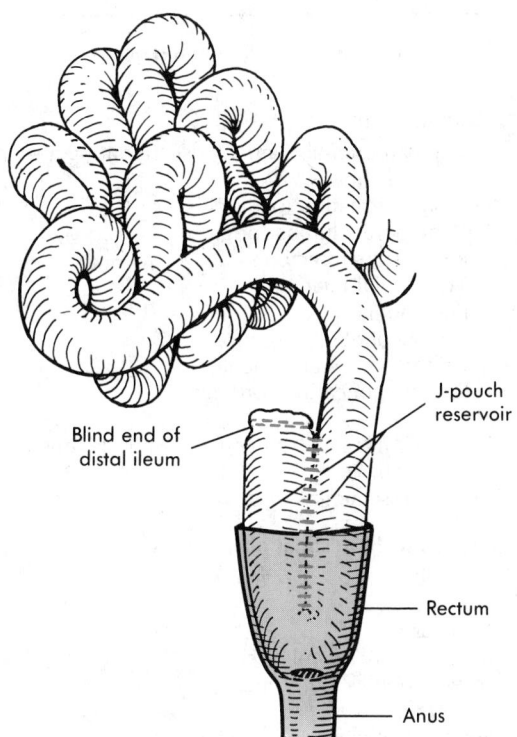

Fig. 31-20   Ileoanal anastomosis with a valveless ileal reservoir. Side-to-side anastomosis of a J-loop of terminal ileum is incised at apex and anastomosed to anal sphincter; remaining rectal mucosa provides support. Defecation occurs through anus.

Labels on figure: Blind end of distal ileum; J-pouch reservoir; Rectum; Anus

---

stool. The terminal ileum adapts to the loss of the colon and begins to reabsorb water. Patients with ileostomies have "toothpaste" consistency stools within 3 to 6 months after the adaptation of the ileum. Drainage usually occurs 2 to 4 hours after a meal, although there may be a small amount of output intermittently throughout the day.

Exceptions to this pattern of ileostomy elimination are seen in patients who have had previous bowel resections or resections of the ileum for Crohn's disease. The more small intestine that is lost, the greater the chance of a high volume of very liquid output with resultant dehydration.

Maintaining fluid and electrolyte balance

An excessive loss of fluid through the ileostomy, usually from 1000 ml to 2000 ml daily, may occur during the initial postoperative period. The amount of fluid output then diminishes to 500 to 800 ml/day.[68] Sodium and potassium losses are greater with an ileostomy than the amounts normally lost in feces. The person with an ileostomy is therefore at greater risk for dehydration, hyponatremia, and hypokalemia during periods of decreased fluid intake or of increased fluid output. Potassium supplements may be necessary. After the initial period, a large amount of output— requiring the pouch to be emptied hourly or more frequently—is considered to be diarrhea. During these periods, monitor the person for signs of fluid and electrolyte imbalance. Teach the patient how to promote fluid and electrolyte balance (see Box 31-17).

Promoting nutrition

The patient may be kept on a low-residue diet for 6 weeks to decrease the amount of bulky and undigested foods as the intestinal tract recovers from the surgical intervention. As the person begins to add foods, it is recommended that only one high-fiber food be added at a time and that the person chew the food well. Foods should not be eliminated from the diet unless the person is unable to tolerate them after two or three trials.

Food blockage (a large mass of undigested food, especially high-fiber foods) may occur with an ileostomy. The food becomes lodged at a kink, or narrowing, in the bowel and blocks the lumen. The result is a mechanical bowel obstruction. Blockage most commonly occurs when a person eats several high-fiber foods in one meal or does not chew the foods properly.

If the ileostomy becomes blocked, the person should get into a knee-chest position and gently massage the area below the stoma. Stomal edema will develop with a food blockage, and the pouch should be changed to accommodate the swelling. Diarrhea usually follows the removal of the obstruction, and the patient will need fluid replacement. Abdominal pain in the peristomal area is generally present for 3 to 5 days after obstruction. If the obstruction is not passed following the use of the knee-chest position, the patient should notify the physician.

DIVERTICULAR DISEASE OF THE COLON

Diverticula, or pouches, form when increased pressure within the colon pushes weakened areas of the colon out-

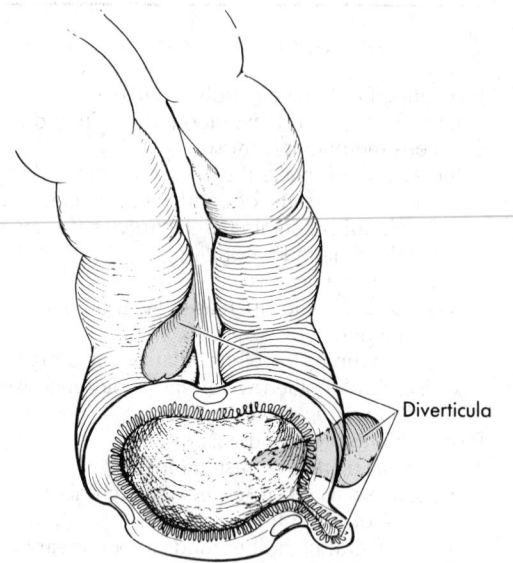

Diverticula

Fig. 31-21 Diverticuli of colon.

ward (Fig. 31-21). The cause is thought to be a low intake of dietary fiber, which is often typical of diets in industrialized societies. Diverticula usually occur after age 40, and the incidence increases with age. The nonsymptomatic condition is called diverticulosis.

Diverticulitis

Symptoms appear when the diverticula become inflamed (diverticulitis), creating painful spasms, or when complications such as perforation, obstruction, or hemorrhage occur. Bowel motility may be slow because of insufficient fiber, leading to constipation, or fast because of the inflammation, leading to diarrhea.

With acute diverticulitis, intravenous fluids or a clear liquid diet may be prescribed to allow the bowel to rest. Antibiotics are also prescribed. Recurrent attacks of diverticulitis or occurrence of complications usually require surgical resection of the involved colon with an end-to-end anastomosis. Bowel surgery is described on p. 973. A temporary colostomy may be necessary for 6 to 8 weeks.

Diverticulosis

When the person is asymptomatic, encourage a diet high in vegetable fiber (fruits and vegetables, whole grain cereals). Patients should avoid foods with seeds and nuts, as these irritate the diverticula. Individuals may add unprocessed wheat bran to foods, but initially only in small amounts that increase slowly to one-fourth cup daily in fruit juices or muffins. Bran initially causes abdominal distention and excess flatus. The purpose of the high-fiber diet is to increase stool bulk and bowel transit time, thus increasing the diameter of the colon and decreasing intraluminal pressure.

Bulk additives such as psyllium seed (Metamucil) and stool softeners such as docusate sodium (Colace) may be prescribed for persons with diverticular disease. Anticholinergic drugs may be given to slow peristalsis and to decrease spasms in the sigmoid colon.[60]

31-18

Causes of intestinal obstruction

Paralytic ileus
Manipulation of abdominal viscera during abdominal surgery
Peritoneal irritation (peritonitis)
Pain of thoracolumbar origin
    Rib or spinal fractures
    Myocardial infarction
    Pneumonia
    Pyelonephritis
    Ureteral or biliary calculi
    Retroperitoneal hemorrhage
Sepsis
Hypokalemia causing decreased muscle tone of bowel
Intestinal ischemia

Mechanical intestinal obstruction
Adhesions
Hernias
Neoplasms
Inflammatory bowel disease
Foreign bodies, gallstones
Fecal impaction
Strictures: congenital, radiation
Intussusception
Volvulus

Because emotional tension often precipitates diverticulitis, the person may need assistance in learning how to reduce emotional tension. Relaxation techniques, planned rest periods, and regular sleeping hours may prove helpful.

INTESTINAL OBSTRUCTION

Etiology

Intestinal obstruction (ileus) occurs when there is impedance to the normal flow of intestinal contents, either because of disturbance to neural stimulation of bowel for peristalsis (paralytic ileus) or because of something interfering with normal flow of bowel contents (mechanical/organic ileus). *Paralytic ileus* results mainly from handling of the bowel during abdominal surgery, from peritonitis, or from pain of thoracolumbar origin (see Box 31-18). *Mechanical obstructions* of the small intestines are primarily adhesions, whereas in the large bowel, neoplasms are the major cause. A *volvulus* is a twisting of the bowel (Fig. 31-22). *Intussusception* is a telescoping of the segment of the bowel within itself. *Hernias* may cause bowel obstruction when a loop of bowel becomes strangulated in the weakened ring or incision (p. 970). In *cancer of the bowel*, the growth narrows the lumen of the bowel. The clinical manifestations and medical therapy of intestinal obstruction are outlined in Table 31-24.

Pathophysiology

When peristalsis ceases, the involved intestinal area becomes distended by gas and fluid. Approximately 7 L of fluid are secreted into the stomach and small intestines per day; most of this fluid is normally reabsorbed in the colon.

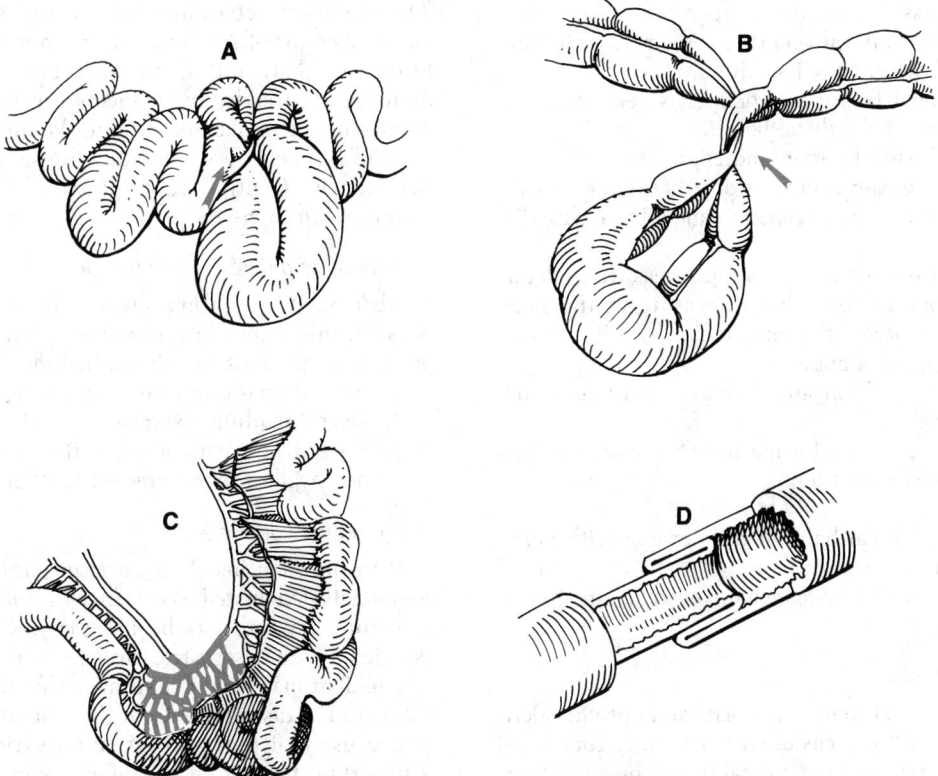

Fig. 31-22   Some causes of intestinal obstruction. **A,** Constriction by adhesions. **B,** Volvulus. **C,** Mesenteric thrombosis. **D,** Intussusception.

REVIEW

Table 31-24   **Obstructive disorders of the intestinal tract**

Disorder	Signs and symptoms	Medical therapy
Paralytic ileus	Continuous abdominal pain, distention, vomiting, obstipation, decreased or absent bowel sounds	Restricted oral intake, IV fluids, GI suction
Mechanical intestinal obstruction	Colicky abdominal pain, vomiting, constipation, high-pitched bowel sounds	Same as above; surgery
Hernia	Lump in weakened area, especially with straining; pain with incarceration	Herniorrhaphy
Cancer of the bowel	Blood in stool, changes in bowel patterns	Resection of bowel, with or without a stoma

When peristalsis ceases, however, much of the fluid remains in the stomach and small intestine. The retained fluid increases pressure on the mucosal wall and, if not removed, results in ischemia, necrosis, bacterial invasion, and eventually peritonitis. Loss of the fluids leads to hypovolemia (shock) and dehydration. Loss of sodium and chloride ions causes a shift of potassium from the cells, leading to hypokalemic alkalosis.

When mechanical obstruction occurs, peristaltic waves proximal to the affected area increase in an effort to move the intestinal contents past the obstruction. These peristaltic movements create a high-pitched abdominal sound.

As the abdomen distends from the distended gut, pulmonary ventilation may become impaired from pressure on the diaphragm. Pressure on the bladder may cause urinary retention. Constipation occurs with mechanical obstruction because some feces usually pass around the obstruc-

tion. When peristalsis ceases completely, as with paralytic ileus or complete organic obstruction, no bowel movement occurs (obstipation).

Nursing Process
Assessment

The following parameters need to be monitored in the patient who is thought to be developing an intestinal obstruction:

1. Bowel sounds: presence and character
   a. Loud, frequent, high-pitched sounds are heard as obstruction is developing.
   b. Bowel sounds are not heard when peristalsis ceases.
   c. Weak bowel sounds and passage of flatus occur as peristalsis returns (flatus is a more significant sign).

2. Vomiting: assess type and frequency
   a. Profuse, nonfecal vomiting is seen with obstruction of the proximal small bowel.
   b. Occasional fecal-type vomitus is seen with obstruction of the distal bowel.
3. Abdominal pain: location and character
   a. Cramping pain occurs as obstruction develops.
   b. Pain becomes more constant and diffuse with distention.
4. Abdominal distention: use a tape measure to determine change in size; always measure at the same site (usually across the umbilicus).
5. Urinary output: amount
   a. Monitor total output (decrease seen with dehydration).
   b. Monitor amount of urine at each voiding for signs of urinary retention.
6. Vital signs
   a. Fever, tachycardia, and hypotension with dehydration.
   b. Fever may also indicate more obstruction or peritonitis.

Diagnostic tests

X-ray films of the abdomen (flat plate and upright) identify air- and fluid-filled areas of obstruction. Serum blood tests indicate alterations from normal (hemoconcentration) when dehydration occurs. There will be a decrease in sodium and potassium and an increase in hematocrit, plasma bicarbonate, serum pH, and blood urea nitrogen (BUN).

Data analysis: nursing diagnoses

Nursing diagnoses are determined from analysis of patient data. Possible nursing diagnoses for the person with an intestinal obstruction may include, but are not limited to, the following:

Diagnostic title	Possible etiologies
Fluid volume deficit	Abnormal loss of GI fluids
Ineffective breathing pattern	Abdominal distention
Pain: abdominal	Abdominal distention

Planning: expected patient outcomes

Expected patient outcomes for the person with an intestinal obstruction may include, but are not limited to, the following:

1. Patient is hydrated (moist skin and mucous membranes, good skin turgor).
2. Breath sounds are clear; respirations are easy and regular.
3. Patient states feeling more comfortable.

Implementation
Assisting with achievement of therapeutic goals

Conservative medical therapy consists of oral intake restrictions, parenteral fluids and electrolytes, and gastric or intestinal suctioning until bowel function returns.

Interventions to achieve patient outcomes
Promoting hydration

Give fluids containing electrolytes parenterally in large quantities (3000 to 4000 ml/day) to prevent dehydration.

The physician determines the amount to be given based on the amount of gastric drainage from nasogastric or intestinal intubation; thus it is important to measure gastric drainage accurately. Flow sheets are helpful for careful monitoring of intake and output. Monitor the patient for signs of fluid overload (bounding pulse, neck vein distention, cough). Central venous pressure (Chapter 9) may be monitored in high-risk patients (elderly, cardiac disease).

Promoting pulmonary ventilation

Abdominal distention creates pressure on the diaphragm, inhibiting chest expansion. Nursing measures to promote aeration of the alveoli include the following:
1. Fowler's position to release pressure on diaphragm
2. Deep breathing exercises
3. Encouraging patient to breathe through the nose and not swallow air to prevent further distention

Promoting comfort

Pain and vomiting often leave the patient physically and emotionally exhausted. Assistance in simple activities such as turning in bed may be necessary. Comfort measures associated with nasogastric intubation (p. 954) are helpful. The patient may need reassurance that the decompression will ease the discomfort from the distention.

Because oral fluids are usually restricted, mouth care is important for preventing infection and increasing comfort. If the patient is poorly nourished, measures to keep the skin soft and intact and free from pressure are indicated.

Surgery

Surgery is usually performed to relieve mechanical and vascular obstruction. The operative procedure varies with the cause and the location of the obstruction and the general condition of the patient. If constricting bands or adhesions are found, they are cut, and it may be necessary to resect the occluded bowel and anastomose the remaining segments. Care of the patient undergoing intestinal surgery is described on p. 973.

Evaluation

Evaluation is based on expected patient outcomes. Questions to consider are:
1. Is the patient hydrated?
2. Have pulmonary complications been avoided?
3. Is the patient relatively comfortable?

HERNIAS

Hernias account for a large number of intestinal obstructions. A hernia is a protrusion of an organ or structure from its normal cavity through a congenital or acquired defect. In addition to a loop of bowel, a hernia, depending on its location, may contain peritoneal fat, a section of bladder, or a portion of the stomach.

If the protruding structure of the organ can be returned by manipulation to its own cavity, it is called a *reducible* hernia. If it cannot, it is called an *irreducible* or *incarcerated* hernia. When the blood supply to the structure within the hernia becomes occluded, the hernia is said to be *strangulated*. Some types of hernias are described below.

Table 31-25   Cancer of the colon

Location	Signs and symptoms	Surgery
Ascending	Occult blood in stool, anemia, nausea/vomiting, right upper quadrant pain, palpable mass	Right colectomy with anastomosis
Descending colon	Gross blood in stool, progressive constipation with increased frequency, pencil-shaped stools	Left colectomy with anastomosis
Sigmoid colon and rectum	Rectal bleeding, constipation and increased frequency, sensation of incomplete bowel evacuation	Sigmoid: left colectomy with anastomosis Upper rectum: resection with anastomosis Lower rectum: abdominoperineal resection with colostomy

Types of hernias

Inguinal	
Indirect	Loop of intestine passes through abdominal ring and follows course of spermatic cord into inguinal canal
Direct	Loop of intestine passes through posterior inguinal wall
Femoral	Loop of intestine passes through femoral ring down into femoral canal
Umbilical	Loop of intestine passes through umbilical ring
Incisional	Loop of intestine or other organ protrudes through weakened scar

A hernia that is not incarcerated can very often be reduced by the person lying down with the feet elevated or by lying in a tub of warm water and pushing the mass gently back toward the abdominal cavity.

Surgery is frequently performed for large hernias or when there is a high risk of incarceration. A *herniorrhaphy* consists of suturing the defect in the fascia. In the postoperative period following repair of an *umbilical* or large *incisional* hernia, a nasogastric tube may be used to prevent postoperative vomiting and distention with subsequent strain on the suture line.

Because of postoperative inflammation, edema, and hemorrhage, *swelling of the scrotum* often occurs after repair of an indirect inguinal hernia. This complication is extremely painful, and any movement of the patient causes discomfort. Ice bags help relieve pain. The scrotum is usually supported with a suspensory or is elevated on a rolled towel. Urinary retention may occur because of the discomfort in movement, which produces hesitancy in urination. Ecchymosis of the lower abdominal wall or upper thigh may occur after extensive manipulation during surgery. The ecchymosis fades in a few days. Sexual functioning is not affected.

The patient who has had elective surgery for a hernia should not drive for at least 2 weeks. Physical activities should not include any heavy lifting, pulling, or pushing for at least 6 weeks.

CANCER OF THE BOWEL
Epidemiology

Malignant tumors of the colon and rectum are among the most commonly occurring malignancies in the United States, third following cancer of the lung and prostate in men and second following cancer of the breast in women.[4]

The incidence of bowel cancer is significantly higher in developed countries whose inhabitants are of Northern European descent, and it is lower in Japan, India, Africa, and some Latin American countries. The incidence of bowel cancer also increases with age and reaches a peak in people in their late 70s. Clinical manifestations and types of surgery are outlined in Table 31-25.

Etiology

Although the cause of cancer of the bowel remains unknown, environmental and genetic factors and preexisting disease appear to be influential (see Box 31-19). The high incidence of colorectal cancer in industrial countries relates to a diet high in animal fat, protein, and refined carbohydrates that are low in dietary fiber. Although a direct causative relationship has not been established, high fat and low-fiber diets may be significant causative factors. Low-fiber diets decrease colonic transit time and potentially increase contact of endogenous or exogenous carcinogens with the bowel mucosa. Popular literature often suggests that certain foods are carcinogenic; however, research has not yet identified specific foods as carcinogenic for bowel cancer. Genetically, some "cancer families" have been identified in which cancers of certain body areas, including the bowel, are transmitted as dominant traits.

Prevention and Health Education

Primary prevention for colon cancer includes reducing fat intake to 30% or less of calories and increasing fiber intake to 20 to 30 g/day with an upper limit of 35 g.[17] These guidelines, established by the National Cancer Institute (NCI), correlate with the guidelines for the Year 2000 from the Public Health Service (Chapter 5). Studies show that

---

31-19

Risk factors for colorectal cancer

Age: over 40
Past history
  Colon polyps (adenomas)
  Cancer: colorectal, breast, genital
  Ulcerative colitis
  Polyposis syndromes
  Immunodeficiency disease
Family history: colorectal cancer, polyposis syndromes

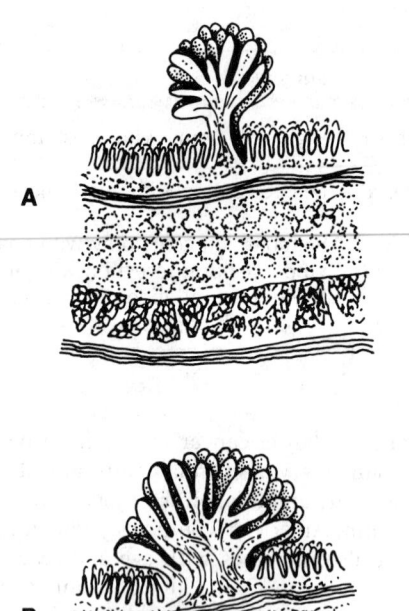

Fig. 31-23 Colon polyps. **A,** Tubular adenoma (note pedicle). **B,** Villous adenoma.

diets high in vegetable fiber offer the most protection. Little is yet known about the mechanisms for cancer protection by fiber; therefore, NCI recommends a fiber intake from a variety of foods (whole grains, vegetables, fruits) rather than fiber supplements.[17]

Secondary prevention involves early detection. Because colorectal cancer develops over time, detection is possible before symptoms appear. Many lives could be saved if everyone followed the following guidelines recommended by the American Cancer Society.

1. Digital rectal examination yearly after age 40
2. Occult blood stool test yearly after age 50
3. Sigmoidoscopy every 3 to 5 years after age 50, following two negative yearly examinations

Many communities have large-scale yearly screenings for colorectal cancer with blood stool tests. Persons can get kits for obtaining stool samples at home and then send the samples to the testing centers. Anyone who develops a change in bowel patterns, a change in the shape of the stool, or the passing of blood should consult a physician.

Pathophysiology

Polyps are *benign* growths (adenomas) on the colonic mucosa; they are considered to be premalignant. The two major types of polyps are the more common *tubular adenoma*, a globelike structure attached to the bowel wall by a "stem" (peduncle), and the *villous adenoma*, a large soft polyp that has several fingerlike projections but no peduncle (Fig. 31-23). Villous adenomas are more likely to become malignant.

Cancer of the colon may develop in one of two ways. In the cecum and *ascending* colon, the lesions tend to develop as polyps that grow as cauliflowerlike masses protruding into the lumen of the colon. These lesions may ulcerate, but obstruction of the colon is uncommon. Eventually, the lesions penetrate the colon wall and extend into surrounding tissue.

In the *descending* colon, especially the rectosigmoid portion, an annular lesion is more common. The early lesion is a small polypoid mass that becomes plaquelike. The plaque grows circumferentially, encircling the colon wall, and then contracts, causing narrowing of the lumen. Obstruction may result from formed stool on the left side that is unable to pass through the narrowed lumen. These lesions also eventually penetrate the colon wall and extend into adjacent tissue.

Cancer of the colon may spread by direct extension or through the lymphatic or circulatory systems, seeding at distant points in the peritoneum or at distant points in the colon. The liver is the major organ of metastasis because the colonic blood vessels empty into the portal vein leading to the liver.

Diagnostic Tests

Diagnosis of cancer of the colon is made by physical examination, sigmoidoscopy, colonoscopy, and barium enema examination (see Table 31-23). Cancer of the rectum can be accurately diagnosed by pathologic examination of a biopsy specimen taken during a proctoscopic examination. Stools are examined for occult blood (p. 963).

Carcinoembryonic antigen monitoring

Carcinoembryonic antigen (CEA) is an antigen seen in fetal life. It was originally isolated from patients with colonic cancer, but it is also seen in persons with ulcerative colitis, cirrhosis, and other forms of cancer and in chronic cigarette smokers.

The CEA test is not useful as a screening test for colonic cancer; however, it is useful as an indicator of the effects of therapy. For example, a drop in CEA level suggests the effectiveness of the therapy. A continued high level or rise in level suggests recurrence or spread of the tumor.

Medical Therapy
Surgery

Treatment of cancer of the colon is always surgical, and the tumor, surrounding colon, and lymph nodes are resected. The amount of bowel resected is based on removal of all tissue supplied by the blood vessel of the diseased tissue. Surgery is performed in one of the following ways: (1) the diseased portion of the bowel is removed (resected), and the remaining ends are joined together in an end-to-end anastomosis (EEA), or (2) the diseased portion of the bowel is removed, and the functioning end is brought out onto the abdominal surface forming a *stoma* (p. 976). Only 10% of persons with rectal cancer require a stoma.

Resection with anastomosis can be performed for cancer of the ascending, descending, or sigmoid colon and upper rectum (Fig. 31-24 *A, B,* and *C*). These surgeries are performed through abdominal incisions, and natural defecation is maintained. The anastomosis may be done by suturing or stapling techniques. A greater amount of rectal

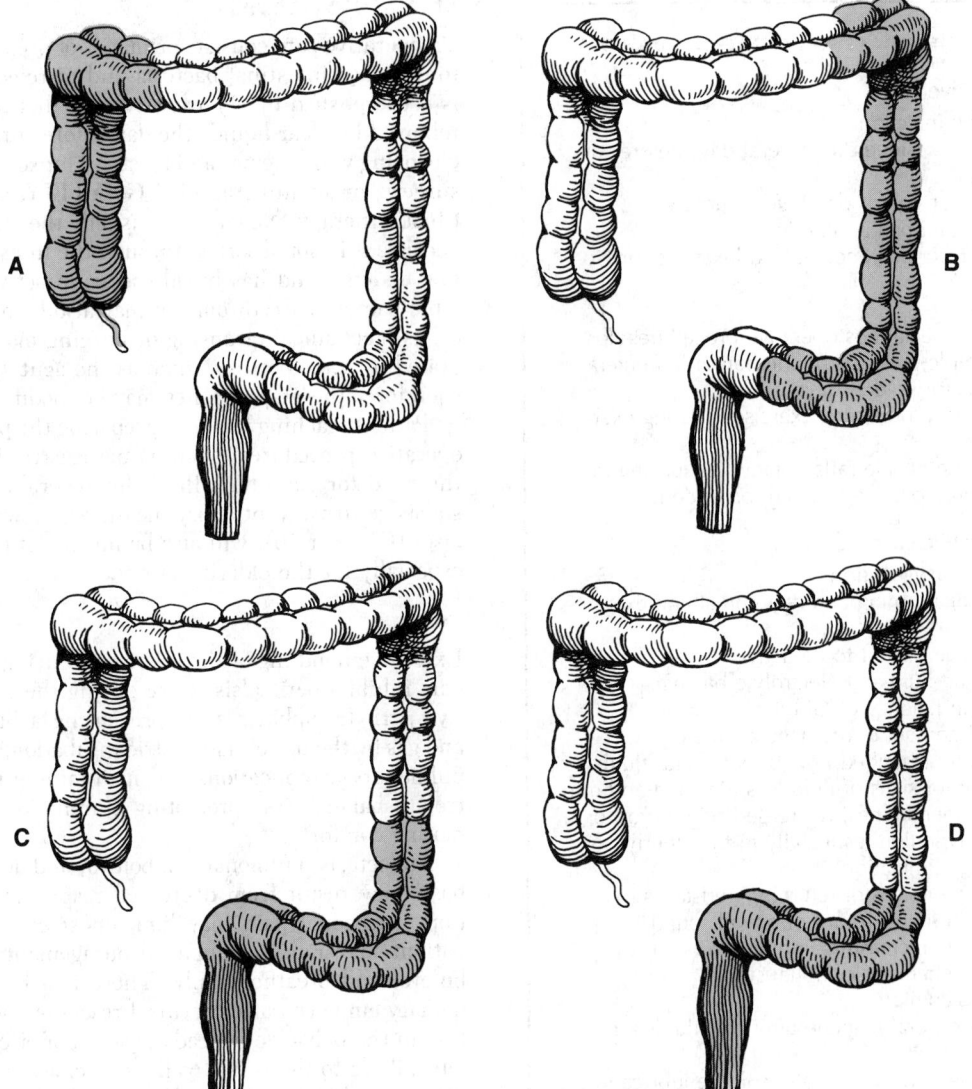

Fig. 31-24 Bowel resection. **A,** Right hemicolectomy. **B,** Left hemicolectomy. **C,** Anterior rectosigmoid resection. **D,** Abdominoperineal resection.

tissue can be removed with the stapling technique for anastomosis.

Growths in the lower rectum require removal of the entire rectum and sigmoid colon by an abdominoperineal resection (p. 974); this surgery requires formation of a stoma. Care of the person experiencing bowel surgery is described below.

Obstruction or perforation of the colon usually requires a temporary colostomy, followed later by closure of the colostomy. Prognosis after surgery depends on the stage and location of growth. Patients with low-lying colorectal stage C cancers have a lower survival rate than those with high-lying colonic cancers.[72] Duke's stages of colorectal cancer are listed below:

Stage A: Confined to bowel mucosa
Stage B: Invading muscle wall
Stage C: Lymph node involvement
Stage D: Metastases or locally unresectable tumor

Other therapies

Radiation therapy is generally ineffective in treating colon cancer but may be used to treat some rectal cancers. It may be used preoperatively in large, locally extensive growths to retard growth; this prevents cells that may accidentally be dislodged during surgery from seeding themselves at other locations. Radiation may be given postoperatively to decrease recurrence.

Chemotherapy is used for metastatic disease and for persons with a high risk of recurrence.[72] It is most effective in preventing liver metastasis. The chemotherapeutic agent of choice is 5-fluorouracil (5-FU), alone or in combination with other agents.

BOWEL SURGERY

Surgery of the bowel may be performed for different reasons, including bowel obstruction, ulcerative colitis, and bowel cancer. The major concern with any type of bowel

The patient undergoing bowel surgery

Preoperative care

Preventing infection
Give low-residue diet several days before surgery.
Give clear liquids day before surgery.
Give prescribed antibiotic.
Give prescribed enemas and laxatives, or GoLYTELY.

Teaching
Explain special postoperative procedures (for example, nasogastric intubation, parenteral fluids for several days).
Teach deep breathing exercises and leg exercises.
Teach use of side rails to facilitate turning in bed without exerting pull on abdomen.

Postoperative care

Promoting oxygenation
Encourage turning and deep breathing exercises.
Encourage patient to be active.

Maintaining fluid and electrolyte balance
Maintain patency of GI tube.
Record amount of drainage accurately.
Maintain prescribed flow of parenteral fluids.
Monitor for signs of fluid loss (dry skin and mucous membranes, decreased skin turgor) or overhydration, especially in the elderly.

Promoting elimination
Monitor for signs of returning peristalsis (passage of flatus, return of bowel sounds).
Encourage increasing ambulation.
Monitor character of initial stools.

Promoting comfort
Give good oral hygiene until oral fluids are taken freely.
Lubricate nares with water-soluble lubricant.
Use measures to maintain moisture of oral mucous membranes (rinse mouth, chew gum, suck hard candy).
Give analgesics on a regular basis during the first 48 hours to minimize severe pain.

Teaching
Drink at least 2000 ml of fluid daily to avoid constipation.
Avoid use of laxatives without medical approval; stool softeners or Metamucil may be used.
Avoid heavy lifting for at least 6 weeks after surgery.

Preoperative Care

Preoperative care consists primarily of preparing the bowel to decrease intestinal bacteria and to remove feces. This is accomplished by (1) a low-residue diet for several days followed by clear liquids the day before surgery, (2) bowel cleansing with enemas and laxatives for several days before surgery, or administration of GoLYTELY, and (3) oral antibiotic therapy. Neomycin is usually the chosen antibiotic because it is not absorbed through the intestinal tract, has low toxicity, and has broad-spectrum activity against colonic bacteria. Erythromycin may also be prescribed. Vigorous mechanical cleansing or purging may be poorly tolerated by some persons, such as the acutely ill or elderly; therefore, these approaches may be modified.

Patient teaching includes preparing the patient for postoperative procedures, such as nasogastric intubation and the need for parenteral fluids for several days until peristalsis returns. Ventilatory measures, as well as leg exercises (Chapter 20), will also be important postoperatively, especially for the elderly patient.

Postoperative Care

Extensive handling of the GI organs during surgery markedly inhibits peristalsis. Care during the early postoperative period emphasizes (1) preventing a buildup of fluid and gas by the use of nasogastric intubation, (2) preventing pulmonary complications, (3) maintaining fluid and electrolyte balance, (4) promoting elimination, and (5) promoting comfort.

Atelectasis, pulmonary embolism, and deep vein thrombosis may result from decreased respiration and circulation. Incisional pain may limit chest expansion and the patient may require much encouragement to move, ambulate, and breathe deeply. There is a high risk of pulmonary embolism after perineal resection. Venous congestion in the pelvic veins leads to stasis of circulation; platelets adhere to the vessel walls, especially at bifurcation of pelvic blood vessels, leading to formation of blood clots with possible embolism.

The length of time required for peristalsis to return depends on the extent of bowel manipulation. Presence of bowel sounds and passage of gas signal the return of function. It is not unusual after a resection of the bowel for diarrhea to occur after peristalsis returns. Usually it is temporary and soon disappears. When stool consistency becomes normal, advise the patient to avoid becoming constipated, because a hard stool and straining to expel it could possibly injure the anastomosis, depending on its location.

The care of the patient experiencing bowel surgery is summarized in Box 31-20.

Abdominoperineal Resection

Malignant growths in the lower two thirds of the rectum are removed by abdominoperineal resection (Fig. 31-24, D). The operation is performed through two incisions: a low midline incision of the abdomen and a wide elliptic incision about the anus. Through the abdominal incision, the sigmoid colon is divided and the lower portion is freed from its attachments and temporarily left beneath the peritoneum of the pelvic floor. The proximal end of the sigmoid is then brought out through a small stab wound on the abdominal wall and becomes the permanent colostomy.

surgery is contamination by fecal contents. Preoperative preparations are directed toward minimizing this problem. Many of the people experiencing bowel surgery are elderly, because the largest number of bowel surgeries are performed for bowel cancer. Elderly persons have a higher risk for postoperative pulmonary embolism and fluid imbalances. If the procedure is performed by laparoscopic surgery, the risks and length of recovery are decreased.

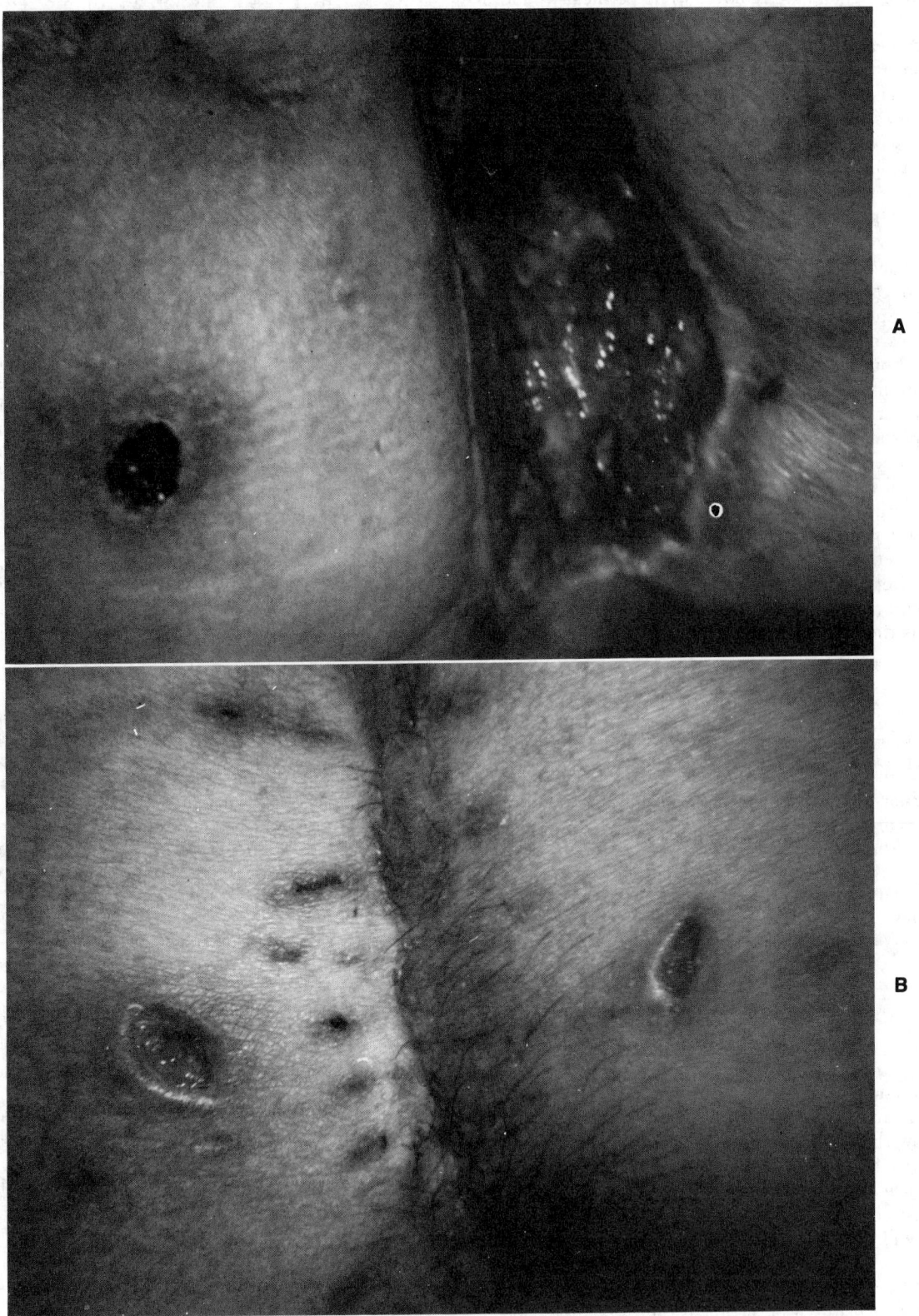

Fig. 31-25   Perineal wound following an abdominoperineal resection for cancer in rectum. **A,** Postsurgical wound; note site of sump drain to left of wound. **B,** Following healing; perineum is completely closed; shape of buttocks looks normal.

Through the perineal incision, the anus, rectum and distal portion of sigmoid are removed. The perineal wound may be closed around Penrose drains, or it may be left wide open to heal slowly from the inside outward (Fig. 31-25). The open perineal wound will take longer to heal than a usual incision. Care of the patient with an abdominoperineal resection is summarized in Box 31-21.

Many patients complain of *phantom rectal sensations* and of feeling the necessity to defecate. An explanation of cortical perception and transmission of nerve impulses often helps the patient cope with these sensations.

Urinary retention is a common occurrence following rectal excision. Factors that influence urinary retention include loss of pelvic support, chronic urinary tract infection, enlarged prostate, or nerve injury. Loss of pelvic support increases problems with micturition when the patient is supine; thus micturition may improve with ambulation. If nerve injury is present, problems with urinary retention and urinary tract infections may persist for several months with partial resolution of retention but with urinary incontinence experienced at night.

Sexual difficulties may occur in about 40% of males following abdominoperineal resection. Difficulty with ejaculation is more commonly seen than impotence (difficulty with erection), but they may occur together. Convalescence after an abdominoperineal resection is prolonged and may require many months. Support is usually needed during this time.

FECAL DIVERSION: STOMAS

Diversion of the fecal stream may be performed for GI diseases or for trauma. Common reasons for ostomy surgery include the following:

Type	Reason
Ileostomy	Ulcerative colitis, familial polyposis
Temporary colostomy	Trauma: gunshot wounds, stab wounds
	Complications of diverticulitis, volvulus, bowel ischemia, perforation
Permanent colostomy	Cancer of colon and rectum

Diversion of the fecal stream may be temporary or permanent. In a *temporary diversion* the fecal stream is rerouted to allow the GI tract an opportunity to heal or to provide an outlet for the stool when an obstruction is present. A *permanent diversion* implies that the intestine cannot or will not be reconnected; thus, a return to a normal elimination mode will not occur.

Surgical Sites

When the small bowel (ileum) is the site of diversion, the ostomy is called an *ileostomy*. The surgical diversion of the large colon will result in a *colostomy*. The anatomic location of the colostomy will determine the name, that is, *ascending colostomy, transverse colostomy,* or *sigmoid colostomy*. The effects are different for each type of ostomy (Table 31-26).

Guidelines for Care　31-21

The patient with an abdominoperineal resection

Preoperative care
Prepare patient as for other bowel surgery.
Prepare patient for a stoma (p. 979).
Prepare patient for a perineal incision: wound may be open and, if so, will take longer to heal.

Postoperative care
Provide care as for other bowel surgery.
Preventing complications
　Shock: monitor for early signs and institute shock measures.
　Hemorrhage
　　Check perineal dressing frequently: initial drainage is profuse and serosanguineous.
　　Reinforce initial dressings as necessary.
　　Report excessive bleeding to physician.
　Thrombophlebitis/pulmonary embolism
　　Encourage leg exercises (Chapter 20) until patient is ambulatory.
　　Encourage use of elastic stockings with elderly patients or those with poor leg circulation.
　　Encourage ambulation when permitted.
Promoting healing
　Maintain low continuous suction of sump catheters, if present.
　Change perineal dressing as frequently as needed after first 24 hours.
　　Record precise directions for dressing change on nursing care plan.
　　Irrigate wound with normal saline solution by use of catheter, hand-held shower massage, or Water Pik.
　　Cover with dry dressings and hold in place with a T-binder (the T "top" is wrapped around the waist and the T strap is brought up between the legs).
　Substitute sitz baths for irrigation when patient is ambulatory; maintain free flow of water on perineal wound in sitz tub (rubber ring may be helpful).
　Provide stoma care (p. 979).
Promoting urinary elimination
　Maintain patency of indwelling catheter.
　Monitor for residual urine when catheter is removed.
　　Keep accurate intake and output records.
　　Monitor for lower abdominal distention, patient discomfort, restlessness.
　Use measures to encourage voiding if patient has inability to initiate stream.
Promoting comfort
　Assist patient to find a comfortable position in bed: side-lying is usually preferred.
　Assist patient to turn frequently.
　Try a foam pad under buttocks for supine position.
　Give narcotics at regular intervals until severe pain decreases (about 3 days postoperatively).
　Give patient/family opportunities to express feelings about the ostomy.

Table 31-26   ## Comparison of ileostomy and colostomies

	Ileostomy	Ascending colostomy	Transverse colostomy	Sigmoid colostomy
Location	Ileum	Ascending colon	Transverse colon	Sigmoid colon
Type of drainage	Liquid-to-paste consistency	Liquid-to-soft	Soft	Soft-to-formed
Bowel regulation	No	No	No	Only with irrigations (if desirable)
Fluid imbalance	Monitor for dehydration if high-output diarrhea	Same	May occur with bouts of diarrhea	Usually not a problem unless there were previous resections
Skin irritation	Occurs easily because of digestive enzymes	Same	Can occur from exposure to stool	Same as transverse colostomy
Other complications	Food blockage Prolapse of stoma Stricture	Prolapse Stricture	Prolapse Stricture	Prolapse Stricture Constipation

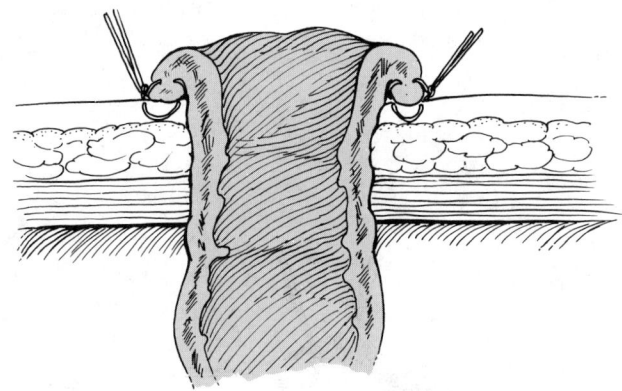

Fig. 31-26   Formation of an end stoma.

The two main types of functioning stomas are the end stoma and the loop stoma. A nonfunctional end stoma is referred to as a *mucous fistula*.

When an *end stoma* is created surgically, the proximal bowel is brought out through an incision in the abdominal wall, folded over on itself (forming a cuff), and sutured. The stomal surface is the mucosal lining or inner layer of the intestinal wall (Fig. 31-26). The remaining *distal* bowel may be surgically removed, oversewn to form a Hartmann's pouch (Fig. 31-27), or brought to the skin surface to form another stoma, the mucous fistula (Fig. 31-28). If the proximal and distal stomas are adjacent (Fig. 31-29), they are referred to as a *double-barreled ostomy*.

The *loop stoma* is created by bringing the bowel through an abdominal incision, sliding a support under the bowel, and opening the upper wall of the bowel (Fig. 31-30). The posterior wall remains intact. There is one stoma, but there are two openings: proximal and distal. The loop ostomy is generally a temporary procedure.

Patients who do not receive adequate bowel preparation before a loop or double-barreled procedure may have a bowel evacuation through the rectum. Patients should be told this may occur. Mucus may continue to be passed through the rectum.

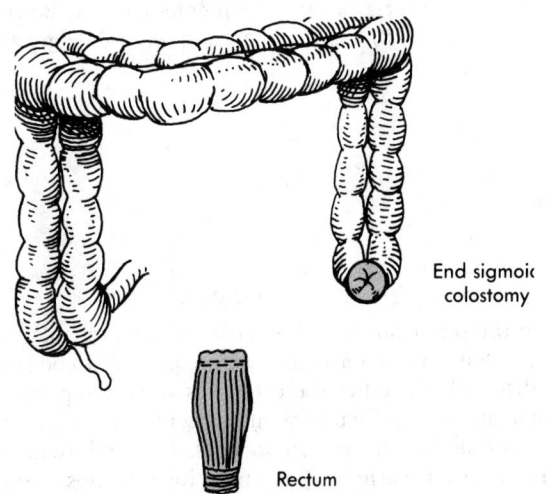

End sigmoid colostomy

Rectum

Fig. 31-27   End sigmoid colostomy with an oversewn rectum left intact (Hartmann's pouch).

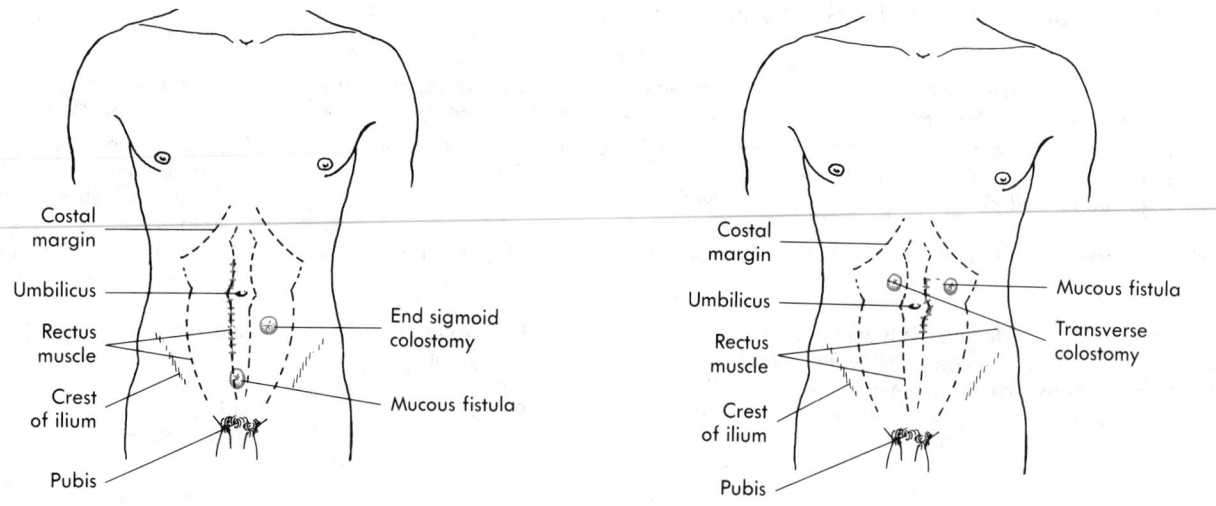

Fig. 31-28   End sigmoid colostomy and mucous fistula.

Fig. 31-29   Transverse colostomy; adjacent mucous fistula.

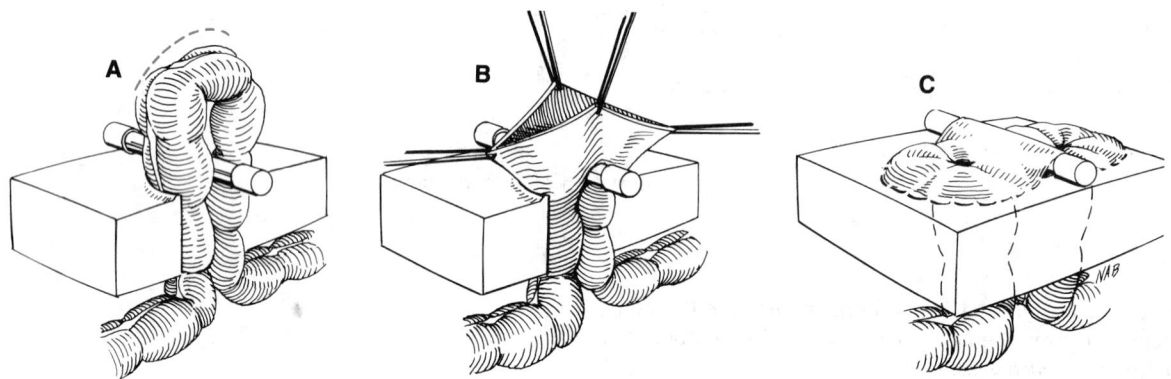

Fig. 31-30   Loop colostomy. **A,** Bowel brought through incision and supported with rod. **B,** Incision in anterior wall. **C,** Edges are folded over to make two openings in one stoma.

Psychologic Response to Ostomy Surgery

When the physician tells the person of the probable need for an ostomy, the immediate reaction is likely to be shock and disbelief. Whether the ostomy is to be temporary or permanent, it is difficult for most people to accept. It is not unusual for the person to be sad, withdrawn, and depressed after learning of the need for ostomy surgery.

Removal of any part of the body involves a sense of loss. Thus, the person facing ostomy surgery may experience grief and mourning over the lost part, which includes shock, denial, anger, and depression. (See Chapter 15 for a discussion of these reactions.) The change in body image may result in feelings of guilt, shame, or disgust. Usually the formation of the stoma is viewed as mutilating surgery, but for some individuals the surgery may be a relief or release from coping with chronic pain, diarrhea, or debility. No matter what reaction is expressed, patients need time and the support of others to work through their feelings.

The patient with a colostomy or ileostomy

Prepare the person for surgery by describing the ostomy, answering questions, and dispelling misconceptions.

Monitor the stoma postoperatively for swelling, color, function, and intactness of mucocutaneous suture line.

Assess the readiness of the person to view the stoma and to begin learning about care of the ostomy.

Promote acceptance of the change in the body through own facial expressions and empathic interactions.

Instruct the person in the care of the ostomy through use of a detailed and individualized care plan.

Provide the person with written instructions and supplies.

Provide necessary follow-up care.

Provide information concerning support services such as the United Ostomy Association and American Cancer Society.

Suggested preoperative teaching for the patient requiring a stoma

Simple explanation with drawings of anatomy of the GI tract

Explanation of surgery
  Areas to be removed
  Effect on bowel function

Definition of terms: colostomy (or ileostomy), stoma, pouch

Explanation of appearance/sensation of stoma and basic management

Availability of nurse/enterostomal therapist after surgery to teach patient the care of the stoma

Availability of Ostomy Visitor (p. 982)

Preoperative Care

The general preoperative and postoperative care for bowel surgery (p. 974) is followed for the person scheduled for ostomy surgery. Guidelines for ostomy care are summarized in Box 31-22.

Counseling and teaching are important aspects of preoperative care. Assist the patient and family and friends to identify their feelings and reactions to the proposed surgery. Assess the patient's knowledge of the surgery, as well as responsiveness to information. Some people are very upset by the impending surgery and want little information. However, it is important for each person to know at least what is meant by ostomy surgery and the type of management it will require. Many people have misconceptions about the ostomy that add to the preoperative anxiety. Dispelling these myths and giving correct information can lessen the fears of an ostomy. Some suggested information is listed in Box 31-23.

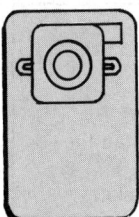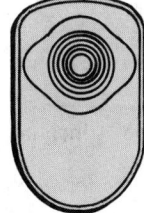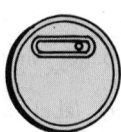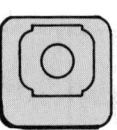

Fig. 31-31 Closed end pouches and patches for regulated colostomies.

Postoperative Care
Stoma drainage

Assess the stoma regularly for color and to ensure intactness of the stoma-skin suture line. A red color denotes viability. A stoma that has impaired circulation will appear dark, dusky, or black.

The stoma secretes mucus immediately following surgery and will continue to do so. During the first 24 to 48 hours, the stomal drainage is mucoid and serosanguineous. As intestinal function returns, flatus will be produced. Fecal drainage is initially liquid for all ostomies. Drainage from a colostomy may then change quickly, depending on its location (Table 31-26).

Protecting the skin

Fecal drainage from the stoma can be very irritating to the skin surrounding the stoma; therefore, the skin needs protection. *Skin barriers* are substances that are applied to protect the skin. The most commonly used barriers are 4 × 4 inch squares or pectin-based *wafers* that are cut to fit snugly around the stoma. *Pastes* are useful to fill in creases or folds in poor locations and to supplement wafers for a longer seal. Powders must be covered with a *sealant* (spray, liquid, gel, wipe) before a pouch can be applied.

Peristomal skin infections may be bacterial or fungal. The most common is a yeast infection from *Candida albicans*. The skin becomes bright red with papular lesions in an irregular area; secondary skin changes occur as the process continues, and dry, scaling areas develop. Treatment involves the use of nystatin (Mycostatin) powder sealed with a skin sealant.

Changing the pouch

Products for ostomy care are available in a variety of styles, shapes, and sizes. Pouches are available in clear and opaque plastics, and covers are designed to make the wearing of a pouch more comfortable (Fig. 31-31).

An effective pouching system protects the skin, contains the stool, molds to the body contour, allows comfortable bending and movement, and is inconspicuous and odorproof. Selection of an effective pouching system is crucial to the rehabilitation process.

Preparing the patient to care for the stoma facilitates incorporation of the body changes into the new body image. Most persons do not wish to look at the stoma immediately. Do not push them to look at the stoma, but gently encourage them to look at it as they show interest in doing so.

31-24

Changing the pouch

Pattern

1. The pattern should be ⅛ inch larger than the stoma.
2. Always label the pattern for "top" or "skin" side.

Skin barrier (Stomahesive, Hollihesive, Reliaseal, Colly-Seel)

1. Use either a fourth, a half, or a full wafer, depending on the size of the stoma and the abdomen.
2. Round the corners to conform to the shape of the adhesive on the pouch.
3. Trace the pattern on the paper side.
4. Cut hole on pattern line (line will not be visible when it is cut).
5. Smooth sides of the opening with your finger.

Pouch

1. Pouch opening should be slightly larger than the opening of the skin barrier (paper can cut the stoma).
2. Trace pattern on the paper side of the pouch (use the opening from the skin barrier that has already been cut).
3. Cut the hole larger than the line of the pattern (cut outside the line).
4. Smooth edges around the opening.
5. Remove paper backing from the pouch, center the openings, and apply the shiny side of the skin barrier to the pouch.

Applying the system

1. Remove the old pouch and skin barrier carefully.
2. Cleanse the skin with warm water.
3. Pat the skin dry.
4. Warm the skin barrier (the pouch is already attached).
5. Remove the backing; save this paper (it can be used as a pattern in the future).
6. Center opening with stoma; press and seal to the skin; hold hand against the pouch to help seal the skin barrier to the skin.
7. Close the bottom of the pouch.

From Broadhurst BB, Broadwell DC: Ostomy care for children, Unpublished material, 1981.

A patient may be unable (or may refuse) to participate in self-care, which creates a management problem. The patient, family member or friend, nurse, and physician need to discuss the problem openly. Someone must be prepared to care for the stoma after the patient is discharged from the hospital. If the patient is unwilling to assume an active role, an early consultation with a psychiatric nurse clinician may be helpful.

Teach the patient the steps of changing the pouch (Box 31-24) and give written instructions before discharge. A minimum of three lessons are generally needed. Lessons should begin when the patient is receptive to instruction.

During the first lesson, the patient observes the steps of the procedure. The nurse informs the patient that the stoma has no touch sensation, and the red color means the stoma has healthy blood supply. Address questions and concerns. During the second lesson, the patient assists with preparing the pouch, cleansing the skin and stoma, and centering the pouch around the stoma. The patient changes the pouch with supervision as needed for the third lesson. Some persons need more practice, and additional sessions are scheduled. A visiting nurse referral may be needed for assessment of the patient's ability to adapt to the ostomy in the home environment.

Before discharge, the patient needs a supply of pouches and skin barriers, a list of what supplies to order, and the names of local suppliers. A prescription for ostomy supplies may be needed for insurance reimbursement.

Promoting regular elimination: colostomy irrigation

Persons with descending or sigmoid colostomies may decide to manage the colostomy with regular irrigations. The purpose of regular colostomy irrigations is to stimulate emptying of the colon at a convenient and regular time.

A patient who is free of stool between irrigations can wear a closed-end pouch with a gas-relief valve or stoma "cap," a small square pouch with an absorbent dressing. The stoma will continue to secrete mucus and expel flatus between irrigations, so an ostomy covering with a gas filter is desirable (Fig. 31-31). Some persons are unable to regulate the colostomy with irrigations and decide to wear drainable pouches instead of irrigating.

Persons who have irrigated their colostomies successfully for years may develop irregular results with irrigation secondary to aging. As one ages, there is a decrease in mucus production and peristalsis. This is often frustrating for patients who may feel they have failed because the elimination pattern is unpredictable.

Various types of commercial irrigation sets are available, and they all require similar supplies: an irrigation sleeve that fits over the stoma and is long enough to drain into the toilet, a cone tip for the insertion of water into the stoma (Fig. 31-32), an enema bag to contain the solution, and clips to close the top and bottom of the sleeve.

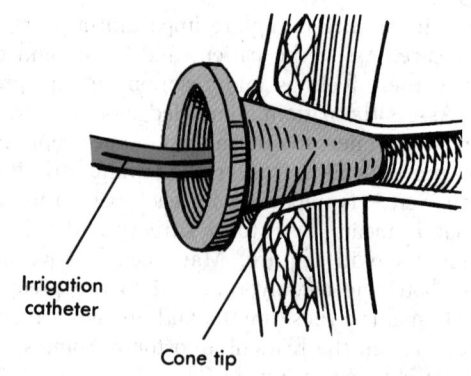

Irrigation catheter

Cone tip

Fig. 31-32 Cone irrigating tip inserted in stoma.

31-25

Colostomy irrigation

1. Remove old pouch.
2. Clean skin and stoma with water.
3. Apply irrigating sleeve and belt.
4. Fill bag with desired amount of tepid water (250 to 1000 ml).
5. Hang bag so bottom of bag is at shoulder height.
6. Remove air from tubing.
7. Gently insert irrigating cone snugly into stoma, holding it parallel to floor.
8. Let water run in slowly until patient identifies need to expel stool.
9. Remove cone and allow solution to drain into container.
10. When most of stool is expelled (about 15 minutes) rinse sleeve with water and close up bottom end.
11. Encourage activity to complete bowel emptying (about 30 to 45 minutes).
12. Remove sleeve and apply clean pouch.

When prescribed, irrigations are begun after the bowel has begun to function and the stool is beginning to become soft, usually about the seventh postoperative day. The procedure for irrigation is outlined in Box 31-25.

The irrigation procedure is usually performed in the bathroom. The patient may wish to sit on a chair on a pillow and face the commode until the perineal wound heals. Subsequently the patient sits on the toilet (Fig. 31-33). Cramping during an irrigation may be caused by inserting the water too rapidly or from water that is too cold. Rate of flow varies with the pressure (height of the bag) and caliber of the tube.

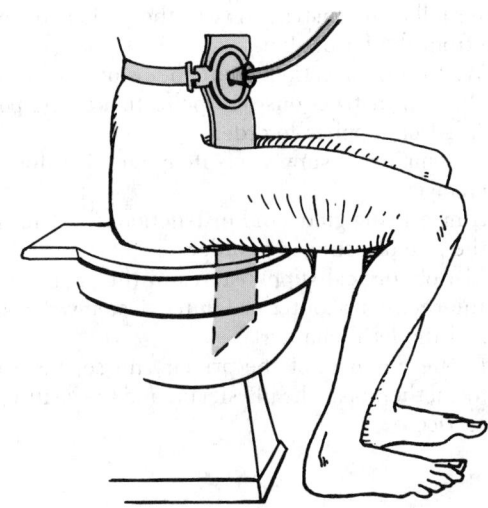

Fig. 31-33   Colostomy irrigation with person sitting on toilet; irrigating sleeve drains into toilet.

Promoting nutrition

Anyone with an ostomy should eat balanced meals at regular intervals, and chew foods slowly and thoroughly. Patients need to be informed that certain foods such as seeds, kernels, and other undigested residue will be visible in the stool.

Persons with a *colostomy* do not need a restricted diet, although many persons develop their own food preferences. They should be informed which foods tend to cause gas in order to avoid these foods as desired. Most pouches are odor-proof, and some are available with gas-relief valves that make gas less of a problem.

Persons with an *ileostomy* need to avoid high-fiber or high-residue foods for 4 to 6 weeks after surgery. High-fiber foods can then be added one at a time in small amounts. If the person is unable to tolerate the food after two or three trials, the food can be eliminated from the diet.

Promoting return to normal activity

Most persons achieve optimal recovery within 3 months, and they can return to their normal activities, including work. Discuss questions about activities before the patient goes home. Traveling is possible for the ostomate. Preparations to be considered are listed in Box 31-26. With careful planning the person with an ostomy can participate in activities enjoyed before the surgery.

Promoting sexuality

The opportunity for the patient and significant other to ask questions regarding the return to normal sexual functioning needs to be provided. It is most often the nurse who hears cues such as, "I guess I'll never be able . . . ," or, "I wonder what my spouse . . . ." The nurse takes this opportunity to clarify this concern with the person. Arrangements can be made, if desired by the patient, for the significant other to be present when the nurse or physician frankly discusses sexual functioning. Many persons will not verbalize their concerns about sexuality so that a deliberate meeting must be planned to facilitate expression of these concerns. The patient and sexual partner can be assisted to consider sexual positions that may be more facilitating and less problematic if a bag is worn.

About 15% of men with ostomies have decreased sexual activity that may be related either to nerve injury or to psychologic reasons. The successful return to sexual activity depends on psychosexual functioning before surgery and adaptation and coping following surgery. Other ways of expressing affection may be considered. Counseling may be helpful if nerve injury is not present and sexual difficulties are being experienced. Women have a decreased incidence of nerve injury because of the larger pelvis. Ostomy surgery does not interfere with contraception, pregnancy, or delivery. A pamphlet entitled *Sex and the Ostomate* is available from the United Ostomy Association.*

---

*United Ostomy Association, 36 Executive Park, Irvine, CA 92714.

The patient with a stoma

Promoting nutrition and elimination

Eat a balanced diet. Avoid foods that cause diarrhea or constipation.

Drink at least 2500 ml of fluids daily (6 glasses).

Avoid foods that cause flatus, as desired.

Promoting return to normal activities

Participate in activities enjoyed before surgery.

Avoid direct contact sports such as football. Activities such as swimming, tennis, and planned exercise programs are all possible.

When traveling:

Wear seat belt above or below stoma.

Hand-carry regular ostomy supplies to facilitate care if baggage is misplaced.

Use disposable bags.

Carry plastic bags for disposal of used supplies.

Take extra supplies for unexpected events requiring extra days.

Eat moderately. Use restraint when eating new foods.

Use caution about water intake in areas where "traveler's diarrhea" is a high risk.

Promoting sexuality

Allow time to ease into sexual relations.

Resume sleeping in bed with partner if this was habit before surgery.

Talk with partner about the stoma.

Empty the pouch before intercourse.

Use an attractive cover over the pouch.

Tape pouch to abdomen or groin.

Experiment with different positions.

Preventing complications

Report the following symptoms to physician or nurse enterostomal therapist:

Changes in configuration, color, consistency, or odor of stool

Bleeding through stoma or rectum

Persistent diarrhea or lack of stool evacuation despite medications, treatment, fluids, diet, and exercise program

Persistent skin irritation despite treatment

Changes in contour of stoma (prolapse, inversion)

Persistent leakage around appliance

Signs of dehydration and electrolyte imbalance

Community resources

During and after hospitalization, the patient and significant others have additional resources available to assist in adapting and coping with the ostomy. A representative from the local chapter of the United Ostomy Association can be requested to visit the patient either preoperatively or postoperatively. This visitor can share how he or she has learned to live well with the ostomy. The patient may wish to become a member of the Association and through meetings learn how others in the community are effectively dealing with the ostomy.

The enterostomal therapist, a nurse with additional education in providing ostomy care, should be consulted (if available) to assist or coordinate instruction. Consult the social worker, clinical nurse specialist, dietitian, and clergy as needed.

The American Cancer Society in certain locations will assist with providing ostomy supplies to persons with financial need. It also can provide assistance with information about home supplies, medications, and transportation.

Closure of Colostomy

If the colostomy was created to relieve obstruction or to divert the fecal stream to permit healing of a portion of the bowel, the person will be readmitted to the hospital at a later date for a further examination and for possible resection of any diseased portion of the bowel. The ostomy subsequently may be closed.

In preparing to resect the bowel and close the colostomy, the physician may order irrigation of the colostomy and probably both openings of a loop colostomy. The irrigation fluid, usually normal saline solution, is instilled into each opening as ordered. For irrigation of the distal stoma, the patient should sit on the bedpan or the toilet. Unless the distal bowel is obstructed, the solution instilled into the distal loop will be expelled through the rectum. The returns are inspected before being discarded.

Requirements Before Discharge

Give the following instructions to the patient before discharge from the hospital:

1. Written information about the ostomy
2. Written instructions for application of the pouch
3. A list of supplies to order
4. A temporary supply of items needed for pouch changes
5. A measuring guide and instructions for determining the size of pouches to order
6. List of surgical supply stores in the area
7. Information about the United Ostomy Association and the local chapter
8. Phone numbers of the primary nurse, the enterostomal therapist, the physician, and the visiting nurse service

Table 31-27   **Common anal lesions**

Lesion	Description	Symptoms	Treatment
Anal fissure	Slitlike ulceration in epithelium of anal canal	Pain with defecation; bleeding; constipation	Stool softeners; analgesic ointments; sitz baths; surgical removal of fissure if medical therapy ineffective
Anal abscess	Abscess in tissue around anus	Persistent throbbing anal pain with walking, sitting, defecation; systemic signs of infection	Incision and drainage of abscess
Anal fistula	Hollow track leading through anal tissue from anorectal canal through skin near anus	Purulent discharge near anus	Fistulectomy or fistulotomy
Hemorrhoids	Varicosities of lower rectum and anus	Bleeding with defecation; pain if thrombosed	Analgesic ointments for mild discomfort; injection, ligation, or hemorrhoidectomy for severe discomfort

ANORECTAL DISORDERS

Pathophysiology

The anorectal area may develop fissures, abscesses, or fistulas (Table 31-27). A *fissure* is usually the result of trauma caused by passage of hard-formed stool that overstretches the anal lining. It does not heal readily. An *anal abscess* may develop in an anal fissure, and if the sinus tract draining the abscess does not close, a chronic draining *fistula* may develop.

Hemorrhoids occur frequently as a result of congestion in the veins of the hemorrhoidal plexus. Heredity, occupations requiring long periods of standing or sitting, the erect posture assumed by human beings, structural absence of valves in the hemorrhoidal veins, increase of intraabdominal pressure caused by constipation, straining at defecation, and pregnancy are factors that predispose to development of hemorrhoids. Hemorrhoids may be internal (above the internal sphincter) or external (outside the anal sphincter). Many persons have both internal and external hemorrhoids.

Nursing Process
Assessment

Pain, bleeding, and itching are the major symptoms of hemorrhoids. Data to be collected include the following:
1. Pain
   a. Onset: with defecation, sitting, or walking
   b. Character: constant or episodic; sharp or throbbing
2. Bleeding: presence, amount, color (bright or dull red)
3. Stool: consistency (hardness), streaked with blood or pus
4. Itching: frequency, onset

Bleeding is usually bright red because of proximity of the bleeding site. Internal hemorrhoids often bleed with defecation, whereas external hemorrhoids rarely bleed. Rectal bleeding must not be confused with menstrual bleeding in women.

Data analysis: nursing diagnoses

Nursing diagnoses are determined from analysis of patient data. Possible nursing diagnoses for the person with an anorectal lesion may include, but are not limited to, the following:

Diagnostic title	Possible etiologies
Constipation	Anal discomfort
Pain: rectal	Anal surgery

Planning: expected patient outcomes

Expected patient outcomes for the person with an anorectal lesion may include, but are not limited to, the following:
1. Stool is soft and formed.
2. States feeling more comfortable after surgery.

Implementation
Assisting with achievement of therapeutic goals
Anorectal surgery

Preoperative care. Give the patient a laxative if needed and encourage a full, normal diet until a few hours before administration of local anesthetic. Stool softeners are often given to facilitate passage of the stool through the rectum postoperatively, and a bulk laxative such as psyllium (Metamucil) may be given to increase the bulk of the stool. An enema may be prescribed 1 to 2 hours before surgery.

Postoperative care. Because the operations are often considered minor, there may be a tendency to minimize anorectal surgery. In reality, the surgery may cause as much discomfort as many major surgeries. The pain, which results from rectal spasms, may inhibit urination and defecation. Patients worry considerably about passing the first stool, which can be uncomfortable. Pain can be minimized by the use of analgesics, sitz baths, and stool softeners.

Table 31-28 Treatment of hemorrhoids

Procedure	Description	Comments
Injection	Sclerosing solution injected into submucosal area	Bleeding stops in 24 to 48 hours
Ligation	Constriction of hemorrhoids by rubber bands	Destroyed tissue sloughs off within 1 week
Infrared photocoagulation	Radiation for 1.5 sec by an infrared photocoagulator probe	Tissue becomes necrotic and sloughs off
Hemorrhoidectomy	Excision of hemorrhoids	Preoperative: stool softener Postoperative: dressings may be omitted; stool softeners; first defecation is painful; monitor for excessive bleeding.

Guidelines for Care 31-27

The patient following anorectal surgery

Assessment
Monitor vital signs every 4 hours for 24 hours.
Monitor for signs of restlessness, thirst.
Inspect rectal area or dressing every 2 to 3 hours for 24 hours.
Monitor urinary output.

Promotion of comfort
Assist patient to a position of comfort; side-lying is often preferred.
Use floatation pad under buttocks for sitting.
Give analgesic medications as needed during first 24 hours.
Use moist heat after first 12 hours: rectal compresses or sitz baths 3 to 4 times/day.

Promotion of elimination
Give stool softener as prescribed.
Give an analgesic shortly before first bowel movement, if possible.
If an enema is prescribed, use a well-lubricated catheter or small rectal tube.

Patient teaching
Take a sitz bath after each bowel movement for at least 1 to 2 weeks after surgery.
Eat adequate dietary fiber; drink at least 2000 ml of fluids/day, and exercise moderately.
A stool softener may be desired every day or every other day until healing is completed.
Report the following symptoms to physician: rectal bleeding, continued pain on defecation, suppurative drainage.

During the first 12 hours after surgery, hemorrhage is a possibility. Blood may collect in the anal canal and not be expelled; therefore, monitor other signs of hemorrhage (vital signs, restlessness, thirst). Avoid moist heat (sitz baths) during this period, as moist heat will encourage further bleeding by dilating the blood vessels. The postoperative care of the patient experiencing anorectal surgery is summarized in Box 31-27.

Interventions to achieve patient outcomes
Promoting normal stools

Chronic constipation may precipitate anal lesions. Once the lesion is present, defecation may initiate rectal spasms, causing the person to delay defecation. This leads to formation of a hard stool as water is reabsorbed in the colon, causing further discomfort. Therefore, institute measures to promote passage of a soft stool, including activity, adequate fluids (at least 2000 ml/day), and dietary fiber. A stool softener may be prescribed.

Promoting healing

Abscesses are incised and drained. Dressing containing purulent drainage must be changed frequently to protect the skin. Hemorrhoids may be injected, ligated, coagulated, or excised (see Table 31-28).

Evaluation

Evaluation is based on the expected patient outcomes. Questions to consider include:
1. Is stool soft and formed?
2. Is the patient comfortable?

FECAL INCONTINENCE
Pathophysiology

Voluntary emptying of the rectum occurs when the external anal sphincter (under cortical control) relaxes and the abdominal and pelvic muscles contract. Conditions that interrupt transmission of messages to and from the brain (cortical lesions, spinal cord lesions) cause injury to the sphincter (trauma, fistulas, abscess) or cause perineal muscle relaxation (childbirth, perineal surgery, aging) and may lead to fecal incontinence.

Assessment

Fecal incontinence is characterized by involuntary passage of stool. Data to be collected include the following:
1. Frequency of defecations
2. Nature of the stool
3. Awareness of need to defecate
4. Ability to contract abdominal and perineal muscles
5. Willingness of person to participate in exercise or bowel control program.

Implementation

1. Assisting with bowel control
   a. Provide a high-fiber diet to facilitate a formed stool.
   b. Provide a fluid intake of about 3000 ml/day to promote a soft stool.
   c. Administer a stool softener daily, if necessary.
   d. Plan a bowel training program to prevent incontinence if control is not feasible. Within a few days the patient will probably defecate only once a day when stimulated. If the stool remains soft, the program may be changed to every other day. Consistency in carrying out the plan is important for success (see Box 31-28).
   e. If fecal incontinence is uncontrollable, identify the defecation pattern. Place the patient on the toilet or commode at the time that defecation is anticipated. Protective disposable pants are available to provide the person with a sense of security and dignity. A rectal pouch may be used to collect liquid stools.[29]
2. Assisting with comfort. Assist the person to cleanse the anal and perineal areas as soon as possible after fecal incontinence to eliminate odor and prevent skin breakdown.
3. Counseling and teaching
   a. Provide empathic communication. The person may have feelings of regression, inadequacy, or uncleanliness as a result of the loss of control. The person needs to feel accepted as an adult and accept the condition as a situational physical condition and not personal inadequacy.
   b. Encourage patients to participate in all or some of their own management to the extent that is possible, thus providing them with a sense of control.
   c. Teach perineal exercises for weak perineal muscles (Chapter 33).

31-28

Bowel training program

1. Include patient and family/friend in the planning.
2. Determine when bowel evacuation usually occurs (most frequent times are after breakfast or dinner).
3. Determine whether a morning or evening program is more suitable for patient.
4. Insert glycerine or bisacodyl (Dulcolax) *suppository* 30 minutes before expected time of defecation; give suppository at *same time every day.*
5. Have patient sit on toilet if possible for defecation.
6. If necessary, massage abdomen toward the sigmoid area (left lower quadrant) to encourage defecation; digital rectal stimulation may also stimulate defecation.

SUMMARY

1. GI signs requiring immediate medical follow-up include (1) a sore that bleeds easily and does not heal, (2) a lump or thickening or a persistent red or whitish patch in the mouth, (3) persistent heartburn or indigestion, (4) abdominal pain accompanied by nausea and vomiting, and (5) a change in bowel habits or the presence of blood in the stool.
2. Obesity is defined as more than 20% over established height and weight standards; morbid obesity is 45 kg (100 lb) above the standard. Protein-calorie malnutrition is less than 90% of desirable weight.
3. Without behavior modification, most persons who lose weight by weight control programs return to or surpass their original weight within 5 years.
4. Surgery for obesity includes gastroplasty and gastric bypass.
5. Protein-calorie malnutrition leads to decreased muscle mass, decreased vital capacity, edema, malabsorption, and risk for infection. Special therapies include tube feedings, total parenteral nutrition, or gastrostomy feedings.
6. Complications of tube feedings include aspiration, tube dislodgement, tube clogging, nausea, bacterial contamination, dehydration, diarrhea, and hyperglycemia.
7. TPN solutions are deposited into the superior vena cava to provide greater dilution of the highly concentrated solutions.
8. TPN solutions must be prepared and given under strict aseptic conditions to prevent bacterial contamination.
9. Complications of TPN include infection, air embolism, lung injury from tube dislodgement, thromboembolism, electrolyte imbalances, overhydration, hyperglycemia, hypoglycemia, vitamin D deficiency, and vitamin A excess.
10. A gastrostomy is insertion of a feeding tube directly through the abdominal wall into the stomach; feedings consist of blenderized foods or special formulas.
11. Factors placing the person at high risk for inflammatory mouth disorders include poor oral hygiene, stress, nutritional deficiencies, debilitating diseases, heavy smoking, and chemotherapy.
12. Common inflammatory disorders of the mouth include aphthous or herpetic stomatitis, Vincent's angina, thrush, gingivitis, and periodontitis.
13. Contributing factors to cancer of the mouth and esophagus include alcohol and heavy smoking or chewing tobacco.
14. Swallowing is impaired by common esophageal disorders including achalasia (aperistalsis of esophagus), esophageal stricture, esophageal diverticulum, or gastroesophageal reflux.
15. Esophageal disorders of motor origin produce dysphagia for both solids and liquids; with paralysis of neurologic origin, the dysphagia is mainly for liquids, and with obstruction, there is dysphagia for solids.

16. A hiatal hernia consists of herniation of the upper part of the stomach through the diaphragm, causing heartburn.

17. Heartburn is relieved by taking antacids; eating a high-protein, low-fat diet in small frequent feedings; avoiding smoking; avoiding lifting, bending, or lying down immediately after eating; and sleeping with upper body elevated.

18. Acute gastritis is a common occurrence; stress erosions (or ulcers) are a form of gastritis resulting from stress; chronic gastritis may lead to pernicious anemia or gastric cancer.

19. Gastric ulcers result from increased back diffusion of gastric acid into the tissues; gastric acid and emptying rate are normal. Duodenal ulcers result from increased gastric acid emptied more rapidly into the duodenum.

20. The major therapy for peptic ulcers is drug therapy, primarily antacids, histamine H_2 antagonists, and sucralfate.

21. Teaching the person with a peptic ulcer includes information about medications, suggestions for eating, and avoidance of smoking and stress, if possible.

22. Surgery for peptic ulcer may include a Billroth II (gastrojejunostomy, the most common), Billroth I (gastroduodenostomy), or vagotomy (with or without pyloroplasty).

23. Complications of peptic ulcer include hemorrhage, perforation, or pyloric obstruction.

24. Dumping syndrome occurs from entrance of a hyperosmolar mixture directly into the jejunum after gastric surgery.

25. Malabsorption syndrome is a group of disorders resulting from inadequate absorption of fat in the small intestine; common malabsorption syndromes include lactase deficiency and celiac sprue.

26. Inflammation of the intestines (enteritis) may result from viruses, bacteria, or parasites. Common parasitic infections include amebiasis (from fecally contaminated food or water) or trichinosis (from improperly cooked pork).

27. Although symptoms of appendicitis may be atypical, a common site of abdominal pain is McBurney's point (halfway between the umbilicus and right iliac crest).

28. If appendicitis is suspected, avoid heat (increases pressure within appendix leading to rupture); also avoid enemas (increased intraluminal pressure may also lead to a ruptured appendix).

29. Ulcerative colitis affects primarily the left colon with a continuous area of mucosal involvement; the liquid stools contain blood, but not fat. Crohn's disease affects segmental areas of the ileum, cecum, and right colon, involving submucosal layers; the frequent semisoft stools contain fat but not blood. Surgery may be useful for ulcerative colitis and sometimes for Crohn's disease.

30. Care of the person with ulcerative colitis or Crohn's disease includes a low-residue, high-protein, high-calorie diet, medications (corticosteroids, sulfasalazine), comfort measures following diarrhea and to protect skin, and promotion of sexuality.

31. Diverticular disease involves outpouching of the colon wall; diverticulitis is the inflammatory condition, diverticulosis the quiescent phase. Encourage a high-fiber diet to increase bowel transit time and stool bulk.

32. Intestinal obstruction may result from inhibition of peristalsis (paralytic ileus) or from mechanical obstruction, such as by adhesions, volvulus, intussusception, hernias, or cancer. Therapy consists of inserting a nasogastric tube, restricting oral intake, and removing the source of obstruction, if possible.

33. Hernias may occur in the inguinal, femoral, or umbilical areas from mural defects or in weakened scars from previous abdominal surgeries. Of concern is the possible entrapment (incarceration) of a loop of bowel. The treatment is surgical.

34. Recommendations for early detection of colorectal cancer include a digital rectal examination yearly after age 40; occult blood stool test yearly after age 50; and proctosigmoidoscopy every 3 to 5 years after age 50, following two negative yearly examinations.

35. Colon polyps (adenomas) are benign growths that are premalignant; the villous adenomas are more likely to become malignant than the pedunculated tubular adenomas.

36. Cancers of the ascending colon are of the cauliflowerlike mass type, and because the chyme is liquid, there is less probability of obstruction. Cancer of the descending colon is usually an annular lesion that may narrow the lumen and obstruct the more solid feces.

37. Surgery for cancer of the colon and upper rectum usually consists of resection with anastomosis; surgery for the lower rectum consists of an abdominoperineal resection with a colostomy.

38. Types of stomas include an end stoma (end of bowel brought out abdominal wall to form a single stoma), loop stoma (loop of bowel brought out abdominal wall and opened, creating one stoma with two openings), and double-barreled ostomy (ends of both proximal and distal ends of resected colon brought out to form two stomas).

39. Stoma care includes cleaning the skin to prevent skin breakdown, early treatment of excoriated skin, and application of pouches to prevent leakage.

40. Persons with a sigmoid colostomy may be able to regulate elimination by colostomy irrigations.

41. Teaching the person with a colostomy includes promoting nutrition and elimination, promoting return to normal activities and sexuality, and preventing complications.

42. Inflammatory anorectal lesions include anal fissures, anal abscesses, and anal fistulas; hemorrhoids are varicose veins of the rectum.

43. Relief of discomfort from anal lesions may include measures to prevent constipation (which irritates the lesions) and sitz baths.

STUDY QUESTIONS

- What types of tissue changes occur in obesity and in protein-calorie malnutrition? What are the results in each?
- Gastrointestinal disorders alter function of the GI tract. What changes can occur in functioning? What general effects can result from the altered functioning?
- What are the differences in electrolyte and acid-base imbalances resulting from loss of gastric secretion versus loss of intestinal secretions? Explain the rationale.
- What are the differences and similarities among the infections of the mouth, stomach, and intestines?
- What types of obstructions can occur in the GI tract? What are the effects?
- Compare and contrast cancer of the mouth, esophagus, stomach, and bowel in terms of occurrence, incidence in males and females, methods of prevention (if any), and types of surgery performed.

REFERENCES AND SELECTED READINGS

1. * Alterescu V: Colostomy, *Nurs Clin North Am* 22:281-290, 1987.
2. * Alterescu V: The ostomy: What do you teach the patient? *Am J Nurs* 85:1250-1253, 1985.
3. Altman DF: Gastrointestinal diseases in the elderly, *Med Clin North Am* 67(2):1250-1253, 1985.
4. American Cancer Society: *Cancer facts and figures 1991*, New York, 1991, The Society.
5. * Atkins JM, Oakley CW: A nurse's guide to TPN, *RN* 49(6):20-24, 1986.
6. Atkinson RL: Low and very low calorie diets, *Med Clin North Am* 73(1):203-214, 1989.
7. * Backer CL, LoCicero J: Surgical management of esophageal disorders, *CCQ* 9(3):12-19, 1986.
8. Bates B: *A guide to physical examination*, ed 5, Philadelphia, 1991, JB Lippincott.
9. * Beck ML: Nutritional support: percutaneous endoscopic gastrostomy, *Nursing 89* 19(4):76-77, 1989.
10. * Becker KL, Stevens SA: Performing in-depth abdominal assessment, *Nursing 88* 18(6):59-63, 1988.
11. * Benedict P, Haddad A: Postop teaching for the colostomy patient, *RN* 52(3):85-90, 1989.
12. Binder V, Riis P: Lifelong control with inflammatory bowel disease patients, *Med Clin North Am* 74(1):219-227, 1990.
13. * Bockus S: Troubleshooting your tube feedings, *Am J Nurs* 91(5):24-28, 1991.
14. Bongiovanni GL: *Essentials of clinical gastroenterology*, ed 2, New York, 1988, McGraw-Hill.
15. * Broadwell D: Peristomal skin integrity, *Nurs Clin North Am* 22:321-322, 1987.
16. * Bruckstein DC: Percutaneous endoscopic gastrostomy, *Geriatr Nurs* 9(2):32-33, 1988.
16a. * Bryant GA: When the bowel is blocked, *RN* 55(1):58-67, 1992.
17. Butrum RR, Clifford DK, Lanza E: NCI dietary guidelines: rationale, *Am J Clin Nutr* 48:888-895, 1988.

18. * Carr P: When the patient needs TPN at home, *RN* 49(6):25-30, 1986.
19. * Cerrato PL: How safe are modified fasts, *RN* 52(11):79-81, 1989.
20. * Dalton-Loehman D, Connor PA: Beyond ileostomy: surgery for a normal life, *RN* 52(7):29-34, 1989.
21. * DiIorio C, Price ME: Swallowing: an assessment guide, *Am J Nurs* 90(7):38-41, 1990.
22. * Dobkin KA, Broadwell DC: Nursing considerations for the patient undergoing colostomy surgery, *Sem Oncol Nurs* 2:249-255, 1986.
23. * Doughty DB: Colorectal cancer: etiology and pathophysiology, *Sem Oncol Nurs* 2:235-241, 1986.
24. Eisenberg P: Enteral nutrition: indications, formulas, and delivery techniques, *Nurs Clin North Am* 24(2):315-337, 1989.
25. * Erickson P: Ostomies: the art of pouching, *Nurs Clin North Am* 22:311-320, 1987.
26. * Feickert DM: Gastric surgery: your crucial pre- and postop role, *RN* 50(1):24-35, 1987.
27. * Feickert DM, Jillson E, Palazzo T: Gastrectomy for stomach carcinoma, *AORN J* 47:1396-1406, 1988.
28. * Foltz AT: Nutritional factors in the prevention of gastrointestinal cancer, *Sem Oncol Nurs* 4:239-245, 1988.
29. Freedman P: The rectal pouch: a safer alternative to rectal tubes, *Am J Nurs* 91(5):105-106, 1991.
29a. * Fritsch DE, Klein DG: Ludwig's angina, *Heart Lung* 21:39-47, 1992.
30. * Greitzu S: Closeup on cancer care: colorectal cancer, when a polyp is more than a polyp, *RN* 49(9):22-30, 1986.
31. Groer MW, Shekleton ME: *Basic pathophysiology: a conceptual approach*, ed 3, St Louis, 1989, Mosby–Year Book.
32. * Hennessy K: Now TPN therapy begins at home, *RN* 51(6):81-84, 1988.
33. Hennessy K: Nutritional support and gastrointestinal disease, *Nurs Clin North Am* 24(2):373-380, 1989.
34. * Irwin M: Managing leaking gastrostomy sites, *Am J Nurs* 88:359-360, 1988.
35. * Joachim G et al: Inflammatory bowel disease: effects on lifestyle, *J Adv Nurs* 12:483-487, 1987.
36. * Johndrow PD: Making your patient and family feel at home with TPN, *Nursing 88* 18(10):65-69, 1988.
36a. * Johns JL: When the patient has an ulcer, *RN* 54(11):44-50, 1991.
37. * Johnson S: A safer gastrostomy for the high-risk patient: percutaneous endoscopic gastrostomy, *RN* 49(3):29-32, 1986.
38. Kennedy-Caldwell C: The morbidly obese surgical patient, *Crit Care Nurs* 7(5):87-89, 1987.
39. Kohn CL, Keithley JK: Enteral nutrition: potential complications and patient monitoring, *Nurs Clin North Am* 24(2):339-351, 1989.
40. * Konopad E, Noseworthy T: Stress ulceration: a serious complication in critically ill patients, *Heart Lung* 17(4):339-348, 1988.
41. McConnell EA: Auscultating bowel sounds, *Nursing 90* 20(5):106, 1990.
42. McCrae AD, Hall NH: Current practices for home enteral nutrition, *J Am Dietetic Assoc* 89:233-239, 1989.
43. * Medvec BR: Esophageal cancer: treatment and nursing intervention, *Sem Oncol Nurs* 4:246-256, 1988.
44. * Meize-Grochowski AR: When the diagnosis is Crohn's disease, *RN* 54(2):52-55, 1991.

* Recommended for student reading.

45. Mendeloff AI: Diet and colorectal cancer, *Am J Clin Nut* 48:780-781, 1988.
46. Metheny NM: *Fluid and electrolyte balance: nursing considerations*, Philadelphia, 1987, JB Lippincott.
47.* Moore MC: Do you still believe these myths about tube feedings? *RN* 50(5):51-55, 1987.
48.* Neufeldt J: Helping the inflammatory bowel disease patient cope with the unpredictable, *Nursing 87* 17(8):47-49, 1987.
49.* Olender L: Why tube feedings may be the wrong answer, *RN* 52(6):43-45, 1989.
50. O'Toole MT: Advanced assessment of the abdomen and gastrointestinal problems, *Nurs Clin North Am* 25(4):771-776, 1990.
51. Pagana KD, Pagana TJ: Diagnostic testing and nursing implications: a case study approach, ed 3, St Louis, 1989, Mosby—Year Book.
52. Petrosino BM et al: Implications of selected problems with nasoenteral feedings, *Crit Care Nurs Q* 12(3):1-18, 1989.
53. Podiasky P, Budzinski HM: Percutaneous endoscopic gastrostomy, *AORN J* 45:1403-1411, 1987.
54.* Price ME, DiIorio C: Swallowing: a practice guide, *Am J Nurs* 90(7):42-46, 1990.
55. Price SA, Wilson LM: *Pathophysiology: clinical concepts of disease processes*, ed 3, New York, 1986, McGraw-Hill.
56. Rakel RE: *Conn's current therapy 1989*, Philadelphia, 1989, WB Saunders.
57.* Rideout BW: The patient with an ileostomy: nursing management and patient education, *Nurs Clin North Am* 22(2):253-262, 1987.
58. Ruderman WB: Newer pharmacologic agents for inflammatory bowel disease, *Med Clin North Am* 74(1):139-154, 1990.
59. Schreiber H, Guyton DP: Gastric bubble: therapy for obesity, *Ohio State Med J* 82:476-479, 1986.
60. Schroeder SA et al: *Current medical diagnosis and treatment 1991*, ed 30, Norwalk, Conn, 1991, Appleton & Lange.
61.* Schulmeister L: Join the fight against oral cancer, *Nursing 87* 17(5):66-67, 1987.
62.* Shipes E: Psychosocial issues: the person with an ostomy, *Nurs Clin North Am* 22:291-302, 1987.
63. Sleisinger M, Fordtran JS: *Gastrointestinal disease: pathophysiology, diagnosis, and management*, ed 4, Philadelphia, 1989, WB Saunders.
64.* Smith CE: Assessing bowel sounds, *Nursing 88* 18(2):42-44, 1988.
65. Smith DB: Continent diversions: an overview, *Dimens Oncol Nurs* 3(4):18-23, 1990.
66.* Starkey JF, Jefferson PA, Kirby DF: Taking care of a percutaneous endoscopic gastrostomy, *Am J Nurs* 88:42-45, 1988.
67. Turnball GB: Dealing with sexuality after ostomy surgery, *Progressions* 1(1):15-18, 1989.
68. Way LW: *Current surgical diagnosis and treatment*, ed 9, Norwalk, Conn, 1991, Appleton & Lange.
69. Wang JF: Stomach cancer, *Sem Oncol Nurs* 4:257-264, 1988.
70. Williams SR: *Essentials of nutrition and diet therapy*, ed 5, St Louis, 1990, Mosby—Year Book.
71. Worthington PH, Wagner BA: Total parenteral nutrition, *Nurs Clin North Am* 24(2):355-369, 1989.
72. Wyngaarden JB, Smith LH: *Cecil's textbook of medicine*, ed 18, Philadelphia, 1988, WB Saunders.
73.* Young CK, White S: Preparing patients for tube feedings at home, *Am J Nurs* 92(4):46-53, 1992.

32

The Patient with Biliary and Pancreatic Problems

Virginia L. Cassmeyer
Dorothy R. Blevins

After studying this chapter, the learner should be able to:

- Describe the anatomy and physiology of the biliary system and pancreas.
- Describe the nature of cholecystitis, cholelithiasis, and cancer of the biliary system.
- Discuss the treatment approaches for cholecystitis, cholelithiasis, and cancer of the biliary system.
- Explain the nursing care of the patient experiencing problems of the biliary system.
- Contrast the pathophysiological basis for signs and symptoms of acute and chronic pancreatitis and pancreatic tumors.
- Describe the treatment for acute and chronic pancreatitis and pancreatic tumors.
- Contrast the nursing care of the patient experiencing acute and chronic problems of the pancreas.

The biliary system and pancreas are affected by various pathologic processes that alter normal metabolism. Some of the disorders are chronic and require that the patient make changes in life-style to keep the disorder under control. Patients with biliary system or pancreatic problems need nursing support to deal with acute problems as well as chronic health problems.

ANATOMY AND PHYSIOLOGY

Biliary System

The gallbladder, a pear-shaped organ, lies on the inferior surface of the liver. The biliary system consists of the gallbladder and its associated ductal system (Fig. 32-1). The ductal system provides a pathway for the bile that is formed in the liver to be transported to the gallbladder or to the intestine and also functions to regulate bile flow. The liver produces up to 1 L of bile per day. As it is formed, bile is excreted into the hepatic ducts, where it passes into the cystic duct to be stored in the gallbladder.

The capacity of the gallbladder is usually 50 ml but can increase under normal conditions. In the gallbladder, bile is concentrated to a solution that is 5 to 10 times as concentrated as that produced in the liver.

Bile contains cholesterol, phospholipids, bile salts, bilirubin, and a very small amount of protein and electrolytes; 97% of bile is water. Some toxins, drug metabolites, and hormones are excreted in bile. Because bile can be released directly into the duodenum through the common bile duct, the removal of the gallbladder has no long-term consequences.

Neural and hormonal mechanisms control the secretion of bile from the gallbladder. Food, particularly lipids in the duodenum, causes the release of *cholecystokinin* (CCK), also sometimes still called cholecystokinin-pancreozymin, from the mucosa of the duodenum. CCK is released into the blood and travels to the gallbladder. One of its activities is to stimulate the gallbladder musculature to contract. At the same time it causes the muscle of the sphincter of Oddi (at the end of the common bile duct) to relax and permit entry of bile into the duodenum. Gastrin, another gastrointestinal hormone, and vagal stimulation can also cause the gallbladder to contract.

Bile acids are predominantly composed of a cholesterol derivative, and they function in intestinal metabolism of fats and other substances as follows:

1. Facilitate fat digestion by emulsifying fats for action by intestinal lipases
2. Facilitate absorption of fats, fat-soluble vitamins, iron, and calcium
3. Activate the release of pancreatic and intestinal enzymes

Most of the bile salts secreted into the duodenum are reabsorbed into the enterohepatic circulation from the terminal ileum or other parts of the intestines. These bile salts are recirculated two to three times per meal. The reabsorption from the intestinal tract is so efficient that only 15% to 25% of the bile salts need to be replaced per day.

Pancreatic Exocrine System

The pancreas, an elongated flattened organ, is located in the posterior abdomen with its head lying in the curvature of the duodenum and its tail resting against the spleen. The pancreatic exocrine system includes the exocrine glands of the pancreas (acinar cells) and a ductal system (Fig. 32-1). (The endocrine functions of the pancreas are described in Chapter 28.) Acinar cells release their secretions into ducts that converge to form the main pancreatic duct (duct of Wirsung). Lining the ducts are cells (ductal cells) that secrete a bicarbonate-rich fluid. In most persons, the pancreatic duct merges with the common bile duct at the entry into the duodenum, but in some persons the common bile duct and pancreatic duct do not merge.

The acinar cells of the pancreas secrete multiple digestive enzymes.

1. Proteolytic enzymes: trypsinogen, chymotrypsinogen, and procarboxypeptidase
2. Amylolytic enzyme: amylase
3. Lipolytic enzymes: lipases
4. Nucleolytic enzymes: ribonuclease and deoxyribonuclease

The pancreatic exocrine secretions are released under the influence of the *vagus nerve, secretin, cholecystokinin* (CCK), and *gastrin* during digestion. Gastrin is released during the gastric phase and stimulates the release of bicarbonate-rich solution. The entry of chyme and acids into the small intestines stimulates the release of secretin and cholecystokinin. *Secretin* then *stimulates* further secretion of the pancreatic *bicarbonate-rich solution*, and *cholecystokinin stimulates* the release of the *pancreatic enzyme-rich* solution.

Physiologic Changes with Aging

The gallbladder and ductal system do not show changes with aging. The composition of bile is increasingly lithogenic, which may be related to an increase in biliary cholesterol.[24] Cholelithiasis and cholecystitis increase in the aged. The pancreas shows anatomic and physiologic changes with aging. Ductal hyperplasia and fibrosis occur. These anatomic changes are not always associated with altered physiologic function, although the volume of stimulated pancreatic secretion decreases after age 40 and the enzyme output and the activity of lipase decrease.[24] One last change in pancreatic function noted in the elderly is an increase in pancreatitis after surgery.[34]

PREVENTION AND HEALTH EDUCATION

Primary Prevention

Gallstones

Preventing gallstones, the most prevalent disorder of the biliary tract, is not currently possible. Populations at higher risk are those who are obese and those with certain metabolic and hemolytic disorders. Patients who tend to form stones in the ducts are usually advised to be careful of their fat intake and to drink generous amounts of fluids unless contraindicated for some reason.

Pancreatic disease

A major cause of chronic pancreatitis is alcoholism. Thus a major focus of primary prevention for pancreatic disease is preventing or controlling alcoholism. This is a very difficult undertaking. Interventions appropriate for the prevention and control of alcoholism are discussed in Chapter 13. The second major cause of pancreatitis is gallbladder disease. Thus measures helpful in decreasing gallstone formation would also help to prevent pancreatitis.

Secondary Prevention

Early detection of disease allows for the most beneficial treatment. Many disorders of the biliary system and pancreas are associated with vague, persistent, nonspecific gastrointestinal symptoms long before more specific or severe symptoms occur. Nurses can encourage persons who complain of vague but persistent symptoms to seek medical evaluation and can discourage the use of home remedies and over-the-counter preparations that delay the seeking of professional help.

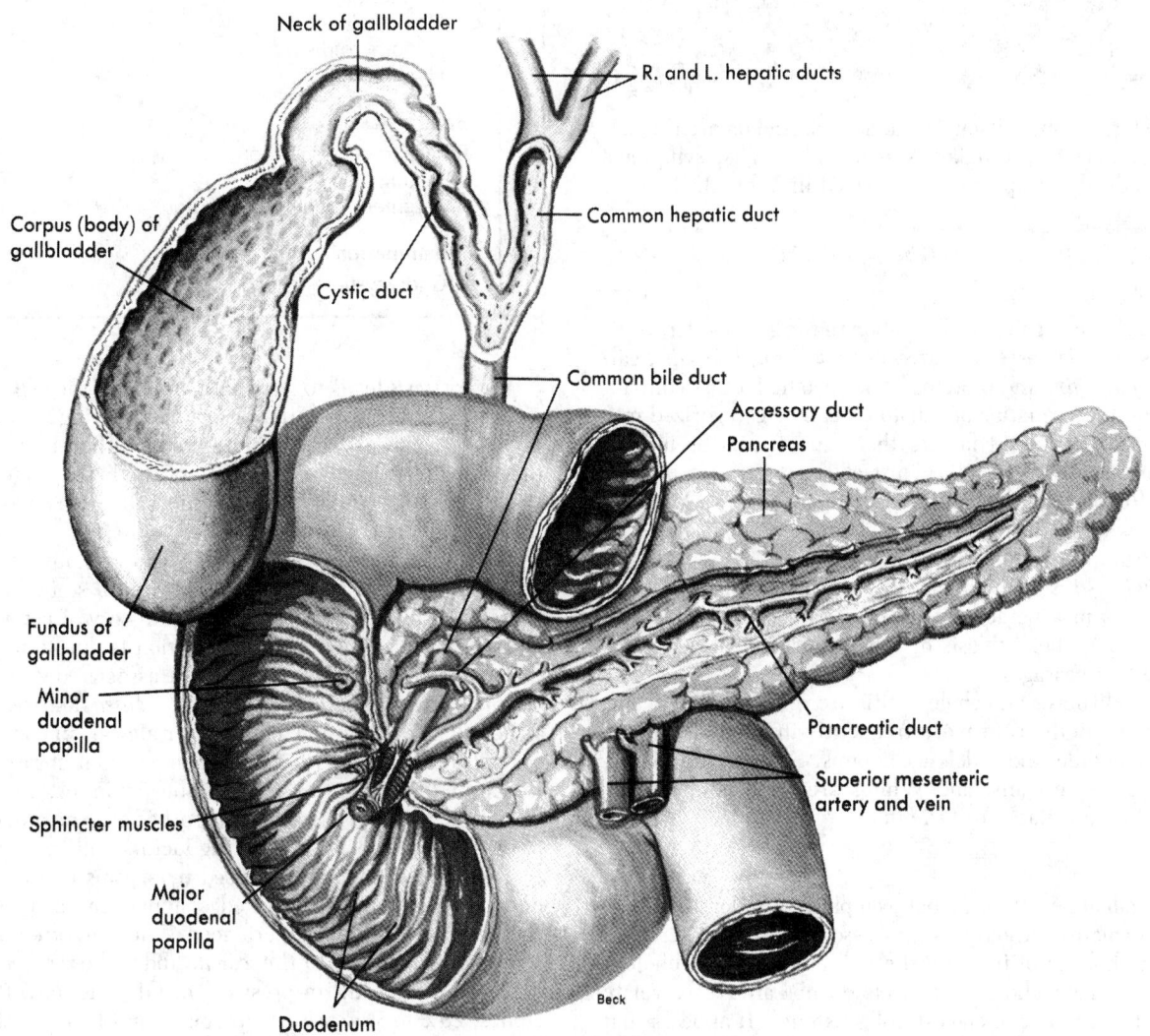

Fig. 32-1   Anatomic schemata of biliary and pancreatic ductal systems. Note head of pancreas surrounds common bile duct. (From Thibodeau GA: *Anthony's textbook of anatomy and physiology,* ed 13, St Louis, 1990, Mosby–Year Book.)

Disorders encountered in the biliary system and pancreas include obstruction and inflammatory problems as well as tumors. The disorders to be discussed include:

The biliary system
1. Cholecystitis
2. Cholelithiasis
3. Carcinoma

The pancreas
1. Pancreatitis
2. Tumors of the pancreas

The nursing process that relates to the above disorders concludes the discussion of biliary system and pancreatic disorders respectively.

DISORDERS OF THE BILIARY SYSTEM

Stone formation, inflammation, and carcinoma are the major disorders of the biliary system. The signs, symptoms and medical therapy are summarized in Table 32-1.

CHOLELITHIASIS/CHOLECYSTITIS
Etiology/Epidemiology

Cholelithiasis is gallstone formation in the gallbladder. Gallstones are composed primarily of *cholesterol, bile salts,* calcium, *bilirubin,* and proteins. The specific factors contributing to the formation of gallstones can be categorized into *metabolic factors* and factors that cause stasis or inflammation. See Box 32-1 for a list of factors increasing the risk of cholelithiasis. About 75% of gallstones in Western cultures are cholesterol stones. The remaining 25% consist of bilirubin pigment stones.

Cholecystitis is inflammation of the gallbladder. The symptoms may be acute or chronic and usually are associated with cholelithiasis or other causes of obstructions of the bile passages.

Cholelithiasis and cholecystitis are very common health problems. Both occur more frequently in women who are in the middle and older age groups. American Indians, Mexican Americans, and Whites are affected more frequently than Blacks or Orientals.

Pathophysiology

Why gallstones form is not completely understood. Although many pathologic states associated with increased serum cholesterol increase the risk of developing cholelithiasis, serum cholesterol levels do not always correlate with the presence of cholesterol gallstones. It appears that a proper relationship among lecithin (a phospholipid), bile salts, and cholesterol is necessary for cholesterol to be soluble in bile. A reduction in the bile salt pool (reabsorbed in the terminal ileum) decreases the amount of bile salts and thereby the solubility of cholesterol.

Increased serum bilirubin associated with various pathophysiologic states can change the relationship between bile salts, cholesterol, and lecithin and result in stone formation.

32-1	Factors increasing the risk of cholelithiasis

Metabolic
Biliary cholesterol saturation
  Estrogens
  Oral contraceptives
  Obesity
  Terminal ileal disease or resection
Increased levels of serum bilirubin
  Hemolytic anemias
  Cirrhosis
Increased serum cholesterol
  Obesity
  Pregnancy
  Diabetes mellitus
  Hypothyroidism
  Hyperlipidemia

Biliary stasis
Biliary tract obstruction
  Fasting
  Parenteral hyperalimentation

Inflammation
  Cholecystitis

Biliary stasis leads to stagnation of bile in the gallbladder and to excessive absorption of water, allowing the salts to precipitate easily. Fasting states reduce the normal stimulation of bile flow. *Inflammation* of the biliary system results in the absorption of more of bile salts with a reduction in the solubility of cholesterol.

Gallstones may be present for years without signs and symptoms, which may only occur when a stone becomes lodged in a biliary duct. However, a history of *postprandial indigestion* is common. The indigestion is due to impaired metabolism of fatty foods and may be associated with *flatus, diarrhea, abdominal distention,* and *nausea* and *vomiting.* Eructations occur immediately after a meal, in contrast to several hours later with gastric ulcers. If fat absorption is impaired for some time, fat-soluble vitamins, including vitamin K, will not be properly absorbed and the production of vitamin-K–dependent clotting factors will be impaired.

Biliary colic, which is caused by spasms of the biliary ducts as they attempt to dislodge stones, can cause one of the most severe pains experienced. The pain often *radiates through to the back under* the *scapula* and to the *right shoulder.* The pain can result in prostration. Of patients with gallstones, 20% to 50% are asymptomatic and 18% have biliary pain.

Stones may lodge anywhere along the biliary tract (Fig. 32-2). If they lodge in the small bile ducts, hepatic duct, or common bile duct (choledocholithiasis), the stones obstruct bile flow, serum bilirubin levels are elevated, and the patient becomes jaundiced (see p. 995). Obstruction of the common bile duct prevents bile from getting to the GI tract and clay-colored (grayish-white) stools will result.

Table 32-1   Biliary tract disorders

Disorder	Signs and symptoms	Therapy
Cholecystitis	History of intolerance of fatty foods, gaseous eructations after meals, flatus, diarrhea, abdominal distention Nausea, vomiting Pain: right upper quadrant, referred to right scapula Fever, tachycardia Leukocytosis	Conservative: NPO, nasogastric intubation, IV infusions, meperidine hydrochloride, spasmolytics (papaverine, amyl nitrate), anticholinergics (chronic condition), antibiotics for acute episode, surgery
Cholelithiasis Choledocholithiasis	As for cholecystitis Biliary colic: intense spasmodic pain with diaphoresis, tachycardia and prostration Jaundice, grayish-white stools Elevated serum bilirubin Prolonged prothrombin time	First pain control; stabilize hemodynamically; surgery; endoscopic retrieval of stones; shock wave lithotripsy; chemodissolution of stones
Carcinoma	Jaundice, weight loss, pain, right upper quadrant mass	Pain control; surgery for comfort

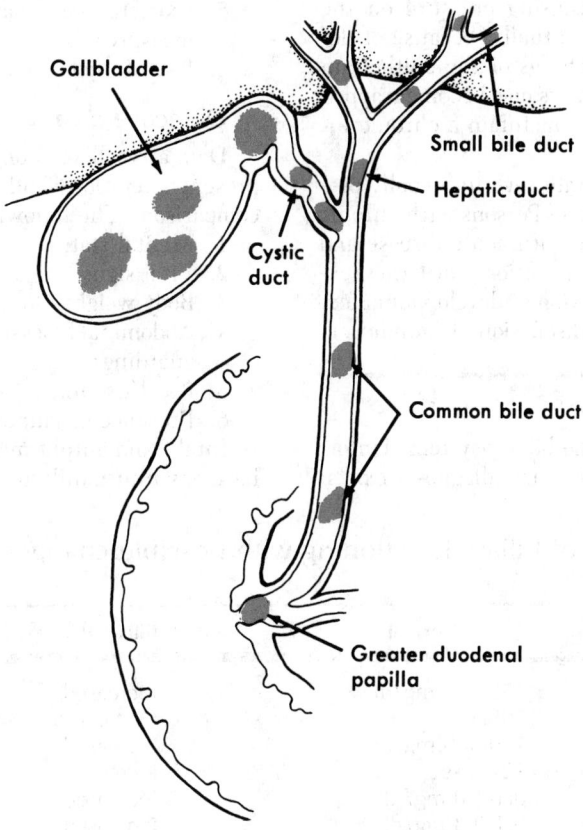

Fig. 32-2   Common sites of gallstones.

Stones may also cause pressure and subsequent necrosis and infection of the walls of the biliary ducts. Occasionally a stone, because of its location, blocks the entrance of pancreatic fluid and bile into the duodenum. This condition is difficult to differentiate from obstruction caused by malignancy. Cholelithiasis may precede or follow cholecystitis. Complications are similar to those for cholecystitis.

Cholecystitis may be acute or chronic and is usually associated with gallstones or other obstructions of the biliary tract system. In acute cholecystitis, the gallbladder is usually very enlarged and resembles a distended sac. Inflammation occurs, and the wall of the gallbladder becomes thickened and edematous. The inflammation results in leukocytosis (increased production of white blood cells) and fever. Impaired circulation, edema, and distention of the gallbladder produce ischemia, which can lead to necrosis and gangrene. Perforation of the gallbladder may occur, leading to biliary peritonitis, pancreatitis, and fistula formation. Bacterial invasion can lead to empyema of the gallbladder, ductal cholangitis, abscess formation, and sepsis.

Chronic cholecystitis may produce a variety of structural changes whether or not stones are present. The structural changes are not the result of an infectious process but are related to a diseased gallbladder wall with inefficient emptying. Chronic cholecystitis is caused by chemical or mechanical irritation from stones causing pressure on the mucosa or from biliary stasis. Eventually, because of destruction of the mucosa, outpouchings of the epithelium may form. Bacteria and other irritants may become trapped in these outpouchings, which may maintain a chronic inflammatory process.

Several acute attacks of moderate severity usually precede the chronic form of the disease. Persons with chronic disease may not be as ill as those with acute disease and therefore may not seek medical attention until they experience pain from biliary obstruction or develop jaundice. (See p. 877 in Chapter 30 for a discussion of jaundice.)

CARCINOMA OF THE BILIARY SYSTEM

Cancer can occur anywhere in the biliary system. Unfortunately, at present no method of early diagnosis exists.

Identification is often made during surgery. Jaundice may be the first sign and indicates that the lesion has developed sufficiently to obstruct bile passage at some point. Spread by direct extension to the liver resulting in hepatic dysfunction or to the peritoneal surface resulting in peritonitis may be the initial manifestation. The prognosis is usually one of rapid deterioration with death ensuing within a few months. Surgery is only done for palliation. Drainage of the biliary tract or surgical bypass of the area of obstruction can improve the patient's comfort. (See Chapter 11 for a general discussion of cancer.)

Nursing Process
Assessment
Subjective data

Some patients with biliary tract disease will be admitted for surgery while their disease is quiescent, whereas others will be in an acute stage of the disease. Thus the actual problems present in individual patients vary. Minimum data to collect include the following:
1. Presence of discomforting signs and symptoms (pain, jaundice, vomiting, diarrhea): onset, severity, location, factors that aggravate or alleviate signs and symptoms
2. Food and fluid intake patterns
3. Understanding of disease
4. History of respiratory problems
5. Expectations related to diagnostic or therapeutic measures
6. Use of medications

Objective data

Data are collected on admission to determine extent of present alterations and to serve as a baseline for future comparison. The following data are collected:
1. Mental status
2. Vital signs
3. Body weight
4. Abdominal assessment for distention, tenderness, or guarding
5. Breath sounds
6. Presence of jaundice

Intake and output measurements are started if patients have any unusual fluid losses or are acutely ill. Urine and

Table 32-2 Laboratory tests of biliary functioning with possible changes in hepatocellular and biliary disease

Test	Normal	Biliary disease	Hepatocellular disease
Serum total cholesterol	150-200 mg/dl	Increased	Decreased
Cholesterol ester	70%	Decreased	Decreased
Serum phospholipids	150-380 mg/dl	Increased	Decreased
Serum prothrombin time	12-15 sec	Increased	Increased
Total bilirubin	0.1-1.0 mg/dl	Increased	Increased
Conjugated (direct)	0.1-0.3 mg/dl	Increased	Increased
Unconjugated (indirect)	0.2-0.8 mg/dl		Increased
Urine bilirubin	None	Increased	Increased
Urine urobilinogen	0.1-1.0 Ehrlich U/dl	Decreased	Increased
Fecal urobilinogen	90-280 mg/day	Decreased	
Alkaline phosphatase	30-85 IU/L	Increased	Increased (slightly)

Table 32-3 Types of jaundice

Category	Pathology	Possible findings
Obstructive		
Intrahepatic	Suppression of bile flow in canaliculi or small biliary ductiles (chole-stasis)	Direct* bilirubin elevated; alkaline phosphatase elevated; no enlargement of bile ducts seen on scan or ultrasound
Extrahepatic (biliary tract obstruction)	Obstruction of bile flow in large bile ducts	Direct* bilirubin elevated; alkaline phosphatase elevated; enlargement of bile ducts documented by scan, ultrasound; absence of urobilinogen in urine; prolonged prothrombin time
Hepatocellular	Hepatocyte injury from toxins, viruses (hepatitis) or as part of syndrome of cirrhosis	Transaminases (ALT, AST) elevated 10-fold to 15-fold; both direct* and indirect† bilirubin may be elevated (direct more than indirect); prolonged prothrombin time
Hemolytic	Excessive amounts of bilirubin are released from RBCs; liver is unable to excrete bilirubin as rapidly as it forms	Usually mild elevation of total bilirubin (indirect more than direct)

*"Direct" measures conjugated bilirubin.
†"Indirect" measures unconjugated bilirubin.

stool are examined for color changes. Dark brown urine, caused by the presence of bilirubin, and clay–colored (grayish-white) stool, resulting from an absence of bile, may be noted. A dipstick test on urine for bilirubin can be done quickly and easily.

Diagnostic tests

Most persons with signs and symptoms of biliary tract disease will have an ultrasound to assist in the diagnostic process. Also, it is not unusual for patients with signs and symptoms of biliary tract disease to have diagnostic tests performed on the liver, pancreas, and biliary tract. See Table 32-2 for tests of serum bilirubin, urine bilirubin, urine urobilinogen, fecal urobilinogen, and other tests related to the biliary system and Table 32-3 for findings of these tests in obstructive and hepatocellular jaundice. The absence of urinary urobilinogen is a highly significant finding, suggesting the presence of obstructive jaundice (a history of antibiotic therapy may influence the test results).

Other diagnostic tests that may be used with persons with biliary tract disease are listed in Box 32-2. A common test of the biliary tract is an oral cholecystogram. If the gallbladder is not visualized on the first set of x-rays, the test may be repeated the next day. Barium studies, if necessary, should follow gallbladder studies to prevent a barium-filled colon from obscuring the gallbladder.

Some patients find the oral dye of the oral cholecystogram very irritating. Diarrhea is not uncommon, and nausea and vomiting can occur. If vomiting soon after ingestion of the tablets is reported, directions are sought about further dosage. Intravenous injection of the dyes may cause allergic reactions such as dyspnea, chills, diaphoresis, faintness, and tachycardia in susceptible patients. Patients are queried about past allergies or reactions to x-ray examinations involving dye. Some patients report temporary dysuria after the test.

Data analysis: nursing diagnoses

Nursing diagnoses are determined from analysis of patient data. Possible nursing diagnoses for the person with biliary tract disease before definitive medical treatment may include, but are not limited to, the following:

Diagnostic title	Possible etiologies
Pain	Biliary colic and jaundice
Knowledge deficit: diagnostic and therapeutic measures	Lack of exposure to information
Altered nutrition: more than body requirements	Excessive intake in relation to metabolic needs, lack of knowledge

Possible nursing diagnoses after laser laparoscopic cholecystectomy may include, but are not limited to, the following:

Diagnostic title	Possible etiologies
Pain	6-inch to 8-inch incision
Knowledge deficit: needs immediately after treatment and at discharge	Lack of exposure to information

Possible nursing diagnoses after abdominal cholecystectomy or shock-wave lithotripsy treatment may include, but are not limited to, the following:

Diagnostic title	Possible etiologies
Breathing pattern, ineffective	High surgical incision, abdominal distention
Fatigue	Surgical or lithotripsy procedure; malnourishment before surgery or lithotripsy
Fluid volume deficit, high risk for	Nausea and vomiting after surgery, bleeding, loss of fluids through external drainage tubes
Injury, high risk for	Obstruction of T-tube after surgery or obstruction of bile duct by fragment of stone after lithotripsy

32-2

Radiographic and endoscopic studies for biliary disorders

Cholecystography (gallbladder series)
Explanation

A normal liver removes radiopaque dyes from the bloodstream and concentrates them in the gallbladder. The dye-filled functioning gallbladder shows up as a dense shadow on the x-ray film. Nonvisualization of the gallbladder suggests nonfunctioning. If a fatty meal is taken, the normal gallbladder contracts and expels the dye. An x-ray at this time outlines the bile ducts. Stones that are not radiopaque show up as dark patches on the film.

Patient preparation

1. Procedure is explained to patient.
2. Presence of iodine allergy is assessed because the dye contains iodine.
3. If an oral cholecystogram is to be done, administer the Bilopaque or Telepaque tablets as ordered (usual dose is 3 g but is determined by weight).
4. If an intravenous cholecystogram is to be done, the dye will be administered just before examination in the radiology department.
5. Diet
   a. A low-fat meal is eaten the evening before the test.
   b. No further foods may be taken after the evening meal.
   c. Black coffee, tea, or water may be taken for breakfast.
6. Laxatives or enemas are given as prescribed.

Cholangiography
Explanation

Test used to visualize the bile ducts and demonstrate presence of stones, strictures, or tumors, or the patency of the common bile duct after surgery. In *percutaneous transhepatic cholangiography*, the dye is injected through skin and abdominal wall into a blood vessel or bile duct; in *surgical cholangiography*, the dye is inserted through a needle or catheter into the common bile duct.

Patient preparation

1. Explain procedure to patient.
2. Omit meal before test.
3. Decrease patient's fluid intake.
4. Give laxative, if prescribed.

Endoscopy
Peritonoscopy

Direct visualization of peritoneum and liver, sometimes combined with liver biopsy; air sufflation, which may be painful, may be used.

Endoscopic retrograde cholangiopancreatography (ERCP)

Use of fiberscope to visualize and obtain a biopsy of the biliary and pancreatic tracts; the fiberscope is passed through the oral pharynx to the duodenum and into the biliary and pancreatic ducts. Contrast media may be injected through the endoscope and dilation or sphincterotomy may be used to remove gallstones or enlarge the sphincter.

Patient preparation

1. Written consent is required.
2. Procedure is explained to patient.
3. Nothing by mouth is allowed after midnight.
4. Skin is prepared before peritonoscopy.
5. Sedatives are given as prescribed.

Knowledge deficit: needs immediately after treatment and at discharge	Lack of exposure to information
Nutrition, altered: high risk for less than body requirement	Nausea and vomiting after treatment
Pain	Incisional; spasms of ductal system associated with obstruction of T-tube or of cystic or common bile ducts from stone fragments
Skin integrity, impaired	Incision, potential long-term drainage tubes; potential bile drainage irritating the skin

Planning: expected patient outcomes

Expected patient outcomes for the patient with biliary tract disease before definitive medical treatment may include, but are not limited to, the following:

1. States pain is controlled and does not demonstrate behaviors associated with discomfort.
2. Describes the purpose of diagnostic and therapeutic measures.
3. Describes ways to reduce caloric and fat content in the diet.

Expected patient outcomes for the patient after laser laparoscopic cholecystectomy may include, but are not limited to, the following:

1. States pain is controlled and does not demonstrate behaviors associated with pain.
2. Describes care needs after discharge, signs and symptoms to report immediately, and follow-up care.

Expected patient outcomes for the patient after abdominal cholecystectomy or shock-wave lithotripsy treatment may include, but are not limited to, the following:

1. Breath sounds are clear and present in all lobes.
2. States fatigue is gradually improved and rates fatigue as lessened on a 1 to 5 scale (1 = no fatigue, 5 = severe fatigue).
3. Maintains normal fluid volume as evidenced by stable weight, moist mucous membranes, adequate skin turgor, and balanced intake and output.
4. Has no undetected obstruction of T-tube drainage; reports immediately recurrence of severe pain, jaundice, nausea and vomiting, or fever.
5. States immediate care needs, pain relief methods, activity allowed, dietary requirements, signs and symptoms to report immediately, and follow-up care.
6. Consumes a balanced diet with food from all food groups and restricted in fat if the patient had lithotripsy.
7. States pain is controlled; activity not inhibited because of pain.
8. Incision heals without complications.

Implementation
Assisting with achievement of therapeutic goals
Conservative management

A variety of treatment measures are used in biliary tract disease (see Table 32-1). Conservative treatment of acute cholecystitis/cholelithiasis usually will effect improvement within 1 to 7 days. Food is withheld until acute symptoms subside. If vomiting persists, a nasogastric tube is inserted and attached to suction. Meperidine hydrochloride may be given for pain and is preferred because its spasmogenic effect on the biliary tract is less than that which occurs with opiates. The inhalation of amyl nitrite may diminish intestinal and biliary spasms. When food is tolerated, a reducing diet (if appropriate) and careful avoidance of fat usually are recommended until definitive treatment is implemented. Definitive treatment will be recommended because recurrent attacks are common and may result in more severe problems such as pancreatitis.

Surgery

After stabilization of the patient's physical status, diagnostic tests are initiated to determine the best definitive treatment. The most common treatment for cholecystitis and cholelithiasis is laparoscopic cholecystectomy (LC) using a laser or cautery to remove the gallbladder. The first LC was performed in the United States in 1988. LC offers several advantages over the common abdominal cholecystectomy including: (1) less invasive and thus less chance of wound infection or respiratory impairment, shorter healing time, and shorter recuperative time; (2) no unsightly scar; and (3) less pain and thus much more rapid return to normal activities. Importantly, the mortality and morbidity associated with LC is no greater than that associated with the traditional cholecystectomy, which is very low. Most patients are discharged on the day of surgery or on the first postoperative day.

Surgeries of the biliary tract
Cholecystectomy Removal of gallbladder
Cholecystostomy Creation of an opening into gallbladder for drainage
Choledochotomy Incision into common bile duct
Choledocholithotomy Incision into common bile duct to remove a stone
Choledochoduodenostomy Anastomosis of common bile duct with duodenum
Choledochojejunostomy Anastomosis of common bile duct with jejunum
Cholecystogastrostomy Anastomosis of gallbladder with stomach

LC involves preprocedure preparation of the patient similar to any patient having abdominal surgery, including NPO after midnight, an enema to reduce the mass of the colon, and an antibiotic given with any premedications for anesthesia. In the operating room, the patient receives a general anesthetic, has a nasogastric tube and foley catheter inserted, and has intravenous fluids started.

The surgery is carried out using video monitors and instrumentation through four cannulas introduced by trocars into the peritoneal cavity via four small (5 mm to 10 mm) incisions. These incisions are made at the umbilicus, midline in the epigastric region and in the right upper quadrant at the midclavicular line and at the anterior axillary line. After the first incision is made at the umbilicus, carbon dioxide is introduced to insufflate the abdominal cavity, which allows for the insertion of the instruments. The carbon dioxide is removed at the end of the surgery.

An LC is not the surgery of choice for everyone. Persons who have had extensive abdominal surgery may have too many adhesions to allow for this procedure. Gallstones within the common bile duct cannot be removed with this procedure. Of course, persons who cannot tolerate general anesthesia cannot be treated with this procedure. Potential complications of the procedure include injury to the hepatic or common bile duct, injury to the bowel, wound infection, abdominal abscess formation, and retained stones in the common bile duct.

The alternative surgical approach to LC is removal of the gallbladder through an abdominal incision. An abdominal incision may be used for other types of surgery on the gallbladder or duct system. Other types of surgical procedures that may be carried out are defined in Box 32-3. The terminology used to indicate specific biliary tract surgery is self-explanatory once common terms are understood. *Cholecyst* refers to the gallbladder, *choledocho* refers to the common bile duct, and *lith* refers to a stone (see Box 32-3). Biliary tract anastomoses are palliative operations to provide biliary drainage to the intestine by bypassing an obstructed area.

Dissolution agents and gallstone lithotripsy

Persons with gallbladder problems who are not candidates for surgery because of the presence of other health problems that make anesthesia too risky may be treated with dissolution agents or shock wave lithotripsy. Shock wave lithotripsy and dissolution therapy are currently used in 10% of patients with cholelithiasis.[11] Gallstone lithotripsy is still being implemented under strictly defined protocols.

Chenodeoxycholic acid and ursodeoxycholic acid (UDCA) now are being used to dissolve small (≤20 mm in diameter) cholesterol stones. These compounds are bile acids and increase cholesterol solubility. The drugs, which are taken daily for up to 2 years, can cause elevated hepatic enzymes and diarrhea. Also, gallstones can reoccur after the drugs are discontinued.

Lithotripsy involves the use of shock waves to disintegrate gallstones. Shock waves are applied to the gallstones located in the gallbladder or common and hepatic bile duct, which are located by use of ultrasound. The shock waves are usually passed through a water medium, although some machines are "dry" lithotripters and use liquid couplers contained by membranes between the shock wave source and the patient's skin.[2] Approximately 1500 shocks are delivered over 1 to 2 hours. The fragments of the disintegrated stones are excreted through the common bile duct into the small intestines.

Use of lithotripsy for patients with bile duct stones requires that the patient have an endoscopic spincterotomy or percutaneous transhepatic catherization at least 5 days before the lithotripsy.

At this time lithotripsy can be used only: (1) on patients who have fewer than three stones that are <3.0 cm in diameter, (2) in patients with no acute complications of gallstone disease, (3) in patients with no acute cholecystitis, (4) in patients with no allergy to iodine or bile acids, (5) in patients with normal coagulation profiles, (6) in patients with normal liver and pancreatic function tests, and (7) in patients with no pacemakers or artificial heart valves.[2,11,16] The gallstones must be located so that the shock waves, which disintegrate the gallstones, do not penetrate the lung or head of the pancreas.[16] Lithotripsy is usually used in combination with dissolution agents. Modifications in the lithotripters have altered the body surface area over which the shock wave enters the patient. Some lithotripters allow the waves to penetrate a larger skin area, decreasing the pain.[2] Also, lithotripters vary in the actual pressure delivered to the second focus.[2] Currently, most lithotripters can be applied to patients using no anesthesia or only light IV sedation.[2]

Biliary drainage

External biliary drainage is used in empyema, for fistula, when chronic decompression of the biliary tract is required, and often after abdominal cholecystectomy when the common bile duct has been explored. Drainage is provided by a catheter inserted into the gallbladder (cholecystostomy) or by a T-tube inserted into the common bile duct (choledochostomy) (Fig. 32-3). Usually stab wounds are used to bring these tubes through the skin.

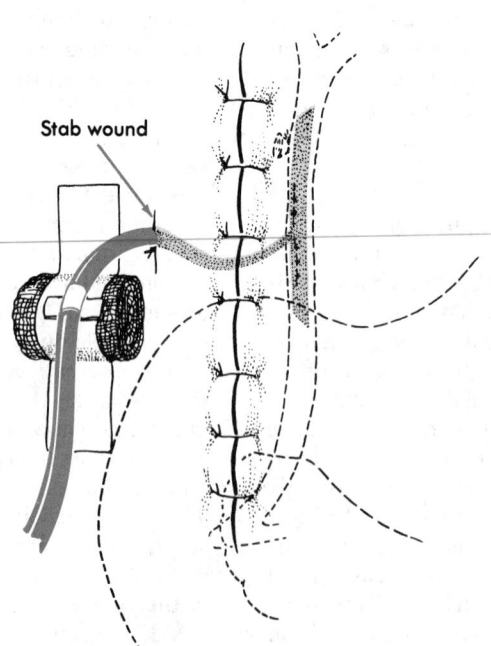

Fig. 32-3 Section of T tube emerging from stab wound may be placed over roll of gauze anchored to skin with adhesive tape to prevent lumen from being occluded by pressure.

The T-tube is inserted to maintain patency of the common bile duct and to ensure drainage of bile out of the body until edema in the common duct has subsided enough for bile to drain into the duodenum normally. (For some patients with extensive ductal disease, the T-tube may be used for long periods of time.) Cholangiograms (op-grams) are commonly performed in the operating room to ensure patency of the common bile duct; radiopaque dye is inserted through the T-tube.

When a T-tube is used after exploration of the common bile duct, at first the entire output of bile (normally 500 to 1000 ml/day) may flow through the T-tube, but within several days most of the bile will be flowing into the duodenum. If bile is not flowing out the tube or into the duodenum, it can be assumed that drainage is obstructed and that bile is being forced back into the common bile duct into the liver. The patient is observed closely for jaundice, particularly in the sclerae.

Before the T-tube is removed, the patency of the common bile duct must be assessed. The tube is clamped for variable intervals and the patient monitored for signs of distress. If distress occurs, the tube is unclamped immediately and the physician is informed. A cholangiogram is usually performed to confirm patency of the duct before the tube is removed. After removal of the T-tube, the patient may have chills and fever caused by edema and a local reaction to the bile; these symptoms usually subside within 24 hours.

Interventions to achieve patient outcomes
Promoting comfort

Pain control is a need of all persons with biliary tract disease before definitive treatment. Analgesics such as meperidine will be needed to control the pain from biliary colic adequately and should be freely administered. Measures to decrease nausea and vomiting, such as maintenance of an NPO status or dietary fat restriction, will be necessary.

Pain control remains a need in the posttreatment period regardless of the treatment, although pain is much less after laparoscopic cholecystectomy. For the patient who has an abdominal cholecystectomy, pain remains a problem for up to 6 weeks. Immediately after surgery injectable analgesics are necessary. After the person is ambulating well and eating well, oral analgesic are usually satisfactory. For patients who had lithotropsy treatment, pain may continue for some time until the disintegrated stones are passed into the duodenum. Pain control is necessary to allow for adequate ambulation, deep breathing, and nutritional intake after definitive treatment.

Dressings, such as those present after abdominal surgical treatment of biliary tract disease, are monitored for moisture, which is uncomfortable and increases the risk of infection. Moist dressings are changed immediately. Additionally, great care is taken to avoid tension on biliary drainage tubes, another source of discomfort.

Teaching

The time available for preoperative or prelithotripsy teaching is often limited because patients may be acutely ill and undergoing diagnostic procedures and treatments to prepare them for surgery or lithotripsy within a short time. Or, conversely, the patient scheduled for elective surgery or lithotripsy may come to the hospital the morning of treatment 1 to 2 hours before the treatment. The nurse must be prepared to give essential information in the brief period that is available, as well as to address the patient's expressed concerns.

After treatment, carefully assessing the patient's understanding of treatment care measures is important.

Patients who have had an LC will be discharged on the day of surgery or the first day after surgery. Before discharge, patients should be eating without difficulty, walking, and have no abdominal distention, evidence of bleeding, or bile leakage. They are instructed to report immediately any severe pain, any tenderness in the right upper quadrant, any increase in abdominal girth, any leakage of bile-colored drainage from the puncture sites, any increase in pulse, or any symptoms of low blood pressure. Patients are instructed that they usually can return to work in 3 days and can resume full activity after 1 week. Patients should know that oral analgesics control incisional pain and a heating pad usually relieves shoulder pain, which results from insertion of carbon dioxide into the abdomen during surgery.

Patients who have an abdominal cholecystectomy are discharged 5 to 7 days after surgery. They need to know that recovery at home takes 3 to 6 weeks. The patient is instructed to increase activities gradually as tolerated, but to limit heavy lifting (nothing greater than 10 pounds) until full recovery is achieved at about 6 weeks. The patient also is taught how to monitor for signs and symptoms of infection, jaundice, or bile leakage and to report any signs or symptoms immediately. The nurse teaches the patient that oral analgesics should control any pain.

32-4

Patient Teaching

The patient with a chronic biliary system disorder

Dietary restrictions
  Low-fat diet if fat is poorly tolerated
  Low-calorie diet if weight reduction is necessary
Drug therapy, if appropriate
  Medication: importance in preventing recurrence of symptoms
  Medications: when and how to use
Dressings or drainage tube
  Biliary drainage: expected amount
  Dressing change or emptying of drainage bag: how to do and frequency
  Dressings: need to keep dry and skin clean (soap and water is sufficient by time of discharge); a daily shower may be permitted
  Dressing change: technique and availability of supplies
  Signs to report to physician: excessive drainage, leakage, obstruction (jaundice, grayish-white stools)
Follow-up care
  Signs and symptoms to report to health care provider (pain, fever, jaundice, dark urine, grayish-white stools, pruritus, tube dislodgement)
  Follow-up care: plans

The patient undergoing abdominal surgery to treat biliary tract disease

Preoperative

Carry out actions used in preparing any patient with abdominal surgery (see Chapter 31).

Pay particular attention to improving respiratory function, because the high incision and right upper quadrant (RUQ) pain predispose the patient to *atelectasis* and *right lower lobe pneumonia*.

Explain the types of biliary drainage tubes that are anticipated.

Provide care required because of severity of acute symptoms or the presence of jaundice.

Administer intravenous fluids and antibiotics as prescribed.

Administer analgesics (usually meperidine) as prescribed and required.

Provide comfort measures for pruritus, nausea and vomiting, and pain.

Administer vitamin K as prescribed.

Postoperative

Place patient in low-Fowler's position, assist to change position frequently.

Urge patient to deep breathe at regular intervals (every 1 to 2 hours) and to cough if secretions are present until ambulating well.

Monitor frequently for signs of hemorrhage (shock) the first few hours postoperatively (hemorrhage is rare, but may occur when the inflamed gallbladder was adherent to the liver and difficult to remove).

Give analgesics fairly liberally the first 2 to 3 days.

Maintain a dry, intact dressing; usually a drain is inserted near the stump of the cystic duct; some serous fluid drainage is normal initially.

Encourage progressive ambulation when permitted.

Increase diet gradually to regular with fat content as tolerated when appropriate (appetite and fat tolerance may be diminished if there is external biliary drainage).

Biliary drainage

Connect any biliary drainage tubes to closed gravity drainage.

Attach sufficient tubing so the patient can move without restriction.

Explain to patient the importance of avoiding kinks, clamping, or pulling of the tube.

Monitor the amount and color of drainage frequently; measure and record drainage at least every shift.

Report any signs of peritonitis (abdominal pain, rigidity, or fever) to the physician immediately.

Monitor color of urine and stools; stools will be grayish-white if bile is flowing out a drainage tube, but the normal color should gradually reappear as external drainage diminishes and disappears.

Patients who have had lithotripsy treatment need to know how to control pain with analgesics and low-fat diets and the importance of maintaining an adequate fluid intake to assist with the passage of the disintegrated stones. Patients should know that nausea, vomiting, and hematuria may be present for 24 hours and are treated symptomatically. The patient is instructed to report reoccurrence of fever, jaundice, prolonged nausea and vomiting, or pain, all of which indicate obstruction of the biliary tract. Patients who have had lithotripsy treatment are monitored by ultrasound and laboratory tests for passage of stones 6 weeks, 3 months, and 6 months after the procedure.

Persons with prolonged illness, as with biliary tract fistulas or metastatic carcinomas, need supportive care and instructions related to specific symptoms including fatigue and activity intolerance. They may need instructions on dealing with chronic biliary drainage and dietary restrictions. They also need to know signs and symptoms to report. Important teaching points for patients with chronic biliary system disorders are summarized in Box 32-4.

Promoting physiologic stability

The patient who has had an abdominal cholecystectomy or lithotripsy have needs for various interventions to promote oxygenation, maintain fluid volume status and nutritional status, and prevent infection. See Box 32-5 for a summary of nursing care for the patient undergoing abdominal surgery to treat biliary tract disease and promote physical stability.

Evaluation

Evaluation is based on expected patient outcomes. Questions to ask may include the following:

1. Is the patient comfortable?
2. Can the patient explain the purpose of the diagnostic tests and the expected outcomes of the therapeutic measures?
3. Can the patient explain how to reduce calorie and fat intake?
4. Does patient know when and what to report to the physician?
5. Did the patient remain free of atelectasis or pneumonia in the right lower lobe?
6. Is jaundice decreased?
7. Are all incisions healing?
8. Does the patient know how to care for self at home, for example, how to take medications and care for any drainage systems or dressings?

DISORDERS OF THE PANCREAS

Acute and chronic pancreatitis and benign and malignant tumors are the major problems of the pancreas. Table 32-4 summarizes the signs, symptoms, and medical therapy for these problems.

PANCREATITIS

Pancreatitis is a serious inflammatory disorder of the pancreas that can be *acute* or *chronic*. Acute pancreatitis can

REVIEW

Table 32-4   Disorders of the pancreas

Disorder	Signs and symptoms	Medical therapy
Acute pancreatitis	*Acute pancreatitis:* Epigastric pain, abdominal tenderness Nausea, vomiting Shock, dehydration Fever, tachycardia Jaundice Abdominal rigidity Hyperglycemia Hypocalcemia Serum amylase greater than 300 Somogyi units	Fluid deficit: hydrating fluids, albumin, blood or plasma, electrolyte replacement Inhibition of pancreatic activity: NPO, nasogastric suction, antacids, histamine$_2$ receptor blockers Pain: meperidine hydrochloride Paralytic ileus: Miller Abbot intubation, electrolyte balance restored
Chronic pancreatitis	*Chronic pancreatitis:* Recurring episodes of signs and symptoms associated with acute pancreatitis, diarrhea, steatorrhea, weight loss, malnutrition, jaundice, diabetes mellitus	Treatment similar to that for acute pancreatitis Nutritional deficit: high calorie, high protein, low fat diet Malabsorption: pancreatic enzyme replacement: pancreatin, (Viokase), pancrelipase (Cotazym, Pancrease) Obstruction/cysts: fiberoscopy with cannulization and sphincterotomy of sphincter of Oddi, surgery
Tumors	Anorexia, nausea and vomiting, weight loss Pain Jaundice Hyperglycemia Peptic ulcer, diarrhea, steatorrhea	Tumor/complications: pancreatic-duodenal resection (Whipple), cholecystojejunostomy or other bypass operation, pancreatic resection, chemotherapy, symptomatic treatment Chemotherapy Pancreatic resection Pancreatic resection and gastrectomy, cimetidine

occur as a single episode or as recurrent attacks (recurrent acute pancreatitis). The unique morphologic feature of acute or recurrent acute pancreatitis is that, except in cases of alcohol-induced pancreatitis, the pancreas returns to normal after successful treatment.[31]

In chronic pancreatitis permanent and progressive destruction of the pancreas occurs, with normal tissue being replaced by fibrous tissue. Chronic pancreatitis can eventually lead to chronic insufficiency of pancreatic hormones (insulin).

Etiology/Epidemiology

The causes of pancreatitis are numerous. Biliary disease is a common cause of acute pancreatitis. Many times in acute pancreatitis the cause is unknown. The principal cause of chronic pancreatitis in adults in the United States is alcoholism. A major cause in children is cystic fibrosis; approximately 85% of patients with cystic fibrosis have impaired pancreatic exocrine function.[12] See Box 32-6 for a summary of causes of pancreatitis.

Pathophysiology

Although many causes of pancreatitis are known, the manner in which they result in acute inflammation is unknown. The currently favored pathologic factor leading to the acute inflammation is *autodigestion*. This theory proposes that proteolytic enzymes, particularly trypsinogen, are activated within the pancreas itself. Once activated to trypsin, trypsinogen can activate itself and other enzymes. The activated proteolytic enzymes digest pancreatic and surround-

---

32-6

Causes of pancreatitis

Alcoholism
Biliary tract disease
Postoperative—abdominal or nonabdominal surgery
Postretrograde cholangiopancreatography
Cystic fibrosis
Blunt abdominal trauma
Metabolic problems (increased serum calcium [hyperparathyroidism and postrenal transplant patients] hypertriglyceridemia)
Cancer of pancreas
Infections (especially viral)
Connective tissue disease with vasculitis such as systemic lupus erythematosus
Drugs (antihypertensives, diuretics, antimicrobials, immunosuppressives, and oral contraceptives)
Intestinal diseases such as regional enteritis and penetrating duodenal ulcers
Unknown
Malnutrition

Adapted from Toskes PP, Greenberger NJ: Acute and chronic pancreatitis, *Disease-a-Month* 29:5-81, 1983; and Toskes PP: Recurrent acute pancreatitis, *Hosp Pract* 20:85-88, 90-92, 1985.

ing tissues and cellular membranes. This autodigestion results in edema, interstitial hemorrhage, vascular drainage, coagulation necrosis, fat necrosis, and parenchymal cell necroses. The injured tissue releases histamine and bradykinin, which increase vascular permeability, cause vasodilation, and cause more edema. The initiation of activation of the proteolytic enzymes is thought to result from reflux of bile into the pancreatic duct, obstruction of the pancreatic duct or ampulla of vater, ischemia, anorexia, trauma, endotoxins, and exotoxins.

Regardless of the cause, the acute inflammatory process and autodigestion result in a spectrum of physiologic alterations that can cause mild to very critical events. Pain may result from distention of the pancreatic capsule, from obstruction of bile flow caused by compression of the common bile duct, and from peritoneal irritation. The pain may radiate to the back, flanks, and substernal area and may be more intense when the person is lying supine. Difficulty in breathing may accompany the severe pain.

Ascites and ileus distend the abdomen and lead to hypoventilation. Vomiting at first relieves pain, but continued vomiting worsens it. The patient often assumes a flexed posture to relieve pain.

Fluid and electrolyte abnormalities result from vomiting, local edema, ascites, or calcium precipitation into the inflamed pancreas. Hypovolemic shock may ensue if fluid loss is severe. Shallow respirations may reflect metabolic alkalosis (induced by loss of gastric contents), limited diaphragmatic excursion, or ascites. Decreased breath sounds may be the result of atelectasis or pleural effusion. Crackles may be present.

Multiple complications can occur as a result of acute pancreatitis. These complications can affect all systems. Box 32-7 lists some of the major complications.

Acute pancreatitis may be divided into three stages, edematous or interstitial, hemorrhagic, and necrotizing. The majority of patients (80% to 90%) with acute pancreatitis recover without any residual dysfunction. The mortality rate is approximately 10%.[5] The occurrence of the following factors increases the risk of death from acute pancreatitis:

1. Hypotension
2. Need for massive fluid and colloid replacement
3. Respiratory failure associated with adult respiratory distress syndrome
4. Hypocalcemia

The organ destruction that occurs in chronic pancreatitis is caused by the same factors as those described for acute pancreatitis, that is, autodigestion. In chronic pancreatitis caused by alcohol abuse, the pancreatic juices secreted contain decreased bicarbonate, increased protein, and a decreased amount of substances that inhibit trypsin activation.[26] In addition, the pancreatic juices of persons with chronic pancreatitis may be altered in other ways that allow for calcium precipitation. The changes described above would allow for formation of protein plugs that block the pancreatic ducts and precipitate autodigestion, inflammation, fibrosis, and stenosis with loss of normal cell function. The changes in tissue mass and function result in:

1. Diminished secretion of enzymes and pancreatic hormones
2. Obstruction, stasis of flow, and secondary infection of pancreatic ducts
3. Malnourishment from poor food absorption
4. Steatorrhea, weight loss
5. Hyperglycemia

Pain may be very severe during acute flare-ups of chronic pancreatitis, and for some patients, pain may be chronic. For other patients with chronic pancreatitis, between acute attacks the pain may disappear or may be only a vague discomfort.

Distention and distortion of the ductal system in chronic pancreatitis may lead to the development of pseudocysts (collections of liquefied necrotic tissue). These cysts may contain digestive enzymes. Large pseudocysts are a serious complication of pancreatitis because of the possibility of rupture, bleeding, and erosion into nearby tissue or into the peritoneal cavity. Infection, abscess formation, and fistula formation may occur. Although small pseudocysts may resolve over time, large ones are surgically removed.

32-7

Major complications of acute pancreatitis

Cardiovascular
Hypotension/shock from hypovolemia or hypoalbuminemia

Hematologic
Leukocytosis from generalized inflammation or secondary infections, anemia from blood loss, disseminated intravascular coagulation (DIC) from unknown causes

Respiratory
Atelectasis, pneumonitis, pleural effusion, adult respiratory distress syndrome (ARDS) from hypotension/shock and DIC

Gastrointestinal
Hemorrhage from peptic ulcers, gastritis

Pancreas and liver
Hemorrhage from varices; pancreatic pseudocysts or abscesses from structural changes; ascites from destruction of pancreatic capsule and the generalized inflammatory process that increases capillary permeability

Renal
Oliguria and increased blood urea nitrogen (BUN) from hypovolemia (resulting in prerenal or acute renal failure)

Metabolic
Increased blood glucose from decreased insulin release associated with the stress response or destruction of beta cells of pancrease; increased triglycerides from the stress response and changes in insulin release or secretion; decreased calcium associated with low albumin, precipitation of calcium to free fatty acids to form soaps, and unknown causes.

Neurologic
Encephalopathy: alterations in cognitive functions from increased metabolic byproducts (BUN), altered tissue perfusion (hypovolemia and shock), pain, multiple stressors, or unknown causes

TUMORS (NEOPLASMS) OF THE PANCREAS

Pancreatic tumors may be benign or malignant. Benign tumors are usually adenomas or cystadenomas and are relatively rare. Malignant tumors occur more frequently and are most often found in the head of the pancreas. Men are affected far more often than women, usually after middle age. Cancer of the pancreas is the fourth most common cause of cancer mortality in men.

Most malignant tumors of the pancreas appear to begin in the ductal areas, causing eventual blockage and resulting in chronic pancreatitis. Direct extension of the lesion may cause its spread to the posterior wall of the stomach, duodenum, colon, and common bile duct. The tumor may be diffusely spread over the entire gland, or it may be a well-defined growth. It usually grows rapidly, is highly invasive, and metastasizes frequently. Many patients live only 3 to 6 months after diagnosis is confirmed. Symptoms usually occur late in the course of the disease. Pain occurs in about 85% of patients. Jaundice occurs from common bile duct obstruction but is seldom a primary sign.

Islet cell tumors give rise to particular syndromes that are important in the differential diagnosis of hypoglycemia and peptic ulcer. These tumors may be benign or malignant. *Beta-cell pancreatic adenoma (insulinoma)* results in hyperinsulinism and episodes of hypoglycemia. Fasting or exercise precipitates attacks, and glucose ingestion or infusion relieves symptoms. *Non–beta-cell tumors* that produce gastrin result in peptic ulceration of the duodenum or jejunum. Hypersecretion of gastric acid is extremely severe in this Zollinger-Ellison syndrome (see Chapter 31). The patient often gives a history of severe diarrhea and steatorrhea.

Nursing Process
Assessment
Subjective data

The nursing history should be thorough and should carefully document the course of symptoms, particularly pain and vomiting. The use of any medications, alcohol, and home remedies are explored. When alcohol use is a factor in pancreatitis, data are collected about the person's present perception of drinking as a problem for which help is needed (see Chapter 13). Baseline data about food intake patterns and likes and dislikes can help the nurse and dietitian plan for patients with anorexia and malnutrition. Information about measures the patient found useful in promoting pain control should also be obtained.

Objective data

A complete physical examination is necessary. Special attention is directed to the abdomen to elicit signs of ascites, guarding, or tenderness. Dehydration is usually found in acute pancreatitis. Although unusual, hypocalcemia may occur, therefore the patient is monitored for the presence of Chvostek's sign and Trousseau's sign. Baseline abdominal girth can help determine further abdominal distention in either acute or chronic pancreatitis. A brief listing of important data for persons with any type of pancreatic problem includes the following:

General appearance and posture
Mental status
Body weight
Vital signs
Breath sounds
Abdomen: girth, bowel sounds, tenderness, muscle
  mass, guarding
Chvostek's and Trousseau's signs
Intake and output

Diagnostic tests

Of the greatest value in establishing a diagnosis of acute pancreatitis are measurements of enzyme levels (Table 32-5). With pancreatic trauma, a peritoneal tap may reveal an increased amylase level in the peritoneal fluid. When elevations of AST, alkaline phosphatase, and bilirubin occur, obstruction of the common bile duct or liver disease is usually present. Laboratory findings consistent with acute inflammation (leukocytosis) may be present. Serum electrolytes, blood glucose, and urinary ketones also are assessed.

Radiography, scans, ultrasound, and ERCP are used to diagnose chronic pancreatitis, carcinoma, and complications of acute pancreatitis.

Data analysis: nursing diagnoses

Nursing diagnoses are determined from analysis of patient data. Possible nursing diagnoses for the person with pancreatic disorders may include, but are not limited to, the following:

Diagnostic title	Possible etiologies
Pain	Inflammation of peritoneum, stretching of capsule of pancreas, or spasms of ducts; diagnostic tests, improper positioning
Fluid volume deficit	Vomiting, lack of intake, hemorrhage
Self-care deficit: variable	Generalized weakness
Altered health maintenance	Substance abuse, perceptual/cognitive impairment, lack of knowledge
Hopelessness	Long-term stress, failing physical condition, abandonment
Altered nutrition: less than body requirements	Anorexia, inability to obtain food, noncompliance with enzyme replacement
Knowledge deficit: illness, self care, follow-up	Lack of previous exposure; not attentive to instructions

Planning: expected patient outcomes

Expected patient outcomes for the person with pancreatic disorders may include, but are not limited to, the following:
1. States comfort level is increased.
2. Fluid status returns to normal and is maintained at normal as evidenced by weight, intake and output, vital signs, and skin turgor.
3. Gradually increases participation in self-care activities.
4. States goal and methods of treating substance abuse.
5. Has access to supportive services for long-term alcoholism control or hospice services when prognosis for pancreatic carcinoma is poor.

Table 32-5   Diagnostic tests for nonendocrine (exocrine) pancreatic disease

Laboratory tests	Normal	Interpretation
Blood tests		
Amylase, serum	60 to 150 Somogyi units	Serum and urinary enzyme levels are increased when there is cellular injury. (There are other causes of increased serum enzymes, however.) Lower levels may be seen in advanced chronic state of pancreatitis.
Lipase	0 to 1.5 U/ml	Levels parallel amylase levels
Calcium	4.5 to 5.75 mEq/L; 9 to 11 mg/dl	Serum calcium levels are lowered as calcium is deposited into inflamed and necrotic pancreatic tissue.
Bilirubin (direct, conjugated)	0.1 to 0.3 mg/dl	Bilirubin levels are elevated when biliary obstruction exists.
Glucose	90 to 120 mg/dl	A transient hyperglycemia may occur in acute pancreatitis; permanent carbohydrate intolerance may occur if beta cells are destroyed in chronic pancreatitis.
Urine tests		
Amylase (urine, 24 hour specimen)	35 to 260 Somogyi U/hour	Increased levels are found in acute pancreatitis.
Radiographic tests		
Flat plate of abdomen	No calcification of pancreas visualized	See serum calcium above.
CAT; ultrasonography	Normal structures visualized	These tests are used to detect calcification, masses, enlargement, and ductal distention.
Other procedures	See Box 32-2	These tests are used to detect ductal obstruction and pseudocysts.
Endoscopic retrograde cholangio-pancreatography	See Box 32-2	See Box 32-2
Other tests		
Pancreatic secretion test (secretin given IV; analysis of duodenal contents)	Volume 117-392 ml/80 min HCO$_3$ 16-33 mEq/80 min Amylase 439-1921 U/80 min	Decreased release of bicarbonate and/or enzymes are found in chronic pancreatitis. Increased acid secretion is found in Zollinger-Ellison syndrome.
D-xylose test (25 g D-xylose given orally)	5-8 g excreted in urine/5 hours 25-40 mg serum levels in 2 hours	Lowered blood or urinary level indicates malabsorption conditions. Used to help identify causes of malnutrition.
Quantitative fecal fat	7 g/24 hours	Elevated levels show steatorrhea.

6. Expresses less apathy and identifies one example of improvement in situation.
7. Takes replacement enzymes with bland food.
8. Explains how to implement medical regimen and other self-care needs on discharge.

Implementation
Assistance with achievement of therapeutic goals
Acute pancreatitis

Medical treatment is directed toward (1) decreasing secretions of the pancreas, (2) resting the pancreas, (3) preventing and treating complications (see Box 32-7), and (4) controlling pain.

Rest of the pancreas during the acute phase is achieved by measures that reduce stimulation of the exocrine secretions such as the following:

1. Nothing-by-mouth (NPO) status
2. Nasogastric suction

3. Histamine$_2$ receptor blockers
4. Antacids

These measures decrease stimulation of the vagus nerve, and thus decrease secretion of hydrochloric acid, and decrease secretion of the pancreatic enzymes and fluid and electrolyte secretions stimulated by secretin, gastrin, and CCK. Antibiotics are not usually administered in the edematous stage or in the absence of complications.

Pain relief is usually achieved with meperidine hydrochloride rather than morphine or codeine, because it is less spasmogenic on the sphincter of Oddi. Some patients find that pain is decreased if they assume a sitting position with the trunk flexed or lie on their sides with their knees drawn up to the abdomen.

The following nursing interventions are used depending on the presence or extent of fluid and electrolyte deficit and the presence of complications of acute pancreatitis:

1. Maintain intravenous fluid replacement (blood, albumin, plasma, fluids) and electrolytes as ordered.

2. Monitor vital signs and central venous pressure every 1 to 4 hours, or even more frequently if necessary.
3. Monitor intake and output every 1 to 4 hours.
4. Administer vasopressors and other measures for shock.
5. Maintain patency of the gastrointestinal tube.
6. Monitor for elevated glucose levels, Chvostek's and Trousseau's signs, and increasing abdominal girth.
7. Encourage deep breathing.
8. Administer as prescribed for complications: insulin, calcium, antibiotics, vitamin K.

As soon as the acute attack passes, oral fluids and foods are started.

Chronic pancreatitis

Therapy for the acute attack of chronic pancreatitis includes the therapies discussed above (NPO, nasogastric suction, antacids, and other medications, and IV fluids). In addition, as the acute attack subsides, medical attention will turn to confirming the diagnosis, to treating the malabsorption, and, in some instances, to surgery. Pancreatic enzyme replacement drugs contain amylase, lipase, and trypsin. They are taken at mealtimes to aid digestion and to facilitate the absorption of nutrients and fat-soluble vitamins. The patient should observe stools for steatorrhea, which should decrease when fat intake is lowered and enzymes improve absorption.

Surgery

An exploratory laparotomy may be performed in acute pancreatitis when a diagnosis cannot be established and the possibility of general peritonitis, perforation of an organ, or a bowel obstruction cannot be excluded. If biliary obstruction is present, a surgical or endoscopic procedure may be done to divert or increase bile flow at the sphincter of Oddi and thereby reduce regurgitation of bile into the pancreatic duct.

For the treatment of pseudocysts the surgeon may employ external drainage, construct anastomoses between the pancreas and gastrointestinal tract (for example, pancreatojejunostomy), or resect part or all of the pancreas.

Exploratory surgery is often necessary to diagnose pancreatic tumors. Various techniques may be used to treat pancreatic tumors or to relieve pancreatic duct obstruction. Procedures to relieve obstructive jaundice are sometimes helpful in providing comfort (cholecystostomy, choledochojejunostomy). Often malignant tumors of the pancreas are inoperable by the time diagnosis is made.

Pancreatoduodenal resection (Whipple's procedure) is sometimes done when the carcinoma is localized with no evidence of metastasis. Whipple's procedure involves resection of the antrum of the stomach, duodenum, varying amounts of pancreas, and often the gallbladder. Anastomoses are constructed between the stomach, common bile duct and pancreatic ducts, and the jejunum. Malabsorption syndrome follows total pancreatectomy (protein, fat, iron, calcium, phosphate, vitamin B_{12} deficiencies occur), as does carbohydrate intolerance.

The patient with extensive pancreatic surgery or disease may have a prolonged postoperative course. Malnourishment, postoperative complications (hemorrhage, fistulas, anastomotic leak, infection) and metabolic derangements may occur. Hemorrhagic and hypovolemic shock can lead to renal failure. Wound care must be meticulous. Drains are usually employed, and dressings should be inspected frequently and changed as often as necessary to maintain dryness. If a pancreatic fistula develops, severe tissue breakdown can occur from digestion of skin and underlying tissues by the pancreatic enzymes. Measurement of biliary or pancreatic drainage is carefully recorded.

Interventions to achieve patient outcomes

The patient with acute pancreatitis may be acutely ill and require intensive care. The priorities of care are controlling pain, managing fluids and electrolytes, and monitoring for complications. The patient with chronic pancreatitis and pancreatic tumors needs care to control pain, nutritional support, and help dealing with the potential hopelessness. The person with chronic pancreatitis often needs help to deal with substance abuse. All patients have teaching needs.

Controlling discomfort

Control of pain is a major priority. Meperidine hydrochloride, 75 to 100 mg every 3 to 4 hours, may be necessary to reduce pain. As stated in the preceding section, some patients find that the pain is decreased if they assume a sitting position with the trunk flexed or a side-lying, knee-chest position with their knees drawn up to the abdomen.

The measures used to rest the pancreas (NPO status, nasogastric suctioning, and medications) will also assist with pain control by decreasing the continual autodigestive process and associated edema and inflammation. In addition, the nurse should help the patient initiate relaxation techniques (deep breathing, imagery, and distraction techniques such as music, TV, and sewing) to help with pain control (see Chapters 6 and 10). These measures should be introduced after the patient has adequate pain control from the analgesic. If the patient is highly distressed, these techniques are not easily used. Comfort measures such as backrubs and purposeful touch are important and should be implemented.

Maintaining fluid and electrolyte balance

As soon as the patient is admitted, the nurse should institute monitoring related to fluid and electrolyte status, cardiac output, and renal status. This is a critical need. Monitoring includes intake and output; vital signs; daily weights; daily electrolytes; and blood urea nitrogen (BUN), creatinine, and hemodynamic measurements as necessary. An indwelling catheter may be necessary in acute pancreatitis because decreased renal function can occur in association with the hypotension and shock. Monitoring parameters and frequency of monitoring depend on the stability of the patient's condition. Fluids, electrolytes, colloids, or blood are given as necessary. The nurse is responsible for administering these and for monitoring the patient's response to them. Frequent adjustments in therapy may be necessary in relation to the patient's response to fluid therapy. If the patient develops shock, all the care described in Chapter 9 will be necessary.

<table>
<tr><td>

The Elderly with Biliary or Pancreatic Problems

Assessment

Assess elderly person for changes in ability to tolerate dietary fats; pancreatic secretions decrease with age.

Assess acutely ill elderly patients, especially after surgery, for signs of pancreatitis.

Intervention

Teach elderly persons to avoid overweight and to exercise regularly within their capabilities to help decrease gallstone formation.

Teach persons to report changes in ability to tolerate dietary fats and any sudden unrelieved abdominal pain suggestive of gallstones or pancreatitis.

Assist persons who have gradual development of dietary fat intolerance to plan a low-fat diet.

Common disorders in elderly

Cholelithiasis

Cholecystitis

Pancreatitis after surgery or major organ failure

</td><td>

Patient Teaching 32-8

The patient with pancreatic disorders

After pancreatic surgery
  Self-care as to dressings, tubes, medications
  Need for low-fat, high-calorie diet, as appropriate
  Need for continued medical follow-up care
After pancreatitis
  Prevention of further attacks (avoidance of alcohol, narcotics, and abdominal injury; medical care when ill)
  Reporting symptoms indicating relapse or complications
    Pain
    Nausea and vomiting
    Abdominal distention
    Steatorrhea
    Polyuria, polydipsia, polyphagia
    Weight loss
    Fever
  Maintaining low-fat, bland diet with several small feedings per day and vitamin supplements
  Avoiding rich foods to keep pancreatic secretions at a minimum
  Continuing medication therapy (pancreatic enzymes, bile salts, oral hypoglycemic agents, or insulin)—scheduling, rationale, dose, side effects
  Need for continued medical follow-up care
Pain management
  Avoidance of pain stimulants
  Timing of food and enzyme replacements
  Use of antacids, histamine$_2$ receptor blockers

</td></tr>
</table>

Providing self-care

During the acute phase of the illness the patient will need assistance with all care. Dehydration and potential malnutrition make the patient particularly prone to skin breakdown.

Promoting healthy lifestyle patterns

If unhealthy lifestyle patterns such as alcoholism are indicated as a cause of pancreatitis, the nurse must work with the patient on this problem. This care will be instituted after the patient is stabilized, but it must be introduced before the patient leaves the hospital. See Chapter 13 for further information on coping with alcoholism.

Counseling

Patients with chronic pancreatitis and their families require much support. Long-term illness, physical deterioration, and chronic pain combined with alcohol, and, sometimes, narcotic addiction often result in apathy and hopelessness. These factors and the patient's affect or behavior may evoke the same feelings of apathy and hopelessness in health care providers.

The nurse who has developed self-awareness about perceptions and the responses evoked by apathetic patients may be more able to exhibit hopefulness in patient interactions. Patients can be helped to maintain hope by nurses who do the following:

1. Promote self-esteem.
2. Make referrals for treatment of substance abuse.
3. Reinforce the notion that the patient can control pain by prescribed measures.

Promoting nutrition

The patient is NPO and often has a nasogastric tube in place during the acute phase of the illness. Institution and maintenance of NPO status is a major intervention. Good oral hygiene is necessary to decrease discomfort from the NPO status and from the nasogastric tube. When the acute symptoms decrease (3 to 5 days), oral fluids and food are restarted. The patient is started on clear liquids and then advanced to a low-fat, bland diet, distributed over five to six small feedings daily. When refeeding starts, the patient is observed carefully for pain, nausea, and vomiting, all of which indicate continuing inflammation. If these occur, the physician is notified and the methods described previously for inhibition of pancreatic activity are reinstituted. If food is restricted for long periods, parenteral hyperalimentation may be necessary. After discharge from the hospital, patients are advised to avoid alcohol and other gastric stimulants, such as caffeine, and to remain on a low-fat, bland diet with several small feedings daily. The patient needs to know how to take the pancreatic enzyme supplements. The dietitian may need to work with the patient to help plan an appropriate diet.

Teaching the patient

Teaching the patient and significant others is ongoing. At the beginning of hospitalization, the patient and significant others need basic instructions about the disease, the diagnostic tests, and the treatment. Because of the pain and the distress it causes and because of potential fluid status and cardiovascular instability, the patient and family experience tremendous stress and anxiety. Therefore explanations and instructions should be brief and as simple as possible and may need to be repeated. Support and continuity of care are also instituted to help decrease anxiety. Long-term education is directed toward prevention of future attacks by avoiding alcohol, maintaining a nutritious diet, and continuing medications as prescribed. The patient must report immediately any recurrence of signs and symptoms. Follow-up care is explained in detail. See Box 32-8 for summary of priority teaching points.

Evaluation

The expected patient outcomes serve as the basis for evaluating the extent to which patient status was improved. Questions to ask may include the following:

1. Was discomfort relieved?
2. Was detection and treatment of complications prompt?
3. Did serum amylase return to normal?
4. Were self-care needs met?
5. Were patient and family referred to appropriate supportive services?
6. Did the patient identify examples of improvement?
7. Was patient adequately prepared to manage the treatment regimen at home?

SUMMARY

1. The gallbladder can store and concentrate bile; it can release bile under neural (vagal) and hormonal stimulation (cholecystokinin, gastrin).
2. The secretions of the pancreas are necessary for absorption of nutrients and neutralization of acid chyme. Acinar cells secrete several kinds of enzymes, and ductal cells secrete a bicarbonate-rich fluid into the pancreatic ducts.
3. The incidence of cholelithiasis and cholecystitis increases with age.
4. In the elderly, pancreatitis after surgery occurs more frequently.
5. Prevention of alcoholism is a major way to decrease the occurrence of pancreatitis.
6. Cholecystitis (often associated with cholelithiasis) can be an acute or chronic inflammatory process.
7. Cholecystography is a common test of gallbladder filling, concentration, and emptying. Not all stones are visualized by this test.
8. In cholecystitis conservative treatment (NPO, pain control, intravenous fluids) may allow later elective surgery.
9. Laparoscopic cholecystectomy is the treatment of choice for cholelithiasis.
10. Nursing priorities for the patient having an LC are teaching and control of pain.
11. Nursing priorities for patients having abdominal cholecystectomies include measures to prevent RLL complications, to control pain, and to promote wound healing and biliary tube drainage.
12. Acute pancreatitis involves autodigestion of pancreatic tissue. Treatment includes measures to reduce pancreatic secretions (nothing by mouth, nasogastric drainage, H_2 receptor blockers, antacids).
13. Acute attacks of pancreatitis may be seen in relapsing acute pancreatitis or in chronic pancreatitis.
14. Chronic pancreatitis is characterized by permanent structure changes, diminished exocrine and endocrine secretions, malnourishment, and the development of pseudocysts.
15. Pancreatic surgery may be used in patients with pseudocysts and other complications of pancreatitis and in patients with pancreatic tumors or biliary obstruction.
16. Pain control is very complex in chronic pancreatitis.
17. The nurse can promote hope by supporting measures of pain relief, making referrals to resources for chemical addiction, and affirming the patient's self-esteem.

STUDY QUESTIONS

- How would you explain the differences between laparoscopic and abdominal cholecystectomy to a patient as you counsel him or her?
- How do the needs differ in a patient with acute pancreatitis as compared with the patient with chronic pancreatitis?
- How would you explain to a patient's family why pain is sometimes so severe in biliary disease? In pancreatitis?

REFERENCES AND SELECTED READINGS

1.* Adinaro D: Liver failure and pancreatitis: fluid and electrolyte concerns, *Nurs Clin North Am* 22(4):843-852, 1987.
2. Adwers JR: Clinical trials of gallstone lithotripsy, *Hosp Pract* 24(7):83-90, 1989.
3.* Bagg AM: Whipple's procedure: nursing guidelines, *Crit Care Nurse* 8(5):34-45, 1988.
4.* Birdsall, C, Fiore-Lopez N: How do you manage pancreatic sump tubes, *Am J Nurs* 87:770-771, 1987.
5.* Blake RL: Acute pancreatitis, *Prim Care* 15:187-199, 1988.
6. Bradley EL: Complications of chronic pancreatitis, *Surg Clin North Am* 69:481-497, 1989.
6a.* Brown A: Acute pancreatitis: pathophysiology, nursing diagnoses, and collaborative problems, *Focus Crit Care* 18:121-130, 1991.
7. Crist D, Cameron JL: The current management of acute pancreatitis, *Adv Surg* 20:69-124, 1987.
8. DiMagno EP: Early diagnosis of chronic pancreatitis and pancreatic cancer, *Med Clin North Am* 72:979-992, 1988.
9. Fain JA, Amato-Vealey E: Acute pancreatitis: a gastrointestinal emergency, *Crit Care Nurse* 8(5):47-63m, 1988.
9a.* Farha GJ, Beamer L: New options for treating gallstone disease, *Am Fam Physician* 44:1295-1304, 1991.
10. Frazee RC, et al: Open versus laparoscopic cholecystectomy, *Ann Surg* 213:651-653, 1991.
11. Glassman JA: *Biliary tract surgery: tactics and techniques.* New York, 1989, Macmillan Publishing.
12. Greenberger NJ: Chronic pancreatitis and exocrine insufficiency, *Hosp Pract* 20(1A):33-38, 40-45, 1985.
12a.* Greifzus, Dest V: When the diagnoses is pancreatic cancer, *RN* 22(9):38-45, 1991.
13.* Haicken BN: Laser laparoscopic cholecystectomy in the ambulatory setting, *J Post Anesth Nurs* 6(1):33-39, 1991.

*Suggested for student reading.

14. Jeffres C: Complications of acute pancreatitis, *Crit Care Nurse* 9(4):38-46, 1989.
15.* Jurf JB, Clements L, Llorente J: Cholecystectomy made easier, *Am J Nurs* 90(12):38-39, 1990.
16. Lancaster S, Biaro-Marshall D: Gallstone lithotripsy, *Am J Nurs* 88:1629-1630, 1988.
17.* Marta MR: Endoscopic retrograde cholangeopancreatography: its role in diagnosis and treatment, *Focus on Crit Care* 14(5):62-63, 1987.
18.* Munn NE: When the bile duct is blocked, *RN* 20:50-57, 1989.
19.* Nurses Clinical Library: *Gastrointestinal disorders*, Springhouse, Pa, Nursing '85 Books, 1985, Springhouse.
20. Potts JR: Acute pancreatitis, *Surg Clin North Am* 68:281-299, 1988.
20a. Richards K: Lasers in general surgery, *Nurs Clin North Am* 25:667-671, 1990.
21. Rottenberg R: An update of pancreatic cancer, *Patient Care* 20(3):144-146, 151, 154-156, 158, 162, 1986.
22. Rowland GA, Marks DA, Torres W: The new gallstone destroyers and dissolvers, *Am J Nurs* 89:1473-1478, 1989.
23. Sabesin S: Countering the danger of acute pancreatitis, *Emerg Med* 19(17):71-73, 81-83, 87-89, 91-92, 95-96, 1987.
24. Sleisenger MH, Fordtran JS, editors: *Gastrointestinal disease: pathophysiology, diagnosis, management*, ed 4, Philadelphia, 1989, WB Saunders.
25. Southern Surgeon Club: A prospective analysis of 1518 laparoscopic cholecystectomies, *N Engl J Med* 324:1073-1078, 1991.
26. Steer ML: Classification and pathogenesis of pancreatitis, *Surg Clin North Am* 69:467-480, 1989.
27. Swazuk KJ, Mueller BG, Daly CJ: Laser cholecystectomy: A perioperative nursing view, *AORN J* 50:998-1001, 1004-1005, 1989.
28. Tilkian SM, Conover MB, Tilkian AG: *Clinical complications of laboratory tests*, ed 4, St Louis, 1987, Mosby–Year Book.
29. Toskes PP: Diagnosis of chronic pancreatitis and exocrine insufficiency, *Hosp Pract* 20(10):97-100, 102-103, 107-108, 1985.
30. Toskes PP: Recurrent acute pancreatitis, *Hosp Pract* 20(7):85-88, 90-92, 1985.
30a. Wolfe BM, Gardiner B, Frey CF: Laparoscopic cholicystectomy, a remarkable development, *JAMA* 265:1573-1574, 1991.
31. Wyngaarden JB, Smith LH, editors: *Cecil textbook of medicine*, ed 18, Philadelphia, 1988, WB Saunders.

Classic

32. Dougherty WM: Serum bilirubin, *Nurs '82* (11):138-139, 1982.
33. Kelber MB: Pancreatic enzymes: deciphering diagnostic studies, *Nurs '82* 12(12):65-67, 1982.
34.* Knudsen F: Gastrointestinal and metabolic problems in older adults. In Steffle B, editor: *Handbook of gerontological nursing*, New York, 1984, Van Nostrand Reinhold.
35.* Taylor DL: Gallstones: physiology, signs and symptoms, *Nurs 83* 13(6):44-45, 1983.
36.* Taylor DL: Jaundice: physiology, signs and symptoms, *Nurs 83* 13(8):52-54, 1983.

33

The Patient

with

Urinary Problems

Roberta Stokes
H. Fred Farley

After studying this chapter, the learner should be able to:

- Describe interventions for urinary retention and urinary incontinence.
- Describe the causes and methods of prevention of urinary tract infections (UTI).
- Explain pathophysiologic differences among, signs and symptoms of, and therapeutic modalities and nursing interventions for glomerular disorders.
- Describe the pathophysiology of obstructive urinary disorders.
- Describe the pathophysiology and interventions for renal calculi.
- Compare different approaches to prostatectomy and the related nursing interventions.
- Describe the care of the person undergoing surgery of the urinary tract.
- Differentiate between acute and chronic renal failure, including pathophysiology, signs and symptoms, medical therapy, and nursing interventions.
- Explain the physiologic principles of dialysis and the types of renal replacement therapies and related care.

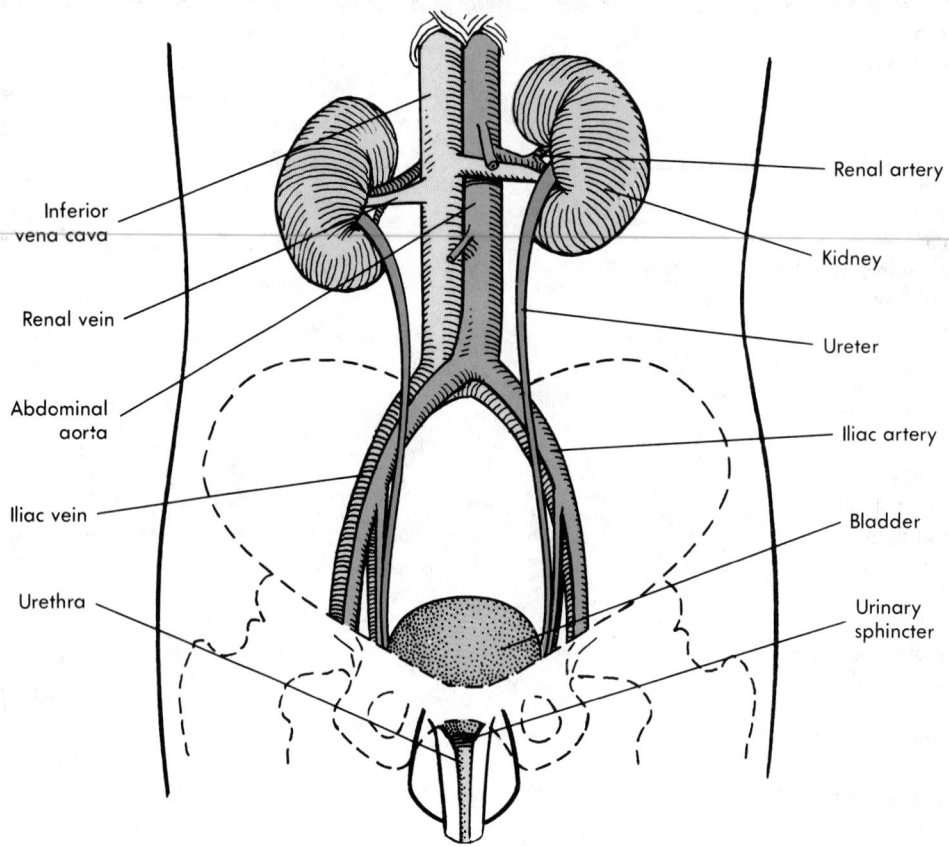

Fig. 33-1 Kidneys and other structures of urinary system.

The maintenance of *homeostasis,* defined as the state of the dynamic equilibrium of the internal environment, is essential for life. The body must regulate blood pressure, acid-base balance, hormonopoiesis (hormone production), fluid volume, and electrolyte composition. Moreover, the body must have a mechanism for eliminating the end products of metabolism.

The kidneys and other structures of the urinary system play major roles in the regulation of the internal environment. Some of the urinary disorders discussed in this chapter may lead to destruction of renal tissue, with subsequent alterations in fluid and electrolyte balance, excretion of body wastes, and regulation of body processes.

This chapter begins with a brief review of the major concepts relating to anatomy and physiology of the urinary system. (For a more intensive review, the reader is referred to a physiology text). The next part of the chapter describes major urinary disorders, some of which may lead to renal failure. The last part of the chapter discusses renal failure, both acute and chronic, and includes renal replacement therapies.

ANATOMY AND PHYSIOLOGY

The urinary system consists primarily of the kidneys, ureters, bladder, and urethra (Fig. 33-1). Although the prostate gland is primarily a male reproductive organ, it is

discussed in this chapter because enlargement or infection of the prostate affects the urinary tract.

Upper Urinary Tract
Kidney anatomy

The kidneys are vital organs for maintaining homeostasis. They have the important task of regulating the composition and volume of the plasma which, in turn, produces similar changes in the interstitial fluid. The kidneys receive about 1 L/min or 25% of the total cardiac output of 4 to 5 L/min. The entire plasma volume is filtered approximately 60 times every 24 hours (or 1200 ml/min). This enables the kidneys to regulate the components of plasma precisely.

Gross structure of the kidney

The kidneys are paired, retroperitoneal, bean-shaped organs located just above the waistline on either side of the vertebral column. The right kidney is usually lower because the right lobe of the liver lies above it. The upper border of the left kidney is protected by the eleventh and twelfth ribs. Each kidney is encased in a hard fibrous capsule (Fig. 33-2) that contains pain receptors. Perirenal fat cushions the kidneys and helps hold them in place. Both the capsule and perirenal fat tend to limit bleeding when the kidney is injured. An adrenal gland is located atop each kidney.

The outer layer, the *cortex,* contains the glomeruli, prox-

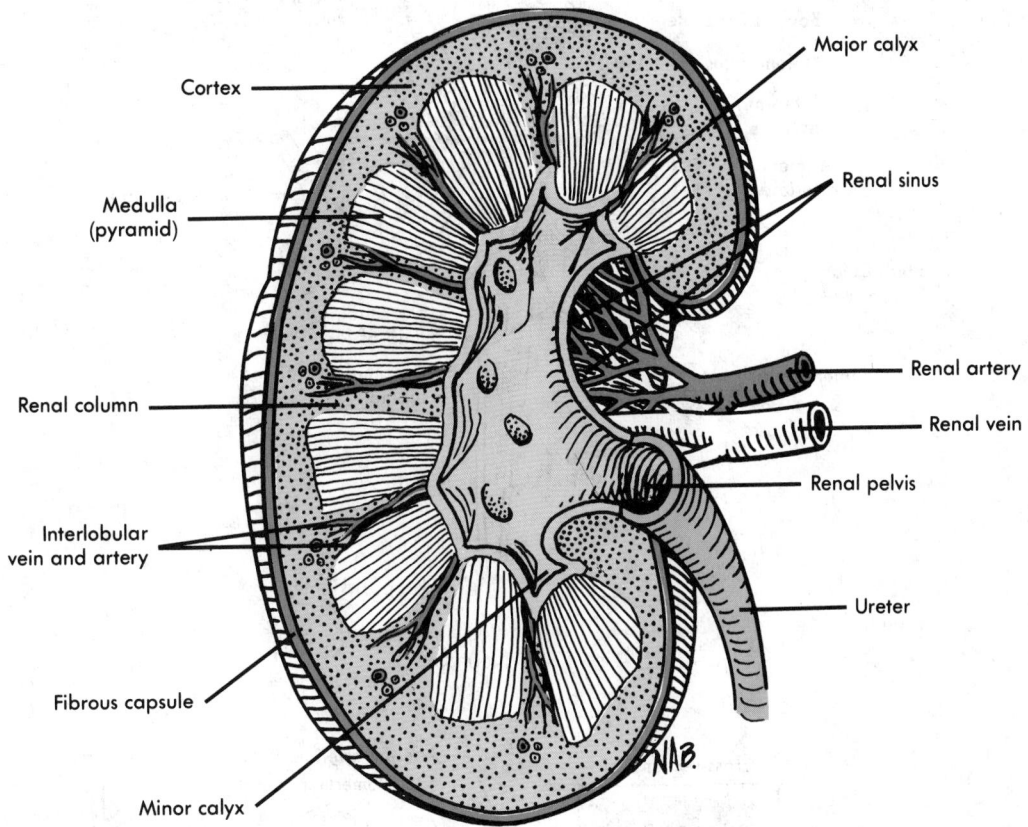

Fig. 33-2 Frontal section of kidney.

imal and distal convoluted tubules, the first portion of the loops of Henle, and the collecting tubules. The inner layer, the *medulla,* contains conical masses or pyramids formed by the loops of Henle and the collecting tubules.

The nephron
Types of nephrons

The nephron is the basic functional unit of the kidney (Fig. 33-3). Each kidney contains approximately one million of these units. Because of its ability to compensate, about 75% to 80% of the nephron can be destroyed without causing harmful effects.

There are two types of nephrons, cortical and juxtamedullary (Fig. 33-4). *Cortical* nephrons are located in the outer two thirds of the cortex and have a high-pressure peritubular capillary network. This network arises from the efferent arteriole and surrounds the proximal and distal convoluted tubules and loops of Henle. This is where filtration occurs and urine is formed. The cortical nephrons also have a low-pressure capillary network that is nutritive, supplies blood to the rest of the nephron, and allows for reabsorption from the tubule back into the blood.

Juxtamedullary nephrons have a more complex vasculature. The efferent arteriole of juxtamedullary nephrons also branches into a second peritubular capillary network that surrounds the proximal and distal tubules of these nephrons. However, this capillary network is located in the deep cortex.

A series of hairpin loops called *vasa recta,* located in the medulla, wrap around and run parallel to the long thin loops of Henle. The vasa recta branch into capillary networks around the loops of Henle and the collecting ducts of both types of nephrons. The presence of the vasa recta results in increased resistance in juxtamedullary nephrons. This resistance leads to a higher filtration rate and less blood flow. Vasa recta also act as a countercurrent exchanger, preventing the interstitial gradient from being dispersed. This action contributes significantly to the kidney's ability to concentrate urine.[53]

Juxtaglomerular apparatus

The juxtaglomerular apparatus is a combination of specialized cells located near the glomerulus at the junction of the afferent and efferent arterioles (Fig. 33-5). Juxtaglomerular cells contain granules of inactive renin. The juxtaglomerular apparatus is believed to secrete renin and to play a role in both autoregulation of the glomerular filtration and renal control of extracellular fluid volume through the renin-angiotensin-aldosterone system (p. 1015).[53]

Flow of blood and urine

The nephron contains two types of microscopic structures, those for blood flow and those for urine flow.

Blood flow

Blood flow through the kidneys begins in the *renal artery,* which arises from the abdominal aorta. Blood then flows

Bowman capsule
Glomerulus
Efferent arteriole
Afferent arteriole
Interlobular artery
Interlobular vein
Distal convoluted tubule
Collecting tube
Descending limb of loop
Proximal convoluted tubule
Ascending limb of loop
Loop of Henle

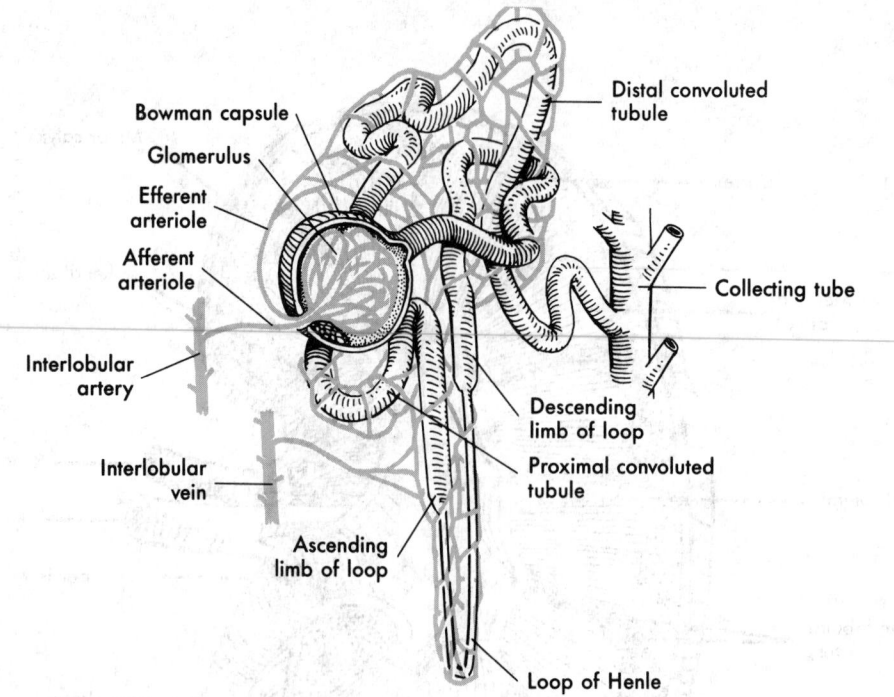

Fig. 33-3 Nephron.

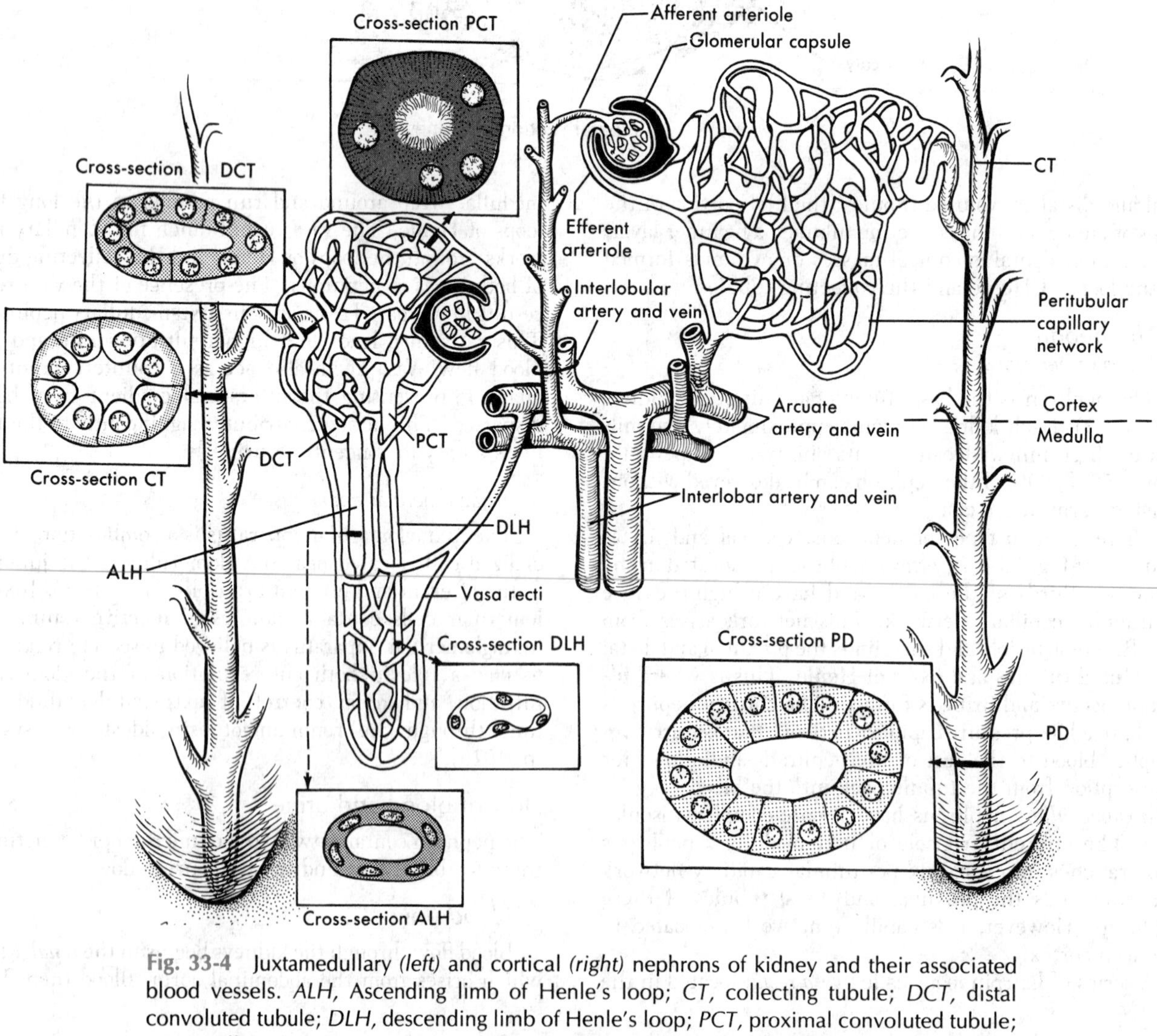

Cross-section PCT
Afferent arteriole
Glomerular capsule
Cross-section DCT
CT
Efferent arteriole
Interlobular artery and vein
Peritubular capillary network
Cross-section CT
Arcuate artery and vein
Cortex
Medulla
DCT
PCT
Interlobar artery and vein
DLH
ALH
Vasa recti
Cross-section DLH
Cross-section PD
PD
Cross-section ALH

Fig. 33-4 Juxtamedullary *(left)* and cortical *(right)* nephrons of kidney and their associated blood vessels. *ALH,* Ascending limb of Henle's loop; *CT,* collecting tubule; *DCT,* distal convoluted tubule; *DLH,* descending limb of Henle's loop; *PCT,* proximal convoluted tubule; *PD,* papillary duct. (From McClintic JR: *Human anatomy,* St Louis, 1983, Mosby–Year Book.)

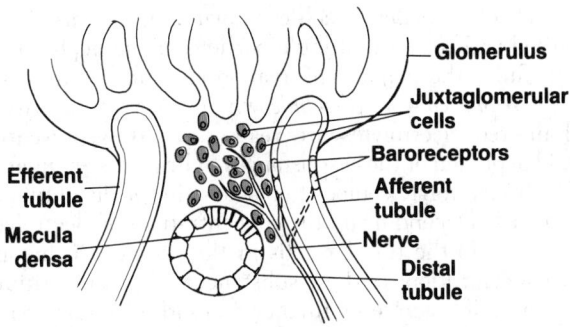

Fig. 33-5   The juxtaglomerular apparatus.

33-1	**Major functions of the kidneys**	
	Urine formation	Glomerular filtration, tubular reabsorption and secretion
	Fluid and electrolyte control	Maintain correct balance of fluid and electrolytes within a normal range by excretion, secretion, and reabsorption
	Acid-base balance	Maintain pH at normal range by directly excreting H^+ ions and forming bicarbonate for buffering
	Excretion of waste products	Direct removal of metabolic waste products contained in the glomerular filtrate
	Blood pressure regulation	Regulate blood pressure by controlling circulating volume and renin secretion
	RBC production	Erythropoietin secreted by kidneys stimulates bone marrow to produce RBCs
	Regulation of calcium-phosphate metabolism	Vitamin D activation regulated by kidneys

through increasingly smaller arteries: the *interlobar, arcuate,* and *interlobular* arteries. The interlobar arteries divide into the *afferent arterioles* located in the cortex. These arterioles subdivide into a tuft of capillaries or glomeruli, which are finely coiled within Bowman's capsule. The distal ends of the glomeruli are connected to *efferent arterioles,* which divide to form peritubular capillaries that surround the tubules (as described earlier); this allows material to be selectively transferred between the tubules and peritubular capillary network. After passing through the capillaries, blood returns to the *venules,* and then to the *renal vein,* which leaves the kidney through the hilum and joins the inferior vena cava.

Urine flow

Urine is filtered from the glomerulus into Bowman's capsule. From there it flows through a long tubule subdivided into the proximal convoluted tubule, loop of Henle, distal convoluted tubule, and collecting tubule (see Fig. 33-3). The latter joins other collecting tubules. Urine empties through papillary ducts into the calyces (see Fig. 33-2) and into the renal pelvis. Urine then flows down the ureter into the urinary bladder and is excreted through the urethra via the urinary meatus.

Renal Physiology

The functions of the kidney are summarized in Box 33-1. These functions, accomplished during the formation of urine, are described in succeeding paragraphs.

Urine formation
Glomerular filtration

The first process involved in urine formation is called *glomerular filtration.* It is defined as the movement of water and select substances through the glomerular capillaries into Bowman's capsule.

The glomerular filtrate arising from the glomerular capillaries approximates 180 L/day. The amount of glomerular filtrate in a given time period is called the *glomerular filtration rate* (GFR). The GFR in an average-sized man is approximately 125 ml/min (7.5 L/hr). The average GFR in a woman is about 10% less. The same forces that affect fluid transport between vascular and interstitial spaces in other parts of the body (see Chapter 7) also affect filtration in the glomerular capsule. The GFR is affected by changes in hydrostatic pressure. Such changes can be caused by

(1) diminished renal perfusion from hypovolemia, (2) occlusion of the glomeruli from diabetic nephropathy, (3) alteration in the plasma protein concentration from hypoproteinemia, (4) alterations of the basement membrane from an autoimmune disorder, and (5) arteriolar constriction from sympathetic stimulation or medication.

The blood supply to the kidneys is basic to the formation of glomerular filtrate, or beginning urine, and to the nutrition and respiration requirement of kidney cells. Severe and prolonged problems with maintaining cardiac output and renal perfusion have profound effects on the formation of urine and the viability of the cells responsible for maintaining consistency in the internal environment.

Tubular phase

The second process in urine formation involves the selective alteration and reduction of the glomerular filtrate. When blood enters the glomerular capillaries at a pressure not less than 60 to 70 mm Hg, an ultrafiltrate of plasma is formed. This *ultrafiltrate* (primitive urine) contains approximately the same concentration of the elements of plasma minus the proteins. The ultrafiltrate then passes through the tubular system and is modified into actual urine. During this process, there is a constant movement of particles and fluid between the tubule lumen, interstitium, and peritubular capillaries. The ultrafiltrate is altered by the processes of reabsorption, secretion or both (Fig. 33-6). *Reabsorption* is the transport of substances that the body needs, such as sodium, chloride, potassium, bicarbonate, and water from the tubular lumen into the interstitium and blood. *Secretion* is the transport of sub-

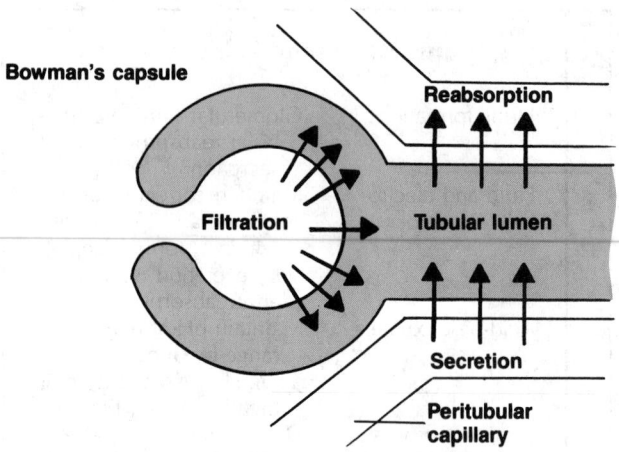

Fig. 33-6 Processes of filtration, secretion, and reabsorption in the formation of urine. (From Richard C: *Comprehensive nephrology nursing*, Boston, 1987, Little Brown & Co.)

stances not needed by the body from the blood and interstitium into the tubule lumen.

Fluid and electrolyte control

Were it not for some conserving mechanism in the kidneys, a person would be depleted of fluid and salts within 3 to 4 minutes. The *proximal convoluted tubule* reabsorbs up to 85% to 90% of water in the ultrafiltrate; up to 80% of filtered sodium; and the majority of filtered potassium, bicarbonate, chloride, phosphate, glucose, and protein.

Dehydration would still occur if the body did not have an additional mechanism within the kidneys to conserve filtered water. This mechanism allows urine to be concentrated to less than 1% of the daily filtered volume. The kidneys can vary the amount of fluid excreted so precisely that intake over that required for normal fluid balance is excreted and intake under that required for normal fluid balance leads to further concentration of the urine. The mechanisms responsible for this increased urine concentrating ability and precision in excreting appropriate urine volume exist in the loop of Henle and the distal convoluted and collecting tubules. The *loop of Henle* reaches into the medullary portion of the kidney, which is highly hypertonic in comparison to the filtrate. In the *descending* portion of the loop, sodium diffuses into the filtrate as the tubule passes deeper into the medullary area, and water moves out of the primitive urine in response to the high sodium concentration. The result is a reduction in volume of the glomerular filtrate and a dramatic increase in its osmolality. In the *ascending* limb of the loop of Henle, sodium is reabsorbed into the interstitium, but the loop is impermeable to the movement of water either into or out of the tubule. The primitive urine now presented to the *distal convoluted* and *collecting tubules* is greatly reduced in volume but hypotonic because of the reabsorption of sodium. The influence of antidiuretic hormone (ADH) on these last two segments of the tubule allows water to be reabsorbed into the interstitium in an amount compatible with maintenance of proper fluid balance. The reabsorption of water from the forming urine increases osmolality and results in the excretion of a hypertonic urine.

Electrolyte balance is achieved mainly in the distal convoluted and collecting tubule portions of the nephron. As with fluid, the major conservation site for electrolytes is the *proximal convoluted tubule* where the vast majority of all filtered electrolytes are reabsorbed, thus preventing rapid depletion of these substances. The precise regulation of body electrolyte composition occurs in the distal tubular segments. Depending on the concentrations of electrolytes presented to the tubular cells in the primitive urine and the concentrations of these substances in the interstitium, tubular cells secrete or further reabsorb electrolytes into the urine (Table 33-1).

Regulation of acid-base balance

The kidney maintains the blood at the slightly alkaline pH of 7.35 to 7.45. The alkalinity of blood is controlled by the rate at which bicarbonate ions are excreted from the body and by the rate at which bicarbonate ions are restored to the buffering system. The secretion of hydrogen ions is accomplished by the cells of the proximal and distal convoluted tubule and the thick portion of the loop of Henle. Secretion of hydrogen ions is accompanied by the restoration of bicarbonate ions.

The most abundant buffer in the extracellular fluid is the sodium bicarbonate-carbonic acid system (see Chapter 8). Remember that strong acids react with sodium bicarbonate and convert into a weak acid (carbonic acid). Carbonic acid then dissociates into carbon dioxide and water. The carbon dioxide is eliminated by the lungs. During the process one mole of bicarbonate is lost from the extracellular fluid for each mole of acid reacting with the buffer system. The buffering system is replenished by the kidney.

Two processes result in the restoration of bicarbonate: regeneration and reabsorption. For every filtered bicarbonate ion that combines with a hydrogen ion, a filtered sodium ion is reabsorbed along with a bicarbonate ion. Bicarbonate ions are also formed when carbon dioxide combines with water in the tubular cell. The net result is excretion of hydrogen ions with the return of bicarbonate to the peritubular capillaries.

Excretion of waste products

Metabolic wastes are excreted in the glomerular filtrate. Creatinine is little modified in its passage through the nephron; creatinine contained in the glomerular filtrate is excreted unchanged in the urine. Other wastes, such as urea, are excreted unchanged in the glomerular filtrate but undergo reabsorption during passage through the nephron. The amount of waste material excreted in urine in such an instance is only a fraction of that originally contained in the glomerular filtrate.

Excretion of drugs by the kidneys occurs through both filtration at the glomerular level and secretion into the urine by distal tubular cells. Penicillin is an example of a drug secreted by tubular cells.

Blood pressure regulation

Renal regulation of blood pressure is controlled by the renin-angiotensin-aldosterone system. *Renin* is a hormone released by the juxtaglomerular apparatus (adjoining the glomerulus) in response to sodium depletion, renal artery hypoperfusion, or stimulation of the renal nerves through

Table 33-1   Fluid and electrolyte control by kidney

Site	Function	Effect	Physiologic basis
Glomerulus	Filtration of water and electrolytes	Beginning of urine formation	Hydrostatic pressure
Proximal convoluted tubules	Reabsorption of large amounts of water, sodium, potassium, bicarbonate, chloride, phosphate	Conservation of fluid and electrolytes	Reabsorption by active and passive transport Bicarbonate reabsorption controlled by acid-base imbalance
Loop of Henle			
Descending limb	Diffusion of sodium into tubule Reabsorption of water	Reduction in urine volume; urine is hypertonic	Medulla of kidney is hypertonic
Ascending limb	Reabsorption of sodium	Urine becomes hypotonic	Water remains in loop because membrane is impermeable to water
Distal convoluted tubule and collecting tubule	Reabsorption of water Secretion of potassium, hydrogen and ammonia ions as needed Reabsorption of sodium	Fluid and electrolyte control depending on body needs	Water is reabsorbed as needed by effect of ADH Extra potassium is secreted Hydrogen and ammonia ions are secreted, depending on acid-base imbalances Sodium is reabsorbed by effect of aldosterone

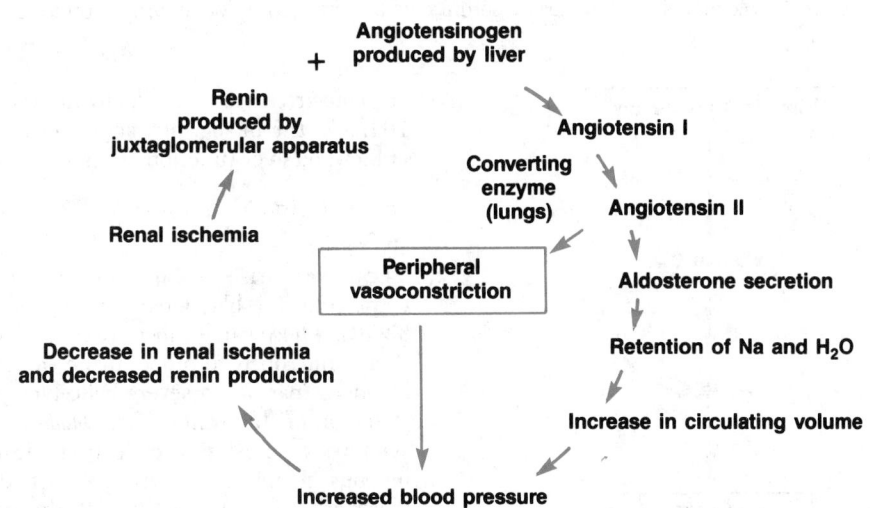

Fig. 33-7   Diagram of the renin-angiotensin system. (From Lancaster LE: Renal failure: pathophysiology, assessment and intervention, *Crit Care Nurse* 2(1):38-55, 1982.)

the sympathetic pathways. *Angiotensinogen*, which is produced in the liver, is activated to *angiotensin I* in the presence of renin. An enzyme in the lungs converts angiotensin I to the active form, *angiotensin II*. Angiotensin II is a powerful *vasoconstrictor* that also stimulates the release of aldosterone by the adrenal glands. *Aldosterone* increases sodium reabsorption by the kidney; water follows the sodium, leading to an increase in blood volume (see Fig. 33-7). A low GFR, seen with numerous kidney diseases (such as glomerulonephritis, nephrotic syndrome, polycystic disease, renal trauma, renal failure) usually leads to hypertension by activation of the renin-angiotensin-aldosterone system. (See Chapter 26 for a discussion of hypertension.)

Stimulation of red blood cell production

Red blood cell (RBC) production is primarily controlled by the kidneys. *Erythropoietin* is a hormone that is secreted by the kidneys. Erythropoietin stimulates bone marrow to produce RBCs. Persons with chronic renal failure often have serum hematocrit values of 18% to 30% (normal values are 42% to 47%). This decrease in hematocrit values is the result of decreased secretion of erythropoietin from the diseased kidneys compounded by bone marrow toxicity, decreased life span of RBCs and increased bleeding, all of which are associated with the altered metabolic state present in chronic renal failure.

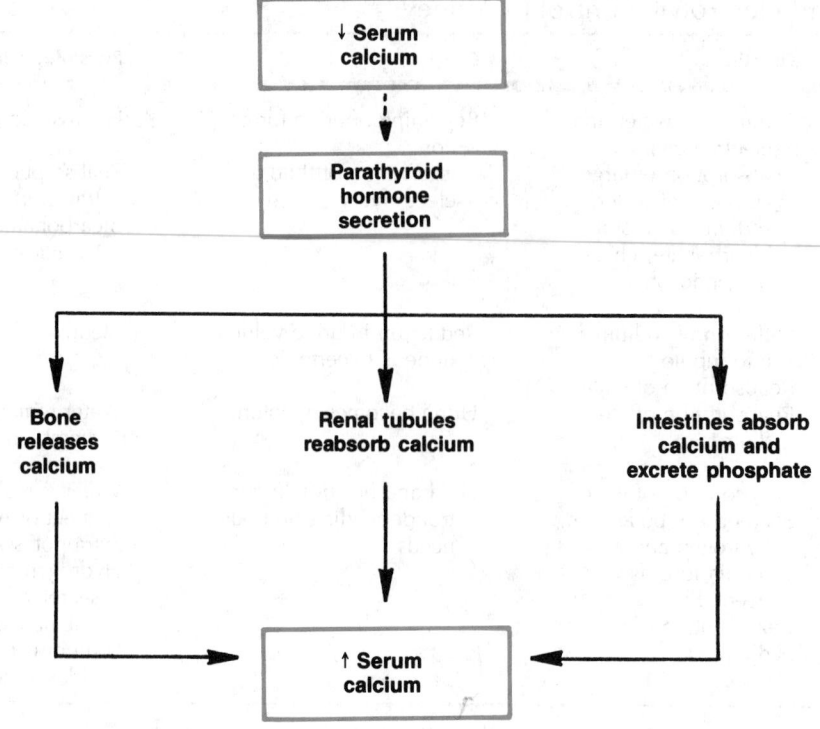

Fig. 33-8   Mechanism of increasing serum calcium effected by parathyroid hormone.

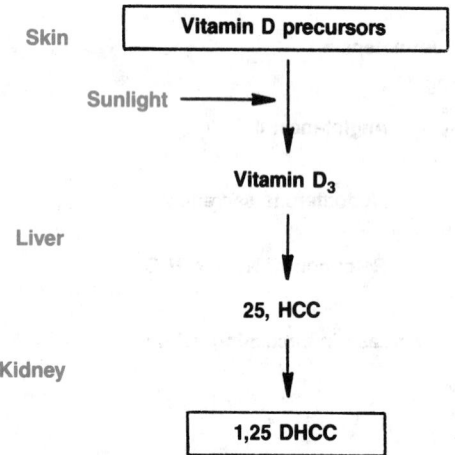

Fig. 33-9   Vitamin D metabolism. 25-Hydroxycholecalciferol (25-HCC) is an intermediate stage in the development of the active form of 1,25-Dehydroxycholecalciferol.

Regulation of calcium-phosphorus metabolism

Calcium-phosphorus metabolism is controlled by the kidneys. Most of the reabsorption of calcium (65%-70%) occurs at the proximal tubule with the rest occurring at the loop of Henle (20%-25%) and the distal tubule (10%). The amount of calcium reabsorption is primarily determined by parathyroid hormone (PTH) and vitamin D. The effect of PTH is shown in Fig. 33-8.

Vitamin D (cholecalciferol), which is classified as a hormone, facilitates intestinal absorption of calcium. Vitamin D itself is not the active substance; instead, vitamin D precursors must undergo a series of metabolic changes to

be converted to 1,25 dehydroxycholecalciferol (1,25-DHHC), the biologically active form (Fig. 33-9). Normal kidney and liver function are essential for the conversion.[22]

Lower Urinary Tract
Anatomy

The *ureters* arise as extensions of the kidney pelves and empty into the bladder in an area called the *trigone* (Fig. 33-10). These small tubes are composed of smooth muscle; their function is to propel urine from the kidney into the bladder. Spasm and severe colic-type pain result from obstruction of the ureters. The *bladder*, situated behind the symphysis pubis, is a collecting bag for the urine. The mucous membrane is arranged in folds called *rugae* that, together with the elasticity of the muscular walls, can distend the bladder considerably to hold large amounts of urine. A layer of skeletal muscle encircles the base of the bladder, forming the *external urinary sphincter*. The bladder is innervated by both the sympathetic and parasympathetic nervous system, whereas the ureters receive fibers only from the sympathetic nervous system.

The *urethra* transports urine from the bladder to the external meatus. Male and female urethras differ in length and accessibility of reproductive organs. The female urethra is short (about 4 cm long), exits anterior to the vagina (see Fig. 35-1), and is separate from the reproductive organs. The male urethra (see Fig. 35-3) is 18 to 20 cm long and transports semen as well as urine. The urethra is innervated by both the sympathetic and parasympathetic nervous systems.

The *prostate gland* is a male reproductive gland about the size of a walnut that encircles the upper portion of the male urethra (Fig. 33-10). It is shaped like a doughnut

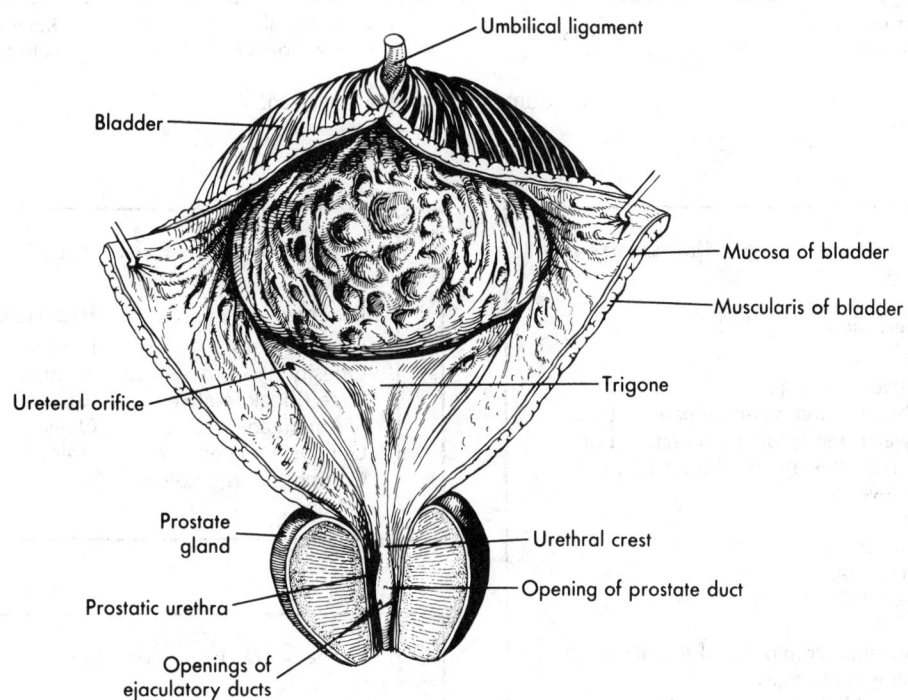

Umbilical ligament

Bladder

Mucosa of bladder

Muscularis of bladder

Trigone

Ureteral orifice

Prostate gland

Urethral crest

Opening of prostate duct

Prostatic urethra

Openings of ejaculatory ducts

Fig. 33-10   Interior of urinary bladder and some associated structures. (From McClintic JR: *Human anatomy*, St Louis, 1983, Mosby—Year Book.)

with the urethra passing through the "hole." When the prostate is enlarged, the urethra is squeezed, causing obstruction of urinary flow. Numerous prostatic ducts empty into the urethra. Bacteria from urinary tract infections may travel up these ducts, causing prostatic infection.

Micturition

Urine flows out the kidney pelves and is propelled through the ureters by peristaltic action. About 200 to 300 ml of urine can collect in the bladder before the urge to void is initiated. Baroreceptors in the bladder wall are triggered by the stretching of the bladder walls, which causes reflex stimulation of parasympathetic nerves to the bladder, resulting in bladder contractions. When the motor nerves to the external urinary sphincter are inhibited, the muscle relaxes, opening the sphincter and permitting urine to be expelled. Stimulation of the sphincter muscles can keep the sphincter contracted against strong bladder contractions. Voluntary control over micturition can be exerted by stimuli transmitted over descending spinal pathways from the brainstem.

Use of a large balloon (30 ml) in-dwelling catheter (such as after a transurethral resection of the prostate) can stimulate the parasympathetic nerves, causing uncomfortable bladder contractions. Pressure on the sphincter by the balloon can also create an urge to void, although the bladder has been emptied by the catheter.

Physiologic Changes With Aging

A direct relationship exists between blood supply to the kidneys and renal function. The rate of blood flow to the kidneys is about 5 to 10 times greater than that to the heart, liver, and brain. Glomerular capillary pressure,

which is the force that promotes ultrafiltration, is controlled by blood flow to the kidneys. Therefore, physiologic alterations in the vascular bed can lead to age-related changes in renal function.

Arteriosclerotic changes in renal arteries are the most common form of renal vascular pathology.[1] Arteriosclerotic changes occur to some extent in most normal individuals with aging. The degree of morphologic change experienced depends on the specific arteries affected and the extent of involvement.

Aging is also known to cause predictable increases in both systolic and diastolic blood pressure.[40] This slow increase in blood pressure begins at birth and continues through adulthood. Untreated hypertension further accelerates the development of atherosclerosis, which can lead to renal failure.

Changes also occur in kidney structure and function with aging. About 40% of glomeruli are lost by age 70. The glomerular and tubular basement membranes thicken, leading to a 46% decrease in GFR from age 20 to 90.[1] If heart failure is also present with compensatory vasodilation, renal ischemia is increased further and the risk of renal failure is increased.

The ability to concentrate urine and sensitivity to ADH stimulation also decreases with age. Elderly persons have greater difficulty eliminating heavy solute loads and are slower to conserve fluids with fluid restriction.[29] Electrolyte imbalance may occur more readily from a decreased ability to conserve sodium, excrete potassium, and form and excrete ammonia.

Urinary incontinence may occur in acutely ill elderly persons who lack energy for voluntary control or who may be confused or disoriented. Stress incontinence may be

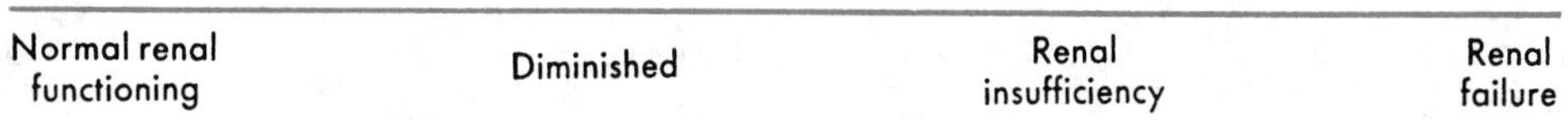

Normal renal functioning	Diminished	Renal insufficiency	Renal failure

Fig. 33-11   Continuum of renal function.

33-2

Conditions and substances that can result in kidney damage

Inadequate perfusion

Hypovolemia
Blood loss (surgery, trauma)
Plasma loss (burns, surgery, acute pancreatitis)
Sodium and water loss (prolonged diarrhea or vomiting, gastrointestinal tract drainage, sustained high fever)
Cardiac failure
Myocardial infarction
Cardiac dysrhythmias
Congestive heart failure
Septic shock
Infections (untreated streptococcal throat, untreated urinary tract sepsis)
Vascular changes (diabetes mellitus, hypertension, renal artery stenosis)

Toxic substances

Solvents (carbon tetrachloride, methanol, ethylene glycol)
Heavy metals (lead, arsenic, mercury)
Antibiotics (kanamycin, gentamicin, polymyxin B, amphotericin B, colistin, neomycin, phenazopyridine)
Pesticides
Poisonous mushrooms

33-3

Risk factors for diabetes and hypertension

Diabetes	Hypertension
Familial history	High sodium intake
Obesity	Familial history
Race (Black, Native American)	Advanced age
Gender (female)	Obesity
Corticosteroid medications	Stress

33-4

Urinary tract infections

Primary prevention

1. Cleanse perineal area properly; a shower is more desirable than a bath.
2. Drink adequate volume of fluid, 3 to 4 L/day.
3. Void frequently during waking hours, every 2 to 3 hours during day.

Secondary prevention

1. Seek prompt medical attention for symptoms.
2. Continue with drug therapy even though symptoms abate.
3. Follow steps 1 through 3 listed above.
4. Follow-up care with repeated urine cultures is essential.

---

noted in women with relaxed perineal muscles or in males following prostatectomy. Benign prostatic hypertrophy (p. 1051) occurs in more than half of all men over age 50 and 75% of men over age 70; the enlarged prostate presses on the urethra, resulting in urinary symptoms.

PREVENTION AND HEALTH EDUCATION

Primary Prevention

Two measures can be effective in reducing the incidence of renal failure: (1) identification of individuals at risk and (2) identification and control of environmental factors that can result in renal failure. Box 33-2 summarizes conditions and substances that can result in injury to the kidneys.

Secondary Prevention

Renal dysfunction can be somewhat elusive. Renal function can be described as being on a continuum (Fig. 33-11)—at one end of the continuum is normal renal function, whereas at the other end is renal failure. It is when persons near the point of renal failure that they begin to exhibit signs and symptoms. Two other points on this continuum are decreased renal reserve and renal insufficiency.

Decreased renal reserve exists when renal function has diminished to the point at which additional physiologic stress results in signs and symptoms. This stress could result from intercurrent illness, infection, or dietary overindulgence. Signs and symptoms of decreased renal reserve usually resolve once the stress is removed. *Renal insufficiency* is defined as the reduced capacity of the kidney to perform its functions. Renal insufficiency is generally experienced when the GFR is 20% to 40% of normal. The person with renal insufficiency typically requires symptomatic management by the physician. It is important to follow these two points on the renal function continuum, because proper management can prevent the loss of more renal functioning and eliminate the need for more aggressive therapy. Regular physical examination, including serum chemistry evaluation can aid in the detection of changing renal status.

Diabetes mellitus is the most common cause of end-stage renal disease (ESRD) in the United States.[52] Hypertension and glomerulonephritis follow closely. Early detection and prompt treatment of these conditions can either prevent or slow the progression of nephron damage. Persons at risk for developing diabetes and hypertension (Box 33-3) should be screened regularly.

Urinary tract infections (UTI) are a significant source of morbidity in the United States. These infections contribute to illness during the active stage but also can lead to the development of chronic renal failure. Although the vast majority of UTIs clear spontaneously, there remains a portion significant enough to warrant consideration as a health problem. Early detection and treatment of a UTI decrease the probability of renal complications. Box 33-4 summarizes health care practices helpful in prevention and treatment of a UTI.

Tertiary Prevention

Tertiary prevention in persons with urinary disorders focuses on helping them adapt as fully as possible to limitations imposed by their illness. For example, for patients with chronic renal failure requiring dialysis, it is the domain of nursing to assist patients and their families adjust to the treatment regimen and changes in life-style.[22] Another example is assisting patients who have had urinary diversion procedures to adapt to changes in urinary patterns and body image. Overall, tertiary prevention involves preventing further urinary disability and reduced functioning.

MAJOR HEALTH PROBLEMS OF THE URINARY SYSTEM

The major health problems of the urinary system can be categorized in a number of ways. The following common disorders will be discussed in this chapter.
1. Urinary dysfunction
   a. Urinary retention
   b. Urinary incontinence
2. Urinary tract infections
   a. Pyelonephritis
   b. Lower urinary tract infection
3. Glomerular disorders
   a. Glomerulonephritis: acute, chronic
   b. Nephrotic syndrome

4. Obstructive disorders
   a. Urinary calculi
   b. Benign prostatic hypertrophy
   c. Urethral strictures
   d. Neoplasms: renal, bladder, prostate
5. Other urinary disorders
   a. Polycystic disease
   b. Vascular disorders
   c. Diabetic nephropathy
   d. Trauma

Another major health problem of the urinary system is congenital disorders. Congenital disorders include structural malformation, lack of or poor development of one or both kidneys, dysplasia, and polycystic disease. Any of these conditions can result in morbidity in adults. (For more information about congenital disorders refer to a pediatric nursing text.)

Any of the preceding disorders can lead to loss of renal function resulting in what is called *renal failure*. Renal failure is classified as (1) acute or (2) chronic. Acute and chronic renal failure are discussed at the end of this chapter.

URINARY DYSFUNCTION

URINARY RETENTION
Etiology

Under normal conditions, a person consuming an adequate diet, including adequate fluid intake, has a urinary output approximately equal to fluid intake. Inadequate urinary output may occur either when the kidneys are not producing urine or when urine is retained in the bladder (*urinary retention*). Causes of urinary retention include urethral obstruction, decreased sensory activity to and from the bladder, surgery, medications, and muscle tension.[59] Causes of urinary retention can be categorized as either mechanical or functional (Box 33-5).

33-5

Major causes of urinary retention

Type of retention	Cause
Mechanical obstruction	
	Urethral stricture
	Urinary tract malformation
	Spinal cord malformation
Acquired	Calculus
	Inflammation
	Trauma
	Tumor
	Hyperplasia
	Pregnancy
Functional obstruction	Neurogenic bladder dysfunction
	Ureterovesical reflux
	Decreased peristaltic activity of the ureter
	Detrusor muscle atrophy
	Anxiety, such as fear of pain after surgery
	Medications, for example anesthetics, narcotics, sedatives, and antihistamines

Pathophysiology

A mechanical obstruction exists when urine flow is blocked. This blockage can exist anywhere within the urinary system from the collecting ducts to the urinary meatus. Most obstructions in adults are acquired. A functional obstruction exists when there is an obstruction that cannot be attributed to a mechanical problem.

A key symptom of urinary retention is inability to void. The bladder becomes distended with urine and is sometimes displaced to either side of the midline. Percussion over a full bladder produces a "kettledrum" sound. Discomfort occurs from pressure of the bladder on other organs and the person has an urge to urinate. Restlessness and diaphoresis may also occur with a full bladder.

Voiding 25 to 50 ml of urine at frequent intervals often indicates *retention with overflow*. The intravesicular pressure increases as the bladder continues to fill with urine and overcomes the sphincter's restraining capability. A small amount of urine flows out of the bladder to reduce the intravesicular pressure to the level where the sphincter can control the flow of urine once again. The patient may state that the bladder continues to feel full. The bladder fills again and the cycle is repeated. The specific gravity of the person's urine is normal or high in retention with overflow because the kidney's ability to produce urine is not impaired.

Nursing Process

Assessment

Subjective data

The patient is asked questions to provide data on the following:

1. Understanding of the disorder
2. Voiding patterns, including absence of voiding or voiding frequently in small amounts without relief of bladder distention
3. Dietary habits, including fluid intake
4. Presence of suprapubic pain
5. History of urinary problems

Objective data

Objective data should include intake and output, assessment of level of hydration, palpation for bladder distention, and visual inspection of urine for color, clarity, sedimentation, and odor.

Data analysis: nursing diagnoses

Nursing diagnoses are determined from analysis of patient data. Possible nursing diagnoses for the person with urinary retention may include, but are not limited to, the following:

Diagnostic title	Possible etiologies
Urinary retention	Obstruction, position for voiding, immobility, effects of medications (narcotics, anesthetics, sedatives, antihistamines)
Knowledge deficit	Lack of information

Planning: expected patient outcomes

Expected patient outcomes for the person with urinary retention may include, but are not limited to, the following:

1. Voids 200 to 400 ml at each voiding.
2. Demonstrates home care of catheter to prevent infection.

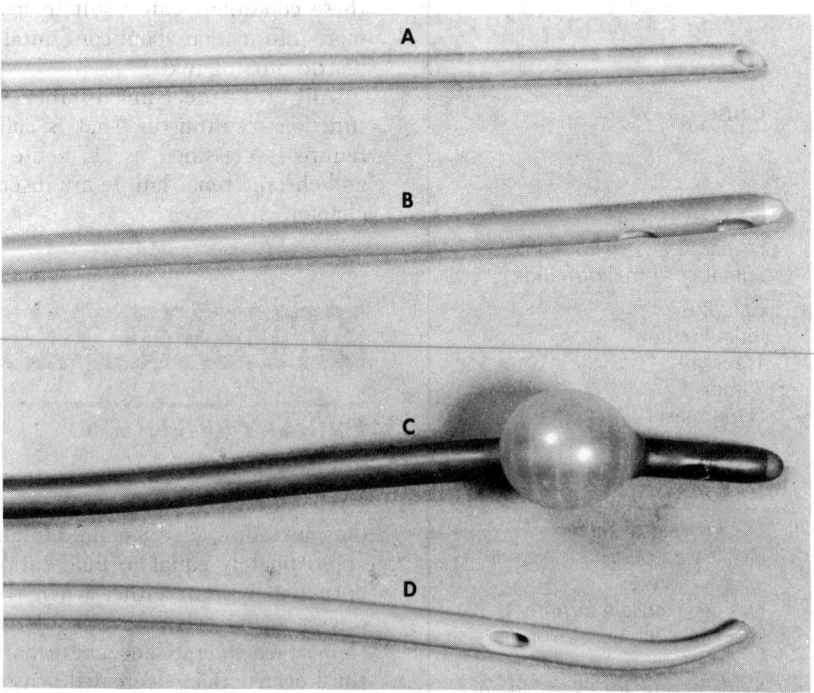

Fig. 33-12   Urethral catheters. **A,** Whistle-tip catheter. **B,** Many-eyed Robinson catheter. **C,** Foley catheter. **D,** Coudé catheter.

3. Describes signs of retention or UTI (for in-dwelling catheter) to be reported to physician.

Implementation
Assisting with achievement of therapeutic goals

Interventions for urinary retention are aimed at reestablishing urine flow. Some mechanical obstructions must be corrected by surgical intervention; others, such as that caused by an enlarged prostate, may require temporary urethral catheter drainage.

Promotion of micturition

If the person is having difficulty eliminating urine from the bladder in the absence of mechanical obstruction, measures that encourage voiding are attempted before catheterization is instituted. These measures may include ensuring a position that facilitates voiding (positional stimuli), running water or blowing bubbles in water (auditory stimuli), or pouring water over the perineum or placing the hands in water (tactile stimuli). Having the person sit in lukewarm water may help to relax the urinary sphincters.

Cholinergic medications, such as bethanechol chloride or neostigmine, may be given to initiate voiding by stimulating the bladder detrusor muscle to contract. However, these medications must never be given if a mechanical obstruction is either present or suspected.[9] Persons with long-term problems may be taught to carry out intermittent catheterizations (p. 1022) rather than maintaining an indwelling catheter.

Catheter usage and types

Assisted urinary drainage is used in a variety of clinical situations in both acute and chronic care. Major reasons for catheter drainage include the following:

1. Relieve temporary anatomic or physiologic urinary obstruction.
2. Permit healing of various parts of the urinary system postoperatively.
3. Permit accurate measurement of urinary output in severely ill patients.
4. Relieve inability to void.
5. Achieve continence.
6. Prevent retention of urine in certain types of persons with neurogenic bladder dysfunction.
7. Permit irrigation to prevent obstruction of urine flow.

Reestablishment of the flow of urine is an immediate treatment goal. The type of catheter used to provide drainage in the presence of obstruction depends on the location of the blockage.

Straight catheters (Fig. 33-12) are used for single catheterizations. The various catheters have different uses:

1. Robinson—intermittent catheterization (ease of insertion)
2. Coudé—prostatic hypertrophy (avoid trauma to gland)
3. Whistle-tip—presence of hematuria and blood clots (less chance of blockage)
4. Filiform (thin, stiff catheter)—urethral stricture

The *Foley catheter* is the most frequently used self-retaining catheter; it is used when continuous drainage is required. The Foley catheter has a double lumen with an inflatable balloon at the distal end. The balloon is inflated with either normal saline or sterile water after it has been placed well within the bladder (Fig. 33-13). In-dwelling urethral catheters must be securely anchored to prevent accidental dislodging of the catheter (Fig. 33-14). Proper anchoring will prevent accidental traction (possible injury to the bladder or urethra) and yet keep the catheter from moving in and out of the urethra (possible irritation and

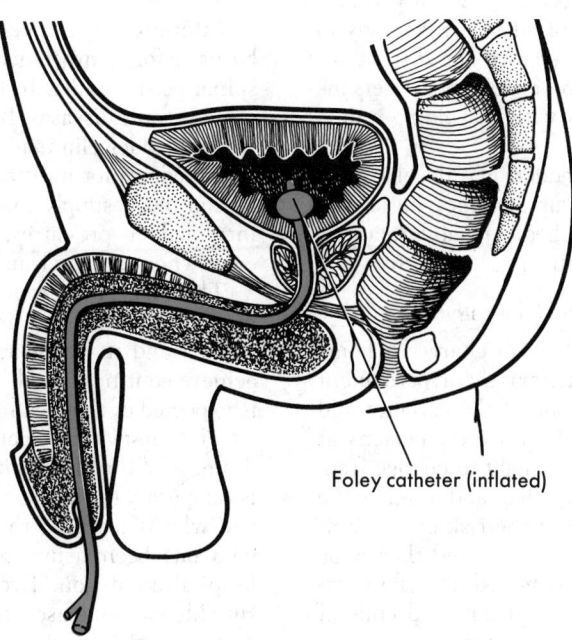

Fig. 33-13   Foley catheter in place with balloon inflated.

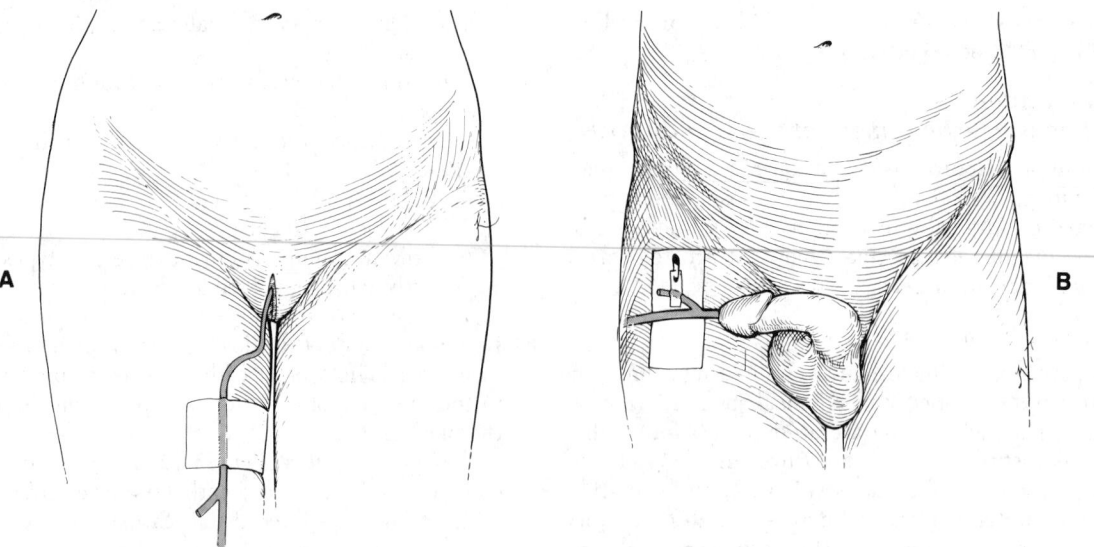

Fig. 33-14   Anchoring of Foley catheter. **A,** In female. **B,** In male. Proper anchoring prevents accidental traction that could result in injury to bladder or urethra but keeps catheter from moving in and out of urethra.

infection). Guidelines for maintenance of an in-dwelling urinary drainage system are listed in Box 33-6.

Difficulties following catheter removal

It is normal to note some dribbling of urine for a few hours after an in-dwelling urethral catheter has been removed because of dilation of the sphincter muscles by the catheter. Dribbling of urine that persists longer than a few hours is reported to the physician; this symptom may indicate damage to the sphincters. Stress incontinence may persist for several months if the catheter has been in place for more than a few days.

Inability to initiate voiding may occur when the catheter is removed. The person is encouraged to drink fluids to stimulate the sphincters and is assessed for distention. Measures to promote voiding are encouraged. Persons should not go longer than 8 hours without voiding unless fluid intake has been restricted.

Cystitis (inflammation of the bladder) may develop after catheter removal because of imcomplete emptying of the bladder as muscle tone is reestablished. Any abnormalities in color, odor, or sediment in the urine are reported.

Home care for persons with in-dwelling catheters

It is not uncommon for persons to be discharged to home requiring catheter drainage on a temporary or permanent basis. Ideally, frequent disconnection of the catheter and drainage tubing should be avoided. However, persons at home must disconnect the tubing at night to change from a leg bag to the overnight drainage bag and reverse the procedure in the morning. To lessen the risk of contamination, the person should wash the hands and then wipe the catheter and tubing with povidone iodine before disconnection and reconnection. The disconnected ends of the drainage bags are protected with a connector cap or with a sterile gauze secured in place with a rubber band.

A shower or tub bath with a catheter in place is generally permitted unless there is an unhealed surgical incision. The adhesive tape holding the catheter in place will need to be replaced after bathing.

There is no need for men or women to remove an indwelling catheter before intercourse, a question persons may be hesitant to ask. The man can fold the in-dwelling catheter over the penis to facilitate insertion during intercourse. Questions pertaining to resumption of usual lifestyle are encouraged so the person can be as well prepared as possible for self-care at home.

Intermittent catheterization

Intermittent catheterization of the urinary bladder may be used for neurogenic bladder dysfunction secondary to spinal cord trauma, birth defects, urinary retention, and some chronic diseases. Because periodic complete emptying of the bladder eliminates residual urine (an excellent culture medium for multiplication of bacteria) and maintains a good blood supply to the bladder wall by avoiding high intrabladder pressures, infections are often decreased, even when only a clean technique is used.

The goals of intermittent catheterization may vary from patient to patient but are generally to prevent urinary retention and its sequelae (UTI and renal damage) and to achieve continence. The patient should know exactly what is expected of the treatment plan to elicit full cooperation.

The *hospitalized* patient with intermittent catheter drainage of the bladder may be one for whom the treatment is temporary (as in the early phases of spinal cord trauma), one who is learning the technique for home use, or one who has been using intermittent catheterization before hospital admission. Even though the clean technique is suitable for home use, sterile technique is necessary during hospitalization to decrease the possibility of hospital-acquired (nosocomial) infection when the catheterization is

---

Maintenance of drainage system

Action	Rationale
Never disconnect the catheter except to irrigate	Prevent introduction of bacteria
Collect urine samples by inserting a small-bore needle into the drainage port that has been cleansed with alcohol or povidone-iodine.	Maintain closed system and prevent introduction of bacteria
Never elevate drainage bag above level of the patient's bladder or cavity being drained; suspend bag from the bed frame when the patient is recumbent and from below the knee when the patient is ambulatory.	Prevent reflux of urine back into bladder; drainage bags are available with antireflux valves
Drainage bags and tubing should never be allowed to rest on the floor.	Prevent contamination of system
Observe tubing for kinks and loops.	Obstructions result in reflux of urine
Empty drainage bag into a measuring container that is used only for that particular patient; cleanse measuring container regularly.	Prevent cross-contamination of drainage system
Cultures of urine are usually ordered at regular intervals when a patient has an in-dwelling catheter.	Provides data on changing numbers and types of organism present in urine before symptoms appear
Observe collecting system daily for sedimentation and leaks.	Replace when sediment or leaks are present

---

performed by hospital personnel. When hospitalized, the patient who customarily performs self-catheterization may continue to use clean technique if this method is used at home, but preferably a sterile catheter will be used each time or special precautions will be taken to store the reusable catheter in a closed container. Specimens for culture must be obtained by the usual sterile catheterization technique to avoid contamination of the specimen. The patient is informed about the reasons why sterile precautions are necessary in the hospital setting.

A No. 14 Fr Robinson catheter is generally used for an adult. The volume of urine obtained with each catheterization is recorded to ensure that schedule adjustments can be made if necessary. The adult bladder should not be permitted to hold more than 300 ml at any time, because greater amounts lead to overdistention of the bladder with greater susceptibility to infection. The frequency of catheterization is determined by the amount of residual urine (more than 200 ml means that more frequent catheterization is necessary). Usually such individuals will need catheterization every 4 to 6 hours. A small amount of residual urine (less than 200 ml) after voiding means that the person will only need to do self-catheterization every 8 to 12 hours. Some individuals may also have to catheterize themselves at night if they have a large output of urine during these hours. It is important to realize that the person who normally does not perform self-catheterization at night at home may need to do so during periods where the fluid intake is greater than usual, as with intravenous fluid administration.

In some instances the physician will prescribe the frequency of catheterizations; in other instances, adjustment of the schedule may be a nursing judgment. If the nurse notes that excess volumes of urine are being obtained with a prescribed schedule, the physican is consulted about the need to alter the schedule.

Color, clarity, and odor of the urine are noted, and any symptoms of a UTI are reported. Periodic urine specimens are obtained and sent for culture and sensitivity. Some individuals are given long-term antibiotic therapy prophylactically.

In most cases, clean (not sterile) catheterization technique is prescribed for *home use.* Hand washing is advised before each catheterization, and the meatal area is cleansed with soap and water. After inserting the catheter and draining the bladder, the catheter is removed and washed with soap and water before being stored in a clean, closed container for the next use. The catheter is reused until it becomes either too soft or too hard to be directed properly.

Most individuals require much support during the actual teaching but very quickly become comfortable with the procedure. Initially, a mirror is used to teach women where to place the catheter. The woman should learn to catheterize while sitting on the commode, using palpation to locate the urethral meatus. Men may sit or stand to catheterize themselves. It is important that men use generous amounts of lubricant to avoid urethral irritation; women generally do not require lubrication of the catheter.

If sterile catheterization technique is needed for home use, more time and practice will be required to learn good sterile technique. Careful explanation of sterilization of equipment must be provided, and planning for adapting sterile intermittent self-catheterization to the individual's usual life-style must be worked out with the person.

If teaching of self-catheterization is performed on an outpatient basis or if hospitalization is short, follow-up for adjustment of schedule and other concerns of adaptation to home routine should be provided. This may be done by the primary nurse, by the physician, or by referral to a home health care nurse. Ongoing urologic care with periodic urine cultures is essential.

Table 33-2 **Types of incontinence**

Type	Definition	Related factors
Stress	Involuntary loss of <50 ml urine with increased abdominal pressure	Relaxed pelvic muscles associated with age, obesity, incompetent bladder outlet
Reflex	Involuntary loss of urine when a specific volume is reached, occurring at somewhat predictable intervals	Neurologic impairment such as spinal cord lesion
Urge	Involuntary loss of urine occurring soon after a strong sense of urgency to void	Decreased bladder capacity, bladder infection, increased fluid intake, increased urine concentration, overdistention of bladder
Functional	Involuntary unpredictable loss of urine	Sensory, cognitive, or mobility deficits
Total	Continuous and unpredicable loss of urine	Neurologic dysfunction; independent contractions of detrusor muscle as a result of surgery, trauma, or disease affecting spinal cord nerves; fistulas

Interventions to achieve patient outcomes
Relieving urinary retention

Provide the patient with privacy. If a bedpan is used, place the patient in a sitting position to enlist the aid of gravity and increase intraabdominal pressure; this may help stimulate the bladder sphincter. Warm the bedpan for comfort before offering it. Run water from the faucet and flush the toilet; the sound of running water offers the power of suggestion and may facilitate voiding. If the patient is tense and can sit in warm water, the warmth may help relax the internal sphincter and perineal muscles. If these measures in addition to administrating cholinergic medications fail, catheterization may be indicated.

Facilitating patient learning

Specific patient teaching depends on the underlying cause of urinary retention and the need for an in-dwelling catheter or intermittent catheterization. Teaching may include the following:

1. Rationale for type of care required.
2. Use of Credé method of emptying bladder (if appropriate): place hands flat against abdomen below umbilicus; make firm downward strokes toward bladder six times, then apply direct pressure over bladder to force out urine.
3. Maintenance of adequate fluid intake to prevent UTI.
4. In-dwelling urethral catheter: maintenance of catheter patency, caring for equipment, dealing with catheter problems, procurement of supplies, need for ongoing care.
5. Intermittent catheterization: techniques, frequency, adaptation of catheterization routine to life-style, procurement of supplies, need for ongoing care.
6. Signs or retention or UTI to be reported to physician.

Evaluation

Evaluation is based on expected patient outcomes. Questions to consider may include the following:

1. Has the person urinated at least 200 to 400 ml with each voiding? Is the bladder no longer palpable?
2. Does the patient know home care use of catheter, measures to prevent UTI, where to purchase supplies, and signs to report to physician?

URINARY INCONTINENCE

Urinary incontinence, the involuntary expulsion of urine, may be encountered in a number of temporary and permanent conditions. Inability to control urination is a problem that frequently leads to emotional distress and can seriously impair an individual's socialization patterns if not managed either by the person or by others in a way that makes the person feel physically and emotionally comfortable and socially acceptable. Urinary incontinence occurs most frequently in persons over the age of 65. Several types of incontinence have been identified (Table 33-2).

Etiology

The five major causes of urinary incontinence and the nature of the incontinence they cause are outlined in Table 33-3.

Cerebral confusion is most common in the aged. In many instances the elderly person is incontinent because of a lack of awareness of the need to empty the bladder. This type of incontinence is often not associated with any definite pathologic problem at the cerebral level. Cerebral clouding also occurs in acutely ill persons, who may be so ill that cerebration is dulled. They may not be able to think or may not have the energy to exercise voluntary control. Likewise a person who is comatose is incontinent because of loss of the ability to control voluntarily the opening of the external sphincter. As soon as urine is released into the posterior urethra, the bladder contracts and empties. This is the reason why voiding sometimes occurs under anesthesia.

Infection anywhere in the urinary tract may lead to incontinence because bacteria in the urine cause irritation of the mucosa of the bladder and stimulate the urethro-bladder reflex abnormally.

Disturbance of the central nervous system pathways may occur in diseases such as cerebral embolus, cerebral hemorrhage, brain tumor, meningitis, or traumatic injury of

Table 33-3   Major causes of urinary incontinence

Cause of urinary incontinence	Awareness of need to void	Cortical ability to inhibit voiding	Reflex arc	Bladder response to filling	Result
	Factors involved				
Cerebral confusion	Impaired	Impaired	Intact	Normal	Uncontrolled voiding because of reflex response
Infection	Intact	Intact, but overcome by strong reflex response	Abnormally stimulated	Heightened	Voiding because of strong reflex response (urgency)
Disturbance of CNS pathways (cortical lesions)	Diminished	Impaired	Intact	Heightened	Voiding because of reflex response
Disturbance of urethrobladder reflex					
Upper motor neuron lesion	Destroyed	Destroyed	Intact but deranged	Heightened	Voiding because of reflex response
Lower motor neuron lesion	Destroyed	Destroyed	Destroyed or impaired	Diminished to absent	Distention or incomplete emptying
Tissue damage	Intact	Intact, but not functional because of poor muscle response	Intact	Normal	Loss of control of voiding because of muscular impairment

the brain. Adequate voluntary (cortical or cerebral) control of bladder function is prevented in these situations. Urgency incontinence may be present as a result of the inability to inhibit completion of the urethrobladder reflex by the higher centers.

Disturbance of the urethrobladder reflex may result from lesions of the spinal cord or damage to peripheral nerves of the bladder. This form of incontinence may be seen in persons with spinal cord malformations, injuries, or tumors, and those with compression of the cord caused by fractures of the vertebae, herniated disk, metastatic tumor, or postoperative edema of the spinal cord. The person has a *neurogenic* bladder (see the following discussion) and may have either reflex or overflow incontinence. The person has no way of knowing when voiding is occurring.

Tissue damage to the sphincters of the bladder from instrumentation, surgery, or accidents, scarring following urethral infections, lesions involving the sphincter, or relaxation of the perineal structures may cause urinary incontinence. The latter cause of incontinence is seen occasionally following childbirth. The problem is local in nature and does not involve the nervous system.

Pathophysiology

Persons with urinary incontinence often present baffling management problems. Solutions require understanding of the physiologic basis of incontinence.

Bladder and sphincter control are necessary to have urinary continence. Such control requires normal voluntary and involuntary muscle action coordinated by a normal urethrobladder reflex. As bladder filling occurs, the pressure within the bladder gradually increases. The detrusor muscle (the three-layered bladder wall) responds by relaxing to accommodate the greater volume. When a certain point of filling is reached, usually 150 to 200 ml of urine, the parasympathetic stretch receptors located in the bladder wall are stimulated. The stimuli are transmitted through afferent fibers of the reflex arc to the reflex center for micturition. Impulses are then carried through the efferent fibers of the reflex arc to the bladder, causing reflex contraction of the detrusor muscle. The internal sphincter, which is normally closed, reciprocally opens, and the urine enters the posterior urethra. Relaxation of the external sphincter and perineal muscles follows, and the bladder content is released. Completion of this reflex act can be interrupted and voiding postponed through release of inhibitory impulses from the cortical center, which results in voluntary contraction of the external sphincter. If any part of this complex function is upset, there is apt to be urinary incontinence.

Neurogenic bladder

A neurogenic bladder may be one of two types, upper motor neuron, or lower motor neuron. The *upper motor neuron* or *automatic* bladder occurs with lesions above the S2 spinal cord level or impairment of the cerebrocortical center.

These lesions do not destroy the reflex arc for voiding (although they may derange it); they destroy the potential for cortical control to inhibit the reflex. The bladder is *hypertonic* and has a small capacity (less than 150 ml). The increased detrusor tone and increased sensitivity to small amounts of urine present in the bladder result in precipitous *reflex* voiding and the potential for vesicoureteral reflux.

Damage to nerves in the cauda equina or sacral segments of the spinal cord may cause destruction of the reflex arc by interruption of its afferent, efferent, or central components. The result is a *"lower motor neuron"* or *"flaccid"* bladder. The bladder is *hypotonic* with capacities of 500 ml or more. Overflow incontinence, retention of residual urine, and the potential for vesicoureteral reflux are problems imposed by a hypotonic bladder.

Overflow incontinence is considerd to be caused by pressure exerted on the distended bladder by the abdominal muscles. Residual urine, urine remaining in the bladder after incomplete emptying, provides a medium for the growth of bacteria, and a UTI is common.

Stress incontinence

Urinary incontinence that occurs during coughing, straining, or heavy lifting is termed *stress incontinence*. It is seen primarily in women who have relaxed pelvic musculature, but it may also occur in men following prostatectomy. When bladder pressure is suddenly increased, urine enters the proximal third of the urethra then returns to the bladder when the pressure is decreased after exertion. Some of the urine escapes through the urethra. Usually the person is continent at night because bladder pressure is decreased in the recumbent position.

Nursing Process
Assessment
Subjective data

The following questions are asked when assessing incontinence:

1. Is there a total inability to control urination?
2. What is the frequency of incontinence?
3. Can anything be associated with precipitating incontinence (stress, fear, laughing, exercise)?
4. Is pain or burning present with incontinence?
5. Is there a state of awareness to void before incontinence?
6. Does dribbling occur?

Objective data

Important objective data to obtain include the following:
1. Volume of urine output
2. Characteristics of urine
3. Palpation of bladder to identify residual urine
4. Patient's level of consciousness to determine ability to cooperate
5. Patient's ability to follow directions
6. Is there a physiologic reason for incontinence (for example, spinal cord injury)

Diagnostic tests

Normally the bladder contains little or no urine after voiding; however, certain disease states inhibit the bladder from emptying completely. Some common conditions in which incomplete emptying of the bladder occurs are benign prostatic hypertrophy, urethral strictures, and interruptions in bladder innervation. Urine left in the bladder after voiding is called *residual urine*.

One way to determine the amount of residual urine is to *catheterize* the person immediately after voiding. This may be ordered by the physician on a one-time or on a repeated basis. Before catheterizing the person, the physician is consulted regarding the plan for establishing urinary drainage. If a large amount of residual urine is suspected, the physician may wish the catheter to be left in place in the bladder. *Residual urine volumes of 50 ml or less indicate near normal or returning bladder function.*

To avoid passing a catheter to measure residual urine volumes, x-ray examination of retained urine may be performed. In this procedure a radiopaque substance excreted by the kidneys is injected intravenously. As the dye is excreted in the urine, it passes into the bladder. A sufficient amount of urine containing the radiopaque material is allowed to accumulate in the bladder before the person is instructed to void. Immediately after voiding an x-ray film is taken. Any urine retained in the bladder will be visualized on the radiograph. This means of determining residual urine is used in conjunction with other studies requiring visualization of the urinary tract.

Cystometric examination is performed to evaluate bladder tone. In general, the examination is indicated when incontinence is present or when there is evidence of neurologic dysfunction of the bladder. An in-dwelling catheter is inserted before the examination. After the person assumes a supine position, a liter bottle of normal saline or sterile distilled water and a cystometer are connected to the catheter. Fluid is instilled at a constant and specified rate; measurements of the pressure exerted on the fluid by the bladder musculature are recorded after the instillation of every 50 ml of fluid. The person is asked to report feelings of fullness, the need to void, and any urgency or discomfort. Fluid is instilled until urgency occurs or it is determined that the sensation is absent. During cystometric examination, bethanechol chloride (Urecholine) may be administered to determine its effect on enhancing the tone of a flaccid bladder, or an anticholingeric medication may be given to assess relaxation in a hyperactive bladder. There is no specific care required after cystometric examination.

Electromyography may be used to evaluate sphincter tone and intactness of nerve pathways.

Data analysis: nursing diagnoses

Nursing diagnoses are determined from analysis of patient data. Possible nursing diagnoses for the person with urinary incontinence may include, but are not limited to, the following:

Diagnostic title	Possible etiologies
Incontinence (specify type)	Altered environment, sensory deficit, neurologic impairment, relaxed pelvic muscles, overdistention, decreased bladder capacity
Skin integrity, impaired, high risk for	Urine irritation

Diagnostic title	Possible etiologies
Body image disturbance	Loss of body functions, change in life-style, change in social involvement
Knowledge deficit	Lack of information

Planning: expected patient outcomes

Expected patient outcomes for the person with urinary incontinence may include, but are not limited to, the following:

1. Achieves optimal urinary control
2. Skin remains intact
3. Verbalizes feelings and frustrations without self-deprecating statements
4. Describes actions to control incontinence (as appropriate), measures to maintain skin integrity, and plans for follow-up care

Implementation

Assisting with achievement of therapeutic goals

Control of urinary incontinence is largely dependent on its cause. Measures include surgery, treatment of associated conditions, programs of bladder retraining (p. 1029), or the use of drainage devices.

Surgery for stress incontinence

Surgery may be indicated for severe stress incontinence. A *vesicourethropexy* (Marshall-Marchetti-Krantz operation) consists of fixation of the urethra to the fascia of the rectus muscle of the abdomen with support given to the neck of the bladder. A suprapubic incision is usually made, but a transvaginal repair may be carried out if there is scar tissue around the urethra from vaginal surgery. A urethral catheter is inserted postoperatively and maintained for 5 to 6 days. The urine may be pink, but the urethral catheter is not irrigated as a rule. It is not uncommon for difficulty in voiding to be experienced immediately after the in-dwelling catheter is removed. The woman is observed for signs of vaginal bleeding. Straining and use of Valsalva's maneuver should be avoided until healing has occurred, and mild laxatives may be given to prevent straining from constipation. Surgeons differ in the amount of activity permitted in the early postoperative period.

A surgical procedure that is less invasive is the *Stamey procedure,* a suspension of the bladder neck by sutures passed adjacent to the ureterovesical junctions.[13] A small incision is made above and lateral to the symphysis pubis. The needles are introduced suprapubically and the positions are checked by cystoscopy (a bulge can be noted at the junction wall) before suturing. The procedure is then repeated on the opposite side. A percutaneous suprapubic catheter is inserted following the suturing; the catheter is removed when spontaneous voiding occurs, which may take several days. There is minimal postoperative discomfort. Antibiotics are given for 2 weeks postoperatively. The patient should refrain from sexual activity until permitted (usually 1 to 2 months).

Sphincter dysfunction

Repair of a sphincter that has been cut is almost impossible. When the *external sphincter* has been damaged, the person will be incontinent on urgency. A voiding schedule can be planned so that voiding occurs before the bladder is full enough to exert sufficient pressure to open the internal sphincter involuntarily. When the *internal sphincter* is damaged, there may be no acute feeling of the need to void. Here the problem is not one of incontinence but of retention. To ensure regular emptying of the bladder, a regular voiding schedule is necessary. If both sphincters are damaged, there will be total incontinence.

Urge incontinence

Incontinence caused by urinary tract infection (UTI) is generally temporary, responding to treatment of the infection by systemic antibiotics. Specific causes of infection such as obstruction must be identified and corrected when possible. Provision must be made for adequate fluid intake of 3000 ml or more per day unless contraindicated by the person's medical condition. Because of heightened bladder sensitivity to even small amounts of urine, urgency to void demands rapid response by the nurse to the request for help to void.

The person who has a brain tumor, meningitis, or traumatic injury to the brain that prevents adequate voluntary control of bladder function and causes urgency incontinence by inhibiting cortical control over the urethrobladder reflex may also respond to a bladder retraining program (p. 1029). If the person's condition or response prohibits such a program, a drainage device should be used.

Neurogenic bladder dysfunction

Persons with injuries of the spinal cord experience a transitory period of "spinal shock" in which urinary retention occurs. This is treated with continuous or intermittent catheter drainage that aims to prevent a UTI and overdistention of the bladder. Following this acute stage, further management depends on the exact nature of any residual neurogenic bladder dysfunction. Persons with a lesion *above the sacral segments* and who have an intact urethrobladder reflex may initiate voiding by pinching or stroking trigger areas of the thighs or suprapubic area. In persons with a *lower motor neuron* lesion, the use of the *Credé method,* which consists of exerting manual pressure over the bladder, (p. 1024), may be ordered to provide for more complete bladder emptying. The appropriateness of this technique must be determined by the physician as based on the person's complete urologic status. An increasing number of persons with neurogenic bladder dysfunction are being taught intermittent self-catheterization using clean technique to prevent infection and manage incontinence. Maintenance of a regular schedule is stressed, and the frequency of catheterization is determined on an individual basis.

Certain medications are sometimes used alone or in conjunction with an intermittent catheterization program in the management of incontinence related to neurogenic bladder dysfunction. Alpha adrenergic drugs such as ephedrine sulfate are used to increase urethral resistance. Anticholinergic drugs such as propantheline are prescribed to control the reflex bladder activity.

Urinary drainage for incontinence

Occasionally there are justifications for the use of an in-dwelling catheter for the incontinent patient. Such rea-

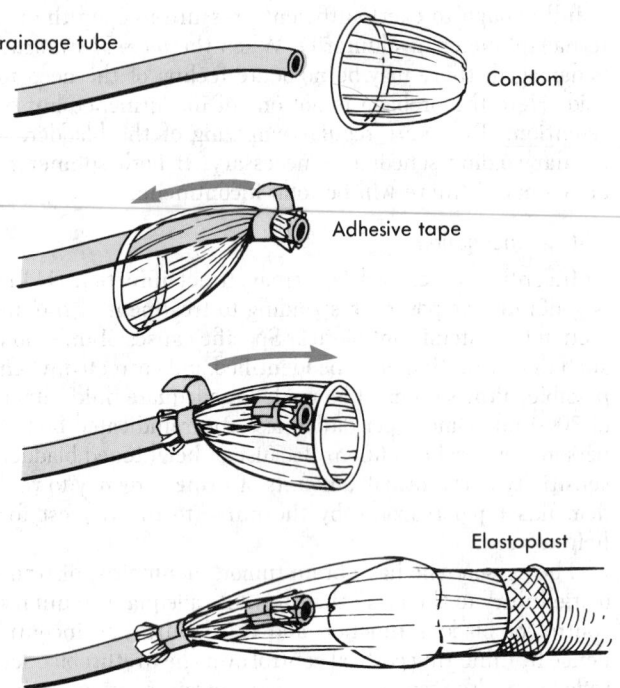

Fig. 33-15   One method of making external drainage apparatus.

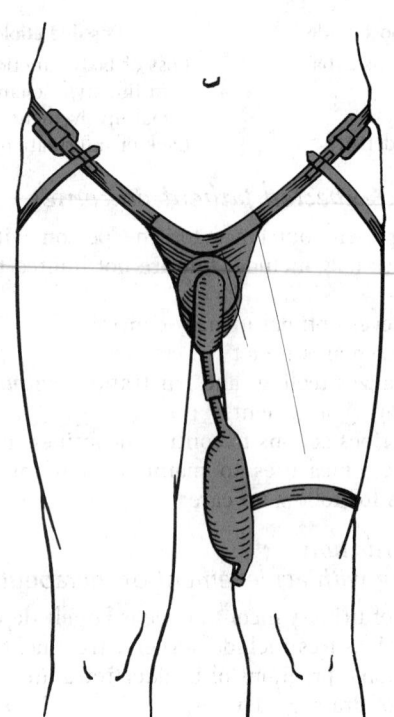

Fig. 33-16   Rubber urinary appliance. Bag is emptied by drain valve at bottom of bag.

sons include the need to protect a surgical incision or to permit healing of a decubitus ulcer in the area. In-dwelling catheterization, however, presents many potential dangers, such as UTI, urethritis, epididymitis, and urethral fistulas. All other means to manage incontinence should be tried before resorting to catheterization. Proper catheter management is essential.

In males, *external drainage* can be easily accomplished by applying a watertight apparatus to the penis. The following is one method. Select a condom of the correct size. Puncture a hole in the closed end of the condom with an applicator stick. Attach the punctured end of the condom to a firm rubber or plastic drainage tube with either a 33 mm (⅛-inch) piece of rubber tubing or a strip of adhesive tape (Fig. 33-15). Before applying the condom, clean and dry the penis thoroughly and check it for edema, skin breaks, or discoloration. Invert the condom and roll it onto the penis. There should be no roll at the top that could cause constriction. At least 2.5 cm (1 inch) of the condom should remain between the meatus and drainage tube to allow for penile erection. There should not be so much slack as to cause twisting and subsequent interference with drainage. Elastoplast is then applied over the condom and around the penis (never touching the skin). *Under no circumstances should adhesive tape be used.* The Elastoplast must not be constricting.

The external catheter should be removed daily, and the skin washed and checked. Frequent checking is necessary to determine whether edema or irritation is present and to ensure proper drainage. This is especially important in men

with loss of sensation. The external device is attached to straight drainage or to a leg bag.

For persons who need external catheter drainage indefinitely, a rubber urinary appliance (sometimes called an *incontinence urinal*) may be used (Fig. 33-16). There are several models available, and the one best suited to the person's needs is selected. Two appliances are recommended to allow for cleaning and drying. They should be washed with mild soap, turned inside out, and thoroughly dried before using.

Most persons prefer to manage their own incontinence if they are at all able to do so. The nurse supports and encourages this, offering assistance as necessary and instruction in basic principles of skin care, equipment selection, and maintenance. The choice of management method should take into account the person's ability to manage as independently as is possible.

Implantation of an *artificial urinary sphincter* can be used to achieve continence when other methods have failed. In this procedure a hydraulically activated sphincter mechanism is placed around the urethra or bladder neck. The sphincter is made to open and close at will by squeezing one of two bulbs implanted under the skin of the labia or scrotum (Fig. 33-17). Postoperative nursing care of the person with such an implant includes observation for and reporting of fever or pain on inflation of the device, swelling of the genitalia, and recurrence of incontinence. Complications of the procedure include erosion of the urethra, abscess, cellulitis, and mechanical malfunctions in the system. Men have had more success with the artificial sphincter than have women.

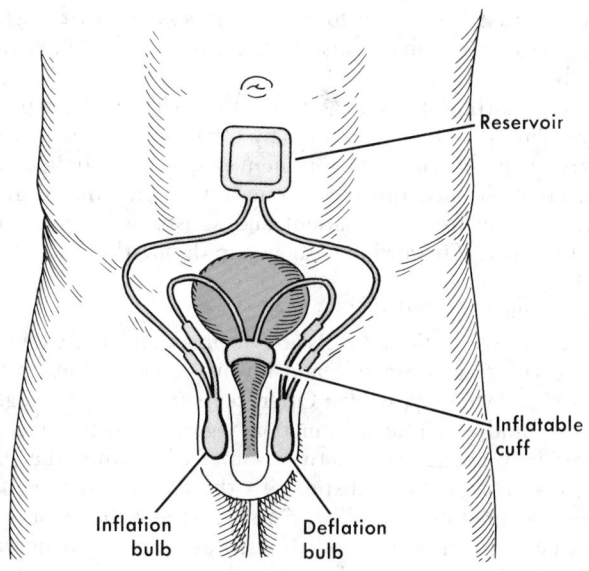

Fig. 33-17 Artificial bladder sphincter. Compression and re-ease of inflation pump bulb inflates cuff surrounding urethra stopping urine flow. Compression and release of deflation pump bulb deflates inflatable cuff, returning fluid to storage reservoir. This releases urethral constriction, permitting urine to flow.

Inteventions to achieve patient outcomes
Assisting with urinary control

Because the person who experiences incontinence may at times have bladder control, respond immediately when assistance to toilet is requested. Offer assistance to toilet shortly after each meal, a time when urination is most frequent because of ingested fluids. Lack of prompt assistance may lead to episodes of incontinence that further frustrate the person and may lead to the belief that nothing can be done. No program of bladder retraining or management can be successful without the person's cooperation. Encourage self-care of incontinence whenever possible. Be supportive of the patient by providing a relaxed atmosphere when providing care for incontinence.

When incontinence is caused by dulled cerebration in the elderly, by confusion, or by acute illness, control can usually be established if a persistent *bladder retraining* schedule is carried out (see Box 33-7). A voiding schedule is developed and must be strictly adhered to until the person gradually relearns to recognize and react appropriately to the feeling of having to void. A successful program of this type, leading to complete rehabilitation, or continence, requires mental competence of the individual. Otherwise someone else must always remind the person to follow the schedule. However, with proper support, bladder retraining is possible even when the incontinent person is not fully mentally competent.

People ordinarily void on awakening, before retiring, and before or after meals. If a diuretic such as coffee has been taken, it is usually necessary to void about 30 minutes later. Using this knowledge, the nurse can begin to set up

---

33-7

Bladder retraining

Establish patient's usual voiding patterns.
Plan toileting based on the patient's usual pattern; assist patient as necessary.
If no voiding pattern can be determined, plan toileting for every 1 to 2 hours.
Encourage patient to use normal toileting position.
Encourage patient to empty bladder completely.
Provide for a fluid intake of 3000 ml/day for adequate urine volume.
Schedule most fluids to be taken before 4 PM.

---

a schedule for placing the person on a bedpan or taking the person to the toilet. Then if a record is kept for a few days of the times the person voids involuntarily, it is usually possible to determine the normal voiding pattern. If the schedule based on the pattern of incontinence is not successful, toileting every 1 to 2 hours should be carried out on a 24-hour basis.

During the retraining program, *mobilization* of the individual, attention to the *position* assumed for voiding, and adequate *fluid intake* contribute to reduction of the possibility of infection. Complete emptying of the bladder eliminates the possibility of residual urine acting as a medium for bacterial growth; a high fluid intake provides for internal bladder irrigation.

Elderly persons isolated from their families and familiar surroundings, confused by institutionalization, or suffering feelings of loss of self-esteem frequently respond well to mobilization in bladder retraining programs. Their circulation is enhanced by the imposed mobility, their awareness is increased, and they respond to the attention given them. In instances in which nurses believe that it is easier to change bed linen than it is to establish an appropriate bladder retraining program, a disservice is done to the individual and more work is actually created for the nurse. The person becomes subject to UTI and skin breakdown, and feelings of worthlessness are increased. For those who can be continent, incontinence is an indignity.

When possible, toileting should be carried out in surroundings that remind the person of the voiding function. Take the person to the bathroom to use the toilet; if this is not possible, a bedside commode can be an adequate substitute. A bedpan is unfamiliar and most people find using one distasteful. Many men can void into a urinal more easily if allowed to stand at the bedside. For women who must remain in bed, voiding into a bedpan can be facilitated if the head of the bed is elevated, a position more consistent with normal voiding and one that facilitates complete bladder emptying. Few persons can void adequately in the supine position.

Providing adequate amounts of fluids, a minimum of 3000 ml per day, is necessary to ensure that there will be adequate amounts of urine produced and present in the bladder to stimulate the voiding reflex at the proper times. Fluids may be given at scheduled times, the largest portion

The Elderly with Urinary Problems

Assessment

Determine urinary habits, especially if patient has any difficulty with urinary control.

Assess for mobility problems, diuretics, or mental changes that may contribute to functional (environmental) incontinence.

Assess for signs of urinary tract infections, commonly experienced by elderly women and men. Usual signs of fever and pain or burning with urination may be minimal or absent; confusion and anorexia may be the only symptoms.

Monitor kidney function when elderly undergo extensive testing that may lead to dehydration, which can compromise marginal kidney function in some elderly persons.

Intervention

Refer person with incontinence to a physician for further work-up; this condition is *not* a normal concommitant of aging.

Give diuretics early in day so patient will not need to use toilet frequently after bedtime.

Arrange environment to facilitate toileting, such as moving furniture, using bedside commode, ensuring grab bars by the toilet (or raised seat), and keeping call light within reach.

Schedule fluid intake to match toileting time, about every 2 hours while awake.

Maintain patient's usual routines as much as possible.

Limit stimulants such as coffee and tea.

Plan for increased need for toileting if patient is receiving intravenous therapy.

Try to avoid use of urinary catheters; if catheter is necessary, use good aseptic technique to prevent urinary tract infection.

Teach patient to report to health care provider any change in the urine or presence of blood; be aware that the patient may not be able to monitor own urine if vision is diminished.

Common disorders in Elderly

Urinary incontinence
Urinary tract infections
Benign prostatic hyperplasia
Cancer of kidney, bladder, or prostate
Renal failure

---

being given during the day before 4 PM to decrease the frequency of voiding through the night. Persons on fluid restriction because of medical problems should, of course, receive no more fluids than the amount prescribed.

Maintaining skin integrity

Meticulous skin care is absolutely essential when caring for the person with urinary incontinence. Without proper cleansing, the person will be subject to skin breakdown, which, as a result of continued incontinence, is extremely difficult to heal. When a person who is incontinent also has a diminished level of consciousness, he or she should be assessed frequently to ensure dryness. A person who has been incontinent must be cleaned and dried immediately.

Low airflow beds help to control skin breakdown in immobile patients. This therapy offers some hope in the care of the bedridden incontinent person. The protective cover of the bed provides a one-way barrier that draws water away from the patient and assists in keeping the patient dry. The airflow also aids in drying the skin.

Facilitating positive body image

Encourge patient to discuss feelings and frustrations concerning incontinence and involve family members in activities when possible. Offer reassurance, encouragement, and concrete information regarding management, especially about those activities that are within the patient's control. Be realistic with the patient. If incontinence cannot be controlled, reassure patient that odor and discomfort can be controlled, such as by maintenance of good hygiene, use and frequent changes of incontinence pads, and frequent changes of undergarments as necessary.

Scheduling fluids to decrease probability of incontinence at selected times, such as social activities or when a toilet is not readily available, also helps to maintain a positive body image. Fluids can be limited before the desired times and increased at other periods of the day so that the desired 3000 ml of fluids are ingested in the 24-hour period.

Teaching patient and family

Because the patient, often with family assistance, is usually involved in control of urinary continence, teaching is an important aspect of patient care. Explanation of the rationale for activities such as toileting schedule, mobility, and fluid requirements will increase the probability of the person following through with the activities.

Persons can be taught *perineal exercises* to help control mild stress incontinence. The exercises consist of tightening and relaxing perineal and gluteal muscles and can be performed in a number of ways. Much of the problem of incontinence caused by a relaxed perineum in women can be prevented if perineal exercises are taught before and following childbirth. These exercises also may be included as part of the health teaching of any woman. Following are different methods for performing perineal exercises.

1. Tighten the perineal muscles as if to prevent voiding. Hold for a count of 10, then relax (Kegel exercises, see Chapter 35).
2. Inhale through pursed lips while tightening perineal muscles.
3. Bear down as if to have a bowel movement. Relax then tighten perineal muscles.
4. Hold a pencil in the fold between the buttock and thigh.
5. Sit on toilet with knees held wide apart. Start and stop the urinary stream.

Additional teaching includes care of any drainage systems, measures to maintain skin integrity, and signs and symptoms of urinary tract infection (frequency, dysuria) that should be reported to the physician.

Evaluation

Evaluation is based on expected patient outcomes. Questions to consider may include the following:

1. Is the patient achieving optimal urinary control?
2. Is the patient's skin free of any excoriation?
3. Is the patient making comments that suggest a more positive body image?
4. Can the patient describe maintenance of any necessary equipment, bladder retraining or how to do perineal exercises (if appropriate), measures to maintain skin integrity, and plans for follow-up care?

URINARY TRACT INFECTION

Etiology/Epidemiology

Urinary tract infection (UTI) is a significant source of morbidity in the United States and plays a significant role in the development of chronic renal failure. Infection occurs in both acute and chronic stages in all portions of the urinary tract. Females appear more predisposed to UTI than males. Factors postulated in their higher infection rates include a shorter urethra that is closer to the rectum and the lack of the prostatic fluid protection that is present in the male. Infection rates for females approximate 1% of school-aged girls and 4% of women through the childbearing years.[15] Incidence of infection in females increases directly with sexual activity and with aging. Pregnancy does not seem to increase infection rates, although spontaneous clearing of infections is decreased during pregnancy, and there is a higher incidence of acute kidney infections progressing upward from the lower urinary tract.

Factors contributing to UTI are summarized in Table 33-4. Structural and functional abnormalities of the urinary tract, obstruction of the flow of urine, and impaired bladder innervation promote UTI. Mechanisms involved include stasis of urine, which provides a culture medium for bacteria, reflux of infected urine higher into the urinary tract, and increasing hydrostatic pressure.

Urinary tract infections may occur in the upper portion of the urinary tract (pyelonephritis) or in the lower urinary tract (cystitis, urethritis). Most infections in the lower urinary tract result from gram-negative organisms, such as *Escherichia coli*, *Klebsiella*, *Proteus*, *Enterobacter*, *Pseudomonas*, or *Serratia*, that originate in the person's own intestinal tract and ascend through the urethra to the bladder. *Staphylococcus saprophyticus* is a gram-positive organism that appears to affect young women, particularly in summer and autumn. The yeast *Candida albicans* tends to affect persons who are debilitated by other disease or who are taking immunosuppressive medications. *Candida* found in the urine is significant because this organism is associated with sepsis and death.

Escherichia coli is the most common organism identified with pyelonephritis. Acute pyelonephritis is usually caused by bacterial infection but may also develop as a result of seeding of bacteria from the bloodstream. Chronic pyelonephritis also results from a bacterial infection; however,

Table 33-4   Risk factors associated with development of UTI

Risk factor	Common examples
Female	Short urethra
Structural abnormality	Strictures
	Incompetent ureterovesical junction anomalies
Obstruction	Tumors
	Prostatic hypertrophy
	Calculi
	Iatrogenic causes
Impaired bladder innervation	Congenital spinal cord malformation
	Spinal cord injury
	Multiple sclerosis
Chronic disease	Gout
	Diabetes mellitus
	Hypertension
	Sickle cell disease
	Chronic renal disease
Instrumentation	Catheterization
	Diagnostic procedures

other factors such as urinary reflux and urinary tract obstruction also play a part.

Prevention
Primary prevention

Three considerations are important in preventing infection of the urinary tract: (1) preventing or minimizing morbidity that can accompany these infections, (2) preventing recurrence of the infection, and (3) preventing renal damage from untreated or inadequately treated ascending infection. Certain chronic health problems predispose persons to UTI by changing the metabolism of tissues, creating extrarenal obstructions, and altering the function and structure of kidney tissue. Common among these health problems are diabetes mellitus, gout, hypertension, polycystic kidney disease, and glomerulonephritis. Control of these disorders decreases the potential for UTI.

Instrumentation of the urinary tract is associated with high rates of infection. Catheterization, even when performed without breaks in asepsis, results in significant infection of the bladder. *Nosocomial infections* account for a sizable percentage of all UTIs. Drug-resistant strains of *Staphylococcus* and *Psuedomonas*, along with various other organisms commonly found in hospitals, are frequently involved in nosocomial UTIs. Prevention and control of all urinary infections can be influenced most significantly by lowering this nosocomial infection rate.

Primary prevention of UTI also includes teaching females the importance of wiping the perineal area from front to back to minimize the risk of introducing fecal flora into the urinary tract. Uncircumcized males should clean the glans of the penis daily to reduce the risk of accumulation of bacteria under the foreskin.

Secondary prevention

Although the great majority of noncomplicated urinary infections are asymptomatic and clear spontaneously, there

Table 33-5 Urinary tract infections

Disorder	Signs and symptoms	Medical therapy
Pyelonephritis	Sudden fever, chills Costovertebral tenderness Leukocytosis WBCs in urine	Antibiotics Bed rest for acute episode Hydration
Cystitis/urethritis (lower UTI)	Urgency Frequency Dysuria Suprapubic discomfort Cloudy urine with WBCs	Antibiotics Hydration
Prostatitis	Fever Chills Low back pain Perineal pain Urgency Frequency Dysuria Tender prostate Urethral discharge	Antibiotics Bed rest for acute episodes Sexual abstention Analgesics Stool softeners Sitz baths

remains a portion significant enough to warrant consideration as a health problem. There is no controversy among those practicing preventive health care regarding the question of the need for screening of asymptomatic infections; however, there exists difficulty in identifying the specific risk groups in which the detection and treatment of these infections yield significant improvement in the person's health. As health care becomes more oriented toward prevention, specific target populations will be better defined and the number of screening programs for asymptomatic UTI will increase.

Anyone with symptoms of dysuria, cloudy urine, or frequent small voidings should be examined for UTI and treated appropriately to prevent extension of a lower UTI into the kidney. Persons complaining of fever and costovertebral tenderness should be encouraged to seek medical attention for early treatment of pyelonephritis, thus preventing further kidney damage.

Pathophysiology
Pyelonephritis

Infection usually begins in the lower urinary tract and ascends into the kidneys. After the bacteria reach the kidney, they begin to multiply in the medullary interstitial tissue and renal tubules. As infection develops, an inflammatory exudate accumulates in the interstitium. The renal tubules become necrotic and the renal cortex may also become inflamed. The glomerular capillaries, however, are usually spared from the inflammatory process. Pockets of infection (renal abscess) develop and are distributed throughout the renal medulla or the entire kidney. After the acute inflammation subsides, healing begins through the formation of scar tissue.[43]

The clinical manifestations of acute pyelonephritis are those of inflammation and range from no symptoms to a sudden onset of fever, chills, costovertebral (flank) pain, and suprapubic tenderness (Table 33-5). Because acute pyelonephritis may cause symptoms similar to cystitis, it is extremely difficult to identify renal involvement solely on the basis of symptoms. Differentiation between upper and lower UTIs is essential for therapeutic management.[43]

Chronic pyelonephritis destroys renal tissue permanently through repeated inflammation and scarring. The process of developing chronic renal failure from repeated kidney infections occurs over a number of years or after several extensive and fulminant infections. It is estimated that pyelonephritis represents the original diagnosis in one third of all persons with chronic renal failure.

Lower urinary tract infection

Whenever stasis of urine occurs, such as with incomplete emptying of the bladder, renal calculi, or genitourinary obstructions, the bacteria have a greater opportunity to grow and a more alkaline media, which favors their growth and multiplication.

UTI occurs primarily when host resistance is impaired. The major factors in preventing a UTI are tissue integrity and blood supply. A break in the surface of the mucous membrane lining permits the bacteria to invade the tissue and cause infection. Breaks in tissue integrity result from erosions caused by tips of in-dwelling catheters or rough-edged renal stones, from neoplasms, or from invasion of the tissue by parasites such as Schistosoma. In the bladder, blood supply to the tissues can be compromised when the pressure within the bladder is markedly increased, as may occur with overdistention of the bladder, contracture of the bladder neck, or obstruction of the urethra by an enlarged prostate, metastatic growth, or urethral stricture.

The symptoms that bring the person to medical attention typically include urinary urgency, burning on urination (dysuria), and slight to gross hematuria. Most persons, however, are asymptomatic or minimally symptomatic, the infection being identified only on routine examination of the urine. Bacteriuria and positive urine cultures serve as

Table 33-6   Urinalysis

Test	Normal	Abnormal
Color	Amber-yellow	Red indicates hematuria (possible urinary obstruction, renal calculi, tumor, renal failure)
Clarity	Clear	Cloudy: debris, bacterial sediment (urinary infection)
pH	4.6-8 (average 6)	Alkaline on standing or with UTI
		Increased acidity with renal tubular acidosis
Specific gravity	1.003-1.035	Usually reflects fluid intake; the less the fluid intake, the higher the specific gravity
		If specific gravity remains low (1.010-1.014), renal disease is suspected
Protein	0-8 mg/dl	Proteinuria may occur with high-protein diet and exercise (particularly prolonged)
		Seen in renal disease
Sugar	0	Glycosuria occurs after a high intake of sugar or with diabetes mellitus
Ketones	0	Ketonuria occurs with starvation and diabetic ketoacidosis
Red blood cells	0-4	Injury to kidney tissue (see hematuria)
White blood cells	0-5	Urinary tract infection (UTI)
Casts	0	UTI, renal disease

the basis for diagnosing a lower UTI. Growth of a single pathogen in excess of 1×10^5 organisms/ml of urine in a properly obtained and stored midstream specimen indicates infection.

Nursing Process
Assessment
Subjective data

Specific questions are directed at eliciting presence of abnormal findings. *Dysuria* is often described as "burning with urination" and is usually associated with *frequency* and *urgency* (see Box 33-8) when a UTI is present. Ask the patient about the approximate amount of urine at each voiding: small amounts may be caused by infection whereas large amounts may be the result of increased fluid intake or a diuretic. Frequency associated with suprapubic discomfort and sense of fullness is more likely to be caused by retention with overflow (p. 1020). *Nocturia* may accompany frequency; if present, ask the number of times this occurs per night, amount of fluid taken over 24 hours (especially during the evening), and if this is a change from the usual pattern.

Pain resulting from urinary disorders is located in different areas depending on the organ involved. Pain from the kidney is usually experienced in the flank over the kidney site in the back between the twelfth rib and the iliac crest (costovertebral angle). Pain from the ureters may begin over the kidney area but then radiates to the front along the course of the ureter and down into the groin. Pain from the bladder is usually suprapubic.

Additional data seen with pyelonephritis include history of chills and fever, nausea or vomiting, and fatigue and anorexia.

Objective data

Assess body temperature for fever because fever is indicative of infection. Although fever caused by pyelonephritis can spike to high temperatures, this may not occur in older persons. Inspect the urine for color and clarity, which can indicate the presence of bacteria. The urine

33-8	**Urinary symptoms**	
	Dysuria	Painful urination
	Frequency	Voiding at frequent intervals
	Urgency	Need to void immediately
	Hesitancy	Difficulty initiating voiding
	Nocturia	Awakening at night with need to void

will generally be cloudy from precipitate of phosphate salts in an alkaline urine or from bacterial growth. A urinary or vaginal discharge may also give the urine a cloudy appearance.

Diagnostic tests
Urinalysis

Ideally, the urine specimen is collected from the first voiding of the day. This sample is preferable because it is concentrated and abnormal constitutents are more likely to be present. Cleansing the meatus before collecting the specimen decreases the likelihood of external contamination; mild soap followed by water or a special antiseptic solution may be used. About 50 to 100 ml of urine is sufficient to determine specific gravity in addition to microscopic analysis (see Table 33-6). WBCs, bacteria, and pus may be identified with UTI. Protein may be noted with pyelonephritis, especially with chronic infection. If the urine cannot be analyzed immediately, the specimen must be refrigerated to retard bacterial growth.

Urine culture

Urine cultures are used to confirm suspected infections, to identify causative organisms, and to determine appropriate antimicrobial therapy. Cultures are also obtained for periodic screening of urine when the threat of UTI persists.

A sample of urine that has been properly collected and

33-9

Directions for collecting a midstream urine specimen

Equipment needed

Sterile container for the urine
Three sponges (cotton or gauze) saturated with
   cleansing solution

General directions

Only outside of collecting container is touched
Urine is collected in container well after urinary
   stream is started

Special directions
Female

Labia are kept separated throughout procedure
Meatus is cleansed with one front-to-back motion
   with each of the three cleansing sponges

Male

Foreskin is retracted if man is uncircumcised
Glans is cleansed with each of the three cleansing
   sponges

stored is considered to be normal if it contains 10,000 or fewer organisms per milliliter. Organisms of this magnitude are the result of normal urethral flora and do not signify UTI. A UTI is diagnosed when bacterial counts in a properly collected and stored sample reach *100,000 or more organisms per milliliter* and the organisms are of one or very largely one bacterial type.[47] Contamination of the urine specimen during collection is most likely when bacterial counts include predominant colonies of *Staphylococcus, Streptococcus,* and diphtheroids, when two or more organisms contribute significantly to the total bacterial count, or when repeated cultures yield differing results. All these results indicate a need to repeat the culture, with particular attention to the collection of the specimen and to its handling.

Specimens for urine culture may be obtained either by catheterization or by midstream voiding (see Box 33-9). It should be made clear, however, that *urethral catheterization should never be used routinely in collecting urine for culture because of the risk of introducing additional bacteria into the bladder.* Catheterization may be necessary to obtain a sterile urine specimen when the person is unable to void after being adequately hydrated or if the person is incontinent of urine. When a catheter is passed, meticulous attention is given to nontraumatic aseptic technique. After urine flow from the catheter is established, 5 to 10 ml of urine should be collected directly into a sterile specimen container. Care must be taken to ensure that the rim and the inside of the container are not touched by the catheter or by the hands. If a culture tube with a cotton plug is used as specimen container, care must be taken to keep the tube upright to prevent moistening the cotton and thereby contaminating the specimen. Cultures may also be ordered on the urine taken from the renal pelvis during ureteral cath-

eterization or when ureterostomy or nephrostomy tubes are in place.

In collecting a voided specimen for culture, the nurse must decide if the patient is capable of independently obtaining the specimen or if nursing or medical personnel will need to collect a midstream specimen. Most persons who are ambulatory and are given precise and unhurried direction will be able to collect their own midstream urine specimen.

The first voided specimen of the day should be used whenever possible because bacteria will be more numerous. If the specimen is not cultured immediately, refrigeration is mandatory to prevent growth of organisms in the specimen.

Other tests

A noninvasive technique used in localizing the *precise* site of infection involves determining the presence of antibody-coated bacteria (ACB) in the urine of patients with UTI. The existence of ACB in urine correlates closely with the incidence of upper UTI; persons with lower UTI do not show ACB in their urine. *Blood cultures* may also be necessary to identify the source of infection.

Renal function tests (Table 33-7) may be performed to determine the effect of kidney infection on renal function. If renal damage is extensive with chronic pyelonephritis, BUN and serum creatinine will be elevated. *Radiologic examinations* and *renal biopsy* (p. 1037) may be required to make a differential diagnosis in chronic pyelonephritis.

A more extensive urologic workup, including intravenous pyelogram (IVP) and voiding cystogram, may be performed for men and young children after a repeated or even first UTI, or when infection does not abate. This workup is performed on women when infection occurs repeatedly or cannot be cleared up with treatment. The rationale for this extensive workup is that a UTI is not common in men and young children and that a significant portion of infections in these populations involve abnormality of the urinary tract.

Data analysis: nursing diagnoses

Nursing diagnoses are determined from analysis of patient data. Possible nursing diagnoses for the person with UTI may include, but are not limited to, the following:

Diagnostic title	Possible etiologies
Infection, high risk for	Catheterization, alkaline urine
Pain: costovertebral, suprapubic, perineal	Urinary tract infection
Knowledge deficit	Lack of information

Planning: expected patient outcomes

Expected patient outcomes for the patient with UTI may include, but are not limited to, the following:

1. Further infection has been avoided.
2. Verbalizes relief of symptoms.
3. States feeling comfortable.
4. Describes antibiotic regimen, need for high fluid intake, symptoms to report to physician, and plan for follow-up care as indicated.

Table 33-7   **Selected renal function tests**

Test	Normal results	Purpose/significance	Nursing implications
Specific gravity of urine	1.010-1.026	Measures ability of kidneys to concentrate urine	First morning void is usually in the high normal range in healthy individual. False high is caused by presence of radiographic dyes
Osmolality of urine	400-600 mOsm/kg	Excellent indication of renal function. Osmolality is total concentration of particles in solution	No special preparation
Urine chemistries	Sodium: 130-220 mEq/L Potassium: 39-90 mg/24 hrs Calcium: 100-300 mg/24 hrs	Urine electrolytes reflect ability of kidney to excrete and reabsorb electrolytes	Abnormal results may be caused by disease processes other than renal disorders, for example, elevated urine calcium in hyperparathyroidism or prolonged immobilization
Creatinine clearance	Men: 100-150 ml/min Women: 85-125 ml/min	Clearance is rate at which a substance is excreted in terms of plasma concentration. Because diet and metabolic state have little influence on it, serum creatinine is excellent for determining glomerular filtration rate.	Procedure 1. Patient empties bladder and time is noted 2. *All* urine is saved for 24 hours 3. Exactly 24 hours after start of procedure the patient voids and specimen is saved 4. Total urine volume and urine creatinine is measured 5. Serum creatinine is determined at end of 24-hour period 6. Creatinine clearance is then calculated by formula: $$\text{Clearance: } \frac{UV^*}{P^*}$$ *U = Urine creatinine concentration *V = Urine volume *P = Plasma creatinine concentration
Serum creatinine	Men: 0.85-1.5 mg/dl Women: 0.70-1.25 mg/dl	Indicates ability of kidneys to excrete nitrogenous wastes	No specific preparation for test. Diet and metabolic rate have little effect on serum creatinine
Blood urea nitrogen (BUN)	5-20 mg/dl	Indicates ability of kidneys to excrete nitrogenous wastes. BUN gives a rough estimate of GFR	BUN can be affected by high-protein diet, blood in GI tract, catabolic state (injury, infection)

Implementation

Assisting with achievement of therapeutic goals

Monitoring

Monitor the vital signs of a person with pyelonephritis every 4 hours; chills and fever associated with hypotension and tachycardia can be indicative of sepsis and bacteremic shock. Report increased flank or suprapubic pain, or foul-smelling or cloudy urine to the physician immediately.

Administering antibiotics

Medications commonly used in the treatment of UTI include antibiotics such as ciprofloxacin (Cipro) and trimethoprim-sulfamethoxazole (Bactrim). Administer antibiotics on time as prescribed to maintain adequate blood levels. If given intravenously, have prescribed antibiotic serum levels drawn at the correct times to ensure reliable results. Most antibiotics are measured at peak levels (30-60 minutes after infusion) and trough levels (30-60 minutes before the next dose).

Maintaining hydration

Encourage fluid intake of at least 3000 ml/day unless contraindicated by oliguria or other symptoms of renal failure. Increased fluids dilute the urine, which (1) prevents crystallization of sulfonamides, (2) provides a continual flow of urine to discourage urine stasis with multiplication of bacteria, (3) helps wash away ascending bacteria, and (4) lessens dysuria.

Interventions to achieve patient outcomes

Preventing further infection

Use urinary catheterization *only* when mandatory. If needed, use meticulous sterile technique during insertion and irrigation. Follow guidelines for maintaining drainage (p. 1023) to prevent reflux of urine. Provide perineal care at least every shift and as needed. Offer the patient cranberry, plum, or prune juices, which acidify the urine; bacteria do not grow in an acidic medium.

Promoting comfort

Medicate as prescribed for flank or suprapubic pain. Sitz baths may provide some relief from urethritis. Back massages often provide short-term relief. High fluid intake can help relieve the urinary "burning" feeling of a lower UTI.

Facilitating patient learning

Patient teaching is important and includes the following:
1. Take the antibiotics for the prescribed period, even after symptoms abate; infection may still be present even if asymptomatic. The course of antibiotic therapy may extend over weeks.
2. Report for urine cultures as instructed (usually 2

weeks after drug therapy is discontinued and possibly every month thereafter for several months).
3. Maintain a fluid intake of at least 3 quarts or L/day.
4. Monitor urinary output and report decreased output (may indicate decreased renal function).
5. Report signs of recurrence to physician (flank pain, chills, and fever for pyelonephritis; dysuria, frequency, and urgency for lower UTI).

Evaluation

Evaluation is based on expected patient outcomes. Questions to consider may include the following:
1. Has further infection been avoided?
2. Is the patient free of fever and pain?
3. Can the patient explain the reason for a fluid intake of at least 3000 ml/day and describe plans to follow this?
4. Can the patient describe the antibiotic regimen, need to continue taking the medication, and report for follow-up urine cultures?

33-10

Classification of glomerular diseases

Primary glomerulonephritis

Acute diffuse proliferative glomerulonephritis
Rapidly progressive glomerulonephritis
Membranous glomerulonephritis
Minimal change disease
Membranoproliferative glomerulonephritis
Chronic glomerulonephritis

Secondary to systemic diseases

Systemic lupus erythematosus
Goodpasture's disease
Wegener's granulomatosis
Bacterial endocarditis
Diabetes mellitus

GLOMERULAR DISORDERS

Glomerular disorders, which are a group of diseases that result from injury to the glomeruli, are termed *glomerulonephritis*. The glomerulus plays an essential role in the functioning of the kidneys; therefore, any injury to the glomerulus is likely to result in some change in renal functioning.

There are several different diseases of the glomerulus resulting in a number of classification systems to assist in defining glomerulonephritis[1] (see Box 33-10). For purposes of discussion, in this chapter glomerulonephritis is discussed as either acute or chronic; the nephrotic syndrome is described as a component of glomerulonephritis. Table 33-8 provides a summary of the major glomerular disorders, including etiology, signs and symptoms, and medical therapy.

REVIEW

Table 33-8   **Glomerular disorders**

Disorder	Signs and symptoms	Urine Characteristics	Medical therapy
Acute glomerulonephritis	Headache, malaise, facial edema, mild fever, flank pain, oliguria, shortness of breath, elevated BUN and creatinine	Protein 1-3+, casts, blood	No specific therapy; antibiotics for residual streptococcus, bed rest, dietary protein and sodium restriction as needed
Chronic glomerulonephritis	Usually asymptomatic initially, hypertension; may progress to renal failure	Albumin, casts, blood	No specific therapy; treatment for exacerbation of acute episodes
Nephrotic syndrome	Massive edema with anorexia, fatigue, shortness of breath, hypoalbuminemia, hyperlipidemia	Large amount of protein, casts	No specific therapy; bed rest and corticosteroids for severe edema

ACUTE GLOMERULONEPHRITIS

Etiology/Epidemiology

Glomerulonephritis (GN) is a disease that affects the glomeruli of both kidneys. Etiologic factors are many and varied; they include immunologic reactions (lupus erythematosus, streptococcal infection), vascular injury (hypertension), metabolic disease (diabetes mellitus), and disseminated intravascular coagulation (DIC). Glomerulonephritis exists in acute, latent, and chronic forms. The most common form of *acute glomerulonephritis* occurs 1 to 2 weeks after a streptococcal infection. Common sites of infection include the throat (tonsillitis, strep throat) and the skin (impetigo).

School-aged children and adolescents are most likely to develop the illness. The prognosis of acute poststreptococcal glomerulonephritis (APSGN) is generally good; however, some patients develop chronic GN and end-stage renal disease, requiring dialysis or transplantation.[22]

Pathophysiology

Normal glomerular membranes consist of three types of cells: epithelium, basement membrane, and endothelium. Any or all three of these cells may be affected by glomerulonephritis. Acute glomerulonephritis is the result of an antigen-antibody reaction with glomerular tissue that produces swelling and death to capillary cells. The antigen-antibody reaction activates the complement pathway, resulting in chemotaxis of polymorphonuclear (PMN) leukocytes with release of lysosomal enzymes that attack the glomerular basement membrane (GBM). (Leukocytosis is a common symptom.) The response in the GBM is an increase in the three types of glomerular cells. The various disease entities tend to attack specific cells, therefore, differential diagnosis is usually made by renal biopsy. The ability to make a differential diagnosis has been greatly aided by the tremendous increase in knowledge about the immune system.

Signs and symptoms reflect *damage to the glomeruli* with leaking into urine by protein (proteinuria) and red cells (hematuria). As the disease process continues, scarring occurs, leading to *decreased glomerular filtration* producing oliguria and retention of water, sodium, and nitrogenous wastes (increased BUN and serum creatinine level). This results in fluid overloading, edema, and azotemia as noted by shortness of breath, edema, hypertension, headache, weakness, and anorexia. Elevated antistreptolysis O (ASO) titers are encountered in APSGN; however, no relationship exists between the rise in ASO titer and the incidence or severity of APSGN.[43]

Nursing Process

Assessment

Subjective data

The person with acute glomerulonephritis is likely to present with some signs and symptoms of renal failure, and should be assessed for changes in voiding patterns and presence of headaches and flank pain. The person may complain of recent flulike symptoms and a sore throat.

Objective data

Objective data include evaluation of the extent of fluid retention and characteristics of the urine, as a baseline for ongoing assessment and evaluation:

1. Breath sounds, for signs of rales (crackles)
2. Edema of legs, sacrum, periorbital areas
3. Body weight: weigh daily for increase
4. Blood pressure, for elevations
5. Urine, for signs of increased blood, cloudiness, casts, increased specific gravity

Diagnostic tests

The most important immediate diagnostic test is urinalysis to determine presence of proteinuria, hematuria, and cellular debris. BUN and serum creatinine are obtained to determine renal function. Immunologic tests such as antigen-antibody titers, immunoelectrophoresis and ASO may be obtained.

A composite urine for creatinine clearance and protein can also provide important information. Instructions for obtaining a composite urine specimen are provided in Box 33-11.

Renal biopsy

The differential diagnosis for glomerulonephritis can often be difficult to establish. A renal biopsy may be necessary to assist in diagnosis and establishing a definitive treatment plan. The biopsy can be performed either through a skin puncture (closed biopsy) or through an incision (open biopsy). The use of a fluoroscopic guided needle biopsy now allows for most renal biopsies to be obtained by the closed method.

Inherent in taking a biopsy specimen of this vascular tissue is the potential threat of hemorrhage. Throughout the procedure, care is taken to prevent and to detect early loss of blood. Before biopsy is performed, a thorough med-

---

33-11

Instructions for composite urine specimen

1. The bladder is emptied and the urine *discarded* at the time appointed to start the test.
2. Urine from *all* subsequent voidings is saved.
3. Specific directions for storing the urine should be given. Some specimens need to be kept cold during the collection period, some need preservatives added, some need no special care.
4. The person should void into a separate receptacle before defecation to prevent contamination of the specimen.
5. The bladder is emptied and the urine *added* to the collection at the appointed time to end the test.
6. The designated amount (properly labeled) is sent to the laboratory.
7. If an aliquot (5-10 ml sample of the total specimen) is the designated amount, the total amount collected is (1) measured and recorded on the specimen requisition and (2) mixed well before the aliquot is selected.

ical evaluation with particular attention to detection of any abnormality in bleeding or coagulation time is carried out. The patient's blood is usually typed and cross-matched with 2 units of blood; the blood is held for the patient until any threat of bleeding has passed.

An open biopsy carries less risk of hemorrhage and provides better visualization of the kidney; however, the risk of infection is increased, and a longer period of recovery is required.

Preprocedure care. Preparation before biopsy includes discussing the procedure with the patient. Topics covered include the necessity for the examination, the procedure itself, the care to be anticipated, and any questions of concern to the patient. The preparation of the patient is shared by the physician and nurse. In most institutions it is necessary to have the patient sign a special permit before having the biopsy performed. The biopsy may be carried out in the patient's room, in the radiology department, or in the operating room.

Procedure. Before *percutaneous (closed) biopsy*, the patient is taken to the radiology department for localization of the kidney by a plain film, a dye contrast film, or fluoroscopic location. The position of the kidney in relation to body landmarks is marked on the skin in ink. The lower pole of the kidney is located for biopsy site because it contains the fewest number of large vessels. The patient is then transported to the area where the biopsy will be performed. Sedation is usually not required except for children or adults who are restless and unable to relax sufficiently to follow necessary instructions during the test. The patient is placed prone over a sandbag or firm pillow and an additional soft pillow. The body is bent at the level of the diaphragm, with the shoulders on the bed and the spine in straight alignment. The physician identifies the location for biopsy, and a local anesthetic agent is injected. As the biopsy is being taken, the patient is instructed to hold his or her breath. Pain may be felt in the kidney region as the tissue sample is taken. The needle is withdrawn immediately, and direct pressure is applied to the site for 20 minutes. A pressure bandage is then applied.

Postprocedure care. After the procedure the patient is turned supine and is kept flat and motionless for 4 hours. One small pillow may be used under the head. Coughing and other activity that increases abdominal venous pressure is to be avoided during this time. Blood pressure and pulse are taken each 15 minutes for 1 hour, every 30 minutes during the next hour, and every hour for an additional 2 to 3 hours to assess for hemorrhage. The patient should remain in bed for at least 24 hours following the procedure.

Liberal intake of fluids is encouraged to help maintain a dilute urine and prevent intrarenal clot formation. Serial urine specimens should be obtained to evaluate hematuria.[22] Bed rest is maintained until the urine is clear. Initially, the urine is likely to demonstrate blood, but this rarely continues after a 24-hour period.

Complications include persistent hematuria, perirenal or intrarenal arteriovenous fistula, aneurysm, and laceration of organs or blood vessels adjacent to the biopsied kidney.[22]

Data analysis: nursing diagnoses

Nursing diagnoses are determined from analysis of patient data. Possible nursing diagnoses for the person with acute glomerulonephritis may include, but are not limited to, the following:

Diagnostic title	Possible etiologies
Fluid volume excess	Compromised regulatory mechanism, excess fluid intake, excess sodium intake
Infection, high risk for	Decreased immune response
Knowledge deficit	Lack of information

Planning: expected patient outcomes

Expected patient outcomes for the person with acute glomerulonephritis may include, but are not limited to, the following:
1. Maintains fluid balance as near normal as possible.
2. Maintains stable weight from day to day.
3. Maintains vital signs close to normal limits.
4. Does not acquire any infection.
5. Describes nature of illness, therapeutic regimen, signs and symptoms indicating medical attention, and need for follow-up care.

Implementation
Assisting with achievement of therapeutic goals

The care of the person with acute glomerulonephritis can be complex because of the overall ramifications of the disease.

Control of infection

Persistent infection is treated promptly to help further decrease antigen-antibody complex formation. Persons with poststreptococcal glomerulonephritis are given a prophylactic antibiotic; the drug of choice is penicillin. Rationale for this therapy is based on preventing futher infections that could reactivate the nephritis. Prophylactic therapy may be continued for months after the acute phase of illness.

Activity

Bed rest is instituted until clinical signs disappear; this may involve a period of several months. Ambulation is allowed when blood sedimentation rates and blood pressure are normal and edema abates. If ambulation causes an increase in proteinuria or hematuria, bed rest is reinstituted. Because the period of bed rest may be long and the person usually does not feel ill, the nurse may need to continue reinforcing the importance of bed rest and assist in planning diversionary activities. When bed rest is reinstituted after periods of ambulation, the person may become depressed. Helping the person to express concerns and feelings can serve as a basis for helping to make realistic plans about the illness and its sequelae.

Maintenance of fluid balance

Edema and fluid overloading are anticipated and treated initially with dietary sodium restrictions. Remember that water follows sodium; restricting sodium decreases fluid retention. The amount of restriction depends on the severity of fluid retention, and it is maintained until dependent edema and circulatory overload are no longer a problem. Diuretics are generally reserved for managing severe fluid overload and pulmonary edema. The nurse is constantly alert for signs of fluid overload. Blood pressure elevation is treated with antihypertensive drugs only after fluid control has proved unsuccessful in controlling hypertension. Dietary protein is reduced only when BUN and creatinine levels are elevated. The diet should contain sufficient carbohydrate to prevent catabolism and thus maintain nitrogen balance.

Interventions to achieve patient outcomes
Preventing fluid volume excess

Keep strict records of fluid intake and output. Calculate the difference between fluid intake loss and determine the net fluid change.[43] Fluid restrictions must be maintained.

It is important to weigh the patient at least daily. Use a metric scale, if possible, because it is easier to calculate fluid changes. Balance the scale before each use and weigh the patient at the same time each day with the same clothing. Teach the patient how to obtain a correct weight, if necessary.

Take vital signs at least twice daily, including apical pulse. Listen for presence of a dysrhythmia. Assess for neck vein distention indicating fluid overload and congestive heart failure. Assess for periorbital, pretibial, pedal, and sacral edema. Measure edematous legs.

Administer diuretics when prescribed. Evaluate their efficacy and monitor for complications such as hypokalemia. Monitor the serum potassium levels closely, especially for those diuretics that eliminate potassium (see Chapter 25).

Preventing infection

Exposure to any infection must be avoided because even mild infections may reactivate nephritis. The patient must avoid contact with any persons with upper respiratory infections (URI). The patient should know to seek prompt medical treatment for sore throats and URIs. Cultures should be obtained and, when indicated, appropriate antibiotics should be prescribed.

Facilitating patient learning

Because of the long-term nature of glomerulonephritis, patient teaching is important. Proteinuria, hematuria, and cellular debris may exist microscopically even when other symptoms subside. Although fatigue may be present, these persons usually feel well; therefore, they often must be convinced of the need to continue prescribed treatment and to return for follow-up care. Teaching includes the following:

1. Nature of the illness and effect of diet and fluids on fluid balance and sodium retention.
2. Diet teaching regarding prescribed sodium and fluid restrictions (provide written information regarding sodium content of foods, as necessary).
3. Medication regimen (dose, frequency, side effects, need to continue as per physician instructions).
4. Need to pace activities with rest if fatigue is present.
5. Avoidance of trauma and infection (may exacerbate the illness).

6. Signs and symptoms indicating need for medical attention (hematuria, headache, edema, hypertension).
7. Importance of follow-up health care.

Evaluation

Evaluation is based on expected patient outcomes. Questions to consider may include the following:

1. Are signs of fluid retention decreased?
2. Is the person eating a balanced diet according to prescribed guidelines (low salt, sufficient carbohydrate)?
3. Has the person been following prescribed fluid restrictions?
4. Are there any signs of other infections?
5. Does the patient know the nature of the illness, therapeutic regimen, and need for follow-up health care?

CHRONIC GLOMERULONEPHRITIS
Etiology/Epidemiology

Although chronic glomerulonephritis (CGN) may follow the acute disease, the majority of persons give no history of the disease. In most instances no evidence of predisposing infection can be found. The course of chronic glomerulonephritis is extremely varied. Some persons with minimal impairment in renal function continue to feel well and show little progression of disease. With other individuals the progression of renal deterioration may be slow but steady and end in renal failure. In still other individuals the progression of disease is rapid.

Pathophysiology

CGN is characterized by slow progressive destruction (sclerosis) of glomeruli and gradual loss of renal function. The glomeruli have varying degrees of hypercellularity and become sclerosed (hardened) as the disease progresses. This results in decreased renal function and increased presentation of signs and symptoms of renal failure. The kidneys decrease in size; eventually there is tubular atrophy, chronic interstitial inflammation, and arteriosclerosis. The underlying pathophysiologic changes are the immune responses described for acute glomerulonephritis.

Various symptoms of *failing renal function*, none of which may seem severe, may lead the person to seek health care. There may be a slow onset of recurrent dependent *edema*, or there may be mild *headache*, especially in the morning. *Dyspnea on exertion* or difficulty sleeping in a flat position may be noted. *Blurring of vision* may lead the person to an ophthalmologist, who may be the first to suspect chronic renal disease based on ocular vascular changes. Occasionally, chronic nephritis is discovered during routine physical examination or may be discovered by a school nurse who observes marked visual changes and lassitude in a student. Early in the disease urinalysis shows the presence of albumin, casts, and blood. At this point renal function tests may be normal. The ability of the kidneys to regulate the internal environment will begin to decrease as more and more glomeruli become scarred and the amount of functional renal tissue is reduced. Finally, when few intact nephrons remain, hematuria and proteinuria decrease, the specific gravity of the urine becomes fixed, and the non-protein nitrogen level in the blood increases. Although the process is insidious and slow, CGN eventually results in end-stage renal disease. This may take 10 to 15 years.

Nursing Process
Assessment
Subjective data

General questions to ask include: (1) Have you experienced shortness of breath, headaches, weakness, or anorexia? (2) Have you noticed any change in your pattern of urination, either frequency or volume? and (3) Do you recall a recent infection of symptoms of a virus? It is also important to determine if there is a history of renal problems in the past.

Objective data

It is important to establish baseline vital signs including temperature, pulse, respirations, and blood pressure. Vital signs are assessed frequently, at least every 6 hours, until stable. The person is assessed daily for edema. Daily weighing is one of the best means of assessing the person's fluid status. Intake and output should be assessed at least every 8 hours until stable. The urine is assessed for color, clarity, specific gravity, and odor.

Diagnostic tests

Urinalysis is essential to determine the presence of proteinuria, hematuria, and cellular debris. BUN and serum creatinine are obtained to determine renal function. Immunologic tests such as antigen-antibody titers and immunoelectrophoresis may also be obtained. A composite urine for creatinine clearance and total protein can also provide important data about renal function. Renal biopsy (p. 1037) may be necessary to make the differential diagnosis.

Data analysis: nursing diagnoses

Nursing diagnoses are determined from analysis of patient data. Possible nursing diagnoses for the person with chronic glomerulonephritis may include, but are not limited to, the following:

Diagnostic title	Possible etiologies
Activity intolerance	Generalized weakness, electrolyte imbalance
Knowledge deficit	Lack of exposure/recall

Planning: expected patient outcomes

Expected patient outcomes for the patient with chronic glomerulonephritis may include, but are not limited, to the following:

1. Maintains bed rest as prescribed.
2. Obtains adequate rest.
3. Resumes usual activities within tolerance when permitted.
4. Describes medication and dietary regimen and need for follow-up care.

Implementation
Assisting with achievement of therapeutic goals

No specific therapy exists to arrest or reverse the disease process. With some forms of CGN, steroids and cytotoxic agents may be attempted, although results of these therapies in arresting disease are not well documented. Treatment of renal failure begins when the illness destroys so much kidney tissue that the individual's kidneys are no longer able to control the internal environment independently.

With any exacerbation of hematuria, hypertension, and edema, the person is put to bed, and treatment similar to that for acute glomerulonephritis is instituted. Signs of pulmonary edema and congestive heart failure (resulting from fluid retention) are monitored. Treatment is symptomatic and supportive.

Interventions to achieve patient outcomes
Promoting activity tolerance

During the period of enforced bed rest, assist the patient with ADL as necessary. Coordinate assessments and interventions to minimize interruptions and maximize rest. Place objects well within the patient's reach to avoid undue exertion. Provide bed exercises within the prescribed activity limitations to promote muscle strength and tone. After bed rest is no longer necessary, establish a progressive but gradual activity regimen that will help increase physical endurance.

Facilitating patient learning

The teaching for the person with chronic glomerulonephritis is the same as for acute glomerulonephritis (p. 1039). Care involves teaching the person to live healthfully, to avoid infections, to eat a balanced diet with moderate sodium intake if prescribed, to appropriately administer medication, and to maintain follow-up health care visits and report to the physician any exacerbations in signs and symptoms.

Women with CGN who become pregnant appear to be susceptible to toxemia and to spontaneous abortion. The woman who has had nephritis of any nature should be urged to see a physician if she plans on pregnancy. When pregnancy does occur, she should remain under close health supervision.

The person also needs to know what resources are available in the community to assist with chronic renal disease. The National Kidney Foundation is organized at the local level to assist in locating resources.

Evaluation

Evaluation is based on expected patient outcomes. Questions to consider may include the following:

1. Has the person participated in bed activities within activity prescription without expressing fatigue?
2. Did the person resume usual ADL when permitted without fatigue?
3. Can the person describe health regimen and need for follow-up care?

NEPHROTIC SYNDROME
Etiology

Nephrotic syndrome is not a single disease entity but a constellation of symptoms. In nephrotic syndrome there is damage to the glomeruli and quantities of protein are lost in the urine. This condition has been associated with allergic reactions (insect bites, pollen, acute glomerulonephritis), infections (herpes zoster), systemic disease (diabetes mellitus, sickle cell disease, amyloidosis), circulatory problems (severe congestive heart failure, chronic constrictive pericarditis), selected drugs and chemicals, and pregnancy. Known glomerular disease is the most common precipitating event in adults; in children the syndrome appears frequently with no evidence of a causative factor. In approximately 25% of children and 50% to 75% of adults who develop nephrosis the disease progresses to renal failure within 5 years.[43] In other individuals (particularly children) there may be remissions or nephrosis may exist in a chronic form. Other than treating the underlying illness, little can be done to prevent a recurrence of nephrosis.

Pathophysiology

The initial change in nephrotic syndrome is a derangement of cells in the glomerular basement membrane, resulting in increased membrane porosity with loss of large amounts of protein into the urine (proteinuria). As protein continues to be excreted, serum albumin is decreased (hypoalbuminemia), thus decreasing the serum osmotic pressure. The capillary hydrostatic fluid (push) pressure in all body tissues becomes greater than the capillary osmotic (pull) pressure, and generalized edema results (Fig. 33-18). As fluid is lost into the tissues, the plasma volume decreases, stimulating secretion of aldosterone to retain more sodium and water and decreasing the glomerular filtration rate to retain water. This additional fluid also passes out of the capillaries into the tissue, leading to even greater edema. Altered renal function and development of symptoms of renal failure occur as a result of progressing glomerulonephritis. Loss of appetite and fatigue are common. Women usually have amenorrhea or other disturbances in their reproductive cycle.

In many instances of nephrotic syndrome, there is an elevation of serum total lipids, cholesterol, phospholipids, and triglycerides.[56] The low-density lipoproteins (see Chapter 25) are usually increased. The mechanism that causes the disturbance in lipid metabolism is not clear.[43]

Nursing Process
Assessment
Subjective data

The person with nephrotic syndrome displays the signs and symptoms of acute glomerulonephritis (p. 1037). General questions for the person with nephrotic syndrome include the following:

1. Have there been changes in voiding patterns?
2. Is the person experiencing headaches or nausea?
3. Has appetite changed? Any anorexia?
4. Is fatigue present?

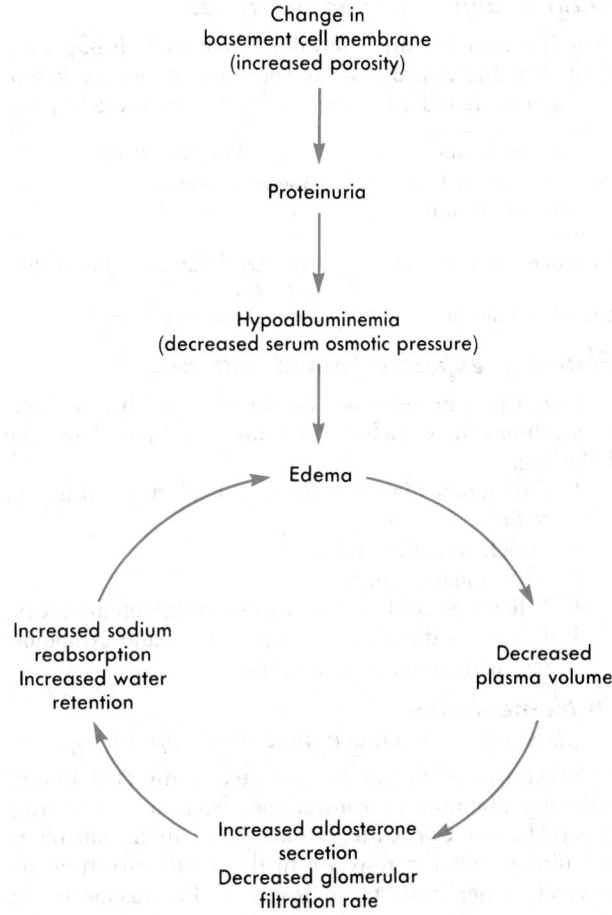

Fig. 33-18 Pathophysiologic changes in nephrotic syndrome.

Objective data

The person with nephrotic syndrome is assessed for signs of fluid retention and infection:

1. Edema: amount, location, degree of pitting
2. Intake and output: monitored every 8 hours until stable
3. Daily weights and abdominal girths
4. Condition of skin: assess frequently as severe edema may lead to skin breakdown
5. Respiratory status: monitored at least each shift (as renal failure progresses, pulmonary edema may develop)
6. Signs and symptoms of infection

Diagnostic tests

The diagnosis of nephrotic syndrome is made on the basis of proteinuria, hypoalbuminemia, and hyperlipidemia. It is essential that serum albumin, cholesterol, and triglycerides be obtained. Urinalyses and a composite urine specimen (p. 1037) for total protein are collected. A renal biopsy is sometimes used as a means of definitive diagnosis.

Data analysis: nursing diagnoses

Nursing diagnoses are determined from analysis of patient data. Nursing diagnoses for the person with nephrotic syndrome may include, but are not limited to, the following:

Diagnostic title	Possible etiologies
Nutrition, altered, less than body requirements	Anorexia, edema
Infection, high risk for	Decreased nutrition, immobility, edema
Knowledge deficit	Lack of exposure/recall

Planning: expected patient outcomes

Expected patient outcomes for the person with nephrotic syndrome may include, but are not limited to, the following:

1. Eats a diet high in protein and calories and low in sodium.
2. Weight remains stable.
3. Skin remains intact.
4. Follows prescribed measures when infection occurs.
5. Describes dietary and drug therapy and symptoms requiring immediate attention.

Implementation
Assisting with achievement of therapeutic goals

Treatment of nephrotic syndrome is directed toward reducing albuminuria, controlling edema, and promoting general health. Corticosteroids may be useful in controlling the illness, but the response to them will vary from remission of nephrosis to no response. Prednisone is the steroid preparation most frequently prescribed. The diet should contain normal to increased amounts of protein (1 g/kg body weight per day) and be high in calories. Periodic determination of proteinuria and measures of renal function enable the physician to monitor response to treatment and level of kidney function.

To control edema, sodium intake is reduced and diuretics may be employed to increase excretion of fluid. When diuretics are administered over prolonged periods, hypokalemia usually results. Potassium may be supplemented through dietary intake. Medication supplements should be initiated only after attempts to increase serum potassium through dietary means have failed. Close monitoring of oral and parenteral fluid is necessary. Bed rest is usually ordered when edema is severe; however, immobility is contraindicated for prolonged periods.

Interventions to achieve patient outcomes
Promoting nutrition

Appetite may be diminished as a result of fluid retention. Sodium intake is restricted, which further reduces palatability of foods and leads to a decreased nutritional intake. Use measures to promote food intake (Chapter 5). Develop a diet plan together with the patient, family, and dietitian to include foods the patient likes. The diet should be high in calories to provide energy, low in sodium to reduce fluid retention, and contain the maximum allowable protein that can be tolerated by the kidney, yet replace lost protein. Whenever possible, the protein should be of high biologic value (lean meat, fish, poultry, and dairy products).

Offer oral hygiene at regular intervals. Good mouth care can help to reduce the unpleasant metallic taste and breath odor that is partially responsible for the anorexia of renal failure.

Preventing infection

Persons with nephrosis need to direct particular attention toward preventing infection, because body defenses are impaired by urinary protein losses. When infection is suspected, it is important to attend to the problem immediately. Obtain specimens for culture and sensitivity according to established protocols. Administer antibiotics at prescribed times to maintain blood levels. Inform the patient of the importance of prescribed medications and the need to take all the antibiotic as directed.

Edematous tissue are particularly susceptible to injury and infection. During periods of severe edema, meticulous skin care is essential to prevent skin breakdown. As edema increases, the patient becomes increasingly uncomfortable. Careful positioning and frequent changes in position may increase comfort while also protecting the skin. If the scrotum becomes very edematous, a sling to support it not only provides comfort but also aids in reducing swelling (see Chapter 35).

Facilitating patient learning

As the patient begins to convalesce, the teaching plan includes the following:

1. Medication regimen: type, dosage, side effects, and need to finish antibiotic prescription (as appropriate)
2. Nutrition teaching
3. Self-assessment of fluid status: weight, presence of edema
4. Signs and symptoms requiring immediate attention (increase in edema, fatigue, headache, infection)
5. Need for follow-up care.

Evaluation

Evaluation is based on expected patient outcomes. Questions to consider may include the following:

1. Is the person eating the prescribed diet in sufficient quantities?
2. Has weight remained stable?
3. Is skin intact without signs of infection?
4. Can the person describe dietary and drug therapy and symptoms requiring follow-up?

OBSTRUCTIVE DISORDERS

Obstructive disorders are a significant source of morbidity. Obstruction of the urinary tract can occur in any portion of the urinary tract from the urinary calyces to the meatus. The signs and symptoms that a person displays are usually characteristic of the location and extent of the obstruction. Box 33-12 summarizes the locations and major causes of the common urinary tract obstructions.

Obstruction of the urinary tract produces pathophysiologic changes leading to symptoms of obstruction. Therapy consists of reestablishing drainage and relieving the acute discomfort. In the following pages, the pathophysiology of

<table>
<tr><td colspan="2">Location and causes of urinary tract obstruction</td></tr>
</table>

Location	Major causes
Kidney	Calculi
	Ptosis
	Polycystic disease
Ureteral obstruction	Calculi
	Trauma
	Nephroptosis ("floating" or dropped" kidney)
	Enlarged lymph nodes
	Lymphosarcoma
	Reticulum cell sarcoma
	Hodgkin's disease
Lower urinary tract	Bladder neoplasm
	Urethral strictures
	Trauma
	Chronic inflammation
	Calculi
	Tumors
	Benign prostatic hypertrophy (BPH)

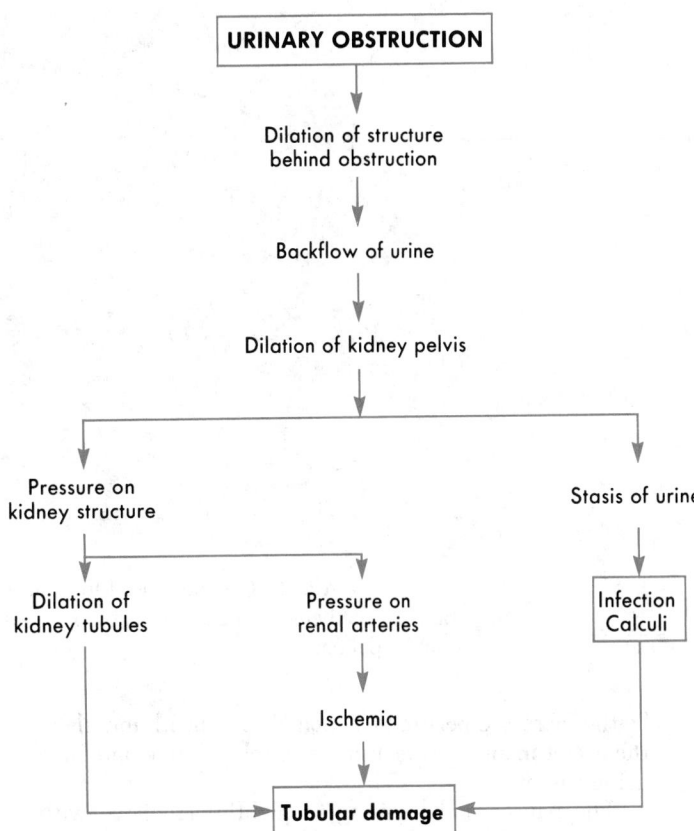

Fig. 33-19 Pathophysiology of uncorrected urinary obstruction.

and therapy for urinary obstruction will be discussed. Several major causes of urinary obstruction are then described in more detail; these topics include the following:

1. Urinary calculi
2. Benign prostatic hypertrophy
3. Urethral strictures
4. Neoplasms: renal, bladder, prostate

Pathophysiology of Urinary Obstruction: Hydronephrosis

Obstruction of any part of the urinary system from the kidney to the urethra will generate pressure that may cause functional and anatomic damage to the renal parenchyma (Fig. 33-19). When any part of the urinary tract is obstructed, urine collects behind the obstruction producing a dilation of the structure. Muscles of the affected areas contract in an effort to push the urine around the obstruction. Partial obstruction may produce slow dilation of structures above the obstruction without functional impairment. As the obstruction increases, however, pressure builds up in the tubular system behind the obstruction causing a backflow of urine and dilation of the ureter (*hydroureter*). The urine backup eventually reaches the kidney, causing dilation of the kidney pelvis (*hydronephrosis*). Pressure buildup in the renal pelvis leads to destruction of kidney tissue and eventual renal failure.

With obstruction urine flow is decreased even to the point of stagnation. This stagnant urine provides a good culture medium for bacterial growth, and rarely is obstruction seen without some infection. The specific effects that occur with obstruction depend on the location of the obstruction, the extent of obstruction (partial or complete), and the duration. Obstruction in the *lower* urinary tract causes bladder distention. If this is prolonged, muscle fibers become hypertrophied and *diverticuli* (herniated sacs of bladder mucosa) develop between the hypertrophied

muscle bands. Because the diverticulum holds stagnant urine, infection often occurs, and bladder stones may form.

Obstruction of the *upper* urinary tract leads even more quickly to hydronephrosis because of the small size of the ureters and kidney pelvis. Increased pressure causes partial ischemia of arteries between the renal cortex and medulla and dilation of the renal tubules leading to tubular damage. Stasis of urine in the dilated pelvis predisposes to infection and calculi, which add to the renal damage. Some urine can flow back up the renal tubule into the veins and lymphatics as a compensatory mechanism to prevent kidney damage. The unaffected kidney then takes on increased elimination of waste products. With prolonged obstruction the unaffected kidney hypertrophies and may function as effectively alone as both kidneys did before the obstruction. Obstruction of both kidneys leads to renal failure.

Hydronephrosis can occur without any symptoms as long as kidney function is adequate and urine can drain. An acute upper urinary tract obstruction will cause pain, nausea, vomiting, local tenderness, spasm of the abdominal muscles, and a mass in the kidney region. The pain is caused by the stretching of the tissues and by hyperperistalsis. Because the amount of pain is proportional to the rate of stretching, a slowly developing hydronephrosis may cause only a dull flank pain, whereas a sudden blockage of the ureter such as may occur from a stone causes a severe stabbing (colicky) pain in the flank or abdomen. The pain may radiate to the genitalia and thigh and is caused

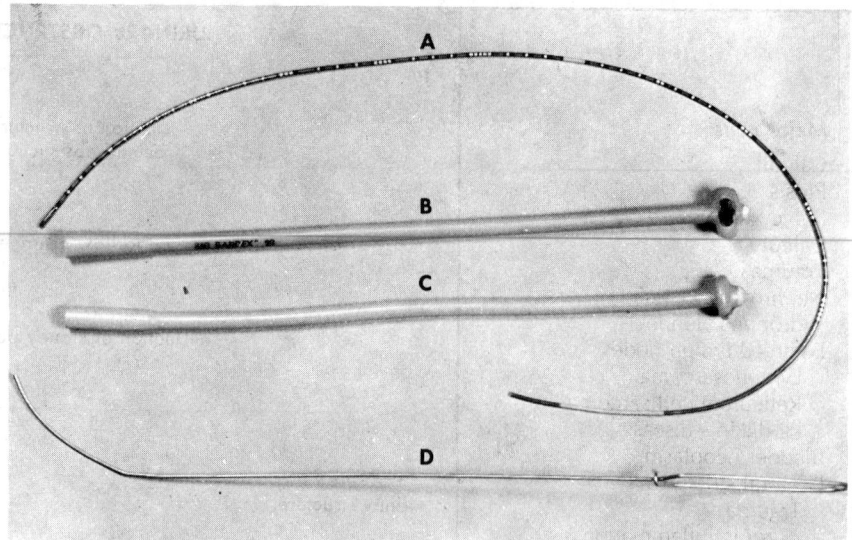

Fig. 33-20   A to **C,** Catheters used to drain renal pelvis. **A,** Ureteral catheter. **B,** Malecote (batwing) catheter. **C,** Pezzer (mushroom) catheter. **D,** Stylet used to insert urethral catheter in male patient.

by the increased peristaltic action of the smooth muscle of the ureter in an effort to dislodge the obstruction and force urine past it.

The nausea and vomiting frequently associated with acute ureteral obstruction are caused by a reflex reaction to the pain and will usually be relieved as soon as pain is relieved. A markedly dilated kidney, however, may press on the stomach causing continued GI symptoms. If the renal function has been seriously impaired, nausea and vomiting may be symptoms of impending uremia.

When the bladder is distended from lower urinary tract obstruction, the person will experience lower abdominal discomfort and a feeling of the need to void although voiding may not be possible. The bladder may be palpated above the symphysis pubis. With partial obstruction such as by benign prostatic hypertrophy the patient first complains of increasing urinary frequency because the bladder fails to empty completely at each voiding and therefore refills more quickly to the amount that causes the urge to void (usually 250 to 500 ml). Nocturia may also be present.

Therapy for Urinary Obstruction

The person with a sudden obstruction is usually acutely ill and may have severe colic but will not be able to remain in bed until the pain has been relieved. It is not unusual to see a person with acute renal colic walking the floor doubled up and vomiting. Narcotics such as morphine and meperidine and antispasmodic drugs such as propantheline bromide (Pro-Banthine) and belladonna preparations are usually necessary to relieve severe colicky pain. After narcotics have been given, the patient will be dizzy and must be protected from injury. As the pain eases, the patient can usually be made relatively comfortable in bed. As soon as the nausea subsides large amounts of fluids are urged.

If a *ureter* becomes obstructed, a catheter must be placed directly into the renal pelvis. This prevents renal damage

that otherwise would occur as pressure in the kidney increases because of continued urine formation. When there is complete obstruction of a ureter, a *nephrostomy* or *pyelostomy* tube may be inserted surgically into the renal pelvis. The surgical incision is located laterally and posteriorly in the kidney region. Catheters used as nephrostomy or pyelostomy tubes are usually of the Pezzer (mushroom) or Malecot (batwing) types (Fig. 33-20). An alternate form of drainage for a ureteral obstruction is the surgical placement of a ureterostomy tube (a whistle-tip or many-eyed Robinson catheter, No. 6 or No. 8 Fr) that is passed through an incision in the upper outer quadrant of the abdomen into the ureter above the obstruction. The catheter is then passed through the ureter to the renal pelvis.

If the ureter is unobstructed or partially obstructed, the *renal pelvis* may be drained by a ureteral catheter, which is passed up the ureter to the renal pelvis by a cystoscope (p. 1052). Ureteral catheterization is performed before gynecologic and lower abdominal surgery when there is danger of not recognizing and accidentally injuring the ureter during the operation. Ureteral catheterization is also used after surgery involving the ureters to prevent stricture as the ureter heals. When used for this purpose, the catheter is referred to as a *splinting catheter* (Fig. 33-21). Whether it is expected to drain urine will depend on its relation to other catheters used.

Adequate anchorage of nephrostomy catheters must be provided to prevent accidental dislodgement and trauma to the tissues in which they lie. The openings made for these tubes are essentially fistulas that rapidly decrease in size on removal of the catheter. Even 30 minutes after removal of this type of catheter it is often impossible to reinsert a similar-sized tube. When a catheter is inserted during surgery, it is usually sutured in place. In this case, additional anchorage consists of affixing the tube to the skin with adhesive tape after the skin has been cleansed. When

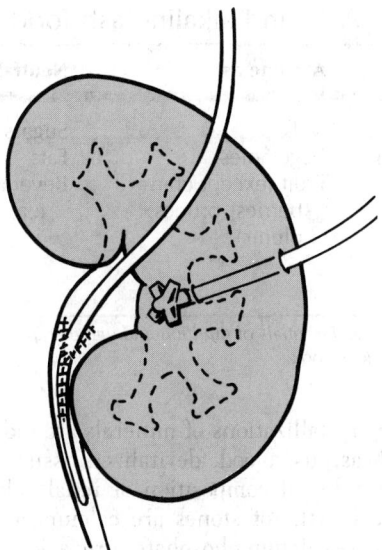

Fig. 33-21   Placement of splinting catheter after repair of ureteropelvic stricture. Note use of nephrostomy tube for drainage of urine during healing of anastomosis.

Renal calculus composition and contributing factors

Composition of stone	Factors contributing to stone formation
Calcium (oxalate and phosphate)	Hyperphosphaturia and/or hypercalciuria resulting from Hyperparathyroidism Vitamin D intoxication Multiple myeloma Immobilization Severe bone disease Renal tubular acidosis Prolonged intake of steroids
Uric acid	High purine diet Gout
Cystine	Cystinuria resulting from genetic disorder of amino-acid metabolism

the tube is not sutured in place, it should be anchored to the skin at *two points* using adhesive—with some slack in the tubing between the anchor points.

Free drainage of catheters leading to the renal pelvis is of the utmost importance. Because the normal renal pelvis has only a 5- to 8-ml capacity, great pressure can be exerted on renal structures even when these catheters are obstructed for only a few minutes. Care must be taken to prevent kinking of the tubes while the patient is in the side-lying position in bed.

In some cases nephrostomy tubes may be left in place for several months, with the patient returning to the hospital later for their removal. Occasionally, the nephrostomy tube serves as a form of urinary diversion for long-term use. The person at home with a catheter draining the kidney pelvis must know how to obtain medical assistance quickly should the catheter become obstructed or dislodged.

When obstruction occurs below the *bladder*, constant drainage must be provided to prevent renal damage, which may occur because of inadequate emptying of the lower urinary system. One means of providing drainage is by the use of a *cystostomy* tube (usually a Foley, Malecot, or Pezzer catheter), which is placed directly into the bladder through a suprapubic incision. This method is usually used when the urethra is completely obstructed or when the prolonged use of a urethral catheter is to be avoided in a male patient. During some operative procedures both a cystostomy tube and a small urethral catheter will be inserted to drain the bladder. Both catheters must be monitored for patency. If patency is assured, it is not necessary to record the output from each catheter separately, because both tubes drain the bladder. The catheters will not necessarily drain equal amounts of urine. As is true with nephrostomy and ureteral catheters, secure anchorage of these catheters.

URINARY CALCULI

Etiology/Epidemiology

Urinary stones, which are termed *urolithiasis* ("lith" refers to stones), may develop at any level in the urinary system, but are most commonly found within the kidney (nephrolithiasis). Fig. 33-22 illustrates the most common locations of urolithiasis. Supersaturation of urine is believed to be the major cause of urinary calculi. When concentrations of the stone-forming substance exceeds its solubility in urine, stone growth can occur. No demonstrable cause can be found for over half of the urinary stones that occur (idiopathic). A major predisposition is urinary tract infection. Other factors are listed in Box 33-13.

It is estimated that 1% to 5% of Americans will develop urolithiasis. About one third of the individuals who have recurrent upper urinary tract calculi will eventually need to have the affected kidney removed.

Prevention

Measures can be taken to decrease the potential for renal stones in persons at high risk. Adequate hydration (intake of 2500 ml/day or more unless contraindicated) will help to prevent urinary stasis that can lead not only to stone formation but also to a UTI. Persons restricted to bed should be encouraged to turn and move frequently, exercising their arms if the legs are immobilized. Changing the body position of a bedfast patient by means of a Circ-Olectric bed or tilt table or by sitting up in a wheelchair (if permitted) can help to prevent urinary stasis. Even with exercises and the use of a wheelchair, however, paraplegics and quadriplegics often develop urinary calculi. *Persons with in-dwelling catheters need scrupulous aseptic technique in catheter care to prevent infection and require adequate hydration*

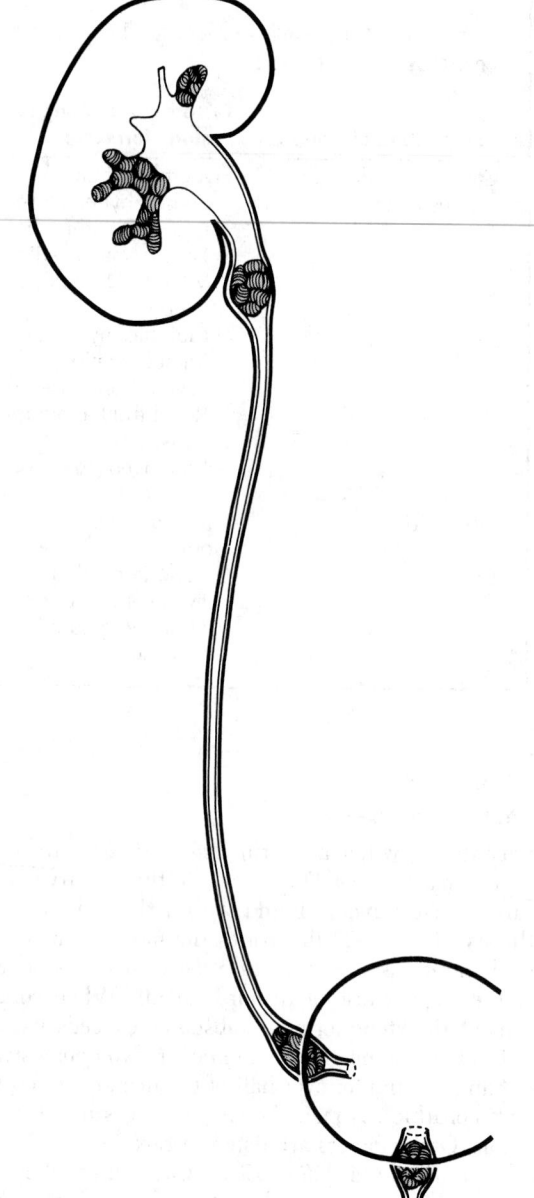

Fig. 33-22 Common locations of renal calculus formation.

Table 33-9	Acid and alkaline ash food groups		
Acid ash	**Alkaline ash**	**Neutral**
Meat	Milk	Sugars
Whole grains	Vegetables	Fats
Eggs	Fruit (except cran-	Beverages (coffee,
Cheese	berries, prunes,	tea)
Cranberries	plums)	
Prunes		
Plums		

From Williams SR: *Essentials of nutrition and diet therapy,* ed 5, St Louis, 1990, Mosby–Year Book.

(stones) are crystallizations of minerals around an organic matrix such as pus, blood, devitalized tissue, tumors, or urates. The mineral composition of renal calculi varies. About three fourths of stones are calcium and oxalates; other stones are calcium phosphate, uric acid, and cystine. Increased concentration of urine solutes, resulting from low fluid intake, as well as increased organic matter from urinary tract infections or urinary stasis, may provide the nidus for stone formation. In addition, infection increases the alkalinity of the urine (by the production of ammonia), resulting in precipitation of calcium phosphate and magnesium ammonium phosphate.

Nursing Process
Assessment
Subjective data

Pain *(renal colic)* is the primary symptom in an acute episode of renal calculi. The location of the pain depends on the location of the stone. If the stone is in the pelvis of the kidney, the pain is caused by hydronephrosis and is more dull and constant in character, occurring primarily in the costovertebral angle. As the stone moves along the ureter, the pain can be excruciating and is intermittent in character. It is caused by spasm of the ureter and anoxia of the wall of the ureter from the pressure of the stone. Pain follows the anterior course of the ureter down to the suprapubic area and radiates to the external genitalia. Often a stone is "silent" causing no symptoms for years; this is especially true of very large renal stones. Extremely small smooth stones may be passed without the person's awareness. Nausea and vomiting often accompany renal colic.

Objective data

The urine is monitored for the presence of blood. *Gross hematuria* may occur if the stone has rough edges, and microhematuria is usually present. Whenever a stone is suspected, all urine is strained to determine the presence of stones that are frequently passed during voiding. Patterns of urination are also noted because frequency or voiding in small amounts may be experienced. The acidity or alkalinity of the urine can be determined with pH paper.

Diagnostic tests

Urinalysis, to determine the urine pH, presence of casts, crystals, and blood cells, and urine culture, to identify UTI, are performed. A 24-hour urine collection is made to measure calcium oxalate, phosphorus, and uric

and good catheter drainage to wash away minerals that can be deposited at the tip of the catheter.

Persons at risk for developing calcium oxalate or phosphate or magnesium ammonium phosphate stones may be placed on an acid ash diet (Table 33-9) to promote excretion of an acid urine.

Pathophysiology

Urinary calculi result in obstruction of the urinary tract; the obstruction may be partial or complete. Complete obstruction leads to *hydronephrosis* with its associated signs and symptoms.

The pathophysiologic processes associated with urinary stones tend to be mechanical in nature. Urinary calculi

cid levels. A nitroprusside urine test may be performed o check the presence of cystine.

BUN and serum creatinine tests are important to deermine the level of rénal function. Because urinary stones re frequently composed of calcium, phosphorus, and uric cid, these serum levels are usually obtained.

Calcium stones are radiopaque and can be noted with KUB (kidney, ureter, bladder) x-ray examination; uric cid stones usually cannot be seen in radiographic studies. An intravenous pyelogram (IVP) (Table 33-10) may also be btained. IVP may demonstrate dilation of the ureter above n obstructing stone. Very small stones, however, may be vashed away during radiographic studies. Ultrasound of he kidneys may also be ordered to detect hydronephrosis.

Data analysis: nursing diagnoses

Nursing diagnoses are determined from analysis of patient lata. Possible nursing diagnoses for the person with uriary calculi may include, but are not limited to, the folowing:

Diagnostic title	Possible etiologies
Pain	Visceral inflammation
Knowledge deficit	Lack of exposure/recall

Planning: expected patient outcomes

Expected patient outcomes for the patient with urinary calculi may include, but are not limited to, the following:
1. Describes feeling more comfortable.
2. Describes measures to prevent urinary calculi recurrence and symptoms of recurrence to be reported.

Implementation
Assisting with achievement of therapeutic goals

About 90% of urinary calculi are passed spontaneously. therefore, *the urine of all patients with relatively small stones should be strained.* Urine can be strained easily by placing two opened 4-inch × 8-inch gauze sponges over a funnel. The urine from each voiding is strained, and one needs to

Table 33-10   Common radiologic examinations of the urinary tract

Test	Purpose	Procedure	Nursing implications
Retrograde pyelography	Visualization of urinary tract	1. Ureteral catheterization required 2. Radiopaque material (Hypaque, Renografin) gently injected 3. Radiographs are taken of the renal collecting structures	Patient may experience discomfort in region of kidneys as dye is injected Pain may be experienced if too large a volume of dye is injected and renal pelvis becomes distended
Intravenous pyelography (IVP)	Determine size and location of kidneys Demonstrate presence of calculi, cysts or tumors Outline filling of renal pelvis Outline ureters and bladder Determine anatomic abnormalities of urinary tract	1. Radiograph of abdomen (KUB) is taken to identify size and position of kidneys 2. Radiopaque dye is given intravenously 3. Radiographs of the kidneys are taken at 3-, 5-, 10-, and 20-minute intervals	Bowel cleansing required Fluids are often withheld for up to 8 hours to produce slight dehydration The patient is informed that a feeling of warmth, flushing of the face, and a salty taste in the mouth may occur as the dye is injected The patient is observed for signs and symptoms of a reaction to the dye including respiratory distress, diaphoresis, urticaria, instability of vital signs, or unusual sensations Cardiopulmonary resuscitation equipment and emergency medications should always be available for immediate use
Kidney, ureters, and bladder (KUB) radiograph	Gross visualization of kidneys, ureters, and bladder Calcifications and stones can be located	Radiograph of abdominal region obtained	Bowel cleansing may or may not be ordered
Urethrography	Visualization of urethral size and shape	Radiography of urethra taken after instilling 20 ml of radiopaque water-soluble lubricant	No special preparation
Computed tomography (CT)	Visualization of kidneys and renal circulation	Whole body CT scanner segments kidneys Can be done with IV contrast dye	If dye is used, same implications apply as for IVP

Continued.

Table 33-10 Common radiologic examinations of the urinary tract—cont'd

Test	Purpose	Procedure	Nursing implications
Renal angiography	Visualization of renal circulation Particularly useful in evaluating renal artery stenosis	Procedure is similar to IVP; however, the contrast dye is often injected directly into the femoral artery by passing a catheter through the artery to the level of the renal arteries	Nursing implications are the same as for IVP Patient must be observed for bleeding at arterial puncture site, especially within first 4 hours; the pressure dressing is checked for fresh bleeding; the puncture site is checked for tenderness or swelling; vital signs and distal pulses must be assessed frequently (q 15 min × 4 hours); bed rest should be maintained for 8 hours after the procedure
Renography	Visualization of urinary tract Measures renal bloodflow Measures renal tubular and excretory function	Involves scintillation scanning or photography Radioactive isotope such as iodohippurate sodium tagged with I^{131} or I^{125} is injected intravenously Scintillating probes placed over the kidneys record the photographs	Because only trace doses of bound isotopes are used, no special precautions are necessary
Ultrasound	Used to distinguish between abnormal fluid collections and solid masses. Used to identify obstructions and detect abscesses. Often used to diagnose abscesses, ureteral leaks, and obstructions in renal transplant recipients	Sound waves are used to outline internal body structures. The procedure is accomplished by computer interpretation of tissue densities	Procedure is painless and noninvasive. A full bladder assists in outlining structures

watch closely for the stone because it may be no bigger than the head of a pin and the patient may not realize that it has been passed.

Stones smaller than 5 mm have a good chance of being passed. If there is no infection or obstruction, the stone may be left in the ureter for several months. The person is observed closely but permitted to carry out usual activities. A person who is up and about is more likely to pass a stone than one who is in bed. Fluids should be taken freely (3000 ml/day or more) to promote passage of the stone and prevent infection.

Patients frequently have two or three attacks of acute renal colic before the stone passes. This is probably because the stone gets lodged at a narrow point in the ureter, causing temporary obstruction. The ureters are normally narrower at the ureteropelvic and ureterovesical junctions and at the point where they pass over the iliac crest into the pelvis. If the stone is to pass along the ureter by peristaltic action, the patient will have some pain. The patient is involved in determining when pain medication is needed.

If the stone fails to pass, one or two ureteral catheters may be passed through a cystoscope up the ureter and left in place for 24 hours. The catheters dilate the ureter, and when they are removed the stone may pass into the bladder.

If there are *signs of infection*, an attempt is made to pass a ureteral catheter past the stone into the renal pelvis. If such an attempt is successful, the catheter is left as a drain, because pyelonephritis will quickly follow if adequate urinary drainage is not reestablished. When there is a catheter in each ureter, each catheter is labeled and should drain into a separate drainage bag. Check the catheters frequently to see that they are draining. Patients with ureteral catheters are usually confined to bed to prevent possible dislodgement of the catheters.

If the stone has passed to the lower third of the *ureter* it can sometimes be removed by *manipulation*. Special catheters with expanding baskets and loops are passed through the cystoscope, and an attempt is made to "snare" the stone. This procedure is performed with the patient under anesthesia. The aftercare of a patient on whom manipulation has been carried out is the same as that following cystoscopy. Watch for any signs suggestive of peritonitis or a decreased urinary output because the ureter occasionally is perforated during manipulation.

Bladder stones may be crushed with a lithotrite (stone crusher) that is passed transurethrally. This procedure is known as a *litholapaxy*. Following bladder stone removal, the bladder may be irrigated (intermittently or constantly) with an acid solution such as magnesium and sodium citrate (G solution), or Renacidin to counteract the alkalinity caused by the infection and to help wash out the remaining particles of stone.

Percutaneous nephrolithotomy

Until the early 1980s surgery was usually required to remove a urinary stone. Percutaneous nephrolithotomy (endourology) is now a common method for urinary stone removal. A small nephrostomy tract is made through a skin incision over the kidney region. An endoscope is then passed through the tract and a snare basket is used to retrieve the calculi. If the calculi cannot be removed, ultrasonic lithotripsy (breaking up of the stone by ultrasound) is used. If infection is present, the area may be irrigated with an acidifier, such as Renacidin. Local anesthesia may be used and recovery is rapid. The person may experience renal colic pain postoperatively, which is usually relieved with meperidine. There may be copious drainage of urine or serous fluid from the tract for 3 to 4 days postoperatively. Dressings are changed frequently to prevent infection and aid in patient comfort. A 2-week course of antibiotics is prescribed after surgery. Complications are rare but may include hemorrhage or sepsis; the patient should report signs of urinary bleeding, pain, or unexplained fever to the physician immediately.

Extracorporeal shock wave lithotripsy

Extracorporeal shock wave lithotripsy (ESWL) is another recent development in the treatment of urinary stones. It is usually accomplished by submerging the patient in a large tub of warm water and aiming ultrasonic waves over the area of the urinary calculi. The water bath is used to allow the passage of shock waves into the body. Repeated firing of the ultrasonic waves results in the disintegration of the calculi. It may require more than 1500 shock waves to break up a large stone. The small particles pass spontaneously over 2 to 5 days. Because the procedure is uncomfortable general, regional, or local anesthesia may be used. Aiming the sound waves is best accomplished when the patient is able to control both breathing and movement while in the water bath.

A newer method of ESWL omits the water bath. A membrane coupling device is applied to the skin over the kidney.[47] Because this approach requires less energy, intravenous sedation may be all that is necessary.

The patient may experience renal colic pain for several days after ESWL when passing the stone fragments. Pain is controlled by narcotic analgesics. Occasionally, urinary obstruction may occur as a result of stone fragments blocking urine flow. The patient is instructed to observe the volume of urine output for several days following discharge. Flank pain may indicate urinary retention. When these symptoms occur, the patient should contact the physician immediately.

Open surgical removal of urinary calculi

Open surgery to remove renal calculi is performed less often since the advent of percutaneous nephrolithotomy and ESWL. The stone may be removed through the renal pelvis (pyelolithotomy), through the renal tissue (nephrolithotomy), or directly into a ureter (Fig. 33-23). Large bladder stones may be removed through a suprapubic incision. Care of the patient undergoing urologic surgery is discussed on p. 1050.

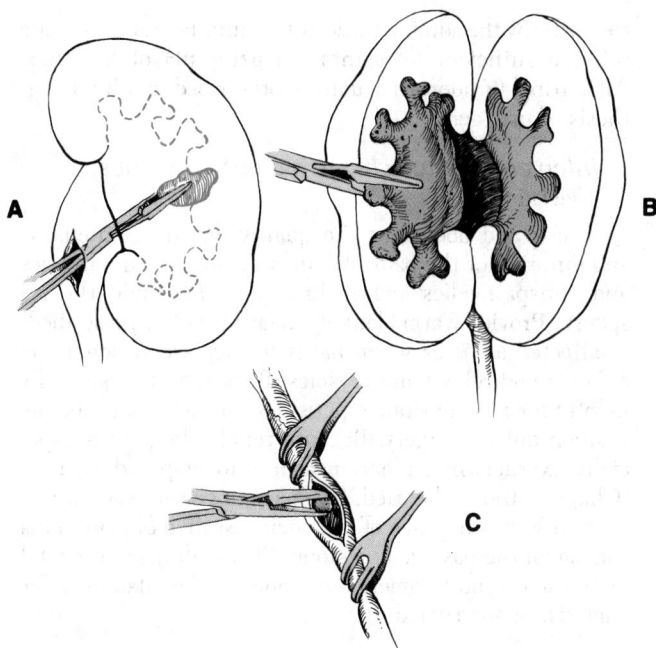

Fig. 33-23   Surgical removal of renal calculi from upper urinary tract. **A,** Pyelolithotomy, removal of stone through renal pelvis. **B,** Nephrolithotomy, removal of staghorn calculus from renal parenchyma (kidney split). **C,** Ureterolithotomy, removal of stone from ureter.

Long-term care

Persons who have recurrent urinary calculi benefit from ongoing prophylactic therapy, which is determined by the type of stone being produced. *All* persons with recurrent renal stones should drink fluids in sufficient quantity to produce very dilute urine and nocturia (unless contraindicated as with CHF). This may amount to a daily intake of up to 4 L of fluid. The purpose of the increased fluid intake is to rinse away any precipitates that can serve as a nidus for stone formation.

Any underlying identifiable cause of calciuria is treated to prevent recurrence of calcium stones. Hydrochlorothiazide (HCTZ) in doses of 50 mg twice a day may be prescribed for persons with hypercalciuria to decrease urinary excretion of calcium. Persons receiving HCTZ therapy must be monitored carefully for signs of electrolyte imbalances, especially hypokalemia.

As previously stated, more than 50% of calcium stones are idiopathic. Foods high in calcium are sometimes restricted, but a very low-calcium diet is usually unsatisfactory because it is unpalatable. The solubility of oxalate salts is not pH dependent; therefore manipulation of pH is not useful. Sodium or potassium phosphate, 1.5 to 2 g/day, may be prescribed to decrease levels of urinary calcium.

Phosphatic calculi develop in alkaline urine; thus their prevention depends on keeping the urine acid and preventing a UTI. Medications such as ascorbic acid or ammonium chloride may be given for a time to increase urine acidity.

Prophylaxis for *uric acid* stones consists of alkalinizing

the urine by the administration of sodium-potassium citrate solution sufficient to maintain a urine pH of 6 to 6.5. Allopurinol (Zyloprim) usually is prescribed to inhibit synthesis of uric acid.

Interventions to achieve patient outcomes
Alleviating pain

Assess and document the quality, location, intensity, and duration of the pain. Administer prescribed narcotics and antispasmodics and evaluate and document the response. Provide warm blankets, heating pad (if prescribed) to affected area, or warm baths to increase regional circulation and relax tense muscles. Back rubs are especially helpful for a postoperative patient who was in a lithotomy position during surgery. Because renal colic pain is especially excruciating, other measures to help reduce pain (Chapter 10) may be tried, but may not be very successful.

Notify the physician of a sudden cessation of pain. This can signal the passage of a stone. Strain all urine for solid matter and send fragments or stones to the laboratory for analysis, as instructed.

Facilitating patient learning

Teaching focuses on methods to prevent recurrence of urinary calculi and symptoms of recurrence to be reported to the physician.
1. Methods to prevent UTI (which may lead to stasis and deposition of crystals leading to stone development):
   a. Drink at least 3000 ml of fluids each day.
   b. Avoid situations that lead to urinary stasis whenever possible (such as long periods of inactivity).
   c. Practice good perineal hygiene.
2. Dietary prescriptions, including a variety of menus that include necessary dietary restrictions (acid or alkaline ash diets, p. 1046).
3. Prescribed medication regimen: names, dosages, side effects.
4. Need to report signs and symptoms of calculi recurrence (flank pain or pain radiating down into the groin).

Evaluation

Evaluation is based on expected patient outcomes. Questions to consider may include the following:
1. Does the patient have signs and symptoms of flank pain or pain radiating down into groin?
2. Has the medication been effective in relieving the patient's pain?
3. Can the patient describe measures to prevent recurrence of urinary calculi and signs of recurrence to be reported to physician?

UROLOGIC SURGERY

Surgery of the urinary tract may be performed for various reasons, such as renal calculi, tumors, multiple cysts, trauma, congenital defects, "floating" kidney (nephroptosis), or renal hypertension. The types of surgeries are described in Table 33-11.

Table 33-11   Types of urologic surgery

Site	Surgery	Description
Kidney	Nephrectomy	Removal of a kidney
	Partial nephrectomy	Removal of part of a kidney
	Pyelolithotomy	Incision into renal pelvis for removal of calculi
	Nephrolithotomy	Incision into kidney parenchyma for removal of calculi
	Nephropexy	Fixation of a floating kidney
	Pyeloplasty	Plastic repair of ureteropelvic junction
Ureters	Ureterolithotomy	Incision into ureters for removal of calculi
	Ureterectomy	Excision of a ureter
	Ureterostomy	Creation of a new outlet for a ureter
Bladder	Cystectomy	Removal of the bladder
	Segmental bladder resection	Partial removal of the bladder

Preoperative Care

General preoperative preparation for surgery (Chapter 20) is appropriate for the urologic patient. Patient concerns may be focused not only on the diagnosis but also on possible changes in urinary elimination. For many patients, interruption in urinary elimination is temporary. If one kidney is removed, adequate waste removal can be maintained by the remaining kidney or by even less than half of one kidney remaining functional. The remaining kidney may grow to handle the extra load.

Partial removal of the bladder will decrease capacity of the bladder to about 60 ml immediately postoperatively, but the elastic tissue of the bladder will regenerate so that the person is able to retain from 200 to 400 ml of urine within several months. If the entire bladder is removed, diversion of the urinary tract is necessary.

Instructions in effective deep breathing exercises are crucial after kidney surgery because of the high flank incision interfering with ventilation.

Postoperative Care

The basic needs of the patient requiring urologic surgery are the same as those of any other surgical patient. Special emphasis is placed on promotion of ventilation and adequate urinary output, prevention of distention and hemorrhage, and attention to drainage tubes and dressing (see Box 33-14).

Promoting ventilation

Surgery of the kidney or upper ureters usually involves a flank incision that can influence respiratory status. Because the incision is directly below the diaphragm, deep breathing is painful and the patient is reluctant to take deep breaths. Splinting of the chest is common, and therefore atelectasis or other respiratory complications must be guarded against. In addition, because of the placement of the incision there is a greater incisional pull every time the person moves, as compared with an abdominal incision. The patient is often reluctant to turn in bed or to get up to ambulate. Most patients will be more comfortable turning themselves if they are given time, side rails to hold onto, and encouragement. Incisional pain usually requires a narcotic every 3 to 4 hours for 24 to 48 hours after surgery. Turning, ambulation, and deep breathing exercises can be planned so that these activities occur at the time the analgesic has the greatest effect. Patients may lie on the affected side unless a nephrostomy tube is in place. Even then they can be tilted to the affected side with pillows placed at the back for support. Ascertain that the tube is not kinked and that there is no traction on it.

Promoting adequate urinary output

Monitor urinary output carefully for several days postoperatively to ascertain adequate renal functioning and drainage. The output should be at least 50 ml/hour, preferably greater, to prevent urinary stasis and subsequent infection. A urinary output of 20 to 30 ml/hour in a patient with satisfactory fluid intake (at least 1200 ml/day) and in the absence of signs of urinary retention is reported immediately to the physician. Urinary output includes drainage from nephrostomy or cystostomy tubes, urethral or ureteral catheters, and an estimate from urine-soaked dressings. Daily weights are compared with the preoperative weight and with each other to identify fluid retention.

Relieving distention

Following kidney surgery most patients have some abdominal distention that may result in part from pressure on the stomach and intestinal tract during surgery. Patients who have had renal colic before surgery frequently develop paralytic ileus postoperatively. This condition may be related to the reflex GI tract symptoms caused by postoperative pain. Because of the problem of abdominal distention following renal surgery, food and fluids by mouth are often restricted 24 to 48 hours postoperatively. By the fourth postoperative day most patients tolerate a regular diet. Fluids are then usually forced to 3000 ml/day.

Preventing hemorrhage

Hemorrhage may follow such operative procedures as prostatectomy, nephrolithotomy, or nephrectomy. It occurs most often when the highly vascular parenchyma of the kidney has been incised. The bleeding may occur on the day of surgery, or it may occur 8 to 12 days postoperatively, during the period when tissue sloughing normally occurs with healing. The presence of bright red blood on the dressing or in the urine is reported immediately to the physician. The patient is observed for signs of shock. Because many patients with urologic disease have hypertension, the blood pressure may be relatively high but still represent a marked drop for the individual. Comparisons should therefore be made with baseline data.

If hemorrhage occurs, a pressure dressing is applied over the incision while the physician's arrival is awaited.

33·14

Guidelines for Care

The patient following urologic surgery

Promote ventilation:
  Encourage breathing exercises.
  Encourage frequent self-turning in bed.
  Encourage ambulation.
Monitor output and maintain patency of urinary catheters.
Prevent complications:
  Change wet dressings to protect skin.
  Restrict food and oral fluids if paralytic ileus is present.
  Encourage fluids to 3000 or more ml/day when permitted.
  Monitor for bright red blood on dressing or in urine.

Measures to prevent shock are instituted. Several liters of sterile physiologic saline solution for irrigation should be available.

Changing dressings

There may be large amounts of urinary drainage following urologic surgery, except after nephrectomy. The drainage may be pink or dark red but should not be bright red. If the surgery involves a flank incision, drainage is usually the heaviest on the posterior edge of the dressing because of gravity flow. It is important therefore to turn the patient on the side opposite the surgery to examine the posterior edge of the dressing. When a suprapubic incision is present, drainage is heaviest on the side and in the inguinal region.

The dressings are usually held in place by Montgomery straps and must be changed frequently. Urinary drainage irritates the skin, has an unpleasant odor, and leads to discomfort. If a drain is present, the end of the drain should be placed over dressings, then covered with additional dressions to absorb the drainage. If a drainage tube is present, presence of large amounts of drainage on the dressing with little drainage coming from the tube indicates blockage of the tube. If a large amount of drainage is present, a disposable drainage bag used for urinary stomas may be applied over the drainage site.

A catheter is usually inserted during surgery to drain urine from the operative area and permit healing to occur. Different types of drainage tubes may be inserted, and each tube is connected to a separate drainage system. It is important to know the purpose of the catheter and the area to be drained.

BENIGN PROSTATIC HYPERTROPHY
Etiology/Epidemiology

Benign prostatic hypertrophy (BPH) is an adenomatous enlargement of the prostate gland. More than half of all men over 50 years of age and 75% of men over 70 have some symptoms of prostatic enlargement. The cause is not known but appears to be related to changing hormone levels that are experienced during the aging process.

Pathophysiology

The prostate is an encapsulated gland, weighing about 20 g, that encircles the male urethra below the bladder neck. The signs and symptoms associated with BPH are the result of the enlargement of the prostate causing a partial or complete obstruction of the lower urinary tract.

One of the early symptoms of benign prostatic hypertrophy is *nocturia* (awakening at night to void) and urinary *frequency* in general. The man notices that the urinary stream is smaller and more difficult to start *(hesitancy)*. The bladder muscle must contract more forcibly to push the urine past the partial obstruction, and the overworked muscles hypertrophy. Stagnant urine is held in trabeculae, or cellules, formed by sagging of the atonic mucous membranes between hypertrophied muscle bands. The bladder will not empty completely at each voiding (residual urine). This urine becomes alkaline from stasis and is a fertile medium for bacterial growth. The man will then complain of symptoms of cystitis (frequency, urgency), and bladder stones may occur. Some men develop hematuria from rupture of blood vessels that have become overstretched. Destruction of renal function can eventually occur from back pressure up the ureter to the kidney. Acute urinary retention is not uncommon.

Assessment

Subjective data

The most frequent and disturbing symptoms of BPH include dysuria and nocturia. The man is asked about urinary patterns, including the presence of frequency, hesitancy, dribbling, number of times he must get up at night to void, and the force of the urinary stream. *Hesitancy* refers to difficulty in initiating voiding that is often accompanied by a decrease in the force and flow of the urinary stream. The man is asked if he has to strain to start or maintain urinary flow.

Because urinary tract infection may occur as a result of stasis of urine, the man is assessed for chills and pain or burning on urination.

Objective data

Patterns and amounts of urination are noted. The bladder is distended and, when percussed, elicits a "kettle drum" sound.

Diagnostic tests

Urinalysis is performed to determine the presence of casts, crystals, and blood cells, and a urine culture is obtained to assess for infection. BUN and serum creatinine tests are important to determine the level of renal function. An IVP (p. 1047) is usually obtained to evaluate the functions and structure of the kidneys and urinary tract.

Enlargement of the lateral lobes of the prostate gland may be palpated by digital rectal examination. Enlargement of the middle lobe is diagnosed by signs of partial obstruction of the urethra, and the obstruction and bladder trabeculae are visualized by cystoscopy.

Cystoscopy

Cystoscopy is the direct examination of the bladder using an instrument called a *cystoscope* (Fig. 33-24). The cystoscope relies on a flexible optic fiber to provide illu-

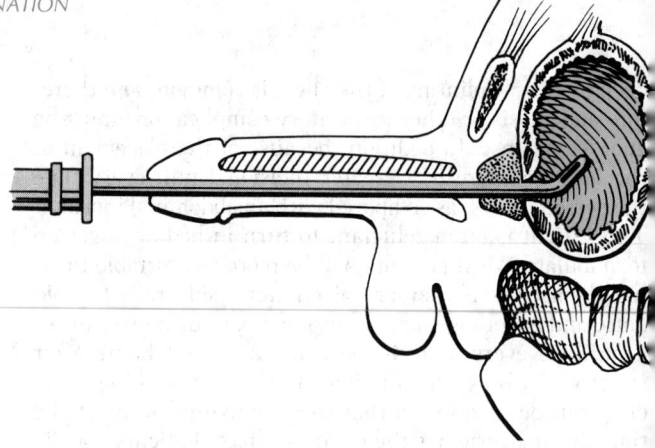

Fig. 33-24   Cystoscope inserted for examination of bladder.

mination into the urinary tract. The instrument is attached to the illuminating source then slowly passed through the urinary tract, thus enabling direct visualization of the urethra, ureteral orifices, and bladder.

Preprocedure care

Fluids are forced for several hours before the procedure. This ensures a continuous flow of urine, in the event that specimens need to be collected, and aids in preventing multiplication of bacteria that may be introduced during the procedure. If radiographs are to be taken during the procedure, bowel preparation may be ordered.

Method

If the patient is relatively comfortable and relaxed, the cystoscope can be passed with little discomfort, provided there is no obstruction in the urethra. A local anesthetic such as procaine may be instilled into the urethra before insertion of the cystoscope. Any discomfort felt during this procedure is the result of contraction or spasm of the bladder sphincters; this can be decreased through deep-breathing exercises and general relaxation on the part of the patient. A sedative such as diazepam may be given to the anxious person. General anesthesia is required when the person is overly apprehensive or when much manipulation is anticipated. In these instances, anesthesia reduces the possibility of trauma to the urethra or perforation of the bladder caused by sudden vigorous movement of the patient during the examination.

When the patient is awake, passing the instrument will be followed immediately by a strong desire to void. This occurs as a result of the pressure the instrument exerts against the internal sphincter. During the examination the bladder is distended with distilled water to make visualization more effective. As the bladder becomes increasingly distended, the urge to void increases.

During cystoscopy a number of tests may be performed on the urinary system. *Cystography* involves the injection of a radiopaque dye such as methiodal (Skiodan) or air as a contrast medium to visualize the bladder and determine its size, shape, and any irregularities. Bladder capacity may be measured through instillation of distilled water. A *voiding cystourethrogram* can reveal reflux of urine into the ureters on voiding, a bladder malfunction that can lead to pyelonephritis.

Ureteral catheterization (with a nylon, radiopaque, No. 4 to 6 Fr catheter) can be performed through the cystoscope. The catheter is inserted into the ureteral opening in the bladder, into the ureter, and into the renal pelvis (Fig. 33-25). This procedure may involve one or both ureters. It is performed (1) when culture and analysis of urine from individual kidneys is required; (2) when tests of renal function are to be performed on the kidneys separately;

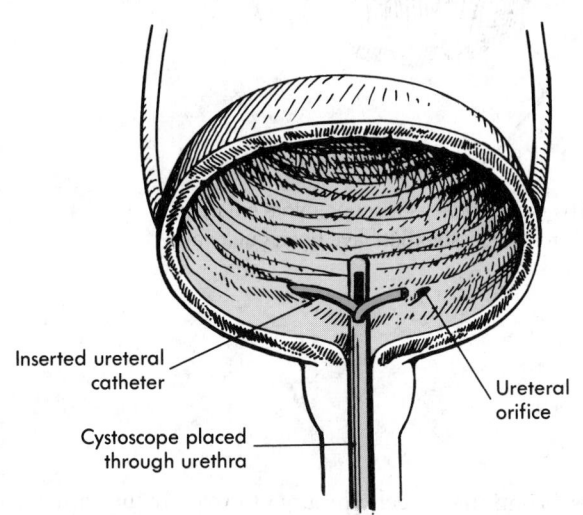

Inserted ureteral catheter

Cystoscope placed through urethra

Ureteral orifice

Fig. 33-25 Ureteral catheterization through cystoscope. Note ureteral catheter inserted into left orifice. Right ureteral catheter is ready to be inserted.

and (3) when visualization of the urinary tract is desired and intravenous pyelogram visualization has been inadequate, obstruction is present, or sensitivity to intravenous radiopaque material is noted.

Postprocedure care

Care should be taken that the person does not stand or walk alone immediately after cystoscopy. Blood that has drained from the leg while the person is in the lithotomy position will flow back into the vessels of the feet and legs as the person stands. Accidents caused by dizziness and fainting can occur from the sudden change in distribution of blood.

Three complications of cystoscopy that need to be monitored are bleeding, perforation of the bladder, and spread of infection throughout the urinary tract or into the bloodstream (sepsis). Observation for frank bleeding (pink-tinged urine is normal) is necessary. Monitor urinary output and voiding pattern to detect obstruction, and increase fluid intake to prevent stasis. Administer mild analgesics for discomfort, and provide warmth if the patient complains of being chilly. Monitor vital signs as necessary.

Interventions

If urinary retention is present, the man is catheterized to relieve the retention. If the obstruction is severe, an indwelling catheter is inserted. Urinary tract infection is treated with antibiotics. Surgery is the primary treatment for BPH. During surgery the capsule of the prostate gland is left intact, and the adenomatous soft tissue is removed by one of four surgical routes: transurethral, suprapubic, retropubic, or perineal (Table 33-12).

Table 33-12 Comparison of types of prostatic surgery

	Transurethral resection	Suprapubic resection	Retropubic resection	Perineal resection	Total perineal resection
Reason for surgery	Enlargement of medial lobe surrounding urethra	Extremely large mass of obstructing tissue	Large mass located high in pelvic area	Large mass located low in pelvic area	Cancer of prostate gland
Location of incision	No incision; removal by way of urethra	Low midline abdominal incision through bladder to prostate gland	Low midline abdominal incision into prostate gland (bladder not incised)	Incision between scrotum and rectum	Large perineal incision between scrotum and rectum
Drainage tubes	Three-way Foley catheter with 30-ml bag in urethra, constant irrigation for 24 hr	Cystotomy tube or drain through incision; Foley catheter with 30-ml bag in urethra	Foley catheter with 30-ml bag in urethra, constant irrigation for 24 hr	Foley catheter with 30-ml bag in urethra	Foley catheter with 30-ml bag in urethra; drain in incision
Bladder spasms	Yes	Yes	Few	Few	Few
Dressing	None	Abdominal dressing easily soaked with urinary drainage	Abdominal dressing; no urinary drainage	Perineal dressing; no urinary drainage	Perineal dressing; urinary drainage
Complications	Hemorrhage; water intoxication; incontinence	Hemorrhage; wound infection	Hemorrhage; wound infection	Hemorrhage; wound infection	Urinary incontinence; wound infection; impotence; sterility

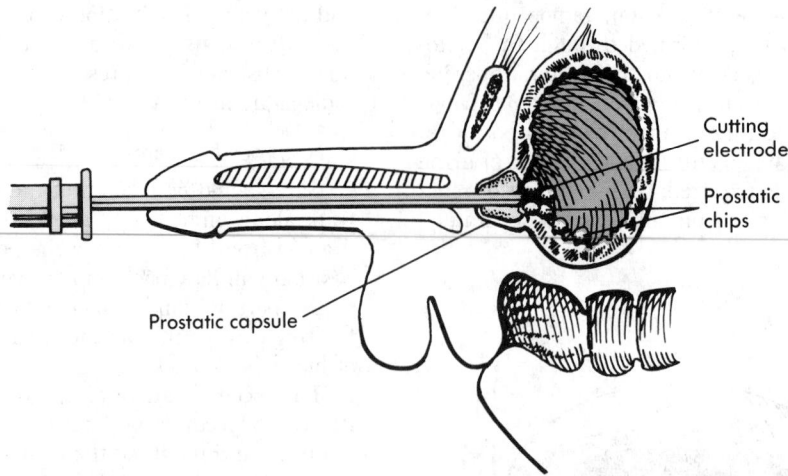

Fig. 33-26 Transurethral resection of prostate gland by means of resectoscope. Note enlarged prostate gland surrounding urethra and tiny pieces of prostatic tissue that have been cut away.

Two newer approaches include *balloon dilatation* of the prostate under endoscopy, and *transuretheral incision of the prostate* (TUIP) at the bladder neck. These measures break the prostatic capsule and allow for decompression of the prostate.[54]

Transurethral prostatectomy

Transurethral prostatic resection (TURP) is performed when the major enlargement exists in the medial lobe that directly surrounds the urethra. There must be a relatively small amount of tissue requiring resection so that excessive bleeding will not occur and the time required to complete the surgery will not be prolonged. A resectoscope (an instrument similar to a cystoscope but equipped with a cutting and cauterization loop attached to electric current) is passed through the urethra. The bladder is irrigated continuously during the procedure. Tiny pieces of tissue are cut away, and the bleeding points are sealed by cauterization (Fig. 33-26). A transurethral prostatectomy may be performed with the patient under general or spinal anesthesia.

Urinary drainage

Following a TURP, a large (No. 24 Fr) three-way Foley catheter with a 30-ml balloon is usually inserted into the urethra. After the retention balloon of the catheter is inflated, the catheter is pulled down so that the bag rests in the prostatic fossa and provides hemostasis. Traction may be applied to the Foley catheter to increase pressure on the operative area to control bleeding. The large-size catheter (No. 24 Fr) is used to facilitate removal of clots from the bladder. Because the catheter retention balloon exerts pressure on the internal sphincter of the bladder, the pa-

tient continually feels the urge to void. If the catheter is draining properly, the strongest of these sensations usually passes momentarily. Attempting to void around the catheter causes the bladder muscles to contract and results in a painful "bladder spasm."

Discuss the physiology of the "need to void" with the patient preoperatively so that spasms will be seen as an expected event and not an abnormal complication. Teach the patient that the catheter produces the sensation of fullness and that *not* straining to pass urine around the catheter and drinking large amounts of fluids reduces irritation and spasm. Narcotics are given to lessen the pain sensation; belladonna and opium (B & O) suppositories are prescribed to relieve bladder spasms. As the nerve endings become fatigued, the frequency and severity of spasms decrease, usually in 24 to 48 hours.

The bladder is constantly irrigated initially by a three-way drip with normal saline or other prescribed solution. The purpose of constant irrigation is to keep the bladder free of clots that would block urinary drainage. Constant bladder irrigation is usually discontinued after 24 hours if no clots are draining from the bladder. The catheter may then be irrigated manually as necessary.

The patient may not be able to void after removal of the catheter because of urethral edema, and the catheter may have to be reinserted. There may also be some urinary incontinence after catheter removal because the internal and external sphincters, which lie above and below the prostate gland, may have been disturbed during surgery. Continence usually returns. The time, amount, and control of voiding is recorded until normal urinary elimination patterns return.

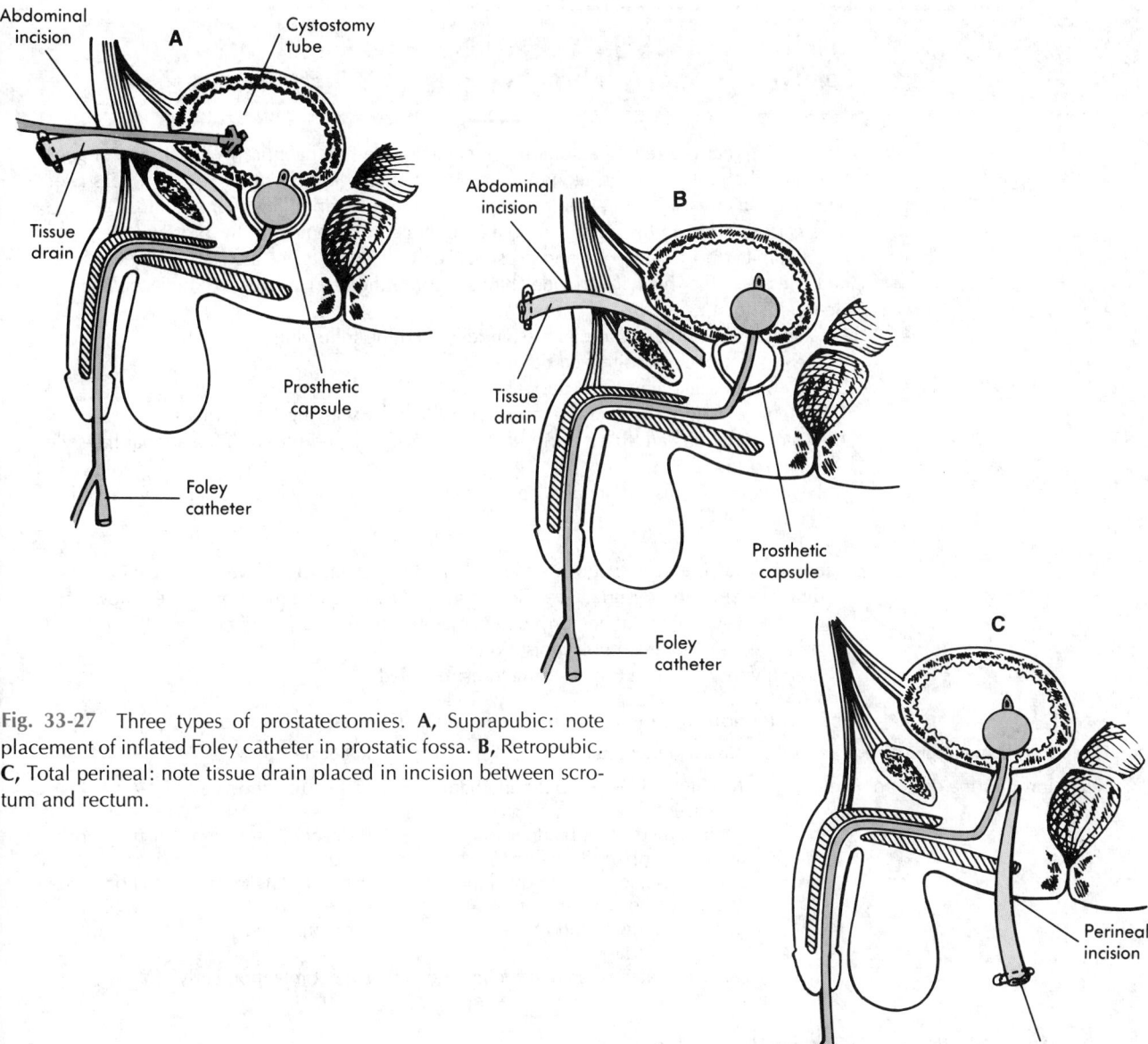

Fig. 33-27   Three types of prostatectomies. **A,** Suprapubic: note placement of inflated Foley catheter in prostatic fossa. **B,** Retropubic. **C,** Total perineal: note tissue drain placed in incision between scrotum and rectum.

Complications

Persistent bladder discomfort, bladder spasms, or failure of a catheter to drain properly usually signifies one of several serious complications that require immediate medical attention: (1)hemorrhage and clot retention, (2) catheter displacement, or (3) unsuspected *bladder perforation* during surgery as evidenced by severe abdominal pain.

Bleeding may result from a full bladder causing pressure on the outside of the prostatic fossa, "milking" the bleeding vessels. Straining to have a bowel movement may also cause prostatic hemorrhage, as can enemas, rectal tubes, and rectal thermometers, all of which are avoided for about a week postoperatively. About 2 weeks after TURP, when desiccated tissue is sloughed out, there may be a secondary hemorrhage. Instruct the patient to report any bleeding to the physician.

Patients now rarely develop *water intoxication* as a result of excessive irrigating solution being absorbed into the venous sinusoids during surgery, but it may occur. Cerebral edema may result, and patient confusion and agitation may be the first signs of this condition.

Suprapubic prostatectomy

The alternate methods of prostatectomy are open operations. In the *suprapubic resection* the prostate gland is removed from the urethra by way of the bladder; this type of resection is performed when a large mass of tissue must be resected. The usual method of draining urine following surgery is illustrated in Fig. 33-27, A. There will be some type of hemostatic agent placed in the prostatic fossa and urine will be drained by Foley catheter or cystotomy tube or both.

Nursing Care Plan	**Man with transurethral resection prostatectomy for benign prostatic hypertrophy**

DATA: Mr. S. is a 72-year-old retired automobile mechanic. He had been in his usual state of good health until about 4 months ago when he started to develop nocturia. Several weeks later he noted difficulty initiating voiding. He also noted mild dribbling after voiding. On physical examination his physician noted moderate enlargement of his prostate. He is being admitted for cystoscopy and possible TURP. His vital signs are stable. He is married and states that his wife provides him support at home. He lives in a two-story, single-family home.

The nursing history obtained on admission identified the following:
1. He has not been hospitalized before.
2. He does not take any medications.
3. He enjoys outdoor activities and exercises daily by walking 2 to 3 miles.
4. His expectations are that he will have the procedure and return to his normal life-style within a few days.
5. His wife is in constant attendance and tends to answer any questions that are asked of the patient.

Collaborative nursing actions include those to monitor for postoperative complications, including bleeding and dysuria. Specific nursing actions include monitoring the following:
1. Signs and symptoms of hemorrhage: hematuria; increased pulse; decreased blood pressure; restlessness; cool, moist skin
2. Inability to void once urinary catheter is removed

Nursing diagnosis: Urinary retention, high risk for: related to obstruction secondary to TURP

Expected patient outcomes	Nursing interventions	Rationale
Retention of urine does not occur	Monitor urinary output and characteristics	Detect retention early
	Maintain constant bladder irrigation as prescribed during first 24 hours	Prevent clots from obstructing urine flow
	Maintain patency of in-dwelling urinary catheter by irrigating	Prevent clots from obstruction catheter
	Encourage high fluid intake (2500 to 3000 ml/day)	Promote urinary flow
	After catheter is removed, continue to monitor for signs of retention	Detect retention early

Nursing diagnosis: Pain: related to bladder spasm

Expected patient outcomes	Nursing interventions	Rationale
Mr. S. states feeling more comfortable	Teach Mr. S. not to try to void around catheter	Reduce likelihood of spasm
	Monitor for pain at regular intervals for 48 hours to identify early signs of bladder spasm	Identify presence of spasms so that medication may be administered
	Give prescribed medications (analgesics, antispasmodics)	Relieve pain
	Tell Mr. S. spasms will decrease in intensity and frequency within 24 to 48 hours	Decreased anxiety will decrease pain

Nursing diagnosis: Injury, high risk for: hemorrhage or infection related to surgery

Expected patient outcomes	Nursing interventions	Rationale
Infection does not occur Bleeding is minimized	Monitor vital signs, report signs of shock or fever	Prevent shock before it occurs
	Monitor appearance of urine for persistent bright red color rather than expected dark red beyond first few hours postoperatively	Urine should change from cherry pink to amber in the first 2 to 3 postoperative days

Nursing diagnosis: Injury, high risk for: hemorrhage or infection related to surgery—cont'd

Expected patient outcomes	Nursing interventions	Rationale
	Teach Mr. S. to avoid Valsalva maneuver	May initiate prostatic bleeding during initial postoperative period because of pressure
	Avoid use of rectal thermometers, rectal examinations, or enemas for at least 1 week	May inititate prostatic bleeding
	Maintain strict asepsis of urinary drainage system, irrigate only when necessary	Minimize potential of introducing organisms that could cause infection
	Encourage high fluid intake to 3000 ml/day	Increase urinary output that will reduce potential of infection

Nursing diagnosis: Incontinence, stress or urge: related to catheter removal following surgery

Expected patient outcomes	Nursing interventions	Rationale
Mr. S. achieves urinary control	Assess Mr. S. for dribbling after catheter is removed	Detect incontinence
	If dribbling occurs:	
	a. Tell Mr. S. this is common occurrence and continence will return	Patient needs to be reassured this is normal
	b. Teach perineal exercises	Assist in bladder control

Nursing diagnosis: Sexual dysfunction: high risk for, related to TURP

Expected patient outcomes	Nursing interventions	Rationale
Sexual functioning is maintained	Give Mr. S. opportunity to discuss feelings about effects of prostatectomy on sexual intercourse	This is a difficult subject for many patients to raise
	Provide information as necessary	Lack of knowledge may create anxiety and lead to sexual dysfunction
	a. Probable return of previous level of functioning	
	b. Occurrence of retrograde ejaculation (urine may have a milky appearance)	
	Avoid sexual intercourse for 3 to 4 weeks after surgery	Bleeding and discomfort may occur

Nursing diagnosis: Knowledge deficit: related to TURP

Expected patient outcomes	Nursing interventions	Rationale
Mr. S. describes activity restrictions and need for medical follow-up	Teach Mr. S.:	
	a. Avoidance of heavy activites for 3 to 4 weeks (check with physician regarding resumption of long walks)	May initiate bleeding
	b. Avoidance of straining at stool for 4 to 6 weeks; use of stool softeners or laxatives as necessary	Straining may initiate bleeding; stool softeners will reduce the need to strain at stool
	c. Fluid maintenance of at least 2500 ml to 3000 ml/day	Will reduce potential of infection and clot formation
	d. Instructions for medical follow-up	Follow-up is essential to ensure no complications have developed

Hemorrhage is a possible complication, and the precautions are the same as those taken following TURP. Because there is some oozing of blood from the prostatic fossa, continuous bladder irrigations are usually ordered for the first 24 hours.

Cystotomy tubes are usually removed 3 to 4 days postoperatively; urethral catheters generally remain until the suprapubic wound is healed. After the urethral catheter has been removed, the nursing care of the patient is similar to that for the patient undergoing transurethral resection. If the suprapubic wound should reopen and drain, a urethral catheter is usually reinserted.

Retropubic prostatectomy

In a retropubic prostatectomy a low abdominal incision similar to that used for suprapubic prostatectomy is made, but the bladder is not opened. Rather, it is retracted and the adenomatous prostatic tissue is removed through an incision in the anterior prostatic capsule (Fig. 33-27, *B*).

Sphincter muscles are seldom damaged by retropubic prostatectomy, and there is no urine fistula. A large Foley catheter is inserted postoperatively, but bladder spasms are not usually a problem. When the Foley catheter is removed, the patient seldom has difficulty voiding. Hemorrhage from the prostatic fossa and wound infection may complicate the surgery; therefore, precautions to prevent bleeding as discussed under TURP are taken. There should be no urinary drainage on the abdominal dressing. If urinary drainage on the abdominal dressing, purulent drainage, fever, or increased pain with ambulation occurs, notify the physician because these symptoms may indicate deep wound infection or pelvic abscess.

Perineal prostatectomy

The perineal approach is used primarily for confirmed or suspected cancer of the prostate (Fig. 33-27, *C*). The incision is made between the scrotum and rectum. In addition to removal of the adenomatous prostate tissue, adjacent tissue may be excised when cancer is confirmed. Preoperative and postoperative care is similar to that given a patient having radical perineal surgery.

Postoperative counseling and teaching

Common to all patients undergoing prostatectomy are concerns regarding *sexual functioning* and the *ability to be continent of urine*. The nurse may need to provide an opportunity during interactions with the patient to promote expressions of these concerns by the patient. Impotence may occur physiologically if the perineal nerves are cut during a radical perineal prostatectomy, not with the other types of prostatectomies. If the man believes that the surgery will or may produce impotence, however, this may occur because of psychologic influences. Temporary urinary incontinence frequently follows transurethral or suprapubic prostatectomy. Most men have some difficulty with continence after any type of prostatectomy. The patient should understand that this is normal for a period after surgery, and he should be taught perineal exercises to hasten recovery of control over voiding.

The following points should be included in preparing the patient for discharge from the hospital: (1) Vigorous exercises, heavy lifting, and sexual intercourse should be avoided for about 3 weeks after returning home. (2) Driving during this period is also not advised. (3) Straining with defecation should be avoided; stool softeners or mild cathartics may be prescribed as home-going medication. (4) Fluids are encouraged to prevent stasis and infection and to keep stools soft. (5) The patient is instructed to notify his physician should his urinary stream diminish. The urinary stream also will be checked on the patient's postoperative visit to the physician. This is important because urethral mucosa in the prostatic area is destroyed during surgery and strictures may form with healing.

URETHRAL STRICTURES

A urethral stricture is a narrowing or constriction of the lumen of the urethra. Urethral strictures can be congenital or acquired. Congenital urethral strictures can occur in isolation or in combination with other urinary tract anomalies. Acquired urethral stricture can result from trauma secondary to accident or instrumentation, infection, muscular spasm, or pressure from the outside, by adjacent structures, or by growing tumors. Urethral strictures occur more often in men than women, primarily because of the length of the urethra. A common cause of strictures in the past was the instillation of silver nitrate in the male urethra for the treatment of gonorrhea.

Urethral strictures are repaired by transurethral visual urethrotomy or by urethroplasty with end-to-end anastomosis or with an inlay graft. Care of the person after transurethal visual urethrotomy is similar to that after a TURP (p. 1054). The urethroplasty is open surgical repair through a lower abdominal approach; the care of the patient is similar to that following other urologic surgeries (p. 1050).

NEOPLASMS

Neoplasms of the urinary system are a significant source of morbidity. The major neoplasms are found in the kidney and bladder. Cancer of the prostate causes urinary problems by pressure on the urethra, leading to obstruction (Table 33-13). Tumors growing anywhere within the abdominal cavity can result in renal involvement through metastasis or invasion, or by pressure of the tumor creating urinary obstruction. Urinary diversion (p. 1061) may be required in treating urinary neoplasms.

RENAL NEOPLASMS

Malignant renal tumors, primarily adenocarcinomas, account for 2% of all cancers. Small benign renal tumors (adenomas) may occur without causing significant damage or symptoms. Renal cell carcinomas rarely occur before the age of 40 years, are more commonly seen in the 50- to 70-year age range, and occur twice as often in men as in women.[47]

Hematuria is the most frequent symptom of renal cell carcinoma. Unfortunately, the hematuria is often intermittent, lessening the person's concern and causing pro-

REVIEW

Table 33-13   Tumors of the urinary tract

Site	Incidence	Signs and symptoms	Medical therapy
Kidney	2%	Hematuria Dull flank pain Flank mass Unexplained weight loss Fever Polycythemia	Nephrectomy Radiation
Bladder	5%	Intermittent hematuria Anemia Cystitis Suprapubic pain RBCs, WBCs, and bacteria in urine	Transurethral fulguration or excision of small papillomas Segmental or total cystectomy Intravesicular chemotherapy if the bladder is not removed Palliative chemotherapy
Prostate	20%	Urethral obstruction Low-back pain Hematuria Anemia	Radical resection of prostate Radiation Hormonal therapy

crastination in seeking medical care. Any person with hematuria should have a complete urologic examination, because it is only by immediate investigation of the first signs of hematuria that there is any hope of cure. Other symptoms may include dull flank pain, flank mass, weight loss, fever, hypercalcemia, increased sedimentation rate, and polycythemia. Hypertension may result from stimulation of the renin-angiotensin system.

An IVP may show a distortion of renal outline suggesting a kidney tumor. Small tumors in the parenchyma may not be apparent on a routine pyelogram but may be identified by ultrasound or CT scan. A CT scan is also useful in differentiating between renal cell carcinoma and renal cyst. Angiography may also be performed to differentiate a cyst from a tumor.

Unless the person is a poor surgical risk or has extensive metastases, the diseased kidney is removed (*nephrectomy*) through a transabdominal, thoracoabdominal, or retroperitoneal approach. The first two approaches are preferred to secure the renal artery and vein and prevent any spread of malignant cells. (See p. 1050 for care of the person requiring urologic surgery.)

Following surgery for a malignant tumor that is radiosensitive, the patient may be given a course of x-ray therapy. Hospitalization may not be necessary during this time. Chemotherapy has not yet proved of value in the treatment of renal cell carcinomas. The survival rate after therapy depends on the extent of metastasis. The 10-year survival rate is very low, especially because many persons do not seek initial treatment until the disease is far advanced.

TUMORS OF THE BLADDER
Etiology/Epidemiology

The most common site of cancer in the urinary tract is the bladder. It occurs four times more often in men than women, more often in whites than blacks, and more often in persons over the age of 50. Bladder cancer occurs twice as often in *smokers* than nonsmokers, and it is estimated that smoking is responsible for deaths from bladder cancer in 47% of men and 37% of women.[3] Other risk factors include aniline dye and schistosomiasis.

Pathophysiology

Almost half of bladder tumors involve the trigone of the bladder, and most of the remainder are found on the posterior and lateral walls. Tumors range from small benign papillomas to large invasive carcinomas. Most of the neoplasms begin as papillomas; therefore, all bladder papillomas are considered premalignant and are removed when identified. Squamous cell carcinoma occurs less frequently and has a poorer prognosis.

Grades I (well differentiated) and II (medially differentiated) bladder tumors are usually superficial, while grades III (poorly differentiated) and IV (anaplastic) tumors are usually invasive. Bladder cancers are *staged* according to the depth of invasiveness:

Stage O:	Mucosa
State A:	Submucosa
Stage B:	Muscle
State C:	Perivesical fat
State D:	Lymph nodes

Painless *hematuria* is the first symptom in the majority of bladder tumors. It is usually intermittent, and the individual may fail to seek treatment. Painless hematuria occurs also in nonmalignant urinary tract disease and in cancer of the kidney; therefore, any hematuria should be investigated. Cystitis may be the first symptom of a bladder tumor because the tumor may act as a foreign body in the bladder. Renal failure from obstruction of the ureters sometimes is the reason given for seeking medical care. Vesicovaginal fistulas may occur before other symptoms develop. The last two conditions indicate a poor prognosis because usually the tumor has infiltrated widely.

Diagnostic tests

Cytologic examination of the urine may identify malignant cells before the lesion can be visualized by cystoscopy. The diagnosis is established by cystoscopic visualization of the bladder with biopsy. Clinical determination of the invasiveness of the tumor is important in establishing a therapeutic regimen and in predicting the prognosis. Any person who has had a papilloma removed should have a cystoscopic examination every 3 months for 2 years and then at less frequent intervals if there is no evidence of a new lesion. The necessity for frequent examination should be fully explained by the urologist, and the explanation should be reinforced by the nurse. Emphasize the need for repeated cystoscopies because papillomas tend to recur without symptoms until they are far advanced tumors.

Interventions
Surgery

Small tumors with minimal tissue layer involvement may be adequately treated with transurethral fulguration or excision. A Foley catheter may or may not be inserted after surgery. Nd:YAG-lasers may be used for low-grade tumors. The urine may be pink tinged, but gross bleeding is unusual. Burning on urination may be relieved by forcing fluids and applying heat over the bladder region by means of a heating pad or a sitz bath.

If the tumor involves the dome of the bladder, a *segmental resection* of the bladder (p. 1050) may be carried out. Over half of the bladder may be resected. A *cystectomy*, or complete removal of the bladder, usually is performed only when the disease appears curable. Complete removal of the bladder requires permanent urinary diversion (p. 1061).

Radiation

External cobalt radiation of large invasive tumors may be given before surgery to retard tumor growth. Supervoltage irradiation can be given when the patient physically cannot tolerate surgery. Radiation is not curative and has little value in patient management if the tumor is deemed inoperable. Internal radiation (radioisotopes or radon seeds) are rarely used since the introduction of better methods of external radiation.

Chemotherapy

Chemotherapy is primarily palliative. Thiotepa may be instilled into the bladder as a topical treatment. The patient is dehydrated 8 to 12 hours before thiotepa treatment, and the drug remains in the bladder for 2 hours.

CANCER OF THE PROSTATE

The prostate gland is the second most common site of cancer among men. There is a familial tendency for the disease. Prostate cancer is responsible for 10% of all deaths from cancer in men. It rarely occurs before age 50 and the incidence increases with age. The younger the man at the age of onset, the more lethal is the disease. Although cancer may start anywhere within the prostate gland and may be multifocal in origin, it usually arises in the peripheral lobes resulting in a palpable nodule. Early detection of nodules on palpation can lead to early treatment and improve the prognosis significantly. For this reason all men over age 40 should have an annual rectal examination.

Prostate specific antigen (PAS) is elevated in the serum of about 60% of men with prostate cancer and serves as a tumor marker.[47] It is not a useful tool for prostate cancer screening, because up to 30% of men with BPH can have false-positive levels and 30% of men with prostatic cancer can have false-negative levels.[54] However, the PAS serum level drops sharply with complete response to treatment, which makes it helpful for determining effectiveness of therapy. Prostatic biopsy is performed for palpable prostate nodules.

Prostate cancer usually begins with changes in voiding patterns, including frequency, urgency, and nocturia because of the enlarged gland pressing on the urethra. Complete urethral obstruction can develop. Hematuria can occur resulting in anemia. Treatment is surgery or radiation.

Total Prostatectomy

Total prostatectomy is usually curative in patients in whom a diagnosis of prostatic cancer is made before local extension of the cancer or distant metastasis. The entire prostate gland, including the capsule and adjacent tissue, is removed. The remaining urethra is then anastomosed to the bladder neck. The perineal approach is the favored approach, but a retropubic route may also be used (see p. 1058). Because the internal and external sphincters of the bladder lie close to the prostate gland, urinary incontinence may occur in about 4% of patients after prostatectomy.

Preoperative care

If a perineal approach is planned, the patient is given a bowel preparation similar to that for bowel surgery (Chapter 32) and only clear fluids the day before surgery to prevent fecal contamination of the operative site. Postoperatively, when food is permitted, a low-residue diet may be given until the wound has healed.

Total prostatectomy results in physiologic sexual dysfunction from disruption of genital innervation in 20% of men.[54] Most of these patients lose emission, ejaculation, and erectile potency. Both the man and his sexual partner are alerted to the potential for sexual dysfunction before surgery, but it can be stressed that 80% will not experience sexual difficulties.

Postoperative care

The patient returns from surgery with an in-dwelling urethral catheter. A large amount of urinary drainage on the dressing for a number of hours is not unusual. This can be managed by use of an ostomy bag around the dressing. Urinary drainage should decrease rapidly. There should not be the amount of bleeding that follows other prostatic surgery.

Because the catheter is not being used for hemostasis, the patient usually has few bladder spasms. The catheter is used both for urinary drainage and as a splint for the urethral anastomosis; therefore, care is taken that it does not become dislodged or blocked. The risk of blockage is greatest during the first hour. The catheter may be irrigated intermittently or continuously as ordered by the physician. The catheter is usually left in the bladder for 2 to 3 weeks.

Fecal incontinence may occur after surgery as a result

f relaxation of the perineal musculature. Control of the ectal sphincter usually returns readily. Return of function an be facilitated by perineal exercises (p. 1030) started vithin a day or two after surgery and continued after rectal phincter control returns, to strengthen bladder sphincters unless the bladder sphincters have been permanently damged).

The patient who experiences sexual dysfunction or in-ontinence after total prostatectomy is often very de-pressed. At times the man may have difficulty talking to his sexual partner about his concerns and the effect of his impotence on their relationship. The nurse can encour-ge each person to share his and her feelings separately, hen gently encourage and facilitate mutual sharing by the artners.

Radiation

Radiation may be used in place of surgery, especially with lder men with curative lesions or in the absence of me-astasis. The 15-year results are better with surgery than adiation for patients with localized lesions. External beam adiation or interstitial radiation with implantation of I-25 seeds may be used.

Palliative therapy

atients with metastatic disease may be given androgen herapy in the form of diethylstilbesterol (DES) or orchiec-omy (removal of the testes). Luteinizing hormone-releas-ng hormone (LHRH) agonists may be given to suppress H and serum testosterone.[47] Corticosteroids may be given or bone pain.

URINARY DIVERSION

Urinary diversion procedures are surgical procedures that ivert the urinary flow from its normal flow patterns to a ewly created opening, usually on the abdominal wall. lthough urinary neoplasms are one of the major reasons or urinary diversions, these procedures may also be per-ormed for neurogenic bladder dysfunction, chronic pro-ressive pyelonephritis, urinary birth defects, or irrepa-able urinary tract trauma.

Urinary Diversion Procedures

he most common urinary diversion procedures include reterostomy, ileal or colonic conduits, and continent uros-omies (see Box 33-15). These procedures require place-ent of an external abdominal stoma.

A *cutaneous ureterostomy* is used when the physical con-ition of the person prohibits more extensive surgery. This s usually temporary therapy followed by more extensive reatment. The ureters drain directly through the stoma; here is no reservoir. Initially the ureterostomy stoma ap-ears pink, but it turns pale in several weeks. Stricture of ne ureter at the stoma may occur and is treated with ilation; untreated strictures can result in hydronephrosis rom urine backup. UTI is also a common complication.

The *ileal conduit (ileal loop)* is the most common per-anent urinary diversion. A section of the ileum is resected ith the mesentery and blood supply intact, and the ileum

---

33-15

Types of urinary diversions

Cutaneous ureterostomy

Ureters excised from bladder and brought out through skin in one or two stomas.

Conduit urostomies

Ureters drain into reservoir; urine flows freely through reservoir and out through stoma into a drainage bag
  Ileal conduit (ileal loop): a section of ileum is used to form a reservoir (Fig. 33-28)
  Colonic conduit: a section of the colon is used for the conduit reservoir

Continent urostomies

Ureters drain into a reservoir that has a valved stoma; stoma is catheterized to remove urine (drainage bag not required)
  Kock continent ileal reservoir: reservoir is formed from loops of small intestine (Fig. 33-29)
  Cecoileal continent urinary reservoir (Indiana pouch): reservoir formed from portion of large intestine and ileum

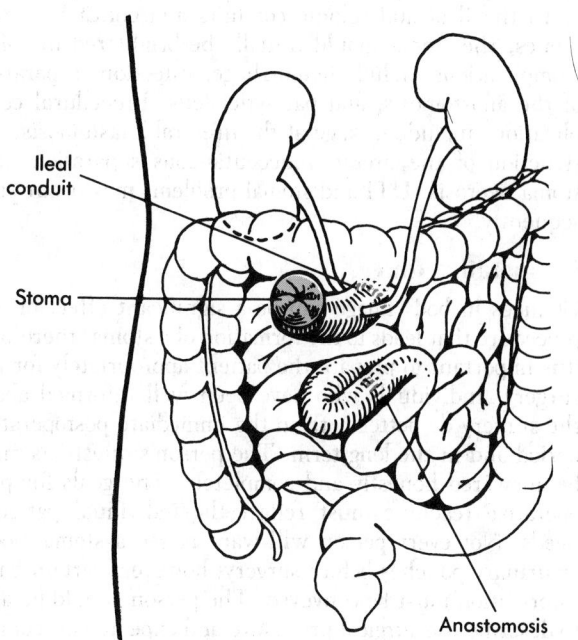

Fig. 33-28   Ileal conduit or ileal loop.

---

itself is then anastomosed (Fig. 33-28). The ureters are excised from the bladder and anastomosed to one end of the resected ileal portion; that end is then sutured closed to form a pouch that serves as a conduit reservoir. The open end of the resected ileal portion is then brought through the abdominal wall to the skin to create a stoma. The urinary bladder may be left intact or resected, de-pending on the reason for the diversion. The *colonic conduit* is preferred by some surgeons because it has been shown to reduce the incidence of urinary reflux in some people.[6]

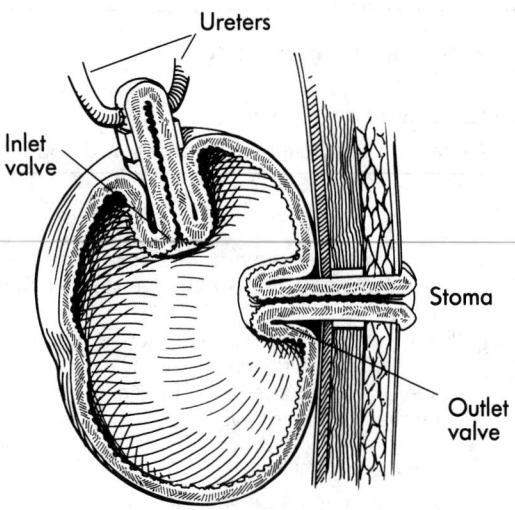

Fig. 33-29 Kock continent ileal urinary reservoir.

Continent urostomies, which are newer procedures, differ from the ileal and colonic conduits by formation of a "valved" stoma (Fig. 33-29). The urine remains in the reservoir until removed by catheter; thus an external drainage bag is not required.

In the ileal and colonic conduits and continent urostomies, the stoma should initially be bright red in color. Complications include hemorrhage, infection, separation of the anastomosis, and paralytic ileus. Procedural complications include leakage at the ureteral anastomosis, obstruction of the ureter, mucocutaneous separation, and stoma necrosis. UTI and stomal problems may occur subsequently.

Preoperative Care

Changes in body image can be a significant effect of any procedure that leads to the formation of a stoma, therefore, it is important to prepare the patient appropriately for the surgery. Individuals who have been well informed about the surgery do better both in the immediate postoperative period and in the long term. The person's questions must be answered honestly and completely. The goals for preoperative teaching must reflect the individual patient's needs. Not every person will want to see a stoma model or urinary pouches before surgery; however, certain basic information must be conveyed. The person should be able to describe the surgical procedure and expected outcomes.

The person is instructed concerning the appearance of the stoma. Anatomic charts, models, and simple drawings are ways of explaining the placement of the stoma. It is stressed that work, hobbies, physical activities, diet, and clothing should not change significantly after surgery.

A patient who is willing may be given an opportunity to handle a urostomy appliance to dispel any misconceptions. Patients can be reassured that stoma care will be provided immediately after surgery and that they will be assisted in mastering self-care before hospital discharge.

When the nurse perceives that it is appropriate, a visit from a person who has mastered the care of a urostomy can be reassuring to the patient. Many local cancer societies have volunteers available to provide this support. Preoperative preparation for ureterostomy is similar to that for other bowel procedures (Chapter 31).

Location of the stoma on the abdomen depends on the procedure. Ideally, the determination of the exact location of the stoma is made before surgery and includes an evaluation of the person's body when lying, sitting, and standing. The reason for this careful evaluation is to ensure that the location of the stoma allows for a smooth, even skin surface surrounding the stoma, for optimal adherence of the appliance.

Postoperative Care
Immediate care

Following a *cutaneous ureterostomy*, the patient generally returns from surgery with catheters (stents) inserted through the ureters to drain the renal pelves. The stents are usually left in place for 7 to 14 days. Patency of the catheters must be maintained because hydronephrosis can ensue rapidly if obstruction occurs.

After an *ileal or colonic conduit*, stents are usually left in place in the stoma for 7 to 10 days to promote urinary drainage. The person with a *continent urostomy* will usually have a catheter in the stoma sutured in place to allow drainage from the reservoir. Another drain tube may be placed into the pelvic area. These catheters prevent overdistention of the reservoir that may cause anastomosis leakage. A nasogastric tube with suction is also used for 2 to 3 days postoperatively to allow for the return of effective intestinal peristalsis and healing of the intestinal anastomosis. Nothing is permitted by mouth until the return of bowel sounds or passing of gas; the diet is then gradually advanced from small amounts of fluids to a normal diet.

During the immediate postoperative period, urinary output is monitored closely; decreased urinary output could signal obstruction of urinary drainage or complications such as dehydration or renal failure. Urine is tested for presence of blood. Blood in the urine is expected in the immediate postoperative period; however, it should clear within the first few postoperative days.

The abdominal incision is assessed daily for healing and signs and symptoms of infection. Care of the abdominal incision is sometimes complicated by the leakage of urine into it; this complication is minimized by using appropriate drainage bags postoperatively.

Skin care

In any type of urinary diversion care must be taken to prevent urine leakage onto the surrounding skin and the abdominal incision. For the ureterostomy and the conduit procedures, a transparent pouch is placed around the stoma in the operating room. This allows visualization of the stoma, catheter or stents, and stoma sutures. Any evidence of gray or black discoloration, indicating stomal necrosis, is reported to the surgeon. The pouch is changed in 24 to 48 hours postoperatively to allow for better visualization and assessment of the stoma and peristomal skin.

In the early postoperative period, the pouch is positioned to drain to the side of the bed, facilitating drainage and emptying of the pouch. The urostomy pouch has a valve at the bottom that permits emptying. Drainage tubing and

Table 33-14   Therapy for skin problems with urinary stomas

Problem	Therapy
Rash around stoma or under pouch	Dry and powder skin (except under adhesive)
	Use a skin barrier under pouch until skin is healed
Macerated skin around stoma	Dry skin and apply a hydrophobic skin barrier
	Decrease size of pouch opening
Crystals on or around stoma	Apply vinegar compresses on stoma and inside pouch for acidification
	Use pouch with antireflux valve
Ulcerated stoma	Enlarge pouch opening
	Consult enterostomal therapist if healing does not occur in 1 week
Monilial infection following antibiotic therapy	Dry skin and apply nystatin powder
	Encourage drinking of extra fluids to increase urine flow
	Consult enterostomal therapist if healing does not occur in 1 week
Folliculitis	Trim hair around stoma at regular intervals to prevent pulling hair follicles during pouch changes
Hyperplasia of skin around stoma	Decrease pouch opening size

a collection bag can be attached to the valve of the pouch to allow continuous drainage in the postoperative period. The procedure for changing the pouch is outlined in Box 33-16.

The skin is examined closely whenever the pouch is changed or if signs of skin problems are noted. Teach the patient to take action to correct problems that occur (Table 33-14).

Use and care of pouches

The stomal edema begins to subside within 7 days, but the stoma continues to decrease gradually in size for the next 6 to 8 weeks. The patient should be taught how to measure the stoma before going home, and how to adjust the pouch size to accommodate the smaller stoma. Too large an opening is a frequent cause of skin problems for persons with an ileal or colon conduit. Too small an opening in the pouch may restrict circulation or cause trauma to the stoma.

Several types of pouches are available (Figs. 33-30 and 33-31). All have two things in common: a pouch to collect the urine and an outlet or valve at the bottom for easy emptying every 3 to 4 hours. The basic types of pouches are (1) permanent pouches that can be washed and reused, (2) semidisposable pouches that fit onto a permanent disk or faceplate, and (3) one-piece or two-piece disposable pouches that are discarded after use. All adhere to the body with some form of adhesive to form a watertight seal. The type of pouch selected depends upon the patient's preference, body build, and special needs, such as physical or visual impairment. The enterostomal therapist can assist in the assessment and selection of the appropriate pouch for the patient.

Most persons can wear a pouch for 3 to 5 days between changes. An interval longer than 7 days should be discouraged because of potential odor, crystallization problems, or risk of infection. An appropriate schedule that eliminates leakage and provides the best skin protection needs to be determined based on patient adaptation.

Proper cleaning of reusable equipment is essential for odor control, general hygiene, and prevention of stomal complications. Manufacturers include cleaning instruc-

---

33-16

Changing a urinary pouch

1. Assemble needed supplies before starting.
2. Empty the pouch and gently remove the appiance from the skin.
3. Cleanse the skin surrounding the stoma with mild soap and water. Rinse and pat dry. Wash any mucous secretions from the stoma gently.
4. Place a rolled piece of gauze or cotton balls over the stoma opening to absorb draining urine while reapplying the pouch.
5. Measure the diameter of the stoma and cut a corresponding opening in the skin barrier (if used) and the pouch or select the corresponding size of precut pouch.
6. Apply skin sealant around the stoma if desired. Allow the area to dry completely.
7. Attach the pouch to the skin barrier. The pouch and skin barrier may be applied to the skin separately or together. In the early postoperative period it is easier to attach the pouch to the skin barrier and then to apply the system in one piece to the skin.
8. Apply the pouch and skin barrier around the stoma, keeping the adhesive area free of wrinkles or creases. Press gently but firmly into place and hold for approximately 30 seconds.
9. The valve at the bottom of the pouch must be closed or attached to drainage tubing and a collection bag.

---

tions with their equipment. The following are the principles for proper cleaning of reusable urinary appliances:

1. Clean equipment promptly.
2. Use adhesive remover as necessary to remove residue.
3. Avoid soaking equipment for prolonged periods of time (20 to 30 minutes in soap and water is sufficient). Longer soaking speeds deterioration of many appliances.

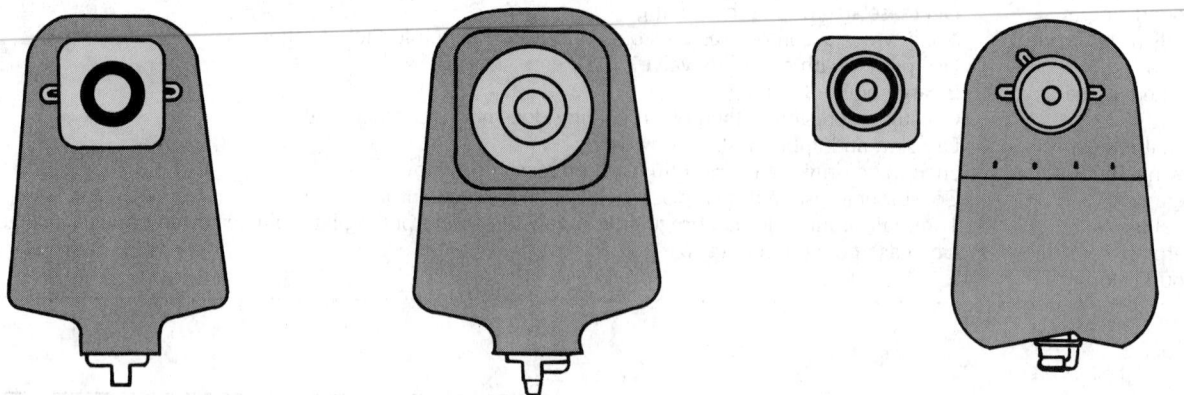

Fig. 33-30   Disposable one- and two-piece pouches.

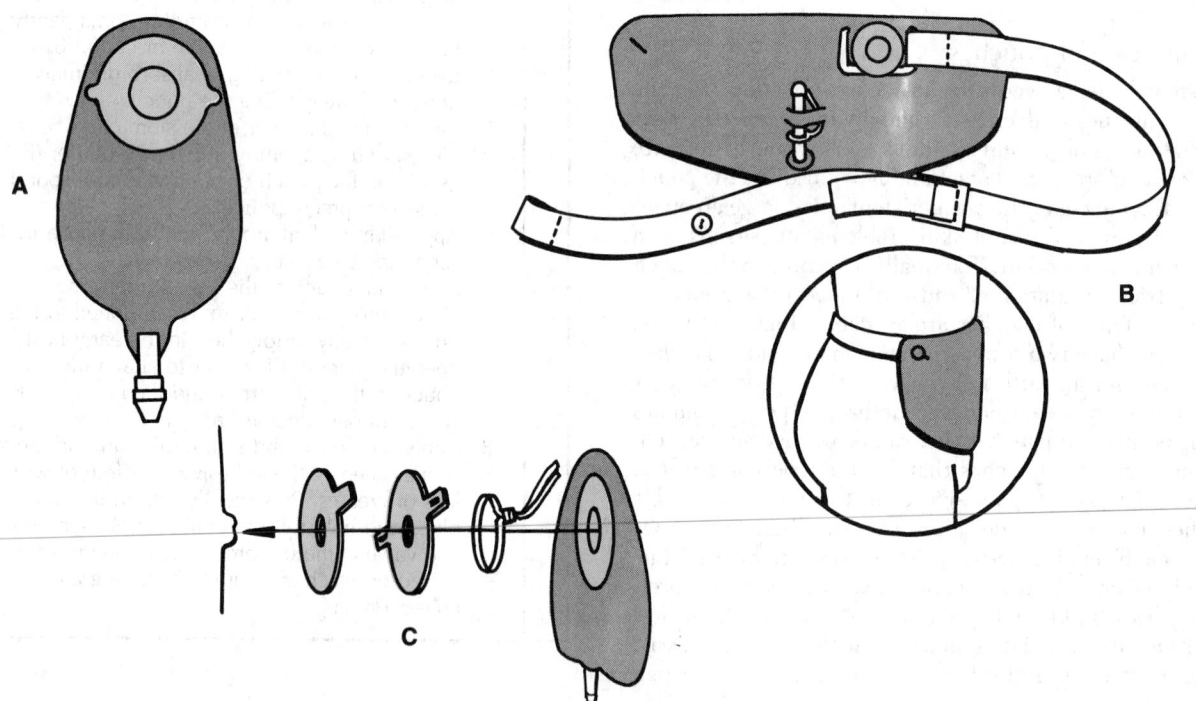

Fig. 33-31   Reusable pouches. **A,** One-piece pouch. **B,** One-piece nonadhesive pouch. **C,** Two-piece reusable faceplate and reusable or disposable pouch.

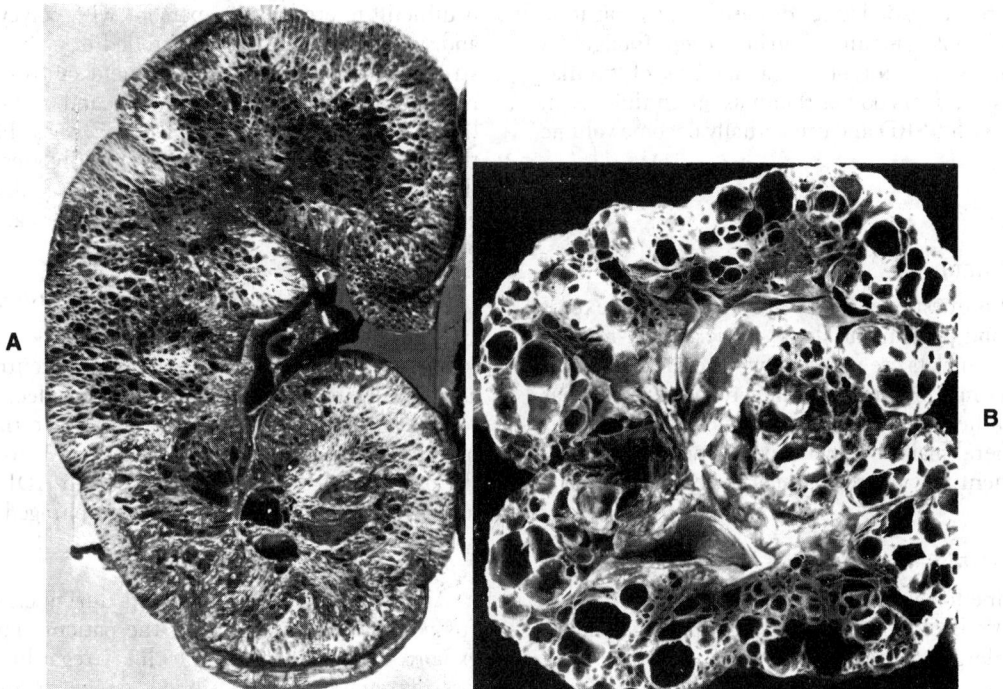

Fig. 33-32   Polycystic disease of kidney. **A,** Newborn infant. **B,** Adult. (From Kissane JM: *Anderson's pathology,* ed 9, St Louis, 1990, Mosby–Year Book.)

4. For odor problems, soak appliances in half-strength vinegar water for an additional 20 to 30 minutes.

Patient teaching

A teaching plan for the person with a urinary diversion includes the following:

1. Nature of the urinary diversion
2. Assessment of stoma appearance and changes that require medical attention
3. Methods to protect the skin
4. Use and care of pouches
5. Signs and symptoms of UTI
6. Community resources to obtain supplies and for ongoing support
7. Need for follow-up care

OTHER URINARY DISORDERS

Several disorders of the urinary tract do not fit into the classifications discussed thus far. These disorders, polycystic disease, vascular disorders, diabetic nephropathy, and trauma are discussed in this section.

POLYCYSTIC DISEASE

Etiology/Epidemiology

Polycystic disease is an inherited defect that involves the kidneys bilaterally. It is categorized into two groups, infantile and adult. The infant usually develops symptoms and dies within a few months after birth. In adults, the disease is inherited as an autosomal dominant trait, and affects about 1 of every 500 adults. Symptoms usually develop between the ages of 20 to 50. It is evenly distributed between the sexes and accounts for 5% to 8% of adults with end-stage renal disease (ESRD), which is usually reached 10 to 15 years after symptoms arise.

There is no preventive care for polycystic disease. However, early detection and medical care can prevent and control infection of the diseased kidneys and retard the development of ESRD.

Pathophysiology

The kidneys are usually enlarged and filled with cysts (Fig. 33-32). In adults, the collecting tubules are usually involved. At first only segments of the nephrons are cystic, but gradually the cysts increase in number and size. As the cysts enlarge, they distort the calyces and pelves and compress surrounding tissue causing ischemia. Both kidneys can become large, grossly appear to be full of variously sized bubbles, and feel bumpy. The cysts can be filled with tubular fluid (urine), serous fluid, blood, or a combination of fluids.

Signs and symptoms relate to loss of tubular function and tissue destruction (hematuria, calculi, polyuria, proteinuria, and hypertension) and increased kidney size (abdominal fullness and palpable abdominal mass). Also, the kidneys often become infected and lose their ability to concentrate urine or regulate sodium. Patients with polycystic kidney disease are not as anemic as other patients with ESRD because the site of erythropoietin production is not affected. Therefore, the energy level of these patients may be slightly higher than that of other patients with ESRD.

Patients with polycystic kidney disease usually continue to excrete a variable amount of urine, even though its quality is poor as a result of a gradual loss of tubular function. These patients do not retain as much fluid as an anuric patient with ESRD and can actually become volume depleted.

Nursing Process
Assessment
Subjective data

The patient is questioned about the presence and extent of discomfort and pain in the flank. Colicky pain may be experienced when clots are passed down the ureter. Symptoms of uremia may be present when renal function has deteriorated to the point of end-stage renal disease. Fever, chills, and general malaise may be experienced by the patient. The patient may express concerns about the failing kidney.

Objective data

Monitor urine for blood. Monitor vital signs and report repeated elevations of blood pressure. On physical examination, the enlarged kidneys appear as large palpable abdominal masses.

Diagnostic tests

Serum and urine electrolytes and creatinine clearance tests provide accurate data about renal function. A urine culture is obtained to determine the presence of UTI. Although a retrograde pyelograph and KUB can give valuable data about the size of the kidneys, the intravenous pyelogram (IVP) (p. 1047) is most often used to confirm the diagnosis.

Data analysis: nursing diagnoses

Nursing diagnoses are determined from analysis of patient data. Possible nursing diagnoses for the person with polycystic disease may include, but are not limited to, the following:

Diagnostic title	Possible etiologies
Pain	Renal inflammation
Grieving, anticipatory	Loss of renal function
Coping, ineffective individual	Situational crisis, personal vulnerability
Knowledge deficit	Unfamiliarity with information sources

Planning: expected patient outcomes

Expected patient outcomes for the person with polycystic disease may include, but are not limited to, the following:
1. States feeling more comfortable.
2. Verbalizes feelings about potential loss of renal function and shares feelings with family members.
3. Uses other support systems as appropriate.
4. States symptoms of infection and hematuria to report to physician, and plans for follow-up care.

Implementation
Assisting with achievement of therapeutic goals

Interventions for the patient with polycystic disease center largely on preventing infection and bleeding. Infection is difficult to eradicate in persons with polycystic kidneys, and when infection is uncontrolled it leads to further destruction of kidney tissue. Frequent culture of the urine is performed and instrumentation and catheterization of the urinary tract are avoided whenever possible. Antibiotic therapy is often instituted. When antibiotics are ordered, they should be given on time and on a regular schedule to ensure adequate blood levels. Monitor the patient's urinary output closely.

Interventions to achieve patient outcomes
Promoting comfort

Analgesic drugs may be necessary to control flank pain associated with enlarged kidneys. When bleeding from ruptured cysts becomes severe enough to turn the urine from pink to red, bed rest is usually instituted. At these times, the patient will require assistance with ADL. Otherwise, independence in ADL should be encouraged.

Facilitating anticipatory grieving

Approaches to helping patients during grieving are discussed in Chapter 15. Offer the patient opportunities to explore and communicate feelings regarding anticipated loss of renal function. Provide an open and supportive environment for both patient and family or significant others. Anticipate tears, anger, and regressive behavior and explain to family that the patient's behavior is not directed at them personally. Provide an atmosphere of trust and concern. Explore the need to restructure short- and long-term goals. Provide opportunities for patient and family to discuss these concerns alone.

Assisting with coping

The emotional overtones of this illness can be severe for both the individual and the family. Challenges exist in helping the person deal with an illness on an individual basis when relatives have died of the same disease and children have not yet developed symptoms. Counseling regarding family health care and the individual's role in passing on a potentially fatal disease to children will, at times, be required. Assist patient to find supportive persons, such as family or friends, clergy, and support groups.

Facilitating patient learning

The patient should know how to perform the following:
1. Monitor for signs of infection and hematuria (fever, increased flank pain, blood in urine) and report signs to physician.
2. Monitor urinary output and report changes to physician.
3. Report for diagnostic tests as instructed to identify early signs of kidney tissue destruction.
4. Take antibiotics as instructed.
5. Report to physician for follow-up care as instructed.

Evaluation

Evaluation is based on expected patient outcomes. Questions to consider include the following:
1. Is the patient comfortable?
2. Have patient and family had opportunities to verbalize and share feelings regarding anticipated loss of renal function?

3. Has patient identified appropriate sources of support, such as clergy and support groups?
4. Does patient know signs of infection and hematuria to report to physician?
5. Does patient state plans for follow-up care?

VASCULAR DISORDERS

Renal diseases resulting from vascular disorders are caused by one of two processes: *renal artery stenosis*, which is a narrowing of the main renal artery, or *nephrosclerosis*, which is sclerosis of renal arterioles. *Diabetic nephropathy* is also a vascular disorder that occurs as diabetes progresses.

Renal Artery Stenosis
Etiology/epidemiology

Stenosis of the renal arteries is usually classified as either arteriosclerosis or fibromuscular dysplasia. Atheromatous plaques may produce narrowing of the renal artery or arteries at the origin, main trunk, or one of the main branches. It is more common in men, especially those over age 50, and in patients with diabetes mellitus. Fibromuscular dysplasia involves the layers of the renal arteries and their branches. It occurs more commonly in young women. The end result of the stenosis is narrowing of the lumen of the arteries supplying the kidneys. Obstruction of the renal arteries can also be caused by aneurysms, thromboses, and emboli.

Pathophysiology

Renal stenosis results in a major reduction in circulation to the kidneys. This change in perfusion causes increased secretion of renin and activation of the renin-angiotensin-aldosterone system (Chapter 26). The end result is accelerated hypertension, which, if left untreated, leads to further pathologic changes in the kidneys. These changes include nephrosclerosis.

The signs of renal artery stenosis are:
1. Hypertension
2. Disparity in size of kidneys
3. Delayed appearance of contrast medium in renal arteriograph
4. Hyperconcentration of contrast medium in calyceal system on IVP.
5. Lesion evidenced on renal arteriograph.

Interventions

Medical treatment includes vigorous antihypertensive therapy to control blood pressure. When a well-defined lesion exists in the renal artery, vascular surgery may be performed to remove the affected area.

Nursing interventions are the same as those for hypertension (Chapter 26). The patient should know the importance of medical follow-up for identification of renal insufficiency.

Nephrosclerosis
Etiology

Renal disease associated with hypertension is called *nephrosclerosis*. *Benign nephrosclerosis* is associated with chronic, mild, or moderate hypertension and slowly developing renal insufficiency. *Malignant nephrosclerosis* is associated with marked hypertension, diastolic pressure greater than 140 mm Hg, rapidly developing renal failure, headaches, blurred vision, and congestive failure.

Pathophysiology

The renal vasculature is affected in *benign* nephrosclerosis. The renal arterial vessels show thickening and narrowing of their lumens and some glomerular capillaries are sclerosed and collapsed. Renal blood flow can be reduced as a result as these vascular changes. The renal tubules can also be affected, resulting in tubular atrophy. Signs and symptoms are usually mild and include mild proteinuria from glomerular damage. Nocturia may occur from moderate loss of tubular concentrating ability. There may be casts in the urine from tubular injury. Although the renal insufficiency is relatively mild, these patients are at risk for acute renal failure.

In *malignant* nephrosclerosis, the major changes are necrosis and thickening of the arterioles and glomerular capillaries and diffuse tubular loss and atrophy. There is gross hematuria with red cell casts, heavy proteinuria, and elevated plasma creatinine. Malignant nephrosclerosis is a medical emergency, and the high blood pressure must be lowered to prevent permanent renal damage as well as damage to other vital organs.

Interventions

Treatment of both benign and malignant nephrosclerosis is directed toward early detection and treatment of hypertension. Antihypertensive therapy is initiated.

For hypertensive emergencies, potent vasodilators such as diazoxide and sodium nitroprusside are used. These intravenous medications usually act rapidly. Diazoxide is given as an intravenous bolus by a physician. Monitor the patient closely for tachycardia, hypotension, hyperglycemia, and marked sodium and water retention. Sodium nitroprusside is given as a continuous intravenous drip by the nurse. It is titrated on the basis of patient response, as prescribed. Monitor the patient continuously for headache, hypotension, muscle twitching, tachycardia, restlessness, and retrosternal or abdominal pain.

When significant renal damage exists, stabilizing the person's current level of renal function or slowing deterioration of renal tissue is the treatment goal. Control of hypertension is continued, and management of end-stage disease and uremic symptoms provides for comfort and increased independence in daily living, although renal function may not improve.

Diabetic Nephropathy

Diabetic nephropathy is the leading cause of end-stage renal disease (ESRD). Approximately 30% of patients who begin treatment for ESRD are diabetic, and 50% with type I diabetes develop renal failure within 15 to 18 years of disease onset.

Diffuse glomerulosclerosis is the most common lesion seen in the kidneys of patients who have had diabetes for more than 2 years. There is glomerular basement thick-

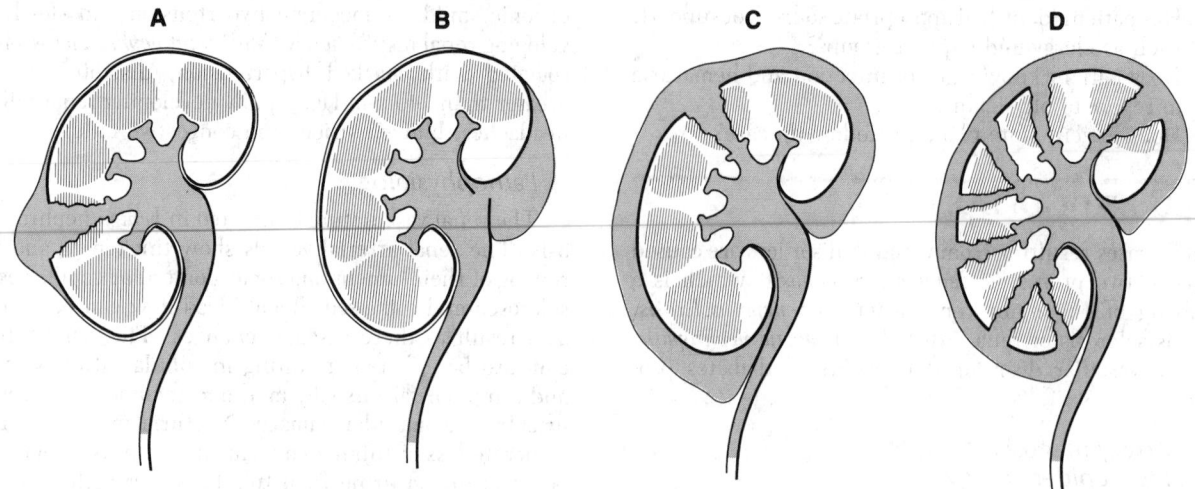

Fig. 33-33   Four degrees of renal trauma. **A,** Urine is extravasating from split in renal parenchyma but confined under renal capsule. **B,** Urine is extravasating through tear in renal pelvis. **C,** Urine is extravasating through rent in kidney and capsule and surrounds kidney and renal pelvis. **D,** Kidney is shattered and urine is extravasating in all areas. (From Winter CC, Morel A: *Nursing care of patients with urologic diseases,* ed 4, St Louis, 1977, Mosby–Year Book.)

ening and mesangial cell proliferation. Although the cause is unknown, it is thought that it may be secondary to complement-mediated tissue injury.

Spherical masses called Kimmelstiel-Wilson lesions are observed in about 50% of patients and are thought to arise from the thickened capillary wall of the glomerulus. As nodule size increases, the adjacent capillaries are compressed until the entire glomerulus becomes ischemic. Progressive diabetic nephropathy is characterized by proteinuria leading to nephrotic syndrome (p. 1041) and finally ESRD. Dialysis is of limited value but renal transplantation shows promising results.

TRAUMA TO THE URINARY TRACT

Assessing intactness of the urinary tract structures must be a part of the evaluation of any person with traumatic injury to the lower trunk. Injuries that are particularly conducive to urinary tract damage include fractures of the pelvis and sharp blows to the abdomen or flanks.

Trauma of the Lower Urinary Tract

Pelvic fractures may result in *bladder perforation* and *ureteral* and *urethral tearing.* After bladder perforation or ureteral or urethral injury, urinary output may be scant or absent, the urine may be bloody, and symptoms of peritonitis may appear. Treatment is directed toward stabilizing the patient and surgically repairing the perforation or laceration. After stabilizing the patient, a cystotomy may be performed to provide urinary drainage when the injury involves the bladder or urethra. When the ureters are involved, splinting catheters may be required. When injury is extreme, urinary diversion may be required (p. 1061). The immediate treatment goal is to provide for adequate urinary drainage to prevent damage to the kidneys.

Kidney Trauma

A sharp blow to the body, particularly to the lower back or flanks, may result in contusion, tearing, or rupture of a kidney (Fig. 33-33). Signs and symptoms of trauma to the kidneys include frank bleeding from the urinary meatus, hematuria, pain, and tenderness of the upper abdominal quadrant and flank on the involved side. Signs of shock may be present if hemorrhage is extensive. Treatment includes controlling bleeding, preventing shock, and promoting drainage of the urinary tract. Vital signs, fluid balance, and hematocrit levels are monitored to assess hemostasis. Complaints of pain may indicate development of ureteral colic, signifying obstruction of the ureter by a clot. Surgical intervention is required to control severe hemorrhage; spontaneous healing of the kidney is otherwise permitted. Nephrostomy with catheter placement may be required to permit adequate urinary drainage. Bed rest is maintained until gross hematuria clears; thereafter, activity is progressed according to continued absence of hematuria. In the presence of extensive damage a nephrectomy may be required.

A kidney may become loosened and "float" or become displaced (*nephroptosis*). If symptoms of obstruction occur in the presence of nephroptosis, the kidney may be sutured to its anatomic site (*nephropexy*) to eliminate kinking of the ureter. Postoperatively, the patient is positioned with hips elevated to prevent tension on the suture line.

RENAL FAILURE

Renal failure is the inability of the kidneys to function. *It is a state of total or nearly total loss of the kidneys' ability to excrete waste products, to maintain fluid and electrolyte balance (including acid-base balance), and to control blood pressure.*

Table 33-15   Common causes of acute renal failure

Classification	Causes: conditions or substances
Prenal ARF	
Hypoperfusion	Hemorrhage, dehydration, burns, diarrhea, vomiting, third spacing, cirrhosis, peritonitis, nephrotic syndrome, renal artery/vein thrombosis or stenosis, renal infarction, diuretic abuse
Vasodilatation	Sepsis and anaphylaxis
Decreased cardiac output	Cardiogenic shock, dysrhythmias, severe congestive heart failure, pericardial tamponade, acute pulmonary embolism
Intrarenal ARF	
Glomerular damage	Acute poststreptoccal glomerulonephritis and SLE, Goodpasture's syndrome, bacterial endocarditis
Vascular disease	Polyarteritis nodosa, periarteritis, vasculitis, hypersensitivity angiitis, scleroderma, hypertension
Other disease	Interstitial nephritis, papillary necrosis, acute pyelonephritis, allergic nephritis, hypercalcemia, uric acid nephropathy, kidney myeloma
Ischemia (ATN)	Hypovolemia, cardiogenic shock, severe prolonged ARF
	Circulation to kidney interrupted less than 30 minutes (surgical cross-clamping above renal arteries)
	Procurement of cadaveric kidneys for transplantation
Nephrotoxicity (ATN)	Heavy metals and ions: mercuric chloride, copper sulfate, gold
	Organic solvents: carbon tetrachloride, ethylene glycol
	Antibiotics: aminoglycosides (gentamicin, tetramycin, kanamycin, amikacin). Other antimicrobials: vancomycin, amphotericin-B, methacillin, tetracycline, some cephalosporins
	Analgesics: phenacetin, acetaminophen, NSAIDs (ibuprofen)
	Immunosuppressive agent: cyclosporine A
	Chemotherapeutic agents: cisplatin, methotrexate, carmustine, lomustine, streptozocin, mitomycin, bleomycin, cyclophosphamide
	Radiologic contrast media: iodine-based dyes
Postrenal ARF	
Obstruction	Ureteral: fibrosis, calculi, crystals, clots, accidental ligation
	Bladder: neoplasms
	Urethral: stricture, prostatic hypertrophy

The person in renal failure cannot independently sustain life.

Renal failure may be acute in onset or may develop slowly and progressively over several years. When renal failure occurs suddenly, such as within a few days, biochemical changes are often dramatic and the person has little time to adjust to these changes. The person becomes very ill and usually requires care in a critical care unit.

When renal failure occurs as the end result of a chronic kidney illness in which kidney tissue is destroyed progressively over the course of several months or years, control of symptoms and preservation of functional abilities are achieveable goals. Dietary adjustment, medications, and attention to preventing additional illnesses compensate for loss of kidney function in early stages of progressing renal failure. As renal function continues to deteriorate, dialysis or transplantation becomes necessary to support life.

ACUTE RENAL FAILURE

Acute renal failure (ARF) is defined as a sudden impairment or decline in renal function associated with an increase in the serum concentration of urea (*azotemia*) and creatinine. It is often associated with *oliguria* (urine output less than 400 ml/24 hours), hyperkalemia, and sodium retention.

ARF is often reversible; however, prolonged episodes may lead to irreversible kidney failure, which requires either dialysis or transplantation.

Etiology

Acute renal failure generally follows an identifiable trauma that is either toxic or ischemic in nature. The health of the individual before the insult is usually good to adequate. Conditions that can precipitate acute renal failure include the following:

1. Ischemia
2. Nephrotoxicity
3. Acute glomerular disease
4. Acute severe kidney infection
5. Bilateral occlusion of the renal arteries
6. Mechanical obstructions of the urinary tract
7. Hemoglobinemia and myoglobinemia

All these conditions can lead to massive and rapid destruction of kidney tissue. ARF has been organized into three classifications depending upon the etiology or physiologic location of the renal insult: prerenal, intrarenal, and postrenal ARF (see Table 33-15).

Prerenal acute renal failure

Prerenal factors are directly related to *hypoperfusion* states (decreased amount of blood flow to the kidneys). Conditions

Table 33-16   Symptoms caused by physiologic changes in acute renal failure

Symptoms	Physiologic effects	Findings
Oliguric phase		
Nausea, vomiting, drowsiness, confusion, coma, GI bleeding, asterixis, pericarditis	Inability to excrete metabolic wastes	Increased BUN and creatinine levels
Nausea, vomiting, cardiac dysrhythmias, Kussmaul's breathing, drowsiness, confusion, coma	Inability to regulate electrolytes	Hyperkalemia, hyponatremia, acidosis
Edema; congestive heart failure; pulmonary edema; hypertension	Inability to excrete fluid loads	Fluid overload, hypervolemia
Diuretic phase		
Urinary output of up to 4 to 5 L/day, postural hypotension, tachycardia	Increased production of urine	Hypovolemia, loss of sodium and potassium in urine
Increasing mental alertness and activity	Slowly increasing excretion of metabolic wastes	Initially, high BUN (fluid loss greater than solute loss), gradual return of BUN to normal

that result in decreased cardiac output, vasodilatation, or decreased circulating blood volume can result in decreased blood flow to the kidneys.

Intrarenal acute renal failure

Intrarenal (parenchymal) ARF results from injury to renal tissue. It is typically associated with intrarenal ischemia, toxins, or prolonged prerenal ARF. Damage may be to the glomerulus, or more commonly to the tubular system. ARF resulting from tubular damage is termed *acute tubular necrosis* (ATN). Ischemia or nephrotoxicity are the two most common conditions that cause ATN.

Ischemic kidney injury occurs when kidney perfusion is obliterated or reduced below a mean arterial pressure of 60 or 70 mm Hg in the afferent arteriole. Below this critical level the ability of the afferent and efferent arterioles to maintain glomerular filtration is lost. As a result, the glomerular filtration rate decreases. Ischemia also occurs when kidney circulation is interrupted for longer than 30 minutes. Prolonged or severe prerenal ARF is a common cause of ATN. Ischemic injuries damage not only the tubular epithelial cells but also the basement membrane cells, which, unlike tubular cells, do not regenerate. Therefore, ATN resulting from ischemia may cause permanent nephron damage and irreversible renal failure.

Nephrotoxicity can be caused by a wide variety of substances (Table 33-15) injurious to renal tubules. The substances include heavy metals, ions, organic solvents, contrast media, pesticides, poisonous mushrooms, and medications. The most common nephrotoxins are medications, especially aminoglycosides belonging to the antibiotic group. Aminoglycosides bind to the cells of the proximal tubule where they have a very prolonged half-life. This causes damage to the tubules, leading to ARF. The basement membrane cells are not damaged; therefore, the chances of reversibility of ATN resulting from nephrotoxicity are good.

Postrenal acute renal failure

Postrenal ARF usually results from *obstruction* to the outflow of urine from the renal calyces to the urethral meatus.

For renal failure to develop the obstruction must be bilateral below the level of the bladder or unilateral in the person with only one functioning kidney. Postrenal ARF is frequently reversible; however, prolonged obstruction may result in intrarenal damage and irreversible renal failure.

Pathophysiology

The course of acute renal failure is usually characterized by an initial oliguric phase followed in a number of days to a few weeks by a diuretic period. Major problems during the *oliguric* phase include inability to excrete fluid loads, to regulate electrolytes, and to excrete metabolic waste materials (Table 33-16). During the *diuretic* phase large amounts of fluid and electrolytes are lost.

Oliguric phase

The oliguric phase of ARF is the period during which the patient's urinary volume is less than 400 ml in 24 hours. It usually lasts 1 to 2 weeks. If the oliguric phase is prolonged beyond 2 weeks, the prognosis for recovery decreases.

Inability to excrete fluid loads

Because of the decreased kidney function, fluids are retained in the body, resulting in fluid overload and edema (Chapter 7). When fluid overload is excessive, congestive heart failure and pulmonary edema may occur. Hypertension accompanies acute renal failure when the person is hypervolemic, although this is usually not a finding when fluid balance is controlled.

Inability to excrete fluid loads leads to decreased urinary output. Either *oliguria* or *anuria* (urinary output below 100 ml in 24 hours) may be present, although oliguria is more common. Classically, the patient in acute renal failure shows a fall in urinary output within 1 to 2 days to between 50 and 400 ml in 24 hours. The urine *specific gravity is low* (1.010), and the osmolality of the urine approaches that of the person's serum (280-320 mOsm). Specific gravity and urine osmolality remain within this fixed range and reflect tubular damage with loss of concentrating ability.

Electrolyte imbalances

The three major electrolyte problems are hyperkalemia, hyponatremia, and acidosis.

Potassium imbalance. In the normal individual the potassium ion is exchanged in the distal convoluted tubule of the nephron for either sodium or hydrogen ions; for the healthy person there is no mechanism in the body to conserve the potassium ion. However, in the individual with acute renal failure in whom a large number of tubular cells are no longer functional, no mechanism exists to remove potassium from the body. *Hyperkalemia* is said to exist when the serum concentration of this ion reaches a level of 5.5 mEq/L or higher. Serum concentrations of 7 to 10 mEq/L can be quickly reached in acute renal failure and are incompatible with normal cardiac function and life.

In monitoring for signs of potassium toxicity, electrocardiography and laboratory determinations of serum potassium are the most reliable indicators. Rarely does the patient become symptomatic, and pulse changes must not be relied on to indicate the degree of rise of potassium in the patient's system.

Sodium imbalance. *Hyponatremia* in acute renal failure most commonly develops with overhydration of the patient. The oliguric patient cannot excrete large volumes of urine; when the administration of sodium-free or low-sodium intravenous or oral fluids continues in such an individual, the serum is diluted and the serum concentration of sodium falls.

In this situation hyponatremia is accompanied or caused by hypervolemia. In the very acutely ill, the situation commonly occurs when the patient receives numerous drugs and fluids in an attempt to treat coexisting life-threatening problems. When the volume of drugs and fluids cannot be reduced to a safe level, dialysis is required to remove the excess fluid and restore sodium balance.

Signs and symptoms of hyponatremia include warm, moist, flushed skin; muscle weakness, muscle twitching; and behavioral changes involving confusion, delirium, coma, and convulsions. Serum sodium concentrations will be below 130 mEq/L. The hematocrit and hemoglobin values fall suddenly without evidence of bleeding; this is caused by hemodilution.

Increases in total body content of sodium also occur in acute renal failure. This commonly occurs when the patient is receiving medications high in sodium content and excess sodium in the diet. Edema and increasing blood pressure indicate retention of sodium and fluids even though the serum sodium concentration is normal or below normal.

Metabolic acidosis. Acidosis develops when hydrogen ion secretion and bicarbonate ion production diminish in the tubular cells. The pH of the blood decreases, the carbon dioxide content decreases, and central nervous system symptoms of drowsiness progressing to stupor and coma may appear. Although the lungs are unable to compensate totally for the increasing acid load, they help determine the rate at which acidosis develops and the frequency or need for dialysis. In compensating for increased metabolic acid loads, the lungs attempt to excrete more carbon dioxide. Kussmaul's breathing is noted.

Inability to excrete metabolic wastes

Decreased kidney function alters the body's ability to get rid of metabolic waste materials, producing typical signs and symptoms referred to as *uremia.* BUN and serum creatinine values rise sharply. In the person who has already sustained illness and trauma, BUN values may increase at a rate of 30 mg/100 ml/day. Signs and symptoms include neurologic manifestations such as confusion, convulsions, coma, and asterixis. GI bleeding may result from uremic gastritis or colitis. Serum uric acid and phosphate levels also rise. Decreased cellular immunity causes an increased tendency for infections to develop. Bruising and bleeding result from changes in blood coagulation factors. Pericarditis (Chapter 25) is thought to develop as a result of pericardial irritation from uremic toxins.

Diuretic phase

The diuretic phase begins when the 24-hour urine volume exceeds 400 ml and ends when blood urea nitrogen (BUN) and serum creatinine levels begin to fall. Increased output indicates that the damaged nephrons are healing and are able to begin excreting urine. At first daily urine volume increases slowly, although within 1 to 2 days diuresis up to or exceeding 4 to 5 L/day may occur. Although fluid can be excreted, the kidneys are not yet healed. Often there is inability to excrete proportional amounts of waste materials, and BUN may rise or remain elevated as urine volume increases. At times excessive excretion of sodium and potassium occurs during diuresis. Complete recovery of renal function is slow and requires anywhere from days to several months. Return of the renal function to normal or near-normal levels is evidenced when the kidney can both conserve and dilute urine and when serum electrolytes and nonprotein nitrogen levels become normal.

Prognosis

Recovery from an episode of ARF depends on the underlying illness, condition of patient, and careful supportive management given during the period of kidney shutdown. The leading cause of death is infection, such as of the urinary tract, lungs, and peritoneum. Infection develops in approximately 80% of patients with ARF. The incidence of GI bleeding, the second most frequent cause of death, is about 25%. Mortality from fluid overload and acidosis has been reduced as a result of dialysis and other forms of therapy. There is potential for recovery of renal function in patients who survive the acute episode of tubular insufficiency. Although kidney tissue may regenerate more completely after toxic injury than ischemia, both forms usually show return to normal or near-normal renal function.

For those in whom acute renal failure has been caused by glomerular disease or severe infection of kidney tissue, the prognosis may not be as favorable. Return of renal function is determined by the extent of scarring and obliteration of functional renal tissue that has occurred during the acute episode of kidney failure. A significant number of adults who develop acute glomerulonephritis show some decrease in renal function, which may remain at a level at which biochemical abnormalities are not produced, or may progress to a chronic form of renal failure.

Prevention and Health Education
Primary prevention

The most important nursing intervention associated with ARF is primary prevention. The incidence of ARF can be reduced through identification and observation of individuals at risk for ARF, control of environmental factors, a thorough understanding of the pathophysiology of ARF, strategic planning of nursing interventions, and continued evaluation of those interventions. It is important for nurses to monitor urinary output and laboratory values of patient receiving antibiotics (especially aminoglycosides) and cyclosporine A.

The greatest incidence of ARF occurs in persons who have undergone major trauma, extensive burns, aortic surgery, massive blood loss, or severe myocardial infarction. ARF also frequently occurs in patients with sepsis and in those having abnormal intravascular coagulation, such as DIC, because these acutely ill persons are prime candidates for inadequate kidney perfusion. Frequent monitoring of urinary output and detection of excessive fluid losses helps to identify instances of inadequate renal perfusion before renal failure develops.

Significant factors in preventive care for the general population include control of nephrotoxic drugs, increased medical supervision of persons with sore throats and upper respiratory tract infections, and increased case finding and treatment of individuals with bacteriuria and obstructive disease of the urinary system. Attempts to control the distribution and identification of nephrotoxic drugs and chemicals is largely accomplished through the Food and Drug Administration (FDA). Identification of nephrotoxic drugs and chemicals, enforced labeling of these substances, and drug dispensing by prescription only are examples of this agency's attempts to promote public health. Proper labeling and storage of potentially toxic drugs and chemicals in the home can reduce further the number of accidental ingestions of nephrotoxic substances.

Secondary prevention

Early detection and prompt diagnosis is essential to prevent permanent damage to renal tissue. Encourage persons who complain of persistent symptoms to seek prompt medical evaluation. All possible measures to optimize patient survival can be taken if the patient's condition is diagnosed early in the course of ARF.

Medical Therapy for Acute Renal Failure

Before the early 1980s there were basically three treatment options for ARF: conservative management, hemodialysis (HD), and peritoneal dialysis (PD). Conservative management with pharmacologic and diet therapy still remains the primary approach to stabilize the patient with ARF. This approach, however, may be ineffective in some situations. Therefore, HD (p. 1086) and PD (p. 1089) have been the standard aggressive therapies for invasive intervention.

Hemodialysis is often a difficult procedure to perform when the patient is hemodynamically unstable, has bleeding complications, or needs more than a prescribed 3- to 4-hour treatment to correct underlying fluid overload, acid/base imbalance, and uremia associated with ARF. For many years clinicians have had to use aggressive HD once or twice daily because of threatening conditions that must be reversed immediately, such as hyperkalemia, severe acidosis, or pulmonary edema.

Although peritoneal dialysis is considered less taxing than HD, it may be problematic in the critically ill patient. History of abdominal surgery, abdominal trauma, certain diseases, or lack of surgical support for catheter placement may eliminate PD as an option of ARF management.

In 1982 the FDA approved a safer, gentler modality for the management of ARF called *continuous renal replacement therapy* (CRRT), which is now the invasive intervention of choice for the critically ill ARF patient. HD and PD continue to be used to treat ARF, but whenever possible they are reserved for hemodynamically stable patients or those with end-stage renal disease.

Continuous renal replacement therapy

CRRT provides continuous (8-24 hours or more) *ultrafiltration* (filtration as a result of hydrostatic pressure) of extracellular fluid and clearance of uremic toxins. This technique uses a highly porous, extracorporeal hemofilter that is perfused continuously by blood flowing from the cannulation of a large artery and returning through a large vein. The goal of CRRT is to remove fluid from the patient either by gravity drain system or by a suction-assisted fluid collection system. The removed fluid contains dissolved noncellular components of the patient's plasma, such as urea, creatinine, and electrolytes.

There are three variants of CRRT: slow continuous ultrafiltration (SCUF), continuous arteriovenous hemofiltration (CAVH), and continuous arteriovenous hemofiltration dialysis (CAVHD).[42] *SCUF* provides a slow ultrafiltration that decreases the patient's fluid volume over several hours to days of therapy. No fluid replacement is prescribed, and solutes such as creatinine and urea are minimally removed. SCUF is usually used for patients with congestive heart failure or myocardial infarction accompanied with low renal perfusion secondary to decreased cardiac output.[42]

CAVH is often the preferred therapy when a patient's clinical status requires moderate fluid removal and solute clearance. The ultrafiltration rate ranges from 500 to 800 ml/hour. However, a hemodynamically compromised patient cannot tolerate aggressive fluid shifts, so fluid replacement is administered by means of continuous infusion. The replacement fluid amount is based on the hourly net fluid loss goal of 50 to 400 ml/hour. CAVH is also prescribed when the serum chemistries are high, especially potassium and urea, or when the serum bicarbonate is low, which indicates metabolic acidosis. Replacement fluids may be standard fluids, such as lactated Ringer's solution or normal saline. However, solutions used most often include half-normal saline with calcium glucepate or chloride, or quarter-normal saline with two ampules of sodium bicarbonate.[42]

CAVHD is used when the patient's volume status is excessive and the uremia is severe. With CAVHD, either peritoneal dialysate (hypertonic dialyzing fluid) or a custom dialysate is infused countercurrent to the patient's blood flow through a *hemofilter*. The countercurrent flow increases the diffusibility toxins from the patient's uremic plasma. The dextrose contained in the dialysate enhances fluid removal by the osmotic effect across the semipermeable membrane of the hemofilter. CAVHD is different from standard HD in that the flow rate of the dialysate is reduced, which is better tolerated by the critically ill ARF patient.

Nursing Process
Assessment
Subjective data

Assessment should include questions that ascertain the following:
1. Voiding patterns, including any recent changes
2. Unexplained weight gain
3. Presence of nausea and anorexia
4. Family history of renal disease
5. Recent history of flulike symptoms
6. Presence of nephrotoxins, including those in environment, at work, and in medications
7. Preexisting diseases, especially cardiac disorders, vascular disease, urinary diseases, and systemic conditions (such as diabetes mellitus and SLE) known to affect renal function
8. Recent surgeries or acute illnesses

Objective data

Objective data must include the measurement of fluid intake and urine output in a 24-hour period. Daily weighings are essential because they provide the best measure of fluid status. Blood pressure, including postural changes, is measured frequently until stable, and the pulse rate and rhythm are also recorded. Fluid status is assessed by observing for skin turgor and peripheral edema and auscultating breath sounds. The person is assessed for the presence of halitosis that can result from acidosis and from ammonia secretion. The person is observed carefully for any changes in mental status.

Diagnostic tests

Diagnostic tests include urinalysis and creatinine urinary clearance to monitor changes in kidney function. Serum creatinine and BUN are also obtained. Serum chemistries must be followed closely to ensure that the person is maintaining homeostasis (see Table 33-17). Specific tests used to assist in making the diagnosis and identifying the cause of acute renal failure include KUB, IVP, cystoscopy, and renal ultrasound. In some cases a renal biopsy may be performed to provide the differential diagnosis.

When oliguria or rising serum creatinine and BUN values are noted, the physician must determine whether the decreased output and decreased renal function are the results of inadequate renal perfusion or of frank renal failure. This distinction directs treatment. In instances of poor kidney perfusion, restoring circulating volume by adding fluids and otherwise increasing cardiac output prevents the death of kidney tissue and subsequent renal failure. In contrast, the treatment of true renal failure is supportive and is based on careful balance of input and output of fluid, electrolytes, and wastes.

In addition to the urine sodium concentration as a diagnostic sign, the physician may wish to challenge the patient's ability to excrete fluid. In this instance usually 100 to 500 ml of fluid is given as rapidly as possible intravenously. A poorly perfused but intact kidney should respond with increased urinary output. During this treatment the patient must be closely monitored for signs and symptoms of congestive heart failure and pulmonary edema. The kidney in acute failure will be unable to produce a greater urine flow in response to this fluid challenge. The physician may give furosemide, 40 to 80 mg intravenously, in an attempt to produce a greater flow of urine. The test may be repeated if there is no response to the initial trial, although subsequent attempts to produce urine in this manner are contraindicated.

Table 33-17   Comparison of serum laboratory values in acute renal failure (ARF)

Serum component	Normal value	Change in ARF
Sodium	135-145 mEq/L	Increases (with some variance)
Potassium	3.5-5.0 mEq/L	Increases
Chloride	96-106 mEq/L	Increases (with some variance)
BUN	8-20 mg/dl	Increases
Creatinine	0.5-1.5 mg/dl	Increases
Calcium	8.5-10.5 mg/dl	Decreases
Phosphorous	2.0-4.5 mg/dl	Increases
Carbon dioxide combining power	24 mEq/L	Decreases
Magnesium	1.5-2.5 mEq/L	Increases (or stays normal)
Alkaline phosphatase	25-100 U/ml	Increases (or stays normal)
Osmolality	280-295 mOsmol/kg H_2O	Increases (with some variance)
Hematocrit	40%-50%	Decreases
Hemoglobin	12-16 g/dl	Decreases
White blood count	4000-10,000/m³	Varies

Data analysis: nursing diagnoses

Nursing diagnoses are determined from analysis of patient data. Possible nursing diagnoses for the person with acute renal failure may include, but are not limited to, the following:

Diagnostic title	Possible etiologies
Injury, high risk for	Sensorimotor deficits, lack of awareness of environmental hazards, bleeding tendency
Infection, high risk for	Urinary stasis, decreased immune response
Nutrition, altered: less than body requirements	Anorexia, nausea, and vomiting
Coping, ineffective individual	Changes in health status, situational crisis
Knowledge deficit	Cognitive limitations, lack of interest in learning, unfamiliarity with informational sources

Planning: expected patient outcomes

Expected patient outcomes for the person with acute renal failure may include, but are not limited to, the following:

1. Does not become injured or sustain bleeding.
2. Displays no signs of infection.
3. Eats prescribed diet.
4. Describes alternative ways of coping.
5. Describes nature of illness, diet therapy, signs to report to physician, and plans for follow-up care.

Implementation

Assisting with achievement of therapeutic goals
Oliguric phase

During the oliguric phase of acute renal failure, development of hyperkalemia, severe acidosis, severe fluid overload and pulmonary edema, infection, convulsions, or pericarditis indicate need for immediate intervention. Nursing care of the patient with ARF in the oliguric phase is summarized in Box 33-17.

Control and excretion of metabolic waste buildup. Because the patient's ability to excrete metabolic wastes (nonprotein nitrogen products and acids) cannot keep pace with production of these substances, alternative routes of excretion and control over production of these materials must be found. Means available to accomplish this include providing carbohydrate to spare protein stores, preventing additional tissue trauma, and increasing excretion of wastes through the lungs and through dialysis.

Decreasing the production of metabolic wastes can be influenced through dietary means. Calories in the form of carbohydrates and fats provide energy and spare body protein stores, thus decreasing nonprotein nitrogen production. The body recycles urea to synthesize amino acids for protein building so that some regeneration of tissues can occur even though protein intake is curtailed.

In compensating for increased metabolic acid loads, the lungs attempt to excrete more carbon dioxide. To maximize this pathway for acid excretion, pulmonary hygiene should be carried out. Preventing atelectasis and maintaining maximal lung expansion are goals of nursing care.

33-17

Guidelines for Care

The patient in oliguric phase of acute renal failure

Control and excretion of metabolic waste buildup
  Provide carbohydrate to spare protein stores
  Prevent additional trauma
  Give pulmonary hygiene to prevent atelectasis
Maintain fluid and electrolyte balance
  Maintain fluid restrictions
  Keep accurate records of intake and output
  Weigh patient daily
  Monitor vital signs frequently, including postural signs
  Assess patient's fluid status
  Administer phosphate-binding medications as prescribed
  Monitor serum electrolytes
Maintain nutrition
  Monitor intravenous fluids
  Take measures to relieve nausea (antiemetics, comfort measures)
  Give fluids in frequent small amounts, when permitted
  Provide a diet high in carbohydrates during protein restrictions
  Provide a diet low in potassium during hyperkalemia and high in potassium during hypokalemia
Prevent injury
  Assess orientation; orient confused patient
  Maintain bed rest during acute phase
  When patient is ambulatory, assess motor skills and monitor ambulation
  Protect patient from bleeding: instruct patient to use soft toothbrush, administer stool softeners, perform guaiac tests on stools and emesis
Prevent infection
  Assess for signs and symptoms of infection
  Maintain strict asepsis for any intrusive procedures
  Provide pulmonary hygiene
  Protect skin when patient is on bed rest
  Turn weak or immobile patient frequently
  Protect patient from others with infections

Control of fluids. The oliguric or anuric patient is unable to excrete more than minimal amounts of fluid. Nursing care is directed toward three broad objectives: (1) monitoring for signs of fluid overload, (2) maintaining the patient's energy expenditure at a level compatible with the individual's state of health, and (3) controlling or helping the patient to control fluid intake.

All observations regarding the patient's state of hydration need to be recorded so that hour-to-hour and day-to-day comparisons can be made. Any finding indicating retention of fluids is reported to the physician. Edema can first be noted in dependent areas such as the feet and legs, in the presacral area, and around the eyes. The patient is observed carefully for signs of pulmonary edema and congestive heart failure. Central venous or arterial monitoring lines will help to provide data for short-term comparisons in managing the fluid balance of the critically ill person. Accurate recording of intake and output is extremely important as are daily weight records.

The patient in renal failure is unable to excrete fluid loads, and much energy is expended just to maintain current functional status. Positioning and activity are determined daily based on assessment of the energy level and ability to ventilate adequately.

Controlling fluid intake is essential when the ability to excrete fluid is limited. All fluid (parenteral and oral) must total only slightly more than daily output if severe overhydration is to be avoided. When the patient is neither to gain nor lose additional body fluid, the physician will calculate the patient's fluid replacement using the following as a guide: intake will approximate 500 ml/day plus urinary output and adjustments for additional fluid lost through fever, diarrhea, and wound drainage. Fortunately, when sodium intake is controlled, extreme thirst does not develop.

Devices that allow 50 to 150 ml of fluid to be isolated from the main intravenous solution container and drip chambers that allow precise control of fluids through administration of smaller drops of fluid are added safety measures when giving fluids parenterally to anuric or oliguric individuals. Accuracy in fluid balance records is essential. For the patient who is unable to take medications with small amounts of fluid, medications may be given in soft foods such as applesauce.

Interventions for hyperkalemia. Interventions to control the rise of serum potassium and to prevent cardiac arrest include those that (1) decrease the intake of potassium, (2) protect the cardiovascular system, and (3) assist in removal of potassium from the body by nonrenal means.

Decreasing the intake of potassium is achieved by administering intravenous feedings or a diet in which the potassium content is very low or absent. All fluids and drugs that the patient receives intravenously should be checked for potassium content. Some medications (for example, most penicillin preparations) contain large amounts of this ion.

Protecting the cardiovascular system from high levels of extracellular potassium (K^+) *is essential.* When high K^+ levels occur and the patient is exhibiting cardiovascular effects, renal dialysis is required. Because it takes several hours to get the dialysis treatment under way and for the K^+ to be reduced to safe levels, other therapy is instituted. Hypertonic glucose (25%) may be given with 1 unit of regular insulin per 2 g of glucose. Over a 30-minute period, 200 to 300 ml of fluid is given to promote the movement of K^+ back into the cells. This lowers the serum K^+ level and reduces cardiac instability resulting from the high serum K^+ levels. The K^+ levels will begin to fall in 1 hour and will remain lowered for 4 to 6 hours.[15] In addition to hypertonic glucose, calcium gluconate may be given intravenously to reduce the irritability of cardiac cells caused by the hyperkalemia.

To *promote the excretion of potassium* from the body when the kidneys are nonfunctional, an exchange resin such as sodium polystyrene sulfonate may be ordered for the patient as a temporary measure before a dialysis treatment when (1) the serum K^+ level is high and rising rapidly; (2) the serum K^+ level is rising, although at a controlled rate, and other metabolic disturbances do not necessitate dialysis; or (3) control of a rising serum K^+ is required before a patient's transfer to an acute-care area where dialysis can be provided. This drug reduces serum potassium by exchanging sodium for potassium ions in the intestinal tract. It can be administered orally, through a nasogastric tube, or by enema. The medication is given orally when the patient's condition permits; oral daily doses range from 15 to 60 g/day. When sodium polystyrene sulfonate is administered in enema form, the usual dose is 50 g of exchange resin for each enema. It may be repeated daily or as necessary to lower serum potassium. Typically, sodium polystyrene sulfonate induces an osmotic fluid shift into the bowel producing diarrhea, which helps to expel the medication, additional K^+, and additional fluid from the GI tract. If spontaneous bowel movements do not occur, a laxative or cleansing enema can be given to ensure the elimination of potassium from the bowel.

Diuretic phase

Medical therapy during the diuretic phase is symptomatic. Electrolyte imbalances are likely to persist and are treated as in the oliguric phase. When polyuria is present, dehydration can become a problem and fluid replacement then becomes necessary. Assess patient for adequate hydration. Detection of fluid losses and electrolyte imbalances (sodium and potassium) continue to be important. Assess for changes in mental status indicative of low serum sodium levels. Monitor for hypokalemia (serum potassium less than 3.5 mEq/L, muscle weakness, and constipation). Encourage early ambulation and independence in ADL as tolerated. Place patient in a room with a bathroom nearby or provide a bedside commode to avoid fatigue from frequent voiding.

Interventions to achieve patient outcomes
Preventing injury

The confused, agitated, or restless patient must be protected from injury. Keep siderails elevated at all times and pad them if necessary. To allay patient anxiety, explain the rationale for the mental status change (electrolyte or acid/base imbalance, uremia). Offer reassurance and support. Accompany an ambulatory patient to the bathroom and monitor closely to prevent accidents. Reorient patient to person, place, and time at regular intervals. Facilitate orientation by placing a calendar, television, or radio, and familiar objects nearby. Involve family members in the reorientation process.

Bleeding may occur from changes in blood coagulation factors. Use measures to prevent bleeding (see Box 33-17). Further information on protection from bleeding can be found in Chapter 27. Use meticulous skin care to prevent skin breakdown from edema.

Preventing infection

Preventing infections and tissue breakdown decreases production of metabolic wastes. Aseptic technique should be rigorously pursued in all treatments performed on the patient. In-dwelling lines and catheters are a common source of infection and are to be avoided when possible. *The patient should be isolated from anyone with an infection, including other patients, health care personnel, and visitors.* Detecting existent infections early so that treatment can be instituted promptly decreases tissue breakdown. When the patient is extremely weak and immobile, frequent turning and repositioning to prevent decubiti must be performed. Skin care for patients with edematous tissues should include observation and prevention of pressure and trauma; these tissues are particularly prone to breakdown.

Pruritus commonly occurs and may lead to skin lesions from scratching. Measures to relieve pruritus include bathing patient every day (or more often if necessary) using superfat soap. Administer prescribed antipruritics.

Maintaining adequate nutrition

Most persons in acute renal failure are too ill to tolerate oral feedings either initially or for sustained periods. Some patients who are able to tolerate fluids orally find that eating food compounds their nausea as a result of an altered biochemical environment and accompanying GI tract irritation. Intravenous hypertonic glucose in amounts of 100 g/day or more provides a temporary source of energy that slows the burning of the body's own protein stores. Maintaining a positive nitrogen balance is not feasible when the patient is severely ill or nauseated. During this period, administer antiemetics as prescribed. Rinsing the mouth frequently helps to keep lips and mouth moist. Use meticulous mouth care to protect teeth and mucous membranes.

When the patient can tolerate oral fluids, provide fluids frequently in small amounts; ginger ale and other effervescent soft drinks are often tolerated better than other fluids. When oral feedings are started, dietary protein and potassium are avoided unless dialysis has been initiated.

In this case, modest amounts of protein and potassium are allowed to increase protein available for tissue building and to increase the palatability of the diet. Foods high in carbohydrate and fat are encouraged. A total intake of 2000 calories per day is desired but often not achieved because of anorexia.

Avoid giving the hyperkalemic patient potassium-rich foods, such as bananas, cantaloupes, potatoes, chocolate, and nuts. Conversely, encourage the hypokalemic patient to eat these foods. In both situations, monitor the patient closely and administer medications (either an exchange resin or potassium supplement) as indicated. As potassium levels become normalized in the diuretic phase, a more normal diet is permitted. Protein restrictions are continued until BUN and serum creatinine levels decline.

Facilitating coping

The person with ARF faces the reality of renal failure at a time when energy resources for coping are at a low level. Encourage development of a nurse-patient relationship that assists the patient in expressing perceptions of illness. When patient begins to feel stronger during the diuretic phase, assist him or her to explore various coping methods (see Chapter 6). Involve significant others in patient care. Promote patient independence when patient begins to feel better.

Facilitating patient learning

During the diuretic phase, the patient is usually ready for learning about kidney disease and measures to prevent recurrence of renal failure. Teaching includes the following:

1. Cause of renal failure and problems with recurrent failures.
2. Identification of preventable environmental or health factors contributing to the illness (such as hypertension, nephrotoxic drugs).

Table 33-18   States of chronic renal failure

Stage	Clinical features
Stage I Decreased renal reserve	Residual renal function 40% to 75% of normal Asymptomatic: normal BUN and plasma creatinine levels Excretory and regulatory renal functions are intact Homeostasis is maintained At least 50% to 60% loss of renal tissue required before signs are evident; no symptoms are evident until loss of renal tissue is at least 80%
Stage II Renal insufficiency	Residual renal function 20% to 40% of normal Decreased glomerular filtration rate, solute clearances, ability to concentrate urine, and hormone secretion Symptoms: rising BUN and serum creatinine, mild azotemia, polyuria, nocturia, and anemia Signs and symptoms can become more severe if kidneys are stressed, such as with fluid volume depletion or exposure to a nephrotoxic substance Decreased ability to maintain homeostasis
Stage III End-stage renal disease (ESRD)	Residual renal function less than 15% of normal Excretory, regulatory, and hormonal renal functions severely impaired Unable to maintain homeostasis (fluid, electrolyte, and pH imbalances) Markedly elevated BUN and plasma creatinine, anemia, hyperphosphatemia, hypocalcemia, metabolic acidosis, hyperuricemia, hyperkalemia, fluid overload (usually oliguric with urine osmolality similar to plasma osmolality) Uremic syndrome develops; all body systems are affected from renal failure Last stage of progressive chronic renal failure

3. Prescribed dietary and medication regimen.
4. Explanation of risk of hypokalemia and reportable symptoms.
5. Signs and symptoms of infection and of returning renal failure to be reported to physician.
6. Need for ongoing follow-up care.

Evaluation

Evaluation is based on expected patient outcomes. Questions to consider may include the following:

1. Is the patient free of injury and infection?
2. Is the patient oriented to person, time, and place?
3. Has the patient's potassium level returned to normal range?
4. Is the patient eating a well-balanced diet?
5. Is the patient coping with the illness?
6. Does the patient know the nature of the illness, dietary and medication regimen, reportable symptoms, and need for follow-up care?

CHRONIC RENAL FAILURE

Chronic renal failure (CRF) exists when the kidneys are no longer capable of maintaining an internal environment consistent with life and when return of function is not anticipated. For the majority of individuals the transition from health to a state of chronic or permanent disease is a slow one extending over a number of years (Table 33-18). Recurrent infections and exacerbations of nephritis, obstruction of the urinary tract, and destruction of vessels from diabetes and long-standing hypertension lead to scarring of kidney tissue and progressive loss of renal function. Some individuals, however, develop total irreversible loss of renal function acutely; such loss of renal function usually develops in a matter of a few hours or days and follows a direct traumatic insult to the kidneys.

Prognosis

The individual with CRF can to some extent control and manage the symptoms of the disease. Although renal function that has been lost as a result of destruction of kidney tissue cannot be recovered, the life of the person can be maintained by limiting the intake of substances that require renal excretion and by providing alternative routes of excretion for waste products and electrolytes. By adhering to a prescribed management routine, albeit quite strict and demanding, life may be sustained. For some individuals medication and diet therapy alone may control uremic symptoms; other individuals may require dialysis or transplantation to control the symptoms of their disease.

Prevention and Health Education
Primary prevention

Obstruction and infection of the urinary tract and hypertensive disease are common and often asymptomatic causes of renal damage and renal failure. A significant reduction in the incidence of renal failure can be affected through increasing attention to general health promotion. Yearly physical examinations in which blood pressure is determined, urinalysis is performed, and the person is questioned about dysuria or pain in the urinary tract assist in early detection of diseases that may lead to renal failure.

Secondary prevention

General health maintenance can reduce the number of individuals progressing from renal insufficiency into frank renal failure. Care is aimed toward adequately treating medical problems and closely supervising the person's health status in times of stress (infection, pregnancy).

Etiology

CRF can be caused by a variety of conditions, including renal disorders (glomerular, tubular, infection, obstruction) and systemic diseases (see Box 33-18).[22]

Pathophysiology and Clinical Manifestations

During chronic renal failure, some of the nephrons (including the glomerulus and tubules) are thought to remain intact while others are destroyed (intact nephron hypothesis). The intact nephrons hypertrophy and produce an increased volume of filtrate with increased tubular reab-

---

33-18

Causes of chronic renal failure

Congenital or developmental disorders
  Malformations of urinary tract
  Medullary cystic disease
  Polycystic kidney disease
  Hereditary glomerulonephritis with deafness
Glomerulonephritis
  Glomerulopathies
    Diffuse: involves all glomeruli
    Focal: involves some glomeruli
    Segmental: involves portions of individual glomeruli
    Membranous: glomerular capillary wall thickens
    Proliferative: number of glomerular cells increased
    Acute: changes occur over days or weeks
    Chronic: Changes occur over months or years
  Acute streptococcal glomerulonephritis
Tubular disorders
  Renal tubular disorders
  Fanconi syndrome
  Heavy metal poisoning (lead, mercury)
Renal neoplasms: benign, malignant, Wilms' tumor
Infectious renal diseases: pyelonephritis, renal tuberculosis
Obstructive renal disorders: nephrolithiasis, retroperitoneal fibrosis
Renal disorders and systemic disorders
  Diabetes mellitus
  Diabetes insipidus
  Primary hyperparathyroidism
  Hepatorenal syndrome
  Gout
  Amyloidosis
  Scleroderma
  Goodpasture's syndrome
  Systemic lupus erythematosus
  Nephrotic syndrome
  Hypertensive nephropathy
Renal problems in pregnancy

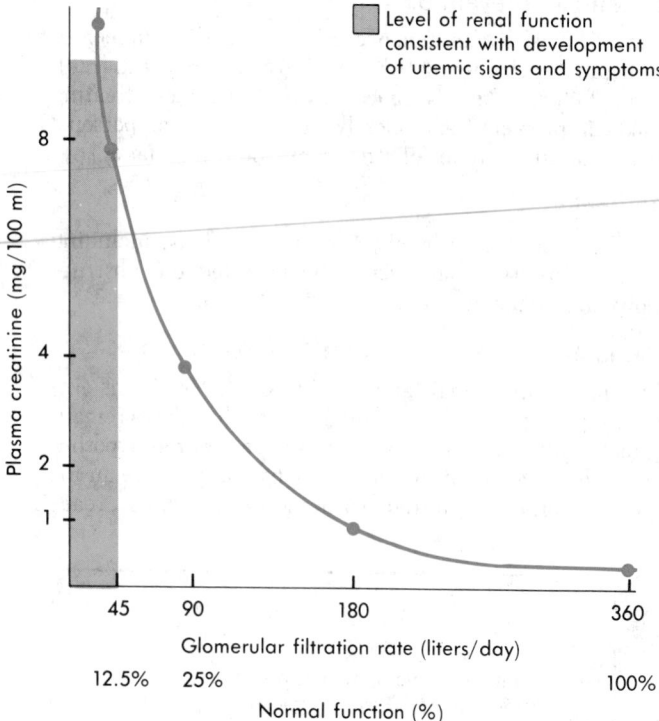

Level of renal function consistent with development of uremic signs and symptoms

Fig. 33-34 Glomerular filtration and plasma creatinine levels.

sorption in spite of a decreased GFR. This adaptive method permits the kidney to function until about three fourths of the nephrons become destroyed. The solute load then becomes greater than can be reabsorbed, producing an osmotic diuresis with polyuria and thirst. Eventually, as more nephrons are damaged, oliguria occurs with retention of waste products.

The point at which the patient becomes obviously symptomatic and displays signs of typical renal failure occurs when approximately 80% to 90% of renal function has been lost (Fig. 33-34). At this level of renal function, creatinine clearance values will fall to 15 ml/minute or less.

The symptoms of uremia usually develop so slowly that the patient and family often do not recall the time of onset of the illness. Common symptoms include the following:
1. Early symptoms—lethargy, headaches, physical and mental fatigue, weight loss, irritability, depression.
2. Later symptoms—anorexia, persistent nausea and vomiting, shortness of breath on either mild or no exertion, and pitting edema; pruritus may be absent, mild, or severe

As renal function deteriorates, *all organ systems are affected* (see Table 33-19). Every aspect of the patient's physical, social, and psychologic functioning is affected by the disease.

Integumentary system

Patients with end-stage renal disease (ESRD) have a characteristic yellowish, gray-bronze skin hue from retained pigments[53] and an underlying pallor from anemia. The patient usually complains of dry skin and pruritus caused

by the depressive effect of the uremic toxins on the oil and sweat glands and calcium or phosphate deposition on the skin surface. Uremic frost, a white dustlike material, is rarely seen today, because dialysis is usually initiated promptly for treatment of severe azotemia.[22]

As a result of protein wasting, the patient's nails are brittle, thin, and easily broken; ridges are typically visible on the nail surface. The hair tends to be coarse and dry and may fall out easily.

Cardiovascular system

Five major cardiovascular conditions occurring with CRF include hypertension, accelerated atherosclerosis, myocardial dysfunction, pericarditis, and hyperkalemia.

Hypertension. Hypertension is the most common cardiovascular problem observed in CRF. It results chiefly from sodium and water retention and from malfunction of the renin-angiotensin system (p. 1015). Sodium and water retention occur when the kidneys lose their ability to filter and excrete salt and water. The patient with CRF often produces excessive amounts of renin.[53] Renin is converted to angiotensin II, which is a potent vasoconstrictor and a substance that stimulates aldosterone secretion. Both peripheral vasoconstriction and aldosterone elevate blood pressure. Normally an increase in blood pressure reduces renin production; however, in CRF, renin is often produced despite an elevated blood pressure. Antihypertensive drugs, such as captopril, inhibit the action of the enzyme that converts angiotensin I to angiotensin II, thus reducing the effects of chronic renin secretion in the ESRD patient.[11]

Accelerated atherosclerosis. Patients with CRF have an increased incidence of atherosclerosis. The reasons for this are not well understood. Hyperlipidemia, commonly seen in this patient population, is a possible contributing factor.[11]

Myocardial dysfunction. Left ventricular hypertrophy with CRF is often a result of hypertension, atherosclerosis, and anemia. Excessive myocardial hypertrophy decreases myocardial contractility because there is insufficient blood supply for the increased muscle mass. Additionally, fluid overload may cause congestive heart failure in a patient whose myocardial function is compromised.

Hyperkalemia. Hyperkalemia is a life-threatening complication of renal failure (p. 1071). High serum potassium levels change the balance between intracellular and extracellular potassium. The membrane potential is altered, affecting the electrical activity of the heart. Potentially lethal cardiac dysrhythmias may result in cardiac arrest and death.[11]

Pericarditis. Pericarditis is a frequent cardiovascular complication of CRF. If it is not treated, it may lead to hemorrhagic pericardial effusion and cardiac tamponade (see Chapter 25). The pericardium may become inflamed by uremic toxins, bacteria, or viruses. Signs include a pericardial friction rub (from harsh rubbing of pericardial

Table 33-19 Manifestations of chronic renal failure

System	Manifestation	Etiology
Integumentary		
Skin	Yellow, gray, bronze pigmentation	Retained pigments
	Pallor	Anemia
	Dryness, scaliness	Decreased size of sweat glands and activity of oil glands
	Pruritus	Dry skin, phosphate crystals
Nails	Thin, brittle	Protein wasting
Hair	Dry	Decreased oil gland activity
	Coarse	Protein wasting
Cardiovascular	Hypertension	Fluid overload, sodium/water retention
	Accelerated atherosclerosis	Hyperlipidemia
	Myocardial dysfunction	Left ventricular hypertrophy
	Congestive heart failure	Fluid overload, hypertension
	Hyperkalemia	Decreased excretion of potassium by kidney
	Pericarditis	Uremic toxins in pericardial fluid; increased pericardial membrane permeability
Respiratory	Uremic lung or pneumonitis	Decreased macrophage activity
	Pulmonary edema	Fluid overload
	Uremic pleuritis, pleural effusion	Increased permeability of pleural membrane because of uremic toxins
	Kussmaul's respirations	Compensatory mechanism for metabolic acidosis
Neuromuscular	Somnolence, confusion, coma	Fluid/electrolyte and acid/base imbalance, uremic toxins
	Peripheral neuropathy "restless leg" and "burning feet" syndromes	Decreased nerve conduction, both motor and sensory, because of uremic toxins
Gastrointestinal		
Oral cavity	Halitosis, stomatitis	Urea converted to ammonia by saliva
Stomach	Anorexia, nausea, vomiting	Decomposition of urea in stomach releases ammonia, which produces small ulcerations and bleeding
Bowel	Diarrhea	Hypermotility from electrolyte imbalance, particularly hyperkalemia
	Constipation	Hypomotility from electrolyte imbalance, particularly hypokalemia; decreased fluid intake; decreased bulk in diet and decreased activity
Hematopoeitic	Anemia	Decreased erythropoeitin secretion; loss of RBCs through GI tract and dialysis; decreased RBC survival time; uremic toxins interfering with folic acid activity
	Platelet dysfunction	Decreased cell surface adhesiveness
	Susceptibility to infection	Decreased neutrophil phagocytosis and chemotaxis
Metabolic	Carbohydrate intolerance	Decreased sensitivity to insulin in peripheral tissues; decreased production of insulin
	Hyperlipidemia	Increased production of serum triglycerides; increased liver output of glycerides from increased insulin levels; reduction in lipase activity
	Protein wasting	Accumulation of end products of protein metabolism with decreased renal function; decreased protein intake
Skeletal	Hypocalcemia	Decreased GI reabsorption because of decreased renal conversion of vitamin D; response to elevated serum phosphatase
	Hyperphosphatemia	Decreased renal excretion
	Metastatic calcifications	Deposition of calcium phosphate crystals in soft tissue and other structures
	Bone dissolution and demineralization	Secondary parathyroidism
Reproductive	Diminished fertility, changes in menstruation	Hormonal changes because of uremic toxins

layers), low-grade fever, hypotension, and chest pain. The heart may become significantly compressed by pleural effusion between the pericardial layers (cardiac tamponade), requiring pericardial fenestration or pericardiectomy to maintain cardiac output and prevent death.[11]

Respiratory system

Respiratory problems in CRF include pulmonary edema, pleural effusions, uremic pleuritis, and a condition referred to as *uremic lung* or *uremic pneumonitis*. The sputum is tenacious and the cough reflex is depressed. Susceptibility to infection is increased because of the reduction in pulmonary macrophage activity that occurs in uremia. A superimposed bacterial infection in the "wet" uremic lung is common. The respiratory system tries to compensate for the metabolic acidosis by increasing the respiratory rate (Kussmaul's respirations) to eliminate carbon dioxide in an effort to decrease the carbonic acid concentration of the body.[11]

Neuromuscular system

Changes in mental functioning are a profound result of CRF. Patients may exhibit confusion, decreased memory, short attention span, and inability to think clearly. Somnolence, stupor, coma, and seizures may also occur in severe cases. These changes are related to fluid/electrolyte and acid/base imbalances and uremic toxin accumulation. Also as a result of the latter a slowing of peripheral nerve conduction occurs, which leads to peripheral neuropathy. Symptoms include bilateral paresthesia and a burning sensation beginning in the toes and spreading up the legs. Painful leg cramps, and crawling, prickling, and itching sensations of the legs develop, usually at night. This syndrome is often relieved by movement and thus is called "restless leg" syndrome. Symptoms of "burning feet" syndrome may also occur and include bilateral painful, burning, prickling, and tingling sensations in the feet. If dialysis is initiated before motor nerve dysfunction develops, these neuropathic changes may be prevented.[11]

Gastrointestinal system

The accumulated uremic toxins and ammonia resulting from the decomposition of urea are irritating to the mucosal lining of the GI tract. These irritants cause anorexia, nausea, and vomiting, which interfere with nutrition. If the patient cannot ingest an adequate amount of calories, catabolism occurs to provide the necessary energy, further accelerating and aggravating the uremia.[11]

In the oral cavity small painful ulcerations occur (stomatitis). Often the patient experiences the taste of blood as a result of the mouth lesions. In addition, as urea decomposes, it emits a distinctive odor that resembles urine. This causes halitosis, which is not only foul smelling but also alters the patient's taste sensations. These changes in the oral cavity further impede nutritional intake.

The gastric mucosa also becomes irritated by the decomposing urea, causing small gastric ulcerations. Bleeding that results from these ulcerations and from increased capillary fragility produced by the uremic toxins is usually manifested as slow GI oozing rather than full GI bleeding.

Bowel function is rarely normal. Hyperkalemia is frequently accompanied by hypermotility and diarrhea. Hypokalemia produces hypomotility and constipation. In addition, decreased fluid intake, activity level, and dietary bulk, and ingestion of phosphate binders serve to aggravate the constipation.

Hematopoietic system

The three major hematopoietic manifestations of CRF are anemia, platelet dysfunction, and increased susceptibility to infection.

Anemia. Anemia, one of the most debilitating effects of CRF, is caused by the following: (1) decreased erythropoietin secretion by the dysfunctional kidneys, (2) loss of RBCs through the GI tract or hemodialysis, (3) decreased RBC survival time from the effect of uremic toxins, (4) production of crenated cells by the hypertonic serum resulting from action of uremic toxins, and (5) decreased folic acid activity because of interference of the uremic toxins. Epoetin alfa, the recombinant form of human erythropoietin, plays a critical role in regulating erythropoiesis; the patient treated with this hormone has increased hematocrit, decreased need for transfusions, and less fatigue.

Platelet dysfunction. The uremic toxins adversely change the surface of the platelets, decreasing adhesiveness or aggregation capabilities, which results in bleeding. Bruises and petechiae are often seen on the skin. The patient is also at increased risk for bleeding as a result of platelet dysfunction.

Metabolic dysfunction

The three aspects of endocrine dysfunction in CRF are carbohydrate intolerance, hyperlipidemia, and protein imbalance.

Carbohydrate intolerance. Carbohydrate intolerance in CRF results from an insensitivity of peripheral tissues to insulin, delayed production of insulin by the pancreas, and an increased half-life of insulin. The serum insulin level is often elevated in uremia because of slowed insulin degradation by the kidney; however, the insulin cannot be effective because of peripheral resistance. These changes do not typically result in hyperglycemia or ketoacidosis. Adequate insulin is released to prevent these conditions in most instances.[22]

Hyperlipidemia. Serum triglyceride levels are elevated in uremia because of increased production and decreased removal of triglycerides. The increased production is related to the peripheral resistance to insulin, and to elevated serum insulin, which cause an increased output of glycerides by the liver. Reduction in activity of the enzyme lipoprotein lipase contributes to the abnormality.[22]

Protein imbalance. There is an accumulation of end products of protein metabolism with decreased renal function, as evidenced by an elevated blood urea nitrogen (BUN).

Skeletal system

Calcium, phosphorus, vitamin D, the parathyroid glands, the skeletal system, and the kidneys exist in an intricate and balanced relationship; renal failure inevitably disrupts this balance. Individuals with renal failure will develop one or more of the following problems: hyperphosphatemia, hypocalcemia, hyperparathyroidism, inadequate vitamin D metabolism, osteodystrophies, or metastatic calcifications. Abnormalities of calcium, phosphorous, or vitamin D metabolism are among the earliest changes to occur with progressive loss of renal function. Early recognition and treatment can prevent the significant damage to the skeletal system that can result from these imbalances.[11]

Reproductive system

Multiple problems related to sexual and reproductive functioning occur in the patient with renal failure. The causes are multifactorial and include hormonal abnormalities, psychologic problems, anemia, antihypertensive medications, and malnutrition. Dialysis may result in some improvement. Transplantation often results in normalization of sexual functioning.[11]

Testosterone is markedly decreased in males and ovarian hormone secretion is suppressed in females. There appears to be end-organ resistance to follicular-stimulating hormone in both sexes. These changes can result in decreased spermatogenesis in males, and amenorrhea and infertility in females.[11]

Nursing Process
Assessment
Subjective data

The nursing assessment of the person in chronic renal failure is extremely complex, particularly because of the multisystem involvement and chronicity of the disorder. Subjective data to be collected include the following:

1. Perception of illness
   a. Reason for coming to the hospital initially
   b. Understanding of proposed plan of care
   c. Expectations of results of therapy
2. History of past illness
   a. Illnesses associated with renal disease
   b. Other illnesses and hospitalizations
   c. Medication regimen
   d. Other therapies
3. Activity
   a. Ability to ambulate, climb stairs, and get in and out of a chair
   b. Presence of bone pain
   c. Fatigue: presence, extent
   d. Usual daytime activities
   e. Recent employment history
   f. Recreational interests
4. Rest and sleep
   a. Nightly sleeping pattern
   b. Activities that induce sleep at night
   c. Daytime napping pattern
   d. Presence and extent of pruritus
5. Nutrition
   a. Present dietary prescription and ability to follow diet
   b. Daily eating patterns
   c. Fluid intake in 24 hours
   d. Impediments to eating (anorexia, nausea and vomiting, bad taste in mouth)
6. Elimination
   a. Frequency and difficulties with urination
   b. Usual amount voided in 24 hours
   c. Color of urine
   d. History of UTI
   e. Usual bowel habits and use of laxatives or enemas
   f. Occurrence of diarrhea or constipation
7. Reproductive system
   a. Menses pattern (females)
   b. Recent changes in sexual functioning
   c. Concerns about reproductive or sexual functioning
8. Social
   a. Persons living at home; relationships
   b. Support persons called upon for help
   c. Type of dwelling and presence of stairs
9. Psychologic: other concerns

Objective data

Objective data to be collected for the patient with chronic renal failure includes the following:

1. Height and weight
2. Vital signs: temperature, pulse (radial, apical, peripheral), respirations and breath sounds (adventitious sounds, friction rub), blood pressure, heart sounds
3. Signs of fluid retention: edema (peripheral, periorbital), neck vein distention, obvious difficulty with breathing, cough with frothy sputum
4. Status of vascular access for dialysis (if present)
5. Neuromuscular difficulties
   a. Muscle tone and strength, symmetry
   b. Weakness or loss of function in extremities
   c. Balance
   d. Loss of sensation, tremors
   e. Senses: vision, touch, taste/smell
   f. Ability to speak
   g. Orientation
   h. Level of alertness and responsiveness
6. Skin: color, turgor, temperature, lesions, condition of nails
7. Urine: color, specific gravity

Once the initial data is obtained, it must be continuously updated. All subsequent assessments are determined by the medical regimen and nursing interventions. Some areas of ongoing assessment are listed in Box 33-19.

Diagnostic tests

A wide variety of diagnostic tests is required once the diagnosis has been made. Many tests will be required to confirm the initial diagnosis. As renal failure progresses, the person will continue to have serum chemistries monitored to ensure that treatment is adequate. Serial creatinine clearance, serum creatinine, and BUN are monitored.

> **Monitoring parameters for the person with chronic renal failure**
>
> 1. Intake and output every 8 hours
> 2. Fluid excess: palpating for edema, auscultating breath sounds, checking blood pressure at least every 8 hours, daily weight records
> 3. Cardiac rhythms every 8 hours
> 4. Level of consciousness every 8 hours
> 5. Signs of electrolyte imbalances
> 6. Presence of fatigue and shortness of breath
> 7. Signs of GI bleeding (bleeding gums, guaiac-positive stools)
> 8. Presence of pruritus and evidences of skin excoriations
> 9. Presence of discomfort: muscle cramping, headaches, ocular irritations
> 10. Insomnia
> 11. Anorexia, bad taste in mouth, daily dietary intake
> 12. Signs of infection

Data analysis: nursing diagnoses

Nursing diagnoses are determined from analysis of patient data. Possible nursing diagnoses for the person with chronic renal failure may include, but are not limited to, the following:

Diagnostic title	Possible etiologies
Fluid volume excess	Compromised regulatory mechanism
Nutrition, altered: less than body requirements	Electrolyte imbalances, protein imbalance, anorexia, bad taste in mouth
Oral mucous membrane, altered	Decomposing urea
Infection, high risk for	Compromised immune response
Injury, high risk for	Neurologic changes, bleeding potential, hyperkalemia
Skin integrity, impaired, high risk for	Pruritus, dry scaly skin
Fatigue	Uremia, anemia, insomnia
Pain: muscle cramps, ocular irritation	Uremic toxins
Coping, ineffective, individual	Situational crisis
Knowledge deficit	Lack of exposure, cognition limitations

Planning: expected patient outcomes

Expected patient outcomes for the patient with chronic renal failure may include, but are not limited to, the following:

1. Does not show signs of additional fluid retention.
2. Eats a balanced diet within prescribed limits.
3. States mouth feels comfortable and bad taste is lessened.
4. Does not show signs of infection.
5. Does not incur any injury.
6. Is free of skin lesions.
7. States feeling more rested and less fatigued.
8. States muscles and eyes are not uncomfortable.

9. Describes feelings about illness and plans for activities that facilitate social interactions.
10. Develops trusting relationship with health care professionals.
11. Describes nature of CRF, rationale for therapy, therapeutic regimens, and need for follow-up care.

Implementation
Assisting with achievement of therapeutic goals

The treatment goals for the person with CRF are listed in Box 33-20. Conservative therapy consists of controlling fluid, sodium, and protein intake. Medications are given to control hypertension, decrease serum phosphate, replace calcium, manage congestive heart failure, decrease potential for GI irritation, and control anemia.

Medications

When kidney function is impaired, drugs are not excreted effectively, thus their efforts may be prolonged. Persons with CRF must therefore be monitored closely for signs of side effects of toxicity. These persons must have the necessary information to monitor themselves at home. Because hypertension commonly occurs with CRF, antihypertensive drugs may be prescribed (Chapter 26).

Measures to decrease hyperphosphatemia help to protect the bones and kidney from further damage. Medications such as calcium carbonate and calcium acetate bind phosphorus in the intestinal tract and allow it to be eliminated. These drugs should be taken at meals to bind the phosphates in the food. The drugs should not be taken with other medications because they also bind drugs in the intestinal tract.

The major electrolyte requiring replacement in a patient with renal failure is *calcium.* Calcium requires vitamin D for absorption; therefore it is not sufficient to administer calcium preparations alone. The active form of *vitamin D* must be given in order for the calcium to be absorbed, either ergocalciferol (least active) or 1.25 dihydrocholecalciferol (most active) (see p. 1016).[22] Examples of calcium supplements include those used for hyperphosphatemia as well as calcium gluconate and calcium lactate.

Cardiotonics are used to manage congestive heart failure that often occurs. Examples include digoxin and digitoxin; digoxin is the preferred cardiotonic because of its greater margin of safety.

Diuretic agents are prescribed to increase the formation of urine and enhance the excretion of fluids and solutes. The major contribution of diuretics lies in their ability to potentiate the effect of the antihypertensive agents. Furosemide, bumetanide, metolazone, and spironolactone are commonly used.

Histamine H_2 receptor antagonists, such as ranitidine or cimetidine, are used to decrease the potential of gastric irritation, ulceration, and bleeding occurring secondary to renal failure.

Anemia is treated with *epoetin alfa (EPO),* a recombinant human erythropoietin (p. 1080) and an *iron supplement.* Transfusions are avoided unless the patient has been refractory to EPO or iron therapy or has experienced significant blood loss, because transfusions depress the patient's stimulus to RBC production, and may cause transfusion reactions.

Vitamin supplements frequently given patients with CRF include the B complex vitamins, vitamin C, folic acid, and vitamin B$_6$. These vitamins are water soluble and are lost during hemodialysis. It may be appropriate to administer vitamin K to the patient receiving antibiotics.

Interventions to achieve patient outcomes
Promoting fluid balance

It is important to adhere to the fluid prescriptions. Fluid intake must be sufficient to maintain renal function without producing diuresis or fluid retention. The person needs to understand the effects of excessive or inadequate fluid intake and signs indicating fluid retention or dehydration in order to maintain the fluid prescriptions both during hospitalization and at home. During hospitalization, monitor the patient's fluid intake and output carefully. Weigh the patient daily at the same time of day with the same wearing apparel.

Facilitating nutrition

Although severely restricted *sodium* diets are *not* now usually prescribed, most persons with CRF require some salt restrictions. If a no-added salt (NAS) diet is prescribed, a normal diet is followed except that no extra salt is added to prepared foods, and obviously salted foods are omitted. For more restricted diets, the specific amount of sodium permitted is prescribed; the dietitian can be especially helpful to patients in planning meals that meet the sodium restriction. *Salt substitutes should be avoided* by all persons with CRF because these substitutes contain large amounts of potassium.

Potassium intake may need to be restricted. If severe hyperkalemia is present, measures to remove the excess serum potassium must be taken (p. 1075). If hyperphosphatemia is present, dietary restriction of *phosphates* will be necessary. Food high in phosphorus include meat, poultry, fish, eggs, milk and cheese, and legumes.

Protein intake is reduced to decrease azotemia, acidosis, and hyperkalemia, and to relieve distressing GI symptoms. Some protein is needed to help maintain nitrogen balance. The preferred proteins are those of high biologic value that contain more essential amino acids, such as fish, poultry, eggs, milk. A newer approach to protein replacement that promotes positive nitrogen balance is the use of mixtures of essential amino acids and ketoacid analogs. *Carbohydrates* are encouraged to provide energy without placing an undue load on the kidneys.

Because the patient is frequently anorexic and may have a bad taste in the mouth, it requires creativity on the part of nurse and family to encourage the patient to eat the prescribed diet (see Chapter 5). Decreased salivary flow and ammonia from breakdown of urea can lead to irritation of the oral mucous membranes. Provide *oral hygiene* several times a day, especially before meals. Mouth care can help remove the taste of blood and urea. Lip emollients can help keep lips moist.

Preventing infection

Persons with CRF are at greater risk for infection than the general population because of decreased neutrophil phagocytosis and chemotaxis. Prevention and control of

---

33-20

Treatment goals for the person with chronic renal failure

1. Stabilization of the internal environment as demonstrated by the following:
   a. Mental alertness, attention span, and appropriate interaction with the environment
   b. Absence or control of peripheral edema, absence of pulmonary edema
   c. Control of electrolyte balance:

Sodium	125 to 145 mEq/L
Potassium	3 to 6 mEq/L
Bicarbonate	>15 mEq/L
Calcium	9 to 11 mg/dl
Phosphate	3 to 5 mg/dl

   d. Serum albumin   >2 g/dl
   e. Control of protein catabolism and protein breakdown products

Urea nitrogen	<100 mg/dl
Creatinine	<15 mg/dl
Uric acid	<12 mg/dl

   f. Absence of joint inflammation and pain
2. Infection and abnormal bleeding are not present.
3. Blood pressure is controlled at less than 160/100 mm Hg sitting, less than 30 mm Hg postural change on standing.
4. Anorexia, nausea, and pruritus are absent or controlled.
5. Intercurrent illness is resolved or controlled (heart failure, infection, dehydration).
6. There is no toxicity from inadequately excreted medication.
7. Nutrient intake is sufficient to maintain positive nitrogen balance.
8. Fluid restrictions are maintained.
9. Adjustment to life-style changes is adapative.
10. Coping mechanisms are appropriate.
11. Trusting relationship is established between patient and nurse.

---

infection is similar to that for acute renal failure (p. 1075). Counsel the person to avoid exposure to individuals with known infections and to avoid extreme fatigue, which lowers body resistance. Encourage the patient to seek medical attention for early signs of infection.

Promoting safety and maintaining skin integrity

Significant rises in serum potassium can be averted by preventing tissue breakdown. Potassium is largely an intracellular cation, and extensive tissue damage can liberate a lethal amount of this ion into the system of the person with CRF. Edema also adds to poor nutrition of the skin. Carry out measures to prevent undue pressure on the skin. Because uremia retards wound healing, instruct patient to monitor scratches for evidence of infection.

Most persons with end-stage renal disease develop pruritus. Patients say that itching is of a deep sensation. Factors that appear to exacerbate the itching include increasing levels of serum phosphorus, dry skin, and warm moist heat. Itching is largely symptomatic, and measures that are effective in controlling it vary. Keeping the skin moist and supple through use of lotions and bath oils, controlling the room temperature during sleep to prevent excessive warmth, and bathing with a vinegar solution are measures that, used alone or in combination, may provide some relief from itching. Antipruritic medications may be prescribed. Injury to the skin from vigorous scratching may lead to skin infections. Fingernails can be trimmed closely, and a soft cloth rather than the fingernails should be used to scratch the skin.

Mild or unfatted soaps should be used to avoid excessive skin dryness. Pruritus often decreases with a reduction in BUN and improved phosphorus control. Encourage the use of phosphate binders and the reduction of dietary phosphorus if elevated phosphorus is a problem.

GI bleeding needs to be diminished when possible. Urea is broken down to ammonia by the action of intestinal bacteria. Because ammonia is a mucosal irritant, ulcers and bleeding can occur. Administer prescribed antacids (every 2 to 4 hours) and H_2 receptor antagonists to prevent bleeding. Suggest that the patient use a soft toothbrush to decrease bleeding of the gums. Instruct the patient to look for and report signs of melena.

Neurologic changes can also lead to injuries from decreasing patient alertness or vision, or from muscle weakness. Assess the patient's awareness to the environment. At times the person may need to be helped in limiting activities to a level commensurate with mental processes and level of awareness. Individuals caring for the patient need to be aware of the possibility of seizure activity and take appropriate precautions. Correction of abnormal body chemistries will help to decrease the potential for injury.

Promoting rest

Fatigue is a common complaint of persons with CRF because of the effects of uremia, anemia, and recurring thoughts concerning the disease state and resultant changes in life-style. Treatment for uremia and anemia will help to decrease fatigue. Plans for daily activities should include provision of rest periods. Naps are best taken early in the day; late naps interfere with the quality of sleep. Measures to promote sleep are appropriate.

Promoting comfort

Muscle cramping in the lower extremities and hands may be temporarily relieved by heat and massage in some persons. *Ocular irritation* in CRF is caused by hyperphosphatemia leading to calcium deposits in the conjunctiva, which cause burning and watering of the eyes. Methylcellulose (artificial tears) placed in the conjunctival sac every few hours helps to reduce irritation.

Facilitating coping

Numerous alterations in life-style, group membership, and feelings regarding the self occur for the person with CRF. The numerous physical changes that occur often make it difficult to carry on activities that were once normally pursued. Chronic fatigue may make it impossible for the person to continue to be employed. Because the patient is often tired and not feeling well, it may be difficult to plan in advance for social events. The former roles of the sick member of the family must often be taken on by another. When roles cannot easily be changed or assumed by other members of the family, serious threats to the organization of the family group occur. Physical appearance also changes and is of much concern to most persons. As uremia progresses, the individual often becomes thin and weaker and appears sallow. Thoughts concerning death and the quality of life are common.

Denial often becomes a chief defense mechanism for the patient. With it the individual can periodically forget the constant threat to life. The use of this mental mechanism for the person with CRF can be quite appropriate as long as it is not manifested by maladaptive or harmful behavior. Inappropriate uses of denial involve continuous dietary indiscretion and failure to take prescribed medications.

Patients with chronic renal failure need the hope and encouragement that with treatment discomfort will be lessened and they will be allowed to pursue what seems most productive and important to them. Hope should not be focused on cure, but on learning to manage a new style of life. In managing the changes that occur as a result of CRF, patients should be encouraged to be as independent and as active as possible. They should be taught to manage the treatment and should be given the responsibility of doing so. Nursing care should be provided as part of the team approach that assists patients in identifying problems and resources to meet them, and helps patients and their families adjust to the changes in their life-style.

Facilitating patient learning

To promote self-care, every aspect of health care promotion pertaining to end-stage renal disease must be conveyed to the patient and significant others who may be participating in care (see Box 33-21). Education about *medications*, concerning prescribed, over-the-counter, and folk medicines, is carried out with the person. The use of popular medications that are sold without prescription must be discouraged. All medications should be prescribed by the physician. Aspirin may be hazardous because it is normally excreted by the kidneys and may rapidly build to toxic levels and prolong bleeding time. Many cold preparations contain large amounts of sodium. Remembering to take prescribed medications can be a problem for the person who may have many pills to take each day, especially if the person is confused. Correlating pill-taking times with major activities of the day or use of mechanical devices to separate the daily allotment of pills may be helpful. Patient teaching includes the following:

1. Nature of chronic renal failure
2. Diet regimen, including fluid restrictions
3. Medication regimen, including action, dosage, frequency, and side effects
4. Relationships between diet, fluid restriction, medication, and blood chemistries
5. Relationships between symptoms and their causes
6. Need for rest periods, and need to pace activities to prevent fatigue
7. Availability of community resources
8. Symptoms that must be reported to the physician (changes in urinary output, edema, weight gain, dyspnea, infection, behavioral changes)
9. Need for continued medical follow-up

The patient with chronic renal failure

Administer prescribed medications (antihypertensives, calcium products, vitamin D preparations, cardiotonics, diuretics, histamine H$_2$ receptor antagonists, epoetin alfa, iron supplements, and vitamin supplements).

Encourage the person to remain within prescribed fluid restrictions.

Encourage a diet high in carbohydrates within the prescribed limits of sodium, potassium, phosphorous, and protein.

Administer phosphate-binding agents with meals, as prescribed.

Provide oral hygiene at frequent intervals, especially before meals.

Protect the patient from infection.

Assess the environment and protect the patient from injury.

Provide rest periods to decrease fatigue.

Use measures to decrease pruritus, muscle cramping, and eye irritation.

Provide patient with opportunities to discuss feelings about chronicity of disease.

Provide counseling if denial interferes with therapy.

Encourage hope by helping the person learn how to manage the new life-style.

Teach the person about the nature of CRF, rationale for therapy, therapeutic regimens, and need for follow-up care.

Evaluation

Evaluation is based on expected patient outcomes. Questions to consider include the following:

1. Is the patient following the required fluid and diet prescription?
2. Does the patient state that mouth feels comfortable and bad taste is lessened?
3. Have infection and injury been prevented?
4. Has skin integrity been maintained?
5. Does the person describe feeling more comfortable and less fatigued?
6. Has the patient planned for activities to facilitate social interactions and developed a trusting relationship with health care professionals?
7. Can the person describe the nature of CRF, rationale for therapy, therapeutic regimen, and symptoms to be reported?

RENAL REPLACEMENT THERAPIES

Dialysis

Dialysis involves the movement of fluid and particles across a semipermeable membrane. It is a treatment that can help restore normal fluid and electrolyte balance, control acid-base balance, and remove waste and toxic material from the body. It can sustain life successfully in both acute and chronic renal failure where substitution for or augmentation of normal renal function is needed. Specifically, dialysis is used to remove excessive amounts of drugs and toxins in poisoning of both an intentional and accidental nature, to correct serious electrolyte and acid-base imbalances, to maintain kidney function when renal shutdown occurs as a result of transfusion reactions, to temporarily replace renal function in persons with acute renal failure of various origins, and to permanently substitute for loss of renal function in persons with chronic end-stage renal disease.

Physiologic principles of dialysis

Dialysis is based on three principles: diffusion, osmosis, and ultrafiltration (Fig. 33-35). *Diffusion* involves the movement of *particles* from an area of greater concentration to an area of lesser concentration. In the body this usually occurs across a semipermeable membrane. Diffusion is involved in the clearance of solute from the patient's body in both hemodialysis and peritoneal dialysis. Diffusion results in the movement of urea, creatinine, and uric acid from the patient's blood into the dialysate solution. This solution contains fewer particles to be removed from the bloodstream and higher concentrations of particles to be added to the blood (Fig. 33-36). Because the dialysate contains no protein waste products, the concentration of these substances in the blood will decrease because of random movement of the particles across the semipermeable membrane into the dialysate. The same principle applies to the movement of potassium ions. Although the concentration of red blood cells and protein is high in blood, these molecules are quite large and do not diffuse through the membrane pores; hence they are not lost from the blood.

Osmosis involves the movement of *fluid* across a semipermeable membrane from an area of lesser to an area of greater concentration of particles. Osmosis is responsible for movement of extra fluid from the patient, particularly in peritoneal dialysis. Fig. 33-36 shows that glucose has been added to the dialysate to make its particle concentration greater than that of the patient's blood. Fluid will then move through the pores of the membrane from the patient's blood to the dialysate.

Ultrafiltration involves the movement of fluid across a semipermeable membrane as a result of an artificially created pressure gradient. Ultrafiltration is more efficient than osmosis for removal of fluid and is used in hemodialysis for this purpose. During dialysis, osmosis and diffusion or ultrafiltration and diffusion occur simultaneously.

Hemodialysis
Procedure

Hemodialysis involves shunting the patient's blood from the body through a dialyzer in which diffusion and ultrafiltration occur and back into the patient's circulation. To perform hemodialysis there must be access to the patient's blood, a mechanism to transport the blood to and from the dialyzer, and a dialyzer (area in which the exchange of fluid electrolytes and waste products occurs). Presently there are five major means for gaining access to the patient's bloodstream. These include the following:

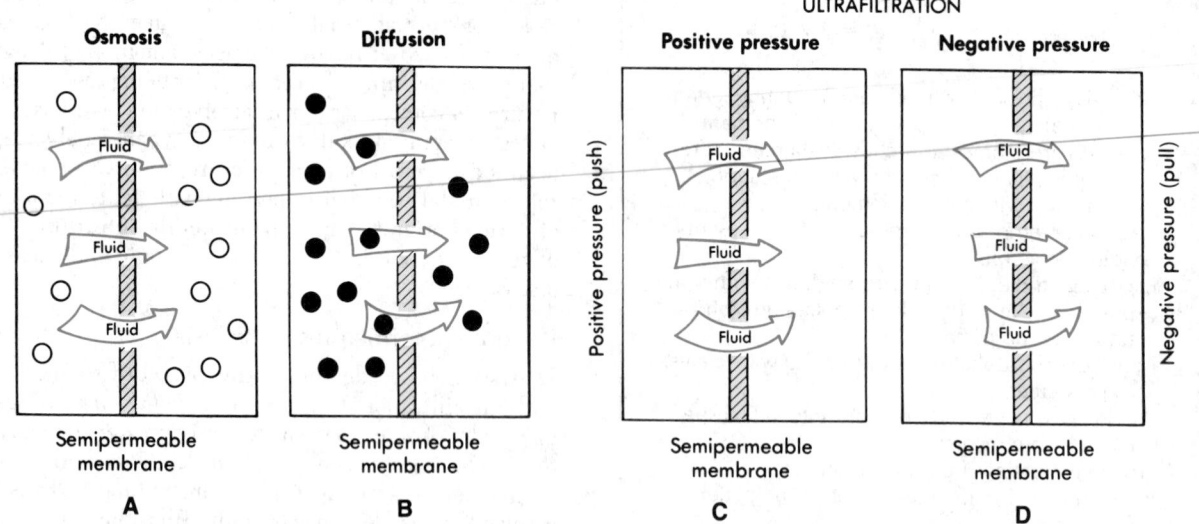

Fig. 33-35 Dialysis is based on principles of **A**, osmosis, and **B**, diffusion and ultrafiltration. Ultrafiltration occurs when either **C**, positive pressure or **D**, negative pressure is placed on the system. Ultrafiltration can be maximized by exerting both positive and negative pressure on system simultaneously.

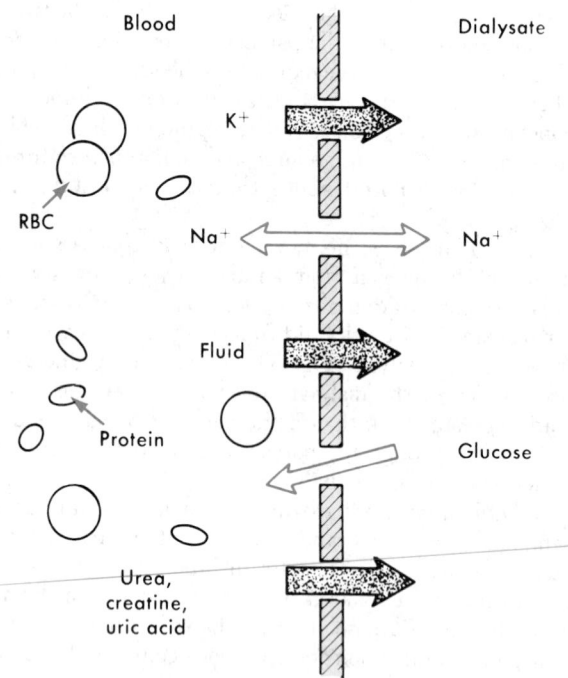

Fig. 33-36 Osmosis and diffusion in dialysis. Net movement of major particles and fluid is illustrated.

1. Arteriovenous fistula (Fig. 33-37, A)
2. Arteriovenous graft (Fig. 33-37, B)
3. External arteriovenous shunt (Fig. 33-37, C)
4. Femoral vein catheterization (Fig. 33-37, D)
5. Subclavian vein catheterization (Fig. 33-37, E)

The indications and nursing implications for each access is summarized in Table 33-20.

Many persons expect to leave the dialysis treatment with a feeling of well-being. Few persons feel this way; most experience some minor discomfort that diminishes within several hours after dialysis. The greatest feeling of well-being seems to occur the day after dialysis.

Dialysis for an acute problem may be carried out daily or as often as the condition of the patient warrants. Hemodialysis for chronic renal failure is usually performed two or three times a week.

Nursing care of the patient during hemodialysis should center around (1) monitoring the physical status of the patient before and during dialysis for evidence of physiologic imbalance and change, (2) comfort and safety needs of the patient, and (3) helping the patient to understand and adjust to the care and changes in life-style. This latter objective involves educating the person as to the specifics of the treatment program (diet and medications in particular) and how these relate to altered kidney function. The person is encouraged to express concerns and feelings, and attempts must be made to help the individual work through these feelings. If dialysis is performed at home, the patient and back-up person must be able to institute all the care described.

The environment must provide protection from conditions that would promote infection. Because there is the potential for blood spills as a result of the treatment, all equipment must be easy to clean. Great care must also be taken to dispose properly all soiled articles to prevent cross-contamination between patients.

Because the person spends a great deal of time at the dialysis center, the environment should be warm and inviting. Activities should be available to assist the person in using the time on dialysis as fully as possible. Art and music therapy both provide effective and productive diversion.

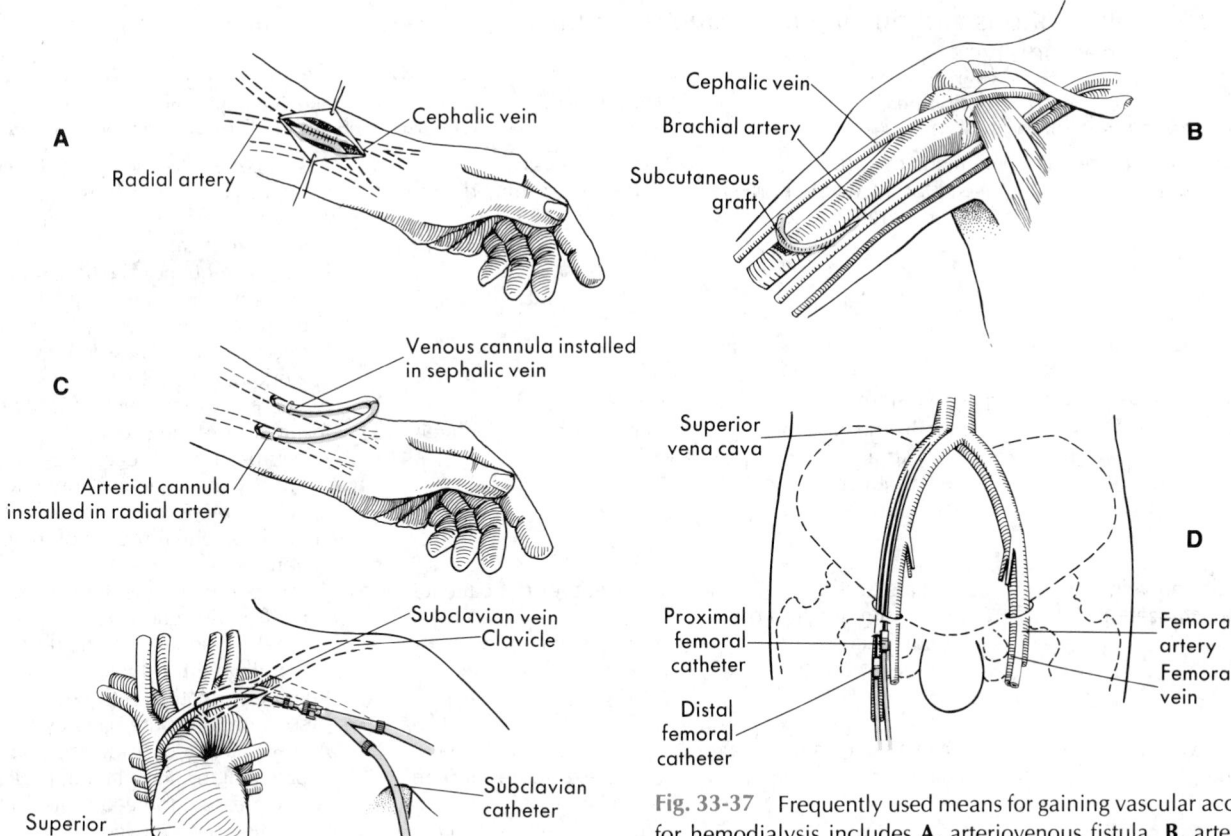

Fig. 33-37 Frequently used means for gaining vascular access for hemodialysis includes **A,** arteriovenous fistula, **B,** arteriovenous graft, **C,** external arteriovenous shunt, **D,** femoral vein catheterization, and **E,** subclavian vein catheterization.

Predialysis care

Before the procedure, patients should have an opportunity to become familiar with the dialysis unit. They should be given an explanation of what will happen and what will be expected of them during the treatment. Patients often want to know (1) what types of pain will be experienced during the treatment, (2) how long and how often the dialysis will be, (3) what they should feel like during and after the treatment, (4) what they will be allowed to do during dialysis, and (5) if family members may be present during the therapy. Monitoring activities include the following:

1. Record current weight and compare to patient's dry weight (estimated weight with no excess fluid and near normal blood pressure).
2. Obtain baseline vital signs.
3. Assess patient for fluid overload (pedal edema, periorbital edema, neck vein distention, adventitious breath sounds).
4. Assess vascular access for patency and infection.

A blood sample is drawn to determine the level of serum electrolytes and waste products, and the patient's physical status is assessed.

Patients should be told that they may experience some headache and nausea during the treatment and for a few hours afterward. Headache and nausea result from change in fluid, acid-base, and waste balance during dialysis. The symptoms should never be extreme, and relief should be attained from rest and sleep, mild analgesics, or antiemetics. Postural hypotension may also occur following dialysis; it is transitory in nature and caused by a relative depletion of intravascular volume secondary to fluid removal. The hypotension may produce dizziness and faintness. Relief should be obtained within a few hours with rest. The patient is assured that all of these symptoms will abate and that frequent monitoring during the procedure will help to control the degree of change that occurs during dialysis and the development of these symptoms.

Hemodialysis equipment

The *dialyzer* or artificial kidney contains the semipermeable membrane and a means for blood and dialysate to flow in a single compartment divided by the membrane. Membranes are made of regenerated cellulose acetate, polymethylmethacrylate, or polyaerylonitrile. These membranes allow for increased rate of diffusion of molecules in the middle molecule range (2000-5000 daltons) and higher ultrafiltration rates.

Dialysate has a composition similar to plasma and has two functions as it flows opposite uremic plasma. First, it carries away waste materials and fluids removed from the blood. Second, it prevents the removal of essential electrolytes and prevents excessive water depletion.

The *hemodialysis machine* automatically mixes dialysate concentrate with *purified* water, heats the dialysate, delivers it to the dialyzer, and then discards the "spent" dialysate

Table 33-20   Indications and nursing implications for the major types of vascular access for hemodialysis

Type	Indications	Advantages	Nursing implications
Femoral vein catheterization	Immediate access Need for access seen as short duration	Ease of access Can be used immediately	Assess patient frequently for bleeding from insertion sites Apply pressure for 5 to 10 min after pulling catheter Requires frequent irrigation with heparin solution to maintain patency Sterile technique is essential when working with catheters
External shunt	Long term (weeks to months) needed for vascular access Access required within a few hours	Ease of access Can be used immediately	Assess patient frequently for bleeding at insertion site Assess patency of access frequently by observing continuous flow of blood through shunt Shunt is potential source of infection
Subclavian vein catheterization	Immediate access Short or long duration of vascular access	Does not restrict patient's activity Requires only one catheter	Assess patient frequently for bleeding from insertion site Sterile technique is essential when working with catheter Requires irrigation with heparin solution to ensure patency
Arteriovenous fistula and graft	Permanent access required	Is least likely of all the accesses to develop an infection Once maintained it provides easy access	Assess patency of fistula or graft by palpating or auscultating bruit Apply pressure to needle site after needles are removed Instruct patient to avoid compression of fistula by tight clothing or carrying objects with arm bent Patient must be instructed to assess fistula for signs and symptoms of infection including pain, redness, swelling or excessive warmth

down the drain after contact with the uremic plasma. The standard for dialysate mixture is 34 parts purified water to 1 part dialysate concentrate.

The *blood pump*, located on the hemodialysis machine, is used to circulate the blood from the patient to the dialyzer and back. Blood flows of 200-350 ml/min are required to achieve an adequate dialysis in a short time (3-5 hours). The blood pump is a simple roller-type device.

The *heparin pump* provides the heparinization required to prevent dialyzer clotting. The pump holds a syringe of heparinized saline and delivers the solution through the bloodline to the patient. The *air detector* detects air in the extracorporeal system to prevent air emboli. It is an important safety device.

Care during hemodialysis

When the patient has an external shunt used for temporary situations only, no pain should be experienced during initiation of dialysis. However, pain of a moderate degree may be present when venipuncture is performed in an arteriovenous fistula. A local anesthetic is used in most

dialysis centers before insertion of the needles.

Nursing care includes measures to increase the patient's physical comfort. Lying relatively immobile for even a few hours can produce pressure over bony prominences and general restlessness. Changing the patient's position increases tolerance to limited movement. Mouth care is required if the patient is nauseated and vomiting. Because an upper extremity is generally kept immobile during dialysis, the patient may need help with activities requiring the use of both hands.

Activity during dialysis is largely a matter of individual preference. Some persons sleep throughout their treatment; others read or carry on various activities.

Eating during dialysis is largely a matter of individual preference. Some individuals may become quite hungry, whereas for others the smell of food causes nausea. Patients may ask that they be allowed to eat foods not generally allowed during dialysis. Practice indicates that either allowing or discouraging eating freely during dialysis is a matter of individual unit philosophy. Because of the frequency of nausea, vomiting, and disequilibrium many patients experience during hemodialysis, it may be best to discourage eating to decrease the potential of aspiration.

Hypovolemia

Most physical problems that occur during dialysis are related to hypotension from removal of fluid and disequilibrium from a rapid reduction in extracellular electrolytes and wastes. Hypovolemia and shock can occur during dialysis as a result of rapid removal of *fluid* from the intravascular compartment. Because this can occur faster than reequilibration of intracellular and intravascular volume relationships, the person may appear edematous and yet exhibit signs of shock. Signs and symptoms that indicate that the intravascular volume is being rapidly depleted are anxiety, restlessness, dizziness, nausea and vomiting, diaphoresis, tachycardia, and hypotension. Activities to prevent hypovolemia include the following:

1. Check blood pressure and pulse every 30 to 60 minutes (more frequently if signs of shock present); blood pressure should show only a slight increase.
2. Monitor blood flow and dialyzer pressure settings carefully to prevent too-rapid blood flow.
3. Withhold rapid-acting antihypertensives the morning of dialysis (unless person is severely hypertensive).
4. Evaluate need for withholding medications that predispose to hypovolemia (analgesics, tranquilizers, hypnotics, nitroglycerin).

In treating a patient who shows signs of hypovolemia, initial nursing measures include placing the head of the bed in a flat position, and raising the patient's feet. Administration of normal saline solution may be necessary to restore blood pressure. Throughout a hypotensive episode vital signs, level of consciousness, and any complaints offered are closely monitored. Vomiting frequently accompanies hypotension. Because of upper-extremity immobility, it may be difficult for the patient to clear the mouth if vomiting should occur. The patient is helped to a safe position so that aspiration is avoided.

When the weight losses of several dialysis treatments are correlated with the patient's blood pressure, pulse, and other indications of hypovolemia, an individual pattern of the patient's tolerance to fluid removal can be determined. This trend or pattern can be used to help adjust the rate and overall effect of the dialysis in keeping with the patient's physiologic tolerance.

Disequilibrium phenomenon

A disequilibrium phenomenon occurs for many dialysis patients toward the end of or after dialysis. Disequilibrium results when excess *solutes* are cleared from the blood more rapidly than they can diffuse from the body's cells (particularly those of the central nervous system) into the vascular compartment. Hence, disequilibrium exists in the concentration of solute inside and outside the cells. Because particle content is greater inside the cells, water is taken in and edema results. Intracellular pH changes are also present. To some degree this process occurs with all patients with each dialysis procedure and helps to explain why patients do not feel their best immediately after treatment. *Severe disequilibrium*, or *disequilibrium phenomenon*,

is most likely to be seen in the person whose blood chemistry values are exceptionally high before dialysis. Signs and symptoms of disequilibrium include *headache, restlessness, mental confusion,* and *nausea* and *vomiting.* Severe disequilibrium may result in convulsions, especially in children when BUN levels exceed the concentration of 100 mg/ml.

Treatment includes anticipation of severe disequilibrium. Often when a patient is beginning dialysis treatments, the procedures are kept short and may be spaced more frequently than normal during the first week. This allows solute to be cleared from the body without producing the extremely wide swings in body chemistry that would result in severe disequilibrium. Keeping the patient quiet, reducing environmental discomfort such as temperature extremes and bright lights, and closely supervising the patient to ensure physical safety are nursing care requirements. Mild analgesics may help to relieve headache. If disequilibrium becomes severe and the patient is still on dialysis, the therapy may be discontinued.

Blood loss

To prevent the patient's blood from clotting as it flows through the dialyzer, heparin is administered. Protamine sulfate is not generally given to the patient to counteract the effect of heparin. The patient is watched for signs of bleeding anywhere in the body. At the end of the treatment when dialysis needles are removed from the fistula, manual pressure is held until bleeding or oozing ceases. Pressure dressings are applied to the puncture sites. The sites are observed at frequent intervals to detect hemorrhage or oozing. During and shortly after dialysis, treatments that cause tissue trauma such as venipuncture or intramuscular injections should not be performed. The patient who has had recent surgery, dental extractions, or recent trauma to soft tissues will have clotting times monitored frequently during dialysis to prevent hemorrhage. These patients need to be closely observed for signs of bleeding.

Postdialysis care

Following dialysis, the person's weight is recorded again to determine the amount of fluid loss during treatment and postural vital signs are assessed.

Facilitating patient learning

A sample teaching plan is described in Box 33-22. Major teaching points specific to hemodialysis include the following:

1. The process of dialysis and relationship to the person's own body needs.
2. Care of the vascular access, including monitoring for complications (absent thrill or bruit over artery indicating no blood flow, constriction of fistula, infection, hemorrhage).
3. Where to obtain care if complications occur.
4. Common complications of hemodialysis.
5. Changes in medication schedule required before and after dialysis treatments.
6. Ways to schedule dialysis treatments for minimal interference with life-style.
7. Alternative modes of treatment for end-stage renal disease.

33-22

Patient Teaching

The patient on hemodialysis

Orientation to hemodialysis and visit to the unit
  when appropriate
Nature of renal failure
  Normal kidney function
  Kidney failure specific to patient's pathophysi-
    ology (types, causes)
Dietary reinforcement, including rationale: restric-
  tion of protein, potassium, sodium, and fluids,
  and increase in calories
Review of medication regimen
  Purpose of each prescribed medication
  Common side effects
  Dosage and times of each medication
  Prescription filling procedure
Care of vascular access (if appropriate)
  Procedure for assessing presence of thrills and
    bruits and who to notify if these signs are ab-
    sent
  Guarding against constriction of fistula (such as
    sleeping on affected arm or wearing tight
    clothing)
  Hygiene and removing dressing after dialysis
  Signs and symptoms of infection
  Measures to control hemorrhage should it de-
    velop when away from dialysis unit
Hemodialysis process
  Principles of dialysis (teach on basis of patient's
    learning level)
  Sequence of activities during hemodialysis
  Common sights and sounds of dialysis unit
  Common complications and their treatments:
    hypotension, nausea, vomiting, cramping
Laboratory data: types, meaning, and effects of
  hemodialysis, diet, and medications on each
  value
Alternative modes of treatment of ESRD: free-
  standing hemodialysis centers, home dialysis,
  peritoneal dialysis, kidney transplantation

Peritoneal dialysis

In peritoneal dialysis the dialyzing fluid is instilled into the peritoneal cavity and the peritoneum becomes the dialyzing membrane (Fig. 33-38). In comparison with hemodialysis treatments, which last 3 to 6 hours, peritoneal dialysis is maintained continuously for up to 36 hours. The procedure, once instituted, is largely a nursing responsibility. Peritoneal dialysis is used in treating acute and chronic renal failure. It can be performed in the hospital or at home.

The major advantages of peritoneal dialysis include the following:

1. The procedure provides a steady state of blood chemistries.
2. Any location can be used, and machinery is not needed.
3. The process can be easily taught to patient or family.
4. Few dietary restrictions are required; because of the loss of protein across the peritoneal membrane into the dialysate, the patient is usually placed on a high-protein diet.
5. The patient has more control over daily life.
6. The procedure can be used for persons who are hemodynamically unstable.

Procedure

Access to the peritoneum is gained through introduction of a catheter into the peritoneal space. For acutely ill patients, and those who are chronically ill and require sporadic dialysis, a sterile catheter is inserted for each procedure. For the chronically ill person treated on a routine basis, a special catheter can be placed into the peritoneal space, the catheter remains until it malfunctions or another form of treatment is selected for the patient. These catheters present a continued potential entrance for organisms into the peritoneum.

To insert a peritoneal catheter, the physician cleanses the abdomen and anesthetizes a small area in the midline of the abdomen about 5 cm (2 inches) below the umbilicus. A small incision is made, and a many-eyed nylon catheter is inserted into the peritoneal cavity (Fig. 33-38).

A dressing is placed around the protruding catheter. Dialysis is initiated for the person with a permanent catheter by carefully cleansing the catheter and surrounding skin with a bactericidal agent before the catheter is connected to the dialysate line. Approximately 2 L of sterile dialysate warmed to body temperature is attached by tubing to the catheter and allowed to run into the peritoneal cavity as rapidly as possible. This usually takes about 10 minutes. The tubing is then clamped, and 10 to 30 minutes are allowed for osmosis of fluid and diffusion of particles into the dialyzing solution. This is called a *dwell time*. At the end of the dwell time the tubing is unclamped and the fluid is allowed to flow by gravity from the abdomen.

Fluid should drain in a steady stream. Drainage time should average about 10 to 15 minutes. The first drainage may be pink tinged as a result of the trauma of catheter insertion; however, this should clear with the second or third drainage. At no time should fluid draining from the abdomen appear grossly bloody. After fluid has drained from the abdomen, another cycle is started immediately. After the dialysis has been completed, the permanent catheter is again cleansed and a sterile cap is applied to the tip; the temporary catheter is removed, and the incision is covered with a dry sterile dressing. The small abdominal wound from the catheter should heal completely in 1 to 2 days.

Preprocedure care

Weight, blood pressure, and pulse are recorded before the procedure is initiated. These values serve as baseline information to assess changes in the patient's condition. For persons undergoing insertion of a peritoneal catheter before dialysis, assessment should be made of their knowledge of the procedure and their anxiety level. A mild sedative may help the severely anxious person to better tolerate the insertion of the catheter. It is important that these patients void just before catheter insertion; this decompresses the bladder and prevents accidental puncture during catheter placement.

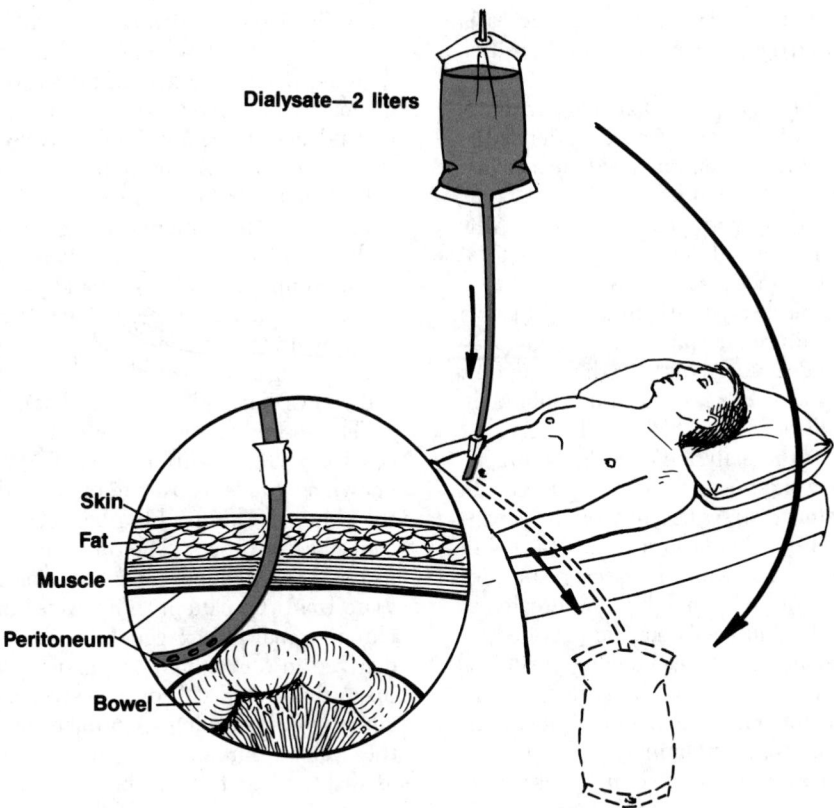

Fig. 33-38   Patient receiving peritoneal dialysis. Dialysis fluid is being inserted into peritoneal cavity.

Care during peritoneal dialysis

The person undergoing acute peritoneal dialysis may be confined to bed during the treatment as a result of general fatigue and the constant fluid exchanges that take place. Comfort measures and diversionary activities should be of high priority. During the dialysis, the patient is able to turn from side to side and move about in bed as desired as long as the catheter remains undisturbed. The patient is provided assistance with hygiene care as needed. If peritoneal dialysis is carried out at home, the patient and a backup person need to be able to do all steps of the procedure to ensure that therapy is not interrupted when the patient is too ill to perform dialysis alone.

Nursing activities during peritoneal dialysis include the following:

1. Maintain strict aseptic technique to prevent infection.
2. Monitor vital signs frequently.
3. Maintain strict intake and output records.
4. Assess catheter site for signs of infection.
5. Assess patient for edema.
6. During cycles maintain accurate record of each cycle, including the following:
   a. Type of dialysate
   b. Amount of dialysate infused
   c. Amount of dialysate recovered
   d. Time dialysate was left in-dwelling
   e. Characteristics of returned dialysate (effluent)

Complications of peritoneal dialysis

Complications most commonly associated with peritoneal dialysis include hypotension and hypovolemia, inadequate drainage of fluid from the peritoneal space, pain, atelectasis, respiratory distress, and peritonitis. As with hemodialysis, *hypotension* is most likely to result from rapid removal of fluid from the intravascular space. In addition to checking vital signs and observing the patient's behavior, records of fluid balance are crucial in determining the amount of fluid that has been removed. The net gain or loss of fluid from the abdomen should be determined at the completion of each cycle. To decrease the amount of fluid that is being removed from the vascular space, the physician may decrease the hypertonicity of the dialysate and may increase the rate at which fluid is administered through an intravenous line.

Drainage of fluid from the abdomen can be slow or impossible to start. Generally, this problem results when the tip of the catheter has become lodged against abdominal tissues. It may also result from plugging of the catheter with blood or fibrin that has accumulated as a result of tissue trauma. A small amount of heparin may be added to the dialysate to decrease the chance of a clot forming in the catheter. When the dialysate does not drain freely from the abdomen, the patient should turn from side to side in an attempt to reposition the catheter in the peritoneal cavity. In addition, firm pressure may be applied to the abdomen with both hands and the head of the bed may be raised. If the flow of the dialysate does not increase, the physician is called to irrigate the catheter or reposition it.

Severe *pain* should not be experienced during peritoneal dialysis. Moderate levels of pain are often experienced as fluid is instilled and withdrawn from the peritoneal cavity. Procaine hydrochloride may be instilled with the dialysate in an attempt to control the patient's discomfort. Mild analgesics may be ordered for administration at 3- to 4-hour intervals during the procedure.

When the patient is markedly overhydrated and shows evidence of congestive failure and pulmonary edema, *respiratory difficulty* may be encountered as the dialyzing fluid infuses. The quality and rate of respiration should be closely observed. The head of the bed can be raised to decrease the pressure of the dialysate on the diaphragm. The amount of dialyzing fluid used for each cycle may be decreased when respiratory distress becomes prolonged and severe. The patient, although encouraged to eat while being dialyzed, may find that this increases respiratory difficulty. To help overcome additional pressure created by a full stomach, frequent small meals may be provided.

Peritonitis is an ever-present threat during peritoneal dialysis. Aseptic technique must be rigidly maintained during insertion of the catheter and throughout the procedure. Care should be taken to avoid contaminating the solution or the tubing when dialysate solution is hung. Cultures of the dialysate fluid are performed routinely to ensure continued attention to asepsis and to identify organisms if peritonitis should develop subsequently. The patient should be observed for signs of peritonitis. These include an elevated temperature, tenderness or pain of the abdomen, and cloudy effluent. In more severe cases, the patient may have fever, nausea, vomiting, chills, and diarrhea.[16]

Other approaches to peritoneal dialysis

Several advances in the management of patients with chronic end-stage renal disease have led to two variations of peritoneal dialysis. These technologies emphasize home-

and self-dialysis. *Continuous ambulatory peritoneal dialysis* (CAPD) is one development that is leading to safe self-dialysis that is practical and relatively inexpensive when compared to hemodialysis and that promotes patient independence. Basically, CAPD involves continuous contact of dialysate with the peritoneal membrane. Approximately 2 L of dialysate are maintained interperitoneally and exchanged by the patient through a permanent peritoneal catheter 4 to 5 times a day.[22] No special equipment is required for the exchanges, and the patient can therefore lead a fairly normal life-style. Exchanges can take place at home or at work by connecting an empty bag to the catheter and opening a clamp to allow drainage. A full dialysate bag is then instilled and the patient has completed an exchange.

The second method is *continuous cyclic peritoneal dialysis* (CCPD). CCPD differs from CAPD in that a machine known as a *cycler* is used to instill and drain dialysate from the patient. The machine has a series of clamps that are controlled by timers. The timers open and close the clamps in sequence to allow for instillation and drainage of dialysate from the patient. The cycle times for patients with chronic renal failure generally allow for the patient to be dialyzed in 6 to 8 hours. A patient can therefore connect up to the cycler at bedtime, set the machine, and be dialyzed while sleeping. A number of alarms are built into the cycler to protect the patient from such malfunctions as dialysate that is too hot or cold, long or short dwell times, improper return of fluid, and changes in catheter pressures. The greatest advantage of CAPD and CCPD over other forms of dialysis is that both offer patients unprecedented freedom in managing their own care.

Facilitating patient learning

The teaching requirements for the patient undergoing peritoneal dialysis are consistent with the teaching plan for hemodialysis. However, the patient will need to be instructed in the specifics of the process of peritoneal dialysis. If CAPD is planned, training should be accomplished in a home training center that is equipped to assist the patient in dealing with home care.

Kidney Transplantation

A kidney transplantation is performed to prolong the life of a person with chronic renal failure. It is not a cure for CRF but rather an ongoing therapy with its own side effects and potential complications. Kidneys may be obtained from related donors (preferred approach) or from cadavers.

During surgery the transplanted kidney is placed in the iliac fossa (Fig. 33-39). Generally, the peritoneal cavity is not entered. The patient's own kidneys are not disturbed unless they are infected or are the cause of significant hypertension, in which case the recipient undergoes bilateral nephrectomy before transplant surgery. The recipient's kidneys are left intact whenever possible to maintain erythropoietin production, blood pressure control, and prostaglandin synthesis and metabolism. The donor ureter is used to the extent that is possible. If long enough, the donor ureter is connected to the bladder in such a way as to prevent reflux of urine. If the ureter is short, a ureteroureterostomy may be performed. Care of the patient experiencing organ transplant is described in Chapter 42.

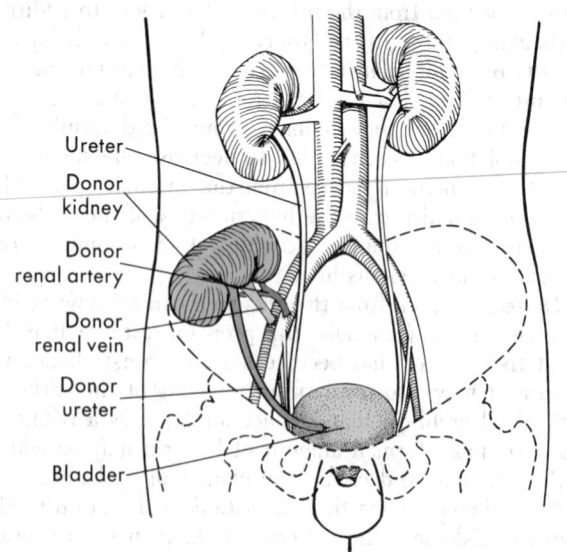

Ureter
Donor kidney
Donor renal artery
Donor renal vein
Donor ureter
Bladder

Fig. 33-39 Location of transplanted kidney showing anastomosis or renal artery, renal vein, and ureter.

SUMMARY

1. The kidneys are essential for the following reasons:
   a. Regulate electrolytes
   b. Eliminate wastes
   c. Regulate fluid volume
   d. Maintain acid-base balance
   e. Regulate blood pressure
   f. Stimulate production of RBCs
   g. Regulate calcium-phosphate metabolism
2. The kidneys regulate blood pressure by contolling fluid volume as well as mediating the renin-angiotensin-aldosterone system.
3. Diabetes mellitus is the leading cause of end-stage renal disease.
4. Hypertension is another leading cause of renal disease that could be minimized by early detection and adequate treatment.
5. Urinary retention can result in hydronephrosis that leads to permanent damage to the kidneys.
6. Control of urinary incontinence is largely dependent on its cause. Accurate diagnosis of the cause of the incontinence is therefore essential before a program to reestablish continence is developed.
7. Females are more likely to develop UTI than are males. Approximately 1% of all school age girls and 4% of all women in their childbearing years are diagnosed as having UTI.
8. If untreated, lower UTIs can migrate to the kidneys, resulting in pyelonephritis.
9. Untreated streptococcal infections can lead to the development of acute glomerulonephritis.
10. The clinical manifestations of the nephrotic syndrome include the following:
    a. Severe generalized edema
    b. Pronounced proteinuria
    c. Hyperalbuminemia
    d. Hyperlipidemia
    The presence of these findings defines nephrotic syndrome.
11. Corticosteroids are usually prescribed for the treatment of the nephrotic syndrome because of their antiinflammatory effect.
12. Obstruction of any part of the urinary system from the kidney to the urinary meatus may lead to hydronephrosis and may cause functional and anatomic damage to the renal parenchyma.
13. Lithotripsy is fast becoming the treatment of choice for renal stones because of its noninvasive nature and the short recovery period.
14. An alkaline-ash diet is often effective in preventing the recurrence of renal stones.
15. A transurethral prostatectomy is the treatment of choice for prostatic hypertrophy but can only be employed if there is a relatively small amount of tissue to be removed; otherwise bleeding can be excessive.
16. An essential component of the preoperative teaching plan for the person about to undergo any urostomy surgery is preparation for the presence of the ostomy and a drainage appliance.
17. Major components of the treatment of a person with polycystic disease are prevention, early detection, and treatment of any infections that devleop so that renal function can be preserved.
18. Proteinuria is never considered a normal finding.
19. Causes of acute renal failure may be prerenal (hypofusion, vasodilatation, decreased cardiac output), intrarenal (damage to kidney tissue, primarily ischemia or nephrotoxicity), or postrenal (lower urinary tract obstruction).
20. The oliguric phase of ARF is characterized by inability to excrete fluid loads (oliguria), hyperkalemia, hyponatremia, metabolic acidosis, and uremia. In the diuretic phase there is excessive diuresis with loss of sodium and potassium.
21. Nursing care during the oliguric phase includes controlling the buildup of metabolic waste, maintaining fluid and electrolyte balance and nutrition, and preventing injury and infection. During the diuretic phase, monitoring fluids and electrolytes continues, coping is facilitated, and patient teaching is instituted.
22. The three stages of chronic renal failure are decreased renal reserve, renal insufficiency, and end-stage renal disease.
23. All body systems are affected by CRF.
24. ARF and CRF can be treated by conservative medical management, hemodialysis, or peritoneal dialysis and its variations. Continuous renal replacement therapy is an option for the patient who is critically ill with ARF. Kidney transplantation may be considered with end-stage renal disease.
25. Nursing interventions for CRF include administering medications, promoting fluid balance and nutrition, preventing infection and injury, maintaining skin integrity, promoting rest and comfort, facilitating coping, and teaching the patient.
26. Dialysis involves movement of fluid and particles across a semipermeable membrane by diffusion, osmosis, and ultrafiltration. Hemodialysis involves shunting the patient's blood through a dialyzer to exchange fluids, electrolytes, and waste materials. With peritoneal dialysis, the peritoneum becomes the dialyzing membrane.
27. Kidney transplantation is not a cure for renal ~ but rather an ongoing therapy with it~ and potential complications

STUDY QUESTIONS

- What are the major causes of urinary incontinence? What measures can the patient take to reduce incontinence? How would you go about planning a bladder retraining program?
- What are the differences between upper and lower urinary tract infections in terms of causative organisms, clinical manifestations, and treatment? Why is it important to stress prevention of UTIs to patients who are at risk for infection?
- What is the effect of obstruction of urinary flow from the kidneys? How would you explain this to the patient? What conditions can cause urinary obstruction?
- In what ways do the four types of prostatectomy surgeries differ? How would patient teaching differ for each type?
- How do acute and chronic renal failure differ in terms of course of the disease, outcomes, medical management, and nursing interventions?

REFERENCES AND SELECTED READINGS

1. Abuelo IG: *Renal pathophysiology: the essentials*, Baltimore, 1988, Williams & Wilkins.
2. * Alt B, Balduf R, Thompson E: When a vascular access site complicates care, *RN* 49(10):36-39, 1986.
3. American Cancer Society: *Cancer facts and figures—1991*, Atlanta, 1991, The Society.
3a. * Baer CL, Lancaster LE: Acute renal failure, *CCNQ* 14(4):1-21, 1992.
4. * Barat M: Correcting electrolyte imbalances, *RN* 50(2):30-33, 1987.
5. * Bristoll S, et al: The mythical danger of rapid urinary drainage, *Am J Nurs* 89:344-345, 1989.
6. * Brogna L, Lakaszawski ML: The continent urostomy, *Am J Nurs* 86:160-163, 1986.
7. * Chambers J: Save your diabetic patient from early kidney damage, *Nursing 85* 15(5):58-63, 1985.
8. Chambers JK: Fluid and electrolyte problems in renal and urologic disorders, *Nurs Clin North Am* 22:815-826, 1987.
9. Clark JB, Queener SF, Karb VB: *Pharmacologic basis of nursing practice*, ed 3, St Louis, 1990, Mosby–Year Book.
10. * Conti MT, Eutropius L: Preventing UTIs: what works? *Am J Nurs* 87:307-309, 1987.
11. Crandall BI: *Chronic renal failure*. In Ulrich BT: *Nephrology nursing: concepts and strategies*, Norwalk, Con, 1989, Appleton & Lange.

12. Eschback JW, Adamson JS: Recombinant human erythropoietin: implications for nephrology, *Am J Kidney Dis* 11:203-209, 1988.
13. Fowler JE, Crowley JL: Stress urinary incontinence: endoscopic suspension of the vesical neck, *AORN J* 45:922-933, 1987.
14. Gillenwater JY: *The 1991 year book of urology*, St Louis, 1991, Mosby–Year Book.
15. Goldberger E: *A primer of water, electrolyte and acid-base syndromes*, ed 7, Philadelphia, 1986, Lea & Febiger.
16. Graham-Macaluso MM: Complications of peritoneal dialysis: nursing care plans to document teaching *ANNA J* 18(5):479-483, 1991.
17. Guyton AC: *Textbook of medical physiology*, ed 8, Philadelphia, 1991, WB Saunders.
18. * Harwood C: Pulverizing kidney stones: what you should know about lithrotripsy, *RN* 48(7):32-37, 1985.
19. Jacobson JR: *The principles and practice of nephrology*, St Louis, 1990, Mosby–Year Book.
20. * Kadas N: Reducing fluid overload without dialysis, *RN* 49(5):27-31, 1986.
21. Klake S, Schreener G, Ichikawa I: The progression of renal disease, *N Engl J Med* 318(25):1657-1665, 1988.
22. Lancaster LE: *Core curriculum for nephrology nursing: 1991 edition*, Pitman, NJ, 1990, American Nephrology Nurses Association.
23. Leadbetter GW, Gillenwater JY: Contempo 1991: Urology, *JAMA* 265(23):3175-3176, 1991.
24. Levinsky NG, Rettig RA: The medicare end-stage renal disease program, *N Engl J Med* 324(16):1143-1148, 1991.
25. Lu I: Incontinence stress index: measuring psychological impact, *J Gerontol Nurs* 3(7):18-25, 1987.
26. * Martin JP: Transrectal ultrasound: a new screening test for prostate cancer, *Am J Nurs* 91(2):69, 1991.
27. Massry SG: Contempo 1991: Nephrology, *JAMA* 265(23):3135-3137, 1991.
28. McCormick KA, Scheve AA, Leahy E: Nursing management of urinary incontinence in geriatric inpatients, *Nurs Clin North Am* 23:231-264, 1988.
29. Metheney N: *Fluid and electrolyte balance: nursing considerations*, Philadelphia, 1987, JB Lippincott.
30. Moriarity MB: The NIH puts the spotlight on incontinence *RN* 52(3):44-45, 1989.
31. Newman D, Smith D: Incontinence: the problem patients won't talk about, *RN* 52(3):42-43, 1989.
32. Newman DK, et al: Restoring urinary continence, *Am J Nurs* 91(1):28-34, 1991.
33. * Niel JV: What's wrong with this peristomal skin, *Am J Nurs* 91(12):44-45, 1991.
34. Nolph K, Linblad A, Novak J: Continuous ambulatory peritoneal dialysis, *N Engl J Med* 318(24):1595-1599, 1988.

*Recommended for student reading.

35.* Norris MK: Dialysis disequilibrium syndrome, *Nursing* 19(4):33, 1989.

36.* Palmer MH: Incontinence: the magnitude of the problem, *Nurs Clin North Am* 23:139-158, 1988.

37.* Percutaneous lithotripsy for renal calculi, *Am J Nurs* 85:772-773, 1985.

38.* Petillo MH: The patient with a urinary stoma: nursing management and patient education, *Nurs Clin North Am* 22:263-280, 1987.

39.* Plawecki HM, et al: Chronic renal failure, *J Gerontol Nurs* 13(12):14-17, 1987.

40. Porth C: *Pathophysiology*, ed 3, Philadelphia, 1990, JB Lippincott.

41. Prevention and treatment of kidney stones. (Kidney Stone Consensus Conference), *JAMA* 260:977-981, 1988.

42. Price CA: Continuous renal replacement therapy: the treatment of choice for acute renal failure, *ANNA J* 18(3)239-244, 1991.

43. Richard C: *Comprehensive nephrology nursing*, Boston, 1986, Little, Brown & Co.

44. Rowland RG, Mitchell ME, Bihrle R: Alternative techniques for a continent urinary reservoir, *Urol Clin North Am* 14(4):797-804, 1987.

45.* Ruge CA: Shock (wave) treatment for kidney stones, *Am J Nurs* 86:400-401, 1986.

46. Schrier R: *Renal and electrolyte disorders*, ed 3, Boston, 1986, Little, Brown & Co.

47. Schroeder SA et al: *Current medical diagnoses and treatment*, ed 30, Norwalk, Conn, 1991, Appleton & Lange.

48.* Smith DAJ: Continent restoration in the homebound patient, *Nurs Clin North Am* 23:207-218, 1988.

49.* Solomon J: Does renal failure mean sexual failure? *RN* 49(8):41-43, 1986.

50.* Strangio L: Believe it or not: peritoneal dialysis made easy, *Nursing 88* 18(1):43-46, 1988.

51. Tanagho EA, McAninch JW: *Smith's general urology*, ed 13, Norwalk, Conn, 1991, Appleton & Lange.

51a.* Tootla J, Easterling AD: Current options in bladder cancer management, *RN* 55(4):42-49, 1992.

52. Trusler LA: Simultaneous kidney-pancreas transplantation, *ANNA J* 18(5):487-491, 1991.

53. Ulrich BT: *Nephrology nursing: concepts and strategies*, Norwalk, Conn, 1989, Appleton & Lange.

54. Way LW: *Surgical diagnosis and treatment*, ed 9, Norwalk, Conn, 1991, Appleton & Lange.

55. Williams SR: *Essentials of nutrition and diet therapy*, ed 5, St Louis, 1990, Mosby–Year Book.

55a.* Willis D: Taming the overgrown prostate, *Am J Nurs* 92(2):34-40, 1992.

56.* Wiseman K: Nephrotic syndrome: Pathophysiology and treatment, *ANNA J* 18(5):473-474, 1991.

Classic

57. Hadley E, et al: Bladder training and related therapies for urinary incontinence in older people. Proceedings of the National Institute of Aging workshop, Bethesda, Md, April 26-27, 1983.

58. Lancaster L: *The patient with end-stage renal disease,* ed 2, New York, 1984, John Wiley & Sons.

59. McConnell MF, Zimmerman MF: *Care of patients with urologic problems,* Philadelphia, 1983, JB Lippincott.

Sexual and Reproductive Problems

Unit Nine

34

Sexuality in Health and Illness

Nancy Fugate Woods
Donald D. Kautz

After studying this chapter, the learner should be able to:

- Describe physiologic changes that occur during the phases of human sexual response.
- Describe changes in sexuality that occur with aging.
- Appreciate the variety of sexual expression.
- Identify ways in which illness and environment affect sexuality.
- Relate types of alterations in sexual health and appropriate nursing interventions.
- Describe methods of prevention of sexual problems.
- State approaches that facilitate assessment of sexual health.
- Describe nursing interventions for persons with alterations of sexual health.

This chapter discusses content basic to considering sexual concerns of medical-surgical patients. Content includes the relationship of sexuality to health and to illness; sexual concerns, difficulties, and dysfunctions; prerequisites for nursing intervention (including awareness of own value system); nursing assessment; and roles of the nurse in providing sexual health care.

It is difficult to estimate how many nurses include sexual assessments as a routine part of their practice, but it is believed that many yet do not do so. In one study, nurses stated they believed (1) discussing sexual issues was not a priority, (2) most hospitalized patients were too ill to discuss sexual concerns, (3) talking about sex would make the patients anxious, and (4) most patients had only minor sexual concerns.[27] However, several studies have shown that 75% to 85% of patients wanted to discuss sexual concerns yet would not initiate the discussion. These patients indicated that they felt it was the nurse's responsibility to initiate the subject. Some health problems discussed in this text have been found to create sexual problems. It is currently estimated, for example, that 50% of all men with diabetes experience difficulties attaining erections.[23] Thus at least one out of every two men with diabetes may have sexual problems. Nurses can include a 5-minute to 10-minute assessment of sexuality as a routine part of their care and can assist patients to prevent or overcome sexual problems that are a result of or exist concurrently with their illness.

SEXUALITY AND HEALTH

Human sexuality is not merely a biologic phenomenon, but one that pervades the total person. A complex interrelationship exists among biologic, psychologic, and sociocultural aspects of our sexuality. The very complexity of human nature makes it difficult to define sexuality, much less sexual health. Nevertheless, the recognition of the importance of sexuality as a component of health has led the World Health Organization to suggest the following definition[78]:

> Sexual health is the integration of the somatic, emotional, intellectual, and social aspects of sexual being, in ways that are positively enriching and that enhance personality, communication, and love.

Sexual function, sexual self-concept, and sexual roles and relationships are important dimensions of sexual health. *Sexual function* refers to the ability of an individual

34-1	Definition of terms	
	Biologic sex	Female or male
	Gender identity	Person sees self as man or woman
	Gender role	Outward manifestations of masculinity or femininity

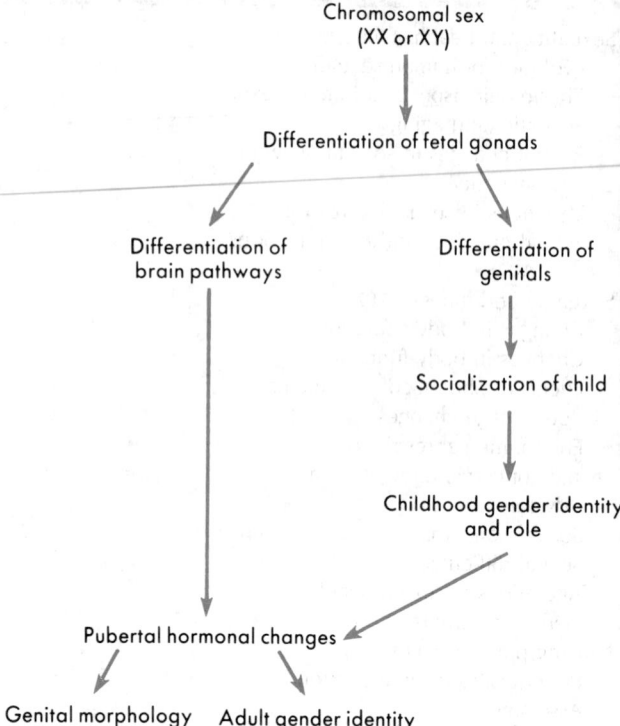

Fig. 34-1 Evolution of sexuality.

to give and receive sexual pleasure. *Sexual self-concept* refers to the image one has of oneself as a man or a woman and the evaluation of that image as masculine or feminine. Sexual self-concept includes body image and the evaluation of one's body and self within the context of the culture. *Sexual relationships* are the interpersonal relationships in which one's sexuality is shared with another.

Evolution of Human Sexuality

The evolution of our sexuality illustrates the complexity and interrelationship of the dimensions of our sexuality. From the moment of conception a variety of factors come into play to influence our sexuality, not only as children but also as adults. In early embryonic life the X or Y chromosome from the paternal sperm sets in motion a process analogous to a relay race; that is, each component has control of the process for a time, eventually yielding control to another[74] (Fig. 34-1). The chromosomes tag the undifferentiated fetal gonads as male or female, thus setting in motion another process by which hormonal secretions of the testes in turn affect not only the appearance of the genitals but also pathways in the brain.

The appearance of the infant's genitals at birth initiates another series of events, those primarily dependent on socialization of the child. The behavior of other persons during infancy and early childhood and the appearance of the child's external genitals are instrumental in the evolution of childhood gender identity and role (Box 34-1). In fact, gender identity seems to be well established by the time a person is 18 months of age. At puberty, biologic influences again come to the fore as hormones influence the genital structure and eroticism.

Thus from conception we are all sexual beings subject

Table 34-1   Significant developmental experience related to sexual function, sexual self-concept, and sexual relationships

	Sexual function	Sexual self-concept	Sexual role-relationship
Infancy	Orgasmic potential present Erectile function present	Gender identity reinforced Association of sexuality and good-bad Distinction between self and others	
Childhood	Genital pleasuring and explanation Engages in sensual activity (e.g., hugging)	Core gender identity solidified (by age 3)	Sex role differences learned Discrimination between male and female role models Learns sexual vocabulary
Preschool	Sex play Exploration of own body and those of playmates Self-pleasuring (masturbation)		Learns about sex roles Parental attachment and identification
School age		Curiosity about sex Sexual fears and fantasies Interest in aspects of sexual development Self-awareness as sexual being	Same-sex friends
Adolescent, prepubertal	Menarche Seminal emissions	Concerns about body image	Same-sex sexual experiences as part of friendship
Early adolescence	Awkwardness in first sexual encounter (50% not sexually active) Masturbation, petting	Sexual thoughts, fantasies Anxiety over inadequacy, lack of partner, virginity	Beginning appropriate sex friendships Dating Learning
Late adolescence	May or may not be sexually active	Responsibility for sexual activity	Learning intimacy in relationship Sex role behaviors, lifestyles explained
Young adult	Experimentation with sexual positions, expression Explanation of techniques	Responsibility for sexual health, e.g., contraception, STD prevention Development of adult sexual value system, tolerance for others	Learning to give and receive pleasure Long-term commitment to relationship
Middle adult	Adaptation to altered sexual function, e.g., vaginal dryness of menopause, slower erections	Accept body image changes related to aging	Adjustment of relationship as roles change
Late adult	Slower sexual function	Accept slowed sexual response cycle without ending sexual aspects of relationship	Develop new ways for sharing sexual pleasure and intimacy with aging Adaptation to loss of partner or illness of partner

From Woods NF: Human sexuality, an overview. In Mitchell PH et al: *AANN's neuroscience nursing: phenomena and practice*, Norwalk, Conn, 1988, Appleton & Lange.

to multiple influences throughout life. If the previous processes proceed without interference, the person's biologic sex is congruent with gender identity and gender role.

This complex set of biologic and psychosocial variables begun at conception has a pervasive influence on the remainder of our lives. The biologic component of sexuality (sexual function or expression) constantly interacts with the psychologic components (gender identity, thoughts, and feelings), as well as with social factors (such as sanctioned role, mores, and folkways regulating sexual expression). Such complexity mandates a holistic approach to conceptualizing a person's sexual problems and concerns.

Sexual development continues throughout the life span, with each component of sexuality being influenced by biologic development as well as sociocultural forces. Some of the significant developmental experiences related to sexual function, sexual self-concept, and sexual relationships are outlined in Table 34-1.

Physiologic Aspects of Human Sexuality
Phases of the human sexual response

Masters and Johnson, pioneers in the scientific study of the physiologic aspects of sexual behavior, demonstrated that sexual response is a cyclic phenomenon consisting of four phases[71] (Box 34-2). The physiologic changes seen during human sexual response (Table 34-2) depend on two main principles: myotonia and vasocongestion. It is through the congestion of pelvic blood vessels and involuntary muscular contractions in the pelvic organs and other parts of the body that changes supportive of orgasmic experience are attained.

Excitement phase

The excitement phase is the initial component of the cycle. It develops from sexually arousing stimuli such as touch. An increase in sexual tension is observed during this phase. Vasocongestive changes are seen in the external genitals and the breast in both women and men. In addition, a sex flush, which looks like a red, maculopapular rash, appears over the chest in some persons. An increase in both the heart rate and blood pressure is evident, paralleling the level of sexual excitement.

Plateau

The plateau phase is a consolidation period during which sexual tension becomes intensified. Vasocongestion continues. The uterus continues to elevate in the pelvis, which creates a tenting effect in the innermost portion of the vagina. The sex flush continues to spread, sometimes involving the neck, face, and arms. Hyperventilation occurs in both sexes, along with heart rates of 100 to 175 beats per minute. There is elevation of systolic blood pressure (20 to 60 mm Hg for women, 20 to 80 mm Hg for men) and diastolic blood pressure (10 to 20 mm Hg for women, 10 to 40 mm Hg for men).

Orgasm

Orgasm, the involuntary climax of sexual tension, involves only a small portion of the sexual response cycle. The climactic release of sexual tension is evident in contractions throughout the body. Uterine contractions are also noted in women with orgasm, much like those characteristic of labor.

Resolution

During the resolution phase, the changes involving the blood vessels, sexual organs, and muscular tension are reversed. The uterus and testes return to their normal positions. Cardiovascular and respiratory rates quickly return to normal. Occasionally, a thin film of perspiration may appear over the entire body. Women may at this time begin another sexual response cycle immediately; men have an obligatory period during which they cannot be restimulated to higher levels of sexual tension.

Triphasic concept of human sexual response

Kaplan[66] has suggested a triphasic concept of human sexual response. She delineates three phases—desire, excitement, and orgasm—that are related components of sexual response but are governed by separate neurophysiologic systems. This notion is useful for understanding not only the physiology of sexual response, but also the consequences of pathophysiologic conditions, the etiology of sexual dysfunction, and appropriate therapies.

Desire phase

The desire phase refers to the experience of a sexual appetite or drive produced by the activation of a neural system in the brain. Sexual desire is experienced as sensations that move the person to seek sexual experiences. It is likely that the sexual centers of the brain have either neural or chemical connections with the pleasure and pain centers of the brain. The pleasure centers are stimulated when we have sex, which accounts for the pleasurable quality of sexual behavior. On the other hand, the pain centers can inhibit the sexual system. Some persons suggest that the pleasure center is stimulated by release of endorphins in sexual behavior. If a sexual object or situation produces pain, then it will cease to evoke desire.

Testosterone is important in mediating sexual desire in both men and women. Luteinizing hormone and the neurotransmitters serotonin and dopamine also may be important in mediating sexual desire. Bonding to another person and love are powerful stimuli to sexual desire. Many

---

34-2

Phases of the human sexual response

Phase	Description
Excitement	Increase in sexual tension evidenced by swelling of genitalia and vaginal lubrication
Plateau	Intensification of sexual tension with more pronounced genital swelling
Orgasm	Involuntary climax and release of sexual tension evidenced by muscle contraction
Resolution	Dissipation of muscle tension and swelling

stimuli seem to be capable of evoking sexual desire, such as sight, smell, and other sensory cues, and some of these are conditioned by culture. Fear and pain, however, are potent inhibitors.

The connections between the sex center and other parts of the brain also make it possible for people to "turn off" sexual desire when other stimuli are more important or when it is not to the individual's advantage to pursue sexual activity. Hypoactive desire and inhibited sexual desire are common problems of the sexual desire phase.

Excitement phase

The excitement phase is similar to the excitement and plateau phases described by Masters and Johnson and is produced by reflex vasodilation of the genital blood vessels. This vasodilation causes the genitalia to swell and changes their shape to adapt to their reproductive function. The vasocongestion is primarily a parasymphathetically mediated response, and an intense sympathetic response such as that produced by fear and anxiety can instantly lead to loss of erection. It is believed that erection is governed by two spinal reflex centers. The thoracolumbar center (psychogenic) appears to respond more to psychic stimuli, whereas the sacral center is stimulated from tactile input to the genitalia. It is believed that the spinal reflex centers and the higher neural connections are analogous in men and women. Disorders of the excitement phase include difficulty in attaining or maintaining erection in men and difficulty with swelling and lubrication in women.

Orgasm phase

The orgasm phase corresponds to orgasm as described by Masters and Johnson. It is also a genital reflex governed by spinal neural centers, but it consists of reflex contractions of certain genital muscles. Disorders of the orgasm phase include inadequate ejaculatory control (premature

ejaculation), retarded ejaculation in men, and orgasmic dysfunction in women. Other disorders include painful intercourse and sexual phobias.

Requirements for sexual response

The requirements for the physiologic sexual response include intact sexual organs, adequate vasculature to support the vasocongestive changes, functional innervation of the genital organs, and the appropriate hormonal milieu.[58] The changes of myotonia and vasocongestion are thought to be mediated by the autonomic nervous system. Perception of the sexual experience at cortical levels requires intact sensory pathways from the genitals and other peripheral structures to the cortex. The capacity to stimulate oneself or a partner sexually depends on the presence of intact motor pathways from higher centers to the effector muscles involved. It should also be noted that thoughts and feelings or visual, auditory, and olfactory-gustatory stimuli alone may result in arousal to orgasmic experience even in the absence of tactile perception.

Adequate hormonal milieu, with appropriate hormonal release, influences both the structure and function of the genitals; for example, the decreased estrogen levels during menopause are believed to be responsible for a decreased amount of vaginal lubrication. Finally, the presence of intact genital structures is usually thought to be a requisite for sexual response, but substitution of prosthetic devices for sexual organs is an option beginning to be explored. Although each of these components is important in sexual response, it is possible for humans to have profound sexual pleasure even when one or more of these is absent.

Sexuality and Aging

Changes in sexual function become accentuated during middle age (see Box 34-3), although their onset is gradual and they probably begin long before they are perceived.

Table 34-2 Sex organ changes during sexual response

Phase	Changes in female	Changes in male
Excitement	Vaginal lubrication Vagina becomes longer and wider Uterus begins to elevate in pelvis Clitoris becomes longer and wider Labia minora extend outward Nipples enlarge, areolae become engorged, breast size increases	Penis becomes erect Scrotal sac tenses Testes begin to rise toward perineum Nipples enlarge
Plateau	Clitoris retracts Labia and outer part of vagina (orgasmic platform) become congested Uterus continues to rise in pelvis	Diameter of penis continues to increase Testes increase in size 50% and elevate close to perineum
Orgasm	Orgasmic platform contracts rapidly (throbbing sensation) Uterine contractions Rectal sphincter contractions	Expulsive contraction along entire urethra to expel semen Internal bladder sphincter contractions (prevent semen from entering bladder) Rectal sphincter contractions
Resolution	Vasocongestion decreases rapidly from vagina/labia and slowly from clitoris and breasts Uterus descends to usual position	Rapid loss of penis size to 1 to 1.5 times usual size Slower resolution of penis size to usual size Testes descend into scrotum

34-3	Factors that influence sexual interest and activity in middle and old age	
	Women	**Men**
	Marital status: availability of a partner	Past sexual experience
	Age	Age
	Enjoyment of sex in earlier years	Objective and subjective health ratings
		Social class

Men need more time to attain an erection, and once attained, it is likely to be less full than in earlier years. The testes elevate more slowly with sexual excitement, and vasocongestive changes in the scrotum and testes are less noticeable. With prolongation of the plateau phase, middle-aged men actually achieve much better control over ejaculation than they had as young adults.

Orgasm is perceived as happening more quickly, and feelings of ejaculatory inevitability may disappear entirely. Resolution of sexual tension becomes more rapid with age, and the obligatory refractory period (a period during which the man cannot be restimulated to orgasm) becomes longer. With aging, men actually gain better control of ejaculation, and because of reduced ejaculatory demand, they may be satisfied not to ejaculate with each intercourse.[25]

In women, menopausal changes may lead to delay in production of vaginal lubrication and diminished expansion of the vaginal barrel. Changes in external genitals and the breasts are apparent. The woman's orgasmic experience becomes shorter, and resolution occurs more rapidly.[25]

Studies of healthy aging individuals indicate that a decline in overall interest and activity is seen with age. However, men from each age range tend to report greater interest and activity than women in each respective age range. Several factors can influence sexual interest and activity in middle and old age. Level of sexual activity in youth appears to be related to that in older years.[40,43,54]

As men age, an interest-activity gap appears; that is, they desire more sexual activity than they are able to experience. This gap grows as men age; however, it remains small for women. Women without a socially acceptable partner may adaptively inhibit their sexual interest. The wider interest-activity gap for men may reflect their socialization to express more interest in sex. Other social factors, such as the role loss associated with children leaving the parents' home and retirement, are likely to influence the older person's sexual interests.

In spite of these changes, many older adults remain sexually active. Kaplan[25] estimates that 50% of healthy persons over age 60 remain sexually active. However, there is a tendency among health professionals to ignore sexuality in the aged, possibly because of two reasons. First, health professionals may assume that elders would be too embarrassed to discuss sexual concerns. In response to a caution that the nursing assessment was going to include some potentially embarrassing questions regarding sexuality, one 70-year-old woman responded, "Honey, I've been having sex longer than you've been alive; you're not going to embarrass me." Second, health professionals may assume that elders would not be interested. Yet, in their study of women with heart disease, Baggs and Karsh[4] found that all of the separated and divorced women wanted to be asked about sexual activity, as did 76% of widows, including their oldest participant, age 88. These examples illustrate the need to conduct sexual assessments with people of all ages, regardless of marital status.

In addition, most older adults have chronic illnesses. Diabetes, hypertension, arthritis, heart disease, and chronic obstructive lung disease are examples of chronic illnesses prevalent in older adults and known to cause sexual problems. Some elders maintain sexual interest and activity in spite of physiologic changes, whereas others do not.[35]

Recent Changes in Societal Views of Sexuality

Most people who write about sexuality agree there has been a sexual revolution in America. Many believe this revolution began in the 1960s, but the beginning can probably be traced to publications by Kinsey and his associates on sexuality in the human male and female in 1948[67] and 1953.[68] In D'Emilio's and Freedman's recent history of sexuality in America,[15] they postulate that the combination of the gay rights movement, the women's movement, the Supreme Court legalization of abortion, relaxation of the ban on pornography, and the availability of the birth control pill created an atmosphere that drastically changed the way sexuality was viewed. Magazines, television, and other media portrayed a societal consensus that sexuality was good, sexual expression was a right of every individual, and "if it feels good, do it." It is important to remember that not everyone thought this way, but the media message was strong. During this time, nursing texts began to include chapters on sexuality; in 1979, the first edition of Phipps, Long, and Woods *Medical-Surgical Nursing* included a chapter on sexuality.

Several political and social events occurred in the 1980s, however, that have changed this view of sexuality. Teenage pregnancy rates rose; AIDS became epidemic; Reagan, a conservative, was elected president; and the new conservative right gained political power. These trends were contrary to the views of the seventies.

The 1990s are likely to bring even more changes. In 1991, the U.S. Congress continued to debate the issues of the legality of abortion, funding or permitting exhibition of sexually explicit art, and the status of sex education in the schools. Another issue was the routine testing of health care workers for HIV infection. Those in favor of this practice believe that the public has a right to know; those against it believe that the risk of a health care provider transmitting the HIV virus to a patient is extremely low.

Differing viewpoints exist within nursing as well. For example, some nurses believe that nurses should include an assessment of every patient's knowledge of safe sex practices, whereas others believe that this is inappropriate for the majority of patients. Nurses are encouraged to keep an open mind, to consider both sides of issues related to sexuality, and to recognize that patients may have different opinions.

Variations in Sexual Expression

Sexual behavior is a product of society and culture and our biology. Each culture has a set of norms that prescribes which behaviors are sexual and which are acceptable. In cross-cultural comparisons of sexual behavior, a wide variety of sexual expression is found. In Western society, sex is frequently equated with penis-in-vagina intercourse. Yet a wide range of behaviors exists encompassing sexual meaning (for example, talking, sharing thoughts and feelings, or just touching another person). This wide range of behaviors causes us to question what is "normal." Yet normal can refer to prevalence of a behavior, optimal function, a statistical distribution, or fashionable or socially acceptable behavior. Comfort[63] suggests that as professionals we not restrict our definition of normal to what we, personally, admit to enjoying. Instead he recommends that we consider the following questions:

1. What does the behavior mean to the individual?
2. Does the behavior enrich or impoverish the sexual life of the individual and those persons with whom sexual relations are shared?
3. Is the behavior tolerable to society?

Variation in sexual behavior is bounded only by one's imagination and to some extent by the culture. Different types of sexual expression are described in Box 34-4.

Sexual intercourse may be restricted to marriage or to a similar relationship in some societies. In others, there may be legitimized extramarital rights, and in some, premarital sexual freedom is encouraged. The position for intercourse varies between cultures and within cultures. Usually the position assumed for intercourse reflects other aspects of the culture; for example, in cultures where families sleep in the same quarters, often side-to-side positions are used to afford some privacy from other occupants of the room.

Culture also dictates whether the woman plays an active or passive role in sexual activity and the duration of the act of intercourse. Precopulatory stimulation may be brief or lengthy, and the type used, such as kissing, painful acts, and manipulation of the breasts or genitals, varies with the culture. Sexual frequency may also be governed by norms, and in some cultures is prohibited during menses, lactation, or pregnancy, or before hunts or battles.

Heterosexuality is the most prevalent form of sexual expression among adults of known societies, but it is rarely the only type of sexual behavior in which humans engage. Homosexual behavior is found in most species of mammals; in humans it is most common among adolescents and males. Since "normal" sexual response may be determined by cultural norms as well as physiologic, phylogenetic, legal, statistical, moral, and social standards, it is impossible to state a hard and fast definition of what constitutes the "normal state."

Homosexuality

Homosexuality is the most common sexual variation, yet it is poorly understood by health professionals. It has been viewed as an illness, a criminal offense, and a lifestyle in Western society. Recently the American Psychiatric Association removed homosexuality from the "illness" classification; however, the social climate remains less liber-

34-4	**Sexual variations**	
	Heterosexuality	Choice of adult sexual partner of opposite sex
	Homosexuality	Choice of adult sexual partner of same sex
	Bisexuality	Choice of adult sexual partners of same and opposite sex
	Transvestism	Sexual satisfaction achieved by dressing in clothing of opposite sex
	Incest	Sexual relations with close relative, for example, child
	Zoophilia	Choice of sexual object is an animal
	Fetishism	Sexual object is an inanimate object
	Voyeurism	Sexual satisfaction achieved by watching others
	Exhibitionism	Sexual satisfaction achieved by exposing genitals
	Sadism	Sexual satisfaction achieved by inflicting pain
	Masochism	Sexual satisfaction achieved by receiving pain

ated. Although the majority of society still seems to subscribe to the definition of homosexuality as an illness, most homosexuals do not classify themselves as ill. The association of HIV infection and AIDS with homosexual and bisexual men has contributed to the perception of homosexuality as an illness.

Kinsey[67,68] estimated that 13% of women and 37% of men had had at least one homosexual experience leading to orgasm. The extent to which these persons engaged in homosexual behavior varied greatly. Thus Kinsey suggested that a continuum existed on which the two poles represented exclusive heterosexuality (0) and homosexuality (6), and the five remaining categories (1 through 5) represented a combination of the two. Individuals in categories 1 and 5 had predominant heterosexual or homosexual orientations. Those in categories 2 and 4 still had a clear preference for heterosexual or homosexual relations, but retained an active interest in the other form. Category 3 represented persons who had equal heterosexual and homosexual interests.

The Institute for Sex Research[62] conducted a large-scale study of the sexual dimensions of homosexual experience in the San Francisco Bay area. Although the authors of the report are careful to point out that their results may not mirror the entire homosexual population, the study did include men and women, both white and black. Results revealed that homosexuality encompasses more than the person's sexual tendencies. Although there was variability on the homosexual-heterosexual continuum for both male and female homosexuals, there was more heterosexuality in the feelings and behaviors of homosexual women than men.

Most of the homosexual men and women were relatively covert about their homosexuality. The mother and siblings were more likely to be aware of the individual's homosexuality than other family members. Families were more likely to be aware of the person's homosexuality than other members of society. In most cases friends, employers, and colleagues were aware of the person's homosexuality.

Homosexual men or women could not be stereotyped as sexually hyperactive or inactive; instead, the amount of activity varied with each individual. Public cruising (purposive search for a sexual partner) was infrequent among lesbians. Of those homosexuals involved in public cruising, most conducted their sexual activity in their own homes. Gay bars were the most popular cruising locales.

Homosexual men had many more sexual partners than did lesbians. There seemed to be more emphasis placed on sexual activity among males. This may be a function of

---

34-5	**Risk of HIV infection from sex practices**

No risk (no exchange of HIV-infected body fluids)

Analingus with barrier
Body-to-body rubbing
Cunnilingus with barrier
Erotic bathing/showering
Exhibitionism
Fellatio with condom
Kissing (dry/wet)
Massage, touch
Mutual/solo masturbation
Nibbling/biting (with no blood)
Nipple stimulation
Nonmucosal body licking/kissing
Sadomasochistic activity with no blood drawn
Unshared sex toys

Low risk (exchange of HIV-infected body fluids may occur)

Analingus without barrier
Cunnilingus without barrier (higher risk during menstruation)
Fellatio without condom without ejaculation
Ingestion of urine or feces
Penile-vaginal/rectal intercourse with condom (risk of leakage)
Sadomasochistic activity with blood drawn but precautions used

High risk (exchange of HIV-infected body fluids)

Coitus interruptus without condom
Penile-vaginal/rectal intercourse without condom
Shared sex toys

Modified from Chateauvert M, Duffie A, Gilmore N: HIV antibody testing: counselling guidelines from the Canadian Medical Association, *Patient Educ Counsel* 18:35-49, 1991.

---

lesbians' preference for relationships based more on emotions than on sex, or it may merely be a function of the problems male homosexuals have in meeting partners. For both male and female homosexuals, a relatively steady relationship with a love partner was a meaningful event.

The male homosexual subculture seemed to place more emphasis on youth than did women. Social prestige did not seem to be a major determinant in sexual appeal.

A variety of sexual techniques was used. Male homosexuals most frequently employed fellatio, hand-genital stimulation, and anal intercourse. Female homosexuals most frequently engaged in masturbation with their partners and in cunnilingus. Men and women both specified receiving oral-genital sex as a preferred technique.

Sexual problems encountered included difficulty in meeting a suitable sexual partner, maintaining affection for the partner, and meeting the other's sexual request. There was a lower incidence of these problems among lesbians. Almost two thirds of the male homosexuals had at some time contracted a sexually transmitted disease from homosexual sex, but only one of the lesbians had done so. More women than men had considered stopping their homosexuality, but only a minority in each case had done so. At interview, more men than women regretted their homosexuality.

About 20% of the homosexual males had been married, and more than 33% of the white lesbians and almost 50% of the black lesbians had been married once. They did not perceive their homosexuality as having a particular effect on their children.

Homosexual men and women seemed to have more friends than their heterosexual counterparts. Their friends included both homosexuals and heterosexuals. Lesbians were more involved in activities outside the home or with others than were homosexual males. Men were more likely than women to have had social difficulties, but few had been arrested because of their homosexuality.

When homosexual respondents were compared with their heterosexual counterparts in terms of adult psychologic adjustment, it appeared that the dysfunctional and asexual homosexuals were less well off than those in the heterosexual group. However, homosexual adults who have come to terms with their homosexuality are no more distressed psychologically than heterosexual men and women.[62] Thus therapists would do well to consider why a person's homosexuality is problematic and examine ways to enhance the person's life rather than direct therapy at changing the person's sexual orientation.

Sexual Practices and HIV Infection/AIDS

The AIDS epidemic has led to frank and open discussion of sexual practices. Many publications, newspapers, and magazines have published discussions of sexual practices linked with HIV infection.

Although AIDS is a disease of heterosexual as well as homosexual and bisexual men, the onset of the AIDS epidemic has had a profound effect on the sexual lifestyles of homosexual men, particularly in California and New York, where the incidence of AIDS is the highest. Two sexual practices that have been found to transmit HIV infection are unprotected anal intercourse and sex with multiple partners. Before the onset of AIDS, these practices were common in homosexual and bisexual men. In efforts to reduce the incidence of HIV infection, particularly in homosexual and bisexual men, campaigns to teach safer sex practices have been instituted in all states. In addition to these educational programs, anonymous testing for HIV infection is offered in most major cities. Professionals who care for people with AIDS agree that these preventive programs have been effective with the general population of gay men, and that these men now practice safe sex. Some persons, however, still continue to place themselves at risk.[49] This may be because some gay men may not perceive themselves as being at risk.[69] Investigators from the Multicenter AIDS Cohort found that heavy drinking, drug use, and younger age were associated with an increased number of sexual partners and failure to use condoms among 644 men who engaged in anal intercourse.[45]

These data illustrate the need for nurses working in all settings to have a basic understanding of safe sex practices to answer patients' questions and for health teaching. The guidelines in Box 34-5 rank sexual activities by risk, ranging from no risk to high risk for HIV infection; these recommendations are for all people, regardless of sexual orientation. (For additional information regarding HIV infection, see Chapter 19.)

SEXUALITY AND ILLNESS

People today seem to be more comfortable in expressing their concerns about their sexual health than has previously been the case. As a result of this increased comfort, nurses are increasingly expected to provide accurate information about sexuality and health, as well as to listen with comfort and understanding to the sexual concerns patients describe. Although many persons can openly describe their problems, others are too embarrassed or lack the vocabulary necessary to do so. For this reason it is important that nurses have a frame of reference to help them identify persons at risk for sexual problems or concerns.

There are many ways in which illness may affect sexuality and sexual function. Illness may influence sexuality through changes in body structure or function, use of certain medications, or alteration in the person's body image.

Changes in Body Structure

Changes in the structure of the nervous system, circulatory system, or genital organs may result in sexual health problems. Many examples of these structural changes and the probable mechanism by which they interfere with sexual health are given in Table 34-3. Anatomic disruptions are probably best exemplified by the spinal cord–injured per-

Table 34-3   Changes in body structure and sexual health

System	Probable mechanism of interference
Central and peripheral nervous systems	
Spinal cord injury	Disrupts integrity of peripheral nerves and spinal cord reflexes involved in sexual response (for example, erection)
Spinal cord tumors	
Herniated disk	
Multiple sclerosis	
Spina bifida	
Amyotrophic lateral sclerosis	
Tumors of frontal or temporal lobes	May interfere with function of centers controlling sexual drive
Cerebrovascular accident	
Trauma to frontal or temporal lobes	
Cardiovascular system	
Thrombus formation in vessels of penis	May interfere with blood supply to penis, thus interfering with erection
Leriche's syndrome	
Sickle cell disorders	
Leukemia	
Trauma to vasculature supplying sexual organs	
Reproductive/sexual system	
Prostatectomy, radical perineal	May destroy nerve supply, interfering with sensory and motor aspects of sexual response
Abdominal perineal resection	
Lumbar sympathectomy	May result in disturbed ejaculation
Rhizotomy	May result in impotence, as well as disturbed ejaculation
Absence of penis or penile injury	Precludes or discourages intromission
Penectomy	
Imperforate hymen	
Congenital absence of vagina	
Pelvic exenteration	
Vaginectomy	
Obstetric trauma or poor episiotomy	Leaves gaping vaginal opening or painful scarring, thus discouraging intercourse
Damage to pubococcygeus muscle	

son who has sustained irreversible damage to neural pathways that interferes with some methods of sexual function (Chapter 37).

Changes in Body Function

Many illnesses alter physiologic processes essential to the sexual response, including nervous transmission, vasocongestion, hormonal metabolism myotonia, and perception of pleasurable sensation. Table 34-4 illustrates some illnesses that have the potential to interfere with sexual response and the hypothesized mechanisms by which they affect sexual response.

In general, it appears that the extent of a physiologic disorder and its chronicity determine relative frequency of sexual problems. Women with diabetes have a higher rate of difficulty with lubrication than do nondiabetic women, particularly women who have been diabetic for 6 years or longer and who have neuropathy.[28,51] This relationship between chronicity and dysfunction is also observed in men with diabetes. A high incidence of problems with erection, however, is found among men with diabetes during the first year after diagnosis. It is believed in this instance that the lack of diabetic control (physiologic derangement) is responsible for the sexual dysfunction.[31] For chronic illnesses as a group, it is easy to hypothesize a relationship between perception of health status, degree of fatigue, metabolic derangements, altered roles, fear of dying, and the demands of a chronic illness on the partner and changes in the sexual relationship.

Although some medical-surgical conditions do not interfere directly with sexual functions, their perceived seriousness or the presence of symptoms discourages persons from engaging in their usual sexual practices. One very common example is associated with cardiac disease, more specifically myocardial infarction. Although marital sex probably does not demand a great energy expenditure, many persons are fearful of attempting intercourse after having a heart attack. One study of married men who had had myocardial infarctions demonstrated that heart rates with orgasm were much lower in this group than among the younger group studied by Masters and Johnson.[64] An active physical conditioning program did produce significant improvements in the frequency and quality of sexual activity for men who had had a myocardial infarction. This energy expenditure associated with sex seemed to be better tolerated by those who exercised regularly.

In general, the literature indicates that the postmyocardial infarction patient may return to regular sexual ac-

Table 34-4   Influence of changes in body function on sexual health

Physiologic interferences	Hypothesized mechanism of action	Physiologic interferences	Hypothesized mechanism of action
Systemic diseases		Trauma to penis	
Pulmonary disease	Debility, pain, and depression probably interfere with sexual desire and expression	Vaginal infections	
Renal disease		Senile vaginitis	
Malignancies		Vulvitis	
Infections		Leukoplakia	
Degenerative diseases		Bartholin's cyst	
Some cardiovascular diseases		Allergic response to vaginal sprays and deodorants	
		Vaginitis after radiation therapy	
Metabolic disruptions		Pelvic inflammatory disease	
Cirrhosis	Hepatic problems in men result in estrogen buildup from inability of liver to conjugate estrogens; similar processes occur in women along with general debility	Fibroadenomas	
Mononucleosis		Endometriosis	
Hepatitis		Uterine prolapse	
		Anal fissures, hemorrhoids	
		Pelvic masses	Local irritability, damage to genitalia, and consequent interference with reflex mechanisms involved in erection and ejaculation
Hypothyroidism	By depression of CNS function, general debilitation, and depression, libido may be decreased, and impaired erectile abilities in men may result	Ovarian cysts	
Addison's disease		Prostatitis	
Hypogonadism		Urethritis	
Hypopituitarism			
Acromegaly			
Feminizing tumors			
Cushing's disease		**Medical or surgical castration**	
Diabetes mellitus		Orchiectomy	Lowered androgen levels depress libido and lead to impotence, retarded ejaculation, or impaired sexual responsiveness
		Radiation therapy	
Diseases of the genitalia		Oophorectomy, adrenalectomy	
Priapism	Each of these problems involves damage to genital organs, which may result in painful intercourse		
Peyronie's disease			
Balantitis			
Phimosis			
Genital herpes			

Modified from Kaplan HS: *The new sex therapy,* New York, 1974, Quadrangle Press.

tivity provided there are no symptoms of congestive heart failure. However, certain conditions that increase energy expenditure during intercourse are to be avoided. These include having intercourse shortly after a meal or soon after alcohol consumption, because both increase the heart rate and metabolic demands. Extremes in temperatures and anxiety-provoking or secretive situations should also be avoided. The energy expenditure in climbing two flights of stairs appears to produce a greater increase in heart rate than does orgasm.[42]

Effects of Pharmacologic Agents

Pharmacologic agents that may affect sexual drive as well as performance are listed in Table 34-5. The relationship between extent of physiologic problems and degree of sexual dysfunction may be demonstrated by pharmacologically induced changes. For example, alcohol induces transiently positive changes; in small doses it initially promotes relax-

ation and release of inhibitions, as do other psychoactive drugs. However, in larger doses, alcohol has negative effects on sexual function, leading to central nervous system depression and interference with motor activity.

Several categories of drugs have demonstrably negative effects on sexual function. These include antihypertensives, antidepressants, antihistamines, antispasmodics, sedatives, tranquilizers, ethyl alcohol, some sex hormone preparations, and some narcotics and psychoactive drugs.

Patients who take medications that have negative effects on sexual function should be informed that there may be alternative medications. For example, those who are taking the antidepressant Amoxapine (Asendin) might not experience sexual dysfunction with Imipramine (Tofranil). Those taking one antihypertensive may experience less sexual side effects with another. Thus nurses should recommend that patients talk with their physician about sexual side effects, to see if an alternative drug is available.[53]

Table 34-5   Drug effects on human sexual behavior

Drug or drug category	Effect	Probable mechanism of action
Oral contraceptives	Positive	Permits separation of sexual activity from concern about conception
Antihypertensives Clonidine (Catapres) Guanethidine (Ismelin) Methyldopa (Aldomet) Propranolol (Inderal) Reserpine (Serpasil) Trimethaphan (Arfonad)	Negative	Peripheral blockade of nervous innervation of sex glands
Antidepressants Amitriptyline (Elavil) Desipramine (Norpramin, Pertofrane) Imipramine (Tofranil) Nortriptyline (Aventyl) Pargyline (Eutonyl) Phenelzine sulfate (Nardil) Protriptyline (Vivactil) Tranylcypromine sulfate (Parnate)	Negative	Central depression; peripheral blockade of nervous innervation of sex glands
Antihistamines Chlorpheniramine (Chlor-Trimeton) Diphenhydramine (Benadryl) Promethazine (Phenergan)	Negative	Blockade of parasympathetic nervous innervation of sex glands
Antispasmodics Glycopyrrolate methobromide (Robinul) Hexocyclium (Tral) Methantheline (Banthine) Poldine (Nacton)	Negative	Ganglionic blockade of nervous innervation of sex glands
Sedatives and tranquilizers Benperidol Chlordiazepoxide (Librium) Chlorpromazine (Thorazine, Megaphen) Chlorprothixene (Taractan) Diazepam (Valium) Mesoridazine (Serentil) Methaqualone (Quaalude) Phenoxybenzamine (Dibenzyline) Prochlorperazine (Compazine) Thioridazine (Mellaril)	Negative and positive	Central sedation; blockade of autonomic innervation of sex glands; suppression of hypothalamic and pituitary function Tranquilization and relaxation

Continued.

Table 34-5 Drug effects on human sexual behavior—cont'd

Drug or drug category	Effect	Probable mechanism of action
Ethyl alcohol	Negative Transiently positive	Central depression; suppression of motor activity; diuresis Release of inhibitions; relaxation
Barbiturates	Negative	Central depression; suppression of motor activity; hypnosis
Diuretics Bendroflumethiazide (Naturetin) Chlorthiazide (Diuril) Spironolactone (Aldactone)	Negative	Diuresis
Sex hormone preparations Cyproterone acetate Methandrostenolone (Dianabol) Nandrolone phenpropionate (Durabolin) Norethandrolone (Nilevar)	Negative	Antiandrogenic effects on sexual function; loss of libido; decreased potency
Methadone	Negative	Suppresses secondary sex organ function in men
Potassium nitrate (saltpeter)	Questionable	Diuresis
Cantharis (Spanish fly)	Negative	Irritation and inflammation of genitourinary tract; systemic poisoning
Yohimbine	Questionable	Stimulation of lower spinal nerve centers
Strychnine	Questionable	Stimulation of neuraxis; priapism
Narcotics and psychoactive drugs Amphetamines Cocaine	Negative	Central depression; decreased libido and impaired potency
Heroin LSD Marijuana Methadone Morphine	Transiently positive	Release of inhibitions; increased suggestibility; relaxation
L-Dopa and p-chlorophenylalanine (PCPA)	Questionable	Improvement of well-being
Amyl nitrite	Questionable	Vasodilation of genitourinary tract; smooth muscle relaxation
Caffeine	Questionable	Central nervous system stimulant
Vitamin E	Questionable	Supports fertility in laboratory animals
Selenium	Questionable	Supports fertility in laboratory animals
Lithium carbonate	Questionable	Produces broad endocrine changes; diuresis
Clomiphene citrate (Clomid)	Questionable	Stimulates gonadotropic hormones; enhances expectations of achieving pregnancy
Bromocriptine (Parlodel)	Questionable	Stimulates gonadotropic hormones
Cimetidine (Tagamet)	Negative	Unknown
Clofibrate (Atromid S)	Questionable	Unknown
Disulfram (Antabuse)	None by itself; negative with alcohol	Blocks alcohol metabolism; produces aldehyde syndrome

Pharmacologic agents are now being used as one option to treat erectile dysfunction. Pharmacologic erection programs (PEP) are offered by urologists who specialize in the treatment of impotence. As a part of an extensive educational program, men are taught to self-inject the penis with doses of vasoactive drugs in order to achieve an erection that lasts from 30 to 40 minutes and is sufficiently hard to permit intercourse. Papaverine HCl, used alone or in combination with phentolamine mesylate, have a reported success rate of 65% to 100%, with the incidence of side effects as low as 2% to 13%. These agents affect only the ability to get an erection; they do not affect orgasm or ejaculation. PEP programs are widely used by men with impotence from diabetes, hypertension, pelvic trauma, and arteriosclerosis who want to continue intercourse and do not wish to have a penile implant.[57]

Body Image Changes

The extent to which distortion of body image influences sexuality often depends on the perceptions of two persons: oneself and a significant other. Multiple variables may influence the body image of a woman who has had a mastectomy. Although one might suspect that the extent of surgery and pain in the operative area would be most important, the value she assigned to her breasts, her preoperative body image, and social factors such as the quality of her preoperative sexual relationship are also influential. In one study the quality of the relationship the woman had with her husband before the surgery was the most important determinant of her return to sexual functioning after surgery.[77]

The visibility of a defect plays an important role in sexual adaptation. Visibility of a disability seems to be just as disruptive of marital and family relations as it is of other social relationships.[79]

Finally, the meaning and significance one attaches to the changed body part may interfere with sexual behavior. The amputee who views the loss as castration, the woman who sees her hysterectomy as a neutering surgery, and the person who equates an ostomy with loss of adult control are likely to experience problems with self-image and, in turn, sexual adjustment. Thus both society's perception of the person and the individual's concept of self can interfere with sexual health. Some common health problems resulting in body image change are listed in Box 34-6.

Several authorities believe that the interpersonal components of sexual problems are of primary importance. They advise that both partners be involved in the treatment of sexual problems.

Environmental Restrictions

Environmental factors such as privacy, competing stimuli, and segregation interfere with sexual expression. Institutionalization rarely affords sufficient privacy for sexual expression. Many institutions segregate persons on the basis of sex. For whatever reason this may be done, the act of segregation may elicit a range of adaptation, including masturbation, homosexual activity, or withdrawal from human warmth. Often these adaptive behaviors are punished, and those who resort to them are stigmatized. In some institutions staff members may assume an in loco parentis stance, treating even aging persons as if they required protection from their sexual desires.

SEXUAL CONCERNS, DIFFICULTIES, AND DYSFUNCTIONS

People have a variety of sexual problems ranging from concerns about sexual phenomena to alterations in sexual health. Each type of problem usually is the consequence of antecedents, and each requires somewhat different therapeutic approaches.

Sexual Concerns

Sexual concerns constitute a source of worry, dissatisfaction, or discomfort but do not produce difficulty in sexual function, profound problems in the sexual relationship, or a greatly altered sexual self-concept. Sexual concerns arise because of misinformation or lack of information, conflicting values, difficulty communicating about sexual issues, and anxiety or guilt about sexual phenomena.

These concerns are usually amenable to sex education strategies, such as permission giving, provision of limited information, values clarification exercises, rehearsal of communication, validation of normalcy, and provision of anticipatory guidance.

Sexual Difficulties

Sexual difficulties create discomfort in the sexual relationship, may occasionally interfere with sexual function, and sometimes may challenge the person's sexual self-image. Sexual difficulties include the following:

1. Inability to relax
2. Disinterest in sexual activity
3. Sexual dissatisfaction

34-6

Some health problems resulting in body image changes that may raise sexual concerns

Surgically induced
Mastectomy
Ostomy
Hysterectomy
Amputation of limb or limbs
Vulvectomy

Traumatically induced
Burns
Lacerations, scarring
Amputations
Pelvic irradiation

Others
Dermatologic disorders
Obesity
Congenital anomalies of sexual organs (for example, absence of penis, hypospadias)
Unusual breast size, including immaturity or hypertrophy

---

4. Inability to please or be pleased by a partner
5. Disagreement about when to engage in sexual behavior

These difficulties are amenable to counseling approaches, including relaxation training, exploration of alternatives in the sexual repertoire, provision of specific suggestions, and training in communication skills.

Alterations in Sexual Health

Contemporary systems for classification of *sexual dysfunction* include desire phase, arousal phase, and orgasm phase dysfunctions, coital pain, and dissatisfaction with sexual frequency.[66] Although this schema addresses the functional dimension of sexual health, it does not address the dimensions of self-concept and relationships. The following paragraphs describe alterations in sexual function, sexual self-concept, and sexual relationships as a basis for a diagnostic taxonomy for nursing practice.

Alterations in sexual function
Alterations in sexual desire

Alterations in sexual desire include low sexual desire and sexual aversion. Low sexual desire reflects lack of interest in sex. Low frequency of self-stimulation and activity with a partner and diminished desire for sexual activity, incidence of fantasy, erotic dreams, or seeking erotic stimulation define this alteration. Low sexual desire and aversion are part of a continuum on which aversion includes a clearly negative response to the idea of sex.

Physiologic and psychosocial factors contribute to alterations in sexual desire. Depression, severe stress, certain pharmacologic agents, low androgen levels, and certain illnesses can interfere with sexual desire. Pharmacologic agents such as narcotics, sedatives, and alcohol, centrally acting antihypertensives (such as reserpine and methyldopa), and testosterone antagonists are associated with low sexual desire.

Illness-associated malaise, thought processes, and fear and anger produced by interpersonal conflicts, as well as concerns about intimacy or sexual self-concept, can also inhibit sexual desire. Anxiety and guilt linked to childhood experiences such as sexual abuse, pressure to have sex, and repeated unpleasant experiences may also interfere with sexual desire. Common diagnoses in nursing practice include the following:

Low sexual desire related to chronic pain, medication regimen, partner's poor health and inability to have intercourse, or depression

Sexual aversion related to rape trauma

Therapies for low sexual desire and sexual aversion relate to underlying causes when this can be determined. When low sexual desire is related to chronic pain, the strategies may include identification of positions of maximum comfort and alternative stimulation that does not intensify pain. Sexual aversion typically is treated in the context of intensive sex therapy or psychotherapy.[66]

Alterations in sexual arousal/excitement

Many alterations in sexual arousal exist for men and include decreased subjective arousal, difficulty attaining an erection, difficulty maintaining an erection, and decreased subjective arousal combined with difficulty in some aspect of attaining or maintaining an erection. Alterations in women's sexual arousal include decreased physiologic arousal and decreased physiologic subjective arousal. Diminished vasocongestion is a symptom of diminished physiologic arousal, whereas loss of erotic sensation is a symptom of diminished subjective arousal.[66]

Alterations in sexual arousal typically reflect body-mind-social interaction. Transient episodes of alterations in arousal are common. Pharmacologic agents such as certain antihypertensives, sedatives, and tranquilizers may interfere with physiologic sexual arousal in both men and women. Diseases affecting vascular function, such as diabetes, can impair vasocongestion.[53] As people age, vasocongestive responses to sexual stimuli and vaginal lubrication appear more slowly, and the response may be less intense than in younger years. Anxieties about sexual performance and fear of failure are commonly associated with alterations in sexual arousal.

Alterations in sexual arousal commonly encountered in nursing practice include the following:

Decreased vasocongestion and vaginal lubrication related to diabetic neuropathy

Decreased vaginal lubrication related to anxiety about pain with intercourse

Difficulty attaining an erection related to a medication

Difficulty maintaining an erection related to fear of failure.[76]

Strategies for treating alterations in sexual arousal include reducing anxiety about the problem and correcting or transcending the physiologic problems if possible. Anxiety can be reduced through desensitization exercises in which the person is instructed to use erotic imagery to approximate sexual situations evoking anxiety.

Structuring sexual encounters so they are not demanding is a second strategy. Exercises that emphasize pleasure rather than pressure to perform often begin by refocusing the person's attention on sensual aspects of touch without genital touching for a period of time. After the person has pleasure in sensual experiences without anxiety, sexual activity is gradually reintroduced.

Physiologic problems can sometimes be modified to restore sexual function. Drug regimens can be modified and strategies can be introduced to persons to amplify erotic sensations in parts of their bodies not affected by disease. A penile prosthesis may be implanted in men as a method of treatment for organic erectile dysfunction.

Alterations in orgasm

Alterations in orgasm in men include problems with ejaculation and orgasm and with the perception of pleasure associated with orgasm. Ejaculatory problems include premature ejaculation and inhibited ejaculation. *Premature ejaculation* occurs when men ejaculate too rapidly for their own or a partner's pleasure. Often men with premature ejaculation do not perceive erotic sensations that occur before orgasm and progress rapidly from very low to very high levels of arousal. Anxiety about sex is common, and many men have learned to make their sexual encounters quick. *Inhibited ejaculation*, sometimes referred to as retarded ejaculation, implies the inability to ejaculate during sexual activity or the need for an extended period of time to ejaculate, even with adequate stimulation. Inhibited ejaculation is often associated with anger or lack of trust. Physiologic alterations and medications can interfere with ejaculation.[67,76]

Alterations in orgasm for women include *anorgasmia*, a global inability to have orgasm, and situational anorgasmia, the inability to have orgasm in certain situations. Anorgasmia with intercourse is common. Inadequate stimulation, self-observation, and fear of loss of control over sexual or aggressive impulses often produce these alterations.

Both physiologic and psychosocial mechanisms can produce orgasm phase alterations. Because a person has a physiologic problem does not justify attributing the alteration to the disease; instead, an emotional or cognitive process may be involved.

Therapeutic strategies for anorgasmia include structuring situations for sexual activity that reduce anxiety. Distraction from self-observation through the use of fantasy and imagery along with self-pleasuring exercises often reduce anxiety sufficiently to enhance awareness of erotic sensation and orgasm.

Strategies for premature ejaculation include the use of the start-stop techniques (p. 1116), in which stimulation is withdrawn intermittently, or the source of stimulation is stopped intermittently to increase awareness of erotic sensations and to increase tolerance of pleasure associated with arousal. Retarded ejaculation is treated with a combination of relaxation and stimulation techniques, and these are sometimes enhanced by the use of imagery.

Pain with coitus

Vaginismus is a relatively rare sexual problem characterized by an involuntary, conditioned spasm of the vaginal outlet, thus causing it to shut tightly. This problem precludes sexual intercourse, but vaginismic women may be orgasmic with alternative methods of sexual stimulation.

Dyspareunia, or painful intercourse, may be attributable to a number of factors ranging from a full lower bowel to feelings of aversion toward sexual intercourse. It is sometimes felt by women with steroid alterations, for example, the postpartum mother and postmenopausal women.

Alterations in sexual self-concept

An individual's sexual self-concept can be changed dramatically because of developmental transitions or health-related events. In response to surgery or injury that produces changed body image or in response to taking on the identity of a disease, sexual self-concept may change. Embarrassment and shame associated with bodily changes can produce anxiety about sexual relationships.

Nursing diagnoses commonly associated with alteration in sexual self-concept include the following:

Altered sexual self-concept related to identification with an illness

Anxiety about sexual encounters related to changed body image (for example, after ostomy surgery)

Anxiety about sexual encounters related to feelings of inadequacy as a man or woman

Altered sexual self-concept related to a partner's lack of acceptance of change in one's body

Strategies for enhancing sexual self-concept include those directed at accepting and transcending alterations in body image, transcending the sick role, obtaining support from a partner, and enhancing perception of one's sexual self-concept as positive.

Alterations in sexual relationships

Sexual relationships can be changed by developmental transitions and changes in health status. Value conflicts about sexual activity, difficulty communicating about sexual issues, dissatisfaction with sexual frequency, a partner's inability to provide sexual stimulation, inability to please a partner, and conflicts about the timing of sexual activity may all occur as people experience ill health.

Some examples of nursing diagnoses related to alterations in sexual relationships include the following:

Value conflicts related to using alternative forms of sexual expression required by the illness, by partner's inability to reconcile roles as caretaker/lover, by partner's lack of acceptable sexual outlet, or by partner's inability to provide sexual stimulation because of reduced mobility

Adjustment, impaired sexual related to dissatisfaction with decreased sexual frequency

Strategies for promoting healthy sexual relationships include facilitating involvement that is mutually acceptable to both partners. Communicating clearly and comfortably about concerns and problems, negotiating mutually acceptable solutions to conflicts, obtaining adequate information about the consequences of health problems for sexuality, and clarifying sexual values can enhance the quality of sexual relationships.

Gender Disorders

Although many gender disorders exist, they are encountered less often in nursing practice than the problems discussed earlier.

Transsexualism refers to the condition of people who are convinced that they are "trapped in the body of the wrong sex." This gender identity problem may be encountered in some medical-surgical services. Transsexuals believe that they belong to the opposite sex and desire the body, appearance, and social status of the opposite sex. Many actually live in the role of the opposite sex before treatment. Male-to-female transsexuals are usually treated initially with hormonal therapy, and later surgical revision of the genitals is performed. The surgery involves removal of the male genitals and revision of the scrotal and neighboring tissue to resemble the female genitals. Usually the surgery is cosmetically successful, and an artificial but functional vagina can be created. These women are, of course, sterile, since they have neither ovaries nor uterus.

The female-to-male transsexual has a less cosmetically effective and functional surgical transformation. In a series of procedures, the breasts and vulva are revised and a phallus is created. Hormonal therapy is also used to effect the transformation. Often the creation of the penis requires extensive grafting and surgical revision, and the female-to-male transformation is consequently more difficult and usually less satisfactory. After the transformation these men are also sterile.

Both men and women electing transsexual surgery require considerable emotional support. They usually have careful psychologic assessments before and after the surgery. Because of their cultural conditioning, nurses sometimes find it difficult to relate appropriately to the transsexual. Often it is necessary to analyze one's attitudes and values carefully to be accepting of these patients.

Transsexualism should not be confused with *tranvestism,* the act of dressing in the clothing of the opposite sex. Additionally, transsexuals are not homosexuals.

Hermaphroditism is a congenital condition in which the reproductive structures appear ambiguous. Early life experiences seem to have profound effect on our gender identities. It is important, therefore, that sexual assignment be correctly established early in life to prevent gender confusion later.

NURSING PRACTICE
Prerequisites for Intervention

Three prerequisites are important before practitioners can help individuals with their sexual problems:
1. A knowledge base
2. Awareness of own value system
3. Ability to communicate genuinely and therapeutically with patients

Knowledge base

The knowledge base that is required is listed in Box 34-7. Without such knowledge the nurse has no basis for the interpretation of patient's concerns and thus no basis for intervening.

Awareness of own value system

In addition to an adequate knowledge base, an awareness of one's own value system, including the biases and beliefs about appropriate and inappropriate sexual behavior, is also

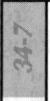

	Knowledge base prerequisite for addressing sexual concerns
34-7	Understanding of sexual response Knowledge of the variety of sexual behaviors that exist in our society and their prevalence Understanding of the types of sexual dysfunctions Awareness of the relationship between age, life events, pathologic conditions, behavioral problems, pharmaceutic agents, and sexual function

---

	Principles that facilitate obtaining a sexual history	
34-8	**Action**	**Effect**
	1. Obtain sexual history early in nurse-patient relationship	Legitimizes sexuality as part of health Provides permission for patient to discuss sexual concerns
	2. Avoid overreaction or underreaction to patient's comments	Facilitates truthful data gathering
	3. Use language patient understands	Facilitates accurate data gathering
	4. Move from less sensitive to more sensitive areas	Facilitates patient-nurse comfort
	5. Terminate sexual history by inquiring if patient has additional questions or concerns	Conveys a willingness by nurse to further explore sexual matters

---

important. Unless professionals can accept their own sexuality and are comfortable with their own behavior, it is difficult to convey comfort to others. Self-acceptance is seen as prerequisite to the development of a nonjudgmental and tolerant approach. Just as individuals have belief systems related to sexual phenomena, so do professionals. This does not imply that the sex educators or counselors must condone every variety of sexual activity. Rather, it is essential that they be aware of their own feelings and values and attempt to keep them in perspective by acknowledging them. This assists them in maintaining a supportive climate that encourages sharing of feeling by patients and simultaneously permits professionals to acknowledge the validity of their own beliefs.

Furthermore, there may be some issues about which the professional has such strong beliefs that these values would interfere with effective intervention. An example encountered in practice is the health professional whose basic conviction is that homosexuality is an illness or deviation rather than a variation in sexual expression or orientation. No matter how extensive the professional's training, knowledge base, and therapy skills, such a strong basic belief is likely to interfere greatly with the ability to relate objectively to a homosexual's sexual problems. Often professionals need to acknowledge their inability to deal with sexual problems because of their own value systems. Topics likely to elicit biases among health professionals include abortion, alternative lifestyles, and sexual variations.

One strategy that may be helpful in discussing sexual topics is to practice presenting opposing viewpoints on a sexual issue. For example, being able to discuss both pro-choice and pro-life stands on abortion may facilitate discussing other topics in a nonjudgmental manner.

Therapeutic communication

Finally, the professional needs to be able to communicate genuinely and therapeutically with patients. Often this involves using the person's own language, which may be different from that of the health professional. Without the ability to interact accurately and empathetically with individuals, the most sophisticated knowledge base and objective attitudes are of little benefit.

Nurses frequently encounter behavioral problems that involve the individual's sexuality. One common problem is the patient who acts out sexually, for example, by making inappropriate sexual gestures, using explicit sexual lan-

guage, or exposing the sexual organs. Two general principles are helpful in coping with such a situation:
1. Analyze what meaning this behavior might have for the patient.
2. Assert the right as a human being to establish limits that protect the nurse's integrity.

In responding to a patient who has exhibited sexual behavior that is deemed inappropriate, one can analyze why the behavior occurs and share this observation with the patient. Is the patient attempting to gain control in a situation in which he or she has little or no control? Is the patient trying to obtain validation of his masculinity or her femininity? Is the patient unaware that the behavior has sexual overtones or is making the nurse uncomfortable?

Nurses have the right to establish limits with patients to protect their own integrity. Violation of certain bodily boundaries, for example, touching the breasts or buttocks of the nurse or exposing one's genitals, is not behavior that nurses must tolerate to be "accepting of patients." Nurses' responses, however, can address three important points:
1. The inferred meaning of the behavior can be shared—"I know you feel helpless right now. . ."
2. The boundary can be established—"That's not acceptable behavior."
3. The patient's sexuality can be validated—"You're a good looking guy, but that's just not acceptable behavior."

Some patients cannot respond appropriately to these strategies, and in some instances the nurse may need to believe that not working with this patient is permissible.

Assessment
Sexual history

Many health care providers may not be experienced in eliciting a sexual history and at first may be uneasy. No doubt this uneasiness is conditioned by social prohibition about discussing intimate matters such as sexual experiences or behavior. However, health professionals are expected to be informed, willing to discuss sexual matters openly with patients, and prepared to educate and counsel them appropriately. Nurses who are hesitant to deal with sexual matters with patients are helped by working through their own feelings about sex and sexual matters. Seeking counsel from other nurses or health professionals who are comfortable with the topic is often helpful. Some nurses may find it helpful to attend a workshop on sexuality for nurses.

Although there is no single approach to taking a sexual history, application of certain principles facilitates both the patient's and the nurse's comfort. Absolute requirements for history taking include the following:

1. Provision of privacy, such as in a closed room
2. An atmosphere of trust between patient and nurse, such as assurance of confidentiality for the patient
3. Comfort on the part of nurses with their own sexuality

Some principles for promoting patient-nurse comfort are listed in Box 34-8. The sexual history itself may be therapeutic. Within the context of obtaining the data, the nurse can provide permission for the patient to discuss concerns, provide limited information or suggestions, or validate the normalcy and acceptability of the patient's concerns and practices.

It may be necessary for both patient and nurse to define their terms. Street language may be unfamiliar to the nurse, and highly technical language may be confusing to the patient. The nurse may need to become familiar with some commonly used street language to be sure of what the patient is reporting.

The technique of moving from less sensitive to more sensitive areas paves the way for both the patient and nurse. For example, the nurse may explore a woman's sexual role before discussing her ability to have orgasm, her menstrual history before her experience with sexual variations, and her personal experiences with sex education before her actual sexual experiences. In all of these situations, the decision to pursue the topics depends on the cues presented by the patient that sexual concerns are present.

Brief sexual assessment

A brief assessment can be incorporated in the nursing history by means of three questions (see Box 34-9). The first of these questions deals with the person's role, the next with the affective-cognitive elements of sexuality, and the last with biologic aspects of sexual function. The questions may be modified to deal with illness, hospitalization, life events, or any other relevant entity that may influence or interfere with sexual health.

The questions may also be adapted to elicit the patient's expectations of changes resulting from procedures or hospitalization that he or she is about to experience. These brief items invite the patient to explore sexual concerns. Often it is unnecessary for the nurse to ask the second and third questions, because many patients proceed to state their concerns about masculinity, femininity, and sexual functioning without further prompting.

Brief sexual history

1. Has your (illness, pregnancy, or hospitalization) interfered with your being a (husband, wife, father, mother)?
2. Has your (abortion, heart attack, etc.) changed the way you see yourself as a (woman, man)?
3. Has your (colostomy, hysterectomy, etc.) changed your ability to function sexually (or your sex life)?

Self-help organizations that publish sexuality pamphlets

National Multiple Sclerosis Society: *Sexuality and MS*
American Arthritis Foundation: *Living and Loving*
American Cancer Society: *Sexuality for the man with cancer, Sexuality for the woman with cancer*
American Diabetes Association: publishes several pamphlets and articles for men and women with diabetes

---

Roles of the Nurse in Providing Sexual Health Care

Nurses may intervene with sexual problems among patient populations through four strategies: educating patient groups likely to have sexual concerns, providing anticipatory guidance throughout the life cycle, promoting a milieu conducive to sexual health, and validating normalcy about sexual concerns.

Providing patient education

Several self-help groups and other organizations publish easy-to-read pamphlets on sexuality (see Box 34-10). These pamphlets can often be purchased for a nominal fee and given to patients. Most pamphlets can be obtained directly from state or local chapters. Chapters of other self-help groups can be contacted about availability of sexuality resources for patients. Some groups publish newsletters that address sexuality, such as *"Sex over Forty,"* a monthly publication from PHE, Inc.*

Nurses can also write their own pamphlets for patients. Although this requires some effort, it may provide additional incentive for staff to address sexuality. Once developed, these pamphlets can be made available to others. For example, Kautz developed a series of pamphlets for patients undergoing microscopic diskectomies that included how the operation may affect sexuality; copies may be obtained.†

---

*PHE, Inc, PO Box 1600, Chapel Hill, NC 27515.
†Finance Dept, Dept of Nursing, University of Kentucky Hospital, 800 Rose St, Lexington, KY 40536-0084.

Nurses can also assist patients by providing specific information relating to conditions conducive to optimal sexual functioning, specific approaches to sexuality for patients with certain diseases or surgeries, and directives for coping with some sexual dysfunctions. One specific suggestion often incorporated in sexual education is that a couple having difficulties with intercourse abstain for a specified period. This admonition is designed to reduce the "pressure to perform" perceived by a member of the dysfunctional couple.

Patients with ostomies, who often have concerns about appliance leakage during intercourse, can be given specific suggestions (see Box 31-26 in Chapter 31).

Nurses can offer some simple directives for coping with specific sexual dysfunction. The man whose problem is premature ejaculation can be taught to use the squeeze technique or the partner may learn to apply it. The technique consists of applying pressure over the coronal ridge of the glans, exerting enough pressure for 3 to 4 seconds to relieve the feeling of ejaculatory inevitability during intercourse. The squeeze technique is used three to four times during one session of intercourse. Often the technique must be used several times over a 2-week to 3-week period to produce results. (For additional information consult reference 56.)

Another area of health promotion is in the correct use of condoms. For condoms to be effective in preventing the spread of STDs and AIDS, the Centers for Disease Control (CDC) guidelines must be followed (see Chapter 18).

Patient education implies more than mere dissemination of information. Just as nurses learn to examine their own values and to communicate with others, patients may also need assistance in exploring the attitudes and values that shape their sexual behavior and in developing the ability to communicate comfortably about sexual phenomena. Thus providing accurate information about sex and sexuality is not synonymous with education for a healthy sexuality.

Providing anticipatory guidance

Nurses are often in strategic positions to provide anticipatory guidance at sensitive points in the life cycle. Adolescence and middle age are two life periods during which anxiety about sexuality is likely to surface. By informing individuals about the usual changes experienced at these points (for example, nocturnal emissions or concerns about masturbation in adolescents or worry about effects of menopause on the ability to function sexually among middle-aged persons), nurses can assist individuals to cope realistically with major changes in their bodies. Adults with young children can also benefit from anticipatory guidance regarding their children's sexuality. Planned Parenthood publishes a book, *How to talk with your child about sexuality,* to assist parents in anticipating sexual concerns of their children. Other books on this subject are available in bookstores.

Anticipatory guidance can also be given to patients who have been admitted to the hospital, to assist them with sexual concerns that are likely to arise when they return home. For example, a woman who has a mastectomy can be advised that she may not feel like having sex until her incision heals. Both she and her partner may have concerns about how her body will look. She will be given information about specially designed bras and breast prostheses (see Chapter 36). Finally, she may benefit from being advised that friends and family will be curious about how she looks, and she may find them staring at her breasts. One woman confided that while attending church services a few weeks after her mastectomy, she was shocked at the number of people, including the minister, who stared at her breasts when talking with her. While she was aware that these people had a natural curiosity, she was not prepared for their reaction. While the nurse cannot prevent this reaction from occurring, the patient can be assisted to think through how she will handle this situation if and when she experiences it.

Promoting a milieu conducive to sexual health

The first step in promoting a milieu conducive to sexual health is to give patients permission to ask about intimacy and sexual concerns. By including sexuality as a routine part of a comprehensive nursing assessment, the nurse is saying, "It's okay to talk about sensitive issues."

Another approach is providing time for privacy and intimacy for patients and their partners while in the hospital or other health care institution. Patients and families experience tremendous crises during hospitalizations and often need time alone to help each other cope effectively. A young man who had recently become a quadriplegic in a motor vehicle accident became very anxious at night in the intensive care unit. The nursing staff became concerned that his anxiety might prevent him from being weaned from the ventilator. His girl friend also became extremely anxious at night and was having difficulty sleeping in the waiting room knowing he was anxious in the ICU. The staff elected in this situation to allow her to sleep with him in the ICU bed. This anxiety-reducing intervention benefited the patient, his partner, and the staff, and he was weaned from the ventilator within a few days.

Other approaches include minimizing guilt felt in conjunction with sexual thoughts, feelings, and behavior. This may be accomplished by assisting persons in examining objectively the consequences of their activities within a reality-oriented framework. Reduction of performance anxiety (for example, concern about how well one is able to function) can be facilitated by helping individuals understand the relationship between being attentive to their own performance and losing touch with their sexual feelings. "Spectatoring" refers to the habit of watching oneself or a partner perform. Just as in athletics, one cannot be both spectator and performer without minimizing the effectiveness of the performance.

Often individuals need to be advised to modify their environments to reduce competing stimuli. Use of anxiety-provoking settings or those settings prone to interruption may establish dysfunctional patterns. The relationship between anxiety and orgasmic dysfunction and premature ejaculation has been well established.

Finally, maintenance of good general health facilitates optimal sexual functioning. Fatigue, pain, and malaise are stimuli that compete with sexual pleasure.

Validating normalcy

Validating normalcy is a function that nearly all health professionals perform but sometimes undervalue. Often the focus is on finding out what is wrong, what the pathophysiologic process is, and what therapy to prescribe to correct the malfunction. Often family members approach health professionals to find out whether they are normal, acceptable, and not perverted. They seek out the health professional for validation of their sexual normalcy. People may be concerned about their thoughts, fantasies, dreams, and feelings, as well as overt sexual behavior. In the process of validating normalcy, nurses often help patients exchange labels. Often labels bearing negative connotations such as "dirty," "perverted," or "abnormal" are exchanged for labels such as "healthy" and "okay."[61] Although most sexual acts could be considered normal in some sense, patients do need to be made aware of the consequences of their behavior. The health professional cannot ignore patients' ethical codes or the legal code.

One situation sometimes encountered in nursing practice is the adolescent questioning whether it is "normal" not to be sexually active. For example, a young woman came to a clinic requesting a prescription for an oral contraceptive. The physician who saw her did a pelvic examination and gave her the prescription. The nurse, who had been with her during the examination, noted that she was quite anxious about the procedure and was very hesitant to leave the examining room. After pursuing the reason for her obvious discomfort with the situation, the nurse found that the woman was seeking a prescription at her boyfriend's insistence; furthermore, she was *not* convinced that she wanted to become sexually active, but she feared that the relationship would end if she did not meet the young man's demands. She wanted some reassurance that she was "normal" for having these reservations and that *not* being sexually active was okay.

Another occasion for validating normal sexual attitudes is during the physical examination. Many nurses who perform pelvic examinations make these an educational experience for their patients. At the beginning of the examination, the examiner asks the woman whether she would like a mirror so that she can watch the examination as it is being performed. As the examiner inspects the external genitals, it is possible to identify the anatomic parts, pointing out how healthy the genitals appear. The examiner using a lighted speculum can identify the woman's internal pelvic structures. For many women, this is the first time they have been able to see their external genitals, to say nothing of their cervices and other internal structures.

Families often encounter disabling diseases or injuries that interfere with usual forms of sexual expression. Couples may ask nurses to validate the normalcy or health of the adaptations they make, such as the exploration of new types of sexual expression.

Using sexual information to promote health in other areas

Addressing sexual concerns may promote the adoption of other health habits by patients. For example, nurses teach patients with chronic obstructive pulmonary disease to

---

34-11

Common sexual concerns of patients with strokes and their partners

Changes that occur with sexual function

Interferences with desire: A patient who is aphasic will have difficulty communicating sexual feelings and desires. Both partners may fear lack of ability to perform and so may not initiate sex. If sex is not initiated, there is no proof of erectile dysfunction or vaginal dryness.

Interferences with excitement and orgasm: Most people are "sexually conditioned" to use only certain positions or certain sex acts. After a stroke, a couple may need to try other "unusual" positions to be successful.

Changes in sexual self-concept

Depression, dementia, and emotional lability are all common to stroke. Depression severely reduces desire, which then can make the depression worse. Stroke survivors may have perceptual problems and not realize how disabled they are, which interferes with forming realistic expectations about sex and intimacy. Dementia interferes with understanding what is happening. Emotional lability is very difficult to deal with during sex; making love while crying or laughing uncontrollably is not very romantic.

Changes in sexual roles and relationships

If the person who had the stroke needs some physical care, this will change the roles of each person in the relationship. One of the most common concerns of spouses is the "loss" of part of their partner and whether the spouse will be the "same person I've been married to for the last 40 years." The partner of a person with dementia may have ethical concerns about whether the stroke survivor can continue to consent to participate in a sexual relationship. People who have strokes who have not been involved in relationships for a long time due to death of a spouse may respond inappropriately to "intimate" touching as part of routine nursing care by the staff.

Recommendations and nursing interventions

Always ask if patients have sexual concerns, no matter how old they are. Encourage the expression of feelings of both partners. Patients have reported an overwhelming need for information that was completely ignored by health professionals.[39] Recommend making slow changes in sexual activities, spending time talking with their spouse, just being together, and not trying to have sex too quickly after hospital discharge. Recommend they try different coital positions. A man who is hemiplegic will probably not be able to support himself in a superior position, and thus the couple may need to try a side-lying or other position for intercourse.[8,33,39]

maintain optimal levels of endurance with low levels of exercise, stopping smoking, using pursed lip and abdominal breathing techniques, and complying with medications and breathing treatments. All of these activities not only serve to stabilize the disease and increase the ability to perform ADLs, but they also can potentially increase their sexual performance. In addition, the nurse can suggest these patients wear their nasal oxygen cannula and use proper breathing techniques during lovemaking.

Sexual concerns may motivate self-care. A woman with multiple sclerosis (MS) sought out home health services to assist her in learning to perform her own intermittent catheterization for bladder management. Even though her MS had caused visual problems, poor hand and wrist strength, and paraplegia, the home health nurse and occupational therapist were able to teach her to catheterize herself with the use of a "cock up" wrist splint, "labia spreader," lighted magnifying mirror, hard rubber catheters, and a urinal. The patient expressed her gratitude that her husband would no longer need to perform this activity for her.

Burgener and Logan[8] report that a 64-year-old male with a stroke described his distress at his wife's helping him to toilet. This distress affected his sexual self-concept, as well as his relationship with his wife. The nurse assisted him to become independent in toileting, and he became confident in resuming a more sexual relationship, rather than a patient-caregiver relationship, with his wife.

Putting It All Together

This chapter has outlined some skills and knowledge useful for nurses in addressing sexual concerns. Box 34-11 illustrates some typical sexual concerns of stroke patients and their partners, and interventions the nurse can use to prevent or assist to overcome sexual problems.

SUMMARY

1. Human sexuality is a complex of interrelating biologic and psychosocial variables that begin at conception and continue through life; components include biologic (sexual function or expression), psychologic (gender identity, thoughts, and feelings), and social factors (such as sanctioned role, mores, and folkways regulating sexual expression).

2. The physiologic phases of human sexual response may be divided into four categories (excitement, plateau, orgasm, resolution) or three categories (desire, excitement, orgasm).

3. The excitement and plateau phases are characterized by vasocongestion of pelvic blood vessels leading to swelling of genitalia and by vaginal lubrication, the orgasm phase by myotonia (involuntary muscle contractions in the pelvic organs and other parts of the body), and the resolution phase by muscle relaxation and return of normal blood flow.

4. Although generally a decline in overall interest and sexual activity is seen with age, many persons continue with an active sexual life into old age; the level of activity appears related to the extent of sexual activity during youth.

5. Sexual expression varies and includes heterosexuality, homosexuality, bisexuality, transvestism, incest, zoophilia, fetishism, voyeurism, exhibitionism, sadism, and masochism; social norms influence expected sexual expressions.

6. Illness may affect sexuality and sexual function through changes in body structure, changes in body functions, effects of pharmacologic agents, body image changes, or environmental restrictions (privacy, competing stimuli, partner segregation).

7. Sexual concerns and difficulties generally do not produce profound problems in sexual response although they may temporarily interfere with sexual functioning; sexual concerns and difficulties are usually amenable to sex education and counseling.

8. Alterations in sexual health include alterations in sexual function (desire, arousal, orgasm), in sexual self-concept, and in sexual relationships.

9. Alterations in sexual desire include low sexual desire and sexual aversion. Therapy is directed toward underlying causes; intensive sex therapy or psychotherapy is often required for sexual aversion.

10. Alterations in sexual arousal reflect body-mind-social interaction and may result from drugs, diseases affecting vascular function, age, and anxiety about sexual performance. Transient episodes of alteration in arousal are common. Therapies include anxiety-reducing approaches and exercises that emphasize pleasure rather than pressure to perform.

11. Alterations in orgasm include ejaculatory problems in men and anorgasmia in women; both physiologic and psychologic mechanisms can produce orgasm phase alterations. Therapies include anxiety-reducing strategies for anorgasmia and relaxation-stimulation techniques for ejaculatory problems.

12. Alterations in sexual self-concept may result from disease or injury. Therapies include strategies toward accepting and transcending body image changes, transcending the sick role, obtaining partner support, and enhancing a positive self-concept.

13. Alterations in sexual relationships during illness result from value conflicts about sexual activity, problems with communication, or difficulties in sexual functioning. Therapies include promoting communication and providing education to resolve conflicts and promote sexuality.

14. Nursing interventions for persons with sexual concerns, sexual difficulties, and alterations in sexual response include awareness of the nurse's own value system, therapeutic communication, prevention of sexual problems through education, anticipatory guidance, and promotion of a milieu conducive to sexual health.

STUDY QUESTIONS

- What instances in your own life shaped some of your feelings about yourself as female or male?
- What nursing behaviors would increase your comfort in describing your own sexual history?
- Examine your beliefs about homosexuality. In what ways

might your beliefs help or hinder working with homosexual patients who have sexual concerns?

▸ Examine the list of diseases in Table 34-4 and the list of medications in Table 34-5. Have any of these conditions existed for patients for whom you have provided care recently? How might their sexual response have been affected? Did they express any concerns about their sexuality or sexual response? Discuss the nursing care that could have been offered.

REFERENCES AND SELECTED READINGS

1. * Allen M: A holistic view of sexuality and the aged, *Holistic Nurs Pract* 1(4):76-83, 1987.
2. Andersen BL, LeGrand J: Body image for women: conceptualization, assessment, and a test of its importance to sexual dysfunction and medical illness, *J Sex Research* 28:457-477, 1991.
3. * Bachers E: Sexual dysfunction after treatment for genitourinary cancers, *Semin Oncol Nurs* 1(1):18-24, 1985.
4. * Baggs J, Karch AM: Sexual counseling of women with coronary heart disease, *Heart Lung* 16:154-159, 1987.
5. Bernhard L: Sexuality expectations and outcomes in women having hysterectomies, *Chart* 83(10):11-15, 1986.
6. * Bernhard L, Dan A: Redefining sexuality from women's own experiences, *Nurs Clin North Am* 21:125-136, 1986.
7. Brink P: Cultural aspects of sexuality, *Holistic Nurs Pract* 1(4):12-20, 1987.
8. Burgener S, Logan G: Sexuality concerns of the post-stroke patient, *Rehab Nurs* 14:178-181, 195, 1989.
9. * Campbell M: Sexual dysfunction in the COPD patient, *DCCN* 6(2):70-74, 1987.
10. Chateauvert M, Duffie A, Gilmore N: HIV antibody testing: counselling guidelines from the Canadian Medical Association, *Pat Educ Council* 18:35-49, 1986.
11. Cochran SK, Peplau LA: Sexual risk reduction behaviors among young heterosexual adults, *Soc Sci Med* 33:25-36, 1991.
12. * Cohen J: Sexual counseling of the patient following myocardial infarction, *Crit Care Nurse* 6(6):18-29, 1986.
13. * Cooley M, et al: Sexual and reproductive issues for women with Hodgkin's disease: overview of issues, *CA Nurs* 9:188-193, 1986.
14. Donlou J, et al: Psychosocial aspects of AIDS and AIDS-related complex: a pilot study, *J Psychosoc Oncol* 3(2):39-55, 1985.
15. D'Emilio J, Freedman EB: *Intimate matters, a history of sexuality in America*, New York, 1988, Harper & Row.
16. * Fischman S, et al: Changes in sexual relationships in postpartum couples, *JOGNN* 15(1):58-63, 1986.
17. Fogel CI, Lauver D: *Sexual health promotion*, Philadelphia, 1990, WB Saunders.
18. * Frank-Stromberg M: Sexuality and the elderly cancer patient, *Semin Oncol Nurs* 1(1):49-55, 1985.
19. Friend R: Sexual identity and human diversity: implications for nursing practice, *Holistic Nurs Pract* 1(4):21-41, 1987.
20. Gloeckner M: Perceptions of sexuality after ostomy surgery, *J Enterost Ther* 18:36-38, 1991.
21. * Grunbert K: Sexual rehabilitation of the cancer patient undergoing ostomy surgery, *J Enterost Ther* 13:148-152, 1986.
22. * Heinrick K: Effective response to sexual harassment, *Nurs Outlook* 35(2):70-72, 1987.
23. Kaiser FE: Sexuality and impotence in the aging man, *Clin Geriatr Med* 7:63-72, 1991.
24. Kansky J: Sexuality of widows: a study of the sexual practices of widows during the first fourteen months of bereavement, *J Sex Marital Ther* 12:307-321, 1986.
25. Kaplan HS: Sex, intimacy, and the aging process, *J Am Acad Psychoanal* 18:185-205, 1990.
26. * Katzin L: Chronic illness and sexuality, *Am J Nurs* 90(1):55-59, 1990.
27. Kautz DD, Dickey CA, Stevens MN: Using research to identify why nurses do not meet established sexuality nursing care standards, *J Nurs Qual Assur* 4(3):69-73, 1990.
28. Koch PB, Young EW: Diabetes and female sexuality: a review of the literature, *Health Care Women Int* 9:251-262, 1988.
29. * Kus R: Sex, AIDS, and gay American men, *Holistic Nurs Pract* 1(4):42-51, 1987.
30. * Lamb M: Sexual dysfunction in the gynecologic oncology patient, *Semin Oncol Nurs* 1(1):9-17, 1985.
31. Leese DL: An overview of urologic complications in diabetes mellitus, *Urol Nurs* 11:17-20, 1991.
32. Lichtenberg PA, Strzepek DM: Assessments of institutionalized dementia patients competencies to participate in intimate relationships, *Gerontologist* 30:117-120, 1990.
33. Litz BT, Zeiss AM, Davies HD: Sexual concerns of male spouses of female Alzheimer's disease patients, *Gerontologist* 30:113-116, 1990.
34. Lloyd EE, Toth LL, Perkash I: Vacuum tumescence: an option for spinal cord injured males with erectile dysfunction, *SCI Nurs* 6:25-28, 1989.
35. LoPiccolo J: Counseling and therapy for sexual problems in the elderly, *Clin Geriatr Med* 7:161-179, 1991.
36. * MacElveen-Hoehn P: Understanding sexuality in progressive cancer, *Semin Oncol Nurs* 1(1):56-62, 1985.
37. Mason DR: Erectile dysfunctions: assessment and care, *Nurse Pract* 14:23-24, 1989.
38. Mason JO, McGinnis JM: Healthy people 2000: an overview of the national health promotion and disease prevention objectives, *Pub Health Rep* 105:441-446, 1989.
39. McCormick GP, Riffer DJ, Thompson MM: Coital positioning for stroke afflicted couples, *Rehab Nurs* 11(2):17-19, 1986.
40. McCracken AL: Sexual practice by elders: the forgotten aspect of functional health, *Sex Marital Ther* 14:13-18, 1988.
41. McCusker J, et al: Responses to the AIDS epidemic among homosexually active men: factors associated with preventive behavior, *Pat Educ Council* 13:15-30, 1989.
42. * McCann ME: Sexual healing after heart attack, *Am J Nurs* 89:1133-1140, 1989.
43. Mulligan T, Palguta RF: Sexual interest, activity, and satisfaction among male nursing home residents, *Arch Sex Behav* 20:199-204, 1991.
44. * Papadoupolous C, et al: Sexual activity after coronary bypass surgery, *Chest* 90:681-685, 1986.
45. Penkower L, et al: Behavioral, health and psychosocial factors and risk for HIV infection among sexually active homosexual men: the Multicenter AIDS Cohort Study, *Am J Pub Health* 81:194-196, 1990.
46. * Persaud D: Assessing sexual functions of the adult with traumatic quadriplegia, *J Neurosurg Nurs* 18(1):11-12, 1986.
47. * Price J: Promoting sexual wellness in head-injured patients, *Rehab Nurs* 10(6):12-13, 1985.
48. * Schain W: Breast cancer surgeries and psychosexual sequelae: implications for remediation, *Semin Oncol Nurs* 1:200-205, 1985.
49. Schechter MT, et al: Patterns of sexual behavior and condom use in a cohort of homosexual men, *Am J Pub Health* 78:1535-1538, 1988.

* Recommended for student reading.

50. Siegel K, et al: Factors distinguishing homosexual males practicing risky and safer sex, *Soc Sci Med* 28:561-569, 1989.

51. Slob AK, et al: Sexuality and psychophysiological functioning in women with diabetes mellitus, *J Sex Marital Ther* 16:59-69, 1990.

52. Smedley G: Addressing sexuality in the elderly, *Rehab Nurs* 16:9-11, 1991.

53. Steele D: Drugs causing sexual dysfunction and their alternatives: a reference tool, *Urol Nurs* 9:10-12, 1989.

54. Turner BF, Adams CG: Reported change in preferred sexual activity over the adult years, *J Sex Res* 25:289-303, 1991.

55. Waterhouse J, et al: Development of the sexual adjustment questionnaire: impact of cancer and surgery, *Oncol Nurs Forum* 13(3):53-59, 1986.

56. Williams CB: Controlling premature ejaculation: patient guide, *Med Asp Hum Sexual* 25(3):15-16, 1991.

57. Williams L: Pharmacologic erection programs: a treatment option of erectile dysfunction, *Rehab Nurs* 14:264-268, 1989.

58.* Woods NF: Toward a holistic perspective of human sexuality: alteration in sexual health and nursing diagnoses, *Holistic Nurs Pract* 1(4):1-11, 1987.

59. Woods NF: Human sexuality: an overview. In Mitchell PH, et al: *AANN's neuroscience nursing: phenomena and practice,* Norwalk, Conn, 1988, Appleton & Lange.

60. Zapka JG, et al: HIV antibody test result knowledge, risk perceptions and behavior among homosexually active men, *Pat Educ Council* 18:9-17, 1991.

Classic

61. Annon J: *The behavioral treatment of sexual problems,* Honolulu, 1974, Enabling Systems.

62. Bell A, Weinberg M: *Homosexualities,* New York, 1978, Simon & Schuster.

63. Comfort A: The normal in sexual behavior: an ethnological point of view, *J Sex Ed Ther* 2:1-7, 1975.

64. Hellerstein H, Friedman FH: Sexual activity and the postcoronary patient, *Arch Intern Med* 125:987-999, 1970.

65. Kaplan HS: *Disorders of sexual desire and other new concepts and techniques in sex therapy,* New York, 1979, Simon & Schuster.

66. Kaplan HS: *The new sex therapy,* New York, 1974, Brunner/Mazel.

67. Kinsey AC, Pomeroy WB, Martin CW: *Sexual behavior in the human male,* Philadelphia, 1948, WB Saunders.

68. Kinsey AC, et al: *Sexual behavior in the human female,* Philadelphia, 1953, WB Saunders.

69. Larson J: *Heart rate and blood pressure responses of coronary artery disease patients during sexual activity and a two-stair climbing test,* Master's thesis, Seattle, 1978, University of Washington.

70. Masters W, Johnson V: *Homosexuality in perspective,* Boston, 1979, Little, Brown.

71. Masters W, Johnson V: *Human sexual response,* Boston, 1966, Little, Brown.

72. Masters W, Johnson V: *Human sexual inadequacy,* Boston, 1970, Little, Brown.

73. Mims F: A model to promote sexual health, *Nurs Outlook* 26:121, 1978.

74. Money J, Ehrhardt A: *Man and woman, boy and girl,* Baltimore, 1972, The Johns Hopkins University Press.

75. Rubin A, Babbott D: Impotence and diabetes mellitus, *JAMA* 168:498-500, 1958.

76.* Woods NF: *Human sexuality in health and illness,* ed 3, St Louis, 1984, Mosby–Year Book.

77. Woods NF, Earp JA: Women with cured breast cancer: a description of women's experiences four years after mastectomy, *Nurs Res* 27:279-285, 1978.

78. World Health Organization: *Education and treatment in human sexuality: the training of health professionals,* Tech Rep Series, No 572, Geneva, 1975, The Organization.

79. Zahn MA: Incapacity, impotence, and invisible impairment: their effects upon interpersonal relations, *J Health Soc Behav* 14:115-123, 1973.

80. Zalar MK: Role preparation for nurses in human sexual functioning, *Nurs Clin North Am* 17:351-363, 1982.

The Patient
with
Reproductive
Problems

Barbara C. Long
Greer Glazer

After studying this chapter, the learner should be able to:

- Describe the primary and secondary prevention for genital infections and malignancies.
- Carry out health teaching regarding menstruation and menopause and alterations in sexual functioning.
- Describe approaches used for sterilization and infertility.
- Differentiate types and effects of inflammatory and structural disorders of the reproductive tract in females and males.
- Identify the incidence and therapeutic approaches for cancer of the reproductive tract in females and males.
- Plan nursing care for persons experiencing surgery of the reproductive tract.

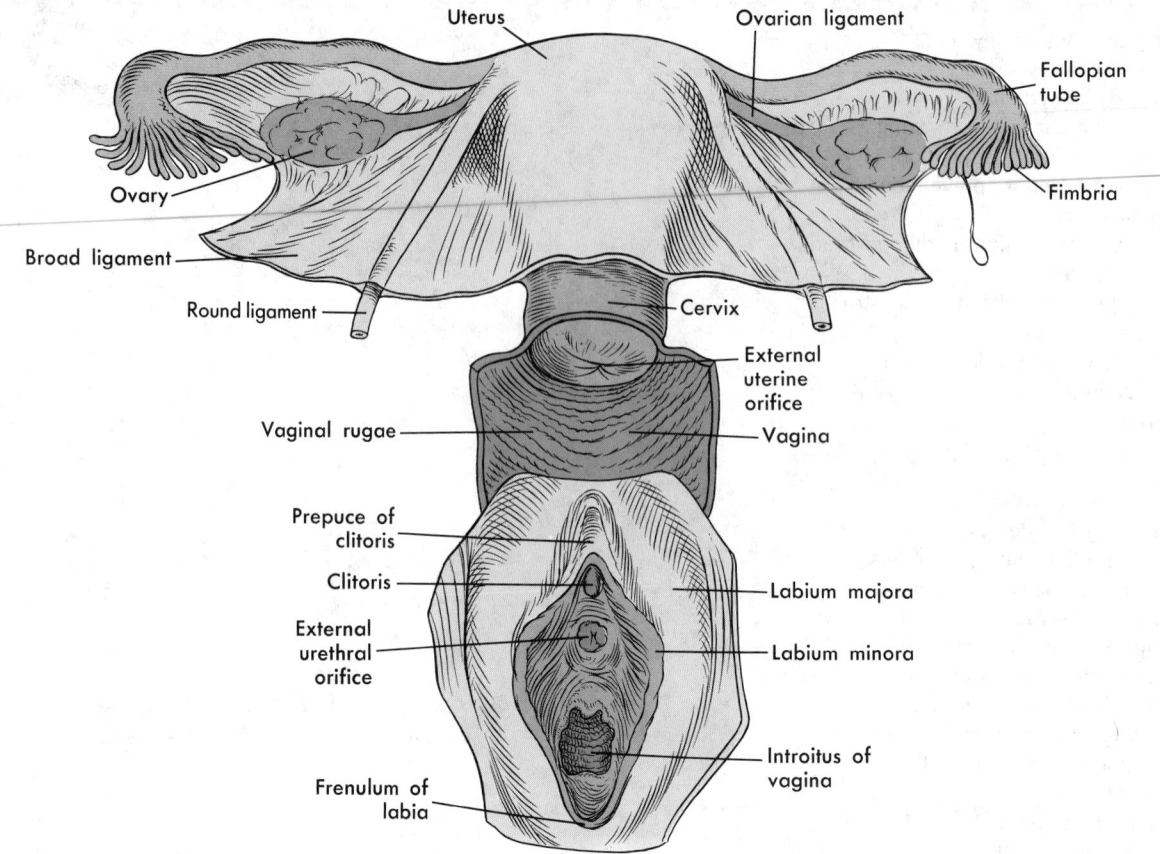

Fig. 35-1 Female internal organs of reproduction. Major ligaments are shown.

Nurses and lay people have become more enlightened about the prevention of problems of the reproductive system. This increased awareness has led many persons to initiate requests for information about or treatment of reproductive system problems. Although men and women are better informed today about matters relating to reproductive health, many neglect preventive measures and ignore signs or symptoms of illness because of embarrassment and the special significance that they attach to the reproductive organs.

In spite of advances in medicine, nursing, science, and technology, diseases and disorders of the genital system continue to threaten the lives and the physical and emotional health of men and women, sometimes needlessly. Many of these problems are preventable; many of them can be treated and cured.

ANATOMY AND PHYSIOLOGY
Female Genital System
External structures

The external genitalia, or vulva, of the female consist primarily of the labia majora, labia minora, and clitoris (Fig. 35-1). Two glands are located in this area: Skene's glands (paraurethral), opening into the urethral orifice, and Bartholin's glands, situated at each side of the vaginal opening near the base of the labia. These glands are common sites of infection.

Internal organs

The female internal reproductive organs, consisting of the vagina, uterus, uterine fallopian tubes, and ovaries, are shown in Fig. 35-1. These organs are located within the cavity of the true pelvis unless their size is increased by disease or pregnancy.

Vagina

The vagina leads from the external structures to the uterus. The length of the vaginal canal varies, and the posterior wall is longer than the anterior wall. The uterine cervix protrudes into the upper vagina, creating recesses (fornices) around the margins of the cervix.

The vagina is lined with pink mucous membrane arranged in folds called *rugae*. Physiologic events such as pregnancy and pathologic conditions such as infections often alter the color of the vaginal mucosa because of congestion with blood. The membrane is lubricated by vaginal secretions that are normally acidic during the years of ovarian function; neutral or alkaline secretions are normally found in postmenopausal women. An alkaline medium promotes growth of bacteria.

Uterus

The uterus consists of three portions: the fundus (upper crest), the main body (corpus), and the neck (cervix). In adult females the position of the uterus may vary. It is usually anteverted (tipped forward) and slightly anteflexed bent forward at an angle), but it may also be retroverted, retroflexed, or in midposition. During menopause the uterus decreases in size.

The uterus has three functional layers: parametrium or outer layer, myometrium or middle muscular layer, and endometrium or mucous membrane lining. The outer surface of the uterus is covered by the peritoneum. Reflection of the peritoneum posteriorly between the uterus and rectum creates a space known as the *cul-de-sac of Douglas.* This space is a common entry site for endoscopy or for surgical drainage of the peritoneal cavity.

Uterine tubes

The uterine or *fallopian* tubes are two narrow muscular canals 8 to 14 cm long. They extend outward from the uterine corpus near the fundus (Fig. 35-1). The uterine tubes serve as a site for union of the sperm and ovum and transport of the fertilized ovum to the uterus. Strictures of the fallopian tubes prevent passage of the ovum.

Ovaries

The ovaries are endocrine glands as well as reproductive organs. Their functions are to store follicles, to produce mature ova, and to produce and secrete estrogen, progesterone, and androgens. Ovarian functions are readily disturbed by acute and chronic diseases. These functions can also be altered or interrupted by surgery, radiation, and the ingestion of drugs such as oral contraceptives. After menopause the ovaries undergo rapid regressive changes and decrease in size.

Endocrine functions

The major hormones produced by the ovaries are estrogen and progesterone. *Estrogen* is the hormone responsible for the development of secondary sex characteristics at the time of puberty. After puberty the primary function of estrogen is to cause development of the endometrium in preparation for implantation of a fertilized ovum. Estrogen causes the retention of calcium and phosphorus and thus promotes bone growth. After menopause the decline of estrogen levels may account for some of the symptoms that sometimes occur, such as hot flashes, osteoporosis (loss of calcium from bone), and vaginal atrophy. *Progesterone* enhances the action of estrogen on the endometrium. It also prevents muscular contractions of the myometrium as an aid for maintaining pregnancy should the ovum become implanted.

Secretion of ovarian hormones is cyclic, with each cycle requiring an average of 28 days. Unless stimulated by pituitary hormones, however, the ovaries do not fulfill their hormone-secreting and ovum-producing functions.

The phases of the menstrual cycle are illustrated in Fig. 35-2 and described in Box 35-1. The secretory (luteal) phase is the least variable part of the menstrual cycle. Irregular menstrual cycles are most frequently related to longer or shorter menstrual or proliferative (follicular) phases.

On the day of ovulation, about 25% of women experience pain in the lower abdomen on the side of ovulation. This pain (mittelschmerz) is probably a result of peritoneal irritation from follicular fluid or blood released from the ovary with the ovum. This sign rarely occurs with every

---

35-1

Menstrual cycle

Menstrual phase (menstruation): Day 1 to day 4
Estrogen and progesterone withdrawn before onset of menstrual flow
Shedding of endometrial lining

Proliferative (follicular) phase: Day 5 to day 14
Regrowth of endometrial tissue
Secretion of follicle-stimulating hormone (FSH) by the pituitary gland
Development in ovary of a mature graafian follicle containing a mature ovum
Secretion of increasing amounts of *estrogen* by graafian follicle
Suppression of FSH when estrogen level becomes high, leading to secretion of luteinizing hormone (LH) by pituitary gland

Secretory (luteal) phase: Day 15 to days 25 to 28
Rupture of graafian follicle releasing ovum (ovulation) starts the secretory phase
Movement of ovum through fallopian tube to uterus
Formation of corpus luteum at site of ruptured graafian follicle
Production of *progesterone* by corpus luteum
Stimulation by progesterone of endometrial cell growth
Significant decrease in progesterone level if implantation does not occur; menstrual phase then begins again

---

cycle and is therefore an unreliable indicator of ovulation. If the pain occurs on the right side and is severe, it may be mistaken for appendicitis.

Male Genital System

The male reproductive organs and associated structures are shown in Fig. 35-3. The male reproductive organs produce sperm, suspend the sperm in a liquid, and deliver the sperm into the vagina to fertilize an ovum. Another important function is secretion of male hormones, the androgens. Sperm are produced in the testes and are conveyed through the vas (ductus) deferens to the urethra. Semen consists of sperm with fluids from the seminal vesicles and the prostate gland. The prostate gland is important clinically because of its affinity for congestive, inflammatory, hyperplastic, and malignant disease. Because the prostate gland encircles the urethra, even benign enlargement (hypertrophy) may lead to obstruction of the urethra.

The male hormone *testosterone* is produced by the interstitial cells of the testes and is responsible for development of the genitalia during puberty and for maintaining the genitalia in a functional state during life. Androgenic hormones are also responsible for the development of secondary sex characteristics including growth of body hair and thickening of the vocal cords. Testosterone secretion is closely related to pituitary gland function, and the rate of secretion is determined by levels of luteinizing hormone (LH) in the blood. Secretion of testosterone decreases slowly with age.

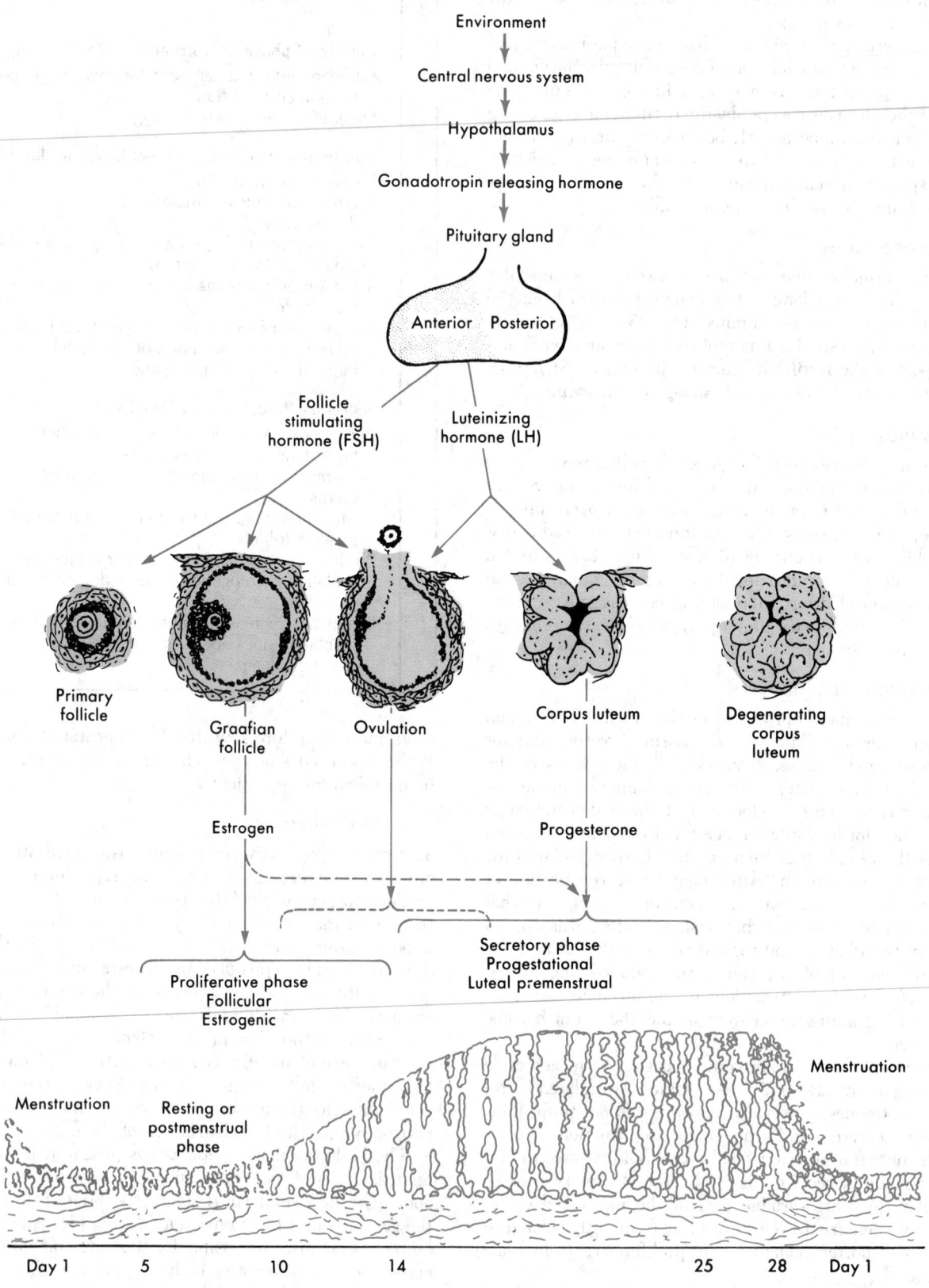

Fig. 35-2 Hormone control of menstrual cycle.

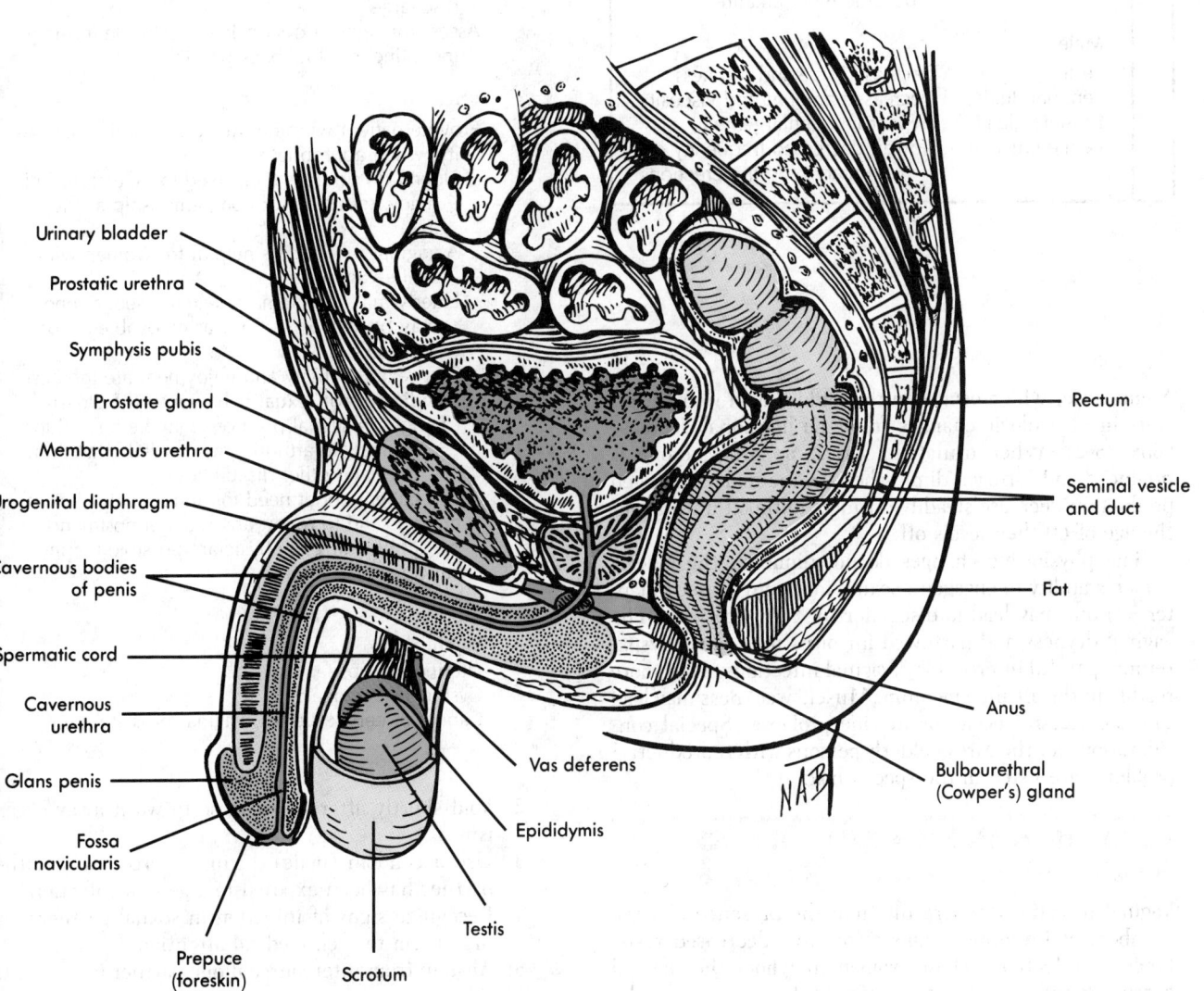

Urinary bladder

Prostatic urethra

Symphysis pubis

Prostate gland

Membranous urethra

Urogenital diaphragm

Cavernous bodies of penis

Spermatic cord

Cavernous urethra

Glans penis

Fossa navicularis

Prepuce (foreskin)

Scrotum

Testis

Epididymis

Vas deferens

Rectum

Seminal vesicle and duct

Fat

Anus

Bulbourethral (Cowper's) gland

Fig. 35-3   Male organs of reproduction.

<table>
<tr><td colspan="2">

35-2

Physiologic changes in reproductive tract with aging

</td></tr>
</table>

Female	
Uterus	Decreased size
Ovaries	Atrophy, with decreased size
Vagina	Decreased width and length
	Vaginal entrance (introitus) narrowed
	Vaginal secretions decrease and become more alkaline
Male	
Testes	Decreased size and firmness
Seminal fluid	Decreased amount and viscosity
Prostate gland	Hypertrophy (enlargement)
Penile erection	Slower, decreased frequency of involuntary morning erections

Physiologic Changes With Aging

Menopause, which occurs in the middle-aged woman, results in physiologic changes from the hormonal decrease (Box 35-2). When ovulation ceases, no progesterone is produced and estrogen diminishes. In the male, androgen production decrease steadily during adulthood until about the age of 60 then levels off.

The physiologic changes do not diminish the elderly person's ability to engage in sexual intercourse (see Chapter 34) but may lead to discomfort or complications. The vaginal dryness and narrowed introitus may cause dyspareunia (painful intercourse). Vaginal infections occur more readily in the alkaline medium. Muscle weakness may lead to cystocele, rectocele, or uterine prolapse. Special considerations for the care of elderly persons with reproducti problems are listed in the special box.

PREVENTION AND HEALTH EDUCATION
Primary Prevention: Prevention of Infection

Vaginal infections may result from the presence of large numbers of invading organisms or from decreased resistance to infection. Those women in whom the natural barriers to infection are at a minimum (low estrogen levels, thinness of the vaginal epithelium, or reduced acidity of the vagina) are at greatest risk (Box 35-3).

Large numbers of organisms may invade the vagina or urethra from inadequate personal hygiene, from another person during sexual intercourse, or from use of unclean articles such as douche nozzles. Decreased resistance to infection may result from vaginal secretions becoming more alkaline, providing a more suitable medium for bacterial growth. Vaginal yeast infections may be a side effect of drugs such as the tetracyclines or oral contraceptives. Preventive measures include the following:

1. Wipe from front to back (female) after bowel movements

The Elderly with Sexuality and Reproductive Problems

Assessment

Determine meaning of sexuality to patient; age does not imply loss of sexuality.

Assess for problems engaging in sexual intercourse because of disability or disease.

Determine frequency of regular gynecologic examination in elderly women; some women are not aware that these examinations should be continued after menopause.

Assess for signs of vaginitis (vaginal pruritus and discharge).

Assess for signs of cystocele or rectocele (urinary incontinence, low back pain).

Intervention

Provide patient with information regarding sexuality, when appropriate.

Elderly do not lose their need for affection, intimacy, touching, or companionship as they age.

A vaginal lubricant is helpful for women with senile vaginitis.

Elderly male and female sexual responsiveness may be slower, but just as enjoyable as for younger adults.

Past sexual activity and enjoyment are the best indicators of sexual behavior in the elderly.

Changes in sexual positions may be helpful for patients with arthritis, myocardial infarction, stroke, and other disabilities.

Teach patient about need for annual pelvic examinations and to report any signs of postmenopausal bleeding to physician (possible uterine cancer).

Common disorders in elderly

Vaginitis
Uterine prolapse
Cystocele, rectocele
Cancer of cervix, uterus, vagina, prostate, penis

2. Void shortly after intercourse to wash away organ isms

3. Use a condom (male) during intercourse if eithe partner has been exposed to a genital infection

4. Recognize signs of infection in sexual partners an urge them to seek medical attention

5. Abstain from intercourse if one partner has a genit infection

6. Avoid douching (which may alter vaginal pH) unles advised by a physician for treatment

7. Seek immediate medical attention for early signs vaginal infection (abnormal vaginal discharge, vag nal itching), especially in persons at high risk.

Secondary Prevention: Early Detection of Cancer

Dramatically decreased rates of death from cancer are a sociated with early detection and treatment. Persons high risk for cancer of the cervix include women who wer sexually active at an early age and those with multiple se partners. Sexually transmitted diseases (STDs) that ar associated with cervical cancer include human papillo

---

35-3

Risk factors for vaginal infections

Aging
Diabetes
Pregnancy
Malnutrition
Inadequate perineal hygiene
Excessive douching
Use of vaginal inserts
Oral contraceptives
Broad-spectrum antibiotics
Intercourse with infected partner

35-4

Risk factors for uterine cancer

Cancer of the cervix
First sexual intercourse at early age
Multiple sexual partners
Cigarette smoking
Certain STDs

Cancer of the endometrium
History of infertility
Failure of ovulation
Prolonged estrogen therapy without added progestin
Late menopause
Combination of diabetes, high blood pressure, and obesity

35-5

Examinations for prevention of uterine cancer as recommended by the American Cancer Society

1. After three or more consecutive annual Pap tests with normal findings, test may be performed less frequently at discretion of physician.
2. More frequent Pap tests for persons at high risk
3. Endometrial tissue sample at menopause for persons at high risk for endometrial cancer

---

35-6

Patient Teaching

Menstruation

Knowledge of the physiologic process
Factors that may alter the menstrual cycle: stress, fatigue, exercise, acute and chronic illness, changes in climate or working hours, pregnancy
Personal hygiene
  Wear pads during early period of heavy flow
  Change tampons frequently to decrease risk of toxic shock syndrome
  Consult a physician if tampons cause discomfort
  Take a daily bath for comfort (warm bath may relieve slight pelvic discomfort)
Exercise
  Exercise is not contraindicated and may help prevent discomfort
  Modify exercise if fatigue occurs
Diet
  Restrict salt intake if fluid retention is present
  Consult physician if fluid retention persists after menstruation
Discomfort (dysmenorrhea)
  For mild discomfort take aspirin, acetaminophen, or ibuprofen (Motrin), apply warmth, rest
  For prolonged severe discomfort, consult physician.

---

mavirus (HPV) and *Herpesvirus hominis* type 2 (HVH-2) (see Chapter 18). High-risk factors for endometrial cancer include early problems with menstruation or ovulation or late menopause, lack of progestin with prolonged estrogen therapy, and obesity[1] (Box 35-4).

The decline in deaths from cervical cancer is primarily the result of increased use of the Papanicolaou (Pap) smear for mass screening, combined with more frequent and more thorough gynecologic examinations. Cancer of the cervix is easier to detect through Pap smear than is cancer of the endometrium.

Health teaching for prevention of uterine cancer includes regular pelvic examinations that include a Pap smear. Recommendations of the American Cancer Society to detect cancer early are listed in Box 35-5.

Health Teaching Related to Menstruation and Menopause

Menstruation

Menstruation occurs on an average of every 28 days; the normal range is 26 to 34 days. The menstrual flow usually lasts for 3 to 7 days (average 4 days). Normally 30 to 180 ml (average 50 ml) of menstrual fluid is lost during the period. One half to three fourths of the fluid is blood, and the remainder is mucus, fragments of endometrial cells, and desquamated vaginal epithelium.

Normally menstrual fluid does not clot unless it is retained in the uterus or vagina for a prolonged time. It is believed that the endometrium produces an anticoagulant that prevents clotting of blood in the uterus. An occasional very small clot may occur during the first 24 hours, and this is probably a particle of endometrial tissue. Large clots or pus in the menstrual flow are never normal.

During pregnancy menstruation ceases, and then returns within 6 to 8 weeks after delivery, although lactation suppresses the menses for varying periods of time. Unless disease occurs, the menstrual periods recur during adult life until menopause.

Menstruation is a manifestation of normal body function and should be treated as such. The "period" and "monthly period" are accurate terms to use if the woman does not wish to say "menstruating." Terms such as "being sick," "on the rag," or "having the curse" are to be avoided because of their negative connotation. Suggestions for health teaching related to menstruation are listed in Box 35-6.

Table 35-1 Activities to modify PMS discomfort

PMS symptoms	Activity
Behavioral changes	Increase intake of foods rich in vitamin B₆ (yeast, wheat germ, whole-grain cereals, liver, legumes); decrease dairy products intake; increase outdoor exercise
Water and sodium retention	Restrict salt intake; restrict intake of coffee, tea, cola, chocolate; increase intake of foods rich in vitamin B₆ (see above)
Increased appetite, (especially for sweets), headache, fatigue	Restrict free sugar, sodium, and animal fat intake; substitute complex carbohydrates for simple sugars
Depression	Increase intake of green leafy vegetables, legumes, and whole-grain cereals (high in B vitamins)

Adapted from Abraham G: Nutritional factors in the etiology of the premenstrual tension syndrome, *J Reprod Med* 28:446-464, 1983.

To become knowledgeable about the patterns of their menstrual cycles, women are encouraged to keep a written record. Establishing this habit makes it possible to predict the onset of the next menstrual period and to determine the range of cycles and duration of flow. Should it be necessary to seek the attention of a health professional for any reason, it is helpful to know the date of onset of the last menstrual period (LMP).

Premenstrual syndrome

Premenstrual syndrome (PMS), which occurs in approximately 10% of all menstruating women, is the presence of symptoms in the premenstruum or early menstruation with the absence of postmenstrual symptoms. Identical symptoms must occur in three consecutive cycles to confirm a diagnosis of PMS. Symptoms vary considerably among women and may include behavioral changes (tension, irritability, mood swings, anxiety, crying, depression, insomnia), fatigue, signs of water and sodium retention (edema, weight gain, breast enlargement and tenderness, and abdominal bloating), palpitations, increased appetite, headache, and backache.[27] The cause is unknown although many factors have been suggested.

The nurse can assist women with PMS by acknowledging the existence of the syndrome and its attendant symptoms, which may be severe for some women. Encourage women to keep a menstrual symptom calendar to document the cyclic nature of the symptoms.[27]

Simple measures to relieve PMS symptoms include dietary changes, not smoking and drinking, and participating in planned exercise. A diet high in complex carbohydrates, moderate in protein, and low in refined sugar and sodium should be eaten, especially during the premenstrual interval. The consumption of caffeine (in tea, coffee, caffeine-containing beverages), chocolate, and alcohol, and smoking should be reduced or eliminated. Regular exercise

---

35-7

Causes of dysmenorrhea

Primary dysmenorrhea
High concentration of uterine prostaglandins

Secondary dysmenorrhea
Pelvic inflammatory disease
Endometriosis
Malpositioned uterus
Cervical stenosis

---

three to four times a week for 30 minutes is encouraged, especially during the premenstrual interval. Because fatigue may exaggerate PMS symptoms, adequate rest, sleep, and relaxation are helpful. Additional activities are listed in Table 35-1. Information can be obtained from PMS Action, Inc.*

Dysmenorrhea

Although menstruation is a normal physiologic process, some women experience varying degrees of discomfort (menstrual cramps). Dysmenorrhea is the greatest single cause of absenteeism by women from school or work. Dysmenorrhea may result from various causes (Box 35-7). An intrauterine device (IUD) may also cause menstrual discomfort. Primary dysmenorrhea often disappears after pregnancy or by age 25.

Women who are consistently unable to engage in usual activities because of pain associated with menstruation should be urged to seek health care for diagnosis and treatment of any existing secondary dysmenorrhea.

Treatment of secondary dysmenorrhea is aimed at the organic cause. Surgical and pharmacologic interventions may be appropriate depending on the severity and type of pathology. If the uterus is found to be in an abnormal position and can be manually returned to a normal position, a pessary may be inserted for a trial period to learn whether malposition is the cause of dysmenorrhea. Dilation of the cervical canal is done when a cervical stricture is found and thought to be the cause of dysmenorrhea.

If no organic cause of dysmenorrhea can be found, the woman is advised to try rest, moderate exercise, and avoidance of constipation. Local application of heat and mild analgesics are usually prescribed. Aspirin is a prostaglandin antagonist. Heat causes vasodilation of blood vessels, thereby increasing the blood flow and relieving ischemia, increasing elimination of the menstrual flow, and decreasing muscle hypertonus.

Because protaglandins cause uterine contractions, medications that usually give the best relief of discomfort are the prostaglandin inhibitors. These drugs include ibuprofen (Motrin, Rufen), mefenamic acid (Ponstel), naproxen (Naprosyn, Anaprox), and fenoprofen calcium (Nalfon). Motrin can be obtained without a prescription. These drugs are effective when started at the onset of bleeding. Encourage taking prostaglandin inhibitors with milk or

*PO Box 16292, Irvine, CA 92713.

food to prevent side effects. Oral contraceptives have also been used to suppress ovulation by inhibiting prostaglandin levels.

Other measures that may be explored include systematic relaxation, exercise, muscle toning, massage, effleurage, breathing techniques, manual pressure on the abdomen, and orgasm. Biofeedback and autogenic training have also been used. Positive attitudes toward menstruation and alternative interventions from which to select the most useful interventions are helpful for the woman experiencing dysmenorrhea.

Menopause

The *climacteric* is the transitional phase between reproductive and nonreproductive ability. Menopause is said to have occurred when there has been no menstrual flow for 1 year (although some women have periods even after 1 year of amenorrhea). During the climacteric, which usually lasts for 12 to 18 months, there is a gradual decline in ovarian function. The ovaries gradually cease to produce ova and estrogen, and as a result the menses become scanty, irregular, and further apart, until they stop altogether.

Natural menopause may occur between 35 and 60 years of age (average age 51 years). Cigarette smoking and living at high altitudes are associated with early menopause.

Menopause may be artificially induced by such procedures as irradiation of the ovaries, surgical removal of both ovaries, or hysterectomy. Each of these has one common consequence, namely, cessation of menstruation. However, surgical removal or irradiation of the ovaries results in menopause with all its physiologic changes, whereas ovaries left intact after hysterectomy will continue to function provided the age of climacteric has not yet been reached.

Physiologic factors in menopause

Physiologic changes in the genital organs as a result of loss of hormonal functioning are listed in Box 35-2, p. 1126. Because sexual functioning does not depend on the release of ova or hormones, women can enjoy sexual activity during the climacteric and after the menopause.

Many women go through the climacteric with little awareness of its occurrence. Some women, however, experience *hot flashes (flushes),* which are felt as waves of warmth accompanied by flushing of the skin, especially the face, neck, and arms, and perspiration. The hot flash is the perception of the spread of heat from an anatomic point of origin on the body to other areas of the body. Hot flashes may be so mild that they are hardly noticed or so severe that they produce distress. Estrogen may be prescribed by the physician for severe discomfort. During estrogen therapy women should be seen at least every 6 months for examination because of increased risk of endometrial cancer and for review of menopausal symptoms. The examination should include the breasts and reproductive organs, Pap smear, and blood pressure.

Vaginal changes (vaginal dryness, burning, itching, and occasional bleeding after menopause) result from thinning of the vaginal mucosa because of decreased estrogen. Vaginal infections occur more frequently because vaginal secretions are more alkaline. Estrogen therapy helps decrease vaginal difficulties.

Patient Teaching 35-8

Menopause

Knowledge about menopause
  Cessation of ovarian function with cessation of menstruation over 12 to 18 months
  Changes in reproductive ability
    Conception still possible during the period of change
      Contraception should be used for 1 year after last menstrual period
      Rhythm method unreliable contraceptive method during this period
    Ability to conceive ceases when menopause completed
  Sexual ability still present
  Physical symptoms vary from mild to severe; estrogen therapy may be given to relieve severe symptoms
Promotion of health and physical appearance
  Moderate exercise to maintain muscle tone and help prevent osteoporosis
  Dietary control to prevent weight gain
  Calcium supplement to prevent osteoporosis
  Activities that encourage self-esteem and interest outside of self
  Peer support groups during menopause, if necessary
Prevention of discomfort
  Relief of vasomotor reactions (hot flashes)
    Moderation of factors identified by the person as exacerbating hot flashes (excitement, alcoholic beverages, heavy eating, excessive clothing, impairment of heat loss in hot weather)
  Vitamin E or B complex vitamins
  Prevention of dyspareunia (painful intercourse): local application of lubricant or vaginal cream
  Relief of vaginal itching: vitamin E or estrogen therapy

Skeletal changes may also occur from lack of estrogen. About 25% of postmenopausal women develop *osteoporosis* characterized by decreased bone mineral content and bone calcium. Osteoporotic problems include back pain, decreased height and mobility, and fractures of the spine, arm, upper femur, and ribs (Chapter 40). A significant factor in the development of osteoporosis is a low calcium/high phosphorus imbalance. Many women ingest inadequate amounts of calcium; an intake of 1200 mg of calcium daily is desirable (1500 mg for postmenopausal women). For absorption of calcium, 400 IU of vitamin D a day is needed. Estrogen replacement therapy is protective against osteoporosis for as long as it is administered.

Counseling and teaching

Most women have heard of the "change of life." The negative image of menopause is reinforced by the media, books, health professionals, and the general public. Depending on the climate in which they were reared and on their own changes in attitude toward normal functions of the reproductive organs, women may feel more or less free to discuss menopause and their feelings and concerns during this period of life. Because many problems related to the reproductive organs occur in this age group, and because it is important for mental health that women be helped to make menopause as comfortable as possible, it is important for nurses to identify women who can profit from interventions.

Feelings of depression and uselessness may occur, particularly among women who have been highly invested in the maternal role. Peer support groups may be very helpful in these situations.

Education regarding menopause should precede its onset (Box 35-8). Women approaching menopause, regardless of whether it is an event of normal aging or is artificially induced, need to know what menopause is, why it occurs, the effects menopause has on reproductive and sexual ability, what can be done to make menopause more comfortable, and those symptoms that require medical attention.

INTERFERENCES WITH REPRODUCTION

The ability to have children may be modified either to prevent conception or to terminate a pregnancy (Box 35-9). Some persons are unable to procreate. The topics of contraception and abortion are covered in maternity nursing texts and are not repeated here.

Sterilization

Voluntary sterilization has become increasingly acceptable to both men and women as a method of preventing pregnancy. It is the most commonly used method of fertility control for married couples older than 30 years. Sterilization may also be performed in selected instances where pregnancy would create risks to the health or life of the woman or infant (for example, heart disease, severe diabetes, probable genetic defects to the infant).

Because sterilization may be a permanent method of contraception, it is absolutely necessary to obtain voluntary, informed consent. Patients receiving federal funds for sterilization must be at least 21 years old and mentally competent.

Methods of sterilization

Methods of sterilization are described in Table 35-2. The abdominal approaches are favored by some physicians be-

cause they are familiar with the female pelvic anatomy as viewed from the abdomen and because the fallopian tubes are free and suspended in this position, which makes them easy to see, manipulate, and ligate or cauterize. The vaginal approach is favored by some physicians and women because of the absence of a visible scar, ease of peritoneal entry, and rapid postoperative recovery; however, because of its higher complication rate, it is less frequently used today.

Successful sterilization (conception prevented) is dependent on the technique used and the surgeon's experience in performing the procedure. The main causes of failure in the female are recanalization of the fallopian tube, erroneous ligation, and pregnancy resulting from tuboperitoneal fistula. In the male spontaneous recanalization (reanastomosis) may occur; the cause is unknown but duplication of the vas deferens has occasionally been noted.

Effects of sterilization
Physiologic effects

Although tubal sterilization usually terminates a woman's ability to bear children, ovarian hormones and menstrual functioning are not altered and artificial menopause is not induced. Ability to derive satisfaction from sexual intercourse should not be impaired, and some women may experience greater enjoyment from intercourse free from fear of pregnancy.

Because vasectomy interrupts the continuity of the vas deferens, sperm are prevented from being ejaculated with other components of the semen. However, sperm are still produced and the ejaculate is not noticeably diminished in amount. Residual fertility lasting for a variable period is present because of sperm in the semen beyond the point of occlusion of the vas. Sperm *gradually* disappear from the ejaculate; thus conception is possible in the immediate

---

35-9

Interferences with reproduction	
Contraception	Process of temporary prevention of impregnation or conception
Sterilization	Process of making an individual incapable of reproducing, either permanently or until the process is reversed
Abortion	Termination of a pregnancy before the fetus is viable
Infertility	Inability to achieve a pregnancy within a stipulated time (at least 1 year) of unprotected sexual intercourse

---

35-10

Informed consent guidelines (federal) relating to sterilization

Choice is made by patient, without pressures (for example, loss of welfare benefits, wrath of health care provider).
Benefits and risks of sterilization are described:
  Benefits: permanent, no further costs or decision making.
  Risks: usual surgical risks, possibility of future pregnancy (not 100% effective).
Alternative contraceptive methods are described.
Patient is encouraged to ask questions.
Patient may decide not to undergo sterilization without penalty.
Explanations are given about the entire sterilization procedure, costs, and possible side effects (effects on hormones, weight changes, menstrual changes, sexual response).
Written instruction and risk factors are explained to patient.
Written consent to the procedure is signed by patient and witnessed; husband's consent is optional.
  After consent, a 30-day waiting period must precede the sterilization.

postoperative period. Semen analysis will determine when sperm have finally disappeared.

Psychologic effects

Men and women who elect sterilization seem to have little or no regret after surgery if they understand what to expect during and after the procedure and are able to express their feelings and have questions answered before the procedure. Persons with preexisting emotional problems have reported depression, loss of self-esteem, guilt, and difficulty in sexual adjustment after surgery.

Preoperative care

Preoperative counseling is indicated to identify men and women before surgery who may later have strong regrets and emotional problems. One aim of counseling before surgery is to confirm that the decision for sterilization is made as objectively as possible. Previous experience with other methods of contraception can be explored and reasons for dissatisfaction with the methods determined. There may be lack of knowledge about contraceptive methods, and with adequate information the couple might choose a means other than sterilization. Young persons and those who are unhappy about pregnancies or who have marital problems are poor candidates for sterilization because they may change their minds at a later date. The discussion of sterilization methods should be based on the federal government's informed consent guidelines (Box 35-10).

Postoperative care

Many sterilization procedures are performed on an outpatient basis, and the patient can be discharged when the effects of general anesthesia have worn off and vital signs are stable. If the patient expresses feelings of guilt or regret about having been sterilized, a review of the reasons for sterilization and positive effect on sexual relationships may need to be repeated. Teaching guidelines following a sterilization procedure are described in Box 35-11.

Patient Teaching   35-11

The patient who has had a sterilization procedure

Woman

Rest for 24 to 48 hours after procedure
No heavy lifting or strenuous exercise for 1 week
Abstain from sexual intercourse
   Abdominal method: until wound is healed and no discomfort is present
   Vaginal method: 1 week
Report to physician signs of fever, persistent abdominal pain, or bleeding from incision

Man

Apply ice to scrotum, take sitz baths for minor discomfort and swelling
Wear scrotal support for 48 hours
Rest for 48 hours after procedure
No heavy lifting or strenuous exercise for 1 week
Abstain from sexual intercourse for 3 days
Use an alternate method of contraception until physician reports semen no longer contains sperm
Report to physician signs of fever, persistent scrotal pain, or profuse incisional bleeding

---

Table 35-2   Methods of sterilization

Method	Description	Comments
Female		
Tubal sterilization		
Abdominal		
Minilaparotomy	Ligation or cutting of fallopian tubes under direct vision through small abdominal incision	Local or general anesthesia Complications: wound infection, hematoma, bladder injury Advantages: good chance for sterility reversal
Laparoscopy	Electrocoagulation and sectioning of segment of fallopian tubes by laparoscopy through small abdominal incision	Local or general anesthesia Advantages: minimal discomfort, short procedure
Vaginal		
Culpotomy	Ligation or cutting of fallopian tube through small incision in cul-de-sac of Douglas	Local, spinal, or general anesthesia Higher complication rate than laparoscopy (infection, hemorrhage)
Culdoscopy	Electrocoagulation of segment of fallopian tubes by culdoscope through small incision in cul-de-sac of Douglas	Local anesthesia Higher complication rate than laparoscopy
Male		
Vasectomy	Removal of a segment of vas deferens through small incision in scrotum	Local anesthesia Complications rare Bruising, mild edema, and mild discomfort common

Causes of infertility

Disorder	Effect
Female	
Obstructions of fallopian tubes	Interfere with transport of ovum
Diseases of body or cervix of uterus	Inhibit passage of active sperm
Hormonal deficiencies	Inhibit release of ovum
	Inhibit development of endometrium for implantation
Male	
Obstruction of vas deferens	Interfere with transport of sperm
Diseases of testes, undescended testes, hormonal deficiencies	Inhibit development of sperm
Sperm-bound immunoglobulins	Inhibit sperm penetration of ovum

Sterilization reversal

Requests for reversal of previous sterilization may be made because of divorce and remarriage, death of children or change in economic status, as well as for other reasons. The chances of reversing the effects of sterilization are improving as a result of refinement of microsurgical techniques.

Reconstruction of the fallopian tubes involves an end-to-end anastomosis of the ligated or dissected tubes. Success of restoration of tubal function is partly dependent on the original surgery performed, especially regarding the length of the tubal portion excised. Ligation of the tubes produces adhesions that must be dissected away to the point of tubal patency; this reduces the amount of remaining tubal structure. Also the length of the fallopian tube remaining after reconstruction may play a role in permitting adequate time for the fertilized ovum to undergo maturational changes in preparation for implantation. Reports of success after microsurgical reversal are reported to be 40% to 75%.[22]

In the male, reconstruction consists in attempting to rejoin the severed ends of the vas deferens (vasovasostomy). Success is measured by the presence of sperm in the semen after reconstruction. Reports of success in restoring fertility range from 29% to 85%.[22]

Infertility

It has been estimated that 10% to 15% of all couples in the United States are infertile. Approximately 50% of couples who undergo assessment and treatment for infertility are likely to conceive. Although infertility is most often attributed to women, in about 40% of infertile marriages the man is infertile.[22]

The fertility of a couple is affected by coital frequency and the age of the man and the woman. Increased coital frequency enhances fertility. Frequent ejaculation improves sperm motility unless ejaculation is excessive, which results in depletion of available sperm. Fertility peaks at age 24 years in women and age 25 years in men.

Cause and prevention

There are many causes of infertility in men and women (Box 35-12). Some are preventable or correctable, others are not. There is no known cause in 10% to 20% of infertility cases.

One of the most common preventable causes of infertility in women is infection of the pelvic organs (PID), especially as a result of gonorrhea and chlamydia, which cause obstruction of the fallopian tubes. Such serious consequences are preventable through prophylactic use of penicillin for women exposed to gonorrhea and through early diagnosis and treatment of all vaginal and cervical infections. Gonococcal cultures should be obtained every 6 months for women with multiple partners. If infection is present and the woman has an IUD, the device should be removed. Barrier contraceptives reduce the risk for infections and PID.

Many of the ovarian and hormonal problems that cause infertility produce symptoms such as menstrual irregularities and ill health before a problem with conception is ever recognized. Many of these problems can be managed with hormone therapy, provided women seek help at an early age or as soon as deviations are noticed. Birth control pills should be avoided by women who have not established normal menses.

In males, bilateral undescended tests (cryptorchidism) should be corrected surgically before puberty. The incidence of testicular cancer in undescended testes is 30% to 50% higher than in descended testes.[58] In later life cryptorchidism may produce sterility because of failure of the testes to develop their sperm-producing function, even if the condition is surgically corrected. Destruction of testicular tissue by infectious processes can be prevented through prompt treatment when symptoms first appear.

Assessment

It is important that couples who wish to have children seek medical advice if they are unsuccessful after about a year of trying to achieve pregnancy. Infertility evaluation often requires a long time.

Attempts to correct infertility are based on data obtained through a detailed history and physical examination as well as from laboratory tests and clinical studies. A sexual history is taken and sexual practices are reviewed. Suggestions about sexual intercourse are given if this seems to be the problem. The couple should attempt to be at the first interview together because they share responsibility for infertility, information is needed by both partners, and this

35-13

Examination for infertility

Tests	Data obtained
Male	
Multiple semen examination	Determine presence, number, and motility of sperm
Testicular biopsy if sperm count low or absent	Presence of sperm indicates obstruction of vas deferens
Female	
Basal body temperature chart	Determines that ovulation is occurring
Postcoital test of cervical secretions	Measure ability of sperm to penetrate cervical mucus and remain active, and quality of the mucus
Endometrial biopsy, serum progesterone and estradiol levels, laparoscopic inspection of ovaries	Determine whether ovulation is occurring (if in question)
Laparoscopy	Determine patency of fallopian tubes
Hysterosalpingography (x-ray after insertion of contrast media)	Determine patency of uterus and fallopian tubes
Hormonal tests for males and females	Determine whether the problem is hormonal

may be their first opportunity to confront their feelings about being infertile.

Examination of the man

Many physicians prefer to carry out examination of the man first, because it is more easily accomplished and less time consuming. Stricture and varicoceles (dilated veins of the spermatic cords) may be corrected by surgery.

If sperm count and motility of sperm are low, thyroid extract and vitamins may be prescribed along with a well-balanced diet, rest, and moderate exercise. A lack of vitamins A and E in the diet may cause some atrophy of the sperm-producing structures. The couple is advised to have intercourse every other day during the fertile period (usually 12 to 16 days before the beginning of the next menstrual period). When the man is completely aspermatic, conception is impossible, and the couple should be counseled regarding the alternatives available to them.

Examination of the woman

If the man is found to be fertile, examination of the woman is carried out (Box 35-13). If sperm are being destroyed by vaginal and cervical secretions, smears from these sites are studied. If the secretions are too acid or too alkaline, medicated douches may be prescribed. A douche with sodium bicarbonate (15 ml to 1L water) performed just before intercourse has been found to increase the motility of sperm in many cases. Tubal strictures or obstructions are sometimes repaired by microsurgery. Underlying metabolic diseases are corrected if possible.

Coping with infertility

Couples who wish to have children but find themselves unable to do so experience immeasurable emotional distress. Feelings of inadequacy are common, as are anger and guilt. The infertile couple must confront feelings about lack of control, self-image, self-esteem, and sexuality. Couples who are informed that they will never be able to have children experience a life crisis with all of its ramifications,

and they have a strong need to grieve. Those who are told that they are a normal and fertile couple, but for whom pregnancy does not result despite months or years of tests, studies, examinations, and advice, commonly have feelings of frustration alternating with hope.

All these couples require emotional support, including encouragement to grieve, to express their anger and other feelings in order to regain objectivity and to avoid premature decisions and actions about alternatives. The urgent need for such support is reflected in the emergence of support groups organized by infertile individuals and couples.

Alternative infertility approaches

Among the alternatives available to infertile couples are adoption, remaining childless, artificial insemination, in vitro fertilization, and surrogate motherhood.

Artificial insemination is the placement of a few drops of donor semen in the cervicovaginal, intracervical, or intrauterine (more painful) area. It is simple, safe, inexpensive, and highly successful. The major indication for artificial insemination is male infertility. Previous loss of children because of Rh or ABO incompatibility or severe hereditary defects transmitted by the man are other indications. Therefore, artificial insemination is not reserved exclusively for infertile couples.

Artificial insemination is homologous (AIH) when the partner's semen is used and heterologous (AID) when donor semen is used. Criteria for donor selection is based on semen analysis as well as on a complete history and physical examination. Donor candidates with venereal disease, diabetes, hepatitis, blood diseases, prostatic infection, AIDS, and a family history of hereditary disorders are excluded. Fertility of donors must be proved by semen analysis.

In vitro fertilization (IVF) involves recovering one or more of the woman's ova from her ovarian follicles through laparoscopy and fertilizing the ova with the partner's sperm in a petri dish. If fertilization and cleavage occur, the resulting embryos are transferred into the woman's uterus about 48 hours after the ova retrieval has taken place. This procedure is indicated for women with complete blockage of the fallopian tubes, for oligospermia of the male, for immunologic causes of infertility, and for unexplained infertility. The chance of a successful pregnancy is about 20% per IVF attempt, so the odds are very much against any one couple achieving a pregnancy.

Gamete intrafallopian transfer (GIFT) consists of aspirating oocytes from follicles by laparoscopy or minilaparotomy, or by vaginal aspiration. The oocyte is mixed with washed sperm and then placed in the fallopian tube by laparoscopy or minilaparotomy. The preembryo travels to the uterus for implantation 4 days after ovulation on a natural timetable. Higher pregnancy rates have been obtained with GIFT than with IVF.

Zygote intrafallopian transfer (ZIFT) consists of aspirating oocytes transvaginally guided by ultrasound, mixing the oocytes with sperm, then placing the fertilized ova (zygotes) in the uterine end of the fallopian tube.

Surrogate mothers are women who contract to conceive by artificial insemination and give the baby to the semen donor after delivery. There are many social, moral, psychologic, and legal implications surrounding this approach.

MAJOR HEALTH PROBLEMS OF THE REPRODUCTIVE SYSTEM

The major problems of the reproductive system include inflammation, structural disorders, tumors, and sexually transmitted diseases. The first three types of disorders are discussed separately in this chapter for women and men because of the inherent anatomic differences. Sexually transmitted diseases are discussed in the Infection Unit (Chapter 18). The various disorders that fall within the cited categories are as follows:

1. Female disorders
   a. Inflammatory disorders: vaginitis, cervicitis, pelvic inflammatory disease, toxic shock syndrome
   b. Structural disorders: relaxed vaginal outlet, uterine displacement, uterine prolapse, fistulas
   c. Tumors: ovarian tumors and cysts, endometriosis, uterine fibroid tumors, cervical polyps, and cancer of the cervix, endometrium, and ovary
2. Male disorders
   a. Inflammatory disorders: urethritis, prostatitis, epididymitis, orchitis
   b. Structural disorders: hydrocele, spermatocele, varicocele, torsion of spermatic cord
   c. Tumors: cancer of the testes, prostate gland, penis

INFLAMMATORY DISORDERS IN WOMEN

Types of Inflammatory Disorders

Inflammations of the female reproductive tract are seen most commonly in the vagina, cervix, or fallopian tubes and adjacent areas (Table 35-3). Many of these infections can be prevented (p. 1126).

Etiology and Pathophysiology
Vulva and vagina

Normally the vagina is protected from infection by its pH and the presence of *Döderlein's bacilli*. If the vaginal pH is altered, if the invading organisms are numerous, or if the women's resistance is decreased by aging, malnutrition, stress, or disease, the risk of infection is increased. Yeast organisms grow best in an acid pH less than 4.7, whereas *Trichomonas* and organisms causing nonspecific vaginitis thrive in a pH greater than 5 (more alkaline).

Organisms causing infection of the vulva and vagina are most often introduced from outside sources such as clothing, hands, douche nozzles, or other contaminated articles or during intercourse. In sexually active women reinfection may occur after treatment unless their sexual partners are also successfully treated.

Women of menopausal and postmenopausal age often develop vaginitis (sometimes referred to as *atrophic* or *senile vaginitis*). Increased alkalinity of the vaginal secretions is a contributing cause, and the pyogenic bacterial invasion of the thin vaginal mucosa produces symptoms of burning, pruritus, and *leukorrhea* (whitish-yellow vaginal discharge).

Inflammation may also occur in Bartholin's glands or less frequently in Skene's glands. The infection is usually unilateral but may be bilateral. With infection the duct from the gland becomes partially or completely obstructed, resulting in severe redness, enlargement of the gland, and edema of the surrounding tissues. The area becomes tender, and walking may become painful. The usual result of the infectious process is an abscess. Occasionally, acute bartholinitis subsides, leaving fibrotic or scar tissue. When this occurs, a Bartholin's cyst develops. The cyst may vary in size, from a few centimeters in diameter to the size of a hen's egg and is mobile. Pain occurs with large cysts and with infection.

Cervix

Cervicitis, infection of the cervix, is the most common gynecologic disorder, affecting more than half of all women. There are two forms of cervicitis, acute and chronic, of which the chronic is the most frequent. Cervicitis usually progresses from the acute to the chronic form if not treated and it may go undetected for a long time. In fact, the cervix may heal and appear quite healthy after the disease has spread upward. This condition presents few symptoms, and those symptoms that occur do not ordinarily lead women to seek medical attention. If the vaginal discharge is slight, the women may not become concerned.

Cervicitis may follow childbirth or abortion or it may be caused by infection of a cervical laceration or erosion. In untreated cervicitis the tissues are constantly irritated, and there is some evidence that this irritation predisposes to cancer.

REVIEW

Table 35-3   Inflammatory disorders of the female reproductive tract

Disorder	Causative organisms	Signs and symptoms	Medical therapy
Vulvitis/vaginitis	*Candida, Trichomonas, Gardnerella,* coliform bacteria, *Gonococcus,* herpes simplex	Itching of vulva or vagina, vaginal discharge, dyspareunia	Antifungal agents, antibiotics (oral, topical, douches), sitz baths
Cervicitis	*Gonococcus, Chlamydia,* Streptococcus, Staphylococcus, herpes virus	Mucopurulent discharge, red, edematous cervix, low back pain	Antibiotics, cauterization of cervix (if eroded)
Pelvic inflammatory disease (salpingitis)	*Gonococcus, Chlamydia,* coliform bacteria, *Streptococcus, Mycoplasm,* anaerobic bacteria	Severe abdominal pain, lower abdominal cramps, intermenstrual spotting, dyspareunia, fever and chills, malaise, nausea and vomiting, foul-smelling purulent vaginal discharge	Cefoxitin with doxycycline, tetracycline; rest; heat to abdomen, analgesics, sexual abstinence until recovery
Toxic shock syndrome	Toxin from *Staphylococcus aureus*	High fever, vomiting, watery diarrhea, sore throat, myalgia, erythematous rash with desquamation; if severe, impaired renal, hepatic, cardiopulmonary function	Antibiotics, rapid hydration, supportive therapy for septic shock

Fallopian tubes

Inflammation of the fallopian tubes, *salpingitis,* may be local or more often may spread to the ovaries, pelvic peritoneum, pelvic veins, or pelvic connective tissue. This widespread inflammation is termed *pelvic inflammatory disease* (PID). The pathogens may invade the pelvic organs during sexual intercourse, childbirth or the postpartum period, or after abortion. Risk factors for PID include young age at first sexual intercourse, multiple sex partners, high frequency of sexual intercourse, and use of IUDs.[7] Contraceptive barrier methods *decrease* the risk of PID.

Pathogenic organisms are usually introduced from outside the body and pass up the cervical canal into the uterus. They seem to cause little trouble in the uterus but pass into the pelvis by way of the fallopian tubes, through thrombosed uterine veins, or through the lymphatics of the uterus (Fig. 35-4). The invaded structures become host to an acute or chronic inflammatory process.

Many of the pathogens causing PID lodge in the fallopian tubes. Purulent material collects in the tubes, adhesions form, strictures may occur, and sterility is a frequent result. Adhesions resulting from inflammation may cause such distress that complete removal of the uterus, fallopian tubes, and ovaries is necessary. Although generalized peritonitis can occur, the infection usually remains confined to the lower abdomen and pelvis. A severe inflammatory process may lead to dehydration, electrolyte imbalances, and prostration.

Toxic shock syndrome

Toxic shock syndrome (TSS), although not exclusively a reproductive disorder, occurs most commonly in menstruating females, especially among those using superabsorbent tampons. These tampons provide a milieu favorable to bacterial growth because they can contain a large amount

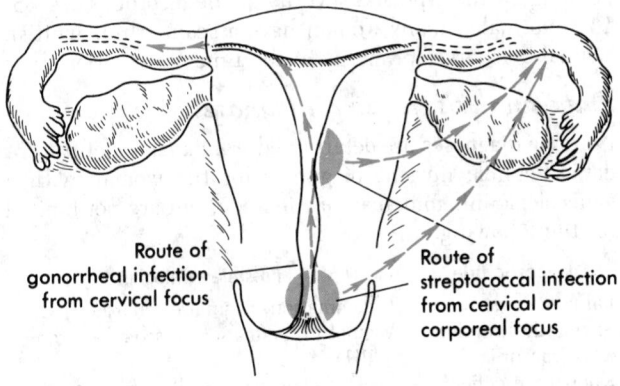

Fig. 35-4   Two chief routes of pelvic infection. (From Novak ER, Jones GH, Jones HW Jr: *Novak's textbook of gynecology,* ed 9, Baltimore, 1975, Williams & Wilkins.)

of menstrual blood and may be left in place more than 6 hours. Women at increased risk for TSS are those who insert tampons with their fingers instead of the applicator, and those who have a chronic vaginal infection or herpes genitalis. TSS has been associated with toxins produced by *Staphylococcus aureus* that result in sepsis. Septic shock is discussed in Chapter 9.

Nursing Process
Assessment
Subjective data
Itching

Itching is a major symptom of vulvular or vaginal infection. The itching may result from irritation from the vaginal discharge or from end products of the inflammatory response. The degree of itching experienced is monitored for signs of decreasing intensity as the inflammation subsides. Itching is most intense with *Trichomonas* infections.

Causes of vulvar or vaginal itching other than infection include epithelial changes seen with menopause, high urinary sugar content as in diabetes mellitus, pediculosis pubis, scabies, allergies, pinworms, or cancer of the vulva. With severe pruritus there are usually excoriations of the skin caused by scratching, and secondary infection may result. Dysuria may occur as a consequence of local irritation of the urinary meatus.

Pain

Pain is primarily a symptom of PID. In *acute* PID there is usually severe cramping lower abdominal pain; in chronic PID the pain is typically dull and aching and may be located in the lower back as well as the lower abdomen. Occasionally women have been thought neurotic because of ongoing reports of the diffuse pain, only to have chronic PID diagnosed later.

Objective data

Vaginal discharge is a major finding in most inflammations of the female genital tract. The *character* and *amount* of the discharge are monitored because these differ depending on the type and severity of the disorder (Box 35-14). Normally, many women have a scant, thin, whitish vaginal discharge, primarily at the time of ovulation.

Data analysis: nursing diagnoses

Nursing diagnoses are determined from analysis of patient data. Possible nursing diagnoses for the woman with a gynecologic inflammation may include, but are not limited to, the following:

Diagnostic title	Possible etiologies
Pain: itching	Inflammation, vaginal discharge
Sexual dysfunction: dyspareunia	Vaginal inflammation, discomfort from PID
Knowledge deficit	Lack of exposure/recall, information misinterpretation

Planning: expected patient outcomes

Expected patient outcomes for the woman with a gynecologic inflammation may include, but are not limited to, the following:

1. States feeling more comfortable.
2. Describes how infections of the reproductive organs occur and spread.
3. Describes potentially undesirable effects of infections of the reproductive tract.
4. States signs that indicate improvement or lack of response to therapy.
5. Describes methods to prevent infection of sexual partner and reinfection of self.
6. Describes plans for sexual abstinence until inflammation subsides.
7. States that intercourse is no longer painful.

Implementation

Usual methods for medical therapy are given in Table 35-3. Some alternative therapies developed by women are included in Table 35-4.

Assisting with achievement of therapeutic goals
Medications

The major types of prescribed medications are antibiotic, antifungal, or amebicidal agents (Box 35-15). The medications should be used by the patient for the prescribed number of days. They may be prescribed to be taken orally, used topically, or as a suppository (to be placed in the vagina) or douche. Douching is also used to apply heat to promote healing by increasing circulation and for comfort. If both heat and topical medications are prescribed, the topical medication is applied after the douche.

Supportive therapy

Patients with severe PID are usually hospitalized for intensive therapy. They are usually placed on bed rest in mid-Fowler's position to provide dependent drainage so that abscesses will not form high in the abdomen where they might rupture and cause generalized peritonitis. Fluids are given intravenously to correct dehydration and acidosis.

Table 35-4   Alternative therapies for vaginitis

Infection	Intervention	Dosage	Administration
Candida (Monilia)	Gentian violet	Few drops/qt water 0.25% to 2% (over-the-counter drug)	Douche or local application
	Vinegar (white)	1 tbsp/1 pt water	Douche every day for 5 to 7 days; twice daily for 2 days
	Acidophilus culture	2 tbsp/1 pt water	Douche twice daily
	Acidophilus yogurt Plain yogurt	1 application to labia hourly and as needed for symptom relief	
Trichomonas	1 handful chapparel chamomile	Steep in 1 qt water for 20 min	Douche 2 to 3 times/wk for 2 wk
Nonspecific vaginitis	Vinegar douche	5 tbsp/2 qt water	Every other day for 1 wk
	Salt (sea)	1 tbsp/1 qt water	Every other day for 1 wk
	1 tsp goldenseal and 1 clove minced garlic	Steep in 1 qt boiling water	Douche every day for 1 wk
	1 tsp goldenseal	Steep in 1 pt water; strain through cloth	Douche every day for 1 wk
	Povidone-iodine (Betadine) gel		Twice daily for 1 wk

From Fogel CI, Woods NF: *Health care of women: a nursing perspective*, St Louis, 1981, Mosby–Year Book.

35-14

Types of vaginal discharges with inflammation

Inflammation	Discharge
Vaginitis	
Candida	White, curdlike, cheesy, sweetish odor
Trichomonas	Yellow to green, frothy, foul odor, copious
Gardnerella	Grayish white, fishy or foul odor, scanty
Cervicitis	Whitish yellow (mucopurulent), amount varies

35-15

Drugs commonly prescribed for inflammations of the female reproductive tract

Drugs	Route
Antibiotic	
Ampicillin	Oral
Procaine penicillin G	Oral
Tetracylcline	Oral
Antifungal	
Clotrimazole (Gyne-Lotrimin)	Vaginal, topical
Micronazole (Monistat)	Vaginal, topical
Nystantin (Mycostatin, Nilstat)	Vaginal, topical, oral
Amebicidal	
Metronidazole (Flagyl)	Oral

Surgical procedures

Surgical intervention may be necessary in selected instances as described below.

Incision and drainage of abscess. An abscess of a Bartholin's gland may need to be incised and drained (I & D). After I&D a small amount of purulent drainage tinged with blood is expected, but any active, bright red bleeding should be reported to the physician. Relief from pain occurs almost immediately after I&D. The woman may experience soreness or mild pain for about a day. Sitz baths serve the purpose of cleansing and giving comfort. Warm water can be used to cleanse the involved area after each voiding or bowel movement.

Cauterization of cervix. When cervical lacerations or erosions are present, the area is usually cauterized. Silver nitrate sticks may be used to remove very small lesions. For larger areas requiring cauterization, an electric or thermal cautery unit is used. The woman is informed that a small, lubricated sheet of lead will be placed against the skin under the lumbar areas as a safety device for grounding electrical charges and that there will be slight bleeding,

which will be controlled by a tampon or packing inserted by the physician. The odor of burning tissue when cautery is used is distressing to some patients. They are told to expect an odor but that the odor is insignificant and that the procedure is over quickly. Slight discomfort may be experienced.

Instructions for follow-up care vary, but usually include the following:

1. Leave the tampon or packing in place as long as the physician advises (usually 8 to 24 hours).
2. Report to the hospital or physician's office if bleeding is excessive (more than occurs during a normal menses).
3. Do not douche or have sexual relations until the next visit to the physician unless specific instructions have been given for resumption of intercourse.
4. An unpleasant discharge caused by sloughing of destroyed cells may appear 4 to 5 days after cauterization; frequent warm baths will help this condition.

Removal of reproductive organs. If a tubal abscess develops with PID, a salpingectomy (removal of the fallopian tubes) may be necessary. In severe chronic PID more reproductive organs may also need to be removed. Surgery of the reproductive tract is discussed on p. 1143.

Interventions to achieve patient outcomes
Assisting with comfort

Itching is the primary discomfort with inflammations of the vulva and vagina. Frequent bathing and Sitz baths may be helpful. Soothing lotions may be prescribed. Vinegar douches that decrease the alkalinity of the vagina may also relieve the pruritus.

Pain is the primary discomfort with PID. Heat (hot water bottle or electric heating pad) applied to the abdomen may promote circulation and comfort. Analgesics are often necessary to relieve the pain.

35-16

Patient Teaching

The woman with an inflammation of the reproductive tract

Knowledge of spread of infection and its effects
Application of vaginal medication
1. Wash hands before and after procedure
2. Lie on back for 10 minutes after insertion to facilitate distribution of medication in vagina
3. Do not douche after insertion of medication
4. Wear a minipad
Sexual intercourse
 Abstain, if possible, to prevent discomfort and spread of infection to partner
 If abstention not feasible, advise male to use a condom
If repeated infections have occurred:
 Use an alternative brand of birth control pill or alternative method of control
 Use only clean equipment if douches are used
 Restrict frequency of sexual intercourse
 Encourage sexual partner(s) to seek medical attention
Report signs of further infection (increased vaginal discharge, bleeding, pain, fever).

Dyspareunia (discomfort with intercourse) may be present as a result of inflammation. Abstinence is advised until the inflammation subsides.

Counseling and teaching

Women with PID are usually of childbearing age. If severe or chronic PID is present, infertility may result from adhesions in the fallopian tubes or from removal of reproductive organs. The woman needs opportunities to identify her feelings regarding potential or actual infertility. Many women with inflammations of the reproductive tract can be treated on an ambulatory basis. Women who are hospitalized will require further therapy at home. The woman needs to know the nature of the inflammation, how to apply vaginal medications, and how to prevent reinfection (Box 35-16).

Evaluation

Evaluation is based on expected patient outcomes. Questions to consider may include the following:

1. Does the patient state the she feels more comfortable including during intercourse?
2. Can the patient describe how infections of the reproductive organs occur and spread?
3. Can the patient describe potentially undesirable effects of infections of the reproductive tract?
4. Can the patient state signs that indicate improvement or lack of response to therapy?
5. Can the patient describe methods to prevent infection of her sexual partner?
6. Does the patient describe plans for sexual abstinence until inflammation subsides?

STRUCTURAL DISORDERS IN WOMEN

Types of Structural Disorders

Women may experience problems with relaxation of the vaginal outlet, displacement or prolapse of the uterus, or fistulas that may develop between the bladder or rectum and the vagina (Table 35-5).

Etiology and Pathophysiology

Most of the structural problems of the reproductive tract experienced by women result primarily from stretching and weakening of the ligaments supporting the uterus or of the muscles of the perineum. Structural problems rarely occur in nulligravidas. When the pelvic-supporting tissues are *relaxed,* the urinary bladder may sag below the uterus and press against the vaginal wall *(cystocele)* (Fig. 35-5). This leads to stress incontinence (see Chapter 33). Similarly the posterior vaginal wall may weaken and the rectum may herniate into the vagina *(rectocele).* The weakened rectal wall predisposes to constipation and hemorrhoids. Causes of cystocele and rectocele include unrepaired childbirth lacerations, loss of pelvic muscle tone from repeated pregnancies, or congenital weakness.

The uterus itself may be *displaced,* either flexed forward (anteflexion) or backward (retroflexion) or tilted backward (retroversion) (Fig. 35-6). A displaced uterus may be congenital or may be caused by PID, endometriosis, pregnancy, pelvic tumors, or trauma. In addition the uterus may lose its support because of childbirth injuries or muscle relaxation due to age, and descend *(prolapse)* into the vaginal canal. With complete uterine prolapse, the cervix protrudes beyond the vaginal orifice. Cystoceles, rectoceles, and uterine prolapse are more commonly seen in older women.

Fistulas are abnormal passageways between two organs. *Vesicovaginal fistulas* are openings between the bladder and vagina and lead to leakage or urine through the vagina. Because the vagina does not have a sphincter, urinary incontinence results. *Rectovaginal fistulas,* which are less common, are passageways between the rectum and vagina. These lead to fecal incontinence and uncontrollable flatus expulsion. Causes of fistulas include radiation of the cervix, gynecologic surgery, or trauma during childbirth. Both types of fistulas may close spontaneously but frequently need to be repaired surgically. If so, 4 to 6 months are required for the inflammation to subside before surgery can be attempted.

REVIEW

Table 35-5   Structural problems of the female reproductive tract

Disorder	Signs and symptoms	Medical therapy
Relaxed vaginal outlet	Dragging pain in back of pelvis, stress incontinence, constipation, hemorrhoids	Plastic surgery
Uterine displacement	May be asymptomatic; dysmenorrhea, backache	Postural exercises, vaginal pessary
Uterine prolapse	Bearing down sensation, backache	Vaginal pessary, hysterectomy
Fistulas	Vaginal leakage of urine, gas, or feces	Surgical removal of fistula (fistulectomy)

Nursing Process
Assessment

Women with structural disorders of the reproductive tract often experience low-grade discomfort in the pelvic area and back. In addition, problem with urinary or fecal control may be present. Data to be collected if incontinence is present include the following:

1. Extent of incontinence
2. Pattern of incontinence: incontinence from a cystocele is intermittent, occurring most during stress (such as laughing or crying); incontinence from fistulas is continual seeping
3. Usual methods of coping (for example, use of pads, plastic pants, avoidance of fluids before social occasions)
4. Feelings regarding incontinence

Data analysis: nursing diagnoses

Nursing diagnoses are determined from analysis of patient data. Possible nursing diagnoses for the woman with a gynecologic structural disorder may include, but are not limited to, the following:

Diagnostic title	Possible etiologies
Pain: backache	Vaginal or uterine structural disorder
Incontinence, stress	Relaxed pelvic muscles
Knowledge deficit	Lack of information

Planning: expected patient outcomes

Expected patient outcomes for the woman with a gynecologic structural disorder may include, but are not limited to, the following:

1. States feeling comfortable.
2. Performs self-care measures to remain continent.
3. Describes care following surgery.

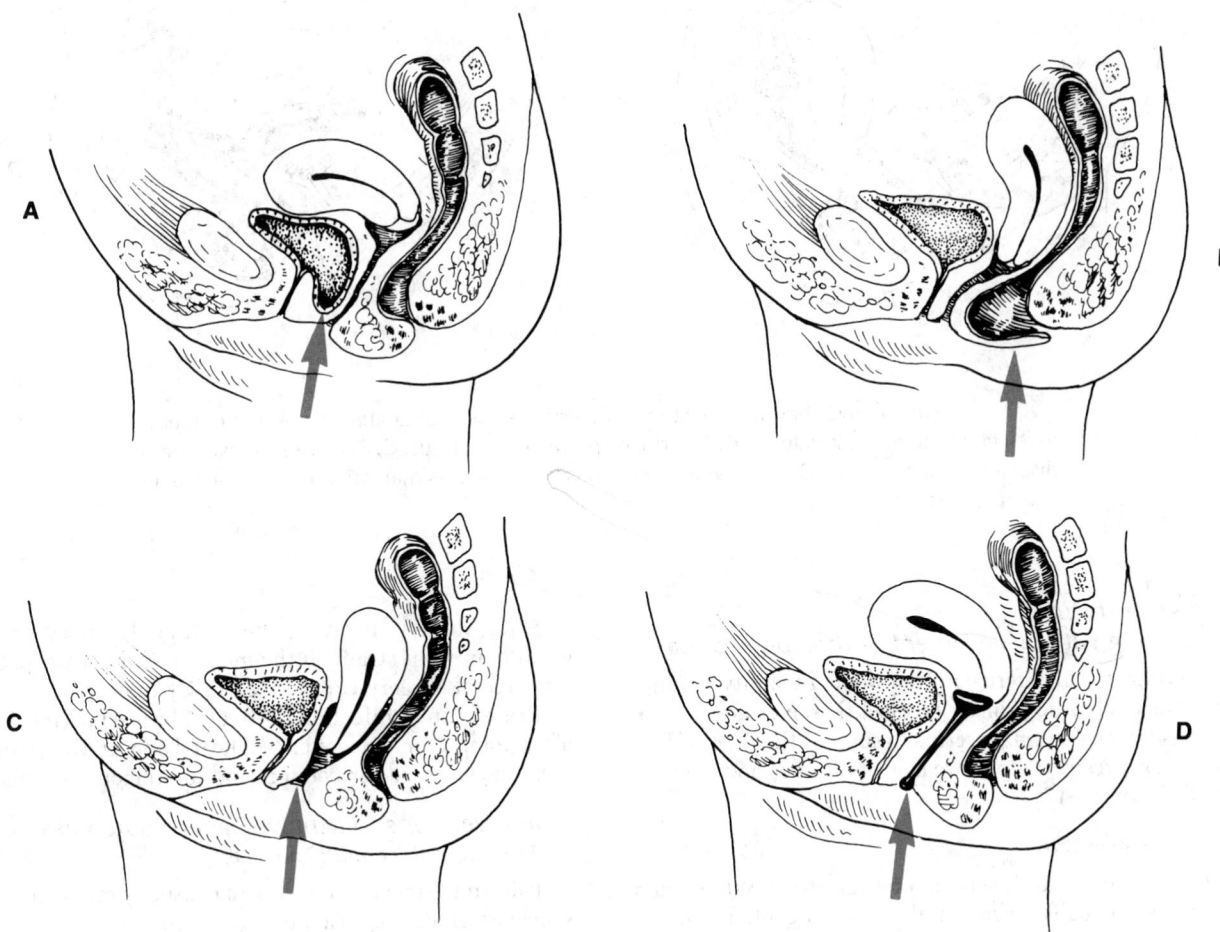

Fig. 35-5 Abnormalities of vagina. **A,** Cystocele: downward displacement of bladder toward vaginal orifice. **B,** Rectocele: pouching of rectum into posterior wall of vagina. **C,** Prolapse of uterus into vaginal canal. **D,** Stem pessary in place to maintain normal anatomic position of uterus.

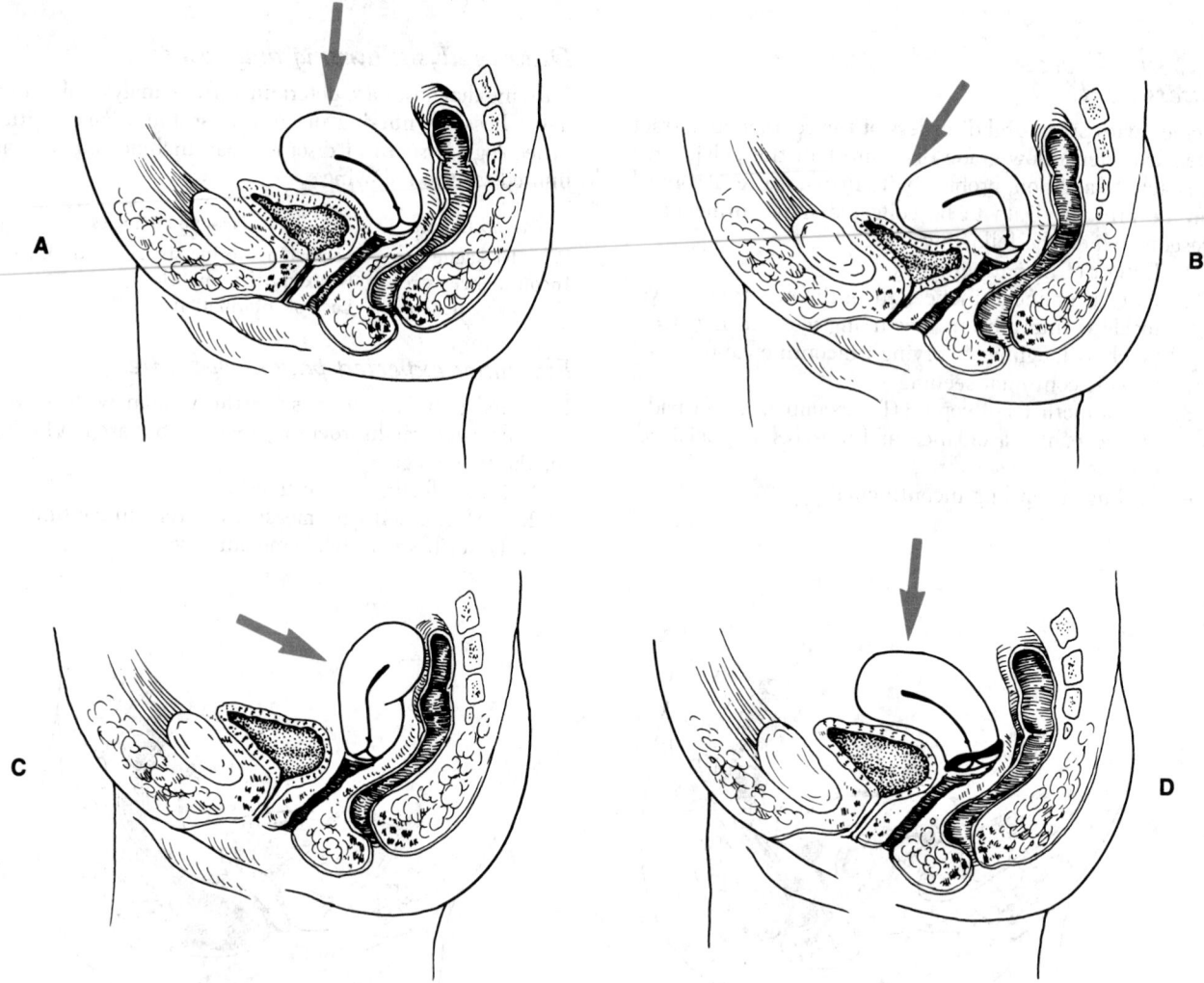

Fig. 35-6   Normal and abnormal positions of uterus. **A,** Normal anatomic position of uterus in relation to adjacent structures. **B,** Anterior displacement of uterus. **C,** Retroversion (backward displacement) of uterus. **D,** Normal anatomic position of uterus maintained by use of rubber S-shaped pessary.

Implementation

Assisting with achievement of therapeutic goals

If symptoms interfere with the woman's ability to function effectively, the primary medical therapies are the use of a *pessary* (plastic ring inserted to support the uterus [Fig. 35-7]), or *surgery* to repair weakened muscles and walls or fistulas (Box 35-17).

Preoperative care

If the rectum is involved, preoperative laxatives and enemas are usually given to reduce bowel contents. Clear liquids are given 24 hours before surgery.

Postoperative care

Repair may be accomplished vaginally or through a suprapubic incision. In the latter method, a suprapubic tube may be inserted and maintained for several days to permit healing (see Chapter 33). An indwelling urethral catheter is inserted after anterior colporrhaphy to keep the bladder empty and to allow edema to subside to prevent pressure on the incision.

After surgery involving the rectum, laxatives may be given to prevent strain on the incision. Care of the patient after rectal surgery is described in Chapter 31.

Prevention of infection is effected by good perineal care after voiding or defecation. A heat lamp at the perineal area may be used for comfort and to promote healing.

Interventions to achieve patient outcomes
Assisting with comfort and ADL

Pain from structural disorders is usually minimal. Nonsalicylate analgesics usually provide comfort.

Psychologic discomfort related to incontinence is usually more of a problem. The woman can be helped to explore her feelings about the incontinence and possible effects on social life and sexual functioning. Before surgery is planned, alternative methods of keeping dry can be explored. For a vesicovaginal fistula, a menstrual rubber cap (Tassette) may be attached to a catheter and leg bag urinal. For stress incontinence, menstrual pads or padded plastic pants may be helpful.

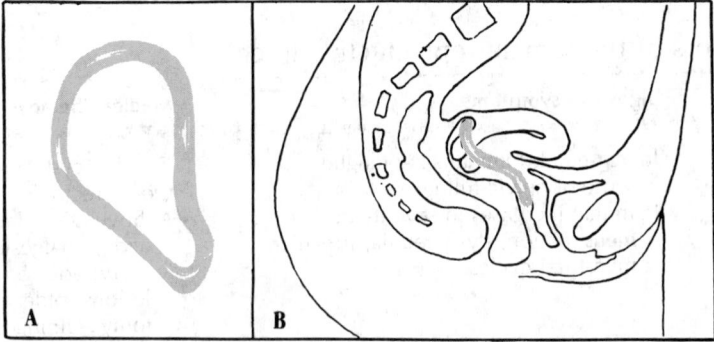

Fig. 35-7 A, Albert Smith pessary. **B,** Pessary in place to hold posterior vaginal fornix, and with it attached cervix, well backward and upward in pelvis. (From Beacham DW, Beacham WD: *Synopsis of gynecology,* ed 10, St Louis, 1982, Mosby—Year Book.)

Dribbling of fecal matter into the vagina from the rectovaginal fistula is particularly distressing and may be temporarily lessened by a high enema; this is useful before social situations. Constipating diets to decrease fecal leakage are not useful because they eventually cause pressure that may aggravate the condition and increase the size of the fistula.

Counseling and teaching

Kegel exercises can be learned by women to help prevent stress incontinence and prolapse of the uterus, bladder, or rectum. The Kegel muscle is a major support muscle for the pelvic floor. The muscle surrounds the urethra, vagina, and rectum; it may be felt by placing a finger along the upper vagina wall while tightening the perineum. Because the muscle may lose tone if not exercised, women are encouraged to do Kegel exercises 100 times a day for life. Kegel exercises consist of tightening the perineum (as if to prevent voiding) and holding the contraction for a count of 10, then relaxing; it is repeated 100 times.[23]

Preoperative and postoperative teaching include the following:

1. Preoperative
   a. Do Kegel exercises as instructed.
   b. Do pelvic exercises to assist in repositioning of uterus:
      (1) Knee-chest position for 5 minutes three times a day
      (2) Lie on abdomen 2 hours a day
   c. Seek medical consultation for symptoms of lower abdominal pain or incontinence.
2. Postoperative
   a. Use douches or mild laxatives as prescribed (gently inserting douche nozzle).
   b. Avoid heavy lifting, prolonged standing, or sexual intercourse until permitted (usually about 6 weeks).
   c. Expect loss of vaginal sensation for several months (normal response).
   d. Avoid enemas after rectal surgery until healing is complete.
   e. Report signs of infection or increased pain to physician.

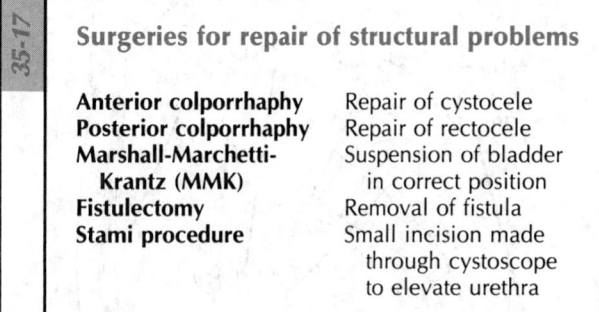

35-17	**Surgeries for repair of structural problems**	
	Anterior colporrhaphy	Repair of cystocele
	Posterior colporrhaphy	Repair of rectocele
	Marshall-Marchetti-Krantz (MMK)	Suspension of bladder in correct position
	Fistulectomy	Removal of fistula
	Stami procedure	Small incision made through cystoscope to elevate urethra

Evaluation

Evaluation is based on expected patient outcomes. Questions to consider may include the following:

1. Does the woman feel more comfortable?
2. Does she have better control of her incontinence?
3. Does she know what to do after she goes home?

BENIGN TUMORS IN WOMEN

Type of Tumors

Many different types of benign neoplasms affect the female reproductive tract. The more common sites for these tumors are the ovaries or myometrium of the uterus (Table 35-6).

Ovarian tumors

Most ovarian tumors are benign and are often asymptomatic. There are numerous types depending on the site and tissue involved. Ovarian cysts occur frequently. Simple cysts are thin-walled structures containing serous fluid and often occur during menopause. Corpus luteum cysts result from an exaggeration of the process of formation and resorption of the corpus luteum. Follicle cysts arise during the evolution or involution of the graafian follicle. Cysts do not become malignant. Severe pain may result if a cyst becomes twisted on its pedicle, and the symptoms may resemble appendicitis.

Polycystic ovarian disease (Stein-Levanthal) is characterized by enlargement of the ovaries, with numerous cystic follicles encased in a fibrotic capsule. Effects of these tu-

Table 35-6 **Benign tumors of the female reproductive tract**

Type	Signs and symptoms	Medical therapy
Ovarian tumors and cysts	Increased abdominal size; fatigue; sense of pelvic fullness	Ovarian cystectomy Oophorectomy
Endometriosis	Pain that increases in severity during menstruation, dyspareunia, irregular menstrual cycles	Antiovulation drugs (oral contraceptives, danazol), analgesics Surgery: younger than 35 years, resection of lesions; older than 35 years, total hysterectomy, salpingectomy, oophorectomy
Uterine fibroid tumors	Menorrhagia, low back pain, dysmenorrhea, constipation, irregular enlarged uterus	Small tumors: no treatment Severe symptoms or rapidly growing tumors: myomectomy or hysterectomy
Cervical polyps	Leukorrhea, abnormal vaginal bleeding	Surgical removal (polypectomy)

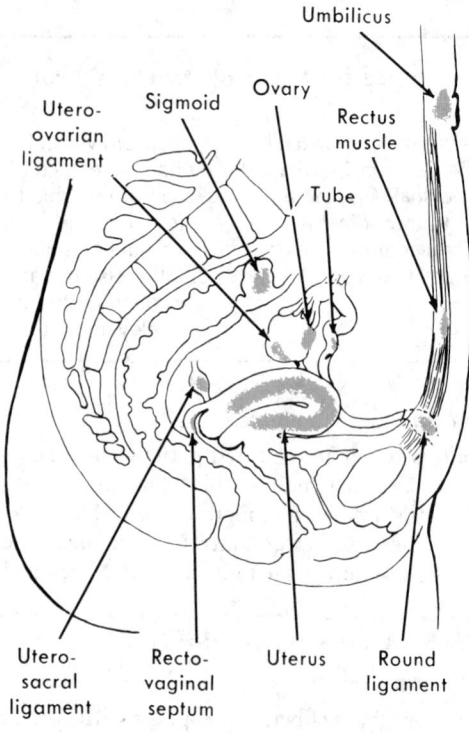

Fig. 35-8 Sites of endometrial implants.

often occur on the ovary and are known as *chocolate cysts.* Occasionally these cysts rupture and spread endometrial cells still farther throughout the pelvis.

Endometriosis begins with dysmenorrhea, then progresses to pain felt several days before menstruation. Rupture of a large endometrial cyst produces a severe peritoneal reaction requiring surgery.[58] Approximately half of the women with endometriosis are infertile, and endometriosis is sometimes first detected when a woman complains of inability to conceive.

If the woman is young and wants children, the treatment for endometriosis is usually as conservative as possible. Pregnancy is beneficial, because menstruation ceases during this time. If a young woman has endometriosis, she and her husband usually are advised to have their family early, because the fertility rate is low, sterility caused by adhesions may occur, and a hysterectomy may have to be done within a reasonable period of time. Nursing the infant is also recommended because it delays the onset of menstruation after delivery. Menopause stops the progress of this condition.

Uterine fibroid tumors

Fibroid tumors are the most common tumors of the female genital tract. They are discrete benign tumors of the uterine muscle and connective tissue. The sizes of myomas are variable. Most are found in the body of the uterus (corporeal) but some occur in the cervix or may involve the broad ligament. Submucous tumors may impinge on the blood vessels of the endometrium and produce bleeding. As they grow larger they may impinge on the opposite uterine wall and distort the cavity of the uterus. In some instances submucous tumors develop pedicles and may protrude through the vagina or cervix, resulting in infection or ulcerations.

Fibroid tumors of the uterus tend to disappear spontaneously with menopause. They rarely become malignant. Infertility may result from a myoma that obstructs or distorts the uterus or fallopian tubes. Myoma in the body of the uterus may cause spontaneous abortions, and those near the cervical opening may make the delivery of a baby difficult and may contribute to hemorrhage postpartally. Myomectomy is the procedure of choice during childbearing years.

mors are often not noted unless there is compression of a neighboring organ or blood supply, a menstrual disorder, or infertility.

Endometriosis

Endometriosis is a condition in which endometrial cells that normally line the uterus are seeded throughout the pelvis and occasionally extend to as distant a location as the umbilicus (Fig. 35-8). With each menstrual period the endometrial cells are stimulated by the ovarian hormones and bleed into the surrounding areas, causing an inflammation. Subsequent adhesions may be so severe that pelvic organs become fused together, occasionally causing a stricture of the bowel or interference with bladder function. Encased blood may lead to palpable tumor masses, which

Cervical polyps

Cervical polyps form when an area of the mucosa proliferates. These growths are usually visible at the cervical os as bright red, vascular, fragile areas. They are most often pedunculated and appear to protrude from the cervical canal. Polyps may occur singly or in clusters.

Because of the vascularity of the polyp, bleeding is a common symptom. The bleeding is small in amount and occurs between menstrual periods and closely resembles that of early cancer of the cervix. Especially characteristic is the contact bleeding produced by coitus, douching, or vaginal examination.

The pedicle by which the polyp is attached is usually quite small, and the polyp can easily be removed by twisting the pedicle at its base or by biopsy. Tissue examination of removed polyps is essential because epidermoid cancer arises from cervical polyps in a small percentage of cases.

Surgery of the Reproductive Tract

Minor surgical procedures are performed primarily for diagnostic purposes. Major surgery involves removal of one or more reproductive organs (Box 35-18). Most major surgeries require hospitalization although a vaginal hysterectomy may be performed at an ambulatory surgical center. Laparoscopically-Assisted Vaginal Hysterectomy (LAVH) is a newer procedure; the uterus is detached laparoscopically then removed vaginally. The patient is scheduled to undergo surgery early in the morning and then goes home late the same day.

Minor procedures
Preoperative care

Dilation and curettage (D and C) is the standard procedure for investigating any irregular bleeding. In addition it may be performed to correct a cervical stricture or to treat dysmenorrhea. Cervical biopsy and conization of the cervix are done to test for the presence of malignancy. All these procedures may be performed as ambulatory surgery. Cervical biopsy does not require anesthesia, whereas local or general anesthesia may be used for D and C or conization. The usual preoperative preparation is given; shaving is rarely required.

Postoperative care
Monitoring vaginal bleeding

Bleeding is monitored every 15 minutes for 2 hours and then as necessary thereafter. The blood loss is best recorded in estimated milliliters. A blood loss of at least 60 ml is required to saturate a perineal pad. It is important to record each pad change as well as blood loss. Any excessive bleeding is reported to the physician. More blood is lost by conization of the cervix than with the other procedures, and oozing may be controlled by packing inserted at the time of surgery.

Promoting comfort

Mild abdominal cramping may be experienced postoperatively. Mild analgesics such as codeine sulfate and nonsalicylate analgesics are usually ordered to relieve pain. Abdominal pain after D and C that is continuous, sharp, and not relieved by analgesics should be reported immediately to the surgeon; this type of pain may indicate perforation of the uterus.

35-18

Surgeries of the female reproductive tract

Minor procedures

Dilation and curettage (D and C)
  Dilation of the cervix and scraping of uterine walls
Cervical biopsy
  Punch biopsy of the cervix
Conization of cervix
  Removal of cone-shaped portion of cervix

Major procedures

Oophorectomy
  Removal of ovaries
Salpingectomy
  Removal of fallopian tubes
Hysterectomy (vaginal, abdominal)
  Removal of uterus, either through the vagina or abdomen
Radical hysterectomy
  Removal of uterus, upper vagina, and parametrium
Pelvic exenteration
  Removal of pelvic viscera (bladder, rectosigmoid) and all reproductive organs

---

Teaching the patient

1. If vaginal packing is in place, remove when instructed (usually 8 to 24 hours).
2. Do not douche or wear tampons until instructed.
3. Report the following to the surgeon:
   a. Soaking 3 or 4 pads a day with bright red blood
   b. Excessive pain
   c. Temperature greater than 38° C (100° F)
4. Resume sexual intercourse as instructed (usually when the woman feels comfortable)
5. Resume normal activities as instructed (usually in 1 week)
6. Avoid vigorous exercise for 3 to 4 weeks.

Major procedures
Preoperative care

Preparation of the patient for gynecologic surgery is similar to that for major abdominal surgery. Function of other systems within the pelvis (urinary, intestinal) is evaluated, particularly if there are any symptoms of dysfunction.

Psychologic preparation

Removal of reproductive organs can significantly affect the woman emotionally, and time may be needed to help her adjust to the proposed changes. The reproductive organs are a major component of "womanhood," and loss of these organs creates a change in body image. Many women see menstrual functioning as a symbol of femininity; therefore, with sudden cessation of menstruation some women

A woman undergoing major gynecologic surgery

Preoperative care

1. Identify patient's understanding of planned surgical procedure and correct misunderstandings
2. Encourage and support self-exploration of feelings related to proposed surgery
3. Provide support stockings for persons at high risk for thromboembolism
4. Teach breathing and leg exercises

Postoperative care

1. Monitor
   a. Fluid and electrolyte balance
   b. Breath sounds and respiratory excursion
   c. Abdominal distention
   d. Pain in abdomen
   e. Pain in thighs
   f. Dressing
   g. Signs of urinary tract infection
2. Encourage breathing exercises every 2 to 4 hours until patient becomes active
3. Provide urinary drainage
   a. Maintain patency of indwelling urinary catheter
   b. When catheter is removed, monitor for leakage of urine in vagina (sign of urinary fistula)
4. Provide pain medication (see Chapter 10)
5. For gas pains, apply heat (hot water bottle, electric heating pad) to abdomen, encourage ambulation, try a rectal tube
6. Prevent thrombophlebitis
   a. Teach patient to avoid sharp flexion of knee or thighs; no pillows under knees
   b. Continue support stockings for patients at high risk
   c. Encourage leg exercises every hour while awake until ambulating freely
   d. Lower head of bed to flat position for a short time every 2 hours for 24 hours, then every 4 hours until ambulating freely
   e. Encourage walking, increasing distance
   f. Encourage deep breathing (enhances venous return)
7. Continue providing emotional support
8. Teach patient
   a. Resume home activities gradually
   b. Avoid douches or tampons until instructed by physician
   c. Avoid heavy lifting (over 20 lbs) or vigorous activity (tends to cause pelvic blood congestion) for 6 weeks
   d. Resume driving in 3 to 4 weeks as desired
   e. Resume preoperative sexual activities such as cuddling or closeness immediately; sexual intercourse in 6 weeks
   f. Report immediately to physician any signs of thromboembolism

state feelings of being "less of a woman." Significant other may also be dealing with disturbed feelings.

Feelings of sexuality in terms of sexual relations are also threatened. Some women worry that sexual relations may be hindered or be less satisfactory. In actuality, many women find that sexual relations after hysterectomy are enhanced because fear of pregnancy has been removed. Except in rare instances of pelvic exenteration, sexual intercourse is possible after healing has occurred.

Women who experience some difficulties in adjusting may be those of childbearing age and those at menopause. The latter are still adjusting to life's changes and may be at a crisis period in their life. The nurse's role is to help the woman and her significant other explore feelings and to correct myths or misunderstandings before surgery to facilitate an easier recovery.

Physiologic preparation

Close proximity of the urinary tract and bowel to the reproductive organs requires measures to prevent infection. Preoperative measures are also taken to prevent postoperative thromboembolism:

1. Antibiotics to treat or prevent infection
2. Bowel preparation if bowel will be involved
   a. Mechanical cleansing (laxatives, enemas) or GoLYTELY (see Chapter 31)
   b. Liquid diet for 24 hours
3. Medicated douches if risk of infection is high
4. Persons at high risk for thrombophlebitis (varicose veins, obesity, diabetes mellitus, history of venous thrombosis or pulmonary embolus)
   a. Low-dose heparin
   b. Support stockings
   c. Discontinuation or oral contraceptives 3 to 4 weeks preoperatively.

Postoperative care

General care of the patient after major gynecologic surgery is essentially the same as that after abdominal surgery. Measures to prevent respiratory complications are important. Fluid and electrolyte balance is monitored carefully.

Preventing thromboembolism

Thrombophlebitis and pulmonary embolism are major postoperative complications after pelvic surgery as a result of venous stasis in the major pelvic veins. Symptoms may be absent until signs of pulmonary embolism occur (chest pain, hemoptysis) 1 week later. Because the involved veins are usually deep in the thigh, the only local symptoms may be pain and swelling in the thigh and a positive Homan's sign (pain with dorsiflexion of foot). Preventive activities are described in Box 35-19.

Promoting urinary function

Urinary *retention* is a common occurrence after gynecologic surgery as a result of handling of the bladder during surgery. An indwelling urinary catheter is usually inserted at least 24 hours postoperatively until muscle function returns. Urinary *fistula* may result despite careful surgical technique. It is identified by leakage of urine through the vagina. Many such fistulas close spontaneously.

Table 35-7   Cancer of the female reproductive tract

Site	Incidence	Usual age (yr)	Signs and symptoms	Medical therapy
Cervix	2.5%	30 to 50	Early: may be asymptomatic, vaginal discharge, spotting between menses Late: dark, foul vaginal discharge, pain	Conization of cervix for cancer in situ in young women; hysterectomy, radiation (internal, external)
Endometrium	6%	50 to 70	Early: postmenopausal bleeding Late: uterine enlargement, pain	Hysterectomy and bilateral salpingo-oophorectomy, radiation (internal, external), progestin for metastases
Ovary	4%	All ages	Early: asymptomatic Late: ascites, edema of legs, pain	Salpingo-oophorectomy; hysterectomy may also be necessary; chemotherapy, radiation

Promoting gastrointestinal function

Gastrointestinal function usually returns 24 to 72 hours after surgery, depending on the extent of handling of the intestines. Persistent nausea and vomiting with severe abdominal distention may indicate ileus, and all oral intake is stopped and a nasogastric tube is inserted. Most patients, however, have return of function. Abdominal distension with abdominal cramping may result from collection of gas in the sluggish bowel. Ambulation and heat encourage expulsion of the gas (see Chapter 31).

Counseling and teaching

Postoperatively, many women feel depressed for several days. The patient often is unable to explain why she is depressed and crying. Grieflike responses to loss of a body part may appear as they do after loss of other body parts. Feelings of guilt, shame, and remorse are common. Encouraging the woman to continue activities associated with being feminine, such as using makeup, arranging her hair, and wearing her own clothing, often helps her regain her feminine perspective. During this time she needs understanding and empathic care. Significant others may need help in understanding the woman's need for reassurance of continued love and affection. Postoperative teaching includes home care, resumption of activities, and follow-up care (Box 35-19).

Operative Endoscopy

Surgery may also be performed in some instances through a laparoscope. Examples of operative endoscopy are ovarian cyst enucleation, oophorectomy, salpingectomy, endocoagulation of endometriotic implants, and enucleation of myomas or extrauterine fibromas. Recovery after operative endoscopy is longer than incisional surgery because of longer duration of anesthesia and greater manipulation. Women require the same nursing interventions as those for major gynecologic surgery. There is a higher incidence of postoperative bleeding and bowel and urinary problems.

CANCER IN WOMEN
Epidemiology

Malignancies in the female reproductive tract occur primarily in the uterus (cervix and endometrium) and in the ovaries (Table 35-7); they may also occur, although less frequently, in the vagina or vulva. Cancer of the reproductive tract now ranks third to cancer of the breast and colorectum in females.[1]

The death rate from cancer of the *cervix* has fallen steadily over the past 40 years. This decline has been attributed to early detection through annual examinations (including a Papanicolau smear) and improved surgical and radiotherapeutic techniques. Cancer of the cervix identified and treated early at the preinvasive stage is 100% curable, thus *early detection* (p. 1127) *is vitally important.* The incidence of *endometrial* cancer is not decreasing significantly partly because it is primarily a disease of postmenopausal women and women are living longer.

Cancer of the *ovary* has had a steady slow *increase* in incidence but appears to be leveling off.[1] Because it is asymptomatic in the early stages, it is often far advanced before diagnosis is made. The only effective means of ensuring early diagnosis is a pelvic examination every 6 months, including careful ovarian palpation, and surgical exploration of any questionable ovarian growth. The Pap test does *not* reveal ovarian cancer.

Pathophysiology
Cancer of the cervix

Most cervical cancers are squamous carcinomas that arise in the intraepithelial layers (preinvasive stage or carcinoma in situ). This stage is classified as cervical intraepithelial neoplasia (CIN). Predisposing factors include human papillomavirus (HPV) (Chapter 18), early sexual activity, multiple partners, and chronic inflammation. It usually takes 2 to 10 years for squamous cell carcinoma to become invasive beyond the basement membrane. Spread usually occurs by direct extension or by means of the lymph system. Therapy depends on the stage (extent of spread) (Table 35-8).

Cancer of the endometrium

Cancer of the endometrium is primarily a slow-growing adenocarcinoma. Because it occurs mostly in postmenopausal women, estrogen stimulation unopposed by progesterone is thought to be implicated. Prolonged use of estrogen without added progestin during menopause increases the risk of endometrial cancer. Cancer of the

Table 35-8   Stages of cancer of female reproductive tract

Stage	Cervix	Endometrium	Ovary
0	Confined to epithelium (CIN)	Confined to epithelium	–
I	Confined to cervix	Confined to corpus	Confined to ovary
II	Extends outside cervix but does not involve pelvic wall or lower third of vagina	Involves corpus and cervix	Involves ovaries with pelvic extension
III	Involves pelvic wall and lower third of vagina	Involves pelvic and vaginal wall (but not bladder or rectum)	Intraperitoneal metastases
IV	Involves bladder, rectum, or metastatic spread	Involves bladder, rectum, or metastatic spread	Involves metastatic spread

---

35-20

Guidelines for Pap tests

1. Schedule Pap tests:
   a. Premenopausal: first half of menstrual cycle before ovulation
   b. Postmenopausal, not taking combined hormone therapy: at any time
   c. Postmenopausal, taking combined hormone therapy: at first part of cycle (not when taking progesterone)
2. Avoid douching, coitus, tampons, or vaginal medications for 48 hours before examination.
3. Slight vaginal bleeding (spotting) may occur after the examination; excessive bleeding should be reported.

---

endometrium is usually diagnosed when the postmenopausal woman seeks medical care for vaginal bleeding.

Cancer of the ovary

Ovarian cancer causes more than twice as many deaths as cancer of the uterus because the patient with ovarian cancer may be asymptomatic until the cancer is far advanced. The pathophysiology of ovarian cancer is complex, and there are a great variety of tumors. The ovaries may be a site of metastasis from the gastrointestinal tract, breast, pancreas, or kidneys. The risk for ovarian cancer increases with age.

Diagnostic Tests
Pelvic examinations

Pelvic examinations are useful for visualization of changes in the vulva, vagina, and cervix; for palpation of internal organs, especially the ovaries and surface of the uterus; and for obtaining Pap smears.

Women are advised to avoid douching and applying any vaginal preparation (medicinal or deodorant) for at least 24 hours before examination. They should void immediately before the examination, because an empty bladder makes palpation of the pelvic organs easier, decreases patient discomfort, and eliminates possible distortion of the position of pelvic organs caused by a full bladder. The technique for performing pelvic examinations is described in most physical examination texts.

After the pelvic examination a woman may need assistance in removing her legs from the stirrups and getting down from the table. Elderly women merit careful assistance after the pelvic examination because unnatural positions, such as the knee-chest and lithotomy positions, may alter the normal circulation of blood sufficiently to cause faintness.

Papanicolaou (Pap) test

The Pap test is a cytologic test that makes it possible to detect abnormal cells, not all of which are cancerous. However, the Pap test has made is possible through routine use to detect precancerous conditions and cancer of the cervix early enough to make treatment of these conditions almost 100% successful. For detection of atypical cells, the Pap test is 95% accurate. False-negative reports are most frequently the result of an inadequate sample or improper technique. Guidelines for Pap tests are listed in Box 35-20.

The Pap test involves microscopic examination of cells collected from the vaginal pool, exocervix, and endocervical canal. Samples of cells are obtained by using a cytology brush, applicator, spatula, or vaginal irrigation. Secretions containing exfoliated cells are preferably obtained from the cervix or external os. The secretions are collected, smeared on the slide, and immediately fixed with cytologic spray or liquid. The slide may also be placed in a 95% alcohol fixative for 15 to 30 minutes, then allowed to dry.[20] The slides are labeled and sent to the laboratory.

Do-it-yourself Pap tests are available. These can be used by women who are reluctant or unable to visit a physician for examination. Women who have had subtotal hysterectomy in which the cervical stamp was left intact should continue to have regular Pap testing.

Obtaining endometrial cells for study

The Pap test is not ideal for detecting endometrial cancer, although samples may be obtained by cervical aspiration when performing a Pap test. Less than half of women with uterine cancer have an abnormal Pap test result at the time of routine Pap test screening. Probably the main reason the Pap test is inadequate is that cells rarely exfoliate from the endometrium in the early stages of uterine cancer.

One method of obtaining endometrial cells for study is by *vacuum curettage*. The procedure and apparatus used for vacuum curettage are similar to those used in suction cu-

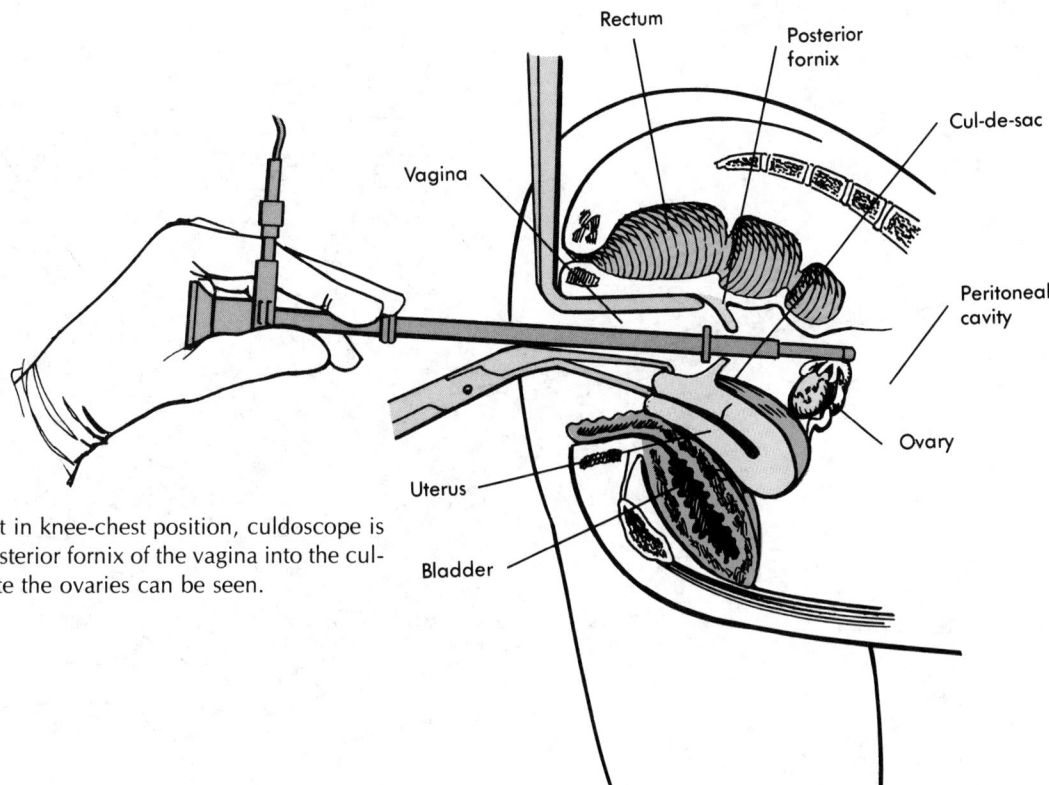

Rectum
Posterior fornix
Cul-de-sac
Vagina
Peritoneal cavity
Ovary
Uterus
Bladder

Fig. 35-9   With patient in knee-chest position, culdoscope is inserted through the posterior fornix of the vagina into the cul-de-sac of Douglas. Note the ovaries can be seen.

Endoscopic procedures for visualization of pelvic organs

Colposcopy
Visualization of vagina and cervix under low-power magnification
Culdoscopy
Insertion of a culdoscope through posterior vaginal vault into cul-de-sac of Douglas for visualization of fallopian tubes and ovaries (Fig. 35-9)
Hysteroscopy
Insertion of a hysteroscope through the cervix for visualization of inside of the uterus
Laparoscopy
Insertion of a laparoscope (under local anesthesia) through small incision in abdominal wall (inferior margin of umbilicus), which is insufflated with carbon dioxide; permits visualization of all pelvic organs (Fig. 35-10)

An *endometrial biopsy* is performed by presenting a small curette into the uterus and obtaining several strips of endometrial tissue. The specimens are taken from several sites of the uterine cavity to increase the chances of obtaining malignant cells. For diagnosis of endometrial cancer, the biopsy method is considered to be about 90% accurate.

Endoscopy

The pelvic organs and surrounding tissues can be directly visualized by endoscopy. Endoscopic procedures include colposcopy, culdoscopy (Fig. 35-9), peritoneoscopy (laparoscopy), and hysteroscopy (Box 35-21). The most common procedure is the laparoscopy (Fig. 35-10). Depending on the organs and structures inspected, these methods are valuable for determining the cause of abnormal bleeding, in evaluating the stage of malignancies, and for inspecting organs for size, shape, and position.

Most of the procedures used for visualizing the pelvic organs can be performed on an outpatient basis; this allows the physician to schedule the procedure at the appropriate time of the menstrual cycle.

Maintaining asepsis throughout any of the endoscopic procedures is important in preventing infection. Air may enter the abdominal cavity during the procedures and cause discomfort; a prone position with a pillow under the abdomen may increase comfort. Douching and intercourse should be avoided for about 1 week following a culdoscopy. Complications such as hemorrhage and infection are rare, but women should be cautioned to report fever or pain in the lower abdomen.

rettage for performing an abortion, except that the curette is much thinner. With the patient under general anesthesia, the cervix is dilated and the suction tip is inserted through the cervix into the uterus. Suction is applied and the entire uterine cavity is suctioned to secure specimens. Vacuum curettage is considered to be at least as good as conventional endometrial biopsy for diagnosing endometrial cancer.

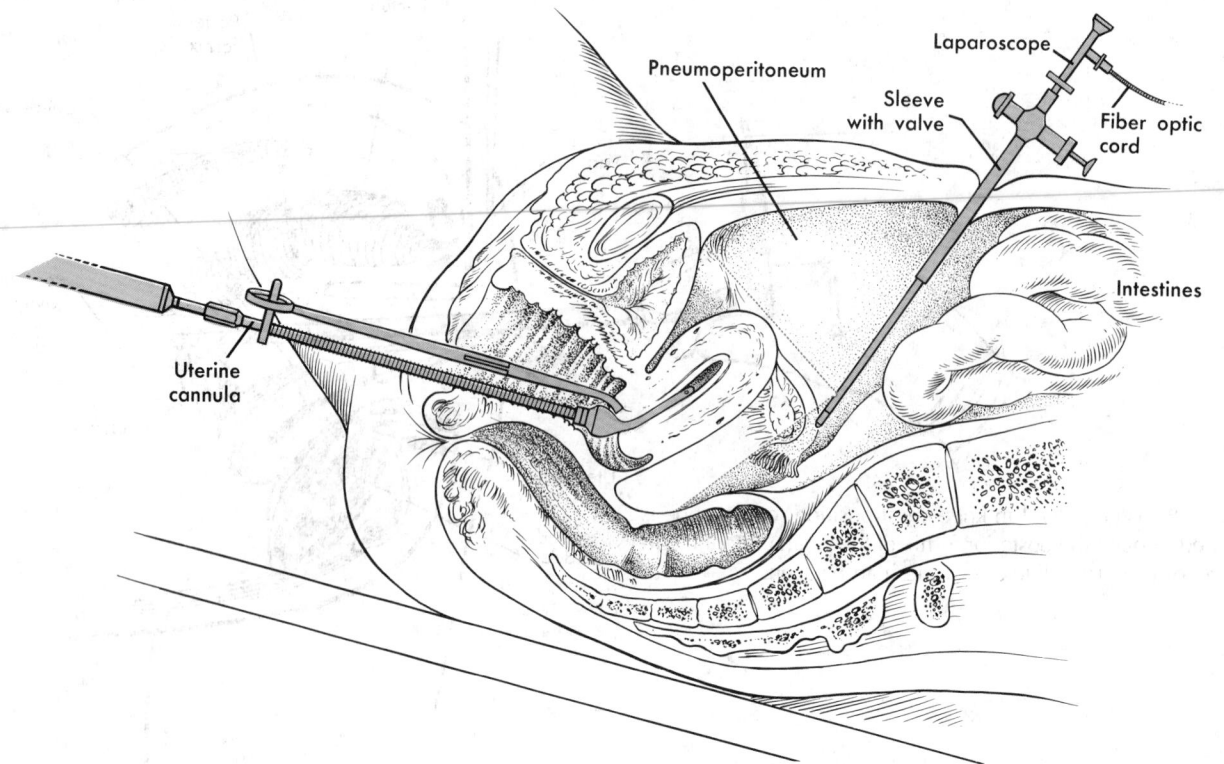

Fig. 35-10   Schema of gynecologic laparoscopy. (From Cohen MF: *Laparoscopy, culdoscopy and gynecography: techniques and atlas,* vol 1, Philadelphia, 1970, WB Saunders.)

Other diagnostic approaches

Ultrasound has become a useful diagnostic tool for gynecologic problems. It can be used to locate pelvic masses, displaced IUDs, and ectopic pregnancies. Uterine fibroids can be located and measured. *Computed tomography* (CT) and *magnetic resonance imaging* (MRI) provide better indirect visualization of masses and affected lymph nodes, especially in obese women and those with abdominal distention.

Treatment Modalities
Surgery

Total abdominal hysterectomy (TAH) with or without bilateral salpingo-oophorectomy (BSO) is the most common treatment for gynecologic cancer (Box 35-18, p. 1143). A unilateral *salpingo-oophorectomy* may be performed for women of childbearing age who have stage I ovarian cancer. The woman with cancer not only experiences the same feelings associated with loss of her reproductive organs as other women but at the same time faces the concerns related to cancer (Chapter 11). Anxiety is commonly experienced, and the woman requires considerable empathy and emotional support as she works through her feelings.

Radical hysterectomy (Box 35-18, p. 1143) may be recommended for stage II cervical or endometrial cancer. Radical hysterectomy usually requires a longer hospitalization than TAH. Retroperitoneal drains are inserted and connected to low-pressure suction. The drains are removed when drainage is less than 50 ml/day (usually in 3 to 5 days). Because the bladder is usually atonic as a result of

nerve damage, either an indwelling or suprapubic catheter is required for 2 to 3 weeks. The woman is taught care of the catheter before hospital discharge. The catheter is removed when the woman can void with less than 100 ml of residual urine. Additional care of the patient with hysterectomy is discussed on p. 1144.

Pelvic exenteration (Box 35-18) may be performed for selected patients with recurrent or persistent cancer of the cervix. The procedure is done only when there is no lymphatic involvement and there is chance of cure. Nursing care includes care following hysterectomy as well as care following abdominoperineal bowel resection (Chapter 31) and urinary diversion (Chapter 33). Because of the great extent of the surgery, the woman may be overwhelmed psychologically. She usually experiences changes in body image, sexual relations, and social life-style, in addition to dealing with the fears pertaining to cancer recurrence and death. Both the woman and her significant other need ongoing supportive nursing care.

Radiotherapy

Intracervical, intrauterine, or external whole pelvic irradiation may be given preoperatively to shrink the tumor to facilitate safety of the operation. Radiation may also be used as adjunct therapy postoperatively. Guidelines for radiation therapy are described in Chapter 11. Premenopausal women who receive pelvic irradiation will lose their ovarian function.

Radiation of the pelvic organs may create problems in sexual functioning, including lack of libido, marked pain

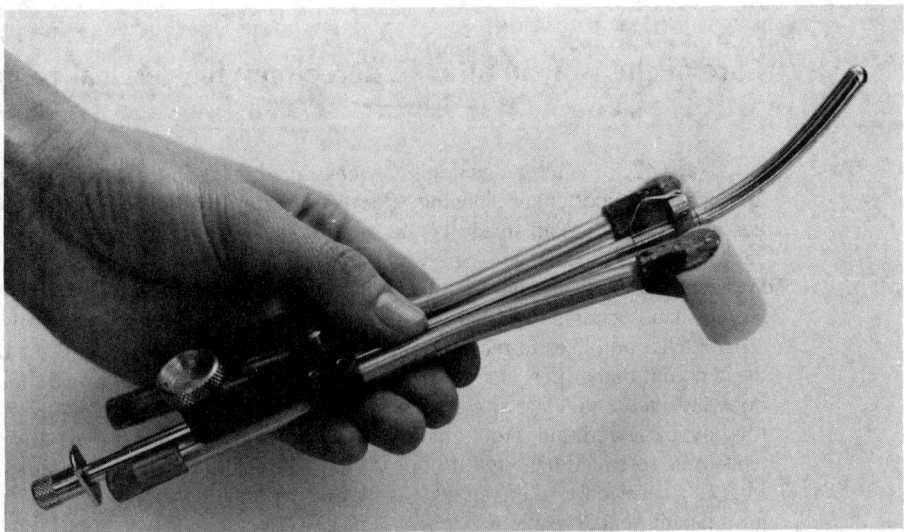

Fig. 35-11   Assembled configuration of tandem and colpostat before placement.

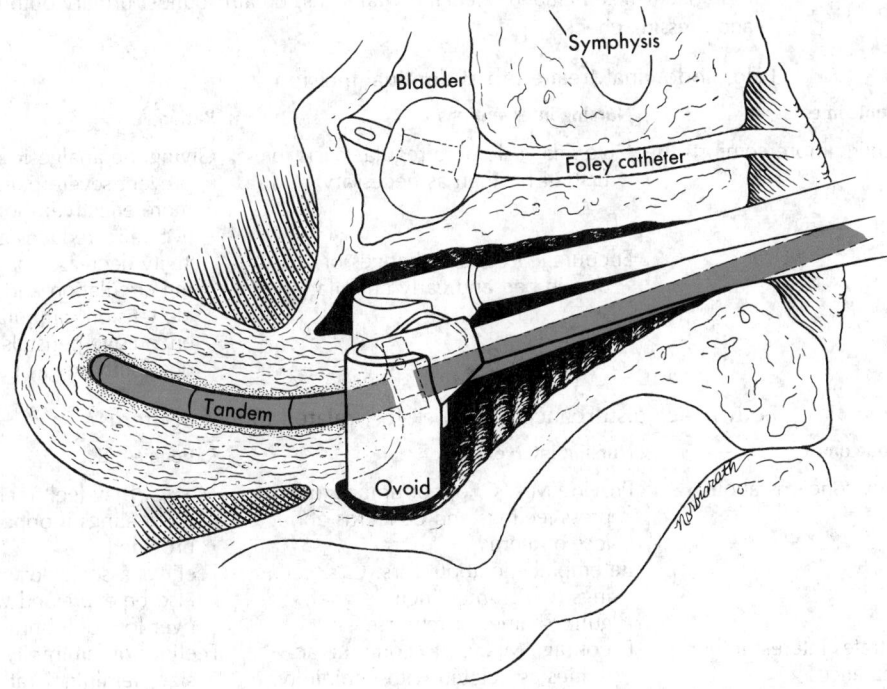

Fig. 35-12   Placement of tandem and colpostat before vaginal packing.

or discomfort with intercourse, and feelings of a narrow or shortened vagina. These problems may add to the woman's feelings of sexual inadequacy from interferences with reproductive function.

Intracavitary implant

Radium or cesium may be inserted through a tandem placed in the uterine cavity (Figs. 35-11 and 35-12). During an intracavitary implant, it is important that all normal tissues remain in their natural position. Gauze packing is usually inserted into the vagina to push both the rectum and the bladder away from the area being irradiated. A

urinary catheter is inserted before therapy to prevent bladder distention. Low-residue diet and cleansing enemas are given before therapy, and the enema is repeated after therapy to prevent bowel distention.

Nursing care consists of the following guidelines:

1. Keep patient flat in bed; may turn side to side
2. Provide analgesics for severe uterine contractions from dilation of cervix
3. Provide good perineal care; there will be foul-smelling vaginal discharge from cell destruction; a room deodorizer is helpful
4. Encourage fluids to 3000 ml/day to maintain urinary adequacy

Nursing Care Plan	**Care of the woman after hysterectomy for cervical cancer**

DATA: Mrs. C., age 42, saw her gynecologist 2 weeks ago because of bleeding between periods and occasional postcoital bleeding. The result of her Pap smear 5 years previously had been negative. The Pap smear this time was positive and a cervical biopsy confirmed cancer of the cervix, stage I. She was admitted yesterday for a total hysterectomy.

Admission notes indicate that Mrs. C. is married and has two teenagers, a boy and a girl. Her husband accompanied her to the hospital and appeared to be supportive. Mrs. C. is a bank teller and likes to read, knit, and watch TV. She has varicose veins but states these do not bother her. Her preoperative concerns centered mainly on the cancer: "I hope they get it all." She also stated, "Well, at least I hadn't planned any more children. My boy joked and said, 'You're going to be neutered like our cat was!' I wonder how it feels to be so-called neutered. I hope it won't affect my sex life." The nurse explored Mrs. C.'s knowledge of the surgery and explained that the surgery would not prevent her from having sexual relations.

Mrs. C. returned from the recovery room alert with an IV running and stable vital signs. The dressing was dry. She had an order for morphine sulfate (MS) 10 mg IM q3h PRN. Monitoring activities included checking vital signs, breath sounds, urinary output, fluid intake, and dressing checks.

Nursing diagnosis: **Pain, abdominal, related to abdominal incision**

Expected patient outcomes	Nursing interventions	Rationale
Mrs. C. states feeling more comfortable	Give analgesic on a regular basis for first 24 hr, then as necessary	Giving the analgesic regularly will prevent severe pain and thus be more effective; morphine sulfate (MS) also reduces anxiety
	Encourage frequent changes of position in bed and early ambulation	Activity decreases pain by increasing circulation and reducing muscle tension; ambulation will also encourage peristalsis, decreasing possibility of gas pains

Nursing diagnosis: **Body image disturbance: high risk for, related to loss of uterus**

Expected patient outcomes	Nursing interventions	Rationale
Mrs. C. verbalizes concerns about loss of uterus	Provide Mrs. C. opportunities to express feelings and concerns about loss of uterus	Mrs. C. may feel freer to talk about her feelings if opportunities are provided
	Be empathetic about Mrs. C.'s feelings, which may include grief, guilt, shame, or remorse	Feelings associated with grief may also be expressed when grieving over loss of a body part
Mrs. C. demonstrates interest in her personal appearance	Encourage Mrs. C. to continue activities associated with femininity, such as fixing hair, using makeup, wearing own apparel	Feelings of femininity will emphasize "feminine" rather than "neuter," and that she herself has not changed
Mrs. C. verbalizes plans to resume former activities	Help Mrs. C. make plans for resumption of former activities	If life pattern is not changed, her thoughts about her body changes may diminish

Nursing diagnosis: **Constipation: high risk for, related to pelvic surgery**

Expected patient outcomes	Nursing interventions	Rationale
Stool is soft and formed	Monitor stool characteristics and frequency	Peristalsis may be decreased from handling of pelvic viscera
	Encourage oral fluids when permitted	Hydration will promote a soft stool
	Encourage ambulation	Ambulation promotes peristalsis

Nursing diagnosis: Urinary elimination, altered patterns related to pelvic surgery

Expected patient outcomes	Nursing interventions	Rationale
Mrs. C. voids in sufficient quantities	Monitor urinary output until she voids sufficiently Monitor for distention above symphysis pubis and for lower abdominal discomfort other than incisional pain	Handling of bladder during pelvic surgery may decrease bladder muscle tone, leading to urinary retention (Mrs. C. did not have an indwelling catheter)

Nursing diagnosis: Tissue perfusion: altered peripheral, high risk for, related to pelvic venous stasis from surgery

Expected patient outcomes	Nursing interventions	Rationale
No leg or thigh pain occurs	Monitor discomfort in legs/thighs	Early detection will ensure early treatment of thrombophlebitis
	Encourage leg exercises and frequent turning in bed until ambulating well	Exercises promote venous return (muscle pumps)
	Avoid use of knee gatch or pillows under knees; encourage Mrs. C. to keep knees flat when in bed	Pressure on popliteal veins or sharp knee flexion may increase venous stasis
	Encourage to lie completely flat in bed for short periods q2hr for 24 hr then q4hr until ambulating well	Lying flat for periods of time will help blood return from the pelvic veins
	Encourage ambulation	Ambulation promotes venous return (muscle pumps)
	Provide antiembolic stockings	Mrs. C. is at higher risk for thrombophlebitis because of varicose veins (sluggish circulation) and sedentary life pattern

Nursing diagnosis: Knowledge deficit, related to surgery

Expected patient outcomes	Nursing interventions	Rationale
Mrs. C. describes self-care	Teach Mrs. C. When activities can be resumed (see text)	Activities are resumed gradually to permit healing; heavy activities are avoided for 6-8 weeks
	Signs of thrombophlebitis to be monitored and reported	Thrombophlebitis may occur 7-10 days postoperatively, after patient goes home
	Signs of vaginal bleeding to be reported	Bleeding could indicate impaired healing
	Need for medical follow-up	To ensure that metastasis has not occurred
	Reinforce the preoperative explanations of the surgery and effect on sexual relationships	Preoperative anxiety may have decreased her awareness; hysterectomy does not interfere with satisfactory sexual relationships
	Find out what she has told her daughter about regular Pap smears	Regular Pap smears enhance early detection of cervical cancer
	Suggest she use support hose in her job as a bank teller	Preventive measure for thrombophlebitis because of her varicose veins

Table 35-9 Inflammatory disorders of the male reproductive tract

Disorder	Causative organisms	Signs and symptoms	Medical therapy
Urethritis	Chlamydia trachomatis, urea-plasma, urealyticum	Urgency, frequency, and burning with urination, purulent urethral discharge	Antibiotics
Prostatitis	Chlamydia trachomatis, Neisseria gonorrhoeae	Perineal pain, fever, dysuria, urethral discharge	Antibiotics, rest, hydration, analgesics, stool softener, Sitz baths
Epididymitis	Same as for prostatitis	Sudden scrotal pain, scrotal edema	Antibiotics, injection of procaine around spermatic cord, bed rest with scrotal elevation, analgesics
Orchitis	Pyogenic bacteria, gonoccoci	Same as for epididymitis; nausea and vomiting, pain radiating to inguinal canal	Same as for epididymitis

5. Follow general guidelines for internal radiation (Chapter 11)
6. Plan care that includes measures to decrease social isolation.

Radiation sickness may result as a systemic reaction to the breakdown and reabsorption of cell proteins. Local reaction may include cystitis and proctitis. Vaginal discharge will continue for some time after termination of therapy, and the patient may need to take douches for as long as the odor and vaginal discharge persist. Some vaginal bleeding may occur for 1 to 3 months after irradiation of the cervix. The woman who is at home should report persistent rectal irritation to the physician. The patient is usually discharged from the hospital within a day or two after the applicators are removed, but may return for another course of radiation.

Complications to watch for after radiation of the uterus are vesicovaginal fistulas, ureterovaginal fistulas, cystitis, phlebitis, and hemorrhage. Each is caused by the radiation or by extension of the disease process. The patient is urged to report even minor symptoms to her physician.

Chemotherapy

Chemotherapy has not significantly improved cancer of the uterus and therefore is rarely used in this situation. Chemotherapy is used more often for cancer of the ovaries. Combinations of drugs such as cisplatin, doxorubicin, and cyclophosphamide may be given. The drugs are not curative, but some long-term remissions may result.[58] If cancer of the ovaries has spread to peritoneal surfaces throughout the abdomen, a more effective method of giving chemotherapy is by the intraperitoneal route. Higher drug concentrations can be given than by the intravascular route.[10]

INFLAMMATORY DISORDERS IN MEN

Nonspecific pyogenic organisms as well as specific organisms such as the gonococci and tubercle bacilli may cause stubborn infection of the male reproductive system. Urethritis, prostatitis, epididymitis, and orchitis are the most common infections (Table 35-9). Infecting organisms may reach the genital tract by direct spread through the urethra, or they may be borne by blood or lymph.

Etiology and Pathophysiology
Prostatitis

Prostatitis is commonly associated with urethritis. It may be acute or chronic; recurrent episodes of acute prostatitis may cause fibrotic tissue to form. The fibrosis causes a hardening of the prostate gland that may initially be confused with carcinoma. In the granulomatous form of prostatitis, the enlargement may take 3 to 6 months to resolve.

Epididymitis

Epididymitis is one of the most common inflammations of the male reproductive system. It is frequently a complication of gonorrhea or the first indication of tuberculosis of the genitourinary tract. It may follow instrumentation or prostatectomy.

Traumatic or chemical epididymitis is a sterile inflammation caused by direct injury or reflux of urine down the vas deferens. The chemical form is frequently seen in military recruits during basic training as a result of straining with a full bladder, which causes urinary reflux.

Bilateral epididymitis usually causes sterility. Untreated epididymitis leads rather rapidly to necrosis of testicular tissue and septicemia, which can be fatal.

Orchitis

When mumps are contracted after puberty, approximately 18% of the cases are complicated by orchitis (inflammation of the testes). Orchitis may also be caused by bacteria, trauma, or surgical manipulation, or it may follow septicemia or tuberculosis. Usually both testes are involved, and if it is bilateral, sterility often results. Sterility does not occur with unilateral involvement.

Prevention

Because urethral infection spreads so readily to the genital organs, men should not be catheterized unless it is absolutely necessary. Some trauma to the urethral mucosa is likely to accompany catheterization or the passage of instruments, such as a cystoscope, because of the length and curvature of the male urethra. The distal part of the urethra is not sterile, and trauma makes the urethra susceptible to attack from bacteria. Fluids should be given liberally after passage of instruments through the urethra.

Any postpubertal male who is exposed to mumps usually

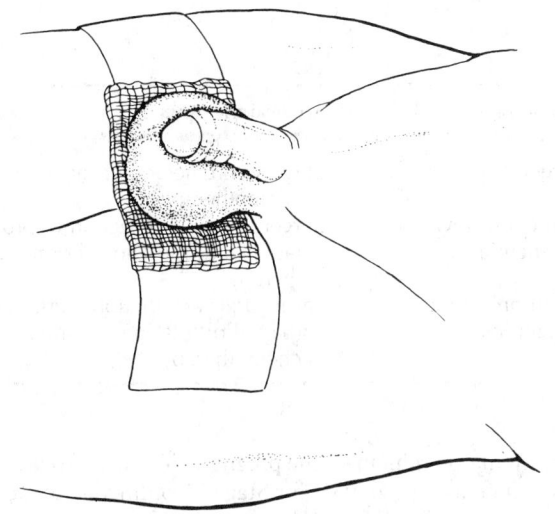

Fig. 35-13   Bellevue bridge.

is given gamma globulin immediately unless he has already had the disease. If there is any doubt about exposure, globulin usually is given. Although gamma globulin may not prevent mumps, the disease is likely to be less severe, with less likelihood of orchitis developing and subsequent sterility.

Diagnostic Tests

The site of the infection will influence treatment. The physician may obtain segmented bacteriologic localization cultures to make the determination. Four sterile culture tubes are used for collection. The patient must be well hydrated, have a full bladder, and be able to cooperate.

1. The first 5 to 10 ml of a voiding is collected.
2. After approximately 200 ml have been voided, a 5- to 10 ml midstream specimen is collected.
3. The patient is asked to stop voiding, and the prostate gland is massaged rectally until prostatic secretions are collected.
4. The next 5 to 10 ml of urine are collected, and the bladder is then emptied.
5. If not cultured immediately, the specimens are refrigerated and taken to the laboratory for culture within 4 hours.

Intervention
Assisting with comfort

Mild to moderate discomfort may be experienced by the man with an inflammation of the genital tract. *Heat* may be applied for prostatitis by means of sitz baths, but is *contraindicated for epididymitis or orchitis* because of possible destruction of sperm cells. *Cold* is applied in the latter cases for relief of swelling and discomfort. If an ice cap is used, it should be placed under the scrotum and should be removed for short intervals every hour to prevent ice burns. A plastic glove may be filled with crushed ice and placed with the palm of the glove under the scrotum; the fingers provide cold to the sides.

Swelling and discomfort of the scrotum can also be re-

35-22	Male reproductive disorders that may affect sexual functioning
Sterility	**Impotence**
Bilateral epididymitis	Radical prostatectomy
Severe bilateral orchitis	External radiation of
Torsion of testes	pelvic floor
	Total penectomy

lieved by elevation of the scrotum, either on a folded towel or with adhesive strapping known as a Bellevue bridge (Fig. 35-13).

Counseling and teaching

Female nurse must be particularly sensitive to the reaction and feelings of male patients who have diseases of the reproductive system. The patient may feel more comfortable discussing his problems with a male nurse. However, it is incumbent on all nurses to provide a comfortable environment in which these patients can verbalize their concerns and feelings.

Patient comments with subtle sexual connotations may reveal concerns the patient has regarding his sexuality, and he often must be given permission to discuss these concerns. The patient may "try out" his sexuality on a female nurse. Rejections from her may be perceived by the patient as less threatening than rejection by a loved one would be.

Certain reproductive disorders in the male are accompanied by a high incidence of sexual dysfunction. The patient may be worrying needlessly about possible sterility (inability to conceive a child) or impotence (inability to have an erection). If the patient does have a condition in which the incidence of sexual dysfunction is high, the nurse needs to know the specific patient situation, because these dysfunctions do not always occur in each disorder (Box 35-22).

Teaching includes the need to continue antibiotic therapy for the prescribed length of time (which may be lengthy in chronic prostatitis).

STRUCTURAL DISORDERS IN MEN

Structural disorders of the testes and scrotum that may occur in males include hydrocele, spermatocele, varicocele, or torsion of the spermatic cord (Box 35-23). Immediate medical attention should be sought for any swelling of the scrotum or the testes within it. Any acute swelling of sudden onset must be considered twisting (torsion) of the spermatic cord until proved otherwise.

Hydrocele is treated by aspiration of the fluid and injection of a sclerosing drug. Usually no therapy is needed for *spermatocele*, although aspiration or surgical excision may be done. *Varicocele* is often seen in men with low fertility. Ligation of the spermatic vein has been shown to improve semen quality.

Torsion of the spermatic cord interrupts the blood supply, leading to ischemia and severe pain that is not relieved and may be aggravated by scrotal elevation. Absence of pain indicates infarction and necrosis. *Immediate surgery* is nec-

Table 35-10   Cancer of the male reproductive tract

Site	Incidence	Usual age (yr)	Signs and symptoms	Medical therapy
Testes	0.1%	18 to 35	Painless enlarged testis, gynecomastia	Surgery: orchiectomy; radiation, chemotherapy
Prostate gland	22%	>60	Urethral obstruction, low back pain, anemia	Surgery: radical resection of prostate gland, radiation, hormonal therapy
Penis	0.01%	40 to 60	Nodular growth on foreskin, fatigue, weight loss	Laser surgery, radiation, surgery (partial or total penectomy), chemotherapy

---

35-23

Structural disorders of testes and scrotum

Hydrocele
Benign nontender collection of clear amber fluid within the outer covering of the testes, leading to scrotal swelling
Spermatocele
Benign nontender cystic mass attached to epididymis containing milky fluid and sperm
Varicocele
Dilation of spermatic vein, primarily on left side (because of increased retrograde pressure of left renal vein)
Torsion of spermatic cord
Kinking and twisting of spermatic cord and artery

---

essary and the infarcted testis is removed to minimize an immune reaction to antigenic sperm that may cause infertility.[58] The contralateral testis is usually fixed prophylactically to the scrotal wall (orchiopexy) to prevent torsion of its spermatic cord with subsequent infertility.

Body image disturbances may include fears of castration, loss of masculinity, sterility, and impotence. The possibility of these fears being justified depends on the degree of insult to the testis and the functioning of the remaining testicle.

TUMORS IN MEN

Tumors of the male reproductive tract are usually malignant. The more common tumors involve the testes, prostate gland, and penis (Table 35-10).

Pathophysiology
Cancer of the testes

Cancer of the testes is the second most common malignancy in men between the ages of 18 and 35 years and is the second most common cause of death from cancer in this age group. The most common type of testicular cancers is seminomas, which usually spread slowly through the lymphatics. Embryonal tumors invade the spermatic cord and metastasize early to the lungs.[51]

Removal of the testis, with examination of the nodes, is indicated for testicular cancers. *Biopsy of the testis is contraindicated* because of the highly metastatic character

of testicular carcinoma. The prognosis following treatment of seminomas is good: 95% for Stage I (confined to testicle), 70% to 90% for Stage II (metastasis to retroperitoneal nodes), and 50% to 70% for Stage III (distal metastases).

Cancer of the prostate gland

The prostate gland is the second most common site of cancer among men; it is responsible for 12% of all deaths from cancer in men. It rarely occurs before the age of 60 years, incidence increases with age, and there is an increased familial risk. (Prostatic cancer is discussed in Chapter 33).

Cancer of the penis

The incidence of penile cancer is highly dependent on hygienic standards as well as cultural and religious practices. It almost never occurs in a male who was circumcised at birth. Circumcision after puberty does not decrease the risk of cancer when compared with the incidence among uncircumcised males. Circumcision removes the prepuce or foreskin, which provides a haven for bacteria. The bacteria act on desquamated cells producing smegma, which is irritating to the tissue of the glans penis and the prepuce. This chronic irritation is considered to be carcinogenic. Trauma and sexually transmitted diseases are felt to be coincidental to penile cancer rather than causative. Most penile malignancies are squamous cell carcinomas. The lesion may cause erosion through the prepuce with a foul odor and discharge.

Prevention and Health Education

Regular testicular self-examination (TSE) is recommended to detect cancer of the testes in its early stages when it is most likely to be localized and most curable. *All young men should be taught testicular self-examination* (Box 35-24). By performing TSE routinely, each man can get to know what is normal for him and more readily identify any lumps or abnormalities. Any swelling that is not normal should be examined by a physician. Nine of ten testicular cancers are detected by the patient or his sexual partner.

Diagnostic Tests

The prostate can be palpated by digital examination. A newer screening tool is transrectal ultrasound. Because prostatic tissue is rich in acid phosphatase, there is usually an increase in serum acid phosphatase with cancer of the

Testicular self-examination (TSE)

Perform TSE after a bath or shower when scrotum
  is warm and most relaxed
Grasp testis with both hands and palpate gently
  between thumb and fingers (Fig. 34-14)
    The testis should feel smooth, egg-shaped, and
      firm to touch
    The epididymis, found behind the testis, should
      feel like a soft tube

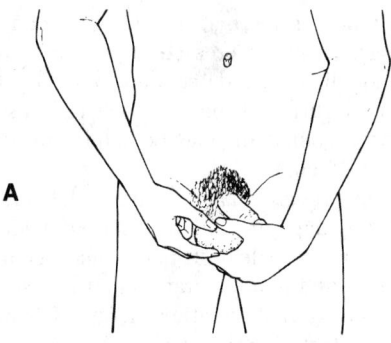

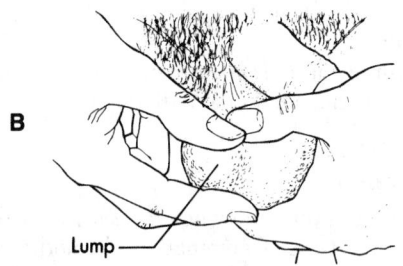

Fig. 35-14 Testicular self-examination. **A,** Grasp testis with both hands; palpate gently between thumb and fingers. **B,** Abnormal lumps or irregularities are reported to physician. (Modified from Fred Hutchinson Cancer Research Cancer Control Program: Self testicular exam, Seattle, 1980, Cancer Control Program.)

prostate. Diagnosis of cancer of the prostate gland is confirmed by *prostatic biopsy.* If the transrectal route is used for biopsy, no bowel preparation is required. There is no discomfort because the prostate has no nerves. Vital signs are monitored for possible hemorrhage because of the high vascularity of the gland. Bleeding may be from the urethra or the bladder and may be internal. The man is observed for fever, acute urinary retention, rectal bleeding, and pain or swelling of the scrotum.

Surgery

Surgery of the prostate gland is discussed in Chapter 33.

Surgery of the testicle

Orchiectomy consists of en bloc excision of the spermatic cord, the contents of the inguinal canal, and the testis with the tunica attached. The adjacent area is explored for metastases.

Preoperative care

In addition to usual preoperative care, psychologic preparation for surgery is important. The man will usually be concerned about the effects of castration. *Unilateral* removal of a testis will *not* demasculinize him or cause sterility. Prostheses are available to replace the removed testis.

Postoperative care
Activity

Bed rest may be instituted for 24 to 48 hours after extensive removal of tissue, but ambulation usually is begun within 12 hours after surgery. Leg exercises are important if bed rest is to be maintained. The scrotum is elevated on a rolled towel, or the man may wear an athletic supporter while in bed. An athletic supporter or tight undershorts should be worn for support when the patient is ambulating.

Postoperative complications

The two major problems after scrotal surgery are edema and intrascrotal hemorrhage. *Edema* may be controlled by ice bags for the first 12 hours and a compression dressing for 3 to 5 days. Ice is best applied by filling a rubber glove with crushed ice. Signs of hemorrhage or complaints of increasing discomfort are reported to the physician.

Teaching

1. Avoid prolonged standing, which increases scrotal edema.

2. Wear athletic supporter or tight undershorts until healing is complete.
3. Take 20-minute tub baths three times per day for 1 week after discharge.
4. Avoid heavy lifting for 4 to 6 weeks.

Penile surgery

Small noninvasive tumors may be removed by laser surgery. Large lesions without deep infiltration require partial penectomy, removing the penis at a point 2 cm beyond the tumor.[58] The remaining penis must be long enough for the man to void standing, direct the stream, and not void on himself. If this is possible, sexual function will probably be retained. Large deep infiltrating tumors require total penectomy with perineal urethrostomy (the urethra is redirected to an opening between the scrotum and the anus). Sexual counseling is indicated for the man with a total penectomy. Some men with urethrostomy have experienced orgasm and ejaculation following stimulation of the perineal, scrotal, and testicular regions. Counseling may also be helpful for the significant other.

Radiation

Testicular seminomas respond to radiotherapy whereas nonseminomas do not. External beam radiation is given to the abdomen following orchiectomy.

Although the normal testis is shielded during external radiation of an involved testis, it does receive radiation scattered from the abdomen. A period of 70 days is required to determine whether spermatogenesis has been affected. Spermatogenesis may be decreased for 7 months to 5 years or more. Although genetic defects are possible after irradiation, there is currently no evidence to cause serious concern. Genetic counseling may be helpful for those couples desiring children.

Radiation for *prostatic* cancer may be delivered by external beam or by implant. The testes are shielded during external radiation. Erectile dysfunction may occur. Iodine-125 retropubic prostatic implantation may be used initially or after failure of external radiation therapy. Complications of iodine-125 implantation include blood loss from multiple needle punctures during implantation, deep vein thrombosis, pulmonary emboli, hematomas, and abscesses. Potency is retained.

Small noninfiltrating *penile* tumors can be treated with external beam radiation. Nodal radiation is not as effective as surgery.

Chemotherapy

Chemotherapy is given following *orchiectomy* for those patients with metastases. Combination chemotherapy with cisplatin, vinblastine, and bleomycin is effective. For *prostatic* or *penile* cancer, chemotherapy is given only for palliative effect with deep distant metastasis.

Hormone Therapy

Estrogen therapy may be used for advanced prostatic cancer when metastasis has occurred, especially to the bone. Bilateral orchiectomy to eliminate androgen may be combined with estrogen therapy. Estrogen may also be given prophylactically following surgery or radiation therapy. In males, estrogen frequently causes gynecomastia (enlargement of the breasts), loss of libido, arrest of spermatogenesis, and testicular atrophy.

Estrogen helps to decrease pain and reduce tumor size. The use of hormone therapy provides a longer symptom-free period but makes palliation more difficult when symptoms recur. If endocrine therapy is delayed, symptoms recur earlier but longer palliation is possible.

SUMMARY

1. Premenstrual syndrome (PMS) consists of behavioral changes, fluid retention, fatigue, headache, backache, or increased appetite, which occurs repeatedly in many women before and during menstruation.

2. Dysmenorrhea is a common cause of absenteeism from work or school. Interventions include prostaglandin inhibitors, rest, heat applications, and moderate exercise.

3. Methods of sterilization include tubal ligation in the female and vasectomy in the male; although sterilization may be reversed in some cases, this is not always successful.

4. Infertility may result from obstructed fallopian tubes or vas deferens, from uterine or testicular disorders, or from hormonal deficiencies. Couples who are assessed as infertile need support in coping with the infertility and in examining alternative strategies (remain childless, adopt, artificial insemination, in vitro fertilization, GIFT, ZIFT, and mother surrogate).

5. Genital infections occur most often in females with low estrogen levels, who are malnourished, who have alkaline vaginal secretions, or who have been exposed to large numbers of organisms. Good personal hygiene, protection from infected sexual partners, and avoidance of unprescribed douching can help to prevent genital infections.

6. Pelvic inflammatory disease (PID) is a widespread inflammation of female pelvic organs; spread is up the genital tract. Chronic PID may cause adhesions requiring removal of some of the organs.

7. Toxic shock syndrome, which occurs mostly in menstruating females who use superabsorbent tampons, is associated with toxins from *Staphylococcus aureus*. Treatment consists of antibiotics and supportive care similar to that given for septic shock.

8. In the male, the common genital inflammatory disorders are urethritis, prostatitis, epididymitis (most common), and orchitis. Bilateral epididymitis usually causes sterility.

9. Common structural disorders in the female are a relaxed vaginal outlet leading to stress incontinence, displacement or prolapse of the uterus, or fistulas; the treatment is primarily surgical. Perineal (Kegel) exercises may help prevent stress incontinence by strengthening the Kegel muscle.

10. Common structural disorders in the male are hydrocele, spermatocele, varicocele, or torsion of the spermatic cord.

11. Common *benign* genital tumors in the female include ovarian cysts and tumors, uterine fibroid tumors, cervical polyps, and endometriosis (seeding of endometrial cells in the pelvis). Cervical polyps are removed for biopsy. Uterine fibroid tumors are removed only when growth is rapid or when size is causing other difficulties.

12. Removal of the uterus (hysterectomy) ends menstruation but does not lead to menopausal symptoms if the ovaries are left intact.

13. The most common genital cancer in females is cancer of the endometrium, occurring primarily in postmenopausal women. However, ovarian cancer causes more deaths than uterine cancer. The incidence of cancer of the cervix has decreased because of better screening by means of Pap smears.

14. Women should have a Pap test at least every 3 years after two initial negative tests 1 year apart. Persons at high risk for cervical cancer (early sexual activity, multiple sex partners) should have more frequent Pap tests.

15. Most genital cancers in males are prostatic cancers occurring primarily in men over age 60. Young men have a higher incidence of cancer of the testes, that can be detected early by testes self-examination (TSE).

STUDY QUESTIONS

What effect does frequent douching have on the vagina? Why is douching *not* recommended following gynecologic surgery?

What is the difference between sterility and infertility?

What is the main purpose of sterilization? How do the different approaches to infertility compare and contrast?

What are the similarities and differences between genital inflammations in women and in men in terms of method of infection, types of organisms, and usual therapy? What is a serious side effect of PID and of bilateral orchitis?

Compare the incidences of the different types of genital cancers in both sexes. Which cancers occur more frequently? Why are cervical cancers identified earlier than ovarian cancers? What effect does this have?

Why do body image disturbances occur frequently after genital surgery in women and men? What implications does this have for nursing?

REFERENCES AND SELECTED READINGS

1. American Cancer Society, *Cancer facts and figures, 1991*, Atlanta, 1991, The Society.
2. Barbo DM, editor: Symposium on the postmenopausal woman, *Med Clin North Am* 71(1):1-148, 1987.
3.* Berger PH et al: Radical hysterectomy: treatment for advanced cervical carcinoma, *AORN J* 52:1212-1218, 1990.
4.* Boarini JH, Bryant RA, Ingang SF: Fistula management, *Semin Oncol Nurs* 2:287-292, 1986.
5. Boyd AS: Varicoceles and male infertility, *Am Fam Physician* 37:252-258, 1988.
6.* Cashavelly BJ: Cervical dysplasia: an overview of current concepts in epidemiology, diagnosis, and treatment, *Cancer Nurs* 10:199-206, 1987.
7. Centers for Disease Control: Pelvic inflammatory disease: guidelines for prevention and management, *MMWR* 40(RR-5):1-25, 1991.
8. Chamorro T: Cancer of the vulva and vagina, *Semin Oncol Nurs* 6(3):198-205, 1990.
9. Davis DC, Dearman CN: Coping strategies of infertile women, *J Obstet Gynecol Neonatal Nurs* 20(3):221-227, 1991.
10.* Doane LS, Fischer LM, McDonald TW: How to give peritoneal chemotherapy, *Am J Nurs* 90(4):58-64, 1990.
11. Dodek OI: The infertile couple, *Am Fam Physician* 38:101-112, 1988.
12.* Dulaney PE, Crawford VC, Turner G: A comprehensive education and support program for women experiencing hysterectomies, *J Obstet Gynecol Neonatal Nurs* 19(4):319-325, 1990.
13. Eriksson JH, Walczak JR: Ovarian cancer, *Semin Oncol Nurs* 6(3):214-227, 1990.
14. Feldman JE: Ovarian failure and cancer treatment: incidence and interventions for the premenopausal woman, *Oncol Nurs Forum* 16:651-657, 1989.
15.* Fehring RJ: Methods used to self-predict ovulation: a comparative study, *J Obstet Gynecol Neonatal Nurs* 19(3):233-237, 1990.
16.* Fehring RJ: New technology in natural family planning, *J Obstet Gynecol Neonatal Nurs* 20(3):199-205, 1991.
17. Frank DI: Factors related to decisions about infertility treatment, *J Obstet Gynecol Neonatal Nurs* 19(2):162-167, 1990.
18.* Frank EP: What are nurses doing to help PMS patients? *Am J Nurs* 86:136-140, 1986.
19. Fullerton JT: Papanicolaou smear: an update on classification and management, *J Am Acad Nurse Pract* 1(3):84-90, 1989.
20.* Ginsberg CK: Exfoliative cytologic screening: the Papanicolaou test, *J Obstet Gynecol Neonatal Nurs* 20(1):39-46, 1991.
21.* Hampton BG: Nursing management of a patient following pelvic exenteration, *Semin Oncol Nurs* 2:275-286, 1986.
22. Hatcher RA et al: *Contraceptive technology 1988-1989,* ed 14, New York, 1989, Irvington.
23.* Henderson JS, Taylor KH: Age as a variable in an exercise program for the treatment of simple urinary stress incontinence, *J Obstet Gynecol Neonatal Nurs* 13:266-272, 1987.
24.* Higgs DJ: The patient with testicular cancer: nursing management of chemotherapy, *Oncol Nurs Forum* 17(2):243-249, 1990.
25.* Hubbard JL, Holcombe JK: Cancer of the endometrium, *Semin Oncol Nurs* 6(3):206-213, 1990.
26.* Jenkins B: Patients' report of sexual changes after treatment of gynecologic cancer, *Oncol Nurs Forum* 15(3):349-354, 1988.
27. Keye WR: Premenstrual symptoms: evaluation and treatment, *Compr Ther* 14:19-26, 1988.
28. Kirkpatrick MK, Brewer JA, Stocks B: Efficacy of self-care measures for perimenstrual syndrome (PMS), *J Adv Nurs* 15:281-285, 1990.
29.* Lamb MA: Psychosexual issues: the woman with gynecologic cancer, *Semin Oncol Nurs* 6(3):237-243, 1990.
30.* Lasater SJ: Testicular cancer: a perioperative challenge, *AORN J* 51(2):513-523, 1990.
31. Lavy G: Hysteroscopy as a diagnostic aid, *Obstet Gynecol Clin North Am* 15:61-72, 1988.
32.* Lincoln R, Roberts R: Continence issues in acute care, *Nurs Clin North Am* 24(3):741-754, 1990.
33.* Lindow KB: Premenstrual syndrome: family impact and nursing implications, *J Obstet Gynecol Neonatal Nurs* 20(2):135-138, 1991.
34. Lindsay R: The menopause: sex, steroids, and osteoporosis, *Clin Obstet Gynecol* 95:963-972, 1987.
35.* Martin FL: When the solution is a prosthesis, *RN* 53(3):32-35, 1990.
36.* Martin JP: Transrectal ultrasound: a new screening tool for prostate cancer, *Am J Nurs* 91(2):69, 1991.
37.* McKeon VA: Cruel myths and clinical facts about menopause, *RN* 52(6):52-59, 1989.
38.* Menken J, Trussell J, Larsen V: Age and infertility, *Science* 233:1389-1394, 1986.
39.* Milne BJ: Couples' experience with in vitro fertilization, *J Obstet Gynecol Neonatal Nurs* 17:347-351, 1988.
40.* Moore J: Vaginal hysterectomy: its success as an outpatient procedure, *AORN J* 48(6):1114-1120, 1988.
40a.* Moore S et al: Nerve sparing prostatectomy, *Am J Nurs* 92(4):59-64, 1992.
41.* Nolte S, Hanjani P: Intraepithelial neoplasia of the lower genital tract, *Semin Oncol Nurs* 6(3):181-189, 1990.
42. O'Laughlin KM: Changes in bladder function in the woman undergoing radical hysterectomy for cervical cancer, *J Obstet Gynecol Neonatal Nurs* 15:380-385, 1986.
43.* Pace-Owen S: Gamete intrafallopian transfer (GIFT), *J Obstet Gynecol Neonatal Nurs* 18:93-97, 1989.
44. Persinger C: Carcinoma of the penis, *J Urol Nurs* 7(2):398-407, 1988.
45. Pernoll ML, Benson RC: *Current obstetric and gynecologic diagnosis and treatment,* ed 7, Norwalk, Conn, 1991, Appleton & Lange.
46.* Reznichek CG, Reznichek R: The problem most men won't talk about: impotence, *RN* 54(3):28-32, 1990.

*Recommended for student reading.

47.* Rubin D: Gynecologic cancer: cervical, vulvular and vaginal malignancies, *RN* 50(5):56-63, 1987.

48.* Rubin D: Gynecologic cancer: uterine and ovarian malignancies, *RN* 50(6):52-57, 1987.

49. Sampselle CM: Changes in pelvic muscle strength and stress urinary incontinence associated with childbirth, *J Obstet Gynecol Neonatal Nurs* 19(5):371-377, 1990.

50. Schover LR et al: Sexual dysfunction and treatment for early stage cervical cancer, *Cancer* 63(1):204-212, 1989.

51. Schroeder SA et al: *Current medical diagnosis and treatment*, ed 30, Norwalk, Conn, 1991, Appleton & Lange.

52.* Secor RMC: Bacterial vaginosis: a comprehensive review, *Nurs Clin North Am* 23:865-875, 1988.

53. Shattuck JC: Pelvic inflammatory disease: education for maintaining fertility, *Nurs Clin North Am* 23(4):899-906, 1988.

54. Speroff L, Glass RH, Kase N: *Clinical gynecologic endocrinology and infertility*, ed 4, Baltimore, 1989, Williams & Wilkins.

55.* Thompson LJ: Cancer of the cervix, *Semin Oncol Nurs* 6(3):190-197, 1990.

56.* Tinkle MB: Genital human papillomavirus infection: a growing health risk, *J Obstet Gynecol Neonatal Nurs* 19(6):501-507, 1990.

57. Velduis JD: Management of amenorrhea, *Hosp Pract* 23(11A):40-56, 1988.

58. Way L: *Current surgical diagnosis and treatment*, ed 9, Norwalk, Conn, 1991, Appleton & Lange.

59. Yoder LH: The epidemiology of ovarian cancer: a review, *Oncol Nurs Forum* 17(3):411-415, 1990.

60.* Zion AB: Resources for infertile couples, *J Obstet Gynecol Neonatal Nurs* 17:255-258, 1988.

36

The Patient with Problems of the Breast

Barbara C. Long

After studying this chapter, the learner should be able to:

- Evaluate breast self-examination (guidelines, techniques).
- Differentiate between benign and malignant breast disorders.
- Describe the pathophysiology and interventions for women with benign breast disorders.
- Explain the risk factors and pathophysiology of breast cancer.
- Describe the types of surgery for breast cancer, most common procedures, and postoperative care.
- Describe types of breast reconstruction and required care.

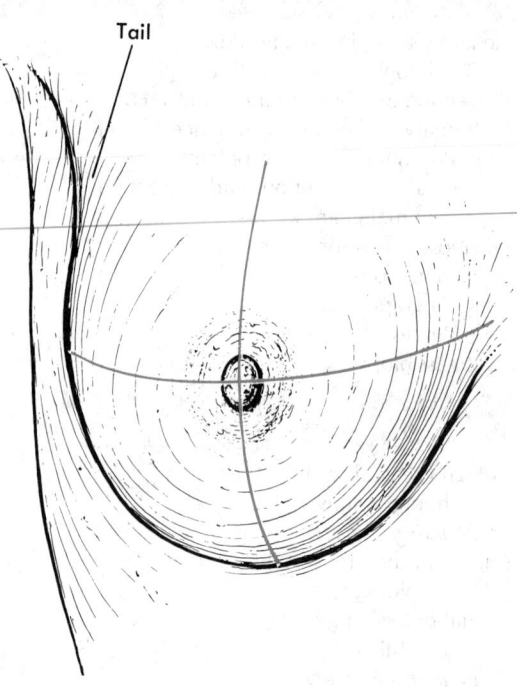

Fig. 36-1 Breast mass includes "tail" that extends from upper, outer quadrant toward axilla. (From Malasanos L, et al: *Health assessment,* ed 4, St. Louis, 1990, Mosby–Year Book.)

36-1

Guidelines for Care

Guidelines for breast self-examination

1. Perform BSE regularly each month
   a. Premenopausal women: 7 to 8 days after conclusion of the menstrual period
   b. Postmenopausal women: at a set time each month (such as the first day of the month)
2. Use a systematic approach (one of the three listed here)
   a. Palpate in concentric circles beginning at outer rim of breast tissue and move toward nipple
   b. Divide breast into quadrants and examine area in each quadrant from outer perimeter toward nipple
   c. Palpate inner half then outer half of breast
3. Examine the entire breast tissue, including the tail (Fig. 36-1) and the nipple
4. Carry out examination in both the horizontal and vertical body positions (Fig. 36-2)
5. Use the flat parts of the fingers for palpation

The breasts are associated with feelings of sexuality and are an integral component of sexual behavior. The development of the breasts in the female adolescent indicates her approaching womanhood and emphasizes her femininity. The breast, especially the nipples, which are erectile tissue, are erogenous areas in sexual activity. The advertising media emphasize the desirability of the female breast; femininity is typified by a fashion model's breasts, whereas masculinity is typified by the flat, expansive chest of the lifeguard. Diseases of the breast, therefore, evoke varied feelings and cause fears and concerns that influence the practice of breast self-examination or the seeking of diagnostic and therapeutic care.

ANATOMY AND PHYSIOLOGY

The breasts lie over the pectoralis muscles of the chest. Each breast is composed of 12 to 20 lobes of glandular tissue separated by connective tissue. The lobes are held in place by suspensory ligaments connected both to the skin and to the underlying fascia. The milk gland ducts in each lobe join to form a larger duct that terminates in a small hole in the nipple. The glandular tissue is surrounded by fat that determines the size of the breasts. Lymphatic drainage of the breasts is primarily to the axillary nodes but some lymph also drains toward substernal and diaphragmatic nodes.

The breasts are associated functionally with the reproductive system as an organ for milk production in the postpartum woman. The female sex hormones influence the development of the breasts and the production of milk.

Physiologic Changes With Aging

As fat decreases and tissue atrophies with age, the breasts generally become smaller and hang more loosely. The nipples become smaller and flatter. The breasts may feel more granular with palpation.

PREVENTION AND HEALTH EDUCATION

Primary Prevention: Avoidance of Common Breast Problems

Premenstrual breast discomfort

Tenderness, discomfort, and swelling of the breasts before menstruation are normal functional changes in the breasts that respond to monthly cyclical changes in estrogen and progesterone. Water retention contributes to the swelling. Women who experience some of these problems can be taught to reduce dietary salt intake during the immediate premenstrual period. Increased physical activity during this time will improve cardiovascular dynamics and help reduce the tight, puffy feeling.

Breast discomfort during physical activity

Bras provide support for the breasts and help prevent sagging and pulling on the underlying muscles. All but small-breasted women may find physical activity uncomfortable unless a bra is worn. A *jogbra,* which does not contain metal clips or fasteners and which has seams on the outside of the fabric away from the skin, may provide greater comfort for physical activity.

Secondary Prevention: Early Detection of Malignancy

Examination of the breast

Mortality from breast cancer can be prevented in many instances through early diagnosis and treatment. The American Cancer Society recommends examinations of the breast as follows:

1. Monthly breast self-examination by *all* women over 20 years of age

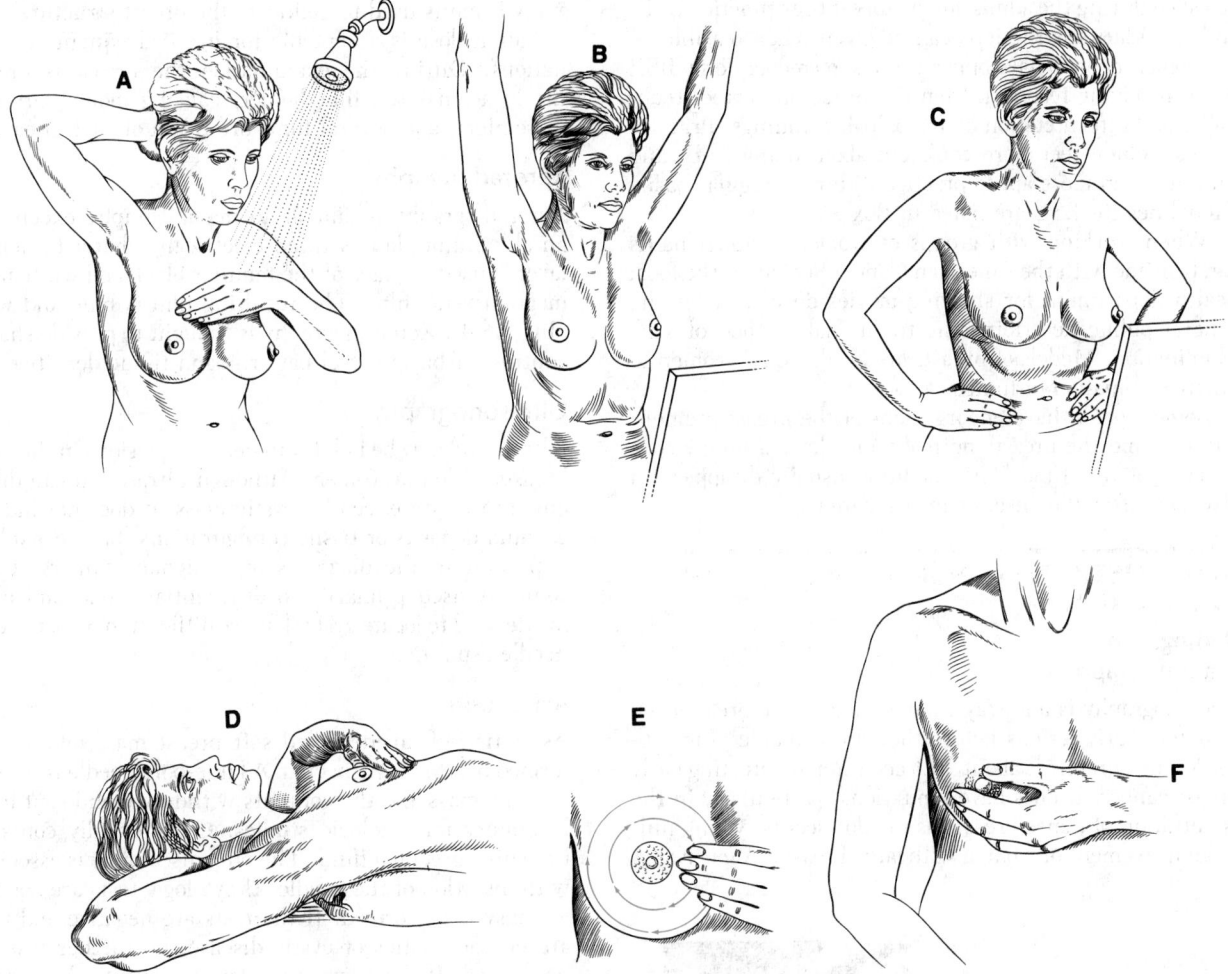

Fig. 36-2 Breast self-examination. **A,** Examine breasts during bath or shower, since flat fingers glide easily over wet skin. Use right hand to examine left breast and vice versa. **B,** Sit or stand before a mirror. Inspect breasts with hands at sides, then raised overhead. Look for changes in contour or dimpling of skin. **C,** Place hands on hips and press down firmly to flex chest muscles. **D,** Lie down with one hand under head and pillow or folded towel under the scapula. **E,** Palpate that breast with other hand using concentric circle method. It usually takes three circles to cover all breast tissue. Include the tail of the breast and the axilla. Repeat with other breast. **F,** End in a sitting position. Palpate the areola areas of both breasts, and inspect and squeeze nipples to check for discharge.

2. Women at high risk before age 50: mammography yearly; breast examination by physician every 2 years
3. Women 20 to 40
   a. One baseline mammogram between ages 35 to 40
   b. Breast examination by physician every 3 years
4. Women 40 to 49: breast examination by physician and mammography every 1 to 2 years (the newest recommendations are mammography yearly after age 40)
5. Women over 50: breast examination by physician and mammography yearly

Studies have shown that the groups of women who are least likely to have regular breast examinations by a physician are elderly, poorly educated, low-income, and black. Some of the reasons are as follows:

Lack of knowledge
Low priority set on preventive measures
Lack of income

Fear of finding a tumor
Concern over possibility of breast removal
Fear of death
Possible life changes if breast cancer is found
Embarrassment
Examination is considered too trivial for a busy physician

Most breast cancers (about 90%) are discovered by self-examination. Breast cancer is usually curable when discovered early and treated immediately. All women, beginning at high school age, should know how to carry out breast self-examination.

Breast self-examination (BSE)

Nurses working in the hospital or community settings have the responsibility of teaching women how to examine their breasts and of explaining why it is necessary. Patients can be asked during the admission history if they practice BSE, and necessary instructions can be given when feasible.

Women need to have opportunities to *practice* doing BSE while receiving feedback from the nurse on correct technique and interpretation of any palpable findings. Practice makes women feel more confident about doing BSE, and they are then more apt to practice BSE on a regular basis. Guidelines for BSE are listed in Box 36-1.

When working with groups of women, arrangements can be made with the American Cancer Society or the local health department for showing movies developed for the general public describing the traditional method of self-examination. Models of breasts are available for women to practice palpation of lumps.

Some women have engorgement of the breast premenstrually, and the breasts normally may have a lumpy consistency at this time. The condition usually disappears a few days after the onset of menstruation.

DIAGNOSTIC TESTS FOR BREAST EVALUATION

Radiographs

Mammography

Mammography is an x-ray examination of the breast used to detect early lesions before they are palpable (Fig. 36-3). Mammography is about 90% accurate in detecting early breast cancer. It does have limitations, particularly in the penetration of dense breasts as in adolescents, young nulliparous women, or women with large breasts. A *low-energy*

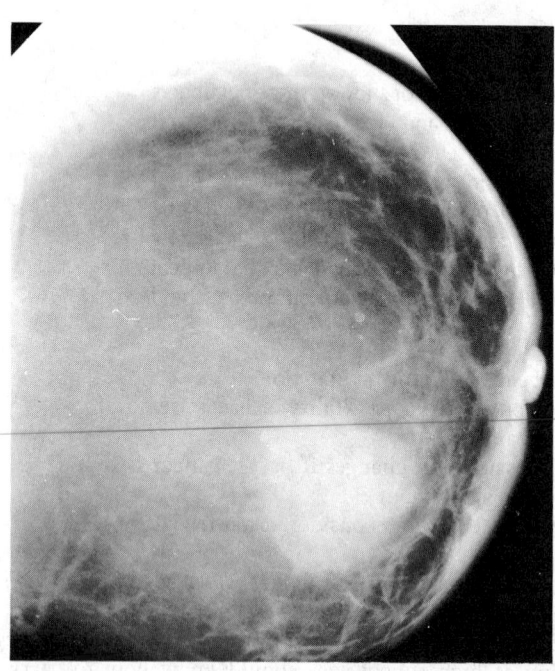

Fig. 36-3 Mammogram of patient with area of density indicating carcinoma. (From Cramer LN, Lapayowker MS: *Applied anatomy of the female breast: surgical, radiographic, and thermographic.* In Masters FW, Lewis JR Jr: *Symposium of aesthetic surgery of the face, eyelid, and breast,* vol 4, St Louis, 1972, Mosby–Year Book.)

x-ray beam is used to delineate the breast structures; thi radiation dose is acceptable for use in frequent reexami nations. During the examination the breast is presse firmly against the film holder, causing momentary mil discomfort, and several films are taken of each breast.

Xeroradiography

Xeroradiography is similar to mammography except tha an aluminum plate with an electrically charged seleniun layer is used in place of the familiar black and white mam mogram x-ray film. The resulting film is blue and white (Fig. 36-4). Xeroradiography is thought to provide sharpe contrast of blood vessel patterns and tissue densities.

Ultrasonography

Ultrasound may be helpful in detecting lesions in the dens breasts of young women. Although ultrasound can differ entiate the presence of a cystic mass, it does not indicat calcium deposits or tissue configurations, facts considere important in the diagnosis of malignant tumors. Ultra sound is used primarily to differentiate solid and cysti masses and to locate cysts that are difficult to palpate befor needle aspiration.

Aspiration

Aspiration of an identified soft breast mass may be per formed if a cyst is suspected. A large-bore needle is inserte into the mass and the contents withdrawn and sent to th laboratory for cytologic studies. Cysts usually contain brownish-greenish fluid. The only discomfort is associate with insertion of the needle. If cytologic tests are positive a biopsy is performed. If the tests are negative and ther are characteristics of cystic disease, no further tests ar performed. If there are some doubts, despite the negativ results, further radiographic studies may be performed.

Breast Biopsy

Biopsy is the only way to determine conclusively whethe a tumor is benign or malignant. Most lesions (80%) ar found to be benign.

The procedure is usually performed with a patient un der local or general anesthesia in an ambulatory surgica suite. An incision is made and a portion of the mass (o the entire mass if it is very small) is removed and sent t the laboratory for examination. Following the procedur the patient may experience mild discomfort. Results wil be available immediately if a frozen section is done, o within 48 to 72 hours.

Sometimes the small lesion size makes location of the lesion difficult or uncertain when biopsy is attempted. Therefore, to locate areas for surgical biopsy, a small methylene blue dye mark is made within the area of the breas using a syringe and needle during mammographic monitoring (needle localization). This is done in the x-ray department a few hours before the surgical biopsy, and the mark is made while the patient is under local anesthesia. No color disfiguration is apparent on the breast surface as a result of this procedure, but the mark ensures that the biopsy tissue corresponds to the site identified by mammogram. This procedure requires preinstruction to the patient and support in the x-ray department.

MAJOR HEALTH PROBLEMS OF THE BREAST

Breast lesions may be benign or malignant. Although benign lesions are more common, cancer of the breast is a major type of cancer in women and requires much more nursing care. Therefore, cancer of the breast is discussed in more detail. Breast disorders occur primarily in women, but *they can also occur in men.*

BENIGN BREAST DISORDERS

The major benign breast disorders are fibrocystic in nature (mammary dysplasia, cysts), benign tumors (fibroadenomas), or infections (mastitis with or without breast abscess) (Table 36-1). The most common disease of the breast is mammary dysplasia.

Pathophysiology

Benign breast disorders are usually characterized by one or more movable breast masses, often seen bilaterally (Fig. 36-5). The nodularity may be discrete or diffuse. If tenderness is present, it usually occurs or is increased premenstrually. Any nipple discharge, which may be clear, green, or brownish (but not bloody), is usually spontaneous, especially just before menstruation. Women who take oral contraceptives may experience some nipple discharge that ceases when the pill is discontinued.

Males may have overdevelopment of breast tissue (gynecomastia) as a result of estrogen production during puberty or older age, adrenal or gonadal tumors, or certain drugs, for example, amphetamines, antidepressants (tricyclic), antihypertensive agents, antineoplastic agents, cimetidine, diazepam, digitalis, estrogen, human chorionic gonadotropin, isoniazid, and phenothiazines.

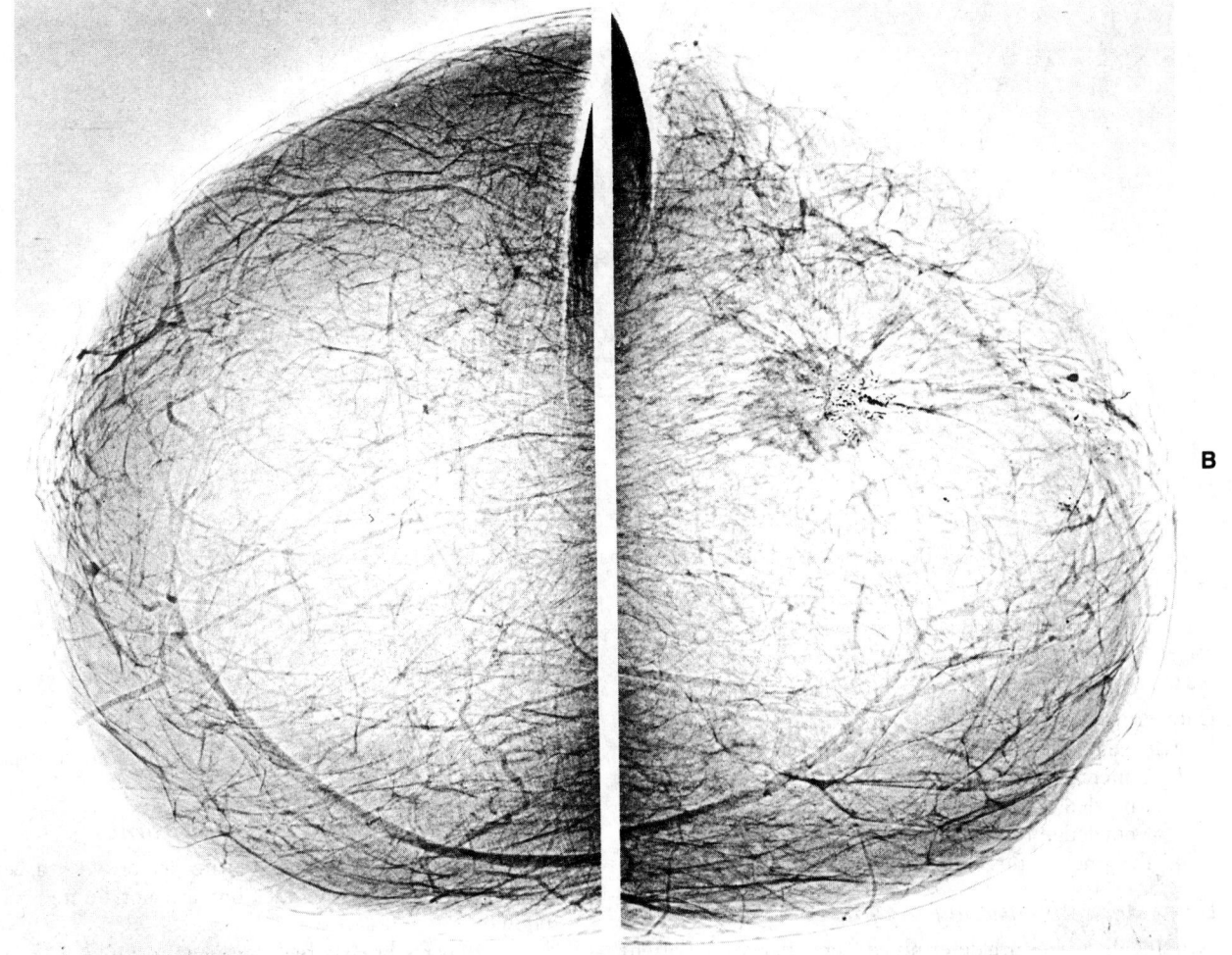

A   **B**

Fig. 36-4   Xeroradiographs. **A,** Normal left breast. **B,** Right breast shows mass with spiculated margins characteristic of neoplasm. (Courtesy University Hospitals of Cleveland, Ohio.)

REVIEW

Table 36-1 Benign breast disorders

Disorder	Characteristics	Signs and symptoms	Medical therapy
Mammary dysplasia (fibrocystic disease)	Refers to several cystic nodular disorders of the breast that become painful during menstruation; seen mostly in women age 30 to 50; estrogen hormone a causative factor	Painful, often multiple and bilateral soft masses in breast; may increase in size or remain the same	Aspiration of probable cyst biopsy of doubtful cyst to confirm diagnosis; yearly mammograms; intermittent diuretics for premenstrual breast engorgement; symptomatic pain relief
Fibroadenoma	Fibroplastic tumors commonly seen in young women under age 25	Firm, round, freely movable, nontender mass in breast	Surgical excision with patient under local anesthesia on outpatient basis
Mastitis	Inflammation of breast, usually from cracked or infected nipples	Pain, redness, swelling of breast, fever	Systemic antibiotics; incision and drainage if an abscess forms; symptomatic pain relief

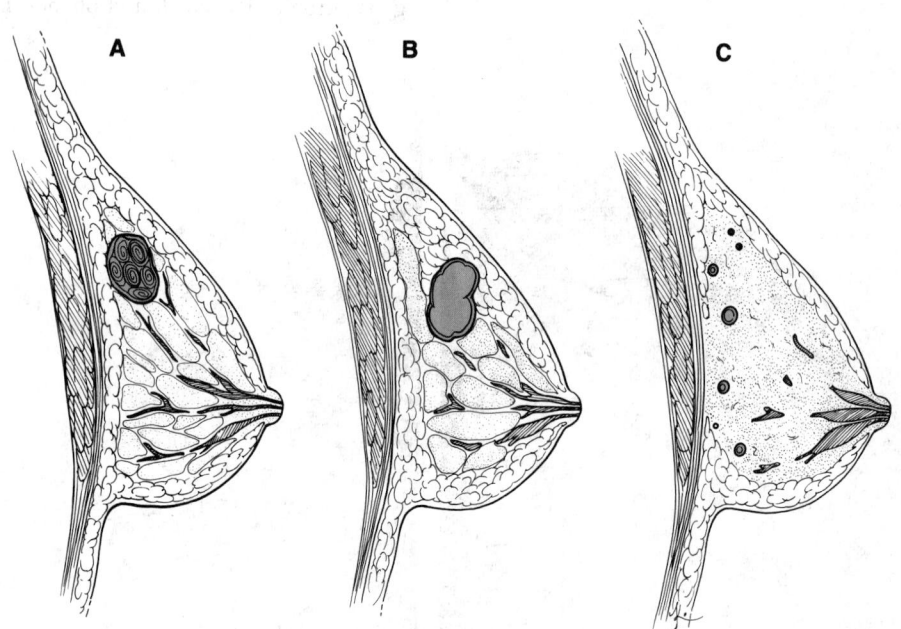

Fig. 36-5 Benign breast disorders. **A,** Fibroadenoma. **B,** Cyst. **C,** Adenosis (mammary dysplasia).

Nursing Process
Assessment

Data are collected concerning the person's feelings and knowledge about the disorder, including the following:

1. Concerns about the mass
2. Knowledge of benign versus malignant tumors
3. Knowledge regarding breast self-examination
4. Presence of discomfort

Data analysis: nursing diagnoses

Nursing diagnoses are determined from analysis of patient data. Possible nursing diagnoses for the person with a benign breast disorder may include, but are not limited to, the following:

Diagnostic title	Possible etiologies
Pain	Breast disorder
Anxiety	Fear of cancer
Knowledge deficit	Lack of information/recall, information misinterpretation

Planning: expected patient outcomes

Expected patient outcomes for the person with a benign breast disorder may include, but are not limited to, the following:

1. Reports breasts feel more comfortable.
2. Signs of anxiety are decreased.
3. Demonstrates correct technique for BSE.
4. Describes:

Table 36-2   Differences between benign and malignant breast masses

Benign	Malignant
Usually bilateral; may be unilateral	Unilateral
Found often in outer quadrants but may occur anywhere	Found most often in upper outer quadrant and tail or in central nipple portion
Single or multiple	Usually single
Well-circumscribed	Irregular
Soft or firm	Firm
Movable	Nonmovable
Usually have cyclic tenderness; may be nontender	Nontender
No skin changes	Later findings: skin thickened; dimpling
	Very late: ulceration
No palpable lymph nodes	Palpable lymph nodes except in early period
No nipple retraction; discharge usually bilateral, serous, or greenish	Nipple retraction; discharge usually unilateral and may be bloody

   a. Difference between benign and malignant breast disease

   b. Plans to do monthly BSE

   c. Plans for yearly medical follow-up

Implementation
Interventions to achieve patient outcomes
Assisting with comfort

Breast discomfort may be decreased by mild analgesics (such as aspirin or acetaminophen), by application of heat or cold, or by breast support. Heat may be applied by application of a warm damp washcloth covered by a dry towel and heating pad or hot water bottle. Some women experience relief from an ice bag or a washcloth wrung out in cold water (especially for mastitis).

Wearing a firm brassiere both day and night may also help to relieve breast discomfort. The brassiere should fit well and give good support, especially for the upper outer breast quadrant.[65]

Reducing anxiety

Most women who identify a breast mass immediately think of cancer and are, therefore, usually very anxious until the diagnosis is verified. Spouses or significant others may also experience anxiety. Even after being told that the condition is benign, some women continue to have some anxiety. *Mild* anxiety is useful as this acts as a stimulus for continuing medical follow-up.

The woman who is moderately or severely anxious needs an opportunity to express her concerns to an empathic listener. As the anxiety decreases, the woman is better able to deal with any discomfort and continue her usual activities.

Facilitating learning

The risk of breast cancer in women with mammary dysplasia is twice that for women in general. It is *very important*, therefore, that these women know how to perform accurate breast self-examination and how to recognize masses that differ from the masses of their dysplasia (Table 36-2). More frequent medical follow-up than that specified for asymptomatic people is indicated.

The role of methylxanthines in the reduction of symp-

toms in benign breast disorders is controversial. Omission of coffee, tea, and chocolate from the diet may help some people and is worth a try.

Evaluation
Evaluation is based on expected patient outcomes. Questions to consider may include the following:

1. Is breast discomfort lessened?
2. Does the patient appear less anxious?
3. Does the person know:
   a. The difference between benign and malignant disease?
   b. The method and frequency of breast self-examination?
   c. The frequency of medical follow-up?

CANCER OF THE BREAST
Epidemiology
The breast is the leading site for cancer in women but is now second to lung cancer in the number of deaths from cancer in women. It is estimated that 1 out of 9 women in the United States will develop cancer of the breast, and this probability increases with age.[1] The incidence of breast cancer has been increasing (especially in blacks) in the United States at about 3% per year since 1980; some of this increase is believed to result from early detection during screening programs.[1] Mortality rates have remained about the same.

Numerous risk factors have been identified for breast cancer (see Box 36-2). A major factor that places the woman at risk is a long uninterrupted time period of cyclic hormone changes, that is, early menarche, late menopause, and no pregnancy. Epidemiologic studies have supported the hypothesis that high fat consumption is positively associated with a higher incidence of breast cancer.[5] It must be noted, however, that 75% of women with breast cancer are *not* in the high risk group; therefore *all* women should be considered at risk for breast cancer.

Pathophysiology
Breast cancer is not one disease but many, depending on the tissue of the breast involved, its estrogen dependency,

Table 36-3 TNM classification of breast cancers

Stage	Tumor size	Nodal involvement	Metastasis
I	Less than 2 cm (T1)	None (N0)	None (M0)
II	Less than 5 cm (T1 or T2)	Movable axillary nodes (N1)	None (M0)
III	Greater than 5 cm with invasion of skin or attached to chest wall	Movable or fixed axillary nodes (N1 or N2)	None (M0)
IV	Any size (any T)	Any nodes (any N)	Yes (M1)

36-2

High-risk factors associated with breast cancer

Sex	Female (99% in women)
Age	80% are over age 35; mean and median age is 60
Familial history	Mother/sister, especially with premenopausal or bilateral breast cancer
Menstrual history	Menarche before age 11; menopause after age 50
Pregnancy	First live birth after age 30; or nullipara
Medical history	Primary breast cancer (risk increased 7 times for a second primary breast cancer); uterine endometrial cancer; mammary dysplasia
Diet	High fat intake

---

and the age of onset. Most breast tumors at the time of diagnosis are infiltrating tumors of the ducts. About 6% to 8% are invasive lobular, and 4% to 6% are noninvasive.

Malignant breast tumors differ from benign tumors (Table 36-2). They are usually solitary, irregularly shaped, firm, nontender, nonmobile masses with a tendency to adhere to the pectoralis muscles and to the skin, causing retraction or dimpling of the skin. The skin may become thickened, giving it an "orange peel" effect. Involvement of the lymph nodes is present in about two thirds of the women at the time of diagnosis. Even when the lymph nodes are negative, it is believed that micrometastasis is present. Favored sites for metastasis are the lungs, bone, liver, brain, adrenal glands, and ovaries.

Breast cancers are classified using the TNM classification (described in Chapter 11). *T* refers to tumor size, *N* to nodal involvement, and *M* to metastasis. The classification of breast cancer (Table 36-3 and Fig. 36-6) serves as a basis for prognosis and direction for treatment.

The stage of breast cancer is the most reliable indicator of prognosis. Stage I tumors have 75% to 90% cure rate with the accepted forms of therapy.[65] Stage III tumors are more poorly differentiated and have a high rate of recurrence. Patients with negative hormone receptors and negative lymph nodes have a higher recurrence rate that patients with positive hormone receptors and negative lymph nodes.

Medical Therapy

Because two thirds of patients with breast cancer eventually show metastasis, breast cancer is now considered to be a *systemic* rather than a local disease.[65] Even when the lymph nodes are negative it is thought that micrometastasis has already occurred by the time of diagnosis. Medical therapy, therefore, has now changed from primarily local therapy (surgery of the breast) to include additional therapies (radiation, chemotherapy, hormone therapy).

Surgery of the breast

Eighty to ninety percent of breast cancers are operable. The type of surgery depends on the extent of the growth and patient choice. Because breast cancer is being identified at earlier stages than in the past (as a result of BSE and mammography screening), surgical procedures are less radical than in the past. The two most commonly used procedures are lumpectomy with axillary dissection and modified radical mastectomy.

Lumpectomy

Lumpectomy is a type of segmental mastectomy in which only the tumor and a margin of surrounding clear tissue are removed, not the entire breast (as in mastectomy). *Cryolumpectomy* consists of freezing and thawing the tumor several times before removing it. *Quadrantectomy* is another form of segmental mastectomy in which the quadrant of the breast in which the tumor is located is removed. In most instances, axillary nodes are dissected through a separate incision to examine the nodes for metastasis, to determine further treatment, and as a preventive method for spread of metastasis.

Lumpectomies are an option when the tumor is small (less than 4 cm) and can be totally removed. When lumpectomy is combined with a course of radiation, the long-term results are similar to those following a modified radical mastectomy. Although the breast is not removed, breast appearance does change because of loss of tissue through biopsy and surgery, and from skin changes with radiation. Hospital stays generally average 1 to 2 days.

Modified radical mastectomy

The entire breast tissue, axillary lymph nodes, and fascia underlying the breast are removed with a modified radical mastectomy. The pectoralis major muscle remains

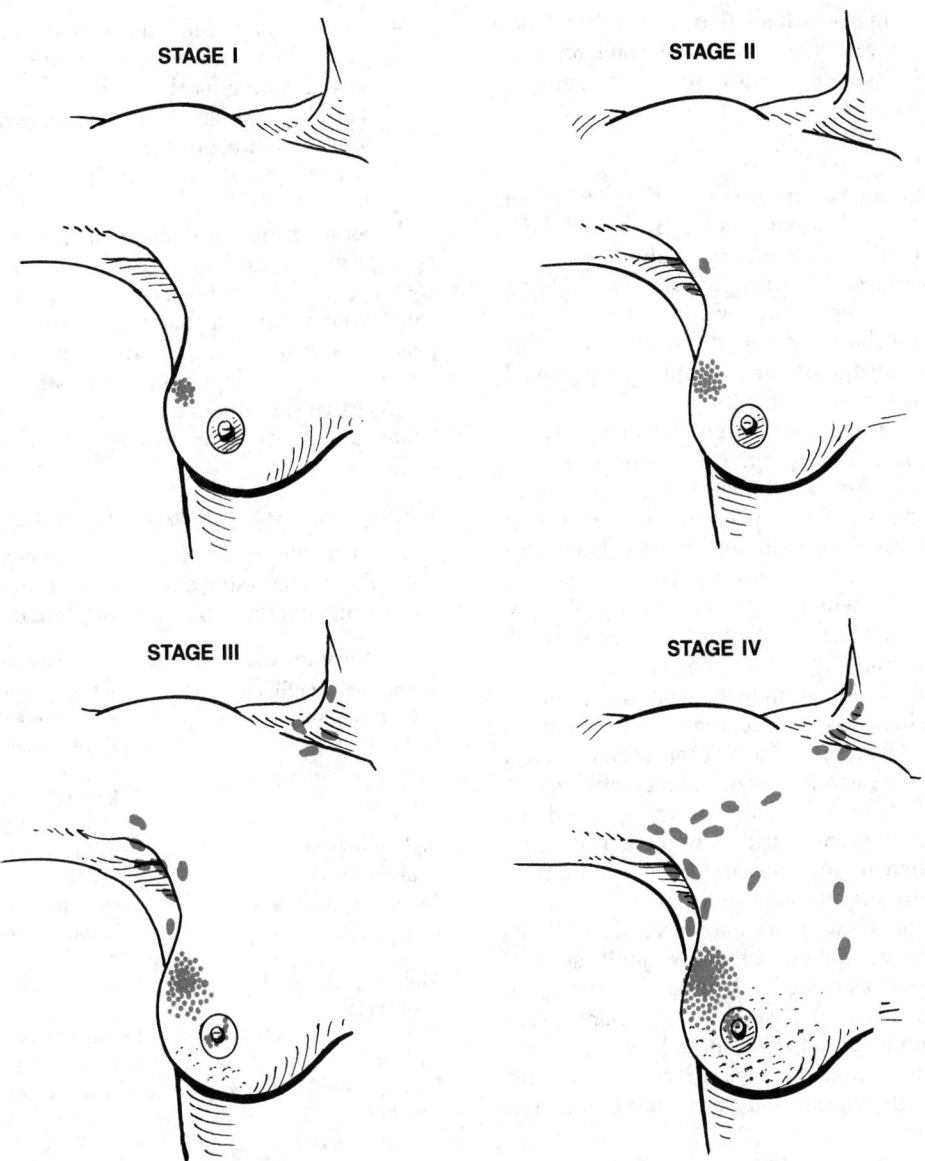

STAGE I

STAGE II

STAGE III

STAGE IV

Fig. 36-6   Stages of breast cancer. Note that in Stage I the tumor is small and there is no nodal involvement. As the tumor progresses to Stage IV, tumor size increases, nodal involvement is more extensive, and the skin finally dimples.

intact. Because the majority of breast cancers are ductal and the ducts lead to the nipple, the nipple is removed, but as much skin as possible is retained. Following removal of early cancers, breast reconstruction (p. 1177) may be done at this time if the patient so desires. Hospital stays generally average 3 to 5 days, but may be longer if reconstruction has been done.

Radiation therapy

Radiation therapy alone, without surgery, is not an effective therapy for breast cancer. Radiation may be used with far advanced cancer to contain the tumor before surgery. After lumpectomy, radiation is very useful to prevent recurrence. The entire breast is radiated 5 days a week for 5 weeks, followed by a boost to the tumor bed, either by external beam therapy or by interstitial implants (brachytherapy). For *brachytherapy*, a hospital stay of 2 to 3 days is necessary. Hollow catheters are placed (with the patient under anesthesia) in parallel rows under the skin over the affected breast area. The patient then returns to a private room on the division, where radioactive strands are threaded by the physician into the tubes and fastened with "buttons". If Iodine-125 is used, a low-energy radioisotope, a thin rubberized lead shield, is placed over the dressing to minimize radiation exposure; more extensive shielding is necessary if Iridium-192 is used.[41] There is generally little discomfort except a dull aching sensation that can be relieved by analgesics. The implant is usually removed in 24 hours. Except for a pulling sensation, there is little discomfort with removal. The patient should not shower while the implant is in place. Radiation of the breast tissue continues for several weeks and may cause some mild discomfort. (Care of the patient with internal radiation is discussed in Chapter 11).

Adjuvant therapy

Because micrometastases occur even in patients with normal axillary nodes, the National Cancer Institute (NCI) in 1988 issued a clinical alert recommending that all patients with breast cancer receive adjuvant therapy.[46] Beneficial effects have been noted in prevention of recurrence, but no effects have yet been noted on survival.[65] All patients are now being evaluated after surgery and appropriate adjuvant therapy is being recommended.

Hormonal therapy, usually tamoxifen (Nolvadex), is recommended for women with positive hormone receptors, except for the premenopausal woman with positive lymph nodes. *Chemotherapy* is recommended for all women with negative hormone receptors and for the premenopausal woman with positive lymph nodes and positive estrogen receptors. Combined chemotherapy, especialy CMF (cyclophosphamide, methotrexate, fluorouracil) is more effective than single drugs.[65]

Every patient is considered individually. Factors in deciding therapy include risk of recurrence and benefits of therapy as compared with side effects. Tamoxifen is usually well tolerated but is relatively expensive. Side effects may include hot flashes, vaginal discharge or dryness, and loss of menstrual cycles in premenopausal women. With chemotherapy, most women experience mild weight gain, nausea, mild fatigue, hair thinning or loss, loss of menstrual cycles (in premenopausal women), and decreases in WBC and RBC counts. Some women experience vomiting, total hair loss, infection, and stomatitis. During chemotherapy, women are encouraged to eat well, get sufficient sleep, drink plenty of liquids (to help prevent side effects of cyclophosphamide), remain involved, and report signs of illness or stomatitis. In general, chemotherapy is well tolerated by most women.

A new approach for the patient with *advanced* breast cancer is high-dose chemotherapy with autologous bone marrow transplantation (ABMT). Bone marrow is removed before chemotherapy, purged of any remnants of cancer, then reintroduced after chemotherapy to regenerate new bone marrow. This procedure results in higher frequency of complete remissions in patients with metastatic breast cancer, and may keep some patients disease-free for extended periods of time.

Nursing Process
Assessment

If a malignant breast tumor is suspected or diagnosed as such, the following *subjective data* are obtained as a baseline for planning:

1. Concerns about the diagnosis and forthcoming therapy
2. Feelings and thoughts about sexuality and the relationship of the breast to these feelings
3. Thoughts about feelings of the sex partner (if appropriate) concerning the forthcoming potential therapy options

4. Future goals, life expectancies, zest for living, and actual or perceived responsibility to others
5. Usual coping mechanisms
6. Family relationships and the existence and availability of support persons
7. Knowledge about BSE (for examination of other breast)

If possible, data are obtained from the sex partner (if appropriate) regarding attitudes about the forthcoming therapy. This identifies possible conflicts in perceptions, the degree of support that can be anticipated from the sex partner, and the potential effects of the partner's feelings on the woman's adaptation and relationships.

Objective data include observations about the woman's behavior and vital signs, which might indicate signs of high anxiety.

Data analysis: nursing diagnoses

Nursing diagnoses are determined from analysis of patient data. Possible nursing diagnoses for the person with breast cancer may include, but are not limited to, the following:

Diagnostic title	Possible etiologies
Decisional conflict (treatment options)	Unclear values, lack of information, support system deficit
Anxiety	Fear of surgery, cancer, removal of breast, change in family relationships; decision making about surgery
Body image or self-esteem disturbance	Loss of breast, difficulty making decisions
Infection, high risk for	Loss of skin intactness, decreased immune response (node removal)
Mobility, impaired physical	Restricted shoulder movement
Pain	Incision, loss of breast tissue
Fatigue	Surgery, adjuvant therapy
Coping, ineffective individual	Fear of cancer recurrence, death
Sexuality patterns, altered	Loss of breast
Knowledge deficit	Lack or misinterpretation of information

Planning expected patient outcomes

Expected patient outcomes for the patient with cancer of the breast may include, but are not limited to, the following:

1. Participates in making decisions concerning therapy, as possible.
2. Demonstrates signs of decreased anxiety.
3. Demonstrates femininity, such as by applying makeup, fixing hair, putting on own nightgown.
4. Incision does not become infected.
5. Participates in arm exercises.
6. States feeling more comfortable.
7. Rests between activities.
8. Looks at incision.
9. Interacts with others appropriately, especially with spouse or significant other.
10. Describes:
    a. Plans for breast prosthesis (if appropriate)
    b. Ways to prevent infection and edema in affected arm

c. Plans for monthly BSE
d. Personal and community support resources, as needed

Implementation
Interventions to achieve patient outcomes

Because surgery is the primary therapeutic approach for patients with breast cancer, nursing care focuses on preoperative and postoperative care. Care of the patient following mastectomy is summarized in Box 36-3. Patients having lumpectomy and axillary node dissection require similar care except for the type of exercises and not requiring information on breast prostheses.

Preoperative care
Assisting the patient with decision making

Patients report that the period from the time of tumor identification until surgery is a one of high anxiety. Making decisions when anxiety is high is very difficult. Providing necessary information and support can facilitate the decision-making process.

When the diagnostic work is completed and the tumor has been classified, the physician, often after consulting the hospital tumor board members (medical, surgical, and radiation oncologists) and plastic surgeon, discusses and proposes treatment options. The patient and spouse/friend are involved at this point in the treatment decision plan. If the malignancy is in stage I or II, the woman usually has several options for therapy that offer her a comparable prognosis. The choices are usually lumpectomy with radiation, or mastectomy. Two pamphlets that may be helpful for the patient in decision making are "Breast care: understanding treatment options" and "Mastectomy: a treatment for breast cancer" available from NCI.* Up-to-date and accurate information about cancer treatment can also be obtained from NCI. Women may be influenced by magazine articles and may need help in acquiring accurate information and in sorting out what is best for them from their standpoint. She is the one making the final decision and it should be an educated decision. Female nurses have the advantage of facilitating decision making because of their expertise as health professionals while taking into consideration the subjective hesitations of the woman. The nurse can help the woman work through the steps of the decision-making process. Providing structure for the process can help decrease the anxiety about making a "wrong" decision.

For the patient with stage III cancer there are fewer options and greater consequences. Mastectomy is generally the treatment of choice from a medical standpoint. The woman may feel a sense of *powerlessness* at this point. Letting her make decisions about other aspects of her life and activities of daily living, when possible, helps her hold onto a sense of control of her life.

Women having a mastectomy usually have the option of choosing immediate or delayed breast reconstruction (p. 1177). This information often helps to decrease the concerns of the woman who fears deformity from loss of a

*National Cancer Institute, Building 31, Room 10A24, Bethesda, Md 20892 (1-800-4-CANCER).

36-3 **Guidelines for Care**

The patient who has had a mastectomy

Preoperative care
1. Help patient explore feelings about loss of breast and fears related to cancer
2. Provide simple explanations; repeat as necessary
3. Teach patient:
   a. Expectation of catheter to drain wound
   b. Need for postoperative exercises

Postoperative care
1. Give immediate care
   a. Place patient in semi-Fowler's position
   b. Wound care:
      (1) If Hemovac suction is used, empty when halffull to maintain suction
      (2) Check dressing and bed for signs of drainage
   c. Elevate arm on pillow
   d. Monitor circulation of arm on affected side; report signs of swelling and numbness of lower arm or inability to move fingers
   e. Avoid blood pressure readings, blood testing, IVs, or injections in affected arm
   f. Teach patient to sit up in bed by *pushing* up on elbow of *unaffected* side, rather than pulling up with arm
   g. Encourage deep breathing exercises
   h. Give analgesics for comfort
2. Encourage postmastectomy arm exercises
   a. Start gentle exercises early (see p. 1171)
   b. Start special mastectomy exercises (see p. 1171) when prescribed
3. Encourage rest periods; monitor for fatigue
4. Provide emotional support
   a. Continue to help patient explore feelings
   b. Prepare patient in advance concerning size of incision and be with her, if possible, when she looks at incision
   c. Encourage patient to identify feelings about resuming sexual activities (if appropriate) and to discuss these feelings with sexual partner
5. Teach patient
   a. Wear a brassiere padded with a soft fluffy filling or temporary soft prosthesis until incision is healed (if appropriate)
   b. Substitute a regular breast prosthesis later
   c. Avoid clothing that constricts the underarm
   d. Avoid injections, blood drawing, and blood pressure measurements in affected arm
   e. Report symptoms indicating need for immediate medical attention:
      (1) Edema of affected arm
      (2) Redness of infection of scar
      (3) Breakdown of scar tissue
      (4) Mass in other breast or axillae
   f. Plan to do monthly breast self-examination on remaining breast

breast and may facilitate making the decision regarding therapy.

Assisting with coping with preoperative anxiety

The preoperative period has been reported by patients as a time of high anxiety. After finding the lump, the first concern is whether or not it is malignant. Couples often have to wait 3 days after the biopsy for the report and they describe this waiting period as being very difficult. The major concern of the woman after receiving the diagnosis is *survival;* this includes the extent of the cancer, fear of recurrence, and worry about a shortened life span.[49] Other concerns include ability to return to previous life style, concerns about children, coping ability, treatments, and appearance.[49]

The nurse provides opportunities for the woman to explore her feelings. Simple explanations with repetition may decrease fears of the unknown. If the woman does not fully comprehend the physician's explanation, the nurse can repeat the explanation and report this to the physician, who in turn can talk with the woman again and clarify any misconceptions, alleviating needless anxiety. Because attention span, memory, and perception are limited when anxiety levels are high, it is helpful if the nurse can be present when information is given the patient. The nurse can then repeat, reinforce, or clarify the information.

The American Cancer Society sponsors a volunteer program called *Reach to Recovery* in which the patient has an opportunity to visit with a carefully selected and trained volunteer who has had breast surgery. This assures the woman that she will receive practical help from someone who has made a satisfactory adjustment to the same operation. Although most of the patient visits by the volunteer occur during the postoperative period, preoperative visits can be requested and may be very helpful to some women.

Spouses also report feelings of stress and anxiety in the preoperative period, both during the diagnostic period and on the day of surgery.[49] Nurses having contact with spouses can provide the same support given the woman.

Promoting self-esteem

Because much emphasis is placed on the breast as a symbol of attractiveness, the thought of losing a breast becomes almost intolerable to many women. This is particularly true of those who depend largely on physical attractiveness to hold the esteem of others and to secure gratification of their emotional needs. Psychologists have pointed out that there is a symbolic connection between the breasts and motherhood that is severely threatened when a breast must be removed. In addition, cancer of the breast often occurs at menopause or soon after when some women feel that they have lost much of their sexual attractiveness. Surgical removal of the breast may save a woman's life, but it also may make her feel less feminine.

The woman may be coping with feelings of "being less than a woman," disfigurement, sexual acceptance, or social isolation. Although these feelings are experienced more often by the woman who will have a mastectomy, some of the same feelings occur even when only part of the breast is removed. Some women preoperatively have been unable to discuss their concerns and feelings with those close to them, including their spouse. The nurse can help the patient express feelings and understand what breast surgery means to her as a person. It may be helpful to assist the woman to share her concerns about sexual acceptance with her spouse/significant other. The woman who is having breast surgery, be it a lumpectomy or a mastectomy, has a special need to feel understood and accepted by all persons who are providing care.

Preoperative teaching

Preoperative teaching includes the following information if a mastectomy or lumpectomy with axillary dissection is planned:

1. A catheter attached to suction will be used to drain the incision.
2. The arm on the affected side will be elevated.
3. Sitting up and turning in bed should be done by *pushing* up on the unaffected side rather than pulling, to prevent strain on the incision.
4. Postoperative exercises will be started early.

Postoperative care
Preventing infection of incision

Following the completion of surgery and closure, a stab wound may be made and a catheter inserted and attached immediately to a low, constant suction, such as with a Hemovac or other low suction system. The purpose of the catheter is to remove blood and serum that may collect under the skin that would prevent healing and predispose the tissue to infection. There is usually no drainage from around the incision when a catheter is draining correctly. The catheter is usually removed within 3 to 5 days or when the amount of drainage is less than 5 to 10 ml in 24 hours.

The dressing is checked often for the first few hours to detect hemorrhage or excessive serous oozing. The bedclothes under the patient must be examined for blood that may flow down from the surgical site. Any evidence of bleeding is reported to the surgeon. After 24 hours, the incision may be left covered or uncovered. Because the incision is not healed by the time of hospital discharge, the patient is taught signs and symptoms of infection to be reported immediately to the physician.

Facilitating shoulder range of motion

When the patient returns from surgery, after axillary nodes have been removed, she is placed in a semi-Fowler's position to decrease venous oozing. The arm is elevated to enhance circulation and prevent edema. The pillows are arranged so that the hand is higher than the arm and the arm is above the level of the right atrium. *No blood pressure readings, injections, or blood testing* should be done on the *affected* arm because of the risk of circulatory impairment or infection (to prevent lymphedema). A sign or tape should be placed on this side of the bed with this message.

Exercises are essential to prevent shortening of muscles, stiffness, and contracture of the shoulder girdle, and to preserve muscle tone so that the affected arm can be used without limitations. To prevent additional deformities, exercises should be bilateral ones with the patient using both arms simultaneously. The time to start specific postoperative exercises depends on the extent of the operation.

Postmastectomy arm exercises

Exercise: climbing the wall

1. Stand facing wall with toes 6-12 inches from wall.
2. Bend elbows and place palms of hands against wall at shoulder level.
3. Move both hands parallel to each other up the wall as far as possible until incisional pull or pain occurs.
4. Move both hands down to starting position.
5. Goal is complete extension with elbow straight.
6. Activities that use the same action: reaching top shelves, hanging out clothes, washing windows, hanging curtains, setting hair.

Exercise: elbow pull-in

1. Extend arms sideways to shoulder level.
2. Clasp hands behind neck.
3. Pull elbows forward until they touch.
4. Return to position 2.
5. Unclasp hands and extend arms sideways at shoulder level.
6. Lower arms to side.

Exercise: back scratch

1. Place hand of unoperated side on hip for balance.
2. Bend elbow of affected arm, placing back of hand on small of back.
3. Work hand up the back slowly until fingers reach opposite shoulder blade.
4. Lower arm and straighten both arms.

Exercise: rope pull

1. Attach a rope over a shower rod, hook, or over top of an open door.
2. Sit on a chair (with door between legs if using a door) and grasp each end of rope.
3. Alternately pull on each end, raising affected arm to a point of incisional pull or pain.
4. The goal is to raise the affected arm almost directly overhead.

Postlumpectomy arm exercises[54]

Straight arm raising: while lying flat, raise arm straight back along side of head
Elbow push: while lying flat, place hands behind neck and push elbows back against surface
Shoulder rotation: raise shoulders and rotate in a forward direction
Fist clenching: while sitting, raise arm forward level with shoulder, then clench and unclench fist
Climbing wall: see Box 36-4

The patient is encouraged under close supervision to exercise each day more and more to the limits of incisional pulling and pain. A specific exercise schedule planned by nurse and patient together is imperative. It is an important aspect of nursing care for the patient.

Continuing exercises after mastectomy are as recommended by the American Cancer Society (see Box 36-4). Exercises are begun with 5 repetitions, working up to a maximum of 20 repetitions unless otherwise specified. The woman is instructed to move slowly and rest when pain occurs. With exercise, full range of motion will return; that is, both arms can be extended equally high above the head. This will not be achieved for 2 to 3 months; therefore, the patient must learn and be motivated in the hospital so she will continue to exercise at home on a regular basis. Exercise to help regain full range of motion after *lumpectomy* are described in Box 36-5.

Promoting comfort

Pain in the operated area may be referred to the affected arm or shoulder. Sensations of numbness and tingling over the chest that are painful may cause the patient to take short, shallow breaths in the early postoperative period. She is kept comfortable with analgesics, and a deep breathing routine is started. Each chest excursion may painfully discourage compliance, and the patient may need considerable encouragement.

Phantom symptoms of the missing breast occur in those women who had painful breasts or nipples before the surgery. This can be very disconcerting to the woman, and reassurance may be needed that these sensations will eventually disappear.

Promoting rest

The body requires increased energy for healing and for coping with the grief over the loss of the breast. *Fatigue* occurs not only in the early postoperative period but often for up to 6 weeks after surgery. The woman needs to know that this is a normal reaction and that she should plan for rest periods.

Patients with advanced breast cancer usually experience *asthenia*, a combination of physical and mental fatigue. These patients need to know that this sense of fatigue is normal and that rest periods should be planned before and after activities. Support by family and friends in facilitating rest is helpful.

Slings are usually avoided. Gentle exercises started early in the postoperative course help to decrease muscle tension as well as to regain muscle function more quickly.

Early exercises for postmastectomy patient

Surgical day	Flex and extend fingers; pronate and supinate forearm
First postoperative day	Squeeze rubber ball
As soon as tolerated	Brush teeth and hair

The patient must know what motion is intended in each exercise, such as shoulder abduction. For example, the patient may brush her hair with the arm on the affected side, but she may lower her head and hunch her shoulders in such a way that she does not get normal use of the shoulder girdle. The whole intent of the exercise may, therefore, be lost.

Nursing Care Plan	Patient following mastectomy for cancer

DATA: Mrs. L., age 35, discovered a lump in her right breast quite accidentally while bathing. She is not familiar with breast self-examination. Mammography and a breast biopsy confirmed the diagnosis of cancer. In a conference with the surgeon and plastic surgeon, Mrs. L. elected to have a modified radical mastectomy with consideration of breast reconstruction in 6 months.

Mrs. L. was very quiet during the admission procedure. The primary nurse talked with her the evening before surgery, and Mrs. L. stated that her major concern was "whether they would get it all." She is glad to know that breast reconstruction can be done in the near future because she doesn't think she wants to go through life with a deformed chest. She also said her husband had supported the surgery, and they both feel it will not affect their relationship. Mr. L. accompanied his wife to the hospital for admission and spent the evening with her. Her mother is caring for their 3- and 6-year-old daughters while Mrs. L. is hospitalized.

After surgery, Mrs. L. returned to the division with intravenous fluids and wound catheter attached to a Hemovac suction. Vital signs were stable.

Collaborative nursing actions included monitoring the dressing and catheter for wound drainage and observing the arm for signs of enlargement (lymphedema). Medical orders included keeping her right arm elevated on pillows to prevent lymphedema. A sign was placed on her door reminding others to avoid blood pressure readings, starting IVs, and injections, or taking blood samples from Mrs. L.'s right arm.

Nursing diagnosis: **Pain: related to surgical incision**

Expected patient outcomes	Nursing interventions	Rationale
States feeling more comfortable	Give prescribed narcotic on a regular basis for first 24 hr; then re-evaluate	Expected incisional pain is better controlled if not allowed to become severe; Mrs. L. will participate in exercises earlier if comfortable
	Encourage deep breathing exercises every 2-4 hr	Narcotic will ease discomfort from deep breathing; these exercises will prevent lung problems that would increase Mrs. L.'s discomfort

Nursing diagnosis: **Mobility, impaired physical: related to shoulder immobility**

Expected patient outcomes	Nursing interventions	Rationale
Participates early with arm exercises	Demonstrate early exercises (keep instructions simple) Visit Mrs. L. every 2 hours to provide encouragement	Because of discomfort and narcotic, Mrs. L. may have difficulty concentrating
	Explain rationale for exercises to Mr. L. so he can encourage Mrs. L.	Exercises will help prevent stiffness and contractures of shoulder from disuse

Nursing diagnosis: Body image disturbance: related to loss of breast

Expected patient outcomes	Nursing interventions	Rationale
Begins to look at incision and to talk about loss of breast	Spend planned time talking with Mrs. L. Give Mrs. L. opportunities to talk about her feelings Don't push Mrs. L. but listen to what she says Observe for signs of her touching dressing and use this as an opening to discuss Mrs. L.'s thoughts about her surgery	Mrs. L. may need to deny her feelings initially As Mrs. L. begins to think about her surgery, she may need reassurance that the nurse is interested and willing to listen to her concerns
	Check with Mrs. L.'s surgeon about a Reach to Recovery volunteer visitor and then explain the program	Interacting with someone who has been through the experience is often helpful in adjustment
	Encourage Mrs. L. to put on makeup and wear her own clothes as soon as possible	Mrs. L. may need reassurance of her femininity

Nursing diagnosis: Knowledge deficit: related to lack of information

Expected patient outcomes	Nursing interventions	Rationale
States plans to do BSE regularly on other breast and to teach her daughters when older	Teach BSE: demonstration with return demonstration	Women who have a chance to practice BSE under supervision are more confident about doing BSE
	Explain high risk of daughters for breast cancer and need for continued monitoring	Mother's breast cancer is a high risk factor for daughter
States plans to continue exercises until full shoulder ROM returns	Demonstrate exercises to be done later; give Mrs. L. booklet from American Cancer Society with instructions	Seeing and returning a demonstration and having written material for reference will promote follow-up of the activity
States plans for rest periods at home	Explain reason for expected fatigue after surgery and help Mrs. L. to plan her day to include rest periods	Care of young children is tiring and Mrs. L. still needs additional energy for healing; rest will give her additional energy for coping
Identifies where to obtain breast prostheses, if needed	Encourage visit by Reach to Recovery volunteer; if not, discuss types of prostheses and where to obtain them	Mrs. L. may postpone reconstructive surgery or may want to use a soft prosthesis before surgery
Describes symptoms to be reported to physician	Instruct Mrs. L. to report signs of arm edema, redness or infection of incision, or any mass in other breast	Lymphedema and incisional breakdown are better treated if identified early; Mrs. L. is at high risk for cancer in other breast
States ways to prevent edema and infection	Discuss ways to prevent infection and edema of right arm	Mrs. L. is at risk for infection and edema of right arm because right axillary lymph nodes were removed

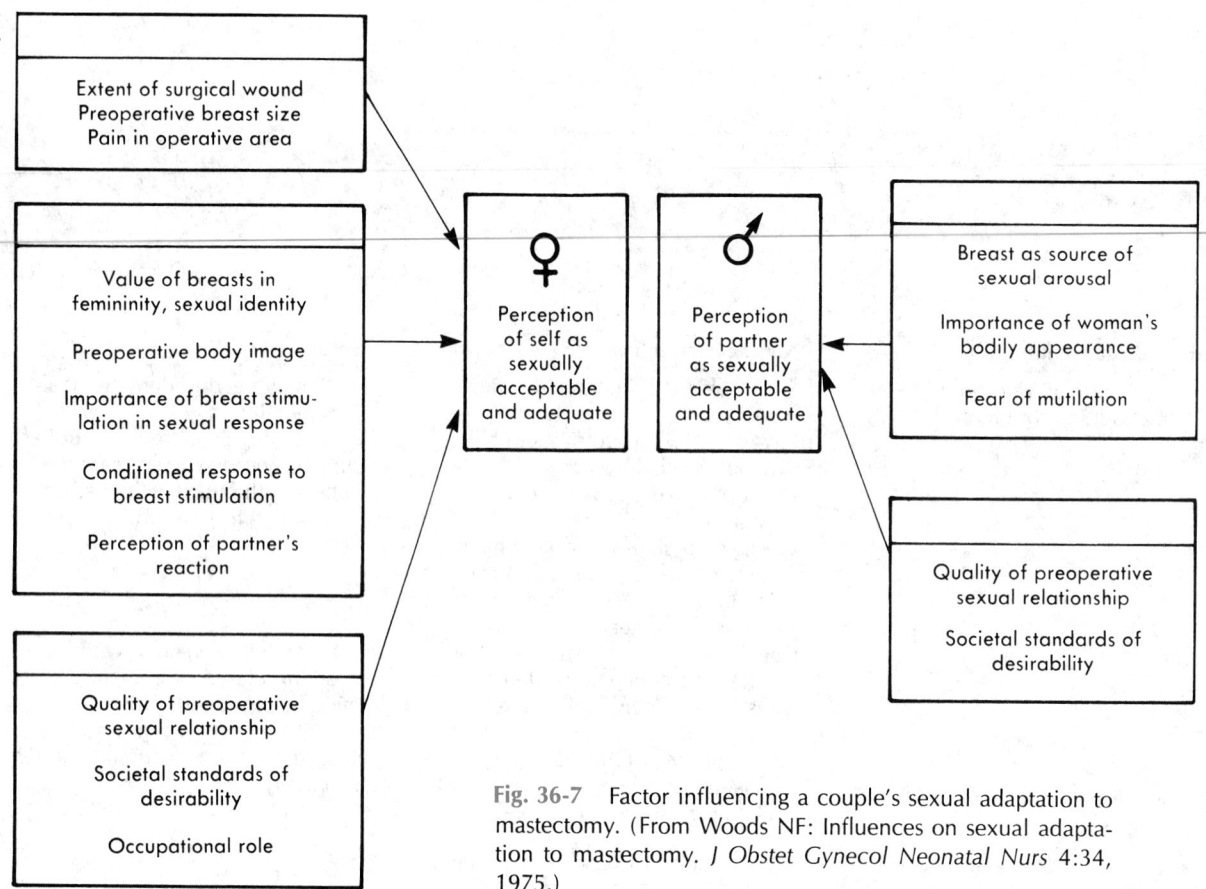

Fig. 36-7   Factor influencing a couple's sexual adaptation to mastectomy. (From Woods NF: Influences on sexual adaptation to mastectomy. *J Obstet Gynecol Neonatal Nurs* 4:34, 1975.)

Facilitating coping

After surgery, denial of the changes in body image may take the form of the woman speaking about "the cancer" and "the mastectomy" but never dealing with her loss or her fears on an emotional level. Denial here is a conservation of energy. If she is to express herself on an emotional level, she must have someone who is capable and responsible to support her according to *her* need. If she does not receive this professional assistance, the impact of her loss occurs at a later date when support systems may not be available.

Not looking at the dressing or incision can be expected initially from both the patient and spouse. The incision is large, and the feeling experienced by most women is that of mutilation. Postponing looking at the incision delays the impact of the realization that the breast is indeed gone. Preparing the woman in advance concerning the appearance of the incision is helpful, but she still needs considerable support when viewing the incision and her new image. She is usually physically capable when she feels stronger and begins to respond socially to others. She is encouraged to look at the incision several times before discharge from the hospital while health professionals are available for support.

Feelings of anger and resentment may occur and, if present, frequently are projected onto female staff or friends. Families may also express anger or anxiety and may complain without cause about the care the patient is receiving. Feelings of decreased self-worth and self-esteem on the part of the patient plus increased dependency needs often produce depression.

The feeling of being isolated and alone during this experience can be helped by interaction with others who have had the same experience such as visitors from the Reach to Recovery program. Reach to Recovery volunteers hold the potential of motivating the patient, extending hope, and providing visible evidence that femininity, personality, and activity can be retained. They can be good resource people as the patient moves from the hospital to the community. Often whether the patient has the opportunity to use this resource depends on a nurse initiating the contact.

Patients often experience periods of depression for weeks to months after breast surgery, especially after mastectomy. Emotions are more labile and the woman may cry more easily. It is helpful for her to know in advance that this may occur. She may have difficulty sleeping or concentrating if she is still acutely grieving with little recognition or little support. She usually will be unable to express her needs; significant others can be told of her continuing need for support and patience and can help to extend the kind of support needed. Women who have *immediate* breast reconstruction generally have fewer episodes of depression. The patient can be encouraged to use community support groups (p. 1177).

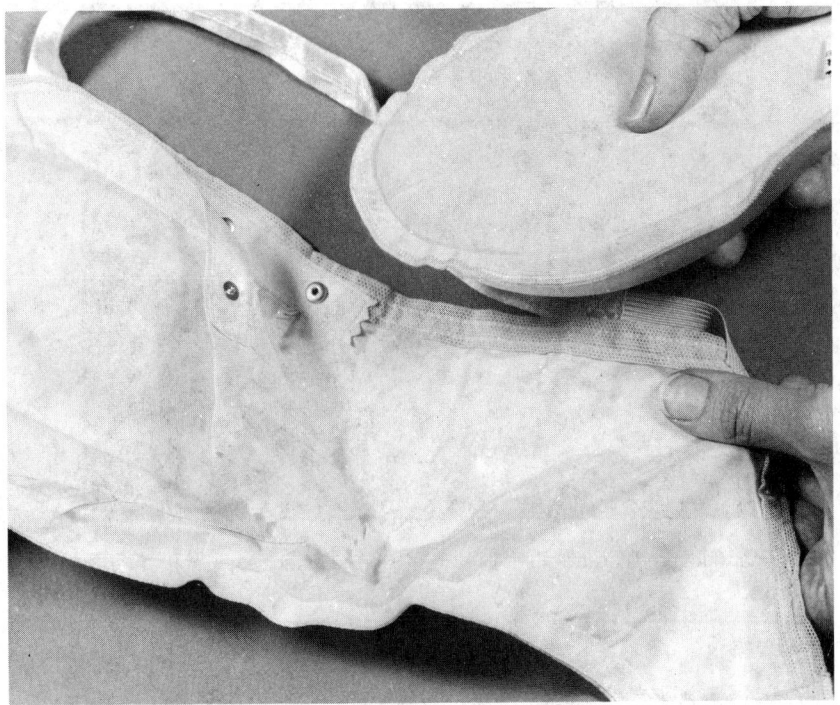

Fig. 36-8   Inner pocket can be made in patient's own brassiere that holds padding or prosthesis securely. Note that snaps simplify removal of padding.

Facilitating sexual adaptation

Woods[69] has identified a number of factors that can influence sexual adaptation following mastectomy (Fig. 36-7). Women with very small or very large breasts may have long-unresolved feelings about breast size and may also experience more difficulty in obtaining a satisfactory breast prosthesis. They may perceive the surgery as mutilating, and withdraw from the sexual relationship, fearing rejection from their partner. Women who felt sexually inadequate before surgery may find these feelings enhanced postoperatively and use the surgery as a reason for withdrawing from sexual relationships.

The nurse can initiate a discussion with the patient concerning her thoughts and feelings about return to sexual activity (if appropriate) and can encourage the patient to talk about her concerns with her sexual partner. Sexual and marital counseling is helpful for couples who are unable to communicate their feelings openly with each other.

Facilitating learning
Breast prosthesis

Unless a breast reconstruction has been done immediately following breast removal, information about breast prostheses is given to the patient whenever she asks about them or appears interested. The Reach to Recovery volunteer is a good resource person for current information and suggestions concerning prostheses and clothing. She may accompany the patient as she shops for her first prosthesis, serving as a support person. Breast prostheses are not fitted until at least 6 weeks postoperatively or until the incision has healed and is no longer tender. Suppliers are also listed under "Prosthetic devices" in the Yellow Pages.

Until the incision is well healed, the woman is advised to wear one of her own brassieres, which can be lightly padded with a soft, fluffy filling (Fig. 36-8) or a temporary soft prosthesis, available from Reach to Recovery, that will not shift and embarrass her. Opaque, loose-hanging gowns are usually most acceptable to the patient.

Breast prostheses vary in price, type, and weight (Figs. 36-9 and 36-10). Women want prostheses to make them look symmetric and *feel* bilaterally weighted. Even small-breasted women will change posture if weighting is not balanced. Firm, molded prostheses have a disadvantage of remaining elevated when the woman is lying supine, whereas fluid types have a more natural look.

Preventing infection in affected arm

When axillary nodes are removed the affected arm is more susceptible to infection because of decreased lymph drainage. Instructions to the patient to prevent infection include the following:

1. Avoid injections and blood drawing in the affected arm.
2. Wear a thimble when sewing.
3. Use a soft cloth to push back cuticles.
4. Shave affected axilla with an electric razor with a narrow head to reduce nicks or scratches.
5. Wear gloves when gardening or using strong detergents.
6. Use insect repellent to avoid stings or bites.
7. Avoid burns and sunburns.
8. Wash cuts well on affected arm, apply an antibacterial ointment, and cover with a sterile bandaid or dressing. Check often for signs of infection.

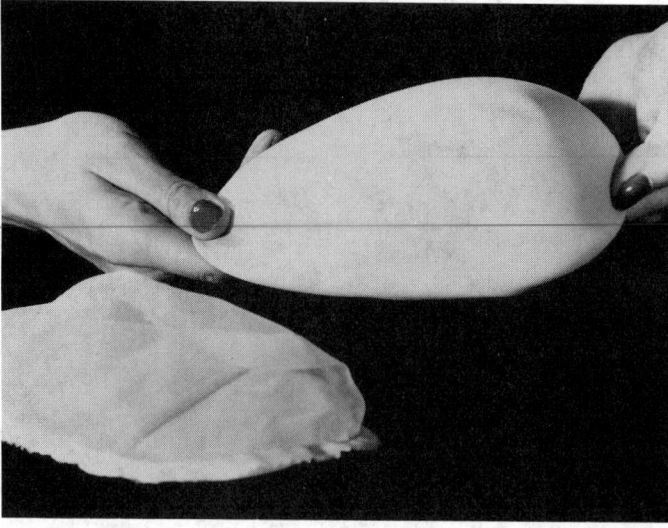

Fig. 36-9 Foam-covered, liquid-filled breast prosthesis. (Courtesy Camp International, Jackson, Mich.)

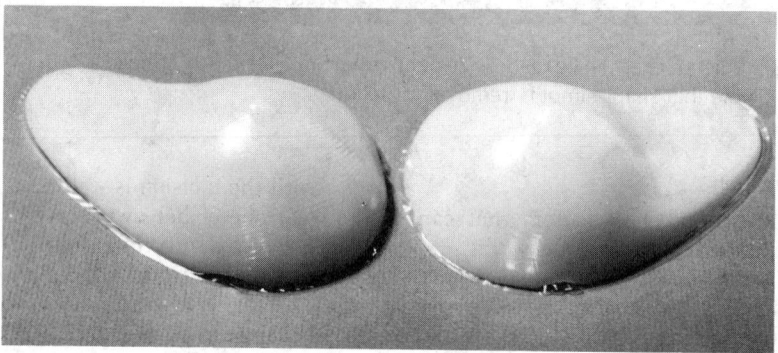

Fig. 36-10 Silicone-filled breast prostheses. (Courtesy Camp International, Mich.)

9. Consult physician if infection of the affected arm occurs; treatment is antibiotics, heat, rest, and elevation of the arm.

Preventing lymphedema

Many patients develop a slight edema of the affected upper arm that disappears within a week. A few patients, however, develop severe edema that persists, that may become permanent, and that is caused by surgical interruption of lymph channels when the axillary nodes are dissected. The incidence is greater in persons who are obese, develop infections, or are subjected to radiation. Some surgeons order an elastic sleeve (similar to an elastic stocking) that should extend from the wrist to the shoulder. It may be removed when the patient is in bed.

Measures to help prevent edema include:
1. Avoid blood pressure measurements in affected arm.
2. Avoid injuries and infection of affected arm.
3. Wear clothing that does not restrict the underarm or wrists (avoid elastic cuffs).
4. Wear watch and bracelets on unaffected arm.
5. Carry heavy packages or handbags using unaffected arm.
6. Consult physician if edema occurs.

Early identification of recurrence

Over half of breast cancer recurrences are seen within the first 3 years and another 20% within the next 2 years. Therefore, the woman needs to carry out SBE on the remaining breast tissue and opposite breast *regularly* every month. Ask the woman to demonstrate BSE and teach her any aspects that she is not performing correctly. If the woman has daughters, they are at increased risk for breast cancer and need to practice BSE regularly also. Encourage the patient to carry out follow-up visits to the physician as instructed and to have yearly mammograms.

Use of community resources

After patients return home from the hospital, they often feel isolated and alone. Many women find it helpful to attend support groups for breast cancer patients or for cancer patients in general. If additional information about therapy is desired, the person can contact societies that offer information on breast cancer (Box 36-6). Local hospitals, the American Cancer Society, and the YMCA may also provide local support groups for persons with cancer.

Evaluation

Evaluation is based on expected patient outcomes. Questions to consider when evaluating the care of women who have had therapy for breast cancer may include the following:

1. Did the patient participate in making decisions concerning therapy?
2. Does the patient appears less anxious?
3. Has the patient had an opportunity to discuss her feelings and begin dealing with the change in her body image?
4. Does the patient know ways to prevent infection and edema of the arm?
5. Has the patient been exercising during her hospital stay, and does she know the home exercises?
6. Does the patient state that she feels more comfortable?
7. Is the patient aware that she will tire easily for at least 6 weeks after therapy is completed and needs to plan rest periods?
8. Has the patient identified people to turn to for support when she feels depressed or needs help?
9. Is the patient interacting with others, especially her spouse or significant other, appropriately?
10. Does the patient know where to obtain a breast prosthesis, if appropriate?
11. Can the patient perform breast self-examinations, and does she plan to carry them out monthly?
12. Is the patient aware of the need for yearly follow-up by a physician?

Breast Reconstruction

Since 1980 improvement in plastic surgery techniques have made breast reconstruction a viable alternative to breast prostheses for many women. There is no evidence that breast reconstruction changes the course of the disease or masks recurrence.[65] For some women, however, breast reconstruction is not essential to their positive self-image and self-esteem, femininity, or sexual experience. Some do not want the added surgery and accompanying anesthesia, the cost in terms of time and money, or the pain. Other women consider breast reconstruction necessary for their self-esteem and continuing relationships with others. Breast reconstruction is contraindicated when there is an aggressive tumor, a probability that metastasis has occurred, or a concern about adequate healing.

The benefits of breast reconstruction include avoidance of an external prosthesis that has potential for slipping, greater choice of clothing (including lower necklines), and loss of self-consciousness about appearance. Women say they feel better about themselves and experience fewer periods of depression following breast reconstruction.

The *original* nipple is no longer "saved" because there is always a question about the possible spread of cancer cells into the nipple. Creation of a new areola and nipple is performed as ambulatory surgery at a later date. The

---

36-6

Support services for patients with breast cancer

American Cancer Society: informational services, Reach to Recovery, I Can Cope (local support groups). Check telephone book for local office or contact national headquarters (1599 Clifton Rd NE, Atlanta, GA 30329; 1-404-320-3333).

YWCA: ENCORE—a program for postoperative breast cancer patients (exercises to music, water exercises, discussion periods). Check local YWCA office.

National Cancer Institute: information services, free publications, referral services (Building 31, Room 10A24, Bethesda, MD 20892; 1-800-4-CANCER).

National Lymphedema Network: provides information and guidance about lymphedema, counseling hotline, and referral services. (Suite 3, 2215 Post St., San Francisco, CA 94115; 1-800-541-3259).

National Alliance of Breast Cancer Organizations: provides information to assist with decisions about therapy (1180 Avenue of the Americas, New York, NY 10036; 1-212-719-0154).

---

areola is formed by free grafting of tissue, either from part of the other areola (if it is large) or from skin of the upper thigh just below the pubic hair. The nipple is more difficult to fashion; the more common approach is to create folds of tissue with local skin and fat flap grafts.

Timing of breast reconstruction

Breast reconstruction can be performed immediately after surgery or at a later time. An increasing number of women are electing immediate reconstruction; this may prolong the initial hospitalization, but eliminates the need for a second hospitalization and contributes to self-esteem from the beginning.

The decision for reconstruction should be made in combination with the surgeon, plastic surgeon, and patient. The goal of reconstruction is a breast mound and nipple-areola complex that is similar to the remaining breast. The new breast will not have the exact contours of the natural breast; it is generally a little rounder and flatter and will not sag. The opposite breast can be altered to match the reconstructed breast.

Types of breast reconstruction

The two major approaches to breast reconstruction are the submuscular insertion of an *implant* to provide breast form or a *muscle flap graft* (Table 36-4). The implant is used when the pectoralis major muscle is intact and there is good skin cover. Muscle flap grafts are used when muscle and skin are inadequate; the grafts may be obtained from the back (latissimus muscle) or from the abdomen.

Breast implant

If the skin is sufficient to cover an implant, surgery may consist of placing a permanent silicone implant under the pectoralis muscle. The newer silicone gel implants are

Table 36-4   Types of reconstruction breast surgery

Surgery	Description	Comments
Implants		
Silicone implant	Implant inserted into a pocket beneath the pectoralis major muscle	Simplest procedure but may lead to complications Ambulatory surgery or overnight hospital stay Requires ample residual skin Result is less symmetric than in other surgeries No ptosis
Tissue expansion	Temporary or permanent expandable bag inserted in submuscular pocket; bag is expanded slowly over time by saline injections in subcutaneous port	Common procedure Ambulatory surgery or overnight hospital stay Useful following modified radical mastectomy if enough tissue present Requires frequent office visits
Flap grafts		
Abdominothoracic	Flap graft advanced from area below breast	Three-day hospital stay Provides better breast detailing than implants More prominent abdominal scar
Latissimus dorsi	Flap graft advanced from latissimus dorsi muscle (lateral upper back)	Five-day hospital stay Useful following radical surgery when tissue lacking Implants may be needed Horizontal back scar
Transabdominal	Flap graft using rectus abdominus muscle tunneled from lower abdomen to breast area	Seven-day hospital stay Useful following radical surgery when tissue lacking Horizontal scar on lower abdomen Removes some abdominal fat (lipectomy)

soft and flexible, better approximating breast tissue than the older models. Possible complications of silicone implants include infection in the early postoperative period, deflation, a hard round breast, false mammography results, and silicone leaks.

It has also been suggested that the silicone filling or the implant covering can lead to autoimmune or connective tissue disease. Although most surgeries have not resulted in complications, differing opinions regarding the safety of breast implants led the Food and Drug Administration (FDA) in early 1992 to issue some recommendations. Breast implants were permitted following breast cancer surgery (because of the offsetting positive contributions to recovery), but a moratorium was imposed on breast implants solely for cosmetic purposes until data establishing safety could be provided.

If the skin covering the breast is tight, the skin can be stretched (like stretching of the abdomen during pregnancy) by gradually expanding the area below the skin. An all-saline sac or a combination saline/silicone gel sac is implanted under the muscle; the sac is then slowly expanded over a 3-month period by adding saline by injection into a receiving port placed subcutaneously below the axilla. When the desired volume has been achieved, the temporary sac is surgically removed and the permanent silicone implant is inserted into the enlarged space, or the injection port is removed from the permanent implant. The woman will experience minimal discomfort with this procedure.

The woman is asked not to smoke for at least 1 week before surgery because complications occur more frequently among smokers.[9] Postoperative teaching includes the following:

1. Report signs of drainage, fever, or other signs of infection.
2. Wear a bra continuously until healing occurs to maintain the implant position and alignment.
3. Avoid raising arms (such as to wash hair or reach cupboards) for 1 to 3 weeks, as instructed.
4. Avoid hard pushing movements, for 1 to 3 weeks in order to avoid separation of the pectoralis muscle where the implant has been inserted and to avoid pulling out the sutures.
5. Avoid heavy lifting for 6 weeks.

Latissimus dorsi flap graft

A latissimus dorsi graft is a free flap graft in which an "island" of latissimus muscle, fat, and skin (Fig. 36-11) is transferred to the breast area where it provides adequate cover for an implant. Care of the person with a flap graft is discussed in Chapter 43.

Transabdominal island flap

The transabdominal island flap (TAIF) method creates a breast that better approximates breast tissue than the silicone implant. TAIF surgery involves transferring a section of abdominal skin and fat and part of the rectus abdominis muscle to the breast area by tunneling under the skin. The tissue is then shaped as a new breast.

TAIF involves more extensive surgery than the implant procedure and usually requires a week-long hospital stay. Following surgery, the patient will experience abdominal discomfort, tightness, and paresthesia. The abdomen will be flatter (tummy tuck) but the waistline may be temporarily larger.[29] Possible complications after TAIF surgery

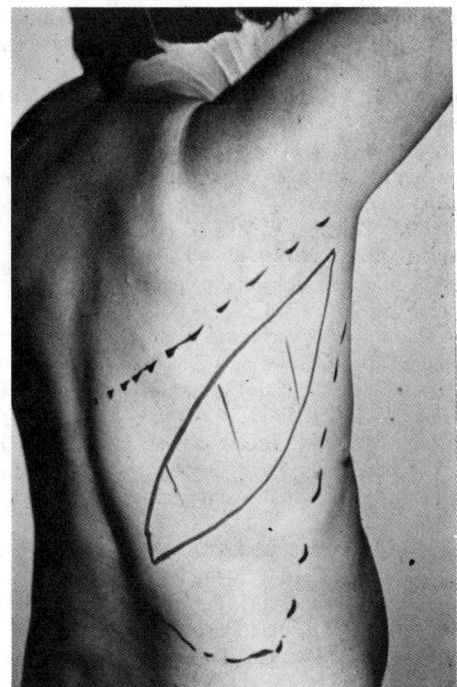

Fig. 36-11 Free latissimus flap. Flap has been outlined on patient before removal. (From Meeker MH, Rothrock JC: *Alexander's care of the patient in surgery*, ed 9, St Louis, 1990, Mosby–Year Book.)

include hematoma/seroma, infection, or flap necrosis in the early postoperative period. Fat necrosis is identified by the appearance of a local indurated area. Hernias and abdominal-wall weakness may occur later.

Preoperatively, a liquid diet is prescribed for 24 hours to aid bowel decompression, which is necessary for a relaxed abdominal wall. Postoperative care includes the following:

1. Position patient with head elevated and knees flexed, to prevent pull on abdominal incisions.
2. Monitor and empty suction drains from breast and abdomen every 30 minutes for 24 hours; notify physician if drainage is less than 50 ml/hr.
3. Monitor color and temperature of new breast tissue (it should be paler and cooler than surrounding tissue but not mottled or cold).
4. Give prescribed isoxsuprine (Vasodilan) and oxygen by nasal cannula to aid flap oxygenation.
5. If nausea is present, give prescribed antiemetic to prevent pull on abdominal incision from vomiting.
6. Clean umbilicus and tape over incision with cotton swab saturated with hydrogen peroxide to prevent infection.
7. Suggest patient ambulate during first week by leaning slightly forward with knees flexed, to ease pull on abdominal incisions.
8. Teach the patient to do the following;
   a. Avoid raising arms above shoulder level for 4 weeks.
   b. Avoid heavy lifting for 6 weeks.

The Reach to Recovery program of the American Cancer Society has a program of volunteers who have had breast reconstruction because of cancer. This is an additional resource for patients and professionals.

Metastatic Disease

Metastases from the breast is primarily by way of the intramammary lymphatics to regional nodes and then to systemic dissemination. Spread may also be from the primary mass to extension of local structures (skin, ribs). As stated earlier, the most common metastases are to bone, lung, liver, and brain. Bone metastases have a better prognosis whereas multiple sites of metastases and short disease-free intervals have a worse prognosis.[25]

Treatment is primarily palliative and includes radiation, hormone therapy, and chemotherapy. Hormone therapy may include ablation of the ovaries or tamoxifen. Chemotherapy with autologous bone marrow transplantation (p. 1168) is now being used. The care of the patient with advanced cancer is discussed in Chapter 11.

SUMMARY

1. A baseline mammogram should be obtained by a woman between 35 and 40 years of age, then repeated every 1 to 2 years until age 49, and yearly thereafter.
2. Most breast cancers are discovered by BSE; therefore, BSE should be performed by all women over age 20.
3. Lumps from benign breast disorders are usually seen bilaterally and are discrete, tender, and freely movable. Lumps from malignant tumors are usually solitary, irregularly shaped, nontender, and nonmobile.
4. Common benign breast disorders include fibrocystic disease, fibroadenomas, and mastitis.
5. Breast discomfort from benign breast lesions may be decreased by mild analgesics, heat or cold, or by breast support.
6. Radiologic tests for breast cancer include mammography and xeroradiography. The only way to determine conclusively whether a tumor is malignant is by breast biopsy.
7. High-risk factors for breast cancer are a mother or sister with breast cancer (especially premenopausal), menarche before age 11, menopause after age 50, or first live birth after age 30; however, *all* women are considered at risk.
8. The most common surgical procedures for stages I and II are lumpectomy with axillary dissection and radiation, and modified radical mastectomy. The choice is made by patient and spouse based on the surgeon's recommendations.
9. Adjuvant therapy is recommended to prevent recurrence. Chemotherapeutic regimens are more effective for premenopausal women, whereas hormonal therapy for estrogen receptor-positive tumors is more effective in postmenopausal women.
10. Loss of a breast is a traumatic experience for many women and may lead to feelings of decreased femininity and self-worth. Women need considerable support during this time.
11. Reach to Recovery, sponsored by the American Cancer

Society, consists of specially trained volunteers who can provide support and information to women having mastectomies.

12. Shoulder exercises following a mastectomy are started early and continued until the shoulder regains full movement.

13. Breast prostheses of various types may be purchased to wear in a bra after the incision has healed.

14. Lymphedema (swelling of the upper arm) may result after axillary node removal because of interference with lymphatic drainage. Elevating the arm after surgery and starting exercises early can help to prevent lymphedema.

15. Infection of affected arm may be prevented by avoiding trauma and bites, and treating all lesions early.

16. New advances in breast reconstruction have made this an option for many women who are not satisfied with a breast prosthesis. Types of breast reconstruction include a breast implant, latissimus dorsi flap, and a transabdominal island flap.

STUDY QUESTIONS

- What are some reasons why many women do not practice BSE? What implications does this have for patient teaching?
- What are the factors that can influence the type of surgery selected by women with stage I or II breast cancer?
- Mrs. Smith has stage III breast cancer. She has just read an article about lumpectomy with radiation and says she does not understand why the surgeon said this would be ineffective for her. How would you reply?
- Ms. Jones asks you why she needs radiation after her lumpectomy when a friend of hers had her breast removed without needing radiation. How would you reply?
- What screening and support resources are available in your community for persons with breast cancer?

REFERENCES AND SELECTED READINGS

1. American Cancer Society: *Cancer facts and figures: 1991*, New York, 1991, The Society.
2. American Cancer Society, Reach to Recovery: *Exercises after mastectomy, patient guide*, New York, 1983, The Society.
3.* Brown-Daniels CJ, Blasdell A: Early breast cancer: adjuvant drug therapy, *Am J Nurs* 90(11):32-33, 1990.
4. Bruera E et al: Asthenia in breast cancer, *Am J Nurs* 89(5):737-741, 1989.
5. Butrum RR, Clifford CK, Lanza E: NCI dietary guidelines: rationale, *Am J Clin Nutr* 48:888-895, 1988.
6.* Cawley M, Kostic J, Cappello C: Informational and psychosocial needs of women choosing conservative surgery/ primary radiation for early stage breast cancer, *Cancer Nurs* 13(2):90-94, 1990.
7.* Chavez A: Conservation surgery with radiotherapy: an alternative in breast cancer, *Semin Oncol Nurs* 1:195-199, 1985.
8. Clark JC et al: Reintegration and maintenance of employees with breast cancer in the workplace, *AAOHN J* 1989 37(5):186-196, 1989.
9. Cohen IK, Turner D: Immediate breast reconstruction with tissue expanders, *Clin Plast Surg* 14:491-498, 1987.

10. Culver J et al: Implementing the American Cancer Society Breast Cancer Awareness program in the workplace, *AAOHN J* 37(5):166-170, 1989.
11.* d'Angelo TM, Gorrell CR: Breast reconstruction using tissue expanders, *Oncol Nurs Forum* 16(1):23-27, 1989.
12.* Dietrick-Gallagher M et al: Teaching patients to care for drains after breast surgery for malignancy, *Oncol Nurs Forum* 16(2):263-265, 1989.
13.* Dinner M, Coleman C: Breast reconstruction: use of autogenous tissue, *AORN J* 42:490-496, 1985.
14. Ediken S: Mammography and palpable cancer of the breast, *Cancer* 61:263-265, 1988.
15.* Eich SJ: Promising early breast cancer treatment without mastectomy, *Cancer Nurs* 8:51-58, 1985.
16.* Ellerhorst-Ryan JM et al: Evaluating benign breast disease, *Nurs Pract* 13:13-29, 1988.
17.* Ellerhorst-Ryan JM: Breast cancer: saving lives through early detection, *Ohio Nurses Rev* 64(3):8-9, 1989.
17a. FDA nears decision on breast implants, *Am J Nurs* 92(1):11-12, 1992.
18.* Feather BL, Lanigan C: Looking good after your mastectomy, *Am J Nurs* 87:1048-1049, 1987.
19. Feather BL, Wainstock JM: Perceptions of postmastectomy patients, part I: The relationships between social support and network providers; part II: Social support and attitudes towards mastectomy, *Cancer Nurs* 12(5):293-300, 301-309, 1989.
20.* Fernsler JI: Employee counseling with respect to lifestyles, life events, and breast cancer risks, *AAOHN J* 37(5):158-164, 1989.
21. Fowble B et al: *Treatment of breast cancer,* St Louis, 1991, Mosby–Year Book.
22.* Fox K: Ellen's going home: can she manage without you? Preparing your postmastectomy patient for discharge, *Nursing 89* 19(5):80-81, 1989.
23.* Greitzu S: Breast cancer: the risks and options, *RN* 49(10):26-32, 1986.
24.* Gottschalk LA, Hoigaard-Martin J: The emotional impact of mastectomy, *Psychiatry Res* 17:153-167, 1986.
25. Harris JR et al: *Breast diseases,* ed 2, Philadelphia, 1991, JB Lippincott.
26. Hellman S et al: *Cancer of the breast.* In DeVita V: *Cancer: principles and practices of oncology,* ed 3, Philadelphia, 1989, JB Lippincott.
27. Hery M et al: Conservative treatment (chemotherapy/radiotherapy) of locally advanced breast cancer, *Cancer* 57:1744-1749, 1986.
28. Holmberg K et al: Psychosocial adjustment after mastectomy and breast-conserving treatment, *Cancer* 64:969-974, 1989.
29.* Hutcheson HA: TAIF: new option for breast reconstruction, *Nurs 86* 16(2):52-53, 1986.
30.* Hutcheson HA: Breast reconstruction using abdominal tissues: a nursing diagnosis approach. *Plast Surg Nurs* 7(1):11-16, 1987.
31.* Jussak PF: Male breast cancer, *Innovations Oncol Nurs* 2(1):1-5, 1986.
32.* Knobf MT: Primary breast cancer: physical consequences and rehabilitation, *Semin Oncol Nurs* 1:214-224, 1985.
33.* Knobf MT: Early-stage breast cancer: the options, *Am J Nurs* 90(11):28-30, 1990.
34. Leffall LD: Breast cancer in black women, *Cancer* 31:4-6, 1987.
35. Levitt SH: Primary treatment of early breast cancer with conservation surgery and radiation therapy, *Cancer* 55:2140-2148, 1985.
36.* Lewis RM, Ellison ES, Woods NF: The impact of breast cancer on the family, *Semin Oncol Nurs* 1:206-213, 1985.

37. Lippmann ME, Lichter AS, Danforth DN: *Diagnosis and management of breast cancer,* Philadelphia, 1988, WB Saunders.

38. Love RR et al: Side effects and emotional distress during cancer chemotherapy, *Cancer* 63:604-612, 1989.

39. Love SM: Fibrocystic diseases, *Patient Care* 24(7):65-82, 1990.

40.* Mach E: Most breast lumps aren't cancer, *RN* 53(12):20-23, 1990.

41.* Mast DE, Mood DW: Preparing patient with breast cancer for brachytherapy, *Oncol Nurs Forum* 17(2):267-270, 1990.

42. McGee RF, White CH: Helping employees and families cope with breast cancer treatment, *AAOHN J* 37(5):178-185, 1989.

43.* McKann CF: The changing role of surgery in the treatment of breast cancer, *Semin Oncol Nurs* 1:176-180, 1985.

44.* Morra ME: Breast self-examination today: an overview of its use and its value, *Semin Oncol Nurs* 1:170-175, 1985.

45.* Nash JA: Breast cancer: screening detection and diagnosis, *Semin Oncol Nurs* 1:163-169, 1985.

46. National Cancer Institute: *Clinical alert,* Bethesda, Md, May 16, 1988, The Institute.

47.* Nielsen BB, East D: Advances in breast cancer: implications for nursing care, *Nurs Clin North Am* 25(2):365-375, 1990.

48.* Northouse LL: A longitudinal study of the adjustment of patients and husbands to breast cancer, *Oncol Nurs Forum* 6(4):511-516, 1989.

49.* Northouse LL: The impact of breast cancer on patients and husbands, *Cancer Nurs* 12(5):276-284, 1989.

50.* Norwood SL: Fibrocystic breast disease: an update and review, *J Obstet Gynecol Neonatal Nurs* 19(2):116-121, 1990.

51. Owen P et al: Facilitating adherence to ACS and NCI guidelines for breast cancer screening, *AAOHN J* 37(5):153-157, 194-196, 1989.

52. *Radiation therapy and you: a guide to self-help during treatment,* No 80-2227, Washington, DC 1985, National Institutes of Health.

53.* Relfsnider E: Educating women about benign breast disease, *AAOHN J* 38(3):121-126, 1990.

54.* Rush DL, Kloppenborg EM: Don't underestimate the lumpectomy patient's needs, *RN* 53(3):58-65, 1990.

55.* Sawyer RF: Breast self-examination: hospital-based nurses aren't assessing their clients, *Oncol Nurs Forum* 13(5):44-48, 1986.

56.* Schain WS: Breast cancer surgeries and psychosexual sequelae: implications for remediation, *Semin Oncol Nurs* 1:200-205, 1985.

57.* Schain WS: The sexual and intimate consequences of breast cancer treatment, *Cancer* 38:154-161, 1988.

58. Schroeder SA et al: *Current medical diagnosis and treatment,* ed 30, Norwalk, Conn, 1991, Appleton & Lange.

59.* Solomon J: The good news about breast reconstruction, *RN* 49(11):47-48, 1986.

60. Systemic sclerosis following breast implants, *Nurses Drug Alert* 13(11):86-87, 1989.

61. Taplin S et al: Breast cancer risk and participation in mammographic screening, *Am J Pub Health* 79:1494-1497, 1989.

62. Tackenberg JN: Cryolumpectomy: another option for breast cancer, *Nursing 90* 20(5):32J, 32L, 1990.

63.* Vogel CL: Systemic therapy for breast cancer, *Semin Oncol Nurs* 1:188-194, 1985.

64.* Ward S et al: Factors women take into account when deciding upon type of surgery for breast cancer, *Cancer Nurs* 12(6):344-351, 1989.

65. Way LW: Current surgical diagnosis and treatment, ed 9, Norwalk, Conn, 1991, Appleton & Lange.

66.* Wellisch DK: The psychologic impact of breast cancer on relationships, *Semin Oncol Nurs* 1:195-199, 1985.

67. Willis MA et al: Interagency collaboration: teaching breast self-examination to black women, *Oncol Nurs Forum* 16:171-177, 1989.

68.* Zenmore R, Shepel LF: Effects of breast cancer and mastectomy on emotional support and adjustment, *Soc Sci Med* 28:19-27, 1989.

Classic

69. Woods NF: Influences on sexual adaptation to mastectomy, *J Obstet Gynecol Neonatal Nurs* 4:33-37, 1975.

Problems of Cognition, Sensation, and Motion

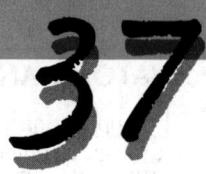

37

The Patient with Neurologic Problems

Elizabeth Schenk

After studying this chapter, the learner should be able to:

- Explain the difference in types of neurons and how they transmit impulses.
- List the divisions of the central nervous system, peripheral nervous system, peripheral nervous system, and autonomic nervous system.
- List four physiologic changes in the nervous system that occur with aging.
- Explain three components of the neurologic assessment.
- Explain the importance of primary, secondary, and tertiary prevention of problems of the nervous system.
- State five symptoms of increased intracranial pressure.
- List five nursing actions to decrease intracranial pressure.
- Explain the pathophysiology involved in two degenerative diseases and three infection-related diseases of the nervous system.
- Define cerebrovascular accident, cerebral thrombosis, cerebral embolism, transient ischemic attack, and cerebral hemorrhage.
- State two complications of brain surgery and their treatment.
- Describe two characteristics of circulation in the brain.

ANATOMY AND PHYSIOLOGY

The application of the nursing process to patients with neurologic problems requires knowledge of the structure and function of the nervous system. The nervous system works as an electrical conductance system. It coordinates and controls all activities of the body. These activities can be divided into the following four kinds of functions:

1. Receiving information (stimuli) from the internal and external environment over sensory (afferent) pathways
2. Communicating information between distant parts of the body (periphery) and the central nervous system
3. Computing or processing the information received at various reflex (spinal cord) and conscious (higher brain) levels to determine responses appropriate to existing situations
4. Transmitting information rapidly over varied motor (efferent) pathways to organs for body action control or modification

Neuroglia cells

While the basic structural and functional unit of the nervous system is the neuron, *neuroglia cells* serve as an adjunct. Neuroglia cells make up almost half of the micro-

scopic structures of the spinal cord and brain. They provide nourishment, support, and protection for the neurons. Four different types of neuroglia cells have been identified. These cells and their functions are listed below:

1. Astrocytes
   a. Maintain chemical environment for conduction and transmission of impulses
   b. Meet nutritional needs of neurons
   c. Store information
   d. Support structures of neurons
   e. Participate in the blood-brain barrier
2. Ependyma
   a. Produce cerebrospinal fluid (CSF)
3. Microglia
   a. Take part in phagocytosis
4. Oligodendroglia
   a. Produce lipid-protein complex that forms myelin sheaths around axons

All of the cells, except microglia, arise from the embryonic ectoderm. Because they can divide and multiply by mitosis, they serve as a source for tumors of the nervous system (Fig. 37-1).

Neuron

The basic structural and functional unit of the nervous system is the *neuron*. It is a highly specialized and differ-

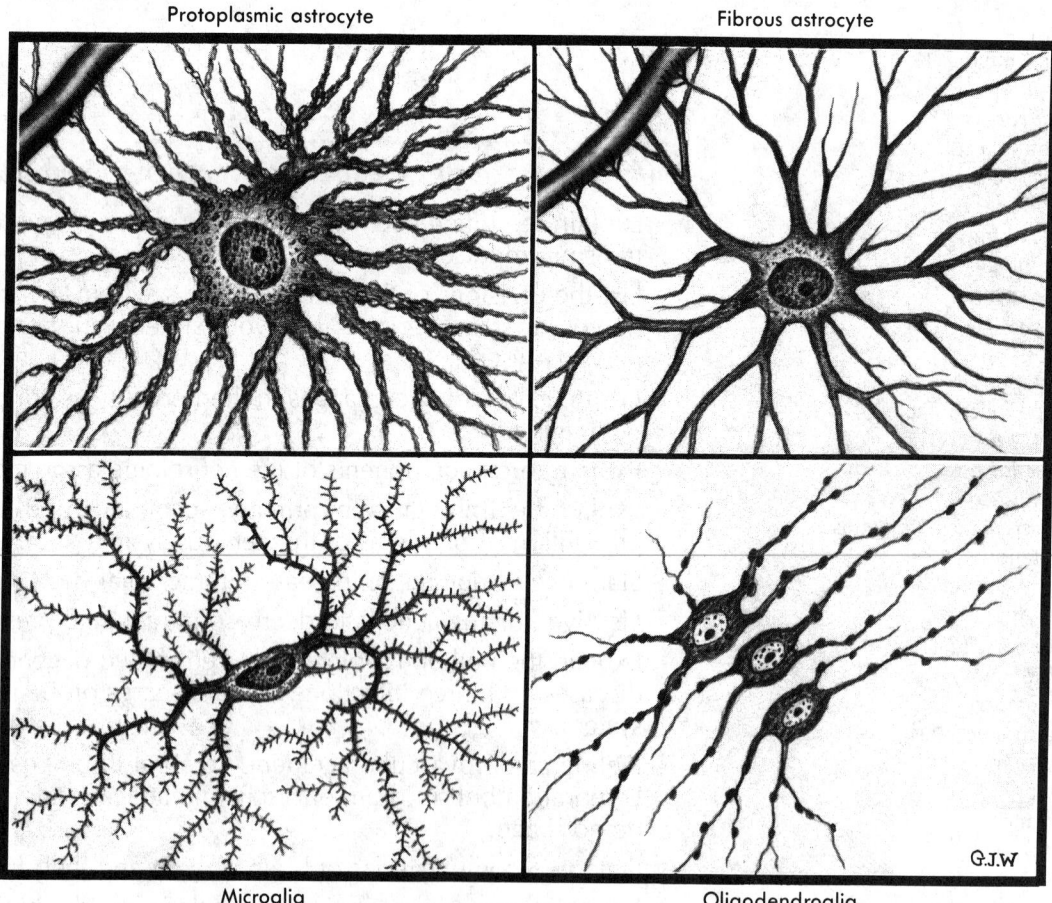

Fig. 37-1   Types of neuroglia cells. (From Thompson JM, et al: *Mosby's manual of clinical nursing*, ed 2, St Louis, 1989, Mosby—Year Book.)

entiated cell, but it has all the basic biologic and biochemical properties of other body cells. The single neuron acts as a miniature nervous system and has properties specific for its electrical function. Its specialized properties are excitation and electrical-chemical conduction. The neuron consists of a *cell body* (soma, or perikaryon) with two extensions: *dendrites*, which receive information from axon terminals at special sites called *synapses*, and *axons*, which transmit information away from the cell body to adjacent neurons (Fig. 37-2). A cell membrane encloses the outer boundary of the soma, dendrite, and axon (Fig. 37-2 and 37-3).

One centrally located nucleus is typically found in each neuron. This nucleus is the repository for deoxyribonucleic acid (DNA). Inside the nucleus is a *nucleolus* containing ribonucleic acid (RNA) (Fig. 37-4). *Cytoplasm*, granular in nature, surrounds the nucleus and contains other organelles such as *mitochondria, neurofilaments, microtubules,* the *Golgi complex,* and *Nissl bodies*. Each carries out a specific function related to the neuron.

Neurons can be classified according to structure and function. Structurally, the divisions include the number of processes. *Unipolar neurons* have only one process or pole; the general sensory neuron is an example of a unipolar

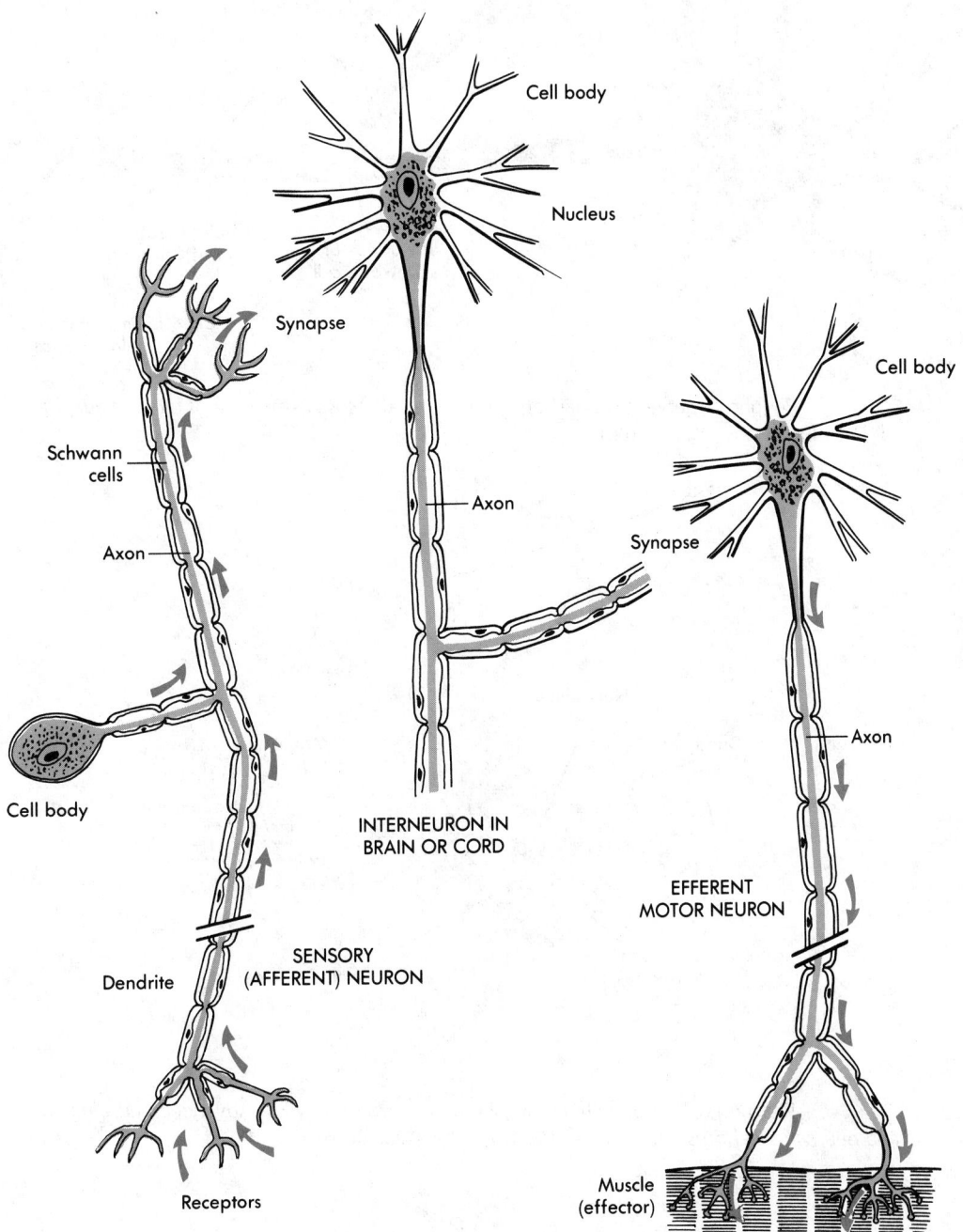

Fig. 37-2   Diagram of neurons showing the cell body (soma), dendrites, and axon. Direction of impulse conduction indicated by arrows.

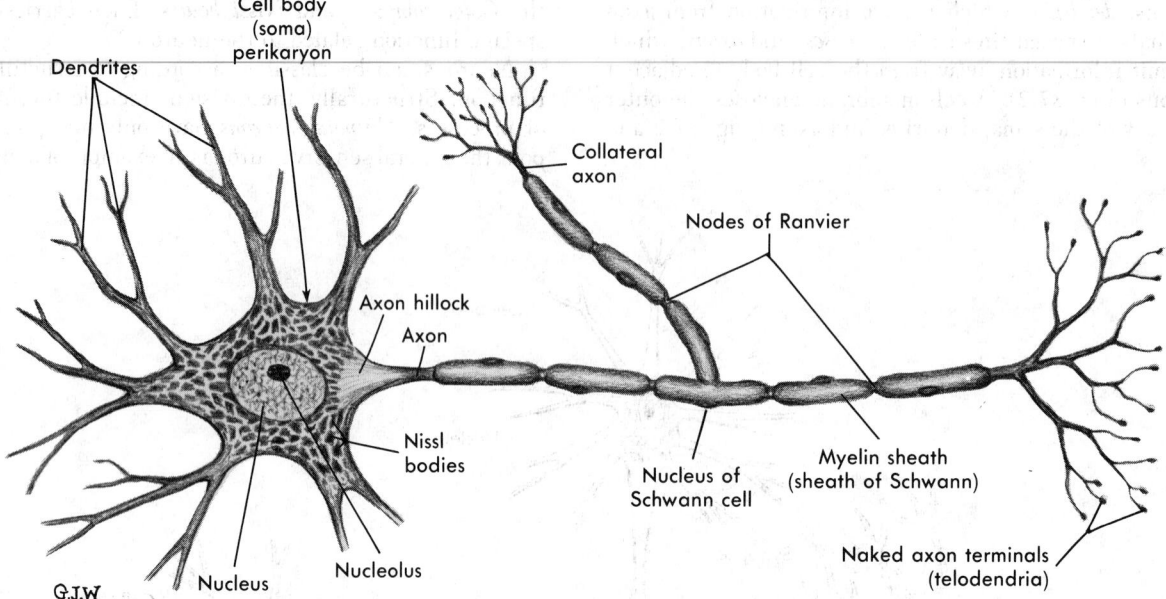

Fig. 37-3 Peripheral nerve. (From Thompson JM, et al: *Mosby's manual of clinical nursing* ed 2, 1989, Mosby–Year Book.)

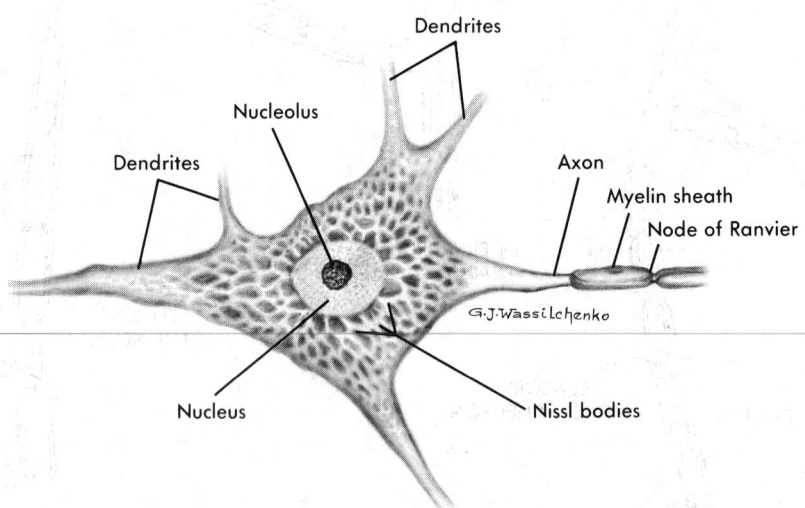

Fig. 37-4 Diagram of neuron with composite parts. (From Rudy EB: *Advanced neurological and neurosurgical nursing,* St Louis, 1984, Mosby–Year Book.)

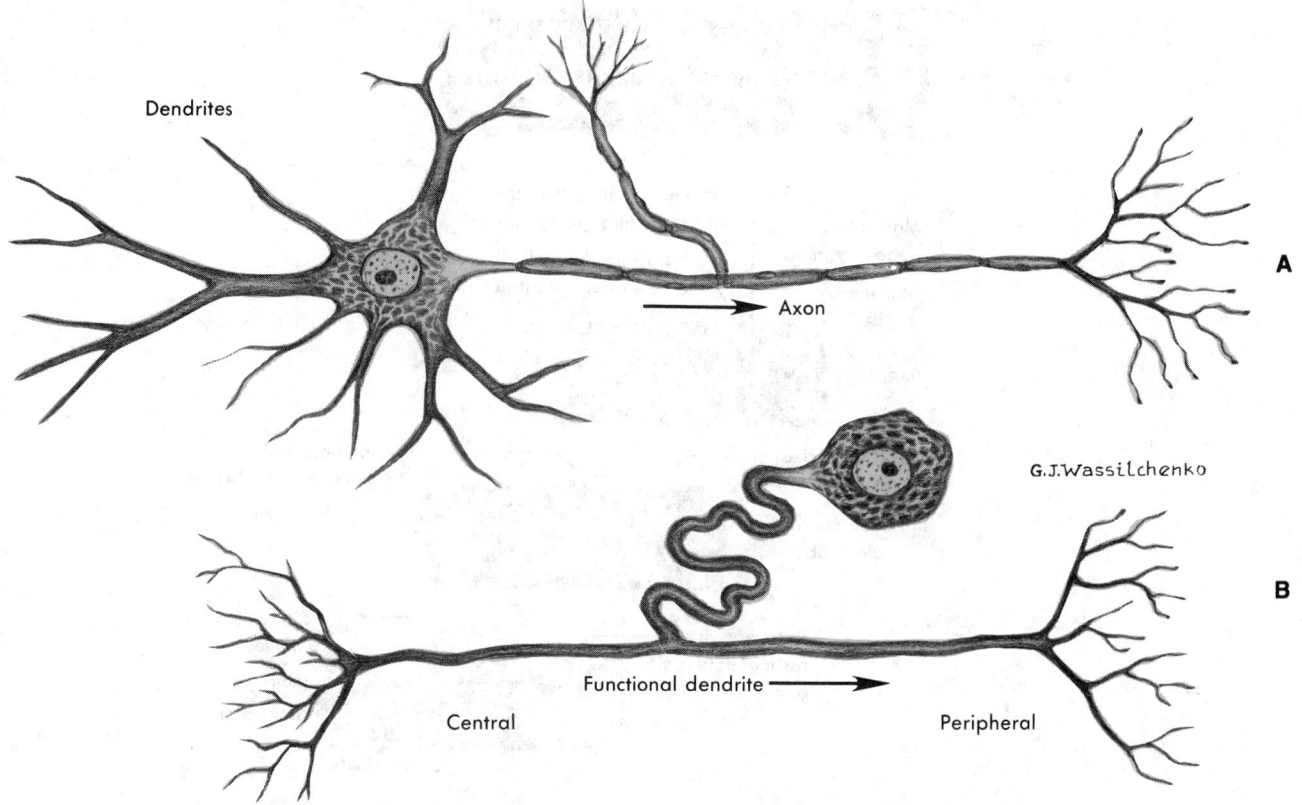

Dendrites

Axon

A

G.J.Wassilchenko

B

Functional dendrite

Central

Peripheral

Fig. 37-5   Types of neurons. **A,** Multipolar. **B,** Unipolar. (From Thompson JM, et al: *Clinical nursing*, St Louis, 1986, Mosby–Year Book.)

neuron. The *bipolar neuron* contains two poles: one dendrite and one axon. These neurons are found in the rods and cones of the retina, the mucous membrane of the nose, and other special sensory areas. The multipolar neuron consists of one axon and one or more dendrites (Fig. 37-5).

Neurons may also be classified by the length of the axon. *Golgi type I neurons* are large and have long axons. They make up the long fiber tracts of the spinal cord, cerebellum, and cerebral cortex. *Golgi type II cells* are smaller cells that are found in the brain and spinal cord. They have short axons that branch repeatedly. The purpose of these neurons is to establish complex circuits in the nervous system.

Neurons are functionally known as *afferent, internuncial,* or *efferent*. Afferent neurons are sensory neurons that conduct impulses from the periphery *to* the central nervous system. Internuncial neurons are found in the central nervous system and assist in impulse conduction. Efferent or motor neurons transmit impulses *from* the central nervous system to the periphery.

Neurons are grouped in chains in the peripheral nervous system to form *nerves*. These collections are called *fiber tracts* in the central nervous system.

Collections of neurons are connected in complex ways. The connection determines what each collection of neurons is capable of doing. The neurons are organized into circuits, some of which are simple and made up of relatively

few neurons and others that are very complicated. A single neuron may be a part of several different neurologic circuits and thus may have a role in several functions.

Many of the important functional properties of the neuron lie within the *cell membrane*. The membrane is permeable to oxygen, carbon dioxide, and certain inorganic ions, and it is impermeable to organic compounds (proteins) and other inorganic ions. This characteristic of the membrane is called *differential permeability*.

The neuron also can be characterized by the property of *excitability*. Excitability means that the resting potential of neurons is unstable under certain conditions, as when the membrane of the neuron is stimulated. This unstable condition gives rise to *action potentials*. Action potentials can only arise from excitable cells. All nervous system functions occur from the phenomenon of the action potential (Fig. 37-6).

Action Potential

Two phases occur within the action potential—*depolarization* (positive state) and *repolarization* (return to the more normal resting potential). When resting, the nerve fiber is charged, with the inside of the cell membrane negatively charged in relation to the outside. A high concentration of sodium exists extracellularly, and a high concentration of potassium exists intracellularly. When the nerve fiber is stimulated, there is an influx of sodium and a loss of intracellular potassium by diffusion. The cell becomes pos-

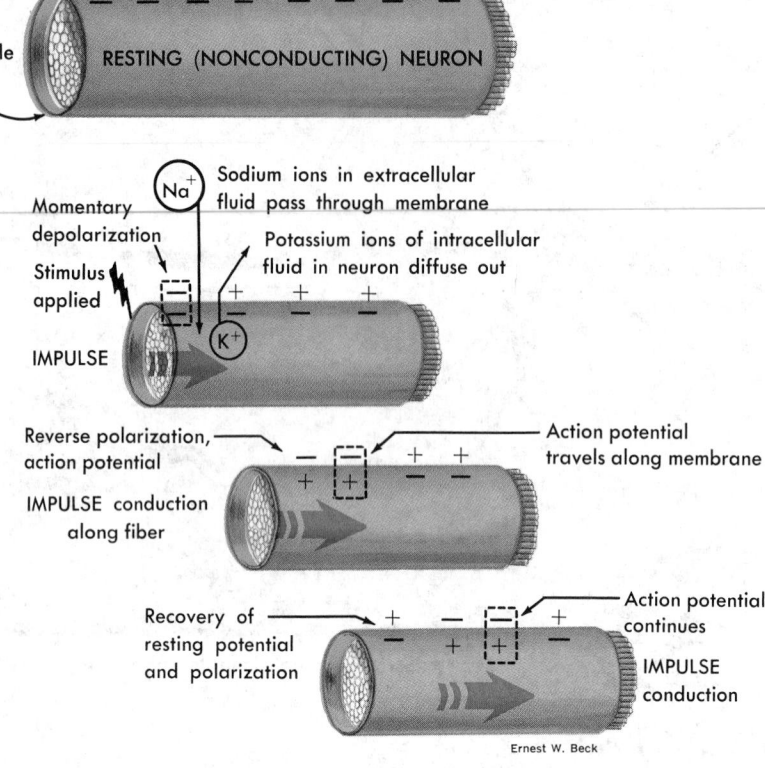

Fig. 37-6 Upper diagram represents polarized state of membrane of nerve fiber when it is not conducting impulses. Lower diagrams represent nerve impulse conduction: a self-propagating wave of negativity or action potential travels along membrane. (From Thibodeau GA: *Anthony's textbook of anatomy and physiology*, ed 13, St Louis, 1990, Mosby–Year Book.)

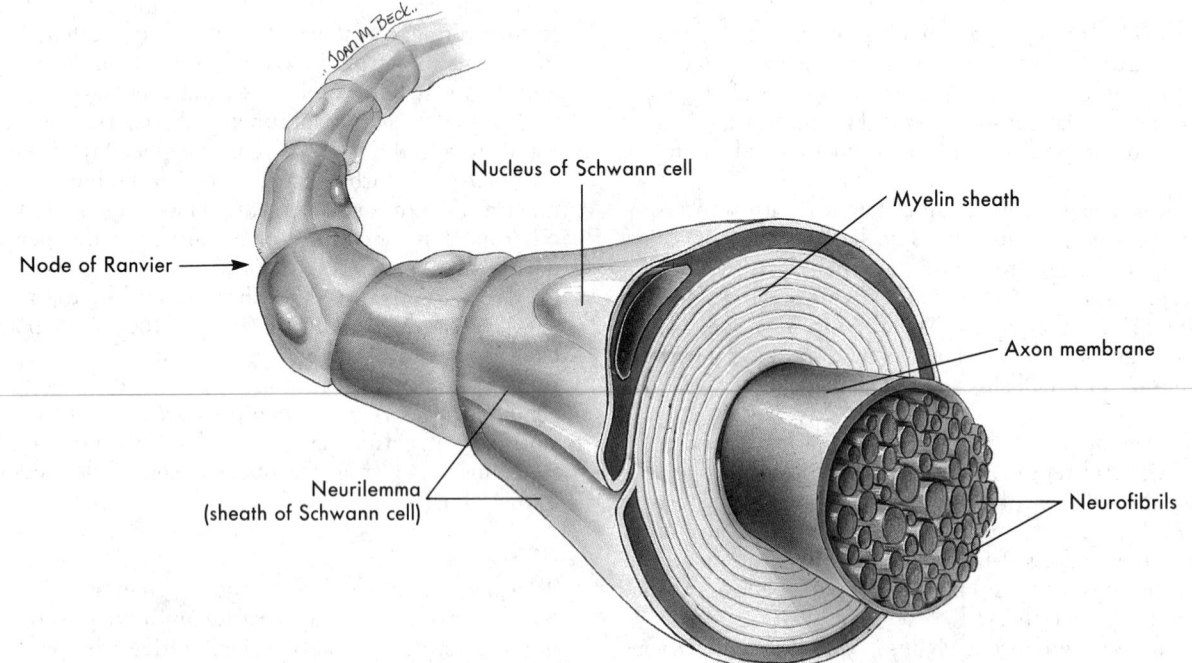

Fig. 37-7 Diagram of a nerve fiber and its coverings. This myelinated axon is located outside the central nervous system. Myelin is produced by the concentric layers of the Schwann cell. The neurilemma is the outer sheath of the Schwann cell and is indented by successive nodes of Ranvier. (From Christensen BL, Kockrow EO: *Foundations of nursing*, St Louis, 1991, Mosby–Year Book.)

itive, and the action potential (depolarization) occurs. After depolarization, the ion flow is reversed and the membrane is returned to its resting state. During depolarization and part of the repolarization process, there is a time interval called the *absolute refractory period.* During this time the nerve cannot be restimulated. This prevents repetitive excitation of the nerve.

When an action potential is generated it proceeds automatically to completion regardless of the type of stimulus that started the depolarization. This means that a strong stimulus does not cause a larger action potential. The action potential also spreads over the entire membrane without a decrease in velocity. The velocity is related to the size of the axon (velocity is higher with a larger diameter) and whether myelin is present.

Myelin is an excellent insulator of axons. The myelin sheath is deposited around the axons by Schwann's cells, and this layer may be as thick as the axon itself. Myelin prevents almost all ion flow across the axon and its membrane. However, at distances of approximately 1 mm, the sheath is interrupted by *nodes of Ranvier.* At these small, uninsulated areas, ions can flow easily between the extracellular fluid and the axon (Fig. 37-7).

The presence of myelin causes such fibers to be called *large fibers;* those without myelin are called *small fibers.* Large fibers have a greater conduction velocity because (1) the jumping effect allows depolarization to proceed quickly and (2) energy is conserved, because only the nodes depolarize. Large fibers appear white because of the myelin; the *white matter* of the nervous system is made up of myelinated fibers.

Many action potentials of neurons originate in a receptor neuron where internal and external stimuli are normally received. A receptor is like a transducer and can change one form of energy into another form. A receptor, however, responds or depolarizes to *only one* type of stimulus. For example, the retina of the eye responds only to the stimulus of light, which is converted to electrical energy and travels over the optic nerves to the visual cortices for perception.

Synapses

Neurons make contact with one another at sites called *synapses.* Transmission occurring across a synapse is a chemical process that occurs because of the release of neurotransmitters. The synapse consists of the *presynaptic terminal,* the *synaptic cleft,* and the *postsynaptic membrane.* Three types of interneuronal synapses occur. When the axon of one neuron synapses with the cell body of another neuron, it is called *axosomatic. Axodendritic* synapses occur between the axon of one neuron and the dendrites of another. Finally, *axoaxonic* synapses occur when one axon connects with another axon.

The end of the axon contains a chemical substance that is released by the action potential. The substance diffuses across the synapse to the adjacent cell membrane. *Synaptic transmission* is both *excitatory* and *inhibitory* in nature. Excitatory neurotransmitters react with receptor sites on the postsynaptic membrane to enhance permeability to sodium, chloride, and potassium ions. Inhibitory neurotransmitters decrease the postsynaptic membrane permeability to sodium while increasing the permeability to potassium and

chloride ions. The membrane becomes *hyperpolarized.* The amount of neurotransmitter released depends on the amount and speed of impulses stimulating the presynaptic terminal. Whether a neuron fires depends on the sum of the excitatory and inhibitory inputs.

At least 30 different neurotransmitters can affect transmission of an impulse at the synapse.

These actions include the following:
1. Acetylcholine—plays role in speeding impulse transmission
2. Norepinephrine—maintains arousal (awakening from a deep sleep, dreaming, and regulation of mood)
3. Dopamine—involves gross subconscious movement of the skeletal muscles and character of emotional responses
4. Serotonin—induces sleep, affects sensory perception, controls temperature, and has a role in controlling mood

In the past few years another group of chemical messengers, known as *neuropeptides,* has been discovered. Some of these function as neurotransmitters themselves, but most often they increase or decrease the response of the other neurotransmitters. In 1975 *enkephalins* were discovered; they act as a natural painkiller. Enkephalins are thought to inhibit pain impulses and bind with the same receptors in the brain with which chemicals such as morphine bind.

Chemical endorphins have been isolated in the pituitary. They are thought to suppress pain and are linked with memory, learning, and sexual activity.

Chemicals allowing excitatory transmission are *acetylcholine, norepinephrine, dopamine,* and *serotonin.* Those inhibiting transmissions are *gamma aminobutyric acid* (GABA) in brain tissue and *glycine* in the spinal cord.

Divisions of the Nervous System

Macroscopically, the nervous system has two major divisions. These are the *central nervous system* and the *peripheral nervous system* (Fig. 37-8).

Central nervous system

The central nervous system (CNS) is made up of collections of neurons and their connections into the brain and spinal cord. All the basic informational processes occur within the CNS. Areas of the brain and spinal cord are distinguished where cell bodies are concentrated into *nuclei* and groups of axons run in *tracts* that interconnect the parts. Collections of neurons are connected in complex ways. The connections determine the capability of each collection of neurons. The brain and spinal cord are structurally continuous. The brain is housed in the skull and the spinal cord in the vertebral column.

Skull

Surrounding the brain is the skull, a bony structure that encloses and protects it (Fig. 37-9). The skull is divided into two primary sections: the *cranium* and the *bones of the face.* Only the former will be discussed here.

The cranium is made up of eight bones that are joined by a series of fixed joints called *sutures.* The bones are made up of three layers that are called the *outer table,* the

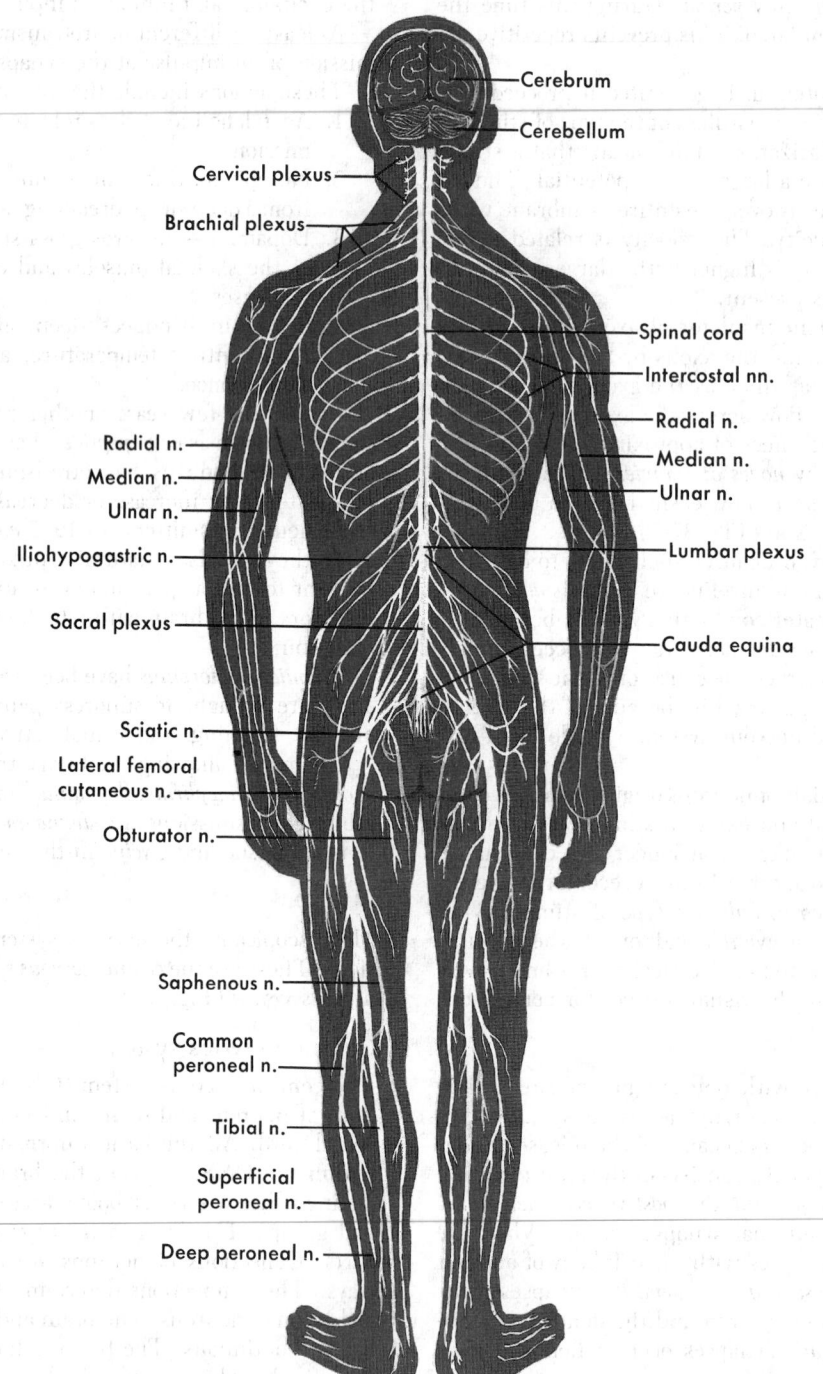

Fig. 37-8 The central and peripheral divisions of the nervous systems. The central nervous system (CNS) consists of the brain and spinal cord. The peripheral nervous system is composed of the cranial and spinal nerves. (From Christensen BL, Kockrow EO: *Foundations of nursing,* St Louis, 1991, Mosby–Year Book.)

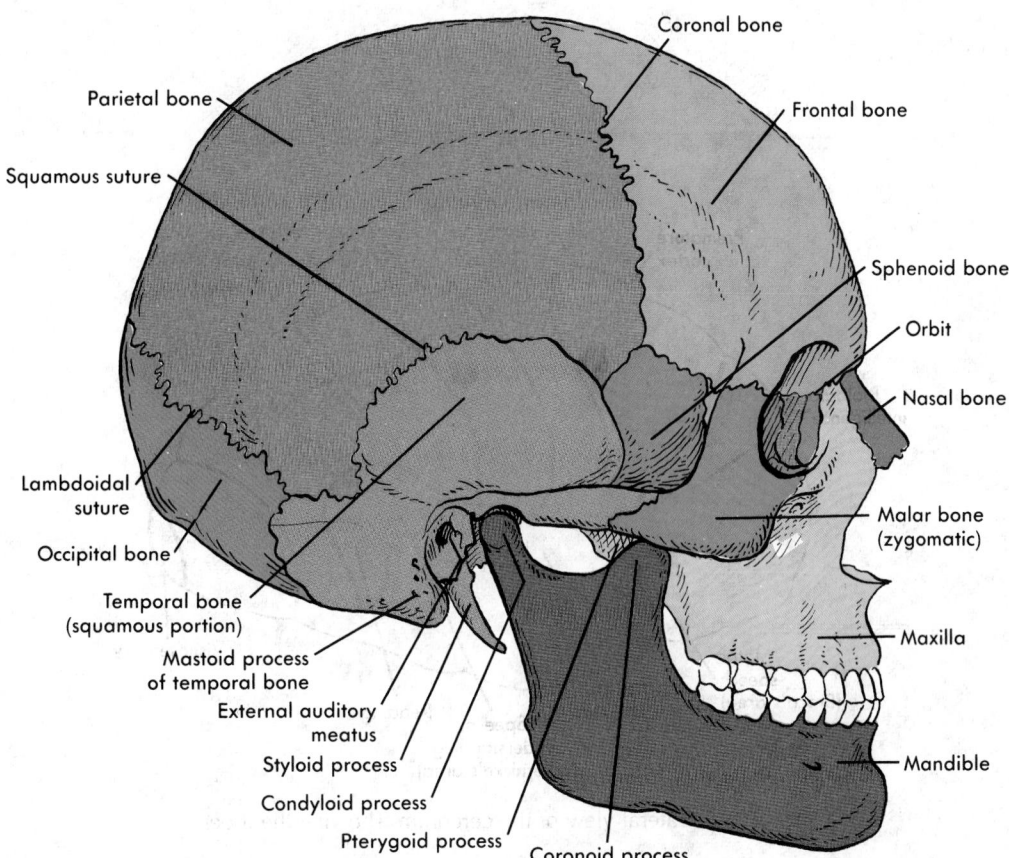

Fig. 37-9   Lateral view of skull. (From Thibodeau GA: *Anthony's textbook of anatomy and physiology,* ed 13, St Louis, 1990, Mosby—Year Book.)

diploe, and the *inner table.* The outer and inner table are solid, whereas the diploe is spongy. The inner table forms an inner cavity that is divided as follows:

1. Anterior fossa—contains frontal lobes
2. Middle fossa—contains temporal, parietal, and occipital lobes
3. Posterior fossa—contains brainstem and cerebellum

The *foramen magnum* is a large oval shaped opening at the base of the skull. It is at this level that the spinal cord and brain connect.

Brain

The brain weighs about 3 pounds and is divided grossly into the following three main areas: (1) the cerebrum, (2) the brainstem, and (3) the cerebellum.

Cerebrum

The cerebrum of each hemisphere (right and left) is composed of the following four major lobes: the *frontal, parietal, temporal,* and *occipital.* The cerebrum is the largest part of the brain and is covered on the outside by the cerebral cortex, which is approximately ¼ inch thick and contains more than 14 billion neurons. It receives and analyzes all impulses, controls voluntary movement, and stores knowledge of all impulses received.

The cerebrum is longitudinally divided into right and left hemispheres. The major folds of the cortex divide each hemisphere into four lobes. Each cerebral lobe, named for

the overlying cranial bone, carries out specific functions such as general sensation, perception, special senses, and speech (Figs. 37-10 and 37-11).

Deep within the cerebrum are the *basal ganglia.* These are masses of gray matter (cell bodies) and include the caudate nucleus, putamen, and globa pallidus. The basal ganglia function as part of the extrapyramidal system and control postural adjustment and fine voluntary movements, especially those of the hands and lower extremities.

One function of the cerebrum deserves special mention—that of speech. Speech is a function of the dominant hemisphere, which is on the left side of the brain for all right-handed people and most left-handed people. The two identified speech centers are Broca's area and Wernicke's area. *Broca's area* is in the frontal lobe adjacent to the motor cortex and controls verbal, expressive speech. *Wernicke's area* is in the posterior part of the temporal lobe and may extend to adjacent parts of the parietal lobe. It is responsible for reception and understanding of language. An area in the frontal lobe governs ability to write words, and an area in the occipital lobe controls ability to understand written material. The specific functions of the cerebral cortexes are listed in Box 37-1.

Brainstem

The *brainstem* lies deep in the center of the hemisphere and connects with the spinal cord at the level of the medulla (Fig. 37-12). It carries all nerve fibers passing between

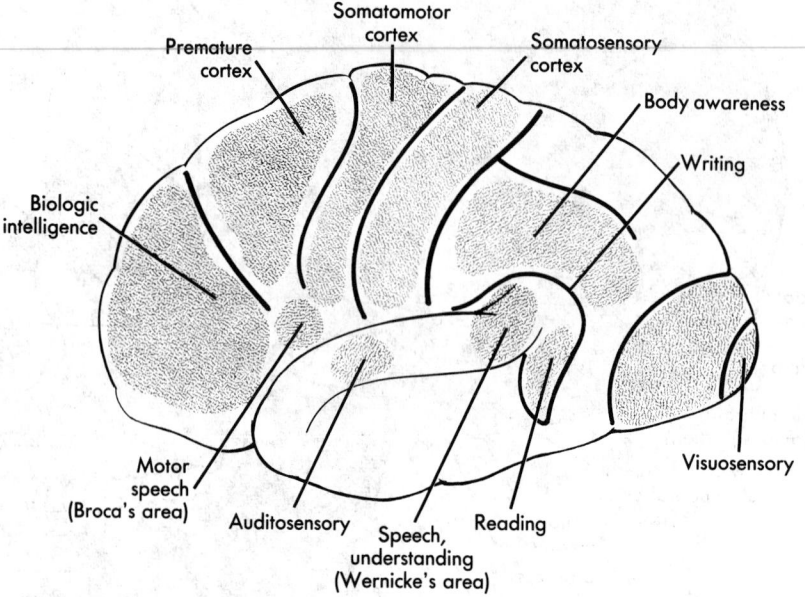

Fig. 37-10 Lateral view of the cerebrum, showing the lobes.

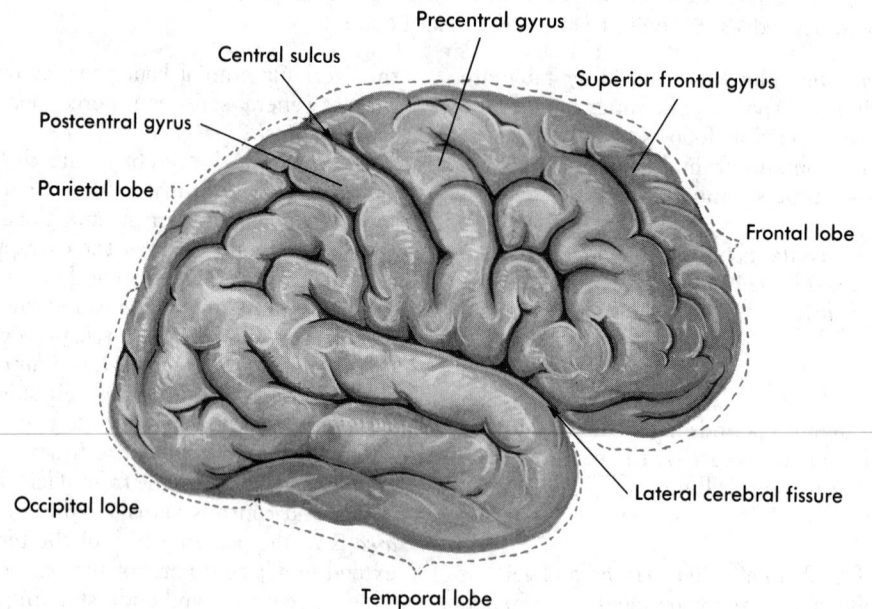

Fig. 37-11 Lateral view of the skull, showing the cranial bones and sutures that separate them.

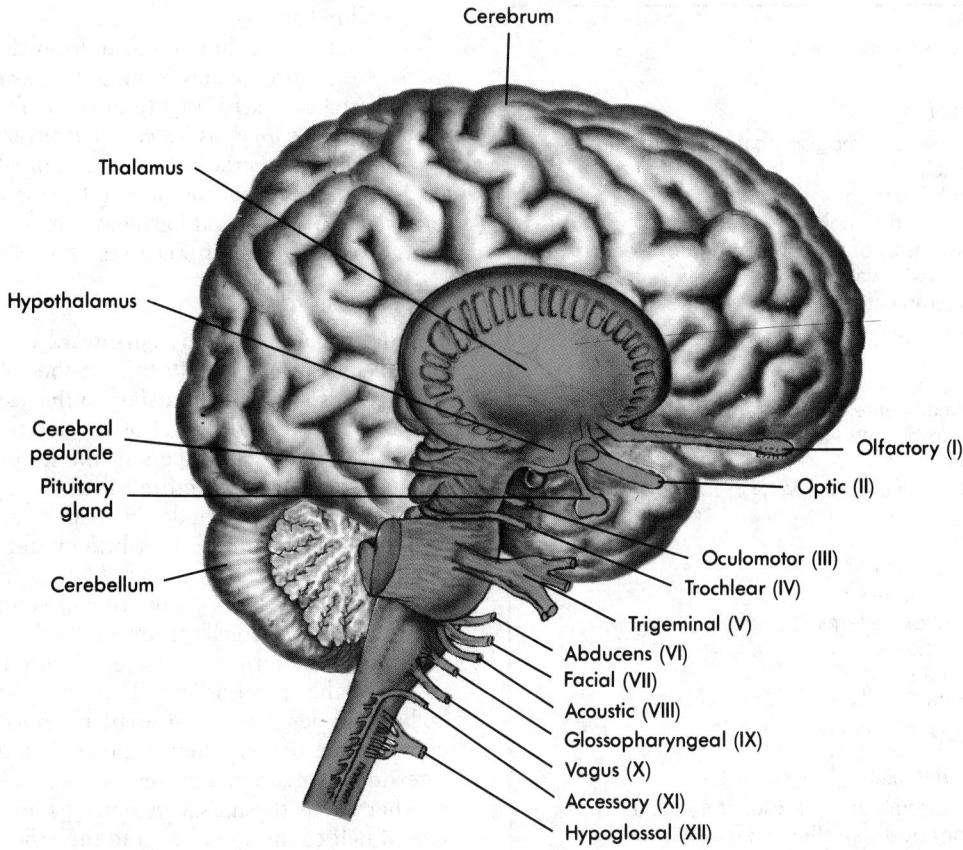

Fig. 37-12   Lateral view of the brain, showing the brainstem. Also shown are the cranial nerves, which arise from it. (From Rudy EB: *Advanced neurological and neurosurgical nursing*, St Louis, 1984, Mosby—Year Book.)

Specific functions of cerebral cortexes

Frontal cortex	Conceptualization
	Abstraction
	Judgment formation
	Motor ability
	Ability to write words
	Higher level centers for autonomic functions
Parietal cortex	Highest integrative and coordinating center for perception and interpretation of sensory information
	Ability to recognize body parts
	Left versus right
	Motor movement
Temporal cortex	Memory storage
	Auditory integration
	Hearing
Occipital cortex	Visual center
	Understanding of written material

the brain hemisphere and the spinal cord; additionally, all cranial nerves except cranial nerve I arise from it. Several structures are contained in the brainstem. These include the diencephalon, the midbrain, the pons, and the medulla oblongata. The diencephalon is often called the innerbrain because it lies directly beneath the cerebrum. It contains the thalamus and the hypothalamus. The thalamus, an oval structure with two lobes, is approximately 1 inch (3 cm) in diameter; it composes four fifths of the diencephalon. The thalamus serves as a relay station for some sensory impulses while interpreting other sensory messages, such as pain, light touch, and pressure.

The *hypothalamus*, which lies below the thalamus, plays a vital role in the *control of body temperature*, *fluid balance*, *appetite*, and *certain emotions*, such as *fear, pleasure,* and *pain*. Both the sympathetic and parasympathetic divisions of the autonomic nervous system are under the control of the hypothalamus, as is the pituitary gland. Thus the hypothalamus influences the heartbeat, the contraction and relaxation of the walls of blood vessels, and hormone secretion.

The specific functions of each of the structures that are located in the brainstem are listed in Box 37-2.

Of special importance is the core of tissue that extends throughout the entire brainstem called the *reticular for-*

Brainstem functions

Diencephalon

Receives sensory impulses (pain, temperature, and touch)
Acts as relay station
Controls pain threshold
Acts in synthesis of vasopressor and oxytocin
Helps maintain wakeful state
Controls temperature
Generates emotional response

Pons

Pneumotaxic center (rhythmicity of respirations)
Connection between medulla, midbrain, and cerebellum
Origin of cranial nerves V, VI, VII, and VIII

Midbrain

Motor movement
Relay of impulses
Postural reflex patterns
Auditory reflexes
Righting reflex
Some control of vision
Origin of cranial nerves III and IV

Medulla oblongata

Cardiac, vasomotor, and respiratory center
Center for cough, swallowing, and hiccuping
Role in reticular activating system
Origin of cranial nerves IX, X, XI, and XII

---

mation or the *reticular activating system* (Fig. 37-13). This interconnecting network of cells is the integrating center for respiration, cardiac function, motor systems, and states of consciousness. Stimulating these cells leads to wakefulness, and decreasing stimulation results in sleepiness (as in anoxia caused by increased intracranial pressure).

Cerebellum

The cerebellum is located below the posterior cerebrum and is about one fifth the size of the cerebrum. It has two lateral hemispheres and a medial part called the *vermis*. It controls skeletal muscles to produce coordinated movement, equilibrium, and erect posture. It acts with the cerebrum to coordinate muscle activity and produce skilled movement. Voluntary movements can proceed without the cerebellum, but they are clumsy and incoordinated (as in *asynergia* and *cerebellar ataxia*). The cerebellum receives both sensory and motor impulses, and it can detect errors in muscle synergy and adjust muscular control within the body.

Spinal vertebrae

The vertebral column is divided into these five regions: *cervical*, *thoracic*, *lumbar*, *sacral*, and *coccygeal*. The total number of vertebrae is 33 and is divided as follows:

1. 7 cervical
2. 12 thoracic
3. 5 lumbar
4. 5 sacral vertebrae fused to form the sacrum
5. 3 to 5 fused bones forming the coccyx

Each vertebra is separated from those above and below by *cartilage* and *fibrous tissue* called *intervertebral discs*. The *vertebral foramen* is the center of the spinal cord and is part of the vertebral canal containing the spinal cord and spinal meninges. Muscles and ligaments are attached to the vertebrae at the vertebral processes (Fig. 37-14).

Spinal cord

The spinal cord is the downward continuation of the medulla oblongata. It is 17 to 18 inches (45 to 48 cm) long and extends from the brainstem to the second lumbar vertebra. It starts at the level of the foramen magnum and ends at L2. The cord tapers in the lower thoracic region into a cone-shaped structure called the *conus medullaris*.

The spinal cord includes H-shaped central gray matter (cell bodies) surrounded by white matter composed of ascending and descending tracts. The gray matter resembles a butterfly (Fig. 37-15). The front or ventral horn consists of multipolar neuronal structures such as cell bodies and dendrites that form the efferent neurons of the ventral roots and the spinal nerves. The dorsal horn contains cell bodies and dendrites of afferent neurons and sensory receptors from the periphery. The gray matter also contains internuncial neurons that send impulses from one level to another, from the dorsal to ventral horns, and from one lateral half of the spinal cord to the other. The ascending pathways transmit sensory information from receptors in the periphery to the spinal cord and brain. The descending pathways transmit impulses from the brain to the motor neurons in the spinal cord (*upper motor neurons*) or to the peripheral nervous system (*lower motor neurons*). Some examples of ascending and descending spinal cord tracts are found in Fig. 37-15. See Table 37-1 for a list of the tracts of the spinal cord.

The spinal cord is also the site of reflex pathways. Reflexes do not require relay to the brain level for action—they are an example of the simplest neural circuit. A reflex action consists of a specific stereotyped motor response to an adequate sensory stimulus. The response may involve skeletal muscle movement. A reflex may involve only one spinal cord level, or it may involve more spinal cord levels (segmental reflex). One example of the simple reflex arc is the knee jerk (Fig. 37-16).

Circulation of the brain and spinal cord

The arterial system of the brain includes the larger conducting arteries and the penetrating smaller vessels that enter the brain at right angles after branching off from the conducting vessels. The smaller vessels supply nutrients to the neurons. The conducting arteries and the areas they supply include the following:

1. Internal carotid arteries—80% of blood supply
   a. Anterior cerebral arteries
      (1) Medial surface of the frontal and parietal lobes
      (2) Basal ganglia
      (3) Portions of the internal capsule and corpus callosum

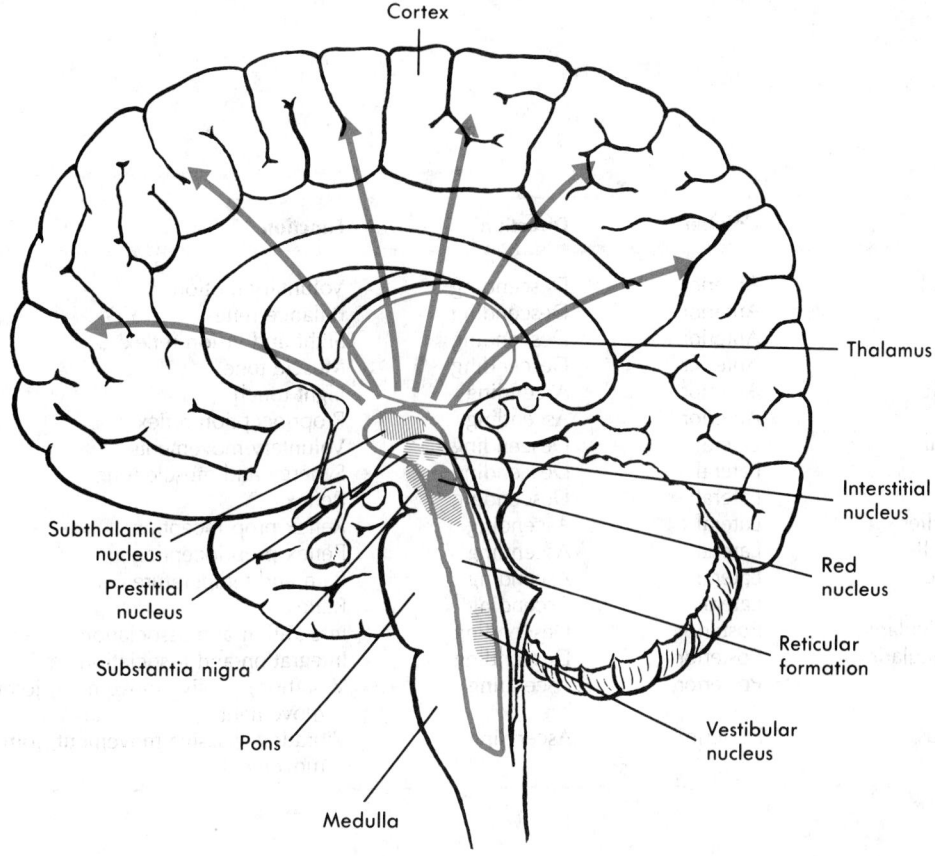

Fig. 37-13 Reticular activating system. (From Thompson JM, et al: *Mosby's manual of clinical nursing*, ed 2, St Louis, 1989, Mosby–Year Book.)

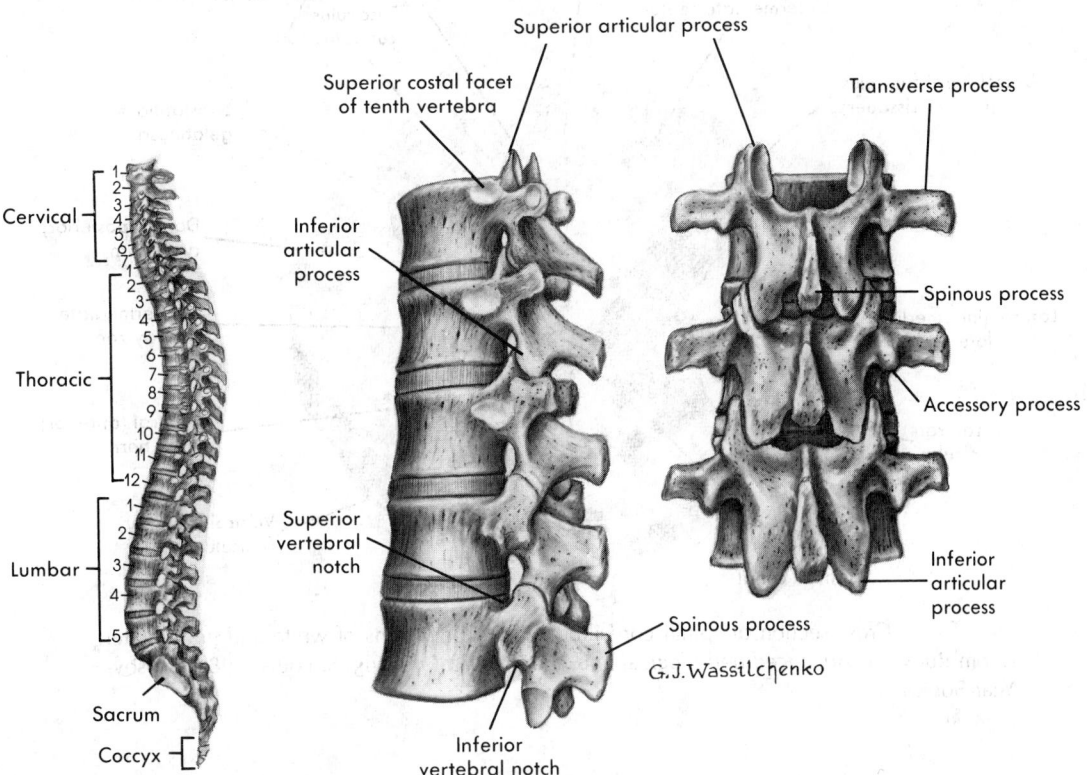

Fig. 37-14 Vertebral column and anatomical structure of vertebrae. (From Rudy, EB: *Advanced neurological and neurosurgical nursing*, St Louis, 1984, Mosby–Year Book.)

Table 37-1

Tract	Column	Direction	Function
Ventral corticospinal	Anterior	Descending	Voluntary motion
Vestibulospinal	Anterior	Descending	Balance reflex
Tectospinal	Anterior	Descending	Sight and vision reflex
Reticulospinal	Anterior	Descending	Muscle tone
Ventral spinothalmic	Anterior	Ascending	Light touch
Spinoolivary	Anterior	Ascending	Proprioception reflex
Lateral corticospinal	Lateral	Descending	Voluntary movements
Rubrospinal	Lateral	Descending	Synergy and muscle tone
Olivospinal	Lateral	Descending	Reflex
Dorsal spinocerebeller	Lateral	Ascending	Reflex proprioception
Ventral spinocerebeller	Lateral	Ascending	Reflex proprioception
Lateral spinothalmic	Lateral	Ascending	Pain and temperature
Spinotectal	Lateral	Ascending	Reflex
Fasciculus interfascicularis	Posterior	Descending	Integration and association
Septomarginal fascicularis	Posterior	Descending	Integration and association
Fascicularis gracilis	Posterior	Ascending	Vibration, passive movement, joint, and two-point movement
Fascicularis cuneatus	Posterior	Ascending	Vibration, passive movement, joint, and two-point movement

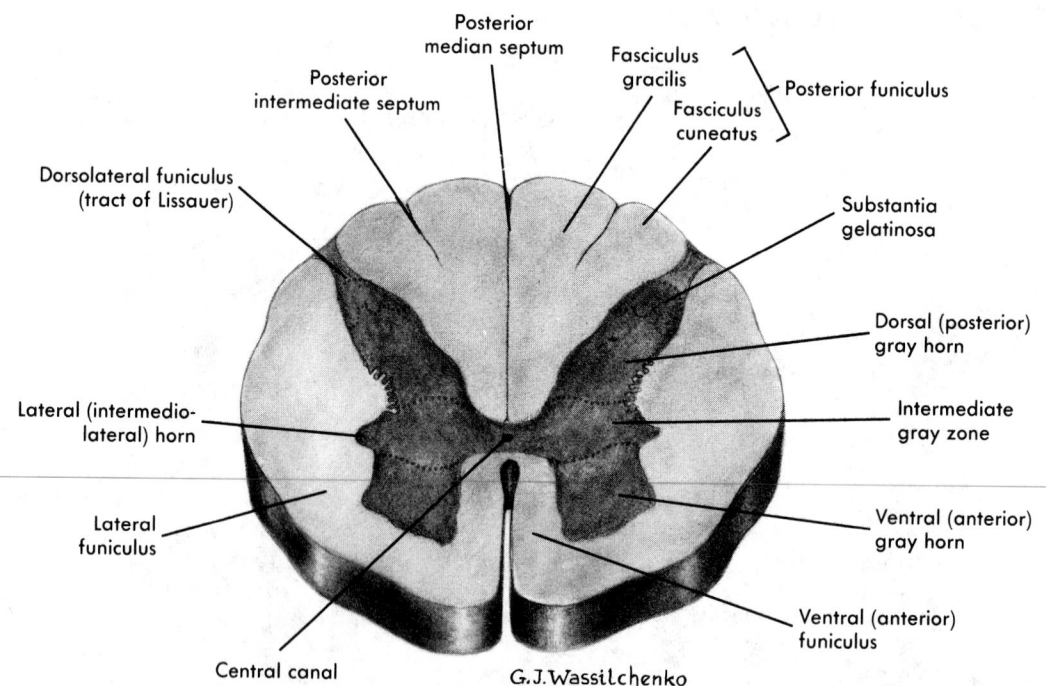

Fig. 37-15 Cross section of spinal cord illustrating subdivisions of white and gray matter. (From Rudy EB: *Advanced neurological and neurosurgical nursing*, St Louis, 1984, Mosby–Year Book.)

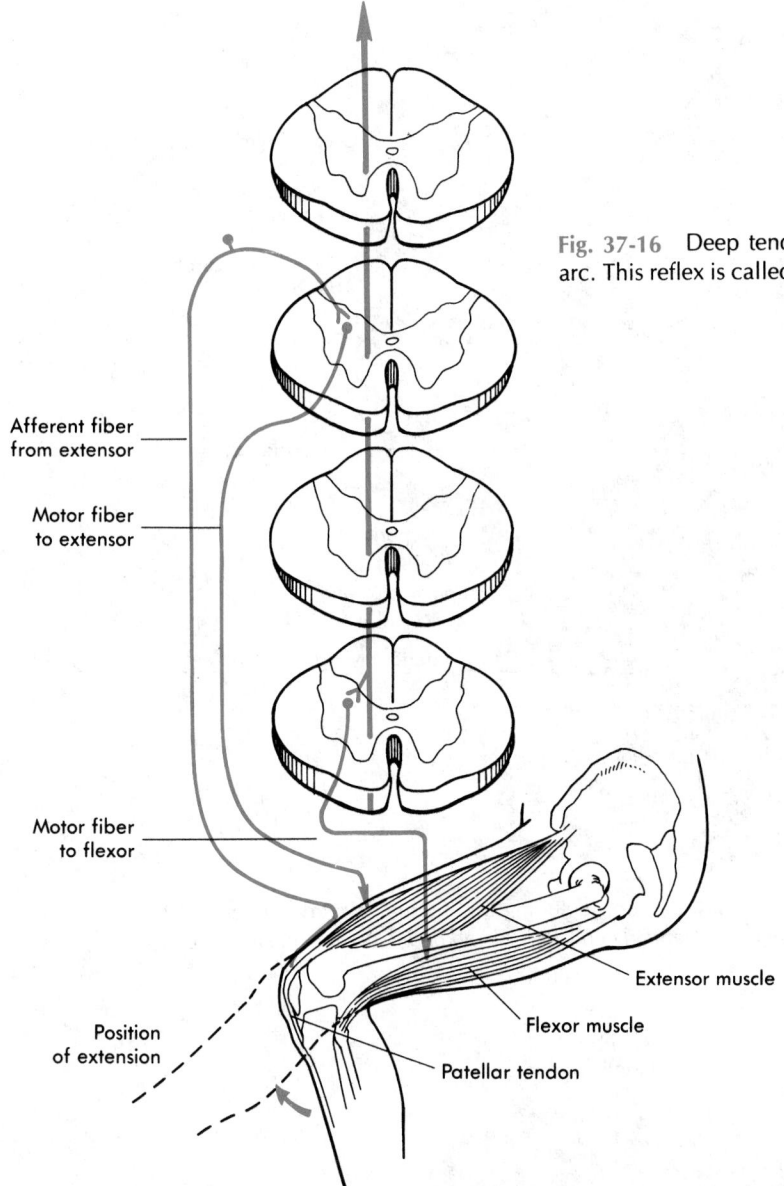

Fig. 37-16   Deep tendon reflex that demonstrates the reflex arc. This reflex is called the knee jerk or patellar tendon reflex.

Afferent fiber from extensor

Motor fiber to extensor

Motor fiber to flexor

Position of extension

Extensor muscle

Flexor muscle

Patellar tendon

  b. Middle cerebral arteries
    (1) Lateral surfaces of parietal, frontal, and temporal lobes
    (2) Precentral (motor) gyri
    (3) Postcentral (sensory) gyri
  2. Vertebral arteries—20% of blood supply
    a. Basilar artery
      (1) Brainstem
      (2) Cerebellum
    b. Posterior cerebral arteries
      (1) Portions of temporal and occipital lobes
      (2) Vestibular organs
      (3) Cochlear apparatus
The posterior cerebral artery connects to the middle cerebral artery by the posterior communicating branches. The anterior cerebral arteries connect through the anterior communicating branches. The purpose of this connection in the Circle of Willis is to ensure circulation in case of

a problem in any of the four main arteries. Branches of cerebral arteries reach all parts of the brain (Figs. 37-17 and 37-18).

Circulation to the brain has several unique characteristics. Systemic circulation favors the CNS overall, balancing parts to assure a constant supply of nutrients (glucose and oxygen) to the brain. The brain is also able to change its blood flow to respond to changes in blood pressure. In the presence of increasing blood pressure, cerebral vessels constrict, whereas they dilate when blood pressure falls. Vasodilation also occurs with elevated carbon dioxide content, hypoxia, and an elevated hydrogen ion concentration.

Cerebral veins have no valves. All veins of the brain terminate in sinuses created by the dura mater. They empty into the superior vena cava via the jugular vein.

The blood supply to the spinal cord comes from the spinal artery and two radicular arteries. The spinal artery

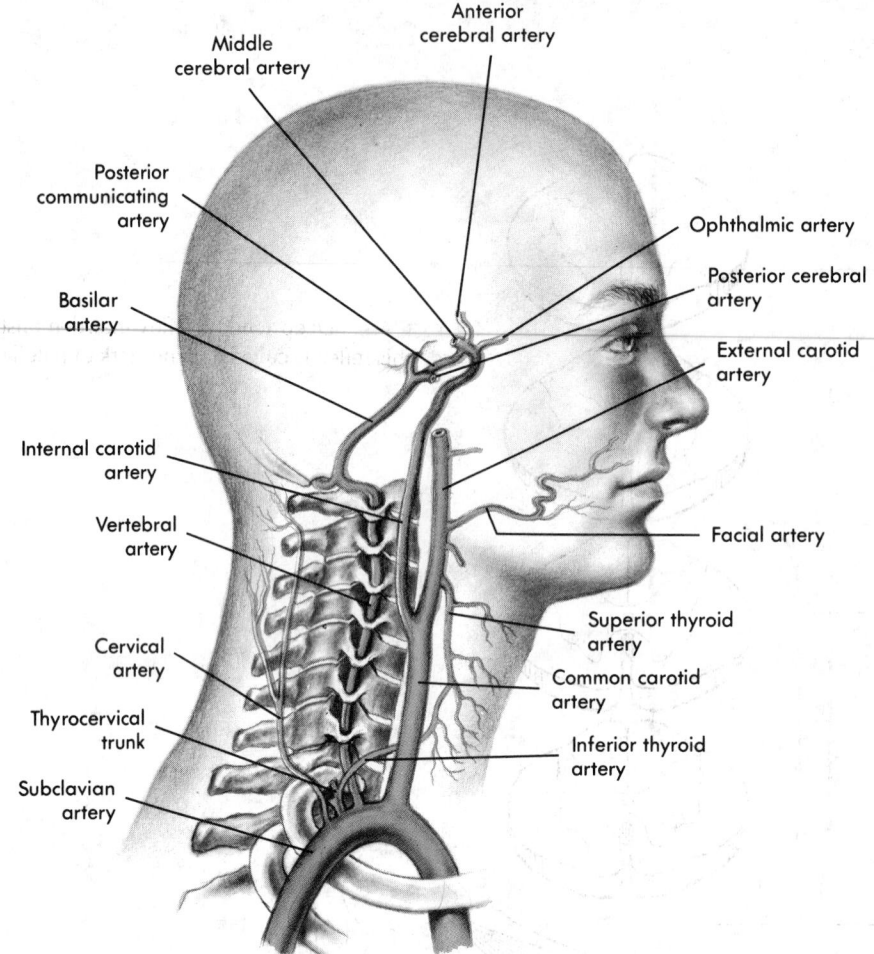

Fig. 37-17 Conducting arteries of the brain, including the internal carotid arteries and the vertebral arteries. (From Rudy EB: *Advanced neurological and neurosurgical nursing*, St Louis, 1984, Mosby–Year Book.)

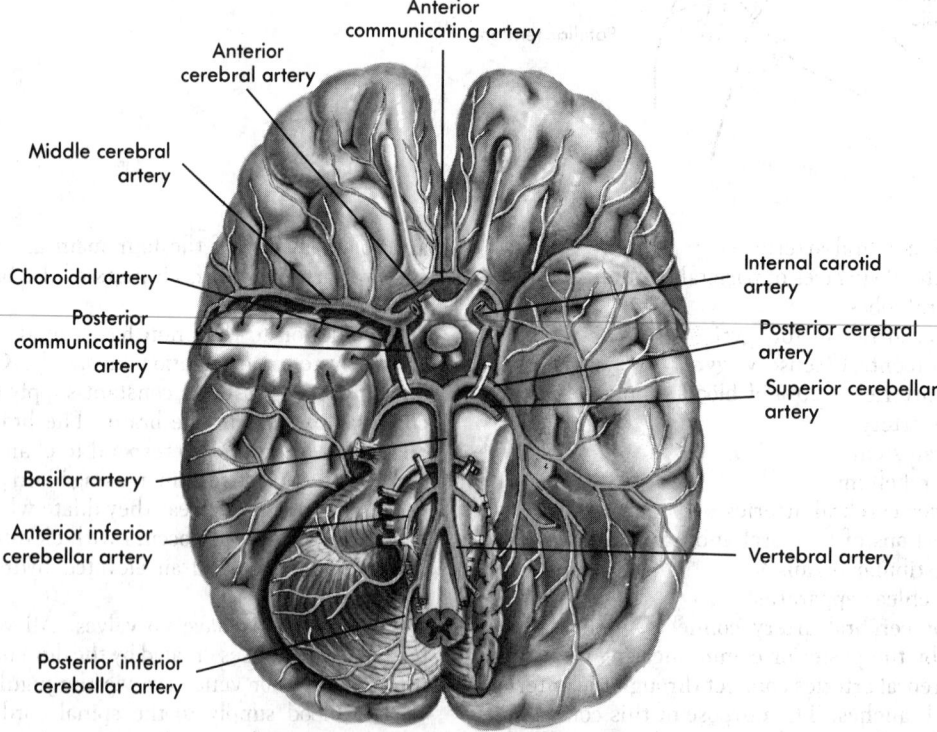

Fig. 37-18 Blood supply of the brain showing the penetrating vessels and the Circle of Willis. The internal carotids and the vertebral arteries anastomose at the Circle of Willis. (From Rudy EB: *Advanced neurological and neurosurgical nursing.* St Louis, 1984. Mosby–Year Book.)

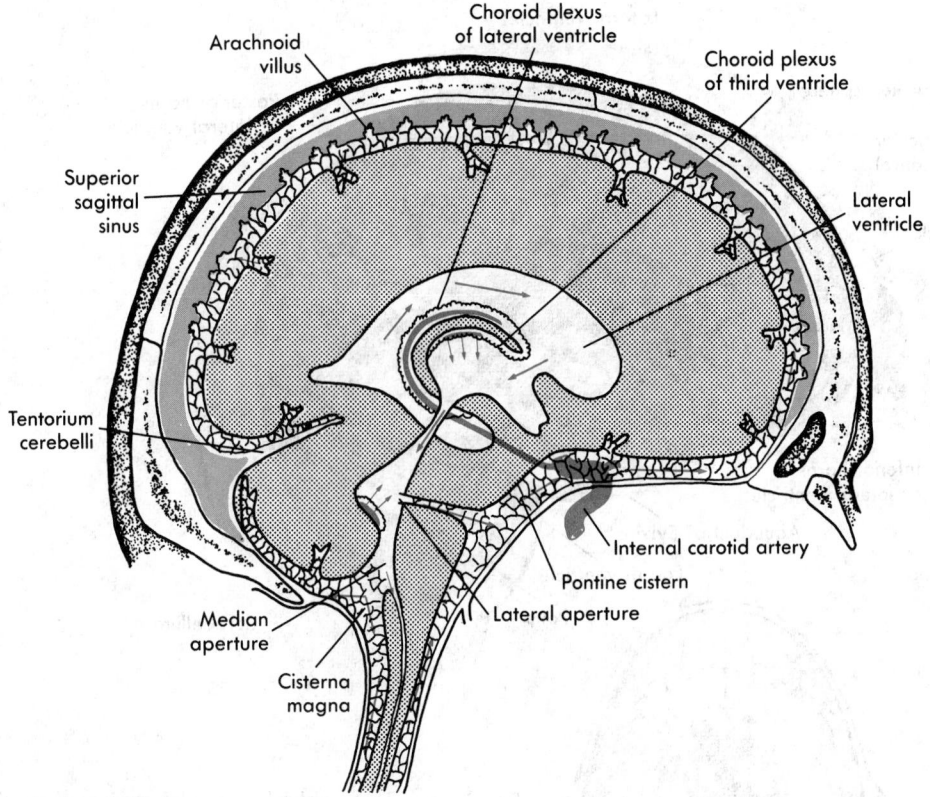

Fig. 37-19   Path of circulation of cerebrospinal fluid from its formation in the ventricles to its absorption into the superior sagittal sinus. (From Nolte J: *The human brain*, ed 2, St Louis, 1988, Mosby–Year Book.)

arises from the vertebral arteries, whereas the radicular arteries arise from the aorta.

Blood-brain barrier

The blood-brain barrier is a physiologic mechanism that aids in maintaining the homeostasis of the brain through selective permeability. Normally, substances enter the blood by way of capillaries into the cerebrospinal fluid or by the capillaries into the extracellular fluid. The barrier is permeable to O_2, CO_2, and water. It is slightly permeable to electrolytes but is impermeable to fixed acids and bases and most drugs.

Cerebrospinal fluid (CSF)

Cerebrospinal fluid (CSF) is found in the ventricles of the brain, in the central canal of the spinal cord, and in the subarachnoid space. It serves as a fluid cushion for the tissue of the nervous system and helps support the weight of the brain. Cerebrospinal fluid is formed in the vessels of the choroid plexus. In a 24-hour period the choroid plexus secretes approximately 500 to 570 ml of CSF. However, only 125 to 150 ml is circulating at any one time. After circulating around the brain and spinal cord, the fluid returns to the brain and is absorbed from the subarachnoid space through the arachnoid villi. The cerebrospinal fluid then enters the venous system and follows the pathway through the jugular vein to the superior vena cava into the systemic circulation (Fig. 37-19).

37-3	Normal characteristics of cerebrospinal fluid (CSF)	
Specific gravity	1.007	
pH	7.35 to 7.45	
Chloride	120 to 130 mEq/L	
Glucose	50 to 80 /100 ml	
Pressure	50 to 200 mm water	
Total volume	80 to 200 ml (15 ml in ventricles)	
Total protein	15 to 45 mg/100 ml (lumbar) 10 to 25 mg/100 ml (cisternal) 5 to 15 mg/100 ml (ventricular)	
Gamma globulin	6% to 13% of total protein	
Cell count		
RBC	none	
WBC	0-5 0-10 cells (all lymphocytes and monocytes)	

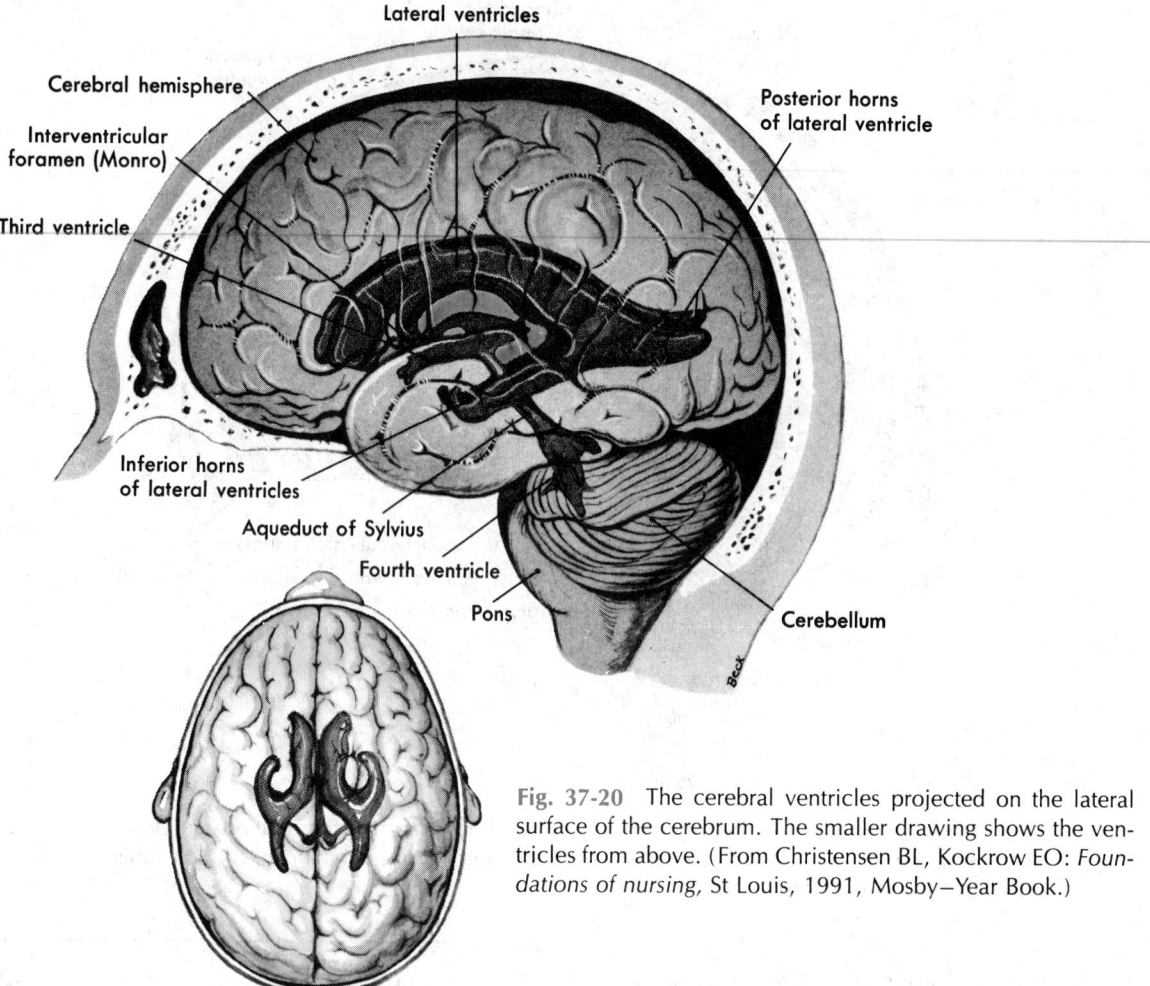

Fig. 37-20 The cerebral ventricles projected on the lateral surface of the cerebrum. The smaller drawing shows the ventricles from above. (From Christensen BL, Kockrow EO: *Foundations of nursing*, St Louis, 1991, Mosby–Year Book.)

Normally there are up to 8 lymphocytes/ml of spinal fluid. An increase in the number of cells may indicate an infection, such as tuberculosis or a viral infection. Bacterial infections such as tuberculous meningitis often lower the blood sugar level, as well as the chloride levels. Spinal fluid protein is increased in the presence of degenerative disease and/or brain tumor. Blood in the spinal fluid indicates hemorrhage from somewhere in the ventricular system. See Box 37-3 for normal characteristics of CSF.

Ventricles

The ventricular system is made up of four cavities. The two lateral ventricles are found within each cerebral hemisphere and are the largest cavities. They are separated by a thin layer called the *septum pellucidum*. Each of the lateral ventricles communicates with the central ventricle, which communicates with the fourth ventricle (Fig. 37-20). Parts of the lateral, third, and fourth ventricles are lined with a dense layer of capillaries called the *choroid plexus*.

Meninges

The coverings of the nervous tissue in the brain and spinal cord are called the meninges. These coverings help support, protect, and nourish the vital tissues below. The

outermost is the *dura mater*. It is a very tough membrane with two layers. One of these meningeal layers sends four processes deep into the brain. These processes form fibrous compartments for protection of the brain. The *arachnoid* is a delicate membrane that lies beneath the dura and closely covers the brain. Projections called *arachnoid villi* extend into the overlying dura. The innermost of the meninges is the *pia mater*, which is a vascular membrane with many minute plexuses of blood vessels. The same three meninges are also found in the spinal cord.

Three potential spaces are associated with the meninges. These include the following:
1. Extradural (external to the dura)
2. Subdural (between the dura and the arachnoid)
3. Subarachnoid (between the arachnoid and the pia mater (see Fig. 37-21).

Peripheral nervous system

The peripheral nervous system (PNS) is basically a set of common channels located outside the CNS. *Peripheral nerves are individual nerves or bundles of nerves that are motor, sensory, or "mixed"* (both sensory and motor fibers). The peripheral nervous system consists of *12 pairs of cranial nerves*, which carry impulses to and from the brain, and

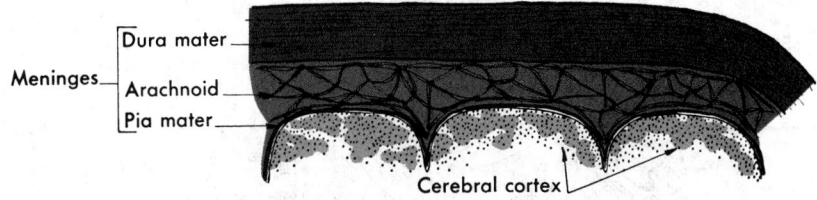

Fig. 37-21   Schematic drawing showing the structure of the meninges around the brain. (From Christensen BL, Kochrow EO: *Foundations of nursing,* St Louis, 1991, Mosby–Year Book.)

Table 37-2   Parasympathetic and sympathetic nervous system influence

Organ system	Parasympathetic influence	Sympathetic influence
Heart	Decreases rate	Increases rate
Blood vessels	Dilates visceral and brain vessels	Constricts
Lung	Constricts bronchi	Dilates bronchi
Gastrointestinal	Increases peristalsis	Decreases peristalsis
Anal sphincter	Opens	Closes
Urinary	Contracts bladder	Relaxes bladder
	Opens sphincter	Closes sphincter
Eye	Constricts pupil	Dilates pupil
	Accommodates for near vision	Accommodates for far vision
Skin	Not applicable	"Goose flesh"
Gastric and salivary secretions	Increases	Decreases
Liver	Not applicable	Stimulates glycogen
Adrenal medulla	Not applicable	Stimulates production of epinephrine

31 pairs of spinal nerves, which carry impulses to and from the spinal cord. Each spinal nerve innervates a specific part of the body for sensation; these parts are called *dermatomes.* Several spinal nerves may also join together to form a complex network of nerve fibers called plexuses.

Peripheral nerves that transmit information toward the CNS are *afferent* or sensory in nature, and peripheral nerves that transmit information away from the CNS are *efferent* or motor in nature. In the peripheral nervous system the motor and sensory nerves usually travel together but separate at the cord level into a *posterior* or *sensory root* and an *anterior* or *motor root.*

The peripheral nervous system is divided into the *somatic* and *autonomic nervous systems.* The somatic nervous system innervates skeletal (striated) muscles. Fibers of axons liberate the neurotransmitter *acetylcholine* at the skeletal muscle cells; this produces an action potential and movement.

Autonomic nervous system

Body functions regulated by the autonomic nervous system include those of the *cardiovascular, respiratory,* and *endocrine systems.* Regulatory efforts have the goal of preserving homeostasis. Fibers of the autonomic nervous system synapse once after leaving the CNS at a site called the *ganglion.* The neurotransmitter is *acetylcholine.* The autonomic nervous system can be subdivided into the *sympathetic nervous system* and the *parasympathetic nervous system.* The sympathetic system functions to maintain homeostasis and to provide defense against stressors. During stress, sympa-

thetic responses include an *increase* in blood pressure and heart rate and *vasoconstriction* of peripheral blood vessels. The parasympathetic system conserves and restores regulatory functions (see Table 37-2).

Sensory System Pathways

Stimulation of receptor neurons in the body is the first step in sensation. These receptor neurons provide the brain with information about the internal and external environments. The general sensory system includes the following:

1. Receptor neurons, which respond to specific stimuli
2. Posterior roots of the peripheral or afferent sensory nerves, which carry nerve impulses (action potentials) toward the CNS
3. Ascending or sensory tracts within the spinal cord and brain
4. Sensory area of the cerebral cortex, in which stimuli are perceived and interpreted

From the receptor neuron, the sensory impulse travels to the spinal cord along the afferent fibers of the nerve involved. These fibers enter the spinal cord through the posterior root and proceed along either the *spinothalamic tracts* or the *posterior columns.* The pathway followed is specific to the sensation.

Motor System Pathways

After sensation has been perceived by the brain, corrective action or response is initiated. This action is conveyed by the descending motor pathways, which include the *corticospinal (pyramidal) tracts,* the *extrapyramidal system,* and

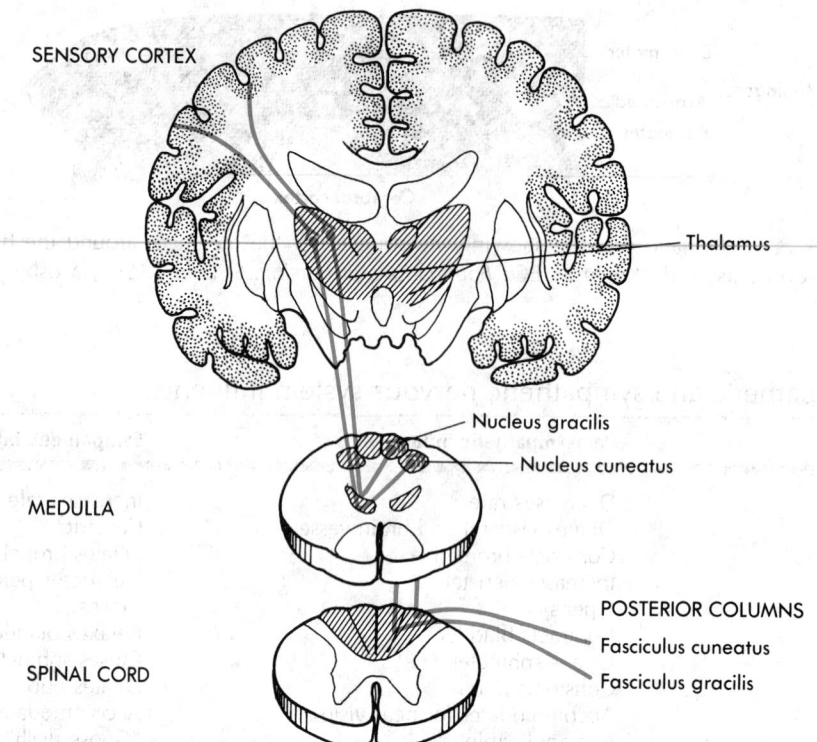

Fig. 37-22 Pathways for fine touch, deep touch and pressure, vibration, and proprioception. Note how stimuli entering through dorsal route (posterior) travel on same side as posterior columns to medulla where they cross to opposite side, ascend to thalamus, and end in somasthetic area where perception occurs.

the *cerebellar system.* The corticospinal system is primarily concerned with skilled, voluntary movement of skeletal muscle. Fibers that combine to form the corticospinal tracts arise from the upper motor neurons, which are located in most areas of the cerebral cortex.

After fibers leave the cerebral cortex they travel to the medulla, in which the majority of fibers *decussate* (cross over) to the opposite side. These fibers eventually synapse with the anterior horn cells, which are in the spinal cord and the motor nuclei in the brainstem. These cells are the *lower motor neurons* and are the final communication pathway with muscles via the *myoneural junction* (Fig. 37-22).

The *extrapyramidal tracts* provide *separate pathways* between the *cortex,* the *basal ganglia,* the *brainstem,* and the *spinal cord.* These include all descending motor pathways other than the corticospinal tracts, and they are named for their points of origin and termination. Generally, the extrapyramidal tracts help maintain muscle tone and control of gross autonomic skeletal muscle movement.

Visceral efferent pathways from the spinal cord control the action of involuntary or smooth muscles located within the walls of hollow organs, tubes, the heart, and glands.

Effectors

Effectors are cells of the body that "do something." They interact with the internal and external environments in some way and carry out the commands of the nervous system. The two classes of effectors are muscles and glands. They are both transducers and are capable of converting one form of energy into another. *Effectors,* like nerve tissue, are *excitable tissues* and are *able to generate action potentials.* The nervous system controls muscles and glands by directly turning them on or by altering the level of spontaneous activity.

Physiologic Changes With Aging

Studies have shown that the nervous system does change with aging. The effect of these changes is variable. The brain itself significantly *decreases in weight* with aging, along with a substantial loss of neurons. Those cells not destroyed undergo structural changes. Brain cells are lost at a rate of 1% a year after 50 years of age.[30] The loss is inconsistent, so that some parts of the brain lose cells at a faster rate. The cortex generally loses cells at a faster rate than the brainstem. There may be a general decline in interconnections of dendrites. Also senile plaques and neurofibrillary plaques, as well as the age pigment lipofuscin, are found in neuronal cells. In addition, there is a significant *reduction of cerebral blood flow, a decrease in brain metabolism, and a decrease in oxygen utilization.*

The aged may also experience an altered *sleep/wakefulness ratio* and a *decreased ability to regulate body temperature.* These suggest changes in the function of the hypothalamus in the aging.

The control of the autonomic nervous system over various functions of the body is unpredictable and labile in the elderly, but some changes do occur. Additionally, sensory and motor conduction *decreases in velocity of nerve impulses* occur with aging, sensory conduction decreasing faster than motor. This occurs especially in peripheral nerves and more often in females. In the spinal cord the blood supply to the white matter has been found to be decreased, leading to diminished reflexes in the lower (distal) extremities.

It is important for the nurse to realize that normal changes that occur with aging in the nervous system cannot be equated with senility, Alzheimer's disease, or organic brain disease. These conditions occur in a small number of older persons, and many aged persons reach advanced ages without any deterioration in the ability to think.

PREVENTION AND HEALTH EDUCATION

Problems that occur in the nervous system can have devastating results. These results often have impact on almost every body system and produce changes that are chronic and debilitating. Problems in other body systems, if discovered and treated in a timely fashion, can have much more satisfactory results than those in the nervous system.

Primary Prevention: Prevention of Disease

Many of the problems of the nervous system have no known cause and thus cannot be prevented. For other problems, however, preventive measures can be emphasized. Neurologic problems can be divided into several main categories in terms of prevention as follows.

Problems resulting from vascular disease

Neurovascular diseases can at times be prevented, or their results can at least be minimized. Many of the cerebrovascular diseases are thought to occur more frequently as a result of the presence of certain risk factors. These same factors also increase the risk of cardiac disease:

1. Cigarette smoking
2. Hypertension
3. Hypercholesteremia
4. Obesity
5. Stress-related occupations and a hectic pace of life

Problems resulting from metastasis

Cigarette smoking has been identified as a major cause of lung cancer. This is significant to the nervous system because neoplasms of the lung often metastasize to the brain. In fact, a significant number of lung malignancies are discovered after signs and symptoms of brain metastasis occur.

Problems resulting from trauma

Some actions can play an important role in preventing head injuries and spinal cord injuries. Factors that can influence the outcome include the following:

1. Use of seat belts in automobiles
2. Use of helmets while riding motorcycles or snowmobiles
3. Practice of firearm safety—keeping guns away from children
4. Minimal use of drugs and alcohol
5. Not driving after drinking or taking drugs
6. Safe use of motor vehicles—no showing off or speeding
7. Use of precautions while swimming and especially not diving into shallow water

Problems resulting from infections

Neurologic diseases resulting from infections can sometimes be prevented. Because ear or sinus infections can be a source of brain abscess or meningitis, it is important that these infections be treated. Also, because several of the neurologic diseases related to infections are spread through sexual contacts, such as AIDS and syphilis, the practice of responsible sex is important. This may include abstinence, monogamy, or the use of latex condoms.

Secondary Prevention: Early Detection

Early detection of neurologic diseases often is difficult. Many initial symptoms are so vague that it is easy to deny or minimize their importance. Also, some changes may occur over such a long period of time that adaptation to them occurs. Certain *warning symptoms* can be found in such vague patterns that patients may be thought at first to be suffering from hysteria. The symptoms that are significant include the following:

1. Headaches that first occur after middle age or change in character, especially ones that are worse in the morning or awaken a person from sleep
2. Clumsiness or loss of function in an extremity
3. Changes in visual acuity
4. Any new or worsened seizure activity
5. Numbness or tingling in one or more extremities
6. Pain that is neurologic in nature
7. Galactorrhea
8. Cessation of menses
9. Personality changes

Tertiary Prevention: Prevention of Complications

It is important to mention the issue of tertiary prevention for the patient with neurologic dysfunction. Unfortunately, many of these patients are *prone to iatrogenic complications*, as well as *functional disabilities*. These occur secondary to the neurologic problems and include contractures, decubiti, and eye damage, as well as other hazards of immobility.[102] It is extremely important for the nurse working with neurologically impaired patients to be aware of rehabilitative concepts and apply them in nursing care. Many patients with neurologic dysfunctions may also benefit from formal inpatient rehabilitative care after an acute hospitalization.

Looking to the Future

The U.S. Department of Health and Human Services has published goals for the United States for the year 2000. One goal is to reduce the number of deaths from strokes to no more than 20 per 100,000 persons from a baseline of 30.3 per 100,000 in 1987. Although stroke mortality has declined by more than 50% since 1972, there is still room for improvement. Stroke mortality also continues to be higher for Blacks than Whites. (In 1987 the age-adjusted death rates for Black men and women were 57.1 and 46.7 per 100,000 respectively, compared with 30.3 and 26.3 for White men and women). To help narrow this gap, a special population target proposing a greater proportional reduction in stroke deaths has been established for blacks. Special efforts will also be focused in areas such as the southeastern United States (often called the Stroke Belt), where deaths from strokes are higher than in any other part of the country.[83]

Table 37-3 **Cranial nerves**

Nerve	Origin	Function	Assessments
Olfactory (I)	Olfactory	Sensory—smell	Identification of odors
Optic (II)	Lateral genic- ulate body	Sensory—vision	Visual acuity: inspection of fundi; determination of visual fields.
Oculomotor (III)	Midbrain	Motor—pupil constriction, eleva- tion of upper eyelid, extraocular movements	Tested together for extraocular movements (Fig. 37-31); also pupil reflex for CNIII
Trochlear (IV)	Midbrain	Motor—downward/inward eye movements	
Trigeminal (V)	Pons	Motor—jaw movement Sensory facial sensation	Jaw strength; facial sensation; corneal reflex
Abducens (VI)	Pons	Motor—lateral eye movements	
Facial (VII)	Pons	Motor—facial muscles Sensory taste on anterior two thirds of tongue	Facial movements; identification of tastes
Acoustic (VIII)	Pons	Hearing—cochlear division Balance—vestibular division	Whisper; caloric test
Glossopharyngeal (IX)	Medulla	Sensory—pharynx and posterior tongue, with taste Motor—pharynx	Identification of tastes
Vagus (X)	Medulla	Sensory—pharynx and larynx Motor—palate, pharynx and larynx	Gag reflex; uvula motion; soft palate movement; hoarseness
Spinal accessory (XI)	Medulla	Motor—sternocleidomastoid, up- per part of trapezius	Shoulder and neck motion
Hypoglossal (XII)	Medulla	Motor—tongue	Tongue motion

Adapted from Bates B: *A guide to physical examination,* ed 2, Philadelphia, 1979, JB Lippincott.

COMMON NEUROLOGIC MANIFESTATIONS

The practice of neurologic nursing is concerned with problems of the nervous system that have a variety of causes. Whatever the cause, various symptoms occur, at times related to both organic and functional causes. Because of the nature of the anatomy and physiology of the nervous system, *organic lesions or trauma result in clinical manifestations related to the site affected, regardless of the underlying pathologic condition.* Other manifestations result not from the damaged site itself, but from other parts of the nervous system that are affected by the damaged site. One example of this is a lack of control or regulation. The nurse must realize that patients with neurologic problems may have to make significant changes in lifestyle and adaptation. The psyche and the body are one in the person; often there is no clear-cut distinction of symptoms. A person is an open system in which many subsystems interplay.

In this section, we will discuss neurologic manifestations resulting from alterations in neurologic function and structure that are common to many pathologic conditions. A brief review of neurologic assessment is helpful in this discussion.

NEUROLOGIC ASSESSMENT

Complete neurologic assessment is usually performed in phases and depends on the condition of the patient and the urgency in collecting the data. It includes a history and neurologic examination.

Neurologic examination of the conscious adult includes physical examination of the following:

1. Mental status
   a. Level of consciousness
   b. Orientation
   c. Mood and behavior
   d. Knowledge
   e. Vocabulary
   f. Memory
2. Cranial nerve function (Table 37-3)
3. Language and speech
4. Meningeal signs
5. Sensory status
   a. Touch
   b. Pain
   c. Temperature
   d. Proprioception
6. Motor status
   a. Gait and stance
   b. Muscle strength
   c. Muscle tone
   d. Coordination
   e. Involuntary movements
   f. Muscle stretch reflexes

Table 37-4   Commonly used states of awareness and associated behaviors

	State					
	Conscious-aware		**Semiconscious-semicomatose**		**Unconscious-comatose**	
Level	Alert	Confused	Obtunded, drowsy	Stupor	Light coma	Deep coma
Behaviors	Normal activity Aware, mentally functional	Poor coordination Delirium Hallucinations Restlessness Excitable May be combative Short attention span Inappropriate actions and judgments Decreased awareness Disorientation	Sleepy Very short attention span Ready arousal Responds appropriately when aroused Ability to respond verbally Fends off painful stimuli with purposeful movement	Apathetic Slow moving Blank expression Drooping head Staring Arousal only to vigorous stimuli Incomplete arousal to painful stimuli No verbal response or moaning Response to verbal communication is inconsistent and vague	Not oriented to time, place or person Response is only by grimace or withdrawing limb from pain Primitive and disorganized response to painful stimuli	Absence of response to even the most painful stimuli

From Phipps W and others: Medical-surgical nursing, ed 4, St. Louis, 1991, Mosby-Year Book.

More detailed descriptions of selected portions of the examination will be covered in specific parts of this chapter. The reader is also referred to a neurologic nursing text for additional information.

In clinical settings, it is not feasible or essential to completely repeat the total neurologic exam during the shift-to-shift assessment of the patient. In many settings, such as intensive care units, the neurologic checks are performed every hour. Certain features have been identified as most important and should be emphasized when one is doing these checks. Generally these include the following:

1. Orientation
2. Level of consciousness (Table 37-4)
3. Ability to speak
4. Muscle strength
5. Involuntary movements
6. Any abnormal posturing

GLASGOW COMA SCALE

One way to standardize observations of patients is the Glasgow Coma Scale. It was developed in 1974 and consists of assessment of three parts of the neurologic assessment. These include the following:

1. Eye opening
2. Best motor response
3. Best verbal response

37-4

Glasgow Coma Scale

	Stimuli	**Score**
Eyes open	Spontaneously	4
	To speech	3
	To pain	2
	None	1
Best verbal response	Oriented	5
	Confused	4
	Inappropriate words	3
	Incomprehensible	2
	None	1
Best motor response	Obeys commands	5
	Localizes to pain	4
	Flexes to pain	3
	Extends arm to pain	2
	None	1

The stronger the stimulus needed to obtain a response, the lower the score assigned to the part (see Box 37-4). The number value assigned to each parameter is added to yield an objective score. The score for normal persons who are not neurologically impaired is 14. The lowest possible score is 3. Any score of 7 or less is commonly accepted as a definition of coma (Fig. 37-23).

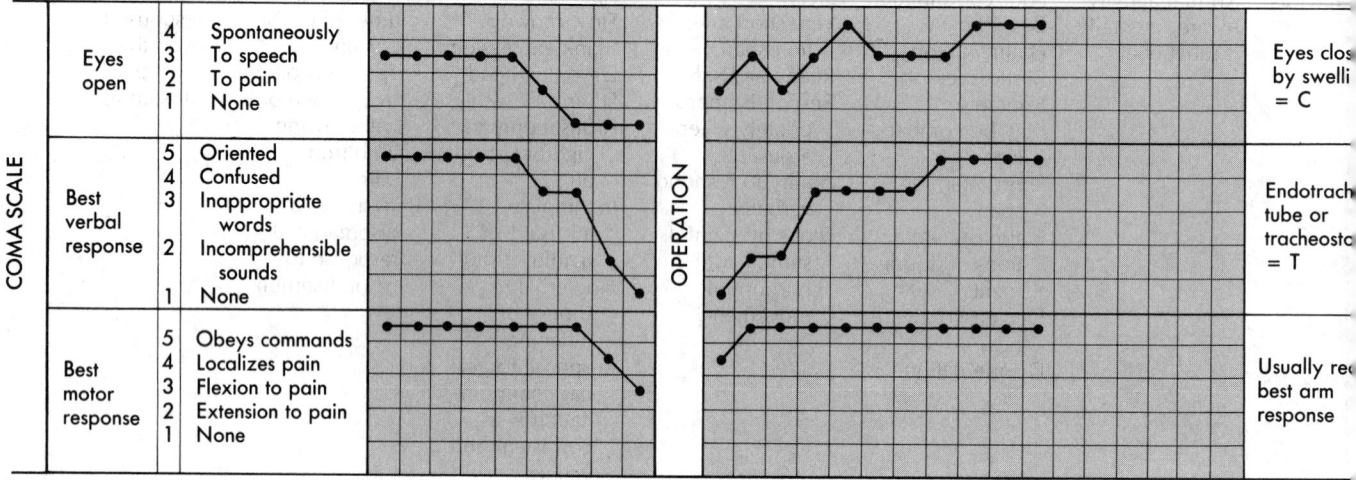

Fig. 37-23   Glasgow Coma Scale, demonstrating measurement of level of consciousness. Notice change in patient's condition just before and after surgery.

37-5

Levels of cognitive functioning
(Rancho Los Amigos Scale)

I.   **No response**
     Patient is completely unresponsive to any stimuli.

II. **Generalized response**
     Patient reacts inconsistently and nonpurposefully to stimuli in nonspecifc manner.

III. **Localized response**
     Patient reacts specifically but inconsistently to stimuli.

IV. **Confused—agitated**
     Patient is in heightened state of activity with severely decreased ability to process information.

V.   **Confused—inappropriate**
     Patient appears alert and is able to respond to simple commands fairly consistently.

VI. **Confused—appropriate**
     Patient shows goal-directed behavior, but depends on external input for direction.

VII. **Automatic—appropriate**
     Patient appears appropriate and oriented within hospital and home setting, goes through daily routine automatically, with minimal to absent confusion and has shallow recall of actions.

VIII. **Purposeful—appropriate**
     Patient is alert and oriented, is able to recall and integrate past and recent events, and is aware of and responsive to culture.[100]

RANCHO LOS AMIGOS SCALE

Another scale that has been developed is the Rancho Los Amigos Levels of Cognitive Functioning.[100] It was developed as a behavioral rating scale to aid in assessment and treatment of the head-injured person. It represents the progression of recovery of cognitive abilities as demonstrated through behavioral change. The tool is used to assess the patient and to give some structure to interventions. See Box 37-5 for the levels of cognitive functioning.

In this tool, eight levels of cognitive functioning are grouped in four basic recovery phases. These include the following:

Level	Recovery phase
II, III	Decreased response
IV	Agitated response
V, VI	Confused response
VII, VIII	Autonomic response

HEADACHE

Headache is a common symptom experienced by many patients. It can result from many pathologic processes, and its significance also is variable. *The source of recurring headache should be determined through careful physical examination with appropriate neurologic assessment.* Persons have been known to self-treat headaches for months, believing them to be nothing to worry about, only to learn later that the pain was caused by a more serious problem such as a brain tumor. Because of the site of some tumors in the brain, headache may be the only symptom for many months.

Pathophysiology

Headache may have many causes. Some of these are as follows:

1. Expanding brain masses such as neoplasms
2. Intracranial bleeding
3. Inflammation of the meninges as in meningitis
4. Other infections of the brain and spinal cord
5. Head trauma
6. Cerebral hypoxia
7. Dilation of the cerebral blood vessels
8. Psychologic factors such as stress
9. Systemic disease including eye, ear, and sinus problems
10. Allergies

The exact pathophysiology of head pain is not known. Although the skull and brain tissues are not capable of sensory pain, pain arises from the scalp and its blood vessels and muscles, from the dura mater and its venous sinuses, from the blood vessels at the base of the brain, and from some cervical cranial nerves. Blood vessels dilate and become congested with blood. Headaches are divided into the following three categories:

1. Vascular
   a. Migraine
   b. Cluster
   c. Hypertensive
2. Tension
   a. Psychogenic problems (tension or stress)
   b. Medical problems (cervical arthritis)
3. Traction-inflammatory
   a. Infection
   b. Intracranial or extracranial
   c. Occlusive vascular structures
   d. Arteritis

Efforts have been made to make the classification of headache more meaningful for the neuroscience nurse.[84] See Table 37-5 for details about and comparison of three specific types of headache.

Table 37-5   Comparison of migraine, cluster, and tension headaches

Type	Onset	Frequency	Duration	Nature	Prodromal symptoms/associated symptoms	Treatment
Migraine headaches	Occur at any age. Strongly hereditary. More common in women than men	Episodic, tend to occur with stress or life crisis. May occur with menstruation	Hours to days	Occur slowly; pain becomes severe, with one side of head affected more than other	Prodromal: visual field defects, confusion, paresthesias. Associated: nausea, vomiting, chills, fatigue, irritability, sweating, edema	Ergotamine tartrate. Methysergide maleate. Inderal. Nonnarcotic analgesics. Relaxation techniques. Application of heat or cold. Avoidance of dietary tyramine, nitrate, and gluconate
Cluster headaches	Early adulthood; precipitated by alcohol or nitrates. More common in men	Episodes clustered together in quick succession for few days or weeks with remissions that last for months	Few minutes to few hours	Pain intense: throbbing, deep, often unilateral; begin in infraorbital region and spread to head and neck	Prodromal: uncommon. Associated: flushing, tearing of eyes, nasal stuffiness, sweating swelling of temporal vessels	Narcotic analgesics during acute phase, often intramuscularly
Tension headaches (muscle contraction)	Often in adolescence; related to tension or anxiety. No family history	Episodic; vary with stress	Variable, can be constant	Dull, constant, uncommon aggravating pain, vary in intensity; usually bilateral and involve neck and shoulders; pain may be poorly defined	Prodromal: uncommon. Associated: sustained contraction of head and neck muscles	Nonnarcotic analgesics. Relaxation techniques. Amitriptyline (Elavil)

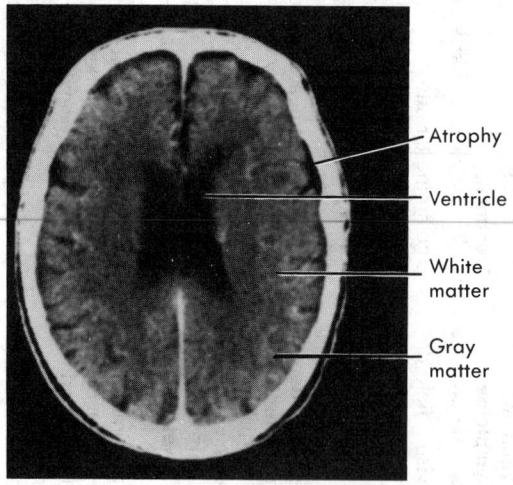

Fig. 37-24 CT scan printouts. CT brain scan differentiates between gray and white brain matter. (From Ballinger PW: *Merrill's atlas of radiographic positions and radiologic procedures,* ed 7, St Louis, 1991, Mosby–Year Book.)

Nursing Process
Assessment

Both subjective and objective data are important in determining more about the cause and nature of the headache.

Subjective data

1. Patient's understanding of headache and possible causes
2. Awareness of any precipitating factors such as stress
3. Measures that relieve symptoms, including medications
4. Location, frequency, pattern, and character of head pain, including site of return, time of day, and intervals between headaches
5. Initial onset of headache
6. Presence of any prodromal symptoms
7. Presence of associated symptoms
8. Family history of headaches (especially important with migraine)
9. Situations that make headache worse
10. Presence of allergies

Objective data

1. Behavior: signs indicating stress or anxiety or pain
2. Change in ability to carry on daily activities
3. Abnormalities on physical assessment part of neurologic examination
4. Temperature
5. Sinus drainage

Information about the patient's understanding of the nature and precipitating factors is helpful for planning necessary teaching. It is not unusual for the patient to manifest little objective data in the presence of subjective complaints.

Headache pain may be made worse by stress or tension. Knowledge of the patient's perception of the effect of stress on the symptoms is important in planning for measures that relieve or reduce effects of stress.

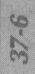

Computed tomography (EMI, CT, or CAT scan)

Purpose

Detection of cerebral and spinal cord pathology using a technique of scanning without radioisotopes

Preparation of patient

1. No special physical preparation
2. Patient teaching
   a. Explain procedure
   b. Time: Approximately 20 to 30 minutes for CT scan without contrast medium; 60 minutes if scans with and without contrast medium are done
   c. Sensation: Procedure is painless, except for slight discomfort when IV is started for injection of contrast medium. Also, there is some discomfort in lying still and possible feelings of claustrophobia as a result of head being positioned in head holder
   d. Patient must maintain motionless position until scan is completed

If contrast medium is used, history of allergy to iodine (seafood) is determined before medium is given

Procedure

1. Patient lies supine with the head positioned within a rubber head holder to prevent air gaps between the machine and scalp.
2. Head is scanned in two planes simultaneously and at various angles. Each image is a specific layer of brain tissue.
3. The computer calculates tissue absorption in contiguous layers of brain tissue and diplays a printout. Selected photographs of the printouts are taken.
4. Tumor densities are compared with the normal brain tissue. (Tumors, infarctions, bone displacement, and the ventricles are well visualized.)
5. If a contrast study is desired, the patient receives the contrast medium and the scanning process is repeated.

After procedure

1. No adverse effects except the risk of transient increased intracranial pressure in patients with masses or other brain pathology.
2. Plan period of rest as needed for the patient.

Migraine headaches are unusual in that there are *prodromal signs* and *symptoms* that occur before the acute attack. These may include the following:

1. Visual field defects
2. Confusion
3. Paresthesias
4. Paralysis in rare cases

During the actual attack, signs and symptoms may include nausea, vomiting, sensitivity to light, chilliness, fatigue, irritability, sweating, edema, and other autonomic signs.

Magnetic resonance imaging (MRI)

Purpose
Detection of cerebral and spinal cord pathology using a technique of scanning using magnetic forces to image body structures

Preparation of patient
1. No special physical preparation
2. Patient teaching
   a. Explain procedure
   b. Time: approximately 45 to 60 minutes
   c. Sensation: Procedure is painless, except for discomfort in lying still and possible feelings of claustrophobia as a result of head being positioned in head holder
   d. Patient must maintain motionless position until scan is completed
   e. Machine makes different noises during procedure that could startle patient
   f. Because scan involves a magnetic force, patient should remove all credit cards, watches, or other metal from clothing before entering scan room
3. Patient should be questioned about presence of metal in body (orthopedic appliances, aneurysm clips, pacemakers)

Procedure
1. Patient lies supine with the head positioned in a head holder.
2. Machine slowly scans parts of the brain or spinal cord. Images appear on a monitoring screen.
3. Magnetic field is used to measure the activity of the tissues.

After procedure
1. No adverse effects

Positron emission tomography (PET scan)

Purpose
Detection of cerebral and spinal cord pathology using radioactive fluorine

Preparation of patient
1. No special physical preparation
2. Patient teaching
   a. Explain procedure
   b. Time: Approximately 45 minutes
   c. Sensation: Procedure is painless, except for slight discomfort when fluorine is injected; also, there is some discomfort in lying still
   d. Patient must remain motionless until the scan is completed

Procedure
1. Patient is injected with or inhales radioactive fluorine
2. Patient lies supine with head immobilized
3. Head is scanned
4. A color composite picture is obtained. Various shades of colors indicates level of glucose metabolism

After procedure
1. No adverse effects
2. Patient may need period of rest

In assessing headache several key points are considered. These include the following:

1. Localized type of head pain is usually associated with migraine headaches or an organic disorder.
2. Generalized headache is usually related to psychologic causes or the presence of increased intracranial pressure.
3. Migraine headaches may change from one side of the head to the other but affect only one side of head at one time.
4. Headaches that occur with increased intracranial pressure usually are present on awakening and may awaken the person from sleep.
5. Sinus headaches typically occur early in the morning and increase in intensity as the day progresses.
6. Many headaches are related to stress.
7. Pain described as dull, nagging, aggravating, and ever present often occurs with psychogenic headaches.
8. Organically caused pain tends to be constant and progressive in nature.
9. Migraine headaches may be associated with menstruation.
10. Headaches may be precipitated by eating foods containing monosodium glutamate, sodium nitrate, or tyramine, as well as by alcohol.
11. A family history of headache is important, especially with migraine headaches.
12. Sleeping too long, fasting, or inhaling toxic fumes in work situations with inadequate ventilation can cause headaches.
13. Oral contraceptives may make migraine headaches worse.
14. Any secondary gains that patients receive from headaches must be assessed.

Diagnostic tests

It is important to evaluate headaches that are not slight and transient. Usual testing includes a neurologic examination, including a CT scan. The CT or EMI scan is becoming more available as a way to easily and safely detect abnormalities in the CNS (Fig. 37-24). It has replaced many invasive and painful procedures that neurologic patients previously were subjected to during a diagnostic workup. See Box 37-6.

The MRI scan may also be performed.[69] See Box 37-7 for information. Another scan that is similar to the CT and the MRI is the PET (positron emission tomography) scan (see Box 37-8). In this scan the patient receives an injection of deoxyglucose with radioactive fluorine. The head is scanned and a color composite picture is obtained. Various shades of colors indicate levels of glucose metabolism.

A lumbar puncture may also be performed. A lumbar puncture is not done, however, if there is evidence of increased intracranial pressure or if a brain tumor is sus-

Lumbar puncture

Purpose
To obtain cerebrospinal fluid (CSF) for examination or relief of pressure.

Preparation of patient
1. Usually a permit is signed by patient or family member.
2. Occasionally sedation is given before procedure.
3. Patient teaching
   a. Explain procedure
   b. Time: approximately 10 to 15 minutes
   c. Sensation: slight pain and pressure may be felt as the dura is entered. A sharp shooting pain down one leg may be felt, caused by the needle coming close to a nerve.
   d. Other: Remind patient to lie still and not to move suddenly.

Procedure
1. Patient is usually positioned on the side with both knees and head flexed at an acute angle to allow maximum lumbar flexion and separation of interspinous spaces. Occasionally patients may be positioned sitting up and leaning over the bedside table.
2. Local anesthetic is usually used to anesthetize the lumbar area.
3. Under strict aseptic technique the needle is inserted below the level of the spinal cord at the L4-L5 or L5-S1 interspace (Fig. 37-24).
4. Inner needle is removed to allow drainage and measurement of spinal fluid.
5. Level of fluid column in manometer used to measure pressure is read.
6. Fluid is collected for various tests or to relieve pressure. Occasionally the first specimen of spinal fluid contains blood from slight bleeding at the site of puncture. This specimen should not be sent for cell count.
7. *Queckenstedt's test* may be performed to test for subarachnoid block. The jugular veins are compressed for 10 seconds, first on one side, then on the other side, and then on both sides at the same time. Any change in spinal fluid pressure during the compression is noted.
8. Needle is withdrawn.

After procedure
1. Patient lies flat in bed for several hours. Caution patient not to lift head.
2. Site of puncture should be observed for any leakage of CSF.
3. Headache is fairly common and is thought to be caused by the loss of spinal fluid through the dura mater. The sharpness and size of the needle, the skill of the physician, whether the patient lies flat, and the patient's emotional state may determine whether a headache occurs.
4. Headaches are usually treated with bed rest, analgesics, and ice applied to the head.

Cisternal puncture

Purpose
To obtain CSF for examination, or for instillation of contrast medium for diagnostic studies

Preparation of patient
1. Usually a permit for surgery is signed.
2. Back of patient's neck may be shaved.
3. Procedure is performed in the patient's bed or in treatment room.
4. Patient is positioned in a side-lying position at the edge of the bed or treatment table with the head bent forward.
5. Patient teaching
   a. Same as for lumbar puncture.
   b. Procedure may be more frightening to the patient because of the close proximity of the procedure to the brain.

Procedure
1. Same as for lumbar puncture except for different site (between C1 and base of skull).
2. Head of patient should be held firmly during procedure so it does not rotate.

After procedure
1. Patient observed immediately for dyspnea, apnea, or cyanosis.
2. Headache occurs less frequently than with lumbar puncture.

pected, because the quick reduction in pressure produced by removal of the spinal fluid may cause brain herniation. In this situation a CT scan must be done first. Box 37-9 outlines the procedure for lumbar puncture (see Fig. 37-25).

At times, because of anatomic abnormalities or other causes, a lumbar puncture may not be possible. At these times a cisternal puncture may be attempted. The cisternal puncture is made between the first cervical vertebra and the base of the skull (Fig. 37-26) (see Box 37-10).

Other tests that may be done include a brain scan (Fig. 37-27) and plain skull films (see Box 37-11 for preparation for brain scan).

The skull x-ray films will demonstrate bony abnormality as well as congenital changes, but will not yield the information that more sophisticated procedures do.

Data analysis: nursing diagnoses

Nursing diagnoses are determined from analysis of patient data. Possible nursing diagnoses for the person with headache may include, but are not limited to, the following:

Diagnostic title	Possible etiologies
Sleep pattern disturbance	Pain/discomfort, anxiety
Anxiety	Threat/change in health status/role functioning/situational/maturational crisis
Pain	Headache
Coping, ineffective individual	Situational crises

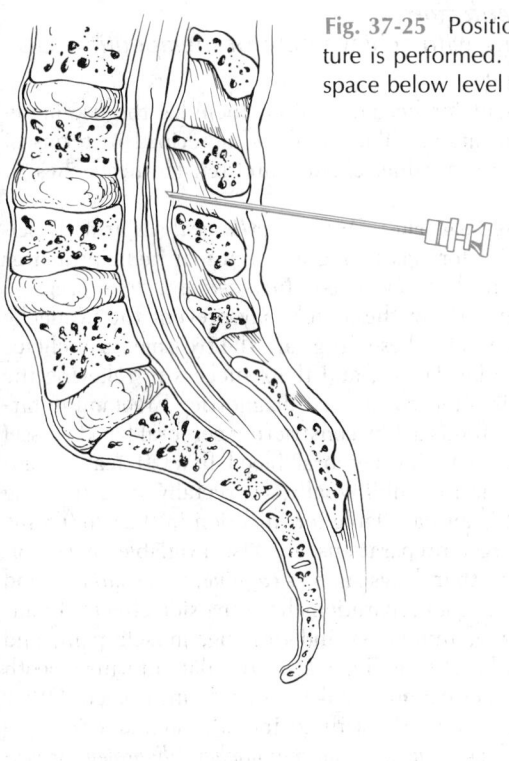

Fig. 37-25   Position and angle of needle when lumbar puncture is performed. Note that needle is in fourth lumbar interspace below level of spinal cord.

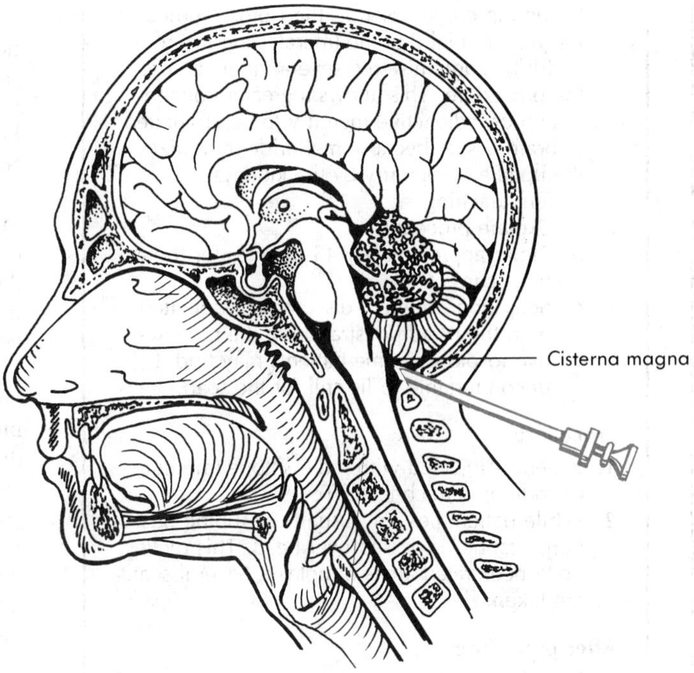

Cisterna magna

Fig. 37-26   Cisternal puncture. Position of needle when cisternal puncture is performed. Note needle length and short bevel.

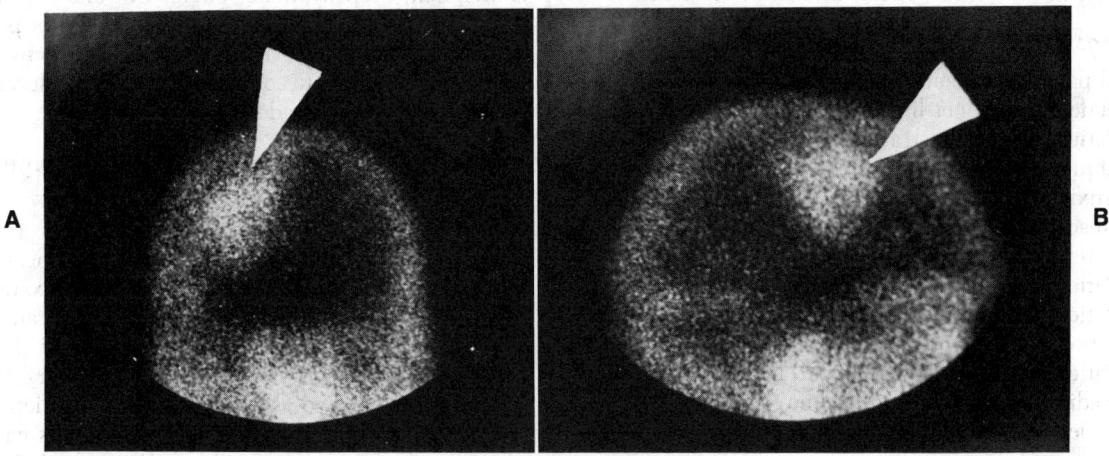

A   B

Fig. 37-27   Brain scans. **A,** Anteroposterior view. **B,** Lateral view. White pointers indicate tumor seen in both views. (From Pagana KD, Pagana TJ: *Diagnostic testing and nursing implications: a case study approach,* ed 3, St Louis, 1990, Mosby–Year Book.)

37-11

Brain scan

Purpose
Detection of cerebral pathology using radioactive isotopes and a scanner

Preparation of patient
1. No physical preparation of patient
2. When mercury is used as the isotope indicator, a mercurial diuretic (meralluride [Mercuhydrin]) is administered several hours before the procedure. This allows a greater concentration of radioactive mercury to be circulated to brain tissue, because melluride minimizes the uptake of mercury by the kidneys.
3. Patient teaching
   a. Explain procedure.
   b. Time: approximately 45 minutes for the actual scan
   c. Sensation: minimal discomfort associated with the IV administration of the radioactive iosotope. Some patients may find it uncomfortable to lie still for the scan.

Procedure
1. Patient is injected with radioisotope (mercury or sodium pertechnetate Tc 99m)
2. While patient lies still, usually in supine position, scanner is passed over head. This picks up concentrated areas of uptake. Several scans are taken.

After procedure
1. No adverse effects.
2. Plan period of rest as needed for the patient.

Diagnostic title	Possible etiologies
Knowledge deficit	Lack of exposure, information misinterpretation, cognitive limitation
Self-care deficit	Pain/discomfort, depression

Planning: expected patient outcomes

Expected patient outcomes for the person with headache may include, but are not limited to, the following:

1. Patient can demonstrate prescribed relaxation techniques.
2. Anxiety is decreased.
3. Headache pain is decreased.
4. Patient can carry out ADL with minimal difficulty.
5. Patient demonstrates improved coping mechanisms.
6. Patient can explain prescribed medication (dosage, action, side effects, and frequency).
7. Patient can explain the importance of continuing medical supervision for chronic headache.
8. Patient can identify any factors that trigger headache.
9. Patient can explain the danger of continued use of over-the-counter drugs for chronic, recurring headache.
10. Patient is able to sleep at least 6 hours per night.

Implementation
Assisting with achievement of therapeutic goals
Medications

Treatment for headache often includes the use of selected medications. These will be described in terms of their use for migraine, cluster, and tension headaches.

Migraine headaches. *Acetylsalicylic acid* (aspirin) is seldom effective for classic migraine but may be helpful after the headache has developed. *Ergotamine tartrate* preparations taken early in the attack may prevent the headache from developing. These drugs are the treatments of choice in migraine headaches, and their success in relieving the headache is often considered diagnostic. Ergotamine tartrate preparations act by constricting cerebral blood vesssel walls, thus reducing cerebral blood flow. It may be administered orally, sublingually, or rectally in 2 to 4 mg dosages. It is also available for injection in 0.25 to 0.5 mg dosages. Ergot preparations are also available in combination with other drugs such as *caffeine, phenobarbital,* and *belladonna.* Ergot preparations have the side effects of nausea, vomiting, numbness and tingling, muscle pain, and changes in heart rate. They also stimulate uterine smooth muscle, so they cannot be taken by pregnant women. Other drugs that may be substituted include nonnarcotic analgesics, such as *phenacetin, acetaminophen, ibuprofen,* or *propoxyphene (Darvon),* as well as narcotics, such as *codeine. Propranolol hydrochloride (Inderal)* has been used to prevent migraine headaches with limited success. Methysergide maleate (Sansert) has been used in the prophylactic treatment of migraine and other vascular headaches.

Cluster headaches. Because the pain associated with cluster headaches is so severe, narcotic analgesics are often prescribed during the actue attack. Often these must be administered intramuscularly for optimal relief.

Patients with cluster headaches usually feel fine between attacks, so no analgesia is needed during these times.

Tension headaches. The nonnarcotic analgesics are often prescribed for tension headaches. These include acetaminophen, propoxyphene, phenactin, and acetylsalicylic acid. Narcotic analgesics such as codeine may be prescribed along with diazepam (Valium) for relief of tension. It is far better, however, to counsel the patient to develop other ways to relieve the headache.

Interventions to achieve patient outcomes
Promoting rest and relaxation

Because stress and emotional upsets may precipitate some headaches and make others worse, measures are taken to facilitate relaxation and rest. Relaxation techniques (Chapter 10), planned sleeping hours, and rest periods as needed may prove helpful. Because alcohol has been found to be significant in causing cluster headaches, it should not be used as a way to relieve tension.

Some patients who have tension headaches have found relaxation by regular physical exercise to be helpful.

Decreasing anxiety

Patients with chronic headaches may respond to psychotherapy. It may be used to help the patient develop awareness of stressors, as well as to deal with feelings about being the victim of headache pain.

Assisting with comfort and ADL

Other treatments that have been found to be helpful with headache include cold packs applied to the forehead or base of the brain. Pressure applied to the temporal and carotid arteries may be helpful depending on the cause of the headache. Patients who are having migraine headaches, especially, may be most comfortable lying in a dark room with minimal auditory stimulation.

Identifying triggering factors

Discovery of triggering factors associated with severe recurring headaches will need to be made through ongoing assessment of the person's personality, habits, and ADL. Clues may be obtained from seeking information about the person's goals and aspirations, work habits, family relationships, coping mechanisms, and relaxation patterns. The person may be asked to keep a diary of activities and the occurrence of headaches, as well as the nature of the headaches and how they were treated.

Triggering factors may include the following:
1. Fatigue
2. Alcohol
3. Stress
4. Climatic changes
5. Hunger
6. Menstruation
7. Allergies

Facilitating learning

Teaching is an important part of nursing care of the patient with head pain. Box 37-12 lists appropriate teaching activities.

It may be helpful to educate the patient about foods that may cause headaches or make them worse. These include those containing tyramine, nitrates, or glutamate. For example, monosodium glutamate (MSG) is often used in Chinese cooking. Other foods that may provoke headaches are included in the following list:
1. Vinegar
2. Chocolate
3. Yogurt
4. Alcohol
5. Fermented or marinated foods
6. Ripened cheese
7. Herring
8. Cured sandwich meats
9. Excessive caffeine
10. Pork

Evaluation

Evaluation of headaches is based on the expected patient outcomes and should be done in conjunction with the patient. Questions to consider may include the following:
1. Is the patient able to sleep?
2. Has the patient's anxiety decreased?
3. Is pain decreased?
4. Is the patient functioning optimally?
5. Does the patient demonstrate improved coping mechanisms?

Patient Teaching **37-12**

The patient with headache

1. Avoid factors found to trigger or increase headache.
2. Use relaxation measures (such as biofeedback) when emotional tension is present.
3. Maintain regular sleep patterns.
4. Take medications as ordered—be aware of their side effects and report these to physician.
5. Follow up with medical care as indicated.
6. Allow others to assist with activities during headaches.
7. Structure home and work environment to keep stressors at a reasonable level.

---

6. Is the use of medication within medical guidelines?
7. Is the patient following medical advice?
8. Is the patient keeping follow-up appointments?

NEUROLOGIC PAIN

Pathophysiology

Neurologic pain other than headache is commonly seen in nursing. It is sometimes difficult to distinguish between pain produced by lesions within the nervous system that cause objective sensory abnormalities and peripherally produced, somatic pain in a distant organ (see Box 37-13). Although in practice pain may be viewed from the standpoint of neural transmission, the transmission of pain impulses is not fully understood. Neurologic pain may arise from lesions involving peripheral cutaneous nerves, the sensory nerve roots, the thalamus, and the central pain tract (spinothalamic) at some level (Fig. 37-28). Pain receptors are not adaptable. Pain impulses continue at the same rate as long as the stimulus is present. They are specific for pain only. Pain receptors can be activated by the following:
1. Cellular damage
2. Certain chemicals such as histamine
3. Heat
4. Ischemia
5. Muscle spasms
6. Sensations of heat, cold, and itching that go beyond a specific level of intensity

Pain that is described as unbearable and does not respond to treatment is classified as *intractable*. It is chronic and often disabling.

Nursing Process
Assessment

Both subjective and objective data are important to assess in the patient with neurologic pain. Again, it should be remembered that pain is highly subjective, and there may not be a great deal of objective data to accompany the subjective complaints.

37-13

Site of problem and resulting neurologic pain

Site of problem	Results	Characteristics of pain
Peripheral cutaneous nerves	Pain usually limited to anatomic area supplied by affected nerve or nerves	Often described as burning sensation, but can be described as sharp or dull and aching
		Pain may be constant or permanent
		Often described as severe
		Also called local pain
Root pain	Limited to dermatomes supplied by affected sensory nerve roots (pain from lesion arising from deep somatic and visceral stimulus may radiate beyond dermatomes) (Fig. 37-8)	Aggravated by anything that causes direct or indirect movement of spinal cord (sneezing, coughing, or straining)
Central lesion within thalamus	Pain confined to contralateral side of body	Pain described as burning, pulling, and swelling
		Often aggravated by emotional stress and fatigue
		Influenced by cutaneous stimulation
Central spinothalamic tract	Pain sensation distributed to level of tract involved	May be similar to thalamic pain, but less disturbing
	Hemisection of spinal cord produces loss of pain and temperature sensation on contralateral side at a level one or two segments below injury	

37-14

Types of pain sensation

Paresthesia	Abnormal sensation
Hyperalgesia	Increased pain sensation
Hypoalgesia	Decreased pain sensation
Analgesia	Blocked pain sensation
Dysesthesia	Pain sensation caused by stimulus that normally would not be painful
Referred pain	Pain that occurs in a site other than its origin
Causalgia	Intense, continuous, burning pain
Local pain	Occurring as a result of direct stimulation of pain receptors

Subjective data

1. Patient's understanding of the pain
2. Any precipitating factors
3. Measures that relieve symptoms, including medication
4. Site, frequency, and nature of pain
5. Usual coping patterns when under stress
6. Presence of associated symptoms
7. Measures that make pain worse

Objective data

1. Behavior: signs indicating pain or stress
2. Change in ability to carry out ADL
3. Muscle weakness or wasting
4. Vasomotor responses (flushing, for example)
5. Spinal reflexes and sensory examination

The quality of pain and its distribution are important factors to assess. Pain may vary from mild to excruciating. Terms with which the nurse should be familiar include those listed in Box 37-14.

As stated earlier, neurologic pain may arise from lesions involving peripheral cutaneous nerves, the sensory nerve roots (posterior), the thalamus, and the central pain tract. Each of these sources produces characteristic pain.

Diagnostic tests

It is extremely difficult to evaluate pain objectively. Electrical stimulation may be attempted to define the pain to a greater extent. The person with intractable pain may undergo psychologic testing as part of the workup. Tests to rule out causes of the pain may be indicated, including the myelogram (see Box 37-15). This is commonly done when back pain is present (Fig. 37-29).

Data analysis: nursing diagnoses

Nursing diagnoses are determined from analysis of patient data. Possible nursing diagnoses for the person with neurologic pain may include, but are not limited to, the following:

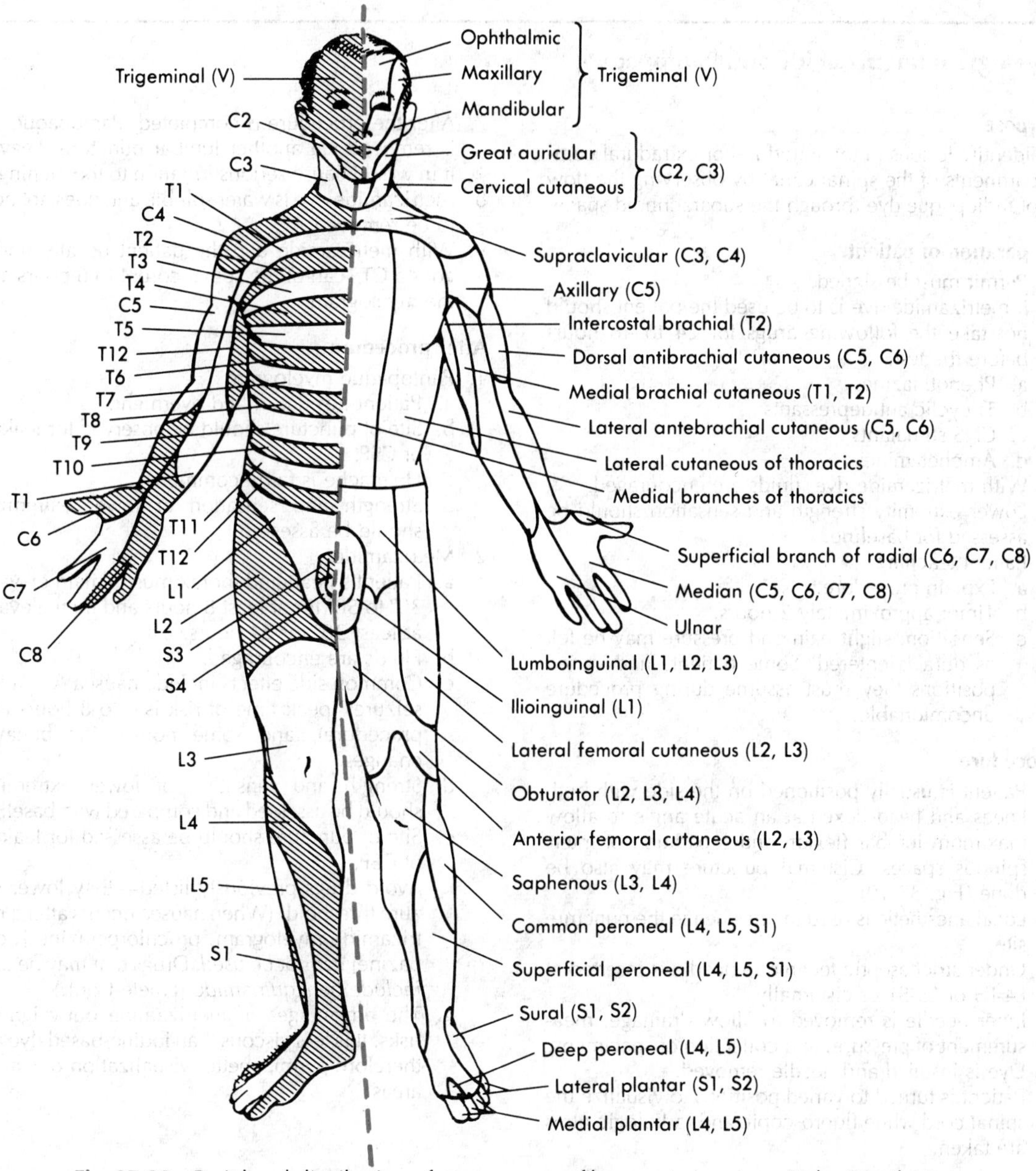

Trigeminal (V)

Ophthalmic
Maxillary } Trigeminal (V)
Mandibular

C2

C3

Great auricular
Cervical cutaneous } (C2, C3)

T1
C4
T2
T3
T4
C5
T5
T12
T6
T7
T8
T9
T10

Supraclavicular (C3, C4)

Axillary (C5)

Intercostal brachial (T2)

Dorsal antibrachial cutaneous (C5, C6)

Medial brachial cutaneous (T1, T2)

Lateral antebrachial cutaneous (C5, C6)

Lateral cutaneous of thoracics

Medial branches of thoracics

T1
C6

T11
T12

Superficial branch of radial (C6, C7, C8)

Median (C5, C6, C7, C8)

Ulnar

C7

C8

L1
L2
S3
S4

Lumboinguinal (L1, L2, L3)

Ilioinguinal (L1)

L3

Lateral femoral cutaneous (L2, L3)

Obturator (L2, L3, L4)

L4

Anterior femoral cutaneous (L2, L3)

Saphenous (L3, L4)

L5

Common peroneal (L4, L5, S1)

Superficial peroneal (L4, L5, S1)

S1

Sural (S1, S2)

Deep peroneal (L4, L5)

Lateral plantar (S1, S2)

Medial plantar (L4, L5)

Fig. 37-28 Peripheral distribution of sensory nerve fibers, anterior view. *Right,* Distribution of cutaneous nerves. *Left,* Dermatomes *(shaded areas)* and segmental distribution of cutaneous nerves.

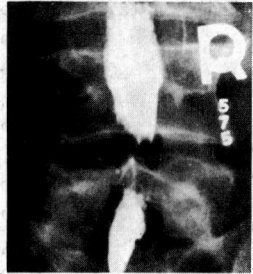

Fig. 37-29 Myelogram showing almost complete block in interspace between fourth and fifth lumbar vertebrae. (From Moseley HF, editor: *Textbook of surgery,* ed 3, St Louis, 1959, Mosby–Year Book.)

37-15

Myelogram (metrizamide and Pantopaque)

Purpose

To identify lesions in the intradural or extradural compartments of the spinal canal by observing the flow of radiopaque dye through the subarachnoid space.

Preparation of patient

1. Permit must be signed.
2. If metrizamide dye is to be used the patient should not take the following drugs for 24 to 48 hours before the test:
   a. Phenothiazines
   b. Tricyclic antidepressants
   c. CNS stimulants
   d. Amphetamines
3. With metrizamide dye, fluids are encouraged.
4. Lower extremity strength and sensation should be assessed for baseline.
5. Patient teaching
   a. Explain procedure.
   b. Time: approximately 2 hours.
   c. Sensation: slight pain and pressure may be felt as dura is entered. Some patients find varied positions they must assume during procedure uncomfortable.

Procedure

1. Patient is usually positioned on the side with both knees and head flexed at an acute angle to allow maximum lumbar flexion and separation of interspinous spaces. Cisternal puncture may also be done (Fig. 37-10).
2. Local anesthetic is used to anesthetize the puncture site.
3. Under strict aseptic technique needle is inserted at L4-L5 or L5-S1 or cisternally.
4. Inner needle is removed to allow drainage, measurement of pressure, and collection of specimens.
5. Dye is instilled and needle removed.
6. Patient is turned to varied positions to visualize the spinal cord while fluoroscopic and radiologic films are taken.

7. After the procedure is completed, Pantopaque dye is removed via another lumbar puncture. Leaving it in would cause serious irritation to the meninges.
8. Metrizamide dye is water soluble and does not need to be removed.
9. With metrizamide dye the patient usually undergoes a CT scan of the spinal cord 4 to 6 hours after the myelogram.

After procedure

1. Pantopaque myelogram
   a. Patient lies flat in bed overnight.
   b. Site of puncture should be observed for leakage of CSF.
   c. Headache is fairly common.
   d. Strength and sensation of lower extremities should be assessed.
2. Metrizamide
   a. Patient's head and thorax must remain elevated 30° to 50° for at least 8 hours and then elevated at least 30° for 24 hours.
   b. Fluids are encouraged.
   c. Common side effects include nausea, vomiting, seizures (peak time of risk is 4 to 8 hours after procedure), and some nonspecific behavior changes.
   d. Strength and sensation of lower extremities should be assessed and compared with baseline.
   e. Site of puncture should be assessed for leakage of CSF.
   f. Avoid drugs previously listed—they lower seizure threshold. (When nausea occurs after a metrizamide myelogram, prochlorperazine [Compazine] *cannot be used*. Drugs that *may be used include benzquinamide* [Emete-Con].)
   g. The advantages of metrizamide outweigh the risks. It is less viscous than iodine-based dye and therefore permits better visualization of smaller areas.

Diagnostic title	Possible etiologies
Anxiety	Threat/change in health status
Coping, ineffective individual	Chronic physical/psychosocial disability
Sleep pattern disturbance	Pain/discomfort
Mobility, impaired physical	Pain/discomfort
Self-care deficit	Pain/discomfort
Knowledge deficit	Lack of exposure/recall, information misinterpretation

Planning: expected patient outcomes

Expected patient outcomes for the person with neurologic pain may include, but are not limited to, the following:

1. Patient demonstrates minimal anxiety.
2. Patient demonstrates improved coping mechanisms.
3. Patient demonstrates good management of sleep and rest patterns.
4. Patient explains the relationship between pain and emotional upsets.
5. Patient's pain is decreased.
6. Patient demonstrates physical methods including proper positioning that can be used for pain control.
7. Patient demonstrates minimal difficulty in carrying out ADL.
8. Patient has minimal restrictions in physical mobility.
9. Patient demonstrates ability to maintain home.

The patient with neurologic pain

1. Avoid factors that increase pain
2. Use relaxation measures such as biofeedback and meditation when emotional tension is present
3. Maintain regular rest and sleep pattern
4. Take medication as prescribed
5. Be aware of physical methods of controlling pain (such as positioning) and use them
6. Follow up with medical care as indicated
7. Structure home and work environment to keep stressors at a minimum

10. Patient states the plan for follow-up care.
11. Patient explains medications to be taken, including dosage, action, side effects, and frequency.

Implementation
Assisting with achievement of therapeutic goals
Medications

Treatment for patients with neurologic pain may include the use of medications. These often include the nonnarcotic analgesics—acetaminophen, propoxyphene (Darvon), phenacetin, ibuprofen and acetylsalicylic acid. Narcotic analgesics such as codeine may be prescribed along with diazepam (Valium) or amitriptyline hydrochloride (Elavil). The emphasis should be on helping the patient learn other measures to control pain.

Nonsurgical methods of pain relief

Neurologic pain has been found to respond to other methods of pain control. These include transcutaneous electrical nerve stimulators and spinal cord stimulators. Both use electrodes applied near the site of pain or on or around the spine. The goal is to modify the sensory input by blocking or changing the painful sensation with a stimulus that is perceived to be less painful or nonpainful.

Acupuncture has also been used to treat patients with neurologic pain. See Chapter 10 for a further explanation of these procedures.

Nerve block

A nerve block involves the injection of a substance such as a local anesthetic or alcohol or phenol close enough to a nerve to block the conduction of impulses. It is used to treat chronic pain that may result from trigeminal neuralgia, cancer, or peripheral vascular disease.

Surgery

In cases of intractable pain that does not respond to medical and nursing actions, surgery may be necessary to reduce or abolish pain. Neurosurgical procedures that may be done include the following:

1. Neurectomy—interruption of the peripheral or cranial nerve supplying a specific part of the body. The nerve fibers to the affected area are severed from the cord. Fibers controlling movement and position sense are also interrupted. Cannot be used to control pain in the lower extremities.

2. Rhizotomy—resection of a posterior nerve root just before it enters the spinal cord. Cannot be used with pain in the lower extremities because position sense is lost. Involves a laminectomy.

3. Cordotomy—pain pathways in spinothalamic tract (anterior and lateral aspect of the cord) on the side opposite the cord are severed. This results in a wide sense of analgesia, while other sensory and motor functions are preserved. In a percutaneous cordotomy, a spinal needle is inserted laterally between C1 and C2. A wire electrode is inserted into the lateral cord, and a lesion is made to destroy ascending pain fibers.

These procedures all have potential complications that must be considered before the decision is made to do surgery. For example, with cordotomy, the patient may expect to have problems with postural hypotension, temperature sensation, and possibly bladder and motor function. Also, patients may have a temporary paralysis or leg weakness and loss of bowel and bladder control that results from edema of the cord. Usually this disappears in several weeks.[104]

Interventions to achieve patient outcomes
Promoting rest and relaxation

As with headache, stress and emotional upsets may precipitate neurologic pain or make it worse. Rest and relaxation should be facilitated. Relaxation techniques, planned sleeping hours, and rest periods throughout the day may be helpful. Relaxation techniques used include biofeedback and meditation.

Some patients with pain, especially pain defined as intractable, may respond well to psychotherapy. It can help the patient develop awareness of stressors and how they influence the perception of pain.

Assisting with mobility and ADL

A patient having neurologic pain may be extremely uncomfortable. The nurse should help the patient attain a position of comfort. For example, the patient with root pain should avoid movements that cause direct or indirect movement of the spinal cord. Significant nursing activities include the following:

1. Patient should not lie in a horizontal plane for long periods, as this causes tension or traction on the thoracic and sacral nerve roots.
2. Sitting may help to relieve tension on the nerve roots.
3. When moving a person with root pain, sharp flexion of the neck and extension of the legs should be avoided as much as possible.
4. Straining during bowel movements can intensify pain—stool softeners are often indicated.

The identification of any triggering factors of neurologic pain is important. This can be done by a thorough assessment of personality, habits, and ADL. The person may be asked to keep a diary of ADL and the occurrence of the pain.

Facilitating learning

Teaching is an important part of nursing care for the patient with neurologic pain. Appropriate teaching activities are listed in Box 37-16.

Causes of increased intracranial pressure

Space-occupying lesions that increase tissue volume
Cerebral contusions
Hematomas
Infarctions
Abscesses
Intracranial tumors

Cerebrospinal problems
Increase in production of cerebrospinal fluid
Blockage in ventricular system
Decreased absorption of cerebrospinal fluid

Cerebral edema
Use of contrast dye that changes homeostasis of brain
Overhydration with hypotonic solution
Aftereffects of trauma to brain

Levels of consciousness

Alert	Responds appropriately to auditory, tactile, and visual stimuli
Loss of ability to abstract	Inattentiveness, slowed thinking, difficult to arouse
Confusion	Disorientation, inability to follow simple commands
Stupor	Responds to verbal commands with moaning or groaning, if at all
Semicomatose	Loss of ability to cooperate, responds only to pain—response may range from purposeful to decerebrate or decorticate
Comatose	Loss of ability to respond to any external stimuli and loss of all brain functions[16]

Evaluation

Evaluation of the patient with peripheral nerve or intractable neurologic pain considers how the person is functioning in spite of the pain. Questions to consider may include the following:

1. Is the patient showing little anxiety and good coping strategies?
2. Is the patient sleeping at least 6 hours a night?
3. Is the patient using physical methods to control the pain in a correct way?
4. Is the patient able to carry on normal ADL?
5. Is the patient's mobility improved?
6. Is the patient able to manage home maintenance activities?
7. Is the patient following up with appointments?
8. Is the use of medications within guidelines?
9. Is the patient cooperating with medical advice?
10. Is the patient's pain improved?

INCREASED INTRACRANIAL PRESSURE

Pathophysiology

Increased intracranial pressure is a complex manifestation that is the consequence of multiple neurologic conditions. It often occurs suddenly and requires surgical intervention.

The contents of the skull, or cranial contents, are brain tissue, vascular tissue, and cerebrospinal fluid. The brain makes up 80% of the intracranial content, blood volume makes up 10% and the cerebrospinal fluid makes up the remaining 10%. Any increase in the volume of one of the cranial contents results in increased intracranial pressure, because the cranial vault is rigid, closed, and nonexpandable. Specific causes of increased intracranial pressure are listed in Box 37-17.

An increase in any one of the cranial contents is usually accompanied by a reciprocal change in the volume of one of the others. Brain tissue cannot expand without serious effects in the flow and amount of cerebrospinal fluid and cerebral circulation. Space-occupying lesions displace and distort the brain and vascular tissues as pressure increases. The buildup of pressure may occur slowly (days or weeks) or rapidly, depending on the cause. At first, one hemisphere of the brain will be more involved, but eventually both hemispheres will be affected.

As the pressure increases within the cranial cavity, it is at first compensated for by venous compression and cerebrospinal displacement. As the pressure continues to rise, the cerebral blood flow decreases and inadequate perfusion occurs. This inadequate perfusion initiates a vicious circle causing the P_{CO_2} to increase and the P_{O_2} and the pH to fall. These cause vasodilation and cerebral edema. The edema further increases the intracranial pressure, causing increased compression of neural tissue and an even greater increase in intracranial pressure.

When the pressure exceeds the brain's ability to compensate, pressure is exerted on surrounding structures where the pressure is lower. This movement of pressure is called *supratentorial shift* and can result in two kinds of herniation. *Central* or *transtentorial herniation* is the downward displacement of the cerebral hemispheres through the tentorial notch. This compresses the diencephalon and brainstem. The other type of herniation is called *uncal herniation* and occurs when expanding masses in the middle fossa or temporal lobe shift over the lateral edge of the tentorium, pushing the uncus toward the midline. As a result of herniation, the brainstem is compressed at variable levels, which in turn compresses the vasomotor center, the posterior cerebral artery, the oculomotor nerve, the corticospinal nerve pathway, and the fibers of the ascending reticular activating system (Fig. 37-30). The life-sustaining mechanisms of consciousness, blood pressure, pulse, respiration, and temperature regulation fail.

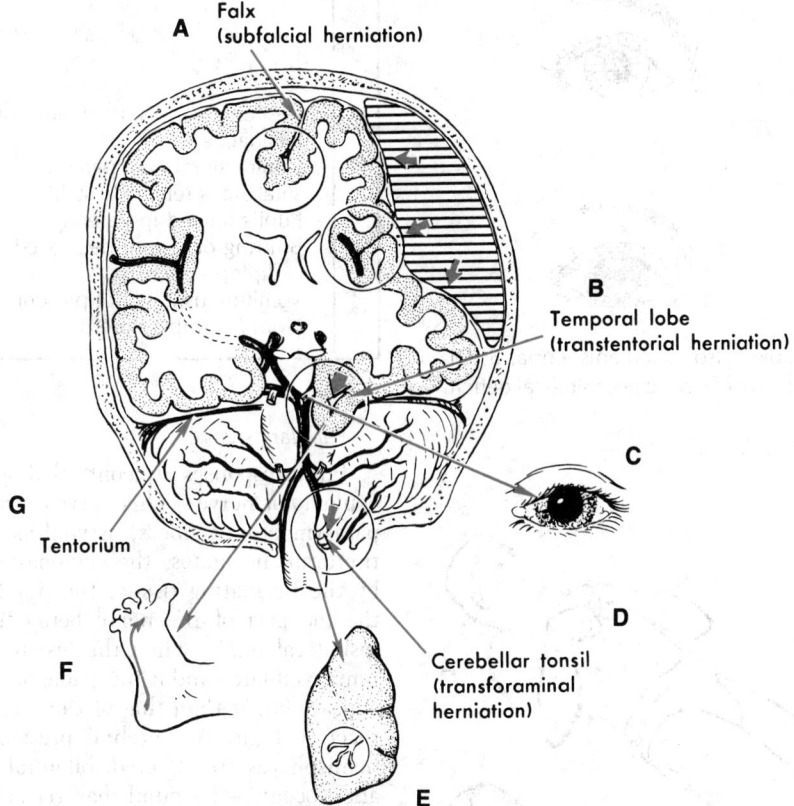

Fig. 37-30 Consequences of increased intracranial pressure. Expanding temporoparietal epidural hematoma with medial and downward pressure has produced subfalcial, transtentorial, and transforaminal internal herniations. Note distortion of falx, *A*, bulging of medial temporal lobe at tentorial edge, *B*, and herniation of cerebellar tonsil with descending pressure on brainstem, *D*. Also note how major blood vessels are collapsed in encircled areas. Some consequential effects of continuing and/or expanding pressure on neural structure with alterations in body functions are detailed: *C*, homolateral dilation and fixation of pupil with ptosis of eyelid; *E*, life-threatening respiratory arrest through indirect effects on respiratory centers in brainstem; *F*, contralateral Babinski sign showing extension of view of brainstem.) (Modified from an original painting by Frank H Netter, MD; from Clinical symposia. Copyright by Ciba Pharmaceutical Co, Division of Ciba-Geigy Corp, Summit, NJ. All rights reserved.)

Nursing Process
Assessment
Subjective data

1. Patient's understanding of condition
2. Presence of visual changes: diplopia or blurred vision
3. Ability to think
4. Presence of pain, especially headache
5. Ability to carry on daily activities
6. Presence of nausea

Objective data

1. Level of consciousness
2. Pupillary signs
3. Vital signs
4. Focal motor or sensory signs
5. Presence of vomiting or hiccuping
6. Eye changes including papilledema
7. Speech patterns

The detection of increased intracranial pressure must occur early when it is still reversible and before the stage of decompensation. The ability to make accurate observations, to interpret observations intelligently, and to record observations carefully is the most important part of nursing care for patients with increased intracranial pressure.

Level of consciousness

A decreasing level of consciousness is an early sign of increased intracranial pressure. *Any change in the level of consciousness is one of the most important observations for the nurse to make, report, and record.* Restlessness, disorientation, and lethargy may be the first signs seen.

The observations are recorded in terms of *behaviors* and *symptoms* and not in terms of labels. Flow sheets that document neurologic changes in an objective way are helpful, especially when frequent neurologic checks are being done.

The Glasgow Coma Scale is another way to document the neurologic patient's condition.[98] See p. 1207 for a description of this tool. A description of levels of consciousness is presented in Box 37-18.

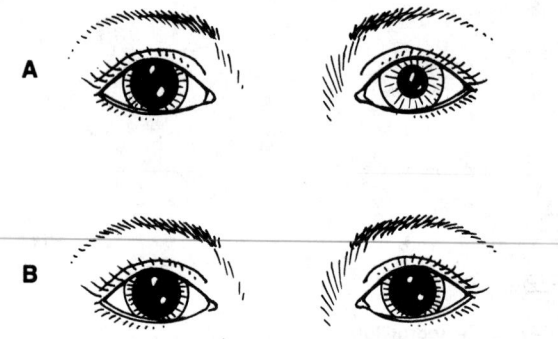

Fig. 37-31 **A,** Unequal pupils, also called anisocoria. **B,** Dilated and fixed pupils, indicative of severe neurological deficit.

37-19	**Classic signs of early increased intracranial pressure**
	Restlessness, disorientation, or lethargy
	Headache
	Contralateral hemiparesis
	Vital signs relatively stable
	Pupils dilated ipsilaterally
	Blurring of vision, decreased visual acuity, or diplopia
	Vomiting usually not present
	Normal temperature

Pupillary signs

Pupil responses are controlled by cranial nerve III (the oculomotor nerve). This nerve carries sensory, motor, and parasympathetic fibers, as well as sympathetic fibers. As the brain herniates, the oculomotor nerve is compressed by the herniating tissue, the pupilloconstrictor fibers in the top part of the nerve being the first affected. The ipsilateral pupil (when the lesion is in one hemisphere remains dilated and is incapable of constricting. The pupil appears larger than that of the affected side and does not react to light. As cerebral pressure increases and both hemispheres are affected, bilateral pupil dilation and fixation occur—the pupil may respond to light slowly. Dilating pupils are a sign of impending tentorial herniation. When pupils dilate or change in ability to react, the physician should be notified immediately. A pupil that is fixed and dilated is sometimes referred to as a "blown pupil" and is an ominous sign[49] (Fig. 37-31).

Visual disturbances

Another sign of increased intracranial pressure that occurs fairly early is some type of visual distrubance. These may include *diplopia* or *blurring* or *decreased visual acuity*. Diplopia usually results from paralysis or weakness of one of the muscles that controls eye movement.

Vomiting usually occurs in patients who have lesions below the tentorium. This vomiting usually occurs without the presence of nausea.

Blood pressure and pulse

The effect of increased intracranial pressure on pulse and blood pressure is variable. Compensatory changes occur in the cerebral vasculature relative to hypoxia. Herniation, however, causes ischemia of the vasomotor center. This excites the vasoconstrictor fibers, causing the systolic blood pressure to rise. If the intracranial pressure continues to increase, blood pressure may fall, especially the diastolic blood pressure. An increased systolic blood pressure followed by a sharp drop in blood pressure is often seen as the patient's condition deteriorates.

Pressure in the vasomotor center also increases the transmission of parasympathetic impulses through the vagus nerve to the heart; as a result the pulse rate slows. Slowing of the pulse rate in conjunction with a rising systolic blood pressure is a significant observation that should be reported. For consistency, blood pressure and pulse should be taken in the same arm.

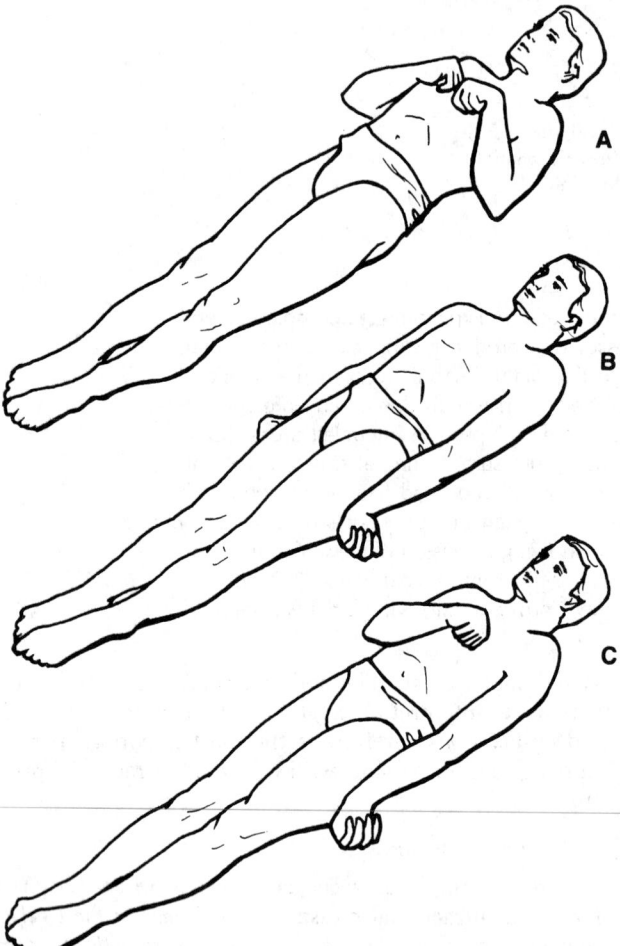

Fig. 37-32 Decorticate and decerebrate responses. **A,** Decorticate response. Flexion of arms, wrists, and fingers with adduction in upper extremities. Extension, internal rotation, and plantar flexion in lower extremities. **B,** Decerebrate response. All four extremities in rigid extension, with hyperpronation of forearms and plantar extension of feet. **C,** Decorticate response on right side of body and decerebrate response on left side of body. (From Zschoche D: *Mosby's comprehensive review of critical care,* ed 3, St Louis, 1985, Mosby–Year Book.)

Table 37-6   Altered respiratory patterns in coma

Respiratory pattern	Characteristics	Indications
Cheyne-Stokes	Periods of hyperventilation that gradually diminish to apnea of variable duration; respirations then resume and gradually build up to hyperventilation	Bilateral deep hemispheric and basal ganglionic dysfunction; the upper brain stem may be involved
Central neurogenic hyperventilation (CNHV)	Continuous rapid and deep respirations at a rate of 25/min	Systemic acidosis and hypoxemia should be excluded; has no segmental localizing influence; increasing regularity correlates with increasing depth of coma
Apneustic breathing	Prolonged inspiratory phase followed by apnea (inspiratory cramp)	Indicates lower pontine damage
Cluster breathing	Closely grouped respirations followed by apnea	Indicates lower pontine damage
Ataxic breathing	Chaotic respirations	Indicates damage to medullary centers; can precede respiratory arrest
Gasping breathing	Characterized by gasps followed by apnea of variable duration	Indicates damage to medullary centers; can precede respiratory arrest
Depressed breathing	Shallow, slow, and ineffective breathing	Usually caused by medullary depression

A widened pulse pressure, increased systolic blood pressure, and bradycardia are together referred to as *Cushing's response*. It is considered an important diagnostic characteristic of late-stage increased intracranial pressure.[3]

It is important to assess the trend of blood pressure and pulse. Indications of Cushing's response should be reported immediately.

Headaches

The patient with increased intracranial pressure (ICP) may complain of a headache. It is thought to result from *venous congestion* and the *tension in the intracranial blood vessels* as the cerebral pressure rises. The location and duration of the headache should be elicited from the patient. Headache that occurs with increased intracranial pressure usually increases in intensity with coughing, straining at stool, or stooping. *Headache is usually present in the early morning and may awaken the patient from sleep.*

It is important to realize that patients do not always complain of headache. Even if they do, the complaints may be vague and uncertain (see Box 37-19 for signs of ICP). As the intracranial pressure increases, the headache usually becomes worse.

Respiration

Herniation produces respiratory dysrhythmias that are variable and related to the level of the brainstem compression or failure. The breathing pattern may be deep and stertorous or periodic (Cheyne-Stokes) respirations. See Table 37-6 for description of respiratory patterns. Another breathing pattern found with increased intracranial pressure is *ataxic breathing.* This is an irregular and unpredictable breathing pattern with random shallow and deep breaths and occasional pauses. This type of breathing is seen in patients with medullary damage.[29] As intracranial pressure increases to fatal levels, respiratory paralysis occurs. The beginning of periods of apnea is significant. It is important to remember that the patient with a decreased level of consciousness will require assistance in keeping the airway clear. Persons with acute increased intracranial pressure require supplemental oxygen to prevent hypoxia, which can further increase intracranial pressure.

Controlled mechanical hyperventilation may be used to lower increased intracranial pressure. Increasing the tidal volume setting on a ventilator lowers the $PaCO_2$ to a significant degree. During hyperventilation, arterial blood gases and tidal volumes are monitored. This type of therapy should not be used for more than 48 hours because the brain may adapt to the lower $PaCO_2$ levels, leading to local ischemia. The patient must be weaned from the hyperventilation because an abrupt stop may lead to swelling of the brain.

Temperature

Failure of the thermoregulatory center because of compression occurs later with increased intracranial pressure and gives rise to high, uncontrolled temperatures. Hyperthermia must be controlled because it increases the metabolism of brain tissue.

Focal motor and sensory symptoms

Compression of the *upper motor neuron pathway* (corticospinal tract) *interrupts transmission* of *impulses* to the *lower motor neuron,* and *progressive muscle weakness* occurs. This often begins with the presence of drift and may progress to hemiparesis and hemiplegia. *Drift* is tested by asking the patient to close the eyes and extend the arms straight out in front for about 30 seconds. If one arm is weakened, it will drift downward without the patient being aware of it. Testing of the lower extremities includes the ability to push and pull against the tester, the ability to dorsiflex and plantar flex the feet, and the ability to do straight leg raises.

The presence of the *Babinski sign, hyperreflexia,* and *rigidity* are *additional signs of decreased motor function.* Seizures may occur. Herniation of the upper part of the brainstem produces *decerebrate rigidity* (fixed posture with arms, legs, and trunk extended and with flexion of the palms and plantar joints) or decorticate rigidity (fixed posture with flexion of the arm, wrist, and fingers, with adduction of the arm and extensors and internal rotation of the legs) (see Fig. 37-32). The worsening of existing motor defects is significant, and such signs should be reported to the physician.

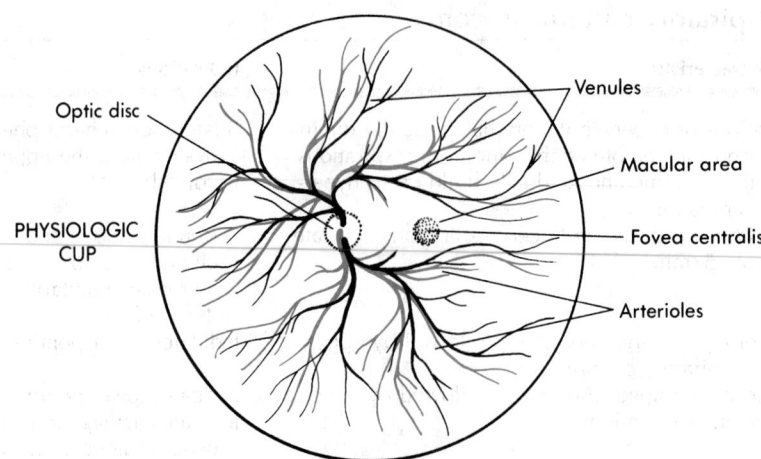

Fig. 37-33 Structures of the left eye as visualized through the funduscope.

Papilledema

The *blind spot* of the retina measures the size and shape of the optic papilla or optic disk. As intracranial pressure increases, the pressure is transmitted to the eyes through the cerebrospinal fluid and to the optic disk. Because the meninges of the brain reflect out around the eyeball, they permit the direct transmission of pressure along the spaces through the cerebrospinal fluid. As the optic disk swells, the retina is also compressed. The damaged retina cannot detect light rays. Visual acuity is lessened as the blind spot enlarges (Fig. 37-33).

Papilledema is also referred to as choked disk, which is caused by the engorgement of the retinal veins.

Vomiting

Projectile vomiting may be associated with increased intracranial pressure. The significance of vomiting and its frequency and character must be associated with other clinical signs.

Hiccuping

Compression of the vagus nerve (cranial nerve X) causes spasmodic contraction of the diaphragm. This compression occurs as brainstem herniation occurs. *Hiccuping in a patient who is at risk for increased intracranial pressure or who has other symptoms should be reported to the physician immediately.*

Diagnostic tests

The diagnosis of increased intracranial pressure can be made with the CT scan, which can show actual structural herniation and shifting of the brain. The displacement of the brain to the right or left occurs at a relatively late stage of increased intracranial pressure. Most of the time, however, *acute increased intracranial pressure is a medical emergency,* and there is little time for diagnostic tests. The diagnosis must be made on the basis of observation and neurologic testing. Although the frequency of "neuro checks" is often ordered by the physician, the nurse should use judgment to decide whether more frequent assessments and recordings are indicated. The presence of even subtle changes may be very significant.

In some postoperative or critically ill patients internal measuring devices are used to diagnose increased intracranial pressure. One of the most common requires the placement of a hollow screw through the skull into the subarachnoid space. The screw is attached to a Luer-Lok, which is connected to a transducer and oscilloscope for continuous monitoring. The transducer is fastened level with the screw for accurate readings. A manometer may be attached for intermittent readings, or constant monitoring is available with the monitor.

It has become evident that the traditional *clinical signs of increased intracranial pressure do not always correlate with the actual pressure changes as seen on the monitor.* Many of the classic signs of increased pressure do not appear until the pressure has reached extremely high levels, and the chance to reverse the rising pressure and prevent permanent brain damage has already passed.

Data analysis: nursing diagnoses

Nursing diagnoses are determined from analysis of patient data. Possible nursing diagnoses for the person with increased intracranial pressure may include, but are not limited to, the following:

Diagnostic title	Possible etiologies
Injury, high risk for	Sensory/motor deficits
Sensory/perceptual alteration	Altered sensory reception/transmission/integration
Mobility, impaired physical	Neuromuscular impairment
Pain	Increased intracranial pressure
Tissue perfusion, altered cerebral	Decreased cerebral blood flow
Airway clearance, ineffective	Perceptual/cognitive impairment
Breathing pattern, ineffective	Neuromuscular impairment
Hyperthermia	Illness/trauma

Planning: expected patient outcomes

Expected patient outcomes for the person with increased intracranial pressure may include, but are not limited to, the following:

1. Patient does not have an injury resulting from trauma.

2. Patient has minimal problems as a result of sensory-perceptual alterations.
3. Patient maintains optimal levels of mobility.
4. Patient has minimal pain.
5. Cerebral tissue pressure is adequate.
6. Cerebral edema is reduced.
7. Patient's airway is patent.
8. Patient's breathing pattern is effective.
9. Patient's temperature returns to normal.

Implementation
Assisting with achievement of therapeutic goals

The prevention of increased intracranial pressure may not be possible, but prevention of further rises in pressure and resulting damage to brain tissue is crucial. The detection of early signs is important to prevent irreversible effects.

The medical treatment of patients with increased intracranial pressure depends on the cause of the pressure. For example, if it is caused by an intracranial tumor, the tumor is removed surgically (p. 1289). If surgery is not possible (or not indicated), efforts are made to reduce the pressure through the use of drug therapy or direct physical measures.

Mechanical decompression

Rapidly rising intracranial pressure is often relieved by mechanical decompression. This may include a craniotomy, in which a bone flap is removed and then replaced or a craniectomy, in which the bone flap is removed and not replaced. This latter procedure is commonly performed to decompress the brain when pressure is high.

Other means of decompression may include continuous ventricular drainage or drainage of any subdural hematoma.

Medications

The three types of drugs usually administered to patients with increased intracranial pressure are *osmotic diuretics, corticosteroids,* and *anticonvulsants.* Osmotic diuretics are also referred to as *hyperosmolar drugs.* They draw water from the edematous brain tissue. Fluid is also drawn from uninjured tissue and can lead to fluid and electrolyte imbalance. The traditional osmotic diuretic is mannitol in a 15% to 25% solution. The usual dose is 1.5 to 2 g^m/kg of body weight administered over 30 to 60 minutes. It starts to reduce increased intracranial pressure within 15 minutes and its effects last for 4 to 6 hours. It is important for the patient receiving this drug to have a Foley catheter in place because of the large amounts of urine that usually are produced. Glycerol is another osmotic diuretic that is sometimes given, but it has the disadvantage of causing rebound swelling of brain tissue and must be given orally.

The corticosteroid most likely to be given is dexamethasone. An antacid may be given with it. Monitoring blood glucose levels is important because steroids can affect carbohydrate metabolism and glucose utilization.

Anticonvulsants are given to prevent seizures. Phenytoin (Dilantin) is the most commonly prescribed drug. It can be given intravenously but is not recommended to be given intramuscularly.

Narcotics and other drugs that cause respiratory depression are avoided.

Internal monitoring devices

Internal monitoring devices are being used more frequently to diagnose and monitor increased intracranial pressure. *Three basic monitoring systems* are used. These include the following:
1. *Ventricular catheter*—consists of cannula that is implanted through burr holes into the anterior horn of the lateral ventricle of the nondominant cerebral hemisphere. The catheter is connected to a transducer and recording device.
2. *Subarachnoid bolt or screw*—one of earliest methods. It is inserted through skull into the subdural or subarachnoid space. The screw is attached to a transducer and oscilloscope so that continuous monitoring may be done.
3. *Epidural sensory*—placement of a fiberoptic sensor in the epidural space through a burr hole in the skull. The sensor cable is connected to the monitor.

Monitoring produces pressure waves that can be evaluated to indicate pathology (Fig. 37-34).[50]

Interventions to achieve patient outcomes
Preventing injury

Numerous nursing activites are geared toward providing a safe environment for the patient with increased intracranial pressure. The patient may have altered sensory/perceptual reception and this can lead to increased confusion and agitation. The nurse should be aware that the *patient is at risk for seizures* and take necessary precautions.

Promoting mobility

Any patient at risk is discouraged from doing isometric exercises. Passive range of motion exercises are appropriate and will not increase systemic blood pressure because they are not resistive. Spacing of nursing activities is important in maintaining lower pressure levels.[3,10,61,101]

Maintaining comfort

The patient with increased intracranial pressure may experience headache. Narcotics and other drugs that cause respiratory depression are avoided. The use of cool cloths may help headache pain. The patient may be sensitive to light and noise. If this occurs, keeping the patient in a darkened, quiet environment may help ease discomfort.

Maintaining cerebral perfusion

Conservative measures to reduce venous volume may be implemented. The head of the bed is elevated to 30 to 45 degrees to promote venous return, and the neck is kept in a neutral position. Positioning to avoid flexion of the hips, waist, and neck is important. Rotation of the head, especially to the right, has been found to increase intracranial pressure. Nursing care is planned to cause the least distress to the patient. Care is grouped to allow adequate rest. Keeping the patient comfortable will help in maintaining cerebral blood flow.

Fluid intake may also be restricted. When osmotic diuretics are administered, urine output must be carefully

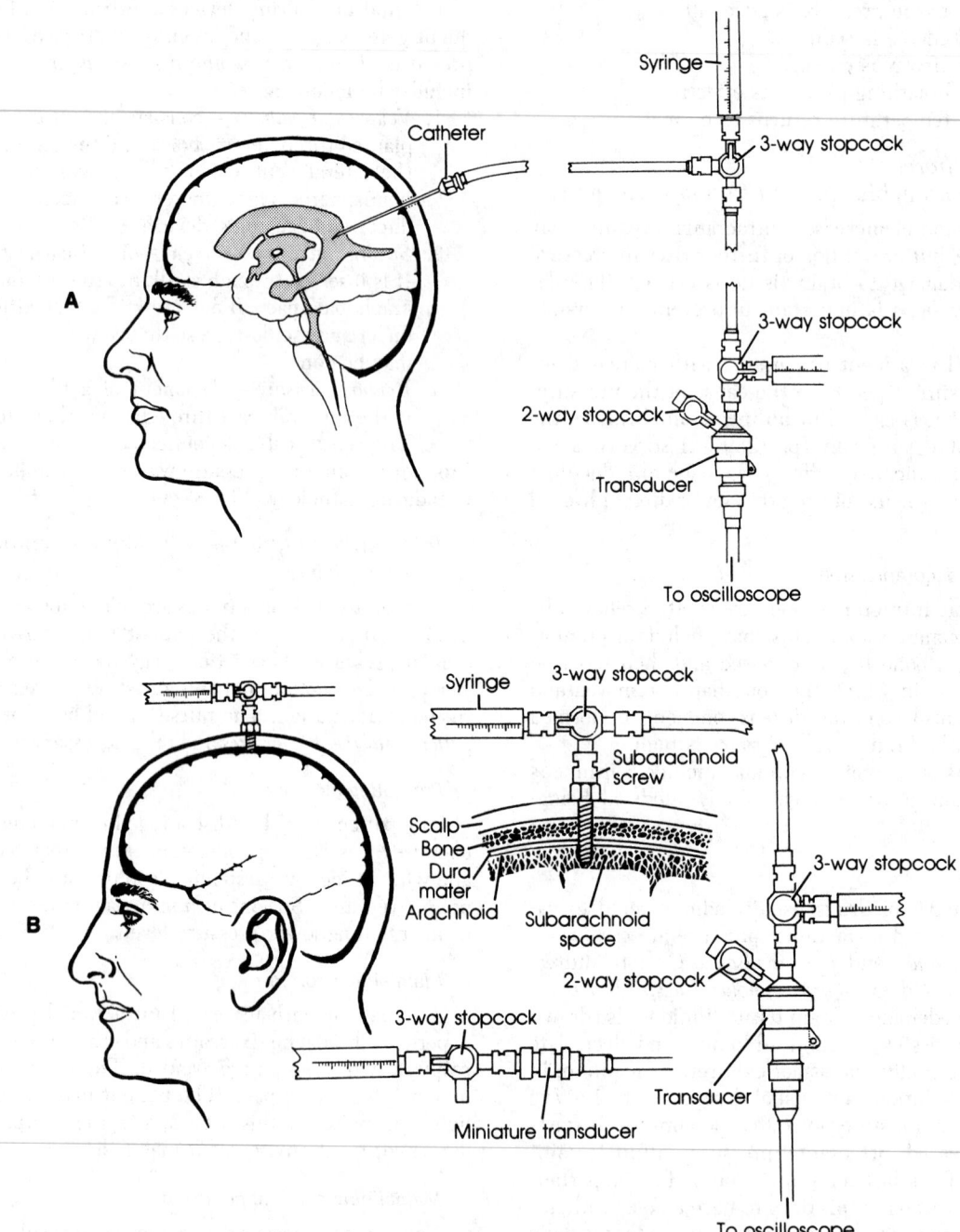

Fig. 37-34 Equipment for pressure monitoring. **A,** Ventricular pressure monitoring. Catheter is inserted through burr hole in skull into lateral ventricle and attached to transducer and oscilloscope to monitor intracranial pressure. **B,** Subarachnoid screw pressure monitoring. The subarachnoid screw is inserted through a burr hole in the skull and attached to a transducer and oscilloscope for continuous monitoring. (From Rudy EB: *Advanced neurological and neurosurgical nursing,* St Louis, 1984, Mosby—Year Book.)

monitored. An indwelling catheter is often used. The Valsalva maneuver is eliminated to the extent it is possible because it causes increased intrathoracic pressure, which indirectly increases intracranial pressure. This includes not allowing the patient to become constipated or to strain during defecation.

Maintaining effective respirations

Suctioning should be performed only when necessary (and then with the patient well preoxygenated) because it causes coughing and gagging. Suctioning should not be performed at the same time as other procedures that could cause increased intracranial pressure.

Oxygen therapy via mask or cannula is administered to improve brain oxygenation. Endotracheal intubation may be necessary. With the use of controlled ventilation, the P_{CO_2} can be lowered to below normal, which causes a slightly alkalotic pH. The decrease in the P_{CO_2} and the increase in the pH will decrease vasodilation and thereby decrease intracranial pressure.

Lidocaine may be given via an IV line or an endotracheal tube to suppress the cough reflex if cough is a problem.

Preventing hyperthermia

A hypothermia blanket may be necessary to control the patient's body temperature. Increased temperature may lead to accelerated brain damage. Care must be taken when using the blanket not to bring the patient's temperature down too quickly or to leave the blanket on for too long a period of time. The temperature of a neurologically impaired patient will tend to continue to decrease after the blanket is turned off.[23]

Evaluation

Evaluation of the patient with increased intracranial pressure includes frequent checks to evaluate neurologic status. Questions to consider may include the following:
1. Is the patient's safety monitored and in good control?

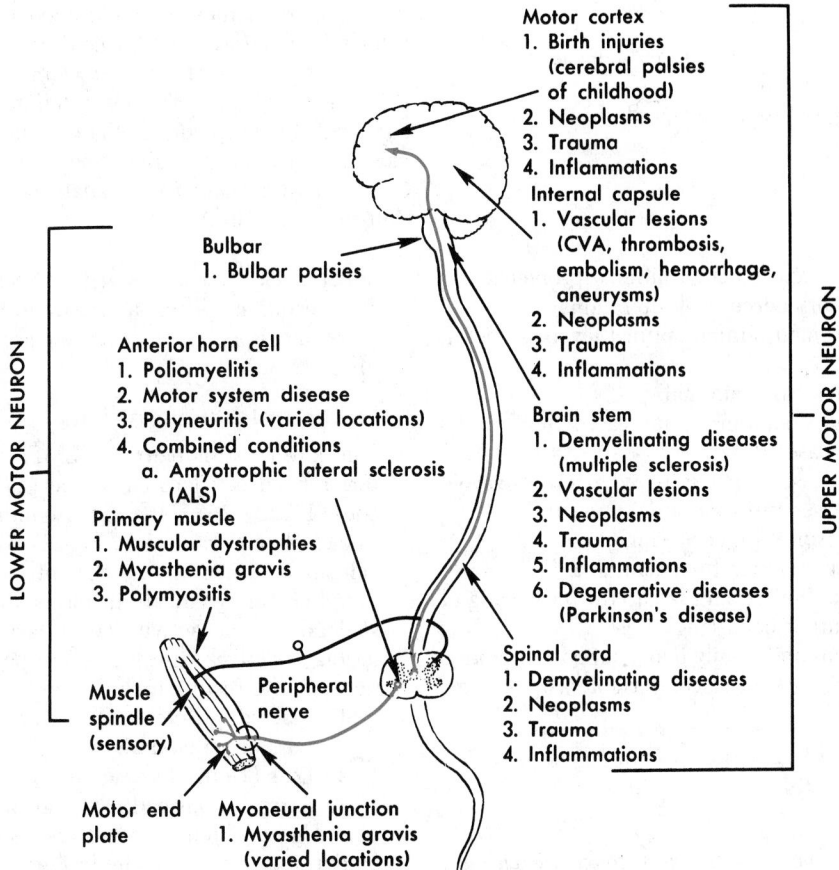

Fig. 37-35   Disturbances in motor function are classified pathologically along upper motor neuron (UMN) and lower motor neuron (LMN) structures. It should be noted that the same pathologic condition occurs at more than one site in UMN area shown on right. A few pathologic conditions involve both UMN and LMN structures, as in amyotrophic lateral sclerosis. Other lesion sites include myoneural junctions and primary muscles, making it possible to classify conditions as neuromuscular and muscular, respectively. (Modified from Chusid JG: *Correlative neuroanatomy and functional neurology,* ed 15, Los Altos, Calif, 1970, Lange Medical Publications.)

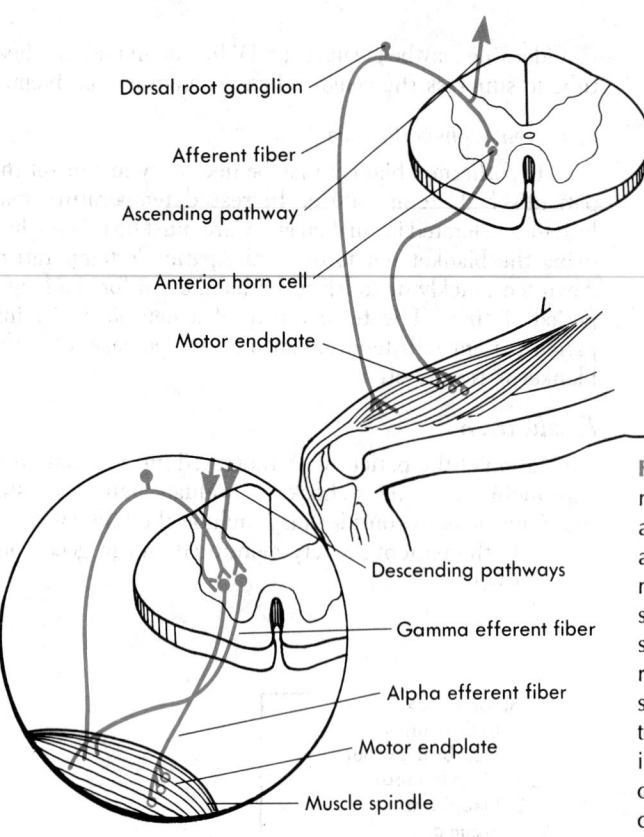

Dorsal root ganglion
Afferent fiber
Ascending pathway
Anterior horn cell
Motor endplate

Descending pathways
Gamma efferent fiber
Alpha efferent fiber
Motor endplate
Muscle spindle

Fig. 37-36 Structures making up lower motor neuron including motor (efferent) and sensory (afferent) elements. Shown on left is anterior horn cell in anterior gray column of spinal cord and its axon terminating in motor end-plate as it innervates extrafusal muscle fibers in quadriceps muscle. Detailed in enlargement are sensory and motor elements of γ-loop system. γ-Efferent fiber is shown innervating polar or end region of muscle spindle (sensory receptor of skeletal muscle). Contraction of muscle spindle fibers stretch central portion of spindle and cause afferent spindle fiber to transmit impulse centrally to cord. Muscle spindle afferent fibers in turn synapse on anterior horn cell and are transmitted by way of α-efferent fibers to skeletal (extrafusal) muscle, causing it to contract. Muscle spindle discharge is interrupted by active contraction of extrafusal muscle fibers. (Modified from Truex RC, Carpenter MB: *Human neuroanatomy*, ed 6, Baltimore, 1969, Williams & Wilkins.)

2. Is the patient experiencing minimal problems as a result of sensory-perceptual alterations?
3. Is the patient maintaining optimal levels of mobility?
4. Is the patient's pain minimal?
5. Are signs and symptoms of increased intracranial pressure decreased?
6. Are nursing measures being spaced in a way to avoid further increases in intracranial pressure?
7. Is effective respiration occurring?
8. Is the patient's temperature maintained?
9. Is fluid intake limited and is careful measuring of intake and output occurring?
10. Are the patient and family being supported, and is the patient being kept as comfortable as possible?

ALTERATIONS IN MUSCLE TONE AND MOTOR FUNCTION

Pathophysiology

Motor function disturbances are the *most commonly encountered neurologic symptoms.* Because the nervous system is designed primarily for the movement of the body in space and of the various parts in relation to each other, damage to it often causes serious problems in mobility. A loss of function, either motor or sensory, is called *paralysis.* A lesser degree of paralysis is called *paresis.* Damage to sensory pathways that are concerned with motor function may occur at the same time as the loss of motor function.

Injury or disease of motor neurons results in *alterations of muscle strength,* *tone,* and *reflex activity.* The specific clinical manifestations differ according to whether the lesion involves an upper motor neuron or a lower motor neuron (Fig. 37-35).

Lower motor neuron signs

The lower motor neurons (LMNs) consist of a large anterior horn cell located in the gray matter of the spinal cord (Fig. 37-36). They are also found in the motor cranial nuclei of the brainstem (Fig. 37-37). This anterior horn cell, in conjunction with the anterior spinal nerve and the peripheral nerve involved, forms a motor unit that affects skeletal muscle activity (voluntary and reflex). When a lesion selectively involves some part of the lower motor neuron, the results include the following:

1. Flaccid muscle weakness or paralysis
2. Loss of reflex activity
3. Loss of muscle tone
4. Atrophy confined to the involved muscle or muscles

The degree of muscle weakness is directly related to the extent and severity of the lesion.

The involved muscles become *flaccid* because the motor unit has been damaged and normal reflex activity has been interrupted. This flaccidity also is manifested in *hypotonia* and *hyporeflexia* and/or *areflexia* (reduced or absent muscle stretch reflexes). This interruption of the motor unit results in localized muscle atrophy or wasting. This atrophy also increases with nonuse of the muscle. In some LMN lesions, the affected muscle exhibits small localized, spontaneous, and involuntary contractions called *fasciculations.*

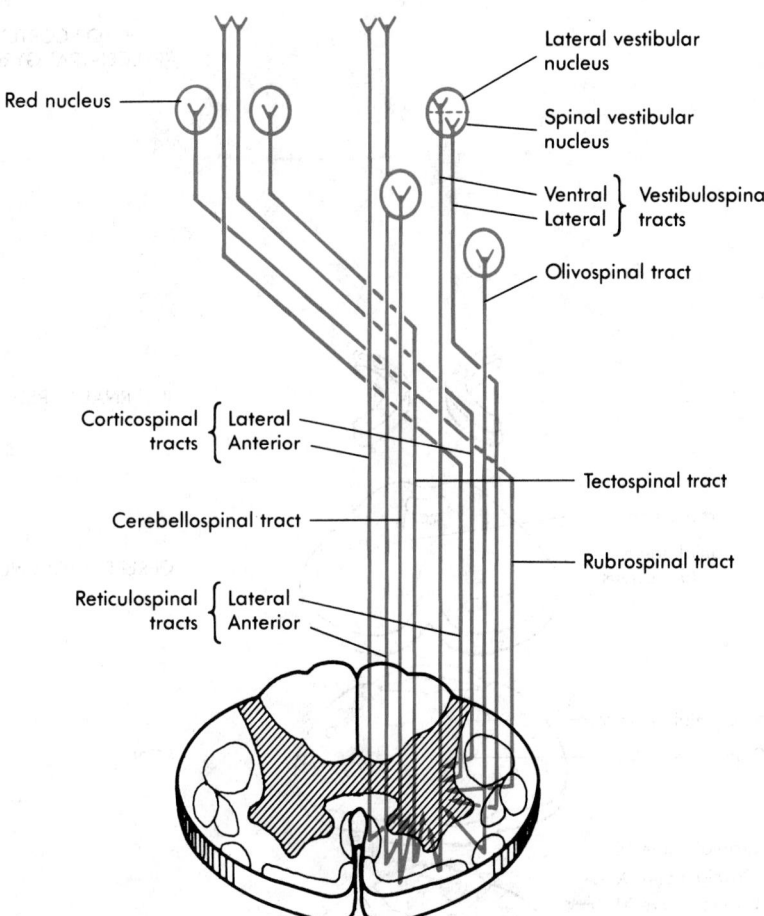

Red nucleus

Lateral vestibular nucleus

Spinal vestibular nucleus

Ventral ⎱ Vestibulospinal
Lateral ⎰ tracts

Olivospinal tract

Corticospinal ⎰ Lateral
tracts ⎱ Anterior

Cerebellospinal tract

Reticulospinal ⎰ Lateral
tracts ⎱ Anterior

Tectospinal tract

Rubrospinal tract

Fig. 37-37   Nuclei and their respective pathways descend and terminate around the LMN in the ventral column of the spinal cord.

Upper motor neuron signs

Upper motor neurons (UMNs) originate in the motor strip of the cerebral cortex and in multiple brainstem nuclei (Fig. 37-38). These axons then pass through the brainstem, deccusate (cross) in the medulla, and descend in the spinal cord via the corticospinal tracts. These fibers synapse with LMNs in the spinal cord. The collective working of both the UMN and LMN is essential for fine, orderly, and smooth muscle movements.

When a UMN lesion is rostral to the medulla, as in a cerebrovascular accident, deficits will occur contralateral to the lesion and will result in *hemiplegia*. The distribution or degree of paralysis is not always equal within hemiplegic distribution. The following are upper motor neuron signs:

1. Paresis or paralysis of voluntary muscle tone and spasticity
2. Hyperreflexia
3. Late atrophy from disuse
4. Increased muscle tone

Initially, the muscles affected by an upper motor lesion are *flaccid (hypotonic)* and *hyporeflexic*. Gradually, and with variability, the reflex arcs become increasingly hyperreactive. Then paresis, or paralysis of voluntary muscle movement, occurs with increased tone and spasticity. The spasticity is characterized by *increased resistance* to *passive move-*

ment, hyperreflexia, and *clonus.* (Clonus can be defined as a forced series of alternating contractions and partial relaxation of a muscle that occurs in some neurologic diseases.) A unilateral Babinski sign is present on the hemiparetic side.

Upper motor neuron lesions caudal to the medulla produce deficits ipsilateral to the lesion. Spinal cord injury is an example of this. If the cord is transected, the lesion extends into both halves of the spinal cord; deficits will be demonstrated as quadriplegia, or paraplegia, with loss of motor function, muscle tone, and reflex activity, as well as somatic and visceral sensations below the level of injury. Box 37-20 lists clinical syndromes of UMN and LMN lesions.

Nursing Process
Assessment

Both subjective and objective data are important in determining more about any abnormal muscle movements.

Subjective data

1. Patient's understanding of the problem and possible causes
2. Initial onset of problem
3. Measures that improve symptoms

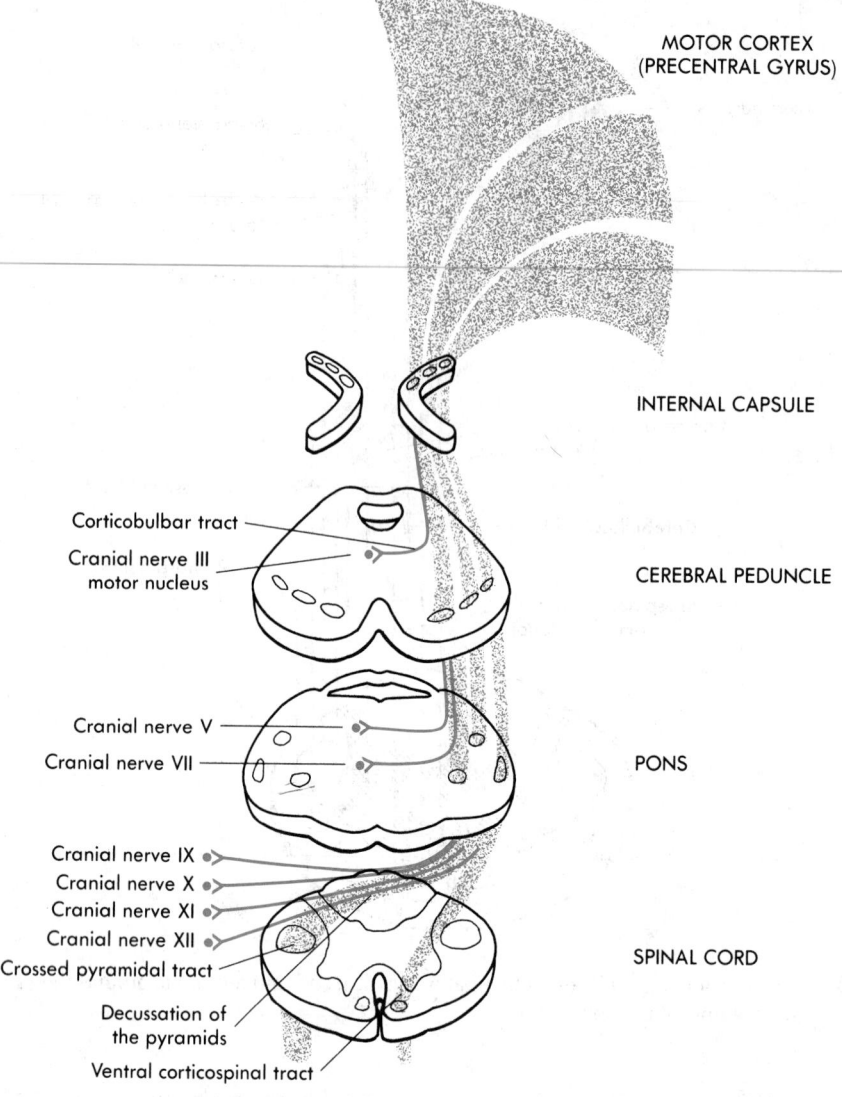

MOTOR CORTEX (PRECENTRAL GYRUS)

INTERNAL CAPSULE

Corticobulbar tract
Cranial nerve III motor nucleus

CEREBRAL PEDUNCLE

Cranial nerve V
Cranial nerve VII

PONS

Cranial nerve IX
Cranial nerve X
Cranial nerve XI
Cranial nerve XII
Crossed pyramidal tract
Decussation of the pyramids
Ventral corticospinal tract

SPINAL CORD

Fig. 37-38   Structures making up upper motor neuron, or pyramidal system. Pyramidal system fibers are shown to originate primarily in cells in precentral gyrus of motor cortex; converge at internal capsule; descend to form central third of cerebral peduncle; descend further through pons, where small fibers are given off to cranial nerve motor nuclei along the way; form pyramids at medulla, where majority of fibers decussate; and then continue to descend in lateral column of white matter of spinal cord, where they synapse with anterior horn cells at all segments of cord. A few fibers descend without crossing at medulla level. (Modified from original painting by Frank H Netter, MD: Reproduced with permission from The Ciba Collection of Medical Illustrations. Copyright 1983 by the Ciba-Geigy Corp. All rights reserved.)

37-20

Clinical syndromes of UMN and LMN lesions

Motor component	UMN characteristics	LMN characteristics
Reflex	Hyperreflexia, extensor toe sign (Babinski's sign)	Hyporeflexia or areflexia
Muscle tonus	Hypertonia, clasp-knife spasticity, clonus	Hypotonia, flaccidity
Muscle movement	Paralysis or paresis of movements in hemiplegic distribution, etc.	Paralysis or paresis of individual muscles in peripheral nerve distribution
Muscle wasting	Late atrophy from disuse	Early atrophy or denervation
Muscle fasciculations	Not present	Present

4. Presence of clumsiness or incoordination
5. Presence of any abnormal sensation

If the lesion occurs suddenly, such as in spinal cord injury from trauma or a cerebrovascular accident, subjective symptoms of the muscle weakness may be minimal. Frequently, subjective symptoms occurring early in an illness involving abnormal muscle movements or sensations are ignored.

Objective data

1. Coordination
2. Muscle strength
3. Muscle tone
4. Any atrophy of muscles
5. Presence of clonus or fasciculations
6. Ability to move muscles, abnormal gait
7. Abnormal reflexes
8. Change in ability to carry on daily activities

Diagnostic testing

One of the *most common diagnostic procedures to evaluate muscle dysfunction* is *electromyography* (see the box on p. 1231). In motor disease, electrical activity of various types and abnormal patterns appear in resting muscle. An electromyogram (EMG) provides direct evidence of motor dysfunction and can be used to detect a dysfunction located in the motor neuron, the neuromuscular junction, or muscle fibers (see Box 37-21). It is particularly helpful in the diagnosis of lower motor neuron disease, primary muscle disease, and defects in the transmission of electrical impulses at the neuromuscular junction.

Diagnostic title	Possible etiologies
Injury, high risk for	Sensory/motor deficits
Skin integrity, impaired, actual or high risk for	Immobility
Disuse syndrome, high risk for	Immobility, weakness
Mobility, impaired physical	Neuromuscular impairment
Activity intolerance	Bed rest, immobility
Nutrition, altered: less than body requirements; actual or high risk for	Chewing or swallowing difficulties
Swallowing, impaired	Neuromuscular impairment
Incontinence, bowel	Neuromuscular impairment
Incontinence, total	Neurologic dysfunction/disease
Self care deficit: feeding, bathing/hygiene, dressing/grooming, toileting	Neuromuscular impairment
Body image disturbance	Loss of body functions
Knowledge deficit	Lack of exposure/recall

Planning: expected patient outcomes

Expected patient outcomes for the person with alterations in muscle tone and motor function may include, but are not limited to, the following:

1. Patient remains free of traumatic injury.
2. Patient's skin will remain intact and free of breakdown.
3. Patient describes measures to prevent skin breakdown.

37-21

Electromyogram (EMG)

Purpose

To measure the contraction of a muscle in response to electrical stimulation.

Preparation of patient

1. No special preparation.
2. Patient teaching
   a. Explain procedure.
   b. Time: approximately 45 minutes for one muscle study.
   c. Sensation: some discomfort when electrodes are inserted—persons with sensory neuropathies may have more intense pain. Some discomfort when electrical current is used.
   d. Muscle may ache for a short time after the procedure.

Procedure

1. Electrodes are inserted into selected skeletal muscle.
2. Electrical current is passed through electrodes.
3. Machine graphs the variations of muscle potentials (voltage).

After procedure

1. Observe for signs of bleeding at site of electrode insertion.
2. Plan rest period for patient.
3. Medicate patient as needed for discomfort.

---

4. Patient lists signs of skin breakdown that require professional assessment.
5. Patient remains free of infection.
6. Patient's mobility will be at optimal level without contractures.
7. Patient describes and demonstrates range of motion.
8. Patient demonstrates measures to prevent muscle or joint deformities.
9. Patient demonstrates safe swallowing mechanism.
10. Patient directs bowel and bladder program.
11. Patient has regular bowel evacuations without diarrhea or constipation.
12. Patient demonstrates ADL that can be done alone and can describe methods of assistance for those functions that are dependent.
13. Patient verbalizes positive self-concept.
14. Patient states plans for follow-up care.
15. Patient describes dosage, function, side effects, and toxic effects of medications to be taken.

Implementation

Successful nursing care of the patient with motor dysfunction includes those activities that prevent complications such as decubitus ulcers or joint contractures, as well as those that develop the person's optimal level of functioning.

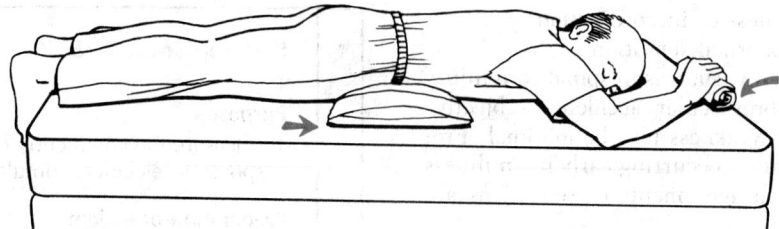

Fig. 37-39   Patient lying prone with feet extending over end of mattress. Note small pillow under midsection and hand is flexed around rolled towel.

Assisting with achievement of therapeutic goals
Medications

Patients having ongoing problems with spasticity may be given skeletal muscle relaxants to decrease tone and involuntary movements and to help relieve anxiety and tension. Common side effects include drowsiness and dizziness, which are potentiated when the medications are used in combination with alcohol, barbiturates, sedatives, hypnotics, or tranquilizers. Some commonly prescribed medications are the following:

1. Baclofen (Lioresal)—a derivative of GABA (an inhibitory neurotransmitter). Acts on the spinal cord.
2. Dantrolene sodium (Dantrium)—acts directly on skeletal muscle by impairing Ca^{++} release from the sacroplasmic reticulum. Can cause additional side effects of muscle weakness, slurred speech, drooling, and anuresis.
3. Diazepam (Valium)—centrally acting muscle relaxant and antianxiety agent.[22]

Interventions to achieve patient outcomes
Preventing injury

Patients with paralysis have significant safety needs. Protection of the patient from falling is a major one. When left alone, hemiplegic patients need to have the side rail raised on the side of the bed next to their affected side. A chair restraint may be helpful when the patient is up in a chair.

Also, the eye on the affected side of the body should be protected when the lid remains open and there is no blink reflex. If this is not done, damage to the cornea will occur, leading to corneal ulcers and blindness. Irrigation with a physiologic solution of sodium chloride, followed by artificial tear solution (methylcellulose) is sometimes used. An eye pad may be used to keep the eye closed. If a pad is used, it must be changed daily and the eye cleaned and carefully examined for signs of infection or drying of the cornea. Eye shields are preferable to pads, because there is no danger of lint entering the eye.

Maintaining skin integrity

Skin over bony prominences needs to be inspected regularly for signs of pressure. Paralyzed persons are at risk for decubitus formation. The following factors account for this:

1. Muscles are not being used.
2. Interference with autonomic reflexes that monitor and maintain vasomotor tone may result in altered circulation to the paralyzed areas.
3. Accompanying sensory loss may prevent the individual from perceiving pain and pressure, the warning symptoms of tissue injury.

Persons who are physically capable of activity are taught to turn themselves in bed and to reposition themselves independently. Paraplegics are taught how to shift their weight in bed; for the quadriplegic patient these activities are done by the staff. Weight shifts while in a wheelchair or other chair are also important. These may include controlled leaning from one side to another or push-ups done by the patient to relieve pressure for a short time every hour or so. Most patients are taught to do a weight shift for 5 minutes every hour. If the patient is not able to independently do a weight shift, then the staff must do it. However, patients are taught to take the responsibility to remind the staff when it is time for the weight shift. If the person also has a loss of sensation, no external heat such as hot water bottles or heating pads should be used (the heat may not be felt and a burn could result). Paralyzed or weakened areas should be inspected daily for any signs of skin irritation; a mirror or other device to assist in this assessment is imperative so that all areas can be visualized.

Maintaining mobility and activity

The limbs of a person who has acute hemiplegia, as with the person who has paraplegia or quadriplegia, are often flaccid at first. Spasticity with a tendency to muscle contracture develops gradually. The joints then become flexed and fixed in useless positions with deformity unless preventive measures are taken by the nurse. Joint capsules and ligaments around the immobile joint shorten, and the limb may be drawn into a flexor or an extensor contracture with or without muscle spasm.

Based on assessment of the joints that are vulnerable to contracture and deformity formation, the nurse should carefully place the limbs in a normal anatomic position to prevent deformity. Counterpositioning may be used. In hemiplegia, for example, the affected upper limb is pulled inward at the shoulder joint and the wrist drops; in the lower limb the knee flexes and the foot drops. In *counter-*

positioning the nurse positions the patient so that the shoulder and upper arm are in abduction, the elbow is flexed, the wrist is dorsiflexed, the knee is in a neutral position, and the foot is dorsiflexed. If the person is supine, a pillow can be placed between the upper arm and body to hold the arm in abduction. Hand splints are often used to prevent hand deformity. Footboards may be used to prevent footdrop, although some feel that these contribute to increased spasticity and should not be used routinely for patients with UMN lesions. A sling may be useful for shoulder subluxation.

Physical therapists and occupational therapists can provide splints, braces, and casts that can be an adjunct to positioning.

The prone position is excellent for patients who are able to tolerate it. Not only is the chance of skin breakdown decreased with this position, but the position also causes extension of the hip and knee joints by means of gravity. Many patients are able to comfortably assume this position. A pillow placed under the chest may make the patient more comfortable and make breathing easier (Fig. 37-39).

Positioning of the paralyzed person is extremely important. Knee flexion and foot-drop are serious complications that must be prevented. The development of a flexion contracture at the knee joint interferes with the person's ability to bear weight in an upright position and to transfer independently. As a result, the level of self-care and independence may be diminished. Subluxation of a shoulder joint in a person with hemiplegia, related to inadequate support of the joint when in an upright position, causes pain and limits therapy. Keeping the paralyzed person upright or semiupright for long periods of time results in hip deformities. Most joint deformities in a paralyzed person are preventable with early and continuing nursing interventions.

In addition to positioning, interventions for the person with paralysis include range of motion (ROM) exercises to all joints. These may be passive (carried out by the nurse) or active (carried out by the patient). Passive ROM is indicated at least three times daily for all joints that the person cannot voluntarily move.

Promoting nutrition

Patience and persistence are necessary in giving food and fluids to the person with hemiplegia. So much difficulty may be encountered in swallowing food and fluids because of paralysis that the patient may believe that effort is not worthwhile. Important nursing measures are listed in Box 37-22.

Some patients may have severe dysphagia and require prefeeding and feeding exercises. This activity often is shared by nurses, speech therapists, and occupational therapists. In patients at severe risk of aspiration, a *video fluoroscopy with barium may be used to rule out aspiration.* This procedure requires the patient to swallow small amounts of liquid or semisolid barium while fluoroscopy is being done.

Self-help devices for feeding are available. These include utensils with universal cuffs (Fig. 37-40), covered plastic cups, plate guards, and the Asepto syringe.

37-22

Nursing measures to improve nutrition

1. Make patients feel that problem is not overwhelming.
2. Give positive feedback to patient when any improvement is noted.
3. Avoid foods that cause choking, such as mashed potatoes.
4. Check affected side of mouth for accumulation of food and subsequent poor mouth hygiene—it may be helpful to irrigate mouth after eating.
5. Encourage patient to feed self as soon as possible.
6. Dentures should be used if at all possible.
7. Make sure patient is sitting up at 90 degrees.
8. Keep patient's head up and chin slightly tucked. Head should not be extended.
9. Encourage patient to tip head toward unaffected side while swallowing.
10. Do not mix liquids and solid foods.
11. Encourage patient to take small bites.
12. Have patient swallow completely before taking another bite.

Maintaining elimination

The person with paralysis from a UMN or LMN lesion may have problems with bowel and bladder control. These are discussed in Chapters 31 and 32.

Promoting self-care

During the rehabilitative and acute phases, patients with paralysis are taught how to carry out ADL to the extent that they are able. A variety of self-help devices are available that assist with dressing with one hand, for example. The occupational therapist becomes involved in many of these activities, including homemaking. It is important to stress the concept of the rehabilitative team in managing these patients. Volunteers may also be included in helping the patient find meaningful diversional activities.

Promoting acceptance of body image

The person with paralysis will need assistance in adjusting to the change in the body. The loss of the ability to function independently when paralyzed is traumatic. The person also may have fears of rejection by loved ones, concerns about the future, and loss of self-esteem. A grief reaction similar to that described for the stages of death and dying may occur. At times, persons may relate to the paralyzed portion of the body as though it were not a part of them. Nursing interventions to help the patient cope with the loss of function and change in body image are essential.

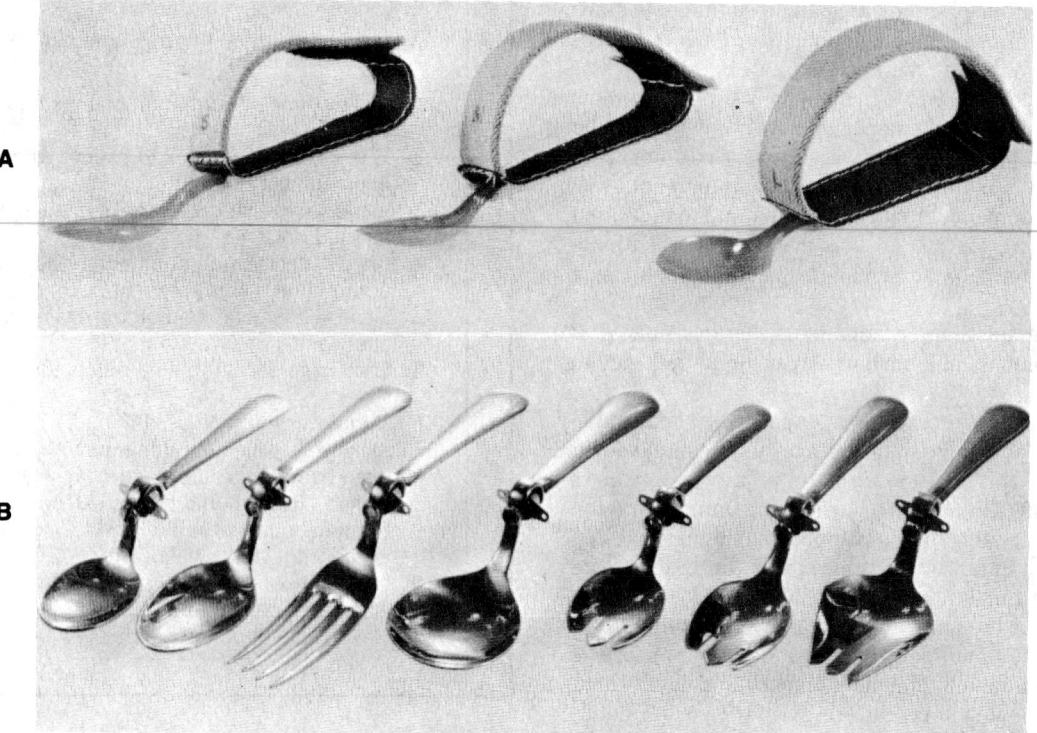

Fig. 37-40 Self-help devices for quadriplegic. **A,** Spoons with small, medium, and large universal cuff attachments that fit over hand. **B,** Swivel spoons, forks, and sporks (combination spoon and fork, last three on right), which are used with universal cuff. (Courtesy Fred Sammons, OTR, Chicago.)

Facilitating learning

Teaching is an extremely important part of caring for the person with motor problems. Appropriate teaching activities are outlined in Box 37-23.

Evaluation

Evaluation of the patient with motor dysfunction is made based on the perception of the patient and measurement against the defined patient outcomes. Questions to consider may include the following:

1. Does the patient remain free of traumatic injury?
2. Is the patient's skin intact?
3. Is the patient doing skin checks or asking staff to do them?
4. Is the patient knowledgeable about range of motion?
5. Are the joints freely moveable?
6. Is the patient receiving adequate nutrition?
7. Is the patient swallowing without difficulty?
8. Is the patient's fluid intake adequate?
9. Does the patient assume control of bowel and bladder program?
10. Is the patient as independent in ADLs as possible?
11. Does the patient verbalize a positive self-concept?
12. Can the patient state plans for follow-up care?
13. Does the patient verbalize knowledge of the medication regime?

ALTERATIONS IN SENSORY FUNCTION
Pathophysiology

The presence of a lesion anywhere within the sensory system pathway, from the receptor to the sensory cortex, alters the transmission or perception of sensory information. The parietal lobe cortex is of major importance in interpretation of sensation with the exception of sight, hearing, smell, taste, and thermoregulation. Loss, decrease, or increase in sensation of pain, temperature, touch, and proprioception, singly or in combination, results in difficulty in daily living. Because these sensations normally help the person to be aware of alterations in the internal and external environments, any alteration in sensation lessens the ability to be completely and accurately protected.

One specific loss is that of *proprioception,* or *the ability to know the position of the body and its parts without looking directly at the part.* Lack of control of body temperature, or *hyperthermia,* is another dysfunction and occurs as a result of malfunction in the thermoregulatory center in the brain, such as that which occurs after brain surgery near the hypothalamus or from head injury.

The patient with motor or sensory dysfunction

1. Always lock wheelchair when transferring patient
2. Check condition of affected eye frequently
3. Be aware of placement of affected extremities before movement
4. Protect paralyzed limbs from injury
5. Have patient wear shoes (*not* slippers) that fit well for ambulating or transferring

Skin care

1. Regular inspection of skin surfaces, using mirror or other device
2. Need to turn frequently
3. Weight shifts
4. No use of heating pads, hot water bottles, or excessively hot water for bathing

Activity needs

1. Range of motion
2. Proper positioning
3. Frequent changes in position

Medications

1. Use of medication, side effects, dosage, and timing
2. Reporting of side effects to physician
3. Importance of not combining medication with other mood-altering drugs or alcohol

Nutrition-diet

1. Foods that can be easily tolerated
2. Measures to decrease swallowing difficulty
3. Use of special appliances to assist with eating

ADL

1. Teaching techniques of bathing, grooming, dressing
2. Importance of having meaningful recreational activities
3. Bowel and bladder care

Other teaching

1. Importance of good fluid intake
2. Follow-up care—where to procure equipment, supplies
3. Methods for relieving feelings of frustration

Fig. 37-41 presents common patterns of sensory loss. A cerebral lesion results in various alterations in sensation contralateral to the lesion. This distribution results because all sensory fibers have decussated (crossed) before reaching the sensory cortex of the cerebrum. On the other hand, transection of the spinal cord results in total bilateral sensory loss distal to the lesion, because all pathways have been severed. The characteristic distribution of deficits with Brown-Sequard syndrome is ipsilateral (same side) loss of proprioception and vibratory sense and contralateral (opposite side) loss of pain, temperature, and crude touch sensation.

Nursing Process
Assessment

The sensory examination is the most difficult part of the neurologic examination. Subjective data are collected as follows.

Subjective data

1. Patient's understanding of the sensory disturbance
2. Measures that relieve symptoms, including medications
3. Site of sensory abnormality
4. Onset of sensory problem
5. Presence of associated symptoms
6. Alteration in sensation
   a. Pain
   b. Touch
   c. Temperature
   d. Proprioception
   e. Stereognosis

Data analysis: nursing diagnoses

Nursing diagnoses are determined from analysis of patient data. Possible nursing diagnoses for the person with sensory dysfunction may include all those listed under Alterations in Muscle Tone and Motor Function (p. 1231), with the addition of the following:

Diagnostic title	Possible etiologies
Sensory/perceptual alteration	Altered sensory reception/ transmission/ integration

Planning: expected patient outcomes

Expected patient outcomes for the person with sensory dysfunction may include, but are not limited to, the expected patient outcomes listed under Alterations in Muscle Tone and Motor Function (p. 1231), as well as the following:

1. Patient can demonstrate how to compensate for each sensory deficit or loss.
2. Patient can explain safety factors needed in ADLs to protect against injury.
3. Patient can demonstrate how to inspect the affected body parts for injury.
4. Patient can state signs and symptoms that would indicate worsening of the condition and the need to seek medical assistance.
5. Patient demonstrates minimal anxiety.
6. Patient's discomfort or pain is minimal.

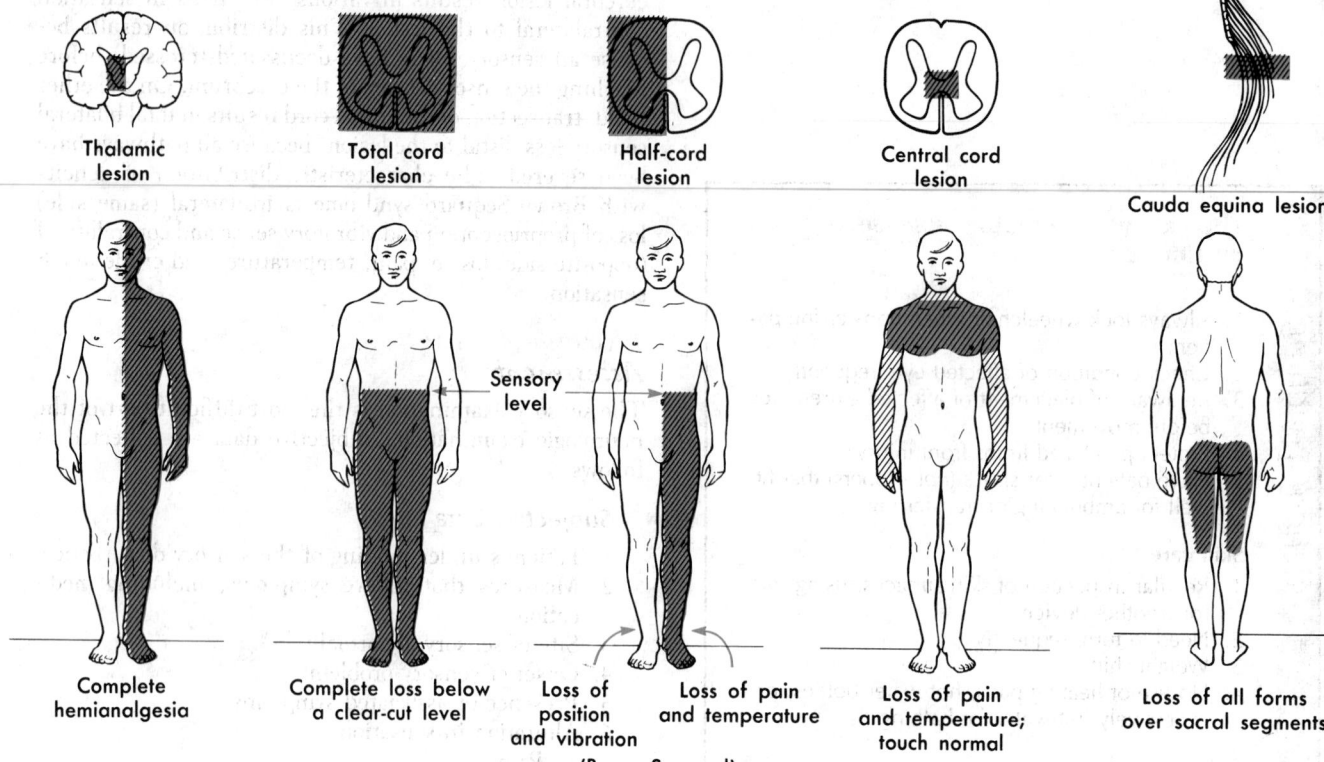

Fig. 37-41 Common patterns of sensory abnormality. Upper diagrams show site of lesion; lower diagrams show distribution of corresponding sensory loss. (Modified from Bickerstaff, ER: *Neurology for nurses*, ed 2, London, 1971, English Universities Press Ltd, and Hodder & Stoughton, Ltd.)

Implementation

Interventions to achieve patient outcomes

Facilitating learning

The most important nursing intervention for the patient with sensory dysfunction is teaching the person and family protective measures in relation to the sensory deficit or alteration (see Box 37-23). Teaching the person to use noninvolved senses to an increased extent helps to avoid injuries. For example, teaching the person with hypoesthesia (lessened touch) to visually inspect involved body parts regularly will help to prevent injuries.

Evaluation

Evaluation of the patient with sensory dysfunction involves the patient and family. Questions to consider may include those listed under Alterations in Muscle Tone and Motor Function (p. 1234), as well as the following:

1. Is the patient carrying out ADL in a safe manner?
2. Is the patient successfully compensating for sensory deficits?
3. Is the patient inspecting affected body parts for injury?
4. Can the patient state signs and symptoms that indicate the need to notify the physician?
5. Is the patient free of pain or discomfort?

MAJOR HEALTH PROBLEMS OF THE NEUROLOGIC SYSTEM

Functioning of the neurologic system can be interrupted for a variety of reasons. These include the following:
1. Interference with impulses because of conduction of impulses
2. Interference because of degenerative changes
3. Interference because of vascular problems
4. Interference because of infection
5. Interference because of trauma
6. Interference because of tumors

Some common neurologic disorders are listed in Box 37-24.

37-24

Health problems of the neurologic system

1. *Interference with function because of problems with conduction of impulses*
   a. Epilepsy or seizures
   b. Myasthenia gravis
2. *Interference with function because of degenerative diseases*
   a. Multiple sclerosis
   b. Parkinson's disease
   c. Amyotrophic lateral sclerosis (ALS)
   d. Alzheimer's disease
   e. Neurofibromatosis
3. *Interference with function because of vascular conditions*
   a. Cerebrovascular accident (CVA)
   b. Intracerebral hemorrhage
4. *Interference with function because of infection/inflammation*
   a. Meningitis
   b. Encephalitis
   c. Brain abscess
   d. Poliomyelitis
   e. Guillain-Barré syndrome
   f. Neurosyphilis
   g. AIDS
5. *Interference with function because of trauma*
   a. Craniocerebral
   b. Spinal cord
   c. Peripheral nerve
6. *Interference with function because of tumors*
   a. Intracranial
   b. Intraspinal

INTERFERENCE WITH FUNCTION BECAUSE OF PROBLEMS WITH CONDUCTION OF IMPULSES

EPILEPSY OR SEIZURES

Epilepsy (convulsive disorder) is one of the oldest diseases known to humans. (For purposes of this text the terms *epilepsy, seizure disorder,* and *convulsive disorder* will be used interchangeably.) Seizures occur in all races and affect males and females equally. There is no apparent geographic distribution. Epilepsy can begin at any age, but in many the onset is before the age of 20. The incidence is about 1 in every 200 to 300 persons. Between 2 and 4 million persons in the United States are affected by epilepsy. Many of these are children.

There are numerous ways to classify seizures. One common way is the International Classification of Epileptic Seizures. In this classification, seizures are identified as partial (beginning locally), generalized (bilaterally symmetric and with no local onset), unilateral, or unclassified. Another way to classify seizures is based on the clinical features of the attack. The five groups in this type of classification are the following:
1. Grand mal (major or generalized)
2. Petit mal
3. Psychomotor
4. Jacksonian and focal
5. Miscellaneous (myoclonic, akinetic)

Table 37-7 shows the characteristics of each type of seizure.

Pathophysiology

Epilepsy may be defined as a transitory disturbance in consciousness or in motor, sensory, or autonomic function with or without loss of consciousness. It is associated with sudden, excessive, and disorderly electrical discharges in the neurons of the brain that result in the sudden, violent, involuntary contraction of a group of muscles. The patterns or forms of seizures vary and depend on the area of the brain from which the seizure arises. The pattern is stereotyped in the individual, although variations may occur with progression of cerebral lesions (Fig. 37-42).

Seizures can involve essentially all parts of the brain at once, as in the generalized type, or only a minute focal spot. In the first type, the excessive neuronal discharges are thought to originate in the brainstem portion of the reticular activating system; these then spread throughout the CNS including the cortex and the deeper parts of the brain. The process may last from a few seconds to as long as 3 to 5 minutes, or it may stop immediately, as in a *petit mal seizure.* Stoppage of a seizure is thought to result from fatigue of the neurons involved in precipitating the seizure or by inhibition of certain structures within the brain. The excessive neuronal discharges may result in a *tonic convulsion,* with the contraction of all muscles at once, or a *clonic convulsion,* with alternate contraction and relaxation of opposing muscle groups. This gives the characteristic jerking movements of the body. Seizures are followed by inhibition of cerebral function with a variable length. This is called the *postictal period.*

When recurrent generalized seizure activity occurs at such frequency that full consciousness is not regained between seizures, it is called *status epilepticus.* This is a medical emergency and requires intensive medical and nursing

Table 37-7   Characteristics of seizures

Type of seizure	Etiology	Characteristics	Clinical signs	Aura	Postictal period
Grand mal	Most common	Generalized, characterized by loss of consciousness for several minutes	Aura Cry Loss of consciousness The fall Tonic-clonic movements Incontinence	Present Flashing lights Smells Spots before eyes Dizziness	Present Need for sleep 1 to 2 hrs Headache common
Petit mal	Usually occur during childhood and adolescence Frequency decreases as child gets older	Sudden impairment in or loss of consciousness with little or no tonic-clonic movement Occurs without warning Has tendency to appear a few hours after arising or when person is quiet	Sudden vacant facial expression with eye focused straight ahead All motor activity ceases except perhaps for slight symmetric twitching about eyelids Possible loss of muscle tone Consciousness returns	Not present	Not present
Psychomotor	Occur at any age	Sudden change in awareness associated with complex distortion of feeling and thinking and partially coordinated motor activity Longer than petit mal	Behaves as if partially conscious Often appears intoxicated May do antisocial things such as exposing self or carrying out violent acts Autonomic complaints may occur Chest pain Respiratory distress Tachycardia Gastrointestinal distress Urinary incontinence	Present Complex hallucinations or illusions	Present Confusion Amnesia Need for sleep
Jacksonian-focal	Occur almost entirely in patients with structural brain disease	Depend on site of focus May or may not be progressive	Commonly begin in hand, foot, or face May end in grand mal seizure	Present Numbness Tingling Crawling feeling	Present
Myoclonic	May antedate grand mal by months or years	May be very mild or may have rapid, forceful movements	Sudden involuntary contraction of muscle group, usually in extremities or trunk No loss of consciousness	Not present	Not present
Akinetic	Not common	Peculiar generalized tonelessness	Person falls in flaccid state Unconscious for minute or two	Rarely present	Not present

Frontal motor

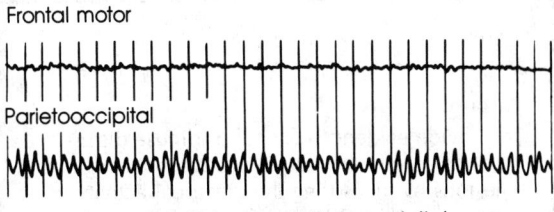

Parietooccipital

Normal adult, 10/sec. activity in occipital area.

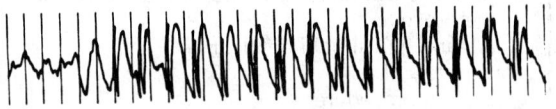

Absent attacks (petit mal seizures).
Synchronous 3/sec. spikes and waves.

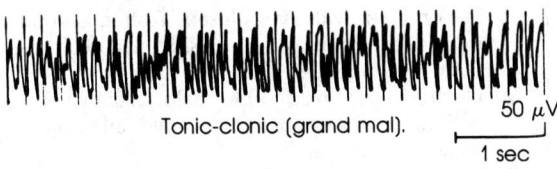

Tonic-clonic (grand mal).   50 μV
                                 1 sec

Right temporal

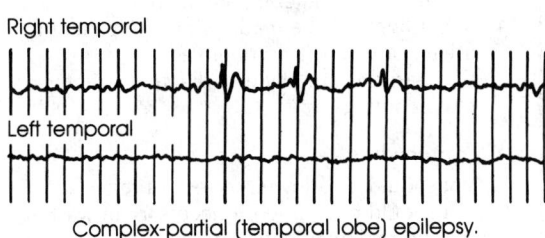

Left temporal

Complex-partial (temporal lobe) epilepsy.
Right temporal spike focus.

Right frontal

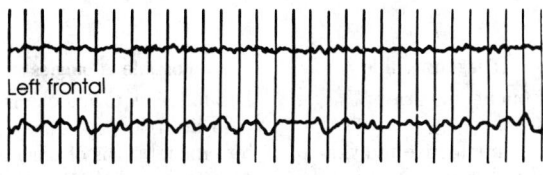

Left frontal

Brain tumor. Left frontal slow wave focus.

Right frontal

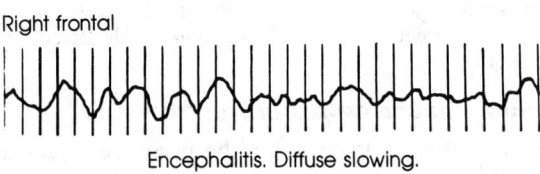

Encephalitis. Diffuse slowing.

Fig. 37-42 Tracings of electroencephalogram. The normal tracing is demonstrated as are several pathologic states.

care to prevent death from brain damage secondary to prolonged hypoxia and exhaustion.

Seizures occur in many childhood and adult illnesses. Causes include the following:

1. Cerebral anoxia
2. Hypoglycemia
3. Disturbance of calcium balance
4. Electrolyte imbalances
5. Disturbance in hydration
6. Injection of drugs and poisons with convulsive activity
7. Numerous metabolic disturbances and disorders
8. Infections that cause high temperature elevations
9. Generalized inflammatory processes
10. Degenerative tissue disorders
11. Hysteria

In many patients with epilepsy, a localized organic lesion serves as the focus for the abnormal neuronal discharges from the damaged brain tissue. These organic lesions include the following:

1. Neoplasms
2. Inflamed areas or abscesses
3. Sclerosis
4. Vascular formations or hematomas
5. Congenital malformations
6. Trauma
7. Other space-occupying lesions

Nursing Process
Assessment

Assessment of both subjective and objective data is important in the patient who is having a seizure (see Box 37-25).

Subjective data

1. Patient's understanding of the seizure disorder and what might be causing it
2. Awareness of precipitating factors
3. Presence of an aura
4. Postictal feelings
5. Presence of amnesia

An *aura* is defined as the set of symptoms that occurs before the seizure. An aura occurs in about 50% of all patients with *grand mal seizures* and usually includes a change in sensation or a change in affect. The exact character of the aura varies from person to person but may include numbness, flashing lights, dizziness, tingling of the arm, smells, or spots before the eyes. The patient may not be able to describe the aura precisely, but it gives conclusive evidence of the impending seizure and allows the patient to seek privacy and safety before it occurs.

During the postictal phase the individual is groggy and acts confused. Complaints of headache or muscular pain are common. A deep sleep usually follows. During this phase the pupils may remain dilated and plantar reflexes may be abnormal. After a variable period of time the patient awakens and is frequently unaware of the occurrence of the seizure. A dull headache and depression are common.

37-25

Observations to be made about a person having a seizure

Aura

Presence or absence; nature if present; ability of patient to describe it (somatic, visceral, psychic)

Cry

Presence or absence

Onset

Site of initial body movements; deviation of head and eyes; chewing and salivation; posture of body; sensory changes

Tonic and clonic phases

Movements of body as to progression; skin color and airway; pupillary changes; incontinence; duration of each phase

Relaxation (sleep)

Duration and behavior

Postictal phase

Duration; general behavior; ability to remember anything about the seizure; orientation; pupillary changes; headache; injuries present

Duration of seizure

Length from aura to relaxation phase

Level of consciousness

Length of unconsciousness if present

Presence of injury

Injury to mouth, lips, tongue, or soft tissues from seizure
Injury to extremities

37-26

Electroencephalogram (EEG)

Purpose

To provide evidence of focal or diffuse disturbances of brain function produced by organic lesions by measuring the electrical activity of the brain (Fig. 37-42).

Preparation of patient

No special preparation beforehand
Patient is encouraged to be quiet and rest before the procedure
Scalp and hair should be clean
Patient teaching
    Explain procedure
    Time: 1 hour or more
    Sensation: not painful—electrodes are applied to scalp with collodion

Procedure

1. Patient usually sits in a comfortable chair or lies on a cot with eyes closed. Testing is done in a special room where outside electrical activity is eliminated
2. Electrodes are fixed to the scalp, usually with collodion, in a set pattern to cover all scalp areas
3. The basic resting rhythm is affected by opening the eyes or altering attention
4. Recordings can be made while the patient is asleep or when sleep deprived
5. Comparisons are made of different patterns of the recordings

After procedure

Patient should be allowed to rest if tired
Patient should be assisted if necessary in washing hair and removing collodion from scalp

---

Objective data

1. Number of seizures occurring within a specific time
2. Behavior: signs of stress or fatigue
3. Character of seizure
4. Injuries sustained

Diagnostic tests

By far the most common test used to evaluate seizure disorders is the electroencephalogram (see Box 37-26). It is safe and noninvasive and allows for more specific diagnosis.

Data analysis: nursing diagnoses

Nursing diagnoses are determined from analysis of patient data. Possible nursing diagnoses for the person with seizures may include, but are not limited to, the following:

Diagnostic title	Possible etiologies
Anxiety	Threat/change in health status
Adjustment, impaired	Disability requiring change in lifestyle
Coping, ineffective individual	Situational crisis of diagnosis
Social isolation	Alteration in behavior during seizures
Oral mucous membrane, altered	Treatment with phenytoin
Injury, high risk for	Seizures
Knowledge deficit	Lack of exposure/recall
Noncompliance with medications	Treatment side effects

Planning: expected patient outcomes

Expected patient outcomes for the person with seizures may include, but are not limited to, the following:

1. Seizures are reduced or at least do not increase in severity or number.
2. Patient shows a low level of anxiety.
3. Patient shows social participation.

Table 37-8   **Anticonvulsants used to prevent seizures**

Drug	Use related to seizure type	Average daily dose	Toxic effects
Phenytoin sodium (Dilantin)	Grand mal, focal, psychomotor	0.4-0.6 g (divided dose)	Ataxia, vomiting, nystagmus, drowsiness, rash, fever, gum hypertrophy, lymphadenopathy
Phenobarbital (Luminal)	Grand mal, focal, psychomotor (adjunctive)	0.1-0.4 g (divided dose)	Drowsiness, rash
Primidone (Mysoline)	Grand mal, focal, psychomotor	0.5-2.0 g	Drowsiness, ataxia
Mephenytoin (Mesantoin)	Grand mal, focal, psychomotor	0.3-0.5 g	Ataxia, nystagmus, pancytopenia, rash
Ethosuximide (Zarontin)	Petit mal, psychomotor, myoclonic, akinetic	750-1500 mg	Drowsiness, nausea, agranulocytosis
Trimethadione (Tridione)	Petit mal	0.3-2.0 g (divided dose)	Rash, photophobia, agranulocytosis, nephrosis
Diazepam (Valium)	Status epilepticus, mixed	8-30 mg	Drowsiness, ataxia
Carbamazepine (Tegretol)	Grand mal, psychomotor	0.3-2.0 g	Rash, drowsiness, ataxia
Valproic acid (Depakene)	Petit mal, absence of seizures	5-35 mg/kg body weight (at least tid dosage)	Nausea, vomiting, indigestion, sedation, emotional disturbance, weakness, altered blood coagulation
Clonazepam (Clonopin)	Petit mal, akinetic, myoclonic	5-20 g	Grand mal seizures, drowsiness, ataxia, hypotension, respiratory depression

4. Patient remains free of traumatic injury.
5. Patient can describe medication to be taken, including action, side effects, toxic effects, and dosage schedule.
6. Patient can explain the importance of avoiding alcohol while taking anticonvulsant drugs.
7. Patient explains how to use available community resources.
8. Patient and significant other can explain the necessary measures to carry out if a seizure does occur.
9. Patient can explain the importance of taking medication regularly even when the seizures are controlled.
10. Patient wears medical alert tag.
11. Patient demonstrates a patent airway.

Implementation
Assisting with achievement of therapeutic goals
Medications

Treatment of patients with a seizure disorder almost always includes the use of one or more of the anticonvulsant drugs (see Table 37-8). The choice of medications depends on the type of seizure. Anticonvulsant medications act generally on the cerebral cortex and are not selective in acting on the part of the brain involved in abnormal neuronal discharges.

The dosages of anticonvulsant drugs are difficult to establish and regulate because of the high incidence of side effects and the toxicity of the drugs. The drug of choice is introduced in an average therapeutic dose, and the dose is increased until seizure control is reached. If toxicity is reached before control of the seizures, the dose is decreased to the previous nontoxic or tolerated dose. Additional secondary drugs may be introduced at this time to aid in seizure control.

Failure to take the prescribed medication or to take an adequate dose is often the cause of failure in treatment. Tests to determine the blood level of the anticonvulsant are helpful in providing an accurate check on the therapeutic and toxic levels of the medications taken.

Surgical treatment

Surgical treatment of seizures is becoming less common, but it may still be used in some cases in which medical therapy is not effective. *Cortical resection* is one surgical approach. It involves removal of the brain tissue in which the focus of electrical discharge is located. The localization of tissue must occur in a part of the brain that is easily accessible to surgery and that can be removed without leaving the person with a serious disability.

Another surgical approach involves *stereotactic* procedures using electrical stimulation. This technique is used to interrupt the pathways of seizure activity, to destroy the foci, or to alter the actions of the cortical nerve cells.

Interventions to achieve patient outcomes
Promoting adjustment and socialization

Because most persons with seizures do not have symptoms between attacks and because a majority of seizures can be controlled by medication, the person with seizures should be encouraged to lead as normal a life as possible. Until seizures are controlled, however, the person should avoid dangerous activities such as driving a car, working on or about machinery, or swimming. Once the person has achieved seizure control for a significant period and has learned the importance of taking the medication regularly

Nursing actions during a seizure

1. Never leave the person alone.
2. If patient is in upright position, lower to floor or bed and move adjacent articles and equipment away to prevent injury.
3. Loosen constricting clothing, especially around the neck.
4. Turn head to one side to aid with airway.
5. No effort should be made to restrain the person manually or with restraints.
6. If the jaws are not already clenched when seizure is first observed, a padded tongue blade may be inserted between the back teeth to prevent injury to the tongue and mouth tissues. The mouth should not be pried open—this may cause injury to the patient or to self.
7. Pad side rails if the patient is confined to bed or has seizures during sleep. Pillows should not be used for padding because of danger of suffocation.
8. Accurate observations should be made and recorded.

The patient with a seizure disorder

1. Use of medication, including side effects, dose, timing; reporting side effects to physician
2. Importance of avoiding the use of alcohol with anticonvulsants
3. Safety measures to avoid injury in case of seizures
4. Good oral hygiene if patient is taking phenytoin
5. Importance of adequate rest and diet
6. Importance of taking medication even when free of seizures
7. Community resources
8. Restrictions concerning driving
9. Importance of follow-up care
10. Importance of verbalizing feelings
11. Need to avoid excessive stress
12. Importance of wearing medical alert bracelet
13. Importance of not overprotecting self

and avoiding alcoholic beverages, these restrictions can be relaxed. Maintaining adequate rest and nutritional intake is also important. Family members need to be assisted to discuss their attitudes and feelings about the individual's illness.

The issue of driving a car is one that often poses a problem. Epilepsy does impose driver limitations. Usually 1 year without seizures should elapse before the person is eligible to drive and then only if seizures are completely controlled.

Promoting good oral hygiene

The patient who is taking Dilantin is especially prone to developing gingival hyperplasia. Good mouth care, utilizing a soft toothbrush, is essential. The teeth should be brushed in a gentle fashion to prevent excessive bleeding. Regular visits to the dentist are important.

Preventing injury

The primary goals of the nurse and family caring for a patient having a seizure are protection from injury and observation and recording of the seizure activity. Specific actions are listed in Box 37-27.

Facilitating learning

Teaching is an important part of the care of the patient with seizures. This includes the patient, as well as members of the family, who should learn to care for the person during and after a seizure. Involvement of the family or significant other during the hospitalization is essential. One of the more important things for the family to learn is the need to be calm and accept the family member's seizures.

Teaching for the patient with a seizure disorder includes the actions defined in Box 37-28.

Evaluation

As with other conditions, evaluation of the patient experiencing seizures is made using the feelings and input of the patient. Questions to consider may include the following:

1. Is the number of seizures decreased?
2. Is the patient verbalizing feelings?
3. Is the patient socializing with others?
4. Is the patient refraining from dangerous activity?
5. Can the patient explain daily routine that includes adequate rest?
6. Is the patient able to identify available community resources?
7. Is follow-up care occurring as prescribed?
8. Is the patient wearing a medical alert bracelet?
9. Is the patient taking the medication as prescribed?
10. Are blood levels of the prescribed anticonvulsants within normal limits?
11. Is the patient coping well?
12. Is the patient receiving regular dental care?

MYASTHENIA GRAVIS

Myasthenia gravis is a neuromuscular disease that affects the lower motor neurons and muscles. Excessive fatigue occurs along with weakness of muscles, especially those involved with the face, eyes, larynx, and pharynx and the process of respiration. The fatigue and weakness worsens with exercise and is improved with rest. It affects about 1 in 20,000 persons.

The cause of myasthenia is unknown, although it is thought to be an autoimmune disease. It characteristically starts between the ages of 20 and 30 or in late middle age. In younger persons, women are affected more than men, but in older persons men are affected to a greater extent. Familial occurrence is rare.[68]

Pathophysiology

No structural change in the muscle or nerve is observed in cases of myasthenia gravis. Nerve impulses fail to pass to muscles at the myoneural junction. It is not known

Comparison of myasthenia gravis and Eaton-Lambert syndrome

	Myasthenia gravis	Eaton-Lambert syndrome
Onset	Slow and insidious	Slow and insidious
Vision	Diplopia common	Diplopia not as common
Muscle involvement	Cranial nerves; arms and hands; trunk and lower limbs affected (difficulty with walking and sitting); distal muscles not as affected as proximal muscles	Muscles of trunk as well as those of pelvis and shoulder girdle are most commonly involved
Weakness	Weakness and generalized fatigue that comes on quickly	Increased weakness with exertion, but there may be temporary increase in muscle power at first

specifically why the motor nerve impulses fail to pass to the muscle and cause it not to contract. This is believed to be caused by a *decrease in the release of acetylcholine* from the presynaptic terminals or a *blockage of or a reduction in the number of postsynaptic membrane receptor sites.* It is known that circulating antibodies to the acetylcholine receptor (AChR) are present and are believed to cause the myasthenic weakness.

About 10% of patients with myasthenia have been found to have a thyoma, and nearly 70% have changes in the cellular structure of the thymus gland (usually hyperplasia). The role of the thymus gland in the pathophysiology of myasthenia gravis is unclear.

In severe cases, the respiratory muscles and bulbar cranial nerves may be involved, leading to severe respiratory infection and possible death. However, sensation is not lost and the involved muscles usually do not atrophy.

Nursing Process
Assessment
Subjective data
1. Patient's understanding of disease
2. Fatigue—when it occurs and where it occurs
3. Profound muscle weakness
4. Presence of diplopia
5. Difficulty in keeping eyelids open and mouth closed or chewing and swallowing
6. Effect of stress on the symptoms
7. Patient's perception of muscle weakness

Objective data
1. Documented muscle weakness on neurologic testing
2. Presence of ptosis of eyelids
3. Documented weight loss
4. Breath sounds
5. Muscle atrophy

Exacerbation of the disease occurs with upper respiratory infections, emotional tension, and menstruation. Because of the slow and insidious onset of myasthenia gravis and the occurrence of symptoms with stress, patients with this disease are sometimes misdiagnosed as suffering from neurosis or hysteria.

It is important to differentiate between myasthenia gravis and Eaton-Lambert syndrome, a condition associated with cancer that has many of the same symptoms as myasthenia gravis. Because the onset of Eaton-Lambert syndrome may precede the discovery of the cancer by months or years it is important that the patient be checked thoroughly for malignancy. *Cancers associated with Eaton-Lambert syndrome are* the following:

1. Oat cell carcinoma of the lung (most common)
2. Rectal carcinoma
3. Cancer of the stomach
4. Cancer of the prostate
5. Cancer of the breast

The clinical differences between myasthenia gravis and Eaton-Lambert syndrome are described in Box 37-29.

Diagnostic tests

Diagnosis of myasthenia gravis is partially made on the basis of EMGs that rule out other muscle disorders. A specific diagnostic test that is used is the edrophonium chloride (Tensilon) test. Edrophonium is a very short-acting anticholinesterase drug. The procedure for the test is as follows:

1. Edrophonium and normal saline are drawn up in separate syringes.
2. Each is injected intravenously separately.
3. It is important that the patient not be aware which solution is being given.
4. Increased strength in a predetermined muscle group with the administration of edrophonium is a positive test.

The results occur in 30 seconds to 1 minute and usually last only a few minutes.

A chest x-ray examination or CT scan of the chest may be done to determine the presence of a thyoma. The curare test may be done if all other tests are normal or questionable. Because curare causes respiratory paralysis, equipment and personnel to intubate the patient should be available. The curare test may be definitive when other tests are not.[68]

Data analysis: nursing diagnoses

Nursing diagnoses are determined from analysis of patient data. Possible nursing diagnoses for the person with myasthenia gravis may include, but are not limited to, the following:

Diagnostic title	Possible etiologies
Airway clearance, ineffective	Decreased energy/fatigue
Nutrition, altered: less than body requirements	Chewing or swallowing difficulties
Activity intolerance	Generalized weakness
Self-care deficit: bathing/ hygiene, dressing/ grooming	Intolerance to activity/ fatigue
Knowledge deficit	Lack of exposure/recall

Planning: expected patient outcomes

Expected patient outcomes for the person with myasthenia gravis may include, but are not limited to, the following:

1. Patient has a patent airway.
2. Patient demonstrates an effective pattern of breathing.
3. Patient maintains optimal nutrition.
4. Patient maintains an optimal level of mobility.
5. Patient demonstrates minimal self-care deficits.
6. Patient and family verbalize adequate knowledge of myasthenia gravis.
7. Patient can explain the action, side effects, and toxic effects of each anticholinesterase or cholinergic drug.
8. Patient can explain the reason for taking the medication at the exact time.
9. Patient can explain the need to monitor effects of medication on respiration, swallowing, and general muscle strength.
10. Patient can list drugs that act on the neuromuscular junction and are contraindicated.
11. Patient can explain the need to avoid overexertion and emotional tension.

Implementation
Assisting with achievement of therapeutic goals
Medications

Two medications that are used in myasthenia gravis are neostigmine (Prostigmin) and pyridostigmine (Mestinon). These drugs block the action of cholinesterase at the myoneural junction and allow acetylcholine to act. Atropine or other anticholinergic agents that block the effects of acetylcholine can be used to treat the side effects of neostigmine and pyridostigmine. Treatment is planned so that the patient receives the drug in the amount tolerated without side effects and yet is able to carry out activities essential for normal living. Usually, the patient is allowed to adjust the dosage. Ambenonium chloride (Mytelase) may also be given in doses of 10 to 25 mg orally 3 or 4 times daily. Corticosteroids such as prednisone are sometimes used as an adjunct to other drug therapy.

It is often difficult to distinguish between *myasthenic crisis* (too little drug) and *cholinergic crisis* (too much drug), because both conditions cause severe muscle weakness. Administering edrophonium (Tensilon) intravenously differentiates between the two conditions. A positive test (increase in strength) indicates underdosage of the drug. An increase in weakness is a sign of overdosage.

Interventions to achieve patient outcomes
Maintaining an effective airway

Respiratory complications are common for the patient with myasthenia gravis, and for this reason they are usually advised not to live alone. They are also cautioned to avoid crowds or other circumstances where infections are common. Upper respiratory infections are seen because patients may not have the energy needed to cough effectively and may develop pneumonia or airway obstruction. Aspiration is common. Many patients have airway equipment at home.

During acute episodes of the disease, the following are important:

1. Tracheostomy set at bedside, because respiratory status may change rapidly
2. Serial determinations of vital capacity, minute volumes, and tidal volumes

---

37-30

Patient Teaching

The patient with myasthenia gravis

1. Medications
   a. Importance of taking medication at time prescribed
   b. Dose individually determined and related to the activity of the person
   c. How to adjust dose to maintain muscle strength
   d. Side effects and how to monitor
   e. Medications to avoid
   f. Importance of not taking medications with fruit, tomato juice, coffee, or other medications
   g. Importance of not taking over-the-counter drugs without checking with physician
2. Respiratory care
   a. Avoid crowds during peak times for upper respiratory infections
   b. Eat only when sitting up
   c. Importance of seeking medical treatment at first sign of upper respiratory infection
3. Pattern of activity
   a. Activities planned around time of day when fatigue is lessened
   b. Importance of frequent rest periods
   c. Plan so that minimum amount of energy is used in activities that are essential to remaining relatively self-sufficient, and conserve energy for other activities the patient wishes to take part in
   d. Activity and exercise to tolerance should continue
   e. Need for diversional activities
   f. Independence and socialization encouraged
4. Nutritional concerns
   a. Importance of maintaining adequate nutrition
   b. Importance of eating only when sitting up
   c. Adequate fluid intake (at least 2,000 ml/ day)
5. Other considerations
   a. Importance of expressing fears
   b. Need to wear Medic-Alert tag
   c. How to avoid constipation

3. Suction as necessary
4. Nasogastric tube if swallowing is too dangerous (patient will not be able to cough to indicate if tube is in trachea, so careful assessment of the position of tube is important)
5. With severe impairment in respiratory function, the patient will probably require endotracheal intubation and ventilator assistance (see Chapter 24 for further discussion of the patient on mechanical ventilation)

Maintaining activity

Patients with severe symptoms of myasthenia gravis may be too weak to do anything for themselves. The nurse may have to turn and position the patient in addition to doing most of the other ADL. It is important to remember that the patient with myasthenia gravis will remain alert and will often be very frightened. Psychologic support and reassurance are essential.

Facilitating learning

The patient with myasthenia gravis often has a great deal of control over his/her medication schedule and can do much to prevent respiratory problems. A well-informed patient is more likely to stay healthy. Teaching should include the points listed in Box 37-30.

Evaluation

Evaluation of the patient with myasthenia gravis is important. Involving the patient in this process is essential. Questions to consider may include the following:

1. Is the patient free of respiratory infection?
2. Is mobility maintained at optimal levels?
3. Is the patient able to carry on ADL independently?
4. Is the patient taking medication as ordered?
5. Can the patient explain the action, time element, and side effects of the medication?
6. Does the patient know what drugs to avoid? (See Box 37-31)
7. Does the patient demonstrate knowledge of any necessary equipment?

INTERFERENCE WITH FUNCTION BECAUSE OF DEGENERATIVE DISEASES

The term *degenerative diseases* is used to refer to neurologic diseases in which there is a premature senescence of nerve cells, there is a known or suspected metabolic disturbance, or the cause of the disease is unknown. Included in this section are five such diseases. They are the following:

1. Multiple sclerosis
2. Parkinson's disease
3. Amyotrophic lateral sclerosis (ALS)
4. Alzheimer's disease
5. Neurofibromatosis (Von Recklinghausen's disease)

See Table 37-9 for a comparison of these five diseases.

37-31

Drugs to be avoided by persons with myasthenia gravis
1. Muscle relaxants
2. Barbiturates
3. Morphine sulfate
4. Tranquilizers
5. Neomycin (potentiates muscle weakness because of effect on myoneural junction)

Table 37-9   Comparison of degenerative neurologic diseases

Disease	Pathologic signs	Effect	Medical treatment
Multiple sclerosis	Multiple foci (patches) of nerve degeneration throughout the brain and spinal cord	Demyelination causes nerve impulses to be interrupted (blocked) or distorted (slowed)	No specific treatment Symptomatic treatment Judicious use of ACTH or corticosteroids
Parkinson's disease	Destruction of nerve cells of basal ganglia of brain	Decreased dopamine (neurotransmitter substance with anticholinergic effect)	Anticholinergic alkaloids Synthetic anticholinergic drugs Levodopa Carbidopa-levodopa Surgery in selected cases
Amyotrophic lateral sclerosis	Destruction of myelin sheath of motor neurons of lateral tracts of spinal cord and brain	Demyelination causes nerve impulses to be interrupted (blocked) or distorted (slowed)	No specific treatment Symptomatic and supportive care
Alzheimer's disease	Degeneration of neurofibrils and presence of plaque in brain	Destruction of neurons leading to impairments in intellectual functioning	No specific treatment Symptomatic and supportive care
Neurofibromatosis (Von Recklinghausen's disease)	Numerous fibromas of spinal or cranial nerves and skin, café au lait spots on the skin, and developmental anomalies	Tortuous interfacing of tissue cords that result in multiple tumors	No medical treatment except supportive care Tumors removed surgically Genetic counseling

Another degenerative disease is syringomyelia. This is a destruction of the gray and then white matter of the spinal cord that occurs as a result of the development of *syrinxes* (cysts filled with CSF). As a result, nerve pathways in the spinal cord are destroyed and nerve impulses are interrupted. This disease will not be discussed in further detail, but the nurse should be aware of it.

MULTIPLE SCLEROSIS

Etiology/Epidemiology

Multiple sclerosis is a common degenerative neurologic disease. At least 250,000 persons in the United States suffer from it.[76a] The cause remains unknown despite research. Several hypotheses have been advanced as to the cause:

1. Genetic—it has been found that relatives of persons with multiple sclerosis have a much higher incidence of the disease than the general population. Several studies have demonstrated an increased incidence of multiple sclerosis among siblings and even distant relatives. A person with an identical twin with the disease has a 20% risk of having the disease.[106]
2. Epidemiologic—the disease is rare between the equator and latitudes 30 to 35° north and south.[106] When they move to another region, they retain the same risk.
3. Viral—the serum and cerebrospinal fluid of patients with multiple sclerosis has been found to contain antibodies to many viruses, including measles, mumps, herpes simplex, and influenza.
4. Immunologic—most persons with multiple sclerosis have been found to have abnormalities of the spinal fluid indicative of autoimmune disease.

The onset of symptoms usually occurs between the ages of 20 and 40. The course of the disease is estimated to be 12 to 25 years. The highest number of persons with multiple sclerosis live in the Great Lakes area, the Pacific Northwest, and the north Atlantic states. There has been no evidence to suggest a sexual mode of transmission.

Pathophysiology

Multiple foci of demyelination are distributed randomly in the white matter of the brainstem, spinal cord, optic nerves, and cerebrum. During the demyelination process (primary degeneration), the myelin sheath and the sheath cells are destroyed, but there is early sparing of the axon cylinder. The outer myelin sheath destruction causes interruption or distortion of the impulse so that it is slowed or blocked. There is evidence of partial healing in areas of degeneration, which accounts for the transitory nature of early symptoms. In later stages the degeneration may extend to gray areas of the cord and limit healing. Although the outer surface of the brain appears normal, brain weight may be decreased and the ventricles may be enlarged.

Because of the wide distribution of areas of degeneration, the variety of signs and symptoms in multiple sclerosis is greater than in other neurologic diseases. It is a chronic, remitting, and relapsing disease. The majority of persons recover from their early episodes, with remissions lasting for a year or more. Exacerbations of multiple sclerosis may be aggravated or precipitated by fatigue, chilling, and emotional disturbances. In rare cases the disease may terminate in death within a few years of onset.

Nursing Process
Assessment

Early symptoms of multiple sclerosis are usually transitory. Many persons may be considered neurotic because of the wide variety and temporary nature of symptoms and the emotional instability produced by the disease. Subjective symptoms are important in making the diagnosis.

Subjective data

1. Patient's understanding of disease
2. Presence of eye problems
   a. Diplopia
   b. Scotomas (spots before the eyes)
   c. Blindness
3. Presence of weakness or numbness of part of the body such as hand
4. Presence of unusual fatigue
5. Presence of tremor
6. Presence of emotional instability
7. Presence of bowel and bladder problems
8. Presence of impotence in men
9. Loss of joint sensation and proprioception
10. Presence of vertigo

Objective data

1. Documented abnormalities in neurologic testing
   a. Nystagmus
   b. Scanning speech
   c. Muscle weakness and spasms
   d. Changes in coordination
   e. Spastic ataxic gait
2. Behavior: presence of euphoria, emotional, lability, mild depression
3. Urinary incontinence, frequency, or retention
4. Difficulty in swallowing
5. Intentional tremors of upper extremities

It is suspected that the presence of euphoria is caused by patient's attempts to reassure themselves that their condition is not serious. Motor signs associated with multiple sclerosis have UMN characteristics. Pain is not a common symptom.

Diagnostic tests

Examination of the cerebrospinal fluid usually shows elevated gamma globulin level and an increased white blood cell count. An electroimmunodiffusion determination is done. A CT scan may demonstrate enlargement of the ventricles. Cerebral atrophy is present in advanced disease.

Even in early stages of multiple sclerosis, abnormal visual and brainstem evoked potentials are present. The visual evoked response will show optic atrophy in the majority of cases. Evoked potentials are electrical measurements of physiologic maturation of the human nervous system. They provide information about the primary sensory areas of the cortex.

Data analysis: nursing diagnoses

Nursing diagnoses are determined from analysis of patient data. Possible nursing diagnoses for the person with multiple sclerosis may include, but are not limited to, the following:

Diagnostic title	Possible etiologies
Incontinence, total or urge	Neurologic dysfunction
Incontinence, bowel	Neuromuscular impairment
Nutrition, altered: less than body requirements or more than body requirements	Chewing or swallowing difficulties
Skin integrity, impaired, actual or high risk for	Immobility, mechanical forces
Activity intolerance	Generalized weakness
Mobility, impaired physical	Neuromuscular impairment
Self-care deficit: feeding, bathing/hygiene, dressing/grooming, toileting	Neuromuscular impairment
Pain	Immobility, spasticity
Adjustment, impaired	Disability requiring change in lifestyle
Knowledge deficit	Lack of information about MS

Planning: expected patient outcomes

Expected patient outcomes for the person with multiple sclerosis may include, but are not limited to, the following:

1. Patient has minimal complications because of urinary incontinence.
2. Patient remains free of infection.
3. Patient's bowel patterns are continent to the degree possible, and complications of any incontinence or constipation are minimal.
4. Patient maintains adequate nutrition.
5. Patient's skin is intact.
6. Patient maintains optimal mobility.
7. Patient has minimal deficits in self-care activities.
8. Patient has minimal discomfort.
9. Patient verbalizes a positive self-concept.
10. Patient demonstrates minimal anxiety.
11. Patient/family can verbalize knowledge of disease.
12. Patient can explain the action, side effects, and toxic effects of prescribed medications.
13. Patient can state plans for follow-up care.
14. Patient can state how to secure community help.

Implementation
Assisting with the achievement of therapeutic goals
Medications

At present there is no specific treatment for multiple sclerosis. Favorable results seem to occur with the use of adrenocorticotrophic hormone (ACTH) and the corticosteroids. Their efficacy remains controversial. Some physicians prefer oral prednisone or intramuscular or oral dexamethasone (Decadron). ACTH may be given intramuscularly or intravenously. The effects of ACTH and the steroids on the demyelinating process is unknown. It is known from testing that (1) nothing is gained from long-term treatment, and (2) some gain is possible from taking high doses of steroids at the start of an exacerbation, because the episode then seems to resolve more rapidly.

Interventions to achieve patient outcomes
Preventing bladder problems

Urinary frequency and urgency may respond to timed doses of propantheline bromide (Pro-Banthine). Prevention of urinary tract infection remains a problem, and such infections are a major cause of death. Cholinergic drugs such as bethanechol (Urecholine) may be helpful for the patient with atonic bladder. Oxybutynin chloride (Ditropan) is used to treat neurogenic bladder. It acts by exerting a direct antispasmodic effect on smooth muscles. Some patients are given prophylactic doses of medications such as trimethoprim and sulfamethoxazole (Bactrim, Septra) or nitrofurantoin (Macrodantin). Cystometric studies can be helpful in defining the specific bladder problem.[76a]

The patient should be encouraged to drink adequate fluids. Several glasses of cranberry juice a day may be helpful in decreasing urinary tract infection.

Preventing bowel complications

Constipation is common for patients who have multiple sclerosis. It is important that the diet include foods high in roughage, as well as adequate fluids. The use of prune juice may be helpful, as well as stool softeners that are prescribed by the physician. Laxatives should be used judiciously, so as not to cause dependence on them.

If bowel incontinence is a problem, assessment of the patient's usual bowel habits is important. A bowel training protocol may be instituted. See Chapter 31 for further discussion of this topic.

Maintaining adequate nutrition

A well-balanced diet with plenty of high-vitamin foods is important. Obesity should be avoided because it makes it more difficult for the patient to maneuver and to meet daily needs. High-fiber foods and prune juice may help reduce constipation.

Preventing skin breakdown

Many persons with multiple sclerosis have motor involvement that prevents them from moving about freely and changing position readily. Also, they may have sensory disturbances that affect how they sense pressure. As a result, decubiti can easily develop. Patients must be taught the importance of turning at least every 2 to 3 hours. Other devices such as air mattresses or special beds may also be helpful.

Promoting activity and mobility

Persons with multiple sclerosis should have a daily routine for rest and activity. They are usually advised to exercise regularly but never to the point of extreme fatigue. During an acute exacerbation, patients are often kept as quiet as possible, bed rest is maintained, and all activities are limited.

One side of the body is usually affected more than the other. The patient may learn to stabilize the gait by leaning

37-32

Nursing Research

Buelow J: A correlational study of disabilities, stressors and coping methods in victims of multiple sclerosis, *J Neurosci Nurs* 23(4):247-252, 1991.

Patients admitted to the hospital for an exacerbation of their multiple sclerosis were asked to identify the stressors in their daily lives. These 20 patients were also asked to identify the coping mechanisms they used to deal with the stressors. The Barthel scale was used to measure the overall stress, with the overall mean stress score for the 20 patients of 1.49 on a scale of 1 to 3. The most stressful items identified were feeling tired, inability to walk, and uncertainty about the future. The most common coping theme was self-reliance. Coping mechanisms used most frequently included a sense of humor and trying to learn more. No relationship was found between the degree of disability and stressors. A negative correlation was found between depression and optimistic coping. Uncertainty about the future and fatalistic coping were positively correlated.

37-33

Patient Teaching

The patient with multiple sclerosis

1. Use of medications, including side effects, dose, timing; importance of reporting side effects to physician
2. Importance of good fluid intake
3. Importance of spacing activities so that time is left for relaxation and fun activities
4. Range of motion exercises, as well as other exercises
5. Good, balanced diet
6. Emotional reactions of persons with multiple sclerosis
7. Safety factors to prevent injury
8. Positioning for prevention of decubiti
9. Importance of skin inspection
10. Importance of avoiding temperature extremes
11. Community resources and how to obtain them
12. Disease process
13. Compensatory techniques for visual problems

toward the uninvolved side. Having the foot slap forward in taking a step may sometimes be overcome by putting the heel down in a pronounced fashion and rolling the weight forward on the side of the foot.

The judicious use of passive and active exercises, when the person is not in acute exacerbation, can be useful in maintaining function. Drugs such as diazepam (Valium) and dantrolene sodium (Dantrium), as well as baclofen (Lioresal), have been used to prevent spasticity.

Effort is made to maintain activity and work or school as long as possible. Patients can be helped to plan their activities so that they may continue to function even when the disease is well advanced.

Controlling the environment

Hot baths should be avoided because the heat can increase weakness in the person with multiple sclerosis. Traveling in hot weather should be carefully planned to prevent travel during the warmest part of the day.

Promoting adjustment

Persons with multiple sclerosis need a peaceful, relaxed environment. They may have slowness of speech and slowness in the ability to respond. Members of the family may need help in understanding this problem and meeting it calmly. The person may have sudden explosive emotional outbursts of crying or laughing. Reminding the patient of something sad may stop the laughing, and holding the patient's mouth open may stop the crying. Box 37-32 discusses a research study of persons with multiple sclerosis.

Facilitating learning

Teaching is important for both the patient with multiple sclerosis and his/her significant others. In late stages of the disease all functions of care usually have to be assumed by someone other than the patient. Teaching needs are listed in Box 37-33.

Evaluation

Evaluation should include the patient and caregivers. Questions to consider may include the following:

1. Is the patient infection free?
2. Is elimination occurring without difficulty?
3. Is patient able to maintain weight at a desired level?
4. Is the skin free of pressure sores?
5. Is an exercise program being followed?
6. Can daily functions be accomplished?
7. Is discomfort kept to a minimum?
8. Does the patient verbalize a positive adjustment?
9. Is the patient's anxiety minimal?
10. Is the patient taking medication as ordered?
11. Can the patient explain the use of the medication?
12. Is the patient reporting for follow-up care?
13. Can the patient explain how community agencies may be of assistance?

PARKINSON'S DISEASE

Epidemiology

Parkinson's disease is one of the more common diseases of the nervous system. It is also referred to as idiopathic Parkinson's and paralysis agitans. The disease was first described in 1817 by James Parkinson. It affects both men and women in their middle and late years (50 to 70 years old). The mean age at onset is 60 years of age, and the prevalence of the disease increases with age. It has been increasing as a cause of mortality in the elderly in the past 20 years.[40] The incidence is about 130 per 100,000 population. It affects all races and classes of persons. The course of Parkinson's disease varies from person to person.

The cause of Parkinson's disease includes viral, toxic, vascular, and genetic etiologies, as well as some unknown factors. The characteristic symptoms are also sometimes found in arteriosclerotic patients, leading some to believe that arteriosclerosis may be a causative factor. Drug-in duced parkinsonian syndromes occur with drugs that interfere with the synthesis or storage of dopamine or interfere with the striatal dopamine receptors. These drugs include the following:

1. Reserpine (Serpasil)
2. Phenothiazines
3. Butyrophenones (e.g., haloperidol)

Pathophysiology

The pathologic process that occurs with Parkinson's disease is basically a *depigmentation* of the *substantia nigra of the basal ganglia.* The loss of neurons in the substantia is severe. Also, selective depletion of dopamine occurs and can be correlated with the degree of striatal degeneration. Without dopamine inhibitory influence is lost and excitatory mechanisms are unopposed.

Nursing Process
Assessment

Like many of ther other neurologic diseases, Parkinson's disease starts with subtle symptoms and progresses slowly. The person may not be able to recall the onset of symptoms.

Subjective data

1. Patient's understanding of disease
2. Complaints of fatigue
3. Presence of incoordination
4. Defects in judgment and emotional instability
5. Heat insensitivity

Objective data

1. Presence of tremor (pill-rolling motion of the fingers or resting tremor)
2. Muscular response to movement (bradykinesia)
3. Postural reflexes
4. Appearance of face (masklike facies)
5. Presence of drooling
6. Shuffling gait
7. Trunk forward extension
8. Sensory testing
9. Inability to carry out daily activities
10. Presence of dementia (in about 30% of cases)
11. Presence of constipation, sometimes severe
12. Abnormal swallowing
13. Presence of scaly erythematous eruptions of skin, particularly near the ears and eyebrows and in scalp and nasolabial folds

The tremor is the outstanding sign of Parkinson's disease. Two other frequent signs are muscular weakness with rigidity and loss of postural reflexes. It is essentially a problem of motion. Muscle rigidity prevents normal response and results in characteristic changes. These changes include a masklike appearance of the face and slowed, monotonous speech; drooling; shuffling gait that is propulsive and may not be able to be stopped until an obstruction is met; and moist and oily skin.

Diagnostic tests

No test is diagnostic of Parkinson's disease. The clinical examination and history, along with the response of the patient to administration of medication used to treat Parkinson's disease, confirms the diagnosis.

If there is a history of chronic dementia, the CT scan may show cerebral atrophy. The EEG may show minimal slowing, or it may be normal. Upper GI studies may show delayed emptying of the stomach and hypomotility.

Data analysis: nursing diagnoses

The list of nursing diagnoses for Parkinson's disease is the same as for multiple sclerosis (p. 1247)

Planning: expected patient outcomes

The expected patient outcomes for Parkinson's disease are the same as for multiple sclerosis (p. 1247).

Implementation
Assisting with achievement of therapeutic goals
Medications

Treatment for Parkinson's disease is palliative and symptomatic and depends on pharmacologic manipulation of the disease. The severity of symptoms and the presence of associated disease processes determine the drugs to be used. Particular drugs and their characteristics can be found in Table 37-10. These drugs have had a dramatic effect on the course of the disease. With proper medications many of the symptoms never develop.

After prolonged treatment with some of the drugs, there may be an increased appearance of side effects as well as a decrease in the effectiveness of the medication. It has been found helpful to admit some patients to the hospital for a *drug holiday,* during which all medications are withdrawn for a period of time. The medications are then restarted, and often much smaller doses are able to produce favorable results. *This type of drug holiday must take place in the hospital.* Complications such as aspiration pneumonia can occur because immobility, rigidity, and other symptoms will return when the drugs are withdrawn.[18]

Surgery

A surgical procedure has been used with some success in the treatment of selected patients with Parkinson's disease. It includes destroying portions of the globus pallidus (to relieve rigidity) or the thalmus (to relieve tremor) in the brain by stereotactic methods through the use of cautery, removal, or injection of alcohol. Operative techniques involving cooling or freezing with liquid nitrogen have been attempted with good results in selected cases. Medications used to control rigidity and tremor are discontinued several days preoperatively so that symptoms will be at their maximum during the surgery. Preoperative and postoperative care are the same as for the patient undergoing cranial surgery and will be discussed later in this chapter. Many patients cannot be treated surgically. Results seem best in younger patients with unilateral involvement following other diseases and who have marked tremor and rigidity.

A relatively new and still experimental treatment for Parkinson's disease is the adrenal medullary transplant. In this procedure tissue from the adrenal medulla is placed in contact with the substantia nigra with the hope of restoring the balance of dopamine and acetylcholine. The

Table 37-10 **Medications used in Parkinson's disease**

Medication	Action/effects	Side effects	Comments
Anticholinergic alkaloids Scopolamine hydrochloride Hyoscyamine sulfate	Act against cholinergic excitatory effects More effective in lessening muscle rigidity than in controlling tremor	Central and peripheral cholinergic actions Blurring of vision Dryness of mouth and throat Constipation Urinary retention or urgency Ataxia Dysarthria Mental disturbances	Optimal results depend on dosage that provides compromise between improvement and development of side effects
Synthetic anticholinergic drugs Trihexyphenidyl hydrochloride (Artane) Benztropine mesyulate (Cogentin) Procyclidine hydrochloride (Kemadrin) Biperiden hydrochloride (Akineton)	Some degree of CNS anticholinergic action, but incapable of restoring striatal balance	Same as above	Same as above
Antihistamine drugs Diphenhydramine hydrochloride (Benadryl)	Exert mild central anticholinergic properties	Sleepiness Dry mouth	Do not affect underlying process of Parkinson's disease
Levodopa	Assists in restoring striatal dopamine deficiency	Kidney, liver damage Nausea, vomiting Orthostatic hypotension Insomnia Agitation and mental confusion	Side effects common
Amantadine hydrochloride (Symmetrel)	Acts by blocking the reuptake and storage of catecholamines and allowing accumulation of dopamine in extracellular or synaptic sites	Mental confusion Visual disturbances Seizures	May not be effective for longer than 3 months
Carbidopalevodopa (Levodopa with inhibitor of the enzyme dopa decarboxylase)	Inhibitor limits metabolism of levodopa peripherally and provides more levodopa to brain	Same as levodopa	Fewer side effects than levodopa used alone

procedure is difficult because the patient undergoes three major surgeries at the same time: (1) stereotactic localization of the caudate nucleus, (2) craniotomy, and (3) laparotomy for the adrenalectomy. Results so far have been somewhat encouraging.[18]

Another new treatment approach for Parkinson's disease involves human fetal dopamine cell transplants. Beginning studies suggest that this procedure may be more effective than adrenal medullary transplants. The subject of using fetal tissue, however, is filled with controversy.

Interventions to achieve patient outcomes
Maintaining elimination

The patient with Parkinson's disease may feel urgency and hesitancy in voiding. Measures appropriate for the patient with multiple sclerosis also apply to those with Parkinson's disease. Fluids are forced to at least 2000 ml per day. Cranberry juice is encouraged to acidify urine. Medications such as methenamine mandelate may be prescribed.

Chronic constipation may be a real concern. The patient should be on a diet high in residue and roughage. Fluids are encouraged and stool softeners, suppositories, and prune juice are often helpful. Mild cathartics such as milk of magnesia are used if other measures are not helpful.

Maintaining adequate nutrition

Feeding the patient becomes a real problem when the disease is far advanced because of the danger of aspiration; aspiration pneumonia may be fatal. Unless the disease is well controlled by medication, drooling can be a problem and increases with general excitement. A bib can be used to protect the clothing during naps. When patients are dressed, garments with generous pockets for tissues will help them be less conspicuous and more comfortable.

Promoting activity and mobility

Special attention should be paid to posture. Lying on a firm bed without a pillow may help to prevent the spine rom bending forward. Lying in the prone position also helps. Holding the hands folded behind the back when walking may help to keep the spine erect and prevent the arms from falling stiffly at the sides. The tremor is often less apparent when persons are sitting in an armchair, because they can grip the arms of the chair and partially control the tremor in their hands and arms.

Facilitating learning

Teaching is important for the caregiver and the patient with Parkinson's disease. The teaching is the same as that for the patient with multiple sclerosis (p. 1248).

Evaluation

The evaluation of the care of the patient with Parkinson's disease is based on the expected patient outcomes and is the same as for the patient with multiple sclerosis (p. 1248).

AMYOTROPHIC LATERAL SCLEROSIS

Amyotrophic lateral sclerosis (ALS) is a degenerative motor neuron disease that affects upper or lower motor neurons lying within the brain or spinal cord or a combination of the two. At first, the characteristic disability involves atrophy of the muscles of the hands, forearms, and legs. In later stages of the disease all muscles are involved. It is sometimes called Lou Gehrig's disease because the famous New York Yankee baseball player died of ALS.

Epidemiology/Etiology

ALS affects men more than women and usually first appears in middle age, between the ages of 40 and 70. It also may occur in younger or older persons. There may be a familial element to the disease. Death usually occurs within 2 to 3 years from the time of diagnosis, but some patients may live 5 to 20 years.

The cause of ALS is unknown. Genetic or external agents, metabolic disturbances, inappropriate nutrition, and systemic infection or trauma have been suggested as possible causative agents.

Pathophysiology

In ALS the myelin sheaths are destroyed and replaced with scar tissue. There is direct involvement of the lateral tracts of the spinal cord, with possible involvement of the medulla and the ventral tracts, and loss of large motor neurons. The nerve impulses are distorted or blocked. Symptoms depend on which motor neurons are affected.

Nursing Process
Assessment
Subjective data

1. Patient's understanding of disease
2. Presence of fatigue
3. Dysphagia
4. Difficulty with tasks involving fine finger movements

Objective data

1. Inability to carry out ADL
2. Muscle testing on neurologic examination
3. Evidence of involvement of brainstem and medulla

4. Weight loss
5. Serum CPK elevation

In ALS progressive muscle weakness, atrophy, and fasciculations are present. Spasticity of the flexor muscles is common. With involvement of the brainstem and medulla dysphagia, dysarthria, jaw clonus, tongue fasciculations, and respiratory difficulty occur. As the disease progresses, disability relative to both upper and lower limbs occurs, and one side of the body becomes more involved. The person remains alert, and there is no sensory loss. Death usually occurs within 5 years of diagnosis because of respiratory problems or bulbar paralysis.

Diagnostic tests

Initial testing may include an EMG (p. 1231) to rule out other muscle disease. A muscle biopsy may also be helpful in establishing the diagnosis of ALS.

Data analysis: nursing diagnoses

The nursing diagnoses for the patient with ALS are the same as those for the patient with multiple sclerosis (p. 1247).

Planning: expected patient outcomes

The expected patient outcomes for ALS are the same as for multiple sclerosis (p. 1247).

Implementation
Assisting with achievement of therapeutic goals

Treatment is directed toward relieving the symptoms of the disease. Prostheses are often supplied to support the weakened muscles. As the disease progresses, respirations are affected. At this time constant nursing attention is required. Providing adequate nutrition to the patient is a real challenge, and a nasogastric or gastrostomy tube may be necessary. A cervical esophagostomy also may be used. In some cases, mechanical ventilation may be instituted, although this is an action that needs to be well considered by the patient and the family. Some patients may elect not to be placed on a respirator. Attention to prevention of skin breakdown and contractures is important.

Interventions to achieve patient outcomes
Maintaining function

Nursing interventions include assistance with ADL as limb defects occur. Emotional support is extremely important. Patients and their families should be involved in making decisions about the types of interventions that will be used as the disease progresses. Some patients will decide to use ventilators at home as respiratory muscles become involved, whereas other patients will decide not to use any supportive devices. Because the patient remains alert until death, nurses should remember that they are dealing with someone who is probably very afraid.

Evaluation

Because the outcomes in ALS are similar to those of multiple sclerosis, refer to that part of the chapter for the appropriate questions to consider (p. 1248). An additional reference question is whether the patient is maintaining his or her weight.

Clinical stages of Alzheimer's disease

Stage one
Mild mental impairment
Forgetfulness
Impairment in judgment
Decrease in initiative
Lack of spontaneity

Stage two
Confusion
Agitation
Irritability
Extreme restlessness
Incontinence of urine and stool
Need for constant supervision

Stage three
Total inability to care for self
Inability to communicate
Total incontinence

ALZHEIMER'S DISEASE

Alzheimer's disease is a degenerative disorder that affects the cells of the brain and causes impairment of intellectual functioning. It is recognized as the *most common cause of dementia in the older adult*. It affects men and women equally. Most newly diagnosed persons are in late middle age, but the disease has been documented in some persons as young as 40 years old.

One of the difficulties in making a definitive diagnosis of Alzheimer's disease is that evidence is often obtained only from an autopsy.

Pathophysiology

The changes in the brains of patients with Alzheimer's disease are visible in the cerebral cortex. The first change is the presence of microscopic "plaques" found in brain tissue. These plaques consist of a core surrounded by strands of fiberlike material. In addition, there is degeneration of some of the small fibers (neurofibrils) that run through the body of the nerve cells. These changes were first discovered in 1907 by the German neurologist Alzheimer.[24]

Nursing Process
Assessment
Subjective data

1. Patient's understanding of disease
2. Mental status part of neurologic examination
3. Onset of symptoms

Objective data

1. Inability to carry on ADL
2. Behavior: evidence of agitation, restlessness
3. Presence of incontinence

The patient with Alzheimer's disease goes through three rather distinct stages. These stages are described in Box 37-34.

The diagnosis of Alzheimer's disease is made after ruling out conditions in which there is memory loss. These include the following diseases:

1. Pernicious anemia
2. Drug reactions
3. Hormonal imbalances
4. Depression
5. Drug or alcohol abuse
6. Brain tumor
7. Chronic meningitis
8. Head trauma
9. Pick's disease
10. Parkinson's disease with dementia

The signs and symptoms of Alzheimer's disease occur progressively, but the rate at which they occur varies between individuals. In a few cases, the decline may be very rapid, but in most cases deterioration is gradual. Cause of death is often pneumonia or other infections.

One author cites *four* stages involved with Alzheimer's disease[24].

Stage 1—mild memory lapses, difficulty with attention span, little interest in immediate surroundings or personal affairs

Stage 2—obvious short-term memory lapses, great hesitancy in verbal responses with confabulation to hide memory problems, disoriented to time, frequent losses of objects

Stage 3—disintegration of personality; disoriented to self, time, and place; apraxia; wandering behavior

Stage 4—terminal stage with severe physical and mental deterioration, incontinence, loss of ability to communicate, no recognition of family or self, swallowing problems

Diagnostic tests

No diagnostic test is specific for Alzheimer's disease. A CT scan is used to rule out other abnormalities. Often neuropsychologic testing can reveal characteristic changes in the ability to think. A family history of Alzheimer's aids in the diagnosis.

Data analysis: nursing diagnoses

The possible nursing diagnoses for the patient with Alzheimer's disease are the same as for the patient with multiple sclerosis (p. 1247), with the following additions:

Diagnostic title	Possible etiologies
Injury, high risk for	Sensory/motor deficits
Sleep pattern disturbance	Confusion
Violence, high risk for: self-directed or directed at others	Sensory-perceptual alteration

The violence that sometimes occurs in the patient with Alzheimer's disease occurs most often when the patient does not understand what is happening or what nursing care is being done. It is not an intentional harmful act but an effort to avoid that which is not understood.

Planning: expected patient outcomes

The expected outcomes for the patient with Alzheimer's disease are the same as those for the patient with multiple sclerosis with the addition of:

1. Injury and violence are avoided.
2. Accommodations are made to manage sleep pattern disturbances.

One difference between the two diseases is that in many cases the person with Alzheimer's disease is mentally incompetent, so that the caregiver needs to have major involvement in planning for the outcomes. The patient may not be able to have real input into them.

Implementation

Assisting with achievement of therapeutic goals

No treatment can cure, reverse, or stop the progression of Alzheimer's disease. Nursing care is directed toward maintaining nutrition, continence, hydration, and safety. Emotional support of both the patient and family is important. Appropriate drugs can sometimes be used to lessen anxiety, agitation, and unpredictable behavior.

Interventions to achieve patient outcomes
Preventing injury

One large area for intervention concerns safety. Because of forgetfulness, patients with this condition often do dangerous things. This includes walking outside without appropriate clothing, turning on burners, getting lost, and setting things on fire. The family must make plans to protect the patient from these hazards. This includes removing burner controls from the stove at night, double-locking all doors and windows, and keeping the person under supervision at all times.

Adapting to sleep pattern disturbances

One very frustrating part of Alzheimer's disease is that many of the patients sleep for only short periods of time and are awake most of the night. This must be worked out if the caregiver is to get any rest.

Preventing violence

The violence that sometimes occurs in the patient with Alzheimer's disease occurs most often when the patient does not understand what is happening or what nursing care is being given. It is not an intentional harmful act but an act to avoid that which is not understood.

Efforts to control this violence center most often on controlling the environment. It is important to approach the patient with calmness and unhurried motions. Excessive stimulation is kept to a minimum. Routines should not be changed unless absolutely necessary. *Medications and restraints should be used only when all other approaches have failed.*

Evaluation

Evaluation of the patient with Alzheimer's disease focuses on the patient outcomes. Refer to the evaluation section for multiple sclerosis for appropriate questions to ask (p. 1248). Additional questions to consider may include the following:

1. Is the patient safely carrying out daily activities?
2. Has violence been avoided?
3. Is caregiver getting sufficient rest?

NEUROFIBROMATOSIS

Neurofibromatosis is a genetic disorder transmitted as an *autosomal dominant trait* by either parent. It is also called *multiple neuroma* or *neuromatosis*.

The disease affects one of every 3,000 births and can occur with spina bifida, meningocele, or seizures. About half of the patients with neurofibromatosis have no family history of the disease. Malignant degeneration occurs in a small number of cases, and mental retardation occurs in about one tenth of persons affected with the disease. Men are more commonly affected than women. The clinical symptoms usually appear in later childhood or adolescence and continue to develop with advancing age.

Neurofibromatosis is characterized by the following:
1. Numerous fibromas of spinal or cranial nerves and skin.
2. Café au lait spots on the skin.
3. Developmental disorders of bone, muscle, and viscera.

Neurofibromatosis can be classed as *central* (affecting the intraspinal and intracranial nervous system), *peripheral* (primarily affecting peripheral nerves), or *visceral* (involvement of the viscera and autonomic nervous system).

Pathophysiology

With neurofibromatosis there is proliferation of *fibroblasts*, or *Schwann cells*. This results in interlacing of tissue cords to form tumors in multiple areas. The size of the tumors varies from very small to several centimeters in size. The majority of the tumors occur as nodules along the course of involved nerves. Superficial dermal tumors may also occur, mainly over the trunk; these are asymptomatic. Other tumors such as meningiomas and glioblastomas may also occur.

Café au lait spots are composed of melanin located on the epidermis of the skin. They are pale brown macules, usually uniform in color and round or oval and range in size from 0.5 to 15 cm in diameter. The presence of 5 or more spots that are at least 1.5 cm in diameter is called *Crowe's sign* and is considered sufficient evidence to make the diagnosis of neurofibromatosis. The macules are usually found in the axilla, over the trunk, and over the pelvis.

Nursing Process
Assessment
Subjective data

1. Complaints of facial numbness or weakness
2. Family history of disease
3. Onset of symptoms
4. Understanding of the disease

Objective data

1. Presence of multiple cutaneous neurofibromas
2. Presence of café au lait spots
3. Presence of associated problems, including endocrine or skeletal
4. Presence of visual loss or deafness
5. Limitations in ADL

Diagnostic tests

Analysis of the cerebrospinal fluid of patients with neurofibromatosis will show elevated protein levels. A myelogram will indicate whether spinal cord tumors are present, and the CT scan will be used to determine whether intracranial tumors are present. Skull films may be used to determine if cerebral tumors have caused bone erosion.

Data analysis: nursing diagnoses

Nursing diagnoses are determined from analysis of patient data. Possible nursing diagnoses for the person with neurofibromatosis may include, but are not limited to, the following:

Diagnostic title	Possible etiologies
Anxiety	Threat/change in health status
Body image disturbance	Change in body appearance
Knowledge deficit	Lack of exposure/recall
Pain	Immobility

If the patient suffers the effects of a spinal cord tumor or brain tumor, the nursing diagnoses applicable to those diagnoses will apply. The reader is referred to the section "Interference with Function because of Tumors" in this chapter (p. 1285).

Planning: expected patient outcomes

Expected patient outcomes for the person with neurofibromatosis may include, but are not limited to, the following:

1. Patient expresses minimal anxiety.
2. Patient verbalizes a positive self-concept.
3. Patient maintains social contacts.
4. Patient can verbalize knowledge of the disease and symptoms to watch for.
5. Patient has minimal discomfort.

Implementation
Assisting with the achievement of therapeutic goals

The care of the patient with neurofibromatosis consists mainly of excision of the tumors. There is no medical treatment known to be effective. If the patient develops increased intracranial pressure, monitoring may be indicated. A shunt may be done if hydrocephalus is present.

Supportive care includes genetic counseling and psychosocial support.

The patient should be encouraged to live as normal a life as possible. This includes interacting with others. If the disease causes deformities, these should be discussed openly and the patient is encouraged to verbalize feelings about these. Counseling may be helpful to handle anxiety or feelings of low self-esteem.

Discomfort caused by the disease should be managed by non-narcotic analgesics if at all possible. The reader is referred to the section earlier in this text on neurologic pain (p. 1215).

Interventions to achieve patient outcomes
Facilitating learning

Teaching for the patient with neurofibromatosis includes education about the disease, as well as its hereditary nature.

Evaluation

Evaluation of the patient with neurofibromatosis considers how the patient is able to function within the confines of the disease. Questions to consider include the following:

1. Is the patient verbalizing minimal anxiety?
2. Is the patient verbalizing a positive self-concept?
3. Is the patient involved socially with other people?
4. Is the patient knowledgable about the disease?
5. Is the patient free of pain?

INTERFERENCE WITH FUNCTION BECAUSE OF VASCULAR CONDITIONS

Interference with function because of vascular conditions is common in neurologic nursing. In this section of the chapter the following two conditions will be discussed:

1. Cerebrovascular accident
2. Intracranial hemorrhage

CEREBROVASCULAR ACCIDENT

Cerebrovascular accident (CVA) is the most common disease of the nervous system and is ranked as the third leading cause of death in the United States. Approximately 200,000 deaths occur annually, with another 200,000 persons having residual effects. Stroke affects persons in all age groups, but the greatest number occurs in persons between 75 and 85 years of age. In this section, the term cerebrovascular accident (CVA) will be discussed as a general term. Most neurologists and neurosurgeons, however, refer more specifically to the cause of the CVA. These causes are as follows:

1. Thrombosis
2. Embolism
3. Hemorrhage (discussed on p. 1261)

The medical and nursing care may differ for each, depending on the specific cause (see Box 37-35). Stroke is another term used when referring to CVA; clinically, stroke refers to the sudden and dramatic development of focal neurologic deficits.

CVAs can be precipitated by many underlying factors and are frequently associated with other chronic diseases that cause vascular problems. These include heart disease, hypertension, kidney disease, peripheral vascular disease, and diabetes mellitus. Other risk factors for stroke include obesity, high serum cholesterol, cigarette smoking, stress, and a sedentary lifestyle. Women who use oral contraceptives are also at increased risk. The presence of more than one risk factor increases the risk of stroke and hemiplegia. See Box 37-36 for comparison of right and left hemiplegia.

Pathophysiology

The brain is very dependent on oxygen and has no reserve oxygen supply. When anoxia occurs, as in CVA, cerebral metabolism is promptly altered, and cell death and permanent damage can occur within 3 to 10 minutes. Any condition that alters cerebral perfusion will cause hypoxia or anoxia. Hypoxia first leads to cerebral ischemia. Short-term ischemia (less than 10 to 15 minutes) causes temporary deficits but no permanent deficits. Long-term ischemia causes permanent cell death and results in cerebral infarction, with accompanying cerebral edema.

The type of permanent focal deficits will depend on the area of the brain that has been affected. The area of the

Conditions causing CVA

Thrombosis

Atherosclerosis in intracranial and extracranial arteries

Adjacency to intracerebral hemorrhage

Arteritis caused by collagen (autoimmune) disease or bacterial or arteritis

Hypercoagulability such as in polycythemia

Cerebral venous thromboses

Embolism

Valves damaged by rheumatic heart disease (RHD)

Myocardial infarction

Atrial fibrillation (this arrhythmia causes variable emptying of left ventricle; blood pools, and small clots form, and then at times the ventricle will be emptied completely with release of small emboli)

Bacterial endocarditis and nonbacterial endocarditis causing clots to form on endocardium

Hemorrhage

Hypertensive intracerebral hemorrhage

Subarachnoid hemorrhage

Rupture of aneurysm

Arteriovenous malformation

Hypocoagulation (as in patients with blood dyscrasias)

Generalized hypoxia

Severe hypotension, cardiopulmonary arrest, or severe depression in cardiac output caused by arrhythmias

Localized hypoxia

Cerebral artery spasms associated with subarachnoid hemorrhage

Cerebral artery vasoconstriction associated with migraine headaches

---

brain affected depends on which cerebral vessels are involved. The vessel most commonly affected is the middle cerebral artery; the second most commonly affected is the internal carotid artery. Permanent focal deficits may be unknown when the patient is first seen because of generalized cerebral ischemia that may later resolve.

Cerebral thrombosis

Thrombosis is the most common cause of a CVA, and the *most common cause of cerebral thrombosis is atherosclerosis*. Additional disease processes commonly found with thrombi are hypotension and other types of vascular injury such as arteritis. CVA secondary to thrombosis is seen most often in the 60- to 90-year-old group. Thrombi usually occur in larger vessels and are associated with damage to the vessel wall at the point where the occlusion occurs. The internal carotid arteries are a common source of thrombi.

The onset of symptoms of CVA secondary to thrombosis tends to occur during sleep or soon after arising. This is thought to be related to the fact that elderly persons have decreased sympathetic activity, and recumbency causes a lowering of blood pressure, which can lead to brain ischemia. These persons often also have postural hypotension and poor reflex response to changes in position. Neurologic signs and symptoms very frequently worsen for the first 48 hours after thrombosis.

Cerebral embolism

Embolism is the second most common cause of CVA. Patients who have CVAs secondary to embolism are usually younger, and most commonly the emboli originate from a thrombus in the heart (mural thrombi). The myocardial thrombus is most commonly caused by rheumatic heart disease with mitral stenosis and atrial fibrillation.

Emboli usually affect small vessels and are commonly found at points of bifurcation where the vessels narrow. They most frequently occur in the middle cerebral artery. Another type of emboli is called septic and originates from bacterial endocarditis.

Comparisons of left and right hemiplegia

	Left hemiplegia	Right hemiplegia
Language	Usually intact	Receptive or expressive aphasia in varying degrees
Speech	Dysarthria	Dysarthria
Sensation	Left sensory loss Left homonymous hemianopsia	Right sensory loss Right homonymous hemianopsia
Perception	Decreased awareness of left side of body Other perceptual problems	Normal awareness of right side of body
Movement	Left-sided paralysis or paresis Apraxia	Right-sided paralysis or paresis Less often apraxic
Behavior	Impaired judgment Increased emotional lability	Judgment intact Increased emotional lability
Memory	Deficit of new spatial information	Deficit of new language information

Transient ischemic attack

The term *transient ischemic attack* (*TIA*) refers to transient cerebral ischemia with temporary episodes of neurologic dysfunction. The neurologic dysfunction can be profound with complete loss of consciousness and loss of all sensory and motor function, or there may only be focal deficits. *The most common deficit is contralateral weakness of lower face, hands, arms, and legs, transient dysphasia, and some sensory impairment.* Ischemic attacks may occur over days, weeks, or months—between attacks the neurologic examination is normal. *TIAs most commonly precede cerebral thrombotic attacks.* They can be caused by any of the causes of CVA.

The *major importance of TIAs is that they warn the patient and health care professional of the existence of an underlying pathologic condition.* At least one third of patients who have TIAs will have a CVA in 2 to 5 years. A person with a TIA needs to be aggressively assessed to determine if preventive measures can be taken.

Nursing Process
Assessment
Subjective data

1. Patient's understanding of disease or symptoms
2. Characteristics of onset of symptoms
3. Presence of headache—nature and location
4. Any sensory deficits
5. Visual ability—presence of diplopia, blurred vision
6. Ability to think clearly
7. Any other concomitant symptom

Objective data

1. Motor strength—paresis or plegia is common
2. Change in level of consciousness, including unconsciousness
3. Signs of increased intracranial pressure
4. Respiratory status
5. Ability to verbalize—presence of aphasia

The exact clinical picture varies depending on the area of the brain affected. The most common focal signs and symptoms are caused by disruption of flow through the midcerebral artery. These symptoms include the following:

1. Contralateral paralysis or paresis
2. Contralateral sensory loss
3. Sensory and motor loss most noticeable in face, neck, and upper extremities
4. Dysphasia or aphasia; occurs if dominant hemisphere is affected (left hemisphere in right-handed persons and most left-handed persons)
5. Spatial-perceptual problems, changes in judgment and behavior, neglect of paralyzed side, and inability to recognize paralyzed extremity as own (*anosognosia*) if nondominant hemisphere is affected
6. Contralateral *homonymous hemianopsia*

Aphasia is a disorder of language caused by damage to the speech-controlling areas of the brain. It includes all areas of language, including speech, reading, writing, and understanding.[42,88,89] These abnormalities can occur in a variety of ways as follows:

1. *Sensory aphasia*—inability to comprehend spoken word (also called receptive aphasia)
2. *Motor aphasia*—inability to use the symbols of speech (also called expressive aphasia)
3. *Global aphasia*—inability to understand the spoken word, as well as to speak[88,89]

Diagnostic tests

A lumbar puncture (p. 1212) is usually performed and may reveal increased spinal fluid pressure. If the CVA is caused by hemorrhage, blood will be present in the spinal fluid. The CT scan may show an area of decreased density. The MRI scan will visualize this pathology also. A brain scan can demonstrate diminished perfusion.

After TIAs, a cerebral angiogram may be used to discover blocked or occluded vessels. In some cases a digital subtraction angiogram (DSA) is used instead. See Boxes 37-37 and 37-38 for details of the procedure.

Data analysis: nursing diagnoses

Nursing diagnoses are determined from analysis of patient data. Possible nursing diagnoses for the person with a stroke may include, but are not limited to, the following:

Diagnostic title	Possible etiologies
Mobility, impaired physical	Perceptual/cognitive impairment
Nutrition, altered: less than body requirements	Chewing or swallowing difficulties
Swallowing, impaired	Neuromuscular impairment
Activity intolerance	Generalized weakness
Incontinence, bowel	Neuromuscular impairment
Incontinence, urge or total	Neurologic dysfunction/disease
Disuse syndrome, high risk for	Immobility, weakness
Injury, potential for	Sensory/motor deficits
Adjustment, impaired	Disability requiring change in lifestyle
Sensory/perceptual alteration	Altered sensory reception/ transmission/integration
Self-care deficit: feeding, bathing/hygiene, dressing/grooming, toileting	Neuromuscular impairment
Communication, impaired verbal	Aphasia
Knowledge deficit	Lack of exposure/recall

Planning: expected patient outcomes

Expected patient outcomes for the person who has had a stroke may include, but are not limited to, the following:

1. Patient's skin is intact.
2. Patient can explain the importance of frequent position changes and can demonstrate such positioning.
3. Patient or caregiver can demonstrate exercises to maintain function.
4. Patient can maintain an adequate nutritional status.
5. Patient's swallowing is intact.
6. Patient has minimal complications as a result of incontinence.
7. Patient's continence is improved.
8. Patient remains free of traumatic injury.
9. Patient verbalizes minimal anxiety.

37-37

Cerebral arteriogram (angiogram)

Purpose
To visualize the cerebral arterial system by injecting radiopaque material. Allows detection of
arterial aneurysms, vessel anomalies, ruptured
vessels, and displacement of vessels by mass
lesions

Preparation of patient
1. Patient is given clear liquids morning of procedure.
2. Patient must be assessed for allergy to iodine.
3. If femoral approach is to be used, it is helpful
   to assess and mark the locations of the bilateral pedal pulses.
4. If the carotid artery is used, the neck circumference is measured as part of the baseline
   data.
5. Sedation may be given the night before and
   just before the procedure.
6. If the femoral approach is used, the groin site
   may be shaved the night before.
7. Immediately before the procedure, baseline vital signs, pulses, and neurologic checks should
   be done and recorded.
8. Patient teaching
   a. Explain procedure.
   b. Time: approximately 2 to 3 hours.
   c. Sensation: some discomfort in lying still for
      several hours. At the time of dye injection,
      most patients complain of feeling extremely
      hot and seeing flashes of light.

Procedure
1. Patient is positioned supine on the x-ray table.
2. Local anesthetic is used to anesthetize the area
   of puncture site.
3. Catheter is introduced percutaneously.
   a. In a four-vessel study, catheter is inserted
      into the femoral, innominate, carotid, and
      vertebral arteries.
   b. Each vessel is injected with the contrast
      dye as serial x-ray films are taken.
   c. Carotid or vertebral vessels may be used
      directly.
4. Catheter is withdrawn and pressure is applied
   to puncture site for at least 5 minutes.

After procedure
1. Patient is usually kept in bed overnight.
2. Vital signs are checked frequently (may be as
   often as every 15 minutes for a period of several hours), as well as neurologic checks with
   each vital sign check.
3. Site of puncture is assessed frequently for presence of hematoma.
   a. Femoral: check pulses distal to site for evi-
      dence of arterial occlusion.
   b. Carotid: check for difficulty breathing or
      swallowing; measure neck girth frequently.
   c. Dye used in angiogram may raise intracra-
      nial pressure and cause decreased extrem-
      ity strengths or change in
   d. Level of consciousness.

37-38

Digital subtraction angiography (DSA)

Purpose
To identify abnormalities of the cerebrovascular
system, using a process that removes overlying
structures in an image, so that the clinically significant details can be displayed with enhanced
visibility.

Preparation of patient
1. Permit must be signed.
2. Food may be restricted before procedure.
3. Patient should be asked about allergy to iodine.
4. Patient teaching
   a. Explain procedure.
   b. Time: approximately 45 to 60 minutes
   c. Sensation: some discomfort associated with
      the start of the IV. Injection of the dye may
      be uncomfortable. Some patients may find
      need to lie still uncomfortable.

Procedure
1. Patient is positioned supine on the x-ray table.
2. Local anesthetic may be used to anesthetize
   the area of puncture site.
3. Catheter is introduced into vein, usually in the
   arm for cerebral studies.
4. Dye is injected as films are taken.
5. Catheter is withdrawn.

After procedure
1. Vital signs are checked on return to floor.
2. Circulatory status of arm is assessed.
3. Injection site is checked for presence of hematoma.
4. Usually no activity restrictions—procedure
   can be done on an outpatient basis.
5. The computer performs the subtraction, a process that removes underlying structures in an
   image, so that the clinically significant details
   can be displayed with enhanced visibility.

10. Patient has minimal problems because of altered verbal communication.
11. Patient develops alternative means of communication.
12. Patient safely compensates for visual field cuts, perceptual, motor, and sensory losses.
13. Patient shows optimal ability to manage activities of daily living and home maintenance.
14. Patient or caregiver can explain medication regimen—side effects, times, doses, and route.
15. Patient can state plans for follow-up care.
16. Patient has an effective breathing pattern.
17. Patient has minimal discomfort.

Implementation

Assisting with achievement of therapeutic goals: care in the initial phase

Goals in the initial phase are directed toward survival needs and preventing further brain damage. Care must take into account that some patients may be unconscious. Neurologic assessment is performed at regular intervals to detect changes in status, as well as any complications. Any indication of rising intracranial pressure should be reported at once. Drugs to reduce intracranial pressure, such as dexamethasone (Decadron) may be given. The patient may have an intracranial monitoring device in place. See p. 1225 for a description of these devices.

The use of anticoagulants is controversial. In an attempt to prevent further thrombosis or emboli, heparin may be given if it is certain that the cause of the CVA is cerebral thrombosis or emboli and not cerebral hemorrhage.

Interventions to achieve patient outcomes: care in the acute phase

Goals for the care in the acute phase are directed toward preventing complications from the original CVA, from the immobility and dependency it causes, and from the loss of function caused by focal deficits.

Promoting mobility

Because the CVA frequently results in some paralysis, refer to p. 1228 for a discussion of the care of the person with loss of motor function.

Maintaining adequate nutrition

Fluids may be restricted for the first few days after a CVA in an effort to prevent edema of the brain. In patients who are comatose or who have swallowing difficulties, it may be necessary to use intravenous fluids, or a nasogastric tube may be inserted and tube feedings started. When patients are more alert, food and fluids are offered in small amounts. Returning as soon as possible to a regular diet and a normal fluid intake is desirable.

Promoting activity

Rest and quiet are important even if the CVA has not been serious enough to cause complete loss of consciousness. The length of time the patient remains in bed depends on the type of CVA and the judgment of the physician in regard to early mobilization.

Prevention of joint deformity is initiated during the acute stage. This includes positioning of affected limbs in anatomic position and ROM exercises. There should be a regular schedule for turning the patient to avoid the danger of circulatory stasis, hypostatic pneumonia, and decubitus ulcers.

Maintaining elimination

Urinary output should be noted carefully and recorded for several days after a CVA. Retention of urine may occur, but it is more likely that the patient will be incontinent. If urinary incontinence occurs, the patient should be told that control of elimination should improve day by day. Offering a bedpan or urinal immediately after meals and at other regular intervals is a start to bladder training. A retention catheter may be used for the first several days. In the male patient who is not retaining urine, an external catheter may be very helpful.

Fecal incontinence also is a fairly common occurrence after a CVA. Some patients develop constipation, and impaction can develop rapidly. Elimination must be noted carefully because diarrhea may develop in the presence of an impaction, thus causing it to go unnoticed. Suppositories such as bisacodyl (Dulcolax) may be prescribed, along with stool softeners. Warm oil–retention enemas are sometimes given when impactions occur. The patient must be cautioned not to strain at the stool (valsalva maneuver). The patient also usually needs assistance in getting on and off the bedpan. Side rails that can be held onto while turning or a trapeze that can be reached with the unaffected arm and hand will help the patient move independently.

Interventions to achieve patient outcomes: care in the rehabilitation phase

The greatest challenge for the nurse in care of the patient who has had a CVA comes after the patient is past the point of danger, because then the long, slow process of learning to use whatever abilities remain or can be relearned must be faced. Also, adjustments to limitations must be faced and made if meaningful life is to continue.

The nurse is an important member of the rehabilitation team. Three nursing goals are:
1. Prevention of further impairment
2. Maintenance of existing abilities
3. Restoration of as much function as possible

Knowledge of the physical arrangements for after-hospital care is important in setting priorities and planning care.

Promoting return of function

Return of motor impulses and movement in involved extremities occurs in stages. These stages can last from hours to months. Recovery may also halt at a specific stage and progress no further. Brunnstrom has defined these recovery stages in degrees of *synergy*. *Synergy has been defined as muscles acting together as a bound unit in stereotyped movement patterns.* See Box 37-39 for these stages.

Return of motor function and impulses is significant for the future use of the affected part but presents new problems. Muscles that draw the limbs toward the midline become very active, and the arm may be held tightly adducted against the body. The affected lower limb may be held inward and adducted to, or even beyond, the midline. Muscles that draw the limbs into flexion are also stimu-

Recovery stages

Flaccidity	No voluntary motion, lack of muscle tone
Partial synergy	Muscle tone develops and muscles contract either voluntarily or with spasticity. Patient can move extremities in part of synergy pattern.
Synergy	Spasticity moderate to severe. Patient can move joints through all or most of synergy pattern.
Breaking out of synergy	Spasticity decreased. Patient can perform combinations of movements that are out of synergy.
Partially isolated	Less influence of spasticity. Movement combinations are less like stereotyped patterns.
Isolated	Near normal movement with good control of voluntary movement and little spasticity.

37-39

lated, with the result that the heel is lifted off the ground, the heel cord shortens, and the knee becomes bent. In the arm, flexor muscles draw the elbow into the bent position, the wrist is flexed, and fingers are curled in palmar flexion.

Persistent nursing efforts must be directed toward prevention of further impairment. It is important that no part of the body remains in a position of flexion long enough for the occurrence of muscle shortening and joint changes that might interfere with free joint action. Appropriate interventions include the following:

1. Passive exercise—stimulates circulation and may help to reestablish neuromuscular pathways
2. Active exercise started as soon as possible
3. Attention to the unaffected limbs to maintain strength—includes keeping unaffected leg in position of slight internal rotation
4. Early ambulation—facilitates vasomotor tone and has positive psychologic effects on the patient and family members

The *Bobath technique* is a treatment approach designed to normalize muscle tone. This is accomplished by providing as many sensations of normal muscle tone, posture, and movement as possible. The *goal of the treatment* is to *redirect short-term memory toward an appreciation of normal movement of the paralyzed side by incorporating techniques of weight bearing, counter-rotation,* and *protraction of the shoulder girdle and pelvis.* The reader is referred to a rehabilitation nursing text for further description of this technique.

Preventing injury

When patients begin to move about and try to help themselves, they may have several problems that can affect their ability to proceed. This predisposes them to injuries. They may have loss of position sense, so that it is awkward for them to handle their bodies normally, even when they

have the muscular coordination to do so. They may have dizziness, spatial-perceptual deficits, diplopia, and alteration of skin sensations. They may also have to work harder to receive a normal amount of air on inhalation because the involved side of the chest does not expand easily.

Facilitating emotional adjustment

If the patient who has had a CVA survives the first few days, consciousness usually returns, and some of the paralysis may disappear. It is then that great understanding is needed to help the patient accept his or her limitations. Using quiet assurance, a nurse can help the patient feel that progress toward recovery and self-sufficiency has begun and will continue.

The patient who has sustained a CVA may be overly emotional, and this reaction, combined with the fear and frustration on becoming aware of his or her condition, may be upsetting to the family. Crying for no apparent reason is common in these patients. Family, staff, and sometimes other patients need reassurance that they are not the cause of the patient's crying.

Facilitating communication

The role of the nurse is very important in dealing with the patient with an impairment in verbal communication. A number of principles have been found to be helpful in working with the aphasic patient. The first is to make communication statements as simple as possible. This includes introducing one idea at a time and using short sentences with common words. It is important to limit choices given to the patient and allowing ample time for response.

The patient should be commended for positive steps. The nurse should avoid correcting errors that will discourage the patient from making further attempts to communicate. It is important for the nurse not to talk down to the patient or to treat the patient like a child. Frustration on the part of the patient should be accepted as part of the problem. It is not unusual for the patient to be able to sing songs or to verbalize other automatic speech. This may include swearing.

When attempting to communicate with an aphasic patient, the environment should be as free of distractions as possible. The patient should be comfortable. The nurse should not communicate a sense of urgency or impatience if at all possible—this only worsens communication problems. Stress felt by the patient will decrease the ability to talk. For patients who can manage its use, a communication board is helpful. These boards include either the alphabet or pictures of common objects. The patient can point to the item that is needed or can spell out the necessary word.

For patients with receptive problems, the nurse should be sure that the patient comprehends what is needed. This may include demonstrations of functions to the patient. The family of the patient with aphasia should be educated about the problem and encouraged to interact with the patient.

Maintaining perceptual ability

After a stroke, persons may have difficulty relating to themselves and their environment. After the acute stage, a multibed environment is advocated, because the sensory input from others is helpful. *Hemianopsia,* or decreased

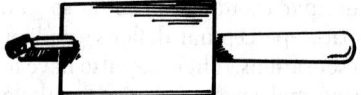

Fig. 37-43   Long-handled skin inspection mirror. (From Dittmar SS: *Rehabilitation nursing*, St Louis, 1989, Mosby—Year Book.)

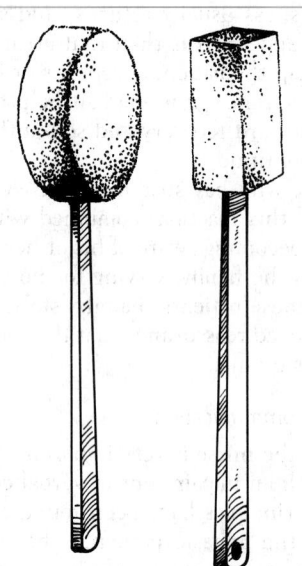

Fig. 37-44   Long-handled bath sponge. (From Dittmar SS: *Rehabilitation nursing*, St Louis, 1989, Mosby—Year Book.)

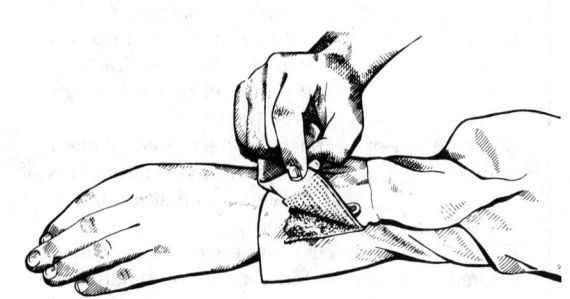

Fig. 37-46   Velcro shirtsleeve to facilitate closure. (From Dittmar SS: *Rehabilitation nursing*, St Louis, 1989, Mosby—Year Book.)

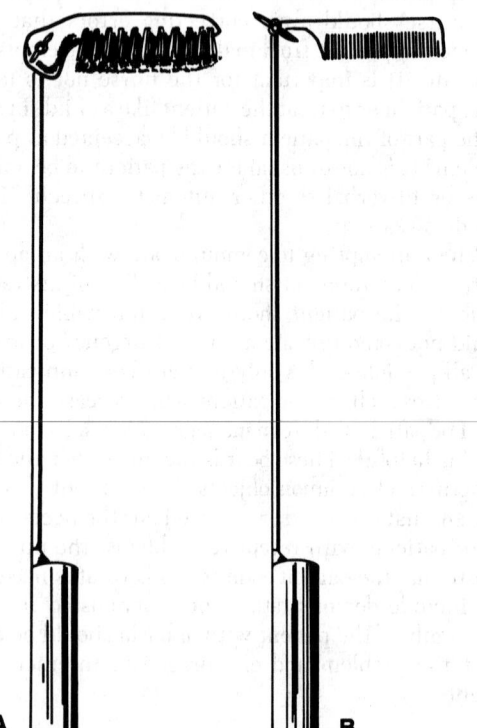

Fig. 37-45   Adapted hairbrush **(A)** and comb **(B).** (From Dittmar SS: *Rehabilitation nursing*, St Louis, 1989, Mosby—Year Book.)

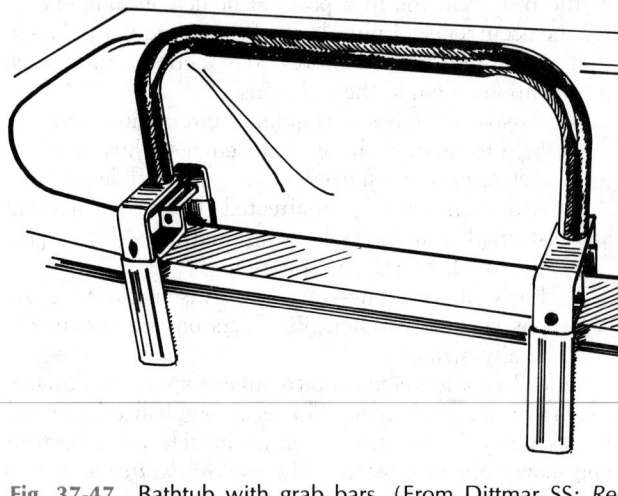

Fig. 37-47   Bathtub with grab bars. (From Dittmar SS: *Rehabilitation nursing*, St Louis, 1989, Mosby—Year Book.)

visual field, occurs commonly. Approaching patients from the side of intact vision and teaching them to scan with their eyes will help make them more aware of stimuli and help prevent injury. Diminished awareness or denial of the affected side (*anosognosia*) can occur and can be a safety hazard. This possibility should be considered when the patient runs into objects or allows the affected arm or leg to drag behind.

Promoting activities of daily living

The patient is evaluated regarding his or her ability to carry out the usual ADL and is assisted by the occupational therapist or nurse in becoming independent in each activity to the extent possible. Rehabilitation in this way is essentially a teaching-learning process in which the patient is actively involved. Many assistive devices are available commercially (see Figs. 37-43 to 37-47).

Facilitating learning

The teaching for a patient with CVA is the same as that for the patient with an alteration in motor function (p. 1235).

Evaluation

See p. 1234 for the evaluation questions for the patient with an alteration in motor function and p. 1236 for evaluation questions for the patient with an alteration in sensory function. In addition to those questions, questions to consider for the patient with CVA may include the following:

1. Can the patient explain the importance of frequent position changes and demonstrate various positions?
2. Is the patient's continence improved, and have minimal complications resulted from incontinence?
3. Has the patient developed alternative means of communication?

Surgery

After the patient's condition is stable (with a CVA), or after one or more TIAs, surgery may be used for selected patients. If the symptoms are associated with an atherosclerotic lesion in the extracranial system (internal carotid artery or common carotid artery), a carotid endarterectomy may be performed.

A carotid endarterectomy involves the reaming out of the diseased vessel under either local or general anesthesia. *Postoperative care* includes the following:

1. Close attention to neurologic signs (changes in strength, mentation, speech, and level of consciousness)
2. Observation for bleeding in the incisional area
3. Observation for swelling of the neck or complaints of dysphagia
4. Availability of tracheostomy tray in case of severe respiratory distress

Revascularization procedures are now possible with the use of stereoscopic microscopes. Commonly, the superficial temporal artery is anastomosed to an artery within the brain such as the midcerebral artery. Other vessels can be used. The purpose is to provide for greater blood flow. The surgery usually does not resolve any permanent deficits, but it may prevent further problems. The *care of the patient*

preoperatively and postoperatively is similar to that for any patient with cranial surgery, but it also includes the following:

1. Checking for pulse in anastomosed vessel
   a. Doppler
   b. Gentle palpation
2. Keeping graft areas free of pressure
   a. Eyeglass frames bent out so as not to occlude vessel
   b. No other restricting bands around head

The patient will have a postoperative angiogram to assess the patency of the vessel.[56]

INTRACRANIAL HEMORRHAGE

Intracerebral or intracranial hemorrhages include bleeding into the subarachnoid space or into the brain tissue itself. These hemorrhages cause damage to the brain by destroying and replacing brain tissue. Nursing and medical treatment of a patient with an aneurysm and intracranial hemorrhage can be significantly different from that of a patient with a CVA.

Intracranial hemorrhages are the third most common cause of CVAs. The peak incidence of aneurysms is in the 35- to 60-year-old age group. Women are affected slightly more often than men. A ruptured cerebral aneurysm is the most common cause of subarachnoid hemorrhage not related to trauma. Bleeding may be from a vessel on the surface of the brain, and the bleeding may be limited to the subarachnoid space. Bleeding from a vessel in the brain substance may form a cerebral hematoma and extend through the brain tissue to the ventricles.

The most common causes of cerebral hemorrhage are as follows:

1. Berry aneurysms—usually congenital defects
2. Fusiform aneurysms—from atherosclerosis
3. Mycotic aneurysms—from necrotic vasculitis and septic emboli
4. Arteriovenous malformations—tangled, interconnected vessels that allow blood to pass directly from the artery to the vein[70]
5. Rupture of cerebral arterioles—from hypertension, which causes thickening and degeneration

Pathophysiology

Any of the causes listed can result in subarachnoid hemorrhage, intracerebral hemorrhage, or a combination of the two. The most common site for berry aneurysms is the anterior portion of the Circle of Willis at the junction of the internal carotid and posterior communicating arteries. Multiple aneurysms are found in many persons.

Aneurysmal rupture occurs when a small hole occurs in a part of the aneurysm. The hemorrhage spreads rapidly, producing localized changes and irritation to the cerebral vessels. The bleeding is usually halted by the formation of a plug consisting of fibrin-platelets and by tissue compression. Within 3 weeks the hemorrhage begins to undergo resorption. Recurrent rupture is a serious risk 7 to 10 days after the initial hemorrhage. The rupture of a vessel causes disruption of the blood flow to a selected area, focal ischemic changes, and infarction of brain tissue. In addition,

The Elderly with Neurologic Problems

Assessment

1. Assess for changes in cognitive function, such as confusion, disorientation, changes in judgment, and difficulty in concentration, abstract thinking, and problem-solving.
2. Monitor for new onset of confusion. Many factors can affect mental status of hospitalized elderly, such as medications, dehydration, pain, need to toilet, or strange equipment.
3. Assess availability of home support persons.

Intervention

1. Provide cues to help maintain orientation; with each contact, remind patient who you are, the time of day, and procedures or routines that will be occurring.
2. Orient the person to unfamiliar equipment, tubings, or changes in the environment.
3. Decrease chances of sensory deprivation by making certain eyeglasses and hearing aids are functioning and properly fitted.
4. Provide opportunities for problem-solving; include person in all aspects of decisions regarding treatments and procedures, no matter what the cognitive ability.
5. Keep structured, familiar routines as much as possible (such as bathing, eating, physical therapy, nighttime rituals).
6. Teach significant others approaches to facilitate patient orientation. If spouse is providing home care, provide resources for obtaining assistance with care and for "time off" periods for spouse.

Common disorders in elderly

Transient ischemic attacks
Cardiovascular accidents
Parkinson's disease
Alzheimer's disease

Nursing Process
Assessment

The assessment for intracerebral hemorrhage includes the factors identified in the subjective and objective assessment for the patient who has had a CVA. Symptoms of an intracranial hemorrhage include the following:

1. Sudden, explosive headache
2. Photophobia
3. Neck rigidity
4. Nausea and vomiting
5. Loss of consciousness
6. Convulsions
7. Respiratory distress
8. Shock

Data analysis: nursing diagnoses

Possible nursing diagnoses for the patient with an intracerebral hemorrhage are the same as for the patient who has had a CVA (p. 1256) with the addition of:

Diagnostic title	Possible etiologies
Tissue perfusion, altered cerebral	Decreased cerebral blood flow

Planning: expected patient outcomes

In addition to those patient outcomes defined for the patient with a CVA (p. 1256), these additional outcomes are important:

1. Patient does not develop signs of increased ICP.
2. Patient does not develop complications from the immobility.
3. Patient can explain the need for surgery and relevant factors.
4. Patient can explain any restrictions in activity.

Implementation
Assisting with the achievement of therapeutic goals

The immediate treatment for intracranial hemorrhage is to keep the person absolutely quiet to prevent additional bleeding. An antifibronolytic agent (aminocaproic acid [Amicar]) may be used to seal the clot. Other nursing actions to be used may include those listed in Box 37-40.

Surgery

The only satisfactory treatment for aneurysm is surgery. Surgery is not usually performed to repair arteriovenous anomalies or hypertensive vascular disease. If an intracerebral hematoma has formed, it may be evacuated after the patient's condition is stable. Before surgery can be performed, angiography must be performed to determine location of the aneurysm. The time after the acute rupture until the surgery is performed varies with the person, their age, the intensity and kind of symptoms present, and the judgment of the surgeon to determine when surgery will be recommended. (See Box 37-41 for postoperative care of the patient with intracranial surgery).

Surgery consists of a craniotomy and location of the aneurysm. When found, the aneurysm may be obliterated by ligation at its neck with the application of a silver clip. If the base of the aneurysm is too large for ligation to be

the sudden release of blood has the effect of a concussion, and unconsciousness occurs. It also causes a rapid rise in cerebrospinal fluid pressure with displacement of the brain. Bleeding into brain tissue itself can cause damage by dissecting the brain along the fiber tracts. In addition, hemorrhage may produce a filling of the ventricular system or produce a hematoma that distorts brain tissue.

Blood itself is a noxious agent, and as it is hemolyzed it irritates the blood vessels, the meninges, and the brain. The presence of the blood and the release of vasoactive substances promote arterial spasms, which can further decrease cerebral perfusion. This arterial spasm, or vasospasm, usually occurs from 4 to 10 days after the hemorrhage and causes constriction or narrowing of the cerebral arteries. These vasospasms are serious complications: They can cause focal neurologic decline, ischemia of the brain, and infarction.

About 50% of the patients with rupture of an aneurysm recover from the initial episode, but at least 50% of these persons will have recurrences of hemorrhage if untreated. Recurrence may occur within 2 weeks, and the danger of death increases with each bleeding episode.

Guidelines for Care

The patient with an intracranial hemorrhage

1. Use gentleness in moving patient.
2. Keep room darkened.
3. Keep patient resting in bed—head of bed is usually elevated 30 degrees. Occasionally bathroom privileges are allowed.
4. Give patient no ice water.
5. Initiate a bowel program to prevent constipation and straining at stool.
6. Allow few visitors.
7. Decrease stimuli in room—no TV or radio in severe cases.
8. Take no rectal temperatures.
9. Encourage patient to seek assistance for change in position.

Guidelines for Care

Postoperative care of the patient with intracranial surgery

1. Assess neurologic status including ability to move, level of orientation, and alertness and pupil checks.
2. Assess degree and character of drainage.
   a. Amount of drainage and bleeding should be minimal.
   b. Initial head dressing can be reinforced as necessary.
   c. Often incision is left open to air after first several days.
3. Promoting mobility
   a. Turning to either side is permitted except when large brain tumors have been removed. If this is the case, patient is not turned to affected side as gravity may cause displacement of brain structures.
   b. For supratentorial surgery, the head of the bed is elevated at least 30 degrees.
   c. If infratentorial surgery was performed, the bed is flat or elevated only slightly and a small pillow is placed under the nape of the neck. Neck flexion is avoided.
   d. Early ambulation is encouraged to prevent complications of bed rest. Observe carefully for signs of postural hypotension and raise head of bed gradually; patient should always sit before standing.
4. Promoting decreased ICP
   a. Space nursing activities to allow patient to rest between them.
   b. Coughing and vomiting should be avoided.
   c. Suctioning should be done only as necessary, and then gently and cautiously.
5. Protecting safety of patient
   a. Use of soft hand restraints if restraints are necessary.
   b. Use of mittens as alternative to restraints; make sure fingers are separated and fingers are placed around large roll. Change mitt at least daily—give range of motion to hand at this time.
   c. Keep side rails up at all times.
6. Promoting electrolyte balance
   a. Accurate intake and output with measurement of specific gravity. Frequent testing for sugar and acetone if patient is taking steroids.
   b. Resumption of diet as soon as possible; assess for difficulty in swallowing or absence of gag reflex.
   c. Monitor electrolytes for evidence of abnormalities.
7. Promoting comfort
   a. Medicate for comfort with codeine sulfate or nonnarcotic analgesic.
   b. Ice cap to head for headache may be helpful.

practical, it may be coated with a liquid, adherent, plastic substance that hardens to form a firm support about the weakened vessel wall or it may be wrapped.[70] If the aneurysm has not ruptured but has produced symptoms, attempts may be made to produce thrombosis by use of an electrical current and other means.

The goal of this immobility is to prevent increased intercranial pressure. Nursing actions to prevent problems of immobility need to be initiated. The reader is referred to the section concerning motor problems (p. 1228).

Other procedures

Not all aneurysms can be treated surgically at the site of the lesion. If surgery is not feasible, the common carotid artery in the neck may be completely or partially obliterated to lessen the flow of blood to the site of the aneurysm and reduce the chances of hemorrhage. This is contingent on whether sufficient blood can be supplied from collateral vessels to preserve brain function. The procedure usually is performed in stages over several days. A clamp (Silverstone or Salibi) with a detachable screw stem that can be tightened gradually is used. Usually the surgeon adjusts it each day, and the nurse assesses the patient closely and is instructed to release the clamp at once if there is evidence of inadequate blood supply, as shown by decreased neurologic status. Immediate removal of the clamps may prevent irreversible complications such as hemiplegia, aphasia, and loss of consciousness. If complete occlusion can be tolerated, the vessel may be permanently ligated. Serial embolizations of blood vessels that "feed" the aneurysm may also be performed via the femoral or axillary route. The procedure is similar to a cerebral angiogram, and the postoperative care is the same. Thrombus formation with resultant cerebral embolism may complicate the patient's postoperative course after any surgery for a cerebral aneurysm.

Interventions to achieve patient outcomes
Facilitating learning

If the patient with an intracranial hemorrhage has neurologic deficits consistent with a CVA, the teaching is the same. Additionally, the points listed in Box 37-42 are important.

The patient with intracranial hemorrhage

1. Importance of following activity restrictions
2. Importance of keeping as free of stress as possible
3. Very specific teaching about what activities are restricted
4. Use of medication and what it does
5. Information about preoperative and postoperative care will be useful

Evaluation

In addition to the questions that should be considered in the evaluation of a patient who has had a CVA, questions to consider when evaluating a patient with intracranial hemorrhage may include the following:

1. Is the patient's neurologic status stable?
2. Does the patient verbalize understanding of surgery planned?
3. Is the patient cooperating with the activity restrictions?
4. Does the patient verbalize understanding of the restrictions?
5. Is the patient relatively calm?

INTERFERENCE WITH FUNCTION BECAUSE OF INFECTION/ INFLAMMATION

Interference with function because of infection/inflammation is a fairly common occurrence. Specific conditions to discuss include the following:

1. Meningitis
2. Encephalitis
3. Brain abscess
4. Poliomyelitis
5. Guillain-Barré syndrome (polyneuritis)
6. Neurosyphilis
7. Herpes zoster
8. Acquired immunodeficiency syndrome (AIDS)

Because these conditions contain many common characteristics, they will be discussed together.

The nervous system may be attacked by a variety of organisms and viruses and may suffer from toxins of bacteria and viruses. These toxins reach the nervous system through a variety of routes. Untreated chronic otitis media and mastoiditis, chronic sinusitis, and fracture in any bone adjacent to the meninges may be the source of infection. Some organisms such as the tubercle bacillus reach the nervous system by means of the blood or lymphatic system. Meningitis can occur as a complication of an invasive procedure such as a lumbar puncture. The exact route of some other organisms is not known.

MENINGITIS
Etiology and Pathophysiology

Meningitis is an acute infection of the meninges. It is usually caused by one of the following organisms:

1. Pneumococci
2. Meningococci
3. Staphylococci
4. Streptococci
5. *Haemophilus influenzae*
6. Aseptic agents (usually viral)

The effect of the bacteria or other organisms in the subarachnoid space is an inflammatory reaction in the pia, arachnoid, and CSF. Pus accumulates in these areas. The bacteria or its toxin, if not treated in a timely manner, may injure cranial and spinal nerves and other structures. In addition, the purulent material that occurs may obstruct the flow of CSF, resulting in hydrocephalus. The longer the infectious process occurs before it is treated, the more complications and neurologic sequalae that can occur.

Meningitis can be classed as bacterial (leptomeningitis) or aseptic. The term *aseptic meningitis* was introduced in 1925 and was first thought to refer to a specific disease. It is now recognized as a complex of symptoms that result from many infective agents, the majority of which are viral. *Herpes simplex* is an example of a virus that can cause aseptic meningitis. Any other pathogenic organism, such as the tubercle bacillus, that gains access to the subarachnoid spaces can also cause meningitis. The incidence of bacterial meningitis is higher in fall and winter when upper respiratory tract infections are common. Children are more often affected than adults because of frequent colds and ear infections.

Pathologic changes that occur include any or all of the following:

1. Hyperemia of the meningeal vessels
2. Edema of brain tissue
3. Increased ICP
4. Generalized inflammatory reaction with exudation of white blood cells into the subarachnoid spaces
5. Associated hydrocephalus caused by exudate blocking the small passage between the ventricles

Nursing Process
Assessment

Subjective and objective assessment are important in any patient with an infection of the nervous system. This assessment includes characteristics that are common to all the infections/inflammations discussed in this section.

Subjective data

1. Patient's understanding of process and possible causes
2. Any history of infection such as upper respiratory infections
3. Measures that relieve symptoms
4. Presence of discomfort, including headache or stiff neck

5. Initial onset of symptoms
6. Presence of difficulty in thinking
7. Presence of muscle weakness, soreness, or incoordination

Objective data

1. Behavior: signs indicating discomfort or disorientation
2. Change in ability to carry out daily activities
3. Abnormalities on physical assessment part of neurologic examination
4. Elevated temperature
5. Presence of vomiting
6. Pulse and blood pressure
7. Increased respirations
8. Abnormal CT results
9. Meningeal irritation
10. Evidence of presence of seizures

The onset of meningitis is usually sudden and characterized by severe headache, stiffness of the neck, irritability, malaise, and restlessness. Nausea, vomiting, delirium, and complete disorientation develop quickly. Temperature, pulse rate, and respirations are increased. Two pathologic signs that occur with meningitis are the following:

1. *Kernig's sign*—the inability of the patient to extend the legs completely without extreme pain
2. *Brudzinski's sign*—flexion of the hip and knee when the neck is flexed

Diagnostic tests

Most of the infections affecting the nervous system can be diagnosed by examining the cerebrospinal fluid. A CT scan and an EEG may also be used. These procedures were discussed earlier in this chapter.

Data analysis: nursing diagnoses

Nursing diagnoses are determined from analysis of patient data. Possible nursing diagnoses for the person with meningitis may include, but are not limited to those for a patient who has had a CVA (p. 1256) or motor dysfunction (p. 1231).

Planning: expected patient outcomes

Expected patient outcomes for the person with meningitis may include, but are not limited to, those for a patient who has had a CVA (p. 1264) or motor dysfunction (p. 1234).

Implementation
Assisting with achievement of therapeutic goals

Treatment of meningitis consists of massive doses of the antibiotic or antibiotics specific for the causative organism. Treatment with multiple antibiotics is common. Culture and sensitivity studies demonstrate the most effective antibiotic. Usually a course of at least 10 days of parenteral administration is needed. The antibiotic may also be given directly into the spinal canal (intrathecally). Hyperosmolar agents or steroids may be necessary to decrease cerebral edema. Anticonvulsants may be given to prevent seizures.

Nursing care for the patient with meningitis includes the following:

1. General care given a critically ill patient
2. Darkened room, with noise kept to a minimum, because sensory stimulation can cause seizures
3. Careful neurologic checks at frequent intervals
4. Padded side rails

Residual damage from meningitis includes deafness, blindness, paralysis, and mental retardation. These complications are usually the result of chronic arachnoiditis. Hydrocephalus may also develop, requiring a shunting procedure.

Isolation of the patient depends on the causative organism. Check the infection control manual of your institution for specific guidelines.

Evaluation

Evaluation of the patient with meningitis includes those points considered in the evaluation of the person with a CVA (p. 1264).

If the patient has motor dysfunction, appropriate evaluation questions can be found on p. 1234.

ENCEPHALITIS
Etiology and Pathophysiology

Encephalitis is an inflammation of the brain tissues and its covering. Occasionally, the meninges of the spinal cord are also involved. It can have a variety of causes, including the following:

1. Syphilis
2. Exogenous poisoning such as that which follows the ingestion of lead or arsenic or inhalation of carbon monoxide
3. Reaction to toxins produced by infections such as typhoid fever, measles, and chickenpox
4. Reaction to vaccination
5. Various viruses, including arbovirus (those transferred by biting arthropod to humans)

Encephalitis caused by a virus and occurring in epidemic form was first described by von Economo in Austria, and the name *von Economo's disease* is still used to identify the widespread epidemic in the United States that followed the influenza epidemic in 1918. Von Economo's disease was also called *sleeping sickness*, a term still used by laypersons. The demonstration that viruses can affect the central nervous system after a prolonged incubation period has resulted in considerable search for viral agents in many chronic neurologic diseases.

Nursing Process
Assessment

The subjective and objective data for encephalitis are the same as for meningitis (p. 1264). The onset of encephalitis is often abrupt, with a high fever, headache, meningeal signs, nuchal rigidity, and vomiting. Drowsiness or coma and focal or generalized convulsions usually develop within 24 to 48 hours after onset of symptoms. Focal neurologic signs develop, such as hemiplegia and cranial nerve palsies. There are typical findings in the CSF. Mortality may be as high as 60%.

Data analysis: nursing diagnoses

The reader is referred to the nursing diagnoses in the discussion of CVA on p. 1256.

Implementation

Nursing care consists of symptomatic or supportive care and careful observation. Any change in appearance or behavior should be reported because the progress of this disease sometimes is extremely rapid. Bed rest is advocated. If disorientation is present, the patient must be attended constantly. During the time when temperature is increased, sponge baths or other hypothermia methods are used.

No specific medical treatment for this disease is available. No isolation is necessary because encephalitis is not transmitted from person to person. Prevention of arboviral infections includes destruction of larvae and elimination of breeding places such as pools of stagnant water. Control includes avoiding bites of the mosquito or tick vectors.

Evaluation

Evaluation includes those questions listed under the evaluation section of CVA on p. 1261.

BRAIN ABSCESS

The frequency of abscesses in the areas of the brain is site specific, with most found in the cerebrum (75%) and cerebellum (25%). Some abscesses, as many as 20%, have multiple foci. Of patients with brain abscesses, 30% to 60% may die and those surviving may have different types of residual deficits, including paralysis and seizures.

A brain abscess is almost always secondary to a foci of infection somewhere else in the body, such as extension of chronic middle ear, sinus, or mastoid infections. The bacteria gain access to the cranial vault directly through bone, through the dura mater, across the subarachnoid and subdural spaces, or along venous routes. Common sites of the primary infection include the following:

1. Ear
2. Sinus or mastoid
3. Lung
4. Heart
5. Pelvic organs
6. Teeth
7. Skin

The three most common organisms involved are the streptococci, staphylococci, and pneumococci. Brain abscesses are most common in older children and young adults but may be seen at any age.

Complications from ear infections account for almost 50% of all brain abscesses. These abscesses are often found in the frontal lobe. Abscesses originating from infections in the frontal, ethmoid, and sphenoid sinuses are also found in the frontal lobe. The sphenoid sinuses may also seed into the temporal lobe. If the abscess is disseminated through the blood stream, the abscesses are multiplied and found in the white matter. Penetrating head injuries, compound fractures, and osteomyelitis of the skull lead to the formation of brain abscesses.

> **37-43**
>
> **Symptoms of brain abscess**
>
> 1. Constant and severe headache
> 2. Drowsiness
> 3. Confusion
> 4. Mental slowness
> 5. Focal or generalized seizures
> 6. Fever with bradycardia
> 7. Signs and symptoms of increased ICP
> 8. Nuchal rigidity

Pathophysiology

The first stage of brain abscess is characterized by local edema, hyperemia, infiltration by leukocytes, and softening of the parenchyma. Septic thromboses of some vessels occur, and the surrounding brain tissue becomes necrotic and edematous. Days to weeks after the beginning stages, there is a process of central liquefaction and necrosis of brain tissue with the formation of a cystic wall of pus. This becomes encased by a wall that is thinner on the ventral side with a predisposition to rupture. If rupture occurs, the infection extends through the entire brain, leading to meningitis.

Nursing Process
Assessment

The questions to ask in collecting data from the patient with a brain abscess are the same as for the patient with meningitis (p. 1264). With a brain abscess, there may be a history of infection. The most common symptom is a constant or intermittent headache that is not relieved by medication and that is increased by straining (see Box 37-43 for other symptoms).

The evolution of symptoms is variable. In some patients there may be a rapid progression of symptoms ending in death, whereas in others the course is more benign. Generally, however, the mortality is high with brain abscess, and residual disability often results.

Diagnostic tests

The diagnosis of brain abscess is made primarily on the basis of the history and examination of the CSF. EEG changes are present (significant slowing at the site of the abscess), and there will be areas of increased uptake on the CT scan. The brain scan is able to locate abscesses that are over 1 cm in size. Arteriography can be helpful in locating temporal lobe abscesses or cerebellar abscesses. The lumbar puncture is contraindicated when intracranial pressure is increased because of the danger of causing herniation of the brain.

Data analysis: nursing diagnoses

The nursing diagnoses and the expected patient outcomes are the same for the patient with brain abscess as for the patient with a CVA (p. 1256).

Implementation

Assisting with the achievement of therapeutic goals

Nursing care consists of administering the appropriate antibiotics, often for extended periods of time. Combined antibiotics along with broad-spectrum antibiotics may be used. Antibiotics that are used include penicillin, chloramphenicol (Chloramycetin), and nafcillen (Unipen). If anaerobic bacteria have been identified, metronidazole (Flagyl) may be used. Agents to reduce ICP may be necessary. Ongoing assessment for signs and symptoms of increased ICP is important. These patients often must undergo long hospitalizations and periods of treatment; as a result, they may need a great deal of psychologic support.

Surgical treatment consists of aspiration or complete excision and evacuation of the abscess. The method of evacuation depends on the site and accessibility.

Evaluation

For the evaluation of a patient with a brain abscess, consider the evaluation questions listed for the patient with a CVA (p. 1261).

POLIOMYELITIS

Poliomyelitis is an acute febrile disease caused by poliomyelitis virus types 1, 2, and 3. Paralysis is more common with type 1. With discovery of the Salk vaccine, its wide use since 1956, and the availability of the Sabin vaccine, this disease has become rare. At one time it was a serious crippler of children and young adults.

Pathophysiology

The incubation period for poliomyelitis is from 7 to 21 days. The virus attacks the anterior horn cells of the spinal cord where the motor pathways are located and may cause motor paralysis. Sensory perception is not affected, because posterior horn cells are not attacked. Poliomyelitis sometimes takes a somewhat different form and attacks primarily the medulla and basal structures of the brain, including the cranial nerves. This is called *bulbar paralysis*. If the medulla is involved, the patient will need respiratory assistance.

GUILLAIN-BARRÉ SYNDROME (POLYNEURITIS)

Guillain-Barré syndrome is also known as *acute inflammatory polyradiculoneuropathy* and *postinfectious polyneuritis*. It is often serious because of the extent to which the nervous system is involved. It involves an acute type of peripheral nerve syndrome resulting in widespread inflammation and demyelination of the peripheral nervous system. The disease affects persons of all ages and is seen equally in men and women. It is the most common demyelinating neuropathy, affecting 1.5 people per 100,000 each year.[57a] The cause is unknown, but it is thought to be either a viral agent or the result of an autoimmune reaction.

Pathophysiology

In Guillain-Barré syndrome, patchy demyelination occurs in peripheral nerves, nerve roots, root ganglia, and spinal cord. Axons are generally spared so recovery may occur early, although they may be affected in severe cases.

Variations in the pattern of onset of weakness occur, as well as in the rate of progression of symptoms. The progression may stop at any point. If cranial nerves VII, IX, and X are involved, the patient may have difficulty in swallowing, speaking, and breathing. The vital centers in the medulla may be affected.

The pathophysiology also is related to infiltration of the peripheral nervous system with mononuclear cells. It is thought that sensitized lymphocytes have a part in the demyelination because more than half of the individuals affected have had a nonspecific infection 10 to 14 days before the onset of the disease. Many persons developed symptoms of Guillian-Barré after receiving swine flu vaccine in the early 1980s.

Symmetric muscle weakness and lower motor neuron paralysis (flaccidity) are present with Guillain-Barré syndrome. The paralysis usually starts in the lower extremities and moves upward to include the thorax, upper extremities, and face. Paresthesias may occur. Respiratory failure is possible if the intercostal muscles are affected; without mechanical ventilation, mortality is 10% to 20%. Autonomic symptoms, such as fluctuating blood pressure, also occur. The bowel and bladder are rarely affected.

Of the persons suffering from Gullain-Barré syndrome, 85% will regain complete function. The recovery period is variable, ranging from weeks to years. Those not recovering completely will have some degree of permanent neurological deficit. Generally, recovery from the disease occurs in the *reverse order* of how paralysis or weakness occurred.

Nursing Process

Assessment

Subjective data

1. Patient's understanding of the disease
2. History of an infection in recent past
3. Initial onset of symptoms and nature of symptoms
4. Presence of muscle weakness

Objective data

1. Abnormalities found in the physical assessment part of the neurologic examination
2. Presence of increased temperature
3. Presence of muscle weakness
4. Abnormalities found with arterial blood gases
5. Presence of dyspnea
6. Blood pressure abnormalities

Data analysis: nursing diagnoses

See section on the patient with a CVA (p. 1256).

Planning: expected patient outcomes

See section on the patient with a CVA (p. 1256).

DATA: Mr. D. is a 45-year-old married auto mechanic with a history of progressive weakness that began in his feet and legs. For the past day he has not been able to walk. He is also complaining of shortness of breath. He gives a history of an upper respiratory tract infection 2 weeks before admission. On admission he demonstrated weakness of all four extremities. His tidal volume was decreased and his respiratory rate was 32. He complained of discomfort in his lower extremities. The sensory examination was WNL. He was alert and oriented ×3. He was admitted to the neurologic unit for observation. He was started on corticosteroids and his respiratory rate closely monitored. The day after admission the patient demonstrated paralysis of muscles below the waist.

The nursing history identified the following:

1. He is unsure about what has happened to him and the reason for his weakness.
2. He expresses anxiety about what to expect.
3. He seems to have a close relationship with his wife.
4. Leisure activities are mainly sports activities.

Collaborative nursing actions include those to prevent further complications caused by muscle weakness and respiratory weakness. Immediate reporting may prevent serious effects (respiratory arrest, clot formation). Nursing actions include monitoring for the following:

1. Signs of respiratory compromise: decreased tidal volume, increased shortness of breath, tachypnea, cyanosis, restlessness.
2. Signs of pulmonary embolism: chest pain, hemoptysis.
3. Signs of DVT (deep vein thrombosis): difference in leg girth, positive Homan's sign, leg pain, difference in temperature of legs.

Nursing diagnosis: Anxiety related to change in health status

Expected patient outcomes	Nursing interventions	Rationale
Mr. D. verbalizes minimal anxiety	Explain to Mr. D. procedures being done	Explanations will help minimize anxiety
	Allow Mr. D. time to verbalize feelings	Expression of fears will lessen anxiety
	Encourage Mr. D.'s wife to spend time with him	Family members are an important source of support

Nursing diagnosis: Breathing pattern, ineffective: related to neuromuscular impairment

Expected patient outcomes	Nursing interventions	Rationale
Mr. D. will have adequate breathing pattern	Assess respiratory rate, tidal volume, and color frequently	Ongoing assessment will detect critical changes
	Notify physician of any changes immediately	Changes in respiratory status can occur quickly
	Keep head of bed at 30 degrees	Position helps respiratory effort
	Give supplemental oxygen as ordered	Lowered oxygen levels in blood are common with impaired respiratory efforts

Nursing diagnosis: Pain related to Guillain-Barré syndrome

Expected patient outcomes	Nursing interventions	Rationale
Mr. D. states that leg pain is improved	Position for comfort	Positioning may relieve pain
	Administer mild analgesic such as acetaminophen	Pain relief
	Teach relaxation measures as appropriate	Promotes rest and eases pain

Nursing diagnosis: Disuse syndrome, high risk for: related to immobility and weakness

Expected patient outcomes	Nursing interventions	Rationale
Contractures do not develop	Position Mr. D. with limbs in normal anatomic position	Will prevent flexion contractures
	Change position q2h	
	Perform passive or active ROM to all extremities several times a day	Activity stretches muscles and keeps joints moveable

Nursing diagnosis: **Disuse syndrome, high risk for: related to immobility and weakness—cont'd**

Expected patient outcomes	Nursing interventions	Rationale
	Assist out of bed at least daily	Change in position helps prevent complications of immobility
	Apply elastic stockings and keep legs elevated when up in chair	Assists with venous return and helps prevent stasis

Nursing diagnosis: **Knowledge deficit: related to lack of exposure to information**

Expected patient outcomes	Nursing interventions	Rationale
Mr. D. can describe nature of disease and possible complications	Review nature of disease with frequent reinforcement	Teaching can raise Mr. D.'s level of cooperation
		Reinforcement of earlier teaching helps promote retention

Nursing diagnosis: **Mobility, impaired physical: related to neuromuscular impairment**

Expected patient outcomes	Nursing interventions	Rationale
Mr. D. has minimal impairments in mobility	Allow Mr. D. to do as much for self as possible	Active exercise has positive effect on Mr. D.
	See actions under "Disuse syndrome," high risk for	

Nursing diagnosis: **Self-care deficit: related to neuromuscular impairment**

Expected patient outcomes	Nursing interventions	Rationale
Mr. D. carries out ADL at highest ability level	Provide basic ADL needs as necessary but encourage Mr. D. to do what he can	Self-care will promote positive self-concept
	Provide sufficient time to do ADL	Doing ADL with deficits often takes more time
	Work with therapists to optimize patient's learning	Team work can accentuate care

Nursing diagnosis: **Body image disturbance, personal identity disturbance: role performance related to loss of body functions and immobility**

Expected patient outcomes	Nursing interventions	Rationale
Mr. D. verbalizes positive self-concept	Provide information about disease and expected progress	Understanding of disease will improve self-concept
	Provide privacy	Mr. D. may be embarrassed by need for physical care
	Provide care but encourage Mr. D. to do as much for self as possible	Ability to care for self will improve self-concept
	Encourage family to visit	Visitors will cheer Mr. D.
	Give family chance to share their concerns	If family concerns are met, they can be more supportive of Mr. D.
	Encourage family to maintain previous role relationships, if possible	There is comfort in knowing that role in family is intact
	Identify Mr. D.'s strengths and weaknesses	Can assist nurse in planning care with patient

Nursing diagnosis: **Skin integrity, impaired, high risk for: related to mechanical forces and pressure**

Expected patient outcomes	Nursing interventions	Rationale
Skin remains intact	Monitor pressure areas for signs of skin breakdown	Early detection of pressure can allow time for measures to prevent breakdown
	Use turning sheet when turning Mr. D. to prevent shearing effect	Shearing forces lead to skin breakdown
	Turn Mr. D. q2h	Turning prevents pressure areas
	Keep skin clean and dry	Moisture leads to skin breakdown
	Use air mattress, water mattress, or special bed	Can assist with relief of pressure areas

Implementation
Assisting with achievement of therapeutic goals

A priority goal is the maintenance of respiratory function. Close monitoring of respiratory function is necessary. Observation should include serial measurements of the patient's vital capacity, tidal volume, and minute volume. Patients who develop respiratory failure require mechanical ventilation and may require tracheostomy. Arterial blood gas monitoring is common. The patient may also require nutritional maintenance intravenously or through a nasogastric tube. If the patient has severe paralysis and is expected to have a long recovery period, a gastrostomy tube may be inserted. Special eye care is important to prevent corneal damage.

Adrenocortical steroids are used at times to treat symptoms. Convalescence may require many months. Attention to the prevention of iatrogenic complications, such as contracture, decubitus ulcers, muscle atrophy, and loss of range of motion, is imperative to allow complete recovery.

Evaluation

The questions listed under Evaluation for the patient with a CVA (p. 1261) also apply to the patient with Guillain-Barré syndrome.

NEUROSYPHILIS
Pathophysiology

In the late or chronic stage of syphilis, infection may involve the brain and spinal cord. The oculomotor nerves may be involved, causing inability of the pupil to react to light (*Argyll Robertson pupil*). *Tabes dorsalis* is the name given to the involvement of the posterior columns of the spinal cord and the posterior nerve roots. Sensory symptoms predominate. The patient may have severe paroxysmal pain anywhere in the body, the most common location being in the stomach (*gastric crisis*). Patients may have areas of severe paresthesia. A common finding in tabes dorsalis is loss of position sense in the feet and legs. The patient is unable to sense where the feet are placed, resulting in a highly characteristic slapping gait. Walking in the dark is increasingly difficult because the person relies on vision in placing the feet. Visual loss or blindness also can occur. Tabes dorsalis can cause trophic changes in the joints so that stability is lost (*Charcot's joint*).

General paresis is the term used to designate another late manifestation of syphilis characterized by degeneration of the brain and deterioration of mental function, as well as evidence of other neurologic disease.

HERPES ZOSTER

Herpes zoster, also known as *shingles*, is a common disease, occurring at higher rates among the old and patients with lymphomas, cancer, and Hodgkin's disease.

Etiology and pathophysiology

The causative organism is the varicella virus, similar to the one that causes herpes simplex. It may occur as a result of a reactivation of the viral infection that lies dormant in the ganglion after a primary case of chickenpox. It is not communicable, except to persons who have not had chickenpox. An acute inflammatory reaction takes place in the spinal or cranial sensory ganglions, the posterior gray matter of the cord, and the meninges.

The rash seen in herpes zoster consists of a vesicular, cutaneous eruption within a dermatome. It may be preceded by severe itching, pain in the area, fever, and malaise. Segmental weakness and atrophy may exist in the same area as the sensory changes. A small percentage of patients first seek medical attention for ophthalmic herpes, with the rash and pain occurring along the distribution of the trigeminal nerve.

Nursing process
Assessment
Subjective data

1. Complaints of pain
2. Any sensory changes
3. Complaints of malaise
4. Complaints of itching

Objective data

1. Fever
2. Presence of rash—vesicular cutaneous eruption within a dermatome
3. Presence of weakness or atrophy in the area of sensory changes

Data analysis: nursing diagnoses

Nursing diagnoses are determined from analysis of patient data. Possible nursing diagnoses for the person with herpes zoster may include, but are not limited to, the following:

Diagnostic title	Possible etiologies
Infection, high risk for	Decreased immune response
Knowledge deficit	Lack of exposure/recall
Pain	Nerve root inflammation
Skin integrity, altered, actual or high risk for	Irritation from the rash of herpes zoster

Planning: expected patient outcomes

Expected patient outcomes for the person with herpes may include but are not limited to the following:

1. Patient remains infection free.
2. Patient can explain prescribed medication (dosage, action, side effects, and frequency).
3. Patient has minimal discomfort.
4. Patient is able to sleep at least 6 hours per night.
5. Patient's skin integrity improves.

Implementation
Assisting with the achievement of therapeutic goals

Treatment for herpes zoster consists mainly of supportive care with medication for control of pain. The pain may persist for some time after the rash disappears. Some persons have pain along the affected nerve root for 1 to 2 years after the initial infection. Phenytoin (Dilantin) and carbamazerine (Tegretol) may be helpful for control of persistent pain. Steroid therapy started early in the disease course is believed to shorten the course but is not recmmended for patients with suppressed immune responses.

A newer treatment for herpes zoster is Capsaicin (Zostrix). Generally the lesions are kept covered until all drainage ceases. The nurse should assess the skin of the patient to monitor healing of the lesions and to detect any signs of infection.

Interventions to achieve patient outcomes
Preventing infection

Isolation may be necessary for staff who have not had chickenpox. This is especially true for the pregnant employee. Also, patients with malignancies, lymphomas, or Hodgkin's disease who have not had chickenpox should be protected from exposure to the patient.

Because the virus is spread by direct contact and airborne routes, strict isolation is often necessary, at least until drainage from any lesions stops. The protective measures are listed in Box 37-44.

Facilitating learning

It is important to educate the patient about the risk of spreading herpes zoster to others. The importance of good hand washing is stressed. The prescribed medications should be reviewed with the patient as to dosage, action, side effects, and schedule for administration.

Evaluation

Evaluation of the patient with herpes zoster includes the following questions:
1. Is the patient free of infection?
2. Is the patient able to state the required medications including dosage, side effects, times, and expected results?
3. Is the patient having minimal pain?
4. Is the patient's rash improving?

ACQUIRED IMMUNODEFICIENCY SYNDROME

Acquired immunodeficiency syndrome (AIDS) is a disease that has serious effects on the nervous system. About 40% of AIDS patients have neurologic symptoms; in fact, with approximately 10% of all AIDS patients the initial presenting problem is neurologic. See Chapter 19 for more information on AIDS. Only the neurological problems associated with AIDS will be discussed in this chapter.

Etiology and Pathophysiology

Patients develop neurologic symptoms either as a result of infection with HIV itself or as a result of associated infections. They may have ADC (AIDS dementia complex), which is also known as subacute encephalitis. Patients with ADC may manifest early signs of difficulty in concentrating or recent memory loss. This progresses to a global cognitive dysfunction with confusion, a vacant stare, and little spontaneous or verbal behavior.[62]

Other neurological problems that may occur include acute inflammatory demyelinating sensorimotor polyradiculopathy (AIDP), chronic inflammatory demyelinating

---

37-44	Isolation measures for patient with herpes zoster

1. Private room with private toilet facilities
2. Gown, masks, and gloves required of caregivers
3. Strict hand washing
4. Linen handled as isolation linen
5. Double-bagging of dressings
6. Disposable dishes if possible
7. Transport patients only as necessary
8. Isolation procedure for visitors

---

polyneuropathy (CIDP), or distal sensory polyneuropathy (DSPN). Mononeuritis multiplex is an inflammation of random individual spinal, cranial, or peripheral nerves. The inflammation leads to sensory or motor deficits. Myopathies such as polymyositis may also occur.[62,73]

Opportunistic infections seen with AIDS include the following:
1. Aseptic meningitis
2. Herpes simplex or herpes zoster
3. Cytomegalovirus
4. Progressive multifocal leukoencephalopathy (PML): a demyelinating disorder
5. Toxoplasmosis
6. Cryptococcal fungal infections: cryptococcal meningitis

Finally, patients with AIDS may develop neoplasms of the CNS; these include primary malignant lymphomas.

Nursing Process
Assessment

The reader is referred to the assessment section for patients with meningitis for assessment factors (p. 1264). The neurologic symptoms of AIDS vary because the neurologic problems vary.

Diagnostic tests

CT scans are helpful in the diagnosis of neurologic problems related to AIDS. The MRI may also be used and often provides imaging, which facilitates diagnosis. Biopsies of brain tissue have also been used to diagnose specific problems.

Data analysis: nursing diagnoses

The reader is referred to the section on CVA (p. 1256).

Planning: expected patient outcomes

The reader is referred to the section on CVA (p. 1256).

Implementation

Treatment of the patient with neurologic problems related to AIDS depends on the nature of the infection. Unfortunately, no treatment is available for many of the problems, such as AIDS dementia complex.

Infections that result from the herpes virus may be treated by acyclovir (Zovirax). Brain abscesses may be treated with pyrimethamine (Daraprim), an antimalarial agent, and sulfadiazine. Cryptococcal infections are usually treated with antifungal agents such as ampho-tericin-B.[62]

Evaluation

The reader is referred to the section on CVA (p. 1261).

INTERFERENCE WITH FUNCTION BECAUSE OF TRAUMA

Interference with neurologic function can occur as a result of trauma. Parts of the nervous system commonly subjected to trauma include the craniocerebrum, the spinal cord, and the peripheral nerves. Traumatic lesions usually result from direct physical force or from sustained compression.

CRANIOCEREBRAL TRAUMA

Craniocerebral trauma, or head injury, causes death or serious disability in people of all ages. Head injury is the second most common cause of major neurologic deficits and the major cause of death between ages 1 and 35. About 77,000 persons die each year in the United States from craniocerebral trauma. Another 50,000 persons survive yearly with mild to severe permanent disabilities.

Brain injury causes more deaths than does injury to any other organ. Causes of head injury include motor vehicle accidents, falls, industrial accidents, assaults, and sports-related accidents. In some states the repeal of laws requiring motorcyclists to wear helmets has resulted in an estimated threefold increase in death and injury from damage to the brain sustained in motorcycle accidents.

Pathophysiology

Craniocerebral trauma may result in injury to the scalp, skull, and brain tissues, either singly or collectively. Some of the variables that may modify the extent of the injury to the head include the following:

1. Location and direction of the impact
2. Rate of the energy transfer
3. Surface area of the energy transfer
4. Status of the head at the time of the impact

Injuries vary from minor scalp wounds to concussion and open fractures of the skull with severe damage to the brain. The amount of obvious damage is not indicative of the seriousness of the trouble. General effects of moderate to severe head injury include *cerebral edema*, *sensory and motor deficits*, and *increased intracranial pressure*. Later damage can occur as a result of *brain herniation*, *cerebral ischemia*, and *hypoxemia*.

Injuries to the brain can result from direct or indirect trauma to the head. Indirect trauma is caused by *tension strains* and shearing forces transmitted to the head by stretching of the neck. Direct trauma occurs when the head is directly injured. This results in *acceleration-deceleration* with *cavitation* (release of dissolved gases from the CSF, blood, or brain tissue). The release of gases damages nervous tissue. Direct trauma also results in rotation of the skull and its contents. These forces can occur at the same time or in succession and can damage the brain by compression, shearing, or tension.

Acceleration injuries occur when the head is struck by a moving object and set in motion. As a result of acceleration forces, *bruising* or *contusion* of the occipital and frontal lobes, brainstem, and cerebellum may occur.

Deceleration injuries occur when the head strikes a solid immovable object with a rapid deceleration of the skull. The brain decelerates more slowly.

Acceleration-deceleration movements that occur with lateral flexion, hyperflexion, hyperextension, and turning cause the cerebrum to rotate about the brainstem, resulting in *shearing*, *stretching*, and *distortion of neural tissue*. The stretching or tension causes fracture of the axons.

Head injuries can be *open* or *closed*. Open head injuries result from skull fractures or penetrating wounds. The amount of injury with this type of wound is determined by the velocity, mass, shape, and direction of the impact. Usually there is some type of skull fracture. These include:

1. Linear—simple break in bone
2. Comminuted—two or more common breaks that divide the bone into more than two fragments
3. Depressed—bone forced below the line of normal contour
4. Compound—can be linear, comminuted, or depressed

37-45 Damage to brain tissue caused by trauma

	Characteristics	Structural alteration	Effects
Concussion	Characterized by immediate and transitory impairment of neurologic function caused by mechanical force	No	May be loss of consciousness that is instant or delayed—usually reversible
Contusion	Likened to bruising with extravasation of blood cells	Yes	Injury may be at site of impact (coup) or at opposite site (contrecoup) Often damage to cortex
Laceration	Tearing of tissues caused by sharp fragment or shearing force	Yes	Hemorrhage is serious complication

Fractures at the base of the skull are usually serious because of their location. When one is sustained, vital centers, cranial nerves, and nerve pathways may be permanently damaged. Trauma and the resulting edema may obstruct cerebrospinal fluid flow directly or indirectly, with resultant increased intracranial pressure. If the injury has caused a direct communication between the cranial cavity and the middle ear or the sinuses, meningitis or a brain abscess may develop. Bleeding from the nose and ears suggests a basal fracture. Serosanguineous drainage from these orifices may contain cerebrospinal fluid and should be noted.

Closed head injuries include concussions, contusions, and lacerations. See Box 37-45 for a comparison of these injuries.

The effect of a blow on the cranium to the brain tissues within the skull is one of sudden movement. This effect can be likened to what happens as one stops suddenly when moving quickly with an open dish of fluid—some of the fluid spills. The only difference is that instead of spilling in the closed cavity, the brain tissue strikes the bony covering forcibly. A contusion or laceration directly below the site of the cranial impact is called a *coup* lesion. A lesion opposite the impact site is called *contrecoup,* which occurs when the brain hits the cranium on the opposite side of the blow. Damage to the brain tissues may include concussion, contusion, or laceration.

Lacerations of the scalp bleed profusely because of its large blood supply. Hemorrhage resulting from craniocerebral trauma may occur at the following sites:

1. Scalp
2. Epidural
3. Subdural
4. Intracerebral
5. Intraventricular

Two of these, *epidural* and *subdural hematomas,* require careful and continuous observation by the nurse and pose special problems to the patient with a head injury. Epidural hematomas form as blood collects rapidly between the dura and skull. Bleeding in this area is commonly caused by laceration of the middle meningeal artery, which is capable of producing rapid clot formation. Common sites for bleeding include sites of basal and temporal skull fractures. If lethargy or unconsciousness develops after the patient regains consciousness, an epidural hematoma may be suspected. Bleeding needs to be controlled promptly and the blood removed.

A subdural hematoma forms as venous blood collects below the dural surface. Because the bleeding is under venous pressure, the hematoma formation is relatively slow. The clot formation will, however, cause pressure on the brain surface and may eventually displace brain tissue. If the expanding clot is not evacuated it can cause increased ICP with compression of vital areas. The focal neurologic signs of clot formation are related to the site of the clot. If a patient who has been conscious for several days to weeks after a head injury becomes unconscious or develops neurologic symptoms, a *subdural hematoma* should be suspected. Subdural hematomas can be classed as follows:

1. Acute—occurs within 24 to 48 hours
2. Subacute—occurs within 48 hours to 2 weeks

3. Chronic—can occur weeks or months after the injury. These occur most commonly in the 60-70 year age range. At times, the cause of hematoma is uncertain.

Intracerebral hemorrhage usually occurs in the frontal or temporal regions.

Most deaths from head injury are from cerebral edema caused by damage rather than the actual primary destruction of vital centers. Brain edema is a major cause of increased ICP. Along with the swelling, local and systemic disturbances in circulation occur with resulting anoxia. The brain damage may be severe and not related to the demonstrated structural damage.

Nursing Process
Assessment
Subjective data

1. Patient's understanding of injury and resulting pathology—also patient's ability to understand
2. Information about nature of the injury—how it happened
3. Presence of headache, nausea, or vomiting
4. Presence of diplopia or other visual problems
5. Unusual sensations (paresthesias, ringing in ears)
6. History of bleeding from ear, nose, eye, or mouth
7. History of loss of consciousness
8. Use of alcohol or drugs
9. Time of most recent food intake

Objective data

1. Respiratory status (presence of patent airway, need for suctioning, need for intubation and mechanical ventilation)
2. Arterial blood gases
3. Level of consciousness and alertness
4. Pupils: size, equality, reactivity
5. Orientation
6. Motor status
7. Vital signs
8. Presence of bleeding
9. Presence of vomiting
10. Speech patterns—abnormalities
11. Presence of increased intracranial pressure

Because many persons with head injury, especially from motor vehicle accidents, have sustained other injuries, the intrathoracic and intraabdominal areas are checked carefully and the limbs are examined for fractures and injuries to nerves or arteries.

Diagnostic tests

Diagnostic tests performed for patients with head injury include skull x-ray films, CT scan, MRF, and possibly cerebral angiography. These procedures were described earlier in this chapter. Other diagnostic tests such as skull and chest films rule out other injuries.

Data analysis: nursing diagnoses

Nursing diagnoses are determined from analysis of patient data. Possible nursing diagnoses for the person with craniocerebral trauma may include, but are not limited to, the following:

Diagnostic title	Possible etiologies
Tissue perfusion, altered cerebral	Decreased arterial cerebral blood flow
Airway clearance, ineffective	Perceptual/cognitive impairment
Breathing pattern, ineffective	Neuromuscular impairment
Injury, high risk for	Sensory/motor deficits
Thermoregulation, ineffective	Trauma/illness
Infection, high risk for	Decreased nutrition
Incontinence, bowel	Neuromuscular impairment
Incontinence, urge or total	Neurological dysfunction
Coping, ineffective individual	Situational crises
Activity intolerance	Immobility, generalized weakness
Mobility, impaired physical	Neuromuscular impairment
Self-care deficit: feeding, bathing/hygiene, dressing/grooming, toileting	Neuromuscular impairment
Skin integrity, impaired, actual or high risk for	Pressure, immobility
Knowledge deficit	Lack of exposure or recall

Planning: expected patient outcomes

Expected patient outcomes for the patient with craniocerebral trauma may include, but are not limited to, the following:

1. Cerebral edema is decreased.
2. Patient can maintain a patent airway.
3. Patient can maintain an effective breathing pattern.
4. Patient remains free of injury.
5. Patient's temperature remains normal.
6. Patient remains free of infection.
7. Patient has minimal complications as a result of incontinence.
8. Patient has regular bowel movements without diarrhea or constipation.
9. Patient regains bowel and bladder continence if able.
10. Patient demonstrates increased independence.
11. Patient maintains optimal mobility and activity.
12. Patient has minimal deficits in ADL.
13. Patient's skin remains intact.
14. Patient can explain and demonstrate prescribed therapy to follow at home.
15. Patient can explain homegoing medication regimen (side effects, desired effects, time, dose, and route) to be followed at home.

Implementation

Assisting with the achievement of therapeutic goals

Medications

Medications are used to reduce cerebral edema and increased ICP, which are common problems in patients with head injuries. These medications include the following:

1. Osmotic diuretics that penetrate the brain slowly
   a. 30% solution of urea
   b. 20% mannitol
2. Dexamethasone

If the patient is receiving one of the diuretics and is not alert, a Foley catheter should be inserted to enable accurate accounting of output. Large amounts of urine can be anticipated.

Electrolyte imbalance

Careful monitoring of electrolytes is necessary. Several types of imbalance may occur with a head injury including the following:

1. Natriuresis (increased urinary excretion of sodium)
2. Inappropriate ADH syndrome (increased plasma levels of ADH, serum hyponatremia, and hypotonicity)
3. Hypernatremia
4. Cerebral sodium retention
5. Elevated plasma cortisol levels

Interventions to achieve patient outcomes

Immediate care is directed toward lifesaving measures and the maintenance of normal body function until the time when recovery is assured. The major aims of medical and nursing management are as follows:

1. To be constantly alert for changes in the patient's condition, especially changes that indicate any increase in ICP
2. To sustain the patient's vital functions until recovery allows the functions to resume
3. To manage complications that will be life threatening and interfere with full recovery

Promoting effective airway clearance and breathing patterns and improved cerebral perfusion

It is extremely important to maintain a patent airway and ensure adequate oxygenation. Anoxia with a buildup of carbon dioxide can produce cerebral hypoxia and subsequent cerebral edema, which can lead to altered cerebral perfusion. It is important to assess the ability to clear the airway. Blood or mucus from injuries may block the airway, or the patient may have vomited and suctioning may be necessary. Inability to clear the airway can lead to airway obstruction, as well as aspiration pneumonia. Oxygen should be given to the patient with a head injury, and if the patient cannot clear the airway an endotracheal tube is inserted. Arterial blood gas levels are checked frequently to determine whether respiratory exchange is adequate. Suctioning should be done as necessary.

Preventing injury

The patient should be kept as quiet as possible. No vigorous effort should be made to "clean the patient up" during the first few hours after the accident. Side rails should always be on the bed because restlessness may come on suddenly or convulsions may occur. The head of the bed is usually elevated 30 degrees. Restlessness may be caused by the need for a change of position, pain, or the need to empty the bladder. Codeine or other analgesics that do not depress the respiratory system are used for pain control. Anticonvulsants may be given to prevent seizures.

Maintaining thermal regulation

The blood pressure, pulse, and respiratory rate are taken frequently until they have stabilized and remain within safe limits. A sudden sharp rise in temperature,

which may go to 42° C or higher, and a sudden drop in blood pressure indicate that the regulatory mechanisms have lost control. The prognosis is poor. Measures are used to reduce temperature to normal because hyperthermia increases brain metabolism, resulting in brain damage. These measures include the following:
1. Administration of aspirin
2. Tepid sponge baths
3. Ice bags to the groin and axilla
4. Reducing temperature of patient's room
5. Electrically controlled cooling mattress

Preventing infection

The patient's ears and nose are checked carefully for signs of blood and serous drainage, which would indicate that the meninges have been torn and that spinal fluid is escaping. No attempt should be made to clean out the orifices. Loose sterile cotton may be placed in the outer openings only. This procedure is performed with caution so that the cotton does not act as a plug to interfere with the free flow of fluid. The cotton should be changed whenever it becomes moist. If there is evidence of drainage of CSF from the nose, the patient should not cough, sneeze, or blow the nose. These activities may enable air to enter the cranial cavity where it may increase symptoms of increased ICP. If there is question about whether drainage from the nose is CSF, a Tes-Tape is used to test for the presence of sugar, which is normally found in CSF.

Meningitis is a possible complication when communication with the nose and ears occurs. With basal skull fracture, antibiotics are commonly used because of the high rate of infection after this type of fracture.

Maintaining elimination

The patient's intake and output should be carefully measured and recorded. The specific gravity of the urine is also measured and can yield clues to electrolyte imbalance. In acute situations these measurements are repeated hourly.

The urinary output should be approximately 0.6 to 1 ml/kg of body weight/hour. If osmotic diuretics have been given, this amount will be greater. An indwelling catheter may be necessary; if so, catheter care to prevent infection should be used (see Chapter 33 for details). The person with cranial trauma should also be assessed for symptoms of diabetes insipidus, a common occurrence.

Bowel evacuation is not encouraged for several days after a head injury. Mild bulk laxatives, bisacodyl suppositories, or oil-retention enemas may be used. A stool softener is often prescribed, and the patient is taught not to strain at stool. When the patient is receiving dexamethasone or other steroids, it is important to check the stool for the presence of occult blood. This will also give a clue to the presence of stress ulcers, which are somewhat common after head injury. The ulcers are apparently caused by autonomic imbalances associated with the injury. Cimetidine (Tagamet) and antacids are routinely given if the patient with a closed head injury is receiving steroids.

Supporting coping ability

It is not uncommon that the patient with a head injury manifests loss of memory and loss of initiative. Behavioral problems associated with lack of judgment and restlessness may also occur. These patients need firm but gentle care, with specific guidelines for what behavior is allowed. It is not helpful to argue with the patient. It may be helpful to redirect their attention to another subject or task. Memory aids such as a log book or written schedule can be very useful in assisting with reorientation. The patient and family need to have gains in functioning pointed out, as it is easy to become frustrated and depressed when progress is slow.[52]

Promoting activity and mobility

The length of convalescence will depend on the amount of brain damage and how rapid the recovery has been. Patients are usually urged to resume normal activity as soon as possible. Headache and dizziness may be present for some time after a head injury. Some persons require intensive and lengthy rehabilitation in a rehabilitation center. Many brain-injured patients recover physically but have behavioral and psychologic problems that make it difficult for them to function completely independently.[52,64]

Some patients are left with serious deficits including hemiplegia. They will need to be taught compensatory techniques so that they can perform self-care measures. The nursing care of these patients is described in the section on patients who have had a stroke (p. 1258).

Maintaining skin integrity

Patients who have experienced craniocerebral trauma may be prone to develop skin problems. The care for the patient who has motor difficulties or is comatose is the same as for the patient with paralysis. The reader is referred to p. 1236 for a discussion of maintaining skin integrity.

Facilitating learning

Patients with head injury may be seen in an emergency room but not admitted to the hospital. These patients need teaching about observations for complications. A sample set of instructions is found in Box 37-46.

Teaching for the patient with a head injury who is left with deficits severe enough to require extended rehabilitation is similar to that for the patient with a motor problem. See p. 1235 for a description of this teaching. In addition, the following points are important:
1. Causes of increased ICP
2. Factors that can increase or decrease intracranial pressure
   a. No sneezing
   b. No heavy lifting, bending, or straining
   c. No straining at stool
3. Signs and symptoms to report to the physician

It is essential that the family be present at the teaching sessions.

Evaluation

Evaluation of the patient with a head injury is based on the expected patient outcomes. Questions to consider may include the following:
1. Are there symptoms of increased ICP?
2. Does the patient have a patent airway and effective breathing pattern?

37-46

Instructions for the patient with a head injury

Patient should be awakened periodically through the first 24 hours to be sure he or she can wake up easily.

Also, for the first 24 to 48 hours, the family should watch carefully for the following warning signs:

1. Vomiting—often with force behind it
2. Unusual sleepiness, dizziness, and loss of balance or falling
3. Complaint of seeing two of everything or blurry objects, jerking movement of the eyes
4. Bleeding or discharge from nose or ears
5. A slight headache may be expected; however, if it gets worse and the patient complains of feeling even worse when moving about, it should be reported
6. Convulsions (fits)—any twitching or movements of arms or legs that the patient is not able to stop
7. Any behavior or symptom that is not normal for the individual

Call a doctor at once if any of these signs are observed by the family.

Call either your personal physician or the emergency services.

Courtesy Department of Nursing, University Hospitals of Cleveland, Cleveland, Ohio.

3. Is the patient able to swallow safely and maintain an adequate diet?
4. Is the patient practicing safety techniques?
5. Is the patient afebrile?
6. Has infection been avoided?
7. Is the patient continent of bowel and bladder?
8. Is the patient demonstrating a positive self concept?
9. Is the patient compensating for sensory-perceptual difficulties?
10. Is the patient functioning in a socially acceptable way?
11. Is the patient's mobility functioning at optimal levels?
12. Does the patient have minimal difficulties in carrying out ADL?
13. Is the patient's skin intact?
14. Is the patient able to verbalize follow-up care and discharge regimen?
15. Is the patient taking medication accurately?

SPINAL CORD TRAUMA

Spinal cord injury from accidents is a common and increasing cause of serious disability and death in the United States. Approximately 10% of traumatic injuries to the nervous system involve the spinal cord. It has been estimated that more than 100,000 persons in the United States are paralyzed as a result of spinal cord injury and that 10,000 more are injured every year. Most persons involved

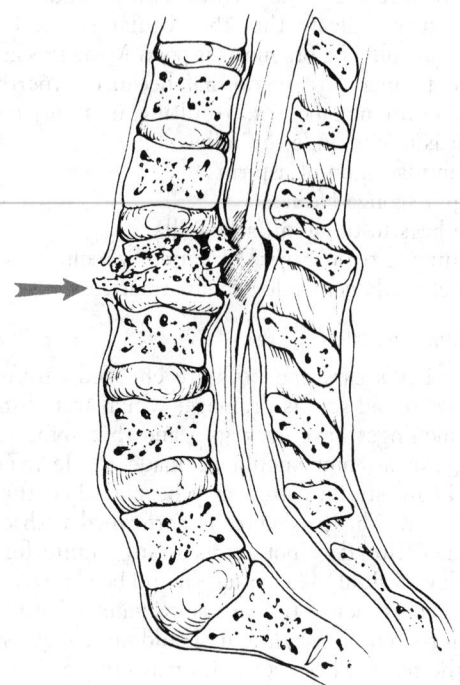

Fig. 37-48   Damage to spinal cord and distortion of adjacent structures that may occur in traumatic injuries to spine.

with spinal cord injuries are males between the ages of 18 and 25. Automobile, motorcycle, diving, surfing, and other athletic accidents and gunshot wounds are major causes of spinal cord injuries. The largest number of spinal cord injuries are caused by vehicular accidents.

The most common sites of injury are the lower cervical region and the junction of the thoracic and lumbar region.

Pathophysiology

The spinal cord may be damaged by lesions arising outside the cord or by lesions within the cord itself. The latter are a less common cause and are usually the result of tumors. Trauma to the spinal cord can result in *concussion, contusion, laceration, complete* or *partial transection, hemorrhage,* or loss of blood supply to a part of the cord (Fig. 37-48).

The soft tissue of the spinal cord is protected by the vertebral column. This column can be injured by various mechanisms, including the following:

1. Hyperextension—also called whiplash. These occur most often in the cervical region and result from the forces of acceleration-deceleration and the reduction of diameter of the spinal cord.
2. Hyperflexion—results in overstretching, compression and deformity of the spinal cord.
3. Vertical compression—primarily occurs in the area of T12 to L2. Injuries result from a force applied downward from the cranium that often results in a burst vertebra.
4. Rotation injury—can involve all parts of the vertebrae.

Injuries that occur to the vertebrae include the following types:

Muscle function after spinal cord injury

Spinal cord injury	Muscle function remaining	Muscle function lost
Cervical above C4	None	All, including respiration
C5	Neck	Arms
	Scapular elevation	Chest
		All below chest
C6-C7	Neck	Some arm, fingers
	Some chest movement	Some chest
	Some arm movement	All below chest
Thoracic	Neck	Trunk
	Arms (full)	All below chest
	Some chest	
Lumbosacral	Neck	Legs
	Arms	
	Chest	
	Trunk	

1. Simple fracture—single break affecting the spinous or transverse process of the vertebra. The spinal cord is not usually compressed and the alignment of the vertebrae is not altered.
2. Compressed or wedged fracture—occurs when the vertebral body is compressed anteriorly. Cord compression may be present.
3. Comminuted or burst fractures—vertebral body shatters into many fragments, any of which may injure the cord.
4. Dislocation of vertebrae—may result in nonalignment of vertebral column with injury to the spinal cord. Partial dislocation is called subluxation.

Severe traumatic lesions of the spinal cord may result in total transection of the spinal cord or a tearing of the cord from side to side at a particular level, with a complete loss of spinal cord functions. This total transection is also referred to as a "complete cord injury." With the complete injury all voluntary movement below the level of the lesion is lost. A partial transection or "incomplete injury" involves a partial transection or injury of the cord. Quadriplegics are patients who sustain injuries to one of the eight cervical segments of the spinal cord. Paraplegics are those whose lesions are confined to the thoracic, lumbar, or sacral regions of the spinal cord. The symptoms of incomplete injuries can vary depending on the nature of the injury and the resultant syndrome. Resultant syndromes can include the following:

1. Anterior cord syndrome
2. Central cord syndrome
3. Brown-Séquard syndrome
4. Herniated disc syndrome

The *anterior cord syndrome* most often results from a *flexion injury* to the *cervical vertebrae. It is the most common type of cord syndrome* and *damages the anterior spinal artery, as well as the spinal cord.* Upper and lower motor function is lost. The *central cord syndrome* results from *flexion or hyperextension injuries.* There is resultant compression of the anterior horn cells and edema of the central spinal cord, causing mixed upper and lower motor neuron loss

and spasticity below the level of the injury. Usually more impairment occurs in the upper extremities.

Another syndrome is the *Brown-Séquard syndrome,* which results from *rotation-flexion injuries where subluxation or dislocation of the fracture fragments occurs.* There is ipsilateral paresis, loss of proprioception, and contralateral loss of pain and temperature sensation.

The last syndrome is the *herniated disc syndrome,* which is very common. In this syndrome, there is *displacement of discs with the escape of cartilage.* It occurs spontaneously or in response to activity or slight injury.

All of these injuries are more common in older persons because of degenerative changes with aging. The lower lumbar and lumbosacral areas are affected most often.[8]

Spinal shock

Initially, in most spinal cord injuries there is a period of flaccid paralysis and a complete loss of reflexes below the level of the lesion. Sensory and autonomic functions are also lost. This is called spinal or neural shock, or areflexia, and it is a transitory event. Spinal shock results from the loss of inhibition of the descending tracts. During this period persons may require temporary respiratory assistance until recovery begins.

Within hours, days, or weeks the involved muscles gradually become spastic and hyperreflexic with the characteristic signs of an upper motor neuron lesion. These changes are thought to represent the release of the muscle stretch reflexes from the inhibitory influence of the damaged pyramidal tract, resulting in hyperactive responses.

The amount of disability that results from spinal cord injury depends on the level of injury. See Box 37-47 for specifics of muscle function after spinal cord injury.

Voiding

The center for micturition is located in the conus medullaris (S2-S4) and is linked to the detrusor muscle of the bladder by parasympathetic sensory and motor fibers that run in the pelvic nerves. Spinal cord injuries that occur at levels above the conus result in a bladder that is capable

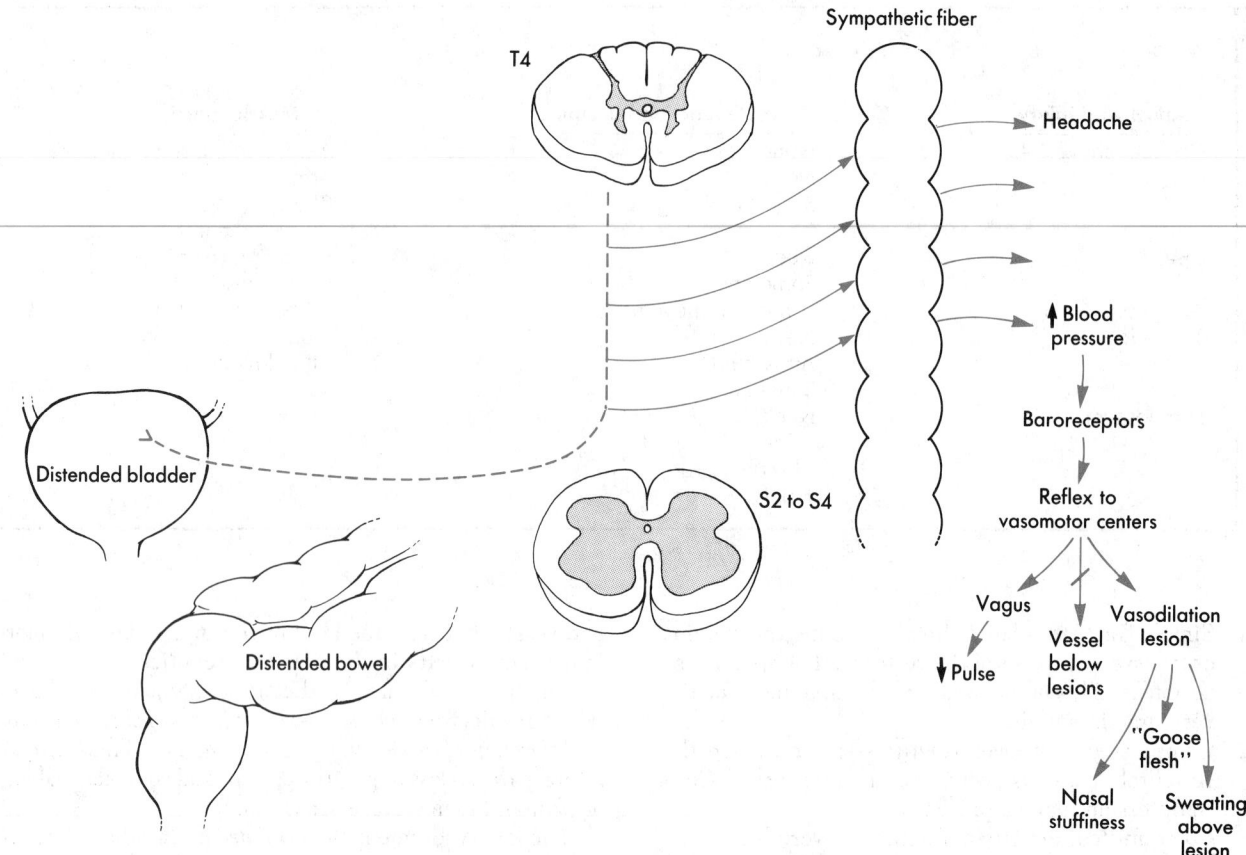

Fig. 37-49 Pictorial diagram of cause of autonomic hyperreflexia and results.

of emptying itself reflexly or involuntarily after the spinal shock phase. The bladder is hypertonic and it is variously known as an "upper motor neuron bladder" and "reflex neurogenic bladder." The emptying occurs spontaneously or automatically. The patient has no control over the act of micturition. Voiding may occur at intervals of 3 to 4 hours; there may be frequency, urgency, and incontinence. The reflex arc is intact in this type bladder. When the cord lesion is at or below the micturition center, the center or the sacral nerve roots are destroyed; the reflex arc is no longer intact. This type of bladder condition is known as a "lower motor neuron bladder" or an "autonomous neurogenic bladder." Contractions of the bladder muscle are the result of impulses transmitted through a mechanism within the bladder wall but are not of sufficient strength or duration to empty the bladder. Abdominal straining or manual compression is necessary for this to happen. *Retention of urine and infection are common complications.*

Autonomic dysreflexia

One complication of spinal cord injury that is extremely important to understand is *autonomic dysreflexia*, or hyperreflexia. It occurs in patients with cord lesions above the sixth thoracic vertebra and most commonly in patients with cervical injuries (Fig. 37-49). Autonomic dysreflexia occurs as a result of abnormal cardiovascular response to stimulation of the sympathetic division of the autonomic nervous system. The clinical signs include the following:

1. Bradycardia
2. Paroxysmal hypertension
3. Sweating
4. "Goose flesh"
5. Severe headache
6. Nasal stuffiness

Patients tend to develop individual symptoms of this condition and are soon able to recognize them.

The most common cause is visceral distention, which can include a distended bladder or impacted rectum. *It is a medical emergency that requires immediate treatment, because it can lead to cerebrovascular accident, blindness, or death.* Treatment is discussed later in this chapter (p. 1282).

Sexual function

In most cases, men experience impotence, decreased sensation, and difficulties with ejaculation. Impairment of fertility is common. The act of erection is under the control of sensory and parasympathetic fibers, while ejaculation requires sympathetic and parasympathetic innervation. Lesions above S2 leave the parasympathetic reflex arc intact; patients may be able to have an erection, but ejaculation is not usually possible. Lesions in the S2 to S4 area usually prevent erection and ejaculation. The higher the level of injury, the more likely a man with complete cord injury is able to perform sexually. The experience of orgasm is described as different from before the injury. Women with spinal cord injury are able to continue to perform sexually, although perception of sexual pleasure is usually altered.

Nursing Process
Assessment

Assessment of the patient with spinal cord injury includes both subjective and objective data.

Subjective data

1. Patient's understanding of injury and resulting deficit
2. Information about nature of injury—how it happened
3. Reports shortness of breath
4. Unusual sensations (paresthesias, and so on)
5. History of loss of consciousness
6. Presence of pain
7. Absence of sensation—sensory level

Objective data

1. Respiratory status
2. Level of alertness and consciousness
3. Orientation
4. Pupil size, equality, and reactivity
5. Proper alignment of body in neutral alignment
6. Motor strength
7. Temperature, blood pressure, and pulse
8. Skin integrity
9. Bowel and bladder status and distention
10. Presence of other injuries

As with the patient with a head injury, the patient with a spinal cord injury should be assessed carefully for the presence of other injuries, primarily fractures or head injury.

Diagnostic tests

It is most important to first detect if there has been any cervical vertebra fracture or displacement. X-ray films are always taken to detect any fracture-dislocations. These often occur before the patient is moved from the backboard or stretcher. A spinal tap or myelography may also be used to detect blockage. It can be carried out also without moving the patient if the dye is injected at the junction between the first cervical vertebra and the base of the skull. CT scanning may also be very helpful in ruling out spinal cord injury. The MRI can detect spinal cord compression and edema. These procedures were discussed earlier in this chapter.

Data analysis: nursing diagnoses

Nursing diagnoses are determined from analysis of patient data. Possible nursing diagnoses for the person with spinal cord injury may include, but are not limited to, the following:

Diagnostic title	Possible etiologies
Infection, high risk for	Spinal cord injury
Injury, high risk for	Sensory/motor deficits
Mobility, impaired physical	Neuromuscular impairment
Activity intolerance	Immobility
Urinary retention	Inability to initiate stream of urine
Incontinence, reflex or total	Neurologic impairment
Incontinence, bowel	Neuromuscular impairment
Dysreflexia	Distended bladder, impacted rectum
Breathing pattern, ineffective	Neuromuscular impairment
Skin integrity, impaired, actual or high risk for	Immobility
Coping, ineffective individual	Situational crisis
Knowledge deficit	Lack of exposure/recall
Self-care deficit: feeding, bathing/hygiene, dressing/grooming, toileting	Neuromuscular impairment
Adjustment, impaired	Disability requiring change in lifestyle
Sexual dysfunction	Physiologic limitations

Planning: expected patient outcomes

Expected patient outcomes for the patient with spinal cord injury may include, but are not limited to, the following:

1. Patient remains infection free.
2. Patient remains free of further injury.
3. Patient's function is preserved to the extent possible with no increase in the level of injury.
4. Patient demonstrates an optimal level of mobility.
5. Patient can demonstrate exercises to maintain function.
6. Patient can explain importance of frequent position changes, including the use of the prone position and weight shifts in the wheelchair.
7. Patient demonstrates minimal complications of bowel and bladder incontinence.
8. Patient evacuates bowel on a regular schedule without diarrhea or constipation.
9. Patient can carry out or direct own bowel and bladder program, including possible intermittent catheterization and use of suppositories and digital stimulation.
10. Patient can explain autonomic dysreflexia, characteristic symptoms, and the actions to be taken when it occurs.
11. Patient's airway is maintained.
12. Patient maintains an effective breathing pattern.
13. Patient remains free of respiratory complications.
14. Patient can explain the need for assisted coughing if required and have caregiver demonstrate.
15. Patient's skin is intact.
16. Patient can do skin inspection or direct others in the inspection of the skin.
17. Patient verbalizes a positive self-concept.
18. Patient is able to direct own care and his involvement in plan of care.
19. Patient demonstrates optimal coping skills.
20. Patient makes a reasonable choice for living arrangements.
21. Patient has minimal limitations in ADL.
22. Patient can explain the medication regimen (side effects, desired effects, time, dose, and route).
23. Patient can explain plans for follow-up care.
24. Patient can explain how to obtain community re-

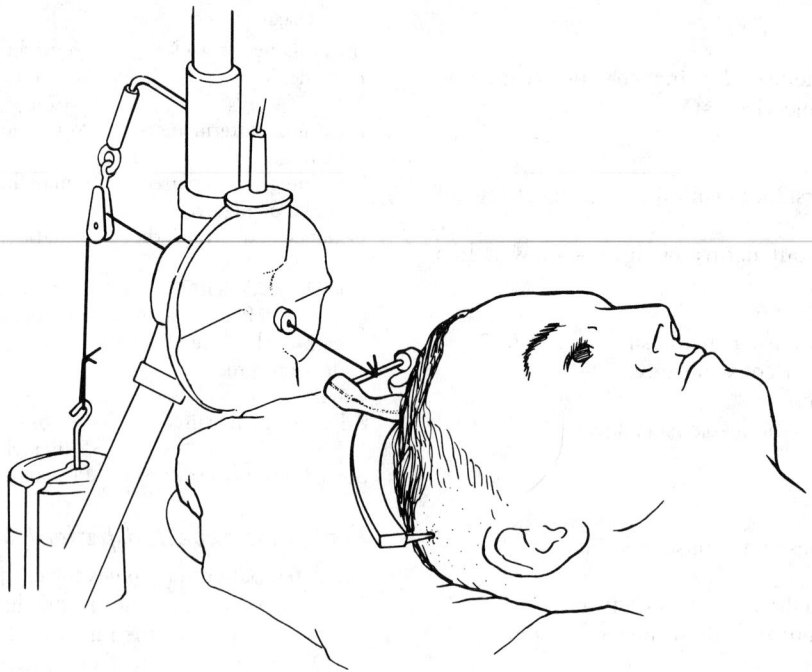

Fig. 37-50 Patient with Crutchfield tongs inserted into skull to hyperextend head and neck.

sources, including the Bureau of Vocational Rehabilitation.

25. Patient remains sexually active, if so desired.

Implementation
Assisting with achievement of therapeutic goals
Immediate stage

Cervical injuries. Immediate care after spinal cord injury is directed toward realignment of the cervical bony column in the presence of demonstrated fractures or dislocations. These measures include the following:

1. Simple immobilization
2. Skeletal traction
   a. Crutchfield tongs (Fig. 37-50)
   b. Halo traction
   c. Stryker or Foster frame
3. Surgery for spinal decompression

It is important to maintain strict body alignment, with the body kept straight and the head flat. Sandbags may be used to maintain alignment.

With Crutchfield tongs it is important to check the traction and orthopedic frame frequently (usually every 4 hours). The tongs should be secure, and the weights should hang freely. The sites where the tongs enter the head are cleansed with hydrogen peroxide, and povidine iodine solution is applied. Usually this is done every shift. When halo traction is used it is also important to check the pin sites and cleanse them as described previously. The traction is attached to a fiberglass body jacket, which should be checked for proper fit. The nurse should be able to insert a finger between the cast and skin. If the nurse cannot insert a finger, the cast is too tight and the physician should be notified.

With the use of a frame (Foster or Stryker), it is important to check pressure points before and after the patient is turned. At least two persons should turn the patient, and all bolts on the frame should be tightened securely before turning. Padding may be used for comfort but care must be taken to maintain body alignment. It is important to assess the patient for any respiratory or cardiovascular difficulty when on the frame.

Often surgical decompression is not performed until after a period of skeletal traction. This allows the patient's condition to stabilize and some initial swelling of the cord to subside. The beginning spontaneous healing of the fracture site provides more stability. With the introduction of the anterior surgical approach to the cervical spinal column, surgical intervention is safer and can be attempted earlier in the hospitalization. The primary advantage of the anterior surgical approach is that it provides immediate stabilization of the spinal cord by techniques of interbody cervical fusion and the direct removal of any extruded disc materials. See Box 37-48 for care of the patient who has had surgical decompression.

Intubation and respiratory assistance may be required in the immediate stage after upper cervical cord injury. Any patient with a cord lesion at the C4 level probably will require permanent ventilatory support. Careful monitoring of blood gas levels and regular pulmonary toilet are essential.

Thoracic and lumbar injuries. Less immediate attention to thoracic and lumbar fracture immobilization is necessary for the patient with limited neurologic deficits. The patient is often treated with bed rest, hyperextension, and bracing. Stabilization of the spine may occur early in the recovery course or may be delayed until some healing has occurred.

Medications. The use of adrenal corticosteroids for the prevention and alleviation of spinal cord edema is widespread. It is believed that the steroids assist in the reestablishment of membrane stability and in the control of central nervous tissue stability.

Intermediate stage

Throughout all stages of hospitalization of the patient with a spinal cord injury, nursing and medical interventions are directed toward restoration of structural or body integrity. All efforts are taken to ensure that the following occur:

1. Contractures do not develop.
2. Range of motion is maintained to the greatest degree possible.
3. Muscle tone is consistent with pathologic condition.
4. Bowel and bladder function are maintained.
5. Skin is intact.

The reader is referred to the section on care of the patient with a motor dysfunction (p. 1231). Most of the care described there applies to the patient with a spinal cord injury. Additional care is described below.

Position and movement. In addition to frequent positioning, the patient with a spinal cord injury is usually placed on a bed with a firm surface or on a specially designed bed that maintains support of the spine.

Early mobilization of the patient is important. When patients, especially quadriplegics, begin to sit up, it may be necessary to wrap their legs with elastic wraps to encourage venous return. Slowly increasing the angle of sitting is essential to prevent hypotension. For this reason a newly quadriplegic patient should use a recliner wheelchair until he or she is able to sit at a 90-degree angle for several hours.

Before the patient is permitted to be up after a spinal injury, a brace may be prescribed. All braces and corsets must be custom made; they are usually expensive, and the cost depends on the type of material used. The brace or corset should be applied before the patient gets out of bed. Some patients are placed in a halo brace (see Chapter 40, Fig. 40-37). The patient should wear a thin, knitted undershirt next to the skin to keep the brace clean and to protect the skin. For some paraplegics, leg braces may permit them to stand and ambulate. Many find, however, that the effort to walk is not justified.

Urinary elimination. Because there is no sensation of needing to void in the patient with spinal cord injury, distention occurs easily. Usually a Foley catheter is inserted initially. Later, bladder training is started. Measures important in this training can be found in Chapter 33.

The presence of an indwelling catheter makes the patient highly susceptible to urinary infection, which can include bladder or kidney infections. These are major causes of death in patients with spinal cord injury, so it is imperative that infection be avoided, if at all possible. The best means of preventing infection is maintenance of fluid intake (3 to 4 L a day) and meticulous aseptic technique. Drinking cranberry juice several times a day has been found helpful in preventing infection, along with prophy-

---

Guidelines for Care 37-48

The patient undergoing spinal decompression

Preoperative care

1. Clarify patient's knowledge of surgery and expected changes.
2. Explain expected postoperative measures (including positioning, bed rest).
3. Encourage patient and family to verbalize fears.
4. Baseline neurologic and physiologic data should be assessed and recorded.

Postoperative care

1. Monitoring
   a. Assess ability to move legs; ask patient to do straight leg raises, dorsiflexion, and plantar flexion. Assess ability to move arms and hands if cervical decompression has occurred.
   b. Assess degree and character of drainage.
      (1) Amount of drainage and bleeding should be minimal.
      (2) Initial dressing can be reinforced as needed.
   c. Assess ability of patient to swallow; observe for swelling of neck.
2. Promoting mobility
   a. Patient can be turned side to side and onto back.
   b. If decompression is in lumbar area, sitting is usually not permitted.
   c. If decompression is in thoracic area, patient should not use arms to pull or push; no trapeze on bed.
   d. Patient is encouraged to do active range of motion and leg exercises such as quadriceps setting.
3. Promoting psychologic comfort
   a. Patient is encouraged to verbalize fears and reactions.
   b. Time should be spent with patient other than when giving direct care.
   c. Information about daily activities, tests, and procedures should be shared with patient.
   d. Medicate as needed for pain.
4. Preventing infection
   a. Incisional area kept clean and dry.
   b. Temperature checked frequently for first several days; report any elevation to physician.
   c. Report any redness, drainage, or induration (hardness) of wound.
   d. Incision often left open to air after first several days.

37-49 The patient with autonomic dysreflexia

1. Place patient in sitting position to decrease blood pressure.
2. Check patency of catheter for kinking. If catheter is plugged, insert new catheter immediately.
3. Check rectum for impaction.
4. If it is necessary to remove impaction, dibucaine (Nupercaine ointment) should be instilled in the rectum for its anesthetic effect.
5. Send urine for culture if no other cause is found; urinary infection can lead to symptoms of autonomic dysreflexia.
6. Administer ganglionic blocking agent such as hexamethonium chloride or a vasodilator such as nitroprusside (Nipride) if conservative measures are not effective.

37-50 Sexual functioning in patients with spinal cord injury

1. Reflexogenic erections occur not only as a result of stimulation of the genitalia, but also as a result of stimulation of "trigger points."
   a. Stroking the thigh
   b. Stimulating the rectum with a finger
   c. Manipulating the catheter
2. Male patients with catheters can either remove the catheter just before sexual activity or turn it back on the penis where it provides extra support.
3. Bowels should be emptied before intercourse to prevent incontinence.
4. Female patients who have a catheter can keep it in place if desired.
5. Female patients should realize that they maintain the ability to conceive—birth control should be practiced if pregnancy is not desired.

lactic antibiotic therapy such as nitrofurantoin or sulfamethoxazole and trimethoprim (Septra, Bactrim).

Autonomic dysreflexia is one complication associated with urinary elimination in the patient with spinal cord injury. It is a medical emergency, and the nurse should be aware of the actions to take in preventing and alleviating the symptoms. The care required with the presence of symptoms is outlined in Box 37-48.

Bowel elimination. Patients are started on a bowel program early in the recovery period. At first, bisacodyl (Dulcolax) suppositories are given at regular intervals—usually every other night. This is followed by digital stimulation to further stimulate peristalsis. The goal is to eliminate the need for the suppositories. Other aids to bowel programs are the use of adequate fluids, stool softeners, and prune juice.

Respiratory function. Generally, patients with cervical injuries below C4 are able to breathe without ventilatory support. However, they do not have normal control of chest muscles or the diaphragm, which makes them prone to respiratory complications. Care of the patient may include use of the inspirometer to increase tidal volume. Other breathing exercises may also be prescribed. The patient may require assisted coughing in which the caregiver exerts upward and inward pressure on the fleshy part of the stomach just below the diaphragm while the patient attempts to cough. This action is similar to the Heimlich maneuver but less force is used. The patient should also be encouraged to avoid situations where respiratory infections may be transmitted. Respiratory infections are often the cause of death in patients with spinal cord injury, especially those with high cervical injury.

If a patient is ventilator dependent, attempts are made to have the patient use a portable ventilator, which allows for mobility. Diaphragmatic pacemakers may be inserted. This is still an uncommon procedure, but it has been effective in allowing patients time off the ventilator.

Skin integrity. Another problem that occurs with spinal cord injury is decubitus ulcers. Every effort should be made to avoid skin breakdown, which is a major cause of morbidity in the patient with spinal cord injury.

Facilitating learning

Teaching of the patient with spinal cord injury encompasses all of the points covered in teaching the patient with a motor dysfunction and sensory dysfunction (Box 37-21, p. 1235). In addition, the patient needs assistance in learning about the effects of the injury on sexual functioning (see Box 37-50). The important thought to keep in mind is that most patients with a cooperative partner are able to engage in a satisfying sexual relationship. The limitation depends on the site of the lesion and whether the cord injury is complete or incomplete. Generally, the higher the lesion, the more normal sexual function is likely to be. Males with sacral lesions are the only patients with spinal cord injuries who are not able to have erection and ejaculate. Education of the patient in the area of sexual function includes the points outlined here.

Evaluation

Evaluation is based on expected patient outcomes. When evaluating the care of the patient with spinal cord injury, questions to consider may include the following:

1. Is the patient free of injury and has further injury been avoided?
2. Does the patient demonstrate an optimal level of mobility and exercises to maintain function?
3. Can patient explain the importance of frequent position changes?
4. Does the patient assume control of bowel and bladder program?
5. Is the patient's airway maintained?
6. Does the patient maintain an effective breathing pattern?

7. Does the patient remain free of respiratory complications?
8. Can the patient explain the need for assisted coughing if required and can caregiver demonstrate it?
9. Is the patient's skin intact?
10. Is the patient doing skin checks or asking staff to do them?
11. Does the patient verbalize a positive self-concept?
12. Is the patient directing and involved in own plan of care?
13. Does patient demonstrate optimal coping skills?
14. Has patient made a reasonable choice for living arrangements?
15. Is the patient as independent in ADL as possible?
16. Can patient explain medication regimen, plans for follow-up care, and how to use community resources?
17. Does the patient remain sexually active, if desired?

PERIPHERAL NERVE TRAUMA

The peripheral nerves that lie outside the brain and spinal cord include the cranial nerves and spinal nerves and their branches and plexuses. *The disorders involving the peripheral nerves are similar to those that affect the central nervous system and are the result of traumatic, degenerative, vascular, inflammatory, neoplastic, and metabolic causes.* Important terms are listed in Box 37-51.

Traumatic causes of peripheral nerve injuries include gunshot and knife wounds, fragmented fracture wounds, and surgical transections, as in denervation surgery and amputation. They result in stretching, laceration, and compression of the peripheral nerve. The degree of injury is variable. Recovery is also variable—axons of peripheral nerves are capable of regeneration under favorable conditions.

Pathophysiology

After trauma (or disease) the axon undergoes secondary or *wallerian degeneration* distal to the lesion and for several segments proximal. The axon and myelin sheath degenerate and undergo fragmentation. The fragmented particles are completely ingested within several weeks; the axis cylinder remains. Schwann's cells and fibroblasts begin to proliferate, covering the degenerated fibers. During the regenerative phase, new axoplasm forms at the proximal edge of the injury and the regenerating fibers now grow distally and enter the empty neurolemmal sheath, which has in the meantime proliferated. Myelin then forms around the regenerated axon. When a nerve has been severely damaged and fibrous tissue is abundant, regeneration is interfered with by a tangled mass known as a *traumatic neuroma;* this may have to be removed surgically.

Nursing Process
Assessment

Assessment includes both subjective and objective data.

Subjective data

1. Patient's understanding of condition
2. Alteration in sensation
   a. Pain

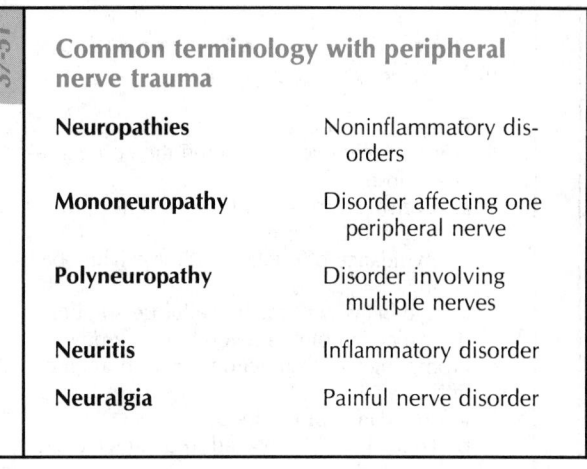

37-51

Common terminology with peripheral nerve trauma

Neuropathies	Noninflammatory disorders
Mononeuropathy	Disorder affecting one peripheral nerve
Polyneuropathy	Disorder involving multiple nerves
Neuritis	Inflammatory disorder
Neuralgia	Painful nerve disorder

   b. Touch
   c. Temperature
   d. Proprioception
3. Site of sensory problems
4. Onset of problem
5. Presence of associated symptoms

Objective data

1. Presence of motor alterations.
2. The clinical signs and symptoms resulting from peripheral nerve lesions depend on the exact location of the lesion and the specific function of the involved nerve or nerves. Because peripheral nerves contain both sensory and motor components, there may be deficits in both components distal to the site. Alterations will occur in pain, touch, temperature, proprioception, and stereognosis. Motor alteration includes *lower motor neuron signs* such as *flaccid paralysis* and *muscle wasting in the muscles innervated by the affected nerves.*

Data analysis: nursing diagnoses

The nursing diagnoses and expected patient outcomes are the same as those for the patient who has sensory (p. 1235). or motor dysfunction (pp. 1231).

Planning: expected patient outcomes

See Expected Patient Outcomes for Alterations in Muscle Tone and Motor Function (p. 1231) and Alterations in Sensory Function (p. 1235).

Implementation

Nursing care is specific on the areas of the body affected by the sensory and motor deficits. Plans for care include measures found in the section on motor dysfunction and sensory dysfunction. Promotion of good health habits in general assists in the creation of conditions favorable to nerve regeneration.

Evaluation

The evaluation for the patient with peripheral nerve dysfunction is the same as for the patient with motor (p. 1234) and sensory problems (p. 1236).

37-52	**Postoperative concerns for the patient with trigeminal neuralgia**

	1. Preservation of eye function (if the upper branch is completely severed the corneal reflex is lost)
	   a. Eye shield to prevent dust or lint from getting into the cornea
	   b. Avoidance of contact with eye while bathing
	   c. Eye baths with methylcellulose solution
	   d. Inspection of eye several times a day
	2. Promoting mouth function (lower branch of fifth cranial nerve)
	   a. Avoidance of hot food
	   b. Food should be placed in unaffected side of mouth
	   c. Mouth care after each meal
	3. Safety concerns
	   a. Electric razor should be used for shaving

37-53	**Comfort measures for patients with tic doloreaux**
	1. Keep room free of drafts 2. Avoid walking briskly to bedside of patient 3. Place bed out of traffic area to prevent jarring of bed 4. Avoid touching the patient's face 5. Patients should not be urged to wash or shave the affected area or to comb the hair 6. Avoid hot or cold liquids that trigger pain 7. Diet may have to be pureed and lukewarm and taken through straw

TRIGEMINAL NEURALGIA

Trigeminal neuralgia is one specific kind of peripheral nerve problem. It is also called *tic doloreaux*. It usually affects persons in middle or late adulthood and is slightly more common in women.

Assessment

Assessment is basically the same as for any patient with peripheral nerve trauma. Trigeminal neuralgia is characterized by excruciating, burning pain that radiates along one or more of the three divisions of the fifth cranial nerve (Fig. 37-51). The second and third divisions are most commonly affected. The pain typically only extends to the midline of the face and head, because this is the extent of the tissue supplied by the offending nerve. There are areas along the course of the nerve known as trigger points, and the slightest stimulation of these areas may initiate pain. Persons with trigeminal neuralgia try desperately to avoid triggering them.

Implementation
Assisting with the achievement of therapeutic goals
Medication

Carbamazepine (Tegretol) is the drug of choice for the treatment of trigeminal neuralgia pain. Drugs such as nicotinic acid, thiamine chloride, analgesics, and even cobra venom have been tried with little success. Absolute alcohol may be injected into the peripheral branches of the trigeminal nerve. This provides relief for weeks to months.[1]

Surgery

Permanent relief of pain is obtained only by surgery that consists of either inserting a fine needle through the cheek and injecting an alcohol solution or by surgical resection of the sensory root of the trigeminal nerve. This is not always successful. Preoperative care includes the following:

1. Measures of comfort
2. Allowing patient to voice questions or concerns
3. Teaching about procedure and what to expect

Postoperative care includes the measures listed in Box 37-52.

Within 24 hours after a fifth nerve resection, many patients develop herpes simplex (cold sores) about the lips. Usually the lesions heal in about a week.

Interventions to achieve patient outcomes
Maintaining comfort and ADL

It is not uncommon for patients with trigeminal neuralgia not to have eaten properly for some time, because eating causes pain. They may be undernourished and dehydrated. They may not have washed or shaved or combed the hair for some time. Oral hygiene often has been neglected.

Measures to increase comfort preoperatively or of patients being treated nonsurgically are found in Box 37-53.

Facilitating learning

Teaching for the patient with trigeminal neuralgia is found in Box 37-54.

BELL'S PALSY (PERIPHERAL FACIAL PARALYSIS)
Pathophysiology

Bell's palsy is thought to be caused by an inflammatory process involving the facial nerve (VII) anywhere from the nucleus in the brain to the periphery. Other theories of causation include local ischemia and edema or emotional trauma with resultant vasoconstriction. Any of the three branches of the facial nerve may be affected. The disorder can be unilateral or bilateral. Most patients (80%) recover spontaneously over a period of a few weeks, although recovery may take as long as a year.

Assessment

Subjective and objective data are the same as for the patient with peripheral nerve trauma (p. 1283). With Bell's palsy there is usually an abrupt onset of numbness or a feeling of stiffness or drawing sensation of the face. *Unilateral weakness of the facial muscles usually occurs, resulting in inability to wrinkle the forehead, close the eyelid, pucker the*

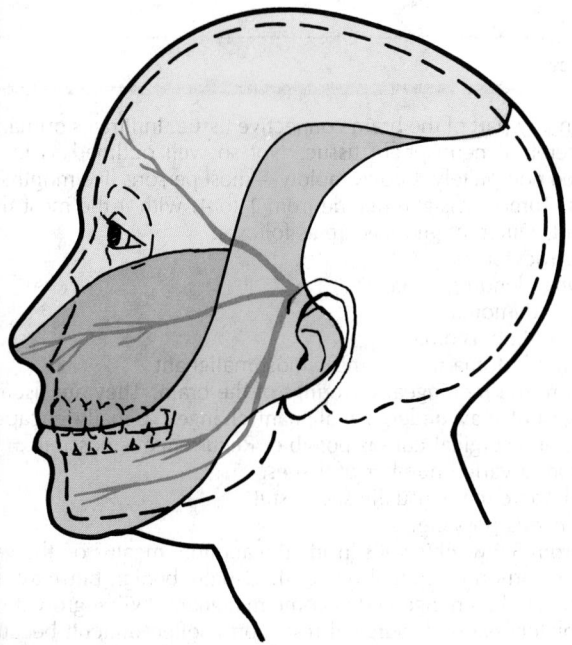

ig. 37-51 Pathway of trigeminal nerve and facial areas in-ervated by each of the three main divisions of this nerve.

ips, or *retract the mouth on that side. The face appears asym-netric with drooping of the mouth and cheek.*

Other symptoms that may occur with Bell's palsy in-lude the following:

1. Loss of taste
2. Reduction in saliva on affected side
3. Pain behind the ear
4. Ringing in ear or other hearing loss

Data analysis: nursing diagnoses

See appropriate section in the discussion of the patient with peripheral nerve trauma (p. 1283).

Implementation

There is *no specific therapy for Bell's palsy.* Electrical stim-lation or warm moist heat along the course of the nerve may help. Steroids given early in the course may speed recovery. Protection of the eyes when the eyelid does not lose is important. Massage of the affected areas is some-imes recommended. Exercises may be prescribed for 5 minutes three times a day. These include wrinkling the row and forehead, closing the eyes, and puffing out the heeks.

INTERFERENCE WITH FUNCTION BECAUSE OF TUMORS

INTRACRANIAL TUMORS

Pathophysiology

ntracranial tumors include both benign and metastatic esions. All areas and structures of the brain can be af-fected. Primary intracranial tumors, or neoplasms, arise from the intrinsic cells of brain tissues and the pituitary and pineal glands. Secondary or metastatic tumors are also a frequent contributing type of intracranial tumor. The prognosis for patients with an intracranial tumor depends on early diagnosis and treatment because as the tumor grows it exerts pressure on vital centers and causes brain damage and death. Although approximately one half of all tumors are benign, they may also cause death by exerting pressure on vital centers.

Brain tumors are named for the tissues from which they arise. The more frequently encountered ones are described in Table 37-11. The brain, in addition, is also a frequent site for secondary tumors from other organs.

The symptoms of intracranial tumors result from both local and general effects of the tumor. Locally, the effects are from infiltration, invasion, and destruction of brain tissues at a particular site. Direct pressure is also exerted on nerve structures, causing degeneration and interference with local circulation. Local edema develops, and ICP in-creases. The increased ICP is then transmitted throughout the brain and the ventricular system. Eventually, the ven-tricular system is distorted and displaced sufficiently to cause partial ventricular obstruction (Fig. 37-52). Papil-ledema results from the general effects of the increased ICP. Death is usually from brainstem compression re-sulting from herniation.

Nursing Process
Assessment

It is important to assess both subjective and objective data in the patient with an intracranial tumor. Box 37-55 on p. 1287 contains a comparison of the symptoms of tumors in specific brain lobes.

Subjective data

1. Patient's understanding of diagnosis
2. Changes in personality or judgment
3. Presence of abnormal sensations (paresthesia or an-esthesia)
4. Visual problems—loss of visual acuity or diplopia
5. Complaints of unusual odors (often accompanies tumors of temporal lobe)
6. Presence of headache

Table 37-11   Types of brain tumors

Type	Incidence	Pathology
Glioma	Accounts for one half of brain tumors	Arises in any part of the brain connective tissue. Infiltrates primaril the cerebral hemisphere tissue. Not so well outlined as to b incised completely. Grows rapidly—most persons live months years. Tumors assigned grade from 1 to 4, with 4 the most m. lignant. Different gliomas are as follows: 1. Astrocytomas 2. Oligodendrogliomas 3. Ependymomas 4. Medulloblastoma 5. Glioblastoma multiforme—most malignant
Meningioma	13% to 18% of all primary tumors in intracranial cavity	Arise from the meningeal coverings of the brain. They are usual benign but may undergo malignant changes. Usually encapsu lated, and surgical cure is possible. Recurrence is possible.
Pituitary tumor	Occurs in all age groups but more often in women	Arise from a varied number of tissues. Surgical approach is usually successful. Recurrence is possible.
Neuroma (schwannoma, neurofibroma)	Acoustic neuroma is most common	Arises from Schwann's cells inside the auditory meatus on the ve tibular portion of cranial nerve III. Usually benign but may u dergo cellular change and become malignant. Will regrow if n completely excised. Surgical resection is often difficult becau of location.
Metastatic tumors	From 2% to 20% of all patients with cancer have metastasis to the brain	Cancer cells spread to the brain via the circulatory system. Surgic resection is very difficult; even with treatment prognosis is ve poor. Survival beyond a year or two is uncommon.

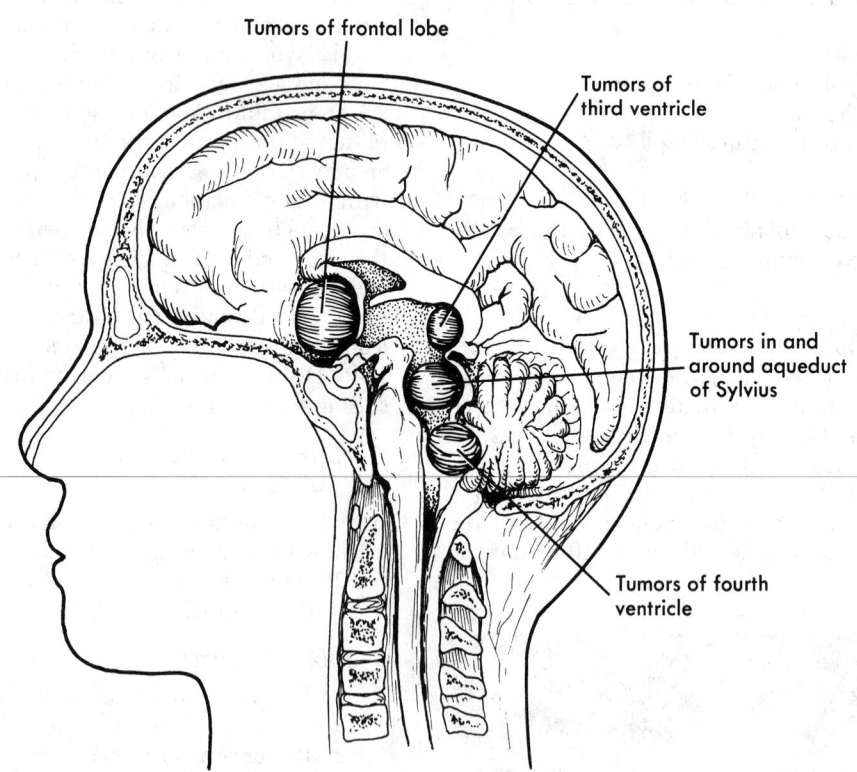

Fig. 37-52   Sites of brain tumors adjacent to ventricular system. Note how developing tumor at varied sites with extension distorts, compresses, and obstructs ventricular system at some point so that increased intracranial pressure occurs early. (From Yahr WD: *Hosp Med* 9:8, 1973.)

Comparison of symptoms of tumors found in specific brain lobes

Area of the brain	Symptoms
Frontal lobe	Personality disturbances (range from subtle personality changes to frank psychotic behavior)
	Inappropriate affect
	Indifference of bodily functions
Precentral gyrus	Jacksonian seizures
Occipital lobe	Visual disturbances preceding convulsions
Temporal lobe	Olfactory, visual, or gustatory hallucinations
	Psychomotor seizures with automatic behavior
Parietal lobe	Inability to replicate pictures
	Loss of right-left discrimination

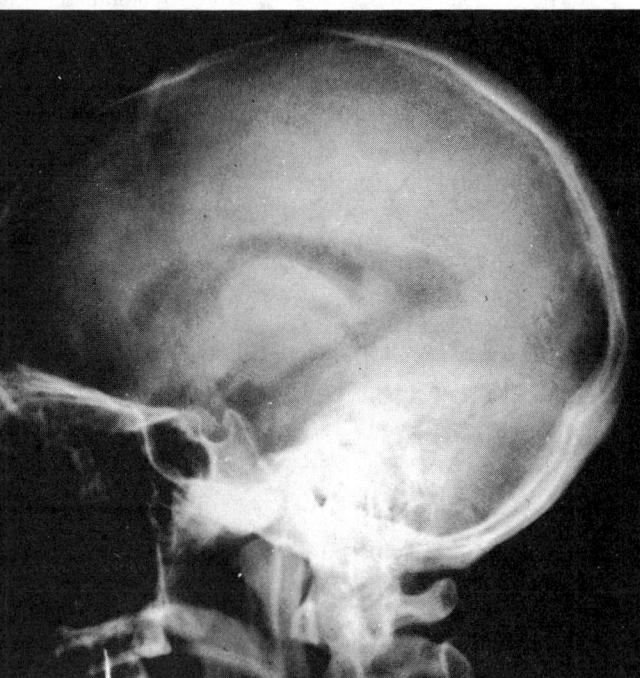
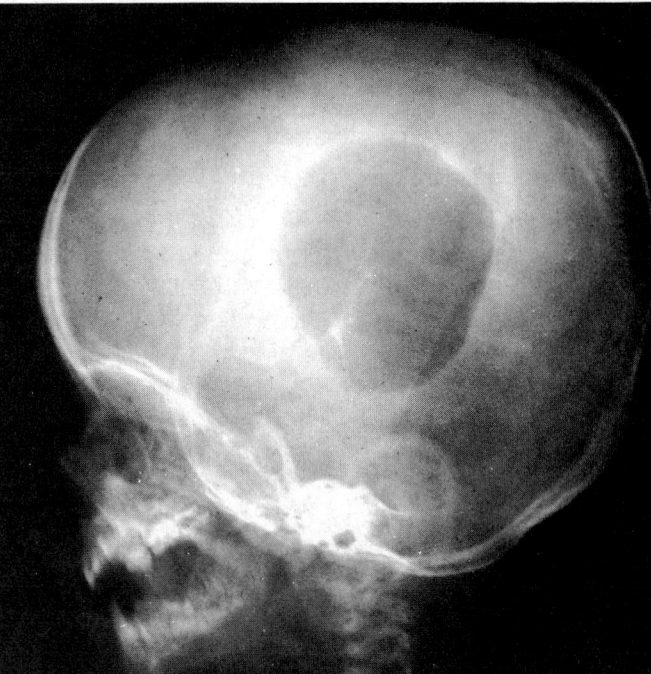

B

Fig. 37-53 Pneumoencephalogram. **A,** Lateral view showing outline of normal ventricle. **B,** Lateral view showing marked distention of ventricle with cerebrospinal fluid (caused by hydrocephalus).

7. Hearing loss
8. Inability to carry on daily activities

Objective data

1. Motor strength
2. Gait
3. Level of alertness and consciousness
4. Orientation
5. Pupils: size, equality, and reactivity
6. Vital signs
7. Fundoscopic examination for evidence of papilledema
8. Presence of seizures
9. Speech abnormalities
10. Cranial nerve abnormalities
11. Symptoms of increased intracranial pressure

Seizures occurring for the first time after middle age are very suggestive of a brain tumor in the cerebrum or its coverings. Intracranial tumors occuring within the cerebral lobes present disturbances that can be related to the function of the specific part of the brain.

Signs and symptoms of increased ICP resulting from intracranial tumors usually occur after localized signs and symptoms have been present for varying periods. See the previous discussion of increased ICP (p. 1220). Headache is at first transitory and later becomes constant; it increases in intensity with straining, coughing, stooping, and change of position. The headache is present in the morning and often awakens the person from sleep. Nausea and vomiting usually occur as the headache increases.

Diagnostic tests

No one procedure is entirely diagnostic of brain tumors, but the CT scan is often the basis of the diagnosis. Other tests that may be used include the brain scan and the EEG. These are discussed on p. 1210 and p. 1240. Another test that is used less frequently since the introduction of the CT scanner is the pneumoencephalogram (Fig. 37-53). See Box 37-56 for details about a pneumoencephalogram.

Other tests that may be helpful in locating the tumor are *arteriography* or *ventriculography* (see Box 37-57 for details about a ventriculogram). Arteriography is described on p. 1257. The ventriculogram is used when the suggested diagnosis is such that a spinal or lumbar puncture is contraindicated because of the presence of increased ICP. Fig. 37-54 shows an aneurysm found on a cerebral angiogram.

Data analysis: nursing diagnoses

Nursing diagnoses are determined from analysis of patient data. The nursing diagnoses for the patient with an intercranial tumor are the same as for the patient with increased intracranial pressure (p. 1224) or motor dysfunction (p. 1231).

Planning: expected patient outcomes

Expected patient outcomes for the person with an intracranial tumor may include, but are not limited to those found in the sections for increased intercranial pressure (p. 1220) and motor dysfunction (p. 1228).

Implementation

Assisting with the achievement of therapeutic goals

The general methods of treatment for intracranial tumors include surgical removal when feasible, radiotherapy, and chemotherapy. The choice of therapy is determined by the tumor type and site of the tumor. A combination of methods is often necessary.

When gliomas are located in areas that are not critical to vital functions, they are usually removed surgically. Most gliomas, however, infiltrate and are difficult to completely excise and treat. Surgery is often combined with radiotherapy and chemotherapy. When the tumor is located in a more critical area where removal would leave the patient with impaired function, a biopsy of the tumor is performed, it is "debrided" if possible, and the patient is treated with radiotherapy or chemotherapy.

Meningiomas are commonly treated by complete excision of the tumor (and overlying bone if infiltrated), because they are usually located in areas that permit removal. Meningiomas are often encapsulated, which aids in their removal.

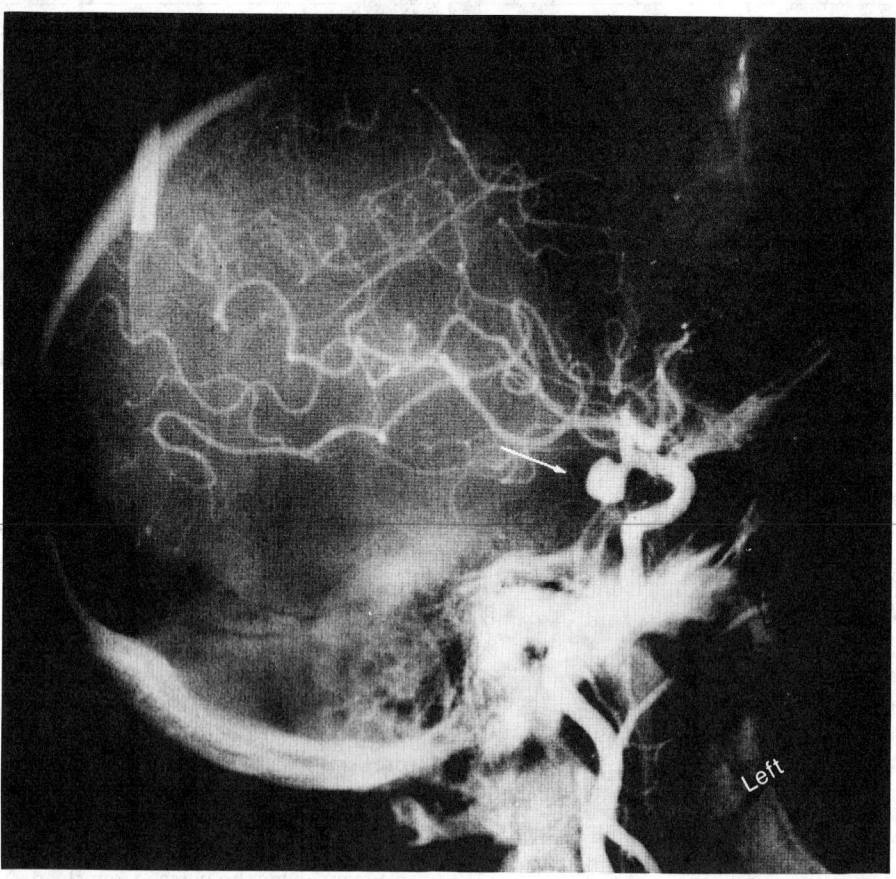

Fig. 37-54 Cerebral angiography showing location of aneurysm at posterior communicating artery. (From Tortorici M: *Fundamentals of angiography,* St Louis, 1982, Mosby–Year Book.)

Surgery

Intracranial surgery is commonly used for all types of pathologic conditions of the brain, including the relief of increased ICP and removal of tumors.

A surgical opening through the skull is known as *craniotomy*. It is a basic preparatory procedure for intracranial surgery. A series of burr holes is made first, and then the bone between the holes is cut with a Gigli saw to permit removal of the bone. Bone is then removed in such a way that it can be replaced if desired. Brain surgery may be performed with the patient under hypothermia to lessen bleeding during the procedure. Drugs to treat hypotension may be used, such as norepinephrine bitartrate (Levophed). Patients may also be placed in a barbiturate coma during the surgery and for several days after it to lessen brain activity, metabolism, and oxygen needs. This may help to prevent worsening of deficits because of hypoxia.

When the brain lesion is in the supratentorium (above the tentorium or in the cerebrum), the incision is usually made behind the hairline. When the incision is into the infratentorium (below the tentorium or in the brainstem and cerebellum), it is made slightly above the nape of the neck.

After craniotomy and removal of the bone, an incision is made into the meninges and the tumor is removed or other cranial surgery performed. The removed bone is carefully saved or preserved and may be replaced at the end of the surgery if there is no indication of infection or increased ICP. If it is not replaced, a bone prosthesis may later be placed over the deficit. *The removal of part of the skull without replacement is called craniectomy. Cranioplasty is the repair of a cranial defect through use of a substitute bone material such as plastic or methylmethacrylate cement.*

37-56

Pneumoencephalogram

Purpose

To detect lesions of the ventricles and cisternal system using air as contrast.

Preparation of patient

1. Prepare as if for surgery.
2. Permit must be signed.
3. Sedative may be given evening before procedure and just before test.
4. General anesthesia may be used.
5. Patient teaching:
   a. Explain procedure.
   b. Time: approximately 2 hours.
   c. Sensation: patient is usually very uncomfortable. Headache is usually severe during procedure; nausea and vomiting are common.

Procedure

1. Patient is positioned as for lumbar puncture or cisternal tap (p. 1212).
2. After the tap is done and pressure measured, the contrast medium (air or oxygen) is injected in amounts of 25 to 30 ml. Patient is watched carefully for headache, nausea, vomiting, or any change in vital signs or color.
3. Head of the table is gradually raised, and head may be rotated to assist air in filling ventricles.

After procedure

1. Patient is placed in bed with head flat. May be in bed 24 to 48 hours.
2. Constant attention with frequent vital signs and neurologic checks is needed until the patient is awake and alert.
3. Severe headache is common and may last for 48 hours.
4. Seizure precautions should be maintained if patient has history of seizures.
5. Tracheostomy set at bedside.
6. Reactions to procedure may be severe and include vomiting, shock, respiratory difficulty, and other signs of increased ICP.

Other

Pneumoencephalogram is now used less frequently because of the availability of the CT scanner. It is never done in the presence of increased ICP because of the danger of herniation.

37-57

Ventriculogram

Purpose

To detect pathology within the ventricular and cisternal system.

Preparation of patient

1. Procedure is performed in the operating room.
2. Surgical permit must be signed.
3. Patient is prepared as if for surgery.
4. Top or back of head is partially shaved.
5. Intravenous or general anesthesia is commonly used.
6. Patient teaching
   a. Explain procedure.
   b. Time: variable. Often patient has craniotomy for tumor removal immediately after test.
   c. Sensation: none during procedure because of anesthesia.

Procedure

1. Patient is positioned, usually supine.
2. Trephine openings (burr holes) are made into the lateral ventricles.
3. Air is introduced directly via the ventricles.
4. X-ray films of the brain and ventricles are taken at intervals.

After procedure

1. Same as for pneumoencephalogram.
2. Observe site of burr hole for bleeding or drainage.
3. Observe for signs of neurologic deterioration that would indicate formation of intracerebral clot.

37-58

Preoperative care of the patient undergoing intracranial surgery

1. Baseline data of neurologic and physiologic status should be recorded.
2. Patient and family should be encouraged to verbalize fears.
3. Treatments and procedures are explained fully, even if unsure whether patient understands.
4. If head is shaved, it is usually done in the operating room.
5. Antiseptic shampoo may be ordered night before surgery and may be repeated in morning.
6. If hair is shaved, it is saved and given to patient or family.
7. Prepare family for appearance of patient after surgery.
   a. Head dressing
   b. Edema and ecchymosis of face common
   c. Temporary decreased mental status (possible).

37-59

Guidelines for Care

Postoperative care of the patient after a shunting procedure

1. Monitoring
   a. Assess neurologic status frequently for any decrease in mental status.
   b. Observe for symptoms of subdural hematoma, one of the possible side effects of the surgery.
   c. Monitor for symptoms of overdrainage, as evidenced by headache, especially when patient is sitting upright or standing.
   d. Assess degree and character of drainage.
      (1) Amount of drainage and bleeding should be minimal.
      (2) Reinforce dressing as needed.
      (3) Often incisional areas are left open to air after several days.
2. Maintain gastrointestinal status
   a. Check frequently for signs of paralytic ileus, because the manipulation of the bowel that occurs with the placement of the peritoneal part of the shunt can predispose the patient to this.
   b. Patient is usually kept NPO for first day, and then clear liquids are started.
   c. Regular diet is resumed as soon as good bowel sounds are present and patient tolerates liquids.
3. Maintaining comfort
   a. Patient may need more frequent pain medication because of involvement of abdominal area.
   b. Keep pressure off incisional sites.
4. Promoting mobility
   a. Turning to either side is permitted.
   b. Raise head of bed gradually when mobilizing patient.
   c. Patient is encouraged to ambulate as much as possible to encourage adaptation to decreased ICP.

Tumors involving the pituitary gland that do not extend outside the sella turcica are usually removed using a transsphenoidal approach. After the surgery, packing is placed inside the nose and remains for 3 to 4 days. A muscle graft from the thigh is used to close the defect in the dura. With this type of surgery, recovery is relatively rapid and the patient has no loss of hair or external cranial incision.

Preoperative preparation of both the patient and family is important. They both are usually very threatened by the prospect of brain surgery. Specific fears may be related to those of a permanent change in appearance, dependency, or both. Preoperative care includes the points listed in Box 37-58.

During the postoperative period the patient is observed regularly for signs of increased ICP. The frequency of making and recording specific observations depends on the patient's condition. A device to measure ICP is often inserted during the surgery (p. 1225). Any change in the patient's vital signs, state of consciousness, pupillary response, or ability to move muscles is reported at once. Restlessness, often secondary to tissue hypoxia, may be the first warning of increased ICP. See p. 1221 for specifics about ICP.

Postoperative care is determined by the patient's condition. Most patients spend at least 1 or 2 nights in an intensive care unit, where arterial monitoring and close nursing observation is possible. Other details of postoperative care are found in the section on intracerebral hematomas.

Hydrocephalus

Occasionally a catheter is placed in a ventricle of the brain to drain excess spinal fluid and to prevent hydrocephalus and increased ICP. The catheter is usually attached to a drainage system. *The tubing and drainage receptacle should be sterile, and care must be taken to prevent kinking of the tubing.* If drainage seems to have stopped,

the neurosurgeon should be notified. At times, the nurse may adjust the level of the drainage device to facilitate drainage, using specific parameters ordered by the neurosurgeon. For example the physician may order that the patient should drain 30 ml every 4 hours. The catheter is usually left in place for 24 to 48 hours and then is removed by the surgeon.

Hydrocephalus of a more permanent nature also occurs in the presence of intracranial tumors and is manifested by symptoms of increased ICP. Hydrocephalus can be communicating or noncommunicating. In communicating hydrocephalus an obstruction exists outside the ventricular system. The ventricles contain an excessive amount of CSF because fluid is not adequately absorbed from the cerebral subdural space. In noncommunicating, or intraventricular hydrocephalus CSF is accumulated secondary to a blockage of the normal flow at some point in the ventricular system. The cerebral ventricle proximal to the blockage then dilates.

Treatment consists of a shunting procedure. The different types of shunt procedures are named for their point of origin and termination and include the following:

1. Cyst to peritoneal
2. Lumbar-peritoneal
3. Ventricular-jugular
4. Ventricular-peritoneal

In this type of surgery excessive CSF is shunted away from the central nervous system and into either the peritoneal cavity (where it is absorbed) or the jugular vein. At times a Ryckham reservoir is placed through a burr hole into the ventricle. This device can easily be palpated through the skin. Some of the shunts have an on-off valve, as well as a part that may be pumped to facilitate drainage. Valves that are inserted can be set for a specific pressure with some control over the amount of fluid drained.

Preoperative care is the same as for any patient having intracranial surgery. Key points of postoperative care are listed in Box 37-59.

Normal pressure hydrocephalus (NPH) does not result in ICP. Persons with NPH have dilated ventricles with normal tissue mass and a normal intracranial pressure. The cause of NPH is unknown.

Radiation therapy and chemotherapy

In some patients with intracranial tumors surgery may not be possible or indicated. In these cases radiation therapy and/or chemotherapy may be used. They are also used at times after intracranial surgery. See Chapter 12 for the care of the patient undergoing these treatments.

Hyperthermia

The use of heat may be combined with chemotherapy. Often, cancer cells have been found to be heat sensitive. The hyperthermia catheter is inserted percutaneously under a stereotactic approach guided by CT. The area is then heated to 105° to 107.6°F for a period of time. Side effects that may occur during treatment are seizures or an embolus.

Interventions to achieve patient outcomes
Maintaining comfort and ADL

Some patients who have had cranial surgery will have residual physical and mental limitations. The patient may have hemiplegia, aphasia, and personality changes. The rehabilitative care and planning are the same as for other patients with chronic and permanent neurologic disease (see sections on the patient with motor dysfunction and the patient with a CVA). Regardless of the eventual prognosis and the diagnosis of the tumor, each patient should be helped to be as independent as possible for as long as possible.

Evaluation

Evaluation of the patient with an intracranial tumor involves both the patient and the family. It is based on the expected patient outcomes. The reader is referred to the sections concerning increased intercranial pressure (p. 1220) and motor dysfunction (p. 1228) for appropriate questions to consider.

INTRAVERTEBRAL TUMORS
Pathophysiology

The pathologic condition that results from spinal cord tumors is caused by spinal cord destruction and infiltrates, displacement and compression of the cord, and disruption of the blood supply or CSF circulation. The severity of symptoms depends on the degree of compression and the speed with which it develops. Adaption can occur with slow-growing tumors. Eighty-five percent of spinal cord tumors are benign.

Primary neoplastic tumors occur *either extramedullary* (outside the cord) or *intramedullary* (within the cord). Secondary or metastatic tumors may also involve the spinal cord, its coverings, and the vertebrae.

Extramedullary tumors of the *intradural type* may at first cause *subjective nerve root pain.* With tumor growth there will be motor and sensory deficits related to the level of the root and spinal cord involvement. As the tumor enlarges, it compresses the cord. Eventually, the patient loses all motor and sensory function below the level of the tumor.

An intramedullary tumor, beginning within the spinal cord, often initially appears as a central cord syndrome including segmental loss of pain and temperature function. In addition, anterior horn cell function is often lost, especially in the hands. Most of the central long tracts next to the gray matter become dysfunctional. Loss of pain and temperature sensations and motor weakness are gradual, progressive, and descending. Caudal motor and sensory functions are the last to be lost, including loss of bowel and bladder function.

Assessment

The subjective and objective data for the patient with an intravertebral tumor are the same as for the patient with spinal cord injury (p. 1279).

Implementation
Assisting with the achievement of therapeutic goals
Surgery

A spinal decompression is commonly used even when complete removal of the tumor is not considered possible. As much of the tumor as possible (and possibly bone) is removed to reduce the obstruction for a time. It can be performed at any level of the vertebral column and may include several vertebrae. The operation is sometimes palliative. Care of the patient undergoing spinal decompression is found in the section on spinal cord injury (p. 1280).

Interventions to achieve patient outcomes
Maintaining comfort and ADL

Convalescent care and rehabilitation depend entirely on the type of tumor and whether it has been successfully removed. The decompression operation may give relief of symptoms for months and sometimes for years. If the tumor is a slow-growing one, radiation therapy may be given while the patient is in the hospital and continued after discharge.

Evaluation

The evaluation of the care of the patient with an intravertebral tumor is the same as for the patient with a motor dysfunction (p. 1234) or spinal cord injury (p. 1282).

SUMMARY

1. The neuron is the basic structural and functional unit of the nervous system.
2. Afferent neurons are sensory neurons that conduct impulses from the periphery to the central nervous system, and efferent or motor neurons transmit impulses from the CNS to the periphery.
3. Impulses travel across neurons as a result of action potentials.
4. Contacts between neurons occur at synapses, where neurotransmitters are released.
5. The nervous system is divided into two major divisions—the central nervous system and the peripheral nervous system.
6. The brain is composed of the cerebrum, the brainstem, and the cerebellum, each of which has specific functions.
7. Systemic circulation favors the CNS overall, balancing parts to assure a constant supply of nutrients to the brain.
8. The general sensory system is made up of receptor neurons, posterior roots of the afferent or posterior sensory nerves, ascending sensory tracts in the spinal cord and brain, and the sensory area of the cerebral cortex.
9. The descending motor systems include the corticospinal system (pyramidal tracts), the extrapyramidal system, and the cerebellar system.
10. Normal changes that occur in the nervous system cannot be equated with senility, Alzheimer's disease, or organic brain disease.
11. The Glasgow Coma Scale is one tool that is useful in standardizing observations of neurologic patients.
12. The source of headache should be determined through careful assessment because it may be a symptom of serious neurologic pathology.
13. The CT scan is an important diagnostic tool in the assessment of brain pathology.
14. The lumbar puncture is not done if there is a question of increased intracranial pressure because the puncture may result in brain herniation.
15. Drugs commonly prescribed for patients with migraine headache include ergotamine tartrate, propranolol hydrochloride (Inderal), and methysergide maleate (Sansert).
16. It is extremely difficult to evaluate neurologic pain objectively.
17. Any increase in the volume of one of the cranial contents (brain tissue, vascular tissue, and cerebrospinal fluid) results in increased intracranial pressure because the cranial vault is rigid, closed, and nonexpandable.
18. As intracranial pressure rises, it is first compensated for by venous compression and cerebrospinal displacement.
19. Classic signs of increased intracranial pressure include restlessness, disorientation, headache, contralateral hemiparesis, an ipsilaterally dilated pupil, and visual changes that include blurring of vision or diplopia.
20. Nursing care measures can significantly influence intracranial pressure.
21. Mannitol is given in the presence of acute increased intracranial pressure.
22. Three types of intracranial monitoring devices include the ventricular catheter, the subarachnoid bolt or screw, and the epidural sensor.
23. Lower motor neuron (LMN) lesions result in flaccid muscle weakness, loss of reflex activity, loss of muscle tone, and atrophy confined to the involved muscles.
24. Upper motor neuron (UMN) lesions result in spasticity and paresis of voluntary muscle tone, hyperreflexia, late atrophy from disuse, and increased muscle tone.
25. Epilepsy is a transitory disturbance in consciousness or in motor, sensory, or autonomic functions with or without loss of consciousness caused by sudden, excessive, and disorderly electrical discharges of the brain.
26. The aura is a set of symptoms that occurs before a seizure and varies from person to person.
27. The mouth of a person having a seizure should never be pried open to insert an airway or tongue blade.
28. Respiratory complications are common in patients with myasthenia gravis.
29. Early symptoms of multiple sclerosis are usually transitory.
30. The use of adrenocorticotrophic hormone (ACTH) and corticosteroids has shown favorable results in the treatment of multiple sclerosis.
31. Drug-induced parkinsonian syndromes occur with drugs that interfere with the synthesis or storage of dopamine or interfere with the striatal dopamine receptors.
32. Death usually occurs within 5 years from the diagnosis of amyotrophic lateral sclerosis (ALS) because of respiratory problems or bulbar paralysis.
33. Alzheimer's disease is a degenerative disorder, usually of older adults, that affects the cells of the brain and causes impairment of intellectual functioning.
34. Neurofibromatosis is a genetic disorder transmitted as an autosomal dominant trait that causes numerous fibromas of the spinal or cranial nerves and skin, café au lait spots on the skin, and developmental disorders of bone, muscle, and viscera.
35. Cerebrovascular accident (CVA) is the most common disease of the nervous system and can be caused by thrombus, embolus, or hemorrhage.
36. The incidence of bacterial meningitis is higher in fall and winter, when upper respiratory infections are common.
37. More than half of the persons affected with Guillain-

Barré syndrome have had a nonspecific infection 10 to 14 days before the onset of the disease.

38. Respiratory isolation is necessary for the patient with herpes zoster until drainage from the lesions stops.

39. Approximately 40% of AIDS patients have neurologic symptoms that result from infection from HIV itself or from associated infections.

40. General effects of moderate to severe head injury include cerebral edema, sensory and motor deficits, and increased intracranial pressure (ICP).

41. Injuries to the brain result from direct or indirect trauma to the head.

42. Direct trauma to the head causes acceleration-deceleration injuries.

43. Contusion or laceration directly below the site of the cranial impact is called a coup lesion, whereas one opposite the impact site is called a contrecoup injury.

44. Subdural hematomas can occur from hours to months after the initial head injury.

45. Many patients with head injury may recover physically, but they will have behavioral and psychologic problems that make it difficult for them to function completely independently.

46. The amount of disability that results from spinal cord injury depends on the level of injury.

47. Autonomic dysreflexia is a complication of spinal cord injury that occurs as a result of abnormal cardiovascular response to stimulation of the sympathetic division of the autonomic nervous system and is considered a medical emergency.

48. The symptoms of intracranial tumors result from both local and general effects of the tumor.

49. A surgical opening through the skull is called a craniotomy, the removal of part of the skull without replacement is called a craniectomy, and the repair of a cranial defect through the use of substitute bone material is called cranioplasty.

50. Increased intracranial pressure (ICP) is one of the most common complications of intracranial surgery.

51. Hydrocephalus may occur after intracranial surgery; it can be treated with a shunt.

52. The pathologic conditions that result from spinal cord tumors are caused by spinal cord destruction and infiltrates, displacement and compression of the cord, and disruption of the blood supply or CSF circulation.

STUDY QUESTIONS

• Explain how medical and nursing treatment varies with patients suffering from a cerebrovascular accident depending on the cause.

• What nursing interventions would be helpful in facilitating the adjustment of a young spinal-cord-injured patient?

• What nursing interventions can increase intracranial pressure?

• How would you assist a patient with apraxia in getting dressed?

• A mother wants to shelter her teenage son with epilepsy. How would you work with this overprotective mother?

REFERENCES AND SELECTED READINGS

1. Adler R: Trigeminal glycerol chemoneurolysis: nursing implications, *J Neurosci Nurs* 21:337-341, 1989.
2. Ake J, Perlstein L: AIDS: impact on neuroscience nursing practice, *J Neurosci Nurs* 19:300-304, 1987.
3.* Andrus C: Intracranial pressure: diagnosis and nursing management, *Neurosci Nurs* 23:85-92, 1991.
4.* Arsenault L: Selected postoperative complications of cranial surgery, *J Neurosurg Nurs* 17:155-163, 1985.
5.* Aumick J: Head trauma: guidelines for care, *RN* 54(4):27-31, 1991.
6. Baggerly J: Epidural catheters for pain management: the nurse's role, *J Neurosci Nurs* 18:290-295, 1986.
6a.* Barker E, Moore K: Neurological assessment, *RN* 55(4):28-35, 1992.
7.* Barker E: Action stat SCI, *Nurs 90* 20(11):33, 1990.
8.* Barker E, Higgins R: Managing a suspected SCI, *Nurs 89* 19(3):52-59, 1989.
9. Beckham M, Rudy R: Acquired immunodeficiency syndrome: impact and implications for the neurological system, *J Neurosci Nurs* 18:5-10, 1986.
10.* Boortz-Marx R: Factors affecting intracranial pressure: a descriptive study, *J Neurosurg Nurs* 17:89-94, 1985.
11. Boss B: The neuroanatomical and neurophysiological basis of learning, *J Neurosci Nurs* 18:256-264, 1986.
12.* Buelow J: A correlational study of disabilities, stressors and coping methods in victims of multiple sclerosis, *J Neurosci Nurs* 23:247-252, 1991.
13. Campbell C: Acoustic neuroma: nursing implications related to surgical management, *J Neurosci Nurs* 23:50-56, 1991.
14. Christ M, Hohloch F: *Gerontologic nursing: a study and learning tool*, Springhouse, Pa, 1988, Springhouse Publishing.
15. Cooper P: *Head injury*, Baltimore, 1986, Williams and Wilkins.
16. Daly B: *Intensive care nursing*, ed 2, Garden City, NY, 1985, Medical Exam Publishing.
17.* Davenport-Fortune P, Dunnum L: Professional nursing care of the patient with increased intracranial pressure: planned or "hit or miss," *J Neurosurg Nurs* 17:367-370, 1985.
18.* Delgado J, Billo J: Care of the patient with Parkinson's disease: surgical and nursing interventions, *J Neurosci Nurs* 20:142-150, 1988.
19. Dittmar S: Rehabilitation nursing: process and application, St Louis, 1989, Mosby–Year Book.
20. Edwards D et al: Hyperthermia treatment for malignant astrocytomas: nursing implications, *J Neurosci Nurs* 23:34-38, 1991.
21. Emich-Herring B, Wood P: A team approach to neurological based swallowing disorders, *Rehab Nurs* 15:242-247, 1990.
22. Ferido T, Habel M: Spasticity in head trauma and CVA patients: etiology and management, *J Neurosci Nurs* 20:17-22, 1988.
23. Fickel V: Acoustic neuroma: postoperative deficits and the role of the neuroscience nurse, *J Neurosci Nurs* 23:57-60, 1991.
24.* Finocchiaro D, Hersfeld S: Understanding Alzheimers disease, *AJN* 90(9):56-60, 1990.
25. Flaskerud J: *AIDS-HIV infection: a reference guide for nursing professionals*, Philadelphia, 1988, WB Saunders.

*Recommended for student reading.

26.* Fode N: Subarachnoid hemorrhage from ruptured intracranial aneurysm, *AJN* 88:673-680, 1988.

27.* Franges E, Beideman M: Infections related to intracranial pressure monitoring, *J Neurosci Nurs* 20:94-103, 1988.

28.* Friedman D: Taking the scare out of caring for seizure patients, *Nurs 88* 18(2):52-60, 1988.

29. George M: Neuromuscular respiratory failure: what the nurse knows may make the difference, *J Neurosci Nurs* 20:110-117, 1988.

30. Gioiella E, Bevil C: *Nursing care of the aging client: promoting healthy adaptation,* Norwalk, Conn, 1985, Appleton-Century-Crofts.

31. Grabbe L, Brown L: Identifying neurologic complications of AIDS, *Nurs 89* 19(5):66-73, 1989.

32. Gryfinski J: Intramedullary spinal cord abscesses, *J Neurosci Nurs* 20:34-38, 1988.

33.* Haight K: What you should know about epidural analgesia, *Nurs 87* 17(9):58-59, 1987.

33a.* Hall G: This hospital patient has Alzheimer's, *Amer J Nurs* 91(10):45-52, 1991.

34. Hansberry J et al: Managing chronic pain with a permanent epidural catheter, *Nurs 90*(10):53-57, 1990.

34a.* Hickey J: Myasthenic crisis—your assessment counts, *RN* 54(5):54-59, 1991.

35. Hickey J: *The clinical practice of neurological and neurosurgical nursing,* ed 2, Philadelphia, 1986, JB Lippincott.

36. Hinkle J: Nursing care of the patient with minor head injury, *J Neurosci Nurs* 20:8-16, 1988.

37. Hodges K, Root L: Surgical management of intractable seizure disorder, *J Neurosci Nurs* 23:93-100, 1991.

38.* Jess L: Investigating impaired mental status: an assessment guide you can use, *Nurs 88* 18(6):42-50, 1988.

39. Jones A et al: Side effects following metrizamide myelography and lumbar laminectomy, *J Neurosci Nurs* 19:90-94, 1987.

40. Joynt R: Neurology, *JAMA* 265:3134-3135, 1990.

41. Kalbach L: Unilateral neglect: mechanism and nursing care, *J Neurosci Nurs* 23:125-129, 1991.

42. Keller C et al: Psychological responses to aphasia: theoretical considerations and nursing implications, *J Neurosci Nurs* 21:290-294, 1989.

43. Kim T: Hope as a method of coping in amyotrophic lateral sclerosis, *J Neurosci Nurs* 21:342-347, 1989.

44. Kirk E, Bradford L: Effects of alcohol on the CNS: implications for the neuroscience nurse, *J Neurosci Nurs* 19:326-335, 1987.

45.* Konikow N: Alterations in movement: nursing assessment and implications, *J Neurosurg Nurs* 17:61-65, 1985.

46. Krause E et al: Radiosurgery: a nursing perspective, *J Neurosci Nurs* 23:24-28, 1991.

47. Lamb C, Barbaro N: Neurosurgical approaches to the management of chronic pain syndrome, *Orthop Nurs* 6(1):23-29, 1987.

48.* Larsen P: Psychosocial adjustment in MS, *Rehabili Nurs* 15:242-247, 1990.

49. Lord-Feroli K, Maguire-McGinley M: Toward a more objective approach to pupil assessment, *J Neurosurg Nurs* 17:309-312, 1985.

50. Luchka S: Working with ICP monitors, *RN* 54(3):34-37, 1991.

51. Maher M, Strong S: Organ donation: a nursing perspective, *J Neurosci Nurs* 21:357-361, 1989.

52.* Mahon D, Elger C: Analysis of posttraumatic syndrome following head injury, *J Neurosci Nurs* 21:382-384, 1989.

53.* Mauser G: Neuromuscular respiratory failure—what the nurse knows makes a difference, *J Neurosci Nurs* 20:110-117, 1988.

54.* McBride E, DiStefano K: Explaining diagnostic tests for MS, *Nurs 88* 18(2):68-72, 1988.

55. McCaffery M, Beebe A: Giving narcotics for pain: a problem solver handbook, *Nurs 89* 19(10)L161-168, 1989.

56. Mitchell S, Yates R: Extracranial/intracranial bypass surgery, *J Neurosurg Nurs* 17:288-292, 1985.

57.* Mocsny N: Slow virus diseases of the central nervous system, *Rehab Nurs* 14(3):130-132, 1989.

57a.* Morgan S: A passage through paralysis, *Amer J Nurs* 92(4):54-58, 1992.

58.* Muswaswes M: Increased intracranial pressure and its systemic effects, *J Neurosurg Nurs* 20:217-222, 1988.

59. Nikas D: Critical aspects of head trauma, *Crit Care Nurs Q* 10(1):19-44, 1987.

59a.* North B et al: Living in a halo, *Amer J Nurs* 92(4):54-58, 1992.

60.* Olson E et al: The hazards of immobility, *Am J Nurs* 90(3):43-48, 1990.

61. Palmer M, Wyness M: Positioning and handling: important considerations in the care of the severely head-injured patient, *J Neurosci Nurs* 20:42-49, 1988.

62. Perlstein L, Ake J: AIDS: an overview for the neuroscience nurse, *J Neurosci Nurs* 19:296-299, 1987.

63.* Pettibone K: Management of spasticity in spinal cord injury: nursing concerns, *J Neurosci Nurs* 20:217-222, 1988.

64. Plylar P: Management of the agitated and aggressive head injury patient in an acute hospital setting, *J Neurosci Nurs* 21:353-356, 1989.

65.* Pollack-Latham C: Intracranial pressure monitoring: Part II. Patient care, *Crit Care Nurs* 7(6):53, 1987.

66. Price M, DeVroom H: A quick and easy guide to neurological assessment, *J Neurosurg Nurs* 17:313-320, 1985.

66a.* Purath J: Assessing headache pain, 54(10):26-31, 1991.

67. Raney D: Malignant spinal cord tumors: a review and case presentation, *J Neurosci Nurs* 23:44-49, 1991.

68.* Rhynsburger J: How to fight Myasthenia's fatigue, *AJN* 89:337-341, 1989.

69. Rudy E: Magnetic resonance imagery: new horizons in diagnostic testing, *J Neurosurg Nurs* 17:331-337, 1985.

70. Rutledge B: Aneurysm wrapping: principles applicable to the neuroscience nurse, *J Neurosci Nurs* 21:370-375, 1989.

71. Santilli N, Sierzant T: Advances in the treatment of epilepsy, *J Neurosci Nurs* 19:144-157, 1987.

72.* Schaefer S: Relieving pain—an analgesic guide, *Am J Nurs* 88:815-827, 1988.

73.* Scherer A: How HIV attacks the CNS, *AJN* 90(5):66-71, 1990.

74. Selcher D: Helping your patients dress for success, *RN* 43-45, 1991. August.

75. Sherburne E: A rehabilitation protocol for the neuroscience intensive care unit, *J Neurosci Nurs* 18(3):140-145, 1986.

76.* Sherman D: Managing an acute HI, *Nurs 90* 20(4):46-51, 1990.

76a. Snyder M: ed A guide to neurological and neurosurgical nursing, ed 2, New York, 1991, Delmar Publishers.

77. Stevens S, Becker K: A simple, step-by-step approach to neurological assessment—part 1, *Nurs 88* 18(9)53-61, 1988.

78. Stevens S, Becker K: A simple, step-by-step approach to neurological assessment—part 2, *Nurs 88* 18(10)51-58, 1988.

79. Stone N: Amyotrophic lateral sclerosis: a challenge for constant adaptation, *J Neurosci Nurs* 19:166-173, 1987.

80.* Sullivan J: Neurologic assessment, *Nurs Clin North Am* 25:795-809, 1990.

81. Tosch P: Patients' recollection of their posttraumatic coma, *J Neurosci Nurs* 20:223-228, 1988.

82. Turner H et al: Comparison of nurse and computer recording of ICP in head injured patients, *J Neurosci Nurs* 20:236-239, 1988.
83. U.S. Dept. of Health and Human Services: *Healthy people: national health prevention disease prevention objectives,* Public Health Service, Washington, DC 1990.
84. Whitney C, Daroff R: An approach to migraines, *J Neurosci Nurs* 20:284-289, 1988.
85.* Whitney F: Relationship of laterality of stroke and emotional and functional outcome, *J Neurosci Nurs* 19:158-165, 1987.
86. Wilton L: Thalamic pain syndrome, *J Neurosci Nurs* 21:362-365, 1989.

Classic

87. Ballenger M: The neurological system and level of consciousness, *Emergency* 16:52-55, 1984.
88. Boss B: Dysphasia, dyspraxia, and dysarthria: distinguishing features, part I, *J Neurosurg Nurs* 16:151-160, 194, 1984.
89. Boss B: Dysphasia, dyspraxia, and dysarthria: distinguishing features, part II, *J Neurosurg Nurs* 16:211-216, 1984.
90. Brunnstrom S: *Movement therapy in hemiplegia,* New York, 1970, Harper and Row, Publishers.
91.* Burnside J: Alzheimer's disease: an overview, *J Gerontol Nurs* 5:14-20, 1979.
92. Byers V, Gendell H: Using metrizamide for lumbar myelography: adverse reactions and nursing implications, *J Neurosurg Nurs* 14:315-317, 1982.
93. Carlson C: Psychological aspects of neurologic disability, *Nurs Clin North Am* 15:309-320, 1980.
94. Chui L, Bhatt K: Autonomic dysreflexia, *Rehab Nurs* 8:16-20, 1983.

95.* Hart G: Strokes causing left versus right hemiplegia: different effects and nursing implications, *Geriatr Nurs* 4:39-43, 1983.
96. Hendrickson S: Psychological care of the patient with neurological dysfunction, *J Neurosurg Nurs* 16:202-207, 1984.
97. Hummelbard AB et al: Prognostic value of brainstem auditory evoked potentials in head injury, *J Neurosurg Nurs* 16:181-187, 1984.
98.* Jones S: Glasgow coma scale, *Am J Nurs* 79:1551-1554, 1979.
99. King R et al: Symposium on rehabilitative nursing: rehabilitation of the patient with a spinal cord injury, *Nurs Clin North Am* 15:225-243, 1980.
100. Malkmus D et al: *Rehabilitation of the head injured adult-comprehensive cognitive management,* Downey, Calif, 1980, Professional Staff Association of Ranchos Los Amigos Hospital.
101.* Mitchell P et al: Moving the patient in bed: effects on increased intracranial pressure, *Nurs Res* 30(4):212-218, 1981.
102. Olson E et al: The hazards of immobility, *Am J Nurs* 67:779-797, 1967.
103.* Ozuna J, Friez P: Effects of enteral tube feedings on serum phenytoin levels, *J Neurosurg Nurs* 16:289-290, 1984.
104. Terzian M: Neurosurgical intervention for the management of chronic intractable pain, *Top Clin Nurs* 1:75-88, 1980.
105. Warren J, Peck E: Factors which influence neuropsychological recovery from severe head injury, *J Neurosurg Nurs* 16:248-252, 1984.
106. Wintrobe M et al: Harrison's principles of internal medicine, New York, 1970, McGraw Hill.
107.* Young M: A bedside guide to understanding the signs of increased intracranial pressure, *Nurs 81* 11(2):59-62, 1981.

38

The Patient with Eye Problems

Wilma J. Phipps

After studying this chapter, the learner should be able to:

- Describe measurement and alterations in visual acuity and types of corrective lenses.
- Identify eye safety measures.
- Identify nursing interventions for the newly blind person.
- Describe major eye inflammations and appropriate nursing interventions.
- Compare the nature of cataracts, glaucoma, and retinal detachment and appropriate interventions for each.
- Write a nursing care plan for an 80-year-old woman having cataract surgery in an Ambulatory Surgery Center.

ANATOMY AND PHYSIOLOGY

Accessory Eye Structures

The eye is protected from dirt and foreign bodies by the eyebrow, eyelashes, and eyelids. The *conjunctiva* is a thin membrane that lines the eyelids (palpebral conjunctiva) and most of the anterior portion of the eye (bulbar conjunctiva) except for the pupil. The palpebral conjunctiva folds back on itself where it joins the bulbar conjunctiva, forming a saclike recess (conjunctival sac). Although the conjunctiva is transparent, the palpebral portion appears pink, reflecting the underlying blood vessels. Small blood vessels may be noted in the bulbar conjunctiva over the sclera of the eye. The conjunctiva protects the eye and prevents it from drying. Inflammation of the conjunctiva (conjunctivitis, p. 1307) gives a reddened appearance to the eye.

The *lacrimal gland* is located above and lateral to the eyeball (Fig. 38-1). Lacrimal fluid (tears) is secreted by the lacrimal gland. The tears provide moisture to lubricate the cornea; excessive secretion drains into the lacrimal sac, on the nasal side of the eye, and through the nasolacrimal ducts into the nose. Eye medications that are dropped into the inner canthus rather than the conjunctival sac drain out into the nose and thus lose their effectiveness on the eye.

Eyeball

Layers of the eye

The eyeball is composed of three coats or layers of tissue: the sclera, the choroid, and the retina (Fig. 38-2). The tough outer coat, or *sclera,* is opaque (white) but becomes transparent anteriorly over the iris and pupil to form the *cornea.* The middle layer, the *choroid,* contains blood vessels and is modified anteriorly into the ciliary body, which is attached to the suspensory ligament and to the iris. The inner coat, the *retina,* which does not have an anterior portion, contains the photoreceptors (rods and cones). These photoreceptors synapse in the retina with bipolar neurons and then with ganglion neurons, and these become the fibers of the optic nerve. The cones, which are less numerous than the rods, are found mostly near the center of the retina and are considered to be the receptors for bright daylight and color vision. The rods, found mostly in the periphery of the retina, are receptors for dim or night vision. Rods contain rhodopsin, a photosensitive protein that becomes rapidly depleted in bright light. The slow regeneration of rhodopsin, which is dependent on the presence of vitamin A, explains the time needed for the eyes to adjust from bright to dim light. Vitamin A deficiency affects night vision.

Chambers of the eye

The interior of the eyeball is divided into two cavities, the anterior and the posterior. The *anterior cavity,* in front of the lens, is further subdivided into two *chambers, an anterior chamber (between the cornea and the iris) and a posterior chamber (between the iris and the lens).* The anterior cavity is filled with a clear liquid, the aqueous humor, which is produced in the ciliary body, drains into the posterior chamber, passes through the pupil into the anterior chamber, and drains out the canal of Schlemm at the junction of the iris and cornea (anterior chamber angle). Obstruction of this drainage leads to glaucoma (p. 1316). The

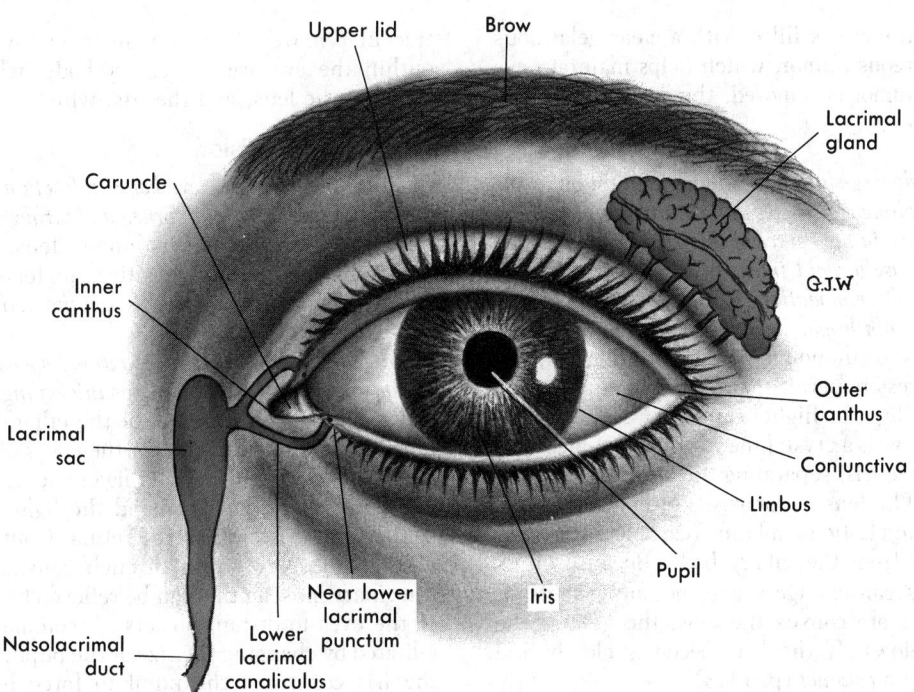

Fig. 38-1 External eye structures. (From Thompson JM, et al: *Clinical nursing,* St Louis, 1986, Mosby–Year Book.)

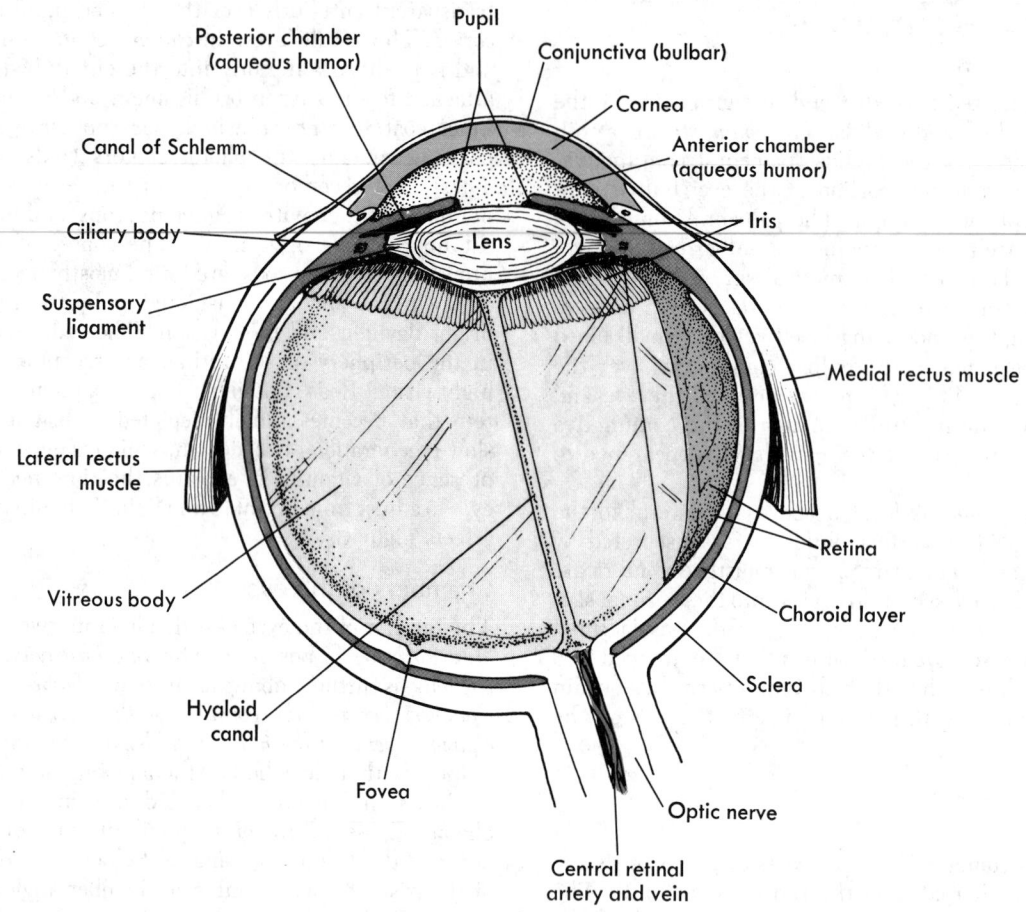

Fig. 38-2   Horizontal section through left eyeball.

posterior cavity of the eye is filled with a clear gelatinous substance, the vitreous humor, which helps maintain eye body. If vitreous humor is removed, the eye collapses.

Iris and lens

The iris is a colored, ring-shaped membrane containing involuntary dilator and sphincter muscles that control pupillary size. The pupil is the space in the center of the iris. The size of the pupil varies in response to light intensity and to focusing from far to near objects (accommodation) to enhance visual acuity; the pupil constricts with bright lights or for near vision. The pupil also responds to autonomic nervous stimulation; pupils dilate with stress to permit more light to enter to see better during the "fight or flight" response.

The lens of the eye is a crystalline, transparent biconvex structure behind the iris, separating the anterior and posterior chambers. The lens is composed of epithelial cells and is covered by an elastic membrane (capsule). It is held in place by fibers from the ciliary body. Because of its elasticity, the lens can change shape, becoming more or less convex. The more convex the lens, the greater the refraction (see below). If the lens becomes cloudy and opaque, it is called a *cataract* (p. 1313).

Muscles of the eye

Eye muscles are of two types, extrinsic and intrinsic. The extrinsic voluntary muscles outside the eyeball control ex-

traocular movement. The intrinsic involuntary muscles within the eye are the ciliary body, which controls the shape of the lens, and the iris, which controls pupil size.

Physiology of Vision

Light rays entering the eye bend (refraction) as they pass over the curved surfaces of the cornea and through various structures of the eye (cornea, aqueous humor, lens, vitreous humor), which have different densities, to focus on the retina. When light rays do not focus on the retina, it is called a refractive error.

The eyes adjust (accommodation) so as to see objects at various distances by flattening or thickening of the lens. Near vision requires contraction of the ciliary body, which decreases the distance between the edges of the ciliary body, thus relaxing the suspensory ligament attached to the lens. The lens then bulges to bend the light ray more acutely so that the rays focus on the retina. Continual close vision may produce eye strain through constant contraction of the ciliary muscle; this can be relieved by frequent shifting of the eyes to distant objects. Accommodation is also facilitated by changing the size of the pupil. With near vision the iris constricts the pupil to force light rays to pass through the shortened but thicker lens.

Light rays are absorbed by the photoreceptors on the retina and are changed to electrical activity to transmit the image to the cortex. The fibers of the optic nerve (cranial nerve II) divide at the optic chiasm, the medial portion of each nerve crosses to the opposite side, and the impulses are then transmitted to the visual cortex (see Fig. 38-5). *Bilateral vision provides depth perception.*

Intraocular Pressure

Intraocular pressure (IOP) is maintained by the balance between the production and drainage of aqueous humor. Drainage can be impeded by blockage of the trabecular meshwork (which filters the aqueous humor as it enters the canal of Schlemm) or by increasing pressure in the episcleral veins into which the canal of Schlemm empties.[28] Some aqueous humor may also drain into ciliary muscle spaces, then into the suprachoroidal space. The trabecular meshwork and entrance to the canal of Schlemm can be blocked by the iris. The Valsalva maneuver, which increases venous pressure, increases the pressure in the episcleral veins, permitting less aqueous humor to drain out and thus increasing IOP.

The normal range of IOP is 10 to 21 mm Hg, with a mean value of 16 mm Hg. The pressure may vary up to 5 mm Hg as a result of diurnal changes. Temporary increases in IOP may occur with emotional stress.

Physiologic Changes With Aging

Visual acuity declines rapidly, often by the middle 40s or early 50s. By age 70 most persons use visual aids. Structural changes occur in the retina, pupil, lens, and cornea; the retina loses cells, the pupils decrease in size, the lens becomes less elastic and may become more opaque, and the cornea flattens (Table 38-1). Farsightedness results from the decreased elasticity of the lens *(presbyopia).* Astigmatism may occur from the irregular curvature of the flattened cornea. *The smaller pupil permits less light to reach the retina and, in addition to a decrease in rhodopsin in the rods, night vision is decreased. Older people, therefore, require more light for seeing objects,* especially for near vision, than do younger persons. The lens also yellows with age, leading to increased difficulty distinguishing among colors, especially at the blue end of the spectrum.

Peripheral vision decreases with age. It is uncertain, however, which of the above factors leads to this problem.

Secretions of the eye also decrease with age. Fewer tears are produced and those that are produced tend to evaporate more quickly, producing a feeling of scratchiness or dryness of the eyes. Artificial tears may be required. Tearing may occur, despite the decreased quantity, if the tear ducts become blocked. Aqueous production is diminished, but because the anterior chamber becomes smaller, a relatively stable intraocular pressure is maintained.[10] Older persons, however, have an increased chance of developing glaucoma from increased pressure in the anterior chamber (p. 1316).

A common eye change noted in older persons is a hazy gray ring around the periphery of the cornea resulting from fat deposits.

PREVENTION AND HEALTH EDUCATION

Vision is one of the most important senses. It orients us to the world around us. It provides pleasure through beautiful sights. It provides data to promote safety and effective interaction with others. Vision also contributes to our self-

---

38-1	Persons who specialize in eye problems or corrective lenses	
	Ophthalmologist	Physician who specializes in diagnosis and treatment of eye diseases; may also prescribe lenses
	Oculist	Same as ophthalmologist
	Optometrist	Professional with special preparation in assessment of vision and in treatment of visual problems (for example, prescribes lenses, visual training, or orthoptic exercises); is not a physician and does not treat eye diseases
	Optician	Person who grinds and fits lenses according to prescriptions written by ophthalmologist or optometrist

Table 38-1   Physiologic eye changes with aging

Problem	Etiology
Farsightedness	Decreased elasticity of lens
Astigmatism	Flattened cornea
Decreased vision, especially at night	Decreased pupil size, decreased rhodopsin
Decreased peripheral vision	Cause unknown
Difficulty distinguishing colors	Yellowed lens
Dryness and scratchiness of eyes	Decreased tear production
Corneal gray ring	Corneal fat deposits

---

concept and feeling of personal worth and well-being. People should therefore be encouraged to have their eyes tested for any problems encountered with visual acuity when young, about every 5 years as a young adult, and every 2 years after age 40. Box 38-1 differentiates among eye specialists.

Because nurses come into contact with persons of all ages, they have opportunities to become involved in many activities that promote good vision and help to prevent injury or further impairment. This is accomplished by participation in promotion of visual acuity, promotion of safety measures, and detection of possible eye disorders.

Promotion of visual acuity

Interference with visual acuity may result from refractive errors or disturbances in visual fields.

Refractive errors

Bending of the light ray (refraction) depends on the shape and condition of the eye. If the anteroposterior dimension of the eye is abnormally long, the light rays will focus in

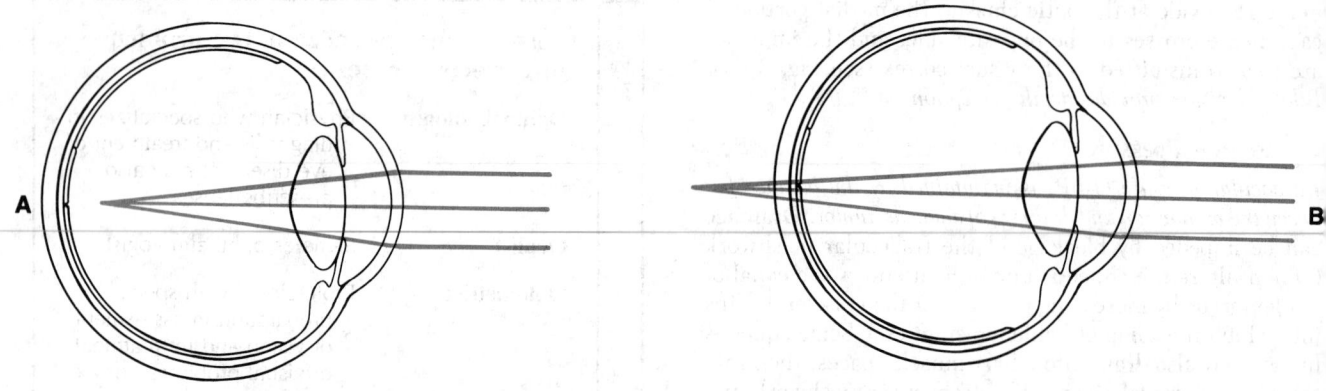

Fig. 38-3   A, Myopia (nearsightedness); image is focused in front of retina. **B,** Hyperopia (farsightedness); image is focused behind retina.

38-2	**Terms describing visual acuity**	
	Accommodation	Ability to adjust for far and near objects
	Emmetropia	Normal eyesight; light rays focus on retina
	Ametropia	Refractive error; light rays do not focus on retina
	Myopia	Nearsightedness; light rays focus in front of retina (Fig. 38-3)
	Hyperopia	Farsightedness; light rays focus behind retina
	Presbyopia	Hyperopia from loss of lens elasticity because of age
	Astigmatism	Irregular curvature of cornea; light rays do not focus at same point

front of the retina (*myopia*). Conversely, if the anteroposterior dimension is abnormally short, the rays will focus behind the retina (*hyperopia*) (Fig. 38-3). As noted earlier, decreased elasticity of the lens occurring with age (presbyopia) also produces hyperopia. The curvature of the cornea may also be asymmetric or irregular so that rays in the horizontal and vertical planes do not focus at the same point (astigmatism). *Refractive errors account for the largest number of impairments of good vision.*

Measurement of visual acuity

Distance vision is usually determined by use of a Snellen chart (Fig. 38-4). The person sits or stands 20 feet from the chart, covers one eye with a piece of stiff paper or a plastic occluder, and reads the line specified by the examiner. The eyes are tested with and without distance lenses. Some experts recommend that the right eye be tested first, followed by the left eye. Adhering to this procedure ensures that recording errors will not be made.

Visual acuity is expressed as a fraction; a reading of 20/20 is considered normal. The upper figure refers to the distance at which the person can read the chart, and the lower figure indicates the distance at which a normal eye can read the line. For example, if an individual is able to read at 20 ft only the line that should be readable at 70 ft, he or she has 20/70 vision in the eye tested.

Near vision is tested by reading small print, such as newsprint, held 35 cm (14 in) from the eye. Any person with vision less than 20/30 in either eye is referred to an ophthalmologist or optometrist for further testing.

Some terms related to acuity are defined in Box 38-2.

Visual fields

The visual field is that portion of the environment that the eye can perceive. The field of vision thus includes peripheral or indirect vision. Normality depends on intactness of all parts of the visual pathways of the eye. Lesions of the retina, optic pathways, and central nervous system affect sections of the field of vision. *Damage to the optic disk (retina) or to the optic nerve anterior to the optic chiasm, as seen with glaucoma, affects only the field of the involved eye* (Fig. 38-5, B1). Lesions at the chiasm or posterior to it produce bilateral visual field defects of a wide variety. For example, a pituitary gland tumor compressing the optic chiasm damages the crossing fibers from the nasal retina and classically causes *bitemporal hemianopsia*, or the *loss of vision in the temporal halves of each eye* (Fig. 38-5, B2). *Loss of vision in the corresponding halves of both visual fields produces homonymous hemianopsia* (Fig. 38-5, B3) and can be further designated as right or left. For example, patients with *right cerebrovascular accidents often experience hemianopsia with left field loss.*

Measurement of visual fields

Visual fields can be tested by various means. One method (confrontation test) is to ask the person *to cover one eye and focus on a point directly ahead.* An object, such as *a pencil,* is *placed peripherally beyond the person's vision,* then *advanced*

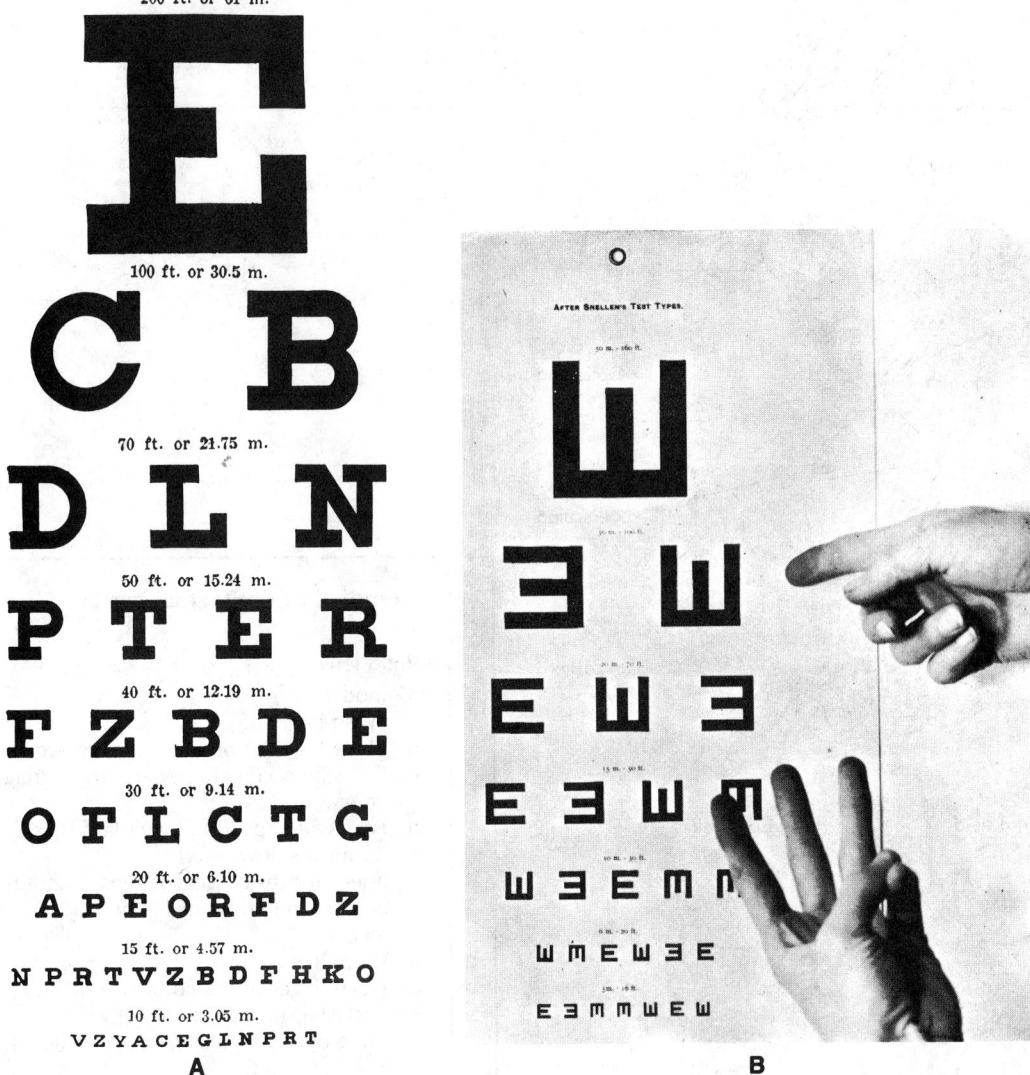

Fig. 38-4 **A,** Snellen chart used in testing vision. **B,** Modified Snellen chart, called "E" game, for testing vision of small children and persons unfamiliar with English alphabet.

centrally until the person first indicates that the object is seen. Normally, the *person should see* about *60 degrees nasally, 90 degrees temporally, 50 degrees superiorly, and 70 degrees inferiorly.*

Types of lenses

Lenses may be worn as glasses or contact lenses (Table 38-2). Glasses may have one focus (for near or far vision), *bifocal* (upper part for distance, lower part for near vision) or *trifocal* (for distance, intermediate, and near vision).

Contact lenses are usually chosen for cosmetic reasons or for sports activities because they do not fog or break easily. Persons who have lenses removed because of cataracts (but without lens implants) achieve better vision with contact lenses than with glasses. Some industrial occupations prohibit use of contact lenses because of irritation of the cornea by dirt or dust trapped under the lens.

Contact lenses are small corrective lenses made of different types of ground plastic worn over the cornea of the eye or between the cornea and sclera (scleral lens). The *lenses may be of various types: rigid, gas permeable (rigid), soft, or extended-wear (soft)* (Table 38-2). The rigid lenses are commonly used because they are cheaper and easier to maintain; they cannot be worn for long periods (usually not over 12 to 24 hours).

The disadvantages of soft-type lenses may include a higher initial cost and more frequent replacement. They are also more difficult to clean and maintain. The use of extended-wear soft contact lenses has increased in the United States. Although some of these lenses can be left in place for as long as a month, the current trend is to limit wear to 1 week before removal for cleaning and disinfection. Persons who use extended-wear lenses must be educated and prepared for the extra care required for these lenses. Scleral lenses are more difficult to wear than corneal lenses and are less frequently prescribed.

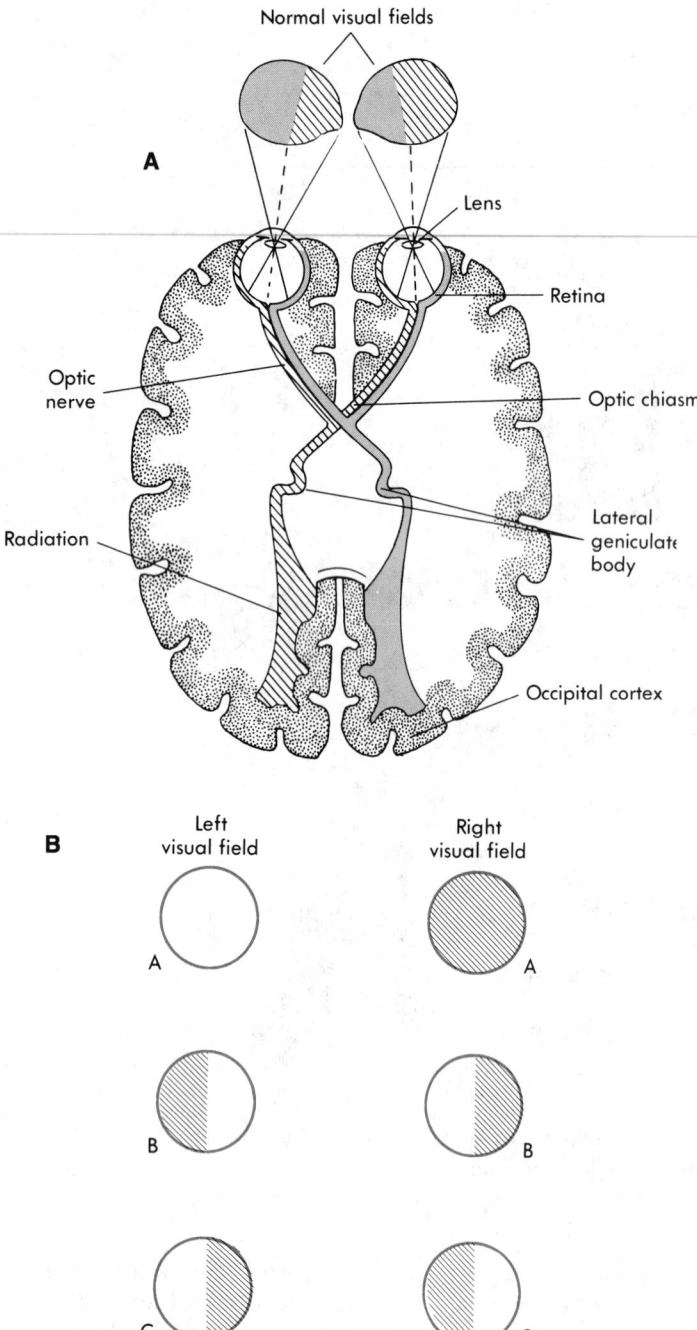

Fig. 38-5 **A,** Visual pathways showing partial decussation at optic chiasm. Normal visual fields show reversal of light rays from the temporal and nasal sides to receptors in the retina. **B,** Abnormal visual fields. *A,* Normal left field of vision with loss of vision in right field as a result of complete lesion of right optic nerve. *B,* Loss of vision in temporal half of both fields as a result of lesion of optic chiasm. This is called bitemporal hemianopsia. *C,* Loss of vision in nasal field of right eye and temporal field of left eye caused by lesion of the right optic tract. This is called homonymous hemianopsia.

38-3

Removal of contact lenses

Rigid lens
Method 1
a. Wash hands
b. Place finger at outer canthus of eye.
c. Pull skin obliquely upward, then straight down.
d. Lens will appear on lower lashes as the upper lid moves downward.
e. If lens moves off center, reposition it by gentle pressure on lid or lens itself.
Method 2
a. Wash hands
b. Place finger or thumb of each hand at base of eyelashes (upper and lower).
c. Bring eyelids together, trapping the lens (the lens will eject).
d. If lens moves off center, reposition it by gentle pressure on lid or lens itself.
Method 3
a. Wash hands
b. Using eye irrigation set, gently flush eye with sterile normal saline solution.
c. Retrieve lens in curved basin.
Method 4
a. Wash hands
b. Use small suction device shaped like a miniature "plumber's helper."
c. Place over center of lens and pull lens off gently.

Soft lens
a. Wash hands
b. Pull upper lid up with one thumb.
c. Be sure lens is in place before attempting removal.
d. Move lens over conjunctiva before grasping it, if possible. If lens does not move freely, put several drops of sterile saline solution in eye, close lid, and wait 1 minute before trying again.
e. Grasp lens with thumb and forefinger of other hand and pinch the soft lens (it will pop off).

Table 38-2   Types of corrective lenses

Lens	Characteristics	Benefits	Disadvantages
Glasses	Impact-resistant material (plastic or glass)	Plastic lenses are lighter in weight than glass	Plastic lenses are more expensive than glass and scratch easily
Contact lenses			
Rigid	Hydrophobic, rigid plastic Usually tinted Cover only the cornea	Least expensive Easy to clean Good optical quality	Easily lost Cannot be worn for long periods
Gas permeable	Rigid plastic, permeable to oxygen and other gases Cover only cornea	Good optical quality Comfortable Can be worn longer than hard lenses	Expensive
Soft	Hydrophyllic, flexible plastic Cover cornea and part of sclera	Can be worn longer (up to 18 hours) Comfortable	Higher initial cost, need frequent replacement Must be kept wet to prevent damage More difficult to clean Absorb atmospheric pollutants
Extended wear	Same as soft lenses but contain more water	Can be worn continuously for several weeks	Expensive Require medical supervision Tear easily

Newer contact lenses with the optical qualities of the rigid lenses and the comfort of the soft are now available. Because of their special properties, along with specially developed contact lens solutions, some of the complications associated with both the rigid and soft lenses can be avoided.

Contact lenses are inserted after being cleaned thoroughly and immersed in a wetting agent such as methylcellulose. Conjunctival secretions provide the lubrication needed for the lenses to be worn in comfort. The lenses are held in place by capillary attraction and by the upper lid. *If the person is injured or unconscious, the nurse removes the contact lenses* (see Box 38-3). Lenses are stored separately in special containers, labeled left or right lens. Soft lenses are kept wet at all times with special solution or sterile saline solution.

Lenses should not be worn longer than the prescribed length of time. Overwearing can cause edema and abrasion of the cornea. All contact lenses can cause problems; most problems are minor and can be managed by changes in routine or lenses. However, problems should not be ignored, because they may lead to or be indicative of more serious problems.

Primary Prevention
Promoting eye safety

Everyone should know how to protect their eyes from injury (see Box 38-4). Many people keep unused eye medications and then use them for self-treatment at a later date. This is hazardous because it not only may lead to eye injury but may delay necessary treatment. Ophthalmic drugs may deteriorate, become more concentrated from evaporation of liquid, or become contaminated with bacteria or fungi.

In the United States there are 1.3 million eye injuries yearly. This includes approximately 1000 occupational eye injuries daily or about 350,000 per year. Over 100,000 persons are permanently disabled by such injuries. Nine out of 10 eye injuries could have been prevented if safety practices and protective eyewear had been used.[20]

38-4

Eye safety measures

1. Avoid frequent rinsing of eyes with unprescribed solutions.
2. Discard any ophthalmic solution that is cloudy, discolored, has been open for ≥3 months, or contains particles.
3. Avoid self-treatment of an eye inflammation with a medication prescribed for a previous eye disorder.
4. To avoid eye strain:
   a. Use a good light for reading or doing work that requires careful visual focus.
   b. When reading or focusing eyes for long periods, look at distant objects for a few minutes at repeated intervals to rest eyes.
5. Avoid rubbing eyes.
6. Wash hands before touching eyes.
7. Wear safety glasses when engaging in activities that could injure the eyes (occupations, sports)
8. Wear dark glasses for prolonged exposure to very bright light (such as sunlight on snow or water)
9. Flush eyes with copious amount of water when any irritating substances are accidentally introduced.
10. Do not attempt to remove foreign bodies from the cornea; cover eye and seek medical attention.
11. If a speck of dust blows in eye, pull upper lid over lower lid and let the tears wash the speck to the inner canthus or lower lid, where it may be safely removed.

Table 38-3 **First aid for eye injuries**

Injury	Interventions
Burns: chemical, flame	Flush eye immediately for 15 minutes with cool water or any available nontoxic liquid seek medical assistance
Loose substance on conjunctiva: dirt, insects	Lift upper lid over lower lid to dislodge substance, produce tearing; irrigate eye with water if necessary; do not rub eye; obtain medical assistance if above interventions fail
Contact injury: contusion, ecchymosis, laceration	Apply cold compresses if no laceration present; cover eye if laceration present; seek medical assistance
Penetrating objects	Do not remove object; place protective shield over eye (e.g., paper cup); cover uninjured eye to prevent excess movement of injured eye; seek medical assistance

Table 38-4 **Symptoms suggestive of eye disease**

Symptom	Eye disease
Conjunctival redness	Conjunctivitis, blepharitis, sty
Crusting discharge	Conjunctivitis, blepharitis, sty
Ocular pain	Foreign body, sty, acute lid infection, glaucoma, keratitis, uveitis
Foreign body sensation ("something in eye")	Foreign body, corneal erosion, blepharitis, chronic conjunctivitis
Blepharospasm	Keratitis, corneal ulcer
Multiple spots ("floaters")	Retinal detachment, intraocular hemorrhage, diabetic retinopathy
Photophobia	Uveitis, keratitis, glaucoma, corneal abrasions
Vision changes	
Blurred vision	Refractive error, cataract, glaucoma, uveitis, retinal detachment
Double vision	Strabismus
Halos around lights	Glaucoma
Blind spots	Hemorrhage, choroiditis
Sudden vision loss	Central retinal artery or vein occlusion

Preventive goggles and break-resistant corrective lenses should be worn by persons who engage in very active physical activities such as sports and selected occupations. Prompt and appropriate care of an injured eye may prevent serious vision impairment or loss of the eye (Table 38-3).

Secondary Prevention

Early detection of eye disease is imperative for protection of vision. Inflammations of the eye are more easily detected than other eye disorders; the person usually complains of discomfort, and redness and discharge are easily observed. Glaucoma is the greatest threat to vision in older persons; the permanent vision loss it causes is preventable if the condition is identified early. Mass screening programs for glaucoma detection have been instituted in many communities, and everyone is urged to participate. All persons with symptoms suggestive of eye disease (Table 38-4) are urged to seek medical assistance.

Diseases of other parts of the body may also affect the eye (Table 38-5). Early detection and treatment of these diseases can help to prevent loss of vision.

VISUAL IMPAIRMENT: BLINDNESS

Vision is essential to most employment and necessary in countless experiences that make life enjoyable and meaningful. Yet, in the United States 8 to 10 million persons suffer from visual impairment that cannot be corrected by eyeglasses or contact lenses. Of these, 2 million cannot read ordinary newsprint.[20] The National Eye Institute estimates that the cost of visual disorders and blindness costs the United States more than $16 billion annually in direct medical care and costs such as days lost from work.

In developing countries there is a high incidence of blindness from preventable causes such as malnutrition and eye infections. The visually impaired population includes not only those who are legally blind. There are well over a million people who, although unable to see well enough to read a newspaper, have vision better than 20/200. Also, there are over 3 million who are monocularly blind, with a small proportion having a defective but not blind second eye. Most persons in this visually impaired but not legally blind population are between the ages of 25 and 64. Nearly 13% of persons over the age of 65 have some form of visual impairment: blindness in both eyes or inability to read newsprint even with eyeglasses. For persons between 20 and 44 years of age, the leading cause of new blindness is diabetic retinopathy. In persons between 45 and 74 years of age, the leading causes of new blindness are glaucoma and diabetic retinopathy.[20]

Although there has been a reduction of blindness in the United States from infections and certain diseases and injuries, *blindness from diseases that occur most frequently among older persons*, including *diabetic retinopathy, glaucoma,*

Table 38-5   Eye manifestations of systemic disorders

Disorder	Effect on eye
Diabetes mellitus	Senile cataracts occur earlier and progress more rapidly
	Diabetic retinopathy; retinal changes lead to decreased vision
	Vitreous hemorrhages
	Retinal detachment
Persistent systemic hypertension	Retinal hemorrhage, retinal edema, and retinal exudate lead to loss of sight
Cerebral vascular accident	Loss of sight in one half of visual field (hemianopsia)
	Emboli may occlude retinal vessel
Demyelinating neurologic disorders (multiple sclerosis)	Nerve damage to eye
Increased intracranial pressure	Papilledema (swelling of optic disc)
Nutritional disorders	
Lack of vitamin A and B	Changes in conjunctiva, cornea, and retina
	Tears reduced
	Eyes and lids become reddened and inflamed
	Night blindness
Excess of vitamin A	Retinal damage
AIDS	Cytomegalovirus (CMV) retinitis

cataract, and *retinal degeneration, has increased.* It is likely that the incidence of blindness will continue to increase because of the steady growth in the number of persons aged 65 and older.

In this regard, *Healthy People 2000* has set the following goals for the year 2000: to reduce visual impairment to no more than 30 per 1000 people from a baseline of 34.5 per 1000 during 1986 to 1988. The special target population for this goal is people age 65 and older. The year 2000 target for this age group is 70 per 1000 as compared with 87.7 in 1986 to 1988.[20]

Impaired Vision

Vision impairment ranges from refractive errors correctable with lenses to total blindness, in which the person may not even be able to perceive light. For legal purposes blindness is defined very precisely in order to determine eligibility for assistance of various kinds (see Box 38-5). *Although many nonseeing persons now prefer to be called visually handicapped, the term blindness is still in common usage.*

Responses to Loss of Vision
Impact of visual loss

People who are born blind or develop blindness very early in life and who are raised as if they could see, and are neither overprotected or rejected, frequently are self-confident persons able to lead active productive lives.

Loss of vision may affect self-esteem and the ability to interact with others and with the environment. The adult who becomes blind fairly rapidly usually has greater difficulty adjusting to the handicap. The impairment may cause a decrease in self-confidence and self-concept. Communication with others is affected, and a sense of isolation may develop. Familiar hobbies that require vision, such as reading, sewing, or crafts, may no longer be possible. Even listening to television creates problems when gaps in sound occur. Mobility or ability to carry out activities of daily living may be restricted or at least modified. Career options, job opportunities, and financial security may be affected.

> **38-5**
>
> ### Legal criteria of blindness
>
> A person is considered legally blind when either of the following conditions exist:
> Visual field no greater than 20 degrees
> Central distance vision in better eye 20/200 or less with use of corrective lenses (eye can see at 20 ft what the normal eye can see at 200 ft)
>
> Report of the National Advisory Eye Council, US Department of Health, Education and Welfare, No. (NIH) 75-664, 1975.

Blindness may influence the person's ability to remain independent, to feel socially adequate, or to feel that he or she is a contributing member of society.

Limitations in the range and variety of experiences are related to the fact that a person who cannot see must use touch and kinesthetic experience to gain knowledge of the world. Objects too large or too small to handle are not perceivable. Many blind persons feel that the restriction in mobility resulting from blindness is its most serious effect. Blind persons cannot move about as quickly, as securely, or as easily as sighted persons. These individuals need to rely on canes, seeing-eye dogs or other persons, particularly when they are in unfamiliar areas.

Coping with visual loss

After a person has been told that blindness will result, there is a *normal reaction* described as *a period of mourning for the "dead" eyes. Grief and mourning over the loss of vision can cause emotional reactions such as denial, anger, guilt, resentment, hopelessness, helplessness, loneliness, and depression.* These strong emotional feelings interfere with the blind person's ability to plan new ways of accomplishing tasks of living.

Fluctuating vision, a common occurrence for many visually impaired persons, *leads to frustration and difficulties*

Guidelines for communicating with blind persons

1. Talk in a normal tone of voice.
2. Do not try to avoid common phrases in speech, such as "See what I mean?"
3. Introduce yourself with each contact (unless you are well-known to the person).
4. Explain why you are in the room.
5. Announce when you are leaving the room so the blind person is not put in the position of talking to someone who is no longer there.

Facilitating independence in ADL for blind persons

Place clothing in specific locations in drawers or closets to facilitate clothing selection.

Keep furniture in specific places to facilitate mobility.

Encourage use of cane when walking in unfamiliar areas.

When assisting a blind person in walking, let the person take *your* arm (Fig. 38-6).

Provide descriptions of food on plate in terms of a clock face, for example, "The peas are at 7 o'clock."

Provide privacy while the newly blind person is learning to cope with eating unless they ask that someone stay.

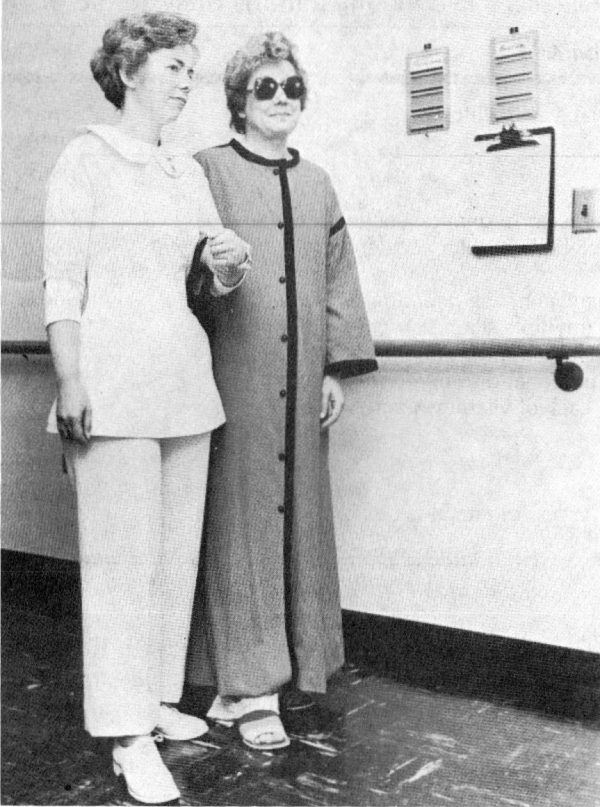

Fig. 38-6 Ambulation of patient who cannot see. Note that patient holds nurse's arm and is led without being held.

in planning or implementing tasks. Fears and uncertainties about the progression of visual impairment can lead to concern about the ability to cope with further deterioration of vision or the necessity of preparing for the future.

The ability to cope with the loss depends on the extent and duration of the handicap, the age at which it occurs, how the person has successfully coped in the past, and the presence of available support systems (family and friends).

Over time, persons with visual losses appear to be able to compensate for their deficit by an increase in sensitivity of the other senses. For example, *many blind people compensate by increasing auditory acuity, tactile acuity, sense of smell, or kinesthetic awareness.*

Role of the Nurse in Working With the Newly Blind

Counseling

Newly blind persons who are trying to cope need an opportunity to talk about their feelings, concerns, and anxieties about the future. Once they have identified these feelings and concerns, they can be helped to identify their strengths and resources and to consider different approaches to dealing with tasks of everyday living. Alternate forms of recreation and pleasurable activities can also be explored. For example, the person who enjoyed reading may be interested in learning Braille or listening to "talking books."

Some persons need assistance in developing a new self-image. It is not unusual for the person to reject initially any aids that officially identify them as "blind," such as the white cane. Patience is required; it sometimes takes a long time to change self-image.

Persons who become blind do not develop impaired hearing or intelligence, yet some sighted persons insist on speaking loudly. Communication should be as it would be for a sighted person (see Box 38-6).

The Americans With Disabilities Act, which was signed by President Bush in 1990, should improve job opportunities for persons with limited vision. The law ensures that employers cannot discriminate against qualified individuals with disabilities. The Americans With Disabilities Act is discussed in greater detail in Chapter 14.

Assisting with ADL

Given time, most blind persons develop ways of coping with activities of daily living (ADL) (see Box 38-7). One elderly blind lady was able to take her many medications accurately by devising a system using rubber bands and strings around the medication bottles to provide clues as to when they were to be taken.

Referring to community services

Many federal, state, and local agencies provide services to persons with severe visual impairment. The health professional can refer these persons and their families to a social worker familiar with services and facilities available in their home area. Community health nurses often have this information readily available. *Services to visually impaired persons include mobility training, personal counseling, vocational rehabilitation, relearning independent self-care, special education, and financial assistance in some instances.* "Talking books" and other tapes are available from public libraries, as well as from organizations for the blind.

Some organizations for the blind loan tape players to blind persons. They mail tapes or records, which are returned in special containers postage free. The U.S. Library of Congress also supplies tapes and records to blind persons; these are returned in special postage-free containers.

Government Assistance

Legal blindness entitles a person to certain federal assistance based on need. Blind persons are entitled to an extra personal deduction in reported income. Counseling and placement services are available through the Social and Rehabilitation Service (SRS) of the U.S. Department of Health and Human Services.

MAJOR HEALTH PROBLEMS OF THE EYE

The most common disorders of the eye in adults include the following:

1. Inflammatory disorders of the eyelid, conjunctiva, cornea, choroid, ciliary body, and iris
2. Cataracts: opaqueness of the lens
3. Glaucoma: increased intraocular pressure
4. Retinal detachment

Each of these is discussed in this chapter.

INFLAMMATORY EYE DISORDERS

Inflammations and infections may occur in any of the eye structures (Table 38-6), and *account for more than half of eye disorders.*

Etiology and Pathophysiology

Most eye inflammations are caused by microorganisms, mechanical irritation, or sensitivity to some substance. Fortunately, a large percentage of inflammations are self-limiting, with no permanent scars. Severe corneal inflammation or ulceration can damage the cornea, causing visual impairment. Complications from uveitis can lead to formation of adhesions, secondary glaucoma, and loss of vision.

The *most common eye inflammations* are *styes and conjunctivitis.* Styes are relatively mild infections of the follicle of an eyelash or gland at the lid margins. Staphylococci are often the infecting organisms. These infections tend to occur in crops because the infecting organism spreads from one hair follicle to another. Poor hygiene and excessive use of cosmetics may be contributing causes. Persons should be taught not to squeeze styes because the infection may spread and cause cellulitis of the lids.

Conjunctivitis is the most common eye disease and may be acute or chronic. Acute bacterial conjunctivitis is usually transmitted by direct contact; the person touches the eyes following finger contact with contaminated objects such as towels or tissues. The *most common infecting organisms* are *staphylococci* and *adenoviruses.* Simple conjunctivitis is usually self-limiting.

Infection by *Chlamydia trachomatis* leads to *trachoma,* a form of conjunctivitis that is rare in the United States, but is the leading cause of blindness worldwide, particularly in low-income persons living in the dry, hot Mediterranean countries and the Far East. Following the acute conjunctivitis stage in trachoma, the eyelids become scarred, and granulations form on the inner surface of the lids and invade the cornea. The entire cornea may eventually become involved with subsequent loss of vision. Secondary bacterial infection is common. Trachomas can be arrested in the early stages with topical and oral tetracycline. Hygienic measures are important in the prevention and treatment of trachoma. Corneal scarring may require corneal transplantation.

Allergic conjunctivitis is commonly associated with hay fever. It is usually chronic and recurrent.

Nursing Process
Assessment
Subjective data

Persons with inflammations of the eye may complain of itching, pain (mild to severe), lacrimation, sensitivity to light (photophobia), or spasms of the eyelids (blepharospasms).

Objective data

The external structures of the eye are routinely inspected during the physical examination. *Inflammations are identified by* the presence of *redness, edema of the lids, and pus or discharge from the eye.* When *considerable discharge* is present, the *lids may become stuck together during sleep.*

Corneal ulcers may be identified by instilling sterile fluorescein, *a yellow-green harmless dye.* Because fluorescein harbors the growth of microorganisms such as *Pseudomonas,* only a new, unopened bottle should be used. Also available are *single-use fluorescein-impregnated paper strips that are gently touched to the inside of the lower lid.* The ulcer is then assessed by shining a penlight obliquely across the eye from the side. If pain and blepharospasm interfere with examination, a drop of anesthetic such as 0.5% proparacaine can be used.

Data analysis: nursing diagnoses

Nursing diagnoses are determined from analysis of patient data. Possible nursing diagnoses for the person with an eye inflammation may include, but are not limited to, the following:

Table 38-6 Inflammatory disorders of the eye

Disorder	Description	Signs and symptoms	Medical therapy
Hordoleum (stye)	Staphylococcal infection of gland at eyelid margin	Localized abcess at base of eyelash, edema of lid, pain	Hot compresses to hasten pointing of abcess, topical antibiotic
Chalazion	Cyst from obstruction of sebaceous gland at eyelid margin	Initial edema and discomfort; later, painless mass in lid	Warm compresses and topical antibiotic initially; surgical removal if large and pressing on cornea
Blepharitis	Inflammation of lid margins, usually by staphylococci	Itching, redness, lid pain, lacrimation, photophobia; crusting ulceration; lids become glued together during sleep	Warm compresses followed by erythromycin or bacitracin eye ointment; steroid eye drops may be prescribed
Conjunctivitis (pink eye)	Inflammation of conjunctiva by viruses, bacteria (highly infectious), chlamydia, allergy, trauma (sunburn)	Redness of conjunctiva, lid edema, crusting discharge on lids and cornea of eye; itching with allergies	Cleansing of lids and lashes, warm compresses; topical antibiotics; steroid eye drops for allergies (contraindicated for herpes simplex virus); no eye patch
Keratitis	Inflammation of cornea by bacteria, herpes simplex virus, allergies, vitamin A deficiency	Severe eye pain, photophobia, tearing, blepharospasm, loss of vision if uncontrolled	Warm compresses; topical antibiotics for bacterial infections; atropine sulfate; idoxuridine for herpes simplex; eye patch, rest; corneal grafting if cornea injured
Corneal ulcer	Necrosis of corneal tissue from trauma, inflammation; may be superficial or may penetrate deeper tissue	Pain and blepharospasm may occur; ulcer may be outlined by fluorescein dye	Superficial ulcer: antibiotic eye drops, eye patch Deep ulcer: topical and systemic antibiotics, atropine sulfate, warm compresses, eye patch; cauterization; corneal transplant if necessary
Uveitis	Inflammation of iris and ciliary body (anterior) or choroid (posterior); the cause is often unknown	*Anterior:* eye pain, photophobia, lacrimation, blurred vision, small pupil *Posterior:* blurring, decreased vision, mild eye discomfort	Scopolamine or atropine to dilate pupil (rests pupil, prevents adhesions), moist eye compresses, corticosteroids

Diagnostic title	Possible etiologies
Pain	Edema of the eye, secretions, photophobia
Infection, high risk for infection of nonaffected eye	Lack of information about how eye infections are spread
Knowledge deficit	Lack of exposure to information

Planning: expected patient outcomes

Expected patient outcomes for the person with an eye inflammation may include, but are not limited to, the following:

1. Patient states pain is decreased.
2. Infection does not spread to opposite eye.
3. The patient can:
   a. State name, dosage, and frequency of eye medication to be taken and the need to discard unused ophthalmic medications after therapy.
   b. Describe method and frequency of eye compresses to be used.
   c. Describe measures to prevent spread of infection to the uninvolved eye and to others in the household.
4. If corneal grafting has been performed, the person can:
   a. Describe the medication program.
   b. Describe activities and movements to be avoided.
   c. Describe the need for medical follow-up.

Implementation

Nursing interventions for the person with an eye inflammation consist primarily of giving eye treatments and medications to hasten healing and decrease pain, and helping prevent the spread of infection (see Box 38-8).

Guidelines for Care

Care of the patient with an eye inflammation

1. Wash hands
2. Apply warm moist compresses as prescribed for healing and to decrease pain.
3. Irrigate eye, if prescribed, to remove discharge.
4. Administer prescribed eye medications.
5. Use eye pads only for inflammations without infection.
6. Dim bright lights if photophobia is present.
7. Give prescribed analgesics for pain.
8. Prevent spread of infection by:
   a. Using separate medication bottles or tubes for each eye if infection is present.
   b. Washing hands before and after touching eye.
   c. Using face cloths and face towels only once if infection is present.

Guidelines for Care

Application of warm moist eye compresses

1. Use sterile technique when infection or ulceration is present; clean technique may be used for allergic reactions.
2. Use separate equipment for bilateral eye infections.
3. Wash hands before treating each eye.
4. Temperature of compresses should not exceed 49° C (120° F).
5. Change compresses frequently over 10 to 20 minutes.
6. Do not exert pressure on eyeball.
7. Sterile petrolatum may be used on skin *around* eyes, if desired, to protect skin.
8. If sterility is not necessary, moist heat may be applied by means of a clean wash cloth.

Assisting with achievement of therapeutic goals
Eye compresses

Warm moist compresses (see Box 38-9) *help relieve pain, promote healing, and help to cleanse the eye, which is normally cleansed by tears.* Treatment is repeated two to four times a day.

Cold moist saline compresses may be ordered to prevent or control edema and severe itching of the eyes and to help control bleeding immediately after eye injury. A small basin of sterile solution may be placed in a bowl of chipped ice at the bedside. *Sterile forceps are used to wring out and apply the compress. If the compress does not need to be sterile, a washcloth or compress may be placed on pieces of ice in a basin.* A rubber glove or small plastic bag packed with finely chipped ice may be applied to the eye and requires fewer compress changes.

Guidelines for Care

Eye irrigation

1. Wash hands.
2. Place patient lying toward side to be irrigated to prevent fluid from flowing into other eye.
3. A plastic squeeze bottle is used unless very large amounts of fluid are needed.
4. Direct the irrigating fluid along the conjunctiva from the *inner* to the outer canthus (Fig. 38-7).
5. Avoid directing a forceful stream onto the eyeball.
6. Avoid touching any eye structures with irrigation equipment.
7. A piece of gauze may be wrapped around the index finger to raise upper lid for better cleaning if heavy discharge is present.
8. Place an emesis basin at side of face to collect irrigating fluid. An alternative is to collect the solution in a folded towel held at the side of the face.

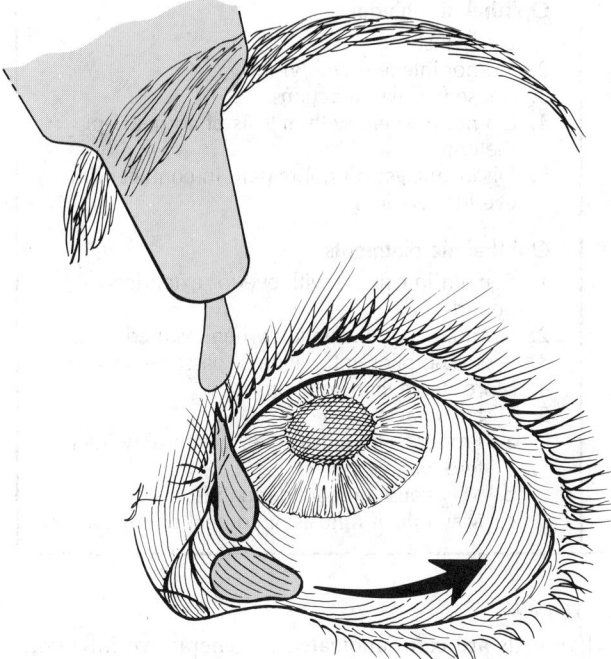

Fig. 38-7   Irrigating the eye. Fluid is directed along conjunctiva and over eyeball from inner to outer canthus.

Eye irrigation

Irrigation is used to remove secretions, discharge, foreign bodies, and chemical irritants from the eye (see Box 38-10). Physiologic saline solution or lactated Ringer's solution is commonly used because these isotonic solutions do not remove the electrolytes necessary for normal eye action. If only a small amount of fluid is needed, sterile cotton balls may be used to drip fluid into the eye.

Table 38-7   Types of ophthalmic drugs

Type	Action	Uses
Mydriatic	Dilates pupil	Examination of interior of eye Prevents adhesions of iris with cornea in eye inflammations
Cycloplegic	Dilates pupil Paralyzes ciliary muscle and iris	Decreases pain and photophobia and provides rest in inflammations of iris and ciliary body and diseases of cornea Eye examinations
Miotic	Contracts pupil Permits better drainage of intraocular fluid	Glaucoma
Osmotic	Decreases intraocular pressure	Acute glaucoma Eye surgery
Secretory inhibitor	Decreases production of intraocular fluid	Glaucoma
Topical anesthetic	Decreases sensation (pain)	Surgery, treatments Eye inflammations
Topical antibiotic	Antiinfective	Eye inflammations
Steroid	Antiinflammatory	Eye inflammations and allergic reactions

---

38-11

Forms of eye medications

Ophthalmic solutions
1. Easily instilled
2. Do not interfere with vision
3. Cause few skin reactions
4. Do not interfere with mitosis of corneal epithelium
5. Disadvantage: do not remain in contact with eye for very long

Ophthalmic ointments
1. Remain in contact with eye for extended periods
2. Do not cause discomfort when instilled
3. Less absorption into lacrimal passageways
4. More stable than solutions
5. Disadvantages:
   a. Produce film across eye, which may interfere with vision
   b. May cause contact dermatitis
   c. May inhibit mitosis of corneal epithelium

Eye pads

Eye pads are contraindicated in general eye infections because they enhance bacterial growth. They may be used for photophobia when the inflammation is *not* caused by bacteria and to protect the eye when corneal ulceration is present.

Eye medications

Accuracy and safety in the administration of eye medications is essential to prevent irreparable damage to the eye. The correct eye to receive the medication must be identified. Labels must be checked carefully, and all medications with labels that are smeared or obliterated are discarded. Solutions that have changed color, are cloudy, contain sediment, or are outdated are also discarded. Elderly persons are particularly susceptible to side effects of medications.

Ophthalmic medications may be instilled as eyedrop solutions or as an ointment (see Box 38-11).

All patients should have their own bottles of eyedrops or tubes of ointment to prevent cross-infection. If an eye infection is being treated with an antibiotic and the same drug is being given prophylactically in the other eye, separate bottles or tubes are used for each eye. Methods for instilling eyedrops and ointments are described in Box 38-12.

Different types of drugs are used for treatment of eye diseases (Table 38-7). The most commonly used drugs for eye inflammations are antibiotic, steroid, and cycloplegic drugs (Tables 38-8 and 38-9).

Drugs applied topically to the eye can be absorbed and may cause systemic side effects. To avoid undesired systemic reactions, care should be taken with topically applied medications to give exactly what is ordered and no more.

Corneal surgery

When the cornea is so damaged from corneal inflammation (keratitis) or from a corneal ulcer, corneal transplantation (keratoplasty) may be performed. Corneal grafts are taken from healthy donor eyes, preferably from young donors (ages 25 to 35) who have died from an acute disease or from injury.[28] The corneas need to be obtained within 5 hours of death. Until recently, the donor cornea had to be transplanted within 24 to 48 hours. Newer corneal preservation media make it possible to use the cornea up to 7 or more days after the death of the donor. By adding insulin and growth factors to the preservation media, it is hoped that the number of endothelial cells transplanted will increase; this should increase the chance of graft success.[4] Another advantage of this new medium is that the increased time of preservation allows the corneal transplant to be planned in advance by the regular surgical team, which increases the chance of a successful outcome.[4]

Persons wishing to donate their eyes for use in keratoplasty can write to the Eye Bank Association of America*

---

*1511 K Street NW, Suite 830, Washington, DC 20005-1401.

Table 38-8   Mydriatic and cycloplegic drugs

Drug	Maximal effect	Duration
Mydriatic action (dilates pupil)		
Phenylephrine (Neo-Synephrine)	20 min	3 hr
Epinephrine (Epitrate)	3 to 5 min	—
Cycloplegic and mydriatic action (dilates pupil; paralyzes ciliary muscle and iris)		
Atropine sulfate (Atropisol, Isopto-Atropine)	30 to 120 min	2 wks
Cyclopentolate (Cyclogyl)	15 to 45 min	2 days
Homatropine (Isopto-Homatropine)	10 to 90 min	2 to 3 days
Scopolamine hydrobromide	15 to 45 min	5 to 7 days
Tropicamide (Mydriacyl)	20 to 35 min	4 to 6 hrs

Table 38-9   Other ophthalmic drugs

Ophthalmic drug	Use and effect
Antiinfectives	
Polymyxin B, neomycin, bacitracin (Neosporin) Neomycin sulfate (Myciguent) Gentamicin sulfate (Garamycin) Chloramphenicol (Chloromycetin, Chloroptic) Erythromycin (Ilotycin) Tetracycline hydrochloride (Achromycin) Chlortetracycline hydrochloride (Aureomycin) Sulfacetamide sodium (Sodium Sulamyd, Isopto-Cetamide) Sulfisoxazole diolamine (Gantrisin) Natamycin (Natacyn) Idoxuridine (Herplex, Dendrid, Stoxil) Acyclovir (Zovirax)	Antibiotic agents may be given for acute inflammatory conjunctivitis, styes, eyelid infections, keratitis, and uveitis; natamycin is antifungal; idoxuridine and acyclovir are antiviral, especially for herpes simplex eye infections
Adrenocorticoids	
Dexamethasone (Decadron phosphate) Fluorometholone (FML Liquifilm) Hydrocortisone (Hydrocortone, Cortamed) Medrysone (HMS Liquifilm) Prednisolone (Pred Forte, Pred Mild, Metimyd)	Topical ophthalmic steroid therapy is indicated for allergic conjunctivitis, nonpyogenic eye inflammations, and for eye trauma (burns, foreign body penetration); chronic therapy may cause increased IOP, susceptibility to fungus infections, glaucoma, and cataracts
Tears substitutes	
Hydroxypropyl methylcellulose (Tears Naturale, Isopto-Tears, Tearisol)	Artificial tears provide lubrication when tears are deficient (age, heredity, connective tissue disorders, environment); also used for lubrication with contact lenses and artificial eyes

tor information. Some states use driver's licenses for potential donors to signify their intent. Nurses need to be alert to situations where corneas may be obtained and to offer the suggestion to the family of a recently deceased person.

Either total or partial replacement of the cornea may be performed (Fig. 38-9). The total penetrating graft is the most frequently used type and is the most effective. A second transplant may be performed if the first is unsuccessful.

Keratoplasty may be *performed* with *local or general anesthesia* or *a combination of both.* The new cornea is sutured in place, and an antibiotic is injected subconjunctivally. An eye shield is applied, remains in place until the day after surgery, and is reapplied at night to prevent inadvertent injury during sleep. Postoperative care of the person having eye surgery is discussed on p. 1314. Glasses may be worn during the day to protect the eye and the patient can expect that some vision will be restored immediately. Vision continues to improve over the next 6 to 12 months.

Corneal grafts heal very slowly because of the lack of blood vessels in the cornea. The patient is advised to avoid bending, lifting, or straining for 1 month to prevent increased intraocular pressure or suture strain; strenuous activities should be avoided for 3 months.

The graft is never totally integrated into the eye; therefore, the person must check his or her eye for the remainder of life for signs of rejection (redness, photosensitivity, pain, vision loss).[37] Any symptoms that persist or increase in severity in a 24-hour period are reported to the physician.

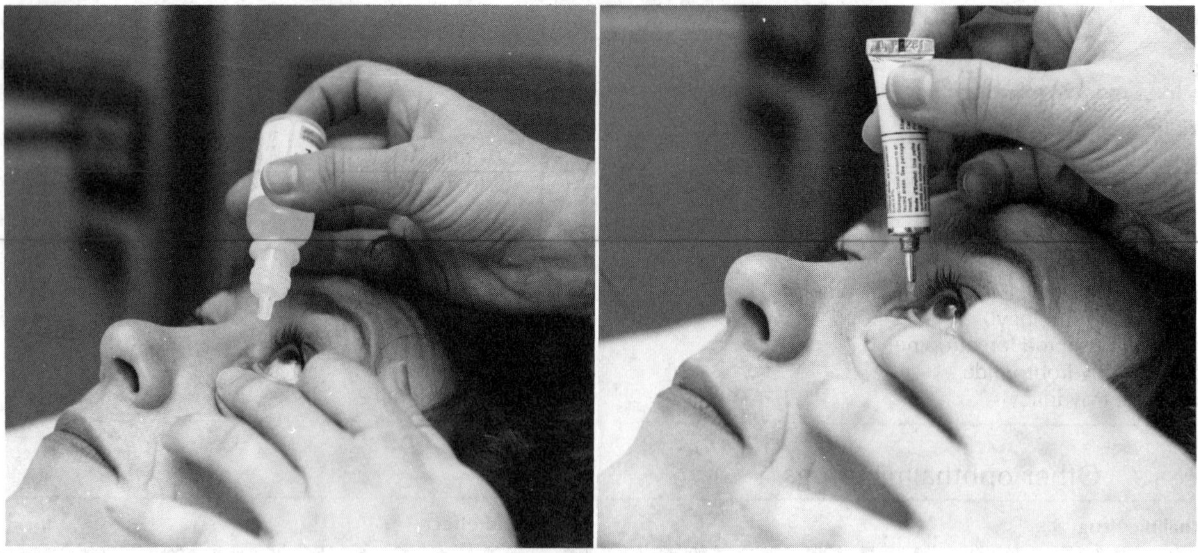

A

B

Fig. 38-8   **A,** Ophthalmic solution is dropped onto conjunctiva of lower lid. **B,** Ophthalmic ointment is squeezed onto conjunctiva of lower lid.

38-12

Guidelines for Care

Instilling eye medications

Eyedrops
1. Wash hands before touching eyes.
2. Clean eyes before instilling eyedrops if crusting or discharge is present.
3. Ask patient to tilt head back and look up (Fig. 38-8).
4. Evert lower lid by pulling down gently on skin below eye.
5. Approach eye from side (not directly from front).
6. Place drops on *center* of conjunctival sac of lower lid.
7. Avoid touching eye with tip of dropper.
8. Ask patient not to squeeze eye shut (loss of medication down cheek).
9. Provide patient with a tissue.

Ointment
1. Follow first four steps above.
2. Press the ointment from the tube directly onto exposed conjunctival sac.
3. Avoid touching eye tissue with tube.

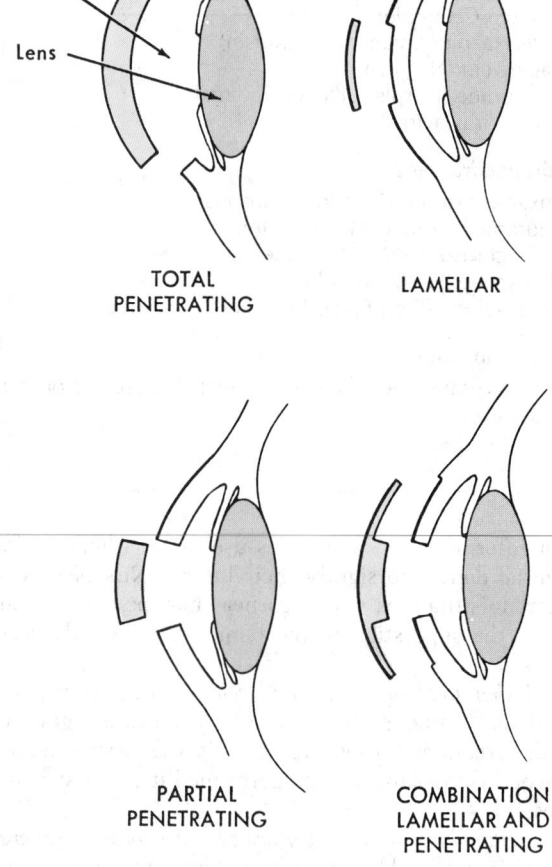

Cornea

Aqueous

Lens

TOTAL PENETRATING

LAMELLAR

PARTIAL PENETRATING

COMBINATION LAMELLAR AND PENETRATING

Fig. 38-9   Types of corneal grafts now being used. Note that in lamellar graft, defect does not penetrate entire thickness of cornea.

Interventions to achieve patient outcomes
Assisting with comfort

Pain from eye inflammations can be reduced by applying warm moist compresses several times each day and by instilling prescribed eyedrops (particularly cycloplegic drugs, which put the iris and ciliary body at rest). If photophobia creates discomfort, the patient's room is kept semi-dark. Avoid using overhead lights that would shine in the patient's eye when he or she is lying in bed. Mild analgesics such as aspirin or acetaminophen (Tylenol) usually suffice, but if pain is severe (as may occur with uveitis) a narcotic may be required.

Preventing spread of infection

When a highly infectious eye condition, such as acute bacterial conjunctivitis, is present, precautions need to be taken to prevent the spread of infection to others. Individual washcloths and towels should be used and discarded after each use. Hands should be washed before and after any contact with the infected eye.

Facilitating learning

The patient needs to be taught how to care for the inflamed eye and how to prevent further episodes of inflammation. Teaching includes instruction about medications and their proper use.

Evaluation

When providing care for the patient with an eye inflammation or infection, questions to consider may include the following:

1. Is the patient comfortable?
2. Is the uninvolved eye free of signs of infection?
3. Does the patient know how to carry out prescribed treatments after discharge?
4. If corneal surgery has been performed, does the patient know about activity limitations and need for continued medical follow-up?

CATARACT
Etiology and Epidemiology

A cataract is a clouding or opacity of the lens that leads to gradual painless blurring of vision and eventual loss of sight (Fig. 38-10). The most common cause of cataract formation is aging (senile cataract). By 80 years of age, about 85% of persons have some clouding of the lens. These *senile cataracts are the most common cause of blindness in the elderly*. Other causes of cataract include trauma, other eye diseases (for example, uveitis), systemic diseases (diabetes mellitus), or congenital defects (either hereditary or as a result of prenatal viral infections such as German measles).

Pathophysiology

The lens of the eye is normally transparent, so that light rays can pass through. Biochemical changes may occur within the lens, or trauma may cause fiber changes that cause the lens to become cloudy and finally opaque, thus blocking the light rays from reaching the retina. A *mature cataract is a developed cataract that separates easily from the lens capsule*. It was previously thought that a cataract had

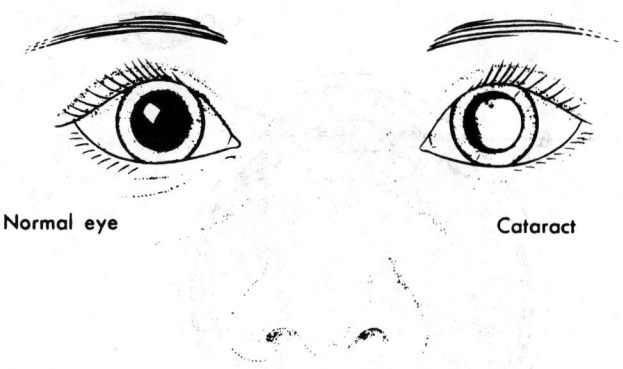

Fig. 38-10   Cataract visible in left eye as white opacity of lens seen through pupil.

to be mature ("ripe") before it could be extracted. Now cataracts are removed whenever the decreased vision interferes with the person's activities of daily living. Cataracts may develop in both eyes, such as with senile cataracts, but usually they do not develop at the same time.

Assessment

Subjective data and *objective data* include the following: Acquired cataracts, either from aging or disease, usually develop gradually. The predominant symptom is progressive loss of vision; the degree of loss depends on the location and extent of the opacity. Persons with an opacity in the center portion of the lens can generally see better in dim light, when the pupil is dilated. The person with presbyopia may find that reading without glasses is possible in the early stages because of resulting myopia. Persons who wear glasses may clean them frequently thinking that dirty glasses are the reason they cannot see as well as usual. In fact, this is a common complaint for which the elderly may seek medical assistance.

If the cataract results from trauma, blurring of vision may be immediate.

Cataract surgery

Surgery is the only method for treating cataracts, although only a small percentage of senile cataracts progress to the point where surgery is required. The decision to remove the cataract depends on the degree of visual impairment, general health, and the use made of the eyes.

Because surgery is usually indicated only for advanced cataracts, elderly persons may believe that they should wait until vision loss is far advanced before consulting an ophthalmologist. Delaying medical examination of the eye can lead to permanent vision loss if there is glaucoma, either alone or in combination with cataracts.

Cataract surgery has changed in recent years as a result of the use of the operating microscope, better instrumentation, improved suture material, and refinement of the intraocular lens.[38] Even patients who are in their nineties can often be operated on with good results. Between 90% and 95% of all cataract operations are successful. Cataracts are usually removed under local anesthesia. The most popular method of cataract removal is the extracapsular cat-

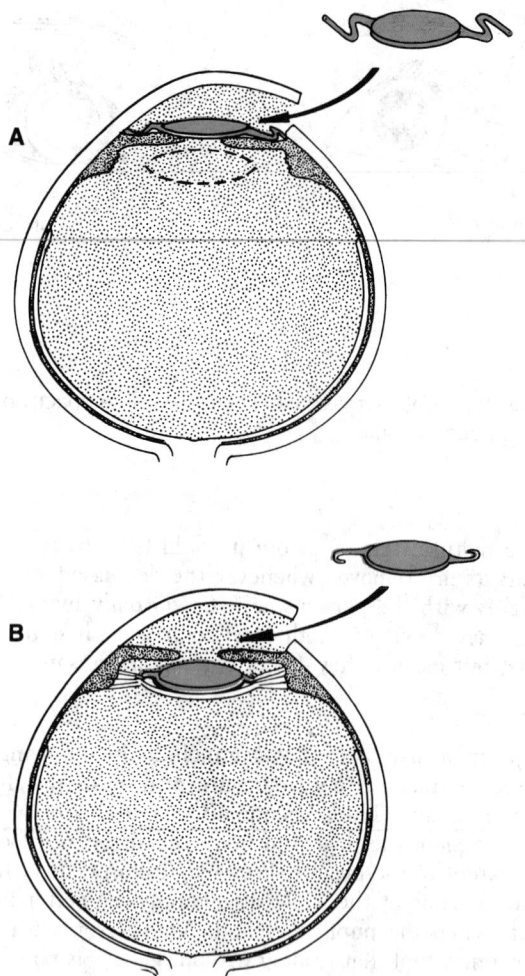

Fig. 38-11 Intraocular lens. **A,** Anterior lens implant in front of iris. **B,** Posterior lens implant behind iris.

aract extraction (ECCE). In this method, only the anterior portion of the lens capsule plus the capsule contents are removed. *Phacoemulsification using ultrasonic vibrations is used to break up the lens, which is then aspirated in small pieces.*

Cataracts can also be removed within their capsule (intracapsular extraction). In this method a freezing *(cryo)* probe that adheres to the surface of lens is used to extract the cataract.

Preoperative care

Preparation of the eye includes instillation of eyedrops, such as a mydriatic/cycloplegic and a local anesthetic (tetracaine, proparacaine) on the day of surgery. A tranquilizer or mild sedative may also be prescribed. If a topical anesthetic is given before surgery, the eye can be protected by an eye pad or glasses.

Intraoperative care

Most eye surgery is now being performed as ambulatory surgery except when complications are present preopera-

tively. Local anesthesia is used for most of the procedure in adults; a general anesthetic (such as thiopentalsodium) may be used briefly for initial eye injections and incision. Because the pupil is widely dilated during surgery, the patient can see only light but not the surgeon's actions. The patient's head is positioned so as to avoid movement during surgery.

Postoperative care

The *goals of postoperative care* are to *prevent* (1) *increased intraocular pressure,* (2) *stress on the suture line,* (3) *hemorrhage into the anterior chamber,* and (4) *infection.* When intraocular pressure (IOP) is increased, pressure is placed on the suture line and bleeding may occur. Anterior flexion of the head not only increases IOP but also may cause anterior synechia (adhesion of the iris to the cornea) because of decreased fluid in the anterior chamber and inflammation from the trauma of surgery. Thus activities that increase IOP, such as straining and leaning over, are contraindicated after surgery because a sudden increase in pressure places stress on the suture line. Protection (eye shield, glasses) of the eye prevents injury. Infection is prevented by the correct use of eye drops and eye pads; topical antibiotics may be given prophylactically.

Specific instructions regarding activities to avoid, eye drops to be instilled, and symptoms to be reported are provided to the patient by the surgeon and nurse. The instructions may include those listed in Box 38-13.

Corrective lenses
Intraocular lens

More than 75% of cataract surgery in the United States now involves intraocular lens implantation at the time of surgery.[38] The intraocular lens provides binocular vision and better optical results than external lenses. It restores vision to near 20/20. There are different styles of lenses but all the lenses consist primarily of two parts: the lens (usually made of polymethylmethacrylate), and the attached flexible loops to hold the lens in position. *The lenses may be implanted in the anterior chamber in front of the iris or in the posterior chamber behind the iris* (Fig. 38-11). *The posterior lens implant, suitable for an extracapsular lens extraction, is used in the majority of patients.*

External lenses

If an intraocular lens is not inserted during surgery, the person must wear an external lens (Table 38-10). Cataract glasses are the least desirable but are used if the person cannot use contact lenses. Loss of depth perception and some peripheral vision make walking difficult. The final pair of glasses is not prescribed until vision has stabilized several months after surgery.

Contact lenses correct some of the problems encountered with cataract glasses but not entirely.[28] The extended-wear soft contact lens (p. 1301) is commonly used. Interruption of the nerve supply to the cornea from surgery usually facilitates the wearing of a contact lens.[28] Persons with rheumatoid arthritis, hemiplegia, parkinsonism, or Alzheimer's disease may have difficulty inserting and maintaining contact lenses.

38-13

Patient Teaching

The patient following eye surgery

1. Sleep on unaffected side for the prescribed time (3 to 4 weeks) to prevent pressure on operated eye.
2. Wash hands before instilling eye drops (p. 1312) or changing eye pad.
3. If an eye pad is required:
   a. Use two oval eye pads, to provide snug, but gentle pressure to prevent blinking against resistance.
   b. Apply tape (paper or silk) diagonally from above nose to lower cheek.
4. Apply metal eye shield at night or when napping to protect eye.
5. Use glasses indoors and sunglasses with side sections outdoors to protect eyes from foreign substances and ultraviolet light until healing occurs.
6. Avoid rubbing or pressing on the eye (creates pressure and may dislodge sutures).
7. Avoid showers and shampooing hair (soap may irritate eye) for specified period as instructed; the time period differs from 1 day to up to 2 weeks.
8. Avoid bending at the waist or lifting heavy objects for at least 1 month to prevent increased IOP or adhesions of the iris.
   a. To pick up objects from floor, kneel while keeping head erect.
   b. To put on stockings or to tie shoes, sit and raise foot to reach hand while keeping head erect.
   c. Long pick-up "reachers" can facilitate picking up small objects from the floor without having to bend over.
9. Avoid straining with bowel movements or with other activities and avoid violent coughing (increases IOP).
10. Limit reading (back and forth movement may loosen stitches); television viewing is usually permitted.
11. Report signs of swelling, discharge, or pain to physician (may indicate infection or hemorrhage).

The Elderly with Eye Problems

Assessment
Assess all older patients for problems with distance and close vision, seeing in dim light, color perception, and glare.
Check on availability and cleanliness of vision aids.

Interventions
Obtain low-vision aids for visually impaired older patients: large-print instructional materials, magnifying glasses, and talking books.
Set up meal tray according to clock face and instruct patient accordingly.
Provide plenty of light during meals, toileting, and ambulation because vision of elderly is decreased in dim light.
Post a sign at bedside of older patient alerting other personnel of patient's visual impairment.
Provide nonambiguous large-type signs at eye level with important instructions and names; for example, TOILET.

Common disorders in elderly
Cataracts
Glaucoma
Diabetic retinopathy

Table 38-10   Corrective lenses after cataract surgery

Type	Advantages	Disadvantages
Lens implant	Cannot be lost or broken Better binocular vision No handling required	Possible complications: vitreous loss, inflammation
Contact lenses	Better visual correction than glasses Better cosmetic appearance Better binocular vision if only one lens removed	Awkward for some elderly persons to manage Easy to lose Difficult adjustment for some persons May cause irritation
Cataract glasses	More acceptable to some elderly persons No physical complications	Magnify objects by 25%; objects appear closer than they actually are Distort peripheral images and colors Heavy lenses May cause visual distortion if poorly positioned

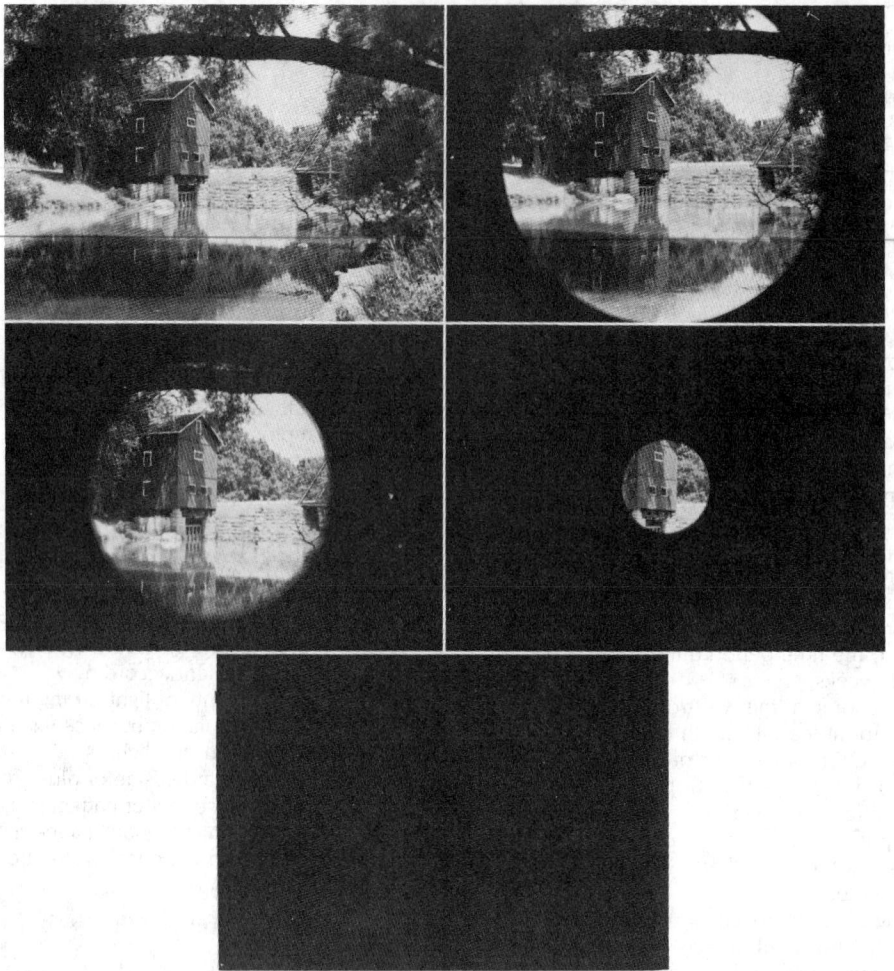

Fig. 38-12 Gradual loss of sight from glaucoma so insidiously destroys vision that person is unaware of impending blindness until extensive and irreversible damage is already present. (From Saunders WH, et al: *Nursing care in eye, ear, nose, and throat disorders,* ed 4, St Louis, 1979, Mosby–Year Book.)

GLAUCOMA

Etiology and Epidemiology

Glaucoma is a group of eye disorders characterized by increased intraocular pressure (IOP) and loss of vision (Fig. 38-12). *It is the second leading cause of irreversible blindness in the United States, affecting nearly 2 million persons.* The incidence of glaucoma is increasing as the number of older persons increases. Less than 1% of persons with glaucoma are under age 70, with the prevalence being 2% to 4% in those over age 75.

Glaucoma may be either primary or secondary to other eye disorders. *Primary glaucoma* has a *genetic predisposition. Primary open-angle glaucoma (the most common form) is six to eight times more common in Blacks than in Whites.* The reason for the increased incidence of glaucoma in Blacks is not known. A recent study suggests that older Black Americans do not receive potentially sight-saving care for open-angle glaucoma at the same rate as older White Americans do.[21] Because early signs may be absent in some forms of glaucoma, *many persons are unaware that they have glaucoma until loss of vision occurs.*

In addition to age and race, other risk factors include diabetes, myopia, and a family history of glaucoma. Early diagnosis and treatment are essential to prevent loss of vision.

Pathophysiology

IOP is maintained by ongoing production and drainage of aqueous humor in the anterior cavity (p. 1299) (Fig. 38-13, A). Glaucoma results when there is interference with the outflow of aqueous humor, leading to a higher-than-normal IOP (normal range is 10 to 22 mm Hg). The pressure may vary as much as 5 mm Hg as a result of diurnal changes. *If the pressure remains elevated, eye damage occurs.* The *optic nerve degenerates* at its origin (has a "cupping" appearance), and the *ganglionic and nerve cells of the retina degenerate. These changes produce loss of vision, first peripheral vision, then eventual blindness if the condition is untreated. The two major types of glaucoma are primary in origin*

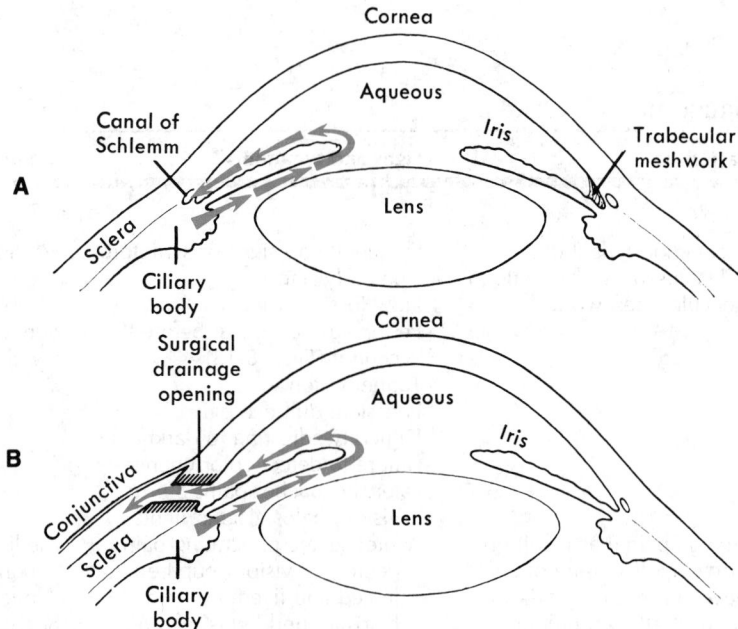

Fig. 38-13 A, Originating from ciliary processes, aqueous flows through pupil into anterior chamber and normally leaves eye by way of canal of Schlemm. **B,** Glaucoma surgery creates new channel through which aqueous can leave eye. (From Havener WH: *Synopsis of ophthalmology*, ed 5, St Louis, 1979, Mosby—Year Book.)

open-angle and angle-closure (closed-angle). Secondary glaucomas may result from eye disorders that block aqueous outflow or increase vitreous pressure (lens changes, uveitis, melanoma of the uveal tract), eye trauma or surgery, or long-term topical steroid therapy.

Open-angle glaucoma

Most glaucomas (90% to 95%) are *primary open-angle glaucomas*. Both eyes are involved. *The onset is insidious and the disorder is slowly progressive. It is termed open-angle because the aqueous humor has open access to the trabecular meshwork.* However, drainage is impeded by degenerative changes in the trabecular meshwork, canal of Schlemm, and adjacent canals.[38] Degenerative changes in the optic nerve may also occur. Early signs are usually absent, but the disorder can be diagnosed by the increased IOP and the normal anterior chamber angle. The pressure may eventually lead to dull eye pain (Table 38-11).

Angle-closure (closed-angle) glaucoma

Closed-angle glaucoma usually occurs as an acute episode, although it may be subacute or chronic. It is termed angle-closure because the anterior chamber is anatomically narrow allowing the iris to be pushed forward, adhering to the trabecular meshwork and impeding aqueous humor flow to the canal of Schlemm. The forward movement of the iris may result from increased vitreous pressure, buildup of fluid in the posterior chamber, or thickening of the lens with age. Intraocular pressure is normal when the angle is narrow but open and the drainage is not blocked. Symptoms result from sudden closure, with an increase in IOP, and include severe eye pain, blurred vision, and halos seen around lights. The adhered iris produces a dilated pupil. If untreated, a blind painful eye results.

Nursing Process
Assessment
Subjective data

Subjective data include the following:
1. Assess discomfort
   a. Eye pain: dull, severe
   b. Headache: severity
   c. Nausea and vomiting
2. Assess report of halos around lights

Objective data

Objective data include the following:
1. Vision: note changes
   a. Visual acuity: Snellen chart if available, reading distant signs, close reading
   b. Visual fields: confrontation test (p. 1300)

Diagnostic tests

Intraocular pressure is measured by means of *tonometry*. In an ophthalmologist's office, an applanation tonometer is generally used. With the use of a slit lamp, a small area of the cornea is flattened to counterbalance a spring-loaded measuring device that measures the pressure (Fig. 38-14). A less accurate direct method, but useful because the instrument is cheaper and portable, is the Schiøtz tonometer. The eye is anesthetized and the tonometer is placed directly on the cornea (Fig. 38-15). The amount of indentation

Table 38-11   Types of glaucoma

Type	Characteristic	Signs and symptoms	Medical therapy
Primary			
Open-angle (chronic, simple)	Most common type (90%) Usually caused by obstruction in trabecular meshwork	Frequently no signs or symptoms in early stages Slow loss of vision Peripheral vision lost before central (Fig. 38-13) Tunnel vision Persistent dull eye pain Difficulty adjusting to darkness Failure to detect color changes Later: headache, pain, blurred vision, halos around lights	Medical: miotics, beta-blockers, carbonic anhydrase inhibitors Surgical: trabeculectomy, trabeculoplasty
Angle-closure (narrow-angle, acute)	Outflow impaired as result of narrowing or closing of angle between iris and cornea Intermittent attacks, pressure normal when angle open; if persistent, acute ocular emergency	Acute: severe prostrating pain, decreased vision, pupil enlarged and fixed, colored halos around lights, eye red, steamy cornea Permanent blindness if marked increase in IOP for 24-48 hours	Medical: osmotic diuretics, carbonic anhydrase inhibitors, miotics Surgical: peripheral iridectomy, iridotomy
Congenital	Abnormal development of filtration angle Can occur secondary to other systemic eye disorders Rare (0.05%)	Enlargement of eye, lacrimation, photophobia, blepharospasm	Goniotomy (incision into region of trabecular meshwork) Trabeculotomy
Secondary	Can result from ocular inflammation, blood vessel changes, trauma	May be similar to open-angle and angle-closure, depending on cause	Directed at cause as well as at decreasing IOP

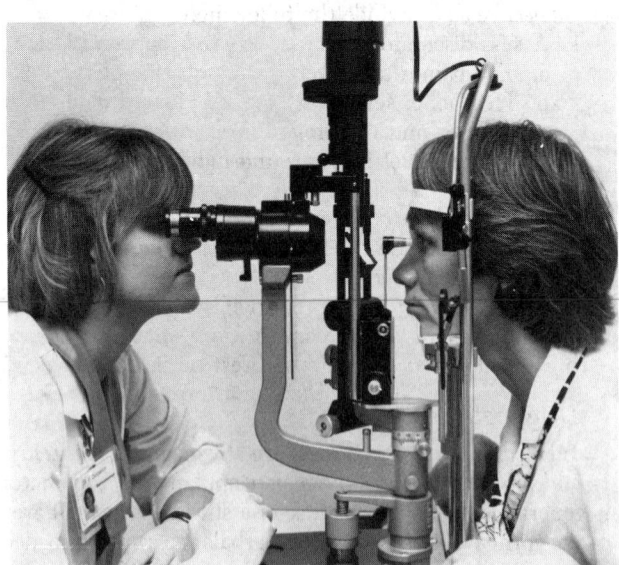

Fig. 38-14   Measurement of intraocular pressure with applanation tonometer.

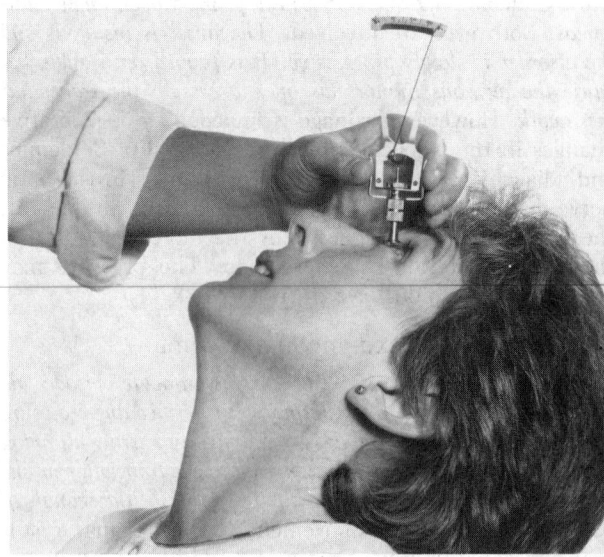

Fig. 38-15   Measurement of intraocular pressure with Schiø tonometer.

that the instrument plunger makes on the cornea is measured on the attached scale. Noncontact tonometers measure IOP by deformation of light reflex from the cornea from a puff of air.[28] Readings greater than 24 mm Hg may suggest glaucoma.

Because of concern that some cases of glaucoma were not diagnosed by measurement of IOP alone, the *National Eye Institute made the following recommendation in December 1991: Eye examinations of the elderly should include dilation of the pupil and examination of the optic nerve. This recommendation was made because some elderly persons with IOPs within normal limits demonstrated changes in the optic nerve that were indicative of glaucoma on further examination.*

The anterior chamber angle can be visualized using a contact lens and special lens *(gonioscopy)*. This technique distinguishes open-angle from closed-angle glaucoma. Visualization of the optic disk by ophthalmoscopy will show cupping of the disk; visual field testing may show decreased peripheral vision.

Data analysis: nursing diagnoses

Nursing diagnoses are determined from analysis of patient data. Possible nursing diagnoses for the person with glaucoma may include, but are not limited to, the following:

Diagnostic title	Possible etiologies
Health maintenance, altered	Impairment in vision, difficulty in doing ADL independently
Knowledge deficit about glaucoma	Unfamiliarity with information resources
Pain	Increased IOP
Sensory/perceptual alteration: visual	Altered sensory reception/transmission

Planning: expected patient outcomes

Expected patient outcomes for the person with glaucoma may include, but are not limited to, the following:

1. Vision is not decreased further.
2. Patient is able to perform ADL more independently.
3. Patient can state recognition of lifetime need for eye medication.
4. Patient can state name, dosage, frequency, and side effects of prescribed eye medications.
5. Patient can describe measures to prevent complications.
6. Patient can list signs or symptoms indicating need to report immediately to ophthalmologist.
7. Patient states discomfort is decreased.
8. Patient can walk independently.

Implementation

Assisting with achievement of therapeutic goals
Medications

It is vital in the control of glaucoma that eye medications be given as prescribed. Drugs used in treatment of glaucoma are listed in Table 38-12. The purpose of pharmacologic therapy is to keep the pupil constricted to permit better drainage of the aqueous humor and to decrease the amount of aqueous humor produced.

Pilocarpine is the miotic drug of choice in the treatment of open-angle glaucoma. Pilocarpine may be given in solution (eye drops) or by membrane-controlled delivery system (Ocusert). The Ocusert is placed in the upper or lower conjunctival sac, preferably at night so the miotic effect reaches a stable level by morning; the effect lasts for 1 week. A pilocarpine gel, Piloplex, decreases the need for the more frequent insertion of pilocarpine eye drops. Miotics frequently decrease vision for 1 to 2 hours after instillation and may cause eye spasms in younger persons.

Beta-adrenergic blocking agents can be used alone or in combination with other drugs. A newer drug, Betaxolol, has an added advantage of decreased pulmonary side effects. Pressing the lacrimal duct for 1 minute after insertion of eye drops helps to prevent rapid systemic side effects.

In severe acute conditions, osmotic agents are given to lower the IOP by drawing fluid from the eye. If the oral osmotic agent is ineffective or produces nausea, mannitol is given intravenously.

Mydriatics and cycloplegic agents are *contraindicated* in persons with glaucoma because these drugs may further restrict drainage of aqueous humor.

Surgery

Surgical intervention is indicated when conservative treatment fails to control the IOP. Two common procedures are trabeculoplasty and trabeculectomy. *Trabeculoplasty is the application of a laser beam (argon) on the trabecular meshwork. This produces a nonpenetrating thermal burn that changes the configuration of the meshwork and leads to increased outflow of aqueous humor. Trabeculectomy is a filtering procedure in which an opening or fistula is made at the limbus under a partial-thickness scleral flap* (Fig. 38-13, *B*). The new opening circumvents the obstruction and aqueous humor flows into the subconjunctival spaces.

Trabeculectomy usually requires overnight hospitalization. *Trabeculoplasty*, however, is frequently performed on an ambulatory basis, and the person usually remains for 3 to 4 hours following the procedure so that the IOP can be checked. A complication of the procedure is a sudden rise in the IOP immediately after surgery. It takes 4 to 8 weeks to see if the procedure is effective. However, glaucoma medications usually must be continued.

Postoperative care

Nursing care for the patient following *trabeculectomy* includes:

1. Routine postanesthesia care
2. Protection of operative eye with patch, shield, positioning patient on back or unoperative side, and safety measures such as side rails
3. Maintaining comfort in the operative eye
4. Assessment, as appropriate, of the IOP, appearance of the bleb, and anterior chamber depth
5. Administration of medications such as a cycloplegic, a mydriatic, and a combination antibiotic and steroid

Interventions to achieve patient outcomes
Monitoring health maintenance

As the patient adjusts to visual changes, he or she may need assistance with activities of daily living. The patient will also need to learn how to modify his or her daily activities so that they can be performed safely and independently.

Table 38-12   Drugs used in treatment of glaucoma

Drug*	Effect with glaucoma
Cholinergic agents (miotics)	
Pilocarpine	Stimulates cholinergic receptors; contracts iris muscle constricting pupil and
Carbachol (Carbacel)	decreasing resistance to aqueous humor outflow; also constricts ciliary muscle to increase accommodation
Cholinesterase inhibitors (miotics)	
Physostigmine (Eserine)	Inhibits destruction of acetylcholine, producing same effects as cholinergic
Isoflurophate (Floropryl)	drugs. DO NOT USE CHOLINESTERASE DRUGS WITH ANGLE-
Demecarium bromide (Humorsol)	CLOSURE GLAUCOMA (increases pupillary block)
Echothiophate iodide (Phospholine iodide)	
Adrenergic agents	
Epinephryl borate (Eppy)	Decreases production of aqueous humor and increases aqueous outflow.
Epinephrine hydrochloride (Glaucon, Epifrin)	DO NOT USE WITH ANGLE-CLOSURE GLAUCOMA
Epinephrine bitartrate (Epitrate, Murocoll)	
Dipivefrin (Propine)	
Beta-adrenergic blockers	
Timolol maleate (Timoptic)	Blocks the adrenergic (sympathetic) impulses, which normally produces my-
Betaxolol hydrochloride (Betoptic)	driasis; mechanism by which the IOP is decreased is unclear
Levobunolol hydrochloride (Betagan)	
Carbonic anhydrase inhibitors	
Acetazolamide (Diamox)	Slows production of aqueous humor
Ethoxzolamide (Cardrase)	
Dichlorhenamide (Daranide)	
Methazolamide (Neptazane)	
Osmotic agents	
Glycerine (Glycerol, Osmoglyn)	Increases blood plasma osmolarity, enhancing fluid flow from aqueous hu-
Mannitol (Osmitrol)	mor into the plasma

*NOTE: The miotics, beta blockers, and adrenergic agents are given by eye drops; carbonic anhydrase inhibitors and osmotic agents are given orally or intravenously (as appropriate).

Assisting with comfort

Pain usually decreases as the IOP decreases. Analgesics may be prescribed. Cold eye compresses may be helpful for painful eye spasms.

Facilitating learning

Glaucoma is a chronic condition, and the patient with newly diagnosed glaucoma needs assistance in understanding and learning to live with the disease. Despite explanations from the physician, the person frequently hopes that an operation will provide a cure, that no further treatment will be necessary, and perhaps that the lost sight will be restored. *It should be explained that lost vision cannot be restored but that further loss can usually be prevented and normal activities can be pursued if the person continues medical care.* There usually is no restriction on the use of the eyes (see Box 38-14 for teaching guidelines).

Evaluation

Evaluation is based on the expected patient outcomes. Questions to ask include the following:
1. Can the patient perform ADL independently?
2. Does the patient know the chronic nature of the disease and treatment?
3. Does the patient understand the need for lifetime eye medication?
4. Can the patient state name, dosage and so on of prescribed medications?
5. Can the patient describe how to avoid complications?
6. Can the patient state signs and symptoms that need to be reported to the ophthamologist?
7. Is the patient comfortable?
8. Can the patient walk independently?

RETINAL DETACHMENT

Etiology and Pathophysiology

The retina is the part of the eye that perceives light; it coordinates and transmits impulses from receptor nerve cells to the optic nerve. It consists of two layers. Retinal detachment occurs when the two retinal layers separate as a result of accumulation of fluid or traction produced by contraction of the vitreous body (Fig. 38-16). As the detachment extends and becomes complete, blindness results. Myopic degeneration, trauma, and aphakia (absence

Nursing Care Plan	**Person with open-angle glaucoma**	

DATA: Mr. M. is a 76-year-old man with a history of open-angle glaucoma. His peripheral vision is markedly decreased. He was admitted for prostate surgery, but his primary nurse elicited the following information during the admission history: he has prescribed eye drops (pilocarpine 1% qid, timolol 0.5% bid) that he uses periodically. He states the drops blur his vision. He knows that his "eye pressure is high" but says he thinks it's getting better because his eyes don't bother him. His wife notes that he bumps into objects more frequently.

Nursing diagnosis: Knowledge deficit: related to lack of recall and misinterpretation of information

Expected patient outcomes	Nursing interventions	Rationale
Mr. M. describes chronicity of glaucoma and need for continued treatment	Ask Mr. M. to explain understanding of glaucoma: What it is Result if untreated Symptoms to be reported Need for medical follow-up	Start teaching at Mr. M.'s level of knowledge. Because glaucoma is a chronic condition, he needs to know the effects of nontreatment (painful blind eye) and how to prevent it
Mr. M. states symptoms requiring reporting to physician	Teach him about glaucoma and need for lifetime eye medication	
Mr. M. or wife demonstrates correct instillation of eye drops	Ask him or wife to demonstrate instilling eye drops; correct his technique as necessary	If his vision is decreasing, he may be having difficulty instilling his eye drops and wife will do it for him

Nursing diagnosis: Noncompliance with medications: related to drug side effects and lack of knowledge about need for lifetime medication

Expected patient outcomes	Nursing interventions	Rationale
Mr. M. states plans to use eye drops at correct times	Explore other reasons for not using eye drops	Mr. M. may have difficulty reading the labels or remembering
	Ask Mr. M.'s wife to bring in the eye drop vials and role play with him use of vials and how to remember to use the eye drops	Role playing will help to identify problems he may be having reading the labels
	Enlist him and his wife in developing a plan to help remember how and when to take the eye drops (such as after meals and at bedtime)	Mrs. M. participation in planning ensures greater probability of carrying out plan; connecting of carrying out plan; connecting the eyedrops with an activity helps the person remember
	Explain relationship of blurred vision with pilocarpine; suggest he consult physician and not plan specific activities for about 1 hr after instilling eye drops	Blurred vision is a side effect of pilocarpine; it usually improves in 1 to 2 hrs

Nursing diagnosis: Injury, high risk for: related to decreased peripheral vision

Expected patient outcomes	Nursing interventions	Rationale
Mr. M. describes measures to prevent injury	Explain nature of decreased peripheral vision and relate it to bumping into objects	Knowledge of rationale may increased probability of actions to prevent injury
	Suggest Mr. M. turn head to see each side	Increases field of vision
	Suggest couple consider clearing wider walk areas in living quarters	Reducing clutter will decrease chance of falls, and injury caused by bumping into things
	Suggest that Mr. M. consider not driving	Loss of peripheral vision makes Mr. M. less aware of cars approaching from side.

The patient with glaucoma

1. Medical follow-up and eye medication will be required for the rest of life.
2. Eye drops *must* be continued as long as prescribed, even in the absence of symptoms
   a. Blurred vision decreases with prolonged use
   b. Avoid driving for 1 to 2 hours after administration of miotics.
3. To prevent complications:
   a. Press lacrimal duct for 1 minute after eye drop insertion to prevent rapid systemic absorption
   b. Have reserve bottle of eye drops at home
   c. Carry eye drops on person (not in luggage) when travelling
   d. Carry card or wear Medic-Alert bracelet identifying glaucoma and the eye drops solution prescribed.
4. Bright lights and darkness are not harmful.
5. There is no apparent relationship between vascular hypertension and ocular hypertension.
6. Report any reappearnce of symptoms immediately to ophthalmologist.
7. If admitted to hospital for a different medical condition, alert the staff of continued need for prescribed eye drops.
8. Avoid the use of mydriatic or cycloplegic drugs (for example, atropine) that dilate the pupils.

of the crystalline lens) are the most frequent causes of retinal detachment. Detachment may follow sudden severe physical exertion, especially in persons who are debilitated. Most often, however, there is no apparent cause. Retinal detachment may occur suddenly or develop slowly.

Nursing Process
Assessment

Subjective and *objective* data include the following: The person first notices flashes of light, followed by floating spots before the eye and progressive loss of vision. The floating spots are blood and retinal cells that are freed at the time of the tear and cast shadows on the retina as they seem to drift about the eye. The area of visual loss depends entirely on the location of the detachment. Usually there is a superior retinal detachment and inferior visual loss. When the detachment is extensive and occurs quickly, the patient may have the sensation that a curtain has been drawn before the eyes. The diagnosis is confirmed by ophthalmoscopic appearance of the retina.

Ongoing nursing assessment includes the patient's subjective statements concerning changes in vision and observations related to signs of anxiety. The person with both eyes patched is assessed for ability to carry out activities of daily living.

Data analysis: nursing diagnoses

Nursing diagnoses are determined from analysis of patient data. Possible nursing diagnoses for the person with retinal detachment may include, but are not limited to, the following:

Diagnostic title	Possible etiologies
Anxiety	Threat of loss of vision, threat to self-concept, threat of change in role functioning
Injury, high risk for	Sensory deficit, lack of awareness of environmental hazards
Knowledge deficit regarding condition, surgery, preoperative and postoperative care, and self care at home	Lack of experience with retinal detachment and its treatment
Pain	Inflammation, increased IOP
Sensory/perceptual alteration, visual	Altered sensory reception/transmission

Planning: expected patient outcomes

Expected patient outcomes for the person with retinal detachment may include, but are not limited to, the following:

1. Anxiety is decreased.
2. No further vision loss occurs.
3. No injuries occur.
4. Patient can describe
   a. Correct use of eye medications
   b. Signs and symptoms indicating further retinal detachment and for immediate medical care
   c. Plans for dealing with limitation of activity.
5. Patient states pain is absent or improved.
6. Patient adjusts to alteration in vision by walking independently.

Implementation preoperatively
Assisting with achievement of therapeutic goals
Promoting eye rest

Immediate care for the person with detachment of the retina includes keeping the eye at rest and in position to prevent further detachment until surgery can be performed to repair the detachment. Bed rest with monocular or bilateral eye patches is usually prescribed. The head is positioned so the retinal hole is in the most dependent position (gravity may help prevent the first retinal layer from pulling further away from the second coat).

Although most surgeons do not use binocular patches, some do patch both eyes preoperatively and for 2 or 3 days postoperatively. Safety precautions, such as side rails, are essential if binocular patching is used. Call signals are placed within easy patient reach. Activities that facilitate communication with blind persons are employed.

Providing emotional support

Anxiety frequently results from concern over possible loss of vision and feelings about having eyes bandaged. Generally, the person has lost vision rapidly and is afraid of losing more vision. Patients need an opportunity to discuss their concerns. Although the promise of restoration of vision cannot be made, it can be comforting to the person to know that with care most retinal detachments can be repaired by surgery.

Retinal surgery

Intraoperative care. Surgery may be performed under either local or general anesthesia. Cyclopentolate or phenylephrine is used to keep the pupils widely dilated so that tears in the retina may be identified during the operation. The surgical procedure may include draining the fluid from the subretinal space so that the retina returns to its normal position, thereby closing the opening in the retina. To drain the fluid from the subretinal space, the sclera and choroid are perforated at the time of the operation.

The retinal breaks are sealed off by various methods that produce an inflammatory reaction *(chorioretinitis)* in the area of the tear so that adhesions will form between the edges of the break and the underlying choroid to obliterate the opening (see Table 38-13). When the retinal tears are small or of recent origin, diathermy may be applied through the sclera with needlepoint electrodes to produce the inflammatory process. An intense beam of visible light directed to the area by means of an elaborate ophthalmoscope may be used to close a retinal tear when the retina is not elevated *(photocoagulation)*. The *laser beam* is used by some surgeons as a source of intense energy to produce chorioretinitis. Subfreezing temperatures ($-40°$ to $-60°$ C) may be applied to the surface of the sclera in the area

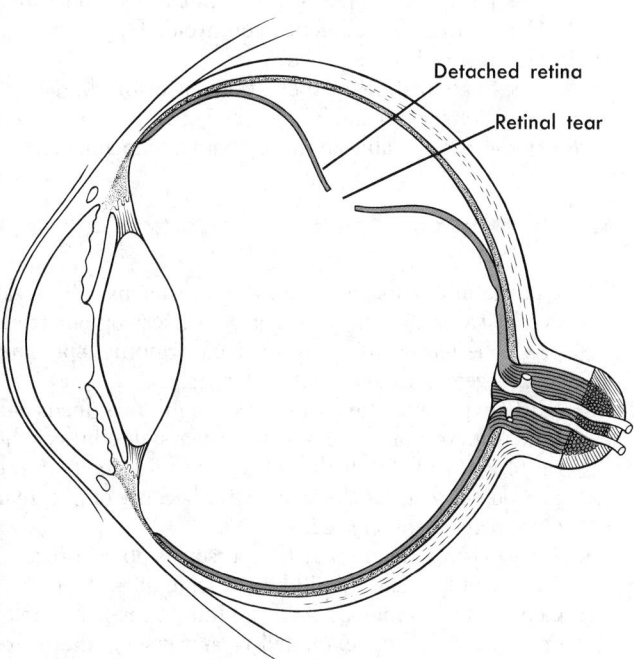

Fig. 38-16   Retinal detachment.

Detached retina

Retinal tear

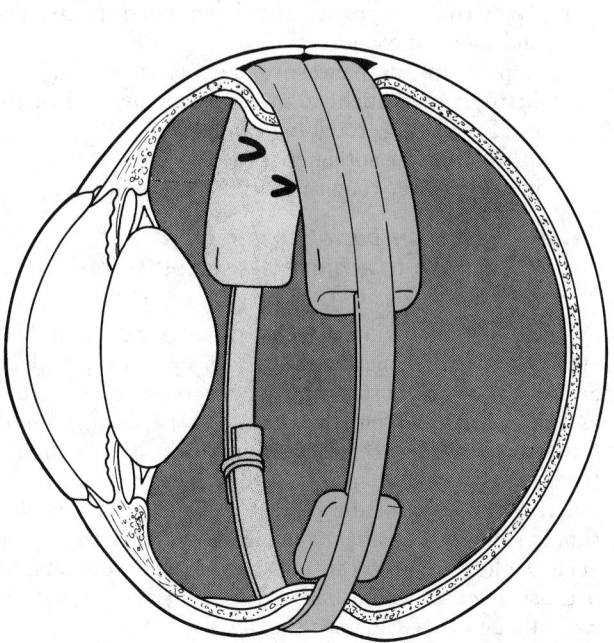

Fig. 38-17   Scleral buckle.

Table 38-13   **Surgical procedures for retinal detachment**

Purpose	Procedure	Method
Removal of fluid from sub-retinal space	Drainage	Needle insertion
Sealing of retinal tear by creating inflammation to adhere retina to choroid	Cryosurgery	Supercooled probe applied to scleral surface over tear
	Diathermy	Application of diathermy (heat) to scleral surface over tear
	Photocoagulation	Strong light focused through pupil onto retinal tear
	Laser	Laser beam focused through pupil onto retinal tear
Splinting of choroid to retina until choroidal scar can seal tear	Scleral buckling	Tuck taken in sclera (to indent sclera and choroid) and sutured; buckle held in place with a piece of silicone held by a strap (Fig. 38-17)

of the hole to produce the inflammatory reaction (cryotherapy). Nitrous oxide or carbon dioxide under pressure, flowing through a tube attached to a delicate instrument, is used to produce these low temperatures.

For most retinal detachments, *scleral buckling* procedures are used. In this procedure, the sclera and choroid are indented (buckled) toward the retinal break. Buckling is accomplished by placing silicone of various shapes and sizes in the region of the break (Fig. 38-17). In addition an encircling tape of silicone can be placed around the entire eye. By these procedures, the choroid is pushed into contact with the retinal tear during healing, and vitreous adhesions that have exerted traction, or pull, on the retinal break are relaxed as the size of the scleral shell is decreased.

Postoperative care. The postoperative care for the person with retinal detachment includes the following:
1. Position and ambulate the patient as ordered.
2. Assist with activities of daily living, as required.
3. Administer eye medications as ordered (mydriatics, cycloplegics, and combination steroid/antibiotic).
4. Apply cold compresses as ordered to reduce swelling and promote comfort.
5. Implement safety measures such as side rails.
6. Instruct the patient to avoid jerking motions of the head (sneezing, coughing, vomiting).
   a. Administer antiemetics, as required.
   b. Administer cough medication, as required.

Implementation postoperatively
Interventions to achieve patient outcomes
Promoting safety

As mentioned earlier, most surgeons do not patch both eyes (binocular) some do patch both eyes preoperatively and for 2 or 3 days postoperatively. Safety precautions such as side rails are essential if binocular patching is used. Call signals need to be kept within reach. Explanation of the immediate environment is also indicated. Everyone entering the room of the patient with both eyes patched should call out the patient's name to announce their presence. Failure to do so can make the patient very anxious because he or she can usually sense that someone is in the room though they can't see them.

Facilitating coping

Patients are usually anxious and apprehensive when admitted to the hospital. Generally there has been a rapid loss of vision, and patients fear losing more vision. Restoration of sight will depend on the extent and duration of the detachment and the success of the surgery. Opportunity to discuss concerns needs to be provided. The nurse caring for the patient should schedule time to sit down and listen to the patient's concerns. Nurses can do much to allay apprehension by answering questions honestly and instilling realistic hope.

Facilitating learning

Patient teaching for persons with retinal detachment includes:
1. Report to ophthalmologist any signs of redetachment (increase in floaters, flashes of light, decreased vision).
2. Use appropriate techniques for administration of eye medications.
3. Limit activities to sedentary work for 1 to 2 weeks.
4. Check with physician about resumption of activities such as active sports or heavy lifting.
5. Discuss plan for medical follow-up (appointment with ophthalmologist and so on).

Evaluation

Evaluation is based on expected patient outcomes. Questions to consider may include the following:
1. Has patient had opportunities to express concerns?
2. Has further detachment been avoided?
3. Has injury been avoided?
4. Does patient know expectations after discharge?
5. Is patient comfortable?
6. Is the patient able to move about independently?

SUMMARY

1. Ophthalmologists (oculists) are physicians who treat eye diseases and may prescribe lenses; optometrists prescribe lenses and provide visual training; opticians make eyeglasses and contact lenses.
2. With hyperopia (farsightedness) light rays focus behind the retina; with myopia (nearsightedness) the rays focus in front of the retina; with astigmatism the rays do not focus at the same point because of irregular curvature of the cornea.
3. 20/40 vision means that the person is able to read at 20 feet only what should be readable at 40 feet.
4. Contact lenses may be rigid (including gas-permeable) or soft (including extended-wear lenses); there are advantages and disadvantages of each type.
5. Eye safety measures include early medical care of eye problems, avoidance of use of previously prescribed eye medications, protecting eyes against foreign objects or bright lights, and removing nonembedded foreign objects immediately by rinsing with water or by carefully removing from the conjunctival sac.
6. Activities for the newly blind person consist of facilitating their independence in ADL and providing counseling to facilitate coping.
7. Inflammation of the eye can occur in the external structures, cornea, and uvea (iris, ciliary body, and choroid); the most common inflammations are styes and conjunctivitis.
8. Treatments for eye inflammations include eye compresses, eye irrigations, and ophthalmic antibiotics (steroids may be given for allergic but not pyogenic inflammations).
9. If the cornea becomes damaged, corneal grafts (keratoplasty) may be performed using donor corneal tissue.
10. A cataract is an opacity of the lens. A cataract that interferes with vision may be removed either extracapsularly (leaving the posterior capsule intact) or intracapsularly (lens and entire capsule). Most persons

now have an intraocular lens implanted at the time of surgery.

11. Most eye surgery is performed as ambulatory surgery. Preoperative care includes insertion of mydriatic or cycloplegic (dilates pupil and relaxes ciliary muscle) and local anesthetic eye drops.

12. Postoperative care centers on preventing increased IOP, stress on the suture line, hemorrhage into the anterior chamber, and infection.

13. The characteristic sign of glaucoma is increased IOP. Most glaucomas are of the primary open-angle type in which aqueous outflow is blocked because of degenerative changes in the trabecular meshwork, canal of Schlemm, and adjacent channels; the disorder is insidious in onset, slowly progressive, and usually lacks symptoms in the early stage.

14. Closed-angle glaucoma occurs in a person with a narrow anterior chamber when the iris falls forward, blocking entrance to aqueous fluid outflow; it is often sudden in onset and requires immediate medical attention; symptoms include severe eye pain, blurred vision, and halos seen around lights.

15. Conservative treatment for glaucoma includes medications to decrease the IOP (miotics and beta-blockers that constrict the pupil, adrenergic agents and carbonic anhydrase inhibitors that decrease production of aqueous humor, and osmotic agents that enhance fluid flow out of the eye). Surgery consists of opening up the trabecular meshwork, opening a channel between the anterior and posterior chambers, or opening a channel between the anterior chamber and subconjunctival space.

16. Persons with glaucoma require continued treatment for life to prevent buildup of IOP; lost vision cannot be restored.

17. Retinal detachment results when the two retinal layers separate, interfering with vision; symptoms include flashes of light, floating spots before the eye, and progressive loss of vision. Persons with retinal detachment require immediate medical treatment.

18. Surgery is performed to return the retina to its original position and adhere the first layer to the bottom layer by means of an inflammatory process. Postoperative care includes avoiding jerking movements of the head and limiting exertional activities until healing has occurred; eye drops are required during this period to rest the eye and prevent infection.

STUDY QUESTIONS

• Examine the chart of a patient with an eye problem. Explain the rationale for the drug therapy.

• Write a care plan for a patient with limited vision. How would a care plan for a person who has recent loss of vision compare with that of a person blinded from childhood?

• Consider bandaging your eyes for one day and carry out all your usual activities. What problems did you encounter? What did you find helpful?

• Describe how you would respond to a person who says, "I don't see as well as I used to. I don't have to go to an eye doctor; he'll only tell me I need glasses, and I already have a pair."

• What services and facilities are available to persons in your community who have limited vision? How are these financed?

• Pretend for 2 days that you have had eye surgery and are instructed not to bend at the waist or lift any heavy objects or to strain with any activity. What problems did you encounter? Now consider that your knees are crippled with arthritis: how would that affect an activity such as putting on pantyhose, given the same restrictions?

REFERENCES AND SELECTED READINGS

1. American Foundation for the Blind: *directory of services for the blind and visually impaired in the US,* ed 23, New York, 1988, The Foundation.

2. Arentsen JJ: The dry eye, *J Ophthal Nurs Technol* 6:134-137, 1987.

3. Bentz LN: Caring for and communicating with blind and visually impaired persons, *J Visual Impair Blindness* 81:472-481, 1987.

4. Binder PS: Ophthalmology, *JAMA* 265(23):3143-3144, 1991.

5. Bishop VE: Visually handicapped people and the law, *J Visual Impair Blindness* 81:53-58, 1987.

6. Bocking H et al: Artificial eyes, *Nurs Times* 86(8):40-41, 1990.

7.* Boruchoff SA: Ophthalmic surgery: risks and benefits, *Emerg Med* 19(11):59-62, 1987.

8.* Boyd-Monk H: Eye trauma in the workplace, *AAOHNJ* 38(10):487-491, 1990.

9. Boyd-Monk H, Steinmetz CG: *Nursing care of the eye,* Norwalk, Conn, 1987, Appleton & Lange.

10.* Boyd-Monk H, Starita RJ: Surgical intervention to stop glaucoma, *JONT,* 4(3):12-15, 1985.

11. Capeno D et al: The elderly patient with cataracts, *Hosp Pract* 22(3):19-24, 1987.

12.* Carver JA: Cataract care made plain, *Am J Nurs* 87:626-630, 1987.

13. Contact lens allergy: the new conjunctivitis, *Am J Nurs* 87:11-12, 1987.

14. Danyluk AW, Paton D: Diagnosis and management of glaucoma, *Clin Symp* 43(4):2-32, 1991.

15.* DeBlase R et al: Postintraocular lens implants, *Geriatr Nurs* 9(6):342-343, 1988.

16.* Ehrenberg M: Blindness prevention, *AAOHN J* 35-243-245, 1987.

17. Frank A, Werfel N: ECCE with pharmacoemulsion, *J Ophthalmic Nurs Technol* 5:103-105, 1986.

18. Gottsch JD et al: Cataracts: diagnosis and treatment, *Hosp Med* (suppl) 23(4):21-29, 1987.

19. Hamrick S et al: Therapeutic ultrasound, *AAORN J* 47:950-960, 1988.

20. Healthy People 2000 National Health Promotion and Disease Prevention Objectives, U.S. Department of Health and Human Services, Public Health Service, Washington D.C., 1990.

21. Javitt JC et al: Undertreatment of glaucoma among black Americans, *N Engl J Med* 325(20);1418-1422, 1991.

22. Karb VK, Queener SF, Freeman JB: *Handbook of drugs for nursing practice,* St Louis, 1989, Mosby–Year Book.

23. Lawlor MC: Common ocular injuries and disorders, *J Emerg Nurs* 15(1):36-43, 1989.

*Suggested for student reading.

24.* Lent-Wunderlich E et al: Helping your patient through eye surgery, *RN* 49(6):43-47, 1986.

25. Lindstrom RL: Advances in corneal transplantation, *N Engl J Med* 315(1):57-59, 1986.

26. Mason G et al: Postanesthesia care of the ophthalmic patient, *J Post Anesth Nurs* 1:23-25, 1986.

27.* Misuse of steroid eye medications, Nurses' Drug Alert, *Am J Nurs* 87:71-1987.

28. Newell F: *Ophthalmology: principals and practice,* ed 7, St. Louis, 1992, Mosby–Year Book.

29. Nowell P: Lasers in ophthalmology, *Nurs Clin J North Am* 25(3):635-643, 1990.

30. Pasby T: Eye injuries in sports, *J Ophthalmic Nurs Technol* 8:99-101, 1989.

31. Seddon JM: The differential burden of blindness in the United States, *N Engl J Med* 325(20):1440-1442, 1991.

32. Shingleton JF: Eye injuries, *N Engl J Med* 325(6):408-413, 1991.

33.* Smith S: Day-care cataract surgery: the patient's perspective, *J Ophthalmic Nurs Technol* 6(2):50-56, 1987.

34. Soll DB et al: Drugs and glaucoma, *Am Fam Physician* 34(1):181-185, 1986.

35. Spencer RE: Transitions, being blind in a sighted world, *J Ophthalmic Nurs Technol* 7:220-222, 1988.

36. Traynar M: Day care eye surgery, *Nurs Time* 86(39):54-56, 1990.

37.* Tooke MC, Elders J, Johnson DE: Corneal transplantation, *Am J Nurs* 86:685-687, 1986.

38. Vaughan D, Asbury T: *General ophthalmology,* ed 11, Los Altos, Calif, 1986, Lange Medical Publications.

39.* West K: ABCs of cataract surgery preparation: assessment, briefing, and counseling, *J Ophthalmic Nurs Technol* 6:156-158, 1987.

40. York S, Proud G: Ophthalmic triage, *Nurs Time* 86(8):40-42, 1990.

CLASSIC

41. Boyd-Monk H: Examining the external eye: I, *Nurs 80* 10(5)58-63, 1980.

42. Boyd-Monk H: Examining the external eye, II, *Nurs 80* 10(6):58-63, 1980.

43.* Boyd-Monk H: Retinal detachment and vitrectomy: nursing care, *Nurs Clin North Am* 16:433-451, 1981.

44.* Gallagher MA: Corneal transplantation, *Am J Nurs* 81:1845, 1981.

45.* Osguthrope NC: If your patient has contact lenses, *Am J Nurs* 84:1255-1256, 1984.

46.* Sullivan N: Vision in the elderly, *J Gerontol Nurs* 9:228-235, 1983.

47.* Todd B: Using eye drops and ointments safely, *Geriatr Nurs* 4:53, 56-57, 1983.

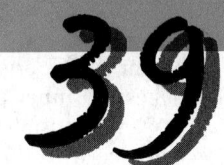

The Patient

with

Ear Problems

Wilma J. Phipps

After studying this chapter, the learner should be able to:

- Describe the mechanics of sound waves and hearing.
- Describe measures to prevent hearing loss.
- Describe the pathophysiology and nursing requirements for persons with ear infections.
- Describe the pathophysiology and care of the person with a balance disorder.
- Describe care of the person having ear surgery.
- Differentiate between conductive and sensorineural hearing loss.
- Describe methods of assessment for conductive and sensorineural hearing loss.
- Describe methods of aural rehabilitation and communication with hearing impaired persons.

The ear is the organ of hearing and equilibrium. Sound reaches the inner ear where it is converted to neural activity and transmitted to the brain for interpretation. Interference with this process leads to impaired hearing. In addition, structures in the inner ear maintain an individual's sense of equilibrium; interference with this mechanism leads to vertigo, producing dizziness and loss of balance.

The root word for the ear is *oto-*, such as in *otology* (science of the ear) or *otosclerosis* ("hardening of the ear"). In some instances the second "o" is dropped, such as in *otitis* (inflammation of the ear).

Nurses are involved primarily in prevention and detection of hearing and vestibular disorders. In addition, nurses participate in health teaching for hearing-impaired persons, in facilitating communication when hearing-impaired persons are hospitalized, and in providing care for persons receiving treatment for disorders of the ear.

ANATOMY AND PHYSIOLOGY

The ears are normally placed on each side of the head at eye level; an imaginary line parallel to the floor can be drawn from the outer canthus of the eye to the top of the outer ear. A lower placed ear may indicate chromosomal or congenital renal abnormalities. The ears are located in the temporal bone, which provides protection for the organs of hearing and equilibrium. Each ear is divided into the following parts: the external ear, the middle ear and mastoid, and the inner ear.

External Ear

The external ear consists of two parts, the pinna (auricle) and the external auditory canal. The *pinna* is composed primarily of cartilage and skin with little subcutaneous fat except for the lobule (lower tip). The external ear is innervated by cranial nerve V (trigeminal), a branch of cranial nerve X (vagus), and cervical nerves.

The ear canal provides a channel along which sound travels to the eardrum. The canal is an S-shaped curve about 2.5 cm (1 inch) long through the temporal bone in an inward, forward, and downward slope in an adult. There are constrictions in the canal close to the midpoint and the eardrum. The canal and outer ear drum are covered by thin sensitive skin. Numerous fine hairs protect the canal from foreign debris, and sebaceous glands in the distal third of the canal provide cerumen (wax) for lubrication.

The *tympanic membrane* (eardrum) separates the external ear from the middle ear. The eardrum is a thin, tough, translucent membrane, nearly oval in shape and directed obliquely downward. The malleus ossicle of the middle ear generally can be seen through the membrane. The tympanic membrane protects the middle ear and vibrates with incoming sound waves for hearing.

Middle Ear

The middle ear lies directly behind the eardrum and is a small air-filled space located in the petrous portion of the temporal bone (toward the face). It contains the ossicles, oval and round windows, and the eustachian tube (Fig.

39-1). The *ossicles* are three movable small bones that transverse the middle ear; these three bones are called the *malleus* (hammer), *incus* (anvil), and *stapes* (stirrup) because of their shapes. The malleus is attached at one end to the tympanic membrane and at the other end to the incus. The incus is connected to the *stapes which is fixed in the oval window*. The stapes is in direct contact with the perilymph of the inner ear. The ossicles mechanically transmit sound vibrations to the fluid in the inner ear. The *oval window* is not a true window because it is covered by the footplate of the stapes. The *round window* located beneath the oval window provides an exit for sound vibrations from the inner ear.

The *eustachian tube* (auditory tube) is a channel extending from the middle ear into the nasopharynx. It allows air to enter and leave the middle ear to equalize pressure on both sides of the eardrum. Swallowing or yawning can move air in and out of the middle ear to change air pressure in the middle ear. Portions of the facial nerves that control movement of the face and supply taste to the tongue are located in the middle ear.

The *mastoid* portion of the temporal bone is located posterior to the external ear and includes the mastoid air cells and mastoid antrum (cavity) that connects to the middle ear. Because of this direct connection infection of the middle ear may lead to mastoiditis. The mastoid process is a conical-shaped portion of mastoid bone that protrudes behind the lower portion of the pinna. The mastoid assists the middle ear in adjusting to pressure changes and lightens the mastoid bone.

Inner Ear

The inner ear (labyrinth) contains both the organs for hearing (cochlea) and the organs of balance (semicircular canals and vestibule) (Fig. 39-2). The bony labyrinth is a rigid capsule. The membranous labyrinth (consisting of three semicircular canals, vestibule, and cochlea) lies within the bony labyrinth but does not completely fill it. Position and balance are maintained by the semicircular canals (rotational movement) and by the membranous utricle and saccule in the vestibule (linear movements).

Two separate fluids are found in the labyrinth, the *perilymph* between the bony and membranous laybrinths and the *endolymph* within the membranous labyrinth. The endolymph is in a contained closed system; the perilymphatic spaces connect to the subarachnoid space containing cerebrospinal fluid.

The *cochlea* is a spiraling bony tube resembling a snail shell. The tube is separated into two compartments by a membranous tube called the *cochlear duct*, which contains endolymph and the organ of Corti. The two compartments of the cochlea contain perilymph; the upper compartment (scala vestibuli) leads from the oval window of the middle ear to the apex of the cochlea, and the lower compartment (scala tympani) from the apex of the cochlea to the round window to permit the sound vibrations to escape.

The organ of hearing, the *organ of Corti*, lies on the basilar membrane of the cochlear duct for its entire length. The organ of Corti has thousands of tiny "hair cells" that project into the endolymph; these hair cells are the most fragile elements in the inner ear and are crucial for hear-

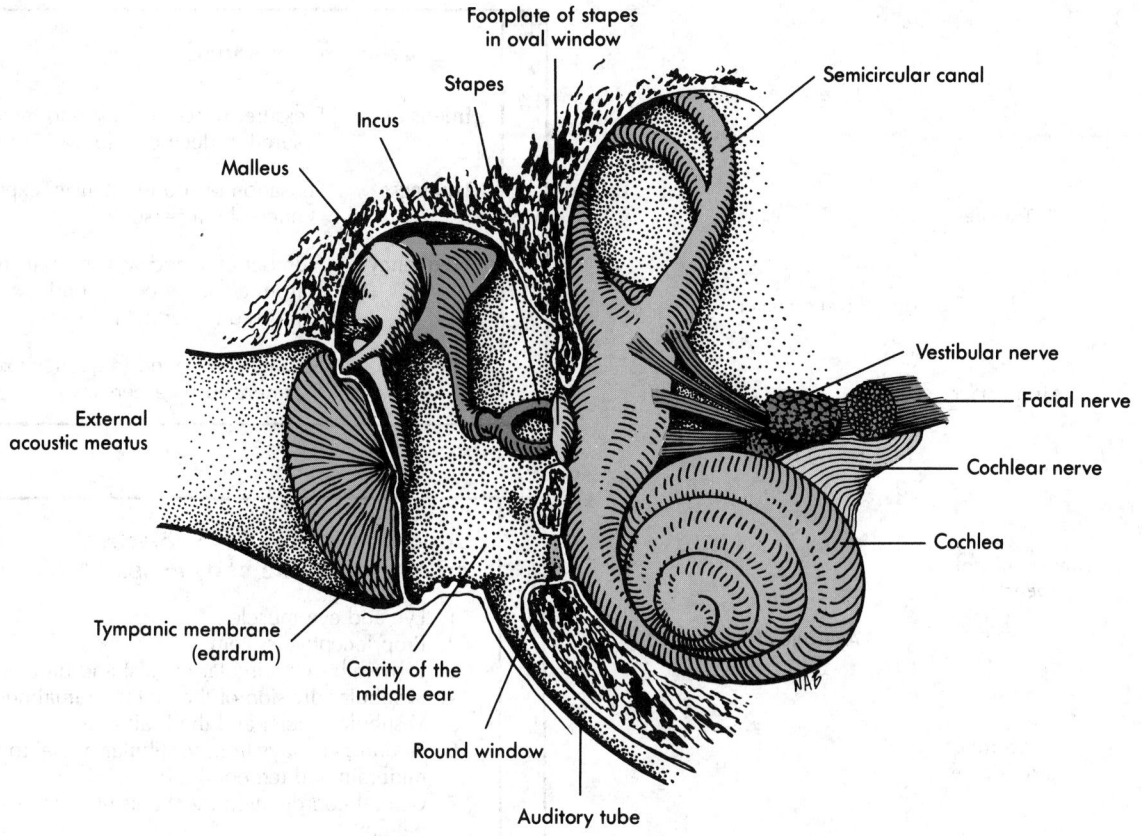

Footplate of stapes
in oval window

Stapes

Incus

Malleus

Semicircular canal

External
acoustic meatus

Vestibular nerve

Facial nerve

Cochlear nerve

Cochlea

Tympanic membrane
(eardrum)

Cavity of the
middle ear

Round window

Auditory tube

Fig. 39-1   Structures of the ear.

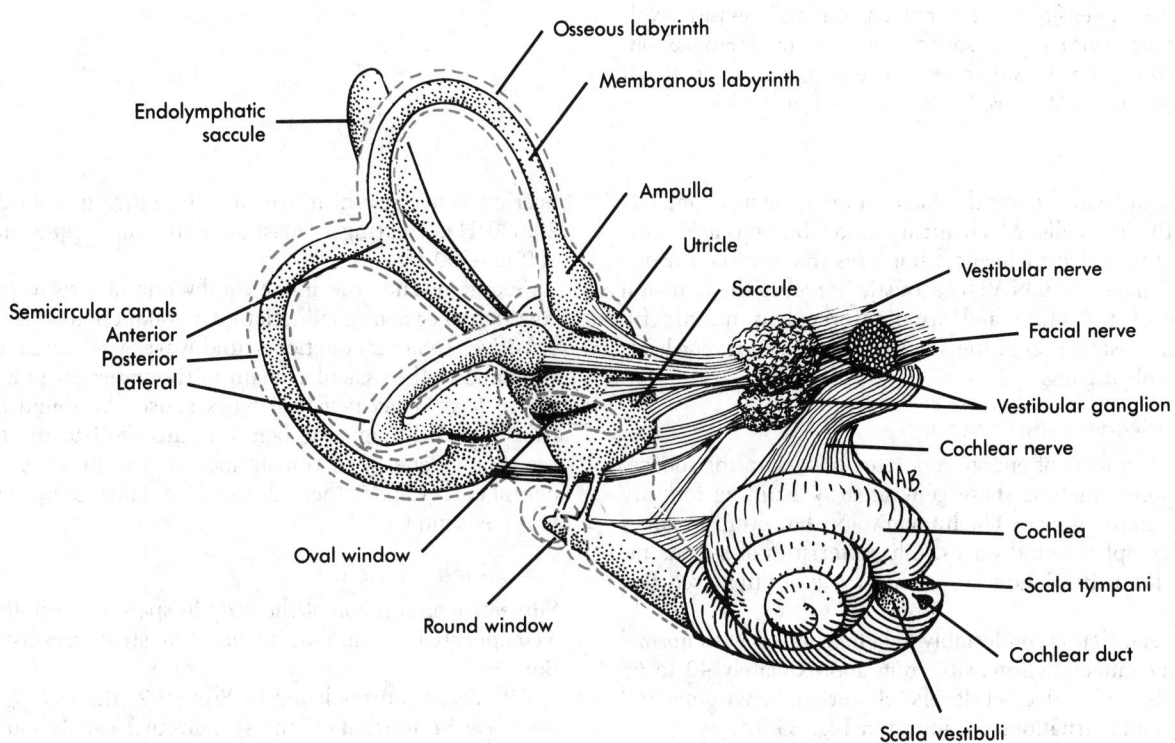

Osseous labyrinth

Membranous labyrinth

Endolymphatic
saccule

Ampulla

Utricle

Saccule

Vestibular nerve

Facial nerve

Semicircular canals
Anterior
Posterior
Lateral

Vestibular ganglion

Cochlear nerve

Cochlea

Scala tympani

Cochlear duct

Oval window

Round window

Scala vestibuli

Fig. 39-2   Structures of the inner ear.

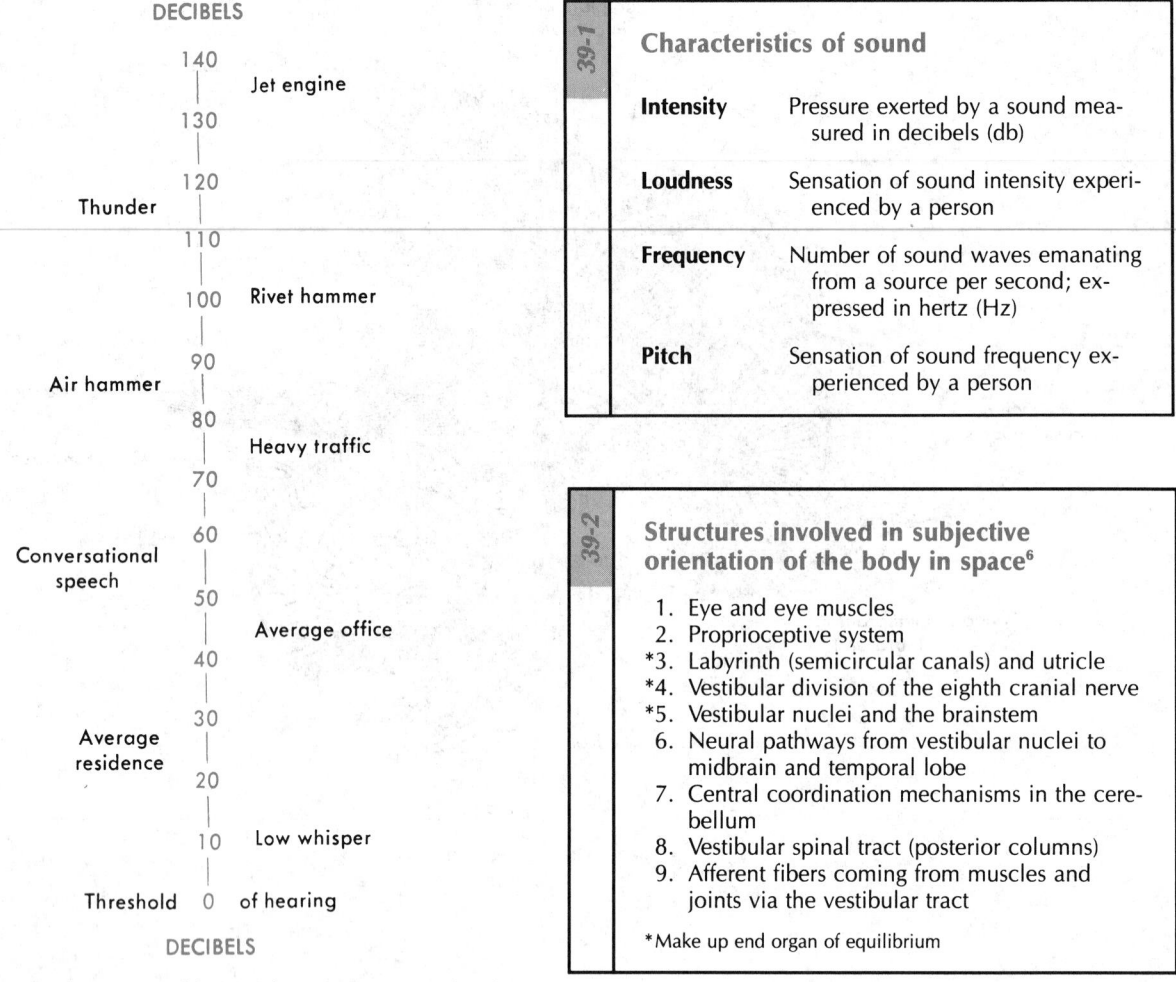

140	Jet engine
130	
120	
Thunder 110	
100	Rivet hammer
90	
Air hammer 80	
	Heavy traffic
70	
60	
Conversational speech 50	
	Average office
40	
30	
Average residence 20	
10	Low whisper
Threshold 0	of hearing

DECIBELS

Box 39-1

Characteristics of sound

Intensity   Pressure exerted by a sound measured in decibels (db)

Loudness   Sensation of sound intensity experienced by a person

Frequency   Number of sound waves emanating from a source per second; expressed in hertz (Hz)

Pitch   Sensation of sound frequency experienced by a person

Box 39-2

Structures involved in subjective orientation of the body in space[6]

1. Eye and eye muscles
2. Proprioceptive system
*3. Labyrinth (semicircular canals) and utricle
*4. Vestibular division of the eighth cranial nerve
*5. Vestibular nuclei and the brainstem
6. Neural pathways from vestibular nuclei to midbrain and temporal lobe
7. Central coordination mechanisms in the cerebellum
8. Vestibular spinal tract (posterior columns)
9. Afferent fibers coming from muscles and joints via the vestibular tract

*Make up end organ of equilibrium

Fig. 39-3 Intensity range of human hearing. Intensity levels of various environmental sounds and situations. (From Saunders WH et al: *Nursing care in eye, ear, nose, and throat disorders*, ed 4, St Louis, 1979, Mosby—Year Book.)

ing. Sound waves enter the cochlear duct and mechanically bend the hair cells. Mechanical sound vibrations are transformed into electrochemical impulses that are then transmitted along the CN VIII (acoustic nerve) to the temporal cortex of the brain and are interpreted as meaningful sound. Destruction of the acoustic nerve by a tumor leads to loss of hearing.

Sound Waves and Hearing

Sound is a form of energy generated by a vibrating source. Pure tones such as those generated by a tuning fork are simple sound waves. The human voice, however, produces more complex sound waves. Characteristics of sounds include intensity, loudness, frequency, and pitch (see Box 39-1).

Speech that is comfortably loud to a person with normal hearing ranges in intensity from approximately 40 to 65 decibels. The decibel levels of various environmental sounds and situations are found in Fig. 39-3.

A sound with a low frequency is perceived as a tone low in pitch, whereas a sound with high frequency is perceived as a high-pitched tone. A child or young adult with normal

hearing can often hear frequencies ranging from 20 to 20,000 Hz. Hearing is most sensitive for frequencies of 500 to 4000 Hz.

Sound reaches the inner ear by one of two ways: air conduction or bone conduction. Air conduction is the most sensitive. In air conduction sound waves pass through the ear canal to the ossicular chain to the inner ear (Fig. 39-4). In *bone conduction* hearing is caused by sound being transmitted through the bones of the skull to the inner ear. Sound energy is transformed in the inner ear into neural energy and is then "decoded" and interpreted by the brain as sound.

Statokinetic System

Subjective orientation of the body in space is controlled by a complicated system that includes the structures listed in Box 39-2.

Of the structures listed in Box 39-2, the *end organ of equilibrium consists* of (1) the semicircular canals and utricle, (2) the vestibular division of the eighth cranial nerve, and (3) the vestibular nuclei. Together these three structures are referred to as the *statokinetic system.*[6]

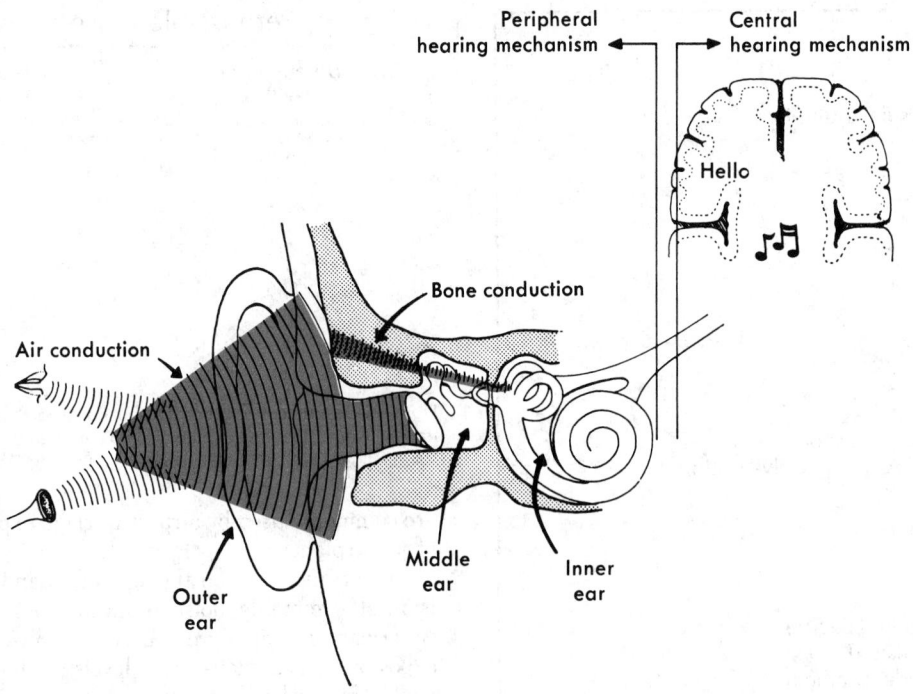

Fig. 39-4   Schema depicting functions of hearing mechanism as it translates sound waves into meaningful sensations. (From Saunders WH et al: *Nursing care in eye, ear, nose, and throat disorders*, ed 4, St Louis, 1979, Mosby—Year Book.)

PREVENTION OF HEARING LOSS

Hearing problems may begin at any age. Understanding the many causes of hearing loss is important for all health team members in all settings. Because nurses occupy a unique position in the health care system, they have the opportunity to teach people how to protect their hearing.

Preventing Ear Disease/Trauma

A certain amount of cerumen in the ear canal is normal, and persons who have no wax have itching and scaling in the ear canal. Usually it is not necessary to clean the ears to remove wax. Occasionally, when the wax becomes impacted and causes pain or temporary deafness, it must be removed by the physician or person instructed in the procedure.

The outer ear may be washed with soap and water during bathing, although this is often unnecessary as the ear canal is generally self-cleaning. If necessary, a cotton-tipped applicator moistened with alcohol may be inserted into the ear canal *only the length of the cotton tip,* which is more than enough to clean the short external canal without causing further problems.

During upper respiratory tract infections, the nose should be blown with both nostrils open. Excessive pressure from nose blowing can force infected secretions up the eustachian tube into the middle ear, leading to middle ear infection.

Persons having ear pain, swelling, drainage, prolonged feelings of plugged ears, or decreased hearing are referred to a physician for treatment. *Chronic problems such as perforated ear drums and necrotic ossicles may result from inattention to early signs of ear disorders.*

The following activities may lead to ear infection or trauma and should be *avoided:*

1. Inserting foreign objects into the ear (such as a hard object to remove wax or to scratch the ear canal if itching)
2. Swimming in stagnant water or in water identified as polluted
3. Instilling outdated medicated solutions into the ear

Monitoring Ototoxic Drugs

Some drugs are ototoxic (see Box 39-3); that is, they have adverse effects on the cochlea, vestibule, or acoustic nerve. Before an ototoxic drug is prescribed a diagnostic audiogram may be obtained. This audiogram provides a baseline for comparison with later audiograms. Persons taking ototoxic drugs need to know the side effects of these drugs so that they can be discontinued before they cause loss of hearing. If symptoms of dizziness, decreased hearing acuity, or tinnitus (ringing in the ears) occur, the next dose of the drug is omitted and the physician is consulted. Audiometric testing may be necessary.

Monitoring Noise Pollution

A major cause of hearing loss is occupational exposure to hazardous noise levels. Exposure to *industrial noise* levels greater than 85 to 90 db for months or years causes cochlear damage. Nurses working in industry can help prevent deafness caused by noise of high intensity by teaching employees why they should wear earplugs or other protective ear devices. Courses are available to familiarize nurses with industrial hearing conservation requirements.

The Occupational Safety and Health Administration

Selected ototoxic drugs

Aminoglycoside antibiotics
Streptomycin
Neomycin
Kanamycin
Gentamycin
Tobramycin
Netromycin
Amikacin

Other antibiotics
Vancomycin
Viomycin
Polymyxin B (Aerosporin)
Polymyxin E (Colistin/Coly-Mycin)
Erythromycin
Minocycline
Capreomycin

Diuretics
Ethacrynic acid (Edecrin)
Furosemide (Lasix)
Acetazolamide (Diamox)

Other drugs
Quinine
Chloroquine
Nitrogen mustard
Bleomycin
Quinidine
Cisplatin
Salicylates

Table 39-1 Permissible noise exposures

Duration per day (hr)	Sound level (dbA, slow)
8	90
6	92
4	95
3	97
2	100
1½	102
1	105
½	110
¼	115

From US Department of Labor, Occupational Safety and Health Administration: *Noise: the environmental problem, a guide to OSHA standards,* Washington, DC, 1979, US Government Printing Office.

are commonly used by airport workers exposed to the noise of jet airplanes.

In persons between the ages of 35 and 65, hearing loss is most commonly noise induced. More than 8 million Americans are at increased risk because of occupational exposure to hazardous noise levels (factory, maintenance, and farm workers). In younger persons, noise from amplified music, motorcycles, snow mobiles, firecrackers, cap guns, and rifle fire in ROTC programs can affect high-frequency hearing.[6] It is important to educate persons so that they understand that noise-induced hearing loss is often preventable and that once hearing is lost it cannot be regained.

Environmental exposure to noise in the workplace is monitored by the Occupational Health and Safety Administration (OSHA), which sets acceptable levels of noise pollution. Since the passage of The Hearing Conservation Amendment in 1982, OSHA requires yearly audiometric testing of noise-exposed workers.

A risk reduction objective from *Healthy People 2000* relates to prevention of hearing impairment in the workplace. The objective is to reduce to no more than 15% the proportion of workers exposed to average daily noise levels that exceed 85 db.[10] There was no baseline data available for this objective. See Fig. 39-3 for levels of environmental sounds by decibels. To reduce the number of people exposed to noise levels that exceed 85 db to no more than 15% may be difficult because it is estimated that 8 million workers in U.S. manufacturing industries are exposed to potentially hazardous average daily levels of noise at 80 db and above. Another 3 million workers in other occupations are exposed to average daily levels above 85 db.[10]

One in four workers exposed to 90 db and over for a working lifetime will develop a hearing impairment. Workers exposed to industrial noise may not show a hearing loss for as many as 10 years after initial exposure. The hearing loss results from progressive destruction of sensory cells in the ear. Once damaged, these cells can neither repair themselves nor be medically restored. Noise-induced hearing loss becomes more severe with continued exposure to noise.[10]

Healthy People 2000 has set the following goals for the year 2000 in regard to hearing impairment: Reduce significant hearing impairment to a prevalence of no more

(OSHA) has established acceptable levels of noise in work environments. *Unprotected* exposure to noise levels in excess of 90 db over an 8-hour day is considered excessive and should be avoided (Table 39-1).

Other causes of noise-induced hearing loss include *firearms* and *high-intensity music*. With an M16 rifle or sport rifle, hearing loss tends to be greater in the ear opposite the dominant hand. With revolvers, hearing loss is equal in both ears. A person firing guns who develops tinnitus, sensation of fullness in the ear, or temporary hearing loss should stop firing guns or wear suitable ear protectors.

Sound in front of a rock band can reach 120 db, and hearing losses of up to 50 db have been measured in some members of rock bands. In the early stage, there is a loss of hearing *at* or *near* frequencies of 4000 Hz. Later the damage extends to both higher and lower tones, with the lower tones affected least.

If *proximity to the high noise level cannot be avoided, ear protectors or earplugs should be worn.* The earplugs are inserted into the external auditory canal and can reduce the noise reaching the middle ear by 10 to 30 db. Usually standard plugs are effective, but custom-made plugs molded to the person's ear canal may be obtained. *If the noise level is extremely high (sound levels may reach 140 db or higher), individuals are not adequately protected with earplugs alone and must wear specially made ear muffs.* Ear muffs

than 82 per 1000 people from a baseline of 88.9 per 1000 in 1986 to 1988. The special target population for this objective is people aged 45 and older. The goal for the year 2000 is to reduce hearing impairment in this population to 180 per 1000 people from a baseline of 203 per 1000 people in 1986 to 1988.[10]

Healthy People 2000 also set a service and protection objective related to care for older Americans. This objective is to increase to at least 60% the proportion of providers of primary care for older adults who routinely evaluate people aged 65 and older for impairment of hearing and functional status.[10]

Major Health Problems of the Ear

Ear disorders may occur in any part of the ear. The more common ear disorders are discussed in this chapter under three headings because of the commonalities in the required care. Disorders included in each category are as follows:

1. Infections of the external/middle ear
   a. External otitis
   b. Otitis media: serous, purulent (acute, chronic)
   c. Chronic mastoiditis
2. Disorders affecting balance
   a. Labyrinthitis
   b. Menière's disease
   c. Acoustic neuroma
3. Disorders affecting hearing
   a. Conductive hearing loss: otosclerosis
   b. Sensorineural hearing loss
   c. Presbycusis

INFECTIONS OF THE EXTERNAL/MIDDLE EAR

The most common disorders of the external and middle ear are infections (Table 39-2). Although many of these infections occur in children, they may also occur in adults.

Etiology and Pathophysiology

Organisms may enter the external ear by way of the external orifice or the middle ear via the eustachian tube, resulting in infections. Infection of the labyrinth (inner ear) may result from extension of middle ear infections, but the effect is primarily on balance (See Box 39-2).

Infections of the external ear, *external otitis*, are primarily bacterial (staphylococci or gram-negative organisms) or fungal. A form of seborrheic dermatitis (Chapter 43) may result from extensive use of objects such as earphones. Infection develops in the skin lining the ear canal, and swelling and debris may lead to closure of the canal. Furuncles may also develop. Pain results from pressure on the sensitive skin lining and can be severe because there is no room for expansion in the bony canal. *Activities leading to water retention in the ear such as swimming, especially in contaminated water, promote external otitis.*

Infection of the middle ear, *otitis media*, is the most common disorder of the middle ear. The infection may be serous or purulent and acute or chronic. *Serous otitis media develops from collection of sterile serum in the middle ear when the eustachian tube becomes blocked because of previous infection or allergy* (Fig. 39-5). *Purulent otitis media* develops from bacterial infection and may be acute or chronic. Chronic infection may spread into the mastoid (chronic mastoiditis) or cause necrosis of the tympanic membrane or ossicles, leading to hearing loss. Acute mastoiditis is rare because of antibiotic treatment of acute otitis media. With chronic mastoiditis, a *cholesteatoma* (benign growth) may develop. It is a skin-lined sac with debris and is often infected. The cholesteatoma may recur when removed.

Nursing Process
Assessment

A person with an ear infection is usually diagnosed and treated on an ambulatory basis. *Early detection and treatment are important to prevent development of chronic infections with subsequent loss of hearing.*

Subjective data

The major symptoms of external and middle ear infections are *pain* and *loss of hearing*, and data are collected about the onset, duration, and severity of these symptoms. *Pain results from pressure on the sensitive skin lining the external canal or pressure on the eardrum from fluid buildup in the middle ear.* Loss of hearing is the result of a blocked external canal or fluid in the middle ear that interferes with passage of sound waves. Persons with ear infections should be questioned about their knowledge of preventive measures.

Objective data

The external ear is inspected for signs of drainage, either serous or purulent. The auricle is also inspected for signs of redness, scaliness, and crusting. When assessing the external ear, manipulation of the ear is important. If the patient complains of pain when any part of the ear is palpated, a *furuncle, lesion,* or some kind of inflammatory process *of the ear canal is suspected*. Water in the ear canal from showering or swimming may aggravate the symptoms.

When an otoscopic examination is performed, care must be taken not to cause the person unnecessary pain. A furuncle may be close to the opening of the canal, causing increased pain from the pressure of the speculum.

Otoscopic examination of the external ear canal and eardrum

The eardrum is important in physical assessment of the ear because it serves as a translucent window through which disease processes in the middle ear can be inferred. The normal tympanic membrane has a wide range of colored hues, the most common being pearly gray. Located in the membrane or seen through it are certain landmarks (Fig. 39-6). For visualization of the external ear canal and

Table 39-2   Infections of the external/middle ear

Disorder	Description	Signs and symptoms	Medical therapy
External otitis	Inflammation of the external ear; may be acute or chronic	Pain with movement of auricle, redness, scaling, itching, swelling, watery discharge, crusting of external ear	Cleaning to remove debris; antibiotic drops or ointment, systemic antibiotics if necessary
Serous otitis media	Collection of sterile serum in middle ear; may be acute or chronic	Sense of fullness in ear, hearing loss, low-pitched tinnitus, earache	Removal of eustachian obstruction by aspiration or insertion of tubes for drainage
Acute purulent otitis media	Infection of middle ear, usually by pneumococci, streptococci, staphylococci, or *Haemophilus influenzae*	Sense of fullness in ear, severe throbbing pain, hearing loss, tinnitus, fever	Antibiotics If severe, bed rest, analgesics, nasal vasoconstrictors Myringotomy if necessary
Chronic otitis media	Chronic inflammation of middle ear; sequela of acute otitis media	Deafness, occasional pain, dizziness, chronic discharge from ear	Local debridement; topical and systemic antibiotics; mastoidectomy and tympanoplasty may be necessary
Chronic mastoiditis	Spread of infection into mastoid from repeated otitis media	Middle ear drainage	Mastoid irrigation; antibiotics; may need mastoidectomy

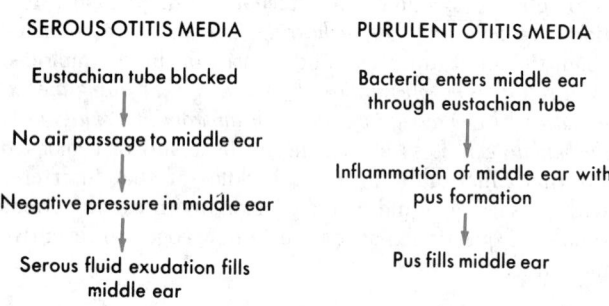

Fig. 39-5   Pathogenesis of otitis media.

eardrum, an otoscope (Fig. 39-7) is used; it has an ear piece (speculum) that can be placed into the ear canal, has illumination to visualize the eardrum, and may have magnification for a more accurate assessment. Otoscopy is performed by persons (including nurses) who are specially prepared to use an otoscope.

Operating microscopic examination

The binocular-operating microscope is found in the offices and clinics of most otologists. With specialized instruction the nurse may learn to use the microscope and manipulate instruments inserted through a speculum into the external ear. The speculum holds open the outermost portion of the external ear canal and allows the passage of both light and instruments. The appropriate speculum size for adults is from 4 to 7 mm in diameter. The microscope provides the examiner with excellent illumination, increased depth perception, and three-dimensional vision.

Most operating microscopes allow changes in magnification to be made. The specially prepared nurse can use the microscope to distinguish normal from abnormal, remove cerumen, and suction drainage.

Data analysis: nursing diagnoses

Nursing diagnoses are determined from analysis of patient data. Possible nursing diagnoses for the person with an external ear problem may include, but are not limited to, the following:

Diagnostic title	Possible etiologies
Pain	Pathophysiologic ear pain caused by infection, inflammation, and swelling
Knowledge deficit about problem	Lack of exposure to information: unfamiliarity with information sources.
Sensory/perceptual alteration, auditory	Decreased hearing caused by debris and infection in ear canal

Planning: expected patient outcomes

Expected patient outcomes for the person with an external ear problem may include, but are not limited to, the following:

1. The patient states discomfort in the ear is decreased.
2. The patient can describe measures for prevention of external ear problems.
3. The patient can describe symptoms requiring medical attention.
4. The patient demonstrates correct technique in application of eardrops and ear ointment.
5. The patient is prepared for the possibility of minor surgery.
6. The patient's hearing is improved.

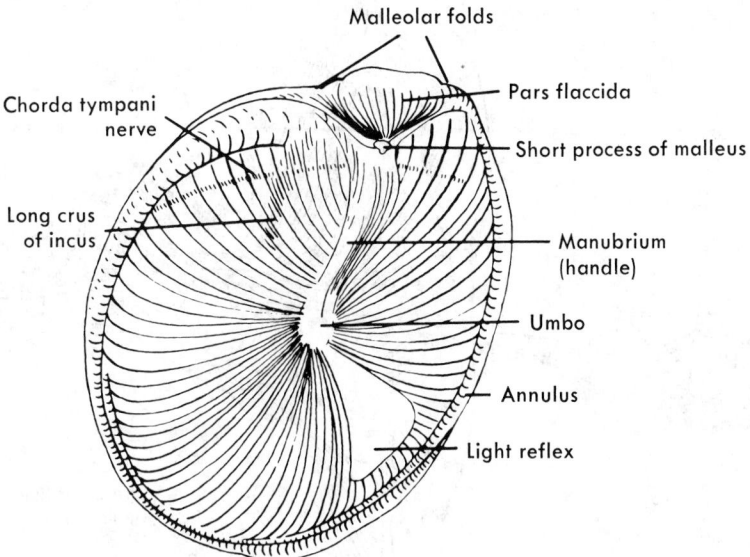

Fig. 39-6 Right tympanic membrane. (From Prior JA, Silberstein JS, Stang JM: *Physical diagnosis: the history and examination of the patient*, ed 6, St Louis, 1981, Mosby–Year Book.)

Implementation

Assisting with achievement of therapeutic goals

Manipulation of the ear during treatments requires gentle handling to maintain comfort. Cross-contamination is prevented by good medical asepsis, including washing hands before and after treatments.

Ear wash

A solution of boric acid and alcohol (which can be obtained at the drugstore) may be used to clean the external ear and provide a drying effect. Ear wash is contra-indicated if the eardrum is perforated. A small (2 to 3 oz) syringe is used to instill the fluid, and the solution is warmed to body temperature to prevent discomfort or dizziness. The person places the affected ear upward. The pinna is pulled up, back, and out, and the tip of the syringe is placed in the ear canal. The warmed solution is pumped vigorously and repeatedly in and out of the canal. The patient then leans over and lets extra solution run out into a small basin or a folded towel. An ear wash is usually prescribed for twice a day until the ear stops draining. Dryness is checked by inserting a cotton-tipped applicator into the ear canal (no farther than the cotton tip).

Ear irrigation

The ear may be irrigated to remove wax, drainage, or debris. A larger amount of solution is used than for an ear wash. *Irrigations are avoided if the eardrum is perforated (causes further inflammation) or if the foreign body to be removed is of vegetable origin or an insect (moisture will cause object or insect to swell).* Tap water is generally used; hydrogen peroxide may be used to help dislodge wax. A large syringe is used, but the technique for insertion of the syringe tip is similar to an ear wash. The person's clothes are protected with a plastic cape, and a kidney-basin is placed below the ear to catch the solution. The fluid is

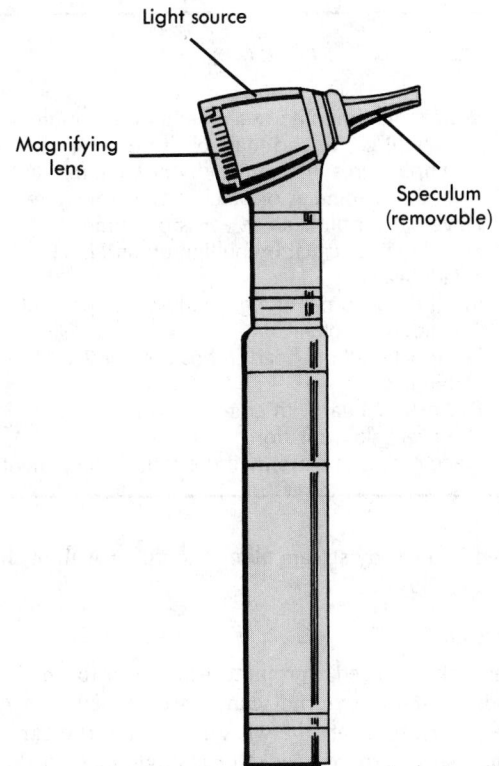

Fig. 39-7 Otoscope.

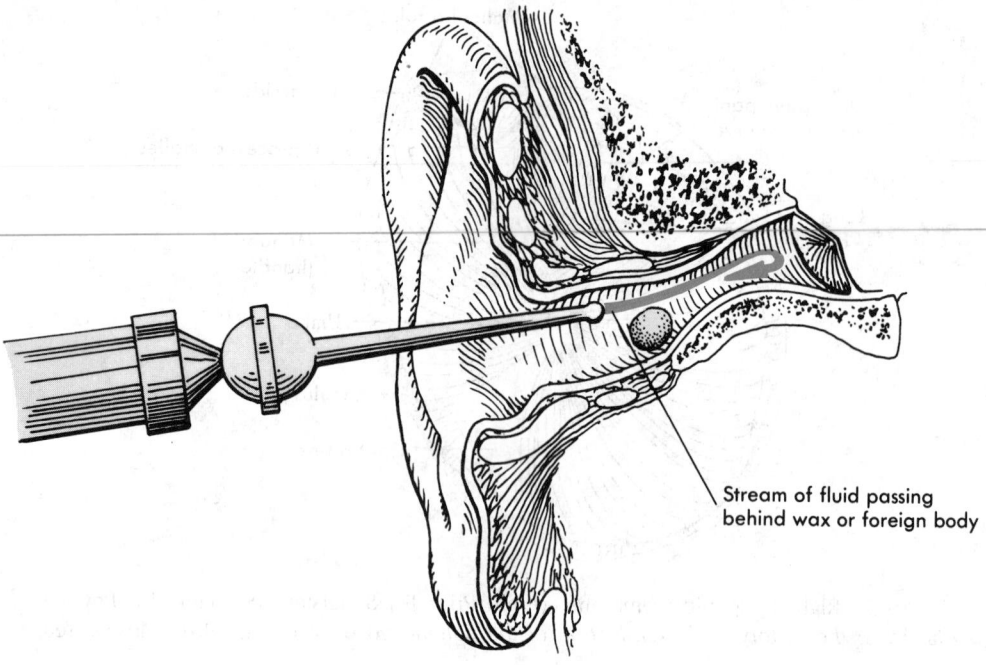

Stream of fluid passing
behind wax or foreign body

Fig. 39-8 Ear irrigation. Note that fluid is directed toward upper canal wall so that stream passes behind the wax or object.

Guidelines for Care

39-4

Instillation of eardrops

Warm solution to body temperature (no more than 38°C); vertigo may result from high or low temperatures. (Warm vial by holding in hand for a few minutes or placing in warm water.)

Have patient tilt head so ear is uppermost.

Straighten ear canal by pulling up and back (adults).

Instill drops to run along canal wall to prevent entrapment of air.

Have patient hold head in position for 2 to 3 minutes.

Dry external ear with cotton balls thoroughly to prevent skin irritation.

Place cotton in ear only if desired by the patient.

---

directed in a steady stream along the upper wall of the ear canal (Fig. 39-8).

Ear wicks

Ear wicks are used to promote drainage or for instillation of eardrops if the external canal is occluded. A bayonet forcep is used to insert the wick gently into the ear canal. Commercially prepared wicks or a single piece of ¼-inch gauze about 2 cm long may be used.

Eardrops

Antibiotics and antiinflammatory agents may be prescribed locally as eardrops, especially for external otitis. Guidelines for instillation of eardrops are listed in Box 39-4.

Ear ointment

Use a cotton-tipped applicator to apply ear ointment. Insert the applicator no farther than the cotton end, and use a new one for each application. Allergic reactions to the medication can occur. Itching, redness, or a feeling of fullness in the ear are common symptoms of allergy.

Surgery

Surgery may be performed on the eardrum to relieve fluid pressure or to repair a perforation (Table 39-3). If it is desirable to keep the eardrum open for fluid drainage, transtympanic tubes can be inserted in a myringotomy incision; the tubes usually drop out by themselves in several months. Surgery of the ear is performed under high power magnification. If mastoidectomy in indicated, a simple procedure is preferred, if possible, as this maintains hearing. Tympanoplasty may follow mastoidectomy if the ossicles are removed. Care of the person after ear surgery is described on p. 1340.

Interventions to achieve patient outcomes
Assisting with comfort

Because ear pain results from the fluid exudate of the inflammatory process, pain usually begins to subside with adequate antibiotic therapy and drainage measures. Analgesics may be helpful. External heat such as a hot water bottle or heating pad set on low may be comforting to some patients.

Monitoring hearing

The patient's hearing is assessed before and after surgery. See Box 39-12 for suggestions for facilitating communication with the person with a hearing loss.

Table 39-3   Surgeries of the eardrum, middle ear, and mastoid

Type of surgery	Description
Myringotomy	Removal by suction of middle ear fluid through an incision made in eardrum
Myringoplasty	Repair of a tympanic membrane perforation
Tympanoplasty (ossiculoplasty)	Reconstruction of ossicles of middle ear
Mastoidectomy	
Simple (closed)	Removal of mastoid air cells
Radical (open)	Removal of mastoid air cells, ossicles, eardrum, wall of ear canal, and middle ear mucosa
Modified (open)	Less extensive than radical mastoidectomy; preserves middle ear structures

Facilitating learning

Ear infections may recur and become chronic; therefore, persons with ear infections need to know how to prevent chronic infection. Teaching includes prevention of further infection, care of the infected ear, and signs requiring further medical attention (see Box 39-5 for more information).

Evaluation

Evaluation is based on expected patient outcomes. Questions to consider may include the following:
1. Is the patient comfortable?
2. Can the patient describe care required at home?
3. Can the patient describe measures to prevent recurring infection?

DISORDERS OF BALANCE
Pathophysiology

Disturbance of the function of the *statokinetic system* (semicircular canals, vestibular portion of the eighth cranial nerve, and vestibular nuclei) results in a subjective sensation of whirling or spinning or of being propelled or tilted in space. These sensations of true whirling or motion of the body are called *systematized vertigo* (Box 39-6). Three of the conditions causing vertigo—labyrinthitis, Ménière's disease, and acoustic neuroma—are disorders of the inner ear involving the *statokinetic system*[6] (see p. 1330).

Labyrinthitis is the most common cause of *vertigo*. There are two major types of labyrinthitis, *suppurative* and *acute toxic* (Table 39-4). Suppurative labyrinthitis is caused by an invasion of the internal ear by infection. Acute toxic labyrinthitis is caused by acute febrile illnesses such as pneumonia, cholecystitis, or influenza; toxic reactions to drugs; overindulgence in alcohol; food or drug allergy; or extreme fatigue. Hearing loss usually does not accompany acute toxic labyrinthitis, but total hearing loss and a nonfunctioning labyrinth are the results of suppurative labyrinthitis. *If the suppurative type of labyrinthitis is inadequately treated with antibiotics or if the diagnosis is delayed, meningitis*

39-6

Causes of systematized vertigo

Ear
External ear
   Wax or foreign bodies
Middle ear
   Retracted tympanic membrane
   Acute disease
      Acute suppurative otitis media
      Otitis media with effusion
   Chronic disease
      Labyrinthitis
      Cholesteatoma (fistula reaction)
Internal ear
   Acute toxic labyrinthitis
   Vascular episodes
   Trauma
   Allergy
   Hydrops of the labyrinth (Ménière's disease)
   Motion sickness
   Postural vertigo

Eighth cranial nerve
Infection
Trauma
Tumors (acoustic neuroma)

Brainstem nuclei
Infections
Trauma
Hemorrhage
Thrombosis of posteroinferior cerebellar artery
Tumors
Multiple sclerosis

Table 39-4 Disorders affecting balance

Disorder	Signs and symptoms	Medical therapy
Suppurative labyrinthitis	Severe, whirling vertigo Tinnitus Sensorineural hearing loss *Results in:* total hearing loss and non-functional labyrinth	Hospitalization High-dose antibiotics IV Drugs to treat symptoms, such as antimotion and antihistamine drugs
Acute toxic labyrinthitis	Whirling vertigo reaching its maximum in 24 hours Nausea and vomiting Incapacity for 3-5 days Any movement of the head causes whirling vertigo No hearing loss	Bed rest in supine position until symptoms abate Avoid movement of head Reassurance that attack will subside in 3-5 days
Ménière's disease	Triad of: 1. Attacks of whirling vertigo, 2. Tinnitus 3. Fluctuating sensorineural hearing loss	Low-salt diet (1.5 g/day) Drug therapy 1. Diuretics 2. Peripheral vestibular suppressant: meclizine, diphenhydramine 3. CNS vestibular suppressant: diazepam 4. Antiemetic: promethazines 5. Anticholinergic: scopolamine
Acoustic neuroma	First symptom is tinnitus, hearing loss that may not occur for months or years Hearing loss, usually to high-frequency sounds Unsteadiness if tumor is large. Vertigo is unusual but may occur. Facial paralysis if seventh and eighth cranial nerves are compressed into internal auditory canal	Diagnosis: MRI will detect early tumors lying within internal auditory canal and is the best diagnostic tool Treatment: Surgical removal of the neuroma

can result. Certain drugs, especially streptomycin, are toxic to the eighth cranial nerve and can destroy the vestibular portion of the nerve.

Ménière's disease is thought to be caused by an overproduction of endolymph in the middle ear. This is why the disease is classified as endolymphatic hydrops, although it is most commonly called Ménière's disease.

Whirling vertigo, in which the body seems to be whirling when the eyes are closed or the environment seems to be turning when the eyes are open, is found in Ménière's disease. Any sensation of movement, up and down or side to side, suggests that the statokinetic system is involved.[6] A triad of symptoms is seen in Ménière's disease. In addition to attacks of whirling vertigo, tinnitus and fluctuating sensorineural hearing loss occur.

Early in the disease one or two symptoms may occur without the third. In two thirds of patients, vertigo is the primary symptom. The diagnosis of Ménière's disease is *not made until all three symptoms are present.*

Ménière's disease is most common is persons between the ages of 30 and 50. Hearing loss is present initially in only one ear. However, 25% to 40% of patients develop bilateral hydrops resulting in deafness in both ears. The therapy for Ménière's disease is outlined in Table 39-4. Surgical treatment may become necessary when medical therapy has failed to relieve the severe attacks of vertigo.

Less than 10% of patients require surgery. Several surgical procedures can be used, but none of them is considered the "perfect" surgical therapy for Ménière's disease.[6]

The person with Ménière's disease usually has recurrent attacks at varying intervals. During an attack, the person is unable to sit or walk and must lie with the head absolutely still to prevent further vertigo. In *most cases, loss of hearing is progressive until deafness results in that ear. There is no cure for the disease, but control is possible.*

An *acoustic neuroma* is a slow-growing, benign tumor of the vestibular portion of cranial nerve VIII causing signs and symptoms listed in Table 39-4. The neuroma can be removed easily without side effects if identified early. If allowed to grow, however, it encroaches on the brain and more extensive surgery is necessary with loss of hearing.

Nursing Process
Assessment
Subjective and objective data

When the examiner is attempting to evaluate vertigo, six basic questions should be asked[6]:

1. Does the patient experience true whirling? The direction and character of the motion are not important, but whether the patient feels that he or she is in motion.
2. What is the pattern of dizziness? Are there parox-

ysmal attacks with intervals of no attacks? Onset, course, severity, duration, time of day, and relationship to menstrual periods, occupation, and trauma should be determined.

3. Are there associated symptoms such as nausea and vomiting? If nausea and vomiting accompany vertigo and there is absence of signs of CNS disease, the cause is usually labyrinthine disease.

4. Is there hearing loss or tinnitus? When either accompanies dizziness, it helps to localize the disorder.

5. Is there history of motion sickness or vestibular sensitivity? When the patient has no history of motion sickness and experiences true whirling vertigo, this indicates significant vestibular abnormalities. Patients who have motion sickness require a less severe ocular, proprioceptive, or vestibular abnormality to elicit symptoms of vertigo.

6. What is the drug history? This is very important because so many classifications of drugs can cause symptoms of dizziness. See Box 39-7.

Subjective data are collected initially from a patient subject to vertigo. Data include knowledge of the disorder, patterns of the episodes (frequency, duration), accompanying symptoms, and safety measures taken. Because of the discomfort of vertigo, many persons fear the attacks; therefore the person's feelings concerning the vertigo are explored. Initial *objective data* include an assessment of the person's hearing ability (p. 1344) because of the close relationship between balance and hearing in the inner ear.

During an attack of vertigo, the following additional data are collected:

1. Onset and duration of the attack.
2. Presence of nystagmus (involuntary jerky movements of the eyes); note if nystagmus occurs in one eye or both eyes and the rapidity of the movement.
3. Reports of tinnitus (ranges from buzzing sounds to painful, loud ringing noises).
4. Color and moisture of skin (pallor and diaphoresis from an autonomic nervous system response).
5. Occurrence of vomiting (also an autonomic nervous system response).

Diagnostic tests

Specific diagnostic tests include *electronystagmography* (ENG) and a caloric stimulation test. ENG is a test used to measure nystagmus. It records the position and movement of the eyeball by recording the changes in the electrical field around the eye when there is a change in position of the eye. Electrodes are placed on the face around the eye; no discomfort is involved.

In the *caloric stimulation test*, cold water or air is irrigated in the external auditory canal. When the vestibular portion of the eighth cranial nerve is intact, labyrinthine function is normal, and the person experiences vertigo and nystagmus. In labyrinthine disorders, the response is hyperactive or absent.

Audiometric testing (p. 1346) is performed to identify concurrent hearing loss. With many labyrinthine disorders, the test initially reveals low-tone sensorineural hearing loss. Neurologic consultation is usually obtained to rule out neurologic disease.

39-7	**Classes of drugs causing vertigo**
	Antibiotics
	Anticonvulsants
	Antihistamines
	Antihypertensives
	Antiinflammatories
	Diuretics
	Muscle relaxants
	Sedatives
	Tranquilizers

Data analysis: nursing diagnoses

Nursing diagnoses are determined from analysis of patient data. Possible nursing diagnoses for the person with a balance disorder may include, but are not limited to, the following:

Diagnostic title	Possible etiologies
Injury, high risk for	Loss of balance during attack of vertigo
Sensory/perceptual alteration: auditory	Inner ear disorder
Anxiety	Concern about future attacks
Knowledge deficit	Lack of exposure/recall, information misinterpretation of information

Planning: expected patient outcomes

Expected patient outcomes for the person with a balance disorder may include, but are not limited to, the following:

1. Injury from loss of balance does not occur
2. Attacks of vertigo and tinnitus occur less frequently
3. Patient states he or she is less anxious about an attack of vertigo
4. The person describes:
   a. The nature of the disorder
   b. Circumstances that precipitate an attack and what to do when an attack occurs
   c. Safety precautions to take
   d. Prescribed medication regimen
   e. Symptoms requiring medical intervention

Implementation
Assisting with achievement of therapeutic goals
Medications

Most persons with a vertiginous disorder receive therapy on an ambulatory basis. Medications may be prescribed to decrease the incidence or severity of the vertigo and consist primarily of *antivertiginous drugs,* such as meclizine (Antivert), demenhydrinate (Dramamine), or diphenhydramine (Benadryl). A *diuretic* such as ammonium chloride or hydrochlorodiazide (Hydrodiuril) may be prescribed to help decrease fluid volume of the endolymph. A *low-salt diet* (1.5 gm/day) is usually prescribed for the same reason as a diuretic. A *vasodilator* such as nicotinic acid is helpful for some persons.

Surgery of the ear

Types of surgery. Surgery may be performed for Ménière's disease if the attacks are incapacitating and cannot

Table 39-5   Surgery for Ménière's disease

Procedure	Description	Results
Conservative procedures		
Endolymphatic shunt	Insertion of tube into endolymphatic sac. Tube is brought laterally into mastoid cavity or is placed medially in subarachnoid space. There is less risk of meningitis and spinal fluid leak when the tube is placed in mastoid cavity.	Vertigo controlled in 60% to 70% of patients; hearing stabilized in 50% to 60% of patients
Vestibular nerve section	Used for uncontrolled Ménière's disease. The superior and inferior vestibular nerves are sectioned, preserving cochlear and seventh nerve. Approach is via middle fossa or by retrolabyrinthine approach.	95 + % control of vertiginous attacks; increased risk to seventh nerve and cochlea; about 10% will have increase in hearing loss
Destructive procedures		
Transmastoid labyrinthectomy	Simple mastoidectomy with removal of enough mastoid cells to uncover the three semicircular canals; canals widely opened and membranous labyrinth removed. Used when symptoms persist after other surgical procedures or when ear function is considered useless.	Control of vertigo is 100%; hearing loss is total.

Adapted from DeWeese DD et al: *Otolaryngology—head and neck surgery,* ed 7, St Louis, Mosby–Year Book, 1988.

be controlled by medication. About 5% to 10% of persons with the disorder require surgery. The types of surgery are described in Table 39-5.

Surgery is required for removal of acoustic neuromas. A translabyrinthine or mastoidectomy approach is preferred, although a suboccipital approach may be needed. Very large tumors may require resection of the facial nerve.

Preoperative care. Ear surgery is often performed with local anesthesia, with the person receiving sedation to relieve anxiety and provide relaxation. The following instructions are given about what to expect in the postoperative period:

1. Minor earache can be expected, but pain is not usually a problem
2. Hearing is decreased because of the ear packing
3. Noises such as crackles or pops may be heard
4. Swelling of the ear will occur
5. Extent of postoperative vertigo depends on the nature of the procedure (more extensive with inner ear surgery)

Postoperative care
1. Position patient with operative ear up for 4 hours after surgery
2. Medicate as necessary for discomfort or vertigo
3. Keep side rails up when patient is in bed (when vertigo is present)
4. Supervise patient during ambulation if vertigo/dizziness is present
5. Monitor patient for:
   a. Changes in hearing, tinnitus, or vertigo
   b. Headache
   c. Bleeding (rare)
   d. Signs of facial paralysis if extensive inner ear surgery is performed (asymmetry when frowning, smiling, closing eye, baring teeth, or blowing through lips)
6. Instruct patient to keep mouth open if sneezing or coughing and to blow nose gently one side at a time, if necessary (prevents increased middle ear pressure and transmission of organisms into middle ear)
7. Reassure patient that improvement in hearing may not be immediate because of edema and packing in ear.

Most ear surgeries require only a cotton ball in the ear after surgery because only small amounts of serosanguineous drainage are expected. Dressings may be used for surgeries other than transcanal approaches. Hospital stays range from 1 to 4 days. Guidelines for patient teaching are listed in Box 39-8.

Interventions to achieve patient outcomes
Promoting comfort and safety

During an attack of vertigo, the person either feels as though the room is spinning around or that he or she is spinning in a stationary room. To prevent falling and to decrease the vertigo sensation, the person has to lie down, avoiding all head movements that aggravate the spinning sensation. If tinnitus is severe, the person may cover the ears in an attempt to lessen the sound. Measures must be taken to protect the person from falling at the onset of the attack. The acute manifestations may last from 1 to 3 hours.[21] After an attack the person is exhausted and requires rest and sleep.

Measures that help reduce vertigo or dizziness include the following:

39-8

The patient after ear surgery

1. Change cotton in ear daily as prescribed
2. Open mouth when sneezing or coughing and try not to sneeze or blow nose for 1 week. If must blow nose, blow gently one side at a time (to prevent increased ear pressure and infection)
3. Keep ear dry for 6 weeks (to prevent infection)
   a. Do not wash hair for 1 week
   b. Protect ear when outdoors using two pieces of cotton (use petroleum jelly on outer ball)
   c. Protect ear with shower cap when bathing
4. Wear ear protectors as necessary for exposure to loud noises
5. Follow activity guidelines
   a. No physical activity for 1 week or until deep external packing is removed
   b. No exercises or active sports for 3 weeks
   c. Return to work in 1 week (3 weeks for strenuous work)
6. Avoid exposure to persons with upper respiratory tract infections
7. Avoid airplane flights for at least 1 week (to prevent effects of pressure changes)

Patient Teaching

The patient with vertigo

1. Nature of the disorder
   a. Physiologic basis for the vertigo
   b. Avoidance of any known precipitating factors
   c. Rationale for a low-salt diet
2. Actions to take during an attack
   a. Lie down immediately and call for help if necessary at the first sign of an attack
   b. If driving when an attack occurs, pull over immediately to the curb
   c. Lie immobile and hold head in one position until vertigo lessens
3. Ask for assistance when ambulating if dizzy
4. Take prescribed medications as instructed, even if no recent attacks have occurred; check with physician before discontinuing any medication
5. Symptoms requiring medical attention: changes in symptoms or nature of attacks

Patient Teaching

39-9

---

1. Stand directly in front of person when speaking so person does not have to turn head
2. Encourage person to move *slowly*
3. Avoid bright, glaring lights
4. If bed rest is prescribed:
   a. Assist with ADL as needed
   b. Keep side rails up
5. Assist with ambulation as needed to prevent falls
6. If vertigo occurs when person is ambulating, have person lie down immediately and hold head still

Supporting coping

The threat of vertigo usually leads to anxiety. The person may dread the experience of an attack or may be embarrassed by the concurrent side-effects such as vomiting. Give the person opportunities to explore feelings and concerns. Anxiety may be decreased by awareness of measures to decrease vertigo occurrences or to minimize the effects.

Facilitating learning

Teaching for the patient with vertigo includes the nature of the disorder, actions to take during an attack, measures to prevent injury, the prescribed medication regimen, and symptoms requiring medical attention (see Box 39-9).

Evaluation

Evaluation is based on the identified patient outcomes. Questions to consider may include the following:
1. Has injury from falls been prevented?
2. Does the patient ask for assistance in ambulating if dizziness is present or if vertigo is imminent?
3. Have signs of anxiety decreased?
4. Does the patient know the nature of the disorder, the medication regimen, and what to do if an attack occurs?

5. Does the patient plan for ongoing medical supervision?

HEARING LOSS

Most ear disorders interfere with hearing to a lesser or greater extent. Inflammations may plug the ear canal or fill the middle ear with fluid, interfering with transmission of sound waves. If the ossicles become fixed, they are less able to transmit the sound vibrations. Inner ear disorders also interfere with the sound vibrations reaching the organ of Corti. Growth of acoustic neuromas places pressure on the cochlear division of the eighth cranial nerve.

Implications of Impaired Hearing

More than 21 million persons in the United States have some kind of hearing impairment. Of these persons, 90.8 per 1000 have hearing impairments and 7.5 per 1000 are deaf in both ears. People with hearing impairments often have less desirable jobs and lower incomes than those without hearing impairments. It is estimated that the group of people with hearing impairments has an annual loss of earnings that totals $1.25 billion.[10]

Hearing is as important as speech in our daily lives. Sound helps keep us in touch with reality and our environment; it adds esthetic pleasure, as well as warnings of danger, to our world. The sense of hearing is critical to normal development and maintenance of speech. Infants learn to speak by imitating others and listening to the sounds they make in relationship to the sounds of others. Congenitally deaf persons lack aural stimulation, which affects their development of speech and conceptual ability. This severe handicap can affect both personality development and responses on intelligence tests.

As hearing diminishes, the effect of not understanding others and not being understood may make people withdraw from social situations, and they may become anxious and insecure. Fear of inadequacy and inferiority may make

Nursing Care Plan

Person with Ménière's disease

DATA: Mrs. B. is a 59-year-old schoolteacher. During the past 6 months, she has had three attacks of "whirling in space" or vertigo, fluctuating hearing in the left ear, noise or tinnitus in the left ear, nausea and vomiting, and a sense of fullness or pressure in the left ear. Two attacks have occurred during class, and one attack occurred at home, where she lives alone. Embarrassment, fear, anxiety, and uncertainty are some of her feelings. Mrs. B. made an appointment at an otology office where diagnostic tests were performed.

These tests included an audiogram, tympanometry, electronystagmography, electrocochleography, a nursing assessment, and physical examination. A diagnosis of Ménière's disease was made. A 1500 mg sodium-restricted diet, Dyazide po qd, labyrinthine compensatory exercises, and Niacin 100 mg tid were prescribed to control the incapacitating attacks of vertigo.

Nursing diagnosis: Anxiety related to effects of disorder

Expected patient outcomes	Nursing interventions	Rationale
Signs of anxiety are decreased	Encourage Mrs. B. to explore concerns about decreased hearing and effects of dizziness attacks and to take action in relation to the concern Explore Mrs. B.'s knowledge of the disorder and correct misunderstandings Encourage realistic hope about expected hearing ability as described by physician Refer Mrs. B. to necessary support services, such as social worker or audiologist	Expressing concerns and receiving realistic counseling and support reduce helplessness and apprehension

Nursing diagnosis: Sensory perception, alteration in vestibular, auditory

Expected patient outcomes	Nursing interventions	Rationale
Mrs. B. describes actions to avoid dizziness Mrs. B. interacts with others accurately	Help Mrs. B. identify avoidable actions that precipitate dizziness attacks Encourage Mrs. B. to move slowly and not turn head suddenly when dizziness is present If tinnitus is distressing, increase background noises such as music If hearing is decreased: 1. Use measures to facilitate communication with hearing impaired (see text) 2. Refer Mrs. B. to audiologist, if appropriate	Understanding cause of dizziness and measures to reduce it may lessen occurrence

Nursing diagnosis: **Injury, high risk for, trauma related to dizziness**

Expected patient outcomes	Nursing interventions	Rationale
Injury does not occur	Keep side rails up when Mrs. B. is dizzy and in bed Assist with ambulation as needed Encourage Mrs. B. to sit or lie down and to remain immobile if signs of dizziness occur Teach Mrs. B. to stop car at side of road and turn ignition off immediately at first signs of dizziness while driving	Knowledge of safety measures reduces possibility of injuries

Nursing diagnosis: **Self-care deficit, high risk for**

Expected patient outcomes	Nursing intervention	Rationale
ADL needs are met Mrs. B. functions as independently as condition permits	Provide desired foods and fluids if nausea is present Assist with hygiene as needed while encouraging independence; place hygiene supplies so that Mrs. B. does not have to turn head Provide sufficient time for ADL so Mrs. B. can move slowly	Assistance with ADL makes it possible for Mrs. B. to function independently and feel in control of situation

Nursing diagnosis: **Coping, ineffective individual**

Expected patient outcomes	Nursing intervention	Rationale
Mrs. B. identifies coping pattern and resultant effects Mrs. B. describes alternative coping behaviors	Make decisions regarding safety of Mrs. B. and others when patient is unable to do so Assist Mrs. B. to identify usual coping behaviors and the consequences of the behaviors Assist Mrs. B. to identify personal strengths Teach Mrs. B. alternative coping behaviors	Support and understanding by caregivers improve coping Discussing possible coping behaviors assists Mrs. B. to choose behaviors that are most functional for her

Nursing diagnosis: **Knowledge deficit about pathophysiology of Ménière's disease related to lack of exposure to information**

Expected patient outcomes	Nursing intervention	Rationale
Mrs. B. describes nature of disorder, therapy, and safety measures	Teach Mrs. B. about the disorder, therapy, and need for medical follow-up (see text) Teach Mrs. B. ways to protect self from injury and to prevent dizziness attacks when possible	Need for information regarding disease increases learning, which assists Mrs. B. to care for self and to live as independently as possible

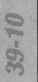

Causes of specific types of hearing loss

Conductive hearing loss—occurs when sound cannot reach cochlea

Obstruction of the external ear canal by cerumen, foreign body, etc.
Tympanic membrane perforation
Serous otitis media
Adhesive otitis
Ossicular discontinuity—trauma, infection, cholesteatoma
Tympanosclerosis
Otosclerosis
Ossicular fixation

Sensorineural hearing loss—occurs when cochlea or eighth cranial nerve is damaged

Presbycusis
Occupational hearing loss (noise-induced)
Head trauma
Drug toxicity—ototoxic drugs
Endolymphatic hydrops (Ménière's disease)
Tumor—neuroma of eighth cranial nerve
Perilymphatic leak

From DeWeese DD, Saunders WH: Textbook of otolaryngology, ed 7, St Louis, Mosby–Year Book, 1988.

them suspicious and depressed. When hearing is completely gone, they may find the silent world almost intolerable.

People who are hard of hearing or deaf are not easily recognized; they appear quite normal. When they fail to respond or respond inappropriately to oral communication, their actions are interpreted as slow or odd, and the speaker may withdraw. This withdrawal response of others may be perceived as rejection by the aurally handicapped person and may further increase isolation and withdrawal. The person who is hard of hearing or deaf may experience varying degrees of stress, depending on personality, the extent and type of loss, the age at onset of loss, and the reaction of family and friends to the loss of hearing.

Older adults with hearing impairment may suffer from reduced interpersonal communication, social isolation, depression, reduced mobility, and exacerbation of coexisting psychiatric conditions.[10]

The Americans With Disabilities Act, which President Bush signed in 1990, should improve job opportunities for persons with impaired hearing. The law ensures that employers cannot discriminate against qualified individuals with disabilities. The act is discussed in greater detail in Chapter 14.

Classification of Hearing Loss
Conductive hearing loss

Any interference with conduction of sound impulses through the *external ear canal*, the *eardrum*, or the *middle ear produces a conductive hearing loss*. The inner ear is not involved and sound amplification will reach the inner ear.

Causes of conductive hearing loss are listed in Box 39-10.

The external auditory canal can be obstructed by cerumen, foreign bodies in the canal, tumors, and swelling from infection. The most common cause is impacted cerumen.

Damage to the eardrum and middle ear can be caused by thickening (tympanosclerosis), scarring, perforation, or retraction of the ear drum. In the middle ear, hearing loss is caused by the presence of liquid (pus, serum, or blood), absence or increase in mobility of the ossicles (tympanosclerosis or otosclerosis), adhesions, tumors, or dislocated or absent ossicles (congenital or acquired).[6]

Otosclerosis is the most common cause of conductive hearing loss in people between the ages of 15 and 50 years. It is a hereditary condition of unknown cause, and it is more common in whites. About 10% of whites have otosclerosis on postmortem examination. Women are affected more than men. Hearing loss may first be noticed in the late teens or early twenties. It may progress more rapidly during or after pregnancy, but no causal relationship has been established for this. If cochlear function is normal or near normal, the hearing loss can be improved by microsurgery with a stapedectomy and replacement with a prosthesis or by a stapedotomy alone.[6]

Sensorineural hearing loss

Sensorineural hearing loss results from damage to the cochlea or the eighth cranial nerve. It can be present at birth (hereditary deafness) or develop later in life. The hearing loss may result from a known disorder (see Box 39-10), it can be a functional hearing loss (no organic cause), or it may be the result of aging (presbycusis). Hearing loss may fluctuate initially, but further progressive hearing loss occurs. Most disorders of the inner ear produce some hearing loss, and a characteristic of severe loss is the inability to discriminate words. Amplification of sounds often causes sound distortion and increases the hearing problem.

Cochlear implants are now available for persons with complete hearing loss. An external device consisting of a small computer changes spoken words to electrical impulses. The impulses are transmitted across the skin to an implanted coil that carries the impulses to an electrode inserted through the round window into the cochlea (Fig. 39-9). Single channel implants are available, but newer multichannel implants that increase speech discrimination are being employed.

Other types of hearing loss

Mixed hearing loss is a combination of both sensorineural and conductive hearing loss. Both elements of air and bone conduction hearing loss occur.

Central hearing loss is a form of sensorineural hearing loss resulting from some type of damage to the brain's auditory pathways or auditory center, such as with a cerebral vascular accident. Sounds may be conducted normally through the ear to the neural pathways, but the person is deaf.

Presbycusis is the term used to describe hearing loss associated with aging. The degenerative changes in this type of hearing loss are similar to the degenerative changes occurring in other body tissues. In many cases, there is

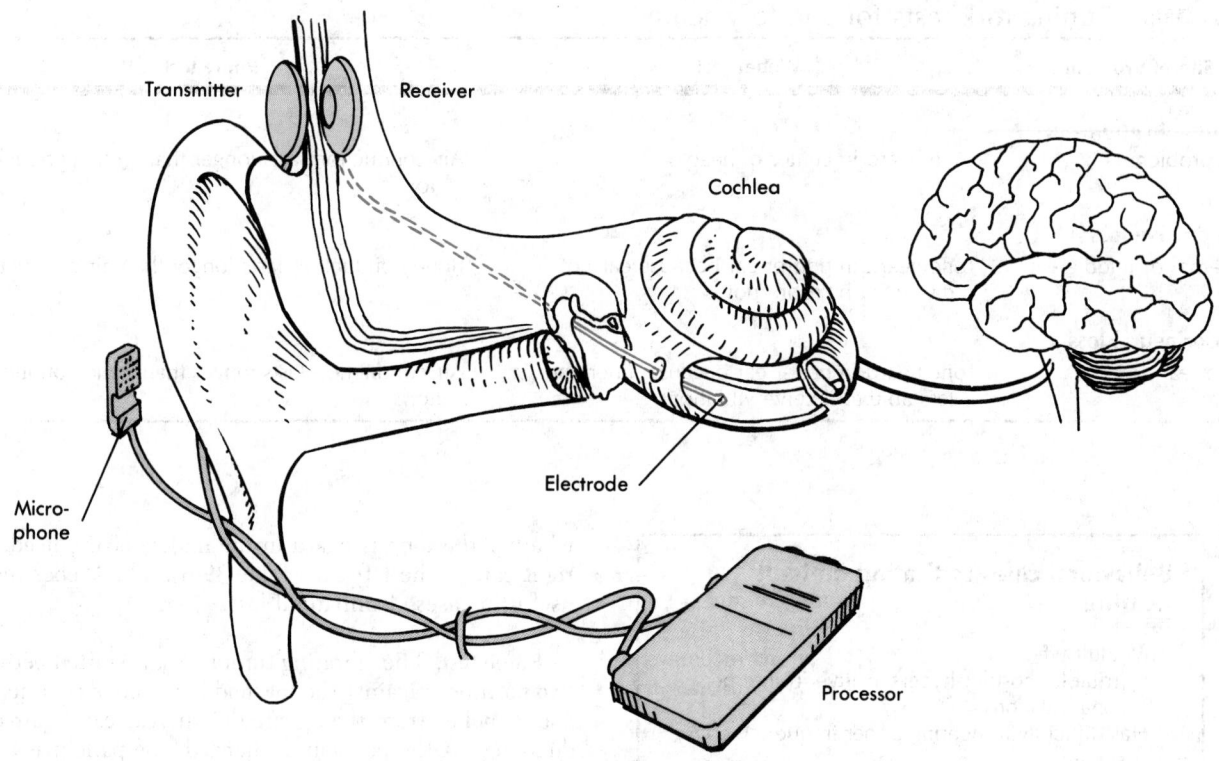

Fig. 39-9 Cochlear implant.

atrophy of the ganglion cells in the cochlea or changes in the basilar membrane. Presbycusis accounts for the majority of neurosensory hearing loss in the elderly. There are three major characteristics of presbycusis: (1) gradual progressive development, (2) loss of higher frequencies, manifested by loss of discrimination in noise, and (3) a narrow range of tolerance to sound intensity. There is no treatment for presbycusis, but hearing can be improved by hearing aids.[6]

Presbycusis becomes increasingly common after age 50. It is reported in 23% of people between ages 65 and 74, 33% of people aged 75 to 84, and 48% of people 85 and older. These figures are believed to underestimate the number of persons affected. When the older person also has a visual problem, it impairs his or her ability to use visual cues for speech-reading and further exacerbates the hearing impairment.[10]

Nursing Process
Assessment

The extent of assessment of auditory acuity by nurses depends on the nurse's preparation and focus of care. All nurses, however, should be prepared to carry out an inspection of the outer ear and at least a gross assessment of hearing ability for all persons entering a health care setting, regardless of the presenting problem. Gross assessment of hearing may be accomplished by evaluating the logical sequences of replies the patient makes during the admission history. One method is to turn one's head away from the individual when asking a simple question that cannot be answered by a yes or no response.

Subjective data

If the person has been identified as having hearing loss, the following data are obtained:
1. Onset, nature and progression of the hearing loss
2. Noticed differences in hearing in right or left ear
3. Family history of hearing loss
4. Presence of other ear symptoms: pressure or pain in ears (middle ear), or ringing in ears or dizziness (inner ear)
5. History of head trauma or exposure to noise (past, present)
6. Current medications with known ototoxic effects (See Box 39-3, p. 1332)
7. Any neurologic symptoms, including visual or speech disorders

Objective data

The person who begins to have difficulty hearing usually demonstrates some behavioral clues indicating that hearing is decreased (see Box 39-11). Persons who exhibit any of these behavioral clues should have their ears examined by an otolaryngologist, who will perform a complete evaluation.

Auditory acuity

Each ear must be tested separately to estimate the hearing. One of the patient's ears is occluded with a finger. While standing 1 to 2 feet away, the nurse whispers two-syllable numbers softly toward the unoccluded ear, and the patient is asked to repeat the numbers. The intensity of the nurses voice can be increased from a soft, medium, or

Table 39-6 Tuning fork tests for auditory acuity

Site of problem	Weber test	Rinne test
Normal hearing		
No problem	Tone heard in center of head	Air conduction lasts longer than bone conduction.
Conductive loss		
External or middle ear	Tone heard in poorer ear because ear not distracted by room noise	Bone conduction lasts longer than air conduction
Sensorineural loss		
Inner ear	Tone heard in better ear because inner ear less able to receive vibrations[1]	Air conduction lasts longer than bone conduction.

39-11

Behavioral clues indicating difficult hearing

Any adult who
  Is irritable, hostile, hypersensitive in interpersonal relations
  Has difficulty in hearing upper frequency consonants
  Complains about people mumbling
  Turns up the volume on television
  Asks for frequent repetition and answers questions inappropriately
  Loses sense of humor; becomes grim
  Leans forward to hear better; face serious and strained
  Shuns large- and small-group audience situations
  May appear aloof and "stuck-up"
  Complains of ringing in the ears
  Has an unusually soft or loud voice
  Repeatedly states, "What did you say?"

---

loud whisper to a soft, medium, or loud voice. If the nurse suspects that the patient is speech-reading, the nurse's face should be turned away. The patient is asked if hearing is better in one ear than in the other ear. If the auditory acuity is different, the ear that hears better should be tested first. Then noise is produced in the better-hearing ear by rapidly but gently moving the finger in the patient's ear canal while testing the other ear.

A watch tick can also be used to test hearing. However, a watch tick is a higher-pitched sound and less relevant to functional hearing than the voice test.

The tuning fork also provides a general estimate of hearing loss. The three major tuning fork tests date from the nineteenth century and are named after their originators: Weber, Rinne, and Schwabach.

Weber test. The tuning fork is set into vibration by striking the tines on the examiner's knuckles or knee. The rounded tip of the handle is placed on the patient's forehead or teeth. Placement on the teeth (even if the patient has false teeth) is generally more reliable. The patient is asked whether the tone is heard in the middle of the head, the right ear, or the left ear (Table 39-6). The Weber test is useful in cases of unilateral loss.

Rinne test. The vibrating tuning fork is shifted between two positions: against the mastoid bone (bone conduction) and 2 inches from the opening of the ear canal (air conduction). As the position is changed, the patient is asked to indicate which tone is louder (in front of the ear or behind the ear) or is asked to indicate when one of the tones is no longer heard (Table 39-6). The Rinne test is useful to differentiate between conductive and sensorineural hearing losses.

With conductive hearing loss, the pathways of normal sound conduction are blocked. However, vibrations against the mastoid bone can bypass the obstruction; therefore bone conduction lasts longer than air conduction. With sensorineural hearing loss, the acoustic nerve has decreased ability to perceive vibrations from either route; therefore normal patterns are reported by the patient.

Schwabach test. This test is also used to differentiate between a conductive and sensorineural hearing loss. The Schwabach test compares the hearing of the examiner (who must have normal hearing) with the patient. However, the Rinne test has replaced this test.

These aforementioned tests can be performed at the bedside by the nurse to give some indication of the amount of hearing. More elaborate and specific hearing tests are performed in a soundproof room.

Audiometric testing

Functional examination for sensitivity (ability to hear sounds) and for speech discrimination (ability to distinguish different speech sounds) is done by audiometry. The graph of the hearing levels of both of these is called an *audiogram. Hearing threshold is defined as the lowest intensity of sound at which an auditory stimulus can be heard.*

Audiologists (specialists in administering hearing tests) have developed audiometric tests to determine not only whether a hearing loss is present, but also the frequency of the loss, how well the person can understand speech, and whether the problem site is in the middle ear (con-

Table 39-7   Types of audiometric testing

Test	Method	Use
Pure-tone audiometry	Person wears earphone; signals when sound is heard	General screening to identify persons requiring further testing
Impedance audiometry	Probe inserted in ear canal; measurements of middle ear pressure are obtained; does not require response from person	Assess presence or absence of abnormality of conductive mechanism of middle ear
Speech audiometry	Speech reception threshold: lowest intensity level in decibels at which person can correctly repeat selected bisyllabic words 50% of time; also a test of speech discrimination	Determine how well person can hear and understand speech
Electrocochleography; evoked-response audiometry	Response on EEG recording to clicks played to ear	Determine if central (brain) portion of hearing is intact or determine location of the lesion interfering with the transmission of sound
Tuning fork tests	Identification of sound made by tuning forks placed on head	Test hearing acuity and discriminate conductive vs. sensorineural hearing losses

ductive loss), or inner ear or auditory nerve system (sensorineural loss) (Table 39-7).

Pure-tone audiometry must be performed in a specially constructed soundproof booth for best results. To test the sound intensity by air conduction, persons wear earphones and are instructed to signal (usually with a finger) when they first hear the tone and when they no longer hear it. The middle frequencies are tested first, and the operator alternately increases and decreases the intensity of the sound until the dial setting is found at which the person being tested can just perceive sound (threshold). In audiometric testing the frequencies 125, 250, 500, 1000, 2000, 4000, and 8000 Hz are commonly employed to assess the hearing sensitivity of an individual.

Hearing loss is identified as the number of decibels reached before the person hears the sound for each specific frequency. Zero loudness is calibrated for that sound barely heard by a person with normal hearing. Up to 20 db loss is considered to be within the normal range.

Data analysis: nursing diagnoses

Nursing diagnoses are determined from analysis of patient data. Possible nursing diagnoses for the hard-of-hearing person may include, but are not limited to, the following:

Diagnostic title	Possible etiologies
Sensory/perceptual alteration: auditory	Altered sensory transmission from loss of hearing
Knowledge deficit	Lack of exposure/recall, information misinterpretation about hearing
Coping, ineffective individual	Situational crises, personal vulnerability

Planning: expected patient outcomes

Expected patient outcomes for the person who is hard of hearing may include, but are not limited to, the following:
1. Patient indicates by facial expression, gestures, or answers that oral communications are heard
2. Patient can explain:
   a. The basis for the hearing loss and any appropriate therapy
   b. Care of hearing aid, if appropriate
   c. Available community resources

3. Patient exhibits coping ability by actively seeking aural rehabilitation appropriate to level of hearing loss

Implementation
Interventions to achieve patient outcomes

Activities for the hearing impaired person include facilitation of communication and aural rehabilitation. It is not uncommon for persons who are beginning to lose their hearing to deny that changes are occurring and that an evaluation of hearing and follow-up of rehabilitative methods are important. Much support and encouragement to explore methods to improve hearing may be necessary.

Facilitating communication

Specific actions to facilitate hearing or speech-reading for persons with impaired hearing are listed in Box 39-12.

Additional activities can be used if the person is hospitalized. Patients are helped to use visual cues by placing them in a bed where they can observe activity and anticipate others approaching them. They will be easily startled if people suddenly enter the unit if the vision is obscured. Because hearing-impaired persons are often sensitive to light changes, they can easily be awakened by turning on a light. Many patients feel less isolated if the nurse touches them lightly on the arm to gain attention and wakes them by touching them on the arm. Special efforts must be made to communicate information about hospital routines and diagnostic tests.

Promoting aural rehabilitation

If hearing loss is irreversible or not amenable to surgical intervention or if the person elects not to have surgery, aural rehabilitation may increase communication. The purpose of aural rehabilitation is to maximize the hearing-impaired person's communication skills.

The auditory sense is our primary mode of communication, and rehabilitation is directed toward teaching the person more effective use of the senses of vision, touch, and vibration plus maximizing the use of any remaining hearing ability. Rehabilitation is affected by the person's

Facilitating communication for persons with impaired hearing

1. Get the person's attention by raising an arm or hand.
2. Stand with a light on your face; this helps the person speech read. Do not stand with your back against a window.
3. Face the person when speaking.
4. Speak clearly, but do not overaccentuate words.
5. Speak in a normal tone; do not shout. Shouting overemploys normal speaking movements and may cause distortion and be too loud for the person with sensorineural damage. If the person has conductive loss only, sometimes making the voice louder without shouting is helpful.
6. If the person does not seem to understand what is said, express it differently. Some words are difficult to "see" in speech reading, such as *white* or *red*.
7. Move closer to the person and toward the better ear if the person does not hear you.
8. Write out proper names or any statement that you are not sure was understood.
9. Do not smile, chew gum, or cover the mouth when talking to a person with limited hearing.
10. Observe for inattention that may indicate tiredness or lack of understanding.
11. Use phrases to convey meaning rather than one-word answers. State the major topic of the discussion first and then give details.
12. Do not show annoyance by careless facial expression. Persons who are hard of hearing depend more on visual clues for acceptance.
13. Encourage the use of a hearing aid if the person has one; allow the person to adjust it before speaking.
14. If in a group, repeat important statements and avoid asides to others in the group.
15. Avoid the use of the intercommunication system as this may distort sound and cause poor communication.
16. Do not avoid conversation with a person who has hearing loss.

Modified from Conover M, Cober J: *Nurs Clin North Am* 5:497, 1970.

Table 39-8   Types of hearing aids

Type	Effective for hearing loss (db)	Placement
Postauricular aid	25-80	Behind ear
In-the-ear aid	25-55	Totally in ear canal (least noticeable)
Eyeglass aid	25-70	In eyeglass temple
Body-worn aid	40-110	Placed in a shirt or specially made pocket (most powerful)

auditory training exercises is to help the person concentrate on the speaker. For some persons, only gross differences between sounds may be recognized.

Speech reading is the current term used for lip reading and is an important means of communication. Speech training is the process of understanding vocal communication by the integration of lip movements with facial expressions, gestures, environmental clues, and conversation contexts. Speech reading is very difficult, however, without auditory cues. Many movements for speech are very rapid, many sounds are very similar (b, m, p), and certain sounds of any language are invisible (the h in English). The hearing impaired person must guess at a high percentage of the words. Knowledge of this fact alone will help the nurse be more understanding of the person who is speech (lip) reading.

Because of reduced auditory feedback (the inability of hearing-impaired persons to monitor their own speech) the clearness, pitch quality, or rate of their speech may deteriorate. These abnormal effects alter the efficiency of communication and reduce the intelligibility of speech. *The goal of speech training is to conserve, develop, or prevent deterioration of speech skills.*

Hearing aids. Hearing aids are instruments made up of miniature parts working together as a system to amplify sound in a controlled manner. They are used by both hard of-hearing persons (slight or moderate hearing loss) and deaf persons (severe or profound hearing loss). *Hearing aids make sound louder* but *do not improve the ability to hear.* Therefore persons with decreased discrimination (the ability to understand what is spoken) benefit less from a hearing aid. Appropriate aural rehabilitation will ensure successful adjustment of most problems. The hearing aid amplifies all background noises such as hospital machinery, footsteps, and department store noises, as well as speech. These noises may mask conversation or confuse the hearing-impaired person, especially the elderly.

Types of hearing aids. Hearing aids vary according to size and location to be worn (see Table 39-8). Regardless of the type of aid, the hearing aid consists of the following parts:
1. Microphone to receive sound waves from the air and change sounds into electrical signals
2. Amplifier to increase the strength of electrical signals
3. Battery to provide the electrical energy needed to operate the hearing aid

background and by the severity of impairment. As with other forms of rehabilitation, success depends on the degree of the patient's motivation.

Types of aural rehabilitation. Aural rehabilitation includes *auditory training, speech reading, speech training,* and the *use of hearing aids.* The use of instruments and training are involved. *Auditory training* is an approach to enhance listening skills. The hearing-impaired person is initially exposed to gross differences in sound and then gradually "fine tuned" so that subtle differences in discrimination of two similar sounds can be made. The primary purpose of

Assessment

1. Assess all elderly for hearing loss of high-pitched sounds, sensitivity to background noise, loss of sibilant consonants, and use of hearing aids.
2. Assess function of hearing aid and identify availability of extra batteries.

Intervention

1. Modify communication skills when speaking to person with hearing impairment:
   a. Face person with light on your face.
   b. Get person's attention. Touch lightly on arm, if necessary.
   c. Speak slowly and distinctly but do not exaggerate lip movements.
   d. Use short phrases and punctuate with body language.
   e. Be aware that vision may also be diminished.
2. Place a note at nurses' station intercom that patient is hard of hearing.
3. Post a sign at bedside alerting personnel that patient is hard of hearing.
4. Try to obtain pocket amplifier for patient if hearing aid is not available.
5. Determine if patient sees otologist regularly so that ears are checked for wax.

Common disorders in elderly
Presbycusis

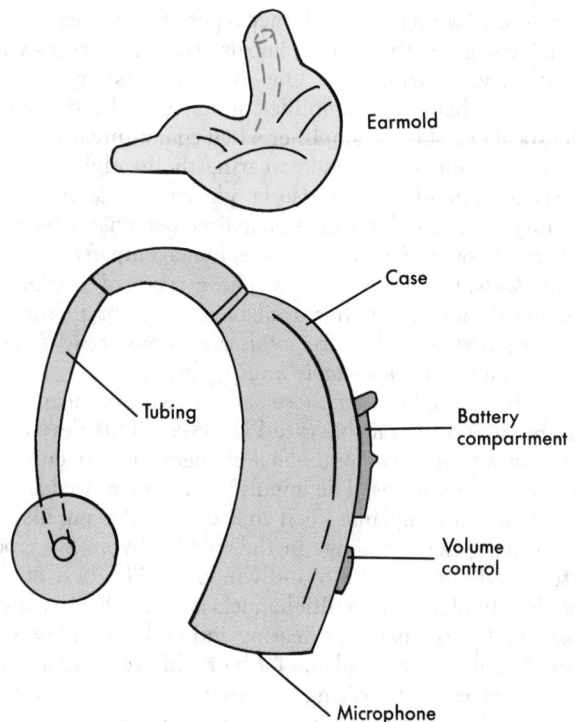

Fig. 39-10 Parts of a hearing aid.

39-13

Care of a hearing aid

1. Turn the hearing aid off when not in use.
2. Open the battery compartment at night to avoid accidental drainage of the battery.
3. Keep an extra battery available at all times.
4. Wash the earmold frequently (daily if necessary) with mild soap and warm water with the use of a pipe cleaner to cleanse the cannula.
5. Dry the earmold completely before reconnecting it to the receiver.
6. Do not wear the hearing aid during an ear infection.

39-14

What to do if hearing aid fails to work

1. Check the on-off switch.
2. Inspect the earmold for cleanliness.
3. Examine the battery for correct insertion.
4. Examine cord plug for correct insertion.
5. Examine cord for breaks.
6. Replace battery, cord, or both, if necessary. The life of batteries varies according to amount of use and power requirements of the aid. Batteries last from 2 to 14 days.
7. Check the position of the earmold in the ear. If the hearing aid "whistles," the earmold is probably not inserted properly into the ear canal, or the person needs to have a new earmold made.

4. Receiver (loudspeaker) to change the electrical signals back into sound waves

On all types of hearing aids but the body-worn type, all four components are housed in one small case. The louder sounds are then directed into the ear through a custom-fitted earmold (Fig. 39-10).

Assisting the person with a hearing aid. The person with a hearing aid should know how to care for the aid (see Box 39-13) and what to do if the aid does not work (see Box 39-14). The nurse must also have a basic knowledge of the hearing aid to assist the person unable or unwilling to care

for the aid when ill. The person is encouraged to use the hearing aid and to store it safely in its case when it is not in use.

Persons who are reluctant to wear their hearing aids (often for cosmetic reasons) need counseling about the benefits of wearing the aid and the improvements in their ability to speak more distinctly. The aid may also serve to notify others to speak more distinctly. When a person with a hearing aid is hospitalized, it is important to encourage use of the aid during hospitalization and its safe storage when not in use.

Assistive hearing devices. Other types of technologies are available to assist the hearing-impaired or deaf persons who do not have hearing aids. One type of assistive hearing device is a hand-held amplifier attached to headphones. The speaker holds the amplifier when communicating with the hearing-impaired person wearing the headphones.

Special amplifiers can also be placed in telephones to magnify the sound for hearing-impaired persons; these amplifiers are obtained from the telephone company.

Implantable hearing devices. Three types of implanted hearing devices are either available for use or in the investigation stage. They are *cochlear implants, bone hearing devices,* and *semi-implantable hearing devices.*

Cochlear implants for those patients with no hearing at all are currently available (see Fig. 39-9). This device incorporates a small computer that changes the spoken word to electrical impulses. The impulses are transmitted across the skin to an implanted coil that carries the impulse to the hearing nerve endings in the cochlea by an electrode introduced through the round windows. The best of the cochlear implants use multichannels and are able to return about half of the patient's hearing and understanding. Cochlear implants are available for both children and adults.

In some cases of hearing loss, sound can be transmitted through the skull to the inner ear. Patients with a conductive hearing loss can use a device in which the receiver is implanted under the skin into the skull. The external device transmits the sound through the skin. This device is worn above the ear and not in the ear canal.

Patients who already use a hearing aid will gain the most from the implantable device. Clinical research has shown that a magnet implanted in the middle ear can be stimulated by an ear canal driver that changes sound to a magnetic force. This system eliminates several bothersome problems of hearing aids, such as feedback and difficulties with hearing in noisy environments. A semiimplantable hearing device is the first step to a totally implantable device that would eliminate any external device. However, many challenges have yet to be met before a workable device is available.

Referring to special services

Special services for persons with a hearing loss are offered by audiology clinics sponsored by universities, hospitals, community programs, local or state departments of health, or the Veteran's Administration, National organizations available to give information and counseling include the following:

1. American Academy of Otolaryngology—Head and Neck Surgeons, 1 Prince St., Alexandria, VA, a professional society for physicians specializing in diseases of the ear and related areas; it can provide information on hearing and balance disorders.
2. American Annals of the Deaf, 5034 Wisconsin Ave., NW, Washington, DC 20016. The April issue every year lists a directory of programs and services for the deaf available by state and includes information about the type of facilities.
3. American Federation of the Physically Handicapped, Inc., 1370 National Press Building, Washington, DC 20004; provides counseling and information.
4. American Speech-Language-Hearing Association, 10801 Rockville Pike, Dept AP, Rockville, MD 20852. This association can answer questions or mail information on hearing aids or hearing loss and communication problems in the elderly and provide a list of certified audiologists in each state.
5. Gallaudet College, 7th and Florida Ave, Washington, DC 20002; the only liberal arts college for the deaf in the world.
6. National Association of Hearing and Speech Agencies, 919 18th St NW, Washington, DC 20006; provides counseling and information.
7. Office of Scientific and Health Reports, National Institute of Neurological and Communicative Disorders and Stroke Bldg 31, Rm 8A06, Bethesda, MD 20205; a focal point for research on hearing loss and other communication disorders. (Pamphlet: Hearing loss: hope through research.)
8. Self-Help for Hard-of-Hearing People (Shhh), 4848 Battery Lane, Dept E, Bethesda, MD 20814; a nationwide organization for the hard-of-hearing; publishes a bimonthly magazine that includes experiences of the hard-of-hearing and new developments in the field of hearing loss; publications and reprints available.
9. Society of Otorhinolaryngology and Head–Neck Nurses, Inc., 439 N Causeway, New Smyrna Beach, FL 32069; a professional nursing society for nurses specializing in caring for patients with problems of the ear, nose, or throat; information on hearing and balance disorders.
10. State Office of Vocational Rehabilitation (in each state); provides vocational training and placement services.
11. Veterans Administration; provides audiology clinics and rehabilitation services for veterans.

Evaluation

Evaluation is based on expected patient outcomes. Questions to consider may include the following:

1. Does the person respond appropriately during interactions?
2. Does the person know (1) the nature of the disorder, (2) care of the hearing aid (if worn), and (3) where to seek appropriate assistance?
3. Has the person obtained appropriate aural rehabilitation?

SUMMARY

1. Sound reaches the inner ear by air conduction through the ear canal and ossicles of the middle ear and by bone conduction through the skull bones to the inner ear. In the cochlea of the inner ear the sound waves are transformed into neural energy and transmitted to the brain for interpretation.
2. Balance is affected by changes in the inner ear involving the semicircular canals, the eighth cranial nerve, and the vestibular nuclei.
3. Disorders that plug the outer ear, add fluid to the middle ear, make the ossicles unmovable, destroy the hair cells of the organ or Corti, or interfere with nerve stimulus transmission over the acoustic nerve will lead to decreased hearing.
4. Hearing can be preserved by preventing infection or trauma of the ear, by using ototoxic drugs with caution and seeking medical attention if symptoms occur, and by preventing frequent exposure to loud noises (or using ear protection for constant loud noises).
5. Ear infections are the most common disorders of the external and middle ears; pain results from pressure by fluid buildup within the enclosed spaces.
6. Serous otitis media develops from collection of serous fluid in the middle ear when the eustachian tube becomes blocked. Purulent otitis media develops from bacteria entering the middle ear through the eustachian tube; pus collects in the middle ear.
7. Ear infections are treated with antibiotics, given by eardrops, by ear ointments, or systemically. Treatments to remove drainage may include ear wash, ear irrigation, or surgery of the eardrum.
8. The person with an ear infection should avoid getting water in the ear (care during showering and shampooing and avoiding swimming).
9. Vertigo is the primary symptom of disorders (such as labyrinthitis, Ménière's disease, acoustic neuroma) affecting the statokinetic system. Tinnitus (ringing in the ears) often accompanies vertigo. Potential for injury is a major problem for the person with vertigo.
10. The uncomfortable sensation of vertigo can be minimized by lying down and holding the head absolutely still.
11. Most ear surgeries are microsurgeries performed through the ear canal. After surgery, hearing will be temporarily decreased because of the swelling and ear packing; crackling noises may be heard. The patient is instructed postoperatively to avoid actions that may increase intraaural pressure or that may lead to infection.
12. Conductive hearing loss, a problem of decreased amplification, is the result of problems of the external or middle ear; it responds well to aural rehabilitation. Otosclerosis (immobility of the ossicles) produces conductive hearing loss.
13. Sensorineural hearing loss results from interference with hearing in the inner ear or neural pathways; it may result from a known disorder or be idiopathic.
14. Presbycusis (hearing loss resulting from aging) is a form of sensorineural hearing loss. The hearing loss is primarily that of sound discrimination, and amplification may further distort the sound.
15. Aural rehabilitation includes the use of hearing aids or other assistive hearing devices, auditory training (improving listening skills), speech-reading (lipreading), or speech training (improving speech clarity).

REFERENCES AND SELECTED READINGS

1. Alberti PW, Ruben RJ, editors: *Otologic medicine and surgery,* vol 1, New York, 1988, Churchill Livingstone.
2. Alberti PW, Ruben RJ, editors: *Otologic medicine and surgery,* vol 2, New York, 1988, Churchill Livingstone.
3. Bates B: *A guide to physical examination,* ed 4, Philadelphia, 1987, JB Lippincott.
4. Bulechek GM, McCloskey JC: *Nursing interventions, treatments for nursing diagnosis,* Philadelphia, 1985, WB Saunders.
5.* DeBlase R, Kucler M: Assistive hearing device aids patient-staff communication, *Geriatr Nurs* 6:223-224, 1985.
6. DeWeese DD, Saunders WH: *Textbook of otolaryngology,* ed 7, St Louis, Mosby–Year Book, 1988.
7. Fairbanks DNF: *Antimicrobial therapy in otolaryngology–head neck surgery,* ed 5, Washington, DC, 1989, AAO-HNS Foundation.
8. Fountain D: Hearing aids and their care, *Geriatr Nurs Home Care* 7(2)12-14, 1987.
9. Gardner G: Ménière's disease. In Rakel RE, editor: *Conn's current therapy 1990,* Philadelphia, 1990, WB Saunders.
10. Healthy People 2000: *National health promotion and disease prevention objectives,* US Dept of Health and Human Services, Public Health Services, Washington, DC, 1990, Government Printing Office.
11.* Jackson J: Don't shout nurse!: hearing problems in the elderly, *Geriatr Nurs* (Oxford) 6(3):12-13, 1986.
12. Lee JC: Deafness: the next ten years, *J Rehab* 51(4):79-83, 1985.
13.* Levene B: Sorry nurse, I can hear you but I can't understand you, *Nurs 85* (Oxford) 2(41):1221-1225, 1985.
14. Mitchell VL: Cochlear implantation: a nursing perspective, *J Soc Otorhinolaryngol Head Neck Nurs* 5(2):11-15, 1987.
15. Reiner A: *Manual of patient care standards,* Rockville, Md, 1988, Aspen Publishers.
16. Plan of the National Institute on Deafness and Other Communication Disorders, Bethesda, Md, 1989, Institute of Health.
17. Riley MAK: *Nursing care of the client with ear, nose and throat disorders,* New York, 1987, Springer Publishing.
18.* Rubin W: Noise-induced deafness: major environmental problem, *Hosp Med* 23(7):19-21, 25-27, 1987.
19. Serra AM, Bailey CM, Jackson P: *Ear, nose and throat nursing,* England, 1986, Blackwell Scientific Publications.
20. Tortora ML: Noise-induced hearing loss: prevention in the work environment, *AAOHN J* 35:271-273, 1987.
21. Wolfson RJ, et al: Vertigo, *Clin Sympt* 38(6):2-32, 1986.

Classic

22. Becker G, Nadler G: The aged deaf: integration of a disabled group into an agency serving elderly people, *Gerontologist* 20:214-221, 1980.
23. Berger KW: *The hearing aid: its operation and development,* ed 3, Livonia, Mich, 1984, The National Hearing Aid Society.
24.* Caruso VG: When the patient has otitis externa, *Geriatrics* 35(5):35-42, 1980.

---

* Recommended for student reading.

25. Chung DY, Gannon RP: Hearing loss due to noise trauma, *J Laryngol Otol* 94:419-423, 1980.
26. Conklin JM, Subtelny JD: Effect of speech training upon speech-reading in hearing-impaired adults, *Am Ann Deaf* 125:442-448, 1980.
27.* Connolly P: Growing up with deafness, *Comm Outlook* 9:290-293, 1980.
28.* Conover M, Cober J: Understanding and caring for the hearing impaired, *Nurs Clin North Am* 5:497-506, 1970.
29. Heller BR, Baynor EB: Hearing loss and aural rehabilitation of the elderly, *Top Clin Nurs* 31(1):21-29, 1981.
30.* Holder L: Hearing aids: handle with care, *Nurs 82* 12(4):64-67, 1982.
31.* Holm C: Deafness: common misunderstandings, *Am J Nurs* 78:1910-1912, 1978.
32. Holm C: How to test your patient's hearing acuity, *Nurs 80* 10(7):60-61, 1980.
33. Hughes GB: *Textbook of clinical otology*, New York, 1985, Thieme-Stratton.
34. Kamenir S, Fothersill R: Hands-on-skill for dealing with hearing aids, *Cancer Nurs* 78(11):44-45, 1982.
35.* Koch KJ: The deaf and hard of hearing: some hints, *Nurs Times* 77(32):Suppl 19-20, 1981.
36. Malkiewicz J: The fine art of giving a physical: how to assess the ears and test hearing acuity, *RN* 45(3):56-63, 1982.
37.* Mamaril AP: Sudden deafness, *Am J Nurs* 76:1992-1994, 1976.
38. McCormick GP, et al: Artificial speech devices, *Am J Nurs* 82:121-122, 1982.
39. Moore JC: Establishment of an outpatient ENT clinic, *AORN J* 31:620-626, 1980.
40.* Programmed instruction: patient assessment: examination of the ear, *Am J Nurs* 75:457-476, 1975.
41. Tortorelli B: Acoustic neuroma: an overview of the disorder and nursing care of these patients, *J Neurosurg Nurs* 6:170-171, August 1981.
42. Voke J: Aspects of hearing, physiology of the ear. Part 1, *Nurs Time* 80(33):28-30, Aug 15-21, 1984.
43. Voke J: Aspects of hearing, functions of the cochlea, Part II, *Nurs Time* 80(34):60-62, Aug 22-28, 1984.
44. Wilson WR, Nadol JR: *Quick reference to ear, nose and throat disorders*, Philadelphia, 1983, JB Lippincott.

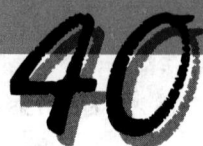

The Patient with Musculoskeletal Disorders

Wilma J. Phipps

After studying this chapter, the learner should be able to:

- Describe three measures to prevent musculoskeletal dysfunction.
- Describe four conservative health measures for persons with joint and muscle disorders.
- Describe the pathophysiologic changes and therapy for rheumatoid arthritis, SLE, degenerative joint disorders, and scoliosis.
- Describe the nursing care of the patient undergoing a total hip or total knee replacement.
- Discuss the care of the patient undergoing spinal fusion.
- Identify different types of fractures and their treatment.
- Explain the pathophysiology of bone healing.
- Describe problems that may occur with immobilization.
- Describe care of the patient after closed and open reduction of hip fractures (including cast care and traction).

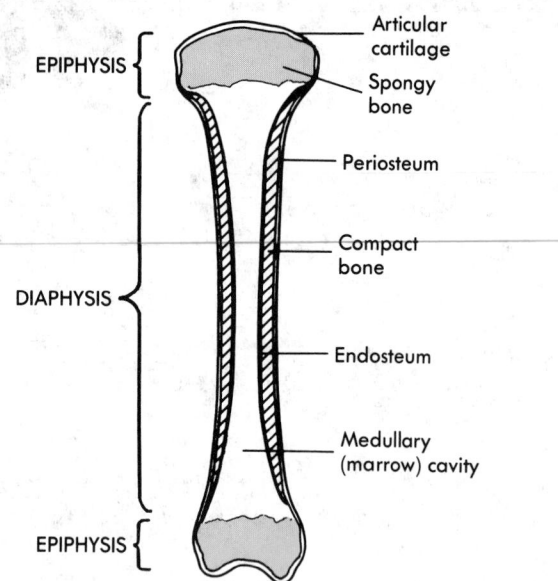

EPIPHYSIS
Articular cartilage
Spongy bone
Periosteum
Compact bone
DIAPHYSIS
Endosteum
Medullary (marrow) cavity
EPIPHYSIS

Fig. 40-1   Structure of long bone as seen in longitudinal section.

ANATOMY AND PHYSIOLOGY

Among the characteristics that distinguish man as a species is the ability to maintain an erect posture and to move about. The individual's posture and movements depend on the proper functioning of the musculoskeletal system. The *musculoskeletal system* is composed of bones, muscles, cartilage, ligaments, tendons, fascia, bursae, and joints.

Components of the Musculoskeletal System
Bones

Bones are composed of both living cells and nonliving intracellular material. They are derived from embryonic hyaline cartilage that undergoes *osteogenesis* to become bone. This process is accomplished by cells called *osteoblasts*. The hard quality of the bone is the result of the deposits of calcium salts.

The functions of the bones are as follows:
1. *Support* body tissues and provide the skeletal framework of the body
2. *Protect* body organs (for example, the bony casing of the skull protects the brain)
3. Provide for *movement* (muscles are attached for contraction and motion)
4. Be a *storehouse* for mineral salts (for example, calcium)
5. Provide for *hematopoiesis* (formation of red blood cells in red bone marrow)

Bones are classified into four groups according to their shape:
1. *Long bones* (femur, humerus) consist of a shaft and two epiphyses (see Fig. 40-1). The shaft is formed mainly of *compact* bone tissue. The epiphyses are formed from spongy (cancellous or trabecular) bone. Trabecular bone provides strength to bone while reducing its weight.

2. *Short bones* (carpals) are irregularly shaped and have an inner core of *cancellous* (spongy) bone with an outer layer of compact bone.
3. *Flat bones* (skull) consist of two outer plates of compact bone with an inner layer of cancellous bone.
4. *Irregular bones* (vertebrae) are similar to short bones.

Muscles

Muscles are divided into three major groups, with the principal function to contract and produce movement of parts of the body or of the entire body. The grouping of muscles is as follows:
1. *Skeletal (striated)* muscle: found in the skeletal system; provides controlled movement, maintains posture, and produces heat
2. *Visceral (smooth)* muscle: found in the digestive tract, urinary tract, and blood vessels; innervated by the autonomic nervous system; contractions not under voluntary control
3. *Cardiac* muscle; found only in the heart; contractions not under voluntary control

Skeletal muscles are organs; they vary in size and shape from long and thin to broad and flat, or they may form bulky masses. Skeletal muscles contract only if they are stimulated. The energy for muscle contraction is supplied by the breakdown of adenosine triphosphate (ATP) and the action of calcium. Fig. 40-2 illustrates the mechanism of skeletal muscle contraction. Muscle fibers that are adequately oxygenated will contract more forcefully than those not adequately oxygenated.

Movements are produced by muscles pulling on bones that serve as levers and joints that serve as fulcrums.

Skeletal muscle is highly vascular. During muscle contraction chemical changes occur, resulting in the formation of waste products. Muscle fatigue and pain result when insufficient oxygen is delivered to the muscle and when waste products are not removed.

Cartilage

Cartilage is composed of fibers embedded in a firm gel. It is strong but flexible, and it is avascular. Nutrients reach the cartilage cells by the process of diffusion through the gel from capillaries located in the *perichondrium* (fibrous covering of the cartilage) or, in the case of articular cartilage, through the synovial fluid. The number of collagenous fibers found in the cartilage will determine its type: fibrous, hyaline, or elastic. *Fibrous* (or fibrocartilage) has the most fibers and therefore the greatest tensile strength. Fibrocartilage composes the intervertebral disks. *Articular* (hyaline) cartilage—smooth, white, shiny, and resilient—covers the articular surfaces of the bone and serves as a cushion. *Elastic* cartilage has the fewest fibers and may be found in areas such as the external ear.

Ligaments

Ligaments are *bands of dense fibrous connective tissue* that are flexible and tough. They connect the articular ends of bones and provide stability. Examples are the medial and lateral collateral ligaments of the knee, which provide mediolateral stability to the knee joint, and the anterior and posterior cruciate ligaments within the joint capsule of the

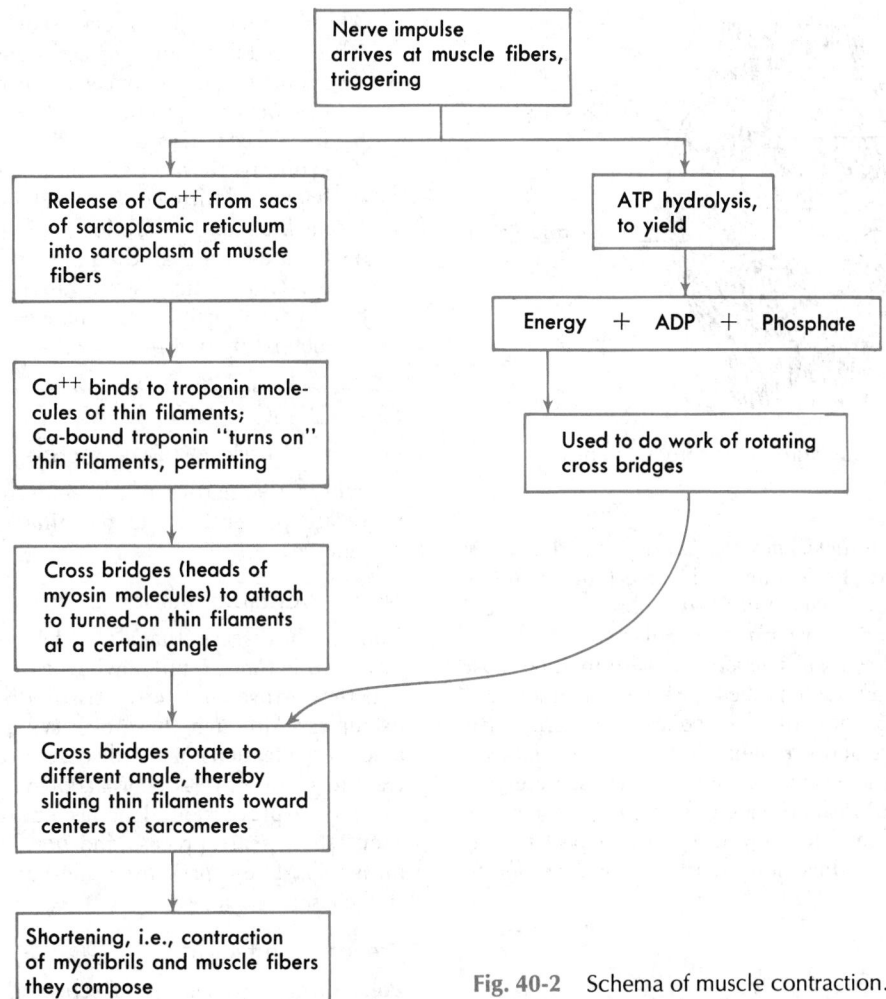

Fig. 40-2 Schema of muscle contraction. (From Anthony CP, Thibodeau GA: *Textbook of anatomy and physiology,* ed 12, St Louis, 1987, Mosby–Year Book.)

knee, which provide anteroposterior stability. Ligaments may also attach to soft tissue to suspend structures. An example of this is the suspensory ligament of the ovary that passes from the tubal end of the ovary to the peritoneum.

Tendons

Tendons are *bands of dense fibrous tissue* that form the termination of a *muscle* and serve to *attach it to a bone.* The tendon is an extension of the fibrous sheath that envelops each muscle and is continuous with the periosteum at its other end. *Tendon sheaths* are tubular structures of connective tissue that enclose certain tendons, especially in the wrist and ankle. These sheaths are lined with synovial membrane that provides lubrication for easy movement of the tendon.

Fascia

Fascia is a *sheet of loose connective tissue* that may be found directly under the skin as *superficial fascia* or as a sheet of dense, fibrous connective tissue making up the sheath of muscles, nerves, and blood vessels. The latter is known as *deep fascia.*

Bursae

Bursae are *small sacs of connective tissue* located wherever pressure is exerted over moving parts. They may, for example, occur between skin and bone, between tendons and bone, or between muscles. Bursae are lined with *synovial membrane* and contain synovial fluid. They serve as cushions between moving parts. Such a bursa, the *olecranon bursa,* is located between the olecranon process and the skin.

Joints

Movement would not be possible unless some flexibility was provided within the skeletal framework. This flexibility is provided by *joints,* or places where the bones come together. The shape of the joint determines the amount and type of movement that is possible, and the classification of joints is based on the amount of movement they allow.

Classification of joints

There are three major classes of joints:
1. *Synarthroses* or *immovable joints:* Bones connected by fibrous tissue or cartilage, such as the bones of the skull that allow no movement.

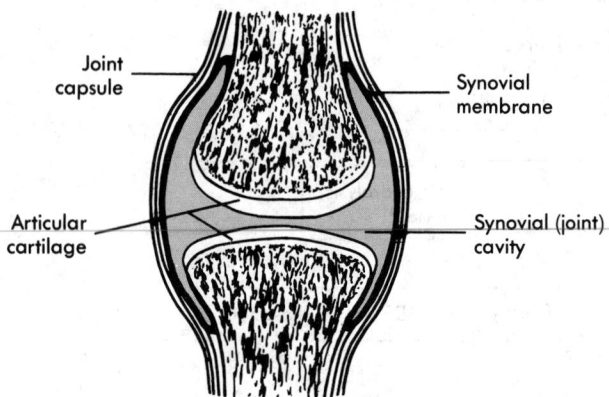

Fig. 40-3 Structure of diarthrodial joint.

2. *Amphiarthroses* or *slightly movable joints:* Joints that allow little movement (for example, intervertebral joints). There is no joint cavity, but tissue (fibrous, cartilage, or bone) is found between the articular surfaces.

3. *Diarthroses* or *freely movable joints:* These include most joints in the body, such as the hip, knee, shoulder, and elbow. The adjacent ends of the bones are covered with hyaline cartilage and surrounded by a fibrous *joint capsule* lined with a synovial membrane that secretes synovial fluid to lubricate the joint (Fig. 40-3). Ligaments and tendons of muscles play an important part in stabilizing the joint. Movements permitted by these joints are as follows:
   a. Flexion
   b. Extension
   c. Adduction
   d. Abduction
   e. Rotation
   f. Circumduction
   g. Special movements, that is, supination, pronation, inversion, eversion, and protraction

Physiologic Changes With Aging

There are periods in the life span when individuals are most vulnerable to musculoskeletal changes. These changes may occur during childhood and adolescence because of rapid growth and development or from the onset of maturity to old age. Changes in musculoskeletal structure and function vary among individuals during the aging process.

Changes that occur with aging constitute a continuation of the decline that began in the middle years. The total number of body cells diminishes, resulting in evident connective tissue changes, decrease in the amount and elasticity of subcutaneous tissue, and loss of muscle bulk, tone, and strength. Total body fat is decreased and redistributed from the periphery to the center of the body and especially on the abdomen. Other physiologic changes are as follows.

1. There is a general decrease in stature of 6 to 10 cm from onset of maturity to old age.
2. Shoulder width decreases.
3. Flexion occurs at the knees and hips.

4. A narrowing of the intervertebral disk causes diminished size of the intervertebral and intercostal spaces.
5. The following occurrences are common:
   a. Compression fractures of the vertebrae.
   b. Increased curvature of the thoracic spine (senile kyphosis, dowager's hump, or widow's hump).
   c. Backward tilting of the head and a shortening of the neck to compensate for the kyphosis deformity.
   d. Greater arm span than height, thus giving the older person a "gangly" appearance.
   e. Unsteady gait, with changes in the muscles and motor function.

PREVENTION AND HEALTH EDUCATION
Persons at Risk and Risk Factors

Whatever the nature of the musculoskeletal disability, there are prevention and teaching factors that must be considered.

Nonpreventable factors

Many of the diseases that affect the musculoskeletal system have at this time an unknown cause. Rheumatoid arthritis and the diffuse connective tissue diseases are but a few examples. Although these diseases are not now preventable, complications of the diseases are preventable—contractures, atrophy, skin breakdown, and others. In these instances, prevention depends on teaching the patient about the disease process and how to employ preventive measures. These preventive measures will be covered in this chapter.

Preventable factors

Polio vaccine, screening of school-aged children for scoliosis, and screening tests for streptococcal infections with early treatment of the infection to prevent rheumatic fever are examples of preventive measures that can be employed on a community-wide basis in combating illnesses that cause musculoskeletal disability. Early attention to posture; good dietary habits; genetic counseling for individuals with sickle cell anemia and hemophilia; teaching of good body mechanics for individuals whose jobs entail lifting or carrying heavy objects; and concern and attention to the recommendations of the National Safety Council to help avoid accidents at home, on the job, and on the road are all examples of preventive measures that may be employed to decrease musculoskeletal disability within the general population.

Preventive Health Teaching
Promotion of safety

For those individuals who have limitations of motion or mobility, a variety of precautions and protective or safety devices can be employed in the hospital or the home. Examples would be grab bars that can be mounted on a wall near a tub or toilet, safety arms that fit around a toilet, and rails that fasten onto the side of a bathtub. These devices provide the person with both a stable place to hold onto and a point of leverage for assuming a standing or sitting position. Throw rugs and obstacles should be re-

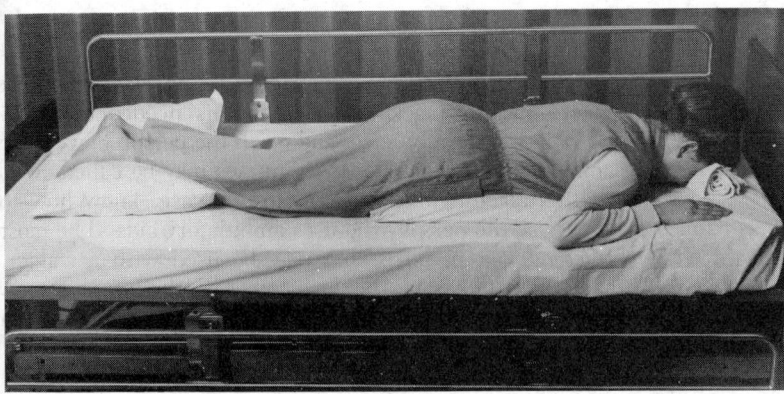

Fig. 40-4 Prone position. (From Rantz M, Courtial D: *Lifting, moving, and transferring patients: a manual,* ed 2, St Louis, 1981, Mosby—Year Book.)

moved from areas used by individuals with ambulatory difficulties, and floors should not be highly waxed. Wheelchairs should have adequate locking devices, and patients who must use wheelchairs should be taught how to lock and unlock the chair. Nurses should know where in the community needed equipment can be obtained.

Prevention of muscle and joint complications
Maintenance of joint mobility

For the individual with limited motion or mobility, range of motion exercises should be carried out to prevent joint stiffness or contracture from disuse. Whenever it is possible, except in conditions where acute joint inflammation is present, range of motion exercises should be performed several times a day. *Active range of motion* is most beneficial for the patient. Encouraging patients to do as much of their own care as they are able to do within the restrictions of their disability will often satisfy active range of motion requirements.

Several precautions should be mentioned. *Passive range of motion* exercises should not be performed past the point of the complaint of pain. Particularly in individuals with pathologic skeletal conditions (gross deformity, osteoporosis), fractures can result if a joint is forced through "normal" range of motion. Also, acutely inflamed, painful, or septic joints should be rested, because harm can be done by moving the joint before inflammation has subsided. The person who has pain is also likely to resist movement to avoid further pain.

Maintenance of posture

Although maintenance of good posture is important for all persons, it is especially important for the patient with chronic arthritis. Poor posture exerts further strain on already damaged joints and not only may cause pain and fatigue but predisposes to increased deformity.

The person who must remain in bed for a long period of time in traction or in a cast should be in a bed with a firm mattress, and a bed board should be placed under the mattress. A firm bed lessens pain by preventing motion and consequent pull on painful joints and helps to keep the spine in good alignment. Boards should be long enough and wide enough to rest firmly on the main side and end rails of the bed, not on the bedsprings. The person with

arthritis should either use no pillow or should use one small pillow that fits well down under the shoulder so that forward flexion of the cervical spine is not encouraged. Knees should not be flexed on pillows, and all patients who must be confined to bed most of the day should lie prone with a pillow under the abdomen for a part of each day to relieve supine pressure areas (inferior scapular areas, sacrum, coccyx, and ischial tuberosities) (Fig. 40-4).

Careful positioning with *trochanter rolls* (rolled towels or bath blankets to brace an extremity in the desired position), supportive pillows, attention to avoiding extreme flexion of joints, and care to avoid compressing nerves or arteries (the result of which can be neurologic or circulatory compromise) are all important considerations for both skin care and general maintenance of the patient.

The unaffected foot (or feet) should rest against a footboard at least part of the day. This helps to maintain the foot in a neutral position for a more normal walking position, prevents the weight of bedclothes from contributing to foot-drop, and provides a firm surface against which the person can do resistive foot exercises. Patients should be taught to check the position of their lower limbs when at rest. If their problem is nonneurologic, they should "toe in" to prevent external rotation contracture of the hip and pronation of the foot. These complications cause serious difficulty when walking is resumed.

For the general public, it should be remembered that *poor posture* throughout life may contribute to *hypertrophic arthritis.* Molding the pelvis correctly with a posterior pelvic tilt will help prevent increased curvature of the lower back with its resultant strain on muscles and joints. Holding the head up with the chin in takes a great deal of strain from the joints of the upper spine. It is surprising how many older persons can benefit from posture improvement even though damage may date from childhood. Nurses should teach patients good body mechanics to prevent muscle strain that could pull a joint out of alignment just enough for musculoskeletal changes to develop or to cause symptoms.

Teaching the person with joint and muscle disorders

The following are *conservative measures* for individuals with joint and muscle disorders. They can be *restorative, preventive,* or *analgesic in nature.*

Activity

Because many musculoskeletal disorders are problems of activity limitation, teaching is directed toward improving activity. Absolute rest of a limb, joint, or part of the body may be ordered to prevent further tissue destruction and pain. As symptoms subside, activity will be gradually increased.

The patient needs to recognize that clues such as pain, tiredness, and progressive loss of dexterity indicate a need for rest. The most frequent indicator that a joint has been overused or misused is an increase in pain or fatigue. Joint *protection techniques* that can be helpful, particularly for chronic inflammatory joint disorders, are as follows:

1. *Energy conservation techniques:* Examples are sliding rather than lifting objects and moving dishes, utensils, or equipment on a cart rather than carrying them.
2. *Avoiding positions of possible deformity:* Because flexor muscles are stronger than extensor muscles, joints tend to become deformed in a position of flexion. For example, avoid sitting for long periods, keeping the knees or elbows bent to avoid pain, and twisting motions to turn doorknobs or remove a lid.
3. *Learning to avoid holding muscles or joints in one position for a long time:*
   a. Activities need to be varied (as just mentioned)
   b. Active range of motion exercises are encouraged.
4. *Learning to use the strongest joints for activities:*
   a. Use good posture when sitting and standing.
   b. Work at a comfortable height.
   c. Stoop and use the knees and not the back when lifting objects.

Assistive, supportive, and safety devices

Although the occupational therapist may recommend specific assistive devices and teach the patient how to use them, the nurse needs to understand the need for them and encourage their use in self-care activities.

Supportive devices or ambulatory aids (walkers, canes, crutches) permit part of the person's weight to be transferred to the upper extremities. The physical therapist determines the specific device that is needed. Physical therapists generally select and teach the person how to use ambulatory devices. However, nurses may be called on to do this teaching. They must, in any case, know how to supervise the person who uses ambulatory aids. The most common gait patterns that may be used with a walker, cane, or crutches are the *three-point gait*, the *two-point gait*, and the *four-point gait*. These gait patterns are covered in Chapter 26.

Examples of *safety devices* used include the following:

1. Grab bars around toilets, tubs, and showers
2. Elevated toilet seats
3. Skid-proof mats or adhesive strips on tub floors
4. Hand rails along hallways and staircases
5. Nonskid wax applied to floors

Use of heat and cold

1. Moist heat is often used for relaxation of muscles and for sedative and analgesic effects.
2. Cold is often used to reduce or prevent swelling after trauma and to reduce pain and stiffness in some cases.
3. Precautions when using heat or cold:
   a. Apply with care to persons with decreased sensation.
   b. Check skin frequently for evidence of redness or burning.
   c. Moist compresses must be left on for 15 to 20 minutes to achieve maximal effectiveness.
   d. Dry heat must have a control device to maintain the heat at a low level.
   e. Do not use heat on joints that are or may be *infected*.
   f. Ice packs must be wrapped in toweling to protect the skin.

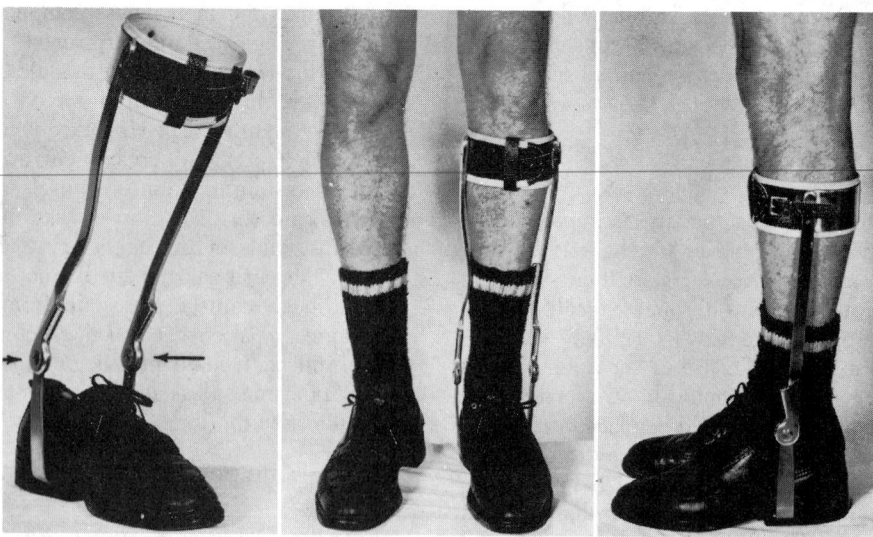

Fig. 40-5   Spring-loaded brace. (From Brashear H, Raney R: *Handbook of orthopaedic surgery,* ed 10, St Louis, 1986, Mosby–Year Book.)

Splinting and bracing

Splints and braces (orthoses) are used to stabilize or support a joint to protect it from improper use or external trauma.

1. *Spring-loaded braces* are designed to oppose the action of unparalyzed muscles and to act as partial functional substitutes for the paralyzed muscles (Fig. 40-5).
2. *Resting splints* are designed to maintain a limb or joint in a functional position while permitting the muscles around the joint to relax (Fig. 40-6). They are used by the patient with rheumatoid arthritis to decrease muscle spasms that contribute to joint deformity.
3. *Functional splints* maintain the joint or limb in a usable position such as in the case of a drop wrist or foot-drop (Fig. 40-7).
4. *Dynamic splints* permit assisted exercise to joints, particularly after surgery to finger joints (Fig. 40-8).

Special considerations for splinting and bracing include the following:

1. Corrective shoes may be ordered for the feet to provide support and safety. These should be oxford type with laces.
2. Observations of the patient's skin should be made after an orthosis has been worn, even for short periods, for areas of skin irritation. Adjustment may be needed by the *orthotist* (brace maker).
3. Patients must learn how to apply and remove braces or splints and how to care for them.
   a. Metal braces should be stored upright.
   b. Splints of molded materials should be stored away from sources of heat.
   c. Leather materials should be treated with Neatsfoot Compound or other leather preservative to prevent drying and cracking.
4. The brace should be adjusted if there is a change in weight (loss or gain).

Positioning and transfer

Principles of positioning (Fig. 40-9) can be found in most fundamentals of nursing texts. However, because pain accompanies nearly all musculoskeletal problems, preventing or minimizing pain must be taken into consideration when positioning the patient. Nurses should be aware that patients in the acute stages of their disorders require the greatest care and gentleness when they must be moved. *Fear of pain often causes irritability and can lead to muscular resistance, which increases pain.* Care must be taken not to jar the bed. Heavy bedclothes over painful extremities may

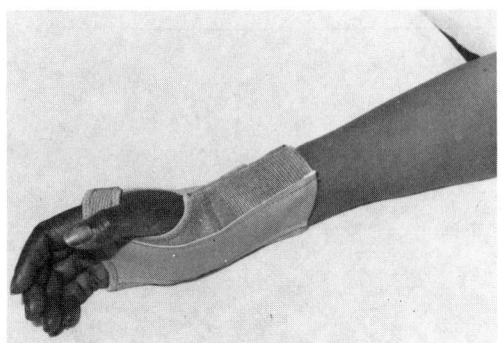

Fig. 40-6   Resting splints.

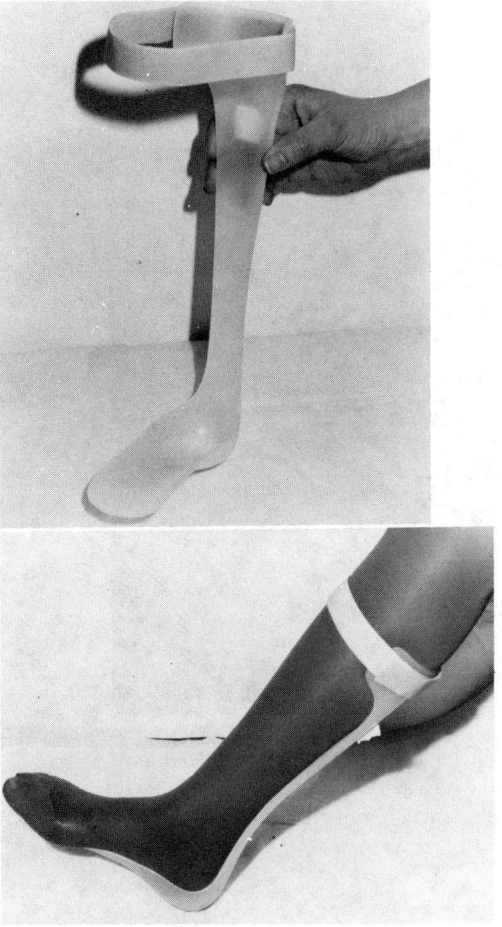

Fig. 40-7   Functional splints.

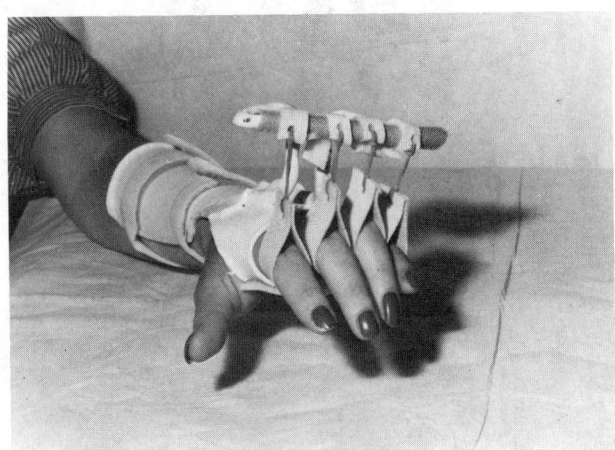

Fig. 40-8   Dynamic hand splint.

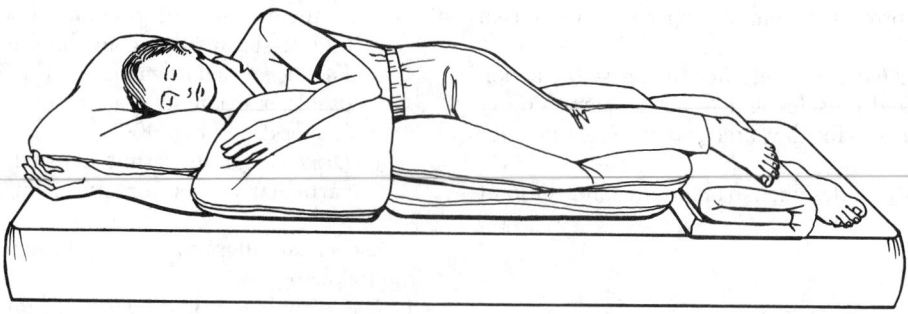

Fig. 40-9 Side-lying position with extremities properly supported with pillows and rolled blankets.

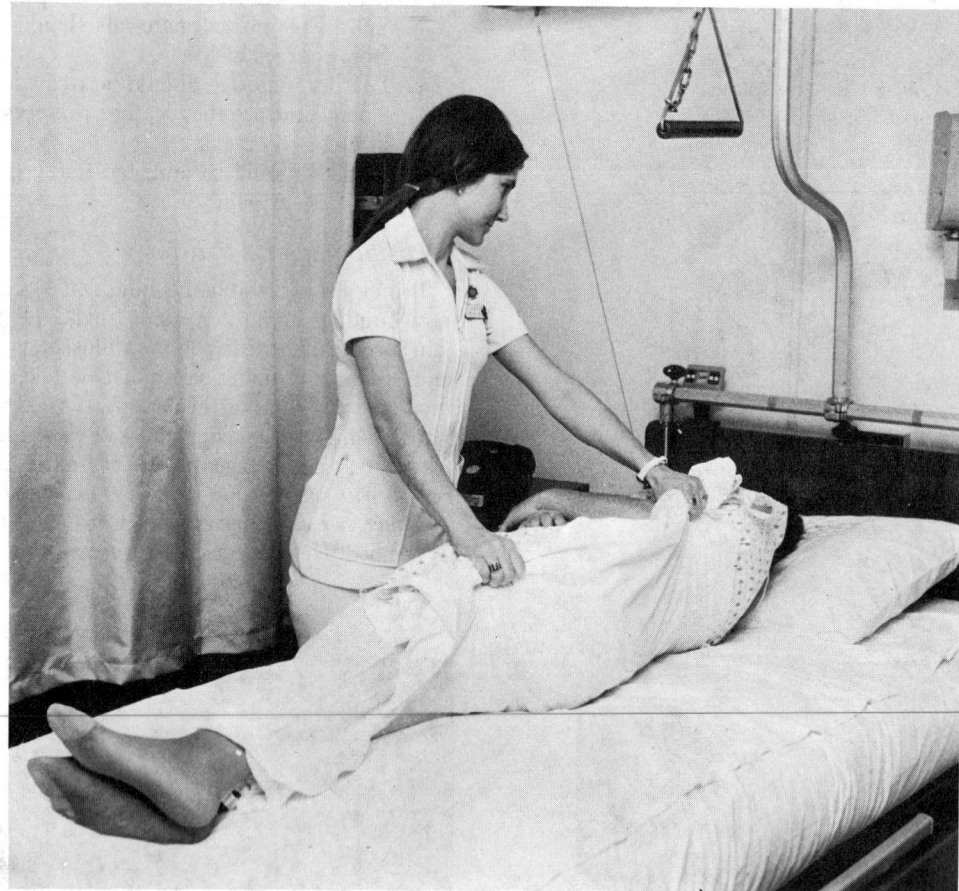

Fig. 40-10 Use of turning sheet. Sheet is held taut with one hand at level of patient's shoulder and other hand below patient's buttocks, providing patient with a sense of support and control. A sheet so placed may also be effectively used as a pull sheet when moving patient from bed to cart.

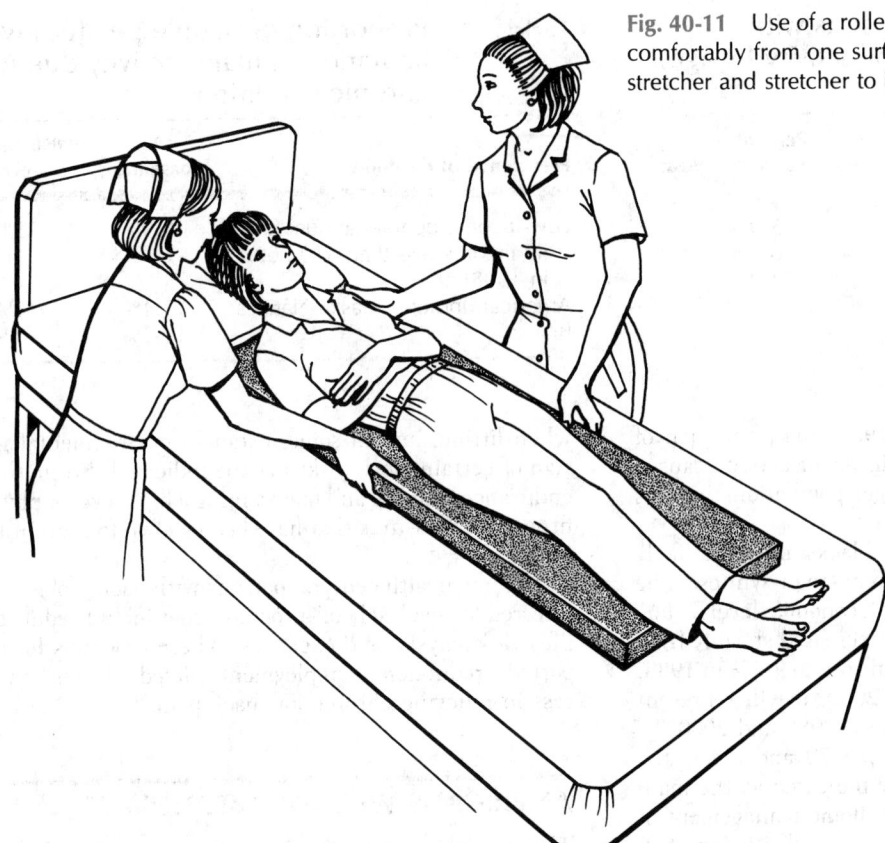

Fig. 40-11   Use of a roller board, effective in moving patients comfortably from one surface to another, such as from bed to stretcher and stretcher to bed.

cause added pain. If bed cradles are used to support linen, caution must be taken not to accidentally bump an involved part of the body when adjusting or removing the cradle. Placing a very painful joint or extremity on a pillow or pillows to move it can reduce pain. Moving patients off the bed using a pull sheet (Fig. 40-10) or a roller board (Fig. 40-11) also facilitates comfort through the move. Frequently, patients prefer to move themselves rather than risk pain from having someone else move them; when it is safe for the patient to do so, the nurse should permit it.

If the patient must use a wheelchair, it should be adjusted to fit that individual. No wheelchair should be purchased for permanent use by a patient unless someone knowledgeable about wheelchairs, preferably a physical therapist, has evaluated the patient and determined what special equipment is needed. Chairs poorly fitted to the patient's needs can be unsafe and encourage poor posture. Principles of transfer are summarized in Box 40-1.

FOCUS ON THE FUTURE

Goals for the Year 2000

Limitation in major activity

According to Healthy People 2000,[81] in 1988 about 9.4% of the total population had some limitation in a major activity, such as working or keeping house, and an additional 5.4% were limited in the amount or kind of major activity they could perform. Limitation in major activity goes up with advancing age as shown in Table 40-1.

The goal for the year 2000 is to reduce to no more than

40-1

Guidelines for Care

Moving and transferring the patient

If one side of the body is stronger than the other, *the patient should always be moved toward the strong side.* This guideline correlates with the principle that it is easier to move objects by pulling them than by pushing them. If the patient moves toward the strong side, the strong side is being used to pull the weak side through the required movement. The person assisting with the move should *support the strong side* to make it more effective.

If there is any question regarding the patient's ability to cooperate with the transfer, a second person should be standing by for assistance if needed.

If the person helping with the transfer has any doubt about his or her ability to accomplish the transfer safely, help should be obtained before attempting it.

The transfer should be accomplished using the strong muscles of the legs rather than the weak muscles of the back.

If lifting is required, adequate help should be available. If adequate help is not available, the transfer should be postponed until help is available.

Whenever possible, pull sheets or a sliding board should be used to move the patient rather than trying to slide the patient (for example, from bed to cart) (Fig. 40-10).

Table 40-1 **Percentage of persons with limitation in major activity by age, 1988**[81]

Age	Percent
Under 18	3.9
18-44	5.9
45-64	16.9
65 and older	22.9

Table 40-2 **Proportion of people per 1000 with limitation in major activity due to chronic conditions**[81]

Prevalence of disability	1988 baseline	2000 Target, % decrease
Low-income people (annual family income less than $10,000 in 1988)	18.9%	15%
American Indians/Alaska Natives	13.4%	11%
Blacks	11.2%	9%

8%, from a baseline of 9.4% in 1988, the proportion of people who experience limitation in major activity caused by chronic conditions. Special target populations for this objective appear in Table 40-2.

Overall, Native Americans and blacks are more likely to report limitations in major activity than whites. The difference is largely explained by economic levels. The prevalence of limitation in activity decreased steadily from 9.9% in 1983 to 9.2% in 1987, then rose to 9.4% in 1988. If the target of 8% is achieved by 2000, it will represent a 15% reduction in disability between 1988 and 2000.[81]

Among noninstitutionalized people 70 and older, the chronic conditions most frequently indicated as the main reason for need for assistance with home management of activities or activities of daily living were arthritis (18.1%), heart disease (13.8%), visual impairment (10.5%), senility (7.2%), and cerebrovascular disease (6.9%). In addition, persons reporting limitations in activity were more likely to have multiple health problems.[81]

Back problems are a major cause of activity limitation. In 1983-88, chronic back conditions rivaled arthritis and heart disease as a major cause of activity limitation.[81]

Chronic back pain is both common and debilitating. The incidence of low back pain is 5% to 14%, and the lifetime reported prevalence ranges from 60% to 90%. In 1983-85, the prevalence of chronic back conditions was 77.5 per 1000 people, 17 per 1000 for disk disorders, 19.7 per 1000 for curvature of back or spine, and 4.0 per 1000 for other impairments of the back.[81]

Low back pain disables 5.4 million Americans and costs at least $16 billion each year. For this reason, one of the objectives for year 2000 is to reduce activity limitation caused by chronic back conditions to a prevalence of no more than 19 per 1000 from a baseline average of 21.9 per 1000 during 1986-88. To achieve this objective, the emphasis is on prevention. Interventions to prevent low back injury include education, physical conditioning, weight loss, teaching persons to squat and bend from the knees when lifting, and in some instances environmental redesign of certain work tasks may be indicated. Strength and endurance training and maintaining a high level of physical fitness are measures that have been shown to prevent back injuries.

In some health centers, persons with back problems are referred to "back school" programs that include education, lifestyle analysis, and exercises. These programs have reported a reduction in employment-related injuries and success in relieving chronic low back pain.[81]

AMERICANS WITH DISABILITIES ACT

The Americans with Disabilities Act, which is discussed in detail in Chapter 14, should assist persons with musculoskeletal problems to be more independent in employment and mobility.

The act addresses four main areas: employment, public services such as bus and rail transportation, public accommodations, and telecommunication services. The employment portion of the act forbids discrimination in hiring or promotion against a qualified person with a disability. Public accommodations such as restaurants, hotels, and retail stores have to remove physical barriers such as steps. This means adding ramps, assuring that doorways are wide enough to accommodate wheelchairs, and providing accessible toilet facilities with grab bars in toilet stalls. Additionally, curbs have to have cut-aways to accommodate wheelchairs, and handicapped parking spaces must be provided.

Unless one has a mobility problem it is hard to appreciate how barriers can interfere with a person's independence. Nurses, in particular, should be sensitive to the needs of those with disabilities and should survey public accommodations in their communities for their accessibility to the handicapped. If barriers exist, these should be brought to the attention of those in charge of the facility.

MAJOR HEALTH PROBLEMS OF THE MUSCULOSKELETAL SYSTEM

The disorders and injuries of the musculoskeletal system are vast in scope. They range from those that cause the patient minor discomfort and inconvenience to those that are life threatening. Among the more troublesome are the inflammatory or rheumatic diseases. These diseases, though they may involve many systems, very often have an arthritic component. There are more than 100 arthritic diseases. One in every seven people in the United States has some form of arthritis. One in every three families in the United States is somehow affected by arthritis. The total economic cost of arthritis in the United States in the late 1980s, including both direct (medical care) and indirect cost (lost wages), was estimated to be more than $13 billion. In addition, it is estimated that another $1 billion is spent on unproven and fraudulent remedies.

Listed here are some common musculoskeletal disorders that will be covered in this chapter.

1. *Inflammatory disorders:* rheumatoid arthritis, systemic lupus erythematosus, polymyositis (dermatomyositis), ankylosing spondylitis
2. *Nonarticular rheumatism:* bursitis, carpal tunnel syndrome, Dupuytren's contracture
3. *Degenerative disorders:* degenerative joint disorders and degenerative joint disorders of the spine
4. *Restrictive disorders:* scoliosis
5. *Other disorders:* gout, bacterial arthritis
6. *Trauma:* fractures of bone and soft tissue injuries

RHEUMATOID ARTHRITIS

Etiology/Epidemiology

Rheumatoid arthritis is a chronic systemic disease. The disease process, although most prominent as a nonsuppurative inflammation in the diarthrodial joints, may also be manifested by lesions of the vasculature, lungs, nervous system, and other major organs of the body.

Rheumatoid arthritis is more prevalent in women than men by a ratio of 2:1 or 3:1. Usually it appears during productive years of life when career and family responsibilities are greatest. Although the cause of this disease is unknown, several theories of causation are under investigation. Areas of study include (1) immune mechanisms, such as the interaction of the IgG class of immunoglobins with the rheumatoid factor (RF) that appears to play a role in perpetuating rheumatoid inflammation; (2) metabolic factors; and (3) infection, with particular attention to viruses.

The signs and symptoms and medical therapy appear in Table 40-3.

Pathophysiology

The disease process within the joints (intraarticular) begins as an inflammation of the synovium with edema, vascular congestion, fibrin exudate, and cellular infiltrate. The inflammatory process is set off by some sort of irritation or damage to joint tissue. This is called a "triggering" event. White blood cells rush into the area, releasing chemicals (including superoxide radicals and hydrogen peroxide)

REVIEW

Table 40-3   Inflammatory disorder: rheumatoid arthritis

Signs and symptoms	Medical therapy
Local	**Goals**
Generalized joint aching with stiffness and limitation in motion	Relief of pain
	Maintenance of joint function
Gradual swelling, warmth, redness, and tenderness	Prevention and correction of deformities
Changes in appearance of hands	Correction of other health problems
Fusiform or spindle-shaped swelling of fingers (Fig. 40-12, A, B)	**Rest**
	Complete bed rest during acute periods; otherwise 2 to 4 hr daily; rest for joints with splints
Swan-neck deformities of fingers	
Ulnar deviation of the hands (Fig. 40-12, C)	**Physical therapy**
All joints can become involved: hips, knees, wrists, elbows, shoulders, and jaw	Active-assistive exercises to regular program of active exercises to preserve function
	Moist heat packs or baths for muscle relaxing and relief of pain
Systemic	
Fatigue, malaise, fever, tachycardia, weakness, loss of weight, anemia; gradual bilateral, symmetric polyarthritis of small and large joints in all extremities	**Medications**
	Table 40-4 lists medications prescribed to reduce inflammation and pain
	Surgery
	Reconstructive surgery may be necessary

useful in destroying bacteria, but also harmful to tissue cells. Also released are prostaglandins (chemicals that mediate inflammation), leukotrienes (producers of inflammation), and digestive enzymes. Particularly damaging to joint tissue is the *enzyme collagenase* because it breaks down collagen, the main structural protein of connective tissue. *The presence of these substances within the joint attracts still more white blood cells, and in rheumatoid arthritis, the process becomes chronic. Continued inflammation leads to thickening of synovium, particularly where it joins the articular cartilage.* At these junctures, granulation tissue forms a *pannus*, or mantle, that covers the surface of the cartilage. The pannus also invades subchondral bone (bone underlying the cartilage). As the amount of granulation tissue from inflammation increases, it interferes with normal nutrition of the articular cartilage and the cartilage becomes necrotic. The degree of erosion of the articular cartilage determines the amount of articular disability. If large areas of cartilage are destroyed, adhesions form between the joint surfaces, and fibrous or bony union (ankylosis) develops

Table 40-4 Medications prescribed in the treatment of rheumatoid arthritis

Medication	Action	Side effects/toxic effects	Precautions
Salicylates			
Examples: acetyl-salicylic acid, choline salicylates	Analgesic, antipyretic, antiinflammatory	Gastric irritation; dose-related salicylism; skin rash; hypersensitivity	Take with food, milk, or antacid; space q 4-6 hr to maintain antiinflammatory effect
Nonsteroidal antiinflammatory agents (NSAIAs)*			
Indomethacin (Indocin)	Analgesic, antiinflammatory	Headache; dizziness; insomnia; confusion; gastrointestinal irritation	Take with food, milk, or antacid; discontinue if CNS symptoms develop and notify physician
Ibuprofen (Motrin)	Same as indomethacin	Same as indomethacin but believed less irritating to GI tract; fluid retention	Delayed absorption if taken with food
Tolmetin sodium (Tolectin)	Same as ibuprofen	Same as ibuprofen	Take with food or milk
Naproxen (Naprosyn)	Same as ibuprofen	Same as ibuprofen; also drowsiness	Take with food, milk or antacid; avoid driving until dosage effect established
Fenoprofen calcium (Nalfon)	Same as ibuprofen	Same as naproxen	Delayed absorption if taken with food; avoid driving until dosage effect established
Sulindac (Clinoril)	Same as ibuprofen	Same as ibuprofen; also skin rash	Take with food, milk, or antacid; not to be used with acetylsalicylic acid
Diflunisal (Dolobid)	Analgesic, antiinflammatory	Gastric irritation; headache; dizziness; skin rash; tinnitus; fluid retention	Take with food or milk; not to be used with salicylates or other antiinflammatory medications
Piroxicam (Feldene)	Analgesic, antiinflammatory	Gastric irritation; anemia; skin rash; fluid retention; dizziness; headache	Take with food or antacid
Diclofenac sodium (Volteran)	Analgesic, antiinflammatory	Possible intestinal irritation, headache, drowsiness, fatigue	Enteric coated: may be taken with food or milk
Nabumetone (Relafen)	Analgesic, antiinflammatory	Gastric irritation, diarrhea, dyspepsia, abdominal pain	Take with food or milk
Potent antiinflammatory agents			
Adrenocorticosteroids (for example, Prednisone)	Interfere with body's normal inflammatory response	Fluid retention, sodium retention, potassium depletion; hypertension; decreased healing potential; increased susceptibility to infection; gastrointestinal irritation; hirsutism; osteoporosis; fat deposits; diabetes mellitus; myopathy; adrenal insufficiency or adrenal crisis if abruptly withdrawn	Take with food, milk, or antacid; dosage not to be increased or decreased without physician supervision; take in morning if taken on a once-a-day basis

*Note: Acetylsalicylic acid (aspirin) is the drug of choice in the initial treatment of rheumatoid arthritis. Nonsteroidal antiinflammatories are aspirin-like drugs. Many patients prefer the NSAIAs over aspirin because they tend to produce less gastric irritation and some of them need be taken only once or twice a day.
†It should also be noted that the immunosuppressive agents azathioprine (Imuran), cyclophosphamide (Cytoxan), chlorambucil (Leukeran) have been used on an investigational basis in patients with severe disease that has not responded to the conventional medications. These are used with great care because of their severe side effects and the attendant risks of the development of neoplasms.

Table 40-4   Medications prescribed in the treatment of rheumatoid arthritis—cont'd

Medication	Action	Side effects/toxic effects	Precautions
Potent antiinflammatory agents—cont'd			
Phenylbutazone (Butazolidin)	Antiinflammatory; analgesic at subcortical site in brain	Gastrointestinal irritation; hematologic toxicity; hypertension; impaired renal function	Used for a short term (7-10 days); take with food or milk
Slow-acting antiinflammatory agents† *Antimalarials*			
Hydroxychloroquine (Plaquenil)	Antiinflammatory (mechanism unknown); effect not expected to be noted for 6-12 mo after beginning therapy	Gastrointestinal disturbances; retinal edema that may result in blindness	Eye examination before beginning therapy and every 6 mo thereafter
Chloroquine (Aralen)	Same as hydroxychloroquine	Same as hydroxychloroquine	Same as hydroxychloroquine
Quinacrine (Atabrine)	Same as hydroxychloroquine	Same as hydroxychloroquine but may be better tolerated; yellow discoloration of skin	May be stopped periodically to prevent deepening of skin discoloration
Gold salts—IM Gold sodium Thiomalate (Myochrysine) Gold thioglucose (Solganal) Gold—oral Auranofin (Ridaura)	Antiinflammatory; effect not noted for 3-6 months after beginning therapy	Renal and hepatic damage; corneal deposits; dermatitis; ulcerations in mouth; hematologic changes	Urinalysis and CBC before each injection; report dermatitis, metallic taste in mouth, or lesions in mouth to physician Oral gold may produce fewer side effects than injectable, but periodic laboratory tests are required
Penicillamine (Cuprimine)	Antiinflammatory (mechanism unclear); effect not expected to be noted until several months after beginning treatment	Fever; skin rash; nephrotic syndrome; hematologic changes; gastrointestinal irritation; lupus-like syndromes; allergic reactions (33% probability if allergic to penicillin); retarded wound healing	Urinalysis, CBC, differential, hemoglobin and platelet count at least weekly for 3 mo, then monthly; report skin rash, fever to physician; food interferes with absorption— take on empty stomach between meals
Methotrexate	Mechanism of action unclear; believed to be immunosuppressive and antiinflammatory in patients with RA	Hepatotoxic; nausea, stomatitis, cytopenia, pulmonary dysfunction	Some evidence that folic acid supplements (1 mg/d) reduce toxic effects

between what were previously free-moving surfaces. Destruction of cartilage and bone, in addition to some weakening of tendons and ligaments, may lead to subluxation or dislocation of joints. Invasion of the subchondral bone may cause eventual regional osteoporosis.

The early manifestations of the disease may include fever, weight loss, fatigue, and generalized aching. *Early morning stiffness* lasting a few minutes to an hour or more is characteristic. The person may describe the location of aching and stiffness in general terms as opposed to naming specific joints. *This kind of discomfort, commonly referred to as fibrositis, is poorly localized.* Such discomfort may be the patient's earliest complaint. These symptoms may be present for some time before they are replaced by more specific, or localized, problems (that is, frank articular inflammation with joint swelling, pain, redness, warmth, and tenderness). In other persons, fibrositis and joint inflammation occur together at the onset. Table 40-3 summarizes signs and symptoms and medical therapy.

Nursing Process
Assessment
Subjective data

The early manifestations of rheumatoid arthritis may lead the person to describe the location of aching and stiffness "in my arms," "in my hands," or "in my legs" as opposed to naming specific joints. This kind of discomfort is more common in the morning ("early morning stiffness") and may be present for some time before the person begins to see and feel the joint changes.

Objective data

1. Inspection and palpation: check same joints on *both sides of body* for symmetry, skin color, size and shape, tenderness, and swelling
2. Evaluate passive range of motion of synovial joints
   a. Note any deviation from normal (limited joint movement most important)
   b. Note presence of crepitation (*crepitus*), which is an audible grating sound made by movement of bony surfaces within the joint
   c. Note pain with range of motion
3. Inspect and palpate skeletal muscles bilaterally
   a. Note atrophy, tone, and tenderness
   b. Test muscle strength by having the person move the muscle against resistance.

Diagnostic tests

1. Serologic tests
   a. Erythrocyte sedimentation rate: will be elevated
   b. Red and white blood cell count: will reveal anemia and leukocytosis
   c. Rheumatoid factor (RF) (present in 50% to 90% of patients, depending on duration and severity of disease): serum will show presence of large antibody-like protein molecules
   d. Latex fixation test is positive
2. Roentgenographic examinations
   a. Periarticular osteoporosis: joint surface erosion
   b. Later: narrowing of joint space, subluxation, and ankylosis

3. Joint aspiration: samples of synovial fluid from within the joint cavity will determine the presence of an aseptic inflammatory process; synovial fluid is cultured and examined microscopically. Commonly there is increased turbidity and decreased viscosity of synovial fluid.

Data analysis: nursing diagnoses

Nursing diagnoses are determined from analysis of patient data. Possible nursing diagnoses for the person with rheumatoid arthritis may include, but are not limited to, the following:

Diagnostic title	Possible etiologies
Self-care deficit; bathing/ hygiene, dressing/ grooming, toileting	Musculoskeletal impairment, inability to use certain joints/ limitations in motion
Pain, chronic: joint	Pathologic changes caused by RA
Injury; high risk for	Loss of muscle strength, pain and stiffness in joints
Knowledge deficit about rheumatoid arthritis	Lack of information regarding RA or misinterpretation of information
Body image disturbance	Change in body appearance; swollen, deformed joints; change in posture

Planning: expected patient outcomes

Expected patient outcomes for the person with rheumatoid arthritis may include, but are not limited to, the following:
1. Patient demonstrates improved ability to perform ADL.
2. Patient is more comfortable; patient states joint pain is decreased.
3. Patient has improved active joint range of motion, and risk of injury is reduced.
4. Patient can explain the disease process and follow-up care including prescribed therapy (exercises, medications) and plans established for follow-up by the physician.
5. Patient has a more positive self-concept.

Implementation
Assisting with achievement of therapeutic goals

1. Give prescribed medications on time and in prescribed doses (Table 40-2).
2. Assist with selection of foods; assist with feeding if necessary; encourage small, frequent meals.
3. Encourage patient to maintain normal weight.

Interventions to achieve patient outcomes
Promoting mobility and preventing injury

1. *Avoid* positioning joints in such a way as to encourage contracture (for examaple, pillows under knees when supine, pillows forcing neck into forward flexion).
2. Encourage regular active range of motion of joints to greatest degree possible.
3. Encourage patient to assist with own ADL to greatest degree possible, with assistive aids if necessary.
4. Encourage patient to perform prescribed exercises on a regular basis.
5. Prevent injury by providing appropriate ambulatory

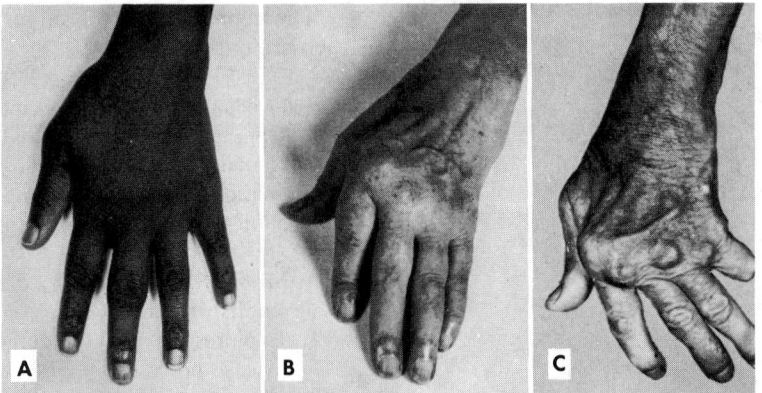

Fig. 40-12   Rheumatoid arthritis of hand. **A,** Early stage. Note fusiform swelling of proximal interphalangeal joints, especially that of middle finger. **B,** Moderate involvement. Note swelling from chronic synovitis of metacarpophalangeal joints and early ulnar drift. **C,** Advanced stage. Noted marked ulnar drift and subluxation of metacarpophalangeal joints with extension of proximal interphalangeal joints and flexion of distal joints. Note also deformed position of thumb. Hand has wasted appearance. (From Brashear H, Raney R: *Handbook of orthopaedic surgery,* ed 10, St Louis, 1986, Mosby–Year Book.)

devices and encouraging patient to wear *shoes,* not slippers, for ambulation.

Assisting with comfort and ADL

1. Assist with self-care while promoting independence as much as possible.
2. Keep patient free of pain with prescribed medications.
3. Apply heat or cold to joints as prescribed.
4. Promote frequent position changes; often patient is more comfortable changing own position.
5. Provide for adequate rest periods.
6. Encourage use of resting splints.

Facilitating learning

When teaching persons about rheumatoid arthritis (and other rheumatic diseases) nurses may find it helpful to use some of the patient teaching material that has been prepared by the Arthritis Foundation.* Booklets, such as *Arthritis: the basic facts,* are written in such a way that most patients can understand and learn from them.

Patient teaching should include information about the following[8]:

1. Proper balance of rest and activity
2. Joint protection and energy conservation techniques
3. Proper use of medications—names of drugs, dosages, precautions in administration, and side effects or toxic effects
4. Plans for implementation of exercise program prescribed by the physician or physical therapist
5. Proper application of heat and/or cold packs

6. Proper use of walking aides and other assistive devices
7. Safety measures to prevent injury
8. Application, appropriate use of, and care of splints, braces
9. The basics of good nutrition and the importance of avoiding weight gain
10. The importance of regular follow-up with the physician
11. The risks of following non-medical programs that promise a "cure"
12. Information about local arthritis support groups and programs, services of the Arthritis Foundation

In teaching the patient it is helpful to understand the following biomechanical principles.

1. Using a cane (in the contralateral hand) can alleviate pain, and the force across a hip can be reduced by 60% by the use of a cane.[46]
2. Arising from a chair or toilet seat may be greatly assisted by raising the level of the seat, because the highest pressures on the hip and knee joints are produced during flexion and pushing off.[46] For this reason, persons with arthritis of the hip or knee can arise best from a firm (not overstuffed) chair with arms.

Promoting a positive body image

1. Compliment patient on each improvement in mobility and self-care.
2. Allow time to listen to patient's concerns about body image.
3. Encourage patient to dress self in street clothes before beginning the day's activities.
4. Encourage self-grooming, combing hair and shaving for men and combing hair and applying makeup for women.

*3400 Peachtree Dr. N.E., Atlanta, GA 30326.

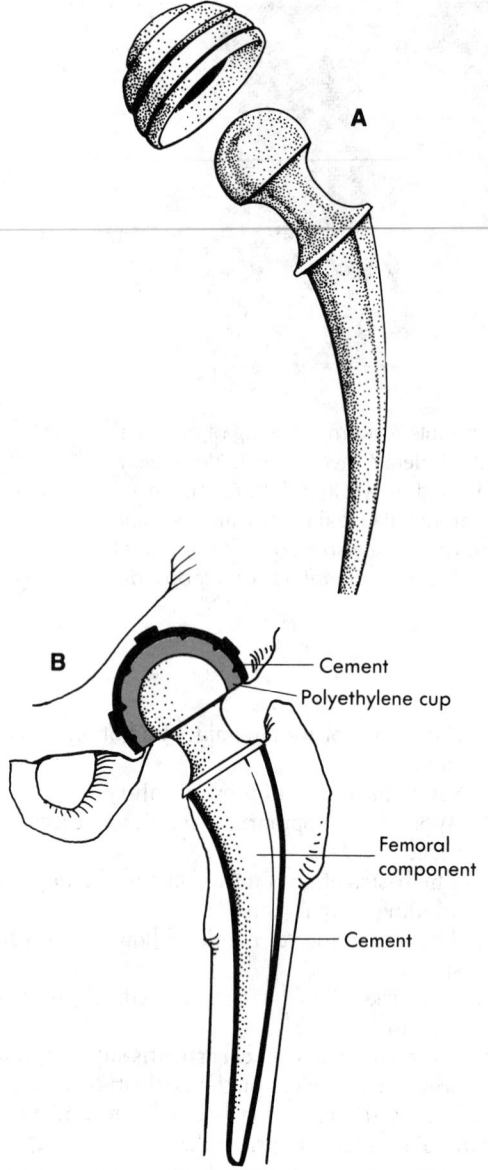

Fig. 40-13 **A,** Acetabular and femoral components of total hip prosthesis. **B,** Total hip prosthesis in place.

Evaluation

Evaluation is based on the expected patient outcomes. Questions to be asked include the following:
1. Is the patient better able to carry out ADL?
2. Is patient comfortable?
3. Is the potential for injury lessened?
4. Can the patient explain the need for follow-up care, medications, the program of exercises, and alternating rest and activity?
5. Does the patient exhibit a more positive attitude about body image?

Reconstructive Surgery

When rheumatoid arthritis is progressive or has caused severe joint destruction, surgery may be indicated to relieve pain and improve function.

The common types of surgery and the indications for each are outlined below.

Synovectomy. The early removal of synovial tissue to arrest the course of rheumatoid arthritis in a particular joint, to maintain joint function, and to prevent recurrent inflammation. The knee and the wrist are the joints most often subjected to this procedure.

Arthrotomy. Opening into a joint. The procedure is used to accomplish the following:
1. Explore the joint to determine the presence of a disease process
2. Drain the joint
3. Remove damaged tissue or foreign bodies within the joint
4. Most often performed on the knee

Arthrodesis. Surgical fusion of a joint. Commonly performed on knee, wrist, or ankle. The procedure is used to accomplish the following:
1. Eliminate painful motion
2. Provide stability

Arthroplasty. Resurfacing of one or both sides of a diseased joint.
1. Purposes
   a. Restore motion of the joint
   b. Relieve pain
   c. Correct deformity
2. Types
   a. Replacement of part of the joint with a prosthesis made of metal or other material such as the "cup" or "mold" arthroplasty of the hip joint.
   b. Surgical reshaping of the bones of the joint, which are then covered with soft tissue used as an interposition device.
   c. Total joint replacement where both sides of the joint are replaced by metal or polyethylene implants.

Replacement arthroplasty

Replacement arthroplasty is available for the shoulder, wrist, elbow, phalangeal joints of the fingers, hips (Fig. 40-13), knee (Fig. 40-14), and ankle. The *hip* and *knee* are the *most commonly replaced joints.* The total cost of these replacements in the United States is estimated to be $4 million dollars annually. The discussion that follows will be limited to these two joints.

Rheumatoid arthritis, degenerative joint disease, and *avascular necrosis* are the *major reasons for performing total joint or replacement arthroplasty. Avascular necrosis* of the bone, or bone death, is caused by inadequate blood supply. It can be a *complication of bone fractures,* corticosteroid treatment for rheumatoid arthritis, and systemic lupus erythematosus. Pain (even at rest), restricted motion, and gait disturbances are characteristic. Surgery in the form of total joint replacement is performed to alleviate pain and increase motion.

The knee replacement consists of a femoral and tibial component and a patellar button (Fig. 40-14). The hip prosthesis consists of an acetabular portion (cup) and a femoral component. The designs of the various prostheses

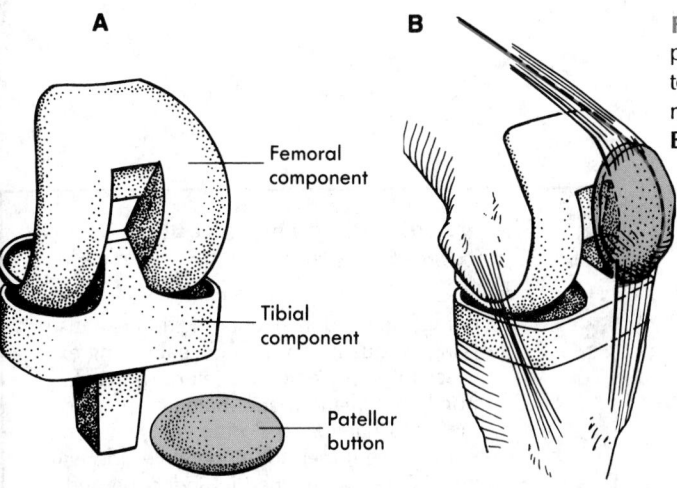

A, Tibial and femoral components of total knee prosthesis. Patellar button, made of polyethylene, protects posterior surface of patella from friction against femoral component when knee is moved through flexion and extension. **B,** Total knee prosthesis in place.

Fig. 40-14

vary in size of the femoral head, shape and length of the femoral shaft, and design of the acetabular component. The care of the patient undergoing total hip replacement is outlined in Box 40-2. The care of the patient undergoing total knee replacement is outlined in Box 40-3 and in the Nursing Care Plan on p. 1373.

Replacement prosthesis may be either *cemented* (held into bone with polymethylmethacrylate) or *uncemented* (treated with a special porous coating that promotes ingrowth of new bone). The uncemented knee replacement may be held in place with short-leg "studs" placed into holes in the recipient bone.[62] The long-term survival of hip and knee replacements is discussed next.

Long-term survival of joint implants
Hip replacement

From the first use of replacement joints, there was concern about how long the implant would survive. In 1989, the first results were published of a 15-year follow-up of patients with hip replacement. This study reported that 78% of the implants were good or excellent and 88% were still functioning after 15 years.[60] Autopsy reports of persons who had had total hip replacement indicated that the polymethylmethacrylate, the cement used to fix the joint in place, was well tolerated. Thus polymethylmethacrylate will continue to be used to fix some, if not the most, hip replacements.

Knee replacement

Research has focused on the presence and significance of wear debris, especially in the patellar component (Fig. 40-9) of the knee prosthesis. Because of wear debris, some orthopedic surgeons have discontinued use of the patellar component of the knee joint.[60] Patients who have considerable wear debris may have pain and/or a squeaking of the knee with movement as the debris rubs against the underside of the patella. Such patients may require a patellectomy (removal of the patella) along with removal of the patellar component and the debris in the knee joint.

SYSTEMIC LUPUS ERYTHEMATOSUS
Etiology/Epidemiology

Systemic lupus erythematosus (SLE) is a chronic inflammatory disease of unknown cause. It affects women, par-

REVIEW

Table 40-5   Inflammatory disorder: systemic lupus erythematosus (SLE)

Signs and symptoms	Medical therapy
General complaints: Moderate to severe—fever, weakness, fatigue, weight loss, sensitivity to sun, erythematous rash ("butterfly" pattern over bridge of nose and cheeks)	Rest: when disease active
Polyarthralgia and arthritis with pain and swelling	No specific treatment; therapeutic program is ordered for the specific problems of the patient
Polyserositis (pleurisy and pericarditis)	Medications (Table 40-2): adrenocorticosteroid therapy to control active manifestations of SLE; salicylates for joint pains; antimalarial drugs (Chloroquine) for cutaneous lesions; cytoxic agents if other drugs fail
Anemia, thrombocytopenia and renal, neurologic, and cardiac abnormalities	
Alopecia (hair loss) possible during periods of active systemic disease	

ticularly adolescents and young adults, 8 to 10 times more often than men. The disease was named after its characteristic rash on the face, the erosive nature of the rash being "likened to the damage wrought by a hungry wolf."

Once thought to be relatively rare and always fatal, better techniques for recognition of the disease have demonstrated it to be fairly common, and its course can be controlled by corticosteroids. Some patients do, however, die as a result of lesions affecting major organs or from secondary infections.

The cause of the disease is unknown, although two major areas are being investigated as possible causes. One possibility is that an aberration of the immune system causes immune complexes containing antibodies to be deposited in tissue, thereby causing tissue damage; the second possibility is the presence of a viral infection caused by or resulting from some immunologic abnormality. A third pos-

The patient undergoing total hip replacement

Preoperative care
Skin care
  Preparation of the skin will follow the hospital's written procedure or the surgeon's written orders.
  The area must be kept free of contamination.
  The patient's environment must be as free as possible from potential sources of contamination.
Reassurance and education
  Patient needs to understand about the surgical procedure, postoperative care, and expectations after discharge.
  Patient is to sign the operative permit and have an understanding of its importance (informed consent).
  Patient may have both hips replaced at one surgery.

Postoperative care
Positioning
  Position will depend on the design of the prosthesis and the method of insertion.
  Restrictions designed to avoid dislocation of the prosthesis usually include the following:
  Flexion limited to 60 degrees for 6-10 days, then 90 degrees for 2-3 months
  No adduction beyond midline for 2-3 months, therefore no sidelying on operative side. Leg is maintained in abduction when lying supine or on the nonoperative side.
  No extreme internal or external rotation.
Wound care: Drains are placed in the wound to prevent formation of a hematoma.
  Maintain constant suction through the self-contained vacuum of the Porto-Vac.
  Note amount and type of drainage. Keep area free of contamination. (Infection at the site of the prosthesis results in total failure of the surgery.)
Activity
  Observe flexion restrictions when elevating head of bed.
  Encourage periodic elevation and lowering of head of bed to provide motion at hip.
  Instruct patient in use of overhead trapeze to shift weight and lift for bedpan, change of linen.

The patient undergoing total hip replacement—cont'd

Encourage active dorsi-plantar flexion exercise of ankles, quadriceps and gluteal setting exercises to promote venous return, prevent thrombus formation, and maintain muscle tone (see Chapter 22).
Patient may be turned to unoperative side with operative leg maintained in abduction and extension.
Begin ambulation as early as the first postoperative day, if tolerated.
  Observe flexion and adduction restrictions.
  Observe weight-bearing restrictions prescribed by surgeon (usually partial weight bearing assisted with walker or crutches).
  Increase amount of walking each day according to patient's tolerance.
Begin sitting when patient demonstrates sufficient control of leg to sit within flexion restrictions (usually requires elevation of sitting surfaces, including use of raised toilet seat).
Medications
  Prophylactic anticoagulant drugs (acetylsalicylic acid, low-dose heparin, or coumadin) may be prescribed to decrease risk of thrombus formation.
  At first, control pain by positioning; use narcotics, gradually tapered to nonnarcotic analgesics according to patient's tolerance. Many patients will have patient controlled analgesia (PCA).
Discharge instructions
  Patient must use ambulatory aid, avoid adduction, and limit hip flexion to 90 degrees for about 2 to 3 months.
  A raised toilet seat is to be obtained and used at home until flexion restrictions are removed.
  Patient may need a long-handled shoe horn and reacher to facilitate ADL within flexion restriction.
  Patient must be made aware of the life-long need for antibiotic prophylaxis to protect the prosthesis from bacterial infection during dental work, intrusive procedures, or surgery.

The patient undergoing total knee replacement

Preoperative care
Same as for total hip replacement.

Postoperative care
Positioning
The operative leg(s) is (are) elevated on pillows to enhance venous return for the first 48 hours. Pillows are placed with caution not to flex the knee (Fig. 40-15). Many patients have bilateral total knee replacements at one surgery.
The patient may be turned from side to back to side.
Wound care
Care of drains as for total hip replacement.
Patient is assessed for systemic evidence of loss of blood (hypotension, tachycardia) if bulky compression dressing is used because it may hold large quantities of drainage before drainage becomes visible.
Bulky dressings are removed before the patient begins active flexion.
Activity
Passive flexion in a continuous passive motion machine (CPM) within prescribed flexion-extension limits may be started in the recovery room. Patient's leg should remain in machine as much as tolerated (up to 22 hours per day) to facilitate even healing of tissue.
Patient is encouraged to perform active dorsiplantar flexion of the ankles, quadriceps setting, and, after the drain is removed, straight leg raising exercises.
Patient begins active flexion exercises three to four times a day about the fifth postoperative day.
Light weight bearing with an assistive device may be started as early as first postoperative day and increased as patient tolerates.
Sitting in a chair with the leg(s) elevated may be started on the first postoperative day.
Patient is encouraged to wear a resting knee extension splint (immobilizer) on the operated leg until able to demonstrate quadriceps control (independent straight leg raising).
Pain control
Initial control of pain with narcotics, positioning; gradual decrease of medication to nonnarcotic analgesics, as patient tolerates.
Patient is encouraged to use ice to knee(s) for 20-30 minutes before and after active flexion. Ice is very effective in reducing pain.
Discharge instructions
Patient must observe partial weight-bearing restriction and use ambulatory aid for approximately 2 months after discharge.
Patient should continue active flexion and straight leg raising exercises at home.
Patient must be made aware of the life-long need for antibiotic prophylaxis as explained in Box 40-2.

---

sibility is that both of these factors combine to produce the disease. Some drugs, notably procainamide (Pronestyl), isonicotinic acid hydrazide (INH, Isoniazid), and penicillin are known to induce lupus-like syndromes.[87] The signs and symptoms and medical therapy are summarized in Table 40-5.

Pathophysiology
Pathologic manifestations of the disease include the following:
1. Synovial involvement as a fibrous villous synovitis
2. Severe vasculitis with necrosis of the walls of the small arteries
3. Renal involvement with thickening of the basement membrane of the glomerular tufts and necrosis of the glomerular capillaries
4. Lymph node necrosis
5. Development of small white spots in the retina called *cytoid bodies*
6. Lesions of the nervous system

The initial manifestation of SLE is often arthritis. In many instances the joint symptoms are transient and respond to treatment. Weakness, fatigue, and weight loss may be present. The patient may complain of sensitivity to the sun, developing a rash and at times fever or arthritis on exposure to sunlight. *Erythema*, usually in a *butterfly pattern*, appears over the *cheeks and bridge of the nose*. The margins of these lesions are bright red, and the lesions may extend beyond the hairline with partial alopecia (loss of hair) above the ears. Lesions may also occur on the exposed part of the neck. Lesions spread slowly to the mucous membranes and other tissues of the body, or they may originate there. These lesions do not ulcerate but cause degeneration and atrophy of tissues.

Depending on the organs involved, the patient may have findings of glomerulonephritis, pleuritis, pericarditis, peritonitis, neuritis, or anemia. Renal and neurologic manifestations are among the more serious manifestations of the disease.

Nursing Process
Assessment
Subjective data

1. Note that patients may express vague symptoms or simply say that they are "always tired."
2. Ask patients about generalized weakness, loss of appetite, loss of weight, skin rashes, and specific joint discomfort (even at rest).
3. Identify the presence and extent of discomfort or stiffness of muscles or joints.
4. Identify the presence of sensitivity of eyes and skin to the sun.
5. Ask patients about hair loss, which occurs during acute episodes.

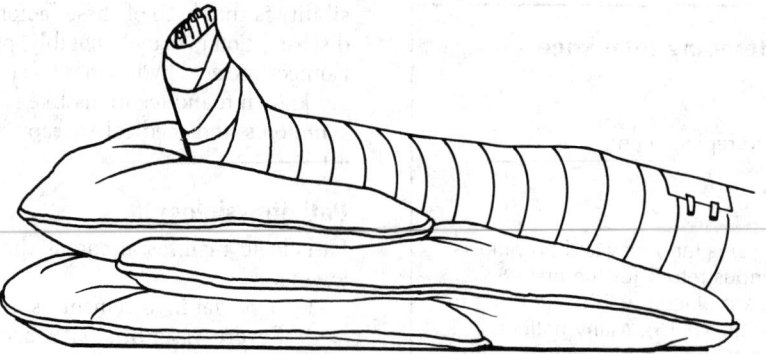

Fig. 40-15 Leg properly elevated on pillows, avoiding knee flexion.

Objective data

1. Observe for erythema over the cheeks and bridge of the nose, above the ears, on exposed part of the neck, and over other body areas
2. Examine for loss of hair or partial loss at normal hairline
3. Check for muscle strength and range of motion of joints

Diagnostic tests

As mentioned above, many organs may be involved. Laboratory findings may be specific to the organs involved, as with proteinuria, abnormal cerebrospinal fluid, or roentgenographic evidence of pleural reactions. A positive lupus erythematosis (LE) cell reaction and positive antinuclear antigen and immunofluorescent studies to identify the antibody responsible for LE cell reaction are helpful in making the diagnosis of the disease. Laboratory findings may also show the presence of anemia, thrombocytopenia, leukocytosis, or leukopenia. A *skin biopsy* is taken of the rash and studied for histopathologic evidence of the disorder.

Data analysis: nursing diagnoses

Nursing diagnoses are determined from an analysis of patient data. Possible nursing diagnoses for the patient with systemic lupus erythematosus may include, but are not limited to, the following:

Diagnostic title	Possible etiologies
Activity intolerance	Fatigue/weakness, painful joints
Pain	Joint pain
Impaired skin integrity; high risk for	Altered immune system
Knowledge deficit	Lack of information, unfamiliarity with information source/not a commonly known disease
Anxiety	Change in health status; uncertainty about outcome; change in status/role/lifestyle
Altered nutrition: less than body requirements	Weakness/fatigue make eating difficult, loss of appetite

Planning: expected patient outcomes

Expected patient outcomes for the person with systemic lupus erythematosus may include, but are not limited to, the following:

1. Patient has less fatigue and weakness, and activity tolerance is improved.
2. Patient states feeling more comfortable and pain is under control.
3. Patient's skin is intact.
4. Patient can explain prescribed therapy and plans for follow-up care.
5. Patient appears less anxious.
6. Appetite improves, and nutrition is improved.

Implementation
Assisting with achievement of therapeutic goals

1. Medications: administer as prescribed
   a. Antiinflammatory analgesics to control arthritic pain
   b. Antimalarial drugs, particularly if rash is extensive
   c. Corticosteroids for severe neurologic and renal involvement
   d. Cytotoxic agents if other drugs fail
   e. Ointments or skin creams for rash
2. Kidney dialysis or transplant for uncontrolled lupus nephritis (Chapter 33)
3. Total hip replacement for avascular necrosis consequent to high-dose steroid therapy (p. 1368)

Intervention to achieve patient outcomes
Improving activity tolerance

1. Encourage planned program of muscle strengthening and range of motion exercises.
2. Allow additional time for patient to complete activities.
3. Pace activities and provide rest periods as needed.

Assisting with comfort and ADL

1. Administer medication for pain of joints and muscles.
2. Help patient with gradual independence in ADL.
3. Provide rest periods as necessary.

Nursing Care Plan	**Patient with total knee replacement**

DATA: Mr. K. is a 59-year-old married office manager with osteoarthritis of the right knee. Over the past 8 months he has had increased pain in his knee with only minimal relief from the nonsteroidal antiinflammatory medications prescribed by his internist. He reports that he must now ambulate with a cane when his pain is severe. He can no longer participate in many activities he used to enjoy because of his discomfort and limited mobility. After consulting his internist and an orthopedic surgeon he has decided to undergo elective total knee replacement. Mr. K. is admitted to the nursing division on the morning of surgery.

The nursing history identified the following:
1. He and his wife reside in a two-story colonial house with their bedroom upstairs.
2. He plans to return home after this hospitalization and has received a 6-week leave of absence from his job.
3. He is not taking any medications other than his "arthritis pills" and has no other preexisting medical problems.
4. He was last hospitalized 18 years ago for a cholecystectomy.

Nursing diagnosis: Knowledge deficit: related to lack of exposure to total knee replacement surgery

Expected patient outcomes	Nursing interventions	Rationale
Mr. K. states he understands the teaching provided by the nurse Mr. K. will have less anxiety related to fear of the unknown and/or misconceptions regarding the surgery and recovery period	*Preoperative: one week before admission* 1. Assess need for instruction and provide as necessary 2. Provide written materials pertaining to total knee replacement (TKR) surgery if available in the institution 3. Review preoperative instruction with patient and family on day of surgery 4. Evaluate patient's understanding of the information taught *Postoperative:* By discharge Mr. K. should be instructed in and able to demonstrate: 1. Independent transfer and ambulation on level surfaces with appropriate ambulatory aid (walker or crutches) 2. Exercises to be performed at home and frequency (straight leg raising and active flexion) 3. Activity restrictions to be observed for approximately 2 months or until follow-up with physician. These include no kneeling or jarring activities 4. Rationale for antibiotic prophylaxis for dental procedures and procedures requiring instrumentation or surgery. Give Mr. K. written direction regarding antibiotic prophylaxis, which he can carry in his wallet. 5. Use of knee immobilizer as resting splint	Understanding about surgical procedure and postoperative care should lessen anxiety and promote desired behaviors for recovery from surgery

Care Plan by Kyle Paskert, MSN, RN.

Continued.

Collaborative nursing actions postoperatively include those to identify possible complications of the surgery. Immediate reporting of and treatment of early signs may prevent serious effects. Nursing actions include monitoring for the following:

a. Neurocirculatory compromise—perform neurocirculatory checks q 2h for the first 24 to 48 h; notify physician of any changes from preoperative status

b. Dislocation of the prosthesis—notify physician if patient complains of sudden onset of increased (severe) pain, joint deformity

c. Impaired skin integrity and/or incision healing—monitor pressure areas for signs of redness; monitor temperature; assess incision for signs or symptoms of infection and excessive drainage

d. Atelectasis/respiratory infection—monitor breath sounds; encourage deep breathing and coughing until ambulatory

e. Problems with elimination—assess for urinary stasis and constipation

f. Fluid and electrolyte imbalance—monitor intake until patient is taking oral fluids equal to at least 1200 ml output; monitor IV fluid flow; assess patient for fluid volume excess or deficit

The following nursing diagnoses are especially pertinent for persons who have undergone TKR surgery. Implementation and evaluation of the related nursing interventions will help to prevent postoperative complications.

Nursing diagnosis: Pain: related to total knee replacement surgery

Expected patient outcomes	Nursing interventions	Rationale
Mr. K. states feeling more comfortable Mr. K. is able to perform necessary postoperative routines/exercises because pain is adequately managed	Assess Mr. K.'s pain and evaluate response to comfort measures provided	Subjective and objective data are important in ascertaining the nature of the patient's postoperative pain and in determining its management
	Patient may be on patient-controlled analgesia (PCA); if not, administer prescribed analgesics (usually narcotic) at timely intervals during the initial postoperative period (especially before physical therapy)	It is usually necessary to administer a narcotic the first 48-72 h after surgery Analgesics have a greater effect if they are administered before pain becomes severe
	Teach relaxation techniques as appropriate	Relaxation facilitates rest and may modify the response to pain
	Use other pain-relieving techniques as pertinent, for example, back rubs, repositioning knee, ice to knee for 30 minutes before and after active flexion exercises	A change in type of cutaneous stimulation may result in pain relief. Ice packs can reduce inflammation
	As pain decreases use milder analgesics	As pain lessens in severity it may be controlled by less potent analgesics (with fewer untoward side effects)

Nursing diagnosis: Impaired physical mobility: related to alterations in lower limb S/P TKR surgery

Expected patient outcomes	Nursing interventions	Rationale
Mr. K. demonstrates optimal level of mobility with adaptive devices by time of discharge	Cough and deep breathe with incentive spirometer q 1-2 h until fully ambulatory	If carried out correctly and at appropriate intervals, pulmonary exercises can effectively prevent atelectasis and pneumonia
No injury occurs during hospitalization	Turn Mr. K. side to back to side q 2 h and prn while bedrest is prescribed	Turning and repositioning frequently provides for better ventilation of the lungs

Expected patient outcomes	Nursing interventions	Rationale
	Encourage Mr. K. to perform active dorsi-plantar flexion, isometric quadricep sets, and after the drain is removed, straight leg raises q 2 h until ambulatory, then qid	Exercises of the lower extremities will prevent venous stasis and promote muscle-strengthening
	Elevate the operative leg on pillows in bed and in chair for the first 48 h. Place the pillows under the calf to avoid knee flexion (Fig. 40-15)	Elevation of the operative leg on pillows enhances venous return. Flexion contracture is to be avoided
	Sitting in a chair with the leg elevated may be started as early as the first postoperative day	The exercise of getting in and out of bed is one means of increasing activity in the early postoperative period; the patient accrues numerous physiologic benefits from such activity
	Assist out of bed to chair two to three times/day, especially for meals	
	Begin light weight-bearing ambulation with assistive device when patient can straight leg raise independently, and flex operative leg to 45 degrees (may be started first postoperative day)	Early ambulation is a significant factor in hastening recovery and preventing postoperative complications
	Increase frequency and distance of ambulation as tolerated	
	If continuous passive motion machine (CPM) is used, patient's leg should remain in the machine as tolerated (up to 22 h/day) within the prescribed extension-flexion limits	Passive flexion of the knee may prevent excessive swelling and bruising around the prosthesis and promote greater ease with active flexion
	Begin active flexion exercises approximately second postoperative day, 4 times/day	Active flexion of the knee is necessary to promote return of function; it is desired that the patient achieve approximately 90 degrees of flexion before discharge from the hospital
	Mr. K. should wear knee immobilizer on operative leg until able to demonstrate quadriceps control (independent straight leg raising) except when flexing; the knee immobilizer may also be worn at night as resting splint	The knee immobilizer provides support of the operative leg and prevents incorrect positioning

Nursing diagnosis: Impaired home maintenance management: high risk for, related to numerous discharge needs

Expected patient outcomes	Nursing interventions	Rationale
Mr. K. and his family will express satisfaction with arrangements made to manage self-care at home	Discuss with Mr. K. and his family their plans upon discharge from the hospital	Adequate discharge planning will foster successful completion of rehabilitation at home
	Determine with them information needed to be taught and learned for home care (refer to knowledge deficit, postoperative)	
	Determine the type of equipment needed, for example, crutches, walker, elevated toilet seat, and consult appropriate department or agency for securing these supplies	
	Ensure that Mr. K. can climb stairs or plan with family for first floor sleeping room	

Preventing skin injury

1. Protect skin when in sunlight by doing the following:
   a. Using skin protector of at least 15 SPF whenever going out in sun.
   b. Wearing long sleeves when going out in sun.
   c. Wearing wide-brimmed hat when going out in sun.

Facilitating learning

1. The nature, course, and treatment of the disease
2. Appropriate balance of rest and activity
3. Appropriate exercise
4. How to avoid exposing skin to sunlight; for example, wearing long-sleeved blouses or dresses, slacks, broad brimmed hats, cotton gloves
5. Appropriate use of prescribed medications—dose, frequency, precautions, potential side effects
6. Application of cosmetics (hypoallergenic, approved by physician) to mask skin lesions, and/or wigs to mask hair loss
7. Information about lupus support groups (if available in patient's area)

Providing emotional support

1. Monitor patient's anxiety level.
2. Provide time for patient to discuss fears and concern.
3. Provide realistic reassurance.
4. Refer patient to social service or another service or agency when it appears anxiety is caused by concerns that can be alleviated with appropriate assistance.

REVIEW

Table 40-6 **Inflammatory disorder: polymyositis (dermatomyositis)**

Signs and symptoms	Medical therapy
Activities involving movement and lifting become difficult or impossible: Climbing stairs Arising from a chair Combing the hair Getting out of bathtub	Symptomatic treatment Medications (Table 40-2): corticosteroids and mild analgesics
Weakness can lead to contractures and atrophy	Physical therapy to prevent contractures, preserve muscle strength
Difficulty with swallowing and presence of reflux esophagitis	Frequent small meals Antacids for reflux esophagitis
Decreased peristalsis	May need complete bed rest with head of bed elevated on blocks
Pulmonary function tests: may indicate impaired gas exchange, decreased vital and total lung capacity	Treatment of underlying malignancy if present
Muscle tenderness, transitory joint pain	
Dusky-red, patchy rash over elbows, dorsum of hands, knees, face, neck, shoulders (dermatomyositis)	
Weight loss	

Promoting adequate nutrition

1. Encourage well-balanced diet consisting of major food groups.
2. Offer small frequent feedings that may be better tolerated than three larger meals.
3. Refer to dietitian for further help in planning meals and snacks to help increase weight.

Evaluation

Evaluation is based on the expected patient outcomes. Questions to be asked include the following:

1. Can the patient explain the need for rest periods alternating with periods of activity?
2. Is the patient more comfortable?
3. Has skin integrity been maintained?
4. Can the patient explain the disorder and the need for continued follow-up care?
5. Is patient less anxious about health status and change in lifestyle?
6. Can the patient explain how to maintain adequate diet?

POLYMYOSITIS (DERMATOMYOSITIS)

Etiology/Epidemiology

Polymyositis (dermatomyositis), an inflammatory disease involving striated (voluntary) muscle, occurs two times more frequently in women than men. It may occur at any age and is believed to affect 5 in every 1 million people in the United States. The cause of the disease is unknown; however, it is thought that some reaction of the autoimmune system, perhaps triggered by a virus, is involved. The signs and symptoms and medical therapy appear in Table 40-6.

Pathophysiology

Pathologic findings on histologic studies of biopsied muscle vary, but the alterations found, in order of their frequency, are the following:

1. Primary degeneration of muscle fibers, either focal or extensive
2. Basophilia of some fibers with central migration of the sarcolemmal nuclei
3. Necrosis of parts or entire groups of muscle fibers
4. Inflammation of blood vessels supplying the muscles
5. Interstitial fibrosis varying in severity with the duration and, to some extent, the type of the disease
6. Variation in the cross-sectional diameter of fibers.[7]

The disease usually runs a course of exacerbations and remissions. Often it is first noted in proximal muscles, in particular the pelvic and shoulder girdles. Climbing stairs, arising from a chair, and other activities that involve lifting the body become increasingly difficult or impossible. Lifting the arms becomes progressively more difficult, and combing the hair may be impossible. Other muscles (neck flexors, the muscles of swallowing) may also become involved. Muscle pain or tenderness is present in some instances in the early stages. *The presence of a rash marks the disease as dermatomyositis. A dusky red lesion may be found in the periorbital region, along with periorbital edema. This dusky red rash may extend over the face, forehead, neck, upper shoulders, chest, and upper back.* Lesions on the arms and legs commonly affect the extensor surfaces. These patches are sometimes scaly.

The weakness of myositis, if it persists, can lead to contractures and atrophy. Individuals with the dermatomyositis form of the disease, particularly if they are over 40 years of age, have a 40% to 50% greater chance of having evidence of a malignant neoplasm found during the first 5 years of illness than the population at large. Some physicians believe that routine yearly examinations should be performed to define or exclude the presence of neoplasms in these patients during that 5-year period.

Nursing Process
Assessment
Subjective data

Polymyositis may vary in its mode of onset and in the rate of progression of symptoms, whether muscular, dermal, or articular. The clinical course may be one of spontaneous remissions and exacerbations.

1. Because muscular weakness is present in nearly all patients and particularly in the lower extremities, the patient is asked to describe the weakness and its effect on ADL.
2. Questions are asked about joint and muscle pain, gastrointestinal problems, appetite, and weight loss.

Objective data

1. Weakness of myositis can lead to contractures and atrophy. Test strength of upper and lower extremities against resistance.
2. Observe patient for respiratory difficulty, because diaphragm may be affected by weakness.
3. Palpate muscles and joints for pain or tenderness.
4. Examine for dusky-red, patchy rash over elbows, dorsum of hands, knees, forehead, neck, shoulders, and chest.

Diagnostic tests
Manual Muscle tests

Manual muscle tests are used to determine the degree of muscular weakness from the disorder. They are used also in cases of injury or muscle disuse. The physical therapist rates the strength of muscles in relation to gravity and applied resistance. Muscle testing is helpful in determining which muscle should be chosen for biopsy. When muscle-strengthening exercises are indicated, the test will indicate groups of muscles that require the most therapy.

Muscle biopsy

Biopsy is performed to aid in the diagnosis of specific muscle disorders. The muscle tissue may reveal degeneration, inflammatory reactions, or involvement of specific fibers.

A muscle biopsy is an operative procedure usually performed by a surgeon. A local or general anesthetic may be used. After the procedure the patient will have minor to moderate discomfort in the form of stiffness or pain at the operative site. The patient is encouraged to resume range of motion activity to avoid undue stiffness.

Electromyography

Electromyography measures the electrical activity of muscles; an *electromyogram* (EMG) is a recording of the electrical potential detected by a thin needle electrode inserted into skeletal muscle. The electrical activity can be heard over a loudspeaker and viewed on an oscilloscope and graph. Normal muscles at rest give off no electrical activity.

The EMG provides evidence of *lower motor neuron disease, primary muscle disease,* and *defects in the transmission of electrical impulses* at the neuromuscular junction, such as in myasthenia gravis. The test cannot be used to differentiate *specific* muscle disorders. There is no specific preparation of the patient, except to reassure the patient that the electrode needles will not cause electric shock and the procedure is not dangerous.

Some discomfort will be felt as the needle is inserted and as the muscle twitches or contracts.[62]

Serum enzyme tests

Serum glutamic-oxaloacetic transaminase (SGOT), creatine phosphokinase (CPK), and aldolase levels are elevated in the presence of active polymyositis or dermatomyositis.

Twenty-four hour urine tests

These urine specimens are used to determine if there is an abnormal creatine/creatinine ratio.

Data analysis: nursing diagnoses

Nursing diagnoses are determined from an analysis of patient data. Possible nursing diagnoses for the person with polymyositis may include, but are not limited to, the following:

Diagnostic title	Possible etiologies
Activity intolerance	Generalized weakness because of muscle involvement
Self-care deficit: feeding; dressing/grooming	Musculoskeletal impairment
Injury, high risk for	Motor deficits caused by muscle involvement and weakness
Mobility, impaired physical	Musculoskeletal impairment
Knowledge deficit	Lack of exposure to information about a disease that is not commonly understood
Infection, high risk for	Related to autoimmune response of disease
Nutrition, altered: less than body requirements	Difficulty in swallowing; in some, difficulty lifting head and holding it up
Personal identity disturbance	Change in mobility/musculoskeletal involvement may result in changes in lifestyle

Planning: expected patient outcomes

Expected patient outcomes for the person with polymyositis may include, but are not limited to, the following:

1. Patient performs ADL with assistance.
2. Patient has increased energy for physical activities and self-care.
3. Patient does not sustain an injury.
4. Patient's mobility is improved using an assistive device.

5. Patient understands the disease and need for continuing with prescribed therapy and follow-up medical care.
6. Patient does not develop an infection.
7. Patient maintains nutritional status.
8. Patient demonstrates acceptance of changes in lifestyle.

Implementation

Assisting with achievement of therapeutic goals
Comfort and ADL

1. During acute episodes, assist with frequent changes of position.
2. Administer prescribed analgesics.
3. Assist with ADL.
4. Provide adequate rest.

Interventions to achieve patient outcomes
Improving activity tolerance and self-care deficit

1. Assist patient with activities as necessary.
2. Provide frequent rest periods between activities.
3. Refer to physical and occupational therapy for assistive devices to help with ADL.

Preventing injury

1. During acute episodes
   a. Assist with frequent changes of position to prevent skin breakdown.
   b. Avoid pressures over bony prominences with appropriate protective devices such as sheepskin.
   c. Assist patient with ambulation.

Promoting mobility

1. Elevate sitting surfaces to facilitate transfers
2. Provide appropriate ambulatory device to facilitate comfortable walking
3. Provide for frequent changes of position and range of motion to prevent contractures
4. Encourage patient to gradually resume independent ADL as symptoms subside

Facilitating learning

The patient and significant others are instructed about the following:
1. The nature and course of disease.
2. Appropriate balance of rest, activity.
3. Use of selected ADL devices to enhance function; for example, long-handled comb.
4. Appropriate use of prescribed steroids—how to take them, dosage, side effects, precautions.

Preventing infection

1. Assure that the patient is not exposed to persons with an upper respiratory infection.
2. Maintain skin in good condition to avoid skin breakdown.
   a. Keep skin clean and dry and well lubricated.
   b. Avoid pressure on bony prominences with protective devices such as sheepskin.
   c. Assist patient with dental hygiene at least twice daily.

Maintaining nutrition

1. Provide small, frequent, high caloric feedings.
2. Ensure that patient can swallow correctly. If patient is having trouble swallowing an enteral feeding tube may be required.

Support coping with changes in lifestyle

1. Allow patient to express concerns and fears about the future.
2. Provide patient with factual information as appropriate.
3. Assist patient to look at possible sources of help.
4. Support patient's decisions about how to improve lifestyle.

Evaluation

Evaluation is based on the expected patient outcomes. Questions to be asked include the following:
1. Can the patient perform ADL with greater ease?
2. Does the patient have more energy?
3. Is the patient free of injury?
4. Is the patient's mobility improved?
5. Is the patient able to describe the nature of the disorder and prescribed therapy and why there is a need for continued professional help?
6. Is the patient free of infection?
7. Is the patient maintaining nutritional status?
8. Is the patient more accepting of changes in her/his lifestyle?

ANKYLOSING SPONDYLITIS

Etiology/Epidemiology

Ankylosing spondylitis is a *chronic progressive disorder affecting the joints of the hips and spine that occurs nine times more frequently in men than women, usually between the ages of 20 and 40.* The progression of the disorder usually decreases after age 50, but limitation of the spine persists. The cause of the disease is unknown, and its progression cannot be stopped by any treatment now known. There is a strong genetic link with the genetic marker HLA-B27, and it is thought that a link between the marker and some form of trigger (perhaps an infection) sets off a reaction in the immune system that leads to the inflammatory process. The HLA marker is found in about 90% of persons with ankylosing spondylitis as compared with 8% in the general population. Approximately 400,000 people in the United States have the disease.[75]

The signs and symptoms and medical therapy can be found in Table 40-7.

Pathophysiology

Spondylitis means inflammation of the spine. As a result of inflammation, the bones of the spine grow together, or ankylose (fuse). Inflammation usually begins around the sacroiliac joints (sacrolitis), eventually obliterating articular cartilage of the affected bones. The cartilage is replaced by new bony growth. Inflammation occurs where the tendon or ligament attaches to bone. The inflammatory

REVIEW

Table 40-7   Inflammatory disorder: ankylosing spondylitis

Signs and symptoms	Medical therapy

Initial symptoms: mild with early morning stiffness and aching
Later: intermittent pain and restricted motion of the back
Extraspinal symptoms include:
  Pleuritic-like chest pain
  Achilles tendonitis
  Peripheral arthropathy (especially hips)
  Nonspecific symptoms include:
    Weight loss
    Malaise
    Fatigue
    Mood change
  "Poker-back" deformity or kyphosis at the cervicodorsal junction
	Goals of medical therapy
	  Relieve pain
	  Achieve and maintain best possible alignment of spine
	  Strengthen intraspinal muscles
	  Prevent interference with breathing capacity
	Postural exercises
	Lying prone (extension) three to four times a day for 15 to 30 minutes
	Rest
	Heat
	Antiinflammatory analgesics
	  Salicylates
	  Nonsteroidal antiinflammatory agents
	  Potent antiinflammatory for short term (phenylbutazone)
	Spinal osteotomy or arthroplasty for severe symptoms

process progresses up the spine, eventually resulting in fusion of the entire spine.

Initial symptoms may include low back pain or aching; pain and swelling of the hips, knees, or shoulders; mild fever; loss of appetite; and fatigue. Low back pain flares and subsides intermittently. Over a period of time, pain subsides and motion of the back becomes restricted. Fusion of the sacroiliac joints and spine up through the cervical vertebrae may occur over a period of 10 to 20 years; as a result, the patient may present either a "poker-back" deformity or a kyphosis at the cervicodorsal junction (Fig. 40-16). Knees are flexed as the person attempts to move the head into an upright position.

Nursing Process
Assessment
Subjective data

Many persons with ankylosing spondylitis remain undiagnosed. The patient complains of low backache, stiffness, and alternating or bilateral "sciatica" that lasts for a few days at a time and subsides. They often complain that they wake up every morning in pain. Later the symptoms become more persistent and begin to include evidence of ankylosis of joints, particularly of the spine. The patient should be questioned about changes in body shape and any loss in height.

Objective data

1. Observe for pain on assuming or maintaining an erect position.
2. Examine patient's posture: patient appears bent forward at the waist, often compensating to achieve an erect position by flexing hips and knees.
3. Palpate for tenderness over the spine and sacroiliac region.
4. Note pain on motion and limitation in turning and bending upper body.

Diagnostic tests

Roentgenograms are most helpful in delineating the disorder. Changes in the sacroiliac joints are the earliest and most diagnostic. There is blurring of the bony margins, then sclerosis, and later ankylosis. Bony growths, called *syndesmophytes*, that bridge the adjacent vertebrae give the appearance of a "bamboo spine." The presence in the serum of HLA-B27 helps to establish the diagnosis. HLA refers to the antigen (human leukocyte antigen) and B27 refers to the gene it marks.

Data analysis: nursing diagnoses

Nursing diagnoses are determined from analysis of patient data. Possible nursing diagnoses for the person with ankylosing spondylitis may include, but are not limited to, the following:

Diagnostic title	Possible etiologies
Body image disturbance	Change in body appearance/immobility, change in lifestyle
Gas exchange, impaired	Changes in the spine and in posture change the chest cavity and decrease chest excursion
Mobility, impaired physical	Intolerance to activity because of pain/fatigue and musculoskeletal impairment
Pain	Inflammation of the spine causing pain
Knowledge deficit	Lack of exposure to information about the disease

Planning: expected patient outcomes

Expected patient outcomes for the person with ankylosing spondylitis may include, but are not limited to, the following:

1. Patient is more accepting of change in body appearance.

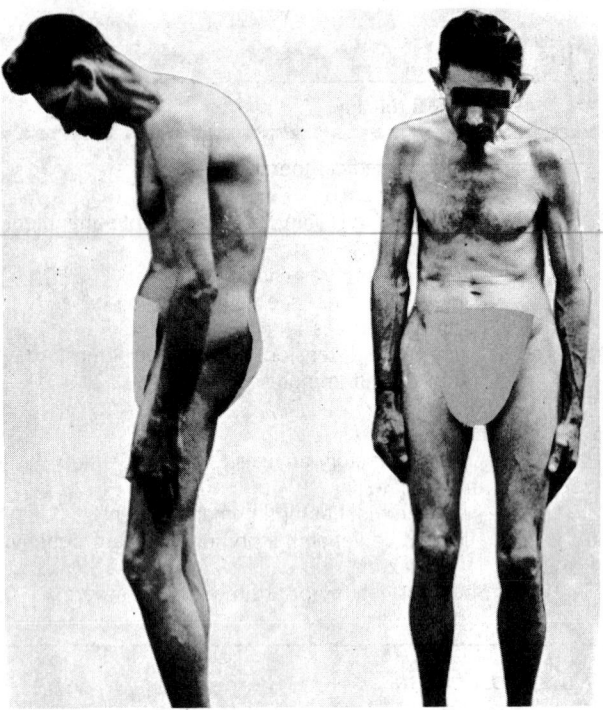

Fig. 40-16 Ankylosing spondylitis in 46-year-old man with ankylosis of entire spine in faulty position. (From Brashear H, Raney R: *Handbook of orthopaedic surgery*, ed 10, St Louis, 1986, Mosby–Year Book.)

2. Patient can demonstrate postural and breathing exercises to minimize interference with breathing capacity.
3. Patient is able to perform ADL with less fatigue and discomfort.
4. Patient states that pain is lessened.
5. Patient knows course of disease, prescribed therapy, and plans for follow-up care.

Implementation
Assisting with the achievement of therapeutic goals

1. Give antiinflammatory analgesics as prescribed. Indomethacin is the most commonly used NSAIA.
2. Provide for rest periods alternating with activity.
3. Provide care for the patient who may have a spinal osteotomy or hip arthroplasty (p. 1386).

Interventions to achieve patient outcomes
Promoting a positive body image

1. Encourage patient to express feelings about changes in body image, if able to do so.
2. Assist patient to express feelings such as anger or depression.
3. Compliment patient on each improvement in mobility.

Improving gas exchange

1. Maintain alignment of the spine
   a. Mattress should be firm.

b. Bed board may be used.
c. Patient should sleep flat without pillow.
d. A back brace may be necessary for support.
2. Postural and breathing exercises
   a. Extension exercises should be performed to maintain erect posture and normal height "thinking tall" and to strengthen paraspinal muscles.
   b. Abdominal lying should be done 3 to 4 times a day for 15 to 30 minutes.
   c. Breathing exercises will help increase breathing capacity.
      (1) Perform deep breathing exercises exhaling through "pursed lips" several times a day.
      (2) Use incentive spirometer 3 times a day to increase vital capacity.

Improving mobility

1. Encourage to do prescribed exercises such as swimming and water walking.
2. Assist with ROM exercises 3 times a day.
3. Maintain alignment of the spine as above.
   a. Firm mattress
   b. Bed board may be used
   c. Patient should sleep flat without pillow under head
   d. Back brace may be necessary for support
4. Offer back massage 3 times daily.

Assisting with comfort

1. Apply heat to painful joints.
2. Apply hydrotherapy by use of Hubbard tank 1 to 2 times daily to entire body; this is best if done just before postural and deep breathing exercises.

Facilitating learning

1. Nature and course of disease
2. Prescribed postural exercises
3. Appropriate use of prescribed medications
4. Methods of applying heat to back and hips
5. Water exercises and swimming are beneficial

Evaluation
Evaluation is based on the expected patient outcomes Questions to be asked include the following:

1. Is the patient more accepting of changes in body appearance?
2. Is the patient able to maintain adequate breathing capacity?
3. Is the patient able to perform ADL with less discomfort?
4. Is the patient more comfortable?
5. Can the patient explain prescribed therapy and plan for follow-up care?

NONARTICULAR RHEUMATISM

Nonarticular rheumatic diseases include those disorders in which the supportive structures and structures located near the joints are inflamed, but the joints themselves are not involved except by the limitations imposed by the supportive structures. *Some of these disorders* are *fibrositis, tenosynovitis, bursitis,* and *carpal tunnel syndrome.*

BURSITIS
Etiology/Epidemiology

Bursitis is inflammation of a bursa, a small fluid-filled sac-like cavity between two articular soft tissue layers. The bursa facilitates joint movements and acts like a pad to cushion joints. The joints affected are the shoulders, elbows, hips, knees, and ankles. In some instances the inflammation of the bursa is preceded by *tendonitis,* that is, inflammation of a tendon, or by *tenosynovitis,* which is inflammation of a tendon and the tendon sheath.

Bursitis may be acute or chronic. It is usually caused by trauma, strain, and overuse of the joint with which the bursa is associated. The shoulder bursa is most often affected. The signs and symptoms and medical therapy are listed in Table 40-8.

Pathophysiology

The synovial lining of the bursal sac becomes inflamed, more fluid is secreted, and the bursa swells. Occasionally, large calcium deposits are present. The swelling is accompanied by pain and limited ability to move the associated joint or the entire extremity.

Nursing Process
Assessment
Subjective data

1. Ask patient to describe location and severity of pain and what preceded present joint pain.
2. Is patient being treated for inflammation of joints resulting from a known cause for the pain?
3. Does the patient have a history of rheumatoid arthritis?
4. Is the patient able to use the joint?

Objective data

1. Palpate the joint for tenderness and swelling of the soft tissues. The swelling will feel "boggy."
2. Observe degree of limited mobility of affected joint.

Diagnostic tests

Affected joint is x-rayed to determine extent of involvement. If a calcified mass of the subdeltoid area is found, surgery may be necessary.

Data analysis: nursing diagnoses

Nursing diagnoses are determined from an analysis of patient data. Possible nursing diagnoses for the person with bursitis may include, but are not limited to, the following:

Diagnostic title	Possible etiologies
Pain	Inflammation of joint space
Mobility, impaired physical, (ROM)	Pain and inflammation limit range of motion
Knowledge deficit	Lack of information about cause and prevention of bursitis

Table 40-8 Nonarticular rheumatism: bursitis

Signs and symptoms	Medical therapy
Deep-seated pain in area of bursa	Antiinflammatory agents are given (Table 40-2)
Pain on movement of involved extremity	Adrenocorticosteroids may be injected into bursa
Passive and active range of motion limited in adjacent joint	Rest of involved area
	Cold compresses during acute phase to help relieve discomfort
	Heat is avoided because it increases fluid exudate in the bursa during inflammatory phase
	Surgical removal of calcium deposits

Planning: expected patient outcomes

Expected patient outcomes may include, but are not limited to, the following:

1. Patient is more comfortable.
2. Patient is able to move affected joint through ROM.
3. Patient can explain what bursitis is, how it is treated, follow-up care, and precautions when taking nonsteroidal antiinflammatory agents (NSAIAs).

Implementation
Assisting with achievement of therapeutic goals

Medications are given as prescribed for inflammation and discomfort:

a. Salicylates
b. Phenylbutazone
c. Indomethacin (NSAIA)

If the above are not effective in relieving pain, the physician may inject adrenocorticosteroids into the bursa.

Interventions to achieve patient outcomes
Promoting comfort

1. Rest of the involved joint may be necessary during the acute phase.
2. Modified joint and extremity exercises may be prescribed to prevent "frozen shoulder," for example.
3. *Cold* (not heat) is applied during acute phase; heat is avoided, as this increases the fluid exudate (additional fluid in the bursa). Heat may be used later.
4. Give analgesics as ordered.

Facilitating learning

1. Patient can state what bursitis is and how it is treated.
2. Patient can describe when to use cold or heat.
3. Patient can demonstrate how to do ROM exercises of affected joint.
4. Patient can state name, dose, side effects, and precautions when taking medications (taking NSAIAs or prednisone with food and never on an empty stomach).

5. Patient can state plans for follow-up care with physician.

Evaluation

Evaluation is based on the expected patient outcomes. Questions to be asked include the following:
1. Is area free of pain?
2. Is full joint range of motion possible?
3. Can patient state medication dosage, side effects, and precautions when taking it (with food, not on empty stomach)?

CARPAL TUNNEL SYNDROME
Etiology/Epidemiology

Carpal tunnel syndrome is caused by pressure being exerted on the median nerve of the wrist. The condition is most common in middle-aged and often obese women and may occur as a result of trauma or of swelling of tendon sheaths caused by processes such as rheumatoid arthritis.

The person will complain of dysesthesia, paresthesia, and hypesthesia of the thumb, index, and middle fingers. Complaints will usually increase when there has been forced flexion of the hand for long periods, such as when typing. The symptoms can be elicited by tapping the median nerve at the wrist (Tinel's sign). The patient may feel that the hand is swollen and may complain of clumsiness when using the hand, especially when grasping or holding onto small objects. Referred pain to the upper extremity is common. Atrophy of the thenar eminence (the padded area of the palm below the base of the thumb) may be present late in the disease.

Pathophysiology

The median nerve passes through a tunnel bounded by the carpal bones dorsally and the transverse carpal ligament volarly (Fig. 40-17). Flexor tendons run through the tunnel parallel to the median nerve. Inflammation and swelling of the synovial lining of tendon sheaths narrow the space available and cause compression of the median nerve.

Nursing Process
Assessment
Subjective data

The symptoms that the patient describes are from the compression of the median nerve and include the following:
1. Episodes of burning pain or tingling in the hands that the patient says are relieved by vigorous shaking or exercising of the hand.
2. Numbness (hypesthesia) affecting the thumb, index, and ring fingers, particularly after prolonged or forced flexion of the wrist, as in knitting or holding a book. Some persons are awakened from sleep by numbness in hand.
3. Feeling of "swelling" in the affected hand.
4. Complaint of difficulty grasping or holding onto small objects; "feels clumsy".

Objective data

1. There is no swelling in the hand, wrist, or fingers.
2. There is a wasting or depressed appearance of the

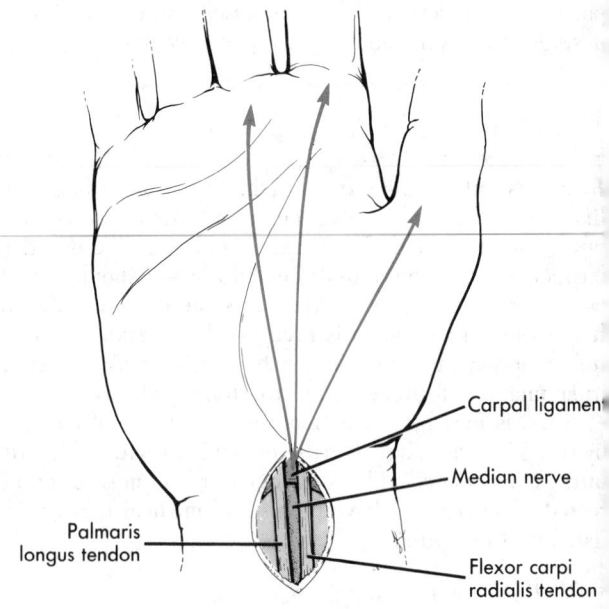

Fig. 40-17 Carpal tunnel syndrome. Volar aspect of wrist retracted to demonstrate position of median nerve. Distribution of median nerve is to thumb and first two fingers. (Adapted from Compere EL: *Orthopaedic surgery*, Chicago, 1974, Year Book Medical Publishers, Inc.)

soft tissue at the base of the thumb on the palmar surface (thenar eminence).

Diagnostic tests

Motor nerve velocity studies that demonstrate a conduction block at the wrist confirm the diagnosis. The equipment and procedure for this test is the same as that used for the electromyogram.[62]

Data analysis: nursing diagnoses

Nursing diagnoses are determined from assessment of patient data. Possible nursing diagnoses for the person with carpal tunnel syndrome may include, but are not limited to, the following:

Diagnostic title	Possible etiologies
Disuse syndrome (hand)	Inflammation and swelling causing compression of the median nerve
Pain	Compression of the median nerve
Knowledge deficit	Lack of information about carpal tunnel syndrome

Planning: expected patient outcomes

Expected patient outcomes for the person with carpal tunnel syndrome may include, but are not limited to, the following:
1. Patient will have maximum function of hand, thumb, and finger.
2. Patient will be free of discomfort.
3. Patient will be able to discuss plans for follow-up care.

Implementation
Assisting with achievement of therapeutic goals
1. Rest
2. Splinting of the wrist
3. Local injections of corticosteroids
4. If pain persists, surgery is required.

Surgery

The surgery involves decompression by surgical release of the transverse carpal ligament and removal of tissues that may be compressing the median nerve. Most patients are operated on in an ambulatory surgery setting and they go home as soon as reacted from anesthesia.

Facilitating learning

Teaching of the patient takes place before the day of surgery, or, if that is impossible, on the day of surgery. Patients should be given written directions about self-care to reinforce the preoperative teaching. The patient is taught the following:
1. Elevate hand and arm on pillows for 24 hours.
2. Perform active thumb and finger motion within limits imposed by the dressing.
3. Take the prescribed analgesic as necessary. Tylenol 3 is frequently prescribed.
4. Check fingers for circulation q 1-2 h; fingers should be warm and pink.
5. Check fingers for sensation and movement q 1-2 h.
6. Ideally, if living alone, patient should have someone at home to assist with meals and other needs for the first 24 hours.
7. Should be able to use hand in normal ADL 2 to 3 days after surgery.

Evaluation

Evaluation is based on expected patient outcomes. Because the patient is not hospitalized, the nurse may call the patient at home within 24 hours of surgery to ask the following questions:
1. Is the patient able to move the fingers on the operative hand?
2. Are the fingers warm and pink?
3. Can the patient feel sensations in the fingers?
4. Is the pain medication helpful in relieving discomfort? How often has the patient taken the pain medication?
5. Can the patient state what she or he is to do until he or she sees the surgeon for a postoperative visit? What is the date and time of the appointment?

DUPUYTREN'S CONTRACTURE
Etiology and Pathophysiology

Dupuytren's contracture is a common problem, particularly in men past middle age. The disorder is caused by a thickening and shortening of the palmar fascia on the ulnar side of one or both hands causing flexion of the ring finger and sometimes the small finger. The bands shorten, and the fingers are pulled into fixed flexion. The skin of the hand is drawn down, forming tight puckers and nodules.

Joints, muscles, tendon, or nervous or vascular tissue do not appear to be involved.

Nursing Process
Assessment
Subjective data

The patient complains of a gradual decrease in the ability to extend the ring and small fingers.

Objective data

The most obvious appearance of the patient's hand is the flexed position of the ring finger and possibly the small finger. The skin of the palm is drawn down, forming tight puckers and nodules. The condition starts in one hand but often occurs in both hands. The patient cannot actively extend the fingers.

Data analysis: nursing diagnoses

Nursing diagnoses are determined from the analyses of patient data. Possible nursing diagnoses for the person with Dupuytren's contracture may include, but are not limited to, the following:

Diagnostic title	Possible etiologies
Disuse syndrome (hand)	Thickening and shortening of palmar fascia
Knowledge deficit	Unfamiliarity with information resources

Planning: expected patient outcomes

Expected patient outcomes for the person with Dupuytren's contracture may include, but are not limited to, the following:
1. Patient will have full use of fingers and hand.
2. Patient will be able to state how to care for self after surgery.

Implementation
Interventions to achieve patient outcomes
Facilitating learning

Most patients will have surgery in an ambulatory care setting. Preoperatively they should be taught the following:
1. Soak hand in warm water and perform finger extension exercises at least twice daily.
2. Avoid activities that require grasping, such as holding a hammer.
3. What to expect on the day of surgery. Time to arrive at ambulatory center, which is usually at least 1 to 1½ hours before scheduled time of surgery. Should be accompanied by someone who will drive them home after surgery.
4. Postoperatively they should plan for the following:
   a. Elevate hand on pillows for at least 24 hours to prevent swelling of hand.
   b. Apply ice packs to hand. A large bag of frozen vegetables covered with towel is an easy and inexpensive way to apply cold packs.
   c. Take prescribed analgesics as prescribed for pain.
   d. Check fingers for sensation, circulation, and finger movements every 1-2 h for 24 hours. Fingers should be warm and pink.

Table 40-9 Degenerative disorder:
degenerative joint diseases (DJD)

Signs and symptoms	Medical therapy
Pain in the movable joints, particularly on weight bearing	Salicylates and nonsteroidal antiinflammatory agents
Mild tenderness to aggravated pain on overuse of joint	Aspirin NSAIAs Intraarticular injection of steroids for severe pain
Joints become enlarged with loss of motion	Adjunctive analgesics (Tylenol, Darvon)
Crepitation	Assistive devices to unload weight bearing from joints (canes, walkers, crutches)
Changes in alignment of affected part with flexion deformity	
Stiffness after periods of rest	Rest Exercise
Changes in certain joints:	Joint protection Surgery
Heberden's nodes— bony protuberances on dorsal surface of distal interphalangeal joints of fingers (Fig. 40-18)	Arthroscopy to remove bits of broken cartilage or bone Realignment (osteotomy) Fusion (arthrodesis) Joint replacement
Bouchard's nodes— on proximal interphalangeal joints of fingers	
Coxarthrosis— a degenerative change presenting with pain in hip with weight bearing; may progress to include pain in groin and medial side of knee	
Knee involvement— varus, valgus (Fig. 40-19), flexion deformity, limited range of motion	

e. Extend fingers every hour while awake.
f. Ideally, if living alone, should have someone with them for 24 hours to assist with meals and other needs.
g. Should be able to use hand in daily activities in 2 to 3 days.

Evaluation

Evaluation is based on expected patient outcomes. The patient should be called within 24 hours of surgery and asked the following questions:

1. Is the patient able to extend fingers and move hand?
2. Are the fingers and hand warm and pink?
3. Is the analgesic relieving discomfort? How often is he or she taking pain medication?
4. Can the patient state what activities he or she can do until he or she sees the surgeon? What is the date and time of his or her appointment with the surgeon?

DEGENERATIVE DISORDERS

Degenerative joint disease
Etiology/Epidemiology

Degenerative joint disease, also known as *osteoarthritis, hypertrophic arthritis, osteoarthrosis,* or *senescent arthritis,* is an extremely common disease that is probably as old as civilization. Almost everyone past 40 years of age has hypertrophic changes in the joints. About 80% of people over age 65 show evidence of osteoarthritic changes on x-ray.[46] Although symptomatic degenerative joint disease is usually noted in the 50- to 70-year age group, it has been observed as early as age 20. It is estimated that 15.8 million people or 12.1% of the United States population has osteoarthritis serious enough to cause pain. There are two forms of osteoarthritis: *primary,* for which the cause is unknown, and *secondary,* a result of trauma, infections, previous fractures, another type of arthritis (such as rheumatoid arthritis), the stress put on weight-bearing joints from long-term obesity, or the "wear and tear" on joints associated with some occupations (for example, coal mining and boxing). There may also be a genetic predisposition to the development of osteoarthritis. See Table 40-9 for signs and symptoms and medical therapy.

Prevention

1. Avoidance of obesity because of the added wear excess weight puts on joints, especially the hips and knees. For example, the knees are subject to peak impacts three to five times greater than total body weight.[46]
2. Avoidance of repeated trauma to joints.
3. Practice of techniques that protect joints in occupations that put joints at risk.

Pathophysiology

Degenerative joint disease (DJD) is a disease of the articular cartilage. Normally this cartilage is white, translucent, and smooth. When affected by the disease, it becomes yellow and opaque. Areas of cartilage soften and the surface becomes rough, frayed, and cracked. This process is thought to occur as a result of digestion of the cartilage by enzymes and alteration of the nutrition of the cartilage. Eventually the cartilage is destroyed, and the underlying subchondral bone goes through a remodeling process. *Osteophytes,* or spurs of new bone, appear at the joint margins and at the sites of attachment of supporting structures. These may break off and appear in the joint cavity as "joint mice." Unlike rheumatoid arthritis (RA), DJD affects only the joints and their surrounding tissue. It is not a systemic disease.

Healthy cartilage is 66% to 78% water, and most of its solid weight is accounted for by collagen and proteoglycans (large water-binding molecules). In osteoarthritis collagen appears unchanged, but the proteoglycan molecules are altered significantly. On microscopic examination healthy proteoglycans have the appearance of fresh Christmas trees, but in osteoarthritis proteoglycans look like scraggly trees. At present, it is not clear whether this change is a cause or a consequence of the disease.[47]

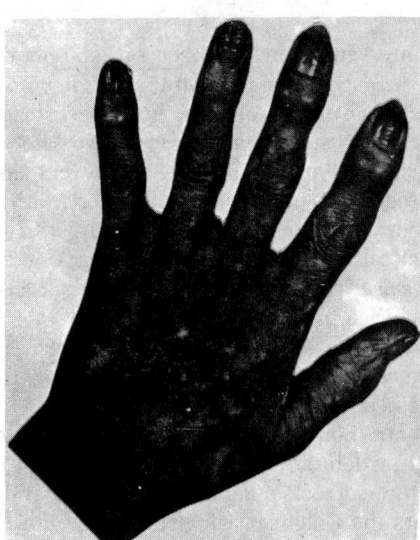

Fig. 40-18   Osteoarthritis of hand. Note enlargement of distal joints of index, middle, and little fingers (Heberden's nodes). (From Brashear H, Raney R: *Handbook of orthopaedic surgery,* ed 10, St Louis, 1986, Mosby–Year Book.)

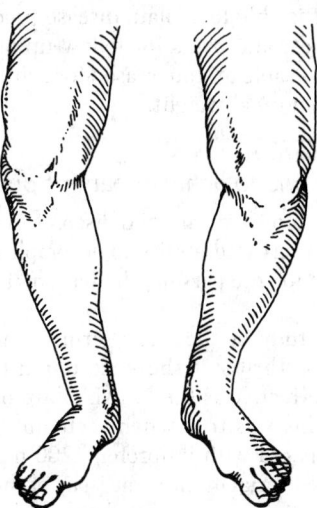

Fig. 40-19   Characteristic valgus deformity (bowing) of knees in degenerative arthritis. This deformity can be corrected by tibial osteotomy or total knee replacement.

Individuals with DJD have pain in the movable joints, particularly the large weight-bearing joints (hips, knees), and the joints of the hand. Inflammation is usually not present, and tenderness is mild; however, the joint may become enlarged. Crepitation may be present on movement, and alignment of the extremity may be changed. The patient usually has stiffness after periods of rest.

Nursing Process
Assessment
Subjective data

The person with degenerative joint disorder is usually in good health. Questions that are asked include the following:

1. When does pain occur?
2. What measures give relief?
3. What joints are involved?
4. What modifications in ADL have been made because of pain or restricted mobility?

Objective data

Because signs and symptoms are usually local, inspection and palpation are the best evaluators.
1. Affected joints may appear normal.
   a. Check for tenderness, grating, and crepitus.
   b. Palpate for enlargement or irregularity in size of joint and flexion or lateral deformities.
2. Observe the person walking. Is there a limp?
3. Evaluate range of motion of major joints.
4. Assess the vertebral column for limitation in cervical or lumbar areas.
5. Does the person have difficulty standing for periods of time or difficulty in arising from chair (particularly one without arms) after sitting for a period of time?

Diagnostic tests

1. X-ray films may be normal if pathologic changes are mild.
2. Progressive changes include the following:
   a. Narrowing of joint spaces
   b. Marginal osteophyte formation
   c. *Eburnation* (sclerosis) of subchondral bone
3. Serologic and synovial fluid examinations will be essentially normal.

Data analysis: nursing diagnoses

Nursing diagnoses are determined from analysis of patient data. Possible nursing diagnoses for the person with degenerative joint disease may include, but are not limited to, the following:

Diagnostic title	Possible etiologies
Pain: in affected joints	Degeneration in affected joints
Mobility, impaired physical	Musculoskeletal impairment caused by degeneration of affected joints
Activity intolerance	Restricted mobility caused by joint involvement
Self-care deficit: ADL	Pain and limited joint movement
Knowledge deficit: DJD	Lack of exposure to sources of information
Nutrition: altered, more than body requirements	Excessive intake in relation to metabolic needs

Planning: expected patient outcomes

Expected patient outcomes for the person with degenerative joint disease may include, but are not limited to, the following:

1. Patient is feeling more comfortable.
2. Patient is able to be more physically active.
3. Patient balances rest and activity.
4. Patient is able to perform self-care activities with less difficulty.

5. Patient is able to explain disease process, treatment measures, and plans for follow-up medical care.
6. Patient is able to state reason for achieving and maintaining normal weight.

Implementation
Interventions to achieve patient outcomes

Measures to relieve pain and discomfort and to promote mobility and increased ability to accomplish ADL are the same as those for the person who has rheumatoid arthritis (p. 1363).

A recent study of the short-term, symptomatic treatment of osteoarthritis of the knee found that acetaminophen was as effective as the NSAIA ibuprofen in relieving symptoms. This was true when acetaminophen 4000 mg/day was compared with ibuprofen 1200 mg/day and 2400 mg/day.[7] An editorial in the same issue of the New England Journal of Medicine points out that the publication of the article presents an opportunity to review the management of degenerative joint disease of the knee and hip, of which medication is only one component.[46]

Supporting weight loss

1. Review reasons why weight loss would improve symptoms.
2. Assess patient's motivation to lose weight.
3. Refer patient to dietitian for dietary assessment and dietary plan.
4. Compliment patient on weight loss no matter how small.
5. Make patient aware of support groups for those attempting to lose weight such as Weight Watchers or Overeater's Anonymous.
6. Make patient aware of good exercises for persons with joint disease, such as water walking, aquacise, and swimming.

Facilitating learning

The teaching plan would include the following:
1. Attention to posture
2. Weight reduction, prevention of weight gain
3. Use of ambulatory aids such as canes, crutches, or walkers to remove weight from painful joints
4. Alteration in ADL to avoid painful activities
5. Use of external measures such as local heat, prescribed exercises, and use of traction (if this is prescribed)

Evaluation

Evaluation is based on the expected patient outcomes. Questions to be asked include the following:
1. Is the patient more comfortable?
2. Is the patient able to be more physically active?
3. Is the patient able to balance rest and activity such as performing prescribed exercises independently?
4. Is the patient able to perform self-care activities with less difficulty?
5. Is the patient able to explain disease process, treatment measures, and follow-up care?
6. Can the patient discuss the reason for achieving and maintaining ideal weight?

Surgical intervention may be necessary to remove damaged bone or cartilage from the joint, realign or change the weight-bearing surfaces of the joint, or resurface the joint. The objectives of surgery are to (1) relieve pain, (2) restore joint function (if possible), and (3) prevent disability or further progression of the disease. Surgery to the knee and hip are most common, but shoulder surgery is becoming more practical and effective. Specific surgeries are:
1. *Debridement* (usually by arthroscopic surgery or arthrotomy): See p. 1368.
2. *Arthrodesis:* Through fusion of the joint, pain is relieved, joint motion is lost, but weight-bearing function is maintained. See p. 1368.
3. *Osteotomy:* Bone is cut to change alignment, thereby correcting deformity in the bone or adjacent joint. The procedure corrects angulation of rotational deformities or alters the weight-bearing surface in a diseased joint (Fig. 40-20). Osteotomy may be thought of as a surgical or intentional fracture, and the extremity is treated the same as after a fracture with the exception that weight bearing may be started earlier. Immobilization of the extremity and nursing interventions are similar to those employed after a fracture (p. 1405).
4. *Arthroplasty:* The two types of arthroplasty are:
   a. Interposition—resurfacing of one side of the joint with metal or other inert material or soft tissue such as fascia.
   b. Replacement—resurfacing of both sides of the joint with metal or polyethylene implants. Replacement implants are available for the hip (see Fig. 40-13), knee (see Fig. 40-14), shoulder, ankle, elbow, wrist, and interphalangeal joints of the fingers. Replacement prostheses may be either *cemented* (held into bone with polymethylmethacrylate) or *uncemented* (treated with a special porous coating that promotes in growth of bone). Care of the patient having an arthroplasty is discussed under rheumatoid arthritis on p. 1368.

DEGENERATIVE DISEASE OF THE SPINE

Degenerative disease of the spine is a common but difficult problem that merits special consideration. The signs and symptoms and medical therapy are listed in Table 40-10.

Pathophysiology

The spine has 23 intervertebral disk joints and 46 posterior facet joints (Fig. 40-21), all of which are subjected to stresses and strains in holding the human body upright and moving it about. The vertebrae in the spinal column are articulated in a series of "couplets" that are able to move through an intervertebral disk joint and two posterior facet joints. The intervertebral disks are composed of an outer layer of cartilage called the *anulus fibrosus* and an inner layer of cartilage called the *nucleus pulposus.* Several common problems arise with these structures in degenerative disease of the spine. They are the following:
1. *Herniated nucleus pulposus* (HNP)—Degeneration and dehydration of the cartilage composing the anulus and the nucleus result in a loss of elasticity. As

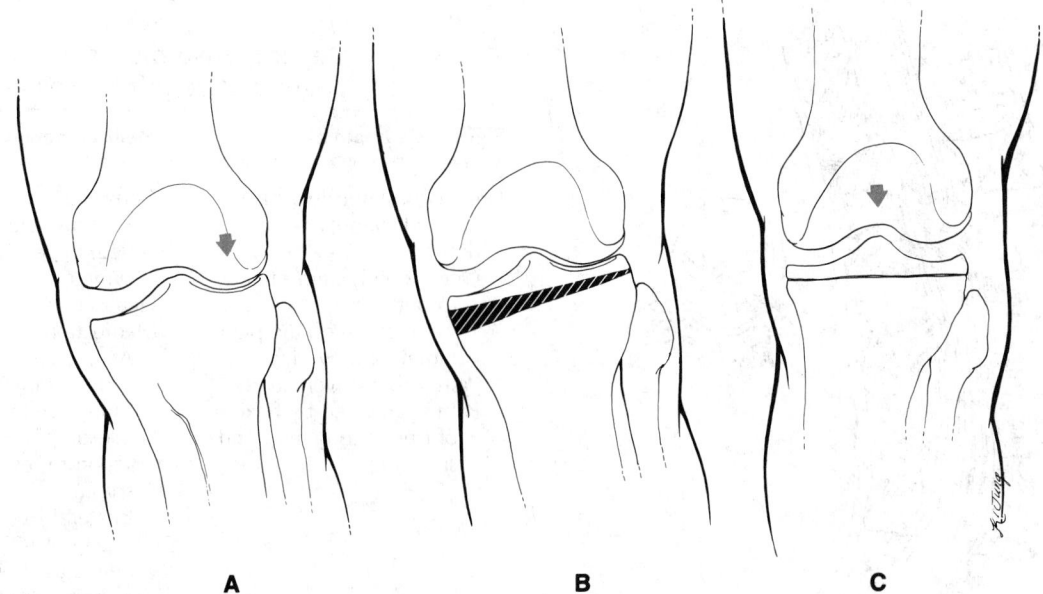

A **B** **C**

Fig. 40-20 Osteotomy of tibia. Genu valgum (anterior view of left knee). **A,** Weight-bearing force is concentrated on one compartment of knee. **B,** Wedge of bone is removed from tibia. Amount of bone removed is determined by amount of correction in angulation necessary. **C,** Distal portion of tibia is swung to proximal portion. Correction of angulation obtained allows weight-bearing forces to be more evenly distributed through both compartments of knee. (Adapted from Hollander JL, McCarty DR Jr: *Arthritis and allied conditions,* ed 8, Philadelphia, 1972, Lea & Febiger.)

the disk loses its resiliency, a strong force exerted across it can result in herniation of the nucleus through the anulus, either posteriorly or laterally. It is commonly referred to as a "ruptured disk." This results in compression of a spinal nerve root and subsequent pain (Fig. 40-22).

2. *Osteophyte* formation along the vertebral column can cause fusion of vertebrae with consequent limitation of motion, usually in the lumbodorsal region.

3. *Spinal stenosis,* or narrowing of the intervertebral foramina at any level of the spine, creates pressure on nerve roots in the involved area, resulting in neurologic symptoms including pain.

4. *Degenerative and/or rheumatoid involvement* of the *hyaline articular surfaces* of *the facet joints* results in *pain and limited motion.* Rheumatoid involvement with consequent loss of vertebral stability is particularly troublesome in the cervical spine.

The *diagnosis* of herniated disk is usually made on the basis of the history and physical examination. A history of low back pain relieved by recumbency and aggravated by flexion of the trunk, coughing, or sneezing is typical. The patient will often complain of sciatic pain radiating down the leg. Some persons, after the initial injury, will have sciatic pain going down the leg but no pain in their back. Deep pressure over the interspace will usually elicit pain. Straight leg raising with the hip flexed and the knee extended (a positive Lasegue sign) will produce sciatic pain. Neurologic signs and symptoms help in determining the level of the disk involved because sensory and motor changes depend on the nerve root involved. The most

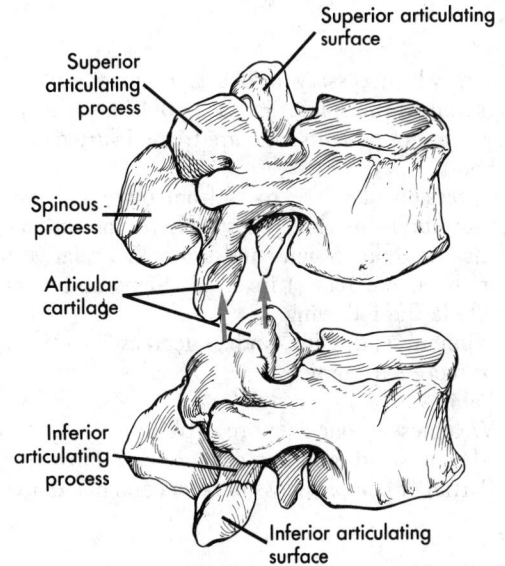

Fig. 40-21 Posterior facet joints of lumbar vertebrae. Each vertebra has four surfaces by which it articulates with its adjacent vertebrae: two on its superior aspect and two on the inferior. Superior articulating surfaces are medially located; the inferior, laterally. These joints are diarthrotic, having a joint capsule with a synovial lining.

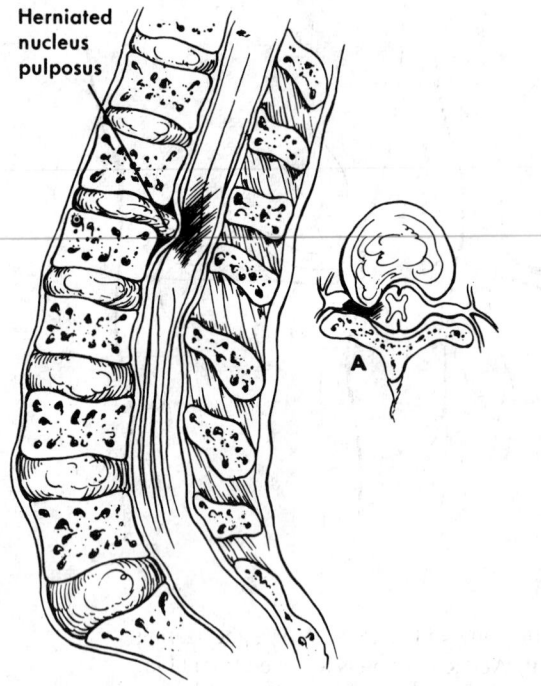

Fig. 40-22 Compression of spinal cord caused by herniation of nucleus pulposus into spinal cord. **A,** Pressure on nerves as they leave spinal canal.

common sites of lumbar herniation are L3-4, L4-5, and L5-S1.

Surgery

Surgery may be necessary to relieve pressure on nerve roots and to stabilize the spine. See Box 40-4 for types of spine surgery. Care of patients who are treated surgically is discussed on p. 1390.

Compression of nerve roots from other causes—stenosis, vertebral instability, osteophyte formation—will also cause neurologic signs and symptoms relative to the level of the nerve root(s) involved. Signs and symptoms may include the following:

1. Numbness, tingling, and/or decreased motion in one or more extremities
2. Pain
3. Weakness of one or more extremities
4. Muscle wasting in one or more extremities
5. Partial or complete loss of bowel and bladder control

Nursing Process
Assessment
Subjective data

The patient seeks help because of pain and inability to walk or to carry on normal activities. Answers to the following questions should be sought:

1. Is low back pain relieved by recumbency?
2. Is pain aggravated by flexion of the trunk, coughing, or sneezing?
3. Is there a history of injury followed by back pain?

REVIEW

Table 40-10 Degenerative disease: degenerative joint disease of spine

Signs and symptoms	Medical therapy
Chief complaint: low back pain relieved by lying down	*Conservative*
Occasionally pain radiates to buttocks	Rest (complete or modified) depending on symptoms
There may be sciatic pain radiating down leg	Heat
Pain follows overactivity	Medications
Pain aggravated by flexion of trunk, coughing, and sneezing	Analgesics and/or antiinflammatory agents
	Muscle relaxants (for example, diazepam)
	Traction to relieve muscle spasm
	Bilateral Buck's traction (Fig. 40-23)
	Pelvic traction
	Corset may be prescribed to support spine

Objective data

1. Observe movements and walking.
   a. Patient appears to guard hips and back.
   b. Patient seeks frequent position changes.
2. Straight leg raising flexing the hip with the knee extended may produce sciatic pain.
3. Palpate for tender areas and spasm of the paravertebral muscles and posterior superior iliac spine.
4. Observe relief of discomfort when patient is supine with head elevated a few degrees and knees flexed.
5. Observe for muscle atrophy; if back problem has been long-standing, changes will be seen in affected leg.

Diagnostic tests
Neurologic examination

1. Neurologic signs and symptoms will help in determining the level of vertebrae involved. Sensory and motor changes depend on the nerve root involved.
2. Roentgenographic evaluation
   a. For those patients whose symptoms are of short duration, the x-ray examination may fail to reveal any abnormlity.
   b. For those patients with long standing disorders, the x-ray examination may show significant narrowing of the disk space.
   c. Myelography, valuable in localizing the lesion, is reserved for confirmation of physical findings before surgery or to exclude conditions such as tumors.
   d. CAT scanning or magnetic resonance imaging (MRI) may be used for diagnosis.

Data analysis: nursing diagnoses and planning: expected patient outcomes

Nursing diagnoses and expected patient outcomes are similar to those for degenerative joint disease (p. 1385).

Types of spine surgery	
Laminectomy	Removal of a portion of the lamina
Diskectomy	Removal of all or part of a herniated intervertebral disk
Foraminotomy	Widening of the intervertebral foramen to allow free passage of the spinal nerve
Spinal fusion	Fusion of two or more vertebrae by insertion of bone grafts with or without the addition of metal rods or wires to achieve vertebral stability Thoracic and cervical vertebrae require fusion because of mobility of the spine in these areas

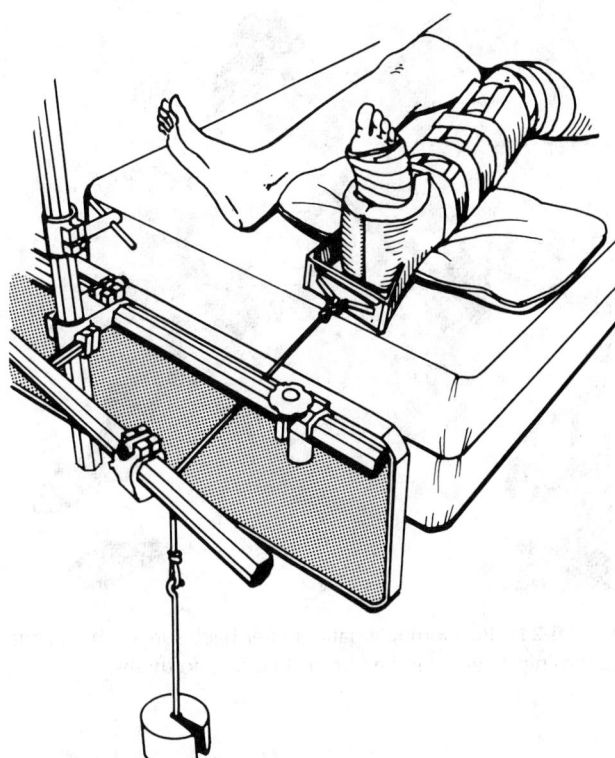

Fig. 40-23 Buck's extension. Heel is supported off bed to prevent pressure on heel, weight hangs free of the bed, and foot is well away from footboard of bed. The limb should lie parallel to the bed unless prevented, as in this case, by a slight knee flexion contracture.

Implementation
Interventions to achieve patient outcomes

For the patient being treated conservatively, the following interventions are appropriate.

Promoting comfort

1. Encourage slight elevation of head of bed and flexion of the knees (pillow under knees) when supine.
2. Roll patient onto bedpan rather than lifting onto pan.
3. Use fracture bedpan or small bedpan.
4. Apply heat as patient desires and tolerates.
5. Remove skin traction for periods of time if it causes patient discomfort.
6. Provide analgesics, antispasmodics at regular intervals as necessary.

Promoting circulation

1. Encourage patient to perform active dorsi-plantar flexion of the ankles at regular intervals.
2. Report any difficulty with brace to physician immediately.
3. Do not drive a car during period that brace must be worn.

Facilitating learning

1. Patients should learn to turn in bed in a *logrolling* fashion to maintain good spinal alignment: *cross the arms over the chest, bend the uppermost knee to the side to which they wish to turn, and then roll over as a unit.*
2. Constipation may be a problem.
   a. Urge patient to drink 3000 ml of fluids daily.
   b. Increase amount of roughage eaten; bran and fresh fruit are helpful.
   c. Give a mild laxative if necessary.
3. If brace or corset is ordered to provide external support for the spine, explain its need and application.
4. Teach principles of body mechanics.
   a. Avoid movements and positions that cause poor alignment of the spinal column and put strain on an injured nerve.
   b. Use a straight chair, not an overstuffed one.
   c. Avoid crossing the legs at the knees.
   d. Elevate the feet but flex the knees.
   e. During acute episodes, avoid stretching of the legs, such as driving a car or climbing stairs.
   f. In picking up items off the floor, bend the knees and keep the back straight.
5. When the acute episode subsides, the physician will order exercises designed to strengthen the back and abdominal muscles.

Evaluation

Evaluation is based on the expected patient outcomes, which are the same as for degenerative joint disease (see p. 1386).

SURGERY OF THE LUMBAR, THORACIC, OR CERVICAL SPINE

A laminectomy and/or spinal fusion may be performed. The nursing care for persons with lumbar, thoracic, or cervical spinal fusion is discussed next.

Care after spinal surgery (lumbar, thoracic, cervical)

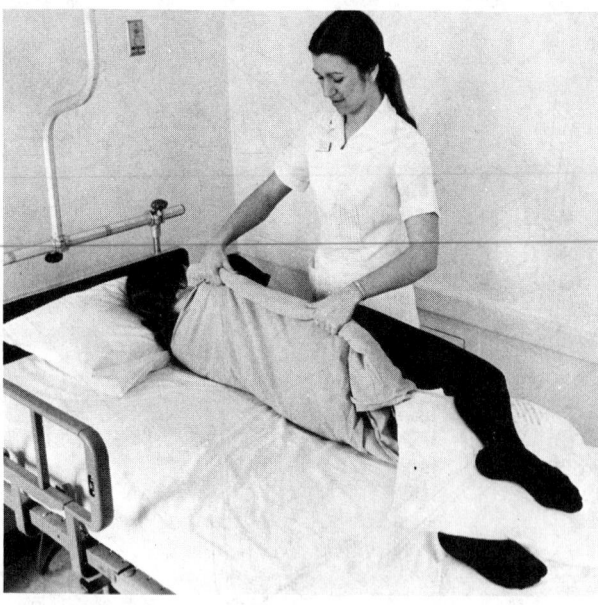

Fig. 40-24 Positioning a patient after back surgery by means of turning sheet extending from shoulders to thighs.

focuses on *positioning* and *mobility, wound care,* and *patient comfort.* Changing position in bed after *lumbar* surgery must be performed by logrolling; assistance is given as necessary, but patients can learn to do this for themselves. *Because patients tolerate sitting less well than walking or lying, sitting is avoided until the person can tolerate it.*

Thoracic spinal surgery may involve entering the chest cavity; if so, nursing care will include chest tube(s) and closed drainage as with other chest surgery (Chapter 24). Mobility restrictions are more prolonged than with lumbar surgery because the thoracic spine is more mobile; consequently, there is greater risk of dislodging grafts through improper motion.

Persons with *cervical spinal surgery* may *require tong* or *halo traction* (Chapter 37) or a halo brace. The person has edema of the throat in the early postoperative period, requiring attention to the person's ability to breathe and swallow.

The care of patients undergoing spinal fusion is discussed below.

Nursing Interventions for Patients Having Surgery of the Lumbar Spine

Preoperative care

1. Instruct patient in logrolling and performance of dorsiplantar exercises
2. Instruct patient about the surgical procedure, postoperative care, and expectations at discharge

Postoperative care

1. Positioning
   a. Head of bed is kept flat.
   b. Patient is encouraged to logroll when changing position from side to back to side.
   c. Use of a turning sheet (Fig. 40-24) is advised until patient can assist with turning.
2. Wound care: drains may be placed in wound to prevent hematoma formation.
   a. Maintain constant suction through drain if required.
   b. Maintain drain free of contamination.
   c. Inspect surgical area frequently for evidence of excess drainage or formation of hematoma (bulging of tissues surrounding surgical site).
   d. In a spinal fusion, inspect donor site (usually iliac crest) for drainage or hematoma.
3. Promoting comfort
   a. Reposition patient frequently.
   b. Narcotics are used initially; may be on patient-controlled analgesia (PCA); then nonnarcotic analgesics as patient tolerates.
   c. Use fracture bedpan or small bedpan.
4. Promoting mobility
   a. Patient with a *simple laminectomy* may be out of bed on the first day after surgery.
   b. Patient with a *laminectomy and fusion* may not be able to be out of bed for 3 to 5 days after the surgery.
   c. Two persons will be required to help patient out of bed. This patient should sit as little as possible while getting up.
      (1) If the patient has a brace or corset, it is applied *before* the patient gets out of bed.
      (2) Assist patient in moving to edge of the bed before turning on side.
      (3) Instruct patient to push off the bed with the uppermost hand and lowermost elbow.
      (4) One person guides the patient's trunk, the other assists the patient's legs over the side of the bed.
      (5) The process is reversed in getting patient back in bed.
   d. Patient may walk as much as tolerated; an assistive aid such as cane may be necessary.
   e. Patient is encouraged to participate in ADL within prescribed limits of mobility.
5. Discharge instructions
   a. May not lift or carry anything heavier than 5 lbs. (2.25 kg).
   b. May not drive car until permitted by surgeon.
   c. Should avoid twisting of the trunk.

Nursing Interventions for Patients Having Surgery of the Thoracic Spine

Preoperative care

Care is the same as for lumbar surgery.

Postoperative care

Care is the same as for lumbar surgery, with the following *additions or exceptions:*

1. Positioning
   a. Head of bed often is ordered to be elevated to 30 degrees.
2. Wound care
   a. If pleural cavity is entered, a chest tube will be inserted and must be managed after surgery (see Chapter 24).

3. Promoting comfort
   a. Assist patient in splinting chest while coughing.
4. Promoting mobility
   a. Encourage and assist patient in vigorous pulmonary toileting.
   b. Assist patient in maintaining bedrest for 1 week or longer with strict attention to avoidance of twisting or bending motions to prevent dislodging grafts.
   c. Discourage patient from vigorous pulling or pushing with the arms, because placing weight on them may dislodge the graft.
   d. Brace is routinely prescribed and must be applied before patient gets out of bed.
   e. Permit patient to perform whatever activities are comfortable within the limitations of the brace.
   f. Encourage participation in ADL within prescribed limits of mobility.
5. Discharge instruction
   a. Teach patient how to apply and remove the brace before getting out of bed for the first time.
   b. Teach patient to wear the brace whenever out of bed.

Nursing Interventions for Patients Having Surgery of the Cervical Spine
Preoperative Care

1. General instructions are the same as for any spine surgery.
2. If *tong* or *halo traction* or *halo brace* is to be used after surgery, familiarize patient with the apparatus before surgery by using pictures or actual tong or brace.

Postoperative care

1. Positioning
   a. Keep head of bed elevated 30 to 45 degrees, particularly if anterior surgical approach was used, to decrease swelling in throat.
   b. If patient is in a cervical brace, position is not restricted except by patient's tolerance.
   c. If patient is in cervical traction, may be turned side to back to side as tolerated.
2. Wound care
   a. Inspect surgical area, including iliac crest donor site, frequently for evidence of excess drainage or formation of hematoma.
   b. If tong or halo traction is being used, pin care may be required (see Chapter 37).
3. Promoting comfort
   a. Provide ice chips to soothe sore throat.
   b. Progress diet slowly because patient will have difficulty swallowing and will be afraid of choking. Full liquids (ice cream, custards, jello, nectars) are often better tolerated than clear juice or broth. However, milk products may increase mucus production.
   c. Medicate with analgesics as for any spine surgery. Donor sites often cause more discomfort than cervical site.
   d. May require aerosol treatments or humidification of air to loosen mucous secretions, facilitate their removal, and make breathing more comfortable.
4. Promoting mobility

a. If patient is in traction, encourage to perform ankle dorsi-plantar flexion exercises and quadriceps-setting 3 times daily to promote circulation, maintain leg strength.
   b. If patient is in brace, may be out of bed and walk as soon as tolerated.
   c. Walker may be necessary if donor site pain restricts mobility.
   d. Encourage participation in ADL to greatest extent possible.
5. Promoting safety
   a. Keep suction equipment and tracheostomy set in patient's room until swelling in throat subsides and patient is swallowing and breathing normally.
   b. Check adjustment screws and straps on brace frequently to ensure there is no loosening of the brace.
   c. When edema decreases brace will need to be readjusted by physician or orthotist.
6. Discharge instruction
   a. Teach patient to wear brace at all times.
   b. Report any difficulty with brace to physician immediately.
   c. Do not drive a car during period of time that brace must be worn.

RESTRICTIVE DISORDERS

Scoliosis

Lateral deviation of the spine from the midline is known as scoliosis. The classifications of scoliosis are the following:

Congenital, acquired, idiopathic (most common), functional (postural) and structural.

Table 40-11 lists the signs and symptoms and medical therapy for scoliosis.

Prevention

Screening programs for school-age children are effective in identifying early indications of scoliosis. Attention to good posture may be effective in preventing the disorder in both children and adults.

Etiology

The causes of scoliosis include the following: rickets, neuromuscular disorders, vertebral disorders, idiopathic (cause unknown), and congenital.

Pathophysiology

Scoliosis may develop in localized areas of the spinal column or involve the whole spinal column. Curves may be S-shaped or C-shaped. The degree of rotation of the curve is important because it determines the amount of impingement on the rib cage. Significant cardiac and pulmonary restrictions may be imposed by curves with a large degree of rotation. The balance of the curve is also important because it affects the stability of the spine and mobility of

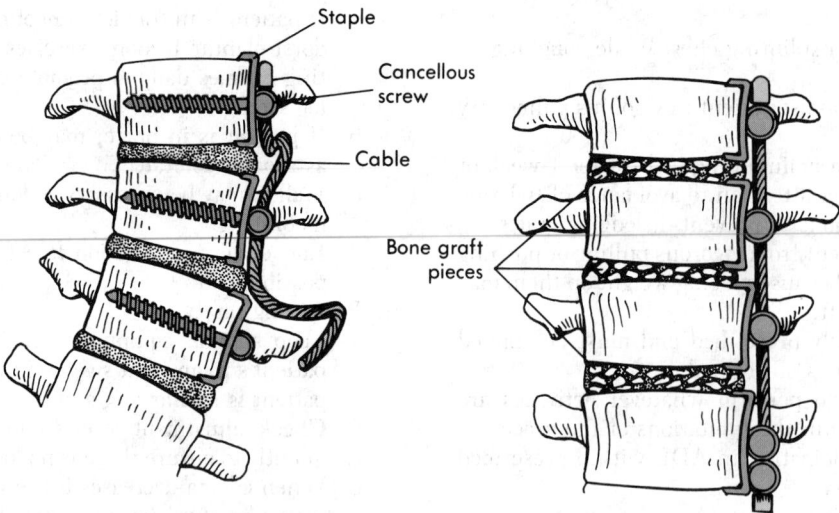

Fig. 40-25   Scoliosis fusion with Dwyer instrumentation. Cable is passed through openings in heads of screws that are embedded in vertebral bodies. Spaces between vertebrae are filled with bone chips as grafting material. Cable is pulled taut to secure and maintain correct alignment of vertebrae.

the trunk. Significant deviations in balance of the curve affect gait patterns.

The individual may initially have slight, mild, or severe deformity. Early deformity may not be obvious except on specific examination. Deformity will increase with growth and age. In the early stages, individuals may note that clothing does not fit correctly or hang evenly. The height of the shoulders is uneven. Pain is not usually an accompanying factor. In advanced scoliosis, when the cardiorespiratory system is affected, respiration is restricted and cardiac output is decreased. The curvature of the spine is confirmed on x-ray.

Nursing Process
Assessment
Subjective data

1. Clothing does not fit correctly or hang well.
2. Patient is unable to breathe comfortably or take a deep breath (pain may not be a problem).
3. Patient complains of progressive difficulty with ambulation.
4. Patient may state negative feelings about appearance.

Objective data

Observation and palpation are most important. Observe the gait, posture, and ability to rise from a chair; compare height of the shoulders. Palpate the spinal column with the patient in an upright position and bending forward. Palpate chest expansion on deep inspiration.

1. Visible curvature in spine and/or a pronounced rib hump when patient bends forward from the waist
2. Palpation of spinal curve with patient in upright position
3. Notable limp
4. Shoulders are uneven in height
5. One arm hangs closer to the body than the other

Data analysis: nursing diagnoses

Nursing diagnoses are determined from analysis of patient data. Possible nursing diagnoses for the persons with scoliosis may include, but are not limited to, the following:

Diagnostic title	Possible etiologies
Activity intolerance, high risk for	Musculoskeletal impairment
Body image disturbance	Scoliosis/change in body image
Breathing pattern, ineffective	Musculoskeletal impairment/ change in shape of thoracic cavity
Knowledge deficit	Lack of exposure to newer methods of treatment of scoliosis
Mobility, impaired physical	Musculoskeletal impairment/scoliosis
Pain, chronic: back	Musculoskeletal impairment/scoliosis

Planning: expected patient outcomes

Expected patient outcomes for the person with scoliosis being treated conservatively may include, but are not limited to, the following:

1. Patient balances rest and activity in terms of activity intolerance.
2. Patients states he or she feels better about body image since learning how to have clothing altered to disguise deformity.
3. Patient can demonstrate how slow controlled breathing pattern is effective.
4. Patient can explain what scoliosis is and her or his role in the following: postural exercises, applying, removing, and caring for brace; maintaining maximal function and independence, and long-range planning.

Table 40-11   Restrictive disorder: scoliosis

Signs and symptoms	Medical therapy

Lateral deviation of spine away from midline (in thoracic spine region)
One shoulder is higher than other
Movement of chest is restricted on deep inspiration
May complain of shortness of breath or difficulty in taking deep breath
	Early or postural scoliosis may be amenable to:
	  Postural exercise
	  Exercise combined with traction (for example, Cotrel's traction)
	In scoliosis where the curve is flexible (less than 40 degrees) and the patient is cooperative, bracing (Milwaukee brace, Risser cast, and a halofemoral or halopelvic traction) in combination with exercise may be sufficient to correct the deformity
	Corrective surgery (realignment of vertebrae and fusion) when curve exceeds 40 degrees and/or bracing has failed; usually accomplished with bone grafting and instrumentation
	Harrington rod instrumentation—series of rods and hooks that apply compression to the posterior spinal elements
	Dwyer instrumentation—titanium cables passed through heads of titanium screws imbedded in the vertebral bodies (Fig. 40-25)
	Luque instrumentation—two L-shaped rods and a series of wires that apply transverse traction to the vertebral bodies

5. Patient demonstrates positive response to impairment in physical ability by emphasizing what she or he can do.
6. Patient is able to control pain by postural exercises and rest periods.

Implementation
Facilitating learning

When patients are being treated conservatively, a major role of the nurse is teaching.
1. Instruct patient how to apply, remove, and care for brace.
2. Instruct and supervise patient in performance of prescribed exercises and use of traction equipment.
3. Advise patient regarding the selection of loose fitting, but attractive, clothing that conceals brace (particularly important for women and adolescents).
4. Advise patient that wearing brace need not restrict normal or desired activities.

Evaluation

1. Is patient able to balance rest and activity?
2. Does the patient state he or she feels better about appearance?
3. Can patient demonstrate a slow controlled breathing pattern?
4. Can patient explain what scoliosis is and his or her role in the conservative measures being used to treat it?
5. Does the patient emphasize what she or he can do instead of what he or she cannot do?
6. Is patient able to control pain by postural exercises and rest periods?

Some forms of scoliosis are not amenable to treatment with bracing or body cast; surgery may be performed to correct

the scoliosis. Most commonly, lumbar fusion is performed through a posterior incision, with the bone for the graft being taken from the iliac crest. Scoliosis fusions involve internal devices such as those listed in Table 40-11.

Expected patient outcomes of surgery

1. Complications of surgery are avoided.
2. Patient is able to explain surgical procedure.
3. Patient can perform prescribed exercises correctly.
4. Patient can explain follow-up program, including appointments with surgeon and physical therapist.

After surgery, the patient may be immobilized in a cast that extends from neck to pelvis. The cast remains on for 6 months. The care of the patient in a cast is covered on p. 1406.

Care of the person after spinal fusion for scoliosis is outlined below. The risk of postoperative pulmonary complications as a result of immobilization is high; therefore, preventive measures are important. Paralytic ileus is a common complication, and nasogastric suction is commonly employed in the first 24 to 72 hours after surgery. Patients with major *spinal procedures* also tend to retain fluid; therefore, they are *at risk for fluid overload* in the early postoperative period.

Nursing care of the patient undergoing scoliosis fusion
Preoperative care

1. Instruct the patient regarding pulmonary function studies (see Chapter 24).
2. Instruct the patient regarding the surgery, postoperative care, and expectations after discharge.

Postoperative care

1. Promoting comfort
   a. Medicate with narcotic analgesics as necessary; gradually decrease to nonnarcotic analgesics as pa-

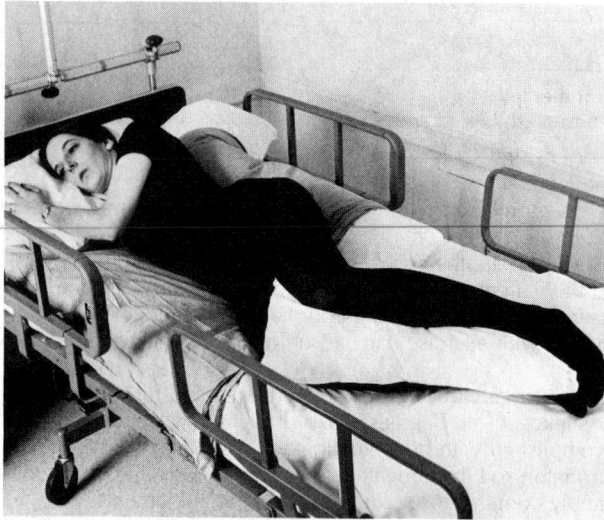

Fig. 40-26 Pillows behind the back provide support. Pillows between legs maintain anatomic alignment and decrease pull on lower back.

tient tolerates. Many patients will have PCA for pain relief.
   b. Turn and position frequently.
   c. Use a small or a fracture bedpan.
2. Positioning
   a. Bed is kept flat from 1 to 14 days, depending on the surgical technique used.
   b. Position patient side to back to side with use of a turning sheet (see Fig. 40-24) and pillows between the legs (Fig. 40-26) to maintain alignment.
3. Promoting safety
   a. Monitor vital signs, motor function, and sensation in the lower extremities frequently.
   b. Monitor closely for respiratory impairment.
4. Promoting mobility
   a. Encourage leg exercise as for other spinal surgery.
   b. Encourage participation in ADL to extent possible within limits imposed by surgery and/or brace, cast.
   c. Begin activity out of bed, in brace or cast if prescribed, as soon as surgeon permits. (Commencement of activity depends on surgical technique.)
5. Preventing complications
   a. To prevent atelectasis encourage breathing exercises including use of incentive spirometer as prescribed.
   b. To prevent paralytic ileus delay administration of oral food and fluid until patient is actively passing flatus.
   c. Monitor intravenous intake and urine output closely to prevent fluid overload until patient has postoperative diuresis (usually 3 to 4 days).
6. Wound care—same as for any spine surgery
7. Discharge teaching
   a. Care of brace or cast if required
   b. Use of bed board under mattress at home
   c. Plans for follow-up with physician and physical therapist.

Evaluation

Evaluation is based on the patient outcomes. Questions to consider may include the following:
1. Have complications of surgery been avoided?
2. Can the patient explain the nature of the surgery that has been performed?
3. Can the patient perform prescribed exercises correctly?
4. Is the patient functioning at the highest possible level?
5. Does the patient understand the reason for the physician's and physical therapist's follow-up program?

OTHER DISORDERS

GOUT
Etiology/Epidemiology

Gout or gouty arthritis is a metabolic disorder that affects men eight to nine times more frequently than women. It can occur at any age, the peak age of onset occurring in the fifth decade. Of all persons with gout, 85% have a genetic or familial tendency to develop the disease. Gout develops as a result of prolonged hyperuricemia (elevated serum uric acid) caused by problems either in synthesizing purines or by poor renal excretion of uric acid. The signs and symptoms and medical therapy are listed in Table 40-12.

Pathophysiology

Urate crystals form in the synovial tissue, causing severe inflammation. The inflammatory process is extremely rapid, occurring over a few hours. Acute symptoms are extreme pain, swelling, and erythema of the involved joints. Typically the great toe is involved (the first metatarsophalangeal joint), but other joints, such as the heel, ankle, and knee, may also be affected. Pain is so severe that the patient may not tolerate even the weight of a sheet over the joint. Renal damage may occur, especially if recurrent uric acid stones have been present. Between attacks of gout, the patient may be asymptomatic, but repeated attacks can occur with gradually increasing frequency if the disease is untreated. Patients with gouty symptoms may develop *tophi*, or deposits of monosodium urate in their tissues. These consist of a core of monosodium urate with a surrounding inflammatory reaction. Patients with tophaceous deposits (Fig. 40-27) tend to have more frequent and more severe episodes of gouty arthritis.

Nursing Process
Assessment
Subjective data

1. Acute episodes: chief complaint will be severe pain in great toe or other joints.
2. Question patient about previous episodes and what brought relief.
3. Has there been weight gain?
4. Is there a history of gouty arthritis in the family?
5. Does the patient take medication for gout?

REVIEW

Table 40-12 Gout

Signs and symptoms	Medical therapy

Acute: rapid onset of severe pain in inflamed joints—most frequently large toe
Presence of swelling and tenderness, malaise, headache, and fever
Chronic: always present in those who have familial tendency
Acute exacerbations occur when not diagnosed or not treated
Deposits of *tophi* (deposits of monosodium urate in tissues) most noticeable in ears, on knuckles, and on great toe
	Medications—acute attack
	 Colchicine (0.6) mg—oral administration of 2 tablets initially, then 1 tablet each hour until nausea, vomiting, or diarrhea occur, or joint symptoms subside; limit is 6.0 to 8.0 mg
	 Colchicine 1.0 to 3.0 mg in saline intravenously over a 10-minute period
	 Phenylbutazone (Butazolidin)
	 Indomethacin (Indocin)
	Absolute rest of the joint
	
	Preventive therapy consists of reduction of the body pool of urates by one of two methods:
	 Enhancing uric acid excretion
	  Probenecid (Benemid)—0.5 g daily for 1 week, then increased by 0.5 g weekly until serum uric acid is in normal range, then 0.5 g daily
	  Sulfinpyrazone (Anturane)—used for patients who do not tolerate Benemid
	 Decreasing uric acid formation
	  Allopurinol (Zyloprim)—100 mg twice a day initially, increased by 100 mg every 2-4 weeks until serum uric acid level is normal; then 500 mg daily

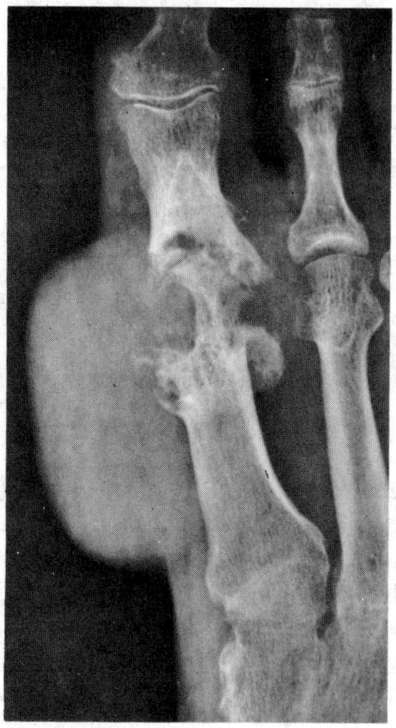

Fig. 40-27 Gout.

Diagnostic tests

1. Serum uric acid level will be elevated (hyperuricemia).
2. The 24-hour urinary uric acid level may be elevated.
3. Synovial fluid from the joint shows presence of monosodium urate crystals.
4. Sedimentation rate will be elevated.
5. X-ray examination will reveal soft tissue swelling.

Data analysis: nursing diagnoses

Nursing diagnoses are determined from an analysis of patient data. Possible nursing diagnoses for the person with gout may include, but are not limited to the following:

Diagnostic title	Possible etiologies
Pain: joint	Inflammation of joints with deposits of urate crystals in synovial tissues
Knowledge deficit	Lack of exposure to information about gout
Injury, high risk for: damage to joints or kidneys	High urinary levels of uric acid/uric acid stones, urate crystals in synovial tissues

Planning: expected patient outcomes

Expected patient outcomes for the person with gout may include, but are not limited to, the following:

1. Patient is free of joint pain.
2. Patient avoids subsequent attacks of gout.
3. Patient understands need to take medication as prescribed. Most patients take uricosuric agents daily for life to prevent injury to kidneys by uric acid kidney stones or to the joints by deposits of urate crystals.

Objective data

1. Patient cannot tolerate anyone touching the joint and will display guarding of the affected joint.
2. The joint is swollen and red (first metatarsal, tarsal joints, ankle, knee, or elbow) (see Fig. 40-27).
3. A low-grade fever is present.
4. Nodular swelling may be visible in the subcutaneous tissues overlying the joints or in the cartilage of the helix of the ear.

REVIEW

Table 40-13   **Bacterial arthritis**

Signs and symptoms	Medical therapy
Pain	Rest or immobilization
Swelling	Antibiotics specific for the organism
Tenderness of joint	Surgical drainage may be necessary
	Resumption of active range of motion when infection subsides

Implementation

Assisting with achievement of therapeutic goals

1. Give medications as prescribed. NSAIAs are frequently prescribed. Salicylates are to be avoided because they affect renal tubular handling of urate, causing increased serum levels.[83a]
2. Ensure that prescribed fluid intake is met.

Interventions to achieve patient outcomes

Promoting comfort

1. Provide absolute rest until pain of acute attack subsides.
2. Avoid touching joint or moving affected extremity until acute pain subsides.

Facilitating learning to prevent kidney and joint damage

1. Instruct patient in nature of disease.
2. Explain that dietary restrictions are not effective in lowering uric acid levels, except in those who are obese.
3. The emphasis is on prophylactic use of medications that decrease uric acid formation or enhance uric acid excretion.
4. Instruct patient in proper use of prescribed medications. Prophylactic medications must be taken daily for life.
5. Instruct patient not to take salicylates and to check over-the-counter medications carefully to ensure that they do not contain solicylates.
6. Encourage patient who is obese to reduce weight because this usually reduces uric acid level.
7. Encourage patient to take sufficient fluid daily to ensure daily output of 2000 to 3000 ml.
8. Encourage patients who are heavy consumers of alcohol to reduce their alcohol intake because alcohol can cause hyperuricemia and precipitate an acute attack of gout.

Evaluation

Evaluation is based on the expected patient outcomes. Questions to be asked include the following:

1. Is the patient free of joint pain?
2. Is the patient able to discuss medications, the need to take medication daily (to prevent joint and kidney damage), and follow-up care with physician.

BACTERIAL ARTHRITIS

Etiology

Bacterial arthritis is inflammation of the synovial tissues caused by bacterial agents, such as gonococci, meningococci, staphylococci, coliforms, salmonella, or *haemophilus influenzae*. Factors that predispose to infection are 1) susceptibility of the patient, 2) recent joint surgery or trauma, 3) intraarticular injections, and 4) rheumatoid arthritis. The joint cavity may become involved. The signs and symptoms and medical therapy are listed in Table 40-13.

Pathophysiology

Synovial tissues respond to bacterial invasion by becoming inflamed and secreting synovial fluid. If the joint cavity becomes involved, pus will be present in the synovial membrane and the synovial fluid. If allowed to progress, the infection will cause abscesses in the synovium and subchondral bone, eventually destroying cartilage. Ankylosis of the joint may result.

Nursing Process

Assessment

Subjective data

1. Ask patient to describe the onset of pain and changes noted in the joints.
2. Is patient being treated for another infection?
3. Is there a history of recent surgery or trauma?
4. Is there a history of recent sexual contact with a carrier of gonorrhea?

Objective data

1. Monitor the affected joint: it will be swollen and warm to touch.
2. Observe patient's resistance to movement of joint.
3. Monitor body temperature; fever may be present.
4. Observe for contractures that may be present if infection is of long duration.

Diagnostic tests

1. Joint may be aspirated to obtain synovial fluid for culture and sensitivity.
2. Joint fluid white cell count will be elevated, and glucose content will be reduced.
3. Roentgenograms may show loss of joint space and lytic changes in bone.

Data analysis: nursing diagnoses

Nursing diagnoses are determined from analysis of patient data. Possible nursing diagnoses for the person with bacterial arthritis may include, but are not limited to, the following:

Diagnostic title	Possible etiologies
Activity intolerance	Immobility; infection of joint
Pain	Infection in joint capsule
Knowledge deficit	Lack of exposure to information about the infection, its prevention, and its treatment

Planning: expected patient outcomes

Expected patient outcomes for the person with bacterial arthritis may include, but are not limited to, the following:

1. Activity improves as infection responds to antibiotics.
2. Patient's pain is lessened.
3. Patient understands need to take medication as prescribed after discharge.
4. Patient understands need to rest joint as prescribed.
5. Patient demonstrates ability to care for own cast or other joint-immobilizing device after discharge.
6. Patient can state plans for follow-up care.

Implementation

Assisting with achievement of therapeutic goals

1. Antibiotics are given as prescribed; reactions to drugs are monitored.
2. Surgical drainage or system of irrigation and drainage may be employed. Drainage is monitored for amount and color.
3. As soon as infection subsides, encourage the patient to move the affected joint to prevent contracture.

Interventions to achieve patient outcomes
Assisting with comfort and ADL

1. Give pain medication as prescribed.
2. During the acute stage, assist patient in resting and immobilizing the joint to help control pain and prevent deformity.
3. Assist patient with self-care.

Facilitating learning

1. Instruct patient in care of cast or other joint-immobilizing device.
2. Encourage active joint motion when motion is permitted.
3. Instruct patient in proper administration of antibiotics if therapy is to be continued after discharge.
4. Assure that patient is aware of plans for follow-up with physician.

Evaluation

Evaluation is based on the expected patient outcomes. Questions to be asked include the following:

1. Has infection of the joint subsided?
2. Can patient demonstrate joint range of motion without discomfort?
3. Can the patient care for cast or other joint-immobilizing device?
4. Can patient state plans for follow-up care?

TRAUMA TO BONE

The person who has suffered trauma to the musculoskeletal system has sustained an interruption in the integrity of one or more components of that system. *Musculoskeletal trauma is most frequently manifested as bone fracture, but it may also include injury to soft tissue, muscle, ligament, meniscus, tendon, or joint.*

FRACTURE OF BONE
Etiology/Epidemiology

Fracture of bone usually occurs as a result of a blow to the body, a fall, or other accident. However, fracture may occur during normal activity or after a minimal injury if the bone is weakened by a disease such as primary or metastatic cancer or osteoporosis. This is called a *pathologic fracture,* or a collapse of the bone. Bone may also fracture when the muscles associated with it are unable to absorb energy as they usually do. This type of fracture is called a *fatigue* or *stress fracture.* Another type of fracture occurs when a strong ligament or tendon attachment pulls a fragment of bone away from the rest of the bone. This is called an *avulsion fracture. Fracture can occur at any age, although older persons, persons with balance or mobility problems, persons who work at high-risk occupations (for example, steelworkers, race car drivers), and persons with chronic degenerative or neoplastic diseases are at higher risk for injury.* The signs and symptoms and immediate medical therapy are listed in Table 40-14.

Primary and Secondary Prevention

One approach to preventing fracture is to make the environment safer. Examples of measures that can be taken include the following:

1. Mounting grab bars on the wall next to a tub or toilet
2. Attaching safety arms around a toilet
3. Removing throw rugs and obstacles from areas used by individuals with locomotor problems
4. Assuring that wheelchairs have adequate locking devices
5. Teaching individuals who must use ambulatory devices and wheelchairs how to use them properly

A *second* approach is to continue to educate the public regarding the following:

1. The dangers of drinking and driving
2. The advisability of using seat belts
3. Attending to safety precautions when climbing ladders, using power tools or heavy equipment
4. Wearing recommended protective clothing (for example, steel-toed shoes, hard hats) for hazardous work at home or on the job
5. Wearing proper protective clothing while engaging in sports (for example, protective padding, well-fitting running shoes)

A *third* approach is to continue to educate women regarding the problem of *osteoporosis.* Individuals most at risk to develop osteoporosis are small-framed, nonobese, menopausal white females who smoke. Contributing factors are diets low in calcium throughout life, smoking, excessive coffee intake, too much protein in the diet, and a sedentary lifestyle. Measures that can be taken to retard osteoporosis include the following:

1. Increasing calcium intake
2. Stopping smoking
3. Decreasing coffee intake
4. Decreasing excess protein in the diet
5. Engaging in regular moderate activity such as walking, bike riding, or swimming at least 3 days a week

Table 40-14 Fractures

Signs and symptoms	Medical therapy
Complete fracture	**Management objectives**
Pain immediate and severe and aggravated by movement and pressure at site	Reduction of fracture by approximating the fracture fragments
Loss of function of injured part	Maintenance of fragments in correct alignment
Obvious gross deformity when compared with normal extremity	Prevention of excessive loss of joint mobility and muscle tone
Loss of rigidity of injured part—motion at site of fracture	**Immediate management**
Movement produces grating sound (crepitus) of bone fragments	Provide splint before moving patient or maintain support above and below fracture site until patient can be moved and immobilization applied with splints for transportation
Soft tissue edema—localized swelling and ecchymosis (may not be apparent for several hours or days)	Elevate extremity to minimize edema
Warmth over injured area resulting from increased blood flow to the area	Transport patient for emergency treatment
	Observe injured part at frequent intervals for local changes in color, sensation, or temperature
Loss of sensation or paralysis distal to injury resulting from nerve entrapment	Tetanus immunization is given if compound fracture is present
Signs of shock related to severe tissue injury, blood loss, or intense pain	Cold applications are used to reduce hemorrhage, edema, and pain
Evidence of fracture on x-ray film	Medication for pain is given
NOTE: Symptoms may be absent in linear compacted fractures.	Monitor for signs of shock—falling blood pressure, weak thready pulse, cold clammy skin, oliguria
There may be little or no swelling	**Secondary management**
Pain is present only when pressure is applied to fracture site or on use of limb or body part	*Simple fracture*
	Optimal reduction (replacing bone fragments in their correct anatomic position)
	Manual manipulation: moving the bone fragments into position by applying traction and pressure to the distal fragment
	Traction
	Open reduction: surgical intervention that may incorporate use of an internal fixation device
	Immobilization
	External fixation: cast or splint
	Traction
	Internal fixation: pins, plates, screws, wires, prostheses
	Combination of the above
	Compound fracture
	Surgical debridement of wound to remove dirt, foreign material, devitalized tissue, and necrotic bone
	Administration of tetanus toxoid
	Culture of wound
	Packing of wound
	Treatment with antibiotics
	Observation for signs of osteomyelitis, tetanus, or gas gangrene
	Surgical closure of wound when there is no sign of infection
	Reduction of fracture
	Immobilization of fracture
	Treatment of complications is discussed in Table 40-16

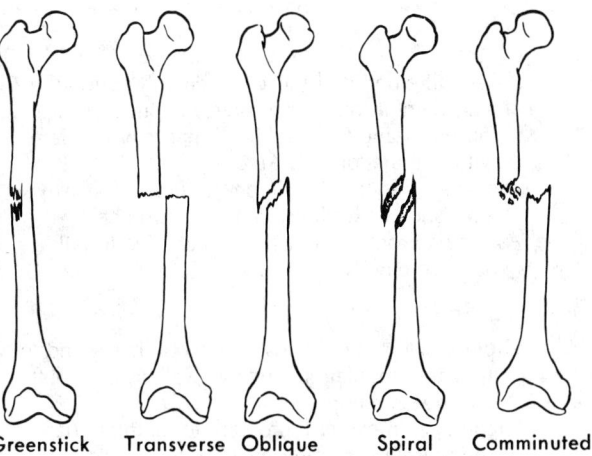

Greenstick   Transverse   Oblique   Spiral   Comminuted

Fig. 40-28   Types of fractures.

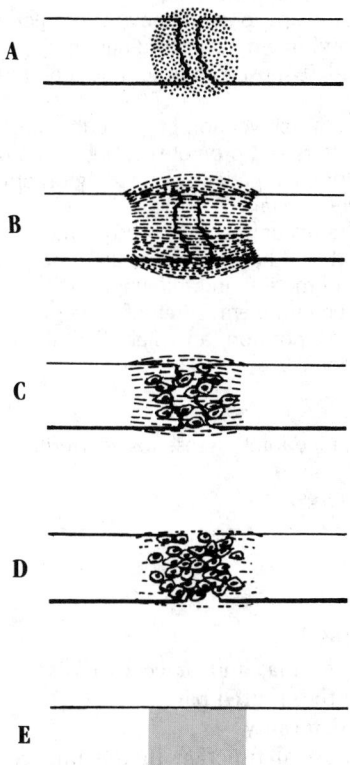

Fig. 40-29 Bone healing (schematic representation). **A,** Bleeding at broken ends of the bone with subsequent hematoma formation. **B,** Organization of hematoma into fibrous network. **C,** Invasion of osteoblasts, lengthening of collagen strands, and deposition of calcium. **D,** Callus formation: new bone is built up as osteoclasts destroy dead bone. **E,** Remodeling is accomplished as excess callus is reabsorbed and trabecular bone is laid down.

40-5

Classification of bone fractures

Classification according to types of fractures

Complete fracture: complete separation of the bone producing two fragments

Incomplete fracture: a partial break in the bone without separation of the bone

Simple or closed fracture: bone is broken; skin is intact

Compound or *open* fracture: the fracture parts extend through the skin

Fracture without displacement: bone is broken; bone fragments are in alignment in normal position

Fracture with displacement: bone fragments have separated at the point of fracture

Comminuted fracture: the bone has broken into several fragments

Impacted ("telescoped") fracture: one bone fragment is forcibly driven into another bone fragment

Classification according to line of fracture (Fig. 40-28)

Greenstick: splintering of one side of the bone (occurs most often in children with soft bones)

Transverse: break across the bone

Oblique: line of fracture at an oblique angle to the bone shaft

Spiral: line of fracture encircles the bone

6. Exploring with one's physician the advisability of estrogen replacement at menopause

Pathophysiology and bone healing

A bone is said to be *fractured* or *broken* when there is an interruption in bone continuity. Commonly, a fracture is accompanied by *soft tissue* injury to surrounding tissues, that is, ligaments, muscle tendons, blood vessels, and nerves.

The classification of bone fractures is given in Box 40-5.

Immobilization of a bone that is fractured is necessary for bone healing. Immobilization takes place by the following means:

1. *Physiologic splintage.* This form of splintage will occur naturally, because guarding, avoidance of use, and muscle spasm will occur as a result of pain on movement.

2. *External orthopedic splintage.* This is accomplished with devices such as plaster casts and traction.

3. *Internal fixation.* In this method the opposing ends of the fracture are held in place by screws, plates, or rods. After immobilization is accomplished, new bone called *callus* begins to form by the following stages of growth (Fig. 40-29):

   a. *Hematoma formation.* Because blood vessels are injured, bleeding occurs at the site of the fracture. The blood collects and fastens the broken ends of bones together.

b. *Fibrin meshwork.* The hematoma becomes organized as fibroblasts invade the area, forming the fibrin meshwork. White blood cells wall off the area, localizing the inflammation.

c. *Invasion by osteoblasts.* The osteoblasts enter the fibrous area to help hold the union firm. Blood vessels develop, establishing a source of nutrients for building collagen. Collagen strands begin to incorporate calcium deposits.

d. *Callus formation.*

i. Osteoblasts continue to lay the network for bone buildup.

ii. Osteoclasts destroy dead bone and help to synthesize new bone.

iii. The collagen strengthens and continues to incorporate calcium deposits.

e. *Remodeling.* In this final step, excess callus is reabsorbed and trabecular bone is laid down along lines of stress.

Factors that impede or prevent callus formation include the following:

1. *Delayed healing or delayed union.* Delayed union occurs when the fracture does not heal within the usual time for healing.

a. Reasons:

(1) Callus is broken or torn apart by too much activity.

(2) Edema at the fracture site impedes flow of nutrients to the area.

(3) Immobilization is inefficient.

(4) Infection is present at fracture site.

(5) Patient is in poor nutritional state.

b. Correction: More complete immobilization or open reduction for surgical measures.

2. *Nonunion.* Nonunion is the term used when healing does not occur even in a much longer period of time.

a. Reasons:

(1) Too much bone loss at time of injury to permit bridging of bone fragments.

(2) Bone necrosis has occurred because of lack of blood supply.

(3) Anemia, endocrine imbalance, or other systemic conditions that interfere with the process are present.

b. Correction:

(1) Crutches may have to be used indefinitely.

(2) A brace may be worn to support the limb.

(3) Surgery may be performed to unite bone fragments with a bone graft.

Nursing Process
Assessment
Subjective data

1. Pain at site of injury
2. Loss of sensation or movement of affected part
3. Description of how trauma occurred
4. Did the person fall? In older persons fracture of hip, ankle, etc., may occur first, causing the person to fall.
5. Understanding how injury sustained (may report having heard bone snap)

The Elderly with Musculoskeletal Problems

Assessment

Assess all elderly for muscle strength and tone, gait, painful joints or muscles, contractures, deformities, and foot problems that may interfere with ambulation and ADL.

Assess availability, condition, and use of assistive aids, such as walkers, canes, or crutches.

Assess environmental factors conducive to falls because elderly are at high risk for falls.

Intervention

Order assistive aids to foster independence and to increase ambulation, such as walker, cane, lift, bedside commode.

Encourage an exercise program to maintain baseline muscle and joint function.

Perform active and passive range of motion for elderly on bedrest.

Obtain orders for progressive ambulation as early in hospitalization as possible.

Position extremities in normal body alignment; elderly are highly susceptible to flexion contractures.

Teach good foot care and importance of well-fitted shoes.

Request physical therapy for patients with gait/mobility problems.

Request occupational therapy for problems with ADL and fine motor coordination.

Teach elderly how to transfer and ambulate safely.

Initiate a fall-prevention program that identifies risk factors and promotes an individualized plan for each patient, depending on ability and tendency to fall.

Use restraints only as a last resort; reevaluate use every 4 to 8 hours; remove them frequently for range of motion and toileting.

Be sure environment is free of clutter; bed is kept in lowest position, and night light illuminates the floor.

Common disorders in elderly

Degenerative joint disease (osteoarthritis)
Osteoporosis
Hip fractures

Objective data

1. Warmth, edema, and/or ecchymosis over and surrounding the injured part
2. Obvious deformity
3. Loss of normal function in the injured part—inability to bear weight
4. Immobilization device(s) applied to the injured part
5. Signs of systemic shock
6. Signs of circulatory, motor, or sensory impairment to the injured part (see Table 40-15)
7. Indicators of apprehension or fear

Diagnostic tests

Radiographs of site to determine extent of injury.

Table 40-15   Observations for signs and symptoms of neurocirculatory impairment

Observation	Interpretation
Tissue color white	Decreased arterial blood supply
Tissue color blue	Venous stasis and poorly oxygenated tissue
Color slow to return to nail bed after application of moderate pressure	Decreased arterial blood supply
Edema	Fluid accumulating in tissues; poor venous return
Tissue cold or cool to touch	Decreased arterial blood supply
Patient unable to move parts distal to cast	Pressure on nerves innervating parts distal to cast
Patient complaint of heightened or decreased sensation or paresthesia in part underlying or distal to cast	Pressure on nerves innervating parts underlying or distal to cast
Patient complaint of extreme pain unrelieved by elevation, analgesic, or repositioning	Pressure on nerve endings in parts underlying or distal to cast

NOTE: Comparison of tissue should be made with contralateral tissue to determine extent of deviation from normal

Data analysis: nursing diagnoses

Nursing diagnoses are determined from analysis of patient data. Possible nursing diagnoses for the person with a fractured bone may include, but are not limited to, the following:

Diagnostic title	Possible etiologies
Tissue perfusion, altered: peripheral	Decreased mobility, pressure, trauma
Mobility, impaired physical	Musculoskeletal impairment, decreased strength and endurance, pain
Self-care deficit	Musculoskeletal impairment, pain/discomfort, intolerance to activity
Powerlessness	Health care environment, decreased mobility
Skin integrity, impaired, actual or high risk for	Decreased mobility, pressure, shearing forces
Infection, high risk for	Tissue trauma, surgical intervention
Nutrition, altered: less than body requirements	Fatigue, pain, chewing or swallowing difficulties
Pain	Injury to bone, injury to soft tissue at fracture site, muscle spasm, immobility, improper positioning, pressure points
Injury, high risk for	Sensory/motor deficits
Knowledge deficit: fracture	Lack of experience with fracture and how it is treated

Planning: expected patient outcomes

Expected patient outcomes for the person with a fracture may include, but are not limited to, the following:

1. Patient's skin is warm and skin and mucous membranes are pink.
2. Patient participates in a program of progressive activity.
3. Patient is able to carry out ADL with minimal assistance.
4. Patient states he or she feels more in control of situation as mobility improves.
5. Patient's skin is intact and free of pressure ulcers.
6. Patient does not develop an infection.
7. Patient is able to maintain weight within 5 lb of preinjury weight.
8. Patient states feeling more comfortable.
9. Patient does not sustain an injury.
10. Patient and/or significant other can explain the following:
    a. Nature of injury and course of treatment that must be followed to prevent injury or infection and to achieve desired result
    b. Limitations of motion and restrictions of activity to be observed and for how long
    c. How to perform or modify ADL within the limitations of activity and motion that must be observed
    d. How to care for cast, pins, or other immobilization devices, if applicable
    e. Safe use of an ambulatory or other ADL assistive device, if necessary
    f. Aseptic technique in carrying out wound care, if necessary
    g. Techniques appropriate to prevent skin breakdown, swelling, and neurocirculatory impairment
    h. Measures that can be taken for relief of pain or discomfort
    i. How to use prescribed medications
    j. Plans for follow-up care

Implementation
Interventions to achieve patient outcomes
Promoting comfort and preventing complications

The purpose of positioning is to promote comfort and prevent complications. Knowledge needed before positioning includes the following:

1. Where is the fracture?
2. What is the nature of the fracture?
3. Has the fracture been reduced?
4. What method was used to reduce the fracture?
5. What are the tolerances of the method used to reduce the fracture?
6. Is the fracture stable?
7. Has the orthopedist requested special precautions?

After this information is obtained, positioning should be carried out with careful attention to the following:

1. Avoid altering the alignment of the fracture
2. Avoid changing the direction of the pull of traction
3. Avoid compromising the integrity of the cast
4. Avoid placing undue stress on the internal fixation device
5. Avoid changing position of patient before fracture has been reduced or splinted
6. After fracture is reduced or splinted, assist patient in changing position at *least* every 2 hours
7. Provide overhead frame and trapeze to assist patient in moving about in bed

Monitoring for neurocirculatory compromise

Monitoring for neurocirculatory compromise must be carried out every hour in the initial stages of fracture. Damage to blood vessels and/or nerves may occur at the time of the fracture or after the fracture or its reduction. Some swelling of a fractured extremity may be expected and is often well controlled by elevating the extremity. However, unrelieved swelling of an extremity that is in a cast or compression dressing can result in tissue damage and/or neurologic impairment. *Evidence of impaired circulation or sensation must be reported to the physician immediately.* Frequency of neurocirculatory checks can usually be reduced if there is no evidence of compromise within 48 hours of the fracture or reduction of the fracture (See Table 40-15).

Monitoring neurocirculatory status of the injured part includes the following:

1. Palpation for warmth
2. Observation of color
3. Application of moderate pressure to the nail bed and subsequent observation of capillary refill
4. Questioning the patient regarding pain or paresthesias in the injured part
5. Touching the injured part to test the patient's ability to discriminate sensation
6. Observation of patient's ability to voluntarily move body part distal to fracture

Promoting mobility and self-care

Encourage the patient to do the following:

1. Move about to the greatest extent possible within the restriction of the fracture reduction and the immobilizing devices
2. Accomplish as much of own self-care as possible
3. Perform muscle toning (isometric) exercises on a regular basis: quadriceps setting, gluteal setting
4. Follow through with exercise program (including ambulation) prescribed by the physician and taught by the physical therapist.
5. Resume normal functioning for all ADL (within limits of immobilization or fixation device) as soon as possible; for example, using bedside commode or toilet instead of bedpan

Decreasing powerlessness

1. Encourage patient to express feeling about his or her injury and immobility.
2. Encourage patient to participate in planning his or her care.
3. Encourage patient to give as much of own care as possible.
4. Give the patient as much control over the daily schedule as possible.
5. Prepare patient for scheduled tests and procedures and try to avoid unexpected events.
6. Compliment the patient on even the smallest gain in being more independent.
7. Provide realistic reassurance.

Maintaining skin integrity

1. Early identification of skin areas at risk, particularly areas over bony prominences (for example, heels, sacrum, elbows, ischial tuberosities)
2. Application of a skin toughening agent, such as tincture of benzoin, two or three times a day to areas identified as being at risk
3. Regular (at least every 8 hours) inspection for signs of pressure (erythema, induration)
4. Regular turning (at least every 2 hours) within the limits of the system of fracture immobilization
5. Turning the patient with a turning sheet (see Fig. 40-24)
6. Moving the patient from one surface to another with a pull sheet or roller board
7. Rolling the patient onto his or her side or lifting them to place them on a bedpan rather than sliding the pan under them
8. For patients who cannot be fully turned because of traction or other limiting factors, consideration should be given to using one or more of the following:
   a. Sheepskin pads
   b. Flotation pads
   c. Alternating air pressure mattress or alternating air pressure system, such as the Lapidus system
   d. Foam mattress
   e. Foam heel and/or elbow pads
   f. Special beds, such as the CircOlectric, Clinitron, or Mediscus bed
   g. Turning frames, such as the Foster or Stryker frames
9. Regular inspection of skin areas in contact with cast edges or traction apparatus and taking appropriate measures to eliminate chafing or rubbing in those areas
10. Assisting the patient with keeping skin clean and dry, especially under casts, slings, traction apparatus

Preventing infection and promoting wound healing

1. Strict attention to aseptic technique during dressing changes
2. Attention to drains to maintain their placement and patency
3. Caring for pin site as ordered
4. Encouraging to eat a well-balanced diet

Promoting nutrition

1. Encourage patient to eat regular meals
2. Give the patient plenty of time to eat

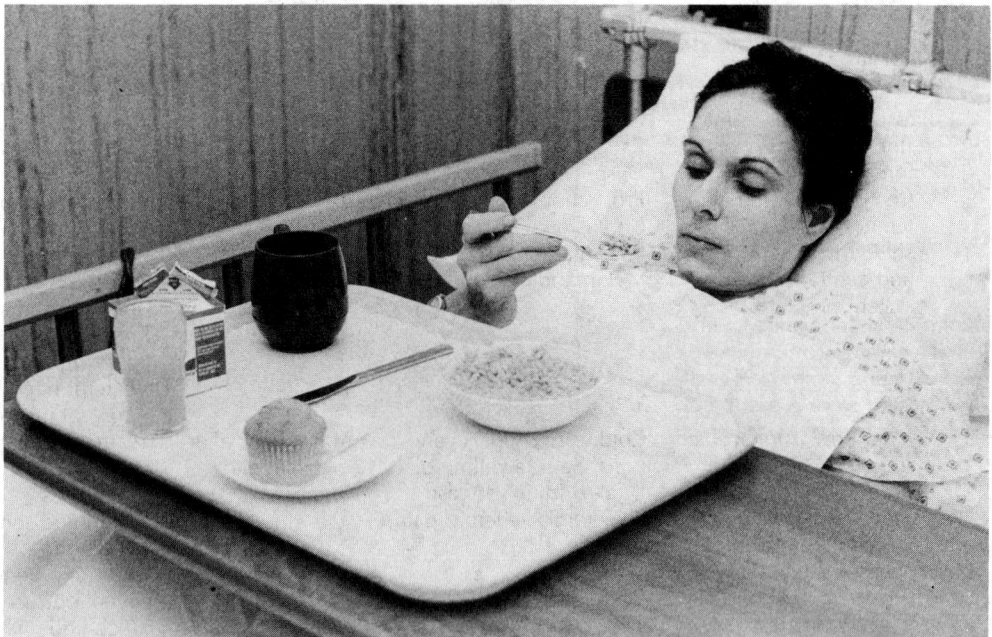

Fig. 40-30 Patient who can neither sit up nor lie on one side to eat meals can still be made comfortable with some elevation of the head and shoulders on pillows. Additional means of elevating patient to a more upright position is to put frame of bed in reverse Trendelenburg's position.

3. Encourage self-feeding, but assist the patient or provide special assistive utensils as necessary
4. Attend to the patient's need for roughage and fluid as noted, and encourage protein intake of 150-300 g per day
5. Position the patient to facilitate comfortable intake of food and fluid (Fig. 40-30)

Maintaining immobilization of the reduced fracture

The purpose of immobilization is to hold the broken bone fragments in contact with each other until healing takes place. Immobilization can be accomplished in the following ways:
1. Externally with
   a. Cast
   b. Splint
   c. Brace
   d. Cast brace
   e. Traction
2. Internally with
   a. Metal plates, pins, screws, nails
   b. Bone grafts with addition of metal plates, pins
   c. Prosthetic implants
3. Externally and internally with combinations of the above

Assisting with comfort and ADL
Managing pain

The person with a fracture will most often have severe pain at the fracture site, pressure from edema in damaged soft tissues adjacent to the fracture, and spasm of muscles in the fracture area. Continued pain and the muscle spasm accompanying it can put undue stress on the fracture fragments and retard efforts both to reduce and maintain reduction of the fracture. Patients who are in severe pain will resist efforts to assist them in carrying out measures designed to prevent complications. If the fracture is repaired by open reduction and internal fixation, the patient will have operative pain.

Measures the nurse can take to help reduce pain include the following:
1. During the initial stages of treatment, administer prescribed narcotic and nonnarcotic analgesics in appropriate dosages at timely intervals unless patient-controlled analgesia (PCA) is being used
2. Administer prescribed agents such as diazepam (Valium) to reduce muscle spasm
3. Apply ice compresses, as ordered, to affected part
4. Reposition the patient frequently within the restrictions of the prescribed treatment
5. Instruct the patient how to use relaxation techniques (deep breathing, imagery) to reduce tension
6. As pain subsides, negotiate with the patient a reduction in the strength and/or frequency of analgesics

It is important, in using analgesics, to try to strike a balance between having the patient comfortable enough to perform required exercises and other activities, and having the patient so overly medicated as to risk potential damage through over-extending activity or being heavily sedated. This is one advantage of PCA, which usually maintains comfort while preventing overmedication.

Table 40-16   Complications of fracture

Complication	Mechanism	Signs	Onset	Treatment
Fat embolism	Pressure changes in interior of fractured bones force molecules of fat from marrow into systemic circulation, resulting in respiratory and central nervous system problems	Chest pain Pallor Dyspnea Prostration Confusion Petechial hemorrhage of skin and conjunctivae	2-3 days after injury	Supportive measures; that is, high Fowler's position, oxygen therapy, blood transfusion to relieve hypovolemic shock, digitalization for heart failure Diuretics Bronchodilators Corticosteroids Proper immobilization and careful handling may help prevent occurrence
Ischemic paralysis (contracture)	Arterial flow is interrupted to injured part by trauma or pressure	Coldness, pallor, cyanosis, pain, swelling distal to injury or cast	At injury or after cast application	Treatment of fracture Release of cast or constricting bandages
Osteomyelitis	Bacteria introduced through wound or from another site in body (for example, boils) Infection of marrow spaces, haversian canals, and subperiosteal space with subsequent destruction of bone by proteolytic enzymes	Hyperemia, edema, pain, pus		Culture and sensitivity testing, antibiotics, surgical drainage, and debridement Prevention: use of aseptic technique when caring for open wound

Preventing injury

1. Monitor the patient's movement in bed to ensure that undue stress is not put on injured part.
2. Supervise patient's exercises while in bed.
3. Monitor mobilization to ensure a safe environment.
   a. Remove unnecessary equipment from patient's room so clutter will not interfere with safe ambulation.
4. Monitor patient's use of ambulatory aid to be sure it is being used correctly and safely.

Facilitating learning

The patient and significant other is taught the following:

1. How bone heals and precautions taken by staff to ensure that nothing is interfering with the healing (frequent neurocirculatory checks and vital signs).
2. About how cast is applied and how it should be cared for.
3. What will be done in surgery and the types of fixation devices that may be used (pins, screws, rods, and so on).
4. About skin or skeletal traction and how it is maintained.
5. The importance of eating a diet that will assist in bone healing. Emphasis is on protein, calcium and vitamins A, B, C and D to aid in the healing process.
6. The need to maintain a fluid intake of about 3000 ml per 24 hours.
7. About the use of an ambulatory aid. The initial teaching may be by the physical therapist, but the nurse will need to understand what has been taught

so she or he can supervise the patient in use of the aid.

8. About how he or she will be gradually mobilized and the exercise program that will need to be followed to regain full use of affected joint(s).
9. The role of the patient in his or her own recovery and rehabilitation.

Monitoring for complications

The complications of bone fractures, their mechanism, signs, onset, and treatment are listed in Table 40-16.

Evaluation

Evaluation is based on the expected patient outcomes. Questions to consider may include the following:

1. Is tissue perfusion normal (skin warm and pink)?
2. Is patient able to be up about by self using an appropriate ambulatory aid?
3. Is patient able to be more independent in self-care?
4. Is patient more in control of situation and expressing confidence in his or her future?
5. Is patient's skin intact?
6. Is the patient free of infection?
7. Is the patient able to eat a well balanced diet?
8. Is the patient free of pain?
9. Is patient free of injury?
10. Can the patient and/or significant other explain the following?
    a. Nature of injury and course of treatment.
    b. Limitations of motion and restriction in activity

c. How to modify ADL to meet prescribed limitations on motion

d. How to care for cast, pins, and other immobilization devices

e. How to use ambulatory aids (walker, crutches, cane) safely

f. How to care for any wounds using aseptic technique

g. Measures to prevent skin breakdown, swelling, and neurocirculatory impairment

h. Measures to relieve pain or discomfort (change of position, elevation of affected part, ice packs, analgesics)

i. How to use prescribed medications

j. Plans for follow-up care

TREATMENT OF FRACTURES WITH EXTERNAL FIXATION DEVICES

Casts

Casts are the most common external fixation device. They are made of plaster of Paris, fiberglass, and plastic, which are available in the form of rolled bandages that are applied over the part to be immobilized in much the same manner as an Ace bandage. *Plaster,* which has to be moistened before application, dries very slowly, is heavy, and loses its strength and integrity if it becomes wet. If a plaster cast requires revision, it generally must be removed and a new one reapplied. However, plaster is less expensive than fiberglass or plastic.

Fiberglass and *plastic* casts are also moistened before application, dry quickly, are light in weight, and may be immersed in water without losing their strength. Plastic casts may be reheated and remolded if revision is necessary. Disadvantages include the fact that some types of fiberglass require drying under special ultraviolet lights, and persons wearing fiberglass or plastic casts may suffer maceration of the skin under the cast after immersion in water unless they dry the skin throughout with a warm air dryer. Specific discussions regarding the advantages and disadvantages of various cast materials can be found in orthopedic texts.

Before a cast is applied, the skin is cleansed and inspected for cuts or abrasions that may become infected. Skin lesions are treated with disinfectant. Normal skin may be treated with tincture of benzoin, then wrapped with cotton padding or stockinette before cast is applied. Bony prominences are padded with sheet wadding or felt to protect them from pressure. For specific techniques of cast application, consult specialized texts.

A cast is removed by splitting it with an electric cast saw. The saw is very noisy; but if it is used properly, it will not damage the skin beneath the cast. Newer cast saws are connected to a cannister vacuum that sucks up plaster dust that results from the sawing. Skin enclosed in a cast for a period of time may be covered with an exudate of built-up secretions and dead skin. To remove this exudate, oil is applied, followed by numerous soaks and bathing with warm water. This process may take several days, but attempts to remove the exudate more rapidly may cause an uncomfortable skin irritation.

Special considerations in caring for the patient in a cast are outlined in Box 40-6.

Traction

Traction is the mechanism by which a steady pull is placed on a part or parts of the body. Traction may be used to accomplish the following:

1. Reduce a fracture
2. Maintain correct position of bone fragments during healing
3. Immobilize a limb while soft tissue healing takes place
4. Overcome muscle spasm
5. Stretch adhesions
6. Correct deformities

Countertraction is a force that counteracts the pull of traction. *Suspension* is the use of traction equipment—frames, splints, slings, ropes, pulleys, weights—to suspend a body part but not exert a "pull" on that part. To suspend the part correctly and continuously, the suspension has to be balanced by weights. Suspension is often referred to as *balanced suspension.* Balanced suspension is often used in conjunction with traction.

There are two types of traction: skin traction and skeletal traction.

Skin traction

Skin traction is achieved by applying wide bands of moleskin, adhesive, or commercially available devices directly to the skin and attaching weights to them. The pull of the weight is transmitted indirectly to the involved bone. Buck's extension and Russell traction are the two most common forms of skin traction used for injury to the lower extremities.

Buck's extension

Buck's extension is the simplest form of skin traction and provides for straight pull on the affected extremity (Fig. 40-23). It is often used to relieve muscle spasm and to immobilize a limb temporarily; for example, after hip fracture before open reduction and internal fixation. If adhesive substances are to be used, the skin of the leg is shaved and tincture of benzoin is applied to protect the skin. Adhesive tape or moleskin is then placed on the lateral and medial aspects of the leg and secured with a circular gauze or elastic bandage. The adhesive material should not cover the malleoli, because skin breakdown would occur over these bony prominences. The tapes are attached to a spreader bar sufficiently wide to pull the tapes away from the malleoli. Rope is attached to the spreader, passed through a pulley on a crossbar at the foot of the bed, and suspended with weights. The maximal weight that should be applied by skin traction is 3.6 kg (8 lb). Greater amounts of weight can cause skin damage. Commercial foam rubber Buck's traction splints are also in wide use and are applied simply with Velcro straps. Contraindications to placing a patient in Buck's traction are stasis dermatitis, arteriosclerosis, allergy to adhesive tape, severe varicosities or varicose ulcers, diabetic gangrene, or marked overriding of bone fragments that would require more than 3.6 kg of weight to reduce the fracture.

40-6

Guidelines for Care

The patient in a cast

Patient education

Explain why the cast is being applied and how it will be applied

Advise the patient that the plaster cast will feel warm as it dries

Explain the extent of immobilization

Explain care of the cast and expectations after discharge

Instruct patient not to insert sharp objects (coat hangers or pencils) under the cast as these may abrade the skin and lead to infection

Handling the new cast

Support wet cast with the flat of the hands or on pillows to avoid indentations that will cause pressure on underlying skin

Place cotton blankets or other absorbent material under the cast to aid drying

Expose the cast to air as much as possible to aid drying

Turn the patient frequently to aid drying

Use a cast dryer or hair dryer on a warm, not hot, setting to circulate air over the cast

Do not apply paint, varnish, or shellac to the cast; plaster is a porous material that allows air to circulate to the skin

Skin care

Inspect skin at edges of cast and underlying cast for redness or irritation; apply petal-shaped strips of adhesive tape or moleskin around rough edges of cast

Remove plaster crumbs from skin with a washcloth moistened with warm water

Use creams and lotions sparingly as they may soften the skin and cause the cast to stick to the skin

Apply waterproof material around perineal area to prevent soiling of and damage to cast and irritation of the skin

Attend to patient's complaint of pain under the cast, particularly over bony prominences, as this may indicate pressure on the skin. If discomfort is not relieved by repositioning, report to physician at once. Cast pressure may need to be relieved by cutting a window in the cast or cutting the cast in two (bivalving)

Turning—turning to any position is generally permitted as long as the integrity of the cast is not compromised and the patient is comfortable

Toileting—for a long leg or hip spica cast

Use a fracture pan with blanket roll or padding as support under the small of the back

Elevate the head of the bed, if permitted, or place the bed in reverse Trendelenburg's position

Abdominal discomfort—cast may be "windowed" (an opening cut into it) to provide relief of abdominal distention or a port for checking bladder distention

Mobilization

Weight bearing is at the discretion of the physician, and the amount of weight bearing will be prescribed

A cast shoe (Fig. 40-31) or a walking heel incorporated into a lower extremity cast will permit weight bearing without damaging the cast

Prevention of neurocirculatory problems

Perform neurocirculatory checks every h for at least 24 hours after cast application to detect difficulty from swelling or pressure of cast on nerves or vessels. Notify physician of color changes, alterations in sensation, or motion unrelieved by position change. Cast may need to be bivalved (cut in two) to relieve pressure (Fig. 40-32)

Elevate affected extremity on pillows until danger of swelling is over (usually 24-48 hours)

After mobilization of patient with lower extremity or upper extremity cast, avoid keeping extremity in dependent position for prolonged periods

After lower extremity cast is removed, encourage patient to wear elastic stocking and elevate affected leg at rest until full mobility is regained

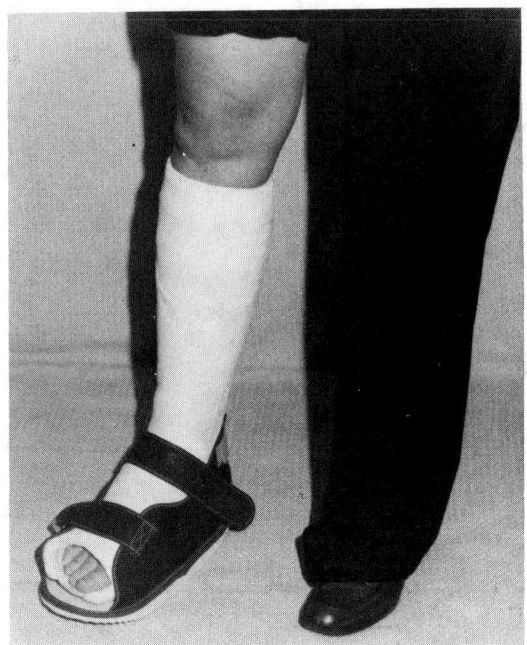

Fig. 40-31   Short leg walking cast with cast shoe.

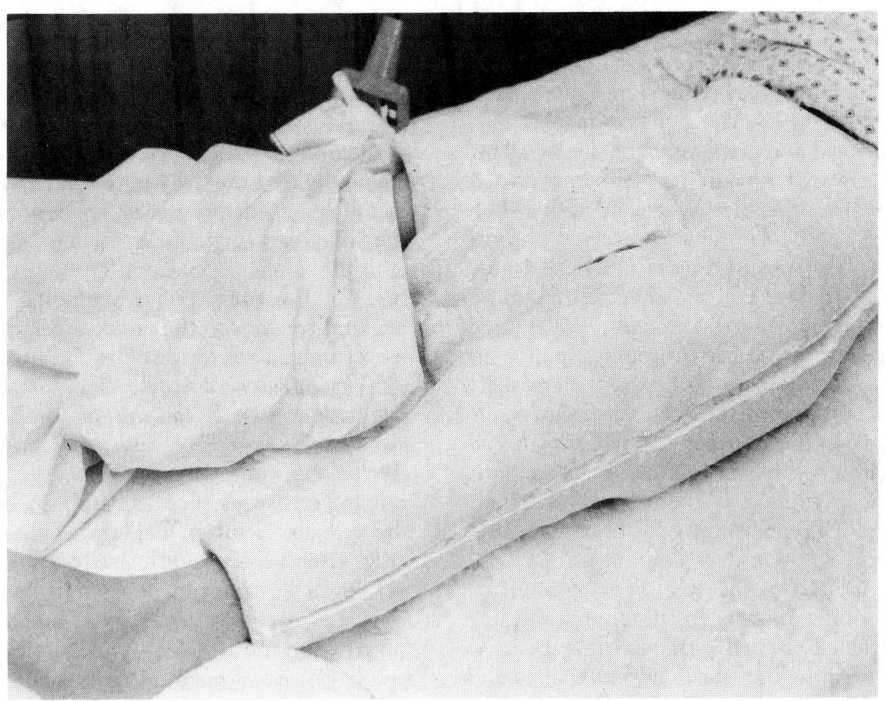

Fig. 40-32   Bivalved cast.

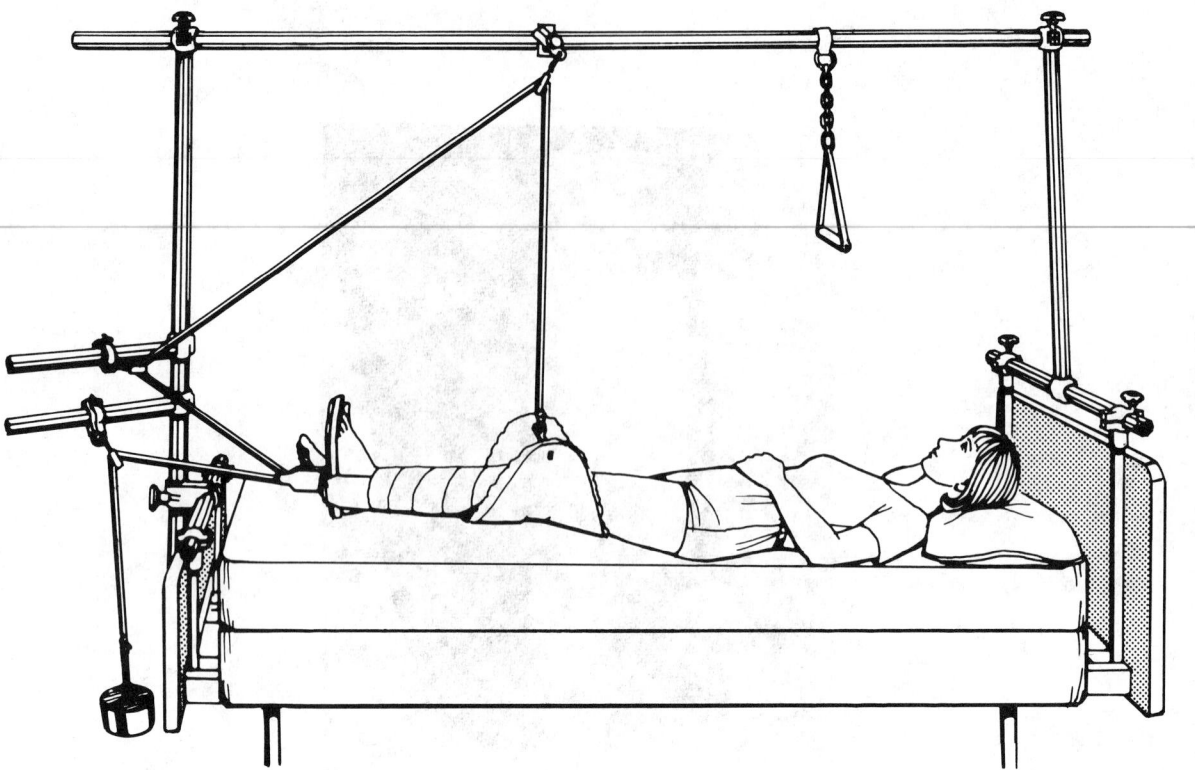

Fig. 40-33   Russell traction. Hip is slightly flexed. Pillows may be used under lower leg to provide support and keep the heel free of the bed.

Russell traction

Russell traction is sometimes used because it permits the patient to move more freely in the bed and it permits flexion of the knee joint (Fig. 40-33). It requires an overhead frame attached to the bed and preparation of the leg as for Buck's traction. A footplate with pulley attachments is used instead of a spreader bar. The knee is suspended in a sling to which a rope is attached. The rope is directed upward to a pulley that has been placed on the overhead frame directly above the tibial tubercle of the affected extremity. The rope is then passed downward through a pulley on a crossbar at the foot of the bed, back through a pulley on the footplate, back again to another pulley on the crossbar, and then suspended with weights. This arrangement effects a double pull from the crossbar to the footplate, so the traction is equal to approximately double the amount of weight used. Usually the foot of the bed is elevated on blocks (or the bed put in Trendelenburg position) to provide countertraction.

Russell traction is used in the treatment of intertrochanteric fracture of the femur when surgery is contraindicated. Bilateral Russell or Buck's traction may be used to treat back pain because they partially immobilize the patient and reduce muscle spasm.

Skeletal traction

Skeletal traction is traction applied directly to bone. Under local or general anesthesia, a Kirschner wire or Steinmann pin in inserted through bone distal to the fracture (the site of insertion varies with the type of fracture) (Fig. 40-34). The pin protrudes through the skin on both sides of the extremity, and the exposed ends of the pin are covered with corks or metal protectors. Small sterile dressings are usually placed over the entry and exit sites of the pin. A metal U-shaped spreader or bow is attached to the pin, and the rope on which the traction weights are hung is tied onto the spreader. Skeletal traction can be used for fractures of the tibia, femur, humerus, and cervical spine. Skeletal traction to the cervical spine is achieved through use of tongs applied to the skull (Fig. 40-35).

When a balanced suspension apparatus is used in conjunction with skin or skeletal traction, the patient is able to move about in bed more freely without disturbing the line of pull of the traction. The use of a balancing apparatus facilitates nursing measures such as bathing, skin care, and placing the bedpan. A full or half-ring Thomas or Hodgen splint (Fig. 40-36) is frequently used for suspension of the lower extremities. Straps of canvas, muslin, or synthetic lamb's wool are placed over the splint and secured to provide support for the leg. The areas under the popliteal space and heel are left open to prevent pressure on these parts. If it is desirable to have the knee flexed or to permit movement of the lower leg, a Pearson attachment is clamped or fixed to the Thomas splint at the level of the knee.

Special considerations in caring for the patient in traction are described in Box 40-7.

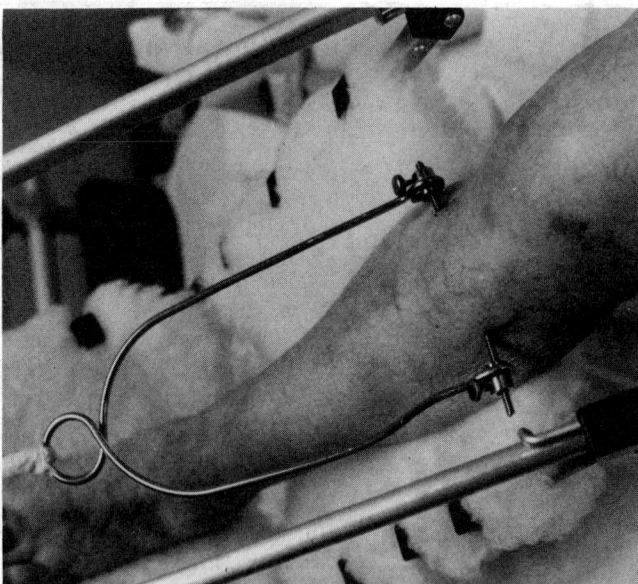

Fig. 40-34 Tibial pin traction with Steinmann pin used in treatment of a distal femoral fracture. The bow attached to the pin provides a place of attachment for the rope that holds the traction weights. The pull exerted by the weight keeps the fracture fragments aligned. Pin sites must be inspected at least daily to detect signs of pin reaction or infection.

Guidelines for Care   40-7

The patient in traction

Patient education

    Explain traction in relation to fracture and physician's plan of treatment

    Explain amount of movement permitted and how to achieve it (for example, how trapeze can be used to assist with movement)

    Explain correct body positioning

Maintaining the traction

    Inspect traction apparatus frequently to assure that ropes are running straight and through the middle of the pulleys; that weights are hanging free; that bedclothes, the bed, or the frame and bars on the bed are not impinging on any part of the traction apparatus

    Check ropes frequently to be sure they are not frayed

    Avoid releasing weights from or altering the line of pull of the traction

    Avoid adding weight to the traction

    Check the position of the Thomas splint frequently; if the ring has slid away from the groin, readjust the splint to its proper position without releasing traction

    Avoid bumping into or jarring the bed or traction equipment

    Be sure weights are securely fastened to their ropes and do not touch the floor

    Avoid manipulation of pins

Skin care

    Encourage the patient to turn slightly from side to side and to lift up on the trapeze to relieve pressure on the skin of the sacrum and scapulae; have the patient lift up for routine skin care

    Avoid padding the ring of the Thomas splint as this will create dampness next to the skin. Bathe the skin beneath the ring, dry it thoroughly, and powder the skin lightly

    Inspect skin frequently to be sure it is not being rubbed, contused, or macerated by traction equipment; readjust splints or the extremity in the splint to free the skin from pressure

    Keep skin areas around pin sites clean and dry; direct care to pin sites (that is, cleansing with cotton applicators and hydrogen peroxide or alcohol) is *controversial,* so check with patient's physician to determine if pin care is to be done routinely and what method the physician prefers

Toileting

    Use a fracture pan with blanket roll or padding as support under the small of the back

    Protect the ring of the Thomas splint with waterproof material when female patients are using the bedpan

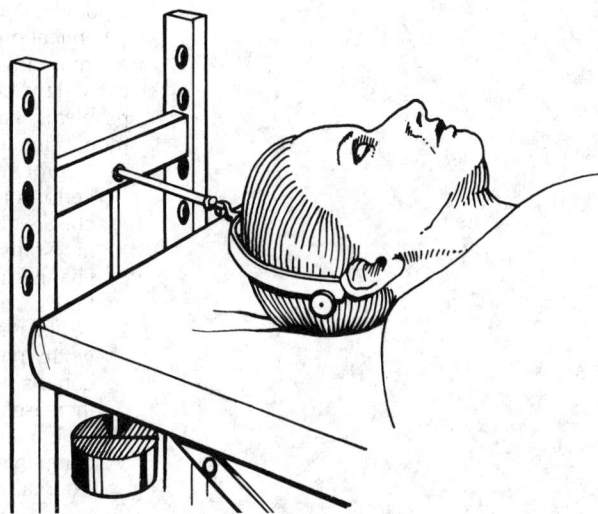

Fig. 40-35 Traction to the cervical spine can be maintained through the use of Crutchfield tongs inserted into the skull.

Nursing Care Plan	**Patient with an intracapsular hip fracture, open reduction, and internal fixation with a prosthetic implant**

DATA: Mrs. W. is an 81-year-old widowed, retired secretary. This evening she tripped and fell on an icy step when leaving her niece's home. She complained of immediate, severe pain in her left hip and was unable to move her leg. Emergency Medical Services was called, and Mrs. W. was accompanied to the hospital by her niece and her niece's husband. In the emergency room it was noted that her left leg was shorter than her right, and it was externally rotated. Her vital signs were stable, and the neurocirculatory status of the left leg was intact. An x-ray examination revealed an intracapsular femoral neck fracture. Intravenous fluids were started. An ECG, urinalysis, CBC, and serum electrolyte study were obtained. She was transferred to the nursing unit with physician's orders for morphine sulfate 4 to 6 mg every 3 to 4 hours as necessary for pain. Buck's extension was applied. Consent was obtained for surgical repair in the morning. Replacement of the femoral head and neck with a regular stem Austin Moore prosthesis is planned.

The nursing history identified the following:
- Mrs. W. lives alone in her own apartment in a senior citizen complex.
- Mrs. W. has no children but has nieces and nephews in the area who see her regularly. They assist with shopping and other errands.
- Mrs. W. would like to return to her own apartment after being discharged from the hospital, but she worries that she might need help at home. Her family is considering hiring a home health aide.
- She takes no medications other than aspirin for occasional "stiffness" on awakening.
- She has never been hospitalized and last saw a physician 2 years ago for "the flu."

Nursing diagnosis: Knowledge deficit related to lack of exposure to surgery

Expected patient outcomes	Nursing interventions (preoperative)	Rationale
Mrs. W. can explain the teaching provided by the nurse about preoperative and general postoperative care. Mrs. W. states that she is experiencing less anxiety related to fear of the unknown and/or misconceptions about surgery and the recovery period.	Assess need for instruction and provide as necessary. Provide written materials pertaining to the surgery, if available in the institution. Review preoperative instruction with Mrs. W. and family before the surgery. Evaluate Mrs. W.'s understanding of the information taught.	Information may reduce anxiety and reduce fear of the unknown.
	Nursing interventions (postoperative)	
	Collaborative nursing actions include those to identify possible complications of surgery. Immediate reporting of and treatment of early signs may prevent serious problems. Nursing actions include monitoring for the following: 1. *Neurocirculatory compromise:* Perform neurocirculatory checks q2h for the first 24-48 hr. Notify physician of any changes from preoperative status. 2. *Dislocation of the prosthesis:* Notify physician if Mrs. W. complains of sudden onset of increased pain, especially groin pain, particularly if accompanied by deformity or external rotation.	

3. *Impaired skin integrity and/or impaired wound healing.* Monitor pressure areas for signs of redness, monitor temperature, and assess incision for signs or symptoms of infection or excessive drainage.
4. *Atelectasis/respiratory infection:* Monitor breath sounds until Mrs. W. is ambulatory.
5. *Urinary retention:* Assess output qh.

Expected patient outcomes	Nursing interventions	Rationale
	6. *Constipation:* Assess bowel status each day until Mrs. W. is able to have a bowel movement. 7. *Fluid and electrolyte imbalance:* Monitor intake and output until Mrs. W. is taking oral fluids without difficulty, monitor IV fluid rates, and assess Mrs. W. for fluid volume excess or deficit. *By discharge Mrs. W. should be instructed in and be able to explain or demonstrate the following:* 1. *Independent ambulation* on level surfaces with appropriate ambulatory aid and independent stair climbing 2. *Activity restrictions to be observed for approximately 2 months* or until follow-up with physician, for example, limiting flexion of the affected hip to 90 degrees, avoiding adduction of the affected leg beyond midline, avoiding extreme internal and external rotation of the affected hip, and maintaining partial weight-bearing status with the walker or crutches 3. *Independent ADL* with assistive devices	

Nursing Care Plan	Patient with an intracapsular hip fracture, open reduction, and internal fixation with a prosthetic implant—cont'd

Nursing diagnosis: Pain related to surgical procedure

Expected patient outcomes	Nursing interventions	Rationale
Mrs. W. states feeling comfortable. Mrs. W. is able to perform necessary postoperative routines/exercises	Assess Mrs. W.'s pain and evaluate response to comfort measures provided.	Subjective and objective data are important in ascertaining the nature of Mrs. W.'s postoperative pain and determining its management.
	Administer prescribed analgesics (usually narcotic) at timely intervals during initial postoperative period.	It is usually necessary to administer narcotics in the first 48-72 hr after surgery. Analgesics have a greater effect if they are administered before pain becomes severe.
	Teach relaxation techniques as appropriate. Use other pain relieving techniques as appropriate, for example, back rubs, repositioning.	Relaxation facilitates rest and may modify the response to pain. A change in type of cutaneous stimulation may result in pain relief.
	As pain decreases, use milder analgesics as prescribed.	Pain may be controlled by less potent analgesics (with fewer untoward side effects) as pain lessens in severity.

Nursing diagnosis: Mobility, impaired physical related to alteration in lower limb status after surgical repair of hip fracture

Expected patient outcomes	Nursing interventions	Rationale
Mrs. W. demonstrates optimal level of mobility with adaptive devices within prescribed limitations of activity by time of discharge. No injury occurs during Mrs. W.'s hospitalization.	Have Mrs. W. deep breathe and cough every 1-2 hr until fully ambulatory.	If carried out correctly and at appropriate intervals, pulmonary exercises can effectively prevent atelectasis and pneumonia.
	Encourage Mrs. W. to perform active dorsiflexion, plantar flexion, isometric quadriceps setting and gluteal setting, and active range of motion of unaffected limbs q2h until ambulatory.	Exercising promotes venous return, prevents thrombus formation, and helps to maintain muscle tone.
	Determine from surgeon the limits of motion and weight bearing permitted, keeping in mind the following guidelines:	Restrictions on positioning are designed to avoid dislocation of the prosthesis.
	1. Hip flexion is usually limited to 90 degrees for 2-3 mo. Adduction beyond midline is prohibited for 2-3 mo.	
	2. Extreme internal or external rotation is prohibited for 2-3 mo.	
	3. Partial weight bearing on affected body part with the aid of a walker or crutches is usually observed for 2-3 mo.	

Nursing diagnosis: Mobility, impaired physical related to alteration in lower limb status after surgical repair of hip fracture—cont'd

Expected patient outcomes	Nursing interventions	Rationale
	Turn Mrs. W. from back to unoperated side q2h and prn. Avoid positioning patient on operative side, and observe flexion restrictions when elevating the head of the bed.	Turning and repositioning frequently promotes circulation, respiratory effort, and muscle activity.
	When turning Mrs. W., hold the operative leg in abduction; use pillows to maintain 30-degree abduction when turning is accomplished.	Prevents adduction of leg.
	Assist Mrs. W. to walk using the appropriate ambulatory aid. Begin walking the first or second postoperative day and increase the frequency and distance of ambulation as tolerated.	Early postoperative activity, including walking, can hasten recovery and prevent postoperative complications.
	Begin sitting when Mrs. W. demonstrates sufficient control of the affected leg to sit within flexion restrictions.	Prepare Mrs. W. for discharge while assuring that Mrs. W. can sit safely within prescribed limits on flexion.
	Elevate sitting surface with pillows to keep angle of hip within prescribed limits.	Limits hip flexion to 90 degrees.

Nursing diagnosis: High risk for impaired home maintenance management related to independent living situation

Expected patient outcomes	Nursing interventions	Rationale
Mrs. W. and family express satisfaction with arrangements made to facilitate self-care at home.	Discuss with Mrs. W. and family their plans for Mrs. W.'s care after discharge from the hospital.	Adequate discharge planning will foster successful completion of rehabilitation at home or will help to identify areas in Mrs. W.'s performance of required functional abilities indicating a need for a skilled nursing facility, rehabilitation hospital, or other form of intermediate care.
	Determine with Mrs. W. what she must do for herself to return to her own home.	
	Determine with Mrs. W. the type of equipment and services needed for return home (for example, crutches, walker, elevated toilet seat, homemaker, companion, physical therapy, Meals on Wheels, and shopping services).	
	Assess Mrs. W.'s progress at regular intervals to determine whether her functional ability will permit carrying out of the above plans.	
	Involve appropriate department (for example, social service department) for assistance in planning, if Mrs. W. is unable to achieve functional levels consistent with the initial plan.	

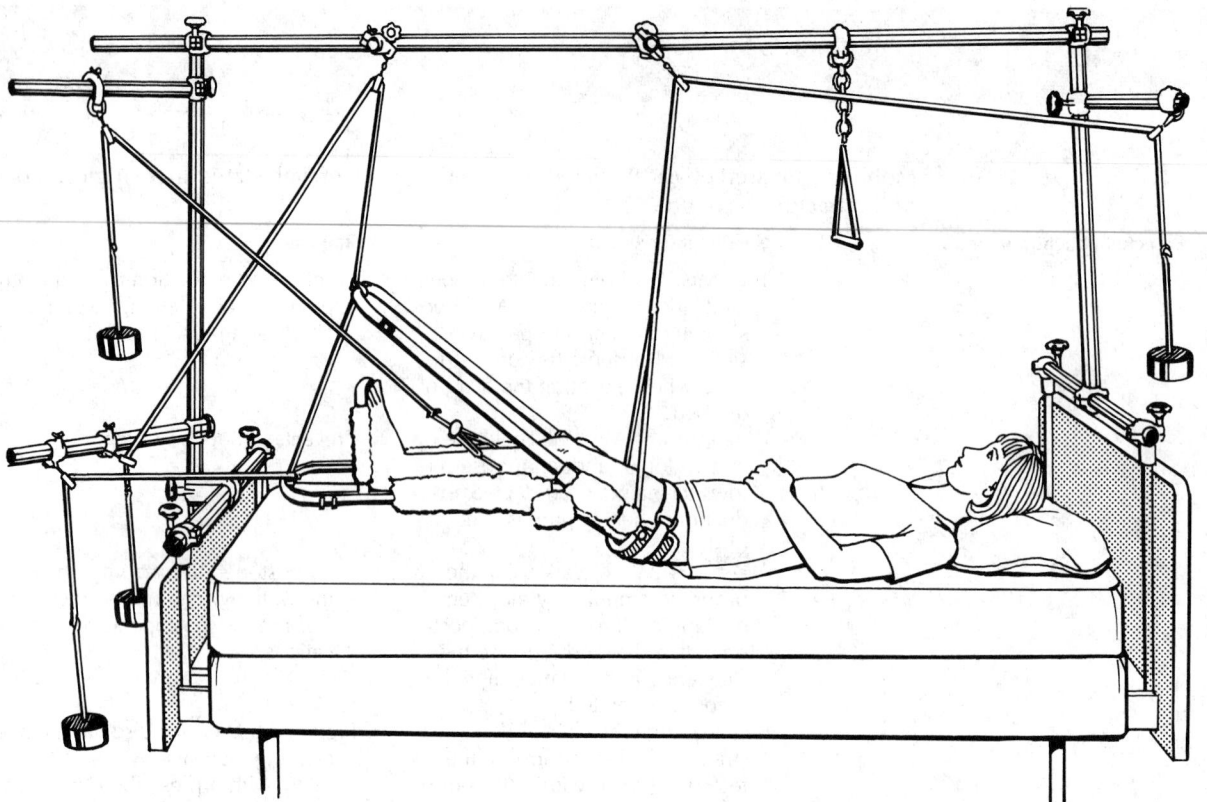

Fig. 40-36   Balanced suspension with Thomas splint and Pearson attachment. This apparatus can be used alone or, as in this case, with skeletal traction.

Other Types of External Immobilization

Other devices for external immobilization of fractures include the following:

1. Braces made of rigid plastic material
2. Plaster or plastic braces that incorporate metal struts attached to pins inserted into bone (for example, a halo brace) (Fig. 40-37)
3. Metal struts attached to pins inserted into bone (for example, the various types of Hoffman or Charnley external fixation devices) (Fig. 40-38).

Devices such as the Hoffman or Charnley may be used in conjunction with plaster or alone. All of these devices provide extremely rigid fixation while allowing the patient some degree of mobility. It is quite possible for the patient in a halo brace to ambulate. The patient with an external fixator on the lower leg can be out of bed in a wheelchair, or even ambulate without bearing weight on the affected leg.

Nursing care for patients in these devices is essentially the same as for patients in casts and/or skeletal traction, with the exception that they may be mobilized earlier.

TREATMENT OF FRACTURES WITH INTERNAL FIXATION DEVICES

Open Reduction

Open surgical reduction of fractures has the advantage of allowing visualization of the fracture and surrounding tissues. It is particularly indicated when soft tissue is caught between bone fragments or when known damage to nerves or blood vessels exists. *The disadvantages of internal fixation are that is requires anesthesia and it carries the risk of infection at the time of surgery. Internal fixation is carried out under the most vigorous aseptic conditions, and patients may receive a short course of prophylactic intravenous antibiotics after surgery.*

The internal fixation devices available include the following:

1. Plates and nails such as the Neufeld nail (Fig. 40-39, *A*)
2. Transfixation screws (Fig. 40-40)
3. Kuntschner nail (intramedullary rods) (Fig. 40-39, *B*)
4. Prosthetic implants such as the Austin Moore prosthesis (Fig. 40-41), which are used when proximal fragment of the fracture is jeopardized

It should also be noted that *bone grafts*, either *autograft* (the patient's own bone) or *allograft* (cadaver bone), may be used either in conjunction with internal fixation devices when excessive bone is lost at the fracture site, or alone, as in spine surgery. It should also be noted that fixation with internal devices does not preclude additional fixation with external devices (casts, braces, or traction), particularly in cases of very complicated fracture or multiple trauma.

In general, the primary objective of care is to protect the fixation device until healing takes place. Metal that

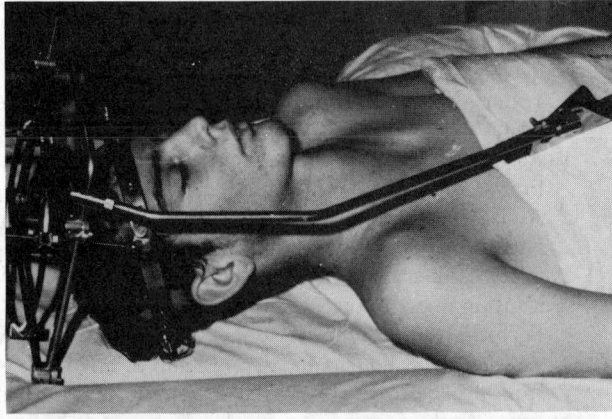

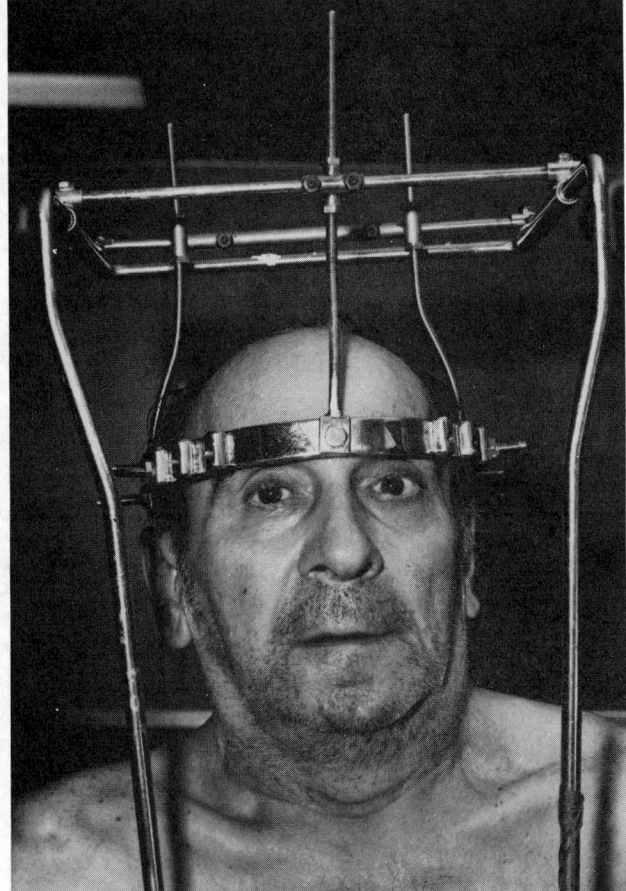

Fig. 40-37   **A,** Halo brace attached to body cast. Metal strut will be anchored firmly into body cast with additional plaster. **B,** Metal ring, or halo, that attaches to skull. (Courtesy Dr. Henry Bohlman, Cleveland, Ohio.)

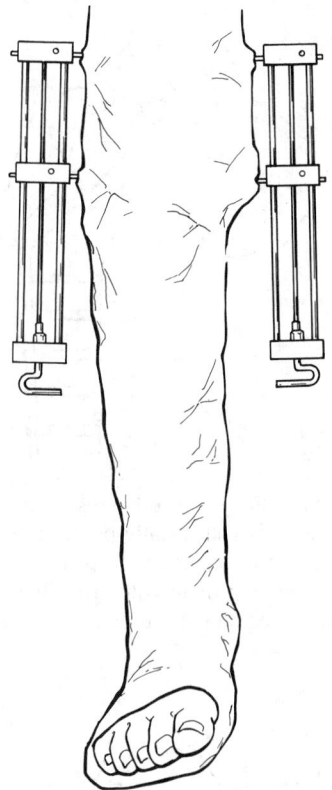

Fig. 40-38   Example of an external fixator, in this case a Charnley compression apparatus. Skeletal pins through bone above and below the area of fracture or repair attach to the external metal supports to maintain rigid fixation. This particular device is equipped with hand screws that allow the pins to be brought closer together, thus providing increased compression.

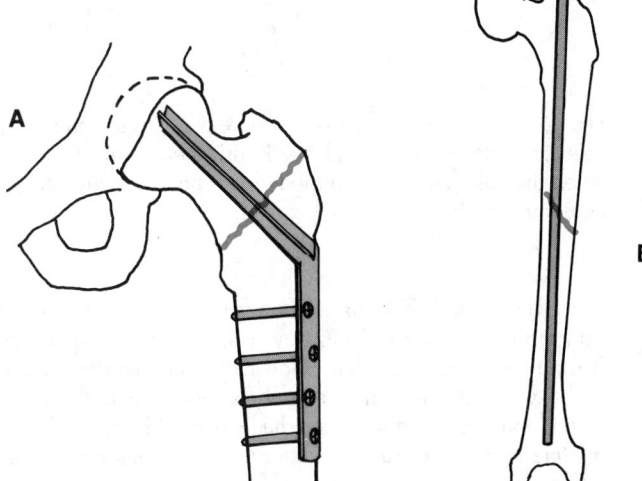

Fig. 40-39   **A,** Neufeld nail and screws, used in repair of intertrochanteric fracture. **B,** Kuntscher nail (intramedullary rod) used in repair of mid-shaft femoral fracture.

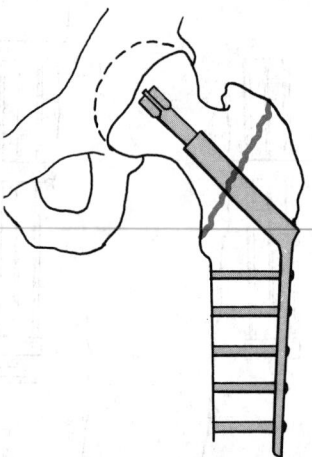

Fig. 40-40   Ken sliding nail used in repair of intertrochanteric fracture. Sliding nails will usually permit the patient to bear weight to some degree as they will "give" slightly when subjected to weight-bearing forces without shifting their placement or "cutting out" (penetrating) through the femur.

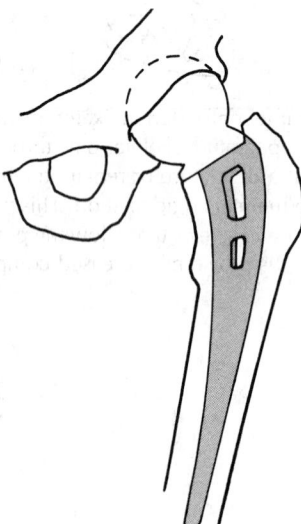

Fig. 40-41   Regular stem Austin Moore prosthesis, commonly used to replace the femoral head and neck in hip fractures when the vascular supply to the femoral head may eventually be compromised.

can fatigue and break cannot be expected to substitute for intact bone. If the fixation device breaks, healing of the fracture will be disrupted. However, mobilization of patients who have had an internal fixation is usually much faster than for those who have had external fixation. *Nursing interventions for patients with internal fixation include the following:*

1. Patient education
   a. Prepare the patient for general anesthesia
   b. Explain the surgical procedure and general nursing care after surgery

c. Postoperatively, explain the limits of motion and weight bearing on the affected part
2. Promoting mobility
   a. Determine, in consultation with the physician, the limits of motion and weight bearing permitted
   b. Assist the patient with turning within the prescribed limits
   c. Assist the patient in transferring and ambulating within the prescribed limits (may be up as early as first postoperative day)
3. Prevention of neurocirculatory problems
   a. Perform neurocirculatory checks every hour for the first 24 to 48 hours; notify physician of any change from preoperative status that may indicate pressure from *swelling, constriction of bandages, or damage to nerves or vessels* during surgery
   b. Maintain elevation of affected extremity
4. Maintenance of immobilization of fracture; considerations for care are the same as for patients in casts or traction (p. 1405) if these devices are used

FRACTURE OF THE HIP

Etiology/Epidemiology

Hip fractures are perhaps the most common fracture seen in the hospital. They occur more frequently in women than in men. Some factors explaining this follow:

1. Women have a wider pelvis with a tendency to coxa vara
2. Women have postmenopausal hormonal changes often accompanied by an increased incidence of osteoporosis
3. Women's life expectancy is greater than that of men

A recent study of hip fracture in women identified several factors that increase the risks of falls associated with hip fracture. These are: lower-limb dysfunction, neurologic conditions, barbiturate use, and visual impairments. The authors' recommendations include the following: aggressive treatment of ocular disease and visual impairment, physical therapy for women with mobility problems, and consideration given to discontinuing medication that affects *cognitive function.*[25]

Primary Prevention

Because most falls occur in the home and the *height of the fall* and *landing on hard surfaces increase risk of fracture*, the authors of the above study recommended several changes in the home. These include: lowering beds, installing wall-to-wall carpeting, and providing grab bars, stair rails, or other aids that would help prevent a falling person from landing on the floor.

The authors also pointed out that several studies have identified that increased body weight decreases the risk of hip fracture. Possible explanations for this are that heavier persons have greater bone mass and their fatty tissue offers protection during a fall.[25]

The following is a review of the hip joint for a clearer understanding of what is involved in a fracture of this area. The hip joint is a ball-and-socket joint formed by the acetabulum, a deep round cavity in the innominate bone, and the rounded upper portion of the femur. The upper part of the femur is composed of a head, neck, greater and lesser trochanter, and shaft. The distal part of the femur ends in two condyles. The head of the femur fits into the acetabulum. The hip joint is surrounded by a fibrous capsule, ligaments, and muscles. The greater trochanter serves as a point of insertion for the abductor muscles and short rotator muscles of the hip, whereas the lesser trochanter serves as a point of insertion for the iliopsoas muscle.

Pathophysiology

Fractures of the hip may be classified into two general categories (Fig. 40-42):

1. *Intracapsular*—occurring within the hip joint and capsule; these include
   a. Subcapital fracture
   b. Transcervical fracture
   c. Basal neck fracture
2. *Extracapsular*—occurring outside the hip joint and capsule to an area 5 cm (2 in.) below the lesser trochanter; these are called *intertrochanteric* fractures

The blood supply to the femoral head is of paramount importance in fractures in or about the hip joint. The blood supply to the femoral head varies with age. The chief source of blood supply to the femoral head in adults is the posterior retinacular artery (Fig. 40-43). The nutrient and periosteal vessels of the femoral shaft extend into the trochanteric region and lower part of the neck.

Blood supply to the head of the femur comes up through the neck of the femur and is often disrupted in an intracapsular fracture. When blood supply is interrupted, death (*avascular necrosis*) of the femoral head may occur.

Assessment
Subjective and objective data

Signs and symptoms of hip fracture include the following:

1. Severe pain at the fracture site
2. Inability to move the leg voluntarily
3. Shortening and external rotation of the leg
4. Other signs and symptoms consistent with signs and symptoms of any fracture such as pain, bruising at site or on other places on body

Medical Management

The choice of fixation device depends on the location of the fracture, the potential for avascular necrosis of the femoral head, and the personal preference of the surgeon. An *impacted intracapsular fracture without displacement* may be treated with bedrest alone. Common choices include the following:

1. *Stable plate and screw fixation;* implies non–weight bearing status for 6 weeks to 3 months
2. *Telescoping nail fixation;* implies minimal to partial weight-bearing status for 6 weeks to 3 months
3. *Prosthetic implant,* usually Austin Moore prosthesis or Bi-Polar prosthesis, to replace femoral head and neck; implies some position restrictions for 2 weeks to 2 months and partial weight-bearing restrictions for up to 2 months
4. *Closed reduction and external fixation* if general medical condition precludes surgery

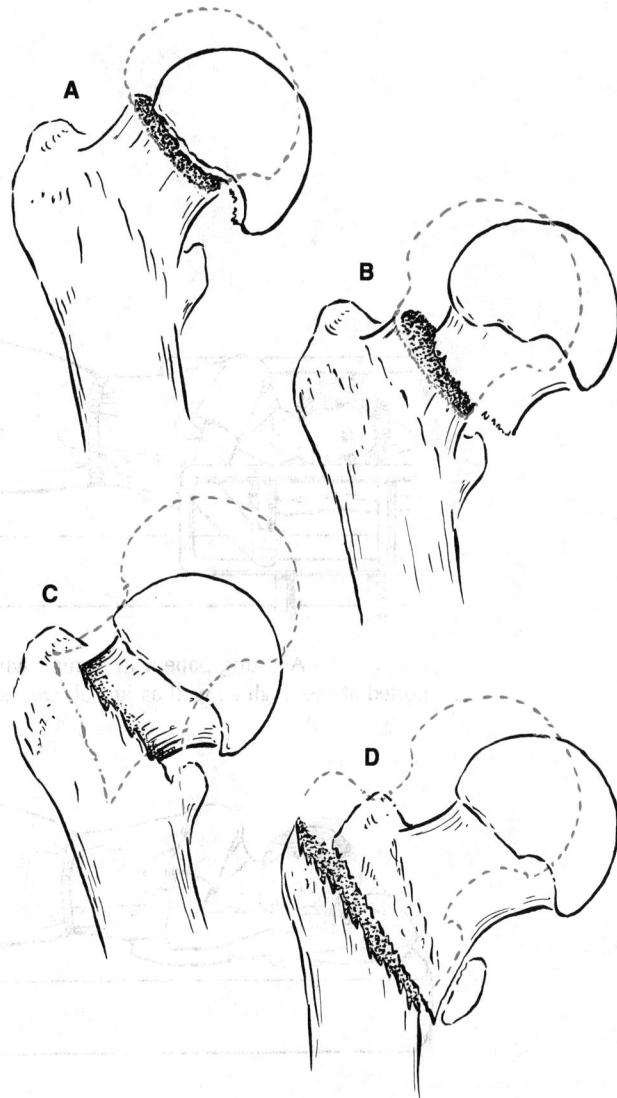

Fig. 40-42   Fractures of hip. **A,** Subcapital fracture. **B,** Transcervical fracture. **C,** Impacted fracture of base of neck. **D,** Intertrochanteric fracture.

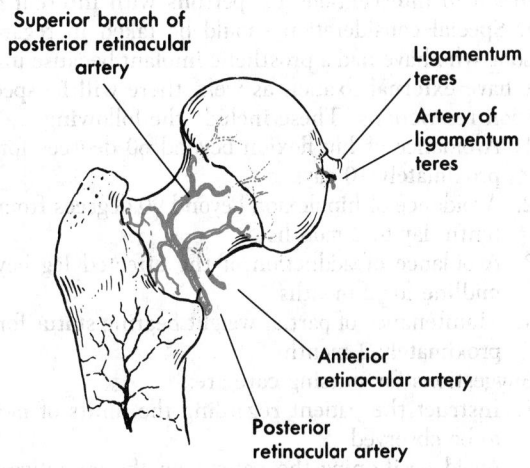

Fig. 40-43   Posterior view of the blood supply to head of femur.

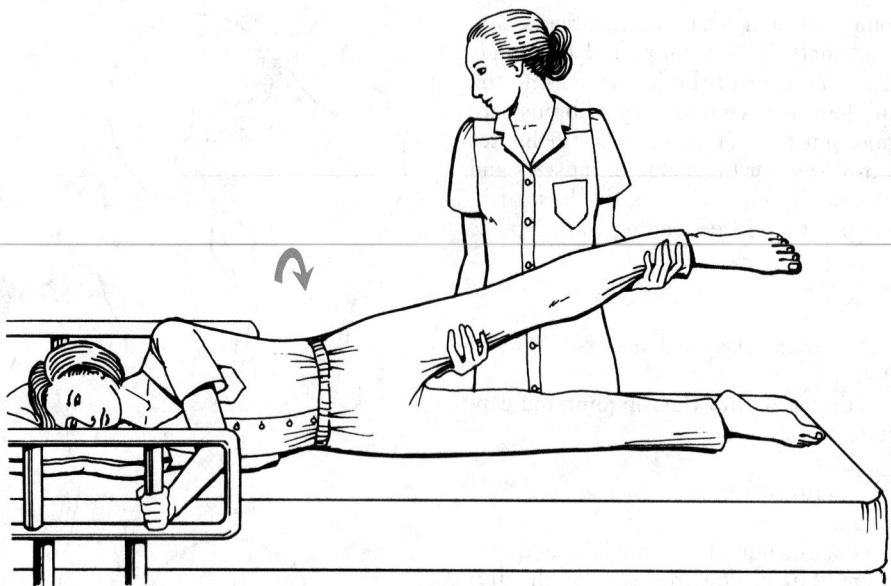

Fig. 40-44 Assisting patient in turning while maintaining abduction of the hip. Leg is supported at the thigh as well as just above the ankle to avoid putting undue stress on the hip.

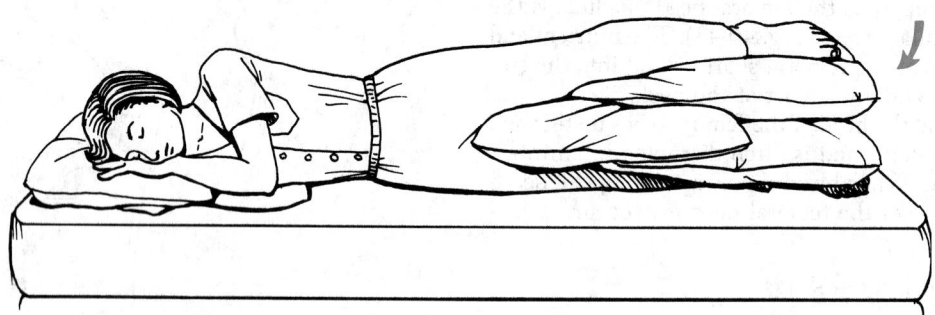

Fig. 40-45 Pillows are staggered in a wedge-shaped arrangement to maintain abduction of the hip.

Nursing Interventions

Nursing interventions should include those already noted for general care of patients with fractures with specific attention to interventions for persons with internal fixation. Special consideration should be taken in regard to persons who have had a prosthetic implant because unless they have external fixation as well, there will be specific position restrictions. These include the following:

1. Avoidance of hip flexion beyond 60 degrees for approximately 10 days
2. Avoidance of hip flexion beyond 90 degrees from the tenth day to 2 months
3. Avoidance of adduction of the affected leg beyond midline for 2 months
4. Maintenance of partial weight bearing status for approximately 2 months

Suggestions for nursing care are:

1. Instruct the patient regarding the limits of motion to be observed
2. Avoid positioning the patient on the operative side in bed
3. Assist patient in maintaining abduction of hip (Fig. 40-44 and 40-45)
4. Carefully monitor the patient's position through transfer, standing, and sitting
5. Provide a chair with a firm, nonreclining seat and arms; elevate the sitting surface as necessary with pillows or foam cushions to keep the angle of the hip within the prescribed limits when the patient is sitting

In general, patients who have had *any* kind of internal fixation for a fractured hip should avoid elevation of the operated leg when sitting in a chair as this puts excessive strain on the fixation device.

FRACTURES OF THE SPINE
Etiology/Epidemiology

Spinal, or vertebral, fractures occur as the result of falls, diving accidents, blows to the head or body by heavy objects, or with increasing frequency, as the result of osteoporosis and metastatic lesions of the spine. Spine fracture can occur at any age.

Pathophysiology

Vertebral fracture may occur with displacement or without displacement. If fracture fragments are displaced, they may place pressure on spinal nerves or injure the spinal cord itself. Such pressure will result in partial or complete dysfunction of the body parts innervated from the level of injury. Depending on the extent of injury to the nervous system structures, dysfunction may be permanent, partially permanent, or temporary. Fracture can occur at any level of the spine, from occiput through the sacrum.

Assessment

Subjective and objective data

Signs and symptoms of vertebral fracture include the following:
1. Pain at the site of injury
2. Partial or complete loss of mobility or sensation below the level of injury
3. Evidence of fracture/fracture dislocation on routine x-ray film, on myelography, or on high resolution CAT scans.

Medical Management

Objectives in management will be stabilization of the fracture, reduction of the fracture, and decompression (that is, removal of pressure from spinal nerves or the spinal cord).

Immediate management

1. Immobilization of the patient with backboard and cervical collar
2. Immediate transport to a hospital

Surgical management

1. Decompression of nerve structures through laminectomy (see Chapter 37) or appropriate reduction of the fracture and removal of fracture fragments
2. Reduction of the fracture through operative procedures, or in some cases, traction (for example, cervical traction through application of tongs to the skull)
3. Stabilization of the fracture with bone grafting and/or internal fixation devices such as Harrington, Jacobs, or Luque rods.
4. Maintenance of stabilization with external fixation devices such as casts, corsets, or braces as necessary

NOTE: Compression fractures of the spine may be treated with bed rest until the patient's pain subsides, then the patient is gradually mobilized, sometimes with stabilization by a corset or brace.

Nursing Interventions

Many of the nursing interventions required by the patient with spinal fracture are identical to those outlined for the patient with spinal cord injury in Chapter 37. Of special concern are interventions designed for the following purposes:

1. Maintaining the stability of the fracture fixation
   a. Pay strict attention to *logrolling* the patient for position changes (Fig. 40-46)
   b. Position the patient with pillows between the legs (see Fig. 40-45) and at the back when side lying to prevent strain on the back.
   c. Observe proper technique when turning the patient on a Stryker frame or Foster bed, (CircOlectric beds are often contraindicated for patients with spine fracture as they load [put weight through] the spine when the patient is in the vertical position)
   d. Avoid elevating the head of the bed beyond the prescribed level (usually only 30 degrees and only on the physician's order)
   e. When the patient is to be mobilized, apply prescribed corsets or braces *before* getting the patient out of bed
2. Preventing neurocirculatory problems
   a. Perform neurocirculatory checks every hour in the first 24-48 hours after surgery; report decrease in neuromotor function to the physician
   b. Perform passive range of motion to involved extremities at least qid
   c. Encourage patient to actively and frequently move noninvolved extremities to the extent possible
3. Promoting comfort—in addition to usual comfort measures
   a. Reposition the patient frequently
   b. Wait a few minutes to ascertain the patient's comfort, because small adjustments may be necessary and may not be immediately recognized
4. Promoting psychologic comfort
   a. Recognize that the patient may have feelings of powerlessness, anger, and/or fear about the situation, particularly if there is neuromotor deficit
   b. Encourage the patient to express such feelings
   c. Encourage the patient to take advantage of psychologic and or social counseling where it is available
   d. If long-term rehabilitation is indicated, prepare the patient for care in a rehabilitation setting

Other nursing interventions are similar to those for any patient who has a fracture (p. 1397), including interventions for individuals in casts or traction (p. 1405).

EFFECTS OF IMMOBILIZATION

Persons who are immobilized after a fracture may have complications related to their immobility. An outline of the effects of immobilization on the various body systems, pathophysiology, nursing assessment, and nursing interventions follows.

Cardiovascular System
Pathophysiology

The common problems associated with the cardiovascular system are as follows:
1. Increased incidence of deep vein thrombosis (DVT) and pulmonary embolus (PE)
2. Increased work load on the heart

Failure of the vessels in the legs to assume or maintain vasoconstriction results in the pooling of venous blood, decreased venous return, and diminished cardiac output.

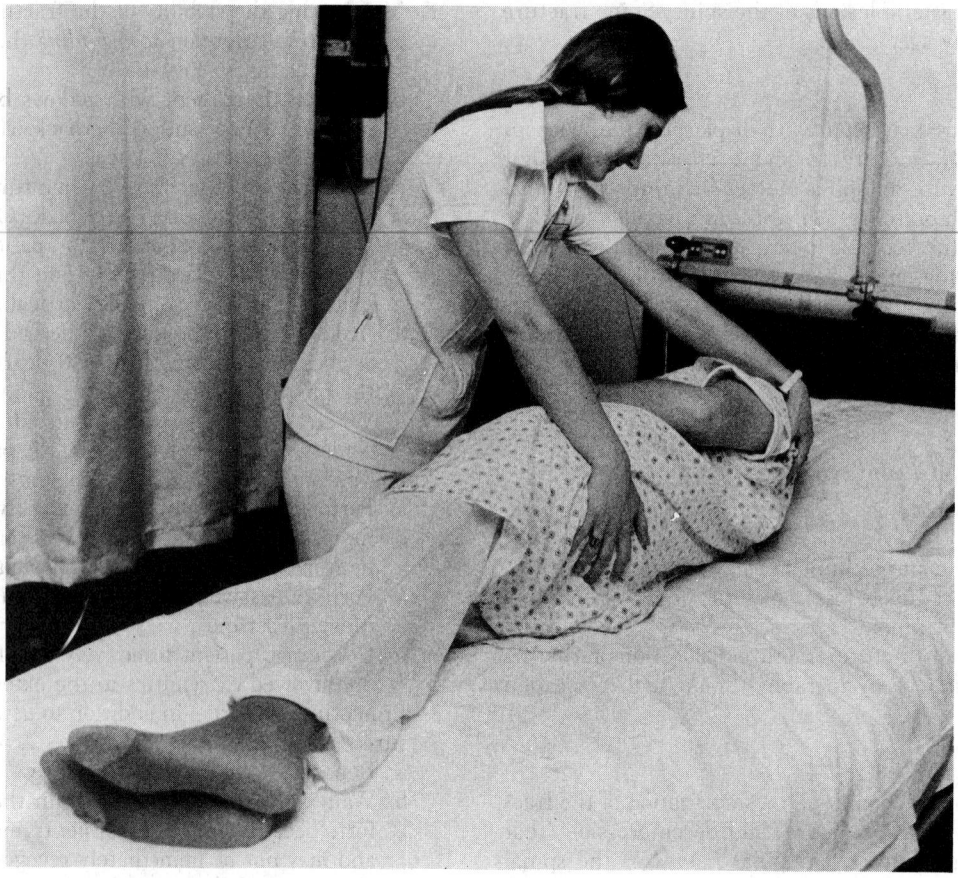

Fig. 40-46   Logrolling patient. Patient crosses arms over chest, holds legs in extension and feet together. Nurse supports patient at level of shoulders and buttocks.

Nursing assessment

Objective data

1. Palpate peripheral pulses.
2. Monitor blood pressure and heart rate and force.
3. Observe for signs and symptoms of DVT (pain in leg) and PE (chest pain, cough).

Nursing interventions

1. Assist patient with active and passive range of motion and isometric exercises of extremities
2. Reposition patient frequently within limitations as directed by physician's orders.

Respiratory System
Pathophysiology

Decreased movement, decreased stimulus to cough, and decreased depth of ventilation all contribute to the pooling of secretions in the bronchi and bronchioles.

Nursing assessment
Objective data

1. Observe for inability to cough and raise secretions.
2. Auscultate for sounds of moisture in the chest.

Nursing interventions

1. Reposition frequently within prescribed limitations.
2. Encourage active range of motion exercises of unaffected joints.
3. Prevent hypostatic pneumonia by having patient cough and deep breathe at regular intervals (at least every 2 hours). An incentive spirometer may be used 3 to 4 times daily.

Skin Integrity
Pathophysiology

Loss of skin integrity (abrasions, decubitus ulcers) is caused by friction, pressure, or tissue layers sliding on each other. The process of restricted circulation and tissue ischemia is intensified by infection, trauma, obesity, sweating, and poor nutritional state.

Nursing assessment
Objective data

1. Observe for *areas of pressure* and *irritation*, as may occur from the plaster cast or traction equipment or from pressure on the sacrum, elbows, and heels.
2. Monitor *body temperature for elevation*, which may indicate infection.

Nursing interventions

1. Prevent decubitus ulceration by keeping skin clean and dry, especially sacrum, elbows, and heels.
2. Turn the patient as permitted to change points of pressure at frequent intervals. Some patients cannot be fully turned, for example, patients in traction. In this instance, other methods must be provided, such as the following:
   a. Flotation pads that distribute pressure equally over large skin areas.
   b. Air pressure mattresses that alternate pressures on the skin.
   c. Sheepskin pads that decrease friction, distribute pressure, and reduce moisture.
   d. Elbow and heel pads.
3. Special beds may be necessary to turn the patient from supine to prone positions.
   a. The Stryker or Foster frame permits movement in a horizontal direction to two positions—supine and prone.
   b. The CircOlectric bed permits more position changes. Movement is vertical and can be stopped at any angle while good body alignment is maintained.
4. If decubitus ulcer results, follow hospital policy for special nursing measures.

Gastrointestinal System
Pathophysiology

Constipation is the most frequent complication of immobility. The change in normal dietary habits and fluid intake, lack of activity, and having to use a bedpan are contributing factors.

Nursing assessment
Subjective and objective data

1. Ask the patient about daily bowel habits.
2. Observe appetite and foods the patient selects.
3. Monitor the fluid intake.
4. Ask the patient what is normally taken for constipation.

Nursing interventions

1. Encourage the patient to be as active as possible within the prescribed limitations (turning, moving).
2. Encourage fluid intake of 2500 to 3000 ml/day unless contraindicated.
3. Assist the patient in selecting foods that are high in roughage or fiber.
4. Give stool-softening agents and suppositories as prescribed.

Urinary System
Pathophysiology

Increased urinary calcium from bone destruction, increased urinary pH (alkaline), increased citric acid (which causes the precipitation of calcium salts), stasis of urine in the bladder, and infection can all cause urinary problems.

Nursing assessment
Subjective and objective data

1. Observe quantity of fluid intake. Ask the patient about normal fluid intake.
2. Has the patient a history of urinary problems?
3. Ask the elderly male patient about urinary problems before admission. Some men will describe hesitancy and frequency because of an enlarged prostate gland.

Nursing interventions

1. Encourage fluid intake.
2. Limit calcium intake (milk) to dietary orders.
3. Monitor urinary output and report difficulties to the physician. (Potential is high for bladder infection and formation of renal stones.)

Musculoskeletal System
Pathophysiology

Atrophy and weakness of the muscles will occur because of disuse. Bone growth (*osteoblastic*) and bone destruction (*osteoclastic*) activity is disrupted by immobility. The osteoclastic activity takes precedence, with the result that bone matrix is destroyed and calcium is released. The end results is *osteoporosis* and renal stones.

Nursing assessment
Objective data

1. Ask patient to demonstrate prescribed exercises.
2. Ask patient to demonstrate movement of unaffected limbs.

Nursing interventions

1. Encourage active and isometric exercises of unaffected limbs.
2. Have patient demonstrate prescribed exercises.
3. Do passive exercises when patient is unable to do active movement.

SUMMARY

1. Bones have several functions. These include the following: (a) *supporting* body tissues *and* providing the *skeletal framework*, (b) *protecting* body organs, (c) *providing* for *movement*, (d) serving as a *storehouse* for mineral salts and, (e) providing for *hematopoesis*.
2. There are four types of bones: *long* bones (femur, humerus); *short* bones (carpals); *flat* bones (skull); and *irregular* bones (vertebrae).
3. Bursae are lined with synovial membrane and serve as cushions between moving parts.
4. Joints provide flexibility at places where bones come together.
5. There are three major classes of joints: (1) synarthroses, or immovable joints, (b) amphiarthroses, or slightly movable joints, and (c) diarthroses, or freely movable joints.
6. Joints permit the following movements:
   a. Flexion
   b. Extension
   c. Adduction

    d. Abduction

    e. Rotation

    f. Circumduction

    g. Special movements such as supination, pronation, inversion, eversion, and protraction.

7. Preventive health teaching requires knowledge about safety devices such as grab bars and safety arms around toilets that can be used by patients in their own homes.

8. Both heat and cold are prescribed in treating persons with musculoskeletal problems, and precautions must be observed with each.

9. Rheumatoid arthritis is more common in women than in men.

10. The cause of rheumatoid arthritis is unknown, but immune mechanisms are considered to be a strong etiologic factor.

11. Persons with rheumatoid arthritis can benefit from being involved in a support group.

12. The primary group of drugs used to treat rheumatoid arthritis are the nonsteroidal antiinflammatory agents (NSAIAs).

13. Replacement arthroplasty can be used to replace a variety of joints. The most commonly replaced joints are the hip and the knee.

14. Persons with artificial joints require protection from bacteremia and must take prophylactic antibiotics before dental procedures, surgery, or instrumentation of the GI or GU tract.

15. Restrictions on movement necessary to prevent dislocation of a prosthesis are prescribed by the surgeon and depend on the design of the prosthesis and method of insertion.

16. Persons with joint replacements must use an ambulatory aid (walker, crutches, or cane) until able to walk securely without aid.

17. Persons with joint replacements will have a prescribed exercise program, which should be followed after discharge.

18. The course of systemic lupus erythematosus (SLE) is believed to be caused by an aberration of the immune system.

19. Polymyositis (dermatomyositis) is an inflammatory disorder of striated muscles of unknown causation.

20. Persons with polymyositis have exacerbations and remissions of their disease.

21. Ankylosing spondylitis causes the bones of the spine to grow together, and the patient may have a "poker-back" deformity or scoliosis.

22. Persons with ankylosing spondylitis may have impaired gas exchange because of change in the chest cavity and decrease in chest excursion.

23. Bursitis refers to inflammation of a bursa. The shoulder joint is the most commonly affected.

24. Bursitis is usually caused by trauma, strain, or overuse of a joint. It is often treated by injection of corticosteroids into the affected joint capsule.

25. Carpal tunnel syndrome causes episodes of burning pain or tingling in the hands. Numbness (hypesthesia) affecting the thumb, index finger, and ring finger occurs after prolonged flexion of the wrist, as in typing.

26. Degenerative joint disease (DJD) is also known as osteoarthritis, hypertrophic arthritis, osteoarthrosis, or senescent arthritis.

27. DJD is very common in persons between 50 and 70 years of age.

28. Prevention of DJD centers on (a) avoiding obesity, (b) avoiding repeated trauma to joints, and (c) protecting joints in occupations that put joints at risk.

29. Treatment of DJD includes agents to relieve pain, assistive devices such as a cane to unload weight from weight-bearing joints, rest, exercise, and surgery including arthroplasty.

30. A herniated disk is an example of a degenerative disease of the spine.

31. Sciatic pain is common in persons with a herniated disk.

32. Persons with a herniated disk can be treated conservatively with rest, heat, analgesics, muscle relaxants, and sometimes traction to relieve muscle spasm.

33. When conservative therapy is not successful in treating a herniated disk, surgery may be necessary to relieve compression on nerve roots.

34. Patients who have spinal surgery must be taught to do logrolling when turning from side to side.

35. Scoliosis causes a visible curvature of spine when the patient leans forward from the waist.

36. Corrective surgery to realign vertebrae and fusion are used to treat scoliosis when the curve of the spine exceeds 49 degrees.

37. Scoliosis surgery usually involves bone grafting and the use of instrumentation such as Harrington rods, Dwyer instrumentation, or Lugue instrumentation.

38. Gout is a metabolic disorder involving the joints.

39. Treatment of gout involves preventive therapy with uricosuric agents, which either enhance uric acid excretion (probenecid [Benemid]) or decrease uric acid formation (Allopurinol [Zyloprim]).

40. Fracture of bones is treated with immobility by splinting, bracing, casting, traction, or surgery.

41. A major complication of fracture is fat embolism, which can be life-threatening and is manifested by chest pain, pallor, dyspnea, prostration, confusion, and petechial hemorrhage of skin and conjunctivae.

42. Monitoring for neurocirculatory status in a patient with a cast includes palpation for warmth, observation of color, application of moderate pressure to nail bed, touching the injured part to test sensation, observing patient's ability to move body part distal to fracture, and questioning patient about pain or decreased or increased sensation distal to the cast.

43. A wet cast is handled with the flat of the hands or on a pillow to avoid indentations and pressure on underlying skin.

34. Because a plaster cast is porous, paint, varnish, or shellac should not be applied to the cast because this will interfere with circulation of air to the skin.

45. Traction is a mechanism that provides a steady pull on part or parts of the body.

46. Traction is used to reduce a fracture, maintain correct position of bone fragments during healing, immobilize a limb while soft tissue healing takes place, overcome

muscle spasm, stretch adhesions, and correct deformities.

47. Maintaining traction requires that ropes run straight and through pulleys, weights hang free, and nothing impinges on any part of the traction apparatus.

STUDY QUESTIONS

- Describe the anatomic structure of bones and the purposes of the skeletal system.
- Discuss the importance of the synovial joint and the composition of the joint.
- Review the range of motion through which a joint such as the shoulder would be exercised.
- Describe the complications that may occur from immobilization of the joint; the complications that may arise from total body immobilization.
- Select a patient who has a form of "arthritis." Write a nursing care plan based on the patient's defined nursing problems.
- Outline the care of the patient immobilized in a spica hip cast.
- What precautions must be taken in the care of a patient in traction?
- What precautions must be taken in the care of a patient with a total hip replacement?

REFERENCES AND SELECTED READINGS

1.* American Nurses' Association and National Association of Orthopaedic Nurses: Orthopaedic nursing practice: process and outcome criteria for selected diagnoses, *Orthop Nurs* 6(2):11-16, 1987.
2. Anderson LP: Carpal tunnel syndrome, *Orthop Nurs* 5(4):40-41, 1986.
3.* Barden RM: Osteonecrosis of the femoral head, *Orthop Nurs* 4(4):45-51, 1985.
4. Blaha JD, Pickett JC (editors): Controversy on total knee arthroplasty, *Clin Orthop Rel Res* 192S:2-112, 1984.
5. Blake SA: Non-cemented femoral prostheses: intraoperative focus, *Orthop Nurs* 4(1):40-41, 1985.
6. Blauvelt C, Nelson F: A manual of orthopedic terminology, ed 4, St Louis, 1990, Mosby–Year Book.
7. Bradley JD et al: Comparison of an antiinflammatory dose of ibuprofen, and analgesic dose of ibuprofen, and acetaminophen in the treatment of patients with osteoarthritis of the knee, *N Engl J Med* 325(2):87-91, 1991.
8. Brashear HR, Ranney RB: *Handbook of orthopaedic surgery,* ed 10, St Louis, 1986, Mosby–Year Book.
9. Brooks PM, Day RO: Nonsteroidal antiinflammatory drugs—differences and similarities, *N Engl J Med,* 324(24):1716-1723, 1991.
10. Burgess S et al: Systemic lupus erythematosus and renal insufficiency, *ANNA J* 13(3):168-171, 1986.
11. Callahan J: Compartment syndrome, *Orthop Nurs* 4(4):11-18, 1985.
12.* Cochran S: Action stat! Open fracture, *Nurs 87* 17(5):33, 1987.
13.* Collier IC: Assessing functional status of the elderly, *Arth Care Res* 1(1):45-52, 1988.
14. Crocker C: Acute postoperative pain: cause and control, *Orthop Nurs* 5(2):11-16, 1986.

15. Crenshaw AH: Campbell's operative orthopaedics, ed 8, St Louis, 1992, Mosby–Year Book.
16.* Coheny MO: Porous coated femoral prosthesis: concepts and care considerations, *Orthop Nurs* 4(1):43-45, 1985.
17.* Doheny MO, Sedlak CA: Body image considerations, for adult scoliosis patient having spinal fusion surgery, *Orthop Nurs* 6(6):18-22, 1987.
18. Enis JE: Total hip arthoplasty in the geriatric patient, *Hosp Med* (suppl) 23(4):44-48, 1987.
19. Falkenburg SA: Choosing hand splints to aid carpal tunnel syndrome recovery, *Occup Health Saf* 56(5):60-64, 1987.
20. Farrell J: Illustrated guide to orthopedic nursing, ed 3, Philadelphia, 1986, JB Lippincott.
21.* Fractured femur with internal fixation (pictorial), *Orthop Nurs* 6(2):38-41, 1987.
22. Fritzler MJ: Antinuclear antibodies in the investigation of rheumatic diseases, *Bull Rheum Dis* 35(6):1-10, 1985.
23.* Gamron R: Taking the pressure out of compartment syndrome, *Am J Nurs* 88(8):1076-1080, 1988.
24. Gardine A: Not another fractured hip, *Can Nurs* 82S(6):34-36, 1986.
25. Grisso JA, et al: Risk factors for falls as a cause of hip fracture in women, *N Engl J Med* 324S(19):1326-1331, 1991.
26.* Hansell M: Fractures and the healing process, *Orthop Nurs* 7(1):43-50, 1988.
27. Hennig LM et al: Keeping up on arthritis meds, *RN* 49(2):32-38, 1986.
28. Hines NA, Bates MS: Discharging the patient in skeletal traction, *Orthop Nurs* 6(4):21-24, 1987.
29.* Hoyt N: Infections following orthopaedic injury, *Orthop Nurs* 5(5):15-24, 1986.
30. Ignatvicius DO: Meeting the psychosocial needs of patients with rheumatoid arthritis, *Orthop Nurs* 6(3):16-21, 1987.
31. Ivey M, Clark RL: Arthroscopic debridement of the knee for septic arthritis, *Clin Orthop Rel Res* 199:201-206, 1985.
32.* Johnson J: Respiratory complications of orthopaedic injuries, *Orthop Nurs* 5(1):24-28, 1986.
33.* Johnson L: Operative management of unstable pelvic fractures, *Orthop Nurs* 8(4):21-25, 1989.
34. Jones Walton P: Effect of pin care on pin reactions in adults with extremity fracture treated with skeletal traction and external fixation, *Orthop Nurs* 7(4):29-33, 1988.
35.* Joseph N: Arthritis medications from A to Z, *Caring* 8(1):14-16, 1989.
36. Karlin L: Musculoskeletal trauma, *Emerg Care Q* 3(1):57-60, 1987.
37.* Kiem HA, Hensinger RN: Spinal deformities: scoliosis and kyphosis, *Clin Symp* 41(4):3-32, 1989.
38.* Klippel JH: Systemic lupus erythematosus, treated related complications superimposed on chronic disease, *JAMA* 263(13):1812-1815, 1990.
39.* Klippel JH, Strober S, Wofsy D: New therapies for the rheumatic disease, *Bul Rheum Dis* 38(4):1-7, 1989.
40. Koffler D: Immunology of systemic lupus erythematosus and related rheumatic diseases, *Clin Symp* 39(2):2-36, 1987.
41. Koopman WSI: Rheumatology, *JAMA* 265(23):3169-3170, 1991.
42.* Lamb K, Miller J, Hernandez M: Falls in the elderly: causes and prevention, *Orthop Nurs* 6(2):45-49, 1987.
43.* Lambert VA, et al: Coping with rheumatoid arthritis, *Nurs Clin North Am* 22:551-558, 1987.
44. Leach RE, editor: *Progress in sports medicine,* Philadelphia, 1985, JB Lippincott.
45.* Levy RN, et al: Progress in arthritis surgery: with special reference to current status of total joint arthroplasty, *Clin Orthop Related Res* 200:299-321, 1985.
46.* Liang MH, Fortin P: Management of osteoarthritis of the

*Recommended for student reading

hip and knee (an editorial), *N Engl J Med* 325(2):125-127, 1991.

47. * Liang MH: Osteoarthritis: a joint endeavor, *Harvard Health Letter,* 17(6):1-4, 1992.

48. * Liddel DR: An in-depth look at osteoporosis, *Orthop Nurs* 4S(3):23-28, 1985.

49. Lin P (editor): Posterior lumbar interbody fusion, *Clin Orthop Related Res* 193:2-132, 1985.

50. Lorish C, Richards B, Brown S: Missed medication doses in rheumatic arthritis patients: intentional and unintentional reasons, *Arth Care Res* 2(1):3-9, 1989.

51. McCarthy DJ, editor: *Arthritis and allied conditions: a textbook of rheumatology,* ed 11, Philadelphia, 1989, Lea and Febiger.

52. McGuire L: Administering analgesics which drugs are right for your patient, Nursing 9020(4):34-41, April 1990.

53. Maher AB: After the emergency is over: delayed and occult injuries in the trauma patient, *Orthop Nurs* 4(2):25-27, 1985.

54. * Maher AB: Early assessment and management of musculoskeletal injuries, *Nurs Clin North Am* 21:717-727, 1986.

55. Malasanos L, et al: Health assessment, ed 4, St Louis, 1990, Mosby—Year Book.

56. Mankin HJ and Treadwell BV: Osteoarthritis: a 1987 update: Bull Rheum Dis 36(5):1-10, 1986.

57. * Marchette L, Marchette B: Back injury: a preventable occupational hazard, *Orthop Nurs* 4(6):25-29, 1985.

58. * Miller B: Osteoarthritis in the primary health care setting, *Orthop Nurs* 6(5):41-46, 1987.

59. Morrey BF, Kavanagh BF: Cementless joint replacement: current status and future, *Bull Rheum Dis* 39(4):1-7, 1987.

60. Morrey BF: Orthopedics, *JAMA* 265(23):3151-3152, 1991.

61. * Mourad L, Droste M: *The nursing process in the care of adults with orthopaedic conditions,* ed 2, New York, 1988, John Wiley & Sons.

62. Mourad L: *Orthopedic disorders, vol IV of Mosby's Clinical Nursing series,* St Louis, 1991, Mosby—Year Book.

63. * Mulvey MA, Sharma PK: Traumatic amputation, *RN* 54(9):26-30, 1991.

64. National Institute of Arthritis and Musculoskeletal and Skin Disease: NIH: osteoporosis: cause, treatment, prevention, *Orthop Nurs* 5(6):29-38, 1986.

65. * Nordby EJ: A comparison of disectomy and chemonucleolysis, *Clin Orthop Related Res* 200:279-283, 1985.

66. * Nussman DS, Poole RC: Rescue and recovery in traumatic hip dislocation, *Am J Nurs* 9(11):34-38, 1991.

67. Omer G: Assessment of hand trauma, *Orthop Nurs* 4(2):29-33, 1985.

68. Osborne LJ, DiGiacomo I: Traction: a review with nursing diagnoses and interventions, *Orthop Nurs* 6(4):13-18, 1987.

69. Peters P: Successful return to work following a musculoskeletal injury, *AAOHN J* 38(6):264-270, 1990.

70. Pfeiffer CA, Wetstone SL: Health locus on control and well-

being in systemic lupus erythematosus, *Arth Care Res* 1(3):131-138, 1988.

71. * Pigg J, Driscoll P, Caniff R: *Rheumatology nursing: a problem-oriented approach,* New York, 1985, John Wiley & Sons.

72. Robinson JE, Marx LO: A nail-safe method, *Am J Nurs* 85(2):158-161, 1985.

73. Rodts MF: Surgical intervention for adult scoliosis, *Orthop Nurs* 6(6):11-17, 1987.

74. Schoen DC: Assessing a fractured hip, *Nurs 87* 17(3):97-98, 1987.

75. Schumacher HR: *Primer on the rheumatic diseases,* ed 9, Atlanta, 1988, Arthritis Foundation.

76. Sheidler V: Patient-controlled analgesia, *Curr Concepts Nurs* 1(1):13-16, 1987.

77. * Shellenbarger T: When you're asked about carpal tunnel syndrome, *RN* 54(7):40-42, 1991.

78. * Sproles KJ: Nursing care of skeletal pins: a closer look, *Orthop Nurs* 4(1):11-20, 1985.

79. Swezey RL, editor: *Straight talk on ankylosing spondylitis,* Sherman Oaks, Calif, 1985, Ankylosing Spondilitis Association.

80. Unkle D, DeLong W: Adominal trauma associated with pelvic fractures, *Orthop Nurs* 8(4):27-29, 1989.

81. United States Dept of Health and Human Services, Public Health Service, Healthy People 2000: *Health promotion and disease prevention objectives,* Washington, DC, 1990, Government Printing Office.

82. * Walsh CR, Wirth CR: Total knee arthroplasty: biomechanical and nursing considerations, *Orthop Nurs* 4(1):29-34, 1985.

83. Wick JL: The role of ergonomics in the elimination and prevention of work-related musculoskeletal problems, *Orthop Nurs* 8(1):41-42, 1989.

83a. Wise CM: *Hypeuricemia and gout.* In Rakel RE, editor: *Conn's current therapy 1991,* Philadelphia, 1991, WB Saunders.

84. * Willey T: High-tech beds and mattress overlays: a decision guide, *Am J Nurs* 89(9):1142-1145, 1989.

85. * Zubay RL: Understanding magnetic resonance imaging from a nursing perspective, *Orthop Nurs* 7(6):17-23, 1988.

Classic

86. * Cave L: Lowering the uncertainties of arthritis with nurse-led support group, *Orthop Nurs* 3(5):39-42, 1984.

87. Moskowitz RW, et al: *Osteoarthritis: diagnosis and management,* Philadelphia, 1984, WB Saunders.

88. * Olson EV (editor): The hazards of immobility, *Am J Nurs* 67:780-797, 1967.

89. * Wagner MM: Assessment of patients with multiple injuries, *Am J Nurs* 72S(10):1822-1827, 1972.

Problems of Defense and Protection

Unit Eleven

41

The Patient with Immunologic Problems

Barbara C. Long
E. Ronald Wright

After studying this chapter, the learner should be able to:

- Identify the immune response in immunodeficiencies, gammopathies, hypersensitivities, and autoimmunities and give examples.
- Describe methods of immunosuppression and the care of the immunodeficient person.
- Compare and contrast the four types of hypersensitivities.
- Describe the pathophysiologic bases of type I hypersensitivities and related interventions.
- Describe blood transfusion and tissue transplant reactions.
- Compare autoimmune diseases based on their immunoresponse.

Immunologic alterations occur in a wide variety of diseases. In some disorders the immunologic basis is clearcut, such as in allergic disorders and immunodeficiency diseases. In other disorders, the role of the immunologic response as the causative agent is less well documented. Because immunologic factors are operative in such a wide variety of disorders, much of the information about the disorders is found elsewhere in the text. This chapter describes the various categories of immune disorders and discusses in more detail those disorders not described elsewhere. HIV infection and AIDS is discussed in Chapter 19.

REVIEW OF THE IMMUNE SYSTEM

The immune system serves to protect the body from invading foreign cells and body-damaging substances. The basic systems and their functions are described in Chapter 16; only the essentials are highlighted here. The immune system distributes through the body a variety of cells and substances that recognize and take action against invading agents. The protective body mechanisms can be divided into nonspecific and specific immune response systems.

Nonspecific Immune Response

Certain cells and proteins in the blood and tissues respond to foreign substances or to damaged self-cells in the same way, regardless of the type of invasion or cell destruction. The degree of response, however, varies in relation to the extent of damage. The outcome of the response is the *inflammatory response* (Chapter 16).

The key cells of the nonspecific immune response are the *phagocytic* cells, including the *granulocytic white blood cells* (WBC), especially the *neutrophils*, and the monocytes. In response to tissue injury or invasion of microorganisms, WBCs are attracted to the site in response to chemical stimulation (chemotaxis). The WBCs migrate from the blood vessel into the affected tissue, where they engulf and destroy foreign materials.

Another major factor in the nonspecific response is the *complement* system. This system is composed of inactive serum proteins that, when activated in a sequential series of steps, have the ability to damage cell membranes and destroy the cell. The system can be activated by the binding of specific antibodies to foreign cell antigens, by certain bacterial cell components, or by materials released from the damaged tissues cells.

Other factors that appear in the body in response to the inflammatory response include the *acute-phase proteins*. These proteins are synthesized by the liver and multiply in the serum to provide materials that mediate the inflammatory response.

Specific Immune Response

The internal specific immune response is designed to recognize and take action against *specific* foreign molecules called *antigens (immunogens)*. The introduced antigen stimulates the production of specifically reactive molecules called *antibodies (immunoglobulins)*, or cells *(cytotoxic lymphocytes)*. The immunoglobulins or cytotoxic lymphocytes bind to the antigens to inactivate or destroy the foreign agent. The system also remembers prior contact with the antigenic material and responds faster and more efficiently to subsequent contact.

There are two types of specific immune responses, the *cell-mediated system,* which provides the cytotoxic lymphocytes, and the *humorally mediated system,* which provides the circulating immunoglobulins.

Cell-mediated immune response

The key cells of the cell-mediated immune response are the *T-cell lymphocytes* that are produced in the bone marrow and mature in the thymus gland. From the thymus the T cells migrate to the medulla of regional lymph nodes and spleen. Each mature immunosensitive T-cell lymphocyte is capable of responding to a specific antigenic signal. When exposed to its specific antigen, the T cell begins to divide, increasing the number of that antigenically responsive cell in the lymph node. Some of the T cells are carried by the lymph into the bloodstream to the specific antigens. The T cells then attack and destroy the antigenic molecules (cytotoxic effect). The T cells also release a number of soluble substances (lymphokines) that activate nonspecifically reactive phagocytes to attack the tissues at the site.

Other T-cell lymphocytes regulate the T-cell function and production of antibodies by the B-cell system. T-cell lymphocytes known as *helper T cells* (T_H or T_4 cells) are

Table 41-1 **Comparison of T cells and B cells**

	T cells	B cells
Immune response	Cell mediated	Humorally mediated
Source	Bone marrow	Bone marrow
Site of maturation	Thymus	Bone marrow, intestinal lymphoid tissue
Storage	Medulla of regional lymph node or spleen	Cortex of regional lymph node or spleen
Functions	Destroy antigenically labeled cells	Synthesize and release immunoglobulins (antibodies)
	Release lymphokines that activate phagocytes	Form memory (B_M) cells
	Regulate T-cell function	
	Regulate production of antibodies by B cells (helper T cells)	
	Prevent or modify B-cell and T-cell activity (suppressor T cells)	
	Form memory (T_M) cells	

necessary to provide a full immunologic humoral (B cell) or cell-mediated (T cell) response. Another type of T cell, known as *suppressor T cells* (T_S or T_8 cells), operates to prevent or modify the function of the two systems. Additional T cells, *memory T cells* (T_M), remember contact with the antigen and on subsequent exposure respond immediately to its presence in the body. The functions of T cells are summarized in Table 41-1.

Humorally mediated immune response

The key cells of the humorally mediated immune response are the *B-cell lymphocytes*. These are produced in the bone marrow, but mature outside the thymus, such as in bone marrow or gut-associated lymphoid tissues. From there the B cells migrate to the cortex of regional lymph nodes and spleen.

As with T cells, the immunosensitive B cells are programmed to respond to a single antigen. When the antigen is present, the B cell begins to proliferate and differentiate into a *plasma cell*. A plasma cell is designed to synthesize and release large amounts of *immunoglobulin* (antibody) that will combine with the antigen that caused its production. These antibody molecules are released into the circulation where they become part of the gamma globulin fraction of the serum. The B cells producing the immunoglobulin remain in the lymphoid tissue and continue to synthesize additional molecules of the specific antibody. Note that this is different from the T-cell response where cytotoxic T cells are released; in this case the B cells remain, and their product is released. Thus the level of active specific antibody begins to rise in the serum fraction (*antibody titer*), as well as in the level of the gamma globulin fraction in general. These antibodies are carried by the blood and other body fluids to where they encounter their specific antigen and bind to it. Upon binding, the antibody may inactivate the antigen, precipitate it, or activate other antigen-damaging processes (such as the complement cascade) to remove the antigen.

The immunoglobulins are subdivided into different classes on the basis of molecular structure and function. The generic symbol for immunoglobulins is Ig, and each of the classes is designated by a letter of the alphabet: IgG, IgM, IgA, IgE, and IgD. The predominant immunoglobulin is IgG (Table 41-2).

The B-cell system is similar to the T-cell system in that it is controlled by helper and suppressor T cells, forms memory (B_M) cells, and is rendered self-tolerant by the same mechanisms.

Physiologic Changes With Aging

The extent of immunologic changes with aging varies among individuals depending on multiple factors, such as genetics, nutritional status, and presence of disorders that deplete the immune system. In general, however, the immune response is decreased with aging.

The thymus gland atrophies with age. Remember that T cells mature in the thymus; therefore, the major change is a *reduction in T-cell function*, including both cytologic and immunoregulatory activities. However, there is no marked change in the total number of T cells or of any T-cell subset. Although the antibody response is also variably reduced by age, this is believed to be the result of T-cell rather than B-cell changes. The resulting deficiency that develops gradually with age is one of cellular immune incompetence and is of clinical importance.[21] The contribution of age-related immunodeficiency, however, is difficult to separate from immunodeficiencies that result from underlying diseases.

The decreased immune response with age can be noted by a decreased response to skin tests by the elderly. Older persons also have fewer signs and symptoms of inflammations, such as lower temperature elevations, than can be expected.

Infections occur more frequently in the elderly, even in the person with no underlying disease. Infections also tend to be more severe.[21] Common infections include influenza and pneumococcal pneumonia. Morbidity and mortality are higher than in younger persons. It is because of the severity of disease commonly experienced that yearly influenza im-

Table 41-2   Immunoglobulin (Ig) mechanisms and functions

Immunoglobulin	%	Mechanisms	Functions
IgG	75-82	Reacts with surface antigen on target cells; causes lysis of cell Enhances phagocytosis Crosses placenta	Destroys antigen-carrying cells Long-term immunity Major memory Ig Passive immunity for fetus
IgM	7-10	Reacts with surface antigen on target cells; causes lysis of cells Agglutination Is predominant early in immune responses	Major control of intravascular antigens
IgA	10-15	Prevents microorganisms from penetrating epithelial cells	Protects mucosal surfaces from bacteria, viruses, and toxins
IgE	trace	Attach to mast cells or basophils; upon binding antigen, releases chemical mediators	Protect against parasitic infections
IgD	trace	Found on surface of B cells in association with IgM	Assists B-cell response to antigen

munizations for the elderly are strongly recommended.
There is an increased *potential for cancer* associated with age. One theory for the increase is decreased immune surveillance (see Chapter 16). Another theory is that older persons, by virtue of living longer, have been exposed to more carcinogens. Although tumors occur more frequently in older persons, the tumors tend to grow more slowly and metastasize less frequently.[21]

MAJOR HEALTH PROBLEMS OF THE IMMUNE SYSTEM

Immunologic disorders occur when the immune response malfunctions. The disorders may be a result of immune deficiencies, abnormal production of immunoglobulins, excessive response to specific antigens, or immune response to self-antigens (Table 41-3). Each of these major categories will be discussed in this chapter. The majority of immunologic problems (other than the great variety of autoimmune diseases discussed throughout the text) are hypersensitivity disorders, so these disorders will be discussed in more detail.

IMMUNODEFICIENCIES

The following discussion of immunodeficiencies pertains to general immunodeficiencies. AIDS, an acquired immunodeficiency disease, is discussed in Chapter 19.

Etiology and Pathophysiology

Protection of the host depends on an intact immune system. Interference with development of cells and tissues of the immune response leads to immunodeficient disorders. Because the cells and tissues of the immune response system develop sequentially, if a defect in that development appears, the severity of the resulting deficiency reflects the stage of development at which the abnormality arose (Fig. 41-1). Deficiencies may exist in immunoglobulin synthesis (B-cell deficiency), cellular immune functions (T-cell deficiency), or phagocyte defects.

Immunodeficiencies may be primary or secondary. Primary immunodeficiencies, those resulting from improper fetal development, are genetic disorders in children. Some primary immunoglobulin deficiencies may not become evident until the person is an adult, and these are termed *common variable immunodeficiencies* (CVI). Persons with CVI develop recurrent virulent infections and display a high incidence of malignancies, hematologic disorders, and autoimmune diseases.

Secondary immunodeficiencies are a nonspecific depression of the immune response as a result of some interference with the immune system. These deficiencies are present to one degree or another in most of the major disease conditions experienced by persons in addition to the normal response to aging. Thus when caring for a person over the age of 60 years or with any acute disease condition, the concepts of immunodeficiency must be considered. Situations in which immunodeficiency plays a major role are listed in Box 41-1.

Major stress of any type may affect immune response as a result of increased corticosteroid production and alterations in protein metabolism. A form of immunodeficiency, immunosuppression, may result from or be deliberately created by the use of radiation, drugs, or antigens and antibodies (Table 41-4).

41-1	**Disorders characterized by immunodeficiencies**

Protein-calorie malnutrition
Alcoholism
Infections (especially viral)
Cancer
Autoimmune diseases
Lymphomas (including Hodgkin's disease)
Allergies
Trauma
Transplantation

Nursing Process
Assessment
Subjective data

Subjective data to obtain from the person with immunodeficiency include the following:
1. Knowledge of the immunodeficiency
2. Knowledge of prevention of infection
3. Occurrence of recurrent infections (type)
4. Concerns related to the immunodeficiency

Recurrent viral or fungal infections are suggestive of T-cell—mediated deficiencies, whereas recurrent bacterial infections may have an underlying B-cell (immunoglobulin) deficiency.

Objective data

Objective data include monitoring for early signs of infection (fever, pain, nasal discharge, cough, and enlarged nodes). Breath sounds are monitored daily for decreased sounds indicating pulmonary infection. The skin is inspected daily for lesions.

Diagnostic tests
T-cell (cellular) deficiency tests

T-cell function can be screened by delayed hypersensitivity skin testing to common antigens. Specific antigens, including purified protein derivative (PPD), *Candida* organisms, mumps antigen, streptokinase, and streptodornase, are injected intradermally. Reactions are read after 24 to 48 hours to determine hypersensitivity. The test is to determine the hypersensitivity, not the presence of disease. A person who does not react to any of these antigens is said to be *anergic*.

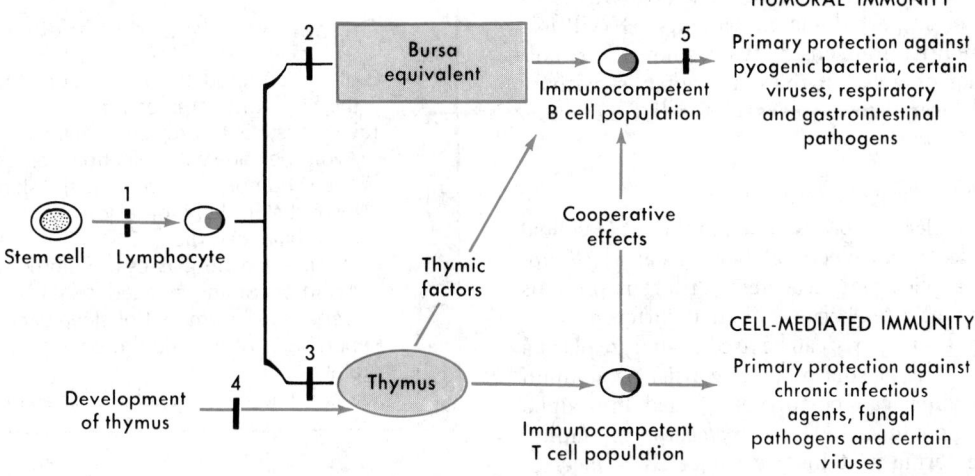

Fig. 41-1   Causes of immunodeficiencies. Abnormalities at *1* result in combined humoral and cell-mediated immunodeficiency. Blockage at *2* produces agammaglobulinemia. Blockage at *3* or *4* results in drastic reduction of T cell-mediated function, and because of cooperative effects on B cell system some reduction in humoral response occurs. Abnormalities in synthesis of specific immunoglobulin classes are reflected by blockage at *5*. Some blockages result in complete deficiency, whereas others show up as reduction in response.

Table 41-3   Classification of immunologic disorders

Category	Immune response	Examples
Immunodeficiencies	Deficiencies in the proper expression of immune response system, part of the system, or specific cells	Primary deficiencies, deficiencies associated with other diseases, acquired immunodeficiency syndrome (AIDS)
Gammopathies	Abnormal production of immunoglobulins	Multiple myeloma, hypergammaglobinemia
Hypersensitivities	Exaggerated or inappropriate response to specific antigen	Anaphylaxis, allergies, transfusion reactions, graft rejections
Autoimmunities	Immunologic attack on self-antigens	Rheumatoid arthritis, SLE, glomerulonephritis

Table 41-4   Induced immunosuppression

Method	Comments	Use
Antigen administration	Specific antigen administered in small amounts over time	Allergy desensitization
Antibody administration	Specific antibody administered to combine with antigen and block contact with immunocompetent cell	Obstetrics: prevent sensitive Rh-negative mother from responding to Rh-positive fetus during pregnancy
Monoclonal antibodies (MoAbs)	Clones of a single immunoglobulin-producing cell; react with receptors on T-cell surface preventing lysis of cells.	Organ transplantation
Irradiation	Destroys lymphocytes, thus fewer cells available for immune response; total body irradiation affects hematopoietic system, gastrointestinal (GI) system, and central nervous system (CNS)	Local irradiation: renal allografts Total body irradiation: organ transplantation
Drugs	Corticosteroids impair T cell function and cause catabolism of immunoglobulins and lymphocytopenia	Diseases where immune disorder is unknown (for example, autoimmunities); tissue and organ transplantation
	Cytotoxic drugs destroy rapidly dividing immunologically stimulated cells	
	Cyclosporine (Sandimmune) acts against T helper cells and facilitates development of T suppressor cells	Organ transplantation

Sensitization with dinitrochlorobenzene (DNCB) is an additional test for suspected anergic patients. DNCB is a chemical to which natural sensitivity does not occur. Following application of DNCB to the skin, contact sensitivity can be elicited after 1 to 2 weeks if T-cell function is present.

B-cell (humoral) deficiency tests

Plasma protein electrophoresis. The movement of colloid (protein) particles in an electrical field is called *electrophoresis*. In an applied electrical field, different proteins migrate at different rates because of their different sizes and shapes, and this property can be used to analyze plasma protein content. The plasma proteins consist of albumin and globulins, which can be further divided into alpha globulins, beta globulins, and *gamma globulins* (immunoglobulins). The serum proteins are subjected to electrophoresis in a medium that stabilizes the migration so that the proteins can be stained and examined.

Quantitative immunoglobulin test. Three of the immunoglobulins—IgG, IgA, and IgM—can be measured quantitatively, whereas IgD and IgE are present in amounts too small to measure. Venous blood is collected; no special preparation is required.

Data analysis: nursing diagnoses

Nursing diagnoses are determined from analysis of patient data. Possible nursing diagnoses for the person with an immunodeficiency may include, but are not limited to, the following:

Diagnostic title	Possible etiologies
Infection, high risk for	Decreased immune response, lack of information
Knowledge deficit	Lack of exposure/recall, information misinterpretation

Planning: expected patient outcomes

Expected patient outcomes for the person with an immunodeficiency may include, but are not limited to, the following:

1. Signs of infection do not occur.
2. Describes measures to avoid infection.
3. Describes signs dictating immediate medical attention.
4. Explains the need for continued medical follow-up.

Implementation

Assisting with achievement of therapeutic goals
Replacement therapy

Specific replacement therapy may be given for primary immunodeficiencies. When B-cell deficiency is present, gamma globulin may be given at monthly intervals. Gamma globulin is a purified concentrated solution of antibodies, mostly IgG, found in normal plasma. Gamma globulin can be given intramuscularly but problems with this approach include pain at injection site, toleration of only small volumes per injection, and degradation of antibody at the injection site. *Intravenous* immunoglobulin (IVIG) is now

---

41-2

Patient Teaching

The patient with immunodeficiency

Explain immunodeficiency, that is, the inability of the body to fight infection.
Take measures to prevent infection
    Avoid persons with infections (especially colds).
    Avoid bumping or breaking the skin.
    Inspect skin daily for lesions.
    Eat a balanced diet.
    Drink at least 6 glasses of fluid per day.
    Avoid becoming fatigued.
    Get a regular amount of sleep each night.
Report signs of infection to physician immediately.
See physician on a regular basis as instructed.

---

more commonly used. Larger doses can be given with fewer side effects and less discomfort. About 3% to 12% of patients experience fever, chills, headache, myalgias, and nausea during infusion.[27] These effects can be prevented by preadministration of acetaminophen, antihistamines, or hydrocortisone. The infusion is started slowly, then increased in rate if no adverse reactions occur. Vital signs are monitored, especially for a drop in blood pressure. If changes in vital signs or other adverse reactions occur, stop the infusion, change to normal saline infusion, and notify physician.[41] Be prepared for anaphylaxis.

Replacement therapy for T-cell–mediated immune deficiencies is more complex. Transfer factor (extracted from lymphocytes of humans who have demonstrated delayed hypersensitivity reactions), thymosin (a thymic hormone), bone marrow transplants, and fetal thymic transplants have been used.

Interventions to achieve patient outcomes
Preventing infection

The most important factor in the care of the immunodeficient or immunosuppressed person is protection from infection. Care differs depending on whether the degree of immunosuppression is minimal, moderate, or severe:

1. Care for minimal immunosuppression
    a. Use good medical asepsis.
    b. Avoid persons with infections.
    c. Remove sources where bacteria may proliferate.
    d. Avoid injections as much as possible.
    e. Maintain nutrition at optimal level (immune response is decreased by malnutrition).
    f. Maintain adequate fluid hydration (intake of more than 1500 ml/day) (hydration helps dilute effects of infection).
2. Care for moderate immunosuppression
    a. If severe leukopenia is present, place person in a single room to decrease infection potential.
    b. If person is acutely ill, give mouth care, perineal care, and pulmonary hygiene to prevent infection.
    c. Use same protective measures as for minimal immunosuppression.

3. Care for severe immunosuppression
   a. Use protective isolation by laminar air flow units (Chapter 11).
   b. Use same protective measures as for moderate immunosuppression.

Facilitating learning

People who are immunosuppressed, as well as their families, need to know the nature of immunosuppression and how to avoid infection (see Box 41-2).

Evaluation

Questions to consider may include the following:
1. Has infection been prevented during hospitalization?
2. Does the person know
   a. The nature of immunodeficiency?
   b. How to prevent and identify infection?
   c. The need for continued medical follow-up?

GAMMOPATHIES

Pathophysiology

Gammopathies, better termed *hypergammaglobulinemias*, are elevated levels of gamma globulin in the serum. The normal synthesis of an immunoglobulin is the result of the proliferation of plasma cell differentiation of a single clone of B cells in response to an antigenic signal. In gammopathies a single clone or multiple clones of plasma cells begin to overproduce immunoglobulin product in response to inappropriate antigenic stimulation.

Monoclonal (M-type) *gammopathies* involve a single B-cell clone and are commonly referred to as *plasma cell dyscrasias*. A common monoclonal gammopathy is multiple myeloma.

Polyclonal gammopathies involve the overproduction of virtually all classes of immunoglobulins. The major causes are infectious diseases (especially chronic bacterial infections such as lung abscess and osteomyelitis), connective tissue diseases (such as SLE and rheumatoid arthritis), and chronic active liver disease. IgG and IgM are the most commonly involved immunoglobulins, and the degree of immunoglobulin level reflects the severity of the disease. The development of high levels of dysfunctional gamma globulins depresses the synthesis of normal immunoglobulins, which renders the person susceptible to infection.

MULTIPLE MYELOMA

Etiology and Pathophysiology

Multiple myeloma is a monoclonal plasma cell malignancy seen in both men and women, occurring in middle and old age. It is characterized by widespread bone destruction, anemia, hypercalcemia, and hyperuricemia. These symptoms are traced to the proliferation of plasma cell tumors from the bone marrow into the hard bone tissue, causing an erosion of the bone. Frequent recurrent infections (especially of the respiratory tract) and spontaneous pathologic fractures occur because of the production of ineffective

The Elderly with Immunologic Problems

Assessment

Assess nutritional status of all elderly persons, especially those living alone. Good nutrition is an important factor in maintenance of the immune system.

Assess carefully elderly patients in nursing homes or those entering hospital from a nursing home for signs of infection. Risk of infection in these persons is high because of high rates of immobility from neurologic or cardiovascular disorders, from high use of invasive catheters, or from malnutrition.[42]

Assess mobility status of elderly patients; immobility may lead to skin breakdown and infection.

Assess patient for changes in mental status, anorexia, claims of "feeling poorly," or comments by family members that the elderly person looks ill. These may be early signs of infection in the elderly, as compared to signs of fever and pain in the younger adult.

Intervention

Consider every elderly patient as partly immunodeficient and take all precautions to prevent infections, especially respiratory infections.

Monitor elderly patients' responses to antibiotic therapy; the incidence of drug reactions is greater because of the older person's greater sensitivity.[42]

Monitor fluid and dietary intake to maintain fluid balance and good nutritional status; this is necessary for maintenance of the immune system.

Common disorders in elders

Infections, especially bacteremic pneumonia, UTI, tetanus, and herpes zoster
Malignancies
Autoimmune disorders

immunoglobulins, which, in turn, depress the production of normal antibodies. Renal failure may result from precipitation of urate and calcium crystals. (For additional information, see Chapter 33).

Medical Intervention

Combination chemotherapy is the major treatment. Alkylating agents, specifically melphalan and cyclophosphamide (Cytoxan), are the drugs most commonly used. Several weeks may elapse between the initiation of therapy and signs of improvement. Periods of remission of 6 years or more have been obtained with chemotherapy. Radiation therapy may be given for palliative treatment of localized bone pain and pathologic fractures.

Supportive Nursing Care

Ambulation and adequate hydration are vitally important to prevent renal complications from the increased amounts of urates and calcium being excreted in the urine. Fluid

Table 41-5   Summary of hypersensitivity reactions

| Property | Hypersensitivity type | | | |
| | Immediate (humoral) | | | Delayed (cellular) |
	I Anaphylactic	II Cytotoxic	III Immune complex	IV Cell mediated
Immune system mediators	IgE (IgG) bound to mast cells	IgG or IgM (+ complement)	IgG or IgM + complement	T cells, macrophages
Allergens	Exogenous antigens	Foreign cells or alteration of cell surface antigens	Soluble antigens	Infectious agent, contact allergens, foreign tissues, cancer cells
Response to intradermal skin test	Wheal and flare within 30 min, edema	Not done	Erythema and edema within 3 to 8 hr	Erythema and induration within 24 to 48 hr
Pathophysiologic effects	Release of histamines, kinins, SRS-A from mast cells, which affect smooth muscle shock organs	Direct cytotoxic destruction of cells	Acute inflammatory reaction; primarily polymorphonuclear neutrophil leukocytes	Tissue destruction, primarily lymphocytes and macrophages
Examples	Systemic anaphylaxis, atopic allergies, hay fever, insect sting reactions	Hemolytic disease of the newborn (Rh), transfusion reactions	Serum sickness, Arthus reaction, glomerulonephritis	Tuberculin reaction, skin graft rejection, poison ivy

---

41-3

Factors influencing hypersensitivity responses

Increased responsiveness of the host
Increased amount of allergen
Nature of allergen
Entrance of allergen through appropriate site
Short time period between contacts

---

intake should be sufficient to ensure a urinary output of a minimum of 1500 ml/24 hr. Ambulation may be difficult because of the skeletal pain and the possibility of fractures. A lightweight spinal brace and analgesics may facilitate ambulation. Be alert for neurologic deficits in the lower extremities as a result of spinal cord compression.

Measures to prevent infection are instituted; they include avoidance of persons with upper respiratory tract infections. Medical attention should be sought for any signs of infection, and antibiotics are often given, because infections are usually caused by gram-positive organisms. Rest periods are planned if fatigue from anemia is present.

HYPERSENSITIVITY REACTIONS

Pathophysiology

The immune response system that has been previously sensitized is designed to provide an immediate, effective, protective reaction to subsequent encounters with the sensitizing antigen. This of course is a positive factor in the provision of immunity; however, under a given set of conditions or because of an idiotypic reactivity to a particular antigen, the response of the immune system may produce

detrimental effects. This *inappropriate response* is usually manifested as a tissue-damaging overreaction to the antigen; thus it is termed *hypersensitivity* or *allergy*. The antigenic stimulants invoking the reactions are referred to as *allergens*. Hypersensitivities, then, are classic expressions of the immune system, but they take place in inappropriate sites, in excessive amounts, or with inappropriate involvement of nonspecific tissues. Whether an allergic response occurs and to what degree depend on a combination of interrelated factors (see Box 41-3).

Hypersensitivities can be broadly divided into two categories based on the components of the immune system involved in mediating the hypersensitivity reaction: humoral or immediate response (B-cell mediated) and cellular or delayed response (T-cell mediated). The humoral response can be further subdivided into type I anaphylactic, type II cytotoxic, and type III immune complex (Table 41-5). Because type I, II, and III hypersensitivities are the result of interactions involving circulating antibodies, these reactions can be transferred from a sensitized host to a nonsensitized host by serum transfer. Type IV cell-mediated sensitivities can be transferred only by lymphocyte exchange.

TYPE I HYPERSENSITIVITIES (ANAPHYLACTIC)

Etiology

The type I hypersensitivities may take different forms depending on the type and amount of allergen and the degree of sensitization (Table 41-6). *Anaphylactic shock* is the most serious, life-threatening form and requires immediate medical intervention. Common antigens include insect bites (especially bee stings), drugs (especially penicillin and heterologous antiserum), food, pollen, and x-ray contrast media. *Urticaria (hives)* can be caused by foods, especially eggs, fish, and nuts, or drugs such as penicillin. Chronic urti

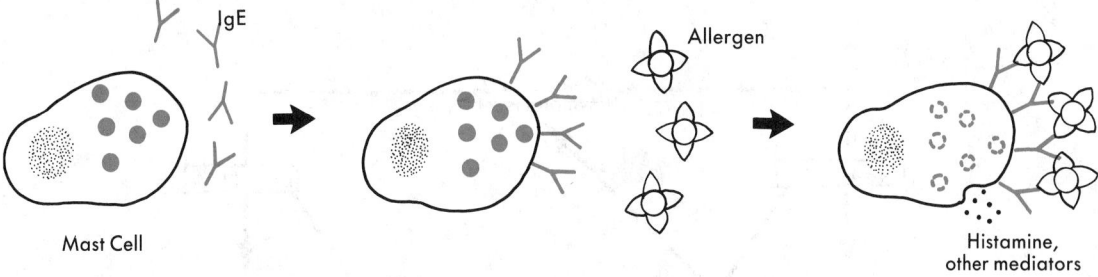

Fig. 41-2 Type I hypersensitivity. IgE binds to mast cell; allergen then binds to IgE, causing degranulation of mast cell with release of histamine and other mediators.

REVIEW

Table 41-6 Type I hypersensitivities (allergies)

Disorder	Signs and symptoms	Medical therapy
Anaphylactic shock	Initial itching and sneezing, apprehension Edema of face, hands, and other body parts; dyspnea, wheezing, shock	Epinephrine subcutaneously; Benadryl intramuscularly; aminophylline to relax bronchial spasm; tracheal intubation for tracheal edema; control of shock
Urticaria (hives)	Skin lesions: pale pink elevated edge on an erythematous background (wheal) Pruritus	Self-limiting; epinephrine or antihistamines may be given
Atopic		
Allergic rhinitis (hay fever)	Sneezing, itching, and watery eyes, running nose	Antihistamines; cromolyn sodium; allergic immunotherapy (Chapter 23)
Allergic asthma	Wheezing, coughing, dyspnea	Epinephrine, bronchodilators (Chapter 24)
Atopic dermatitis	Pruritus; vesicles; oozing and crusting lesions; scaling	Wet dressings, topical steroids (Chapter 43)

...caria may be caused by stress or exposure to heat or cold.

The less severe and more common forms of type I hypersensitivities are the atopic allergies, seen in about 15% of the population. *Atopy* refers to an inherited hypersensitivity. It is the tendency to become hypersensitive that is inherited, not the allergy to a specific substance. What persons become hypersensitive to is determined by the allergens to which they are exposed. Common antigens include *inhalants* (pollens, mold spore, animal dander, house dust) and *contactants* (fibers in wool, furs, and nylon; plant oils; soaps; cosmetics; perfumes; hair dyes; nickel in jewelry or clothing fasteners; occupational chemicals. Changes in temperature and stress may exacerbate symptoms.

Pathophysiology

Type I hypersensitivities are associated with the reactions mediated by the IgE class of immunoglobulins. The IgE immunoglobulins attach to the surface of mast cells and basophils, providing a site for allergens to bind to the cells. This causes the cell to release a variety of vasoactive substances, including histamine (Fig. 41-2).

Thus in type I reactions the detrimental symptoms are not at the site of the antigen-antibody reaction but at the site of the organs or tissues where the histamine and other mediators exert their action. If those mediators remain confined to a local area, the tissue reactions remain localized and are referred to as *local anaphylaxis*. The local hypersensitivity that most people demonstrate to a mosquito bite, the wheal-flare type of reaction, is the classic

example of this type of reaction. The reaction may also become localized in the nose and eyes (hay fever), in the bronchial passages (allergic asthma), or in the skin (atopic dermatitis). If, however, the mediators become released systemically, the response is known as *systemic anaphylaxis*, which can produce *anaphylactic shock* (Chapter 9).

The three main effects of the vasoactive substances are the following:

1. Constricts smooth muscle such as in the bronchi, resulting in bronchial spasm
2. Increases vascular permeability, resulting in urticaria (hives) or tissue edema
3. Increases mucous secretions, as occurs in hay fever and asthma

Symptoms depend on the type of allergy and the organ affected (Fig. 41-3) and include the following:

1. Respiratory: wheezing, sneezing, rhinitis with conjunctivitis
2. Dermal: urticaria, angioedema, rash
3. GI: nausea, vomiting, diarrhea
4. General symptoms: fever, malaise, joint pains, hematopoietic suppression, anaphylaxis

For type I reactions to occur, the hypersensitive individual must initially come into contact with the allergen that triggers the synthesis of the specific antiallergenic IgE antibodies. This primary contact is known as a *sensitizing dose*. On subsequent contact with the allergen (termed the *shocking* or *challenging dose*), the individual exhibits the symptoms of type I sensitivity. Persons who are allergic to

ALLERGY

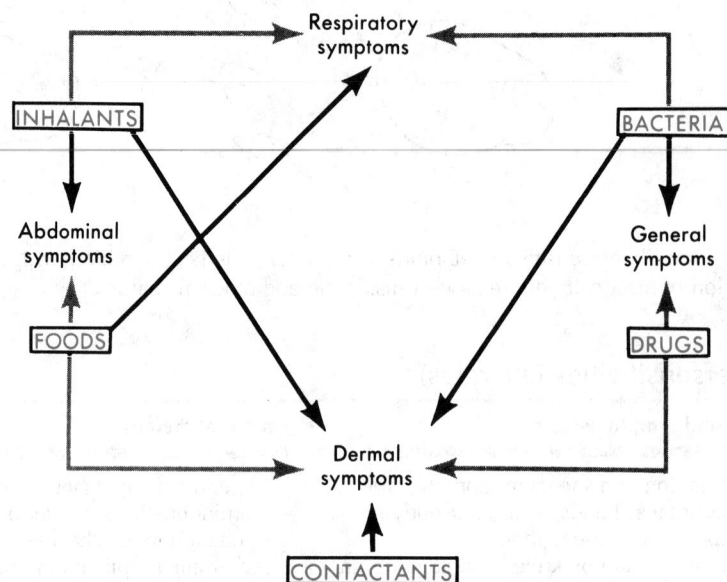

Fig. 41-3 Causes of allergic responses and symptoms produced.

pollenating grasses will have the same symptoms no matter which grass is pollenating. If they move from one geographic area to another, they will become sensitized to whatever grasses are present in that area.

Nursing Process
Assessment

All patients should be questioned about allergies and sensitivities to drugs before drug therapy is initiated. If there is any positive history, the physician is consulted before a new drug is given, and if it is given, the patient is watched closely for allergic responses.

It is usually possible to determine specific allergens to which a person is hypersensitive by taking a history that includes the following:

1. History of allergic reactions in the past (type, frequency, perceived cause)
2. Familial history of allergies
3. Recent exposure to sensitizing substances
4. Changes in living, working, or environmental conditions
5. Characteristics of present environment (house, clothing, plants and trees, or animals)
6. Increased stress in recent past
7. Types of symptoms: respiratory, dermal, or general
8. Alleviating factors, either prescribed by a physician or self-prescribed

Diagnostic tests
Skin testing

Skin tests are often used to determine whether a person has a sensitivity to certain substances in the external environment. Several methods of testing are used (Table 41-7). Occasionally one drop of a test extract is instilled into the eye to test for sensitivity (conjunctival test). Redness

of the conjunctiva and tearing will appear within 5 to 15 minutes in an allergic person. Tests for allergenic substances are usually done in a series.

Radioallergosorbent test

The radioallergosorbent test (RAST) for IgE antibodies provides the same information as skin tests. A blood sample is drawn for the test. RAST is easier to perform, more comfortable for the patient, and safer; but it is less sensitive and more costly than skin testing. RAST is especially useful for detecting IgE antibodies to occupational chemicals or potentially toxic allergens.

Use test

A person with a food allergy is asked to keep a food diary for at least a week. On the basis of this diary, suspect foods such as milk, wheat products, and eggs may be removed from the diet (elimination diet) until symptoms subside and then added one at a time in an attempt to identify the offending foods. Reaction to the use test may be immediate or over a period of time. Some persons become discouraged during the testing and may need encouragement to adhere to the testing schedule.

Data analysis: nursing diagnoses

Nursing diagnoses are determined from analysis of patient data. Possible nursing diagnoses for the person with an allergy may include, but are not limited to, the following:

Diagnostic title	Possible etiologies
Health maintenance, altered	Environmental changes, lack of knowledge
Knowledge deficit	Lack of exposure/recall, information misinterpretation

Table 41-7   Allergy skin tests

Test	Method	Time of reading	Positive signs	Use
Intradermal	Allergens are injected intradermally at spaced intervals on forearm or intrascapular area; control tests with diluent alone done concurrently	15 to 30 min	Wheal with surrounding erythema	Allergies to pollen, feathers, animal dander, dust
Scratch	Skin cleaned with alcohol and allowed to dry; skin scratched superficially (1 to 4 mm long), and extract applied to scratch	30 min	Erythema	Same as for intradermal
Patch	Sensitizing substance applied to small (1-inch) gauze square and covered with tape	48 hr	+Erythema only ++Erythema and papules +++Erythema, papules, and vesicles ++++All of above and bullae or ulceration	Allergies to clothing, detergents, perfumes, cosmetics

Planning: expected patient outcomes

Expected patient outcomes for the person with an allergy may include, but are not limited to, the following:
1. Demonstrates a decrease in symptoms.
2. Describes plans to alter habits or environment.
3. Describes substances that are allergenic and approaches for avoidance.
4. Describes rationale for immunotherapy and need to continue regular injections (if pertinent).
5. Describes need for constant availability of an anaphylaxis emergency kit for self-treatment (if anaphylaxis is a possibility).
6. Describes drug therapy to relieve symptoms.

Implementation
Assisting with achievement of therapeutic goals
Preventing anaphylactic reaction

Persons with a history of allergies are at high risk for developing anaphylactic reactions from drugs or animal sera. Hospitalized persons who are sensitive to certain substances should be identified, and the information posted conspicuously outside of the room, on the medical order sheets of the patient's record, or in both places. In addition, many hospitals use a special color identification bracelet for the person who is sensitive to certain substances.

If immunization is necessary, animal sera should be avoided and another type given, if possible. When it is necessary to use animal serum, the individual should first be tested for sensitivity to the substance. An intradermal skin test preceded by a scratch or eye test is recommended. If animal sera, allergenic extracts, or contrast media containing iodide are given, a syringe containing 1:1000 epinephrine hydrochloride, an antihistamine such as diphenhydramine (Benadryl), and isoproterenol (Isuprel) should be readily available. The patient is kept under surveillance for at least 20 minutes. Any reaction that occurs within a few minutes forewarns of an impending emergency. Persons with known history of anaphylactic reactions should

Drugs commonly prescribed for atopic allergies

Mast cell stabilizer: cromolyn sodium (Nasalcrom or Rynacrom as a nasal spray; Opticrom as eye drops)
Antihistamines: diphenhydramine (Benadryl), terfenadine (Seldane [nonsedating]), hismanal (Astemizole [nonsedating]), chlorpheniramine (Chlor-Trimeton), brompheniramine (Dimetane)
Vasoconstricting agents: epinephrine, pseudoephedrine (Sudafed, Novafed)
Bronchodilators: aminophylline, theophylline, isoproterenol, terbutaline, albuterol
Corticosteroids (for severe reactions):
Oral: prednisone
Nasal spray: Decadron Turbinaire, Vancenase, Beconase, Nasalide

always have ready access to an anaphylactic emergency kit containing oral antihistamine and isoproterenol tablets and a syringe with epinephrine for self-injection.

Therapy for anaphylaxis

At the first signs of *anaphylactic shock,* place the patient in a recumbent position and give 0.3 ml epinephrine hydrochloride (1:1000) (less for children) subcutaneously or intramuscularly. Epinephrine causes vasoconstriction and decreases vascular permeability, thus preventing systemic spread of the allergen with more severe consequences. An antihistamine, such as diphenhydramine (Benadryl), is then given; it does not reverse the effects of histamine but prevents further activation of the histamine. Persons outside health care agencies must seek *immediate* medical attention. Corticosteroids are given to decrease the inflammatory effects of severe anaphylaxis. Aminophylline or theophylline are given for bronchospasms. Tracheal intubation may be necessary for airway maintenance. Shock therapy with intravenous fluids and oxygen therapy are initiated immediately (Chapter 9).

Drug therapy for *atopic* allergies is primarily for symptom relief. Some of the common drugs are listed in Box 41-4.

Allergen immunotherapy

An attempt may be made to slowly desensitize a person by injecting small but increasingly larger doses of the allergen at regular intervals (usually 1 to 4 weeks) over a long period. This treatment may take up to 5 years. It is about 80% effective against pollens causing hay fever but is less effective against asthma or dermatitis. It is essential that the person understand that desensitization is of little value until the environment is controlled; otherwise the constant exposure to allergens will only increase antibody response.

Interventions to achieve patient outcomes
Controlling environment

Persons whose allergies are caused by environmental inhalants will need to avoid dust, animal dander, fungus spores, pollens, and other allergens. Methods of decreasing environmental inhalant antigens include the following:
1. House dust
   a. Use synthetic materials (avoid wool and cotton)
   b. Cover mattresses and pillows with allergy-free covers; place closet garments in plastic bags
   c. Avoid wool carpets or felt rug pads; keep bedroom floor uncarpeted.
   d. Damp dust every day; put away articles that are difficult to dust; do not shake articles
   e. Use air conditioner, if possible
   f. Change furnace filter every month during use
2. Animal dander
   a. Have no fur-bearing pets, if possible
   b. Keep any family fur-bearing pet in outdoor enclosure
   c. Avoid furniture stuffed with feathers or horsehair
3. Pollens and fungus spores
   a. Clean frequently areas of mold buildup, such as shower stalls, shower curtains, damp basements
   b. Minimize number of indoor plants
   c. Use air conditioner, if possible; keep windows closed at night
   d. Keep car windows closed when driving; if using car air conditioner, start car, open windows, and allow air conditioner to run 10 minutes before entering car (spores build up on air conditioner)
   e. Limit being outdoors between sunset and sunrise, especially when windy (highest spore and pollen counts occur between midnight and 8 AM)
   f. Do not hang wash outside to dry (pollen and molds stick to wet wash)
   g. Avoid gardening, raking leaves, mowing lawn, or being near freshly cut grass
   h. If possible, plan vacations in areas that are free of the specific allergen

Facilitating learning

The major nursing responsibility when caring for the person with an atopic allergy is teaching the patient about the nature of the disorder and the methods that can be used to avoid the allergen. The major points for teaching are summarized in Box 41-5.

Evaluation

Evaluation is based on expected patient outcomes. Questions to consider may include the following:
1. Does the person know how to avoid the specific allergens?
2. Have plans been made to decrease contact with the allergen?
3. Does the person know when to seek medical help?

TYPE II HYPERSENSITIVITIES (CYTOTOXIC)
Pathophysiology

The underlying mechanisms of type II hypersensitivities involve the direct binding of *IgG* or *IgM* immunoglobulins to an antigen on the *surface of a cell* (see Fig. 16-7). This antibody labeling then triggers the destruction of the cell by phagocytic attack, nonspecific lymphocytic attack, or cell lysis.

41-5

Patient Teaching

The patient with allergies

Inhalant allergy: control environment (see text).
Drug allergy
  Remind physician of allergy when new medication is prescribed
  Read all labels of nonprescription drugs before taking new drug
  Wear a MedicAlert bracelet indicating the known drug allergy
Food allergy
  Examine labels of new prepared foods for presence of allergen
  Avoid eating unknown foods when traveling
Contact allergy
  Use a nonallergenic soap or detergent and cosmetics and take these when traveling
  Use Ivory soap if allergic to most soaps and detergents
  Coat nickel-containing jewelry or clothing fasteners with clear nail polish
  Use gloves if necessary to handle allergen (such as occupational chemicals)
Allergy to insect stings
  Avoid walking barefoot outdoors (yellow jackets nest in the ground)
  Avoid eating outdoors
  Keep a sting emergency medical kit readily available and know how to use it; teach its use also to significant others
All persons with allergies
  Continue medical follow-up if medications are required
  Report side effects of prescribed medications
  Report severe episodes to physician; as instructed

Table 41-8   Types of blood components

Blood component	Description	Usage	Comments
Red blood cells (RBC)			
Packed RBCs (PRBCs)	RBCs separated from plasma and platelets	Anemia Moderate blood loss	Decreased risk of fluid overload as compared to whole blood
Washed RBCs	RBCs washed with sterile isotonic saline before transfusion	Previous allergic reactions to transfusions	Increased removal of immunoglobulins and protein
Frozen RBCs	RBCs frozen in a glycerol solution; cells are washed after thawing to remove the glycerol	Storage of rare type blood Storage of autologous blood for future use	Relatively free of leukocytes and microemboli Expensive
Leukocyte-poor RBCs	RBCs from which most leukocytes have been removed	Previous sensitivity to leukocyte antigens from prior transfusions or from pregnancy	Fewer RBCs than packed RBCs Washed leukocyte-poor RBC units have more RBCs than nonwashed
Neocytes	RBC units with high number of reticulocytes (young RBCs)	Transfusion-dependent anemias	Fewer problems with iron overload Expensive
Other cellular components			
Platelets:			
Random donor packs	Platelets separated from RBCs by centrifuge; given in 50 ml of plasma	Thrombocytopenia DIC	Plasma base is rich in coagulation factors Platelets preparations can also be packed, washed, or made leukocyte-poor
Pheresis packs	Platelets from an HLA-matched donor, separated by pheresis	Allosensitized persons with thrombocytopenia	Requires specialized techniques
Granulocytes	Granular leukocytes separated by pheresis	Granulocytopenia from malignancy or chemotherapy	Allergen sensitization may occur with chills and fever
Plasma components			
Fresh frozen plasma (FFP)	Freezing of plasma within 4 hrs of collection	Clotting deficiencies Liver disease Hemophilia Defibrination	Preserves factors V, VII, VIII, IX, X and prothrombin Minimizes hepatitis risk
Factor concentrates VIII and IX	Prepared from large donor pools Heated to inactivate HIV	VIII: Hemophilia A IX: Hemophilia B	Increased risk of hepatitis (VIII, IX) and thromboembolism (IX) Given in small volumes
Cryoprecipitate	Precipitated material obtained from FFP when thawed	Hemophilia A Infection of burns Hypofibrinogenemia Uremic bleeding	Contains factors VIII, XIII, and fibrinogen

Serum albumin:
   Normal serum albumin (NSA)
   Plasma protein fraction (PPF)
	Albumin chemically processed from pooled plasma	Hypovolemic shock
		Hypoalbuminemia
		Burns
		Hemorrhagic shock
			No risk of hepatitis
			Does not require ABO compatibility
			Lacks clotting factors
			Hypotension may occur if PPF is given faster than 10 ml/min

Immune serum globulin	Obtained from plasma of preselected donors with specific antibodies	Hypogammaglobulinemia Prophylaxis for hepatitis A	Given intramuscularly or intravenously

Blood Transfusion Reactions
Etiology

The type II hypersensitivity is classically illustrated by the reactions that occur in mismatched blood transfusion reactions. Blood replacement therapy is used when there has been excessive blood loss (whole blood or blood components) or in treatment of diseases of the hematopoietic system. Replacement therapy may be whole blood or one or more of the blood components (Table 41-8). Blood transfusions are not without dangers to the recipient; therefore, the transfusion of 1 unit (500 ml) of blood for minor therapy is not recommended.

Pathophysiology

Many antigens are found on the surface of red blood cells, but in terms of potential immunologic reaction the major clinically significant systems are the ABO and Rh systems.

ABO system

The four major human blood groups are listed in Box 41-6. Because type AB contains both antigens, persons with type AB may receive blood from any type (Fig. 41-4). Persons with type O may donate blood to other types, but because both antigens are absent in type O, they may not receive another type without having a reaction.

Within the serum, individuals possess naturally occurring antibodies to the red blood cell (RBC) surface antigens of the ABO blood groups that are not present on their own RBCs. Thus a person with type A blood will possess anti-B antibodies within the serum. These antibodies, called *isohemagglutinins*, are usually of the IgM class. The antibodies are capable of cross-reacting with the A or B antigens on the surface of the "foreign" ABO types. On transfusion, mismatched blood will be immediately coated by the isohemagglutinins, causing agglutination of the introduced cells and the rapid lysis (breakdown) of the cells. The products released by the lysed cells are then dumped into the bloodstream.

Rh system

The Rh system is more complex because at least 27 different antigens are in this system. The most immunogenic is the D antigen. When the term *Rh positive* is used, the presence of antigen Rh-D is implied; *Rh negative* indicates the absence of antigen D. Approximately 85% of the population has Rh-positive blood.

When the person with Rh-negative blood is first exposed to Rh-positive blood, Rh antibodies are formed. On subsequent exposures to Rh-positive blood, the Rh antibody binds to its corresponding antigen on the surface of the RBCs containing the Rh antigen. The Rh-antigen RBCs are then rapidly broken down by macrophages in the spleen with conversion of hemoglobin to bilirubin resulting in jaundice.

HLA system

Human leukocyte antigens (HLA) are found on many types of tissue cells and on blood leukocytes and platelets. The system is more complex than the RBC antigen systems, and literally thousands of combinations of the antigens can occur. Sensitization may occur through preg-

nancy or through exposure to platelets and white blood cells (WBCs) during transfusions. Repeated transfusions of blood cells may lead to transfusion reactions.

Prevention of transfusion reactions

Prescreening of potential blood donors is essential. Blood received from volunteer donors through the American Red Cross Blood Service or hospital blood banks is preferable to that of paid donors, who may be less likely to report past or present diseases that may affect the recipient.

After the blood has been collected, the blood group and subgroups including Rh typing are identified, and the blood is tested for syphilis, hepatitis, HIV antibodies, and cytomegalovirus (CMV). The blood must be cross-matched with blood from the recipient to determine compatibility and prevent an acute hemolytic reaction. Cross-matching consists of mixing samples of the donor's blood and the recipient's blood and examining for cell clumping or hemolysis.

Most of the serious reactions that now occur during transfusions are the result of human error. Safeguards include the following:

1. Blood must be kept cold until ready to use (warm blood is a good medium for bacterial growth).
2. Blood that has remained at room temperature for more than 30 minutes should not be used or returned to refrigeration for reissue.
3. Do not transfuse a unit of blood longer than 4 hours.
4. The unit of blood must be labeled with the patient's name, and the label must be checked against the patient's wristband before the blood is given.
5. All blood products should be administered through filters to prevent embolism from clots; use the correct filter for the type of blood product.
6. If blood must be warmed (rarely needed), use an in-line blood warmer with a monitoring device only (not water bath, incubator, or microwave oven) to prevent

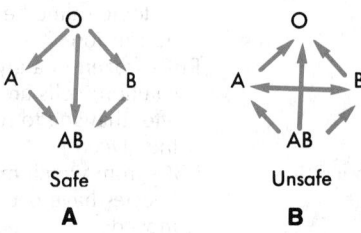

41-6	**Major blood groups**	
A	Antigen A is present
B	Antigen B is present
AB	Both antigens A and B are present
O	Neither antigen A nor B is present

Fig. 41-4 Blood groups and the groups each can receive blood from and give blood to. **A**, Safe. **B**, Unsafe.

Table 41-9   Immunologic reactions to blood transfusions

Reaction	Cause	Mechanism	Symptoms	Occurrence	Action
Acute hemo-lytic	Recipient antibody incompatible with transfused red cells	RBCs agglutinate, rapid hemolysis Capillary plugging (type II hypersensitivity)	Lumbar pain Constriction of chest Pain in vein Fever, chills Hemoglobinuria Signs of shock	Shortly after initiation of transfusion	Stop transfusion Continue IV saline Blood unit and blood sample from patient sent to lab for immediate testing Treat for shock and renal failure
Delayed hemo-lytic	Anamnestic immune response	Slow hemolysis	Jaundice Anemia	Days to weeks after transfusion	Monitor adequacy of urinary output and degree of anemia
Allergic	Transfer of an antigen or a reaginic antibody from donor to recipient	Immune sensitivity to foreign serum protein (type I hypersensitivity)	Urticaria Anaphylaxis (wheezing, dyspnea, shock)	Within 30 minutes after initiation of transfusion	Mild: give antihistamine, continue transfusion Severe: stop transfusion; give aqueous epinephrine (0.4 ml of 1:1000 solution)
Febrile	Reaction of antigen on WBC or platelets Bacterial contamination	Leukocyte agglutination Bacterial pyrogens	Fever, chills, headaches, muscle pains	Within 30-90 min after initiation of transfusion	Stop transfusion Continue IV saline Antipyretics after ruling out hemolytic reaction Transfuse with leukocyte-poor blood or washed RBCs
Graft versus host disease	Immunodeficient person receives lymphocytes	Engraftment of donor lymphocytes, which are then "rejected"	Dermatitis Stomatitis Diarrhea Liver dysfunction	Delayed	Steroids Azathioprine Symptomatic therapy
Noncardiac pulmonary edema	Donor antibodies react with recipient HLA antigen	Infiltration of pulmonary bed by microaggregates, which block blood flow	Fever, chills Urticaria Cough Orthopnea Cyanosis Shock	During transfusion or shortly thereafter	Stop transfusion Continue IV saline Give oxygen as needed Steroids Furosemide

RBC hemolysis from temperatures over 38°C (100.4°F).

7. The patient must be monitored throughout the blood administration.

Complications of blood transfusions
Immunologic transfusion reactions

Immunologic reactions that can occur with blood transfusions include acute hemolytic, delayed hemolytic, allergic, febrile, graft versus host disease, and noncardiac pulmonary edema (Table 41-9). The most serious reaction is the acute hemolytic reaction that occurs during administration of the first 50 ml of blood transfused. Several hours after a hemolytic reaction, the urine becomes red (port-wine urine) and the urinary output is diminished. The urine contains RBCs and albumin. This reaction is thought to be caused by the release of a toxic substance from the hemolyzed blood that causes a temporary vascular spasm in the kidneys, resulting in renal damage, and blockage of the renal tubules by the hemoglobin precipitated out in the acid urine (hemoglobinuria). If the patient receives more than 100 ml of incompatible blood, irreversible shock with complete renal failure may occur, and death may follow.

As blood cells disintegrate (lyse), large amounts of potassium are released into the bloodstream; if renal function is impaired, hyperkalemia will develop. If this occurs, the patient may be treated with renal dialysis. Because fever is a sign of both acute hemolytic reaction and the less serious but more common febrile reaction, the transfusion is stopped until the diagnosis is made.

Nonimmunologic reactions

Complications other than those of immunologic origin include the following:
1. Fluid overload
   a. Occurs mostly in elderly persons and those with congestive heart failure or severe anemia (hemoglobin less than 5 g/dl)

b. Can be prevented by use of packed cells and slower infusion rate for persons at risk

c. If it occurs, slow down or stop infusion (depending on severity of symptoms), administer O_2, place patient in high Fowlers position

2. Air embolism (rare now with use of IV bags rather than bottles)

a. Results when blood is administered under air pressure following severe blood loss

b. If occurs, place patient in left side-lying Trendelenburg position (diverts air away from pulmonary artery)

3. Complications of massive blood replacement (exchange of one blood volume in 24 hours)

a. Thrombocytopenia with abnormal bleeding (from platelet deterioration)

b. Cardiac dysrhythmias (from cold blood)

c. Electrolyte level imbalances

(1) *Hyperkalemia* (potassium released as RBC break down)

(2) *Hypocalcemia* (binding of sodium citrate from donor blood with recipient's serum calcium ions)

4. Transmission of disease

a. Hepatitis: occurs in 5% to 10% of blood transfusions; blood is screened for hepatitis B and non A, non B; hepatitis A is rarely transmitted by transfusion

b. HIV: a rare complication; donated blood is tested but test is not 100% accurate; the number of new infections among blood product recipients has decreased; HIV is inactivated in blood products by heat treatment

c. Syphilis and malaria: incidence is rare

d. Cytomegalovirus: symptoms occur in about 40 days (fever, malaise, splenomegaly); the condition is benign and treatment is symptomatic

5. Transfusion hemosiderosis

a. Defined as an iron overload from chronic transfusions for hematopoietic disorders

b. If it occurs, RBCs or neocytes are given for future transfusions to decrease number of transfusions required

Autologous blood transfusions

One method of preventing immunologic blood transfusion reactions and disease transmission is by using the person's own blood for replacement. There are two approaches for using autologous blood: planned collection and autotransfusion. In *planned autologous transfusion*, blood is collected at regular intervals before the time when usage is anticipated, such as before surgery. The patient's hemoglobin level should be above 11 g/dl (hematocrit above 33%). The blood is then stored until needed. This method is especially useful for persons with a rare blood type, for those whose religious beliefs preclude receiving donor blood, and for those undergoing planned surgeries for which blood transfusions are expected.

A different form of planned autologous transfusion is *acute normovolemic hemodilution* in which one or two units of blood are collected from the patient immediately before

surgery.[37] A concurrent intravenous administration of crystalloid or colloid solution maintains normovolemia. The blood lost during surgery is diluted blood; the full-strength blood is then transfused after surgery.

Autotransfusion consists of collecting, filtering, and immediately reinfusing the person's own blood lost during surgery or in the emergency room following massive trauma. The blood is suctioned into a bag and passed through a filter to remove aggregates of fibrin, RBCs, platelets, and other microaggregates. Anticoagulant is added through a volume control system. When the bag is full, it is disconnected from the system, and the blood is transfused into the patient with an administration set and a standard or a microembolic filter. Blood that has been contaminated by gastrointestinal contents or that is close to a malignant tumor is not autotransfused.

Autotransfusion is safe and cost effective, uses warm blood, and contains more RBCs than stored blood, but platelet, fibrinogen, and clotting factors are decreased. The potential exists for nephrotoxic effect from RBC damage with release of hemoglobin.

TYPE III HYPERSENSITIVITIES (IMMUNE COMPLEX)

Pathophysiology

The type III hypersensitivities result from the union of *soluble* antigens with immunoglobulins of the IgM and IgG classes. The complexes that are formed are too small for phagocytosis, so rather than being removed by the reticuloendothelial system (RES), they are deposited in body tissues. This causes an inflammatory response, usually intravascular. Immune complexes are a common factor of connective tissue (collagen) disorders, especially lupus erythematosus and rheumatoid arthritis (Chapter 40). Complexes may also be trapped in glomeruli, which results in glomerulonephritis (Chapter 33).

Serum Sickness

A type III hypersensitivity of clinical significance is serum sickness, which can develop from 1 to 3 weeks after the administration of a large amount of "foreign" serum (for example, horse serum used with some prophylactic serums). It may also occur with the administration of certain drugs, particularly antimicrobials such as penicillin.

Itching and discomfort at the injection site are usually the first symptoms noted. These are followed by lymphadenopathy, fever, urticaria or erythematous rash, facial edema, and joint pain. Objective signs of arthritis may be present.

Serum sickness is a self-limiting disease. Mild symptoms respond well to antihistamines, salicylates, and topical steroids. More severe symptoms may be treated with a steroid such as prednisone, although this is rarely necessary. Epinephrine is given if an anaphylactic reaction occurs.

TYPE IV HYPERSENSITIVITIES

Pathophysiology

Type IV hypersensitivities are cell mediated (delayed type) involving T cells. Antigens identified as foreign to the body can cause a reaction in two ways, by direct or by indirect action. The T lymphocyte can destroy the antigen directly by attaching itself to the antigen cell wall, breaking down the cell membrane, and causing lysis and death of the cell. This direct action approach appears to be a major factor in transplant rejections. The indirect approach consists of activating nonspecific phagocytic cells (macrophages and polymorphonuclear leukocytes) through release of lymphokines by the sensitized T lymphocytes. Cell mediated reactions occur hours to days after exposure to the antigen.

Clinical examples of type IV hypersensitivities are microbial hypersensitivity reaction, allergic contact dermatitis (Chapter 43), and tissue transplant rejection (Chapter 42).

Microbial Hypersensitivity Reaction

An example of microbial hypersensitivity is the body's reaction to the tubercle bacillus. The body does not react initially when the bacillus invades a nonsensitized host. However, as the cell-mediated response is activated, tissue destruction (cavitation) and general toxemia result (Chapter 24). After the initial sensitization, subsequent contact with the tubercle bacillus will elicit a hypersensitivity reaction. This is the basis of the tuberculin skin test.

Tissue Transplant Rejection

The rejection of foreign cells and tissues by the body is a beneficial function of the immune system primarily mediated by a type IV hypersensitivity. If it were not for this mechanism, the human body would be a haven for the inappropriate establishment of growth of any animal cell that penetrated the external defense mechanisms; however, this process is regarded as a disservice when it operates to prevent the positive aspects of the exchange of tissues between hosts (transplants). The antigenic determinants of the tissues that lead to transplant rejection are primarily found on the surface of cells within the transplanted tissues. These antigens are known as *human leukocyte antigens* (HLA) (p. 1440) or histocompatibility antigens.

Transplant tissue destruction can be prevented by immunosuppressive therapy. Tissue transplantation and the care of patients with organ transplants are discussed in Chapter 42.

AUTOIMMUNE DISEASES

Individuals sometimes respond to some of their own (self) antigens, triggering an immune response. The symptoms of such an attack are referred to as autoimmune disease or *autohypersensitivity*. Autoimmune diseases cannot be explained by a single cause. Multiple mechanisms of autoimmunity usually occur and the underlying causes are unknown.[51]

Self-reactive immunoglobulins are often associated with certain pathologic states in the body but many times can also be isolated from the serum of "normal" persons as well, especially in older persons. The chance that the immune control mechanisms will be lost increases with age. For the most part, these self-reactions are not immuno-

41-7

Some diseases with autoimmune aspects

Type II cytotoxic humoral response
Autoimmune hemolytic anemia
Pernicious anemia
Idiopathic (immune) thrombocytopenia
Grave's disease (toxic goiter)
Pemphigus vulgaris
Myasthenia gravis
Goodpasture's syndrome (glomerulonephritis)

Type III immune complex humoral response
Rheumatoid arthritis
Systemic lupus erythematosus
Sjögren's syndrome
Poststreptococcal glomerulonephritis
Scleroderma
Ulcerative colitis

Type IV cell-mediated response
Systemic lupus erythematosus
Multiple sclerosis
Guillain-Barré syndrome

logically initiated; the causative agent lies outside the immune system, but the immune response serves as the pathogenic mechanism.

In general, the immunologic *responses* in autoimmune diseases fall into three categories that correlate with three of the four hypersensitivity reactions (see Table 41-5). The three responses include the following:

1. *Type II cytotoxic humoral response* in which IgG and IgM antibodies bind to cell membranes, fix complement, and destroy the cells by lysis.
2. *Type III immune complex humoral response* in which IgG and IgM antibodies react with *serum* antigens, producing antigen-antibody complexes that are deposited in body tissues and cause an inflammatory reaction.
3. *Type IV cell-mediated response* in which cytotoxic (killer) T cells attach to cell walls, break cell membranes, and destroy the cells.

Examples of autoimmune diseases characteristic of each of the above three categories are listed in Box 41-7. Care of persons experiencing these diseases is described elsewhere in the text.

SUMMARY

1. Although immunologic changes with aging vary greatly among individuals, the immune response is decreased as evidenced by decreased T-cell function. Older persons experience more severe infections (especially influenza and pneumococcal pneumonia), and have an increased potential for cancer.
2. Major health problems of the immune system may be categorized as immunodeficiencies, gammopathies, hypersensitivities, and autoimmunities.
3. Immunodeficiencies may result from deficiencies in B

cells or T cells or from both cells combined. Most primary immunodeficiencies are genetic; the major secondary immunodeficiencies encountered in general practice are immunosuppression and acquired immunodeficiency syndrome (AIDS).

4. Immunosuppression may be induced by administration of antigen, specific antibodies, or monoclonal antibodies, by radiation, or by drugs (corticosteroids, cytotoxic drugs, and cyclosporine).

5. The major interventions for immunodeficiencies are replacement therapy with gamma globulin and transfer factor, and prevention of infection.

6. Gammopathies are excessive production of immunoglobulins; the most common gammopathy is multiple myeloma (an excess of plasma cells).

7. Hypersensitivity reactions are exaggerated or inappropriate responses to specific antigens (allergens).

8. Type I hypersensitivities are associated with reactions mediated by IgE immunoglobulins that are attached to mast cells; when the allergen binds to the IgE, histamine is released, producing a systemic (anaphylactic shock) or a local allergic reaction.

9. Therapy for anaphylaxis consists of epinephrine to constrict blood vessels and dilate bronchioles, counteracting the effect of histamine. Antihistamines are given to shorten the duration of anaphylaxis; corticosteroids decrease the inflammatory effects. An open airway must be maintained.

10. The most common allergens in adults are seasonal inhalants (pollens, spores, grasses), and environmental inhalants (house dust, animal dander). Patients are taught measures to avoid and control exposure to the specific antigens.

11. Type II hypersensitivities are cytotoxic reactions from the direct binding of IgG or IgM immunoglobulins to the surface of foreign cells to trigger cell destruction; an example is blood transfusion reactions.

12. The major antigens on RBCs are the AB antigens, Rh antigens, and HLA antigens. AB blood group indicates presence of both A and B antigens; O blood group indicates absence of either antigen. Absence of an antigen produces antibodies (isohemagglutins) that will cause agglutination of donor RBCs containing the missing antigen. Therefore, people with type O blood may donate blood to other types but may not receive another type without having a hemolytic reaction.

13. Rh-positive reactions indicate presence of antigen Rh-D; Rh-negative reactions indicate absence of antigen Rh-D.

14. Immunologic reactions to blood transfusions include hemolytic (most serious), allergic, febrile, graft-versus-host disease, and noncardiac pulmonary edema. Diseases that may be transmitted by blood transfusions include hepatitis, AIDS, syphilis, malaria, and cytomegalovirus.

15. Autologous blood transfusions consist of using the person's own blood for replacement, either by stored blood previously collected or by autotransfusion of blood from excessive bleeding.

16. Type III hypersensitivities are characterized by immune complexes formed by the union of IgM or IgG immunoglobulins with soluble antigens; the small complexes get trapped in body tissues causing an inflammatory response. An example is serum sickness that occurs after administration of a large amount of foreign serum.

17. Type IV hypersensitivities are cell-mediated (T cell) reactions, differing from the other three types, which are humoral (B cell) reactions. T cells destroy foreign antigens directly (as in transplant rejections) or they may release lymphokines to activate macrophages.

18. Autoimmune diseases are the result of an immune response to self-antigens, usually as a result of an agent outside the immune system. Immunologic responses seen in autoimmune diseases may be type I, type II, or type III hypersensitivity responses.

STUDY QUESTIONS

- How would you explain to a lay person the difference among immunodeficiencies, gammopathies, hypersensitivities, and autoimmune disease?
- Look at Fig. 41-1. Explain in your own words the immunodeficiencies that would develop at each of the five marked positions.
- A friend who gets allergic rhinitis (hayfever) is coming to visit you this summer. What advance preparations can you make to help decrease the symptoms?
- Examine the chart of a patient who has received a blood transfusion. What safeguards were taken to prevent transfusion reaction? Should additional safeguards have been taken? If a reaction occurred, what actions were taken?

REFERENCES AND SELECTED READINGS

1. Anderson JA, Adkinson NF Jr: Allergic reaction to drugs and biologic agents, *JAMA* 258:2891-2899, 1987.
2. * Baron M, Tafuro PL: The extremes of age: the newborn and the elderly at increased risk for the development of infection, *Nurs Clin North Am* 20(1):181-190, 1985.
3. Barrett JT: *Textbook of immunology*, ed 5, St Louis, 1988 Mosby–Year Book.
4. * Benson ML, Benson DM: Autotransfusion is here, are you ready? *Nursing 85* 15(3):46-60, 1985.
5. * Birdsell C, Carpenter K, Considine R: How is autotransfusion done? *Am J Nurs* 88:108-111, 1988.
6. Blansfield J: Emergency autotransfusion in hypovolemia, *Crit Care Nurs Clin North Am* 2:195-199, 1990.
7. * Bonato J: Blood transfusions: are they safe? *Crit Care Nurs* 9(7):40-45, 1989.
8. Buckley RH: Immunodeficiency diseases, *JAMA* 258:2841-2850, 1987.
9. * Butler S: Current trends in autologous transfusion, *RN* 52(11):44-50, 1989.
10. Committee on Transfusion Practices, American Association of Blood Banks: The latest protocols for blood transfusions, *Nursing 86* 16(10):34-41, 1986.
11. Condemi JJ: The autoimmune diseases, *JAMA* 258:2920-2929, 1987.
12. Costa AJ: Anaphylactic shock: guidelines for immediate diagnosis and treatment, *Postgrad Med* 83:368-373, 1988.

*Recommended for student reading.

13. Creticos PA, Norman PA: Immunotherapy and allergy, *JAMA* 258:2874-2880, 1987.

14. Croman LC: The relationship between nutrition, infection, and immunity, *Med Clin North Am* 69(3):519-531, 1985.

15.* Dickerson M: Anaphylaxis and anaphylactic shock, *Crit Care Nurs Q* 11:68-74, 1988.

16. DiJulio JE: Treatment of B-cell and T-cell lymphomas with monoclonal antibodies, *Semin Oncol Nurs* 4(2):102-106, 1988.

16a.* Drago SS: Banking your own blood, *Am J Nurs* 92(3):61-64, 1992.

17.* Espersen S: Nursing support of host defenses, *Crit Care Nurs Q* 9(1):51-56, 1986.

18.* Freedman S et al: Nursing considerations in the administration of blood component therapy, *Semin Oncol Nurs* 6(2):155-162, 1990.

19.* Gaunder BN: Insect bites and stings: managing allergic reactions, *Nurs Pract* 11(3):16-20, 1986.

20.* Girard NJ, Morgan RG, Orr MD: Autologous salvage of blood: perioperative nursing considerations, *AORN J* 47:492-503, 1988.

21. Graziano FM, Lemanske R Jr: *Clinical immunology*, Baltimore, 1989, Williams & Wilkins.

22.* Griffin JP: Nursing care of the critically ill immunocompromised patient, *Crit Care Nurs Q* 9(1):25-34, 1986.

23.* Gurevich I, Tafuro P: Nursing measures for the prevention of infection in the compromised host, *Nurs Clin North Am* 20(1):257-266, 1985.

24. Gurka AM: The immune system: implications for critical care, *Crit Care Nurse* 9(7):24-35, 1989.

25. Hadden JW: Immunopharmacology: immunomodulation and immunotherapy, *JAMA* 258:3005-3010, 1987.

26.* Hahn K: Monitoring a blood transfusion, *Nursing 89* 19(10):20-21, 1989.

27. Heinzel FP: Infections in patients with humoral immunodeficiency, *Hosp Pract* 24(9):99-130, 1989.

28.* Hotter AN: Wound healing and immunocompromise, *Nurs Clin North Am* 25(1):193-203, 1990.

29. Kaplan AP, Buckley RH, Mathews KP: Allergic skin disorders, *JAMA* 258:2900-2909, 1987.

30. Kaliner M, Eggleston PA, Mathews KP: Rhinitis and asthma, *JAMA* 258:2851-2873, 1987.

31. Kotwas L et al: Blood collection techniques, *Semin Oncol Nurs* 6(2):109-116, 1990.

32.* Martin E et al: Autotransfusion systems, *Crit Care Nurse* 9(7):65-73, 1989.

33.* Mennies JH et al: An overview of adult allergic disorders, *Nurs Pract* 10(6):16-23, 1985.

34. Miller DS: Intravenous immune globulin for treating primary immunodeficiency disease, *MCN* 12:244-248, 1987.

35. Minnefor AB et al: IV immune globulin efficacy and safety, *Hosp Pract* 22(10):171-183, 1987.

36. National Blood Resource Education Program's Nursing Education Working Group: Choosing blood components and equipment, *Am J Nurs* 91(6):42-46, 1991.

37. National Blood Resource Education Program's Nursing Education Working Group: Autologous transfusion, *Am J Nurs* 91(6):47-48, 1991.

38. National Blood Resource Education Program's Nursing Education Working Group: Preventing and managing transfusion reactions, *Am J Nurs* 91(6):48-50, 1991.

39. Norman PS: Immunotherapy of IgE-mediated disease, *Hosp Pract* 25(4):81-86, 1990.

40. Osserman EF, Merlin G, Butler VP: Multiple myeloma and related plasma cell dyscrasias, *JAMA* 258:2930-2937, 1987.

41.* Parsons L, Klopovich PM: Immune globulin therapy, *Semin Oncol Nurs* 6(2):136-139, 1990.

42.* Petrucci KE, Booth-Blaemire E, Watson K: Aging, immunity, and critical care nursing, *Crit Care Nurs Clin North Am* 1(4):787-795, 1989.

43.* Phillips A: Are blood transfusions really safe? *Nursing 87* 17(6):63-65, 1987.

44. Platts-Mills TAE et al: Dust mite allergy: its clinical significance, *Hosp Pract* 22(9):91-100, 1987.

45.* Pluth MN: A home care transfusion program, *Oncol Nurs Forum* 14(5):42-46, 1987.

46.* Querin JJ, Stahl LD: 12 simple sensible steps for successful blood transfusions, *Nursing 90* 20(10):68-81, 1990.

47.* Randall BJ: Reacting to anaphylaxis, *Nursing 86* 16(3):34-39, 1986.

48. Rayfield S et al: Maximizing safe blood transfusions, *Adv Clin Care* 5(5):17-19, 1990.

49.* Recking JB et al: Understanding immune system dysfunction, *Nursing 87* 17(9):34-42, 1987.

50.* Rieger PT: Monoclonal antibodies, *Am J Nurs* 87:469-473, 1987.

51. Schroeder SA et al: *Current medical diagnosis and treatment*, Norwalk, Conn, 1991, Appleton & Lange.

52.* Smith SL: Immunosuppressive drugs used in clinical practice, *Crit Care Nurs Q* 9(1):19-24, 1986.

53. Stites DP, Terr AT: *Basic and clinical immunology*, ed 7, Norwalk, Conn, 1990, Appleton & Lange.

54. Valentine MD et al: Anaphylaxis and stinging insect hypersensitivity, *JAMA* 258:2881-2885, 1987.

55. Widman FK: *An introduction to clinical immunology*, Philadelphia, 1989, FA Davis.

56. Wyngaarden JB, Smith LH: *Cecil textbook of medicine*, ed 18, Philadelphia, 1988, WB Saunders.

42

The Patient with an Organ/Tissue Transplant

Virginia L. Cassmeyer

After studying this chapter, the learner should be able to:

- Describe the criteria used to select candidates for various transplants.
- Describe donor criteria for selected organs or tissues.
- Discuss legislative activity that has been initiated to increase the supply of organs/tissues and to enhance fairness in the distribution of organs/tissues.
- Describe the three types of rejections of allogenic transplants, and the immunology underlying rejection. Discuss the type of histocompatibility testing and matching conducted for various transplants.
- Explain the action and major adverse effects of the five most common drugs used to prevent and treat acute rejection.
- List the major infections for which the immunosuppressed transplant recipient is at high risk.
- Describe the general nursing care diagnoses and care needs of the potential transplant recipient, the patient pretransplant, and the patient posttransplant.
- Design care plans that list the common needs and interventions for persons who have had corneal, renal, liver, pancreatic, heart, lung, or bone marrow transplants.

Organ transplantation has moved from being a medical experiment to being a major therapeutic intervention in selected patients. Persons with certain types of end-stage diseases can now be offered survival and improved quality of life. For many persons the term *transplantation* means whole organ transplants. However, many types of tissues are transplanted. Some common tissue transplants include:

1. Whole blood or components
2. Cornea
3. Tendon, ligament, fascia, dura mater
4. Bone
5. Heart valve
6. Skin
7. Bone marrow

Organs that are commonly transplanted include:

1. Kidneys
2. Livers
3. Hearts
4. Lungs
5. Heart-lungs
6. Pancreases or islet cells of the pancreas

Although various types of transplants can be performed, including autografts, allografts, and xenografts (Box 42-1), this chapter focuses on solid organ and cornea allograft and bone marrow autografts and allografts.

TRANSPLANTATION CRITERIA

Criteria for Recipients

Transplantation of hearts, lungs, kidneys, and pancreases and/or islet cells is considered for patients who have end-stage failure and who do not respond to conventional therapy or whose condition is worsening in spite of careful management. The patient must be free of irreversible infections, unresectable malignancies, or concurrent illnesses that make the risk of surgery unacceptably high. Additionally, there should be no anatomic problems that would make transplantation impossible. Lastly, the therapeutic benefits of the transplantation to the recipient and his or her ability to pay for the transplantation are important criteria in selecting recipients.

Allogenic bone marrow transplantation is used not only when failure of the bone marrow occurs such as in severe aplastic anemia or severe combined immunodeficiency disease, but also in some cases of leukemia and lymphoma to replace the bone marrow after high doses of chemotherapy or irradiation. Autologous bone marrow transplantation also is used after high doses of chemotherapy or irradiation. Both types of bone marrow transplantation are described in this chapter.

Potential factors considered in assessing recipients for transplantations

Because the supply of organs and bone marrow is limited, individual transplant centers may consider various factors besides the disease status and therapeutic benefits in deciding on the best candidates for transplantation. Some of these additional factors include age, functional ability, psychologic status, family support, perceived ability to manage posttransplantation regimen, rehabilitation potential, ability to return to work, and improved quality or length of life. The age range for recipients has been broadened considerably. In a few situations or centers the patient's responsibility for his or her disease involvement such as abuse of alcohol leading to liver failure is considered.[8,19] In the past some centers considered the patient's contributions or benefits to society, but that is not considered at this time. No one center considers all these factors. In some centers the only criteria are disease status, improved quality of life, desire and ability to handle posttransplantation regimen, and available financial reimbursement for the transplantation.

Payment for transplantation

A major issue in relation to transplantation is reimbursement for the procedure. At this writing, before a transplantation is undertaken, the financial reimbursement for that transplant must be clearly identified. Medicare covers the cost of kidney transplantation for anyone who meets social security disability and Medicare requirements. A limited number of transplants are covered by state programs and the Veterans' Administration. Many third-party payers cover the cost of selected extrarenal transplants such as heart, liver, and heart-lung, but consider pancreatic and lung transplants experimental and will not reimburse for these. Third-party payors also cover the non-Medicare covered aspects of renal transplantation or the total coverage, if the person is not eligible for social security disability and Medicare. However, many persons are uninsured, and therefore are not eligible for any type of transplant. The issue of whether organ/tissue transplantations of all types should be available to everyone needing them without regard to ability to pay for them is continually being discussed at public forums as this and other health care concerns are discussed.

Allocation of transplant tissue/organs

Because of the shortage of organs for transplantation, various legislative acts have been passed to (1) increase the supply of organs and (2) to ensure the fair allocation of donated tissues/organs. The present criteria for allocating

> ### Transplant definitions
>
> **Autografts**
> Transplantation of tissue from one part of the body to another; examples include skin, bone, veins, fascia, blood, bone marrow, and adrenal medulla
>
> **Allografts**
> Transplantation of tissue or organs from one member of a species to another member of the same species; examples include all types of tissues and organs
>
> **Xenografts**
> Transplantation of tissue from a member of one species to a member of another species; examples include heart valves and skin

---

42-2

Pointers that may help the nurse in talking with families about donating organs/tissues

Make sure that brain death or death has been discussed with the family

Obtain permission from the primary or attending physician

Contact the local OPO to gain assistance

Try to determine the beliefs of the potential donor, that is, had a donor card been signed

Identify which of the family members to involve; in some instances this may only be the legal next-of-kin, and in other instances this may include a large extended family, stepparents, fiancees, and so on

Approach the family after they have had some time to grieve

Provide a comfortable, private place for discussion with the health team members and family discussion

Ascertain what the family understands about brain death and the hope of recovery

Speak slowly, be sensitive, refer to the potential donor by name, and do not be afraid to refer to the potential donor as dead

Provide adequate, accurate information on the options available to them related to discontinuing life-support on the brain-dead person

Provide adequate, accurate information on tissue and organ donation including the fact that informed consent is necessary, the other evaluation required, and the fact that there is no cost to the family

Assure that the family understands that organ/tissue donation will not interfere with the timing of the funeral service or having an open casket service

Provide time for the family to discuss the request and make the decision

Present consents only after the family has had time to make the decision and has given an affirmative response

---

42-3

Management of the brain-dead patient

Continuous ventilator support and care

Continuous hemodynamic monitoring (arterial [pulmonary and systemic] blood lines, venous pressure lines, cardiac monitoring) with documentation or measurements at least hourly

Measurement of blood pressure, pulse, respiration, intake, output, temperature at least every hour

Measurement of blood gases every 6 hours or as ordered

Assessment of cardiac rate, rhythm, and heart sounds; breath sounds; and skin integrity every 2 to 4 hours

Collection of specimens for serum and urine electrolytes and osmolality, BUN, and blood, urine, and sputum cultures

Maintenance of systolic blood pressure at 100 mm Hg or greater with position, fluids, and vasopressors as ordered

Maintenance of optimal respiratory status and pO_2 at > or equal to 100 mm Hg by suctioning the airway and turning the patient as needed and manipulating the ventilator as ordered

Maintenance of urinary output at 100 ml/hr by replacing fluids as ordered, and assessing for presence of diabetes insipidus (Chapter 29) and assisting with treatment as necessary; monitoring for and treating increased serum glucose; and giving fluid challenges for oliguria if necessary

Maintenance of electrolyte balance by monitoring electrolytes and renal status and administering fluid and electrolyte replacement as ordered

Prevention of infection by use of sterile technique when handling invasive lines and dressings by providing appropriate skin and respiratory care and by continuing or instituting antibiotic therapy as ordered

Maintenance of normal body temperature with warming or cooling blankets. Aspirin is preferred for hyperthermia because of the hepatic toxic effects of tylenol; wrapping the head of the patient can be very helpful if hypothermia is the problem

---

extrarenal transplants are (1) blood type, (2) size, (3) medical urgency, (4) geographic location, and (5) waiting time.[9] The criteria for allocation of kidneys is under debate.[9] Currently, legislation requires that all families or guardians of potential donors be asked to consider donating organs/tissues.

Organ procurement organizations (OPOs) are responsible for organ recovery in the United States. These organizations have offices in major cities and provide services on a local, state, and regional basis. OPOs provide 24-hour assistance to evaluate potential donors and coordinate organ recovery. The organ transplant coordinators of the OPO assist in the recovery of organs and communicate back to donor families and hospitals about the outcomes of transplantations. Guidelines for the sharing of organs and standards for the recovery and transplantation of organs have been developed by the United Network for Organ Sharing (UNOS). UNOS operates under the U.S. Department of Health and Human Services. OPOs are members of UNOS. UNOS has a national waiting list of potential recipients and a system for computer matching potential recipients with donor organs. UNOS, through the OPO, helps to distribute organs. The Organ Procurement Transplant Network (OPTN) is operated by the UNOS and is the central repository for information about all organs procured and distributed. Although the distribution of organs has been centralized, the criteria for allocation are still controversial and subjective in some cases. Overall the guidelines allow an organ to go to a recipient within an OPO's service area before going to someone with higher medical needs outside of the OPO's service area. The philosophy behind this guideline is that keeping organs for recipients within a defined community acts as an incentive for others to donate organs and tissues.

42-4

Additional tests that may be performed to evaluate the status of an organ in a potential donor

Heart
ECG
Echocardiogram
Cardiac consultation
Cardiac enzymes and isoenzymes including CK with MB fraction
Cardiac catheterization may be conducted if there is a questionable history of cardiac disease

Lung
Chest x-ray with measurements
Arterial blood gas analysis at baseline and after intervention with an FiO_2 of 100% and positive-end-expiratory-pressure (PEEP) of 5 mm Hg
Gram stain and culture of sputum

Hepatic
Serum laboratory analysis of liver function including enzymes (transaminases [AST, ALT], alkaline phosphatase, GGTP, LDH); bilirubin (total and direct); hemoglobin, hematocrit, partial thromboplastin time, prothrombin time, total protein, and albumin

Kidney
Serum and urine tests including serum electrolytes, BUN, and creatinine and urine culture and urinalysis

Pancreas
Serum and urine tests including serum electrolytes, BUN, creatinine, amylase, and glucose and urine culture and urinalysis

42-5

Age criteria for specific donors

Organ/tissue	Age
Kidneys	6 months-65 yrs
Liver	Term newborn-55 yrs
Pancreas	1 yr-60 yrs
Heart	Term newborn-55 yrs
Lung	12 yrs-55 yrs
Heart-lung	Term newborn-65 yrs
Bone, fascia, connective tissue, bone marrow	15 yrs-65 yrs
Heart valves	Term newborn-55 yrs
Eyes	No age limit
Saphenous veins	5 yrs-65 yrs
Skin	Maximum age 70; minimum age limited because person needs to be 5 feet tall and weigh at least 100 pounds

Registered nurses can be involved in various ways with the allocation of transplant tissue and organs. They may function as organ transplant coordinators, may be involved politically on the national and state levels, may serve on advisory boards of local organ banks or OPOs, or may serve on various committees that establish policies and guidelines related to organ and tissue retrieval and transplantation within acute-care institutions.

Donor Criteria

The majority of organs used for transplantation are cadaver organs; for these, nurses will be involved in organ donation and recovery. Nurses, particularly those in critical care, assist in identifying potential donors, approach families about donating (see Box 42-2), provide support to families as they make their decisions, care for brain-dead patients (see Box 42-3), assist with laboratory studies and procedures to establish the functioning of specific organs, and assist with testing for brain death.

The typical donor of organs dies from brain death; has no preexisting disease of the organ(s) being recovered; has no transmittable diseases, sepsis, or extracranial malignancy; and has no history of death of unknown etiology.[12]

The potential donor must be hemodynamically salvageable and have relatively normal organ function.[12] Box 42-4 presents a summary of tests that may be used to assess the health status of organs for transplantation. Additionally, the criteria for donors of lungs and heart-lungs include no history of smoking and no chest tubes.[12] Potential donors of *tissues*, *as opposed to organs*, can have died from cardiac death.[12] However, there are other specific criteria for donors of tissues such as no tissue irradiation and no use of chronic steroid therapy.[12] For potential donors of eyes the criteria specifically identifies the transmittable diseases that must not be present including active hepatitis, AIDS, rabies, viral encephalitis, or Creutzfelt-Jakob disease.[12] The age limits or requirements of potential donors varies for different organs/tissues and centers. Because of the age variation, the Midwest Organ Bank[16a] recommends consulting organ procurement centers for any potential donors between the ages of birth to 70. (Box 42-5).

To decrease the risk of transmitting HIV through transplantation, criteria for exclusion of high-risk donors have been established.[1,12] Those excluded include:

1. Persons with clinical or laboratory evidence of HIV infection.
2. Men who have had sex with other men one or more times since 1977.
3. Persons with past or present history of intravenous drug abuse.
4. Persons immigrating since 1977 from countries such as Haiti and Central Africa where HIV is thought to be transmitted mostly by heterosexual activity.
5. Persons with histories of receiving clotting factor concentrates for hemophilia.
6. Sexual partners of any of the persons in groups 1-5.
7. Persons who have engaged in prostitution since 1977 and any of their heterosexual partners from the last 6 months.

IMMUNOLOGY AND TRANSPLANTATION

Successful transplantation of allografts requires manipulation of the recipient's immune system. All cells and tissues in the body have markers or antigens on the cell membrane surface. These antigens allow one cell to be recognized by other cells as either "self" or "nonself". The antigens distributed on the surface of the cells of any one person are unique for that person, except for identical twins, and are controlled by the genes of that person. These cell markers are important in protection of the body from invasion by foreign substances. Because foreign substances have different markers, they can be recognized as foreign (nonself) by the immune system.

The B and T lymphocytes of the immune system are the surveillance cells that can recognize the cell membrane markers as foreign (nonself) or nonforeign (self). When the markers on cell membranes are recognized as foreign (nonself), the B and T lymphocytes are activated, which means that these cells differentiate, proliferate, and clone to be able to attack and control or destroy the foreign substance.

The ability of immune cells to recognize foreign substances is due to the genetic factor that is called the *major histocompatibility complex (MHC)*. The MHC, which regulates the immune responsiveness of tumors, is the *human leukocyte antigen (HLA)* genetic complex located on chromosome 6. The HLA genetic complex encodes cell membrane markers or antigens on almost all cells in the body. The HLA antigenic complex is classified into two groups. *Class I HLA* antigens are encoded by three loci on chromosome 6, loci A, B, and C. *Class II HLA* antigens are encoded at two loci referred to as D and DR. HLA class I antigens are expressed by almost all cells including leukocytes, platelets, and cells of most solid organs. HLA class II antigens are expressed on fewer cells; however, these antigens are found on many of the immune system cells including B and some T lymphocytes, macrophages, and monocytes. Each of the five loci on chromosome 6 can encode for one of many different specific antigenic factors or *alleles*. Over 100 alleles are known or suspected to exist. These individual alleles are identified by a number following the specific loci. For example, HLA-A1 refers to the specific allele numbered 1 of the A loci. If there is uncertainty about whether a specific allele for a loci is unique, it will be distinguished by a lower case "w" placed before the number. For example HLA-Bw4 refers to an allele for the B loci for which some uncertainty exists.

Each person has two number 6 chromosomes and each chromosome will encode for five specific HLA antigens, one for each specific loci. Each person inherits one number six chromosome and thus, one set of five HLA antigens or one *haplotype* from each parent. Therefore, using Mendelian inheritance principles, two siblings have a 25% *possibility* of sharing both haplotypes, a 25% *possibility* of sharing neither haplotype, and a 50% *possibility* of sharing one haplotype (Box 42-6).

A second antigen system important to the acceptance of transplant tissue is the ABO blood typing system. The ABO antigens are on red blood cells and other tissues. Some minor red cell antigens, particularly the Lewis system, are

---

42-6

Inheritance of haplotypes

Father haplotypes		Mother haplotypes	
(F1)	(F2)	(M1)	(M2)
A9	A23	A10	A30
B5	B27	B35	B8
Cw7	Cw1	Cw5	Cw2
Dw1	Dw2	Dw7	Dw8
DR5	DR7	DR5	DR3

		Mother	
		M1	M2
Father	F1	M1F1	M2F1
	F2	M1F2	M2F2

---

important to transplantation rejection or acceptance and are assessed in recipients and donors.[5] The RH antigen system does not seem to have a role in survival or rejection of transplant tissue or organs.

Tissue Typing and Matching Procedures

In preparation for all transplants, some of the tests for tissue typing and matching, typing and matching of red blood cells, and leukocyte cross-matching will be carried out. See Table 42-1 for a description of major tests that may be used in establishing compatibility between the donor organ/tissue and the recipient.

The number of tests and the exact tests used vary for different types of transplants. There are several reasons for this variability. First, although all the antigens discussed have some role in allowing "self" cells to be differentiated from "nonself" cells, and all antigens are on at least some of the immune system cells, the individual loci of the HLA system and the red blood cell antigens may not be equally important in the activation of the immune system to attack the foreign "nonself" transplant tissue. Second, the immunogenicity of transplant tissue varies from most allogenic to least allogenic as follows: bone marrow, skin, islets of langerhans, heart, kidney, and liver.[25] Last, the preservation time of many cadaver tissues and organs is too short to allow the various tests that are now available to be conducted (Table 42-2).

Histocompatibility testing for different types of transplants

Transplantation of tissues and organs from *live donors* is associated with maximum histocompatibility testing. Transplantation of a kidney from a live donor requires establishment of ABO compatibility. Additionally, HLA matching by use of microlymphocytotoxicity testing and MLC are completed. White cell cross-match and mixed lymphocyte cross-match are also conducted. With cadaver kidneys, time does not allow for MLC testing to be performed. Compatibility of the HLA-B and HLA-DR anti-

Table 42-1   Tests used for tissue typing and matching

Test	Explanation
AB compatibility	Tests surface antigens on RBCs and other tissues; compatibility is same as for blood transfusions; recipient would have antibodies to any AB antigens present on donor cells and not on recipient cells.
Minor red cell antigen testing	Test surface antigens on RBCs; transplant recipients who have had multiple transfusions may have antibodies to known minor red cell antigens.
Microlymphocytotoxicity testing	Detects class I HLA antigens (A, B, C) and match of these antigens between recipient and donor.
Mixed leukocyte culture or mixed lymphocyte culture (MLC)	Detects class II HLA antigens (D and DR); takes 4 to 5 days to complete test so only performed with living, related donors; there is a 24-hour HLA-DR typing test that may be used for cadaver kidneys.[18,40]
White cell cross-match	Detects presence of preformed circulating cytotoxic antibodies in the recipient to antigens on the lymphocytes of the donor; positive cross-match is predictor of rejection.
Mixed lymphocyte cross-match	Also detects presence of preformed cytotoxic antibodies in the recipient to antigens on the lymphocytes of the donor; used to test potential recipients against selected panel of donor lymphocytes; tells probability of finding cross-match negative donor; response changes over time so potential renal transplants candidates are screened monthly.[29]

Table 42-2   Recovery and preservation time of tissues and organs

Organ/tissue	Maximum recovery time	Maximum preservation time
Bone marrow	6 hrs	Indefinite; frozen
Cornea	6 hrs	7 days
Heart	Immediate	3-5 hrs
Kidney	Immediate	48 hrs
Liver	Immediate	24 hrs
Pancreas	Immediate	8 hrs

Adapted from LifeLink of Georgia, Atlanta, Ga., 1979 and Hawke D, Kraft J, Smith SL: *Tissue and organ donation and recovery.* In Smith SL: *Tissue and organ transplantation: Implications for professional nursing practice,* St Louis, 1990, Mosby–Year Book.

the ideal transplant comes from an identical ABO donor. However, incompatible matches are acceptable in emergency situations.[30] HLA typing and matching and MLC testing do not seem to be as clinically important in liver transplantation as in other types of transplantations.[30]

Histocompatibility testing, although possible for corneal transplants, is controversial. Sight is restored without HLA matching 90% of the time, and ABO compatibility has not been shown to increase the success of the transplant. However, class I HLA matching may be beneficial for patients who are at high risk for allograft rejection resulting from corneal vascularization.[41]

It is important to remember that research is ongoing to improve histocompatibility testing and to identify the most important antigen matching for the various types of transplants. As new information and technology accumulates, tissue-matching procedures for transplants may change. However, data must be collected over many years and from many recipients of transplants.

Rejection

The major focus of medical and nursing care after transplantation is prevention or early identification of rejection so that appropriate interventions can be initiated. The major reason for transplant failure is rejection.

Rejection can be classified into one of three types: *hyperacute, acute,* or *chronic.* A special type of rejection that occurs in recipients of allogenic bone marrow transplants is *graft versus host disease (GVHD).*

Hyperacute rejection

Hyperacute rejection occurs at the time of transplantation or within 48 hours after the transplant. It is mediated by the humoral immune system. *Preformed circulating cytotoxic antibodies* to incompatible ABO blood group antigens, to antigens on the vascular endothelium, or to histocompatibility antigens are responsible for the hyperacute rejection. The *combination of the preformed antibody with the antigen causes activation of complement, entrapment of formed blood elements* and *clotting factors, massive intravascular coagulation,* and *necrosis of the graft from decreased perfusion.*

gens seems most important, whereas compatibility of HLA-C antigens appears to be of little value.[24]

Successful *allograft bone marrow* transplantation requires maximal compatibility between donor and recipient. This compatibility is identified by microlymphocytotoxicity testing for class I HLA antigens and by MLC testing for class II HLA antigens. ABO and RH compatibility are not necessary. If a transplant with ABO-incompatible bone marrow is planned, the recipient must undergo plasma exchange to eliminate antibodies against the ABO group of the donor.[42]

Because of the very short preservation times of the heart, liver, lung, or pancreas, only minimal histocompatibility testing is currently possible. With a heart transplant, ABO compatibility is established and a mixed lymphocyte cross match is carried out. In liver transplants,

The degranulation of phagocytic cells causes the release of hydrolytic enzymes that also cause tissue destruction.

Currently there are no data showing that hyperacute rejection occurs in nonrenal transplants.[29] The liver seems to be particularly protected from hyperacute rejection, possibly because of the type of blood flow and the large cell mass of the liver. Primary prevention of hyperacute rejection is by ensuring ABO blood group compatibility and avoiding transplantation if positive lymphocyte cross-matches occur (white cell cross-match).[29]

Acute rejection

Acute rejection usually occurs within 1 week to up to 3 months after the transplantation. Acute rejection episodes may reoccur at any time after the first episode, but decrease in frequency over time. Acute rejection is mediated by the *cellular immune system.* In acute rejection, foreign antigens are trapped by macrophages. This macrophage-antigen interaction can stimulate differentiation and maturation of various T-cell lines. These activated T cells cause destruction of the transplanted tissue directly or indirectly through activation of other immune cells. Acute rejection is treated by pharmacologic interventions. A major nursing intervention for all transplants is to assess for and assist with treatment of acute rejection.

A special type of acute rejection is *accelerated acute rejection,* which occurs soon after transplantation and, although treatable, is not as responsive to medications.

Chronic rejection

Chronic rejection occurs from 3 months to longer after transplantation. It is mediated by both the cellular and humoral immune systems and results in slow, progressive loss of graft function. Chronic rejection does not respond to medications.

Chronic rejection of a kidney means the recipient must resume dialysis while chronic rejection of a pancreatic transplant requires the resumption of therapy for insulin-dependent diabetes mellitus. Chronic rejection in other nonrenal transplant recipients is potentially life-threatening unless a retransplantation is performed.

Graft-versus-host disease (GVHD)

Persons who receive allogenic bone marrow are at risk for GVHD depending on the degree to which the donor and recipient are HLA incompatible as identified by microlymphocytotoxicity testing and MLC.[7] In the person who has an allogenic bone marrow transplant, irradiation therapy and chemotherapy are used to destroy the immunocompetent cells of the recipient. The donor's immunocompetent cells, once they engraft in the recipient, recognize other cells of the recipient as foreign and attack them. The tissue/organs most affected are the skin, liver, and gastrointestinal tract.[7] GVHD can occur as an acute or chronic process. Histocompatibility testing and immune suppression are used to prevent or minimize GVHD.

Drug Therapy to Prevent Rejection

Survival of all types of allogenic organ grafts and bone marrow, except for the cornea, requires the use of immunosuppressive agents. The immunosuppresive agents most commonly used include: azathioprine, corticosteroids, cyclosporine, lymphocytic immune globulin, and muromonab CD-3 (OKT-3). Each of these drugs will be briefly discussed. The ideal immunotherapy regimen has not been determined. Most patients, regardless of the type of transplant, will receive over the lifetime of the transplant a combination of cyclosporine, azathioprine, and corticosteroids. Lymphocytic immune globulin and OKT-3 are used to treat acute rejection episodes.

Another immunosuppressive agent discovered in Japan and used experimentally in the United States is 15-deoxyspergualin (DSG). Research is still ongoing on this agent.[37a]

Azathioprine

Azathioprine (Imuran) inhibits RNA and DNA synthesis and decreases the proliferation of immune cells. It is readily absorbed from the GI tract, although it can be given intravenously. Azathioprine is metabolized in the liver and its metabolites are excreted by the kidneys. It may take several days for its effects to be seen. The oral dosage is 1 to 3 mg/kg body weight.[13] The major toxic effect is suppression of the bone marrow. The white blood cell count is used to adjust the dosage. A summary of all side effects and important nursing implications is presented in Table 42-3.

Corticosteroids

Corticosteroids are antiinflammatory and immunosuppressive agents. They include the endogenous glucocorticoid, cortisol, and synthetic glucocorticoids, such as prednisone and methylprednisolone. Corticosteroids cause a decrease in lymphocytes, monocytes, eosinophils, and basophils within 4 to 6 hours after administration. These decreases are due to a redistribution of these cells from circulatory to noncirculatory sites. Of the lymphocytes, T-lymphocytes are affected. Corticosteroids cause an increase in neutrophils because of increased release from bone marrow and decreased migration from the circulation. However, corticosteroids inhibit the ability of neutrophils to adhere to vessel walls, which is necessary for migration to sites of inflammation. Thus, the accumulation of neutrophils at the graft site is actually decreased. Corticosteroids decrease production of interleukin 1 (IL-1) and interleukin 2 (IL-2), which are necessary for full functioning of the immune system. They also decrease production of prostaglandins.

Corticosteroids are readily absorbed from the gastrointestinal tract. They also may be given parenterally. Corticosteroids are metabolized in the liver and excreted by the kidneys. Their side effects from the GI tract are many, and these are listed in Table 42-4 along with a discussion of nursing implications.

Cyclosporine

Cyclosporine is an immunosuppressive agent that is selective for lymphocytes, mainly T lymphocytes. It is not myelotoxic. It acts by inhibiting the expression of receptors for IL-2 on T lymphocytes.[22] Importantly, if T lymphocytes are activated to express IL-2 receptors before immunosuppression is started, cyclosporine is not effective. Cyclosporine also affects macrophage activation.

Table 42-3   Azathioprine therapy: summary of side effects and nursing implications

Side effects	Assessment parameters	Nursing interventions
Cardiovascular: fluid and electrolytes		
Renal toxicity	Serum creatinine, BUN, Creatinine clearance, Urine output, Peripheral edema	Restrict fluids, Administer diuretics, Decrease dosage
Gastrointestinal		
Nausea, vomiting, Anorexia, Diarrhea, Hepatotoxicity, Pancreatitis	Appetite, Elimination pattern, Serum transaminases, phosphatases, bilirubin, coagulation factors, serum amylase, lipase, calcium	Administer oral dose with meals, Consult with dietician, Institute enteral or parenteral nutrition
Hematologic		
Leukopenia, Thrombocytopenia, Macrocytic anemia	WBC count with differential, Platelet count, Red blood cell count, Bleeding (oozing, hemorrhage), Signs/symptoms of infection, Inspect mucous membranes for opportunistic infections	Increase attention to infection control measures, Administer platelets, Administer packed red blood cells, Administer oral antifungal agent, Administer antibiotics, Decrease dosage
Neurologic		
None	None	
Psychologic		
None	None	
Dermatologic		
Stomatitis	Inspect mucous membranes	Maintain good oral hygiene

From Hooks MA: *Immunosuppressive agents used in transplantation.* In Smith SL: *Tissue and organ transplantation: implications for professional nursing practice,* St Louis, 1990, Mosby–Year Book.

Cyclosporine is given orally and parenterally. It is eliminated by hepatic mechanisms. Cyclosporine has many adverse effects; the most important of which is nephrotoxicity. The side effects and appropriate nursing implications are presented in Table 42-5.

Lymphocyte immune globulin

Antilymphocyte sera (ALS) or globulin (ALG) are products from animals that contain heterogenous antibodies to lymphocytes in general or to T lymphocytes in particular. ALS/ALG induces immunosuppression by depleting small lymphocytes from lymph nodes and lymphoid organs. It also coats and opsonizes the lymphocytes so that they can be phagocytized by macrophages. ALS/ALG is given by slow IV infusion. Because it is a foreign substance, the patient is monitored closely for an allergic reaction. An antipyretic and an antihistamine are given first to inhibit allergic reactions. ALS/ALG is used to both prevent allograft rejection and to treat acute rejection. In both instances it is given for 14 to 28 days in fixed doses based on body weight.

Muromonab CD-3

Muromonab CD-3 (Orthoclone, OKT-3) is a monoclonal antibody against mature T lymphocytes. It decreases the level of T lymphocytes by making them incompetent as immune cells. OKT-3 is used primarily to treat acute rejection episodes. It is given intravenously for 10 to 14 days. The effectiveness of therapy is monitored by the T-lymphocyte count and by serum levels of OKT-3.

OKT-3 is a foreign protein and can result in development of antibodies after one course of therapy. It is necessary to test for antibodies before a second course of the drug is administered. Adverse reactions to OKT-3 include chills and fever lasting for up to 1 hour. Respiratory symptoms may occur and be life-threatening if the patient is fluid overloaded.[13] Aseptic meningitis and infection with cytomegalovirus or herpes simplex viruses can occur. Other adverse effects include headache and flulike symptoms. Most side effects occur during the first two doses, if they are going to occur. To decrease some of the side effects patients may be given methylprednisolone, acetaminophen,

Table 42-4   Corticosteroid therapy: summary of side effects and nursing implications

Side effects	Assessment parameters	Nursing interventions
Cardiovascular; fluid and electrolytes		
Sodium retention	Serum electrolytes	Administer low-sodium, high-potassium diet
Potassium wasting	Serum calcium, phosphorus	Administer oral or parenteral electrolyte replacement
Calcium and phosporus wasting	Serum albumin	Administer oral or parenteral calcium, phosphorus replacement
	Intake and output	
Metabolic alkalosis	Acid-base status	Administer antihypertensives
Fluid retention	Peripheral edema	Instruct patient about side effects
Systemic arterial hypertension	Blood pressure	Decrease dosage
	Body weight	
Pulmonary		
Infection	Breath sounds	Deep breathing exercises
		Ambulation
		Avoid persons with respiratory infections
Gastrointestinal		
Peptic ulceration (esophagus, stomach, duodenum)	Guaiac stools and vomitus	Administer oral corticosteroids with food
	Serum amylase, lipase	Administer antacids, H_2 receptor blockers
	Serum calcium	Consult dietition
Pancreatitis	Serum transaminases, phosphatses, bilirubin	Decrease dosage
Hepatitis		
Increased appetite	Coagulation factors	
Diarrhea	Peritoneal signs	
Endocrine		
Impaired glucose tolerance	Serum glucose	Insulin
Diabetes mellitus	Polydipsia, polyuria	Thryoid hormone replacement
Cushing's syndrome	Cushingoid characteristics—moon face, truncal obesity, buffalo hump, straie	Instruct patient about consequences of sudden corticosteroid withdrawal
Hypothyroidism		
Impaired carbohydrate tolerance	T_3, T_4, TSH	Avoid sudden withdrawal from corticosteroids
Hypothalmic-pituitary adrenal suppression	During period of steroid withdrawal or increased stress: headache, lethargy, weakness, hypotension	
Osteoporosis	Assess patient complaints of back or limb pain	Administer calcium and vitamin D supplements
		Institute a weight—bearing exercise regimen
Hematologic		
Neutrophilia, decreased eosinophils, decreased basophils	White blood cell (WBC) count with differential count	Increase attention to infection control measures
		Administer oral antifungal agents
		Administer antibiotics
Lymphocytopenia	Inspect mucous membranes for opportunistic infection	
Opportunistic infections		
Impaired wound healing	Assess for signs/symptoms of infection	
Aseptic necrosis of femoral and humoral heads	Wound healing	
Neurologic/muscular skeletal		
Headache	Neurologic status	Analgesics for headaches
Insomnia	Sleep periods	Provide environment conducive to sleep
Vertigo	Muscle mass/strength	Initiate seizure precautions in susceptible patient
Seizures		Consult physical therapy
Increased intracranial pressure		Decrease dosage
		Give dose in the morning if possible
Muscle weakness/wasting		Encourage ambulation

From Hooks MA: *Immunosuppressive agents used in transplantation.* In Smith SL: *Tissue and organ transplantation: implications for professional nursing practice,* St Louis, 1990, Mosby–Year Book.

Table 42-4   **Corticosteroid therapy: summary of side effects and nursing implications—cont'd**

Side effects	Assessment parameters	Nursing interventions
Psychologic		
Psychosis	Mental status	Consult psychiatrist if necessary
Euphoria		Instruct patient about side effects
Depression		Decrease dosage
Dermatologic		
Thin, fragile skin	Inspect skin	Administer topical antiacne medication
Petechiae, ecchymoses	Inspect mucous membranes	Avoid adhesive tape
Erythema		Avoid skin trauma
Acne		Counsel regarding options for dealing with hirsutism
Hirsutism		Mouth care
Stomatitis		
Other		
Blurred vision		Consult ophthalmology department
Cataracts		

Table 42-5   **Cyclosporine therapy: summary of side effects and nursing implications**

Side effects	Assessment parameters	Nursing interventions
Cardiovascular: fluid and electrolytes		
Nephrotoxicity	Cyclosporine levels	Administer diuretics
Systemic arterial hyperten-sion	Serum creatinine, BUN	Administer antihyptensives, oral or parenteral
	Creatinine clearance	Administer magnesium
Hyperkalemia	Peripheral edema	Decrease dosage
Hypomagnesemia	Blood pressure	Administer IV cyclosporine over 2-6 hours
Anaphylaxis if administered rapidly IV	Serum magnesium	
	Serum potassium	
Pulmonary		
Infections	Breath sounds	Deep breathing exercises
		Ambulation
		Avoid persons with infections
Gastrointestinal		
Hepatotoxicity	Cyclosporine levels	Decrease dosage
	Serum transaminases, phosphatases, bilirubin	
	Coagulation factors	
Endocrine		
None	None	None
Hematologic		
Lymphocytopenia	Cyclosporine levels	Decrease dosage
Lymphoma	CBC with differential count	Increased attention to infection control measures
Opportunistic infection	Inspect mucous membranes for opportunistic infection	Administer oral antifungal agent
		Administer antibiotics
	Bacterial, viral, and fungal cultures	
Neurologic		
Tremors	Cyclosporine levels	Assure patient that tremors and paresthesias are dose related
Paresthesias	Neurologic status	Decrease dosage
Muscle weakness		Provide physical therapy
Increased sensitivity to temperature changes		Administer analgesics for headaches
		Initiate seizure precautions in susceptible patient
		Instruct patient about side effects

From Hooks MA: *Immunosuppressive agents used in transplantation.* In Smith SL: *Tissue and organ transplantation: implications for professional nursing practice*, St Louis, 1990, Mosby–Year Book.

> ## Organisms responsible for infections in transplant recipients
>
> **Bacterial infections**
> Gram-negative organism including *P. aeruginosa,* *Serratia marcesans, Proteus rettgeri, E. cloacae, Legionella pneumophilia,* and various *Nocardia* species.
>
> **Viral Infections**
> Herpes viruses including herpes simplex virus 1 and 2, varicella zoster virus, cytomegalovirus, and Epstein-Barr virus.
>
> **Fungal Infections**
> Candidal species (most commonly *C. albicans*), other fungi including *Aspergillis fumigatoa, Cryptococcus neoformans, Coccidioides immitus,* and *Histoplasma capsulatum.*
>
> **Parasitic Infections**
> Parasitic infections including *Pneumocystis carinii* and *Toxoplasmosis gondii.*

> ## Nursing diagnoses for the patient who is a potential recipient of a transplant
>
> Fear related to
>   Perceived inability to manage self-care
>   Severity of illness
> Ineffective individual coping related to
>   Situational crises
>   Threat of death
>   Change in role with family unit
> Powerlessness related to
>   Lack of control over when transplant will be performed
> Knowledge deficit: pretransplant evaluation, transplantation process, self-care after transplant related to
>   Lack of exposure to information

and an antihistamine before OKT-3 is administered. The patient needs intensive monitoring of vital signs (every 15 minutes for 4 hours is recommended) during the first two doses because of the increased risk for an allergic reaction. If no problems occur during the first 2 doses, less frequent monitoring is required for subsequent doses.

Infections

Immunosuppressive therapy must be taken for the lifetime of the allogenic transplant. This immunosuppressive therapy makes the transplant recipient a prime candidate for infections. Infections, besides occurring more frequently, spread more rapidly from localized sites to the total body and can result in sepsis. Although protective isolation may still be used in some institutions, the primary intervention to decrease exposure is good hand washing and use of aseptic techniques for all invasive procedures. The nurse must also provide care that protects surface barriers from organisms. This care would include mouth care after every meal, upon arising, and at bedtime. The patient's back, perineum, gluteal folds, and other skin folds should be washed daily, well lubricated, and be kept free of moisture. Additional preventive interventions such as deep breathing every 2 hours, and encouraging fluids to flush the urinary system should be instituted as appropriate. Nutritional and fluid status should be assessed and interventions should be initiated to promote adequate nutrition (which will enhance the immune response); adequate fluid intake should be ensured.

Physical assessment of the skin; insertion sites of invasive devices; lungs, mouth, and throat; temperature and pulse should be implemented at least every 8 to 12 hours to allow for early detection of infections. At the same time, information about symptoms related to the presence of any infection should be elicited. Patients will need to institute similar self-care measures to prevent infections and detect them early for as long as they are on immunosuppressive therapy.

Caregivers and others with active infections should avoid contact with the patient while he or she is in the hospital and after discharge. The patient's hospital environment should be cleaned daily. Containers of water such as humidifier bottles, live flowers, and live plants should be eliminated from the environment or, if they are necessary, should be replaced daily. Box 42-7 lists some of the common organisms causing infections in persons with transplants who are on immunosuppressive drug therapy.

NURSING MANAGEMENT
Nursing Management of the Patient Who is a Potential Recipient of a Transplant

Persons with various types of end-stage organ failure, if they meet the criteria for transplantation as described on page 1447, may have to consider whether or not to accept transplantation as a treatment alternative. These persons will have additional nursing needs related to the evaluation of their candidacy for a transplant. Box 42-8 lists some of the nursing diagnoses that can be used to guide care. Of course, the patient still has all the care needs related to the specific organ failure. Choosing transplantation as an alternative is a decision that the patient and significant others make. Nurses provide information, support, and counseling.

A major need of the patient and significant others is education. The patient and significant others need to receive appropriate information about the transplantation, the evaluation necessary before being identified as a candidate, the preoperative and postoperative care requirements, and the continual care that will be required after the transplant. Information about the side effects of immunosuppressive therapy needs to be discussed.

Once the patient decides to have a transplant, he or she will undergo evaluation. The exact evaluation will vary depending on the organ involved, but will include both extensive physical and psychosocial evaluation. Histocompatibility studies as appropriate for the specific transplant will be conducted. Underlying physical problems such as hypertension, ascites, bleeding, and infections must be treated before transplantation.

Nursing Management of the Pretransplant Recipient

Once the patient has been placed on the waiting list for a transplant, nursing care focuses in helping patients:

1. Cope with the waiting period.
2. Manage their end-organ failure as well as possible so that they remain in the best physical condition possible.
3. Implement self-care practices to maximize their physical health so that potential complications of surgery will be minimized.

The two nursing diagnoses: ineffective individual coping and knowledge deficit, along with those dictated by the end-stage organ failure will guide care.

Counseling, assisting patients in identifying coping mechanisms, and helping patients learn new coping mechanisms are the major interventions that will be used to help patients during the waiting period. There should be established routine contact between the pretransplant recipient and the transplant team. Pretransplant recipients should have someone they can contact in case of an emergency or if any questions arise.

Pertinent self-care measures for the end-stage organ failure should be discussed and reviewed. This includes a review of dietary restrictions, fluid needs, medications and planned medical follow-up.

The interventions needed for the last area of care include promotion of adequate pulmonary function. Specific interventions would include abstaining from smoking, as well as treatment of any underlying pulmonary infection. Because the person waiting for a transplant is chronically ill, nutritional status may be impaired and interventions to improve nutrition must be implemented. Adequate nutrition is important for adequate immunity, adequate energy to maintain a good level of activity before and after transplantation, and adequate wound healing.

Any active infection must be treated. The mouth is a common site of infection and patients need to be referred for appropriate dental care to repair teeth and treat gum problems. The patient is taught proper oral care so that a healthy mouth is maintained. Other sites of infection such as the bladder and the dialysis access site are assessed and any infections should be treated promptly.

Nursing Management of the Patient after Transplantation

Many of the nursing diagnoses and much of the care for the person who undergoes transplantation is the same as that for a patient after any type of surgery (See Chapter 22). However, unique aspects of care include evaluating the patient for potential complications associated with his or her transplantation, assessing for and preventing infections, and assessing for rejection. The major complications other than infection, other immunosuppression-related problems, or rejection are listed in Table 42-6. See Box 42-9 for a list of potential nursing diagnoses that would

Table 42-6   Major potential complications associated with specific types of transplants

Kidney

Acute tubular necrosis; fluid and electrolyte imbalance; hemorrhage; occlusion of renal artery or vein; leakage of urine from anastomoses sites.

Heart

Leakage of blood at sites of anastomoses; hemorrhage; cardiac tamponade; hemodynamic instability such as arrhythmias, decreased cardiac output, hypervolemia, or hypovolemia.

Lung

Pulmonary infections; reperfusion edema of lung; hemodynamic instability.

Liver

Hypertension; hypovolemia; electrolyte imbalance; thrombosis of portal vein or hepatic artery; biliary complications; coagulopathy; pulmonary problems.

Pancreas

Thrombosis of vessels; respiratory problems; peritonitis.

Bone marrow

Acute and chronic complications related to radiation and/or chemotherapy given prior to the transplant, including gastrointestinal complications, pancytopenia, venoocclusive disease, and pulmonary complications; lack of engraftment.

guide care to meet the unique needs of persons after a transplantation.

Infection is one of the most common problems facing the posttransplant patient. The patient's temperature is monitored regularly and fever reported immediately. *Sources of fever* are wound, pulmonary, or other nosocomial infections; rejection; hematoma; infarctions; or drug reactions. The search for the source of fever would include collecting sputum, urine, nasal secretions, blood, and wound drainage. Tracheal aspirates and bronchial washings may be collected and biopsies may be performed. The patient may have a chest x-ray to assess for pulmonary infiltrate. Oral mucous membranes, the perineum and between skin folds are assessed for signs of candidal infection. Diagnostic tests to assess transplant organ function will also be conducted to rule out rejection as the cause of the fever. Nursing care to prevent nosocomial infections must be instituted immediately after surgery and build on presurgery care. See pp. 1456 for a discussion of care needs to prevent infection. Invasive devices such as urinary catheters, arterial lines, and intravenous lines should be removed as soon as possible to decrease the risk of infection.

A major posttransplantation need is for the immunosuppressive therapy to be initiated as ordered to prevent rejection and the reoccurrence of signs and symptoms of organ failure. The various agents used for immunosuppression are associated with multiple side effects. These side

<table>
<tr><td>

42-9

Potential nursing diagnoses for the patient after transplantation

High risk for infection related to
  Impaired immune function
  Poor nutritional status
  Loss of skin integrity
  Presence of invasive lines
Altered oral mucous membrane related to
  Infection from immunosuppression
Altered protection related to
  Drug therapies
  Inadequate nutrition
Impaired home maintenance management
  related to
  Reoccurrence of end-stage organ failure from
    rejection
Anxiety related to
  Threat of rejection
  Threat of change in role function
  Threat of death
Fluid volume excess or deficit related to
  Compromised organ function (renal, hepatic,
    cardiac, lung, and pancreatic) from ischemia
    or rejection
  Loss of blood at surgical sites
Impaired gas exchange related to
  Ventilation-perfusion imbalance associated with
    infection or fluid overload
Decreased cardiac output related to
  Electrical abnormalities associated with electro-
    lyte imbalance
  Ineffective contractility associated with fluid
    overload or deficit
Activity intolerance related to
  Generalized weakness associated with fluid and
    electrolyte problems
  Poor nutrition
  Long-term chronic illness
  Corticosteroid therapy
  Imbalance between energy needs and supply
Body image disturbance related to
  Change in physical function
  Change in appearance from corticosteroids
  Change in role in family unit
Knowledge deficit: self-care following transplan-
  tation (diet, physical activity); fluid allotment;
  medicines; signs and symptoms of infection or
  rejection to monitor for and report; other moni-
  toring requirements such as blood glucose,
  body weight, occurrence of dyspnea; and fol-
  low-up care related to
    Lack of previous exposure to information
    Large amount of information to master

</td></tr>
</table>

effects and relevant nursing implications were discussed on pp. 1452-1456. Based on the drug therapy used, this nursing care will need to be implemented.

The patient must be assessed for signs of rejection. Signs and symptoms of rejection include signs and symptoms of organ failure such as increased serum creatinine (kidney), increased serum enzymes (liver), decreased cardiac output (heart), hypoxemia (lung), increased blood glucose levels (islet cells/pancreas), increased serum amylase (pancreas), and so forth. Additionally, signs of increased immune activity are usually present. Early recognition of rejection is essential to allow for the most successful treatment.

General nursing needs of any patient posttransplantation include the following:

1. Assessing for signs and symptoms of infection.
2. Assessing for signs and symptoms of rejection.
3. Assessing for signs and symptoms of dysfunction of the transplanted organ/tissue.
4. Assessing for signs and symptoms of common postoperative complications.
5. Assessing for signs and symptoms of major complications associated with the specific types of transplants (see Table 42-6).
6. Monitoring for overall physical functioning including hemodynamic status, intake and output, daily weight, laboratory values, GI functioning, pulmonary status, and nutritional status.
7. Administering immunosuppressive therapy and other therapy as prescribed.
8. Assessing for signs and symptoms of side effects of immunosuppressive therapy.
9. Initiating care to prevent infections and other complications of surgery.
10. Managing invasive lines, monitoring devices, the surgical incision, and dressings appropriately.
11. Initiating interventions to maintain nutritional status.
12. Initiating measures to control discomfort.
13. Teaching about management of self-care needs:
    Medications and their side effects
    Signs and symptoms of side effects of medications that must be reported
    Ways to deal with the side effects of medications
    Signs and symptoms of rejection to monitor for and to report
    Prevention of infection
    General health promotion measures
    Follow-up care
14. Providing counseling and support to help patients and significant others manage the prolonged hospitalization, role changes, and other stressors.

Nursing Management of Persons with Specific Types of Transplants

Corneal transplantation

When the cornea is so damaged that severe vision impairment occurs, *corneal grafting (keratoplasty)* may be necessary. Loss of vision caused by an opaque or destroyed cornea may be restored by replacing the damaged layers with a corneal graft obtained from a new cadaver or from an eye freshly removed by operation. For best results the donor cornea must be removed within 6 hours of death and should be grafted within 24 to 48 hours. Transplants preserved for longer periods may be used for lamellar grafts, which are discussed later in this chapter. The present practice is to keep a waiting list of persons who need grafts, because eye banks are not able to keep up with the demand. Eye Bank for Sight Restoration, Inc.,* is a nonprofit organization that collects and distributes donated eyes throughout the country.

Corneal transplantation cannot be performed if there is any infection. The kind of corneal graft used depends on the depth and size of the damaged part that must be replaced (Fig. 42-1). Corneal transplants or grafts may involve the entire thickness of the cornea (total penetrating), only part of the depth of the cornea (lamellar), or a combination of these, in which a small part of the graft involves the entire thickness of the cornea (partial penetrating). Obviously, the more penetrating graft is more difficult to establish. For the penetrating graft, the eye surgeon seldom uses a donor eye that is over 48 hours old.

Preoperative nursing care

Persons usually have only a short notice that they are to be admitted to the hospital for surgery. Although they have been waiting for a donor cornea, this short period for actual preparation may result in them feeling hurried and uneasy. They may be anxious about the surgical procedure itself and more specifically about its chances of success. A calm efficient manner on the part of the nurse, along with explanation of the routine preoperative preparation, will help ease this anxiety.

Postoperative nursing care

The person may be permitted out of bed following full recovery from the anesthetic. Discharge from the hospital is usually within 2 to 4 days postoperatively.

The operative eye is covered with a sterile eye pad. A metal or plastic shield is placed over the pad for extra protection. The patient will continue to wear the shield at night for several weeks. Corneal grafts heal very slowly because of the lack of blood vessels in the cornea and require from 12 weeks to 6 months to heal firmly.

Patient teaching

Patient teaching includes instructions about medications and assessment for corneal graft rejection. Patients are frequently sent home on cycloplegic, steroid, and sulfa eye drops (see Chapter 38).

Because the cornea is normally avascular, the recipient's immune cells are not exposed to the cornea and thus, immunosuppression therapy is not used. However, patients are instructed to check for graft rejection daily for the rest of their lives. The eye is checked at the same time each day for redness or increase in redness, irritation, discomfort, or a decrease in vision. Any symptoms that persist or increase in severity in a 24-hour period should be reported to the surgeon.

*210 E. 64th St., New York, NY 10021.

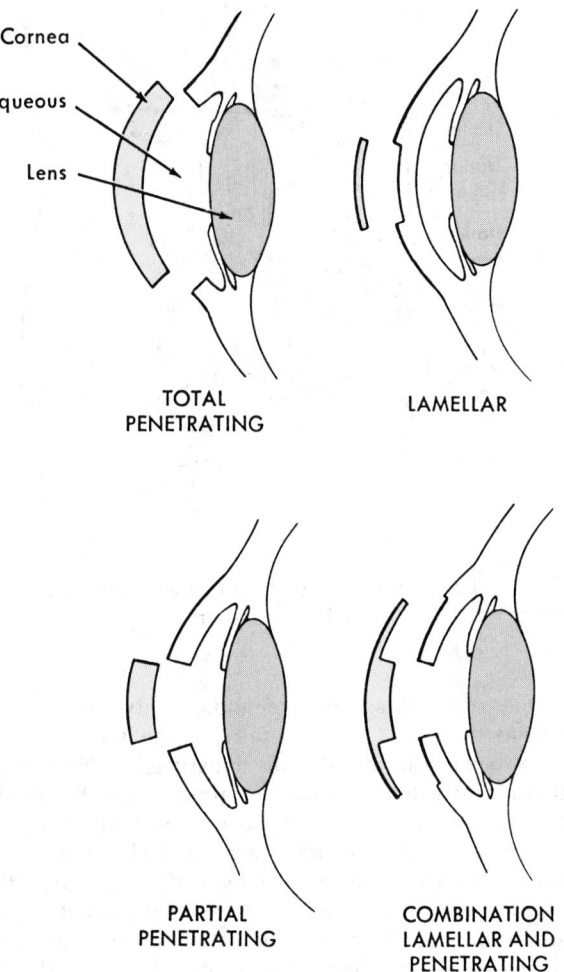

Fig. 42-1   Types of corneal grafts currently in use. Note that lamellar graft defect does not penetrate entire thickness of cornea.

Many persons expect to see immediately following the graft. Vision, however, is sometimes poor while the sutures are in place. Once the sutures are removed, vision usually improves remarkably. The sutures may remain in place for at least a year, and the patient will be scheduled for monthly visits to the surgeon during that time.

Kidney transplantation

Major advances have been made in renal transplantation. In 1988 alone, more than 9000 victims of end-stage renal disease (ESRD) underwent transplantation.[36] Developments in surgical technique, tissue typing, and antirejection drug therapy have made transplantation a reasonable therapy. However, the major block to further use of transplantation as a form of treatment for chronic renal failure remains the availability of donor kidneys for transplantation. It has been estimated that of the 12,500 to 25,000 potential donors, only 10% to 15% will actually give organs.[12]

Kidney transplants are being performed with increasing frequency in an effort to prolong the lives of persons with

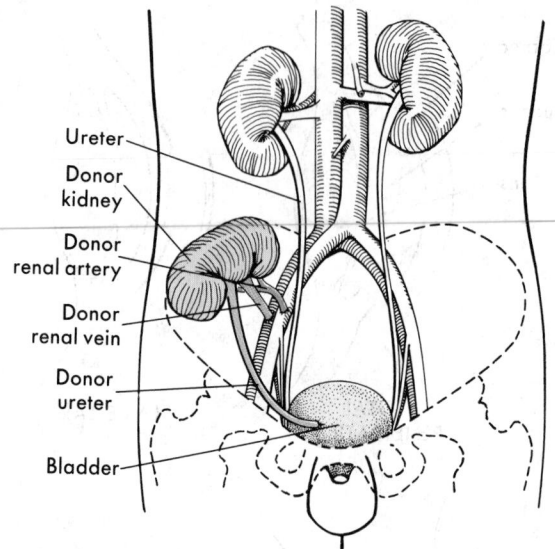

Fig. 42-2 Location of transplanted kidney showing anastomosis of renal artery, renal vein, and ureter.

end-stage renal disease. At present the ability to completely overcome the body's tendency to reject the grafted kidney has not been achieved. Persons undergoing kidney transplantation in essence exchange a program of chronic dialysis and its limitations for a new therapeutic program with new limitations and requirements. Unless the kidney has been donated by an identical twin, the body senses the graft as a foreign tissue and attempts to destroy it (rejection). Kidney allografts may be obtained from cadavers, matched family members, or an identical twin. Although more than 80% of the transplanted kidneys are from cadavers, better results are obtained from related donors. Currently, success rates 1 year after transplantation are about 75% when a cadaveric kidney is used and greater than 90% when a living related organ is transplanted.[33] The major requirement for the donated kidney is histocompatibility between the donor organ and the recipient. The important antigens are the human leukocyte antigens (HLA) and the ABO blood groups.

Living related donors must be in good general health, be highly motivated to be a donor, have good mental health, and not be receiving drugs such as barbiturates, which depress reflexes and electrical brain activity. The donor is given a complete medical evaluation and in some cases may be referred to a psychiatrist for further evaluation. Normally, the living related donor organ is harvested and immediately transplanted to the recipient. Both surgeries can occur simultaneously. Cadaver donor criteria were described on p. 1449.

Surgery

During surgery the transplanted kidney is usually placed in the iliac fossa (Fig. 42-2). Generally, the peritoneal cavity is not entered. The patient's own kidneys are not disturbed unless they are infected or are the cause of significant hypertension for which the recipient might undergo bilateral nephrectomy before transplant surgery. The

recipient's kidneys are left intact whenever possible to maintain erythropoietin production, blood pressure control, and prostaglandin synthesis and metabolism. The donor ureter is used to the extent that is possible. If long enough, it is connected to the bladder in such a way as to prevent reflux of urine. If the donor ureter is short, a ureteroureterostomy may be performed. A catheter is placed in the surgical wound to promote drainage of any accumulating fluid.

Postoperative nursing care

Immediate postoperative care includes maintaining drainage of the urinary bladder and monitoring hourly output, assessing the adequacy of fluid and electrolyte balance, protecting the patient from infection, observing for signs and symptoms of rejection and other complications (see Table 42-6), and identifying the effects of medications that have been administered throughout the entire care cycle. A free flow of communication must be maintained with the patient and significant others regarding the individual's progress.

In the operating room, a Foley catheter is inserted into the bladder to promote drainage of urine and to prevent bladder distention and pressure on the newly anastomosed ureter. If gross hematuria or clots are noted in the drainage system, the physician should be notified immediately.

As with any surgical patient, the possibility of hemorrhage and hypovolemia exists. Hemodynamic monitoring is instituted. Blood pressure and pulse are determined frequently. Because the patient may have little or no urinary output for a number of hours to days after transplantation, fluid and electrolyte balance must be monitored carefully. Parameters indicating disturbed fluid and electrolyte balance are listed in the discussion of care of the patient with renal failure (Chapter 33). Any drainage from dressings or tubes is carefully calculated into the patient's fluid balance record. The care of the patient following renal transplantation is summarized in Box 42-10.

Rejection

Rejection, the leading cause of graft failure, may occur as a hyperacute event, as an accelerated event, as an acute event, or as a slow and progressive decline in renal function (chronic rejection). In a *hyperacute* event, rejection occurs immediately after surgical implantation. Instantly following arterial anastomosis, circulating cytotoxic antibodies infiltrate and infarct the foreign tissue. The kidney undergoing hyperacute rejection is usually removed immediately to prevent further complications. *Accelerated* rejection usually occurs 3 to 5 days after transplant. It presents as a sudden severe episode of graft dysfunction, and it can sometimes be reversed with large doses of potent immunosuppressive-drug therapy. *Acute* rejection typically begins within the first 2 weeks. Most transplant patients undergo at least one episode of acute rejection. The delay in occurrence of the first attack is related to the time it takes for T lymphocytes to become sensitized. Signs and symptoms indicative of acute rejection of the kidney are listed in Box 42-11.

Chronic rejection is a slow, progressive process. The signs and symptoms are similar to those that occur in acute

Guidelines for Care

42-10

The patient who has undergone renal transplantation

Prevention of rejection, infection
  Maintain sterile technique in caring for wound, urinary drainage catheter, and other invasive lines
  Encourage early ambulation
  Administer medications as prescribed
  Assess patient for signs and symptoms of infection both at surgical incision and systemically
  Good handwashing
Fluid and electrolyte balance
  Maintain accurate intake and output
  Weigh patient daily at same time
  Monitor for signs of fluid and electrolyte imbalance
  Monitor and regulate parenteral fluid replacement as prescribed by physician (usually 1 ml replacement for each 1 ml output)
  Encourage oral intake as tolerated
Assisting with comfort and ADL
  Promote rest periods when fatigue is present
  Administer pain medication as prescribed
  Assist with ADL as necessary but encourage independence
Control of environment
  Maintain calm reassuring environment
  Reverse isolation may be used while patient is hospitalized
  Restrict visitors with colds or other infections
  Provide diversional activities as tolerated

42-11

Signs and symptoms of acute rejection of a transplanted kidney

Decrease in urine output
  Oliguria
  Anuria
Fever greater than 37.7° C (100° F); this may be masked by steroid therapy
Pain or tenderness over grafted kidney
Edema
Sudden weight gain; 2 to 3 pounds in a 24-hour period
Hypertension
General malaise
Increase in serum creatinine and BUN values, proteinuria
Decrease in creatinine clearance
Evidence of rejection on renogram or other test

rejection; however, they occur more slowly. In most instances the patient will eventually lose all functioning of the transplanted kidney as chronic rejection progresses.

Treatment of acute rejection usually consists of large doses of SoluMedrol (methylprednisolone) administered intravenously, or the use of lymphocyte immune globulin or OKT-3.

Patient teaching

Thorough teaching is necessary. The following outcomes describe the teaching needs. The person who has undergone a renal transplant or the significant other can state or demonstrate the following:
1. The prescribed diet and how it will be achieved
2. The medication plan including:
   a. Name, dose, frequency, rationale, and side effects of prescribed medications (immunosuppressives, antacids, etc.)
   b. Method of obtaining medications
3. Accurate taking and recording of oral temperature, 24-hour urine specimens, weights, fluid intake, and urinary output
4. Recommended preventive health care measures
   a. State measures useful in preventing infection
   b. State plans for dental and gynecologic health care (if appropriate)
   c. State need to avoid immunization with live virus vaccines

5. A program for continued health supervision
   a. Explain concept of immunosuppression and relate this to health care needs
   b. Describe signs and symptoms requiring immediate medical attention
   c. Relate appropriate information regarding sexual functioning and family planning
   d. State need to preserve dialysis access
   e. State resources available for assistance with illness and rehabilitative concerns and means of contact with resources
   f. Explain specific plans for follow-up care

Heart transplantation

Heart transplantation may be considered for persons who have end-stage cardiac ischemia or cardiomyopathy. The 1-year survival rate is presently 80%, and the 5-year rate 50%.[21] The donor heart is from a person with a comparable body weight and ABO compatibility with the recipient. Surgery consists of removal of the diseased heart (leaving the posterior walls of the recipient's atria to spare the SA node) followed by anastomosis of the atria, aorta, and pulmonary arteries (Fig. 42-3).

Postoperative nursing care

The patient who has a heart transplant will need care similar to that of any patient having open-heart surgery (see Chapter 25). Additionally the patient may have hypervolemia or hypervolemia, decreased cardiac output, rejection, or infections (see Table 42-6) and will need care to prevent these complications and to detect the early onset of any of these complications.

Hypervolemia can result from fluid replacement and corticosteroid therapy. Nursing care focuses on carrying out appropriate assessment including hemodynamic monitoring, intake and output, daily weights, pulmonary status, and so on. The nurse administers diuretic therapy, inotropic agents, and vasodilators as ordered to treat the hypervolemia. Fluids will be restricted along with sodium. Additional care should focus on the protection of skin in-

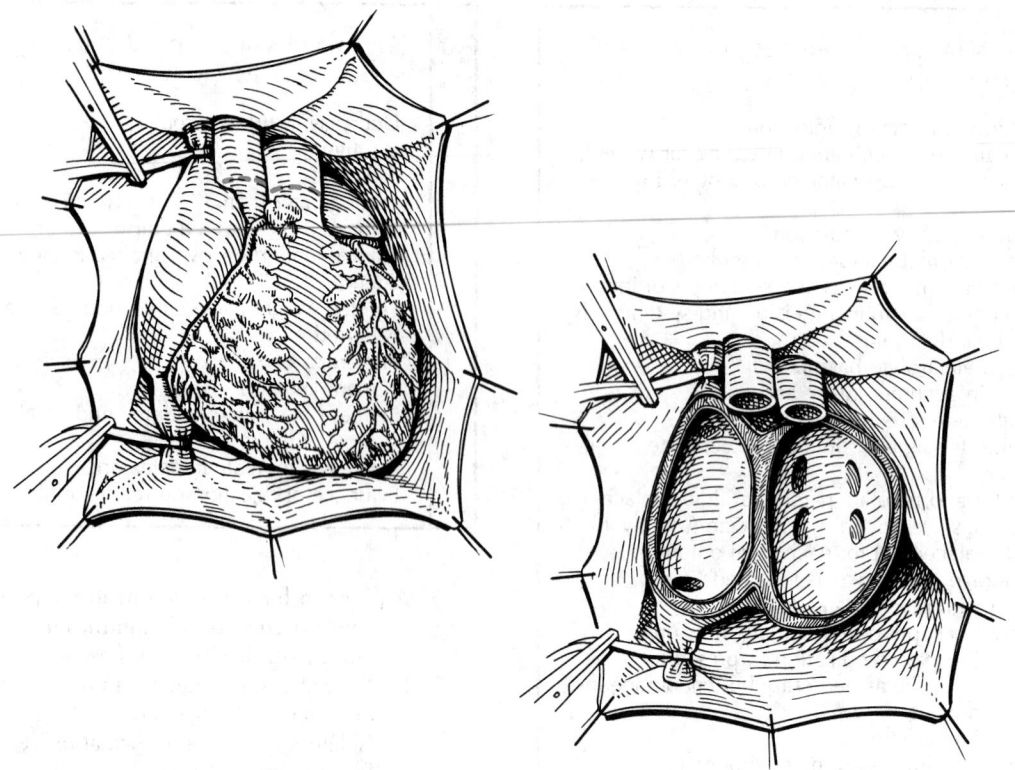

Fig. 42-3 Heart transplantation. The diseased heart is removed, leaving the posterior walls of the atria. The new heart is then anastomosed to the atrial walls and great vessels.

42-12

Signs and symptoms of acute rejection in heart transplant patients

Symptoms
Fatigue, lethargy
Dyspnea
Decreased tolerance for exercise

Signs
Fluid retention, peripheral edema, crackles, jugular venous distention (JVD), S₃ gallop
Pericardial friction rub
EKG changes: arrhythmias and decreased voltage
Decreased cardiac output
Hypotension
Cardiac enlargement

---

tegrity because the hypervolemia and edema will increase the patient's risk for skin breakdown.

Decreased cardiac output can result from rejection, hypovolemia, arrhythmias, or preservation injury. Nursing interventions in the care of the patient who has undergone a heart transplant consist of monitoring the patient's cardiac output, identifying signs and symptoms of decreased cardiac output, and assisting with treatment to improve cardiac output. Treatment is the same as for other patients experiencing decreased cardiac output (see Chapter 25).

Rejection of the transplanted heart can be an acute or chronic process. Acute rejection occurs most frequently in the first 3 months after the transplant. To assess for rejection, an endomyocardial biopsy is the major diagnostic test used. Individual institutions use various protocols for the frequency of biopsies. The biopsies are necessary because other early signs and symptoms of rejection may not be present.

Although some patients may have rejection without early clinical signs and symptoms, the nurse will monitor the patient for the multiple signs and symptoms listed in Box 42-12.

The patient showing signs of rejection may be treated with increasing doses of immunosuppressive agents. Additionally, methylprednisolone boluses, lymphocytic immune globulin, or OKT-3 may be given. The nurse will assist with this therapy. The patient will need considerable support during rejection episodes because of the potential life-threatening nature of rejection.

Chronic rejection is insidious and occurs more than 3 months after transplantation. The process is characterized by graft atherosclerosis. This atherosclerosis can result in myocardial ischemia, myocardial infarction, or cardiac failure. The ischemia and infarction may not be associated with pain because the transplanted heart is denervated. There is no effective treatment to stop the chronic rejection process or the associated atherosclerosis. Treatment focuses on interventions to improve cardiac function as much as possible. Retransplantation may be necessary.

Infection is one of the most severe complications. Pulmonary infection is the most common, but infections can occur anywhere. The organisms causing the infections are listed in Box 42-4. All the care described on p. 1456 to prevent infection will be necessary.

Patient teaching

Patient and family education is an important part of nursing care. The patient will need to be able to manage all medications, administer them correctly, manage any side effects, and report those side effects that need to be reported. The patient will need to manage dietary restrictions, which may include sodium, cholesterol, and calorie restrictions. A diabetic diet may be necessary for some patients who develop hyperglycemia from the corticosteroids. Sometimes the patient will be on fluid restrictions. Health care measures to prevent infections and improve cardiac fitness will need to be taught and patients will need to understand which signs and symptoms of infection and decreased cardiac functions need to be reported. The patient will need to understand the follow-up care, which will include repeat cardiac catheterization and biopsies.

Lung transplantation

Lung transplantation is used to treat persons with interstitial pulmonary fibrosis, sarcoidosis, pulmonary hypertension, emphysema, cystic fibrosis, eosinophilic granuloma, and lymphangiolyomyomatosis. Single- and double-lung transplants may be used, as well as a heart-lung transplant.

Single-lung transplantation has been used for restrictive lung disease because the decreased compliance and increased pulmonary resistance of the recipient's remaining lung results in preferential ventilation and perfusion of the transplanted lung. Double-lung transplants are used in persons with emphysema or cystic fibrosis. Lung transplants are still considered experimental in most instances.

Postoperative nursing care

The patient who has undergone a lung transplantation will be in the intensive care unit after surgery. The most important focuses of care are initiating appropriate immunosuppressive therapy, monitoring for infection and rejection, promoting adequate airway clearance and gas exchange, and instituting care to prevent the major complications associated with lung transplantations (see Table 42-6). Impaired gas exchange is a common complication and may be caused by reperfusion edema of the lung, impaired cough, infections, or rejection.

One difference in immunosuppression in lung transplants from other transplants is that corticosteroids are not used for 7 to 14 days posttransplant. Because corticosteroids jeopardize the healing of the tracheal and bronchial anastomoses, OKT-3 is used instead. Once healing has occurred, corticosteroids replace the OKT-3.

Intensive respiratory care is necessary. This includes frequent position change and deep breathing along with postural drainage and coughing. Supplemental oxygen is necessary. The patient having a lung transplant is prone to cardiovascular complications from hypervolemia or hypovolemia, myocardial irritability, or decreased contractil-

ity. Hemodynamic status must be carefully managed to maintain adequate cardiac output without fluid overload that can result in pulmonary edema. Decreased cardiac output also must be managed carefully to prevent an elevation in pulmonary vascular resistance. The patient is at risk for arrhythmias because of the use of cardiopulmonary bypass. Arrhythmias are treated as they would be in any situation (see Chapter 25).

The use of anticoagulants with cardiopulmonary bypass or excessive replacement of blood products place the patient at risk for bleeding from coagulopathy. Careful monitoring of blood loss from the mediastinal tubes and of coagulation studies is necessary. Administration of platelets or fresh frozen plasma may be necessary. Additional needs include nutritional support, comfort measures, and promotion of adequate sleep.

The patient undergoing a lung transplant is at risk for rejection and infection. Rejection may be acute or chronic in nature. Acute rejection usually occurs before the end of the third postoperative week. Acute rejection is associated with increased hypoxemia, fever, malaise, desaturation with minimal activity, and pulmonary infiltrate. Pulmonary function tests will worsen. The patient will need to be monitored for any of these signs and symptoms so that appropriate therapy can be instituted. Acute rejection usually responds to bolus doses of corticosteroids. Early treatment is the key to maintaining the viability of the transplanted lung.

Infection of the lungs with any of the organisms listed in Box 42-7 is one of the most severe complications following lung transplantation. All of the care for the prevention of infection described on page 1456 is necessary.

Patient teaching

The patient who has a lung transplant will need education about the following:
1. Proper medication administration.
2. Side effects of the medication that need to be reported and ways to handle other side effects.
3. Signs of rejection that should be monitored and reported.
4. Health measures to prevent infections and promote optimum health.
5. Activity regimen to enhance pulmonary functioning.
6. Follow-up care.

Hepatic transplantation

Hepatic transplantation is performed for various reasons, including biliary atresia, chronic active hepatitis, fulminant hepatitis, end-stage cirrhosis with sequelae, metabolic diseases of the liver, and hepatic malignancy. One problem with using transplants in malignancy is the excessively high recurrence rate of the malignancy.[30] Most organs are obtained from brain-dead donors, although organ transplantation from live donors has been performed in children. The recipient of live donor transplant is matched for human lymphocytic antigens and blood group. The recipient receiving a cadaver organ is usually matched for blood group although transplants using cadaver organs have been performed despite the presence of nonidentical blood groups.

Both vascular and biliary drainage system reconstruction is necessary.

Postoperative nursing care

The major physiologic complications postoperatively include rejection, infection, and occlusion of vessels (see Table 42-6). In addition, because of the patient's preoperative illness and the surgery itself, all patients are at increased risk for any of the common postoperative complications described in Chapter 22.

Postoperatively the patient will be in an intensive care unit. Constant monitoring of hemodynamic, cardiovascular, neurologic and respiratory status; fluid and electrolyte balance; and liver function is necessary. Bed rest is maintained for several days. Assessment of liver function with blood tests such as serum transaminases (ALT, AST), bilirubin, albumin, and clotting factors should show improvement immediately (within 24 hours) if a complication does not occur. Immunosuppression therapy is started before surgery and must be continued on a very regular schedule after the operation.

While instituting the tremendous physical care needed, the nurse must deal with the psychosocial needs of the patient and significant others. The patient and significant others must be kept aware of the status of the transplant. They will have been informed of the risks of the procedure before surgery, and keeping them informed will help them deal with the uncertainty. The patient and significant others need time to express their fears and concerns. They also need help coping with the social isolation and the separation that can occur with the long hospitalization (several weeks to a month) that is sometimes involved.

The nurse can help the patient and significant others stay up to date. Short frequent meetings between health team members and the patient and significant others can result in patients and significant others getting answers to many of their questions, and an established time during each day for longer meetings can be set aside as necessary. If significant others cannot visit often, the nurse can decrease the patient's homesickness by encouraging telephone calls and communication via audiotapes or letters. The nurse can help the patient cope with the long separation by encouraging hobbies such as reading, crossword puzzles, needlework, and television.

Rejection

Immunosuppression is usually maintained with cyclosporine and corticosteroids. Because of the nephrotoxicity of cyclosporine, various centers have examined ways to decrease the dosage of cyclosporine. One approach is to include azathioprine, which had been used previously with other types of transplants, so the dose of cyclosporine can be decreased.

The amount of immunosuppressive therapy will be altered on the basis of the appearance of signs of rejection that are listed below:

1. Increased temperature ($\geq$38°C), tachycardia malaise, hypertension, fluid retention
2. Enlargement of the liver
3. Tenderness over the transplant site
4. Recurrence of abnormal liver function tests (serum transaminases [ALT, AST], bilirubin, albumin, and clotting factors)

5. Altered functioning seen on hepatic scan or hepatic perfusion studies or abnormalities on liver biopsy

If signs of rejection occur, the dosage of immunosuppressive agents may be increased, or additional agents, such as lymphocytic immune globulin or OKT-3 are added. The nurse must always be aware that these drugs will increase the risk of infection.

Patient teaching

A major focus of care will be on patient education. The patient and family must receive education before surgery, immediately after surgery, and in preparation for discharge. They will need considerable education about the immunosuppressive agents. They must be taught how the medications are to be taken, the importance of never missing a dose of immunosuppressive therapy, and how to monitor for signs of infection or rejection. The patient must learn ways to avoid infections. Follow-up care must be understood, and there should be a way for the patient to contact some member of the health team (either the nurse or physician) at all times.

Pancreatic transplantation

Pancreatic transplantations have been performed since 1966. Cadaver and live donor pancreas, whole and segmental sections, have been transplanted. Over 1000 transplantations were performed from 1982 to 1988. The graft and patient survival rates have increased. In transplantations performed since 1982, the 1-year patient and graft survival rates were 82% and 46%, respectively.[39]

Pancreatic transplantation poses a unique problem; the exocrine function of the transplant is not needed, but it must be managed in some way. Digestive enzymes released from the exocrine ducts can be very irritating to tissue. Several approaches to solving this problem have been used, including injecting the exocrine duct with synthetic polymer, or anastomosing the exocrine ducts to the bowel or to the bladder. The bowel anastomosis is the most physiologic (i.e., closest to normal) because the GI tract will not be damaged by the digestive enzymes, but the transplanted pancreas is exposed to GI bacteria. The bladder anastomosis can lead to bladder damage from the exocrine secretions, but it does allow for easy assessment of graft function through assessment of urinary amylase.

The major issue about transplantation for treatment of diabetes mellitus is benefits versus risks. The documented benefits of transplantation are its favorable effects on neuropathy and progressive nephropathy. It has no influence on the progression of proliferative retinopathy, however. The risks are because of the immunosuppression necessary to prevent rejection.

Immunosuppressive therapy includes cyclosporine, azathioprine, and prednisone for long-term therapy, and lymphocyte immune globulin or OKT-3 monoclonal antibodies for induction of immunosuppression or rejection. The tremendous risk of infection, the side effects of these drugs, the cost of immunosuppression ($7000/year), the long hospitalization (2 to 3 weeks), and the frequent postdischarge clinic visits (twice a week)[32] must be considered when risks and benefits are weighed.

Currently, some of the risks are eliminated because most

pancreas transplantations are performed on persons who have or are receiving a renal transplantation. Thus, these patients are already undergoing immunosuppressive therapy. Transplantation in a nonrenal transplanted person with IDDM has been performed infrequently. Interestingly, persons who have a renal transplant with the pancreatic transplant have survived the longest.

Another type of transplantation that could be used in IDDM patients is islet transplantation, which is still in an experimental stage of development. Techniques have been developed[37a] to isolate islet cells from adult or fetal pancreatic tissue; the estimated 250,000 islets needed for a single transplantation can be obtained from one human pancreas.[13b] Islet cells have been transplanted into various sites, including the kidney capsule, the liver (by injection into the portal vein), and the spleen. Research about whether the site of transplant influences graft survival is ongoing.

Islet transplantation is believed to offer several advantages over pancreatic organ transplantation. One advantage is that there are no exocrine secretions to be dealt with. However, the major advantage relates to immunosuppression needs. In animal studies, pretreatment of islet cells to destroy leukocytes on the donor tissue allowed for transplantation of the cells into a temporarily immunosuppressed recipient animal, and the graft survived after withdrawal of immunosuppressors.[13b] Transplantations of islets in humans has been limited to persons who are immunosuppressed because of renal transplantation. A clinical trial is now in progress at one center[13b] to transplant islets into persons with long-term IDDM and no kidney damage. The results of this trial and others will provide definitive information on the role of islet transplantation in persons with IDDM. Another area of experimentation in islet cell transplantation is to package the islet cells in a synthetic membrane that allows contact between the islet cells and blood but not between the islet cells and the recipient's immune cells. This type of packaging would prevent the need for immunosuppression.

Postoperative nursing care

Postoperatively these patients are critically ill and need careful monitoring of hemodynamic status, fluid and electrolyte status, immune status, and graft status (see Table 42-6). Any signs of rejection must be identified as quickly as possible so that appropriate additional immunosuppressive therapy can be initiated. The patient also needs all the care any patient would get during the postoperative period (see Chapter 22).

The success of pancreatic and islet transplantations is assessed by analyzing blood glucose response and C-peptide levels. A successful transplantation results in normoglycemia within 2 to 3 days and increased C-peptide levels. Insulin levels can also be measured, but then the patient cannot be on exogenous insulin. If bladder anastomosis of the exocrine pancreatic ducts is used, the success of the transplantation can be analyzed through urinary amylase levels. Rejection results in elevation in blood glucose level, decrease in C-peptide level, and decrease in urine amylase level.

Transplantation as a treatment in IDDM is still a rel-

atively rare procedure, but as advances are made in understanding immunosuppression or with use of islet cells, more may be carried out.

Patient teaching

A major focus of nursing care is to prepare the patient for discharge. The patient must be able to do the required self-monitoring, know signs of infection, rejection, or other complications to report, and know how to manage the immunosuppressive therapy. The patient must be aware of the follow-up care, which consists of twice-weekly visits for some time after the transplant.

Bone marrow transplantation

Bone marrow transplantation (BMT) following treatment with high-dose chemotherapy or radiotherapy is being used in patients with a variety of hematologic malignancies and solid tumors. This is a "rescue" technique that allows administration of what would be toxic doses of drugs and/or radiation when best effect is achieved with high doses.[26]

There are three types of tissue or bone marrow donors: allogeneic, usually from a sibling who has a close human leukocyte antigen (HLA) match; syngeneic, from an identical twin; or the most recent type used, autologous bone marrow transplantation (ABMT) in which patients serve as their own donors. ABMT has been useful because it is frequently difficult to identify a donor that has a close HLA match.

In ABMT the patient's marrow is usually disease free or has been purged of tumor cells before reinfusion. The rationale for ABMT is based on the knowledge that higher doses of chemotherapy or radiation will increase the number of tumor cells killed in a logarithmic fashion; that is, doubling the dose may result in 10 times or more the number of tumor cells killed. Large doses of drugs can be given because ABMT provides a rescue for bone marrow depression.

Autologous bone marrow "harvest" (the term used for donating the bone marrow) is done when the patient is in remission or when the tumor burden is small and bone marrow involvement cannot be microscopically identified. The purpose of the harvest is to collect enough stem cells (pluripotent cells) to reconstitute the hematopoietic system after therapy.

If there is a possibility that malignant cells may be present, autologous bone marrow purging, to remove the residual malignant cells, may be performed by one of three methods: separation of malignant cells from the marrow based on density differences between malignant and normal cells (physical); use of immunotoxic or monoclonal antibodies (immunologic); use of drugs such as mercocyanine 540, mafosfamide, or 4-hydroperoxycyclophosphamide (pharmacologic).

If allogenic BMT is used, a conditioning regimen must be initiated to permit acceptance of the foreign tissue by the recipient's body. Early regimens used with allogenic BMT included total body irradiation in combination with drugs such as cyclophosphamide. New regimens include fractimated or hypofractimated irradiation, total lymphoid irradiation, busulfan, and arabinosylcytosine.[34]

Most autologous or allogenic bone marrow is obtained

42-13

Patient Teaching

The bone marrow harvest procedure

Explain that bone marrow forms special stem cells that produce all blood cells.

Discuss special preparation, for example, shower with antiseptic soap the evening before harvest.

Describe the harvest procedure:

General or spinal anesthesia is used

Needle placed through skin in back side of hip bone

If transplant is autologous, filtered bone marrow is frozen until needed

If transplant is allogeneic or syngeneic, marrow is transferred to blood transfusion bag and given immediately through an intravenous line

Explain what happens after recovery.

Pain in harvest sites can be relieved by medication

Patient is out of bed the night of the harvest

Pressure dressing is removed the day after harvest

Surgical sites are kept clean and covered for 3 days; on each day the sites are cleaned, Betadine ointment is applied, and the sites are covered with an adhesive bandage

---

by multiple needle aspirations from the posterior iliac crest under general or spinal anesthesia, although the anterior iliac crest and sternum may also be used. The amount of marrow extracted ranges from 600 to 2500 ml for the average adult (see Box 42-13).

After processing, the marrow is given to the patient intravenously through a transfusion bag, or it can be frozen at $-140°C$ although $-196°C$ is preferred (cryopreservation). Marrow can be kept for a period of 3 years or more.

Posttransplant nursing care

Acute complications of BMT, whether autologous or allogeneic, are often caused by the high-dose chemoradiotherapy and the toxicity to the gastrointestinal tract, lungs, liver, kidneys, and other organs. A second major set of problems is caused by nonfunctioning bone marrow. Another complication of BMT is venoocclusive disease (VOD) of the liver. This results from the narrowing or fibrous obliteration of the terminal hepatic venules and sublobular veins from reticulin-collagen deposits in the veins. Symptoms of VOD usually occur 1 to 4 weeks after reinfusion and include ascites, hepatomegaly, elevated ALT, alkaline phosphatase and bilirubin levels, jaundice, and coagulation difficulties. Other acute complications include hemorrhagic cystitis and acute graft-versus-host-disease (GVHD) if allogenic BMT is used.

The procedure involves psychologic stress in patient, significant others, and nursing staff who may try to be positive about the outcome. It cannot be overemphasized that hope has a major role with BMT. The involvement of staff and patient is intense in a BMT unit and nurses may be placed in the paradoxic situation of providing hope to dying patients. (See Chapter 15 for discussion of hope.)

Bone marrow transplants are associated with chronic complications that are the result of the high-dose chemotherapy and radiation therapy used in the conditioning regimen and to treat chronic GVHD. Relapse of the primary disease may occur. Chronic problems from the conditioning regimen include restrictive lung disease and leukoencephalopathy.

Chronic GVHD can result in changes in skin, joints, and hair growth; chronic stomatitis; caries; hepatic dysfunction; structural changes in the esophagus or other parts of the GI tract; chronic inflammation and stricture formation with adhesions in the vagina; and changes in the vaginal mucosa. The patient may also experience various types of infection resulting from bacterial, fungal, or viral organisms, as a result of the immunosuppressive therapy used to treat the GVHD. Pulmonary infections, sinus infections, oral candidal infections, and infections with varicella zoster are some of the more frequently occurring ones. The patient is treated symptomatically for each of these problems as well as being placed on methotrexate, cyclosporine, and corticosteroids.

Patient teaching

The patient receiving an allogenic bone marrow transplant has many educational needs. Information the patient must receive and master includes the following:

1. Medications: how to take, expected effects, side effects, and what to report.
2. Health care measures to prevent infections.
3. Signs and symptoms of infection that need to be reported.
4. Ways to deal with the changes caused by the drug therapy and GVHD.
5. Health care measures to promote optimum health.
6. Planned follow-up care.

SUMMARY

1. Transplantation of tissues and organs is a major therapeutic intervention for selected patients.
2. The major criteria for a recipient of transplant is the presence of end-stage disease that is unresponsive to conventional therapy or worsening despite careful management, ability to achieve improvement in quality and quantity of life, and financial means to cover the cost of the procedure. The age range of potential recipients has been broadened in recent years.
3. Medicare covers the cost of renal transplants, some transplants are covered by state programs, and third-party payers cover some transplants, but some persons may be ineligible for any transplant because of lack of financial means.
4. Legislation has been passed to increase the supply of organs and the fair allocation of donated organs; the family or guardians of all potential donors must be approached about donating organs.
5. Donors of organs must die from brain death, have no preexisting disease of the organ(s) being recovered, have no transmittable diseases or sepsis, no history of intravenous drug abuse, no extracranial malignancies, and no death of unknown etiology.

6. The potential donor must have been maintained hemodynamically until the organs are recovered.

7. To decrease the potential transmission of HIV, criteria for the exclusion of high-risk persons have been identified.

8. Successful allogenic transplantation requires manipulation of the recipient's immune system to prevent rejection.

9. Three types of rejections occur: hyperacute, acute, and chronic.

10. Rejection results from activation of humoral and/or cellular immune responses to mismatched HLA class I and II antigens, ABO antigens, and minor red blood cell antigens.

11. Acute rejection is a cellular immune response that occurs from approximately 7 days after the transplant up to 3 months after the transplant. Immunosuppressive therapy is used to prevent and treat acute rejections.

12. Chronic rejection is a slow, progressive process that occurs anywhere from 3 months after the transplant and leads to loss of function of the transplant. It is not treatable.

13. Azathioprine, corticosteroids, and cyclosporine are the immunosuppressive agents that are used in all types of transplants to prevent acute rejections.

14. Bolus doses of corticosteroids, OKT-3, and antilymphocytic immune globulin are used to treat acute rejection episodes.

15. A major focus of nursing care is the prevention or early detection of infections, which the transplant patient is at risk for because of immunosuppression.

16. Once the patient decides to undergo a transplant and is accepted for a transplant, nursing care needs to focus on helping the patient and significant others deal with the waiting period, helping the patient manage the end-stage failure carefully, and helping the patient implement appropriate preventive health practices to maintain as healthy a state as possible.

17. After transplantation all patients must be monitored carefully for rejection and infection. Rejection signs and symptoms are unique for each type of transplant but include signs and symptoms indicative of a decrease in function of the transplanted organ.

18. Other major complications of the postrenal transplant patient include acute tubular necrosis, fluid and electrolyte imbalance, hemorrhage, and occlusion of the renal artery or vein.

19. Heart transplants are associated with the following additional major complications: hemorrhage, cardiac tamponade, and hemodynamic instability.

20. Lung transplant patients are at risk for reperfusion edema of the lung, hemodynamic instability, coagulopathy, and pulmonary infections.

21. Pancreatic transplant patients are at risk for peritonitis and multiple respiratory complications.

22. Patients who undergo allogeneic bone marrow transplants are at risk for acute and chronic complications resulting from the conditioning radiation and/or chemotherapy and acute and chronic GVHD.

23. After any organ or bone marrow transplant, all patients need consistent, detailed monitoring for signs and symptoms of infections, rejections, common complications, side effects of drugs, and overall physical functioning.

24. After any organ or bone marrow transplant, all patients need extensive education about the medications and their side effects, signs and symptoms of rejection to report, general health measures, and prevention of infection.

25. Postcorneal transplant patients do not need immunosuppressive therapy because the cornea is normally avascular.

STUDY QUESTIONS

• What health care measures should be included in the daily care of posttransplantation patients to prevent candidal infections?

• Many posttransplantation patients require treatment for diabetes mellitus. Why are these patients at risk for developing diabetes mellitus?

• Why does a single lung transplant often prove effective in restrictive lung disease but not in emphysema?

• What are the differences in terms of immune response, signs and symptoms, and treatment for hyperacute, acute, and chronic rejection?

• What types of transplants can be performed even if the blood type of the donor and the recipient are not identical?

REFERENCES AND SELECTED READINGS

1. American Federation of Clinical Tissue Banks: *Operational standards*, Richmond, Va, 1989, The Federation.
2.* Balthazor JE: Steroid psychosis and hepatic encephalopathy in liver transplant patients: which is which and what do you do? *Crit Care Nurs Q* 14(3):51-55, 1991.
3.* Bidigare SA, Oermann MH: Attitudes and knowledge of nurses regarding organ procurement, *Heart and Lung* 20:20-24, 1991.
4. Boychuk JE, Malen JI: *Lung transplantation.* In Smith SL: *Tissue and organ transplantation: implications for professional nursing practice*, St Louis, 1990, Mosby—Year Book.
5. Braun WE: *Histocompatibility and renal transplantation.* In Garovy MR, Guttman RD: *Renal transplantation*, New York, 1986, Churchill Livingstone.
6.* Buchsel PC, Kelleher J: Bone marrow transplantation, *Nurs Clin North Am* 24:907-938, 1989.
7.* Clark JC, Webster JS: *Bone marrow transplantation.* In Smith SL: *Tissue and organ transplantation: implications for professional nursing practice*, St Louis, 1990, Mosby—Year Book.
8. Cohen C, Benjamin M, and the Ethics and Social Impact Committee of the Transplant and Health Policy Center, Ann Arbor, Mich: Alcoholics and liver transplantation, *JAMA* 265:1299-1301, 1991.
8a. Cunningham N, Smith SL: Postoperative care of the renal transplant patient, *Critical Care Nurse* 10(9):74-81, 1990.
9. Davis FD: Organ procurement and transplantation, *Nurs Clin North Am* 24:823-836, 1989.
10. Emery RW et al: Treatment of end-stage chronic obstructive

* Recommended for student reading.

pulmonary disease with double lung transplantation *Chest* 99:533-537, 1991.

10a. Goetz FC, Moudry-Munns K, Sutherland DER: Whole organ pancreas transplantation in the 1990s, *Clinical Diabetes* 9(3):33, 36, 39-41, 1991.

10b. Grossman RF et al: Results of single-lung transplantation for bilateral pulmonary fibrosis, *N Eng J Med* 322:727-733, 1990.

11.* Harasyko C: Kidney transplantation, *Nurs Clin North Am* 24:851-864, 1989.

12. Hawke D, Kraft J, Smith SL: *Tissue and organ donation and recovery.* In Smith SL: *Tissue and organ transplantation: implications for professional nursing practice,* St Louis, 1990. Mosby—Year Book.

13.* Hooks MA: *Immunosuppressive agents used in transplantation.* In Smith SL: *Tissue and organ transplantation: implications for professional nursing practice,* St Louis, 1990, Mosby—Year Book.

13a. Kibard MC, Kiberd BA: Nursing attitudes towards organ donation, procurement, and transplantation, *Heart Lung* 21:106-111, 1992.

13b. Lacey PE, Scharp DW: Islet cell transplantation. In Rifkin H, Porte D, editors: *Ellenberg and Rifkin's diabetes mellitus: theory and practice,* ed 4, New York, 1990, Elsevier.

13c. Lange SS, Prevost S, Lewis P, Fadol A: Infection control practices in cardiac transplant recipients, *Heart Lung* 21:101-105, 1992.

14.* Leslie HW, Bottenfield S: Donation, banking, and transplantation of allograft tissues, *Nurs Clin North Am* 24:891-906, 1989.

15.* Macdonald SN, Naucke NA: *Heart transplantation.* In Smith SL: *Tissue and organ transplantation: implications for professional nursing practice,* St Louis, 1990, Mosby—Year Book.

16. Maddrey WC, Thiel DHV: Liver transplantation: an overview, *Hepatology* 8:948-959, 1988.

16a. Midwest Organ Bank: Organ & Tissue Procurement Manual, Westwood Kan, 1991, The Organization.

17. Public health service inter-agency guidelines for screening donors of blood, plasma, organs, tissues, and semen for evidence of hepatitis B and hepatitis C, *MMWR* 40(RR-4):1-17, 1991.

18. Morris PJ: *Renal transplantation: indicators, outcomes, complications, and results.* In Schrier RW: *Diseases of the kidney,* ed 4, Boston, 1988, Little, Brown & Co.

19. Moss AH, Siegler M: Should alcoholics compete equally for liver transplantation? *JAMA* 265:1295-1298, 1991.

20.* Muirhead J: Heart and heart-lung transplantation, *Nurs Clin North Am* 24:865-880, 1989.

21. Painvin G et al: Cardiac transplantation: indications, procurement, operation, and management, *Heart Lung,* 14:484-489, 1985.

22. Palacios R, Moller G: Cyclosporin A blocks receptor for HLA-DR antigen on T cells, *Nature* 290:792-794, 1987.

23. Pereira BJG et al: Transmission of hepatitis C virus by organ transplantation, *N Engl J Med* 325:454-460, 1991.

24.* Perryman JP, Stillerman PU: *Kidney transplantation.* In Smith SL: *Tissue and organ transplantation: implications for professional nursing practice,* St Louis, 1990, Mosby—Year Book.

24a. Pezze JL: RATG: Implications for nursing care in organ transplantation, *Critical Care Nurse* 10(9):18-25, 1990.

25. Roitt IM, Brostoff J, Male D: *Immunology,* ed 2, St Louis, 1989, Mosby—Year Book.

25a. Scharp DW, Lacy PE: The clinical possibility of human islet transplantation, *Clinical Diabetes* 9(3):42-45, 1991.

26. Schryber S, Lacasse CR, Barton-Burke C: Autologous bone marrow transplantation, *Oncol Nurs Forum* 14(4):74-80, 1987.

27.* Shaefer M, Williams L: Nursing implications of immunosuppression in transplantation, *Nurs Clin North Am* 26:291-314, 1991.

28. Sheets L: Liver transplantation, *Nurs Clin North Am* 24:881-890, 1989.

29.* Smith SL: *Immunologic aspects of transplantation.* In Smith SL: *Tissue and organ transplantation: implications for professional nursing practice,* St Louis, 1990, Mosby—Year Book.

30.* Smith SL, Ciferni M: *Liver transplantation.* In Smith SL: *Tissue and organ transplantation: implications for professional nursing practice,* St Louis, 1990, Mosby—Year Book.

31. Starzel TE, Iwatsuke S: *Transplantation of the liver.* In Schiff L, Schiff ER, editors: *Diseases of the liver,* ed 6, Philadelphia, 1987, JB Lippincott.

32. Sutherland DER et al: *Pacreas transplantation.* In Rifkin H, Porte D, editors: *Ellenberg and Rifkin's diabetes mellitus: theory and practice,* ed 4, New York, 1990, Elsevier.

33. Task Force on Organ Transplantation: Organ transplantation: issues and recommendations—Report of the Task Force on Organ Transplantation, Rockville, Md, April 1986, Health Resources and Services Administration (NTIS No HRP 0906976).

33a. Theodore J, Lewiston N: Lung transplantation comes of age, *N Engl J Med* 322:772-774, 1990.

34. Thomas ED: Bone marrow transplantation, *Cancer* 37:291-301, 1987.

35. Trulock EP et al: The Washington University-Barnes Hospital experience with lung transplantation, *JAMA* 266:1943-1946, 1991.

36. UNOS Releases: 1988 transplantation statistics, *United Network for Organ Sharing Update* 5(5):1-2, 1989.

37. Vernale C: Critical care nurses interactions with families of potential organ donors, *Focus on Critical Care,* 18(4):335-339, 1991.

37a. Wakelee-Lynch J: Promise of the future, transplanting islet cells, *Diabetes Forecast* 45(1):28-33, 1992.

38.* Whiteman K et al: Liver transplantation, *Am J Nurs* 90(6):68-72, 1990.

39. Wills BG, Post LC: *Pancreas transplantation.* In Smith SL: *Tissue and organ transplantation: implications for professional nursing practice,* St Louis, 1990, Mosby—Year Book.

40. Wilson LM: *Treatment of chronic renal failure.* In Price SA, Wilson LM: *Pathophysiology: clinical concepts of disease processes,* ed 4, St Louis, 1992, Mosby—Year Book.

Classical

41. Bennett TO et al: Histocompatibility, penetrating keratoplasty, *Acta Ophthamol* 53:403-407, 1975.

42. Bensinger WI et al: ABO-incompatible marrow transplants, *Transplantation* 33:427-429, 1982.

43. Lafferty K, Prowse S, Simeonovic C: Current status of experimental islet transplantation, *Trans Proc* 16:813-819, 1984.

44. Miller WV, Rodey G: *HLA without tears,* Chicago, 1981, American Society of Clinical Pathologists.

45. Scharp DW: Clinical feasibility of islet cell transplantation, *Trans proc* 16:820-825, 1984.

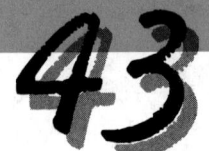

The Patient with Dermatologic Problems

Barbara C. Long

After studying this chapter, the learner should be able to:

- Describe the psychologic effect of skin disorders.
- Differentiate skin inflammations resulting from bacteria, viruses, fungi, and parasites and appropriate therapy.
- Describe correct methods of applying medications to the skin.
- Describe measures for relief of pruritus.
- Differentiate between contact and atopic dermatitis and methods of prevention.
- Explain the pathophysiology of psoriasis and therapeutic measures.
- Differentiate types of skin tumors and surgical interventions.
- Compare and contrast the different types of grafts and measures to promote healing.
- Identify different types of cosmetic surgeries.

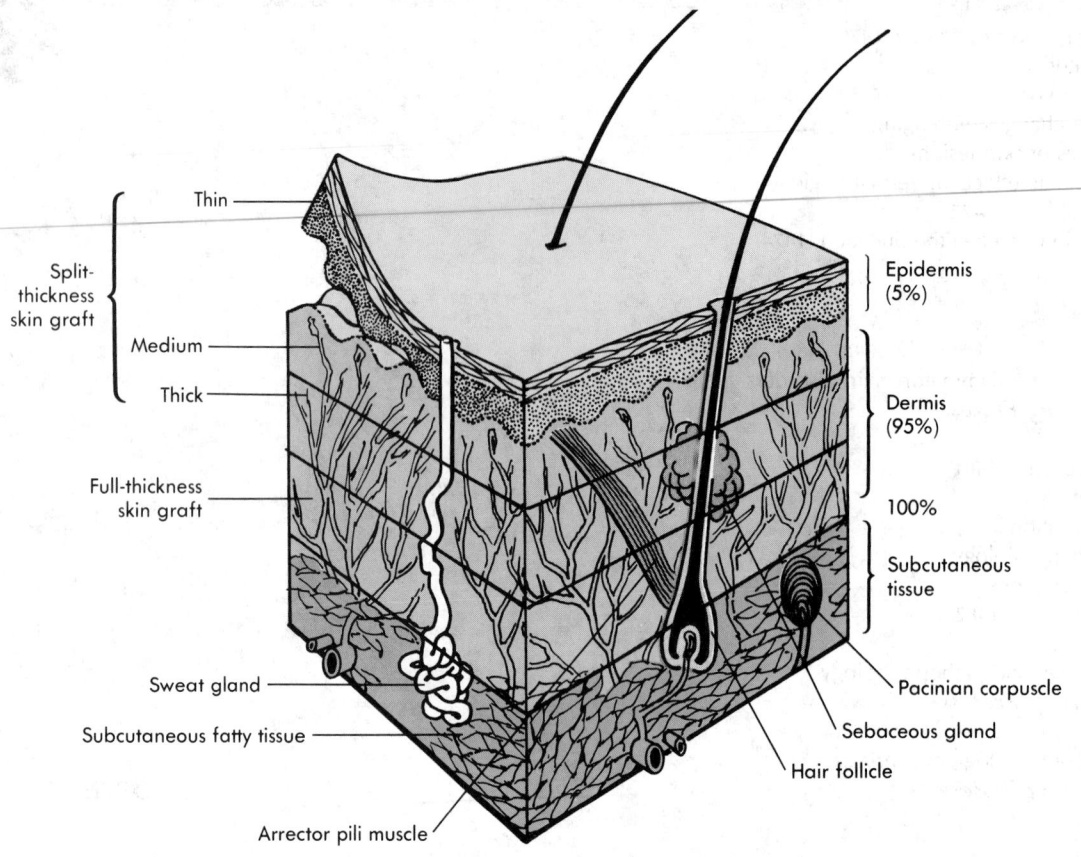

Fig. 43-1   Structures of the skin and skin layers.

The skin is the largest organ of the body. It is exposed to the external environment and provides the first line of defense of the body; at the same time it is affected by changes in the internal environment. General health maintenance requires maintenance of healthy skin. Skin changes may result from environmental changes (such as heat and cold, sunlight, and lack of moisture), from systemic disorders, and from disorders of the skin itself. In this chapter the major health problems of the skin of adults and surgical correction of impairments of the skin and underlying tissue (plastic surgery) are discussed.

ANATOMY AND PHYSIOLOGY

Anatomy

The skin is composed of two main layers, the epidermis and the dermis. The *epidermis* is composed of two parts, a thin layer of closely packed dead squamous cells covering a second layer of cells containing *melanin*, which gives skin its color. The dead cells are constantly being shed and replaced by deeper cells. Blood vessels do not reach into the epidermis (Fig. 43-1).

The second main layer, the *dermis*, is composed of bundles of collagen fibers and elastic connective tissue that act to support the epidermis. It is well supplied with nerves and blood vessels and contains the sweat glands, sebaceous glands, and hair follicles.

Below the dermis is the subcutaneous tissue, consisting of loose connective tissue and fat. It is loosely attached to underlying structures in most body areas.

Physiology

Functions of the skin include protection, heat regulation, sensory perception, secretion, and production of vitamin D (Box 43-1). Fat-soluble substances can penetrate the skin by passing through the hair follicles and sebaceous glands. Atrophic or senile skin contains fewer hair follicles, thus permeability of fat-soluble substances through skin is decreased in the elderly.

The epidermis can be weakened by scraping or stripping the surface, such as by dry razors or by removal of tape. Once the barrier has weakened, permeability to substances such as bacteria or drugs is increased. Large amounts of drugs can be absorbed by extensive denuded skin areas. Epidermis that becomes overdry may crack and lead to breaks in the surface. When the epidermis remains wet for long periods, it becomes macerated and the moisture provides a medium for bacterial growth.

Blood vessels of the skin assist in control of body temperature by constriction in cold environments to promote conservation of heat and by dilation in warm environments to promote loss of heat by radiation. Further loss of heat occurs by evaporation of perspiration from skin surfaces. These mechanisms help maintain a constant internal body temperature.

Table 43-1   Changes from aging in skin, hair, and nails

Parameters	Observable changes	Cause
Skin		
Color	Paleness in white skin	Decreased vascularity of dermis; loss of melanocytes
	Brown spots (senile lentigenes)	Hyperpigmentation
	Purple patches (senile purpura)	Blood leaking from poorly supported fragile capillaries
Moisture	Dry skin, decreased perspiration	Decreased sebaceous and sweat gland activity
Elasticity, turgor	Decreased elasticity	Loss of collagen and elastic fibers
	Loose folds and wrinkles	
	Decreased turgor	
Texture	Some rough areas	Environmental effects over time and decreased moisture
	Thinner, more transparent skin	Thinning of epidermis from decreased vascularity of dermis; loss of underlying tissue
Hair		
Color	Grayness	Decreased number of melanocytes in hair
Consistency	Thinner on head and body	Decreased density and rate of hair growth
	Coarser in nose of men	Increased density of nasal hair
Distribution	Loss of hair on head and body	Decreased rate of hair growth; decreased hormones; decreased peripheral circulation
	Increased hair on face of women	Higher androgen-to-estrogen ratio
Nails	More brittle	Slowing of nail growth; decreased peripheral circulation
	Longitudinal ridges	
	Thickening and yellowing of toenails	

43-1

Functions of the skin

Protection from environment; pathogenic organisms, foreign substances, heat, rays
Heat regulation
  Conduction: transfer of heat by direct contact to other objects or air
  Convection: removal of heat by air currents on skin
  Evaporation: removal of heat by water loss from skin surface
Sensory perception: sensory receptors in skin
Excretion: removal of water and electrolytes
Production of vitamin D: effect of sunlight

Skin Changes With Aging

As people grow older changes occur in the skin and hair (Table 43-1) that make differentiating normal from abnormal changes more difficult. The changes result primarily from loss of subcutaneous tissue, degeneration of collagen and elastic fibers, loss of melanocytes, increased capillary fragility, decreased secretion of sweat glands, hormonal changes, and overexposure to environmental elements. The skin wrinkles and becomes looser, and spotty pigmentation develops on sun-exposed areas (Fig. 43-2).

The elderly person is also more likely to have one or more chronic diseases and to be taking medications that can cause skin changes. Dry skin may cause itching and may lead to skin breakdown if scratched. Skin infections

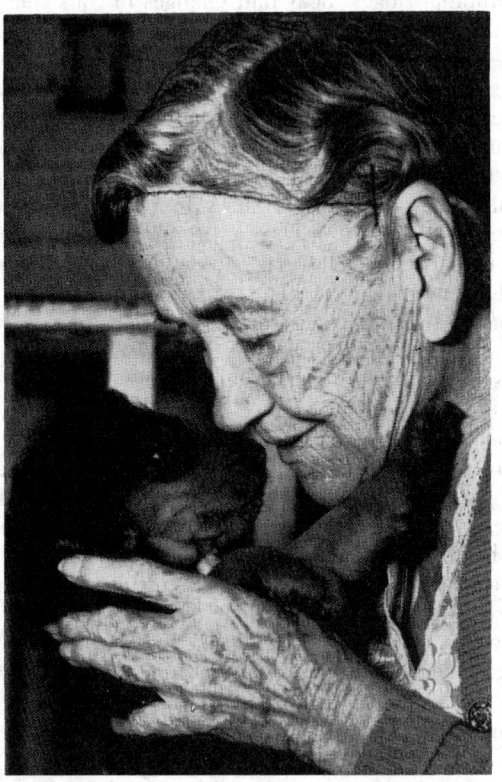

Fig. 43-2   Elderly patients have skin changes. Note discolored spots on skin and tiny raised areas on this woman's eyelid. (VanDerMeid from Monkmeyer Press Photo Service.)

Table 43-2   Skin lesions

Term	Description	Example
Change in color		
Macule	Flat spot less than 1 cm	Freckle
Change in cell growth		
Papule	Raised mass less than 1 cm	Measles spot
Nodule	Raised mass 1 to 2 cm	Mole
Tumor	Raised mass over 2 cm	Epithelioma
Change involving fluid		
Vesicle	Fluid-filled sac less than 1 cm	Small blister
Bulla	Fluid-filled sac more than 1 cm	Large blister
Pustule	Pus-filled sac less than 1 cm	Acne lesion
Wheal	Circumscribed raised skin containing intracellular fluid	Hives
Changes in consistence or integrity		
Plaque	Large raised surface on skin	Psoriasis
Crust	Dry exudate over a lesion	Eczema lesion
Scale	Dry exfoliation of skin cells	Psoriasis
Fissure	Crack in skin surface	Crack in corner of mouth
Ulcer	Erosion of skin surface	Decubitus ulcer
Lichenification	Leatherlike thickening of outer skin layer	Lichen planus

occur more readily because of increased epidermal permeability. Stasis dermatitis may result from circulatory impairment of the legs. Toenails become thicker and difficult to trim; fingernails become more brittle and develop longitudinal ridges. Body hair changes in consistency and distribution.

Types of Skin Lesions

Different types of lesions may be observed on the skin. Changes from normal skin may be in terms of color, cell growth, presence of extra fluid, consistency, or integrity (Table 43-2). Swelling of the skin may result from the presence of fluid in or between tissue cells or from overgrowth of tissue cells (Fig. 43-3). Fluid may appear as fluid-filled sacs on the skin surface or in the tissue. *Interstitial* fluid results from increased extracellular body fluid (Chapter 7) and is termed *pitting edema* because a finger pressed over the swollen tissue leaves a pit on the skin surface. Extra fluid *within* cells causes swelling but is not termed edema and does not pit when pressed. Different terms are used for overgrowth of tissue cells, depending on the size of the growth. The term *tumor* refers to a growth over 2 cm and is not restricted to malignancy; tumors can also be benign.

Lesions may occur singly or in multiples. They may be discrete (separate) or they may coalesce into each other. They may occur in patches located in certain body areas or occur widely distributed in an even or uneven pattern. The use of correct medical terms when describing skin lesions facilitates communication with others.

PSYCHOLOGIC EFFECTS OF DERMATOLOGIC PROBLEMS

There is a certain degree of "beauty orientation" in Western culture. Cosmetics to enhance good looks are extensively used by men and women. It is no wonder that skin disease or physical defects that detract from "good looks" produce psychologic reactions.

Emotional reactions to a deformity or defect must not be underestimated. Pride in oneself, the ability to think well of oneself and to regard onself favorably in comparsion with others, is essential to the development and maintenance of a well-integrated personality. Every person with a defect or handicap, particularly if it is conspicuous to others, suffers some threat to emotional security. The extent of the emotional reaction and the amount of maladjustment that follow depend on the individual's makeup and ability to cope with emotional insults. It is not unusual for the individual to withdraw from a society that is unkind. The defect may be used to justify failure to assume responsibility or to justify striking out against an unkind society.

Skin diseases that produce marked disfigurement of visible body surfaces can therefore result in alterations in body image. Feelings of decreased worth by persons with large draining lesions or with severe disfigurement are reinforced during interactions with others. Some people are repelled by the sight of severe skin diseases or may experience a threat to their own body integrity and physically withdraw to avoid interaction. Some persons may experi-

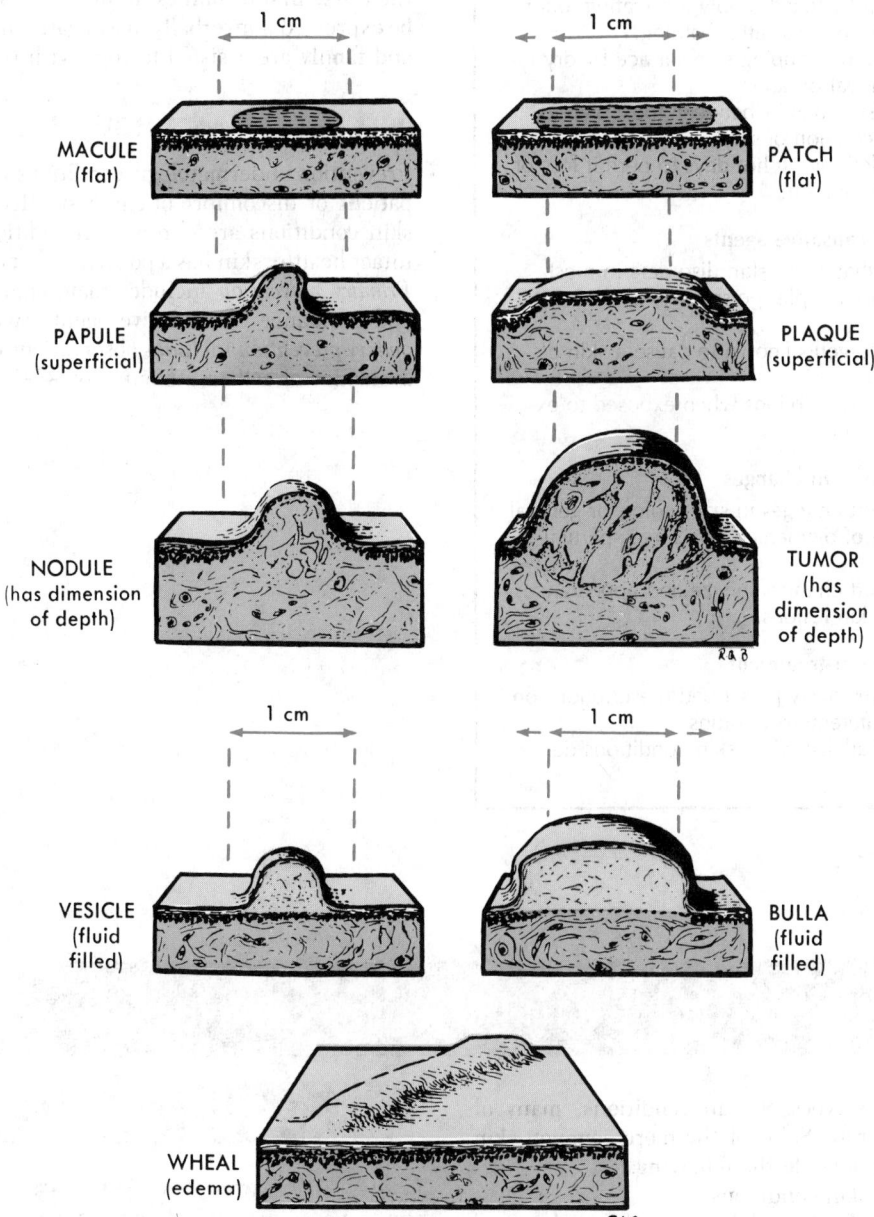

Fig. 43-3 Skin lesions. (From Stewart WD, Danto JL, Maddin S: *Dermatology: diagnosis and treatment of cutaneous disorders*, ed 4, St Louis, 1978, Mosby–Year Book.)

43-2

Prevention of skin disorders

Maintenance of healthy skin

Avoid strong or harsh soaps or detergents.
Keep skin well hydrated; apply lubricating lotion or cream to dry areas after bathing.
Avoid scraping or stripping skin surface by dry razors or removal of tape.
Dry damp areas (such as between toes) well to prevent maceration of skin.
Wear loose clothing on hot days to permit loss of heat by evaporation.

Avoidance of causative agents

Avoid agents that cause skin disorders in most persons, for example, poison ivy, excessive sunlight.
Avoid specific agents known to cause a skin disorder in self.
Use protective skin lotions when exposed to excessive sunlight.

Observation of skin changes

Note and report changes in size, color, or general appearance of pigmented skin areas, particularly moles.
Note and report changes in size and appearance of existing skin lesions.

Avoidance of self-treatment

Do not use previously prescribed prescriptions on new and different skin lesions.
Seek medical advice when skin conditions develop.

ence nonverbal messages of disgust when others view their disfigurement for the first time. This is markedly poignant when those nonverbal messages are sent by significant others or by health professionals.

In working with the person with severe skin disease, the nurse first examines his or her own feelings that could be expressed nonverbally in a negative manner. The patient and family are assisted to cope with their feelings.

PREVENTION AND HEALTH EDUCATION

Prevention of dermatologic conditions not only relieves the patient of discomfort but is cost effective because many skin conditions are chronic. In addition, maintenance of intact healthy skin has a positive effect on one's well-being. *Primary prevention* includes maintenance of healthy skin and avoidance of causative agents (when possible). *Secondary prevention* includes observations of skin changes and avoidance of self-treatment (Box 43-2).

MAJOR HEALTH PROBLEMS OF THE SKIN

There are numerous types of skin conditions, many of which occur only rarely. Some of the more common skin conditions discussed include the following:

1. Inflammatory skin conditions
   a. Bacterial infections: folliculitis, furuncles, and carbuncles
   b. Viral inflammations: herpes simplex, herpes zoster, warts
   c. Fungal inflammation: candidiasis, dermatophytoses
   d. Parasitic infestations: pediculosis, scabies
2. Acne
3. Dermatitis: contact, atopic, or stasis
4. Scaling papular disorders: psoriasis, pityriasis rosea, lichen planus
5. Tumors of the skin: keratoses, hemangiomas, premalignant lesions, malignant lesions
6. Skin disorders in blacks

INFLAMMATORY SKIN DISORDERS

Types of Inflammatory Skin Disorders

The skin may become inflamed from bacteria, viruses, or funguses or by parasitic infestation.

Bacterial skin infections

Most bacteria that normally inhabit the skin are nonpathogenic. Pathogenic bacteria that penetrate the outer skin layer may cause a superficial skin infection or superficial *folliculitis* or they may penetrate deeper, causing a deep folliculitis or a *furuncle* (Table 43-3).

Superficial folliculitis occurs most often with uncleanliness, maceration, exposure to oils and solvents, traction on the hair from tar therapy, or occlusion therapy. Furuncles and carbuncles occur most often in obese, poorly nourished, fatigued, or otherwise susceptible persons with

REVIEW

Table 43-3   Bacterial skin infections

Type	Description	Signs and symptoms	Medical therapy
Folliculitis	Infections of the hair follicles, primarily by *Staphylococcus*; occurs frequently after tar or occlusive therapy	Itching of hairy areas, pustules in hair follicles; abscess may develop	Saline or Burow's solution soaks; topical antibiotics
Furuncles (boil)	Deep folliculitis or nodule around hair follicle	Local swelling and redness; severe local pain; core turns yellow and "points" in 3 to 5 days; may rupture spontaneously	Systemic antibiotics; hot moist compresses (discontinued when drainage starts); incision and drainage (I & D); topical antibiotics after I & D
Carbuncle	Cluster of furuncles		
Cellulitis	Diffuse spreading infection of skin and subcutaneous tissue, usually resulting from cocci	Area is red, warm, swollen, painful with poorly defined borders; fever, malaise, leukocytosis	Hot moist dressings; systemic antibiotics; rest

REVIEW

Table 43-4   Viral skin inflammations

Type	Description	Signs and symptoms	Medical therapy
Herpes simplex (fever blister, cold sore)	Infection by herpes simplex virus; may occur anywhere but seen primarily on lips, mouth, genitalia	Initial burning and itching; appearance of painful, small, grouped vesicles; crust forms, healing within 10 to 14 days	Primarily symptomatic; early application of zinc sulfate solution or moistened styptic pencil may help; analgesics; acyclovir for immunocompromised patients
Herpes zoster (shingles)	Acute vesicular eruption by the V-Z virus along a nerve pathway	Cluster of skin vesicles along course of peripheral sensory nerves; usually one side, primarily on thorax or face; crust develops and drops off in 10 to 14 days; pain, malaise, fever, itching; neuralgic pain may persist	Acyclovir (Zovirax); analgesics; rest; calamine lotion for itching; steroids to decrease incidence of neuralgia. Postherpetic neuralgia: tranquilizers, analgesics, topical capsaicin (Zostrix)
Herpetic whitlow	HSV infection of finger seen most often in health care professionals	Vesicles on finger preceded by intense itching/pain; fever, chills, and malaise may occur	Primarily symptomatic; elevation and immobilization of finger; analgesics
Warts (verruca)	Benign growths from a viral infection; plantar warts on soles of feet grow inward; anogenital warts have a cauliflower appearance	Small, circumscribed, painless, hyperkeratotic papules, usually on hands, may disappear spontaneously; pain with plantar warts; itching with anogenital warts	Removal by electrodesiccation or cryosurgery

poor hygiene, in debilitated elderly people, and in persons with inadequately treated diabetes mellitus.

Viral skin inflammations

Viruses may cause either simple or more serious skin inflammations (Table 43-4). One of the most common viruses found in humans is the *herpes simplex* virus (HSV). It occurs as two similar yet serologically different strands, type 1 and type 2. The type 1 virus is found primarily in lesions of the face and mouth (fever blister, cold sore), eye (keratitis), and brain (encephalitis). Type 2 is associated with lesions of the genitalia that can be transmitted by

sexual contact (see Chapter 18). Factors that may precipitate recurrence of herpes simplex lesions include fever, upper respiratory tract infection, exhaustion, and stress. Lesions are also more common during the menses or after direct exposure to the sun's rays. Depression of immune function may predispose to HSV infection.

Herpes zoster (see Plate 1) is caused by the same virus (varicella zoster, V-Z) that causes varicella (chicken pox). Varicella is believed to be the primary infection in a nonimmune host, whereas herpes zoster is thought to be the response in a partially immune host. Although herpes zoster is far less communicable than chicken pox, persons

REVIEW

Table 43-5 Fungal skin inflammations

Type	Description	Signs and symptoms	Medical therapy
Candidiasis (moniliasis)	Overgrowth of yeastlike fungus, primarily in mouth and vagina	Mouth: white spots like milk curd Vagina: cheesy discharge, itching	Ketoconazole (Nizoral) orally, nystatin (Mycostatin) orally or vaginally, clotrimazole (Mycelex) troches or vaginal cream
Dermatophytoses			
Tinea capitis	Fungal infection of scalp (ringworm of scalp)	Round lesion with erythema, slight scaling and some pustules around edge; temporary alopecia	Antifungal medication by shampoo or topical application
Tinea corporis	Fungal infection of nonhairy parts of body (ringworm of body)	Flat lesions with clear centers and red borders	Oral griseofulvin and topical application of antifungal medication
Tinea cruris	Fungal infection of groin (jock itch)	Brown to red lesion extending outward from groin, itching	Same as for tinea corporis
Tinea pedis (athlete's foot)	Fungal infection between and under toes	Cracks between toes, maceration, vesicular lesions; toenails may become thickened and discolored	Oral griseofulvin for weeks or months, antifungal topical medication
Tinea versicolor	Superficial fungal infection, mostly on trunk	Hypopigmented macules that do not tan; scaling, mild pruritus	Topical Selsun suspension or 50% propylene glycol in water; imidazole creams

who have not had chicken pox may develop it after exposure to the vesicular lesions of persons with herpes zoster. For this reason, susceptible persons should not care for patients with herpes zoster.

Herpes zoster (shingles) can be serious in any adult and may even lead to death from exhaustion in elderly debilitated persons. It is one of the most drawn out and exasperating conditions found in elderly patients and leads to discouragement and demoralization. The lesions follow nerve pathways and never cross the body midline, although nerves on both sides can be affected. Although recurrence is possible, immunity usually occurs after one attack. Herpes zoster often occurs in immunocompromised persons. Acyclovir (Zovirax), an antiviral drug, is given for herpes simplex in immunocompromised persons and for persons with herpes zoster. It only controls the symptoms; it does not affect the disease. Corticosteroids may be given to decrease the incidence of postherpetic neuralgia (PHN). Pain in PHN can be severe and usually lasts less than 1 year, but may persist for years. *Herpetic whitlow* and *warts* are two other commonly seen viral skin inflammations (see Table 43-4).

Fungal inflammations

Fungi are larger and more complex than bacteria. They may be unicellular, such as yeast, or multicellular, such as molds. Fungi may cause common skin disorders (Table 43-5).

Yeasts thrive in warm, moist environments such as the mouth and vagina (*candidiasis*). Problems occur when there is an overgrowth, commonly occurring with pregnancy, use of oral contraceptives, poor nutrition, antibiotic therapy, diabetes mellitus, other endocrine diseases, and immu-

43-3

Facts about athlete's foot

1. It is seen mostly in young men.
2. Walking barefoot in gymnasiums or around swimming pools does not necessarily lead to infection.
3. Prophylactic foot baths are ineffective.
4. Wearing white socks does not affect the course of infection.
5. Susceptible persons will acquire athlete's foot regardless of their activities.

nosuppressed conditions. Oral candidiasis may be the first sign of AIDS or AIDS-related complex (ARC).[29]

The more common fungal infections are the dermatophytoses (tinea). Tinea *capitis* (Fig. 43-4) (inappropriately called *ringworm of the scalp*) is transmitted readily under crowded conditions where poor hygiene exists. Minor scalp trauma facilitates implantation of the spores; hence the infection can be spread by contaminated barber's instruments, combs, or sharp brushes. Tinea *cruris* (jock itch) occurs frequently in men, especially those who have tinea pedis and those who frequently wear athletic supporters or tight shorts, but it is being seen more frequently in women who wear tight pantyhose or slacks. Tinea *corporis* is seen primarily on the face, arms, or trunk, especially on exposed areas.

The most common dermatophytosis is tinea *pedis*, or athlete's foot. There are many misconceptions about prevention and treatment of athlete's foot (Box 43-3). It is often confused with other foot eruptions, such as contact

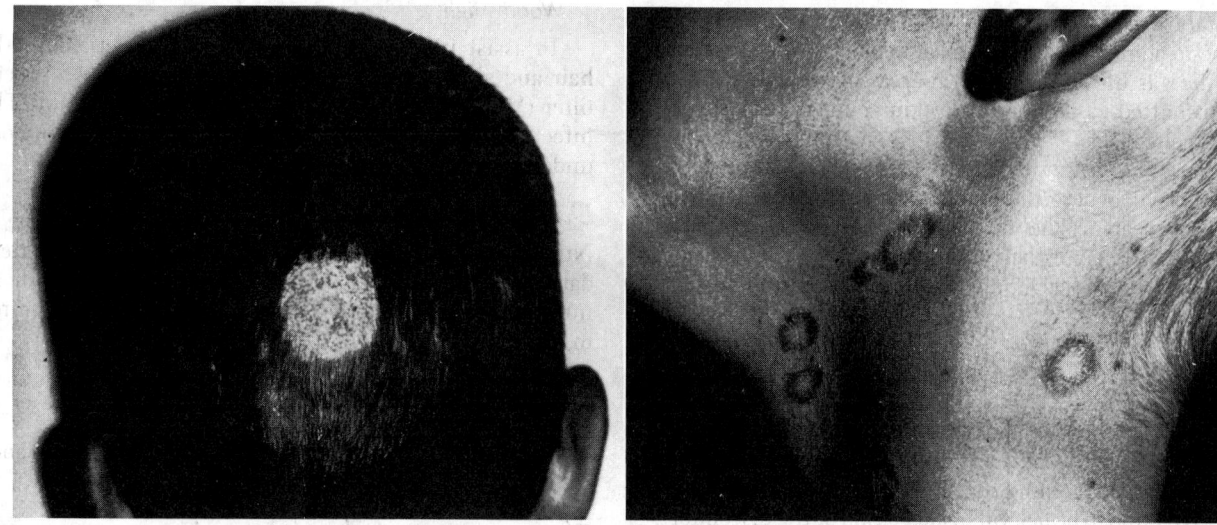

Fig. 43-4   A, Tinea capitis. **B,** Tinea corporis. (From Stewart WD, Danto JL, Maddin S: *Dermatology: diagnosis and treatment of cutaneous disorders,* ed 4, St Louis, 1978, Mosby–Year Book.)

REVIEW

Table 43-6   Parasitic infestations

Type	Description	Signs and symptoms	Medical therapy
Pediculosis			
Head lice	Attach to hair shaft and lay eggs (nits); transmitted by direct contact	Itching of scalp, excoriation of skin, and secondary infection from scratching	Topical application of permethrin (Nix), lindane (Kwell, Scabene), malathion (Prioderm), or pyrethrin (RID) by shampoo, lotion, or cream; combing with fine-toothed comb to remove nits
Body lice	Found in seams of underclothing; transmitted by direct contact, clothing, linens	Same as for head lice	Topical application of lindane, permethrin, or malathion by lotion or cream
Pubic lice	Resemble tiny crabs; nits are visible in pubic hair; transmitted by sexual contact, bed linen, towels	Same as for head lice	Same as for body lice
Scabies	Female itch mite burrows under skin and lays eggs; transmitted by prolonged contact	Severe itching; wavy brownish, threadlike lines seen mostly on hands, arms, and body folds and genitalia; secondary infections	Lindane (Kwell, Scabene), crotamiton (Eurax), or permethrin

dermatitis, psoriasis, or simple intertrigo (chronic bacterial infection of the areas between the toes, or intertriginous areas). Factors that may lessen infection include wearing sandal-type shoes or going barefoot (to decrease tissue moisture) and using good foot hygiene including washing the feet frequently and drying well between the toes.

Tinea *versicolor* is caused by a different fungus than the other types of tinea. It is a common, noncontagious, superficial fungal infection.

Most fungal infections are chronic with periods of exacerbation. Topical agents that are most effective are broad-spectrum imidazoles: clotrimazole (Mycelex), econazole (Spectazole), miconazole (Monistat-Derm), and ketoconazole (Nizoral).

Parasitic infestations

Parasites may live on the body or clothing (lice) or burrow under the skin (itch mite), causing inflammations of the skin (Table 43-6).

Lice obtain their nutrition by sucking blood from the skin. They leave their eggs on the skin surface attached to hair shafts, and this results in the transference from person to person. Control and treatment of pediculosis (lice infestation) can be hampered by persons of all incomes who refuse to admit that the lice exist among family members.

Scabies is highly prevalent in areas of overcrowding. It is transmitted easily by skin to skin contact. It is uncommon among blacks.[44] The itch mite penetrates the skin and lays eggs; the larvae mature in 10 days and move to the skin surface, where the female is impregnated; then the cycle is repeated. The incubation period varies, but often a long period elapses before symptoms are noted. Scabies occurs among all age groups and socioeconomic levels.

Nursing Process
Assessment
Subjective data

Subjective data from persons with inflammations of the skin are centered on the extent of *itching* and *pain*. Data are collected concerning the site, intensity, duration, and methods found to be helpful in alleviation of the discomfort. Data are also collected concerning the person's knowledge of the type of infection, measures to control spread, and prescribed treatments to be carried out at home.

Objective data

The skin is routinely assessed during physical inspection and whenever there is patient contact, such as while providing hygiene care, comfort measures, or prescribed treatments. Changes in previous lesions or occurrence of new lesions are reported and recorded.

Diagnostic tests
Tzanck smear

Vesicular disorders may be differentiated by a Tzanck smear. The top of the vesicle is cut and a smear taken from the base of the vesicle. Examination of the smear may identify a virus (herpes simplex or zoster) or acantholytic cells (pemphigus). The test is negative for vesicles from burns, erythema multiforme, or dermatitis herpetiforme.

KOH test

If the causative factor is believed to be a fungus, a potassium hydroxide (KOH) examination may be carried out. The lesion is scraped with a knife blade, and the scraping is placed on a slide, which is set in a KOH solution before microscopic study.

Culture

If the primary lesion is a pustule, a culture of the pustule contents may be taken to identify the causative organism. Streptococci and staphylococci are commonly seen.

Wood's light

To assist in the diagnoses of fungal infections of the hair and skin (tinea), the hair is illuminated by a special filter (Wood's filter) attached to an ultraviolet lamp. The infected hairs fluoresce a brilliant green or appear luminous under the light.

Data analysis: nursing diagnoses

Nursing diagnoses are determined from analysis of patient data. Possible nursing diagnoses for the person with an inflammatory skin disorder may include, but are not limited to, the following:

Diagnostic title	Possible etiologies
Pain: itching	Skin lesions
Knowledge deficit	Lack of exposure or recall, information misinterpretation

Planning: expected patient outcomes

Expected patient outcomes for the person with an inflammatory skin disorder may include, but are not limited to the following:
1. States feeling comfortable.
2. Describes measures to prevent spread.
3. Describes prescribed treatment measures.
4. Describes plans for medical follow-up for severe inflammatory disorders.

Implementation
Assisting with achievement of therapeutic goals

Inflammatory skin disorders are treated primarily by cleaning the lesions, then applying a topical medication. If pruritus or discomfort is present, antipruritic agents or analgesics may be prescribed.

Topical medications

Topical medications can be prepared in a variety of bases (Table 43-7). *Powders* are effective in reducing friction and moisture in intertriginous areas (between fingers and toes). The powders are first sprinkled into the hand, then applied to the skin to avoid releasing excess powder into the air and causing irritation to the mucous membrane. Powders are used sparingly to prevent caking and are not used on wet surfaces because this leads to caking. Cornstarch is *not* recommended, because it encourages growth of yeast, bacteria, and funguses.

Lotions must be shaken well because the insoluble powder may settle out. Lotions with a water or alcohol base are applied by patting gently. (Alcohol increases the cooling

Table 43-7 Comparison of vehicles for topical medications

Type	Base	Effect
Powder	Dry	Drying by absorbing moisture; cooling by evaporating moisture
Lotion	Powder suspended in water or oil	Protective, cleansing, cooling, antipruritic effect depending on drug and base used
Creams and ointments	Emulsions of oil and water	Occlusive covering over skin to prolong contact of medication with skin, good skin penetration, warming effect
Paste	≥50% powder in ointment base	Holds medication for longer period of time with slower skin penetration

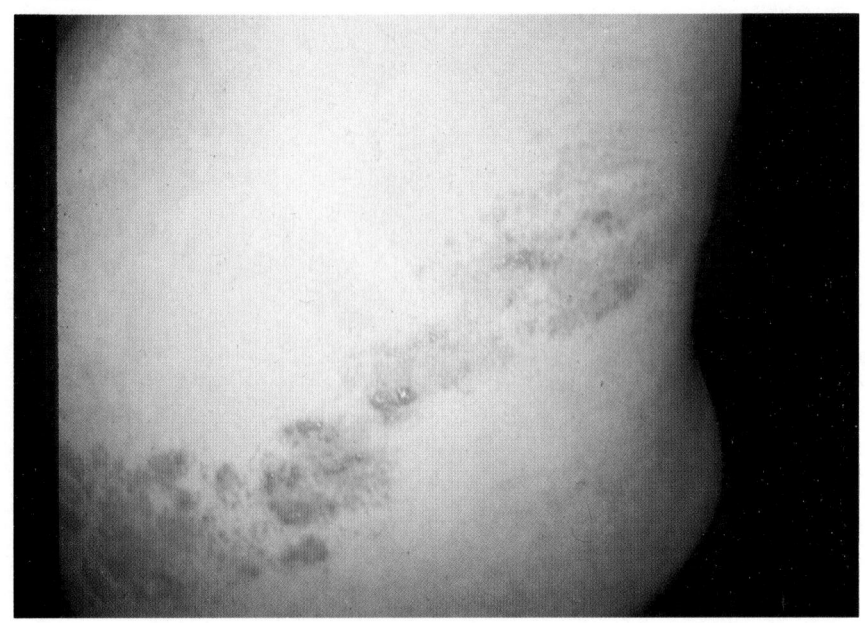

PLATE 1 Herpes zoster.
(Courtesy David Bickers, M.D., Cleveland, Ohio.)

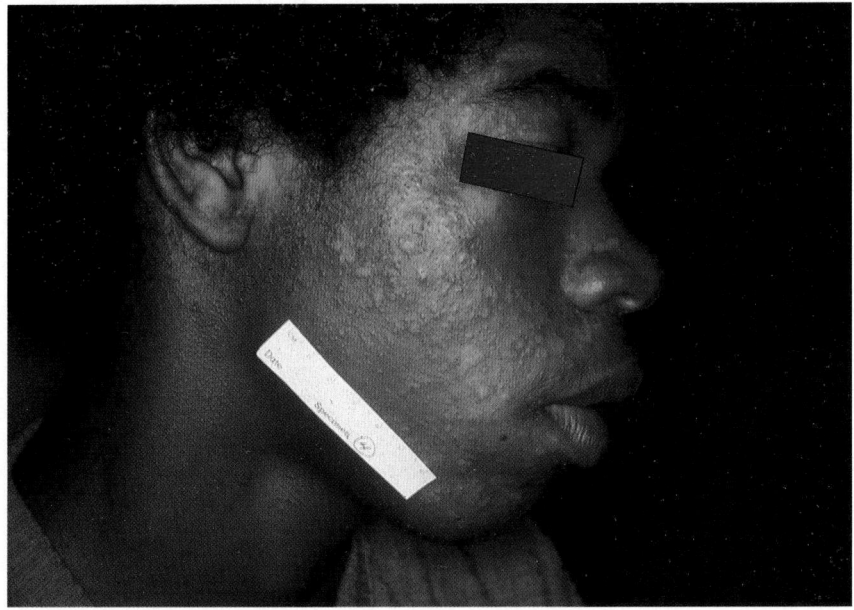

PLATE 2 Contact dermatitis from hair preparations.
(Courtesy David Bickers, M.D., Cleveland, Ohio.)

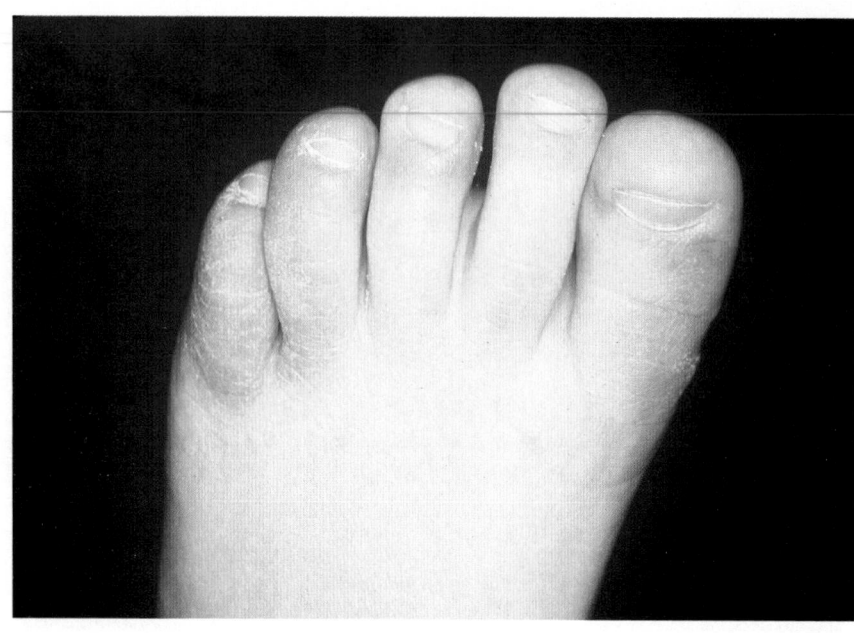

PLATE 3 Dermatitis from shoes.
(Courtesy David Bickers, M.D., Cleveland, Ohio.)

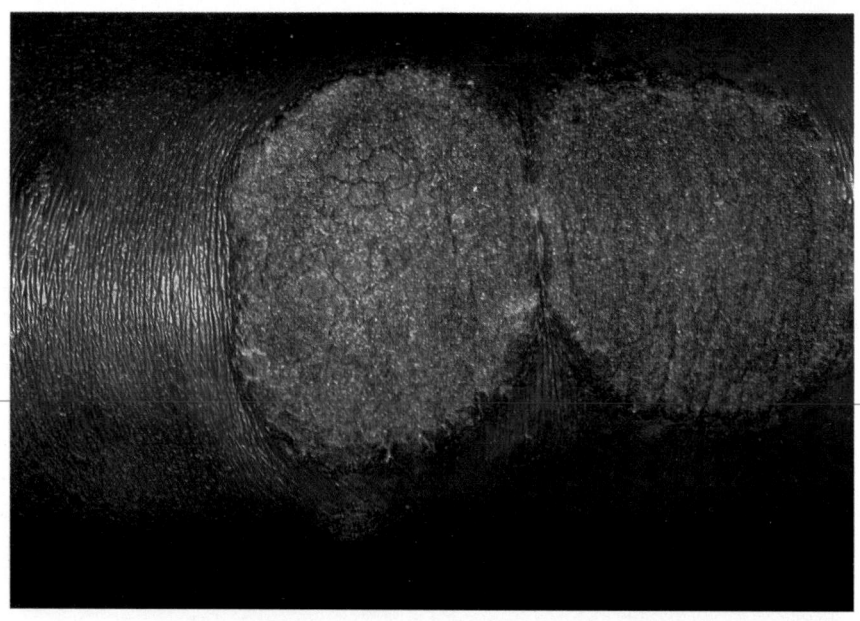

PLATE 4 Scaling lesions of psoriasis.
(Courtesy David Bickers, M.D., Cleveland, Ohio.)

(Plates 5 and 6 courtesy David Bickers, M.D., Cleveland, Ohio.)

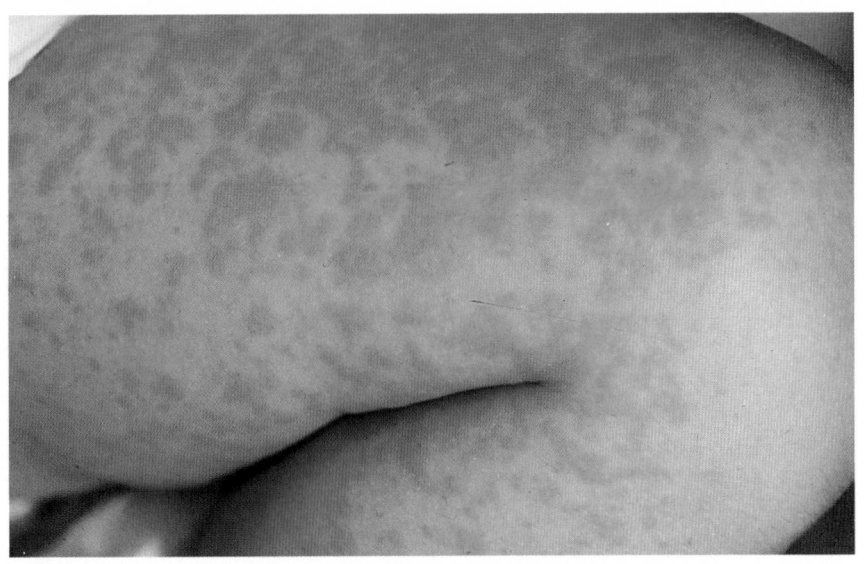

PLATE 5   Maculopapular rash resulting from a drug allergy.

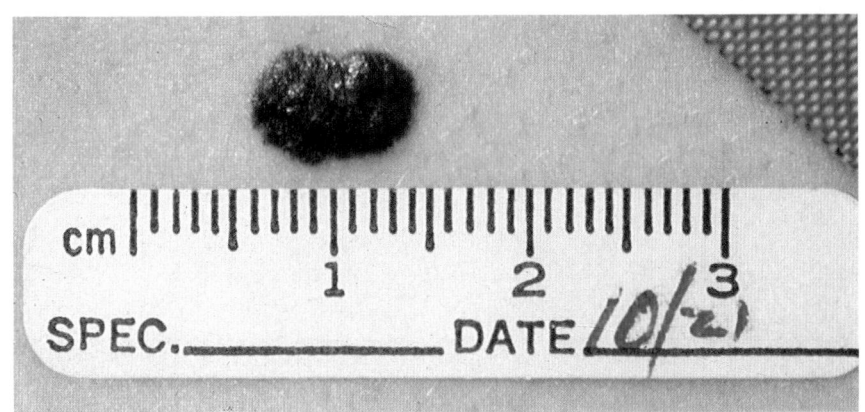

PLATE 6   Malignant melanoma.

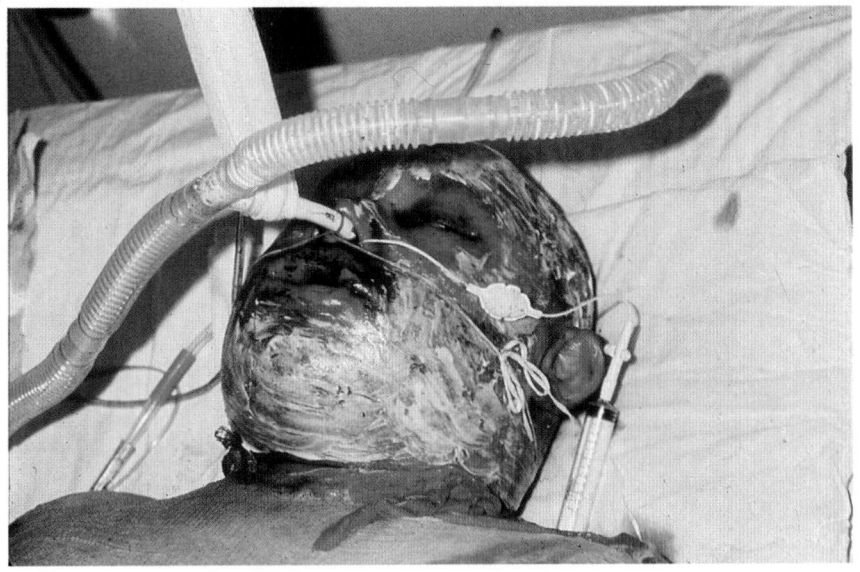

PLATE 7   Endotracheal intubation for patient with severe edema 5 hours postburn. *(Courtesy Burn Center, Cleveland Metropolitan General Hospital.)*

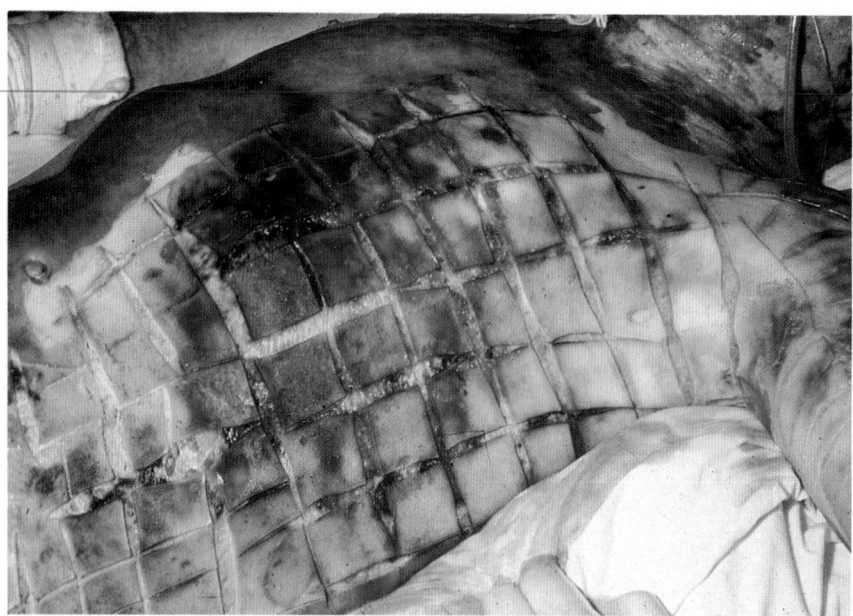

PLATE 8 Grid escharotomy used to alleviate circulatory and pulmonary constriction. *(Courtesy Burn Center, Cleveland Metropolitan General Hospital.)*

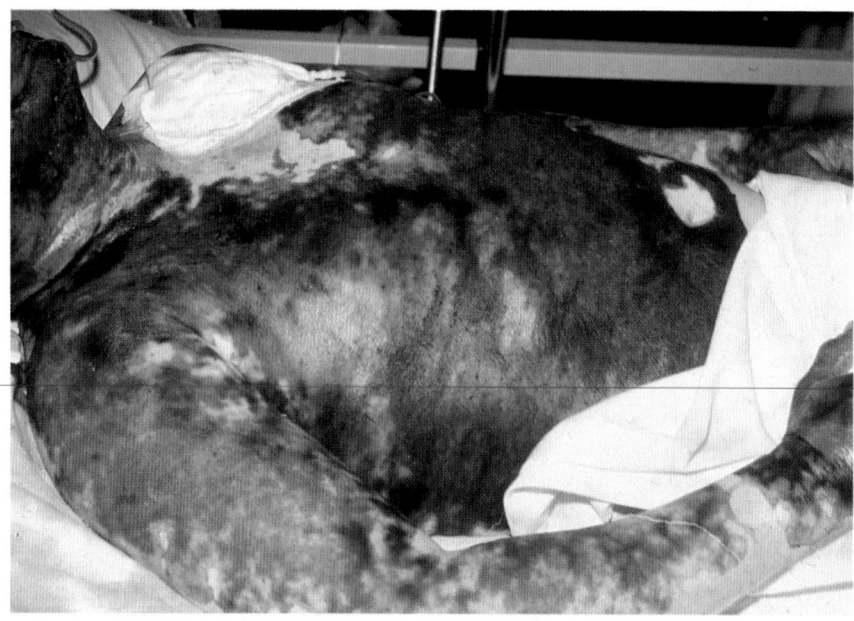

PLATE 9 Postburn *Pseudomonas* infection. *(Courtesy Burn Center, Cleveland Metropolitan General Hospital.)*

effect of the lotion.) A gauze pledget may be used to apply extremely thin lotions. Lotions with an oily base are applied thinly and evenly with the palm of the hand. A small area of skin is often tested to determine whether the cream or lotion will be tolerated over the entire body. The topical medication is applied to a small area, about 4 cm (1.5 in), on the person's forearm. The time and exact location of the trial are recorded, and the skin response to the trial medication is observed after 24 hours.

Ointments do not usually leave an oily residue on the skin unless they have a petroleum base. A nonporous covering such as plastic should not be used over an ointment unless so prescribed, because the heat retention may increase percutaneous absorption of the medication.

Ointments may be applied by the patient with gloved hands or with the bare palm, depending on the type of ointment used (gloves should be used by health care professionals). If a dressing is to be applied, the ointment may be spread on the dressing with a tongue blade before application to the skin. Anthralin may be caustic to normal skin, so gloves should be worn. Crude coal tar is always applied in firm, long, downward strokes to prevent folliculitis, because tar is an irritant. Creams, as opposed to ointments, may be rubbed in. When ointments are applied at frequent intervals (4-6 hours), the remaining ointment is removed before more ointment is applied.

Wet dermatologic dressings

Wet dressings are used frequently over various lesions for cooling, drying, antipruritic, vasoconstricting, or debriding effects. Plain tap water or physiologic saline solution may be used or medications may be added. An astringent effect may be obtained with the use of Burow's solution.

The type of dressing material used for a wet dressing should not have a cotton filling, because cotton leaves particles and a residue on the skin, which may cause irritation. Several layers of fine mesh gauze are ideal, and roller gauze or Kerlix may be used for extremities. A face mask may be designed by cutting openings for the eyes, nose, and mouth from several thicknesses of gauze. At home, muslin-type cotton material such as clean old sheets may be used; the materials need not be sterilized but are washed or discarded every 24 hours.

The best effects of wet dressings are obtained by several treatment periods spaced over the waking hours (Box 43-4). The solution is applied at room temperature to prevent the marked vasoconstriction with subsequent vasodilation that occurs with cold solutions. Although the dressings can be kept wet by adding solution, this usually leads to excessive dripping.

Interventions to achieve patient outcomes

Specific nursing interventions are summarized in Box 43-5. General nursing interventions are described below.

Promoting comfort

Pain with skin inflammations is usually minimal except in selected situations such as herpes zoster. In general, aspirin or acetaminophen usually suffice as analgesics, and the application of wet dressings and topical medications usually relieves most discomfort from pain. Pruritus (itching) is a major discomfort, to one extent or another, with skin inflammations.

Pathophysiology of pruritus. Pruritus is a cutaneous symptom that provokes the desire to scratch and is an underlying symptom of many disorders. It is a modified form of pain but is less tolerable. It occurs only in the skin, certain mucous membranes, and the eyes. The areas most sensitive to itching are the nostrils, mucocutaneous junction, external ear canal, and perineum.

One of the most common causes of pruritus is dry skin, sometimes occurring as a result of excessive bathing, particularly with bubble bath, which has a drying effect. Other causes of pruritus include the following:
Skin irritants: plastic or glass fibers, wool, plant products
Insects
Drug reactions
Psychogenic reactions
Skin diseases: inflammations, dermatitis
Infectious diseases
Systemic diseases: obstructive biliary disease (jaundice), uremia, diabetes mellitus
Neoplasia: Hodgkin's disease, leukemia, lymphoma
Factors that can intensify itching include vasodilation, tissue anoxia, and stasis of circulation. Pruritus leads to the motor response of scratching. Persons with very intense itching may excoriate the skin severely by digging deeply into the skin with their fingernails when trying to alleviate the itch. Persons with generalized itching may be observed to be in almost constant motion—twisting, rubbing, and scratching.

General management for relief of pruritus
1. Apply cold to cause vasoconstriction.
2. Avoid soaps and detergents with dry skin; use a bath oil.
3. Hydrate in a tepid bath followed by immediate application of an emollient lotion.
4. Use cool, light, nonrestrictive clothing or bedclothes.
5. Keep nails trimmed to avoid skin excoriation from scratching.
6. Keep the room cool (about 20° C, or 68° to 70° F) and increase the humidity (30% to 40%).

43-4

Application of dermatologic wet dressings

1. Prepare solution to apply at room temperature. Sterility is not required.
2. Soak dressing thoroughly in solution.
3. Protect bed or clothing with towel or bath blanket.
4. Wring out dressing (should be wet but not dripping).
5. Apply dressings in smooth layers (two to four layers); wrap fingers and toes separately; wrap joints so that they can bend.
6. Remove, soak, and reapply dressings every 3 to 5 minutes.
7. Continue treatment for 20 to 30 minutes.
8. Pat skin dry.

43-5

The patient with an inflammatory skin disorder

Bacterial infections

Cleanse skin well with soap and water or with hexachlorophene.
Use wet compresses to apply heat or as a medium for medication (for example, Burow's solution).
Apply prescribed antibiotic topical medication.
Elevate an extremity with cellulitis.
Teach family members how to prevent spread of staphylococcal infections:
  Avoidance of contamination from drainage
  Cleansing practices
  Disposal of contaminated articles

Viral inflammations

Assist with relief of pain and pruritus:
  Loose clothing to minimize contact
  Analgesics as prescribed
  Warm moist compresses
  Spirits of camphor or camphorated lip ice to oral lesions of herpes simplex
  Neuralgia after herpes zoster:
    Analgesics as prescribed (narcotics are usually avoided)
    Tranquilizers and sedatives as prescribed
    Ethyl chloride spray for possible temporary relief
    Other forms of pain relief measures (see Chapter 10) that might be helpful
  Calamine lotion over vesicular areas to relieve itching

Fungal inflammations

Promote dryness of affected area:
  Area dried well after washing
  Powders applied lightly to prevent maceration and caking
  Clean loose-fitting clothing for aeration
  For athlete's foot, cotton socks, changed at least daily; sandal-type shoes when possible
Promote healing:
  Give prescribed topical medication
  Teach need for continuation of treatment for prescribed time (may be weeks or months)

Parasitic infestations

Wash area well before treatment.
Remove nits with a fine-toothed comb.
Apply a *thin* layer of prescribed lotion or cream.
Shampoo, shower, or bathe thoroughly after prescribed time to remove medication.
If eyelashes are involved, remove nits and apply petroleum jelly to smother lice.
Give analgesics or antipruritic agents as necessary.
Teach prevention of spread to all family members:
  Machine wash clothing and bed linens
  Dry clothing and linens in dryer or iron after line drying
  Dry clean clothing that cannot be washed
  Treat all family members and household linens if one is infested

43-6

Guidelines for baths and soaks

1. The water temperature should be of comfort to patient—usually 32° to 38°C (90° to 100°F).
2. Medication should be completely dissolved while tub is filled.
3. The soak should last 20 to 30 minutes.
4. Persons are assisted out of the water when oils are added, to prevent slipping.
5. A rubber mat will help prevent slipping.
6. Skin is *patted* dry, not rubbed, to avoid skin irritation.
7. Creams or ointments are applied immediately after the bath to retain moisture.
8. After a medicated bath, pour 1 cup bleach into used tub water; let stand 5 minutes; wipe sides and bottom of tub; drain tub and clean as usual.

Baths and soaks

Tub baths or soaks to a specific part of the body are soothing and antipruritic and are an effective means of rehydrating the skin. Substances may be added to the bath for special therapeutic effects (Table 43-8). Guidelines for baths and soaks are listed in Box 43-6.

Facilitating learning
Prevention of spread

Bacterial infections and parasitic infestations may spread to other persons, particularly caregivers and family members, if precautions are not instituted.

For *staphylococcal* infections in hospitalized patients, wound isolation procedures are instituted until drainage subsides. Hands must be washed thoroughly after contact with the patient. Gloves are usually worn when changing dressings.

It is not uncommon for entire families to have some type of staphylococcal infection after one member has had a boil. Teaching includes the following:

1. All family members should bathe and shampoo daily with bacteriostatic soap while infection lasts.
2. Razor blades are discarded after use.
3. Separate bath linens are used by each family member.
4. Bath linens are changed daily while infection lasts.
5. Contaminated wound supplies are discarded in two sealed plastic bags.

With *parasitic* infestations, all family members should take one treatment to prevent spread. Clothing, linen, and towels are washed, then dried in an automatic dryer or ironed after line drying, or are dry cleaned. Garments that have been stored for 1 month will not be infested. No special precautions are needed for other objects, because parasites do not live long away from the host.

When caring for persons with *herpetic* lesions, the Centers for Disease Control (CDC) recommends the use of drainage and secretion precautions (see Chapter 17) until all lesions are crusted. Finger infection (herpetic whitlow, Table 43-4) may result from contact with the herpes sim-

Table 43-8 Preparations commonly used for baths or soaks

Substance	Effect	Suggested actions
Colloids: oatmeal, cornstarch, soybean powder	Antipruritic, drying	Tub surfaces become very slippery; support person to prevent falls
Potassium permanganate	Antifungal, drying, deodorizing	Strain pulverized tablet through cheesecloth to prevent irritation; stains surfaces and linens
Burow's solution (aluminum acetate)	Antibacterial, drying	Commonly used for soaks
Sulfur bath suspension	Antibacterial	Rinse body with tepid water after bath to remove residual sulfur particles
Tar preparations (Balnetar, Zetar, Alma-Tar, Polytar)	Antipruritic, moisturizing	Do not use soap with tar baths
Bath oils: Alpha-Keri, Jeri-Bath, Domol	Antipruritic, moisturizing	Tub surfaces may become slippery

plex virus. To help prevent a disseminated infection, strict isolation precautions are used for protection of the immunocompromised person with a localized herpes zoster infection.

Self-help skills

Many persons with skin inflammations will be carrying out treatments at home and, therefore, may need teaching about therapeutic measures. Written instructions are more likely to be followed correctly. Points to stress in teaching include the following:

1. Use medication only as prescribed.
2. Avoid harsh rubbing of the skin.
3. Avoid nonporous covering over dressing unless prescribed.
4. Dissolve completely all solid medications added to baths and soaks.
5. Apply lotions and powders in thin layers.
6. Use old clean sheets, if desired, for wet dressings.

Evaluation

Evaluation is based on expected patient outcomes. Questions to consider may include the following:

1. Is the person comfortable?
2. Does the person know how to care for the lesions at home?

ACNE

The major form of acne is acne vulgaris seen mostly in adolescents, although it may occur in adults. A different form is acne rosacea seen in adults.

ACNE VULGARIS

Etiology

Acne vulgaris is a common skin disorder, the cause of which is unknown but is thought to be multifactorial. Contributing factors may include free fatty acids, endocrine effects, stress, heredity, and infection. Diet and dirt are not causes of acne.[13] The disorder is more quiescent in summer because of the drying effects of the sun.

Prevention

Actions that contribute to plugging of the pilosebaceous follicles are to be avoided.

1. Keep hair and hands away from face.
2. Shampoo hair and scalp frequently.
3. Wear loose clothing and avoid tight collars.
4. Keep skin clean; avoid greasy, oil-based cosmetics.

Pathophysiology

At puberty sebaceous glands undergo enlargement from androgen stimulation. When sebum is released it passes through the follicular canal, where it is combined with sebaceous gland cell fragments, epidermal cells, and bacteria. The sebum and debris may become plugged in the hair follicle (Fig. 43-5) to form an *open comedo* (blackhead) if it is at the surface, or a *closed comedo* (whitehead) if it is below the surface. The dark color of the blackhead is melanin, not dirt, and results from passage of melanin from the adjoining epidermal cells.

Inflammatory lesions apparently develop from escape of sebum into the dermis; the sebum then serves as an irritant, causing an inflammatory reaction. Free fatty acids may also be an irritant in the follicle itself.

Acne occurs mostly on the face and neck, upper chest, and back, although the upper arms, buttocks, and thighs may also be involved. Comedones are the first visible signs, and the skin is characteristically oily. The inflammatory lesions include papules, pustules, nodules, and cysts. Superficial lesions usually heal without scarring, whereas large lesions often result in scarring if the inflammation has involved the dermis. The typical scar resembles an old volcano (ice-pick scar); however, many other sizes and shapes may result, depending on the depth and extent of the inflammatory lesions.

Interventions

The major medical therapy for acne is drug therapy. *Systemic* therapy includes isotretinoin (Accutane) or antibiotics (tetracycline, erythromycin). *Topical* therapy with tretinoin (Retin-A) is effective. Sulfur-zinc lotion or benzoyl peroxide may also be used. Commercial preparations contain benzoyl peroxide. *Intralesional* therapy with corticosteroids may be given for acute inflamed lesions. Come-

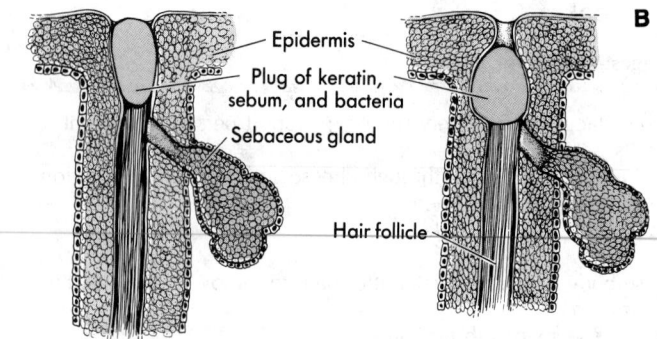

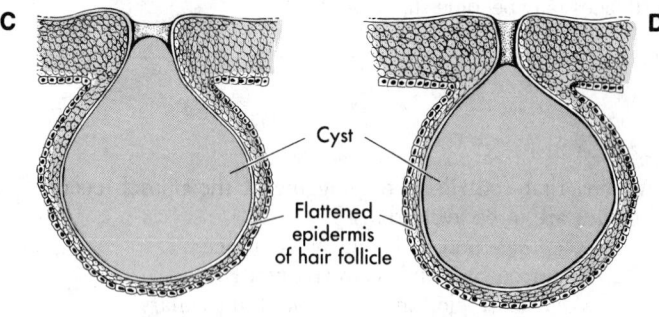

Fig. 43-5 Formation of lesions in acne vulgaris. **A,** Open comedo (blackhead), early stage. **B,** closed comedo (whitehead), early stage. **C,** Cyst formation in open comedo, advanced stage. **D,** Cyst formation in closed comedo, advanced stage. (From Parish JH: *Dermatology and skin care*, New York, 1975, McGraw-Hill.)

dones may be removed with a comedo extractor. Disfiguring scars may be removed by dermabrasion or laser reconstruction (p. 1495).

Counseling and teaching are the major nursing therapies. Stress appears to be one of the causative factors; therefore, the person may be helped by identifying and coping with stressors (Chapter 6). Acne can be a stressor, producing facial disfigurements and sometimes leading to behavior that is hostile, aggressive, and anxious, as well as shy and withdrawn. Psychologic counseling is often desirable. Teaching the person with acne includes the following:

1. General skin care
    a. Keep skin clean; wash face two to three times daily.
    b. Use a medicated soap/cleanser or agent prescribed by physician.
    c. Avoid vigorous rubbing of the skin (prevent further inflammation).
    d. Use cosmetics that are water based rather than cream based and avoid those that contain wax esters.
    e. Never leave cosmetics on face at night.
2. During therapy
    a. Follow the prescribed therapy even when immediate improvement is not noted for 2 to 3 weeks.
    b. Expect skin desquamation during therapy.

c. Avoid using self-remedies during therapy.
d. Remove cosmetics before applying topical medications.
e. Avoid exposure to direct sunlight if using tretinoin or taking tetracycline (photosensitivity).
f. Avoid pregnancy if taking Accutane (possibility of birth defects).

ACNE ROSACEA

Acne rosacea is a skin condition that usually affects persons over 25 years of age. The actual cause is unknown although many causative factors have been suggested. Acne rosacea begins with redness over the cheeks and nose, followed by papules, pustules, and enlargement of superficial blood vessels. Years of acne rosacea lead to an irregular, bulbous thickening of the skin of the distal part of the nose (rhinophyma), with a red-purple discoloration and dilated follicles.

Treatment includes systemic tetracycline, metronidazole, or isotretinoin (Accutane). Topical therapy for papules and pustules may be prescribed: hydrocortisone cream, topical antibiotics, mitronidazol cream (MetroGel), or benzoyl peroxide. Avoiding stimuli that cause vasodilation seems appropriate. Rhinophyma may be treated by plastic surgery.

DERMATITIS

Dermatitis, a superficial inflammation of the skin, refers to several different conditions resulting in the same type of lesions (Table 43-9). The term *eczema* is often used synonymously with dermatitis but frequently refers to the chronic type.

Etiology and Pathophysiology

Contact dermatitis may result from irritation of the skin from the substance itself (*irritant contact dermatitis*) (see Plates 2 and 3) or from a hypersensitivity immune reaction from contact with a *specific* antigen (*allergic contact dermatitis*) (Table 43-10). The sensitizing allergen may reach the site by direct contact; by indirect contact such as transmission by animals, from one part of the body to the other, by the hands, or on clothing; or by the air such as in smoke.

Atopic dermatitis is hereditary hypersensitivity of the skin that lowers the threshold to pruritus so that minor stimuli cause intense itching. Exacerbating factors include sudden changes in temperature or humidity; exercise; psychologic stress; fibers such as wool, fur, or nylon; detergents; and perfumes. There is a marked tendency toward vasoconstriction of superficial blood vessels, and the skin blanches readily. Adults with eczema often have had atopic dermatitis during infancy and adolescence.

Persons with atopic dermatitis are highly susceptible to viral infections, especially herpes, and to bacterial infections such as those caused by *Staphylococcus* or beta hemolytic *Streptococcus*. There is also an increased incidence of fungal infections such as tinea.

Stasis dermatitis results from decreased circulation in the legs. The cause of *sehorrheic* dermatitis (dandruff) is

REVIEW

Table 43-9   Types of dermatitis

Type	Signs and symptoms	Medical therapy
Contact	Site and pattern of lesions depend on exposure pattern; erythema, local edema, vesicles, then oozing, crusting and scaling; pruritus Chronic: skin becomes brownish and thickened	Weeping uninfected lesions: wet dressings with Burow's solution; topical steroids; systemic corticosteroids for acute conditions
Atopic	Pruritus; lesions similar to contact dermatitis; become localized in adults to antecubital and popliteal areas, behind ears, under chin	Same as above
Stasis	Skin reddened and edematous, pruritus, infection from excoriations with scratching	Elevation of legs; wet compresses for weeping lesions, topical corticosteroids
Seborrheic (dandruff)	Erythematous scaly lesions of scalp, face, ears, chest, or back	Selsun Blue shampoo for scalp; topical steroids for severe lesions

Table 43-10   Common causes of contact dermatitis of different areas

Area	Cause
Face	Cosmetics, hair sprays, hair dyes, airborne contactants
Earlobes	Nickel
Ears	
Pinnae	Photosensitizers
Canals	Medications
Eyelids	Cosmetics, airborne sensitizers, transfer by hands
Nose (bridge)	Metal or plastic spectacle supports
Lips and perioral area	Toothpaste, lipstick
Neck	Perfumes, clothing (especially wool)
Axillae	Deodorants, clothing, perfumes
Scapular area	Nickel in clasps on straps
Breasts	Elastic and other brassiere material
Waist	Elastic
Perianal area	Dibucaine (Nupercaine) and other medications, excessive use of cleansers
Arms and legs	Poison ivy and other plants
Wrists	Nickel, etc., in watchbands
Hands	Detergents and other cleansers, gloves
Feet	Medication for "athlete's foot," shoes

From Moschella SL, Hurley HJ: *Dermatology,* ed 3, Philadelphia, 1991, WB Saunders.

basically genetic and is influenced by factors such as hormones, nutrition, infection, and stress.[49]

Nursing Process
Assessment
Subjective data

When acute lesions from contact dermatitis or exacerbation of eczema occur, it is important to identify the causative factors in order to avoid further contacts or to change, if possible, any exacerbating factor. Data to collect initially include the following:

1. Knowledge of causative factors and method of contact
2. Possible contacts with irritants in the home, at work, or during recreational activities
3. History of recurrent infections (possible decreased immune response)
4. New drug prescriptions, especially penicillin or sulfanilamide
5. Increase in stress noted by patient
6. Alleviating factors (physician or self-prescribed)
7. Extent of pruritus and alleviating factors

Objective data

The lesions are inspected daily for changes and presence of infections. Observations are also made concerning the extent of scratching of the lesions by the patient.

Diagnostic tests

Hypersensitivity to specific antigens can be tested in vivo by skin tests or by the use test (Chapter 41). In skin testing, the antigens are administered to the skin either through intradermal, scratch or patch tests, or an allergen may be instilled in the eye.

Data analysis: nursing diagnoses

Nursing diagnoses are determined from analysis of patient data. Possible nursing diagnoses for the person with dermatitis may include, but are not limited to, the following:

Diagnostic title	Possible etiologies
Pain: itching	Skin lesions
Knowledge deficit	Lack of exposure/recall, information misinterpretation

Planning: expected patient outcomes

Expected patient outcomes for the person with dermatitis may include, but are not limited to, the following:
1. States itching is decreased.
2. Describes:
   a. Causative agents (if known), source of the agent, and method of control
   b. Measures to prevent further contact
   c. Problems of self-treatment
   d. Treatment measures to be carried out at home

Implementation
Assisting with achievement of therapeutic goals

Weeping infected lesions respond rapidly to wet dressings with Burow's solution (p. 1479) for 20 minutes four times daily. Crusts and scales are not removed but are allowed to drop off naturally as the skin heals.

The major form of *topical* therapy consists of corticosteroid cream or ointment. Fluorinated corticosteroids may be used for localized lesions in adults but are *never used on the face*. An occlusion wrap over the steroid in adults may enhance the steroid effect but may lead to folliculitis. The occlusion wrap consists of a nonpermeable covering, such as plastic wrap, over the dressing; it is only applied when prescribed by the physician.

Interventions to achieve patient outcomes
Promoting comfort

The focus of care is relief of the pruritus in order to break the itch-scratch cycle that leads to lesions and discomfort. Measures to promote relief of itching are described on p. 1479. Application of the wet dressings and topical steroids helps to reduce the itching. Colloidal baths may be helpful. Sedatives and tranquilizers are used judiciously to help decrease itching but not induce sleepiness.

Facilitating learning

The more the person knows about the condition and what will affect it, the better the person can prevent further contacts and enhance recovery. Teaching includes avoidance of exacerbating factors, positive effects of sunlight, and dangers of self-treatment (see Box 43-7).

Evaluation

Evaluation is based on expected patient outcomes. Questions to consider may include the following:
1. Is itching decreased?
2. Does the person know how to care for the skin at home and how to prevent further recurrence?

SCALING PAPULAR DISORDERS

Papulosquamous disorders are characterized by papular lesions with scaling borders. The most common of these is *psoriasis* (Table 43-11). There are no precipitating factors

---

43-7 · **Patient Teaching**

The patient with dermatitis

Describe nature of the causative agent (if known) and method of contact; avoidance of agent
Avoid extremes of heat and cold
Avoid dry skin:
  No harsh soaps and detergents (use a mild soap such as Ivory)
  Soak in bath water (oil may be added) for 20 to 30 minutes
  Apply steroid cream directly after bath
Avoid wool, nylon, or fur fibers on sensitized skin
Use gloves if necessary to handle irritant or allergenic substance
Limit strenuous exercise, especially in hot weather (leads to itching)
Expose affected areas to sunlight (improves condition)
Describe dangers of self-treatment (may lead to delay in healing and increase in infected lesions or to increased absorption through denuded skin areas)
Avoid other persons with infections (for those with atopic dermatitis)

---

for psoriasis, but some persons may develop exacerbations after climatic changes, stress, trauma, or infection. Pregnant women often see a remission of symptoms. *Pityriasis rosea* occurs mostly in the spring or fall; the cause is unknown. *Lichen planus* may follow exposure to dyes, color film developer, or gold, but usually the cause is unknown.

Pathophysiology of Psoriasis

The turnover time for normal skin is 28 days. After the cells in the basal layer of the skin divide, it normally takes them 14 days to reach the stratum corneum (outer skin layer) and an additional 14 days for the cells to be sloughed off. In psoriasis the time is accelerated to 4 to 7 days. Much of the scaling (see Plate 4) seen in psoriasis is rapid shedding of the cells; treatment is therefore based on slowing the mitotic activity.

Nursing Process
Assessment

Subjective data include the following:
1. Knowledge about the disease
2. Measures used for control at home
3. Concerns about appearance
4. Usual recreational and social activities

Objective data include observations regarding changes in the lesions.

Data analysis: nursing diagnoses

Nursing diagnoses are determined from analysis of patient data. Possible nursing diagnoses for the person with psoriasis may include, but are not limited to, the following:

Diagnostic title	Possible etiologies
Body image disturbance	Change in body appearance
Knowledge deficit	Lack of exposure/recall, information misinterpretation

REVIEW

Table 43-11   Types of papulosquamous disorders

Type	Characteristics	Signs and symptoms	Medical therapy
Psoriasis	Common hereditary chronic disorder; not infectious or contagious; has periods of exacerbation	Elevated, erythematous, sharply circumscribed, scaling plaques; occur mostly on scalp, elbows, and knees; mild pruritus; nails become yellowed and pitted	Wet dressings with acute flare-ups; topical steroids with occlusive wraps; PUVA therapy; coal tar therapy followed by ultraviolet light; anthralin
Pityriasis rosea	Common skin disorder in young adults, especially women; not contagious; lasts 6 to 8 weeks, rarely recurs	Starts with single lesion; oval, thin scaly border, yellowish center; multiple lesions appear later; pruritus	Topical steroids; ultraviolet light, systemic steroids in severe cases
Lichen planus	Common skin disorder; may resolve in 6 to 18 months or become chronic	Shiny flat-topped papules on flexor surfaces of wrists, ankles, trunk, and mucous membranes; severe pruritus; nails become distorted	Topical steroids with occlusive wrap; intralesional or systemic steroids, PUVA therapy; isotretinoin (Accutane) or etretinate (Tegison) orally

Table 43-12   Psoriasis therapy

Type	Action	Comments
Bland emollients (petrolatum, mineral oil)	Hydration of skin	Use for mild lesions Facilitates scale removal
Keratolytics (salicylic acid, ammoniated mercury)	Hydration and softening of skin Antimitotic	Avoid using on face Cover with occlusive wraps May cause skin maceration and folliculitis Not applied to irritated skin
Corticosteroids	Antimitotic Antiinflammatory	Topical use for most lesions; cover with occlusive wraps; may cause folliculitis Intralesional use for plaques Rarely given systemically May produce rebound psoriasis when withdrawn
Coal tar preparations	Action unknown Have keratolytic, antipruritic, and photosensitizing effects	May develop folliculitis with long-term use Avoid direct sunlight for 24 hours after use Avoid use on face Stains skin, hair, and clothing Available as cream, lotion, gel, solution, and shampoo May be used with ultraviolet light therapy (Goeckerman routine)
Anthralin products	Antimitotic Inhibits enzyme metabolism	May cause skin irritation Not applied to open skin areas Petrolatum is used to protect normal skin during therapy Wear gloves during application; stains skin, hair, and clothing Avoid using on face
Photochemotherapy with ultraviolet light	Inhibition of DNA synthesis	May cause pruritus, erythema, vesicles, flare-up of lesions, transient nausea May be carcinogenic for light-skinned persons or those previously exposed to x-ray therapy Avoid direct sunlight for 12 to 24 hours after ingestion of Psoralen
Methotrexate	Antimitotic Inhibition of DNA synthesis	For severe lesions not amenable to other treatment Given orally unless nausea is present Requires close monitoring of hematologic, renal, and liver functioning
Synthetic retinoids	Corrects abnormal cell differentiation	Used for severe pustular psoriasis Side effects: pruritus, lip edema, sore mouth, thirst, fragile skin, peeling of palms and soles May be used with anthralin or ultraviolet therapies

Planning: expected patient outcomes

Expected patient outcomes for the person with psoriasis may include, but are not limited to, the following:

1. Participates in social activities.
2. Describes:
   a. The nature of the disorder (noncurable, recurrence of symptoms).
   b. Problems with self-medication.
   c. The prescribed treatment program.

Implementation
Assisting with achievement of therapeutic goals

Although there are several therapeutic regimens for psoriasis (Table 43-12), the more common treatments are steroids under occlusive wraps, crude tar therapy, and PUVA therapy.

Application of occlusive wrap

Occlusive wraps are usually prescribed over topical steroid therapy for psoriasis. Plastic wrap or plastic bags may be used to cover large areas. The bags should not be rapidly flammable. If large areas must be covered for home therapy, a plastic exercise body suit can be worn, particularly for overnight therapy.

Crude tar therapy

Coal tar preparations may be applied as a topical medication, as a bath (Balnetar), or in combination with ultraviolet light (UVA). In the latter case the tar preparation is applied 12 hours before the UVA treatment. Estar Gel or Fototar are applied to the affected area for 5 minutes, then the excess is removed by patting with tissue to minimize staining. Areas treated with coal tar preparation should be protected from direct sunlight for at least 24 hours after application of the tar product. Folliculitis may result from coal tar therapy.

PUVA therapy

PUVA therapy consists of a combination of orally administered methoxsalen (Psoralen) and long-wave ultraviolet light (UVA), hence the name. Methoxsalen is a photosensitizing agent. The person is exposed to UVA 2 hours after ingestion of the methoxsalen. Some side effects of PUVA therapy include pruritus, erythema, localized blistering, a moderate flare-up of psoriasis, and transient nausea. Because the skin remains photosensitive until methoxsalen is excreted, persons receiving this treatment are warned to avoid exposure to the sun for at least 8 hours after ingestion of the medication.

Interventions to achieve patient outcomes
Counseling and teaching

Because the lesions are commonly found on visible skin areas, persons with psoriasis are faced with a socially disabling disease. They may need help in identifying and coping with their feelings and with changes that may occur in their life-style. Arms and legs can be covered with clothing if the person is sensitive about appearance. Social contacts are encouraged.

Lesions may fade with treatment, only to recur eventually in the same area or elsewhere. The disease is not curable and may wax and wane continuously. Persons who are not aware of this may lose confidence in the physician and seek a quick cure. Because psoriasis is so common and so stubborn in response to treatment, manufacturers of patent remedies find a lucrative field for their products among persons with the disease. Self-treatment may lead to considerable expense for worthless products, increased discomfort, and delay in treatment of acute episodes. Persons with psoriasis are encouraged to consult a dermatologist as needed.

Evaluation

Evaluation is based on expected patient outcomes. Questions to consider may include the following:

1. Is the person planning social activities with others?
2. Does the person know the nature of the disease (incurable)?
3. Does the person plan to follow medical therapy (rather than self-treatment) when exacerbation occurs?

SKIN REACTIONS FROM SYSTEMIC DISEASES

Changes in the skin may result from systemic conditions, most commonly dermatitis medicamentosa, erythema multiforme, and discoid lupus erythematosus.

DERMATITIS MEDICAMENTOSA

Skin lesions may result from toxic, metabolic, or allergic reactions to drugs (Table 43-13). Many of the reactions are hypersensitivity immune reactions and include fever, malaise, and vasculitis in addition to skin changes. The rash is often a bright red color, semiconfluent, maculopapular (see Plate 5), generalized, and bilateral. It can appear at any time, but the onset is usually sudden. Hypersensitivity occurs early when previous sensitization has taken place.

Persons are asked upon hospitalization if they have any allergies. For drug allergies, a sticker indicating the drug is placed on every physician's order sheet to alert the physician or nurse not to order or give the drug to the patient. Sudden skin changes in patients receiving medications are brought to the physician's attention.

Teaching the patient may include the suggestion that the patient wear a Medic-Alert bracelet specifying the drug to which the patient is allergic so that the drug is not administered unknowingly in an emergency situation. Persons who are taking drugs that cause photosensitivity reactions are advised to avoid direct exposure to sunlight.

ERYTHEMA MULTIFORME

Erythema multiforme is a skin condition believed to occur secondary to an underlying systemic disease such as an infection. The skin eruption is characterized by red to purple macules, papules, and vesicles, and may be preceded by fever, chest pain, and arthralgia. The treatment is to

Nursing Care Plan	**Person with psoriasis**

DATA: Mrs. L., age 35, was referred to a psoriasis day-care center for a 6-day Goeckerman regimen therapy (crude tar with exposure to ultraviolet light). Mrs. L. told the nurse that she recently sent away for a new ointment that was supposed to cure her psoriasis, but the lesions began to flare up and itching increased. She also said that her husband has been urging her to go out with him more to social events, but her arms and legs have "looked so bad" that she has not wanted others to see her until she is better.

Nursing diagnosis: Body image disturbance: related to lesions on arms and legs

Expected patient outcomes	Nursing interventions	Rationale
Mrs. L. states plans to go out socially with husband	Help Mrs. L. identify her positive attributes Discuss with Mrs. L. types of clothing that could hide the more obvious lesions	Awareness of positive attributes helps to increase self-esteem Hiding the lesions may help her feel better about herself and increase her desire to interact with others

Nursing diagnosis: Knowledge deficit related to information misinterpretation

Expected patient outcomes	Nursing interventions	Rationale
Mrs. L. describes chronicity of psoriasis and plans to follow only prescribed treatment	Review her understanding of the nature of psoriasis Explain the lack of cure for psoriasis and problems with self-treatment Suggest she discuss with physician lotions or ointments to use after her present treatment when lesions itch or flare up Review with her how to apply ointments	Lesions may fade with treatment only to recur. Self-treatment products are often ineffective and costly Ointment is more effective if spread in thin layer over plaques

Table 43-13 Skin reactions to common medications

Reaction	Medication
Erythematous rash	Antibiotics, sulfonamides, thiazide diuretics, barbiturates, phenylbutazone
Purpura (ecchymosis, petechiae)	Thiazides, sulfonamides, barbiturates, anticoagulants
Mucocutaneous lesions (vesicles, bullae, ulcers)	Sulfonamides, penicillin, barbiturates, phenylbutazone
Urticaria	Penicillin, salicylates
Photosensitivity	Phenothiazines, thiazides, tetracycline, griseofulvin, sulfonamides, chlorpromazine, nalidixic acid, tretinoin (Retin-A), isotretinoin (Accutane), fluorouracil, methotrexate

seek out the underlying cause and eliminate it if possible. Local treatment includes baths, soaks, and dressings. If the lesions appear in the mouth, special mouth care is indicated, including irrigations with warm salt solution.

DISCOID LUPUS ERYTHEMATOSUS

Lupus erythematosus occurs in two forms, systemic (SLE) (see Chapter 40) and discoid (DLE). DLE is a chronic, relatively benign skin condition seen in young adults, rarely after age 50 years. Precipitating factors include physical trauma and stress. There is no cure for DLE.

The lesions of DLE are well demarcated and erythematous, have a characteristic scaly border with an atrophied center, and vary in size. The most common sites are the cheeks (butterfly pattern), scalp, and chest, although other parts of the body may also be involved. In addition to the skin lesions the person may have leukopenia, an increased sedimentation rate, positive response to rheumatoid factor test and serologic test for syphilis (STS), and a low titer of antinuclear factors.

Preventive measures include avoiding physical trauma, such as by using protective lotions to prevent sunburn and wearing warm clothing to protect against cold and wind. If stress is a precipitating factor, measures to reduce stress (see Chapter 6) can be instituted. Palliative measures include topical steroid therapy under occlusive wraps or intralesional steroid therapy.

Table 43-14 Tumors of the skin

Tumor	Description	Medical therapy
Keratoses		
Corn	Thickened skin lesion with a center core that thickens inwardly	Corrective shoes; felt pad with a center hole for relief of pressure
Callus	Thickened horny skin layer in circumscribed lesions often seen on plantar surface of foot	Well-fitting shoes, moleskin and padding; scraping with emery board; salicylic acid plasters
Seborrheic keratosis	Benign tumors; resemble large, darkened, greasy warts	Do not require treatment; may be removed by curettage and electrodesiccation or cryotherapy
Actinic keratosis (senile, solar)	Benign round or irregular tumors; red-brown to gray in color, with a dry scaly appearance; 25% may become malignant	Removal by curettage and electrodesiccation or cryotherapy
Premalignant		
Leukoplakia	Thickened white or reddish patch on mucous membrane of mouth or vagina; may develop into invasive squamous cell carcinoma	Small lesions removed by electrodesiccation; large lesions excised
Pigmented nevi (mole)	Circumscribed pigmented papules; brown moles with hair or evenly colored dark moles are usually benign	Excised for cosmetic reasons or if sudden change in size or color, or bleeding
Malignant		
Squamous cell carcinoma	Malignant tumor of surface epidermis; starts as a firm nodule, becomes indurated with an inflammatory base; may metastasize if on lip or ear (Fig. 43-6)	Removal by surgical excision, curettage with electrodesiccation, irradiation, or chemosurgery
Basal cell carcinoma	Malignant tumor primarily over hairy areas; tumors have a translucent appearance with indurated center; may be ulcerated with crusting; grow slowly and rarely metastasize	Same as above
Malignant melanoma	Most serious but relatively uncommon skin cancer; lesions vary in appearance and rate of growth; often have irregular pigmentation; metastasize frequently; early diagnosis leads to more favorable prognosis	Total wide excision with skin grafts to cover defects in many cases; chemotherapy, immunotherapy
Kaposi's sarcoma	Commonly seen with AIDS; discrete red, purple, or dark plaques or nodules on skin and mucous membranes; slowly progressive	Radiation therapy may be given for palliation

TUMORS OF THE SKIN

Etiology

Over 600,000 cases of skin cancer are diagnosed a year, most of which are basal or squamous cell carcinomas. About 32,000 people are diagnosed yearly with melanoma, the most serious form of skin cancer. The incidence of skin cancer has been increasing at a rate of 4% per year.[1] Tumors of the skin may be benign (keratoses), premalignant, or malignant (Table 43-14).

Pathophysiology

The term *keratosis* refers to any cornification or growth of the horny layer of the skin; keratoses are benign growths. Corns and calluses result from pressure or friction from poorly fitting shoes, faulty weight-bearing, or with neu-

ropathies such as diabetic neuropathy. Seborrheic keratoses are commonly seen in older persons. Actinic keratoses result from exposure of the skin to radiation, primarily solar. They are noted most often on exposed skin areas of persons who work outdoors and on older persons. Light-skinned persons are more vulnerable to skin changes from irradiation. Actinic keratoses may develop into squamous cell carcinomas.

The term *premalignant* does *not* imply that all such lesions become malignant; it does imply that the tendency to become malignant exists. Leukoplakia develop in the mucous membranes of the mouth or vagina; red patches (erythroleukoplakia) have a higher malignancy potential than white patches. External irritants, such as poorly fitting dentures, cheek biting, and pipe or cigarette smoking, appear to have an etiologic relationship to oral leukoplakia. Chronic maceration, friction, and senile atrophy may lead

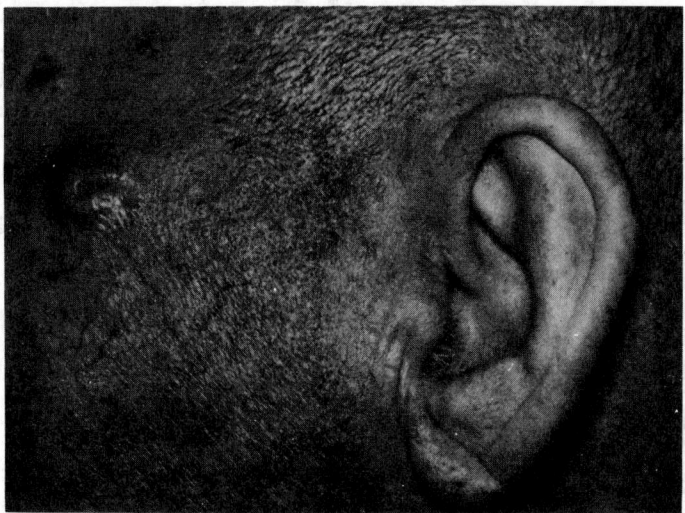

Fig. 43-6   Squamous cell carcinoma in infratemporal area, one of the commonest sites for this tumor. (From Stewart WD, Danto JL, Maddin S: *Dermatology: diagnosis and treatment of cutaneous disorders*, ed 4, St Louis, 1978, Mosby–Year Book.)

to leukoplakia of the vagina. Pigmented nevi are commonly seen in all persons. Benign moles have an even color.

Malignant tumors, with the exception of some tumors such as malignant melanoma, are often of less serious consequence than malignant tumors elsewhere on the body. Skin carcinomas appear mostly on exposed skin or at areas of chronic irritation. Squamous cell carcinomas that develop on hair-bearing skin rarely metastasize, but lesions of the lip or ear frequently metastasize to regional lymph nodes. Basal cell carcinomas grow slowly and rarely metastasize, but untreated tumors can become locally invasive with severe tissue destruction, infection, and hemorrhage.

Prevention

Primary prevention of skin tumors includes protection of the skin from excessive solar radiation and other ultraviolet rays. Preventive measures include the following:

1. Limit sun exposure between 11 AM and and 3 PM (DST) when rays are the strongest (UV rays can pass through clouds and through 3 feet of water).
2. Wear protective clothes when in the sun, such as hats, long sleeves, long pants, and sun glasses.
3. Use a sunscreen with a sun protection factor (SPF) of at least 15. Be sure the sunscreen protects against UVA and UVB rays (benzophenone will do this).
4. Apply sunscreen over all exposed areas 15 to 20 minutes before going outdoors.
5. Avoid tanning lamps (they emit UV rays).

Secondary prevention consists of early detection of skin cancers, especially melanomas. Activities include the following:

1. Do skin self-examination (SSE) monthly after a bath or shower, looking for changes in skin lesions:
   a. Stand before a mirror; examine front, back, and both sides
   b. Check forearms and upper underarms, and backs of legs (may be easier to do this while sitting)

   c. Check back of neck using a hand mirror
   d. Palpate scalp carefully; separate hair to examine any rough surfaces

2. Report the following changes to the physician:
   a. Development of a ring of new pigment around the base of a mole
   b. Development of uneven pigmentation
   c. Sudden growth in size of a mole or tumor
   d. Loss of hair in a mole or sudden growth of hair on a non-hair bearing mole
   e. Bleeding in a mole

Medical Therapy

Methods of therapy for skin tumor include surgery, curettage with electrodesiccation, cryosurgery, or irradiation.

Surgery

Ninety percent of skin tumors are removed by excisional surgery. A punch biopsy may be used for identification of basal cell carcinomas. Superficial lesions can be removed by slicing off the lesion with a sharp blade. This is especially useful for removing flat lesions. *Moh's procedure* removes a malignant lesion in layers, with each layer examined under a microscope to determine where the tumor ends. This produces less loss of underlying healthy tissue.

Curettage with electrodesiccation

The *curet* is a spoon-shaped instrument with sharp edges and is used in a downward scraping motion across a lesion (Fig. 43-7). A local anesthetic is usually first injected around the lesion. Curettage is usually followed by electrodesiccation to stop the bleeding.

In *electrodesiccation* an electric current is used to coagulate the tissue and curtail capillary bleeding. It may also be used to cut tissue under local anesthesia. After most electrosurgical procedures the wound is left exposed to air dry. Dressings may be used if the area is subject to

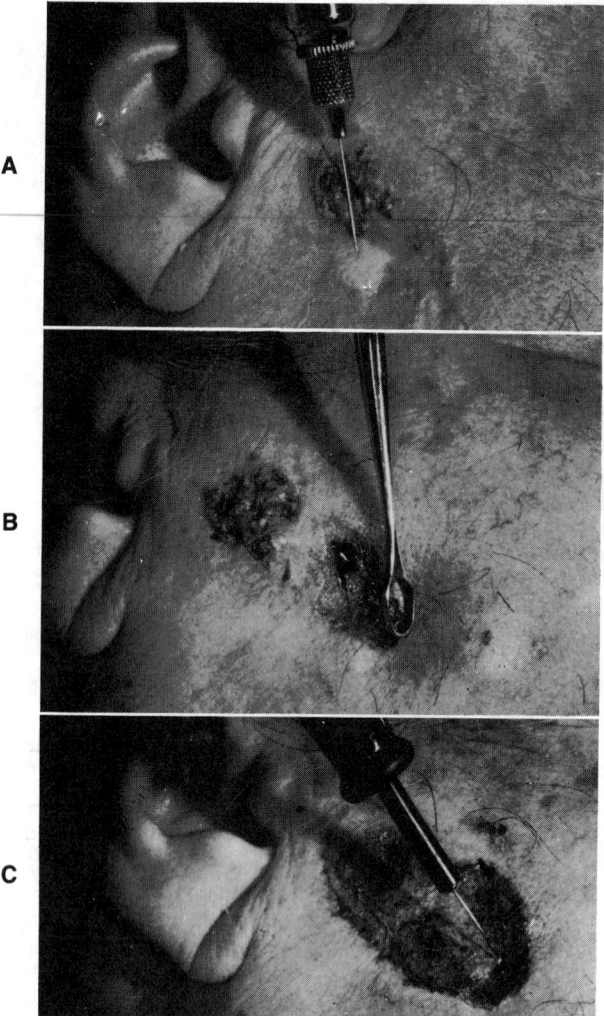

Fig. 43-7 **A,** Infiltration with local anesthesia. **B,** Curettage. **C,** Electrodesiccation for hemostasis. (From Stewart WD, Danto JL, Maddin S: *Dermatology: diagnosis and treatment of cutaneous disorders,* ed 4, St Louis, 1978, Mosby–Year Book.)

frequent trauma or rubbing or if oozing is present. The wound may be wiped with 70% alcohol to hasten drying. A hemostatic nonocclusive dressing may be made by covering the wound with Gelfoam powder and Micropore tape.

Cryosurgery

Cryosurgery is the rapid freezing of tissue with substances such as carbon dioxide snow or liquid nitrogen. The rapid freezing causes formation of intracellular ice, which destroys the cell membranes and produces cell dehydration. Cryosurgery is frequently used for removal of warts and keloids as well as removal of skin tumors (benign and malignant).

Although cryosurgery is not usually painful, a tingling pain occurs when the freezing substance is applied and may be uncomfortable to some persons, particularly if multiple lesions are treated. Local anesthesia may be necessary. Analgesics may be helpful during thawing.

Tissue necrosis may not be evident until 24 hours after cryosurgery. A clear or hemorrhagic bulla forms during the first day, but inflammatory reactions and bleeding are unusual. A serous exudate occurs during the first week, followed by eschar, or crust, formation. The crust drops off in 3 to 4 weeks as the underlying tissue heals. Scarring usually results. Hypopigmentation may occur because melanocytes are highly vulnerable to freezing.

Irradiation

X-ray therapy may be used in the treatment of basal cell carcinoma for selected tumors, especially when there are poorly defined margins or when the tumors are located in structures that are difficult to reconstruct, such as the eyelids or the tip of the nose.[56]

MALIGNANT MELANOMA

Melanomas differ from the other types of skin cancers because of the higher incidence of metastasis and mortality. Most deaths from skin cancer result from melanomas. The incidence of melanomas in the United States has been increasing in recent years, probably because of increased exposure to the sun. Persons with light skin are at increased risk for melanoma.

There are various types of melanomas. Two thirds of the melanomas are *superficial spreading* melanomas, which grow slowly and are slightly elevated, irregularly shaped, notched lesions with variations in color (blue, black, brown, pink, gray) (see Plate 6). Less frequently seen (15%) are the *nodular* melanomas, which are blueberry shaped with variations in color from blue-black to rose-gray. The nodular melanomas grow and metastasize more quickly than other forms. The patient's prognosis is based on the depth of invasion within the skin. The more superficial the growth the better the prognosis. Melanomas on the trunk have a poorer prognosis than those on the extremities.

Although melanomas cannot be prevented, all questionable moles should be examined by a physician so that early treatment can be instituted if malignancy is diagnosed. Warning signals of melanoma are as follows[1]:

A Asymmetry
B Border irregularity
C Color not uniform
D Diameter less than 6 mm

The person who has a newly diagnosed melanoma is usually very anxious and requires considerable emotional support. The nursing approach consists of empathic listening and of promoting hope without giving false reassurance. The importance of immediate therapy is stressed because it improves the prognosis. Surgery often involves a wide lesion, and skin grafting may be necessary. Regional lymph nodes are frequently dissected. Chemotherapy and immunotherapy are reserved for metastatic disease.

KAPOSI'S SARCOMA

Kaposi's sarcoma was a rare malignant disorder in older men in the United States until recently, although it was endemic in young black men of equatorial Africa. The disorder is now seen with increasing frequency as one of the opportunistic disorders occurring in conjunction with acquired immunodeficiency syndrome (AIDS), especially in homosexual men.

Persons with Kaposi's sarcoma develop discrete, red, purple, or dark plaques or nodules scattered widely over the body on the skin and mucous membranes. Some lesions may regress spontaneously. The disorder is slowly progressive and successful treatment of the sarcoma, unfortunately, does not affect survival. Many persons die of an associated opportunistic infection. For additional information, see Chapter 19.

SKIN DISORDERS IN BLACKS

The reported incidence of dermatologic disorders varies among different races. Persons with black skin rarely have skin disorders that are affected by solar irradiation, because the pigment of black skin screens out the sun's rays.

Pigmentary changes more commonly result because of the greater amount of melanin present. *Hyperpigmentation* is commonly seen after acne vulgaris, skin eruptions caused by drugs, lichen simplex chronicus, and pityriasis rosea. *Hypopigmentation* may result from atopic dermatitis and tinea. Some dermatologic disorders that are unique to blacks include traumatic alopecia and pseudofolliculitis barbae. Keloids are common.

TRAUMATIC ALOPECIA

Hair shafts in blacks are highly susceptible to breakage, and hair loss may result from some hair care practices such as tight hair curlers, corn-row braiding, hot combing, or the use of picks. Wetting or "softening" the hair before the use of a pick may help prevent trauma to the hair. The hair usually grows back when the specific practice is discontinued.

PSEUDOFOLLICULITIS BARBAE

Hair follicles in blacks are curved rather than straight; therefore, the hair curls back as it grows. After shaving, the sharpened point of the hair shaft (especially if a straight razor has been used) acts like a hook and reenters the skin, causing an inflammatory response. The most commonly affected areas include the chin and upper anterior neck. The legs and axilla may also develop pseudofolliculitis from shaving.

The lesions consist of papules and pustules, with some postinflammatory hyperpigmentation. Treatment consists of growing a beard or shaving with a safety razor set at a coarse setting. As the beard is growing, a brush or rough washcloth may be used to dislodge ingrowing hairs. A mild depilatory may be used in place of shaving.

KELOIDS

Although keloids are seen in all races, they are much more common in blacks. Keloids are hard, raised, shiny growths of collagen tissue that usually originate from a scar and then grow beyond the wound, often with clawlike projections. Keloids occur most often in young adults but may

---

The Elderly with Dermatologic Problems

Assessment

Assess for presence of dryness and intactness of skin, skin infections, and lesions.

Identify medications currently taken by patient and assess potential for photosensitivity (see Table 43-13). Thiazides and phenothiazines are common medications taken by the elderly.

Intervention

Teach elderly patient to avoid frequent baths, especially hot baths, that cause additional skin dryness. Tell patient to apply lotion to skin immediately following bathing.

Teach patient to report early signs of skin infection to physician. The elderly patient's decreased immune response may delay healing. The elderly person with herpes zoster needs protection from secondary infection, such as pneumonia.

Teach patient to differentiate benign skin lesions commonly seen with aging (brown spots, bruises) from potentially malignant lesions, and to report the latter to physician.

Common disorders in the elderly

Benign skin tumors
Skin cancers
Dermatitis medicamentosa
Skin infections, especially herpes zoster
Stasis dermatitis of legs

---

require many years to reach full growth. Highly susceptible areas for keloid growth include the sternum, mandible, ear, and neck. Keloids may recur after simple excision; therefore surgery is often followed by intralesional steroid therapy, radiation therapy, or electron beam therapy.

PLASTIC SURGERY

Plastic surgery is concerned with correction or reconstruction of deformities of body structures either present at birth or resulting from disease or trauma. Purposes of the surgery include restoration of function and improvement in appearance. Types of plastic surgery are listed below.

Skin grafting
Cosmetic surgery
  Removal of skin marks
    Dermabrasion
    Medical dermatattooing
  Fat removal (liposuction)
  Nose straightening (rhinoplasty)
  Face lifting (rhytidoplasty)
  Breast reconstruction (mammoplasty)

General Care of the Person Having Plastic Surgery
Preparation for surgery

It is believed that any plastic surgery for an obvious defect is justified if it helps people feel they have a better chance for positive recognition. The plastic surgeon may reshape a nose or repair a deformed hand so that an emotionally stable person will feel more confidence. It is foolish to assume, however, that reconstructive surgery alone will correct a basic personality problem. Some people blame an apparently trivial physical defect for a long series of failures in their lives when the major defect lies within their personalities. Because of this possibility, the person is usually studied before surgery is planned. It is necessary to know what the person expects the surgery to accomplish before the physician can decide whether such expectations are realistic and if surgery should be performed.

Before surgery the surgeon will tell the patient what probably can be done and what changes are possible. It is important to know what the patient has been told so that misunderstandings and misinterpretations can be avoided. Preparation is necessary for the normal appearance of skin grafts and reconstructed tissue immediately after surgery. Postoperative tissue reaction may distort normal contours, suture lines may be reddened, and the color of the newly transplanted skin may differ somewhat from that of surrounding skin. The appearance of the surgical area changes as the edema decreases and the suture line becomes less reddened and indurated. The scar will be less noticeable 6 months after surgery than at 6 days or 6 weeks postoperatively.

The patient who is scheduled for plastic surgery may have extensive scarring and deformity and may be exceedingly sensitive to scrutiny. On the other hand, the patient may have little apparent deformity, and it may be difficult to understand why the patient wishes to have surgery. The nurse cannot know what the disfigurement means to the individual and should avoid judgment concerning the necessity of surgery.

Many plastic surgeries are now performed on an outpatient basis at specialized plastic surgery clinics. Procedures that require extensive grafting usually require hospitalization.

Maintaining psychologic comfort

Plastic surgery raises many of the same concerns of other surgeries. Specific concerns may include the following:
1. Economic
   a. Possible long hospitalization and convalescence for skin grafting
   b. Elective cosmetic surgery is usually not covered by medical insurance
2. Physical discomfort
3. Physical appearance in postoperative period
4. Final outcome of surgery

These concerns may result in anxiety and mild depression during the first few days after surgery. Empathic communication by the nurse helps the patient identify and deal with concerns.

SKIN GRAFTING

Skin grafting consists of replacing damaged skin with healthy skin to prevent unsightly scars.

Graft Sources

Skin for grafting may be obtained from various sources (Box 43-8). The most suitable form is the *autograft*, because

43-8	Graft sources	
	Autograft	Tissue moved from one part of the body to another
	Homograft	Tissue transplanted from another person
	Heterograft	Tissue transplanted from another species

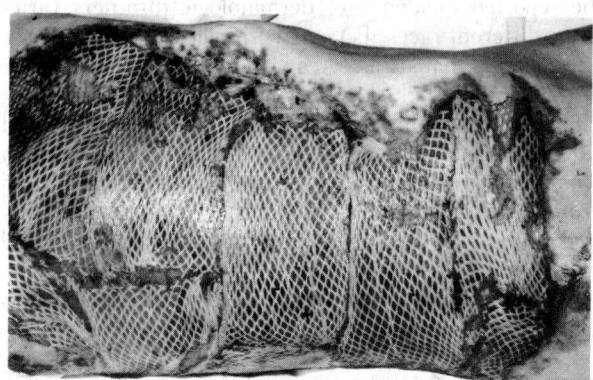

Fig. 43-8 Mesh graft covering full-thickness burn. (Courtesy Burn Unit, Cook County Hospital, Chicago.)

it does not provoke an immune response with rejection of the graft. *Homografts* (which are temporary) may be necessary if the patient's condition is poor and if large areas must be covered, as with burns. The survival time of homografts varies from a few days to a number of weeks. Depending on the tissue used and the recipient site, the transplanted tissue will then die and slough off or be absorbed and replaced by the host's own developing tissues. *Heterografts*, which are rejected quickly by the recipient, are used only in special cases, such as when homografts are not available and covering of the wound is essential.

Types of Grafts

Plastic surgery may be performed by means of *free grafting*, which consists of cutting tissue from one part of the body and moving it directly to another part. It may also be done by leaving one end of the graft attached to the body to provide a blood supply for the graft until blood vessels form at the new place of attachment (*flap graft*).

The surgeon selects skin for grafting that is similar in texture and thickness to that which has been lost, and studies the normal lines of the skin and its elasticity to avoid noticeable scars. Scar tissue contracts with time, and in normal circumstances this is good because it produces a complete closure of the line of injury. However, in some

Table 43-15   Various types of skin grafts

Type of graft	Description	Use	Comments
Free grafts			
Split-thickness: thin	Epidermis and thin layer of dermis (0.25 to 0.30 mm)	Burns	Becomes vascularized quickly Survives transplantation readily Donor sites heal quickly Poor cosmetic results Considerable postgraft contraction Does not withstand trauma
Split-thickness: intermediate or thick	Epidermis and thicker layer of dermis (0.40 to 0.45 or 0.55 to 0.60 mm)	Widely used over large wounds	Less contraction Better cosmetic results Epithelialization of donor site occurs completely but more slowly
Full-thickness	Epidermis and all of dermis	For small areas where matching skin color and texture is important	Best cosmetic results No contraction Donor site must be sutured (no epithelialization) Limited donor sites Lowest transplantation survival
Flap grafts	Skin and subcutaneous tissue; one end remains attached to donor site for vascularization	Large areas of defect; over avascular areas	More complex, requires greater skill Bulky May introduce hair into nonhairy areas
Free flap grafts	Skin, subcutaneous tissue and major blood vessel transferred to recipient site; donor blood vessel anastomosed to recipient blood vessel (microsurgery)	Over bony areas or areas requiring large amounts of tissue (breast reconstruction, head and neck defects, deep decubiti)	Blood flow established immediately; less contraction; more normal skin appearance, but may not match; may introduce hair into nonhairy areas

cases scar tissue may contract in such a way that surrounding tissues are pulled out of normal contour, and distortion may result.

Free grafts

Free grafts are the most commonly used skin grafts. There are several types of free grafts, each with its advantages and limitations (Table 43-15). Split-thickness grafts consist of epidermis and varying thicknesses of the dermis. Full-thickness grafts include the entire dermis and epidermis (Fig. 43-1). The most widely used type is the intermediate or thick split-thickness graft. This can be cut into large pieces with a dermatome set to ensure a uniform thickness of the graft, and these can then be cut into smaller pieces to match the area to be grafted.

Meshed grafts are either thin or intermediate split-thickness grafts that have been placed through a perforating machine that creates a mesh. Meshed grafts are elastic and can be used to cover larger areas than the original size (Fig. 43-8). They also conform more easily to irregular surfaces and can be placed over less clean bases than regular split-thickness grafts. Cosmetic appearance is poor. Meshed grafts are used frequently to cover large burned areas.

In order to survive, full-thickness grafts must develop their own blood supply (which takes 2 weeks). Regeneration of skin at the donor site is not possible because the underlying tissue has been removed. The donor site heals by *secondary* intention (Chapter 22) with scar formation.

Flap grafts

Flap grafts are used to cover larger defects than can be covered by free grafts. Flap grafts are made by cutting along three sides of a flap (two long and one short side). There are basically two major types of flap grafts. The *transposed* graft is slid over to a nearby skin area to be covered and is sutured in place. The *tube pedicle* graft is formed by suturing the long sides of the graft together to form a tube and then suturing the end to another area of the body. An intermediary site may be used, such as the forearm, in a two-step procedure, to permit moving the tube to a farther site on the body. After the graft has taken, the original site is freed and the graft is sutured to the recipient site.

Island flaps are narrow strips of neurovascular tissue from which the skin has been removed. The flap is transferred to a distant site through a tunnel made *under* the skin. The only scars that remain are at the donor and recipient sites.

Free flap grafts

Development of microsurgical techniques has permitted the use of free flaps (Table 43-15). A large amount of tissue can be moved because blood flow is reestablished at the

Patients with skin grafts

Preoperative care
Recipient site:
Apply warm soaks and compresses under aseptic conditions (as prescribed).
Apply prescribed topical antibiotics.
Donor site: clean with germicidal soap as prescribed, usually the night before and the morning of surgery.

Postoperative care of recipient site
Elevate graft site when possible.
Protect graft site from pressure and motion (for example, place graft site uppermost, use cradle over bed).
Instruct patient not to lie on dressing.
Apply warm moist compresses, if prescribed:
Wash hands before changing dressings.
Use meticulous aseptic technique.
Warm compresses to no more than 40.5° C (105° F).
Compresses may sometimes be covered with a sterile petroleum jelly dressing and moistened by gently directing fluid from sterile syringe under edge of dressing.
Report any signs of hematoma or fluid collection under graft.

Postoperative care of donor site
Keep donor site covered for 24 to 48 hours until serum dries.
Apply heat lamp with caution (denuded skin is sensitive) to hasten drying.
Use a bed cradle, if appropriate, to allow more air circulation.
Leave fine-mesh gauze, which is adherent to donor site, in place until it drops off (usually within 3 weeks).
Trim loose edges of mesh gauze as it loosens with healing.
Give analgesics as necessary for discomfort.

Postoperative care after flap grafts
Support body parts placed in awkward position from immobilization of flap graft.
Assess graft as possible for circulatory insufficiency (sharp color demarcation, decreased temperature).
Maintain aseptic technique to prevent infection.
Assist patient to be as self-sufficient as possible with activities of daily living.
If hospitalization is prolonged, help patient plan diversionary activities.

The patient with a skin graft

Keep surface of healed graft moistened daily with a skin lotion for 6 to 12 months. (Grafted skin does not sweat; it dries and cracks easily.)
Protect grafted skin from direct sunlight with a sunscreen lotion for at least 6 months.
Wear a strong elastic stocking for 4 to 6 months with grafts on lower extremities.
Report changes in the graft (hematoma, fluid collection) to physician.

new site by anastomosing the donor blood vessel with a recipient site blood vessel. Some free flaps contain functional nerves that can be reattached to permit sensation at the recipient site. Surgery often takes from 4 to 12 hours. Significant peripheral disease and diabetes mellitus are contraindications for surgery.

Care of the Person with a Skin Graft

Nursing care of patients with skin grafts is summarized in Box 43-9. Four conditions are necessary for a graft to survive.

1. Adequate vascularization of the recipient site
2. Constant contact with the underlying tissue
3. Immobilization
4. Freedom from infection

Anything that comes between the undersurface of the graft and the recipient area, such as a discharge caused by infection, excess serous fluid, or blood, will float the graft away from close contact and may cause it to die. To prevent floating, some surgeons insert drains at strategic spots along the edges of the graft, or a small catheter is inserted on the edge of the graft under the recipient skin and attached to suction to remove the fluid.

The area is inspected frequently to see if the skin is adhering to the underlying tissue. If fluid collects under the skin graft, it is removed by aspiration with a sterile needle and syringe, or the fluid is rolled to the wound edge with a sterile applicator.

A wide variety of materials are used as dressings. The choice depends on the kind of graft and the surgeon's preference. Petrolatum, Adaptic gauze, or Telfa dressings are often selected. Often the graft is covered with a piece of coarse mesh gauze anchored to the adjacent skin edges with an elastic bandage to give firm, gentle pressure and to immobilize the area. The first dressing may be covered with a compress of sterile normal saline solution. Because the compress is moist, it fits the contour of the wound better. Continuous pressure is necessary to keep the graft adherent to the recipient bed, but pressure should not be so firm as to cause death of the graft.

Inner dressings on the recipient site are usually changed by the surgeon 1 to 2 days after surgery, and it is usually possible to know then whether the result of the operation is satisfactory (see Box 43-9).

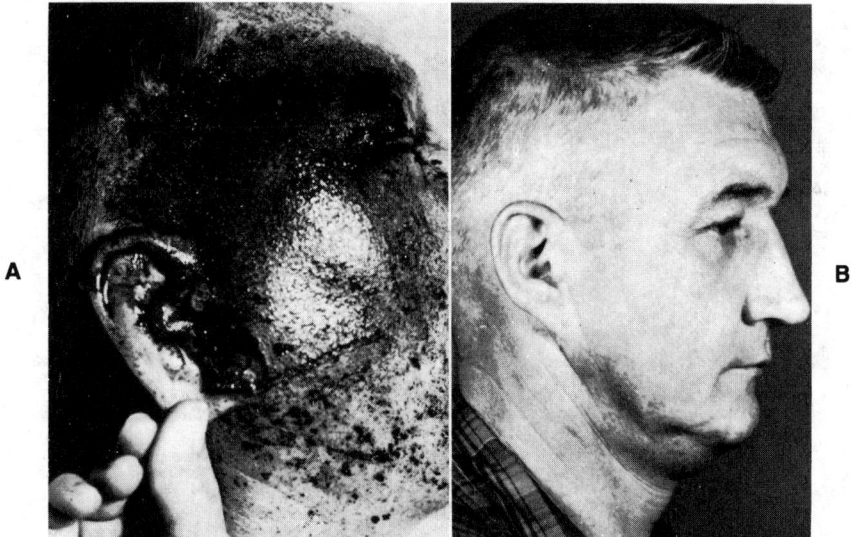

Fig. 43-9   A, Meticulous cleansing and dermabrasion were required to remove impregnated bits of galvanized metal. **B,** Postoperative view of patient 17 years after dermabrasion. (From Saunders WH, et al: *Nursing care in eye, ear, nose, and throat disorders,* ed 4, St Louis, 1979, Mosby–Year Book.)

Before patients with skin grafts are discharged, they need to know how to care for the recipient and donor sites at home until healing has occurred (Box 43-10).

Care of the Patient Undergoing Microvascular Surgery (Free Flaps)

Patients are instructed to refrain from smoking for 1 week before microvascular surgery because of the profound vasoconstrictive effect of nicotine.[54] If trauma has been experienced before surgery, anticoagulant therapy is given to prevent microthrombi in the flap. Following surgery, the patient is transferred to the critical care unit for continuous flap monitoring.

The major complication is necrosis of the transposed tissue, resulting from decreased circulation from arterial or venous thrombosis at the flap site. *Arterial* thrombosis may result in complete flap failure within hours after onset; it is characterized by pallor or coolness of the flap, and no bleeding when the flap is stuck with a needle. *Venous* thrombosis is less critical and occurs more slowly. It is characterized by a warm, mottled flap that oozes dark blood (from continued arterial blood flow); arterial occlusion will eventually occur.[54]

Circulation of the flap may be monitored by a *laser Doppler* that measures the average blood flow from a probe at the flap site. If the postoperative reading falls to below 50% of the preoperative baseline, the surgeon is notified.[16] A second, more precise method of monitoring blood flow is with a photoplethysmographic (PPG) disk. The disk is applied to the flap surface and measures reflected light from pulsatile changes in tissue blood flow.[54] Changes are reflected in waveforms on a monitor.

If the legs are not involved in the surgery, ambulation is started after 24 hours. Involved extremities are elevated to prevent venous engorgement. The patient is given noth-

ing by mouth for 48 hours in case further surgery for flap ischemia is necessary.

COSMETIC SURGERY
Removal of Skin Markings

Disfiguring marks on the skin may be removed by abrasive action (dermabrasion), by changing the color through medical dermatattooing, or by laser facial resurfacing.

Either local or general anesthesia is used for *dermabrasion.* The skin is abraded with a diamond fraise (Fig. 43-9). There is postoperative swelling, discomfort, crusting, and erythema, which may persist for several weeks. The procedure may be done in stages. A hydrogel dressing is applied after surgery. At home, the patient removes the dressing every 12 hours and compresses the surgical area for 15 to 30 minutes with cloths soaked in lukewarm tap water.[34] A new hydrogel dressing is then applied. New skin regenerates in 8 to 10 days.

Medical dermatattooing is performed on an ambulatory basis; no anesthesia is used, although a sedative may be prescribed to be taken 1 hour before surgery. The procedure is done in several stages; pigment is impregnated into the skin with a tattooing needle. The skin is left exposed to air to dry and crust. An ice bag may be applied to relieve postoperative discomfort.

Laser Surface Resurfacing

Done with a CO_2 laser, this technique may be used to remove skin markings or wrinkles and premalignant lesions.[51] The procedure is done with the patient under general anesthesia. The CO_2 laser beam destroys bacteria in addition to tissue, therefore risk of infection is decreased. Nerve endings are also destroyed, leading to minimal post-

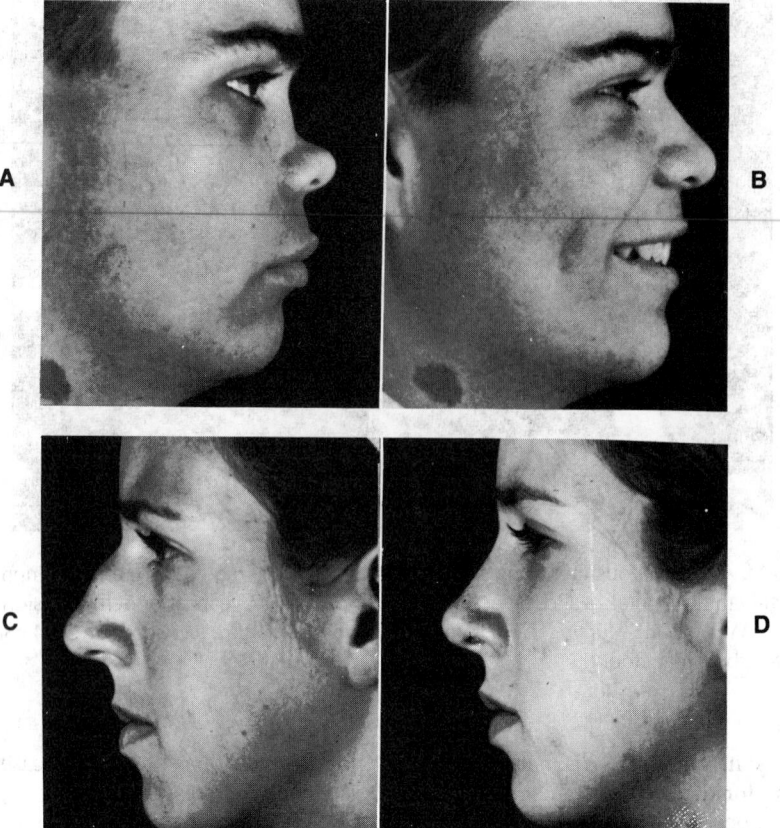

Fig. 43-10 A, Saddle nose after nasal infection at 8 years of age. **B,** The nose is repaired with Silastic nasal implant. **C** and **D,** Nasal convexity and chin retrusion repaired by combined rhinoplasty and chin augmentation. (From Saunders WH, et al: *Nursing care in eye, ear, nose, and throat disorders*, ed 4, St Louis, 1979, Mosby–Year Book.)

operative discomfort. Following surgery, antibiotic ointment is applied to the surgical area and covered with petroleum-based gauze and dry dressings. After 3 days the dressing is removed and the patient applies frequent warm moist compresses as instructed, to soften and remove skin crusts. Sunscreen must be used for at least 6 months after healing.[51]

Fat Removal

Some persons develop excess fatty tissue in areas such as the abdomen, hips ("saddle bags"), thighs, upper arms, or posterior neck ("buffalo hump"). If these persons are of normal weight but have selected areas of excess fat, they may be candidates for liposuction.

Liposuction can be performed as ambulatory surgery. A long, hollow, blunt-tipped cannula is inserted through a small incision and is tunneled through the fat under the skin. The loosened fat is then removed through the cannula by suction. Local anesthetics can be used for small single areas, although general anesthetics may be required for large or multiple areas.

After surgery, the area is taped with an elastic bandage for a period of 1 to 2 weeks. The patient's activity is limited for 48 hours. Nonaspirin analgesics may be taken for discomfort. Complications, though relatively few, may include

bleeding or infection. Initially the skin may be dimpled or hard, but it eventually softens and smooths out.

Fat can also be removed by *abdominoplasty* (dissection of excess skin and fat from the abdomen). This is a more extensive procedure and requires hospitalization for several days.

Rhinoplasty

Reconstructive surgery of the nose can be done either to correct an anatomic problem, or for cosmetic reasons (Fig. 43-10). A local anesthetic is usually used. The incision is usually made at the end of the nose inside the nostril so that it is not conspicuous. A nasal packing is inserted for 24 to 48 hours; the patient is cautioned not to sniff or blow the nose after the packing is removed, to prevent bleeding. A nasal splint may be applied for protection.

There will be ecchymosis (bruising) and swelling around the eyes and nose for 10 to 14 days after surgery; ice compresses and an ice bag may be used to hasten fluid reabsorption. The patient must anticipate waiting several weeks before evaluating the final result of surgery.

Rhytidoplasty

For face lifting, an incision is made at the hairline, and excess skin is separated from its underlying tissue and emoved. The remaining skin is pulled up and sutured at he hairline, thus removing wrinkles and giving firmness and smoothness to the face. A gentle pressure dressing is hen applied and left in place for 24 to 48 hours. The patient frequently needs medication for pain in the postoperative period because of the extent to which the tissue has been undermined. The surgery may be repeated at a ater date.

Blepharoplasty

Excess skin often develops in the upper and lower eyelids n older persons, sometimes interfering with vision. The person's appearance may be altered by large folds of loose skin hanging on the upper cheeks. Blepharoplasty is the removal of the redundant skin. With the patient under local anesthesia, incisions are made in the creases of the upper and lower lids and the excess skin is removed. Steristrips may be used to hold the tissue in place until healing s complete in 4 to 6 weeks. Swelling and ecchymosis usually subsides in 7 to 10 days. Ice compresses are applied to relieve swelling and to prevent further ecchymosis. There is minimal discomfort.

Mammoplasty

Reconstructive breast surgery may be done to replace breast tissue removed by surgery (Chapter 36) or to improve the appearance of the breasts. Some women with conspicuously large and pendulous breasts may wish to have them reduced in size. Large breasts are embarrassing to some women and make it difficult for them to participate in sports, maintain good posture, and buy clothes that fit. Such women often respond to reconstructive surgery remarkably well. Cosmetic surgery of the breast may also be done to make unusually small breasts larger. A variety of approaches may be used for breast enlargement (see Chapter 36). Because of safety concerns however, the Food and Drug Administration placed a moratorium in early 1992 on the use of silicone-filled breast implants solely for cosmetic reasons.

SUMMARY

1. Skin disorders that produce marked visual disfigurement may result in alterations in body image and self-esteem.

2. Bacterial skin infections include folliculitis (infections of the hair follicle), furuncles (deep folliculitis), carbuncles (cluster of furuncles), or cellulitis (diffuse infection of skin and subcutaneous tissue); treatment includes warm soaks or hot moist dressings, and topical or systemic antibiotics.

3. Viral skin inflammations include herpes simplex, herpes zoster, and warts; acyclovir (Zovirax) is given for herpes simplex in immunocompromised patients and for herpes zoster.

4. Fungal skin inflammations include candidiasis and the dermatophytoses (tinea capitis, corporis, cruris, and pedis); treatment includes topical or oral antifungal drugs.

5. Parasitic infestations include those by lice or scabies mite; treatment includes a topical pediculocide/scabicide.

6. Topical medications may be prepared as powders, lotions, creams, ointments, or pastes.

7. Wet dermatologic dressings are given for cooling astringent, antipruritic, vasoconstricting, or debriding effects; the best effects are obtained by several treatments spaced over several hours.

8. Dermatologic baths and soaks are given for soothing, antipruritic, astringent, or medicinal effects; medication should be completely dissolved in the water, and creams or ointments should be applied immediately after the bath.

9. Dermatitis may result from contact with irritants, as an atopic (hypersensitivity) reaction, from stasis of circulation in the legs, or from unknown cause (dandruff). Dressings moistened with Burow's solution and topical steroids may be used for uninfected weeping lesions, and antibiotics may be used for infected lesions.

10. The most common papulosquamous disorder is psoriasis, a chronic condition resulting from rapid cell mitosis. Exacerbations of psoriasis may be treated with occlusive wraps over topical steroid therapy; crude tar therapy, alone or in combination with ultraviolet light; or PUVA therapy.

11. Drugs that may cause photosensitivity reactions include phenothiazines, thiazides, tetracycline, griseofulvin, sulfonamide, nalidixic acid, and chlorpromazine; persons taking these drugs should avoid direct sunlight.

12. Nonmalignant skin lesions are primarily keratoses (corns, calluses, seborrheic keratosis, actinic keratosis) that are characterized by overgrowth and thickening of the epithelium; actinic keratoses result from solar irradiation and may become squamous cell carcinomas.

13. Premalignant lesions include leukoplakia (white or red patches), which may develop into invasive squamous cell carcinoma, and pigmented moles, which may develop into melanoma. Moles that change appearance in color, size, loss of hair, or bleeding should be reported to the physician.

14. Squamous cell carcinoma, which may metastasize, and basal cell carcinoma, which rarely metastasizes, may be removed by surgical excision and curettage with electrodesiccation, cryosurgery, or irradiation.

15. Malignant melanomas have a high incidence of metastasis and mortality; they are treated by radical excision, chemotherapy, and immunotherapy.

16. Free grafts (split-thickness, full-thickness) are sections of epidermis and dermis that are taken from a donor area and transplanted to a distant area. Flap grafts include subcutaneous tissue, and one end remains attached to the donor site. Free flap grafts contain skin, subcutaneous tissue, and a major blood vessel, which are transplanted to a distant site with anastomosis of the blood vessel with a recipient vessel.

17. Care of the person with a graft includes (1) applying firm dressings, to maintain graft contact with the underlying tissue; (2) preventing collection of fluid under the graft, to protect against separation of the graft; (3) protecting the graft site from excess pressure and mo-

tion, to promote vascularization and prevent separation; and (4) using aseptic technique, to prevent infection.

18. Cosmetic surgery includes dermabrasion, medical dermatattooing, or laser resurfacing to remove skin markings; liposuction to remove excess abominal fat; face lifting (rhytidoplasty); and reconstructive surgery of the eyelids (blepharoplasty), nose (rhinoplasty), and breast (mammoplasty).

STUDY QUESTIONS

- Why are counseling and teaching the major nursing strategies for persons with skin disorders?
- Which skin disorders have pruritus as a symptom? What approaches help modify pruritus?
- Mrs. B. tells you that she is thinking about buying a new over-the-counter drug which, although expensive, is being advertised as a cure for psoriasis. Which of the following health teaching approaches would be *most effective*? Explain:
  a. Tell Mrs. B not to waste her money because psoriasis cannot be cured.
  b. Explore her knowledge of psoriasis and experiences she has had with previous therapies.
  c. Suggest she check first with her physician before buying the drug.
- Explain in your own words the differences among the various types of skin grafts. Why is the postoperative care different from free flap grafts than for other types of grafts?

REFERENCES AND SELECTED READINGS

1. American Cancer Society: *Cancer facts and figures 1991*, Atlanta, 1991, The Society.
2. * Berliner H: Aging skin, pt 1, *Am J Nurs* 86:1138-1141, 1986.
3. * Berliner H: Aging skin, pt 2, *Am J Nurs* 86:1259-1261, 1986.
4. Bodey GP: Topical and systemic antifungal agents, *Med Clin North Am* 72:637-659, 1988.
5. Buxton PK: ABC of dermatology: eczema and inflammatory dermatoses, *Br Med J* 295:1112-1114, 1987.
6. * Cohen K: Free-flap surgery: nurses make it work, *RN* 51(3):26-29, 1988.
7. * Crawford E et al: Mohs' chemosurgery: day surgery for cutaneous malignancies, *AORN J* 43:464-468, 1986.
8. * Cuzzell JZ: Clues: itching and burning in skin folds, *Am J Nurs* 19(1):23-24, 1990.
9. * Cuzzell JZ: Clues: recurrent, punched-out lesions, *Am J Nurs* 90(5):21-22, 1990.
10. * Cuzzell JZ: Clues: pain, burning, and itching, *Am J Nurs* 90(7):15-16, 1990.
11. Dolsky RL, Newman J, Fetzek JR: Liposuction: history, techniques, and complications, *Dermatol Clin* 5:313-334, 1987.
12. * Dunn ML, Cockerline EB, Rice MR: Treatment options for psoriasis, *Am J Nurs* 88:1082-1087, 1988.
13. Epstein E: Common skin disorders, ed 3, Oradell, NJ, 1988, Medical Economics Books.
14. Feder HM, Renfro L, Schmidt DD: Common questions about herpes simplex, *Hosp Pract* 24(1A):50-62, 1989.

15. * Goodman T: Grafts and flaps in plastic surgery, *AORN J* 48:650-663, 1988.
16. * Goodman T, White S: Microvascular reconstruction: nursing management, *AORN J* 48:666-676, 1988.
17. Greany D, Goldsmith HS: Cutaneous melanoma: diagnosis and surgical intervention, *AORN J* 42:43-49, 1985.
18. * Gurevich I: Counseling the patient with herpes, *RN* 53(2):22-28, 1990.
19. Habif TP: *Clinical dermatology: a color guide to diagnosis and treatment*, ed 2, St Louis, 1990, Mosby–Year Book.
20. Harber LC, Whitman GB: Photosensitivity: classification, *Dermatol Clin* 4:167-170, 1986.
21. * Hartwig PA: Lasers in dermatology, *Nurs Clin North Am* 25(3):657-666, 1990.
22. * Hetland JR: Scabies: managing an outbreak, *Geriatr Nurs* 8:319-321, 1987.
23. * Hood LM: Scabies: are your patients at risk? *Geriatr Nurs* 8:312-315, 1987.
24. Kaplan AP et al: Allergic skin disorders, *JAMA* 258:2900-2909, 1987.
25. Kleinsmith D, Perricone NV: Common skin problems in the elderly, *Dermatol Clin* 4:485-499, 1986.
26. * Klotz RW: Herpetic whitlow: an occupational hazard, *JAANA* 58(1):8-12, 1990.
27. Kopf AW: Prevention and early detection of skin cancer/melanoma, *Cancer* 62(8):1791-1795, 1988.
28. * Lawler PE: Be sunsensible: steps toward safety in the sun, *Oncol Nurs Forum* 16(3):424-427, 1989.
29. * Lawler PE, Schreiber S: Cutaneous malignant melanoma: nursing's role in prevention and early detection, *Oncol Nurs Forum* 16(3):345-352, 1989.
30. * LeFort SM: Herpes zoster and postherpetic neuralgia: the need for early intervention in the elderly, *Nurs Pract* 14(3):30-41, 1989.
31. Loeser JD: Herpes zoster and postherpetic neuralgia, *Pain* 25:149-164, 1986.
32. * Lombardo BL et al: Group support for derm patients, *Am J Nurs* 88:1088-1090, 1988.
33. * Lynn MM, Holdcroft C: Treatment for fungal skin infections: an update, *Nurse Pract* 14(8):64-71, 1989.
34. * McKinnon CC, Fulton JE: Facial dermabrasion, *AORN J* 51:739-750, 1990.
35. * Moosny J: What's wrong with this patient? . . . scabies, *RN* 52(5):61-63, 1989.
36. Moschella SL, Hurley HA: *Dermatology*, ed 3, Philadelphia, 1991, WB Saunders.
37. * Nichol NH: Atopic dermatitis: the (wet) wrap up, *Am J Nurs* 87:1560-1563, 1987.
38. * Novotny J: Adolescents, acne, and the side-effects of Accutane, *Pediatr Nurs* 15:247-248, 1989.
39. * Parks BR, Smith D: Treatment of head lice and scabies infestations in children, *Pediatr Nurs* 15:522-524, 1989.
40. Pathak MA: Sunscreens: topical and systemic approaches for prevention of acute and chronic sun-induced skin reactions, *Dermatol Clin* 4:321-334, 1986.
40a. Phillips TJ, Dover JS: Recent advances in dermatology, *New Eng J Med* 326(3):167-177, 1992.
41. * Prigel DL: How to spot melanoma, *Nursing 87* 17(6):60-62, 1987.
42. Quan M et al: Management of acne vulgaris, *Am Fam Physician* 38:207-218, 1988.
43. * Reese JL: Nursing interventions for wound healing in plastic and reconstructive surgery, *Nurs Clin North Am* 25(1):223-233, 1990.
44. Reeves JR: Head lice and scabies in children, *Pediatr Infect Dis* 6:598-602, 1987.
45. Rosenbaum M: Pruritus of unknown origin, *Hosp Pract* 23(10A):19-22, 1988.

46.* Roy DJ: Caring for self-esteem of the cosmetic patient, *Plast Surg Nurs* 6:138-141, 1986.

47. Sauer GC: *Manual of skin diseases*, ed 6, Philadelphia, 1991, JB Lippincott.

48. Schaefer DG, Wolf JE: Common dermatologic disorders, *Clin Plast Surg* 14:201-208, 1987.

49. Schroeder SA et al: *Current medical diagnosis and treatment*, Norwalk, Conn, 1991, Appleton & Lange.

50.* Sheahan SL, Seabolt JP: Management of common parasitic infections encountered in primary care, *Nurse Pract* 12(8):19-33, 1987.

51.* Spadoni D, Cain CL: Facial resurfacing: using the carbon dioxide laser, *AORN J* 50:1007-1013, 1989.

52. Stahl S, Hamilton S, Spira M: Surgical treatment of acne scars, *Clin Plast Surg* 14:261-276, 1987.

53.* Stern C: Melanoma, the most lethal skin cancer, *RN* 50(7):12-14, 1987.

54.* Swain D, Shell DH: Microvascular tissue transfer: perioperative nursing considerations, *AORN J* 49:1032-1043, 1989.

55. Toback AC, Anders JE: Phototoxicity from systemic agents, *Dermatol Clin* 4:223-229, 1986.

56. Way LW: Current surgical diagnoses and treatment, ed 9, Norwalk, Conn, 1991, Appleton & Lange.

57. Wyngaarden JB, Smith LH: Textbook of medicine, ed 18, Philadelphia, 1988, WB Saunders.

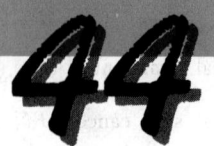

The Patient with Burns

Deborah Goldenberg Klein
Diane E. Fritsch
Lynne C. Yurko

After studying this chapter, the learner should be able to:

- Describe the assessment of burn patient including extent, location, and etiology.
- Differentiate between the three periods of a major burn.
- Describe the emergency care for major burns.
- Describe interventions for replacing body fluids, preventing infection, promoting nutrition and mobility, and providing emotional support.
- Identify learning needs of the patient with burns.

Burn injuries are in many respects the worst of all tragedies an individual can experience. An intensive burn is an overwhelming insult to the patient physically and psychologically, and it is catastrophic in cost and suffering to the family involved.

Approximately 2,000,000 people suffer a thermal injury each year in the United States. Of these victims, 20,000 are admitted to hospitals and 8000 to 12,000 die as a result of burn injury. Burns are caused by flame, scald, direct contact, chemicals, electrical current, and radiation. Injury is frequently a result of the victim's own actions. Eighty-one percent of the elderly population's burn injuries occur in this manner. Scald injuries are the most frequent type of injury, but flame injury is more serious. The annual cost of property and income loss is 13.6 billion dollars. The largest portion is a result of hospitalization costs from major burn injury.

Because of the systemic effects of the burn injury, psychologic implications, and prolonged hospitalization, comprehensive nursing care is required during the acute and long-term recovery phases.

ETIOLOGY, PREVENTION, AND HEALTH EDUCATION

Nurses can help prevent accidental burns by participating in health education programs that emphasize both fire prevention and the consequences of fires, such as burns, deformities, and death. Nurses can promote legislation that would control hazardous practices and make working and living environments safer. Community health nurses are in an unusually advantageous position to recognize unsafe practices in the home and to help families develop safe habits of living.

Prevention programs can be developed to highlight seasonal activities that result in burn injuries (see Box 44-1). Approximately 80% of accidental burns occur in the home and are primarily caused by ignorance, carelessness, and the curiosity of *children*. Infants and children are the most common victims of fires in and about the home. A large number of children have been burned to death or permanently disabled or disfigured by accidental burns.

Death rates from burns are highest in children aged 2 and younger and in persons 60 years and older. Higher death rates are found among men, blacks, American Indians, and the poor.[14] Substandard housing without smoke detectors or with nonworking detectors contributes to the higher death rates. Fires ignited by cigarettes cause about 7% of all residential fires and 17% of fire deaths. Alcohol abuse is not uncommon in cigarette-ignited fires. Burn-related deaths in children under 2 years of age are caused by scalds, playing with matches, lighters, and flammable liquids, and by electrical injuries from contact with power lines.

A high incidence of burn injuries affecting *adults* are related to accidents while cooking, using microwave ovens, smoking, or otherwise using matches. Burns commonly occur when the person is distracted while cooking or falls asleep while smoking.

Each year brings increased demand for careful inspection and regulation of places in which the ill and infirm

---

Seasonal activities resulting in burn injuries

Spring	Barbecuing
	Burning leaves
	Overheated radiators
	Gasoline
	Lawnmowers
Summer	Sun exposure
	Fireworks
	Beach activity
	Sun-heated surfaces (tar, asphalt, sand)
Fall	Hot liquids
	Yard clean-up
	Candles
	Halloween
Winter	Holiday activities
	Fireplaces
	Hot liquids
	Woodburning stoves/space heaters
	Electrical wires

From Lillico S: National burn awareness 1991, Encino, Calif, 1991, The National Burn Awareness Task Force.

---

are housed. Aged persons frequently are housed in old and poorly equipped structures, and many of them have been victims of fire. Nurses can bring pressure to bear to ensure that adequate protection and planned evacuation if a fire occurs. The American Burn Association suggests that all health facilities conduct one mock evacuation drill each year.[31] Attention is being focused on places where large numbers of people congregate. Laws require that doors in public buildings are hinged to swing outward, that draperies and decorations be fireproof, and that stairways with special fire doors be used in new apartment buildings and hotels. Smoke detectors and sprinkler systems are also required in new buildings and residential health care facilities. Nurses working in institutions need to encourage and participate in fire prevention programs.

Rigid enforcement of laws requiring that industrial products be labeled when known to be flammable and that new products be tested carefully for their flammable qualities before being placed on the market is further evidence of government efforts to protect the public from accident by fire. For example, children's night clothes must be flame retardant. Industry can be made safer by constant vigilance by management in cooperation with fire safety officers and health care professionals in identifying hazards and implementing safety programs. All chemicals should be labeled, and antidotes should be identified and available. A core of every work force should be well versed in emergency treatment of all types of burns for the protection of every employee.

Recent statistics indicate a rise in burns associated with microwave ovens. Scalds can occur when the power of the microwave is underestimated. Microwave oven burns are preventable, and users need to be educated about the safe use of these ovens.

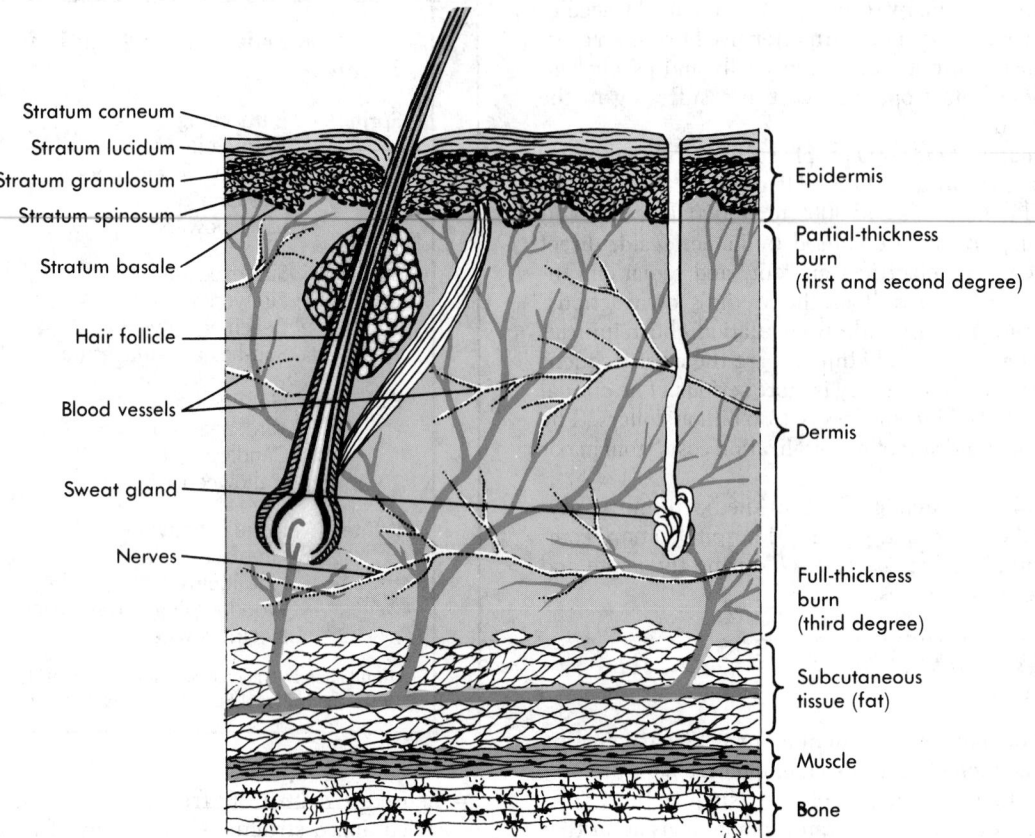

Stratum corneum
Stratum lucidum
Stratum granulosum
Stratum spinosum
Stratum basale

Hair follicle

Blood vessels

Sweat gland

Nerves

Epidermis

Partial-thickness
burn
(first and second degree)

Dermis

Full-thickness
burn
(third degree)

Subcutaneous
tissue (fat)

Muscle

Bone

Fig. 44-1 Levels of human skin involved in burns.

Table 44-1 Goals per 100,000 people for reduction in fire deaths among populations at high risk

Populations	1987 baseline	2000 target
Children age 4 and younger	4.4	3.3
People age 65 and older	4.4	3.3
Black males	5.7	4.3
Black females	3.4	2.6

From Healthy people 2000: *National health promotion and disease prevention objectives*, Public Health Service, Washington, DC, 1990, Government Printing Office.

Sunburn should be cautioned against, because even a relatively mild burn of a large part of the body can cause change of fluid distribution and kidney damage. Camp nurses should keep this in mind in their educational programs for children and camp counselors. Many effective sunscreen products are available and should be used in times of exposure.

The Surgeon General's report on goals to be achieved by year 2000 includes reducing residential fire deaths to no more than 1.2 per 100,000 people from an age-adjusted baseline of 1.5 per 100,000 in 1987.[14] Goals for special populations at high risk appear in Table 44-1.

CLASSIFICATION OF BURNS

Traditionally, burns have been classified as first, second, or third degree. The terms *first*, *second*, and *third degree* are not descriptive of the injury, because they are based only on the visual characteristics of the burn wound. The injury of a burn extends beyond what can be seen. A more accurate description is *partial-thickness* and *full-thickness*, which graphically describes the burn and indicates the depth and severity of the tissue injury (Fig. 44-1).

Partial-thickness burns are characterized by destruction of varying depths from the epidermis (outer layer of skin) to the dermis (middle layer of skin). Partial-thickness burns of the skin involve a part of the epidermis and dermis. The depth of tissue injury is described further as *superficial partial-thickness*, which *involves only the epidermis, and deep partial-thickness*, which *involves the entire epidermis* and *part of the dermis*. Partial-thickness burns are likely to be painful because nerve endings have been injured and exposed. They have the ability to heal because a portion of the epithelial cells has not been destroyed. During the healing phase, dryness and itching are common and are caused by increased vascularization of sebaceous glands, reduction of secretions, and decreased perspiration.

The presence of blisters often indicates a deep partial-thickness injury. The blisters may increase in size as the result of continuous exudation and collection of tissue fluid.

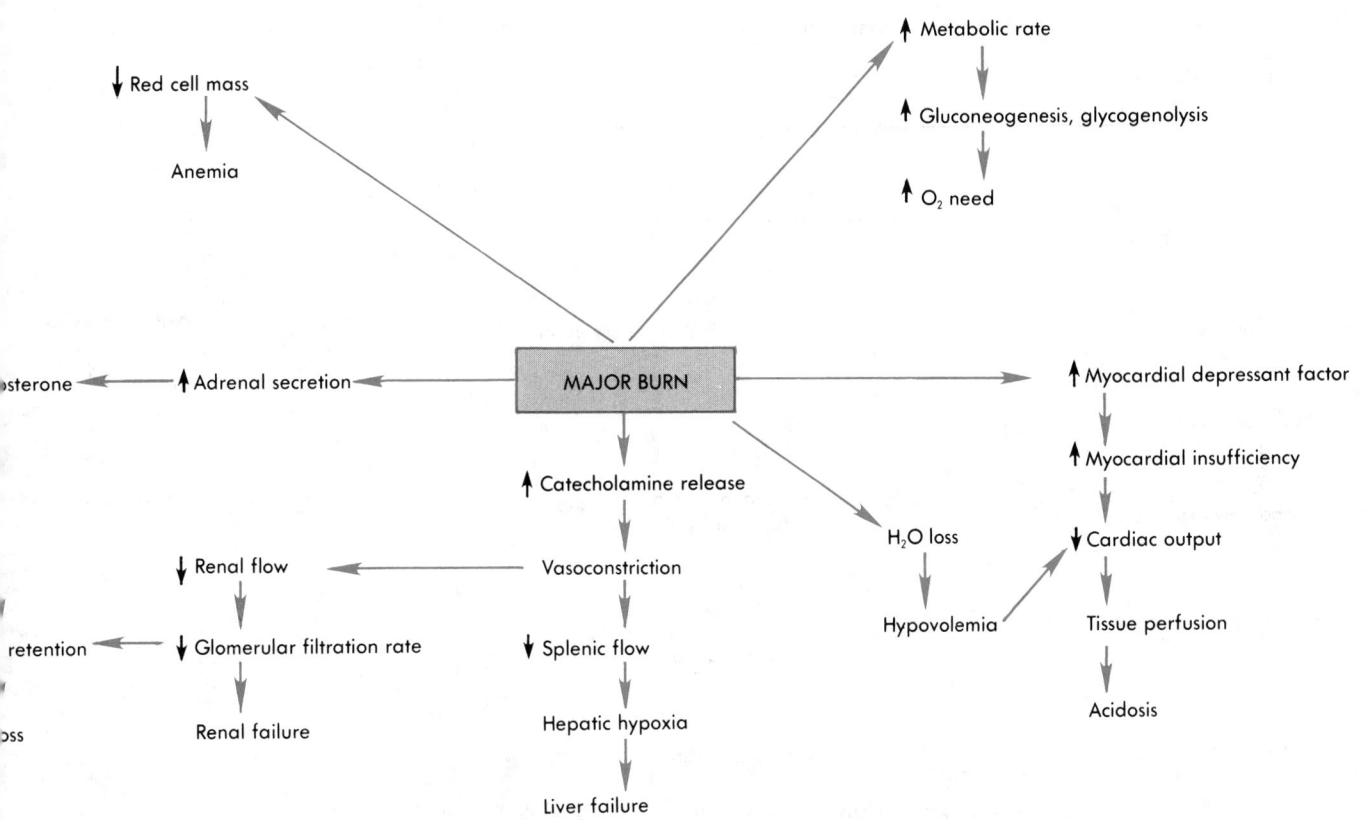

Fig. 44-2   Overview of pathophysiology of a major burn.

Full-thickness burns include destruction of the epidermis and the entire dermis, as well as possible damage to the subcutaneous layer, muscle, and bone. Nerve endings are destroyed, resulting in a painless wound. *Eschar, a leathery covering composed of denatured protein, may form as a result of surface dehydration.* Black networks of coagulated capillaries may be seen. Full-thickness burns require skin grafting because the destroyed tissue is unable to epithelialize. Often a deep partial-thickness burn may convert to a full-thickness burn because of infection, trauma, or decreased blood supply.

PATHOPHYSIOLOGY OF SEVERE BURNS

As a result of burns, normal skin function is diminished, resulting in physiologic alterations. These include (1) *loss of protective barriers against infection,* (2) *escape of body fluids,* (3) *lack of temperature control,* (4) *destroyed sweat and sebaceous glands,* and (5) *decrease in the number of sensory receptors.* The severity of these alterations will depend on the extent of the burn and the depth to which damage has occurred.

Increased knowledge of the physiologic changes that occur during severe burns has led to the saving of many lives. There are *two stages* that occur *following severe burns:* the *immediate hypovolemic stage* and the *diuretic stage.* Fig. 44-2 presents an overview of the pathophysiologic changes seen in a severe burn.

Hypovolemic Stage

The hypovolemic stage begins at the time of burn injury and lasts for the first 48 to 72 hours. It is characterized by a *rapid shift of fluid from the vascular compartment into the interstitial spaces.* When tissues are burned, vasodilation, increased capillary permeability, and changes in the permeability of tissue cells in and around the burn area occur. As *a result, abnormally large amounts of extracellular fluid* (ECF), *sodium chloride,* and *protein pass through the burned area* either *to cause blister formation and local edema or to escape through the open wound.*

Visible fluid loss makes up only a small part of the fluid lost from the circulating blood and other essential fluid compartments. Most of the fluid loss occurs deep in the wound, where the fluid extravasates into the deeper tissues. Burns occurring in highly vascular areas such as muscle tissue or the face are believed to cause a greater fluid shift than comparable burns occurring on other parts of the body. In addition, the greater the percent of injury, the greater the fluid loss. Fully half of the extracellular fluid of the body can shift from its normal distribution to the site of a severe burn. *Hypovolemic shock* occurs, and there is a tremendous drop in blood pressure and inadequate blood flow through the kidneys, which in turn leads to further shock and anuria. Death occurs within a short time if treatment is not given promptly or is inadequate. These changes are summarized in Fig. 44-3.

As a *result of these fluid shifts, dehydration of nondamaged*

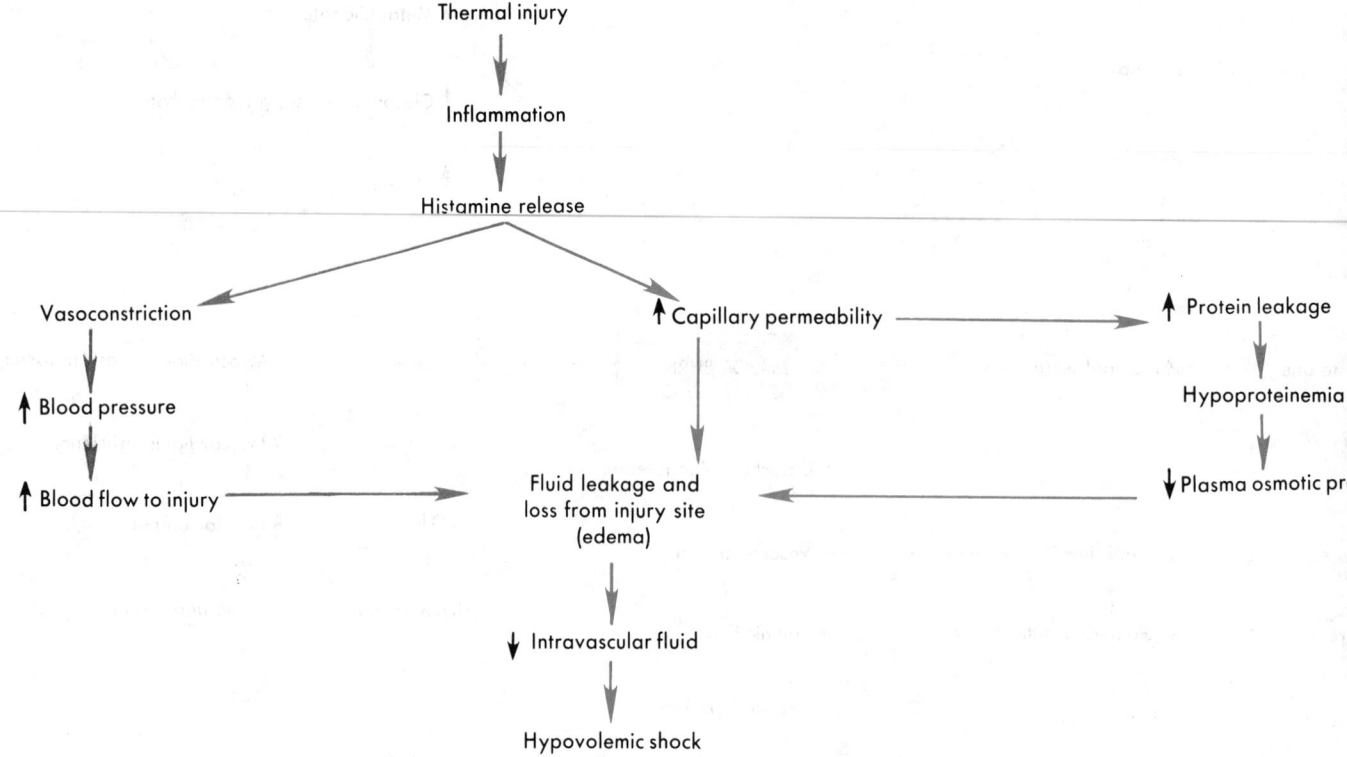

Fig. 44-3 Flow diagram of fluid shifts resulting in hypovolemic shock.

tissue cells may occur. Initially, more fluids and sodium are lost from the capillaries than is protein. This *increases the capillary osmotic pressure, leading to dehydration with pronounced edema in the burned area.* As *protein continues to be lost* into the *burned area because of the increased capillary permeability, hypoproteinemia results.* The *increased amount of protein* in the *tissue spaces leads to edema.* Proteins may be lost through the open wounds. The lymphatic system, which normally functions to remove increased tissue fluid, becomes overloaded and inefficient, thus contributing to edema. *Nitrogen is lost through the kidney from catabolism, leading to significant negative nitrogen balance. Blood urea nitrogen* (BUN) *is elevated when oliguria is present.*

With loss of fluid from the vascular system, *hemoconcentration* occurs and the hematocrit rises. Blood flow becomes sluggish in the burned area and cellular nutrition decreases. Large numbers of red blood cells become trapped in the burned area and are hemolyzed. Renal damage and hematuria may occur as a result of reduced blood volume and passage of the end products of the hemolyzed cells through the glomeruli. The decreased renal blood flow leads to oliguria.

Electrolyte imbalances also occur. *Hyperkalemia* (elevated serum potassium) *results from the release of potassium from damaged tissue cells and red blood cells and from decreased urinary output. Hyperkalemia may lead to heart block and ventricular failure.* Potassium may be encouraged to move back into the cells by the administration of insulin, because potassium is transported back into the cells along with glucose. Sodium is retained by the body as a result of the

endocrine response to stress. Aldosterone is increased leading to increased sodium reabsorption by the kidney However, sodium quickly passes into the interstitial space of the burned area with the fluid shift. Despite the increased amount of sodium in the body, most of the *sodium is trapped in the edema fluid* and a *serum sodium deficit* occurs *Inadequate tissue perfusion results in anaerobic metabolism* and the *acid end products are retained because of the decreased kidney function. Metabolic acidosis may then occur.*

Respiratory distress may result from upper airway obstruction or the effects of hypovolemic shock. Upper-airway obstruction is caused by inhalation of noxious agent or superheated air, causing irritation of the airway, laryngeal edema, and potential obstruction.

Diuretic Stage

Return of vascular integrity begins in approximately 1 hours and rapidly progresses at 18 to 24 hours following the initial burn injury. Although full capillary integrit may not be restored for a number of days, for clinica purposes it may be considered restored at 24 hours. Th *diuretic stage* begins at about 48 to 72 hours after the bur injury as capillary membrane integrity returns and edem fluid shifts back from the interstitial spaces into the in travascular space. Blood volume increases, leading to in creased renal blood flow and *diuresis* unless renal damag has occurred. *Serum electrolyte* and *hematocrit levels* will b *decreased* because of *hemodilution. Fluid overload may occu as a result of the increase in intravascular volume.* The pa tient's vital signs, breath sounds, and urinary output ar

Table 44-2   Physiologic changes with burns

| Change | Hypovolemic stage | | Diuretic stage | |
	Mechanism	Result	Mechanism	Result
Extracellular fluid shift	Vascular to interstitial	Hemoconcentration Edema at burn site	Interstitial to vascular	Hemodilution
Renal function	Decreased renal blood flow from decreased blood pressure and decreased cardiac output	Oliguria	Increased renal blood flow from increased blood volume	Diuresis
Sodium level	Na$^+$ reabsorbed by kidneys *but* Na$^+$ lost in exudate and trapped in edema fluid	Sodium deficit	Na$^+$ loss with diuresis (becomes normal in 1 week)	Sodium deficit
Potassium level	K$^+$ released as result of tissue and red blood cell injury; decreased K$^+$ excretion from decreased renal function	Hyperkalemia	K$^+$ moves back into cells; K$^+$ lost by diuresis (begins 4-5 days after the burn)	Hypokalemia
Protein level	Protein lost into tissues by increased capillary permeability	Hypoproteinemia	Loss of protein during continued catabolism	Hypoproteinemia
Nitrogen balance	Tissue catabolism; protein loss in tissues; more nitrogen lost than taken in	Negative nitrogen balance	Tissue catabolism, protein loss, immobility	Negative nitrogen balance
Acid-base balance	Anaerobic metabolism from decreased tissue perfusion; increased acid end products; decreased renal function (causing retention of acid end products); loss of serum bicarbonate	Metabolic acidosis	Sodium bicarbonate lost in diuresis; hypermetabolism with increased metabolic end products	Metabolic acidosis
Stress response	Occurs because of trauma	Decreased renal blood flow	Occurs because of prolonged nature of injury and psychologic threat to self	Stress ulcers

used to determine the amount of intravenous fluid replacement. Dehydration may occur if rapid urinary output depletes the intravascular reserve. A sodium deficit continues because of the loss of sodium through the burn wound and from an increase in urinary output. *Hypokalemia* (lowered serum potassium) results from potassium moving back into the cells or being excreted in the urine. Protein continues to be lost from the wounds. *Metabolic acidosis remains a possibility because of the loss of sodium bicarbonate in the urine and the increase in fat metabolism secondary to a decrease in carbohydrate intake.*

Following the period of fluid shifts, the patient remains acutely ill. This period is characterized by *anemia* and *malnutrition*. Anemia develops from the loss of red blood cells. *Negative nitrogen balance* begins at the onset of the burn and is the result of tissue destruction, protein loss, and the stress response. It continues throughout the acute period because of continued loss of protein from the wound, tissue catabolism from immobility, and decreased protein intake. Special attention to the nutrition of the patient is important during this time. Increased metabolism from loss of water and heat from the wound, loss of fluid during diuresis, and catabolism during tissue breakdown all lead to *weight loss*.

The differences in changes between the hypovolemic and diuretic stages are summarized in Table 44-2.

PERIODS OF TREATMENT

Three periods of treatment can be identified in the care of the seriously burned patient. These are the *emergent*, the *acute*, and the *rehabilitative periods*.

The *emergent period* refers to the first 48 to 72 hours postburn when the patient is admitted to hospital, the severity of the injury is determined, and first aid and wound care are given. The *acute period* of treatment begins at the end of the emergent period and lasts until all of the full-thickness wounds are covered with skin grafts or partial-thickness wounds are healed. The *rehabilitation period* focuses on returning the patient to a useful place in society. The *two areas of concern* during this phase are: (1) the *restoration of function over joint surfaces that were scarred*, and (2) *the emotional assistance that the patient* and *family will need*. The rehabilitation of the patient actually begins during early hospitalization and is addressed throughout the hospitalization. After discharge, the patient may require emotional assistance and counseling, and may need to be readmitted several times for reconstructive surgical procedures.

Comprehensive Team Approach

Comprehensive care of the burn patient can best be provided by a multidisciplinary team approach. The physician, nurse, respiratory therapist, social workers, physical and occupational therapists, teacher and child-life specialist (if a school-age child), registered dietitian, vocational counselor, clergy, and others all work together to address the needs of the patient. The *nurse's role in the team* is to *coordinate the interactions of the various disciplines* and to *incorporate the team's suggestions and approaches into an effective plan of care.*

Emergent Period

The emergent period of therapy is defined as the time required to resolve the immediate problems resulting from the burn injury. First aid measures are directed toward treating the systemic response to trauma, concurrent injuries, and the burn wound.

Nursing Process
Assessment

Assessment of the person who has sustained a severe burn depends on the severity of the burn injury.

Subjective data

To determine the mechanism of injury information is obtained from either the burn victim or other persons. Data should include the following:

1. How the burn injury occurred
2. When the burn injury occurred
3. Type of burning agent
4. Duration of contact with the burning agent
5. Location (enclosed area suggests possibility of smoke inhalation and/or carbon monoxide poisoning)
6. Presence of an explosion (suggests possibility of other injuries)

The *state of health* and *age of the burn victim are important factors that may modify treatment.* The elderly and very young have a higher mortality than do young adults with the same percentage burn. *Preexisting endocrine, pulmonary, cardiovascular,* or *renal disease or medication history will decrease the person's ability to cope with severe burns. The nurse has the responsibility to learn as much as possible about the patient, including preburn weight,* from relatives and friends.

Objective data

Burns are categorized by the American Burn Association as *major, moderate,* or *minor,* and *on the basis of the size of the burn and the presence of complicating factors* (see Box 44-2).

Assessing the severity of the burn injury
Size and depth of burn

For adults, the *rule of nines* is used in determining the size of the burn. The percentage of body surface burned is estimated by using charts that depict anterior and posterior aspects of the body. In adults, the body is divided into areas equal to multiples of 9% (Fig. 44-4). In clinical

Classification of severity of burns

Major burn injuries

Partial-thickness greater than 25% BSA (greater than 20% in children under 10 years and adults over 40 years of age)
Greater than 10% BSA, full-thickness (children and adults)
Involvement of face, eyes, ears, hands, feet, perineum
Electrical burns
Burns complicated by inhalation injury or major trauma
Burns in patients with preexisting disease (diabetes, congestive heart failure, or chronic renal failure)

Moderate burn injuries

15% to 25% BSA in adults, partial-thickness (10% to 20% BSA in children under 10 years and adults over 40 years of age)
2% to 10% BSA full-thickness
Burns with no concurrent injury
Burns in patients with no preexisting disease

Minor burn injuries

Less than 15% BSA in adults (10% in children or the elderly)
Less than 2% BSA full-thickness injury
Burns in patients with no preexisting disease

practice, the burned area is shaded in on the drawings, and the amount of body surface burned is calculated from the shaded areas. Calculations are modified for infants and children under 10 years of age because of their relatively larger head and smaller bodies (see pediatric textbooks for these figures). The depth of the burn injury is determined by appearance, color, and sensation (Table 44-3).

Age of victim

The severity of a burn also depends on the age of the victim. Infants under 2 years of age and adults over 60 years of age have a higher mortality than persons in other age groups with a similar size injury. Infants have a weak antibody response to infection and in older victims the serious burn may aggravate degenerative processes or exacerbate a preexisting health problem.

Body part involved

The body part involved is an important factor in evaluating the severity of a burn. The anatomic part of the body burned must be considered when estimating the severity of the burn: a 3% burn of the anterior surface of the thigh will probably not be as serious as a 3% burn of the neck, face, or perineal area. Injuries that involve cosmetic and functional areas of the body require a long period of recovery because of both physical and emotional reactions to the burn injury. A *burn of the face, hands,* and *feet will require extensive and meticulous care.* A *burn* of the *head, neck,* and *chest may also involve injury to the respiratory tract*

Table 44-3   Characteristics of depth of burn injury

	Superficial partial-thickness (first-degree)	Deep partial-thickness (second-degree)	Full-thickness (third-degree)
Skin depth	Epidermis	Entire epidermis, dermis Sweat glands, hair follicles intact	Epidermis, dermis Extends to subcutaneous tissue, possibly muscle and bone
Cause	Flash flame, ultraviolet light (sunburn)	Contact with hot liquids or solids Flash flame to clothing Direct flames Chemicals Ultraviolet light	Contact with hot liquids or solids Flame Chemicals Electrical contact
Appearance	Dry, no blisters Minimal or no edema Blanches with fingertip pressure and color returns when pressure removed	Large, moist blisters that will increase in size Blanches with fingertip pressure and color returns when pressure removed	Dry with leathery eschar Charred vessels visible under eschar Blisters rare but thin-walled blisters that do not increase in size may be present No blanching with pressure
Color	Increased redness	Mottled with dull, white, tan, pink, or cherry red areas	White, charred, dark tan, black, red
Sensation	Painful	Very painful	No pain Nerve endings dead

Healing time	2-5 days with peeling
	No scarring
	May discolor
		Superficial: 5-21 days
		  No grafting
		Deep: 21-35 days if no infection
		  May convert to full-thickness and require grafting
			No healing potential
			Requires excision and grafting
			Healing of grafts may take months

and *result in severe respiratory difficulty.* Burns of the perineum are difficult to manage because of the potential for contamination and infection. The *circumferential or encircling burn* of a *limb,* the *neck,* or the *chest has serious consequences.* This type of burn will *cause constrictive contraction of the skin* and *produce a tourniquet effect that may impair breathing and/or circulation.*

Mechanism of injury

Identifying the causative agent is of *prime importance* because the *nature of the agent* has a *direct effect* on *prognosis and treatment.* The *mechanisms of burn injury* are *flame* and flash, *contact, scald, chemical,* and *electric.*

Flame and flash injuries are the second most common type of burn injury and are commonly associated with an inhalation injury if the burn has occurred in a closed space. These injuries may occur from house fires (caused by smoking in bed, children playing with matches) or ignited gasoline or propane. Injuries may be combined-partial and full-thickness burns. The amount and duration of the flame will determine the depth of injury.

Contact burns occur from direct contact with a hot substance, such as hot metal, stoves, hot tar, or irons. The area of burn is usually confined to the area where the substance came into contact with the skin.

Scald burns are the most common burn injury, particularly in children. Scald injury may be caused by steam

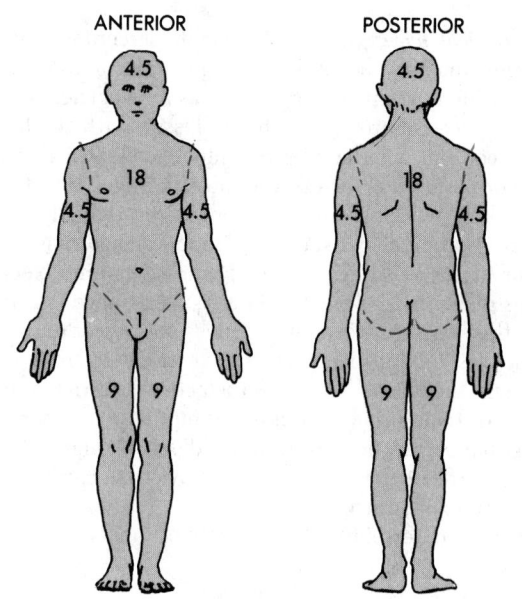

Fig. 44-4   Rule of nines.

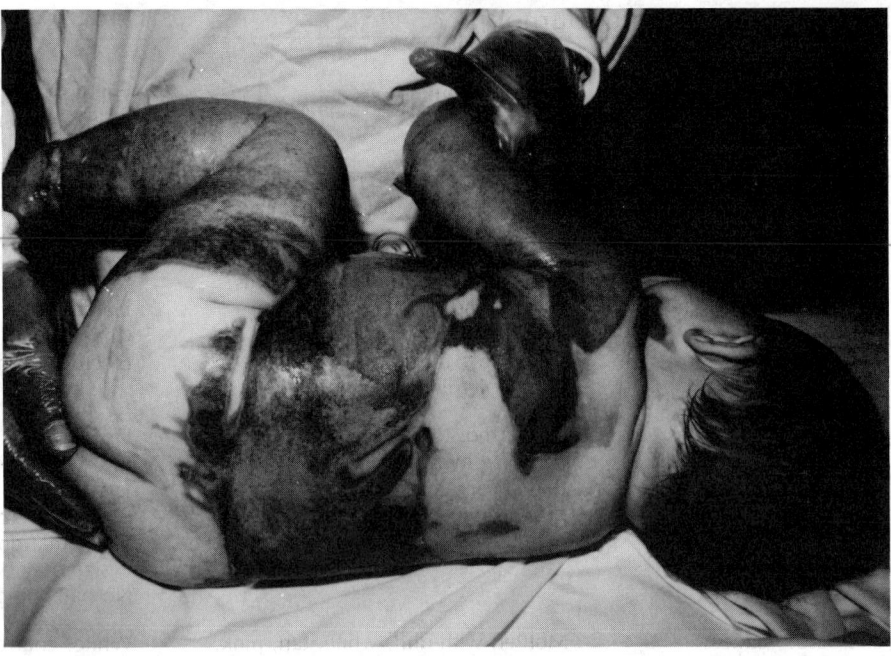

Fig. 44-5 Toddler with scald burn that resulted from being placed in a tub of water that was too hot. (Courtesy of Burn Center, Metro Health Medical Center, Cleveland, Ohio.)

or hot fluids, and may affect a widespread area (Fig. 44-5).

Chemical burns, commonly seen in industry, are caused by strong acids or alkali, such as hydochloric acid and lye (Table 44-4). Household chemical burns may occur from accidental exposure to drain cleaners, paint removers, and disinfectants. Serious burns to the eye may occur when a chemical splashes onto the face. Burns to the upper gastrointestinal tract occur when a noxious chemical is ingested.

Electrical burns consist of a small percentage of burn injuries and may be caused by lightning, or by direct or alternating current. Injury occurs as an electrical current passes directly through the body. Tissue with the highest water content has the least resistance to electrical current and consequently, suffers the most damage. Blood, muscles, skin, tendons, fat, and bones are affected in a decreasing order of resistance. Tissue damage may appear minor at the entrance and exit points, making electrical burns difficult to evaluate. The visual damage is referred to as the "tip of the iceberg" and does not reflect underlying tissue destruction generated as electrical current passes through the body. Victims of electrical burns must be checked frequently for signs and symptoms of hemorrhage, intestinal perforation, and cardiac dysrhythmias. The passage of current through the body may cause cardiac arrest at the time of injury.

Factors determining the severity of burns are listed in Box 44-3.

Medical history

Identifying known and unknown disorders may prevent fatal complications in the burn victim. A prior illness, such as diabetes or renal failure, may become acute during the

44-3	**Factors determining severity of burns**
	Size of burn
	Depth of burn
	Age of victim
	Body part involved
	Burning agent
	History of cardiac, pulmonary, renal, or hepatic disease
	Injuries sustained at time of burn

postburn phase. The physiologic stress seen with the burn may exacerbate a latent disease process or worsen the process if it is active, and thus increase mortality.

Data analysis: nursing diagnoses

Nursing diagnoses are determined from analysis of patient data. Possible nursing diagnoses for the person with burn during the emergent period may include, but are not limited to, the following:

Diagnostic title	Possible etiologies
Airway clearance, ineffective	Laryngeal edema, obstruction, secretions
Impaired skin integrity	Loss of skin from burn injury
Pain	Exposed nerve endings from burn injury, trauma
Fluid volume deficit (1)	Movement of fluid from intravascular to interstitial space (hypovolemic stage), evaporation
Fluid volume deficit (2)	Movement of fluid from interstitial to intravascular space (diuretic stage)

Table 44-4   Agents associated with chemical burns

Chemical agent	Common use	Characteristics	Systemic effects	Agents to remove or dilute chemicals
Oxidizing agents				
Chromic acid	Metal cleansing	Ulcerates, blisters		Water lavage
Potassium perman-ganate	Disinfectant, bleach, deodorizers	Thick, brownish purple eschar		Water lavage Eggwhite solution
Sodium hypochlorite (Clorox)	Disinfectant, bleach, deodorizers	Local irritation, inflam-mation		Water lavage Milk, Eggwhite Starch Paste
Corrosive agents				
Phenol	Deodorizers; sanitizers; disinfectants; manufac-ture of plastics, dyes, fertilizers, explosives	Soft white eschar, brown stain when eschar removed, mild to no pain	Minor exposure: tachy-cardia dysrhythmias	Copious water la-vage Polyethelene glycol solution Vegetable oil
			Significant exposure: CNS depression, hy-pothermia, cardiac depression, respira-tory depression	Lavage with water to debride particles
Phosphorus (white)	Manufacture of explo-sives, insecticides, ro-dent poisons, fertilizers	Necrotic with yellow-ish color Garlic odor Glows in dark Painful	Nephrotoxicity Hepatic necrosis	Lavage with 1% cop-per sulfate (CuSO₄), Cover with castor oil
Pure sodium lye KOH NaOH NH₄OH LiOH Ba₂(OH)₃ Ca(OH)₃	Cleaning agents (washing powders, drain clean-ers, paint removers), urine sugar reagent tablets, Portland ce-ment	Soft gelatinous, brown eschar		Lye; water lavage Pure sodium; oil im-mersion
Protoplasmic poisons				
Salt-formers Tungstic Picric Sulfasalicyclic Tannic Trichloracetic Cresylic Acetate Formic	Industrial	Thin, hard eschar	Hepatic necrosis Nephrotoxicity	Water lavage
Metabolic competi-tor/inhibitor Oxalic acid	Industrial	Chalky white ulcers	Hypocalcemia	Large volume cal-cium salts Copious water la-vage Intravenous calcium
Hydrofluoric acid	Etching of glass	Painful, deep ulcer-ations	Hypocalcemia	Water lavage Subcutaneous cal-cium to area Subcutaneous mag-nesium sulfate

Diagnostic title	Possible etiologies
Hypothermia	Environmental exposure of burn wounds
Infection, high risk for	Loss of protection created by damage to skin
Anxiety: patient and significant other	Threat to self-concept, threat of death, threat/change in health status

Planning: expected patient outcomes

Expected patient outcomes for the person with burns may include, but are not limited to, the following:

1. Patient maintains patent airway, adequate ventilation and oxygenation.
2. No further skin loss occurs.
3. Patient states that pain is controlled.
4. Optimal fluid and electrolyte balance is regained.
5. Patient's body temperature is normal.
6. Patient is free of pathogenic organisms.
7. Patient and family exhibit control of anxiety.

Implementation

During the emergent period of burn injury, the patient's care is provided in a highly collaborative manner between nursing and medicine. These areas include airway management and oxygenation, wound management, fluid resuscitation, and pain control. In addition, the nurse must initiate steps to address the psychosocial aspects of patient care.

Maintaining a patent airway

Persons who are burned on the face and neck or those who have inhaled flame, steam, or smoke should be observed closely for signs of laryngeal edema and airway obstruction. Data indicating potential or existing airway injury are outlined in Box 44-4.

Adequate ventilation and oxygenation may be possible on room air; however, when any inhalation injury has occurred it is best to give oxygen. When smoke is inhaled, carbon monoxide binds with hemoglobin, displacing oxygen. High carboxyhemoglobin levels may result in impaired tissue oxygenation. Providing the victim with 100% oxygen by mask will reverse this condition. If the victim is in respiratory distress or has a suspected inhalation injury, intubation may be necessary (see Plate 7).

Prehospital care

At the scene of a burn injury, the *first action is to remove* the *victim from the hazardous environment.* The length of exposure to the causative agent is directly related to the severity of the injury. *Initial management follows* the ABC's: *airway, breathing, circulation.*

The most common causative agents for burn injury are fire, scald, chemicals, and electricity. Regardless of the cause, the burning process must be stopped. In the case of fire, flames should be extinguished, flammable or hot material removed from the victim, and the victim and rescuer removed from the unventilated or hazardous surroundings. If *clothing is on fire*, the victim's first reaction is to run, which only fans the flame. The *best intervention* is to *stop the person and roll him or her in a blanket, coat,*

> **Factors determining inhalation injury and/ or potential airway obstruction**
>
> Burns to face and neck
> Singed hairs, nasal hair, beard, eyelids, or eyelashes
> Intraoral charcoal, especially on teeth and gums
> Respiratory distress
> Brassy cough
> Hoarseness
> Copious sputum production
> Carbonaceous sputum
> Burn injury occurred in a closed space
> Smell of smoke on victim's clothes or on victim

sheet, or towel on the ground to exclude oxygen and *thereby put out the fire.* The rule is *stop, drop,* and *roll.* The victim should never stand because this will cause the flame and smoke to engulf the facial area, possibly igniting the hair and causing an inhalation injury. Any water source can be used to extinguish flames unless victim is still in contact with an electrical source.

First aid for burn wounds

Once all flame is extinguished, clothing, jewelry, and debris are carefully removed, avoiding removal of clothing that adheres to the burned area. Any clothing removed should be saved for possible analysis of flammability. The *wounds are covered with dressings dampened with normal saline to ease the pain, reduce edema, and prevent evaporation of body water.* The patient is entirely wrapped in a dry cover to prevent heat loss. Ice should never be used because sudden vasoconstriction causes severe shifting of fluids and may increase the depth of injury. Although sterile dressings are preferred, clean, nonsterile dressings can be used because all dressings will be removed at the medical facility. Oils, salves, and ointments should never be used on burns because they hamper treatment at the medical facility.

Scald injury is *related* to the *temperature of the liquid* and *the length of exposure. Initial care* consists of *cooling* the *skin surface with a cool solution.* First aid follows the same treatment plan as for a flame burn.

The *severity* of *chemical burns* is *directly proportional to the length of exposure.* Chemicals cause deep burns over a rather limited area. The chemical should be identified and treatment initiated quickly. The *first priority* is *to remove the chemical agent.* This is accomplished by *copious flushing with water for as long as 20 to 30 minutes to ensure complete removal of the chemical.* Although specific chemical agents have known antidotes, it is best to *flood the exposed area with water to ensure removal of the chemical,* and transport the victim to the nearest medical facility. Burns occurring around the eyes should be lavaged continuously with copious amounts of cool, clean water for up to 30 minutes.

Electrical burns pose *a special hazard to the victim because the total body surface area of the burn* is not *always apparent* and is *often internal. Dysrhythmias* and *neurologic dysfunction are common* in such exposure. Extreme care must be taken in removing the patient from the electrical source to prevent a similar injury to the rescuer.

Initial care for major burns

1. Remove victim from source of burn.
2. Douse with water and remove nonadherent, smoldering clothing to stop the burning process.
3. If chemical burn, carefully remove clothing and flush wound with large amounts of water.
4. If electrical burn and victim is still in contact with electrical source, do *not* touch victim. Remove electrical source with dry nonconductive object (rope).
5. Establish patent airway and assess for inhalation injury. Give oxygen if available.
6. Check peripheral pulses to assess circulatory status.
7. Assess and initiate treatment for injuries requiring immediate attention.
8. Remove tight-fitting jewelry or clothing.
9. Cover burn with moist sterile or clean cover.
10. Cover victim with warm dry cover to prevent heat loss.
11. Transport victim to nearest medical facility.

Pain relief

Pain in extensive burns is best controlled by gentle and minimal handling and by the application of dressings that exclude air from the burned surfaces. The degree of pain is usually inversely proportional to the depth of the burn injury—full-thickness burns cause minimal pain because nerve endings have been destroyed.

In small partial-thickness burns, cool (not cold) compresses on the burn site may provide some relief as long as the victim is kept warm.

Transport

Burns are often more severe than they first appear to be. Therefore, a physician should see all persons with burns, even if the burns appear to be superficial. The hospital or burn center should be notified before a severely burned victim is transported so that preparation can be made for arrival.

For obviously *small burns, fluids may be given by mouth with caution. Large burns* are accompanied by *decreased peristalsis;* therefore, *nothing should be given by mouth. Patients with large burns or smoke inhalation may vomit,* and particular *attention* must be *given to preventing them* from *aspirating vomitus.*

According to the 1991-1992 American Burn Association Directory, 148 hospitals in the United States reported the presence of a specialized burn care service. This represents a 12% reduction in burn beds from 1985 to the present. These burns units are located throughout the United States in major medical centers in or near urban areas. The American Burn Association publishes a list of specialized burn care services every year.[6]

The initial care for major burns is summarized in Box 44-5.

Emergency room management

Rapid and efficient care is essential in the emergency room management of the burn victim. If *respiratory distress is present, an airway is established.* Prophylactic intubation is initiated if heat or smoke has been inhaled, or if the head, neck, or face is involved. *Inhalation injuries are best managed with controlled ventilation because swelling of the upper airway can rapidly cause obstruction* (Plate 7). *Endotracheal intubation is preferred* over a tracheostomy. Edema of the respiratory passages frequently subsides within a few days after the injury; therefore, surgery of the airway should be avoided. *Depending on the severity of symptoms, emergency treatment may include oxygen, suctioning, and postural drainage.*

After an airway has been established, support of circulation is addressed. Burn injuries cause tremendous losses of fluid through the wound as well as into the burn wound and adjacent tissues in the form of edema. *Fluid loss is best replaced through two large-caliber peripheral intravenous catheters.* However, if the burn is large, or complicated by inhalation injuries or preexisting disease, one peripheral line and one central line (for central venous pressure measurement) is preferred. To prevent the introduction of infection, the lines are inserted through unburned areas. An *indwelling Foley catheter is inserted to monitor urine output accurately.* Hourly urine output measurements are used as a guide to the adequacy of fluid (plasma volume) replacement.

Almost every patient who is burned over more than 15% body surface area (BSA) develops thirst and an ileus. Oral fluids will not pass beyond the stomach and they create a threat of regurgitation and aspiration. A *nasogastric tube is inserted* and the *stomach is kept empty by suction* to prevent gastric distention.

Managing pain

Morphine sulfate is the drug of choice for pain relief and is given intravenously in small increments. A morphine sulfate drip can be used (15 mg in 250 ml D5W) and titrated to the patient's pain. The intravenous route is used because of inadequate absorption at peripheral sites. *No medication of any kind should be given intramuscularly or subcutaneously because it may pool and be absorbed later when cardiac output and blood pressure improve.* Large doses of sedatives and analgesics are avoided because of the danger of respiratory depression and the potential masking of other symptoms.

Tetanus prophylaxis is initiated in the *emergency department.* Tetanus toxoid is administered if the patient has been previously immunized but has not received tetanus toxoid in the preceding 5 years. If prior tetanus immunization is not documented, a dose of human tetanus—immune globulin (TIGH) is administered and an active tetanus immunization program is begun.

The treatment of major burns in the emergency room is summarized in Box 44-6.

Replacing body fluids

Replacing fluids and electrolytes is an essential part of the treatment of the burn victim and is *instituted as soon as the severity of the burn and the patient's condition are known.*

44-6 | **Initial treatment of major burns in the emergency room**

1. Establish airway.
2. Initiate fluid therapy by intravenous catheters.
3. Insert indwelling Foley catheter for hourly urine measurement.
4. Insert nasogastric tube to remove stomach contents and prevent gastric distention.
5. Insert central intravenous catheter, if appropriate.
6. Manage pain by intravenous narcotics in small, frequent doses.
7. Provide tetanus prophylaxis.

44-7 | **Indications for fluid resuscitation**

Burns greater than 20% BSA in adults
Burns greater than 10% BSA in children
Patient older than 65 or younger than 2 years of age
Patient with preexisting disease that would reduce normal compensatory responses to minor hypovolemia (cardiac, pulmonary or renal disease, diabetes)

Ideally, fluid therapy is started within an hour after a severe burn to prevent hypovolemic shock. Insertion of two large-caliber peripheral catheters or one large-caliber central venous catheter and one large-caliber peripheral catheter permits the rapid administration of fluids and electrolytes.

Fluids administered during the first 48 hours are given to maintain circulating blood volume. Additional fluids and electrolytes are added to replace losses from vomiting or from nasogastric drainage. *Three types of fluid are considered in calculating the needs of the patient:* (1) *colloids,* including plasma and plasma expanders such as Dextran, (2) *electrolytes,* such as physiologic solution of sodium chloride, Ringer's solution, Hartmann's solution, or Tyrode's solution, and (3) *nonelectrolyte fluids,* such as distilled water with 5% glucose. Medical authorities do not agree about the proportion of colloids and electrolyte fluids needed. Several formulas are described in the medical literature to guide physicians in determining the type and amount of fluids to be administered based on the patient's weight, age, and the percentage of the body burned.[45] The *present trend is to administer balanced salt solutions* (for example, lactated Ringer's), *water,* and *plasma and to use whole blood only if a large number of red blood cells are destroyed* or *if anemia develops.* Indications for the use of fluids are summarized in Box 44-7.

According to the crystalloid resuscitation formula, fluids are administered in three time periods of 8 hours each. In the first three 8-hour periods (24 hours) Ringer's lactate solution (RL) or Hartmann's solution is administered according to the following formula:

4 ml RL × weight (kg) × % BSA burned = ml RL for 24 hr

Because blood volume falls most rapidly and edema increases fastest in the first 8 hours, intravenous replacement must be at a rapid rate. One half of the total amount calculated is given in the first 8 hours after the injury. The time is calculated from the *time of injury,* not from the time emergency care was started. In the second 8-hour period, one fourth of the total amount of calculated Ringer's lactate solution is given, and in the third 8-hour period, the remaining one fourth is given.

Traditionally, the use of colloids in the first 24 hours was avoided because of the leak of protein through the capillaries into the interstitial space. Currently, the use of colloids in the first 24 hours is evaluated on an individual basis. If the patient requires more than 6 ml/kg/% of fluid, colloids may be added.[26]

Patients may complain of moderate to severe thirst during this period. *Frequent oral hygiene* may alleviate patient discomfort. *If oral fluids are permitted, accurate recording of intake is important. Unlimited oral intake and failure to measure and record it may result in water intoxication.*

During the second 24 hours postburn, one half to two thirds of the initial 24-hour volume will be required. Unless started earlier, it is also during this second 24-hour period that colloid solutions are used to replace intravascular volume once capillary permeability significantly decreases.

During fluid resuscitation, adequate volume is assessed by monitoring mental status, vital signs, peripheral perfusion, body weight, and *urine output.* A 15% to 20% weight gain in the first 72 hours of resuscitation is anticipated. Important laboratory tests are serum and urine electrolytes, serum and urine osmolality, and hematocrit. Hourly urine output is generally the most reliable index of adequate fluid replacement. Fluid should be titrated to ensure an output of 30 to 50 ml/hr in the adult and 0.5 to 1 ml/kg/hr in the child. A drop in urine output below 30 ml/hr may indicate insufficient fluid replacement. The most common reasons for this are that the calculated amount of fluid is behind schedule or the severity of the burn has been underestimated. The urine is observed for color and checked for the presence of blood. The physician is notified if hematuria or a positive Hemastix reaction is present.

Data that indicate adequate fluid resuscitation are pulse rate of 120/min or less in the adult, *central venous pressure in low to normal range, pulmonary artery end-diastolic pressure (PAEDP) in low to normal range,* and *mental alertness* (see a summary in Box 44-8).

After the first 48 to 72 hours, the patient enters the *diuretic stage* as edema reabsorption occurs. The urinary output increases dramatically, and it is no longer a reliable guide to fluid needs. Fluid needs are assessed by measuring serum and urine electrolyte levels, and replacement is based on individual assessment using 5% dextrose and water. If dehydration occurs from diuresis, fluid replacement therapy is continued until blood volume is stabilized. Potassium may be added to the intravenous fluid because of potassium losses through the urine. The patient is monitored closely for signs of water intoxication or pulmonary edema.

Wound care

Care of the burn wound can be delayed until all first aid measures have been initiated. Wound care should be carried out carefully and with as little discomfort to the patient as possible. One of the most important factors to be considered is that the patient has lost the ability to withstand infection in the area where the skin is damaged or destroyed. The *goals of the initial wound care* are as follows:

1. Cleanse the wound to eliminate or decrease the dead tissue and debris that serve as the media for bacterial growth
2. Prevent further destruction of viable skin
3. Provide for patient comfort

During the admission procedure, the burn wound and the entire body are washed to remove dirt and debris as well as loose, dead tissue on the burned areas. Detergents (Dreft) or antiseptic preparations are effective cleansing agents. Gentle cleansing with gauze squares is effective in removing dead tissue without causing further tissue damage.

All hair in and around the burn wound is shaved and wiped away because hair attracts and shelters bacteria. Singed hair is clipped short to avoid bacterial contamination of the wound.

Firm, intact blisters are left undisturbed because they are a natural, protective, pain-free dressing. If the blisters are broken and the epidermis is separated, loose tissue must be debrided.

Maintenance of body temperature is a critical factor during cleansing, because the severely burned patient has lost some of the ability to regulate body temperature. The *environment must be heat controlled and kept warmer than usual*. Drafts should be eliminated. A heat lamp or warming lights should be available. Prolonged exposure to air should be avoided. Exposed areas of the body should be covered with sterile sheets and blankets while other areas of the burn are being cleansed.

After the wound is cleaned and before a dressing is applied, cultures of the wound are obtained. Prophylactic systemic antibiotics are usually not indicated. However, wound cultures are obtained to determine which organisms are present in the wounds at the time of admission.

Photographs are taken on admission and at intervals during the patient's hospitalization. They provide a record of the appearance of the burn wound on admission, before the application of topical therapy, and during the healing process.

An early complication of thermal injury is the constricting effect of a *circumferential eschar* of the trunk or extremities. Eschar is a crust or scab that forms over a burn wound. Edema forming rapidly under the constricting eschar of a full-thickness wound on the arms or legs will produce enough pressure to cause occlusion of venous and arterial circulation and may result in *ischemic necrosis,* especially if unburned areas are distal to the constrictive eschar. Circumferential burns of the neck and chest not only occlude circulation but also may result in pressure on the trachea or rib cage, causing respiratory distress. Frequent observations of chest excursions in addition to res-

44-8	Signs of adequate fluid resuscitation	
	Clear sensorium	
	Pulse	< 120 beats/minute
	Urine output	30 to 50 ml/hr (adult)
		0.5 to 1 ml/kg/hr (child)
	Systolic blood pressure	100 mm Hg
	Central venous pressure	5 to 10 mm Hg
	Pulmonary artery end-diastolic pressure	5 to 15 mm Hg
	Blood pH normal range	7.35 to 7.45

piratory rate are necessary to determine whether respiratory restriction is developing. Extremities should be monitored for signs and symptoms of circulatory compromise including diminished peripheral pulses, decreased capillary refill, paleness or cyanosis, temperature decrease, and increase in pain or paresthesias. It may be necessary to monitor circulation every 15 minutes.

Treatment of constrictive eschar is by an escharotomy. The eschar is surgically cut in a linear direction or into squares to alleviate stricture (Plate 8). This is a painless procedure in a full-thickness burn because the nerve endings have already been damaged.

Decreasing anxiety and providing emotional support

Patients with significant burn injuries have received a profound insult to their body and self-image. They are fearful and anxious about possible scarring and disfigurement. They are also aware that they may not survive, and this increases feelings of fear and helplessness. The shock and pain of the accident, the chaos and rush to the hospital, the unknown surroundings and people all intensify the emotional stress.

The nurse is the member of the burn team who spends the most time with the patient and has a considerable influence on the patient's psychologic adjustment. *Interventions that can be used to reassure the patient and alleviate anxiety include the following:*

1. Identify self to patient
2. Orient patient to the surroundings
3. Describe the reasons for physical symptoms (skin loss, pain, cold)
4. Explain the equipment and procedures to be used in treatment

Evaluation

Evaluation is based on the expected patient outcomes. Questions to ask may include the following:

1. Does the patient demonstrate any respiratory distress?
2. Is the patient experiencing pain?
3. Is the patient in optimal fluid and electrolyte balance?
4. Is the patient anxious or fearful?
5. Is the patient free of infection?

Acute Period

The acute period of treatment begins at the end of the emergent period and lasts until the burn wound is healed. The length of this period varies. If the burn is a partial-thickness injury, the acute period extends 10 to 20 days; if the burn is a full-thickness injury over a large percentage of the body requiring surgery for skin grafting, the acute period can last for months.

The nursing care of patients during the acute period of burns is complex. Analysis of data may lead to the identification of numerous nursing diagnoses.

During the *acute period* the *two main principles* of *management* are: (1) *treatment of the burn wound*, and (2) *avoidance, detection*, and *treatment* of *complications*. The *most common complications* are *infection* (septicemia, pneumonia), *renal disease*, and *heart failure*.

Nursing Process
Assessment
Subjective data

Burn patients are often frightened and anxious about their injury and the associated treatments. The intensive care unit (ICU) environment can compound these responses.

Burn patients experience both physical and psychologic pain. Physical pain is usually focused on specific activities such as wound cleansing and debridement, dressing changes, and physical therapy. The patient may react to physical pain in three ways: (1) by ignoring it, (2) by accepting it, or (3) by overreacting to it. The nurse should not judge whether or not the patient is feeling real pain. The nurse must instead assess the patient's reaction to pain and intervene appropriately.

Objective data

The nurse must perform a thorough head-to-toe assessment of the burn patient every shift. Data should include *mental status*, *vital signs*, *breath sounds*, *bowel sounds*, *dietary intake*, *motor ability*, *intake* and *output*, *weight pattern*, *circulatory assessment*, and *observation of burn wounds*, *grafts*, and *donor site*. Purulent drainage, abnormal color, foul odor, redness or swelling in surrounding normal skin, or presence of healing should be noted. Changes in these parameters from shift to shift or from day to day make further investigation necessary.

Metabolism is *increased* following *moderate to severe burns* as a result of *stress*, *fluid loss*, *fever*, and *infection*. Wound healing may be prolonged if adequate nutritional support is not initiated on admission. A nutritional assessment is performed during the first days following burn injury and includes anthropometric measurements (to determine actual weight loss compared to ideal weight), serum electrolytes, liver function tests, and urinalysis.

Data analysis: nursing diagnoses

Nursing diagnoses are determined from analysis of patient data. Possible nursing diagnoses for the person with burns may include, but are not limited to, the following:

Diagnostic title	Possible etiologies
Fear	Long-term illness, death, pain, treatment, life-style changes
Anxiety	Threat to self-concept, threat/change in health status/role functioning, situational crisis
Knowledge deficit	Unfamiliarity with routines and burn healing process
Hypothermia	Environmental exposure of burn wounds
Infection, high risk for	Decreased nutrition, burn wound treatment (dressings, surgery)
Nutrition, altered: less than body requirements	Increased metabolic needs
Pain	Treatment of burn wounds (dressings, surgery)
Skin integrity, impaired	Burn wounds
Social isolation	Alteration in physical appearance, physical isolation (wound/skin)

Planning: expected patient outcomes

Expected patient outcomes for the person with burns may include, but are not limited to, the following:

1. Patient is not fearful (establishes a trusting relationship with his or her primary nurse).
2. Patient will verbalize anxiety.
3. Patient verbalizes understanding of treatments and surgical procedures and participates appropriately in care.
4. Body temperature is normal.
5. Patient is free of pathogenic organisms.
6. Optimal nutritional status is achieved.
7. Patient obtains pain relief.
8. Majority of wounds are closed.
9. Social isolation is decreased.

Implementation
Assisting with achievement of therapeutic goals
Burn treatment methods

Different methods of treating the burned area may be used, depending on the location of the burn, its size and depth, the facilities available, and the patient's response to therapy. One method may be replaced with another during the course of treatment.

Open or exposure method. The exposure method of treatment was accidentally discovered to be effective in 1888 when, during a serious steamboat fire on the Mississippi River, those in attendance ran out of bandages and later observed that the neglected persons fared better than those who received more intensive local treatment.[35] Today the exposure method is used most often in the treatment of burns involving the face, neck, perineum, and broad areas of the trunk. The burned area is cleansed and exposed to air (Fig. 44-6). The exudate of a partial-thickness burn dries in 48 to 72 hours and forms a hard crust that protects the wound. Epithelialization occurs beneath this crust and may be complete in 14 to 21 days. The crust then falls off spontaneously, leaving a healed, unscarred surface. The

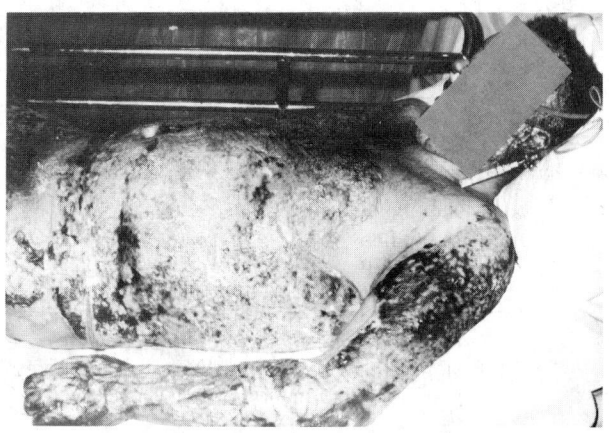

Fig. 44-6   Severly burned man being treated by open method. (Courtesy Burn Center, Metro Health Medical Center, Cleveland, Ohio.)

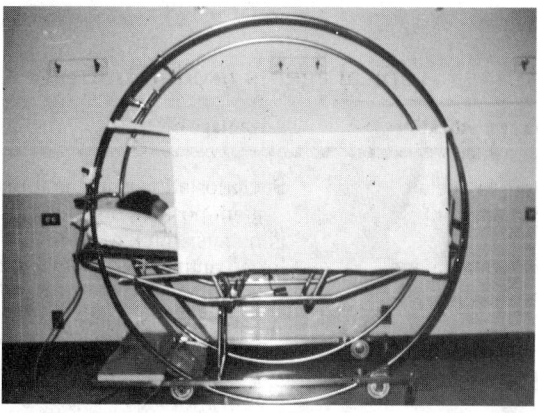

Fig. 44-7   Another exposure method of treating burns. A sheet is draped over CircOlectric bed so that burned areas are not touched. (Courtesy Burn Unit, Cook County Hospital, Chicago.)

dead skin of a full-thickness burn is dehydrated and converted to black, leathery eschar in 48 to 72 hours. Loose eschar may be gradually removed through the use of hydrotherapy and debridement. Uninfected eschar acts as a protective covering. The danger of infection exists as bacteria proliferate beneath the eschar. Spontaneous separation, produced by bacterial action, occurs unless surgical debridement is performed first.

Isolation technique is essential when the exposure method is used. The nurse should wear a sterile gown and mask, and sterile linen may be used on the patient's bed. A cradle may be used on the patient's bed, because no clothing or bed clothes are allowed directly over burned areas. If the burn is extensive, a CircOlectric bed draped with a sheet is an ideal way to care for the patient (Fig. 44-7). The burned person can be kept from embarrassing exposure by wearing a halter and loin cloth. Lights or heat lamps may be used with caution to provide warmth. Advantages of the open method are that the wound is easily inspected and the patient has maximal freedom to perform exercises for the prevention of contractures and the improvement of circulation.

Patients having exposure treatment complain of pain and chilling. Pain may be controlled by administering morphine sulfate, meperidine hydrochloride (Demerol), or salicylates as ordered. Discomfort can be decreased if drafts are avoided and the temperature of the room is kept at 24.4° C (85° F). *Patients lose more heat from burned surfaces than from normal skin surfaces because the vascular bed that normally contracts and retains heat in the body is lost.* The humidity of the room should also be controlled. A humidity of 40% to 50% is usually considered satisfactory. Humidity at this level assists in minimizing fluid loss through the skin. Portable electric humidifiers and dehumidifiers can be used to achieve and maintain this level.

Semiopen method. The semiopen wound care method consists of covering the wound with topical antimicrobial agents and a thin layer of gauze to help keep the agent in

contact with the wound. This method permits the passage of wound exudate through the dressing without the loss of antimicrobial cream. The success of semiopen care depends on cleaning the wound once or twice a day, either at the bedside or in the hydrotherapy tank. Meticulous semiopen wound care speeds debridement, enhances the development of granulation tissue, and enables earlier grafting.

Closed method. In the closed or occlusive method of burn treatment, the wounds are washed and the dressings are changed at least once a day, or in some instances once each shift. Commonly, the dressing consists of gauze impregnated with topical ointments and a gauze wrap. Counterpressure wrappings (elastic bandages) may be applied. When a dressing is in place, nursing observation includes monitoring for signs of impaired circulation (numbness, pain, and tingling) and for signs of infection (odor on dressings, elevated temperature, and elevated pulse rate).

Application of topical agents. The application of topical agents to the burn wound can help to decrease infection and hasten healing. These agents are effective because damage to blood vessels in the burn area prevents systemic antibiotics from reaching the burn wound. Antibiotics may be given prophylactically or may be withheld until an infection occurs. The following is a description of some of the topical drugs currently in use for burn patients.

Mafenide. Mafenide (Sulfamylon) is a white cream containing sulfonamide. It is applied to the wound once or twice daily with a sterile gloved hand in a thin layer, just enough to cover the burn completely. The wound may be left open to air or a single layer of gauze may be used to hold the cream in place. The cream is removed from the wound, and active debriding is performed before the cream is reapplied.

Mafenide is known to inhibit carbonic anhydrase activity, especially in patients with burns of 40% or more of

Table 44-5   Topical agents used in burn therapy

Topical medication	Advantages	Disadvantages
Mafenide acetate (Sulfamylon)	Bacteriostatic against gram-negative and gram-positive organisms Penetrates thick eschar	Metabolic acidosis Pain on application Allergic rash
Silver sulfadiazine (Silvadene)	Broad antimicrobial activity against gram-negative, gram-positive, and candida organisms No electrolyte imbalances Painless and somewhat soothing Not nephrotoxic	With repeated application, skin may develop slimy, grayish appearance, simulating an infection despite negative cultures Prolonged use may cause skin rash and depress granulocyte formation
Povidone-iodine (Betadine)	Broad antimicrobial activity against gram-positive and gram-negative bacteria, fungi, yeasts, viruses, and protozoa	Metabolic acidosis resulting from elevated serum iodine levels Stains clothing and linen Dry, crusting, scabbing wound Skin rash in unaffected area
Silver nitrate	Bacteriostatic effect Lessens pain and eliminates odor Reduces evaporative water loss from burns	Electrolyte imbalances Stains everything it comes into contact with Does not penetrate eschar Pain on application
Nitrofurazone (Furacin)	Inhibits enzymes necessary for bacterial metabolism Broad spectrum of activity Effective against *Staphylococcus aureus* Not absorbed systemically Low incidence of sensitivity	Contact dermatitis on unaffected skin Urine turns a reddish color Overgrowth of fungus and *Pseudomonas* Pain on application
Gentamycin sulfate (Garamycin)	Broad antimicrobial activity Painless	Ototoxicity Nephrotoxicity Development of resistant bacterial strains
Neomycin	Broad antimicrobial activity Causes miscoding in the messenger RNA of bacterial cells	Serious toxic effects Ototoxicity Nephrotoxicity
Scarlet red	Nonantiseptic (applied to gauze soaked with oil-base red dye) Drying agent Applied to donor site Promotes epithelialization	No antimicrobial effects Stains and irritates skin Infection that may have systemic effects may develop beneath scarlet red gauze
Xeroform	Nonantiseptic Debrides and protects donor site Protects graft	Removal may be painful because it sometimes adheres to wound Neither antiseptic nor antimicrobial
Sodium hypochlorite (Dakin's Solution)	Chlorine-based solution that is bacteriocidal Aids in debriding wounds Aids cleaning and draining "soupy" wounds	Dissolves blood clots May inhibit clotting May irritate the skin
Sutilains ointment (Travase)	Topical enzymatic agent Dissolves necrotic tissue by proteolytic action Facilitates removal of eschar and purulent drainage	Mild, transient pain on application Paresthesia, bleeding, dermatitis Dressing must be kept moist at all times
Bacitracin	Prevents drying of wound Keeps eschar soft and pliable Beneficial in facial burns to promote healing Used as open technique Painless on application	No major antibiotic properties Oil based, difficult to wash away
Biobrane	Pain reduced, wound not subjected to daily dressing change Water loss from skin minimized	Cannot be used on eschar or if wound is cleansed with any antiseptic before application

BSA. As a result, metabolic acidosis may occur. The patient is monitored for hyperventilation, which can result from attempts to balance the increased acid load. Other side effects include pain with application of the cream and an allergic rash. Mafenide inhibits epithelial proliferation; therefore, application should be stopped as soon as the wound is clean and there is evidence of healing.

Silver sulfadiazine. Silver sulfadiazine (Silvadene) is a white cream with bactericidal action against many gram-negative and gram-positive bacteria, as well as against *Candida albicans*. It is applied directly to the wound once or twice daily on saturated gauze or with a sterile gloved hand. The wound may be covered with a dressing or left exposed. Silver sulfadiazine does not penetrate as readily as Mafenide acetate; however, patients do not complain of pain with its application.

The patient is observed for side effects common with sulfonamide drugs. The wound may develop a slimy, grayish appearance simulating an infection, despite negative cultures. Silver sulfadiazine should not be used in patients with a history of kidney disease. No electrolyte imbalances are seen with its use; however, prolonged use may lead to toxic symptoms including nausea, vomiting, anemia, leukopenia, granulocytopenia, mental changes, oliguria, anuria, hematuria, jaundice, and skin rashes.

Povidone-iodine. Povidone-iodine (Betadine) ointment is a reddish brown germicidal preparation of 10% povidone-iodine (1% available iodine) with broad-spectrum microbial action. It is applied three times daily. Povidone-iodine can be applied by (1) spreading it with a sterile gloved hand onto the burned surface or (2) impregnating a single-thickness gauze with the povidone-iodine and applying it to the burned surfaces and then spreading additional ointment on top of the gauze layer. Clothing and bedding need to be protected from staining. A dry, crusting wound may be seen as well as skin rashes in unaffected areas. Currently povidone-iodine is used infrequently.

Silver nitrate. Although silver nitrate is used less often than in the past, some physicians still prescribe it. In this treatment, thick gauze dressings are saturated with 0.5% solution of silver nitrate. The dressings are kept wet so that the solution remains in constant contact with the burned surfaces. If the dressing is allowed to dry, the silver nitrate can concentrate and cause tissue destruction. These dressings retain moisture and heat and reduce evaporation. Proponents of this method of treatment believe that it reduces mortality, lessens pain, eliminates odors, and has a bacteriostatic effect. The dressings are removed every 12 to 24 hours, and the patient is placed in a bath of salt solution with the temperature carefully maintained at body temperature. When skin grafts are applied, silver nitrate dressings are placed over the grafts and donor sites on the first postoperative day. Because the silver nitrate is hypotonic, electrolytes are lost into the wound. Therefore, throughout treatment, frequent determinations of blood sodium levels are necessary, and sodium that is lost may need to be replaced. Everything that comes into contact with silver nitrate solution is stained black, so care should be taken when applying the solution to protect skin, clothing, furniture, walls, and floors.

The above treatments and other topical agents used in burn therapy are outlined in Table 44-5.

Wound coverings. The burn wound may be covered with dressings or grafts.

Dressings. Large bulky dressings are rarely used today for large burns except in select instances because infection control is more difficult and partial-thickness burns may develop into full-thickness wounds. The purposes of applying some light covering include prevention of infection from exogenous sources, facilitation of debridement and maximal contact by topical agents, and prevention of fluid evaporation with loss of body heat. The type of dressing that is usually applied consists of a single layer of fine mesh gauze impregnated with a topical medication and held in place by a wrapping of a coarse gauze such as Kerlix.

The dressing change is usually a painful procedure requiring analgesics. Analgesics should be given 30 minutes before the procedure for maximal effectiveness. Most dressing changes are performed after tubbing to facilitate dressing removal and to lessen pain. Additional debridement of eschar and dead tissue may be performed before the new dressing is applied.

Wet dressings may be used with silver nitrate or normal saline applications. Normal saline is applied to clean granulation tissue or to new grafts to maintain moisture or is used with fine mesh gauze to provide for slight debridement. A single layer of fine mesh gauze is usually placed over the wound, covered with thick gauze pads to maintain moisture, and held in place with a gauze wrapping. The dressings must be kept wet. Plastic wrap should *not* be used to cover the dressings; this prevents fluid evaporation, causes increased heat at the wound site, and results in patient discomfort and increased tissue destruction and infection.

Skin grafts. Skin grafts are applied to cover the burn wound and speed healing, to prevent contractures, and to shorten convalescence. Successful grafting reduces the patient's vulnerability to infection and prevents the loss of body heat and water vapor from the open wound. Grafting for cosmetic or functional purposes may be performed during the rehabilitative period. Most skin grafts are applied between the third and twenty-first day after the initial injury, depending on the depth and extent of the burn and the condition of the base.

Grafts are obtained from various sources (Table 44-6). An *autograft* is a graft of skin obtained from the patient's own body. A *homograft* is a graft of skin obtained from a cadaver 6 to 24 hours after death. A *heterograft* is a graft of skin obtained from other animals, such as a pig. Synthetic substitutes for skin are currently being investigated.

The latter three types of grafts afford only temporary coverage. Homografts may grow or "take," but in a matter of weeks they will be rejected by the body and slough off. The advantage of a temporary graft is to reduce water, electrolyte, and protein loss at the burn surface. The covered wound is less painful and allows the patient freedom

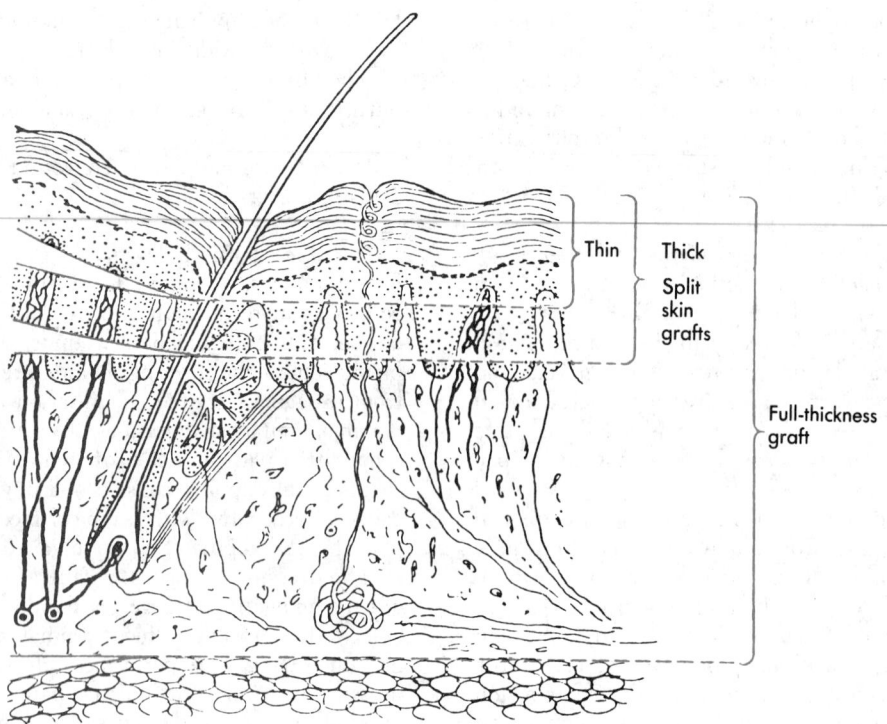

Fig. 44-8 Levels of the skin involved in thin and thick split skin grafts and full-thickness grafts.

Table 44-6 Types of grafts

Graft	Source	Coverage
Autograft	Patient's own skin removed and applied to burn	Permanent
Cultured skin	Patient's skin removed in small squares and grown in Petri dishes to large sizes and then grafted	Permanent
Homograft	Another of the same species (for example, cadaver skin obtained 6 to 24 hours after death) and applied within 5 days	Temporary
Heterograft	Another species (for example, pig skin)	Temporary
Synthetic substitute	Man-made substitute that has properties similar to skin	Temporary

of movement. Temporary grafts are used until the patient is ready for autografts. Often autografting is delayed as a result of complications, such as pneumonia or gastric hemorrhage.

Split-thickness skin grafts are used most frequently in the early stages of wound treatment (Fig. 44-8). The grafts include the two upper layers of skin (epidermis) and part of the middle layer (dermis) but are not taken so deep as to prevent regeneration of the skin at the site from which they are taken (donor site). The grafts are removed with

a dermatone blade from almost any unburned part of the body. The size of these grafts is determined by the sites available and the area to be covered. Grafts may be placed on the recipient bed by two methods—stamping and meshing. Stamping uses "postage stamp" grafts that are stamp-size pieces of donor skin applied over the recipient bed. It is generally used for patients who have large burns and minimal skin that can be used for a graft. Meshing involves taking the sheet of skin after it is removed from the donor and feeding it into a meshing instrument that perforates the sheet with tiny slits. The meshing of the graft makes it more distensible so that it can be stretched to cover wider areas of the body surface (Fig. 44-9).

Full-thickness grafts are composed of layers of skin down to the subcutaneous tissue. They give a better cosmetic appearance than split-thickness grafts when healed and are used early in wound management and if there is a well-defined area of full-thickness burn. Areas that benefit from full-thickness grafts are the hands, neck, and face. Full-thickness grafts can also be used in rehabilitative stages to restore body function and to repair areas of released skin contractures.

Tangential excision and *grafting* is a surgical procedure where the necrotic tissue or eschar is excised down to viable tissue or fascia and immediately covered with autograft or skin substitute. The procedure is best performed between the second and fifth burn day. This technique is used with a well-defined partial-thickness injury where deep epidermal cells remain intact for primary healing. Advantages of tangential excision and grafting are outlined in Box 44-9.

Advantages of tangential excision and grafting

Shortened hospitalization
Prevents potential conversion of burn to full-thickness by removing necrotic tissue before infection occurs
Definitive healing diminishes anxiety and lessens trauma to multiple graftings
Allows early grafting and early restoration of function
Scar formation reduced because of use of full-thickness graft

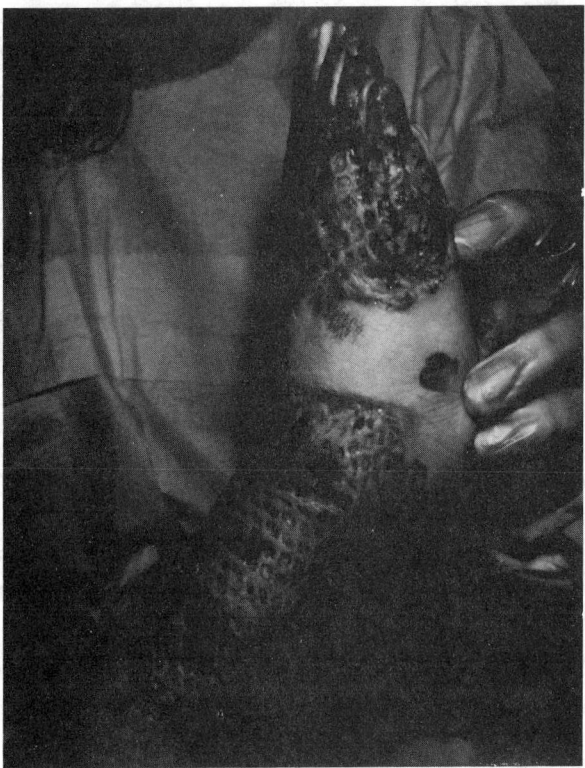

Fig. 44-9   Mesh graft covering a full-thickness foot burn 14 days after placement. (Courtesy Burn Unit, Metro Health Medical Center, Cleveland, Ohio.)

Care of graft sites. Graft sites require skilled nursing management. Autografts are delicate and should not be dislodged. The grafted area may be covered with a large, occlusive, bulky dressing to hold new skin securely in place. Splints may be applied in the operating room to provide immobilization of the graft site and to keep the graft in place.

The dressing remains intact for 48 to 72 hours unless it is found to be purulent and has a strong odor. Dressings are removed slowly and carefully so as not to disturb the graft.

After grafting the donor site represents a wound similar to that of a partial-thickness injury. Care of the donor site is as important as care of the graft itself, because donor sites that fail to heal enlarge the patient's open wound surface. Donor sites may be treated by a variety of methods. One method is covering the exposed surface with fine mesh gauze, with Xeroform, or with a synthetic dressing and leaving it exposed to the air. Exposing the donor site to a heat lamp promotes healing because as the drainage from the wound dries, it serves as a protective covering (Fig. 44-10). The site usually heals within 2 weeks. Another method is to cover the site with sterile gauze and apply a pressure dressing.

Many patients complain of severe pain in the donor site, and the nurse should not hesitate to give medications for pain. The pain should subside in 24 to 48 hours as the wound dries. The wound should be inspected daily for any signs of infection (erythema, purulent drainage, foul odor). If infection develops, antibiotics may be prescribed and the wound treated with wet dressings. Box 44-10 summarizes guidelines for the care of the patient with a burn injury.

Interventions to achieve patient outcomes
Decreasing fear and anxiety

The psychologic responses of the patient in the immediate postburn period are in response to a threat to survival. The fear of death is real as the patient senses the acuity of the situation by experiencing pain, disfigurement, isolation, and dependency from being attached to machines and monitors that maintain vital functions. A variety of behaviors may be seen during the acute and emergent phase (see Table 44-7 for a summary of emotional responses). Patients' reactions are determined by their personality,

their degree of total adjustment to life, and the extent and location of their burns.

The nurse should support and encourage the patient to ease the patient's anxiety. Setting short-term, achievable goals will help to motivate the patient. Providing the family with an explanation of the patient's needs will ease their fears and allow them to encourage the patient.

Facilitating learning

During the period of recovery from a burn injury, the patient and family have enormous learning needs. During the acute period, informational needs are built from the knowledge gained on admission. Explanations of the goals of therapy and expected outcomes must be reinforced frequently because of the stress and overload the patient and family experience.

Preventing hypothermia

As in the emergent period, hypothermia remains a concern. Open burn wounds result in a significant heat loss. The patient's room must be kept at a temperature of 83 to 85° F with a humidity of 40% to 50%. In addition, heat loss can be minimized by exposing only one burned area at a time during dressing changes.

Preventing infection

Infection control begins at the time the patient is admitted to the hospital and continues until healing is com-

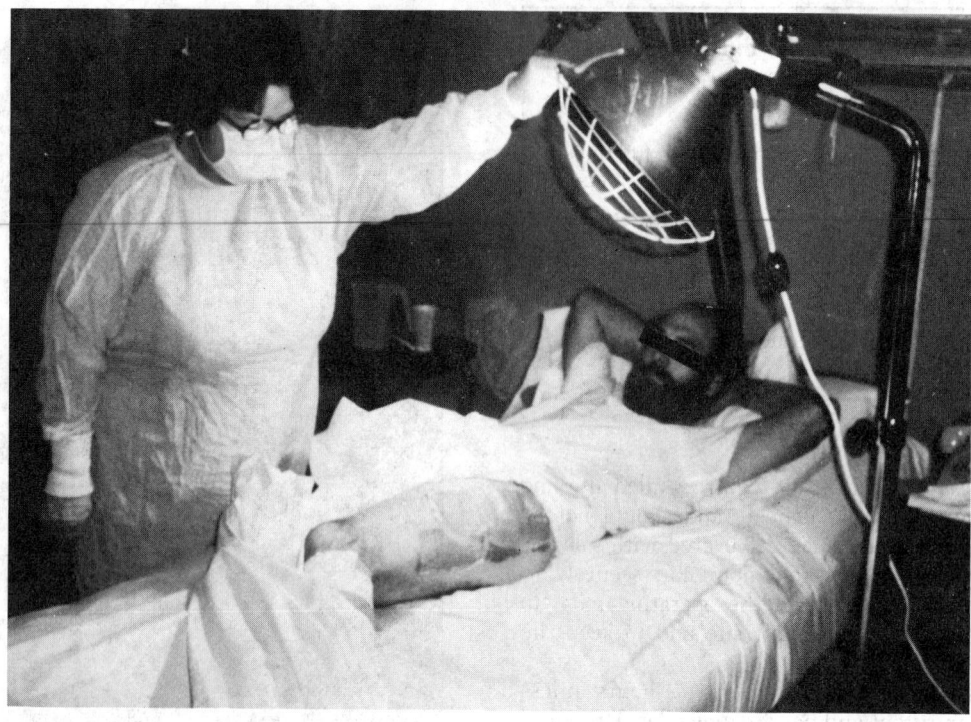

Fig. 44-10 Heat lamp used to dry donor site to promote epithelialization from deep layers and prevent infection. (Courtesy Burn Center, Metro Health Medical Center, Cleveland, Ohio.)

Table 44-7 Emotional responses to severe burns

Patient response	Definition	Behavior exhibited	Nursing approach
Denial	Inability to accept present condition (pain, disfigurement, events of burn accident, hospital environment); buffers impact of overwhelming physical and psychologic crisis	Level of comprehension and understanding in relation to degree of injury is distorted; denial of burn injury: states he or she is "fine"; avoids discussion of injury; may experience period of euphoria	Support patient: allow some degree of denial, but allay patient's fears without distorting truth
Flood reaction	Extreme agitation and concern over multiple issues in a disorganized fashion; problems that existed before the injury are exaggerated	Urgency to settle problems involving employment and finances; family may be gathered at patient's request to discuss patient's concerns	Support patient: orient patient to time and place
Paranoia	Suspicion of intended harm	Confusion; disorientation; lack of trust in caregiver	Acknowledge complaints or manifestations of fear; investigate all complaints; support patient: provide reality orientation
Regression	Adopting behavior of earlier lifetime frame	Infantile, demanding, uncooperative behavior	Acknowledge inability to cope; provide structure: allow patient choice in some instances; reward appropriate behavior
Depression	Withdrawal into self; little or no recognition of external events	Lethargic, stuporous, apathetic, little or no response to painful stimuli	Support patient: encourage verbalization of frustrations; encourage activity within clinical limitations

The patient with a burn injury

1. **Promoting skin integrity**
   Assessment of the severity of injury
   Depth and percentage
   Age and medical history
   Mechanism of injury
   Area of body injured
   Wound care
   Hydrotherapy, cleansing, and debridement
   Application of topical agents
   Assessment of progression of wound healing
   Prevention of scar formation and contractures
   Appropriate positioning
   Application of pressure garments
2. **Monitoring hypovolemia**
   Calculate fluid requirements based on weight and percentage of injury
   Monitor for signs of adequate fluid resuscitation (See "Signs of adequate fluid resuscitation," p. 1513)
3. **Preventing hypothermia**
   Maintain room temperature at 83 to 85° F, 40% to 50% humidity
   Limit wound exposure time during dressing changes
4. **Preventing infection**
   Establish isolation technique based on wound size
   Control visitors and traffic
   Follow strict wound care asepsis
   Do routine wound, nose, throat cultures
   Monitor for signs of wound infection/sepsis
   Use aseptic/sterile technique with invasive lines (intravenous Foley catheters)
   Disinfect patient care equipment thoroughly
5. **Decreasing anxiety**
   Provide consistent information related to treatment and plan of care
   Encourage verbalization of concerns
   Encourage family participation in plan of care
   Provide positive reinforcement of patient's efforts and improvement
6. **Decreasing pain**
   Minimize wound exposure time
   Analgesics
   Medicate 30 minutes prior to dressing change
   Use intravenous narcotics for major burns in emergent phase

Assess patient for pain level
Physiologic indicators of pain
Patient reports according to visual analog scale
Establish diversional activities
Instruct in relaxation techniques
7. **Providing adequate nutrition**
   Assess preburn nutritional status
   Instruct patient concerning current nutritional requirements
   While in hospital
   While on discharge
   Maintain daily calorie counts and weights
   Provide high-calorie, high-protein diet with supplements
   Consult dietitian in planning diet
   Involve patient in choice of diet
   Monitor bowel and bladder function
   Establish appropriate meal environment
   Avoid painful procedures near mealtimes
   Provide a calm, relaxed environment
   Provide positive feedback
   Provide oral hygiene before and after meals
8. **Promoting a positive body image and self-concept**
   Provide emotional support to patient and family
   Determine previous coping strategies
   Assess for readiness to view burned area
   Encourage expression of patient's view of his/her physical appearance
   Provide individual counseling or refer patient to support groups
9. **Encouraging self-care activities**
   Encourage independence in ADL
   Allow patient to assist in wound care procedures
   Include patient in development of plan of care concerning meal selection, time of treatments, rest periods, therapy, and socialization
10. **Promoting mobility**
    Maintain therapeutic positioning (see Table 44-8)
    Proper splint application
    Positioning
    Application of continuous passive motion devices
    Develop activity and exercise schedule
    Adapt environment to patient's current level of mobility

Table 44-8 Therapeutic positioning for the burn patient

Area burned	Description of position
Neck	No pillow
	Towel roll under cervical spine
	Neck splint
Shoulder	90 degrees abduction, neutral rotation
	Elbow splint may be used to aid in maintaining position
Axilla	Abduction with 10 to 15 degrees forward flexion and external rotation
	Support abducted arm by suspending from IV pole, or place on bedside table
	Axilla splint
Elbow	Extension
	Support extended arm on bedside table, foam trough
	Elbow splint
Hand	Hand splint
Dorsal surface	Flexion
Palmar surface	Hyperextension
Hip	Extension with neutral rotation
	Supine with lower extremity extended
	Prone (if medically appropriate)
	Trochanter roll
	Foam wedge along lateral aspect of thigh
	Knee or long leg splint
Knee	Extension
	Prone (if medically appropriate)
	Patient out of bed with lower extremities extended and elevated
	Knee splint
Ankle	Dorsiflexion
	Padded footboard with heels free of pressure
	Ankle splint

plete. Local and systemic infections (septicemia) are the most common complications of burns and are the major cause of death, particularly in burns covering more than 25% of the body. Initially autogenous sources are the primary sources of infection because of bacteria that survive in the hair follicles and sweat glands beneath the burned tissue. However, the patient is also susceptible to infection from exogenous sources.

The organisms that usually infect burns are *Staphylococcus aureus*, *Pseudomonas aeruginosa* (Plate 9), and the coliform bacilli. In recent years, there has been a high incidence of fungal infections resulting from the use of broad-spectrum antibiotics. *Candida albicans*, which is normally found in the gastrointestinal tract, accounts for the majority of the fungal infections. Cultures of the patient's nose, throat, wound, and unburned skin and also a punch biopsy may be taken on admission and at biweekly intervals to determine the presence of bacteria and their sensitivity to antibiotics.

To prevent the introduction of organisms into the wound, all persons who approach the patient should wear gowns, masks, caps, and gloves. Persons with upper respiratory infections should not be permitted near the patient. Surgical aseptic technique and sterile gloves are used when applying dressings. Hydrotherapy tanks and spray tables are used for aggressive cleansing of burn wounds and can be a source of infection. They need particular attention to prevent the spread of infection when the tanks are used by different patients. Care of the severely burned patient in special burn units can contribute to decreased infection because the environment is specifically geared to infection control. If the patient is cared for in a general hospital unit, a private room is essential and all equipment needed by the patient remains in the room. Reverse isolation precautions are initiated if the burn is greater than 25% BSA in an adult or 15% BSA in a child.

Providing nutritional requirements

Pathophysiology. Metabolism is increased following moderate to severe burns as a result of stress, fluid loss, fever, infection, and hypercatabolism. Shivering and the elevated levels of catecholamines, cortisol, and glucagon found shortly after thermal injury increase tissue oxygen consumption and heat production, deplete liver and muscle glycogen stores and fat deposits, and lead to a negative nitrogen balance and weight loss. Protein is broken down, providing amino acids for gluconeogenesis, and amino acids are prevented from incorporating into protein. The diminished rate of protein production prolongs wound healing and increases the patient's susceptibility to infection.

A burn patient remains catabolic until the caloric intake exceeds caloric expenditure. Hypermetabolism continues until the wounds are 90% healed[46] and homeostasis is restored. The patient's total energy and protein requirements include those needed for normal homeostasis plus those required to offset the catabolic state and repair the injury.

Goals of nutritional support. Maintenance of a nutritional support program is critical to survival and is initiated on admission. The goals of the nutritional support program are to establish eating by mouth as soon as possible and to maintain sufficient calorie and protein intake to restore tissue loss. A team approach provides comprehensive input and integrates the efforts of the patient, physician, nurse, pharmacist, dietitian, and occupational and physical therapists.

The protein and caloric needs of the burned patient are highly variable, depending on the extent and depth of injury and the patient's age, sex, preburn nutritional status, and preexisting diseases. *The daily protein requirement is greater than normal as a result of the negative nitrogen balance.* The normal daily protein requirement is 0.8 g/kg of body weight for the adult. The massive mobilization of protein after the burn injury increases the daily requirement by two to four times the amount required before the injury to approximately 1.5 to 3.2 g/kg of body weight. Protein is necessary for tissue repair and healing, not as a source of energy. Therefore, it is important to provide sufficient carbohydrate and fat calories to satisfy energy needs. An appreciable loss of *zinc* generally accompanies a protein and weight loss. Studies indicate that zinc deficiency impairs wound healing and that a zinc deficiency impairs cellular immunity.

The daily *caloric* requirement increases from a normal 1700 to 3000 calories to 3500 to 5000 calories. Because the demand for calories increases with a major burn, appropriate vitamin therapy is essential. *Vitamins and minerals are given at two to three times the recommended daily allowances established for normal healthy adults.* Vitamin C promotes healing, and the daily requirement in the burn patient increases from a normal of 45 mg to 1 to 2 g. B complex vitamins are necessary for the metabolism of the increased protein and carbohydrate intake. Levels of vitamins A, E, K, and folic acid are monitored and supplemented as indicated. Serum levels of calcium, phosphate, and potassium are also monitored and therapeutic levels of iron must be maintained to prevent the anemia associated with burn injury.

Weight loss and gain are monitored to evaluate nutritional status. *Weight gain* occurs initially because of fluid retention; however, following diuresis there is a marked loss of weight. Severe *weight loss* is closely related to protein loss or the loss of body cell mass and the enormous amount of body fluid lost through the burn wound itself. As in other metabolic responses, weight loss depends on the extent of injury: the greater the burn, the greater the weight loss. The weight curve will level out at a point below the preburn weight, and weight gain does not begin until all the wound is nearly healed.

The nutritional supplements given to the severely burned patient in the acute period are aimed at stabilizing cardiovascular function. This is achieved by stabilizing weight and electrolyte balance. Initially, 5% to 10% dextrose solution is used for this purpose.

Feeding methods. Paralytic ileus or gastric dilation is frequently seen in severely burned patients as a result of the neuroendocrine response to stress, hypovolemia, or septicemia. This prevents enteral feeding until the gastrointestinal tract mobility is restored. Total parenteral nutrition (TPN) is indicated once fluid resuscitation is completed. TPN with supplemental fat solutions is used to provide calories.

Oral or tube feeding is the preferred method of providing adequate nutrition and is used as soon as possible. The enteral route is the most natural and convenient means of nutritional support. The burn patient will seldom consume more food from meals after the injury than before the injury; therefore, a combination of parenteral and enteral routes may be necessary to provide the enormous nutritional requirements. Dietary supplements that contain additional calories and protein can be provided by milkshakes, which can be specially made by the hospital dietary department. Patients should be encouraged to drink supplements between meals.

Postburn lactose intolerance may occur in patients being tube fed. Signs of bloating, flatulence, cramps, and diarrhea may be seen. A modification of the strength and type of supplement may be necessary and starting the supplement at half or quarter strength, diluted with water, will often alleviate gastrointestinal complications.

Tube feeding provides a continuous 24-hour infusion of a high-caloric, high-protein commercially prepared supplement. These supplements, containing 1 to 1.5 kcal/ml,

44-11

Nursing Research

Iafrati NS: Pain on the burn unit: patient vs nurse perceptions, *J Burn Care Rehab* 7:413-416, 1986.

The correlation between the pain that the patient feels and the burn nurse's perception of pain was evaluated. Six patients, ages 28 to 74, recovering from burn injury were asked to rate their pain using a visual analog scale after the completion of a daily dressing change. Independently the nurses providing the dressing care were asked to evaluate the amount of pain they felt the patient experienced. The data collected indicated that the nurses misperceived the amount of pain the patient experienced the majority of the time. The burn nurses correctly assessed the patients' pain 31% of the time, overestimated it 34.5% of the time, and underestimated it 34.5% of the time. New graduates, new burn nurses, associate and bachelor graduates, and nurses over the age of 30 tended to overestimate the patient's pain. Veteran nurses, diploma graduates, and nurses under the age of 25 tended to underestimate the patient's pain. The study indicated that patients may not be receiving appropriate analgesia for dressing changes, either being overmedicated or undermedicated.

are hypertonic, and because of the hypertonicity, diarrhea is common. The best means of administering tube feeding is a continuous, slow infusion through a small-diameter, soft, pliable tube inserted through the esophagus into the stomach or duodenum. Diarrhea, nausea, vomiting, and an uncomfortable feeling of fullness may be avoided with a slow, continuous infusion using an infusion pump to regulate the delivery. If diarrhea persists, a kaolin-pectin suspension (Kaopectate) or paregoric may be added to the feeding supplement, or diphenoxylate HCl with atropine (Lomotil) may be prescribed.

The patient is advanced to a regular diet as quickly as possible. However, ingenuity by the nurses and dietitian is needed to motivate the patient to eat the food necessary to meet nutritional requirements. Relatives can suggest favorite foods. All dressing changes and treatments should be timed so they do not immediately precede meals. Milk shakes can supplement the patient's diet and can be taken more easily than solid foods.

Fecal impaction is a common problem in burn patients. Bulk foods and fruit juices must be stressed. Bulk-forming laxatives such as preparations of the psyllium seed (Metamucil) or a fecal softener such as dioctyl sodium sulfosuccinate (Colace) may be prescribed.

Decreasing pain

Psychologic pain may be induced or exaggerated because of loneliness. The patient's complaints of pain may be a call for attention that can be met by the presence and touch of the nurse providing care. Anxiety over anticipated procedures that may or may not be painful may cause a progressive increase in the degree of pain experienced. See Box 44-11 for research about pain in the burn patient. Muscle tension related to fear and apprehension is known

---

44-12	**Nursing interventions that aid in minimizing pain during dressing changes**
	Provide analgesic medications 30 minutes before dressing change.
	Provide clear explanations to gain patient's cooperation.
	Handle burned areas gently.
	Use sterile technique (infection causes increased pain).
	Encourage patient to participate in treatment whenever possible.
	Employ distracting techniques (radio, conversation) and relaxation techniques when appropriate.

to lower the pain threshold. Sleep deprivation, a common occurrence in critical care units, can also make the patient less tolerant of pain. Self-hypnosis or relaxation exercises can be effective in altering the perception of either actual or anticipated discomfort and should be consistently reinforced by the team.[34] Box 44-12 outlines nursing interventions that can aid in minimizing pain during dressing changes. (See Chapter 10 for further information about pain and its management.)

Promoting skin integrity

Eschar is the leathery covering of dead tissue and exudate that forms after the burn injury. It is conducive to bacterial growth because it contains dead tissue, moisture, and warmth. Cleansing and mechanical debridement are performed daily to remove eschar. Washing and friction remove buildup of debris and help to support skin tissue regeneration.

Hydrotherapy is a painless method for removal of dressings and facilitates range-of-motion exercise with minimal energy expenditure and discomfort. The solution used in a hydrotherapy tank may be plain water, normal saline, or an electrolytically balanced solution. To minimize the chance of infection, the nurse should keep the procedure as clean as possible. Use of gowns, masks, gloves, and a plastic, disposable tub liner will decrease the chance of contamination between patients. Tubbing is usually performed once or twice daily and should not exceed 30 minutes to prevent exposure and chilling. Tubbing is started after the patient's vital signs and fluid balance have stabilized. The patient should not be tubbed if there are any sudden changes in body temperature, heart rate, blood pressure, or respiratory rate.

The current trend in wound cleansing is to use a spray table. The patient is placed on a special stretcher that has a drain and is showered with a hose. Patient comfort is enhanced because areas that are not being debrided can be kept covered.

Decreasing social isolation

During the acute period of recovery from a major burn injury, the patient may experience a great deal of social isolation. Extensive bandaging and strict isolation procedures result in separation of the patient from the environment. Measures that bring the environment to the patient can reduce the social isolations. Visitors must be encouraged to look past the bandages and touch the patient. Tape recordings and videos of children or other family members that are unable to visit can be helpful. Other diversional activities, such as music therapy and art therapy, can be started as soon as the patient's condition warrants.

Evaluation

Evaluation is based on the expected outcomes. Questions to ask may include the following:
1. Is the patient able to respond to interventions to decrease fear and anxiety?
2. Is the patient able to achieve pain relief?
3. Can the patient verbalize an understanding of treatments and surgical procedure and participate appropriately in care?
4. Is infection present?
5. Is the patient nutritionally depleted?
6. Is the burn wound healing?
7. Is social isolation improved?

Rehabilitation Period

Rehabilitation begins at the time of admission. However, rehabilitation as the third stage of treatment begins when the patient's burn is reduced to less than 20% of BSA and the patient is capable of assuming some self-care activity. The principles of management are to return the patient to a productive place in society and accomplish functional and cosmetic reconstruction. It is important to remember that rehabilitation does not end when the patient is discharged; it may take from 2 to 5 years after discharge for the patient to reach a maximal level of emotional and physical adjustment.

Preventing limitations of mobility

As the survival rate of patients with large and deeper burns increases, so does the challenge to maintain optimal functioning and cosmetic results. Research indicates that the percentage of patients with joint limitations increases as the degree and extent of burn increases. Although these patients may be critically ill, their rehabilitative needs must be addressed immediately. A comprehensive program of positioning, splinting, exercise, ambulation, and activities of daily living (ADL) must begin on the first or second day after the burn injury and be carried through until after discharge. Any delays in initiating treatment will be detrimental to the patient's ultimate functional outcome. Contractures are among the most serious long-term complications of burns today. They result from muscle and joint stiffening, skin grafting, and prolonged bed rest. Whereas occupational and physical therapists are primarily responsible for addressing the patient's rehabilitation needs during all phases of the patient's recovery, the nurse is responsible for ensuring that all interventions are followed.

Nursing Process
Assessment
Subjective data

The patient must be helped to maintain range of joint motion to prevent scars from forming in positions that would result in deformity. Complaints of pain and pressure should not be ignored, because damage may occur from an improperly applied splint or poor positioning. It is important that patients understand why ambulation or motion is necessary even though it may be painful.

The emotional impact of a severe burn is enormous. The psychologic scars last forever and affect the victim and family for the rest of their lives. The extent to which the family unit adapts depends on how the patient reacts to a new body image and feelings of self-worth.

The hospital environment and hospital personnel influence the adaptation process. In the immediate postburn period, the nurse is primarily concerned with physiologic survival of the patient. At the same time, the nurse must be able to identify psychologic problems and coping mechanisms of the patient and family.

Objective data

The nurse is responsible for assessing the patient's response to positioning, splinting, exercise, and the ability of the patient and family to perform daily wound care after discharge. Correct positioning must be maintained to avoid the development of contractures. The splinted limb is assessed for adequate circulation, cyanosis, temperature, and the presence of pulses. Exercise, ADL, and ambulation must be continuously assessed for patient tolerance both physically and emotionally.

Data analysis: nursing diagnoses

Nursing diagnoses are determined from analysis of patient data. Possible nursing diagnoses for the person with burns in the rehabilitation period may include, but are not limited to, the following:

Diagnostic title	Possible etiologies
Mobility, impaired physical	Intolerance to activity, decreased strength and endurance, pain, severe anxiety
Self-care deficit	Intolerance to activity, fatigue, pain/discomfort, severe anxiety
Body image disturbance	Scarring, contractures, discoloration
Pain	Increasing activity (exercise, ambulation, ADL)
Knowledge deficit	Wound/skin care, exercises, use of adaptive devices
Coping, ineffective family	Inadequate or incorrect information or understanding, prolonged disability of significant person
Coping, ineffective individual	Burn injury, personal vulnerability

Planning: expected patient outcomes

Expected patient outcomes for the person with burns in the rehabilitation period may include, but are not limited to, the following:

1. Patient achieves optimal joint mobility.
2. Patient demonstrates ability to perform ADL.
3. Patient demonstrates a realistic concept of changes in body image and alterations required in daily activities.

4. Patient states pain is controlled.
5. Patient is knowledgeable about self-care and follow-up.
6. Family and patient demonstrate appropriate coping skills.
7. Patient achieves activity tolerance consistent with desired levels.

Implementation
Interventions to achieve patient outcomes
Promoting physical mobility

Therapeutic positioning. Therapeutic positioning, or placing body parts in antideformity positions, is vital to the prevention of burn contractures. Frequent repositioning of the patient in bed (side-lying, supine, prone) is used regularly during the day and night. Correct positioning varies, depending on the area of the body burned (Table 44-8). Positioning can be enhanced by placing patients on a Stryker frame, a Foster bed, a CircOlectric bed, a low-air-loss bed, or a special mattress. These beds facilitate the use of the bedpan and urinal, permit change of position with a minimum of handling, and permit larger skin surfaces to remain free from body pressure than is possible when the patient lies on a regular mattress. These special beds are particularly useful when both the back and front of the trunk, thighs, and legs have been burned. These beds also allow turning of the patient with a minimum of handling and thus help decrease pain.

Prolonged rest in semi-Fowler's position or with pillow pushing the head forward must be avoided even though many patients prefer this position because it enables them to see about the room better.

The bed can often be turned so that the patient can look about without having to assume positions that may lead to the formation of contractures. The bedside table may be changed from one side of the bed to the other at intervals.

Splints. Splints are used to prevent or correct contractures and to immobilize joints after grafting. They are custom made and often molded directly on the patient to ensure optimal conformity (Fig. 44-11). It is the responsibility of the nurse to apply the splint properly and according to an established schedule. An improperly applied splint can promote contractures and lead to additional complications.

Exercises and ambulation. Exercises for prevention and correction of contractures are begun as soon as the patient's condition is stable. Active exercises are preferred, although active assistance and gentle pressure exercises may be more realistic. Supervision by a physical or occupational therapist is desirable. Exercises may be performed more easily in water and may be performed along with dressing changes if the patient is able to tolerate the activity (Fig. 44-12). Continuous passive motion devices (CPM) may be used to prevent contractures of affected joints. When burns are completely covered (by healing or by graft), exercises may be performed more easily in an occupational therapy or physical therapy department where the patient may benefit from a change in environment.

Ambulation decreases the risk of thromboemboli, pro-

DATA: Mr. S. is a 54-year-old businessman, married with two children. He fell asleep while smoking in bed. He woke up after several minutes to discover his bed on fire. He was admitted to the hospital with 25% of his body burned, including his anterior arms, chest, abdomen, and scattered areas on his thighs. Six hours after admission he is receiving 40% oxyen through a face mask. Vital signs are as follows: heart rate 120, respiratory rate 30, blood pressure 140/80, temperature 38.8 C. Two peripheral IVs are placed, each running at 250 ml/hr. A Foley catheter has drained 50 ml the past hour. Mr. S. has a productive cough of gray-tinged sputum and a hoarse voice. Breath sounds clear with coughing. His wounds had been cleansed with Dreft and normal saline and covered with Silvadene dressing. He had complained of nausea and a nasogastric tube was inserted. Antacids were ordered to be administered every 2 hours via tube.

The nursing history identified the following:
1. He smokes 1½ packs/day; he has tried several times to quit.
2. The same day, his wife feared that he would fall asleep while smoking.
3. He owns his own business

Collaborative nursing actions include those to prevent hypovolemia from the movement of fluid from the intravascular to the interstitial compartment, to prevent respiratory distress, and to prevent gastrointestinal distress. Immediate reporting of the early signs of hypovolemia and/or respiratory distress may prevent serious effects (hypovolemic shock, respiratory failure). Nursing actions include monitoring for the following:

1. Signs of hypovolemia: increased heart rate, decreased urine output, decreased blood pressure, decreased sensorium
2. Signs of respiratory distress: increased respiratory rate, shortness of breath, change in patient's color, increased work of breathing, change in ABGs (decreasing pH, decreasing pO_2, increasing pCO_2)
3. Signs of gastrointestinal distress: low gastric pH, heme + nasogastric aspirate, absence of bowel sounds

Nursing diagnosis: **Airway clearance, ineffective: related to laryngeal edema and irritation from smoke inhalation and history of cigarette smoking**

Expected patient outcome	Nursing interventions	Rationale
Mr. S. will maintain adequate ventilation and oxygenation	Assess and document rate, depth, and ease of respirations; note type, amount, color of sputum; observe patient's color	Increased respiratory effort, large amounts of tenacious, gray-tinged sputum and signs of tissue hypoxia indicate the need for endotracheal intubation
		Providing oxygen will increase oxygen supply to body tissues
	Provide respiratory treatment and medications as ordered (pulmonary drainage and clapping, incentive spirometer, bronchodilators)	Respiratory treatments will loosen and thin secretions and will allow Mr. S. to clear his own airway
	Turn Mr. S. every 2 hours	Change in position will help mobilize secretions

Nursing diagnosis: **Fluid volume deficit, high risk for**

Expected patient outcome	Nursing interventions	Rationale
Mr. S. will maintain optimal fluid balance	Provide Mr. S. with IV fluids as calculated	IV fluids will prevent Mr. S. from developing hypovolemic shock
	Monitor and document output hourly	Any deficit or increase in fluid intake or output must be identified quickly to avoid complications of hypovolemia
	Assess Mr. S. for clinical signs of hypovolemia (decreased sensorium; changes in skin from pink to pale, from warm to cool)	These may be the first signs of hypovolemia
	Weigh Mr. S. daily; compare to preinjury weight	Weight is most accurate measure of fluid balance

Nursing diagnosis: Pain: related to exposed nerve endings from burn injury

Expected patient outcome	Nursing interventions	Rationale
Mr. S. will experience minimal pain	Administer Mr. S. with pain medication as ordered; 30 minutes before dressing changes (hydrotherapy and debridement); evaluate and document effectiveness	Decreasing pain will decrease Mr. S.'s anxiety and increase his cooperation during dressing changes
	Assess need for other interventionss that may decrease pain experience (use of the radio, relaxation therapy, hypnosis)	The pain experience is subjective; a variety of pain control techniques may decrease the pain experience
	Assess Mr. S.'s pain history and response to pain	Information about past pain experiences will aid in planning techniques for pain control
	Educate Mr. S. about painful procedures and techniques to reduce pain; encourage him to participate in treatments whenever possible	Information and participation may help decrease the anxiety that is often seen with pain
	Use environmental comfort measures (speak in calm manner, keep Mr. S. warm)	Comfortable environment may decrease anxiety and pain

Nursing diagnosis: Anxiety

Expected patient outcome	Nursing interventions	Rationale
Mr. S. will demonstrate control of anxiety	Gather information about Mr. S.'s background, personality, and level of coping from friends, family, and himself (as appropriate)	Information will assist the nurse in planning interventions to decrease anxiety
	Offer Mr. S. and family simple explanations of his injury and treatments	Too much information may overwhelm Mr. S. and increase anxiety
	Assess Mr. S.'s ability to cope with illness; consult with other services	Social services or pastoral care may be able to provide assistance to Mr. S.

Nursing diagnosis: Infection, high risk for: related to loss of skin from burn injury

Expected patient outcome	Nursing interventions	Rationale
Mr. S. will be free of pathogenic organisms	Document initial appearance of the burn wound (color, dryness, odor)	Early changes in appearance of wound may be the first signs of infection
	Monitor for signs of infection (fever, altered sensorium, increased respiratory rate, foul odor from wound)	Early detection of infection will allow appropriate antibiotics to be prescribed before serious injury occurs
	Implement isolation procedures	To protect Mr. S. from organisms that may cause infection

Nursing diagnosis: Skin integrity, impaired: related to burn injury

Expected patient outcome	Nursing interventions	Rationale
Mr. S. will demonstrate viable healing tissue	Assess need for equipment and supplies and have available before wound care	Adequate supplies should be ordered ahead of time to avoid the problem of discovering halfway through the dressing change that there are not enough supplies available
	Perform prescribed wound care (hydrotherapy and debridement); assess wound during each dressing change	Wound care procedures may change daily, depending on assessment of wound

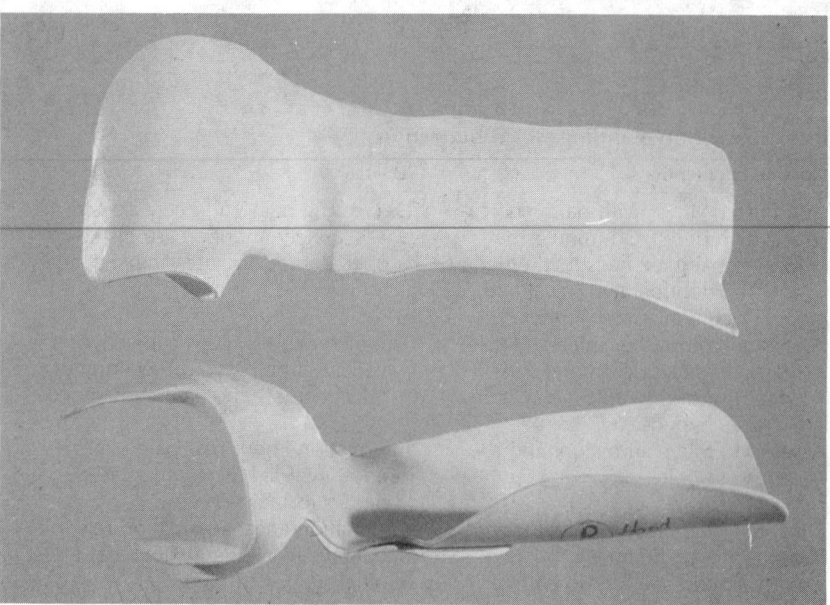

Fig. 44-11   Hand splints for burns. (Courtesy Burn Center, Metro Health Medical Center, Cleveland, Ohio.)

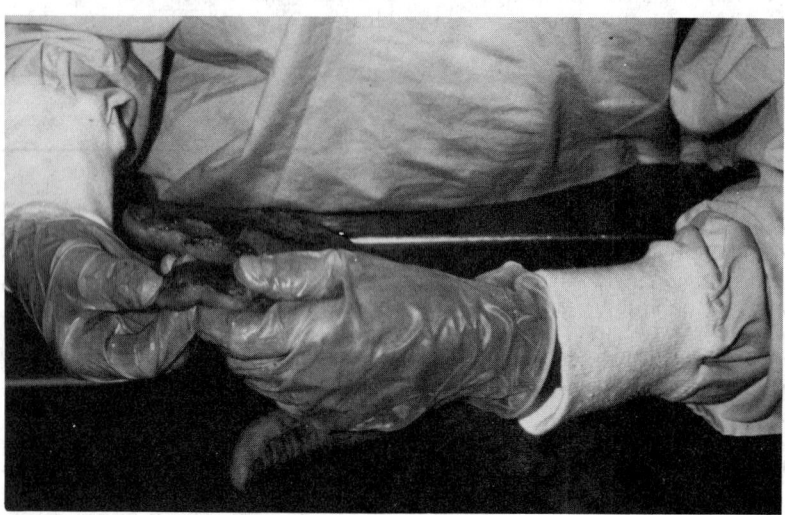

Fig. 44-12   Passive range-of-motion exercise during hydrotherapy. (Courtesy Burn Unit, Metro Health Medical Center, Cleveland, Ohio.)

motes optimal ventilation, helps maintain range of motion and strength in the lower extremities, orients the patient to the environment, and provides a sense of functional independence. Mobilizing the patient requires a progressive approach in those patients with large burns who have less ability to tolerate activity. Initially the patient may need to be transferred with maximal assistance onto a stretcher chair and progress to a sitting position. Gradually the patient may progress to a standing pivot, transfer into a nearby chair, and eventually ambulate with minimal assistance. Before getting out of bed, an elastic bandage support must be applied to the lower extremities to prevent venous stasis, edema, and orthostatic hypotension.

Promoting self-care

One of the ultimate goals in the rehabilitation of a burn patient is to maintain or restore the patient's independence

in performing ADL. The occupational therapist aids in this process by selecting activities that are appropriate to the patient's medical, physical, and mental status. Activities that the nurse can encourage are self-feeding, telephoning, reading mail, and assisting with grooming or burn wound management. The nurse must know what the patient is being taught by the physical and occupational therapists so that progress can be continued in the nursing unit.

After the initial period, the long healing process begins, accompanied by the realization of endless implications for the future. Burns on the face make adjustments difficult. Different kinds of fears include the following: pain, disfigurement, prolonged hospitalization, job security, change in life-style, and reactions of family and friends.

To the adolescent the thought of being different or conspicuous may be unbearable. If possible, the patient should

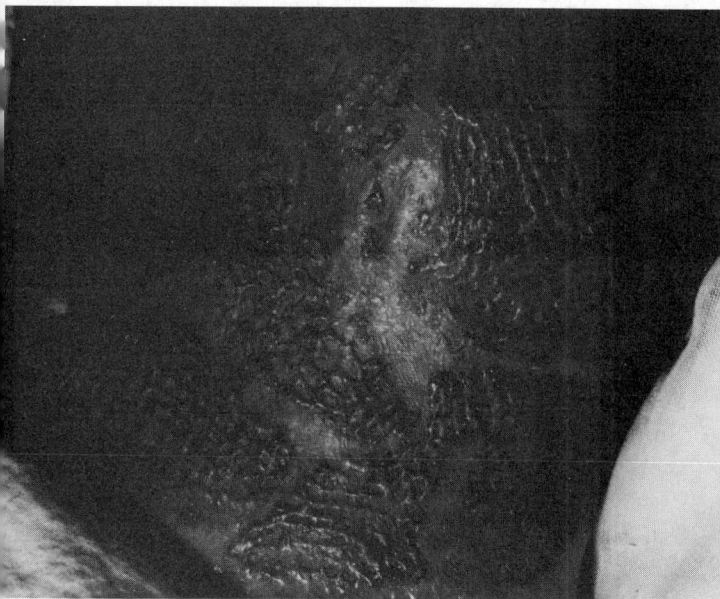

Fig. 44-13   Hypertrophic scarring over chest and abdomen. (Courtesy Burn Center, Metro Health Medical Center, Cleveland, Ohio.)

months. Pigmentation problems are more acute for persons with brown or black skin. Their healed skin may be a different shade, freckled, or whitish in color. Commercial makeup products that help to blend skin tones are available.

Promoting a positive body image

Regardless of its size, a burn injury represents a change in the individual's perception of self. As the burn heals, the patient must deal with a new appearance. The patient must have the opportunity to talk about any concerns or fears. Some patients may discuss these with the nurse when they cannot express them to relatives. The nurse must be prepared to listen actively and help the patient accept changes in appearance. The patient must be allowed to grieve for the loss of the former self. However, the patient should not dwell on the negative, but focus on the positive, productive aspects of self.

Preventing scarring

Whenever a wound of connective tissue heals, hypertrophic scarring occurs unless the skin is adhered to the underlying structure, such as the palm of the hand. Hypertrophic scarring (Fig. 44-13) results from the overgrowth and overproduction of tissue. This occurs especially in areas of stress and movement, such as the hands, legs, and chest. The thickened, rigid scar that results may later cause contractures, especially over a joint.

It has been proved that the application of controlled, constant pressure to the surface of an immature scar will reduce the scar and leave a smooth, pliable tissue. If this pressure is applied to new, healthy tissue, hypertrophic scarring can be prevented (Fig. 44-14). The Jobst garment, a specially designed elastic woven material, provides tridimensional control. It is fitted to each patient and then custom made (Fig. 44-15). Until the garment is completed, ace bandages can be used for a pressure dressing.

Even though the pressure garment helps decrease the formation of thick, disfiguring scars, patient acceptance is

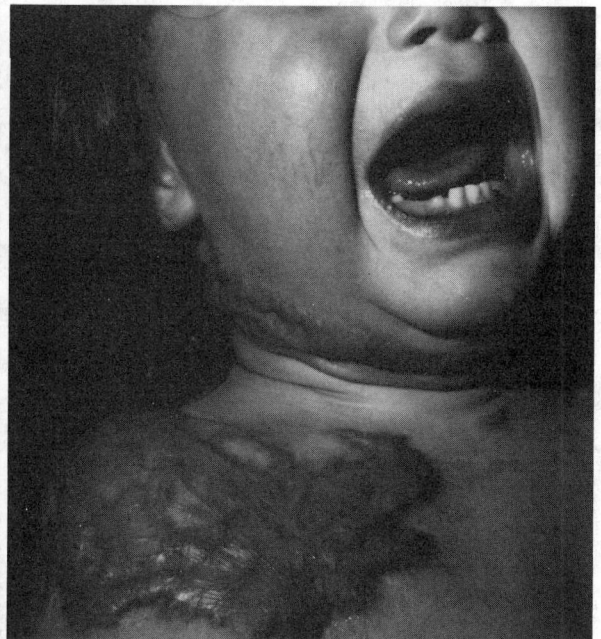

Fig. 44-14   Scar formation occurring from lack of pressure dressing application. (Courtesy Burn Center, Metro Health Medical Center, Cleveland, Ohio.)

see facial burns only after being prepared for the experience. Support and understanding will be needed in order for the patient to cope with what will be seen in the mirror. The patient will exhibit readiness by asking to look in the mirror. Interaction with other burn patients who are further along in their healing process may help the patient feel that recovery is possible. In some instances, the recovery is incredible, and although differences in skin pigmentation remain, the redness that accompanies healed burn wounds often fades considerably within a few

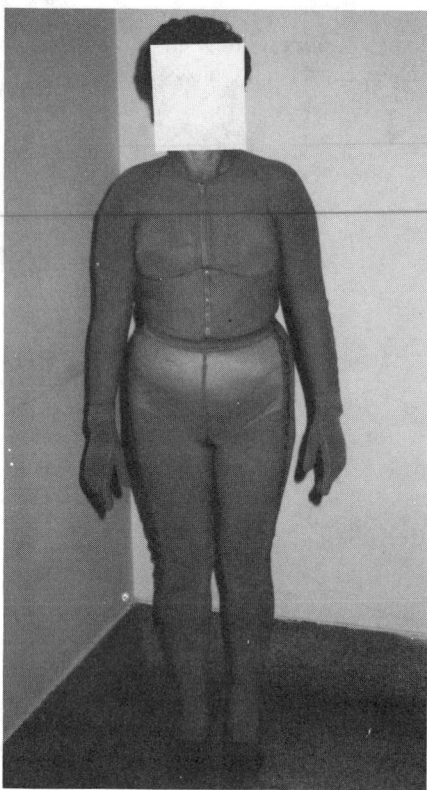

Fig. 44-15 Total body Jobst pressure garment consisting of three separate pieces: jacket, pants, and gloves. (Courtesy Burn Center, Metro Health Medical Center, Cleveland, Ohio.)

a problem. The garment is uncomfortable, especially during hot weather. It must be tight enough to produce the 24 mm Hg of pressure required to exceed capillary pressure, if it is to be effective in reducing edema and scar formation. The patient must wear the garment 23 hours a day for 6 months to a year.

A plan for exercise and splinting must be established before discharge. To prevent scar contracture, daily therapy sessions may be necessary for several weeks or months. Assistive aids can be developed by the occupational therapist to help with ADL.

Promoting comfort

Although less severe, pain remains a problem during the rehabilitation phase. Small areas of skin may remain open and continue to require dressing changes. In addition, newly healed skin is more sensitive. Physical and occupational therapy and increasing activity may result in discomfort. Interventions are focused on appropriate analgesics, diversional activities, and continuing to provide information about what the patient can expect. Daily hydrotherapy is beneficial in helping the patient to relax tense muscles.

Facilitating learning: discharge teaching

Before discharge, burn patients and their families have a great need for education so that they may take increasing responsibilities for their own care. Discharge teaching in-

---

Patient Teaching 44-13

The patient with burns

Patient/significant other verbalizes understanding
  of pathophysiology of burn process
  Depth and percentage of injury
  Functions of the skin
  Need for fluid replacement
Knowledge of healing process
  Nutritional requirements
  Infection control measures
  Rationale for wound management
    Hydrotherapy and debridement
    Topical agents
    Grafting
  Scar formation
    Stages of development
    Use of Ace bandage or pressure garments
    Use of cosmetics and prosthetics
  Purpose of occupational and physical therapy
    toward improved mobility
    Level of activity
    Prescribed exercises
Pain management
  Relation of pain to depth of injury
  Pain control options
    Analgesics
    Diversional activities
    Relaxation exercises
Discharge needs
  Skin care for healed areas
    Protection from sun
    Avoidance of chemical irritants
    Increased sensitivity
    Blister formation
  Skin care for open areas
    Prescribed dressing
    Application
    Abnormal conditions
  Application and care of pressure garments
  Home care needs
    Care of clothing
    Cleanliness of dressing change area, that is,
      shower/bathtub
    Adaptation of home environment, that is,
      handicap rails
  Nutritional needs
    Basic four food groups
    Relationship of dietary intake to healing process
  Emotional readjustment
    To new body image
    Behaviors that may develop at home
      Nightmares/flashbacks
      Grief
      Isolation
      Depression
Dealing with reactions of others
Options for increasing social activity

Discharge instructions for the burn patient

We on the burn team are happy to see that you are able to go home. To ensure that you have the speediest possible recovery, it is important that you are able to care for yourself and recognize problems that may interfere with your complete recovery.

If any of the following occur, please call the hospital and ask for the burn clinic. The nurse will be able to assist you.

1. Healed area breaking open. Cover with clean dressing.
2. Formation of blisters.
3. Signs of infection:
   a. Fever, temperature over 37.2° C (99° F).
   b. Redness, pain, swelling, hardness, or warmth in or around wound or any other part of body.
   c. Increased or foul-smelling drainage from wound.
4. Problems with your Ace bandages or pressure garment such as improper fit, formation of blisters, or opening of healed area underneath.

Your first clinic appointment will be on ___ . A family member can come with you and can register for you and you may go to the burn clinic waiting room.

Skin care for healed burn

These are your guidelines for your daily skin care of a healed burn. When you do your skin care, this is the time to look at the involved areas and note if there are any changes that need to be reported.

1. Wash healed area every day with solution of 2 tbsp Dreft (or Ivory Snow) and water.
2. Wash gently with washcloth to remove dead skin.
3. Rinse skin well after washing.
4. Dry thoroughly.
5. Apply Lubriderm lightly twice a day and more frequently if the skin is dry and flaked.
6. Do not put Lubriderm on open areas.
7. You can purchase Lubriderm at your local drugstore.

Care for burn wound

These are your guidelines for the care of your burn wound. When you perform your care, this is the time to look at the involved areas and note if there are any changes that need to be reported.

Procedure for burn wound care

1. Wash hands.
2. Remove dressing and dispose of in paper bag or wrap in newspaper.
3. Wash hands.
4. Wash open area with gauze using solution of Dreft (or Ivory Snow) and water. Add 1 tbsp Dreft to a basin of water; 2 tbsp Dreft if you use the bathtub. Use a clean towel and washcloth with each dressing change.
5. Rinse skin well.
6. Wash hands.
7. Apply dressing as described below.
8. Wear gloves. Wash basin or bathtub with a disinfectant such as Lysol.
9. Wash hands.

Care of clothing

When you are discharged, you may find that healed burn areas are sensitive to harsh detergents, fabric softeners, and clothing dyes. If you are sensitive, we suggest the following:

1. Before use launder new clothing by machine or hand with Dreft or Ivory Snow.
2. Rinse clothes twice.
3. Do not use fabric softeners.
4. If you have open burns or a healed area that opens, wash all clothes separately from other family members.
5. Scarlet red ointment will permanently stain clothing.
6. If dyes used in clothing cause irritation, wear white articles.

Ace bandages

You have been taught to put on your own Ace bandages while in the hospital, but if you do have a problem with this, please notify the burn clinic. It is also important that you know how to care for them and understand problems that occur.

1. If they are too loose, they will be ineffective and must be rewrapped.
2. If they are too tight, they will cause discomfort, numbness, tingling, and puffiness and must be rewrapped.
3. They must be worn for a long period of time, probably 6-12 months to be effective, so please do not stop wearing them until your doctor tells you.
4. To care for your Ace bandages:
   a. Hand wash with Dreft or Ivory Snow in cold water.
   b. Towel dry.
   c. Lay flat or place over rod or clothesline.
   d. Do not use clothespins.

Pressure garment

You have been taught to put on your pressure garment while in the hospital, but if you have a problem with this, please notify the burn clinic. It is also important that you know how to care for it and understand problems that can occur.

1. If it is too loose, it will be ineffective and you will require a new garment.
2. If it is too tight, it will cause discomfort, numbness, and tingling. Do not wear it if this occurs, but notify the burn clinic as soon as possible.
3. To care for your pressure garment:
   a. Hand wash with Dreft or Ivory Snow in cold water.
   b. Towel dry.
   c. Lay flat or place over rod or clothesline.
   d. Do not use clothespins.

Courtesy Burn Center, MetroHealth Medical Center, Cleveland, Ohio

volves the entire burn team, and because rehabilitation is a gradual process, there should be ample time to plan for the return home in every detail.

Early discharge planning accomplishes two goals. First, it helps solve problems early. For example, if the patient's house burned and needs to be repaired, the family may need to relocate. This could be done before the patient's discharge, thus preventing the added stress of moving after discharge. Second, early discharge planning emphasizes the future. If discharge is discussed, the patient and family will realize that recovery and a return home is possible.

Complete and comprehensive instructions followed by return demonstrations contribute to learning the necessary skills to be independent in self-care activities after discharge. Patients should not be discharged from the hospital until they can care for themselves physically, with assistance if necessary, and are prepared to meet the stresses involved in returning to their former living patterns.

Teaching priorities are summarized in Box 44-13.

A major goal in discharge teaching is to prevent excessive scar formation by exercising, splinting, applying pressure dressings, and, if necessary, undergoing reconstructive surgery. A patient recovering from a major burn may need 12 to 18 months to achieve this goal.

Wound management instructions should include how to care for the healed graft and nongrafted areas. Signs and symptoms of complications, including areas that may blister and break down, and signs of infection are also addressed. Written instructions should include the name and phone number of a physician or nurse that the patient may call with questions or problems concerning follow-up care. (See discharge instructions for the burn patient in Box 44-14.) The Visiting Nurse Association or another home health agency may be of assistance in dressing the patient's wounds at home.

Facilitating individual and family coping

After discharge, the patient has to adjust to temporary or permanent function loss, cosmetic disfigurement, and the reactions of others. The ability to make these adjustments will depend on coping mechanisms before the burn, the severity and site of the burn, and the reactions of others. How well the patient is adapting to these changes can be evaluated during outpatient visits when the burn team and other personnel can discuss the patient's progress.

Follow-up care may not take place at the institution at which the patient was hospitalized if the patient lives several hundred miles away. The burn team members may need to contact their counterparts in the patient's community to plan follow-up care. If possible, a member of the follow-up team should visit the patient in the hospital before discharge.

Job retraining may be necessary if the burn injury caused loss of joint function or other physical limitations that may prevent the patient from returning to a former job. The local office of State Labor and Industry Board can assign a vocational counselor to help the patient return to the work force. Even if retraining cannot begin for several months, contact with the vocational counselor and antic-ipation of retraining may help the patient look beyond immediate problems and think of the future.

Evaluation

Evaluation is based on the expected outcomes. Questions to ask may include the following:
1. Can the patient tolerate increasing activity and mobility as prescribed by the burn team?
2. Has the patient developed contractures?
3. Is the patient able to perform ADL?
4. Is the patient exhibiting a realistic concept of changes in body image?
5. Is pain under control?
6. Is the patient or family able to demonstrate correct dressing changes technique?
7. Is the patient or family demonstrating appropriate coping skills?

SUMMARY

1. The severity of a burn injury depends on the age of the victim, body part involved, burning agent, size and depth of the burn wound, and the victim's medical history.
2. The initial care for a burn includes removing the victim from the source of the burn and dousing the burn with water.
3. The initial systemic response to a burn is the shift of fluid from the intravascular to the interstitial space, creating hypovolemia. This is treated with a calculated dose of lactated Ringer's solution. After 48 to 72 hours the fluid shifts from the interstitial to the intravascular space and hypervolemia occurs.
4. Emotional support of the victim and victim's family is an important role for nurses.
5. Burn wounds must be assessed on a daily basis.
6. Correct splinting and positioning are the best methods for preventing contractures.
7. There is no way to predict how a burn wound will appear after healing.

STUDY QUESTIONS

- Discuss the differences in priorities of care during the emergent and rehabilitative phases of burn injury.
- Differentiate between a partial-thickness and full-thickness burn injury.
- How would you explain to a family member the physiologic changes following burn injury?
- Discuss the differences in fluid resuscitation in the first hours and second 24 hours after a burn injury.

REFERENCES AND SELECTED READINGS

1. Achaver BM, editor: *Management of the burned patient*, Norwalk, Conn, 1987, Appleton & Lange.
2. American Burn Association: Hospital and prehospital resources for optional care of patients with burn injury: guide-

lines for development and operation of burn centers, *J Burn Care Rehab* 11:98-104, 1990.

3.* Bayley EW: Wound healing in the patient with burns, *Nurs Clin North Am* 25:205-221, 1990.

4.* Bayley EW, Smith GA: The three degrees of burn care, *Nursing* 17(3):34-41, 1987.

5. Carrougher GJ et al: Research priorities for burn nursing: report of the wound care and infection control group, *J Burn Care Rehab* 12:272-277, 1991.

6. Committee on Organization and Delivery of Burn Care: *Burn care resources in North America 1991-1992*, Cincinnati, 1991, American Burn Association.

7.* Cooke SS: Major thermal injury—the first 48 hours, *Crit Care Nurs* 6:55-62, 1986.

8. Demling RH, LaLonde C: *Burn trauma*, New York, 1989, Thieme Medical Publishers.

9.* Dotson CH, Kibbee E, Eland JM: Perception of sleep following burn injury, *J Burn Care Rehab* 7:105-107, 1986.

10. Duncan CE, Cathcart ME: A multidisciplinary model for burn rehabilitation, *J Burn Care Rehab* 9:191-192, 1988.

11.* Duncan DJ, Driscoll DM: Burn wound management, *Crit Care Clin North Am* 3:199-220, 1990.

12.* Dyer C, Roberts D: Thermal trauma, *Nurs Clin North Am* 25:85-117, 1990.

13. Gordon M: *Manual of nursing diagnosis*, New York, 1988, McGraw-Hill.

14. Healthy People 2000: National health promotion and disease prevention objectives, US Dept of Health and Human Services, Public Health Service, Washington, DC, 1990, Government Printing Office.

15.* Iafrati NS: Pain on the burn unit: patient vs nurse perceptions, *J Burn Care Rehab* 7:413-416, 1986.

16.* Johnson CL, Cain VJ: Burn care: the rehab guide, *Am J Nurs* 85(1):48-50, 1985.

17. Klein DG, O'Malley P: Topical injury from chemical agents initial treatment, *Heart Lung* 16(1):49-54, 1987.

18. Kravitz M: *Thermal injury*. In Cardona VD et al: *Trauma nursing: from resuscitation through rehabilitation*, Philadelphia, 1988, WB Saunders.

19.* Martin LM: Nursing implications of today's burn care techniques, *RN* 52(5):26-33, 1989.

20. Martyn JAJ: Acute management of the burned patient, Philadelphia, 1990, WB Saunders.

21.* Mechanic HF, Dunn LT: Nutritional support for the burn patient, *Dimen Crit Care Nurs* 5:20-29, 1986.

22. Nowicki CR, Sprenger CK: Temporary skin substitutes for burn patients: a nursing perspective, *J Burn Care Rehab* 9:209-215, 1988.

23.* Roberts D, Appleton V: Psychosocial care of burn-injured patients, *Plastic Surg Nursing* 9(2):62-65, 1989.

24.* Robertson KE, Cross PJ, Terry JC: Burn care: the first crucial days, *American Journal of Nursing* 85(1):30-45, 1985.

25.* Robins EV: Burn shock, *Crit Care Clin North Am* 2:299-308, 1990.

26.* Rue LW, Cioffi WG: Resuscitation of thermally injured patients, *Crit Care Clin North Am* 3:181-190, 1991.

27.* Summers TM: Psychosocial support of the burned patient, *Crit Care Clin North Am* 3:237-244, 1991.

28.* Trofino RB: *Nursing care of the burn-injured patient*, Philadelphia, 1990, FA Davis.

29. Upright JW et al: *Advanced burn life support instructor manual*, Lincoln, 1991, Nebraska Burn Institute.

Classic

30.* Abshagen D: Topical agents and emergency care for minor burn injuries, *Journal of Emergency Nursing* 10:325-331, 1984.

31. American Burn Association: Guidelines for service standards and severity classifications in the treatment of burn injury, *American College of Surgeons Bulletin* 69:24-28, 1984.

32. Andreason NJC et al: Management of emotional reactions in seriously burned adults, *N Engl J Med* 286:65-69, 1972.

33. Artz CP, Moncrief JA, Pruitt BA: *Burns: a team approach*, Philadelphia, 1979, WB Saunders.

34. Bernstein NR: *Emotional care of the facially burned and disfigured*, Boston, 1976, Little Brown.

35. Cockshott WP: The history of the treatment of burns, *Surg Gynecol Obstet* 102:116-124, 1956.

36. Feller I, Archanbeault C: *Nursing the burned patient*, Ann Arbor, Mich, 1973, Institute for Burn Medicine Press.

37.* Freeman JW: Nursing care of the patient with a burn injury, *Crit Care Nurs* Nov/Dec:52-68, 1984.

38.* Heidrich B, Perry S, Amand R: Nursing staff attitudes about burn pain, *J Burn Care Rehab* 2:259-261, 1981.

39.* Jacoby FJ: Care of the massive burn wound, *Crit Care Q* 7(3):44-53, 1984.

40.* Kilbee E: Burn pain management, *Crit Care Q* 7(3):54-62, 1984.

41.* LeMaster JE: *Rehabilitation of the burn-injured patient*. In Wachtel TL, Kahn V, Frank HA, editors: *Current concepts in burn care*, Rockville, Md, 1983, Aspen.

42.* Marvin JA: Planning home care for burn patients, *Nurs 83* 13(8):65-67, 1983.

43.* Nadel E, Kozerefski PM: Rehabilitation of the critically ill burn patient, *Crit Care Q* 7(3):19-33, 1984.

44. Ragiel CA: The impact of critical injury on patient, family, and clinical systems, *Crit Care Q* 7(3):73-78, 1984.

45. Wachtel TL, Frank HA, Fortune JB: *Initial management of major burns*. In Wachtel TL, Kahn V, Frank HA, editors: *Current topics in burn care*, Rockville, Md, 1983, Aspen.

46. Wachtel TL, Yen M, Fortune JB: *Nutritional support for burned patients*. In Wachtel TL, Kahn V, Frank HA, editors: *Current topics in burn care*, Rockville, Md, 1983, Aspen.

47. Williams BP: *The problems and life-style of a severely burned man*. In Bergersen B et al, editors: *Current concepts in clinical nursing*, vol 2, St Louis, 1968, Mosby-Year Book.

48.* Wingate E: Emergent burn care: a time for life-saving measures, *Critical Care Update* 10:49-54, 1983.

Special Environments of Care

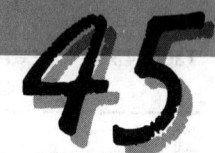

Problems Encountered in Emergencies and Disasters

Barbara C. Long

After studying this chapter, the learner should be able to:

- Identify accident prevention methods.
- Describe the nature of delivery of emergency care.
- Describe parameters of assessment of the injured or unconscious person.
- Identify principles of general management and specific care for accidental injuries or sudden illness (cardiac arrest, MI, near drowning, electrical injuries, poisoning, excess heat or cold, radiation, wounds, and fractures).
- Discuss the nature of rape and appropriate interventions.
- Describe the effects of disasters and appropriate roles of the nurse during disasters.

Table 45-1   Year 2000 national health objective for unintentional injuries[66]

Category	Target rate	1987 rate
Deaths (per 100,000)		
All unintentional injuries	<29.3	34.5
Motor vehicle crashes	<16.8	18.8
Fall or fall-related injuries	<2.3	2.7
Drowning	<1.3	2.1
Residential fires	<1.2	1.5
Hospitalizations (per 100,000)		
Hip fractures (age 65 +)	<607	714
Nonfatal poisoning	<88	103
Nonfatal head injuries	<106	125
Nonfatal spinal cord injuries	<5	5.9
Risk-reduction objectives		
Use of occupant protection systems (seat belts, inflatable safety restraints, child safety seats)	>85%	42%
Use of helmets		
Motorcyclists	>80%	60%
Bicyclists	>50%	8%

Nurses are frequently called on to provide emergency care in the community or in settings where medical help is not immediately available; therefore all nurses need to know the basics of emergency care. In this chapter major points are identified in the delivery of emergency care in the community, in assessment and intervention for common emergencies, and in principles of management in disasters.

ACCIDENT PREVENTION

Accidents in the United States claim almost 100,000 lives each year, half from motor vehicle accidents. Accidents are the leading cause of death in persons younger than 45 years and are the third leading cause in those 45 to 64 years of age.

In terms of morbidity, approximately 60 *million* persons, or about 30 of every 100, are injured in the United States every year. Billions of dollars are spent annually on medical expenses, property damage, and administrative costs related to accidents. Money lost from potential earnings or disability adds to this figure.

Accidents that result in injury or death involve human suffering that cannot be measured in dollars: pain, long-term rehabilitation, disabilities (temporary or permanent), loss and grief, and family disruption.

Unintentional injuries are a major source of morbidity and mortality in the United States; therefore accident prevention is a major public health goal. The Public Health Service and the American Public Health Association (APHA) actively promote accident prevention. National goals for the year 2000, derived under the direction of the Department of Health and Human Services and the Public Health Service, are listed in Table 45-1. Suggestions for approaches to achieve these goals include the following[66]:

45-1

Home safety features for elderly persons

Floors	Large rugs and carpets anchored Small rugs with nonskid backing Avoidance of floor wax (unless nonskid)
Stairs	Uniform height Nonskid treads Risers marked with contrasting color Strong handrails at appropriate heights Adequate lighting
Bathroom	Handrail in tub or shower Skidproof bath mat Treads in tub or on shower floor Seat in shower

---

1. Enact laws in all states requiring vehicle safety belts and motorcycle helmets.
2. Enact laws in all states requiring handguns be designed to minimize likelihood of discharge by children.
3. Enact laws governing installation of sprinkling systems in residences at highest risk of fire.
4. Increase functional smoke detectors to at least one per floor of every residence.
5. Teach injury prevention and control in all schools (grades kindergarten to 12).
6. Require use of effective head, face, eye, and mouth protection for sports that pose risk of injury.
7. Improve signs, signals, markings, and lighting of roads for increased visual stimuli.

Community groups can be helpful in investigating accident statistics in their local area and in disseminating information to encourage accident prevention. Nurses have an important role in accident prevention, both through their roles as professionals and as residents of a community. The influence of nurses can be extended in many areas because nurses work in schools, industry, community nursing programs, and hospitals.

Home

Accidents in and about the home are responsible for almost one fourth of all accidental deaths each year. Falls account for about half the number, and fires and poisoning for most of the remainder. Many aged persons who fall do so when walking from room to room. Some fall because of heavily waxed floors, loose rugs, poor lighting, scattered toys, and other conditions that could have been corrected (Box 45-1). People fall from roofs, windows, high ladders, and steps and are fatally burned or otherwise injured while using solvents and cleansing agents without proper knowledge of their hazards.

The number of electric appliances used in the home has increased the danger of electric shock and fire from over-loaded circuits. Many persons die in fires caused by burning cigarette ashes dropped on furniture or rugs or

---

ges
...ch as Bed

...hen pa-

...cially el-

...rettes that are
...ntion needs to
...older heating
...d other unsafe
features. All ...rsons in ...househ... should know what to
do ... case of fire, and ... ...acuation drills are encourage.... Homes should be e...ipped with smoke alarms
... ...ttic pla... such as the k... hen, bedrooms, hallways,
and basement.

Most accidental poisonings occur in children, but adults
are also at risk. Nonpotable liquids should be kept in original containers, tightly capped, and *never* placed in a soft
drink bottle, drinking glass, or cup. Medications should
never be taken from unmarked or poorly marked bottles.

The community health nurse has an opportunity to assess safety hazards during home visits and to teach the
family general accident prevention as well as specific measures for the safety of the ill person.

Community

Community action can best be effected by group action,
but it often takes persistence to interest and stimulate
group action. Parent-teacher associations, recreational associations, and religious and social groups are usually interested in accident control. Phases of accident prevention
that should be of community interest include the following:

1. Teaching of accident prevention in public schools
2. Better control and inspection of homes for the aged
   and prisons
3. Rigid enforcement of driving regulations
4. Improvement of street lighting and traffic signals at
   busy intersections
5. Periodic inspection of all automobiles
6. Promotion of laws pertaining to fire proofing of buildings
7. Promotion of laws protecting the public from flammable clothing, potentially harmful toys, and similar
   items

Hospitals

Assessing the need for safety in the general environment
and for the safety of specific patients, and taking measures
to prevent injury are important functions of the nurse.
The nurse can participate in policy making and safety
monitoring through membership on hospital safety committees.

> **45-3**
>
> ## Fire safety approaches
>
> 1. Close doors and windows of all patient rooms
>   until evacuation is necessary.
> 2. General precautions
>   a. Do not open a door that feels excessively
>   hot.
>   b. Keep low as possible if air is hot and
>   smoke-filled.
>   c. Use wet cloths around nose and mouth if
>   air is hot (try not to inhale smoke or hot
>   air).
> 3. If evacuation is advisable
>   a. Patients closest to fire are evacuated to op-
>   posite end of corridor (horizontal evacua-
>   tion).
>   b. Downward evacuation is effected (when
>   instructed) by *stairway* (never by elevator).
>   c. Ambulatory patients are evacuated first; pa-
>   tients are led by hospital personnel, if pos-
>   sible.

Falls

Falls are the principal cause of hospital-incurred injuries.
Hospitalized persons are in unfamiliar surroundings with
strange furniture and equipment, and may be weak for
many reasons, or may become confused, all of which can
contribute to falls. Persons at high risk for falls are the
elderly or persons with low grip strength, limited mobility,
or Parkinson's disease.[48] All patients should be assessed for
the potential for falling. Indicators for risk of falling include difficulty in standing up from a chair and tandem
gait.[48] Preventive measures should be instituted (Box
45-2).

The use of side rails is a nursing decision. Side rails
should be kept raised for all unconscious patients. A confused patient may attempt to climb over the side rail and
thus have farther to fall; a vest restraint may be more useful
in this situation. The bed should be in a low position,
placing the patient closer to the floor.

Patients who are weak may need frequent reminders to
seek assistance before ambulating. Some patients do not
want to "bother the nurse" and attempt to walk to the
bathroom unaided, especially at night. All patients should
use supportive slippers or slipper socks with corrugated
soles; paper slippers or elastic stockings without slippers
can be a hazard.

Fire

All hospitals and nursing homes must have established fire
prevention routines, and all personnel must be familiar
with these routines (Box 45-3). Participation in fire drills
should be taken seriously, and evaluation should follow
each drill.

Fires usually occur from smoking or faulty electrical
equipment. Because smoking is also hazardous to health,
many hospitals restrict smoking in patients' rooms and in
many public areas. If smoking is permitted, ashtrays should
be available and the patient and visitors instructed not to
empty them. If patients are careless smokers who may drop

a cigarette or ash, their smoking should be monitored. Faulty electrical equipment should not be used. Any questions about smoke should be investigated and reported immediately. If a fire should occur, the nurse in charge who is most familiar with the patients' conditions should be in charge of any evacuation.

EMERGENCY CARE DELIVERY

Community

The National Safety Act of 1966 requires each county to appoint an emergency medical care committee. The effectiveness of these committees varies greatly, influenced to a large extent by citizen interest and political activity. Every community needs an organized emergency care system with support and input from community health organizations and community political elements.

Many communities have emergency medical technicians (EMTs) or paramedics who respond to emergency calls. EMTs have had preparation beyond basic first aid training but do not carry out invasive procedures. Paramedics have had more training than EMTs and can carry out such skills as starting intravenous fluids, giving medications, defibrillating, and intubating. The preparedness of personnel responding to emergency calls and the responsibilities legally permissible vary among states and communities within each state.

The American Heart Association has been instrumental in developing a program to educate large numbers of persons who are certified to administer cardiopulmonary resuscitation (CPR). This increases the possibility of a trained person being available to initiate resuscitation early in a larger number of emergency situations.

Hospitals

Hospital emergency rooms are often overloaded with persons seeking assistance for nonacute health problems. Newer approaches to delivery of both emergency and nonacute health care, such as urgent care centers in the community, have been initiated.

Many emergency departments have direct radio communication with rescue personnel in the community. Treatment can be initiated at the scene of the accident under medical direction and hospital personnel can be better prepared to receive the injured. This helps to eliminate some of the delays in initiation of care.

Activities of emergency room (ER) nurses include the following:

1. Assessment and triage (sorting patients to determine priority of medical attention)
2. Management of persons with high levels of anxiety
3. Specialized technical skills (initiating parenteral fluids, defibrillation, resuscitation, intubation, operating monitoring devices)
4. Interpreting selected laboratory findings and electrocardiograms and acting on these findings

Legal Aspects of Emergency Care

Nurses who intervene to assist victims in an emergency situation should be aware of the legal ramifications that

---

45-4

Head-to-toe assessment

Head and neck

Assess airway
Assess pupils
Examine ears, nose, mouth for bleeding, other drainage, foreign body
Palpate* cervical spine for pain (do not move head)
Examine head for bleeding, lacerations, contusions, skull depression
Palpate jaw for fracture (pain, deformity)
Ask about neck stiffness (if no history of trauma, assess movement)
Examine neck for distended neck veins, presence of tracheal stoma, tracheal deviation

Chest and spine

Observe chest movements for symmetry of expansion and character of respirations
Palpate clavicles for fracture (pain, deformity)
Examine chest for external injury
Palpate ribs for fracture (pain)
Palpate spine for point tenderness (do not move victim)

Abdomen and pelvis

Palpate pelvis for pain in groin when pressure applied over pelvis
Ask about abdominal pain
Examine abdomen for external injury, rigidity, distention, penetrating objects

Extremities

Examine for signs of external injury
Ask about pain in extremities
If no obvious injury, ask victim to move each limb
Test for sensation in each limb
Assess presence and strength of peripheral pulses

*All palpations should be carried out gently.

---

can ensue as a result of their actions. Many states have enacted Good Samaritan laws in an effort to protect health personnel who aid accident victims. These laws vary in coverage among states as to the classes of people who are protected from liability, types of situations, geographic limits, and extent of immunity.

Good Samaritan laws serve to identify in statutory language those persons or situations that provide some degree of immunity from liability, many of which already exist by common law. Persons are not judged as liable unless they act willfully with gross negligence. Negligence is the key word. Damage must occur if negligence is to be proved, and the actions of the nurse must be the immediate cause of the damage.

"Reasonable care" provided by the nurse at the scene of an accident is usually judged as that care given by another similar nurse *under the prevailing situation*. Thus the

---

45-5

Priority assessment

Airway

Presence of respirations
Presence of foreign body, vomitus, loose dentures
  in mouth

Breathing

Respiration rate, depth, character
Use of accessory muscles for breathing
Tracheal deviation

Circulation

Presence of carotid pulse
Pulse rate, strength, rhythm
Presence of hemorrhage
Skin color, temperature, moisture

Level of consciousness

Response to voice and touch (or painful stimulus)
Pupillary response
If unconscious, presence of Medic-Alert tag

45-6

Possible causes of unconsciousness

Hypoxia (decreased oxygen to brain)
Respiratory insufficiency
  • Airway obstruction from foreign body, secretions
  • Pneumothorax
  • Spinal cord injury
Shock
  • Cardiogenic: cardiac arrest
  • Hypovolemic: hemorrhage

Metabolic (chemical brain depressants)
Extrinsic
  • Drugs: alcohol, narcotics, barbiturates, anti-histamines, tranquilizers
  • Poisons: carbon monoxide, carbon tetrachloride, hydrocarbons, methane gas
Intrinsic
  • Ketones: diabetic ketoacidosis, starvation
  • Glucose: hypoglycemia, hyperglycemia
  • Ammonia: liver failure
  • Urea: kidney failure
  • Hormonal hypofunction: hypothyroidism, Addison's disease
  • Electrolyte imbalance: sodium, potassium, calcium, hydrogen ions

Brain pathologic conditions
Trauma: concussion, brainstem contusion, intracranial hematoma
Seizures: epilepsy, tumors, idiopathology
Cerebrovascular accident: cerebral hemorrhage, thrombosis
Tumors: benign, malignant
Infections: meningitis, encephalitis

---

care provided on a back road on a dark rainy night would not be judged the same as that given in an emergency room.

Nurses who work in hospital emergency departments need to be aware of legal implications of care provided in that setting, such as the care given to minors when parents are not present to give consent.

ASSESSMENT

When an emergency occurs or when a nurse arrives at the emergency scene, it is important to assess the situation, the patient, and the environment before initiating action. Some conclusions can be drawn from the immediate environment. If there is trauma to multiple victims, all should be assessed before any lifesaving interventions are initiated. Overt clues such as an automobile accident, report of falling, or ingestion of poison can give direction to probable types of injuries. A complete head-to-toe assessment is carried out, if possible, before moving the victim so that additional injuries or conditions requiring intervention can be identified (Box 45-4).

Data Collection

A person who is not breathing, who has no palpable pulse, or who is hemorrhaging needs immediate assistance. Obtaining data to identify these circumstances is the first priority in assessment. This is sometimes referred to as the ABCs of emergency assessment (Airway, Breathing, Circulation) (Box 45-5). Assessing the general level of consciousness can be done as the nurse approaches the victim. If pulse and breathing are absent, CPR is initiated (p. 1545). Hemorrhage is treated by direct pressure to the wound.

Before starting the head-to-toe assessment, observe the following and assess those areas first:

1. Victim's general position

2. Obvious signs of deformities or asymmetry
3. Any purposeful movements
4. Signs or symptoms of pain or discomfort

During the overall assessment continue to monitor for changes in level of consciousness and respiratory status. Ask the victim or any relative or friends present to describe the preceding events; the presence of any medical conditions such as heart or lung disease, epilepsy, or diabetes; or any special medications taken by the victim that may have a bearing on the present situation.

If more than one person is on the scene, the nurse or paramedic should remain with the victim while others are given directions to assess the environment for additional signs of danger and call for any needed transportation.

Data Analysis
Level of consciousness

Determine whether the person responds immediately to voice and touch, responds only to painful stimuli, or does not respond. Unconsciousness may be due to many causes (Box 45-6). Pupillary response differs depending on the underlying problem (Box 45-7).

If there has been trauma to the brain it is important to

45-7	**Pupillary response in unconscious patients**	
	Cause	**Pupillary response**
	Shock or respiratory insufficiency	Equal, may be dilated
	Drugs, chemicals	Equal, may be dilated or constricted
	Intracranial hemorrhage, cerebrovascular accident	Usually unequal
	Brain damage	Fixed, no response to light

ascertain level of consciousness at different times. Temporary loss of consciousness followed by alertness and equal pupils usually indicates a concussion. If there is no skull fracture the patient is simply observed for 24 hours. *Alertness after injury followed by increasing loss of consciousness and unequal pupils* usually indicates an intracranial hematoma. Medical attention is urgent if an intracranial hematoma is suspected.

An unconscious person should be placed in a position that facilitates patency of the airway (side-lying position unless contraindicated) and the respiratory status constantly monitored.

Respirations

The rate, depth, and character of respiration provide clues to the presence of ventilatory, central nervous system, or metabolic problems. Most trauma victims breathe a little faster than normal (18 to 24 breaths/min). If the person shows signs of respiratory effort (nasal flaring; suprasternal, intercostal, or substernal retractions), the airway may be partially obstructed. The type of sound accompanying respirations may indicate the degree and location of a partial obstruction. The following findings suggest specific emergency care problems:

1. Rate
   a. Slow (below 10 breaths/min): ventilatory or CNS problem
   b. Rapid (above 26 breaths/min): hypoxia, acidosis, shock
2. Depth
   a. Shallow: shock, chest pain
   b. Deep: hypoxia, hypoglycemia, metabolic acidosis
3. Sound
   a. Inspiratory stridor: upper airway obstruction (above tracheal bifurcation)
   b. Expiratory wheezes or stridor: lower airway obstruction
4. Frothy, blood-tinged sputum: lung injury, pulmonary edema, pulmonary embolus

Shock

In persons who sustain major trauma or a major stressor to the system, such as myocardial infarction, shock usually develops (see Chapter 9). Signs of shock include restlessness, pale cold moist skin, rapid thready pulse, and rapid

shallow respirations. Nausea and vomiting may occur. With anaphylactic shock the victim may complain of itching or burning of the skin, tightness in the chest, and difficulty in breathing. Wheals may develop on the skin and the face and tongue may develop edema.

Sensation

Pain may result from trauma if there is soft-tissue injury, fracture, or visceral damage. Pain may also occur with tissue anoxia, such as with obstruction of blood vessels or frostbite. Data obtained from the patient include location (region), severity, quality, onset and duration, and provoking factors. For a further discussion of pain, see Chapter 10.

Loss of sensation may result from injury to peripheral nerves or injury to nerves in the central nervous system. Peripheral nerve injuries may occur with fractures, lacerations, penetrating wounds, or dislocations. Loss of sensation concurrent with loss of movement and absence of local tissue or bone injury indicates central nervous system injury, for example, spinal cord injury or cerebral hemorrhage.

Other data

Analysis of the data should include the following:
1. Type of injury or medical emergency that has probably occurred
2. Urgency of the need for medical attention
3. Availability of resources for carrying out necessary interventions
4. Availability of transportation
5. Time factor before medical attention can be obtained

GENERAL INTERVENTIONS
Principles of Management

Some principles of management of injuries or sudden illnesses serve as guidelines for giving first aid:
1. Remain calm and think before acting.
2. Identify oneself as a nurse to victim and bystanders.
3. Do a rapid assessment for *priority* data (airway patency, breathing (respiration), and circulation (pulse).
4. Carry out *lifesaving* measures as indicated by the priority assessment.
5. Do a head-to-toe assessment before initiating *general* first aid measures.
6. Keep the victim lying down or in the position in which found (unless orthopnea is present), and protected from dampness and cold.
7. If victim is conscious, explain what is happening; assure victim that help will be given.
8. Avoid unnecessary handling or moving of the victim; move the victim only if danger is present.
9. Do not give fluids if there is a possibility of abdominal injury or if anesthesia will be necessary within a short time.
10. Do not transport the victim until all first-aid measures have been carried out and appropriate transportation is available.

Lifesaving measures (described on succeeding pages) are

carried out first when the initial assessment indicates the presence of breathing or circulatory difficulties. After breathing has been reestablished and excessive bleeding controlled, other interventions are carried out when the head-to-toe assessment is completed.

The victim is kept in a supine or sitting position, depending on symptoms, until all necessary interventions are carried out. Wounds are covered and fractures splinted before the victim is transported. Because shock is a possibility when major injuries occur, the victim should be protected from chilling. On a cold day, protection may be needed underneath the victim, and sufficient covering may be needed to prevent loss of body heat but not to cause vasodilation. Fluids are given orally only to a conscious person showing signs of shock if there will be a considerable delay before medical care can be obtained and if abdominal injury is not present.

Multiple Trauma

Multiple trauma, injury to two or more body systems, occurs with severe injuries, such as crushing injuries, spinal cord injuries, and multiple bone or soft tissue injuries. Motor vehicle accidents are a common cause of multiple trauma. Falls from great heights often cause multiple fractures. Penetrating chest wounds may also involve abdominal organs. Victims of multiple trauma require rapid stabilization at the accident site followed by immediate transfer to an emergency room.

Persons with severe injuries require intravenous fluids initiated as soon as possible to prevent shock. These fluids may be started by paramedics at the accident scene. Shock therapy is started as soon as the patient arrives at the emergency room. The care of accident victims with severe injuries is complex and requires high-quality medical and nursing care by specialized practitioners in both emergency rooms and ICUs.

Psychologic Support

People who experience trauma may have numerous anxieties. It is often easy to overlook the victim's need for emotional support when physiologic needs require immediate attention. Some patient concerns include the following:

Fear of pain
Fear of death
Fear of unknown
Disability
Loss of time from work
Cost of medical care

A calm, interested approach that conveys concern to the victim as a person is helpful. Giving information frequently during all phases of emergency care to both victim and family or friends will help them understand what is occurring and that help is being provided, thus decreasing some of the anxiety.

Varying levels of tolerance to stress are found in different individuals. Highly anxious persons may need someone to stay with them. At the scene of an accident a calm bystander can be helpful. Some hospitals provide selected volunteers for that purpose. All health personnel need to evaluate frequently their own effectiveness in assessing

---

> **45-8**
>
> ### Causes of asphyxia
>
> **Inadequate oxygen in environment**
> Smoke
> Toxic gases
>
> **Obstruction of air passages**
> Foreign bodies in airway
> Tongue falling back in pharynx
> Edema of respiratory tissue
> Laryngospasm
>
> **Secretions in air passages**
> Near-drowning
> Pulmonary edema
>
> **Interferences with respirations**
> Chest trauma
> Depression of respiratory center (drugs)
>
> **Interferences with circulation**
> Electric shock
> Myocardial infarction
> Carbon monoxide poisoning

anxiety and in conveying understanding and emotional support to the victim and family during an emergency.

CARDIOPULMONARY PROBLEMS

For life to be maintained oxygen must be taken in by the lungs and pumped to the tissues; carbon dioxide must be returned from the tissues to the lungs and exhaled. Thus any obstruction that interferes with the diffusion of these gases, failure of the heart to pump, or inadequate blood to carry the oxygen to the tissues is a threat to life and demands immediate emergency intervention. Airway patency, breathing facilitation, and circulation maintenance are the ABCs of emergency care and take first priority in assessment and intervention.

AIRWAY OBSTRUCTION AND BREATHING DIFFICULTIES

Assessment

Asphyxia occurs for various reasons (Box 45-8). Signs of asphyxia are related to the efforts made by the victim to take in air and to the decreasing oxygenation. These signs include the following:

1. Dyspnea and restlessness
2. Use of accessory respiratory muscles (prominent neck muscles, intercostal rib retractions, nasal flaring)
3. Wheezing or stridor from air moving through narrowed passageways
4. Sucking noise on inspiration if an open chest wound is present
5. Coarse rales (crackles) if fluid is present in alveoli

Heimlich abdominal thrust maneuver

1. Stand behind victim.
2. Encircle arms around victim's waist (Fig. 45-1).
3. Place one fist between umbilicus and sternum with thumb against abdomen.
4. Place second hand over fist.
5. Press on abdomen with quick upward thrusts.

Sequence of CPR in adults

Step 1: Assess level of consciousness
1. Shake victim's shoulder and shout, "Are you OK?"
2. If no response, summon help
3. Place victim supine on *firm* surface

Step 2: Open airway
1. Hyperextend neck by jaw thrust maneuver (see Fig. 45-2)
2. Place ear over victim's nose and mouth
   a. Look to see if chest is moving
   b. Listen for air escaping during exhalation
   c. Feel for air movement against face
3. If patient is not breathing, proceed to step 3

Step 3: Initiate artificial ventilation
1. Give two full mouth-to-mouth breaths each lasting 1 to 1½ seconds

Step 4: Assess circulation
1. Palpate carotid pulse
2. If carotid pulse not palpable, proceed to step 5

Step 5: Initiate external cardiac compressions
1. If only one rescuer:
   a. Do 15 cardiac compressions at a rate of 80/min to 100/min
   b. Follow with two artificial ventilations
   c. Repeat sequence
2. If two rescuers:
   a. One person does cardiac compressions, at a rate of 80/min to 100/min without pause
   b. Second rescuer ventilates victim quickly after every five compressions
3. Palpate carotid pulse after four complete cycles to assess effectiveness, and subsequently every few minutes to check for return of spontaneous circulation. CPR is resumed with ventilation.

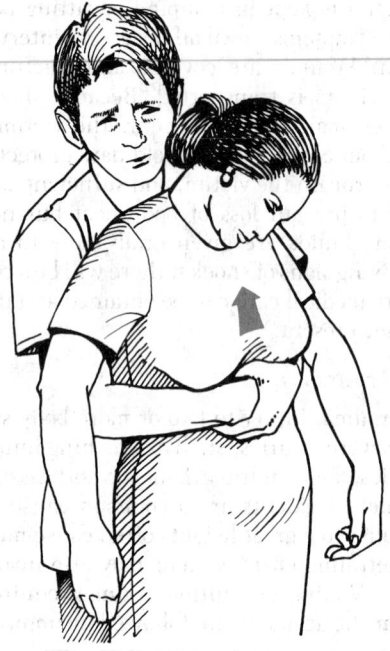

Fig. 45-1 Heimlich abdominal thrust maneuver. Rescuer places fist between umbilicus and xiphoid process with the thumb pressed against the abdomen. Pressure is applied upward.

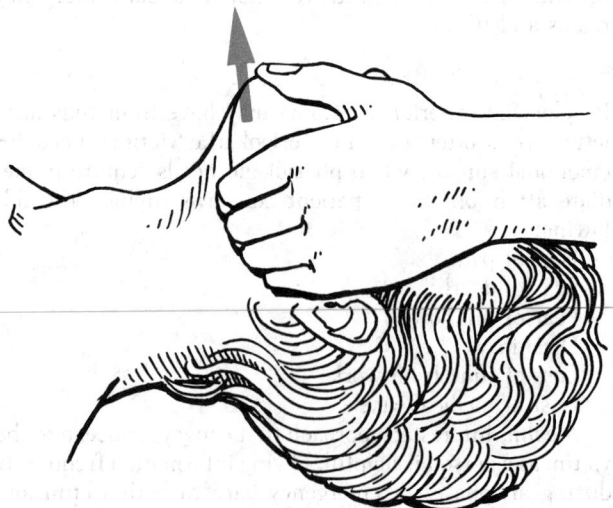

Fig. 45-2 Jaw thrust maneuver for opening airway. Neck remains in straight alignment.

Table 45-2   Life support measures in cardiac arrest

Findings	Action	ABCs of action
No response		
Absence of respirations; cyanosis; dilated pupils	Open airway	A—Open *Airway*
Respirations still absent	Initiate artificial ventilation	B—Restore *Breathing*
Carotid pulse not palpable	Initiate external cardiac compressions	C—Restore *Circulation*
ECG: ventricular fibrillation	Drug therapy; defibrillation	D—Provide *Definitive* treatment

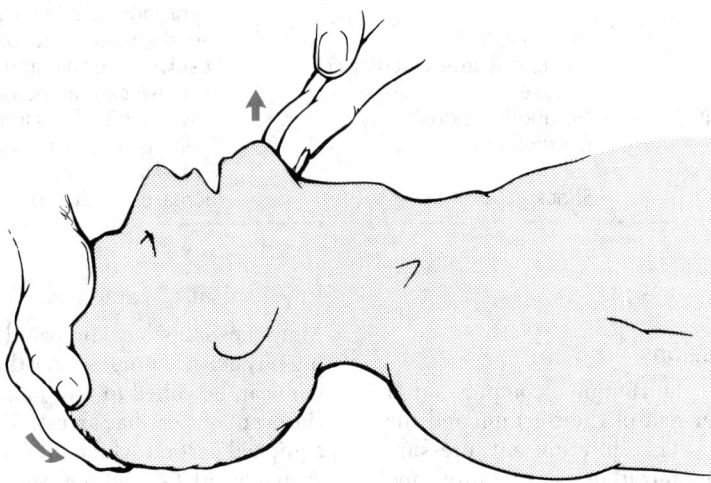

Fig. 45-3   Head-tilt, chin-lift maneuver for opening airway. Place one hand on forehead and place tips of fingers of other hand under lower jaw near chin. Bring chin forward while pressing forehead down.

6. Skin pale (ashen in blacks)
7. Cyanosis (late sign)

Intervention for Asphyxia

The first step in assisting a person who is having extreme difficulty in breathing is to position the person to ensure a maximal airway.

If the airway is obstructed by a *foreign body* the person may need assistance in its removal. The Heimlich abdominal thrust maneuver may be attempted (Box 45-9). If the person is *unconscious* and the tongue is blocking the airway, the jaw can be pulled forward to pull the back of the tongue away from the pharynx (Fig. 45-2). This maneuver alone may be enough to open the airway. If breathing is not initiated, artificial ventilation must be given immediately (see following).

CARDIOPULMONARY RESUSCITATION

Cardiopulmonary arrest is recognized by the cessation of breathing and circulation and signifies a state of clinical death. Immediate and definitive action must be instituted within 4 to 6 minutes after the arrest, or biologic death will occur.

Unresponsiveness, cessation of respirations, development of pallor and cyanosis, absence of heart sounds and blood pressure, loss of palpable pulse, and dilation of the pupils are present. (Pupillary response can be misleading

in patients who are receiving drugs such as atropine or opium derivatives or in the presence of corneal pathologic conditions.) If a hospitalized patient is being monitored by means of an ECG machine or cardiac monitor, the electrocardiographic pattern of ventricular fibrillation or, less commonly, ventricular asystole will appear.

Techniques of Basic Life Support

Basic life support is an emergency procedure that consists of recognizing cardiopulmonary arrest and initiating proper CPR techniques to maintain life until the victim either recovers or is transported to a medical facility where advanced life support measures are available (Table 45-2). The sequence of CPR is in Box 45-10.

Mouth-to-mouth ventilation

Mouth—to—mouth ventilation is performed as follows:
1. Maintain victim in head-tilt chin-lift position (Fig. 45-3).
2. Pinch nostrils.
3. Take a deep breath and place mouth around outside of victim's mouth, forming a tight seal.
4. Blow into victim's mouth.
5. Adequate ventilation is demonstrated by:
   a. Rise and fall of chest (1 to 2 inches)
   b. Hearing and feeling air escape as victim passively exhales
   c. Feeling in own airway the resistance of victim's lungs expanding

Table 45-3 Medications commonly used for cardiac arrest

Medication	Use	Action
Atropine sulfate	Slow pulse after cardiac standstill	Accelerates heart rate
Bretylium tosylate (Bretylol)	Ventricular fibrillation, ventricular dysrhythmias	Suppresses ventricular fibrillation and dysrhythmias
Calcium chloride (10% solution)	Ventricular standstill	Increases myocardial contractility and conduction velocity
Dobutamine HCl (Dobutrex)	Refractory pump failure	Increases myocardial contractility
Epinephrine HCl (Adrenalin) 1:10,000 solution	Ventricular fibrillation	Positive inotropic (force of contractions) and chronotropic (regularity of beat) effect; peripheral vasoconstriction
Isoproterenol HCl (Isuprel)	Asystole, cardiovascular collapse	Positive inotropic and chronotropic effects that increase cardiac output
Sodium bicarbonate (50 mEq)	Metabolic acidosis	Provides bicarbonate to return serum pH to normal
Lidocaine HCl (Xylocaine)	Dysrhythmias	Shortens refractory period, suppresses automaticity of ectopic foci
Dopamine HCl (Intropin)	Shock	Increases cardiac output, causes vasoconstriction

External cardiac compressions

External cardiac massage is the rhythmic compression of the heart between the lower half of the sternum and the thoracic vertebral column. This intermittent pressure compresses the heart, raises intrathoracic pressure, and produces an artificial pulsatile circulation. Correctly performed cardiac compressions can produce a peak systolic blood pressure of >100 mm Hg, but the diastolic pressure is close to zero and the mean blood pressure in the carotid arteries is approximately 40 mm Hg, or one-fourth to one-third normal.

The technique for performing external cardiac compressions is as follows:

1. Position yourself close to victim's sternum.
2. Place heel of one hand on sternum two fingerwidths above tip of xiphoid; and place second hand on top of first hand with fingers parallel and pointing away from body.
3. Position shoulders directly over victim's sternum.
4. Keep elbows locked in a straight position.
5. Depress lower sternum 1½ to 2 inches.
6. Keeping hands in position, release pressure on sternum to allow heart to fill.
7. Repeat, depressing and releasing sternum.
8. Perform compressions regularly and smoothly.

Continuation of CPR

CPR should be stopped for no more than 5 seconds every 4 to 5 minutes to assess the return of spontaneous pulse and respiration. Rescuers should continue CPR until one of the following takes place:

1. Spontaneous circulation and ventilation return
2. Another rescuer takes over basic life support
3. Victim is transported to an emergency facility where qualified personnel assume the responsibility for CPR
4. Victim is pronounced dead by a physician
5. Rescuer is exhausted and unable to continue

In-Hospital Cardiac Arrest

Many hospitals have prepared teams of personnel, including physicians, nurses, anesthesiologists, and technicians, who can be called to give immediate and complete care in the event of a cardiac arrest. Most hospitals have a specially equipped cart on which all necessary emergency items are available: ECG machine, suction device, oxygen, defibrillator, airway and Ambu or other breathing bag, laryngoscope, a variety of endotracheal tubes, cutdown set, fluids for intravenous administration, and tracheostomy set should tracheostomy be necessary.

Medications usually administered during a cardiac arrest (Table 45-3) are generally available on the emergency cart. Supplementary oxygen is given after breathing resumes to treat the resultant hypoxemia. Oxygen is also given for other types of hypoxemia after trauma or stress such as with smoke inhalation, carbon monoxide poisoning, near-drowning, myocardial infarction, or chest injuries.

Complications of CPR

The most common complication of external cardiac massage is fracture of the ribs. This may occur in some individuals even though the technique of external cardiac compressions is performed correctly. Other complications that can occur despite correct CPR techniques include fractured sternum, costochondral separation, lung contusions, and laceration of the liver. Any indication of labored respiration, paradoxical pulse, muffled heart sounds, tachycardia, decreased breath sounds, or drop in blood pressure is reported to the physician immediately.

SPECIAL CARDIOPULMONARY PROBLEMS
Myocardial Infarction

The person suspected of experiencing a myocardial infarction needs immediate attention. The greatest risk of mortality occurs within the first 2 hours after onset. If the heart ceases to beat, CPR is instituted immediately. The patient who is breathing may be more comfortable in a well-supported sitting position. Oxygen is given if avail-

Causes of bleeding	
External	**Internal**
Lacerations	Chest trauma
Crushing injuries	Abdominal trauma, for
Amputations	example, ruptured
Fractures	spleen
Nosebleeds	Thigh trauma
	Esophageal varices
	Peptic ulcers

able. A calm atmosphere is of utmost importance, and the patient should never be left alone before medical help is obtained; fear will add an additional stress to the already overburdened heart (see Chapter 25).

Near-Drowning

Approximately 6000 people die from drowning in the United States every year, over half in home swimming pools. *Near-drowning* refers to asphyxiation or partial asphyxiation from a fluid medium, with the person either recovering spontaneously or resuscitated at least temporarily.[59] *Wet drowning* is the most common type and refers to asphyxiation from the aspiration of fluid into the lungs, inhaled as the person panics and gasps for breath. *Dry drowning* refers to asphyxiation from laryngospasm that prevents both air and water from entering the lungs. *Secondary drowning* is the recurrence of respiratory distress after recovery from the initial incident, and may occur a few minutes to several days later.

If the person has stopped breathing, artificial ventilation is begun as soon as possible, even before the person has been completely removed from the water. Time should not be wasted trying to remove water from the lungs. Persons who have experienced near-drowning should be observed closely for signs of pulmonary edema for at least 24 hours, even if they indicate that they feel all right.

Immersion syndrome is death after submersion in very cold water. It is believed to be caused from dysrhythmias resulting from vagal stimulation.

Electrical Injuries

Electricity can cause injury in a number of ways:
1. Depression of respiratory center
2. Ventricular fibrillation (stimulation of heart at end of refractory period, even by low electric current)
3. Bone fractures and persistent muscle injury (from powerful muscle contractions)
4. Burns at entry and exit points

The extent of injury from electricity depends on the point in the heartbeat cycle that is stimulated by the electricity, the intensity of the current, and skin resistance. Moisture decreases skin resistance, so greater damage occurs when skin is moist from water or perspiration.

The victim must be removed from the source of electricity, with the rescuer being careful to avoid contact with the electric charge. CPR is started immediately if breathing

and pulse are absent, and continued even when there is no evidence of response. Defibrillation is indicated for ventricular fibrillation.

Fluid therapy is given because considerable plasma can pass into extravascular compartments because of the injury, resulting in hypovolemia. The patient is monitored for shock, secondary hemorrhage, respiratory acidosis, and myoglobinuria. Devitalized tissue may eventually require removal and grafting.

HEMORRHAGE

Etiology and Pathophysiology

Considerable blood loss may result from external or internal bleeding (Box 45-11). Internal bleeding is more difficult to identify.

When a blood vessel is severed there is immediate contraction of the vessel wall, reducing the size of the opening and decreasing blood loss. Platelets begin to adhere to the roughened edges until a platelet plug is formed. A clot begins to form in 1 to 2 minutes. By 3 to 6 minutes the clot has filled the end of the blood vessel, blocking blood flow. Arteries have thick walls, and large arteries have musculature that can produce considerable vasospasms. Amputation of a leg, for example, may produce minimal bleeding. Veins and capillaries have thinner walls.

Assessment

External bleeding, if excessive, will saturate the clothing and be readily visible. If the person is wearing bulky outer garments, bleeding may be concealed. The examiner should run the hands quickly over the entire body under the outer clothing, being sure to check underneath the victim. Saturated clothing may need to be cut away so that the area of bleeding can be examined. The scalp is very vascular, and what appears to be considerable bleeding may result from a small scalp laceration.

Three types of bleeding may be observed:
1. Arterial bleeding: spurting bright red blood
2. Venous bleeding: continuous flow of darker blood
3. Capillary bleeding: oozing of blood

Internal bleeding may be difficult to identify. Bleeding into the thorax (hemothorax) may inhibit respirations, and chest pain may be present. Abdominal bleeding may be evidenced by rigidity of abdominal muscles and abdominal pain. Hemoptysis or hematemesis indicate pulmonary or gastrointestinal bleeding.

Shock occurs with severe internal or external bleeding. The victim is assessed for weak rapid pulse, slow shallow respirations, cold clammy skin, anxiety, restlessness, and thirst. The pupils are equal, may be dilated, and respond slowly to light.

Intervention

Actions for control of *external* bleeding include the following:
1. Apply direct pressure over site of bleeding.
2. Apply pressure over a pressure point (Fig. 45-4) if bleeding cannot be controlled by direct pressure.
3. Use tourniquet *only* in selected situations (massive uncontrollable arterial bleeding):

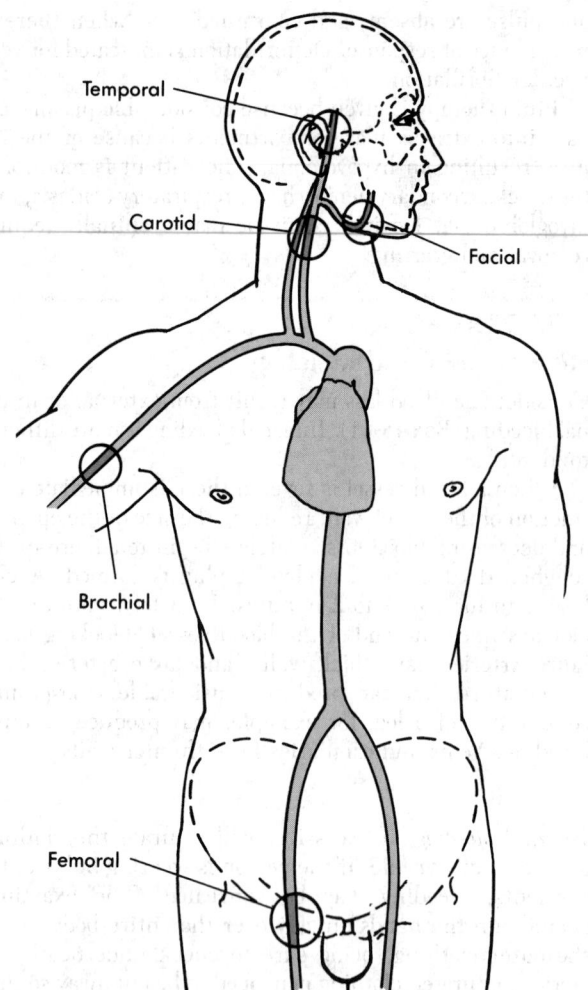

Temporal

Carotid

Facial

Brachial

Femoral

Fig. 45-4 Pressure points: locations at which large blood vessels may be compressed against bone to help control hemorrhage.

    a. Use blood pressure cuff or wide triangular bandage folded six to eight times and wrapped twice around extremity
    b. Use a stick or similar object tied to ends of bandage and twisted *only* to stop bleeding, no further
    c. Do not cover or release tourniquet
    d. Attach a notation to patient giving location of tourniquet and time of application

For suspected *internal* bleeding, keep the person lying down and protected from dampness and cold. Prevent further hypotension and seek immediate medical attention.

POISONING

Poisoning in adults occurs for various reasons:
1. Not checking medication labels (overdose or wrong medication)
2. Lack of knowledge (for example, taking alcohol and sedatives together)
3. Taking an excess amount in an attempt to obtain a desired effect
4. As a suicide attempt

Assessment

A *rapid* assessment is made to determine whether poisoning or overdose has occurred so that immediate action can be taken to prevent or diminish the effects of the poison or drug. It is important to identify clues that indicate that poisoning is a possibility and the type and quantity of the poisonous agent.

The conscious victim is questioned about the type and amount of substance taken or the nature of the poisoning. When the victim is unconscious, not much time should be spent looking for needle marks. Identification of the poison or drug can be facilitated by asking others to look for clues while you examine the victim. Empty containers, spilled fluids, open medication bottles, or syringes may provide needed information. *All* potential agents are gathered in their original containers and taken to the hospital with the victim. The physician may need to know the ingredients of the agent for those situations when an antidote is indicated.

COMMON ACCIDENTAL POISONING

Immediate action is necessary if poisoning is suspected; in some instances delay of a few minutes may make a difference between life and death. An *unconscious* person must be transported *without delay* to the nearest medical facility.

If the person is *conscious* identify the type, method, and estimated amount of poison or drug taken. Have someone call a physician immediately, if possible. Most large cities have poison control centers that maintain an extensive file on the most common substances and drugs. The telephone number is usually easily obtained from a list of emergency numbers in the front of the telephone directory.

Management consists of stopping absorption of the poisonous substance or drug. Poisonous substances can be inhaled, absorbed through the skin or mucous membranes, ingested, or injected. The type of intervention depends on the method by which the poison entered the system (Table 45-4). Families with young children should keep syrup of ipecac in their medicine chests.

If it is known exactly what poisonous substance or drug has been ingested, a specific antidote may be given in some cases by the physician. The use of a "universal antidote" has not proved effective.

INSECT BITES

The most common insect bites that can produce severe reactions are those of wasps or bees. Death can occur either because of multiplicity of bites (especially in young children) or from anaphylactic shock (Chapter 41).

Tick bites can cause tick fever by transmission of a toxin, a virus, as in Colorado tick fever; or rickettsiae, as in Rocky Mountain spotted fever. Ticks carrying a spirochete may cause Lyme disease. Sudden removal of a tick will result in its mouth-piece remaining. Although the

Table 45-4   Types of poisoning

Type	Examples	Therapy
Inhaled	Carbon monoxide, toxic gas	Remove victim from site to fresh air; give oxygen if available; give CPR if indicated; transport to medical center
Contact	Insecticides	Rinse skin with copious amounts of water
Ingested	Drugs, household chemicals, insecticides, lead	1. For noncaustic ingested substances, induce vomiting with syrup of ipecac a. 15 ml for adults b. May be repeated once in 20 minutes c. Follow with 1 to 2 full glasses of water 2. For drugs, follow vomiting with 30 to 50 gm activated charcoal in 60 to 90 ml water 3. For caustic substances a. Give nothing by mouth b. Seek immediate medical attention 4. In the emergency room, lavage may be used to eliminate agent
Injected	Insect bites, drugs	1. Bee stings: a. Remove stinger with scraping motion b. Apply ice c. A paste of sodium bicarbonate and water or weak solution of ammonia may be applied 2. Ticks: a. Remove tick by grasping its head with tweezers and pulling out slowly at 45° angle[55] b. Apply antiseptic after tick is removed 3. Drugs: a. Take victim to medical center b. See Chapter 13 for discussion of substance abuse

Table 45-5   Bacterial food poisoning

Organism	Vomiting	Diarrhea	Fever	Onset (hours)	Duration (days)	Sources
Staphylococcus aureus	Severe	Occasional	—	1-8	8-24 hrs	Meats, poultry, fish, cream-filled foods, mayonnaise
Salmonella	Occasional	+	+	8-48	2-5	Poultry, eggs, meat
Shigella	Occasional	+	+	24-72	3-7	Salads, seafood
Escherichia coli	Rare	+	—	24-72	1-3	Uncooked foods, contaminated water
Campylobacter jejuni	—	Severe	+	1-10 days	2-7	Meat, poultry, fish, mushrooms, contaminated water
Clostridium perfringens	Occasional	Severe	—	8-16	1-4	Rewarmed foods
Clostridium botulinum	Occasional (diplopia, dysphagia, respiratory failure)	Rare	—	24-96	High mortality	Improperly canned foods

traditional method of removing the tick has been applying gasoline or turpentine to the head of the tick or applying the hot end of a previously lighted match to the tick body, this method is *not* recommended in areas in which Lyme disease is endemic. Ticks in these areas should be removed slowly with tweezers, because applying heat to the tick may cause it to inject the spirochete into the host.[55]

Lyme disease occurs mostly in the Northeast states, Wisconsin, Georgia, and California,[40] in some parts of Europe, and in Australia. People living in these areas should wear protective clothing when in wooded or high grass areas. The initial lesion, located primarily in the groin, axilla, or thigh, begins with a reddened area that expands slowly with central clearing. Doxycycline or tetracycline relieves early symptoms and may prevent late manifestations. Arthritic, cardiac, neurologic, and dermatitis symptoms are treated with intravenous penicillin and refractory cases with ceftriaxone (a cephalosporin).

BACTERIAL FOOD POISONING

Food poisoning occurs more frequently than is reported, because the majority of persons recover quickly without treatment. The incidence of food poisoning from commer-

---

Prevention of food poisoning

1. Can low-acid foods (foods other than tomatoes or fruits) under pressure to prevent botulism.
2. Discard any can that bulges.
3. Avoid slow cooling of meat or poultry dishes.
4. Use a meat thermometer when cooking extremely large pieces of meat (especially pork).
5. Keep meats, fish, poultry, mayonnaise, and cream-filled foods refrigerated.

---

cially prepared foods has become relatively uncommon in the United States, but food poisoning from home-cooked foods or improper handling of foods still occurs.

Bacteria such as *Staphylococcus aureus* or *Clostridium botulinum* can produce a toxin that acts as a poison, causing acute gastrointestinal tract upset. Because *S. aureus* toxin (the most common type) does not spread through the body, the symptoms are limited. The *C. botulinum* toxin does spread and can be fatal (Table 45-5). *Salmonella* organisms introduced in food multiply in the intestines, causing acute gastrointestinal tract upset and infection.

Food poisoning is not caused by food that has spoiled or decomposed unless the food happens to contain disease-causing bacteria. Acute food poisoning can be prevented (Box 45-12).

ENVIRONMENTAL INJURIES

HEAT

Three types of general reactions to heat may occur (Table 45-6). *Heat cramps* can be prevented by taking extra salt and water before strenuous exercise in hot weather. The condition is self-limiting. *Heat exhaustion* is vasomotor collapse from the inability of the body to supply vessels adequately with sufficient fluid, usually from loss of sodium through perspiration. This usually occurs after vigorous exercise in hot weather, especially in the unacclimatized person.

Heatstroke is the most serious reaction to heat. It is caused by failure of the perspiration regulating mechanism in the hypothalamus. It is typically seen during a heat wave, and elderly and obese persons are at high risk. The body retains heat rather than dissipating it through perspiration. Without treatment, most heatstroke victims die; the heat permanently damages the entire nervous system. Persons do not recover from heatstroke as quickly as from heat exhaustion, and may have faulty heat regulation for the rest of their lives. These individuals should avoid repeated long exposure to heat. Interventions are listed in Table 45-6.

COLD

Excessive cold can lower body temperature, causing hypothermia, or can injure cells by direct exposure, causing frostbite.

Accidental Hypothermia

Hypothermia may result accidentally from exposure to cold weather. The extent of the cooling effect depends on the temperature and exposure time, the thermal conductivity of the environment, and the amount of air current. Moisture is a good conductor; air is not. Wet clothing therefore contributes to increased cooling of the body. Several light layers of clothing to provide air insulation will keep a person warmer than one heavy layer. Air movement contributes to heat loss; thus lower environmental temperatures can be tolerated better in the absence of wind (windchill factor).

When the body is exposed to cold, shivering occurs to produce heat by increased metabolism. As the cold increases, shivering ceases and heat loss exceeds heat production. The individual becomes listless, apathetic, and sleepy and may become indifferent to the surroundings and not seek adequate protection. Pulse and respirations become slower as metabolism decreases. Freezing of the extremities, unconsciousness, and finally death result if help is not received.

The victim needs to be kept warm while being transferred to a medical facility. Wet clothing is removed immediately and warmed blankets applied. If a tub bath is given, the temperature should be approximately 40° to 42° C (104° to 108° F). Warmer temperatures can cause skin damage from decreased circulation to the skin. Rubbing of the skin is to be avoided because this can also cause skin damage from decreased circulation. Warm liquids may be given if the victim is conscious.

The person experiencing hypothermia is monitored closely during rewarming. Hypovolemic shock can occur from vasodilation. If fluids are given intravenously, overloading of the circulation is a potential complication. Vital signs are monitored for sudden changes. Cardiac monitoring may also be indicated for signs of ventricular fibrillation and cardiac arrest.

Frostbite

Cellular injury occurs with exposure to extreme cold. Cell water freezes, and the resulting ice crystals damage the cell. The degree of injury depends on the depth of freezing. Frostbite occurs most frequently in exposed areas such as the nose, cheeks, ears, and fingers and can be prevented by adequate covering with loose-fitting dry clothing. Toes are also susceptible because of dampness and tight pressure from shoes or boots. Persons with circulatory problems are more prone to develop frostbite.

Superficial frostbite is characterized by soft, whitened, or dull ashen skin that does not redden with pressure. The part can be rewarmed by contact with warm skin, covering, application of warm dry socks if toes are affected, or gently immersing the part in warm, not hot, water.

Deep frostbite is evidenced by hardness of the frozen tissue because of deep subcutaneous tissue injury. After thawing the skin becomes hyperemic and edematous with blister formation. The edema subsides in 24 to 48 hours, and tissue breakdown with necrosis results. The frozen part should be covered to warm it, and the victim should be taken to a medical center as soon as possible. Care is then similar to that for vascular disease of the extremities.

Table 45-6   **Reactions to heat**

Type	Cause	Signs and symptoms	Therapy
Heat cramps	Loss of sodium chloride in perspiration during strenuous exercise in hot weather	Severe cramps; pain in arms or legs	Salty fluids (for example, Gatorade) and food by mouth; extra water; rest in cool place
Heat exhaustion	Sodium and water depletion; fluids are replaced by some water, but inadequate salt	Vasomotor collapse: faintness, weakness; skin pale or ashen, cold, moist	Recumbent position in cool environment; fluids, preferably with salt; transport to medical center if severe
Heatstroke (sunstroke)	Failure of perspiration regulating mechanism; prolonged exposure to heat, especially in elderly, obese, or unacclimated person	Skin dry, hot, flushed; faintness, dizziness; fever; unconsciousness	Reduce body temperature immediately by placing person in air-conditioned room; apply cool moist cloths, use fan; transport immediately to medical center
Burns	Direct heat, chemicals, electricity, radiation	First degree: erythema, pain Second degree: vesicles, pain Third degree: charred, coagulated, white skin	Apply cool water For specific care of severe burns, see Chapter 40

Efforts are made to decrease the oxygen needs of the tissues while healing takes place, to improve blood supply by use of drugs, and to prevent infection of open lesions. Necrotic tissue may have to be debrided for healing to occur.

RADIATION

Radiation injury is caused by exposure to gamma rays and neutrons from radioactive material. Persons can become contaminated directly from unshielded radioactive material, or indirectly by inhaling or swallowing particles of contaminated dust or smoke, or topically by skin contact. The amount of radiation that a person receives depends on various factors:

1. Strength of radiation source
2. Distance from the source
3. Duration of exposure
4. Area of the body exposed to the radiation source
5. Amount and type of shielding (see Chapter 11).

Prevention

Rescue workers who must remove a victim from an area of radioactivity need to protect themselves from radiation exposure. Because radioactive particles can be carried on dust, all skin areas must be covered and a filtering mask worn by rescue workers after an explosion involving nuclear materials. The greater the duration of exposure, the greater the potential for injury; therefore the victim must be removed immediately to a less hazardous environment. Some of the basic principles of emergency care may have to be violated when there is danger of other explosions or when fires occur. The rescue worker should remove all contaminated clothing at the edge of the contaminated area, and any exposed skin areas are washed thoroughly. Rescue workers should take a shower as soon as possible as an additional preventive measure.

Intervention
Local reactions

Radiation can cause a local inflammatory reaction of the skin, similar to a burn. The affected area may be washed gently with soap and water and a dry sterile dressing applied. Further treatment depends on the extent of injury. The person needs to know that continued observation of the skin is important for early detection of skin neoplasms.

Systemic reactions

Systemic reactions to ionizing radiation are primarily cerebral, hematologic, or gastrointestinal (Table 45-7). Cells that are rapidly dividing and differentiating (for example, blood cells and epithelial cells of the skin and gastrointestinal tract) are the most vulnerable. Loss of neutrophils predisposes the person to overwhelming bacterial infection; the loss of platelets results in bleeding. Loss of gastrointestinal epithelial cells leads to rapid fluid and electrolyte loss with severe dehydration and gastrointestinal bleeding. Radiation effects on slow turnover tissues, such as the eye or thyroid, may take several years to develop.

The cerebral syndrome usually results from massive exposure and includes progressive loss of consciousness followed by irreversible cardiovascular collapse.[27] Hematologic effects include decreased blood counts, petechiae, purpura, and bleeding from body orifices. Anorexia, nausea, and vomiting are commonly experienced from gastrointestinal injury. Recovery may be possible with active support of hematologic and gastrointestinal systems. Prolonged weakness, even during convalescence, is common.

The person with acute radiation syndrome is hospitalized. Early nausea and vomiting is usually self-limiting; sedatives and antiemetics may be helpful. Medical therapy is directed toward supportive care; that is, toward fluid and electrolyte replacement, nutrients (TPN may be necessary), and respiratory support as indicated. Various blood

Table 45-7 Effects of radiation on body systems

Organ or effect	Time to onset	Time to maximal effect	Total time from first dose to recovery	Dose required to cause injury (rad)	Major consequences
Cerebral syndrome	Few hours	1-2 days	Usually fatal	3000	Irreversible coma and cardio-vascular collapse
Hematologic syndrome					
Granulocyte depletion	1-2 weeks	4 weeks	6-8 weeks	200-400	Bacterial infection
Lymphocyte depletion	Few hours	1-2 days	4-8 weeks	200-400	Nonbacterial infection (virus, tuberculosis)
Platelet depletion	1-2 weeks	4 weeks	6-8 weeks	200-400	Bleeding
Gastrointestinal syndrome	3-4 days	6-7 days	2 weeks	600-2000	Fluid and electrolyte loss from mucosal sloughing
Skin lesions					
First-degree burn	Few hours	2-3 weeks	6-8 weeks	200	—
Second- or third-degree burn	Few days	1-2 weeks	8-12 weeks	1000	May need skin grafts
Hair loss	—	3 weeks	3-4 months	300	Permanent if greater than 700-800 rad
Sterility	—	Few days to few weeks	—	600-700	Permanent infertility
Hypothyroidism	—	Several years	—	Variable	Myxedema
Cataract	—	Several years	—	300-600	Visual loss
Leukemia	—	5-7 years	—	Unknown	Fatal
Solid tumors (thyroid, bone, breast, lung)	—	Many years	—	Unknown	Usually fatal, except thyroid tumors

From Kaye D, Rose LF: *Fundamentals of internal medicine*, St Louis, 1983, Mosby–Year Book.

Table 45-8 Types of wounds

Type	Description	Therapy
Open wounds		
Abrasion	Scraping of skin surface (brush burn)	Wash well with soap and water; keep clean; no covering necessary
Laceration	Jagged cut through skin and underlying tissue	Wash well with soap and water; edges approximated by "butterfly" adhesive or by suturing
Incision	Straight cut through skin and underlying tissue by sharp knife	Same as for laceration
Puncture	Penetration of skin and underlying tissue by sharp-pointed object; skin quickly seals over when object is removed	Soak wound; encourage bleeding in small wound to wash out bacteria; monitor for signs of infection; tetanus prophylaxis
Stab	Form of puncture wound by large object such as a knife, stick, or piece of glass	Do not remove object; stabilize object to prevent further damage; control bleeding; seek immediate medical attention
Closed wound		
Contusion (bruise)	Injury by blunt object; blood vessels rupture, and blood seeps into tissue; edema from trauma to injured cells	Apply ice or cold compresses for 48 hours; analgesics for pain; rest injured part

elements may be given for hematologic deficiencies. Bone marrow transplantation is frequently necessary. Recombinant granulocyte-macrophage colony-stimulating factor (Chapter 11) has been effective in increasing WBCs and thus decreasing infection potential.[57] Prevention of infection, which takes high priority, includes reverse isolation and prophylactic oral antimicrobial drugs. The same nursing care is required for the person with acute radiation syndrome as for the person receiving radiation therapy (see Chapter 11).

MUSCULOSKELETAL INJURIES

WOUNDS

Injury to soft tissue may result in open wounds, which damage the skin, or in closed wounds, which damage underlying tissue but leave the skin intact (Table 45-8).

Suturing of lacerations and incisions should be carried out within the first few hours after injury to obtain maximal healing with fewer complications or scarring. If the would is grossly contaminated the decision may be made to delay suturing for a few days to permit thorough cleansing. Healing then occurs by tertiary intention.

Puncture wounds are particularly vulnerable to infection, and bacteria such as *Clostridium tetani*, which thrive without air, may infect these wounds. Because anaerobic bacterial infections are extremely serious, a physician should be consulted if the puncture was made by a dirty object.

Tetanus prophylaxis for contaminated wounds depends on the type of the wound and the person's previous tetanus immunization (Table 45-9). (See Chapter 17 for a discussion of active immunization with toxoid or passive immunization with immune serum globulin.) Tetanus (lockjaw) is highly fatal, and the only sure method of prevention is through immunization.

Chest Wounds

Injuries to the chest may result in open chest wounds, fractured ribs, or injuries to the heart (cardiac tamponade) and lung (Table 45-10). These conditions are described in more detail elsewhere in the text.

Table 45-9   Tetanus prophylaxis after injury*

Previous tetanus toxoid injections	Type of wound	Prophylaxis
3 or more	Clean, minor	<10 yr: none >10 yr: tetanus toxoid
	All other	<5 yr: none >5 yr: tetanus toxoid
Less than 3 or none	Clean, minor	Tetanus toxoid
	All other	Tetanus toxoid and TIG (tetanus immune

*Recommended by Centers for Disease Control (CDC).[15]

Table 45-10   Some major injuries affecting chest wall and pleural cavity

Injury	Cause	Signs and symptoms	Initial emergency care
Rib fracture	Blow to chest	Pain on inspiration; local tenderness	Transport
Flail chest	Ribs fractured in more than one place; chest wall becomes unstable	Paradoxical respirations; respiratory distress; chest pain	Apply external pressure: sandbags, pillow, your hand; give oxygen; transport with flail side down
Open pneumothorax (open sucking wound)	Penetrating trauma to chest; loss of negative intrathoracic pressure as air moves in and out of wound	Sucking sound on chest wall during inspiration; tracheal deviation	Cover wound with occlusive dressing during exhalation; give oxygen
Simple pneumothorax	Laceration of lung, hyperinflation (blast injuries, driving accidents), loss of negative intrathoracic pressure	Sudden onset of chest pain; decreased breath sounds of affected area; dyspnea, tachypnea	Semi-Fowler's or Fowler's position; give oxygen
Tension pneumothorax	Complication of other types of pneumothorax; air enters pleural cavity but cannot escape	Respiratory distress; paradoxical chest movements; neck vein distention; tracheal deviation to unaffected side	Maintain airway and breathing; give oxygen (needle thoracotomy by trained person)
Hemothorax	Blunt and penetrating chest injuries; injuries to major blood vessels and heart; blood collects in pleural cavity	Decreased breath sounds; dyspnea (cyanosis and signs of shock if severe)	Treat for shock; give oxygen

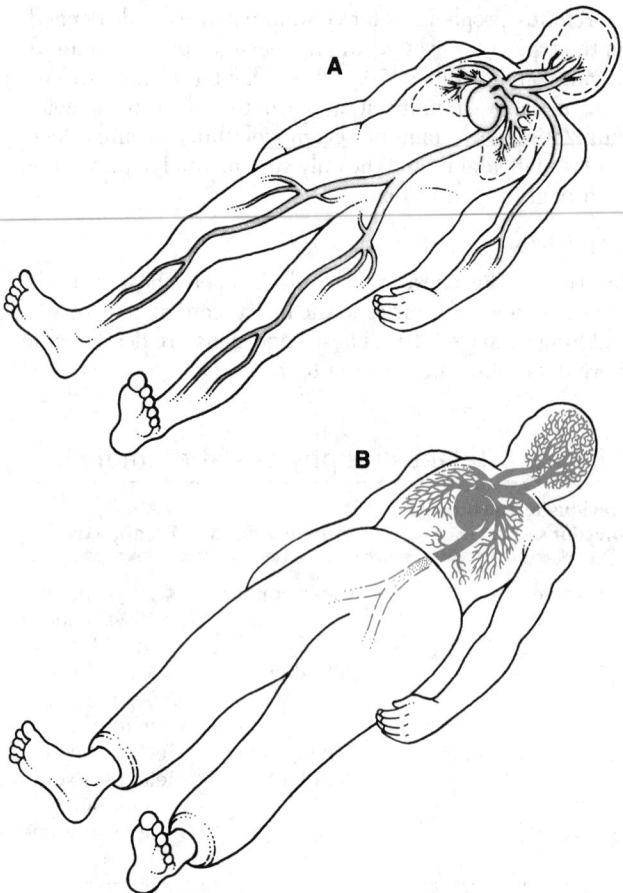

Fig. 45-5 In shock states, perfusion of vital organs is greatly enhanced by a pneumatic antishock garment. **A,** Before application. **B,** After application. (From Sheehy SB, Barber J: *Emergency nursing: principles and practice,* ed 2, St Louis, 1985, Mosby–Year Book.)

Open wounds of the chest create a problem if there is intrusion into the pleural cavity. Air is drawn into the pleural space because of the existing negative pressure. The resultant positive pressure causes pneumothorax (collapse of the lung). A sucking noise is heard as the air is drawn in and respirations are impaired. Immediate action is indicated to cover the opening. A nonporous material must be used, because air can pass through a standard dressing or material. Plastic wrap, which is not only nonporous but tends to cling to the skin, is excellent. If a dressing is used it must be covered with petrolatum to create an air barrier. After the chest wound has been sealed, a pressure dressing is applied. Continual monitoring of respirations is indicated.

Persons with chest trauma are considered to have sustained serious injury until proved otherwise. Primary consideration in emergency management is maintenance of an open airway, breathing, and circulation. Oxygen is adminstered at high flow. Rapid transport after initial emergency measures is essential.

Abdominal Wounds

Blows to the abdomen can rupture underlying organs. The spleen is often lacerated, and the intestines, liver, kidney, and bladder may also sustain injury. Symptoms may include abdominal pain and rigidity, nausea and vomiting, shock, and contusions on the abdominal wall. The victim may assume a position with knees drawn up toward the abdomen. If severe shock is present, a pneumatic antishock garment may be applied before transport. The garment extends from the ankles to below the lowest rib. After application the garment is inflated to apply pressure on the lower half of the body, decreasing the size of the vascular system and redirecting blood flow to vital areas (Fig. 45-5).

If there is an open wound evisceration may occur. If the abdominal organs are exposed to the air and become dry, necrosis can result. The abdominal organs lying outside the abdominal cavity should therefore be covered by a warm, moist, preferably sterile covering. If a sterile dressing is not available it is better to cover the organs with a clean moist cloth and risk infection than not to cover the organs and risk loss of tissue.

Amputations

Traumatic amputations are treated as other wounds by controlling hemorrhage and applying pressure dressings. Severe bleeding does not always occur. The amount of bleeding depends on the extent of trauma that occurs; the greater the amount of trauma, such as the amputation of a limb by a crushing injury, the greater will be the amount of muscle spasm in the arterial walls. This causes the artery to contract, and bleeding is decreased. A limb or appendage that is severed cleanly by a sharp object such as a knife will bleed more profusely. Try to stop the bleeding by applying pressure. If a tourniquet is necessary it should be applied close to the site of the amputation to decrease potential injury to intervening tissue.

The amputated portion should be taken with the victim to the hospital because replantation is sometimes possible. The amputated part should be kept at about 5° C (40° F). It can be transported by placing the part in a dampened dressing inside a plastic bag. Immerse the plastic bag in ice water. The amputated part should never be frozen, cleaned, disinfected, debrided, or perfused before transportation.

FRACTURES

Injury to the musculoskeletal system may result in fractures or dislocations of the bones, strained muscles, or torn ligaments (see Chapter 40 for a complete discussion of these injuries). Emergency care consists of assessment of injury and interventions to prevent further trauma until medical help is available.

Assessment

If pain is localized over a bone or joint it should be considered fractured until a definitive diagnosis is made. Obvious deformity can be either a dislocation (if at a joint) or a fracture. In a compound fracture the bone may protrude through the skin. The ability to move an extremity or digit does not negate a fracture, although the victim usually refrains from movement because of pain. Shock may occur with severe fractures, either from the stress of the trauma or from blood loss, such as the extravasation of blood in the thigh after injury.

Skull fractures may vary from a small linear fracture with few symptoms to severe depression of bone fragments into the brain. Basilar skull fractures may be accompanied by bleeding or draining serous fluid from the nose or ears or both. Fractures of facial bones may interfere with respiration if the air passages become blocked.

Pain or deformity at the *hip* can be caused by either a fracture or dislocation. The leg will be shortened in both instances but turned *outward* if there is a *fracture* and *inward* with a *dislocation.* Fractures of the extremities may be accompanied by loss of circulation or sensation if blood vessels or nerves are pinched by the bone fragment. Circulation distal to the fracture is assessed by observing skin color and presence of pulses. A neurologic check for sensation and circulatory system checks should be repeated after splinting and during transportation.

Intervention

The general management of fractures is listed in Box 45-13.

Fracture of the spine

Any questionable injury to the head, neck, or back is treated as a fracture of the spine. The victim should not be moved when being examined for fracture of the spine (neck or back). The examiner slides a hand under the victim and checks for point tenderness along the length of the spine. Bruises on the head may indicate that a force has been exerted that could cause a neck fracture. Bruises on the shoulder, back, or abdomen are frequently seen with back fractures, but a spinal fracture can be present in the absence of any bruises. If the spinal cord has been damaged there may be loss of movement or sensation to the extremities.

Two problems can occur from a fractured spine: damage to the spinal cord and neurogenic shock (Chapter 9). If the cervical spine is fractured there may be interference with respiration, and respirations must be continually monitored. The victim may use diaphragmatic breathing for a short period but be unable to sustain this. Artificial ventilation is more difficult in that the neck cannot be hyperextended because this can cause further injury to the spinal cord. The head can be extended by gentle traction and the jaw pulled forward to open the airway. Traction must be maintained until the neck can be supported in this position. *The neck should never be flexed, twisted, or hyperextended if a fracture is suspected.* If the victim is not having difficulty with respiration, the neck can be splinted in the position in which it was found.

The person with a potential spine fracture must be transported on a firm base, preferably a back board. *Forward or backward flexion of the spine is to be avoided* to prevent further trauma to the spinal cord. The victim should be slid, not rolled, in straight alignment onto the back board.

45-13

General management of fractures

1. Do not move patient before splinting a fracture (unless there is danger of fire, explosion, or radiation).
2. Cover open wound before splinting.
3. Support fractured bone and move it as little as possible while splinting.
4. Splint fracture in the position it is found.
5. In *severely angulated* fractures of the *shaft* of the extremity bone:
   a. Decrease muscle spasm and prevent damage to blood vessels by straightening severe angulation of bone shaft
   b. Place one hand just below fracture and other hand farther down extremity
   c. Apply gentle traction to straighten extremity
   d. Maintain traction until extremity is splinted
6. *Never* straighten deformities of a *joint* (shoulder, elbow, wrist, knee).
7. Apply splints to include joint above and below fracture.
8. Pad rigid splints (boards) for comfort.
9. Reinforce soft splints (pillows) with a rigid material such as a magazine or board.
10. If using air splint:
    a. Inflate only by mouth to a point where the thumb leaves a slight dent
    b. Keep fingers and toes free for assessment of circulation
11. Handle fractured part gently to prevent pain and shock.

It takes several persons working together to move the victim safely. The victim remains on the back board during the initial diagnostic tests in the emergency room.

SEXUAL ASSAULT: RAPE

Rape is one of the violent crimes for which an increasing number of people, primarily women, are seeking help. Despite the increasing number of rapes reported, it is estimated that the incidence of unreported rape is from 200% to 300% higher.

It is difficult to obtain statistics concerning the sociologic variables relating to rape because of the large number of unreported cases. There are many misconceptions concerning rape; some *facts* include the following:

1. Rape occurs among persons of all social classes.
2. Rape occurs mostly between persons of the same race.
3. A majority of rapes are committed by someone the victim knows.
4. Males, especially young boys, may also be rape victims; the attacker is usually another male.

Rape is a major problem in prisons in the United States. Some prison reform groups are actively addressing this

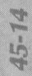

45-14

Rape preventive measures

Prevention of attack

Set house lights to go on and off by timer
Keep light on at all entrances
Place safety locks on windows and doors
Have key ready before reaching door of house or car
Look in car before entering
Insist on identification before letting a stranger in house; check identification with agency if suspicious
Do not list first name on mailbox or in telephone directory
Be alert when walking in street; walk in lighted areas
Walk down center of street if possible
Avoid lonely or enclosed areas

If attacked

Run toward a lighted house; yell, "Fire"
Spit in rapist's face; act bizarre; vomit
Rip off rapist's glasses
Step hard on his foot (instep)
Aim at eyes; try to gouge eyes, scrape face
Hit throat at Adam's apple (larynx)
Use fighting and screaming with caution; this may scare some rapists, encourage others
Try talking to avoid rape
Make close observations about rapist, car, location

---

problem, with the major emphasis on protecting the young and vulnerable from attack.

Rape Crisis Centers

Rape crisis centers are avilable in many large cities. These centers differ in their functions but usually provide one or more of the following:

1. Direct service to the rape victim
2. Service to professional agencies (health, law)
3. Community education

Service to health professionals and education of the community are efforts to help change the system for the rape victim.

The victim service consists of volunteers, many of whom have been raped themselves, who serve as victim advocates throughout the medical examination and police interview. Some form of follow-up service, such as counseling, may be available. Some rape crisis centers have volunteer attorneys who can offer the victim legal advice or representation.

Rape Trauma Syndrome

Rape is a traumatic event for the victim physically, psychologically, and socially. *Physical* force is often used, a weapon may be used either as a threat or to injure the victim, or the hands or fists may be used to beat the victim or threaten choking. Injury can also occur as the victim is attempting self-defense or is struggling on the ground

or floor. The vagina and perineum may be injured by force used during the sexual attack, and the rectum may also be lacerated if anal sex has been attempted, more commonly in rape of males.

Psychologic trauma is usually severe; the rape victim is in a state of crisis. Fear is a dominant theme as the victim perceives the event as life threatening. Other feelings expressed by victims are depersonalization, shame, degradation, defilement, violation, guilt, humiliation, and anger. The victim has not only been under threat of harm but has also been subjected in many instances to multiple sexual assaults by one or more persons. Fellatio (oral sex) is frequently demanded, and some rapists will urinate on the victim before leaving.

The person who has been raped goes through the same phases as any person facing a crisis situation. The initial phase is one of shock and disbelief. After the initial acute phase, there is a period of pseudoequilibrium when the victim rationalizes the event or attempts to suppress thoughts concerning the rape. Later there are periods of depression, phobic reactions, and nightmares.

The rape victim also experiences *sociologic* crisis. If the woman is married, marital relationships may be affected. If she is single she often fears repeated occurrences and may feel the need to move, especially if the attack occurred in her home or apartment. Decisions must be made concerning whom to tell about the incident, because loss of needed support of family and friends may occur. Job security or relationships with co-workers may be threatened. Sociologic problems take considerable time to resolve, but concerns related to these potential problems may occur in the initial emergency period.

Prevention and Health Care

All women need to know the measures they can take to help prevent rape from occurring (Box 45-14). It would also be helpful if every woman learned methods of self-defense. Some communities introduce both issues of rape and self-defense into secondary school curricula. Many YWCAs teach classes in self-defense. Rape crisis centers and police stations may provide information on availability of classes in the community.

Persons who are raped may seek medical help directly or call the police, who will then take the victim for medical examination. Some victims fear reprisal by the rapist or are unwilling to let others know about the rape and therefore do not seek medical attention. Victims need to be encouraged to report the incident.

Most hospitals have developed protocols for care of the rape victim in the emergency department. The protocol may include some of the following:

1. High priority in triage
2. Provision for privacy without leaving the victim alone
3. Provision of a victim advocate (such as a woman from the rape crisis center)
4. Routines to ensure protection and comfort of the victim:
   a. Person(s) designated to have primary contact with the victim
   b. Authority of the primary contact person to make the decision of victim readiness for medical ex-

amination or police interview (if no life-threatening injury is present).

Assessment

Subjective data

The victim will be asked many questions by the examiner to identify the type of assault and potential for injury. If the victim has been threatened she may have succumbed through fear, and this needs to be elicited. Victims often talk freely to the nurse about their feelings; their fears concerning injury, mutilation, or death at the time of assault; or present fears concerning pregnancy or sexually transmitted disease. Other feelings of degradation, feeling "dirty," shame, guilt, and so forth, may be expressed. Anger may be directed at the assailant or projected toward medical care personnel.

Data are collected related to pain or discomfort, either local at the site of assault or general and diffuse. The victim may complain of a sore throat if choking was used as a threat or after oral sex. Nausea may also be reported.

Objective data

Objective behavioral signs are noted. Some women respond emotionally and cry, shake, laugh inappropriately, or are extremely restless. Other victims appear overtly calm and subdued; usually the effect of the experience hits them later.

A head-to-toe assessment for signs of physical trauma is usually carried out by the physician. The clothing will be inspected and described and is often requested by the police for evidence. Clothing should not be washed or discarded. Other data needed by the police usually include samples of the assailant's hair from combing of pubic hair and fingernail deposits for samples of the assailant's tissue.

Diagnostic tests

Papanicolaou smears of the vagina, mouth, or rectum and saline suspensions are done to test for the presence of sperm. An acid phosphate test will demonstrate recency of intercourse. Tests will be inconclusive if the victim has bathed or douched since the rape. Tests for sexually transmitted disease are done at the initial visit to obtain baseline information for future comparison.

A pregnancy test is done initially and repeated if the next menses is missed. Tests for HIV antibody may be done if requested by the patient, and repeated in 2 to 4 months if initially negative.[57]

Intervention

Emotional support

Most victims need to talk with someone who cares about what is happening to them and who is nonjudgmental. The nurse uses crisis intervention theory to decide how best to help the victim (see Chapter 6). Many hospitals have contacts with the rape crisis center, and the victim is given the choice of having a victim advocate from the center to be with her during the entire examination period, both medical and legal. Medical examinations or interviews by the police are not begun until the volunteer arrives.

Preparation for the physical examination is carried out in advance. Having a pelvic examination after a sexual assault can be a traumatic experience especially if the victim has never had a pelvic examination.

Sexuality

The victim has many concerns related to her sexuality. Time is needed to work through these concerns, and long-term counseling is helpful to many victims.

Concern about possible *pregnancy* depends on the circumstances: whether she is in the childbearing years, whether birth control is in effect at the time of sexual assault, and at what point in the menstrual period the rape occurs. If pregnancy is a possibility postcoital hormone contraceptive therapy is initiated immediately.

Concern about *sexually transmitted diseases* (STD) is common. Ceftriazone is given intramuscularly and tetracycline is given orally after the initial examination as a preventive measure. The person needs to know that medical follow-up is important and that she should be retested for STD in about 6 weeks unless symptoms occur earlier. In addition, the woman may experience vaginal discharge, itching, and a burning sensation caused by an acute vaginal infection (vaginitis).

Home discharge plans

The victim should not go home to an empty house or apartment. The volunteer from the rape crisis center, the social worker, or police can all facilitate arrangements for transportation to her home or to the home of family or friends. Frequently the victim goes to the police station after medical care is completed to follow up with the police report. The victim needs to know about the availability of follow-up medical services and counseling services. Some medical centers have psychiatrists who are especially interested in counseling rape victims.

DISASTERS

Disasters are sudden catastrophic events that disrupt patterns of life and in which there is possible loss of life and property in addition to multiple injuries. Disasters can be either natural phenomena or caused by people (Box 45-15).

Effect of Disasters

The effects of disasters are multiple. People are killed or injured and separated from their families. Many become homeless. In mass casualty disasters (Table 45-11) confusion and chaos occur during the early stages. Panic rarely occurs, but when it does it is because the involved persons believe that escape routes are limited and may be closing off. Effective leadership and communication can usually prevent panic.

Transportation difficulties are created as streets and roads become clogged by persons trying to get away from the impact area or others trying to get in. Food and water supplies can become contaminated or nonexistent. Medical supplies may be inadequate to meet the sudden increased need. Utilities can become disrupted. Law enforcement is necessary to prevent looting and other civil disorders. Es-

---

45-15

Causes of disasters

Natural	**Man-made**
Air	**Transportation**
Tornado	Air
Hurricane	Land
Blizzard	Water
Land	**Fire**
Earthquake	Housing
Volcanic eruption	Forest
Avalanches	Explosion
Cave-in	
	Disease
Water	Epidemic
Floods: slow rising and	
flash floods	**Civil**
Tidal wave	Riot
	War (nuclear attack)

45-16

Community groups involved in disaster planning

Governmental	Political, law enforcement, fire department
Health	Hospitals, physicians, nurses, pharmacists, social workers
Official	American Red Cross
Nonofficial	Telephone company, parent-teacher organization, religious organization

---

Table 45-11   **Types of disasters**

Type	Number of people	Cause
Multiple patients	<10	Multiple-vehicle accident, bus accident, bomb, explosion, fire
Multiple casualty	10 to 100	Airplane crash, riot, tornado, hurricane, minor earthquake
Mass casualty	>100	Severe hurricane, major earthquake, war bombing

---

tablishment of a communication system takes first priority to prevent chaos.

Roles of Nurses in Disasters

The actual role assumed by a given nurse at a disaster will depend on the abilities of the nurse and the specific situation. Nurses can participate in many ways. A nurse may be the only health care provider in a given area and be responsible for giving initial first aid treatment or supervising the activities of others. Because of their education and experience, professional nurses can be especially helpful in aiding victims to cope with their emotional reactions to the disaster. Nurses may also be asked to serve at emergency morgues for support of families experiencing the loss of loved ones.

The American Red Cross, which assumes an active role during disasters along with governmental agencies, operates shelters for victims. The agencies provide supplies and food as well as service personnel (shelter manager, nurses, physicians, food helpers). Nurses interested in serving during disasters at home or in other parts of the country may contact the local American Red Cross office. Other services provided by the American Red Cross include emergency services on an individual family basis and aid for recovery.

Prevention

Community planning is necessary to identify and, if possible, prevent disasters, and to educate the public to minimize the number of casualties.

Community planning

Most states have disaster service agencies that act as coordinating units for the local agencies. Every community should have a disaster planning group as part of the local emergency medical committee. There should be representation by all groups who will be active participants if a disaster occurs (Box 45-16). The disaster planning committee has the following functions and responsibilities:

1. Identify the types of disasters that may occur in the local community
2. Organize a disaster plan to be followed for different situations
3. Arrange for simulated drills to test the effectiveness of plans
4. Determine need for education or updating of necessary skills of participants

Nurses need to be active participants in the planning, implementation, and evaluation phases of community disaster preparedness. In addition, nurses need to develop their own nursing response plan to determine roles of community health, institutional, and volunteer nurses in the event of a disaster in their community.[53]

During a disaster local hospitals become actively involved and need their own disaster plan to cope with the sudden influx of persons needing emergency care. Any time a large number of injured persons are in need of emergency care, hospital disaster plans are put into effect. Testing of hospital disaster plans at specified intervals by simulated drills is necessary for determining whether the plans are effective and what changes, if any, are needed.

Public education

Public awareness of potential community disasters is needed for effective community preparedness. Disaster planning committees need support and participation of community members. Individuals need to know what they should do in the event of a disaster. Most radio and television stations regularly notify communities of potential disasters, give directions for preventive actions, and give methods of obtaining further information should the disaster occur. Because electricity may be cut off, battery-operated radios should be available in all homes for continued communication.

All homes should have an emergency food cabinet with sufficient nonperishable foods to meet nutritional needs for several days. Supplies are rotated with current supplies to prevent food from spoiling or becoming outdated.

Assessment
Triage

There are essentially two different approaches to triage during a disaster. The *military* triage system, which may be initiated during a mass casualty disaster, is based on the philosophy of doing "the best for the most with the least by the fewest." Persons with injuries of such a magnitude that there is question of survival are given low priority for transportation. In this system the numbers of critically injured must greatly outnumber the health and transportation personnel available. Victims are reclassified as the emergency situation changes. Priority is then given to those victims with the greatest chance of survival.

The more commonly used *civilian* triage system is used with multiple patients or multiple casualties. Persons with the most critical or life-threatening injuries are given the highest priority for treatment and transportation. Different patient-sorting methods may be used, such as the one listed in Box 45-17.

Disaster syndrome

The behavior of victims after the impact of disaster can be characterized as progressing through phases of shock, awareness, euphoria, and anger. The victims are experiencing loss; therefore the phases are similar to those experienced by others during any kind of loss (grieving).

The *shock phase* may last only a few minutes or for several hours after impact. The victim is dazed and unable to comprehend what is occurring, and cannot follow even simple directions. Persons prepared to function in emergencies are less apt to spend much time in the shock phase.

The *awareness phase* may last up to several days. Victims become aware of survival and try to help others, minimizing their own injuries or losses. During this stage guilt feelings may arise because others died and they survived. The victim is highly suggestible, can follow simple directions, but cannot carry out problem solving effectively.

The *euphoria phase* may last for several weeks. The victim feels a sense of brotherhood with the community and participates willingly in helping others with plans for recovery.

Before resolution, the victim may go through the "Why me?" or *anger phase* that occurs because of the experienced loss. The anger is often projected against helping persons who were not personally affected by the disaster. It is especially important for nurses who may be assisting victims during the recovery phase to understand that the anger is part of the loss experience. As the victim copes with the losses incurred by the disaster and life returns to more normal patterns, the anger will disappear.

45-17

Four-color coded triage system

0—Black: Dead

1—Red: Critical or life-threatening
These victims have a reasonable chance of survival only if they receive immediate treatment. Emergency treatment is initiated immediately and continued during transportation. This category includes victims with respiratory insufficiency, cardiac arrest, hemorrhage, and severe abdominal injury.

2—Yellow: Serious
These victims can wait for transportation after they receive initial emergency treatment. They include victims with immobilized closed fractures, soft-tissue injuries without hemorrhage, and burns on less than 40% of the body.

3—Green: Minimal
Victims in this category are ambulatory, have minor tissue injuries, and may be dazed. They can be treated by nonprofessionals and held for observation if necessary.

From Baker FJ: *Topics Emerg Med* 1:49-157, 1979.

Intervention
Emergency aid stations

The number, size, and staffing of emergency aid stations depend on the type and extent of the disaster. One person in each aid station is designated for triage. One person must be designated the leader and is responsible for making decisions for maximal effectiveness of the unit. In the absence of a physician, a nurse assumes leadership of emergency care.

The types of injuries that occur will depend on the type of disaster. Common injuries and conditions requiring care include soft-tissue and bone injuries, respiratory insufficiency, cardiac arrest, and childbirth.

Victims are not transported until first aid care has been given, as in any emergency. If hemorrhage has not been controlled or fractures splinted, the victim may arrive at the medical center in shock that could have been prevented or minimized; surgical intervention will not take place until measures to treat shock are instituted and the patients's condition is stable. If first aid measures are instituted before transportation, the victim can be taken to surgery at the earliest opportunity. Records of all treatment given at an emergency aid center *must* accompany a victim who is referred or transported to a medical center or any other health care facility.

Shelters

Most shelters are set up in schools, which can house a large number of people. The role of the nurse in a shelter is to assess and provide for health needs of the shelter population. Some nursing functions include the following:

1. Isolate persons with suspected infectious diseases
2. Identify persons with chronic illnesses and ascertain whether prescribed drugs are available
3. Monitor shelter occupants for signs of developing health problems
4. Identify persons having problems coping with the disaster and provide emotional support and guidance as necessary
5. Make arrangement for care of pregnant women and infants
6. Assist with necessary immunizations

Assessment of safety factors in the environment is also a nursing responsibility. The nurse is part of the shelter team and advises the shelter manager of any potential health hazards. The care of victims in a disaster is a team effort, and the nurse is an important member of this team.

Adaptation to loss

Adaptation to loss after large-scale community disasters may differ from adaptation to losses under normal life situations because of the *lack of individual support* systems as a result of (1) death of usual support persons or (2) inability of usual support persons to provide help because of their own personal losses. There may also be a *loss of community support* systems resulting from the disaster.

Immediately after a disaster there is usually an immediate outpouring of material assistance and personnel services from people outside the community. This support diminishes with the passing of time, and the victims are often faced with having to work through their grief with less support than usual and sometimes with visual environmental reminders of loss. It is important that long-term counseling services be made available in these situations to people of all ages. Group therapy can be a useful method of providing support by helping the victim realize that he or she is not alone and that others understand what the victim is experiencing. Group therapy also aids in problem solving through group efforts.

SUMMARY

1. Accidents are the leading cause of death in persons less than 45 years of age and the third leading cause in those 45 to 65 years of age.
2. Accident prevention includes monitoring the home for hazards, equipping homes with smoke alarms, participating in fire drills, and using care while driving.
3. The difference between EMTs and paramedics is that the latter are prepared to carry out invasive procedures, such as starting IVs, defibrillation, and intubation.
4. Persons are not judged as liable unless they act willfully and with gross negligence. Reasonable care is judged on the basis of care given by someone with similar training and under the prevailing situation.
5. The parameters of priority assessment of the injured person are the ABCs (airway, breathing, circulation) and level of consciousness.
6. After the priority assessment, a head-to-toe assessment is made for signs of injury.
7. Shock ususally develops in persons who sustain major trauma or a major stressor to the system.
8. Loss of consciousness after a period of alertness after a head injury may indicate an intracranial hematoma that requires immediate medical attention.
9. The sequence for providing care of an injured person is first the priority assessment with immediate lifesaving measures, followed by the head-to-toe assessment before carrying out general first-aid measures.
10. Keep an injured person lying down and protected from cold (but not heated); the person is not transported until all first aid measures have been carried out.
11. Asphyxia is indicated by dyspnea, adventitious sounds, use of accessory respiratory muscles, skin pallor, or eventually cyanosis.
12. Remove foreign bodies from the airway with the Heimlich maneuver if the person is unable to cough up the object.
13. The sequence of CPR is to assess the level of consciousness, open the airway, initiate artificial ventilation, assess circulation, and initiate external cardiac compressions.
14. The person with a suspected myocardial infarction who is breathing should be placed in a comfortable, well-supported sitting position, given oxygen (if available), be cared for with a calm approach to minimize anxiety, and be transported to a hospital immediately.
15. Drowning may be caused by asphyxiation from the aspiration of fluid into the lungs or from laryngospasm that prevents both air and water from entering the lungs. Persons who have experienced near-drowning should be monitored closely for latent pulmonary edema for at least 24 hours.
16. The best method for stopping external bleeding is to place direct pressure on the bleeding vessel; tourniquets are used only for massive arterial bleeding that cannot be controlled by other means.
17. If poisoning is suspected in an unconscious person, the person should be transported immediately to the nearest medical facilitiy.
18. For ingestion of noncaustic substances, give the conscious person syrup of ipecac followed by 1 or 2 glasses of water; if drugs have been ingested, follow the water with activated charcoal.
19. Heat exhaustion is a shocklike reaction to heat; place the person recumbent in a cool environment and provide salty fluids. Heat stroke results from inability to lose heat by perspiration; the skin is hot and dry and unconsciousness may occur. Heatstroke is more serious and requires immediate medical care.
20. Applying too much heat to persons overexposed to cold may lead to skin injury from the decreased circulation and hypovolemic shock from vasodilation.
21. The skin, gastrointestinal mucosa, and blood cells are the tissues most sensitive to radiation.
22. Pneumothorax may result from open chest wounds; a nonporous dressing is required to prevent air from entering the chest.

23. Suspected fractures must be splinted before the person is moved; severely angulated fractures of the shaft of a long bone may be straightened by traction to prevent severe muscle spasms; deformities of a joint are *never* straightened.
24. Persons with a potential spine fracture are transported on a firm base avoiding spine flexion.
25. Persons who are raped experience physical, psychologic, and sociologic trauma.
26. Nurses participate during disasters by providing triage and first aid at emergency aid stations and hospitals, by providing health care at shelters, and by providing emotional support to persons at emergency morgues.
27. Victims of disasters experience grief and mourning reactions; long-term adaptation may be hampered by lack of usual support systems.

STUDY QUESTIONS

What actions should you take in the following situations?
- You are driving with a non-nurse friend along a country road when you suddenly come upon an automobile accident. A man is standing dazed beside the car. A woman is on the ground, apparently thrown from the car; her right leg is bent underneath her; she is conscious. A man is in the driver's seat of the car with blood on his face; the windshield is cracked. A young girl is sitting on the side of the road screaming. You stop to help.
- Your neighbor phones you; her 3-year-old has just swallowed half a bottle of baby aspirins.
- You are working out at a health club. A man near you suddenly clutches his chest and sits down on the floor. His face is pale and sweating.
- You are a camp nurse. On a very hot day, two boys are brought to you. One boy complains of weakness and headache; his skin is cold and clammy. The other boy is confused; his skin is hot and dry and his temperature is 40° C (104° F).

REFERENCES AND SELECTED READINGS

1.* Adamski DB: Assessment and treatment of allergic response to stinging insects, *J Emerg Nurs* 16(2):77-80, 1990.
2. American College of Surgeons, Committee on Trauma: Early care of the injured patient, ed 4, Philadelphia, 1989, WB Saunders.
3.* Baker HM: Some thoughts on helping grieving families, *J Emerg Nurs* 12:359-362, 1987.
4.* Beaver BM: Care of the multiple trauma victim: the first hour, *Nurs Clin North Am* 25(1):11-21, 1990.
5.* Bomberger AS: Radiation injuries: dealing with nuclear-age disaster, *Nurs 90* 20(4):76,79, 1990.
6. Boyd-Monk H: Eye trauma: a close-up on emergency care, *RN* 52(12):22-30, 1989.
7. Brown LKW: Traumatic amputation: mechanisms of injury, treatment, and rehabilitation, *AAOHN J* 38:483-486, 1990.
8.* Burgess AW: Rape trauma syndrome: a nursing diagnosis, *Occup Health Nurs* 33:405-406, 1985.
9.* Buschiazzo L: What's new in CPR, *Nurs 86* 16(1):34-37, 1986.

10.* Butler S: Out of the water, but not out of the woods, *RN* 51(6):26-29, 1988.
11.* Clegg F: The psychological aftermath of disasters, *Nurs 88* (London) 3(31):5-8, 1988.
12. Cook L: Hospital disaster drill game: a strategy for teaching disaster protocols to hospital staff, *J Emerg Nurs* 16(4):269-273, 1990.
13. Dexter WW: Hypothermia: safe and efficient methods of rewarming the patient, *Postgrad Med* 88(8):55-64, 1990.
14.* DiNitto D, et al: After rape: who should examine rape survivors, *Am J Nurs* 86:538-540, 1986.
15. Diptheria, tetanus and pertussis: guidelines for vaccine prophylaxis and other measures, *MMWR* 34:405-425, 1985.
16. Duffy J: Lyme disease, *Infec Dis Clin North Am* 1:511-527, 1987.
17. Garcia LM: *Disaster nursing: planning, assessment, and intervention*, Rockville, Md, 1985, Aspen Systems.
18.* Halpern JS: Mechanisms and patterns of trauma, *J Emerg Nurs* 15(5):380-388, 1989
19.* Hammond SG: Chest injuries in the trauma patient, *Nurs Clin North Am* 25(1):35-43, 1990.
20.* Hanson C: Disaster preparedness: becoming involved, *J Emerg Nurs* 16(4):74A-75A, 1990.
21.* Hayes G, Goodwin T, Miars B: After disaster: a crisis support team at work, *Am J Nurs* 90(2):61-64, 1990.
22.* Heimlich LB: Care of the female rape victim, *Nurse Pract* 12(11):9-18, 1987.
23. Holloway A: Disaster reduction: what it means for nurses, *Int Nurs Rev* 37(6):369-370, 1990.
24. Hoyt NJ: Host defense mechanisms and compromises in the trauma patient, *Crit Care Nurs Clin North Am* 1(4):753-765, 1990.
25.* Huggins B: Trauma physiology, *Nurs Clin North Am* 25(1):1-10, 1990.
26.* Huston CJ: Hypothermia, *Nurs 90* 20(12):33, 1990.
27.* Jackson DF: Abdominal stab wound, *Nurs 89* 19(12):33, 1989.
28. Jacobs BB, et al: Prehospital resuscitation of the trauma patient, *Top Emerg Med* 9(3):1-19, 1987.
29.* Jamison DW: When emergency care is up to you, *RN* 50(4):26-31, 1987.
30.* Jordan K: Chest trauma: how to detect and react to serious trouble, *Nurs 90* 20(9):34-42, 1990.
31. Kitt S, Kaiser J: *Emergency nursing: a physiologic and clinical perspective*, Philadelphia, 1990, WB Saunders.
32.* Laurent CL: Disaster triage of massive casualties from thermonuclear detonation, *J Emerg Nurs* 16(4):248-251, 1990.
33.* LaVoy K: Dealing with hypothermia and frostbite, *RN* 48(1):53-56, 1985.
34.* Lee BC: Be ready for Lyme disease in your own backyard, *RN* 52(4):26-29, 1989.
35.* Lee G: Transport of the critically ill trauma patient, *Nurs Clin North Am* 21(4):741-749, 1986.
36.* Legge M, Murphy MF: Human bite wounds, *J Emerg Nurs* 16(3):145-149, 1990.
37.* Lenehan GP: Emotional impact of trauma, *Nurs Clin North Am* 21(4):729-740, 1986.
38.* Lewellyn C: Emergency care of the replant patient, *Crit Care Nurs Q* 13(1):13-18, 1990.
39.* Leyendecker M, et al: Rescuing a multiple trauma victim, *Nurs 89* 19(10):54-61, 1989.
40. Lyme disease surveillance, United States 1989-1990, *MMWR* 40(25):417-421, 1991.
41.* Maher AB: Early assessment and management of musculoskeletal injuries, *Nurs Clin North Am* 21(4):717-727, 1986.
42.* Martin JS, et al: Early triage and treatment of the acute

*Recommended for student reading.

myocardial infarction patient: how fast is fast? *J Emerg Nurs* 16(3):195-201, 1990.

43. Matz R: Hypothermia: mechanisms and counter measures, *Hosp Pract* 21(2):45-48, 1986.

44.* Mikhail JN: Acute burn care: an update, *J Emerg Nurs* 14:9-17, 1988.

45. Minden P: The Victim Care Service: a program for victims of sexual assault, *Arch Psychiatr Nurs* 3(1):41-46, 1989.

46. Moore EE, et al: Early care of the injured patient, ed 4, Philadelphia, 1990, BC Decker.

47.* Moser MY: When lightning strikes, *Am J Nurs* 86:802-803, 1986.

48.* Nelson NP: Near drowning, *J Emerg Nurs* 16(2):119-122, 1990.

49. Nevitt MC, et al: Risk factors for recurrent nonsyncopal falls, *JAMA* 261(18):2663-2668, 1989.

50. Newton, et al: General treatment of household poisoning, *J Emerg Nurs* 13(1):12-15, 1987.

51.* Nikas DL: Resuscitation of patients with CNS trauma, *Nurs Clin North Am* 21(4):729-740, 1986.

52.* Northrop CE: How Good Samaritan laws do and don't protect you, *Nurs 90* 20(2):66-68, 1990.

53.* O'Hara MM: Emergency care of the patient with a traumatic amputation, *J Emerg Med* 13:272-277, 1987.

55.* Paparone P: The summer scourge: Lyme disease, *Am J Nurs* 90(6):44-47, 1990.

56.* Parker JG: Thoracic trauma: nursing assessment and management, *Nurs Clin North Am* 21(4):685-692, 1986.

57. Schroeder SA, et al: Current medical diagnosis and treatment, Norwalk, Conn, 1991, Appleton & Lange.

58. Sheehy SB: Mosby's manual of emergency care, ed 3, St Louis, 1990, Mosby–Year Book.

59. Sheehy SB, Barber J: Emergency nursing: principles and practice, ed 2, St Louis, 1985, Mosby–Year Book.

60. Sheehy SB, Marvin JA, Jimmerson CL: Manual of clinical trauma nursing: the first hour, St Louis, 1988, Mosby–Year Book.

61.* Shoven JT, et al: Near drowning, *Am J Nurs* 89:680-696, 1989.

62.* Solursh DS: The family of the trauma victim, *Nurs Clin North Am* 25(1):155-162, 1990.

63. Standards and guidelines for cardiopulmonary resuscitation (CPR) and emergency cardiac care (ECC), *JAMA* 255:2905-2988, 1986.

64.* Stotts NA: Seeing red, and yellow, and black: the 3 color concept of wound care, *Nurs 90* 20(2):50-51, 1990.

65.* Tidelksaar R: Home safe home: practical tips for fall-proofing, *Geriatr Nurs* 10(6):280-284, 1989.

66. US Department of Health and Human Services and Public Health Service: *Healthy People 2000: national health promotion and disease prevention objectives*, 1991, Washington, DC.

67.* Wagner MM: The patient with abdominal injuries, *Nurs Clin North Am* 25(1):45-55, 1990.

68. Way LW: Current surgical diagnosis and treatment, ed 9, Norwalk, Conn, 1991, Appleton & Lange.

69. Welsh MD: Acute radiation syndrome, *DDDN* 5(5):277-286, 1986.

46

Care of the Patient in a Critical Care Unit

Maura Hopkins

After studying this chapter, the learner should be able to:

- Describe the physical and psychologic environment of critical care units.
- Identify the types of data needed for the care of critically ill patients.
- Describe interventions to alleviate physiologic stressors (respiratory, cardiovascular, neurologic, renal, gastrointestinal, musculoskeletal/integumentary) that are specific to the critical care setting.
- Describe interventions to alleviate and prevent psychologic stressors for both the patient and the nurse.

<table>
<tr><td>

46-1

Equipment and resources commonly available within or near the ICU

Monitors
Cardiac
Hemodynamic (intraarterial, pulmonary artery, central venous)
Intracranial pressure
External arterial pressure
Respiratory/apnea
Oximetry, capnography
Body temperature

General equipment
ECG machine
Defibrillator
Intubation equipment
Emergency medications
Oxygen therapy equipment
Arterial blood gas analyzer
Hyper-hypothermia machine
Fluoroscopy
Doppler flow detection device

Bedside equipment
Bed scale
Bed with removable headboard
Oxygen and manual ventilation device
Suction device
Intravenous infusion device

Support services
Pharmacy
Laboratory
Respiratory therapy
Radiology, including CAT, MRI, EEG
Dialysis
Chaplain
Social worker
Psychologist
Nutritionist

</td><td>

46-2

Stressors on patients, families, and staff in the ICU

Patient/family
Unfamiliar environment, new faces
Noise, light levels
Interruption of sleep/wake cycles
Sensory deprivation/overload
Inaccessibility of family, friends
Lack of privacy
Lack of information/understanding of prognosis, care plan
Lack of information/understanding of policies, procedures
Anticipation of painful interventions
Confusion/disorientation related to physiologic factors
Impaired communication related to intubation
Observation of crisis intervention in other patients
Fear related to diagnosis
Fear of death

Staff
Expectations of self
Expectations of peers, supervisors
Intricate machinery and techniques
Closed, crowded work area
Constant contact with seriously ill, dying persons
Continual vigilance over multiple patients
Need for constant emergency readiness
Sustained high activity level
Limited breaks away from the high-stress unit
Limited communication with many patients related to intubation or altered level of consciousness
Limited opportunity to communicate with some families
Isolation from other nurses in the hospital
Ethical conflicts related to issues of resuscitation, aggressive therapy, and use of life-maintenance equipment

</td></tr>
</table>

When "respirator centers" were developed in isolated locations nationally to combat the polio epidemic of the 1950s, the expectation was that the concentration of highly skilled personnel along with sophisticated medical equipment would positively influence the victims' survival. In addition to providing treatment these centers were dedicated to research, education, and training. They were, perhaps, the earliest form of the modern day intensive care unit (ICU).

Through the evolution of the coronary intensive care unit of the 1960s to the current nationwide availability of single-purpose and multipurpose critical care units, the role of the nurse in the care of the critically ill patient has remained the focal point of the success of these units. With vigilant observation of the patient's ever-changing condition, the critical care nurse is uniquely able to identify and initiate appropriate therapies, maintain complex treatment regimens, and intervene to prevent life-threatening situations.

In the 1990s nurses find themselves working in a wide array of adult and pediatric critical care environments.

These may be multipurpose ICUs or units specially designated for patients with a common type of problem, such as medical, surgical, coronary, cardiovascular, neurologic/neurosurgical, pulmonary, transplant, neonatal, burn, and shock/trauma units. In all cases the goal of critical care nursing remains the same: to provide continuous, optimal nursing care to patients in life-threatening situations, remaining alert to the physiologic, psychologic, and social needs of the patient as an integrated being.

This chapter provides an overview of some of the common aspects of critical care nursing and the critical care environment. Effects of the critical care environment on patient, family, and staff are described. Assessment of the critically ill patient is followed by interventions designed to alleviate physical, psychologic, and social stressors experienced by critically ill patients.

The reader is referred to other sections of this text and to the chapter references for a more thorough discussion of the physiologic processes, nursing interventions, and techniques of caring for critically ill patients.

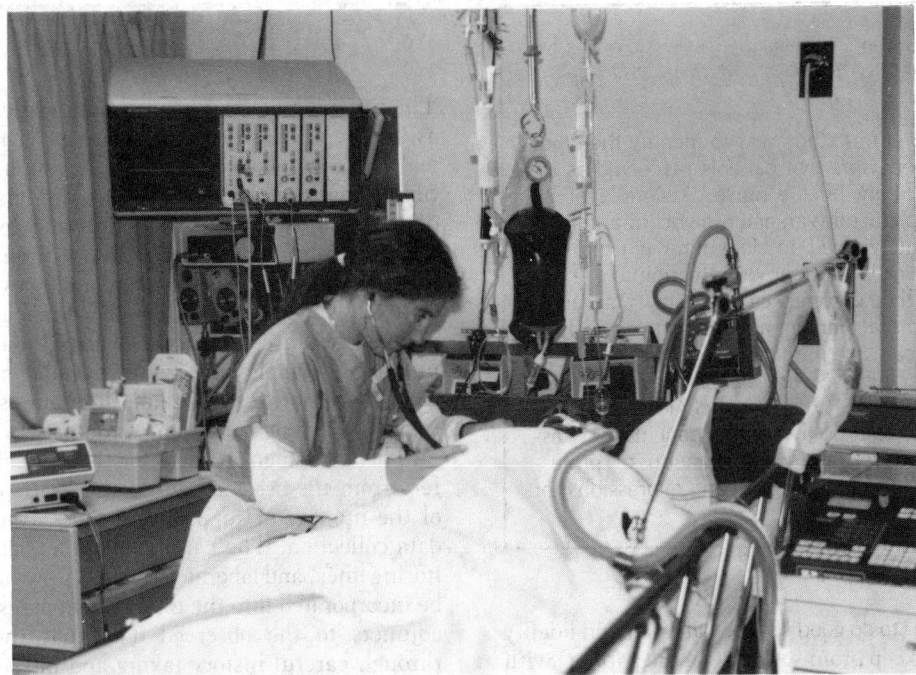

Fig. 46-1 Typical ICU bedside.

ENVIRONMENT IN THE CRITICAL CARE AREA

Physical Environment

The critical care unit is designed, equipped, and staffed to meet the anticipated needs of patients in life-threatening situations. The physical layout is frequently a modified circular design around a central nurses' station, allowing for direct visualization of many or all patients at all times. Patients may be separated in individual rooms or be situated in a large open area with curtains as partitions. The advantage of direct nurse-patient visualization may accompany the disadvantages of limited patient privacy and patient exposure to frequent crisis intervention.

Supplies and equipment in critical care areas are highly sophisticated and must be readily accessible for all patients (see Box 46-1) (Fig. 46-1). Certain pieces of equipment are in constant use at each bedside (for example, cardiac monitor, oxygen, suction equipment), and others must be available within seconds (defibrillator, ventilator, ECG machine, emergency medications). Existing hospital space has often been converted to ICU use, and as the need for more specialized and sophisticated ICU equipment grows the critical care environment often becomes overcrowded.

Psychologic Environment: Stress on Patient and Staff

In the critical care environment advanced forms of technology and medical and nursing therapeutics are used with patients in extended crisis. Although aware of the special nature of this care, the patient and family focus on its appearance: flashing lights; buzzing machines; painful procedures; a noisy, brightly lit, crowded, hyperactive environment permeated by vague fears. The stressors on the patient and family are immense, heightened by those very treatment modalities that may prove lifesaving.

The stress on nursing staff in the critical care area stems in part from very high expectations: advanced knowledge of physiology related to all body systems, astute observation and physical assessment skills, and the technical ability to operate the highly sophisticated equipment. Critical care nurses must have excellent communication skills to deal with the patient's and the family's psychologic and social needs, continually incorporating interventions that the nurse might be tempted to assign a low priority in a critical situation.

Both the patient and the nurse are bombarded by continuous stressors in the critical care environment (see Box 46-2). Low-level stress can be challenging and stimulating and may help to enhance creativity, productivity, and performance in any area. Continuous high-level stress can be devastating, both physically and psychologically. The patient's physiologic response to stress includes neural and hormonal activation that can cause stimulation of target organs (heart, blood vessels, GI tract) already compromised by illness or injury. (Review Chapter 6 on concepts of stress and adaptation for an indepth analysis of the effects of stress.) It is equally important for critical care nurses to understand the psychologic effects of stress on both the patient and family and to recognize that interactions will have to be modified to take this into account. In addition, nurses must be aware of their own stressors and the positive and negative effects of these stressors. They must safeguard their own physical and psychologic health and recognize how insufficient or ineffective coping mechanisms can lead to burnout.

Ethical considerations play a prominent role in the day-to-day nursing care of critically ill patients. Nurses, as patient advocates, find themselves struggling to integrate their own sense of justice (that each patient is treated

Nursing Research

46-3

Cronin SN, Harrison B: Importance of nurse caring behaviors as perceived by patients after myocardial infarction, *Heart Lung* 17(4):374-380, 1988.

The purpose of this study was to identify the types of nursing behaviors that patients perceived as indicators of caring by the nurse. A sample of 22 patients hospitalized with acute myocardial infarction were interviewed to determine what things nurses said or did that conveyed caring to the patients during their coronary care unit stay. Data analysis revealed that nursing actions that focused on the physical care and monitoring of patients, as well as teaching activities, were seen as the most indicative of caring. The authors conclude that critical care nurses should be aware that patients view assessment activities and demonstration of professional competence as significant expressions of caring.

fairly), beneficence (to do good for the patient), and fidelity (to be truthful and keep promises made to the patient) with the needs of the family and other health care providers.

The most complex issues occur in situations in which patients can no longer direct their own care. The determination of who can then best speak for the patient is often very complex in today's diverse social climate; an unrelated friend, lover, or companion may have far more intimate knowledge of the patient's values and wishes than an estranged or distant "next of kin." Not all states recognize such advance directives as the living will, which usually identifies the patient's general wishes regarding resuscitation and prolonged life support. Even more specific and effective is the durable power of attorney for health care (DPA), in which patients have previously named an individual to make health care decisions on their behalf should they become unable. The DPA can be as detailed as the patient desires; it has been upheld in court.

Some of the ethical conflicts most often encountered in the critical care setting include decisions related to (1) withdrawal of life support, (2) withdrawal of food and fluids, (3) do not resuscitate orders, (4) nontreatment of further complications (most notably infections and respiratory failure), and (5) not initiating dialysis. When either family or health care providers do not think that the best interests of the patient are being served, they may seek the opinion of the hospital ethics committee. This group is typically composed of physicians, nurses, administrators, social services professional, a chaplain, and a lay member. The group reviews the specific situation thoroughly and offers a nonbinding opinion to the person requesting the consultation. Ethics committees have provided a safe forum for discussion of differing view points and have assisted families and care givers to view a particular situation within an ethical framework.

The critical care unit is a powerful milieu that must be well understood by nurses who wish to take advantage of its environment to deliver comprehensive, patient-centered nursing care.

ASSESSMENT OF THE CRITICALLY ILL PATIENT

The nursing process is the same in critical care situations as in any other patient care setting. Management of critically ill patients requires establishing a data base, identifying real and potential problems, delineating priorities, defining outcome criteria, determinig goals for intervention, executing the planned intervention, and modifying future goals and plans based on outcomes. Management of critically ill patients differs from management of other patients because of an ever-changing data base, a larger number of complex, interrelated problems, frequent reordering of priorities, and time limitations imposed by the rapidly changing condition of the patient.

The assessment process for the critically ill patient differs from the assessment of other patients only in terms of the number of supportive devices available to assist in data collection. The cardiac monitor, hemodynamic monitoring lines, and laboratory analyses provide data that must be incorporated into the total patient assessment. They are adjuncts to the observed data that the nurse gathers through careful history taking and physical examination. Monitored data is a useless string of unrelated facts and numbers until correlated to physical findings and integrated into a meaningful analysis by the critical care nurse. Assessment activities are also viewed by patients as nurse caring behaviors (for research see Box 46-3).

Nursing History

There are three main sources from which critically ill patients come to an intensive care unit: direct admission, transfer from another patient care division in the same or a different hospital, and postoperatively after certain operations. The patient admitted directly to the ICU (for example, in the case of a myocardial infarction) will often be accompanied by family or friends. Both the patient and family members are useful in obtaining a thorough and accurate history of the current illness, past illnesses/hospitalizations, and a patient profile containing social information and usual coping strategies. Although at the time of admission emphasis is placed on alleviating physiologic threats to survival, one member of the health team may take the opportunity to concurrently interview family members so that crucial facts about the patient's history can immediately be used in patient care. Even in the critical care setting, accurate and thorough history taking is vital to intelligent, individualized care planning and intervention.

When the patient is received in transfer from another nursing division, either directly or after surgery, consultation between the transferring and receiving nursing staff is essential. The ICU nurses benefit from the care plan developed by nurses who have had the opportunity to interact with the patient and family in a noncritical situation. Pertinent history, patient likes and dislikes, coping mechanisms, and family relations can all be relayed to the receiving nurses, enabling them to reduce the initial stress of the unfamiliar ICU environment. This type of pertinent history and care planning is shared among nurse colleagues to promote continuity of care and facilitate the patient's eventual recovery.

Physical Examination

As with the assessment of any patient, history taking is followed by physical examination. The basic skills of inspection, palpation, percussion, and auscultation are used to elicit directly observed data from the patient. As in any other setting, explanations are given and patient cooperation is sought, even if the patient's comprehension of all that is said is questionable. (Refer to a physical assessment textbook for a thorough explanation on the use of these techniques.)

Monitored Data

Nurses in all clinical settings use tools for discrete data collection from patients, for example, stethoscopes, sphygmomanometers, thermometers, and scales. Critical care nurses have the advantage of being able to use additional tools for continuous data collection, for example, cardiac monitors, hemodynamic pressure lines, and intracranial pressure monitoring devices. The explosion in critical care technology in the 1970s and 1980s has provided the critical care nurse with amazing quantities of objective data with minimal time spent in system operation. Computerized monitoring systems are available that occupy less space and provide more capabilities than ever before. The most sophisticated of the "patient data management" systems take information from all the continuously monitored parameters (ECG, dysrhythmias, pulmonary artery pressure, intraarterial pressure, central venous pressure, intracranial pressure, respiration, and body temperature) and combine it with manually entered data such as body weight, height, intake and output, and times of drug administration, and prepare a wide array of hemodynamic calculations and patient response trends for analysis by critical care practioners. Certain types of continuous monitoring devices are in widespread use in nearly all critical care environments.

Cardiac monitoring

Cardiac monitoring is a noninvasive procedure that involves placement on the patient's chest of conductive electrodes that recognize the electrical activity of the heart and relay it to a video display screen. Before electrode placement the skin should be cleansed to remove debris and oils, then very lightly abraded to provide the best contact with the electrode. If necessary excess hair is clipped. Pre-gelled electrodes are applied to the skin in standard three and five lead configurations depending on the leads to be monitored (Chapter 25). The electrodes are connected to the lead wires, then attached to a monitoring cable that is plugged into the bedside monitor (*hardwire monitoring*). Both the actual appearance of the patient's ECG and the numeric representation of the heart rate are displayed on the monitor. Alarm limits are programmed by the nurse so that if the patient's heart rate rises above or falls below a safe range a tone sounds to alert the nurse.

An alternative to hardwire monitoring is *telemetry monitoring*, in which the electrodes placed on the patient's chest

Table 46-1   Normal hemodynamic pressures

Area monitored	Type of measurement	Normal pressure (mm Hg)
Superior vena cava (SVC)	Mean	2 to 6 (3 to 10 cm H_2O)
Right atrium (RA)	Mean	2 to 6 (3 to 10 cm H_2O)
Right ventricle (RV)	Systolic	20 to 30
	Diastolic	0 to 5
	End diastolic	2 to 6
Pulmonary artery (PA)	Systolic	20 to 30
	Diastolic	10 to 20
	Mean	10 to 15
Pulmonary capillary wedge (PCW)	Mean	4 to 12
Left atrium (LA)	Mean	4 to 12
Left ventricle (LV)	Systolic	100 to 140
	Diastolic	0 to 5
Aorta (Ao)	Systolic	100 to 140
	Diastolic	60 to 80
	Mean	70 to 90

are attached to a transmitter worn by the patient in a pocket or pouch. The transmitter sends a radio signal to a receiver, usually located at the nurses' station. The principal advantage of telemetry is that the patient may ambulate freely while cardiac rhythm is monitored. Although sometimes used within a coronary care unit, telemetry patients are most often located on a telemetry or step-down unit where they are in rooms not under continuous direct observation.

Monitoring systems with computerized dysrhythmia analysis also recognize specific rhythm abnormalities, such as single or paired premature ventricular contractions, bigeminal rhythms, runs of ventricular tachycardia, ventricular fibrillation, or asystole. Variations in the audio or visual display of the alarm can alert the nurse to the relative seriousness of the dysrhythmia, even from a distance.

As a noninvasive procedure cardiac monitoring presents low risk to the patient. Nursing interventions of careful skin preparation, electrode placement, and daily skin inspection are directed toward prevention of the potential complication of electrode dermatitis. (Refer to Chapter 25 for a complete discussion of cardiac monitoring and ECG interpretation.)

Hemodynamic monitoring

Hemodynamic monitoring refers to invasive monitoring of the arterial or vascular system via a continuous electronic monitoring device. Table 46-1 lists the normal values of pressures found in the cardiovascular system, many of which are measured via bedside monitoring.

Intraarterial monitoring

Intraarterial monitoring involves placement of a catheter into an artery, usually the radial or femoral artery. The catheter is connected to a high-pressure flush system normally filled with heparinized saline solution. The automatic flush, under pressure, delivers an average of 1 to 3

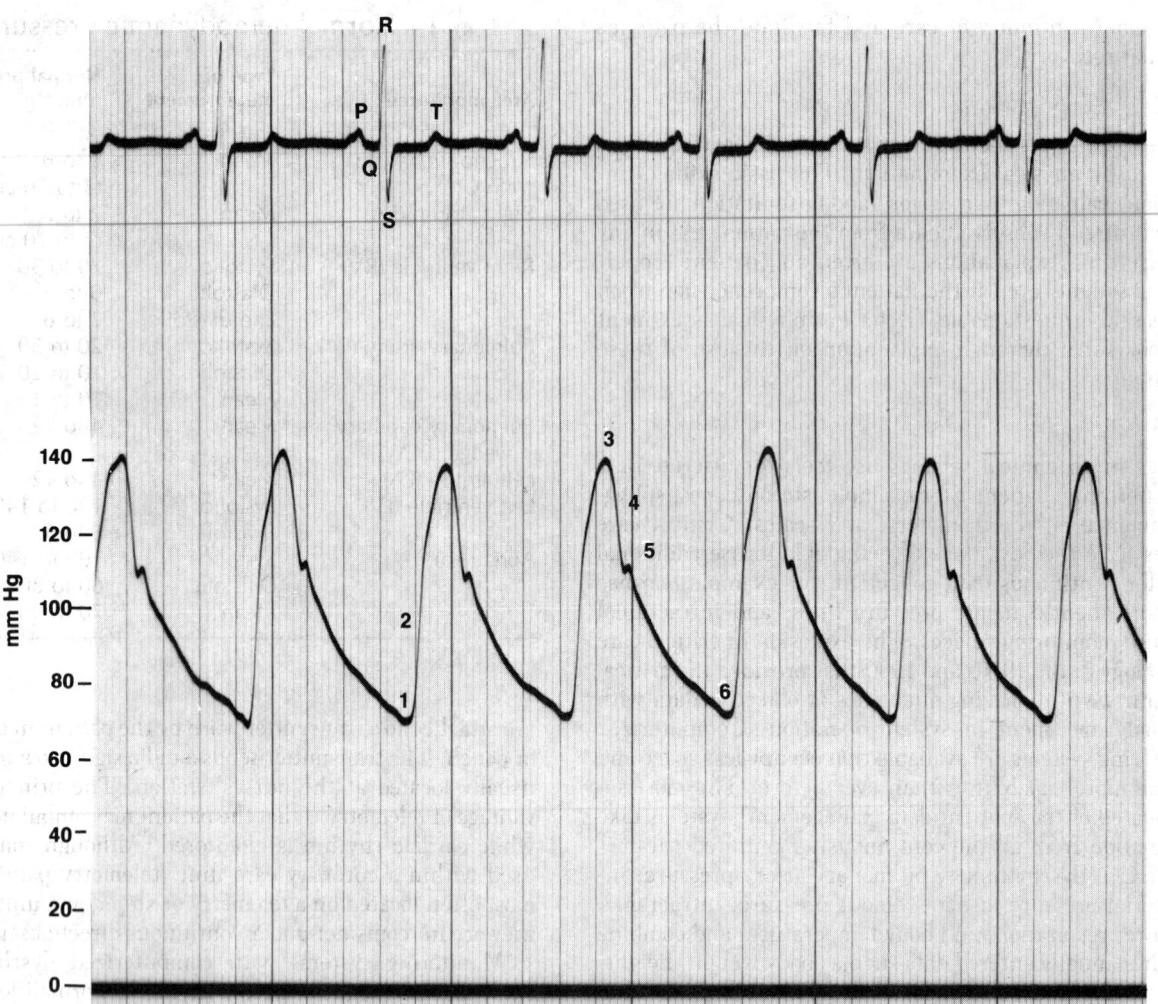

Fig. 46-2 Normal ECG and radial artery waveform. *1,* Aortic valve opens; beginning of systole. *2,* Systolic ejection. *3,* Peak systolic pressure. *4,* Systolic run-off phase. *5,* Dicrotic notch; aortic valve closure; beginning of diastole. *6,* End-diastolic pressure. Note that the upswept wave indicating systolic contraction *(2)* follows ventricular depolarization (QRS). (From Daily EK, Schroeder JS: *Hemodynamic waveforms,* ed 2, St Louis, 1990, Mosby–Year Book.)

ml solution per hour through the catheter just to keep it patent. When an electronic transducer is connected to the system and attached to the bedside monitor a waveform appears on the monitor that represents the fluctuation of the patient's blood pressure in the catheterized artery. A numeric display of the arterial pressure also appears on the monitor; in most patients this direct intraarterial pressure correlates very closely with external cuff pressure measurements. Figure 46-2 shows the relationship between a normal ECG and arterial trace.

Intraarterial pressure monitoring also provides direct access to arterial blood, which can then be easily obtained without further needle punctures for various laboratory tests, including arterial blood gas analysis. However, intraarterial cannulation is not without its problems. Complications of intraarterial monitoring may include the following:

Bleeding
Thrombosis
Inflammation/infiltration
Infection
Air/particulate embolism
Paresthesias
Distal obstruction of the artery

Nursing responsibilities for intraarterial monitoring include the following:

1. Preliminary flush system and transducer set up
2. Assistance with insertion
3. Aseptic maintenance of the flush system and catheter insertion site
4. Maintenance of catheter patency with accurate waveform and pressure readings
5. Continuous patient observation to prevent the immediate life-threatening complication of hemorrhage

Table 46-2   Normal hemodynamic indices

Measurement	Formula	Normal range
Cardiac output (CO)	Heart rate × Stroke volume	4.0 to 8.0 L/min
Cardiac index (CI)	$\dfrac{\text{Cardiac output}}{\text{Body surface area}}$	2.5 to 4.0 L/min/m²
Stroke volume (SV)	$\dfrac{\text{Cardiac output}}{\text{Heart rate}}$	60 to 130 ml/beat
Stroke index (SI)	$\dfrac{\text{Stroke volume}}{\text{Body surface area}}$	35 to 70 ml/beat/m²
Mean arterial pressure (MAP)	2/3 Diastolic + 1/3 systolic pressure	70 to 90 mm Hg
Pulmonary vascular resistance (PVR)	Mean pulmonary artery pressure − mean pulmonary capillary wedge pressure ÷ cardiac output	<2 PVR units
Systemic vascular resistance (SVR)	$\dfrac{\text{Mean arterial pressure} - \text{central venous pressure (in mm Hg)} \times 80}{\text{Cardiac output}}$	900 to 1600 dynes/sec/cm⁻⁵

Pulmonary artery monitoring
Multiple lumen catheter

Pulmonary artery (Swan-Ganz) catheters are used to monitor cardiovascular function in critically ill patients. The catheter is inserted into the superior vena cava via the subclavian, internal jugular, or external jugular vein. The typical pulmonary artery catheter has several openings along its length, and is connected to a high-pressure heparinized flush solution, electronic transducer, and bedside monitor in the same fashion as an arterial line (Chapter 9). The catheter is threaded through the right atrium and right ventricle into the pulmonary artery, where the tip rests (see Fig. 25-42). When the small balloon at the catheter tip is inflated with approximately 1 ml of air, the catheter floats with the blood flow from the pulmonary artery into a pulmonary capillary.

The pulmonary capillary wedge pressure (PCWP) is the same as the pressure in the left atrium because there are no valves to create a gradient between the pulmonary artery and the left atrium. During diastole, when the mitral valve is open, the PCWP represents the filling pressure of the left ventricle (barring mitral valve disease). The pulmonary artery catheter is useful in providing data on both left- and right-sided heart failure and cardiogenic shock (Chapter 25).

The tip of the catheter senses the pressure of the blood at its opening and transmits a representative pressure waveform to the monitor screen, which in turn converts the waveform into a digital value. In this fashion the distinct waveform and pressure of the superior vena cava, right atrium, right ventricle, and pulmonary artery are visualized as the catheter is introduced.

By connecting the pulmonary artery catheter to a cardiac output computer the volume of cardiac output can be determined. A known quantity of injectate (usually 10 ml of NS or D₅W) is injected into the right ventricle via the proximal injectate port of the catheter. Whether iced or

at room temperature, the injectate is cooler than the surrounding blood with which it mixes in the ventricle. The blood plus injectate travel from the ventricle out into the pulmonary artery and flow past the catheter tip. The computer registers the temperature change and calculates the volume of blood that was present to produce the change, and represents this as the cardiac output in liters of blood per minute. Table 46-2 lists the hemodynamic indices that can be calculated from monitored data.

Pulmonary artery pressures are obtained from the distal port when the catheter is not in the wedged position. Central venous pressures (CVP) are obtained from the proximal port, which may also be used for fluid and medication infusions. Some pulmonary artery catheters have two proximal ports to enhance the multipurpose nature of the catheter. Pulmonary artery catheters are used in place of single or multiple central lines in critically ill patients because of the information they provide on left-sided heart function (wedge pressure, cardiac output) that cannot be obtained from a single CVP line.

Alternate approaches

In some cardiovascular ICUs it is common practice to forego using the pulmonary artery catheter and to insert a single line directly into the left atrium during open-heart surgery, allowing direct monitoring of left-sided heart function. Other ICUs are now using a newer type of fiberoptic pulmonary artery catheter that is able to perform continuous monitoring. These special PA catheters have a fiberoptic tip that "reads" the oxygen content of the mixed venous blood (SVO_2) in the pulmonary artery through spectrophotometry. Systemic oxygen saturation reflects the interplay of cardiac output, oxygen transport, and oxygen consumption. Changes in SVO_2 have been directly correlated with changes in cardiac index. Depending on the cause, a drop in SVO_2 may become apparent before other hemodynamic changes, allowing for faster clinical recognition and intervention. Additionally, because of the continuous monitoring, the direct effect on SVO_2 of such nursing interventions as turning, suctioning, and weighing the patient can easily be identified, and care plans modified accordingly. Because of the high correlation between changes in SVO_2 and changes in arterial oxygen saturation, costly arterial blood gas analyses can be reduced. Causes of decreased SVO_2 include the following:

Anemia
Low cardiac output
Arterial oxygen desaturation
Increased oxygen consumption

Risks of pulmonary artery monitoring

As with intraarterial pressure monitoring, pulmonary artery monitoring is not without risk. Nursing responsibilities are similar to those for arterial catheters, with the addition of continuous waveform observation to detect inadvertent catheter tip migration. Complications of pulmonary artery (Swan-Ganz) monitoring include the following:

Dysrhythmias
Infection
Intracardiac knotting
Thrombophlebitis
Balloon rupture with air embolism
Pulmonary artery rupture
Pulmonary infarction

Intracranial pressure monitoring

Intracranial pressure (ICP) is frequently monitored in critically ill patients who have or are suspected of having intracranial disease or secondary increases in intracranial pressure. A catheter placed through the skull into the subarachnoid or intraventricular space is connected to a fluid filled tube, transducer, and pressure monitor (see Chapter 37). The system is set up similarly to other types of hemodynamic pressure monitoring systems but does not use a continuous flush. The ICP wave is transmitted to the monitor screen and converted to a digital value.

Intracranial pressure monitoring allows continuous observation of the patient's response to therapies aimed at lowering intracranial pressure and immediately shows the patient's tolerance of nursing measures that can cause an unsafe rise in ICP (for example, turning, suctioning, changes in bed position). It also allows aspiration of cerebrospinal fluid for analysis or culturing or to relieve excess intracranial pressure unresponsive to other therapies. Nurses are responsible for obtaining accurate pressure measurements, analyzing trends and patient response to interventions, and preventing complications of monitoring. A scrupulously sterile technique is essential in handling the catheter or screw insertion site and all connections in the monitoring tubing system because of the direct avenue for microorganisms into the cerebrospinal fluid.

The preceding are a few of the invasive monitoring techniques available to the critical care nurse for data collection. In all cases the nurse must be knowledgeable about maintaining these lines, about the normal appearance of the waveform associated with each line, of the usual procedures necessary to prevent complications, and

of the signs and symptoms of actual complications. The risk to the patient from invasive monitoring lines is significantly reduced when knowledgeable personnel handle and care for the lines.

Baseline Assessment

The complete history and physical examination is the necessary foundation for further ongoing data collection in the critical care setting, and the importance of accurate and thorough initial information cannot be overemphasized. The multiple sources of data and the continually fluctuating stability of critically ill patients, however, make the constant reordering of priorities a necessity. The critical care nurse uses continuous observation of the patient to update the data base to be able to reformulate short term goals and interventions.

Patient assessment must be thorough yet rapid. It must take into account the physical and psychologic reactions of an entire organism under stress and not be limited by the usual or the expected. It must also be organized and repetitive so that small alterations or deviations from prior findings are noticed. Finally, it must be individualized so that time and attention can be given to particularly significant aspects of the assessment without losing sight of the whole.

Many intensive care units utilize some form of a systems approach to patient assessment. Frequently this consists of a complete head-to-toe systems review at the beginning of the shift, at which time the nurse gathers an initial data base. More time and depth are spent on the systems that present the greatest real or potential threat to the patient. When complete and documented the baseline systems assessment presents an accurate "status report" on the patient's condition and can be updated and compared with previous data. Throughout the rest of the shift, the nurse charts the progress as the patient's condition improves or deteriorates from the baseline, keeping track of vital parameters on an ongoing flow sheet, such as is seen in Fig. 46-3.

Fig. 46-4 shows the outline of a basic beginning of shift assessment guide, which includes the main items to be assessed under each body system. Routine parameters, individualized observations, and specific problems can be noted. The worksheet forms the outline of a consistent repetitive assessment structure, which, once documented in the patient's record, makes information retrieval much easier.

After patient assessment is completed, nursing diagnoses are established and nursing care plans formulated. Nursing interventions for critically ill patients are based on these care plans.

Throughout this text nursing interventions have been described for care of the patient with a particular type of physiologic impairment. These are interventions intended to improve the patient's physiologic functioning before the impairment reaches the critical stage. In some critically ill patients many of these interventions have already been implemented and are ongoing, yet the patient's physiologic condition has deteriorated to the critical level, necessitating acute life-sustaining interventions. In other patients the initial illness is critical in itself (for example, acu-

CRITICAL CARE FLOWSHEET

Adult/Pediatric Glasgow Coma Scale

Pupil Scale (m.m.)
1 2 3 4 5 6 7 8

			Date																							
			Time	07	08	09	10	11	12	13	14	15	16	17	18	19	20	21	22	23	24	01	02	03	04	05	06

PUPILS
- right: Size / Reaction
- left: Size / Reaction

++ = brisk
+ = sluggish
- = no reaction
C = eye closed by swelling

COMA SCALE

Eyes Open:
- 4 Spontaneously
- 3 To speech
- 2 To pain
- 1 None

Eyes closed by swelling = C

Best Motor Response:
- 6 Obey commands
- 5 Localize pain
- 4 Flexion withdrawal
- 3 Flexion abnormal
- 2 Extension
- 1 None

Usually record the best arm response

Best Response to Auditory/Visual Stimulus:

ADULT / **AGE < 2 YRS.**
- 5 Orientation / Smiles, listens, follows
- 4 Confused / Cries, consolable
- 3 Inappropriate words / Inappropriate, persistent cry
- 2 Incomprehensible words / Agitated, restless
- 1 None / No response
- T = Endotracheal tube or tracheostomy

COMA SCALE TOTALS

LIMB MOVEMENT

+ = Present
- = Absent
NT = Not Tested
0 = No Movement
1 = Trace Movement
2 = Movement, but not against gravity
3 = Movement against gravity, but not against resistance
4 = Movement against gravity and some resistance
5 = Full Power

ARMS:
- Voluntary motor (0-5)
- Pronator drift (+)
- Flexion withdrawal
- Flexion Abnormal
- Extension
- No Response

LEGS:
- Voluntary motor (0-5)
- Flexion
- Extension
- No Response

UCSF
The Medical Center at the University of California, San Francisco
San Francisco, California 94143

CRITICAL CARE FLOWSHEET

Fig. 46-3   Sample critical care flowsheet.

Continued.

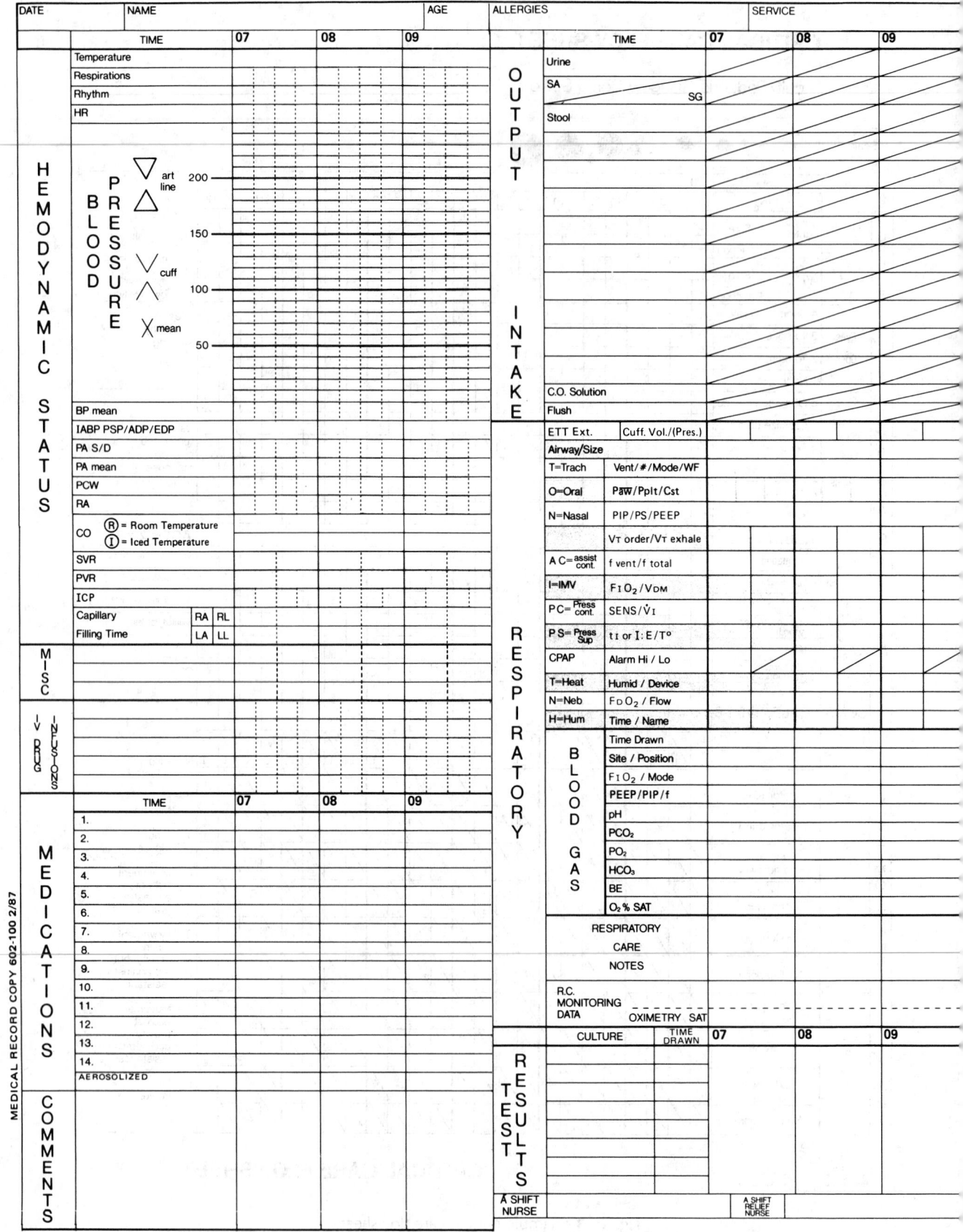

Fig. 46-3, cont'd Sample critical care flowsheet.

CARDIOVASCULAR

Apical HR _____ ECG rhythm _____
BP _____ CVP _____ PAP _____ PCWP __
Pacer: Mode _____ Rate _____ MA _____
Heart sounds: _____
Skin color _____ Temp. _____
Peripheral R: R __ F __ P __ DP __
   pulses   L: R __ F __ P __ DP __
Specifics _____
_____
_____
_____

NEUROLOGIC/PSYCHOLOGIC

LOC _____
Orientation _____
Affect _____
Pupils _____ ICP _____
Motor/sens. _____
Resp. to environment _____
_____
Social/emotional _____
_____
Specifics _____

RESPIRATORY

Rate _____ Quality _____
Breath   R _____
   sounds L _____
FIO$_2$ _____ Source _____
Mech. vent. TV __ Rate __ Mode _____
Chest tube(s) _____
Sputum _____ Cultures _____
Specifics _____

GASTROINTESTINAL

Abdomen _____ Girth _____
Bowel sounds _____
NG _____ Stool _____
Nutrition _____
Incisions/drains/ostomies _____
_____
Specifics _____
_____

FLUIDS/ELECTROLYTES

Last labs done: _____ Time _____
Abnormals: _____
Labs needed _____
   Time _____
IVs infusing (sol., amt., rate, site)
#1 _____
#2 _____
#3 _____
#4 _____
#5 _____

GENITOURINARY

Urine: Amt. _____   Color _____
Appearance _____
S/A _____ S.G. _____ Voids _____
Catheter (type) _____
Skin condition _____
Renal function _____
_____
_____
Specifics _____
_____

INTEGUMENT _____
_____

Fig. 46-4   ICU on-shift assessment worksheet.

myocardial infarction, severe trauma) and critical interventions are necessary immediately to sustain life.

The focus of the remaining three sections of this chapter is on physiologic, psychologic, and social interventions necessary for the individual who is critically ill. Refer to the preceding chapters for an in-depth description of the pathophysiology and nursing interventions involved in individual disease states. The following discussion centers on nursing interventions that are important to or usually found in critical care settings.

INTERVENTIONS FOR THE CRITICALLY ILL PATIENT
Alleviation and Prevention of Physiologic and Physical Stressors

The ultimate goal of nursing intervention for any patient, regardless of the nature of the illness, is to promote, sustain, and restore optimum levels of physiologic, psycho-

logic, and social functioning. However, in a critical care setting the immediate goal of ensuring a patient's survival initially determines the priorities for intervention; physiologic problems must be addressed first. Once life-threatening stressors have been alleviated, priorities are reordered and other problems can be addressed.

Physiologic priorities are determined by the degree of threat to the survival of the individual. Certain body systems are more prone to disorders that require intensive therapeutic interventions, and are frequently encountered in the critical care unit. These disorders are listed by system along with their specific interventions, as well as additional interventions necessary to prevent complications of therapy.

Respiratory system

The highest priority in caring for a critically ill individual is the maintenance of a patent airway and adequate ventilation.

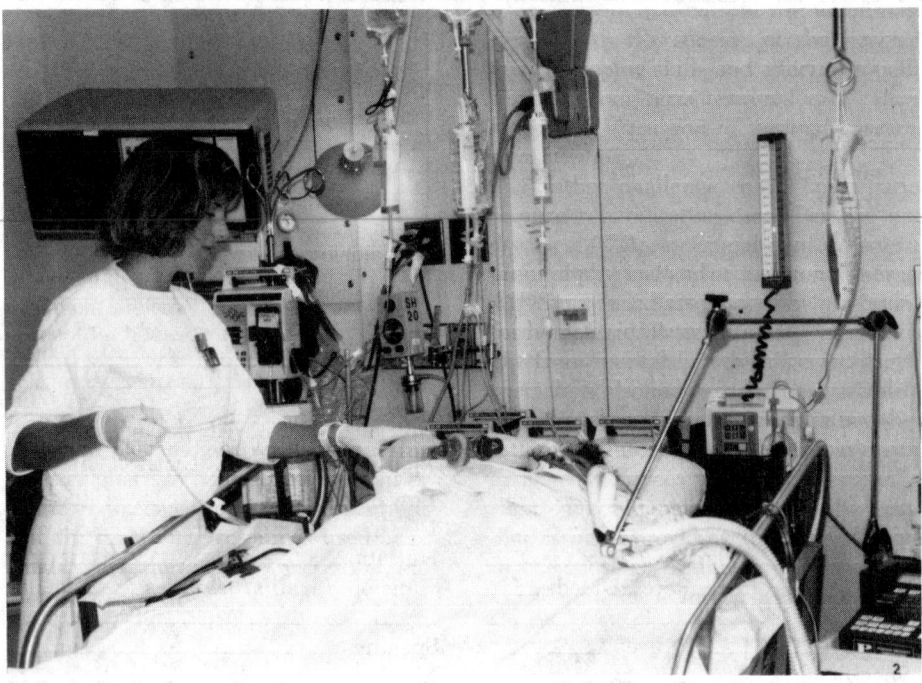

Fig. 46-5 Hand ventilation in a critically ill patient.

Acute respiratory failure

Acute respiratory failure may occur as a primary pulmonary deficit or as a result of a large number of other disorders that can affect the adequacy of ventilation or respiration. Crushing chest injuries, high-level spinal cord injury, neuromuscular diseases, extensive thoracic surgery, end-stage chronic obstructive pulmonary disease, sepsis, severe pneumonia, severe pulmonary edema, pulmonary embolus, congestive heart failure, and shock are just some disorders that may be exhibited by patients in respiratory failure requiring intensive care.

Interventions in respiratory failure are first directed at establishment of an unimpeded airway through endotracheal intubation via the nose or the mouth (see Chapter 24). Assisted ventilation may then be provided by a manual resuscitation device (Ambu or anesthesia bag), followed by continuous mechanical ventilation (Fig. 46-5). Mechanical ventilation devices may be classified by the type of ventilatory support they provide (see Table 46-3).

Patients may require mechanical ventilation for hours, weeks, or months in an acute setting, or may become chronically ventilator-dependent if respiratory failure is irreversible (such as with neuromuscular disease or high spinal cord injury). A tracheostomy is usually performed as soon as the need for permanent support is identified, or when short-term support exceeds 2 to 4 weeks. Mechanical ventilatory support mandates observation of the proper functioning of the equipment, assessment of the effect of the support on the patient's clinical status, and development of alternate communication methods with the patient. When respiratory failure is severe, the patient may require respiratory muscle paralysis with an agent such as pancuronium bromide (Pavulon) to allow for maximum respiratory control. The patient is sedated and otherwise emotionally supported through the terrifying experience of being awake and paralyzed.

Two methods of tracking the systemic effect of the patient's ventilatory status are common in ICUs. Arterial blood gas samples, drawn by direct arterial puncture or via an indwelling arterial line, are analyzed to reveal the patient's arterial pH, P_{CO_2} and O_2 saturation. A noninvasive transcutaneous oximeter (to measure oxygen saturation) or airway capnograph (to measure exhaled carbon dioxide) are also frequently used, and provide differential information on the effectiveness of both oxygenation and ventilation. Pulse oximetry (see Chapter 22) uses transcutaneous plethysmography to analyze the gas concentration in superficial capillary blood. Both direct and indirect methods are frequently used together. Once a relationship is established between the two methods, the risks and high cost of direct sampling can be minimized. Direct arterial sampling would then be indicated when there was an observed change in the surface saturation reading. Changes in mechanical ventilation therapy are usually based on the results of direct arterial sampling.

Mechanical ventilation is a complex therapy and poses major risks for the critically ill patient, including pneumothorax, atelectasis, decreased cardiac output (especially if positive-end expiratory pressure is used), gastrointestinal bleeding from a stress ulcer, and infection. Preventive interventions for the patient receiving mechanical ventilation include frequent assessment, position changes in bed, suctioning to remove secretions, intermittent deep ventilation (bagging or sighing), administration of H_2 antagonists such as cimetidine, administration of sucralfate or antacids via nasogastric or gastrostomy tube, and scrupulous sterile technique in airway management to prevent a respiratory tract infection.

Table 46-3   Types of mechanical ventilation

Type	Comments
Mode variations	
Control mode ventilation (CMV)	Preset tidal volume and preset respiratory rate; not sensitive to patient respiratory effort
	Patient may require paralysis/sedation for control
Assist/control (A/C) ventilation	Preset volume and rate; machine sensitive to patient inspiratory effort; delivers preset tidal volume to patient-initiated breaths
Intermittent mandatory ventilation (IMV)	Preset volume and preset rate for machine breaths; patient breathes spontaneously between machine breaths at own tidal volume; tidal volume stacking can occur
Synchronized intermittent mandatory ventilation (SIMV)	Preset volume and preset rate for machine breaths; patient breathes spontaneously between machine breaths at own volume; patient breaths are synchronized not to compete with machine
Frequency variations	
High-frequency jet ventilation	Jet of gas injected into airway via ET tube; low volume, very high rate (100-140 jets/min)
	Delivers large minute volume without air trapping; indicated in bronchopleural fistula
High-frequency oscillation	Delivers oscillating column of gas within ET; piston pump determines frequency and tidal volume; reduces peak and mean airway pressure; difficult to auscultate breath sounds
Pattern variations	
Inverse-ratio ventilation	Provides increased inspiratory to expiratory time of 2:1 or greater; promotes alveolar stabilization and prevents collapse; useful in severe ARDS unresponsive to high PEEP; very uncomfortable; may require paralysis/sedation
Independent lung ventilation	Allows separate ventilation of each lung via double-lumen endobronchial tube; may be synchronous or asynchronous; indicated in unilateral lung pathology; correct patient positioning is very important
Negative-pressure ventilation	Stimulates ventilation by causing external changes in intrathoracic pressure; indicated in severe muscular disease or nerve impairment; types include chest cuirass, chest shell, pneumobelt, phrenic nerve stimulator; most frequently used outside the critical care unit for long-term support

Adult respiratory distress syndrome

A particularly threatening respiratory complication that is prone to develop in critically ill patients is adult respiratory distress syndrome (ARDS). Also known as shock lung, wet lung, or post-pump lung, the predisposing factors for ARDS include a number of disorders seen in the critically ill: shock, trauma, disseminated intravascular coagulation (DIC), fat embolism, cardiopulmonary bypass, sepsis, cardiac arrest, and multiple blood transfusions. Damage to the alveolar-capillary membrane and increased capillary permeability leads to pulmonary edema and diffuse microatelectasis. ARDS is characterized by severe dyspnea, hypoxemia, diminished lung compliance, and a significant ventilation-perfusion defect.

The primary intervention for ARDS is mechanical ventilation with the addition of positive-end expiratory pressure (PEEP). PEEP aids in reexpanding alveoli and preventing further alveolar collapse, thus improving oxygen transport. Nursing interventions for the patient with ARDS are the same as those for any patient with respiratory failure who is receiving mechanical ventilation, and require a very high degree of skill. (See Chapter 24 for further discussion of respiratory failure, ARDS, and PEEP.)

Cardiovascular system

Cardiovascular problems requiring intensive patient care are so frequently encountered that many institutions have specific ICUs designed for the care of these patients (coronary care unit, postoperative cardiovascular unit). After support of ventilation, maintenance of cardiac function and systemic circulation is the highest priority in life-threatening situations. Disorders of the cardiovascular system that frequently require intensive observation and intervention include acute myocardial infarction, cardiogenic shock, congestive heart failure, open-heart surgery, cardiac transplantation, and major vascular surgery.

Drug therapy

The first line of intervention in severe cardiovascular disorders frequently is *drug therapy* aimed at improving cardiac function until more definitive measures can be instituted. Cardioactive and vasoactive drugs most often administered in a critical care setting are listed in Table 46-4. These highly potent medications often have a very small margin between therapeutic doses and toxic levels. The medications are often ordered in dose ranges that allow the critical care nurse to titrate the amount of drug delivered to create a specific patient response. The critical care nurse must monitor the patient's reaction and administer the amount of drug that, in conjunction with other drugs, fluid, and mechanical therapies, combines to create an optimal patient response.

In addition, the nurse is often responsible for obtaining trough and peak blood samples before and after drug administration, thus tracking the drug's trough and peak levels. The purpose is to maximize the therapeutic response with the minimum necessary dose. This is commonly done with digoxin and certain antiarrhythmics, as well as with many antibiotics.

Table 46-4 Intravenously administered cardiac and vasoactive drugs commonly used in ICU

Drug	Method	Clinical use
Cardiac stimulants		
Atropine sulfate	IV push (diluted or undiluted in 10 ml sterile water)	Symptomatic bradydysrhythmias
Calcium chloride	IV push	Cardiac arrest, systemic hypocalcemia
Digoxin (Lanoxin)	IV push	Congestive heart failure, atrial fibrillation, paroxysmal atrial tachycardia
Dobutamine HCL (Dobutrex)	Diluted in infusion	Low cardiac output states, cardiogenic shock
Epinephrine HCL (Adrenalin)	IV bolus; intracardiac, intratracheal, IV infusion	Asystole, ventricular fibrillation, shock/hypotension, anaphylactic reactions
Antiarrhythmic agents		
Amiodarone HCL (Cordarone)	IV bolus, IV infusion	Ventricular and supraventricular dysrhythmias; atrial flutter and fibrillation
Bretylium tosylate (Bretylol)	IV push, undiluted; may be followed by infusion	Ventricular fibrillation, ventricular tachycardia unresponsive to other agents such as lidocaine
Lidocaine HCL (Xylocaine)	IV bolus followed by IV infusion	To suppress ventricular dysrhythmias or resistant seizure activity (low dose)
Propranolol (Inderal)	IV bolus	Supraventricular and ventricular tachydysrhythmias, angina pectoris
Verapamil (Calan, Isoptin)	IV push	Paroxysmal supraventricular tachycardia
Vasoactive agents		
Dopamine HCL (Intropin)	Diluted in infusion	Shock, hypotension (high dose); improve renal perfusion (low dose)
Isoproterenol HCL (Isuprel)	IV infusion	Heart block, bradydysrhythmias, asystole, shock/hypotension
Morphine sulfate	IV bolus, IV infusion	Pulmonary edema, congestive heart failure, pain management
Nitroglycerine (Nitro-Bid IV)	IV infusion	Hypertensive crisis, congestive heart failure associated with acute myocardial infarction, angina pectoris
Nitroprusside sodium (Nipride)	IV infusion	Hypertensive crisis, congestive heart failure
Norepinephrine (Levophed)	IV infusion	Hypotension, shock
Thrombolytic agents		
Streptokinase, tissue plasminogen activator (TPA)	IV bolus, IV infusion	Pulmonary embolus, immediate therapy for coronary artery thrombosis in myocardial infarction

Reducing myocardial work load

If medication dosage is insufficient to improve the patient's condition significantly, certain *invasive techniques* may be of some benefit. Temporary transvenous pacing of the heart may restore or enhance cardiac function until such time as a permanent pacemaker can be implanted. Intraaortic balloon counterpulsation (IABC) may be necessary for the patient who would benefit from temporary assistance in decreasing the work load on the myocardium (see Box 46-4). A balloon-tipped catheter is threaded into the aorta from a femoral artery; the balloon inflates during ventricular diastole to increase coronary artery filling and deflates just before ventricular systole to decrease afterload and improve left ventricular ejection. Care of the patient with IABC includes critical minute-to-minute assessment of the patient's physiologic response to IABC therapy and intervention to prevent complications (see Chapter 25).

Another advanced technique of myocardial support is the ventricular assist device (VAD). A relatively uncommon therapy, it is reserved for patients with severe left, right, or biventricular failure. It may be used to assist postoperative patients who cannot be weaned from cardiopulmonary bypass. VAD is also used as a temporary support for end-stage patients awaiting cardiac transplantation. The technique involves implanting catheters into the atrium or ventricle to divert blood away from the ventricles into a roller pump located outside the body. The pump returns the blood directly to the aorta, thus bypassing the mitral or aortic valve and reducing the work load on the heart.

Prevention of physiologic stressors to the cardiovascular system is a continual priority of care for all ICU patients. Most preventive measures are aimed at myocardial work load reduction (see Box 46-5).

Prevention of electrical microshock

Finally, in addition to decreasing myocardial work load the myocardium must also be protected from a particular

46-4

Indications and complications of IABC therapy

Indications

Cardiogenic shock with a reversible component
Low cardiac output states
Assist in removing patient from cardiopulmonary bypass
Unstable angina
Acute myocardial infarction
Drug-resistant lethal dysrhythmias with ischemic cause

Complications

Ischemia of catheterized leg
Thrombus formation with eventual embolization
Infection
Aortic damage (aortic wall dissection, intimal laceration)
Balloon rupture with gas embolus (rare)

46-5

Nursing measures to reduce myocardial work load

Enhance oxygenation	Supplemental oxygen, pulmonary hygiene Assisted ventilation
Decrease physical exertion	Bedrest Passive range of motion exercises
Decrease sympathetic stimulation	Reduced environmental stimuli (noise, light) Rest periods Information and reassurance to patient and family

46-6

Nursing interventions to prevent increased ICP in critically ill patients

Maintain patent airway
Minimize arterial blood gas changes
Oxygenate patient before and after suctioning
Limit suctioning to 15 seconds
Elevate head of bed 30° (facilitates venous drainage without impeding arterial supply)
Maintain head and neck in straight alignment
Prevent overly tight tracheostomy ties
Prevent Valsalva maneuver
Assist patient in turning
Prevent coughing, sneezing, constipation
Monitor hydration status, intake and output

hazard of the critical care environment, electrical microshock. The invasive monitoring and therapeutic interventions used in critically ill patients often create a direct pathway to the heart. Direct contact with stray or leaked current could prove fatal, particularly in critically ill patients whose resistance may be further decreased by other breaks in skin integrity and through electrolyte imbalances. Nursing staff in critical care areas are responsible for the safe and proper use of electrical equipment as well as for the implementation of appropriate electrical safety precautions.

Neurologic system

Some neurologic disorders that may require intensive care during an acute phase of illness include the following:

1. Trauma: subdural or subarachnoid hemorrhage, cranial injuries
2. Intracranial neoplasms
3. Intracranial vascular anomalies: massive CVA, intracranial aneurysm rupture
4. Neuromuscular diseases that cause respiratory compromise: Guillain-Barré syndrome, myasthenia gravis

Specialized neurologic interventions for critically ill patients are aimed at maintaining a homeokinetic state of brain metabolism and controlling elevations in intracranial pressure (see Box 46-6). Intracranial monitoring (p. 1570) may be used to assess the extent of potentially dangerous rises in ICP. Meticulous insertion site and tubing care are essential to prevent the devastating complication of intracranial infection. Continuous observation by the critical care nurse is aimed at maintaining patency of the system and detecting changes in ICP.

Removal of cerebrospinal fluid is one method of controlling rising ICP. Other interventions include osmotic diuresis (IV mannitol) to remove excess brain tissue water and mechanical hyperventilation to artificially reduce circulating carbon dioxide (CO_2) levels. Lowered CO_2 levels

cause cerebral vasoconstriction, reducing the potential for progressive interstitial cerebral edema.

Efforts to lower the overall metabolism of the brain reduce the brain's requirements for its natural substrates, oxygen and glucose. This is especially important when transport of these elements is impaired. Interventions to reduce brain metabolism include generalized hypothermia via a cooling mattress and induction of barbiturate coma. Caring for the artificially comatose patient requires the same attentive observations and extensive nursing interventions to prevent complications as are used in the naturally comatose patient, with the addition of mechanical ventilation (see Chapter 37). In addition, complete neurologic assessment must be thoroughly performed at those times when sedation is withdrawn to evaluate patient progress. A lightened level of consciousness at those times necessitates sensitive communication with the patient, even though the ability to comprehend may not be apparent.

Renal system

Acute renal failure in the critically ill patient may result from a primary intrarenal cause, such as acute glomeru-

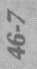

46-7

Comparison of hemodialysis, peritoneal dialysis, and CAVH

Hemodialysis

Rapid, efficient correction of severe serum abnormalities
Short time required
Expensive
Requires highly technical equipment
Poorly tolerated by hemodynamically unstable patients
Risk of hemorrhage

Peritoneal dialysis

Well-tolerated even by very unstable patients
Inexpensive
Technologically simple
Must be performed over several hours or days
Cannot be performed after recent abdominal trauma or surgery
Risk of peritonitis

CAVH

Effective clearance of excess free water
Very well tolerated
Technologically simple to fairly complex
Retains most nutrients and protein-bound medications
Expense depends on filter complexity
Must be performed over several hours or days
Less effective clearance of nitrogen and creatinine
Filtration rate depends on blood pressure and tubing size and height

lonephritis or acute cortical necrosis, or from a structural defect (see Chapter 33). It may be the result of directly nephrotoxic agents such as heavy metal poisoning or pharmacologic agents (for example, aminoglycoside antibiotics). But most commonly, acute renal failure in critically ill patients is the secondary result of any disorder that severely reduces cardiac output and renal perfusion, including cardiac arrest, left ventricular failure, or hemorrhage.

Interventions for the patient with renal failure are intended to provide the regulatory functions the kidneys can no longer maintain. The nurse keeps accurate daily weight and intake/output records so that only the exact amounts of body fluids lost plus a percentage for insensible loss, are replaced. Laboratory values are monitored carefully, with electrolyte intake limited and pharmacologic means of electrolyte removal utilized as necessary, for example, sodium polystyrene sulfonate (Kayexalate). Diuretics are given to increase marginal renal function. Low-dose dopamine hydrochloride may be given intravenously (2 to 4 mcg/kg/min) to enhance renal perfusion and thereby increase urine output. Nutrition is altered through restricted protein intake, because the body cannot appropriately excrete the nitrogen that is produced by amino acid breakdown. The nurse evaluates acid-base balance, anticipating metabolic acidosis from the buildup of acid metabolic wastes (carbonic and lactic acids). All other body systems are affected by the progression of acute renal failure, and continuous interventions are necessary to prevent altered acid-base and electrolyte levels from impairing cardiovascular, respiratory, and neurologic function. Therefore the nurse is alert for such things as ECG changes indicative of increased myocardial irritability and altered contractility, changes in ventilatory pattern such as Kussmaul breathing and acidotic breath, and decreased level of consciousness, altered mentation, or unusual behavior.

As renal failure progresses, an early problem is significant fluid retention. An intervention that may be useful before dialysis is needed is continuous arteriovenous hemofiltration (CAVH). In CAVH a large artery and vein are cannulated, typically at the femoral site. Tubing primed with heparinized saline allows arterial-to-venous blood flow through a highly permeable hollow-filter fiber. The fiber separates plasma water and certain solutes from the blood, passing the ultrafiltrate into a collection bag while the blood returns to the patient. CAVH is a continuous process that uses the patient's blood pressure as the driving force; it is well tolerated even by unstable patients.

When renal failure has reached a level unresponsive to medical intervention, dialysis becomes necessary to mechanically remove the waste products of body metabolism. Hemodialysis, peritoneal dialysis, or CAVH may be initiated in the critically ill patient (see Box 46-7).

Gastrointestinal system

The most common gastrointestinal problem seen in the critical care setting is *acute gastrointestinal bleeding*. This may be the chief complaint of a newly admitted patient, or it may be a complication, such as a stress ulcer, in an already critically ill person. Interventions, such as gastric lavage with saline solution and administration of epinephrine and antacid agents, are intended to control bleeding until its cause and extent are determined. A Sengstaken-Blakemore tube may be used to provide direct compression of esophageal varices to tamponade a serious bleed (see Chapter 30). Administration of blood components and crystalloid fluids is initiated to reverse the hypovolemia of acute hemorrhage. Vasopressor medications cannot be administered to raise systemic blood pressure until the hypovolemic state is corrected. Once the patient's condition has stabilized sufficiently, endoscopic examination to determine the site of bleeding may be performed in the ICU. If indicated, surgical repair may follow.

The primary function of the gastrointestinal system is ingestion and digestion of liquid and solid nutrients. For many critically ill patients this process is interrupted for a long period, during which either enteral or total parenteral nutrition (TPN) may be substituted. TPN solutions contain the essential protein, carbohydrates, and fat necessary to establish a catabolic state in which positive nitrogen balance is maintained. The critical care nurse assesses the adequacy of hydration, albumin level, electrolyte balance, and caloric intake. In addition, the nurse takes active measures to prevent the primary complication of TPN, infection.

Prevention of gastrointestinal complications such as stress ulcers in critically ill patients requires active interventions. Patients at highest risk include those who are receiving no food orally, are receiving mechanical ventilation, have liver dysfunction, are receiving anticoagulants, and have undergone any severe physiologic stress. In addition to the administration of local antacids, sucralfate, and H₂ receptor antagonists (cimetidine), active interventions are required to reduce the psychologic stress inherent in the critical care environment.

Musculoskeletal integumentary system

Although few primary musculoskeletal problems necessitate intensive care, the majority of critically ill patients have severe restrictions placed on their mobility. Unstable hemodynamics, decreased blood flow, bedrest, weakness, and pain, as well as numerous therapeutic and monitoring devices, significantly limit normal motion. Preserving function of weight-bearing muscles, maintaining joint mobility, and preserving continuous skin integrity are significant challenges to critical care nurses. All of the preventive and supportive nursing care techniques used in any patient with restricted mobility are appropriate in the ICU, including aggressive interventions to prevent skin breakdown with reduced-pressure beds (such as bead, air suspension, kinetic). Progress of the ICU patient to the highest level of activity within physiologic capabilities both facilitates continued improvement in physiologic function and visually reassures the patient of an improving condition.

One of the most serious potential complications of immobility is development of deep-vein thrombus, which can embolize and travel to the lungs. *Pulmonary emboli* are found at autopsy in up to 60% of all individuals. Signs and symptoms of pulmonary embolism include dyspnea, pleuritic chest pain, fever, hemoptysis, tachycardia, and pleural friction rub. Preventive interventions can be instrumental in reducing the risk of serious complications (see Box 46-8).

In the past decade the tremendous advances in treating immunocompromised patients has been matched only by the growth of therapeutic interventions that cause secondary immunosuppression. The number of critically ill patients who are compromised hosts increases daily, and routinely includes oncology, hematology, and organ transplant patients. Immunosuppression may be primary (severe combined immunodeficiency disorder), acquired (AIDS), autoimmune (Guillain-Barré, systemic lupus erythematosus), or induced by therapy for a particular disease state (leukemia, solid-tissue tumors, bone marrow or organ transplantation).

In many cases the immunosuppressed patient presents to the ICU in sepsis with accompanying hemodynamic instability and respiratory failure. Nursing interventions are directed at treating the shock state, supporting ventilation, and preventing further infection by scrupulous attention to isolation protocol.

Organ transplantation is an area in which critical care nurses can play a major role in helping turn one family's tragedy into another family's hope. The use of organ transplantation has increased in recent years. Both donors and recipients may receive care in critical care units, and nursing interventions include both exquisite physiologic and psychologic support. (See Chapter 42 for a thorough discussion of organ transplantation.)

	Nursing interventions for prevention of pulmonary embolus
46-8	Elevation of lower extremities Use of antiembolism stockings Hourly active foot dorsiflexion Active/resistive range of motion exercises Observation for Homan's sign Coughing and deep-breathing exercises Administration of low-dose heparin as ordered Inspection of intravenous sites with routine needle changes Use of pneumatic compression devices for lower extremities

Alleviation and Prevention of Psychologic Stressors

Despite the continous attention that the critical care nurse must devote to the assessment of and intervention in physiologic derangements, the nurse must also focus attention on recognizing the psychologic stressors that confront the patient and family. The emotional discomfort and distress that the patient and family must endure will not only affect psychologic health but will have a direct effect on physical recovery as well.

The initial step in preventing or alleviating psychologic stress is to identify the patient's and family's perception of the critical event. Their perceptions will be affected by their individual personalities, cultural heritage, educational level, previous exposure to similar events, either positive or negative, and general level of familiarity with medical interventions and the hospital environment. Following are five specific interventions that nurses in any setting can implement to reduce the psychologic stress of illness on the family.

Acknowledge, accept, and encourage patient and family to air feelings

Because the critically ill person is alienated from familiar surroundings and daily living patterns and depends on others to meet the most basic needs of survival, the patient becomes partially or totally isolated from usual support systems. Feelings of helplessness, powerlessness, loneliness, and depersonalization as well as disturbances in body image are common. Modes of expressing and therefore relieving the frustration, anger, hostility, fear, and depression generated by these feelings are limited by the physical constraints of the critical care environment.

Maintaining an atmosphere of openness and acceptance that encourages expression of feelings can help to provide patients with a means of coping. Talking with patients openly and honestly decreases feelings of depersonalization and anxiety and prevents isolation and alienation. Recognizing that anger and hostility are often indicative of fear, and that depression and withdrawal may mask feelings of hopelessness, loneliness, powerlessness, or loss assist the nurse in accepting these feelings as normal and expected in this situation. Encouraging expression of feelings helps patients identify reasons for feeling or behaving in a way that may seem strange or wrong to them. At the same time it provides protection and permission to feel and act that way. Nurses or other health team members who are helping a patient to talk about feelings must be ready to accept whatever emotionally laden information might be expressed. Nonjudgmental recognition and acceptance of the patient's feelings will help to reinforce the patient's right to the feelings.

Patients who are intubated are unable to freely express their feelings even when alert and oriented, and therefore are particularly vulnerable to psychologic stressors. It is a natural tendency to communicate less with those who cannot talk easily, and the nurse must guard against this. Keeping paper and pencil, a picture board, or a "magic slate" within the patient's reach and providing assistance when necessary will help to reduce the sense of isolation. However, such methods are not convenient for the expression of personal feelings or concerns. The nurse can recognize clues to the patient's emotional state by appearance and behavior and by knowing the types of concerns the patient is most likely to experience. The nurse can verbalize some potential concerns, allowing the patient to validate them as appropriate. Being empathetic with the patient and family conveys acceptance and understanding.

Provide information about physical status, goals of treatment, and interventions

Because it is the patient's *perception* of stress and not the stressor itself that determines the patient's reaction to the illness and the environment, it is essential that the patient and family receive adequate information and simple explanations. Without explanations the critical care environment presents a mysterious and threatening array of noxious stimuli, which may be perceived as extremely unnatural and even magical. The high degree of technical sophistication increases the patient's feelings of vulnerability, and the patient may worry that the cardiac monitor is actually keeping the heart beating, that a blood transfusion indicates hemorrhaging, or that chest physiotherapy indicates pneumonia. A very common misconception of patients after coronary artery bypass is that "open heart" surgery involved cutting the heart wide open and sewing it back together again. Such a perception can lead to a drastic alteration in body image.

Much of what patients learn about their health problems depends on what is taught, both directly and indirectly, by the health care team. Patient teaching in critical care requires establishment of short-term goals. Pain, discomfort, weakness, anxiety, and transient confusion are some of the obstacles to learning that these patients experience. Despite these obstacles, patients and families need simple, repetitive explanations of all procedures and the purpose of each intervention, as well as an introduction to rehabilitation plans and health maintenance strategies. Patients may not understand or believe what they are told the first time, or anxiety and denial may prevent recollection of it. Reinterpretation and reiteration of diagnosis, prognosis, goals of treatment, types of intervention, and expectations of the patient and family may be continually necessary during the entire ICU stay. Keeping the patient and family apprised of the patient's current status as well as of changes in plans helps them to perceive the situation accurately and plan for the future realistically, and promotes cooperation by making them members of the health team.

Encourage and support patient/family involvement in decision making and care

The essence of crisis intervention is to help individuals cope with a major life crisis such as a critical illness might precipitate. Critical care nursing in itself is far broader in scope and more future oriented than crisis intervention alone, but specific situations within the critical care setting may require the immediacy and limited locus of crisis intervention. At that time the patient and family are directed in establishing short-term goals and are given limited choice in acceptable responses. As the crisis situation stabilizes, even though it may be no less critical, the patient and family are given additional information and further responsibility in establishing mutual goals and choosing alternative responses. When the patient and family are knowledgeable about the goals of therapy and understand the patient's diagnosis, current status, and prognosis, they can be involved in many aspects of care planning and can make decisions consistent with the treatment regimen.

Involvement of the individuals who represent the patient's significant support system decreases their feelings of powerlessness, frustration, and anxiety. In addition, when these emotionally important figures, whether family or friends, understand and support the treatment goals and are involved in the patient's care, they are better able to sustain and expand this behavior after the patient leaves the ICU and the hospital. Even when a patient is unconscious, visits by key support figures who talk to and touch the patient may have positive, if unmeasurable, effects and help to decrease the family's feelings of helplessness.

An alert patient can be directly involved in establishing goals of treatment and care planning. One specific mechanism to increase the patient's feeling of personal control is to encourage involvement in structuring the daily schedule of activities. The knowledge that patient preferences are important to the nursing staff and that the person is viewed as capable of making decisions will support self-esteem and reinforce the centrality of the patient's role in recovery.

Promote and maintain a sensory-regulated environment

The environment of the critical care unit is a major stressor with which both the patient and family must cope. (The many sources of external stress are outlined in the first section of this chapter.) In addition, disturbed thought processes and perceptual distortions are often likely to occur in patients receiving narcotics and sedatives, highly anxious patients, patients with multiple interrelated debilitating physical problems, patients with disturbed metabolic and respiratory function, patients deprived of sleep, and older patients. Reality reinforcement on a continuing basis is necessary for these individuals. Although some environmental factors cannot be altered, there are some specific interventions that the nurse can implement to provide a sensory-regulated environment (see Box 46-9).

Prepare the patient and family for transfer from the ICU

Transfer from the critical care unit can represent a significant stress for some patients and their families. The critical care area with its sophisticated electronic equipment and attentive, highly-skilled staff represents security and protection. Patients know that transfer will be to an area where there are fewer nursing personnel per patient, less direct contact with nursing personnel, few automatic monitoring devices, and no direct observation of the bed from the nurses' station. Greater independence and higher patient levels of activity will be expected on the transfer unit, yet the patient will lose the support of the nursing staff who have come to know both patient and family. Patients may have conflicting feelings about the transfer as an indicator of physical improvement if they do not feel as well or as independent as they anticipated they would by transfer time.

The anxiety precipitated by the transfer can be prevented or reduced if the patient and family are taught to interpret particular signs and symptoms and are helped to understand the true purpose of equipment and routines. Signs that indicate progress need to be pointed out continuously, beginning when they first appear. Initiating the discussion of transfer plans with the patient and family as soon as the patient's condition begins to stabilize in the ICU will help them adjust to the idea and prepare for this eventuality. Transfer out of an ICU will frequently occur within several hours to one day after endotracheal extubation.

Along with the projected time of transfer, the patient and family need to know what to expect on the new unit and what will be expected of them. Ideally, a nurse from the receiving unit should meet the patient and family before transfer, especially for patients whose ICU stay has been long and whose remaining hospitalization is expected to be long or challenging. After transfer, visits from members of the ICU staff are helpful in conveying continued concern for the patient's welfare and in providing objective validation of continued progress. With careful planning and execution, transfer from the critical care unit can be a triumphant rather than a traumatic event.

Alleviation and Prevention of Social Stressors

In the critical care setting the patient's physiologic needs often assume priority over psychologic needs, and the patient as a social being may be at risk of being ignored. Limited visiting hours, the strange technical environment, and the aura of danger in the ICU isolate patients from their supportive family and friends and prevent them from assuming their usual social roles. For the most part, a person who is critically ill is narrowly viewed by staff primarily as a patient. The more enduring roles of spouse, parent, child, lover, sibling, friend, or provider may go virtually unrecognized unless nursing staff initiate interventions to provide continuity in these relationships.

Such continuity is fostered through some of the same types of interventions that were used to reduce psychologic stress: increased visiting between patient and family; inclusion of family in discussions of disease process, prog-

---

46-9

Interventions to minimize sensory deprivation/overload

Reduce noise level

Avoid excessive conversation
Avoid raising voice to talk to persons outside conversational range
Use carpeting where feasible
Avoid droning of continuous radio or TV; turn on or off at appropriate intervals
Locate nursing lounge away from patient care area

Maintain day/night orientation

Dim lights at night
Raise/lower shades or open/close window curtains in normal day/night pattern
Reinforce progression of day in relation to specific events, such as meals

Maintain time orientation

Position large-numeral clocks in easy view
Provide wall calendars
Allow wristwatches for certain patients
Provide frequent reorientation to person, place, time

Promote rest and sleep

Schedule most exerting activities before rest period
Coordinate health team activities to provide periods of uninterrupted sleep
Minimize routine cleaning or stocking at night

Provide positive tactile stimuli

Touch or hold patient's hand during conversation
Use soothing physical contact as able (backrubs, face cleansings)
Encourage family to touch patient and hold hands despite dressings

Maintain personal/social integrity

Address patient by name, identify self by name
Provide full and complete information, explanations, and instructions
Avoid discussion over the patient; include the patient in rounds
Encourage visits by family and significant others
Allow important personal belongings at bedside

Reduce pain and discomfort

Administer analgesics appropriately to relieve pain
Reposition immobile patients every 2 hours
Prepare patients for all potentially uncomfortable or painful procedures

Maintain future orientation

Discuss transfer plans early with both patient and family
Initiate teaching regarding rehabilitation and health maintenance strategies as appropriate

nosis, and care plans, and reporting by family of events and activities occurring in the other significant spheres of the patient's life. Relaying telephone messages between the patient and distant friends is one way of maintaining contact with the patient's external world.

Visiting restrictions in critical care units are well known. Originally designed to maximize a patient's rest and minimize outside stressors, they have long been criticized as mechanisms to support nurses' protectiveness of "their" patients and reinforce nurses' reluctance to be observed while providing direct care. Numerous surveys and studies have documented current visiting practices and examined their effects on patient, family, and nurse. The continuing trend is toward more open, flexible visiting hours, which also support unique family needs and constraints. Allowing visits by only immediate family members is also losing support in favor of identifying and encouraging those visitors whom the patient identifies as important, regardless of relationship.

One of the most effective and important ways to prevent disruption in relationships is to prepare the family or friends for their first visit with the patient in the ICU. The patient's physical appearance and the critical care environment should be explained thoroughly before the visitor enters. Visitors need to understand the patient's level of consciousness, ability to communicate, and ability to comprehend communication. They need to be made aware of the importance of their presence to the patient and the patient's need for their support. When the visitor approaches the bedside a staff member should remain with them to facilitate the initial interaction with the patient. At each subsequent visit the nurse caring for the patient meets with the significant others to answer questions and apprise them of the patient's progress.

In addition to supporting the maintenance of the patient's current roles and relationships the critical care nurse must also recognize the inevitability of actual role change for some patients and families during a critical illness. Roles of provider, decision maker, or employer/employee may be altered, reversed, or eliminated. At this point some of the responsibilities of the patient need to be assumed by family and friends.

During the critical phase of illness the family members will be attempting to cope with precipitous role changes and may need assistance in working through problems that arise as family members and friends assume or fail to assume these additional responsibilities. The nurse needs to be aware of how problematic this time is and may need to help the family in requesting professional guidance, such as from a social worker, in assisting the family to reorganize themselves and their resources. The nurse may help the family appoint a temporary leader from among their ranks, one who could be requested to identify the wishes of the family as a whole and who could be contacted in the event of an emergency. The nurse may also help the family to plan visiting schedules that will meet the patient's needs without preventing the family members from maintaining their own responsibilities. It is a period of great emotional stress for both patient and family.

That emotional stress may eventually climax in the death of the critically ill patient. (The reader is referred to Chapter 15 for a complete discussion of dying and death.) The following are some suggestions for the critical care nurse caring for a dying patient:

1. Examine your own feelings about death.
2. Listen to assess the needs of the patient and family.
3. Remain available; be physically and emotionally present.
4. Help with administrative needs such as making telephone calls, obtaining release forms.
5. Provide reassurance of the patient's continued care, even if the patient is not to be resuscitated. Provide information.
6. Respect the person-family relationship, which existed long before the patient-hospital relationship.
7. Attempt to remain nonjudgmental about family or hospital issues.
8. Include the family in care.
9. Provide for patient and family privacy.
10. Provide the opportunity for the family to exercise religious or cultural traditions.
11. Use touch in caring for the patient and family.

The critical care environment is a dynamic milieu intended to maximize the application of critical interventions for the very ill. Knowledgeable nursing care is required to safeguard the patient from its potential hazards while promoting optimum patient outcomes.

SUMMARY

1. The physical layout of an ICU allows for direct observation of all patients at all times, yet provides for as much privacy as possible.
2. ICUs are stressful environments for the patient, family, and nurse. The patient and family are exposed to sensory overload by constant activity and complex equipment, and experience anxieties and fears related to life-threatening situations.
3. The ICU nurse must have a sound knowledge base, astute observational and physical assessment skills, and excellent technical and communication skills.
4. The assessment process for the critically ill patient differs from management of other patients only in terms of the number of supportive devices available to assist in data collection.
5. Common types of monitored data in an ICU include cardiac monitoring, hemodynamic monitoring (intraarterial, pulmonary artery), and intracranial pressure monitoring.
6. The highest priority in caring for a critically ill person is the maintenance of a patent airway and adequate ventilation, followed by maintenance of cardiac function and systemic circulation.
7. Adult respiratory distress syndrome is prone to develop in critically ill patients; maintenance of respiration often requires mechanical ventilation devices.
8. Cardiovascular intervention includes drug therapy to improve cardiac function, measures to reduce myocardial work load, and prevention of electrical microshock. Intraaortic balloon counterpulsation (IABC) or a ventricular assist device (VAD) may be needed to reduce myocardial work load.

9. Neurologic interventions for the critically ill patient include preventing increased ICP and maintaining a homeokinetic state of brain metabolism.

10. Other types of major physical interventions relate to disturbances of kidney function, gastrointestinal bleeding, immunosuppression, and problems of immobility (especially threat of pulmonary embolism).

11. Nursing care of the patient in an ICU must include interventions to alleviate and prevent psychologic stressors; it is sometimes difficult to remember this important aspect of care when so much attention must be paid to monitoring and physical interventions.

12. Interventions to relieve psychologic stressors include providing patients and families with opportunities to express feelings, providing necessary information, supporting decision making, maintaining a sensory-regulated environment, and preparing the patient and family for transfer from the ICU.

13. Interventions to alleviate and prevent social stressors for the patient and family include promoting patient/family relationships and decision making, preparing and supporting the family at their first ICU visit and subsequently as needed, and supporting realistic coping mechanisms.

STUDY QUESTIONS

- Examine the chart of a patient who spent time in a critical care unit. What patient parameters were monitored? What was the purpose of each type of measurement? What implications does each type of measurement have for nursing care of that patient?
- Does the chart identify any psychologic stressors? Were any nursing interventions noted? What other interventions might have been helpful for the patient/family?
- Examine your own beliefs and values about the use of life-sustaining therapies. How would you provide care for a comatose patient whose family insisted on interventions you didn't believe in?

REFERENCES AND SELECTED READINGS

1. Aguilera DC, Messick JM: *Crisis intervention: theory and methodology,* ed 6, St. Louis, 1990, Mosby–Year Book.
2. Alspach JG: *Core curriculum for critical care nursing,* ed 4, Philadelphia, 1991, WB Saunders.
3. Bolgiano KS, Saah ML: Measurement of bedside ventilatory parameters, *Crit Care Nurse* 10(1):60-66, 1990.
4.* Brewer MJ: To sleep or not to sleep: the consequences of sleep deprivation, *Crit Care Nurse* 5(6):35-41, 1985.
5.* Campbell CD, Newsome JA: Detecting life-threatening arrhythmias, *Nursing 90* 20(12):34-40, 1990.
6. Carnevale FA: Transcutaneous O₂ monitoring: assessment techniques, *DCCN* 5(5):264-269, 1986.
7. Charette AL: Bridging the gap between hemodynamics and monitoring, *Crit Care Nurs Clin North Am* 1(3):539-546, 1988.
8.* Coloski D, Mastrianni J, Brown LH: Continuous arteriovenous hemofiltration patient: nursing care plan, *DCCN* 9(3):130-142, 1990.
9. Daily EK, Schroeder JS: *Techniques in bedside hemodynamic monitoring,* ed 4, St. Louis, 1989, Mosby–Year Book.
10. Davidson LJ, Brown S: Continuous SVo₂ monitoring: a tool for analyzing hemodynamic status, *Heart Lung* 15(3):287-292, 1986.
11.* Edler AN: Setting up and using a cardiac monitor, *Nurs 91,* 21(3):58-62, 1991.
12.* Emmanuelson KL, Rosenlicht JM: *Handbook of critical care nursing,* New York, 1986, Fleschner Publishing.
13. English MA: Preventing complications of ventricular assist devices, *DCCN* 8(6):330-336, 1989.
14.* Gahart BL: *Intravenous medications,* ed 7, St. Louis, 1991, Mosby–Year Book.
15. Griffin JP: Nursing care of the immunocompromised patient in the ICU, *Heart Lung* 15(2):179-188, 1986.
16.* Gruppi LA, Killen AR, Rodriguez W: Liver transplantation: key nursing diagnoses, *DCCN* 9(5):272-279, 1990.
17. Hamner JB: Visitation policies in the ICU: a time for change, *Crit Care Nurse* 10(1):48-53, 1990.
18.* Hickey M: What are the needs of families of critically ill patients? A review of the literature since 1976, *Heart Lung* 19(4):401-415, 1990.
19.* Hoffman LA: Airway management for the critically ill patient, *Am J Nurs* 87(1):39-53, 1987.
20. Holloway NM: *Critical care plans,* Springhouse, Penn, 1989, Springhouse.
21. Hudak CM, Gallo BM, Lohr T: *Critical care nursing, a holistic approach,* ed 5, Philadelphia, 1990, JB Lippincott.
22.* Jacquith SM: Continuous measurement of SVo₂: clinical applications and advantages for critical care nursing, *Crit Care Nurse* 5(2):40-44, 1985.
23. Johanson BC, et al: *Standards for critical care,* ed 3, St. Louis, 1988, Mosby–Year Book.
24. Kenner CV, Guzzetta CE, Dossey BM: *Critical care nursing: body, mind, spirit,* ed 2, Boston, 1985, Little, Brown.
25. Kinney MR, editor: *AACN's clinical reference for critical care nursing,* ed 2, New York, 1988, McGraw-Hill Book Co.
26. Konopad E, Noseworthy T: Stress ulceration: a serious complication in critically ill patients, *Heart Lung* 17(4):339-348, 1988.
27. Leske JS: Needs of relatives of critically ill patients: a follow-up, *Heart Lung* 15(2):89-93, 1986.
28. Millar S, Sampson LK, Soukup M: AACN procedure manual for critical care, Philadelphia, 1985, WB Saunders.
29.* Morra L: Troubleshooting pulmonary artery catheters, *RN* 59(2):46-52, 1987.
30.* Mulford E: Nursing perspectives for the patient receiving postoperative ventricular assistance in the critical care unit, *Heart Lung* 16(3):246-247, 1987.
31.* Murphy P: When a nondeath death occurs: helping the family accept the reality of brain death, *Nurs 86* 16(7):34-39, 1986.
32. Ng L, Nuckols OJ: Nursing management of the postoperative cardiac surgical patient in the critical care unit, *Cardiovasc Clin* 16(3):211-233, 1986.
33. Paradiso C: Hemofiltration: an alternative to dialysis, *Heart Lung* 18(3):282-290, 1989.
34. Roberts SL: *Behavioral concepts and the critically ill patient,* ed 2, Englewood Cliffs, NJ, 1986, Prentice-Hall.
35.* Robinet K: Increased intracranial pressure: management with an intraventricular catheter, *J Neurosurg Nurs* 17(2):95-104, 1985.
36.* Shoulders-Odom B: Managing the challenge of IABP therapy, *Crit Care Nurse* 11(2):60-76, 1991.
37.* Smith SL: Liver transplantation: implications for critical care nursing, *Heart Lung* 14(6):617-627, 1985.

*Recommended for student reading.

38. Stanley M: Ensuring a safe ICU stay for your confused, elderly patient, *DCCN* 10(2):62-67, 1991.
39. Weilitz PB: New modes of mechanical ventilation, *Crit Care Nurs Clin North Am* 1(4):689-695, 1989.
40. Wilson T, Broome ME: Promoting the young child's development in the intensive care unit, *Heart Lung* 18(3):274-281, 1989.
41. Zorb SL, Stevens JB: Contemporary bioethical issues in critical care, *Crit Care Clin North Am* 2(3):515-520, 1990.

Classic

42.* Cassem NH, Hackett T, Bascon C: Reactions of coronary patients to the CCU nurse, *Am J Nurs* 70:312-319, 1970.
43. Hay D, Oken D: The psychological stresses of intensive care nursing, *Psychosom Med* 34:117, 1972.
44.* Obier K, Haywood LJ: Enhancing therapeutic communication with acutely ill patients, *Heart Lung* 2:49-53, 1973.
45. Quaal SJ: Comprehensive intraaortic balloon pumping, St. Louis, 1984, Mosby–Year Book.

47

Home Care of the Ill Adult

Carol E. Smith

After studying this chapter, the learner should be able to:

- Describe the trends in health care leading to expansion of home care for medical-surgical patients.
- Discuss the skills used in managing the transition from acute to home care.
- Use the nursing process with home care patients and their families.
- Discuss the home residence as the environment for providing nursing care.
- Evaluate home care through quality assurance.
- Identify issues pertinent to home health care.

In the mid-1980s, approximately the same number of agencies were providing home health care as were hospitals (6500) across the United States.[57] However, forecasters of health care suggest that hospital closures will continue, whereas home care services will increase by as much as 20% annually throughout the 1990s. Medical-surgical nursing home care will be necessary for a large number of adults. Patients may require one or two home visits or around-the-clock nursing care. The nursing process in home care includes expanded assessment of the individual and the home environment, development of nursing diagnoses based on family data, generation of expected outcomes negotiated with the family, and evaluation of effectiveness of care in relation to withdrawing or terminating care. Nurses involved in home health will use many skills to provide care to their medical-surgical patients. These skills and the issues that challenge nurses in home care are discussed in this chapter.

DEFINITIONS AND TRENDS IN HOME CARE

Home care is the provision of nursing care in the person's residence. *Continuity* of *care* is the effective and efficient transition of the patient from hospital to home; it is essential to successful home care. This definition connotes the preparation of the patient for discharge from one health care setting to another as well as coordination of appropriate resources. Congruence between patient and family needs for health care at different stages of illness, together with the nursing care provided, will ensure continuity of care. The goal is to have highly motivated patients and families who know what to expect when patients are discharged to home, manage as much self-care as possible, progress toward the highest level of functioning, and accept help from available resources.

The home health nurse's caseload routinely includes patients with cardiac disease, respiratory disease, diabetes, cancer, and neurologic problems. The home care nurse may be providing or directing nursing services to assist with activities of daily living (ADL), manage wound care, and as the examples in this chapter illustrate, teach families about the technologic aspects of care.

Several principles differentiate home care from medical-surgical care in institutions. One principle is that home care is *continuous* (versus *episodic*) in perspective. In other words, the interrelatedness of the illness to the patient's life-style is considered. The nurse also emphasizes the comprehensive impact of the patient's situation on the whole family. Concern for the effect of environmental factors on the family and patient are apparent in home care practice.

The promotion of patient and family involvement in care is fundamental because self-care may be the only option when the patient has depleted insurance and other benefits. The realities of the economic health care dilemmas dictate that the home care nurse advocate efficient use of professional and family resources.

Trends in health care today have led to an expansion of home care services. Economic trends in health care, technologic innovations, and population demography have resulted in increasing numbers of adult patients requiring medical-surgical care in the home setting. Home care as an alternative to expensive institutional care obtained consumer support in the 1970s.[21] Home care has been documented as cost effective in financial analysis studies conducted by insurance companies, health care professionals, pharmaceutical laboratories, and federal regulatory agencies.[19] The projected insolvency of Medicare and Medicaid, along with the increasing number of older persons in our society, provide the imperative for continued development of home health care delivery systems. Community health organizations, such as the Visiting Nurse Association and other agencies, have established innovative and cost-effective programs of home health care. However, more funding for services of these home care agencies is needed. Home care nursing services are often augmented by private companies that supply equipment as well as specialists for the vast array of technologic care being provided in the home.

Technologic progress has influenced home care greatly. Patients can now be monitored at home through computer linkages to sophisticated diagnostic systems. Technologic innovations, such as small, easily programmed intravenous infusion pumps, have made parenteral home therapies safe and affordable. A variety of respiratory therapies, ranging from oxygen compression tanks to mechanical ventilators, are widely used today with the elderly or patients with multiple chronic illnesses. The continued use of technology and future advances will increase the population of patients dependent on such care at home.

The changing demographics of our population have also influenced the increase in home health care. The number of elderly will more than double by the year 2030, whereas the younger generation is decreasing in numbers.[6] With reduced government programs for the aged, limitations on the amount of skilled nursing services, and decreased availability of nursing home facilities, more elderly persons will need home care. The needs of the elderly may vary significantly, from medical patients dependent on technology to surgical patients requiring short-term home rehabilitation before returning to work. Many individuals can benefit from home care. The combined influences of the patient's physical and psychologic characteristics and the social and economic support available to the family affect the outcome of care provided in the home. In each family, different factors will influence the outcomes of home care. Repeated assessment of these factors is necessary for modifying the home care plan as patient, family, and environmental factors change over time. The home as the environment for nursing care offers a particular challenge to those involved in home care. Nurses will need to manage the transition from acute to home care.

TRANSITION FROM ACUTE CARE TO HOME CARE

The nurse cannot provide nursing care in an individual's home without developing a successful approach or introduction to home care services. Ideally the nurse and other professionals in the acute care setting have initiated discharge planning.

Discharge Planning

The term *discharge planning* is the process of assisting patients and families with their health care needs as they move from one health care setting to another. The overall purpose of discharge planning is to provide continuity of care. Discharge planning includes many activities, from projecting patient needs at discharge to coordinating professionals and volunteers involved in follow-up care. In the mid-1970s, the American Nurses' Association published guidelines for discharge planning for hospitals and community health agencies. Since then, many hospitals have established their own home care agencies.[59] In many of these hospitals and in other situations, the community health nurse meets with the patient and the nurse in the hospital before discharge. In other situations, the nurse caring for the patient in the hospital does the discharge planning.

The discharge planning process encompasses the assessment of the family's needs for teaching, counseling, and nursing care after discharge from the acute care setting. An important component of discharge planning is determining the family's available internal and external resources. Resources range from home health nursing care to equipment rental. Discharge planning may or may not include a referral to a home care agency. If the patient and family are able to meet their own needs after discharge, they may not require any further assistance at home. Families may underestimate the difficulties thay will face when caregiving is necessary 24 hours a day. Assisting families in accepting outside help is a valuable but sometimes difficult task. For some patients, a telephone call by the nurse following discharge can be used to evaluate self-care status and provide continuity of care. The caller should ask specifically about the patient's condition and caregiver fatigue so that follow-up care can be instituted as necessary.

Discharge planning can be either a group process or conducted by one nurse. The group process takes place in a team conference, where personnel from various disciplines and the patient and family discuss the patient's discharge.

The key to either the formal group or the informal discharge planning process is communication with the patient and family. The nurse coordinates the communication and documents the discharge plan on the health care record. Documentation should include both short- and long-range discharge planning goals. For example:

> Ho Chung, a 57-year-old Chinese male of Chinese descent, is hospitalized for neurologic complications of Lyme's disease (an infection from the bite of a deer tick). The short-range goals for Mr. Chung include being able to eat and bathe with assistance as his neurologic function improves. His long-range goals for discharge include being able to perform his ADL with assistance from a home health aide three times a week and his family on the other days.

Discharge planning allows for continuity of care as the patient moves from the acute care setting to home. To be effective, discharge planning begins well before discharge and identifies patients needing home care. See Box 47-1 for characteristics of patients and various aspects of their

---

47-1

Characteristics of patients that influence the need for home care

Patients who cannot manage nursing care on their own
  Comatose or semicomatose patients
  Disoriented, confused, or forgetful patients
  Frail elderly persons
  Patients who live alone
  Patients who do not live alone, but persons at home cannot care for patients adequately
  Patients who have no home, or those whose present home is no longer adequate
Patients who need dressings and wound care
  Patients who have complicated dressings
  Patients who cannot do the dressing themselves
  Patients who will probably not do the dressing unless supervised
Patients who need equipment and transportation (Function shared with social services)
Patients with medication schedules
  Patients with complex schedules or injections
  Patients who are noncompliant
Patients with ostomies (for example, colostomy, ileostomy)
Patients with special teaching needs (for example, new diabetic, complex diet, injections)
Patients who are terminally ill
Patients receiving therapy (occupational, physical, speech)
Patients with tubes (Foley, gastrostomy, suprapubic, nasogastric, tracheostomy)
Patients being transferred
  From another hospital or nursing home
  To another hospital or nursing home (for example, Veteran's Administration hospital)
  The typical patients who need referrals are those with chronic illness, such as arthritis, cancer, cerebrovascular accident, chronic renal failure, congestive heart failure, diabetes mellitus, emphysema, hypertension, or myocardial infarction, and those who are respirator dependent.

Adapted from Rasmusen L: *Nurs Management* 15(5):39-43, 1984.

---

medical-surgical treatment that influence their need for home care. These are not the only criteria, but they are the most common ones. The nurse must be alert for others. Remember that patients may not have any of the characteristics that indicate they will need home care, yet they still need discharge planning.

At the very least, discharge planning should provide the patient and family with (1) instruction in appropriate self-care, (2) identification of family and community resources, (3) awareness of procedures to follow for emergencies, (4) knowledge of follow-up care, and (5) family teaching specific to the patient's concerns. If home care is needed, explanation of home care services, telephone numbers, and, when possible, introductions to home care personnel become part of discharge planning. During hospitalization, as the patient progresses, the nurse collects data or modifies

---

47-2

Financial resources screening checklist

1. Check the government or private resources available to the patient (benefits vary with each plan):
   _____ Medicaid
   _____ Medicare A (home care services)
   _____ Medicare B (home care equipment)
   _____ Blue Cross and Blue Shield Plans/Other Plans
   _____ Employer insurance
   _____ Social Security
   _____ American Cancer Society (free bandages, equipment)
   _____ United Way agencies
   _____ Multiple Sclerosis Society (wheelchair loans)
   _____ Volunteer or charitable organization resources
   _____ Old age assistance
   _____ Supplemental Security Income
   _____ Financial help from family
   _____ Disability payments
   _____ Retirement pensions
   _____ Welfare programs
   _____ Meals on Wheels
   _____ Private insurance
   _____ Savings accounts

2. Do you think that your total income for this year was enough to meet your (the patient and other family members) usual monthly expenses and bills?

   _____ Yes   _____ No

3. In the past 6 months, has money been spent on the patient's physician, hospital, nursing home, or medication bills that has not been reimbursed by insurance?

---

preexisting data, reflecting the change in the patient's health status and ability to function. Discharge planning builds on the patient's strengths and abilities.

Determining discharge planning needs

The initial interview before the patient's discharge includes an assessment of the patient's needs, that is, his or her bio-psycho-social and spiritual needs. The nurse assesses the home environment by asking several questions:

With whom does the patient live?

What are the living arrangements?

Does the patient live in a house or apartment?

Are there stairs to the house or building, or stairs within the premises?

Are all essential rooms on the same floor, such as the bathroom, bedroom, and kitchen?

Is the living environment adequate to meet the patient's needs at the time of discharge?

An adequate living environment includes basics such as running water or indoor plumbing, heating or cooling, and cleanliness. The nurse also asks specific questions pertaining to the patient's medical-surgical care. For example, does the patient receiving intravenous antibiotics have re-

frigeration storage for the medication? Do patients undergoing peritoneal dialysis have a clean area where they can work with their equipment?

The nurse will also want to assess the patient's and family's support systems. Who will be available to the patient when discharged? This includes immediate family or significant others living with the patient. Ask what extended family members, children, friends, or neighbors are part of the patient's support system. What groups have the patient previously engaged in to meet his or her social needs? Will the patient be able to interact with the groups on discharge? What sources of spiritual support does the patient have? Can religious or other groups assist with care or prevent social isolation by visiting or telephoning regularly?

The nurse needs to determine if the patient and family have adequate coping mechanisms to manage the illness and the common stressors of home care. Ask the patient and family what they do to get along during difficult times. Will these coping strategies work for them now, or will they require assistance in developing new coping strategies because of a change in the patient's condition and its subsequent impact on the family? What learning needs do the patient and family have? Can these be adequately met before discharge, or will they require ongoing teaching? Finally, discuss the family's feelings about taking the patient home. Are they fearful of the patient's condition, worried about the extra responsibilites, or overly optimistic about their ability to care for the patient? The more realistic expectations that the family has about home care, the more likely they are to adjust successfully.

Assessing financial needs

Financial assessment must be undertaken before discharge and throughout the home care visits. Financial assistance may be needed because home health care can be expensive and may not be reimbursable.

It is often difficult for nurses to undertake financial assessments. Asking about available financial resources, especially in the person's own home, may seem an invasion of privacy. Nurses need financial data about the patients to ensure they receive the full benefits for which they are eligible under government or private insurance. In today's economic climate, with the high costs of health care, even middle-income families may need assistance because they may be ineligible for government programs or other assistance. Also, identifying the resources currently used by the family allows the nurse to identify other possible sources of financial assistance. Box 47-2 lists financial resources that may be available to patients requiring home care. Referral to a social worker or financial discharge planner who is aware of the current eligibility and reimbursement criteria is essential, especially for the elderly Medicare patient. Each individual will require assessment to identify unique resources. For example, employed individuals may be able to negotiate a special reimbursement plan with their employer, or persons living close to state boundaries may improve reimbursement by moving from one state to another. Financial counseling is available from insurers and specialty support groups.

Lastly, during the initial assessment the nurse determines if the family is currently using any community resources to meet their needs. If so, how many, and how frequently? Are these satisfactory to the patient and family? If the patient and family are using community resources that are satisfactory, the nurse will want to consider these when making a referral, if one is necessary. If possible, the nurse in the acute care setting calls on the skills of the *transition specialist* to help with discharge planning. The *role of the transition specialist* is discussed next.

Transitional Care

Brooten and colleagues[7] developed the concept of *transitional care*. The transitional period is the time from discharge planning to physiologic recovery. A nurse educated as a *transition specialist* can make a difference in both the quality and the cost of care at home. The transition specialist meets with the family while the patient is still in acute care to begin discharge planning. In addition, the transition specialist makes home visits before the patient's discharge to assess the home environment. The transition specialist is then available to the family following discharge. The study of Brooten and co-workers revealed that interventions instituted by transition specialists, including patient education, counseling, home visits, and telephone availability, were successful in terms of quality care.[9] Using discharge planning and home nursing services versus longer hospitalization yielded an average cost saving of 25%.[8]

To manage transition from hospital to home, patients and family members must manage activities ranging from use of sterile techniques to assessment of the adult's psychologic status.[53] To manage home care, the family members must acquire new knowledge and skills, be motivated to help the patient, and adapt to the change created in the roles of family members. The problems typically reported by families who provide home care include the burden of providing daily physical care, financial strain, and difficulty coping with individual role and schedule disruptions.[12] Other problems include the stress of learning the nursing care, unavailability of resources, the difficulty of accepting help from others, and observing any negative changes in the patient such as infection or malnutrition. Further problems noted in long-term home care include equipment failure, the need for home remodeling, and social isolation.[11]

In addition to dealing with these general problems, the nurse transition specialist reviews the literature to identify concerns shared by populations of patients they discharge. The key to providing successful transitional care lies in designing nursing interventions specifically for each family. The interventions for the family of the patient being monitored for cardiac dysrhythmias in the home compared with the patient needing enteral feeding are very different. For example, the problems repeatedly identified in studies of discharged patients receiving mechanical ventilation were initial anxiety followed by depression related to the complexity of the therapy and the constant presence of technology in the home.[53] Several problems experienced by home patients have been documented, including difficulties with finances, body image and sexual relations, social stigma, and issues such as how to arrange the living quarters for safety. These problems have been reported to recur depending on the patient's condition and factors such as the ability to return to work, length of time on ventilator each day, and availability of family support and external resources.

Case-Managed Care

Case-managed care is an approach to providing care that includes an effort to reduce overall costs of services while maintaining the patient's optimum health. *Case-managed care* refers to the supervision and *coordination of paraprofessionals*, consultation with other health professionals, and a direct evaluation of nursing care in the home. Nurses providing case-managed care are referred to as case managers and may not provide any direct patient care themselves, but they coordinate the efforts of all others involved in the home care. Nurses who provide case-managed care may also serve as *transition specialists, service coordinators,* and *quality assurance advocates*. The case manager does a detailed assessment of the patient's needs, discusses options with the patient and family, arranges for selected services to be provided, and then ensures quality care by evaluating patient outcomes on a periodic basis. In the case-managed situation, the nurse may have a caseload of 40 to 50 families.[10]

The nurse who provides case-managed care must develop many skills. The nurse must understand the patient's physical condition and be well versed in the complexity of the patient's insurance or other financial coverage. The case manager needs skill in motivating families toward self-care, recognizing fragmentation of care, facilitating delivery of services on behalf of the family, and advocating for continuing resources when necessary. Arranging long-term services that match the patient's changing acuity level is a key element of case-managed care. Case managers do much of their work by telephone; thus they must be skilled in communication.

Private industries and the federal government support case-managed care as a means of reducing insurance costs and making early hospital discharge to the home safe and less expensive. A home health agency, hospital, health maintenance organization (HMO) discharge program, or an insurance company may employ nurses in case-managed care. Some nurse entrepreneurs have established their own companies that provide case-managed services for Blue Cross/Blue Shield or for large corporations' employees. These nurses have become skilled in matching the patients' needs with the most cost-effective resources available.

The nurse who provides direct care to patients in the home is involved in case management instead of being a case manager. This nurse has a varying caseload of five to seven families daily. The total number of families the nurse manages depends on geographic location, amount of time spent with each family, and the frequency of visits necessary.

The skills needed by the nurse providing direct care to families are similar to those of the nurse acting as a case manager. Both nurses provide teaching and counseling and encourage self-care. The nurse providing the home care performs direct surveillance and monitors the patient's condition. The nurse providing direct care discusses the patient's needs with the case manager, who can assist with resource allocation and help anticipate any problems. Communication with the family is the key element in the success of case management.

SKILLS NECESSARY FOR HOME CARE

The nurse providing direct care to families, the case manager, and any other health professional needs two unique skills to provide home care. First the person needs to gain access to the home so that home care can be provided. Also a primary nursing intervention is family education instead of just individual patient education.

Gaining Access to the Home

Ideally the first visit with the patient and family should be conducted in the hospital before discharge, but often the first visit is to the home. Therefore the initial contact with the patient by the home care nurse is almost always by telephone. When telephoning, identify yourself as a nurse, and the agency from which you are calling. You may need to remind the family that either the hospital discharge team or the physician referred them to your agency. Explain that the purpose of the call is to set up an initial home visit. Establish that the purpose of the initial visit is to discuss the patient and family's home health care needs. Set the time of the visit at the patient's convenience, and state the amount of time it will take. Ask how the family wishes you to enter the home: through the front door or back door possibly with a hidden key. Repeat your name, and have them write down a telephone number where they can reach you. Remember that your tone of voice and the manner in which you conduct the telephone conversation establishes your respect for the patient. Closing with the comment, "I look forward to working with you," accentuates the participatory partnership the nurse seeks to develop.

For the home visit itself, the nurse must obtain the address and check directions to the location. At the first visit the patient's needs are assessed and available home care options are discussed. The nurse must be prepared with all essentials needed for assessment (for example, history-taking forms, stethoscope, other equipment) and supplies necessary for already prescribed treatments (for example, teaching materials, bandages for wound dressing). Typically the home care nurse carries a bag that contains essential equipment but needs to check the contents and add anything necessary for a particular patient. Also, carry charting materials, whether paper, nursing note forms, or tape recorder for dictation. Tell the family you will be taking notes to document the patient's progress during home care. The bag should also contain printed materials that the home care nurse can discuss and then leave with the patient and family. Select the printed materials based on the family's needs for teaching about illness, direct patient care, or other services available.

Have information available on the costs of home care services, insurance reimbursement, and other economic details that the family will need. Options to reduce home care expenditures safely, such as family members providing wound dressing changes 3 days a week or the nurse re-

ducing visits to twice weekly, should be explored. Family members may desire 100% professional care or, on the other hand, may believe they can manage all the care themselves. The nurse must analyze each situation and suggest the best options. The family's caregiving abilities is assessed with regard to the patient's condition. The nurse should note that most insurers have restrictions on the lifetime amount the patient can be reimbursed for home care. Discussing the economics of the health care situation with families can be difficult, but understanding that cost-effective use of their insurance will maintain coverage for them at a later date is essential.

At the first home visit, expect the family to welcome you in a social way, by introducing you to others present, asking you to sit down or have coffee, and so on, just as they would any visitor. Share with the family your pleasure at meeting them and then reiterate the purpose of the visit and the time limits previously set. State simply that you would like to hear how they are managing at home and to check the patient's condition. In this way, you communicate your desire to hear their concerns and also establish that the patient will be examined. Families are often unsure of the nurse's role in the home and need to be able to predict what will happen at each visit. Because the nurse is a guest entering the home, follow normal social protocol. For example, if you will be late, telephone the family as to when they can expect you. When you arrive, do not automatically go to the patient's bedroom, but ask if that is where the patient is to be examined. Explain each of the steps of your examination and the services provided. Acceptance of home care services by the family is essential if the continuity of care is to be maintained.

Family Education

The term *family education* is used to emphasize that the teaching skills employed in home health care involve the entire family or all significant others. In this context the nurse's skill in assessing readiness to learn, providing information, and evaluating outcomes of teaching must be carried out with a group.[50] The home, as the environment for learning, also influences the teaching strategies used. Individual family members often have varying expectations and roles in the education process. The male patient may be interested in learning about the technical aspects of his care but might ask his wife to manage all his medications. In addition, a child might be called on to learn about the financial aspects of insurance, equipment loans, or Medicare benefits. The nurse assists the family in decisions about who should learn what and may even be involved in resolving conflicts between family members who believe other members learned incorrectly. The steps for teaching the family are similar to those for individual patient teaching. Family education, therefore, begins with assessment and diagnosis of learning needs. The final steps include implementing and then evaluating the teaching.

The expected outcome of teaching is learning. Learning has taken place when the person's behavior has changed so that he or she and the nurse agree that the patient's health is enhanced. Thus teaching is not just imparting information, but also ensuring that a *change in behavior* occurs. To assist families to manage home care, they may

Sample interview questions in assessing patients' knowledge about their health care

1. Can you tell me what you have learned about your illness?
2. You have had surgery before. Can you tell me what you remember from that experience?
3. When you spoke with your physician/pharmacist, what did he or she tell you was important to know about your medications?
4. Have you heard about your therapy from anyone else who has had your health problem?
5. Have you read or heard reports about the treatments your physician wants you to undergo?

For patients who have physical limitations, careful assessment of their abilities should be done before determining the type of teaching plans and evaluation to use. For instance, the perception and knowledge of some patients who have had strokes can be evaluated by using picture boards to assist them to identify frequently used articles.

Modified from Smith C: *Patient education: nurses in partnership with other health care professionals,* New York, 1987. Grune & Stratton.

Nursing interventions to enhance willingness or motivation to learn

Provide counseling to reduce patient or family anxieties.
Explore past teaching experiences that created negative attitudes toward learning.
Compliment individuals and groups on information already learned.
Determine what the person wants to learn and teach this first.
Take steps to overcome deficiencies in perceptual skills, such as vision limitations and memory loss.
Complete discharge planning so that financial, housing, or other needed assistance can be found to decrease patient's worries.

Modified from Smith C: *Patient education: nurses in partnership with other health care professionals,* New York, 1987. Grune & Stratton.

need to change routines in daily schedules and responsibilities for household duties. The nurse may need to provide counseling as well as external resources to support these changes in behavior.

Assessing learning needs

Assessing the patient and family's understanding of the illness and its treatment establishes a baseline for teaching. Box 47-3 provides sample interview questions to determine what patients already know about their health care. The nurse can link new knowledge to information the family already has and reinforce behavior change. Any barriers to learning that the patient and family may have, such as reading difficulties or lack of desire to learn, need to be assessed. Attitudes, beliefs, and values influence learning. Attitude or desire to learn varies greatly for each person through the various stages of their home health care. The grieving process as well as beliefs and values affects the desire to learn. Patients and families who are in a stage of denial have difficulty learning. When the family is in denial and unable to learn a procedure such as total parenteral nutrition (TPN), the nurse may need to do the procedure and gradually shift the family to self-care as they are able to cope. Another situation in which a family has difficulty learning is when the family must learn how to change a wound dressing but does not have money to buy bandages. In this situation, before teaching, the home care nurse would obtain dressings from the American Cancer Society, local church organization, and so on. Box 47-4 identifies interventions the nurse may use when enhancing patients' willingness or motivation to learn the necessary home care instruction.

The nurse also must assess the information that family members desire. In addition to information about the patient's biologic condition, family members have personal skills and knowledge needs. The biologic condition and families' personal skill and knowledge needs identified by home care nurses in one study are shown in Figs. 47-1, 47-2, and 47-3. The nursing interventions or skills needed to manage home care are related to each patient's biologic or pathophysiologic condition and to personal skills of the caregiver. Home care nurses indicated in this study that family members needed to be competent in a wide variety of skills including lifting, turning, moving the patient and neurologic checks (Fig. 47-1) and skills to promote health, listening ability, and so on (Fig. 47-2). Along with the above skills, home care nurses recognized the family members' needs for knowledge of depression, grief, and other potential psychologic problems found in home care (Fig. 47-3).

After completing the assessment, the nurse must analyze the data collected to determine nursing diagnoses that clearly indicate the patient's and family's problems or strengths. For example, the nursing diagnosis of *coping, family, potential for growth related to learned management of home care treatments* identifies the family's strengths. Nursing diagnoses that illustrate problems with learning are described in the section on *knowledge deficits* later in this chapter.

Planning and implementing family education

When planning teaching in the home care setting, the three major objectives for the patient and family are (1) comprehension of the illness and its treatment(s), (2) accepting the impact of illness and treatment(s) on life-style, and (3) demonstrating management of treatment procedures and home care. Understanding the patient's and family's life-style helps the nurse to plan with them about how to adapt changes with the least disruption. When a medical regimen causes minimum disruptions in life-style, the patient is more likely to comply with it. Teaching is more effective when it includes not only knowledge of

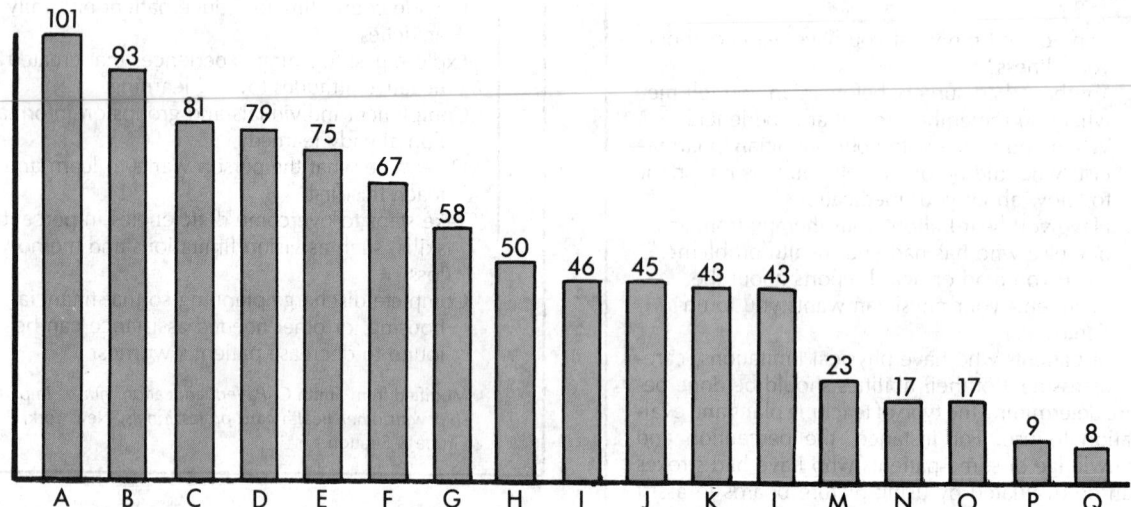

Fig. 47-1 Family members' biologic skill needs for providing home care: as prioritized by registered nurse respondents; number of first prioritized responses. **A,** Lifting, turning, moving. **B,** CPR. **C,** Range-of-motion. **D,** GI—nausea/vomiting. **E,** CV—Apical pulse measurement. **F,** Drug side effects. **G,** Injections. **H,** Sterile dressings. **I,** Constipation. **J,** Diarrhea. **K,** Blood pressure measurement. **L,** Respiratory. **M,** GU—catheter care. **N,** EENT—Sensory-perceptual changes. **O,** Neurotemperature. **P,** Charting. **Q,** Neurologic checks. (From Quiring JD: RN perspective of home health care needs of family members, *Kans Nurs* 59(3):10, 1985.)

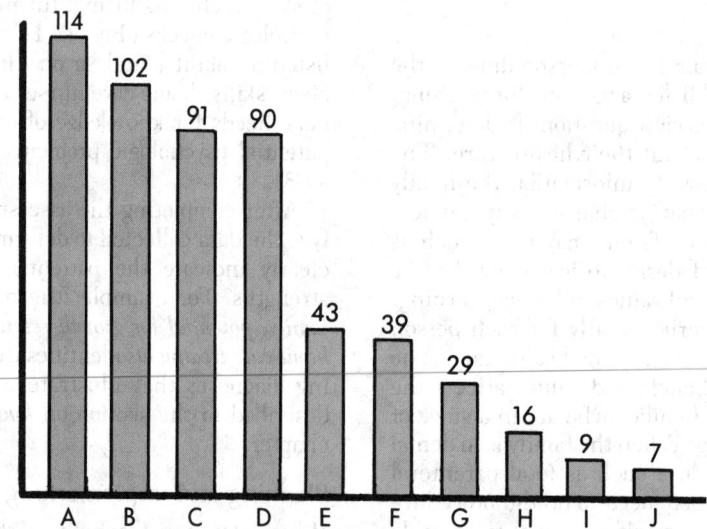

Fig. 47-2 Family members' personal skill needs for providing home care: as prioritized by registered nurse respondents; number of first prioritized responses. **A,** Art of listening. **B,** Promotion of independence/self care. **C,** Attitude toward seriously ill. **D,** Establishing rapport. **E,** Confidentiality/privacy. **F,** Promotion of health. **G,** Interview. **H,** Facilitating development of special abilities. **I,** Life histories. **J,** Avoiding patient abuse. (From Quiring JD: RN perspective of home health care needs of family members, *Kans Nurs* 59(3):10, 1985.)

treatment, but also counseling about scheduling so the patient and family can incorporate home care into their daily routines. The nurse must also plan learning objectives related to symptom control, management of exacerbations, treatment protocols, problem solving, and financial difficulties.

Implementation of teaching plans can take many forms in home health care. The use of computer-assisted instruction and videotapes in the home have been successful. One-to-one demonstration of technical procedures is effective. Also, describing methods of care over the telephone has also ensured learning. Many and varied methods of teaching that incorporate the whole family and emphasize the need to change behavior are most likely to have positive results. Using praise and reinforcement and providing an opportunity to ask questions and to evaluate learning effectiveness are important parts of implementation.

Mazzuca[34] reviewed 320 articles on research conducted to determine what effect patient teaching had on chronic illnesses. The most successful education programs emphasized changing the environment in which patients care for themselves so that home care is easily managed. An example of modifying the home environment might include rearranging furniture so that it is in the field of vision of the patient who is rehabilitating from a cerebrovascular accident (CVA) and has residual hemianopsia. Requiring modification of the environment actively enlists the patient in changing behavior toward desired objectives.

Nurses should list reminders of the new behavior required by patients. For example, suggest to patients that they schedule treatments with meals or other regular activities so they won't forget to do them.

Evaluating outcomes and identifying barriers to teaching in the home

The goal of teaching is to have patients and families incorporate necessary changes in behavior to adapt to illness and its resulting impact. Learning takes place in areas of knowledge, attitude, and behavior. Evaluation, the last step of the nursing process, is essential to patient education. Evaluation is based on what the patient and family believe they need to learn, as well as the learning objectives designed by the home care nurses. *Learning objectives are stated outcomes that are measurable and realistic.* Through the evaluation of the objectives, the nurse helps the patient and family to recognize needs for future learning and identifies success with past learning.

Questioning or listening to patient answers is a common method of evaluating learning. *The method of evaluation used should be acceptable and nonthreatening to the patient and family.* Besides verbal questioning, the nurse should observe for evidence that the patient understands how to incorporate changes brought on by the illness. For instance, the patient should be asked how he or she plans to balance rest and activity during the day.

The nurse must be prepared to address barriers to teaching in the home. The nurse must remember to bring teaching materials for the home visit, even if the patient received hand-outs before discharge. Duplication of materials and information most often reinforces previous teaching.

Families may also state. "We are being taught something

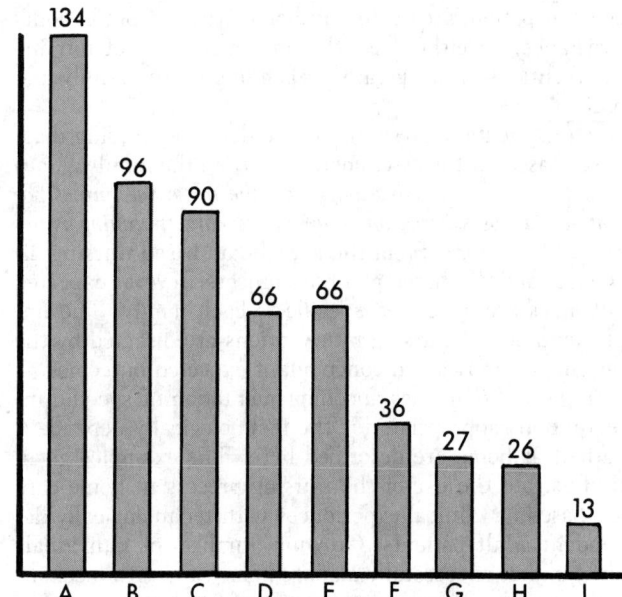

Fig. 47-3 Family members' personal knowledge needs for providing home care: as prioritized by registered nurse respondents; number of first prioritized responses. **A,** Meaning/purpose. **B,** Depression. **C,** Hope. **D,** Dying. **E,** Grief. **F,** Loneliness. **G,** Fulfillment. **H,** Bereavement. **I,** Sexuality. (From Quiring JD: RN perspective of home health care needs of family members, *Kans Nurs* 59(3):10, 1985.)

different now than what the hospital nurse or doctor instructed." The nurse must coordinate patient teaching and clarify consistency of information for the family. Also, duplication of teaching efforts must be avoided. For example, the nurse and physical therapist should decide who is responsible for teaching range-of-motion, thus reducing the cost of education. However, the nurse must remember to reinforce content taught by other health team members.

Another difficulty for home teaching is the wide age variation in patients and families. The home care nurse must consider the developmental, cognitive, and potential learning challenges for children and elders in the family.

Instruction is incorporated into patient care activities, allowing return demonstration and involving the patient and family in evaluating the outcomes. It is also essential to document teaching and the self-care outcomes to illustrate the importance and cost effectiveness of teaching in the home. The Health Care Financing Administration publication no. 11 lists only 12 teaching activities that are considered reimbursable by medicare. Other activities are considered on an individual basis, and having documentation of teaching outcomes increases the likelihood of reimbursement.

NURSING PROCESS IN THE HOME SETTING

The ultimate goal of home care is to assist the patient and family to their maximum level of everyday functioning. In some cases the highest level of function may be the patient's complete recovery and return to work. In other situations the maximum function may be the family's ability to manage the patient's care in the home without professional assistance. In either case the implementation of nursing interventions varies greatly, depending on the family and patient.

During data analysis the nurse develops nursing diagnoses based on the assessment data from the family. *Along with these actual nursing diagnoses, the nurse determines potential diagnoses based on common discharge planning issues seen in home care.* From the actual data-based nursing diagnoses and discharge planning process, several expected outcomes are generated specific to each family. The implementation of nursing interventions are directed by the nursing diagnoses and concomitant expected outcomes.

Expected outcomes and implementation of specific interventions appropriate for the technologically dependent patient at home are described here. The examples given to illustrate the use of the nursing process in home care are based on clinical experiences with technologically dependent adult patients. Growing numbers of individuals and families successfully manage home care with mechanical ventilators, parenteral nutrition infusions, home hemodialysis, intravenous antibiotics or chemotherapy, and other life-sustaining interventions. Using the nursing process with these families supports their adaptive responses to the impact of technologic dependency.

The following discussion outlines the steps of the nursing process employed with adult medical-surgical patients requiring various technical therapies at home. The implementation of highly technical home therapies have been well researched in the adult patient with no disease *complications.* Additional interventions may be necessary when the patient or family experience confounding factors such as multiple illnesses, living alone, lack of a suitable home environment, or inability to accept dependency on technology.

The *man-machine interface* found in technologically dependent patients is a challenge nurses can address through the use of the nursing process. Despite dependence on machines or high-tech equipment, home care allows families to exert control over their lives and maintain their highest level of wellness and functioning. Nurses facilitate home care by advocating patients' independent living, educating families about technologic care, and providing them with resources.

Researchers have verified the efficacy and cost effectiveness of home care for technologically dependent patients. Advantages of home care over institutional care for the patient include *decreased nosocomial infection* and *improved nutritional status.* Home care allows for the *resumption of more normal interactions and routines. More normal daily living* follows adaptation to the noise of the machine and worry about machine failure. Even with these worries, greater *sense of control* and *morale* have been reported by patients receiving home care and their families.

Finally, *financial benefits* of home care versus institutional care have been well documented. Studies have shown that in-home ventilation costs are approximately one-third the cost of hospital care and are even less when skilled services are not needed 24 hours a day. Considering the significance of such advantages, many U.S. institutions have reported discharge preparation protocols for home care of technologically dependent patients.

The combined influences of the physical and psychologic environments of the home impact continuously on the outcomes of care provided. Repeated assessment of these influences is necessary for modifying the care plan as patient and family environmental factors change over time. The home as the environment for nursing care offers a particular challenge to those involved.

Assessment
Assessment of the home as the environment for nursing care

The family home is a unique environment for providing nursing care to the adult patient. Psychologically, the effects of the home territory need to be taken into account when developing the nursing care plan. Physically, the home environment must be assessed for safety, accessibility, and appropriate areas to provide care.

Psychologic factors affecting care planning include motivational as well as financial, patient and family expectations, and developmental, social, and community influences that impact the adaptation to home care. The psychologic factors affecting care in the home are many, varied, and rapidly changing.

Psychologic environment as an influence

The patient's attitude toward discharge to home, family members' reactions to the caregiver role, and the family's ability to accept help from a home care team all influence the outcome of care. Before discharge, the patient's and family's attitudes toward home care are determined. The patient's motivation to return home and the family's willingness to provide and accept home care are important determinants of successful home management. The patient and family's perceptions and concerns about recovery influence acceptance of home care. Besides perceptions, the importance of autonomy and privacy may influence acceptance.

The availability, expense, and type of services considered for home care should be discussed. A *backup plan needs to be negotiated when services become too intrusive or expensive or when friends or others assisting in the home become ill or unavailable.*

Financial influences

Home health care can be a financial burden for families. Cost analyses indicate that home care expenses vary in relation to the type, intensity, and length of services needed. Medicare, Blue Cross/Blue Shield, and an increasing number of other private insurance companies pay for acute, posthospital home care services to reduce the length of hospital stay. For such coverage, however, the care required must be defined as intermittent rather than ongoing. Medicaid and a few insurers pay for longer-term chronic home care services. Supplemental coverage can be obtained in some cases from old age assistance, workers' compensation, disability, welfare, or other financial aid programs. Regardless, the family must pay deductibles and only a percentage is covered; thus most people pay some out-of-pocket costs.

Each of these financial resources varies in the requirements the patient must meet, the length of time benefits are allowed, and the types of equipment or supplies pro-

Table 47-1   Stages of family development

Stages of development	Task
1. Married couple	Establishing a mutually satisfying marriage
	Fitting into the extended family network
2. Childbearing families	Adjusting to parenthood
	Encouraging the development of infants
	Establishing a satisfying home for both parents and infant(s)
3. Families with preschool-age children	Adapting to the critical needs and interests of preschool children in stimulating, growth-promoting ways
	Coping with energy depletion and lack of privacy as parents
4. Families with school-age children	Fitting into the community of school-age families in constructive ways
	Encouraging children's educational achievement
5. Families with adolescent children	Balancing freedom with responsibility as adolescents mature
	Establishing postparental interests and careers as growing parents
6. Families as "launching center"	Releasing young adults into work, military service, college, marriage, and so on with appropriate rituals and assistance
	Maintaining a supportive home base
7. Middle-aged parents	Rebuilding the marriage relationship
	Maintaining kin ties with older and younger generations
8. Aging family members	Coping with bereavement and living alone
	Closing the family home or adapting it to aging
	Adjusting to retirement

Adapted from Duvall E: *Marriage and family development.* Philadelphia, 1977, JB Lippincott Co.

vided. Typically, the complete description of the therapies, equipment, and services covered are included in manuals available from each financial group.

Even with these financial benefits, families incur costs that are not covered. Some uncovered costs can be reduced through using volunteer, charity, community, or religious resources. For example, the local American Cancer Society provides bandages and other supplies free of charge, and some church or volunteer groups provide transportation for clinic appointments. The family member who provides care for the adult at home may have lost time from work, thus increasing the financial burden. The nurse's role is to assess the psychologic impact of the financial situation on the family, coordinate the use of available resources, and refer the family to social workers, case managers, or insurance experts.

Patient and family expectations

Both the patient's and the family's willingness and motivation for home care must be assessed regarding their expectations of home care. Ask the family to describe what they expect from home care. Listen carefully to what the family expects the professionals to do in daily care. Does the family desire around-the-clock service or only availability of a nurse by telephone? Does the patient desire physical care from the family and medication or equipment monitoring from professionals? Does the family recognize the possible changes in their daily schedule that providing home care may bring?

How have the family members reacted to having outside persons coming into their private residence? Can the family obtain support from extended-family members, friends, and religious or community resources? Other long-range expectations of home care, such as the patient or family member becoming self-sufficient so that home services can be terminated or the feasibility of returning to work, can be assessed on a continuing basis. The nurse must realize

that as home care continues, the resources, motivation, and emotional reactions of the family and patient change and must be taken into account when revising the home care plan.

Developmental, social, and community influences

The nurse must take into account other factors when assessing the psychologic environment of the home as the setting for care. One important factor is the family's developmental level. Individuals and families at different developmental levels have different needs, skills, and resources to use in home care management. Family developmental stages and the major tasks associated with each are depicted in Table 47-1.[60]

These stages vary in length, may repeat, may overlap, and may not be sequential. Other tasks may be of prime concern depending on the family, their life-style, and available social and community supports.

Homebound patients often are concerned about other developmental tasks, such as obtaining child care or caring for grandparents. The nurse who assists the family in finding affordable day care for children or live-in help for grandparents can then assist the family to focus on care of the patient at home.

Social and community support for home care also influences the psychologic environment and thus the outcomes of care in the residence. Social support is made up of actions from various sources that assist the person to meet his or her personal goals or manage the demands of a particular situation. Social support has been identified in health care research as significant in affecting a person's adjustment to illness and ability to manage their acute or chronic health problems.[40] Social support is most often received from the persons in the immediate or extended family.

The nurse will find that communities also have resources that can be mobilized to provide the patient and family with social support as part of their home care. Religious denominations, neighborhood associations, community centers, voluntary service groups, and professionally lead support groups can all be sources of social support. These groups can be used so that the patient or family caregiver does not become isolated and overburdened with care. Studies have indicated that social and community support can also lessen the depression of the caregiver that may result from the demands and changes brought on by home care.

Physical environment as an influence

The home is the physical environment for delivery of nursing care. Any physical environment used for patient care requires assessment in terms of *safety, accessibility,* and *appropriateness for care.* The criteria used to assess the safety of the home depend to some extent on the patient's abilities and needs. A patient who is discharged with equipment for hemodialysis may require alterations in the home to provide a safe environment for care. Modifications in the home environment for safety may also be based on the patient's disabilities or physical condition, such as high-rise toilet seats, grab bars in the bathroom, or changing a living room into a bedroom.

Assessment of the physical environment should always include basic information about the home within the community. The location of the residence in relation to necessary home care services and equipment is important. When established home care services are located a long distance away, often an assessment of the community uncovers resources that allows home care to take place safely. Possibly a retired nurse in the rural community can be asked to provide care for the family until they have managed the transition from the hospital. In the urban setting, a hospital-based pulmonary nurse specialist might provide periodic home visits to a ventilator-dependent patient. Another factor related to location of the residence in the community is the availability of transportation to and from needed resources. Arrangements for trips to the grocery, pharmacy, and clinic are part of the safety of home management. Finding community resources to ensure care are frequent challenges for the home care nurse.

The physical environment of the home should always be assessed for basic factors that affect the patient's health and adjustment to home care. Adequacy of heating, cooling, electrical outlets, plumbing and refrigeration, and access to a telephone should be determined. Lack of these resources does not preclude home care unless these are necessary for safety. Some antibiotics that are infused intravenously may require refrigeration. Proper storage would have to be found if no refrigeration was available in their residence. Plumbing and toilet facilities also need to be assessed in relation to the patient's nursing care needs. Another basic factor that affects the patient's adjustment to home care and is influenced by the physical environment is an area where the patient can rest. The patient may be bedridden, unable to climb stairs, or restricted to one area because of medical equipment. Problem solving must be employed to ensure that the family can use the space in their home the way they desire and that the medical equipment does not cause too much noise or interference.

Physical assessment of the patient

Assessment of the adult patient in the home encompasses many of the same data collection procedures appropriate in the acute care setting. In the acute care setting the patient is assessed by other staff around the clock. *In the home setting, the patient and family are the primary data collectors who monitor and provide care.* Thus assessment in the home setting begins with exploring the patient and family's self-management. The patient and family caregivers should be asked to describe the patient's condition and to discuss any concerns. The nurse providing home care may not have seen the patient for a few days and depends on the family's observations or monitoring of specific data. The nurse's questions should illustrate to the patient and family that their information is important.

Assessment in the home proceeds in an orderly fashion. Start by asking the patient and family about their own concerns. The patient and caregiver are asked specific questions about the priority nursing diagnoses, medical problems, or signs and symptoms that the patient is experiencing. For example, a man who is seen at home for a wound infection may report that his incision is sore and tender but that the throbbing pain seems to have decreased. The nurse follows up by asking if anything alleviated the tenderness, such as the warm, moist soaks used twice daily for cleansing the area. The patient is asked if anything aggravated the tenderness or made the symptoms worse, such as wound drainage. If drainage is reported, the nurse asks about the quantity or amount. It helps to obtain specific information by asking the family to describe the size of the drainage area. The type of drainage in terms of color, odor, and presence of blood or exudate is observed by the nurse to obtain objective data. The nurse determines if any signs are associated with the subjective tenderness, such as swelling or elevated body temperature. These signs are measurable and are documented as objective data. Thus, with each problem area, the nurse gathers data from the patient and family that provide detailed characteristics for comparison. The detailed characteristics are used to analyze the symptoms described. By comparing the characteristics from one visit to the next, the nurse monitors the patient's signs and symptoms. The assessment concludes with questions about any other concerns.

Psychologic assessment of the patient

Another essential component of assessment is determining the patient and family's psychologic response to each problem. One man with a wound infection may react to the reduced tenderness and swelling as good news, whereas another may believe he has a serious condition. The patient's psychologic response is influenced by many factors, such as length of illness, presence of multiple symptoms, and reactions of family members.

The primary caregiver's psychologic reactions also should be assessed. The *primary caregiver* is the person who provides the most physical or daily care for the patient. The primary caregiver may be a spouse, sibling, significant other, or grown child. Many individuals may be involved in home care, and their psychologic reactions must also be assessed.

47-5

Checklist for mechanical ventilator equipment*

Checks the ventilator function
Identifies ventilator settings (such as tidal volume, rate)
Sets ventilator settings
Puts the circuit equipment (such as tubing, mist element) together
Connects the circuit
Changes the circuit
Maintains ventilator and equipment
Troubleshoots ventilator (leaks, pressure alarm, and so on)

*A comprehensive equipment check would be conducted using the manufacturer's guidelines for home use.

47-6

Specific assessment of family responsible for care of person on home mechanical ventilation

Emergency procedures
Knows how to use the external battery for the ventilator
Knows how to use the manual resuscitator bag
Knows how to reinsert tracheotomy tube in an emergency
Knows what to do in an electrical power failure
Manages airway problems
Knows what to do if an equipment failure occurs
Has emergency phone numbers of ventilator company with 24-hour services
Manages oxygen in the home
Notifies fire department and emergency services that a ventilator patient is in the home

Home environment
Rearranges or remodels home to accommodate ventilator care
Notifies electric company and establishes appropriate emergency power
Establishes contact with an appropriate home care equipment company
Sets up a patient call system
Orders and obtains supplies
Operates and cares for special medical equipment (ventilator, hospital bed, commode, wheelchair)

Special patient needs
Knows how to communicate with person on ventilator
Has suggestions for diversional activities (hobbies, pastimes, recreation)
Demonstrates techniques to identify signs and symptoms of a respiratory infection
Submits insurance papers or obtains other sources of funds
Knows how to travel with the ventilator
Arranges for respite care

Treatment plan assessment

The treatment plan includes health care professionals' prescriptions for medication, diet, exercise, and physical or psychologic care. Discuss with the patient the specific prescriptions he or she was given and exactly how these prescriptions are being carried out. Ask the patient and family about any difficulties with treatments, obtain their opinion about the benefits or drawbacks of the therapy, and discuss these issues with them.

The treatment plan or therapy prescribed by the patient's health care professional influence the general care of the patient. The treatment plan also dictates any special skills the patient and family must master. Overall assessment of the patient's treatment plan should include questioning about general care, medications, nutrition, home environment, emergency procedures, specific patient needs, and equipment checks. General care assessment includes needs for assistance with hygiene, elimination, communication, rest and activity schedules, transportation, socialization, and continued contact with health care professionals.

Through *medication assessment*, the nurse determines if the patient and caregiver know the purpose of medications and how to give them. Have the patient or family caregiver responsible for giving medications show you the medicines. In the home setting, patients and families must be alert not only to untoward effects and side effects, but also which medications are ineffective. They must anticipate dosage and schedules so they do not run out of medications at times when pharmacies are not open. Assessing actual dose taken versus prescribed dose is critical, since there may be various reasons why patients and families change the dosage, including finances or forgetfulness. They do not want to be labeled as "bad patients," so they may state the prescribed dose as the actual dose. Therefore, ask about daily routine of what is taken and when. Request that the patient count the remaining number of pills in the prescription to determine how many were taken and if that number is correct according to the prescription.

Nutrition assessment includes collection of subjective data that the patient is tolerating foods or special diets, as well as objective data such as weight and calorie counts.

When determining nutritional status, the nurse should also assess the patient's hydration. Family members may have difficulty forcing fluids or restricting intake, if these are necessary. The home health care nurse can support the caregiver in these efforts.

Assessment of knowledge of emergency procedures is necessary with each family. Every family should demonstrate their ability to use the community's emergency telephone system and to call the home health nurse for less serious situations. They can be taught cardiopulmonary resuscitation (CPR) if they desire or need this information. Equipment checks are a very specific and important part of home care assessment. Typically, each piece of equipment comes with a manual that outlines the safety checks, cleaning procedures, and routine maintenance. The family must understand the manuals and incorporate safety checks into everyday schedules. Box 47-5 outlines a checklist for a mechanical ventilator equipment check that is followed by a home care nurse to assess the family's ability to manage the ventilator–dependent patient safely at home. The specific equipment check itself is more detailed and follows specific information provided by the manufacturer. The guidelines for home mechanical ventilation developed by a national commission should be used.[37]

Assessment of specific emergency procedures, home environment, and special patient needs are all based on the patient's particular treatment plan. Box 47-6 lists the assessment required to determine the needs of a family with home care of an adult member who is dependent on mechanical ventilation. The nurse observes the family's and patient's handling of procedures such as suctioning and tracheostomy care to assess their abilities to provide the care correctly. After assessing the patient's specific care needs, as dictated by the treatment plan, the nurse turns to data gathering and resources available to the family.

Family assessment

Family assessment is essential because the success of home care depends on the family members' or significant others' ability to draw on and use internal and external resources. *Internal resources* include the family's or individual's posi-

tive attitude toward home care, ability to solve problems or seek advice, and willingness to accept help or assistance from *external resources*. Accepting help from friends, neighbors, and church or community groups often is difficult for families because of the strong value of independence in U.S. culture. The home health nurse can determine the availability of these and other external resources and then assess the family's willingness to accept such help.

Each family member's reactions to the role he or she carries out in relation to home care influences the family's internal resources. A grown child working full time might not be able to help with the patient's daily physical care but might contribute grocery shopping. The home care nurse may need to assess periodically family members' role responsibilities in home care as these change over time. Also, individuals' reaction to their responsibilities and energy to carry them out vary with the length of time that caregiving continues (see research abstract in Box 47-7). Families also react to changes in the patient's condition, whether improved, declined, or stabilized, during home care. Interview questions that can be used to assess caregiver roles and reactions are listed in Box 47-8. Many times negative reactions to caregiving can be improved by obtaining relief such as *respite care* or financial assistance for the family.

Data Analysis: Nursing Diagnoses

Nursing diagnoses are based on the assessment data collected in the home and on the data gathered from discharge planning. These data are analyzed to identify the patient's and family's human responses to the pathologic condition, medical regimen, treatment plan, and home nursing care. The nursing diagnoses should reflect each family's actual and potential problems and strengths. By diagnosing strengths, the nurse identifies abilities the family can use

---

Nursing Research | 47-7

Smith C, Mayer L, Pingleton S: Caregiver perceptions of managing home ventilation, *Am Rev Respir Dis* 139(suppl)(4):A196, 1989.

This study gathered data on the support services, coping strategies, and perceived knowledge or skill needs of families with an adult receiving home ventilation. Twenty caregivers of ventilated homebound patients were interviewed using four instruments. Patients, aged 17 to 74 years, were receiving 24 hours (8 patients), 14 to 15 hours (4 patients), or 8 to 12 hours (6 patients) of positive-pressure ventilation.

The results revealed that caregivers, all of whom were relatives, provided an average of 7.3 hours per day of direct care, including daily bathing, feeding, or assistance with walking. Nine caregivers could leave the patient alone; six could not. Only two reported using support services. *The Caregiving Inventory* revealed more disrupted schedules, financial strain, increased burden, and negative reaction to caregiving with increasing ventilator hours. *The Family Coping Scales* revealed caregivers and patient used predominantly internal coping skills. The *Family Functioning APGAR* revealed satisfaction with overall family function. Caregivers rated all 57 items on the *Learning Needs Checklist* from needed to very needed. Only three items, ventilator checks, suctioning, and tracheotomy care, were taught to all caregivers. Fourteen needed items were not taught to one third or more of the caregivers.

Conclusions of this study are that (1) greater than 12 hours per day on the ventilator is disruptive to caregivers; (2) caregivers *do* cope but largely use their own internal resources; and (3) survival knowledge and skills are taught, but additional information is needed. Further efforts should be directed toward support and education of caregivers.

47-8

Caregiver role assessment

1. How have the responsibilities of the members of the family changed since the patient has been at home?
2. How do you and other family members feel about these changes in responsibility?
3. Has your health changed since you have been caring for the patient at home? If so, describe how.
4. Family members tell us they have emotional reactions to the changes in the person they are caring for. What has your experience been with these emotional reactions?
5. Family members often state that responsibilities of home care can be overwhelming and difficult. Tell me how you are managing your responsibilities.
6. Family members also have found they have gained strengths or sense that they are successful in caring for the patient at home. Do you find this to be true or not true? Tell me about when you haven't felt successful. Tell me the successes you've experienced.

in dealing with the actual and potential problems they will face. Analyzing the data to determine the coping skills, external resources, and other family strengths is essential because most must eventually manage the home care alone.

The patient and family may be experiencing *translocation syndrome* related to moving from the acute care setting into the home. The stress response to transferring from one health care setting to another has been measured in several studies. Nurses have found that when patients are prepared for transfer well before the relocation takes place, less stress is experienced. In preparing for discharge to the home, the nurse must anticipate the stress or anxiety that the patient or family may experience when leaving the environment of the acute care setting, where health care professionals are readily available. Extensive preparation through teaching and involvement of the patient and family in coordinating resources that are readily accessible and economically feasible lessens the translocation syndrome.

The following nursing diagnoses may be experienced in families who manage home care. The nursing diagnoses presented in this section are based on information from experienced home care nurses, nursing research studies, and data from studies of adults in the home. These diagnoses have been categorized into problem areas of *resource management*, *family dysfunction*, and *knowledge deficits*.

Resource management is the ability to obtain and effectively use resources both inside and outside the family for the patient's home care. Resources may include people, equipment, and monies. Resource management is discussed in more depth under the section on Implementation.

Nursing diagnoses based on resource management
Home maintenance management, impaired

Insufficient financial resources are a common problem reported by families at home. Reimbursements from insurance companies or Medicare vary widely and are constantly changing. The home care nurse must be skilled in understanding government regulations and advocating for the patient's eligibility for coverage. The nurse may enlist the help of a social worker familiar with home care coverage codes and regulations to ensure that information on the costs of home care covered by insurers is made available to the family. In addition, the nurse needs to identify any voluntary sources of financial support for families. Some private agencies, such as the American Cancer Society, may provide bandages, equipment, or other care services free or at a nominal charge.

The nurse must also be concerned about specialty services available to the family. In some instances, the technical support services needed by the patient may be at such a distance that safety is a concern. When this occurs, the nurse must ensure that the family recognizes and can readily manage emergencies such as equipment failure or lack of supplies.

Self-care deficit, bathing/hygiene, dressing/ grooming, feeding, toileting

In many instances the patient requires daily physical care such as feeding, bathing, or assistance with grooming or toileting. Also, technical care, including tracheal suctioning, wound irrigation, or intravenous fluid adminis-

tration, may be required. Family members provide a wide variety of physical care at home for patients undergoing chemotherapy, those debilitated with Alzheimer's disease, or those recovering from a cerebral vascular accident (CVA).

Family members' fatigue and stress are problems the home care nurse must address. The family may be a closed system that does not desire help from the outside or feels shame when they cannot provide care by themselves. When this occurs, the nurse may need to use value clarification strategies with the family to assist them in problem solving with this issue. The nurse employs several other counseling techniques with psychologically related nursing diagnoses.

Decisional conflict related to stress imposed by long-term home care

Dealing with the patient's chronic disability and the home care management creates constraints on family members' daily schedules and use of the home for activities. The family must make many decisions each day about the patient's home care. These decisions may result in conflicts among family members. The patient and family have direct responsibility for managing such conflicts. Patients and families experiencing chronic illness must live with the constraints imposed by the disease and the home care. Therefore, the nurse may use *conflict resolution strategies* to ensure an equitable decision-making process.

Diversional activity deficit

Patients with chronic disease, visible disabilities, or equipment as part of their treatment report experiences of negative *social stigma*. Friends may fear that activities are a physical strain for the patient with a chronic illness. Extended family may believe visiting the home causes the family more grief over the patient's disability. Employers may believe that the presence of medical equipment such as oxygen tubing makes the workplace unappealing to customers. Many people feel uncomfortable around visible changes in the patient and environment and avoid visiting. Potential visitors may feel vulnerable, "If it happens to her, it can happen to me." The patient and family need assistance to anticipate these problems and suggestions on how to deal with such reactions. Patients receiving Medicare must be homebound to have home care. This imposes an additional stigma on the patient who is striving for or needs diversional activity.

Nursing diagnoses based on family dysfunction

When data from home care assessment are analyzed, nursing diagnoses related to family dysfunction may be apparent. Home care puts many demands on families. Meeting these demands can cause physical fatigue of individual members and a variety of psychologic dysfunctions within the family.

Adjustment, impaired

Caring for a family member in the home may alter individual members' everyday activities, interactions, and pattern of social contacts. Participation in religious, leisure, and school activities may be affected. Shifting household responsibilities may make some family members feel overworked. These changes in life-style may be permanent or temporary, depending on the patient's situation and the resources available to the family. The nurse can assist family members to predict the disruptions that home care might create and to support them in adjusting to these disruptions.

Coping, ineffective family: compromised

The length of home care has an effect on the coping within the family. The longer that home care is required, the more the family's coping skills can become depleted. More situational crises arise during prolonged home care, which also challenges families' coping abilities. Other factors that impact family coping abilities, include past experiences and realistic expectations of home care. The family is better able to cope with prolonged home care when positive past experiences such as the length of home care and daily schedule have been predictable.

Family processes, altered

Home care generally disorganizes a family at least temporarily. Communication patterns are altered. Meaningful interactions such as confidential talks, teasing, or humorous exchanges and physical comforting by hugs may decrease. Until the feeling of disruption ebbs and a sense of predictability returns, family processes are disrupted. Ask the family to describe how home care has changed family function. Their own description helps clarify the alterations in communications and personal exchanges they are missing. Steps to rekindle these helpful family processes should be instituted.

Role performance, altered

The spouse may manage the home caregiver role by drastically altering a previously fulfilling role (for example, cook-housekeeper, financial planner). The designated caregiver may perceive home care as an overwhelming burden. The studies of caregiver burden indicate that it is the *perceived* burden more than the actual physical or financial drain that predict role performance problems.[18] Interventions for altered role performance include teaching about new responsibilities and social support. *Social support* in the form of helping with everyday care, contacts with a network of peers, acceptance of caregiving by family members, and provision of emotional concern or praise to the caregiver seem to assist with the perception of burden.

Nursing diagnoses based on knowledge deficits

Nursing diagnoses based on knowledge deficits are frequently seen in home health care.[50] Subjective and objective data from the patient and family must be scrutinized to determine the specific etiologic factor leading to the knowledge deficit. Several common causes of knowledge deficit are discussed here.

Knowledge deficit related to the transfer of learning into the home setting

Patients and families often state that carrying out procedures they were taught or they observed in the hospital seem more complicated once they come home. Health care personnel not immediately available may decrease the per-

son's confidence. Adaptations in procedures may be necessary in the home and such adaptations may be difficult for family members or patients to devise. The complexity of scheduling the total care, including bathing, feeding, and technical treatments, may be difficult. The varied aspects of transferring learning into the home need to be discussed with the family before the patient's discharge. An emphasis on problem solving that incorporates the patient and family environment, including daily routines, is helpful. Make sure the family realizes they can contact the home health agency if they have questions between visits.

Knowledge deficit related to psychologic state (anxiety)

Another personal factor that can make a difference in the patient's and family's learning is their mental or psychologic state. Much has been written about how anxiety affects people's perceptions and behavior. It is generally accepted that individuals who have moderate to severe anxiety may only be able to focus on their immediate concerns. Consequently, the information given when the patient is moderately anxious may be so distorted that the patient may not learn what is intended. Hospitalization may increase a person's anxiety level. Nurses may need to employ methods to reduce anxiety so that the patient and family can attend to learning. For some patients, technical equipment may be overwhelming and create increased anxiety. The nurse initially may need to do the technical care and gradually teach self-care as the patient or family is able to manage it.

Knowledge deficit related to the patient's physiologic state

Physical factors also play a significant part in the patient's knowledge deficit. These factors may include the presence of acute illness or pain, fluid and electrolyte imbalance, altered nutritional states, lack of endurance, or medications, each of which can alter mental alertness. Other physical factors related to treatments may also interfere with motor abilities and learning.

Certain electrolyte and nutritional states also alter the patient's cognitive functioning. The patient may be confused or hallucinate or may simply be too weak to devote the necessary energy to learning. After the electrolyte imbalance is corrected, the patient is better able to concentrate and learn. Patients may lack the physical energy to perform a psychomotor task, such as a dressing change, or they may lack the mental energy to concentrate on learning. Arthritic changes with advancing age may make fingers less functional for fine motor tasks. The tactile perception in the elderly may also be reduced so that manipulation of small objects, such as needles and syringes, can be very frustrating. Nurses must determine any physical changes that might hamper learning and take steps to alleviate these barriers when teaching patients and families.

Knowledge deficit related to cultural and socioeconomic factors

Socioeconomic and cultural factors may also influence the patient's response to teaching. These factors can include a language barrier, cultural background as related to health practices, or lack of finances to purchase necessary home care equipment. The following patient example is used to illustrate how several of these factors impact learning.

> A patient from a mid-Eastern culture had a transverse colostomy and recovered very well. She needed home care because she showed no interest in the colostomy or in performing any of the needed care. In her culture, it was taboo to allow a member of her family to touch her body, yet she could not afford home care services and was uninsured. An interpreter interviewed the patient and it was determined that a neighbor, also of her culture, was willing to learn colostomy care and eventually teach the patient self-care. Once the nurse learned about the taboo her attention was focused on teaching the neighbor, who in turn could instruct the patient at home.

This situation illustrates how important it is to consider all factors affecting patient teaching.

Knowledge deficit related to health beliefs

Folk practices impact home health care, and nurses may include these remedies (when safe) in their teaching. It is always good practice to ask patients what they believe will add to their success in home care management, and try to incorporate folk remedies the families feel necessary. Because the patient controls his or her own care, folk practices may be used and the health care professional may be unaware of it.

Knowledge deficit related to illiteracy

Literacy reports suggest that less than 20% of the adult population reads above the fifth grade level, and that the median literacy of the United States population is approximately at the tenth grade level. Many times the educational materials distributed are above the patient's reading levels. A mismatch of written material with the patient's reading ability can account for unsuccessful learning for the patient.

Both the printed word and the vocabulary used by the nurse should be at an appropriate level for the patient. Results of patient education studies indicated that common "medical words" are not understood by patients. Words such as "hematoma," "secretions," and "post-op" were incorrectly defined by a large majority of those surveyed. How often do nurses use those words in their teaching and assume that the patient understands what they mean? Even for functionally literate patients, the stress associated with illness may reduce their comprehension of spoken words, written materials, and even visual teaching resources. Teaching and reteaching, with opportunities for patients to ask about terms and ideas they do not understand, are important aspects of treating knowledge deficits. Reteaching patients may not be reimbursed, so further education may be included in other care or be charged to the family.

Planning: Expected Patient Outcomes

Planning is directed by the outcomes expected to result from home health care. Statements are made of expected outcomes so that the patient, family, and the home health nurse agree that the outcomes are realistic and measurable. Expected outcomes are based on the patient's condition as reflected in nursing diagnoses, standards of nursing practice, and results from clinical research studies. See the following section for examples of planning home care.

Implementation

Implementation of home care nursing for the adult patient is based on discharge planning, assessment data, nursing diagnoses, and expected patient outcomes *negotiated with the family.* The critical nursing interventions of resource management, counseling, and teaching are implemented with every family. *Resource management includes coordination of services, products, and personnel necessary for cost-effective home care.* The interventions implemented by the home care nurse depends on the internal and external resources available to the family. Coordinating the resources, counseling, and providing information are essential aspects of the nurse's role in home care implementation. See the following section for examples of implementing home care.

Examples of planning and implementing home care

Home intravenous antibiotic therapy

Many clinical studies have established that home intravenous antibiotic therapy (HIAT) is a safe approach for many adult patients. The number of patients dependent on intravenous therapy discharged to home care has increased dramatically. Medical center hospitals and private agencies provide discharge planning and home care for patients receiving HIAT.

Patients are discharged from the hospital when the signs and symptoms of acute infection are under control. Then, when the following expected outcomes have been met, the patient is ready for home teaching:

1. Patient and family agree to manage HIAT.
2. Patient has peripheral vein catheter in place.
3. Family has created a suitable environment in the home for infusion therapy.
4. Arrangements have been made for supplies, medication, laboratory blood studies, and emergency care.

When met, these expected outcomes ensure that the resources necessary for successful HIAT are available to the patient. The first expected outcome of eliciting the patient's and family's agreement to manage HIAT is essential. If the family is not motivated to undertake this complicated therapy, difficulties arise with home care.

Patients receive HIAT *to treat many infections,* including osteomyelitis, endocarditis, urinary tract infections, septic arthritis, cellulitis, pyelonephritis, pelvic inflammatory disease, prostatitis, and complications from medical devices inserted into the body. The National Center for Health Statistics conducted a hospital discharge survey and determined that approximately 51,000 cases of primary and secondary osteomyelitis and 11,000 cases of bacterial endocarditis were diagnosed in 1981.[59] The incidence of such infections, coupled with physician and industry efforts to secure Medicare funding for HIAT, are likely to increase the numbers of patients receiving HIAT.

Researchers have not only documented the efficacy, safety, and cost savings of the infusions in the home, but also that teaching patients and families to manage intravenous antibiotics can be done effectively in the home. Nursing interventions can be determined based on the

	Nursing diagnoses and expected outcomes for the person receiving HIAT	
47-9	**Nursing diagnoses**	**Expected outcomes**
	Coping, ineffective family: compromised, related to ambivalence toward HIAT	Patient or family member (1) state rationale for HIAT, (2) demonstrate readiness to learn by handling equipment or asking questions, and (3) state they agree to undertake HIAT.
	Infection, high risk for acute exacerbation	Patient remains free of high-grade fever and other signs of infection specific to the patient (for example, cough, sputum for pneumonia; painful joint for osteomyelitis).
	Knowledge deficit: management of HIAT related to new treatment	Patient or family member demonstrate each step of HIAT using safe, aseptic technique.

nursing diagnoses and expected patient outcomes (see Box 47-9).

It is helpful to have more than one expected outcome for each diagnosis to provide more than one objective criterion for measuring the results of nursing interventions. The data that need to be gathered to evaluate the results should be readily available and inexpensive. White blood cell (WBC) counts or wound culture laboratory tests may be the most definitive way of determining acute exacerbation of infection, but they are expensive and relatively difficult to obtain and would not be used unless other data (high fever and so forth) indicate that the expected outcomes have not been met. *Expected outcomes used in home care must be simple to use and analyze. The patient and family must collect most of the data needed to judge if expected outcomes are met because they monitor their own home care. If the data collected are difficult for the patient to obtain (for example, unable to read small markings on a thermometer or unable to determine color changes on the chemical strips used to check nitrates indicating urine infection), another person in the home must be taught to gather this information.*

Procedures in implementing HIAT

The overall expected outcome with HIAT is that the patient's infection will be eliminated. However, because HIAT requires complicated technical care, expected outcomes that reflect the patient's and family member's ability to undertake each aspect of HIAT must be carefully written. Box 47-10 lists the 18 steps in the procedure typically used for infusing antibiotics. It is clear from these steps that the terminology the patient must learn just to read these directions can be overwhelming. It is important that instructions not be initiated before patients accept the idea of self-administration and learn some of the common terms.

Before infusions can be undertaken by patients, they need clear understanding of the reasons for the therapy and why it takes place in the home. The presence of an intravenous needle often signifies to the family that the individual is very ill and that the connection to the tubing means the patient should be bedridden with restricted activities. Families may experience anxiety over the patient's condition and may have ineffective coping related to wanting the patient home yet being afraid to manage HIAT. Patients and families need reassurance that continued in-

travenous therapy can be safety conducted in the home. They need to understand that any patient has a potential for an acute exacerbation of infection and may require rehospitalization. The signs of acute infection are listed for them so that they feel confident in deciding when to call for help. The advantages of being mobile and returning to work and household activities are presented to them. Today, most antibiotic home infusions can be given through indwelling catheters.

Home total parenteral nutrition

Estimates[22a] indicate that approximately $500 million per year is spent on reimbursement of nonhospitalized persons receiving home total parenteral nutrition (HTPN). In the late 1980s, at least 14,000 adults were managing TPN at home. Of the patients receiving HTPN, the largest percentage (37.3%) have benign bowel disease such as Crohn's and ischemic bowel disease. Persons with neoplasms and with acquired immunodeficiency syndrome (AIDS) constitute 25% of the patients receiving HTPN. The remaining percentages are spread among patients with other benign illnesses such as motility or swallowing disorders and adhesions.

Most patients (70% to 80%) with benign bowel diseases require lifelong TPN. About three quarters of patients with Crohn's disease and one half of patients with ischemic bowel disease receiving HTPN return to full- or part-time employment. It is generally acknowledged that more patients also might return to work if it were not for Medicare and private insurance stipulations requiring that individuals be unemployed to receive disability payments. Disability payments are necessary because HTPN therapy is very expensive ($40,000 to $200,000 per year).

Resource management

Ideally, the family who is managing long-term HTPN has access to a team of professionals as well as various resources from the community. Many medical centers have a nutritional support team that educates patients about HTPN before discharge.

Commercial agencies have developed teams that give advice on location and storage of products in the home, equipment necessary for implementation, and telephone service for emergencies. Because these agencies are avail-

Procedures expected of patients receiving HIAT

47-10

1. Each morning, review the scheduled times for your medication and plan your activities to allow enough time for the infusion
   a. One-half hour before the scheduled infusion, check your temperature and compare this on the graph to the previous day's level. Check the insertion site of your intravenous (IV) catheter (teach patients to look for signs of infection and irritation and stability of catheter in the vein). If problems exist with the catheter, call the home care nurse, who may be able to provide appropriate instructions.
   b. Draw up antibiotic medication in syringe. (If premixed solutions are not available, several other steps specific to mixing are added here.)
2. Remove the bag of IV solution from the refrigerator 15 minutes before administration to allow it to warm up.
3. Check the expiration date and dosage of any premixed solutions.
4. Draw heparin-saline solution into a syringe if premixed solution is not available and replace the cover on the needle.
5. Hang the IV bag on a hanger above your arm.
6. Squeeze the drip chamber and purge all air from the tubing, making sure fluid is in the drip chamber.
7. Cleanse the rubber stopper of your IV catheter with an alcohol swab for 1 minute.
8. Remove the cap from the needle at the end of the IV tubing.
9. Insert needle into the gummed rubber stopper of your IV catheter.
10. Establish a flow rate by adjusting the flow-control clamp so that solution in the ___ ml bag will take ___ minutes to infuse. That means that ___ drops of solution must fall into the drip chamber every 30 seconds. (Blanks are filled in by nurse.)
11. Check flow rate periodically. When the infusion is completed, remove the needle from the gummed rubber stopper.
12. Replace the cap over the needle.
13. Wipe off the gummed rubber stopper again with an alcohol swab.
14. Remove the cap from the syringe containing the heparin-saline solution and inject it into the gummed rubber stopper.
15. Remove the needle of the syringe from the gummed rubber stopper and replace the cap over the needle.
16. Carefully dispose of needles so that no one will be accidentally injured (use a coffee can with cover; this may be brought to the hospital pharmacy later for proper disposal).
17. Record on your monitoring sheet that infusion was completed and that IV insertion site looks normal.
18. If you have any questions, call the hospital and ask the pharmacist or IV nurse for assistance.

able in many locations across the country, the patient and care giver may travel and arrange for equipment and solutions to be delivered to their destination. Most hospital-based and commercial teams include nurses, physicians, pharmacists, social workers, dietitians, and consulting psychiatrists.

The nurse typically directs the team by calling on the physician and social worker for discharge planning, the pharmacists and dietitians for monitoring the medical and nutrition therapy, and the psychiatrists for counseling the patient and family. Emotional reactions to the dependency on this lifelong technologic care can be overwhelming and may require periodic or long-term psychologic interventions. Unfortunately, not all families have access to such sophisticated teams, so their resources may consist of a nurse from a physician's office, a technician from an equipment company, and the physician.

Counseling for long-term HTPN

The initial psychologic reaction of many patients and family members to HTPN is relief. The relief results from the immediate improvement in the patient's condition. For example, patients with Crohn's disease may be relieved of bowel pain and diarrhea and patients with cancer may be better nourished. Following the initial relief, however, other psychologic reactions require counseling interventions from the nurse.

Psychologic reactions to long-term HTPN

Families often experience anxiety related to learning about complicated technologic care in the home setting. After 3 or 4 months of home care, however, patients may

---

Nursing Research

47-11

Heaphey L: Survey results provide insight into psychosocial issues, *Life Lett Oley Foundation* 9(6):1-2, 1988.

A survey by the Oley Foundation of 172 HTPN families indicates that family members' and patients' perspectives differ on the problems experienced and the resources most helpful in adapting to HTPN.[38] Spouses reported guilt about their ability to eat, distress at social gatherings with food, and concern about eating out. However, patients indicated spouses' ability to eat and eating out were not problems. Body image distortions and sexual difficulties were problems patients ranked as continuing and significant, although spouses did not report these as important issues. This survey highlighted the differences in the patients' and spouses'/caregivers' reactions to HTPN. The third-ranked problem listed by both patient and spouse was "relationships with spouse," especially communication. Yet patients ranked their spouses as their number-one resource for helping with psychosocial problems. The nurse from the physician's office or home care service was ranked second, gastroenterologist third, hospital nurse fourth, and another family member fifth. Very few patients listed another HTPN patient or someone outside the family as a helpful resource. The nurse can assist the patient and spouse to communicate openly about the problems of HTPN.

Table 47-2   Implementation plan for teaching HTPN for up to 10 days

Day	Physical care	Psychologic care	Emergency care
1	If patient has been pretrained and is not overly tired from discharge, have patient demonstrate HTPN. If he/she is too fatigued, have him/her talk about the steps of HTPN while family member carries out procedure.	Give reassurance by pointing out the abilities patient demonstrates or discusses. Describe other families who have succeeded with HTPN.	Demonstrate clamping TPN catheter in emergency; post emergency telephone numbers so family member can call for help.
2	Observe patient set up TPN solution bags, syringes, and medications as taught before discharge.	Decide with patient what aspects of the procedure can be managed independently, and set a calendar for learning the total care.	Describe the signs of water intoxication (confusion, weakness, neck vein distention, puffy eyelids, increased urination) that may occur when TPN is given over 12 hours at home.
3	Make sure patient knows how to weigh self and take temperature daily. Repeat setting up TPN solutions and teach about medications to be taken.	Compliment patient on (1) being able to monitor effects of nutrition therapy by monitoring weight daily, (2) detecting hazards of infection by taking temperature daily, and (3) knowing medication side effects.	Have patient practice with needle caps for appropriate disposal. Reinforce use of aseptic technique and handwashing.
4	Demonstrate use of infusion pump. Have the patient insert the intravenous line into TPN solution bag.	Have the patient review the written instruction manual. Point out how well he/she has followed directions. Encourage patient to write notes in own words in the printed manual.	If signs of water toxicity are present, draw blood laboratory samples for serum sodium, plasma protein, and hematocrit levels.
5 and 6	Have patient set up infusion pump, adjust flow rates, and stop infusion. Discuss timing and scheduling of infusions.	Help family establish an area where TPN supplies can be safely stored and handled. Have the nutrition team, psychiatrist, or clinical nurse specialist telephone to offer support.	Teach patient how to clear air from the tubing. Discuss importance of daily tubing changes to prevent infection.
7	Have patient correct minor problems that may occur with equipment and infusion pumps, such as responding to alarms or troubleshooting back flow of solution.	Begin a record that monitors patient's infusion schedule, need to purchase supplies, daily weight and temperature, medications, laboratory results, and symptoms. Use the records to illustrate patient's self-care abilities.	Use the sign/symptom list (Table 47-3) to identify emergencies that may occur over long-term use of HTPN.
8	Have patient demonstrate catheter care, including inspection of insertion site, dressing changes, catheter cap and extension change, capped heparinization, and connections.	Suggest that family member who is also learning the procedure observe the patient's technique and that they periodically review the manual together.	Demonstrate procedure for repair of a catheter that develops a leak or begins bleeding around inspection site and injection cap, as well as procedure when adapter becomes dislodged.
9	Discuss various side effects and complications of TPN: catheter site infection, solution bag contamination, blood glucose variations, and physical complications.	Emphasize that patient and family member will be the first to recognize metabolic or physical side effects of the therapy and that they then should notify the home care nurse promptly.	Hyperglycemia or hypoglycemia is monitored daily by self-blood glucose monitoring. Serum electrolytes are drawn weekly.
10	Have patient demonstrate each aspect of care following the printed manual.	Review the patient's record keeping and discuss the information. Point out how confident the patient is in managing own home care. Emphasize that telephone contact can be made with home care personnel.	Patient must be prepared for emergencies that occur after long-term use of HTPN, including sepsis, catheter displacement or damage, and psychologic disorders such as anxiety, depression, alcohol or drug addiction problems, and mood disorders related to machine dependency.

Table 47-3 Signs/symptoms and problems experienced by HTPN patients*

Signs/symptoms	Problem	Actions
Swelling of skin over catheter insertion site; sensations of pain, heat, burning near site	Possible leak in catheter at place of swelling	Call home health nurse or physician. Do not use catheter to give fluids. Tape the catheter securely to the skin so that it does not dangle. Avoid rough contact or sports that could dislodge catheter.
Leak of blood from injection cap or catheter	Possible loose cap or leak in catheter	Clamp catheter. Change cap and heparin lock. Go to emergency room for catheter repair or call physician.
Cough, shortness of breath, chest pain	Possible air embolism (air in blood) Air may be drawn into the vein if catheter is not clamped during cap change	If giving fluids, stop and place heparin lock on catheter. Lie on left side. Call physician or go to emergency room.
Redness, swelling, drainage, tenderness at exit site	Skin infection or irritation	Call home health nurse or physician. Change bandage and clean daily. Change the bandage and clean around the catheter if bandage gets wet or soiled.
Chills, fever, fatigue, aches, weakness	Possible infection within the bloodstream	Go to emergency room for tests.

*Patients should always wash hands before starting any procedures and if they have a rash or cuts and scrapes on their hands, gloves are worn for all the procedures. All supplies used on catheter are kept sterile. Aseptic technique is used.

experience depression related to the complexity of long-term or lifelong therapy and the constant presence of technology in their daily lives. Issues of lack of control and dependence, as well as relationship and role changes within the family, typically occur. The research abstract in Box 47-11 describes the spouse's role changes and reactions of the patient receiving HTPN.

Counseling can also involve providing information. Thorough patient teaching about HTPN, as shown in Table 47-2, and discussion of signs and symptoms, problems, and concomitant actions (Table 47-3) can reassure families that they can implement the necessary care.

Evaluation

The last step of the nursing process is evaluation. Evaluation is making a judgment as to whether home care has been successful. This judgment depends on comparison of the patient's and family's status with the expected outcomes of home care.

If expected outcomes have not been achieved, the reasons for this are ascertained. If the patient's physical function falls short of the expected outcomes, the nurse must identify factors contributing to this problem. The nurse may see signs that the patient's pathophysiologic condition is worsening. Referral to the physician or arrangements for transportation to a medical facility may be necessary. Evaluation might reveal that the expected outcomes have not been achieved because of factors other than the patient's physical condition. The patient may have misunderstood what he or she was taught, the resources arranged at discharge may not have been obtained, or the family members may have found home care overwhelming. Another reason expected outcomes are not met is that they may have been unrealistic to achieve in the time allotted.

The nurse reassesses the situation and establishes new outcomes with the patient and family.

Evaluation may also reveal many instances where patients have achieved their expected outcomes. The nurse should acknowledge this with the patient and family. When families are given recognition for their achievements, they feel supported in their efforts. Evaluation data, whether indicative of achievement or not, must be documented, with the rationale related to the outcomes. Evaluation data may be used for justification for reimbursement of extended home care or for the involvement of other home care resources. For Medicare home health benefits to be continued beyond the 2 to 3 weeks of intermittent care allowable, "exceptional circumstances" must be proved. Many patients may qualify for up to 3 months of home care reimbursement when the nurse provides data that document the need for continued home care.

Quality assurance

Quality assurance is another aspect of evaluation. Quality assurance is a formal process of aggregating data to form a basis to evaluate groups of patients and various aspects of care. Examples of quality assurance data obtained about groups of patients are listed in Box 47-12.

These data can be used to project trends in home care services for a particular group of patients. The data from nursing care hours and types of home services used can help identify personnel needed in home health care. Medical and nursing diagnoses help establish appropriate case management. The financial data can be used to plan future services, budget for weekend services, recruit specific types of personnel needed in a home care agency, and justify programs to policymakers.

One of the most interesting aspects of quality assurance

<table>
<tr><td>47-12</td><td>

Quality assurance data for patients receiving home health care

Types and length of nursing and other home services

Nursing and medical diagnoses

Age, sex, income level, and other demographic data

Age and relationship of family members providing care to the patient

Source of the patient's referral

Source of payment for home care services

</td></tr>
</table>

is the use of data from multiple families to evaluate nursing care. The case records or charts of several patients can be reviewed to determine if specific nursing interventions were successful or if the amount of resources used were adequate. Using quality assurance processes, nurses in home care can establish *cost-effective interventions*. Nurses can be leaders in developing home care programs that promote the highest possible level of health and function for a specific adult population. Quality assurance processes and evaluation of individual families can also be used to identify issues and other concerns pertinent to home care. Some of these issues are discussed next.

Issues in home care

Many issues affect how nurses practice home care. These include factors that affect delivery of care such as the cost of nursing services, availability of services, and community resources and patient or family responses to home care. Also, competition often occurs between different home care delivery services. Reimbursement for professional nurses versus home health aides may influence who provides care. Scarcity of services for technologically dependent patients may limit care in some locales. Communities with few resources (free clinics, volunteer agencies, self-care groups) may be unable to provide support for families caring for adults in the home. *Home care nurses can bring the issues of affordable home care, national health insurance, and development of resources for home care of the elderly to legislature or community groups for resolution.*

Many issues arise in everyday care of individuals in the home. As with nursing of adults in any setting, the individual may elect not to follow prescribed regimens. Families may refuse the medical and nursing care available to them. Third-party reimbursement may not pay for professional nursing services. Nurses may observe or suspect abuse or neglect of the patient as family caregivers become overwhelmed with the patient's care. Also, there may be sociocultural or religious conflicts between the family and health care professional's approach to the patient's care. *The home care nurse must identify such conflicts and other issues and discuss these with the patient, family, or other health professionals.*

Caring for various groups of patients also highlights issues particular to each group. Caregiver fatigue, social isolation, and role change are problematic in many cases. The need for custodial or respite care also may be apparent.

Care of dying patients in the home has increased significantly with the success of the hospice movement. The family's coping skills and a focus on palliative care become issues in long-term terminal care. *Home care nurses must be open to discussion of spiritual concerns, life review, and reconciliation.*

Another challenge comes from patients at home who require rehabilitative care. Persons with neuromuscular diseases, CVAs, or spinal cord injuries may require assistance of physical and occupational therapists. Patients with AIDS may need assessment by infection control specialists for home care. Patients with Alzheimer's disease may benefit from mental health or gerontology specialists. Other specialists also may need to be available to patients in their home, such as speech or respiratory therapists. Transportation to clinics and rehabilitation centers may need to be arranged. Services to enhance persons' abilities to manage their own care increase costs but are essential to self-care. The issue of providing the needed services for home care in the most cost-effective manner will continue to be a challenging issue in the 1990s.

SUMMARY

1. Providing nursing care to the ill adult in the home will be an increasing challenge in the decades ahead. In the mid-1980s, there were approximately the same number of agencies providing home health care as there were hospitals. Forecasters of health care suggest that hospital closures will continue, whereas home care services will increase by as much as 20% annually throughout the 1990s. Medical-surgical nursing home care will be necessary for a great number of adults.

2. Patients may require one or two home visits or around-the-clock nursing care. The nursing process in home care includes expanded assessment of the individual and the home environment, development of nursing diagnoses based on family data, generation of expected outcomes negotiated with the patient and family, implementation of appropriate care, as well as extensive evaluation of the effectiveness of care.

3. The acuity levels of individuals requiring care in their homes continues to rise, and the technological aspects of care, including use of mechanical equipment or invasive procedures such as intravenous therapies, increases in home care. These factors, coupled with shorter hospital stays, require increasing sophistication in the area of transition care, starting with discharge planning.

4. The uniqueness of the residence as the environment for care must be taken into account with an adult member requiring home care. The nurse employs special skills in gaining trust so that people allow entry into their home environment.

5. The trends responsible for the increasing need for home care nursing include the emphasis on continuity of care, promotion of family involvement in care, economic limitations on expenses in health care, and the aging population demographics.

6. Skills to manage the patient's transition from acute t

home care include discharge planning and case-managed care, which incorporates supervision of many families and advocates cost reductions in health care services.

7. Discharge planning includes resource management, coordination of hospital and community services, and adequate preparation for home care. Family education is based on the research supporting the use of patient instruction with the added dimension of teaching a group, the family. Transition care incorporates the skills of discharge planning and family education, with emphasis on continuity and self-managed care in the home.

8. The nursing process in home care is an expansion of that used with hospitalized patients. Assessment is broadened to include recognition of environmental, financial, social, and community influences on care. The assessment of the patient's condition, psychologic status, and response to treatment is undertaken with regard to family analysis.

9. Data analysis from assessment in home care has resulted in identification of common nursing problems. These nursing problems can be stated as nursing diagnoses such as self-care deficits, ineffective family coping, and knowledge deficits.

10. Expected patient outcomes and implementation in home care can be readily illustrated through examples of patients at home receiving mechanical ventilation, intravenous antibiotic therapy, or total parenteral nutrition. The technology dependent patient exemplifies the needs of those with high physical acuity, complicated teaching requirements, and family coping challenges. Research suggests these needs can be met in a cost-effective manner with high-quality home nursing care.

11. Evaluation of home nursing care is a complicated process that includes quality assurance and identification of issues related to home management. Specific data are needed to evaluate groups of patients managed at home. Availability of resources and national health insurance are some of the issues impacting home nursing care today.

STUDY QUESTIONS

- How would you care for the patient requiring intravenous antibiotic therapy in the home versus in the hospital?
- What approaches would you consider for a patient who needs daily physical care in the home who has no insurance and an elderly spouse?
- What criteria are issued to determine needs for home care following early discharge from the hospital?
- What advantages do transition skill care and case-managed care offer for home care?
- How do the skills of family education in the home differ from individual patient teaching in the hospital?

REFERENCES AND SELECTED READINGS

1. American College of Physicians: Home health care, *Annals Intern Med* 105:454-460, 1986.
2. American College of Physicians Health and Public Policy Committee: Position paper: home health care, *Annals Intern Med* 105:460, 1986.
3. Baille V, Norbeck J, Barnes L: Stress, social support, and psychological distress of family caregivers of the elderly, *Nurs Research* 37:217-222, 1988.
4. Berger M: The cost and efficacy of home care for patients with chronic lung disease, *Med Care* 36(6):566-571, 1988.
5. Bramwell L: Wives' experiences in the support role after husband's first myocardial infarction, *Heart Lung* 15:578-584, 1986.
6. Branch L, et al: A prospective study of incident comprehensive medical home care use among the elderly, *Am J Public Health* 78:255-259, 1988.
7. Brooten D, et al: Early discharge and specialist transition care, *Image J Nurs Sch* 20(2):64-88, 1988.
8. Brooten D, et al: A randomized clinical trial of early hospital discharge and home follow-up of very-low-birthweight infants, *N Engl J Med* 315:934-938, 1986.
9. Cohen S, et al: Taxonomic classification of transitional follow-up care nursing interventions with low birthweight infants, *Clin Nur Spec* 5(1):31-36, 1991.
10.* Cronin C, Maklebust J: Case managed care: capitalizing on the CNS, *Nurs Manage* 20(3):38-47, 1989.
11.* Eichel CJ: Stress and coping in patients on CAPD compared to hemodialysis patients, *American Nephrology Nurses' Association Journal* 13(1):9-13, 1986.
12. Farce R: Home ventilation: an alternative to institutionalization, *Focus Crit Care* 13(6):28-34, 1986.
13. Fitzgerald J, Moore P, Dittus R: The care of the elderly patients with hip fracture: changes since implementation of the prospective payment systems, *N Engl J Med* 319:1392-1397, 1988.
14. Frederick B, Sharp J, Atkins N: Quality of patient care: whose decision? *J Nurs Qual Assur* 2(3):1-10, 1988.
15. George L, Gwyther L: Caregiver well-being: A multidimensional examination of family caregivers of demented adults, *The Gerontologist* 26:253-259, 1986.
16. Gikon F, Kucharski P: A new look at the community: functional health pattern assessment, *J Community Health Nurs* 4(1):21-27, 1987.
17. Gipson W, Sivak E, Gulledge A: Psychological aspects of ventilator dependency, *Psychiatr Med* 5:245-255, 1987.
18. Given BA, et al: Family caregivers of the elderly: involvement and reactions to care, *Arch Psychiatr Nurs* 2:281-288, 1988.
19. Goldsmith J: A radical prescription for hospitals, *Harvard Bus Rev* 67(3):104-111, 1989.
20. Hagen-Moe D: Training, assessment of learning, and follow-up: three components of an effective home parenteral nutrition training program, *Nutr Clin Pract* 25:30-32, 1986.
21.* Harris M: The changing scene in community health nursing, *Nurs Clin North Am* 23:559-568, 1988.
22. Heaphey L: Survey results provide insight into psychosocial issues, *Life Lett Oley Foundation* 9(6):1-2, 1988.
22a. Howard L et al: Four years of North American registry home parenteral nutrition outcome data and their implications for patient management, *Journal of Parenteral and Enteral Nutrition* 15:384-393, 1991.
23. Jacobs M, Goodman G: Psychology and self-help groups, *American Psychologist* 44:536-545, 1989.

*Recommended for student reading.

24. Jernigan DR: Home management of epidural catheters for pain control, *Caring* 5(10):85-91, 1986.

25.* Johnson EA, Jackson JE: Teaching the home care client, *Nurs Clin North Am* 24(3):687-694, 1989.

26. Joint Commission on Accreditation of Health Care Organizations: Quality assurance in managed care organizations, Chicago, 1989.

27. Kerby G, Mayer L, Pingleton S: Nocturnal positive pressure ventilation via nasal mask, *Am Rev Respir Dis* 135:738-740, 1987.

28.* King F, Figge J, Harman P: The elderly coping at home: a study of continuity of nursing care, *J Adv Nurs* 11:41-46, 1986.

29. Larson S: Home IV antibiotic therapy, the primary care physician's role, *Drug Ther* 11:67-74, 1987.

30. Liebermann A: *Community and home health nursing*, Springhouse, Penn, 1990, Springhouse Corp.

31. Luttrell M: Changes in oxygen reimbursement, *Cont Care* 10:14-16, 1989.

32.* Maraldo P: Home care should be the heart of a nursing sponsored national health plan, *Nurs Health Care* 10:301-304, 1989.

33. Martinson I, Widmer A: *Home health care nursing*, Philadelphia, 1989, WB Saunders.

34. Mazzuca S: Does patient education in chronic disease have therapeutic value? *J Chronic Dis* 35:521-529, 1987.

35. Mitchell M: The power of standards, *Nurs Health Care* 10:307-309, 1989.

36. Moore J: Intravenous amrinone therapy at home, *Focus Crit Care* 15:32-37, 1988.

37. O'Donohue W, et al: Long-term mechanical ventilation: guidelines for management in the home and at alternate community sites, *Chest* 90(1):1S-37S, 1986.

38. Oley Foundation. Oasis system home parenteral nutrition studies, Laura Heaphey, 1987, (personal communication).

39. Pasquale DK: A basis for prospective payment for home care, *Image J Nurs Sch* 19:186-191, 1987.

40. Peters D: Development of a community health intensity rating scale, *Nurs Res* 37:202-207, 1988.

41. Peterson K: Psychosocial adjustment of the family caregiver: Home hemodialysis as an example, *Soc Work Health Care* 10(3):15-32, 1985.

42. Phillips E, et al: DRG ripple and the shifting of burden of care to home health nursing and health care, *Nurs Health Care* 10:325-327, 1989.

43. Quiring J: RN perspective of home health care needs of family members, *Kans Nurse* 59(3):9-12, 1985.

44. Reckling J: Abandonment of patients by home health nursing agencies: an ethical analysis of the dilemma, *Adv Nurs Sci* 11(3):70-78, 1989.

45.* Reinhard S: Case managing community services for hip fractured elders, *Orthop Nurs* 7:42-49, 1988.

46. Rew L, et al: Affirm: A nursing model to promote role mastery in family caregivers, *Fam Comm Health* 9(4):52-64, 1987.

47.* Sabu V, et al: A nursing intervention taxonomy for home health care, *Nurs Health Care* 12(6):296-299, 1991.

48. Select Committee on Aging: House of Representatives: paying the price of catastrophic illness: From accidents to Alzheimers, Washington, DC, 1987, US Government Printing Office.

49.* Smith BA: When is "confusion" translocation syndrome, *Am J Nurs* 86:1280-1281, 1986.

50. Smith CE, editor: Patient education: nurses in partnership with other health care professionals, Orlando, 1987, Grune & Stratton.

51.* Smith C, et al: Adaptation in families with a member requiring mechanical ventilation at home, *Heart Lung* 20(4):349-356, 1991.

52. Smith C, Mayer L, Pingleton S: Caregiver perceptions of managing home ventilation, *Am Rev Respir Dis* 139(Suppl 4):A196, 1989.

53. Smith CE, Shorfheide A, Lackey N: Acute to home care: managing the transition, *Kans Nurse* 59(4):9-11, 1985.

Classic

54. Ballard S, McNamara R: Quantifying nursing needs in home health care, *Nurs Res* 32:236-241, 1983.

55. Cantor MH: Strain among caregivers: a study of experience in the United States, *Gerontologist* 23:597-604, 1983.

56. Chang B: Evaluation of health care professionals in facilitating self-care: review of the literature and conceptual model, *Adv Nurs Sci* 3(1):43-45, 1980.

57. Coleman J, Strauss D: DRGs and the growth of home health care, *Nurs Econ* 2:391-395, 1984.

58. Dickson G, Lee-Villasenor H: Nursing theory and practice: A self-care approach, *Adv Nurs Sci* 3(1):29-40, 1982.

59. Division of Health Care Statistics: National hospital discharge survey, Washington, DC, 1981, US Government Printing Office.

60. Duvall E: *Marriage and family development*, Philadelphia, 1977, JB Lippincott.

61. Rasmusen L: A screening tool promotes early discharge, *Nurs Manage* 15(5):39-43, 1984.

62.* Smith CE: With good assessment skills you can construct a solid framework for patient care, *Nursing* 14(12):26-31, 1984.

63. Sullivan T: *Self-care model for nursing: new directions for nursing in the 80's*, Kansas City, Mo, 1980, American Nurses Association.

64. Trager B: *Home health care national healthy policy*, Home Health Care Services Quarterly, New York, 1980, Haworth Press.

65. Zappacostas A, Peras S: CAPD: *Continuous ambulatory peritoneal dialysis*, Philadelphia, 1984, JB Lippincott.

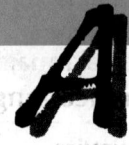

Normal Laboratory Values

Blood, plasma, or serum values

Reference range

Determination	Conventional	SI
Acetoacetate plus acetone	0.3-2.0 mg/100 ml	3-20 mg/l
Aldolase	1.3-8.2 mU/ml	12-75 nmol · s⁻¹/l
Alpha amino nitrogen	3.0-5.5 mg/100 ml	2.1-3.9 mmol/l
Ammonia	80-110 μg/100 ml	47-65 μmol/l
Ascorbic acid	0.4-1.5 mg/100 ml	23-85 μmol/l
Barbiturate	0	0 μmol/l
	Coma level: phenobarbital, approximately 10 mg/100 ml; most other drugs, 1-3 mg per 100 ml	
Bilirubin (van den Bergh test)	One minute: 0.4 mg/100 ml	Up to 7 μmol/l
	Direct: 0.4 mg/100 ml	Up to 17 μmol/l
	Total: 1.0 mg/100 ml	
	Indirect is total minus direct	
Blood volume	8.5-9.0% of body weight in kg	80-85 ml/kg
Bromide	0	0 mmol/l
	Toxic level: 17 mEq/l	
Bromsulfalein (BSP)	Less than 5% retention 45 min after 5 mg/kg IV	<0.05 l
Calcium	8.5-10.5 mg/100 ml (slightly higher in children)	2.1-2.6 mmol/l
Carbon dioxide content	24-30 mEq/l	24-30 mmol/l
	20-26 mEq/l in infants (as HCO₃)	
Carbon monoxide	Symptoms with over 20% saturation	0 (1)
Carotenoids	0.8-4.0 μg/ml	1.5-7.4 μmol/l
Ceruloplasmin	27-37 mg/100 ml	1.8-2.5 μmol/l
Chloride	100-106 mEq/l	100-106 mmol/l
Cholinesterase (pseudocholinesterase)	0.5 pH U or more/h	0.5 or more arb. unit
	0.7 pH U or more/h for packed cells	
Copper	Total: 100-200 μg/100 ml	16-31 μmol/l
Creatine phosphokinase (CPK)	Female 5-35 mU/ml	0.08-0.58
	Male 5-55 mU/ml	μmol · s⁻¹/l
Creatinine	0.6-1.5 mg/100 ml	60-130 μmol/l

Modified from Kaye DA, Rose LF: *Fundamentals of internal medicine*, St Louis, 1983, Mosby–Year Book. Adapted by permission from the New England Journal of Medicine, Vol 302, pages 37-48, 1980.

Abbreviations used: SI, Système international d'Unités (The SI for the Health Professions, World Health Organization, Office of Publications, Geneva Switzerland, 1977); *d*, 24 hours; *P*, plasma; *S*, serum; *B*, blood; *U*, urine; *l*, liter; *h*, hour; and *s*, second.

Continued.

Blood, plasma, or serum values—cont'd
Reference range—cont'd

Determination	Conventional	SI
Ethanol	0.3-0.4%, marked intoxication; 0.4-0.5%, alcoholic stupor; 0.5% or over, alcoholic coma	65-87 mol/l 87-109 mmol/l >109 mmol/l
Glucose	Fasting: 70-110 mg/100 ml	3.9-5.6 mmol/l
Iron	50-150 μg/100 ml (higher in males)	9.0-26.9 μmol/l
Iron-binding capacity	250-410 μg/100 ml	44.8-73.4 μmol/l
Lactic acid	0.6-1.8 mEq/l	0.6-1.8 mmol/l
Lactic dehydrogenase	60-120 U/ml	1.00-2.00 μmol · s⁻¹/l
Lead	50 μg/100 ml or less	Up to 2.4 μmol/l
Lipase	2 U/ml or less	Up to 2 arb. unit
Lipids		
Cholesterol	120-220 mg/100 ml	3.10-5.69 mmol/l
Cholesterol esters	60-75% of cholesterol	
Phospholipids	9-16 mg/100 ml as lipid phosphorus	2.9-5.2 mmol/l
Total fatty acids	190-420 mg/100 ml	1.9-4.2 g/l
Total lipids	450-1000 mg/100 ml	4.5-10.0 g/l
Triglycerides	40-150 mg/100 ml	0.4-1.5 g/l
Lithium	Toxic level 2 mEq/l	2 mmol/l
Magnesium	1.5-2.0 mEq/l	0.8-1.3 mmol/l
5'Nucleotidase	0.3-3.2 Bodansky U	30-290 nmol · s⁻¹/l
Osmolality	285-295 mOsm/kg water	285-295 mmol/kg
Oxygen saturation (arterial)	96-100%	0.96-1.00 l
P_{CO_2}	35-43 mm Hg	4.7-6.0 kPa
pH	7.35-7.45	Same
P_{O_2}	75-100 mm Hg (dependent on age) while breathing room air Above 500 mm Hg while on 100% O_2	10.0-13.3 kPa
Phenylalanine	0-2 mg/100 ml	0-120 μmol/l
Phenytoin (Dilantin)	Therapeutic level, 5-20 μg/ml	19.8-79.5 μmol/l
Phosphorus (inorganic)	3.0-4.5 mg/100 ml (infants in 1st year up to 6.0 mg/100 ml)	1.0-1.5 mmol/l
Potassium	3.5-5.0 mEq/l	3.5-5.0 mmol/l
Primidone (Mysoline)	Therapeutic level 4-12 μg/ml	18-55 μmol/l
Protein: Total	6.0-8.4 g/100 ml	60-84 g/l
Albumin	3.5-5.0 g/100 ml	35-50 g/l
Globulin	2.3-3.5 g/100 ml	23-35 g/l
Electrophoresis	% of total protein	Of total protein
Albumin	52-68	0.52-0.68
Globulin:		
Alpha₁	4.2-7.2	0.042-0.072
Alpha₂	6.8-12	0.068-0.12
Beta	9.3-15	0.093-0.15
Gamma	13-23	0.13-0.23
Pyruvic acid	0-0.11 mEq/l	0.011 mmol/l
Quinidine	Therapeutic: 1.5-3 μg/ml Toxic: 5-6 μg/ml	4.6-9.2 μmol/l 15.4-18.5 μmol/l
Salicylate:	0	
Therapeutic	20-25 mg/100 ml; 25-30 mg/100 ml to age 10 yrs. 3 h post dose	1.4-1.8 mmol/l 1.8-2.2 mmol/l
Toxic	Over 30 mg/100 ml Over 20 mg/100 ml after age 60	Over 2.2 mmol/l Over 1.5 mmol/l
Sodium	135-145 mEq/l	135-145 mmol/l
Sulfate	0.5-1.5 mg/100 ml	0.05-1.2 mmol/l
Sulfonamide	0 mg/100 ml Therapeutic: 5-15 mg/100 ml	0 mmol/1
Transaminase (SGOT) (aspartate amino-transferase)	10-40 U/ml	0.08-0.32 μmol · s⁻¹/l
Urea nitrogen (BUN)	8-25 mg/100 ml	2.9-8.9 mmol/l
Uric acid	3.0-7.0 mg/100 ml	0.13-0.42 mmol/l
Vitamin A	0.15-0.6 μg/ml	0.5-2.1 μmol/l
Vitamin A tolerance test	Rise to twice fasting level in 3 to 5 hr	

Urine values
Reference range

Determination	Conventional	SI
Acetone plus acetoacetate (quantitative)	0	0 mg/l
Alpha amino nitrogen	64-199 mg/d; not over 1.5% of total nitrogen	4.6-14.2 mmol/d
Amylase	24-76 U/ml	24-76 arb. unit
Calcium	150 mg/d or less	3.8 or less mmol/d
Catecholamines	Epinephrine: under 20 µg/d	<55 nmol/d
	Norepinephrine: under 100 µg/d	<590 nmol/d
Copper	0-100 µg/d	0-1.6 µmol/d
Coproporphyrin	50-250 µg/d	80-380 nmol/d
	Children under 80 lb 0-75 µg/d	0-115 nmol/d
Creatine	Under 100 mg/d or less than 6% of creatinine. In pregnancy: up to 12%. In children under 1 yr.: may equal creatinine. In older children: up to 30% of creatinine	<0.75 mmol/d
Cystine or cysteine	0	0
Follicle-stimulating hormone:		
Follicular phase	5-20 IU/d	Same
Mid/cycle	15-60 IU/d	
Luteal phase	5-15 IU/d	
Menopausal	50-100 IU/d	
Men	5-25 IU/d	
Hemoglobin and myoglobin	0	
5-Hydroxyindole acetic acid	2-9 mg/d (women lower than men)	10-45 µmol/d
Lead	0.08 µg/ml or 120 µg or less/d	0.39 µmol/l or less
Phenolsulfonphthalein (PSP)	At least 25% excreted by 15 min; 40% by 30 min; 60% by 120 min.	0.25 l
Phosphorus (inorganic)	Varies with intake, average 1 g/d	32 mmol/d
Porphobilinogen	0	0
Protein:		
Quantitative	<150 mg/24 hr	<0.15 g/d

Steroids:

17-Ketosteroids (per day)

Age (yr)	Male (mg)	Female (mg)	Male (µmol/d)	Female (µmol/d)
10	1-4	1-4	3-14	3-14
20	6-21	4-16	21-73	14-56
30	8-26	4-14	28-90	14-49
50	5-18	3-9	17-62	10-31
70	2-10	1-7	7-35	3-24

Determination	Conventional	SI
17-Hydroxysteroids	3-8 mg/d (women lower than men)	8-22 µmol/d as hydrocortisone
Sugar:		
Quantitative glucose	0	0 mmol/l
Identification of reducing substances		
Fructose	0	0 mmol/l
Pentose	0	0 mmol/l
Titratable acidity	20-40 mEq/d	21-40 mmol/d
Urobilinogen	Up to 1.0 Ehrlich U	To 1.0 arb. unit
Uroporphyrin	0	0 nmol/d
Vanilmandelic acid (VMA)	Up to 9 mg/24 hr	Up to 45 µmol/d

Special endocrine tests

Reference range

Determination	Conventional	SI
Steroid hormones		
Aldosterone	Excretion: 5-19 μg/24 h	14-53 nmol/d
Cortisol		
Fasting	8 a.m.: 5-25 μg/100 ml	0.14-0.69 μmol/l
At rest	8 p.m.: Below 10 μg/100 ml	0-0.28 μmol/l
20 U ACTH	4 h ACTH test: 30-45 μg/100 ml	0.83-1.24 μmol/l
Dexamethasone at midnight	Overnight suppression test: Below 5 μg/100 ml	<0.14 nmol/l
	Excretion: 20-70 μg/24 h	55-193 nmol/d
11-Deoxycortisol	Responsive: Over 7.5 μg/100 ml (after metra-pone)	>0.22 μmol/l
Testosterone	Adult male: 300-1100 ng/100 ml	10.4-38.1 nmol/l
	Adolescent male: over 100 ng/100 ml	>3.5 nmol/l
	Females: 25-90 ng/100 ml	0.87-3.12 nmol/l
Unbound testosterone	Adult male: 3.06-24.0 ng/100 ml	106-832 pmol/l
	Adult female: 0.09-1.28 ng/100 ml	3.1-44.4 pmol/l
Polypeptide hormones		
Adrenocorticotropin (ACTH)	15-70 pg/ml	3.3-15.4 pmol/l
Calcitonin	Undetectable in normals	0
	>100 pg/ml in medullary carcinoma	>29.3 pmol/l
Growth hormone		
Fasting, at rest	Below 5 ng/ml	<233 pmol/l
After exercise	Children: Over 10 ng/ml	>465 pmol/l
	Male: Below 5 ng/ml	<233 pmol/l
	Female: Up to 30 ng/ml	0-1395 pmol/l
After glucose	Male: Below 5 ng/ml	<233 pmol/l
	Female: Below 10 ng/ml	0-465 pmol/l
Insulin		
Fasting	6-26 μU/ml	43-187 pmol/l
During hypoglycemia	Below 20 μU/ml	<144 pmol/l
After glucose	Up to 150 μU/ml	0-1078 pmol/l
Leuteinizing hormone	Male: 6 -18 mU/ml	6-18 u/l
Pre- or postovulatory	Female: 5-22 mU/ml	5-22 u/l
Midcycle peak	30-250 mU/ml	30-250 u/l
Parathyroid hormone	<10 μl equiv/ml	<10 ml equiv/l
Prolactin	2-15 ng/ml	0.08-6.0 nmol/l
Renin activity		
Normal diet	Supine:1.1 ± 0.8 ng/ml/h	0.9 ± 0.6 (nmol/l)h
	Upright: 1.9 ± 1.7 ng/ml/h	1.5 ± 1.3 (nmol/l)h
Low-sodium diet	Supine: 2.7 ± 1.8 ng/ml/h	2.1 ± 1.4 (nmol/l)h
	Upright: 6.6 ± 2.5 ng/ml/h	5.1 ± 1.9 (nmol/l)h
Low-sodium diet	Diuretics: 10.0 ± 3.7 ng/ml/h	7.7 ± 2.9 (nmol/l)h
Thyroid hormones		
Thyroid-stimulating-hormone (TSH)	0.5-3.5 μU/ml	0.5-3.5 mU/l
Thyroxine-binding globulin capacity	15-25 μg T_4/100 ml	193-322 nmol/l
Total tri-iodothyronine by radioimmu-noassay (T_3)	70-190 ng/100 ml	1.08-2.92 nmol/l
Total thyroxine by RIA (T_4)	4-12 μg/100 ml	52-154 nmol/l
T_3 resin uptake	25-35%	0.25-0.35
Free thyroxine index (FT$_4$I)	1-4 ng/100 ml	12.8-51-2 pmol/l

Cerebrospinal fluid values
Reference range

Determination	Conventional	SI	Determination	Conventional	SI
Bilirubin	0	0 μmol/l	Glucose	50-75 mg/100 ml (30%-50% less than blood)	2.8-4.2 μmol/l
Chloride	120-130 mEq/l (20 mEq/l higher than serum)		Pressure (initial)	70-180 mm of water	70-80 arb. u.
Albumin	Mean: 29.5 mg/100 ml ±2 SD: 11-48 mg/ 100 ml	0.295 g/l ±2 SD: 0.11-0.48	Protein:		
			Lumbar	15-45 mg/100 ml	0.15-0.45 g/l
IgG	Mean: 4.3 mg/100 ml ±2 SD: 0-8.6 mg/100 ml	0.043 g/l ±2 SD: 0-0.086	Cisternal	15-25 mg/100 ml	0.15-0.25 g/l
			Ventricular	5-15 mg/100 ml	0.05-0.15 g/l

Hematologic values
Reference range

Determination	Conventional	SI
Coagulation factors:		
Factor I (fibrinogen)	0.15-0.35 g/100 ml	4.0-10.0 μmol/l
Factor II (prothrombin)	60-140%	0.60-1.40
Factor V (accelerator globulin)	60-140%	0.60-1.40
Factor VII-X (proconvertin-Stuart)	70-130%	0.70-1.30
Factor X (Stuart factor)	70-130%	0.70-1.30
Factor VIII (antihemophilic globulin)	50-200%	0.50-2.0
Factor IX (plasma thromboplastic cofactor)	60-140%	0.60-1.40
Factor XI (plasma thromboplastic antecedent)	60-140%	0.60-1.40
Factor XII (Hageman factor)	60-140%	0.60-1.40
Coagulation screening tests:		
Bleeding time (Simplate)	3-9 min	180-540 s
Prothrombin time	Less than 2-s deviation from control	Less than 2-s deviation from control
Partial thromboplastin time (activated)	25-37 s	25-37 s
Whole-blood clot lysis	No clot lysis in 24 h	O/d
Fibrinolytic studies:		
Euglobin lysis	No lysis in 2 h	0 (in 2 h)
Fibrinogen split products	Negative reaction at greater than 1:4 dilution	0 (at >1:4 dilution)
Thrombin time	Control ± 5 s	Control ± 5 s
"Complete" blood count:		
Hematocrit	Male: 45-52%	Male: 0.42-0.52
	Female: 37-48%	Female: 0.37-0.48
Hemoglobin	Male: 13-18 g/100 ml	Male: 8.1-11.2 mmol/l
	Female: 12-16 g/100 ml	Female: 7.4-9.9 mmol/l
Leukocyte count	4300-10,800/mm^3	4.3-10.8 × 10^9/l
Erythrocyte count	4.2-5.9 million/mm^3	4.2-5.9 × 10^{12}/l
Mean corpuscular volume (MCV)	80-94 μm^3	80-94 fl
Mean corpuscular hemoglobin (MCH)	27-32 pg	1.7-2.0 fmol
Mean corpuscular hemoglobin concentration (MCHC)	32-36%	19-22.8 mmol/l
Erythrocyte sedimentation rate (Westergren method)	Male: 1-13 mm/h	Male: 1-13 mm/h
	Female: 1-20 mm/h	Female: 1-20 mm/h
Erythrocyte enzymes		
Glucose-6-phosphate dehydrogenase	5-15 U/gHb	5-15 U/g
Pyruvate kinase	13-17 U/gHb	13-17 U/g

Continued.

Hematologic values—cont'd
Reference range—cont'd

Determination	Conventional	SI
Ferritin (serum)		
Iron deficiency	0-20 ng/ml	0-20 μg/l
Iron excess	Greater than 400 ng/l	>400 μg/l
Folic acid		
Normal	Greater than 1.9 ng/ml	>4.3 mmol/l
Borderline	1.0-1.9 ng/ml	2.3-4.3 mmol/l
Haptoglobin	100-300 mg/100 ml	1.0-3.0 g/l
Hemoglobin studies:		
Electrophoresis for A_2 hemoglobin	1.5-3.5%	0.015-0.035
Hemoglobin F (fetal hemoglobin)	Less than 2%	<0.02
Hemoglobin, met- and sulf-	0	0
Serum hemoglobin	2-3 mg/100 ml	1.2-1.9 μmol/l
Thermolabile hemoglobin	0	0
L.E. (lupus erythematosus) preparation:		
Heparin as anticoagulant	0	0
Defibrinated blood	0	0
Leukocyte alkaline phosphatase:		
Quantitative method	15-40 mg of phosphorus liberated/h/10^{10} cells	15-40 mg/h
Qualitative method	Males: 33-188 U	33-188 U
	Females (off contraceptive pill): 30-160 U	30-160 U
Muramidase	Serum, 3-7 μg/ml	3-7 mg/l
	Urine, 0.2 μg/ml	0.2 mg/l
Osmotic fragility of erythrocytes	Increased if hemolysis occurs in over 0.5% NaCl; decreased if hemolysis is incomplete in 0.3% NaCl	
Peroxide hemolysis	Less than 10%	<0.10
Platelet count	150,000-350,000/mm³	150-350 × 10^9/l
Platelet function tests:		
Clot retraction	50-100%/2 hr	0.50-1.00/2 h
Platelet aggregation	Full response to ADP, epinephrine and collagen	1.0
Platelet factor 3	33-57 s	33-57 s
Reticulocyte count	0.5-1.5% red cells	0.005-0.15
Vitamin B_{12}	90-280 pg/ml (borderline: 70-90)	66-207 pmol/l (borderline: 52-66)

Miscellaneous values
Reference range

Determination	Conventional	SI
Autoantibodies in serum		
Thyroid colloid and microsomal antigens	Absent	
Stomach parietal cells	Absent	
Smooth muscle	Absent	
Kidney mitochondria	Absent	
Rabbit renal collecting ducts	Absent	
Cytoplasm of ova, theca cells, testicular interstitial cells	Absent	
Skeletal muscle	Absent	
Adrenal gland	Absent	
Carcinoembryonic antigen (CEA) in blood	0-2.5 ng/ml, 97% healthy nonsmokers	0-2.5 µg/l, 97% healthy nonsmokers
Cryoprecipitable proteins in blood	0	0 arb. unit
Digitoxin in serum	17 ± 6 ng/ml	22 ± 7.8 nmol/l
Digoxin in serum		
0.25 mg/d	1.2 ± 0.4 ng/ml	1.54 ± 0.5 nmol/l
0.5 mg/d	1.5 ± 0.4 ng/ml	1.92 ± 0.5 nmol/l
Duodenal drainage:		
pH	5.5-7.5	5.5-7.5
Amylase	Over 1200 U/total sample	>1.2 arb. u
Trypsin	Values from 35 to 160% "normal"	0.35-1.60
Viscosity	3 min or less	180 s or less
Gastric analysis	Basal:	
	Females 2.0 ± 1.8 mEq/h	0.6 ± 0.5
	Males 3.0 ± 2.0 mEq/h	0.8 ± 0.6 µmol/s
	Maximal: (after histalog or gastrin)	
	Females 16 ± 5 mEq/h	4.4 ± 1.4 µmol/s
	Males 23 ± 5 mEq/h	6.4 ± 1.4 µmol/s
Gastrin-I in blood	0-200 pg/ml	0-95 pmol/l
Immunologic tests		
Alpha-feto-globulin	Abnormal if present	
Alpha 1-antitrypsin	200-400 mg/100 ml	2.0-4.0 g/l
Antinuclear antibodies	Positive if detected with serum diluted 1:10	
Anti-DNA antibodies	Less than 15 units/ml	
Complement, total hemolytic	150-250 U/ml	
C3	Range 55-120 mg/100 ml	0.55-1.2 g/l
C4	Range 20-50 mg/100 ml	0.2-0.5 g/l

Continued.

Miscellaneous values—cont'd
Reference range—cont'd

Determination	Conventional	SI
Immunoglobulins in blood:		
IgG	1140 mg/100 ml	11.4 g/l
	Range 540-1663	5.5-16.6 g/l
IgA	214 mg/100 ml	2.14 g/l
	Range 66-344	0.66-3.44 g/l
IgM	168 mg/100 ml	1.68 g/l
	Range 39-290	0.39-2.9 g/l
Viscosity	1.4-1.8 expressed as relative viscosity of serum compared to water	
Iontophoresis	Children: 0-40 mEq sodium/liter	0-40 mmol/l
	Adults: 0-60 mEq sodium/l	0-60 mmol/l
Propranolol (includes bioactive 4-OH metabolite) in serum 4h after last dose	100-300 ng/ml	386-1158 nmol/l
Stool fat	Less than 5 g in 24 h or less than 4% of measured fat intake in 3-d period	<5 g/d
Stool nitrogen	Less than 2 g/d or 10% of urinary nitrogen	<2 g/d
Synovial fluid:		
Glucose	Not less than 20 mg/100 ml lower than simultaneously drawn blood sugar	See blood glucose mmol/l
Mucin	Type 1 or 2	1-2 arb. u
	Grades as:	
	Type 1-tight clump	
	Type 2-soft clump	
	Type 3-soft clump that breaks up	
	Type 4-cloudy, no clump	
D-Xylose absorption	5-8 g/5 h in urine	33-53 mmol
	40 mg per 100 ml in blood 2 h after ingestion of 25 g of D-xylose	2.7 mmol/l

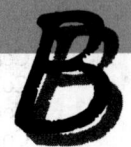

Abbreviations in Common Usage

ā	Before
aa	Of each
ac	Before meals
ad lib	As desired
A/G ratio	Albumin/globulin ratio
AK	Above knee
aPTT	Activated partial thromboplastin time
A/R pulse	Apical/radial pulse
ARDS	Adult respiratory distress syndrome
ASHD	Arteriosclerotic heart disease
ASCVD	Arteriosclerotic cardiovascular disease
AVR	Aortic valve replacement
BaE	Barium enema
b.i.d.	Twice daily
BFT	Biofeedback therapy
BK	Below knee
BMR	Basal metabolism rate
BPH	Benign prostatic hypertrophy
B.R.P.	Bathroom privileges
BS	Bowel sounds
BSP	Bromsulphalein
BUN	Blood urea nitrogen
Bx	Biopsy
c̄	With
CA	Cancer
CABG	Coronary artery bypass graft
CAD	Coronary artery disease
CBC	Complete blood count
cc	Chief complaint
CCK	Cholecystokinin
C.D.	Constant drainage
CDC	Centers for Disease Control
CHF	Congestive heart failure
CNS	Central nervous system
c/o	Complained of
COPD	Chronic obstructive pulmonary disease
CPK	Creatine phosphokinase
CPR	Cardiopulmonary resuscitation
C & S	Culture and sensitivities

Cx	Cervix
Cysto	Cystoscopy
D/C	Discontinue
D & C	Dilation and curettage
Diff	Differential white blood cell count
DIP	Distal interphalangeal joint
DJD	Degenerative joint disease
DM	Diabetes mellitus
DOA	Dead on arrival
DPT	Diphtheria, pertussis, tetanus toxoid
Dx	Diagnosis
DOE	Dyspnea on exertion
ECG	Electrocardiogram
EEG	Electroencephalogram
EENT	Eye, ear, nose and throat
EMG	Electromyogram
ENT	Ear, nose and throat
ESR	Erythrocyte sedimentation rate
FB	Foreign body
FBS	Fasting blood sugar
FH	Family history
FUO	Fever of unknown origin
FWB	Full weight bearing
Fx	Fracture
GI	Gastrointestinal
gtt	Drops
GTT	Glucose tolerance test
GU	Genitourinary
h	Hour
HAV	Hepatitis A virus
HBV	Hepatitis B virus
Hct	Hematocrit
HCTZ	Hydrochlorothiazide
HCVD	Hypertensive cardiovascular disease
HDL	High-density lipoproteins
Hgb	Hemoglobin
HMO	Health maintenance organization
HNP	Herniated nucleus pulposus
HPI	History of present illness

CSF	Cerebrospinal fluid	HTN	Hypertension
CT	Computed tomography	h.s.	At bedtime
CVA	Cerebrovascular accident	Hwb	Hot water bottle
CVA	Costovertebral angle	hx	History
CVP	Central venous pressure	IABP	Intraaortic balloon counterpulsation
ICP	Intracranial pressure	p.c.	After meals
ICS	Intercostal space	PCWP	Pulmonary capillary wedge pressure
ICU	Intensive care unit	P.D.	Postural drainage
IDDM	Insulin-dependent diabetes mellitus	PEEP	Positive end expiratory pressure
IHSS	Idiopathic hypertrophic subaortic stenosis	PERRLA	Pupils equal, round, reactive to light and accommodation
IM	Intramuscular		
IMB	Intermenstrual bleeding	PFT	Pulmonary function test
I & O	Intake and output	PH	Past history
IPPB	Intermittent positive pressure breathing	PI	Present illness
ITP	Idiopathic thrombocytopenic purpura	PIP	Proximal interphalangeal joint
IV	Intravenous	Plt	Platelet
IVC	Intravenous cholangiogram	PMI	Point of maximal impulse
IVP	Intravenous pyelogram	PMNs	Polymorphonuclear leukocytes
LBP	Low back pain	PMP	Past menstrual period
LDH	Lactic dehydrogenase	PND	Paroxysmal nocturnal dyspnea
LDL	Low-density lipoproteins	PNS	Peripheral nervous system
L.E. prep	Lupus erythematosus prep	po	By mouth
LLL	Left lower lobe	POD	Postoperative day
LLQ	Left lower quadrant	PPD	Postpartum day
LMD	Local medical doctor	PPD	Purified protein derivative
LMP	Local medical physician	prn	According to necessity
LMP	Last menstrual period	Pro time	Prothrombin time
LOC	Level of consciousness	PSP	Phenosulphonphthalein
LP	Lumbar puncture	PSRO	Professional standards review organization
LVEDP	Left ventricular end-diastolic pressure	PT	Prothrombin time
L & W	Living and well	P.T.	Physical therapy
lytes	Electrolytes	PTA	Prior to admission
Ⓜ	Murmur	PTT	Partial thromboplastin time
MCH	Mean corpuscular hemoglobin	PVC	Premature ventricular contraction
MCHC	Mean corpuscular hemoglobin concentration	PWB	Partial weight bearing
MCP	Metacarpopharangeal joint	PZI	Protamine zinc insulin
MCV	Mean corpuscular volume	qd	Every day
MGW	Magnesium, glycerin, and water enema	qhs	At bedtime
MRI	Magnetic resonance imaging	qs	As much as necessary
MST	Mean survival time	qod	Every other day
MTP	Metacarpophalangeal joint	qid	Four times a day
MVR	Mitral valve replacement	qh	Every hour
MWB	Minimal weight bearing	qns	Quantity not sufficient
NAD	No acute distress	qoh	Every other hour
NIDDM	Noninsulin dependent diabetes mellitus	qpr	At earliest convenience
NPH	Nonprotein Hagedorn (insulin)	RBC	Red blood cells
NPN	Nonprotein nitrogen	RLL	Right lower lobe
N.P.O.	Nothing by mouth	RLQ	Right lower quadrant
NVD	Neck vein distention	R/O	Rule out
NWB	Nonweight bearing	ROS	Review of symptoms
OD	Overdose	RSR	Regular sinus rhythm
O.D.	Right eye	Rx	Treatment
OOB	Out of bed	s̄	Without
O.R.	Operating room	SBE	Subacute bacterial endocarditis
ORIF	Open reduction internal fixation	sc	Subcutaneous
O.S.	Left eye	Sed rate	Sedimentation rate
O.T.	Occupational therapy	SGOT	Serum glutamic oxidase transaminase
O.U.	Both eyes	SGPT	Serum glutamic pyruvate transaminase
p̄	After	SLE	Systemic lupus erythematosus
P & A	Percussion and auscultation	SLR	Straight leg raising
PAEDP	Pulmonary artery end-diastolic pressure	SOB	Short of breath
PAP	Pulmonary artery pressure	s.o.s.	Administer once if necessary
PAP	Papanicolaou smear	S/P	Status post (occurred in past)
PBI	Protein bound iodine	SR	Systems review

SSE	Soapsuds enema		TPN	Total parenteral nutrition (hyperalimentation)
stat	At once		TSP	Total serum protein
STD	Sexually transmitted disease		TSS	Toxic shock syndrome
STS	Serologic test for syphilis		TURP	Transurethral resection of prostate
T_3	Triiodothyronine		Tx	Traction
T_4	Thyroxine		ung	Ointment
tab	Tablet		URI	Upper respiratory infection
TBC	Tuberculosis		US	Ultrasound
TBG	Thyroxine binding globulin		UTI	Urinary tract infection
TENS	Transcutaneous electrical nerve stimulator		UV	Ultraviolet
THA	Total hip arthroplasty		VC	Vital capacity
THR	Total hip replacement		VDRL	Venereal disease research laboratory test
TIA	Transient ischemic attacks		VNA	Visiting nurse association
t.i.d.	Three times a day		VS	Vital signs
TKA	Total knee arthroplasty		wa	While awake
TKR	Total knee replacement		WBC	White blood count
TM	Tympanic membrane		WNL	Within normal limits
TP	Total protein			

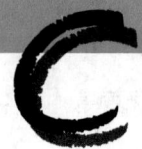

Recommended Daily Dietary Allowances, Revised 1989

Food and Nutrition Board, National Academy of Sciences—National Research Council
Recommended daily dietary allowances, revised 1989
Designed for the maintenance of good nutrition of practically all healthy people in the United States

Category	Age (years) or condition	Weight (kg)	Weight (lb)	Height (cm)	Height (in)	Protein (g)	Fat soluble vitamins Vitamin A (µg RE)*	Vitamin D (µg)†	Vitamin E (mg α-TE)‡	Vitamin K (µg)
Infants	0.0-0.5	6	13	60	24	13	375	7.5	3	5
	0.5-1.0	9	20	71	28	14	375	10	4	10
Children	1-3	13	29	90	35	16	400	10	6	5
	4-6	20	44	112	44	24	500	10	7	20
	7-10	28	62	132	52	28	700	10	7	30
Males	11-14	45	99	157	62	45	1,000	10	10	45
	15-18	66	145	176	69	59	1,000	10	10	65
	19-24	72	160	177	70	58	1,000	10	10	70
	25-50	79	174	176	70	63	1,000	5	10	80
	51+	77	170	173	68	63	1,000	5	10	80
Females	11-14	46	101	157	62	46	800	10	8	45
	15-18	55	120	163	64	44	800	10	8	55
	19-24	58	128	164	65	46	800	10	8	60
	25-50	63	138	163	64	50	800	5	8	65
	51+	65	143	160	63	50	800	5	8	65
Pregnant						60	800	10	10	65
Lactating	1st 6 months					65	1,300	10	12	65
	2nd 6 months					62	1,200	10	11	65

*Retinol equivalents. 1 retinol equivalent = 1 µg retinol or 6 µg β-carotene.
†As cholecalciferol. 10 µg cholecalciferol = 400 IU vitamin D.
‡α-Tocopherol equivalents. 1 mg d-α tocopherol = 1 α-TE.
§1 NE (niacin equivalent) is equal to 1 mg of niacin or 60 mg of dietary tryptophan.

	Water-soluble vitamins						Minerals						
Vita-min C (mg)	Thia-min (mg)	Ribo-flavin (mg)	Niacin (mg NE)§	Vita-min B$_6$ (mg)	Folate (µg)	Vita-min B$_{12}$ (µg)	Cal-cium (mg)	Phos-phorus (mg)	Mag-nesium (mg)	Iron (mg)	Zinc (mg)	Iodine (µg)	Sele-nium (µg)
30	0.3	0.4	5	0.3	25	0.3	400	300	40	6	5	40	10
35	0.4	0.5	6	0.6	35	0.5	600	500	60	10	5	50	15
40	0.7	0.8	9	1.0	50	0.7	800	800	80	10	10	70	20
45	0.9	1.1	12	1.1	75	1.0	800	800	120	10	10	90	20
45	1.0	1.2	13	1.4	100	1.4	800	800	170	10	10	120	30
50	1.3	1.5	17	1.7	150	2.0	1,200	1,200	270	12	15	150	40
60	1.5	1.8	20	2.0	200	2.0	1,200	1,200	400	12	15	150	50
60	1.5	1.7	19	2.0	200	2.0	1,200	1,200	350	10	15	150	70
60	1.5	1.7	19	2.0	200	2.0	800	800	350	10	15	150	70
60	1.2	1.4	15	2.0	200	2.0	800	800	350	10	15	150	70
50	1.1	1.3	15	1.4	150	2.0	1,200	1,200	280	15	12	150	45
60	1.1	1.3	15	1.5	180	2.0	1,200	1,200	300	15	12	150	50
60	1.1	1.3	15	1.6	180	2.0	1,200	1,200	280	15	12	150	55
60	1.1	1.3	15	1.6	180	2.0	800	800	280	15	12	150	55
60	1.0	1.2	13	1.6	180	2.0	800	800	280	10	12	150	55
70	1.5	1.6	17	2.2	400	2.2	1,200	1,200	320	30	15	175	65
95	1.6	1.8	20	2.1	280	2.6	1,200	1,200	355	15	19	200	75
90	1.6	1.7	20	2.1	260	2.6	1,200	1,200	340	15	16	200	75

Daily dietary guide—the basic four food groups

Food group	Main nutrients	Daily amounts*
Milk		
Milk, cheese, ice cream, or other products made with whole or skimmed milk	Calcium Protein Riboflavin	Children under 9: 2-3 cups Children 9-12: 3 or more cups Teen-agers: 4 or more cups Adults: 2 or more cups Pregnant women: 3 or more cups Nursing mothers: 4 or more cups (1 cup = 8 oz fluid milk or designated milk equivalent†)
Meat protein		
Beef, veal, lamb, pork, poultry, fish, eggs	Protein Iron Thiamin	2 or more servings Count as 1 serving 2-3 oz of lean, boneless, cooked meat, poultry, or fish 2 eggs
Alternates: dry beans, dry peas, nuts, peanut butter	Niacin Riboflavin	1 cup cooked dry beans or peas 4 tbsp peanut butter
Vegetables and fruits		4 or more servings Count as 1 serving ½ cup of vegetable or fruit or a portion such as 1 medium apple, banana, orange, potato, or ½ a medium grapefruit, melon Include
	Vitamin A	A dark-green or deep-yellow vegetable or fruit rich in vitamin A at least every other day
	Vitamin C (ascorbic acid) Smaller amounts of other vitamins and minerals	A citrus fruit or other fruit or vegetable rich in vitamin C daily Other vegetables and fruits including potatoes
Bread and cereals		4 or more servings of whole grain, enriched or restored Count as 1 serving
	Thiamin Niacin Riboflavin Iron Protein	1 slice of bread 1 oz (1 cup) ready to eat cereal, flake or puff varieties ½-¾ cup cooked cereal ½-¾ cup cooked pastas (macaroni, spaghetti, noodles) Crackers: 5 saltines, 2 squares graham crackers

*Use additional amounts of these foods or added butter, margarine, oils, sugars, etc., as desired or needed.
†Milk equivalents: 1 oz cheddar cheese, 3 servings cottage cheese, 1 cup fluid skimmed milk, 1 cup buttermilk, ½ cup dry skimmed milk powder, 1 cup ice milk, 1⅔ cups ice cream, ½ cup evaporated milk.

Median Heights and Weights and Recommended Energy Intake

Category	Age (years) or condition	Weight (kg)	Weight (lb)	Height (cm)	Height (in)	REE* (kcal/day)	Multiples of REE	Per kg	Per day‡
Infants	0.0-0.5	6	13	60	24	320		108	650
	0.5-1.0	9	20	71	28	500		98	850
Children	1-3	13	29	90	35	740		102	1,300
	4-6	20	44	112	44	950		90	1,800
	7-10	28	62	132	52	1,130		70	2,000
Males	11-14	45	99	157	62	1,440	1.70	55	2,500
	15-18	66	145	176	69	1,760	1.67	45	3,000
	19-24	72	160	177	70	1,780	1.67	40	2,900
	25-50	79	174	176	70	1,800	1.60	37	2,900
	51+	77	170	173	68	1,530	1.50	30	2,300
Females	11-14	46	101	157	62	1,310	1.67	47	2,200
	15-18	55	120	163	64	1,370	1.60	40	2,200
	19-24	58	128	164	65	1,350	1.60	38	2,200
	25-50	63	138	163	64	1,380	1.55	36	2,200
	51+	65	143	160	63	1,280	1.50	30	1,900
Pregnant	1st trimester								+0
	2nd trimester								+300
	3rd trimester								+300
Lactating	1st 6 months								+500
	2nd 6 months								+500

*Resting energy expenditure.
†In the range of light to moderate activity, the coefficient of variation is ±20%.
‡Figure is rounded.
(From Food and Nutrition Board, National Academy of Sciences–National Research Council, 1989.)

Index